PEDIATRIC RADIOLOGY

Practical Imaging Evaluation of Infants and Children

PEDIATRIC RADIOLOGY

Practical Imaging Evaluation of Infants and Children

Editor

EDWARD Y. LEE, MD, MPH
Associate Professor of Radiology
Chief, Division of Thoracic Imaging
Departments of Radiology and Medicine, Pulmonary Division
Boston Children's Hospital
Harvard Medical School
Boston, Massachusetts

Associate Editors

WINNIE C. CHU, MD, FRCR
Professor of Radiology
Chief, Division of Pediatric Radiology
Department of Imaging and Interventional Radiology
The Chinese University of Hong Kong
Prince of Wales Hospital
Hong Kong, China

JONATHAN R. DILLMAN, MD, MSC
Associate Professor of Radiology
Director, Thoracoabdominal Imaging
Department of Radiology
Cincinnati Children's Hospital Medical Center
Cincinnati, Ohio

ANDREA S. DORIA, MD, PHD, MSC
Professor of Radiology and Associate Vice-Chair of Research
Department of Medical Imaging, University of Toronto
Radiologist and Research Director
Department of Diagnostic Imaging
The Hospital for Sick Children
Toronto, Canada

RICARDO RESTREPO, MD
Professor at Florida International University School of Medicine
Chief, Interventional Pediatric Radiology and Body Imaging
Department of Radiology
Nicklaus Children's Hospital
Miami, Florida

SARA O. VARGAS, MD
Associate Professor of Pathology
Department of Pathology
Boston Children's Hospital
Harvard Medical School
Boston, Massachusetts

Wolters Kluwer

Philadelphia • Baltimore • New York • London
Buenos Aires • Hong Kong • Sydney • Tokyo

Acquisitions Editor: Sharon Zinner
Editorial Coordinator: Lauren Pecarich
Marketing Manager: Dan Dressler
Production Project Manager: Linda Van Pelt
Design Coordinator: Teresa Mallon
Manufacturing Coordinator: Beth Welsh
Prepress Vendor: SPi Global

9 8 7 6 5 4 3 2 1

Printed in China

Library of Congress Cataloging-in-Publication Data
Names: Lee, Edward Y., editor.
Title: Pediatric radiology : practical imaging evaluation of infants and children / editor, Edward Y. Lee ; associate editors, Winnie C. Chu, Jonathan R. Dillman, Andrea S. Doria, Ricardo Restrepo, Sara O. Vargas.
Other titles: Pediatric radiology (Lee)
Description: Philadelphia : Wolters Kluwer, [2018] | Includes bibliographical references.
Identifiers: LCCN 2016039527 | ISBN 9781451175851
Subjects: | MESH: Radiography | Infant | Child
Classification: LCC RJ51.R3 | NLM WN 240 | DDC 618.92/00757—dc23 LC record available at https://lccn.loc.gov/2016039527

LWW.com

RRS1707

To my parents, Kwan-Pyo and Kang-ja, and my family for their constant support and encouragement.
To the trainees and radiologists that I have met during my academic career for sharing their enthusiasm for learning.
To my colleagues in the Department of Radiology, Boston Children's Hospital, for their support and friendship. There is absolutely no better group to be with.

—Edward Y. Lee, MD, MPH

To my family, Allen, Cherie, and Paco for their love and support.
To Faculty of Medicine at the Chinese University of Hong Kong for nurturing me as a medical student, physician, radiologist, teacher, and researcher.

—Winnie C. Chu, MD, FRCR

To the children that I have had the honor to care for.
To my wife, Suzanne, and our three beautiful daughters, Kathryn, Meghan, and Claire.

—Jonathan R. Dillman, MD, MSc

To my father who has been my great mentor, advisor, and friend throughout my life.
To my mother who taught me beautiful lessons of love during the short period of time that I had the privilege to live by her side.
To my husband, son, and extended family accrued throughout the pathway of life, who have taught me values of loyalty, honesty, companionship, and true love.
To Danny Aguilar for providing invaluable illustrations in musculoskeletal chapters.
To my patients whose journeys and battles have been the inspiration of my life.

—Andrea S. Doria, MD, PhD, MSc

To my parents, Jairo and Helena, for providing the inspiration that guided me throughout my career and also for being such incredible physician role models.
To LBS for his support and for constantly reminding me that life is beautiful and to be enjoyed in all aspects.

—Ricardo Restrepo, MD

To my colleagues in pathology, whose great care with their specimens over many years led to the diagnoses depicted herein.
To the young patients of Boston Children's Hospital, whose material enlightens us.

—Sara O. Vargas, MD

The editor and associate editors of this book would also acknowledge that all pathology images, unless otherwise specified, were provided by Sara O. Vargas, MD. Danny Aguilar, medical graphic artist and illustrator, provided schematics for musculoskeletal chapters in this book.

Editors

Editor

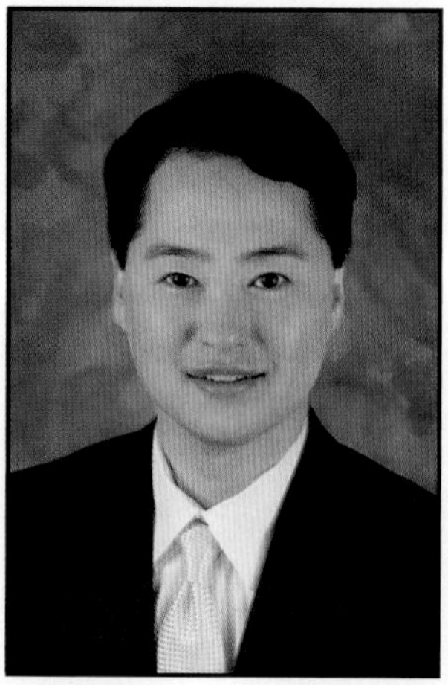

Edward Y. Lee, MD, MPH

Associate Editors

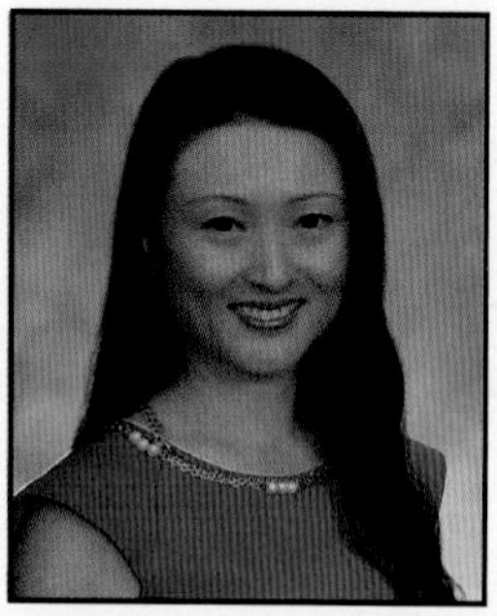

Winnie C. Chu, MD, FRCR

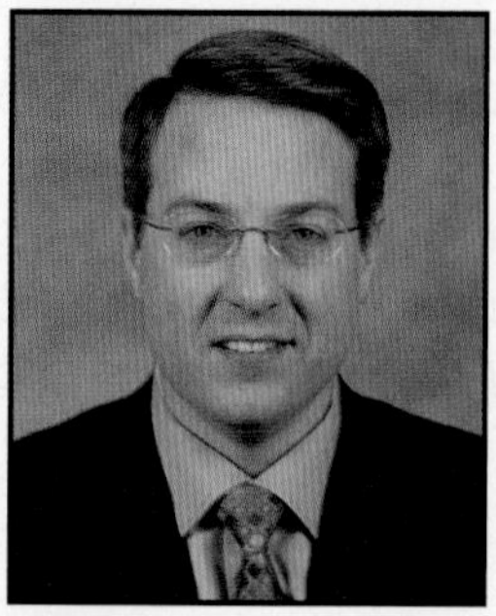

Jonathan R. Dillman, MD, MSc

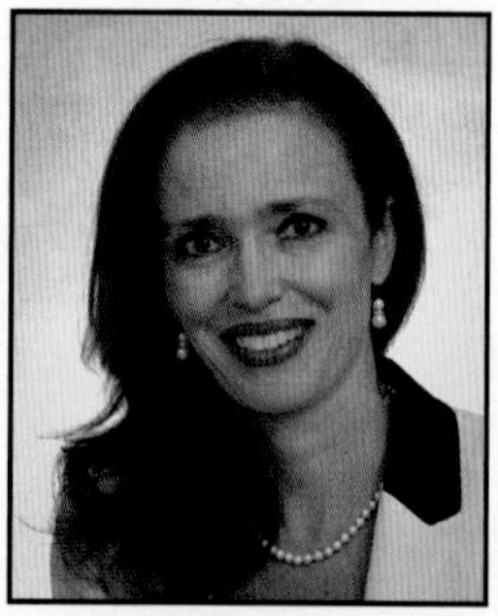

Andrea S. Doria, MD, PhD, MSc

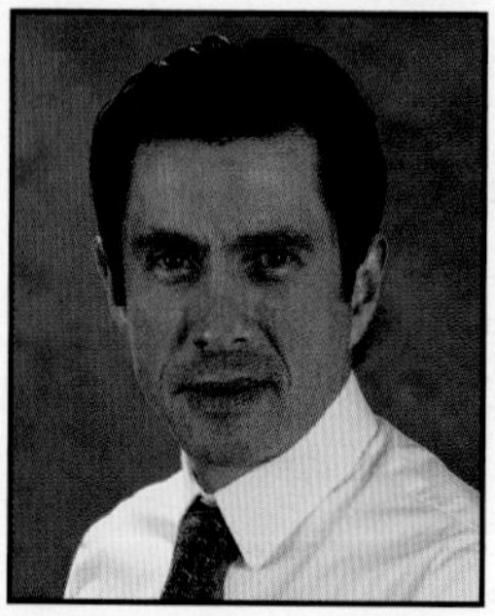

Ricardo Restrepo, MD

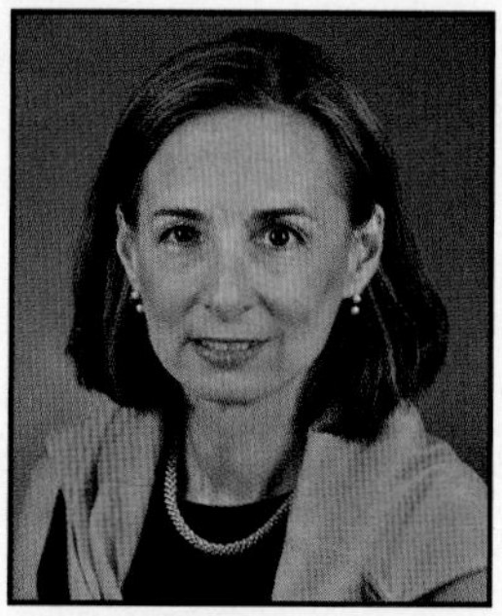

Sara O. Vargas, MD

Contributors

Behrang Amini, MD, PhD
Assistant Professor of Radiology
Department of Radiology
The University of Texas
MD Anderson Cancer Center
Houston, Texas

Savvas Andronikou, MBBCh, FCRad, FRCR, PhD
Professor of Radiology
Department of Radiology
Bristol Royal Hospital for Children
Bristol, United Kingdom

Sudha A. Anupindi, MD
Associate Professor of Clinical Radiology
The Children's Hospital of Philadelphia
Perelman School of Medicine
University of Pennsylvania
Philadelphia, Pennsylvania

Omolola M. Atalabi, MBBS, FWACS, FNPMC, MBA
Associate Professor of Radiology
Department of Radiology
University College Hospital of Ibadan
College of Medicine, University of Ibadan
Oyo State, Nigeria

Fred E. Avni, MD, PhD
Professor of Radiology
Department of Radiology
Jeanne de Flandre Hospital
Lille University Hospital
Lille-Cedex, France

Rama S. Ayyala, MD
Assistant Professor of Radiology
Department of Pediatric Radiology
Morgan Stanley Children's Hospital
Columbia University Medical Center
New York, New York

Paul S. Babyn, MDCM, FRCPC
Professor of Radiology
Chief, Department of Medical Imaging
Royal University Hospital
University of Saskatchewan and Saskatoon Health Region
Saskatoon, Canada

Eric J. Chong Barboza, MD
Professor of Radiology
Chief, Department of Pediatric Radiology
Hospital del Niño Dr. José Renan Esquivel
Panamá City, Republic of Panamá

Mark E. Bittman, MD
Assistant Professor of Radiology
Department of Radiology
NYU Langone Medical Center
New York, New York

Lorna P. Browne, MBBCh, BAO
Associate Professor of Radiology
Department of Radiology
Children's Hospital Colorado
University of Colorado
Aurora, Colorado

Timothy Cain, MBBS, FRANZCR, MBA, FAANMS
Senior Medical Specialist Pediatric Radiologist
Department of Medical Imaging
The Royal Children's Hospital, Melbourne
Melbourne, Australia

Yeun-Chung Chang, MD, PhD
Professor of Radiology
Chairman, Department of Medical Imaging
National Taiwan University Hospital
National Taiwan University College of Medicine
Taipei, Taiwan

Jung-Eun Cheon, MD, PhD
Associate Professor of Radiology
Department of Radiology
Seoul National University Children's Hospital
Seoul National University College of Medicine
Seoul, South Korea

Winnie C. Chu, MD, FRCR
Professor of Radiology
Chief, Division of Pediatric Radiology
Department of Imaging and Interventional Radiology
The Chinese University of Hong Kong
Prince of Wales Hospital
Hong Kong, China

Pierluigi Ciet, MD, PhD
Pediatric Radiologist
Department of Radiology and Nuclear Medicine
Department of Pediatric Pulmonology and Allergology
Erasmus Medical Center–Sophia Children's Hospital
Rotterdam, The Netherlands

Jesse Courtier, MD
Associate Professor of Radiology
Department of Radiology
UCSF Benioff Children's Hospital
University of California, San Francisco
San Francisco, California

Pedro Daltro, MD, PhD
Pediatric Radiologist
Medical Director
Alta Excelência Diagnóstica and CDPI–DASA Corp
Rio de Janeiro, Brazil

Kassa Darge, MD, PhD
Professor of Radiology
Chief, Department of Radiology
The Children's Hospital of Philadelphia
Perelman School of Medicine
University of Pennsylvania
Philadelphia, Pennsylvania

Karuna M. Das, MD
Assistant Professor of Radiology
Department of Radiology
College of Medicine and Health Sciences
Al Ain, United Arab Emirates

Pilar Dies-Suarez, MD
Professor of Radiology
Chief, Department of Radiology
Hospital Infantil de México Federico Gómez
Mexico City, Mexico

Jonathan R. Dillman, MD, MSc
Associate Professor of Radiology
Director, Thoracoabdominal Imaging
Department of Radiology
Cincinnati Children's Hospital Medical Center
Cincinnati, Ohio

Selim Doganay, MD
Associate Professor of Radiology
Department of Pediatric Radiology
Erciyes University Children's Hospital
Kayseri, Turkey

Andrea S. Doria, MD, PhD, MSc
Professor of Radiology and Associate Vice-Chair of Research
Department of Medical Imaging, University of Toronto
Radiologist and Research Director
Department of Diagnostic Imaging
The Hospital for Sick Children
Toronto, Canada

Dawn R. Engelkemier, MD
Pediatric Radiologist
Department of Radiology
Sharp Rees-Stealy Medical Group
San Diego, California

Monica Epelman, MD
Professor of Radiology
University of Central Florida
Vice Chair, Department of Medical Imaging and Radiology
Nemours Children's Health System
Orlando, Florida

Celia Ferrari, MD
Pediatric Radiologist
Chief, Department of Radiology
Hospital de Niños Sor María Ludovica
La Plata, Argentina

Claudio Fonda, MD
Professor of Radiology
Former Head, Department of Pediatric Radiology
Meyer Children's University Hospital
Firenze, Italy

Marielle V. Fortier, MD
Adjunct Associate Professor of Radiology, Duke-NUS
Adjunct Investigator, Singapore Institute for Clinical Sciences
Chief, Department of Diagnostic and Interventional Imaging
K. K. Women's and Children's Hospital
Singapore

Pilar Garcia-Pena, MD
Professor of Radiology
Emeritus of National Health Institutions
Department of Pediatric Radiology
University Hospital Materno-Infantil Vall d´Hebron
Barcelona, Spain

Michael S. Gee, MD, PhD
Associate Professor of Radiology
Chief, Division of Pediatric Radiology
Massachusetts General Hospital
Harvard Medical School
Boston, Massachusetts

Gloria Soto Giordani, MD
Pediatric Radiologist
Department of Radiology
Clinica Alemana
Santiago, Chile

I. Nimala A. Gooneratne, MD
Professor of Radiology
Department of Radiology
Lady Ridgeway Hospital
Colombo, Sri Lanka

Magdalena Gormsen, MD
Pediatric Radiology Consultant
Department of Radiology
Copenhagen University Hospital, Rigshospitalet
Copenhagen, Denmark

Sharon W. Gould, MD
Assistant Professor of Clinical Radiology
Department of Medical Imaging
Nemours/AIDHC Hospital for Children
Thomas Jefferson University
Wilmington, Delaware

Salwa M. Haidar, FFR-RCSI, FPR, FPNR U of T
Pediatric Neuroradiology Consultant
Department of Radiology
Mubarak Al-Kabeer Hospital
Hawalli, Kuwait

Benjamin T. Haverkamp, MD
Assistant Professor of Radiology
Department of Radiology
Children's Mercy Hospital and Clinics
University of Missouri–Kansas City
Kansas City, Missouri

Victor Ho-Fung, MD
Assistant Professor of Radiology
Department of Radiology
The Children's Hospital of Philadelphia
Perelman School of Medicine
University of Pennsylvania
Philadelphia, Pennsylvania

Lisa H. Hutchison, MD, FAAP
Professor of Radiology
Department of Radiology
Children's Mercy Hospital and Clinics
University of Missouri–Kansas City
Kansas City, Missouri

Diego Jaramillo, MD
Professor of Radiology
Department of Radiology
Nicklaus Children's Hospital
Miami, Florida

Amy F. Juliano, MD
Assistant Professor of Radiology
Department of Radiology
Massachusetts Eye and Ear
Harvard Medical School
Boston, Massachusetts

Suma Kannabiran, MD
Resident, Diagnostic Radiology
Department of Radiology
Beth Israel Deaconess Medical Center
Boston, Massachusetts

Khalid Khashoggi, MD
Assistant Professor of Radiology
Head, Department of Radiology
King Abdulaziz University
President, Radiological Society of Saudi Arabia
King Abdulaziz University Hospital
Jeddah, Kingdom of Saudi Arabia

Asef Khwaja, MD
Assistant Professor of Radiology
Department of Radiology
The Children's Hospital of Philadelphia
Perelman School of Medicine
University of Pennsylvania
Philadelphia, Pennsylvania

Tracy Kilborn, MD
Associate Professor of Radiology
Head, Department of Pediatric Radiology
Red Cross War Memorial Children's Hospital
University of Cape Town
Cape Town, South Africa

Hee-Kyung Kim, MD
Assistant Professor of Radiology
Department of Radiology
Cincinnati Children's Hospital Medical Center
Cincinnati, Ohio

Oleksandr Kondrachuk, MD
Radiologist
Department of Radiology
Ukrainian Children's Cardiac Center
Kyiv, Ukraine

Supika Kritsaneepaiboon, MD
Assistant Professor of Radiology
Department of Radiology
Songklanagarind Hospital
Prince of Songkla University
Hat Yai, Thailand

Peter G. Kruk, MD
Volunteer Assistant Professor of Radiology
Rady Children's Hospital San Diego
San Diego, California

Bernard F. Laya, MD, DO
Professor of Radiology
Head, Institute of Radiology
St. Luke's Medical Center–Global City
Taguig City, Philippines

Edward Y. Lee, MD, MPH
Associate Professor of Radiology
Chief, Division of Thoracic Imaging
Departments of Radiology and Medicine, Pulmonary Division
Boston Children's Hospital
Harvard Medical School
Boston, Massachusetts

José Ernesto Lipsich, MD
Professor of Radiology
Chief, Department of Radiology
Juan P. Garrahan Hospital
Buenos Aires, Argentina

Mark C. Liszewski, MD
Assistant Professor of Radiology
Division of Pediatric Radiology
Department of Radiology
Montefiore Medical Center
Albert Einstein College of Medicine
Bronx, New York

Bjorn Lundin, MD, PhD
Associate Professor of Radiology
Section for Musculoskeletal Radiology
Center for Medical Imaging and Physiology
Skåne University Hospital
Lund, Sweden

John D. MacKenzie, MD
Associate Professor of Radiology
Department of Radiology
UCSF Benioff Children's Hospital
University of California, San Francisco
San Francisco, California

Fatma Hamza Makame, MD, MMED
Assistant Lecturer in Radiology
Department of Radiology
Kilimanjaro Christian Medical University of College
Moshi, Tanzania

Zaleha Abdul Manaf, MD
Pediatric Radiologist
Department of Radiology
Kuala Lumpur Hospital
Kuala Lumpur, Malaysia

Peter "Buzz" Marcovici, MD
Pediatric Radiologist
Department of Radiology
Kaiser Permanente Northwest
Clackamas, Oregon

L. Santiago Medina, MD, MPH
Professor of Radiology
Co-director, Neuroradiology and Brain Imaging
Director, Health Outcomes, Policy and Economics (HOPE) Center
Department of Radiology
Nicklaus Children's Hospital
Miami, Florida

Zhu Ming, MD
Professor of Radiology
Chairman, Chinese Society of Pediatric Radiology
Vice Chairman, Chinese Society for Cardiovascular Magnetic Resonance
Department of Radiology
Shanghai Children's Medical Center
Shanghai Jiaotong University School of Medicine
Shanghai, China

Kevin R. Moore, MD
Professor of Radiology
Vice Chair, Department of Medical Imaging
Primary Children's Hospital
Salt Lake City, Utah

Marcia Torre Moreira, MD
Pediatric Radiologist
Department of Radiology
Hospital Infantil Sabará and Fleury Medicina e Saúde
São Paulo, Brazil

John Naheedy, MD
Assistant Professor of Clinical Radiology
Rady Children's Hospital San Diego
San Diego, California

Shunsuke Nosaka, MD, PhD
Clinical Professor of Radiology
St. Marianna University School of Medicine
Director, Department of Radiology
National Center for Child Health and Development
Tokyo, Japan

Clara L. Ortiz-Neira, MD, MSEd
Associate Professor of Clinical Radiology
Department of Radiology
University of Calgary
Red Deer, Canada

Esperanza Pacheco-Jacome, MD, MBA
Associate Professor of Radiology
Co-director, Neuroimaging
Director, Fetal Imaging
Department of Radiology
Nicklaus Children's Hospital
Miami, Florida

Janina M. Patsch, MD, PhD
Assistant Professor of Radiology
Department of General and Pediatric Radiology
Department of Biomedical Imaging and Image-guided Therapy
Medical University of Vienna
Vienna, Austria

Jeannette M. Peréz-Rosselló, MD
Assistant Professor of Radiology
Department of Radiology
Boston Children's Hospital
Harvard Medical School
Boston, Massachusetts

Andrew Phelps, MD
Assistant Professor of Radiology
Department of Radiology
UCSF Benioff Children's Hospital
University of California, San Francisco
San Francisco, California

Daniel J. Podberesky, MD
Associate Professor of Radiology
University of Central Florida and Florida State University Colleges of Medicine
Radiologist-in-Chief
Nemours Children's Health Care System
Orlando, Florida

Tina Young Poussaint, MD
Professor of Radiology
Department of Radiology
Boston Children's Hospital
Harvard Medical School
Boston, Massachusetts

Andria M. Powers, MD
Assistant Professor of Radiology
Department of Radiology
University of Nebraska Children's Hospital
Omaha, Nebraska

Sanjay P. Prabhu, MBBS
Assistant Professor of Radiology
Department of Radiology
Boston Children's Hospital
Harvard Medical School
Boston, Massachusetts

Ricardo Restrepo, MD
Professor at Florida International University School of Medicine
Chief, Interventional Pediatric Radiology and Body Imaging
Department of Radiology
Nicklaus Children's Hospital
Miami, Florida

Cynthia K. Rigsby, MD, FACR
Professor of Radiology and Pediatrics
Department of Medical Imaging
Ann & Robert H. Lurie Children's Hospital
Northwestern University Feinberg School of Medicine
Chicago, Illinois

Richard L. Robertson, MD
Associate Professor of Radiology
Chair, Department of Radiology
Boston Children's Hospital
Harvard Medical School
Boston, Massachusetts

Caroline D. Robson, MBChB
Associate Professor of Radiology
Vice Chair, Department of Radiology
Division Chief, Neuroradiology
Boston Children's Hospital
Harvard Medical School
Boston, Massachusetts

Dilip Sankhla, MD
Pediatric Radiology Senior Consultant
Department of Radiology and Molecular Imaging
Sultan Qaboos University Hospital
Muscat, Sultanate of Oman

Adji Saptogino, MD, PhD
Professor of Radiology
Chief, Department of Radiology
Pondok Indah Hospital Jakarta
Jakarta, Indonesia

Hadeel M. Seif El Dein, MD
Associate Professor of Radiology
Department of Radiology
Pediatric University Hospital
Cairo University
Cairo, Egypt

Sabah Servaes, MD
Associate Professor of Radiology
Department of Radiology
The Children's Hospital of Philadelphia
Perelman School of Medicine
University of Pennsylvania
Philadelphia, Pennsylvania

Abdusamea Shabani, MBBCh, FRCR
Assistant Professor of Radiology
Department of Radiology
Sidra Medical and Research Center
Doha, Qatar

Rahul A. Sheth, MD
Assistant Professor of Radiology
Department of Interventional Radiology
The University of Texas
MD Anderson Cancer Center
Houston, Texas

Ethan A. Smith, MD
Assistant Professor of Radiology
Section of Pediatric Radiology
C.S. Mott Children's Hospital
Department of Radiology
University of Michigan Health System
Ann Arbor, Michigan

Kushaljit S. Sodhi, MD, PhD, MAMS, FICR
Professor of Radiology
Department of Radiodiagnosis
Postgraduate Institute of Medical Education and Research
Chandigarh, India

Jennifer Stimec, MD
Assistant Professor of Radiology
Department of Radiology
The Hospital for Sick Children
Toronto, Canada

Peter J. Strouse, MD, FACR
John F. Holt Collegiate Professor of Radiology
Director, Section of Pediatric Radiology
C.S. Mott Children's Hospital
Department of Radiology
University of Michigan Health System
Ann Arbor, Michigan

Mohamed Issa Tawil, MD
Pediatric Radiologist
Department of Radiology
Sheikh Khalifa Medical City
Abu Dhabi, United Arab Emirates

Paul G. Thacker, MD
Associate Professor of Radiology
Department of Radiology
University of South Carolina
Charleston, South Carolina

Alexander J. Towbin, MD
Associate Professor of Radiology
Department of Radiology
Cincinnati Children's Hospital Medical Center
Cincinnati, Ohio

Donald A. Tracy, MD
Assistant Professor of Radiology
Department of Radiology
Floating Hospital for Children
Tuft Medical Center
Boston, Massachusetts

Andrew T. Trout, MD
Assistant Professor of Radiology and Pediatrics
Department of Radiology
Cincinnati Children's Hospital Medical Center
Cincinnati, Ohio

Sara O. Vargas, MD
Associate Professor of Pathology
Department of Pathology
Boston Children's Hospital
Harvard Medical School
Boston, Massachusetts

Sally A. Vogel, MD, FRANZCR
Pediatric Radiologist
Clinical Director, Department of Pediatric Radiology
Starship Children's Health
Auckland, New Zealand

Daniel B. Wallihan, MD
Pediatric Radiologist
Department of Radiology
Levine Children's Hospital
Charlotte, North Carolina

Peter Winningham, MD
Resident, Diagnostic Radiology
Department of Radiology
Children's Mercy Hospital and Clinics
University of Missouri–Kansas City
Kansas City, Missouri

Edward Yang, MD, PhD
Instructor in Radiology
Director, Neuro MRI
Department of Radiology
Boston Children's Hospital
Harvard Medical School
Boston, Massachusetts

Hye-Kyung Yoon, MD, PhD
Professor of Radiology
Department of Radiology
Kangwon National University Hospital
Gangwon-do, South Korea

Yumin Zhong, MD, PhD
Assistant Professor of Radiology
Department of Radiology
Shanghai Children's Medical Center
Shanghai Jiao Tong University
Shanghai, China

Evan J. Zucker, MD
Assistant Professor of Clinical Radiology
Department of Radiology
Lucile Packard Children's Hospital
Stanford University
Stanford, California

PREFACE

Today, imaging evaluation is an integral component in the daily practice of managing infants and children with a variety of underlying congenital and acquired disorders. Pediatric radiology, unlike other radiology subspecialties, encompasses multiple organ systems and modalities and demands a solid foundation in the imaging of pediatric disease. To this end, the purpose of this book is to provide a comprehensive imaging review of pediatric disorders that are encountered in daily clinical practice.

The idea for this book arose from my interactions with residents, fellows, and faculty members of various specialties that I have encountered as a pediatric radiologist at Boston Children's Hospital, chair of the pediatric radiology section of the Core Examination Committee at American Board of Radiology (ABR), and visiting professor to more than 30 different countries around the world for the past 10 years. Everyone was looking for an up-to-date single volume resource for learning and reviewing the fundamentals and essentials of pediatric radiology. Such a textbook should be practical, covering both common and rare but significant pediatric disorders, while providing international perspectives to broaden its use in any part of the world. However, there was no such book available.

From this came my desire to write a pediatric radiology textbook, which increased every time I felt incomplete after giving pediatric radiology lectures to trainees and practicing radiologists, particularly during the international visiting professorships. It became clear to me that providing essential information about pediatric radiology can be best achieved by creating and organizing the material into a textbook that can reach people in every part of the world. The process of creating this textbook started with formulating an outline with five truly gifted radiology and pathology associate editors on topics that are important for the care of pediatric patients in daily clinical practice. This was later enhanced with exemplary cases that we encountered during our clinical work as well as cases provided by approximately 100 outstanding contributing authors from 40 different countries around the world. The authors who have contributed chapters to this book are recognized experts in their fields from six continents in the world, making this book truly international, current, and comprehensive, providing the most up-to-date information available. Also, many "textbook" images included in this book were given to me by "unknown" radiologists across the world that I have met during my international trips who wanted to share their cases and experience with others. Furthermore, relevant pathology of pediatric disorders is selectively included in order to enhance the understanding of the underlying disease process and radiologic imaging findings.

This book is organized into four main sections based on organ systems, which include pediatric neuroradiology, pediatric thoracic radiology, pediatric abdominopelvic radiology, and pediatric musculoskeletal radiology. The organization and presentation of this book is structured to provide accessibility to both common and less common but important pediatric disorders. Each chapter includes a discussion of practical imaging techniques, normal anatomy and variants, imaging findings, and selected pathologic features of congenital and acquired disorders in a specific section. The discussion of each disorder includes the clinical features, imaging findings, pathologic correlation in some selected cases, and up-to-date management information. Given its focus on disorders affecting the pediatric population, we have emphasized how to differentiate between the normal variants and abnormal pathology and to determine whether a certain radiologic finding is isolated or whether it is related to a genetic or malformation syndrome. In addition, when relevant and possible, differential diagnostic considerations and differentiating features, both clinical and radiologic, between disorders that produce similar imaging findings are also addressed. Every effort was made to cover the broad scope of pediatric radiology practice in a single-volume book without redundancy.

This book is intended primarily for radiology residents, radiology fellows, and practicing radiologists. However, other physicians, such as pediatricians and pediatric specialists, who frequently or occasionally encounter the pediatric patient for diagnostic imaging studies may derive valuable clinical, imaging, and some pathologic information that can be used to manage their pediatric patients.

It is my hope that readers, regardless of level of knowledge, training, and fields of specialties, will be more stimulated and interested in pediatric disorders and imaging after reading this book. If this book helps the readers to better understand the imaging evaluation of infants and children, leading to improvement in care and efficient management of pediatric patients, we will have accomplished our overarching goal. Behind all images that were included in this book, there were living and breathing pediatric patients who were often very sick and close to the end of their promised time in this world. We must recognize that we have an invaluable opportunity to make a true difference in their lives and the lives of their loved ones.

This book has been a journey, not a destination, for me and the associate editors. We invite the readers to join us in this journey of lifelong learning, and we look forward to feedback from readers about what can be improved and added in the next edition. Until then, we hope all the readers will enjoy and learn from this book as much as we did from preparing and writing it.

Edward Y. Lee

Contents

PART I

PEDIATRIC NEURORADIOLOGY

Winnie C. Chu

CHAPTER 1

Skull

Edward Yang • Sara O. Vargas • Tina Young Poussaint

INTRODUCTION

Suspected skull disorders are common indications for imaging in the pediatric age group, being easily identified by caregivers and physicians because of their superficial location. As an osseous structure, the skull manifests many of the pathologies seen elsewhere in the skeletal system, but it does so in the setting of dynamic changes of development and maturation of the skull itself as well as the brain that it protects.

This chapter reviews the radiographic anatomy and disorders affecting the skull as well as its connective tissue covering, the scalp, in the pediatric population. The chapter begins by considering the various modalities for performing an imaging examination of the pediatric skull. Next, normal imaging anatomy and skull development are discussed. Then, an overview is provided of the most commonly encountered diseases of the pediatric skull, including disorders of skull shape and integrity, infectious disorders, diffuse bone diseases, neoplasms affecting the skull and scalp, and features of skull trauma unique to the pediatric population.

IMAGING TECHNIQUES

Radiography

Radiography is the oldest imaging technique available for evaluating the skull and remains widely used because of its low cost, wide availability, and suitability in unsedated patients. In addition, it is associated with relatively low radiation dose compared to computed tomography (CT). Current indications include detection of diffuse bone abnormalities as part of a skeletal survey (e.g., metastatic disease, metabolic bone disease), screening for nonaccidental trauma (child abuse) in a neurologically intact child <2 years, and screening for craniosynostosis. Skull radiographs are also commonly used to assess surgical implants (e.g., shunts, programmable shunt valves, and cochlear implants) and to exclude the presence of radiopaque foreign bodies.

Standard skull radiography technique consists of frontal (usually posteroanterior [PA]), lateral, and Townes projections (Fig. 1.1). Whereas the petrous apices project over the central orbits in the PA projection, they are above the orbits in the Townes view because of angulation used for better visualization of the occipital bone and foramen magnum. An optional view opening up the frontal bone is the Caldwell projection where the petrous apices lie below the orbits. An age-specific dose is delivered with collimation to cover the osseous structures and overlying scalp. Typical delivered skin dose is ~1 mGy, and there is an estimated effective dose of ~0.02 mSv under these conditions.[1]

Ultrasound

Sound waves penetrate osseous structures poorly and therefore ultrasound is not a widely used imaging modality for the skull in most institutions. However, the availability of ultrasound at the point of care and the lack of radiation exposure have prompted the use of ultrasound for selected indications in young (<2 years old) patients who have little hair and relatively sonolucent osseous structures. Specifically, ultrasound has been used to successfully detect skull fractures and sutural synostosis.[2–5] Additionally, ultrasound has long been a first-line tool for evaluating scalp masses.[6,7]

Ultrasound of the skull uses high-frequency (typically >8 MHz) linear transducers coupled with transducing gel. Adjustments are performed to reduce the depth and focus to accommodate the superficial structures being imaged. Typically, stand-off pads are not required. For soft tissue or

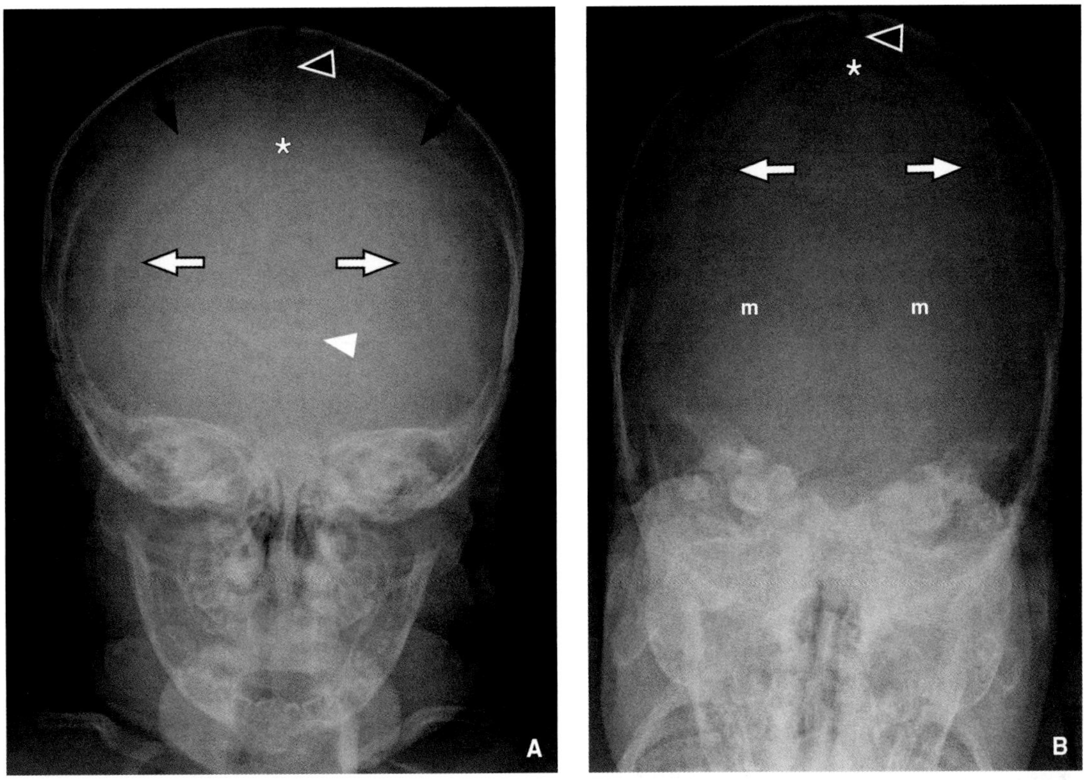

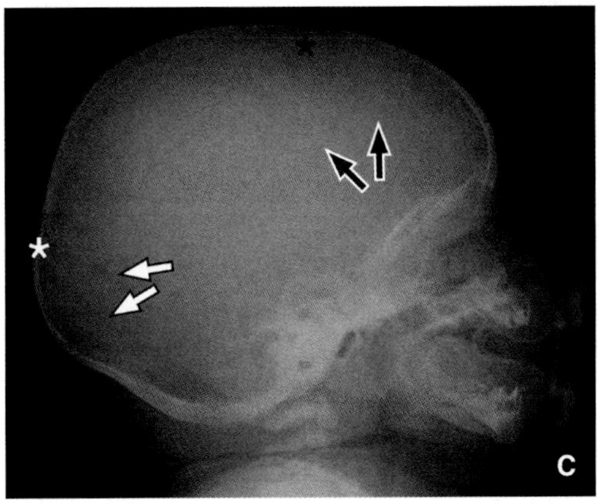

FIGURE 1.1 **Skull radiographs of a normal 3-month-old boy: posteroanterior (PA) (A), Townes (B), and lateral (C) projections.** *Black arrows* indicate coronal sutures, *black arrowhead* the sagittal suture, *white arrows* the lambdoid sutures, *white arrowhead* the metopic suture, *white asterisk* the posterior fontanelle, *black asterisk* the anterior fontanelle, and "*m*" the mendosal sutures.

vascular scalp lesions, color and duplex Doppler are added to demonstrate lesional vascularity and pulsatility of blood flow (i.e., arterial versus venous).

Computed Tomography

As a high-resolution, cross-sectional technique with excellent osseous detail and soft tissue contrast, computed tomography (CT) is the current reference standard for indications such as head trauma, craniosynostosis, and characterization of focal skull lesions. Although some authors have proposed algorithms that omit CT for single-suture synostosis,[8–10] CT has superior sensitivity/specificity for detecting synostosis as it can detect even small areas of osseous bridging that may elude radiography.[11–13] There are also data to suggest that CT becomes increasingly cost-effective for individuals with a high pretest likelihood of synostosis, particularly involving multiple sutures. Regardless of diagnostic strategy for abnormal head shape, common clinical practice is to obtain a head CT with three-dimensional (3D) surface rendering for cases that are scheduled for surgery as the surface model assists procedural planning.[11,14] For reasons discussed later (see "Fractures"), the American College of Radiology Appropriateness Criteria endorses an approach that integrates head CT when imaging is pursued for abusive or nonabusive head trauma.[15,16]

Acquisition of a head CT depends on both the precise hardware available as well as the indication. For most modern multidetector CT instruments, axial acquisition of the head is followed by generation of both submillimeter (isotropic) and 3- to 5-mm-thick data using soft tissue (brain) and bone kernels. The submillimeter data can then be used to create multiplanar reformatted images and surface rendered data, the latter particularly helpful in delineating complex 3D relationships of skull lesions. In our institution, an age-specific dosage scheme[17] compliant with recommendations from both the Society for Pediatric Radiology Image Gently campaign and the ACR CT Accreditation Requirements is used,[18,19] the latter limiting the CT dose index ($CTDI_{vol}$) for a 1-year-old to 40 mGy compared to 80 mGy for an adult. For pediatric patients undergoing evaluation for craniofacial dysmorphism, the field of view is extended below the mandible to capture any facial bone abnormalities, and the dose is reduced to 100 kV and 50 mAs, resulting in a CTDI <5 mGy. The trade-off for this reduced dose is poorer parenchymal detail. Even with these attempts to reduce dose, it is worth noting that a standard head CT still carries an estimated dose that is 20 times a single projection skull radiograph.[20]

Magnetic Resonance Imaging

Magnetic resonance imaging (MRI) has several advantages for imaging of the skull and overlying scalp including superior soft tissue contrast and the ability to suppress fat signal within the skull or scalp. For these reasons, MRI is often used to further characterize soft tissue masses in the scalp and discrete osseous lesions (e.g., primary bone tumors, metastases).[21–24] It also easily depicts communication of scalp/skull lesions with the intracranial contents, a common concern when the differential diagnosis includes lesions such as cephaloceles, sinus pericranii, and dermoid cysts.

The optimal MR protocol for evaluation of a scalp or cranial vault lesion includes at least two planes of fat-suppressed T2-weighted MR imaging (usually, short tau inversion recovery [STIR]) and two planes of contrast-enhanced T1-weighted MR imaging with fat suppression. Advanced imaging techniques such as diffusion-weighted imaging have also been applied to the skull to assess for pathology such as metastatic disease and osteomyelitis.[25,26] In combination with standard brain MRI sequences, these additional sequences make intrinsic marrow signal abnormalities, focal osseous lesions, and soft tissue masses of the scalp conspicuous as the background signal from fat is suppressed. However, erosion of the skull and skull fractures remain poorly seen compared to CT because of the comparatively low spatial resolution of MR.[27,28] New MRI techniques are attempting to address these limitations but are not yet widely used outside of research settings.[29,30]

Nuclear Medicine

Positron and gamma ray emitting radiotracers are rarely used specifically to detect skull pathology. In the case of skull fractures (inflicted or accidental), it is widely accepted that skull fractures do not reliably appear on technetium-based bone scans because of poor callus formation though bone scintigraphy remains commonly performed for detection of fractures elsewhere.[31,32] Whether introduction of ^{18}F-fluorine PET improves sensitivity awaits further investigation.[33] For infections of the skull, there is adult literature that suggests gallium and technetium radiotracers may have some utility particularly for skull base infections,[34–36] but MRI can provide similar information while simultaneously evaluating for intracranial pathology. For oncologic indications, several radiotracers remain in wide use for screening of metastatic disease and can therefore suggest skull involvement. These include staging for tumors common to the cranial vault such as Langerhans cell histiocytosis (technetium 99m methylene diphosphonate [Tc99m-MDP] and ^{18}F-fluorodeoxyglucose [FDG])[37,38] and neuroblastoma (Tc99m-MDP, ^{123}I-metaiodobenzyguanidine [MIBG], and FDG).[39,40]

NORMAL ANATOMY

Major Sutures and Fontanelles

Sutures are fibrous articulations between bones of the cranial vault that develop by intramembranous ossification. The skull base (sphenoid, ethmoid, nonsquamous temporal bone, and occipital bone below the superior nuchal line) develop with enchondral ossification, and therefore the articulations of the skull base ossification centers are called *synchondroses*.[41–44] The major sutures of the cranial vault include the *sagittal suture* separating the paired parietal bones, the *metopic suture* separating the two halves of the frontal bone, the *coronal suture* separating the frontal and parietal bones, and the *lambdoid suture* separating the occipital and parietal bones (Figs. 1.1 and 1.2).

Major openings present at birth include the *anterior fontanelle* at the junction of the coronal/sagittal sutures (called the *bregma* when closed) and the *posterior fontanelle* at the junction of the lambdoid sutures (called the *lambda* when closed).

Accessory/Minor Sutures

A number of minor sutures are seen in the vicinity of the squamous temporal bone, including the *sphenotemporal (sphenosquamous) suture* anteriorly, *temporoparietal (squamous) suture* superiorly, and the *occipitomastoid suture* posteriorly (Fig. 1.2).[45] The H-shaped junction where the sphenoparietal suture meets the coronal/frontosphenoid sutures anteriorly and the sphenotemporal/temporoparietal sutures posteriorly is called the *pterion*. The complexity of occipital bone development (at least eight ossification centers) gives rise to a number of transient sutures in this region (Fig. 1.3). Common transient sutures include midline *superior and inferior occipital fissures* at the lambda and foramen magnum, respectively; *mendosal sutures* including forms dividing the squamous occipital bone transversely; and paired *anterior/posterior intraoccipital synchondroses* that straddle the anterior and posterior extent of the foramen magnum at the skull base.[46–48]

Normal Development and Timing of Suture Closure

The initial ossification of the skull begins at a few months of gestation and is largely complete by term delivery.[49] The

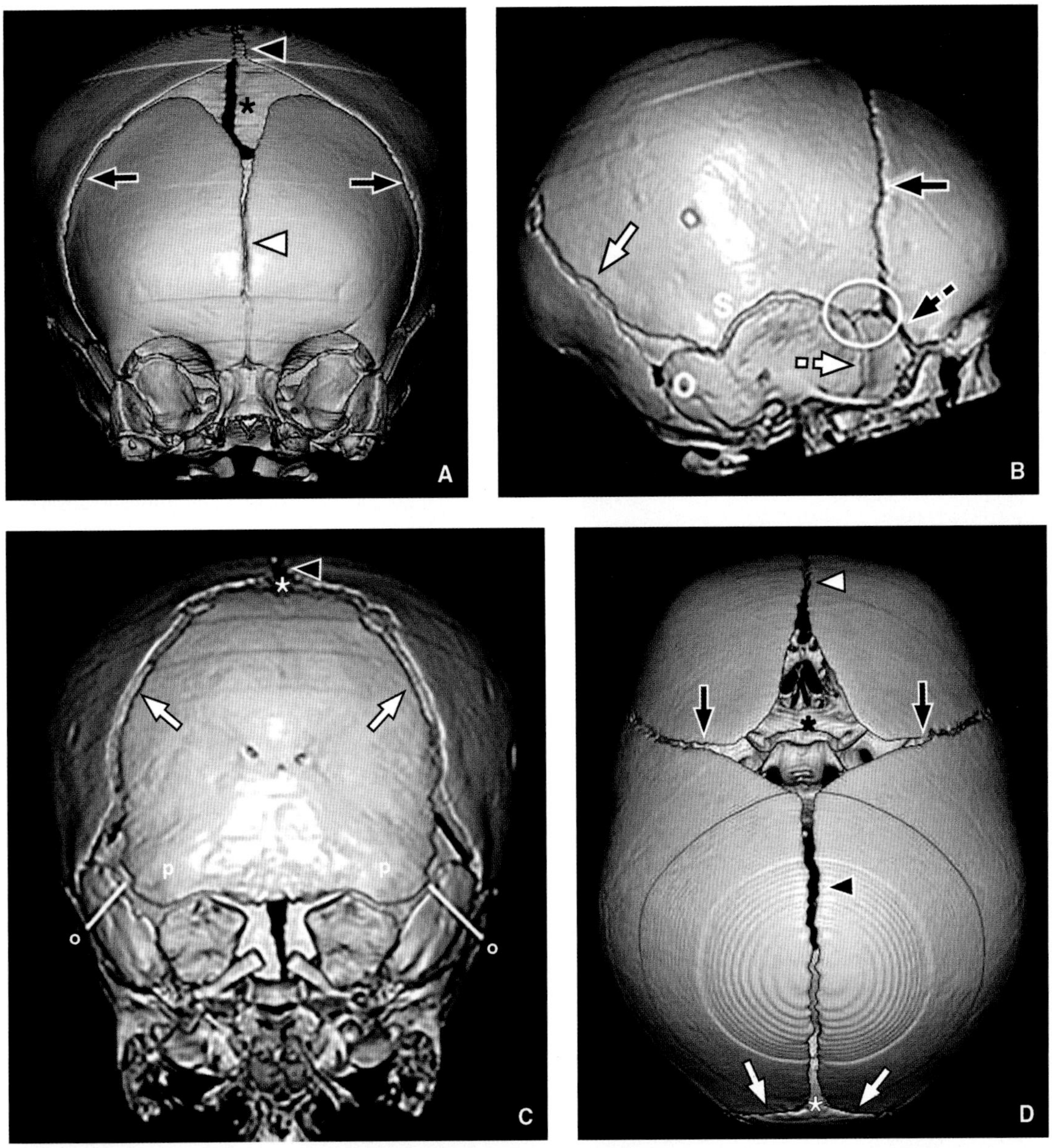

FIGURE 1.2 **Three-dimensional surface renderings of a head CT from a normal 3-month-old boy evaluated for craniosynostosis: frontal (A), lateral (B), posterior (C), and superior (D) views.** Annotations as for Figure 1.1 with additional markings of pterion with a circle, squamous (temporoparietal) suture with "s," sphenotemporal suture with *white dashed arrow*, frontosphenoid suture with *black dashed arrow*, occipitomastoid suture with "o," and posterior intraoccipital synchondrosis with "p."

sutures and skull base synchondroses are patent at birth and then begin to close at variable rates. However, two useful rules of thumb are that no major suture should close in the first year of life and no suture should undergo mature fusion in childhood except for the metopic suture, which normally closes at 3 to 9 months.[44,50–54] As the patient ages, the sutures become more serrated at their outer table though they remain smooth along the inner table.[55,56] For cases where there is subjective narrowing, normative neonatal data have been published for selected sutures based on CT data.[57] Important synchondrosis milestones include closure of frontosphenoid and intersphenoid synchondroses by 1 to 2 years of age and of the sphenoccipital (clival) synchondroses during adolescence.[58] Closure of synchondroses and sutures within the occipital bone follow a more complicated sequence. The synchondroses at the foramen magnum typically close within the first few months of life though other sutures including mendosal sutures and inferior occipital fissure may persist through the first few years of life[47,48,58,59]; variants where these sutures/synchondroses persist into adulthood are occasionally encountered. The anterior and posterolateral fontanelles typically close by the end of the 2nd year. The posterior fontanelle closes much earlier, typically by 3 to 6 months.[60]

Deviations from normal sutural closing (apparent sutural widening) are present in conditions of poor bone

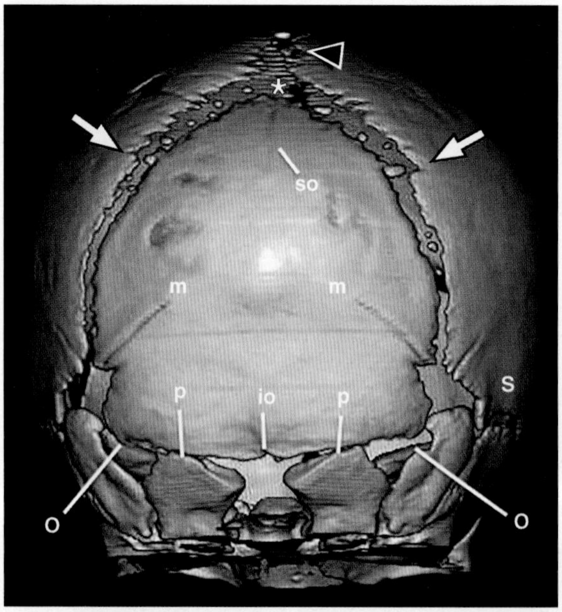

FIGURE 1.3 **Transient sutures of the occipital bone visualized on a three-dimensional surface rendering of a 1-month-old boy's head CT (posterior view).** Markings are as for Figures 1.1 and 1.2 but additional sutures marked include "so", "m", and "io" for superior occipital, paired mendosal sutures, and inferior occipital sutures, respectively.

mineralization (osteogenesis imperfecta, rickets, hypothyroidism) and can be misinterpreted as sutural diastasis from elevated intracranial pressure. Other reported causes of apparent widening of normal sutural width include recovery from chronic malnutrition, in utero renin-angiotensin system disruption (Fig. 1.4), achondroplasia, trisomy 21, and treatment with prostaglandins for prematurity.[61–65]

SPECTRUM OF SKULL DISORDERS

Congenital and Developmental Anomalies

Craniosynostosis

Craniosynostosis refers to premature closure of the cranial sutures (segmental or total) with resultant deformity. Craniosynostoses are usually classified as *primary* or *secondary*, secondary forms representing the consequence of an identifiable cause unrelated to suture development, such as metabolic bone disease, bone dysplasia, or loss of intracranial volume (e.g., shunting, brain injury). The primary craniosynostoses are further divided into *single* versus *multiple suture* forms and *syndromic* versus *nonsyndromic (isolated)* forms.

The overall incidence of craniosynostosis is low, ~3 to 10 cases per 10,000 live births.[13,66] Craniosynostosis typically presents in the neonatal period and occasionally in utero though certain secondary craniosynostoses may present much later in childhood.[67] Upward of 80% of craniosynostosis cases are of the primary nonsyndromic (isolated form), ~75% to 80% being single-suture involvement and 20% to 25% being multiple sutures.[68,69] Excluding rare instances of secondary craniosynostosis, the remaining cases consist of syndromic synostoses that typically involve multiple sutures. Craniosynostosis is seen more commonly with advanced parental age, multiparity, extremes of fetal weight, and (except for unilateral coronal synostosis) male gender.[66,70,71] Although nonsyndromic causes of synostosis are generally viewed as idiopathic/sporadic, it is worth noting that a minority (~10%) of nonsyndromic synostosis has familial transmission (i.e., genetic cause); these familial nonsyndromic cases have a majority (2/3) of bicoronal synostosis compared to the nonsyndromic, nonfamilial cases where unicoronal synostosis constitutes 2/3 of cases.[66,71–73] This

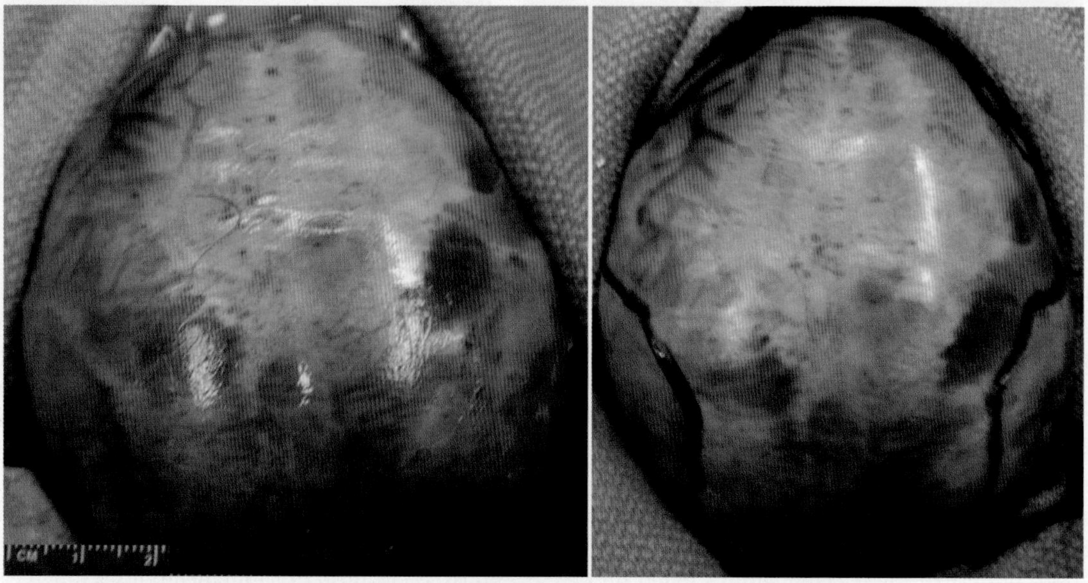

FIGURE 1.4 **Markedly widened cranial sutures (hypocalvarium) in a 1-day-old girl with renal tubular agenesis, pulmonary hypoplasia, and other skeletal anomalies suggesting in utero exposure to renin–angiotensin system blockers or an inborn error in the renin–angiotensin system.** Reflection of the scalp at autopsy shows only a thin membrane covering much of the cerebrum. In the right panel, the margins of the fontanelles are outlined in black ink.

fact may be explained by the increasing detection of mutations responsible for syndromic synostosis in "nonsyndromic" synostosis patients, and therefore many authorities advise genetic screening in coronal synostosis patients.[74–76]

As first recognized by Virchow in the mid-19th century,[77] premature fusion of a suture results in constriction of skull growth in the direction perpendicular to the affected suture and compensatory elongation of the skull in dimensions parallel to the abnormal suture. This simple principle explains the many patterns of deformity seen with craniosynostoses, recently reviewed in detail elsewhere.[78]

Sagittal synostosis is the single most common craniosynostosis, accounting for roughly half of the nonsyndromic cases of craniosynostosis.[66,68,70] Sagittal synostosis causes *scaphocephaly* or transverse narrowing with anteroposterior elongation of the skull, usually with some associated ridging at the site of fusion (Fig. 1.5).

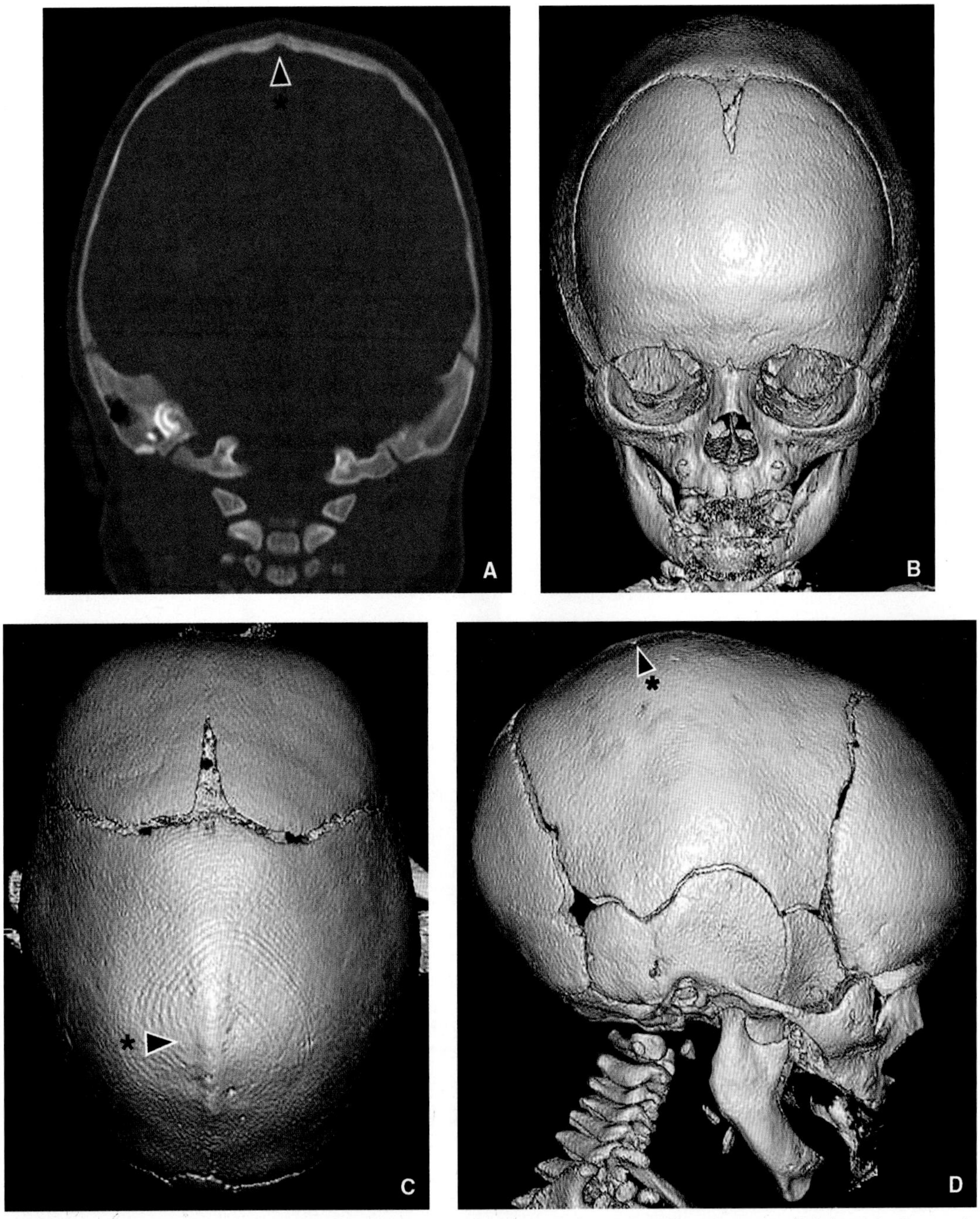

FIGURE 1.5 **Sagittal synostosis in a 3-month-old boy with dolichocephaly and midline osseous ridging. A:** Coronal reformatted bone window CT image shows premature fusion of the sagittal suture accompanied by osseous ridging (*asterisked black arrowhead*). **B–D:** Frontal **(B)**, superior **(C)**, and right lateral **(D)** surface rendering CT images confirm the osseous ridging and depict the elongated AP dimension of the skull consistent with clinical impression of dolichocephaly. When accompanied by osseous ridging, dolichocephaly is called scaphocephaly, a characteristic appearance for sagittal synostosis. Note that the metopic suture has already undergone fusion without deformity, consistent with normal closure.

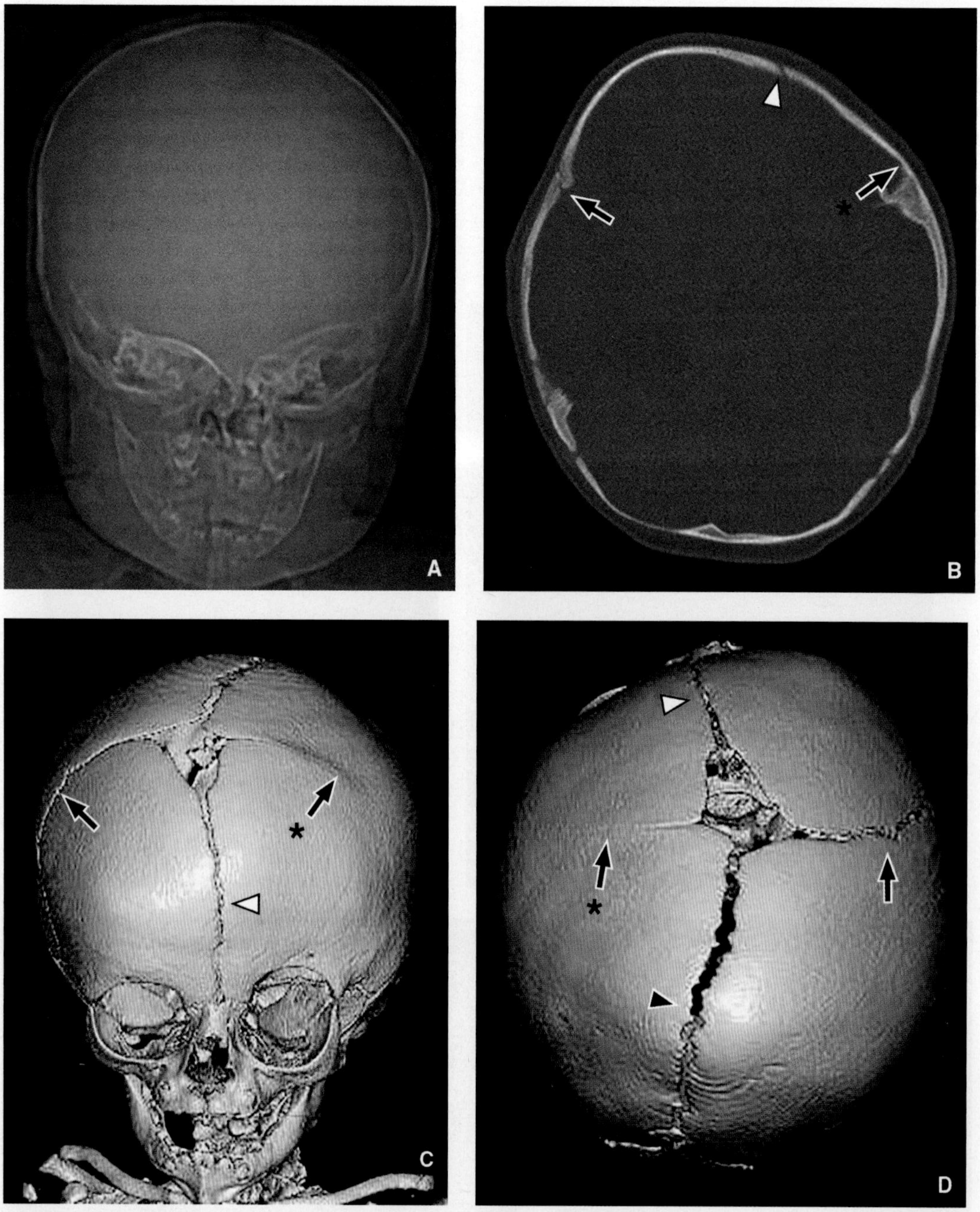

FIGURE 1.6 **Unilateral coronal synostosis in a 4-month-old boy with abnormal head shape. A:** Frontal projection CT topogram demonstrates elevation of the left orbital rim. **B:** Axial bone window CT image demonstrates premature fusion of the left coronal suture (abnormal side *asterisked arrow*). **C and D:** Three-dimensional surface rendering CT images in the frontal **(C)** and superior **(D)** perspective demonstrate left frontal plagiocephaly and right frontal bossing with retraction of the metopic suture to the left. Labeling conventions as for Figure 1.2 with abnormally fused left coronal suture denoted by an *asterisked black arrow*.

Coronal synostosis can be either unilateral or bilateral. For unilateral coronal synostosis, there is flattening of the frontal bone (anterior plagiocephaly) with some compensatory bulging of the contralateral frontal bone and skewing the metopic suture to the ipsilateral side. There is also upward slanting of the lateral orbital rim ("harlequin" deformity) from retraction of the ipsilateral frontal bone and orbital roof (Fig. 1.6). In cases of bilateral coronal synostosis, the harlequin orbit deformity is bilateral and the overall anteroposterior dimension of the skull is reduced, a morphology known as *brachycephaly* (Fig. 1.7).

Metopic synostosis causes narrowing of the frontal bone into a beak-like configuration termed *trigonocephaly*. Historically, metopic synostosis has been thought to be relatively rare at ~5% to 10% of nonsyndromic craniosynostosis, but multiple studies of the past 10 to 15 years have documented an increase of up to 20% of nonsyndromic craniosynostosis.[70,79,80] The

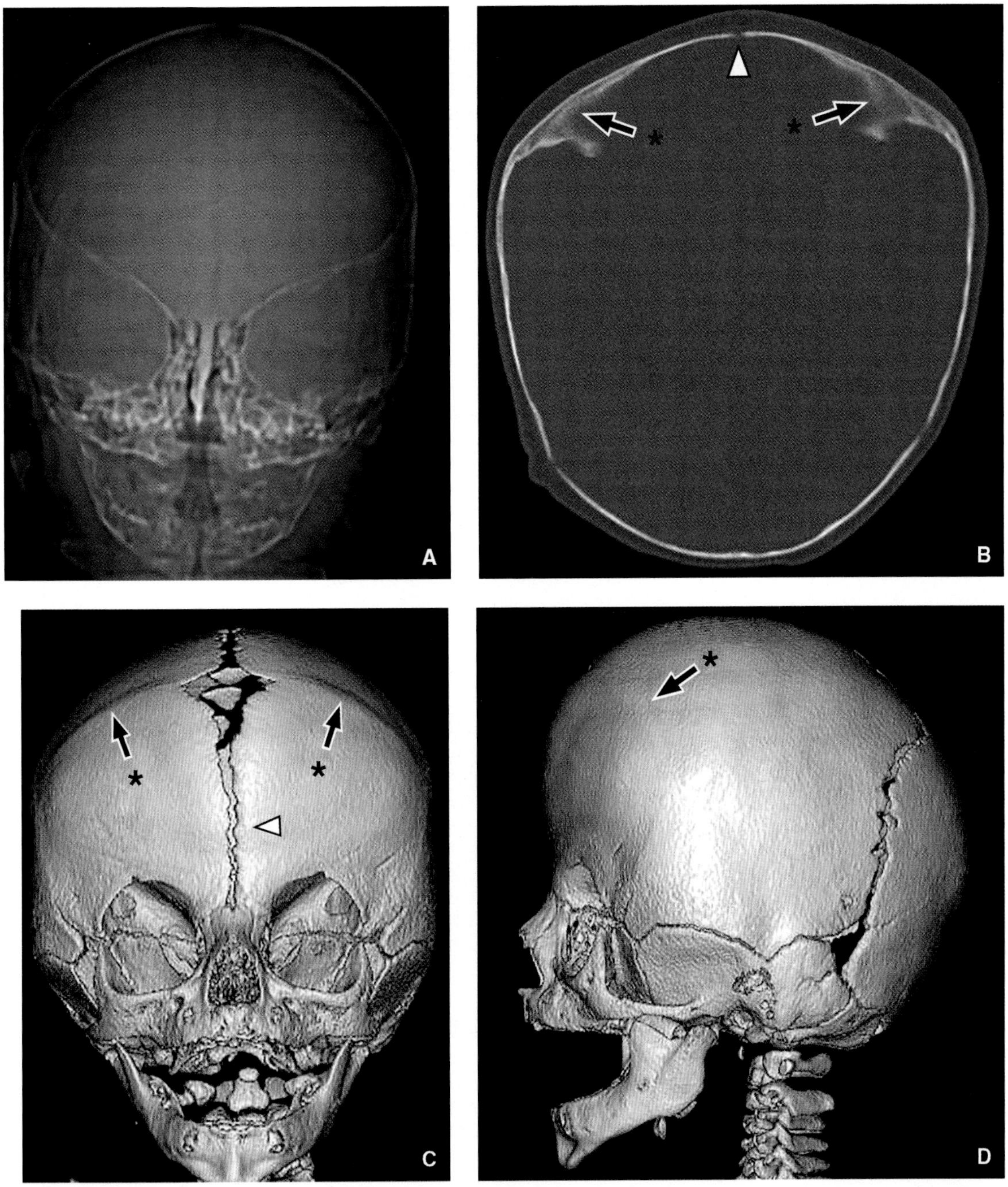

FIGURE 1.7 **Bicoronal synostosis in a 2-month-old boy with skull deformity. A:** Frontal projection CT topogram shows bilateral harlequin deformities of the orbits. **B:** Axial bone window CT image demonstrates bilateral anterior plagiocephaly and premature fusion of both coronal sutures (*asterisked black arrows* with metopic suture denoted by *white arrowhead*). **C and D:** Surface rendering CT images confirm premature fusion and ridging of the coronal sutures with upward retraction of the orbits in the frontal view **(C)** as well as brachycephaly on the lateral view **(D)**.

classic findings of metopic synostosis include retraction of the supraorbital ridges medially, bossing of the parietal bones, hypoplastic ethmoid sinuses, and a W-shaped metopic notch of the endocranial surface of the fused metopic suture (Fig. 1.8).[54,78,81]

Lambdoid synostosis is the most rare of the single-suture synostoses, estimated at <5% of nonsyndromic craniosynostoses.[70] After successful implementation of the "Back to Sleep" program by pediatricians in the 1990s, there was a spike in the diagnosis of lambdoid synostosis, which later proved to be due to misdiagnosis of posterior deformational plagiocephaly (see below).[82,83] In addition to posterior plagiocephaly, true lambdoid synostosis features compensatory enlargement of the ipsilateral frontal bone and contralateral occipital bone as well as skewing of the occipital protuberance towards the side of the synostosis (Fig. 1.9A–C).[84]

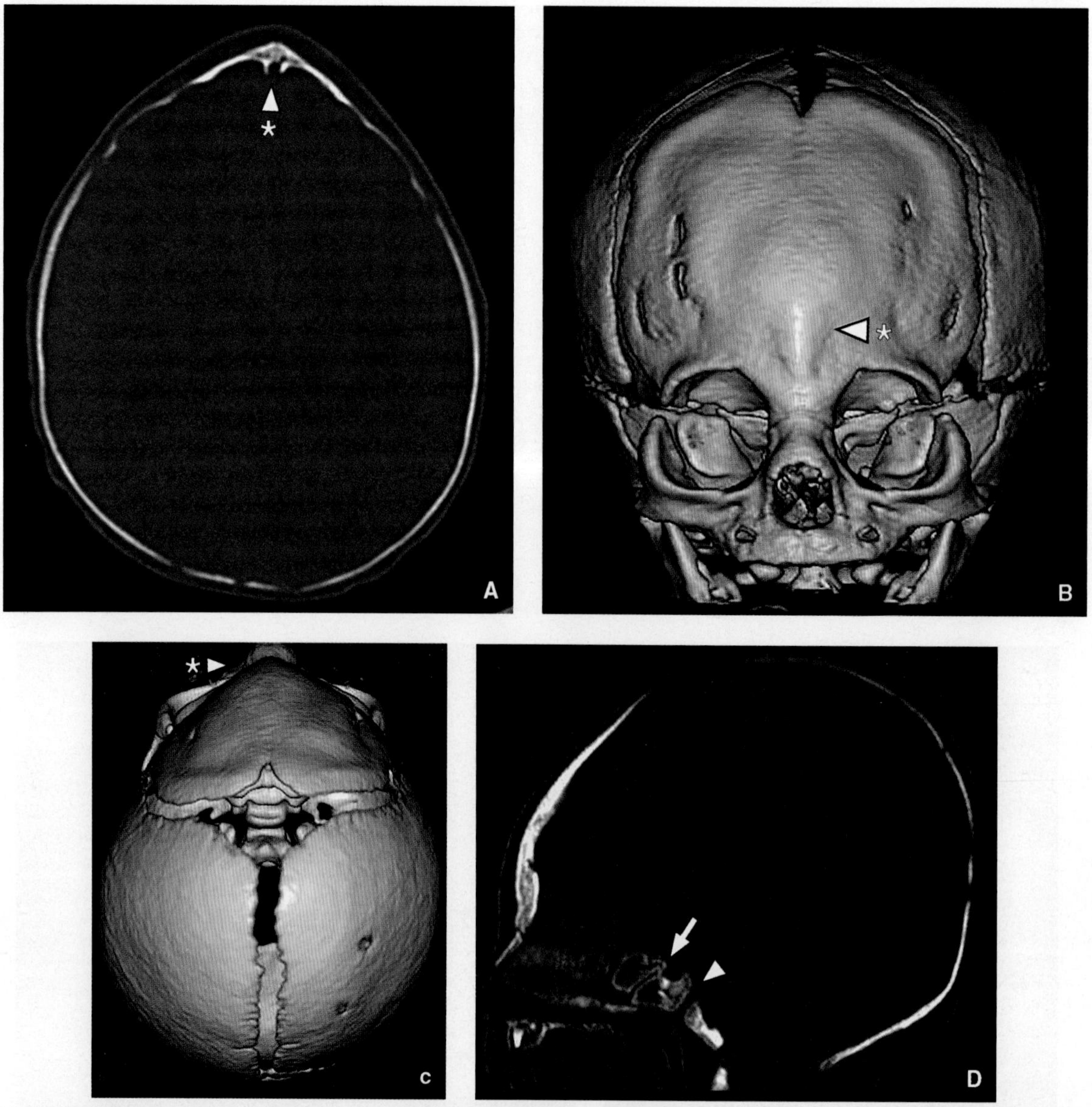

FIGURE 1.8 **Metopic synostosis in a 24-day-old boy with trigonocephaly. A:** Axial bone window CT image confirms trigonocephaly with prominent osseous ridge and metopic notch (*asterisked white arrowhead*) at the site of the prematurely fused metopic suture. **B and C:** Frontal and superior surface rendering CT images **(B and C)** show retraction of the medial orbital, hypotelorism, and the contour deformity of the skull. **D:** Sagittal reformatted CT image demonstrates an incidentally noted persistent craniopharyngeal canal (*arrow*) anterior to the normal spheno-occipital synchondrosis (*arrowhead*).

Craniosynostosis involving multiple sutures can result in unusual shapes.[85] *Turricephaly/oxycephaly* result from bilateral lambdoid synostosis with craniocaudal elongation of the calvaria and bulging at the vertex; this appearance can also be encountered with bicoronal synostosis (Fig. 1.10). When lambdoid, coronal, and sagittal sutures are all fused, there is bulging of the cranial vault where unconstrained by synostosis; this is known as the cloverleaf skull or *kleeblattschädel* (Fig. 1.11).

Syndromic craniosynostosis presents with characteristic additional clinical examination or radiographic findings. The features of the more common syndromic synostoses are summarized in Table 1.1. The major areas of differentiation between the syndromes are the findings outside of the cranial vault, namely findings in the extremities. Bicoronal synostosis (with or without additional sutures), midface hypoplasia, hypertelorism, and varying degrees of exorbitism (proptosis) are commonly seen in all the syndromic craniosynostoses (Figs. 1.10 to 1.12). These similarities are shared at a molecular level as many of the classically recognized syndromes share abnormalities in fibroblast growth factor receptor signaling.

Secondary craniosynostoses are rare, but the most frequent causes in routine clinical practice include overshunting and

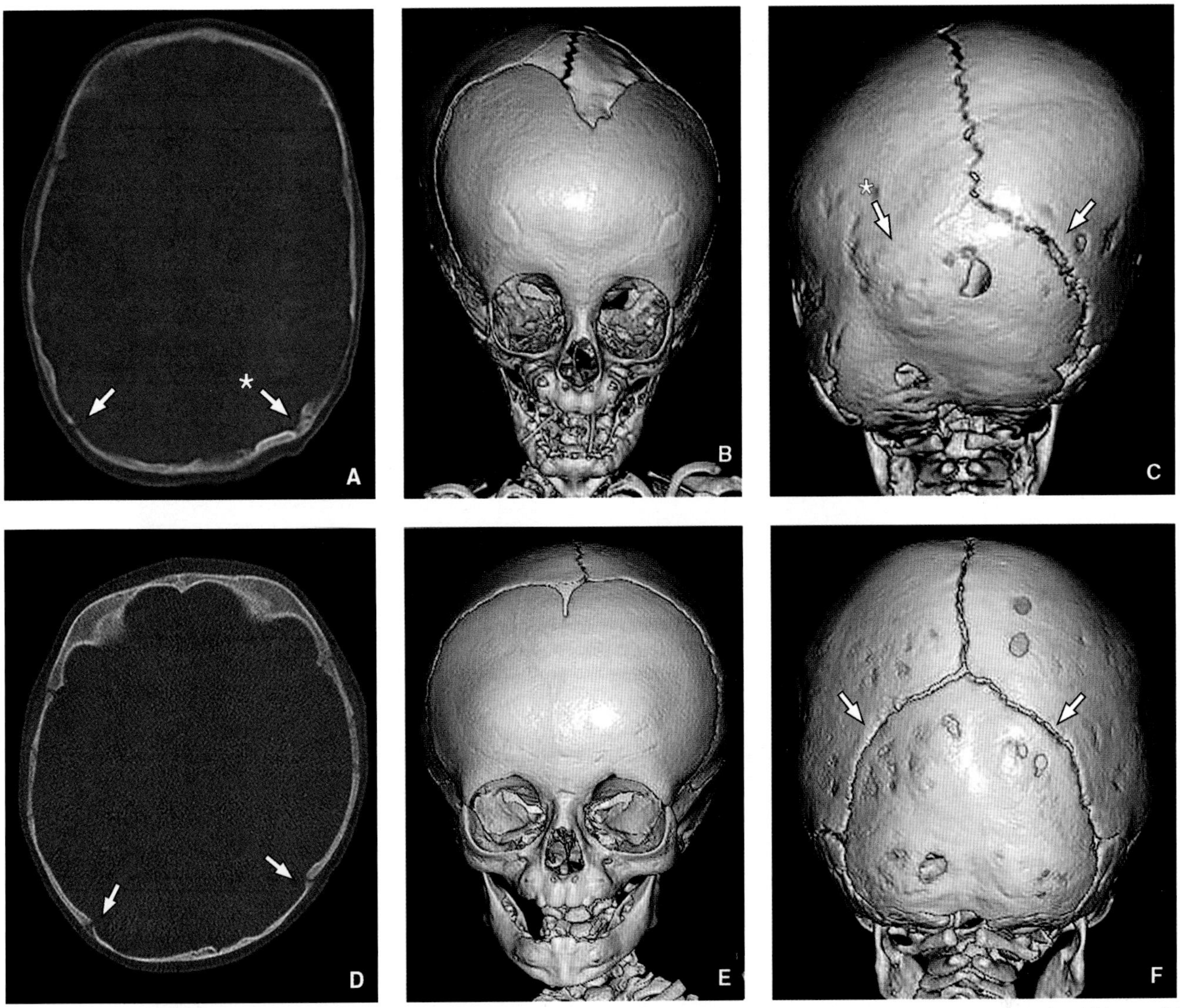

FIGURE 1.9 **Comparison of lambdoid synostosis and posterior deformational plagiocephaly. A–C:** A 6-month-old boy with left posterior plagiocephaly due to left lambdoid synostosis. Axial bone window CT image **(A)** demonstrates fusion and osseous ridging of the left lambdoid suture (*white arrows*, abnormal side *asterisked*). Frontal and posterior surface rendering CT images **(B and C)** show the premature fusion of the left lambdoid suture and also suggest subtle frontal bossing and skewing of the lambda to the left. **D–F:** Comparison case of a 6-month-old boy with deformational left posterior plagiocephaly. Axial bone window CT image demonstrates patency of the lambdoid suture on the affected side **(D)**, confirmed with surface renderings in the frontal and posterior perspective **(E and F)**.

massive brain injury.[86] In both instances, the intracranial volume contracts, resulting in overlapping sutures and premature fusion with osseous ridging (Fig. 1.13). Other reported associations include underlying disorders of bone metabolism, such as rickets; bone dysplasias, such as achondroplasia; metabolic disorders, such as mucopolysaccharidoses; in utero compression; hematologic disorders, such as sickle cell and polycythemia; endocrine disorders, such as hyperthyroidism; and any cause of poor underlying brain growth.[87–96]

Several disorders feature abnormal head shape without fusion of sutures and must be distinguished from true craniosynostosis. Since the institution of the "Back to Sleep" campaign to prevent sudden infant death syndrome, the incidence of *posterior deformational plagiocephaly* has increased by several orders of magnitude and may be seen in up to 13% of infants according to some estimates.[83] Unlike lambdoid synostosis, posterior plagiocephaly does not have associated fusion of the suture (Fig. 1.9D–F) and can usually be managed conservatively with attention to sleeping position. Although it is said that lambdoid synostosis and deformational plagiocephaly pull and push the ipsilateral ear respectively, there is evidence that this physical finding is relatively unreliable.[97,98] A bony ridge along a closed metopic suture, the *metopic ridge*, is present in up to 5% of normal individuals[78] and is distin-

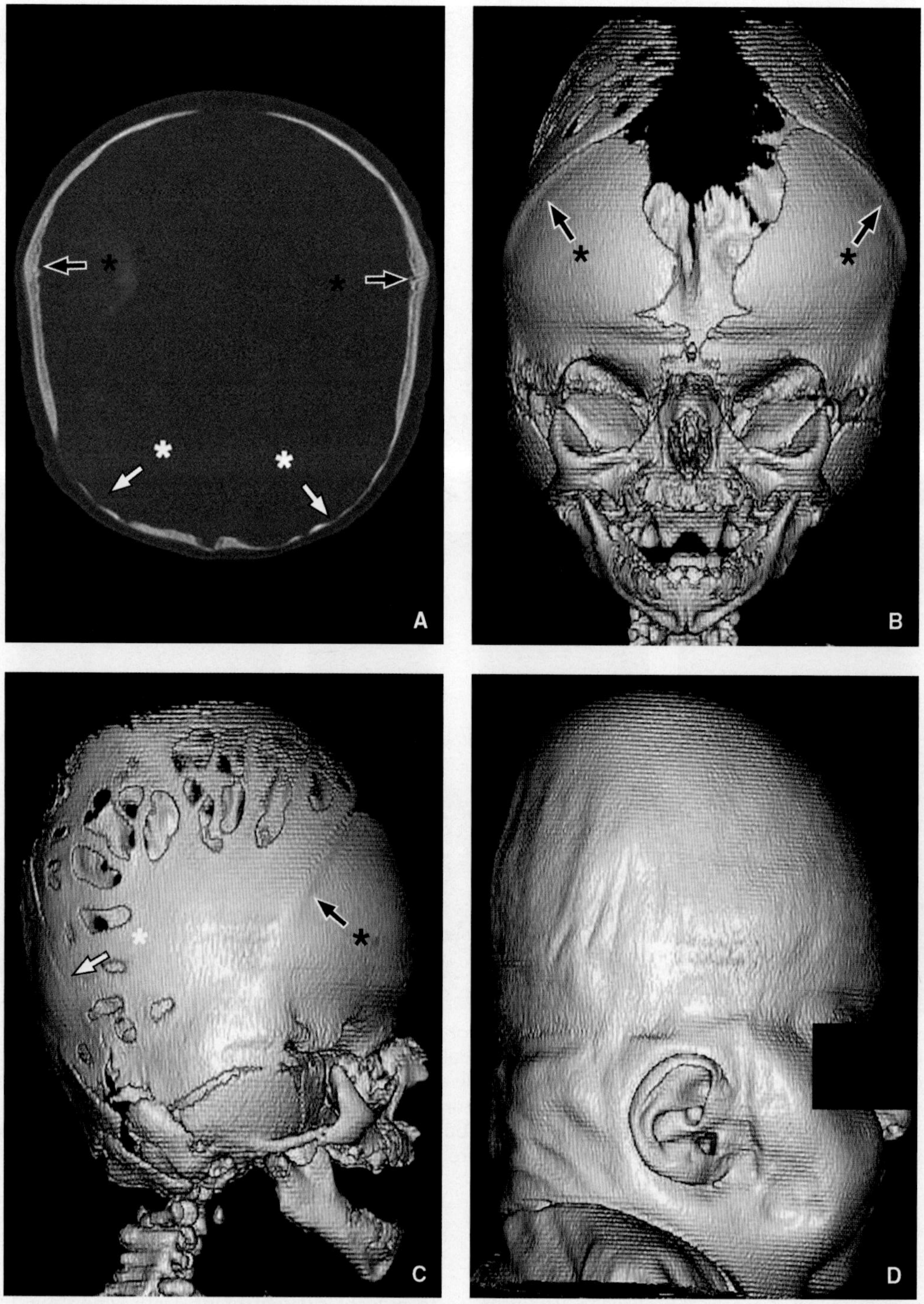

FIGURE 1.10 **Newborn girl with turricephaly and syndactyly at birth, subsequently diagnosed with Apert syndrome. A:** Axial bone window CT image demonstrates bilateral coronal and lambdoid suture synostosis (fused coronal sutures marked with *asterisked black arrows* and lambdoid sutures with *asterisked white arrows*). **B and C:** Frontal **(B)** and right lateral **(C)** perspective surface rendering CT images confirm the synostosis and demonstrate the "towering" appearance of the cranial vault. **D:** Soft tissue windowing of the lateral perspective surface rendered CT image depicts the resulting deformity as viewed externally.

guished from true metopic synostosis by the absence of trigonocephaly.[99] *Dolichocephaly* refers to narrowing of the cranial vault, according to some authors defined as a cephalic index (width:length of skull) <0.75.[100] Dolichocephaly differs from scaphocephaly in that the latter has premature fusion/ridging of the sagittal suture, whereas the former is typically caused by positioning in premature infants.[78,100]

The current surgical approach to craniosynostosis is to perform the initial surgery in the first year of life; some institutions prefer to operate before 6 months and others pre-

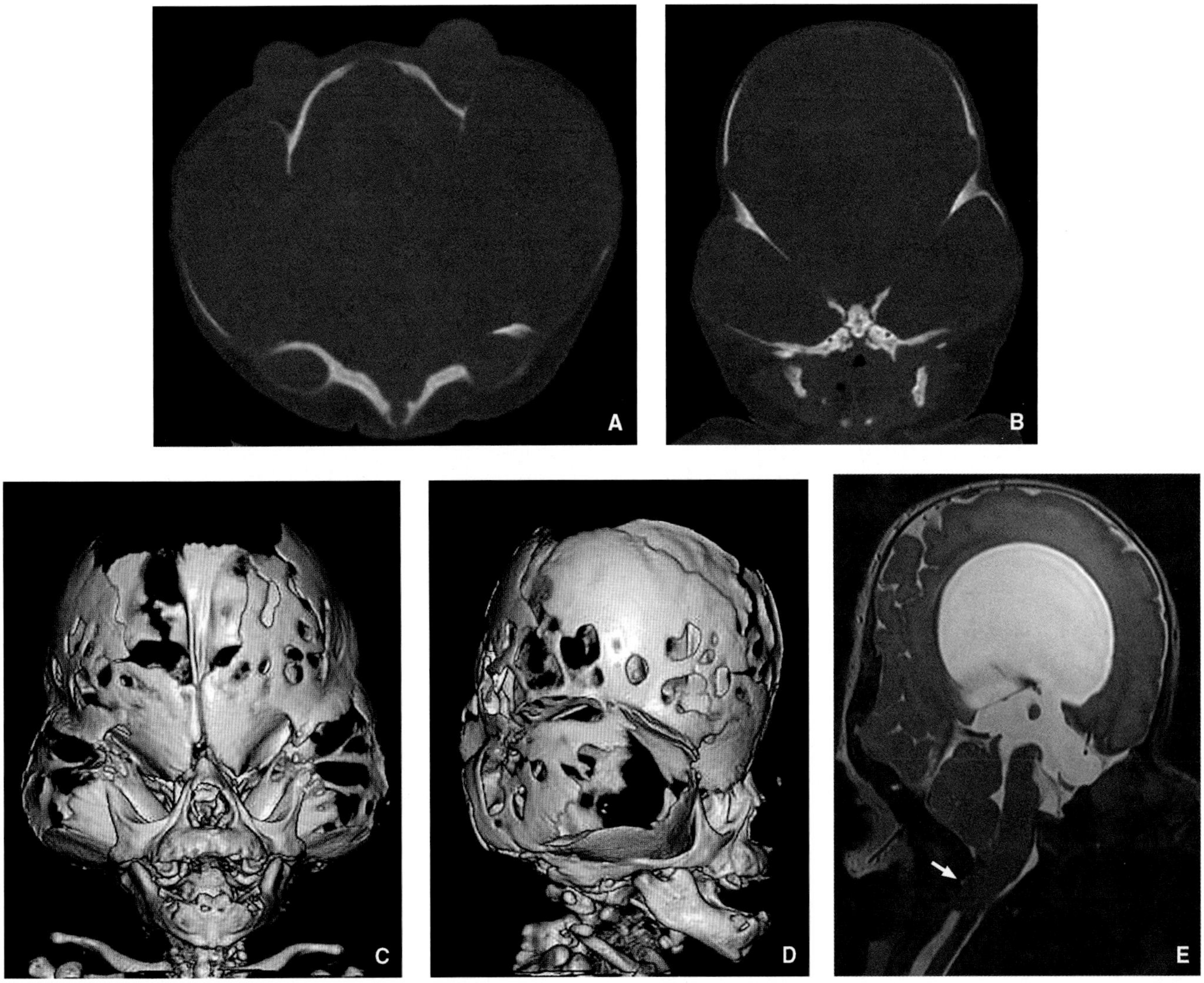

FIGURE 1.11 **Kleeblatschädel or "cloverleaf" skull deformity in a newborn boy with Pfeiffer syndrome and pansynostosis. A and B:** Axial **(A)** and coronal reformatted **(B)** bone window CT images demonstrate constraint along all major (coronal, lambdoid, sagittal) and some minor (squamosal) sutures with bulging of the cranial vault between the abnormally fused sutures. Note also the profound exorbitism. **C and D:** Frontal **(C)** and right lateral **(D)** perspective surface renderings depict the distorted cranial vault in three dimensions as well as the markedly enlarged anterior fontanelle. **E:** Midsagittal T2-weighted MR image demonstrates associated Chiari I malformation (*white arrow*) and hydrocephalus (ballooning of the infundibular recess of the third ventricle).

fer later surgery (better tolerance of blood loss).[101] However, evidence of elevated intracranial pressure (e.g., papilledema or lacunar changes mentioned under the section "Variants") is widely accepted as an indication for early surgery regardless of institutional preference, being uncommon in single-suture synostosis and present in the majority of patients with syndromic, multisuture synostosis.[81,102] Furthermore, a significant minority of syndromic patients require management of additional complications such as communicating hydrocephalus or Chiari I malformations (Fig. 1.11E).[103,104] The syndromic patients also have a high incidence of midface hypoplasia with associated complications of exorbitism/keratitis and respiratory compromise from the midface retrusion.[102,105,106] For single-suture craniosynostosis, surgery generally includes radial and barrel stave osteotomies to remodel the cranial vault and orbitofrontal advancement to normalize the position of the bony orbits.[81] Although simple excision of an abnormal suture has historically been avoided because of poor outcomes, newer endoscopic approaches have found success in patients <6 months when augmented by spacers and postoperative helmeting.[107] In the case of syndromic/multisuture craniosynostosis, it is not uncommon for revision surgeries to be performed later in addition to multistage advancement of the hypoplastic midface through LeFort osteotomies.[102]

TABLE 1.1 Features of the Syndromic Craniosynostoses

Syndrome	Incidence	Transmission	Gene	Clinical Manifestations	References
Apert (acrocephalosyndactyly I)	1:100,000	AD	FGFR2	• Craniosynostosis (bicoronal) • Midface hypoplasia, cleft or high-arched palate, exorbitism, hypertelorism • Syndactyly (2nd–4th digits), symphalangism, radiohumeral fusion • Severe intellectual disability, conductive hearing loss common, cardiac/genitourinary anomalies	75, 102, 105
Crouzon (acrocephalosyndactyly II)	1:65,000	AD	FGFR2	• Craniosynostosis (bicoronal) • Midface hypoplasia, beaked nose, exorbitism, hypertelorism, external auditory canal atresia • No consistent digital abnormality (can have tarsal coalition, clinodactyly, symphalangism) • Chiari I malformation, cognition normal usually, conductive hearing loss	75, 102, 105
Saethre-Chotzen (acrocephalosyndactyly III)	1:50,000	AD	TWIST	• Craniosynostosis (bicoronal or unilateral) • Midface hypoplasia with nasal septum deviation, low set hairline, ptosis • Partial second/third finger second to fourth toe syndactyly, hallux valgus • Normal intellect, sensorineural hearing loss, congenital heart disease	75, 102, 105, 295
Pfeiffer (acrocephalosyndactyly V)	1:100,000	AD	FGFR1 or FGFR2	• Craniosynostosis (bicoronal) • Midface hypoplasia, exorbitism, hypertelorism, choanal atresia/stenosis, low nasal bridge • Broad medially deviated first digits, radiohumeral synostosis, partial second/third syndactyly • Chiari I malformation, conductive hearing loss, more severe variants with intellectual disability, cardiac/genitourinary anomalies	75, 102, 105, 106
Boston-type craniosynostosis	Rare	AD	MSX2	• Craniosynostosis (bicoronal to cloverleaf pansynostosis) • Supraorbital recession without hypertelorism, midface hypoplasia, or proptosis • No consistent extremity findings	296, 297
Carpenter (acrocephalopolysyndactyly II)	Rare	AR	RAB23	• Craniosynostosis (variable sutures) • Low set ears, cardiac defects • Third and fourth digit syndactyly, polydactyly	102
Muencke	1:30,000	AD	FGFR3 (P250R)	• Craniosynostosis (bilateral or unilateral coronal) • Brachydactyly, coned epiphyses, tarsal/metatarsal fusion • Klippel-Feil, sensorineural hearing loss	105
Jackson-Weiss	Rare	AD	FGFR2	• Craniosynostosis (bicoronal) • Midface hypoplasia, exorbitism, hypertelorism • Broad first lower phalanges/metatarsal, tarsal/metatarsal fusions, second and third toe syndactyly	105
Craniofrontonasal	Rare	X-linked Dominant	EFNB1	• Craniosynostosis (unilateral, bilateral coronal) • Hypertelorism, short/bifid nasal bone • Joint laxity, syndactyly • Intellectual disability in half	75

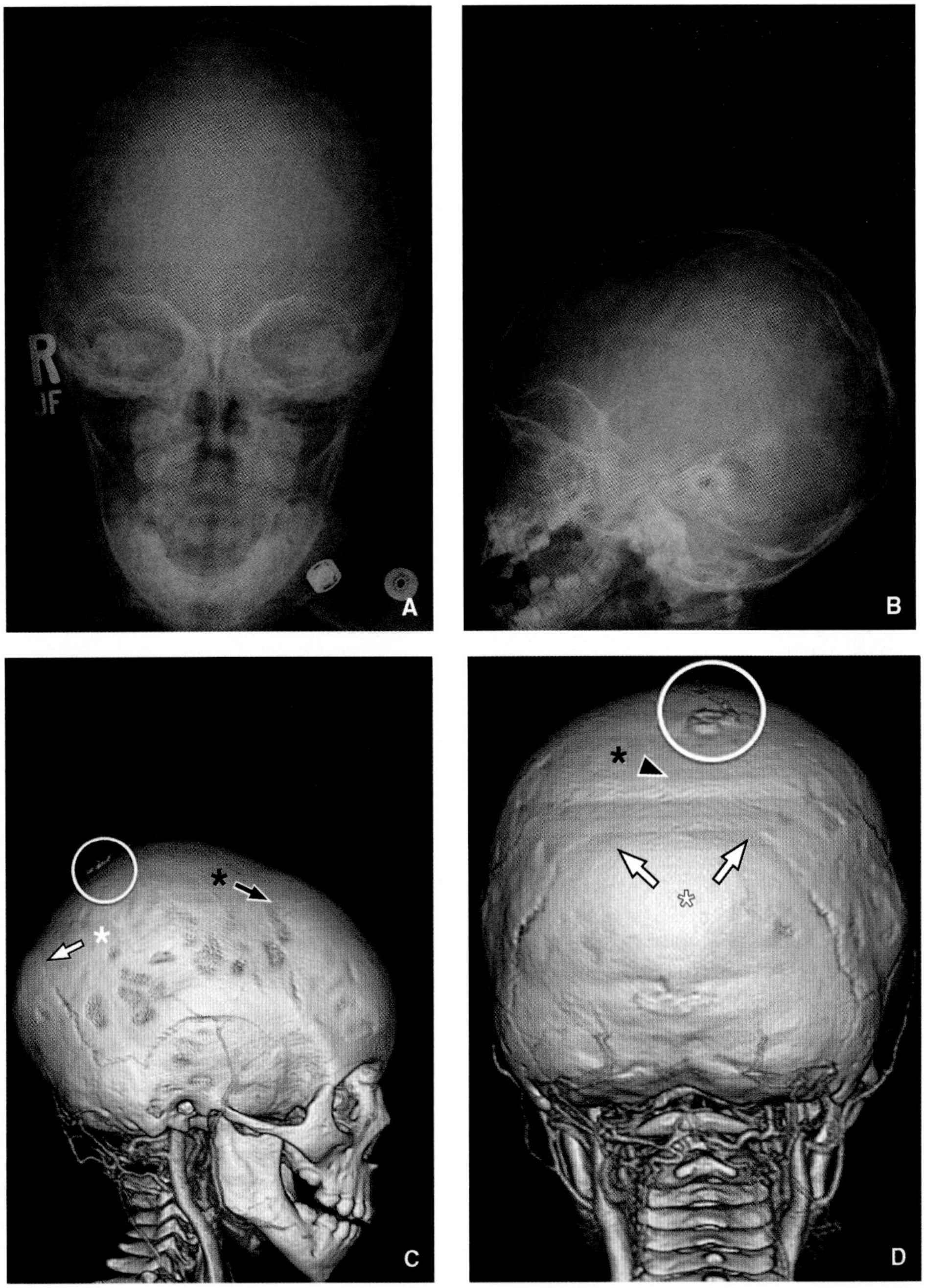

FIGURE 1.12 **Excessive lacunar markings in a 2-year-old boy with multiple suture synostosis and sinus pericranii. A and B:** AP **(A)** and lateral **(B)** skull radiographs demonstrate prominent lacunar changes of the skull and poor visibility of the major cranial sutures. **C and D:** Right lateral **(C)** and posterior **(D)** views of postcontrast surface rendering CT images demonstrate premature fusion of the sagittal suture (*asterisked black arrowhead*) and portions of the lambdoid/coronal sutures (*asterisked white/black arrows*). There is also a tuft of veins along the outer table from a sinus pericranii (*circle*).

Cephaloceles

Cephaloceles are defects of the dura and overlying skull, said to be *primary* when arising in a developmental/congenital context and *secondary* when occurring after trauma or surgery.[108] Cephaloceles are further classified as *meningoceles* when they contain only meninges/cerebrospinal fluid (CSF) or *encephaloceles* when they also contain brain tissue. Collectively, cephaloceles are relatively rare with estimates typically in the range of 1 to 4 cases per 10,000 live births.[109] Although cephaloceles may occur in the setting of a number of syndromes (e.g., trisomies, Walker-Warburg, Dandy-Walker, Meckel syndromes for occipital cephaloceles), 80% of cephaloceles occur in a nonsyndromic, isolated form.[109] Epidemiologic risk factors for cephaloceles are not well understood though there are data to suggest that young maternal age (particularly <20 years old) and race (Hispanic or white more so than African

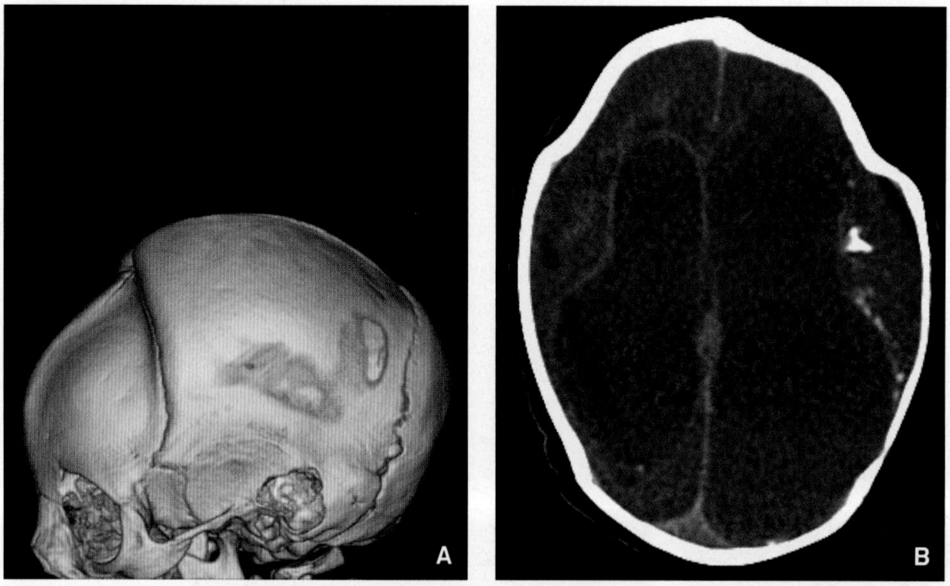

FIGURE 1.13 **Secondary craniosynostosis in a 3-year-old boy with neonatal hypoxic ischemic injury. A:** Left lateral perspective surface rendering CT image demonstrates sutural overlap and fusion. **B:** Axial bone window CT image shows diffuse encephalomalacia underlying the sutural fusion.

American) may represent risk factors.[110] Some authors classify cephaloceles as a defect of neural tube closure, similar to anencephaly or myelomeningocele for the anterior and posterior neuropore, respectively. However, the recurrence rate in siblings and lack of demonstrated decrease with folate supplementation differentiate cephaloceles from classic neural tube disorders.[111,112] Therefore, many authors instead speculate on a variety of other developmental and physical mechanisms to explain the occurrence of these skull defects.

As summarized in Table 1.2, cephaloceles are typically classified according to location, which in turn is associated with slightly different epidemiology and clinical outcome.

Occipital cephaloceles tend to be large with average sac sizes >5 cm,[108,113] and they may therefore encompass brainstem, cerebellum, and dural sinuses as well as the occipital lobe (Fig. 1.14). The largest of these occipital cephaloceles may extend to involve the upper cervical cord, a cervicocranial junction anomaly referred to as inencephaly or a *Chiari III malformation*.[114] In most of the world, occipital cephaloceles are the most common type of cephalocele.[109,115–117] Although a male predominance or equal frequency by gender is reported for other cephaloceles, occipital cephaloceles have a female predominance.[115,118] They are associated with Meckel, Knobloch, and Walker-Warburg syndromes in addition to classic Dandy-Walker malformations. Up to 50% to 65% of affected pediatric patients with occipital cephaloceles require management for hydrocephalus, and up to 27% have microcephaly.[108]

Anterior or *sincipital* cephaloceles involve the frontal bone and/or anterior skull base. Sincipital cephaloceles have complex anatomic relationships because of transient embryologic structures that arise as part of the anterior neuropore. The anterior neuropore transiently extends through the foramen cecum at the anterior skull base and descends into the nasal cavity and nasal soft tissue.[119] When a cephalocele protrudes along this course, it is referred to as a *nasoethmoidal*

TABLE 1.2 Classification Scheme for Cephaloceles Based on Location

Cephalocele Location	Subtype
Occipital	
Parietal	
Temporal	
Interfrontal (split frontal bone only)	
Sincipital	• Nasofrontal (protrusion through fonticulus frontalis, the embryologic frontonasal suture) • Nasoethmoidal (protrusion through foramen cecum) • Naso-orbital (protrusion through anterior skull base and between frontal process of maxilla and lacrimal bone) • Tessier cleft associated
Basal	• Transsphenoidal (craniopharyngeal canal to nasopharynx) • Transethmoidal (cribriform plate to nasal cavity) • Sphenoethmoidal (between sphenoid/ethmoid at planum/cribriform to nasopharynx) • Spheno-orbital (optic canal and superior orbital fissure to orbit) • Sphenomaxillary (superior and inferior orbital fissure to pterygopalatine fossa)

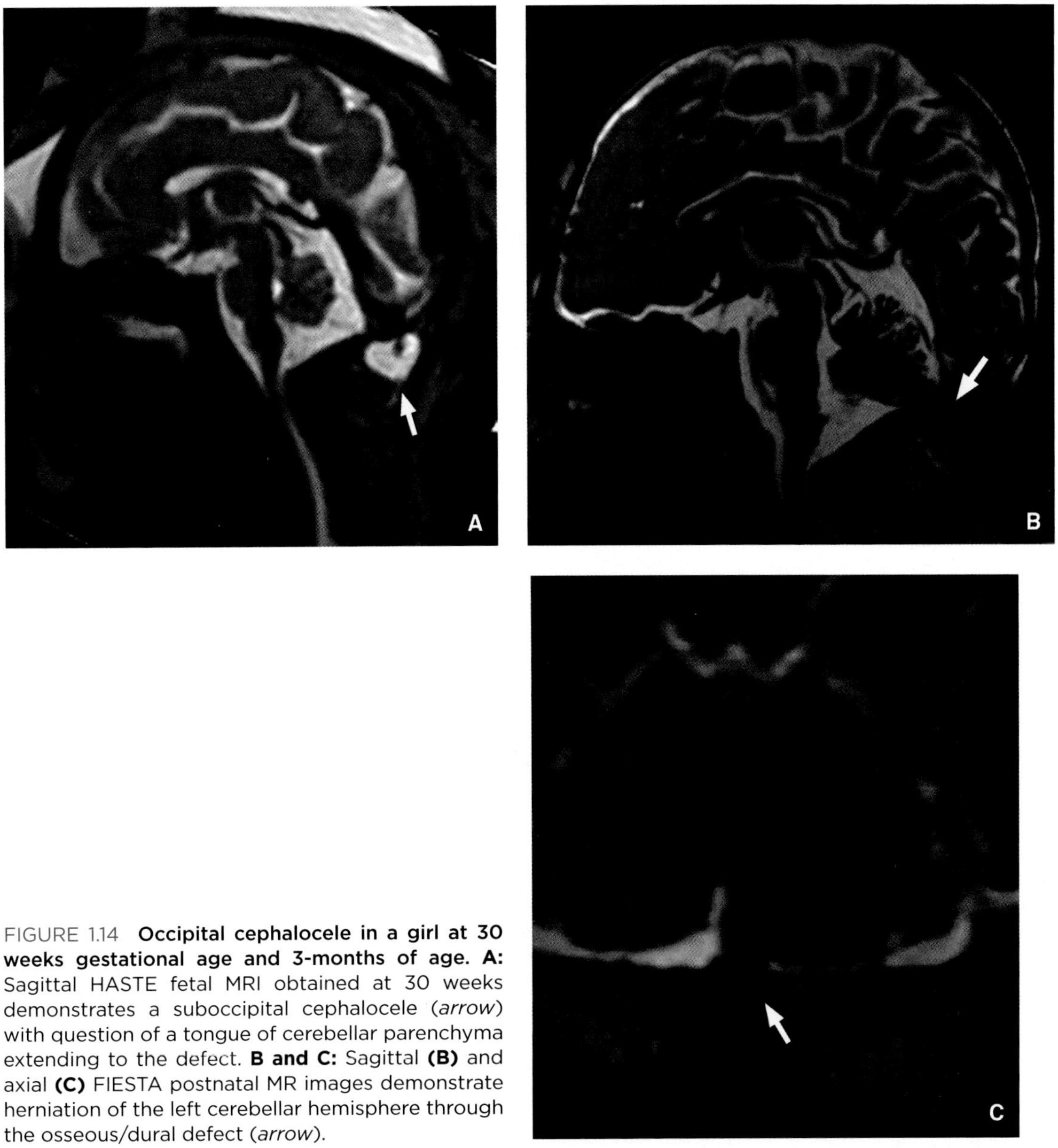

FIGURE 1.14 **Occipital cephalocele in a girl at 30 weeks gestational age and 3-months of age. A:** Sagittal HASTE fetal MRI obtained at 30 weeks demonstrates a suboccipital cephalocele (*arrow*) with question of a tongue of cerebellar parenchyma extending to the defect. **B and C:** Sagittal **(B)** and axial **(C)** FIESTA postnatal MR images demonstrate herniation of the left cerebellar hemisphere through the osseous/dural defect (*arrow*).

cephalocele; caution is required when making this diagnosis in neonates as the cribriform plate does not normally ossify before 6 months.[119] A *naso-orbital* cephalocele takes a similar course but interdigitates between the lacrimal bone and maxilla (frontal process). *Nasofrontal* cephaloceles occur at the primitive nasofrontal suture, known as the *fonticulus frontalis.*[120,121] These sincipital cephaloceles typically present as nasal or orbital masses, frequently disrupting the lacrimal ducts and causing hypertelorism.[108,118] In Southeast Asia, Central Africa, and certain parts of Russia, sincipital cephaloceles constitute the most common type of cephalocele.[108] The spectrum of anterior cephaloceles is depicted in Figures 1.15 to 1.17.

Parietal cephaloceles are the second most common site for cephaloceles in most populations.[116–118] A type of rudimentary cephalocele known as an *atretic cephalocele* is particularly common in this location. These atretic cephaloceles communicate with the scalp through a thin fibrous connection and tiny skull defect. Classically, they are associated with upward deviation of the tentorium, a persistent falcine vein with underdeveloped straight sinus, a divided superior sagittal sinus, and faintly enhancing scalp mass consisting of rudimentary meningeal tissue (Fig. 1.18).[122–124] When some of the classic imaging findings are absent and a skull defect is not appreciated, these atretic cephaloceles may be mistaken for a dermoid cyst or other soft tissue mass of the scalp.[124]

Basal cephaloceles involve the skull base and are further subdivided by location[125,126]: *transsphenoidal, transethmoidal, sphenoethmoidal, transtemporal, spheno-orbital, and sphenomaxillary.* Cephaloceles in this location typically present because of CSF leakage or recurrent infection (Figs. 1.17 and 1.19).[126] Basal and temporal cephaloceles are the rarest cephaloceles encountered, constituting only 5% to 10% of all cephaloceles in most case series.[118,127]

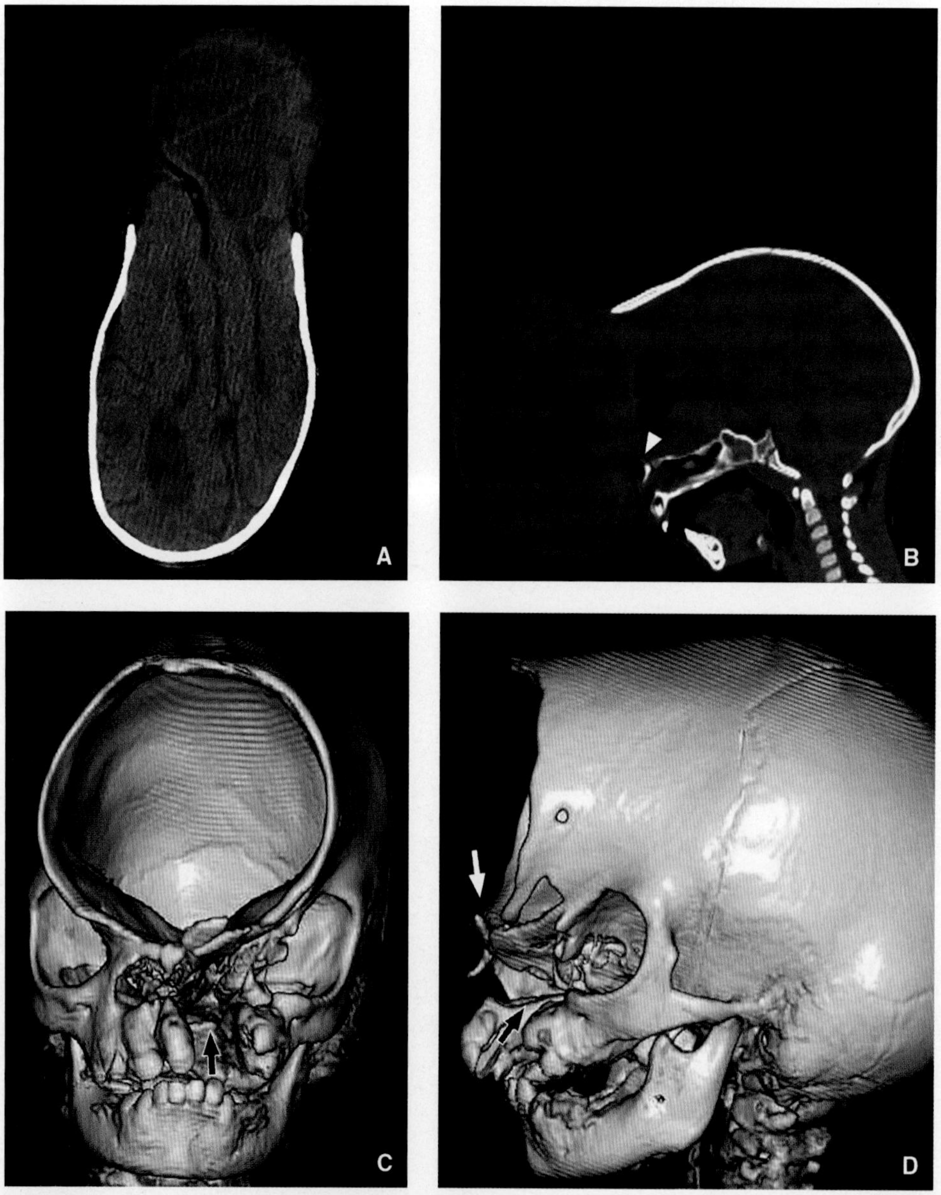

FIGURE 1.15 **Large interfrontal cephalocele and Tessier facial cleft in a 16-month-old girl. A and B:** Axial **(A)** and sagittal reformatted **(B)** CT images demonstrate a large interfrontal cephalocele. The sagittal reformatted CT image demonstrates that the axis of herniation extends above the frontonasal suture (*arrowhead*). **C and D:** Frontal **(C)** and left lateral **(D)** perspective surface renderings of the CT data demonstrate the large frontal bone defect, the presence of the left paramedian Tessier facial cleft (*black arrow*), and some residual bone at the frontonasal suture (*white arrow*).

Cephaloceles are usually appreciated on in utero imaging or by physical examination soon after birth.[116] In some instances, there is an associated "hair collar" that draws attention to the area of abnormality.[128,129] In the rare instance that there is skin breakdown and active CSF leakage, a repair may be attempted emergently.[108,117] Otherwise, the repair is attempted on an elective basis in the early neonatal period. Typically, these repairs involve repairing the dura at the site of defect, usually without attempt at primary repair of the skull defect.[114] In the case of sincipital cephalocele repair, repair of the dural defect occurs in coordination with plastic surgery to repair the facial deformity.[118,120] Although many case series emphasize favorable outcomes of patients with sincipital/anterior cephaloceles where surgical mortalities may be in the single digit percentages,[108,109,118] there are data to suggest that even this population can require surgical management of hydrocephalus and can occasionally have poor developmental outcomes.[116,117]

The degree of disability and overall mortality associated with cephaloceles depends on several factors—quantity of herniated brain tissue, microcephaly (a reflection of extruded CSF and brain matter into the cephalocele), presence of additional congenital anomalies (brain or elsewhere), low birth weight, and hydrocephalus have been consistently found

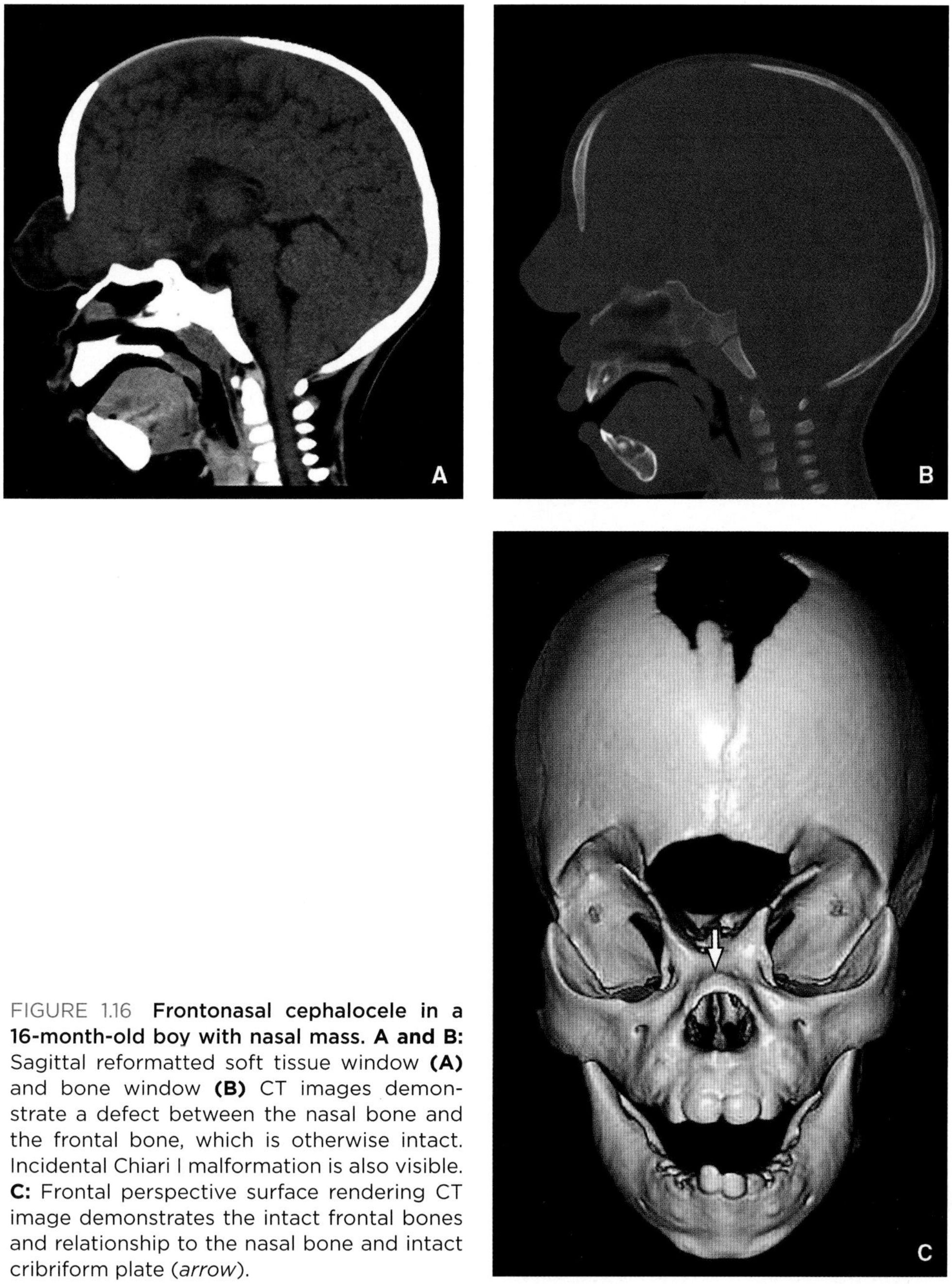

FIGURE 1.16 **Frontonasal cephalocele in a 16-month-old boy with nasal mass. A and B:** Sagittal reformatted soft tissue window **(A)** and bone window **(B)** CT images demonstrate a defect between the nasal bone and the frontal bone, which is otherwise intact. Incidental Chiari I malformation is also visible. **C:** Frontal perspective surface rendering CT image demonstrates the intact frontal bones and relationship to the nasal bone and intact cribriform plate (*arrow*).

to portend a worse prognosis.[109,116,127,130] Taking all cephalocele patients as a group, surgical mortality is variable being reported in the range of 0% to 30%[108,116,117,127,130] and long-term survival (5 years to adulthood) is guarded in the range of 61% to 80%. Only about half of patients surviving surgery attain normal intellectual development.[108,116,127]

Dermal Sinus

A related disease entity to the nasoethmoidal cephalocele is the nasal *dermal sinus*—in this case, there is only a rudimentary (occasionally segmental) sinus tract rather than a true cephalocele sac.[119] Like the dermal sinuses elsewhere, nasal dermal sinuses can serve as a portal for infection and can be seeded with epidermoid (diffusion restricting) or dermoid (T1 hyperintense, nondiffusion restricting) cysts, which can extend to the intracranial compartment.[131] *Nasal glial heterotopias* (nasal gliomas) represent mass-like accumulations of glial (nonneuronal) tissue along the course of a vestigial nasal dermal sinus.[132] Nasal gliomas and nasal dermal sinus tracts/cysts require complete excision including anterior cranial fossa exploration if intracranial extension is present.[132] This topic is discussed in greater depth in the head and neck chapter of this book (Chapter 3).

Sinus Pericranii

Sinus pericranii represent unusually prominent networks of emissary veins that aggregate along the outer table of the skull in the midline, in some cases providing the primary drainage from the underlying brain parenchyma.[133,134] They are rare

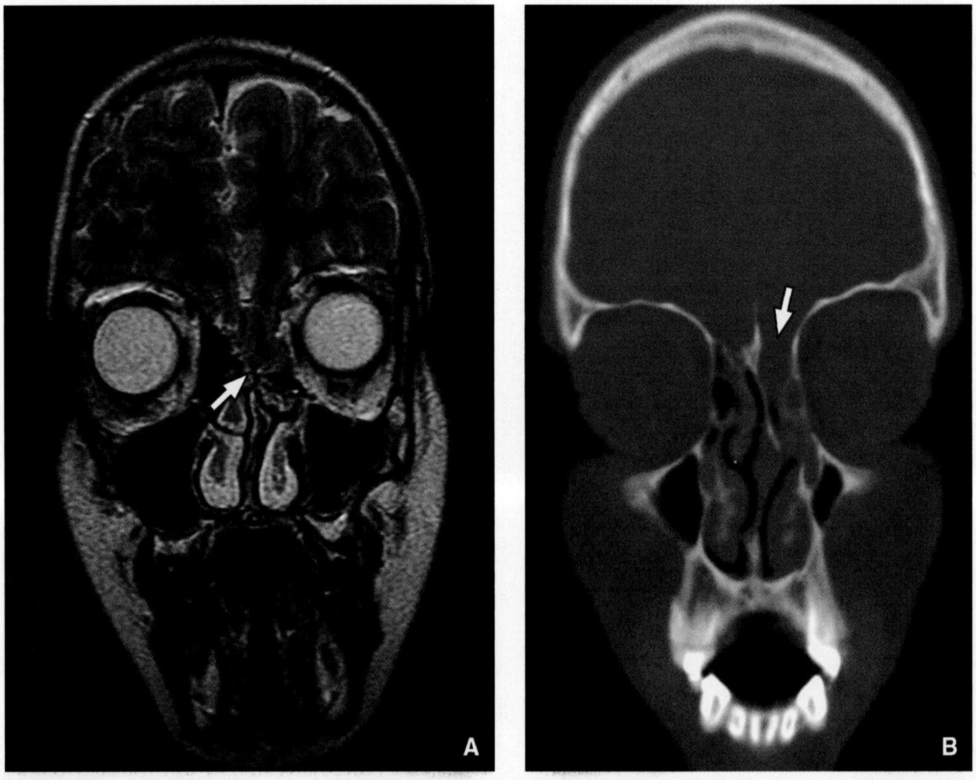

FIGURE 1.17 **Transethmoidal cephalocele in an 8-year-old boy with recurrent meningitis. A:** Coronal T2-weighted MR image demonstrates herniation of left gyrus rectus (*arrow*) through the cribriform plate into the upper ethmoid air cells. **B:** Coronal reformatted bone window CT image shows the corresponding bone deficiency (*arrow*).

and usually reported as small series or single cases. Typical symptoms are those of a soft scalp mass with skin discoloration, occasionally with accompanying headache. They can be mistaken for a soft tissue mass of the scalp but are well depicted by conventional or MR venographic techniques. These techniques demonstrate drainage into the network of scalp veins via the superior sagittal sinus (Fig. 1.20) or directly from the brain parenchyma ("dominant" drainage), the latter often associated with developmental venous anomalies. Provocative maneuvers (i.e., Valsalva) can distend the sinus pericranii at direct visualization or on ultrasound. Sinus pericranii usually do not have associated long-term morbidity, but nondominant lesions can undergo surgical or endovascular obliteration for cosmetic reasons.[134,135] Intervention is contraindicated in dominant sinus pericranii because of the risk of venous hypertension/infarction.

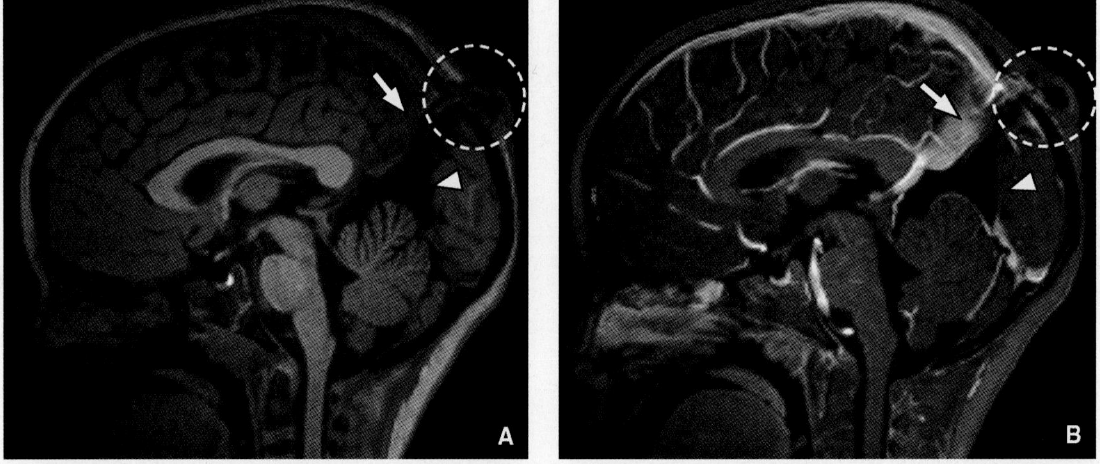

FIGURE 1.18 **Parietal atretic cephalocele in a newborn girl evaluated for persistent midline vertex scalp mass. A and B:** Sagittal T1-weighted MPRAGE precontrast **(A)** and postcontrast **(B)** MR images demonstrate a parietal skull defect with small, faintly enhancing cystic lesion (*circled*) in the overlying scalp. There is associated upward retraction of the tentorium (*arrowhead*), persistence of the embryonic falcine sinus (*arrow*), and deficiency of the straight sinus.

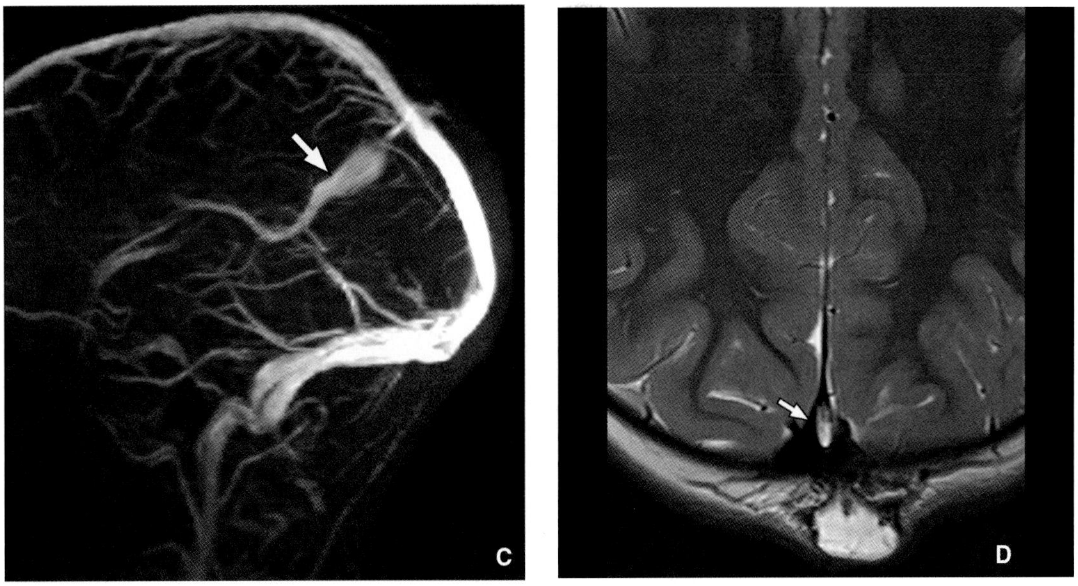

FIGURE 1.18 (*Continued*) **C:** Sagittal MIP of MR venography confirms the anomalous venous drainage (falcine sinus indicated with *arrow*) and suggests sinus pericranii associated with the parietal cephalocele (faint flow-related enhancement). **D:** Axial T2-weighted MR image through the lesion demonstrates the atretic cephalocele sac as well as fenestration of the superior sagittal sinus by stalk of the atretic cephalocele (*arrow*).

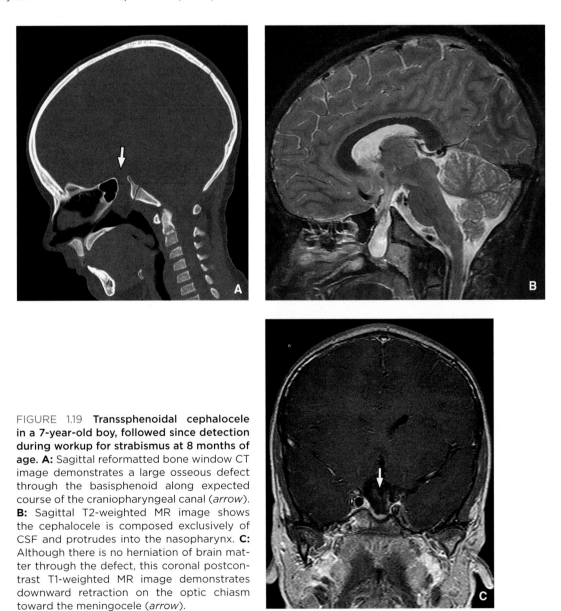

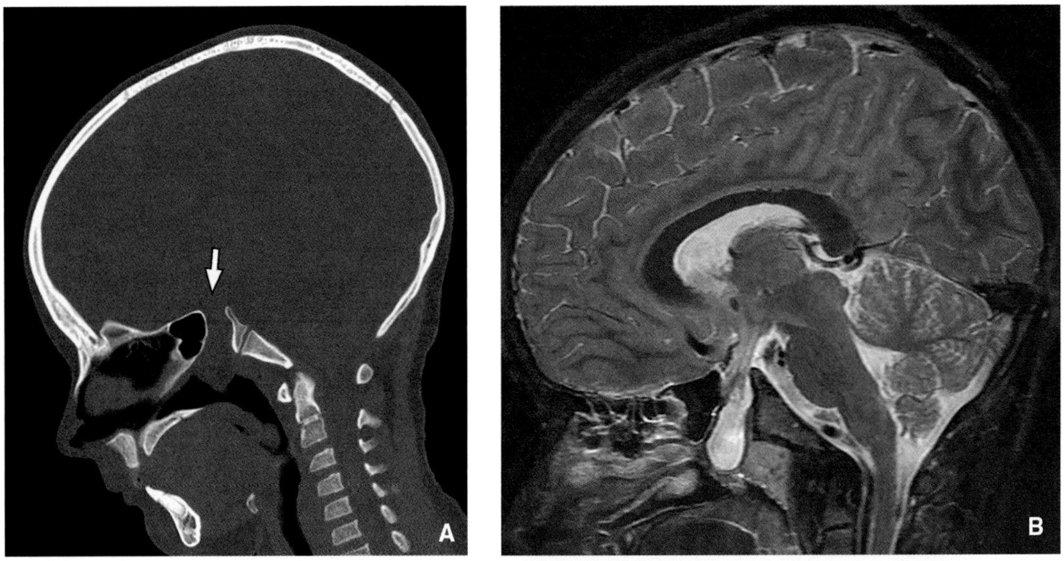

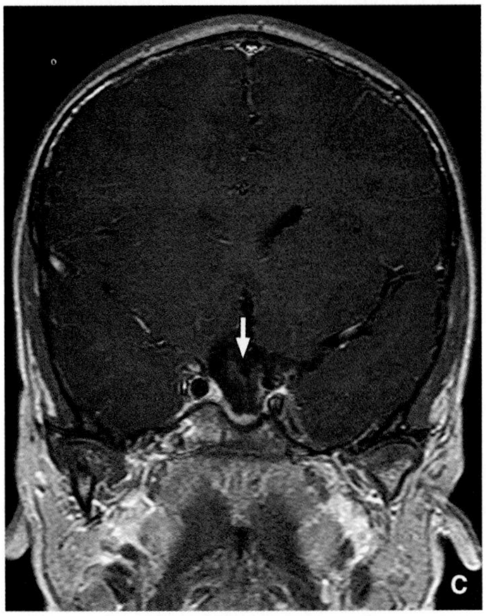

FIGURE 1.19 **Transsphenoidal cephalocele in a 7-year-old boy, followed since detection during workup for strabismus at 8 months of age. A:** Sagittal reformatted bone window CT image demonstrates a large osseous defect through the basisphenoid along expected course of the craniopharyngeal canal (*arrow*). **B:** Sagittal T2-weighted MR image shows the cephalocele is composed exclusively of CSF and protrudes into the nasopharynx. **C:** Although there is no herniation of brain matter through the defect, this coronal postcontrast T1-weighted MR image demonstrates downward retraction on the optic chiasm toward the meningocele (*arrow*).

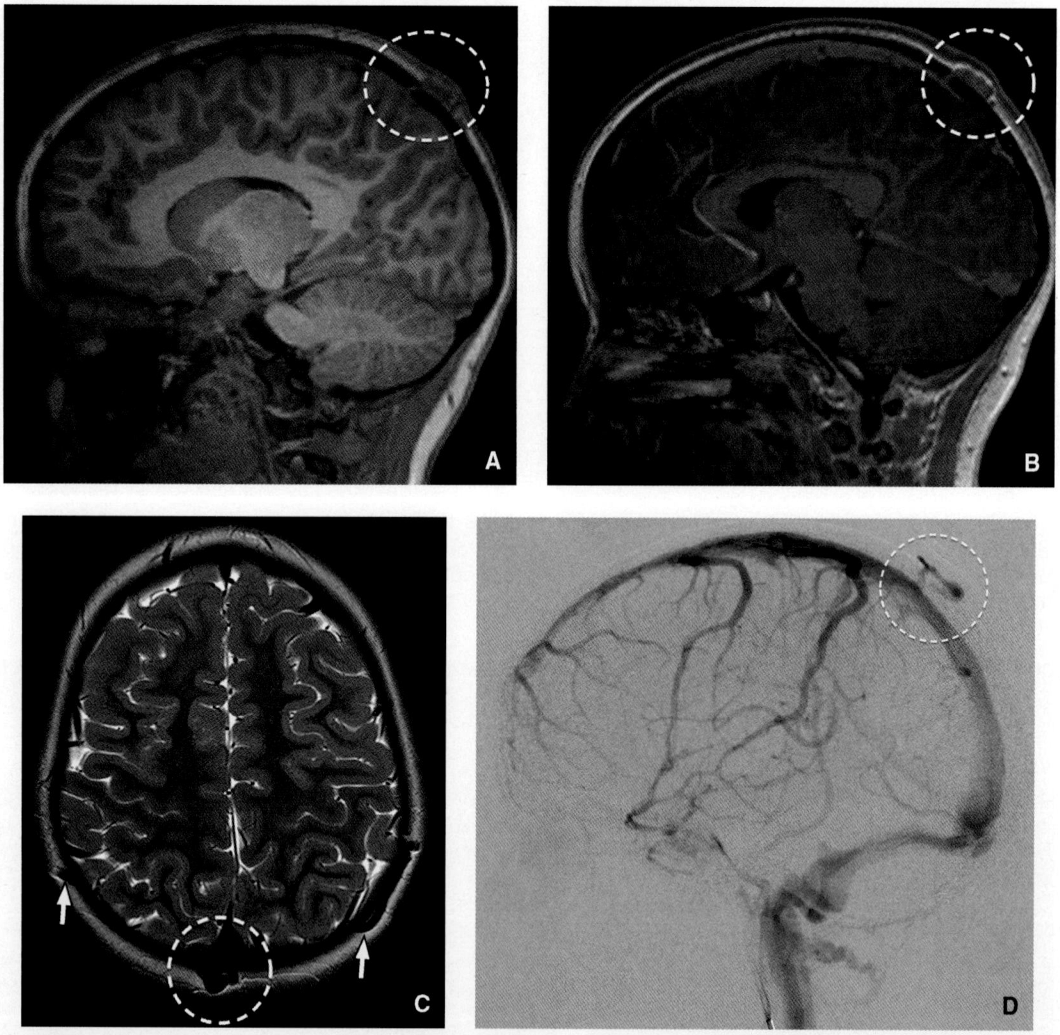

FIGURE 1.20 **Sinus pericranii in a 7-year-old girl. A and B:** Sagittal T1-weighted MPRAGE precontrast **(A)** and postcontrast **(B)** MR images demonstrate a cluster (*circled*) of scalp veins present along the outer table of the parietal bone and in communication with the superior sagittal sinus. **C:** Axial T2-weighted MR image through the sinus pericranii (*circle*) demonstrate prominent scalp veins (*arrows*) draining the lesion. **D:** Conventional angiography (lateral view, right internal carotid injection, venous phase) demonstrates puddling of contrast in the sinus pericranii (*circled*) after traversing a small skull defect.

Normal Variants

Wormian bones are accessory bones of the sutures and fontanelles occasionally encountered in normal individuals, particularly along the lambdoid suture (Fig. 1.21).[136] Extensive wormian bone formation is encountered with metabolic bone disease and bone dysplasia (e.g., Menkes syndrome, osteogenesis imperfecta, cleidocranial dysplasia, hypothyroidism, hypophosphatasia, pyknodysostosis). More than 10 ossicles greater than 6 mm × 4 mm has been suggested as a criterion for distinguishing incidental from pathologic wormian bones.[137]

Within the parietal bones just anterior to the lambdoid suture, *parietal foramina* may be encountered of tiny to moderate size, representing vestiges of emissary veins that typically involute in fetal life; even when fairly impressive sized, they are usually asymptomatic and managed expectantly (Fig. 1.22).[138] *Craniopharyngeal canals* are persistent remnants of the embryologic structures, which allow induction of the pituitary gland (Fig. 1.8D).[139]

Convolutional markings are normal, smooth indentations along the inner table of the skull, primarily along the floors of the anterior and middle cranial fossa where there is contact with brain parenchyma. These indentations are particularly prominent between ages 2 and 7.[140] However, they are distinct from *lacunar changes* that occur more diffusely in conditions of craniocerebral disproportion (Fig. 1.12): this lacunar appearance can be seen transiently in neonates with myelomeningoceles/cephaloceles (luckenschaedel) as well as patients with chronically elevated intracranial pressure.[55,141] The presence of this lacunar skull shape is suspicious for elevated intracranial pressure but is neither sensitive nor specific.[142]

Infection Disorders

Osteomyelitis

Primary infections of the skull are quite uncommon, representing an unusual site of hematogenous colonization by bacteria.[143] However, osteomyelitis still must be considered

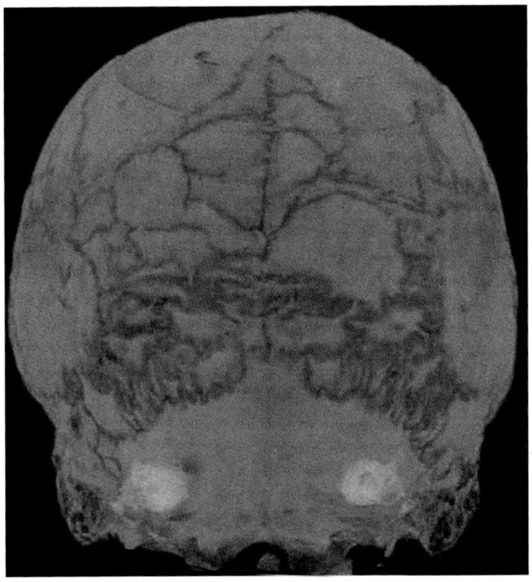

FIGURE 1.21 **Prominent wormian bones in a 27-year-old woman with osteogenesis imperfecta.** Posterior perspective SMIP (surface maximum intensity projection) images demonstrate several accessory sutures/ossicles that obscure the normal lambdoid suture.

as a potential explanation for a pediatric patient with painful scalp mass, fever, and/or bacteremia.[144–146] Although flat bones such as the skull are uncommon sites of tuberculous osteomyelitis compared to the spine and long bones, there does appear to be some tropism for the skull based on limited case series from endemic areas.[147]

More commonly, infections of the cranial vault and skull base are secondary to direct extension from sinus/mastoid infections

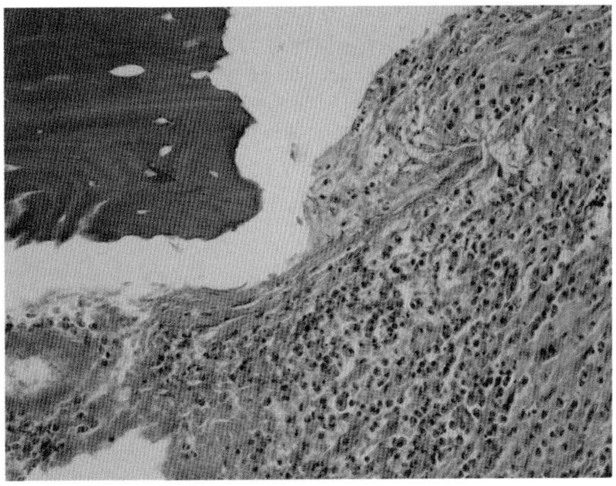

FIGURE 1.23 **Cranial debridement from a 27-year-old woman who developed osteomyelitis following surgical placement of grids and strips.** Purulent material surrounds necrotic bone (hematoxylin and eosin, original magnification, 400×).

or trauma (usually surgery). Although osteomyelitis as a complication of sinusitis or otomastoiditis is relatively rare,[148,149] these disorders occur so commonly that they represent the most frequent etiology of skull osteomyelitis in daily practice. Similarly, osteomyelitis occurs in 2% of craniotomies in historical series, and therefore this postsurgical complication is also occasionally encountered despite perioperative antibiotics.[150]

As with osteomyelitis elsewhere, infection of the skull typically manifests as permeative change and frank destruction of bone, frequently with adjacent phlegmon and abscess (Fig. 1.23). In the case of frontal sinusitis, bone destruction is often accompanied by the more common complications of subperiosteal abscess ("Pott puffy tumor") and empyema

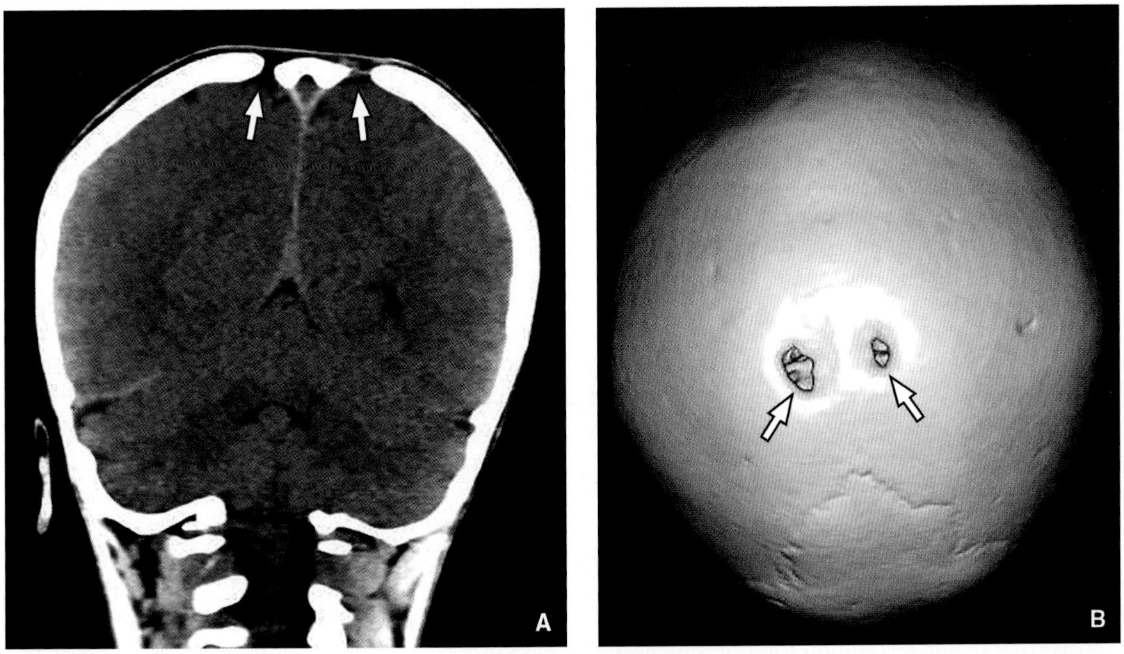

FIGURE 1.22 **Prominent parietal foramina in a 7-year-old boy with Saethre-Chotzen syndrome. A:** Coronal reformatted soft tissue window CT image demonstrates paired defects (*arrows*) in the parietal bone at the vertex consistent with parietal foramina. Note the absence of CSF or parenchymal herniation through the osseous defect implying intact dura. **B:** Superior perspective surface rendered CT image shows typical location of parietal foramina (*arrows*) anterior to the lambdoid sutures. The coronal and sagittal sutures are prematurely fused.

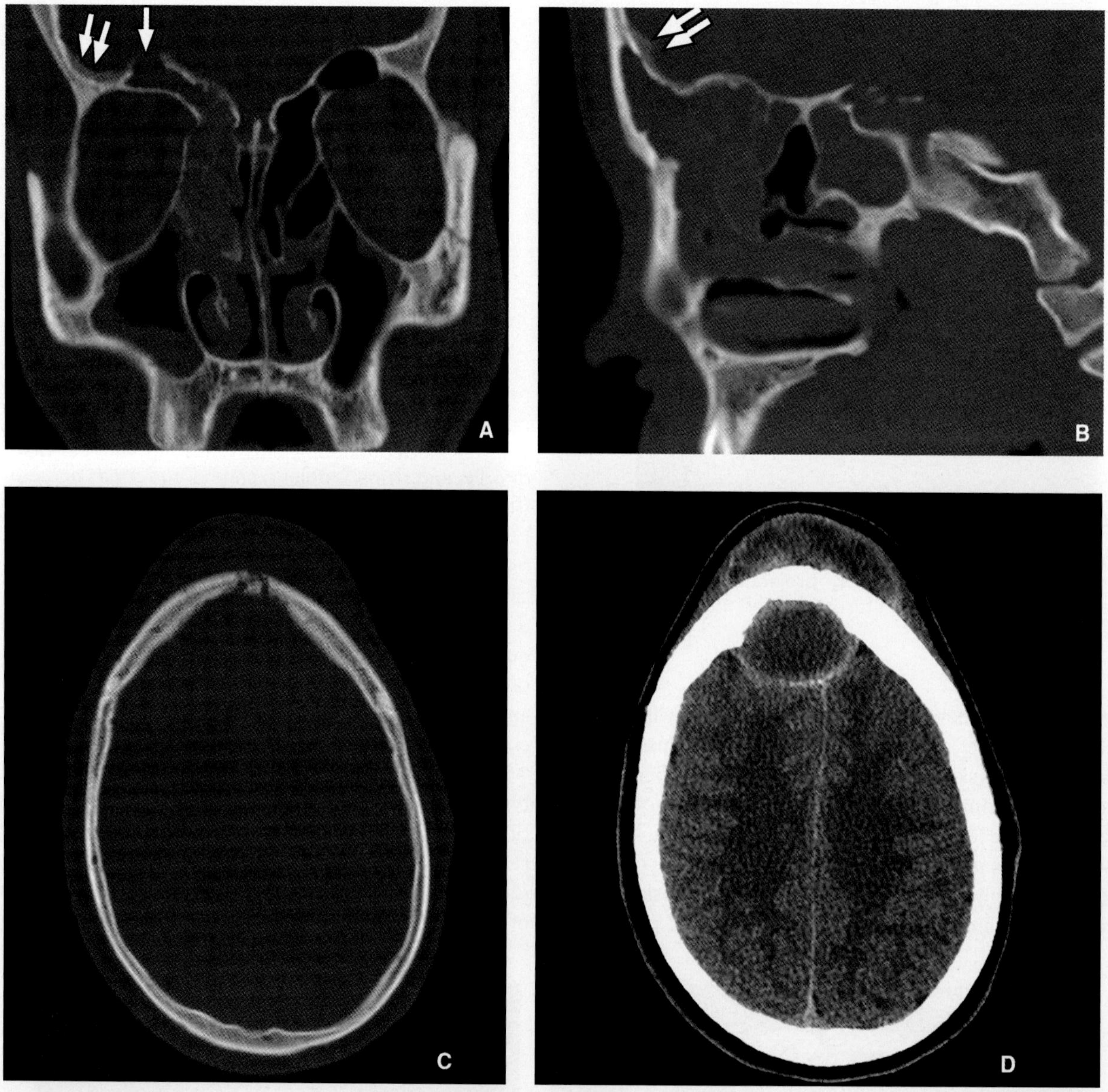

FIGURE 1.24 **Frontal sinusitis complicated by osteomyelitis and subperiosteal abscess (Pott puffy tumor) in a 16-year-old boy. A and B:** Coronal **(A)** and sagittal **(B)** reformatted bone window CT images demonstrate right-sided paranasal sinus opacification. There is erosion through the right frontal sinus (*arrow*) as well as periosteal reaction suggesting osteomyelitis (*double arrow*). **C and D:** Axial CT images through the frontal bone show erosion of bone consistent with osteomyelitis in the frontal bone on the bone reconstruction **(C)** and large subperiosteal abscesses of both the inner and outer table on the soft tissue reconstruction **(D)**.

(Fig. 1.24).[151,152] For sphenoid sinusitis, subtle erosion of the cortex can be an indicator of osteomyelitis of the central skull base and potential extension into the cavernous sinuses (Fig. 1.25). In cases of coalescent otomastoiditis, there is destruction of mastoid air cell septa, but more extensive bone lysis of the temporal bone is occasionally seen.[148]

Whereas otomastoiditis and sinusitis without complicating subperiosteal or subdural abscess can be treated medically, patients with osteomyelitis typically have more extensive disease that requires decompression of the infected cavity (endoscopic sinus surgery, myringotomy with or without incision/mastoidectomy).[153,154] Antibiotic selection usually reflects the predominance of Gram-positive organisms recovered, but polymicrobial and atypical organisms are occasionally also recovered from surgical cultures.[155–157] For infected craniotomy flaps, removal of the infected bony flap is typically performed for extensive infections that cannot be cleared by simple debridement.[150]

Neoplastic Disorders

Palpable abnormalities of the scalp can be due to soft tissue lesions intrinsic to the scalp or abnormality of the underlying cranial vault. Therefore, these growths of the scalp and skull are considered together. The epidemiology of these scalp masses is confounded by differences in terminology

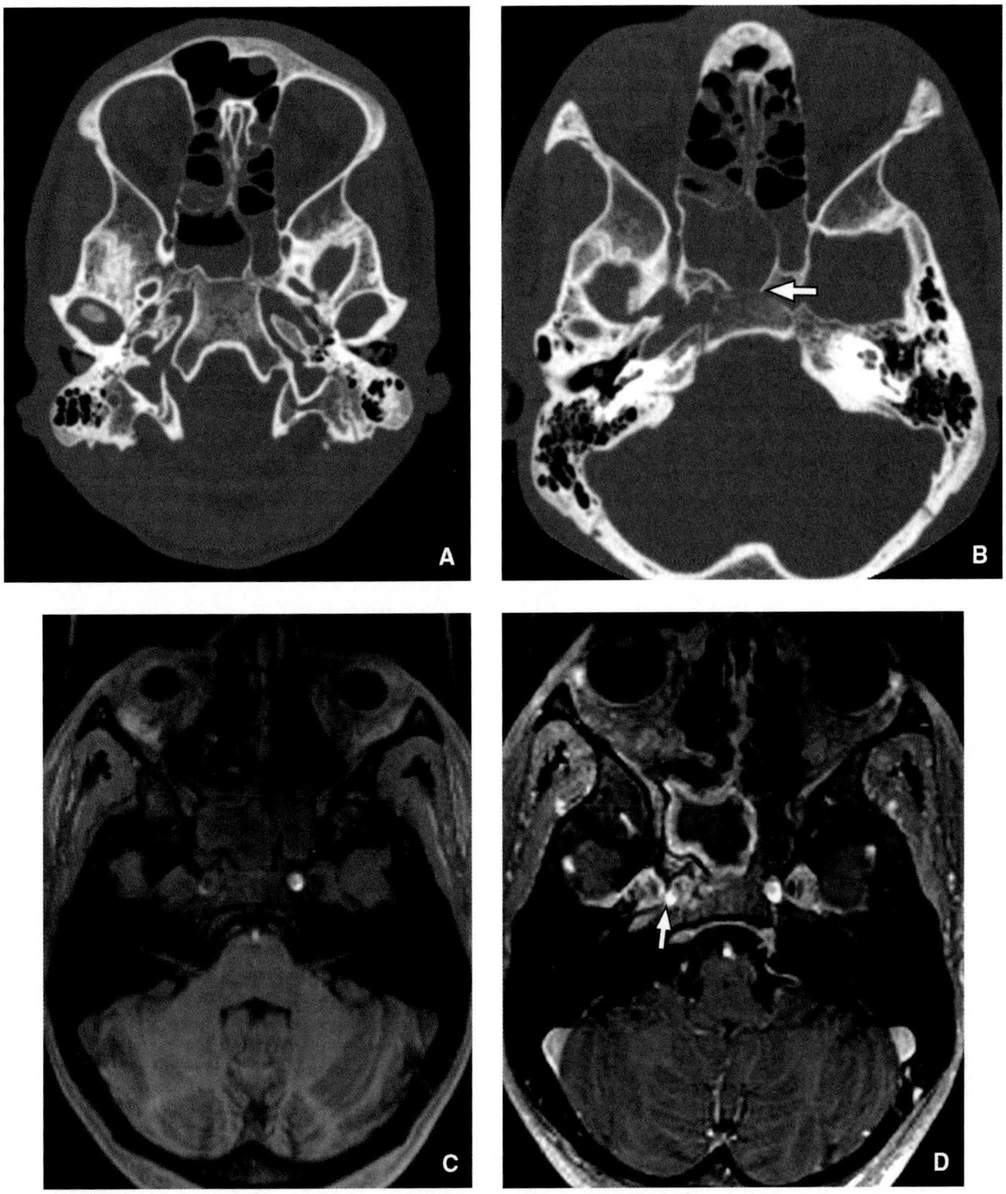

FIGURE 1.25 **Sphenoid sinusitis complicated by osteomyelitis in a 15-year-old boy. A:** Axial bone window CT image shows an air-fluid level in the right sphenoid sinus suggestive of acute sinusitis. **B:** Axial bone window CT image obtained after 2 weeks of symptomatic care (no antibiotics) reveals further opacification of the sphenoid sinuses and interval loss of posterior right sphenoid sinus cortication (*arrow*) suggesting osteomyelitis. **C and D:** Axial T1-weighted SPGR MR images through the skull base before **(C)** and after **(D)** contrast injection demonstrate enhancement of the basisphenoid and attenuation of the right cavernous internal carotid artery (*arrow*). Diffusion imaging was notable for restricted diffusion of sphenoid sinus contents (not shown) consistent with mucopyocele as the inciting cause for the skull base osteomyelitis.

(e.g., heterotopic neural nodules instead of atretic cephalocele) and sampling bias for lesions that are excised versus nonexcised. Nonetheless, several factors appear to consistently influence the pretest likelihood of the histology of any given lesion[158–163]: age of the patient, laterality of the lesion, and aggressiveness of the lesion.

For young pediatric patients (e.g., the first 4 to 5 years of life), the likelihood of a congenital abnormality is intuitively higher. In this group, dermoid/epidermoid cysts, infantile hemangiomas, cephaloceles, sinus pericranii, aplasia cutis, and trauma (e.g., cephalohematoma) are the most likely causes of a palpable scalp abnormality.[161–163] Dermoids and atretic cephaloceles and aplasia cutis are particularly strong considerations when the lesion is midline.[161,163] For older pediatric patients, these congenital lesions are still encountered but at lower frequency. Instead, aggressive lesions become more frequent, especially Langerhans cell histiocytosis, metastases, and primary sarcomas of the skull.[162] Like trauma and infection, these aggressive lesions are often associated with pain.

In the following section, some of commonly encountered mass lesions of the skull and overlying scalp in the pediatric population are discussed. Like extremity lesions, soft tissue and skull lesions can be initially classified as aggressive or nonaggressive, allowing generation of a broad differential. In particular, nonaggressive lesions tend to be circumscribed, relatively homogeneous, and remodel rather than destroy adjacent bone. Conversely, aggressive lesions infiltrate adjacent structures, have heterogeneous signal characteristics, and destroy bone.

Benign Lesions

Dermoid and Epidermoid Cysts

Although not true neoplasms, epidermoid and dermoid cysts are the single most common scalp mass encountered in children, being particularly common in young children. Dermoid/epidermoid cysts are much less commonly encountered in the skull than the scalp, but they are nonetheless the single most common skull mass.[159,163] Dermoid cysts and a subset of epidermoid cysts are congenital malformations, thought to represent sequestrations of primitive ectoderm including squamous epithelium and, in the case of dermoids, dermis with its appendages.[164] A subset of epidermoid cysts (epidermal inclusion cysts) is acquired as a result of misplaced epithelium traumatically introduced into deeper layers later in life. If there is a cutaneous punctum, then dermoid or epidermoid cyst is more properly referred to as a dermoid or epidermoid sinus. Whereas epidermoids tend to occur in the lateral scalp and skull, dermoids have a propensity for periorbital sutures and the midline, the latter site associated with a high frequency of intracranial extension.[165,166] The imaging appearance of an epidermoid is typically that of a cyst on CT and MRI with restricted diffusion (Fig. 1.26).[167–169] Dermoids

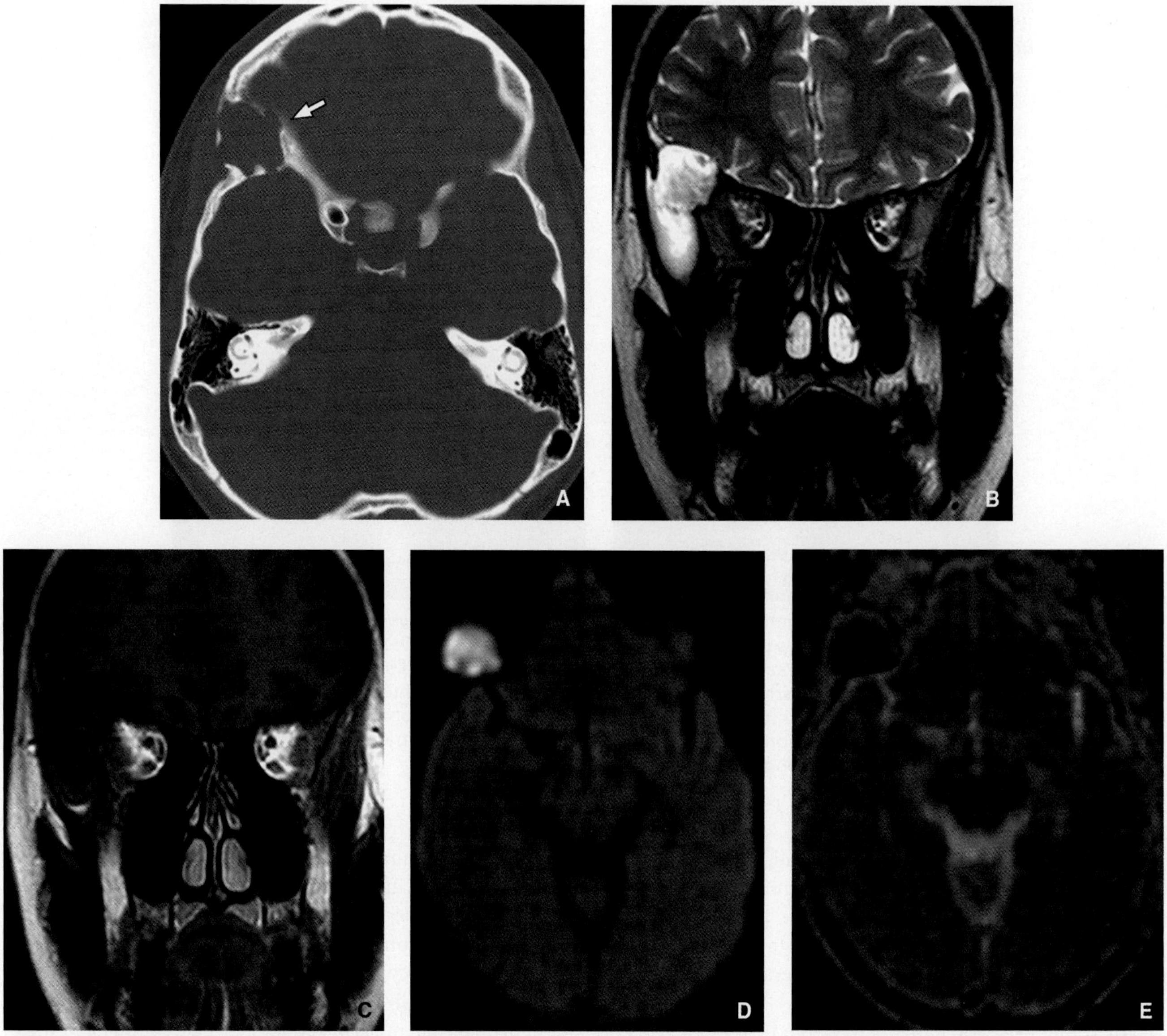

FIGURE 1.26 **Epidermoid cyst incidentally found during evaluation of a 17-year-old girl with headaches. A:** Axial bone window CT image demonstrates a well-circumscribed lucency (*white arrow*) at the confluence of the right frontosphenoid suture and the right sphenoid lesser wing. **B:** Coronal T2-weighted MR image shows the lesion as having high signal approximating CSF. **C:** Coronal T1-weighted postcontrast MR image shows no evidence of enhancement. **D and E:** Diffusion trace **(D)** and ADC **(E)** map MR images show restricted diffusion consistent with an epidermoid cyst.

tend to have more heterogeneous appearance with areas of fat signal (hypodense on CT, T1 shortening on MRI).[164,170] When abutting the skull or located within the diploic space, dermoid/epidermoid cysts smoothly remodel the adjacent bone.[171] Although there is debate about whether some of the intradiploic dermoid/epidermoid cysts may spontaneously resolve,[172,173] excision is both diagnostic and curative in most instances.

Langerhans Cell Histiocytosis

Langerhans cell histiocytosis is a disease of children caused by abnormal proliferation of dendritic (antigen presenting) cells.[37] Although there is a low incidence of this disease (on the order of 1 in 100,000 children), Langerhans cell histiocytosis is one of the two most common skull lesions found in children, particularly older children (juvenile to adolescent).[162,174,175] Old classification schemes attempted to classify Langerhans cell histiocytosis into three separate syndromes: Letterer-Siwe disease (disseminated disease of infancy), Hand-Schüller-Christian disease (skull lesions and pituitary stalk in young children), and eosinophilic granuloma (juvenile to adolescent patients with bone disease only). Because of the extensive clinical overlap between these syndromes, current subtyping of Langerhans cell histiocytosis is by its extent, unifocal, multifocal, or disseminated.[176] Unifocal disease is the most common, constituting upwards of 75% of cases. Upwards of 90% of all cases involve bone, and the skull is involved in over half of cases.[38,175] Only a single site of bone involvement is reported in 33%–67% of cases.[174,175] Skull lesions involve the cranial vault and skull base (particularly temporal bone) in approximately equal proportions.[174,175]

Although a benign tumor, Langerhans cell histiocytosis usually has aggressive features on imaging including destruction of both inner and outer tables of the cranial vault, but the margins are nonetheless sharp ("beveled") (Fig. 1.27).[174] Occasionally, a tiny fragment of bone called a "button sequestrum" may be found within the osseous defect and has been suggested as a specific sign for this disorder.[23] In the skull base and facial bones, the degree of destruction is usually

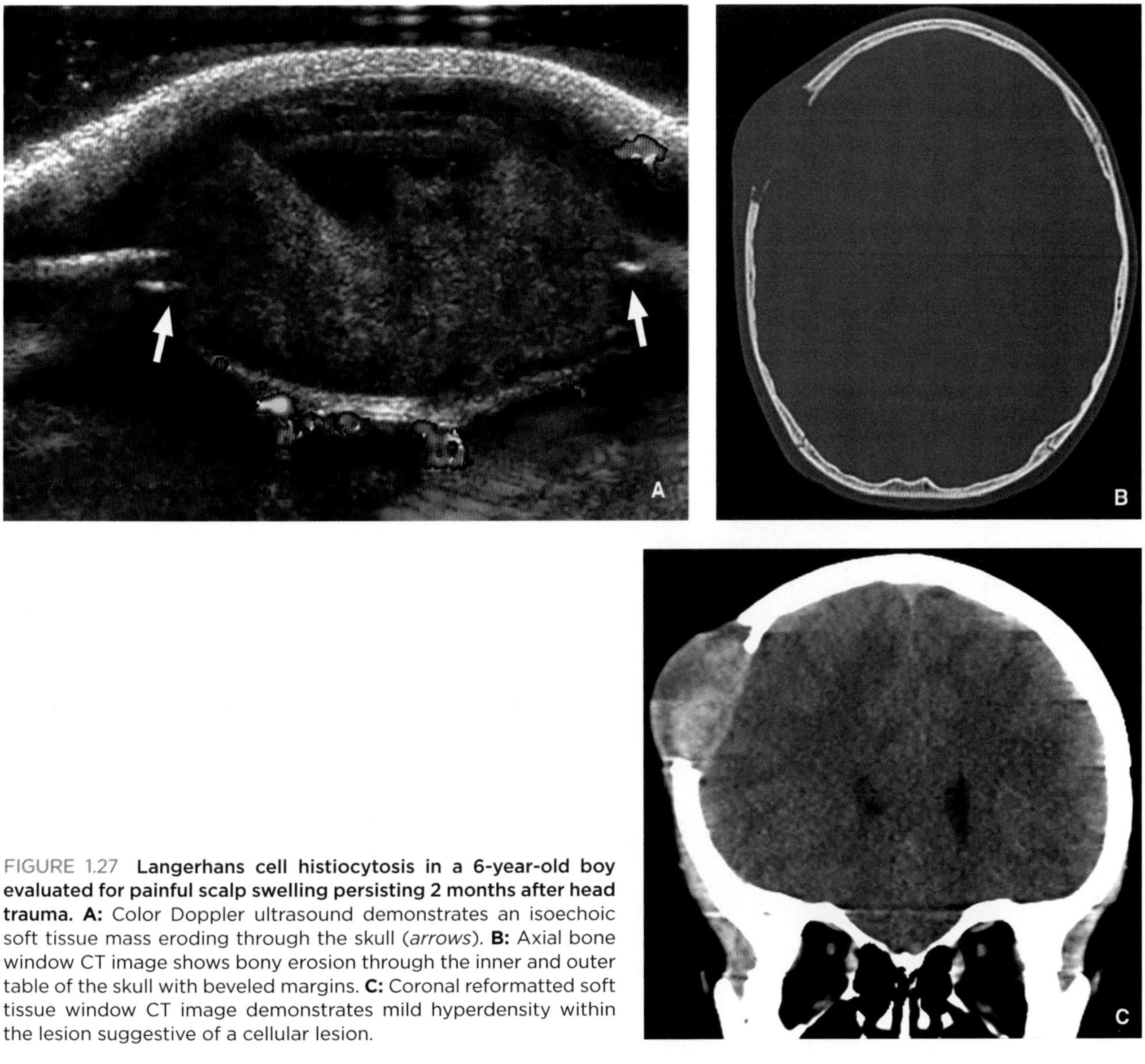

FIGURE 1.27 **Langerhans cell histiocytosis in a 6-year-old boy evaluated for painful scalp swelling persisting 2 months after head trauma. A:** Color Doppler ultrasound demonstrates an isoechoic soft tissue mass eroding through the skull (*arrows*). **B:** Axial bone window CT image shows bony erosion through the inner and outer table of the skull with beveled margins. **C:** Coronal reformatted soft tissue window CT image demonstrates mild hyperdensity within the lesion suggestive of a cellular lesion.

less complete and features small, punched-out lesions of the involved bone.[174] There is often opacification of the adjacent mastoid air cells and paranasal sinuses. Although the osseous findings are best depicted on CT, MRI can better demonstrate soft tissue extension of the skull lesions. In particular, MRI better depicts infiltration into the epidural or even subdural space and involvement of the pituitary stalk, reported in 33% and 10% respectively of Langerhans cell histiocytosis cases involving the skull.[175] Diffusion characteristics are reportedly not striking though mild restricted diffusion has been reported in some cases.[177,178] Unusual manifestations of Langerhans cell histiocytosis include cystic lesions with fluid–fluid levels.[179]

Although single-site Langerhans cell histiocytosis may often spontaneously resolve, surgical curettage of skull lesions is often performed for both diagnosis and treatment. Multisite disease typically requires chemotherapy.[37,180]

Venous Malformation of the Skull (Osseous Hemangioma)
Nonaggressive skull lesions have a narrow zone of transition and benign-appearing bony matrix and typically lack a discrete soft tissue component. An archetype of the nonaggressive skull lesion is the venous malformation of bone (usually referred to by the misnomer "intraosseous hemangioma").[181] Skull venous malformations follow the appearance seen elsewhere in the skeleton, featuring stippled lucency ("sunburst" or "honeycomb" matrix) and modest mass effect on CT with intrinsic T1 hyperintense signal (fatty marrow) and faint enhancement on MRI (Fig. 1.28).[21,182–184] However, it has been suggested that large venous malformations of the skull may have an unusual

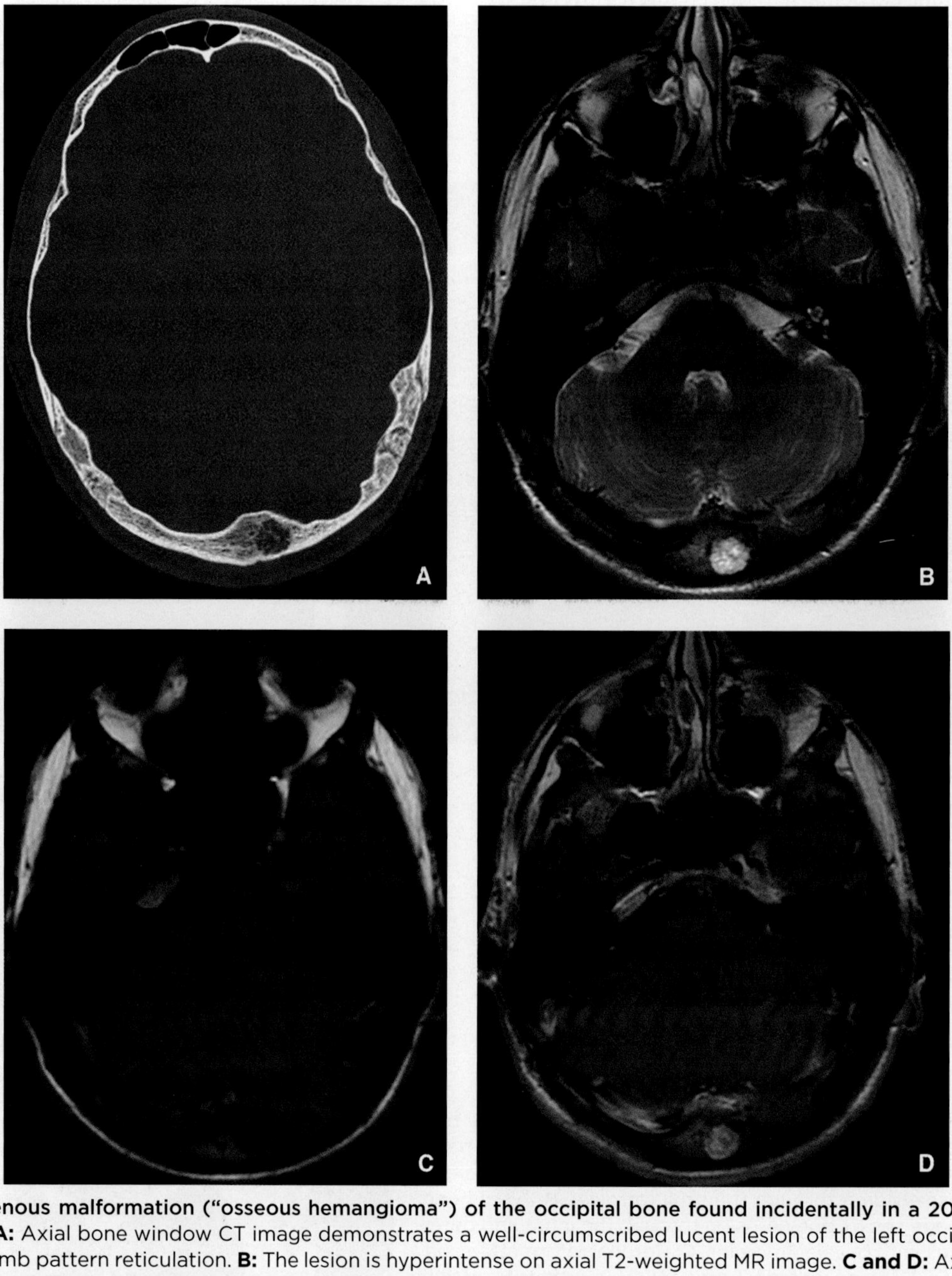

FIGURE 1.28 **Venous malformation ("osseous hemangioma") of the occipital bone found incidentally in a 20-year-old male with headache. A:** Axial bone window CT image demonstrates a well-circumscribed lucent lesion of the left occipital bone with internal honeycomb pattern reticulation. **B:** The lesion is hyperintense on axial T2-weighted MR image. **C and D:** Axial precontrast **(C)** and postcontrast **(D)** T1-weighted MR images show that the lesion enhances. Although cavernous hemangiomas are usually intrinsically T1 hyperintense because of internal fat, the other features of this case are typical of this diagnosis.

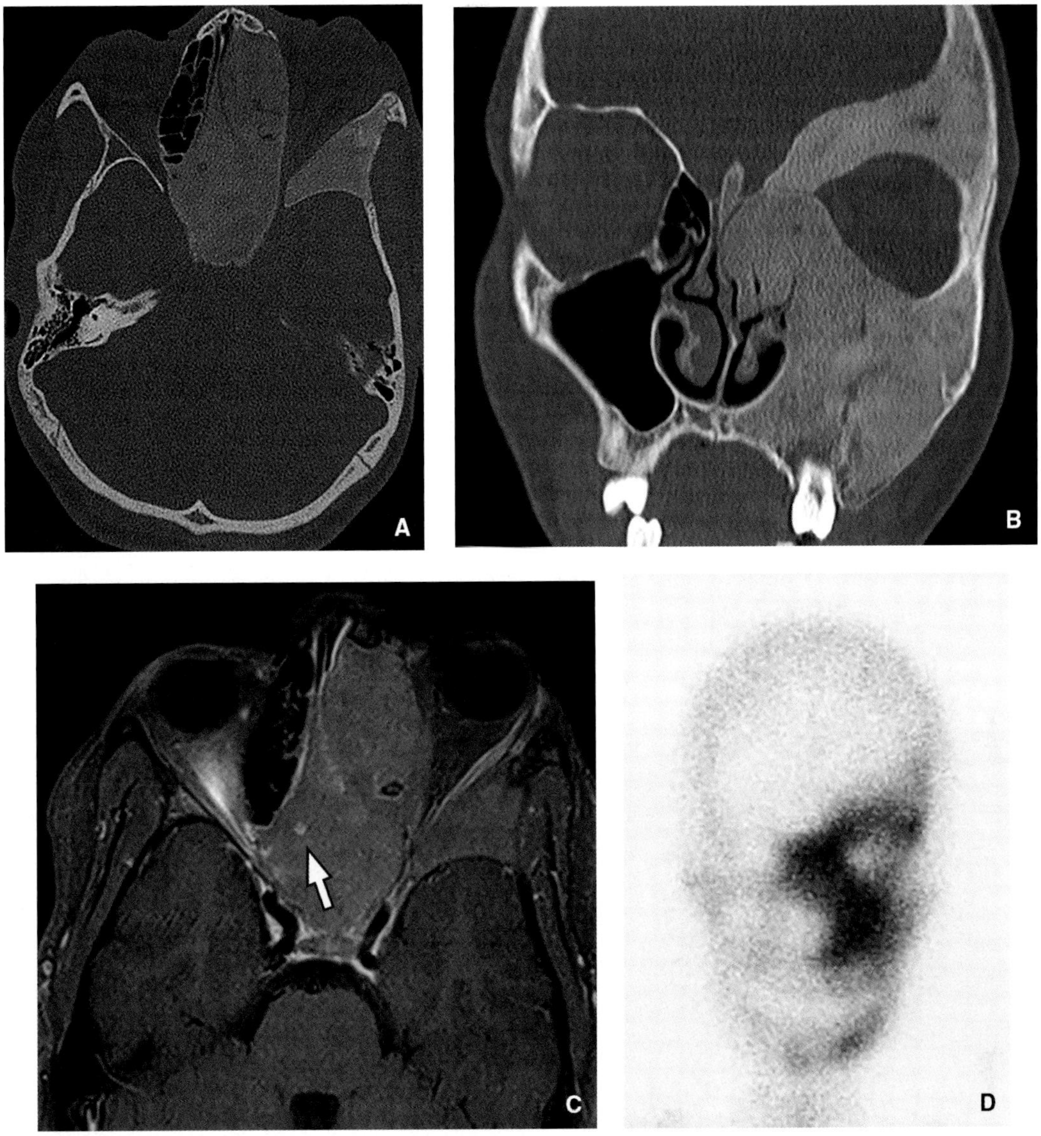

FIGURE 1.29 **Polyostotic fibrous dysplasia in a 13-year-old girl with facial asymmetry. A and B:** Axial **(A)** and coronal reformatted **(B)** bone window CT images show expansile, ground-glass mineralization of the sphenoid, left maxillary, left ethmoid, and left frontal bones typical of fibrous dysplasia. Note mild left proptosis. **C:** Axial postcontrast fat-suppressed T1-weighted MR image shows faint diffuse enhancement of the affected bones with more focal enhancement in a lytic component (*arrow*) of the sphenoid bone. **D:** There is uptake of radiotracer by the fibrous dysplasia on bone scan.

appearance that make them difficult to distinguish from cephalohematomas in infancy.[185] Venous malformations of bone rarely become symptomatic or require treatment (excision with cranioplasty) unless unusually large.[186]

Benign Fibro-Osseous Lesion of Bone

Fibrous dysplasia is a benign fibro-osseous lesion occasionally encountered in the skull, the skull base and facial bones representing a particularly frequent site for the 20% of patients with the polyostotic form.[187,188] As with other sites, an expansile ground-glass appearance is the typical manifestation in the skull with occasional areas of more lucent or sclerotic appearance (Fig. 1.29).[189] However, it is worth noting that these lesions may have a fairly aggressive, enhancing appearance on MRI.[190] Surgery is performed for fibrous dysplasia when it causes neurologic (e.g., visual) or functional (e.g., malocclusion) problems or undergoes rapid growth.[188] Clinically and histologically, fibrous dysplasia may overlap with ossifying fibroma (Fig. 1.30), another benign fibro-osseous lesion common in the skull and gnathic bones.[191]

Malignant Lesions

Malignant Bone Tumors

Compared to the benign tumors of the skull mentioned earlier, malignant primary bone tumors are uncommon and mostly reported in small case series.[192–195] Affected pediatric patients typically present with headache or focal neurologic complaints.

Osteosarcomas involve the skull as the primary site in <7% of cases and account for 0.5% of all head and neck neoplasms.[193] With a peak incidence in the second and

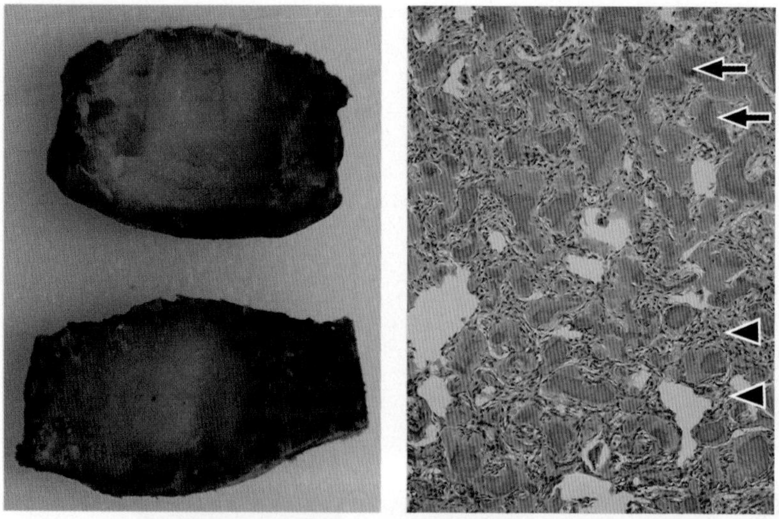

FIGURE 1.30 **This ossifying fibroma of the left parietal skull was resected from a 15-year-old boy who presented with a slowly enlarging mass of the left parietal skull.** Gross examination shows a well-circumscribed gray-white mass expanding the bone but bounded by cortex **(left panel)**. Histologically, a meshwork of round to trabecular pink/eosinophilic osteoid material (*arrows*) is embedded within intervening densely cellular fibrous stroma (*arrowheads*), in a pattern characteristic of the "juvenile psammomatoid" variant (**right panel**, hematoxylin and eosin, original magnification, 200x).

third decade,[196,197] primary osteosarcomas of bone are associated with prior irradiation, fibrous dysplasia, and Paget disease.[193] They are more common in the cranial vault (especially temporal bone) than the skull base and have imaging characteristics of osteosarcomas seen elsewhere: destructive soft tissue mass, permeative change of bone, periosteal reaction, and bone matrix with the exception of telangiectatic forms (Fig. 1.31).[192,193] As with other primary bone tumors,

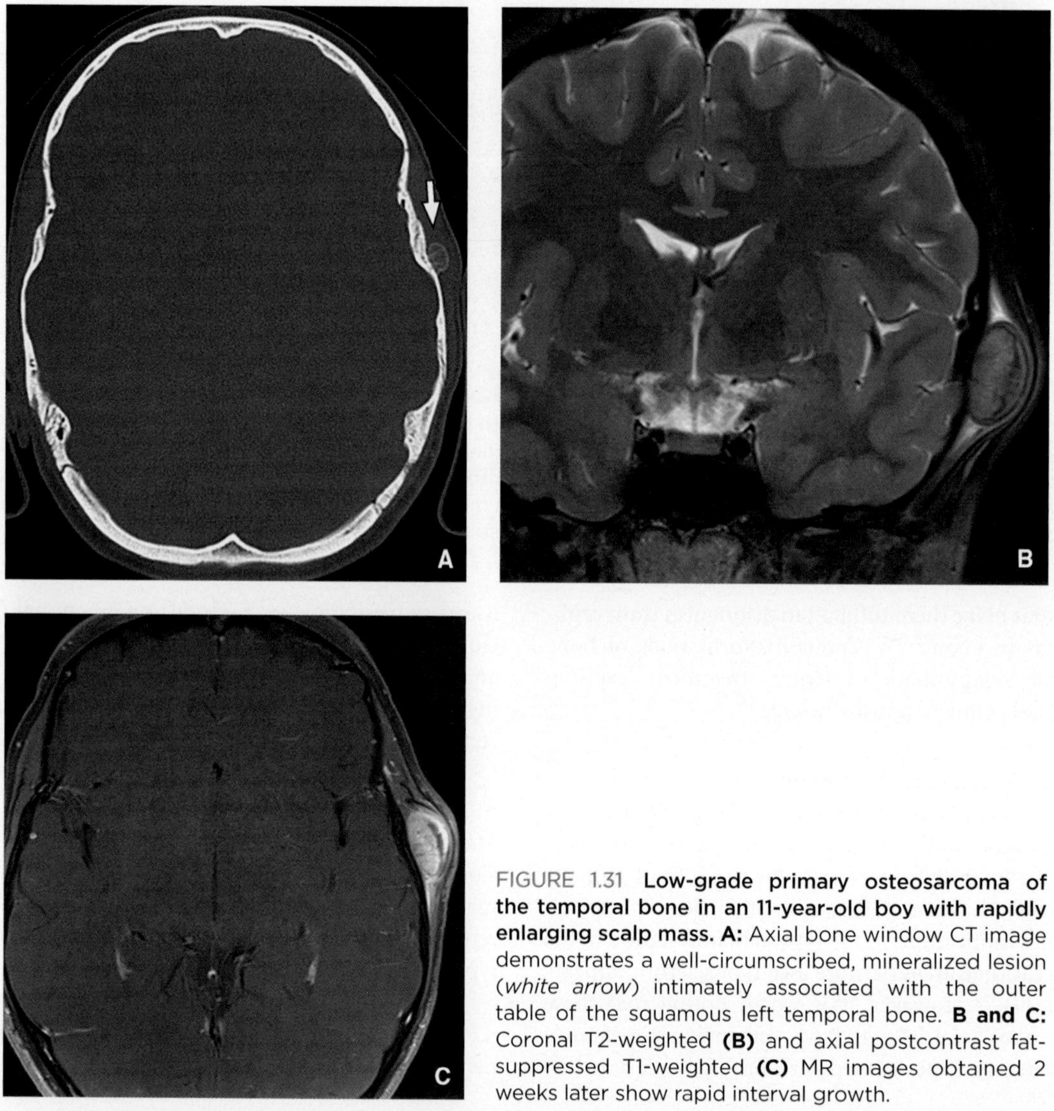

FIGURE 1.31 **Low-grade primary osteosarcoma of the temporal bone in an 11-year-old boy with rapidly enlarging scalp mass. A:** Axial bone window CT image demonstrates a well-circumscribed, mineralized lesion (*white arrow*) intimately associated with the outer table of the squamous left temporal bone. **B and C:** Coronal T2-weighted **(B)** and axial postcontrast fat-suppressed T1-weighted **(C)** MR images obtained 2 weeks later show rapid interval growth.

the treatment consists of excision and adjuvant chemotherapy/radiation. Parosteal forms involving only the outer table have the best prognosis and those violating the dura have the worst outcome.[197]

Ewing sarcoma is the second most common primary bone tumor of children and, like osteosarcoma, involves the skull as primary site rarely, in only 1% to 6% of cases.[194] The most common site of involvement is the cranial vault (temporal bone) though significant numbers of skull base cases are also encountered.[195] In addition to expected bone destruction, the imaging manifestations reflect the hypercellularity of this tumor type with a hyperdense appearance of the soft tissue component on CT and T2 hypointensity with diffusion restriction on MRI.[194,198] Although some retrospective reviews of primary cranial Ewing sarcoma have suggested relatively favorable survival similar to nonmetastatic Ewing sarcoma seen elsewhere, early recurrence and mortality have been reported in cases with violation of the dura.[194,195]

Chondrosarcoma and *chordoma* of the skull in children are very rare and differ from the typical presentation in mid to late life of these tumors. Specifically, it has been suggested that chondrosarcoma of the facial bones is more common in children than in adults, in whom the paramedian skull base is typically involved.[199] For chordoma, the skull base (i.e., clivus) is the most common site of disease unlike adults in whom the remainder of the neuraxis (i.e., sacrococcygeal) is more common.[200] Both these tumors have a similar appearance on imaging in that both have high T2 signal.[201,202] Points of differentiation include the presence of chondroid (arcs and whorls) matrix in chondrosarcomas (Fig. 1.32)

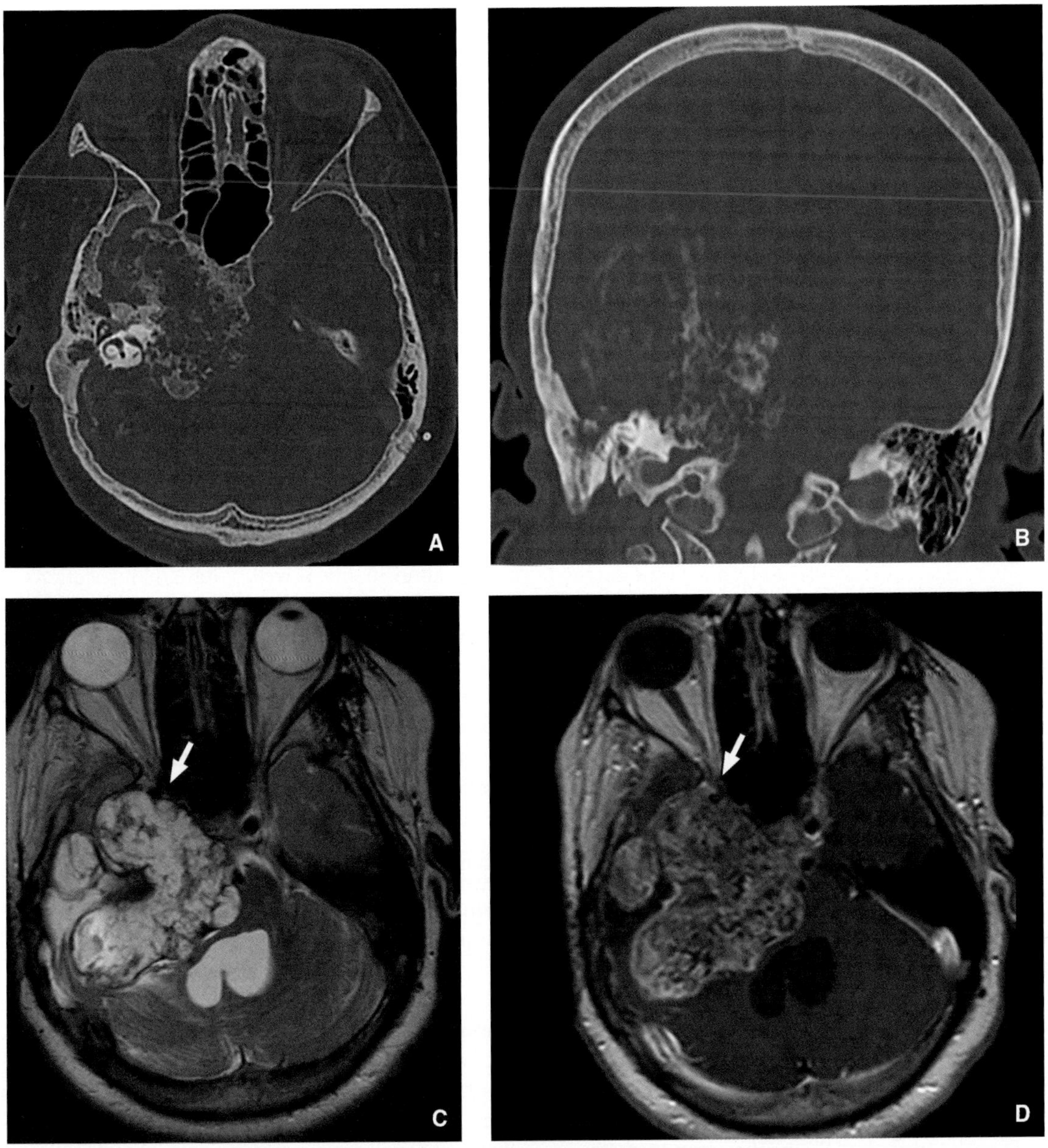

FIGURE 1.32 **Chondrosarcoma in a 15-year-old girl who presented with esotropia. A and B:** Axial **(A)** and coronal reformatted **(B)** bone window CT images demonstrate a large mass with arcs and whorls of mineralization arising from the right petrous apex. **C:** Axial T2-weighted MR image shows the mass as T2 hyperintense. **D:** Axial T1-weighted postcontrast MR image documents heterogeneous enhancement. Note mass effect on the right cavernous sinus and anterior displacement of the right cavernous carotid artery (*arrow*).

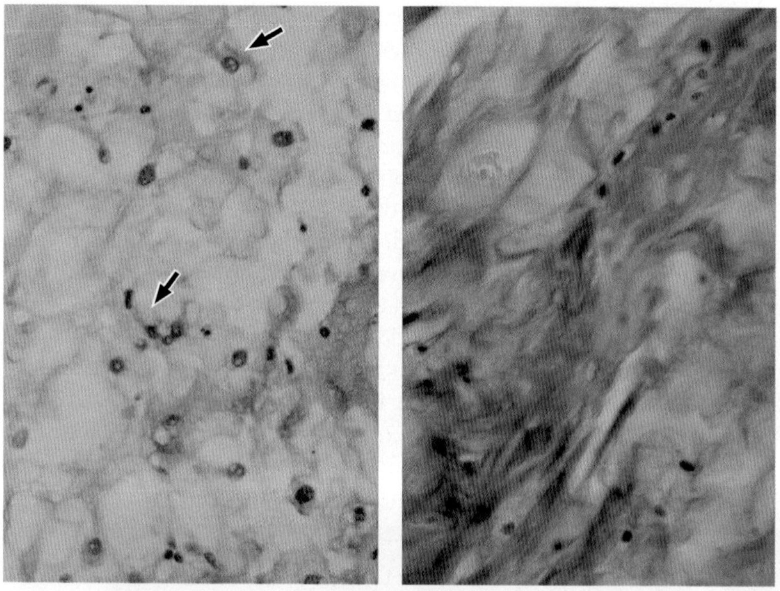

FIGURE 1.33 **Chordoma and low-grade chondrosarcoma, occurring in the skull base of a 12-year-old boy and 14-year-old girl.** The chordoma **(left)** is composed of small cells with bubbly cytoplasm (*arrows*) in an abundant myxoid matrix. The chondrosarcoma **(right)** also has abundant extracellular matrix (hematoxylin and eosin, original magnification, 600×).

and dispersed, destroyed bone fragments in chordomas.[203] Diffusion-weighted MR imaging has also been recently suggested as a means of differentiating between chordoma and chondrosarcoma, the former having lower ADC.[204] Differentiating between these two disease entities is important because of the worse prognosis of chordomas relative to chondrosarcoma. Microscopically, the two tumors can look similar, because chordomas may have an abundant chondromyxoid matrix (Fig. 1.33). Immunostaining for brachyury has been recently identified as a specific marker of notochordal differentiation and can help distinguish the two.[205]

Metastatic Disease Including Neuroblastoma

Hematogenous seeding of tumor can involve the skull, just like other bones. Based on whole body oncologic screening studies, metastatic disease involving the skull is relatively infrequent in pediatric malignancies, constituting ~5% of metastatic bone lesions and affecting 6% to 18% of children depending on the mix of tumors studied.[206–208] However, lesions of the skull and particularly the bony orbits (i.e., greater sphenoid wing producing "raccoon eyes" clinically) are seen in 13% to 25% of pediatric patients with neuroblastoma, the most common nonhematopoietic and non-CNS tumor of children.[209,210] In these metastatic neuroblastoma cases, a variety of patterns have been reported including purely lytic lesions and forms with a productive, blastic component ("sunburst" periosteal reaction).[211,212] In daily practice, some degree of permeative change and periosteal reaction is typically evident, and extension into the adjacent epidural/subgaleal spaces is common (Fig. 1.34). Grossly, neuroblastoma metastasis may look bloody to pale tan and may cause varying degrees of bone destruction and remodeling (Fig. 1.35). Although less frequently encountered, other childhood malignancies that may metastasize to the skull include rhabdomyosarcomas and Ewing sarcoma.[213]

Leukemia and Lymphoma

Hematologic malignancies are the most common forms of cancer in the pediatric population. Leukemia accounts for 30% and lymphoma 11% of cancer in patients <20 years.[214] In the case of leukemia, the marrow is diffusely infiltrated by abnormal cells, and the imaging appearance on MRI is that of red marrow: diffuse T1 hypointensity and enhancement.[215,216] Therefore, leukemic infiltration of the skull and facial bones may cause confusion with cases of profound anemia as well as diffuse metastatic disease (e.g., neuroblastoma).[211] Although lymphoma has a greater propensity for focal lesions, low-grade non-Hodgkin lymphoma can present as diffuse marrow signal abnormality as well.[217] Rare manifestations of hematologic malignancy include destructive lesions of the calvaria from chloroma or lymphoma (Fig. 1.36).[218,219] In these cases, the presence of restricted diffusion may be a helpful clue in suggesting the proper histologic diagnosis.[220] Unless there is diagnostic uncertainty or significant local mass effect, skull involvement by leukemia and lymphoma is treated with systemic chemotherapy.

Traumatic Disorders

Fractures

Pediatric head trauma accounts for an estimated 600,000 emergency room visits in the United States per year,[221] affecting all age groups though more often males than females.[222–224] The vast majority of these injuries occur secondary to falls and traffic accidents. However, abusive or nonaccidental head trauma is often a major concern for children evaluated for head injuries, particularly for infants who are preambulatory. While falls from bed or changing tables account for the majority of head

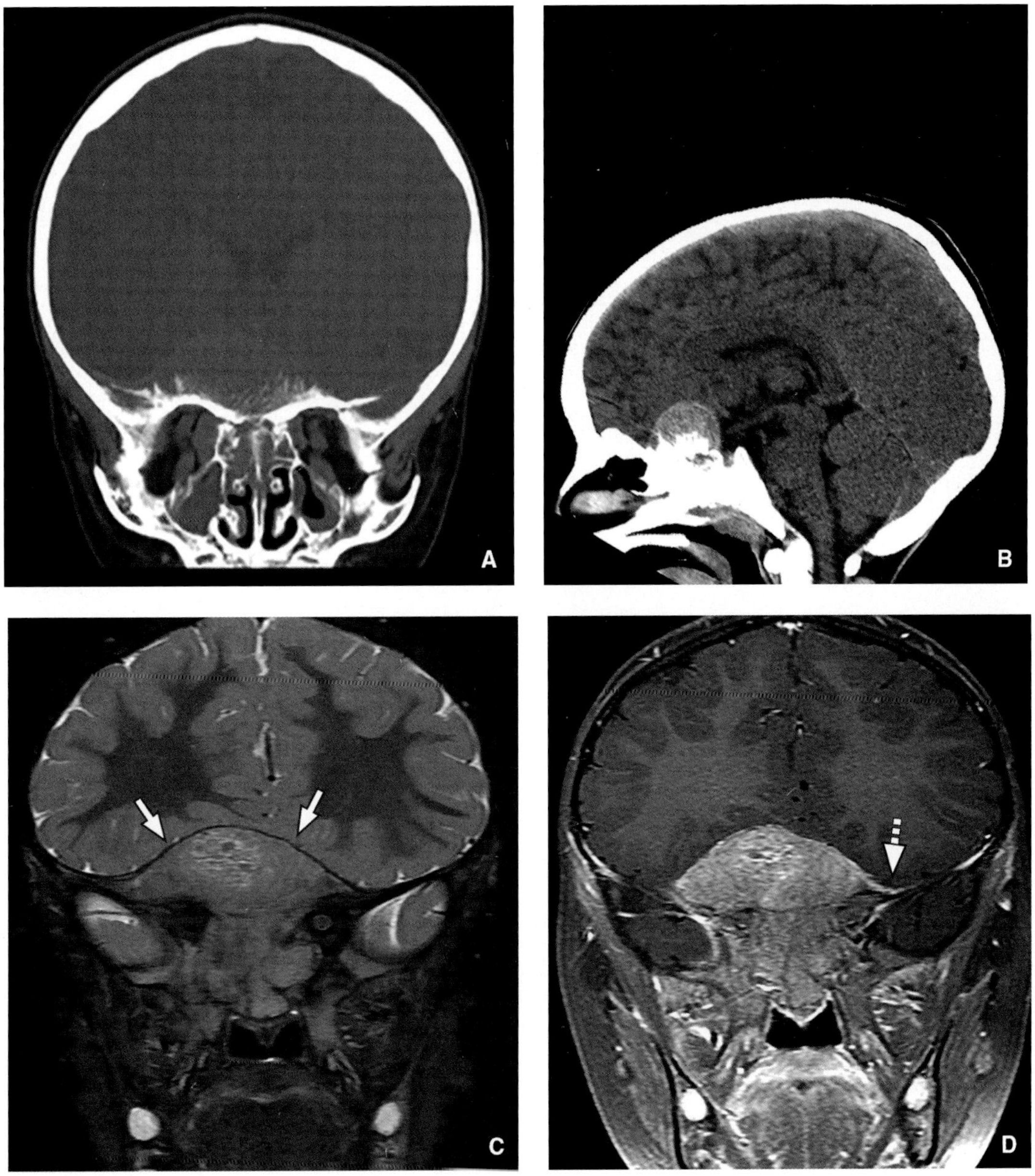

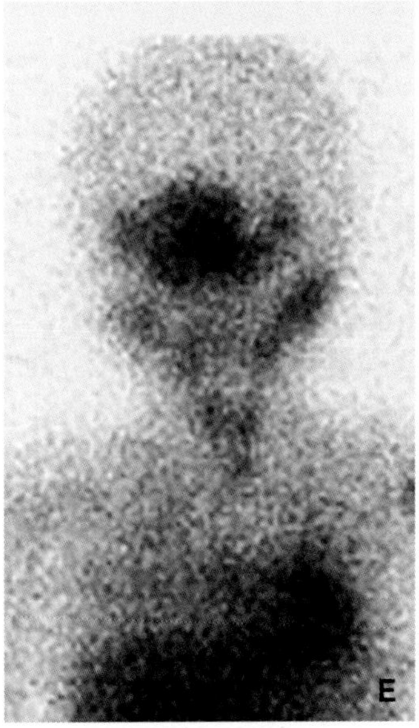

FIGURE 1.34 **Neuroblastoma in a 3-year-old boy who presented with progressive headache. A:** Coronal reformatted bone window CT image shows periosteal reaction of the lesser sphenoid wing and planum sphenoidale. **B:** Sagittal reformatted soft tissue window CT image demonstrates that the spiculation is associated with a hyperdense mass suggesting hypercellular tumor. **C:** Coronal T2-weighted MR image through the affected region also suggests hypercellularity given T2 hypointense signal. **D:** Coronal postcontrast T1-weighted MR image demonstrates avid enhancement of the lesion. Note the dura (*arrows*) is intact in **(C)** though there is dural enhancement/reaction in **(D)** (*dashed arrow*). **E:** Frontal projection I^{131}-MIBG scan shows accumulation of radiotracer within the skull base mass. (Case courtesy of Caroline R. Robson, MB, Boston Children's Hospital and Harvard Medical School, Boston, MA.)

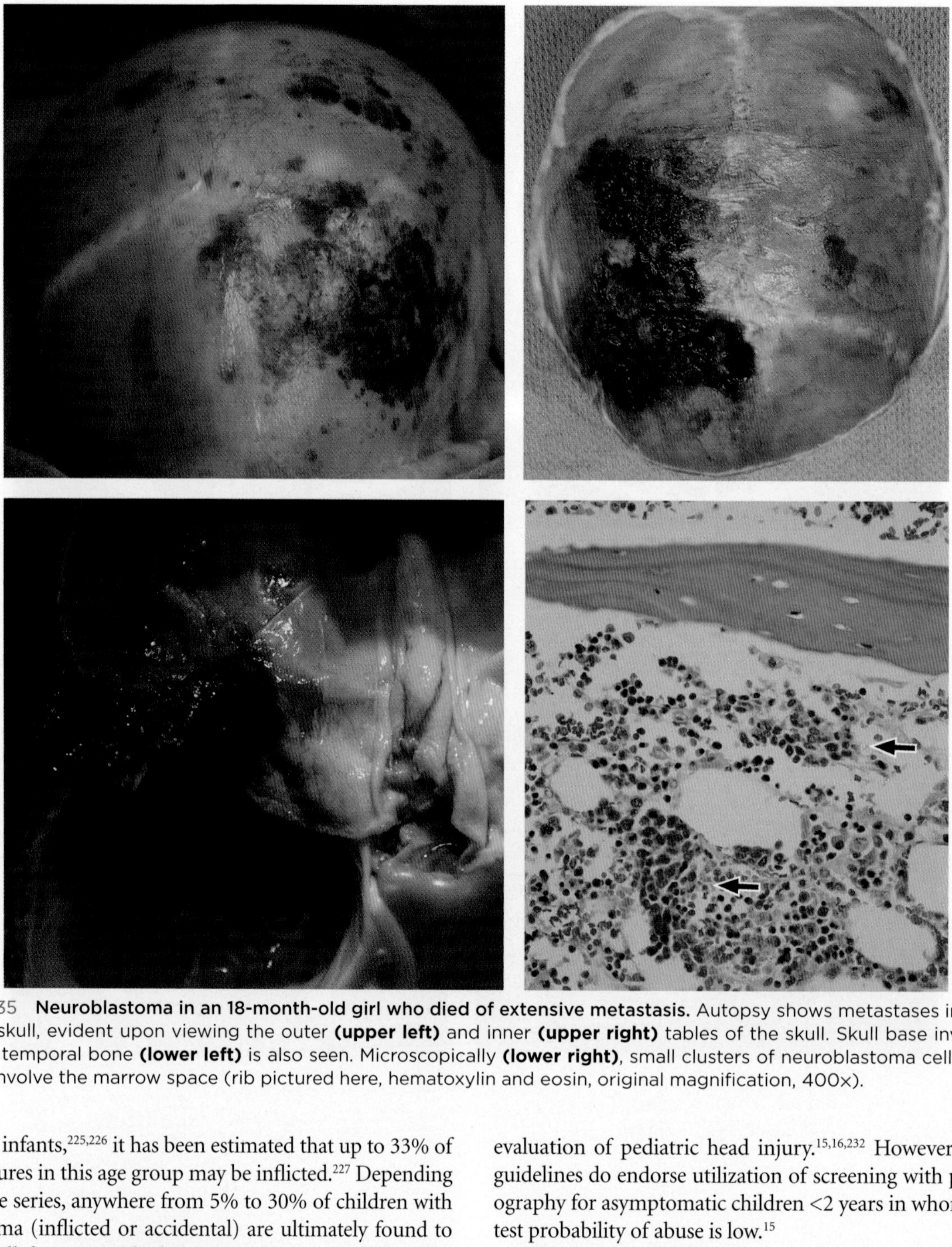

FIGURE 1.35 **Neuroblastoma in an 18-month-old girl who died of extensive metastasis.** Autopsy shows metastases in the right posterior skull, evident upon viewing the outer **(upper left)** and inner **(upper right)** tables of the skull. Skull base involvement in the left temporal bone **(lower left)** is also seen. Microscopically **(lower right)**, small clusters of neuroblastoma cells (*arrows*) diffusely involve the marrow space (rib pictured here, hematoxylin and eosin, original magnification, 400×).

trauma in infants,[225,226] it has been estimated that up to 33% of skull fractures in this age group may be inflicted.[227] Depending on the case series, anywhere from 5% to 30% of children with head trauma (inflicted or accidental) are ultimately found to have a skull fracture with the parietal bone being the most common site.[223,224,228] Although skull fractures increase the risk of intracranial hemorrhage and parenchymal injury, there is abundant literature documenting that children (especially <2 years old) can have significant intracranial injuries without skull fractures, neurologic abnormalities, or symptoms such as vomiting with up to a third of children with intracranial/skull injury clinically normal.[223,229–231] In nonaccidental trauma, detection of these intracranial injuries is especially important because they are the most common cause of death from abuse.[227] Therefore, despite concerns regarding radiation and proposed clinical decision rules, CT remains the preferred modality for evaluation of pediatric head injury.[15,16,232] However, the ACR guidelines do endorse utilization of screening with plain radiography for asymptomatic children <2 years in whom the pretest probability of abuse is low.[15]

Skull fractures are classified as *linear* versus *complex/comminuted* and *depressed* versus *nondepressed*. They have the appearance of fractures seen elsewhere (i.e., sharply marginated lucency), but one unique challenge with very young children is the presence of normal transient sutures (e.g., superior occipital fissure or the mendosal sutures mentioned earlier) and rare accessory sutures/synchondroses in the occipital bone.[46] These minor and variant sutures are best excluded after the review of three-dimension data.[233] Helpful findings suggestive of a fracture rather than a persistent or variant suture include lucencies that do not conform to known ossification centers, sharp linear lucencies without cortication

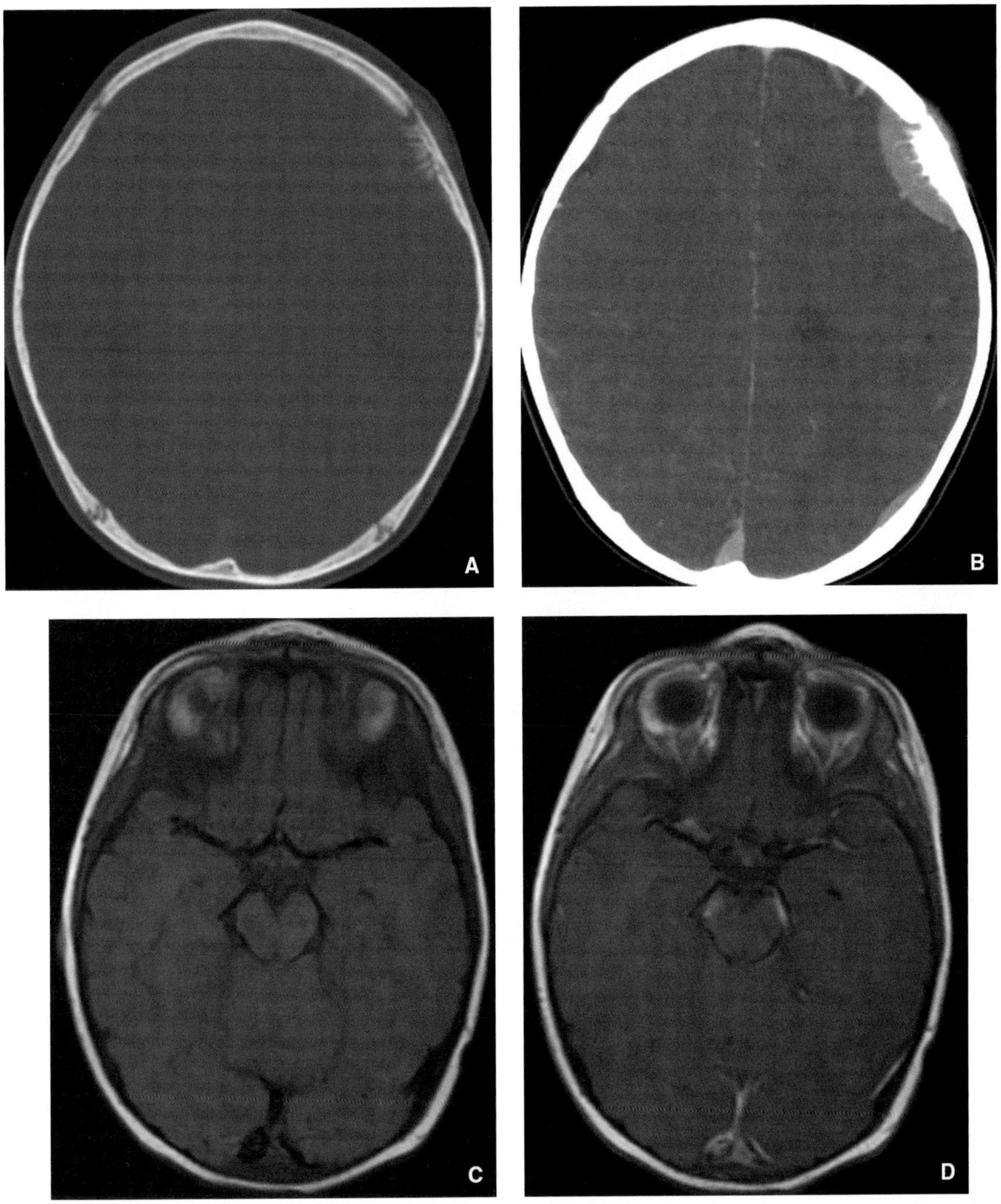

FIGURE 1.36 **Acute myelocytic leukemia initially presenting as scalp swelling and lethargy in a 3-year-old boy. A and B:** Axial bone window **(A)** and postcontrast soft tissue window **(B)** CT images demonstrate spiculation about the diastatic left coronal suture and an associated soft tissue mass. **C and D:** Precontrast **(C)** and postcontrast **(D)** axial T1-weighted MR images show diffusely low marrow signal with faint enhancement elsewhere in the cranial vault, consistent with hematopoietic marrow or neoplastic infiltration. Bone marrow biopsy returned leukemic cells, and the skull lesion was therefore consistent with a chloroma.

(versus the corticated, zigzag appearance of mature sutures), traversal of normal sutures, widening of fracture lines as they approach a suture line, and the presence of adjacent soft tissue trauma (Fig. 1.37).[234] The presence of soft tissue trauma confirms the presence of acute trauma, but it is important to recognize that its absence does not necessarily exclude hyperacute or remote trauma.[227] Although there may be a slightly higher frequency of multiple/bilateral fractures or fractures crossing suture lines in abused children studied as a group, these findings are insufficient to specifically suggest abuse based on the skull fracture appearance.[235] However, the severity of the skull fracture does clearly increase with more severe mechanisms (e.g., increasing height of fall), and therefore discrepant mechanisms of injury should be viewed with suspicion.[226] As mentioned earlier, it is unusual for the skull to produce callus as it heals, making radiographic timing of a skull fracture extremely inaccurate.[227]

The management of head trauma is usually directed towards treating intracranial/parenchymal injury (see "Brain" chapter). Although it has been long suggested that

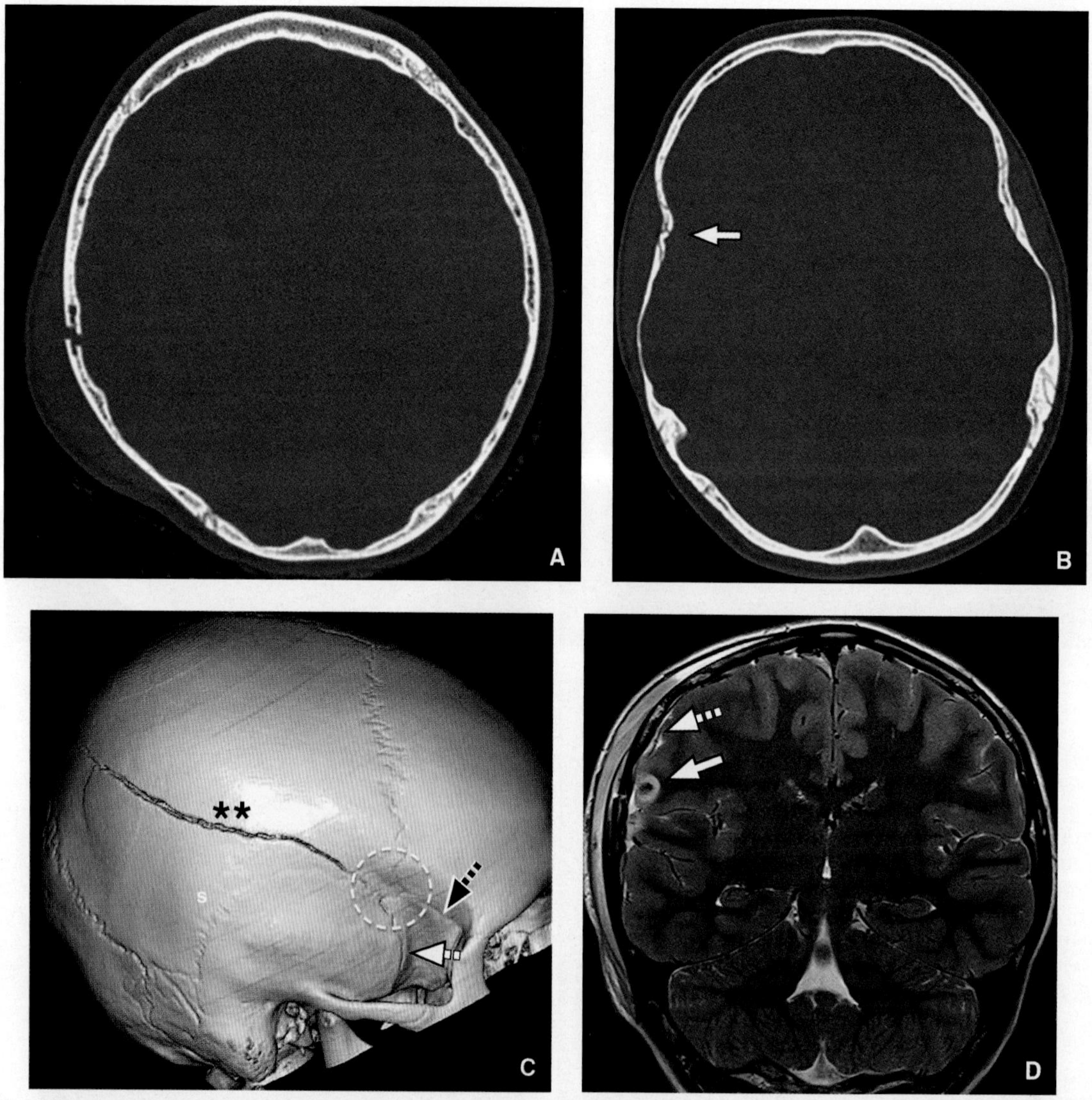

FIGURE 1.37 **Right temporoparietal skull fracture in an 11-year-old boy who fell 20 feet from a tree onto concrete. A and B:** Axial bone window CT images show a right parietal fracture with overlying scalp hematoma, which is difficult to follow into the region of the pterion (*arrow*). **C:** Right lateral projection surface rendering CT image demonstrates the precise course of the fracture (*black double asterisk*) from the parietal bone, across the squamous suture, and posterior to the sphenotemporal suture where the dashed circle represents the pterion, the white dashed arrow represents the sphenotemporal suture, and the dashed black arrow represents the frontosphenoid suture. **D:** Coronal T2-weighted MR image indicates the presence of a small hemorrhagic right parietal contusion (*arrow*) and a thin subdural collection (*dashed arrow*).

neurologically intact children with isolated skull fractures (i.e., no intracranial injury) may be safe to discharge from the emergency room, common practice is to still observe these patients for 1 to 2 days.[224,236,237] Most skull fractures (linear, comminuted, depressed) with intact overlying skin can be managed expectantly. However, cases with foreign bodies or scalp lacerations are usually debrided with approximation of skull fracture fragments and repair of any dural laceration.[238]

Birth-Related Injuries

There are unique patterns of injury that arise in the setting of delivery-related trauma. These injuries have distinct clinical and radiographic findings depending on their precise location within the scalp or cranial vault. As a reminder, several distinct layers are encountered in the scalp as one goes progressively deeper from the skin surface[22]: the subcutaneous fat of the scalp, the *galea aponeurotica* that serves as a point of attachment for frontalis/occipitalis/temporalis musculature, the *subgaleal fascia* that loosely adheres the galeal aponeurotica to the periosteum, and the periosteum itself.

Birth-related hematomas in the subcutaneous fat are known as *caput succedaneum* and have been estimated to occur in up to 25% of normal vaginal deliveries (Fig. 1.38).[239] Hemorrhage into the subgaleal (potential) space causes a *subgaleal hematoma* (Figs. 1.39 and 1.40). This form of neonatal hemorrhage is fairly uncommon but is seen more frequently with vacuum-assisted vaginal delivery.[240] Analogous to epidural hematomas intracranially, *cephalohematomas* arise in the subperiosteal space of the outer table of the cranial vault and are therefore

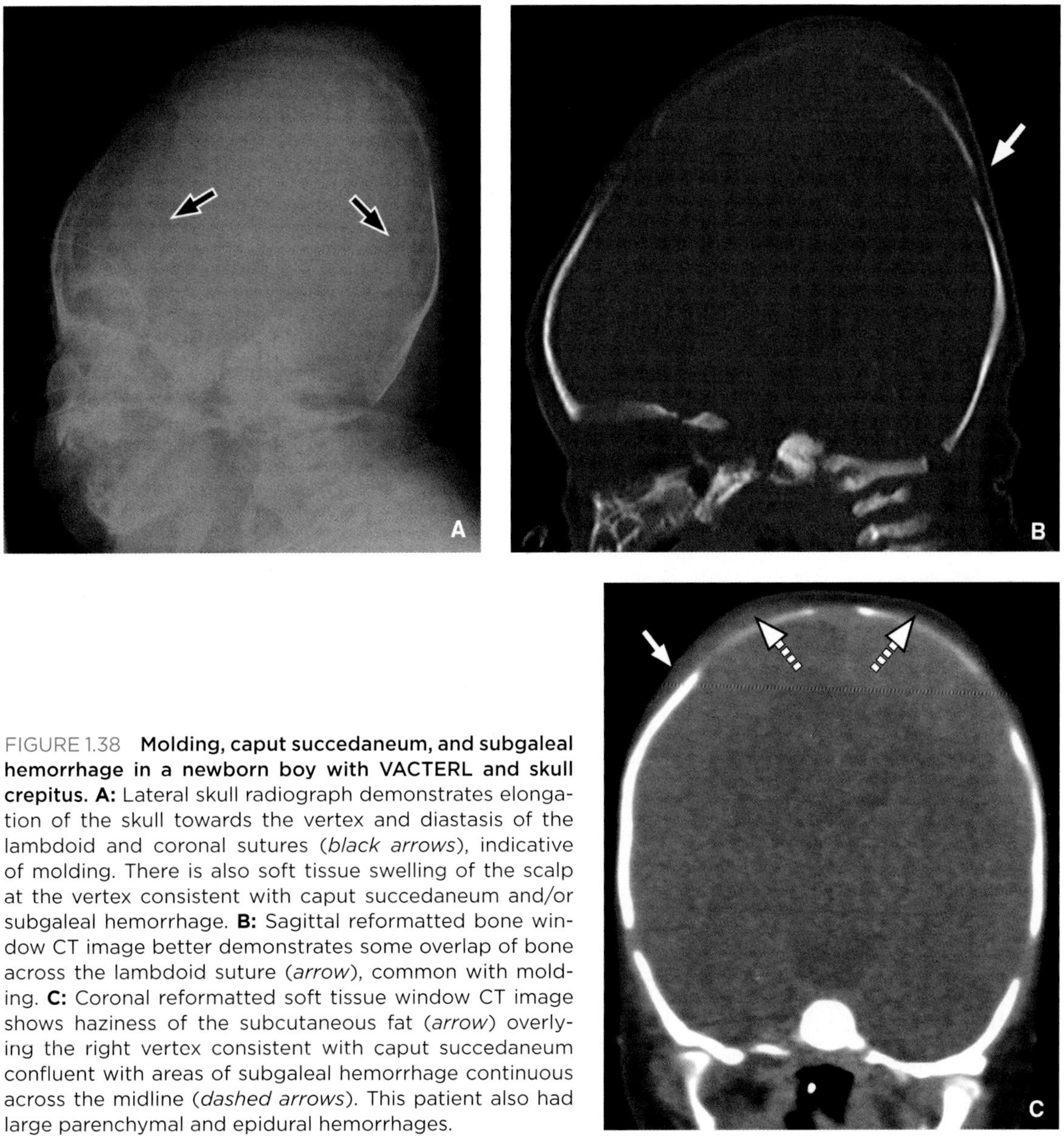

FIGURE 1.38 **Molding, caput succedaneum, and subgaleal hemorrhage in a newborn boy with VACTERL and skull crepitus. A:** Lateral skull radiograph demonstrates elongation of the skull towards the vertex and diastasis of the lambdoid and coronal sutures (*black arrows*), indicative of molding. There is also soft tissue swelling of the scalp at the vertex consistent with caput succedaneum and/or subgaleal hemorrhage. **B:** Sagittal reformatted bone window CT image better demonstrates some overlap of bone across the lambdoid suture (*arrow*), common with molding. **C:** Coronal reformatted soft tissue window CT image shows haziness of the subcutaneous fat (*arrow*) overlying the right vertex consistent with caput succedaneum confluent with areas of subgaleal hemorrhage continuous across the midline (*dashed arrows*). This patient also had large parenchymal and epidural hemorrhages.

bounded by sutures unlike subgaleal hematomas and caput succedaneum (Fig. 1.41). Although having a reported incidence of only ~1% of live births, cephalohematomas frequently elicit concern because of their firmness on physical examination.[161] Therefore, they are the scalp injury most likely to present for surgical and radiological evaluation, constituting more than half of the head and neck trauma evaluated in one series of birth-related trauma.[241] These birth-related hematomas typically follow fluid signal with the precise signal characteristics determined by age of the blood products.[22] The deformities caused by these scalp/skull injuries must be distinguished from *molding*, a normal, transient deformation (craniocaudal elongation) of the cranial vault caused by passage through the birth canal (Fig. 1.38).[242–244]

In the majority of cases, the various forms of delivery-related trauma may be anticipated to resolve uneventfully in the first weeks of life and without residua. When cephalohematomas persist beyond the immediate perinatal period, they can incorporate into the skull as ossified material causing a palpable or radiographic abnormality that can be first detected later in life (Fig. 1.41C).[245,246] Rare complications from these superficial birth traumas include life-threatening exsanguination particularly into the relatively capacious subgaleal space, infection, and skull fractures with significant intracranial hemorrhage.[240,247,248]

Ping-Pong and Growing Fractures

The skulls of neonates and young children are unusually soft leading to patterns of skull fracture not seen in older

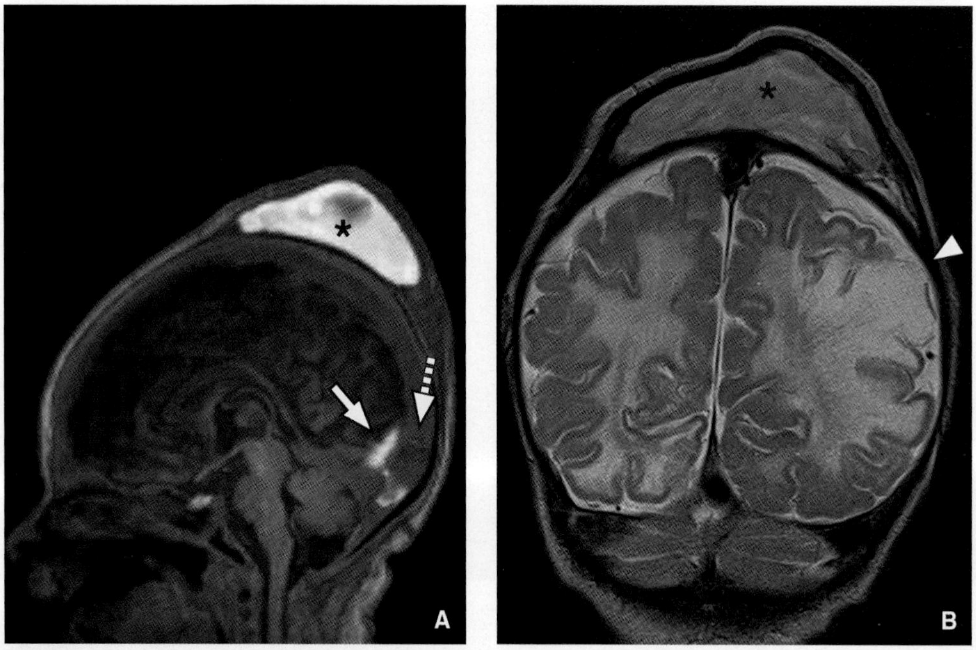

FIGURE 1.39 **Large vertex subgaleal hematoma in a newborn boy with soft tissue mass at the vertex. A:** Sagittal T1-weighted MR image demonstrates large T1 hyperintense hematoma (*asterisk*) at the vertex as well as parturitional subdural hemorrhage (*arrow*) and evolving clot in the torcula (*dashed arrow*). **B:** Coronal T2-weighted MR image shows that the subgaleal hematoma (*asterisk*) extends across the midline and is not confined by sutures. This patient also experienced hypoxic ischemic injury as evidenced by encephalomalacia (*arrowhead*) involving the left parietal cortex.

patients. One peculiar form of skull injury seen in the perinatal period is the so-called *ping-pong (neonatal depressed) fracture,* which is analogous to the incomplete, "greenstick" type of fracture seen in long bones. In this form of skull fracture, there is smooth inward depression without a discrete break in the inner and outer cortex (Fig. 1.42). These injuries are most commonly associated with instrumentation-assisted delivery, but spontaneous vaginal deliveries as well as accidental trauma can produce an identical appearance.[249–251] Ping-pong fractures generally have very good outcome, and while there was once a tendency to perform open repairs of the deformity caused by these injuries, various noninvasive techniques are now being used to repair some of these fractures.[252,253]

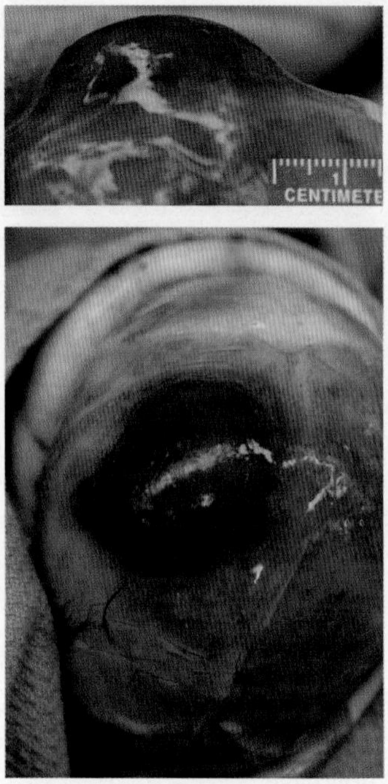

FIGURE 1.40 **Subgaleal hematoma of the parietal region attributed to birth trauma in a 10-day-old premature infant who died of other causes.** This localized red mass has a bulging contour.

Another type of fracture seen uniquely in children is the *"growing" skull fracture* or *leptomeningeal cyst.* In this fracture type, the meninges insinuates itself between a diastatic fracture fragment, causing a progressive enlargement of the osseous gap (Fig. 1.43).[254,255] Like the ping-pong fracture, growing skull fractures are almost exclusively seen in infants. Growing fractures require excision of the protruding meninges and any associated encephalomalacic brain tissue, with or without cranioplasty.[256–258]

Diffuse Bone Disease

As an osseous structure, the skull can be diffusely affected by disorders of bone metabolism, hematopoiesis, and bone dysplasias.[259] The skull manifestations of these diffuse bone disorders are generally asymptomatic or at least require no specific management. However, they are important clues to systemic processes affecting the pediatric patient that may require treatment. Chronic anemia (e.g., thalassemia or sickle cell disease) and other etiologies of extramedullary

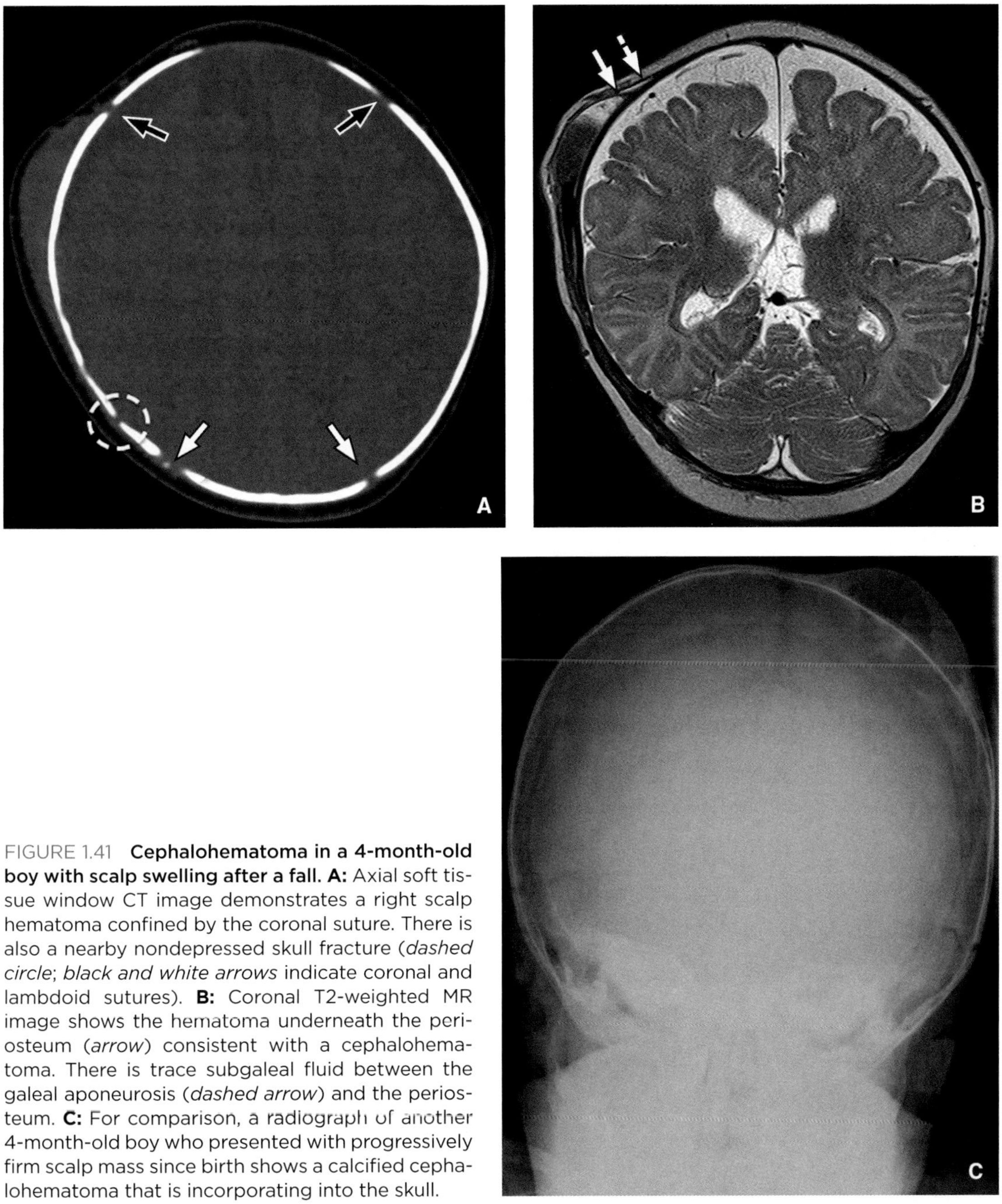

FIGURE 1.41 **Cephalohematoma in a 4-month-old boy with scalp swelling after a fall. A:** Axial soft tissue window CT image demonstrates a right scalp hematoma confined by the coronal suture. There is also a nearby nondepressed skull fracture (*dashed circle*; *black and white arrows* indicate coronal and lambdoid sutures). **B:** Coronal T2-weighted MR image shows the hematoma underneath the periosteum (*arrow*) consistent with a cephalohematoma. There is trace subgaleal fluid between the galeal aponeurosis (*dashed arrow*) and the periosteum. **C:** For comparison, a radiograph of another 4-month-old boy who presented with progressively firm scalp mass since birth shows a calcified cephalohematoma that is incorporating into the skull.

hematopoiesis cause marrow expansion within the diploic space and thickening/sclerosis of the cranial vault.[260–262] In its most exuberant form, these changes can manifest as a "hair on end" appearance due to numerous parallel trabeculae (Fig. 1.44). A similar sclerotic/hyperostotic appearance can be encountered with disorders of bone metabolism such as hereditary hyperphosphatasia,[263,264] pseudohypoparathyroidism,[265,266] and osteopetrosis (Figs. 1.45 and 1.46).[267–269] Inherited bone dysplasias can also have a thickened, sclerotic appearance of the skull in the case of diaphyseal dysplasia (Camurati-Engelmann disease)[270] and pycnodysostosis.[271,272] Lysosomal storage disorders such as mucopolysaccharidoses IH and mucolipidosis II can present with marked skull thickening as well as J-shaped sellae.[92–94] When profound expansion of the skull occurs, these disorders can be rarely associated with hydrocephalus (presumably from venous hypertension), Chiari I malformations, and impingement on the optic nerves. Severe forms of osteopetrosis are also associated with bone marrow failure.

Conversely, there are several bone disorders with thinning and osteopenia as a major feature. Osteogenesis imperfecta, cleidocranial dysplasia (anterior fontanelle delayed closure),

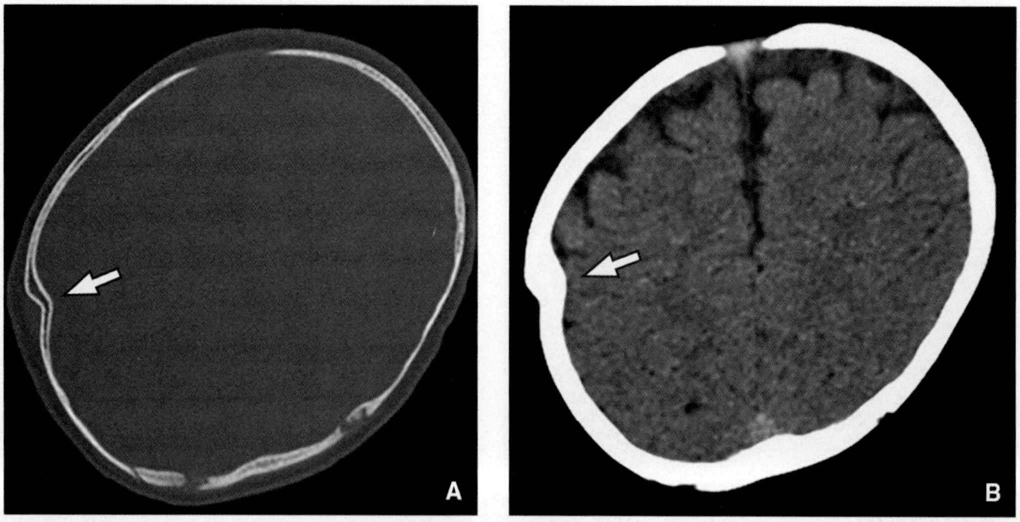

FIGURE 1.42 **Ping-pong (infantile depressed) skull fracture in a 5-month-old girl with head strike against a table and new palpable skull deformity. A and B:** Axial bone window **(A)** and soft tissue window **(B)** CT images demonstrate inward skull deformity (*arrow*) at the point of impact without a discrete fracture line. There was no acute intracranial hemorrhage.

and achondrogenesis type 1A share defective synthesis of proteins necessary for structurally intact bone and therefore have undermineralized, thin calvaria.[273–278] Hypophosphatasia and X-linked hypophosphatemic rickets are inherited disorders of bone metabolism with a similar appearance.[279,280] Although not diffuse, neurofibromatosis can present with multiple foci of dysplastic bone (e.g., sphenoid wing dysplasia, remodeled sella, macrocrania).[281–284]

As a practical matter, the many inherited causes of diffuse skull abnormality are less commonly encountered than acquired problems. For example, sclerosis and thickening of the skull is more commonly encountered in the setting of a minority of individuals with renal osteodystrophy,[285,286] a minority of individuals with primary hyperparathyroidism,[287] compensatory hypertrophy from chronic brain injury (Dyke-Davidoff-Masson syndrome), chronic shunting, and exposure to antiseizure medications such as phenytoin (Fig. 1.47).[288–290] For osteopenia and skull thinning, rickets, hyperparathyroidism (primary or renal osteodystrophy related), and prematurity are more commonly encountered than the mendelian disorders.[286,291–294]

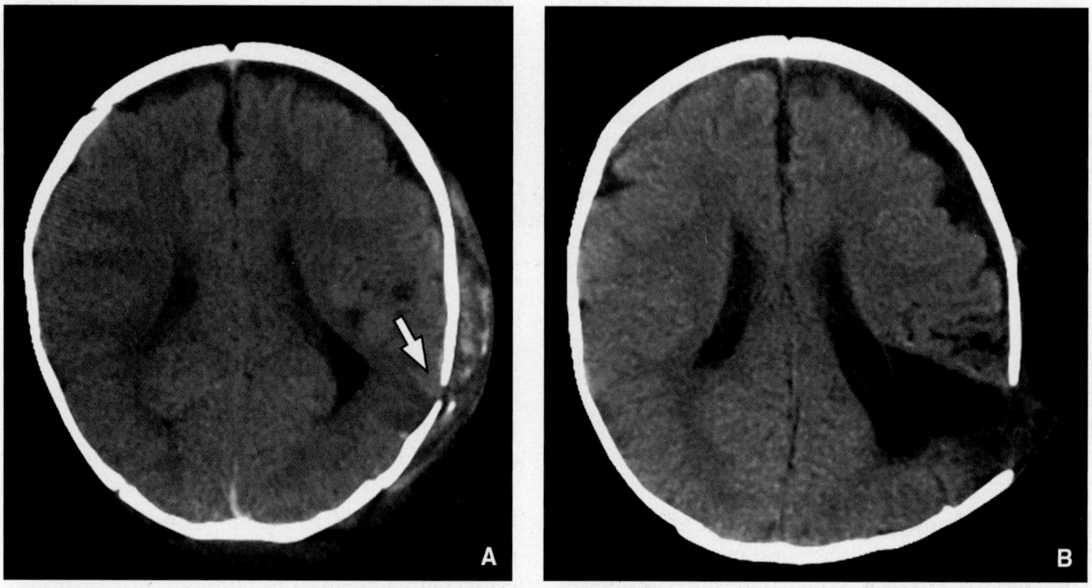

FIGURE 1.43 **Leptomeningeal cyst (growing fracture) in a 4-month-old boy after a 5-foot fall onto a hardwood floor. A:** Axial soft tissue window CT image demonstrates a nondepressed left parietal skull fracture (*arrow*) with overlying scalp hematoma and underlying hemorrhagic contusions (not shown). **B:** One-month follow-up axial soft tissue window CT image documents interval diastasis of the fracture line and protrusion of CSF and encephalomalacic brain through the defect. (Case courtesy of Sanjay Prabhu, MBBS, Boston Children's Hospital and Harvard Medical School, Boston, MA.)

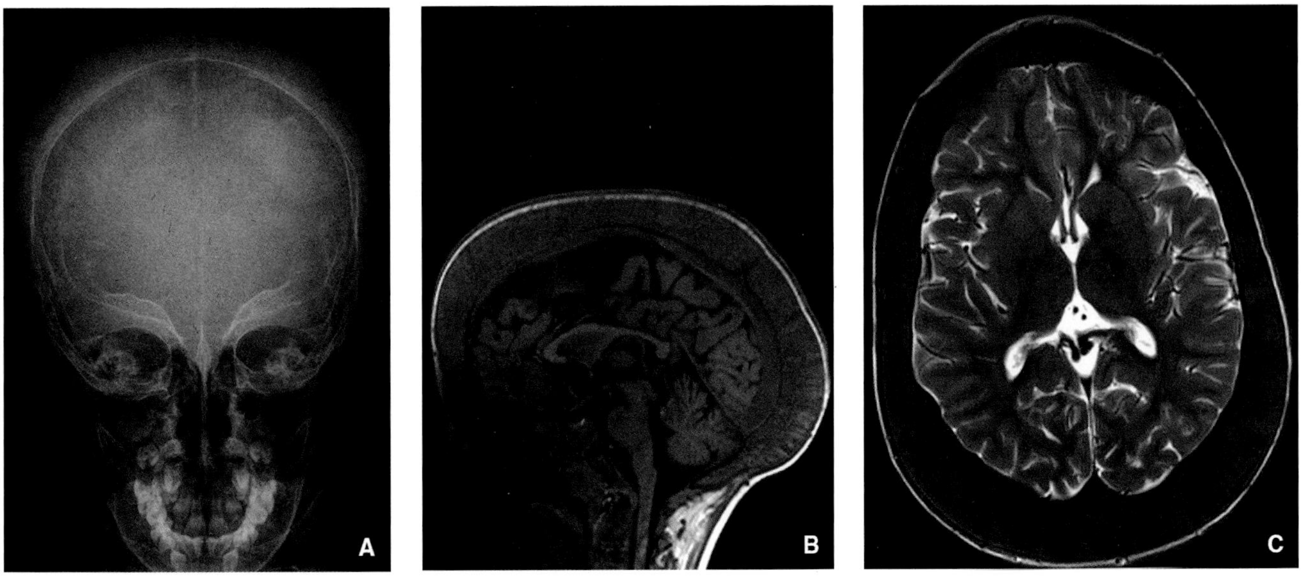

FIGURE 1.44 **Sickle cell anemia in a 10-year-old boy recently adopted from Africa. A:** Frontal skull radiograph demonstrates diffuse calvarial thickening with "hair on end" appearance. **B and C:** Sagittal T1-weighted MPRAGE **(B)** and axial T2-weighted **(C)** MR images demonstrate diffuse decrease in marrow signal accompanying the skull thickening consistent with profound red marrow hyperplasia.

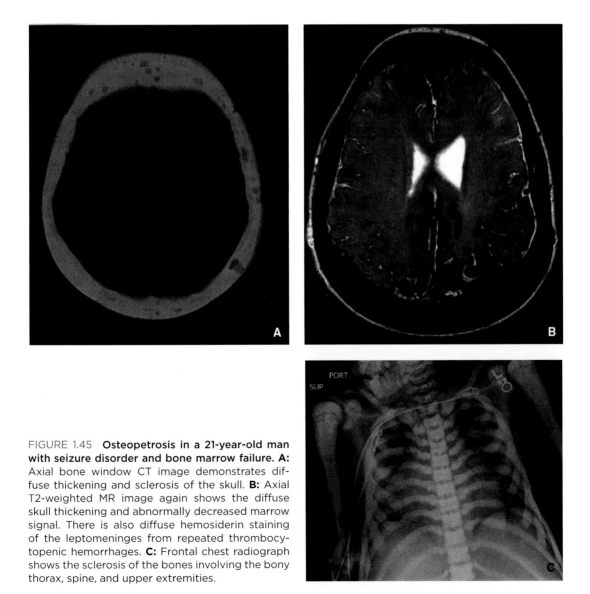

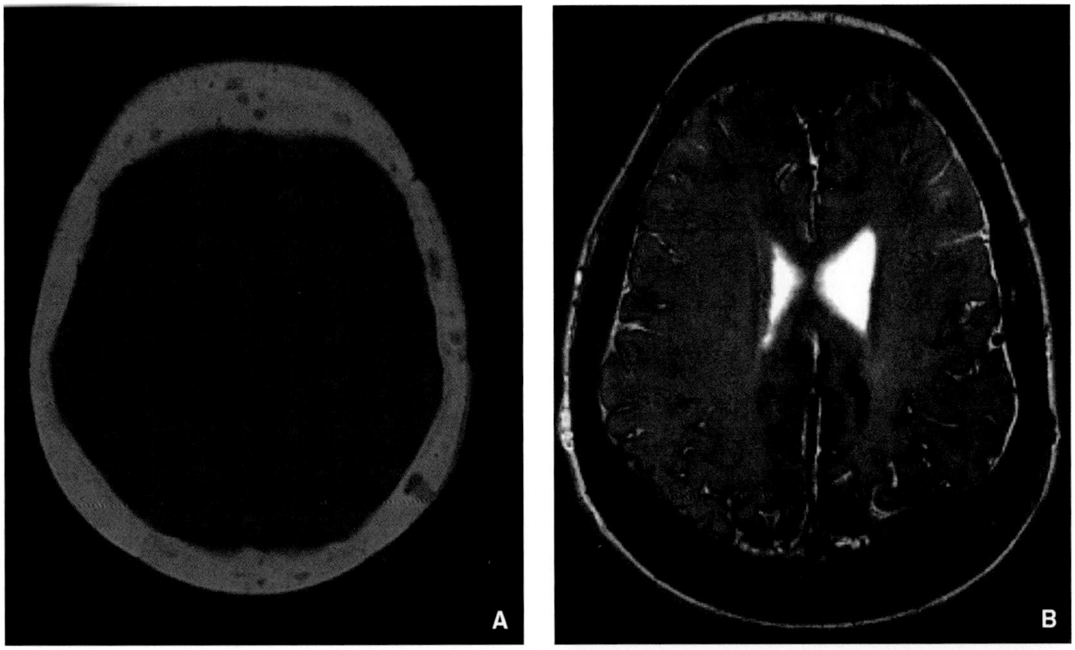

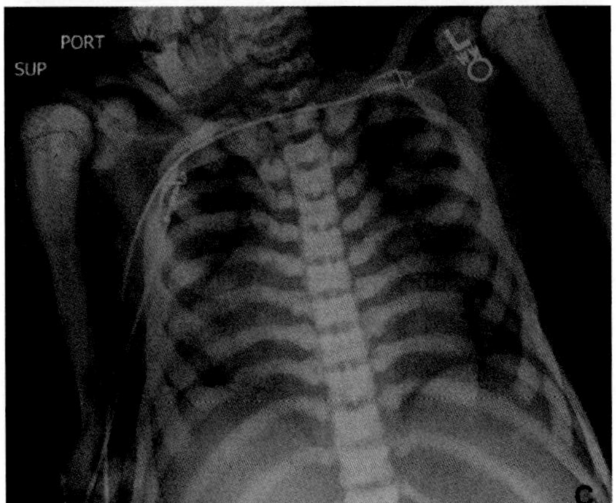

FIGURE 1.45 **Osteopetrosis in a 21-year-old man with seizure disorder and bone marrow failure. A:** Axial bone window CT image demonstrates diffuse thickening and sclerosis of the skull. **B:** Axial T2-weighted MR image again shows the diffuse skull thickening and abnormally decreased marrow signal. There is also diffuse hemosiderin staining of the leptomeninges from repeated thrombocytopenic hemorrhages. **C:** Frontal chest radiograph shows the sclerosis of the bones involving the bony thorax, spine, and upper extremities.

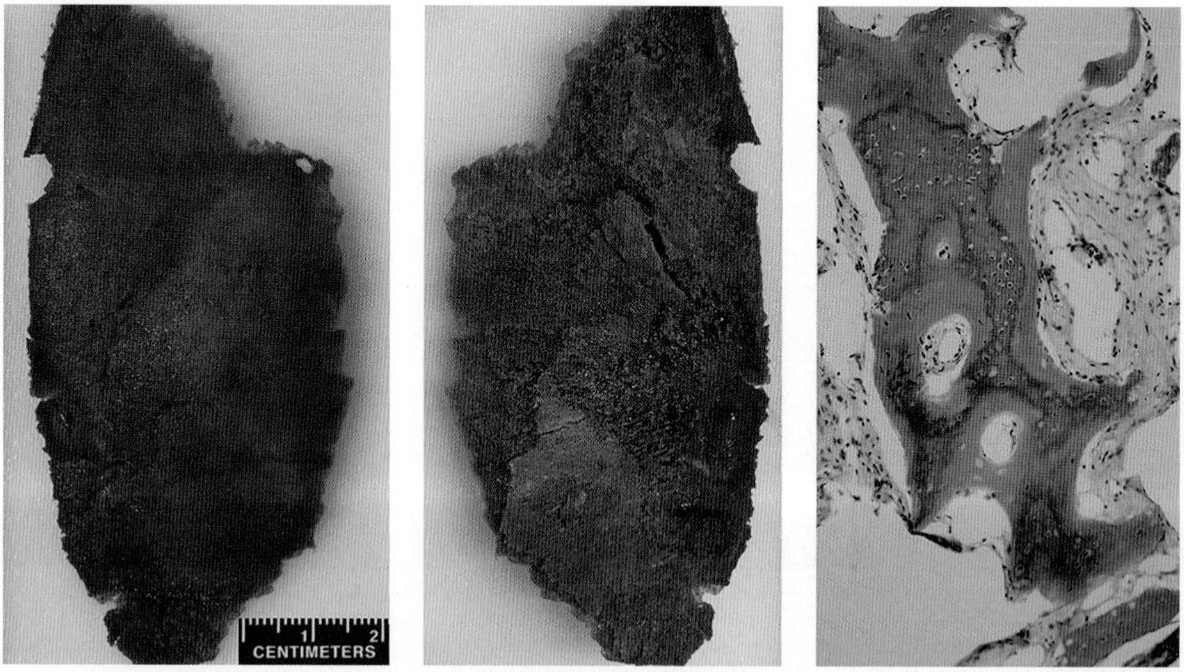

FIGURE 1.46 **This skull fragment was resected during fronto-orbital advancement in a 9-month-old girl with osteopetrosis.** The cortical surface of the bone is smooth **(left)**, whereas the diploic space shows thickened parallel trabeculae **(middle)**. There is deficient mineralization, and prosection could be completed without need for decalcification. Microscopically **(right)**, trabeculae are widened and contain woven bone (hematoxylin and eosin, original magnification, 600×).

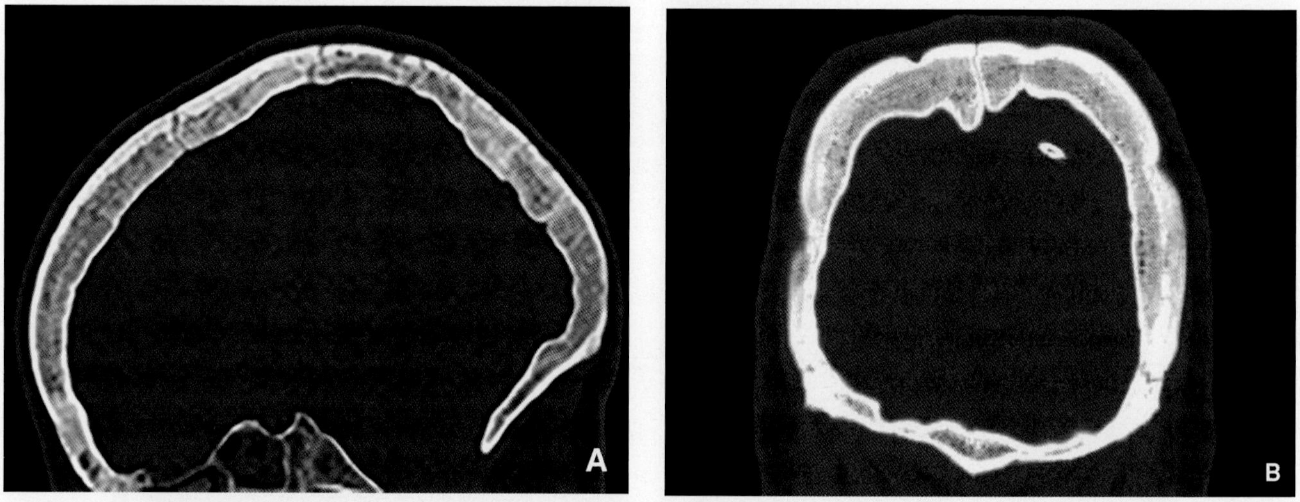

FIGURE 1.47 **Diffuse calvarial thickening secondary to chronic shunting for Chiari II malformation with myelomeningocele in a 19-year-old woman.** Sagittal **(A)** and coronal **(B)** reformatted bone window image CT images demonstrate diffuse thickening of the calvaria attributed to chronic shunting. The shunt tubing is partially visible in **(B)**.

References

1. Mazonakis M, Damilakis J, Raissaki M, et al. Radiation dose and cancer risk to children undergoing skull radiography. *Pediatr Radiol.* 2004;34(8):624–629.
2. Rabiner JE, Friedman LM, Khine H, et al. Accuracy of point-of-care ultrasound for diagnosis of skull fractures in children. *Pediatrics.* 2013;131(6):e1757–e1764.
3. Ramirez-Schrempp D, Vinci RJ, Liteplo AS. Bedside ultrasound in the diagnosis of skull fractures in the pediatric emergency department. *Pediatr Emerg Care.* 2011;27(4):312–314.
4. Regelsberger J, Delling G, Helmke K, et al. Ultrasound in the diagnosis of craniosynostosis. *J Craniofac Surg.* 2006;17(4):623–625; discussion 626–628.
5. Soboleski D, Mussari B, McCloskey D, et al. High-resolution sonography of the abnormal cranial suture. *Pediatr Radiol.* 1998;28(2):79–82.
6. Dubois J, Garel L. Imaging and therapeutic approach of hemangiomas and vascular malformations in the pediatric age group. *Pediatr Radiol.* 1999;29(12):879–893.
7. Luker GD, Siegel MJ. Sinus pericranii: sonographic findings. *AJR Am J Roentgenol.* 1995;165(1):175–176.
8. Agrawal D, Steinbok P, Cochrane DD. Diagnosis of isolated sagittal synostosis: are radiographic studies necessary? *Childs Nerv Syst.* 2006;22(4):375–378.
9. Cerovac S, Neil-Dwyer JG, Rich P, et al. Are routine preoperative CT scans necessary in the management of single suture craniosynostosis? *Br J Neurosurg.* 2002;16(4):348–354.
10. Schweitzer T, Bohm H, Meyer-Marcotty P, et al. Avoiding CT scans in children with single-suture craniosynostosis. *Childs Nerv Syst.* 2012;28(7):1077–1082.
11. Kotrikova B, Krempien R, Freier K, et al. Diagnostic imaging in the management of craniosynostoses. *Eur Radiol.* 2007;17(8):1968–1978.
12. Medina LS, Richardson RR, Crone K. Children with suspected craniosynostosis: a cost-effectiveness analysis of diagnostic strategies. *AJR Am J Roentgenol.* 2002;179(1):215–221.
13. Alderman BW, Fernbach SK, Greene C, et al. Diagnostic practice and the estimated prevalence of craniosynostosis in Colorado. *Arch Pediatr Adolesc Med.* 1997;151(2):159–164.
14. Vannier MW, Hildebolt CF, Marsh JL, et al. Craniosynostosis: diagnostic value of three-dimensional CT reconstruction. *Radiology.* 1989;173(3):669–673.
15. Ryan ME, Palasis S, Saigal G, et al. *American College of Radiology ACR Appropriateness Criteria: Head Trauma-Child.* https://acsearch.acr.org/docs/3083021/Narrative/ accessed August 14, 2016.
16. Meyer JS, Gunderman R, Coley BD, et al. ACR Appropriateness Criteria® on suspected physical abuse-child. *J Am Coll Radiol.* 2011;8(2):87–94.
17. Huda W, Vance A. Patient radiation doses from adult and pediatric CT. *AJR Am J Roentgenol.* 2007;188(2):540–546.
18. Radiology ACo. *CT Accreditation Program Requirements.* http://www.acr.org/~/media/ACR/Documents/Accreditation/CT/Requirements.pdf2013
19. Strauss KJ, Goske MJ, Kaste SC, et al. Image gently: ten steps you can take to optimize image quality and lower CT dose for pediatric patients. *AJR Am J Roentgenol.* 2010;194(4):868–873.
20. Mettler FA Jr, Huda W, Yoshizumi TT, et al. Effective doses in radiology and diagnostic nuclear medicine: a catalog. *Radiology.* 2008;248(1):254–263.
21. Yalcin O, Yildirim T, Kizilkilic O, et al. CT and MRI findings in calvarial non-infectious lesions. *Diagn Interv Radiol.* 2007;13(2):68–74.
22. Sharman AM, Kirmi O, Anslow P. Imaging of the skin, subcutis, and galea aponeurotica. *Semin Ultrasound CT MRI.* 2009;30(6):452–464.
23. Arana E, Marti-Bonmati L. CT and MR imaging of focal calvarial lesions. *AJR Am J Roentgenol.* 1999;172(6):1683–1688.
24. Arana E, Marti-Bonmati L, Ricart V, et al. Dural enhancement with primary calvarial lesions. *Neuroradiology.* 2004;46(11):900–905.
25. Nemeth AJ, Henson JW, Mullins ME, et al. Improved detection of skull metastasis with diffusion-weighted MR imaging. *AJNR Am J Neuroradiol.* 2007;28(6):1088–1092.
26. Ozgen B, Oguz KK, Cila A. Diffusion MR imaging features of skull base osteomyelitis compared with skull base malignancy. *AJNR Am J Neuroradiol.* 2011;32(1):179–184.
27. Yen K, Lovblad KO, Scheurer E, et al. Post-mortem forensic neuroimaging: correlation of MSCT and MRI findings with autopsy results. *Forensic Sci Int.* 2007;173(1):21–35.
28. Eley KA, Sheerin F, Taylor N, et al. Identification of normal cranial sutures in infants on routine magnetic resonance imaging. *J Craniofac Surg.* 2013;24(1):317–320.
29. Eley KA, McIntyre AG, Watt-Smith SR, et al. "Black bone" MRI: a partial flip angle technique for radiation reduction in craniofacial imaging. *Br J Radiol.* 2012;85(1011):272–278.
30. Eley KA, Sherin F, Watt-Smith SR, et al. A novel MRI sequence (black bone) offering an alternative to ionising radiation in the investigation of craniosynostosis. In: *99th Scientific Assembly and Annual Meeting*, Chicago, IL: Radiological Society of North America; December 5, 2013.
31. Nadel HR. Pediatric bone scintigraphy update. *Semin Nucl Med.* 2010;40(1):31–40.
32. Spitz J, Lauer I, Tittel K, et al. Scintimetric evaluation of remodeling after bone fractures in man. *J Nucl Med.* 1993;34(9):1403–1409.
33. Drubach LA, Johnston PR, Newton AW, et al. Skeletal trauma in child abuse: detection with 18F-NaF PET. *Radiology.* 2010;255(1):173–181.
34. Chandler JR, Grobman L, Quencer R, et al. Osteomyelitis of the base of the skull. *Laryngoscope.* 1986;96(3):245–251.
35. Chang PC, Fischbein NJ, Holliday RA. Central skull base osteomyelitis in patients without otitis externa: imaging findings. *AJNR Am J Neuroradiol.* 2003;24(7):1310–1316.
36. Kamarulzaman A, Briggs RJ, Fabinyi G, et al. Skull osteomyelitis due to Salmonella species: two case reports and review. *Clin Infect Dis.* 1996;22(4):638–641.
37. Azouz EM, Saigal G, Rodriguez MM, et al. Langerhans' cell histiocytosis: pathology, imaging and treatment of skeletal involvement. *Pediatr Radiol.* 2005;35(2):103–115.
38. Kaste SC, Rodriguez-Galindo C, McCarville ME, et al. PET-CT in pediatric Langerhans cell histiocytosis. *Pediatr Radiol.* 2007;37(7):615–622.
39. Kushner BH. Neuroblastoma: a disease requiring a multitude of imaging studies. *J Nucl Med.* 2004;45(7):1172–1188.
40. Sharp SE, Shulkin BL, Gelfand MJ, et al. 123I-MIBG scintigraphy and 18F-FDG PET in neuroblastoma. *J Nucl Med.* 2009;50(8):1237–1243.
41. Levi B, Wan DC, Wong VW, et al. Cranial suture biology: from pathways to patient care. *J Craniofac Surg.* 2012;23(1):13–19.
42. Morriss-Kay GM, Wilkie AO. Growth of the normal skull vault and its alteration in craniosynostosis: insights from human genetics and experimental studies. *J Anat.* 2005;207(5):637–653.
43. Srivastava HC. Ossification of the membranous portion of the squamous part of the occipital bone in man. *J Anat.* 1992;180(pt 2):219–224.

44. Cohen MM. Sutural biology. In: Cohen MM, ed. *Craniosynostosis: Diagnosis, Evaluation, and Management.* 2nd ed. New York: Oxford University Press; 2000:11–23.
45. Osborn AG. Scalp and cranial vault. In: Harnsberger HR, Osborn AG, Ross JS, et al., eds. *Diagnostic and Surgical Imaging Anatomy.* Salt Lake City, UT: Amirsys; 2006:I-2–I-7.
46. Choudhary AK, Jha B, Boal DK, et al. Occipital sutures and its variations: the value of 3D-CT and how to differentiate it from fractures using 3D-CT? *Surg Radiol Anat.* 2010;32(9):807–816.
47. Franken EA Jr. The midline occipital fissure: diagnosis of fracture versus anatomic variants. *Radiology.* 1969;93(5):1043–1046.
48. Nakahara K, Utsuki S, Shimizu S, et al. Age dependence of fusion of primary occipital sutures: a radiographic study. *Childs Nerv Syst.* 2006;22(11):1457–1459.
49. Enlow DH. Normal craniofacial growth. In: Cohen MM, ed. *Craniosynostosis: Diagnosis, Evaluation, and Management.* 2nd ed. New York: Oxford University Press; 2000:35–47.
50. Barkovich AJ, Mukherjee P. Normal development of the neonatal and infant brain, skull, and spine. In: Barkovich AJ, Raybaud C, eds. *Pediatric Neuroimaging.* Philadelphia, PA: Lippincott Williams & Wilkins; 2012:20–80.
51. Key CA, Aiello LC, Molleson T. Cranial suture closure and its implications for age estimation. *Int J Osteoarchaeol.* 1994;4:193–207.
52. Sahni D, Jit I, Neelam S. Time of closure of cranial sutures in northwest Indian adults. *Forensic Sci Int.* 2005;148(2–3):199–205.
53. Vu HL, Panchal J, Parker EE, et al. The timing of physiologic closure of the metopic suture: a review of 159 patients using reconstructed 3D CT scans of the craniofacial region. *J Craniofac Surg.* 2001;12(6):527–532.
54. Weinzweig J, Kirschner RE, Farley A, et al. Metopic synostosis: defining the temporal sequence of normal suture fusion and differentiating it from synostosis on the basis of computed tomography images. *Plast Reconstr Surg.* 2003;112(5):1211–1218.
55. Robertson RL, Ball WS, Barnes PD. Skull and brain. In: Kirks DR, ed. *Practical Pediatric Imaging: Diagnostic Radiology of Infants and Children.* 3rd ed. Philadelphia, PA: Lippincott-Raven; 1998:65–200.
56. Slovis TL, Cooper ML. Embryology, anatomy, normal findings, and imaging techniques. In: Coley BD, ed. *Caffey's Pediatric Diagnostic Imaging.* 12th ed. Philadelphia, PA: Saunders; 2013:167–183.
57. Mitchell LA, Kitley CA, Armitage TL, et al. Normal sagittal and coronal suture widths by using CT imaging. *AJNR Am J Neuroradiol.* 2011;32(10):1801–1805.
58. Madeline LA, Elster AD. Suture closure in the human chondrocranium: CT assessment. *Radiology.* 1995;196(3):747–756.
59. Tubbs RS, Salter EG, Oakes WJ. Does the mendosal suture exist in the adult? *Clin Anat.* 2007;20(2):124–125.
60. Popich GA, Smith DW. Fontanels: range of normal size. *J Pediatr.* 1972;80(5):749–752.
61. Beitzke A, Stein J. Pseudo-widening of cranial sutures as a feature of long-term prostaglandin E1 therapy. *Pediatr Radiol.* 1986;16(1):57–58.
62. Capitanio MA, Kirkpatrick JA. Widening of the cranial sutures: a roentgen observation during periods of accelerated growth in patients treated for deprivation dwarfism. *Radiology.* 1969;92(1):53–59.
63. Carter RMS, Anslow P. Imaging of the calvarium. *Semin Ultrasound CT MRI.* 2009;30(6):465–491.
64. De Levie M, Nogrady MB. Rapid brain growth upon restoration of adequate nutrition causing false radiologic evidence of increased intracranial pressure. *J Pediatr.* 1970;76(4):523–528.
65. Gubler MC. Renal tubular dysgenesis. *Pediatr Nephrol.* 2014;29(1):51–59.
66. Boulet SL, Rasmussen SA, Honein MA. A population-based study of craniosynostosis in metropolitan Atlanta, 1989–2003. *Am J Med Genet A.* 2008;146A(8):984–991.
67. Seruya M, Oh AK, Boyajian MJ, et al. Age at initial consultation for craniosynostosis: comparison across different patient characteristics. *J Craniofac Surg.* 2013;24(1):96–98.
68. Di Rocco F, Arnaud E, Renier D. Evolution in the frequency of nonsyndromic craniosynostosis. *J Neurosurg Pediatr.* 2009;4(1):21–25.
69. Cohen MM, Maclean RE. Anatomic, genetic, nosologic, diagnostic, and psychosocial considerations. In: Cohen MM, ed. *Craniosynostosis: Diagnosis, Evaluation, and Management.* 2nd ed. New York: Oxford University Press; 2000:119–143.
70. Kolar JC. An epidemiological study of nonsyndromal craniosynostoses. *J Craniofac Surg.* 2011;22(1):47–49.
71. Lajeunie E, Le Merrer M, Bonaiti-Pellie C, et al. Genetic study of nonsyndromic coronal craniosynostosis. *Am J Med Genet.* 1995;55(4):500–504.
72. Boyadjiev SA, International Craniosynostosis C. Genetic analysis of non-syndromic craniosynostosis. *Orthod Craniofac Res.* 2007;10(3):129–137.
73. Muenke M, Gripp KW, McDonald-McGinn DM, et al. A unique point mutation in the fibroblast growth factor receptor 3 gene (FGFR3) defines a new craniosynostosis syndrome. *Am J Hum Genet.* 1997;60(3):555–564.
74. Wilkie AO, Byren JC, Hurst JA, et al. Prevalence and complications of single-gene and chromosomal disorders in craniosynostosis. *Pediatrics.* 2010;126(2):e391–e400.
75. Agochukwu NB, Solomon BD, Muenke M. Impact of genetics on the diagnosis and clinical management of syndromic craniosynostoses. *Childs Nerv Syst.* 2012;28(9):1447–1463.
76. Lattanzi W, Bukvic N, Barba M, et al. Genetic basis of single-suture synostoses: genes, chromosomes and clinical implications. *Childs Nerv Syst.* 2012;28(9):1301–1310.
77. Cohen MM. History, terminology, and classification of craniosynostosis. In: Cohen MM, ed. *Craniosynostosis: Diagnosis, Evaluation, and Management.* 2nd ed. New York: Oxford University Press; 2000:103–111.
78. Badve CA, K MM, Iyer RS, et al. Craniosynostosis: imaging review and primer on computed tomography. *Pediatr Radiol.* 2013;43(6):728–742; quiz 725–727.
79. Di Rocco F, Arnaud E, Meyer P, et al. Focus session on the changing "epidemiology" of craniosynostosis (comparing two quinquennia: 1985–1989 and 2003–2007) and its impact on the daily clinical practice: a review from Necker Enfants Malades. *Childs Nerv Syst.* 2009;25(7):807–811.
80. Selber J, Reid RR, Chike-Obi CJ, et al. The changing epidemiologic spectrum of single-suture synostoses. *Plast Reconstr Surg.* 2008;122(2):527–533.
81. Shin JH, Persing JA. Nonsyndromic craniosynostosis and deformational plagiocephaly. In: Thorne CH, ed. *Grabb and Smith's Plastic Surgery.* 6th ed. Philadelphia, PA: Lippincott Williams & Wilkins; 2007:226–236.
82. Huang MH, Gruss JS, Clarren SK, et al. The differential diagnosis of posterior plagiocephaly: true lambdoid synostosis versus positional molding. *Plast Reconstr Surg.* 1996;98(5):765–774; discussion 775–766.

83. Laughlin J, Luerssen TG, Dias MS, the Committee on Practice and Ambulatory Medicine, Section on Neurological Surgery. Prevention and management of positional skull deformities in infants. *Pediatrics.* 2011;128(6):1236–1241.
84. Losee JE, Feldman E, Ketkar M, et al. Nonsynostotic occipital plagiocephaly: radiographic diagnosis of the "sticky suture" *Plast Reconstr Surg.* 2005;116(7):1860–1869.
85. Jones MC. Terminology and classification of craniosynostosis. In: Mooney MP, Siegel MI, eds. *Understanding Craniofacial Anomalies: The Etiopathogenesis of Craniosynostosis and Facial Clefting.* Wilmington, DE: Wiley-Liss; 2002:11–15.
86. Kloss JL. Craniosynostosis secondary o ventriculoatrial shunt. *Am J Dis Child.* 1968;116(3):315–317.
87. Cole DE, Carpenter TO. Bone fragility, craniosynostosis, ocular proptosis, hydrocephalus, and distinctive facial features: a newly recognized type of osteogenesis imperfecta. *J Pediatr.* 1987;110(1):76–80.
88. Duggan CA, Keener EB, Gay BB. Secondary craniosynostosis. *AJR Am J Roentgenol.* 1970;109(2):277–293.
89. Higginbottom MC, Jones KL, James HE. Intrauterine constraint and craniosynostosis. *Neurosurgery.* 1980;–(1):39–44.
90. Johnsonbaugh RE, Bryan RN, Hierlwimmer R, et al. Premature craniosynostosis: a common complication of juvenile thyrotoxicosis. *J Pediatr.* 1978;93(2):188–191.
91. Penfold JL, Simpson DA. Premature craniosynostosis-a complication of thyroid replacement therapy. *J Pediatr.* 1975; 86(3):360–363.
92. Patriquin HB, Kaplan P, Kind HP, et al. Neonatal mucolipidosis II (I-cell disease): clinical and radiologic features in three cases. *AJR Am J Roentgenol.* 1977;129(1):37–43.
93. Yamada H, Ohya M, Higeta T, et al. Craniosynostosis and hydrocephalus in I-cell disease (mucolipidosis II). *Childs Nerv Syst.* 1987;3(1):55–57.
94. Schmidt H, Ullrich K, von Lengerke HJ, et al. Radiological findings in patients with mucopolysaccharidosis I H/S (Hurler-Scheie syndrome). *Pediatr Radiol.* 1987;17(5):409–414.
95. Reilly BJ, Leeming JM, Fraser D. Craniosynostosis in the rachitic spectrum. *J Pediatr.* 1964;64:396–405.
96. Shetty AK, Thomas T, Rao J, et al. Rickets and secondary craniosynostosis associated with long-term antacid use in an infant. *Arch Pediatr Adolesc Med.* 1998;152(12):1243–1245.
97. Koshy JC, Chike-Obi CJ, Hatef DA, et al. The variable position of the ear in lambdoid synostosis. *Ann Plast Surg.* 2011;66(1):65–68.
98. Mulliken JB, Enjolras O. Congenital hemangiomas and infantile hemangioma: missing links. *J Am Acad Dermatol.* 2004;50(6): 875–882.
99. van der Meulen J. Metopic synostosis. *Childs Nerv Syst.* 2012; 28(9):1359–1367.
100. Ridgway EB, Weiner HL. Skull deformities. *Pediatr Clin North Am.* 2004;51(2):359–387.
101. Warren SM, Proctor MR, Bartlett SP, et al. Parameters of care for craniosynostosis: craniofacial and neurologic surgery perspectives. *Plast Reconstr Surg.* 2012;129(3):731–737.
102. Bartlett SP. Craniosynostosis syndromes. In: Thorne CH, ed. *Grabb and Smith's Plastic Surgery.* 6th ed. Philadelphia, PA: Lippincott Williams & Wilkins; 2007:237–247.
103. Cinalli G, Sainte-Rose C, Kollar EM, et al. Hydrocephalus and craniosynostosis. *J Neurosurg.* 1998;88(2):209–214.
104. Rich PM, Cox TC, Hayward RD. The jugular foramen in complex and syndromic craniosynostosis and its relationship to raised intracranial pressure. *AJNR Am J Neuroradiol.* 2003; 24(1):45–51.
105. Cunningham ML, Seto ML, Ratisoontorn C, et al. Syndromic craniosynostosis: from history to hydrogen bonds. *Orthod Craniofac Res.* 2007;10(2):67–81.
106. Forrest CR, Hopper RA. Craniofacial syndromes and surgery. *Plast Reconstr Surg.* 2013;131(1):86e–109e.
107. Jimenez DF, Barone CM. Early treatment of anterior calvarial craniosynostosis using endoscopic-assisted minimally invasive techniques. *Childs Nerv Syst.* 2007;23(12):1411–1419.
108. Jimenez DF, Barone CM. Encephaloceles, meningoceles, and dermal sinuses. In: Albright AL, Pollack IF, Adelson PD, eds. *Principles and Practice of Pediatric Neurosurgery.* New York: Thieme; 2008:233–253.
109. Siffel C, Wong LY, Olney RS, et al. Survival of infants diagnosed with encephalocele in Atlanta, 1979–98. *Paediatr Perinat Epidemiol.* 2003;17(1):40–48.
110. Wen S, Ethen M, Langlois PH, et al. Prevalence of encephalocele in Texas, 1999–2002. *Am J Med Genet A.* 2007;143A(18):2150–2155.
111. Copp AJ, Stanier P, Greene NDE. Neural tube defects: recent advances, unsolved questions, and controversies. *Lancet Neurol.* 2013;12(8):799–810.
112. Rowland CA, Correa A, Cragan JD, et al. Are encephaloceles neural tube defects? *Pediatrics.* 2006;118(3):916–923.
113. Baradaran N, Nejat F, Baradaran N, et al. Cephalocele: report of 55 cases over 8 years. *Pediatr Neurosurg.* 2009;45(6): 461–466.
114. Kotil K, Kilinc B, Bilge T. Diagnosis and management of large occipitocervical cephaloceles: a 10-year experience. *Pediatr Neurosurg.* 2008;44(3):193–198.
115. Alexiou GA, Sfakianos G, Prodromou N. Diagnosis and management of cephaloceles. *J Craniofac Surg.* 2010;21(5): 1581–1582.
116. Lo BW, Kulkarni AV, Rutka JT, et al. Clinical predictors of developmental outcome in patients with cephaloceles. *J Neurosurg Pediatr.* 2008;2(4):254–257.
117. Warf BC, Stagno V, Mugamba J. Encephalocele in Uganda: ethnic distinctions in lesion location, endoscopic management of hydrocephalus, and survival in 110 consecutive children. *J Neurosurg Pediatr.* 2011;7(1):88–93.
118. David DJ, Proudman TW. Cephaloceles: classification, pathology, and management. *World J Surg.* 1989;13(4):349–357.
119. Hedlund G. Congenital frontonasal masses: developmental anatomy, malformations, and MR imaging. *Pediatr Radiol.* 2006;36(7):647–662; quiz 726–647.
120. Singh AK, Upadhyaya DN. Sincipital encephaloceles. *J Craniofac Surg.* 2009;20(suppl 2):1851–1855.
121. Suwanwela C, Suwanwela N. A morphological classification of sincipital encephalomeningoceles. *J Neurosurg.* 1972;36(2): 201–211.
122. Morioka T, Hashiguchi K, Samura K, et al. Detailed anatomy of intracranial venous anomalies associated with atretic parietal cephaloceles revealed by high-resolution 3D-CISS and high-field T2-weighted reversed MR images. *Childs Nerv Syst.* 2009;25(3):309–315.
123. Otsubo Y, Sato H, Sato N, et al. Cephaloceles and abnormal venous drainage. *Childs Nerv Syst.* 1999;15(6–7):329–332.
124. Patterson RJ, Egelhoff JC, Crone KR, et al. Atretic parietal cephaloceles revisited: an enlarging clinical and imaging spectrum? *AJNR Am J Neuroradiol.* 1998;19(4):791–795.
125. Kapadia SB, Janecka IP, Fernandes S, et al. Lateral basal encephalocele of the infratemporal fossa. *Otolaryngol Head Neck Surg.* 1996;114(1):116–119.

126. Woodworth BA, Schlosser RJ, Faust RA, et al. Evolutions in the management of congenital intranasal skull base defects. *Arch Otolaryngol Head Neck Surg.* 2004;130(11):1283–1288.
127. Martinez-Lage JF, Poza M, Sola J, et al. The child with a cephalocele: etiology, neuroimaging, and outcome. *Childs Nerv Syst.* 1996;12(9):540–550.
128. Drolet B, Prendiville J, Golden J, et al. 'Membranous aplasia cutis' with hair collars. Congenital absence of skin or neuroectodermal defect? *Arch Dermatol.* 1995;131(12):1427–1431.
129. Drolet BA, Clowry L Jr, McTigue MK, et al. The hair collar sign: marker for cranial dysraphism. *Pediatrics.* 1995; 96(2 pt 1):309–313.
130. Kiymaz N, Yilmaz N, Demir I, et al. Prognostic factors in patients with occipital encephalocele. *Pediatr Neurosurg.* 2010; 46(1):6–11.
131. Huisman TA, Schneider JF, Kellenberger CJ, et al. Developmental nasal midline masses in children: neuroradiological evaluation. *Eur Radiol.* 2004;14(2):243–249.
132. Rahbar R, Resto VA, Robson CD, et al. Nasal glioma and encephalocele: diagnosis and management. *Laryngoscope.* 2003;113(12):2069–2077.
133. Bigot JL, Iacona C, Lepreux A, et al. Sinus pericranii: advantages of MR imaging. *Pediatr Radiol.* 2000;30(10):710–712.
134. Gandolfo C, Krings T, Alvarez H, et al. Sinus pericranii: diagnostic and therapeutic considerations in 15 patients. *Neuroradiology.* 2007;49(6):505–514.
135. Rangel-Castilla L, Krishna C, Klucznik R, et al. Endovascular embolization with Onyx in the management of sinus pericranii: a case report. *Neurosurg Focus.* 2009;27(5):E13.
136. Marti B, Sirinelli D, Maurin L, et al. Wormian bones in a general paediatric population. *Diagn Interv Imaging.* 2013;94(4): 428–432.
137. Cremin B, Goodman H, Spranger J, et al. Wormian bones in osteogenesis imperfecta and other disorders. *Skeletal Radiol.* 1982;8(1):35–38.
138. Griessenauer CJ, Veith P, Mortazavi MM, et al. Enlarged parietal foramina: a review of genetics, prognosis, radiology, and treatment. *Childs Nerv Syst.* 2013;29(4):543–547.
139. Hughes ML, Carty AT, White FE. Persistent hypophyseal (craniopharyngeal) canal. *Br J Radiol.* 1999;72(854):204–206.
140. Macaulay D. Digital markings in radiographs of the skull in children. *Br J Radiol.* 1951;24(288):647–652.
141. Glass RB, Fernbach SK, Norton KI, et al. The infant skull: a vault of information. *Radiographics.* 2004;24(2):507–522.
142. Tuite GF, Evanson J, Chong WK, et al. The beaten copper cranium: a correlation between intracranial pressure, cranial radiographs, and computed tomographic scans in children with craniosynostosis. *Neurosurgery.* 1996;39(4):691–699.
143. Goergens ED, McEvoy A, Watson M, et al. Acute osteomyelitis and septic arthritis in children. *J Paediatr Child Health.* 2005; 41(1–2):59–62.
144. Allison JW, Abernathy RS, Figarola MS, et al. Pediatric case of the day. Tuberculous osteomyelitis with skull involvement and epidural abscess. *Radiographics.* 1999;19(2):552–554.
145. Arnold PM, Govindan S, Anderson KK. Spontaneous cranial osteomyelitis in an otherwise healthy ten-year-old male. *Pediatr Neurosurg.* 2009;45(6):407–409.
146. Prasad KC, Prasad SC, Mouli N, et al. Osteomyelitis in the head and neck. *Acta Otolaryngol.* 2007;127(2):194–205.
147. Shikhare SN, Singh DR, Shimpi TR, et al. Tuberculous osteomyelitis and spondylodiscitis. *Semin Musculoskelet Radiol.* 2011;15(5):446–458.
148. Dudkiewicz M, Livni G, Kornreich L, et al. Acute mastoiditis and osteomyelitis of the temporal bone. *Int J Pediatr Otorhinolaryngol.* 2005;69(10):1399–1405.
149. Hakim HE, Malik AC, Aronyk K, et al. The prevalence of intracranial complications in pediatric frontal sinusitis. *Int J Pediatr Otorhinolaryngol.* 2006;70(8):1383–1387.
150. Decesare GE, Deleyiannis FW, Losee JE. Reconstruction of osteomyelitis defects of the craniofacial skeleton. *Semin Plast Surg.* 2009;23(2):119–131.
151. Blumfield E, Misra M. Pott's puffy tumor, intracranial, and orbital complications as the initial presentation of sinusitis in healthy adolescents, a case series. *Emerg Radiol.* 2011;18(3):203–210.
152. Kombogiorgas D, Solanki GA. The Pott puffy tumor revisited: neurosurgical implications of this unforgotten entity. Case report and review of the literature. *J Neurosurg.* 2006;105(2 suppl):143–149.
153. Chesney J, Black A, Choo D. What is the best practice for acute mastoiditis in children? *Laryngoscope.* 2014;124(5):1057–1058.
154. Wald ER, Applegate KE, Bordley C, et al. Clinical practice guideline for the diagnosis and management of acute bacterial sinusitis in children aged 1 to 18 years. *Pediatrics.* 2013;132(1):e262–e280.
155. Anthonsen K, Hostmark K, Hansen S, et al. Acute mastoiditis in children: a 10-year retrospective and validated multicenter study. *Pediatr Infect Dis J.* 2013;32(5):436–440.
156. Brook I. Fusobacterial infections in children. *Curr Infect Dis Reports.* 2013;15(3):288–294.
157. Munoz A, Ruiz-Contreras J, Jimenez A, et al. Bilateral tuberculous otomastoiditis in an immmunocompetent 5-year-old child: CT and MRI findings (2009: 3b). *Eur Radiol.* 2009; 19(6):1560–1563.
158. Bardales RH, Baker SJ, Mukunyadzi P. Fine-needle aspiration cytology findings in 214 cases of nonparotid lesions of the head. *Diagn Cytopathol.* 2000;22(4):211–217.
159. Gibson SE, Prayson RA. Primary skull lesions in the pediatric population: a 25-year experience. *Arch Pathol Lab Med.* 2007; 131(5):761–766.
160. Kransdorf MJ. Benign soft-tissue tumors in a large referral population: distribution of specific diagnoses by age, sex, and location. *AJR Am J Roentgenol.* 1995;164(2):395–402.
161. Martinez-Lage JF, Capel A, Costa TR, et al. The child with a mass on its head: diagnostic and surgical strategies. *Childs Nerv Syst.* 1992;8(5):247–252.
162. Yoon SH, Park SH. A study of 77 cases of surgically excised scalp and skull masses in pediatric patients. *Childs Nerv Syst.* 2008; 24(4):459–465.
163. Hayden Gephart MG, Colglazier E, Paulk KL, et al. Primary pediatric skull tumors. *Pediatr Neurosurg.* 2011;47(3): 198–203.
164. Smirniotopoulos JG, Chiechi MV. Teratomas, dermoids, and epidermoids of the head and neck. *Radiographics.* 1995;15(6): 1437–1455.
165. Rinna C, Reale G, Calafati V, et al. Dermoid cyst: unusual localization. *J Craniofac Surg.* 2012;23(5):e392–e394.
166. Sorenson EP, Powel JE, Rozzelle CJ, et al. Scalp dermoids: a review of their anatomy, diagnosis, and treatment. *Childs Nerv Syst.* 2013;29(3):375–380.
167. Arana E, Latorre FF, Revert A, et al. Intradiploic epidermoid cysts. *Neuroradiology.* 1996;38(4):306–311.
168. Chen S, Ikawa F, Kurisu K, et al. Quantitative MR evaluation of intracranial epidermoid tumors by fast fluid-attenuated

inversion recovery imaging and echo-planar diffusion-weighted imaging. *AJNR Am J Neuroradiol.* 2001;22(6):1089–1096.

169. Suzuki C, Maeda M, Matsumine A, et al. Apparent diffusion coefficient of subcutaneous epidermal cysts in the head and neck comparison with intracranial epidermoid cysts. *Acad Radiol.* 2007;14(9):1020–1028.
170. Moron FE, Morriss MC, Jones JJ, et al. Lumps and bumps on the head in children: use of CT and MR imaging in solving the clinical diagnostic dilemma. *Radiographics.* 2004; 24(6):1655–1674.
171. Rubin G, Scienza R, Pasqualin A, et al. Craniocerebral epidermoids and dermoids. A review of 44 cases. *Acta Neurochir.* 1989;97(1–2):1–16.
172. Golden BA, Jaskolka MS, Ruiz RL. Craniofacial and orbital dermoids in children. *Oral Maxillofac Surg Clin North Am.* 2012;24(3):417–425.
173. Riebel T, David S, Thomale UW. Calvarial dermoids and epidermoids in infants and children: sonographic spectrum and follow-up. *Childs Nerv Syst.* 2008;24(11):1327–1332.
174. D'Ambrosio N, Soohoo S, Warshall C, et al. Craniofacial and intracranial manifestations of langerhans cell histiocytosis: report of findings in 100 patients. *AJR Am J Roentgenol.* 2008; 191(2):589–597.
175. Prayer D, Grois N, Prosch H, et al. MR imaging presentation of intracranial disease associated with Langerhans cell histiocytosis. *AJNR Am J Neuroradiol.* 2004;25(5):880–891.
176. Paulus W, Perry A. Histiocytic tumors. In: Louis DN, Ohgaki H, Wiestler OD, et al., eds. *WHO Classification of Tumours of the Central Nervous System.* Lyon, France: IARC; 2007:193–196.
177. Lope LA, Hutcheson KA, Khademian ZP. Magnetic resonance imaging in the analysis of pediatric orbital tumors: utility of diffusion-weighted imaging. *J AAPOS.* 2010;14(3):257–262.
178. Okamoto K, Ito J, Ishikawa K, et al. Diffusion-weighted echo-planar MR imaging in differential diagnosis of brain tumors and tumor-like conditions. *Eur Radiol.* 2000;10(8):1342–1350.
179. Nabavizadeh SA, Bilaniuk LT, Feygin T, et al. CT and MRI of pediatric skull lesions with fluid-fluid levels. *AJNR Am J Neuroradiol.* 2014;35(3):604–608.
180. Alexiou GA, Mpairamidis E, Sfakianos G, et al. Cranial unifocal Langerhans cell histiocytosis in children. *J Pediatr Surg.* 2009;44(3):571–574.
181. Greene AK, Rogers GF, Mulliken JB. Intraosseous "hemangiomas" are malformations and not tumors. *Plast Reconstr Surg.* 2007; 119(6):1949–1950; author reply 1950.
182. Bastug D, Ortiz O, Schochet SS. Hemangiomas in the calvaria: imaging findings. *AJR Am J Roentgenol.* 1995;164(3):683–687.
183. Politi M, Romeike BF, Papanagiotou P, et al. Intraosseous hemangioma of the skull with dural tail sign: radiologic features with pathologic correlation. *AJNR Am J Neuroradiol.* 2005;26(8):2049–2052.
184. Sweet C, Silbergleit R, Mehta B. Primary intraosseous hemangioma of the orbit: CT and MR appearance. *AJNR Am J Neuroradiol.* 1997;18(2):379–381.
185. Martinez-Lage JF, Torroba MA, Cuartero Perez B, et al. Cavernous hemangiomas of the cranial vault in infants: a case-based update. *Childs Nerv Syst.* 2010;26(7):861–865.
186. Nasrallah IM, Hayek R, Duhaime AC, et al. Cavernous hemangioma of the skull: surgical treatment without craniectomy. *J Neurosurg Pediatr.* 2009;4(6):575–579.
187. Kransdorf MJ, Moser RP Jr, Gilkey FW. Fibrous dysplasia. *Radiographics.* 1990;10(3):519–537.
188. Ricalde P, Magliocca KR, Lee JS. Craniofacial fibrous dysplasia. *Oral Maxillofac Surg Clin North Am.* 2012;24(3):427–441.
189. Davies ML, Macpherson P. Fibrous dysplasia of the skull: disease activity in relation to age. *Br J Radiol.* 1991;64(763): 576–579.
190. Jee WH, Choi KH, Choe BY, et al. Fibrous dysplasia: MR imaging characteristics with radiopathologic correlation. *AJR Am J Roentgenol.* 1996;167(6):1523–1527.
191. Slootweg PJ, El Mofty SK. Ossifying fibroma. In: Barnes L, Eveson JW, Reichart P, et al., eds. *WHO Classification of Tumours. Pathology and Genetics of Head and Neck Tumours.* Lyon, France: IARC Press; 2005:319–320.
192. Whitehead RE, Melhem ER, Kasznica J, et al. Telangiectatic osteosarcoma of the skull base. *AJNR Am J Neuroradiol.* 1998; 19(4):754–757.
193. Salvati M, Ciappetta P, Raco A. Osteosarcomas of the skull. Clinical remarks on 19 cases. *Cancer.* 1993;71(7):2210–2216.
194. Li WY, Brock P, Saunders DE. Imaging characteristics of primary cranial Ewing sarcoma. *Pediatr Radiol.* 2005;35(6): 612–618.
195. Salunke PS, Gupta K, Malik V, et al. Primary Ewing's sarcoma of cranial bones: analysis of ten patients. *Acta Neurochir.* 2011; 153(7):1477–1485.
196. Bose B. Primary osteogenic sarcoma of the skull. *Surg Neurol.* 2002;58(3–4):234–239; discussion 239–240.
197. Shinoda J, Kimura T, Funakoshi T, et al. Primary osteosarcoma of the skull—a case report and review of the literature. *J Neurooncol.* 1993;17(1):81–88.
198. Maeda M, Matsumine A, Kato H, et al. Soft-tissue tumors evaluated by line-scan diffusion-weighted imaging: influence of myxoid matrix on the apparent diffusion coefficient. *J Magn Reson Imaging.* 2007;25(6):1199–1204.
199. Gadwal SR, Fanburg-Smith JC, Gannon FH, et al. Primary chondrosarcoma of the head and neck in pediatric patients: a clinicopathologic study of 14 cases with a review of the literature. *Cancer.* 2000;88(9):2181–2188.
200. Matsumoto J, Towbin RB, Ball WS Jr. Cranial chordomas in infancy and childhood. A report of two cases and review of the literature. *Pediatr Radiol.* 1989;20(1–2):28–32.
201. Meyers SP, Hirsch WL Jr, Curtin HD, et al. Chondrosarcomas of the skull base: MR imaging features. *Radiology.* 1992; 184(1):103–108.
202. Oot RF, Melville GE, New PF, et al. The role of MR and CT in evaluating clival chordomas and chondrosarcomas. *AJR Am J Roentgenol.* 1988;151(3):567–575.
203. Ginsberg LE. Neoplastic diseases affecting the central skull base: CT and MR imaging. *AJR Am J Roentgenol.* 1992;159(3): 581–589.
204. Yeom KW, Lober RM, Mobley BC, et al. Diffusion-weighted MRI: distinction of skull base chordoma from chondrosarcoma. *AJNR Am J Neuroradiol.* 2013;34(5):1056–1061, S1051.
205. Vujovic S, Henderson S, Presneau N, et al. Brachyury, a crucial regulator of notochordal development, is a novel biomarker for chordomas. *J Pathol.* 2006;209(2):157–165.
206. Daldrup-Link HE, Franzius C, Link TM, et al. Whole-body MR imaging for detection of bone metastases in children and young adults: comparison with skeletal scintigraphy and FDG PET. *AJR Am J Roentgenol.* 2001;177(1):229–236.
207. Goo HW, Choi SH, Ghim T, et al. Whole-body MRI of paediatric malignant tumours: comparison with conventional oncological imaging methods. *Pediatr Radiol.* 2005;35(8): 766–773.

208. Siegel MJ, Acharyya S, Hoffer FA, et al. Whole-body MR imaging for staging of malignant tumors in pediatric patients: results of the American College of Radiology Imaging Network 6660 Trial. *Radiology.* 2013;266(2):599–609.
209. Ahmed S, Goel S, Khandwala M, et al. Neuroblastoma with orbital metastasis: ophthalmic presentation and role of ophthalmologists. *Eye.* 2006;20(4):466–470.
210. D'Ambrosio N, Lyo JK, Young RJ, et al. Imaging of metastatic CNS neuroblastoma. *AJR Am J Roentgenol.* 2010; 194(5):1223–1229.
211. David R, Lamki N, Fan S, et al. The many faces of neuroblastoma. *Radiographics.* 1989;9(5):859–882.
212. Zimmerman RA, Bilaniuk LT. CT of primary and secondary craniocerebral neuroblastoma. *AJR Am J Roentgenol.* 1980; 135(6):1239–1242.
213. Shuper A, Cohen IJ, Mor C, et al. Metastatic brain involvement in Ewing family of tumors in children. *Neurology.* 1998;51(5):1336–1338.
214. Linet MS, Ries LA, Smith MA, et al. Cancer surveillance series: recent trends in childhood cancer incidence and mortality in the United States. *J Natl Cancer Inst.* 1999;91(12):1051–1058.
215. Guillerman RP. Marrow: red, yellow and bad. *Pediatr Radiol.* 2013;43(suppl 1):S181–S192.
216. Jensen KE, Thomsen C, Henriksen O, et al. Changes in T1 relaxation processes in the bone marrow following treatment in children with acute lymphoblastic leukemia. A magnetic resonance imaging study. *Pediatr Radiol.* 1990;20(6):464–468.
217. Vande Berg BC, Lecouvet FE, Michaux L, et al. Magnetic resonance imaging of the bone marrow in hematological malignancies. *Eur Radiol.* 1998;8(8):1335–1344.
218. Porto L, Kieslich M, Schwabe D, et al. Granulocytic sarcoma in children. *Neuroradiology.* 2004;46(5):374–377.
219. Stein-Wexler R, Wootton-Gorges SL, West DC. Orbital granulocytic sarcoma: an unusual presentation of acute myelocytic leukemia. *Pediatr Radiol.* 2003;33(2):136–139.
220. Baur A, Dietrich O, Reiser M. Diffusion-weighted imaging of bone marrow: current status. *Eur Radiol.* 2003;13(7):1699–1708.
221. Dietrich AM, Bowman MJ, Ginn-Pease ME, et al. Pediatric head injuries: can clinical factors reliably predict an abnormality on computed tomography? *Ann Emerg Med.* 1993;22(10):1535–1540.
222. Chan KH, Mann KS, Yue CP, et al. The significance of skull fracture in acute traumatic intracranial hematomas in adolescents: a prospective study. *J Neurosurg.* 1990;72(2):189–194.
223. Guzel A, Hicdonmez T, Temizoz O, et al. Indications for brain computed tomography and hospital admission in pediatric patients with minor head injury: how much can we rely upon clinical findings? *Pediatr Neurosurg.* 2009;45(4):262–270.
224. Harwood-Nash DC, Hendrick EB, Hudson AR. The significance of skull fractures in children. A study of 1,187 patients. *Radiology.* 1971;101(1):151–156.
225. Galarza M, Gazzeri R, Barcelo C, et al. Accidental head trauma during care activities in the first year of life: a neurosurgical comparative study. *Childs Nerv Syst.* 2013;29(6):973–978.
226. Duhaime AC, Alario AJ, Lewander WJ, et al. Head injury in very young children: mechanisms, injury types, and ophthalmologic findings in 100 hospitalized patients younger than 2 years of age. *Pediatrics.* 1992;90(2 pt 1):179–185.
227. Fernando S, Obaldo RE, Walsh IR, et al. Neuroimaging of nonaccidental head trauma: pitfalls and controversies. *Pediatr Radiol.* 2008;38(8):827–838.
228. Rubin DM, Christian CW, Bilaniuk LT, et al. Occult head injury in high-risk abused children. *Pediatrics.* 2003;111 (6 pt 1):1382–1386.
229. Laskey AL, Holsti M, Runyan DK, et al. Occult head trauma in young suspected victims of physical abuse. *J Pediatr.* 2004;144(6): 719–722.
230. Lloyd DA, Carty H, Patterson M, et al. Predictive value of skull radiography for intracranial injury in children with blunt head injury. *Lancet.* 1997;349(9055):821–824.
231. Quayle KS, Jaffe DM, Kuppermann N, et al. Diagnostic testing for acute head injury in children: when are head computed tomography and skull radiographs indicated? *Pediatrics.* 1997;99(5):E11.
232. Maguire JL, Boutis K, Uleryk EM, et al. Should a head-injured child receive a head CT scan? A systematic review of clinical prediction rules. *Pediatrics.* 2009;124(1):e145–e154.
233. Prabhu SP, Newton AW, Perez-Rossello JM, et al. Three-dimensional skull models as a problem-solving tool in suspected child abuse. *Pediatr Radiol.* 2013;43(5):575–581.
234. Sanchez T, Stewart D, Walvick M, et al. Skull fracture vs. accessory sutures: how can we tell the difference? *Emerg Radiol.* 2010; 17(5):413–418.
235. Meservy CJ, Towbin R, McLaurin RL, et al. Radiographic characteristics of skull fractures resulting from child abuse. *AJR Am J Roentgenol.* 1987;149(1):173–175.
236. Greenes DS, Schutzman SA. Infants with isolated skull fracture: what are their clinical characteristics, and do they require hospitalization? *Ann Emerg Med.* 1997;30(3): 253–259.
237. Mannix R, Monuteaux MC, Schutzman SA, et al. Isolated skull fractures: trends in management in US pediatric emergency departments. *Ann Emerg Med.* 2013;62(4):327–331.
238. Ragheb J. Accidental head injuries. In: Albright AL, Pollack IF, Adelson PD, eds. *Principles and Practice of Pediatric Neurosurgery*. New York: Thieme; 2008:803–808.
239. Wisser M, Rothschild MA, Schmolling JC, et al. Caput succedaneum and facial petechiae—birth-associated injuries in healthy newborns under forensic aspects. *Int J Leg Med.* 2012;126(3):385–390.
240. Chang HY, Peng CC, Kao HA, et al. Neonatal subgaleal hemorrhage: clinical presentation, treatment, and predictors of poor prognosis. *Pediatr Int.* 2007;49(6):903–907.
241. Hughes CA, Harley EH, Milmoe G, et al. Birth trauma in the head and neck. *Arch Otolaryngol Head Neck Surg.* 1999;125(2):193–199.
242. Persing J, James H, Swanson J, et al. Prevention and management of positional skull deformities in infants. American Academy of Pediatrics Committee on Practice and Ambulatory Medicine, Section on Plastic Surgery and Section on Neurological Surgery. *Pediatrics.* 2003;112(1 pt 1): 199–202.
243. Oh CK, Yoon SH. The significance of incomplete skull fracture in the birth injury. *Med Hypotheses.* 2010;74(5):898–900.
244. Ortiz MH, Brodie AG. On the growth of the human head from birth to the third month of life. *Anat Rec.* 1949;103(3): 311–333.
245. Firlik KS, Adelson PD. Large chronic cephalohematoma without calcification. *Pediatr Neurosurg.* 1999;30(1):39–42.
246. Wong CH, Foo CL, Seow WT. Calcified cephalohematoma: classification, indications for surgery and techniques. *J Craniofac Surg.* 2006;17(5):970–979.

247. Levkoff AH, Macpherson RI, Wood BP. Radiological case of the month. Unrecognized subaponeurotic hemorrhage. *Am J Dis Child.* 1992;146(7):833–834.
248. Park SH, Hwang SK. Surgical treatment of subacute epidural hematoma caused by a vacuum extraction with skull fracture and cephalohematoma in a neonate. *Pediatr Neurosurg.* 2006; 42(4):270–272.
249. Axton JH, Levy LF. Congenital moulding depressions of the skull. *Br Med J.* 1965;1(5451):1644–1647.
250. Dupuis O, Silveira R, Dupont C, et al. Comparison of "instrument-associated" and "spontaneous" obstetric depressed skull fractures in a cohort of 68 neonates. *Am J Obstet Gynecol.* 2005;192(1):165–170.
251. Ersahin Y, Mutluer S, Mirzai H, et al. Pediatric depressed skull fractures: analysis of 530 cases. *Childs Nerv Syst.* 1996; 12(6):323–331.
252. Mastrapa TL, Fernandez LA, Alvarez MD, et al. Depressed skull fracture in Ping Pong: elevation with Medeva extractor. *Childs Nerv Syst.* 2007;23(7):787–790.
253. Pollak L, Raziel A, Ariely S, et al. Revival of non-surgical management of neonatal depressed skull fractures. *J Paediatr Child Health.* 1999;35(1):96–97.
254. Muhonen MG, Piper JG, Menezes AH. Pathogenesis and treatment of growing skull fractures. *Surg Neurol.* 1995;43(4):367–372; discussion 372–363.
255. Papaefthymiou G, Oberbauer R, Pendl G. Craniocerebral birth trauma caused by vacuum extraction: a case of growing skull fracture as a perinatal complication. *Childs Nerv Syst.* 1996; 12(2):117–120.
256. Zegers B, Jira P, Willemsen M, et al. The growing skull fracture, a rare complication of paediatric head injury. *Eur J Pediatr.* 2003;162(7–8):556–557.
257. de PDV, Njamnshi AK, Ongolo-Zogo P, et al. Growing skull fractures. *Childs Nerv Syst.* 2006;22(7):721–725.
258. Gupta SK, Reddy NM, Khosla VK, et al. Growing skull fractures: a clinical study of 41 patients. *Acta Neurochir.* 1997;139(10):928–932.
259. Reeder MM. Skull and brain. In: Reeder MM, ed. *Reeder and Felson's Gamut's in Radiology.* New York: Springer-Verlag; 2003:1–94.
260. Albert MH, Notheis G, Wintergerst U, et al. "Hair-on-end" skull induced by long-term G-CSF treatment in severe congenital neutropenia. *Pediatr Radiol.* 2007;37(2):221–224.
261. Sebes JI, Diggs LW. Radiographic changes of the skull in sickle cell anemia. *AJR Am J Roentgenol.* 1979;132(3):373–377.
262. Tunaci M, Tunaci A, Engin G, et al. Imaging features of thalassemia. *Eur Radiol.* 1999;9(9):1804–1809.
263. Mazzanti L, Ambrosetto P, Libri R, et al. Involvement of the skull base and vault in chronic idiopathic hyperphosphatasia. *Pediatr Radiol.* 1999;29(1):16–18.
264. Whyte MP, Obrecht SE, Finnegan PM, et al. Osteoprotegerin deficiency and juvenile Paget's disease. *N Engl J Med.* 2002; 347(3):175–184.
265. Kinard RE, Walton JE, Buckwalter JA. Pseudohypoparathyroidism: report on a family with four affected sisters. *Arch Intern Med.* 1979;139(2):204–207.
266. Mackler H, Fouts JR, Birsner JW. Familial pseudohypoparathyroidism; a report of two cases. *Calif Med.* 1952;77(5): 332–334.
267. Cure JK, Key LL, Goltra DD, et al. Cranial MR imaging of osteopetrosis. *AJNR Am J Neuroradiol.* 2000;21(6):1110–1115.
268. Elster AD, Theros EG, Key LL, et al. Cranial imaging in autosomal recessive osteopetrosis. Part II. Skull base and brain. *Radiology.* 1992;183(1):137–144.
269. Elster AD, Theros EG, Key LL, et al. Cranial imaging in autosomal recessive osteopetrosis. Part I. Facial bones and calvarium. *Radiology.* 1992;183(1):129–135.
270. Naveh Y, Kaftori JK, Alon U, et al. Progressive diaphyseal dysplasia: genetics and clinical and radiologic manifestations. *Pediatrics.* 1984;74(3):399–405.
271. Elmore SM. Pycnodysostosis: a review. *J Bone Joint Surg Am.* 1967;49(1):153–162.
272. Shuler SE. Pycnodysostosis. *Arch Dis Child.* 1963;38:620–625.
273. Jaeger HJ, Schmitz-Stolbrink A, Hulde J, et al. The boneless neonate: a severe form of achondrogenesis type I. *Pediatr Radiol.* 1994;24(5):319–321.
274. Lee B, Thirunavukkarasu K, Zhou L, et al. Missense mutations abolishing DNA binding of the osteoblast-specific transcription factor OSF2/CBFA1 in cleidocra nial dysplasia. *Nat Genet.* 1997;16(3):307–310.
275. Smits P, Bolton AD, Funari V, et al. Lethal skeletal dysplasia in mice and humans lacking the golgin GMAP-210. *N Engl J Med.* 2010;362(3):206–216.
276. Spranger J, Cremin B, Beighton P. Osteogenesis imperfecta congenita. Features and prognosis of a heterogenous condition. *Pediatr Radiol.* 1982;12(1):21–27.
277. Tan KL, Tan LK. Cleidocranial dysostosis in infancy. *Pediatr Radiol.* 1981;11(2):114–116.
278. Unger S, Mornet E, Mundlos S, et al. Severe cleidocranial dysplasia can mimic hypophosphatasia. *Eur J Pediatr.* 2002;161(11):623–626.
279. Murthy AS. X-linked hypophosphatemic rickets and craniosynostosis. *J Craniofac Surg.* 2009;20(2):439–442.
280. Rathbun JC. Hypophosphatasia; a new developmental anomaly. *Am J Dis Child.* 1948;75(6):822–831.
281. D'Ambrosio JA, Langlais RP, Young RS. Jaw and skull changes in neurofibromatosis. *Oral Surg Oral Med Oral Pathol.* 1988; 66(3):391–396.
282. Holt JF, Kuhns LR. Macrocranium and macrencephaly in neurofibromatosis. *Skeletal Radiol.* 1976;1:25–28.
283. Jacquemin C, Bosley TM, Liu D, et al. Reassessment of sphenoid dysplasia associated with neurofibromatosis type 1. *AJNR Am J Neuroradiol.* 2002;23(4):644–648.
284. Jacquemin C, Bosley TM, Svedberg H. Orbit deformities in craniofacial neurofibromatosis type 1. *AJNR Am J Neuroradiol.* 2003;24(8):1678–1682.
285. Chang JI, Som PM, Lawson W. Unique imaging findings in the facial bones of renal osteodystrophy. *AJNR Am J Neuroradiol.* 2007;28(4):608–609.
286. Weller M, Edeiken J, Hodes PJ. Renal osteodystrophy. *Am J Roentgenol Radium Ther Nucl Med.* 1968;104(2):354–363.
287. Genant HK, Baron JM, Straus FH, et al. Osteosclerosis in primary hyperparathyroidism. *Am J Med.* 1975;59(1): 104–113.
288. Kaufman B, Weiss MH, Young HF, et al. Effects of prolonged cerebrospinal fluid shunting on the skull and brain. *J Neurosurg.* 1973;38(3):288–297.
289. Lefebvre EB, Haining RG, Labbe RF. Coarse facies, calvarial thickening and hyperphosphatasia associated with long-term anticonvulsant therapy. *N Engl J Med.* 1972;286(24):1301–1302.
290. Sener RN, Jinkins JR. MR of craniocerebral hemiatrophy. *Clin Imaging.* 1992;16(2):93–97.

291. Greer FR. Osteopenia of prematurity. *Annu Rev Nutr.* 1994; 14:169–185.
292. Mitlak BH, Daly M, Potts JT Jr, et al. Asymptomatic primary hyperparathyroidism. *J Bone Miner Res.* 1991;6(suppl 2): S103–S110; discussion S121–S104.
293. Silverberg SJ, Bilezikian JP. Primary hyperparathyroidism: still evolving? *J Bone Miner Res.* 1997;12(5):856–862.
294. Swischuk LE, Hayden CK Jr. Seizures and demineralization of the skull. A diagnostic presentation of rickets. *Pediatr Radiol.* 1977;6(2):65–67.
295. Lee S, Seto M, Sie K, et al. A child with Saethre-Chotzen syndrome, sensorineural hearing loss, and a TWIST mutation. *Cleft Palate Craniofac J.* 2002;39(1):110–114.
296. Jabs EW, Muller U, Li X, et al. A mutation in the homeodomain of the human MSX2 gene in a family affected with autosomal dominant craniosynostosis. *Cell.* 1993;75(3):443–450.
297. Warman ML, Mulliken JB, Hayward PG, et al. Newly recognized autosomal dominant disorder with craniosynostosis. *Am J Med Genet.* 1993;46(4):444–449.

CHAPTER 2

Brain

Sanjay P. Prabhu • Savvas Andronikou • Sara O. Vargas • Richard L. Robertson

INTRODUCTION

Imaging plays a crucial role in the evaluation of neurologic disease in children. During the past several decades, rapid advances in imaging have contributed to a greater understanding of the structural and functional changes that occur in a child's brain throughout childhood. Additionally, imaging provides noninvasive tools to help diagnose the cause of neurologic impairment in pediatric patients. It is important for the radiologist to consider changes of normal brain development from gestation through adolescence when performing and interpreting neuroimaging studies in pediatric patients. Furthermore, it is important to be familiar with age-specific diagnoses and have a clear understanding of the normal appearance and normal variations that characterize each stage of brain development.

This chapter provides an overview of imaging evaluation of pediatric brain disease. First, the role of currently available imaging modalities for assessing the pediatric brain is reviewed. Following this, normal anatomy and development are discussed. Finally, an overview of selected essential pediatric brain disorders is provided with emphasis on the underlying pathophysiology, clinical manifestations, key imaging features with pathologic correlation, and treatment approaches.

IMAGING TECHNIQUES

Radiography

Very few indications remain for performing radiographs to evaluate the brain parenchyma in an acutely ill child. Radiographs, however, continue to have a role in evaluating the skull: (1) as part of a skeletal survey in a victim of suspected child abuse, (2) for detection of osseous abnormalities in metastatic or metabolic disease, (3) as a screening tool for craniosynostosis in a child with an abnormally shaped skull, and (4) for evaluation of shunt catheter integrity and programmable shunt valve settings in pediatric patients with hydrocephalus.

Standard skull radiography technique consists of frontal, lateral, and Townes projections. These views have been discussed in more detail in Chapter 1 of this book.

Ultrasound

Ultrasound (US) of the infant brain is a noninvasive, radiation-free procedure that can be performed at the bedside, in the intensive care unit, or on an intubated, ventilated infant following delivery. It has a number of advantages including ready access, portability, real-time and multiplanar capabilities, and reproducible results.

Currently, US is mainly used in neonates (1) to screen for suspected intracranial hemorrhage and periventricular leukomalacia (PVL) in the premature infant, (2) to monitor progression or resolution of the pathologic process, and (3) to detect the subsequent complications of ventriculomegaly and progressive hydrocephalus. Cranial US also has a role in detecting focal infarcts and hemorrhagic lesions in the term or near-term infant; in screening for congenital midline anomalies, intracranial cystic lesions, vascular malformations, and intracranial calcifications; and in delineating extra-axial fluid collections. Because of its portable nature, it remains the modality of choice for use at the bedside, obviating the need for transportation of the unstable or critically ill child. In older children, transcranial Doppler is used to correlate resistive indices with elevated intracranial pressure in cases of head trauma and assess blood flow in cases of cerebrovascular disease. A sonographic finding or suspected lesion can be further characterized with computed tomography (CT) or magnetic resonance imaging (MRI) when the patient is more stable.

Sonographic scanning in premature infants should be performed using higher-frequency transducers operating between 7 and 10 MHz because of their higher spatial resolution.[1,2] Lower-frequency transducers (3.5 to 5 MHz) are often used in larger infants to obtain adequate penetration of sound waves. Sector transducers with a 120-degree imaging field are ideal to image through the anterior and posterior fontanelles.[3]

To ensure optimal coverage of the brain, scanning should include a series of standardized coronal and sagittal images through the anterior fontanelle (Fig. 2.1). Coronal images are acquired by placing the transducer transversely across the fontanelle and moving it in an arc in an anteroposterior direction to cover the entire brain. The transducer should be carefully positioned to produce symmetrical imaging of both hemispheres. Six to eight angled images should be obtained, with the most anterior image acquired anterior to the frontal horns of the lateral ventricles at the level of the orbits, the second image through the anterior horns of the lateral ventricles at the level of the suprasellar cistern, the third image more posteriorly through the body of the lateral ventricles at the level of the paired foramina of Monro and brainstem, the fourth image with the transducer angled slightly more posteriorly, the fifth image further posteriorly at the level of the prominent paired echogenic choroid plexus in the atria of the lateral ventricles, and the final coronal image posterior to the lateral ventricles.

Sagittal images are obtained by placing the transducer longitudinally along the anterior fontanelle, with one acquired along the midline and two to three acquired on each side by angling the transducer laterally. The true midline-imaging plane is obtained by identifying the comma-shaped fluid-filled cavum septum pellucidum, the curved hypoechoic corpus callosum cephalad to it, and the echogenic cerebellar vermis in the infratentorial region. The cingulate gyrus is located cephalad to the corpus callosum, and the echogenic line between them is the pericallosal sulcus. The cingulate gyrus is separated from the other gyri by the cingulate sulcus. Note that the normal gyri and sulci never extend to the ventricles. The medial aspect of the paired thalamic nuclei, the

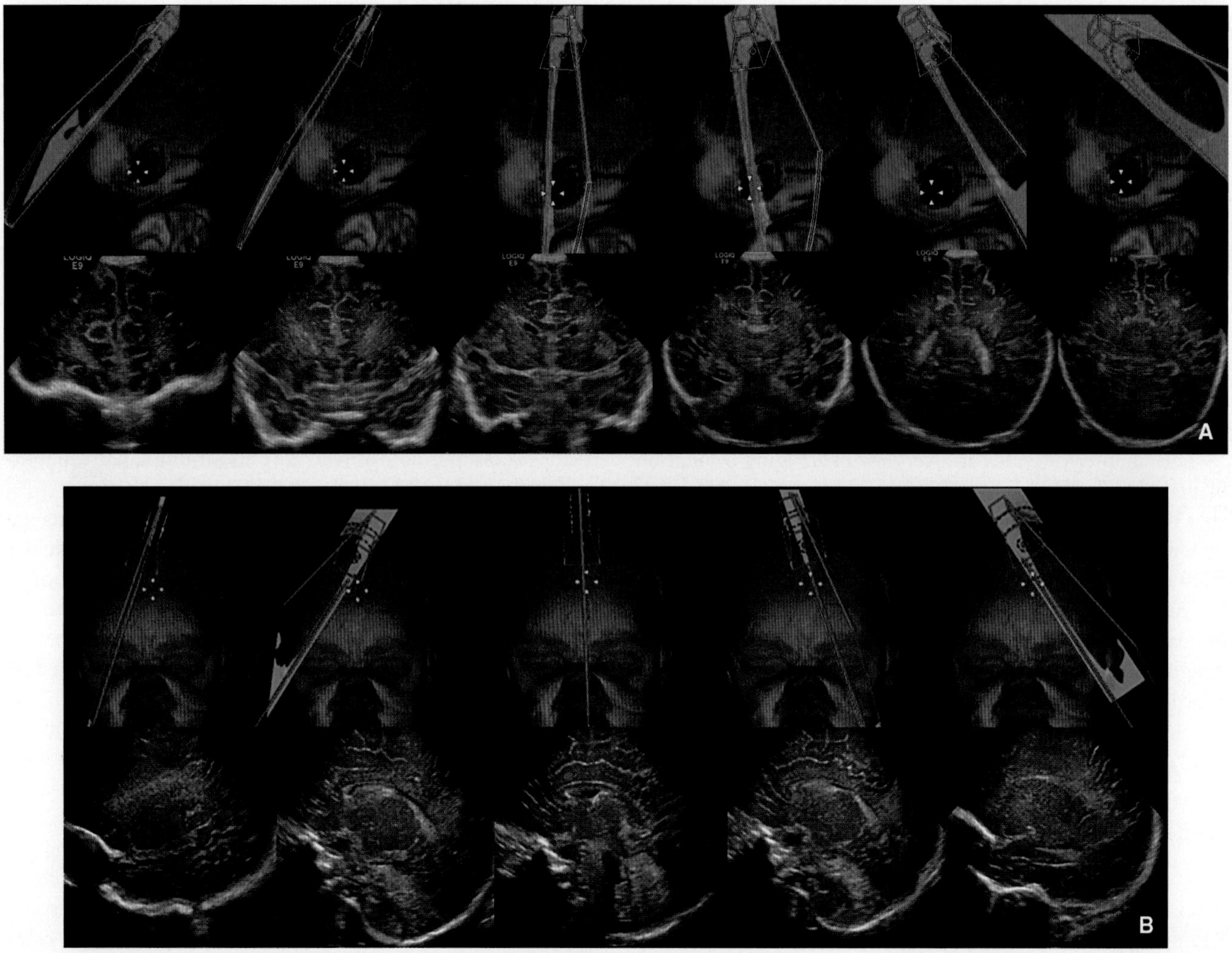

FIGURE 2.1 **A:** Positions of the transducer for coronal ultrasound images through the brain. **B:** Positions of the transducer for sagittal ultrasound images through the brain.

tectum of the midbrain, and fourth ventricle can be identified on this midline image.

The first parasagittal image obtained with the anterior portion of the probe angled more medially than the posterior portion produces a sagittal image showing the frontal horn and body of the lateral ventricle. On this image, attention should be directed in particular to the caudothalamic groove, which is seen as thin echogenic line at the junction of the slightly more echogenic caudate nucleus anteriorly and the relatively less echogenic thalamus posteriorly. The caudothalamic groove is contiguous with the choroid plexus in the roof of the third ventricle. Further lateral angulation provides images through the entire lateral ventricle, and more laterally, through the peripheral brain parenchyma, the Sylvian fissure, and the cerebral convolutions, which increase with gestational age.

In addition to the coronal and sagittal planes, four additional approaches through the midline posterior fontanelle, the squamosal suture, the posterolateral or mastoid fontanelle, and the foramen magnum are used as additional problem-solving tools in some patients with suspected posterior fossa and midbrain anomalies and abnormalities.

Color Doppler is used to investigate the pericallosal segment of the anterior cerebral artery (ACA) in a midline sagittal projection using 7 to 8 MHz vector transducer.[2] Two views are obtained, each for a maximum of 3 to 5 seconds. The first view of baseline Doppler spectrum is obtained without exerting pressure over the fontanelle. Then, the second view is obtained by completely depressing the transducer until further depression of the fontanelle generates no additional pressure. During compression, the Doppler range gate is repositioned over the same portion of the ACA, and a second Doppler spectrum is obtained. Flow velocity and resistive index (RI), which is defined as the peak systolic velocity (PSV) minus the end-diastolic velocity divided by PSV, are the most commonly used spectral Doppler measures used to quantify the cerebral blood flow. All intracranial arteries display a low-resistance flow pattern with continuous forward flow during systole and diastole. Because these arteries usually have a diameter of <5 mm, the spectral lines are broad and the spectral window is filled.[4] In premature babies, the intracerebral RI is high; an RI of up to 1 may be normal.[4] Variations in cerebral blood flow that occur as adaptations to postnatal life are poorly reflected in the RI and PI; hence, they are less informative in the first few months of life. Elevation of RIs is nonspecific, but serial measurements are used to follow pediatric patients with raised intracranial pressures, shunted hydrocephalus, or indomethacin administration.

Computed Tomography

CT remains the neuroimaging modality of choice in the acutely ill child because of its widespread availability and fast image acquisition speeds. Although CT is still used in many institutions around the world for investigation of children with a variety of suspected brain abnormalities, it is best suited for detecting acute intracranial hemorrhage, cerebral edema, hypoxic–ischemic injury (HII), infarction, hydrocephalus/shunt dysfunction, neoplasm, or abnormal collections. Modern multidetector CT scanners can acquire submillimeter thick images, which can be manipulated to produce multiplanar reformats and 3D images, thereby facilitating rapid detection of calvarial and facial fractures. CT remains the modality of choice in the workup of children with suspected craniosynostosis. When performed with iodinated contrast media, CT provides information about inflammatory and infectious lesions and resultant complications such as abscess.

CT angiography (CTA) provides excellent detail of the vascular structures and helps diagnose a variety of arterial and venous abnormalities in the acute setting. CTA also compares favorably with MR angiography (MRA) in evaluating vertebral artery dissection, as shown in a number of adult studies. CT venography (CTV) remains the initial modality of choice in many pediatric centers for assessing pediatric patients with suspected dural venous sinus thrombosis.

However, CT requires use of ionizing radiation, which has the potential to adversely affect tissues in the pediatric patient, particularly when used for multiple studies. Therefore, it is important to consider alternatives to CT, particularly in infants and young children. Once CT is chosen as the imaging modality, the ALARA (As Low As Reasonably Acceptable) principle must be always adhered to. This entails the use of appropriate age- and weight-based dose adjustment parameters available on modern CT scanners and limitation of the scan to the area of concern.

Magnetic Resonance Imaging

More recently, MRI has become the modality of choice for imaging the pediatric brain in almost all elective medical conditions and, more recently, even in the acute setting. The capability of MRI to acquire images in multiple planes with excellent anatomic detail and superb tissue contrast, without the harmful effects of ionizing radiation, makes MRI an ideal tool for imaging the brain in children of all ages. MRI is substantially better than CT for evaluating the brain parenchyma, assessing the posterior fossa, and detecting microhemorrhages. The increasing availability of higher field strength magnets (most commonly 3-Tesla scanners) and multichannel head coils in pediatric institutions provides excellent detail and has improved diagnostic accuracy for many conditions affecting the central nervous system (CNS). MRI can provide vital functional and physiologic information about the brain that cannot be generated by other imaging modalities.

Advanced MR imaging sequences including diffusion-weighted and diffusion tensor imaging (DWI and DTI), susceptibility-weighted imaging (SWI), magnetic resonance spectroscopy (MRS), and perfusion imaging including arterial spin labeling (ASL) are now part of routine pediatric neuroimaging protocols in many institutions.

Two major disadvantages of MRI are longer scan acquisition times and sensitivity to patient motion, which are more relevant in the pediatric age group than in adults. These factors necessitate use of sedation or general anesthesia in a proportion of young pediatric patients. Various techniques have been used to reduce the need for sedation, including mock MRI, which acclimatizes the child to the MRI scanner, and technologies that decrease acquisition times, such as multichannel head coils, parallel imaging, and motion compensation techniques. In order to ensure that the information required to answer the clinical question is acquired in the shortest possible time before lack of patient cooperation becomes problematic, it is important to acquire the most important sequences at the start of the examination and actively monitor the MRI exam in a pediatric patient.

Nuclear Medicine

Nuclear medicine studies are most commonly used to evaluate pediatric epilepsy and brain tumors. In addition, nuclear medicine studies have a role in the assessment of inflammatory brain diseases such as Rasmussen encephalitis and brain death in the pediatric population. Furthermore, nuclear medicine studies have been used to study the pathophysiology underlying various childhood disorders including posttraumatic brain injury, Rett syndrome, and the phacomatoses. As the use of nuclear medicine studies in modern clinical practice primarily involves the evaluation of epilepsy and brain tumors, techniques used in these areas are briefly discussed here.

Radiopharmaceuticals such as ^{99m}Tc-hexamethylpropylene amine oxime (HMPAO) and ^{99m}Tc-bicisate (ECD) are taken up by brain parenchyma in proportion to regional brain perfusion. These agents are used to perform ictal and interictal single positron emission computed tomography (SPECT) studies in pediatric patients with temporal and extratemporal lobe epilepsy. Similarly, ^{18}F-fluorodeoxyglucose–positron emission tomography (^{18}F FDG–PET) is used in the interictal state to highlight the epileptogenic area in the brain. In temporal lobe epilepsy, the sensitivity of ictal SPECT ranges between 60% and 90%, whereas a positive FDG–PET scan can show the epileptogenic focus in up to 85% of cases.[5] Subtraction ictal SPECT coregistered to MRI (SISCOM) is a valuable diagnostic tool used to accurately localize the seizure onset zone in nonlesional and extratemporal epilepsies (Fig. 2.2).

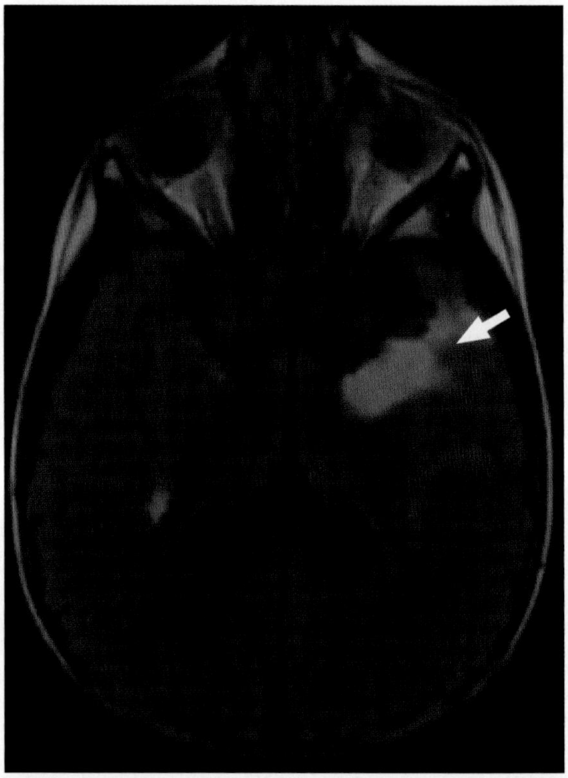

FIGURE 2.2 **A 3-year-old boy with temporal lobe epilepsy.** Axial subtraction ictal SPECT coregistered to MRI (SISCOM) image demonstrates a left temporal lobe epileptogenic focus (*arrow*).

Nuclear medicine studies continue to play an important role in the management of childhood brain tumors. FDG–PET is widely used for metabolic studies of brain tumors. The utilization of FDG–PET in evaluating pediatric brain tumors is based on the assumption that malignant tumors have increased FDG uptake and benign tumors have reduced FDG uptake compared to normal brain parenchyma. Indeed, FDG uptake is increased in the majority of malignant tumors, and the uptake is positively correlated with tumor grade in childhood CNS tumors.

Other tracers such as ^{11}C-methionine PET (MET–PET) have been used in the management of pediatric brain tumors and in the localization of active tubers in pediatric patients with tuberous sclerosis. However, their limited availability has prevented widespread adoption of these tracers in routine clinical practice.

Conventional Cerebral Angiography

Advances in cross-sectional imaging and its ever-increasing availability have improved resolution of angiographic anatomy and led to a progressive decline in the need for diagnostic conventional cerebral angiograms in the pediatric population. However, catheter angiograms are able to resolve small vessels with a spatial resolution of 0.2 mm and temporal resolution of 0.25 seconds, which are superior to CTA and MRA.[6] This technique helps diagnose and plan management of a number of pediatric neurovascular diseases, including intracranial hemorrhage, aneurysms, vascular malformations, dural venous fistulae, trauma, and arteriopathies. Four-vessel catheter neuroangiography remains the "gold standard" modality for the assessment of various disorders including vasculitis, arteriopathies, small aneurysms, arteriovenous malformations (AVMs), and fistulae. The availability of microcatheters has enabled superselective catheterization even in small infants and aids the percutaneous management of various vascular lesions by neurointerventionalists. Catheter size and contrast dose are determined by patient size and age. Disadvantages of this modality include its relatively invasive nature, challenges in obtaining arterial access in children, small risk of lasting neurologic deficits (0.06% to 0.1%), and the small number of trained personnel with pediatric angiographic experience.[7]

EMBRYOLOGY AND NORMAL ANATOMY

Developmental Biology

The change that occurs in the brain from the time of conception to the adulthood is complex, and a detailed discussion of this process is beyond the scope of this chapter. However, a fundamental knowledge of the various steps involved in the development of the brain is essential in order to understand the pathogenesis of various developmental malformations of the pediatric brain and their classification. These steps can be summarized as follows:

In the 3rd week of gestation, the embryo becomes three layered (trilaminar) via a process called gastrulation, following formation of a thick, linear band along the dorsal caudal surface of the epiblast called the primitive streak. The primitive node forms at the cranial end of the streak, and a depression develops along the streak called the primitive groove. As cells begin to migrate between the epiblast and the hypoblast, the layers of the trilaminar embryo are renamed as the ectoderm (epiblast), mesoderm (migrated mesenchymal epiblastic cells), and endoderm (hypoblast). Some mesenchymal cells migrate cranial to the primitive node between the ectoderm and endoderm and form the notochord. The notochord grows in a caudal to cranial direction between 17 and 21 days of gestation. It induces a portion of the ectoderm to become the neural plate. Around 19 to 21 days of gestation, the neural plate differentiates into the neural tube, which gives rise to the CNS, and the neural crest, which gives rise to the peripheral nervous system.

Subsequently, during the 4th week of gestation, the neural tube develops a cranial opening called the rostral neuropore and a caudal opening called the caudal neuropore. Both neuropores normally close by ~24 to 25 days of gestation. Following cranial neuropore closure, the neural tube undergoes segmentation into neuromeres and rhombomeres. The neuromeres then give rise to the prosencephalon (forebrain), which divides into the telencephalon (cerebral hemispheres) and the diencephalon. The rhombomeres give rise to the mesencephalon (midbrain) (Fig. 2.3A) and the rhombencephalon (hindbrain) (Fig. 2.3B and C).

Cerebral cortical formation occurs through a complex process involving a group of neurons that are induced in a neuroepithelial layer and subsequently differentiate, migrate, and organize into a functioning cerebral cortex. This process is controlled by interaction between intrinsic genetic mechanisms and extrinsic information relayed to the cortex by thalamocortical input and other less known factors. Neuronal precursors migrate from the ventricular zone to the cortical plate. Cells begin to migrate centrifugally from the ventricular zone to form the cerebral cortex. Radially oriented glial cells extending between the ventricular margin and the cortex were previously thought to act as scaffolding along which the neurons migrate. More research into this process has helped define that radial glial cells have a more important role in neurogenesis. They have been shown to give rise to cortical neurons as well as glial cells. Once the neurons reach the sur-

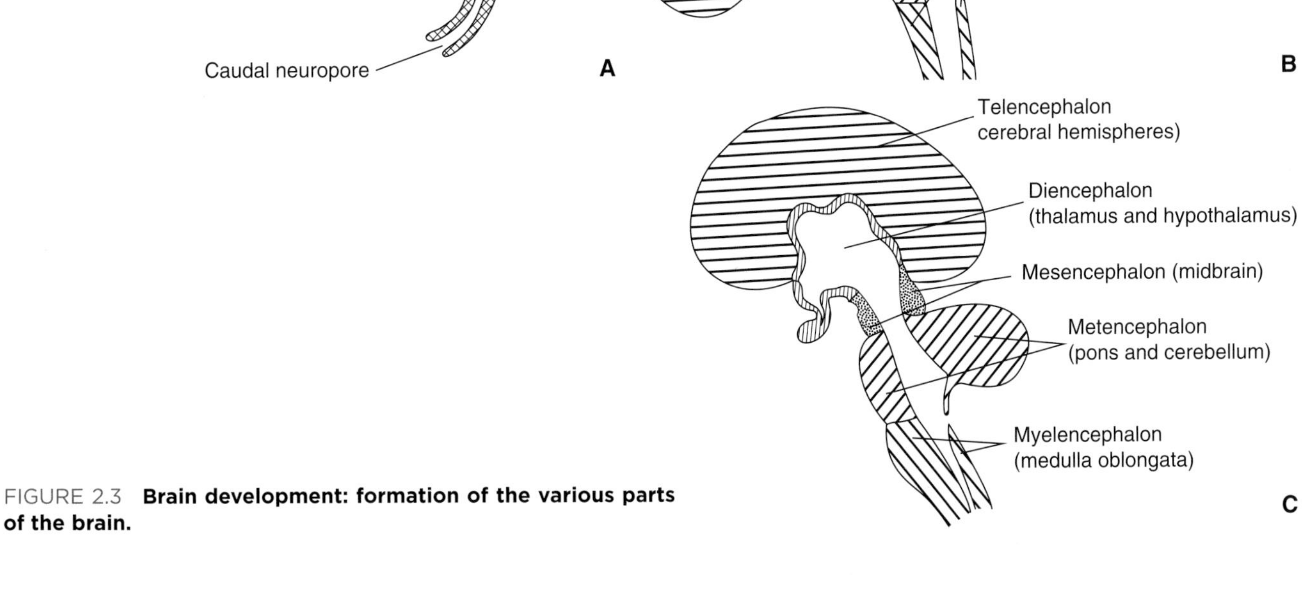

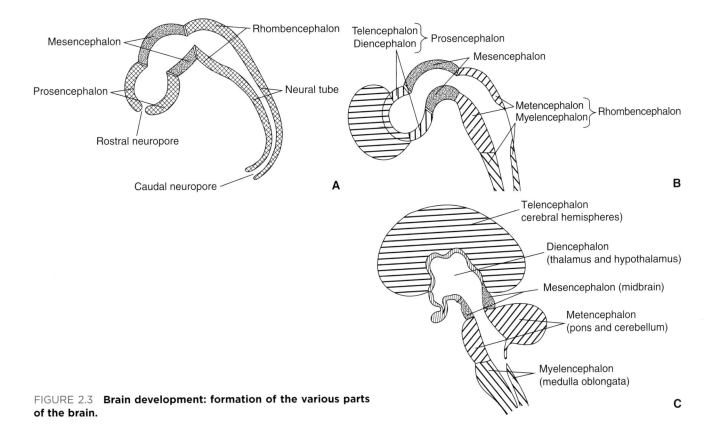

FIGURE 2.3 **Brain development: formation of the various parts of the brain.**

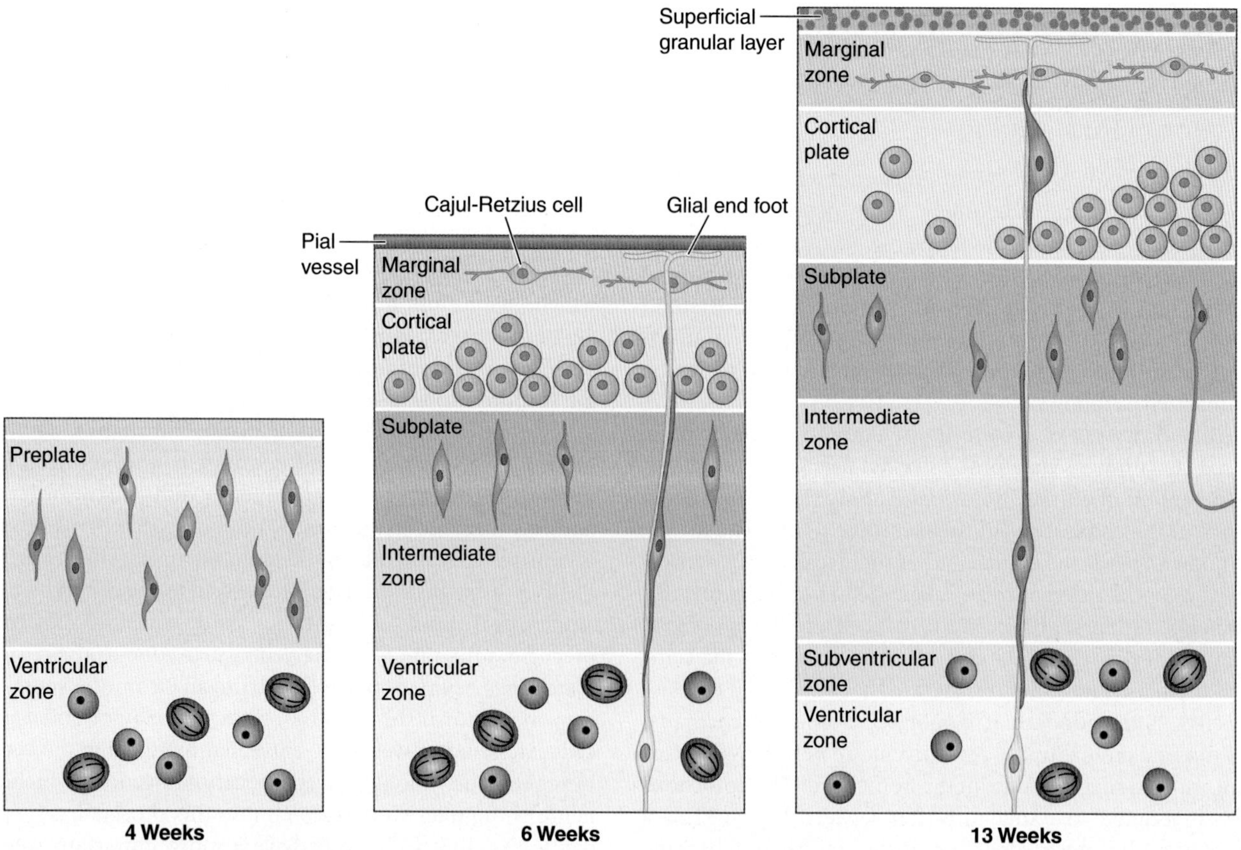

FIGURE 2.4 **Cortical development.**

face, they differentiate to form the normal six-layered cortex (Fig. 2.4).

Based on the patterns of migration, various classifications of malformations of cortical development (MCD) have been proposed. The latest classification by Barkovich et al., describes three primary groups based on the overlapping stages of neuronal migration[8]: (I) malformations caused by abnormal neuronal and glial proliferation, (II) malformations caused by abnormal neuronal migration, and (III) malformations caused by abnormal cortical organization. These disorders are described in a subsequent section of this chapter.

Myelination

The brain parenchyma is composed of gray matter and white matter, which differ in composition (water content and macromolecules) and gross morphology. Although the gray matter consists mainly of neurons, the white matter is composed predominantly of myelinated bundles of axons. The brain of a neonate consists of a large amount of water (89% in gray matter and 82% in white matter), compared to the mature adult brain (82% in gray matter and 72% in white matter).[9]

Myelination of the CNS is primarily a postnatal process. The myelin sheath is a tightly wrapped, multilayered membrane composed of a repeating structure characterized by lipid–cytoplasm–lipid–water surrounding the axons. It is produced by the oligodendroglial cell membranes. Lipid components of myelin in the white matter include cholesterol, galactocerebrosides, sphingomyelin, and phospholipids. They are essential for ensuring stability and strength of the myelin sheath. The other constituents of myelin are a number of proteins including proteolipid protein (PLP), myelin basic protein, myelin-associated glycoprotein, 2', 3'-cyclic-nucleotide 30-phosphodiesterase? and myelin oligodendrocyte glycoprotein. Alterations in the genes controlling the production of these proteins can result in abnormal white matter structure.

Myelination progresses in the human brain in a predictable sequential pattern. Myelination, which starts in the second trimester of gestation, continues postnatally, and lasts into adulthood. The sequence of progression of myelination has been shown to relate to psychomotor development. Certain rules can be used to define the progression of normal myelination. These include progression of myelination in a posterior-to-anterior direction (in keeping with the development of occipital regions and visual areas prior to auditory and speech areas) and in a caudocranial pattern (in keeping with development of the brainstem and cerebellum followed by sensorimotor and higher functions including emotions and abstract thoughts). The corpus callosum also myelinates in a posterior-to-anterior fashion, in keeping with the sequence of myelination in the areas connected by its various sections.

The appearance of the brain parenchyma on MRI changes according to the myelin content. White matter relaxation times, which determine the MR appearance of white matter, are affected by a number of factors, including changes in the structure and chemical composition of the axon and the surrounding myelin and the degree of axonal ensheathment by myelin. Most authors believe that signal changes on T1-weighted MR images correspond with the increase in the certain lipids occurring during myelin formation. The changes on T2-weighted MR images can be explained by myelin sheath maturation and decrease in the water content of the white matter indicated in vitro by thickening and tightening of the spiral of myelin around the axon.

On a practical note, T1-weighted MR images are considered useful for assessment of the state of myelination in the first 6 months of life, and T2-weighed MR images are utilized in older age groups. However, in our experience, on modern 3-Tesla scanners, T2-weighted MR images in the neonate and young infant are as valuable as the T1-weighted MR images to assess myelination. A series of milestones can be used to assess the appropriateness of myelination, as detailed in Table 2.1. As myelination continues well into the teenage years, we do not deem myelination "complete" but prefer to use the term "age appropriate" if the milestones in Table 2.1 are present at a particular age. Myelination is essentially complete by around 2 years of age, except for some areas of persistent nonmyelinated white matter in the parietooccipital regions. These are called the terminal zones of myelination and should not be confused with areas of white matter injury of prematurity, which can have a similar distribution. The various stages of myelination are summarized on Figure 2.5.

TABLE 2.1 Milestones of Myelination

Anatomic Region	Bright Signal on T1-Weighted MR Images	Dark Signal on T2-Weighted MR Images
Middle cerebellar peduncle	At birth	Birth to 2 months
Cerebellar white matter	0-4 months	3-5 months
Posterior limb of internal capsule		
Posterior third	36 weeks of gestation	40 weeks of gestation
Anterior third	0-1 months	4-6 months
Anterior limb of internal capsule	2-3 months	7-11 months
Splenium of the corpus callosum	3-4 months	4-6 months
Genu of the corpus callosum	4-6 months	5-8 months
Occipital white matter		
Deep	3-5 months	9-14 months
Subcortical	4-7 months	11-15 months
Frontal white matter		
Central	3-6 months	11-16 months
Peripheral	7-11 months	11-15 months
Centrum semiovale	2-4 months	7-11 months

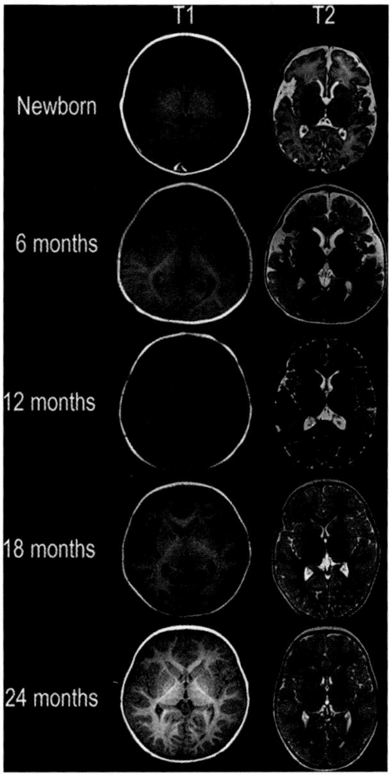

FIGURE 2.5 **Summary of the stages of myelination from the newborn period to 24 months of age on T1- and T2-weighted MR images.**

SPECTRUM OF BRAIN DISORDERS

Congenital and Developmental Anomalies

Several classification systems have been proposed to describe congenital and developmental brain anomalies, in order to incorporate details of morphology, neuropathology, genetics, and clinical findings. Although many of these comprehensive classification systems succeed in incorporating most of the known malformations, they are not always practicable for use in daily clinical practice.

In this section, we use a practical location-based approach that includes the details of morphology and genetics used by some of the more modern classification systems to analyze brain anomalies. Although this is not fully comprehensive, we believe that this is practicable to grasp and use in daily clinical practice. The classification system is summarized in Table 2.2.

TABLE 2.2 Classification of Congenital Brain Malformations

Supratentorial Anomalies
Malformation of cortical development
Lissencephaly (agyria with or without pachygyria)
Pachygyria (isolated)
Polymicrogyria
Schizencephaly
Hemimegalencephaly
Heterotopia
Commissural, midline, and septal anomalies
Corpus callosum anomalies
Holoprosencephaly
Septooptic dysplasia
Infratentorial Anomalies
Cerebellar aplasia or hypoplasia
Rhombencephalosynapsis
Dandy-Walker malformation
Chiari malformation
Mesenchymal Origin Anomalies
Cephalocele/meningocele
Intracranial lipoma
Intracranial cyst (neuroepithelial cyst and arachnoid cyst)
Calvarial and skull base anomalies (discussed in "Skull" chapter)

Supratentorial Anomalies

Malformations of Cortical Development

MCDs encompass a heterogeneous group of cortical lesions resulting from abnormalities during development and formation of the cortical mantle. This process has been summarized in an earlier section in this chapter. The classification of MCDs undergoes periodic revision based upon advances in our understanding of the molecular pathways and genes involved in brain development and the ways in which this complex process can go awry. The latest classification used at the time of drafting this chapter, described by Barkovich et al., is based upon the stage of cortical development that is affected.[8]

The three major stages of cortical development are proliferation, neuronal migration, and postmigrational development. Note that there is temporal overlap between these stages. For instance, neuronal proliferation continues while migration commences and neurons continue to migrate as postmigrational development begins. Further, cells resulting from abnormal proliferation often fail to migrate and organize properly. It is important to recognize that the classification does not encompass every single constellation of abnormalities, but should be seen as a guide.

Using this classification, MCDs are divided into four major groups:

Group I: is defined by abnormalities of neuronal and glial proliferation or apoptosis (resulting in either too many or too few cells) and is divided into three subgroups: (A) reduced proliferation or accelerated apoptosis (resulting in congenital microcephalies), (B) increased proliferation or decreased apoptosis (resulting in conditions such as megalencephalies), and (C) abnormal proliferation (with resultant focal and diffuse dysgenesis and dysplasia).

Group II: is defined by abnormalities of neuronal migration and is divided into four subgroups: (A) abnormalities in the neuroependymal cell (ventricular zone epithelium) during initiation of migration (resulting in periventricular nodular heterotopia), (B) generalized abnormalities of transmantle migration (resulting in lissencephalies), (C) localized abnormalities of transmantle migration (resulting in subcortical heterotopia), and (D) terminal migration anomalies and defects in the pial-limiting membranes (resulting in the cobblestone malformations).

Group III: consists of abnormalities of postmigrational development. These malformations result from injury to the cortex during later stages of development and include late prenatal and perinatal insults.

Group IV: is defined as MCD, not otherwise specified.

This chapter includes some of the more important anomalies that come under this classification with helpful information to identify them on imaging, along with notes about their clinical relevance.

Lissencephaly (Agyria With or Without Pachygyria)

Lissencephaly refers to a "smooth brain" with a paucity of gyri and sulci on the brain surface. Agyria is defined as an absence of gyri with a thickened cortex and is synonymous with "complete lissencephaly." On the other hand, pachygyria refers to the presence of a few broad, flat gyri with thickened cortex and is synonymous with "incomplete lissencephaly."

In classic lissencephaly, the cortex is abnormally thick (12 to 20 mm; normal: 3 to 4 mm) and poorly organized with four layers, namely, a thin outer cortical layer, a thin molecular layer adjacent to the pia, a "cell-sparse zone" medial to the outer cortical layer, and a thickest deep cortical layer.[10] MRI in patients with complete lissencephaly shows a smooth brain surface, with absent gyri and shallow, vertically oriented Sylvian fissures, which results in the "figure-of-eight" appearance on axial images. Callosal dysgenesis with a vertically oriented splenium is seen in severe lissencephaly. The brainstem is usually small.

In patients with incomplete lissencephaly, pachygyria is seen along with agyria or areas of normal brain. Imaging studies show presence of broad gyri and shallow sulci (Fig. 2.6). Gross anatomy demonstrates a paucity of gyri over the surface (Fig. 2.7). Use of high-resolution images helps differentiate between the smooth gray and white matter junction in pachygyria and the irregular, nodular outline in polymicrogyria.

Polymicrogyria

Polymicrogyria is one of the most common MCDs. It refers to the pathologic finding of overfolding and abnormal

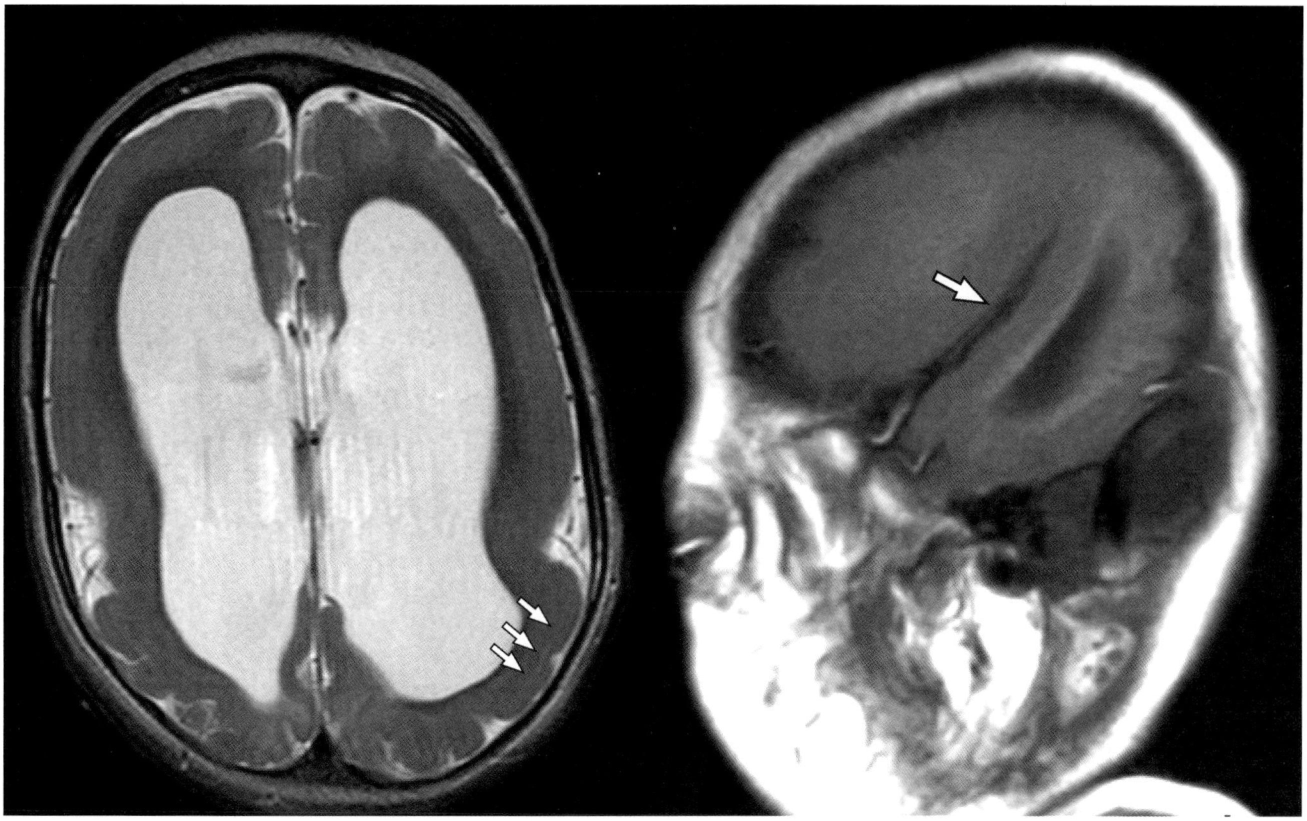

FIGURE 2.6 **Incomplete lissencephaly (pachygyria) in a 3-year-old boy.** Axial T2-weighted MR image (on the **left**) shows lissencephaly characterized by broad gyri and shallow sulci more pronounced in the frontal and temporal lobes. Note the T2 hyperintense cell-sparse zone in the parietal lobes (*white arrows*). Sagittal T1-weighted MR image (on the **right**) shows a vertically oriented Sylvian fissure (*white arrow*).

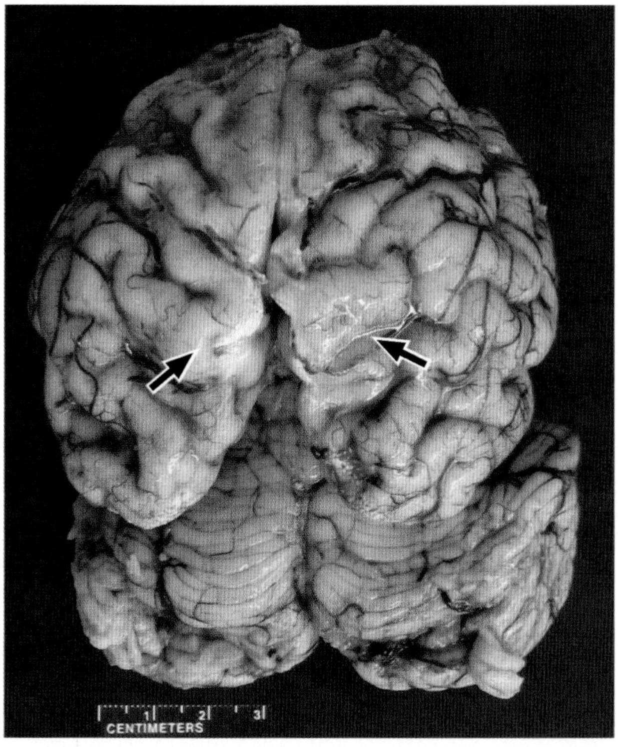

FIGURE 2.7 **Pachygyria in an 11-year-old girl with microcephaly.** The cerebral cortex shows pachygyria, characterized by a paucity of gyri (*black arrows*).

lamination of the cortex. The overfolding is usually microscopic, and the abnormal lamination either unlayered or four-layered in most described cases. Polymicrogyria is most commonly seen in the perisylvian cortex, but almost all cortical regions can be involved. Polymicrogyria is a highly heterogeneous disorder in terms of its pathogenesis, distribution, pathologic appearance, and clinical and imaging features. The clinical presentation is varied, and patients present at all ages from the neonatal period until late adulthood.

Polymicrogyria is classified as an abnormality occurring during late neuronal migration or early cortical organization, with both genetic and nongenetic factors involved in its pathogenesis. Ischemic injury, congenital infections (cytomegalovirus [CMV] being the most common), chromosomal deletion and duplication syndromes (e.g., 22q11.2 deletion), and peroxisomal disorders like Zellweger syndrome are among the common causes implicated in the development of polymicrogyria. Various modes of inheritance, including X-linked and autosomal recessive pedigrees, have been identified. Mutations in genes such as the *TUBB2B* gene have been identified recently. Imaging should be directed toward defining the regional distribution of the polymicrogyria, elaborating additional abnormalities in the white matter, correlating with the head circumference, and identifying clues that point to a possible infective or ischemic etiology such as periventricular calcification or encephalomalacia.[11]

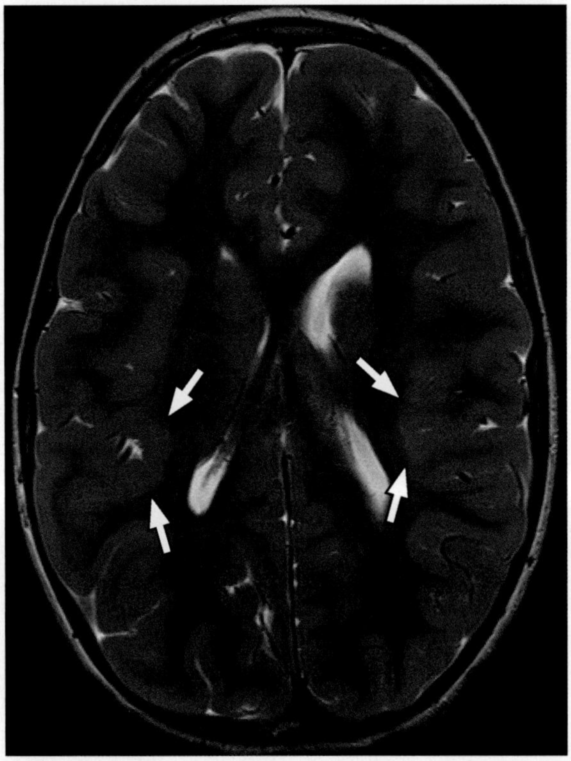

FIGURE 2.8 **Bilateral perisylvian polymicrogyria.** Axial T2-weighted MR image shows the irregular nodular cortical-white matter junction (*arrows*) in the bilateral perisylvian regions, right more than left.

On MRI, polymicrogyria is characterized by an irregular cortical surface and "stippled" gray–white junction with regions of apparent cortical thickening (Figs. 2.8 and 2.9).

Pitfalls to avoid include mistaking deformational changes because of perinatal injury for polymicrogyria and underestimating the abnormality in the cortical outline in patients with incomplete myelination of the white matter.

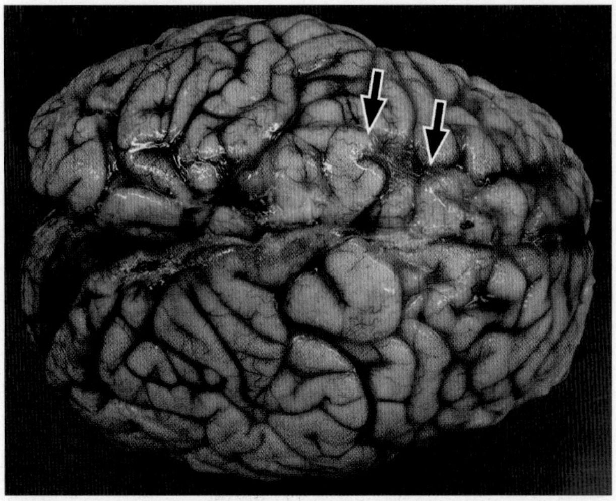

FIGURE 2.9 **Polymicrogyria in a 13-year-old boy with holoprosencephaly.** Superior aspect of the brain shows polymicrogyria of the frontal (right) and anterior parietal lobes (*arrows*).

Schizencephaly

Schizencephaly is a full-thickness cleft lined with gray matter and connecting the subarachnoid cerebrospinal fluid (CSF) spaces with the ventricular system. The cleft is lined by abnormal infolded gray matter extending from the cortex into the ventricles, with associated fusion of the cortical pia and ventricular ependyma within the cleft.[12] Gray matter heterotopias and areas of polymicrogyria are frequently found within and near the cleft. Schizencephaly results from injury to the entire thickness of the developing hemisphere during cortical organization because of prenatal infection, ischemia, or chromosomal abnormalities. Clinical manifestations of schizencephaly most often include varying degrees of developmental delay, motor impairment, and seizures.

On imaging studies, schizencephaly is seen as a full-thickness CSF-containing cleft extending medially from the subarachnoid space into the lateral ventricle. The wall of the cleft is lined with abnormal gray matter, which sometimes extends into the lateral ventricle in the form of subependymal heterotopias. Clefts may be small or large, unilateral or bilateral. The anomaly may be of the open-lip or closed-lip type. In closed-lip schizencephaly, the gray matter–lined lips are in contact with each other. The walls of the cleft in open-lip schizencephaly are separated, and a cleft of CSF can be seen extending to the underlying ventricles (Fig. 2.10).

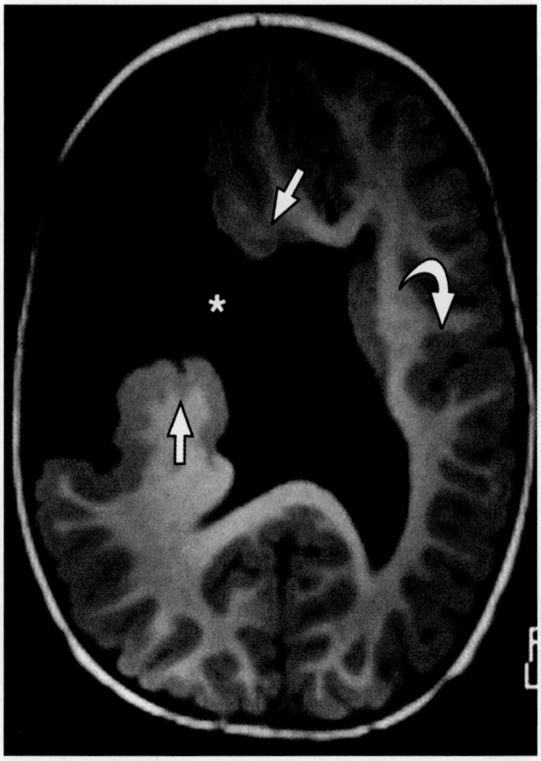

FIGURE 2.10 **Open-lip schizencephaly.** Axial MPRAGE (magnetization-prepared rapid acquisition gradient-echo) MR image demonstrates a large right-sided full-thickness cleft (*asterisk*), lined by abnormal polymicrogyric gray matter (*straight arrows*), that communicates with the lateral ventricle. Also, note absence of the septum pellucidum in this child with septooptic dysplasia and polymicrogyria (*curved arrow*) without schizencephaly in the left cerebral hemisphere.

In addition to defining the schizencephalic cleft, imaging should be directed to identifying additional abnormalities that may coexist in these pediatric patients. The more common associated abnormalities include variable components of septooptic pituitary dysplasia (including optic nerve hypoplasia, absence of septum pellucidum, and ectopic/absent neurohypophysis), pachygyria, polymicrogyria, heterotopia, and arachnoid cysts.

Hemimegalencephaly

Hemimegalencephaly is a rare malformation of cortical development characterized by defective cellular organization and neuronal migration, with resultant hamartomatous overgrowth of a hemisphere. This condition is rare, representing <5% of MCD diagnosed on imaging studies.[13] Affected patients typically present in infancy with macrocrania, developmental delay, and seizures. Hemihypertrophy of part or all of the ipsilateral body may be associated. Seizures are difficult to treat, and severe developmental delay is common.

On imaging studies, hemimegalencephaly is characterized by an enlarged, dysplastic-appearing hemisphere with an abnormal gyral pattern, cortical thickening, and white matter signal abnormalities (Fig. 2.11). The ipsilateral lateral ventricle usually appears enlarged, and the frontal horn points anteriorly on the involved side. Focal or localized type is also described. On CT, there is an enlarged hemisphere and hemicranium, with contralateral displacement of the posterior falx. Dystrophic calcifications are common. On MRI, the dysplastic cortex appears thickened and undulating on T1-weighted MR images. Myelination is accelerated with resultant T1 hyperintensity. Gray matter heterotopias are commonly seen. The ipsilateral ventricle is usually enlarged and deformed. Pachygyria and polymicrogyria are seen in the involved hemisphere. White matter signal is of heterogeneous signal intensity on T2-weighted and FLAIR MR images, with cysts and patchy hyperintensity.

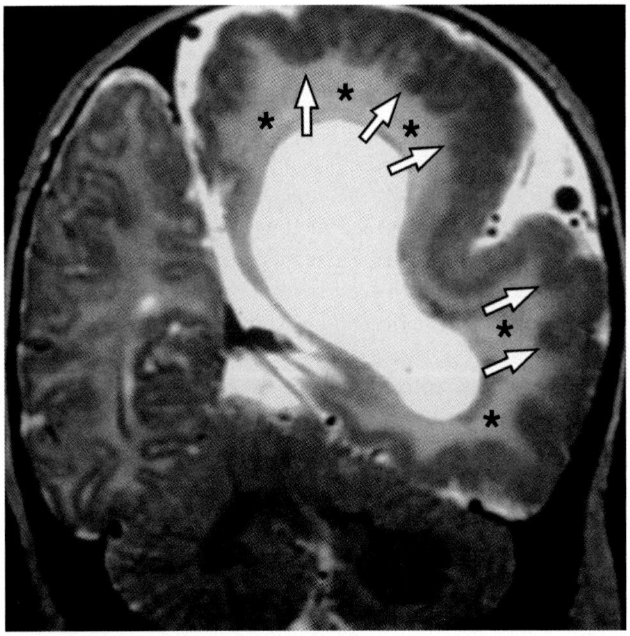

FIGURE 2.11 **Hemimegalencephaly.** Coronal T2-weighted MR image shows the abnormal dysplastic-appearing left hemisphere with an abnormal gyral pattern, cortical thickening, white matter hyperintensity (*asterisks*), and polymicrogyria (*arrows*).

Heterotopia

Gray matter heterotopia is a relatively common form of neuronal migration disorder in which collections of cortical neurons are found in an abnormal location. It results from an in utero arrest of radial migration of neurons from the germinal matrix in the wall of the lateral ventricle to the developing cerebral cortex between 6 and 16 weeks of gestation. It is usually discovered during the evaluation of children or young adults with epilepsy and children with neurodevelopmental abnormalities or as an incidental finding. The pathogenic mechanisms are not fully understood, but they lead to distinct clinicoradiologic syndromes. Based on the location of the ectopically located gray matter, various subtypes are described including band heterotopia, subcortical heterotopia, and subependymal (periventricular) heterotopia.

Band heterotopia is considered the mildest form of classic lissencephaly. It refers to a band of heterotopic gray matter located just beneath the cortex, which lends a typical "double cortex" appearance. The overlying gyral pattern is normal or demonstrates mildly simplified shallow sulci, and a normal cortical ribbon is present. Affected pediatric patients are almost exclusively female. They usually present in childhood with seizure disorders and developmental delay. On imaging studies, band heterotopia is seen as a homogenous band of gray matter between the lateral ventricles and the cerebral cortex separated from the overlying cortex and the underlying lateral ventricles by a layer of normal-appearing white matter (Fig. 2.12).

Subcortical heterotopias are malformations characterized by large, focal, mass-like collections of neurons that are found in the deep cerebral white matter anywhere from the ependyma to the cortex. The involved portion of the affected hemisphere is small, and the overlying cortex is thin with shallow sulci and may be dysplastic.

Subependymal (periventricular nodular) heterotopias are characterized by gray matter nodules lining the ventricular margins and can be divided into two main groups. The first group is characterized by a few scattered heterotopic nodules at the trigones and the temporal and occipital horns. They may be associated with other brain anomalies such as Chiari II malformation, callosal agenesis, and cerebellar hypoplasia. The second smaller group has a large number of nodules that completely or nearly completely line the walls of the lateral ventricles. This group is more likely to be familial, with X-linked and autosomal recessive patterns of inheritance. Mutations in the gene filamin-A (*FLNA*) at chromosome Xq28 have been identified in a subset of these patients.[14]

In other types of heterotopia, focal ectopic masses of gray matter occur in linear or swirling curved columns of neurons that extend through normal-appearing white matter from the

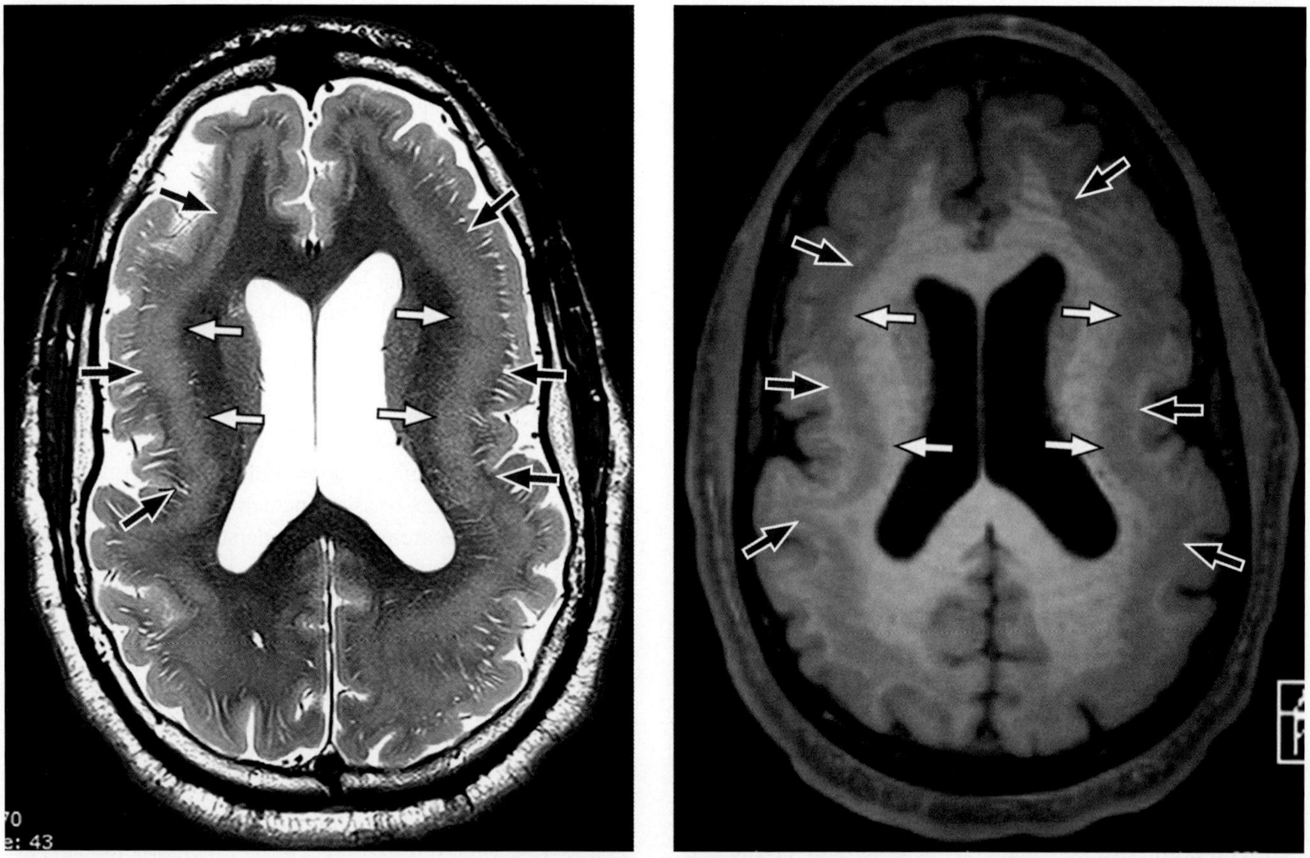

FIGURE 2.12 **Subcortical band heterotopia.** Axial T2-weighted (on the **left**) and axial SPGR (spoiled gradient recalled) (on the **right**) MR images demonstrate the double cortex appearance caused by an inner band of heterotopic gray matter (*white arrows*) separated from the outer cortex by a thin zone of normal white matter (*black arrows*).

ependyma to the pia. The overlying cortex is thin, and the underlying ventricle often appears distorted. These foci follow gray matter on all sequences, do not demonstrate edema, and do not enhance, which differentiates them from glioneuronal tumors like gangliocytomas.

Focal Cortical Dysplasia

Focal cortical dysplasia (FCD) is one of the more common MCDs. It is the most common cause of medically refractory epilepsy in the pediatric population. The most recent classification of FCDs proposed by the International League Against Epilepsy describes three types[15].

FCD type I includes abnormalities of cortical lamination (type Ia), abnormal tangential cortical lamination (type Ib), and abnormal radial lamination (type Ic). FCD type II includes abnormal cortical dyslamination and dysmorphic neurons without balloon cells (type IIa) and with balloon cells (type IIb). FCD type III describes those with an associated lesion. The associated lesion can be hippocampal sclerosis (type IIIa), an epilepsy-associated tumor (type IIIb), vascular malformation (type IIIc), or other lesions (type IIId).[15]

On high-resolution MRI, features of FCD include cortical thickening (which should ideally be confirmed in at least two planes and on two different imaging sequences), blurring of the junction between the white matter and the cortex, T2 and FLAIR hyperintensity in the cortex and adjacent subcortical white matter, T1 shortening in the cortex, and abnormal sulcal/gyral pattern.

In practice, it may be possible to distinguish between type I and type II dysplasias.[16] MRI is able to show abnormalities in the majority of type II dysplasias but only in some of the type I cortical dysplasias. The typical appearance of FCD type IIb (with balloon cells) is a band of hyperintensity on T2-weighted and FLAIR MR images extending from the gray and white matter interface to the surface of the ventricles (Fig. 2.13). In order to visualize this often subtle finding optimally, multiplanar thin-section images should be performed. On modern 3-Tesla MR scanners, a three-dimensional FLAIR sequence with reformats is an excellent method for visualizing these malformations.

Clinical symptoms are more severe in the type II cortical dysplasia usually seen in children. In this type, abnormalities may be seen outside the temporal lobe with predilection for the frontal lobes. New type III is one of the above dysplasias with an additional lesion such as hippocampal sclerosis, tumor, vascular malformation, or pathology acquired during early life.

A complete resection of the epileptogenic zone is required for seizure freedom, or at least seizure control with medications. High-resolution MRI is helpful in identifying those patients who are likely to benefit from surgical treatment in a group of patients with drug-resistant epilepsy. However,

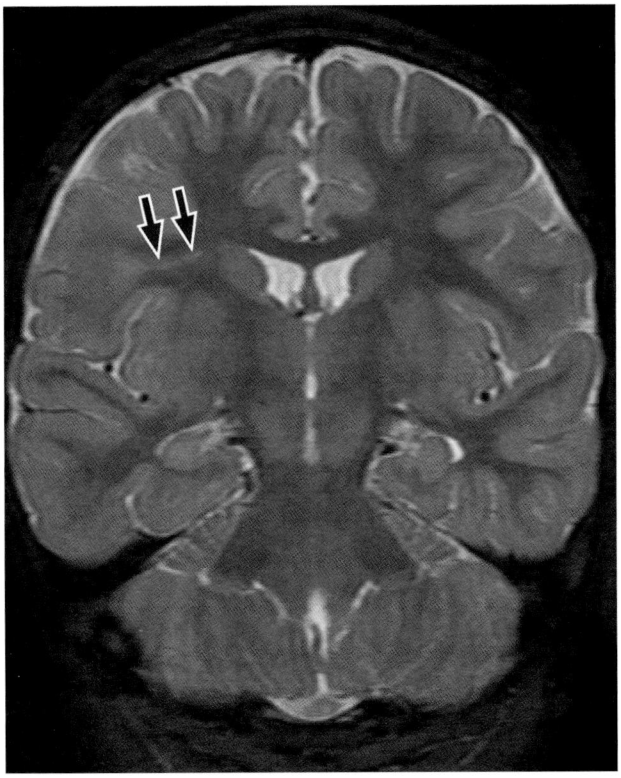

FIGURE 2.13 **Focal cortical dysplasia type IIb.** Coronal T2-weighted MR image shows a band of hyperintensity (*arrows*) extending from the gray and white matter interface to the surface of the ventricles in the right frontal lobe.

the abnormalities may also involve eloquent areas, and resection may not be an option in these cases. Therefore, other diagnostic imaging techniques such as FDG–PET, magnetoencephalography (MEG), DTI, and intracranial electroencephalography (EEG) are widely used to establish the diagnosis and plan management.

Commissural, Midline, and Septal Anomalies

Corpus Callosum Anomalies (Complete and Partial Agenesis). Agenesis of the corpus callosum (ACC) is a relatively frequent malformation. If the normal developmental process of the corpus callosum is disturbed, it may be completely absent (agenesis) or partially formed (hypogenesis).[17] Two types of ACC can be distinguished morphologically: type 1 ACC, in which axons are present but are unable to cross the midline, forming large aberrant longitudinal fiber bundles (Probst bundles) (Figs. 2.14 and 2.15); and the less common type 2 ACC, in which axons fail to form (no Probst bundles).

Callosal dysgenesis is defined as malformation of the corpus callosum as a result of an injury during the formation of its precursors, rather than from an injury to the corpus itself.[17] This failure may result from extrinsic causes (lipoma, interhemispheric cyst, etc.), from disorders in neuronal migration, or an intracortical disposition linked with a gyral anomaly. Formation of most of the cerebrum and cerebellum occurs at the same time as that of the corpus callosum, between 8 and 20 weeks of gestational age. Therefore, callosal anomalies are often associated with other anomalies in the cerebrum and

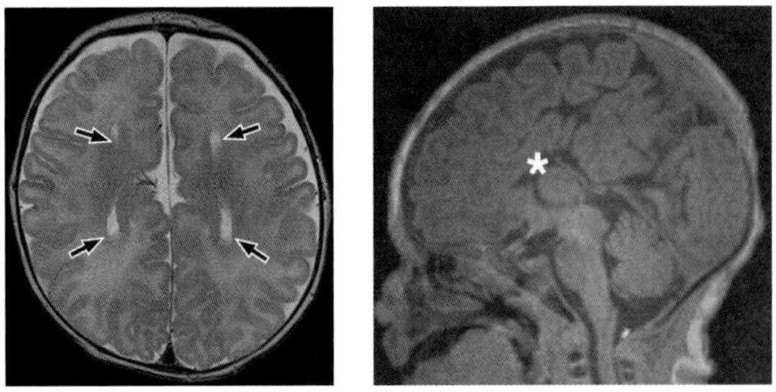

FIGURE 2.14 **Agenesis of the corpus callosum.** Axial T2-weighted (on the **left**) and sagittal MPRAGE (magnetization-prepared rapid acquisition gradient-echo) (on the **right**) MR images show the parallel orientation of the lateral ventricles (*arrows*) in the axial plane and absence of the corpus callosum in its expected position (*asterisk*) in the sagittal plane.

cerebellum, including holoprosencephaly (HPE), encephalocele, and posterior fossa anomalies. HPE shows a spectrum of callosal anomalies from agenesis to the dysgenesis associated with lobar types. This entity is discussed in the next section of this chapter.

Interhemispheric cysts are classified into various types based on morphology and clinical features. Loculated cyst without ventricular communication, known as a type II cyst, is associated more commonly with brain anomalies, including those of the corpus callosum. Intracranial lipomas are congenital malformations resulting from abnormal, persistent maldifferentiation of the formal primordium of the meninges during subarachnoid cistern development. They are associated with up to 40% to 50% of callosal anomalies. Lipomas are most common in the pericallosal area. Anterior pericallosal lipomas are associated with more severe corpus callosal anomalies than posterior pericallosal lipomas.

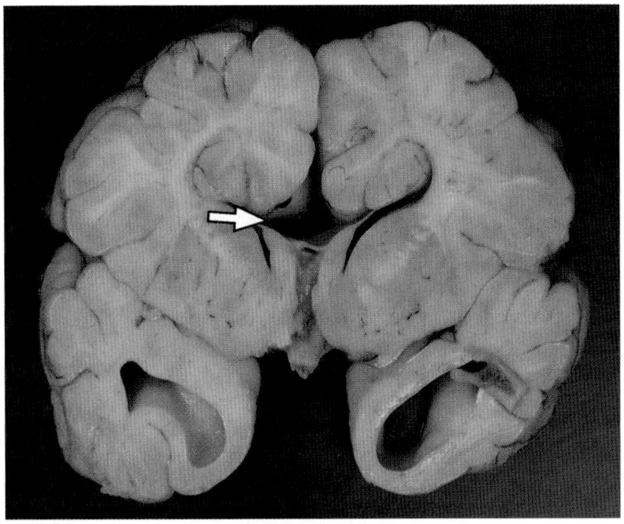

FIGURE 2.15 **Agenesis of the corpus callosum.** Coronal section at the level of the basal ganglia shows an absent corpus callosum (*arrow*) in an 11-month-old boy with Vici syndrome, which is also called immunodeficiency with cleft lip/palate, cataract, hypopigmentation, and absent corpus callosum.

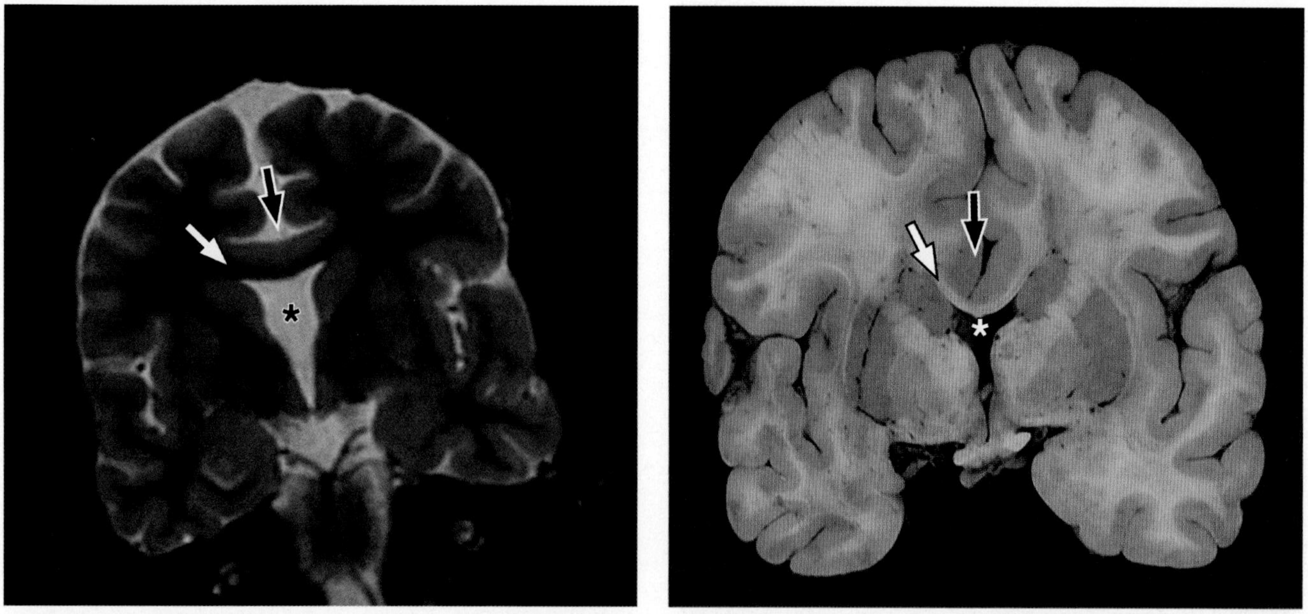

FIGURE 2.16 **Lobar holoprosencephaly in an infant girl.** Coronal T2-weighted MR image (on the **left**) and cut surface of the brain (on the **right**) show fusion of the cortex across the midline (*black arrows*), absent fornices and septum pellucidum (*asterisks*), and a thin corpus callosum (*white arrows*).

Holoprosencephaly. HPE is a complex brain malformation resulting from incomplete cleavage of the prosencephalon, occurring between the 18th and the 28th day of gestation and affecting both the forebrain and the face. It is estimated to occur in 1/16,000 live births and 1/250 fetuses.[18] Three subtypes, in order of increasing severity, are described: lobar (Fig. 2.16), semilobar, and alobar HPE. Another milder subtype of HPE called middle interhemispheric variant or syntelencephaly is also described.

Facial anomalies are seen in a proportion of patients with alobar or semilobar HPE, such as cyclopia, proboscis, median or bilateral cleft lip/palate, hypotelorism, or solitary median maxillary central incisor in minor forms. These midline defects can occur without the cerebral malformations. Clinical features include developmental delay, feeding difficulties, seizures, and an inability to maintain temperature, heart rate, and respiration. Endocrine disorders including diabetes insipidus, adrenal hypoplasia, hypogonadism, thyroid hypoplasia, and growth hormone deficiency are frequent. A number of genes have been implicated in HPE. Gene sequencing and allele quantification are currently available for the four main genes *SHH*, *ZIC2*, *SIX3*, and *TGIF*.[19]

Prenatal diagnosis is based on US and MRI rather than on molecular diagnosis. Treatment is symptomatic and supportive and requires a multidisciplinary management. Outcome depends on the severity of HPE and the medical and neurologic complications associated. Severely affected children have a very poor prognosis. Mildly affected children may exhibit few symptoms and live a normal life.

Septooptic (Pituitary) Dysplasia. Septooptic dysplasia (SOD) is a syndrome characterized by an absence of the septum pellucidum, optic nerve hypoplasia, and varying degrees of pituitary gland dysfunction. In order to avoid emphasis on the absence of the septum and optic nerve hypoplasia, the term septooptic pituitary dysplasia is currently preferred. Only ~30% of SOD cases have complete manifestations, 62% have the complication of hypopituitarism, and 60% have an absent septum pellucidum.[20] The incidence of SOD is 1 in 10,000 live births.[21] SOD can be caused by mutations in *HESX1* and *SOX2*. A genetic diagnosis can currently be made in only <1% of the patients.[22] Affected pediatric patients present with a variety of symptoms including developmental delay, seizures, visual impairment, sleep disturbance, precocious puberty, obesity, anosmia, sensorineural hearing loss, and cardiac anomalies.

MRI findings vary among affected pediatric patients. However, classically, MRI shows hypoplastic optic nerves (unilateral or bilateral) and optic chiasm, partial or complete septum pellucidum agenesis, corpus callosal agenesis or hypogenesis, ectopic or absent posterior pituitary bright spot, and varying degrees of anterior pituitary hypoplasia (Fig. 2.17). Associated lesions to be looked for include schizencephaly and cortical malformations, which can be seen in a substantial proportion of affected patients.

Treatment includes regular ongoing follow-up by a multidisciplinary team, including optimal hormonal replacement for any hormonal insufficiencies, regular ophthalmologic follow-up, and neurodevelopmental support. Close monitoring should be instituted to assess for other associated features such as autism and obesity.

Infratentorial Anomalies

Cerebellar Aplasia, Dysplasia, or Hypoplasia

Cerebellar hypoplasia represents a spectrum of abnormalities ranging from a virtually empty posterior fossa (i.e., cerebellar aplasia) to milder variants with a small hypoplastic

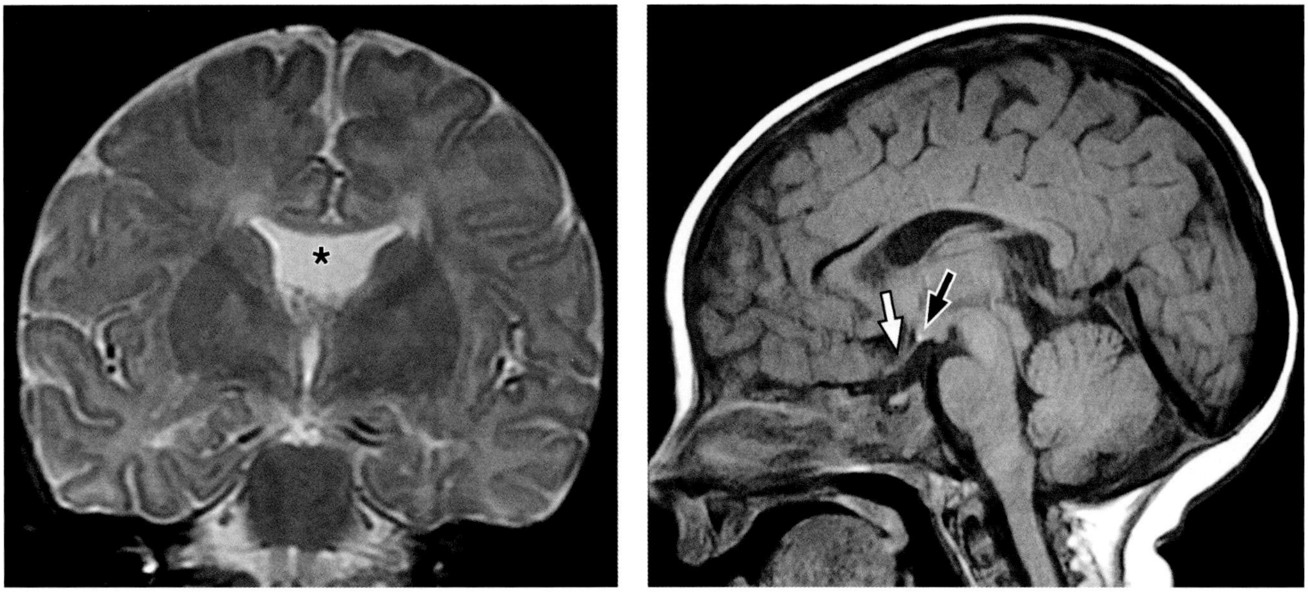

FIGURE 2.17 **Septooptic dysplasia.** Axial T2-weighted (on the **left**) and sagittal T1-weighted (on the **right**) MR images show absent septum pellucidum (*asterisk*), ectopic posterior pituitary bright spot (*black arrow*), and hypoplastic optic chiasm (*white arrow*).

cerebellum (i.e., cerebellar hypoplasia). In the severe variant, both hemispheres and vermis are almost completely absent. The brainstem, particularly the pons, is hypoplastic.

Other unclassified focal or diffuse dysplasias involve the cerebellar hemispheres and/or vermis. They demonstrate asymmetry or focal disruption of cerebellar folia and sulcal morphology. On MRI, a dysmorphic appearance to the cerebellum is seen, with enlarged, vertically oriented fissures or clefts, disordered foliation, abnormal white matter arborization, malformed cortical lining, gray matter heterotopias, and small cyst-like areas in the white matter (Fig. 2.18). It is important to define the difference between cerebellar hypoplasia and atrophy. Cerebellar hypoplasia refers to a congenitally small cerebellum with normal-sized fissures compared

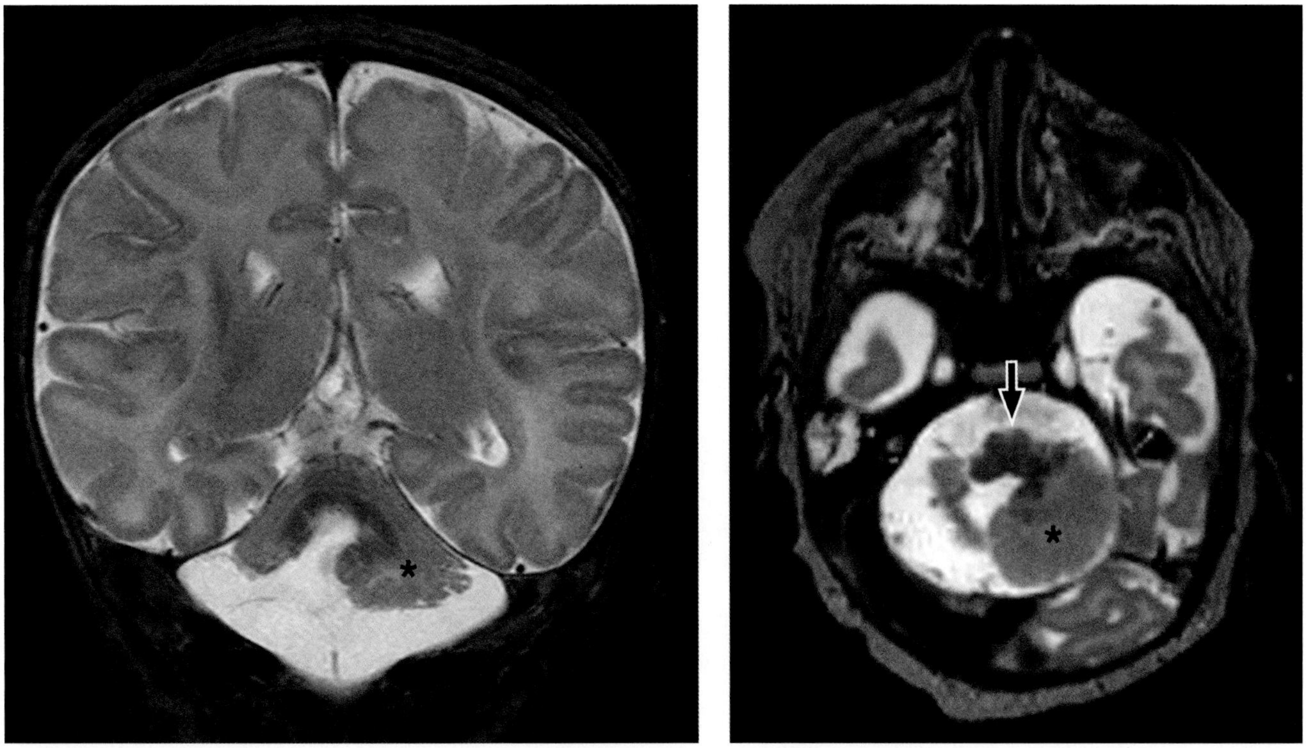

FIGURE 2.18 **Cerebellar hypoplasia.** Coronal (on the **left**) and axial (on the **right**) T2-weighted MR images demonstrate marked right cerebellar hypoplasia, with milder hypoplasia of the left cerebellar hemisphere (*asterisks*) and small inferior vermis with a small flattened pons (*arrow*). Note the abnormal cortical outline in the hypoplastic cerebellar hemispheres.

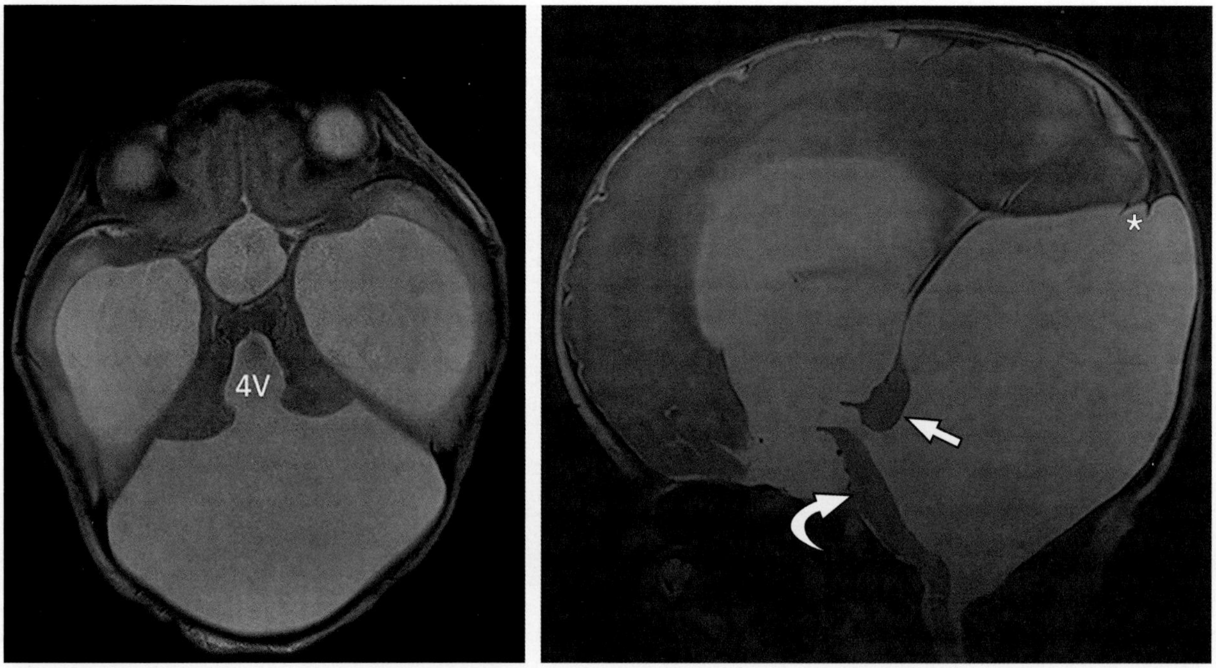

FIGURE 2.19 **Dandy-Walker malformation in a 2-year-old infant boy with severe hydrocephalus.** Axial (on the **left**) and sagittal (on the **right**) T2-weighted MR images show a markedly enlarged CSF-filled posterior fossa, which communicates with an enlarged fourth ventricle (*4V*), upward rotated hypoplastic vermis (*white straight arrow*), high tentorium, hypoplastic brainstem (*curved arrow*), and elevation of the confluence of the venous sinuses (*asterisk*).

to the folia and is usually associated with hypoplasia of the pons. In contrast, cerebellar atrophy refers to a small cerebellum with prominent cerebellar fissures or evidence of progressive volume loss shown on serial imaging.

Dandy-Walker Malformations

Dandy-Walker malformation is a rare congenital malformation characterized by aplasia or hypoplasia of the cerebellar vermis, cystic dilatation of the fourth ventricle, and enlargement of the posterior fossa (Fig. 2.19). A large number of concomitant problems may be present, but Dandy-Walker malformation is recognized whenever these three features are found. Approximately 70% to 90% of affected pediatric patients have hydrocephalus, which often develops postnatally. Dandy-Walker malformation may be associated with atresia of the foramen of Magendie and, possibly, the foramina of Luschka.

Rhombencephalosynapsis

Rhombencephalosynapsis is a rare midline brain malformation characterized by absence of the cerebellar vermis and apparent fusion of the cerebellar hemispheres. The degree of fusion is variable and ranges from partial absence of the nodulus and anterior and posterior vermis in the mild type to complete absence of the vermis on the severe end of the spectrum. Continuity of the cerebellar hemispheres across the midline dorsally is typical.

On MRI, sagittal images show an upwardly convex fastigial recess of the fourth ventricle and absence of the normal midline foliar pattern of the vermis. On coronal MR images, transverse folia are seen with continuity of the cerebellar white matter across the midline (Fig. 2.20). Absence of the vermis is best seen in the axial plane. Aqueductal stenosis and hydrocephalus are common. Partial or complete fusion of the

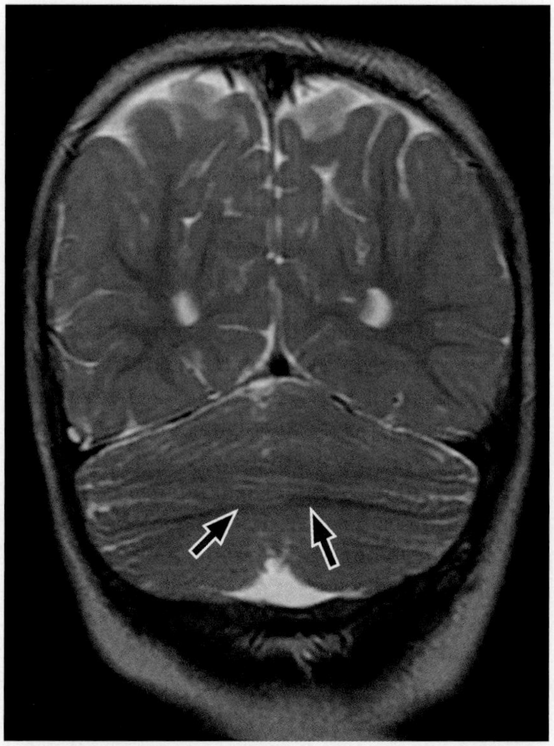

FIGURE 2.20 **Rhombencephalosynapsis.** Coronal T2-weighted MR image shows apparent fusion of the cerebellar hemispheres with transversely oriented folia and continuity (*arrows*) of the cerebellar white matter across the midline.

thalami, fornices, and tectum may be present. Other midline and forebrain anomalies including absent cavum septum pellucidum, absent olfactory bulbs, and corpus callosum dysgenesis can be also seen.

Chiari Malformations

The Chiari malformations are a group of defects associated with congenital caudal "displacement" of the cerebellum and brainstem. Initial descriptions were based on autopsy observations. Three types were described, with a fourth added later. Types II and III are likely to be related to each other.

Chiari I Malformation

Chiari I malformation is the most common type. It is characterized by a peg-like configuration of the cerebellar tonsils, which are displaced into the upper cervical canal through the foramen magnum (Fig. 2.21). Traditionally, the cerebellar tonsillar tips are considered low-lying if they measure at least 5 mm below the foramen magnum. However, recent studies have shown that reliance on a single measurement does not define the malformation or correlate with symptomatology. It is now thought that describing the configuration of the cerebellar tonsils (rounded or peg-like), the amount of CSF around them, the degree of crowding at the foramen magnum, and the configuration of the dens (angled posteriorly or not) is important to define Chiari type I malformations and avoid overdiagnosis. CSF flow studies utilizing cine phase contrast images have been shown to have some value in the assessment of these patients. Many pediatric patients diagnosed with this condition are asymptomatic. When symptoms do occur, affected pediatric patients present with headaches (commonly occipital in location and accentuated by bending forward), neck pain, sleep apnea, and balance problems.

The upper cervical cord should be examined closely for evidence of syringomyelia or presyrinx (potentially reversible edema within the cord caused by alteration in CSF flow dynamics caused by obstruction to CSF flow at the foramen magnum). MRI characteristics of the presyrinx include T2 prolongation, subtle T1 prolongation, and cord expansion without frank cavitation.

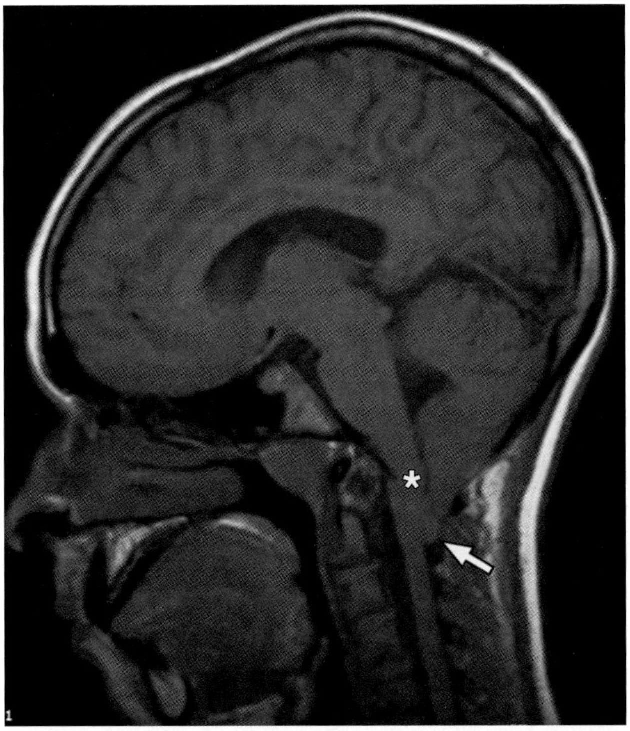

FIGURE 2.21 **Chiari I malformation.** Sagittal T1-weighted MR image shows pointed cerebellar tonsils (*arrow*) extending inferiorly to the mid C2 level, with resultant effacement of the CSF spaces at the level of the foramen magnum and associated kinking (*asterisk*) of the cervicomedullary junction.

Chiari II Malformation

Chiari II malformation is characterized by herniation of the vermis through the foramen magnum, a smooth cerebellar vermis, small brainstem, beaked tectum (due to collicular fusion), absent fourth ventricle, small cerebellum, and crowded posterior fossa (Fig. 2.22). It is almost invariably associated with a lumbosacral spinal myelomeningocele. Approximately two-thirds of affected pediatric patients display a medullary "kink" dorsal to the upper cervical spinal cord, which has been associated with a more symptomatic clinical course. Other features seen on imaging include large massa intermedia, cortical abnormalities including gray matter heterotopia, callosal hypogenesis, and colpocephaly.[23] Interdigitation of the cerebral gyri across the midline is another commonly seen finding. Skull malformations including enlargement of the foramen magnum, scalloping of the petrous pyramid, Luckenschadel, or lacunar skull (round-, oval-, or finger-shaped pits on the inner surface of the membranous part of the skull vault, separated by ridges of bone), and clival shortening are noted on CT performed in these patients.

Given that CM II is associated in almost all cases with myelomeningocele, the initial presenting symptom is an open neural tube defect. A symptomatic CM II is the most common cause of death in patients with myelomeningocele <2 years of age. Around one-third of affected pediatric patients with CM II develop signs and symptoms of brainstem compression by the age of 5 years, and more than one-third of these patients do not survive.

The first consideration in evaluating symptomatic CM II is the degree of hydrocephalus and the shunt, if present. Untreated hydrocephalus or a malfunctioning shunt may increase the intracranial pressure with subsequent downward herniation of an already caudally displaced brainstem and vermis. It is imperative to ensure that the shunt catheter is working optimally and any untreated hydrocephalus is appropriately managed.

Affected pediatric patients younger than the age of 2 years present most frequently with cranial nerve and brainstem signs and must be evaluated urgently, because a symptomatic CM II in these patients can be a neurosurgical emergency. Respiratory difficulties with or without inspiratory stridor are signs of brainstem dysfunction and should prompt

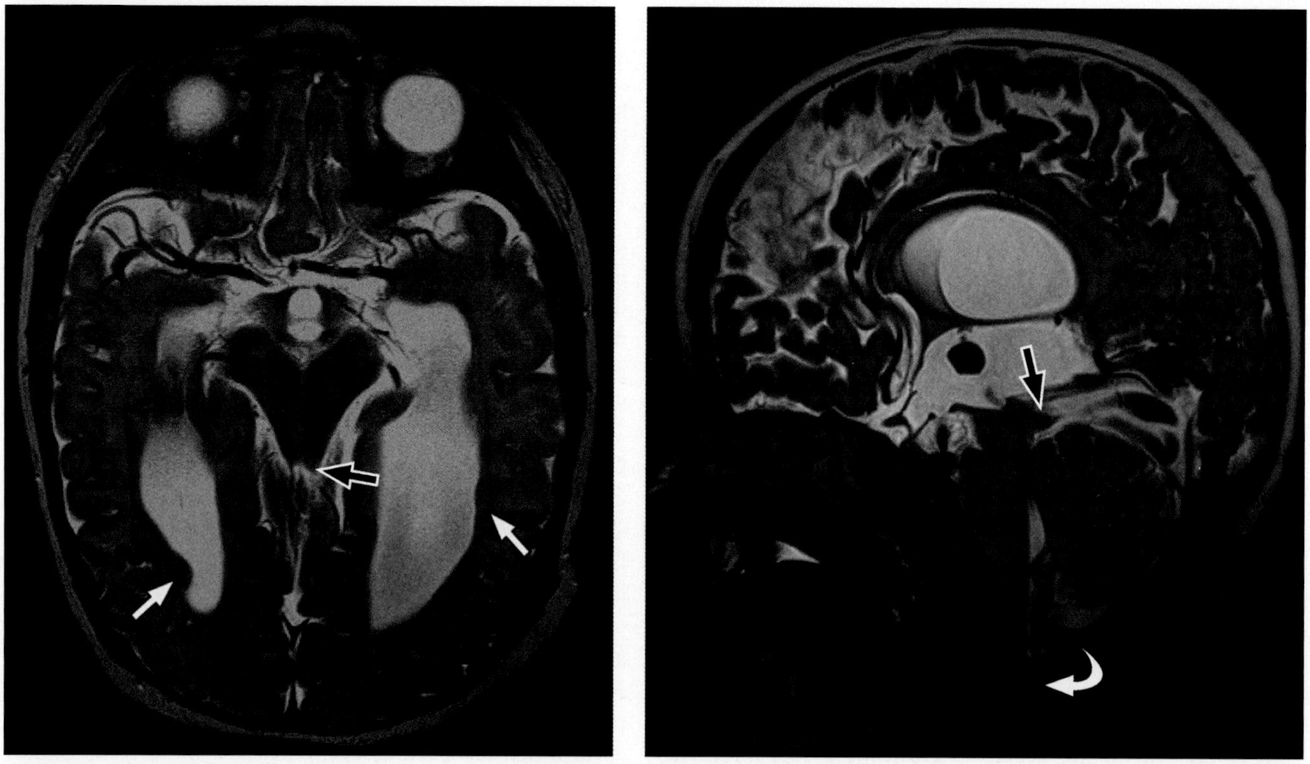

FIGURE 2.22 **Chiari II malformation.** Axial (on the **left**) and sagittal (on the **right**) T2-weighted MR images show a small posterior fossa, herniation of the cerebellar tonsils (*curved arrow*) to the C4 level with mild kinking of the cervicomedullary junction, tectal beaking (*black arrows*), and associated subependymal gray matter heterotopia (*white arrows*).

urgent evaluation. Vocal cord abduction, paresis, or paralysis resulting from dysfunction of the vagus nerve causes the inspiratory stridor. Cranial nerve dysfunction is attributed to various causes including caudal traction on the nerve by the herniated medulla/medullary kink, lower brainstem compression, or an abnormally formed dorsal motor nucleus within the brainstem.

Chiari III Malformation

Chiari III malformation is characterized by features similar to Chiari II, but with an occipital and/or high cervical encephalocele (Fig. 2.23).

Chiari IV Malformation

Chiari IV malformation refers to a constellation of findings including marked cerebellar hypoplasia without displacement of the cerebellum through the foramen magnum. It is considered as a possible variation of cerebellar hypoplasia.

Mesenchymal Origin Anomalies

Cephaloceles (Encephalocele, Meningocele, and Related Malformations)

A cephalocele is defined as an outward protrusion of the intracranial contents through an osseous defect in the cranial vault or skull base (Fig. 2.24). Cephaloceles can be either congenital or acquired lesions and can be open or skin covered. The most common cephaloceles are named according to their location: occipital, parietal, or frontoethmoidal/frontonasal (at the skull base).

Cephaloceles can be subdivided based upon the contents of the lesion into *meningoencephaloceles* (containing brain tissue, meninges, and CSF), *meningoceles* (meninges and CSF, but without brain tissue), *glioceles* (glia-lined outpouching

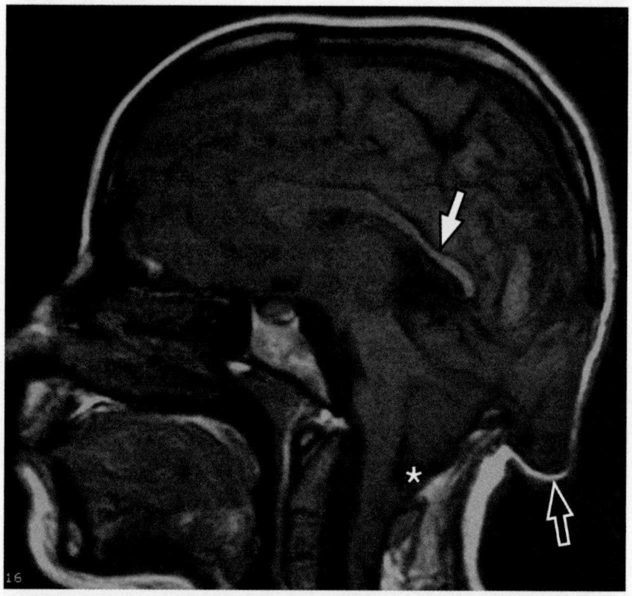

FIGURE 2.23 **Chiari III malformation.** Sagittal T1-weighted MR image demonstrates an occipital encephalocele (*black arrow*), which spontaneously decompressed partially after spinal fusion, low lying cerebellar tonsils (*asterisk*), and thinned posterior half of corpus callosum (*white arrow*).

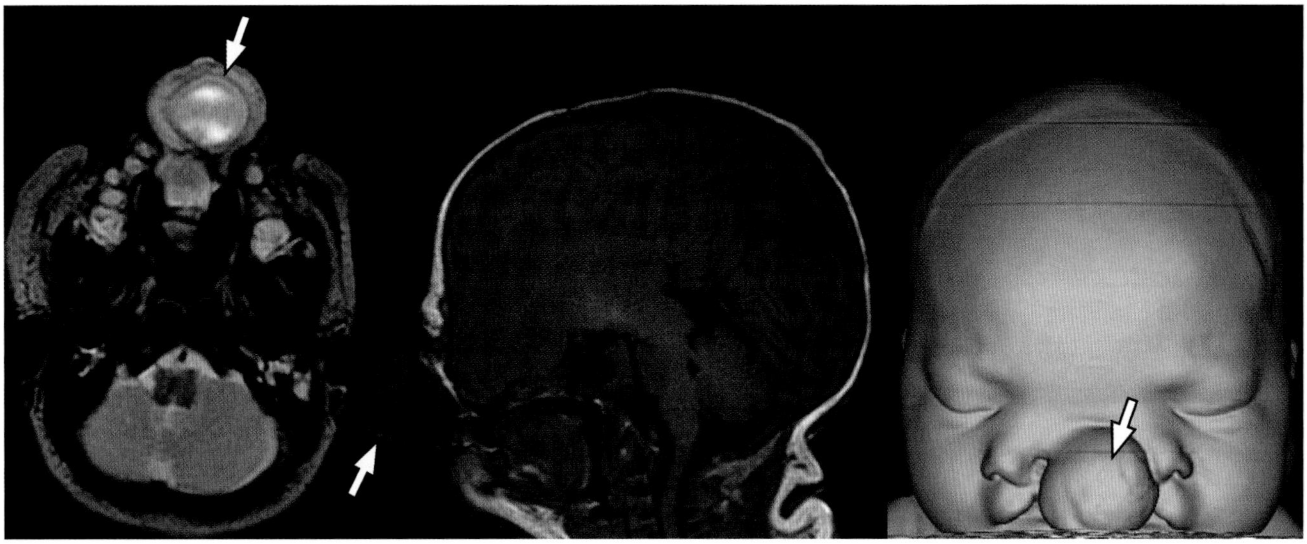

FIGURE 2.24 **Frontoethmoidal encephalocele.** Axial T2-weighted MR (on the **left**), sagittal T1-weighted MR (in the **center**), and 3D reconstructed CT (on the **right**) images show a large frontoethmoidal cephalocele (*arrows*) containing dysplastic brain tissue, associated agenesis of corpus callosum, marked hypertelorism, abnormal nose, and cleft palate and lip.

containing only CSF), and *atretic cephaloceles* (containing dura, fibrous tissue, and degenerated brain tissue).

The role of imaging is to define the osseous defect, delineate the contents, map out the vascular structures within the cephalocele, and assess any coexisting intracranial anomalies. The brain parenchyma within a congenital cephalocele is often abnormal. It is important to recognize that affected pediatric patients may also have extracranial abnormalities such as cleft lip and palate, cardiac abnormalities, and chromosomal anomalies (e.g., trisomies 13 and 18).

Intracranial Lipomas

Intracranial lipomas are rare congenital malformations of the brain parenchyma that are thought to arise from abnormal persistence and maldifferentiation of the meninx primitiva during the development of the subarachnoid cisterns. They are usually found incidentally. They are located most commonly in the pericallosal cistern and are associated with other parenchymal or brain vascular malformations in up to half of cases. Callosal dysgenesis is commonly associated with pericallosal lipomas.

They are usually asymptomatic, but have been associated with seizures (20% to 30%), headaches (25%), and raised intracranial pressure.[24,25] The reported increased incidence of epilepsy in patients with intracranial lipomas may be related to higher incidence of associated intracranial abnormalities and malformations compared with the general population.

Intracranial lipomas have a characteristic appearance on unenhanced CT, with low attenuation values (between −39 Hounsfield Units [HU] and −80 HU) (Fig. 2.25). Calcifications are seen commonly in midline interhemispheric lipomas. On MRI, intracranial lipomas are characterized by T1 hyperintensity and intermediate signal on T2-weighted spin-echo sequences, which nulls on fat-saturated MR images.

Histologically, intracranial lipomas consist of mature adipose tissue. Management is usually conservative and surgical treatment is very rarely needed.

Intracranial Cysts

Primary intracranial cysts are usually benign disorders of development. They may also develop secondarily as a complication of surgery, trauma, or infection. They are often seen as incidental findings on neuroimaging studies, but may occasionally cause focal neurologic deficits. Hemorrhage into the cystic lesions may result in a sudden increase in size and cause obstructive hydrocephalus.

The three most common intracranial cysts are arachnoid cysts, neuroepithelial cysts, and leptomeningeal cysts.

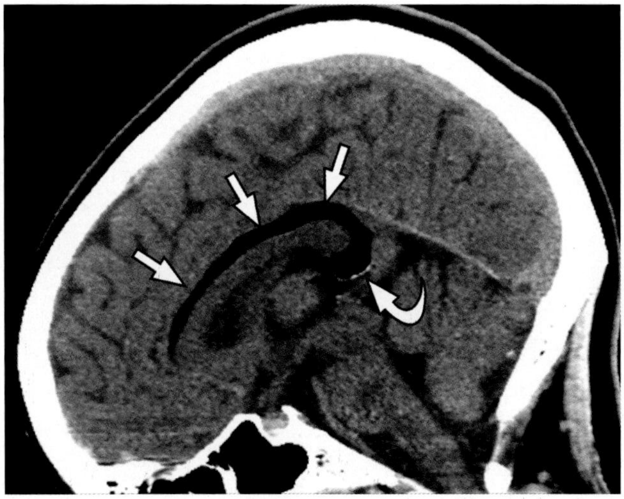

FIGURE 2.25 **Corpus callosum lipoma.** Sagittal reformatted CT image shows a low attenuation (−50 HU) lesion (*straight arrows*) in the midline in the pericallosal cistern with a small amount of calcification (*curved arrow*) along its posterior aspect near the splenium, consistent with a callosal lipoma.

Arachnoid cysts and neuroepithelial cysts are discussed in the following section. The information regarding leptomeningeal cysts is included in Chapter 1 of this book.

Arachnoid Cysts

Arachnoid cysts are benign, fluid-filled lesions located between the dura and the pia mater and lined by a thin layer of the arachnoid membrane. The fluid within arachnoid cysts resembles CSF. These lesions are therefore similar to CSF on all imaging modalities. US demonstrates an anechoic or hypoechoic lesion with well-defined margins and smooth borders. On CT, these lesions are isodense to CSF and may be associated with remodeling and resultant scalloping of the inner surface of adjacent calvarium. MRI is the ideal imaging modality to define the lesion and identify any septations within the lesion. FLAIR MR images may demonstrate a rim of high signal around the lesion, which represents gliosis in the white matter. Suprasellar arachnoid cysts can be challenging to diagnose, especially on CT. Thin-section T2-weighted MR images can be very helpful in defining the thin walls of arachnoid cysts (Fig. 2.26).

The main differential diagnosis is an epidermoid cyst, which characteristically shows decreased diffusion, whereas an arachnoid cyst does not. It is also important to differentiate arachnoid cysts from cephaloceles and a careful evaluation of the surrounding dural and bony outlines should be made, particularly in cases of lesions close to the skull base.

Neuroepithelial Cysts

Neuroepithelial cysts are benign, fluid-filled cysts lined by a single layer of cells resembling ependymal cells that occur in various sites within the brain. They are named based on their location as choroid plexus cysts, intraventricular ependymal cysts, and choroid fissure cysts. They are usually seen as incidental findings on imaging studies and do not cause clinical symptoms. Diagnosis is based on characteristic location and signal intensity that resembles CSF (Fig. 2.27).

Infectious Disorders

Congenital Infections (TORCH)

TORCH (toxoplasmosis, other, rubella, cytomegalovirus (CMV), and herpes) infections result from the transfer of infection to the fetus via the placenta or the birth canal. Congenital malformations result from insults in the first two trimesters, and destructive lesions occur when the infection is transmitted in the third trimester.

Toxoplasmosis

Congenital toxoplasmosis is rare compared to CMV. Hydrocephalus, chorioretinitis, and intracranial calcifications are common presenting features. Infection acquired in early gestation (<20 weeks) causes severe neurologic impairment. Findings seen on imaging studies include intracerebral and periventricular calcifications, with hydrocephalus in some cases (Fig. 2.28).

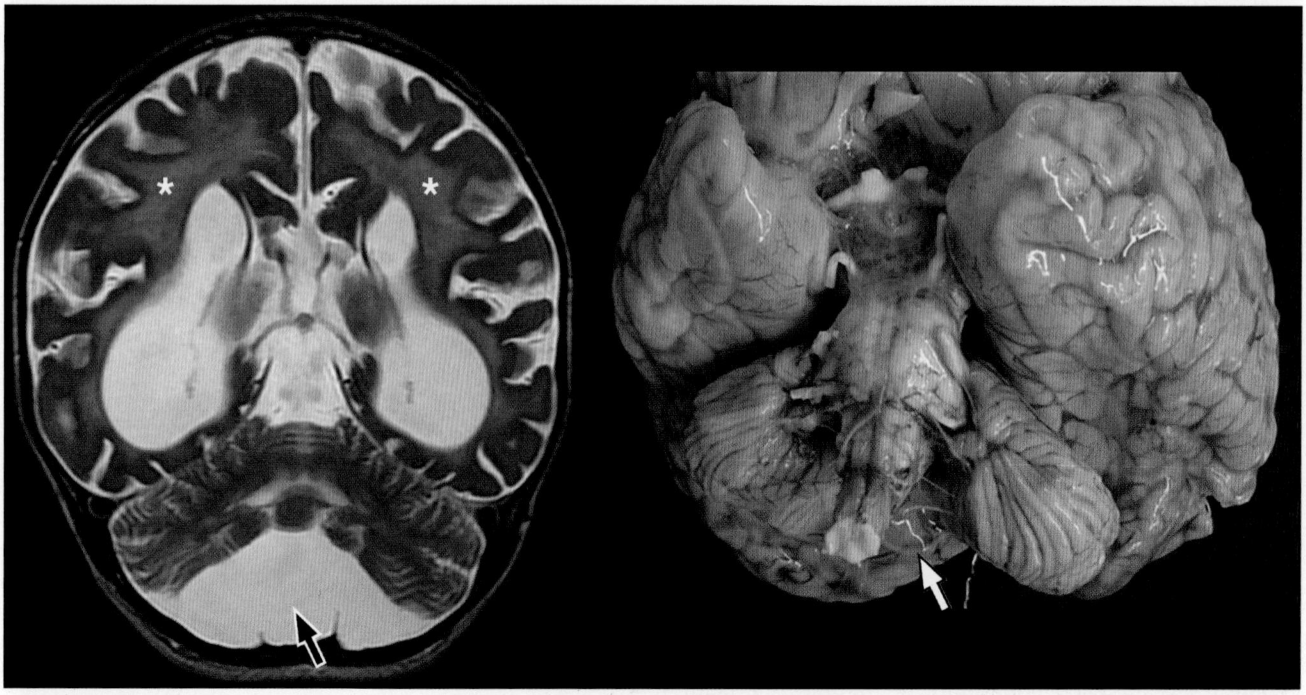

FIGURE 2.26 **Arachnoid cyst in a 3-year-old boy with multiple sulfatase deficiency.** Coronal T2-weighted MR image (on the **left**) and postmortem brain specimen (on the **right**) show a CSF signal intensity thin-walled translucent cyst (*black and white arrows*) overlying the left inferior surface of the cerebellum, with associated cerebellar asymmetry. Note the abnormal diffuse white matter signal intensity (*asterisks*) and volume loss in the supratentorial brain on MR image, which is a manifestation of the underlying metabolic disease.

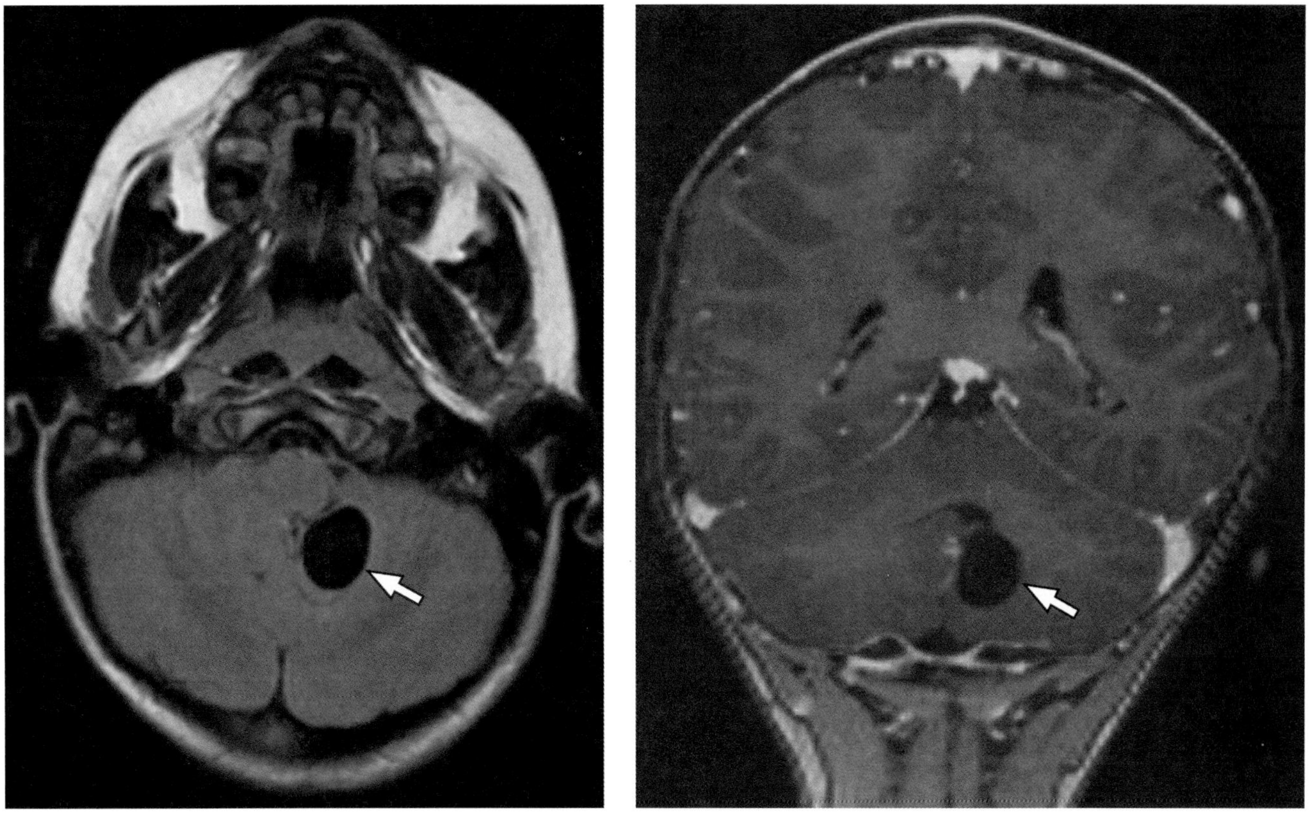

FIGURE 2.27 **Neuroepithelial cyst incidentally found in a 10-year-old boy.** Axial FLAIR MR image (on the **left**) and coronal postcontrast T1-weighted SPACE (Sampling Perfection with Application optimized Contrasts using different flip angle Evolution) MR image (on the **right**) show a cystic CSF signal intensity lesion (*arrows*) in the cerebellum closely related to the margins of the fourth ventricle.

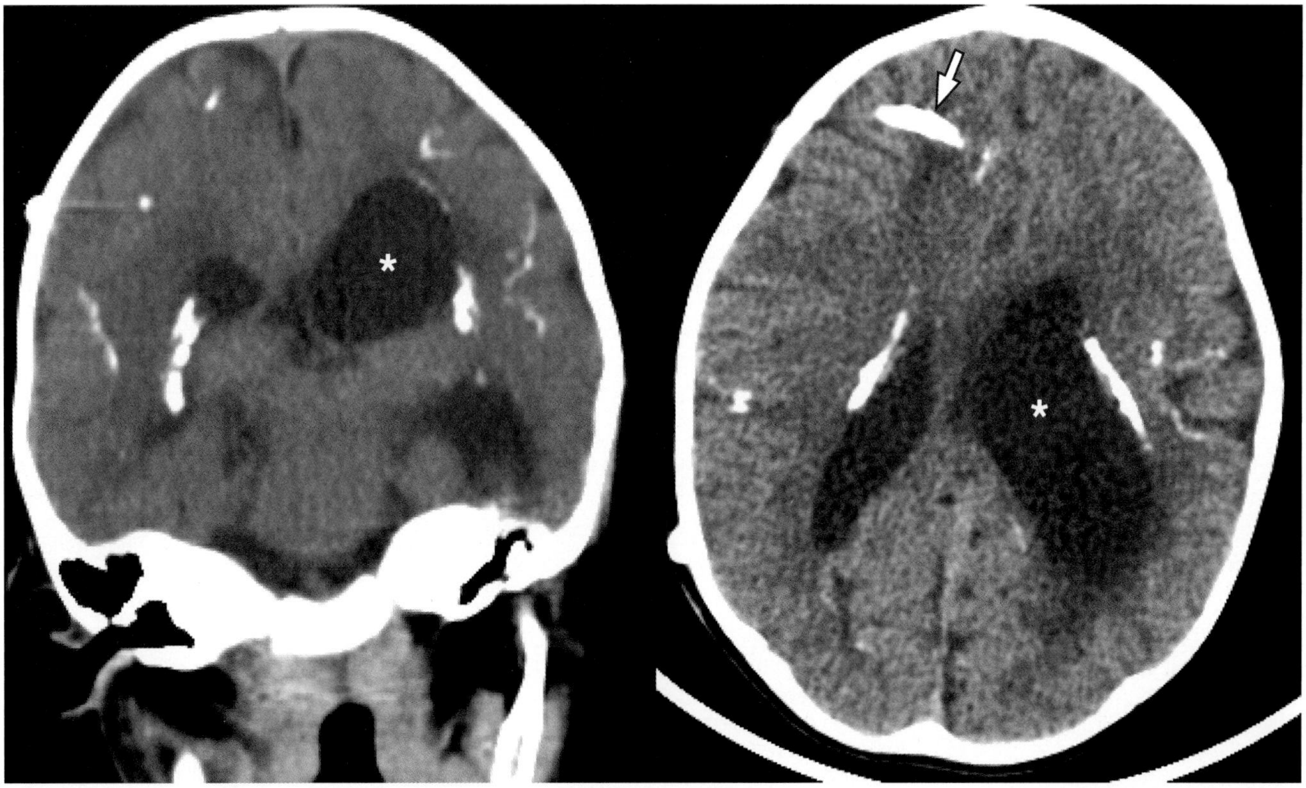

FIGURE 2.28 **Congenital toxoplasmosis in an 11-month-old boy.** Coronal reformatted unenhanced CT image (on the **left**) shows multiple foci of intraparenchymal and subependymal calcification. The child also had hydrocephalus (*asterisk*), which had been shunted by this time. Axial unenhanced CT image (on the **right**) shows a right frontal shunt catheter (*arrow*) and hydrocephalus (*asterisk*).

Other Infections

This category includes a number of organisms that cause congenital infections including Coxsackie virus, varicella (chickenpox), parvovirus B19, chlamydia, HIV, Zika virus, human T-lymphotropic virus, and syphilis. They are relatively less common in the United States and their manifestations are summarized in Table 2.3.

Congenital Rubella

Congenital rubella is rare in the United States. However, during the critical first 12 weeks of pregnancy, the fetal infection rate can be as high as 80%. Features of congenital rubella include congenital heart disease in more than half, deafness in approximately half because of damage to the organ of Corti, and ocular abnormalities such as cataracts in ~40%.[26,27] Further, ~40% of survivors have developmental delay.[28] Some cases of autism have been linked to rubella infection. Neurologic symptoms are related to viral invasion and replication in brain tissue. Rubella appears to have an antimitotic effect on brain cell multiplication with microcephaly being a common outcome of fetal infection. The main brain tissue cell types infected with in utero rubella virus are the astrocyte and, occasionally, the neuron.

Rubella virus preferentially involves the placental and fetal vascular endothelia. Abnormalities of the cerebral vascular system are present on pathologic specimens in more than half of cases. Focal destruction of the vascular walls, with thickening and proliferation, results in luminal narrowing. Imaging findings in survivors include mineralizing microangiopathy with arterial occlusion and stroke. Follow-up studies demonstrate hydranencephaly, microcephaly, cerebellar atrophy, and cerebral parenchymal calcification. Brain ultrasound in neonates with congenital rubella shows a "branched candlestick" appearance of the vessels.

Cytomegalovirus

Of the TORCH infections, CMV is the most common serious viral infection to affect newborns, occurring in nearly 1% of all live births in the United States.[29] The usual route of fetal infection is transplacental, occurring during a primary infection of the mother. Fetal infection results in up to 40% of cases of maternal primary infection.[30] Gestational age at time of infection has little correlation with rate of transmission or severity of disease expression. Of note, maternal antibodies, which protect the fetus in rubella and toxoplasmosis, do not

TABLE 2.3 Other Congenital TORCH Infections

Infection	Clinical Manifestations	CNS Imaging Features
Congenital varicella zoster	Lightning-flash skin lesions in a dermatomal distribution, limb hypoplasia, and weakness following intrauterine damage to the cervical or lumbosacral plexus, segmental spinal cord necrosis, intrauterine growth restriction, cataracts, chorioretinitis, and microphthalmia	Hydrocephalus, porencephaly, hydranencephaly, calcifications, and malformations such as polymicrogyria or focal lissencephaly caused by intracranial vascular injury. Severe microcephaly and cerebellar hypoplasia have also been reported.
Congenital human immunodeficiency virus (HIV)	HIV-related CNS encephalopathy manifests as delay in acquisition of psychomotor milestones. Loss of milestones, acquired microcephaly, and bilateral corticospinal tract involvement follow. CNS symptoms are minor in the first decade. Stable encephalopathy or a subacute slowly progressive course is seen	Progressive mineralizing vasculopathy of the basal ganglia is the most common abnormal finding imaging. Vascular striations seen on US and diffuse hazy hyperdensity of the basal ganglia seen on CT. Strokes occur in 1%–2%, less commonly in the older child than the infected adult and rarely in the infant. Aneurysms of the branches of the circle of Willis have been reported as early as 6 mo of age. MRI is initially normal, and there are no associated brain malformations. Delayed myelination, atrophy, white matter disease particularly involving the subcortical white matter, and progressive multifocal leukoencephalopathy are late findings in the child, along with symptomatic brain involvement by opportunistic infections such as toxoplasmosis and CMV.
Congenital syphilis	Most affected infants are asymptomatic at birth. Latent connatal syphilis (lues tarda) is characterized by hearing loss, saddle nose, and abnormal incisor teeth	Infarcts in meningovascular syphilis, with vascular narrowing on MRA or CTA. Focal or diffuse enhancement as seen in other meningitides. Hydrocephalus on CT and MRI in patients with syphilitic meningitis. Cerebral atrophy and hyperintensities on T2-weighted MR images in late stages.

prevent fetal transmission of the CMV virus, but do play a role in reducing severity of disease. Most infants have silent infections following recurrent rather than primary maternal infection. CMV is considered the leading infectious cause of sensorineural hearing loss in the post-rubella vaccination era. Sensorineural hearing loss occurs in around 10% of infected neonates.[30] Additional clinical manifestations in affected infants include microcephaly, chorioretinitis, and seizures.

Prenatal imaging evaluations may show evidence of atrophy including ex vacuo ventricular dilatation and prominent CSF spaces. Periventricular calcification and subependymal cysts are seen on pre- and postnatal imaging studies. "Ring-like" areas of periventricular lucency have been shown to precede the development of subependymal calcification and are felt to represent foci of subependymal degeneration and inflammation. Subsequent glial scarring and dystrophic calcification occur. Increased echogenicity of the thalamostriate arteries has been described on cranial sonography in the presence of congenital CMV, but this feature is not specific. Periventricular and basal ganglia calcifications are the most common finding on US (Fig. 2.29) or CT performed in the neonatal period and correlate with a poor neurodevelopmental outcome.

On MRI, periventricular foci of signal abnormality can be difficult to differentiate from hemorrhage. Other features of congenital CMV infection on MRI include lissencephaly with a thinned cerebral cortex, enlarged lateral ventricles, white matter volume loss, delayed myelination, and a small cerebellum. These features are thought to result from an insult to the germinal matrix and reflect infection between 16 and 18 weeks of gestation.[29] Localized polymicrogyria with thickened irregular cortices (usually in a perisylvian distribution) and diminished white matter indicates infection late during the phases of neuronal migration or organization between 18 and 24 weeks of gestation (Fig. 2.30). Normal gyral pattern with abnormal white matter hyperintensity indicates infection in the third trimester. However, it should be noted that it is not always possible to predict the pattern of brain abnormality based on the timing of the maternal infection.

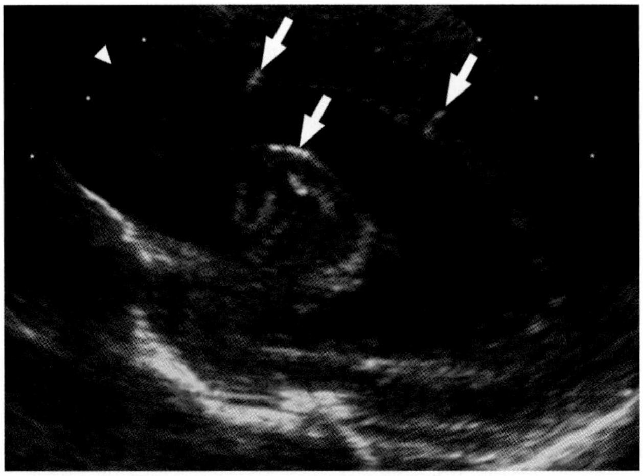

FIGURE 2.29 **Congenital cytomegalovirus infection in a 2-day-old boy.** Parasagittal ultrasound image shows areas of increased echogenicity consistent with periventricular calcifications (*arrows*).

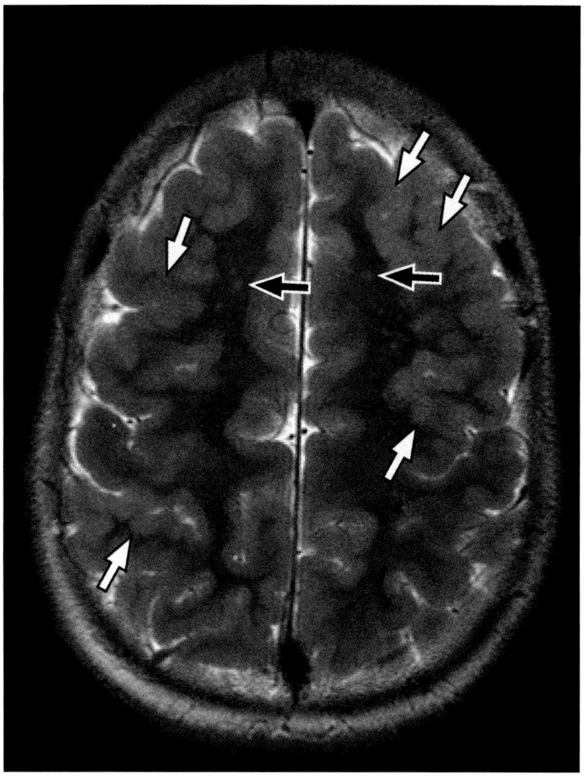

FIGURE 2.30 **Congenital cytomegalovirus (CMV) infection.** Axial T2-weighted MR image shows extensive frontal polymicrogyria (*white arrows*) and subcortical heterotopia (*black arrows*) as a manifestation of congenital CMV.

Herpes Simplex Virus

Neonatal herpes simplex virus 2 (HSV2) occurs usually from transvaginal transmission during passage through the birth canal. Presenting features of HSV2 meningoencephalitis in infants in the first month of life include seizures, lethargy, and fever. It should be noted that HSV1 encephalitis, which affects older children and adults, is different from neonatal herpes infection.

CT in early disease is either normal or demonstrates subtle areas of low attenuation. MRI shows decreased diffusion resulting from infarction in multiple areas and evidence of necrosis, atrophy, encephalomalacia, demyelination, and gliosis (Fig. 2.31). Decreased diffusion may be seen within the brain, predominantly involving the temporal lobes, brainstem, or cerebellum. Later, patchy T2 prolongation may be seen in the white matter, which becomes more pronounced, as the disease progresses. Enhancement of the leptomeninges can demonstrate the disease extent. Increased areas of density in the cerebral cortex are seen on CT, with corresponding T1 and T2 shortening on MRI. Sequela of HSV2 infection includes mental retardation, severe neurologic deficits, or even death secondary to virulent destruction of the brain. Follow-up imaging studies show evidence of encephalomalacia and atrophy of the cerebral parenchyma and cerebellum.

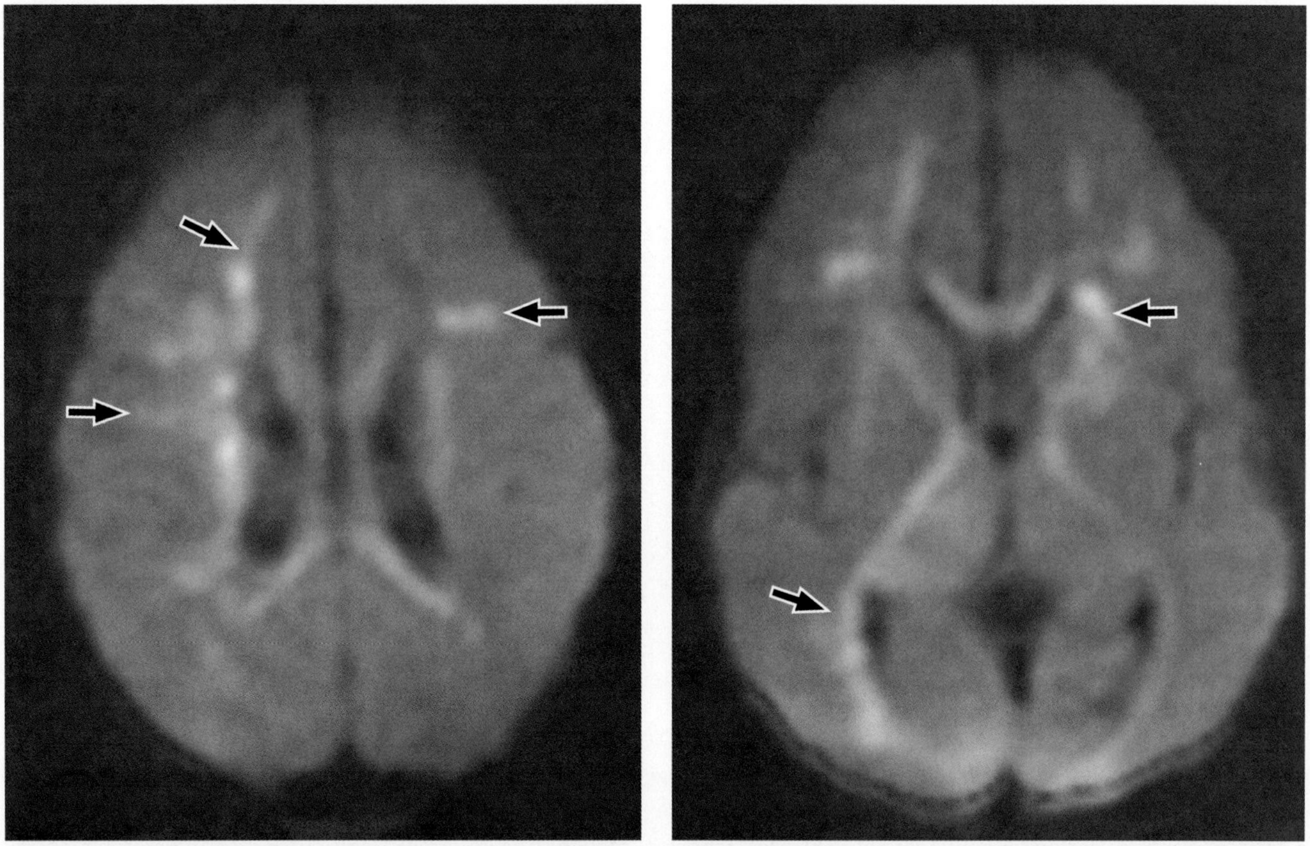

FIGURE 2.31 **Neonatal herpes encephalitis in a 12-day-old girl.** Axial diffusion-weighted MR images show increased signal (indicating decreased diffusion [*arrows*]) in the periventricular and deep frontal white matter (on the **left**), corona radiata, basal ganglia, and internal capsule (on the **right**).

Acquired Infections

Viral Meningitis and Meningoencephalitis

In an immunocompetent child, HSV type 1 is the most common cause of viral encephalitis. Other viruses such as Epstein-Barr virus, influenza viruses, West Nile virus, and Eastern equine encephalitis have emerged as causative viruses in the pediatric population in the United States in recent years. The list of causative viruses is longer in the immunocompromised child.

MRI is the imaging modality of choice in pediatric patients with suspected encephalitis. In the older child with herpes encephalitis, signal abnormalities resulting edema, hemorrhage, and necrosis are seen primarily in the inferomedial temporal lobes (Fig. 2.32). When findings are bilateral, they are usually asymmetric. Signal changes may also be seen in the limbic system, insular cortex, cingulate gyrus, basal ganglia, and parietooccipital cortex. Small petechial foci of hemorrhage are typically seen in HSE in older children. Diffusion-weighted MR images show evidence of cytotoxic edema that resolves over the next 10 to 14 days.[31] Follow-up studies may demonstrate atrophy or ventricular enlargement.[29]

Bacterial Infections

Bacterial Meningitis and Meningoencephalitis

Meningitis refers to inflammation of the subarachnoid space and leptomeninges surrounding the brain and spinal cord (arachnoid mater and pia mater). Most cases of meningitis have an infective etiology. The causative organisms are specific to particular age groups, seasonality, geography, and underlying host factors. After the introduction of the *Haemophilus influenzae* type b (Hib) and pneumococcal conjugate vaccines to the infant immunization schedule, the incidence of bacterial meningitis declined in all age groups except children younger than 2 months. The peak incidence continues to occur in children younger than 2 months. Group B streptococcus remains the predominant bacterial pathogen in the neonatal population. *Streptococcus pneumoniae* and *Neisseria meningitidis* remain relatively common pathogens in older children and adolescents.

Acute bacterial meningitis has two patterns of presentation. In the first type, meningitis develops progressively over one or several days and may be preceded by a febrile illness. The second type is characterized by an acute and fulminant course, with manifestations of sepsis and meningitis developing rapidly over several hours. The rapidly progressive form is frequently associated with severe brain edema.

The primary role of imaging studies in pediatric patients with bacterial meningitis is identifying and monitoring complications including cerebritis, abscess formation, infarcts, subdural empyema, and epidural abscess. The role of a CT at presentation in pediatric patients with suspected bacterial meningitis needs some clarification. Although there may be a role for CT to exclude contraindications for lumbar

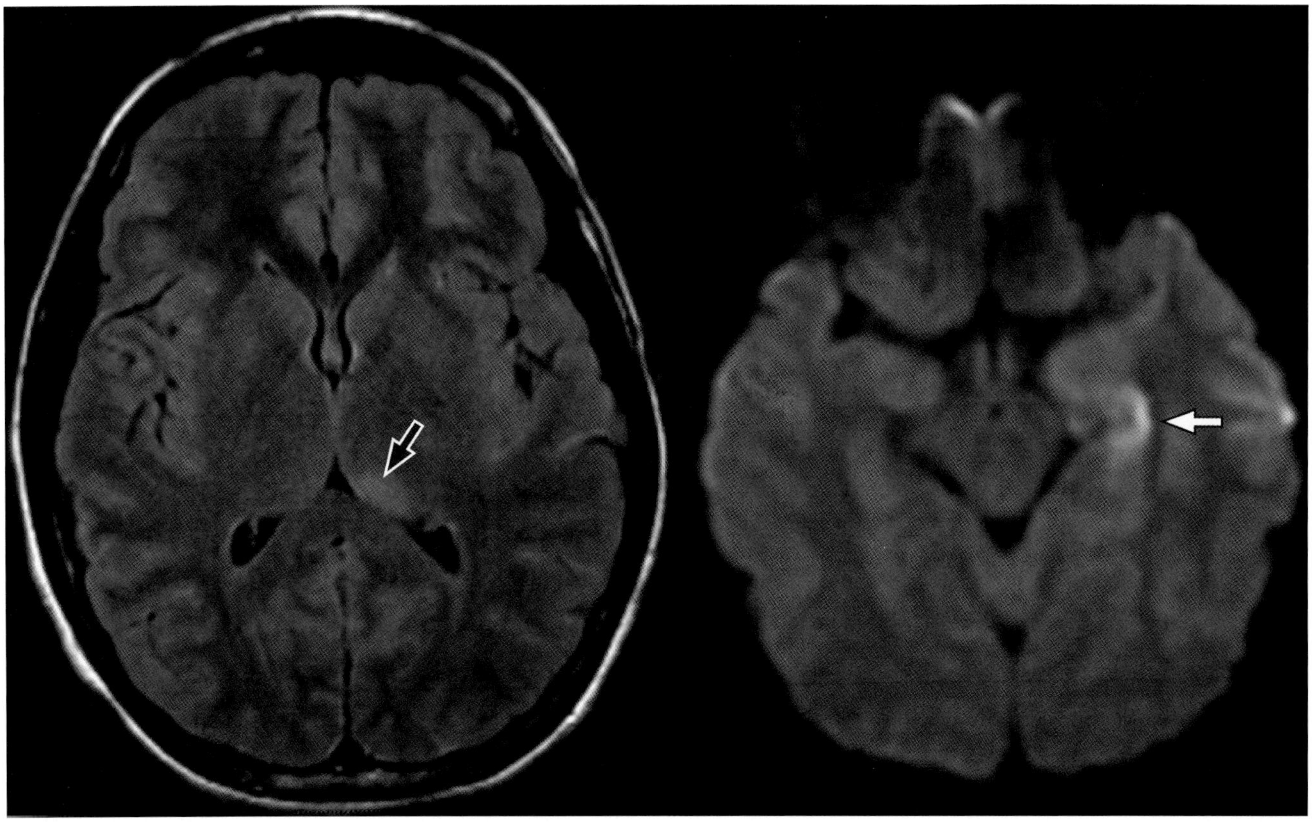

FIGURE 2.32 **Herpes simplex virus encephalitis in a 9-year-old girl.** Axial FLAIR MR image (on the **left**) and axial diffusion-weighted MR image (on the **right**) demonstrate signal abnormality in the left thalamus (*black arrow*) and diffusion restriction in the left hippocampus (*white arrow*). The distribution of findings is most suggestive of herpes encephalitis, which was proven by polymerase chain reaction analysis of CSF.

puncture, it is important to recognize that normal CT findings may not be sufficient to indicate normal intracranial pressure in pediatric patients with bacterial meningitis. Review of the literature indicates that herniation is unlikely in children with bacterial meningitis unless they have focal neurologic findings or coma.[32] In addition, the results of an imaging study do not exclude or prove the presence of acute meningitis. Diagnosis should therefore be made based on clinical history, examination findings, and results of laboratory tests.

CT findings are often normal in the early phase of meningitis. Leptomeningeal enhancement may be seen on contrast administration, a finding that is more pronounced in the later stages of the disease. Imaging studies can help in identifying causes of meningitis. For instance, CT can help identify skull fractures and infections within the paranasal sinuses, mastoid air cells, and the petrous temporal bone, which can spread by direct extension into the brain. Dermal sinus tracts may be the primary source of infection affecting the meninges, leading to intracranial complications (Fig. 2.33).

The diagnostic value of MRI in uncomplicated bacterial meningitis is also low. Findings include leptomeningeal FLAIR hyperintensity and enhancement as well as subarachnoid space distention with widening of the interhemispheric fissure in early meningitis. However, the absence of leptomeningeal enhancement on MRI does not exclude the diagnosis of meningitis. Diffusion-weighted MR images should be utilized, as presence of decreased diffusion can help characterize the fluid within extra-axial collections, differentiate between vasogenic and cytotoxic edema, and reveal early cerebritis and small abscess cavities. The presence of T1 and FLAIR hyperintensity within the sulci suggests protein or pus accumulation.[33]

Tuberculous Infection

Although relatively uncommon in the United States, tuberculous meningitis remains an important cause of morbidity and mortality in children around the world. The pandemic of acquired immunodeficiency syndrome has resulted in an increased incidence of central nervous system tuberculosis worldwide. Infection may occur by either hematogenous seeding of the meninges or release of the organism into the meningeal space. This results in a severe granulomatous inflammatory reaction within the basal cisterns, which can lead to death (if untreated) in a few weeks.

Tuberculomas are space-occupying masses of granulomatous tissue, which form a large percentage of intracranial mass lesions in developing countries. They are single or multiple and can be formed within the meninges, at the gray–white junction, and in the spinal cord, or rarely, in the choroid plexus. Children develop infratentorial tuberculo-

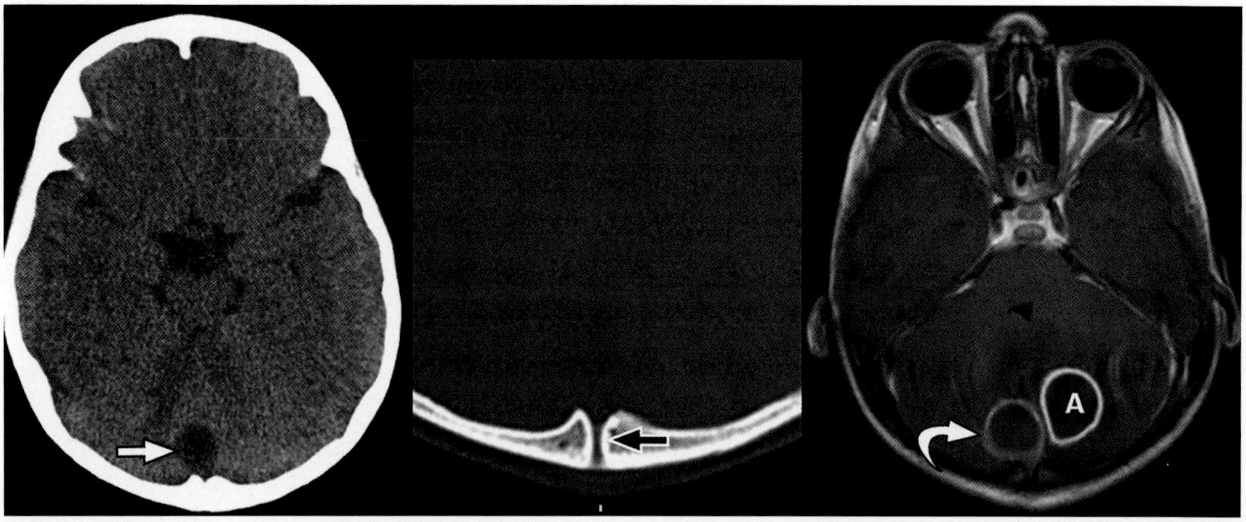

FIGURE 2.33 **Recurrent meningitis in a 3-year-old girl.** Axial CT image (on the **left**) shows posterior fossa dermoid (*white arrow*). A tract (*black arrow*) passing through occipital bone on to the overlying scalp is also seen (in the **middle**). This was not noticed at the time of the CT study, and at a subsequent presentation, axial postcontrast T1-weighted MR image (on the **right**) shows infected material within the dermoid (*curved arrow*) and an adjacent abscess (*A*) in the cerebellar hemispheres.

mas more commonly than adults. Organisms from these foci are released into the subarachnoid space causing meningitis. Meningitis is typically most severe in the basal cisterns and leads to secondary complications, including multiple cranial nerve palsies, vasculitis of the lenticulostriate and thalamoperforating vessels resulting in secondary infarction of the basal ganglia, and hydrocephalus secondary to blockage of the fourth ventricular outlet foramina. It is important to note that hydrocephalus in patients with tuberculous meningitis may need to be treated surgically. This can be determined with an emergent CT at presentation, followed by MRI later.[34] Imaging using diffusion-weighted MRI is important to document the presence of infarcts, which correlates with poor outcome. In particular, bilateral basal ganglia infarcts have a poor prognosis. Border zone necrosis seen in these patients needs to be differentiated from necrosis in older children with herpes, which is most often seen at the insular cortex.[35]

On CT, the presence of hyperdensity within the basal cisterns indicates an exudate resulting from TB meningitis. This is considered a very specific sign for TB meningitis in children.[36] During the initial stages of the disease, noncontrast MRI sequences usually show little or no evidence of meningeal abnormality. As the disease progresses, mild shortening of T1 and T2 relaxation times compared to normal CSF is seen within the affected subarachnoid spaces.[36] Postcontrast T1-weighted MR images show abnormal meningeal enhancement, most marked in the basal cisterns (Fig. 2.34). The interpeduncular fossa, pontine cistern,

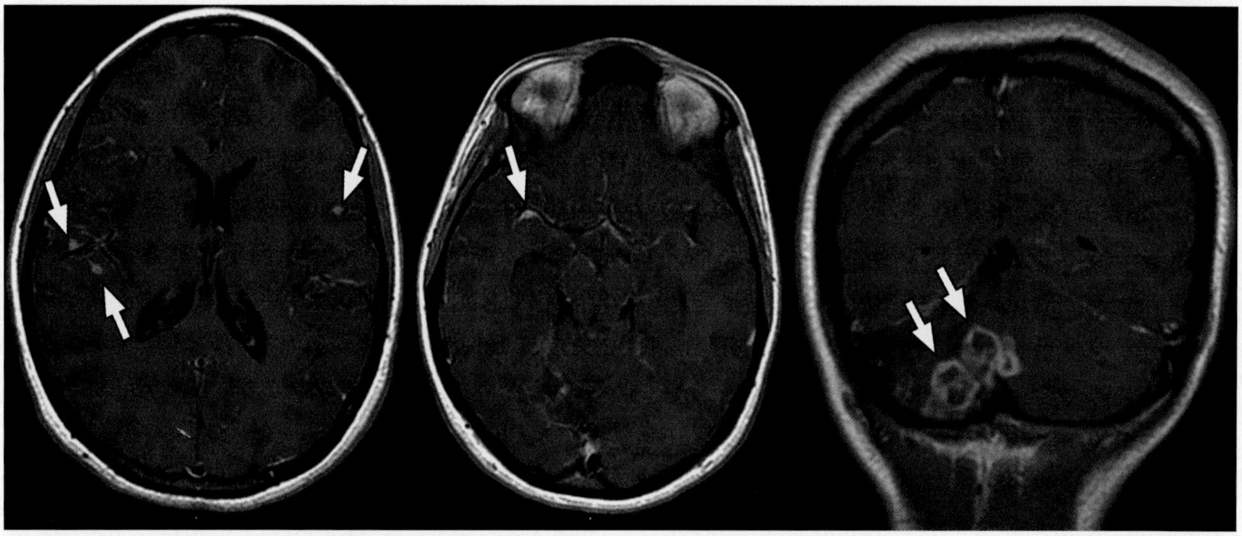

FIGURE 2.34 **Tuberculous meningitis and meningoencephalitis in a 17-year-old girl.** Axial and coronal postcontrast T1-weighted MR images show abnormal linear and nodular meningeal enhancement (*arrows*) in the bilateral temporal lobes and basal cisterns (on the **left** and in the **middle**), and multiple foci of ring enhancement (*arrows*) in the right cerebellar hemisphere with surrounding encephalomalacia (on the **right**).

perimesencephalic cisterns, suprasellar cisterns, and sulci over the convexities are commonly affected.

Intracranial tuberculomas appear as low- or high-density round or lobulated masses with irregular walls showing homogeneous enhancement after contrast administration on CT. They can be either solitary or multiple and are common in the frontal and parietal lobes. The imaging characteristics depend on whether the lesion is noncaseating, caseating with a solid center, or caseating with a liquid center. Edema around the lesion is inversely proportional to duration of the lesion. The presence of the "target sign," a central nidus of calcification with a surrounding ring of enhancement, which was previously thought to be diagnostic of tuberculomas, has been subsequently shown to be nonspecific.[37]

On MRI, intracranial tuberculomas are characterized by hypo- or isointensity or central hyperintensity with a hypointense rim on T2-weighted MR images and isointensity and/or hypointensity on T1-weighted MR images. The appearance of a tuberculoma varies on MRI based on its stage of maturation.[38] A noncaseating tuberculoma usually appears hyperintense on T2-weighted and slightly hypointense on T1-weighted MR images, with homogeneous enhancement after injection of paramagnetic contrast on T1-weighted MR images. Solid caseating tuberculomas appear relatively iso- to hypointense on both T1-weighted and T2-weighted MR images, with an iso- to hyperintense rim on T2-weighted MR images. In the presence of edema, the rim may be difficult to delineate on T2-weighted MR images. Tuberculomas may show rim enhancement on postcontrast T1-weighted MR images.

Differential diagnosis of tuberculomas includes lesions in the healing stage of neurocysticercosis, fungal granulomas, chronic pyogenic brain abscesses, metastases, and lymphoma. Sometimes, large tuberculomas mimic neoplastic lesions on MRI, as they appear predominantly hyperintense on T2-weighted MR images, with mixed intensity on T1-weighted MR images and, possibly, heterogeneous enhancement on postcontrast MR images. Quantitative magnetization transfer imaging and in vivo proton MRS have been shown to be helpful in differentiating tuberculomas from entities like cysticercosis.[39]

Complications of Bacterial Infections

Cerebral Abscess

Cerebral abscess is defined as a focal suppurative process within the brain parenchyma. Pediatric patients with a brain abscess often present with new-onset acute headaches or first-time seizure, with fever and focal neurologic signs on examination. The young infant or neonate with brain abscess usually presents with irritability, a bulging fontanelle, and a rapid increase in head circumference. US in this age group may be used if the child is too unwell to undergo cross-sectional imaging evaluation. Cerebral abscesses are seen as heterogeneous intraparenchymal lesions with surrounding increased echogenicity and sulcal effacement (Fig. 2.35).

Ring-enhancing lesions can be seen on contrast-enhanced CT. However, MRI is the optimal imaging modality in this situation. Abscesses in the brain parenchyma are characterized by central T2 prolongation and T1 hypointensity and

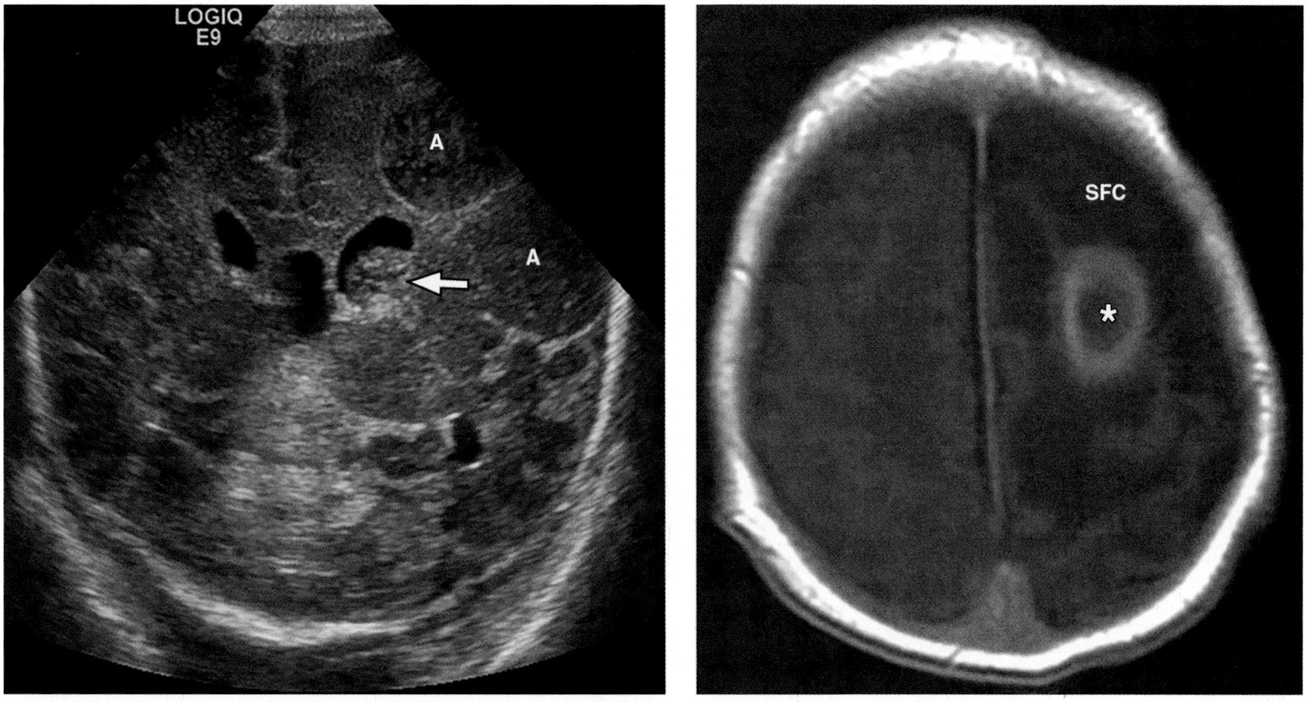

FIGURE 2.35 **Enterobacter cerebral abscess.** Coronal cranial ultrasound image (on the **left**) shows heterogeneous left frontoparietal intraparenchymal lesions (*A*) with surrounding increased echogenicity and sulcal effacement, consistent with cerebral abscess. Also noted is an echogenic lesion (*arrow*) in the left lateral ventricle representing intraventricular pus. Subsequently obtained axial postcontrast MR image (on the **right**) shows a rim-enhancing lesion (*asterisk*) with adjacent subdural fluid collection (*SFC*) overlying the left frontal lobe.

demonstrate enhancement of the walls of the lesion following gadolinium-based contrast administration (Fig. 2.35). Diffusion-weighted MR imaging is helpful to differentiate between an abscess and a necrotic tumor. Therefore, it must be performed in all cases of suspected CNS infection because almost all pyogenic abscesses demonstrate decreased apparent diffusion coefficient (ADC) values, indicating decreased water diffusion compared with nonpyogenic lesions.

Subdural and Epidural Empyema

Subdural empyema is a collection of pus in the subdural space, which is a naturally occurring space between the dura and arachnoid mater. It accounts for ~15% to 25% of pyogenic intracranial infections, and most often results as a complication of head and neck infections like sinusitis, otitis media, or mastoiditis.[40] Abnormal signal in the bone adjacent to empyemas should be recognized on MRI, as this is an early sign of osteomyelitis and needs a longer course of antibiotics.[33]

Epidural empyema is a collection of pus between the dura and the inner table of the skull. Visualization of displaced dura, indicated by a hypointense rim between the collection and brain, suggests that the collection is epidural rather than subdural. Surrounding white matter edema, mass effect, and cortical signal changes can be seen. Empyemas can be identified on CT as fluid collections that are slightly hyperdense compared to CSF; however, it is not always possible to define the exact location and nature of the collection. On MRI, empyemas are slightly hyperintense relative to CSF on T1-weighted MR images and hyperintense relative to CSF and white matter on T2-weighted MR images, with peripheral enhancement after contrast administration (Fig. 2.36). Diffusion-weighted MR imaging can help characterize extra-axial collections as empyemas, typically demonstrating restricted diffusion (Fig. 2.36).

Vascular Complications

Arterial or venous infarcts may be seen on cross-sectional studies in pediatric patients with meningitis, resulting from secondary inflammation of contiguous blood vessels (Fig. 2.37). In pediatric patients with dural venous sinus thrombosis, contrast-enhanced CT venography can show filling defects within the affected sinus and may show hemorrhagic infarcts as areas of low density that do not correspond to an arterial distribution. MR venography used in conjunction with evaluation of flow voids on coronal T2-weighted MR images and postcontrast SPGR or MPRAGE images are used to diagnose dural venous sinus and cortical vein thrombus on MRI. MR angiography can be added to conventional MRI sequences to identify arterial thrombus.

Other Complications

In cases of pneumococcal meningitis, postcontrast imaging of the petrous temporal bones can help detect early labyrinthitis, indicated by enhancement within the labyrinthine structures (Fig. 2.38). In the subacute stage, CT and MRI can

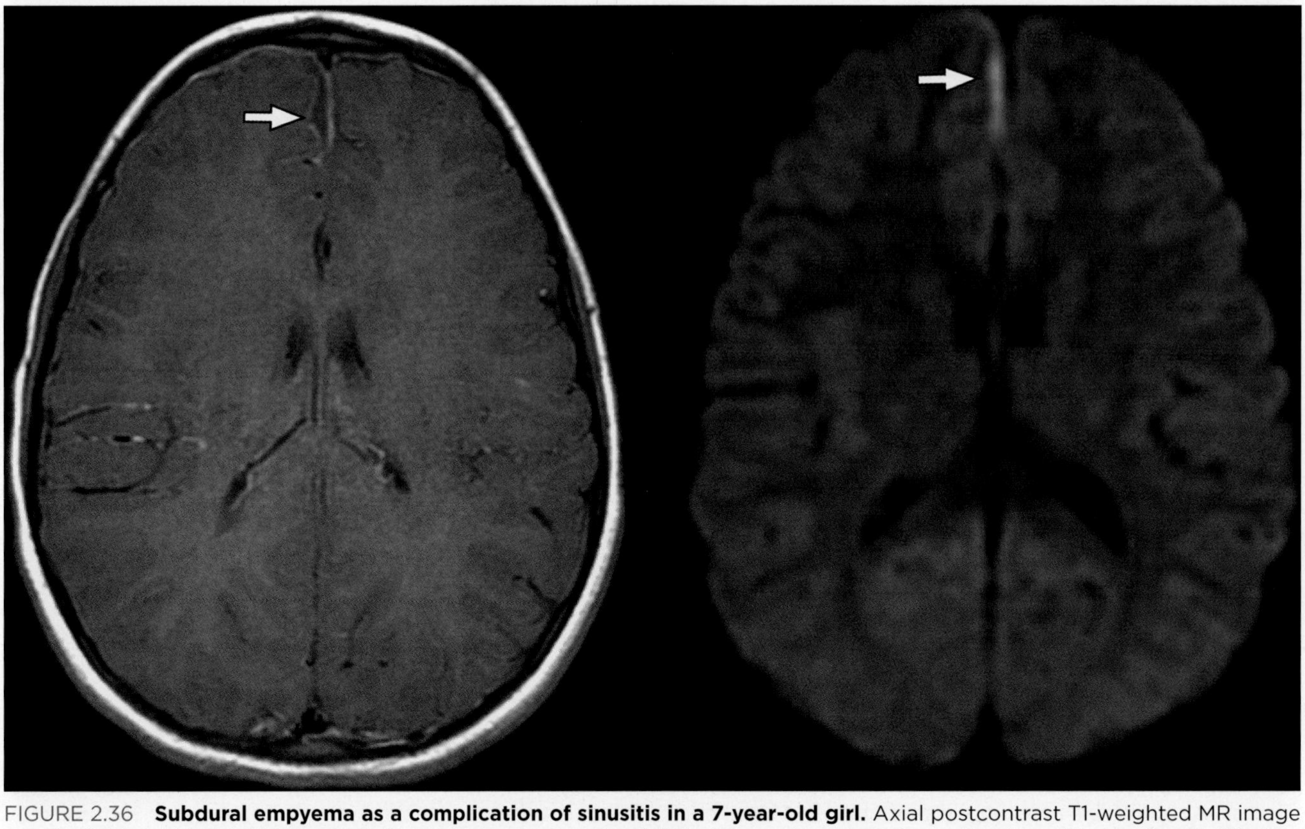

FIGURE 2.36 **Subdural empyema as a complication of sinusitis in a 7-year-old girl.** Axial postcontrast T1-weighted MR image (on the **left**) and axial diffusion-weighted MR image (on the **right**) show a rim-enhancing collection with restricted diffusion, consistent with a right frontal parafalcine subdural empyema (*arrows*).

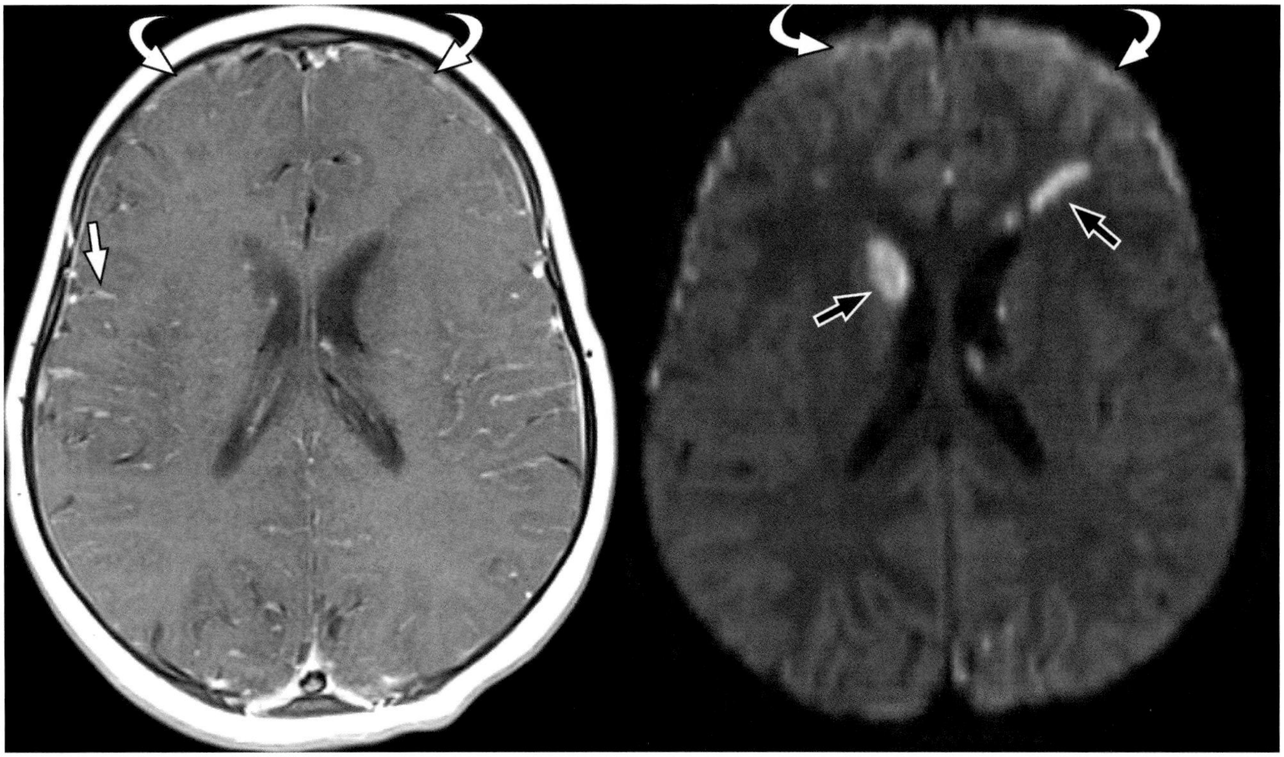

FIGURE 2.37 **Pneumococcal meningitis in a 22-month-old girl.** Axial postcontrast T1-weighted MR image (on the **left**) shows leptomeningeal enhancement (*straight arrow*) and small frontal enhancing subdural collections (*curved arrow*). Axial diffusion-weighted MR image (on the **right**) shows multiple foci of decreased diffusion (*straight arrows*) in the basal ganglia and frontal white matter, without corresponding enhancement on postcontrast MR images, indicating that these are infarcts secondary to meningitis. Note decreased diffusion in the bifrontal subdural empyemas (*curved arrows*).

detect early fibrosis within the inner ear structures and labyrinthitis ossificans[33] (Fig. 2.38).

Fungal Infections

Fungal infection of the CNS is rare in the immunocompetent child. Fungal meningitis or meningoencephalitis must be considered in immunocompromised children (usually chemotherapy-related) presenting with signs of a systemic fungal infection. Manifestations of various fungal infections are summarized in Table 2.4.

Neoplastic Disorders

Brain tumors are the most common solid tumors and are the leading cause of death from solid tumors in the pediatric population.[41] The incidence of all primary brain and CNS

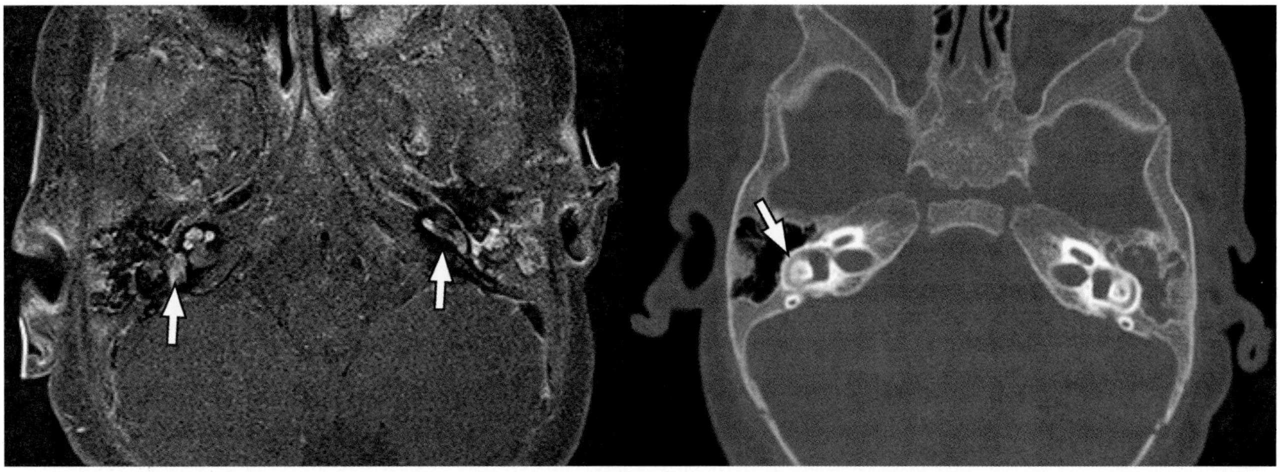

FIGURE 2.38 **Labyrinthine enhancement in an 8-month-old boy with pneumococcal meningitis.** Axial postcontrast T1-weighted fat-saturated MR image obtained at initial presentation (on the **left**) shows enhancement (*arrows*) within the inner ear structures bilaterally. Subsequently obtained CT 2 months later, just before cochlear implantation (on the **right**), shows subtle increased density (*arrow*) in the right lateral semicircular canal, consistent with early labyrinthitis ossificans.

TABLE 2.4 Clinical Manifestations and Central Nervous System Imaging Features of Fungal Infections

Organism	Clinical Manifestations	Central Nervous System (CNS) Imaging Features
Aspergillosis	• Nonspecific symptoms and fever may be absent, making diagnosis challenging. • Signs of meningitis and subarachnoid hemorrhage (SAH) may be present. • In patients with sinus disease, orbital extension with proptosis, ocular palsies, visual deterioration, and chemosis may occur. • In immunocompromised hosts, aspergillosis should be considered in the presence of acute-onset focal neurologic deficits caused by vascular or space-occupying lesions.	• CNS imaging features of aspergillosis infection depend upon immune status of the pediatric patients. • Edematous lesions, hemorrhagic lesions, enhancing solid lesions (referred to as aspergilloma), abscess-like or ring-enhancing lesions, "tumoral form," infarction, and mycotic aneurysm have been described. • Multifocal hypodensities on CT or T2 hyperintensities on MR in the cortex and/or subcortical white matter consistent with multiple areas of infarction are common findings in *Aspergillus* infection. • Superimposed hemorrhage is seen as hyperdensity on CT and hyperintensity on T1-weighted images (T1WI) on MR. • Foci of isointensity or low signal intensity on T2-weighted images (T2WI) on MR may represent fungal hyphae containing paramagnetic elements like manganese, iron, and magnesium, but may also be related to blood breakdown products. • Dural enhancement adjacent to infected paranasal sinuses is due to direct extension of sinonasal disease. • Diffusion-weighted MR imaging (DWI) detects early infarction and can also be beneficial in differentiating these lesions from progressive multifocal leukoencephalopathy and neoplasm. • Lesions in perforating artery territories are more common in hematogenously disseminated aspergillosis.
Cryptococcosis	• Signs of subacute meningitis or meningoencephalitis. • Headache is the most common and sometimes the only symptom of subacute meningitis or meningoencephalitis due to cryptococcosis CNS infection. • Symptoms and signs related to increased intracranial pressure because of hydrocephalus encephalitis may be present. • Meningoencephalitis is associated with high morbidity and mortality, especially among immunocompromised hosts. • Immunocompetent patients present with indolent neurologic disease and more intense inflammatory responses but have better clinical outcome.	• MR and CT abnormalities vary from normal scans to meningeal enhancement, abscesses, intraventricular or intraparenchymal cryptococcomas, gelatinous pseudocysts, and/or hydrocephalus. • Hydrocephalus is the most common finding, although it is nonspecific. • Intraparenchymal and intraventricular mass lesions are less common. • Pseudocysts from cryptococcosis CNS infection are well-circumscribed, round to oval low-density lesions on CT with CSF intensity on both T1WI and T2WI and do not enhance. • Clusters of pseudocysts in the basal ganglia and thalami strongly suggest cryptococcal infection. • Miliary lesions and cryptococcomas may present as variable density masses on CT, with low intensity on T1WI and high intensity on T2WI. • Contrast enhancement of cryptococcomas or the meninges is uncommon in immunocompromised patients because of the underlying immunosuppression and the nonimmunogenic nature of the polysaccharide capsule of the cryptococcal organism. • Immunocompetent pediatric patients are more likely to present with enhancing cryptococcomas.
Mucormycosis	• Immunocompromised children are most at risk for mucormycosis CNS infection. • Common presenting symptoms are headache, fever, sinusitis, facial swelling, and unilateral orbital apex syndrome. • Neurologic deficits resulting from intracerebral abscess formation and thrombosis of major intracranial vessels may be seen.	• CT and MRI show dense opacification with variable mucosal thickening and, usually, lack of fluid levels in the paranasal sinus. • Hypointense to hyperintense contents on T2WI are secondary to the presence of manganese, iron, and calcium. • Osseus erosion is strongly suggestive of the diagnosis in the right clinical setting. • Intracranial findings include infarcts because of vascular thrombosis, mycotic emboli, and frontal lobe abscesses. • Abnormal vascular signal and enhancement in the cavernous sinuses, internal carotid, and basilar artery are seen secondary to thrombus formation.
Candidiasis	• Immunocompromised children and, in particular, premature infants are most at risk for disseminated candida infection involving the CNS. • Premature infants present with irritability, poor feeding, seizures, apnea, and bradycardia. • In older infants and children, *Candida* tends to cause purulent leptomeningitis and ventriculitis similar to bacterial agents. • Hydrocephalus and CSF loculation are common complications.	• Microabscesses are seen as iso- to hypodense lesions on nonenhanced CT and multiple punctate enhancing nodules on postcontrast images. • Granulomas are seen as hyperdense nodules on CT with nodular or ring enhancement. • On MR, granuloma formation and brain abscess may be hypointense on T2W because of the magnetic susceptibility effect of hemorrhage. • Ring enhancement of lesions is seen on postcontrast images. • Features of meningitis, vasculitis, ventriculitis, and infarction may also be seen.

tumors in childhood is ~4.5 cases per 100,000 person-years.[42] In young children <3 years of age, supratentorial tumors are more common than infratentorial tumors.[42] In children between 4 years and 10 years of age, infratentorial tumors occur more frequently. Supra- and infratentorial tumors occur equally after 10 years old age.[42]

Classification of tumors by location in conjunction with the appearance of the lesion on conventional and advanced MR imaging techniques helps limit the differential diagnosis. Table 2.5 summarizes the classification of pediatric brain tumors used to organize this chapter.

TABLE 2.5 Common Anatomic Locations of Pediatric Brain Tumors
Supratentorial Tumors
Tumors of the cerebral hemispheres
• Hemispheric astrocytoma
• High-grade glioma (gliomatosis cerebri and glioblastoma multiforme)
• Oligodendroglioma
• Ependymal tumor
• Embryonal tumor other than medulloblastoma (formerly known as CNS PNET)
Neuronal and neuronal-glial neoplasms
• Ganglioglioma and gangliocytoma
• Desmoplastic infantile ganglioglioma
• Dysembryoplastic neuroepithelial tumor
• Extraventricular neurocytoma
Sellar and Suprasellar Tumors
• Chiasmatic and hypothalamic glioma
• Craniopharyngioma
• Pituitary tumor (macroadenoma and microadenoma)
• Hypothalamic hamartoma
Pineal Region Tumors
• Pineal gland tumor
• Germ cell tumor
• Tectal glioma
Intraventricular Tumors
• Choroid plexus tumor (choroid plexus papilloma and choroid plexus carcinoma)
• Ependymoma
• Central neurocytoma
• Subependymal giant cell astrocytoma
Posterior Fossa Tumors
• Medulloblastoma
• Posterior fossa astrocytoma
• Posterior fossa ependymoma
• Brainstem glioma
• Atypical teratoid/rhabdoid tumor
Miscellaneous Extra-Axial Tumors
• Teratoma
• Meningioma
• Schwannoma
• Lymphoproliferative tumor (leukemia and lymphoma)
• Metastasis

Supratentorial Tumors

Tumors of the Cerebral Hemispheres

Hemispheric Astrocytoma

Astrocytomas are the most common childhood tumors of the CNS, constituting approximately one-third of all pediatric supratentorial tumors. Their peak incidence is between 2 and 4 years of age and during early adolescence. They originate from the cerebral hemispheres, thalamus, hypothalamus, and basal ganglia. As discussed later in this chapter, astrocytomas are more common in pediatric patients with NF1. Most astrocytomas are low-grade and classified as WHO grade I neoplasms. However, high-grade neoplasms also occur, and their imaging characteristics are similar to high-grade primary brain tumors seen in adults. Although most low-grade lesions present with seizures, higher-grade tumors present more acutely with symptoms resulting from mass effect, hemorrhage, and raised intracranial pressure.

On CT, low-grade hemispheric astrocytomas have a mixed solid and cystic appearance, with the solid components typically being hypodense. On MRI, various imaging patterns have been described. These include (1) a mass with a nonenhancing cyst and an intensely enhancing mural nodule (typical of pilocytic astrocytoma), (2) a mass with an enhancing cyst wall and an intensely enhancing mural nodule, (3) a necrotic mass with a central nonenhancing zone, and (4) a predominantly solid mass with minimal to no cyst-like component. Some cyst walls may enhance avidly. However, cyst wall enhancement is not necessarily indicative of the presence of tumor cells. The solid areas are typically hyperintense on T2-weighted MR images relative to brain parenchyma, and vary from homogenous to heterogeneous on contrast-enhanced images (Fig. 2.39). On diffusion-weighted MR images, low-grade astrocytomas have relatively high diffusivity, reflecting the relatively low cell density or nuclear-to-cytoplasmic ratio seen on histology.

Surgical resection is the definitive curative treatment for hemispheric astrocytoma in the pediatric population, although location near eloquent areas may preclude complete resection.

High-Grade Glioma (Gliomatosis Cerebri and Glioblastoma Multiforme)

Gliomatosis cerebri is a rare diffuse infiltrating high-grade glial tumor of astrocytic origin that can rarely occur in the first two decades of life, but is more common in adults. In children, it is nearly always fatal, with a length of survival spanning from 6 months to 3 years after initial presentation. Gliomatosis cerebri can present with a wide variety of symptoms including headaches, vomiting, seizures, and focal neurologic deficits. On CT, it can be difficult to resolve apart from the presence of mild mass effect, especially on noncontrast studies. On MR, gliomatosis cerebri initially presents as T2 and FLAIR hyperintense unihemispheric lesions that progress to become bihemispheric with time. There is general preservation of the anatomic architecture. Mass effect is generally mild, and enhancement is typically absent in the early stage (Fig. 2.40).

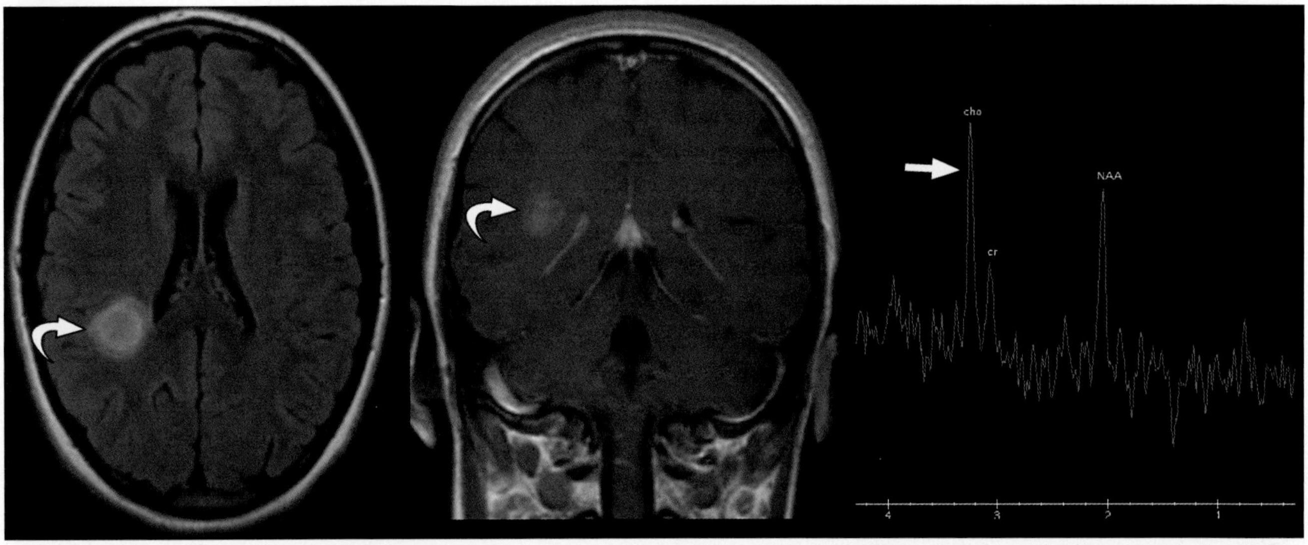

FIGURE 2.39 **Hemispheric pilocytic astrocytoma.** Axial FLAIR MR image (on the **left**), postcontrast coronal T1-weighted MR image (in the **middle**), and single voxel MR spectroscopy image (on the **right**) show a rounded enhancing T2 hyperintense lesion (*curved arrows*) in the right parietal white matter, with elevated choline peak on MR spectroscopy (*straight arrow*).

Glioblastoma multiforme is a highly malignant tumor that comprises ~3% of tumors in children.[43] This tumor typically crosses the midline across the commissural tracts, giving rise to a "butterfly glioma" lesion that involves the contralateral hemisphere (Fig. 2.41). Clinical presentation includes seizures, signs of raised intracranial pressure, and focal neurologic deficits. On MRI, these lesions are hypo- to isointense to white matter on T1- and hyperintense on T2-weighted MR images. Irregular and heterogeneous enhancement of the margins is a common finding. A central necrotic core may

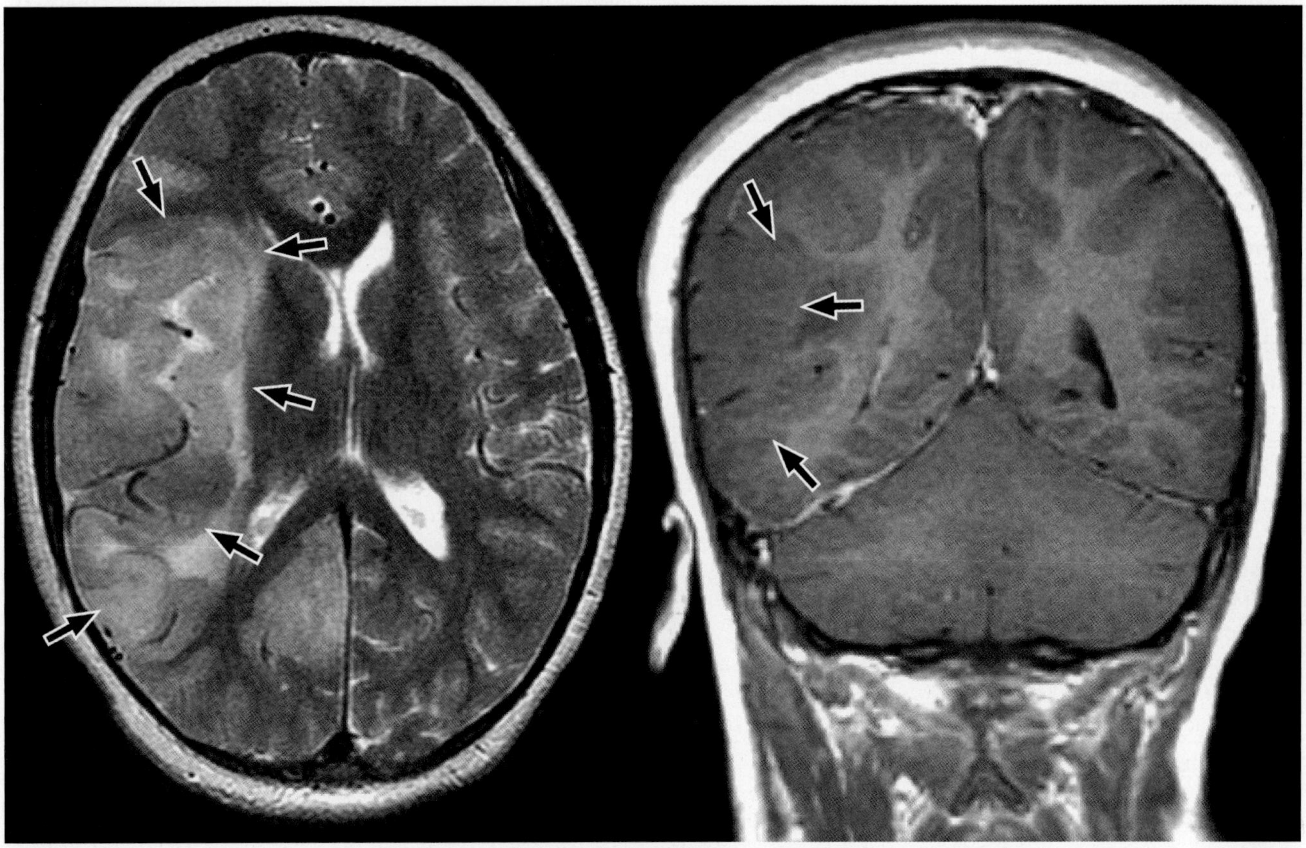

FIGURE 2.40 **Gliomatosis cerebri in a 7-year-old girl who presented with confusion and left-sided weakness.** Axial T2-weighted MR image (on the **left**) and coronal postcontrast T1-weighted MR image (on the **right**) show a large mass (*arrows*) characterized by abnormal T2 signal occupying large portions of the right cerebral hemisphere with mass effect.

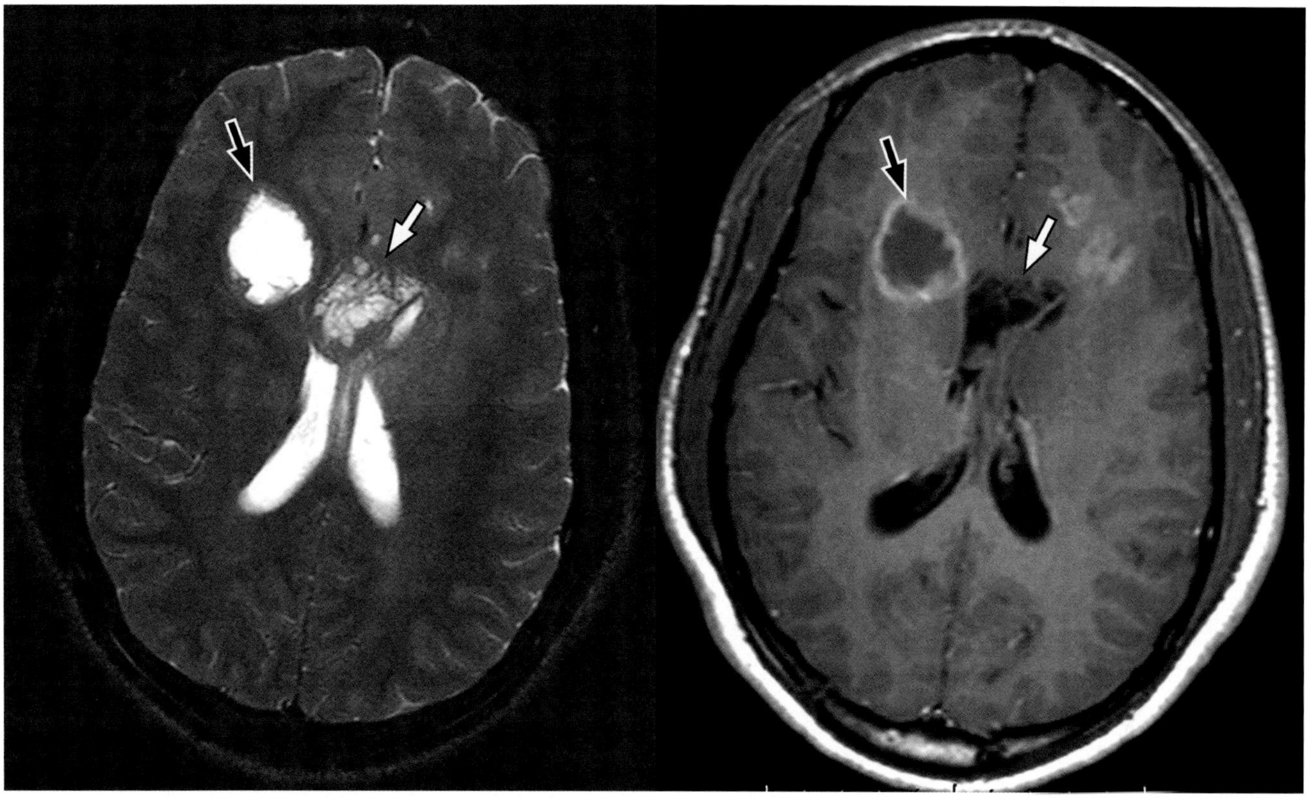

FIGURE 2.41 **Glioblastoma multiforme in a 16-year-old boy.** Axial T2-weighted MR image (on the **left**) and axial postcontrast T1-weighted MR image (on the **right**) show a large frontal lobe mass (*black arrows*) with a T2 hyperintense central necrotic core and enhancing margins. In addition, there is an extensive surrounding T2 hyperintense lesion extending across the midline (*white arrows*), consistent with the "butterfly glioma" characteristic of glioblastoma multiforme.

be seen (Fig. 2.42). Intratumoral bleeding is also common because of the abnormal, rich vasculature that characterizes these tumors. Histologically, glioblastoma multiforme consists of poorly differentiated glial cells, often with pronounced variation in nuclear size and shape (anaplasia or pleomorphism).

The prognosis is poor even when radiotherapy is used in children with glioblastoma multiforme. Two-year survival for GBM in children is ~12%.[44] The median survival time is between 6 months without treatment and 12 months with radiation treatment after initial diagnosis.[44]

Oligodendroglioma

Oligodendrogliomas are glial neoplasms that occur most frequently in adults (peak incidence is in the fourth and fifth decades of life), accounting for only 1% of CNS tumors in the pediatric population.[45] They are slow-growing neoplasms with a peripheral location. Traditional subtyping of oligodendrogliomas based on whether or not they are anaplastic has been supplemented by testing for IDH1 or IDH2 mutation and for codeletion of chromosomal arms 1p and 19q. "Pediatric-type" oligodendroglioma lacks these genetic changes, suggesting that it is a quite different genetic and biologic entity than adult-type oligodendroglioma.

On MRI, oligodendrogliomas are predominantly solid masses located along the periphery of the cerebral hemispheres. The solid components are T2 and FLAIR hyperintense (Fig. 2.43). Presence of prominent cortical thickening is a characteristic feature. Calcification is seen commonly on CT and on susceptibility-weighted sequences on MRI. Chunky nodular calcification is described as a typical feature, but this occurs more commonly in adults. Lesions enhance variably following contrast administration. As with other

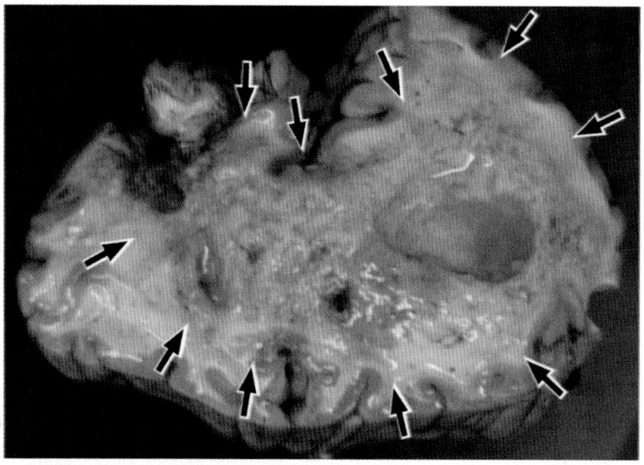

FIGURE 2.42 **Glioblastoma multiforme in a 16-month-old boy who was diagnosed 3 months antemortem.** The cut surface shows a large mass (*arrows*) with multiple areas of yellow-hued necrosis and an ill-defined border.

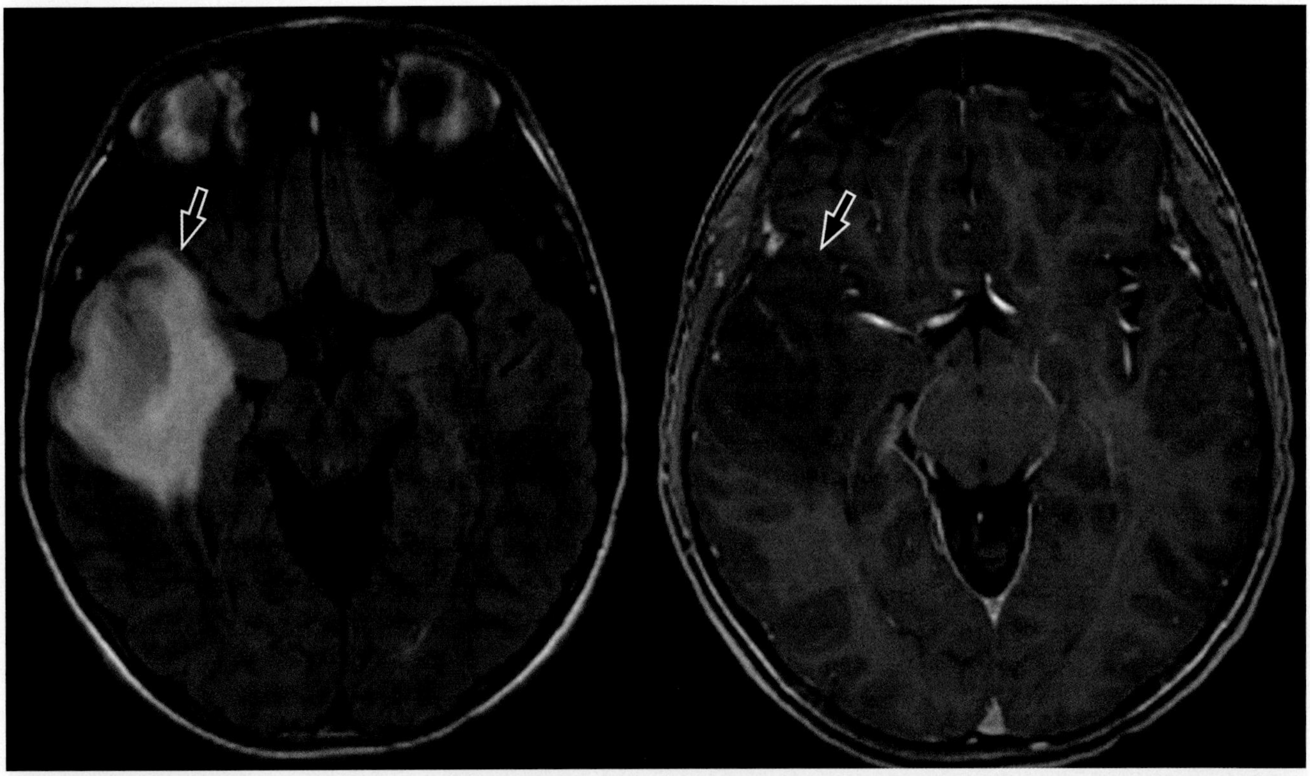

FIGURE 2.43 **Oligodendroglioma in a 15-year-old boy.** Axial FLAIR MR image (on the **left**) and axial T1-weighted SPGR (spoiled gradient recalled) MR image (on the **right**) demonstrate a FLAIR hyperintense lesion in the right temporal lobe that does not enhance following contrast administration (*arrows*). Histology of the resected specimen revealed an oligodendroglioma.

slow-growing peripherally located lesions, remodeling of the inner table of the skull is a common finding.

The current treatment of oligodendrogliomas includes surgical resection with adjuvant radiotherapy and chemotherapy. Local recurrence is common, and close attention should be paid to the resection site on follow-up studies, noting that the recurrent tumors can be nonenhancing, particularly when the presenting lesion was nonenhancing.[46]

Ependymal Tumors

Ependymomas constitute ~6% of all primary intracranial tumors in children.[42] Of these, supratentorial ependymomas typically occur in children <6 years old and account for up to 40% of all ependymomas.[47] These tumors are thought to arise from embryonic rests of ependymal tissue trapped in the developing cerebral hemispheres.

Ependymal tumors are T1 hypointense and isointense to hyperintense to gray matter on T2-weighted MR images, and generally enhance moderately after contrast administration on both CT and MRI (Fig. 2.44). Ependymomas are heterogeneous and often contain calcification and cystic areas. On MRI, there is usually avid enhancement of the soft tissue components of the tumor, intermixed with poorly enhancing or nonenhancing areas.

Grossly, ependymomas are often soft, tan, and distinct from the surrounding normal brain. Microscopically, they consist of cellular collections of round cells within an abundant fibrillary background. The nuclei are often arranged around the fibrillary material in ependymal rosettes or perivascular pseudorosettes (Fig. 2.45).

Embryonal Tumor Other Than Medulloblastoma (formerly known as CNS PNET)

Embryonal tumor other than medulloblastoma, formerly known as central nervous system primitive neuroectodermal tumor (CNS PNET), is relatively rare, accounting for 5% of all supratentorial tumors in childhood.[48] These tumors are more common in the first decade of life, with a peak incidence from birth to 5 years of age. At presentation, supratentorial embryonal tumors are often large and fairly well-defined, occurring either in the cerebral hemispheres or in the lateral ventricles. They may be solid and homogenous or heterogeneous with cyst formation. Calcification is often seen on CT. Following contrast administration, heterogeneous enhancement is seen within regions of necrosis. On MR, solid areas have restricted diffusion and T2-hypointense areas (Fig. 2.46), reflecting high nuclear-to-cytoplasmic ratio and increased cellularity (Fig. 2.47), as well as increased CBV values on perfusion imaging. Hemorrhage can also occur in these lesions. CNS embryonal tumors are a more heterogeneous group of tumors than peripheral PNET and may show differentiation along neuronal, astrocytic, or ependymal lines. They lack the *EWSR1* gene rearrangement characteristic of peripheral PNET/Ewing sarcoma.[49]

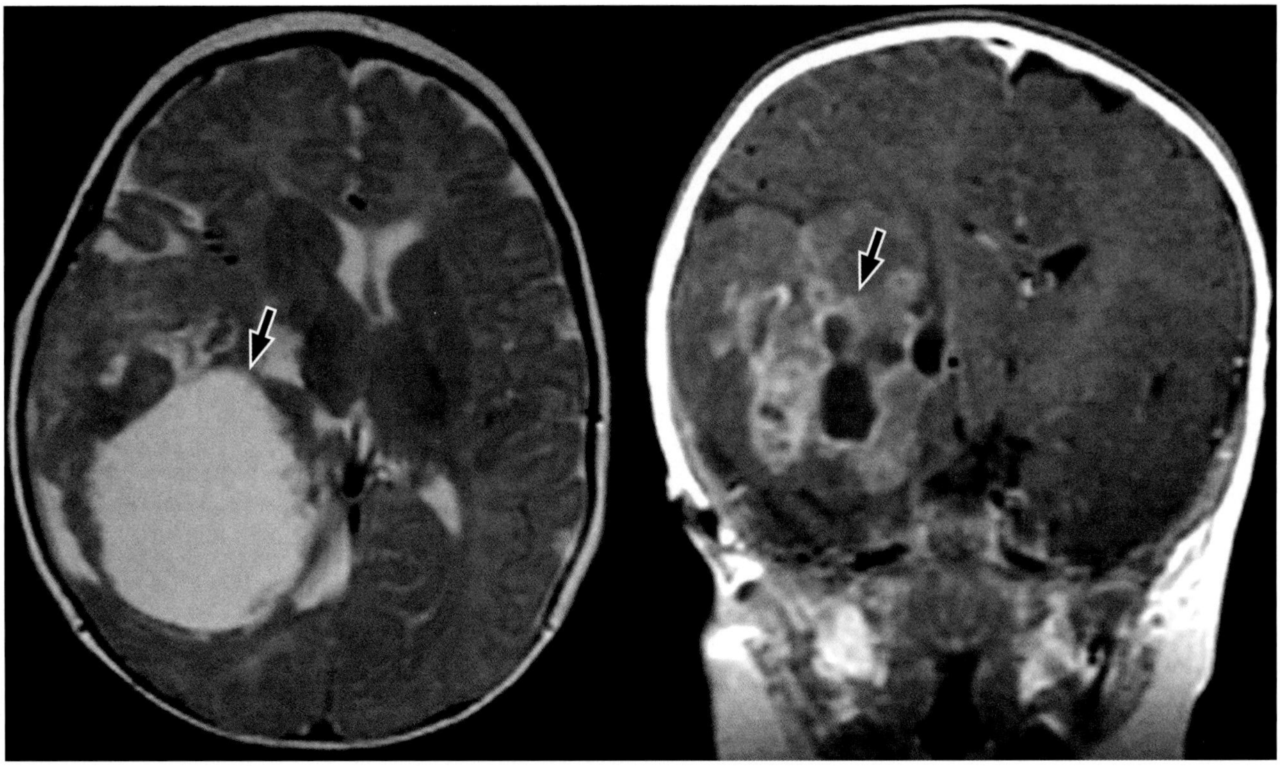

FIGURE 2.44 **Supratentorial ependymoma in a 5-month-old girl.** Axial T2-weighted MR image (on the **left**) and coronal postcontrast T1-weighted MR image (on the **right**) show a large heterogeneous mass (*arrows*) containing a large cystic component and heterogeneous enhancement in the right cerebral hemisphere, with vasogenic edema and marked mass effect on surrounding brain. Histology of the resected specimen was consistent with an anaplastic ependymoma.

Neuronal and Neuronal–Glial Neoplasms

Ganglioglioma and Gangliocytoma

Ganglioglioma and gangliocytoma are both tumors that contain neoplastic mature ganglion cells (neuronal cells). Gangliocytomas are composed solely of neuronal elements, whereas gangliogliomas contain neoplastic glial cells as well (Fig. 2.48). Ganglioglioma and gangliocytoma comprise ~6% of supratentorial tumors in children.[48] Ganglioglioma and gangliocytoma arise most commonly in adolescents and

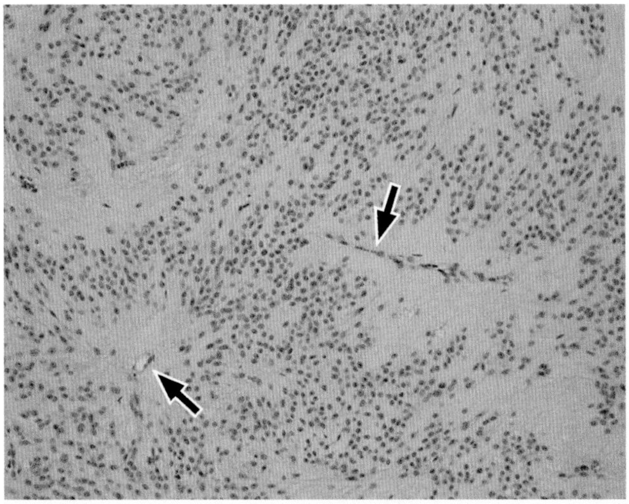

FIGURE 2.45 **Ependymoma in a 6-year-old girl.** Histology from a mass resected from the frontal lobe shows monotonous round cells in a fibrillary background. Tumor cell nuclei are often arranged around hypocellular fibrillary areas with central vessels (*arrows*), forming "perivascular pseudorosettes" (hematoxylin and eosin, original magnification, 200×).

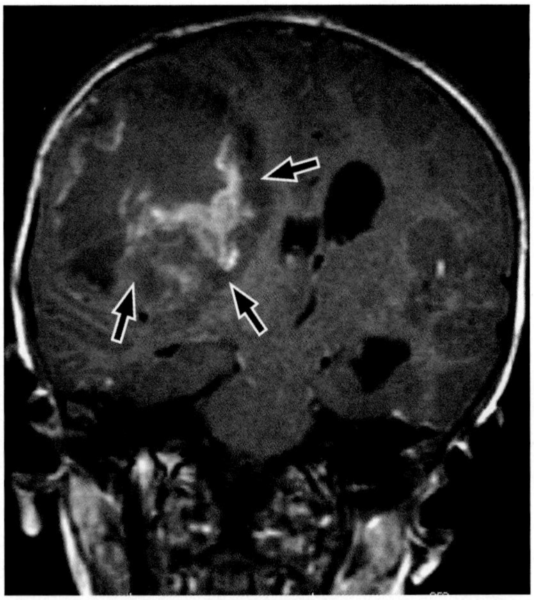

FIGURE 2.46 **Central nervous system (CNS) embryonal tumor (diagnosed as "CNS PNET" before WHO nomenclature was changed) in an 8-year-old boy.** Coronal postcontrast T1-weighted MR image demonstrates a large, partially necrotic, enhancing mass (*arrows*) in the right cerebral hemisphere causing marked mass effect and midline shift.

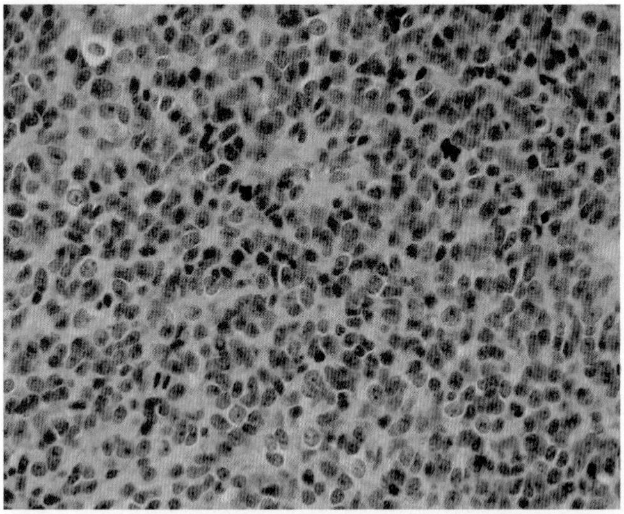

FIGURE 2.47 **Embryonal tumor from the temporal lobe of a 3-year-old girl.** Poorly differentiated densely packed cells with high nuclear-to-cytoplasmic ratio are present (hematoxylin and eosin, original magnification, 400×). Genetic findings may permit specific classification, such as "embryonal tumor with multilayered rosettes, C19MC-altered"; when not further classifiable, the designation "CNS embryonal tumor, not otherwise specified" is appropriate, as the old term "CNS PNET" is now defunct.

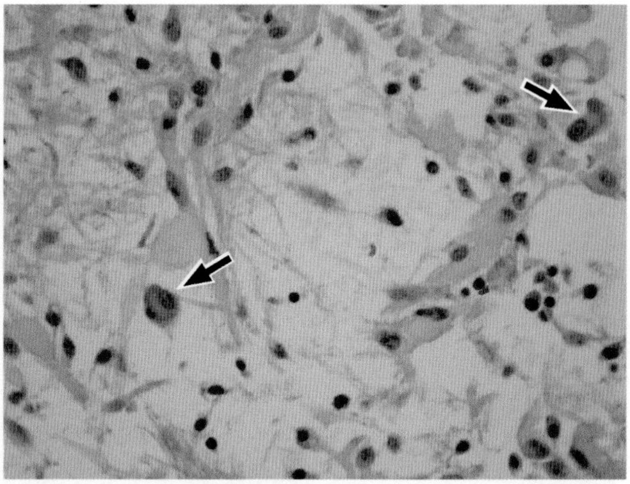

FIGURE 2.48 **Ganglioglioma in a 14-year-old boy.** This mass resected from the parietal lobe is moderately cellular with a spindled glial component and admixed dysplastic, occasionally multinucleate (*arrows*) ganglion cells (hematoxylin and eosin, original magnification, 400×).

in young adults. Both tumors arise in the cerebral cortex, most commonly in the temporal lobe. Presenting symptoms depend upon the size and location of tumors and usually include seizures. In particular, complex partial seizures are commonly associated with temporal lobe tumors.

On imaging studies, the appearance of ganglioglioma and gangliocytoma is virtually identical. Both are seen as intra-axial tumors located peripherally in the cortex with a mixed solid and cystic appearance. The solid components are hyperintense to gray matter on T2-weighted MR images and variably enhance following contrast administration (Fig. 2.49). Presence of mineralization and absence

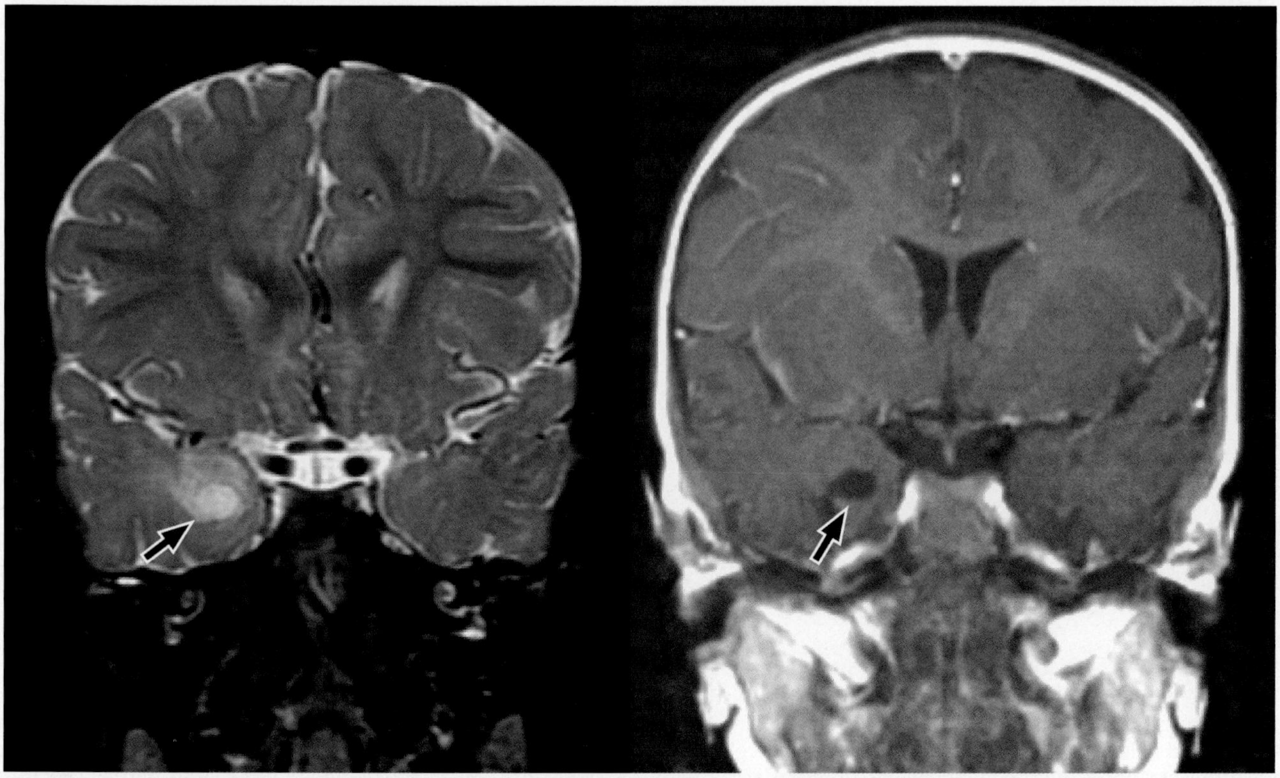

FIGURE 2.49 **Ganglioglioma in an 11-month-old girl who presented with seizures.** Coronal T2-weighted MR image (on the **left**) and coronal postcontrast T1-weighted MR image (on the **right**) show a poorly-defined, nonenhancing, heterogeneous mass (*arrows*) that is hyperintense to gray matter expanding the right temporal lobe, suggestive of a ganglioglioma.

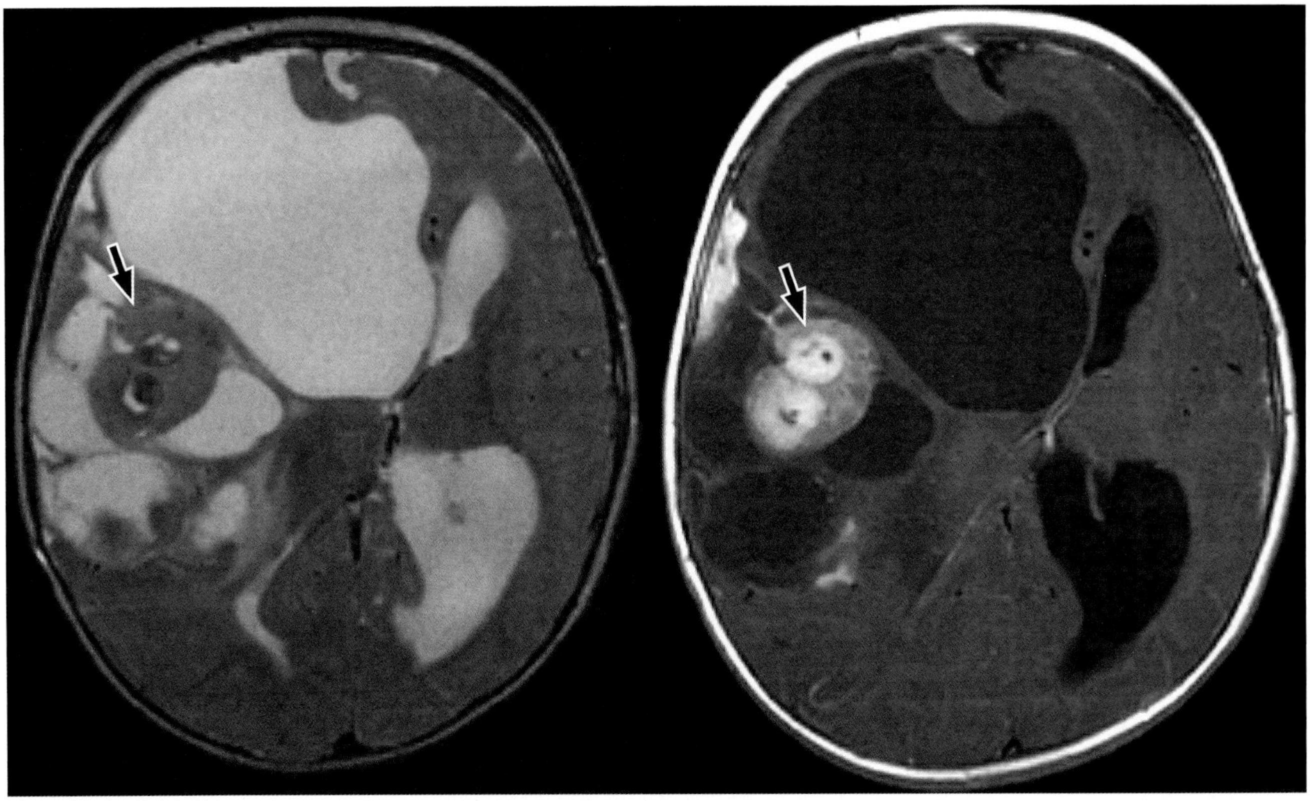

FIGURE 2.50 **Desmoplastic infantile ganglioglioma in an asymptomatic 9-month-old boy who presented with increasing head circumference.** Axial T2-weighted MR (on the **left**) and axial postcontrast T1-weighted MR image (on the **right**) show a large mixed solid and cystic lesion (*arrows*) in the right cerebral hemisphere, with enhancement of some of the solid components. Mass effect from the tumor and leftward midline shift are also present.

of enhancement may suggest the diagnosis of these tumors, although the appearance is still nonspecific.

Surgical resection is the definitive treatment of ganglioglioma and gangliocytoma in the pediatric population.

Desmoplastic Infantile Ganglioglioma

Desmoplastic infantile gangliogliomas (DIG) are rare intracranial tumors that typically occur in the first 2 years of life.[50] They are characterized by both astrocytic and ganglionic differentiation and a prominent desmoplastic stroma. Clinical presentation is usually with rapid and progressively increasing head circumference.

DIGs are typically seen as large mixed solid and cystic masses in the cerebral hemispheres, most commonly in the frontal and parietal lobes. On CT, the solid portion of these large masses is slightly hyperdense compared to normal gray matter and typically located along the cortical margin of the mass. Calcification is not commonly seen. On MRI, the solid components of the lesions are isointense to brain parenchyma on T1- and T2-weighted MR images. As on CT, the solid components enhance avidly following contrast administration on MRI (Fig. 2.50).

Treatment of DIGs is best accomplished by surgical resection, which can often be challenging because of large size and firm attachment to the dura. Chemotherapy may be considered if gross total resection cannot be accomplished. In spite of the aggressive appearance, overall prognosis is good for most pediatric patients.

Dysembryoplastic Neuroepithelial Tumor

Dysembryoplastic neuroepithelial tumors (DNET) are WHO grade I benign, slow-growing mixed neuronal–glial tumors arising from either cortical or deep gray matter (Fig. 2.51). Average age of presentation is 9 years, and most affected pediatric patients present with a longstanding history of often-intractable partial seizures. They comprise <1% of

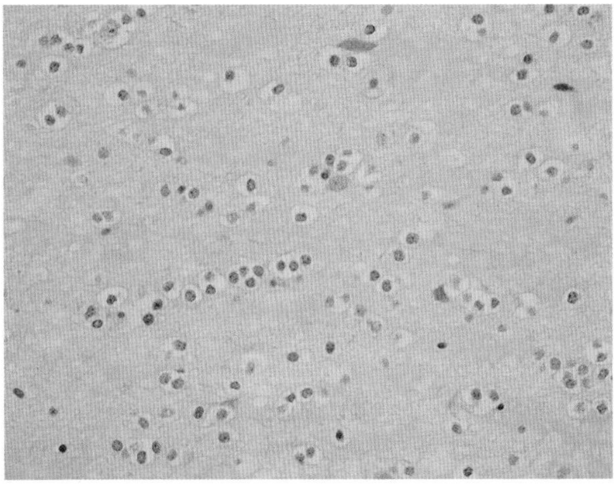

FIGURE 2.51 **Dysembryoplastic neuroepithelial tumor in a 15-year-old boy.** Tumor resected from the temporal lobe shows round oligodendrocyte-like cells with occasional interspersed neurons, present in a pale blue myxoid background (hematoxylin and eosin, original magnification, 400×).

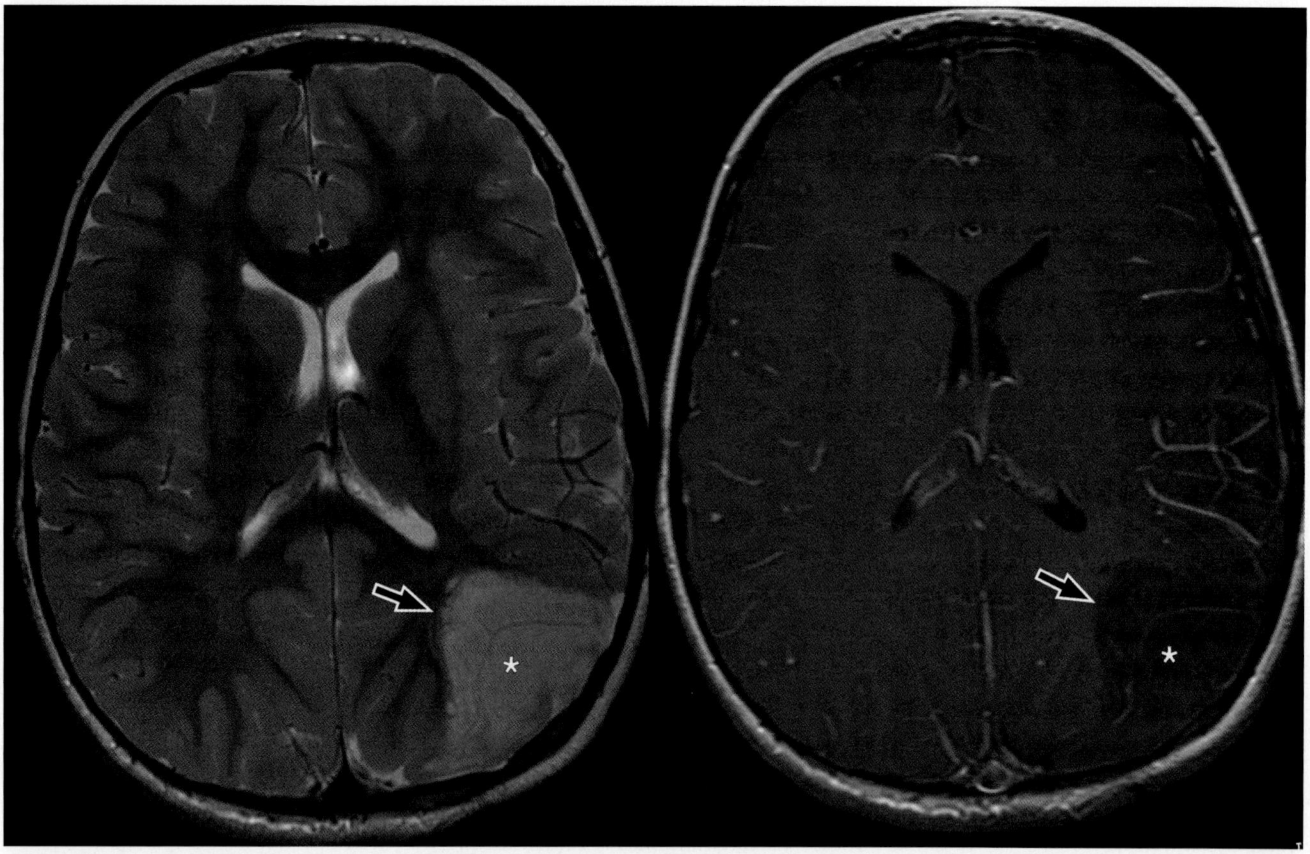

FIGURE 2.52 **Dysembryoplastic neuroepithelial tumor in a 10-year-old boy who presented with seizures.** Axial T2-weighted MR image (on the **left**) and axial postcontrast T1-weighted MR image (on the **right**) show a large cortically based lesion (*asterisks*) with cyst-like areas (*arrows*) along the medial aspect, which does not enhance on the postcontrast MR image.

CNS tumors in childhood.[42] DNETs are located most commonly in the temporal and parietal lobes. Most lesions arise from the cortical gray matter, and associated cortical dysplasia has been reported in more than 80% cases.[51,52]

On CT, the lesion is hypodense to gray matter. On MRI, classic DNETs are seen as cortically based lesions with a gyriform configuration and cyst-like areas on T2-weighted MR images (Fig. 2.52). These areas are hyperintense on FLAIR images. Classic DNETs do not enhance following contrast administration on either CT and MRI. A subtype of DNET involves the subcortical white matter in addition to the cortex and enhances variably following contrast administration. Typically, there is no evidence of surrounding edema or mass effect. Also, their longstanding nature is indicated by the presence of scalloping of the inner table of the calvarium.

Surgical resection is currently the definitive treatment of DNETs.

Extraventricular Neurocytoma

Neurocytomas are rare WHO grade 2 neuroepithelial tumors that account for 0.1% to 0.5% of all CNS tumors.[53] Most neurocytomas are located within the intracerebral ventricular system (in which case they are called "central neurocytomas") in or near the midline, usually attached to the septal leaflets. However, "extraventricular neurocytomas" in cerebral and spinal cord locations have been reported. These tumors are uncommon in childhood and seen most often in young adults in the second to fourth decades.

On CT, neurocytomas are mixed solid and cystic. The solid components are usually hyperdense to the cortex (Fig. 2.53). Calcification is seen in ~50%.[54] Moderate heterogeneous enhancement of solid components is seen following contrast administration. On MRI, these tumors are heterogeneous. They are isointense to the cortex on T1-weighted MR images. On T2-weighed MR images, the lesion has a "bubbly" appearance because of the presence of cysts within the lesion that null on FLAIR MR images. Prominent vascular flow voids may be seen, corresponding to the choroidal vessels supplying the mass. Mild to moderate heterogeneous enhancement of solid components is seen following contrast administration.

Surgical resection is curative in a vast majority of cases. Microscopically, the tumor consists of uniform histologically benign round cells with interspersed areas of neuropil (Fig. 2.54).

Sellar and Suprasellar Tumors

Chiasmatic and Hypothalamic Glioma

Some preferred sites of pilocytic astrocytomas (WHO grade I) include the optic nerve ("optic nerve glioma") and the optic chiasm/hypothalamus. Pilocytic astrocytomas of the optic pathways represent 15% of supratentorial tumors.[55] Moreover,

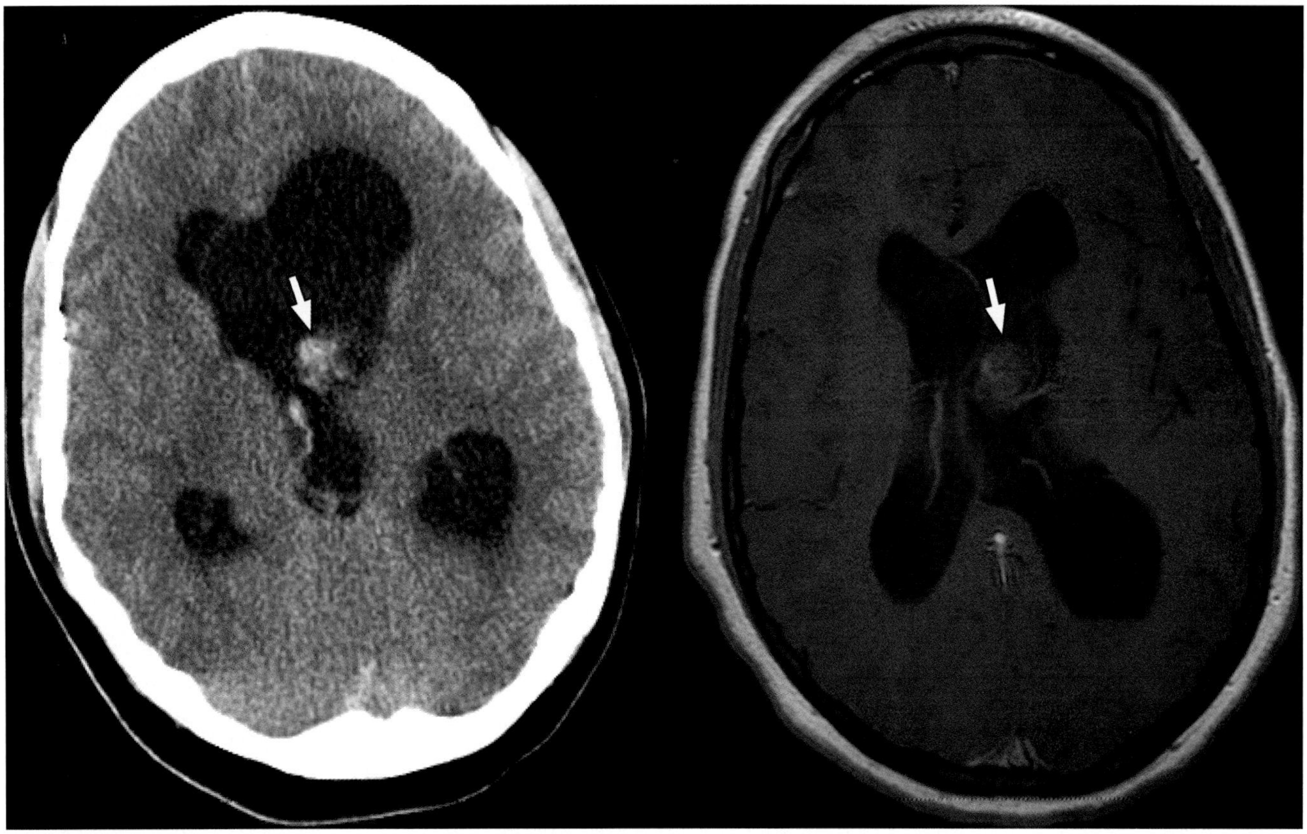

FIGURE 2.53 **Neurocytoma in a 14-year-old girl.** Axial noncontrast CT image (on the **right**) and axial postcontrast T1-weighted MR image (on the **left**) show a hemorrhagic, partially enhancing tumor (*arrows*) arising from the left head of caudate with intraventricular extension.

bilateral optic nerve tumors are virtually pathognomonic of this diagnosis. Optic pathway gliomas may involve the optic nerves, optic chiasm, optic tract, lateral geniculate bodies, and/or optic radiations. Optic gliomas occur with increasing frequency in patients with NF1 (20% to 50%).[56] On the other hand, up to 24% of patients with NF1 have optic pathway gliomas.[57] Tumors in children with NF1 are reportedly less aggressive than those in children without NF1 and tend to be bilateral.

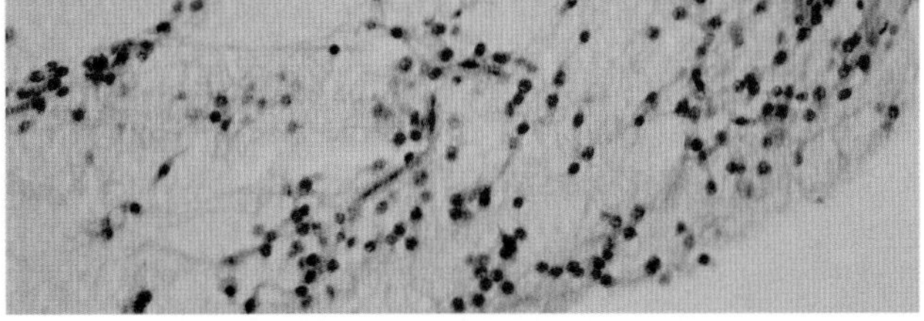

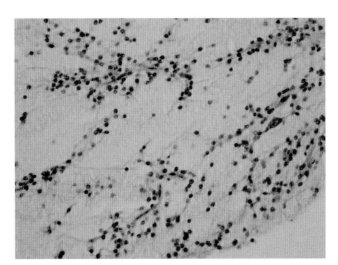

FIGURE 2.54 **Neurocytoma.** This intraventricular mass from the same patient (Figure 2.53) shows round uniform cells interspersed with "nucleus-free" zones of fibrillary neuropil (hematoxylin and eosin, original magnification, 400×).

Optic pathway gliomas are usually T1 isointense to hypointense. On T2-weighted MR images, the lesions demonstrate mixed signal intensity. Intense enhancement is common on postcontrast MR images (Fig. 2.55). The use of axial and coronal postcontrast thin-section T1-weighted fat-suppressed MR images and inversion recovery or T2-weighted MR images with fat suppression enables optimal visualization of the optic pathways. The presence of mass effect and contrast enhancement differentiates tumors from myelin vacuolization seen along the optic tracts in NF1 patients.

Diencephalic syndrome may be seen in pediatric patients with hypothalamic/chiasmatic astrocytomas presenting with failure to thrive. These tumors are often larger, occur at a younger age, are more aggressive than others at presentation, and may seed throughout the CSF pathways.

Craniopharyngioma

Craniopharyngiomas are slow-growing, benign, nonglial tumors arising in the sellar and parasellar regions. They comprise between 3% and 5% of all pediatric brain tumors[58]. Craniopharyngiomas are classified as WHO grade I tumors and arise from ectodermal remnants of the Rathke pouch, with a bimodal incidence in the first and fifth decades of life.

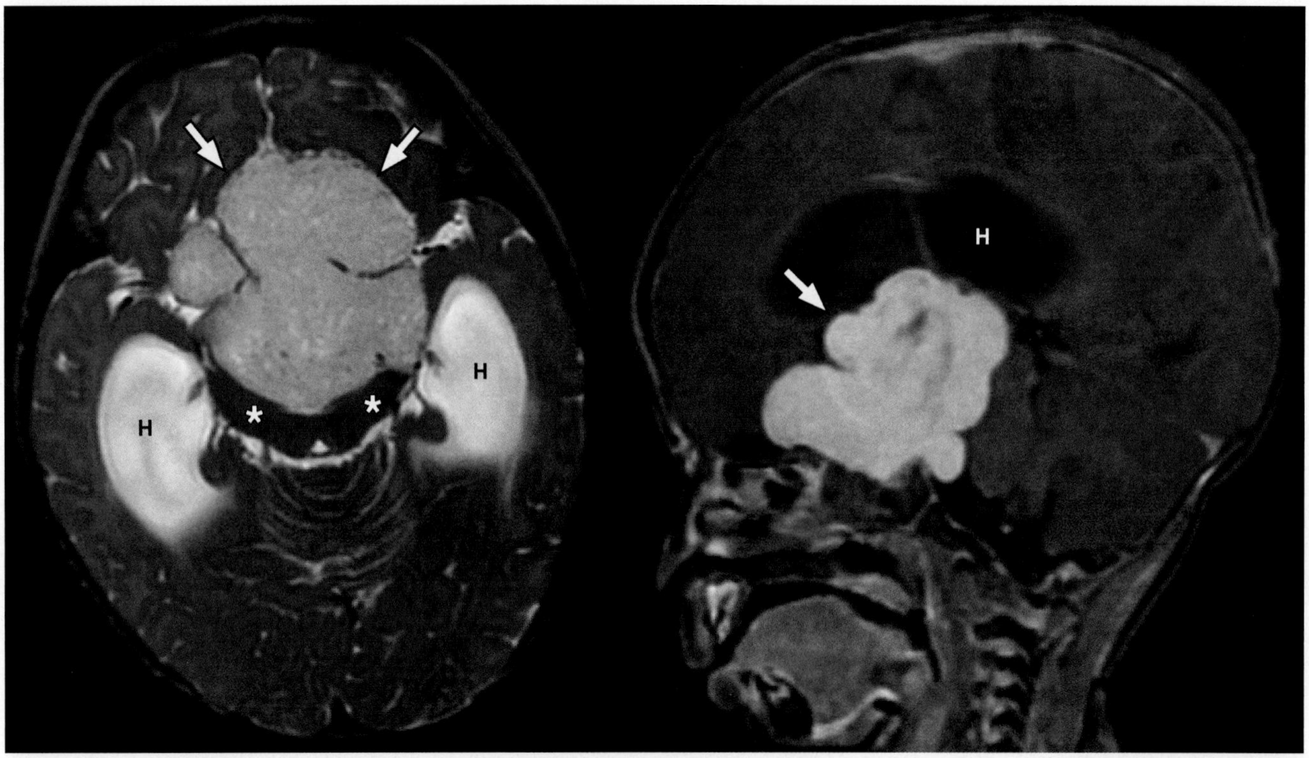

FIGURE 2.55 **Optic pathway glioma in a 6-month-old girl who presented with increased irritability and was diagnosed with diencephalic syndrome.** Axial T2-weighted MR image (on the **left**) and postcontrast sagittal 3D SPGR (spoiled gradient recalled) MR image (on the **right**) show an avidly enhancing suprasellar and sellar intermediate T2 signal intensity lesion (*arrows*) extending to the prepontine region and splaying the cerebral peduncles (*asterisks*) consistent with a large optic pathway glioma with secondary obstructive hydrocephalus (*H*).

The adamantinomatous type is more common in children, whereas the squamous–papillary variant tends to occur in adults.[59,60] Although they are benign, they can invade surrounding structures in the sellar and parasellar regions, eliciting a gliotic response and making resection challenging.

On imaging studies, craniopharyngiomas have a mixed cystic and solid appearance, with 90% of tumors showing calcification and 90% containing cystic areas[61] (Fig. 2.56). On MRI, high signal intensity on both T1- and T2-weighted MR images is seen in areas of lesions with high protein content or in lesions containing subacute hemorrhage.[62] Hypointensity on T1-weighted MR images may reflect the presence of keratin. CT is often used to demonstrate calcification in the lesion, which is important for diagnosis and surgical planning.

Surgical resection remains the mainstay of treatment of craniopharyngiomas, with radiotherapy having a role in cases that are not amenable to gross total resection. Greater than 85% of patients survive 3 years after diagnosis, and subtotal resection and radiation therapy are associated with prolonged survival.[63] The resected specimen is often spongy and variably gritty, and its cysts may contain dark fluid resembling "machine oil." Microscopically, they are composed of squamous epithelium that may, in the adamantinomatous variant, have prominent peripheral palisading and areas of differentiation into stellate reticulum, resembling adamantinomas derived from dental epithelium (Fig. 2.57). Follow-up imaging is directed toward identifying recurrence, second tumors, and associated moyamoya syndrome.

Pituitary Tumor

Macroadenoma and Microadenoma

Pituitary adenomas account for ~3% of all supratentorial tumors in childhood.[64] Clinical presentation is variable and depends on tumor size, hormonal activity, and extrasellar extent. Most adenomas are hormonally active, with most secreting prolactin. Most lesions are microadenomas (<1 cm in diameter) and present with neuroendocrine symptoms. Prolactin secreting or hormonally inactive macroadenomas (>1 cm in diameter) have more variable symptomatology, including neuroendocrine abnormalities, visual field cuts, or headache.

On MRI, adenomas may be isointense or hypointense compared with the normal pituitary gland on T1- and isointense to hyperintense on T2-weighted MR images. On postcontrast images, microadenomas are relatively hypoenhancing compared to normal pituitary tissue (Fig. 2.58). Macroadenomas present as heterogeneous masses that tend to involve the sella and suprasellar region. Hemorrhage into a macroadenoma is a relatively common complication.

Surgical removal is indicated for macroadenomas that cause optic chiasmal compression in children. For macroadenomas without chiasmal compression, surgery is considered for lesions larger than 2 cm and with prolactin levels > 600

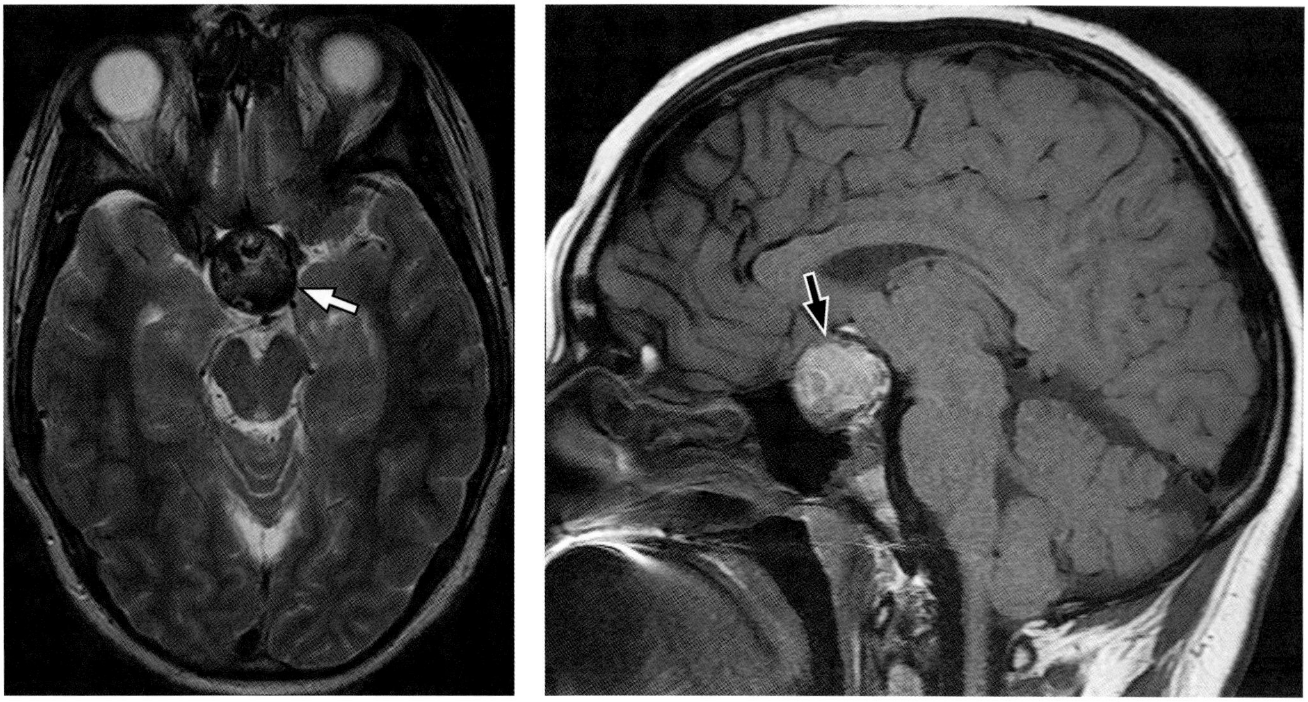

FIGURE 2.56 **Craniopharyngioma in a 17-year-old boy who presented with hypopituitarism.** Axial T2-weighted MR image (on the **left**) and sagittal postcontrast T1-weighted MR image (on the **right**) shows a large, partially calcified, heterogeneous, suprasellar mass (*arrows*) with mass effect upon the optic chiasm and involvement of the pituitary gland.

ng/mL.[65] Functioning microadenomas are usually treated with medical therapy, although some surgeons prefer upfront operative management in pediatric patients. Microscopically, pituitary adenomas may be classified based on their architectural pattern and hormonal content as assessed by immunohistochemical staining (Fig. 2.59).

Rathke Cleft Cyst

Another lesion commonly encountered in the sella or in the suprasellar region is a Rathke cleft cyst. These lesions are congenital, nonneoplastic cysts derived from remnants of Rathke pouch. Rathke cleft cysts are most commonly discovered incidentally, as they are usually not large enough to be symptomatic by compressing surrounding structures. Symptoms result from compression of the optic chiasm, hypothalamus, or pituitary gland and are indistinguishable from those caused by other sellar masses, such as craniopharyngioma or pituitary adenoma.

On MRI, Rathke cleft cysts are typically characterized by high signal intensity on unenhanced T1-weighted

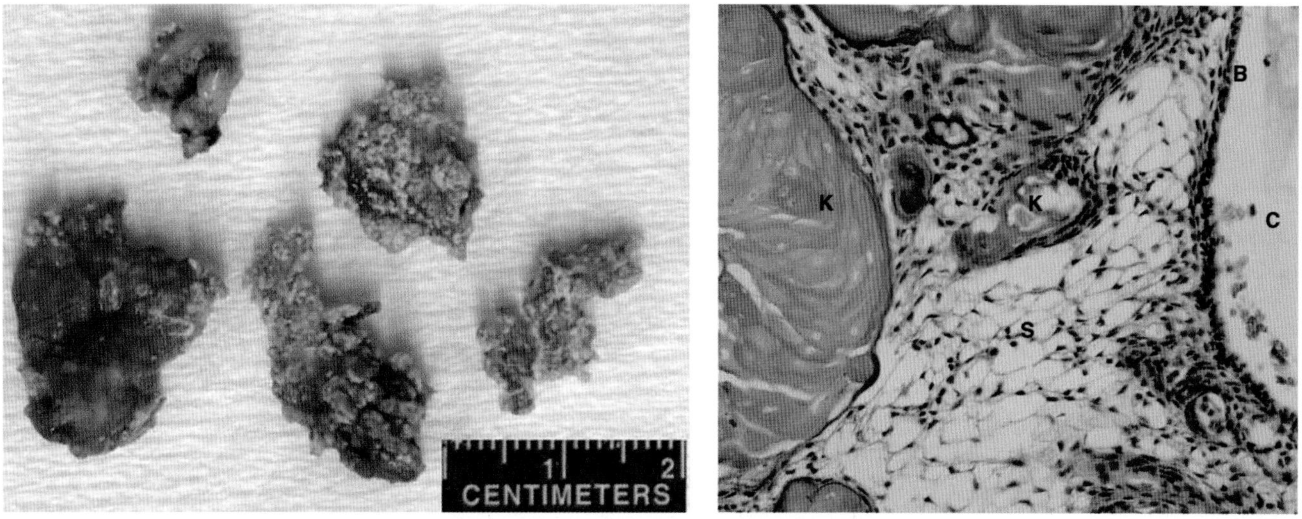

FIGURE 2.57 **Craniopharyngioma in a 3-year-old girl.** This adamantinomatous variant of a craniopharyngioma was a large cystic hypothalamus-centered mass. Gross examination (on the **left**) shows spongy and somewhat chalky pale tan tissue with occasional cysts containing dark, greasy fluid. Microscopically (on the **right**), squamous cells with basal palisading (*B*) and stellate reticulum (*S*) alternate with calcifying keratinous debris (*K*) and cystic spaces (*C*) (hematoxylin and eosin, original magnification, 400×).

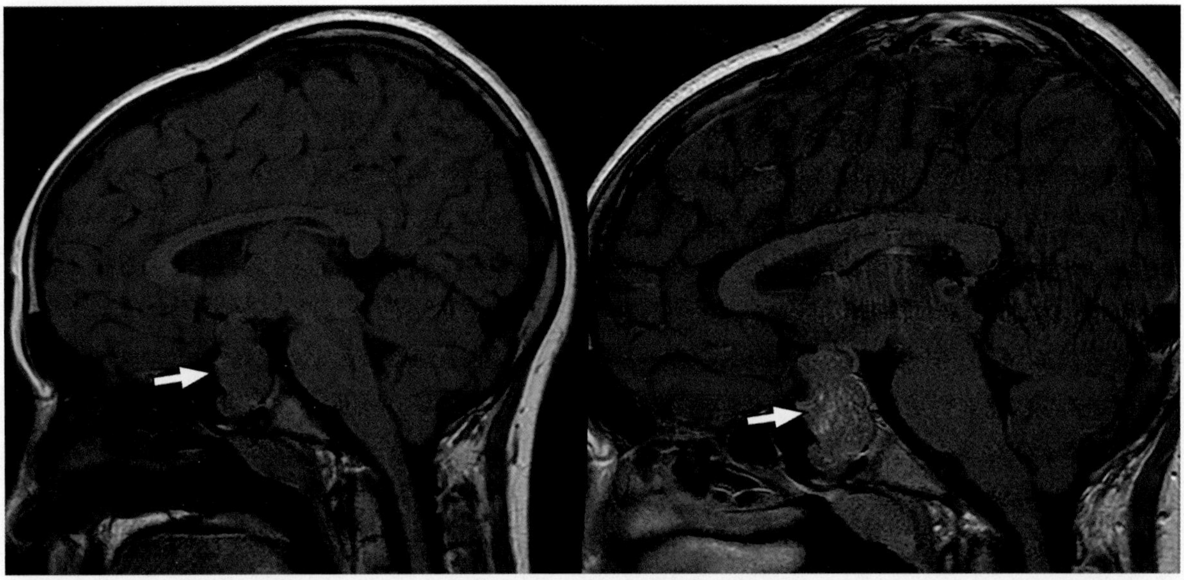

FIGURE 2.58 **Pituitary macroadenoma in a 16-year-old boy who presented with growth hormone deficiency.** Sagittal precontrast T1-weighted MR image (on the **left**) and sagittal postcontrast T1-weighted MR image (on the **right**) through the sella show a large, heterogeneous, partially-enhancing macrolobulated lesion (*arrows*) expanding the sella and extending superiorly into the suprasellar cistern and inferiorly into the sphenoid sinus.

MR images. Intracystic nodules have also been described, but may be difficult to visualize because of similar signal intensity of the cyst fluid and the nodule. Although imaging findings may be helpful for differentiating these lesions from other sellar or suprasellar lesions, radiologic findings can be nonspecific, and features can overlap with cystic craniopharyngiomas or cystic pituitary adenomas. Follow-up imaging is required in many cases, and occasionally, cyst aspiration may be required to establish a diagnosis.

Hypothalamic Hamartoma

Hypothalamic hamartoma (also called hamartoma of the tuber cinereum) is a rare lesion composed of nonneoplastic neuronal tissue, resulting from abnormal migration in the hypothalamus. Affected pediatric patients usually present in

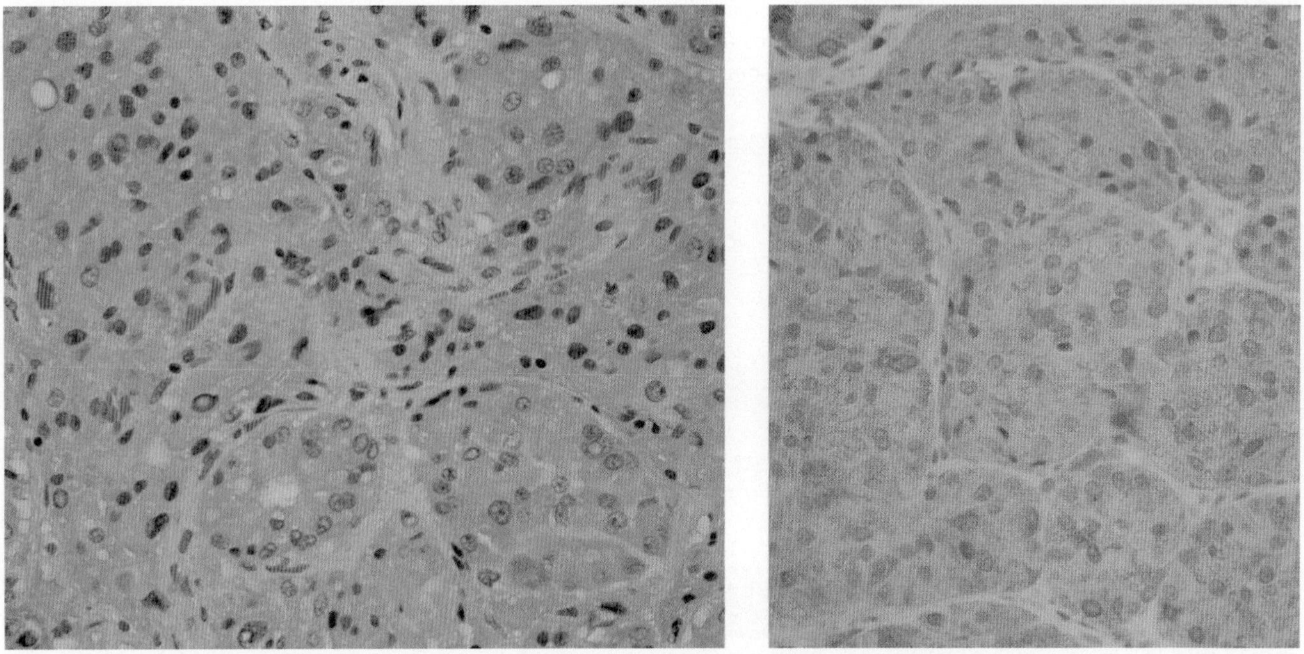

FIGURE 2.59 **Pituitary adenoma in a 13-year-old boy who presented with Cushing disease.** Resected mass demonstrates characteristic nests of cells showing abundant variably granular cytoplasm (**left**, hematoxylin and eosin, original magnification, 400×). Immunohistochemical staining shows brown cytoplasmic reactivity for adrenal corticotropic hormone (**right**, ACTH immunostain, original magnification, 400×).

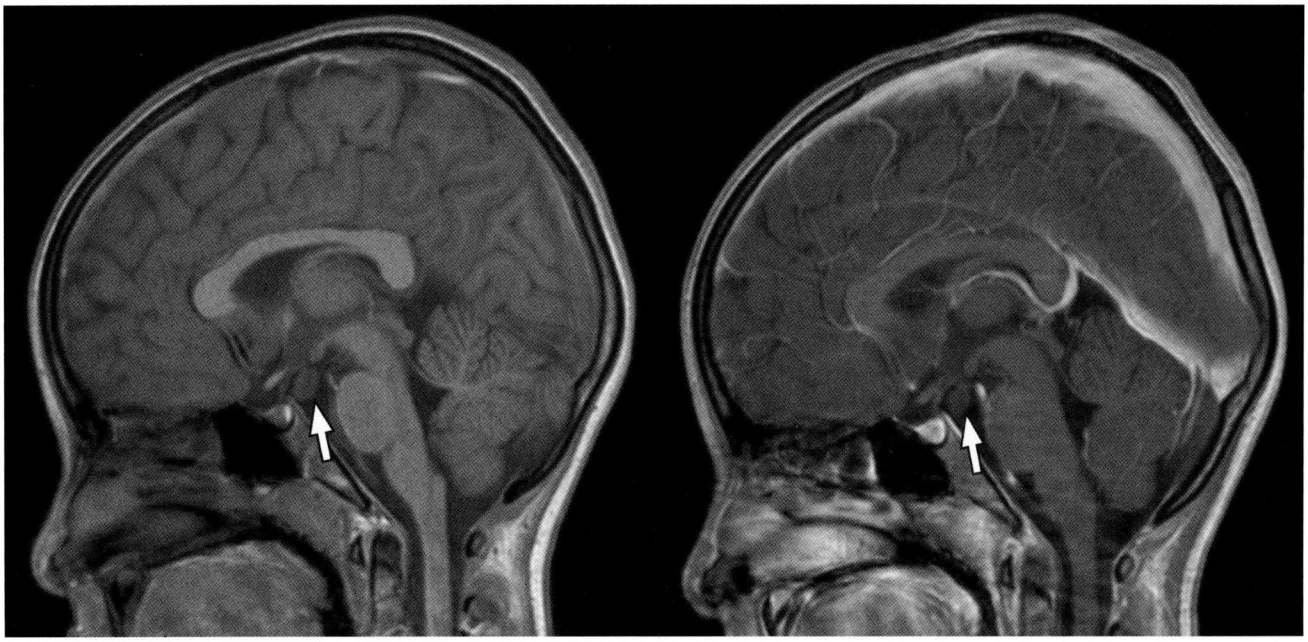

FIGURE 2.60 **Hypothalamic hamartoma in a 4-year-old boy who presented with precocious puberty.** Sagittal precontrast MPRAGE MR image (on the **left**) and sagittal postcontrast T1-weighted MR image (on the **right**) through the sella show a pedunculated, rounded, nonenhancing T1 isointense lesion (*arrows*) originating from the floor of the third ventricle.

the first decade of life, typically with precocious puberty and/or gelastic seizures. In the Pallister-Hall syndrome, there is an association of hypothalamic hamartomas with other associated congenital abnormalities including olfactory bulb hypoplasia, pituitary, thyroid and adrenal gland aplasia, cardiac and renal anomalies, imperforate anus, craniofacial anomalies, syndactyly, and short metacarpals.

On CT, hypothalamic hamartomas appear as gray matter lesions in the suprasellar region. On MRI, they are characterized by a mass centered at or pedunculated from the floor of the third ventricle (Fig. 2.60). The lesions are isointense to gray matter on T1-weighted MR images and isointense or slight hyperintense to gray matter on T2-weighted MR images. Typically, these lesions do not enhance following contrast administration. Presence of enhancement should suggest an alternative diagnosis such as Langerhans cell histiocytosis or germinoma.

Surgical resection is the current management of choice for hypothalamic hamartoma. Options for surgical treatment are complete or partial resection using a transcallosal or other approach, gamma knife radiosurgery, endoscopic disconnection, and, most recently, MRI-guided laser ablation.

Pineal Region Tumors

Pineal Cyst

Pineal cysts are the most common benign findings in the pineal gland, found incidentally on imaging studies. On MRI, they are characterized by hypointensity on T1 and hyperintensity on T2-weighted MR images. Although a thin rim of enhancement of the wall may be seen, there is no nodular enhancement within the cyst. Spontaneous bleeding can occur into the cyst and can cause alteration of the signal intensity so that it does not strictly follow the signal of CSF. There is no need for follow-up in most cases.

Pineal Gland Tumor

Pineoblastomas are rare malignant neoplastic lesions that account for 0.1% of all CNS tumors.[66] They arise in the pineal gland and consist of poorly differentiated small round blue cells (Fig. 2.61). They often differ from other CNS embryonal tumors by showing a greater degree of photosensory differentiation.[67] They are classified as WHO grade IV tumors. On MRI, these lesions are hypointense or isointense on T1-weighted MR images and demonstrate variable low, high, or mixed signal on T2-weighted MR images (Fig. 2.62). Pineoblastomas have lobulated contours and enhance homogenously. Drop metastases are seen throughout the neuraxis in 10% to 20% of patients with pineoblastoma.[68] Therefore, imaging of the entire neuraxis at presentation is imperative in these cases. Peripheral displacement of pineal gland calcification, termed the "exploded pineal pattern" of calcification, is more typical of pineal parenchymal tumors, effectively differentiating them from germ cell tumors.

Pineoblastomas are resected surgically with adjuvant craniospinal radiation and multiagent chemotherapy. Prognosis is relatively poor.

Germ Cell Tumor

Germ cell tumors are the most common pineal region tumors. Sixty-five percent are pure germinomas.[69,70] Other types of CNS germ cell tumor include teratoma (mature and immature variants), embryonal carcinoma, yolk sac tumor, choriocarcinoma, and mixed CNS germ cell tumor.[70]

Pure germinomas are hyperdense on CT and enhance homogenously. On MRI, they are isointense to gray matter

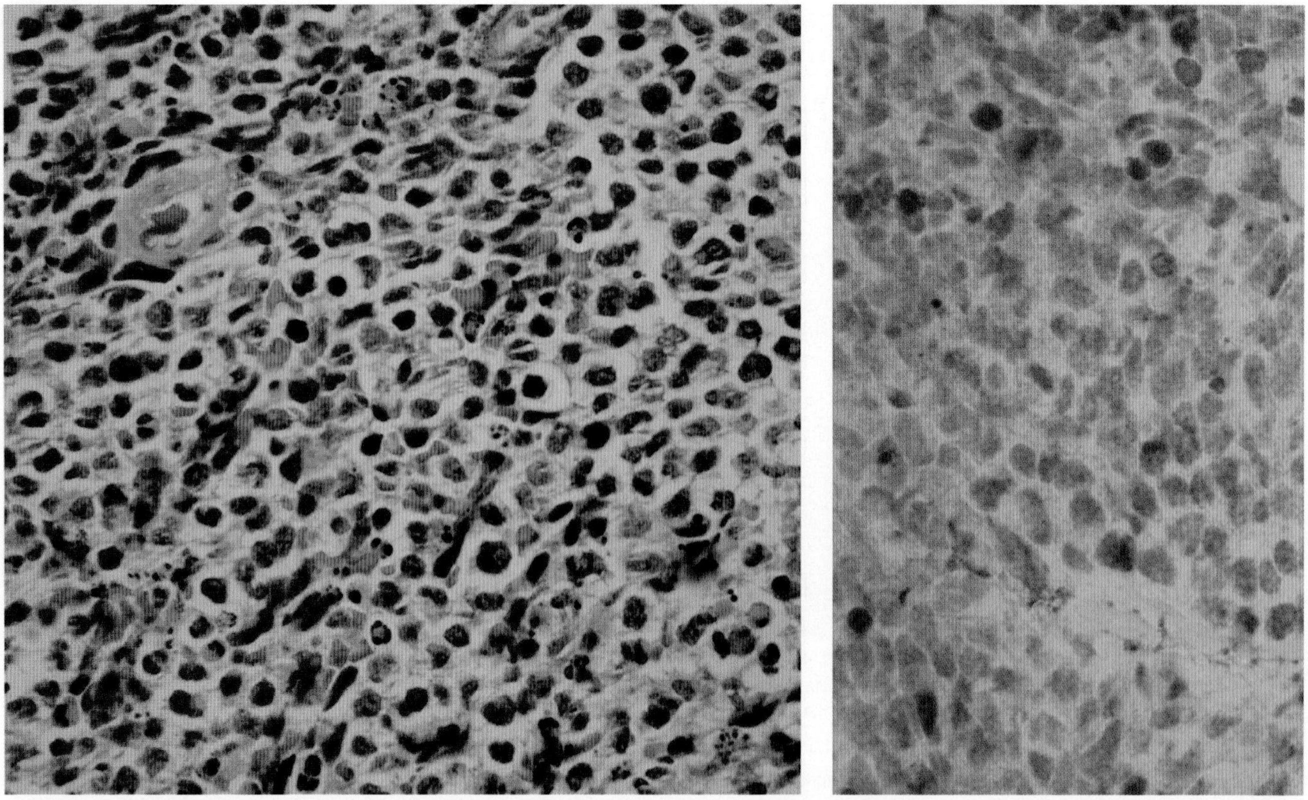

FIGURE 2.61 **Pineoblastoma.** Biopsy specimen from the patient in the preceding image (Figure 2.60) shows the characteristic dense collection of small round blue tumor cells with high nucleus-to-cytoplasm ratios, frequent mitoses, and focal necrosis (**left**, hematoxylin and eosin, original magnification, 600×). Immunohistochemical staining shows strong CRX expression, reflecting photosensory differentiation (**right**, CRX immunostain, original magnification, 600×).

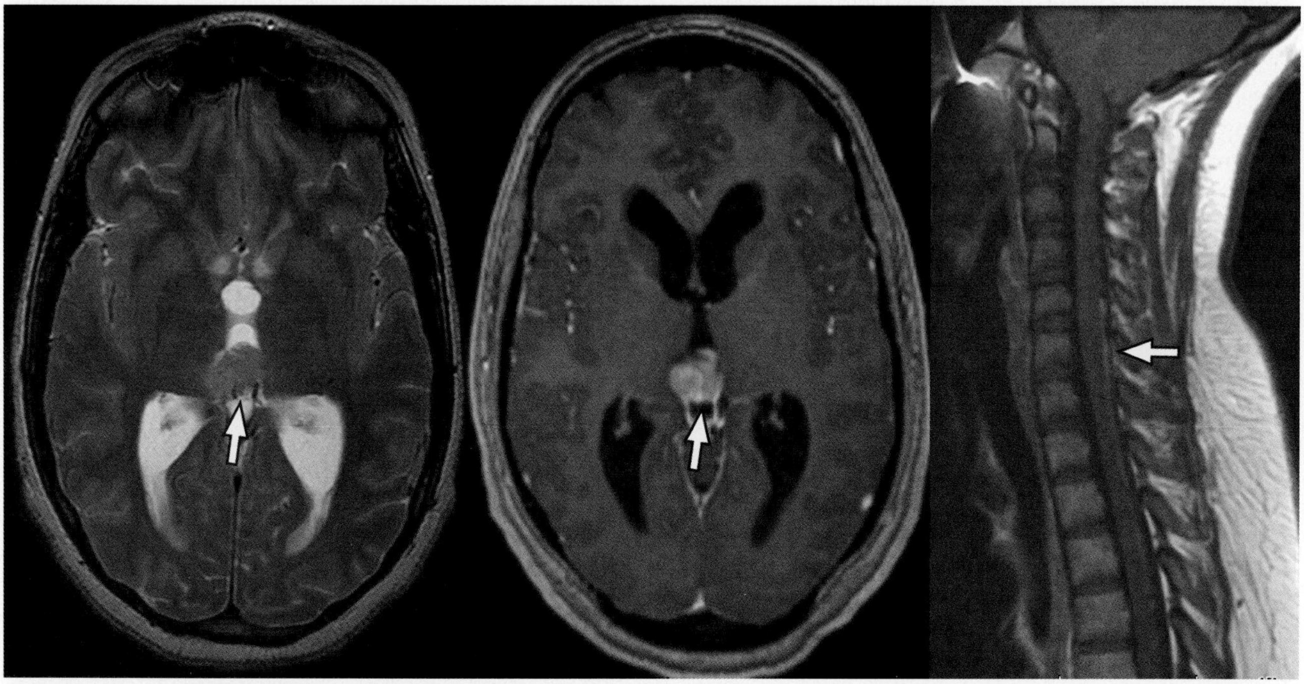

FIGURE 2.62 **Pineoblastoma in a 17-year-old girl.** Axial T2-weighted MR image (on the **left**) and axial postcontrast T1-weighted MR image (in the **middle**) show a T2 hypointense enhancing mass (*arrows*). Sagittal T1 postcontrast MR image (on the **right**) through the cervical spine demonstrates drop metastases (*arrow*) along the surface of the spinal cord.

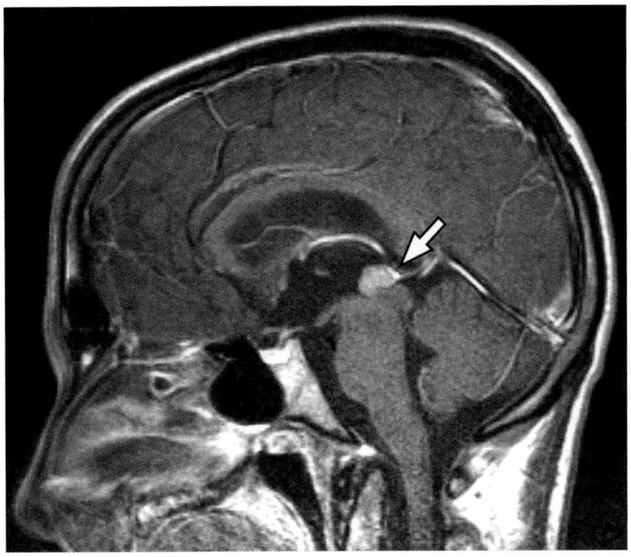

FIGURE 2.63 **Pineal germinoma in a 12-year-old girl who presented with headaches and vomiting.** Sagittal postcontrast T1-weighted MR image shows a homogeneously enhancing pineal mass (*arrow*).

on all sequences and enhance avidly on postcontrast images (Figs. 2.63 and 2.64). They grow anteriorly into the floor of the third ventricle and may infiltrate the thalami and midbrain. Spinal dissemination is relatively common.

Imaging appearances of nongerminomatous germ cell tumors (NGGCTs) are nonspecific. Intratumoral cysts and calcifications are relatively common. Teratomas are heterogeneous and contain fat, cysts, and calcification; they also demonstrate variable enhancement. The presence of hemorrhage suggests a component of choriocarcinoma.

In the past, pediatric patients with imaging findings typical of CNS germinoma were treated empirically with radiation therapy. Today, confirmation of the histologic type prior to treatment is preferred. Stereotactic biopsy is used to acquire tissue with minimal morbidity. Germinomas are highly responsive to radiation therapy. A complete response with a 5-year survival of more than 90% is seen with radiation therapy alone.[71] NGGCTs are less radiosensitive than pure germinomas, with an overall 5-year survival of 30% to 40%.[72] Treatment options for NGGCTs include chemotherapy followed by radiation therapy, with adjuvant surgery or high-dose chemotherapy with stem cell rescue for nonresponsive or high-risk germ cell tumors.[73]

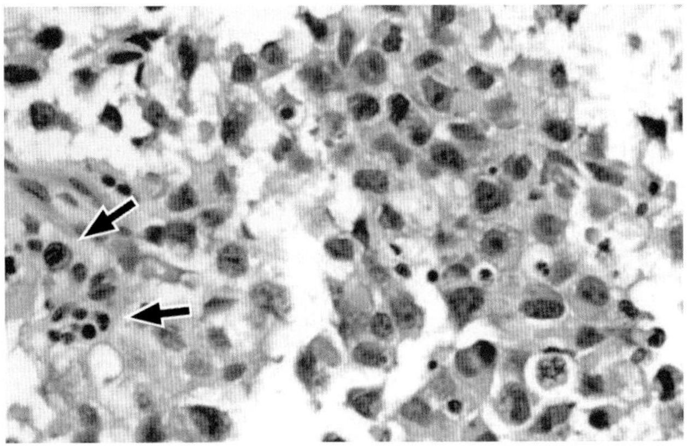

FIGURE 2.64 **Pineal germinoma in a 16-year-old boy.** This biopsy of a pineal region mass shows a pure germinoma, characterized by cells with large round vesicular nuclei and prominent nucleoli; lymphocytes (*lower arrow*) and plasma cells (*upper arrow*) were admixed (hematoxylin and eosin, original magnification, 400x).

Tectal Glioma

Tectal glioma is a tumor centered in the midbrain that can cause obstructive hydrocephalus and raised intracranial pressure as a result of aqueductal stenosis. These tumors present as T1 isointense and T2 hyperintense expansions of the tectum without appreciable enhancement in the initial stages (Fig. 2.65). Most children with these tumors are managed conservatively by treating the hydrocephalus with endoscopic third ventriculostomy or by placement of a ventricular shunt and careful follow-up of the tumor with imaging studies at regular intervals.

Intraventricular Tumors

Choroid Plexus Tumor

Choroid plexus tumors account for ~3% of pediatric brain tumors. Up to 90% of choroid plexus tumors are papillomas, and the rest are choroid plexus carcinomas.[74] More recently, a third type of choroid plexus tumor called atypical choroid plexus papilloma has been described.[75] 70% of all choroid plexus papillomas occur in children younger than 2 years. Rarely, these tumors are diagnosed in the fetal period.[76]

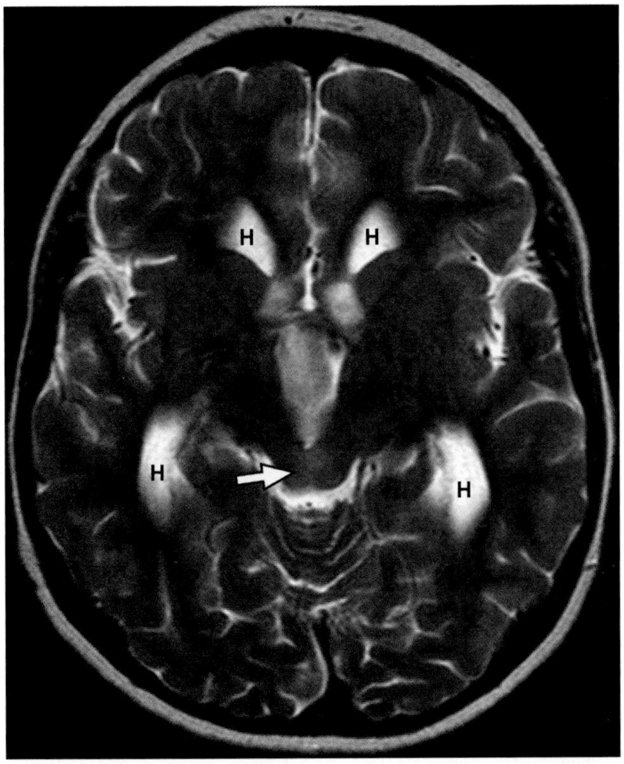

FIGURE 2.65 **Tectal glioma in a 9-year-old boy.** Axial T2-weighted MR image shows a T2 hyperintense lesion (*arrow*) in the tectal region causing hydrocephalus (*H*).

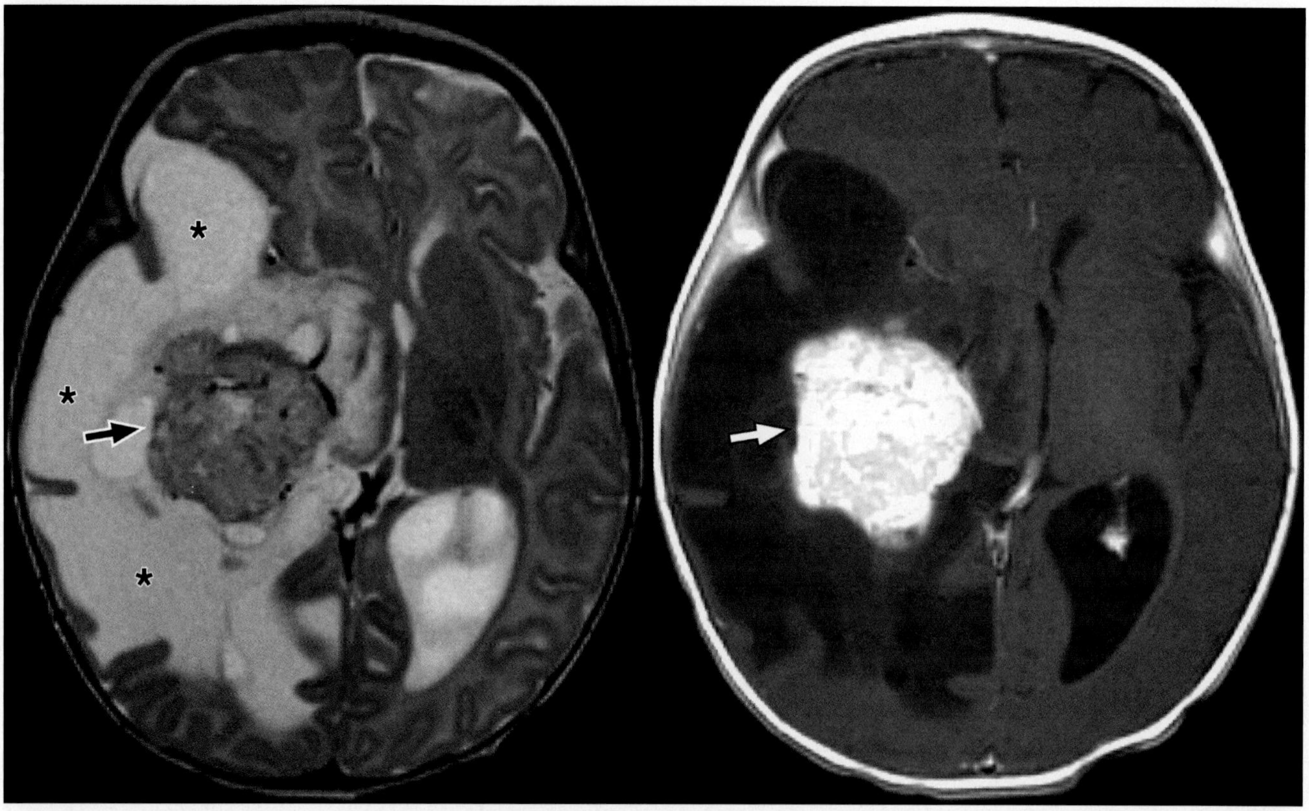

FIGURE 2.66 **Choroid plexus papilloma in a 3-month-old girl who presented with increased head circumference and abnormal gaze.** Axial T2-weighted MR image (on the **left**) and axial postcontrast T1-weighted MR image (on the **right**) show a large lobulated mass (*arrows*) centered within the right lateral ventricle with multiple flow voids and avid enhancement. Note extensive T2 hyperintensity (*asterisks*) in the surrounding brain parenchyma, which reflects CSF secreted from the tumor.

These tumors most commonly occur in the trigone of the lateral ventricles in children, whereas they are most common in the fourth ventricle in adults. On CT, choroid plexus papillomas are typically isodense to hyperdense lobulated masses that homogenously enhance after contrast administration and may have punctate calcifications. On MR, these tumors present as homogeneous, enhancing intraventricular masses that are predominantly hyperintense on T2-weighted MR images and hypointense on T1-weighted MR images (Fig. 2.66). They are characterized by areas of heterogeneous signal intensity on both T1- and T2-weighted MR images because of hemorrhage and necrosis. MRS may help distinguish between papillomas and carcinomas. The myo-inositol (mI) level is significantly higher in choroid plexus papillomas than in choroid plexus carcinomas. On the other hand, carcinomas have significantly elevated levels of choline compared to papillomas (Fig. 2.67). Spinal drop metastases can occur in both choroid plexus papilloma and carcinomas, though are seen more frequently in carcinoma. The entire neuraxis should therefore be imaged in all pediatric patients with suspected choroid plexus neoplasms before surgical intervention.

Histologically, choroid plexus papilloma resembles normal choroid plexus, with a frond-like connective tissue core covered by a single layer of cuboidal epithelium; cytologic atypia is mild and mitotic rate is low (Fig. 2.68). Choroid plexus carcinoma may show frequent mitoses, cellular crowding, nuclear pleomorphism, and necrosis (Fig. 2.69).

Ependymoma

Ependymomas originate from the ependymal cells lining the ventricular system, most commonly from the floor of the fourth ventricle. Imaging features are described subsequently in the section on posterior fossa ependymomas.

Central Neurocytomas

Central neurocytomas have been discussed in a prior section on neuronal and neuronal–glial tumors.

Subependymal Giant Cell Astrocytoma

These lesions are seen almost exclusively in pediatric patients with tuberous sclerosis and will be discussed subsequently in the section on neurocutaneous syndromes.

Posterior Fossa Tumors

Medulloblastoma

Medulloblastoma is an aggressive embryonal neuroepithelial tumor (WHO grade IV) arising from the cerebellum, with a tendency to disseminate throughout the CNS early in its course. It is the most common malignant brain tumor in children, accounting for nearly 40% of all posterior fossa tumors and ~10% to 20% of all pediatric brain tumors.[77]

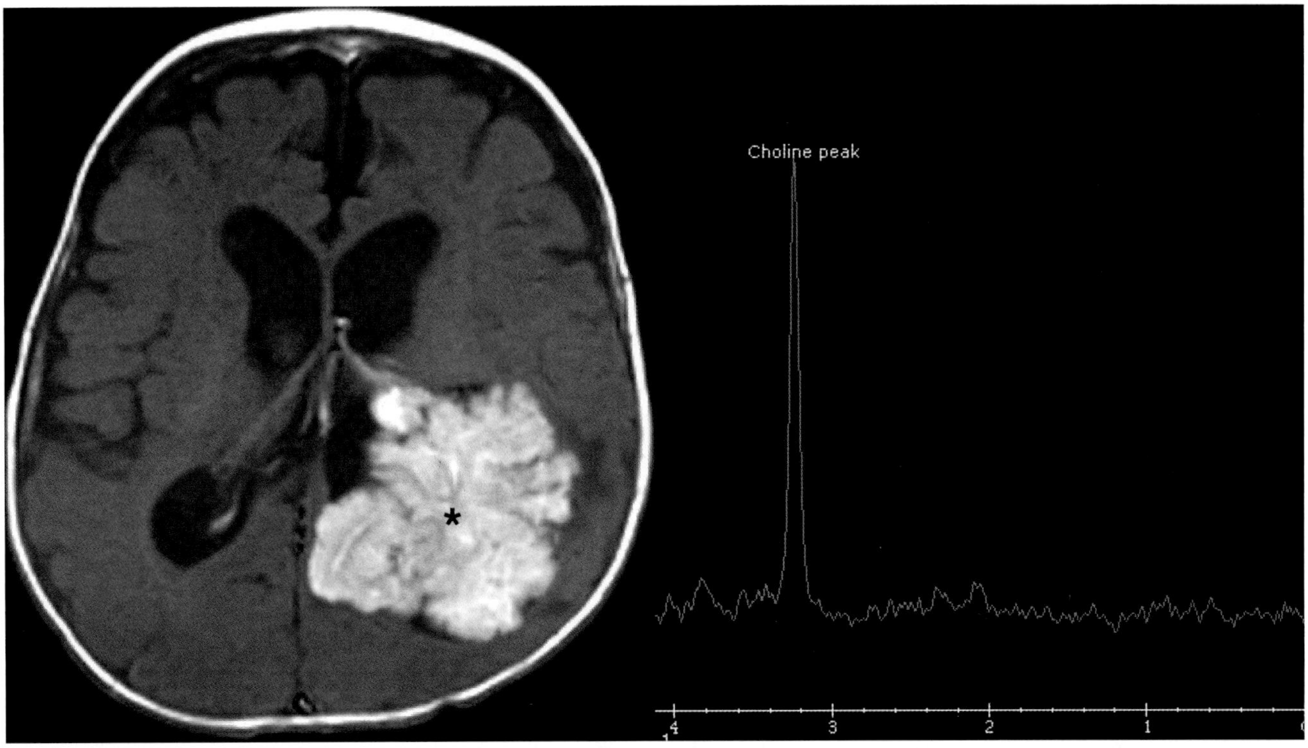

FIGURE 2.67 **Choroid plexus carcinoma in a 4-month-old girl.** Axial postcontrast T1-weighted MR image (on the **left**) shows a large, avidly enhancing mass lesion (*asterisk*) centered within the left lateral ventricle. Single voxel spectroscopy (on the **right**) obtained from the center of the lesion demonstrates a markedly elevated choline peak suggestive of a choroid plexus carcinoma.

Medulloblastomas can be classified based on their histopathologic characteristics into the classic type and four variants including desmoplastic/nodular medulloblastoma, medulloblastoma with extensive nodularity (MBEN), anaplastic medulloblastoma, and large cell medulloblastoma. All types of medulloblastomas are characterized by densely arranged primitive cells with high nucleus-to-cytoplasm ratios (Fig. 2.70). More recently, medulloblastomas have been characterized into major molecular subgroups that are based on various signaling pathways, including the Shh (sonic hedgehog pathway), Wnt (Wingless), ERBB2 (receptor kinase family), and non-Shh/Wnt subtypes. Affected pediatric patients typically present with signs and symptoms of raised intracranial pressure. Cranial nerve dysfunction with difficulty swallowing and nasal speech may also occur.

Medulloblastomas usually arise in the midline within the vermis and grow into the fourth ventricle resulting in obstructive hydrocephalus. In older patients and in those

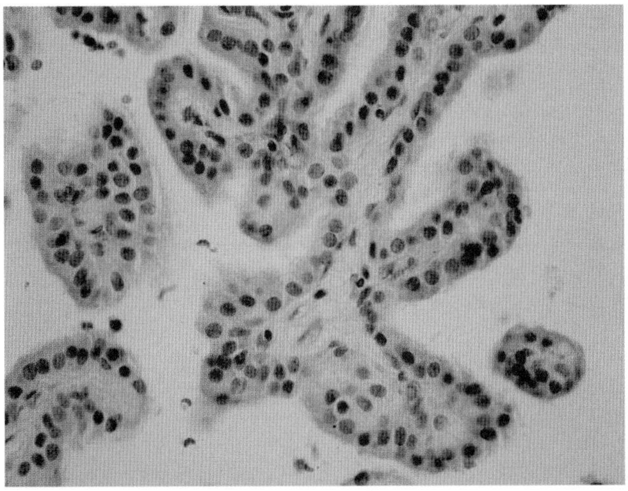

FIGURE 2.68 **Choroid plexus papilloma in a 15-year-old girl.** This intraventricular mass shows a delicate papillary architecture (similar to normal choroid plexus), as well as small and regular nuclei (hematoxylin and eosin, original magnification, 600×).

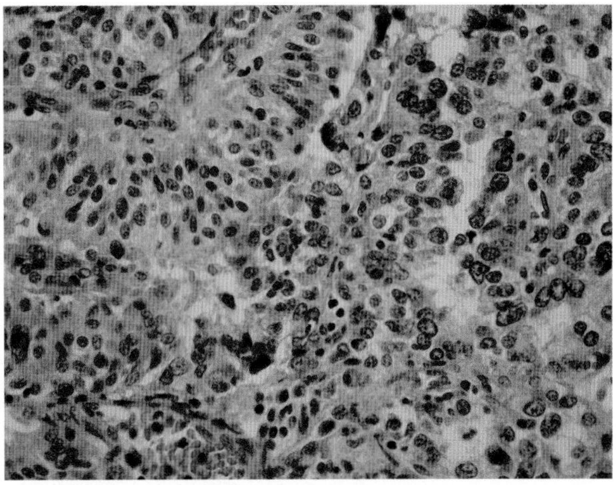

FIGURE 2.69 **Choroid plexus carcinoma in a 1-year-old boy.** This intraventricular mass shows both papillary and sheet-like areas of growth. In areas, there is increased nuclear density, size, and mitotic rate (hematoxylin and eosin, original magnification, 600×).

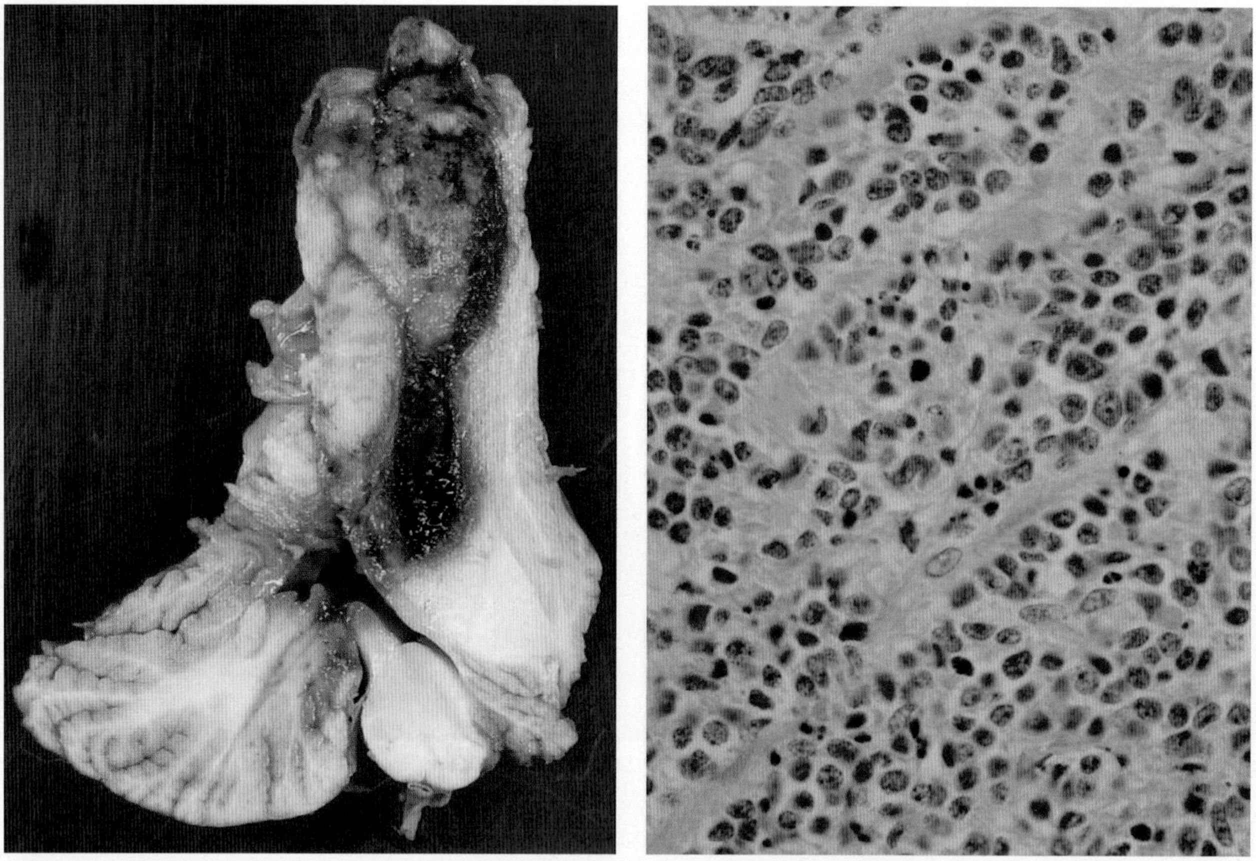

FIGURE 2.70 **Medulloblastoma in a 10-year-old boy who died 6 years after initial diagnosis.** Autopsy specimen (on the **left**) shows the cerebellum and brainstem, which were affected by a large, variegated gray-tan mass with associated hemorrhage. Microscopic examination (on the **right**) showed densely packed primitive small round blue cells (hematoxylin and eosin, original magnification, 600×).

with the desmoplastic subtype, they are localized to the cerebellar hemispheres. On CT, medulloblastomas are hyperdense because of high cellularity, and enhance avidly on postcontrast images. On MRI, they are characteristically hypointense relative to gray matter on both T1- and T2-weighted MR images, with homogeneous enhancement following contrast administration (Fig. 2.71). Imaging of the entire neuraxis should be performed, as the incidence of CSF dissemination at diagnosis is between 20% and 30% at presentation.[78]

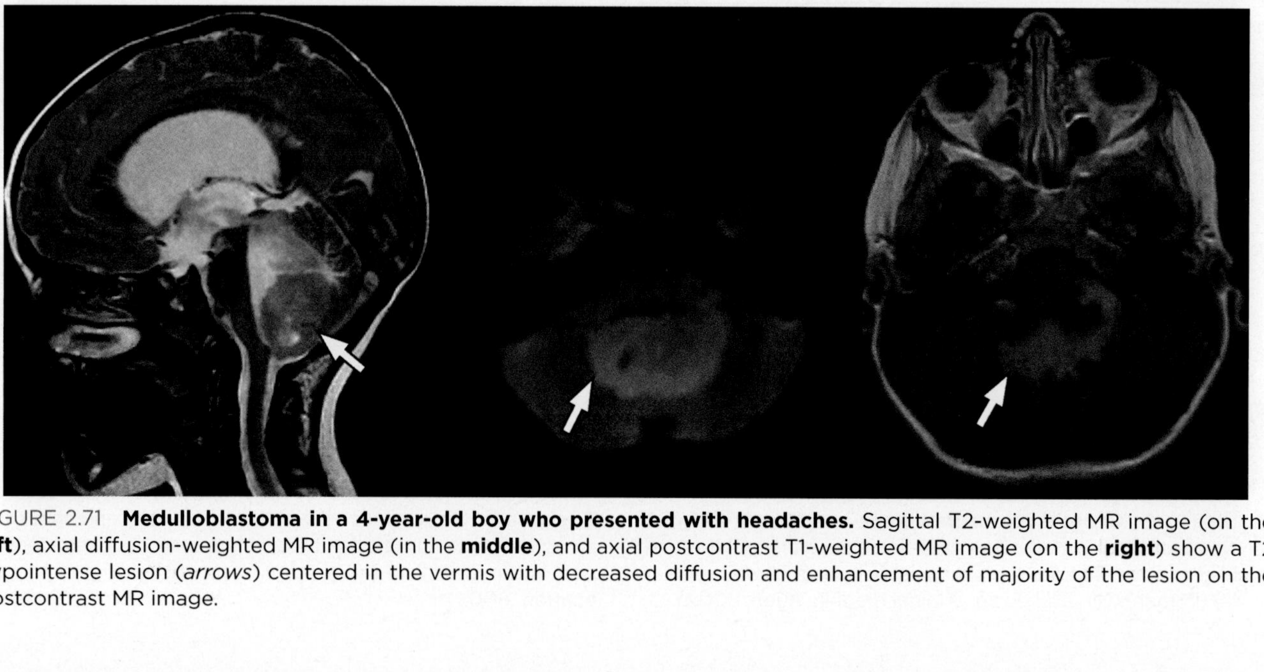

FIGURE 2.71 **Medulloblastoma in a 4-year-old boy who presented with headaches.** Sagittal T2-weighted MR image (on the **left**), axial diffusion-weighted MR image (in the **middle**), and axial postcontrast T1-weighted MR image (on the **right**) show a T2 hypointense lesion (*arrows*) centered in the vermis with decreased diffusion and enhancement of majority of the lesion on the postcontrast MR image.

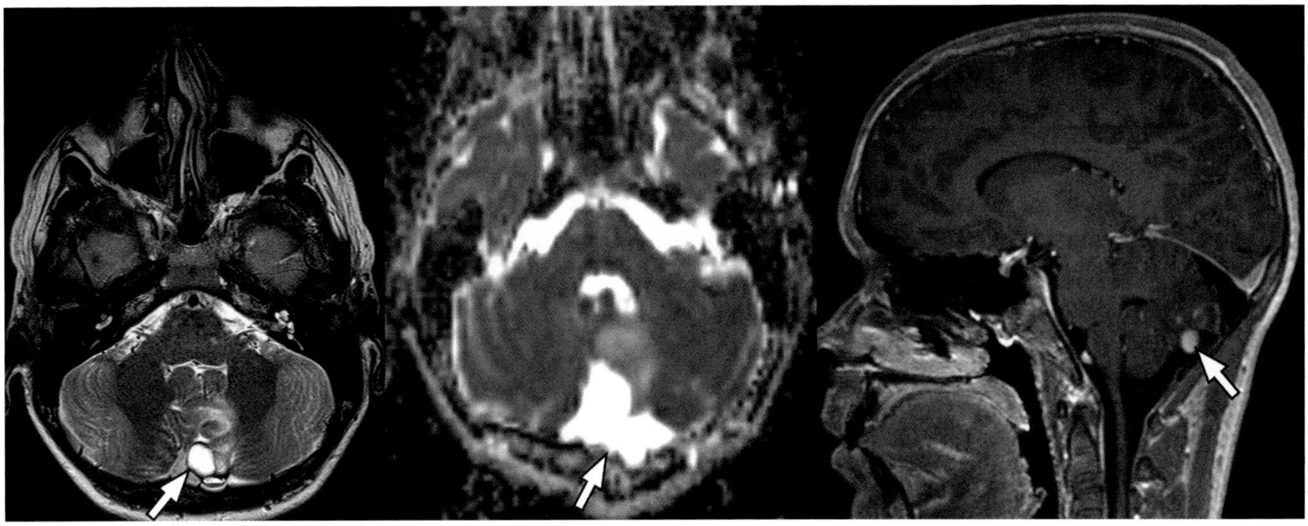

FIGURE 2.72 **Juvenile pilocytic astrocytoma in a 13-year-old boy.** Axial T2-weighted MR image (on the **left**), ADC image (in the **middle**), and sagittal postcontrast MPRAGE (magnetization-prepared rapid acquisition gradient-echo) MR image (on the **right**) show a T2 hyperintense mass (*arrows*) with increased diffusion values and enhancing nodules in the posterior fossa, consistent with a juvenile pilocytic astrocytoma.

Treatment of medulloblastoma consists of a combination of surgery, radiation therapy, and chemotherapy. High-risk features include younger age at diagnosis, incomplete resection or postoperative tumor residuum >1.5 cm^2, and metastatic disease.[79] The integration of histologic subtype with molecular data also permits stratification into low-, standard-, and high-risk tumors for prognostic and therapeutic consideration.[74,80]

Posterior Fossa Astrocytoma

Pilocytic astrocytomas make up the majority of pediatric low-grade gliomas and are classified as grade I WHO tumors. Overall, grade I tumors account for up to 20% to 30% of all childhood brain tumors.[42] Approximately 60% of all pediatric astrocytomas are located in the posterior fossa (including the cerebellum and brainstem). Peak incidence is in the first decade of life, although they remain common in young teenagers. Tumors in older children are more likely to be anaplastic astrocytomas. The most common presentation is of progressively increasing early morning headaches and vomiting over several weeks. Cerebellar signs may be present on examination. Occasionally, more acute presentation is seen with marked obstructive hydrocephalus and brain herniation.

On imaging studies, posterior fossa pilocytic astrocytomas are typically large cystic lesions centered within the vermis or cerebellar hemispheres. Single or multiple enhancing mural nodules may be present (Fig. 2.72). Leptomeningeal spread can be seen in rare cases at presentation. The more recently described pilomyxoid variant of astrocytoma can present with diffuse leptomeningeal spread and diencephalic syndrome. Although pilomyxoid astrocytomas have an indolent course, their propensity for slow-growing, persistent recurrences makes them difficult to treat.

Histologically, pilocytic astrocytomas are moderately cellular neoplasms characterized by two patterns of growth, including more densely packed bipolar cells with Rosenthal fibers and more loosely arranged multipolar cells with associated microcysts and eosinophilic granular bodies (Fig. 2.73). Total surgical resection is often curative.

Posterior Fossa Ependymoma

Ependymomas are tumors that arise from the ventricular ependymal lining. Ependymal tumors represent ~6% of

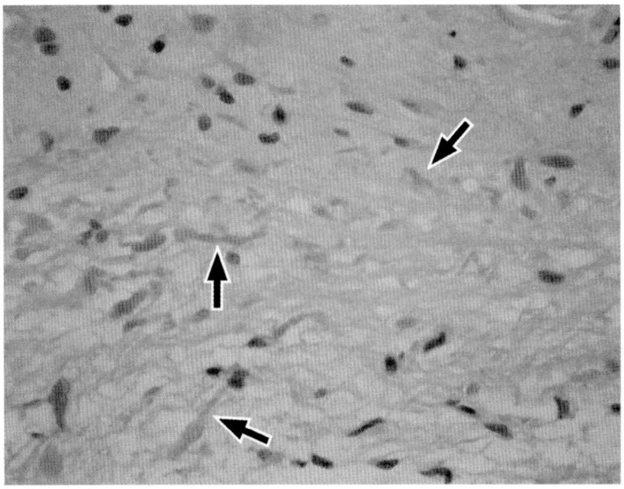

FIGURE 2.73 **Pilocytic astrocytoma resected from the posterior fossa of a 4-year-old boy.** A biphasic pattern is seen; compact areas with elongated, frequently bipolar cells alternate with looser areas showing round to oval cells. The characteristic "hair-like" (piloid) eosinophilic structures called Rosenthal fibers (*arrows*) are admixed (hematoxylin and eosin, original magnification, 600x).

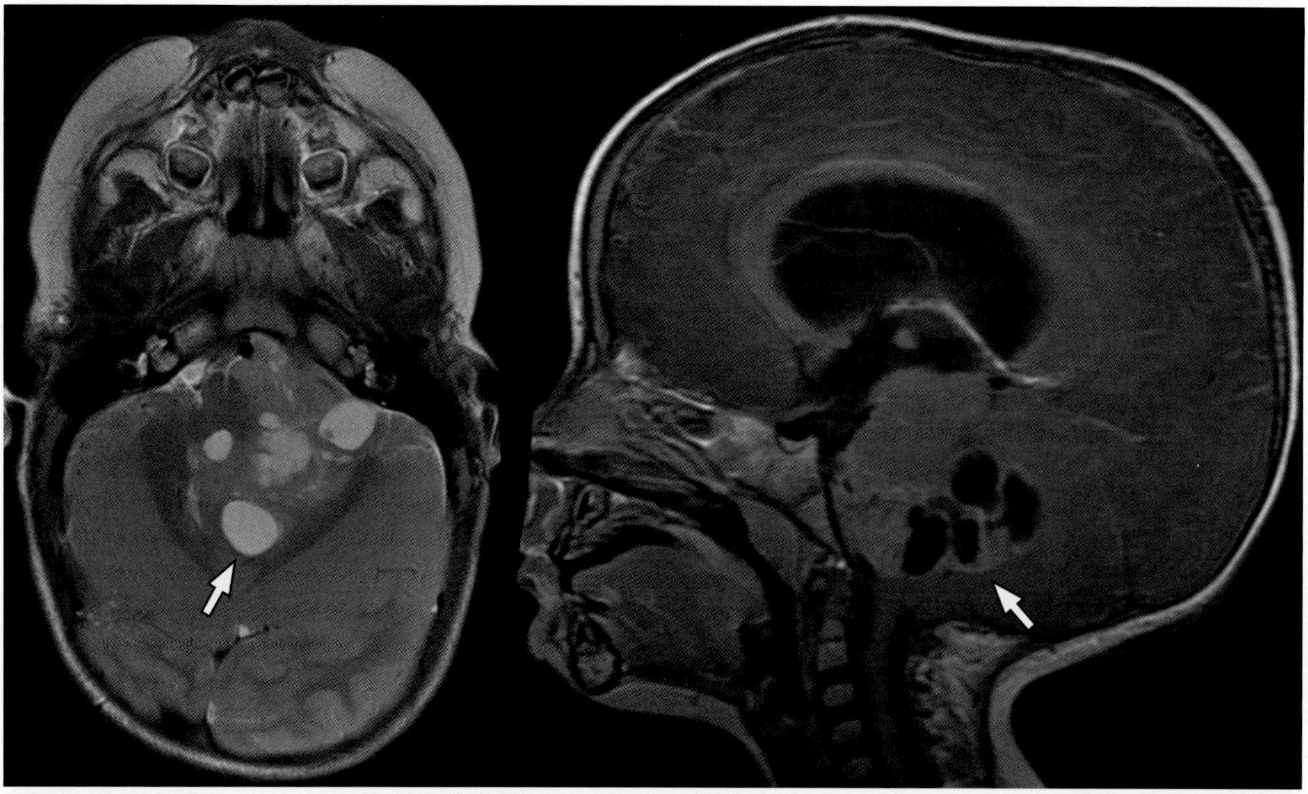

FIGURE 2.74 **Anaplastic ependymoma in the pons and prepontine region.** Axial T2-weighted MR image (on the **left**) and sagittal postcontrast T1 SPACE (sampling perfection with application-optimized contrast using different flip-angle evolution) MR image (on the **right**) demonstrate a heterogeneous lesion (*arrows*) with solid and cystic components extending toward the foramina of Luschka, with enhancement of the solid components following contrast administration.

all childhood intracranial neoplasms.[47] Ninety percent of pediatric ependymomas are intracranial, with 66% to 75% arising from the posterior fossa.[81] Presentation is usually insidious, with progressive development of signs and symptoms related to increased intracranial pressure, including headaches, vomiting, behavioral disturbances, and cerebellar signs like ataxia.

Posterior fossa ependymomas are typically seen as iso- to hyperdense (to gray matter) fourth ventricular masses with punctate calcification, small cysts, and moderate, heterogeneous enhancement on postcontrast images. On MRI, they may be homogenous or heterogeneous masses, isointense to gray matter on T2-weighted MR images and hypointense on T1-weighted MR images. Extension of "tongues" of tumor into the foramina of Luschka and Magendie is helpful in distinguishing these tumors from other posterior fossa masses (Figs. 2.74 and 2.75). Foci of high signal indicating necrosis or cysts and low signal intensity indicating hemorrhage or calcification may be seen. Ependymomas demonstrate significantly higher ADC values than those in medulloblastomas and lower ADC values than those in astrocytomas. Heterogeneous enhancement is seen on postcontrast T1-weighted MR images. Ependymomas are disseminated into the CSF spaces in 8 to 12% of patients at diagnosis, with a lower incidence (<5%) of symptomatic leptomeningeal disease.[82,83]

Complete surgical resection followed by adjuvant therapies has been shown to offer the best prognosis in pediatric patients with posterior fossa ependymomas, who tend to harbor a worse prognosis than adult patients with the same tumor.

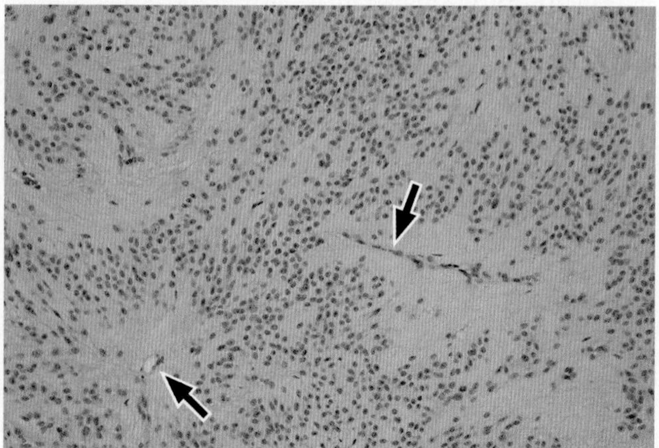

FIGURE 2.75 **Ependymoma in a 6-year-old girl.** Mass resected from the frontal lobe shows monotonous round cells in a fibrillary background. Tumor cell nuclei are often arranged around hypocellular fibrillary areas with central vessels (*arrows*), forming "perivascular pseudorosettes" (hematoxylin and eosin, original magnification, 200x).

Brainstem Glioma

Brainstem tumors can be divided into four types based on their imaging appearances, namely, focal, dorsal exophytic, cervicomedullary, and diffuse intrinsic pontine glioma (DIPG). They account for up to 10% of all brain tumors in children.[47] DIPGs are discussed in more detail, as there are specific imaging and clinical characteristics of these tumors that are important to recognize. Other types of brainstem gliomas have similar characteristics to other gliomas, which are discussed elsewhere in this chapter.

As their name indicates, DIPGs are infiltrative masses that are typically centered in the pons. Presenting signs and symptoms can be varied and include cranial nerve palsies, pyramidal tract signs, and cerebellar dysfunction (nystagmus and ataxia).

On CT, pontine gliomas are hypo- or isodense to gray matter. On MRI, they are isointense to hypointense on T1-weighted MR images and hyperintense on T2-weighted MR images (Fig. 2.76). They typically do not enhance or enhance minimally at presentation. In the later stages of tumor progression, enhancement and necrosis may be seen more frequently. Calcification and hemorrhage are rare.

Because of their location in the brainstem, pontine gliomas were considered inoperable until recently. However, there have been several cases of successful biopsy in recent years using stereotactic and microsurgical neurosurgical techniques.

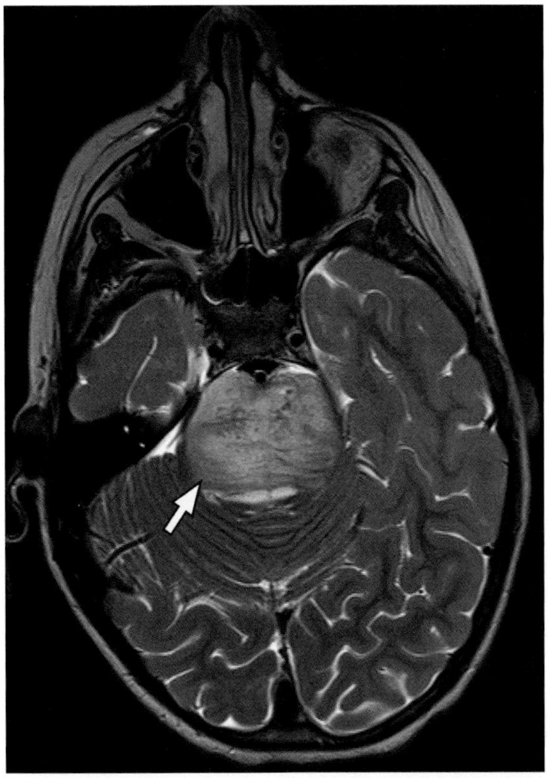

FIGURE 2.76 **Diffuse intrinsic pontine glioma in a 6-year-old boy who presented with swallowing difficulties and signs of cranial nerve dysfunction.** Axial T2-weighted MR image shows an infiltrative lesion (*arrow*) filling and expanding the pons.

Initial response to radiation therapy is good and has improved the median overall survival from weeks to months. Various adjuvant therapies have been tried, but have not resulted in significantly improved patient outcomes.

Atypical Teratoid/Rhabdoid Tumor

Atypical teratoid/rhabdoid tumors (ATRTs) are highly malignant tumors predominantly seen in young children, with a peak incidence between birth and 3 years. These tumors account for ~1% of CNS tumors in children and ~10% of CNS tumors in infants.[84] A majority of ATRTs (60%) are located in the posterior fossa. However, ATRTs are seen at other locations within the CNS including the pineal and suprasellar regions, and the spine.

On T1-weighted MR images, ATRTs are characterized by heterogeneous intermediate signal intensity, admixed with varying areas of low and high signal intensity from cystic change and/or necrosis. On T2-weighted MR images, solid portions of ATRTs have heterogeneous intermediate to slightly high signal intensity with additional zones of T2 hyper- and hypointensity secondary to varying amounts of cystic change, necrosis, edema, prior hemorrhage, and/or calcification (Fig. 2.77).[85] Relative T2-intermediate to hypointense signal seen in the solid areas is attributable to the tumor's highly cellular nature and is associated with restricted diffusion. Imaging of the entire neuraxis is important, because subarachnoid spread throughout the CNS with spinal drop metastases is common, with reported frequency ranging between 25% and 46% (84, 85).

ATRTs are primitive tumors that may show differentiation along epithelial, mesenchymal, neuronal, or glial cell lines. They are a morphologically heterogeneous group; a histologic hallmark is the "rhabdoid" cell, which resembles skeletal muscle because of an intracytoplasmic eosinophilic inclusion, that often indents the nucleus (Fig. 2.78). Nucleoli are usually prominent. ATRTs are characterized by deletion or mutation of the *INI1/hSNF5* gene at chromosome 22q11.2 in ~75% of cases. Loss of expression of the protein INI1 is seen in virtually all ATRTs and is helpful in confirming the diagnosis.[86]

Most patients with ATRTs succumb to their disease. However, in recent years, prognosis for patients with CNS ATRT has improved from historically reported average survival periods ranging from 0.5 to 11 months with the availability of multimodal treatments.[87]

Miscellaneous Extra-axial Tumors

Teratoma

Teratomas are neoplasms consisting of differentiated tissues derived from all three germ layers. They are the most common intracranial tumors occurring in neonates and the second most common germ cell tumors of the pineal region. Benign teratomas have a characteristic heterogeneous appearance on cross-sectional imaging studies, caused by the presence of cystic, solid, fatty, and mineralized tissues (Fig. 2.79). The presence of fat in the lesion is the most useful finding. The presence of a solid, enhancing component

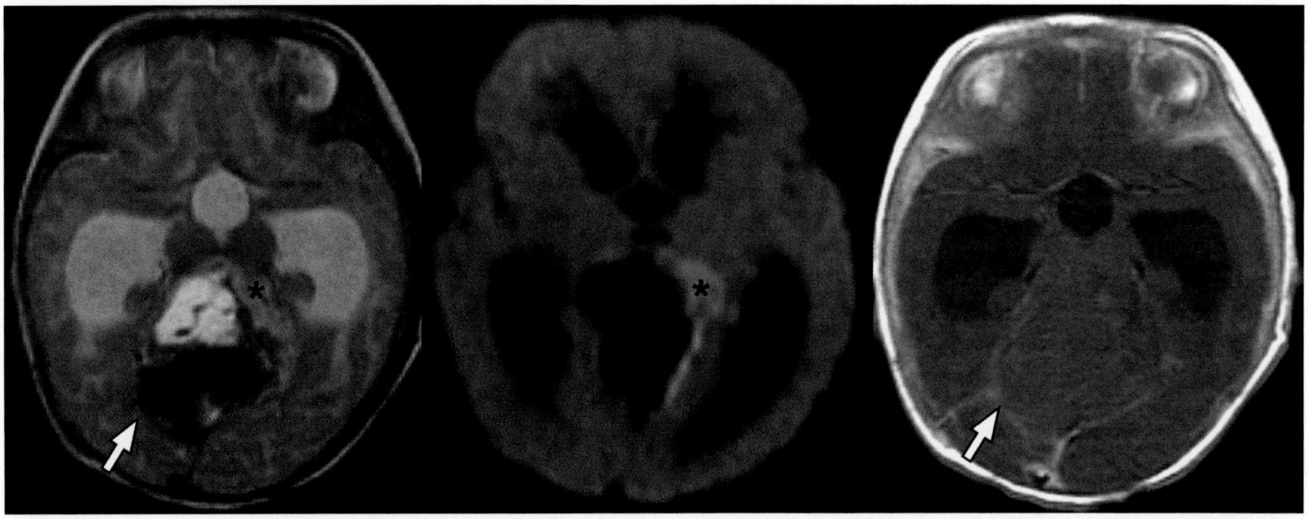

FIGURE 2.77 **Atypical teratoid rhabdoid tumor in an 8-week-old girl who presented with lethargy and bulging anterior fontanelle.** Axial T2-weighted MR image (on the **left**), axial diffusion-weighted MR image (in the **middle**), and axial postcontrast T1-weighted MR image (on the **right**) show a hemorrhagic mass (*arrows*) with solid components (*asterisk*) characterized by decreased diffusion and patchy enhancement following contrast administration.

helps differentiate teratomas from dermoid cysts and lipomas. Teratomas are divided into mature and immature types, depending on whether the tissues in the lesion resemble mature adult tissue or immature embryonic tissue. Malignant teratomas are seen as predominantly solid, enhancing masses without fat or mineralized components.

Meningioma

Meningioma is a rare tumor of childhood and adolescents. In childhood, the presence of a meningioma should raise concern for NF2. On MRI, the appearance of meningiomas in children is identical to that of meningiomas in adults and has been discussed in other parts of this chapter. Radiation-induced meningiomas have been reported following treatment of a number of childhood neoplasms, notably lymphoblastic leukemia (Fig. 2.80). Intense, homogeneous enhancement is characteristic of this tumor, with hyperostosis of adjacent osseous structures being a highly suggestive finding.

Schwannoma

Schwannomas are benign neoplasms arising from the cells that form axonal myelin sheaths. They are rare in childhood, and their presence should raise the possibility of a diagnosis of NF2. They are located most often in the cerebellopontine angle cistern, originating from the vestibular division of the

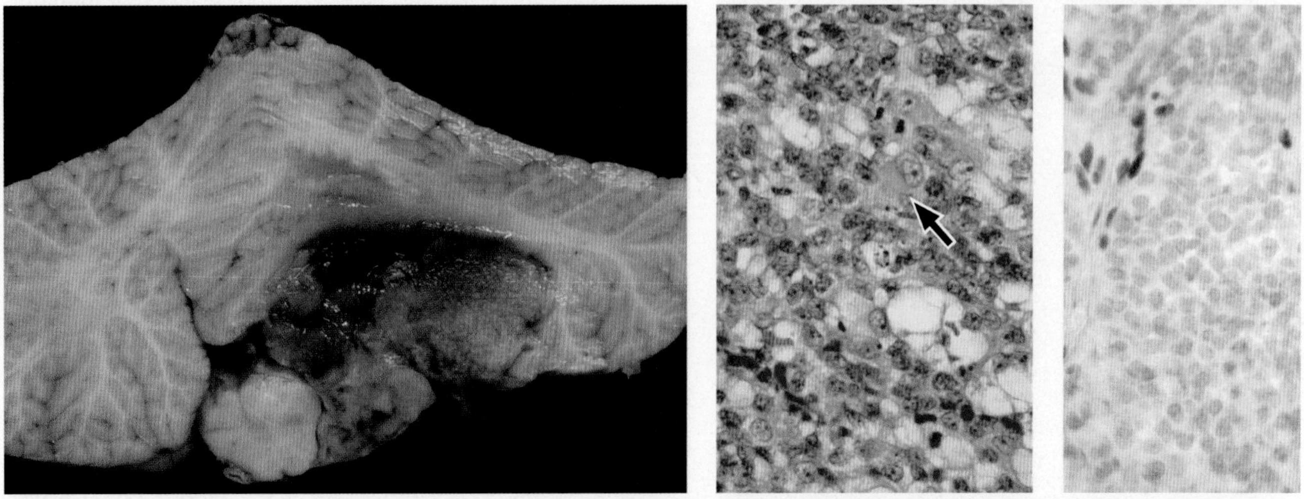

FIGURE 2.78 **Autopsy specimen of a 2-year-old girl who died of atypical teratoid/rhabdoid tumor shows recurrent tumor in the posterior fossa (left panel).** Microscopically, cells are densely packed and primitive in appearance. Variable numbers of rhabdoid cells are characterized by an eccentric pink cytoplasmic inclusion (*arrow*) and a prominent nucleolus (**middle panel**; hematoxylin and eosin, original magnification, 600×). Immunostaining for INI1 shows absent nuclear staining in tumor cells, standing out as pale blue in contrast to interspersed nonneoplastic blood vessels and inflammatory cells, which show strong brown nuclear staining (**right panel**; original magnification, 600×).

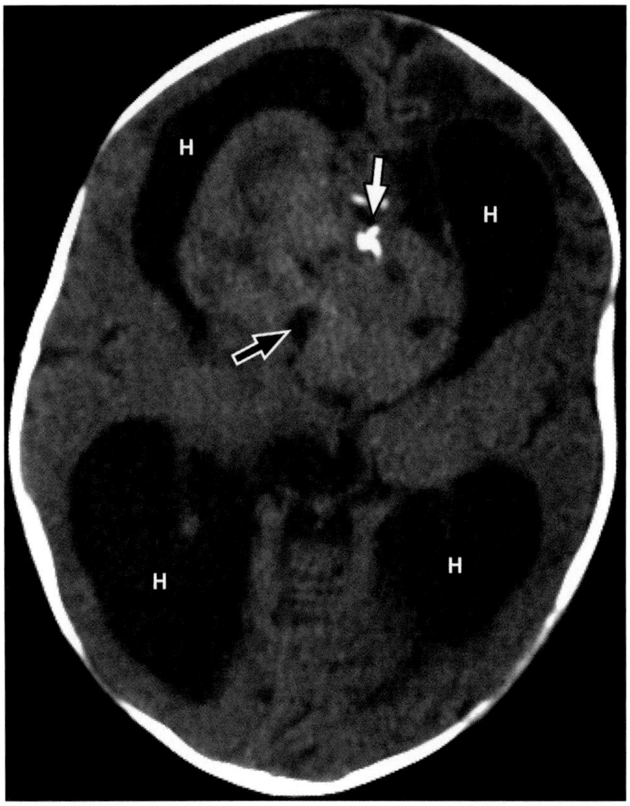

FIGURE 2.79 **Immature teratoma in an 8-week-old girl who presented with hydrocephalus.** Axial CT image shows a large mass centered in the suprasellar region, containing tooth-like elements of calcification (*white arrow*) and low density suggestive of fat content (*black arrow*). Obstructive hydrocephalus (*H*) is also present.

eighth cranial nerve. The next most common site of origin is the trigeminal nerve.

On MRI, schwannomas are seen as enhancing, extra-axial masses that are hyperintense to gray matter on T2-weighted MR images. Relatively, T2 hypointense fibrous components centrally may be identified, lending a "target" appearance to some lesions. Vestibular schwannomas originate from the peripheral portion of the eighth cranial nerve and, therefore, commonly expand the acoustic meatus. Diffuse enhancement is typical in solid portions of tumor. Other schwannomas tend to grow along the course of the nerve of origin, resulting in a characteristic fusiform shape of the affected cranial nerve (Fig. 2.81).

Lymphoproliferative Tumor (Leukemia and Lymphoma)

Lymphoproliferative disorders can involve the pediatric CNS in three forms: (1) solid intra-axial masses, (2) diffuse leptomeningeal infiltration, and (3) focal/multifocal extra-axial masses involving the dura or regional osseous structures. Relapsed acute lymphocytic leukemia of childhood commonly recurs in the CNS.

Primary CNS lymphoma (PCNSL) is extremely rare in children.[88] Most are non-Hodgkin B-cell lymphomas, frequently occurring in the setting of immunosuppression. They may be single or multifocal and usually arise from the deep gray and white matter structures. These lesions are homogeneously hyperdense on CT and isointense to gray matter on T2-weighted MR imaging. Decreased diffusivity is seen on diffusion-weighted MR images because of the high cell density or nuclear-to-cytoplasmic ratio (Fig. 2.82). Tumors diffusely enhance following contrast administration.

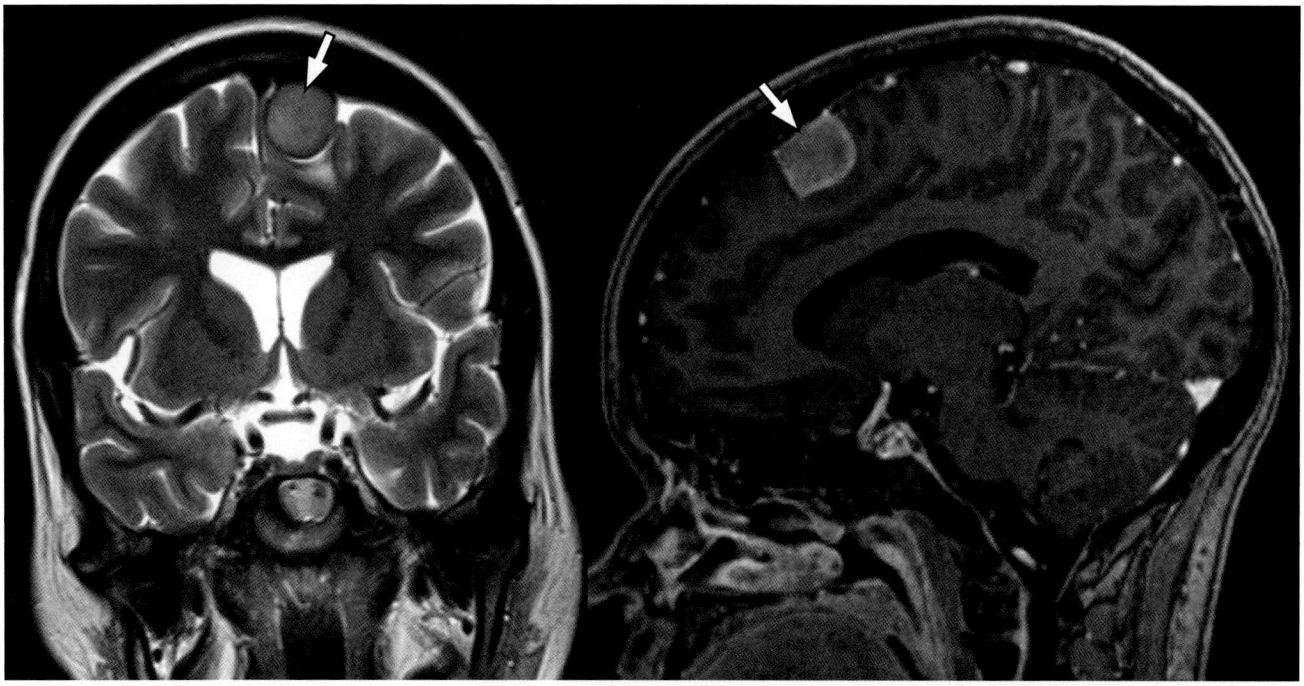

FIGURE 2.80 **Radiation-induced meningioma in an 18-year-old girl with a previous history of cranial radiation for acute lymphocytic leukemia prior to bone marrow transplantation.** Coronal T2-weighted MR image (on the **left**) and sagittal postcontrast MPRAGE MR image (on the **right**) demonstrate a rounded, enhancing, dural-based extra-axial mass (*arrows*) with subjacent subcortical edema in the left superior frontal gyrus.

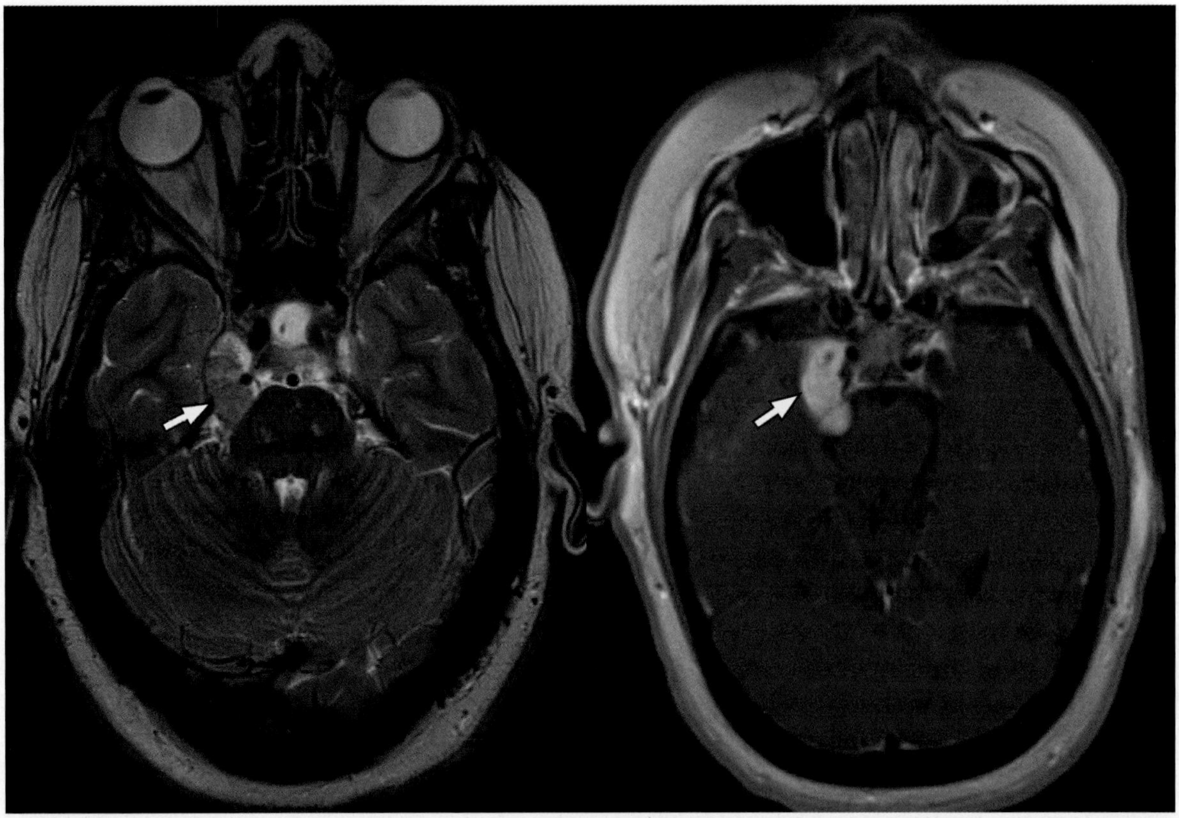

FIGURE 2.81 **Trigeminal nerve schwannoma in a 25-year-old female patient with history of cranial radiation in childhood for the treatment of a suprasellar astrocytoma.** Axial T2-weighted MR image (on the **left**) and axial postcontrast T1-weighted MR image (on the **right**) show an enhancing mass (*arrows*) along the right trigeminal nerve with extension into the right Meckel cave and cavernous sinus.

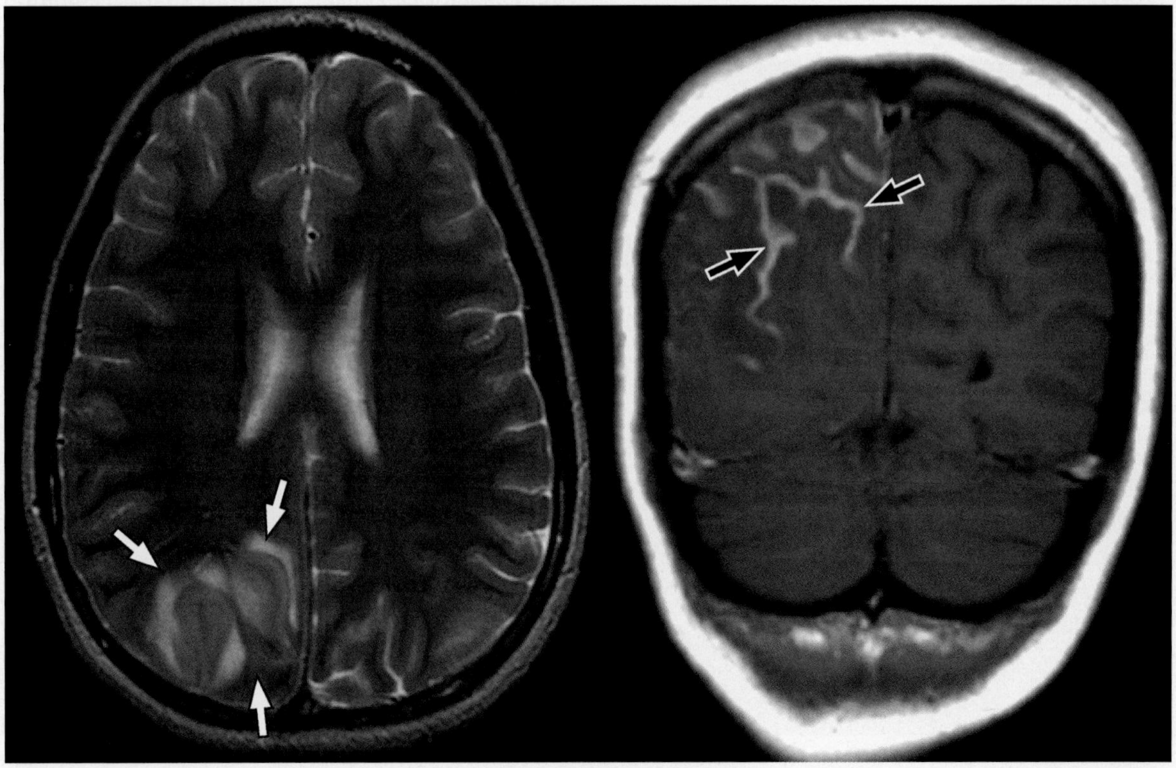

FIGURE 2.82 **Primary CNS B-cell lymphoma in a 17-year-old girl with new onset of seizures.** Axial T2-weighted MR image (on the **left**) and postcontrast coronal T1-weighted MR image (on the **right**) show heterogeneous T2 signal intensity (*white arrows*) in the right parietal lobe, enhancement involving the leptomeninges (*black arrows*), and edema in the adjacent brain parenchyma. The primary consideration was primary CNS lymphoma of the leptomeninges, which was proven by CSF analysis.

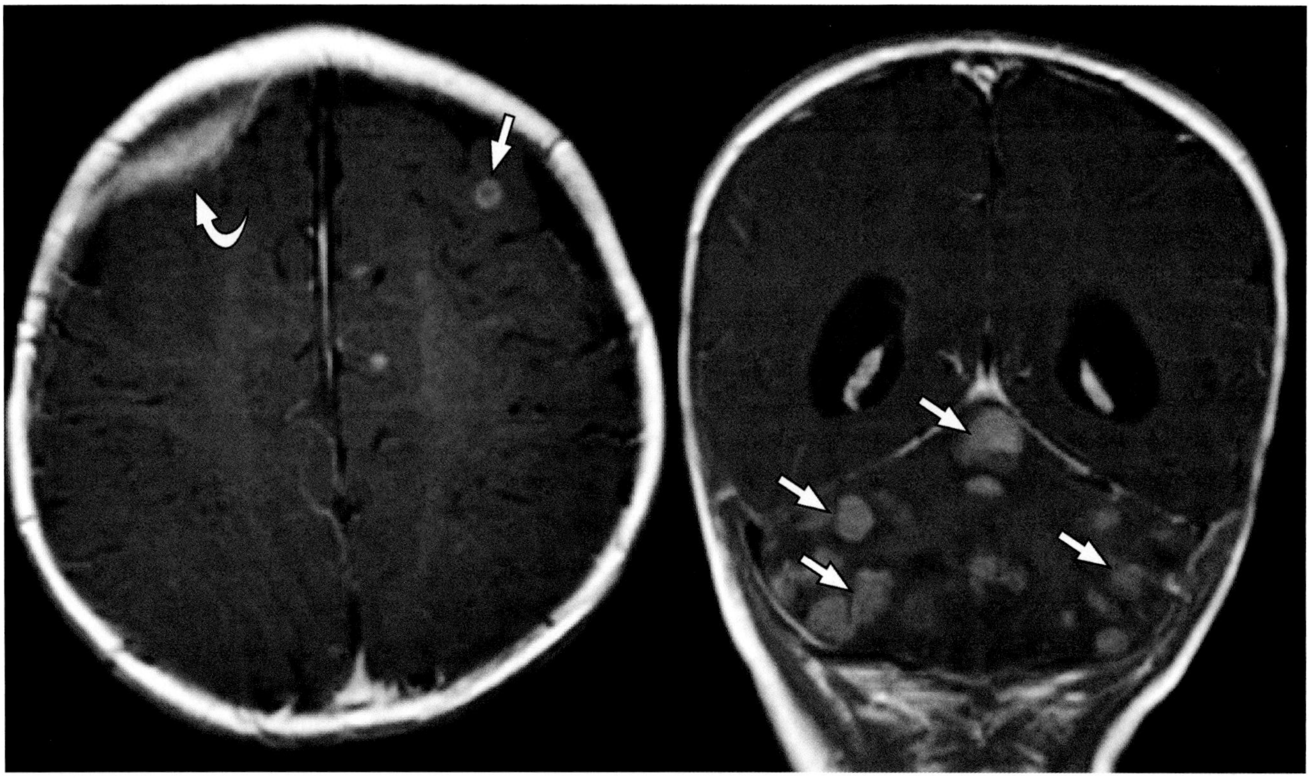

FIGURE 2.83 **Metastatic neuroblastoma in a 7-month-old boy.** Axial (on the **left**) and coronal (on the **right**) postcontrast T1-weighted MR images demonstrate multiple enhancing intraparenchymal masses (*straight arrows*) in the supratentorial and infratentorial compartment. Also, note the calvarial metastasis (*curved arrow*) extending into the epidural space from the right frontal bone.

However, some tumors in immunosuppressed patients are characterized by ring enhancement. The important differential diagnoses in these cases are fungal lesions, tuberculomas, and toxoplasmosis, particularly in immunocompromised pediatric patients with low CD4 counts. Diagnosis of PCNSL is made by the absence of appropriate response to institution of empiric toxoplasmosis therapy.

Lymphomatous involvement of the leptomeninges, dura, and calvarium can occur as a manifestation of PCNSL or in the setting of systemic lymphoma. Granulocytic sarcomas (chloromas) are extra-axial lesions seen in a particular subtype of myelogenous leukemia. They are characterized by high attenuation on CT, low T2 signal, decreased ADC values, and diffuse enhancement after contrast administration.

Metastasis

Metastasis to the CNS may result from hematogenous dissemination, leptomeningeal seeding, or direct extension. Hematogenously disseminated metastases to the brain parenchyma are rare in children. When they do occur, they tend to arise from sarcomatous lesions such as rhabdomyosarcoma and Ewing sarcoma. Cranial or dural metastases also occur via a hematogenous route and most commonly occur in children with neuroblastoma, leukemia, sarcoma, and lymphoma. They are characterized by aggressive lytic calvarial lesions or as nonspecific, enhancing dural masses. Parenchymal metastasis are usually multiple, avidly-enhancing, and located at the gray–white junction (Figs. 2.83 and 2.84). Surrounding vasogenic edema is seen around most lesions.

Leptomeningeal seeding can occur from primary brain tumors such as medulloblastoma, but may also occur in the setting of non-CNS primary tumors and systemic malignan-

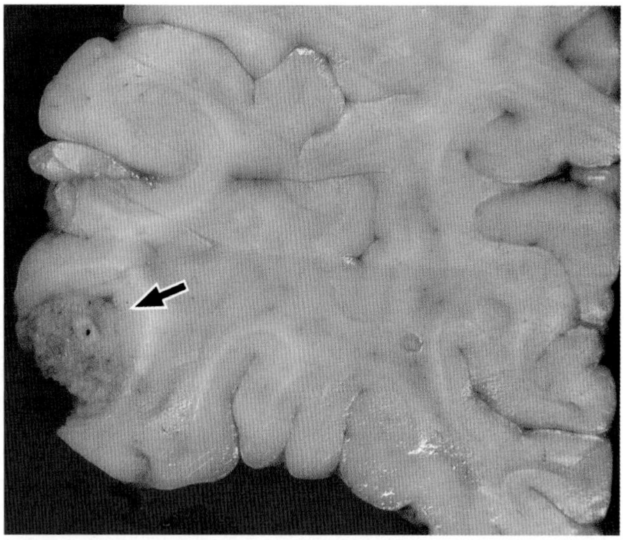

FIGURE 2.84 **Metastatic neuroblastoma in a 7-month-old boy with primary intrathoracic neuroblastoma.** Gross surgical specimen shows a gray nodule (*arrow*) at the gray–white matter junction in the frontal lobe consistent with an intraparenchymal metastatic deposit.

cies. Regardless of the tumor of origin, the imaging appearance is identical and characterized by nodular or smooth enhancement of the leptomeninges. Direct extension into the brain occurs from tumors in the skull base, paranasal sinuses, orbits, and the calvarium.

Traumatic Disorders

Birth Trauma

Birth-related injury occurs more commonly in infants delivered by forceps, vacuum extraction, or cesarean section than those born by spontaneous vaginal delivery. Subdural hematomas (SDHs), most commonly located in the posterior fossa, are the most common intracranial manifestation. SDH results from tentorial tears with rupture of the vein of Galen, straight sinus, or transverse sinus. US may be able show moderate to large SDHs, but smaller hematomas and those located near the convexities can be difficult to visualize. CT demonstrates SDH as a hyperdense extra-axial collection along the tentorium or in the posterior fossa. Some hematomas can be large enough to cause localized mass effect upon the posterior fossa structures including the brainstem. SDH along the convexity may result from rupture of the bridging veins traversing the subdural space.

In the term infant, lobar parenchymal and subpial hemorrhages are occasionally encountered, occurring spontaneously in otherwise healthy neonates in the first few days of life. Spontaneous superficial parenchymal and leptomeningeal hemorrhage also occur in otherwise healthy term neonates. Parenchymal hemorrhage with subpial extension occurs most often in the temporal lobe and in proximity to sutures, often accompanied by minor overlying soft tissue swelling and subjacent decreased diffusion in the brain parenchyma (Fig. 2.85). This pattern suggests local trauma with contusion or venous compression/occlusion as likely causes for these hemorrhages.

Another manifestation of birth-related trauma is calvarial injury, which includes overriding of the calvarial bones at the sutures and depressed fractures (more common in the parietal and frontal bones). Scalp hemorrhage is common following traumatic delivery. Caput succedaneum is hemorrhage in the subcutaneous tissue of the scalp and is seen as hyperdensity crossing the suture lines. Subgaleal hemorrhages occur between the scalp aponeurosis and the periosteum and are seen as hyperdensity in the scalp on CT that cross the midline. They may be compressed by the transducer and difficult to visualize when US is used to define the extent and size. Subperiosteal hematomas, called cephalhematomas, characteristically do not cross the sutures, because of periosteal attachment at the suture lines. Cephalhematomas may demonstrate ossification on follow-up imaging studies.

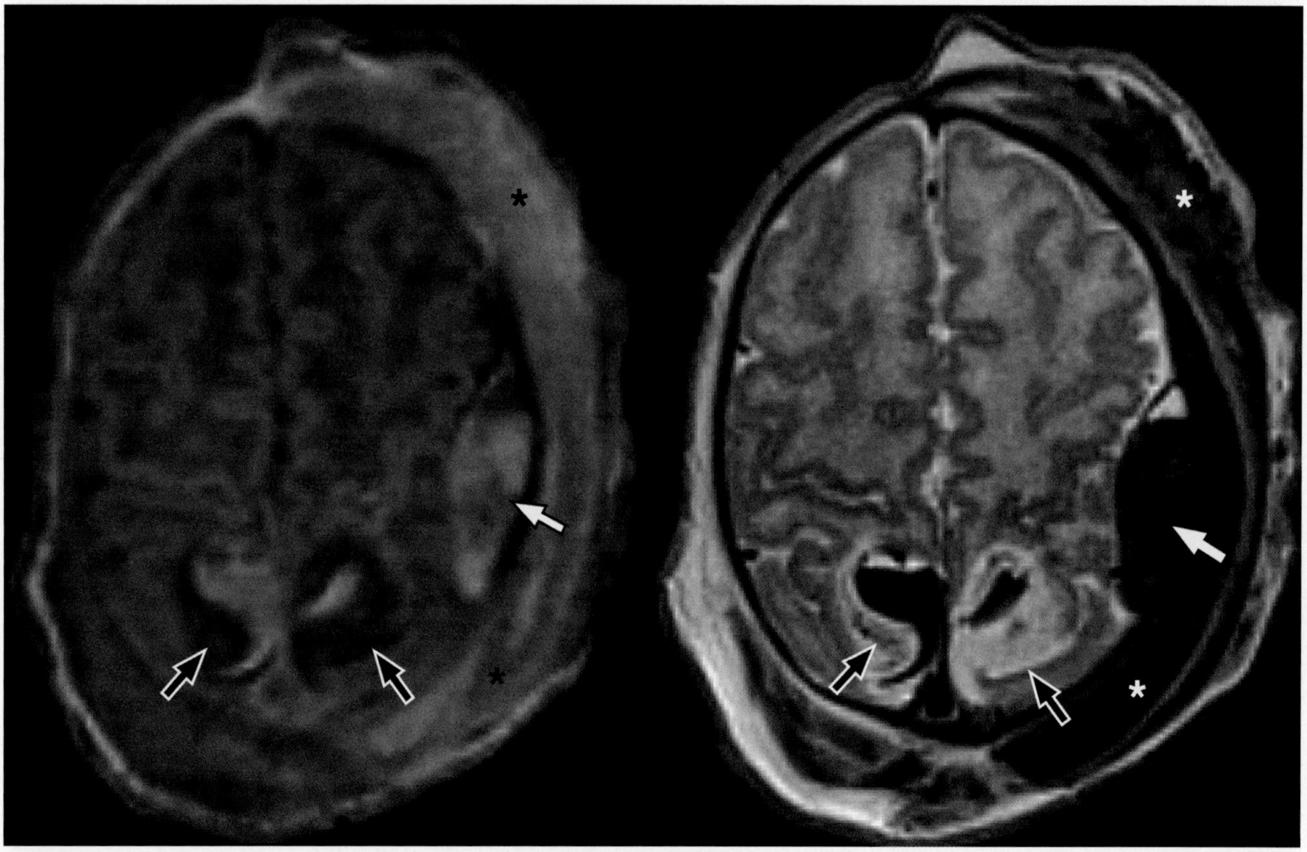

FIGURE 2.85 **Subpial and epidural hemorrhage in a 2-day-old infant boy.** Axial T1-weighted MR image (on the **left**) and axial T2-weighted MR image (on the **right**) show bilateral posterior parietal subpial hemorrhages (*black arrows*) and left frontoparietal epidural hematoma (*white arrows*). Also noted is a large subgaleal and scalp soft tissue hematoma (*asterisks*).

Accidental Trauma

Accidental trauma in young children usually results from falls of distances <3 feet. Fractures in accidental trauma are usually linear. Direct impact can cause so-called ping-pong fractures with buckling of the membranous bone. With increasing severity of trauma, comminuted, depressed calvarial and skull base fractures may occur. Adolescents and young adults commonly present with head injury following motor vehicle accidents and injuries sustained during contact sporting events.

Imaging in accidental trauma is usually carried out initially with a noncontrast CT. Multiplanar reformats and 3D reconstructions help delineate fractures better and help differentiate true fractures from normal variants. Underlying intracranial injuries include extra- and intra-axial hematomas and parenchymal contusions. MRI is used in selected cases, particularly when diffuse axonal injury is suspected or the clinical status of the patient is out of proportion to the abnormalities seen on CT. Diffusion-weighted MR images help assess the degree of parenchymal injury and susceptibility-weighted MR images enable the detection of microhemorrhages not seen on CT or conventional imaging sequences (Fig. 2.86). In addition to the established role in severe brain trauma after accidental trauma, an increasing role for MRI utilizing specialized imaging sequences has been advocated in pediatric patients following mild traumatic brain injury to detect the presence of parenchymal injury not seen on conventional imaging sequences.

Parenchymal Injury

Contusion and Shearing Injury

Parenchymal lesions resulting from head trauma include cerebral contusions and white matter shearing injuries.

Cerebral contusions are defined as bruises of the brain usually caused by deceleration injuries, resulting from contact of the brain with the rough edges of the skull. On the other hand, shearing injuries are caused by rotational impacts to the skull. With rapid rotation of the skull, the brain lags behind; this results in rotational stresses within the brain, producing stretching and disruption of nerve fiber tracts, most commonly at the junction of the gray and white matter, the centrum semiovale, corpus callosum, internal capsule, basal ganglia, and brainstem.[89]

CT is the imaging modality of choice for the evaluation of head injury in acutely ill and unstable pediatric patients. CT can detect large cerebral contusions in the acute phase, indicated by the presence of acute blood products within the brain parenchyma. CT can also delineate any associated extra-axial hematomas or pneumocephalus. MRI is the imaging modality of choice to assess brain parenchymal injury and should be considered in all children with severe head injury or coma. It can detect both contusions and axonal shearing injuries. The presence of restricted diffusion at the junction of the gray and white matter, centrum semiovale, corpus callosum, internal capsule, basal ganglia, and brainstem is characteristic of shearing injury and diffuse axonal injury. Use of susceptibility-weighted images and gradient-echo sequences can detect minute amounts of blood products and should always be employed in MR examination of trauma victims.[90]

MRI is also useful for follow-up of contusion, as chronic manifestations of injuries including encephalomalacia appear as focal hyperintensities on T2-weighted and FLAIR MR images. Subacute and chronic hemorrhages are indicated by the presence of susceptibility on susceptibility-weighted MR images and gradient recalled echo MR images.

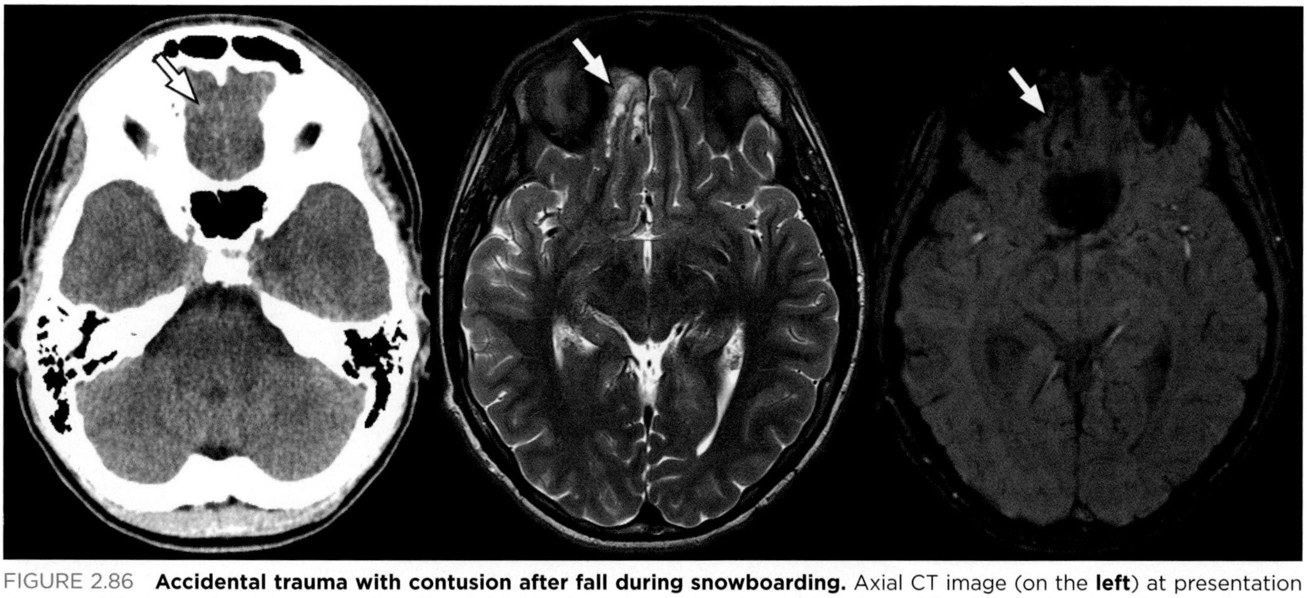

FIGURE 2.86 **Accidental trauma with contusion after fall during snowboarding.** Axial CT image (on the **left**) at presentation shows subtle hyperdensities (*arrow*) in the right inferior frontal lobe. Axial T2-weighted MR image (in the **middle**) obtained 1 month later for evaluation of new onset seizures shows encephalomalacia (*arrow*) in the anteroinferior right frontal lobe with susceptibility artifact (*arrow*) on the susceptibility-weighted MR image (on the **right**).

Long-term follow-up often shows parenchymal volume loss in pediatric patients whose brains have suffered significant injury.

Cerebral Swelling

Generalized cerebral swelling occurs in children more commonly than in adults following similar types of head injury. This is probably caused by a combination of edema and a decrease in cerebrovascular resistance, which in turn leads to vasodilatation and increased cerebral blood volume. Imaging studies (both CT and MR of the brain) show loss of gray and white matter differentiation with slit-like configuration of the lateral ventricles and effacement of the cerebral sulci and basal cisterns. With severe trauma, transtentorial herniation of the temporal lobe may occur. This, in turn, may cause compression of the posterior cerebral artery against the free edge of the tentorium in the ambient cistern and lead to infarcts in the corresponding vascular territory.

Severe swelling of the brain in the setting of trauma or severe hypoxic injury resulting from increased blood volume or axonal shearing injuries is manifested by the presence of the "white cerebellum sign." This term was originally applied to the appearance on CT, but has been defined on DWI on MRI as well. It is used to refer to the diffusely decreased density of the supratentorial brain because of presence of white matter and cortical edema, with relatively increased attenuation of the thalami, brainstem, and cerebellum (Fig. 2.87).

Extraparenchymal Injury

There are three types of extra-axial hemorrhages, which include epidural hematoma, SDH, and subarachnoid hemorrhage.

Epidural Hematoma

Epidural hematoma (EDH), also known as extradural hematoma, refers to hemorrhage into the space between the dura and the overlying calvarium. EDH is seen in ~1% to 3% of pediatric closed head injury admissions, but is a relatively uncommon finding among pediatric patients seen in emergency departments following head trauma.[91] EDH results almost exclusively following craniocerebral trauma. In neonates, EDH may occur following traumatic or instrument-assisted delivery. In young infants and early childhood, falls from heights as low as five feet can result in EDH.

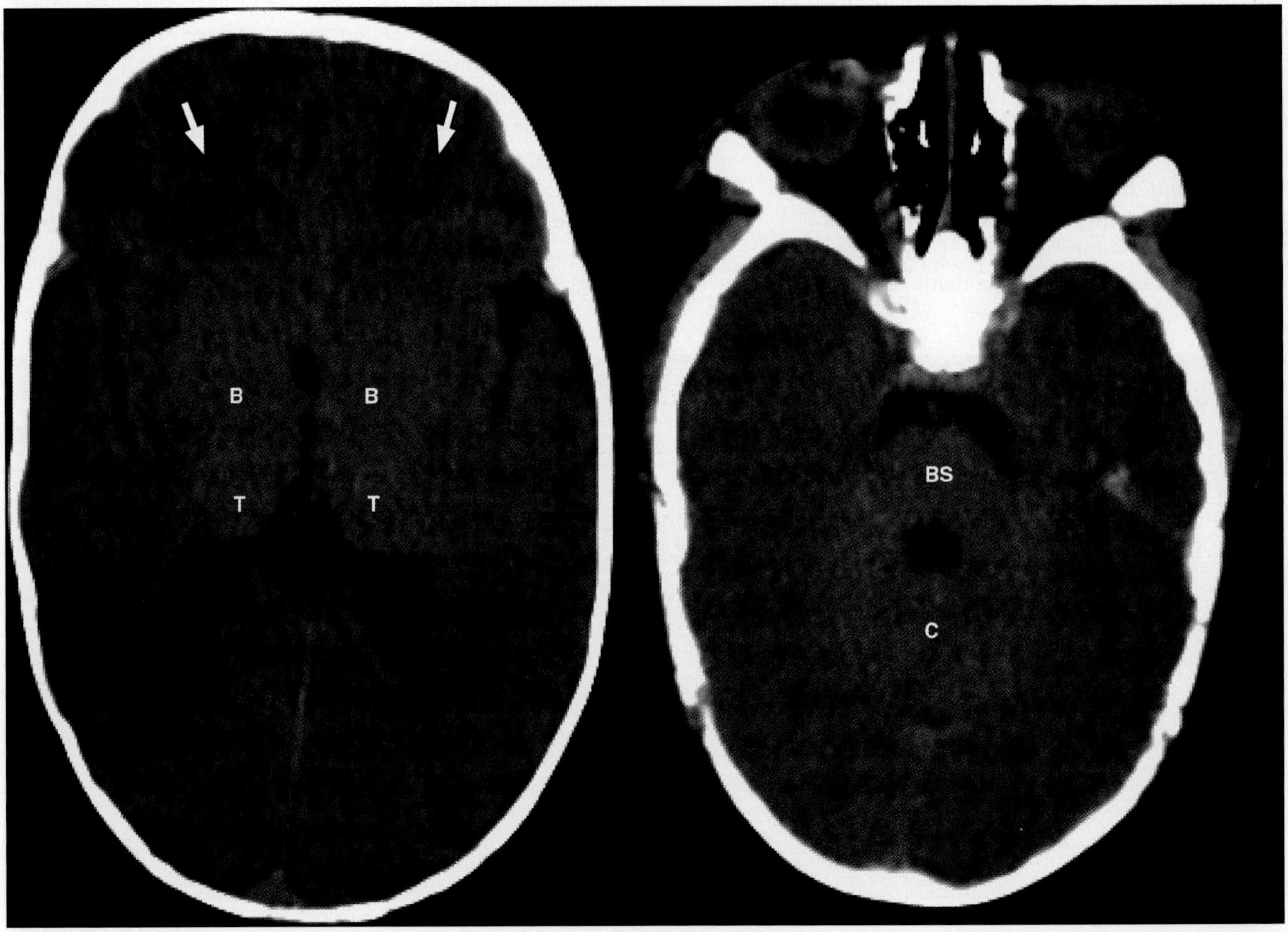

FIGURE 2.87 **Cerebral swelling in an ex-premature 3-month-old infant girl following cardiopulmonary arrest.** Axial CT images show near-total loss of gray–white differentiation (*arrows*) and hypodensity in the supratentorial brain with relative preservation of density within the basal ganglia (*B*), thalami (*T*), brainstem (*BS*), and cerebellum (*C*). This is the "white cerebellum sign" or "reversal sign" indicative of diffuse brain edema and impending infarction.

The incidence of EDH in children following nonaccidental trauma is relatively low (6% to 18%) compared to SDHs.[92] In older children, motor vehicle accidents are the primary cause of EDH.

EDHs are located between the skull and the dura. They occur due to stripping of the dura from the overlying skull surface following direct trauma, which drives the calvarium inward. Blood accumulates in the space between the stripped dura and the overlying bone. The blood does not cross the suture lines of the skull, as the dura is adherent to the suture lines. Unlike in adults, there is a higher frequency of venous than arterial tears as a cause of EDH in infants and younger children.[93] This is attributable to the relative abundance of dural and diploic vasculature in areas of rapid bone growth in young children. In older children and adolescents, EDH typically arises from an injury of the middle meningeal artery because of a squamosal temporal bone fracture. Delayed presentation of EDH following trauma can occur after an initial "lucid interval" as more blood accumulates over time following the initial injury, causing the patient to become more obtunded.

On CT, acute EDH is characterized by a hyperdense, biconvex mass lesion that exerts mass effect upon the adjacent cerebral parenchyma. When mixed hyper- and hypodensity are present within the EDH, active bleeding must be suspected (Fig. 2.88). Brain herniation through the foramen magnum is a life-threatening complication of enlarging EDH in older children. On MRI, acute EDH is seen as a lentiform-shaped mass between the dura and the overlying calvarium. The dura can be identified as a low signal intensity line between the calvarium and the brain. Acute EDH is isointense on T1-weighted MR images and hyperintense on T2-weighted MR images. Late subacute and early chronic EDH is hyperintense on both T1- and T2-weighted MR images. It is worthwhile to note that evolution of blood products on MRI does not follow the same changes as intra-axial blood. Therefore, MRI in patients with extra-axial blood can be an unreliable means of determining the timing of injury.

Treatment of EDH depends on the clinical findings, the size of the EDH, and the degree of mass effect. Signs of raised intracranial pressure, deteriorating consciousness, pupillary abnormalities, hemiparesis, and cerebellar signs indicate a need for emergent craniotomy and evacuation of the hematoma. Evaluation by a neurosurgeon is essential to ensure a good outcome. Small EDHs without significant mass effect may be managed conservatively, but close neurologic observation is required. Larger EDHs (>15 mm in thickness), temporal location, cisternal compression, mixed density of the hematoma (which can indicate active bleeding), or appreciable midline shift (>5 mm) on CT are radiographic indicators of the need for prompt neurosurgical evacuation.[94,95]

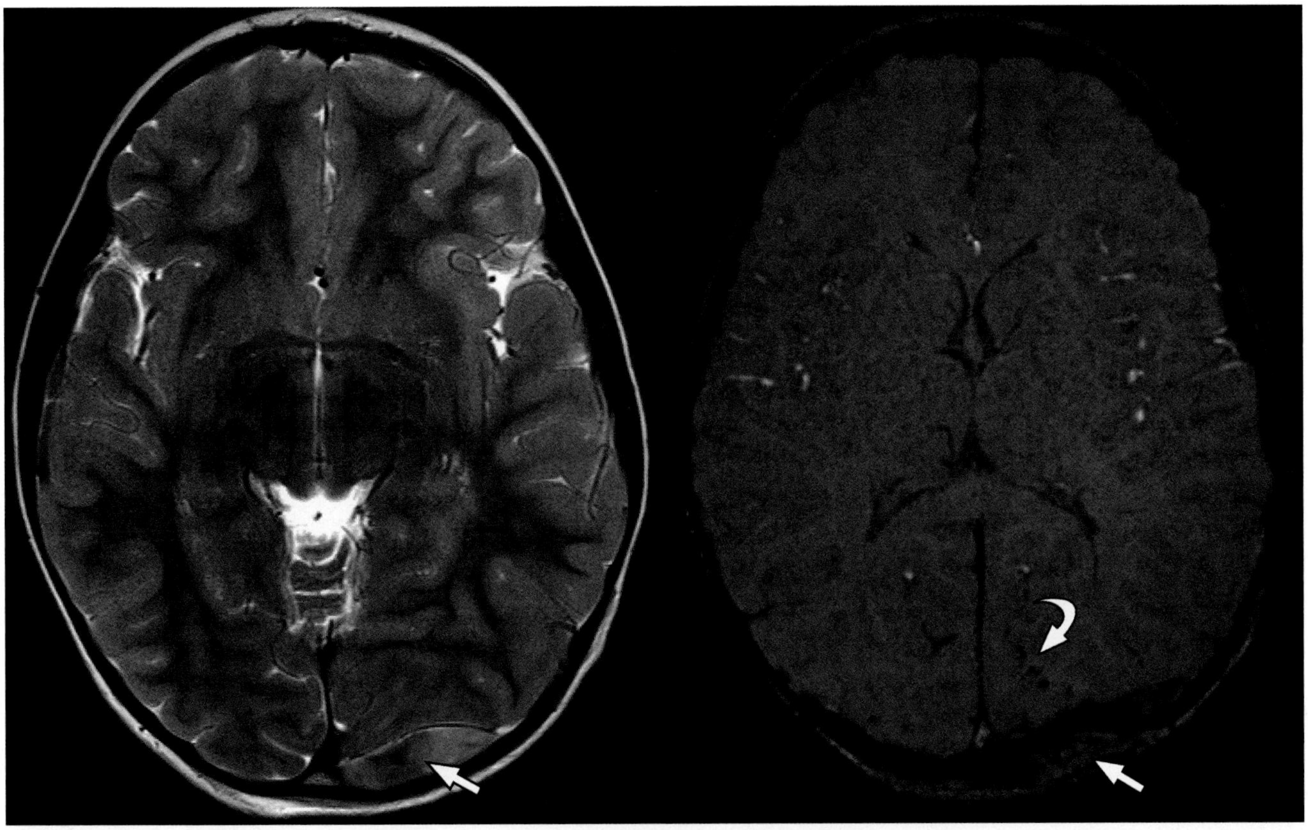

FIGURE 2.88 **Epidural hematoma (EDH) in a 5-year-old girl following motor vehicle accident.** Axial T2-weighted MR image (on the **left**) and susceptibility-weighted MR image (on the **right**) show a biconvex T2 hypointense left parietooccipital EDH (*straight arrows*) with low signal on the susceptibility-weighted MR image and a focal parenchymal occipital contusion (*curved arrow*).

Subdural Hematoma

SDH is defined as hemorrhage into the potential space between the dura and the arachnoid membranes. The etiology of SDH in children is substantially different than that in adults. Abusive head injury is a common etiology of SDH in children, particularly in those <2 years of age.[96] The incidence of SDH varies with age. In neonates, SDH is seen in up to 8% of term deliveries and is more common with instrument-assisted deliveries. In infants and toddlers <2 years of age, SDH occurs in ~12 children per 100,000 child-years with the highest incidence seen in infants of 0 to 4 months of age.[97,98] Nonaccidental, abusive head trauma accounts for the majority of SDH in these children. Among older children and adolescents, other causes of trauma, primarily motor vehicle accidents, account for most cases of SDH.

The cause of SDH is either bleeding from bridging veins that traverse the subdural space or extension of cerebral cortical bleeding caused by traumatic brain injury. Posttraumatic SDH is often located along the frontal, parietal, and temporal convexities, and is caused by tearing of bridging vessels and traumatic impact between the brain and the skull. The presence of SDH in the interhemispheric space or posterior fossa, hematomas in multiple sites, and a disproportionate amount of cerebral swelling and mass effect compared to the size of the SDH are potentially suggestive of nonaccidental trauma as the underlying etiology. However, interhemispheric blood is seen in just as many cases of accidental trauma.

US may be used in neonates and infants with an open anterior fontanelle for evaluation of SDH. The presence of blood vessels coursing through the extra-axial space on color Doppler US helps distinguish between SDH and SAH. On CT, SDH is classically described as a concave extra-axial collection along the surface of the brain that is not restricted by skull sutures (Fig. 2.89). Homogeneous hyperdense SDH is reported to be more frequent in cases of accidental head trauma. Mixed-density SDH may be seen in cases of nonaccidental trauma because of repetitive injuries, but may be observed within 48 hours of single head injury. In addition, it may also occur due to hyperacute bleeding, clot retraction, and leakage of CSF into the subdural space. CT reformats in the coronal plane can be helpful to visualize blood along the tentorium. Blood along the posterior falx cerebri is indicated by a thicker and more irregular appearance of the posterior interhemispheric fissure. MRI is indicated in infants who are clinically stable when abusive trauma is suspected on the basis of history, clinical exam, or skeletal survey, and also as a follow-up study in pediatric patients with an abnormal CT.

The presence of neurologic impairment and midline shift on unenhanced head CT are indicators for surgical evacuation of SDH. Subdural taps and subdural drain placement may be considered in some pediatric patients with chronic SDH and subdural hygromas.

Subarachnoid Hemorrhage

SAH is relatively rare in the pediatric population accounting for 1% to 2% of SAH in patients of all age groups and only 18% of intracranial hemorrhage in children.[99,100] Trauma is the most common cause of isolated SAH in children. Isolated SAH in a child is more likely to be due to accidental trauma, but presence of SAH in association with diffuse axonal injury has been shown in a meta-analysis to have a more significant association with nonaccidental trauma.[101,102] The presence of skull fractures and retinal and/or subdural hemorrhages

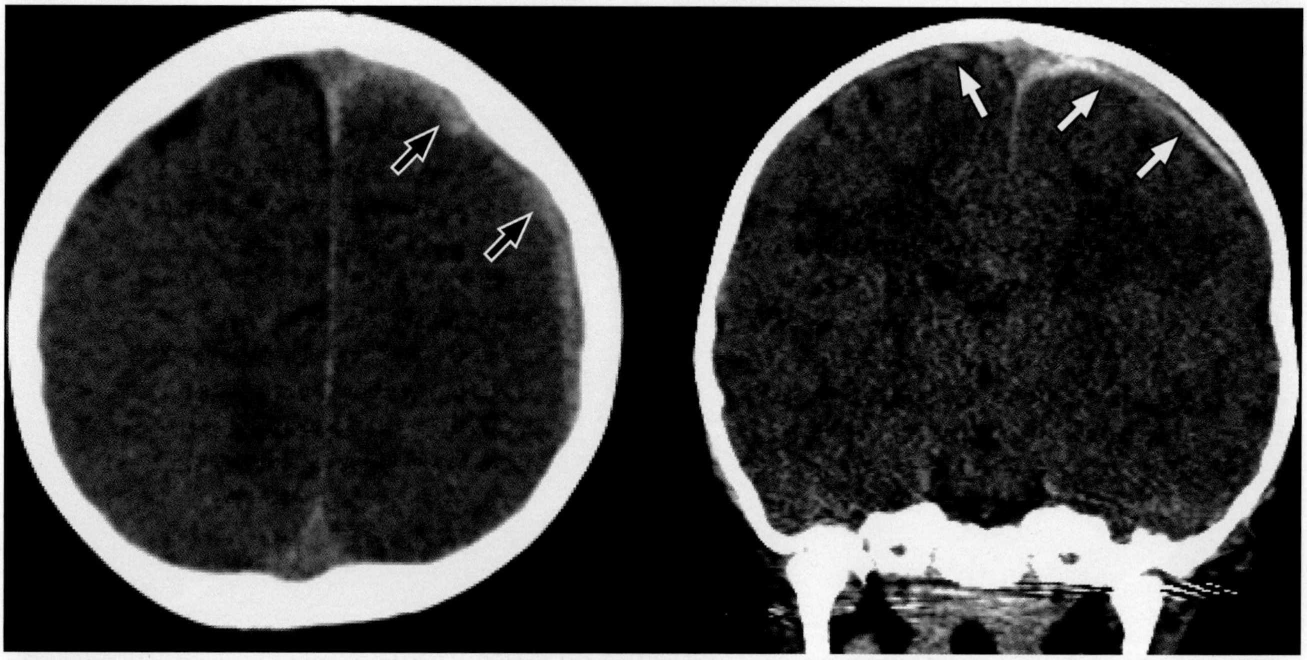

FIGURE 2.89 **Subdural hematoma (SDH) in a 25-month-old boy who was subsequently found to have multiple rib fractures and retinal hemorrhages.** Axial noncontrast CT image (on the **right**) and coronal reformatted CT image (on the **left**) show bilateral acute frontal SDHs (*arrows*), left larger than right, with underlying sulcal effacement.

should raise the suspicion for nonaccidental trauma. As in adults, spontaneous SAH in children is caused most commonly by aneurysm rupture. Other causes include tumors, coagulopathies, AVM hemorrhage, recreational drug use, surgical procedures, and hemorrhagic meningoencephalitis.

The clinical presentation in younger children with SAH is most often increasing irritability and lethargy. Presentation in older children with spontaneous SAH includes a varying combination of severe headaches, nausea and vomiting, decreased level of consciousness, seizures, and focal neurologic deficits.

Noncontrast head CT can detect well over 95% of all SAH within the first 24 hours, regardless of etiology.[103,104] The presence of SAH is indicated by extension of blood within the cerebral sulci (Fig. 2.90), ventricles, and cisternal spaces. On MRI, acute SAH may be difficult to visualize on conventional T1- and T2-weighted MR images because of the relatively lower concentration of hemoglobin in clotted blood and the inhibition of conversion of hemoglobin to deoxyhemoglobin and methemoglobin by the high oxygen tension in CSF. Gradient-echo and susceptibility-weighted sequences are more sensitive to the presence of SAH than standard spin-echo acquisitions. Also, SAH may be indicated by hyperintensity on FLAIR MR images, although the appearance of sulcal high signal on FLAIR MR images is nonspecific and may be due to CSF flow, slow flow in leptomeningeal vessels, increased oxygen tension in the CSF, and elevated CSF protein.

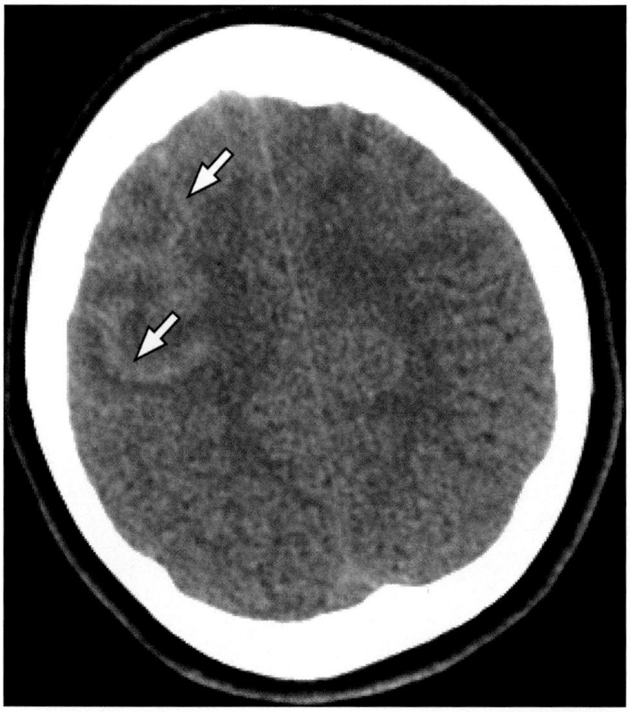

FIGURE 2.90 **Subarachnoid hemorrhage in an 11-year-old girl following accidental head trauma.** Axial noncontrast CT image shows a right frontal SAH (*arrows*). Note the presence of edema indicated by sulcal effacement and hypodensity of the adjacent white matter.

The treatment of SAH is dependent on the underlying cause in the pediatric population.

Nonaccidental/Abusive Head Injury

Nonaccidental, abusive head injury is a leading cause of brain trauma in infants and is associated with high morbidity and mortality.[105] Nonaccidental injury should be suspected in an infant or young child presenting traumatic injury with no given history of injury, when there is a discrepancy between the explanation provided and nature of lesions, injuries of varying ages, multiple injuries, associated retinal hemorrhages, inconsistent or changing clinical history, delay in medical care, repeated injuries, and poor upkeep of the child. Initial presentation varies from relatively minor symptoms to impaired level of consciousness with significant neurologic damage. Neuroimaging findings in children with abusive head trauma also vary and include skull fractures and extra-axial hemorrhages, with or without concomitant brain parenchymal injury.

The decision to perform neuroimaging exams urgently on the child who presents in the emergency department with suspected abuse, but without neurologic findings, can be challenging. Although there is agreement that neuroimaging studies must be performed in all children with overt neurologic symptoms, the decision is less clear for those without obvious CNS involvement. Some authors suggest that children without apparent neurologic signs or symptoms who present with other signs of physical abuse may have intracranial injury and may benefit from neuroimaging.[106] Also, evidence suggests that if one infant twin is injured, the other is at risk and should also undergo a skeletal survey.[107]

Currently, CT is the recommended initial imaging modality for detection of acute blood and fractures when child abuse is suspected. Multiplanar reformatting of multi detector CT images can help identify small extra-axial hemorrhages and parenchymal contusions. Further, 3D reformats can also increase the ability of CT to demonstrate skull fractures and permit differentiation fractures from sutures and normal variants.[108]

Recent literature suggests that MRI (including DWI, MRS, and T2*-weighted MR imaging and/or SWI) should promptly follow the initial CT.[106] MRI is the modality of choice for demonstrating small extra-axial hemorrhages and evaluating parenchymal injury such as contusion, shear injury, and infarction. Additional, significant, or evolving abnormalities are often found on MRI in up to 25% of patients with an abnormal early CT examination.[109,110] The SWI sequence on higher field strength magnets has also increased the sensitivity of MRI for detection of small foci of parenchymal and extra-axial blood.[106,111]

DWI is valuable in the setting of abusive head injury, as it shows HII in the first few hours after the trauma and is more accurate and sensitive in demonstrating hypoxic injury than CT[110] (Fig. 2.91). In addition to the well-described findings of extra-axial hemorrhage, global or focal ischemia, and skull fractures in these infants, the presence of a small SDH

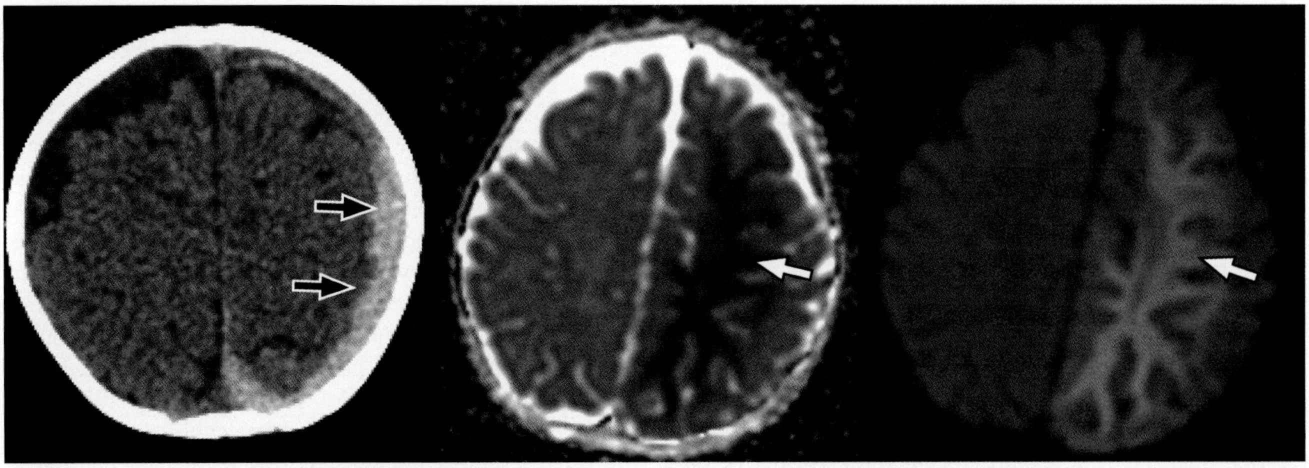

FIGURE 2.91 **Nonaccidental trauma in a 7-month-old girl.** Axial non-contrast CT image (on the **left**) shows acute subdural hematoma (*black arrows*). ADC (in the **middle**) and diffusion-weighted (on the **right**) MR images demonstrate extensive left cerebral hemisphere restricted diffusion (*white arrows*).

with a disproportionately large area of underlying unilateral hemispheric white matter edema is seen more commonly in children with inflicted trauma compared to children with brain injury from accidents. Decreased diffusion may be a sign of head injury related to abuse, arising specifically from cervical vascular compression, whether from kinking during hyperflexion/hyperextension, or from direct strangulation. Follow-up imaging often demonstrates extensive cortical infarction. The role of MRI/DWI in children with a normal early CT and the optimal timing of MRI/DWI after early CT in patients with suspected nonaccidental trauma have not been fully determined.

Elevated lactate, reduced *N*-acetyl aspartate, and elevations in choline-related compounds on MRS following trauma (including nonaccidental trauma) have been reported to correlate with poor outcome.[112,113]

Vascular Disorders

Developmental Variants and Anomalies

Vascular Malformations

Vascular malformations are nonneoplastic lesions that lack proliferative potential but may enlarge over time. The vascular malformations are classified based on their vascular hemodynamics and vascular composition. "Low-flow" lesions include capillary malformations, developmental venous anomalies (DVAs), and cavernomas. "High-flow" lesions include arteriovenous fistulae (AVF) and AVMs.

Developmental Venous Anomaly

A DVA is a radially oriented collection of dilated medullary or subcortical veins separated by normal brain parenchyma and draining into a single, dilated venous collector. DVAs are usually encountered as incidental findings on neuroimaging studies performed for unrelated reasons. Rarely, DVAs may cause headaches, neurologic deficits, or seizures, because of hemorrhage or thrombosis of the draining vein. The appearance of DVA on contrast-enhanced MRI is diagnostic, with a radially arranged group of veins draining into a single vein that in turn drains into a venous sinus (Fig. 2.92). The presence of slow flow or, occasionally, thrombosis in symptomatic cases may result in hyperintensity on noncontrast T1-weighted MR images. DVAs are most commonly located in the frontal and parietal lobes. DVAs are sometimes associated with cavernomas.

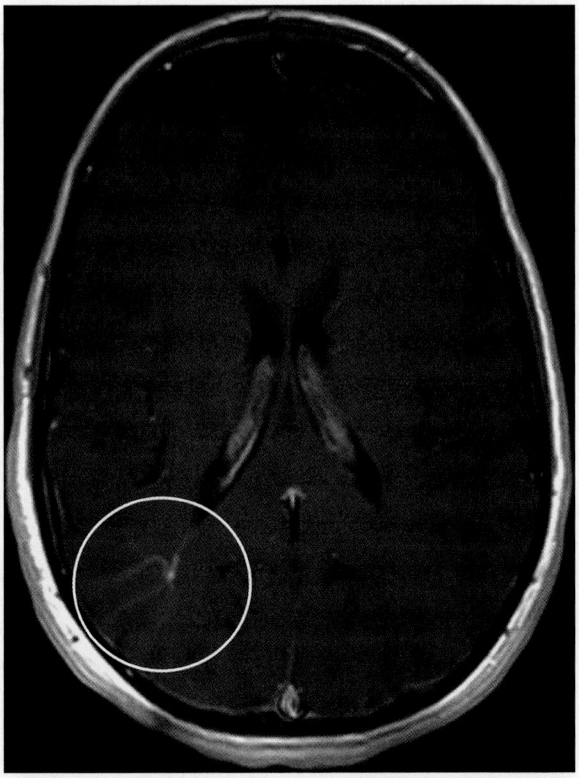

FIGURE 2.92 **Developmental venous anomaly.** Axial post-contrast T1-weighted MR image shows branching, mildly enlarged medullary veins (*circle*) within the right parietal lobe, which extend to the ependymal surface of the right lateral ventricle with a dilated transcortical collecting vein.

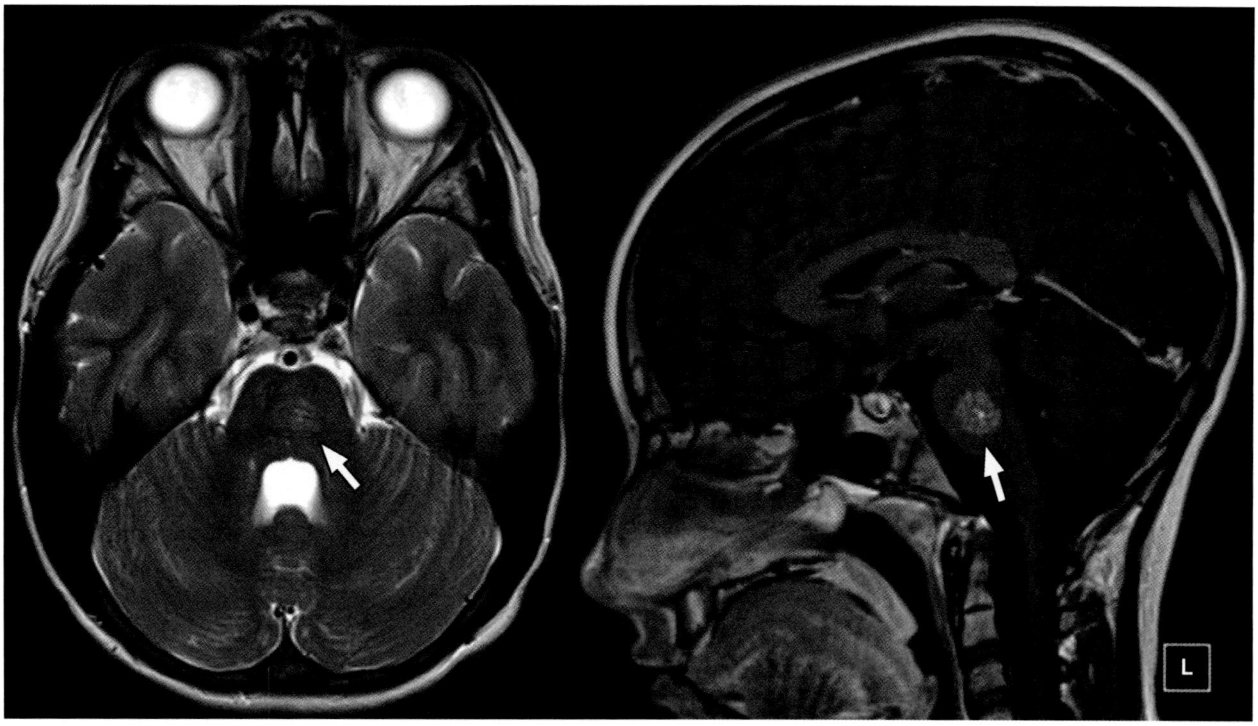

FIGURE 2.93 **Capillary telangiectasia in a 10-year-old boy.** Axial T2-weighted MR image (on the **left**) and postcontrast sagittal T1 SPACE (sampling perfection with application optimized using different flip angle evolution) MR image (on the **right**) show an area of stippled T2 hyperintensity (*arrows*) within the pons with brush-like enhancement. This finding was stable on follow-up studies over 3 years.

Capillary Telangiectasia

Capillary telangiectasias are a type of vascular choristoma usually located in the pons, consisting of a collection of dilated capillaries with intervening normal brain parenchyma. They are usually asymptomatic and seen as incidental findings on neuroimaging studies performed for other reasons or discovered at autopsy. They are usually not visualized on noncontrast images, although subtle T1 hypointensity and T2 hyperintensity may be seen in some cases. Focal hypointensity is seen on susceptibility-weighted and gradient recall echo MR images because of presence of deoxygenated, slow-flowing blood within the constituent vessels. On postcontrast images, capillary telangiectasias demonstrate faint enhancement with fuzzy borders (Fig. 2.93).

Cerebrovascular Malformations

Arteriovenous Fistula and Malformation

Cerebral AVFs and AVMs are high-flow shunts between the arterial and venous system, with enlargement and tortuosity of the involved vessels. AVFs are comprised of direct connections between arteries and veins, whereas AVMs consist of a central interposed network of vessels or nidus connecting the arteries and veins. AVF and AVM are often found together in high-flow vascular malformations in children. High-flow vascular malformations are subdivided, based on location, into dural, subarachnoid (vein of Galen), pial, and parenchymal malformations depending on their arterial supply and venous drainage. Dural AVF/AVM have a meningeal arterial supply and drain into the dural venous sinuses. Vein of Galen malformations (VOGMs) derive their arterial supply from a primitive choroid arcade that drains into the median prosencephalic vein, a persistent embryologic precursor to the vein of Galen. Pial AVF/AVM are supplied by branches of the anterior, middle, or posterior cerebral arteries and drain into cortical veins along the surface of the brain. Parenchymal lesions are most often AVMs; derive their arterial supply from branches of the anterior, middle, or posterior cerebral arteries; and drain into medullary or deep veins. Varices are common in high-flow lesions that drain into veins without surrounding structural support such as the vein of Galen and pial malformations. Although AVMs are considered congenital in origin, it is unclear when they actually develop.

AVFs and AVMs are usually sporadic and solitary. Overall prevalence of high-flow cerebrovascular malformations in children is between 0.014% and 0.028%.[114] Multiple AVMs in children are rare and usually associated with syndromes such as hereditary hemorrhagic telangiectasia (Osler-Weber-Rendu syndrome).

Some high-flow malformations may present soon after birth (e.g., large VOGMs causing congestive cardiac failure). The most common presentation of high-flow malformations in children is intracranial hemorrhage. Seizures are also a common presenting symptom, seen in 20% to 25% of patients with AVMs.[115,116] A small percentage of patients with high-flow malformations presents with other symptoms including headaches, focal neurologic deficits, vascular steal phenomenon, and increased intracranial pressure from venous hypertension.

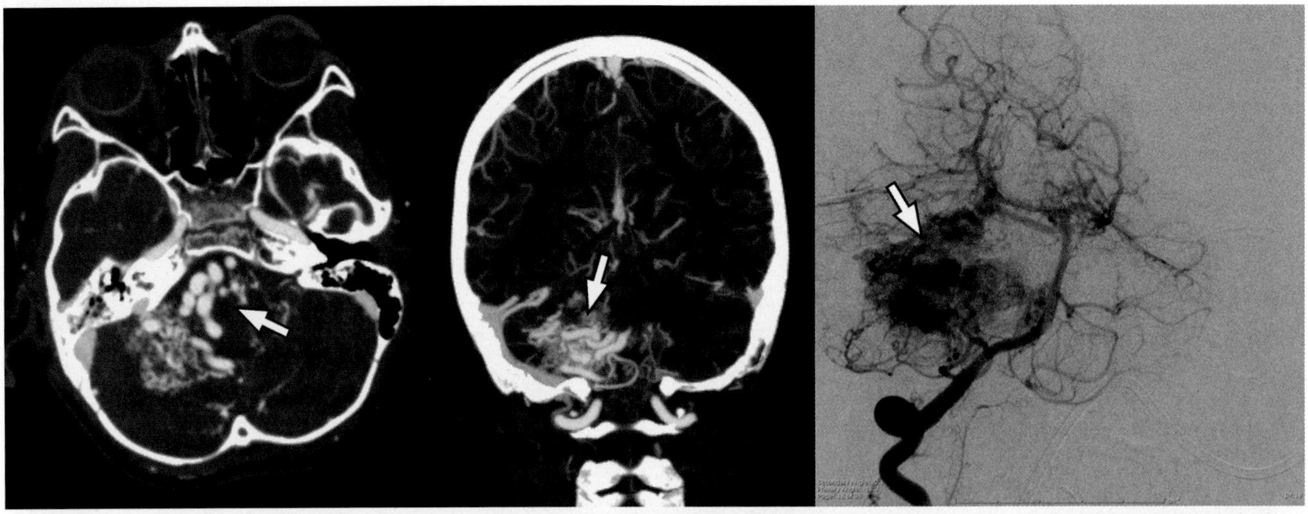

FIGURE 2.94 **Arteriovenous malformation (AVM) in a 12-year-old girl.** Axial (on the **left**) and coronal (in the **middle**) maximum intensity projection (MIP)-reformatted CT images from a CTA and a right vertebral artery injection image (on the **right**) from catheter angiogram demonstrate a large AVM (*arrows*) with a large nidus in the right cerebellar hemisphere.

Imaging of high-flow malformations should define the location of the lesion, identify the arterial and venous components, and assess for complications such as hemorrhage in the acute setting or cerebral atrophy and hydrocephalus resulting from venous hypertension in the chronic setting. In the acute setting, noncontrast CT may be used to demonstrate the presence of hemorrhage. CTA is often used as the initial imaging study of the malformation, although catheter angiography remains the gold standard for assessing high-flow malformations and allows for endovascular treatment of certain lesions.

MRI is used to define the anatomic relationships of the malformation. MRA typically demonstrates a tangle of flow voids with flow-related enhancement on 3D time-of-flight MR angiogram (Fig. 2.94). Temporal resolution of MRA is limited, but the early appearance of draining veins is seen best on dynamic, time-resolved contrast-enhanced MRA. Parenchymal volume loss in children most often occurs due to venous hypertension but may also occur due to an arterial "steal" phenomenon where blood is diverted away from the brain and through the malformation. Occasionally in the acute setting, compression of the malformation by a hematoma may make demonstration of the lesion difficult by CT, MR, and even catheter angiography.

Conventional catheter cerebral angiography remains the gold standard for characterization and delineation of high-flow brain malformations. The technique is used to identify the number and location of feeding arteries and the angiographic location and size of the nidus, assess the degree of shunting, and determine the pattern of venous drainage.

Treatment options include surgical resection, endovascular embolization, and radiation, or a combination of these options.

Cavernous Malformation and Associated Syndromes

Cavernous malformations, also known as cavernomas or cavernous "angiomas," are venous malformations within the CNS characterized by collections of variably sized venous channels, usually containing pockets of clotted and unclotted blood (Fig. 2.95). There is no arteriovenous shunting. The prevalence of cavernomas is ~0.5% in the general population.[117–119] A majority of patients in surgical series of pediatric cavernomas have presented in the second decade of life.[120,121] Cavernomas may occur sporadically or have a familial predisposition with autosomal dominant inheritance. Presence of multiple lesions is more common in familial cases (50%), compared to sporadic cases (1%).[117] A number of genes have been associated with familial cases. In addition, cavernoma-like lesions can occur as sequelae of radiation, usually presenting a few years after brain irradiation.

Cavernomas present following hemorrhage in most cases. Symptoms and clinical features depend upon the lesion's location. These include seizures when the lesion is located in the cerebral hemispheres, and hemiparesis, focal weakness, cranial nerve impairment, and disturbed consciousness when

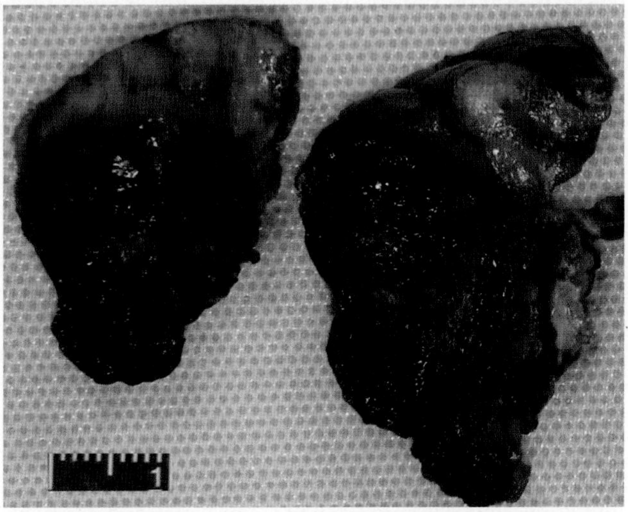

FIGURE 2.95 **Cavernous malformation in a 14-year-old boy.** Surgical specimen shows dilated blood-filled channels with surrounding blood. Microscopically, the channels are ectatic veins (not shown).

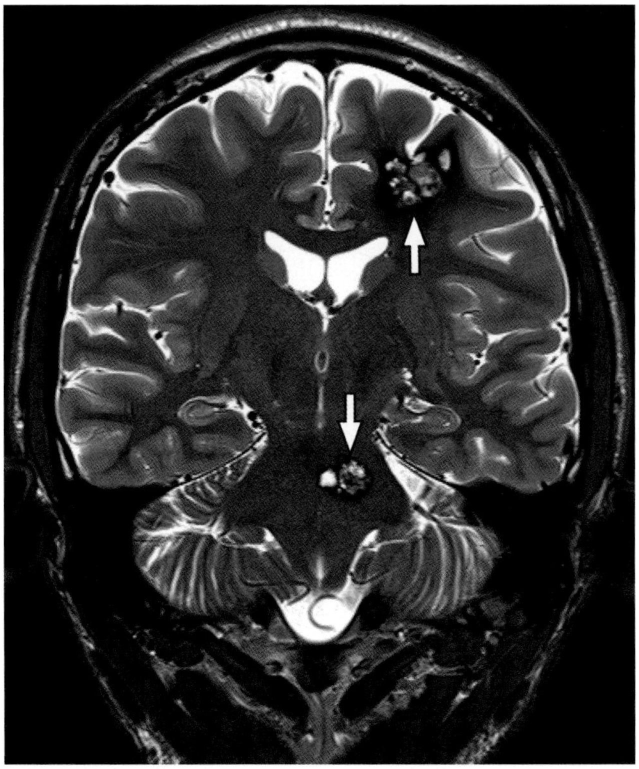

FIGURE 2.96 **Cavernoma in a 3-year-old boy whose father had a history of multiple cavernous malformations with recurrent bleeding.** Coronal T2-weighted MR image shows multiple "popcorn" lesions (*arrows*) with mixed low and high signal intensity foci within them, consistent with blood products of varying ages.

the lesion is in the brainstem. Occasionally, cavernomas are asymptomatic and seen as an incidental finding on neuroimaging studies performed for other reasons.

On noncontrast CT, cavernomas appear as hyperdense masses that may have internal calcifications. Mild enhancement may be present after contrast administration. On MRI, cavernomas are seen as fairly well-delineated, lobulated lesions with varying degrees of mass effect. The presence of blood products of varying ages within the lesion results in combinations of high and low T1 and T2 signal intensities within the lesion (Fig. 2.96). This appearance on unenhanced MRI is rather specific for cavernomas, although other hemorrhagic lesions can occasionally have a similar appearance. If contrast is administered, an associated DVA may be seen.

Vein of Galen Malformation

A VOGM is a form of arteriovenous shunt resulting from development of arteriovenous connections between primitive choroidal vessels and a persistent median prosencephalic vein of Markowski during embryonic life. The median prosencephalic vein fails to regress and becomes aneurysmal because of the high flow through the lesion. VOGM represents 1% of all vascular malformations of the brain. They are classified traditionally into choroidal (type I) and mural (type II) types based on the location and nature of the shunt.[122] However, in reality, there is a spectrum of malformations between the two extremes, and other classifications have also been described.[123,124] More than 80% of VOGMs are of the choroidal type.[124] The mural type of VOGM is characterized by AVF in the inferolateral wall of the median vein of Markowski, with collicular and/or posterior choroidal arteries in the subarachnoid space contributing to the shunt as the arterial feeders.

VOGMs are visualized on either fetal US and/or fetal MRI as midline vascular mass lesions, with increased flow in the supplying arteries and draining veins on color Doppler evaluation. 2D US may show parenchymal changes such as atrophy and encephalomalacia. Cardiomegaly and congestive heart failure with hydrops are seen in some patients, most often those with choroidal malformations. Mural malformations most often come to attention later in infancy when venous hypertension results in hydrocephalus or parenchymal volume loss.

Fetal and postnatal MRI characterizes VOGM well (Fig. 2.97). In addition to directly demonstrating the malformation, MRI shows signs of chronic ischemic brain injury as indicated by hyperintensity in the white matter on T1-weighted MR images. Parenchymal calcifications may be seen due to chronic ischemic injury. The presence of these changes correlates with poor prognosis.

Endovascular therapy is the current treatment of choice. The decision to intervene is based on clinical status, architecture of the constituent vasculature, and intravascular pressure. Neonates with compensated cardiac function may be observed for the first few months of life. Of note, in the presence of severe cerebral parenchymal damage and encephalomalacia, aggressive treatment may not be undertaken because prognosis is poor even if the shunt is successfully closed by embolization.

Extracerebral Vascular Malformation

Dural arteriovenous fistulas (dAVF) and dural AVMs (dAVM) are abnormal shunts that occur between arteries and veins within the dura. Although rare, they do occur in children and may present as a cause of fetal hydrops or postnatal congestive heart failure. The etiology of dAVF/AVM is not fully understood. Theories proposed include recanalization of thrombosed dural venous sinuses and, alternatively, response to venous sinus hypertension. Clinical presentation of dAVF/dAVM may include high-output cardiac failure, headaches, macrocrania, developmental delay, seizures and focal neurologic deficits, hemorrhagic venous infarctions secondary to venous outflow narrowing (a.k.a. "high-flow venopathy"), facial venous prominence, and symptoms of elevated intracranial pressure.

The gold standard for diagnosing dAVF/AVM is catheter angiography. Dural AVF/AVM may be clinically occult, may produce congestive heart failure, or, when between the carotid artery and cavernous sinus, may manifest with dilatation of the superior ophthalmic vein with or without exophthalmos. Although the sensitivity and specificity of CTA and MRA is low for small dAVF/AVM, large malformations can be delineated on MRA, MRV, and postcontrast MR images

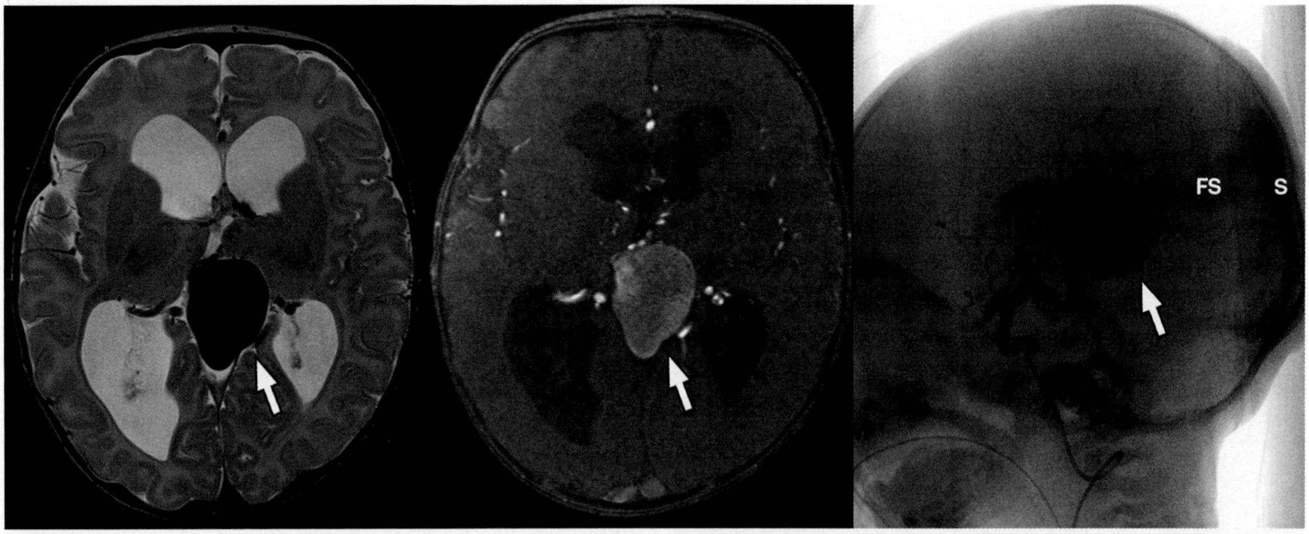

FIGURE 2.97 **Vein of Galen malformation in a neonate boy.** Axial T2-weighted MR image (on the **left**), axial MR image from a 3D time-of-flight MRA (in the **middle**), and catheter angiogram image (on the **right**) show an enlarged median prosencephalic vein of Markowski (*arrows*) draining via a falcine sinus (*FS*) into the superior sagittal sinus (*S*), with arterial feeders from the anterior and posterior circulation.

(Fig. 2.98). Time-resolved MRA has been shown to be better than conventional MRA in evaluation of dAVF/AVM, but can be technically challenging.

Angiographic evaluation of dAVF/AVM is performed using selective injection of both internal and external carotid arteries and the vertebral arteries and following the contrast into the venous phase to visualize the venous drainage. Risk factors for hemorrhage include venous sinus stenosis, partial or total venous occlusion, and venous ectasia. Management is tailored to the individual patient and is based on the anatomic location and hemodynamics of the lesion along with the patient's symptoms.

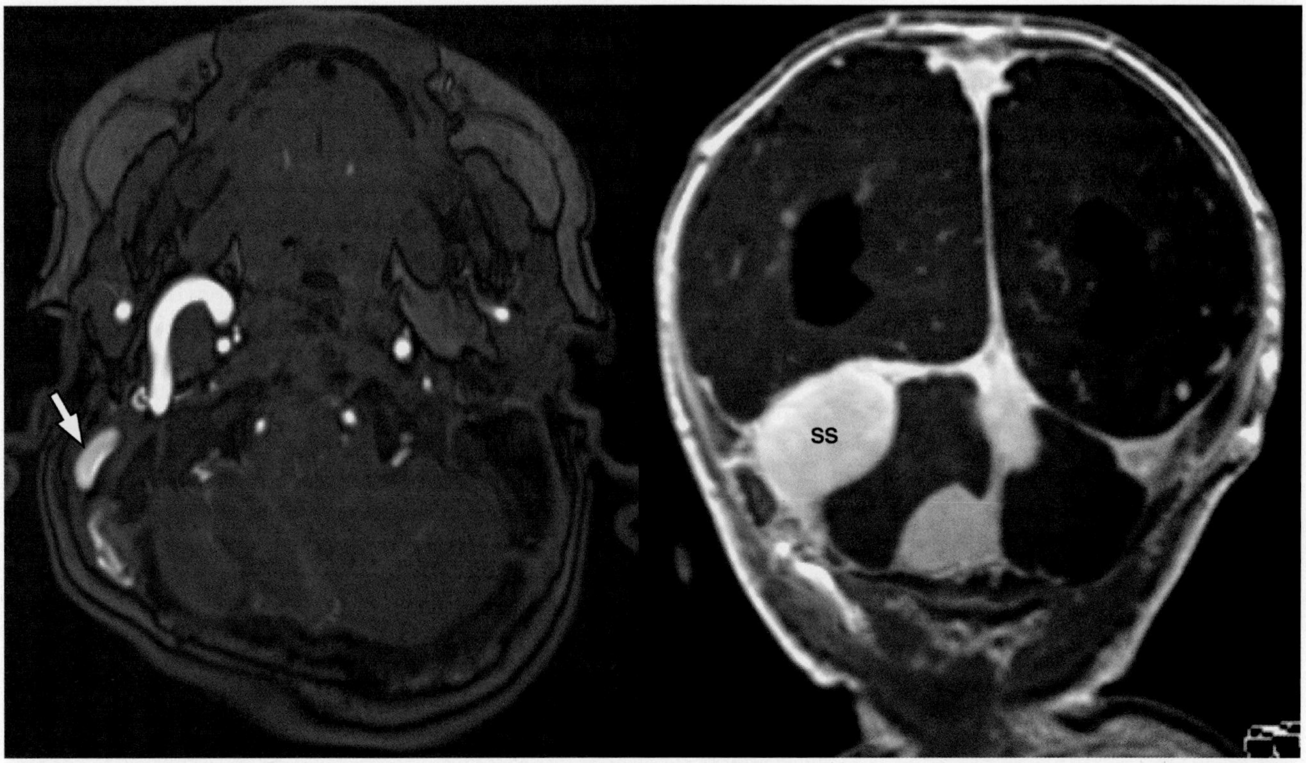

FIGURE 2.98 **Right sigmoid sinus dural arteriovenous fistula in a 7-month-old boy who presented with a marked palpable thrill over the right mastoid.** Axial 3D time-of-flight MRA image (on the **left**) and coronal T1 MPRAGE (magnetization-prepared, rapid acquisition, gradient recalled echo) image (on the **right**) show an enlarged right occipital artery (*arrow*) communicating with the markedly enlarged sigmoid sinus (*SS*).

Most dAVF/AVMs can be treated using an endovascular approach, but some lesions require surgical intervention or a mixed endovascular and surgical approach. Endovascular therapy is often effective in obliterating dAVF/AVM in children, with most affected pediatric patients experiencing substantial and lasting improvement of clinical symptoms, especially when the lesion is comprised of a single-hole fistula. Genetic screening and hypercoagulable workup must be undertaken, particularly when other vascular anomalies or venous sinus thromboses exist.

Intracranial Aneurysm (Congenital and Acquired)

An aneurysm is defined as a localized, pathologic, blood-filled dilatation of a blood vessel caused by a disease or weakening of the vessel wall. Intracranial aneurysms are relatively rare in children, with 0.5% to 4.6% of intracranial aneurysms occurring in patients aged 18 years or younger.[125]

The pathogenesis of intracranial aneurysms in children is different from those in adults; this distinction is important, as the clinical course and prognosis depend on the causative mechanism. Pathogenesis of aneurysms can be related to trauma, infection, inflammation, arteriopathy, excessive hemodynamic stress, metastatic tumor ("oncotic"), and familial and idiopathic causes.[7] Aneurysms presenting during the first two decades of life are usually idiopathic. Nearly 80% of intracranial aneurysms in the pediatric population are idiopathic, posttraumatic, or due to excessive hemodynamic stress such as arteriovenous shunts and hypertension.[126] Congenital aneurysmal arteriopathies and infections account for most of the remainder.

Findings on imaging studies may provide a clue to the pathogenetic mechanism. For example, an aneurysm occurring in a patient with a skull fracture is likely posttraumatic, and the presentation of SAH in an immunocompromised patient favors infection as the etiology. Features of pediatric intracranial aneurysms that have been shown to differ from those affecting adults include male predominance, greater involvement of the posterior circulation and internal carotid bifurcation, and a greater number of giant aneurysms.

Intracranial aneurysms have been divided into four types: fusiform, saccular, traumatic, and infectious. Saccular aneurysms are the most likely to rupture. Traumatic aneurysms are located closest to the skull base and may occur in the anterior and posterior circulations. Intracranial aneurysms in children are most commonly located at the ICA terminus (Fig. 2.99). The next most common locations are the anterior communicating artery and the MCA bifurcation. Aneurysms are usually single in young children. Also, there is a higher frequency of giant aneurysms ($\geq$25 mm in diameter) and fusiform aneurysms in young children under 1 year of age as compared to adults. The presence of multiple synchronous or metachronous aneurysms implies an underlying arteriopathy or predisposition to aneurysm formation.

The initial imaging study is usually a noncontrast CT that is performed in a child presenting with severe headache or meningismus. CT usually demonstrates SAH if there has been rupture of an intracranial aneurysm, but if the CT is normal and the clinical picture is consistent with a SAH, a lumbar puncture may be indicated. The choice of imaging study is based on the age of the child, the availability of imaging options, and personnel trained in interventional treatments. Most institutions perform a CT angiogram or a MR angiogram immediately after detection of SAH on the noncontrast CT to quickly identify the source of the bleeding. A catheter angiogram may be required if the source of the hemorrhage is not demonstrated on noninvasive imaging or when endovascular intervention is contemplated. It is important to note that a noncontrast CT may miss unruptured intracranial

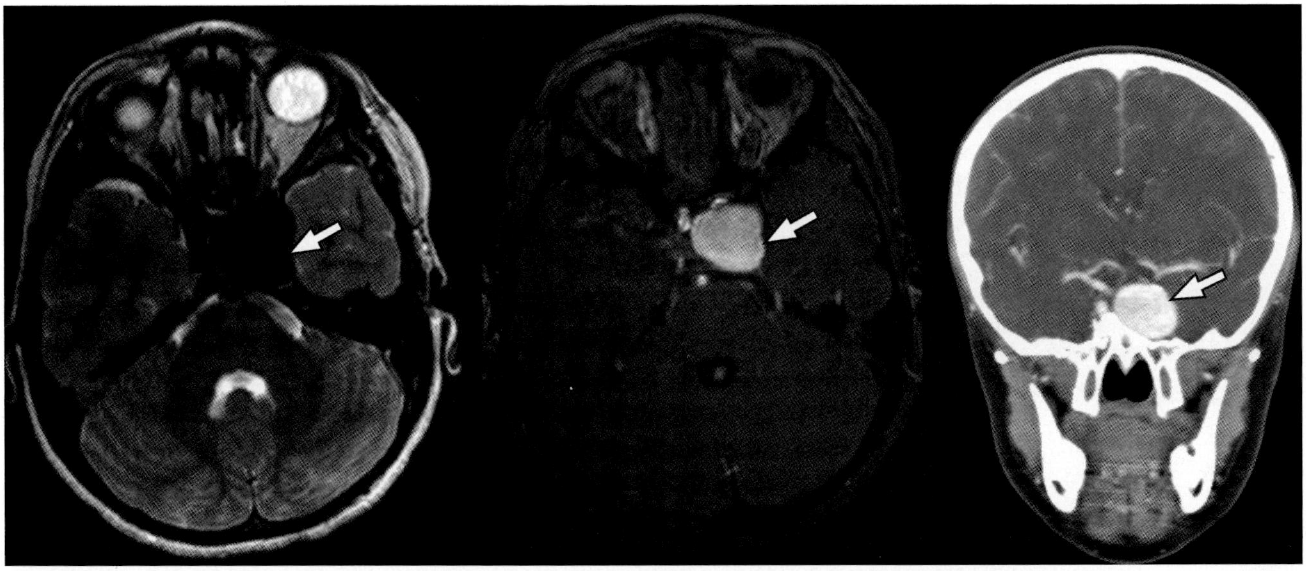

FIGURE 2.99 **Internal carotid artery aneurysm in a 5-year-old boy.** Axial T2-weighted MR image (on the **left**), 3D time-of-flight MRA image (in the **middle**), and coronal reformatted image from CTA (on the **right**) show a 2.5 cm fusiform aneurysm (*arrows*) arising from the cavernous segment of the left internal carotid artery, indicated by the flow void on the T2-weighted MR image, flow-related signal on the MRA image, and contrast enhancement on the CTA image.

aneurysms. MRI with MRA is considered the screening study of choice in pediatric patients with unruptured aneurysms presenting with nonspecific clinical symptoms such as headache or seizure. MRI and MRA are often used for long-term follow-up of children with intracranial aneurysms, to detect enlargement of an untreated lesion, or to look for development of new aneurysms that may warrant more aggressive treatment.

The current treatment options for pediatric intracranial arterial aneurysms include observation, endovascular treatment, and surgical clipping. A multidisciplinary team including neurointerventional radiologists, neurosurgeons, and stroke neurologists is best able to decide upon the most optimal management option for an individual pediatric patient with intracranial aneurysms.

Hemorrhagic, Ischemic, and Thrombotic Disorders

Neonatal Intracranial Hemorrhage

Acute intracranial hemorrhage in the neonate may be epidural, subdural, subarachnoid, subpial, or parenchymal in location. Hemorrhages may be small and noted incidentally on imaging performed for other reasons or may be large and produce acute neurologic symptoms. Birth-related hemorrhage has been discussed in an earlier section of this chapter.

Germinal Matrix Hemorrhage

Parenchymal hemorrhage in preterm infants occurs most often in or around the highly vascular subependymal germinal matrix. Microscopic perivenular hemorrhage in the highly cellular and vascular germinal matrix is thought to be the underlying mechanism, although multiple factors are involved in its causation.

The Papile classification remains the most widely accepted method of grading the severity of germinal matrix hemorrhage (GMH) in the preterm infant. Grade I consists of subependymal hemorrhage only, seen on US as bright echogenic foci in the subependymal area, typically in or anterior to the caudothalamic groove. Grade II is defined as subependymal and intraventricular hemorrhage (IVH) without ventricular dilatation. Grade III is a combination of subependymal and IVH with ventricular dilatation by clot (Fig. 2.100). It is important to distinguish progression of a grade II to a grade III hemorrhage from the development of posthemorrhagic hydrocephalus. Of note, the ventricle is almost completely distended by clot in grade III hemorrhage, whereas the ventricle in posthemorrhagic hydrocephalus is distended mainly with CSF. This difference is important, because ventricular dilatation caused by increasing hemorrhage may have different implications from that associated with posthemorrhagic hydrocephalus. Destruction of the germinal matrix and the precursor glial cells within it has an adverse effect on subsequent brain development.

Periventricular Hemorrhagic Infarction

Periventricular hemorrhagic infarction (PVHI), formerly described as a grade IV GMH in the original Papile classification, is now known to be caused by pressure of the GMH on the periventricular terminal medullary veins that drain the cerebral hemispheres, leading to venous thrombosis and infarction. Between 10% and 15% of very low birth weight infants with IVH develop hemorrhagic necrosis in the periventricular white matter.[127] The most common result of the periventricular hemorrhagic infarction is a large porencephalic cyst, either alone or in combination with other smaller cysts. PVHI may also be seen in utero in the absence of IVH.

US with color Doppler can be used to distinguish extracerebral fluid collections, such as subarachnoid, subdural, or combined hemorrhages, by visualizing the vessels coursing through the extra-axial space. Superficial cortical blood vessels lie within the pia–arachnoid. Fluid in the subarachnoid space lifts the cortical vessels away from the brain surface, whereas fluid in the subdural space approximates cortical vessels to the brain surface and is separated from these vessels by a thin membrane. On CT, acute hemorrhage appears hyperdense relative to the brain parenchyma. Of note, the dural venous sinuses and cortical veins appear relatively dense

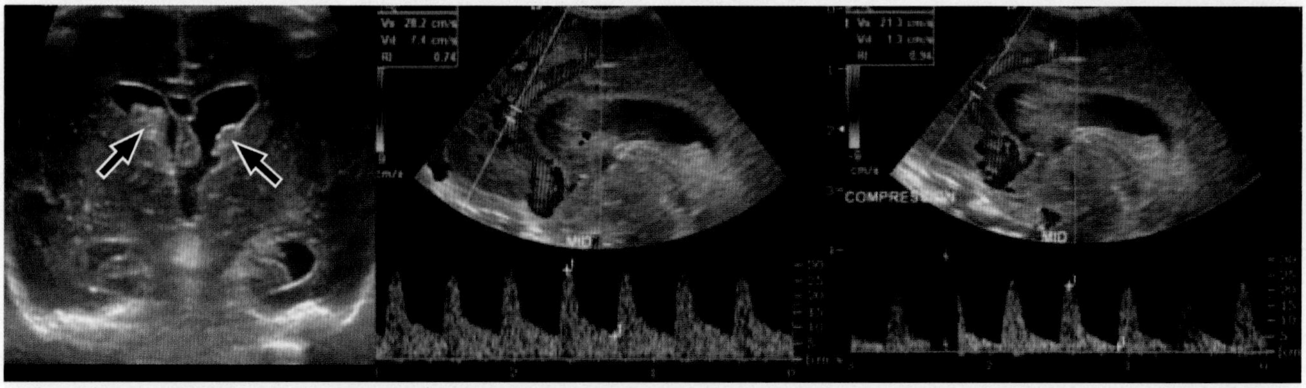

FIGURE 2.100 **Intraventricular hemorrhage in a 4-day-old boy.** Coronal head ultrasound (US) image (on the **left**) shows hemorrhage (*arrows*) within the mildly dilated lateral ventricles. Doppler US evaluation of the anterior cerebral artery without compression (in the **middle**) and with compression (on the **right**) demonstrates the relatively high resistive indices. Of note, the RI increases with compression (RI = 0.91) as compared to without compression (RI = 0.74).

during the first few days of life owing to high hematocrit levels. The low density of the brain parenchyma in this age group further accentuates this finding. This normal density of the venous structures should not be mistaken for subdural bleeding or dural venous sinus thrombosis on CT. In the chronic phase, sites of extra-axial or parenchymal hemorrhage have decreased density relative to the brain parenchyma. On MRI, use of gradient-echo sequences and SWI technique helps delineate significant intracranial hemorrhages in the newborn.

Neonatal Hypoxic Ischemic Injury

Term Infants

Hypoxic ischemic injury (HII) is defined as a clinical syndrome observed in neonates, thought to result primarily from decreased blood flow (ischemia) and oxygen supply (hypoxia) to the brain either before, during, or after birth. Injury is due not only to the initial insult but also hyperemic reperfusion that incites a host of neurotoxic events.

The patterns of brain injury depend upon a number of factors including maturity of the brain, severity and duration of ischemia, and other states including inflammation and infection. It is important to note that the timing of the imaging study also affects the appearance of the brain in these infants. The severity and duration of HII can be divided into two basic types: severe total asphyxia and prolonged partial asphyxia. Severe total asphyxia is characterized by sudden and total loss of blood flow and oxygenation, whereas prolonged partial asphyxia is more sustained, but incomplete loss of blood flow. There is often an overlap between these two types.

Imaging findings of HII also depend on the timing of the imaging study. Early imaging in the first 72 hours may underestimate the ultimate extent of the injury, as the changes resulting from cell death peak around this time after the initial injury.[128] Therapeutic hypothermia may result in the MR being normal or showing a delay in the appearance of the typical imaging features of hypoxia–ischemia.

The central pattern of injury is characterized by damage to the most metabolically active structures, including actively myelinating areas and those containing high concentrations of excitatory neurotransmitters. These areas include the dorsal brainstem, cerebellar vermis, posterior limb of internal capsule, corona radiata, perirolandic white matter, optic radiations, hippocampi, lateral thalami, and posterior portion of the putamen.[128] This deep, central pattern usually results from profound asphyxia caused by sudden interruption of the blood supply, which deprives the brain of oxygen and glucose.[128]

The peripheral pattern of injury is characterized by injury to the cortex and the subcortical white matter, predominantly in the parietooccipital and posterior temporal lobes. It usually results from a period of decreased blood supply (and not complete cessation of blood supply). It is thought to develop as a result of a compensatory shunting of blood to vital brain structures, such as the brainstem, deep gray nuclei, hippocampi, and cerebellum, with relative hypoperfusion of the cerebral cortex and white matter. More prolonged hypoxia results in injury to the watershed zones (borders between vascular territories), which are relatively hypoperfused because of this shunting.

Sensitivity for accurately detecting early ischemia is low on CT and US in the neonate. Because of the requirement for ionizing radiation and the relatively insensitivity of CT for the early manifestations of HII, it is now rarely performed as an initial study in children with suspected HII. On cranial US, ischemic areas of thalamus and basal ganglia may appear focally or diffusely echogenic. However, US findings may be variable in time of onset and US underestimates the extent of injury compared to CT or MRI.

HII typically results in bilaterally symmetric injury, which can make MRI interpretation challenging. The interpretation of MRI in neonates with HII requires knowledge of the normal appearance of the brain for a given stage of development, including the expected myelination pattern, the areas most likely to be affected, and the typical time-course for evolution of injury. It is also important to recognize that the injury from hypoxia–ischemia is, in part, related to energy failure and that other causes of metabolic derangement affecting energy metabolism may produce a similar pattern of injury.

Although there is considerable variability in the MR appearance of HII, some general trends may be observed. Up to 15 to 18 hours following the ischemic event, DWI is often normal.[127,129] Over the next 24 to 48 hours, decreased diffusion develops within the regions of the brain with the highest metabolic requirements. On MRI, T1- and T2-weighted sequences typically also fail to show any abnormality in the first 2 to 3 days. Some studies indicate that ADC values in visibly normal-appearing brain, particularly in the basal ganglia and brainstem, may correlate with outcome. T1 shortening may be seen in the ventrolateral thalami and posterolateral putamina on an MRI performed between 3 and 7 days of life.[129]

The MR signal abnormality is graded as mild if the normal hyperintense signal of the PLIC is preserved. In moderate injury, extension of the T1 shortening anteriorly into the putamen and posteromedially into the thalamus with equivocal or abnormal signal in the PLIC is usually seen, and there is loss of the normal hypointensity of the affected myelinated regions on T2-weighted imaging (Fig. 2.101). In severe injury, the entire thalamus, putamen, and globus pallidus may show T1 hyperintense signal, and the normal hyperintense signal of the PLIC is typically lost on T1-weighted imaging ("absent PLIC" sign). Hyperintense T1 signal is also noted in the perirolandic cortex, and in cases of more severe injury, the insular cortex might be involved. In very severe cases, cortical highlighting is observed throughout, which is a considered a predictor of poor clinical outcome.[127]

On T2-weighted MR images, the deep gray nuclei may become subtly indistinct, and the posterior thalami may become isointense with white matter because of presence of vasogenic edema. When the injury is more severe, the thalami, lentiform nuclei, and caudate head may show

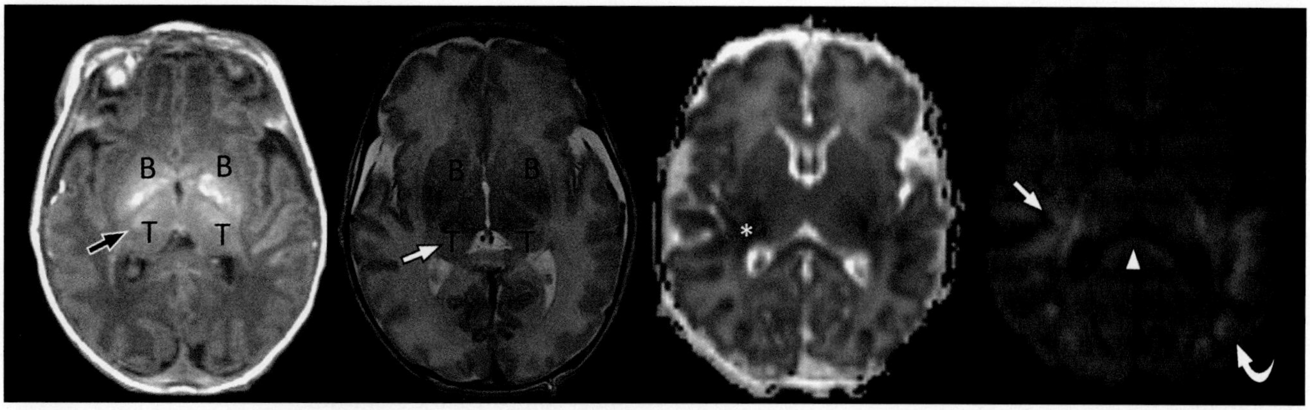

FIGURE 2.101 **Hypoxic-ischemic injury in a term newborn boy with history of perinatal depression.** Axial T1-weighted (*first image* on the **left**), axial T2-weighted (*second image* from the **left**), axial ADC (*third image* from the **left**), and diffusion-weighted (on the **right**) MR images show increased T1 signal (*black arrow*) and loss of normal T2 hypointensity in the ventrolateral thalamus (*T*), basal ganglia (*B*), and internal capsule (*asterisk*), with decreased diffusion in these areas (*white arrow*), perirolandic cortex, the gray and white matter junction (*curved arrow*), and the callosal splenium (*arrowhead*).

T2 hyperintensity, and the normally T2 hypointense PLIC may be "absent." After the first week, in cases with severe injury, T2 shortening develops in the thalami and basal ganglia in either a diffuse or patchy pattern. Hemorrhage, calcification, lipid release from myelin breakdown, myelin gliosis, and paramagnetic effects of free radicals are the proposed causes for this finding. Hemorrhage is considered an unlikely cause for these signal changes because T2 shortening occurs several days after the initial T1 changes, and these regions do not bloom on gradient-echo T2-weighted or susceptibility-weighted MR images. In the chronic stage, atrophy of the injured structures is seen along with T2 prolongation.[129]

Toward the end of the first week, decreased diffusion may be seen in the subcortical white matter in areas that showed normal or even increased diffusion on early examinations. By 10 to 14 days, the diffusion abnormalities typically normalize, and ultimately, increased diffusion may be present. In the longer term, signal abnormalities related to gliosis, mineralization, or hypermyelination associated with variable tissue loss are seen on both T1- and T2-weighted sequences.[127,128]

The abnormalities on MRI evolve over the first 2 weeks after birth. Thus, initially mild injury may evolve to a more severe injury pattern in the first week because of delayed cell death. In chronic stages, a pattern referred to as ulegyria (mushroom-shaped gyri), characterized by shrunken gyri and enlarged sulci, is seen in the cortex. Encephalomalacia is seen in a parasagittal distribution.

Premature Infants

Premature infants are particularly vulnerable to the effects of ischemic injury because of low physiologic cerebral blood flow to white matter, an immature autoregulatory system for cerebral blood flow, vulnerability of premyelinating oligodendrocytes to free radical attack, and increased frequency of events potentially causing hypoperfusion, like respiratory distress syndrome, pneumothorax, patent ductus arteriosus, and neonatal sepsis.

In premature infants, HII predominantly affects the deep gray matter and brainstem nuclei. Accompanying GMH occurs in some, and white matter injury occurs in most affected infants. Profound asphyxia in infants <32 weeks of gestation results in injury to the thalami, basal ganglia, and brainstem. The thalamus is more likely to be injured than the basal ganglia because it myelinates earlier (23 to 25 weeks). As myelinated regions have higher metabolic activity and hence higher energy demands, they are more susceptible to acute profound hypoperfusion.[127] The preterm cortex may be relatively spared, possibly explained by the caudocranial pattern of myelination, and by an increase in cortical glutamate receptors in infants closer to term gestation.

As with term neonates, if MR imaging is performed on preterm infants on the first day of injury, T1- and T2-weighted MR images may be normal or show subtle abnormalities. Diffusion-weighted MR imaging shows decreased diffusion by 24 hours, and in 3 to 5 days, diffusion decrease in the thalami becomes apparent but subsequently pseudonormalizes. T2-weighted MR images show hyperintense signal in the thalami by day 2, and T2 shortening develops after the first week (Fig. 2.102).[127,130,131] T1-weighted MR images show hyperintense signal in injured regions by day 3, and T1 shortening persists into the chronic stage. In the chronic stage, the thalami are small, shrunken, and often calcified, the brainstem and cerebellum are small, the basal ganglia might be small or absent, and the cerebral white matter volume is reduced. The reduction of cerebral white matter is possibly the result of loss of the thalamocortical, corticothalamic, and corticoputaminal axons. On MRI, white matter volume loss is best appreciated by observing the distance between the depths of the sulci and the ventricular margins. If the sulcal depths are close to or abutting the ventricle, this indicates severe white matter volume loss. Also, the corpus callosum shrinks and remains thin when it is expected to thicken, which is around 6 months of age.

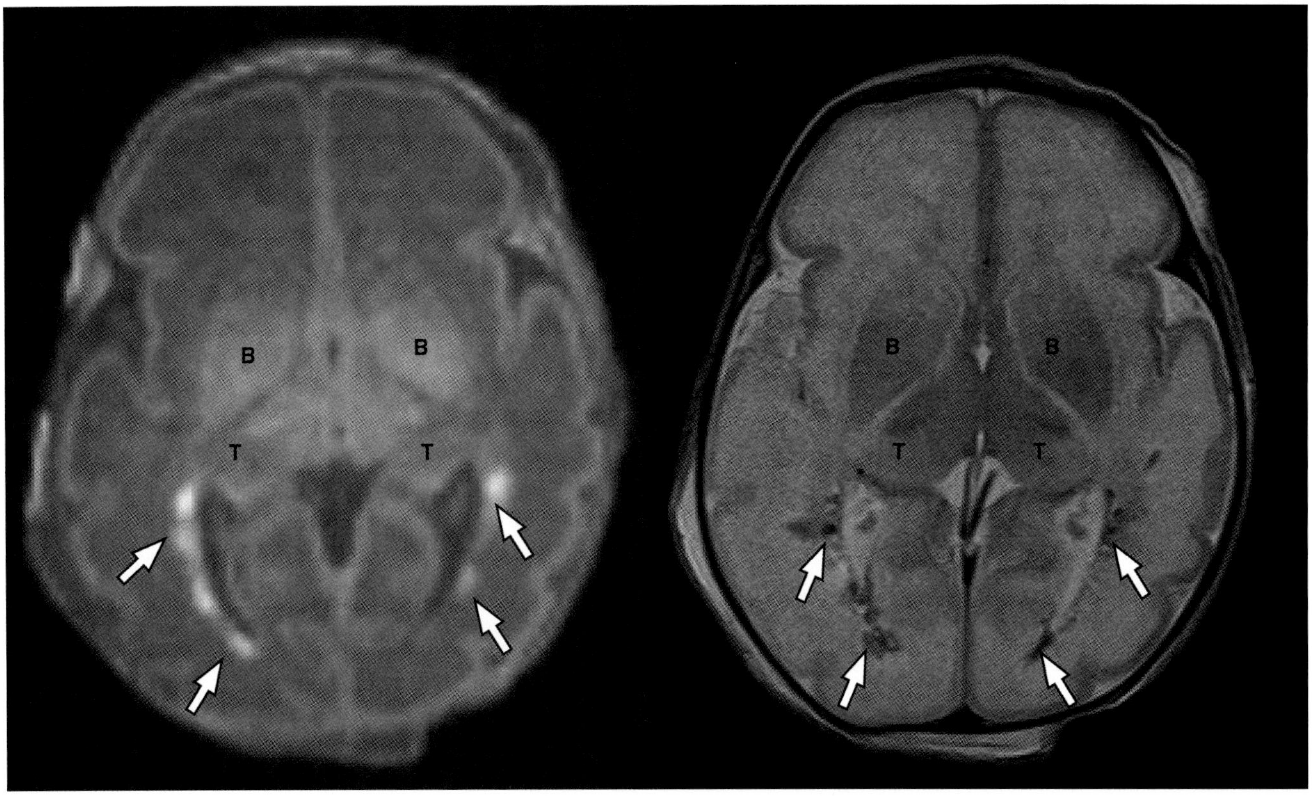

FIGURE 2.102 **Deep medullary vein thrombosis and hypoxic injury in a 30-week gestation preterm newborn infant.** Axial T1-weighted (on the **left**) and T2-weighted (on the **right**) MR images obtained at 14 days of age show hypoxic injury indicated by thalamic (*T*) and basal ganglia (*B*) signal abnormality and T1 hyperintensity and T2 hypointensity consistent with medullary vein thrombosis (*arrows*).

White Matter Injury of Prematurity (a.k.a. Periventricular Leukomalacia)

White matter injury of prematurity, a.k.a. periventricular leukomalacia (PVL), is characterized by focal areas of necrosis in the periventricular white matter, optic radiations, and acoustic radiations, and less prominent, more diffuse cerebral white matter injury. White matter injury of prematurity is characterized in the acute phase by coagulation necrosis and neuroaxonal swelling. A variable amount of hemorrhage may be present. In the subacute stage, cysts may form in the larger lesions. Ultimately, gliosis develops and the cysts become less apparent.

On US, the brain may appear normal initially within the first 2 weeks. After 10 to 14 days, deep white matter echogenicity increases.[129] Echogenic abnormalities are typically located along the trigones of the lateral ventricles but can involve extensive areas of white matter. Encephalomalacia develops subsequently in these areas within 2 to 3 weeks after the initial insult. Encephalomalacia is characterized by single or multiple cysts ranging between 1 mm to 3 cm diameter, occasionally communicating with the ventricular system (Fig. 2.103). Associated dilatation of the adjacent ventricle and prominence of the sulci and interhemispheric fissure are seen. On MRI, heavily T2-weighted thin-section MR images help delineate cystic areas optimally. Associated hemorrhage appears as foci of T1 shortening and hypointensity on T2-weighted sequences. Imaging studies on follow-up show white matter loss and squaring of the ventricles, but the cystic foci become less conspicuous (Fig. 2.104). In general, injury progressing to cyst formation is much less common today than in the past because of advances in care of the premature infant.

Childhood Arterial Ischemic Stroke

Arterial ischemic stroke (AIS) is defined as "rapidly developing clinical signs of focal disturbance of cerebral function, with symptoms lasting 24 hours or longer, or leading to death, with no apparent cause other than of vascular origin." Although this is a clinical definition, the high frequency of stroke mimics in children means that brain imaging is mandatory to distinguish vascular from nonvascular stroke syndromes.

There is a misconception that AIS is a rare childhood disorder. Approximately 2 to 6/100,000 children are affected annually, and it is one of the top ten causes of childhood death.[132] Presenting symptoms and clinical findings vary with the age of the child and usually relate to the site of ischemic injury. Infants typically present with nonspecific signs of seizures, hypotonia, and lethargy. Older children often have a similar presentation to that of adults, although initially the etiology of their symptoms is often unclear, resulting in significant delays in recognition and appropriate investigation.

Focal cerebral arteriopathy of childhood (FCA) accounts for a quarter of the arteriopathies, with moyamoya pattern

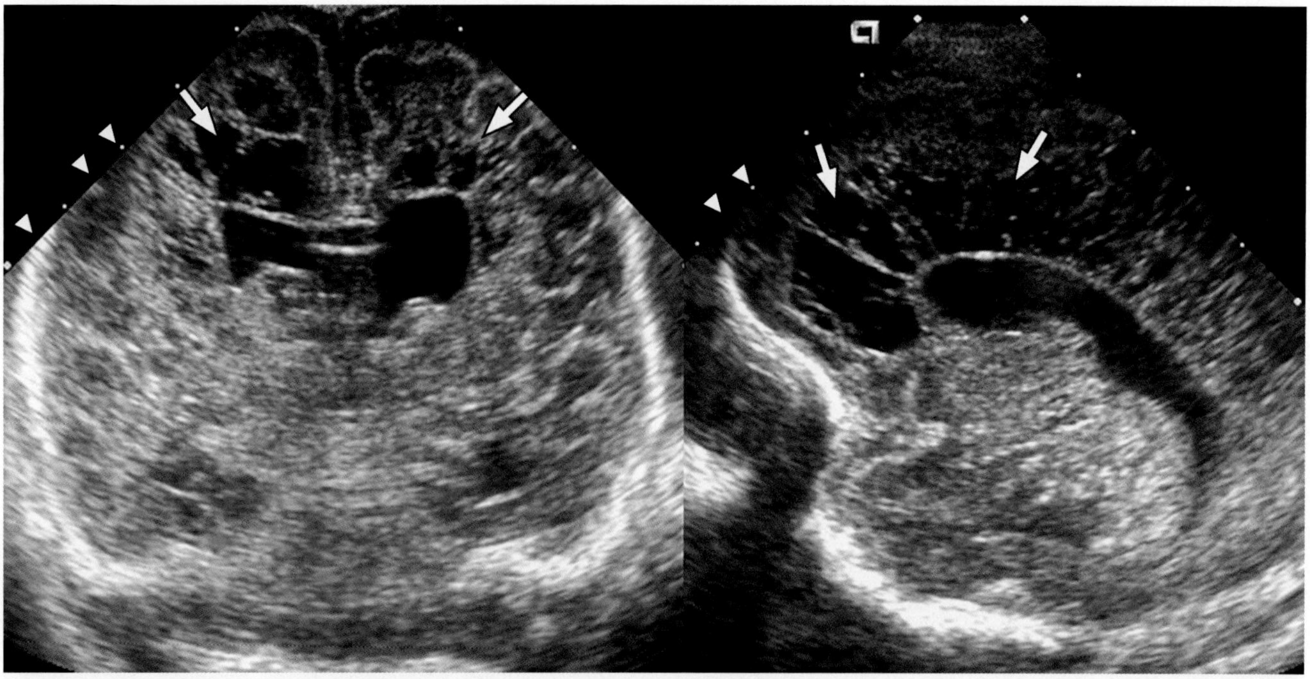

FIGURE 2.103 **Periventricular leukomalacia (PVL) in a premature infant boy.** Coronal (on the **left**) and sagittal (on the **right**) head ultrasound images show cystic changes (*arrows*) in the periventricular white matter, which are characteristic for PVL.

vasculopathies and arterial dissection accounting for 22% and 20%, respectively.[133] Vasculitis, sickle cell disease (SCD), and postvaricella angiopathy (PVA) account for ~25%, although postvaricella vasculopathy is rarely seen in children who have been immunized for chickenpox.[133] Cardiac disease (both congenital and acquired) and hypercoagulable states like protein C and S deficiency, antithrombin III deficiency, and factor V Leiden mutation are potential precipitators of AIS in children.

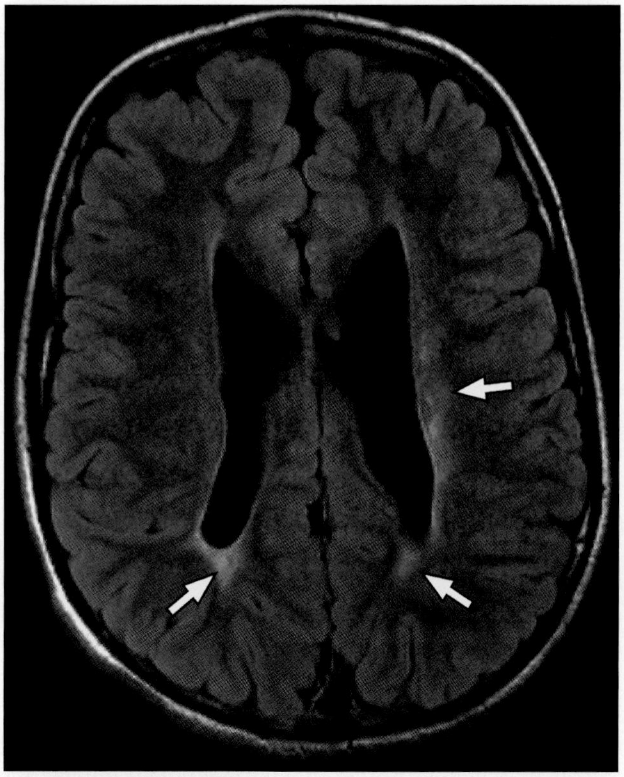

FIGURE 2.104 **Sequelae of periventricular leukomalacia in a 10-year-old boy born at 27 weeks of gestation, with developmental delay, cerebral palsy, and seizures.** Axial FLAIR MR image shows periventricular white matter signal abnormality (*arrows*), white matter loss, and squaring of the lateral ventricles.

MRI is the imaging modality of choice for the investigation of pediatric AIS because of its greater sensitivity and specificity in the diagnosis of stroke and conditions that may cause stroke-like symptoms ("stroke mimics"). Immediate access to an MRI unit is the gold standard but is not universally available. The initial diagnostic imperative is for the confirmation of AIS and exclusion of alternative treatable pathologies. CT may be obtained when MRI is unavailable within the required time for assessment.

The majority of strokes occur within the anterior circulation, predominantly involving the middle cerebral artery (MCA) territories (Fig. 2.105). This is likely because most AIS is due to emboli, which are flow directed, and therefore, most likely to lodge in the MCA , the intracranial vessel with the greatest amount of blood flow. In general, a focal pattern of infarction is seen in nonprogressive arteriopathies and thromboembolic disease. A pattern of infarction involving the watershed areas is seen in the progressive occlusive vasculopathies. Lacunar infarcts are rare in childhood age groups.

Vasculopathy

The pathophysiology and imaging appearances of a number of different types of arteriopathy in childhood are discussed in more detail below.

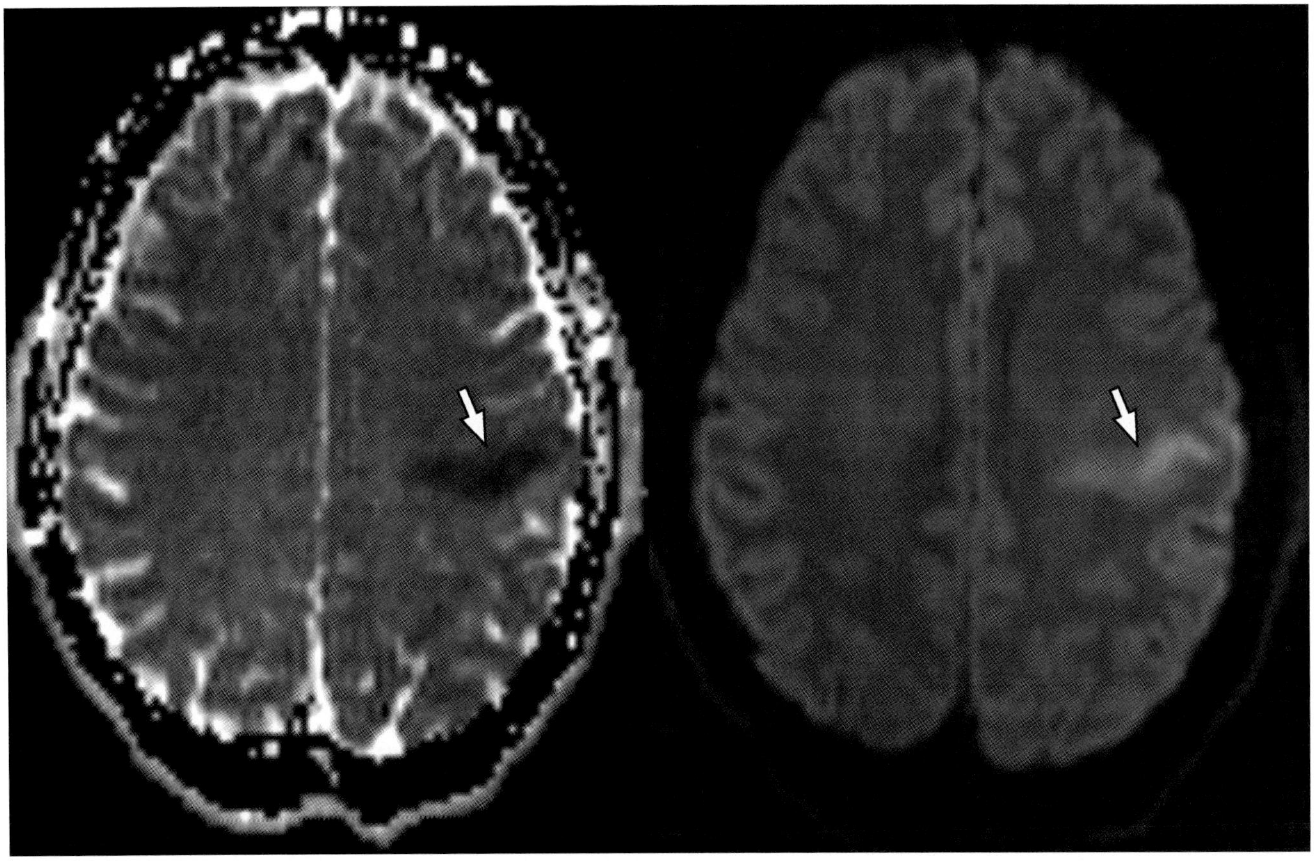

FIGURE 2.105 **Acute arterial ischemic stroke in a 3-year-old boy.** Axial ADC (on the **left**) and diffusion-weighted (on the **right**) MR images show decreased diffusion (*arrows*) in the left postcentral gyrus and adjacent subcortical and deep white matter, consistent with acute infarction.

Focal Arteriopathy of Childhood

Focal cerebral arteriopathy of childhood (FCA) refers to children with idiopathic focal intracranial arterial stenosis. This term includes previously described entities including transient cerebral arteriopathy (TCA) of childhood and nonprogressive CNS vasculitis.

TCA is a monophasic and transient cerebral arteriopathy. A formal diagnosis of TCA may be made after confirming that there is no evidence of additional stenoses nor progression of the original stenosis on follow-up imaging studies performed 6 months after the initial stroke. The presence of unifocal or multifocal symptomatic cerebral arterial stenosis without an identified cause has been called primary nonprogressive CNS vasculitis in children. These labels are provisional diagnoses that do not specify an underlying pathophysiology.

FCA is a descriptive term coined by the International Pediatric Stroke Study (IPSS) investigators that may be applied at baseline (unlike TCA) and does not imply an underlying mechanism (unlike vasculitis).[133] The cause of FCA remains unknown. A preceding viral infection has been shown to be the best predictor of FCA in the IPSS.[133] FCA may be due to post varicella angiopathy if there is a history of varicella infection in the prior 12 months. Hemiplegia is the most common presenting symptom, reflecting the typical location of the infarct in the basal ganglia or internal capsule, areas supplied by the lenticulostriate arteries.

Imaging findings in FCA include typical findings of an infarct including hypodensity on CT (varying with age of the infarct) and restricted diffusion on MRI. The focal arterial lesion may be defined by CTA or MRA. Catheter angiography remains the most reliable modality to define the arterial lesion. Some pediatric patients with presumed FCA will have progressive steno-occlusive disease and prove to have early moyamoya vasculopathy.

Moyamoya Vasculopathy

The term "moyamoya" refers to the characteristic appearance of dilated lenticulostriate perforating vessels on angiography resembling a "puff of smoke" or "moyamoya" in Japanese, resulting from progressive occlusive disease of the distal internal carotid arteries. It is important to understand that the term moyamoya is descriptive only and the vascular pattern may result from a variety of different causes. Idiopathic moyamoya is called "moyamoya disease." The moyamoya pattern, however, can be seen in pediatric patients with other conditions like neurofibromatosis type 1, previous cranial radiation, sickle cell anemia, Down syndrome, Alagille syndrome, and HIV.[134,135] This secondary form is called moyamoya syndrome or vasculopathy. The idiopathic type and secondary types have somewhat similar imaging appearances, although the detailed angiographic pattern is variable, as is the clinical outcome.

Children with moyamoya disease or syndrome most often initially develop headaches. Seizures, transient ischemic attacks, or permanent neurologic deficits and developmental delay or regression may also occur. Unlike in adults with a moyamoya vascular pattern, hemorrhage is very uncommon in children.

The characteristic steno-occlusive changes initially involve the distal intracranial internal carotid arteries at the level of their bifurcation, with extension into the proximal anterior and middle cerebral arteries (Fig. 2.106). Although not part of the original description of moyamoya, which was based on angiography that did not include interrogation of the posterior circulation, steno-occlusive change of the proximal portions of the posterior cerebral arteries is present in up to 25% of children with the vasculopathy. The underlying pathology within the involved arteries includes endothelial hyperplasia and fibrocellular intimal thickening with tortuosity or undulation of the internal elastic lamina and attenuation of the media. There is no evidence of inflammatory change within the vessel wall except in patients with moyamoya syndrome secondary to HIV.

Collateral vessels form in response to the progressive steno-occlusive changes and longstanding cerebral hypoperfusion. These collateral vessels mainly consist of dilated and newly recruited lenticulostriate and thalamostriate perforator arteries, leptomeningeal collaterals from one major vascular territory to another, and dural to pial collaterals. Small flow-related aneurysms occur in <1% of children with moyamoya.

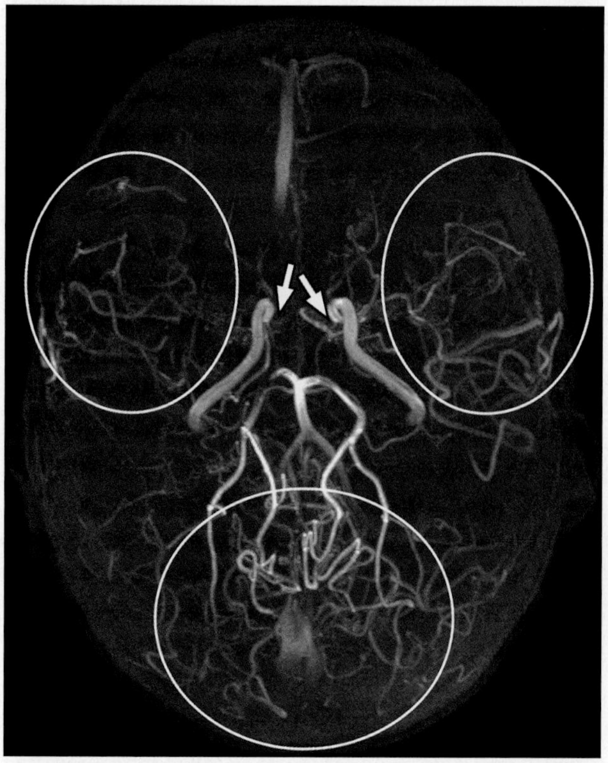

FIGURE 2.106 **Moyamoya disease in previously well 7-year-old boy.** 3D maximum intensity reconstruction from an MRA shows the narrowed bilateral distal internal carotid arteries (*arrows*) and numerous collaterals (*circles*) arising from the posterior circulation and extracranial arteries.

Diagnosis of moyamoya can be made in most cases using a CT angiogram or MRI with MRA, which can demonstrate the occluded or stenotic terminal ICAs and collateral arterial vessels. Findings include decrease in size or loss of the flow voids of the terminal ICA and its proximal branches. The collateral vessels are seen as flow voids within the basal ganglia, thalamus, and basal cisterns on T2-weighted MR images, an appearance that is virtually diagnostic of moyamoya. MRA with three-dimensional maximum intensity projection confirms these findings. Note that the acquisition field of view for the MRA should include the external carotid arteries to visualize the peripheral collaterals in patients with moyamoya. A sensitive but nonspecific sign for moyamoya is the presence of sulcal high signal intensity on FLAIR sequences, known as the "ivy sign."[136] It correlates with vascular enhancement on postgadolinium T1-weighted sequences and is thought to represent engorged pial collateral vessels. DWI sequences allow identification of areas of acute hypoperfusion in pediatric patients presenting with AIS.[137] More recently, arterial spin-labeled images and dynamic susceptibility contrast imaging sequences have been used to detect reduced regional perfusion per vascular territory.[138,139]

The diagnosis of moyamoya vasculopathy is confirmed using conventional catheter angiography, which should include selective injections of both internal and external carotid arteries and at least one vertebral artery to completely map out the steno-occlusive disease, the degree of collateralization, and extent of cerebral hypoperfusion. Angiography is also used to determine the status of vessels that might be used for surgical revascularization, such as the superficial temporal artery, and the existence of spontaneous transdural collaterals from the middle meningeal arteries that would need to be preserved during surgery.

Treatment includes a variety of indirect revascularization procedures using branches of the external carotid artery to supplement blood flow to the brain and direct external carotid–internal carotid arterial bypass operations. Imaging plays an important role in assessing postoperative cerebral revascularization.

Sickle Cell Disease Vasculopathy

SCD is a well-recognized risk factor for both clinical and subclinical AIS. Approximately one in five patients with SCD will have a stroke before the second decade of life.[140] The risk of stroke increases after the age of 2 because of the loss of the protective effects of fetal hemoglobin. A child with SCD has a 250-fold risk of a stroke compared to that of a healthy child.

Typical clinical presentation of affected children includes AIS either during acute vasoocclusive pain episodes and acute anemic crisis or as an isolated phenomenon. The highest rate of stroke in SCD is seen in children between the ages of 2 and 5 followed by those from 6 to 9 years of age. On the other hand, hemorrhagic stroke resulting from rupture of fine moyamoya-like collaterals or flow-related aneurysms predominates in the second and third decades of life.

The causes for AIS in SCD are multifactorial. Nearly 75% of strokes in SCD are related to a large-vessel occlusive vasculopathy. This occlusive vasculopathy results from intimal hyperplasia as consequence of sickle red blood cells directly damaging and adhering to the endothelium. This in turn provokes a proinflammatory state, which is characterized by (1) leukocyte and platelet aggregation, (2) increased vasomotor tone, and (3) proliferation of small myoblasts and fibroblasts within the intimal layer causing progressive luminal narrowing. The supraclinoid ICA is the most affected, followed by the proximal middle and anterior cerebral arteries. The posterior circulation is relatively spared.

The typical MRI appearance includes infarcts at the junctions of the arterial border zones. MRA may show signal dropout in the regions of stenosis, but it is important to remember that both anemia and sickled cells may cause turbulence and signal loss, especially at vessel bifurcations, that may mimic true stenosis. Progressive vasculopathy with moyamoya-type collaterals is seen in up to 40% of patients with SCD vasculopathy. The imaging appearance in these patients is identical to those with idiopathic moyamoya disease. Rarely, strokes result from distal thrombus embolism from aggregates formed at the sites of intracranial stenosis or fat embolism as a result of bone infarction. Although intracranial arterial vasculopathy is the most likely cause of stroke in a patient with SCD, other disorders including infection, cardiac embolism, and venous sinus thrombosis should be considered as well.

The usual initial treatment of acute ischemic infarction resulting from SCD is hydration and exchange transfusion, although there are no controlled studies to prove the value of this approach. Regular blood transfusions have been used in children with SCD for secondary stroke prevention. Limited data suggests that bone marrow transplantation stabilizes the cerebrovascular disease caused by SCD. A number of patients with moyamoya syndrome resulting from SCD have undergone surgical bypass procedures and revascularization procedures in an effort to prevent stroke.[141]

Arterial Dissection

Arterial dissection has been shown to account for up to 20% of childhood AISs.[142] There is significant male predominance for both anterior and posterior circulation dissection. Up to 10% of children with dissection have recurrent dissection and up to 12.5% have recurrent stroke.[143] Cervicocephalic arterial dissections can be either traumatic or spontaneous in origin.

Traumatic dissections may follow direct cranial and cervical trauma. The trauma does not have to be severe to cause vascular injury. Cerebral infarctions are most often due to emboli. Occurrence of dissection following a minor head or neck injury suggests the presence of a defective artery. Intraoral trauma, strangulation, and injury to the neck are all known to cause arterial dissection. Differentiating between spontaneous and traumatic dissection can be difficult, especially when the trauma is minor. Clinical findings are similar, with acute neurologic deficit, headache, and ipsilateral oculosympathetic paresis.

Imaging studies can show the arterial dissection well only if neuroimaging is tailored for this purpose. 3D time-of-flight MRA of the circle of Willis and the cervical arteries should be performed in all suspected cases.[144] More recently, contrast-enhanced 3D MRA has been shown to be useful, especially when there is impaired flow after a dissection, which can adversely affect the time-of-flight acquisition.[145] In addition, precontrast thin-section axial T1-weighted spin-echo MR images with fat suppression with an inferior saturation pulse to suppress flow through the neck is recommended to detect intramural hemorrhage. Catheter angiography remains the gold standard for diagnosis and should be considered whenever there is evidence of an unexplained embolic infarction.

Thrombotic Disorders

Venous Sinus Thrombosis

Cerebral venous sinus thrombosis (CSVT) is an important cause of stroke in neonates and children. The incidence of childhood CSVT varies between 0.4 and 0.7 per 100,000 children per year.[146] The incidence is higher in neonates, with up to 40% of CSVT occurring in the neonatal period.[147] The true incidence is probably higher, with underdiagnosis attributable to older, less sensitive imaging techniques, nonspecific presenting features, anatomical variations of the dural venous sinuses, and rapid recanalization. Presenting features of CSVT are nonspecific and include seizures, altered mental status, encephalopathy, focal neurologic deficits, and other symptoms like headache, nausea, and vomiting. Therefore, clinical diagnosis can be challenging and a high index of suspicion is necessary to achieve early detection and institution of appropriate therapy. CSVT can be particularly challenging to diagnose in neonates, who present more commonly with seizures compared to older children. Also, CSVT can occur in utero and can be detected by US with color Doppler. Predisposing conditions in patients with CSVT include common childhood conditions such as fever, infection, dehydration, and anemia, as well as acute and chronic medical conditions, such as congenital heart disease, nephrotic syndrome, systemic lupus erythematosus, and malignancy. Dehydration is a particularly important risk factor of CSVT in neonates.

US with color Doppler is a useful modality for diagnosing venous thrombosis in the neonatal period (Fig. 2.107). MRI is the preferred imaging modality, although noncontrast CT is sometimes used when MR is unavailable. On CT, linear densities representing thrombus may be seen in the expected locations of the deep and cortical veins, called the cord sign (Fig. 2.108). Direct visualization of thrombosis in a dural sinus may give a "dense clot sign."[9] Venous infarction is the most specific indirect sign on unenhanced CT images. When an infarction does not conform to a major arterial vascular territory (e.g., multiple isolated lesions, involvement of subcortical regions with cortical sparing, and extension beyond one arterial distribution), a venous cause should be strongly suspected. The infarct may be hemorrhagic or nonhemorrhagic. Location of the infarct may give a clue to the venous structure involved. For instance, thrombosis in the sagittal sinus is associated with parenchymal change in the parasagittal region because of

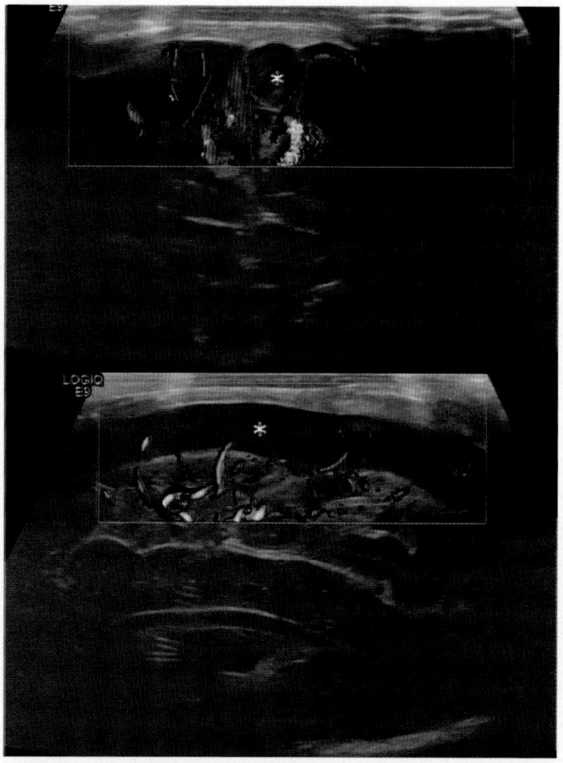

FIGURE 2.107 **Superior sagittal sinus thrombosis in a 2-day-old boy with sepsis and dehydration.** Coronal **(upper image)** and sagittal **(bottom image)** cranial ultrasound images show absence of color Doppler flow and hypoechoic material (*asterisks*) filling the superior sagittal sinus, consistent with superior sagittal sinus thrombosis.

impaired venous drainage. Thrombosis in the vein of Labbé' causes infarction in the ipsilateral temporal lobe. Typical deep gray matter sites of infarction in deep venous thrombosis are the thalami, basal ganglia, and internal capsules.

Contrast-enhanced CT may demonstrate the "empty delta" sign, which is a filling defect in the posterior part of the sagittal sinus. However, the modalities of choice to detect CSVT are CTV or MRI with MR venography because CT with contrast can miss up to 40%.[10] On MRI, acute thrombus can be difficult to differentiate from flowing blood, which is isointense to gray matter on T1-weighted and hypointense on T2-weighted MR images. In this situation, 2D time-of-flight or phase contrast MRV demonstrates absence of flow in the thrombosed venous sinus. Subacute thrombus is of high signal intensity on precontrast T1-weighted sequences (Fig. 2.108). Venous congestion may be visualized on SWI and contrast-enhanced T1-weighted sequences. Postcontrast MR venography is less likely to be affected by complex flow and may offer the best evaluation. Potential false negatives on contrast-enhanced MRV can result from methemoglobin in subacute thrombus, which is bright on T1-weighted MR images, or enhancing chronic thrombus.[11] Diffusion-weighted MR imaging and perfusion sequences can demonstrate venous congestion and help differentiate cytotoxic from vasogenic edema. Parenchymal ischemic injury may be seen in up to two-thirds of children with CSVT, either in a cortical or subcortical location, and may also involve the deep gray matter. The majority of the venous infarcts are hemorrhagic. Primary subarachnoid and subdural hemorrhage may be seen at presentation. IVH in preterm infants is associated with CSVT. Deep venous thrombosis results in hemorrhage into the ventricles as a result of increased pressure within the deep venous drainage system.

Treatment is primarily supportive and directed toward correcting the predisposing condition, but may also include judicious use of anticoagulant and antithrombotic agents after the diagnosis has been established.

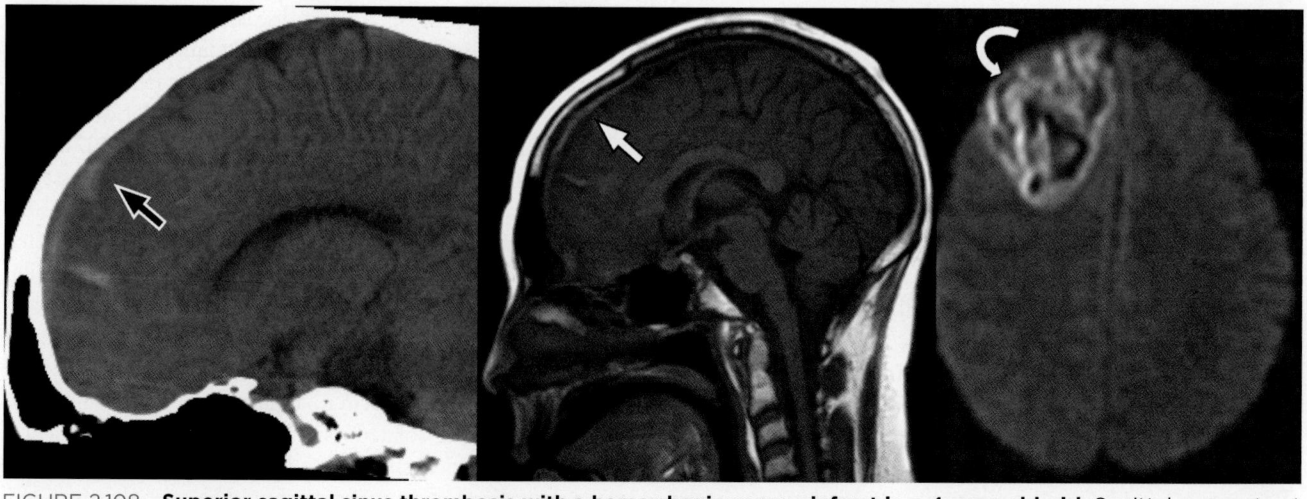

FIGURE 2.108 **Superior sagittal sinus thrombosis with a hemorrhagic venous infarct in a 4-year-old girl.** Sagittal noncontrast CT image (on the **left**), sagittal T1-weighted MR image (in the **middle**), and axial diffusion-weighted MR image (on the **right**) show superior sagittal sinus thrombosis indicated by hyperdensity (*straight black arrow*) on CT, T1 hyperintensity (*straight white arrow*) on noncontrast sagittal T1-weighted MR image, and decreased diffusion and abnormal signal (*curved arrow*) in the right frontal lobe, consistent with a hemorrhagic venous infarct.

Hydrocephalus and CSF Space Disorders

Hydrocephalus

Hydrocephalus can be caused by obstruction of normal CSF flow, decreased CSF absorption, or rarely, because of overproduction of CSF by choroid plexus hyperplasia or a tumor such as choroid plexus papilloma.[11] Obstructive hydrocephalus is divided into two types: communicating and noncommunicating hydrocephalus. Communicating hydrocephalus is due to extraventricular obstruction within the subarachnoid space. In contrast, in noncommunicating hydrocephalus, there is intraventricular obstruction to CSF flow, and there is no communication with the subarachnoid space. More recent classifications based on the effect of pressure flow derangement of CSF dynamics within the circuit diagram of CSF flow are designed to serve as a template for the study of hydrocephalus and its treatments.[11]

Three different categories of hydrocephalus are discussed in the following section, which include (1) noncommunicating hydrocephalus, (2) communicating hydrocephalus, and (3) hydrocephalus secondary to overproduction.

Noncommunicating Hydrocephalus

Noncommunicating hydrocephalus is caused by intraventricular obstruction of CSF flow. Common sites of obstruction are the narrowest channels for CSF flow, namely, the foramen of Monro, cerebral aqueduct, and fourth ventricle and its outflow foramina. In children, neoplastic lesions are a common cause of such obstructions. MRI is the imaging modality of choice in this scenario, although CT often serves as the initial screening test to detect neoplastic lesions and demonstrate the presence and degree of hydrocephalus.

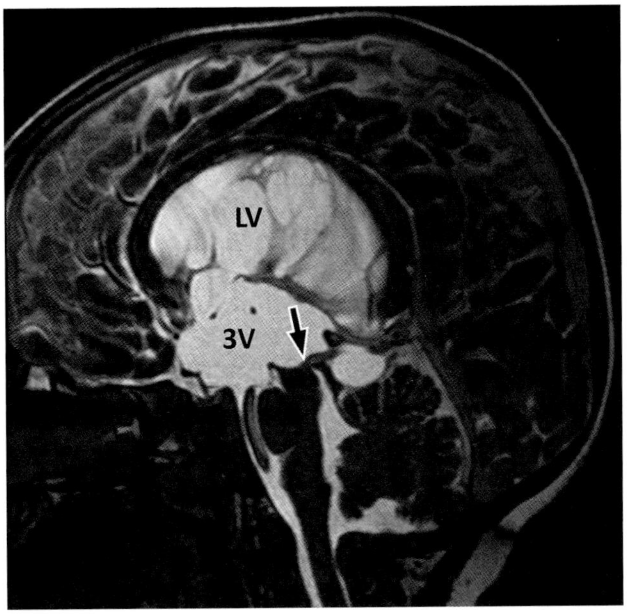

FIGURE 2.110 **Aqueductal stenosis in a 21-month-old boy who presented with increasing head circumference.** Sagittal FIESTA (fast imaging employing steady-state acquisition) MR image shows obstruction of the aqueduct (*arrow*) and absence of normal CSF flow void in the aqueduct, with moderate to severe dilatation of the third (*3V*) and lateral (*LV*) ventricles.

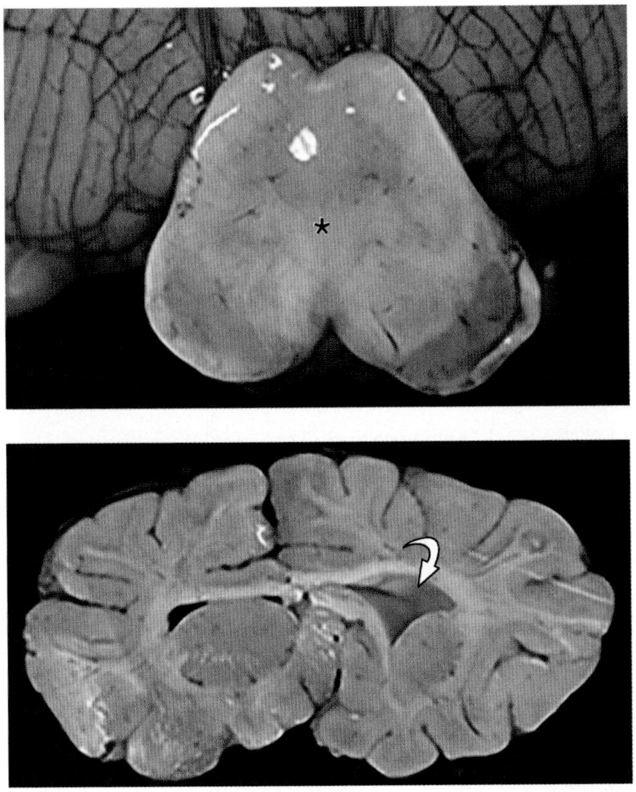
FIGURE 2.109 **Aqueductal atresia in a 9-month-old boy who died in the setting of multiple congenital anomalies.** A cross section of the midbrain shows an absent cerebral aqueduct (*asterisk* in **upper image**); this is associated with hydrocephalus that is most prominent in the lateral ventricles posteriorly, where it takes on a "batwing" appearance (*curved arrow* in **lower image**).

Nonneoplastic causes of noncommunicating hydrocephalus include arachnoid cysts, aqueductal atresia (Fig. 2.109), aqueductal stenosis (Fig. 2.110), aqueductal webs, and IVH. Important sequences to consider in the evaluation of hydrocephalus are heavily T2-weighted 3D sequences like 3D FIESTA (fast imaging employing steady-state acquisition) or CISS (constructive interference with steady state), or the more recently described T2-weighted SPACE (sampling perfection with application-optimized contrast with different flip-angle evolutions) sequence (Fig. 2.110). These sequences can enable detection of septations within the ventricles and arachnoid cysts, and determine patency of the aqueduct.

Communicating Hydrocephalus (Extraventricular Obstruction to CSF Flow)

Extraventricular obstruction to CSF flow can result from a variety of causes, including intracranial hemorrhage, bacterial or granulomatous meningitis (like TB), CSF seeding of tumor, venous hypertension, and skull base abnormalities (e.g., achondroplasia).

Hydrocephalus Secondary to CSF Overproduction

Hydrocephalus in pediatric patients with choroid plexus papillomas and carcinomas has previously been thought to be a result of CSF overproduction. However, this hypothesis has been questioned in more recent literature, and some cases of associated hydrocephalus may be, in fact, a result of obstruction to the arachnoid villi or other CSF outflow channels by high protein levels, hemorrhage into the highly vascular tumor, or intraventricular debris. This is more likely in the case of fourth ventricle tumors, which involve the foramina of Magendie and Luschka. On the other hand, a significant proportion of choroid plexus papillomas is centered within the lateral ventricles in the pediatric population and produces hydrocephalus without obvious ventricular or extraventricular obstruction. It is still thought that hydrocephalus in these pediatric patients is likely to be because of overproduction of CSF. Rare cases of choroid plexus hyperplasia can cause hydrocephalus because of overproduction of CSF.

Investigation and Treatment of Hydrocephalus

The surgical treatment of hydrocephalus typically involves placement of a shunt catheter that diverts CSF from the ventricular system to another region of the body, most commonly the peritoneal cavity. Pediatric patients with intraventricular obstruction may be candidates for a third ventriculostomy, a surgical procedure in which a fenestration is created through the floor of the third ventricle to allow CSF to bypass an obstruction at the level of the cerebral aqueduct. Children with shunts may develop new symptoms if the shunt stops working correctly. Shunt malfunction can be due to intracranial occlusion of the catheter, a break or disconnection in the catheter tubing, or obstruction of the catheter outflow.

Presenting features of shunt malfunction in pediatric patients with shunted hydrocephalus include nausea, vomiting, irritability, fever, altered level of consciousness, or increased seizure frequency. Papilledema, cranial nerve palsies, hyperactive reflexes, and ataxic gait may be found on exam. Infants with shunt malfunction may present with increased head circumference, a bulging fontanelle, or splayed cranial sutures. Neurosurgical consultation is mandatory if shunt malfunction is clinically suspected even if the imaging studies are considered stable compared to prior studies.

US can be considered as the initial imaging study in young infants with large, open fontanelles presenting with clinical features of hydrocephalus. The Levene ventricular index (VI) is the horizontal measurement from the midline falx to the lateral aspect of the anterior horn of the lateral ventricle in the coronal plane obtained at the level of the third ventricle/foramen of Monro.[148] This is most frequently used for monitoring ventricular size following IVH in young infants.[149] As a guideline, the 97th percentile of the VI + 4 mm curve, a curve that has been used as a threshold for intervention for post-hemorrhagic ventricular dilatation, increases from 14 to 15 to 16 mm at 27, 31, and 33 weeks of estimated gestational age, respectively.[148,150] As this increase may be a relatively late sign of increased ICP, the anterior horn width (AHW) is used by some operators and may more accurately reflect early expansion of the ventricles. A normal AHW is <3 mm, with the 95th percentile curve reaching 2 mm at 36 weeks and 3 mm at 40 weeks.[150] An AHW >6 mm is considered abnormal.

Noncontrast CT remains the initial modality of choice in most institutions because of its ready availability, ability to detect changes in ventricular size and configuration and evaluate for the presence of hemorrhage or infarction, shunt catheter discontinuity in the skull and upper neck, and catheter migration. It is particularly important to use low-radiation-dose techniques to minimize radiation exposure to children with ventricular shunts as these patients are likely to require many repeated neuroimaging studies during their lifetime. Of note, no significant loss in diagnostic accuracy is seen when low-dose techniques are employed in this specific clinical setting.

Limited axial T2-weighted MRI in an imaging plane similar to that utilized in prior CT studies can be considered as an alternative in a stable, older child who can lie still for a few minutes in the MR scanner. MRI is the imaging modality of choice to identify the underlying cause of hydrocephalus. Depending on the site of obstruction, the lateral, third, and/or fourth ventricles may be dilated. Periventricular edema is often present with severe obstruction. Occasionally, edema may be seen around the shunt catheter as an early sign of shunt malfunction. Dilatation of the third ventricle typically results in downward displacement of the floor and transverse expansion of the ventricle. The corpus callosum is bowed upward. Depending on the cause and the level of obstruction, the fourth ventricle is normal or small in size (e.g., aqueductal stenosis) or may be dilated (e.g., when the obstruction is at the level of the CSF outlet foramina following IVH or surgery).

It is important to compare the imaging study obtained in a child with hydrocephalus with a baseline study obtained after successful shunt placement.[33] Multiple prior studies should also be reviewed to detect subtle evidence of shunt malfunction. Comparison with prior studies should include those performed with another imaging modality, for instance MRI performed in an interval between two CTs, to avoid missing changes that may have occurred in the interval between the two CTs. Limited ventricular shunt check MRI consisting of T2-weighted MR images is being used increasingly when the study is only intended to evaluate the size of the ventricular system.[151] Use of susceptibility-weighted or gradient-echo images can help with visualization of the shunt catheter tip because blooming can be seen at this location.[151]

A shunt series is a series of plain radiographs performed to differentiate between obstruction and other causes of mechanical shunt malfunction including catheter fracture. When looking at these radiographs, it is important not to mistake the radiolucent areas between the intermittent radiopaque markers seen in some shunts for areas of discontinuity. Shunt mechanism disconnection is seen most commonly at the junction of proximal and distal tubing at the level of the valve (Fig. 2.111). Shunt tubing fracture, however, usually occurs in the neck, likely resulting from its increased mobility. There is also a role for abdominal US and/or CT to evaluate for the presence of ascites or an intra-abdominal mass such as a large CSF pseudocyst (also known as a "CSFoma") in pediatric patients with ventriculoperitoneal shunts. It is worth mentioning again that CT performed in children

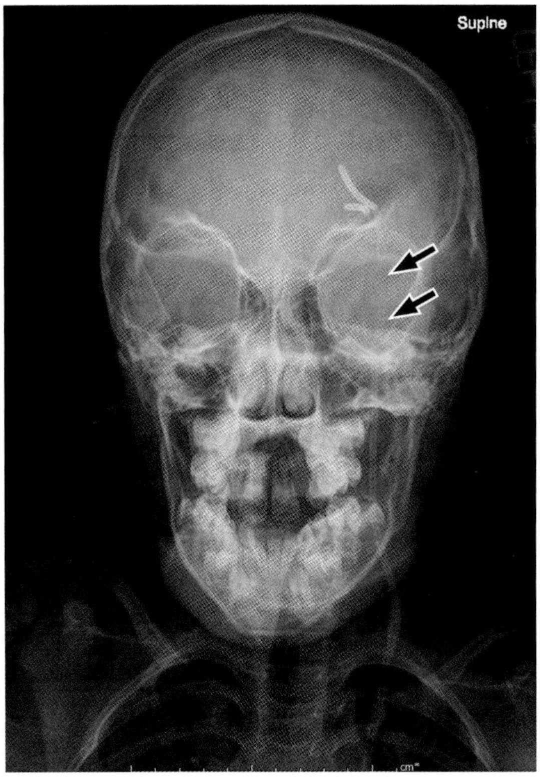

FIGURE 2.111 **Ventriculoperitoneal shunt catheter disconnection in a 10-year-old boy.** Frontal radiograph shows a focal discontinuity (*arrows*) of the shunt catheter.

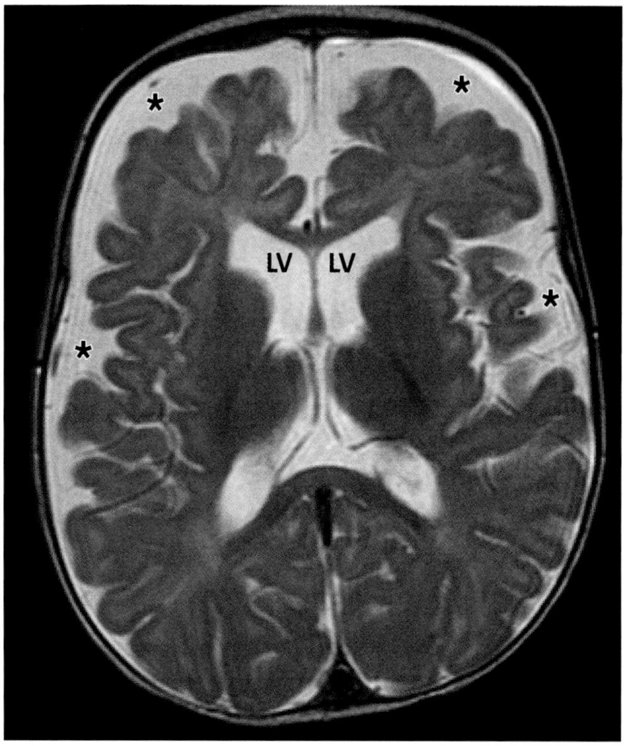

FIGURE 2.112 **Benign extra-axial space enlargement in an 8-week-old boy.** Axial T2-weighted MR image shows moderate enlargement (*asterisks*) of the bifrontotemporal extra-axial spaces with CSF signal intensity fluid. In addition, mildly dilated lateral ventricles (*LV*) are also present.

experiencing true shunt malfunction may be normal, have stable ventriculomegaly, or even show decreased ventricular size compared with prior studies. Therefore, neurosurgical consultation is mandatory if shunt malfunction is clinically suspected, despite normal findings on imaging studies.

Benign Enlargement of Subarachnoid Spaces in Infants

Benign enlargement of subarachnoid spaces in infants is best defined as enlargement of the extra-axial spaces in children <2 years of age with open sutures without significant neurologic problems (Fig. 2.112). These children present with increasing head circumference and mild psychomotor retardation and may have mild axial hypotonia on examination. The exact etiology is still a subject of controversy, but most authors consider this a manifestation of delay in the development of CSF drainage pathways. This theory may explain the phenomenon of spontaneous resolution that occurs in most of these patients.

Cranial US can be the initial modality that shows the enlarged subarachnoid spaces and detects pathologic extra-axial collections (e.g., subdural hematoma) and hydrocephalus as alternative causes of increasing head circumference. MRI is considered in selected cases if the degree of ventricular and extra-axial space enlargement raises the possibility of an obstructive etiology or if the fontanelle is small and does not allow adequate visualization of the posterior fossa structures on US examination.

Treatment is usually conservative. Benign enlargement of subarachnoid spaces usually resolves spontaneously by the age of 2 years, although macrocephaly may persist.

Metabolic Brain Disorders

The term "neurometabolic disorders" refers to inborn errors of metabolism caused by gene mutations that result in the alteration of one or more metabolic pathways, producing brain injury and clinical symptoms. Although they are relatively rare, their incidence is significantly higher in certain ethnic groups.

Although all inborn errors of metabolism result from genetic abnormalities, the onset of symptoms depends on the exact nature of the abnormality. Some metabolic diseases are evident soon after birth, whereas others only become symptomatic later in infancy or childhood. Developmental regression is common among many metabolic disorders, and the loss of developmental milestones previously acquired should prompt consideration of a metabolic abnormality.

Symptoms of an inborn error of metabolism occurring in the newborn are usually nonspecific. Neonates with acute encephalopathy are usually healthy at birth and become ill in the first few days to weeks after birth. Feeding problems, lethargy, irritability, and vomiting usually precede onset of encephalopathy, characterized by decreasing consciousness and/or seizures. Acidosis, hyperammonemia, and tachypnea may also be present. It is important to recognize the possibility of a neurometabolic disorder, as similar symptoms can be present in infants with acute infection, HII, and as sequelae of congenital cardiac anomalies.[152]

Neuroimaging can help aid in narrowing the list of differential diagnoses, provide evidence that enables a firm diagnosis, and help choose the most appropriate test or tests for follow-up and treatment. Characteristic imaging patterns of damage in some of these disorders is explained by the concept of regional selective vulnerability to toxins and ischemia. This concept refers to the fact that a specific cell type is injured by the accumulation or deficiency of a particular metabolite.

Diffusion-weighted MRI and MRS are often useful in narrowing the list of differential diagnoses in acutely ill pediatric patients with suspected neurometabolic disorders, and therefore, must be performed in all cases where there is a possibility of a neurometabolic disease.[152] Characteristic findings on MRS can be diagnostic with certain inborn errors of metabolism in neonates and children.

Many classifications systems of neurometabolic disease exist based on the clinical presentation, enzymatic pathways affected, and the organelle involved. However, a pattern-based approach is most useful when analyzing an imaging study in an affected child.[153] Although many inborn errors of metabolism affect more than one region or cell type within the brain, a useful framework for pattern recognition is division of the neurometabolic disorders into those that predominantly affect gray matter (deep nuclei-predominant or cortex-predominant), predominantly affect white matter (deep white matter, subcortical white matter, hypomyelination/absent myelination), or involve both gray and white matter (with or without thalamic involvement).[154]

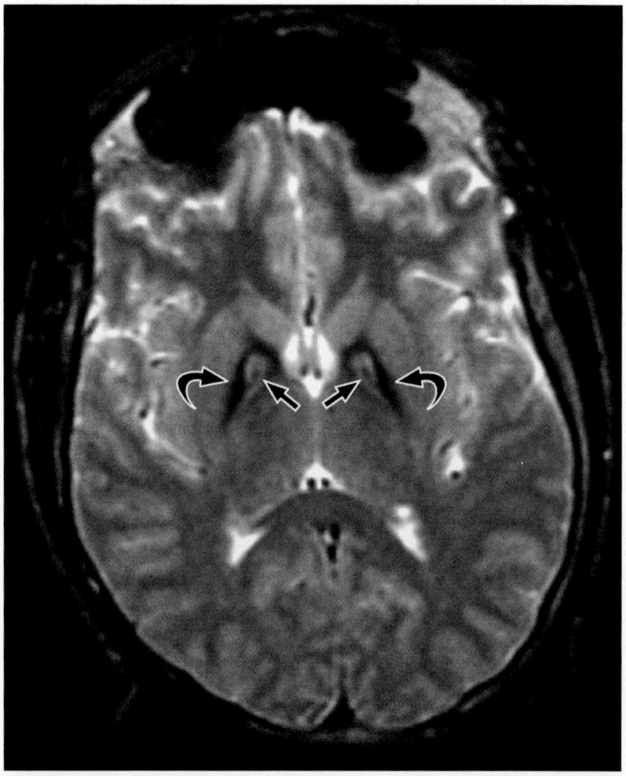

FIGURE 2.113 **Pantothenate kinase-associated neuropathy (PKAN) in a 3-year-old boy who presented with progressive dystonia, spasticity, and athetosis.** Axial T2-weighted MR image shows abnormal T2 hyperintensity (*straight arrows*) with peripheral T2 hypointensity (*curved arrows*) in the globus pallidi bilaterally.

Gray Matter–Predominant Disorders

Deep Gray Nuclei–Predominant Pattern

Iron Accumulation Disorders

Neurodegeneration with brain iron accumulation (NBIA) is the term used to describe a heterogeneous group of conditions characterized by progressive neurodegeneration and abnormally elevated brain iron.[155]

Based on the genetic mutation involved, four subtypes are described:

1. Pantothenate kinase–associated neuropathy (PKAN or NBIA type 1)
2. Neuroferritinopathy (NBIA type 2)
3. Infantile neuroaxonal dystrophy
4. Aceruloplasminemia

The following discussion focuses on PKAN, the most common type of NBIA, and infantile neuroaxonal dystrophy because these two conditions present in the pediatric age group.

Pantothenate Kinase–Associated Neuropathy. Pantothenate kinase–associated neuropathy (PKAN) (previously called Hallervorden-Spatz disease) is a rare autosomal recessive disorder characterized by excessive iron deposition in the globus pallidus and substantia nigra. It is caused by mutations in the pantothenate kinase gene (*PANK2*).

Most affected children present in the first decade or during the early teenage years with progressive gait abnormalities and delayed psychomotor development. Hyperkinesia is seen in a large number of affected pediatric patients. Progressive cognitive impairment leads to dementia.

On MRI, excessive iron accumulation is indicated by marked T2 hypointensity in the GP and SN. The classic "eye of the tiger" sign refers to the small central focus of hyperintensity in the medial aspect of the otherwise hypointense globus pallidus, which is caused by tissue gliosis and vacuolization (Fig. 2.113). This is not seen in all cases of PKAN. There is no contrast enhancement. MRS shows a decreased *N*-acetylaspartate (NAA) peak. DTI has been shown to demonstrate increased fractional anisotropy in both the globus pallidus and substantia nigra because of introduction of local field gradients by iron deposition.[156]

Infantile Neuroaxonal Dystrophy. Infantile neuroaxonal dystrophy (INAD) is a severe psychomotor disorder characterized by psychomotor delay and regression, increasing symmetrical pyramidal tract signs, and spastic tetraplegia. Most affected pediatric patients present between 6 months and 4 years of age.[155] Progressive deterioration occurs, and most affected pediatric patients do not survive beyond the end of the first decade.

On MRI, affected pediatric patients with INAD show striking cerebellar atrophy. T2 hyperintensity in the cerebellum secondary to gliosis is another common finding. T2 hypointensity indicating abnormal iron deposition in the globus pallidus and substantia nigra is seen in up to 50% cases[155] (Fig. 2.114).

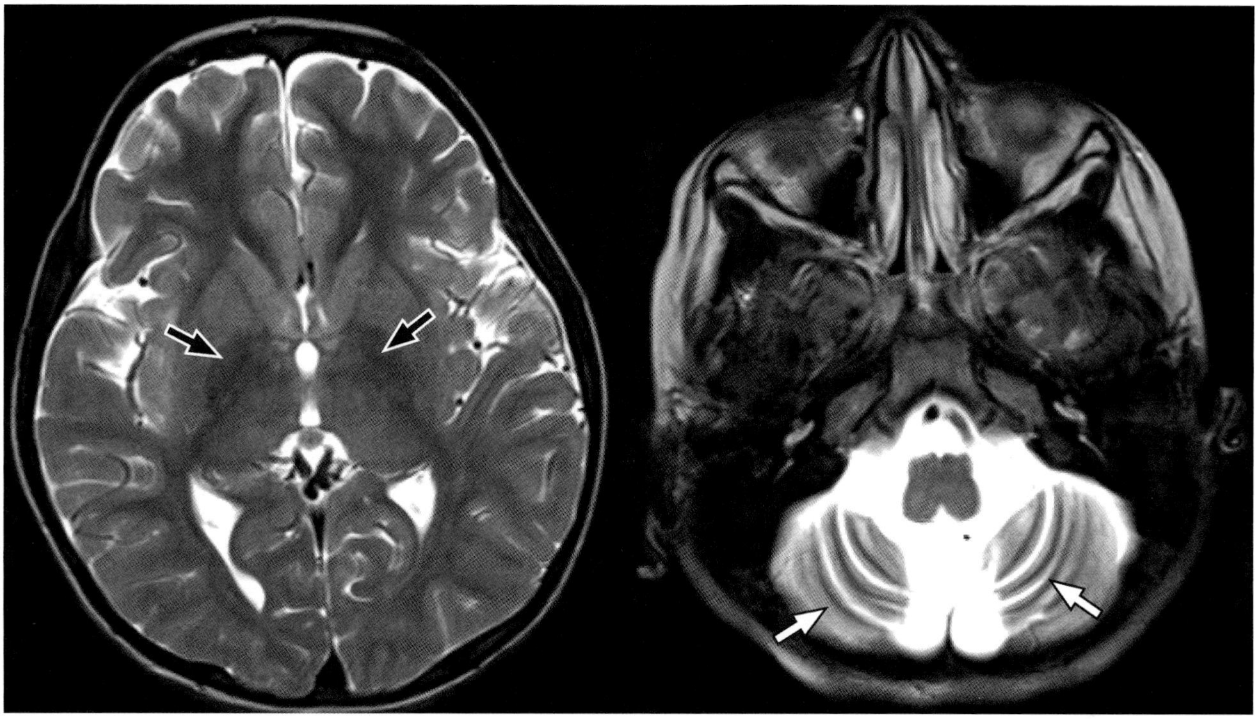

FIGURE 2.114 **Genetically proven Infantile neuroaxonal dystrophy (INAD) in a 5-year-old boy.** Axial T2-weighted MR images show T2 hypointensity (*black arrows*) in the globus pallidi (on the **left**) and marked cerebellar atrophy (*white arrows*, on the **right**).

Creatine Deficiency Syndromes

Creatine deficiency syndromes are autosomal recessive disorders. Creatine and creatine phosphate are required for the storage and transmission of phosphate-bound energy in both muscle and brain. Clinical presentation is with hypotonia and developmental delay caused by creatine depletion. MR may show bilaterally symmetric T2/FLAIR hyperintensity in the globus pallidus. However, the key finding that leads to the diagnosis is a markedly small or absent creatine peak on MR spectroscopy studies (Fig. 2.115). Making the diagnosis on imaging is crucial, as dietary creatine supplementation can partially or completely reverse the symptoms.

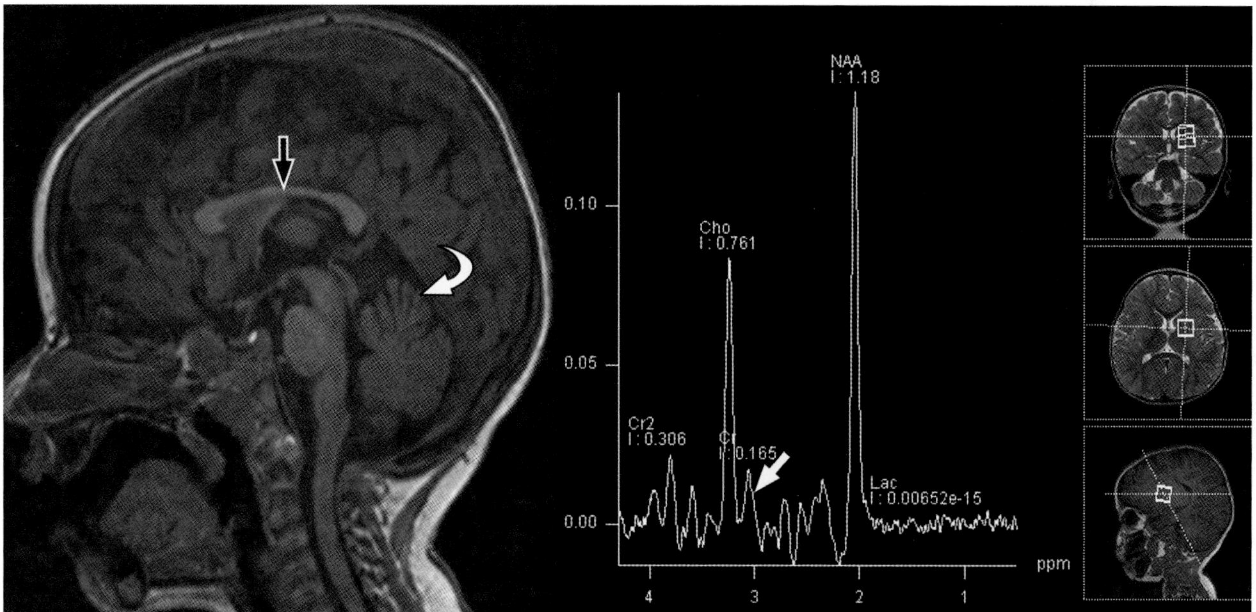

FIGURE 2.115 **Creatine deficiency in a 4-year-old boy with developmental delay who was subsequently proven to have a creatine transporter deficiency.** Sagittal T1-weighted MR image (on the **left**) shows mild thinning of the corpus callosum (*black arrow*) and subtle atrophy of the superior cerebellar hemispheres (*curved arrow*). MR spectroscopy image (on the **right**) demonstrates markedly reduced creatine (*white arrow*).

Copper Metabolism Disorders (Menkes Disease and Wilson Disease)

Menkes Disease. Menkes disease (also known as the "kinky hair" syndrome) is an X-linked recessive disorder caused by an abnormality of copper metabolism. It results in low copper levels and consequent deficiency in copper-dependent mitochondrial enzymes. On physical examination, the hair is characteristically fine, silvery, and brittle. The abnormality in the copper-mediated enzyme pathways leads to defects in connective tissue structure, which manifests as skeletal, vascular, and brain abnormalities. Clinical presentation is characterized by progressive neurologic impairment, seizures occurring in the first few days or months of life, progressive hypotonia, and developmental delay. Some pediatric patients with this condition develop bilateral SDHs and retinal hemorrhages, mimicking nonaccidental trauma.

Neuroimaging findings include progressive parenchymal volume loss involving the supra- and infratentorial compartments, with associated white matter hyperintensities on T2-weighted MR images. T1-weighted MR images may show T1 shortening in the basal ganglia.[157] MRA characteristically demonstrates markedly tortuous and elongated intracranial and cervical arteries (Fig. 2.116). Nonneuroimaging studies that are helpful include plain radiographs that show metaphyseal widening of the femora and ribs, tibial spurs and wormian bones, and abdominopelvic US that may show large bladder diverticula.[157,158]

Treatment is mainly supportive, as the condition is usually lethal in early childhood.

Wilson Disease. Wilson disease or hepatolenticular degeneration is a relatively rare, autosomal recessive, inborn defect in copper metabolism. It is characterized by abnormal accumulation of copper in various tissues, particularly in the liver and the brain. Neurologic symptoms associated with Wilson disease are secondary to copper accumulation in the brain that causes neuronal destruction. Edema, necrosis, and spongiform encephalopathy are seen on histology.

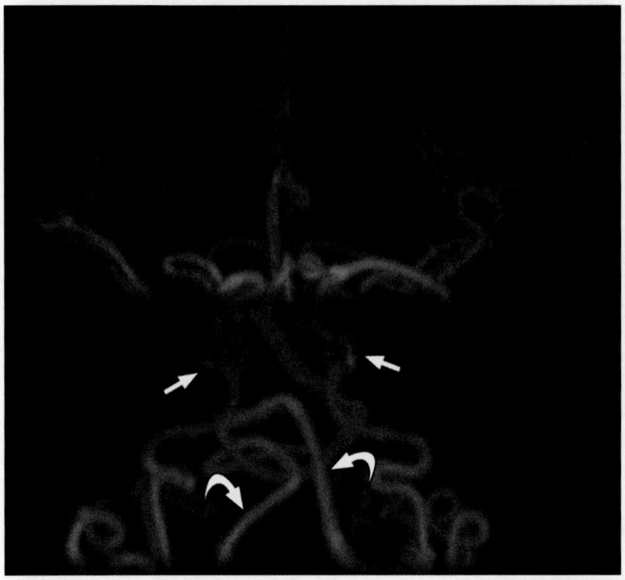

FIGURE 2.116 **Menkes syndrome in a 5-year-old boy.** Maximum intensity projection reformatted image from a MRA demonstrates marked tortuosity of the bilateral internal carotid arteries (*straight arrows*) and vertebral arteries (*curved arrows*).

MRI in patients with Wilson disease demonstrates T1 shortening in the globus pallidus, putamen, and midbrain in patients with hepatic dysfunction.[159,160] In pediatric patients with neurologic symptoms, T2 prolongation is seen in the striatum and the dorsal pons (Fig. 2.117). The "face of the giant panda" sign refers to the high signal intensity on T2-weighted MR images in the tegmentum with sparing of the lateral portion of the pars reticularis and red nuclei, with hypointensity of the superior colliculi.[161] MRI studies following treatment correlate well with improvement in clinical findings.[162] This is helpful in assessing the clinical response to treatment of pediatric patients with Wilson disease.

Management of Wilson disease consists of lifetime therapy aimed at removing or detoxifying copper. This is achieved by the use of chelating agents like D-penicillamine and trientine. In some pediatric patients, zinc is used to block the intestinal absorption of copper.

Cortex-Predominant Pattern

Neuronal Ceroid Lipofuscinoses

Neuronal ceroid lipofuscinoses (NCL) are a group of inherited neurodegenerative disorders characterized by accumulation of lysosomal storage material in neuronal and extraneuronal tissues and loss of neurons in the gray matter.[163] Several types are currently described, including infantile-onset, early and late juvenile, adult, and heterogeneous atypical forms. The infantile and classic juvenile types are the most common types. As expected with cortex-predominant lesions, clinical presentation is with seizures, delayed milestones, ataxia, visual loss, and abnormal behavior.

In young pediatric patients with progressive encephalopathy, the presence of marked atrophy of the cerebrum and cerebellum, thinning of the cerebral cortex, and mild T2 hyperintensity in the cerebral white matter should suggest NCL[164] (Fig. 2.118). The white matter hyperintensity is due to severe myelin loss and gliosis.[165] T2 hypointensity of the thalami is seen in the infantile type. Reduced levels of NAA are seen on MR spectroscopy.

Rett Syndrome

Rett syndrome is a rare neurodegenerative disease caused by mutations in the X-linked methyl CPG–binding protein 2 (*MeCP2*) gene.[166] It is a disorder of neuronal maturation and connections. It is seen predominantly in young females with onset between 4 months and 2 years of age. Affected pediatric patients often present with a decrease in velocity of head growth, ultimately resulting in microcephaly. This is followed by behavioral regression, loss of ability to use words, and onset of motor and cognitive deficits. Hand wringing is a characteristic symptom. Serial imaging studies show a progressive decrease in brain volume.

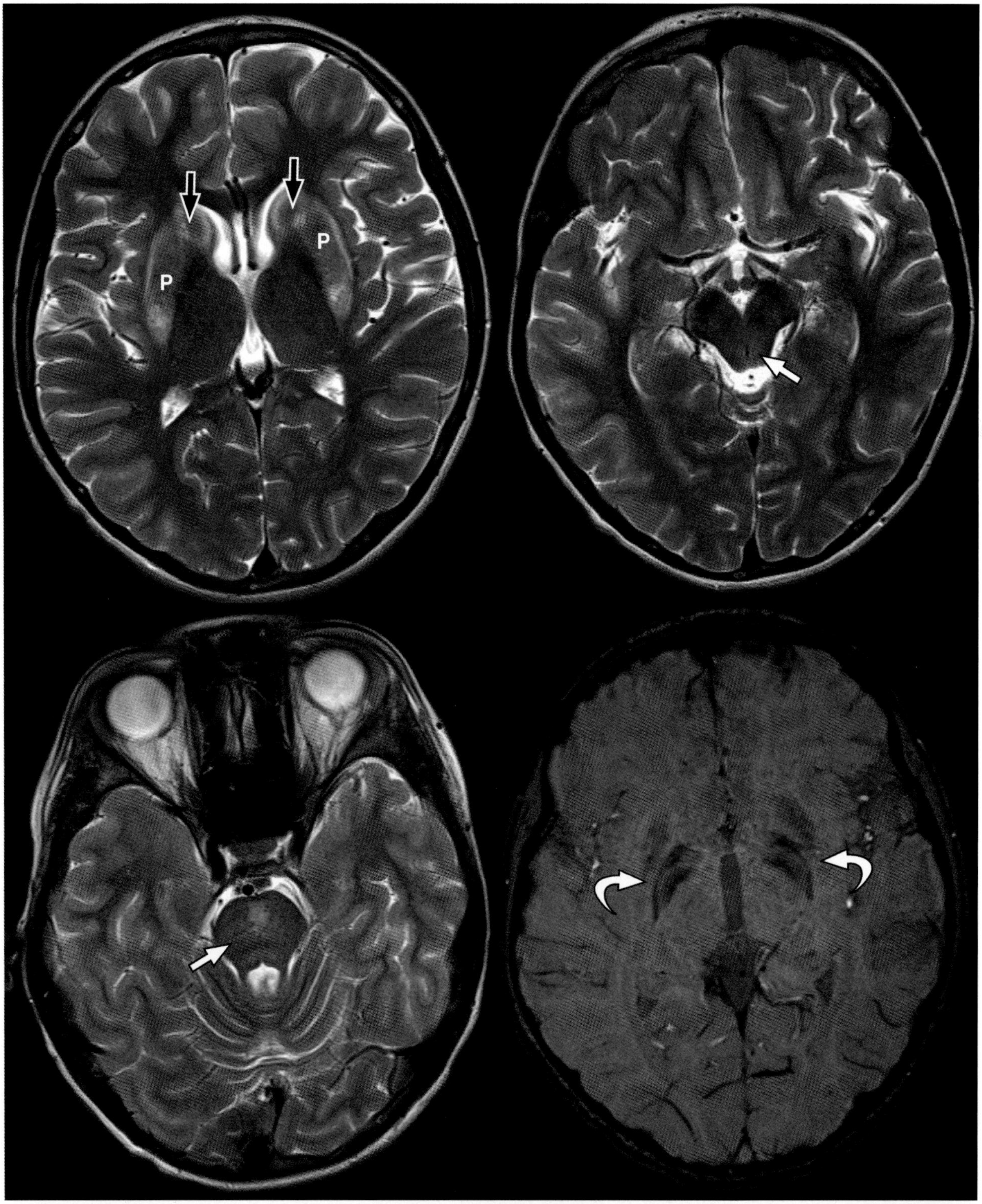

FIGURE 2.117 **Wilson disease in a 12-year-old boy who presented with micrographia.** Axial T2-weighted MR images **(upper panel and bottom left)** show concentric laminar T2 hyperintensity in the putamina (*P*) and caudate nuclei (*black arrows*), abnormal T2 prolongation in the midbrain tegmentum (*white arrows*), sparing the red nuclei and susceptibility (*curved arrows*) on the susceptibility-weighted MR images **(bottom right)** in the caudate and lentiform nuclei (*curved arrows*).

Volumetric analyses suggest that decreased brain volume is a result of global reductions in both gray and white matter.[167] Preferential reduction of the frontal and anterior temporal lobe cortex is seen. DTI shows reduced fractional anisotropy in the corpus callosum, internal capsule, frontal white matter, and anterior cingulate gyrus.[168] Rett syndrome can be difficult to distinguish from other causes of brain volume loss.

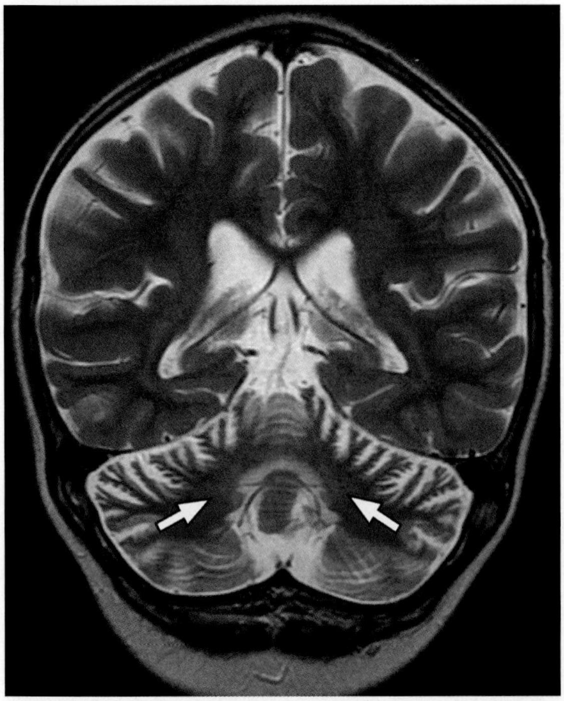

FIGURE 2.118 **Neuronal ceroid lipofuscinoses (NCL) in a 6-year-old girl with developmental delay and seizures.** Coronal T2-weighted MR image shows marked atrophy of the cerebrum and cerebellum, cerebral cortical thinning, and mild T2 hyperintensity (*arrows*) in the cerebral white matter.

White Matter–Predominant Disorders

Deep White Matter–Predominant Pattern

X-Linked Adrenoleukodystrophy

Adrenoleukodystrophy (ALD) is an X-linked recessive disorder caused by mutations of the *ABCD1* gene (Xq28) gene responsible for the peroxisomal membrane transporter required for catabolism of very long chain fatty acids (VLCFA).[154] There is resultant increase in serum VLCFA levels, which causes inflammatory demyelination and adrenal gland atrophy. The disorder presents between 5 and 10 years of age in boys as a mild learning disorder or hyperactivity progressing to dementia and quadriparesis. Most children with this disease have adrenal insufficiency including the "bronzing" or darkening of the skin caused by ACTH hypersecretion. A small group of affected pediatric patients may present solely with adrenal symptoms.

On MRI, childhood X-linked ALD has a characteristic pattern of cerebral white matter involvement, primarily in the parietooccipital lobes and splenium of the corpus callosum. There are typically three zones of abnormality including (1) a T2 hyperintense peripheral zone corresponding to the zone of active demyelination, (2) an enhancing and diffusion restricting rim where active inflammation is occurring, and (3) a central zone of T2 prolongation corresponding to gliosis at pathology[169] (Fig. 2.119). Around 50% of ALD patients present in adulthood.

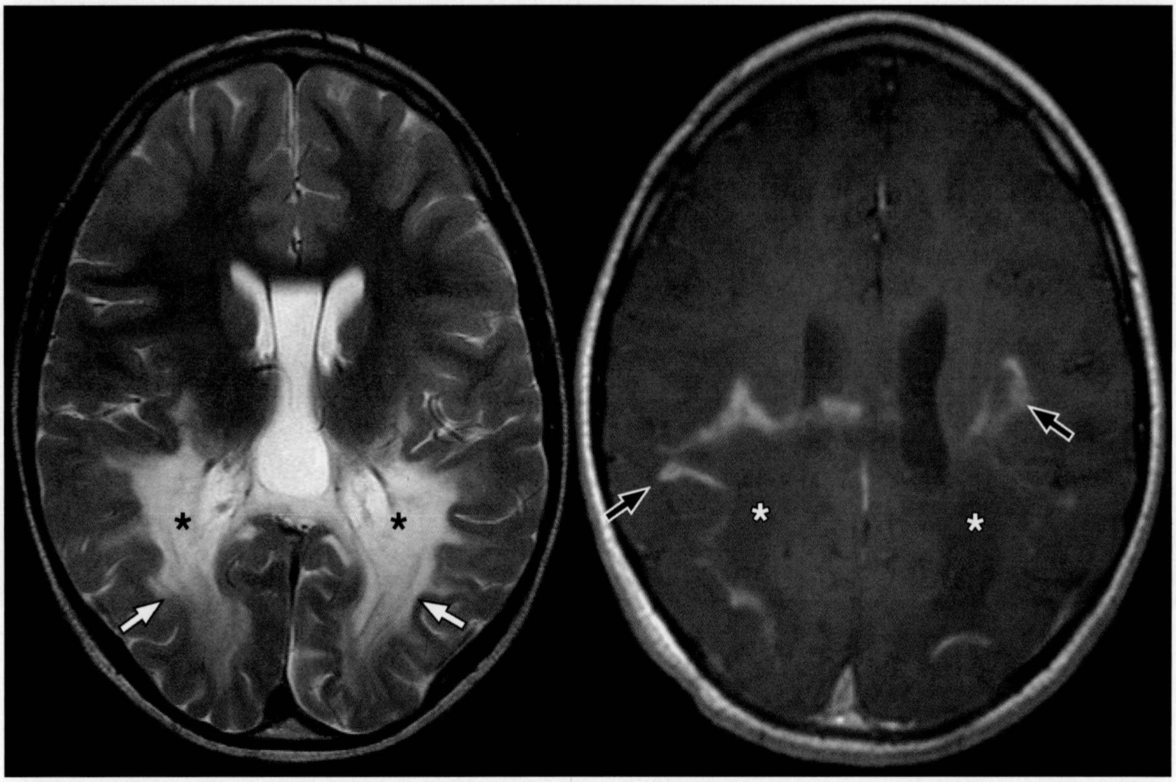

FIGURE 2.119 **X-linked adrenoleukodystrophy in an 8-year-old boy who presented with declining school performance.** Axial T2-weighted MR image (on the **left**) and axial postcontrast T1-weighted MR image (on the **right**) show a central gliotic zone (*asterisks*) and peripheral zone of T2 prolongation (*white arrows*) corresponding to the zone of active demyelination, and an enhancing rim representing regions of inflammation (*black arrows*).

Metachromatic Leukodystrophy

Metachromatic leukodystrophy (MLD) results from mutations affecting the ARSA gene responsible for arylsulfatase A. Late infantile, juvenile, and adult-onset subtypes have been recognized, with the late infantile subtype being the most common. All subtypes present with progressive neurologic deterioration after an initial period of normal development. The late infantile subtype of the disease manifests as a loss of milestones, hypotonia, eventual cognitive impairment, and spastic quadriparesis. On MRI, there is confluent T2 prolongation in the deep and periventricular white matter with sparing of subcortical U-fibers until the end stage of the disease[170] (Fig. 2.120). The diagnosis may be suggested by the presence of cranial nerve or cauda equina enhancement, which is not seen in many other leukodystrophies.[171] Similar appearances can be seen in multiple sulfatase deficiency and saposin B deficiency. The "tigroid" appearance resulting from sparing of the perivascular spaces of the affected white matter is often seen but is not pathognomonic for this disorder.

Krabbe Disease

Krabbe disease is a lysosomal storage disorder caused by β-galactocerebrosidase deficiency, coded by the GALC gene. This leads to buildup of the toxic upstream metabolite psychosine and defective myelin turnover, which is accompanied by proliferation of multinucleated giant (globoid) cells and white matter demyelination.[172] Presentation is in early infancy with progressive neurologic deterioration, irritability, or spasticity with subsequent psychomotor regression. More than 85% of affected pediatric patients die before the age of 2 years. Seizure activity is common with disease progression. Although this is classified in the "white matter predominant" heading, the gray matter is also involved in most of these patients.

On CT in patients with Krabbe disease, there is hyperdensity in the thalamus and other gray matter structures, some of which represents frank calcification.[173] As imaging findings at presentation can be difficult to appreciate on MRI because of lack of myelination, DTI has been suggested to have some value at this age.[174] T2 hypointensity may be seen in the thalami with T2 prolongation in the dentate hila, posterior limb of the internal capsules, and corticospinal tracts in the brainstem (Fig. 2.121). In late-onset Krabbe disease, posterior periventricular white matter and posterior callosal signal T2 signal abnormality become apparent with sparing of subcortical U-fibers. Thinning of the spinal cord is a finding in Krabbe disease also seen in the spinocerebellar ataxias. Additional distinctive features include enhancement and thickening of cauda equina nerve roots and the cranial nerves, particularly the optic nerves.[175–177]

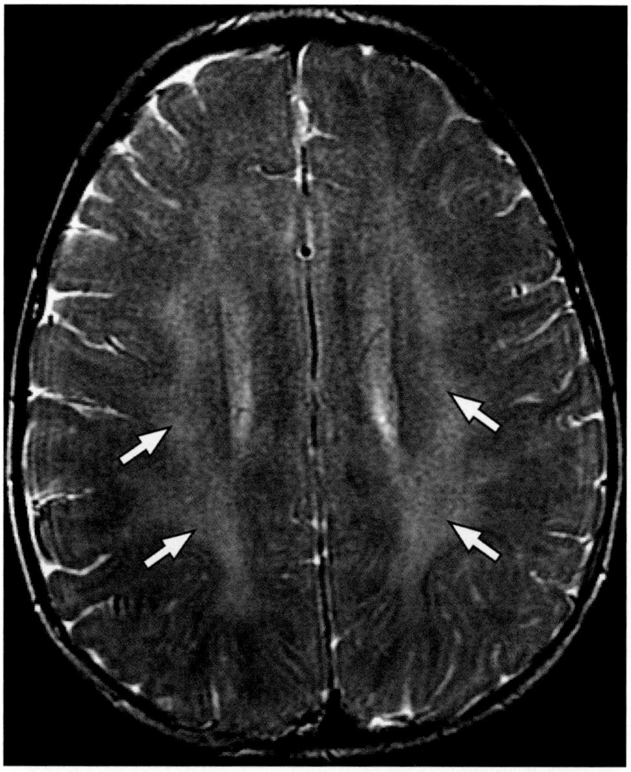

FIGURE 2.120 **Metachromatic leukodystrophy in a 23-month-old girl who presented with developmental delay who was subsequently proven to have arylsulfatase A deficiency.** Axial T2-weighted MR image shows confluent T2 hyperintensity (*arrows*) within the centrum semiovale and corona radiata.

Maple Syrup Urine Disease

Maple syrup urine disease (MSUD) (branched chain ketoaciduria) is a rare autosomal recessive disorder that presents in the early neonatal period with poor feeding, vomiting, ketoacidosis, hypoglycemia, lethargy, and seizures. The infant's urine has a distinctively sweet odor reminiscent of maple syrup. The condition results from mutations in the genes involved in making a protein complex essential for the oxidative phosphorylation of the branched chain amino acids leucine, isoleucine, and valine. Accumulation of these amino acids results in toxicity to the brain and other organs.

Cranial US in MSUD may show increased echogenicity of the deep gray nuclei and periventricular white matter in the acute stage. CT and MRI show diffuse cerebral edema of the white matter. There is decreased diffusion in the areas that are myelinated or actively myelinating at birth including the posterior limbs of the internal capsules, optic radiations, the central corticospinal tracts, hippocampi, dorsal brainstem, cerebellar white matter, and globus pallidi during the acute phase of the disease (Fig. 2.122). The decreased diffusion represents myelin-splitting edema and is believed to be secondary to vacuolating myelinopathy. If treatment is initiated early, most of these changes recover without lasting sequelae. MR spectroscopy may show a peak of branched chain amino acids resonating at 0.9 to 1.0 ppm during a metabolic crisis, which persists on longer echo spectra.

Phenylketonuria

Phenylketonuria is an autosomal recessive disorder caused by mutations of the gene involved in the production of phenylalanine hydroxylase. Deficiency of this enzyme results in the production of compounds like phenylpyruvic acid, phenylacetic acid, and phenylacetylglutamine that are toxic to the

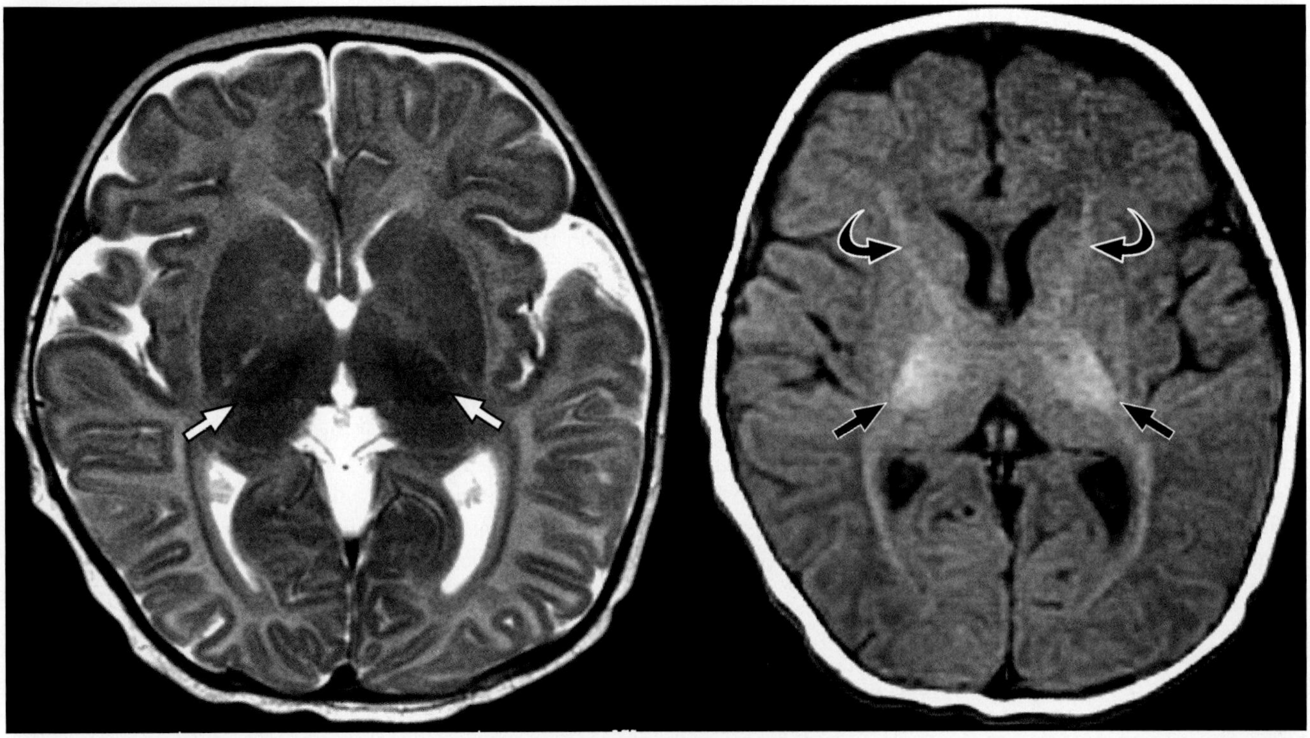

FIGURE 2.121 **Krabbe disease in a 6-month-old boy who presented with flaccidity.** Axial T2-weighted MR image (on the **left**) and axial T1-weighted MR image (on the **right**) show T2 hypointensity (*white arrows*) and T1 hyperintensity (*black arrows*) in the bilateral thalami as well as T1 hyperintensity (*curved arrows*) in the internal capsules.

developing brain. Presenting features include developmental delay, eczematous dermatitis, hypopigmentation, and a peculiar musty odor of the urine, skin, and hair. Imaging features on MRI include T2 prolongation initially in the periventricular white matter of the cerebral hemispheres. This is thought to be due to delayed and defective myelination. Subcortical white matter is involved later in the disease process. Reduced diffusion may be seen in the affected white matter (Fig. 2.123).

Treatment is primarily directed at dietary restriction.

Hyperhomocysteinemia

Hyperhomocysteinemia includes a group of disorders resulting from deficiency from different enzymes involved in homocysteine metabolism. These include cystathionine beta-synthase deficiency, 5,10-methylenetetrahydrofolate reductase deficiency (MTHFRD), errors affecting vitamin B_{12} metabolism, and MET adenosyltransferase deficiency. Imaging features vary depending on the enzyme involved.

Cystathionine beta-synthase deficiency results in multiple small infarcts of varying ages resulting from intimal irregularities in children and young adults.

MTHFRD causes white matter abnormalities resulting from demyelination, which appear as nonspecific areas of white matter T2 prolongation. Errors affecting B_{12} metabolism also result in brain atrophy and destruction of myelin, which manifests as white matter T2 prolongation.

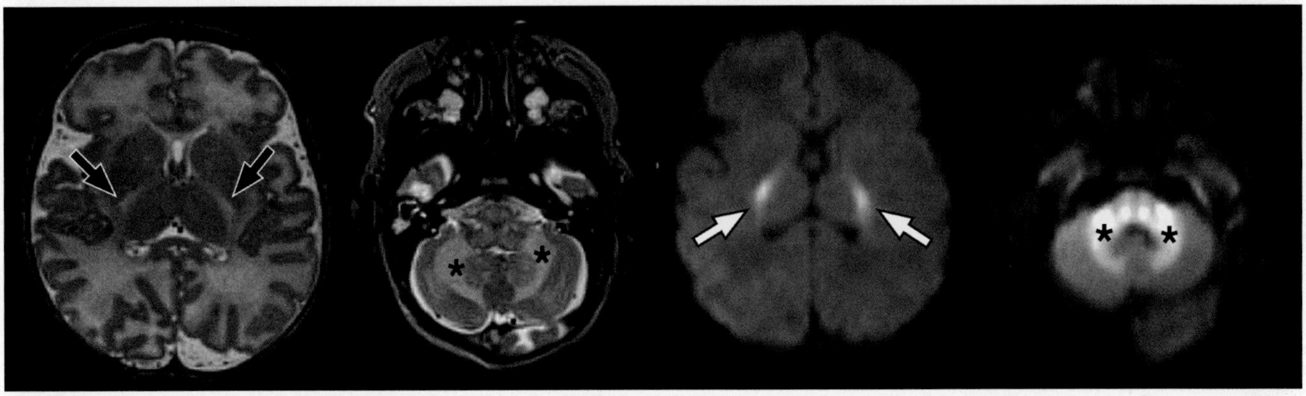

FIGURE 2.122 **Maple syrup urine disease in a newborn girl.** Axial T2-weighted MR images (*first and second images* from the **left**) and axial diffusion-weighted MR images (*third and fourth images* from the **left**) show T2 prolongation (*black arrows*) and decreased diffusion (*white arrows*) in the posterior limbs of the internal capsules as well as the dorsal brainstem and cerebellar white matter (*asterisks*).

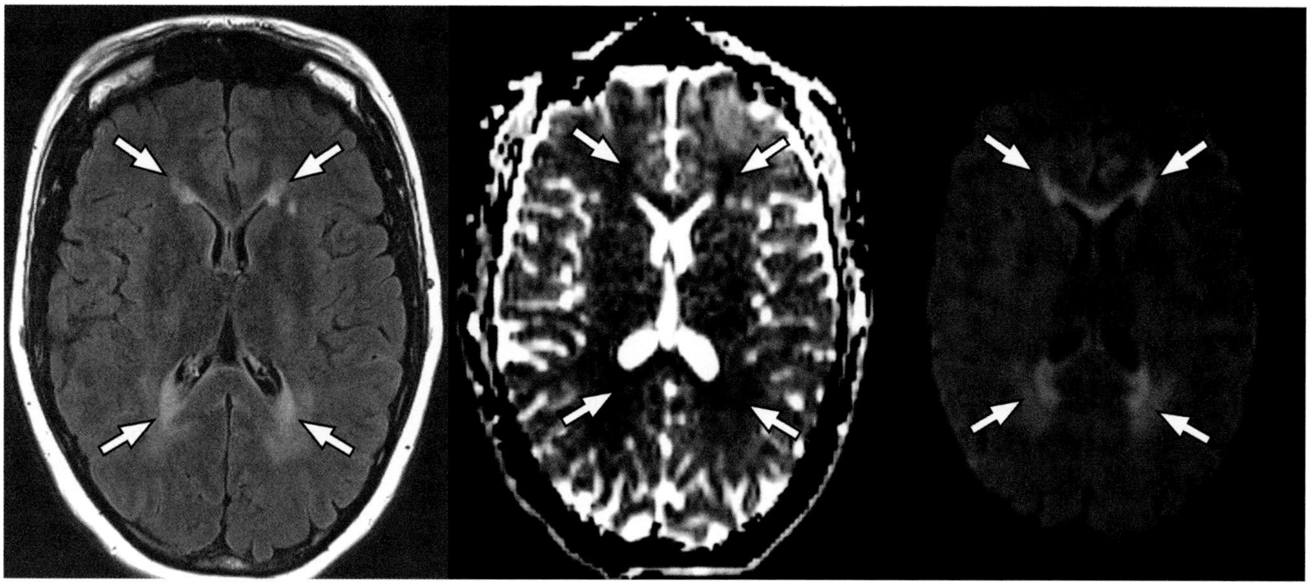

FIGURE 2.123 **Phenylketonuria in a 31-year-old female.** Axial FLAIR MR image (on the **left**), apparent diffusion MR image (in the **middle**), and diffusion-weighted MR image (on the **right**) show decreased diffusion and abnormal T2 hyperintensity (*arrows*) in the periventricular white matter.

Vanishing White Matter Disease

Vanishing white matter disease (VWM) is one of the most prevalent inherited childhood leukoencephalopathies. The basic defect of this striking disease resides in one of the five subunits of eukaryotic translation initiation factor eIF2B, which is essential for the initiation of translation of RNA into protein and is involved under circumstances of stress. Increased glycine in the CSF may be seen as a result of excitotoxic brain damage. Oligodendrocytes and astrocytes are predominantly affected. The classical clinical presentation is early childhood onset of chronic neurologic deterioration, dominated by cerebellar ataxia. A unique feature of VWM is heightened sensitivity to febrile infections, minor head trauma, and acute fright, which may result in rapid neurologic deterioration and unexplained coma. Most affected pediatric patients die a few years after onset of symptoms. There is a wide variety of phenotypes, including antenatal onset and early demise and adult onset with slowly progressive disease. Typical MRI findings are diffuse hyperintensities on T2-weighted MR images in the white matter. Additional lesions in the central tegmental tracts and pons follow CSF signal. MRS shows mildly increased lactate and glucose peaks with decreased NAA, choline, and creatine peaks.

Subcortical White Matter–Predominant Pattern

Galactosemia

Galactosemia is an autosomal recessive condition resulting from mutations in the genes involved in galactose metabolism. Classic or type 1 galactosemia, because of galactose-1-phosphate uridyltransferase (*GALT*) deficiency, is the most common type. This leads to accumulation of galactose-1-phosphate and metabolites like galactitol. The disease presents after the child has been fed milk, with failure to thrive, poor feeding, lethargy, liver dysfunction, and eventually, signs of cerebral edema. Long-term neurologic sequelae, including cognitive impairment, delayed speech, and cerebellar signs (gait, ataxia, coordination problems) may develop even after institution of a galactose-depleted diet. On MRI, T2 prolongation is evident in the subcortical white matter in a pattern resembling delayed myelination. These areas appear slightly heterogeneous on FLAIR MR images (Fig. 2.124). MR spectroscopy can be helpful in

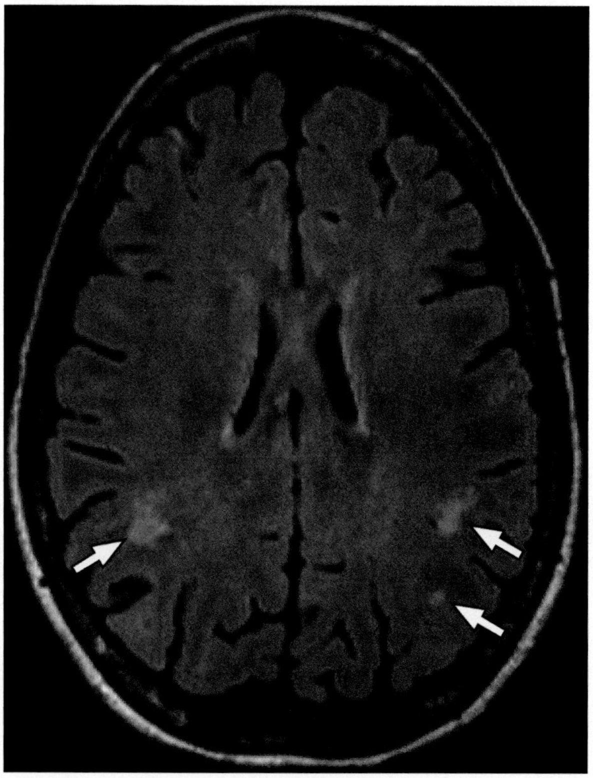

FIGURE 2.124 **Galactosemia in a 16-year-old girl.** Axial FLAIR MR image shows multiple patchy hyperintensities (*arrows*) in the deep and subcortical white matter.

securing a diagnosis, as untreated patients have prominent galactitol peaks in the acute setting. The other types of galactosemia involve the genes for the *GALT* or UDP-galactose-4-epimerase enzymes.

Megalencephalic Leukoencephalopathy with Subcortical Cysts (Van Der Knaap Disease)

Megalencephalic leukoencephalopathy with subcortical cysts (MLC) is a rare condition originally characterized as an autosomal recessive disorder secondary to mutations in a transmembrane gene product involved in regulation of cellular water balance. The resulting disorder is notable for presentation with macrocephaly during infancy. Affected pediatric patients eventually show mild developmental delay in motor and cognitive areas. Deterioration in motor (ataxia, spasticity) and cognitive function occurs over several years, with an increasing incidence of seizures. MRI findings include extensive T2 prolongation in the subcortical and deep white matter, with relative sparing of the periventricular and occipital white matter. There are associated subcortical cysts in the white matter in the temporal lobes and, to a lesser extent, the frontoparietal lobes (Fig. 2.125). Cerebral atrophy occurs over time. A subset of pediatric patients (~25%) has milder clinical and imaging phenotypes, with fewer cysts and less prominent white matter signal abnormality.

Aicardi–Goutières Syndrome

Aicardi–Goutières syndrome (AGS) is caused by gene mutations that trigger an activated immune response with elevated CSF interferon and neopterin levels. This response is thought to be related to the role that the gene products play in metabolizing DNA and RNA strands that then trigger an antiviral response. This results in small-vessel vasculopathy and leptomeningitis. Clinical presentation is in the first few months of life with irritability, pyrexia, truncal hypotonia, extremity spasticity, cognitive impairment, and progressive microcephaly. MRI shows predominantly subcortical white matter signal abnormality, with a frontotemporal predominance and cystic change in patients who present in the first 3 months of life. Other characteristic features are progressive atrophy and presence of parenchymal calcifications in the putamen, dentate nucleus, and deep white matter.

Hypomyelination/Absent Myelination Pattern

Hypomyelination refers to a permanent, substantial deficit in myelin deposition in the brain. The accepted MRI criterion for a diagnosis of hypomyelination is an unchanged pattern of deficient myelination on two successive MRI examinations at least 6 months apart. At least one of the MRI scans should have been obtained at the age of more than 1 year.[178] However, if MRI scan shows significantly deficient myelination in a child older than 18 months of age, permanent hypomyelination is

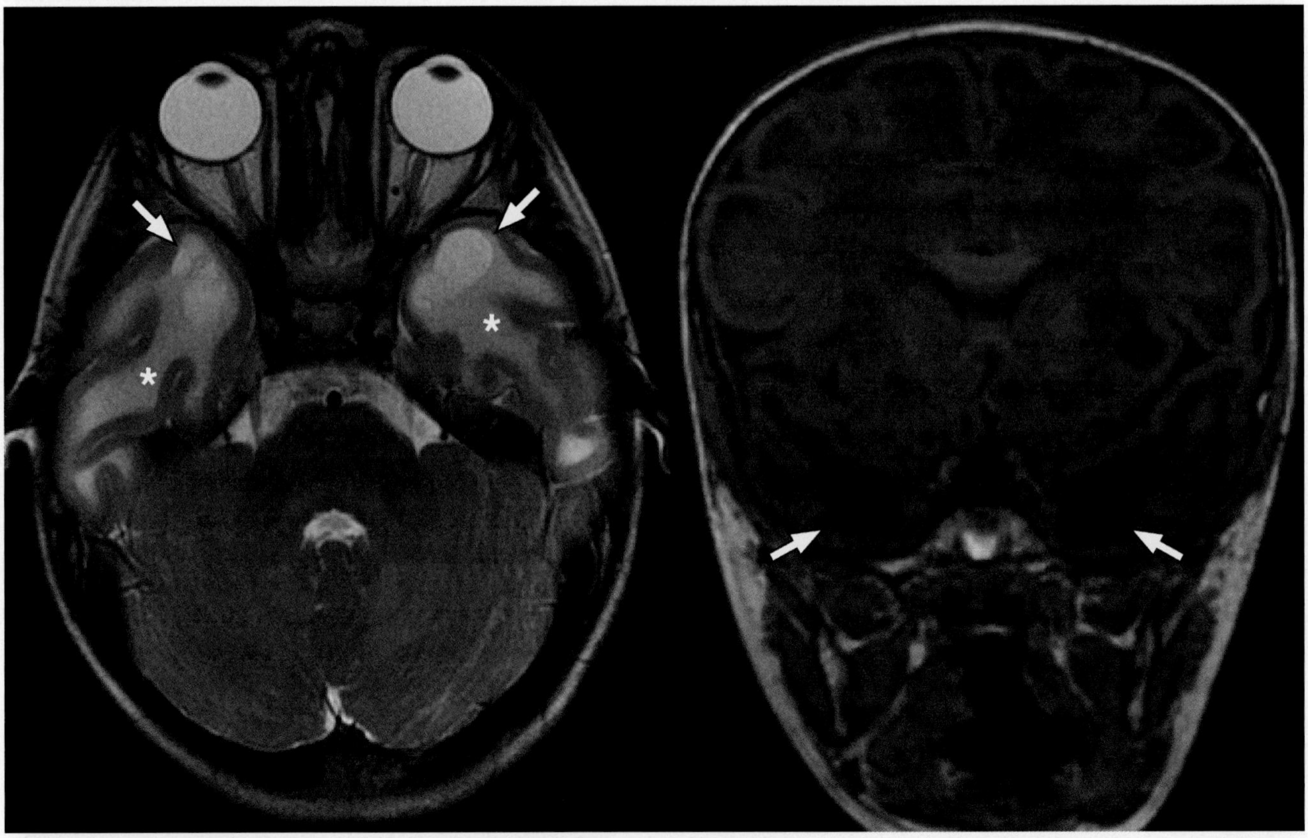

FIGURE 2.125 **Megalencephalic leukoencephalopathy with subcortical cysts.** Axial T2-weighted MR image (on the **left**) and coronal T1-weighted MR image (on the **right**) show extensive T2 prolongation (*asterisks*) in the subcortical and deep white matter with associated cystic changes (*arrows*) in the subcortical white matter in the temporal lobes.

highly likely.[179] Newer hypomyelinating disorders and their genetic defects have been identified in the last few years.[180] In spite of these advances, hypomyelinating disorders of unknown origin still remain the largest single category among the unclassified leukoencephalopathies.

Pelizaeus-Merzbacher Disease (PMD) and PM-Like Disease

Pelizaeus-Merzbacher disease (PMD) is the most typical condition that results in arrested or absent myelination. PMD is caused by abnormalities in the *PLP1* gene locus located on the X chromosome (Xq22), resulting in a predominance of male PMD patients.[181] Clinical features include nystagmus, ataxia, developmental delay (cognitive as well as psychomotor), and hypotonia progressing to spasticity. Patients with the *connatal* form of the disease present at birth and typically succumb in early childhood, whereas patients presenting in infancy (usually by 1 year) are said to have the more common *classic* form of the disease with life expectancy into middle adulthood.[181] Imaging findings are characterized by absent myelination in the connatal form or arrest of myelination in an early infant pattern for the classic form, with some progressive atrophy seen in the classic cases (Fig. 2.126).

4H Syndrome

4H syndrome is a rare disorder characterized by a constellation of hypomyelination, ataxia, hypogonadotropic hypogonadism, and hypodontia. On MRI, the appearance is lack of myelination of the supratentorial white matter with relative sparing of the optic radiations and cerebellar atrophy.[182]

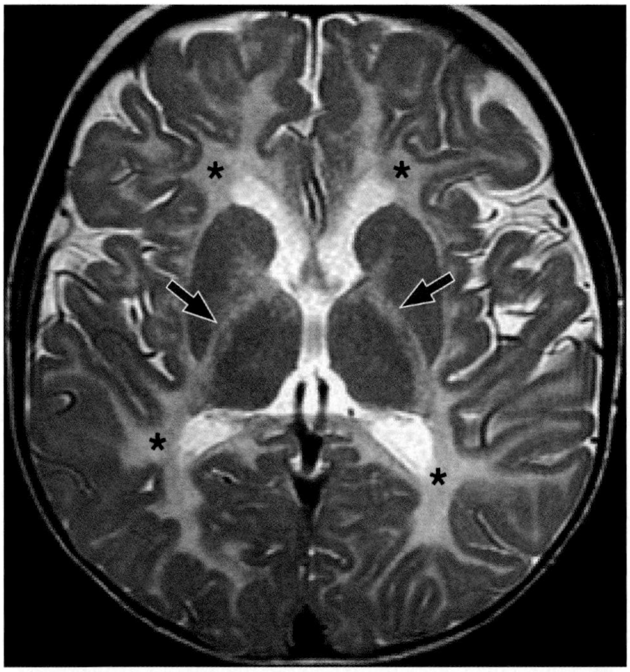

FIGURE 2.126 **Pelizaeus-Merzbacher disease in a 3-year-old boy with developmental delay.** Axial T2-weighted MR image shows complete absence of myelination, indicated by T2 hyperintensity in the white matter throughout the brain (*asterisks*), including internal capsules (*arrows*).

TABLE 2.6 Hypomyelinating Disorders

Pelizaeus-Merzbacher disease (PMD)
Pelizaeus-Merzbacher-like disease (PMLD)
Hypomyelination with hypogonadotropic hypogonadism and hypodontia (4H syndrome)
Tay syndrome (also called trichothiodystrophy with hypersensitivity of the skin to sunlight)
Hypomyelination with congenital cataract (HCC)
18q− syndrome
Hypomyelination with atrophy of the basal ganglia and cerebellum (H-ABC)
Fucosidosis
Salla disease
Cockayne syndrome
Waardenburg-Hirschsprung syndrome with peripheral neuropathy and central hypomyelination
Oculodentodigital dysplasia
Serine synthesis defects
Other early infantile-onset neuronal disorders like infantile GM1 and GM2 gangliosidosis that can present with hypomyelination on MRI

A more comprehensive list of conditions to be considered in cases where hypomyelination is the main syndrome is summarized in Table 2.6.

Disorders Affecting Both Gray and White Matter

Mucopolysaccharidosis

The mucopolysaccharidoses are a collection of disorders resulting from abnormal metabolism of various glycosaminoglycan molecules attached to proteoglycans (glycosylated proteins) within lysosomes. Six major subgroups are recognized (I, II, III, IV, VI, and VII), all transmitted in an autosomal recessive fashion except for type II Hunter disease that is X-linked. Mucopolysaccharidosis (MPS) types I, II, III, and VII are notable for their predominance of CNS morbidity, whereas Morquio (type IV) and Maroteaux-Lamy (type VI) are characterized by musculoskeletal (including spine) abnormalities. There is a wide variation in the degree of abnormal mentation among the CNS-predominant MPS variants. Severe mental retardation is seen in pediatric patients with MPS IH Hurler and MPS IIA Hunter forms of the disease. On the other hand, children with MPS IS (Scheie syndrome) have normal intelligence. Other abnormalities seen in patients with various mucopolysaccharidoses include facial dysmorphism, contractures of the extremities, corneal clouding, airway obstruction, hepatosplenomegaly, dural thickening, and hydrocephalus—symptoms caused by abnormal glycosaminoglycan deposits within tissues.[183]

Neuroimaging studies in MPS patients are characterized by decreased gray and white matter differentiation because of dysmyelination and faint diffuse T2 hyperintensity of the cerebral

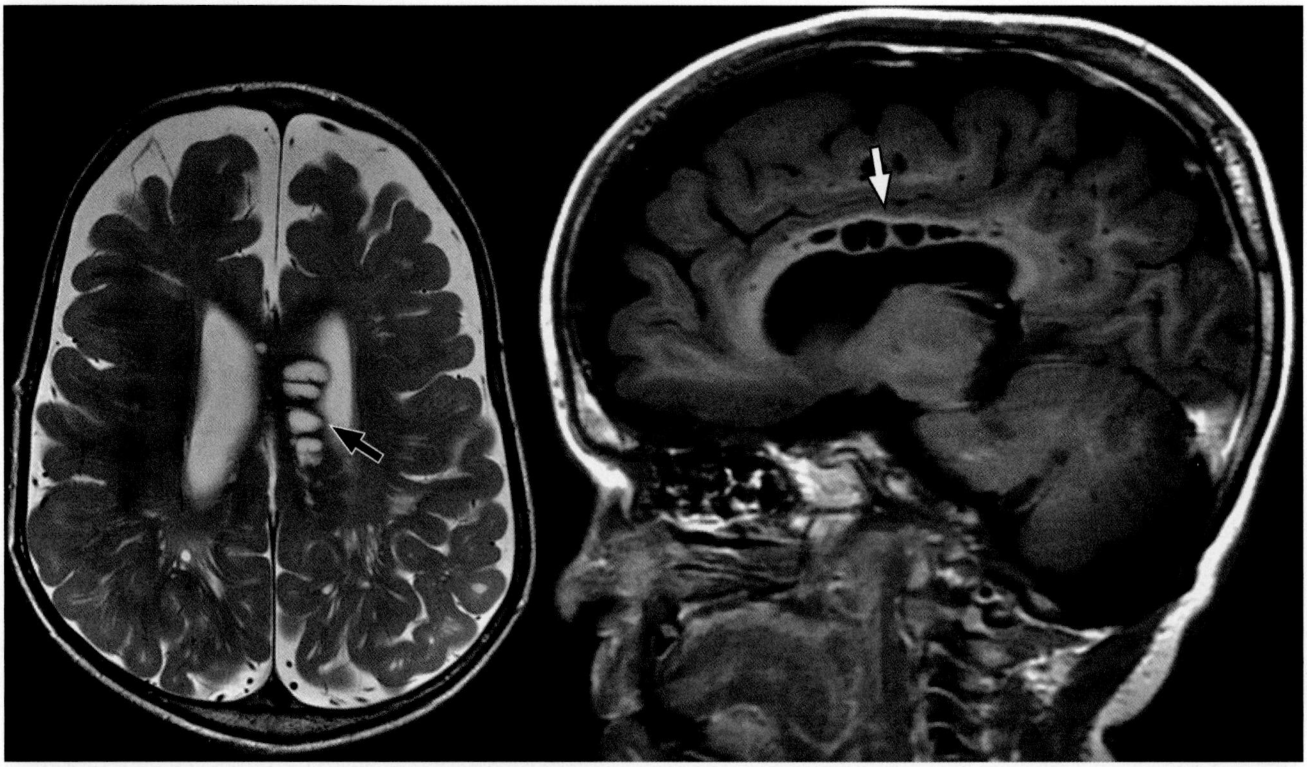

FIGURE 2.127 **Mucopolysaccharidosis in a 6-year-old boy.** Axial T2-weighted MR image (on the **left**) and sagittal MPRAGE (magnetization-prepared rapid acquisition gradient-echo) MR image (on the **right**) show marked perivascular space enlargement (*arrows*) in the cerebral white matter and corpus callosum. Also note presence of mild atrophy, primarily in the frontal lobes.

white matter, including a more pronounced T2 hyperintensity in the periventricular white matter.[184] Presence of markedly prominent perivascular spaces in the cerebral white matter and corpus callosum is a more specific feature that should suggest a diagnosis of MPS[185,186] (Fig. 2.127). Worsening of cognitive impairment seen in at least some MPS patients over time is reflected in imaging studies by progressive white matter signal abnormality and increasing volume loss.[187]

Canavan Disease

Canavan disease is an autosomal recessive disorder resulting from the deficiency of aspartoacylase, an enzyme responsible for degrading NAA. This enzyme deficiency causes buildup of NAA, which causes spongiform changes within the white matter because of osmotic shifts or impaired myelin synthesis. Affected pediatric patients usually present in early infancy with macrocephaly, hypotonia, and irritability followed by spasticity, blindness, and in some cases, seizures. MRI in patients with infantile Canavan disease demonstrates T2 prolongation and decreased diffusion within the subcortical white matter and globus pallidi (with sparing of the corpus striatum) and mild gyral swelling.[188] Occasionally, the brainstem and dentate nucleus may be involved. The decreased diffusion is thought to result from intramyelinic edema caused by NAA accumulation within neurons and increased water migration from the axon into the periaxonal space. Over time, the abnormalities become more widespread and cerebral atrophy occurs.[189] MR spectroscopy is characteristic and shows marked NAA elevation[190] (Fig. 2.128). Treatment is supportive.

Alexander Disease

Alexander disease (AD) is an autosomal dominant disorder caused by missense mutations in glial fibrillary acidic protein (*GFAP*). The decrease in GFAP solubility triggers formation of inclusion bodies such as Rosenthal fibers within neurons, leading to accumulation of abnormal astrocytes and myelin pallor throughout affected brain tissue.[191,192] Historically, three forms of AD have been recognized: infantile form, with typical presentation before 6 months of age, comprising 51% cases; juvenile form, comprising 23% of cases; and adult form, comprising 24% of cases.[193] Earlier onset forms are associated with more severe symptoms. The infantile form is characterized by macrocephaly, failure to thrive, difficulty swallowing, loss of intellectual/motor milestones, lower extremity weakness, ataxia, seizures, and occasionally hydrocephalus. The juvenile and adult forms are dominated more by ataxia, bulbar/pseudobulbar symptoms, and seizures, whereas lower extremity weakness is more frequently seen in the infantile form.[193,194] A small percentage of cases of the juvenile form may also have megalencephaly.[193,194]

Typical imaging characteristics of AD include frontal predominant subcortical to periventricular T2 hyperintensity with swelling of the overlying gyri (Fig. 2.129), swelling of the fornix and optic nerves, periventricular areas of T1/T2 shortening, deep gray matter signal increase or atrophy, dentate hilum signal increase, brainstem (midbrain/medulla) signal increase, and enhancement of involved areas. Progression to atrophy and occasionally white matter cavitation are also common. These findings have been summarized in criteria

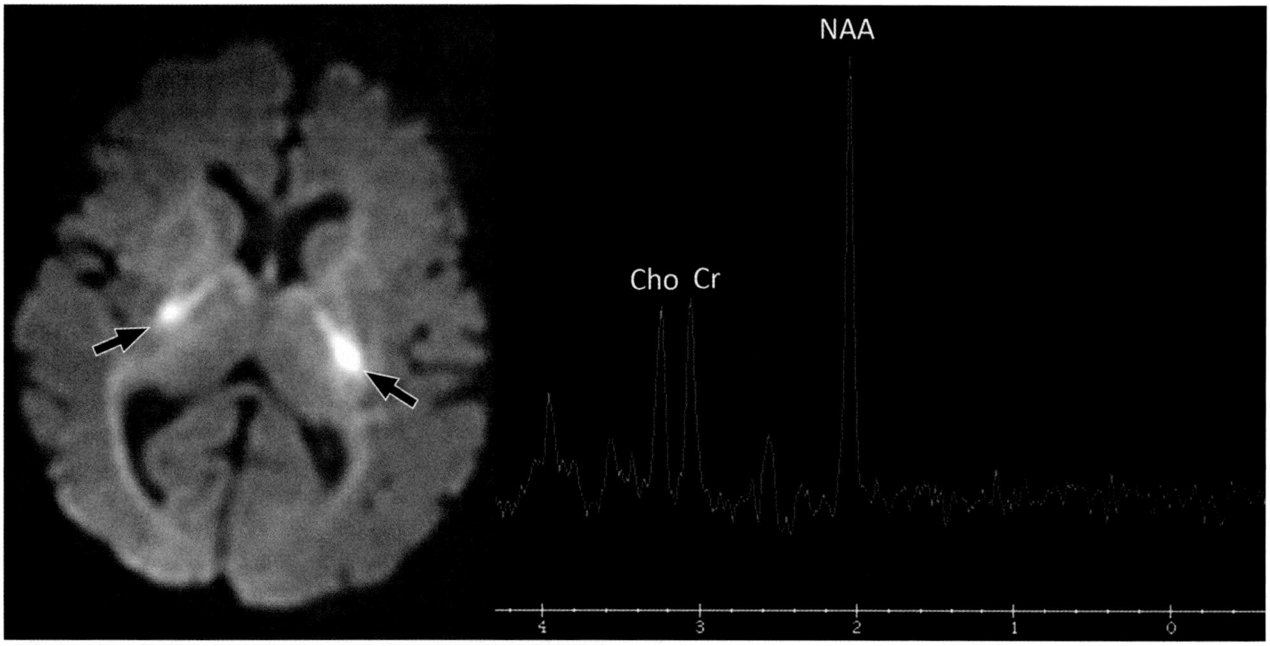

FIGURE 2.128 **Canavan disease in a 5-week-old boy with marked hypotonia and horizontal nystagmus since birth.** Axial diffusion-weighted MR image (on the **left**) and MR spectroscopy image (on the **right**) show decreased diffusion (*arrows*) in the internal capsules and marked elevated *N*-acetyl aspartate (NAA) peak.

used to facilitate diagnosis using MRI in infantile and juvenile AD.[195] However, atypical presentations have been recognized, particularly in juvenile form of the disease. For example, there are well-recognized posterior fossa and brainstem predominant forms of AD including some with tumefactive changes or a ventricular "garland."[196] Adult cases appear to be distinct in appearance, featuring primarily brainstem and cord atrophy with signal abnormality.[197]

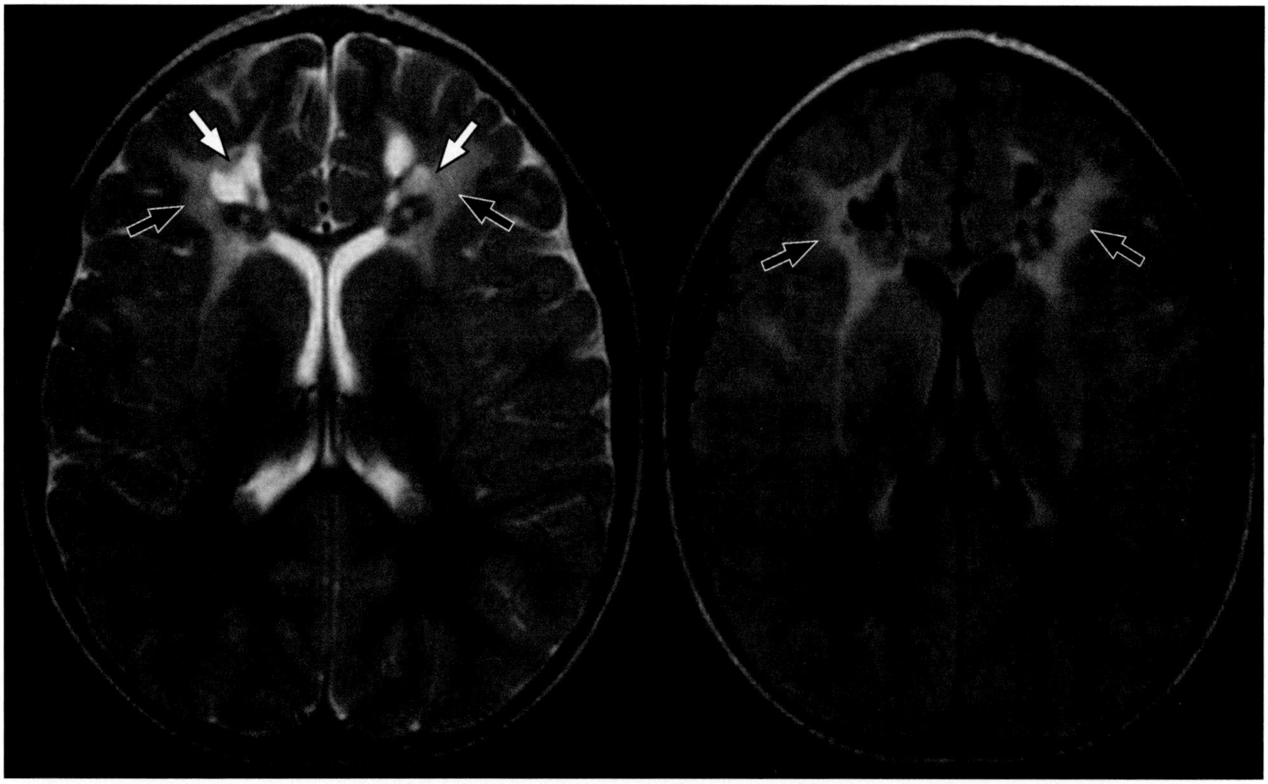

FIGURE 2.129 **Alexander disease in a 4-year-old boy.** Axial T2-weighted MR image (on the **left**) and FLAIR MR image (on the **right**) show rounded cystic lesions (*white arrows*) in the bilateral frontal white matter with adjacent white matter hyperintensities (*black arrows*).

Peroxisomal Disorders

Zellweger Syndrome

Zellweger syndrome (ZSS) is the most severe peroxisomal disorder, with almost all peroxisomal functions being absent. This syndrome of neonatal onset is autosomal recessive in inheritance and is also called cerebrohepatorenal syndrome. Presentation is soon after birth with profound hypotonia or atonia, weak or absent reflexes, and swallowing difficulties. On physical examination, affected pediatric patients have dysmorphic features including a bulging forehead, puffy eyelids, hypertelorism, and epicanthic folds. A variety of ophthalmologic abnormalities are seen, including Brushfield spots, optic atrophy or hypoplasia, glaucoma, corneal clouding, and cataracts.[153] Various limb anomalies are also described, including cubitus valgus, camptodactyly, and talipes equinovarus. Cerebral MRI findings in ZSS include abnormal gyration pattern including bilateral perisylvian polymicrogyria, abnormal T2 hyperintensity in the white matter, germinolytic cysts, and gray matter heterotopia. Brain atrophy and delayed myelination are also seen. A large anterior fontanelle, patellar calcification, hepatomegaly, and renal cysts are other imaging findings of note.

Mitochondrial Disorders

"Mitochondrial disorders" can be described as disorders of the oxidative phosphorylation pathway regardless of clinical syndrome (e.g., Leigh syndrome, MELAS [mitochondrial encephalomyopathy, lactic acidosis, and stroke-like episodes]). These disorders are typically characterized by signal abnormalities of the deep gray matter structures, brainstem (e.g., central tegmental tracts), and in the case of MELAS, cortical gray matter. The finding of abnormal symmetrical T2 and FLAIR hyperintensity in the deep gray matter nuclei is the most helpful and specific MRI finding of a mitochondrial disorder. Varying degree of cerebral and cerebellar atrophy may be present. White matter abnormality may also be seen in mitochondrial disorders, resembling other leukodystrophies. Specific MRI findings associated with specific syndromic phenotypes are described in more detail below.

Pyruvate Dehydrogenase Complex Deficiency

Pyruvate dehydrogenase (PDH) complex is a key mitochondrial multienzyme complex required for the conversion of pyruvate to acetyl-CoA. Most affected pediatric patients with pyruvate dehydrogenase deficiency have a defect in the E1 alpha subunit, associated with mutations in the pyruvate dehydrogenase, alpha-1 (*PDHA1*) gene. The characteristic pattern of brain MRI in patients with PDH complex deficiency is abnormal signal intensity on T2-weighted MR images in the basal ganglia, brainstem, and subtentorial nuclei, with a lactate peak on MR spectroscopy (Fig. 2.130). Cortical atrophy is also a feature as the disease progresses.

Pyruvate Carboxylase Deficiency

Pyruvate carboxylase (PC) deficiency is an autosomal recessive disorder that usually presents with lactic acidemia and severe neurologic dysfunction, leading to death in infancy. Children with PC deficiency present with axial hypotonia and tachypnea during the first hours of life. Abnormal movements (high-amplitude tremor and hypokinesia) and bizarre ocular behavior are the most common findings, whereas epilepsy is infrequent. MRI in complete enzyme deficiency shows cystic PVL. Biochemical findings typically include hypoglycemia, lactic acidosis, and hypercitrullinemia. In the partial enzyme deficiency, leukodystrophy is seen involving the brainstem and subcortical white matter.

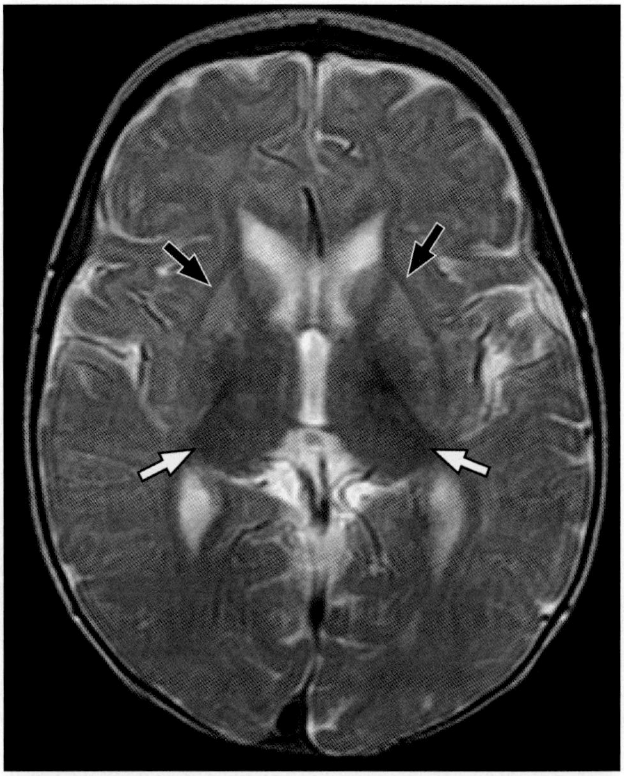

FIGURE 2.130 **Pyruvate dehydrogenase deficiency in a 6-year-old girl with complex 1 deficiency.** Axial T2-weighted MR image shows abnormal signal intensity in the bilateral basal ganglia (*black arrows*) and thalami (*white arrows*).

Leigh Disease

Leigh disease is a progressive neurodegenerative disorder that occurs in young children. It is often referred to as a subacute necrotizing encephalomyopathy. The clinical course can be acute, subacute, episodic, or chronic and progressive. It is a multisystem disease, but is dominated by CNS manifestations. Clinical symptoms include global developmental delay, feeding and swallowing difficulties, vomiting, spasticity, brainstem dysfunction, dystonia, abnormal eye movements, and multiple organ involvement.[198] MRI demonstrates progressive signal abnormalities, most frequency in the lentiform and caudate nuclei, but also variably involving the thalamus, periaqueductal gray matter, tegmentum, red nuclei, and dentate nuclei[198] (Fig. 2.131). Although putaminal involvement is considered as a distinguishing feature of Leigh disease, this finding is seen in other mitochondrial disorders like MELAS.[198] Sometimes, the thalami may be involved as well. Delayed myelination and hypomyelination are commonly

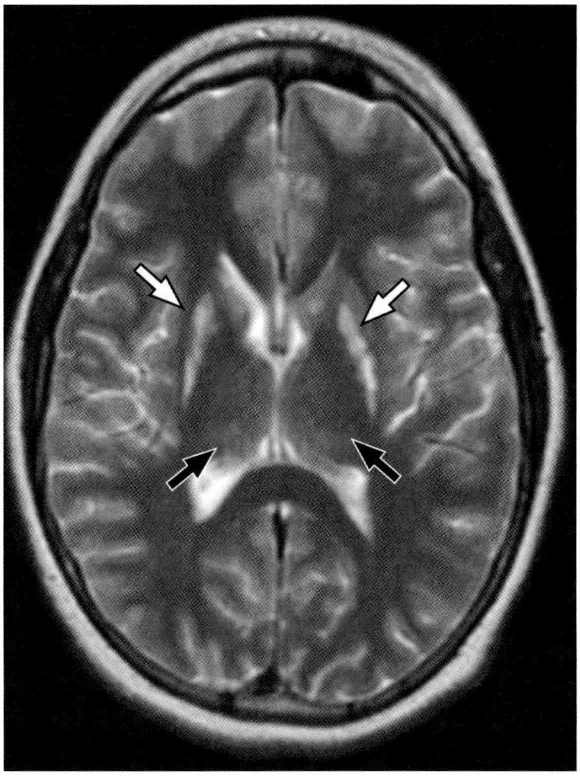

FIGURE 2.131 **Leigh disease in a 3-year-old girl.** Axial T2-weighted MR image shows T2 hyperintensities in the atrophic lentiform (*white arrows*) and caudate nuclei, and less prominent hyperintense foci in the thalami (*black arrows*).

seen MRI findings in pediatric patients with Leigh disease. Diffusion-weighted MR images show restricted diffusion within the lesions in the brainstem, basal ganglia, and dentate nuclei. MR spectroscopy shows lactate elevation, with the highest levels seen in the affected basal ganglia.

Mitochondrial Encephalomyopathy, Lactic Acidosis, and Stroke-like Episodes

Mitochondrial encephalomyopathy, lactic acidosis, and stroke-like episodes (MELAS) is caused by a mutation of maternal mitochondrial DNA. MRI in these pediatric patients shows recurrent stroke-like lesions within the brain, usually involving the cerebral hemispheres. The parietal and occipital lobes are most frequently involved. Progressive atrophy may be detected on follow-up imaging studies. MR spectroscopy shows a very large lactate peak in the infarcted region. Also, elevated lactate can be found even in normal-appearing brain. Findings of MELAS can be nonspecific. However, in a young patient, a diagnosis of MELAS should be considered in the presence of gyriform swelling, strokes of varying ages that predominantly affect gray matter not confined to vascular territories, or an elevated lactate in normal-appearing brain parenchyma.[199]

Kearns-Sayre Syndrome

Kearns-Sayre syndrome is a rare autosomal dominant mitochondrial disorder characterized by onset before 20 years of age, progressive external ophthalmoplegia, pigmentary degeneration of the retina, cerebellar ataxia, and cardiomyopathy. CT of the brain demonstrates calcifications within the globus pallidi and caudate nuclei. MRI findings are varied and can show abnormalities including symmetrical T2 hyperintensity in the basal ganglia (more commonly the globus pallidi and rarely, the caudate nuclei), subcortical white matter, thalami, and brainstem, and cerebral and cerebellar atrophy.[200] The white matter and gray nuclei abnormalities are presumed to result from diffuse spongiform encephalopathy. Of note, the putamina are spared, differentiating Kearns-Sayre from Leigh disease. MR spectroscopy may or may not show lactate elevation with in the brain.

Glutaric Aciduria Type 1

Glutaric aciduria type 1 is an autosomal recessive disorder caused by deficiency of a mitochondrial enzyme called glutaryl-CoA dehydrogenase. This enzyme is involved in the metabolism of the amino acids, L-lysine, L-hydroxylysine, and L-tryptophan. Some affected children present with acute encephalopathy and typically have macrocephaly on imaging examination. In other pediatric patients, gradual neurologic deterioration may be the presenting feature with concomitant hypotonia, dystonia or choreoathetosis, and tetraplegia. Most affected pediatric patients may have an acute encephalopathic crisis by age 12 months.

Imaging studies demonstrate enlarged extra-axial spaces in the frontal and temporal lobes. T2 prolongation is seen in the basal ganglia (predominantly the putamina, less commonly the caudate, and rarely, the globus pallidi), tegmentum, substantia nigra, and periventricular white matter.[201] There is relative sparing of the optic radiations and subcortical U-fibers (Fig. 2.132). MR spectroscopy reveals elevated lactate with decreased NAA levels.[202] Chronic SDHs have been reported in up to 20% to 30% of affected patients. These develop after relatively minor trauma and may be accompanied by retinal hemorrhage. Although the possibility of child abuse may be raised in this clinical situation, it is important to consider glutaric aciduria type 1 in these pediatric patients.[203]

Treatment includes institution of a low lysine diet, carnitine supplementation, and intensified emergency treatment during acute episodes of intercurrent illness. Striatal injury can be prevented in the majority of neonatally-diagnosed patients by combined metabolic treatment introduced and monitored by an experienced interdisciplinary team.

Urea Cycle Disorders

Urea cycle disorders (UCD) are caused by single gene defects involved in the detoxification pathway of ammonia to urea. UCD include deficiency of one of six enzymes (*N*-acetylglutamate synthase [NAGS], ornithine transcarbamylase [OTC], carbamoyl phosphate synthetase [CPS I], argininosuccinate lyase [ASL], argininosuccinate synthetase [ASS], and arginase) and two membrane transporters involved in urea biosynthesis.[204] The most common urea cycle defect is OTC deficiency followed by argininosuccinic acidemia (ASL deficiency) and citrullinemia (ASS deficiency). All urea cycle defects are autosomal-recessively inherited except OTC deficiency, which is X-linked.

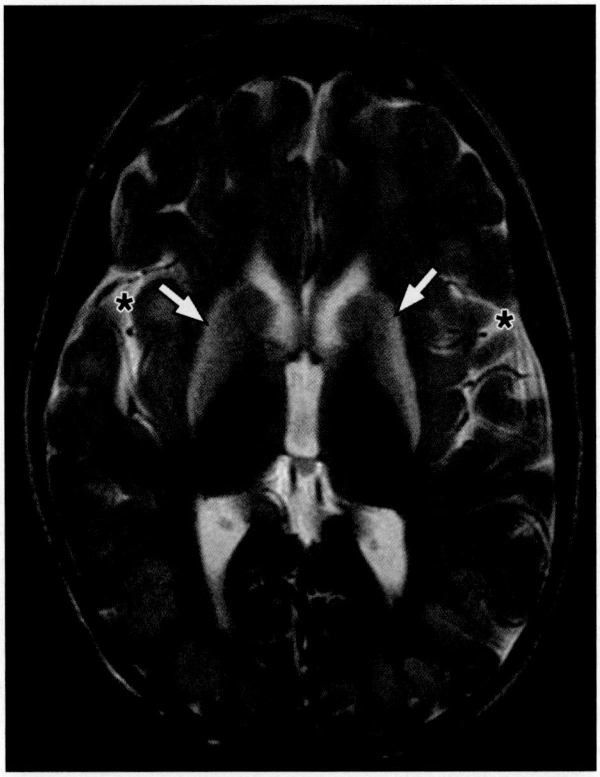

FIGURE 2.132 **Glutaric aciduria type 1 in a 2-month-old infant boy.** Axial T2-weighted MR image shows enlarged extra-axial spaces in the temporal lobes (*asterisks*) and hyperintensity and volume loss in the basal ganglia, predominantly in the putamen (*arrows*).

MRI abnormalities in neonates with urea cycle defects include vasogenic edema and related signal abnormality predominantly affecting unmyelinated white matter. Deep gray matter involvement is also seen including basal ganglia, perirolandic, and insular cortical abnormalities similar to those seen in noninherited causes of hyperammonemia (i.e., hepatic encephalopathy). Four common patterns of UCD include (1) diffuse severe cerebral edema followed by diffuse atrophy (type 1), (2) extensive infarct-like abnormality (type 2) often presenting as acute hemiplegia, (3) presumably-ischemic lesions in cerebral intervascular boundary zones (type 3), and (4) reversible, symmetric cortical involvement of the cingulate gyri, temporal lobes, and insular cortex with sparing of the perirolandic cortex (type 4).[205] Sometimes, the areas of signal abnormality are accompanied by restricted diffusion. MR spectroscopy in these cases shows elevation of glutamine/glutamate reflecting the presence of hyperammonemia. Differentiation from HII can be made based on the predominant lentiform nucleus involvement as opposed to the predominant thalamic injury seen in hypoxic injury.[205]

Propionic and Methylmalonic Acidemia

Both propionic and methylmalonic acidemia are autosomal recessive disorders that cause ketoacidosis and excretion of the respective acids in the urine. Propionic acidemia is caused by mutation in the genes encoding propionyl-CoA carboxylase, PCCA (chromosome 13q32), or PCCB (chromosome 13q21-23). Methylmalonic acidemia is caused by a mutation of the gene (MCM) at chromosome 6p21, which encodes for the methylmalonic-CoA mutase enzyme.

Typical initial clinical presentation is usually in early infancy with episodes of metabolic acidosis, vomiting, tachypnea, lethargy, and seizures, often leading to coma and death. Older pediatric patients present with progressive encephalopathy sometimes associated with movement disorders or dystonia. Neurologic examination usually reveals central hypotonia with pyramidal tract signs at time of crises; dystonia and choreoathetosis are common sequela of basal ganglia involvement.

On CT, there is hypodensity in the putamina and caudate nuclei in propionic acidemia and within the globus pallidi in methylmalonic acidemia. Correspondingly, there is T2 prolongation within these areas on MRI (Fig. 2.133). Periventricular T2 and FLAIR hyperintensity, delay in myelination, and volume loss is seen in later stages of the disease. During the acute phase of clinical decompensation, decreased diffusion may be seen in the affected areas. MR spectroscopy reportedly shows reduced NAA and myoinositol and increase in the glutamine/glutamate complex in the basal ganglia in propionic acidemia.

Treatment is focused on managing the metabolic ketoacidosis in these disorders using vigorous alkali therapy and protein restriction. Hyperammonemia may be treated by drug therapy (*N*-carbamyl glutamate), or in persistent cases, with hemodialysis or hemofiltration.

Gangliosidoses

Gangliosides are minor myelin constituents composed of a glycosphingolipid (ceramide lipid bound to an oligosaccharide) and at least one sialic acid molecule.[154] Gangliosidoses are inherited autosomal recessive disorders of ganglioside metabolism.

In GM_1 gangliosidosis resulting from lysosomal beta-galactosidase deficiency, MRI shows diffuse white matter abnormalities (type 1 GM_1), cerebral atrophy (type 2 GM_1), and basal ganglia abnormalities (type 3 GM_1). GM_2 gangliosidosis results from abnormalities in the hexosaminidase enzyme, and there are three distinct biochemical types, B, O, and AB. The B and O types are each distinguished into infantile, juvenile, and adult types; the AB variant only has an infantile type. Infantile type B GM_2 is the classic Tay-Sachs disease (TSD), and infantile type O GM_2 is the same as Sandhoff disease (SD). Imaging findings include high density in the thalamus on CT, low signal intensity on T2-weighted MRI in the infantile type, and cerebral and cerebellar atrophy in the late-onset type (Fig. 2.134). Neuroimaging findings in GM_2 gangliosidosis are virtually identical to those seen in GM_1 gangliosidosis. However, GM_1 gangliosidoses are somewhat distinct in that they are associated with kyphoscoliosis and hepatomegaly. GM_2 gangliosidoses are distinguished by their higher incidence of cherry red maculae and macrocephaly, though SD also features hepatosplenomegaly.[154]

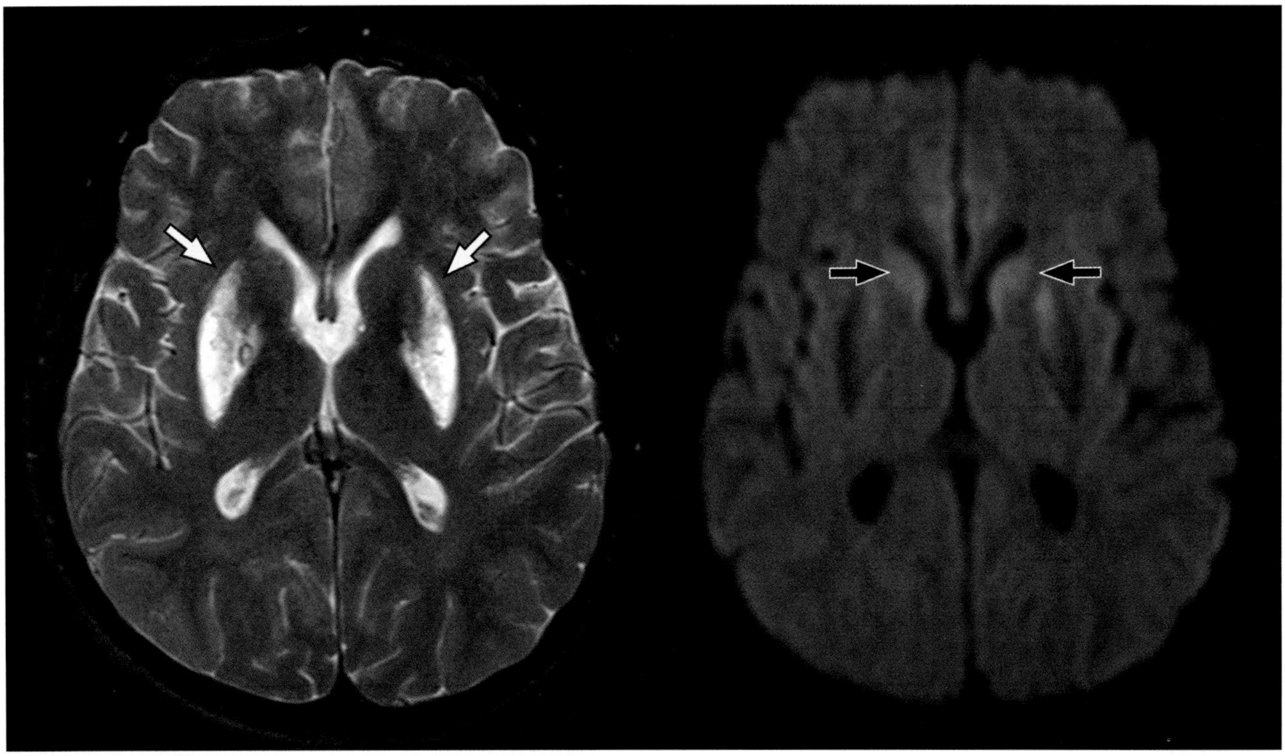

FIGURE 2.133 **Methylmalonic aciduria in a 7-year-old girl.** Axial T2-weighted MR image (on the **left**) and diffusion-weighted MR image (on the **right**) show T2 prolongation (*white arrows*) and decreased diffusion (*black arrows*) in the basal ganglia.

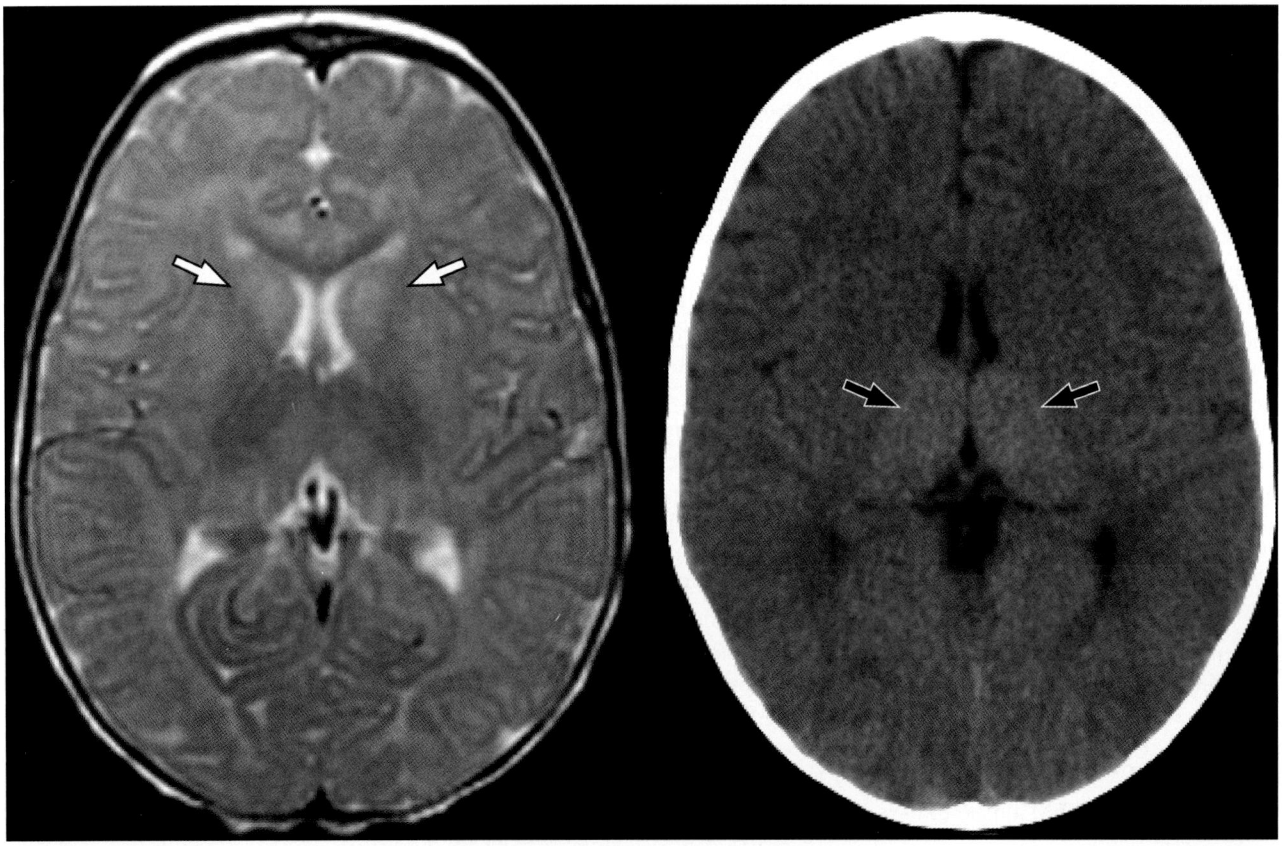

FIGURE 2.134 **Tay-Sachs disease in an 11-month-old boy who presented with hypotonia.** Axial T2-weighted MR image (on the **left**) shows abnormal T2 hyperintensity (*white arrows*) in the bilateral basal ganglia and thalami and delayed myelination characterized by hyperintensity in the white matter that should be myelinated by this stage. Axial CT image (on the **right**) obtained a few weeks later demonstrates bilaterally hyperdense thalami (*black arrows*) suggestive of mineralization.

Acquired Inflammatory White Matter Disorders

Acute Disseminated Encephalomyelitis

Acute disseminated encephalomyelitis (ADEM) is defined as the first episode of inflammatory demyelination associated with multifocal neurologic deficits, involving multiple sites in the CNS, accompanied by encephalopathy (defined as altered behavior or consciousness).[206] Use of this precise definition is important to avoid applying the term "ADEM" to any child with acute demyelination accompanied by multifocal MRI lesions.[206] It is thought that ADEM is usually triggered by an inflammatory response to viral infections and vaccinations, and a history of recent infection or vaccination can be elicited in many cases.

Clinical presentation is of an acute, monophasic illness characterized by one or more of the following symptoms: fever, headaches, meningism, visual/mental status disturbances, or irritability. Ataxia, nystagmus, sensory dysfunction, or weakness may be present if the cerebellum or spinal cord is involved. Also, the deficits may not occur contemporaneously. New deficits within 3 months of onset are considered to be part of the same acute episode.

Imaging findings of ADEM are nonspecific and do not typically allow differentiation of ADEM from multiple sclerosis (MS) or encephalitis. Noncontrast CT is usually nondiagnostic, although faint hypodensities may be seen if lesions are large. Ring-enhancing lesions may be seen on CT obtained a few days after onset of neurologic symptoms.[207,208] On MRI, characteristic findings are multiple, bilateral, asymmetrically distributed, patchy foci of hyperintensity on T2-weighted and FLAIR MR images within the juxtacortical and deep white matter of the cerebral hemispheres (Fig. 2.135). Larger lesions may be T1 hypointense, whereas smaller lesions are not well visualized on precontrast T1-weighted MR images. Contrast enhancement in ADEM on MRI is variable. The lesions may or may not enhance with contrast medium, and a mixture of enhancing and nonenhancing lesions, depending on their age, may be seen.[209] Lesions involving the deep gray matter nuclei (thalami and basal ganglia) and white matter are also seen in some cases. Cortical lesions may be seen in up to 30% of affected patients. Other areas of involvement include the brainstem, middle cerebellar peduncle, and cerebellum. Lesions within the corpus callosum, which are common in MS, are rarely seen in ADEM.

Outcome after ADEM is favorable, with a complete recovery expected in ~70% of cases and residual neurologic deficits persisting in up to one-third of patients 2 years after disease onset. Further ADEM episodes occur rarely and happen in two contexts: recurrent ADEM and multiphasic ADEM. A subset of these pediatric ADEM patients with recurrent disease ends up as MS or neuromyelitis optica (NMO). Those over 11 years with ADEM appear to have a greater risk of MS.

Clinically Isolated Syndrome

Clinically isolated syndrome (CIS) refers to the first neurologic episode lasting at least 24 hours, caused by inflammation/demyelination at one or more sites in the CNS. However, unlike in ADEM, there is no associated encephalopathy. It can also be monofocal and affect a localized part of the CNS (e.g., optic neuritis, transverse myelitis) or be multifocal. Clinically isolated syndromes are more common than ADEM in young children.

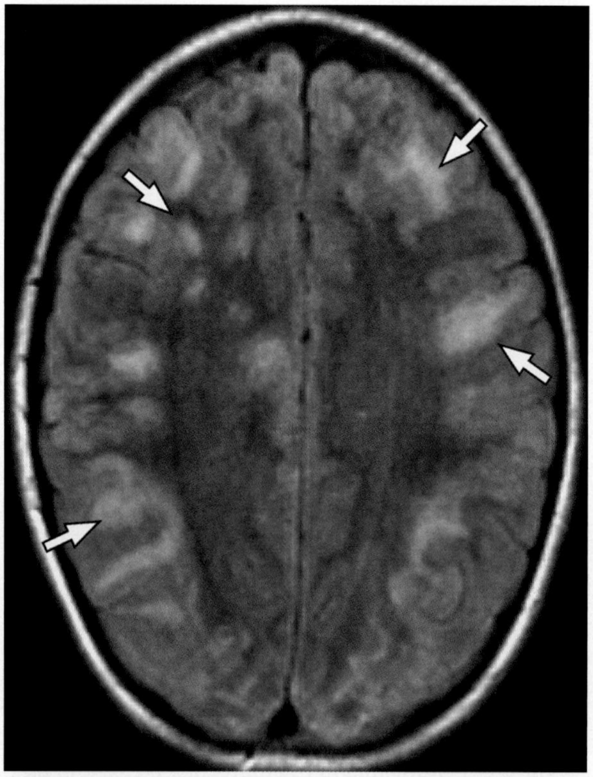

FIGURE 2.135 **Acute disseminated encephalomyelitis in a 9-year-old girl who presented with drowsiness for 2 weeks following viral illness.** Axial FLAIR MR image shows multiple hyperintensities (*arrows*) within the white matter and the cortex of the brain.

Neuromyelitis Optica

Neuromyelitis optica (NMO) refers to sequential or concomitant optic neuritis and transverse myelitis. More recently, this term has been expanded to include pediatric patients with encephalopathy, seizures, intractable vomiting, and brainstem-mediated hiccups. Unlike ADEM, NMO is more common in nonwhite children and may be associated with systemic autoimmune disease. Presence of serum antibodies against aquaporin 4 (NMO-IgG) is moderately sensitive and very specific for pediatric NMO.

Imaging features of CIS and NMO overlap with ADEM, and the differentiation between these entities should be based on clinical assessment. In 10% of patients with NMO, lesions are seen in the periependymal regions including the periaqueductal gray matter and the hypothalamus, which are rich in aquaporin 4 (Fig. 2.136).

High-dose corticosteroids are the current treatment of choice in inflammatory, demyelinating CNS diseases. Other options include the use of anti-inflammatory and

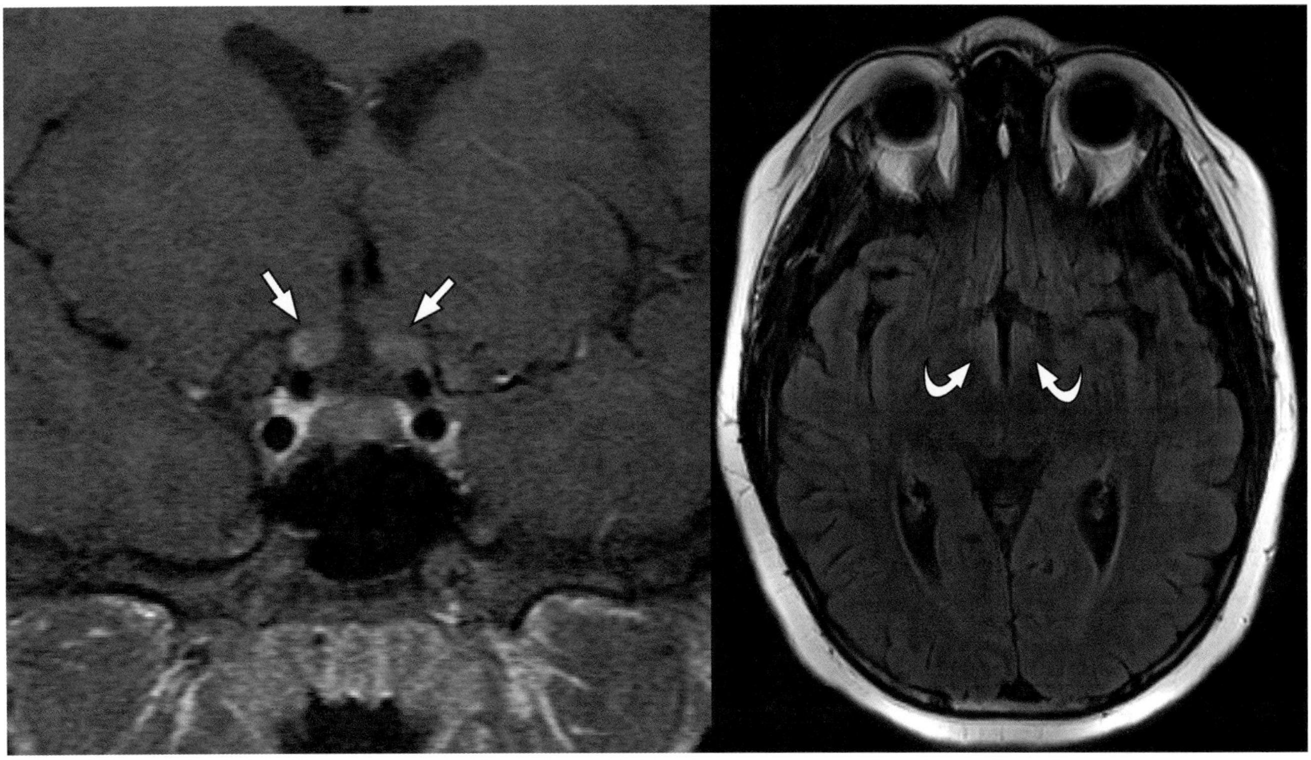

FIGURE 2.136 **Neuromyelitis optica in a 17-year-old boy.** Coronal postcontrast T1-weighted fat-suppressed MR image (on the **left**) shows bilateral optic nerve enlargement and enhancement (*arrows*). Axial FLAIR MR image (on the **right**) demonstrates hyperintensities (*curved arrows*) in the bilateral hypothalamic regions.

immunosuppressive treatments such as IV immunoglobulin (IVIG) and plasmapheresis.

Multiple Sclerosis

An ADEM-like, first demyelinating event can represent the first attack of MS. Currently, there are no absolute clinical features, or radiologic, serum, or CSF biomarkers that can distinguish ADEM from pediatric MS. Diagnosis of MS in children is based on clinical evidence of a second demyelinating event involving new areas of the CNS. Therefore, to diagnose pediatric MS, international consensus definitions require an initial ADEM event followed by two subsequent non-ADEM demyelinating events. Another difference between ADEM and MS is that there is complete or near-complete resolution of lesions in ADEM on repeat MRI, whereas follow-up imaging of MS usually demonstrates new, often asymptomatic, lesions. Many clinical and imaging features of MS in children are similar to those that characterize MS in adults, although important differences may also be noted.

Presence of white matter lesions situated perpendicular to the corpus callosum (Dawson fingers) has been found to be 100% specific for MS during the first episode of demyelination[210] (Fig. 2.137). Recent MRI criteria for pediatric MS suggest fewer total T2 lesions ($\geq$5 vs. $\geq$9) are required to identify children with MS with a high sensitivity (94%).[211] Modification of the McDonald criteria to $\geq$2 lesions in the periventricular region is also considered more sensitive for pediatric MS while maintaining high specificity.[211] Brainstem lesions are also considered as a more specific criterion in children than the broad category of infratentorial lesions.

It is important to note that pediatric-onset MS is characterized by a more significant radiologic disease burden both early and later in the disease course. Despite this, disability is slower to progress in pediatric-onset MS than adult-onset MS.

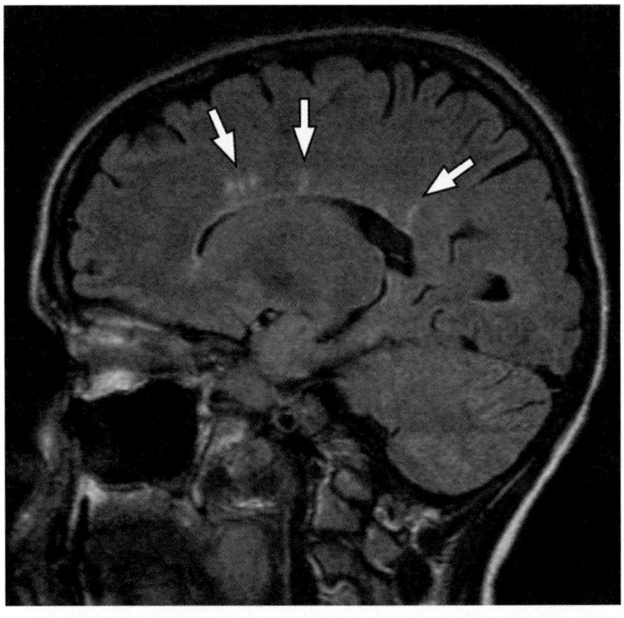

FIGURE 2.137 **Dawson fingers in a 16-year-old girl with multiple sclerosis.** Sagittal FLAIR MR image demonstrates white matter hyperintensities (*arrows*) situated perpendicular to corpus callosum.

Neurocutaneous Syndromes (Phacomatoses)

Neurocutaneous syndromes or phacomatoses are congenital and hereditary disorders characterized by developmental lesions of the neuroectoderm, leading to abnormalities in multiple organ systems, primarily those of ectodermal origin, including the skin, nervous system, and eyes. The four most common phacomatoses are neurofibromatosis (types 1 and 2), tuberous sclerosis, Sturge-Weber disease, and von Hippel–Lindau disease. Imaging of the brain and spine plays an important role in the diagnosis and management of these disorders.

Neurofibromatosis Type 1

Neurofibromatosis type 1 (NF1) is the most common neurocutaneous disorder, with an incidence of 1 in 3,000 to 4,000 persons. It is inherited as an autosomal dominant disorder with variable penetrance, caused by defects in the NF1 gene on chromosome 17 which is responsible for encoding the protein neurofibromin. Neurofibromin is a tumor suppressor, acting as a negative regulator of the Ras family guanine triphosphatases (GTPases). Pediatric patients with NF1 usually present during the first decade of life. NF1 is a complex disorder, affecting multiple cell types and multiple systems of the body, with a wide range of expression and unpredictable behavior.

A list of diagnostic criteria has been defined to enable diagnosis, and two or more criteria must be present for a diagnosis of NF1.[212]

1. Six or more café au lait spots
   a. 0.5 cm or larger in prepubertal individuals
   b. 1.5 cm or larger in postpubertal individuals
2. Two or more neurofibromas of any type or one or more plexiform neurofibromas
3. Freckling of the axilla or groin
4. Optic glioma (optic pathway tumor)
5. Two or more Lisch nodules (benign iris hamartomas)
6. A distinctive bony lesion: dysplasia of the sphenoid bone or dysplasia or thinning of long bone cortex
7. First-degree relative with NF1

Although there are no neuroimaging findings in the diagnostic criteria for NF1, neuroimaging may be the first modality that demonstrates the presence of lesions indicative of NF1, like optic pathway gliomas, sphenoid abnormalities, or plexiform neurofibromas in a young child. Later in life, precocious puberty and learning disabilities may also be manifestations of neurofibromatosis.

Common intracranial manifestations of NF1 include optic pathway tumors, other astrocytomas, and areas of myelin vacuolization ("NF spots").

Tumors

One to three percent of patients with NF1 develop tumors within the CNS.[213] Astrocytomas are the main type of CNS tumor in children with NF1, and pilocytic astrocytoma (World Health Organization grade 1) is the main histologic type. The optic pathways and brainstem are most often affected, but any part of the brain can be involved.

Optic Pathway Tumors

Optic pathway gliomas are the most common tumor of the CNS in NF1, with a reported prevalence ranging between 6% and 24%, depending on whether baseline neurologic imaging or clinical databases were analyzed.[214,215] They represent ~5% of childhood brain tumors, and up to 70% of these are associated with NF1.[216] Optic gliomas can involve any portion of the optic pathway, including one or both optic nerves, the chiasm, the optic tracts, the lateral geniculate bodies, or the optic radiations.

Approximately 50% of affected patients develop symptoms and signs, which include decreased visual acuity, visual field defects, optic atrophy, hydrocephalus, or hypothalamic dysfunction, papilledema, and occasionally, proptosis.[217] Precocious puberty and hypopituitarism may be a presenting feature with hypothalamic involvement of NF1.

MRI is the imaging modality of choice for the evaluation of optic pathway tumors. High-resolution thin-section axial and coronal T1-weighted MR images are obtained through the optic pathway. Optic nerve gliomas manifest as thickening of the optic nerve sheath complex, which may be tubular, fusiform, eccentric, or globular with kinking and tortuosity. Lesions are typically hypointense on T1-weighted MR images and hyperintense on T2-weighted MR images. Enlargement and expansion of the optic chiasm may be seen. Large tumors can have a mixed solid and cystic appearance, with areas of heterogeneous enhancement in the more solid-appearing areas (Fig. 2.138). T2 prolongation extending posteriorly to the lateral geniculate bodies along the optic tracts and radiations is considered a tumor and should not be mistaken for edema.

Spontaneous regression of large optic pathway tumors has been well described in pediatric patients with and without NF1, manifesting as an overall decrease in tumor size on MR imaging and functional improvement in visual function.

Treatment in children with symptomatic tumors includes surgery, chemotherapy, or radiation.

Other Astrocytomas

Other intraparenchymal brain tumors occur in patients with NF1 and are mainly low-grade astrocytomas. These tumors present in the second decade of life. Most of these tumors are pilocytic astrocytomas. High-grade tumors can also occur, but are comparatively rare.

Brainstem Mass Lesions

Brainstem mass lesions have been reported in ~18% of patients with NF1.[218] Most of these lesions in NF1 have a relatively benign course and may regress or stabilize over time.[218] These lesions are isointense on T1-weighted and hyperintense on T2-weighted MR images and demonstrate variable degrees of contrast enhancement. MR spectroscopy may be used to distinguish them from areas of myelin vacuolization.

Tectal Gliomas

These tumors have been discussed in an earlier section. Presentation of tectal gliomas in pediatric patients with

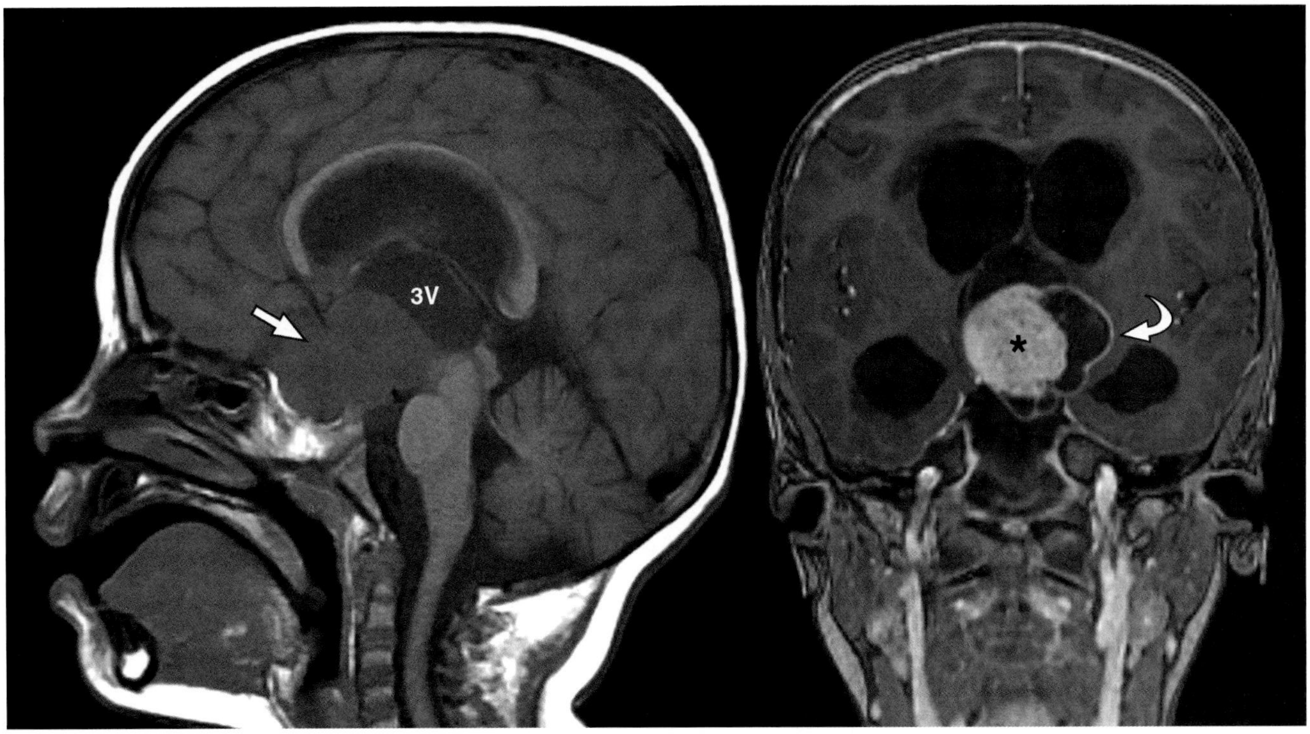

FIGURE 2.138 **Optic pathway glioma in a 4-year-old girl with neurofibromatosis type 1.** Sagittal T1-weighted MR image (on the **left**) and coronal postcontrast MPRAGE MR image (on the **right**) show a large, lobulated suprasellar mass (*straight arrow*) centered at the optic chiasm, extending into the third ventricle (*3V*). Note marked enhancement of the central solid component (*asterisk*) and rim enhancement of the cystic components (*curved arrow*).

NF1 is similar to that seen in other non-NF1 patients, with hydrocephalus resulting from aqueductal obstruction. Note that aqueductal narrowing in patients with NF1 can result from aqueductal stenosis as well, wherein the tectum is not enlarged and the proximal aqueduct may be dilated.

Myelin Vacuolization (Neurofibromatosis Spots)

NF spots are characteristic foci of hyperintense T2 signal intensity seen on MR imaging studies in the basal ganglia, internal capsule, brainstem, and cerebellum in children with NF1 (Fig. 2.139). NF spots occur in 43% to 93% of pediatric NF1 patients.[217] These lesions are not space occupying, appear by age 3 years, and increase in number and size until about 10 to 12 years of age, after which they decrease in size.[217] They are uncommon after the late second decade. NF spots typically do not enlarge, do not enhance, do not cause mass effect or clinical symptoms, and do not require treatment.

In young children under 2 years of age, NF spots are difficult to detect because of incomplete myelination of the white matter in the brain. Although they are typically asymptomatic, at least two studies have suggested that children with learning disabilities and NF1 tend to have a higher number of NF spots.

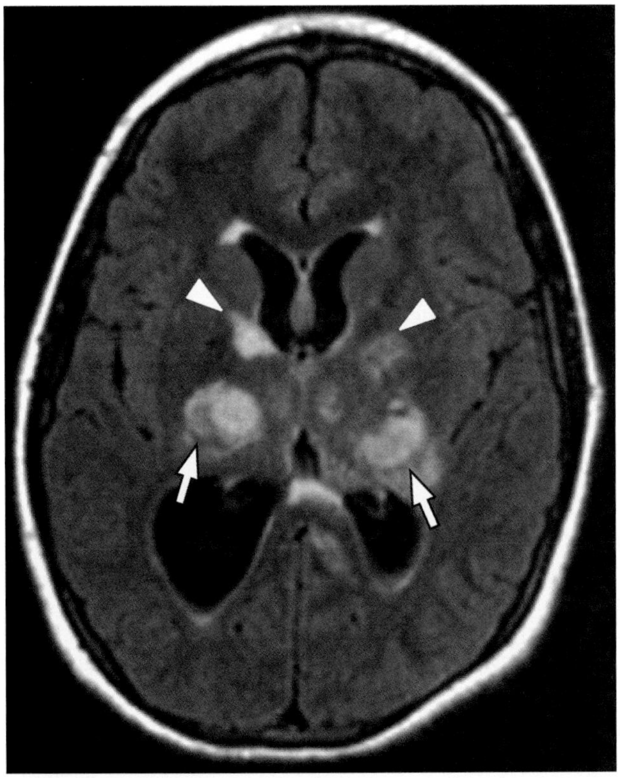

FIGURE 2.139 **Myelin vacuolization in a 13-year-old girl with neurofibromatosis type 1.** Axial FLAIR MR image shows multiple rounded T2 hyperintense areas of myelin vacuolization (NF spots) in the bilateral thalami (*arrows*) and basal ganglia (*arrowheads*) without mass effect on adjacent structures.

Cerebrovascular Abnormalities

Cerebrovascular abnormalities in patients with NF1 are uncommon and include dolichoectasia of the internal carotid arteries, arterial stenoses and occlusions, moyamoya disease, aneurysms, AVMs, and AV fistulae. These are discussed elsewhere in this chapter. Of note, occlusive vasculopathy may also result from radiation for optic pathway gliomas.

Osseous Dysplasias

Sphenoid wing dysplasia is an uncommon manifestation of NF1 and presents as defect in the greater sphenoid wing and enlargement of the middle cranial fossa. A congenital neuroectodermal and mesodermal maldevelopment has been proposed to explain these bone changes. This abnormality can present as pulsatile exophthalmos resulting from temporal lobe herniation into the orbit. Sphenoid dysplasia can be isolated or associated with an underlying trigeminal plexiform neurofibroma (PNF). A modified multifactorial concept of sphenoid dysplasia emphasizing the interaction between neurofibromas and the sphenoid bone during skull development has also been proposed.

Neurofibromas

Neurofibromas are benign peripheral nerve sheath tumors composed of a mixture of cellular elements such as Schwann cells, fibroblasts, mast cells, and perineural cells. They can arise at any site along the nerve from the dorsal root ganglion to terminal nerve branches. They can result in significant morbidity, mortality, and cosmetic disfigurement. Their growth pattern may be plexiform, diffuse, or mixed; plexiform architecture is virtually pathognomonic for NF1. They can grow at an unpredictable rate and demonstrate a variable pattern of growth from childhood through early adulthood.

PNFs are seen in ~30% to 50% of patients with NF1.[219] They are characterized by longitudinal growth along nerves, involving multiple fascicles and branches, and resulting in substantial disfigurement, overgrowth of the underlying bones, and nerve compression. Malignant transformation may occur in parts of the lesions. The risk of developing a malignant peripheral nerve sheath tumor in patients with NF is ~10% to 15%.[219,220]

MRI is the imaging modality of choice to characterize PNFs. These tumors are T1 hypointense and T2 hyperintense. Variable enhancement is seen following contrast administration. Typically, the center of the lesion is T2 hypointense, referred to as the "target sign", corresponding pathologically to a dense central collagen-rich core. The size and irregular shape of these lesions makes it difficult to follow growth or shrinkage in response to treatment. Volumetric MR imaging measurements for PNFs are now used as they have been shown to have high interobserver correlation.

Enlarging or symptomatic PNFs may require surgical resection, which is usually difficult because lesions are large and infiltrative and often recur. Alternative therapies, including drugs like farnesyl protein transferase inhibitors, angiogenesis inhibitors, cytodifferentiating agents, and hormonal modulators, are being investigated. Molecular therapies based on the underlying genetic abnormality are also being studied.

Other CNS Manifestations

Other manifestations of NF1 include macrocephaly, scoliosis, tumors in the spinal cord and canal, paraspinal tumors, vertebral body scalloping from dural ectasia, meningoceles, and arachnoid cysts.

Neurofibromatosis Type 2

NF2 is an autosomal dominant disorder, which accounts for about 3% of all cases of neurofibromatosis. Its incidence is estimated at 1 in 40,000 to 50,000 persons. It results from defects in the NF2 gene on chromosome 22q11.[221] NF2 is characterized by multiple cranial nerve schwannomas, ocular abnormalities, and skin tumors. The diagnostic criteria for NF2 include the following:

1. Bilateral eighth nerve masses confirmed by CT or MRI
2. A first-degree relative with NF2 and either of the following:
   a. A unilateral eighth nerve mass
   b. Two of the following: neurofibroma, meningioma, glioma, schwannoma, or juvenile posterior subcapsular lenticular opacity (cataract)

The acronym "MISME" (multiple inherited schwannomas, meningiomas, and ependymomas) is a useful mnemonic for remembering the disease manifestations of NF2.

Intracranial Manifestations

Schwannomas

Vestibular schwannomas are tumors arising from Schwann cells that form the myelin sheaths around the nerve root axons of the eighth cranial nerve. They are composed of Antoni A tissue (dense areas) and Antoni B tissue (looser areas). They are uncommon in the pediatric age group. They occur in 95% of adult patients with NF2, most commonly in the third decade of life. Presenting symptoms include hearing loss, tinnitus, or balance dysfunction.

Vestibular schwannomas occur in the internal auditory canal or the porus acusticus. On CT, they are hypodense to isodense and may calcify. On thin-section MR imaging through the posterior fossa, vestibular schwannomas are seen as T1 hypointense and T2 hyperintense lesions with homogeneous enhancement following contrast administration (Fig. 2.140). Larger lesions can be more heterogeneous and may be complicated by necrosis or hemorrhage.

Schwannomas can also develop within the fifth nerve and ninth to twelfth nerves. They vary in appearance from fusiform thickening of the nerve to a nodular mass and can enlarge the bony foramina.

Meningiomas

Meningiomas are dural-based extra-axial tumors arising from the meninges. They tend to occur at a younger age and may be multiple in patients with NF2. When a meningioma is present in a child, the possibility of NF2 should be considered.

On CT, meningiomas are typically hyperdense and avidly-enhancing following contrast administration. On MRI, they are isointense to gray matter on both T1- and T2-weighted sequences, with homogeneous enhancement following contrast administration. Hyperostosis or, less commonly, erosion of the adjacent calvarium may be seen. Displacement of the brain parenchyma may also be present.

Other manifestations of NF2 in the CNS include meningioangiomatosis, spinal tumors (including intramedullary ependymomas and schwannomas, intraspinal schwannomas,

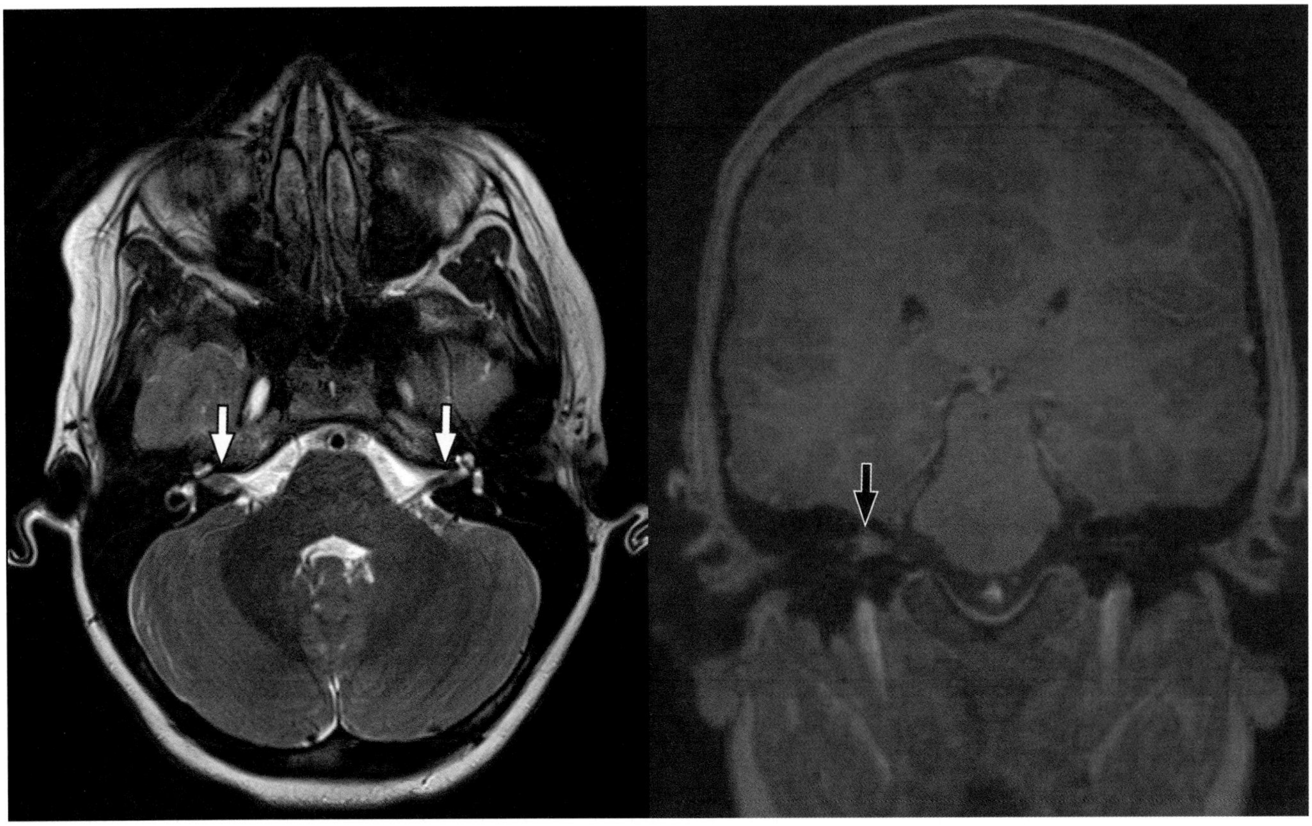

FIGURE 2.140 **Vestibular schwannoma in a 9-year-old boy with sensorineural hearing loss, subsequently diagnosed with neurofibromatosis type 2.** Axial T2-weighted MR image (on the **left**) shows T2 hypointense lesions (*white arrows*) in the bilateral internal auditory canals (IACs). Coronal postcontrast T1-weighted MR image (on the **right**) shows the avid enhancement of the lesion (*black arrow*) in the right IAC.

and meningiomas), and peripheral schwannomas arising from the dorsal nerve roots.

Tuberous Sclerosis

Tuberous sclerosis (TSC) is a genetic, autosomal dominant, multiorgan disorder characterized by the development of hamartomas and benign tumors in the brain, heart, kidneys, liver, lungs, and other sites. It is associated with mutations of the *TSC1* gene on chromosome 9 encoding hamartin or the *TSC2* gene on chromosome 16 encoding tuberin. TSC1 and TSC2 interact physically with high affinity to form heterodimers, an observation that is consistent with the similar clinical features of patients with TSC1 and TSC2 mutations. Loss of the TSC1–TSC2 heterodimer inhibits the mammalian target of the rapamycin (mTOR) cascade. mTOR is a serine–threonine kinase, which plays a major role in ribosome biosynthesis and protein translation. In TSC-associated tumors, loss of TSC1 or TSC2 results in mTOR-dependent phosphorylation of p70S6 kinase, ribosomal protein S6, and 4E-BP1. This results in increased cell growth and proliferation in response to growth factors, amino acids, and nutrients.

The primary manifestations of TSC include hamartomas (defined as disorganized tissue composed of cells normally found in that organ) and benign neoplasms. Hamartomas affect the CNS, skin, nail beds, kidneys, and other organs. TSC patients are also at risk for developing true neoplasms of the brain and kidney.

Diagnostic criteria have been updated by the International Tuberous Sclerosis Complex Consensus conference and are listed here[222]:

Major features

1. Hypomelanotic macules (≥3, at least 5 mm diameter)
2. Angiofibromas or fibrous forehead plaque
3. Ungual or periungual fibroma (>2)
4. Shagreen patch (connective tissue nevus)
5. Multiple retinal hamartomas
6. Cortical dysplasias (≥3, including tubers and cerebral white matter migration lines)
7. Subependymal nodules (≥2)
8. Subependymal giant cell astrocytoma (SEGA)
9. Cardiac rhabdomyoma
10. Lymphangiomyomatosis
11. Renal angiomyolipoma

Minor features

1. Dental enamel pits (≥3)
2. Intraoral fibromas (≥2)
3. Nonrenal hamartoma (histologic confirmation suggested)
4. Retinal achromic patch
5. "Confetti" skin lesions
6. Multiple renal cysts

Definite diagnosis of TSC requires documentation of at least two major features or one major and two minor criteria.

Possible diagnosis requires either one major or ≥2 minor features. However, it should be noted that the above criteria do not integrate genetic testing results.

The intracranial features of TSC are cortical or subcortical tubers, subependymal nodules, SEGAs, and white matter radial migration lines.

The most common clinical manifestations of TSC include epilepsy and cognitive impairment. More recent studies have shown a predisposition of some patients with TSC to develop autism.

Tubers

Tubers (cortical hamartomas) are most commonly found in the cerebral hemispheres, predominantly in the frontal lobes. Clinical features depend on the tuber location. Neurologic findings include abnormalities in cognition, cranial nerve deficits, focal motor or sensory abnormalities, cerebellar dysfunction, and gait abnormalities.

On MR imaging studies, the appearance of cortical tubers changes with age. In neonates, they appear as hyperintense gyri on T1-weighted MR images that are hypointense to white matter on T2-weighted MR images. This signal abnormality may extend through the cortical mantle to the ventricular surface from the cortical tuber. The lesions gradually become isointense as myelination progresses. In older infants, the tubers are hypointense on T1-weighted MR images, with cortical and subcortical areas of T2 and FLAIR hyperintensity (Fig. 2.141). Rarely, they may develop calcification, and a small proportion of degenerated, calcified cortical tubers (3% to 4%) will enhance following contrast administration. Dysmorphic neurons in the tubers can be indistinguishable from those seen in focal cortical dysplasia. Tissue microarray of the tissue may be required to make this distinction.

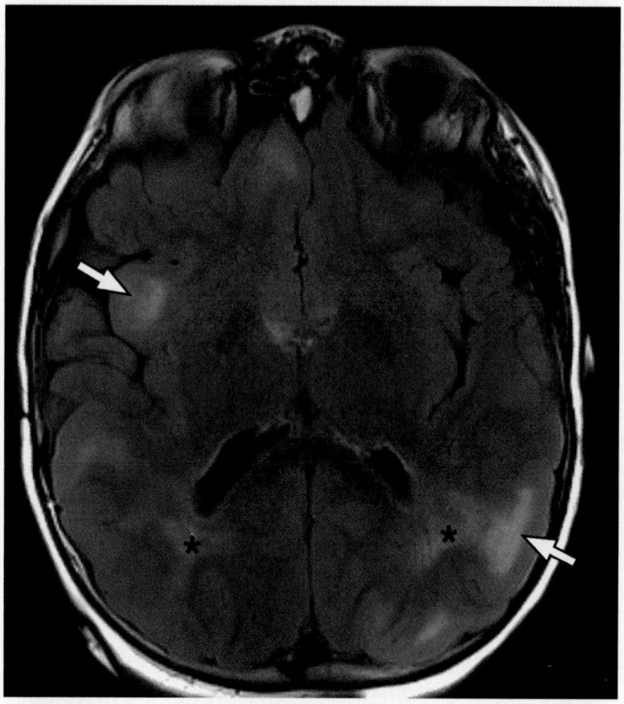

FIGURE 2.141 **Cortical tubers in a 9-year-old boy with tuberous sclerosis.** Axial FLAIR MR image shows multiple cortical hyperintensities (*arrows*) consistent with cortical tubers. Also, note the abnormal signal in the subcortical white matter (*asterisks*) characteristically seen in children with tuberous sclerosis.

Rarely, tubers are present in the cerebellum, brainstem, and spinal cord. Reduction in cerebellar volume has been reported using volumetric analysis in pediatric patients with tuberous sclerosis. This may not be apparent on visual inspection. Cerebellar tubers are usually wedge-shaped and not epileptogenic like cortical tubers.

Treatment includes surgical resection of more epileptogenic tubers in patients with medically-refractory seizures. To identify the tubers with the greatest epileptiform activity, functional studies including arterial spin-labeled MRI, PET (using ^{18}F-FDG or agents like alpha-^{11}C-methyl-L-tryptophan), SPECT, magnetic source imaging, videotelemetry, and subdural grids and strips placement may be required. If seizures can be localized to one or two tubers, the resection of these lesions has been shown to markedly reduce seizure frequency and improve response to medical therapy. Grossly, resected specimens show replacement of the cortical gray matter by an ill-defined area of pallor that obscures the gray–white matter junction (Fig. 2.142); microscopically, there are aggregates of large bizarre cells interspersed with more normal-appearing neurons and astrocytes.

Subependymal Nodules and Subependymal Giant Cell Astrocytomas

Subependymal nodules are benign hamartomatous nodules found along the walls of the lateral ventricles, most commonly at the caudothalamic groove just posterior to the foramen of Monro. They are composed of loosely cohesive clusters of large cells (astrocytes, dysmorphic neurons, and giant cells) with round or oval nuclei and no or minimal atypia. They occur as discrete or roughly confluent rounded foci of tissue, anywhere along the ventricular surface. They are typically benign lesions. Subependymal nodules can enlarge and degenerate into SEGAs

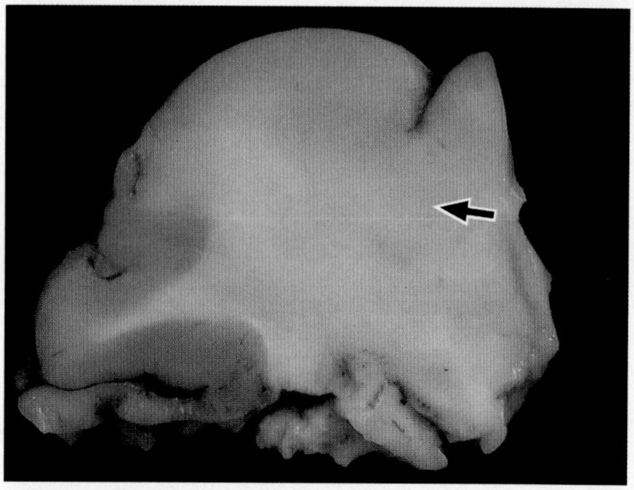

FIGURE 2.142 **Gross specimen of a cortical tuber resected from the temporal lobe of a 2-year-old girl with tuberous sclerosis shows a localized area of pallor (*arrow*) blurring the gray–white matter junction.**

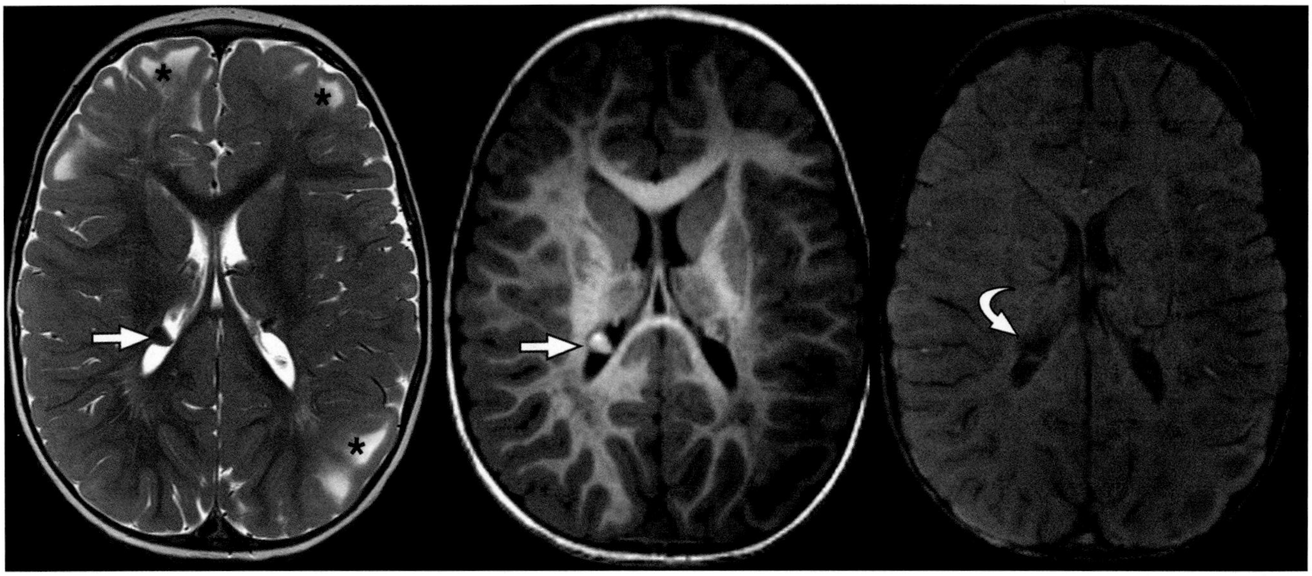

FIGURE 2.143 **Subependymal nodules in a 2-year-old boy with tuberous sclerosis.** Axial T2-weighted MR image (on the **left**), axial MPRAGE MR image (in the **middle**), and axial susceptibility-weighted MR image (on the **right**) show multiple T2 hypointense and T1 hyperintense lesions (*arrows*) along the subependymal surface of the lateral ventricles, with mineralization (*curved arrow*) within some of the lesions indicated by susceptibility on the susceptibility-weighted MR image. Also noted are multiple T2 hyperintense cortical tubers (*asterisks*).

in 10% to 20% of cases, depending on whether pathologic or radiologic criteria are used to diagnose a SEGA.[223]

SEGAs are slow-growing, glial neuronal tumors developing in most cases over 1 to 3 years, although their development can occasionally be more aggressive and involve parenchymal invasion or extensive peritumoral edema. Development of SEGAs is a gradual process that usually occurs within the first two decades of life.

In neonates, subependymal nodules (SENs) appear echogenic on cranial US and can be difficult to differentiate from periventricular gray matter heterotopia. Imaging appearances of SENs on CT and MRI change with age. In the first few years of life, the number of calcified lesions gradually increases. On MRI, they appear as SENs that protrude into the ventricle. They are T1 hyperintense and T2 hypointense in young infants with unmyelinated white matter (Fig. 2.143). As myelination progresses, SENs become more isointense to white matter and may be best visualized on T1-weighted MR images, where their hyperintensity contrasts with low signal intensity of the CSF. Larger nodules may show variable degrees of T2 hypointensity related to the presence of calcification. T2* MR images are ideal to demonstrate the presence of calcification. Both SEGAs and subependymal nodules enhance following contrast administration (Fig. 2.144). The most useful distinguishing imaging feature between SEGAs and hamartomas is growth on serial imaging studies.

Microscopically, SEGA consists of large plump cells with astrocytic and sometimes ganglion cell-like differentiation; abundant eosinophilic cytoplasm is characteristic (Fig. 2.145). Treatment of SEGA includes resection or insertion of a shunt to bypass obstruction caused by lesions at the foramen of Monro. More recently, rapamycin therapy has shown promise by stabilizing growth and reducing the size of SEGAs in some studies.

White Matter Lesions

White matter abnormalities are seen in nearly 100% of patients with TSC using MRI.[224] These include wedge-shaped, tumefactive, and linear or curvilinear lesions in the cerebral or cerebellar hemispheres. These lesions are composed of

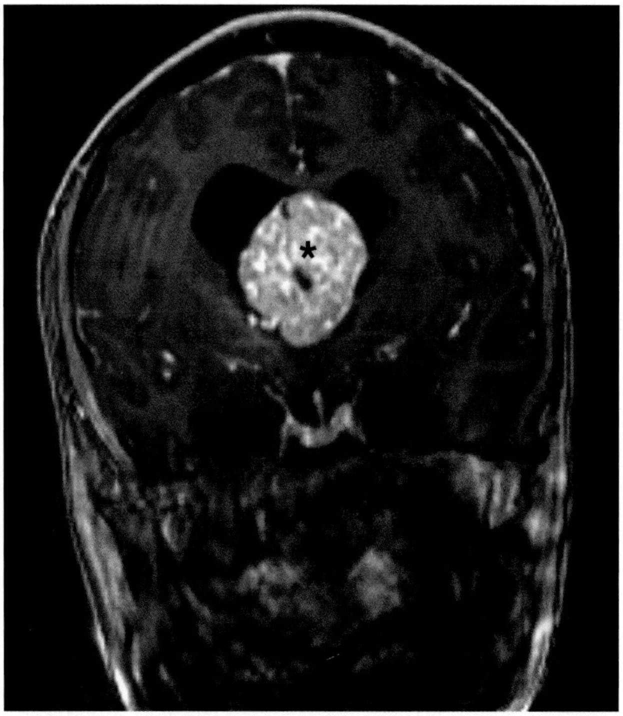

FIGURE 2.144 **Subependymal giant cell astrocytoma (SEGA) in a 12-year-old girl with tuberous sclerosis.** Coronal postcontrast MPRAGE (magnetization-prepared rapid gradient-echo) MR image shows a large enhancing mass (*asterisk*) centered around the foramina of Monro, subsequently shown at surgery and pathology to be a SEGA.

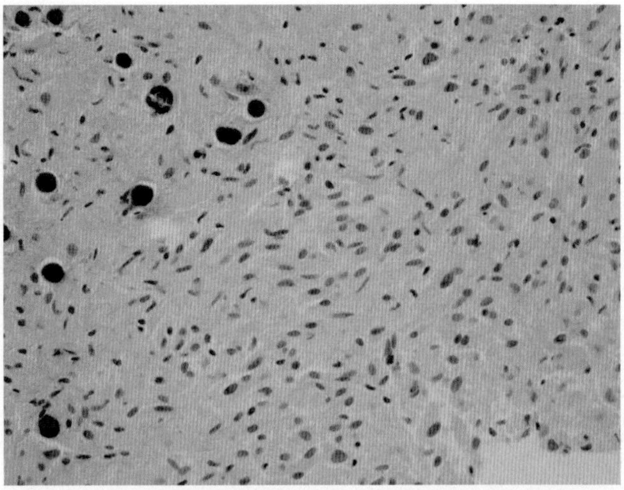

FIGURE 2.145 **Subependymal giant cell astrocytoma in an 8-year-old boy.** This tumor was resected from the subependymal/ventricular region of the brain. The tumor cells have well-defined borders and abundant eosinophilic cytoplasm and peripherally placed round to elongated nuclei, some with prominent nucleoli; frequent microcalcifications are admixed (hematoxylin and eosin, original magnification, 400×).

neurons and glial cells and include giant neurons and balloon cells. The balloon cells are dysplastic cells with characteristics of both neurons and glia. TSC-associated white matter lesions have pathologic and imaging characteristics of both cortical tubers and focal cortical dysplasia with balloon cells.

On CT, they may be seen as low attenuation, well-defined areas within the cerebral white matter that do not enhance after intravenous contrast administration. Calcification may occur within a portion or the entire lesion. On MR, these lesions resemble cortical tubers and can be seen to course through the cerebral mantle from the cortex to the ventricular surface, if imaged in the appropriate plane. They can be difficult to visualize when the white matter becomes myelinated on T1-weighted sequences, but can sometimes be identified in infants as subtle hyperintense foci. On FLAIR and T2-weighted MR images, they are seen as well-defined linear or curvilinear areas of high signal intensity. Some lesions may calcify and appear as linear or curvilinear areas of T1 hyperintensity. Enhancement is only seen in these lesions if they degenerate, and in these cases, calcification is almost invariably present.

Vascular Lesions

Vascular lesions are rare in TSC. Aneurysms in the kidney, liver, aorta, and distal extremities have been described in various studies. Cerebral aneurysms are very rare, but have been reported in children with TSC, mainly in the internal carotid arteries or the ACA distribution. These locations are otherwise uncommon locations for aneurysms in children. Therefore, it has been suggested that the cerebral aneurysms that have been reported in TSC are related to the disease, rather than being incidental. Certainly, an aneurysm should be considered as a likely possibility and a cerebral angiogram performed if a child with TSC presents with subarachnoid or intraparenchymal hemorrhage.

Non-CNS Manifestations

Hamartomas and benign neoplasms in the heart, kidneys, liver, lung, spleen, and other sites are present in a significant proportion of patients with TSC and are discussed elsewhere in this book.

Sturge-Weber Syndrome

Sturge-Weber syndrome (SWS) or encephalotrigeminal angiomatosis is a congenital syndrome that results from failure of development of superficial cortical veins, causing diversion of blood to the leptomeninges and formation of abnormal vascular channels as a consequence. The abnormal vasculature affects the skin of the face, choroid and sclera of the eye, and the brain and leptomeninges. The cutaneous lesion is called a port-wine stain, caused by dilated veins containing deoxygenated blood. SWS is defined by the intracranial abnormality, with or without the facial lesion.[225] Isolated port-wine stain is not considered to be SWS. Port-wine stains occur in 1 in 300 live births.[226,227] Estimated incidence of SWS is 1 in 20,000 to 50,000 live births.[228] The overall incidence of SWS is higher in patients with bilateral facial lesions. Also, involvement of the forehead by the port-wine stain is a strong predictor of neurologic and ophthalmologic sequelae.[229]

Although this is a sporadic disorder, recent research has identified a mutation in the *GNAQ* gene on chromosome 9q21 in patients with SWS and port-wine stains. *GNAQ* encodes Gαq, a member of the q class of G-protein alpha subunits that mediates signals between G-protein–coupled receptors and downstream effectors and increases cell proliferation and inhibits apoptosis because of increased downstream signaling through the RAS effector pathways.[230]

The presenting features include congenital glaucoma caused by alteration in the intraocular pressure by venous hypertension, enlarged globe (buphthalmos or "ox eye") in a neonate caused by intrauterine glaucoma, the port-wine stain at birth, or seizures resulting from the intracranial abnormalities. Seizure onset is usually delayed beyond the neonatal period.

Imaging features on CT include presence of cerebral calcifications in a gyral distribution, cerebral atrophy ipsilateral to the facial nevus, hypertrophy of the skull and sinuses, and enlarged choroid plexus in the involved hemisphere. MRI is the most useful imaging study in the first year of life. An abnormal MRI is the best predictor of all adverse clinical outcomes for these patients. Most authors now agree that a gadolinium-enhanced brain MRI should be obtained within the first 3 months of life, with the caveat that a negative result should not be considered conclusive if neurologic symptoms develop.[229] On MRI, the main findings are cerebral atrophy, white matter abnormalities in the region of the leptomeningeal angiomatosis, hypertrophy of the overlying calvarium, and congested deep cerebral veins (Fig. 2.146). Contrast administration should be always employed when evaluating a child with suspected SWS because this enables visualization of enhancement of the superficial gyri and allows assessment of the extent of leptomeningeal vascular abnormality even

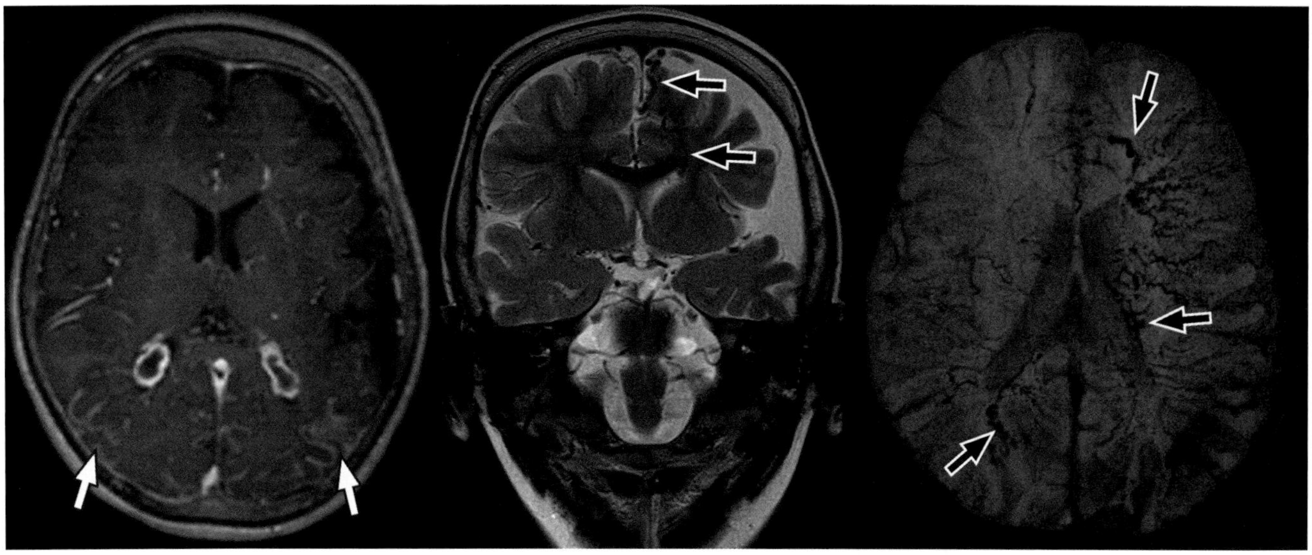

FIGURE 2.146 **Bilateral Sturge-Weber syndrome in a 4-year-old boy.** Axial postcontrast T1-weighted MR image (on the **left**) demonstrates bilateral leptomeningeal enhancement (*white arrows*). Prominent leptomeningeal vessels (*black arrows*) are shown on coronal T2-weighted MR image (in the **middle**) and axial minimum intensity projection from a susceptibility-weighted MR sequence (on the **right**).

before rest of the abnormalities become visible. MRI perfusion studies and SWI are also useful in detecting perfusion defects. Microscopically, the leptomeningeal abnormality is an angiomatosis.

Treatment includes surgical removal of the affected lobe or hemisphere when seizures are medically intractable. Seizure freedom has been seen in up to 81%.[231] Results of limited cortical resection are less dramatic, but relief from seizure activity is seen in these cases as well.

von Hippel–Lindau Disease

von Hippel–Lindau (VHL) disease or CNS angiomatosis is an autosomal dominant disorder with incomplete penetrance, characterized by retinal angiomas, cerebellar and spinal cord hemangioblastomas, renal cell carcinomas, endolymphatic sac tumors, pheochromocytomas, papillary cystadenoma of the epididymis, angiomas of the liver and kidney, and cysts of the pancreas, kidney, liver, and epididymis. The disease is caused by a defect in a tumor suppressor gene called VHL, located at chromosome 3p25-p26.

The diagnosis is established if patients have more than one hemangioblastoma of the CNS, one hemangioblastoma with a visceral manifestation of the disease, or one manifestation of the disease and a known family history. The incidence of VHL is one in every 36,000 live births, with a penetrance of 90% by age 65 years.[232] Twenty percent of patients may present with de novo mutations. Onset of clinical symptoms is usually delayed beyond the early teens, and most patients present in the third or fourth decade. However, occasionally, the disease presents earlier in adolescent patients.

Hemangioblastomas of the CNS are the most common tumor in VHL disease, affecting 60% to 80% of all patients.[233] Although considered benign, they are a major cause of morbidity. They can arise anywhere along the craniospinal axis and are often associated with edema or cysts (associated cysts occur with up to 80% of hemangioblastomas) or both.[234] CNS hemangioblastomas are most commonly seen in the spinal cord and cerebellum, followed by the brainstem, lumbosacral nerve roots, and supratentorial region. Pathologic features of hemangioblastoma are depicted on Page 25 (Spine Chapter). Other intracranial manifestations including papillary cystadenoma of the endolymphatic sac are seen in adult patients with VHL.

On CT, the typical appearance of a hemangioblastoma is a large fluid-filled cyst with an enhancing nodule in the wall. MR imaging is the modality of choice. On MRI, hemangioblastomas appear as sharply marginated cerebellar masses characterized by T2 hyperintensity and T1 hypointensity. When a solid nodule is seen within the cyst wall, it contains small flow voids within it, representing enlarged feeding and draining vessels. The presence of hemorrhage results in increased signal intensity on precontrast T1-weighted MR images. Solid portions of tumor enhance avidly following contrast administration (Fig. 2.147). Angiography may be performed prior to surgical resection to show the location and size of the arteries supplying the tumor and embolize larger vessels if feasible. On angiographic studies, hemangioblastomas are characterized by tangles of tightly packed, wide vessels that become opacified in the early arterial phase.

Visceral manifestations of VHL include cysts in various organs like the liver, pancreas, spleen, adrenal gland, and epididymis; pancreatic neuroendocrine tumors and pheochromocytomas; hepatic adenomas; and renal cell carcinomas. Therefore, complete evaluation of these patients requires imaging of the abdomen and pelvis in addition to imaging of the brain and spinal cord.

Treatment includes resection of larger, symptomatic hemangioblastomas with or without preoperative embolization. Smaller lesions (<3 cm diameter) and those not associated with cysts have been shown to respond to stereotactic radiation.

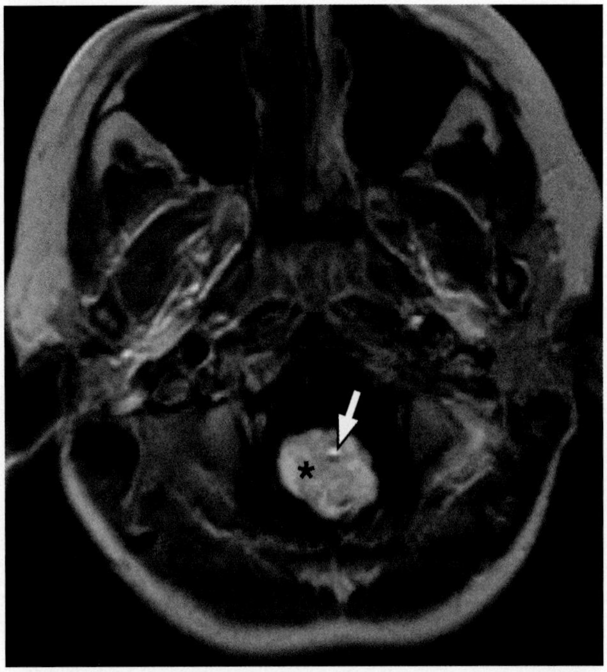

FIGURE 2.147 **Hemangioblastoma in a 6-year-old girl with von Hippel-Lindau disease.** Axial postcontrast T1-weighted MR image shows a sharply-marginated, avidly-enhancing cerebellar mass (*asterisk*) with a blood-fluid level (*white arrow*).

Other Neurocutaneous Syndromes

Other phacomatoses like ataxia telangiectasia, blue rubber bleb nevus syndrome, neurocutaneous melanosis, and incontinentia pigmenti are rare, and a discussion of these entities is beyond the scope of this chapter.

References

1. Veyrac C, Couture A, Saguintaah M, et al. Brain ultrasonography in the premature infant. *Pediatr Radiol.* 2006;36(7):626–635.
2. Yikilmaz A, Taylor GA. Cranial sonography in term and near-term infants. *Pediatr Radiol.* 2008;38(6):605–616; qiuz 718–719.
3. Daneman A, Epelman M, Blaser S, et al. Imaging of the brain in full-term neonates: does sonography still play a role? *Pediatr Radiol.* 2006;36(7):636–646.
4. Chavhan GB, Parra DA, Mann A, et al. Normal Doppler spectral waveforms of major pediatric vessels: specific patterns. *Radiographics.* 2008;28(3):691–706.
5. Spencer SS. The relative contributions of MRI, SPECT, and PET imaging in epilepsy. *Epilepsia.* 1994;35(suppl 6):S72–S89.
6. Kaufmann TJ, Kallmes DF. Diagnostic cerebral angiography: archaic and complication-prone or here to stay for another 80 years? *AJR Am J Roentgenol.* 2008;190(6):1435–1437.
7. Thiex R, Norbash AM, Frerichs KU. The safety of dedicated-team catheter-based diagnostic cerebral angiography in the era of advanced noninvasive imaging. *AJNR Am J Neuroradiol.* 2010;31(2):230–234.
8. Barkovich AJ, Guerrini R, Kuzniecky RI, et al. A developmental and genetic classification for malformations of cortical development: update 2012. *Brain.* 2012;135(pt 5):1348–1369.
9. Koenig SH, Brown RD III, Spiller M, et al. Relaxometry of brain: why white matter appears bright in MRI. *Magn Reson Med.* 1990;14(3):482–495.
10. Barkovich AJ, Koch TK, Carrol CL. The spectrum of lissencephaly: report of ten patients analyzed by magnetic resonance imaging. *Ann Neurol.* 1991;30(2):139–146.
11. Leventer RJ, Jansen A, Pilz DT, et al. Clinical and imaging heterogeneity of polymicrogyria: a study of 328 patients. *Brain.* 2010;133(pt 5):1415–1427.
12. Barkovich AJ, Norman D. MR imaging of schizencephaly. *AJR Am J Roentgenol.* 1988;150(6):1391–1396.
13. Tinkle BT, Schorry EK, Franz DN, et al. Epidemiology of hemimegalencephaly: a case series and review. *Am J Med Genet A.* 2005;139(3):204–211.
14. Parrini E, Ramazzotti A, Dobyns WB, et al. Periventricular heterotopia: phenotypic heterogeneity and correlation with Filamin A mutations. *Brain.* 2006;129(pt 7):1892–1906.
15. Blumcke I, Thom M, Aronica E, et al. The clinicopathologic spectrum of focal cortical dysplasias: a consensus classification proposed by an ad hoc Task Force of the ILAE Diagnostic Methods Commission. *Epilepsia.* 2011;52(1):158–174.
16. Colombo N, Tassi L, Galli C, et al. Focal cortical dysplasias: MR imaging, histopathologic, and clinical correlations in surgically treated patients with epilepsy. *AJNR Am J Neuroradiol.* 2003;24(4):724–733.
17. Schell-Apacik CC, Wagner K, Bihler M, et al. Agenesis and dysgenesis of the corpus callosum: clinical, genetic and neuroimaging findings in a series of 41 patients. *Am J Med Genet A.* 2008;146A(19):2501–2511.
18. Dubourg C, Lazaro L, Blayau M, et al. Genetic study of holoprosencephaly. *Ann Biol Clin (Paris).* 2003;61(6):679–687.
19. Dubourg C, Lazaro L, Pasquier L, et al. Molecular screening of SHH, ZIC2, SIX3, and TGIF genes in patients with features of holoprosencephaly spectrum: mutation review and genotype-phenotype correlations. *Hum Mutat.* 2004;24(1):43–51.
20. Morishima A, Aranoff GS. Syndrome of septo-optic-pituitary dysplasia: the clinical spectrum. *Brain Dev.* 1986;8(3):233–239.
21. Patel L, McNally RJ, Harrison E, et al. Geographical distribution of optic nerve hypoplasia and septo-optic dysplasia in Northwest England. *J Pediatr.* 2006;148(1):85–88.
22. McNay DE, Turton JP, Kelberman D, et al. HESX1 mutations are an uncommon cause of septooptic dysplasia and hypopituitarism. *J Clin Endocrinol Metab.* 2007;92(2):691–697.
23. Miller E, Widjaja E, Blaser S, et al. The old and the new: supratentorial MR findings in Chiari II malformation. *Childs Nerv Syst.* 2008;24(5):563–575.
24. Loddenkemper T, Morris HH III, Diehl B, et al. Intracranial lipomas and epilepsy. *J Neurol.* 2006;253(5):590–593.
25. Yilmaz N, Unal O, Kiymaz N, et al. Intracranial lipomas—a clinical study. *Clin Neurol Neurosurg.* 2006;108(4):363–368.
26. Lindquist JM, Plotkin SA, Shaw L, et al. Congenital rubella syndrome as a systemic infection. Studies of affected infants born in Philadelphia, U.S.A. *Br Med J.* 1965;2(5475):1401–1406.
27. Friedmann I, Wright MI. Histopathological changes in the foetal and infantile inner ear caused by maternal rubella. *Br Med J.* 1966;2(5504):20–23.
28. McLean HQ, Fiebelkorn AP, Temte JL, et al. Prevention of measles, rubella, congenital rubella syndrome, and mumps, 2013: summary recommendations of the Advisory Committee on Immunization Practices (ACIP). *MMWR Recomm Rep.* 2013;62(RR-04):1–34.
29. Vachha B, Rojas R, Prabhu SP, et al. Magnetic resonance imaging in viral and prion diseases of the central nervous system. *Top Magn Reson Imaging.* 2014;23(5):293–302.

30. Manicklal S, Emery VC, Lazzarotto T, et al. The "silent" global burden of congenital cytomegalovirus. *Clin Microbiol Rev.* 2013;26(1):86–102.
31. Obeid M, Franklin J, Shrestha S, et al. Diffusion-weighted imaging findings on MRI as the sole radiographic findings in a child with proven herpes simplex encephalitis. *Pediatr Radiol.* 2007;37(11):1159–1162.
32. Joffe AR. Lumbar puncture and brain herniation in acute bacterial meningitis: a review. *J Intensive Care Med.* 2007;22(4): 194–207.
33. Prabhu SP, Young-Poussaint T. Pediatric central nervous system emergencies. *Neuroimaging Clin N Am.* 2010;20(4):663–683.
34. Buxi TB, Sud S, Vohra R. CT and MRI in the diagnosis of tuberculosis. *Indian J Pediatr.* 2002;69(11):965–972.
35. Omar N, Andronikou S, van Toorn R, et al. Diffusion-weighted magnetic resonance imaging of borderzone necrosis in paediatric tuberculous meningitis. *J Med Imaging Radiat Oncol.* 2011; 55(6):563–570.
36. Andronikou S, Smith B, Hatherhill M, et al. Definitive neuroradiological diagnostic features of tuberculous meningitis in children. *Pediatr Radiol.* 2004;34(11):876–885.
37. Bargallo J, Berenguer J, Garcia-Barrionuevo J, et al. The "target sign": is it a specific sign of CNS tuberculoma? *Neuroradiology.* 1996;38(6):547–550.
38. Kim TK, Chang KH, Kim CJ, et al. Intracranial tuberculoma: comparison of MR with pathologic findings. *AJNR Am J Neuroradiol.* 1995;16(9):1903–1908.
39. Verma R, Gupta R. Multiple ring-enhancing lesions: diagnostic dilemma between neurocysticercosis and tuberculoma. *BMJ Case Rep.* 2014 Apr 7;2014. pii: bcr2013202528. doi: 10.1136/bcr-2013-202528
40. Bhuva P, Nathan B. Subdural empyema. In: Vincent J-L, Hall J, eds. *Encyclopedia of Intensive Care Medicine.* Berlin, Heidelberg: Springer; 2012:2166–2168.
41. Gurney J, Smith M, Bunin G. CNS and miscellaneous intracranial and intraspinal neoplasms. In: Ries LA, Smith M, Gurney J, eds. *Cancer Incidence and Survival Among Children and Adolescents: United States SEER Program 1975–1995 NIH Publication No 99-4649.* Philadelphia, PA: National Cancer Institute SEER Program; 1999:51–63.
42. Ostrom QT, Gittleman H, Fulop J, et al. CBTRUS statistical report: primary brain and central nervous system tumors diagnosed in the United States in 2008–2012. *Neuro Oncol.* 2015;17(suppl 4):iv1–iv62. doi:10.1093/neuonc/nov189.
43. Walker DA. *Brain and Spinal Tumors of Childhood.* London, UK: Arnold; 2004, xx:531. 8 p. of plates p; Distributed in the U.S.A. by Oxford University Press.
44. Broniscer A, Gajjar A. Supratentorial high-grade astrocytoma and diffuse brainstem glioma: two challenges for the pediatric oncologist. *Oncologist.* 2004;9(2):197–206.
45. Fuller GN. The WHO classification of tumours of the central nervous system, 4th edition. *Arch Pathol Lab Med.* 2008;132(6):906.
46. Orkin SH, Nathan DG. *Nathan and Oski's Hematology of Infancy and Childhood.* 7th ed. Philadelphia, PA: Saunders/Elsevier; 2009, xxvi:1841.
47. Dolecek TA, Propp JM, Stroup NE, et al. CBTRUS statistical report: primary brain and central nervous system tumors diagnosed in the United States in 2005–2009. *Neuro Oncol.* 2012; 14 (suppl 5):v1–v49.
48. Paldino MJ, Faerber EN, Poussaint TY. Imaging tumors of the pediatric central nervous system. *Radiol Clin North Am.* 2011; 49(4):589–616, v.
49. Behdad A, Perry A. Central nervous system primitive neuroectodermal tumors: a clinicopathologic and genetic study of 33 cases. *Brain Pathol.* 2010;20(2):441–450.
50. Onguru O, Celasun B, Gunhan O. Desmoplastic non-infantile ganglioglioma. *Neuropathology.* 2005;25(2):150–152.
51. Takahashi A, Hong SC, Seo DW, et al. Frequent association of cortical dysplasia in dysembryoplastic neuroepithelial tumor treated by epilepsy surgery. *Surg Neurol.* 2005;64(5):419–427.
52. Bilginer B, Yalnizoglu D, Soylemezoglu F, et al. Surgery for epilepsy in children with dysembryoplastic neuroepithelial tumor: clinical spectrum, seizure outcome, neuroradiology, and pathology. *Childs Nerv Syst.* 2009;25(4):485–491.
53. Patel DM, Schmidt RF, Liu JK. Update on the diagnosis, pathogenesis, and treatment strategies for central neurocytoma. *J Clin Neurosci.* 2013;20(9):1193–1199.
54. Hassoun J, Soylemezoglu F, Gambarelli D, et al. Central neurocytoma: a synopsis of clinical and histological features. *Brain Pathol.* 1993;3(3):297–306.
55. Burkhard C, Di Patre PL, Schuler D, et al. A population-based study of the incidence and survival rates in patients with pilocytic astrocytoma. *J Neurosurg.* 2003;98(6):1170–1174.
56. von Deimling A, Krone W, Menon AG. Neurofibromatosis type 1: pathology, clinical features and molecular genetics. *Brain Pathol.* 1995;5(2):153–162.
57. Chang BC, Mirabella G, Yagev R, et al. Screening and diagnosis of optic pathway gliomas in children with neurofibromatosis type 1 by using sweep visual evoked potentials. *Invest Ophthalmol Vis Sci.* 2007;48(6):2895–2902.
58. Ostrom QT, Gittleman H, Farah P, et al. CBTRUS statistical report: primary brain and central nervous system tumors diagnosed in the United States in 2006–2010. *Neuro Oncol.* 2013;15 (suppl 2):ii1–ii56.
59. Molla E, Marti-Bonmati L, Revert A, et al. Craniopharyngiomas: identification of different semiological patterns with MRI. *Eur Radiol.* 2002;12(7):1829–1836.
60. Larkin SJ, Ansorge O. Pathology and pathogenesis of craniopharyngiomas. *Pituitary.* 2013;16(1):9–17.
61. Fitz CR, Wortzman G, Harwood-Nash DC, et al. Computed tomography in craniopharyngiomas. *Radiology.* 1978;127(3): 687–691.
62. Ahmadi J, Destian S, Apuzzo ML, et al. Cystic fluid in craniopharyngiomas: MR imaging and quantitative analysis. *Radiology.* 1992;182(3):783–785.
63. Zacharia BE, Bruce SS, Goldstein H, et al. Incidence, treatment and survival of patients with craniopharyngioma in the surveillance, epidemiology and end results program. *Neuro Oncol.* 2012;14(8):1070–1078.
64. Kane LA, Leinung MC, Scheithauer BW, et al. Pituitary adenomas in childhood and adolescence. *J Clin Endocrinol Metab.* 1994;79(4):1135–1140.
65. Zada G, Kelly DF, Cohan P, et al. Endonasal transsphenoidal approach for pituitary adenomas and other sellar lesions: an assessment of efficacy, safety, and patient impressions. *J Neurosurg.* 2003;98(2):350–358.
66. Herrick MK, Rubinstein LJ. The cytological differentiating potential of pineal parenchymal neoplasms (true pinealomas). A clinicopathological study of 28 tumours. *Brain.* 1979;102(2):289–320.
67. Hirato J, Nakazato Y. Pathology of pineal region tumors. *J Neurooncol.* 2001;54(3):239–249.
68. Sung DI, Harisiadis L, Chang CH. Midline pineal tumors and suprasellar germinomas: highly curable by irradiation. *Radiology.* 1978;128(3):745–751.

69. Mufti ST, Jamal A. Primary intracranial germ cell tumors. *Asian J Neurosurg.* 2012;7(4):197–202.
70. Lee D, Suh YL. Histologically confirmed intracranial germ cell tumors; an analysis of 62 patients in a single institute. *Virchows Arch.* 2010;457(3):347–357.
71. Shibamoto Y, Sasai K, Oya N, et al. Intracranial germinoma: radiation therapy with tumor volume-based dose selection. *Radiology.* 2001;218(2):452–456.
72. Robertson PL, DaRosso RC, Allen JC. Improved prognosis of intracranial non-germinoma germ cell tumors with multimodality therapy. *J Neurooncol.* 1997;32(1):71–80.
73. Matsutani M; Japanese Pediatric Brain Tumor Study G. Combined chemotherapy and radiation therapy for CNS germ cell tumors—the Japanese experience. *J Neurooncol.* 2001;54(3):311–316.
74. Louis DN, Ohgaki H, Wiestler OD, Cavenee WK. World Health Organization Histological Classification of Tumours of the Central Nervous System. Lyon, France: International Agency for Research on Cancer; 2016.
75. Osborn AG, Salzman KL, Thurnher MM, et al. The new World Health Organization Classification of Central Nervous System Tumors: what can the neuroradiologist really say? *AJNR Am J Neuroradiol.* 2012;33(5):795–802.
76. Raisanen JM, Davis RL. Congenital brain tumors. *Pathology (Phila).* 1993;2(1):103–116.
77. Packer RJ, Cogen P, Vezina G, et al. Medulloblastoma: clinical and biologic aspects. *Neuro Oncol.* 1999;1(3):232–250.
78. Buhring U, Strayle-Batra M, Freudenstein D, et al. MRI features of primary, secondary and metastatic medulloblastoma. *Eur Radiol.* 2002;12(6):1342–1348.
79. Fisher PG, Burger PC, Eberhart CG. Biologic risk stratification of medulloblastoma: the real time is now. *J Clin Oncol.* 2004; 22(6):971–974.
80. Taylor MD, Northcott PA, Korshunov A, et al. Molecular subgroups of medulloblastoma: the current consensus. *Acta Neuropathol.* 2012;123(4):465–472.
81. Paulino AC, Wen BC, Buatti JM, et al. Intracranial ependymomas: an analysis of prognostic factors and patterns of failure. *Am J Clin Oncol.* 2002;25(2):117–122.
82. Salazar OM, Castro-Vita H, VanHoutte P, et al. Improved survival in cases of intracranial ependymoma after radiation therapy. Late report and recommendations. *J Neurosurg.* 1983; 59(4):652–659.
83. Qian X, Goumnerova LC, De Girolami U, et al. Cerebrospinal fluid cytology in patients with ependymoma: a bi-institutional retrospective study. *Cancer.* 2008;114(5):307–314.
84. Rorke LB, Packer R, Biegel J. Central nervous system atypical teratoid/rhabdoid tumors of infancy and childhood. *J Neurooncol.* 1995;24(1):21–28.
85. Meyers SP, Khademian ZP, Biegel JA, et al. Primary intracranial atypical teratoid/rhabdoid tumors of infancy and childhood: MRI features and patient outcomes. *AJNR Am J Neuroradiol.* 2006;27(5):962–971.
86. Biegel JA. Molecular genetics of atypical teratoid/rhabdoid tumor. *Neurosurg Focus.* 2006;20(1):E11.
87. Chi SN, Zimmerman MA, Yao X, et al. Intensive multimodality treatment for children with newly diagnosed CNS atypical teratoid rhabdoid tumor. *J Clin Oncol.* 2009;27(3):385–389.
88. Jordaan MR, Prabhu SP, Silvera VM. Primary leptomeningeal central nervous system lymphoma in an immunocompetent adolescent: an unusual presentation. *Pediatr Radiol.* 2010;40 (suppl 1):S141–S144.
89. Hesselink JR, Dowd CF, Healy ME, et al. MR imaging of brain contusions: a comparative study with CT. *AJR Am J Roentgenol.* 1988;150(5):1133–1142.
90. Tong K, Holshouser B, Wu Z. *Traumatic Brain Injury. Susceptibility Weighted Imaging in MRI.* Hoboken, New Jersey: John Wiley & Sons, Inc.; 2011:171–190.
91. Kim KA, Wang MY, Griffith PM, et al. Analysis of pediatric head injury from falls. *Neurosurg Focus.* 2000;8(1):e3.
92. Merten DF, Osborne DR, Radkowski MA, et al. Craniocerebral trauma in the child abuse syndrome: radiological observations. *Pediatr Radiol.* 1984;14(5):272–277.
93. Rocchi G, Caroli E, Raco A, et al. Traumatic epidural hematoma in children. *J Child Neurol.* 2005;20(7):569–572.
94. Bullock MR, Chesnut R, Ghajar J, et al. Surgical management of acute epidural hematomas. *Neurosurgery.* 2006;58(3 suppl): S7–S15; discussion Si–Siv.
95. Lee EJ, Hung YC, Wang LC, et al. Factors influencing the functional outcome of patients with acute epidural hematomas: analysis of 200 patients undergoing surgery. *J Trauma.* 1998;45(5):946–952.
96. Reece RM, Sege R. Childhood head injuries: accidental or inflicted? *Arch Pediatr Adolesc Med.* 2000;154(1):11–15.
97. Hobbs C, Childs AM, Wynne J, et al. Subdural haematoma and effusion in infancy: an epidemiological study. *Arch Dis Child.* 2005;90(9):952–955.
98. Squier W, Mack J. The neuropathology of infant subdural haemorrhage. *Forensic Sci Int.* 2009;187(1–3):6–13.
99. Kneyber MC, Rinkel GJ, Ramos LM, et al. Early posttraumatic subarachnoid hemorrhage due to dissecting aneurysms in three children. *Neurology.* 2005;65(10):1663–1665.
100. Meyer-Heim AD, Boltshauser E. Spontaneous intracranial haemorrhage in children: aetiology, presentation and outcome. *Brain Dev.* 2003;25(6):416–421.
101. Piteau SJ, Ward MG, Barrowman NJ, et al. Clinical and radiographic characteristics associated with abusive and nonabusive head trauma: a systematic review. *Pediatrics.* 2012;130(2):315–323.
102. Kemp AM, Jaspan T, Griffiths J, et al. Neuroimaging: what neuroradiological features distinguish abusive from non-abusive head trauma? A systematic review. *Arch Dis Child.* 2011; 96(12):1103–1112.
103. Perry JJ, Stiell IG, Sivilotti ML, et al. Sensitivity of computed tomography performed within six hours of onset of headache for diagnosis of subarachnoid haemorrhage: prospective cohort study. *BMJ.* 2011;343:d4277.
104. Byyny RL, Mower WR, Shum N, et al. Sensitivity of noncontrast cranial computed tomography for the emergency department diagnosis of subarachnoid hemorrhage. *Ann Emerg Med.* 2008;51(6):697–703.
105. Duhaime AC, Gennarelli TA, Thibault LE, et al. The shaken baby syndrome. A clinical, pathological, and biomechanical study. *J Neurosurg.* 1987;66(3):409–415.
106. Ryan ME, Palasis S, Saigal G, et al. ACR appropriateness criteria head trauma—child. *J Am Coll Radiol.* 2014;11(10):939–947.
107. Becker JC, Liersch R, Tautz C, et al. Shaken baby syndrome: report on four pairs of twins. *Child Abuse Negl.* 1998; 22(9):931–937.
108. Prabhu SP, Newton AW, Perez-Rossello JM, et al. Three-dimensional skull models as a problem-solving tool in suspected child abuse. *Pediatr Radiol.* 2013;43(5):575–581.
109. Datta S, Stoodley N, Jayawant S, et al. Neuroradiological aspects of subdural haemorrhages. *Arch Dis Child.* 2005;90(9):947–951.

110. Kemp AM, Rajaram S, Mann M, et al. What neuroimaging should be performed in children in whom inflicted brain injury (iBI) is suspected? A systematic review. *Clin Radiol.* 2009; 64(5):473–483.
111. Hunter JV, Wilde EA, Tong KA, et al. Emerging imaging tools for use with traumatic brain injury research. *J Neurotrauma.* 2012;29(4):654–671.
112. Ashwal S, Babikian T, Gardner-Nichols J, et al. Susceptibility-weighted imaging and proton magnetic resonance spectroscopy in assessment of outcome after pediatric traumatic brain injury. *Arch Phys Med Rehabil.* 2006;87(12 suppl 2): S50–S58.
113. Hunter JV, Thornton RJ, Wang ZJ, et al. Late proton MR spectroscopy in children after traumatic brain injury: correlation with cognitive outcomes. *AJNR Am J Neuroradiol.* 2005; 26(3):482–488.
114. Garza-Mercado R, Cavazos E, Tamez-Montes D. Cerebral arteriovenous malformations in children and adolescents. *Surg Neurol.* 1987;27(2):131–140.
115. Brown RD Jr, Wiebers DO, Forbes G, et al. The natural history of unruptured intracranial arteriovenous malformations. *J Neurosurg.* 1988;68(3):352–357.
116. Wilkins RH. Natural history of intracranial vascular malformations: a review. *Neurosurgery.* 1985;16(3):421–430.
117. Rigamonti D, Hadley MN, Drayer BP, et al. Cerebral cavernous malformations. Incidence and familial occurrence. *N Engl J Med.* 1988;319(6):343–347.
118. Otten P, Pizzolato GP, Rilliet B, et al. 131 cases of cavernous angioma (cavernomas) of the CNS, discovered by retrospective analysis of 24,535 autopsies. *Neurochirurgie.* 1989;35(2):82–83, 128–131.
119. Al-Holou WN, O'Lynnger TM, Pandey AS, et al. Natural history and imaging prevalence of cavernous malformations in children and young adults. *J Neurosurg Pediatr.* 2012;9(2): 198–205.
120. Bhardwaj RD, Auguste KI, Kulkarni AV, et al. Management of pediatric brainstem cavernous malformations: experience over 20 years at the hospital for sick children. *J Neurosurg Pediatr.* 2009;4(5):458–464.
121. Scott RM, Barnes P, Kupsky W, et al. Cavernous angiomas of the central nervous system in children. *J Neurosurg.* 1992;76(1): 38–46.
122. Lasjaunias PL, Chng SM, Sachet M, et al. The management of vein of Galen aneurysmal malformations. *Neurosurgery.* 2006; 59(5 suppl 3):S184–S194; discussion S3–S13.
123. Lasjaunias P, Terbrugge K, Piske R, et al. Dilatation of the vein of Galen. Anatomoclinical forms and endovascular treatment apropos of 14 cases explored and/or treated between 1983 and 1986. *Neurochirurgie.* 1987;33(4):315–333.
124. Gupta AK, Varma DR. Vein of Galen malformations: review. *Neurol India.* 2004;52(1):43–53.
125. Jordan LC, Johnston SC, Wu YW, et al. The importance of cerebral aneurysms in childhood hemorrhagic stroke: a population-based study. *Stroke.* 2009;40(2):400–405.
126. Aeron G, Abruzzo TA, Jones BV. Clinical and imaging features of intracranial arterial aneurysms in the pediatric population. *Radiographics.* 2012;32(3):667–681.
127. Prabhu SP, Grant PE, Robertson RL, et al. Neonatal neuroimaging. In: Gleason CA, Devaskar SU, Avery ME, eds. *Avery's Diseases of the Newborn.* 9th ed. Philadelphia, PA: Elsevier/Saunders; 2012, xx:1498.
128. Barkovich AJ, Raybaud C. *Pediatric Neuroimaging.* Philadelphia, PA: Wolters Kluwer Health/Lippincott Williams & Wilkins; 2012. Available from http://ovidsp.ovid.com/ovidweb.cgi?T=JS&CSC=Y&NEWS=N&PAGE=booktext&D=books3&AN=01438880
129. Volpe JJ. *Neurology of the Newborn.* Philadelphia, PA: Saunders/Elsevier; 2008. Available from http://www.clinicalkey.com/dura/browse/bookChapter/3-s2.0-B9781416039952X1000X
130. Rodrigues K, Grant PE. Diffusion-weighted imaging in neonates. *Neuroimaging Clin N Am.* 2011;21(1):127–151, viii.
131. Takeoka M, Soman TB, Yoshii A, et al. Diffusion-weighted images in neonatal cerebral hypoxic-ischemic injury. *Pediatr Neurol.* 2002;26(4):274–281.
132. Jones BP, Ganesan V, Saunders DE, et al. Imaging in childhood arterial ischaemic stroke. *Neuroradiology.* 2010;52(6):577–589.
133. Amlie-Lefond C, Bernard TJ, Sebire G, et al. Predictors of cerebral arteriopathy in children with arterial ischemic stroke: results of the International Pediatric Stroke Study. *Circulation.* 2009;119(10):1417–1423.
134. Ullrich NJ, Robertson R, Kinnamon DD, et al. Moyamoya following cranial irradiation for primary brain tumors in children. *Neurology.* 2007;68(12):932–938.
135. See AP, Ropper AE, Underberg DL, et al. Down syndrome and moyamoya: clinical presentation and surgical management. *J Neurosurg Pediatr.* 2015;16(1):58–63.
136. Mori N, Mugikura S, Higano S, et al. The leptomeningeal "ivy sign" on fluid-attenuated inversion recovery MR imaging in Moyamoya disease: a sign of decreased cerebral vascular reserve? *AJNR Am J Neuroradiol.* 2009;30(5):930–935.
137. Yamada I, Himeno Y, Nagaoka T, et al. Moyamoya disease: evaluation with diffusion-weighted and perfusion echo-planar MR imaging. *Radiology.* 1999;212(2):340–347.
138. Wang R, Yu S, Alger JR, et al. Multi-delay arterial spin labeling perfusion MRI in moyamoya disease—comparison with CT perfusion imaging. *Eur Radiol.* 2014;24(5):1135–1144.
139. Noguchi T, Kawashima M, Nishihara M, et al. Arterial spin-labeling MR imaging in Moyamoya disease compared with clinical assessments and other MR imaging findings. *Eur J Radiol.* 2013;82(12):e840–e847.
140. Dion J, Bachmeyer C, Favrole P, et al. Moya-moya in an adult with sickle cell anemia. *Presse Med.* 2011;40(4 pt 1):450–451.
141. Smith ER, McClain CD, Heeney M, et al. Pial synangiosis in patients with moyamoya syndrome and sickle cell anemia: perioperative management and surgical outcome. *Neurosurg Focus.* 2009;26(4):E10.
142. Mackay MT, Prabhu SP, Coleman L. Childhood posterior circulation arterial ischemic stroke. *Stroke.* 2010;41(10): 2201–2209.
143. Schievink WI, Mokri B, Piepgras DG, et al. Recurrent spontaneous arterial dissections: risk in familial versus nonfamilial disease. *Stroke.* 1996;27(4):622–624.
144. Provenzale JM. MRI and MRA for evaluation of dissection of craniocerebral arteries: lessons from the medical literature. *Emerg Radiol.* 2009;16(3):185–93.
145. Khan R, Smith JK, Castillo M. False-negative contrast MRA in the setting of carotid artery dissection. *Emerg Radiol.* 2002;9(6):320–322.
146. deVeber G, Andrew M, Adams C, et al. Cerebral sinovenous thrombosis in children. *N Engl J Med.* 2001;345(6):417–423.
147. Ibrahim SH. Cerebral venous sinus thrombosis in neonates. *J Pak Med Assoc.* 2006;56(11):535–537.

148. Brouwer MJ, de Vries LS, Pistorius L, et al. Ultrasound measurements of the lateral ventricles in neonates: why, how and when? A systematic review. *Acta Paediatr.* 2010;99(9): 1298–1306.
149. El-Dib M, Massaro AN, Bulas D, et al. Neuroimaging and neurodevelopmental outcome of premature infants. *Am J Perinatol.* 2010;27(10):803–818.
150. Robinson S. Neonatal posthemorrhagic hydrocephalus from prematurity: pathophysiology and current treatment concepts. *J Neurosurg Pediatr.* 2012;9(3):242–258.
151. Miller JH, Walkiewicz T, Towbin RB, et al. Improved delineation of ventricular shunt catheters using fast steady-state gradient recalled-echo sequences in a rapid brain MR imaging protocol in nonsedated pediatric patients. *AJNR Am J Neuroradiol.* 2010;31(3):430–435.
152. Poretti A, Blaser SI, Lequin MH, et al. Neonatal neuroimaging findings in inborn errors of metabolism. *J Magn Reson Imaging.* 2013;37(2):294–312.
153. Knaap MS, Valk J. *Magnetic Resonance of Myelination and Myelin Disorders*. Berlin, Heidelberg: Springer-Verlag; 2005. SpringerLink (Online Service). Available from http://dx.doi.org/10.1007/3-540-27660-2
154. Yang E, Prabhu SP. Imaging manifestations of the leukodystrophies, inherited disorders of white matter. *Radiol Clin North Am.* 2014;52(2):279–319.
155. Osborn AG. *Osborn's Brain: Imaging, Pathology, and Anatomy*. 1st ed. Salt Lake City, UT: Amirsys Publishing; 2013, xi:1272.
156. Awasthi R, Gupta RK, Trivedi R, et al. Diffusion tensor MR imaging in children with pantothenate kinase-associated neurodegeneration with brain iron accumulation and their siblings. *AJNR Am J Neuroradiol.* 2010;31(3):442–427.
157. Faerber EN, Grover WD, DeFilipp GJ, et al. Cerebral MR of Menkes kinky-hair disease. *AJNR Am J Neuroradiol.* 1989; 10(1):190–192.
158. Harcke HT Jr, Capitanio MA, Grover WD, et al. Bladder diverticula and Menkes' syndrome. *Radiology.* 1977;124(2): 459–461.
159. Trocello JM, Woimant F, El Balkhi S, et al. Extensive striatal, cortical, and white matter brain MRI abnormalities in Wilson disease. *Neurology.* 2013;81(17):1557.
160. Page RA, Davie CA, MacManus D, et al. Clinical correlation of brain MRI and MRS abnormalities in patients with Wilson disease. *Neurology.* 2004;63(4):638–643.
161. Shivakumar R, Thomas SV. Teaching neuroimages: face of the giant panda and her cub: MRI correlates of Wilson disease. *Neurology.* 2009;72(11):e50.
162. Engelbrecht V, Schlaug G, Hefter H, et al. MRI of the brain in Wilson disease: T2 signal loss under therapy. *J Comput Assist Tomogr.* 1995;19(4):635–638.
163. Mole SE. Neuronal ceroid lipofuscinoses (NCL). *Eur J Paediatr Neurol.* 2006;10(5–6):255–257.
164. Vanhanen SL, Raininko R, Autti T, et al. MRI evaluation of the brain in infantile neuronal ceroid-lipofuscinosis. Part 2: MRI findings in 21 patients. *J Child Neurol.* 1995;10(6):444–450.
165. Vanhanen SL, Raininko R, Santavuori P, et al. MRI evaluation of the brain in infantile neuronal ceroid-lipofuscinosis. Part 1: postmortem MRI with histopathologic correlation. *J Child Neurol.* 1995;10(6):438–443.
166. Akbarian S. The neurobiology of Rett syndrome. *Neuroscientist.* 2003;9(1):57–63.
167. Carter JC, Lanham DC, Pham D, et al. Selective cerebral volume reduction in Rett syndrome: a multiple-approach MR imaging study. *AJNR Am J Neuroradiol.* 2008;29(3):436–441.
168. Mahmood A, Bibat G, Zhan AL, et al. White matter impairment in Rett syndrome: diffusion tensor imaging study with clinical correlations. *AJNR Am J Neuroradiol.* 2010;31(2):295–299.
169. Ito R, Melhem ER, Mori S, et al. Diffusion tensor brain MR imaging in X-linked cerebral adrenoleukodystrophy. *Neurology.* 2001;56(4):544–547.
170. Groeschel S, Kehrer C, Engel C, et al. Metachromatic leukodystrophy: natural course of cerebral MRI changes in relation to clinical course. *J Inherit Metab Dis.* 2011;34(5):1095–1102.
171. Maia AC, Jr., da Rocha AJ, da Silva CJ, et al. Multiple cranial nerve enhancement: a new MR imaging finding in metachromatic leukodystrophy. *AJNR Am J Neuroradiol.* 2007;28(6):999.
172. Suzuki K, Suzuki Y. Globoid cell leucodystrophy (Krabbe's disease): deficiency of galactocerebroside beta-galactosidase. *Proc Natl Acad Sci U S A.* 1970;66(2):302–309.
173. Livingston JH, Graziano C, Pysden K, et al. Intracranial calcification in early infantile Krabbe disease: nothing new under the sun. *Dev Med Child Neurol.* 2012;54(4):376–379.
174. Escolar ML, Poe MD, Smith JK, et al. Diffusion tensor imaging detects abnormalities in the corticospinal tracts of neonates with infantile Krabbe disease. *AJNR Am J Neuroradiol.* 2009; 30(5):1017–1021.
175. Bernal OG, Lenn N. Multiple cranial nerve enhancement in early infantile Krabbe's disease. *Neurology.* 2000;54(12): 2348–2349.
176. Jones BV, Barron TF, Towfighi J. Optic nerve enlargement in Krabbe's disease. *AJNR Am J Neuroradiol.* 1999;20(7): 1228–1231.
177. Vasconcellos E, Smith M. MRI nerve root enhancement in Krabbe disease. *Pediatr Neurol.* 1998;19(2):151–152.
178. Barkovich AJ. Concepts of myelin and myelination in neuroradiology. *AJNR Am J Neuroradiol.* 2000;21(6):1099–1109.
179. Schiffmann R, van der Knaap MS. Invited article: an MRI-based approach to the diagnosis of white matter disorders. *Neurology.* 2009;72(8):750–759.
180. van der Knaap MS, Breiter SN, Naidu S, et al. Defining and categorizing leukoencephalopathies of unknown origin: MR imaging approach. *Radiology.* 1999;213(1):121–133.
181. Woodward KJ. The molecular and cellular defects underlying Pelizaeus-Merzbacher disease. *Expert Rev Mol Med.* 2008;10:e14.
182. van der Knaap MS, Naidu S, Pouwels PJ, et al. New syndrome characterized by hypomyelination with atrophy of the basal ganglia and cerebellum. *AJNR Am J Neuroradiol.* 2002;23(9): 1466–1474.
183. Dekaban AS, Constantopoulos G. Mucopolysaccharidosis type I, II, IIIA and V. Pathological and biochemical abnormalities in the neural and mesenchymal elements of the brain. *Acta Neuropathol.* 1977;39(1):1–7.
184. Azevedo AC, Artigalas O, Vedolin L, et al. Brain magnetic resonance imaging findings in patients with mucopolysaccharidosis VI. *J Inherit Metab Dis.* 2013;36(2):357–362.
185. Manara R, Priante E, Grimaldi M, et al. Brain and spine MRI features of Hunter disease: frequency, natural evolution and response to therapy. *J Inherit Metab Dis.* 2011;34(3):763–780.
186. Matheus MG, Castillo M, Smith JK, et al. Brain MRI findings in patients with mucopolysaccharidosis types I and II and mild clinical presentation. *Neuroradiology.* 2004;46(8):666–672.

187. Fan Z, Styner M, Muenzer J, et al. Correlation of automated volumetric analysis of brain MR imaging with cognitive impairment in a natural history study of mucopolysaccharidosis II. *AJNR Am J Neuroradiol.* 2010;31(7):1319–1323.
188. McAdams HP, Geyer CA, Done SL, et al. CT and MR imaging of Canavan disease. *AJNR Am J Neuroradiol.* 1990;11(2):397–399.
189. Janson CG, McPhee SW, Francis J, et al. Natural history of Canavan disease revealed by proton magnetic resonance spectroscopy (1H-MRS) and diffusion-weighted MRI. *Neuropediatrics.* 2006;37(4):209–221.
190. Grodd W, Krageloh-Mann I, Klose U, et al. Metabolic and destructive brain disorders in children: findings with localized proton MR spectroscopy. *Radiology.* 1991;181(1):173–181.
191. Hagemann TL, Connor JX, Messing A. Alexander disease-associated glial fibrillary acidic protein mutations in mice induce Rosenthal fiber formation and a white matter stress response. *J Neurosci.* 2006;26(43):11162–11173.
192. Hsiao VC, Tian R, Long H, et al. Alexander-disease mutation of GFAP causes filament disorganization and decreased solubility of GFAP. *J Cell Sci.* 2005;118(pt 9):2057–2065.
193. Srivastava S, Naidu S. Alexander Disease. 2002 Nov 15 [Updated 2015 Jan 8]. In: Pagon RA, Adam MP, Ardinger HH, et al., editors. GeneReviews® [Internet]. Seattle (WA): University of Washington, Seattle; 1993–2017.
194. Li R, Johnson AB, Salomons G, et al. Glial fibrillary acidic protein mutations in infantile, juvenile, and adult forms of Alexander disease. *Ann Neurol.* 2005;57(3):310–326.
195. van der Knaap MS, Naidu S, Breiter SN, et al. Alexander disease: diagnosis with MR imaging. *AJNR Am J Neuroradiol.* 2001;22(3):541–552.
196. van der Knaap MS, Ramesh V, Schiffmann R, et al. Alexander disease: ventricular garlands and abnormalities of the medulla and spinal cord. *Neurology.* 2006;66(4):494–498.
197. Stumpf E, Masson H, Duquette A, et al. Adult Alexander disease with autosomal dominant transmission: a distinct entity caused by mutation in the glial fibrillary acid protein gene. *Arch Neurol.* 2003;60(9):1307–1312.
198. Saneto RP, Friedman SD, Shaw DW. Neuroimaging of mitochondrial disease. *Mitochondrion.* 2008;8(5–6):396–413.
199. Matthews PM, Tampieri D, Berkovic SF, et al. Magnetic resonance imaging shows specific abnormalities in the MELAS syndrome. *Neurology.* 1991;41(7):1043–1046.
200. Chu BC, Terae S, Takahashi C, et al. MRI of the brain in the Kearns-Sayre syndrome: report of four cases and a review. *Neuroradiology.* 1999;41(10):759–764.
201. Severino M. Glutaric aciduria type 1. In: Rumboldt Z, ed. *Brain Imaging with MRI and CT: An Image Pattern Approach.* Cambridge, UK: Cambridge University Press; 2012:415.
202. Desai NK, Runge VM, Crisp DE, et al. Magnetic resonance imaging of the brain in glutaric acidemia type I: a review of the literature and a report of four new cases with attention to the basal ganglia and imaging technique. *Invest Radiol.* 2003;38(8):489–496.
203. Morris AA, Hoffmann GF, Naughten ER, et al. Glutaric aciduria and suspected child abuse. *Arch Dis Child.* 1999;80(5):404–405.
204. Gropman A. Brain imaging in urea cycle disorders. *Mol Genet Metab.* 2010;100(suppl 1):S20–S30.
205. Takanashi J, Barkovich AJ, Cheng SF, et al. Brain MR imaging in neonatal hyperammonemic encephalopathy resulting from proximal urea cycle disorders. *AJNR Am J Neuroradiol.* 2003;24(6):1184–1187.
206. Krupp LB, Banwell B, Tenembaum S, et al. Consensus definitions proposed for pediatric multiple sclerosis and related disorders. *Neurology.* 2007;68(16 suppl 2):S7–S12.
207. Thajeb P, Chen ST. Cranial computed tomography in acute disseminated encephalomyelitis. *Neuroradiology.* 1989;31(1):8–12.
208. Lukes SA, Norman D. Computed tomography in acute disseminated encephalomyelitis. *Ann Neurol.* 1983;13(5):567–572.
209. Singh S, Alexander M, Korah IP. Acute disseminated encephalomyelitis: MR imaging features. *AJR Am J Roentgenol.* 1999;173(4):1101–1107.
210. Polman CH, Reingold SC, Banwell B, et al. Diagnostic criteria for multiple sclerosis: 2010 revisions to the McDonald criteria. *Ann Neurol.* 2011;69(2):292–302.
211. Rubin JP, Kuntz NL. Diagnostic criteria for pediatric multiple sclerosis. *Curr Neurol Neurosci Rep.* 2013;13(6):354.
212. Szudek J, Evans DG, Friedman JM. Patterns of associations of clinical features in neurofibromatosis 1 (NF1). *Hum Genet.* 2003;112(3):289–297.
213. Korf BR. Malignancy in neurofibromatosis type 1. *Oncologist.* 2000;5(6):477–485.
214. Thiagalingam S, Flaherty M, Billson F, et al. Neurofibromatosis type 1 and optic pathway gliomas: follow-up of 54 patients. *Ophthalmology.* 2004;111(3):568–577.
215. Segal L, Darvish-Zargar M, Dilenge ME, et al. Optic pathway gliomas in patients with neurofibromatosis type 1: follow-up of 44 patients. *J AAPOS.* 2010;14(2):155–158.
216. Kornreich L, Blaser S, Schwarz M, et al. Optic pathway glioma: correlation of imaging findings with the presence of neurofibromatosis. *AJNR Am J Neuroradiol.* 2001;22(10):1963–1969.
217. Rodriguez D, Young Poussaint T. Neuroimaging findings in neurofibromatosis type 1 and 2. *Neuroimaging Clin N Am.* 2004;14(2):149–170, vii.
218. Ullrich NJ, Raja AI, Irons MB, et al. Brainstem lesions in neurofibromatosis type 1. *Neurosurgery.* 2007;61(4):762–766; discussion 6–7.
219. Upadhyaya M. Genetic basis of tumorigenesis in NF1 malignant peripheral nerve sheath tumors. *Front Biosci (Landmark Ed).* 2011;16:937–951.
220. Laycock-van Spyk S, Thomas N, Cooper DN, et al. Neurofibromatosis type 1-associated tumours: their somatic mutational spectrum and pathogenesis. *Hum Genomics.* 2011;5(6):623–690.
221. Evans DG. Neurofibromatosis type 2 (NF2): a clinical and molecular review. *Orphanet J Rare Dis.* 2009;4:16.
222. Northrup H, Krueger DA; International Tuberous Sclerosis Complex Consensus Group. Tuberous sclerosis complex diagnostic criteria update: recommendations of the 2012 International Tuberous Sclerosis Complex Consensus Conference. *Pediatr Neurol.* 2013;49(4):243–254.
223. Adriaensen ME, Schaefer-Prokop CM, Stijnen T, et al. Prevalence of subependymal giant cell tumors in patients with tuberous sclerosis and a review of the literature. *Eur J Neurol.* 2009;16(6):691–696.

224. Baron Y, Barkovich AJ. MR imaging of tuberous sclerosis in neonates and young infants. *AJNR Am J Neuroradiol.* 1999;20(5):907–916.
225. Adams ME, Aylett SE, Squier W, et al. A spectrum of unusual neuroimaging findings in patients with suspected Sturge-Weber syndrome. *AJNR Am J Neuroradiol.* 2009;30(2):276–281.
226. Alper JC, Holmes LB. The incidence and significance of birthmarks in a cohort of 4,641 newborns. *Pediatr Dermatol.* 1983;1(1):58–68.
227. Kanada KN, Merin MR, Munden A, et al. A prospective study of cutaneous findings in newborns in the United States: correlation with race, ethnicity, and gestational status using updated classification and nomenclature. *J Pediatr.* 2012;161(2):240–245.
228. Comi AM. Update on Sturge-Weber syndrome: diagnosis, treatment, quantitative measures, and controversies. *Lymphat Res Biol.* 2007;5(4):257–264.
229. Waelchli R, Aylett SE, Robinson K, et al. New vascular classification of port-wine stains: improving prediction of Sturge-Weber risk. *Br J Dermatol.* 2014;171(4):861–867.
230. Shirley MD, Tang H, Gallione CJ, et al. Sturge-Weber syndrome and port-wine stains caused by somatic mutation in GNAQ. *N Engl J Med.* 2013;368(21):1971–1979.
231. Kossoff EH, Buck C, Freeman JM. Outcomes of 32 hemispherectomies for Sturge-Weber syndrome worldwide. *Neurology.* 2002;59(11):1735–1738.
232. Kim JJ, Rini BI, Hansel DE. Von Hippel-Lindau syndrome. *Adv Exp Med Biol.* 2010;685:228–249.
233. Lonser RR, Glenn GM, Walther M, et al. von Hippel-Lindau disease. *Lancet.* 2003;361(9374):2059–2067.
234. Ho VB, Smirniotopoulos JG, Murphy FM, et al. Radiologic-pathologic correlation: hemangioblastoma. *AJNR Am J Neuroradiol.* 1992;13(5):1343–1352.

CHAPTER 3

Head and Neck

Amy F. Juliano • Sara O. Vargas • Caroline D. Robson

INTRODUCTION

Anatomically, "head and neck" encompasses structures from the skull base to the thoracic inlet: the orbits, face, sinuses and nasal cavity, bony skull base, temporal bones, soft tissues of the neck, and upper aerodigestive tract including the pharynx and larynx. Various congenital and acquired anomalies and abnormalities arise from these structures, and imaging evaluation plays an important role for initial diagnosis and follow-up assessment. In this chapter, imaging techniques for evaluating head and neck in pediatric patients are discussed, and normal anatomy is reviewed. In addition, various commonly and occasionally encountered disorders affecting the pediatric head and neck are presented, including clinical features, characteristic imaging findings, relevant pathologic findings, and current treatment approaches.

IMAGING TECHNIQUES

Radiography

Trauma and inflammatory disease in the sinonasal and orbital regions are sometimes initially evaluated by radiographs. Frontal, lateral, and Waters projections are useful. When obtained in the upright position, air–fluid levels can be appreciated. For mandibular trauma, AP, Towne, oblique, and Panorex views are obtained. Radiographs are also useful when a radiopaque foreign body is suspected. Orbital views are sometimes obtained prior to performing magnetic resonance imaging (MRI) to exclude the presence of a metallic foreign body as a potential contraindication to MRI.

Radiographs are valuable in the assessment of pediatric patients following cochlear implantation. The AP transorbital projection allows visualization of the entire length of the internal auditory canal (IAC) and is useful for confirming appropriate electrode position.[1] A modified Stenvers view (PA oblique with the midsagittal plane forming an angle of 50 degrees with the plane of the film and the central ray 2 cm above and parallel to the horizontal plane) allows visualization of the entire intracochlear electrode array (Fig. 3.1)[2] and can ensure correct positioning and absence of kinking.[3] Postoperative radiographs are recommended when intraoperative radiographs cannot confirm electrode placement, when extrusion is suspected, and for evaluating nonauditory responses.[4]

Lateral radiographs of the neck are valuable for evaluating upper airway abnormalities such as adenoidal hypertrophy, retropharyngeal swelling, epiglottitis, and airway stenosis (Fig. 3.2). Frontal views of the neck are indicated for foreign body ingestion/inhalation, and mass effect on the larynx and upper trachea.[5–9]

Ultrasound

Real-time ultrasound (US) is useful for determining the size, location, and characteristics of lesions in the head and neck.[6,9–12] Ultrasound differentiates solid from cystic lesions and identifies nodal architecture distinguishing nodes from nonnodal masses. Calcification appears hyperechoic with posterior acoustic shadowing, and fat appears moderately hyperechoic. If a cystic structure with echogenic contents is suspected, it is useful to ballot the mass to detect the swirling motion of echogenic particles within. Doppler US provides information about blood flow. US also provides guidance for lesion biopsy, abscess drainage, and injections such as botulinum toxin A.

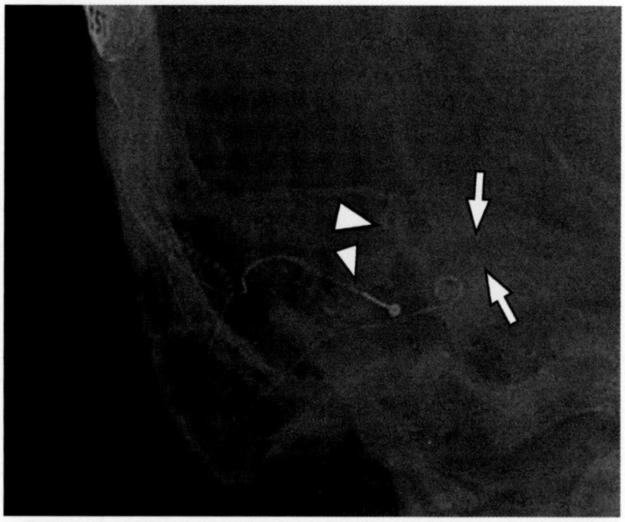

FIGURE 3.1 **Modified Stenvers radiographic view of cochlear implant electrode.** Landmarks include the internal auditory canal (*arrows*), superior semicircular canal (*large arrowhead*), and lateral semicircular canal (*small arrowhead*). The cochlea is located anterior to the semicircular canals and inferior to the internal auditory canal. The tip of the electrode can be seen to form a 360-degree turn in the expected location of the cochlea.

Computed Tomography

Computed tomography (CT) is the primary imaging modality for evaluation of bony architecture and acute inflammatory processes in the head and neck.[6,9,10,12–15] CT provides excellent delineation of soft tissue structures against a background of fat, bony structures against a background of air or fluid; detects calcifications (e.g., phleboliths, sialoliths, and tumoral calcification); and shows bony remodeling or erosion. Contrast-enhanced neck CT is generally obtained using a split bolus technique in which the scout is obtained and the first half of the IV bolus is injected, followed by a 3-minute wait, and then acquisition of helical images during the rapid injection of the second half of the bolus. This technique allows assessment of vessels, abnormal vascularity, and abnormal permeability from inflammation or tumor. The excellent spatial resolution of CT is useful for evaluating small congenital anomalies such as branchial sinus tracts.

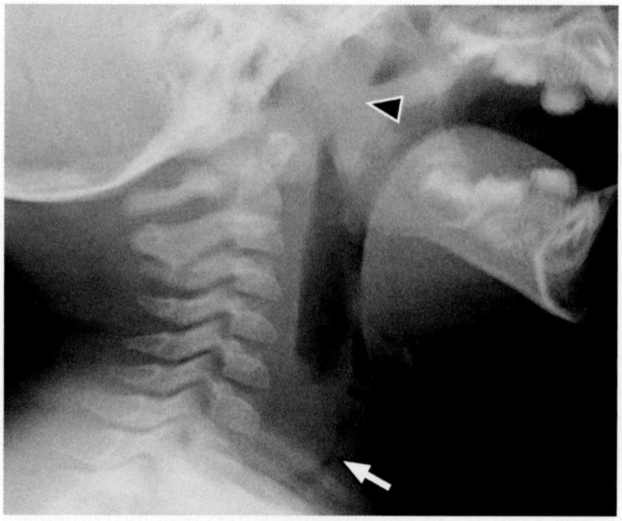

FIGURE 3.2 **Lateral radiograph of the neck in an 18-month-old girl who presented with croupy cough and biphasic stridor.** Radiograph demonstrates severe subglottic stenosis (*white arrow*). A subglottic mass was noted and biopsied during direct laryngoscopy. The mass proved to be ectopic thymic tissue. The child also has adenoidal prominence, focally contacting the soft palate (*black arrowhead*).

For evaluation of small anatomic structures, multiplanar reformatted CT images are helpful. Three-dimensional (3D) CT reconstructions are useful in evaluating traumatic injuries and craniofacial malformations for surgical planning. CT angiography and venography provide details of the arteries and veins of the head and neck for a variety of underlying vascular anomalies and abnormalities

Intraocular lesions are usually evaluated via clinical ophthalmologic assessment and US. CT is mainly used for detection of foreign bodies and intraocular calcification,[9] and in the setting of trauma. For intraocular tumors and other intraocular pathology, MRI is the preferred initial imaging study.[16–20] With increasing awareness and concern regarding the effects of radiation in pediatric patients with hereditary retinoblastoma, in whom there is higher risk of developing second primary malignancies,[21] MRI has now been established as the imaging modality for diagnosis, staging, and treatment monitoring.[22]

Nonenhanced CT is used to evaluate facial and orbital trauma and for preoperative assessment of chronic sinus disease, often providing information that can be used with intraoperative guidance systems. Axial thin sections are obtained, with submillimeter multiplanar bone algorithm reformats. For acute complicated sinonasal and orbital infection and nonocular tumors, contrast-enhanced CT precisely delineates osseous structures. Evaluation of dental lesions and the alveolar processes of the maxilla and mandible is primarily accomplished by CT, increasingly with the use of low-dose cone beam units.

In the temporal bone region, CT is the preferred initial modality for evaluation of congenital external ear and middle ear malformations, conductive hearing loss, suspected retrotympanic mass, suspected jugular dehiscence, vascular variants such as a persistent stapedial artery, and inner ear malformations.[9,10,12–14] Infection and inflammation, including cholesteatoma, and bone destruction are also best evaluated by CT. Suspected coalescent mastoiditis and tumors require the use of intravenous contrast in order to detect intracranial involvement and dural venous sinus thrombosis.

Magnetic Resonance Imaging

MRI is complementary to CT in evaluating head and neck pathology and is sometimes the imaging modality of choice. In general, MRI is a superior technique for delineation of soft tissue elements, vascular components, and intracranial involvement. Skull base evaluation requires a combination of CT for bony involvement and MRI for neurovascular, soft tissue, and marrow involvement. MR angiography (MRA) and MR venography (MRV), Doppler US, and CT angiography are additional techniques helpful for assessment of vascular flow, vessel caliber, and vascular tumors and malformations. Indications for temporal bone MRI include sensorineural hearing loss (SNHL), complicated coalescent mastoiditis, and facial nerve paralysis.

Commonly used MRI techniques for head and neck imaging include fast spin echo (FSE) T1- and T2-weighted imaging, inversion recovery (IR) sequences, fat-suppressed sequences, heavily T2-weighted sequences, diffusion-weighted imaging, flow-sensitive sequences, T1-weighted non–fat-suppressed sequences, and T1-weighted, fat-suppressed, contrast-enhanced sequences. Imaging at 3T with the use of thin-section 3D heavily T2-weighted sequences with submillimeter slice thickness is used for assessment of the membranous labyrinth of the inner ear, cranial nerves, and ocular abnormalities.

Fluoroscopy

Fluoroscopy provides dynamic information not available with radiographs. Video fluoroscopy in conjunction with still images is useful in the assessment of a child with stridor, difficulty feeding, or chronic airway obstruction. Airway caliber and contour in various phases of respiration can be observed, and an airway mass, laryngomalacia, or tracheomalacia may be detected. When performed in conjunction with a barium pharyngogram/esophagogram, vascular rings or slings, mediastinal masses, or esophageal foreign bodies or masses may be detected as well.[9]

Barium pharyngogram may demonstrate pyriform sinus tracts. The exam is performed after resolution of neck inflammation, to reduce false-negative rate related to effacement of the fistulous tract by edema.

Nuclear Medicine

Nuclear medicine is most useful in the head and neck for thyroid gland evaluation. Iodine-123 (I-123) and technetium-99m (Tc-99m) pertechnetate are the main agents used. I-123 is trapped and organified by the thyroid, whereas Tc-99m pertechnetate is trapped but not organified. Common indications for thyroid scintigraphy include identification of ectopic thyroid tissue and evaluation of thyroid nodules.

Octreotide scans may be helpful for identifying paragangliomas, especially in the setting of familial syndromes where there may be multiple tumors. Fluorodeoxyglucose (FDG)–positron emission tomography (PET) CT is used to aid in the diagnosis and staging of head and neck malignancies.

ORBIT AND GLOBE

Embryology and Development

The eye (globe) develops from the neuroectoderm of the forebrain, the surface ectoderm of the head, the mesoderm between these two layers, and neural crest cells.[9,23] The neuroectoderm gives rise to the retina, optic nerve, and smooth muscles of the iris. The overlying surface ectoderm gives rise to the corneal epithelium, conjunctival epithelium, lens, and lacrimal and tarsal glands. The mesenchyme and neural crest cells give rise to the corneal stroma, sclera, choroid, iris, ciliary musculature, part of the vitreous body, and cells lining the anterior chamber.[24]

The optic primordium gives rise to the optic vesicle. The overlying surface ectoderm thickens and forms the lens placode. The outer surface of the optic vesicle then flattens and becomes concave, resulting in the optic cup, whereas the proximal portion of the optic vesicle constricts and forms the optic stalk.[23,24]

In the 5 mm embryo, invagination occurs along the optic stalk, forming a groove. At the distal end, the groove opens into the optic fissure or choroidal fissure, at the inferior edge of the optic cup. Through this fissure, mesenchyme extends into the optic stalk and cup, carrying with it the hyaloid artery, a branch of the ophthalmic artery. Over time, the edges of the fissure approximate and the groove narrows, until the fissure closes and the groove becomes the optic canal, inside the optic stalk. Failure of the fissure to close completely results in a coloboma, which may be seen anywhere along the length of the optic stalk and can affect any of the optic stalk derivatives.

The hyaloid artery travels through the globe within the hyaloid canal during development of the primitive or primary vitreous. Over time, the embryonic hyaloid vascular system involutes. The hyaloid artery and vein become the central artery and vein of the retina, coursing within and along the optic nerve. Persistence and hyperplasia of the embryonic hyaloid system in the globe result in persistent hyperplastic primary vitreous (PHPV).[9]

Normal Anatomy

The globe is embedded in orbital fat and is surrounded by a thin capsule.[9,25–27] The opaque sclera and the transparent cornea form the outer layer of the globe. The middle layer is formed by the uvea, which is vascular and contains pigmented tissue including the choroid, ciliary body, and iris. The retina, the inner layer, is the neural, sensory layer that receives images. The retina is continuous posteriorly with the optic nerve. The refracting media of the eye are the aqueous humor, the crystalline lens, and the vitreous humor. The lacrimal gland is situated in the superolateral orbit. The puncta of the superior and inferior canaliculi are located in the medial aspect of the upper and lower lids. They travel through the superior and inferior canaliculi to the common canaliculus and then enter a small diverticulum of the lateral wall of the lacrimal sac, called the sinus of Maier, and then into the lacrimal sac proper.[9] The nasolacrimal duct (NLD) extends from the lacrimal sac and empties into the inferior meatus of the nasal cavity.

The orbit contains the orbital fascia, extraocular muscles, globe and its appendages, vessels, nerves, and fat.[9,25–27] The optic foramen lies at the orbital apex and transmits the optic nerve and ophthalmic artery. The superior orbital fissure lies inferolateral to the optic foramen and transmits cranial nerves III and IV, the ophthalmic division of cranial nerve V, cranial nerve VI, sympathetic nerves, and the ophthalmic vein. The orbital floor and lateral orbital wall are separated posteriorly by the inferior orbital fissure. This fissure connects the orbit with the pterygopalatine fossa posteromedially and with the retromaxillary fissure and infratemporal fossa anterolaterally.

Except for the inferior oblique, the extraocular muscles originate at the orbital apex and insert on the globe. The inferior oblique muscle arises from the orbital floor just lateral to the opening of the nasolacrimal canal. The orbital fascia forms the periosteum of the orbit. Anteriorly, it forms a circumferential reflection known as the orbital septum. Structures anterior to the septum are termed preseptal; those posterior to it are termed postseptal. The orbital septum provides a barrier to the posterior spread of preseptal inflammation. The postseptal space may be further subdivided by the cone of muscles into intraconal and extraconal compartments.

The orbital cavity grows passively in response to the growth of the globe.[5–9] The globe is 75% of adult size at birth, and its growth is complete by age 7 years. The bony orbit and optic canal have almost reached adult size by age 10 years.

Congenital and Developmental Anomalies

Malformations of the Globe

Anophthalmia

Anophthalmia is congenital absence of the eye, a rare unilateral or bilateral abnormality. By definition, true anophthalmia characterized by complete absence of ocular tissue within the orbit is rare as there is usually a small eye or a dysplastic remnant present. Anophthalmia is associated with infections and congenital syndromes such as trisomy 13 and complex craniofacial malformations.[9,26–29]

Primary anophthalmia results from failure of formation of the optic vesicle. Consecutive anophthalmia is when the optic vesicle forms but then degenerates. Secondary anophthalmia and congenital cystic eyeball are caused by partial or complete failure of the primary optic vesicle to involute early in development. When the cyst is small or nonexistent, anophthalmia results. When the cyst is large, a congenital cystic eyeball results.[30]

On imaging, there is a poorly formed shallow orbit with no globe, and rudimentary orbital tissue is often present (Fig. 3.3). Extraocular muscles are usually seen, and neural tissue related to the optic nerve may be present unless there is true anophthalmia, which is extremely rare.[9]

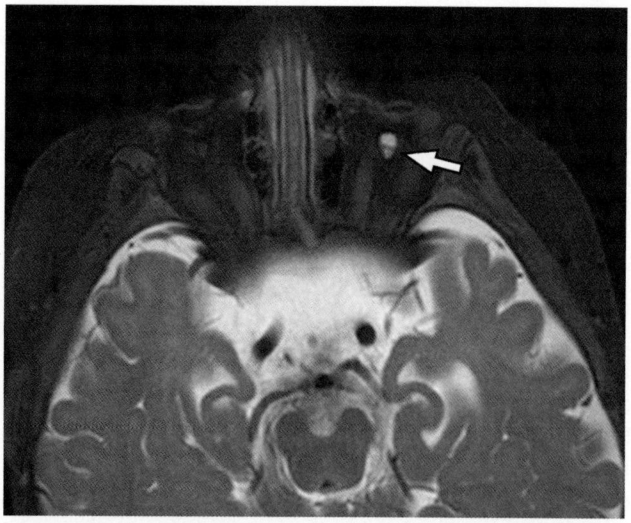

FIGURE 3.3 **Anophthalmia in an 8-month-old girl.** Axial T2-weighted fat-suppressed MR image shows absence of globes with shallow orbits bilaterally. A small cyst on the left may represent dysplastic remnant (*arrow*). The child has *SOX2* anophthalmia syndrome, having esophageal atresia and cryptorchidism as well.

Microphthalmia

In microphthalmia, a small globe and a lens are present, although severe microphthalmia may be difficult to distinguish from anophthalmia clinically and radiologically (Fig. 3.4).[30] A microphthalmic eye that otherwise demonstrates normal architecture is called a nanophthalmic eye. Microphthalmia may exist alone or may be associated with other abnormalities such as glaucoma, cataract, genetic syndromes (e.g., trisomy 13 and holoprosencephaly), and TORCH infections. Microphthalmia with a retrobulbar duplication cyst occurs when ocular tissue prolapses through a coloboma defect (persistent embryonic optic fissure).

Macrophthalmia

A number of conditions can lead to enlargement of the globe. The most common condition is *pathologic axial myopia*, where there is elongation of the globe because of increased anteroposterior dimension of the posterior chamber. Macrophthalmia is sporadic or syndromic in nature (e.g., Stickler syndrome) and may be asymmetric (Fig. 3.5). The abnormal elongation leads to increased risk of retinal abnormalities and staphylomas.

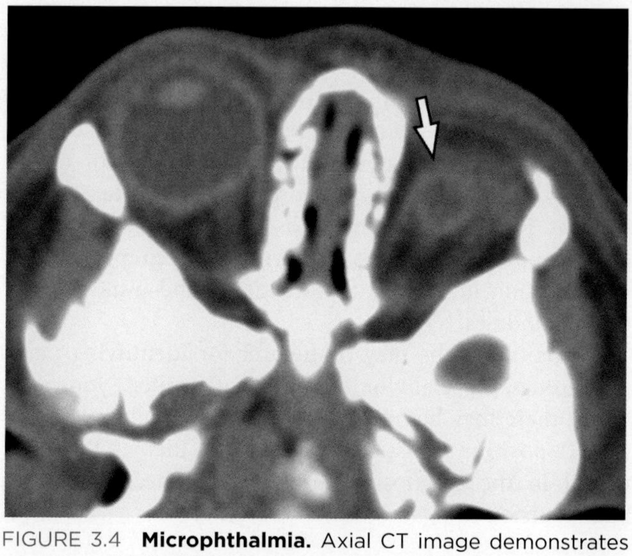

FIGURE 3.4 **Microphthalmia.** Axial CT image demonstrates a very small left globe (*arrow*) and normal-sized right globe.

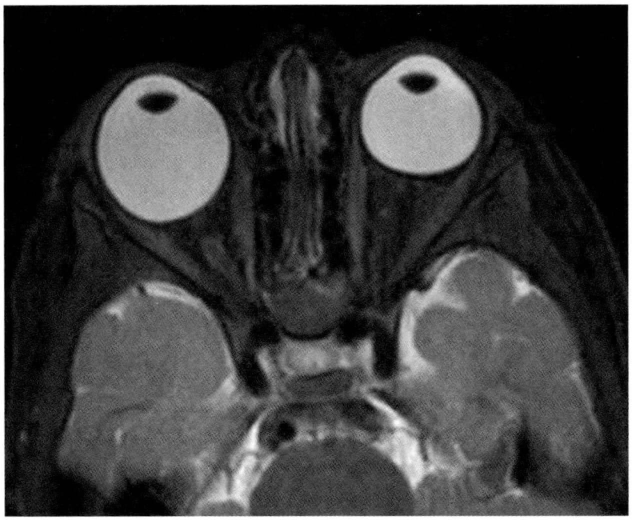

FIGURE 3.5 **Macrophthalmia.** Axial T2-weighted fat-suppressed MR image shows an enlarged right globe. This 14-month-old boy has a developmental defect in the retina and optic nerve with subnormal vision. His poor vision is thought to be related to amblyopia that is a result of restricted movement of the abnormally elongated globe. He does not have elevated intraocular pressure, and therefore this does not represent buphthalmos.

In *buphthalmos*, the globe is enlarged because of increased intraocular pressure at a time when the sclera can be stretched beyond its normal shape and size, as it is prior to age 4 years. There is increased anteroposterior dimension of both the anterior and posterior chambers. The increase in intraocular pressure may be because of congenital primary glaucoma or because of glaucoma related to an underlying condition such as aniridia, neurofibromatosis, or Sturge-Weber syndrome.

Staphyloma

Staphyloma is characterized by thinning and stretching of the scleral–uveal coats of the globe. All the layers are present, and there is no defect in the layers as in coloboma. It usually occurs posteriorly (Fig. 3.6); anterior (corneal) staphyloma is rare. Affected pediatric patients typically present with severe axial myopia. Posterior staphyloma may be seen in high axial myopia, glaucoma, scleritis, and necrotizing infection, or may be from iatrogenic causes. Anterior staphyloma is seen secondary to inflammation involving the scleral–corneal layer.[9]

Coloboma

A coloboma results from incomplete closure of the embryonic optic fissure. A coloboma can involve the cornea, iris, lens, retina, choroid, sclera, and optic nerve, in a continuous or discontinuous fashion, in the inferior aspect. Unlike staphyloma where the uveal–scleral layers are thinned but present, in coloboma, there is a complete structural defect, with a gap through the involved structure(s). Half of all typical colobomas are bilateral.[31] Coloboma is seen as a defect at the posterior globe with focal outpouching of the globe contour at the level of the optic nerve insertion (Fig. 3.7).

In some cases, there may be herniation of dysplastic tissue through the defect.[32,33] A cyst may result, sometimes communicating with the globe, which is small and dysplastic. This is termed microphthalmia with cyst or a colobomatous cyst (Fig. 3.8). The cyst is often larger than the globe, and the cyst content is more similar to cerebrospinal fluid (CSF) than to vitreous.[34] Colobomatous cysts are associated with systemic syndromes such as CHARGE syndrome, VATER association, Warburg syndrome, and trisomies 13 and 18.

Morning Glory Disc Anomaly

Morning glory disc anomaly (MGDA) is a congenital dysplasia of the optic disc/optic nerve, with a funnel-shaped excavation at the optic disc. The appearance resembles a morning glory flower, hence the name. On funduscopic examination, an annulus of chorioretinal pigmentary change surrounds the optic disc excavation, and a central glial tuft overlies the optic disc.[35,36] The condition is usually unilateral and

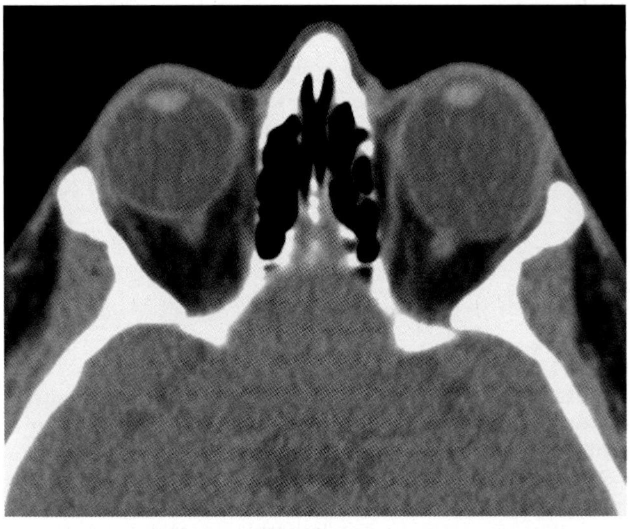

FIGURE 3.6 **Posterior staphyloma.** Axial CT image demonstrates thinning and stretching of the posterior surface of the globe on the left, resulting in elongation of the globe.

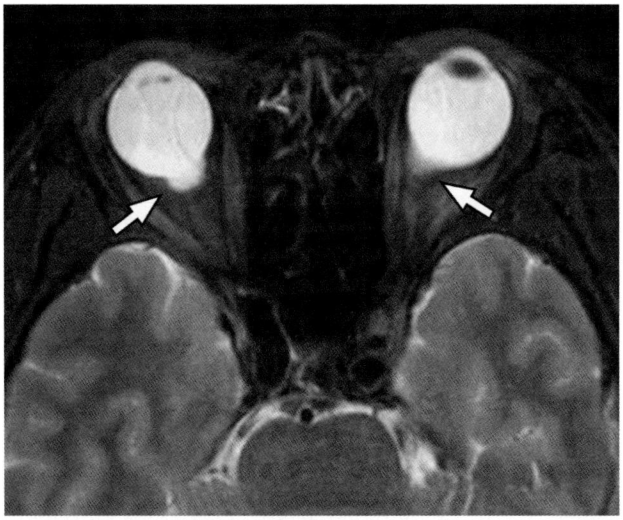

FIGURE 3.7 **Colobomas.** Axial T2-weighted fat-suppressed MR image shows a defect at the posterior right globe at the site of the optic nerve insertion, with a focal outpouching at that location. This is also present on the left (*arrows*).

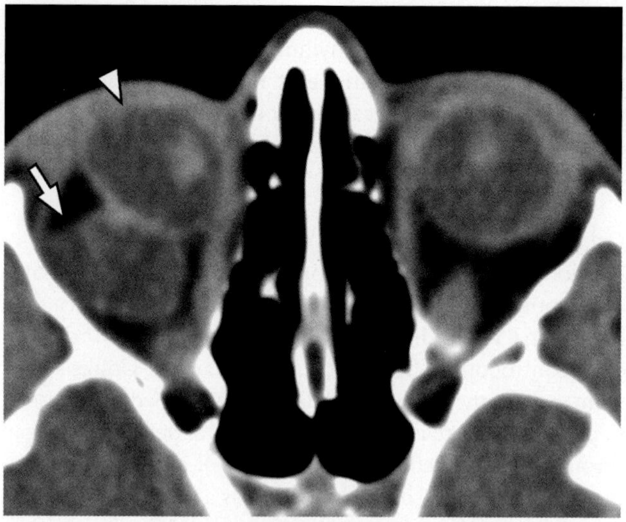

FIGURE 3.8 **Colobomatous cyst in a 3-year-old girl.** Axial CT image demonstrates a colobomatous cyst (*arrow*) posterior to the right globe. The globe is smaller than normal in size and dysplastic (*arrowhead*).

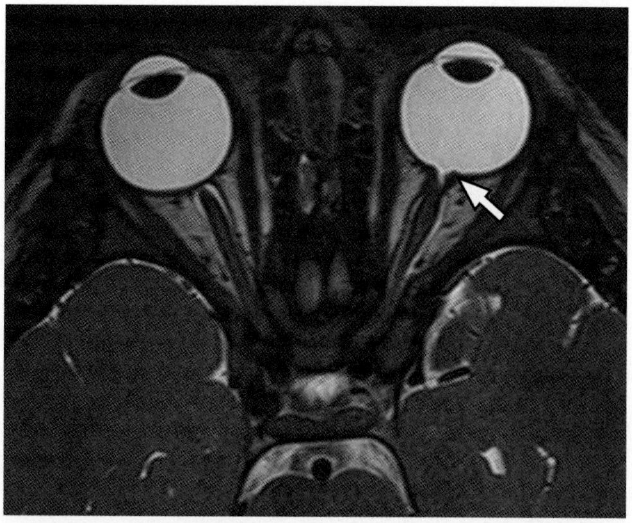

FIGURE 3.9 **Morning glory disc anomaly in a 4-year-old girl.** Axial T2-weighted SPACE MR image shows funnel-shaped morphology of the posterior left globe at the level of the optic disc. Elevated retinal margin can be seen laterally (*arrow*).

sporadic, although there is an association with other ocular and intracranial abnormalities such as midline craniofacial defects, callosal dysgenesis, and basal encephaloceles; vascular abnormalities including segmental aplasia of the circle of Willis and moyamoya disease as seen in PHACES association; and other cerebral malformations.[35,37] Therefore, pediatric patients with MGDA should undergo brain MRI and MRA as part of their imaging workup. To date, the pathogenesis of MGDA is unknown.

On imaging, a funnel-shaped morphology of the optic disc can be seen (Fig. 3.9). In contradistinction to coloboma, elevation of the retinal margins adjacent to the excavation is characteristic. On MRI, one may appreciate abnormal T1 hyperintense soft tissue associated with the distal portion of the optic nerve, representing the glial tissue seen on ophthalmic examination. The ipsilateral optic nerve is sometimes atrophied.[36]

Malformations of the Orbit

Hypertelorism and Hypotelorism

Hypertelorism refers to an increased distance between the medial walls of the orbits.[5–9] This is to be distinguished from telecanthus, where the distance between the apices of the medial canthal ligaments is increased and the eyes appear to be farther apart than normal but the bony interorbital distance is not increased. A combination of telecanthus with lateral displacement of the lacrimal puncta, known as dystopia canthorum, is characteristic of some types of Waardenburg syndrome.[38] Causes of hypertelorism include familial hypertelorism, median cleft face syndrome, cleidocranial dysplasia, syndromic coronal craniosynostosis, cephalocele, trisomy 13, and Hurler disease.

Hypotelorism refers to a bony interorbital distance that is less than normal. Underlying causes of hypotelorism include arhinencephaly, holoprosencephaly, microcephaly, trigonocephaly, sagittal craniosynostosis, and primary developmental abnormalities of the eyes.

Large or Small Orbit

A large orbit may be caused by brain herniation through a mesenchymal bony defect (greater sphenoid wing in neurofibromatosis), cephalocele, or an increase in orbital contents present early in development from, for example, neurofibroma or vascular anomaly.[5–9]

A small shallow orbit is seen in congenital anophthalmia, in microphthalmia, and as a sequela of early insult, for example orbital enucleation and radiation. Exorbitism refers to protrusion of the globe due to a shallow orbit and is characteristic of some forms of syndromic craniosynostosis, or may occur from hyperostotic changes in the orbit as seen in fibrous dysplasia (Fig. 3.10) and osteopetrosis.

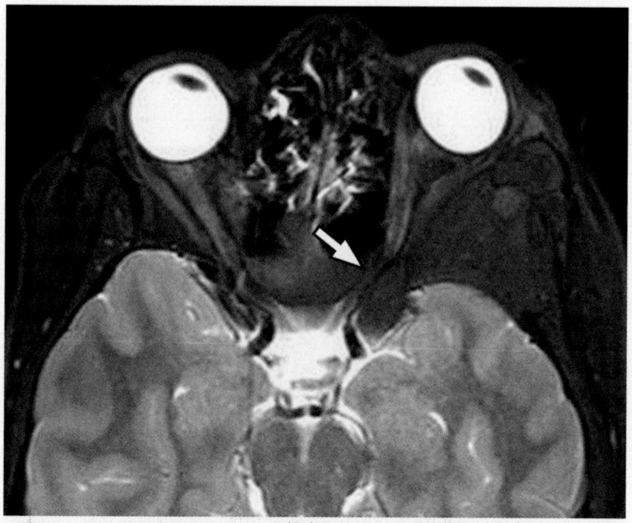

FIGURE 3.10 **Fibrous dysplasia of the sphenoid wing causing narrowing of the optic canal in an 11-year-old girl who presented with left proptosis.** Axial T2-weighted fat-suppressed MR image demonstrates expansion of the greater wing of the sphenoid on the left, including the anterior clinoid process, due to fibrous dysplasia. The left orbit is smaller than normal, and the optic canal is narrowed (*arrow*).

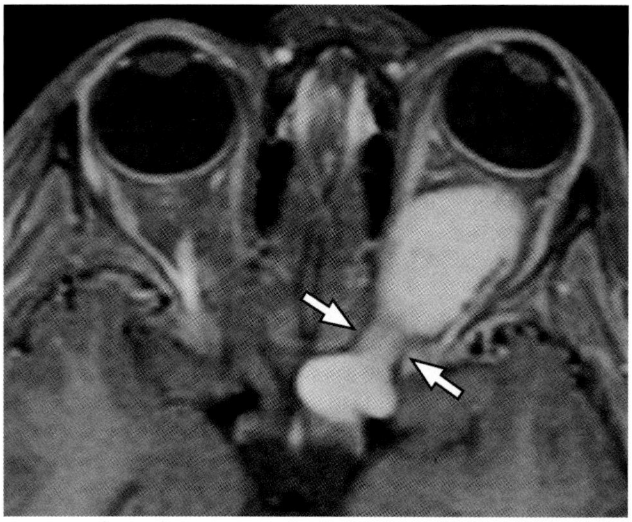

FIGURE 3.11 **Optic nerve glioma in neurofibromatosis type 1.** Axial postcontrast T1-weighted fat-suppressed MR image shows a fusiform enhancing mass along the left optic nerve representing the optic nerve glioma. The left optic canal is expanded as a result (*arrows*).

Large or Small Optic Canal

A large optic canal is almost always due to an intracanalicular optic glioma (Fig. 3.11). Rare causes include other tumors (e.g., neurofibroma, meningioma, hemangioma) and dural ectasia (e.g., in neurofibromatosis). A small optic canal is due to a small optic nerve (e.g., in microphthalmia, optic nerve hypoplasia or atrophy, early orbital enucleation) or bony hyperostosis (e.g., fibrous dysplasia, osteopetrosis) (Fig. 3.10).

Optic Nerve Hypoplasia

Optic nerve hypoplasia, a subnormal number of axons,[26–29] is a frequent anomaly and is often isolated. Particularly when bilateral, it may be associated with ocular, facial, endocrine, or central nervous system (CNS) anomalies, among which are septooptic dysplasia and encephalocele. Although it is primarily a clinical diagnosis, characteristic MR findings are small optic nerves and a small chiasm.

TABLE 3.1 Differential Diagnosis of Leukocoria

Normal-sized Globe	Small Globe
• Retinoblastoma (or could be small or large) • Coats disease • Sclerosing endophthalmitis (*Toxocara*) • Congenital cataract • Vitreous hemorrhage • Total retinal detachment	• Persistent hyperplastic primary vitreous • Norrie disease • Retinopathy of prematurity

Primary Ocular Abnormalities

Persistent Hyperplastic Primary Vitreous

PHPV is caused by failure of the embryonic hyaloid vascular system to regress, resulting in persistence and hyperplasia of the primary vitreous, tunica vasculosa lentis (capillary vascular network covering parts of the lens), and associated embryonic connective tissue. PHPV is usually unilateral and associated with microphthalmia. The typical presentation is unilateral leukocoria (white pupil) with microphthalmia and cataract in a term infant. After retinoblastoma, PHPV is the most common cause of leukocoria in childhood (Table 3.1).[39] The two entities may be differentiated on CT by the presence of microphthalmia and absence of calcification in PHPV. Retinoblastoma usually contains calcifications and involves a normal or large globe. When glaucoma complicates PHPV, it leads to buphthalmos. Other complications include recurrent hemorrhage, retinal detachment, and phthisis bulbi.

On CT, there is increased density of the vitreous chamber (Fig. 3.12A) and enhancement of abnormal intravitreal tissue. Intravitreal densities suggest the persistence of fetal tissue in the Cloquet canal or congenital nonattachment of the retina. Microphthalmia ranges from obvious to subtle, and calcification is absent within or around the globe. The lens may be small and irregular, and the anterior chamber may be shallow.

On MR, there is T1 hyperintensity of the vitreous chamber and enhancement of abnormal intravitreal tissue (Fig. 3.12B).

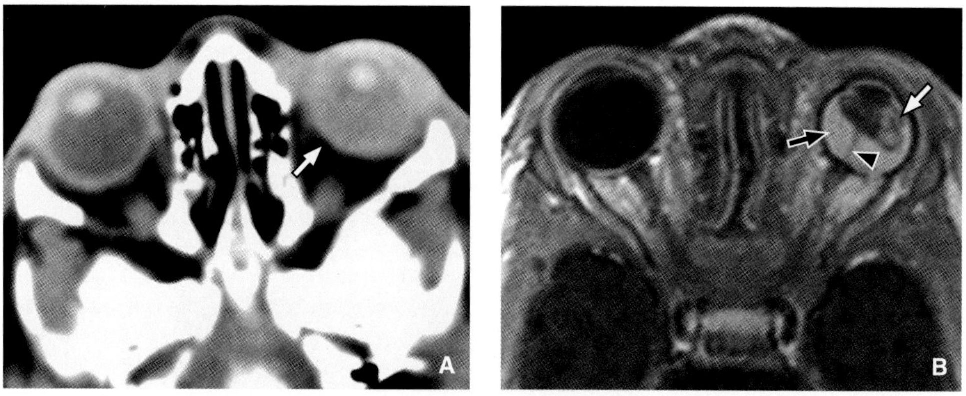

FIGURE 3.12 **Persistent Hyperplastic Primary Vitreous (PHPV) in a 47-day-old infant. A:** Axial CT image shows left microphthalmia, with increased density in the vitreous chamber (*arrow*). **B:** Axial postcontrast T1-weighted fat-suppressed MR image shows T1 hyperintense signal in the vitreous chamber (*black arrow*) and a retrolental mass with enhancing areas (*white arrow*). The Cloquet canal can be seen (*black arrowhead*).

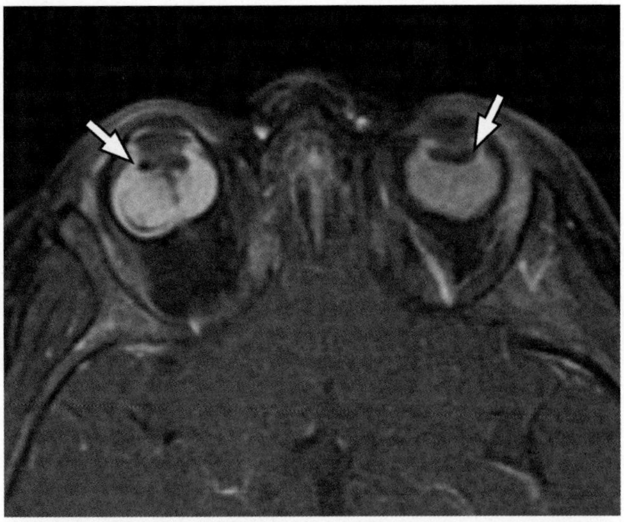

FIGURE 3.13 **Norrie disease.** Axial postcontrast T1-weighted fat-suppressed MR image demonstrates bilateral microphthalmia. The vitreous is T1 hyperintense in signal, and there are retrolental masses (*arrows*).

A discrete linear structure suggestive of the Cloquet canal may be seen. An enhancing retrolental mass may be present. The anterior form of PHPV is characterized by flattening of the lens, a shallow anterior chamber, and enhancement of the anterior segment structures. PHPV is often associated with optic nerve and retinal malformations.[40]

Norrie Disease

Norrie disease, or congenital progressive oculoacousticocerebral degeneration, is a rare, X-linked, recessive disorder consisting of retinal malformation, deafness, and mental retardation or deterioration. Early-onset blindness is due to severe retinal dysplasia. Clinical findings include leukocoria, iris atrophy, retrolental fibroplasia, vitreous hemorrhage, retinal dysplasia, retinal folds, and retinal detachments.[41] The end result is cataracts and opaque corneas, and, eventually, phthisis bulbi.

On imaging, the vitreous chambers are dense on CT and T1 hyperintense on MRI bilaterally (Fig. 3.13). A retrolental mass, retinal detachment, shallow anterior chamber, small dense lens, and optic nerve atrophy and microphthalmia may be seen.[9]

Coats Disease

Coats disease (primary retinal telangiectasias) is a primary retinal vascular anomaly characterized by telangiectatic and aneurysmal retinal vessels, and the accumulation of lipoproteinaceous exudate in the retina and subretinal space, leading to massive exudative retinal detachment.[26–29] Leukocoria may be seen with the occurrence of retinal detachment. The peak incidence is near the end of the first decade, with a higher incidence in males.

Early in the disease, imaging findings may be minimal. Subsequent findings are largely related to retinal detachment. The subretinal exudate of Coats disease is usually hyperintense on T1- and T2-weighted MR sequences (Fig. 3.14) and hyperdense on CT. Coats disease can simulate retinoblastoma, with a mass that should be heterogeneous in density and signal and nonenhancing. Calcification sometimes occurs.

Retinopathy of Prematurity

Retinopathy of prematurity (ROP) (retrolental fibroplasia) is seen in premature low-birth-weight infants who receive prolonged oxygen therapy. Currently, the prevalence of the abnormality has decreased because of judicious use of oxygen in infants.

It is usually bilateral, and may be symmetric or asymmetric. The pathophysiology is not completely understood; excessive oxygen has been implicated. There is proliferation of abnormal peripheral retinal vessels, with subsequent hemorrhage and cicatrization. In the late stage, a dense membrane or vascularized mass is left with tractional retinal detachment and microphthalmos.[9]

In more advanced cases, it may be difficult to differentiate ROP from PHPV and other conditions resulting in microphthalmia with associated retinal detachment.[42,43] A history of prematurity, incubator treatment, low birth weight, bilaterality, and microphthalmia helps confirm the diagnosis of ROP. Calcification is seen in advanced cases.

Congenital Glaucoma

Glaucoma is abnormal elevation of intraocular pressure,[26–29] usually caused by increased resistance to normal outflow of aqueous humor. The increase in intraocular pressure at a young age, when the sclera is still malleable, leads to buphthalmos. Hydrophthalmos refers to the high fluid content

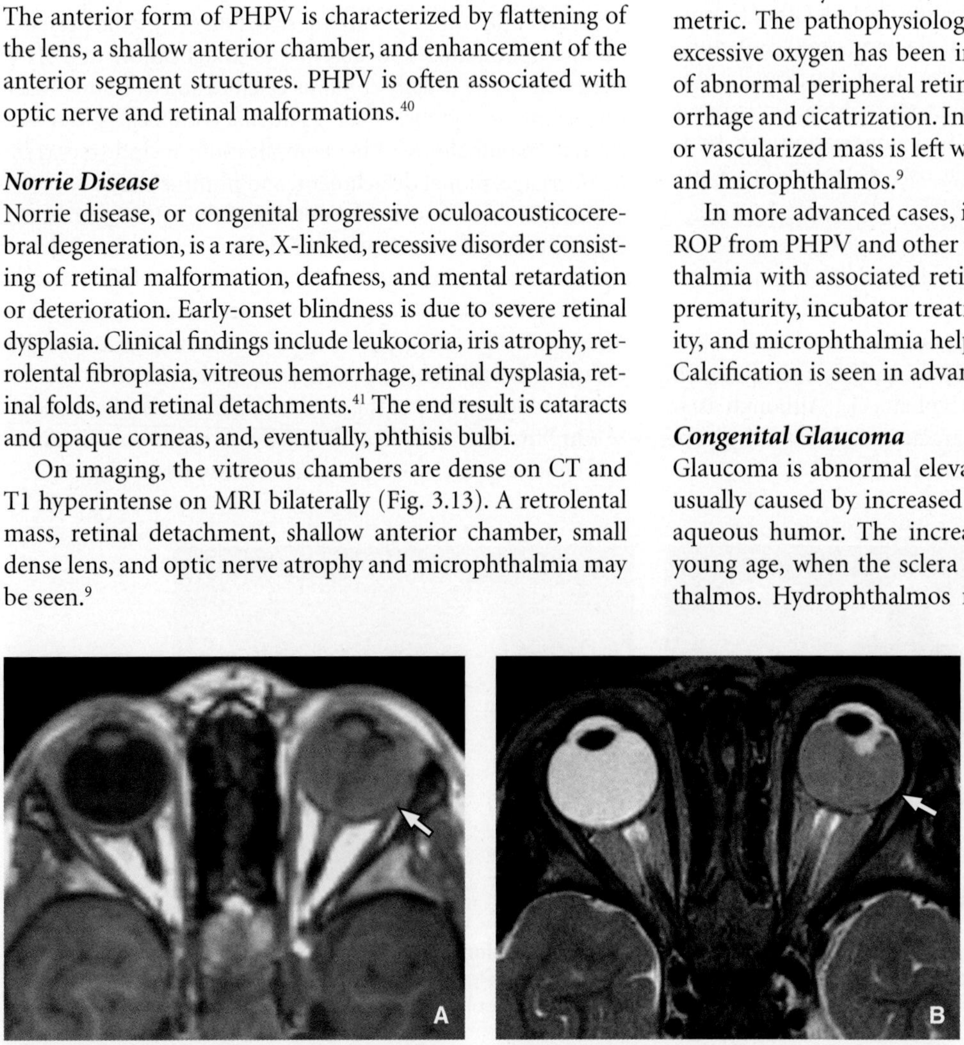

FIGURE 3.14 **Coats disease.** Axial T1-weighted **(A)** and T2-weighted fat-suppressed **(B)** MR images demonstrate a large subretinal exudate occupying most of the vitreous chamber of the left globe, hyperintense to white matter on both sequences (*arrows*).

present with marked enlargement of the eye that is seen in any type of glaucoma present since infancy.[44]

Ocular and Orbital Abnormalities Associated with CNS Malformations

Disorders of neural tube closure in which there may be orbital abnormalities include cephaloceles, dermal sinus and cyst, neuroglial heterotopia, holoprosencephaly, septooptic dysplasia, absence of the septum pellucidum, craniosynostosis, and cranial facial syndromes.[45] Cephaloceles that commonly involve the orbit or optic pathways include sphenoidal, nasoorbital, and frontoethmoidal cephaloceles.[25,46–51] Dermal sinuses, dermoids, and epidermoids are discussed later. Widening of the nasal bridge and hypertelorism should prompt a search for craniofacial anomalies, cephaloceles, and midline intracranial defects such as callosal agenesis.

Midface hypoplasia and hypotelorism are commonly associated with the holoprosencephalies.[45,47,52] Midface and orbital anomalies associated with alobar holoprosencephaly include cyclopia (single midline orbit with proboscis and absent nose), ethmocephaly (median proboscis between two hypoteloric orbits), cebocephaly (rudimentary nose with single aperture and orbital hypotelorism), the rare median cleft lip with hypertelorism, and simple hypotelorism. Septooptic dysplasia anomalies with deficiency of the septum pellucidum and optic hypoplasia are considered a mild form of holoprosencephaly.[45,52,53]

Unilaterally or bilaterally deformed orbits are commonly associated with craniosynostoses, particularly those involving the metopic suture, coronal suture, or multiple sutures.[45,50] Hypertelorism with or without exorbitism is characteristic of syndromic coronal synostosis. Reconstructive craniofacial surgery is often required to improve appearance and preserve vision. Metopic synostosis results in hypotelorism. Treacher Collins syndrome (TCS) (mandibulofacial dysostosis) is as associated with microphthalmia and coloboma.

Neuroophthalmologic involvement often occurs with the neurocutaneous syndromes of childhood such as neurofibromatosis type 1 (NF1) (sphenoorbital dysplasia [Fig. 3.15]), optic glioma (Fig. 3.11), tuberous sclerosis (retinal neuroglial hamartoma), Sturge-Weber syndrome (choroidal venocapillary malformation with buphthalmos), and von Hippel-Lindau disease (retinal hemangioblastoma with retinal detachment and hemorrhage).[45]

Disorders of migration that are often associated with ocular, orbital, or optic pathway abnormalities include dysgenesis of the corpus callosum and the lissencephaly syndromes.[45,54–57]

Malformative Lesions

Malformative abnormalities are neoplastic and nonneoplastic masses that arise from an aberration of development.[26,28,29,45,58] These are usually of neuroectodermal origin (e.g., dermoid or epidermoid) or mesodermal origin (e.g., lipoma). Benign teratomas can also be included in this category,[59] as can vascular anomalies. Malformative lesions are often cystic but may be solid or of mixed consistency. In the orbital region in childhood, malformative lesions include colobomas, duplication cysts of the eye, nasolacrimal duct (NLD) cysts, lacrimal ectopia, dermoids, epidermoids, benign teratomas, and (rarely) arachnoid cysts and lipomas.

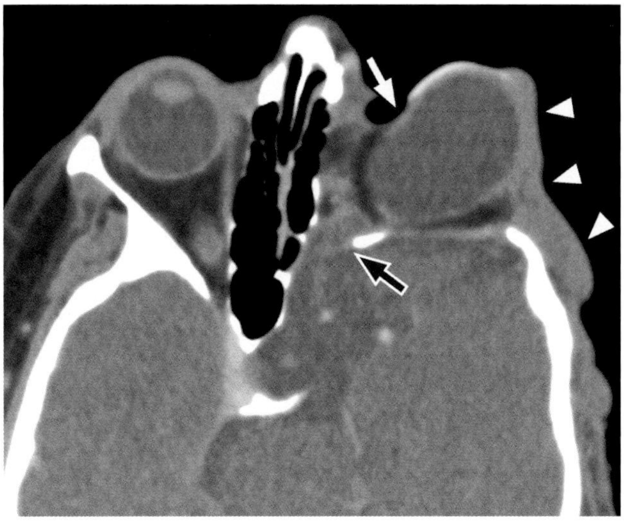

FIGURE 3.15 **Neurofibromatosis type I in a 17-year-old boy.** Axial CT image shows left sphenoid wing dysplasia causing orbital deformity. There is also a meningoencephalocele extending through the deformed orbital apex into the orbit (*black arrow*), macrophthalmia (*white arrow*), and a plexiform neurofibroma overlying the lateral aspect of the left lid (*arrowheads*).

Coloboma

Coloboma and colobomatous cyst have been discussed earlier. See section Malformations of the Globe.

Nasolacrimal Duct Cyst and Mucocele

Congenital NLD cyst and mucocele are the most common abnormalities of the infant lacrimal apparatus.[60–63] They probably result from failure of canalization of the NLD. A residual membrane persists where the duct enters the nasal cavity, leading to partial or complete obstruction of the NLD, usually at the valve of Hasner, located beneath the inferior turbinate. Accumulation of secretions produces cystic NLD dilatation. Affected pediatric patients may present with a medial canthal mass due to a dacryocystocele, epiphora, nasal obstruction, and respiratory distress. It often resolves spontaneously in the early postnatal months; persistence may lead to nasal airway obstruction, infection, or dacryocystitis.

Imaging demonstrates a unilateral or bilateral cystic medial canthus mass in continuity with an enlarged NLD and an intranasal cystic mass (Fig. 3.16). Protrusion beneath the inferior turbinate distinguishes NLD cyst from cephalocele, which lies cephalad to the inferior turbinate.

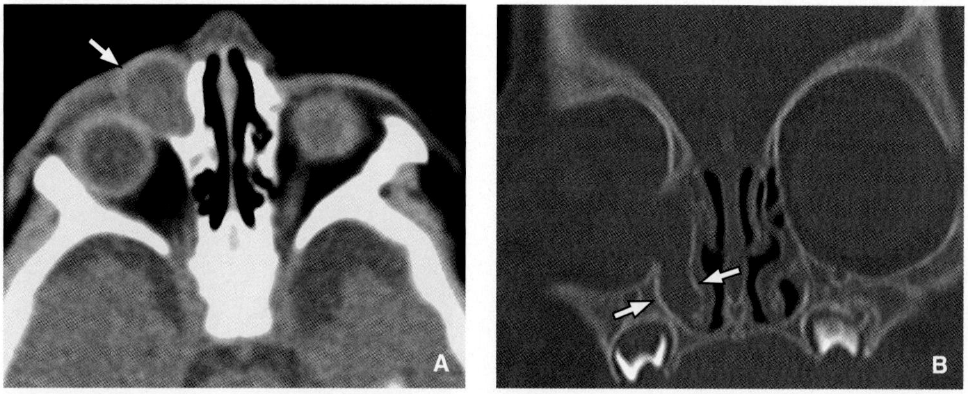

FIGURE 3.16 **Nasolacrimal duct cyst and mucocele in a 3-month-old boy who was born with a "bluish mass" near the right lacrimal sac.** CT images demonstrate a cystic mass (*arrow*) at the right medial canthus **(A)** that is contiguous with an enlarged nasolacrimal duct **(B)**, with the mucocele extending into the inferior meatus of the nasal cavity (*arrows* in **B**).

Lacrimal Gland Ectopia

Ectopic lacrimal gland tissue causes benign solid or cystic lesions of the orbit and may produce proptosis at any age.[64] The ectopic tissue may be located intraconally.

Epibulbar Choristoma, Dermoid and Epidermoid Cysts, Teratoma

Choristoma is a broad term used to denote a congenital maldevelopmental lesion stemming from overgrowth of normal tissue in an abnormal location. The term choristoma can be applied to dermoid cyst, ectopic skin, ectopic bone, or other ectopic tissues. A collection of adipose tissue (lipoma) could be considered a choristoma or a hamartoma if it occurs in an anatomic site where adipose tissue is typically found. Epibulbar choristomas are variable in size, are unilateral or bilateral, and may be associated with the cornea, limbus, or subconjunctival space (Fig. 3.17).[65] Epibulbar choristomas may be associated with ocular anomalies such as staphyloma, aniridia, congenital aphakia, and microphthalmia. They may coexist with choristomas of the eyelid, osseous choristomas of the choroid, orbital dermoids, choristomas of the face and scalp, and preauricular cartilage choristomas (i.e., accessory ear tissue). There is an association with the Goldenhar phenotype of hemifacial microsomia (HFM) and epidermal nevus syndrome.

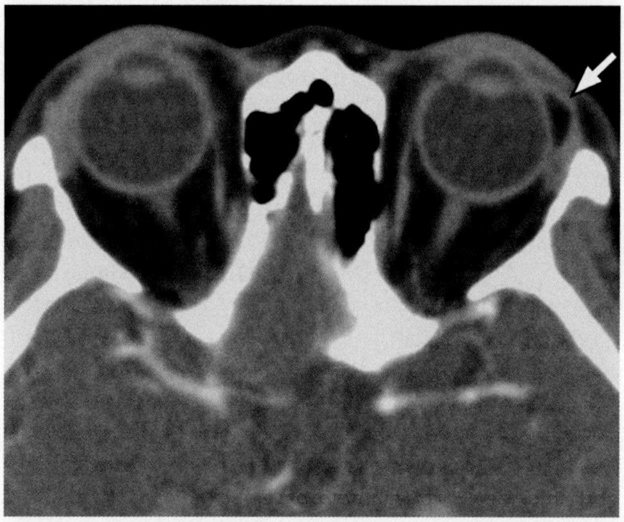

FIGURE 3.17 **Epibulbar choristoma.** Axial contrast-enhanced CT image shows a fat-density lesion (*arrow*) overlying the lateral corneal/conjunctival surface of the left globe.

Dermoid cysts are the most common congenital lesions of the orbit.[28,66–68] They arise from inclusion and sequestration of ectodermal elements, typically in sutures. Dermoids contain dermal adnexal structures such as sebaceous and sweat glands, hair follicles, and sometimes fat (Fig. 3.18), and squamous epithelium (Fig. 3.19). Epidermoid cysts have only keratinizing, stratified squamous epithelium and are rare in the pediatric orbit.[69] In the orbit, dermoids typically occur laterally at the frontozygomatic suture and less commonly medially at the frontoethmoidal or frontonasal suture. Most present as a subcutaneous nodule near the orbital rim (Fig. 3.18B). These lesions demonstrate slow growth, with smooth bony remodeling and displacement of adjacent structures. On CT, they appear sharply defined and hypodense. On MR, they are of variable signal on T1-weighted sequences, are usually hyperintense on T2-weighted sequences, and typically have restricted diffusion and minimal if any peripheral enhancement. Notching of the bony site of origin and bony scalloping are characteristic.

Teratomas contain tissue derived from ectoderm, mesoderm, and endoderm. Orbital teratomas are rarely malignant but can cause significant proptosis in infancy.[26,28,29,58] They are typically cystic and solid and can produce significant mass effect. Imaging reveals fat, soft tissue, calcification, and/or ossification.

Congenital Cystic Eye

A congenital cystic eye results when the optic vesicle does not invaginate normally during embryologic development.[70] There is a large, cystic, often septated structure replacing the normal globe within an enlarged orbit. Incomplete rudimentary fragments of optic nerve and extraocular muscles may be present. On MRI, the fluid within the cystic septated structure exhibits a different signal than does normal vitreous, because it is filled with a more serous fluid.

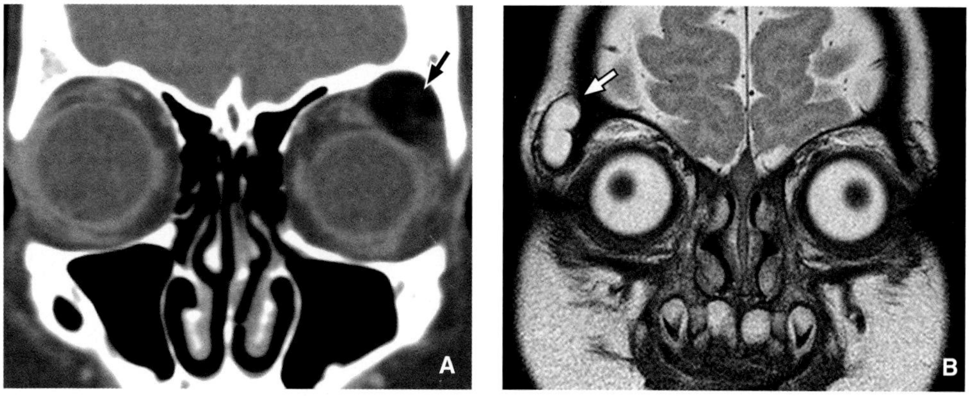

FIGURE 3.18 **Orbital dermoid in a 9-year-old boy. A:** Coronal CT image demonstrates a lobulated mass (*arrow*) that is predominantly of fat density but has some heterogeneous soft tissue in its inferior aspect. It is located in the superotemporal aspect of the orbit abutting the frontozygomatic suture and causes bony remodeling. The mass was surgically removed; pathology revealed a dermoid cyst with sebaceous glands. **B:** Coronal T2-weighted MR image in a different patient shows a well-circumscribed, lobulated cystic mass (*arrow*) overlying the superolateral orbital wall. This mass was also surgically excised and was pathologically confirmed to be a dermoid cyst.

Infectious and Inflammatory Disorders

Preseptal and Postseptal Cellulitis; Orbital Subperiosteal Abscess

Orbital infection is common in children and usually results from acute complicated paranasal sinus infection. Orbital involvement occurs from direct extension via infected intervening bone or via emissary veins (Fig. 3.20), or because of complications of sinusitis such as a ruptured mucocele or mucopyocele (Fig. 3.21). Other sources include trauma, extension of facial or dental infection (Fig. 3.22), and, rarely, hematogenous spread from systemic infection.[30] Infection is most often bacterial in origin, with *Staphylococcus*, *Streptococcus*, and *Pneumococcus* being the primary causative agents.[71,72] Invasive fungal sinusitis can also spread to the orbit, especially in immunocompromised pediatric patients, primarily because of *Mucor* and *Aspergillus*. When infection affects only structures anterior to the orbital septum (skin, eyelids), it is termed preseptal (periorbital) cellulitis. When infection affects structures posterior to the septum, it is termed postseptal (orbital) cellulitis.

Pediatric patients with preseptal cellulitis typically present with rapid-onset soft tissue swelling and erythema, with or without pain, epiphora, and blurred vision. On imaging, there is diffuse soft tissue thickening of the skin and eyelids with adjacent fat stranding. The orbital septum tends to prevent postseptal spread of infection unless there is initiating sinus infection. The clinician should be alerted to sinus opacification, foreign object, or dental infection as a potential source of infection.

Postseptal cellulitis usually results from initiating bacterial sinus infection. Affected pediatric patients typically present with lid edema, proptosis, chemosis, and, if severe, impaired ocular motility. Postseptal extraconal cellulitis or phlegmonous change with or without subperiosteal abscess typically occurs in proximity to the infected sinus and thus occurs medially with ethmoid sinusitis (Fig. 3.20), inferiorly with maxillary antral sinusitis, and superiorly with frontal sinusitis. Contrast-enhanced CT demonstrates hazy increased density of the extraconal fat, with enlargement of extraocular muscles adjacent to extraconal cellulitis/phlegmon. Subperiosteal abscess appears as a low-attenuation, peripherally enhancing elliptical collection. Bone destruction, consistent with osteomyelitis, is sometimes seen. Spread of infection to the intraconal compartment results in orbital cellulitis with stranding of the intraconal fat. Dacryocystitis and dacryoadenitis can complicate or cause orbital infection.

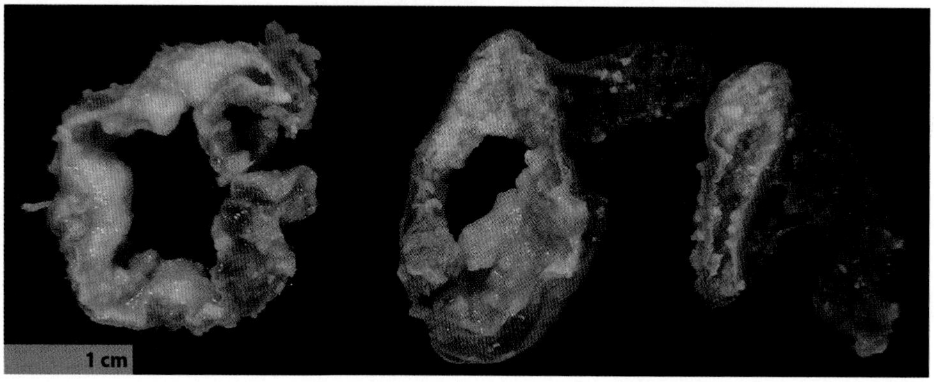

FIGURE 3.19 **Dermoid cyst in a 15-year-old girl.** This dermoid cyst was resected from the floor of the mouth. The cyst was filled with yellow cheesy material, much of which remained stuck to the lining after sectioning. These contents are derived from the keratin debris and sebaceous secretions of the cyst wall, which show a squamous epithelial lining containing adnexal structures (not pictured).

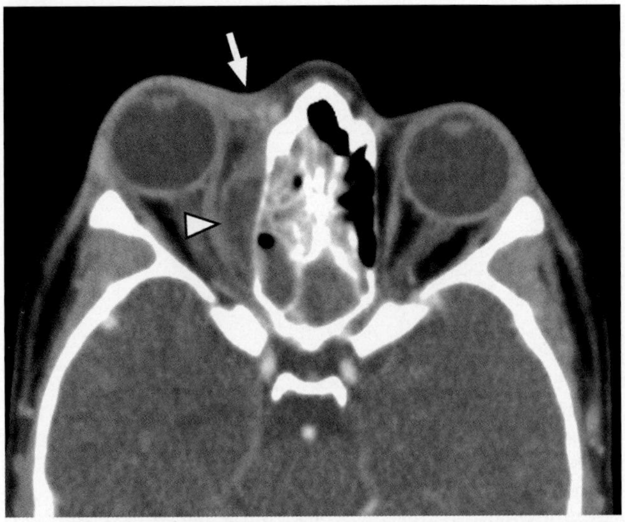

FIGURE 3.20 **Orbital/periorbital cellulitis and subperiosteal abscess secondary to sinusitis.** Axial contrast-enhanced CT image demonstrates ethmoid sinus opacification. There is a subperiosteal abscess (*arrowhead*) laterally displacing orbital contents and causing proptosis, and soft tissue thickening in the preseptal space (*arrow*).

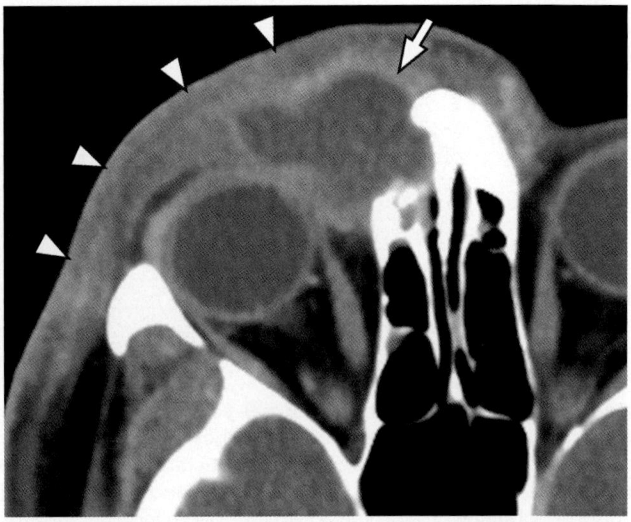

FIGURE 3.21 **Ruptured mucopyocele causing periorbital cellulitis.** Axial contrast-enhanced CT image shows a frontal ethmoid mucocele (*arrow*) that has expanded into the periorbital and orbital region and ruptured, leading to spread of infection to the preseptal/periorbital space (*arrowheads*).

Invasive fungal sinusitis with spread to the orbits is seen predominantly in immunocompromised pediatric patients, with a high mortality of 50% to 80%.[73] The responsible pathogens include Zygomycetes (e.g., *Rhizomucor* and *Mucor*) and *Aspergillus* species. The fungal organisms spread aggressively, with angioinvasion, bone invasion leading to bony destruction visible on CT, and hematogenous dissemination. Tuberculous infection is an important diagnostic consideration for destructive inflammatory sinonasal and orbital disease in endemic areas.

The most frequent vascular complication of orbital infection is thrombosis of the superior ophthalmic vein,[9] which fails to enhance normally on contrast-enhanced CT or MR producing the "tram track" sign. Occasionally, severe postseptal cellulitis with significant infiltration and inflammation of the orbital fat and proptosis causes stretching and, rarely, vascular compromise of the optic nerve.

Complications of postseptal infection include osteomyelitis, epidural abscess, subdural empyema (Fig. 3.23), meningitis, cerebritis, parenchymal abscess, and cavernous sinus thrombophlebitis/thrombosis (Fig. 3.24). MRI is used to detect intracranial complications and osteomyelitis with T2-weighted fat-suppressed MR images, contrast-enhanced T1-weighted fat-suppressed MR images, DWI, and MRV. Rarely, steno-occlusive intracranial arterial complications occur, particularly in the presence of suppurative change and/or thrombophlebitis in the cavernous sinus.

Early treatment consists of appropriate antibiotics and, if necessary, surgical drainage of any abscess or obstructed sinus.

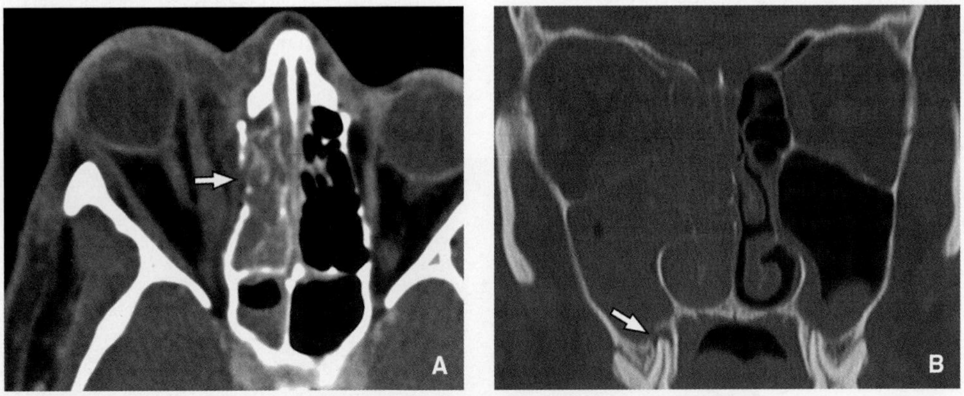

FIGURE 3.22 **Odontogenic sinus infection leading to orbital/periorbital cellulitis. A:** Axial CT image demonstrates extensive ethmoid and sphenoid sinus disease, which spread through the dehiscent lamina papyracea (*arrow* in **A**) into the orbit. **B:** Coronal CT image shows the source of the sinus infection. There is a periapical abscess around the root of a molar that has a dehiscent bony covering (*arrow* in **B**), rendering the abscess contents contiguous with the maxillary antrum. This is also the case on the left side, but there is milder left maxillary sinus disease.

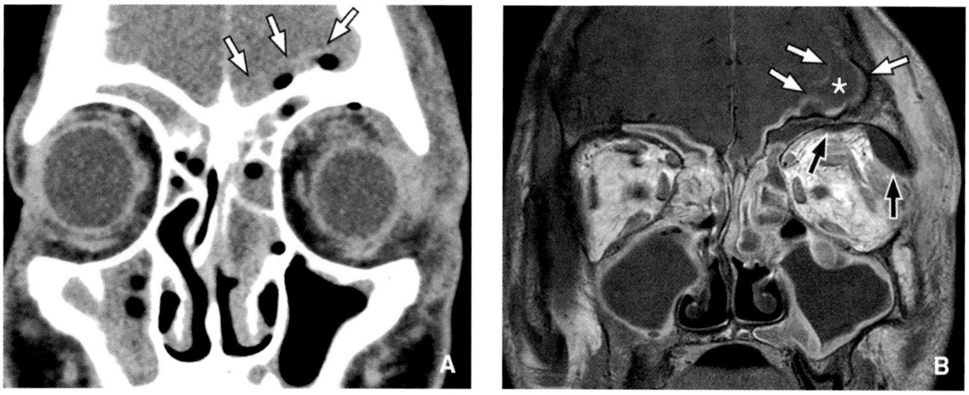

FIGURE 3.23 **Subdural empyema as a result of orbital cellulitis and sinusitis. A:** Coronal CT image shows extensive pansinus inflammation and orbital cellulitis. Foci of gas in the anterior cranial fossa indicate spread of infection intracranially. A dense subdural empyema is seen (*arrows* in **A**). **B:** Coronal contrast-enhanced T1-weighted MR image demonstrates to greater advantage the subdural empyema with rim enhancement (*white arrows* in **B**) and orbital abscesses (*black arrows*). There is also a small subfrontal epidural abscess (*asterisk*).

Idiopathic Orbital Inflammatory Syndrome

Idiopathic orbital inflammatory syndrome (IOIS), commonly referred to as orbital pseudotumor, is a nongranulomatous noninfectious benign inflammatory disease of the orbit with no identifiable cause, responsive to steroid therapy.

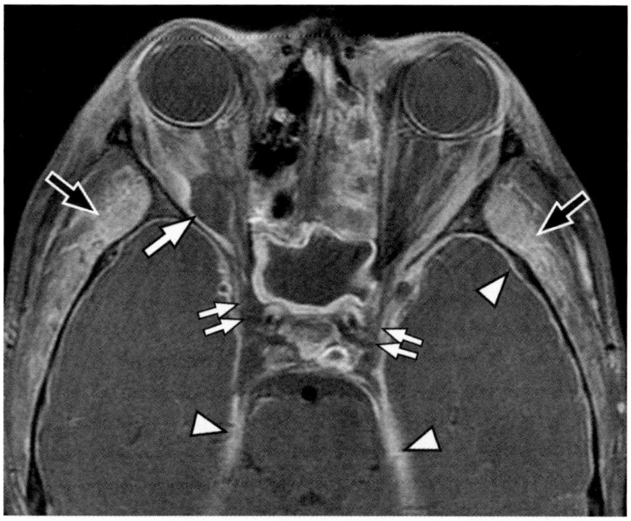

FIGURE 3.24 **Sinusitis, orbital cellulitis and abscess, and bilateral cavernous sinus thrombosis.** Axial postcontrast T1-weighted fat-suppressed MR image shows ethmoid and sphenoid sinus inflammation and fluid, hazy enhancement in the orbital fat from orbital cellulitis, enhancement of the extraocular muscles compatible with myositis, and a focal orbital abscess (*white arrow*) on the right. In addition, there is expansion and nonenhancement of the cavernous sinus (*small paired arrows*), especially on the right, compatible with cavernous sinus thrombosis. There is narrowing of the internal carotid artery flow voids. Tentorial and dural enhancement is related to pachymeningitis (*arrowheads*), and enhancement of the temporalis muscles represents myositis (*black arrows*). This was a 14-year-old boy with a 3-week history of upper respiratory infection and headaches, diagnosed with sinusitis. This progressed to worsening fever, headache, and right eye swelling associated with vision loss. He eventually underwent ethmoidectomy and orbital decompression and was placed on antibiotic and anticoagulation therapy.

IOIS is rare in children.[74] Affected pediatric patients present with pain, swelling, erythema, proptosis, and/or diplopia. The classic finding is "painful ophthalmoplegia." Vision may be impaired if there is optic nerve involvement. Iritis and papillitis are more commonly seen in children than in adults. IOIS is bilateral in up to one-third of pediatric cases without an identifiable underlying systemic condition.[75] This is a diagnosis of exclusion, based on clinical history, disease course, and response to steroids. Histologically, there is an inflammatory/lymphoid infiltrate of orbital tissues acutely; in the subacute or chronic phase, fibroblasts and fibrosis are seen. However, biopsy is rarely performed as the diagnosis can usually be made clinically.

IOIS may be classified according to the primary site of involvement: anterior or diffuse orbital inflammation, orbital myositis, perineuritis and periscleritis, lacrimal adenitis, and apical orbital inflammation (Fig. 3.25). The mass-like

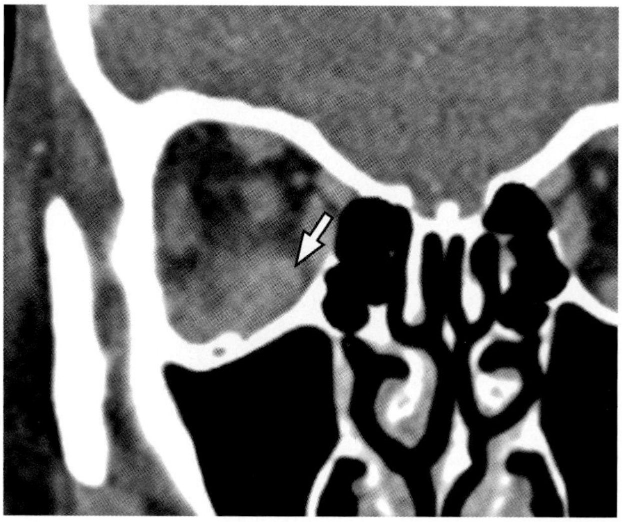

FIGURE 3.25 **Idiopathic orbital inflammatory syndrome (IOIS) in a 17-year-old girl who presented with right orbital pain.** Coronal CT image demonstrates infiltration of the orbital fat and enlargement of the inferior rectus muscle with hazy margins (*arrow*).

manifestation of IOIS is also referred to as "inflammatory pseudotumor." Painful external ophthalmoplegia, also known as Tolosa-Hunt syndrome, is considered a variant of IOIS that involves the orbital apex, superior orbital fissure, and cavernous sinus (Fig. 3.26). The radiographic differential diagnosis of Tolosa-Hunt syndrome includes fungal infection, sarcoidosis, lymphoma, and meningioma.

On CT, depending on the site of involvement, IOIS may be characterized by preseptal soft tissue thickening and edema, orbital fat stranding, an enhancing orbital mass, enlargement of the extraocular muscles including their tendinous insertions, thickening of and stranding around the posterior globe or optic nerve sheath complex, enlargement and enhancement of the lacrimal gland, or soft tissue fullness in the orbital apex and cavernous sinus. MRI is helpful for evaluation of the cavernous sinus region for abnormal enhancement or mass lesions.[76]

Differential diagnosis is broad, because IOIS can affect any structure in the orbit and may be diffuse or mass-like. Orbital cellulitis, neoplasms including lymphoma and leukemia, sarcoidosis (Fig. 3.27), granulomatosis with polyangiitis (Wegener granulomatosis) (Fig. 3.28), and other granulomatous diseases may have similar imaging appearance. In a child, biopsy should be considered if there is an atypical clinical course, if the abnormality is refractory to steroid therapy, or if localized involvement raises the possibility of a malignancy such as lymphoma or rhabdomyosarcoma (RMS).[74]

After infection and other local and systemic causes have been excluded, systemic steroid therapy with a slow taper may be initiated and is considered first-line treatment.[77] Recurrence of symptoms with steroid withdrawal is unusual in the pediatric population.[78]

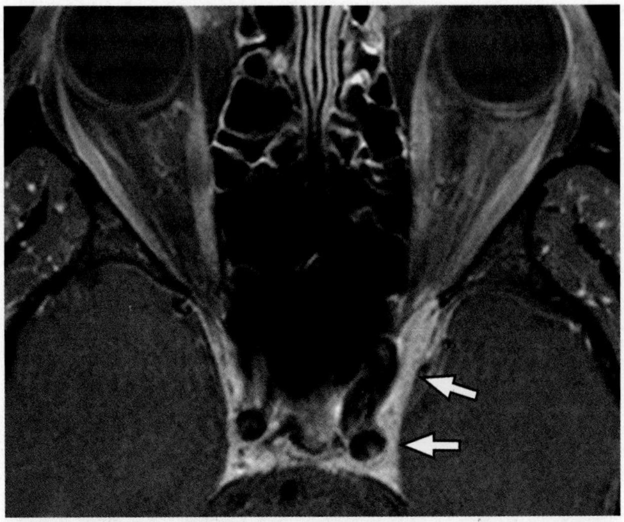

FIGURE 3.26 **Tolosa-Hunt syndrome.** Axial postcontrast T1-weighted fat-suppressed MR image shows thickening and enhancement in the left orbital apex and cavernous sinus (*arrows*). The patient presented with binocular diplopia. Physical examination revealed left third and sixth nerve palsies, Horner syndrome, and pain in the V1 and V2 distribution, indicating pathology involving the left cavernous sinus.

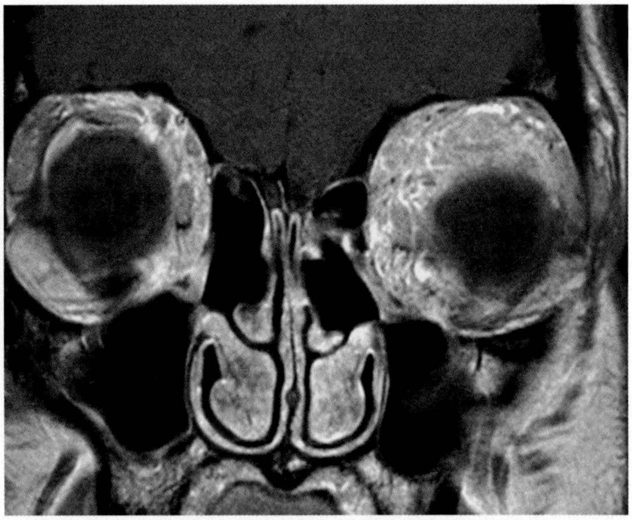

FIGURE 3.27 **Orbital sarcoidosis.** Coronal postcontrat T1-weighted MR image shows ill-defined enhancing soft-tissue in the superior left orbit, causing inferior displacement of the globe. The appearance is nonspecific. This area was biopsied, and pathology revealed noncaseating granulomas compatible with sarcoidosis.

Other Inflammatory Disorders

Chorioretinitis is inflammation of the posterior uvea of the globe. It is usually caused by congenital (TORCH) infections, with cytomegalovirus and congenital toxocara being the most common pathogens in the neonatal age group. On imaging, the vitreous may appear hyperdense on CT and hyperintense on MRI, without a discrete mass.

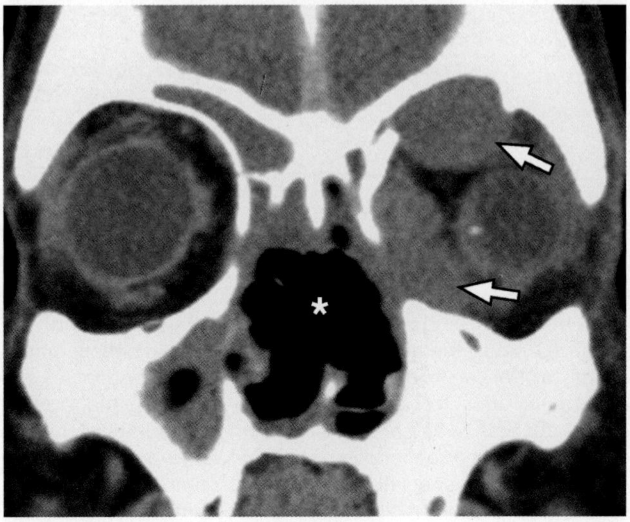

FIGURE 3.28 **Orbital granulomatosis with polyangiitis (Wegener granulomatosis).** Coronal CT image demonstrates soft tissue masses (*arrows*) in the left orbit that are nonspecific in appearance and could be inflammatory, infectious, or neoplastic in etiology. However, note destruction of the nasal septum (*asterisk*), which is compatible with granulomatosis with polyangiitis, that results from a vasculitic, necrotizing, and inflammatory process leading to necrosis of the septum and "saddle-nose deformity."

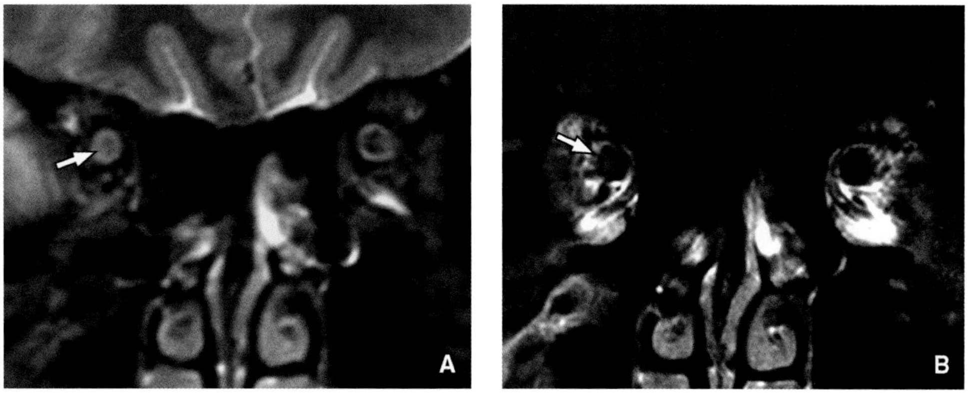

FIGURE 3.29 **Optic neuritis from multiple sclerosis (MS). A:** Coronal T2-weighted fat-suppressed MR image demonstrates abnormally increased signal in the right optic nerve (*arrow* in **A**). Optic nerves should be isointense to white matter on all sequences, because they are essentially extensions of white matter. **B:** Coronal postcontrast T1-weighted MR image demonstrates abnormal enhancement of the right optic nerve (*arrow* in **B**).

Ocular toxocariasis occurs as an intraocular inflammatory response to the death of the larva of the nematode *Toxocara canis*, sometimes leading to sclerosing endophthalmitis. It is usually unilateral and seen in older children.[14] CT findings include homogeneous vitreal density corresponding to a detached retina, organized vitreous, and inflammatory subretinal exudate, similar in appearance to Coats disease and noncalcified retinoblastoma. On MRI, there is variable hyperintensity on T1- and T2-weighted images.

Optic neuritis is not uncommon in children. It is diagnosed using the same clinical criteria used in adults, including subacute vision loss, pain with eye movement, visual field deficits, and a relative afferent pupillary defect. In contrast to adults, children with optic neuritis more frequently have bilateral involvement, profound vision loss, and prominent disc swelling. Etiologies include viral, postviral, granulomatous, postradiation, posttraumatic, demyelinating (Fig. 3.29), neoplastic (e.g., leukemia), and unknown underlying processes.[29] On imaging, the optic nerve appears hyperintense relative to normal white matter on T2-weighted MR images, is variably swollen, and enhances. In one series, the authors found that the risk of multiple sclerosis after a first episode of optic neuritis in children is increased if one or more white matter lesion is seen on a brain MRI performed at the time of initial presentation. None of the patients in their series with a negative brain MRI at presentation were diagnosed with MS for the duration that they were followed (88.5 months).[79] The differential diagnosis includes neuromyelitis optica, in which optic neuritis, hypothalamic signal abnormality, and long-segment spinal cord involvement are MRI features.

Thyroid-Associated Orbitopathy

Graves disease is uncommon in children, and only a minority of pediatric patients have prominent ophthalmic manifestations,[80] termed thyroid-associated orbitopathy (TAO), Graves ophthalmopathy, dysthyroid orbitopathy, or thyroid eye disease, where there is deposition of glycosaminoglycan and fibrosis of the extraocular muscles, and adipogenesis in the orbit.[81]

On imaging, one may see increase in orbital fat, enlargement of the extraocular muscles relatively sparing the tendinous insertions, hypodensity in the muscles (Fig. 3.30), and crowding of the optic nerve at the orbital apex. The inferior and medial rectus muscles are most commonly involved.[30] Coronal images are best for assessing the extraocular muscles, orbital fat, and bony orbital walls for evidence of remodeling. Compressive optic neuropathy at the orbital apex can occur in pediatric patients with significant muscle enlargement. The differential diagnosis for extraocular muscle enlargement includes TAO, IOIS (muscle form), infectious myositis, dural arteriovenous fistula, carotid cavernous fistula, lymphoma/leukemia, metastasis, and acromegaly.[30]

Neoplastic Disorders

Retinoblastoma

Retinoblastoma (RB), a malignant tumor of the immature retina, is the most common primary intraocular tumor in children (80% of all primary ocular cancers), and the third most common intraocular tumor in all age groups. It occurs

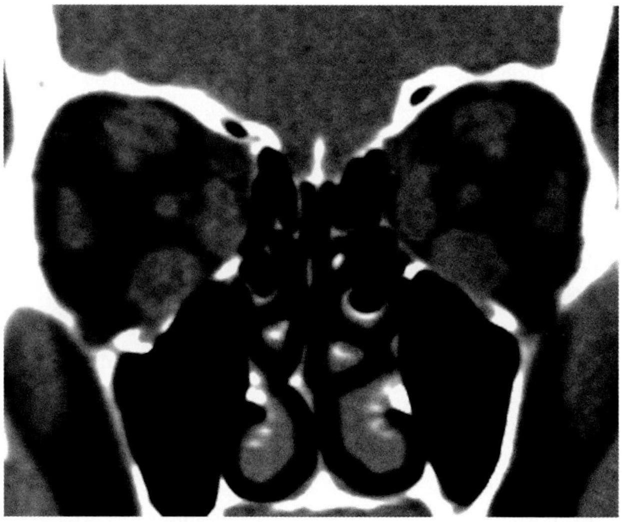

FIGURE 3.30 **Thyroid-associated orbitopathy.** Coronal CT image demonstrates enlargement of all the extraocular muscles and hypodensity in the muscles from glycosaminoglycan deposition.

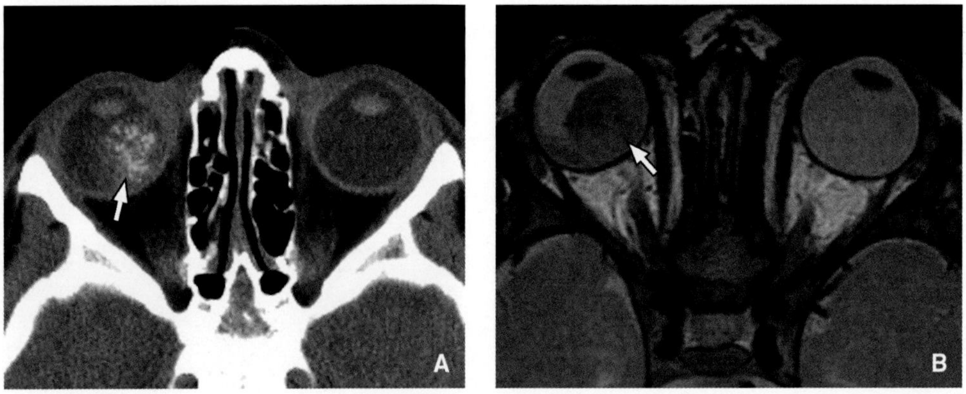

FIGURE 3.31 **Retinoblastoma. A:** Axial CT image demonstrates a soft tissue mass (*arrow*) in the posterior right globe with calcification within it. **B:** Axial T2-weighted fat-suppressed MR image in a different patient reveals a large hypointense right intraocular soft tissue mass (*arrow*).

in infancy, even in utero, with 95% of cases occurring before age 5 years.[82] RB is rarely seen in older children.[83] Tumors may show an endophytic growth pattern, with tumor growing toward the vitreous; it may have an exophytic growth pattern with tumor in the subretinal space, causing an overlying retinal detachment; or it may have a mixed growth pattern. A diffuse infiltrating, plaque-like form occurs less commonly, where the tumor is flat on the surface or beneath the retina, with no obvious mass or calcifications.[83]

RB develops as a result of a "two-hit" oncogenic mutation involving the *Rb1* tumor suppressor gene, occurring between the 3rd month postconception and age 4 years, when retinoblasts are maturing. Both copies of the *Rb1* gene have to be mutated for retinoblastoma to develop. In the familial form (40% of cases, autosomal dominant transmission), all germ cells have an existing mutation of one copy of the gene; tumor develops when the second copy mutates. In the sporadic form, the germ cells are normal, and the somatic retinal cell acquires mutations in both copies of the *Rb1* gene.[84] Affected pediatric patients with the familial form are more likely to have bilateral disease and multiple tumors. The average age of presentation is 7 months for bilateral cases and 24 months for unilateral cases.[85] In pediatric patients with familial RB, second primaries include soft tissue sarcomas, osteosarcomas, carcinomas, CNS tumors, leukemias, uterine sarcomas, lung cancers, and skin cancers. In these patients, the second primary is a greater cause of death than the RB itself.[86,87] Radiation exposure greatly increases the risk of development of a second primary, particularly if occurring before age 1 year.[88] For this reason, CT is no longer recommended for imaging RB.

RB is a major diagnostic consideration in a child presenting with leukocoria, the most common presenting sign (60%), but it is a late sign, with high survival rate but low rate of globe salvage. Strabismus at presentation (20%) is considered an early sign with high survival rate and higher chance of globe salvage.

MRI is used for diagnosis, staging, and treatment monitoring.[22] A combination of ophthalmoscopy, US, and MRI with gradient echo sequences has been shown to effectively detect calcifications. When intraocular calcification within a normal-sized or enlarged globe is present in a young child, RB must be suspected, as very few other simulating lesions contain calcification.[89] The calcific foci are variable in size and number (Fig. 3.31A). The diffuse infiltrating plaque-like form, however, may have very little calcification. The tumor itself appears mildly to moderately hyperintense to vitreous on T1-weighted sequence and hypointense on T2-weighted sequence (Fig. 3.31B). Calcifications appear hypointense on MRI, especially on gradient echo T2-weighted and FSE T2-weighted sequences. There is generally moderate to significant tumoral enhancement.

Optic nerve invasion and orbital invasion increase the risk of metastatic disease.[90,91] Massive choroidal invasion is considered the only other risk factor.[92,93] With orbital extension, tumor can disseminate or extend intracranially. It is therefore important to include imaging of the entire orbit and the brain to evaluate for tumor spread.

Trilateral retinoblastoma refers to a primary midline intracranial tumor, usually in the pituitary or pineal region, in the presence of bilateral retinoblastoma (Fig. 3.32). When there are two midline tumors, the term quadrilateral retinoblastoma is sometimes used.[82]

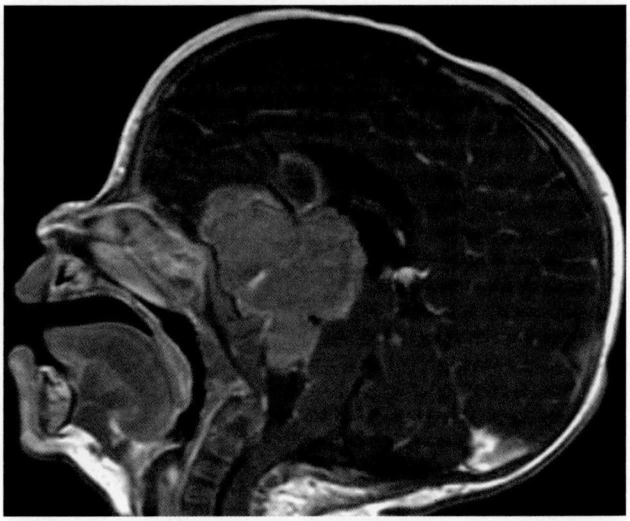

FIGURE 3.32 **Trilateral retinoblastoma in a 2-year-old girl.** Sagittal postcontrast T1-weighted MR image shows a large pituitary tumor in this child who has bilateral retinoblastoma (not shown).

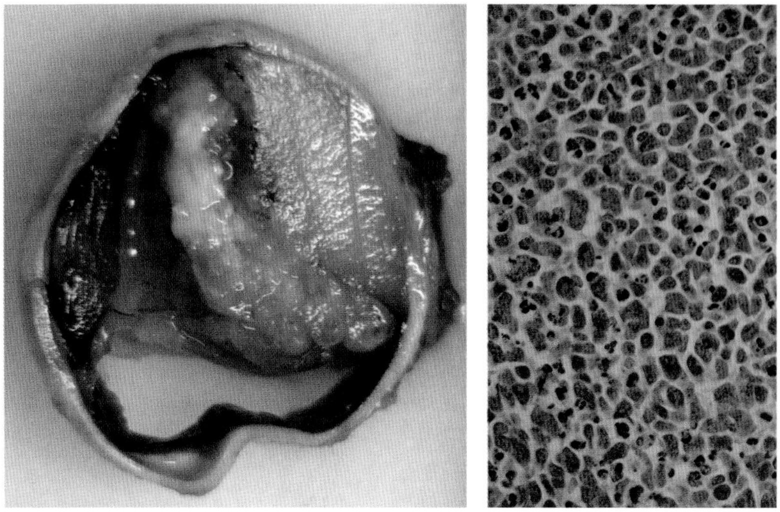

FIGURE 3.33 **Retinoblastoma.** Retinoblastoma, forming a white-gray mass extending from the retina into the vitreous **(left)**; microscopically, the tumor shows poorly differentiated cells with frequent mitotic and apoptotic figures indicating a rapid cell turnover (**right**; hematoxylin and eosin, original magnification, 600×).

Grossly, retinoblastoma is characterized in its early stages by a white-gray nodule on the retina. Later, growth can extend through the retina causing detachment, and involve the vitreous humor. Microscopically, the tumor shows poorly differentiated cells with high nucleus-to-cytoplasm ratios, frequent mitotic figures, and frequent apoptotic cells (Fig. 3.33).

Treatment is best determined by a multidisciplinary team. Options include enucleation, cryoablation, laser photocoagulation, and chemothermotherapy.

Rhabdomyosarcoma

RMS is the most common primary nonocular orbital malignancy in children.[29] RMS accounts for ~50% of all pediatric soft tissue sarcomas and 15% of all pediatric solid tumors. Just over one-third of all RMSs are seen in the head and neck region, with the most common locations being the orbit (Fig. 3.34), masticator space, and paranasal sinuses (Fig. 3.35).[26,29,45,58,68] For orbital RMS, the average age at diagnosis is 7 to 8 years, but it can be seen in older patients. In data collected by the Surveillance, Epidemiology, and End Results (SEER) program, the 5-year survival was found to be highest in children aged 1 to 4 years (77%) and worst in infants and adolescents (47% and 48%, respectively). Orbital site was the most favorable (86%).[94] In children, the embryonal and alveolar subtypes predominate. Affected pediatric patients usually present with rapid-onset unilateral proptosis and globe displacement.

CT, MRI, and PET–CT are used to evaluate and stage RMS. Imaging of the head, chest, and abdomen is obtained for tumor staging. When the tumor is small, the margins are usually well defined; when large, the mass may have irregular margins and appear infiltrative, with surrounding bone and soft tissue invasion. On CT, it is usually isodense to muscle (Fig. 3.34). On MR, RMS is iso- or hypointense on T1-weighted sequence when compared to the brain.[95] Tumors are of variable signal intensity compared to cerebral cortex and demonstrate decreased diffusivity. Internal hemorrhage is uncommon. The degree of enhancement is variable. CT is used to assess osseous involvement or destruction. MRI is superior for soft tissue delineation, for distinguishing tumor from sinus inflammation, for assessing bone marrow involvement, and for detecting intracranial extension or metastasis. Because there are no orbital lymphatics, nodal metastasis is rare except in very advanced cases.[84]

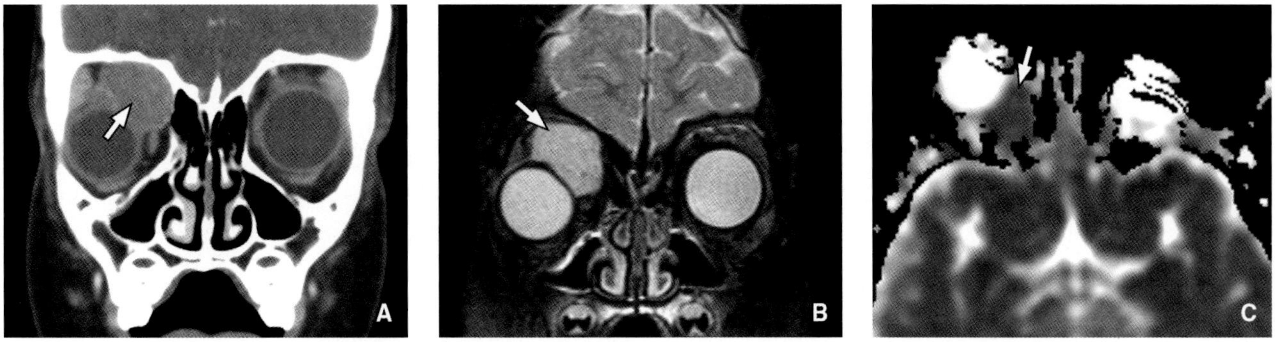

FIGURE 3.34 **Orbital rhabdomyosarcoma, embryonal subtype in a 5-year-old boy with proptosis. A:** Coronal contrast-enhanced CT image reveals a well-circumscribed enhancing mass (*arrow*) located within the superomedial right orbit with inferolateral displacement of the globe. The tumor is located primarily within the extraconal compartment. The superior rectus and superior oblique muscles are indistinguishable from tumor. **B:** Coronal T2-weighted fat-suppressed MR image shows that the tumor (*arrow*) is of lower signal than vitreous but relatively hyperintense compared with cerebral cortex. **C:** ADC map from axial DWI MR image demonstrates the tumor (*arrow*) showing decreased diffusion, attesting to its high grade nature.

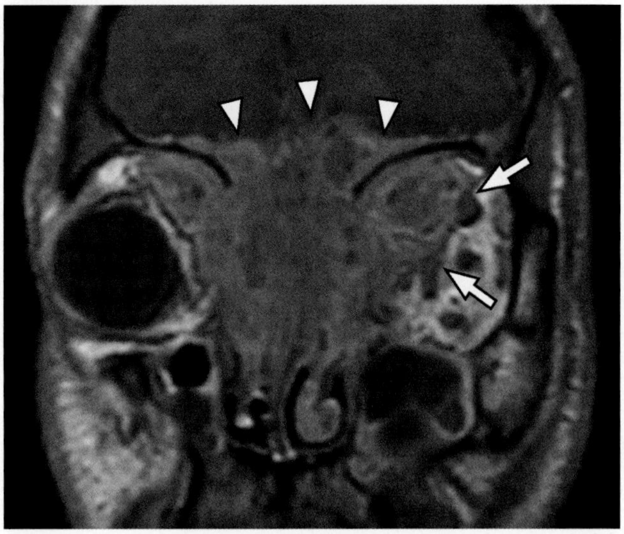

FIGURE 3.35 **Sinonasal rhabdomyosarcoma with orbital extension in a 17-year-old boy who presented with pansinusitis and proptosis.** Coronal postcontrast T1-weighted fat-suppressed MR image shows a large infiltrative mass centered in the nasal cavity and extending into the orbits bilaterally, eroding orbital walls, and displacing and abutting orbital contents such as the extraocular muscles (*arrows*). There is also intracranial invasion (*arrowheads*).

Differential diagnosis includes pseudotumor, lymphoma, leukemic infiltration, and metastatic disease. Neuroblastoma is a relatively common cause of orbital metastatic disease, typically in the first decade of life. Unlike RMS, there are usually multiple extraconal tumor masses with lytic permeative destruction of bone and spiculated periosteal reaction. Ultimately, tissue diagnosis is necessary to distinguish RMS from other noninflammatory solitary orbital tumors, with the exception of infantile hemangioma.

Treatment includes surgery, radiation, and/or chemotherapy. Whereas smaller tumors may be completely excised with a 5-year survival of ≥90%, larger more infiltrative tumors usually require postoperative radiation therapy to control residual disease. When there is significant residual tumor, 5-year survival is ≤35%. Combination chemotherapy helps to improve survival.

Neurofibromatosis Type 1–Related Tumors

NF1 is an autosomal dominant disorder resulting from mutation of the neurofibromin gene on chromosome 17q11.2 and characterized by café au lait spots, axillary or inguinal freckles, neurofibromas and plexiform neurofibromas (PNFs), optic nerve gliomas, Lisch nodules in the eye, sphenoid bone dysplasia, and thinning of long bones.[96] Orbital manifestations include orbital neoplasms (the most common of which is optic glioma [Fig. 3.11]), plexiform neurofibromas, orbital osseous dysplasia (Fig. 3.15), and congenital glaucoma.[97]

PNFs are transpatial and infiltrative. They arise from nerve fascicles, tend to grow along nerves, and may involve multiple nerve branches and plexuses, causing significant morbidity. There may be resultant thickening of periorbital soft tissues (Fig. 3.15), enlargement of the bony orbit, and extensive infiltration of the orbital soft tissues.[98] Although they are more often extraconal,[26] intraconal involvement produces increased density of the intraconal fat; enhancing, irregular nodular thickening of the optic nerve sheath complex; and thickening and enhancement of the uveal/scleral layer, believed to represent PNFs of these structures.[98] PNFs have the potential to transform into malignant peripheral nerve sheath tumors (MPNSTs).

Optic pathway gliomas (OPGs) in NF1 are relatively benign and typically occur in children. Considered low-grade astrocytomas, they are distinct from the extremely rare malignant optic gliomas that are typically seen in adults.[99] On imaging, an optic nerve glioma may be fusiform (Figs. 3.11 and 3.36) or exophytic; the nerve itself is enlarged and may be elongated, with kinking or buckling. On MR, the tumor is iso- to hypointense on T1-weighted sequence and iso- to hyperintense on T2-weighted sequence when compared to normal white matter (Figs. 3.11 and 3.36), with variable enhancement.[100]

Of the OPGs that are low-grade astrocytomas, different imaging features have been noted between those associated with NF1 (NF-OPG) and those not associated with NF1 (non–NF-OPG).[101] In pediatric patients with NF-OPG, the most common site of involvement is the optic nerve, the original shape of the optic pathway is preserved, and cystic components are uncommon. In pediatric patients with

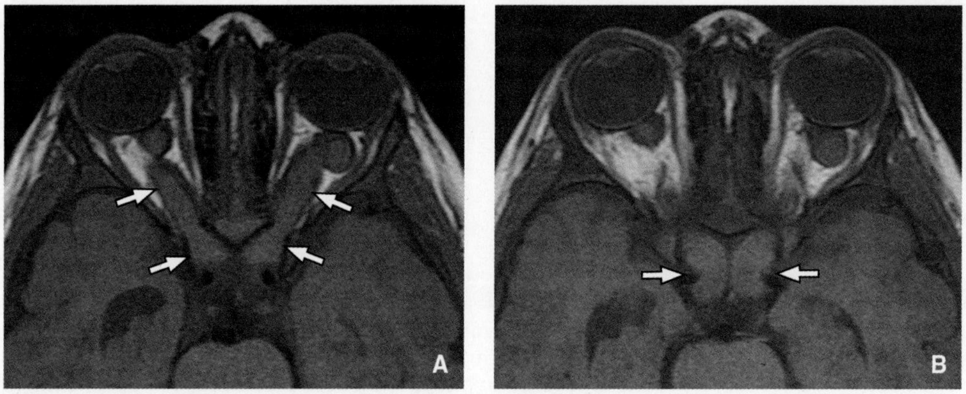

FIGURE 3.36 **Bilateral optic pathway glioma associated with neurofibromatosis type 1 (NF-OPG).** Axial T1-weighted MR images **(A and B)** demonstrate fusiform enlargement of bilateral intraorbital, intracanalicular, and prechiasmatic optic nerves (*arrows* in **A**) with involvement of the optic chiasm and proximal optic tracts (*arrows* in **B**).

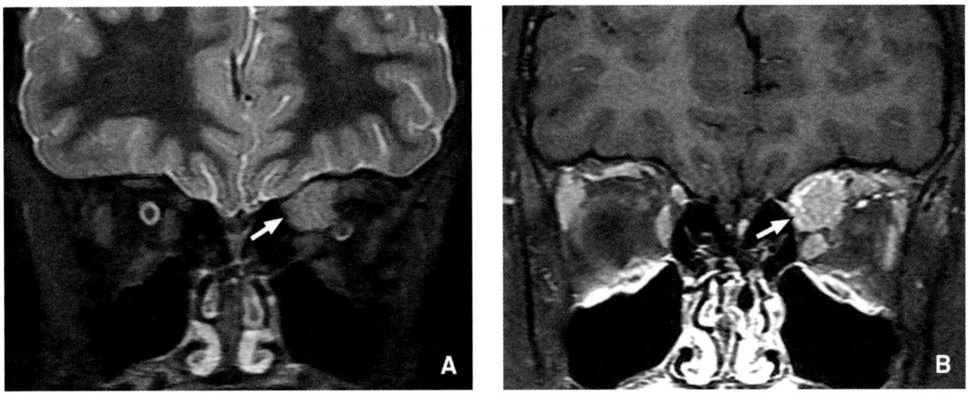

FIGURE 3.37 **Orbital lymphoma in a 9-year-old boy who presented with proptosis. A:** Coronal T2-weighted fat-suppressed MR image shows a homogeneous, hypointense (relative to CSF), left superomedial extraconal mass (*arrow*) involving the left superior oblique muscle. **B:** Coronal postcontrast T1-weighted fat-suppressed MR image shows the homogeneously enhancing mass (*arrow*).

non–NF-OPG, the most common sites of involvement are the chiasm and hypothalamus, the tumor is larger and more mass-like, and cystic components are more common. Pediatric patients with OPG may present with decreased vision or proptosis from mass effect. Additional symptomatology results from intracranial tumor. The differential diagnosis for mild enlargement of the optic nerve without enhancement includes the so-called "NF spot", which is sometimes implicated if the lesion undergoes spontaneous regression.

The prognosis in children with NF-OPG is better than in those with non–NF-OPG, with the tumor often remaining quite stable in imaging appearance over a number of years. The current treatment includes surgery, chemotherapy, and radiation.

Orbital Lymphoma and Leukemia

There is a wide spectrum of orbital lymphoid lesions or lymphoproliferative disorders, ranging from reactive lymphoid hyperplasia to pseudotumor (IOIS) to malignant lymphoma. Reactive lymphoid hyperplasia and orbital lymphoma are essentially indistinguishable from each other on imaging[75] and occur rarely in children. Malignant lymphoma may arise in the orbit, in the sinonasal region with extension into the orbit, or may be a systemic disease that includes an orbital focus. Any orbital structure may be involved, including the lacrimal gland, extraocular muscles, and orbital fat. On MR, lesions have intermediate to low signal on T1-weighted sequences and are isointense to cerebral cortex on T2-weighted sequences, with decreased diffusivity. The globe is rarely deformed by an adjacent lymphoma. Tumors occur in the anterior portion of the orbit, retrobulbar region, or superior orbital compartment (Fig. 3.37).

Leukemia is one of the most common pediatric malignancies and includes acute lymphoblastic leukemia, acute myelogenous leukemia (AML), and chronic myelogenous leukemia.[102] Chronic lymphocytic leukemia is rare in children. Orbital involvement is mainly in the form of deposits of leukemic cells in the bone or soft tissue. These deposits are known as granulocytic sarcomas in the setting of AML, also called chloroma, because of the greenish color of myeloperoxidase on gross examination. Chloromas are usually seen in the subperiosteal region, in the lateral or medial orbital wall (Fig. 3.38). Dural or leptomeningeal disease may be present concurrently.[102]

Differential diagnosis of orbital lymphoma and a focal leukemic deposit includes RMS, Langerhans cell histiocytosis (LCH), and benign lymphoid disorders. The differential diagnosis for diffuse orbital leukemic involvement is metastatic disease, primarily neuroblastoma.

Langerhans Cell Histiocytosis

LCH is a clonal lesion of unknown etiology that is best classified as a neoplasm. LCH is characterized by proliferation and infiltration of abnormal histiocyte-like cells within various tissues. LCH preferentially affects children between the ages of 1 and 4, with disseminated or localized forms of disease that

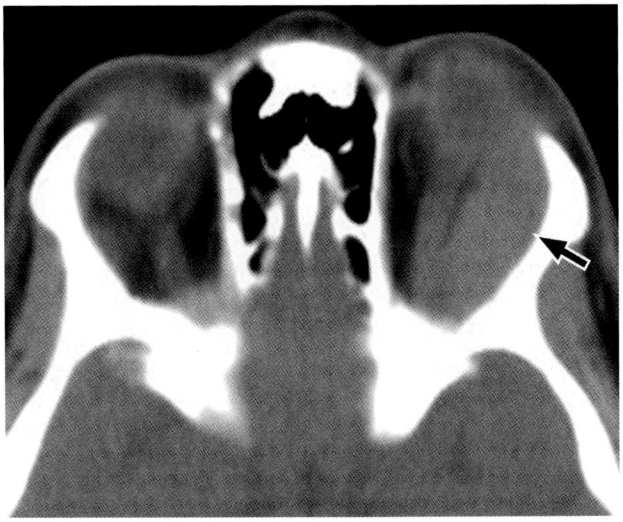

FIGURE 3.38 **Chloroma in the orbit in a 17-year-old girl with a history of acute myelogenous leukema (AML) and chloromas at multiple locations in the body, including the spine and the abdomen.** Axial CT image shows a homogeneous mass (*arrow*) along the lateral orbital wall.

have been variously referred to as Hand-Schüller-Christian disease, Letterer-Siwe disease, and eosinophilic granuloma.[9]

Lesions in children are mostly seen in the bone or bone marrow. Localized orbital involvement is not uncommon. Clinical signs and symptoms include proptosis, edema, erythema, and periorbital pain. Lesions are usually seen in the superior or superolateral orbital wall. Ocular involvement is rare.

On CT, LCH produces sharply defined lytic bone lesions with "punched-out" or beveled margins. On MR imaging, the associated soft tissue mass is of intermediate to low signal intensity relative to cerebral cortex on T2-weighted images with moderate to marked homogeneous or heterogeneous enhancement. There is often intracranial extension, involving the epidural space. Multiple lesions may be seen.[9]

The differential diagnosis for LCH includes ossifying fibroma, giant cell lesion, aneurysmal bone cyst (ABC), lymphoma, and metastasis. Ossifying fibroma is expansile with osseous matrix. Giant cell lesion and ABC are expansile lytic lesions, often with preservation of a thin rim of bone at the margin of the lesion on CT and characteristic fluid–fluid levels on MR.

Vascular Lesions

Orbital vascular lesions include hemangiomas (infantile, congenital, and other), high-flow malformations (arteriovenous malformations [AVMs] and cavernous carotid fistulas [CCFs]), low-flow malformations (venous malformations, lymphatic malformations, and combined malformations), and varices. Only the hemangiomas are considered true neoplasms.[103] The term "cavernous hemangiomas" is a commonly used misnomer for well-encapsulated low-flow venous malformations as determined histopathologically. Vascular malformations and tumors are discussed in detail in other sections of this book. The imaging features of orbital vascular anomalies are briefly discussed and illustrated below.

Infantile Hemangioma

The imaging appearance of infantile hemangiomas depends on the clinical stage. During the proliferative phase, a lobulated, sharply defined, homogeneous, highly vascular soft tissue mass is seen, with intense enhancement. On MRI, proliferating hemangioma is iso- or hypointense to muscle on T1-weighted MR images, moderately hyperintense with vascular flow voids on T2-weighted MR images (Fig. 3.39), and intensely enhancing.[104] During the involuting phase, enhancement and vascularity diminish. After complete involution, a focal region of fibrofatty tissue remains.

A subgroup of patients with infantile hemangiomas has structural anomalies elsewhere in the body, with involvement of the brain, cerebral vasculature, aorta, eyes, and chest wall. In 1978, Pascual-Castroviejo et al., described the association of facial and scalp "hemangiomas" with brain abnormalities, malformations of the extra- and intracranial blood vessels, and congenital heart disease.[105] Subsequently, Frieden et al. coined the acronym "PHACES"[106] denoting the major features of this neurocutaneous association: *p*osterior fossa malformations, *h*emangiomas, *a*rterial anomalies, *c*oarctation of the aorta and cardiac defects, *e*ye abnormalities, and *s*ternal clefting and *s*upraumbilical abdominal raphe. The most common posterior fossa malformation is unilateral cerebellar hypoplasia with a prominent ipsilateral CSF space. Intracranial arterial anomalies include persistent fetal anastomotic connections (e.g., persistent trigeminal artery), aplasia or hypoplasia of the carotid or vertebral arteries, and dilatation and tortuosity of the carotid or cerebral arteries. Steno-occlusive changes with moyamoya collaterals have also been observed.[107] Eye findings include microphthalmia, optic nerve hypoplasia, congenital cataracts, morning glory anomaly, and increased retinal vascularity. The unilateral or bilateral hemangiomas in patients with PHACES tend to be large, regional, and plaque-like, sometimes in a beard-like distribution or in the midline. Therefore,

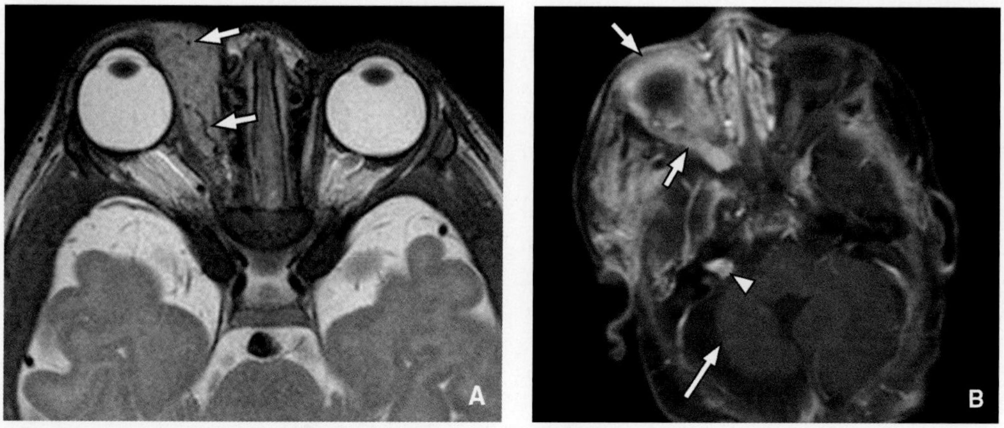

FIGURE 3.39 **Infantile hemangioma in two different pediatric patients. A:** Axial T2-weighted MR image demonstrates a mass in the medial right orbit causing mass effect, displacing the globe laterally and causing proptosis. There are prominent internal flow-voids (*arrows*), which, along with avid homogeneous enhancement (not shown), are diagnostic of a hemangioma. This 2-month-old boy presented with right upper lid swelling that began at age 2 weeks, with the lesion rapidly enlarging over the following weeks. **B:** Axial postcontrast T1-weighted fat-suppressed MR image shows an avidly enhancing preseptal and intraorbital hemangioma (*short arrows*), a large right temporalis muscle hemangioma, and a hemangioma within the right internal auditory canal (*arrowhead*). Note the ipsilateral cerebellar hypoplasia (*long arrow*) in this patient with PHACES association. This 1-month-old boy presented with multiple hemangiomas.

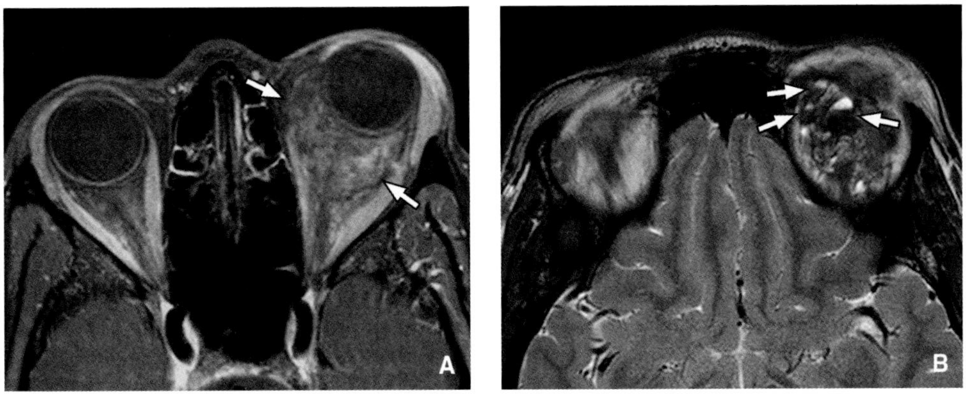

FIGURE 3.40 **Lymphatic malformation. A:** Axial postcontrast T1-weighted fat-suppressed MR image demonstrates a heterogeneous lesion (*arrows*) in the retrobulbar orbit causing proptosis. There are areas of patchy enhancement, corresponding to venous components. **B:** Axial T2-weighted MR image more rostrally shows fluid–fluid levels (*arrows*), characteristic of lymphatic malformations.

pediatric patients with large infantile hemangiomas in the face or head and neck region should undergo brain MRI and MRA to evaluate for PHACES association.[108]

Vascular Malformations

High-flow vascular malformations include AVMs and arteriovenous fistulae (AVF). Low-flow vascular malformations include venous malformations (VMs), lymphatic malformations (LMs), and combined malformations.

VMs are well-defined, transpatial multiloculated cystic masses. The venous lakes typically appear hyperintense on T2-weighted MR images, similar in signal to CSF, with gradual enhancement of the contained venous blood with contrast. The presence of rounded signal voids on MR or calcific foci on CT due to phleboliths is a diagnostic feature of VMs.

Orbital LMs present with proptosis that is sometimes apparent at birth or that manifests subsequently because of rapid enlargement from intercurrent infection or hemorrhage. LMs are typically transpatial lesions. LMs with cysts larger than 1 cm in size are termed macrocystic and are sharply defined. Microcystic LMs consist of small or tiny cysts that are less well defined and sometimes appear more infiltrative. Components of the lesion insinuate within and between normal tissues and structures of the lid and orbit. Cyst contents are hyperintense on T2-weighted MR images unless complicated by hemorrhage, in which case hypointense blood products will be seen. Signal intensity on T1-weighted MR images varies depending on protein content and chronicity of hemorrhage. Macrocystic LMs appear as distinct large locules of fluid spaces separated by enhancing septations. Microcystic LMs may appear to be enhancing without appreciable fluid-filled cystic spaces. Fluid–fluid levels within the cystic spaces related to blood products of various ages are characteristic of LMs (Fig. 3.40).

Many of the orbital low-flow vascular anomalies demonstrate features of both LM and VM and are thus considered combined lesions. Interestingly, these lesions are associated with a significant incidence of intracranial venous anomalies (cavernous malformations and prominent developmental venous anomalies), (Fig. 3.41) and even occasionally AVF.[109]

Orbital AVM and AVF are uncommon high-flow lesions that produce pulsatile proptosis and sometimes a bruit. On imaging, they are characterized by enlarged arterial feeders

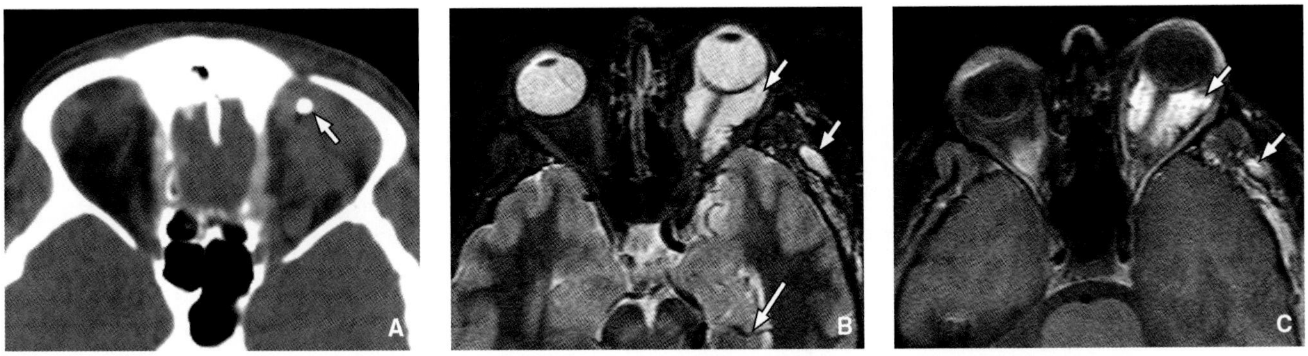

FIGURE 3.41 **Venous malformation (VM) in a 20-year-old woman with multiple venous malformations and a diagnosis of blue rubber bleb nevus syndrome. A:** Axial CT image shows a phlebolith (*arrow*) in the lobulated left orbital mass. **B:** Axial FSEIR image shows hyperintense VMs within the intraconal compartment of the left orbit and within the temporalis muscle and scalp (*short arrows*). Note the associated intracranial developmental venous anomaly (*long arrow*). **C:** The VMs (*arrows*) enhance homogeneously only on delayed postcontrast T1-weighted fat-suppressed MR image acquired several minutes after the administration of contrast.

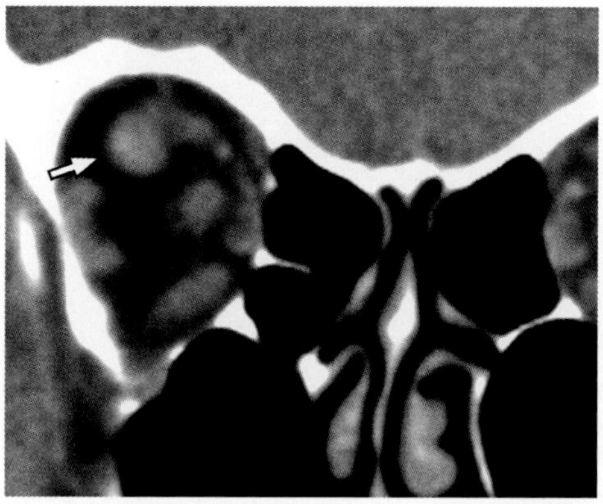

FIGURE 3.42 **Orbital varix.** Coronal contrast-enhanced CT image demonstrates a dilated vascular space that fills with contrast (*arrow*). On axial CT images, this structure can be seen to be contiguous with a vein proximal and distal to it (not shown).

and early draining veins. AVM is distinguished from AVF by the presence of a tangle of small vessels known as a nidus between the feeding and draining vessels.

Orbital Varix

A primary orbital varix presumably occurs as a result of congenital weakness of the venous wall, resulting in dilatation of one or more orbital veins. A tangled mass of venous channels overlaps with the spectrum of VM. With Valsalva maneuver, the varix enlarges and may lead to increased proptosis or globe displacement.[84] Orbital varices may be associated with intracranial vascular anomalies or malformations, including arteriovenous shunts. On CT, calcifications representing phleboliths may be seen. On MR, they are hyperintense on T2-weighted MR images and enhance. Unless thrombosed, they should fill in with contrast at the venous phase (Fig. 3.42).

Cavernous Carotid Fistula

CCF occurs when there is a tear in the cavernous portion of the internal carotid artery, allowing arterial blood to enter the cavernous sinus, leading to increased cavernous sinus pressure and reversal of blood flow in the veins that normally drain into the cavernous sinus. Affected pediatric patients with CCFs present with proptosis, chemosis, pulsating exophthalmos, an auscultable bruit, and/or objective pulsatile tinnitus. On imaging, there is engorgement of the superior ophthalmic vein (Fig. 3.43) and enlargement of the ipsilateral extraocular muscles. Venous thrombosis of the cavernous sinus or superior ophthalmic vein may occur. Mimics of CCF include AVMs and AVFs; isolated dilatation of the superior ophthalmic vein can also occur.[110] Therefore, correlation with clinical history and examination is paramount. Diagnosis of CCF can be confirmed with CTA, MRA, or conventional catheter angiography.

Traumatic Disorders

Orbital injuries can occur from direct blunt or penetrating trauma. Common injuries include traumatic hyphema, globe rupture, vitreous hemorrhage, lens rupture or dislocation, ocular detachments, intraorbital foreign bodies, CCFs, optic nerve injuries, and osseous fractures. Terson syndrome is a vitreous or retinal hemorrhage occurring secondary to a subarachnoid hemorrhage, thought to result from a sudden large increase in intracranial pressure.[111] Retinal hemorrhages are also seen as an important manifestation of inflicted head trauma.

CT is the modality of choice for imaging orbital trauma, demonstrating fractures, hemorrhage, and soft tissue injuries. Radiopaque (e.g., metal) or radiolucent (e.g., wood) foreign objects are also well visualized by CT, whereas MRI is contraindicated if metallic foreign object is suspected. There should be a conscious effort to minimize radiation exposure in children, particularly to the lens, while optimizing the protocol to allow the radiologist to make an accurate diagnosis. CT protocol should consist of thin-section axial scans with multiplanar reformations. US may be useful for evaluating the globe and its contents, but it is contraindicated if there is a possibility of a ruptured globe.[110]

Anterior Chamber Injuries

Traumatic hyphema (posttraumatic bleeding into the anterior compartment) results from disruption of the iris or ciliary body vessels, leading to extravasation of blood into the anterior compartment. On CT, the anterior compartment appears hyperdense. Corneal laceration leads to decreased

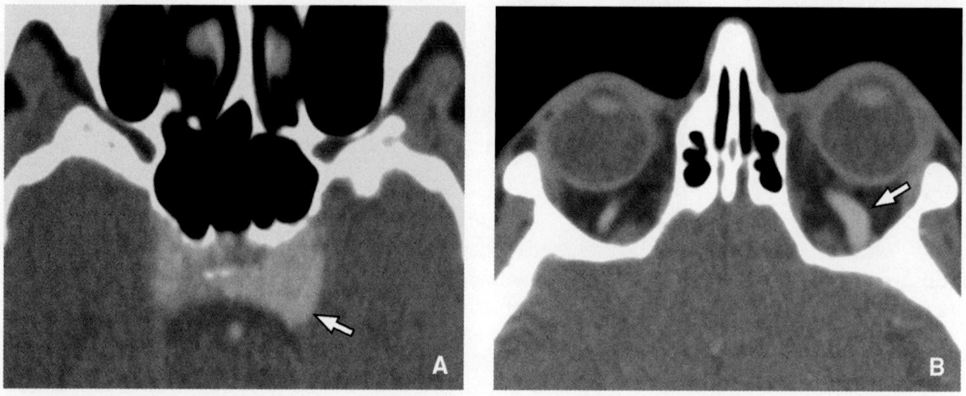

FIGURE 3.43 **Cavernous carotid fistula.** Axial contrast-enhanced CT images demonstrate engorgement of the left cavernous sinus (*arrow* in **A**) and left superior ophthalmic vein (*arrow* in **B**).

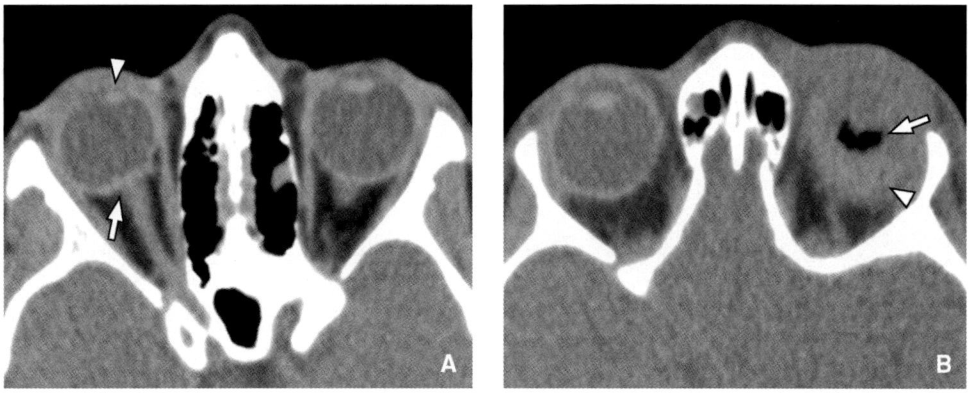

FIGURE 3.44 **Ruptured globe in two different pediatric patients. A:** This patient was a 13-year-old boy who was hit in the eye by glass shards. Axial CT image shows contour deformity to the right globe. The globe is shrunken, with a flattened posterior margin (*arrow*). The lens (*arrowhead*) is also ruptured, appearing foreshortened with loss of the normal biconvex shape. **B:** This 5-year-old girl was sprayed in the eye with a pressure sprayer. Physical examination showed corneal laceration, hyphema, and subconjunctival hemorrhage. Axial CT image demonstrates, intraocular gas (*arrow*) and vitreous hemorrhage (*arrowhead*). The lens is also dislocated, no longer seen in its normal anatomic location.

anterior compartment volume, manifested as decreased anteroposterior dimension of the anterior compartment.

Globe Injuries

Globe rupture, also termed open globe injury, is an ophthalmologic emergency. It is a major cause of blindness, and prompt diagnosis and treatment are crucial to prevent further injury. Unrecognized globe rupture may rarely result in bilateral blindness due to *sympathetic ophthalmia*, a bilateral diffuse granulomatous intraocular inflammation that occurs following unilateral ocular surgery or penetrating trauma.

The injured eye is known as the exciting eye, and the contralateral eye is known as the sympathizing eye.[112] The time from ocular injury to onset of sympathetic ophthalmia ranges from a few days to decades, with 80% occurring within 3 months and 90% within 1 year.[113,114] It is believed to occur as a result of autoimmune inflammatory response to ocular antigens that become exposed to the immune system following loss of globe integrity. Therefore, if the injured globe is nonviable, or if there is little chance of the injured globe regaining visual function following trauma, prompt enucleation may help prevent the occurrence of sympathetic ophthalmia.

On CT, a ruptured globe is suggested by abnormality in the globe contour (Fig. 3.44A), loss of normal globe volume, scleral discontinuity, intraocular gas (Fig. 3.44B), or intraocular foreign objects.[110] Decreased anterior chamber depth suggests an anterior globe laceration. With increased anterior chamber depth, traumatic rupture of the posterior sclera should be suspected. A discontinuity in the posterior sclera allows vitreous to prolapse through the defect, leading to decompression of the vitreous and posterior sagging of the lens.[115] With vitreous hemorrhage, hazy diffuse or mass-like hyperdensity may be seen in the posterior chamber.

Lens Injuries

When there is traumatic deformity of the globe, the zonule fibers of the lens can stretch and tear, resulting in dislocation of the lens. Posterior dislocation is more common than anterior dislocation, in part because the iris prevents the lens from migrating anteriorly. If only some of the fibers are torn, then the lens may remain in position on one side, while angling posteriorly on the opposite side where it projects into the vitreous humor (Fig. 3.45).[110]

With blunt trauma, there may be tearing or rupture of the lens capsule. When that occurs, fluid enters the crystalline lens, normally the least hydrated organ of the body. On CT, therefore, a ruptured lens may retain a relatively normal contour but appear less dense than usual (Fig. 3.46).

Ocular Detachments

There are three main types of detachments in the globe: posterior hyaloid detachment (posterior vitreous detachment), retinal detachment, and choroidal detachment.

In posterior hyaloid detachment, the vitreous body becomes separated from the retina, and vitreous can dissect into the potential space between the posterior hyaloid membrane and the retina.[84] Traction on the retina at points that are still attached increases the risk of subsequent retinal tears and detachment. The detached posterior hyaloid membrane

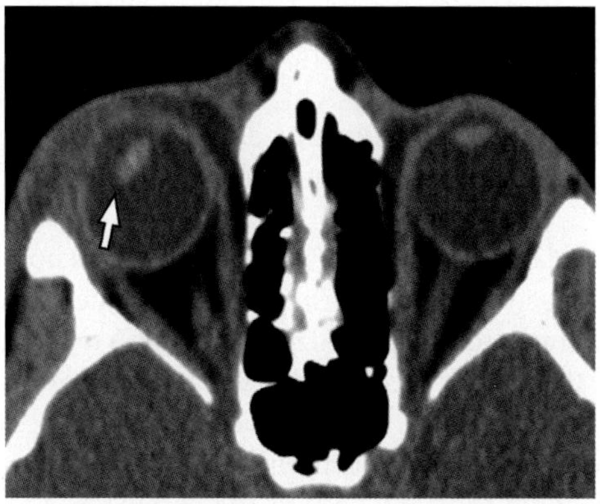

FIGURE 3.45 **Lens dislocation in a 13-year-old boy who was hit in the eye by a paint ball.** Axial CT image shows the lateral portion of the lens dislocated (*arrow*) and angled posteriorly, whereas the medial portion remains anchored.

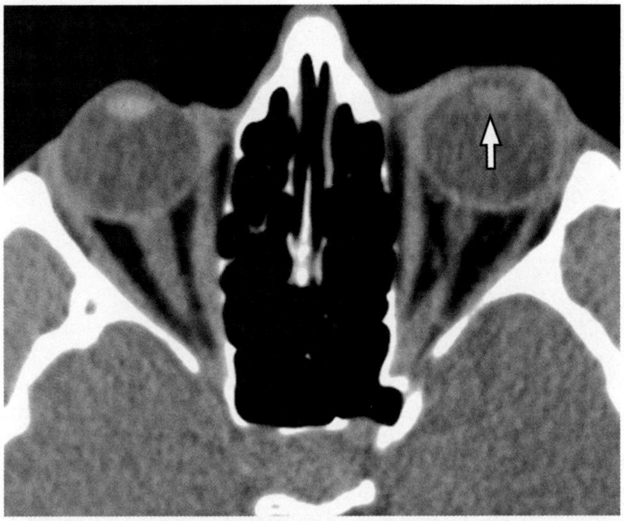

FIGURE 3.46 **Lens rupture in a 9-year-old girl.** Axial CT image demonstrates normal contour of the lenses bilaterally. However, the left lens (*arrow*) is less dense than normal, indicating the presence of fluid that has infiltrated into the lens through a torn capsule.

may be thickened and become visible on imaging. This condition may be seen in children with PHPV.

Retinal detachment is separation of the sensory retina from the retinal pigment epithelium. *Serous* or *exudative detachment* usually occurs as a result of breakdown of the blood–retina barrier due to tumor, inflammation, vasculopathy (e.g., Coats disease), hematologic disorders, or in association with congenital anomalies such as optic nerve colobomas and morning glory syndrome.[116] When there is scarring or another process in the vitreous causing traction of the sensory retina from the pigmented layer, it is referred to as a *traction detachment*. With trauma, there may be subretinal hemorrhage, with or without a tear in the sensory retina. The presence of retinal hemorrhage in a child should raise suspicion for nonaccidental trauma.[110]

The retina is a very thin structure and is not visible per se on imaging. Retinal detachment is diagnosed on imaging based on the difference in appearance of the normal vitreous and fluid accumulated in the subretinal space. The subretinal fluid typically appears homogeneously hyperdense, with a lentiform or V shape, extending from the ciliary body anteriorly to the optic disc posteriorly (Fig. 3.47). If the subretinal fluid happens to be isodense/isointense to vitreous, it may escape imaging detection. US is considered a better modality for imaging retinal detachment than CT or MR.[117]

Choroidal detachment is separation of the choroid from the sclera. Serous or hemorrhagic fluid can then accumulate in the suprachoroidal space. The latter is seen in the setting of trauma; the former occurs in the setting of ocular hypotony, which may result from inflammation, traumatic perforation, or surgery.[110] Suprachoroidal fluid collections appear biconvex, extending from the level of the vortex veins to the ora serrata (Fig. 3.48). Their CT and MR appearance depends on their composition and may be variably dense/intense.

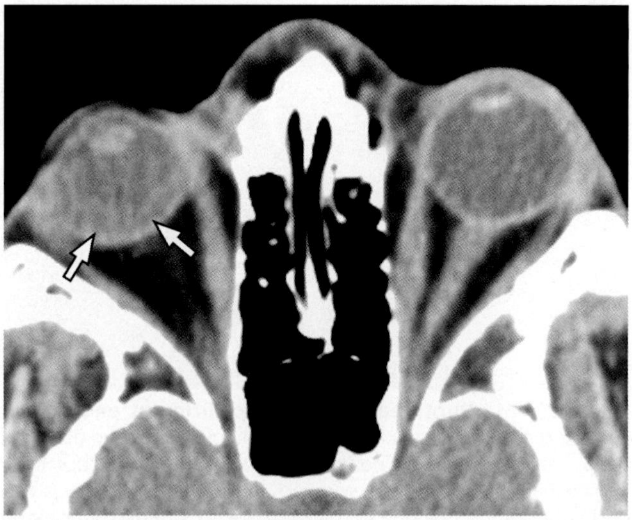

FIGURE 3.47 **Retinal detachment.** Axial CT image demonstrates hyperdense fluid (*arrows*) with a wide V shape in the posterior right globe.

Choroid is thick, and the separated choroid is often visible on CT and MR.

Intraorbital Foreign Objects

MR is absolutely contraindicated if there is any suspicion of a potential intraorbital metallic object, as blindness may result if the patient is subjected to MR scanning because of migration of the object within the magnetic field.

CT is very sensitive for detecting metallic fragments even smaller than 1 mm in size (Fig. 3.49). Glass appears dense on CT but is less reliably detected than metal.[118] Wood appears hypodense and may be mistaken for gas but should have a geometric or linear configuration.

Optic Nerve Injury

The optic nerve can be directly injured in penetrating trauma, by bone fragments causing nerve laceration, or from a nerve sheath hematoma. It can also be indirectly injured from transmission of

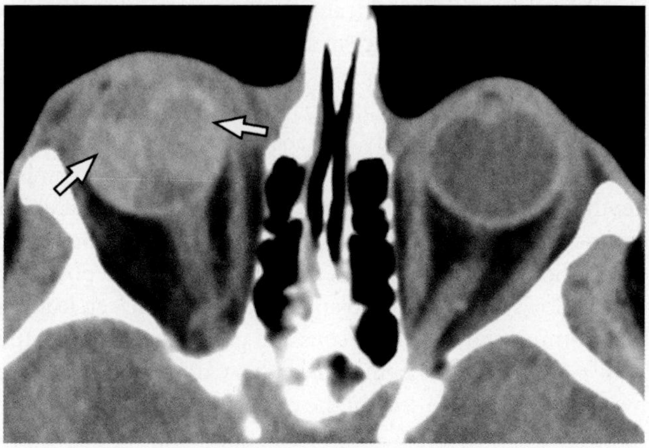

FIGURE 3.48 **Choroidal detachment.** Axial CT image demonstrates biconvex dense fluid collections (*arrows*) on the medial and lateral surfaces of the right globe, not extending to the optic disc.

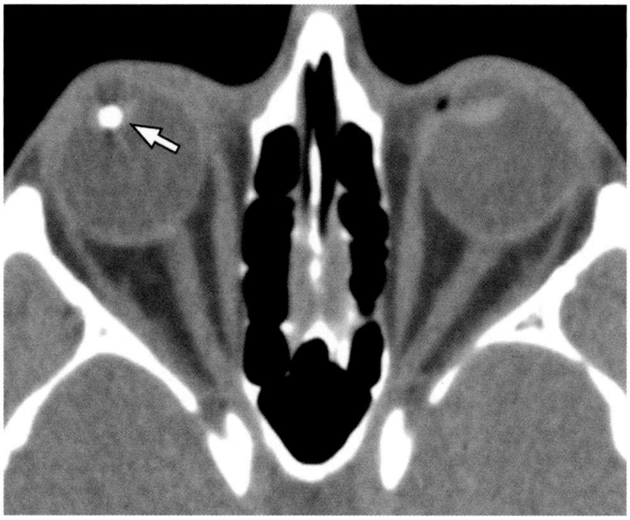

FIGURE 3.49 **Intraocular metallic fragment.** Axial CT image clearly shows a punctate metallic fragment (*arrow*) in the right globe.

forces to the optic nerve following blunt trauma or from vascular compromise. For evaluation of the optic nerve, MRI is necessary, after confirming the absence of any potential intraorbital metallic objects. Normally, the optic nerve should follow white matter signal. If there is disruption of the normal nerve contour, or if there is abnormally hyperintense signal in the optic nerve on T2-weighted sequence, optic nerve injury should be suspected.

FACE, NASAL CAVITY, PARANASAL SINUSES

Embryology and Development

Facial structures develop from several primordia that surround the stomodeum (primitive mouth) at 4 to 5 weeks' gestational age.[119] Between 4 and 8 weeks' gestational age, the nasomedial and maxillary processes fuse to form the upper lip and jaw. The nasomedial processes fuse and give rise to the philtrum of the lip, the premaxillary component of the upper jaw, and the primary palate. The frontonasal prominence gives rise to the forehead, nose, and nasal septum. The maxillary processes form parts of the upper lip, maxilla, and the secondary palate. Between the maxillary process and the nasal primordium is the nasolacrimal groove, which eventually gives rise to the NLD and the lacrimal sac. The bilateral mandibular prominences give rise to the mandible, lower lip, chin, and lower cheek. As basic facial structures are established, mesodermal cells associated with the first and second pharyngeal arches give rise to the muscles of mastication (first arch derivatives, innervated by cranial nerve V) and the muscles of facial expression (second arch derivatives, innervated by cranial nerve VII).

The nasal cavities communicate with the nasopharynx and oral cavity after rupture of the oronasal membrane at the choanae. Turbinates form from the lateral walls of the nasal cavities. Paranasal sinuses form as diverticula of the walls of the nasal cavities and undergo pneumatization after birth.

Normal Anatomy

The nose and paranasal sinuses continue to develop through puberty. The vestibule is the opening to each nasal cavity. The nasal septum consists of cartilage anteroinferiorly and bone (vomer and perpendicular plate of the ethmoid) posterosuperiorly. The superior, middle, and inferior turbinates arise from each lateral nasal wall. Supreme turbinates are variably present in some individuals.

The maxillary and ethmoid sinuses are pneumatized at birth and continue to develop until age 10 to 12 years. The sphenoid sinuses are pneumatized at age 1 to 2 and reach adult size by age 14 years. The frontal sinuses are difficult to distinguish from anterior ethmoid air cells until they become larger and extend above the superior orbital rims at age 8 to 10 years. In some individuals, the frontal sinuses never enlarge and remain nonpneumatized or underpneumatized.

The frontal, anterior and middle ethmoid, and maxillary sinuses drain into the middle meatus via the ostiomeatal complex (OMC). The posterior ethmoid and sphenoid sinuses drain into the sphenoethmoidal recess and superior meatus of the nasal cavity.

Not infrequently, ethmoid air cells expand beyond the confines of the ethmoid bone and encroach into the frontal, maxillary, and sphenoid regions, as well as deep to the lacrimal bone and into the frontal process of the maxilla. These anatomic variants include (1) agger nasi cells—anterior ethmoid air cells pneumatizing the frontal process of the maxilla; (2) supraorbital ethmoid cells—anterior ethmoid air cells pneumatizing the roof of the orbit; (3) Haller cells—infraorbital ethmoid air cells; (4) Onodi cells—posterior ethmoid air cells extending along the sphenoid bone, located superior to the sphenoid sinus and abutting the optic canal; and (5) a posterior ethmoid air cell extending along the maxillary sinus and separated from the maxillary sinus by a bony wall, causing a "double antrum." Variant anatomy must be recognized in order to plan for surgical drainage targeting these particular cells should they be inflamed.

Congenital and Developmental Anomalies

Nasal Obstruction—Complete Nasal Stenosis, Choanal Atresia, Pyriform Aperture Stenosis

Neonates are obligate nose breathers, and obstruction of the nasal passages leads to airway compromise.[120] Congenital causes include pyriform aperture stenosis, nasal cavity stenosis, and choanal stenosis or atresia. Large NLD cysts, craniofacial anomalies, and cephaloceles also cause obstruction. Stenosis of the entire nasal airway is usually bony and may be seen with maxillary hypoplasia.

Choanal atresia is congenital obstruction of the posterior choanae. Incidence has been reported to be between 1 in 5,000 and 1 in 9,000 live births. It is seen more often in females and is more commonly unilateral. Obstruction is invariably bony, with or without a membranous component. Recent literature suggests that mixed bony/membranous choanal atresia occurs in 70% of cases and pure bony obstruction in 30% of cases.[121]

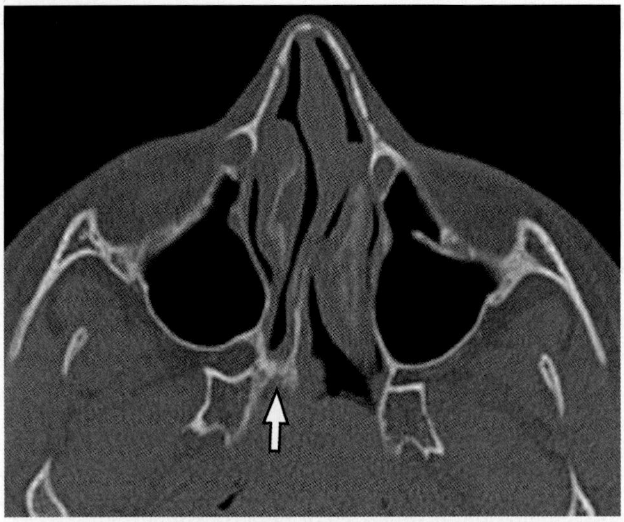

FIGURE 3.50 **Choanal atresia in an 11-year-old boy who presented with chronic sinusitis and obstruction.** Axial bone window CT image demonstrates narrowing of the right posterior choana (*arrow*), with a bony obstruction. The vomer is lateralized (as shown on figure), and the pterygoid plates are medialized (not shown).

There is also medialization of the pterygoid plates and lateral nasal walls (Fig. 3.50).

There are sometimes associated skull base abnormalities or defects.[122] Approximately half of the affected pediatric patients have associated craniofacial anomalies such as CHARGE syndrome. CHARGE is an acronym for *c*oloboma, *h*eart defect, *a*tresia choanae, *r*etarded growth and development, *g*enital hypoplasia, and *e*ar anomalies/deafness. Major criteria (ocular coloboma; choanal atresia; characteristic ear abnormalities—particularly absent or severely hypoplastic semicircular canals (SCCs), hypoplasia of the vestibule, ossicular and other middle ear abnormalities (Fig. 3.51)[123]; cranial nerve hypoplasia/aplasia) and minor criteria (cardiovascular malformations; genital hypoplasia; cleft lip/palate; tracheoesophageal fistula; hypothalamo-hypophyseal dysfunction; distinctive CHARGE facies; developmental delay) have been described. Individuals with all four major characteristics or three out of four major and three out of seven minor characteristics are reported to be highly likely to have CHARGE syndrome.[124]

CT should be performed with the axial plane parallel to the hard palate at the level of the pterygoid plates. CT demonstrates obstruction of the posterior nasal cavity, characterized by medial bowing and thickening of the lateral nasal walls, enlargement of the posterior vomer, and a bony or membranous structure obstructing the choana representing the atretic plate. Bilateral choanal atresia should prompt inspection of the temporal bones for the typical diagnostic inner ear findings of CHARGE syndrome.

Syndromic craniosynostosis, TCS, and other craniofacial syndromes are associated with midnasal cavity stenosis due to midfacial hypoplasia.

Pyriform aperture stenosis is narrowing at the level of the anterior nasal cavity. On CT, there is marked stenosis of the pyriform apertures associated with a triangular morphology of the anterior hard palate. Images should include the maxillary dentition. If there is a single central megaincisor, then there is an association with holoprosencephaly and MR of the brain should be obtained (Fig. 3.52).

Lacrimal Sac Mucocele and Nasolacrimal Duct Mucocele

Lacrimal sac and NLD mucocele is described earlier in the Orbit section. NLD mucocele is common, especially in premature infants, and is an important cause of neonatal nasal obstruction. Most cases resolve spontaneously. Less commonly, pressure buildup may cause the imperforate distal membrane to balloon out into the nasal cavity, leading to an intranasal cystic mass and nasal obstruction. The entire enlarged cystic structure extending from the lacrimal sac to the inferior meatus is referred to as a nasolacrimal mucocele. This is well delineated on CT and MR, which demonstrate a dilated cystic structure at the medial canthal region contiguous with an expanded NLD, terminating in an intranasal submucosal cystic mass that projects beneath the inferior turbinate (Fig. 3.16).

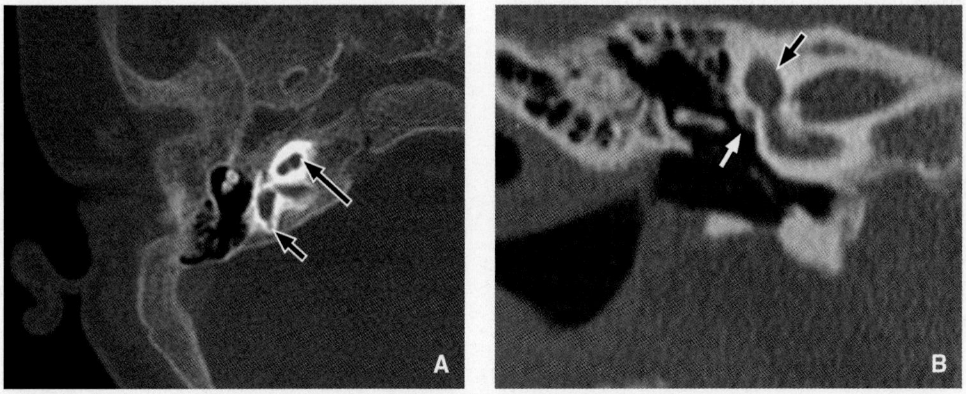

FIGURE 3.51 **Semicircular canal hypoplasia/aplasia in CHARGE association. A:** Axial bone window CT image shows a hypoplastic vestibule with only a rudimentary posterior semicircular canal (SCC) (*short arrow*). The lateral and superior SCCs are absent. There is only a single cochlear turn (*long arrow*), and the cochlear nerve canal is absent, resulting in an "isolated cochlea." **B:** Coronal bone window CT image (different patient) through the middle ear demonstrates oval window stenosis. The tympanic segment of the facial nerve is abnormally inferiorly placed, overlying the stenotic oval window (*white arrow*). The superior semicircular canal is dysplastic, appearing as a bulbous cystic space (*black arrow*). The posterior and lateral semicircular canals were absent and the cochlea formed only 1.5 turns (not pictured).

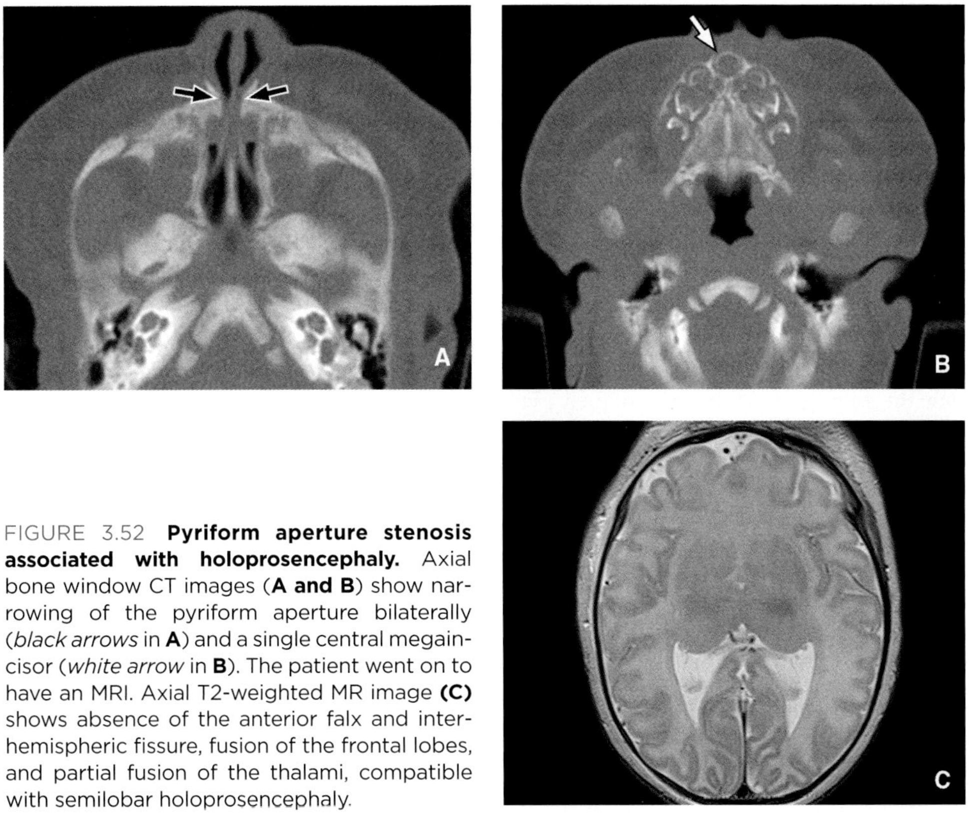

FIGURE 3.52 **Pyriform aperture stenosis associated with holoprosencephaly.** Axial bone window CT images (**A and B**) show narrowing of the pyriform aperture bilaterally (*black arrows* in **A**) and a single central megaincisor (*white arrow* in **B**). The patient went on to have an MRI. Axial T2-weighted MR image **(C)** shows absence of the anterior falx and interhemispheric fissure, fusion of the frontal lobes, and partial fusion of the thalami, compatible with semilobar holoprosencephaly.

Glabellar/Nasal Pit, Dermal Sinus, Dermoid Cyst, Meningoencephalocele, and Nasal Neuroglial Heterotopia

During fetal development, the frontal bone is separated from the nasal bones by a fontanelle called the *fonticulus frontonasalis*. The nasal bones are in turn separated from the underlying cartilaginous nasal capsule by the *prenasal space*. The prenasal space extends up to the base of the brain and down to the nasal tip. Normally, projections of dura around the brain extend through these spaces in the midline and contact the ectoderm, then regress back toward the brain before these spaces are obliterated. By birth, the frontonasal suture is in the location of the obliterated fonticulus frontonasalis, the nasal cartilages and ethmoid bone are in the region of the obliterated prenasal space, and the frontal and ethmoid bones come together around a small ostium at the skull base called the foramen cecum, just anterior to the crista galli. If the embryonic dural projections do not regress properly, anomalies result.

Glabellar/Nasal Pit, Dermal Sinus, and Dermoid Cyst

As the dura regresses, it can bring with it adherent ectoderm, leading to the formation of a dermal tract. The tract can run either (1) from the skin surface of the glabella through the fonticulus frontonasalis (frontonasal suture) toward the foramen cecum or (2) from the skin surface of the nose through the prenasal space (under or through the nasal bones) toward the foramen cecum. Clinical manifestations include cutaneous pits, dermal sinuses, (epi)dermoid cysts, and fibrous cords. Rarely, these sinus tracts, cysts, and cords may extend intracranially and be adherent to the brain. With persistent intracranial communication, recurrent meningitis, abscess, or empyema may result.

Imaging should include the entirety of the potential course of a sinus tract based on embryologic anatomy—the skin surface, nose, and nasal cavity, to the anterior cranial fossa and foramen cecum (Fig. 3.53). The examination of choice is MR, and pulse sequences should include multiplanar thin-section, small field of view, high-resolution T2-weighted

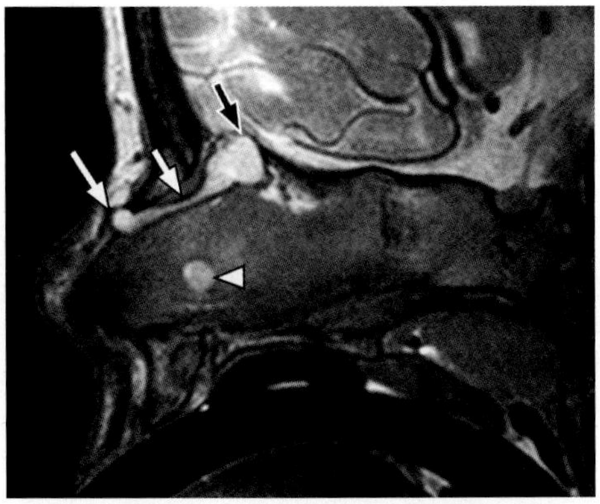

FIGURE 3.53 **Dermoid and dermal sinus (median nasal dermal fistula) in a 9-month-old boy who presented with a small mass overlying the nose.** Sagittal T2-weighted MR image shows a rounded, hyperintense dermoid abutting the nasal bone (*long white arrow*) connected by a tubular dermal sinus tract (*short white arrow*) to a dermoid located at the foramen cecum (*black arrow*) projecting into the epidural space. There is also a dermoid in the nasal septum (*arrowhead*).

fat-suppressed MR images, T1-weighted fat-suppressed MR images, postcontrast T1-weighted fat-suppressed MR images, and DWI. Thin-section axial CT images with multiplanar reformats should be obtained if bony anatomy evaluation is required. CT in infants under 2 years of age should be obtained with contrast in order to demonstrate the enhancing cartilage of the incompletely ossified anterior skull base that could otherwise be mistaken for a bony defect. On CT, the dermoid cyst and/or sinus tract appears as a rounded or tubular hypodense structure. A fibrous channel is difficult to detect. Rim enhancement may occur, but surrounding edema suggests superimposed infection.[125] If a cyst or sinus extends close to or through the foramen cecum, the foramen may appear enlarged, and the crista galli may appear thickened, enlarged, and grooved or bifid.[126] On MR, dermoids appear hypo-, iso-, or hyperintense on T1-weighted MR images, and tend to be hyperintense on T2-weighted MR images with decreased diffusivity. Occasional lesions demonstrate fat suppression. Dermal sinus tracts are usually of similar signal to CSF on all pulse sequences.

Meningoencephalocele and Nasal Neuroglial Heterotopia

The dural projection may fail to regress, resulting in a patent diverticulum that communicates with the intracranial compartment. The diverticulum may contain leptomeninges, CSF, and/or neural tissue, resulting in a meningocele or meningoencephalocele, broadly referred to as cephalocele. A nasofrontal cephalocele protrudes through a persistent fonticulus; a nasoethmoidal cephalocele protrudes through a persistent prenasal space. If the diverticulum becomes closed off and loses its communication with the intracranial compartment, it forms an isolated mass of heterotopic meninges and neural tissue, termed nasal neuroglial heterotopia ("nasal glioma"). Extranasal neuroglial heterotopia comes from tissue that protruded through the fonticulus frontonasalis. Intranasal neuroglial heterotopia comes from tissue that protruded through the prenasal space.

Imaging is helpful for evaluating the location and size of the mass and its relationship with the brain and foramen cecum. On MRI, it is usually hypo- or isointense to gray matter on T1-weighted sequence and iso- to hyperintense on T2-weighted sequence (Fig. 3.54). Hyperintensity on T2-weighted sequence is attributed to dysplastic or gliotic neural tissue and/or CSF. The mass may appear entirely or partly cystic. Enhancement is unusual but may occur if there is significant vascularity or choroid plexus. Sagittal or coronal MR sequences are important to help distinguish nasal neuroglial heterotopia from a cephalocele by showing a lack of communication between the mass and the brain.[127] On CT, the mass is isodense to brain parenchyma or variably hypodense. CT is useful for demonstrating associated bony deformity.

Fissural Cysts

Fissural cysts are cysts that arise along lines of fusion of embryologic facial processes. They include nasolabial cysts, nasopalatine duct cysts, and median palatal cysts.

Nasolabial cyst, also known as nasoalveolar cyst or Klestadt cyst, occurs at the base of the nasal ala and anterior nasal fold and may be bilateral.[128] Its density on CT and signal on MR vary depending on the cyst contents,[129] which may range from serous to mucous to complex if there is superimposed infection. Enhancement is variable.[130,131] When the lesion is large, scalloping of the adjacent bone may be seen (Fig. 3.55).

Nasopalatine duct cysts or median anterior maxillary cysts may be further classified as incisive canal cysts or palatine papilla cysts. The latter are uncommon. The former are thought to arise from nasopalatine duct epithelial remnants.[132] Small incisive canal cysts are not uncommon in children. On CT, the cyst appears as a symmetrical pear-shaped, heart-shaped, or rounded lucent area with a sclerotic rim in the midline of the anterior primary palate (Fig. 3.55B). They develop around vital teeth and can cause splaying of the upper central incisor roots.

A median palatal cyst arises at the junction of the palatal processes in the midline. On CT, it appears as a midline lucent lesion in the hard palate.

Clefts

Clefting results from abnormal development or fusion of facial processes.[133]

- Isolated cleft secondary palate: results from insufficiency of the frontonasal and nasomedial processes or lesions

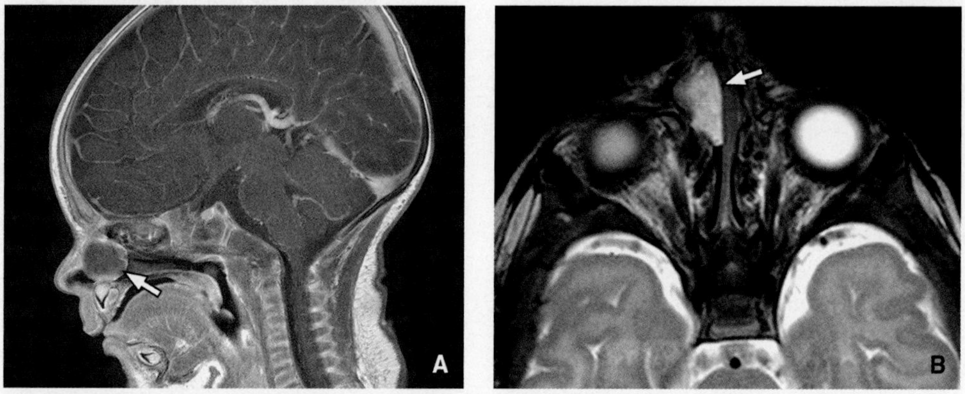

FIGURE 3.54 **Nasal neuroglial heterotopia in a 21-day-old boy who presented with right nasal mass. A:** Sagittal postcontrast T1-weighted MR image demonstrates a nonenhancing hypointense mass (*arrow*) in the nasal cavity. **B:** The mass (*arrow*) is predominantly hyperintense on T2-weighted MR image.

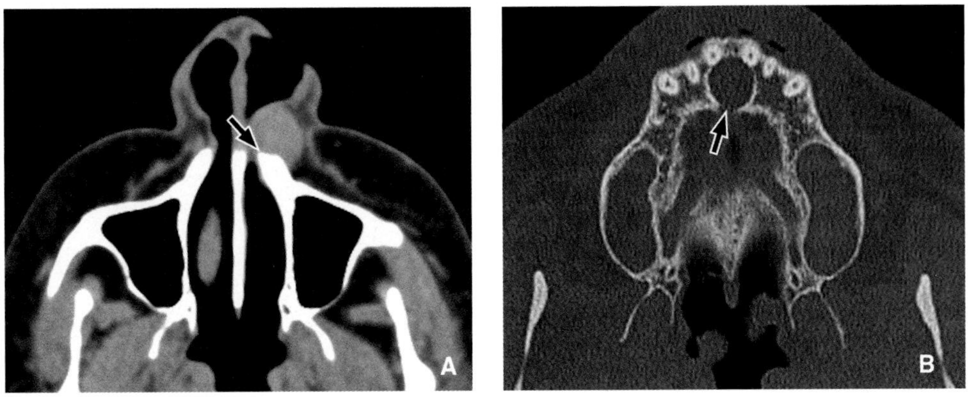

FIGURE 3.55 **Fissural cysts. A:** Nasolabial cyst. Axial CT image shows a proteinaceous cyst at the base of the left nasal ala. Note flattening and scalloping of the underlying frontal process of the maxilla (*arrow*). **B:** Nasopalatine duct cyst. Axial bone window CT image shows a symmetric, expansile, rounded, lucent lesion (*arrow*) at the distal nasopalatine duct in the midline.

that prevent palatal fusion. Fusion of the secondary palatal shelves is prevented by congenital intraoral masses or severe micrognathia. Underdevelopment of the mandible causes backward and upward displacement of the tongue (glossoptosis). This in turn results in a U-shaped cleft of the secondary palate.

- True midline cleft lip and palate: results from failure of fusion of the nasomedial processes. There is hypertelorism when associated with skull base dehiscence and basal cephaloceles. Variable associated hypoplasia or absence of midline structures of the face with hypotelorism should prompt a search for holoprosencephaly.
- Common cleft lip and/or cleft palate: these off-midline clefts result from failure of the nasomedial processes to fuse with the maxillary processes. Bilateral cleft lip and palate is associated with a higher incidence of syndromic anomalies than is unilateral cleft palate or cleft lip.
- Oblique facial cleft: results from failure of the nasolateral process to fuse with the maxillary process. The cleft extends from the medial canthus of the eye to the nose. This may be seen in association with bilateral common cleft lip and/or palate.
- Transverse facial cleft: also termed "wolf mouth" or macrostomia, the transverse facial cleft results from failure of the maxillary and mandibular processes to fuse. This may be unilateral or bilateral. It may be seen in isolation or may be associated with syndromes such as HFM.

Clefts that do not observe lines of embryonic fusion likely result from amniotic band disruption complex.[134] Here, rupture of the amnion leads to generation of fibrous bands that can adhere to and tether parts of the developing fetus. Fetal parts may become disrupted, damaged, or amputated by these bands. Craniofacial deformations are seen in approximately one-third of cases of amniotic band sequence.[135]

Micrognathia

Micrognathia is an abnormally small mandible whereas *retrognathia* refers to a receding chin, but these two findings often coexist. Micrognathia can be sporadic or inherited, isolated or syndromic. Micrognathia is a feature of trisomies 13, 18, and 9.[136] Symmetric micrognathia with hypoplastic and deficient zygomatic arches, malar flattening, and severe anomalies of the external and middle ears is a feature of TCS (Fig. 3.56A) and Nager syndrome. Mildly asymmetric

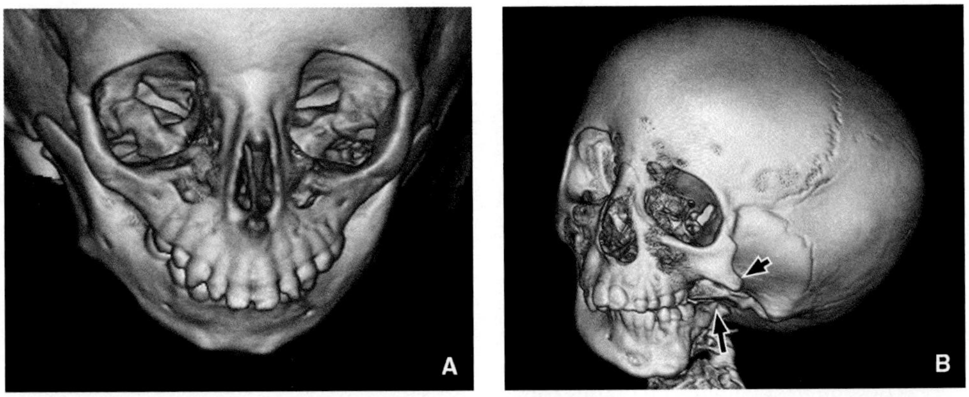

FIGURE 3.56 **Micrognathia. A:** Treacher Collins syndrome in a 21-month-old boy. 3D CT image shows bilateral symmetric micrognathia and malar flattening. The zygomatic arches are absent. **B:** Hemifacial microsomia in a 17-month-old girl. 3D CT image shows underdevelopment of the left hemimandible with absence of the ramus and condyle (*long arrow*). The left zygomatic arch is severely hypoplastic (*short arrow*). There is complete atresia of the external auditory meatus.

micrognathia with external, middle, and inner ear anomalies and branchial apparatus anomalies is the hallmark of branchiootorenal (BOR) syndrome. HFM is characterized by unilateral micrognathia, ipsilateral zygomatic arch deficiency, hypoplastic muscles of mastication, and external and middle ear anomalies (Fig. 3.56B).

Moderate to severe micrognathia is associated with airway obstruction. Mandibular hypoplasia tends to displace the tongue posteriorly and superiorly, which, in turn, prevents normal development of the palate resulting in a palatal cleft, as discussed above. The clinical triad of micrognathia, glossoptosis, and feeding difficulty is known as the Robin sequence, which is a feature of various syndromes, for example, velocardiofacial syndrome and Stickler syndrome.

Imaging of micrognathia is required primarily to assist surgical planning prior to mandibular reconstruction. Axial helical CT images using a low-dose algorithm are used to create multiplanar reconstructed images and a 3D model of the mandible and face.

Infectious and Inflammatory Disorders

Bacterial Sinusitis

The two most common predisposing factors for acute bacterial sinusitis are viral upper respiratory tract infection (URI) and allergy.[137] If symptoms are persistent (longer than 10 days), severe (high fever and purulent nasal discharge), or worsening after initial improvement, acute bacterial sinusitis is suggested. Symptoms beyond 30 days suggest subacute or chronic sinusitis.[137] The most common pathogens are *Streptococcus pneumoniae*, *Haemophilus influenzae*, and *Moraxella catarrhalis*.[138,139] *Staphylococcus aureus* and anaerobic organisms are seen more frequently in children with severe sinus symptoms or with chronic sinusitis (present for over a year).

The ethmoid air cells are separated by thin bony septations; each air cell drains through an independent ostium into the middle meatus.[140] These narrow ostia are readily obstructed by inflamed mucosa. When developed, the frontal sinuses are frequently the conduit for spread of infection to the orbit or brain, the latter related to a rich emissary venous plexus between the posterior frontal sinus mucosa and the meninges. Like the frontal sinus, an infected sphenoid sinus is more prone to the development of intracranial complications.

Pediatric sinusitis occasionally arises as a result of odontogenic infection.[141] A key CT finding is a periapical lucency due to a periapical abscess or granuloma that is dehiscent into the floor of the maxillary antrum (Fig. 3.22B). Perforation after dental trauma or a dental procedure may lead to a tract that then epithelializes to form an oroantral fistula (Fig. 3.57). Congenital bone defects and dental cysts may also act as conduits for spread of infection to the maxillary sinus.

Sinus inflammation and congestion causes increased secretions and accumulation of submucosal fluid with venous congestion.[142] On CT, inflamed sinus mucosa appears as peripheral soft tissue thickening. On MRI, mucosal secretions and submucosal fluid appear hyperintense on T2-weighted sequences

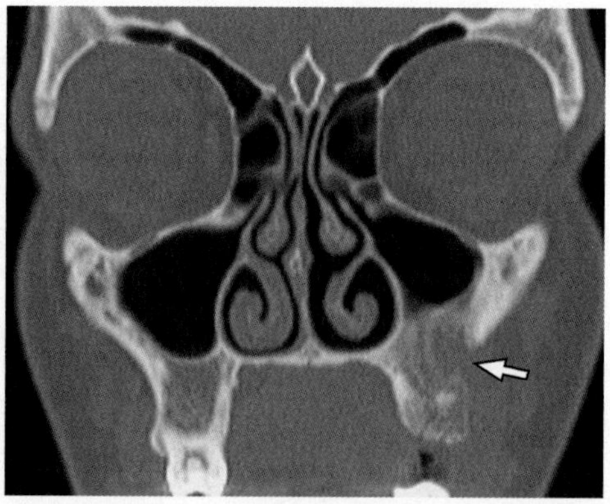

FIGURE 3.57 **Oroantral fistula.** Coronal bone window CT image demonstrates a channel (*arrow*) extending from the left maxillary antrum to the gingival buccal sulcus of the oral cavity. The patient had recently undergone extraction of a tooth and an associated radicular cyst, with persistent pain postoperatively.

and hypointense on T1-weighted sequences. There is a characteristic pattern of a thin rim of enhancement of the inflamed mucosa and nonenhancement of the underlying submucosal fluid (Fig. 3.58). These are findings of sinus inflammation or congestion and not necessarily sinus infection. Sinus CT and MRI often show mucosal thickening in children who do not have signs or symptoms of sinusitis or an URI.[143] Therefore, mucosal thickening and edema seen on imaging should not be reported as "sinusitis" without supportive clinical history. Layering fluid in a sinus (air–fluid level) is more suggestive of an acute infectious sinus process (Fig. 3.58).

Imaging findings of chronic sinusitis include mucosal thickening; lobulated densities representing sinus retention cysts and nasal polyps; loss of sharp mucoperiosteal margins; irregular thinning, demineralization, or dehiscence of bony sinus margins; and/or reactive hyperostosis and sclerosis of the margins (Fig. 3.59).[144] When there is occlusion of a sinus ostium, accumulated secretions can cause increased pressure within the sinus cavity that over time causes expansion of

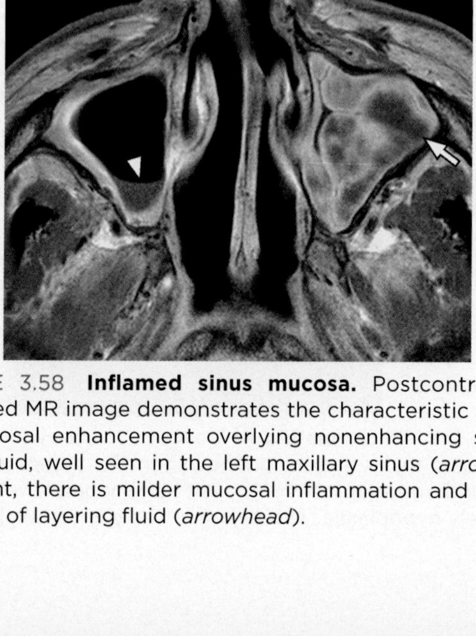

FIGURE 3.58 **Inflamed sinus mucosa.** Postcontrast T1-weighted MR image demonstrates the characteristic pattern of mucosal enhancement overlying nonenhancing submucosal fluid, well seen in the left maxillary sinus (*arrow*). On the right, there is milder mucosal inflammation and a small amount of layering fluid (*arrowhead*).

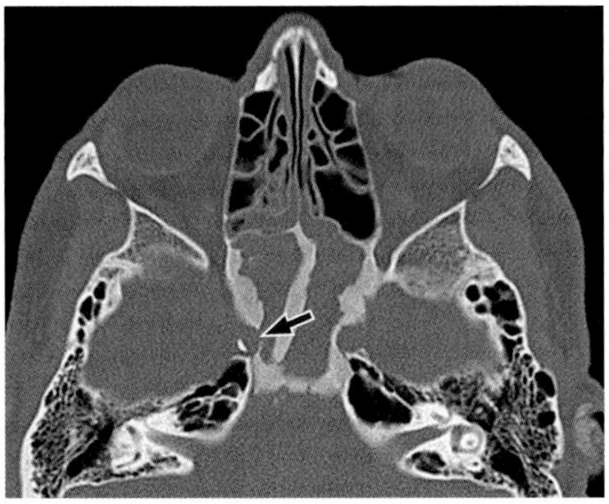

FIGURE 3.59 **Chronic sphenoid sinusitis.** Axial bone window CT image demonstrates hyperostosis and sclerosis of the margins of the sphenoid sinuses, with an area of dehiscence (*arrow*) that borders the right carotid canal.

the sinus cavity with surrounding bony pressure erosion, leading to a mucocele or mucopyocele. On CT, a mucocele is characterized by an expanded and opacified sinus with thinning and/or dehiscence of the bone margins (Fig. 3.60). Mucocele shows minimal peripheral enhancement; this feature helps distinguish a mucocele from an obstructing neoplasm. Because of the low specificity for infectious sinus disease on imaging, CT is usually reserved for the preoperative evaluation of recurrent or chronic sinus infections and for the evaluation of complications of sinusitis, particularly in the orbit. MRI is preferred for imaging intracranial complications.

Complications of sinusitis are usually related to spread of infection to the orbits and the brain. Spread of infection to the orbits most commonly results from ethmoid sinusitis, due to the thin lamina papyracea and the valveless anterior and posterior ethmoidal veins, followed by maxillary and frontal sinusitis. Orbital complications as detailed earlier include periorbital cellulitis, orbital cellulitis, orbital phlegmon, and extraconal subperiosteal abscess, as well as thrombosis of the superior ophthalmic vein. External spread of infection from the frontal sinus to produce a frontal subperiosteal abscess is

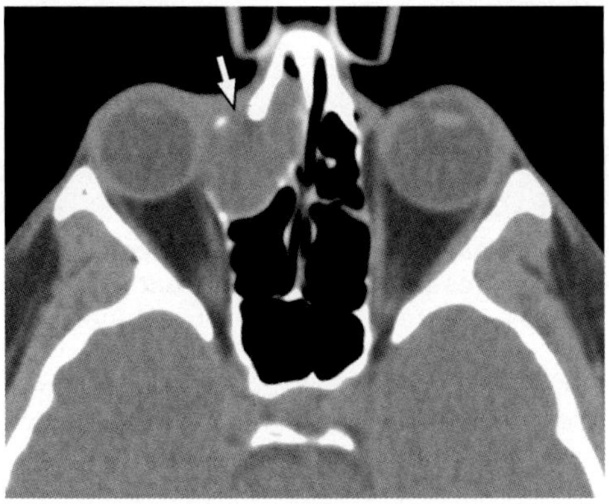

FIGURE 3.60 **Ethmoid mucocele.** Axial CT image demonstrates an expansile opacified right ethmoid air cell, with thinning and dehiscence of the overlying bone (*arrow*). There is lateral displacement of the globe and orbital contents.

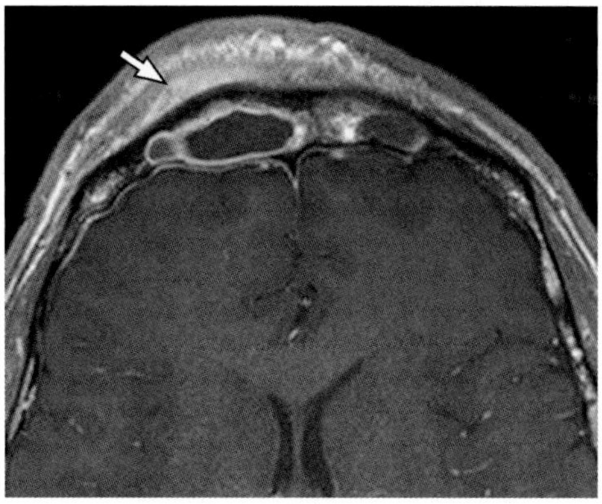

FIGURE 3.61 **Pott puffy tumor.** Axial postcontrast T1-weighted fat-suppressed MR image demonstrates mucosal enhancement and fluid in the frontal sinuses. The infectious process extends through the frontal bone to the subgaleal space, forming a subperiosteal phlegmon (*arrow*) in this patient.

known as Pott puffy tumor (Figs. 3.61 and 3.62). This entity refers to spread of sinus infection via diploic veins anteriorly to the subgaleal space, leading to frontal bone osteomyelitis and subperiosteal abscess.[145] Rarely, a mucocele or mucopyocele can rupture into the orbit causing orbital inflammation (Fig. 3.21). Intracranial complications of acute sinusitis include subdural empyema, epidural or cerebral abscess, cerebritis, meningitis, dural and/or cortical venous sinus thrombosis with venous infarction, cavernous sinus thrombosis, and, rarely, internal carotid artery spasm/thrombosis (Figs. 3.23 and 3.24). As mentioned above, intracranial spread of infection most commonly results from frontal sinusitis, then sphenoid sinusitis, and finally ethmoid sinusitis. Spread of infection can occur via small emissary veins, in which case no bony abnormality is seen, or as a result of osteomyelitis. Osteomyelitis may be initially inapparent on CT or result in only subtle cortical demineralization. However, MRI can reveal abnormal signal intensity and enhancement within the affected frontal or sphenoid bone. Rarely, sphenoid sinusitis may cause optic neuritis.[146]

Persistent sinusitis with inspissated secretions is suggestive of cystic fibrosis, especially if there is concurrent sinonasal polyposis. Other entities to consider with recurrent sinusitis include immune deficiency syndromes, HIV infection, allergic sinusitis, Samter triad (asthma, aspirin sensitivity, nasal polyps), and immotile cilia/Kartagener syndrome. Inflammation of the sinonasal cavities can also occur in granulomatosis with polyangiitis (Wegener granulomatosis) (Fig. 3.27), sarcoidosis, and atopic rhinitis.[137] There is often associated nasal septal destruction.

Silent sinus syndrome describes maxillary sinus atelectasis that causes slow progressive painless enophthalmos.[147] Chronic obstruction of the maxillary sinus ostium results in negative pressure within the antrum, causing inward bowing of the maxillary sinus walls (Fig. 3.63). Depression of the orbital floor leads to increased orbital volume and subsequent enophthalmos and hypoglobus. Patients often present to an ophthalmologist with unilateral ptosis or orbital asymmetry, rather than to an otorhinolaryngologist for sinus evaluation, hence the moniker. Although atelectasis of the sinus is not

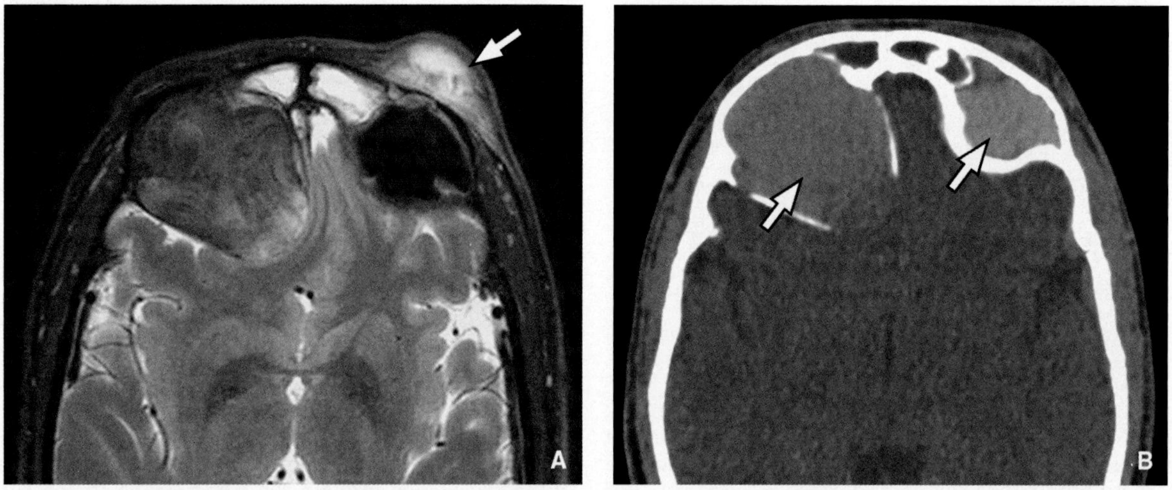

FIGURE 3.62 **Pott puffy tumor and frontal mucoceles causing intracranial mass effect. A:** Axial T2-weighted fat-suppressed MR image demonstrates bilateral frontal mucoceles expanding into the intracranial compartment, causing mass effect on the frontal lobes. There is also a Pott puffy tumor on the left (*arrow*). **B:** Axial CT image at the same level reveals the contents of both mucoceles (*arrows*) to be hyperdense, representing densely inspissated material or fungal colonization. This accounts for the dark signal seen on the MR image. It is important not to assume that dark signal within a sinus on MR images necessarily represents air. In this case, one could easily mistake the lesion on the left for an air-filled hypersinus or pneumosinus dilatans.

uncommon in children, the orbital sequelae are not usually appreciated during childhood.[148]

Finally, it should be mentioned that whenever a "nasal polyp" is seen in the upper nasal cavity against the cribriform plate or ethmoid roof in a small child, the alternative diagnosis of a nasal cephalocele must be considered (Fig. 3.64), as nasal polyps are rare in the first few years of life.

Fungal Sinusitis

Fungal disease of the sinuses may occur in one of five forms: (1) acute invasive fungal sinusitis, (2) chronic invasive fungal sinusitis, (3) chronic invasive granulomatous fungal sinusitis, (4) allergic fungal sinusitis, or (5) fungus ball (mycetoma). The invasive forms are seen mostly in immunocompromised pediatric patients, including bone marrow transplant recipients, with *Mucor* and *Aspergillus* being the usual causative agents.

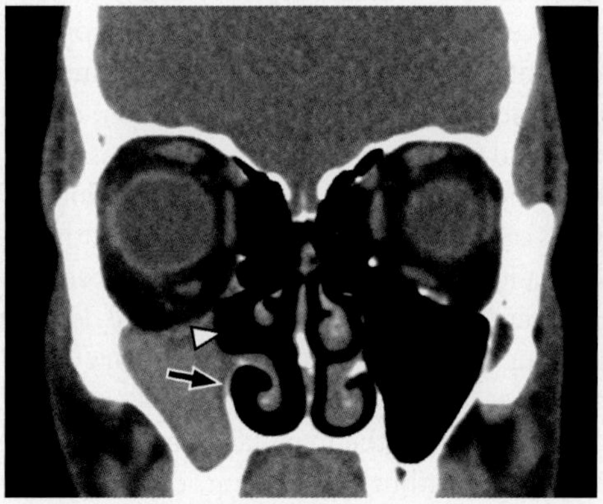

FIGURE 3.63 **Silent sinus syndrome.** Coronal CT image shows depression of the orbital floor, lateral deviation of the lateral nasal wall (*black arrow*), and lateral excursion of the middle meatus (*white arrowhead*), related to negative pressure within the maxillary sinus on the right. The antrum is opacified and filled with inspissated material because of obstructed drainage.

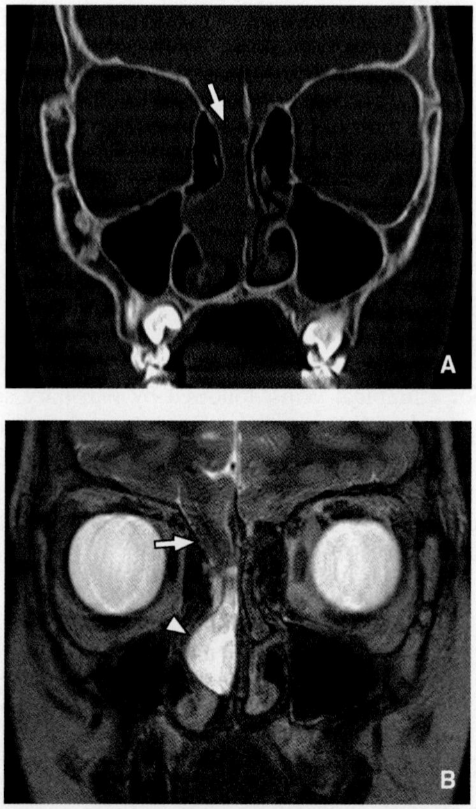

FIGURE 3.64 **Nasal meningoencephalocele in a 13-year-old boy who presented with recurrent rhinorrhea that proved to be related to a cerebrospinal fluid leak. A:** Coronal CT image in bone algorithm demonstrates a polypoid opacity in the right nasal cavity. Note widening and dehiscence of the cribriform plate (*arrow*). **B:** Coronal fat-suppressed T2-weighted MR image confirms the presence of brain parenchyma herniating through the dehiscent cribriform plate into the upper nasal cavity (*arrow*), along with CSF (*arrowhead*).

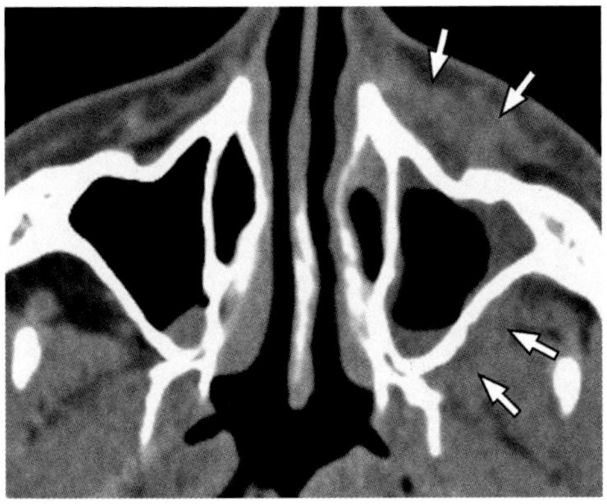

FIGURE 3.65 **Invasive fungal rhinosinusitis.** Axial CT image shows infiltration of the periantral fat (*arrows*). There is a small air-fluid level and mucosal thickening within the left maxillary antrum.

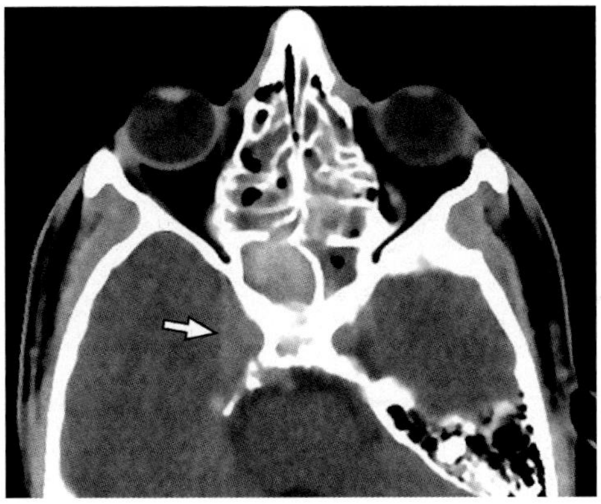

FIGURE 3.66 **Cavernous sinus thrombosis related to invasive fungal sinusitis.** Axial CT image demonstrates expansion and abnormal hyperdensity (*arrow*) in the right cavernous sinus, due to the presence of a dense thrombus. There is extensive ethmoid and sphenoid fungal sinusitis.

The acute invasive form is an aggressive disease, with the organisms demonstrating angioinvasion, bone invasion, and hematogenous dissemination.[73] It is highly associated with nasal infection and is therefore sometimes referred to as invasive fungal rhinosinusitis. Bone erosion and mucosal thickening can range from subtle to severe; extension beyond the sinuses may occur even with intact bony walls.[73] This manifests as soft tissue infiltration of the periantral fat (Fig. 3.65). Sphenoid disease can extend intracranially resulting in cavernous sinus thrombosis or carotid artery invasion, occlusion, or pseudoaneurysm.

On imaging, acute invasive fungal sinusitis is suspected when there is severe unilateral nasal cavity soft tissue thickening. Additional findings include periantral fat infiltration, bone erosion, orbital involvement, and intracranial involvement (leptomeningeal enhancement, cerebritis, granulomas, epidural and cerebral abscess, cavernous sinus thrombosis, and carotid artery compromise) (Fig. 3.66). This is the most lethal form of fungal sinus disease, with mortality of 50% to 80%.[149] Surgical debridement and systemic antifungal therapy are required.

With the chronic invasive form, the involved sinus cavities contain soft tissue that is hyperdense on CT, hypointense on T1-weighted sequence, and markedly hypointense on T2-weighted sequences, resembling air. For this reason, MRI is not as reliable as CT in sinus evaluation and may underestimate the extent of sinus disease if fungal soft tissue is mistaken for air (Figs. 3.62 and 3.67). Chronic granulomatous invasive fungal sinusitis is seen predominantly in Africa and Southeast

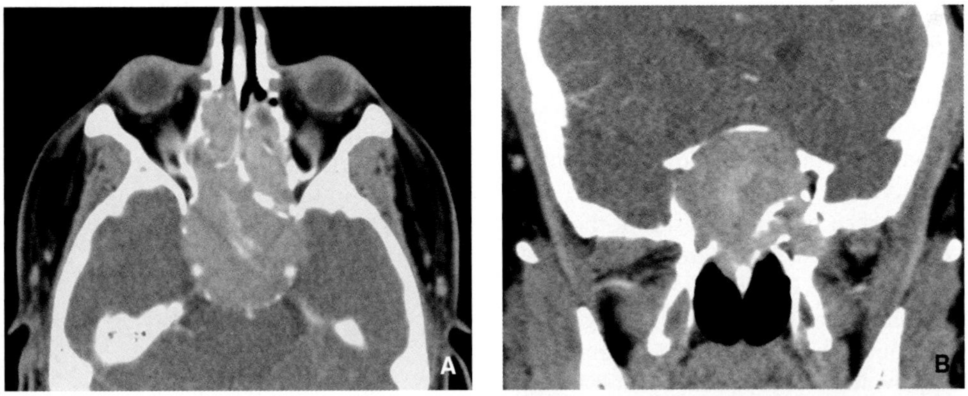

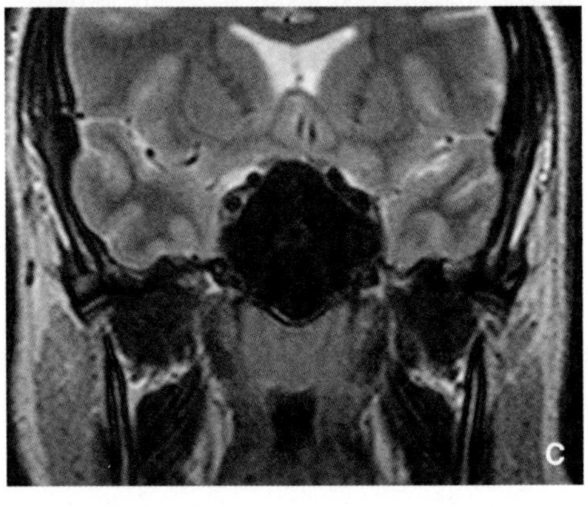

FIGURE 3.67 **Allergic fungal sinusitis.** Axial **(A)** and coronal **(B)** CT images demonstrate complete sinus opacification with expansile margins and hyperdense contents. Coronal T2-weighted MR image **(C)** shows signal dropout within the expanded sphenoid sinus, which could be mistaken for air but is in fact related to allergic mucin and/or metals concentrated by fungal organisms.

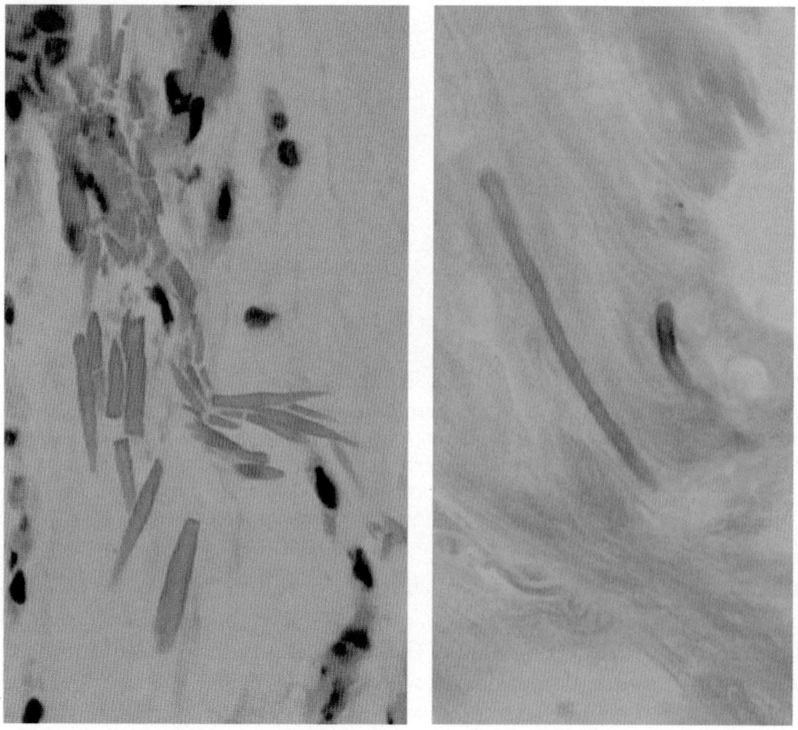

FIGURE 3.68 **Allergic fungal sinusitis in a 10-year-old girl.** The "allergic" mucin shows frequent Charcot-Leyden crystals (**left**, hematoxylin and eosin stain) made up of degranulated contents of eosinophils. Occasional hyphal fungal forms are seen (**right**, Grocott methenamine silver stain, original magnification, 600x for both images).

Asia among the immunocompetent and is relatively uncommon in children.

Allergic fungal sinusitis is the most common form of the five, thought to result from hypersensitivity reaction to inhaled fungus, which generates a chronic noninfectious inflammatory process. It is seen in younger immunocompetent patients. On imaging, there is near-complete pansinus opacification with expansion (Fig. 3.67). The hyperdense sinus contents represent allergic mucin. On MRI, there is characteristic low signal or signal void on T2-weighted sequences; this is related to a high concentration of metals, such as iron, magnesium, or manganese concentrated by the fungal organisms, and a high protein and low water content of allergic mucin (Fig. 3.68).[73]

A mycetoma occurs when fungal organisms in the paranasal sinuses or other confined spaces are not adequately cleared by the mucociliary mechanism, and instead germinate and replicate within the cavity, resulting in a tangled ball of fungal hyphae without an associated tissue inflammatory response. There is no evidence of fungal invasion. It is most commonly seen in the maxillary sinus as a CT hyperdense and T2 hypointense mass. Punctate calcifications within the mass may be seen on CT in mycetomas bearing *Aspergillus* species ("aspergillomas"), which are known for production of calcium oxalate crystals (Figs. 3.69 and 3.70).

Neoplasms and Tumor-Like Disorders

Nasal obstruction, rhinorrhea, and epistaxis constitute a triad of symptoms associated with sinonasal tumors. Tumors in the sinuses may not become symptomatic until there is extension into the nasal cavity.

Juvenile Nasopharyngeal Angiofibroma

Juvenile nasopharyngeal angiofibroma (JNA) is a benign tumor that is presumed to arise from the superoposterior margin of the sphenopalatine foramen on the lateral nasopharyngeal wall.[150] JNA extends from the sphenopalatine foramen into the pterygopalatine fossa and posterior nasal cavity, and frequently erodes into the sphenoid sinus and/or the maxillary sinus. The most common presenting symptoms are nasal obstruction and epistaxis.[151] These biphasic fibrovascular tumors are locally invasive, extremely vascular, and almost always affect adolescent males.

On contrast-enhanced CT imaging, JNA appears as an intensely enhancing mass that originates along the lateral nasal wall in the region of the sphenopalatine foramen and extends asymmetrically into the ipsilateral nasal cavity. As

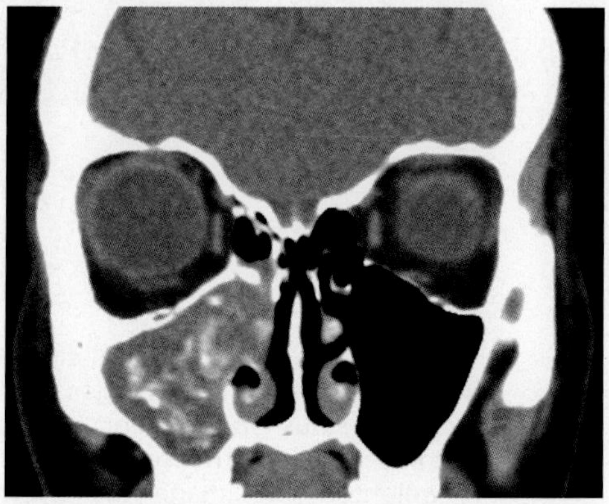

FIGURE 3.69 **Mycetoma in a 16-year-old girl.** Coronal CT image shows a mass with internal calcifications opacifying the right maxillary sinus.

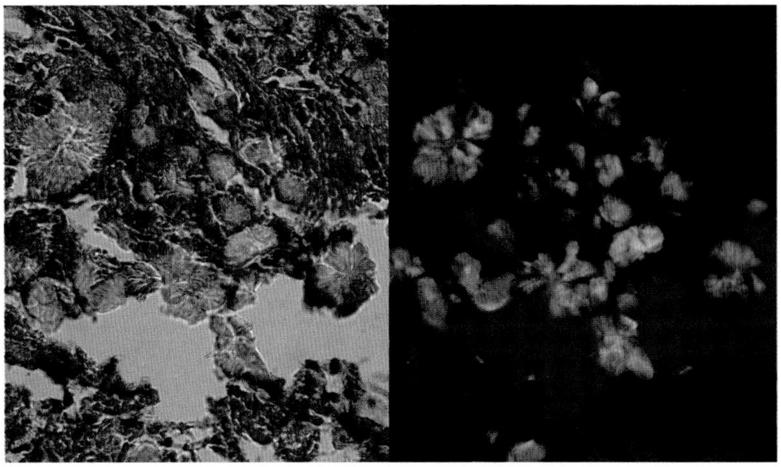

FIGURE 3.70 **Mycotic abscess with calcium oxalate.** Calcium oxalate crystals produced by *Aspergillus* appear as refractile crystals **(left)** that are highlighted with polarized light (**right**; hematoxylin and eosin, original magnification, 600x for both images).

tumor extends into the pterygopalatine fossa, the fossa is expanded and replaced by soft tissue (Fig. 3.71). Tumor may cause anterior bowing of the posterior maxillary wall and, eventually, lytic destruction with antral tumor extension. Tumor can posteriorly displace or erode the pterygoid plates and extend into the sphenoid sinus and central skull base toward the cavernous sinus and middle cranial fossa, or extend laterally through the pterygomaxillary fissure into the infratemporal fossa.[152] Orbital extension also occurs via the superior and inferior orbital fissures. The sphenoid bone around the posterior tumor margin is typically corticated, in contradistinction to the permeative pattern of bony destruction seen with malignant tumors such as RMS.

On MR, JNA is a lobulated tumor that is hypointense relative to brain on T2-weighted MR images because of fibrous stroma. Vascular flow voids are characteristic (Fig. 3.71). The tumor exhibits intermediate signal on T1-weighted MR images and enhances avidly.[153] MR is useful for distinguishing tumor from trapped sinus secretions. Angiography delineates blood supply to the tumor, usually from branches of the external carotid artery, although branches of the internal carotid artery may be recruited as well.[151] Preoperative embolization is often performed to decrease intraoperative blood loss. The tumor consists of fibrous tissue traversed by thin-walled vascular channels (Fig. 3.72). Complete surgical resection is curative.

Rhabdomyosarcoma

RMS is discussed in detail in the Orbit section. Sinonasal RMS is seen more commonly in teenagers, and patients typically present with nasal obstruction, rhinorrhea, epistaxis, and recurrent otitis media.[154] Cervical nodal metastasis occurs in up to 50% of cases. Hematogenous metastasis can also occur, most commonly to the lungs and bones.[155]

CT is useful for assessing bone remodeling and erosion. Skull base foramina may be widened. The mass is usually isodense to muscle, unless complicated by necrosis that leads to a more heterogeneous appearance. On MR, RMS

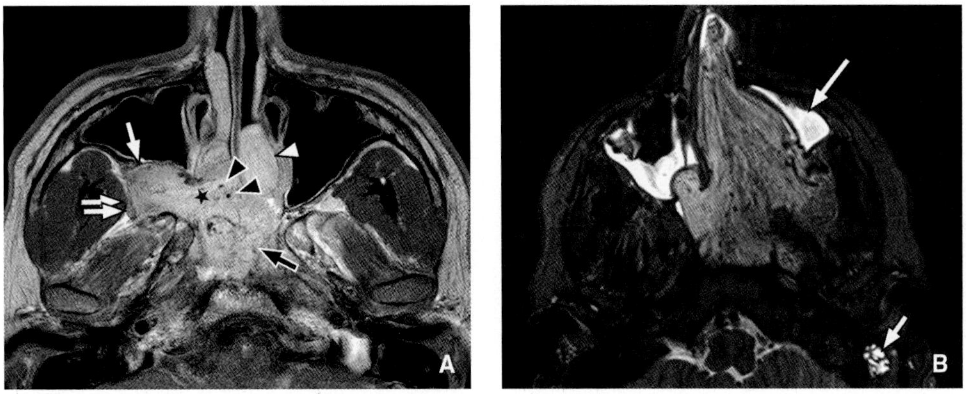

FIGURE 3.71 **Juvenile nasopharyngeal angiofibroma (JNA). A:** Axial postcontrast T1-weighted MR image demonstrates an avidly enhancing mass centered at the sphenopalatine foramen (*black star*), extending to the pterygomaxillary fissure (*single white arrow*), infratemporal fossa (*double white arrows*), sphenoid sinus (*black arrow*), and nasal cavity (*white arrowhead*). Internal flow voids (*black arrowheads*) can be seen. **B:** Axial T2-weighted fat-suppressed MR image of a 17-year-old boy with epistaxis (different patient). This extensive JNA is relatively hypointense because of fibrous content. It is clearly distinguished from the hyperintense secretions within the maxillary antra (*long arrow*). Note the left mastoid air cell secretions (*short arrow*) associated with eustachian tube obstruction by the large tumor.

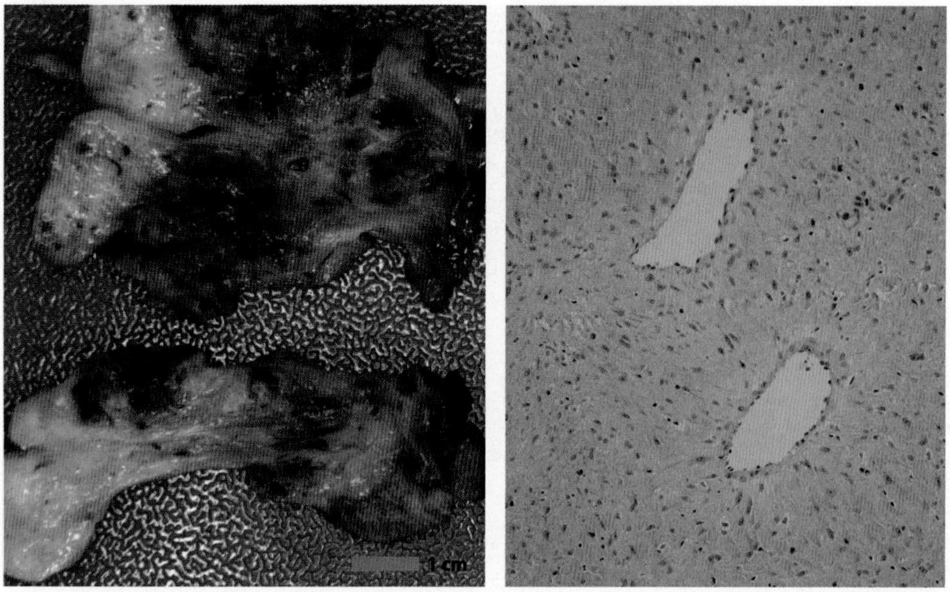

FIGURE 3.72 **Juvenile nasopharyngeal angiofibroma in a 17-year-old boy.** The resected tumor shows tan tissue and blood-filled vascular spaces **(left)**; recent therapeutic embolization accounted for the confluent brownish areas of hemorrhagic necrosis. Microscopically, the tumor shows frequent thin-walled vascular channels embedded in well collagenized fibrous tissue containing plump to stellate fibroblasts (**right**, hematoxylin and eosin, original magnification, 200×).

is isointense to muscle on T1-weighted MR images and hypointense relative to brain on T2-weighted MR images, with decreased diffusivity. MRI is useful for assessment of intracranial extension (parameningeal disease). The tumor enhances heterogeneously (Fig. 3.35).

Lymphoma and sinonasal carcinoma may appear quite similar to RMS on imaging, including the tendency for intracranial extension. However, lymphoma is usually more homogeneous. Sinonasal carcinoma occurs rarely in the sinonasal region in teenagers and is an entity that is distinct from nasopharyngeal carcinoma (NPC). Clinical symptoms and imaging features are indistinguishable from RMS. Sinonasal carcinoma is an epithelial tumor that shows squamous differentiation or may be "undifferentiated." Some harbor the t(15:19) chromosomal translocation of NUT midline carcinoma that portends a rapidly fatal course.[156]

Treatment of RMS includes surgery, radiation, and chemotherapy. Prognosis is better in children than in adults, especially if the patient is younger than age 10 years, gross total resection is possible, the tumor is <5 cm, there is no distant metastasis, and tumor is of the embryonal subtype.[157]

Esthesioneuroblastoma

Esthesioneuroblastoma (ENB) or olfactory neuroblastoma is a rare malignant neuroectodermal tumor that is thought to arise from cells in the olfactory epithelium located in the region of the superior nasal septum, medial portion of the superior turbinates, and cribriform plate.[158] ENB has a bimodal age distribution with one peak occurring during childhood and a second during adulthood. Clinical symptoms are nonspecific and include nasal obstruction, epistaxis, headache, and hyposmia.[159]

CT of ENB reveals a lobulated tumor arising in the sinonasal region with involvement of the ipsilateral nasal cavity and nasal turbinates, maxillary antrum, and ethmoid air cells (Fig. 3.73). There is aggressive lytic destruction of bone, sometimes with spread to the orbit and erosion of the cribriform plate with intracranial spread. The tumor may contain prominent whorls of mineralization (Fig. 3.73A) and shows moderate to marked enhancement. ENB tends to spread to cervical lymph nodes. On MR, the tumor demonstrates variable signal intensity but is generally isointense to cerebral cortex and demonstrates decreased diffusivity and moderate to marked enhancement (Fig. 3.73C). Mineralization results in T2 shortening (Fig. 3.73B). Small cysts along the intracranial margin of a sinonasal mass are said to be highly suggestive of ENB (Fig. 3.73D).[160] ^{18}FDG–PET/CT is a useful adjunct to the initial staging and follow-up of ENB and is used to detect nodal and distant metastatic disease.[161]

Kadish proposed a staging system for ENB as follows[158]:

Type A: Tumor is limited to the nasal cavity

Type B: Tumor is limited to the nasal cavity and paranasal sinuses

Type C: Tumor extends beyond the nasal cavity and paranasal sinuses

Microscopically, ENB resembles neuroblastoma. It consists of uniform cells in a variably prominent background of neurofibrillary material (Fig. 3.74).

Multimodal treatment with chemotherapy, extensive craniofacial resection, and radiotherapy produces significantly improved outcomes especially for patients with advanced disease (Kadish Type C).[159]

Nasopharyngeal Carcinoma

NPC is prevalent in Southeast Asia and the Mediterranean and rarer in North America where it occurs more often in males and African Americans. There is a bimodal age distribution with a first peak in late adolescence/early adulthood

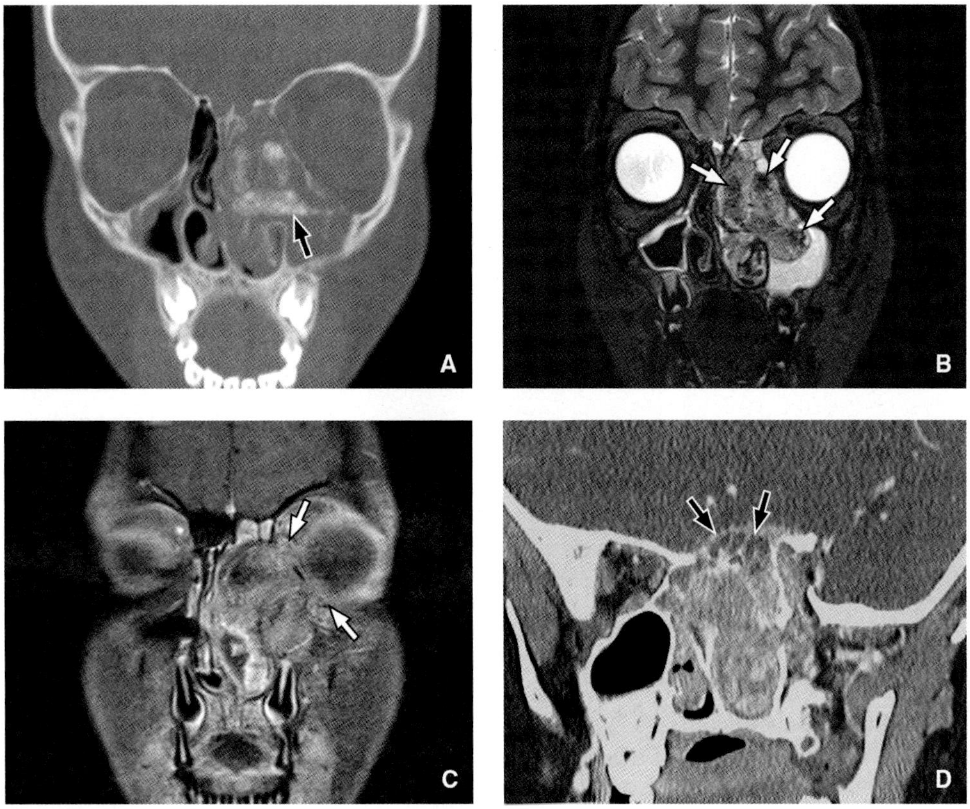

FIGURE 3.73 **Esthesioneuroblastoma (ENB) in two different pediatric patients. A–C:** A 9-year-old boy who presented with left eye tearing and fullness of the left side of the face. Coronal bone window CT image **(A)** demonstrates a lobulated mass involving the left maxillary sinus, ethmoid air cells, nasal cavity, and turbinates, with prominent whorls of mineralization within (*black arrow*). Coronal T2-weighted fat-suppressed MR image **(B)** clearly delineates the margins of the lobulated mass and distinguishes it from trapped fluid in the maxillary and ethmoid sinuses. It is largely isointense with cerebral cortex. Areas of lower signal correspond to mineralized components (*arrows*). Coronal postcontrast T1-weighted fat-suppressed MR image **(C)** shows invasion of the anterior orbit (*arrows*) by this enhancing mass. The patient underwent surgical excision of the mass and proton beam radiation. **D:** A 6-year-old girl who presented with a nasal mass, proptosis, and bloody nasal discharge. Coronal CT image shows small cysts (*arrows*) along the intracranial margin of the sinonasal mass, representing intracranial extension of ENB. The patient was treated with chemotherapy and proton beam radiation.

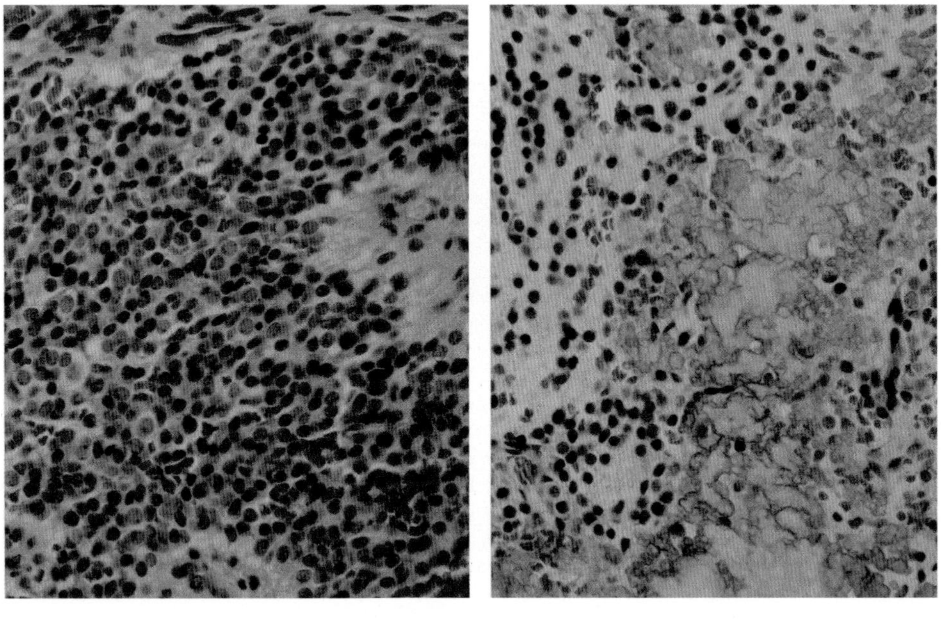

FIGURE 3.74 **Esthesioneuroblastoma in a 9-year-old girl.** This tumor resected from the skull base and nasal region is composed of small round blue cells **(left)**. Areas rich in neuropil and calcification **(right)**, along with low nuclear grade, may portend a favorable prognosis (both hematoxylin and eosin, original magnification, 400×).

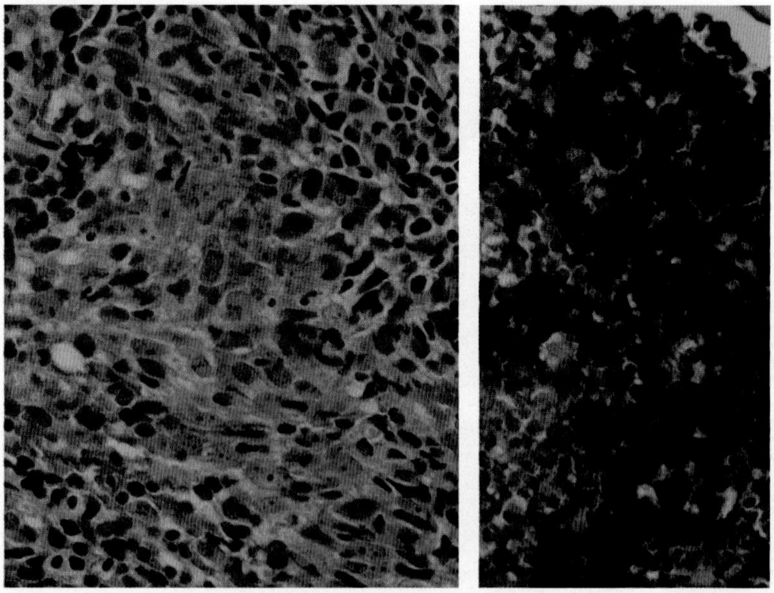

FIGURE 3.75 **Nasopharyngeal carcinoma in a 17-year-old boy.** Large poorly differentiated tumor cells are admixed with small lymphocytes (**left**, hematoxylin and eosin). In situ hybridization for Epstein-Barr virus shows black staining in virtually 100% of tumor cells (**right**, EBER stain; original magnification, 600x for both images).

(ages 15–24 years) followed by a second peak later in life (ages 65–79 years). It is association with Epstein-Barr virus (EBV) (Fig. 3.75). NPCs in children are usually undifferentiated or poorly differentiated. NPCs in children and young adults have better prognosis, especially with high-dose radiation combined with neoadjuvant chemotherapy.[162]

NPC typically arises in the fossa of Rosenmüller. Intracranial extension can occur via extension through the foramen lacerum, direct invasion through the skull base, or spread through foramen ovale (Fig. 3.76A).[163] Metastatic cervical nodes are seen in 80% to 90% of cases at presentation, with 50% having bilateral nodal involvement. Pediatric NPC is usually slightly hyperintense to muscle on T1- and T2-weighted MR images, and necrotic change in cervical nodes is uncommon.[162]

NPC may be difficult to differentiate from RMS and lymphoma based on clinical presentation and imaging appearance (Table 3.2). Intracranial invasion via the skull base can be seen in all three entities. However, if signal intensity and enhancement pattern of the mass appear more homogeneous and bone erosion is absent or mild, lymphoma is favored. Cervical lymphadenopathy is much less common in RMS than in NPC and lymphoma. Nasopharyngeal RMS tends to present in younger patients, whereas NPC is generally seen after age 10 years.

Lymphoma

Lymphoma is the third most common pediatric malignancy in Western countries and accounts for 10% of pediatric solid tumors. In East Asia, there is a high incidence of EBV-related malignancies such as NPC and non-Hodgkin lymphoma (NHL), including the natural killer (NK)/T-cell lymphomas and Burkitt lymphoma subtypes. In equatorial Africa, 50% to 74% of all childhood cancers are lymphomas, related to the high incidence of Burkitt lymphoma.[164,165] However, lymphomas of the head and neck are relatively rare in children in

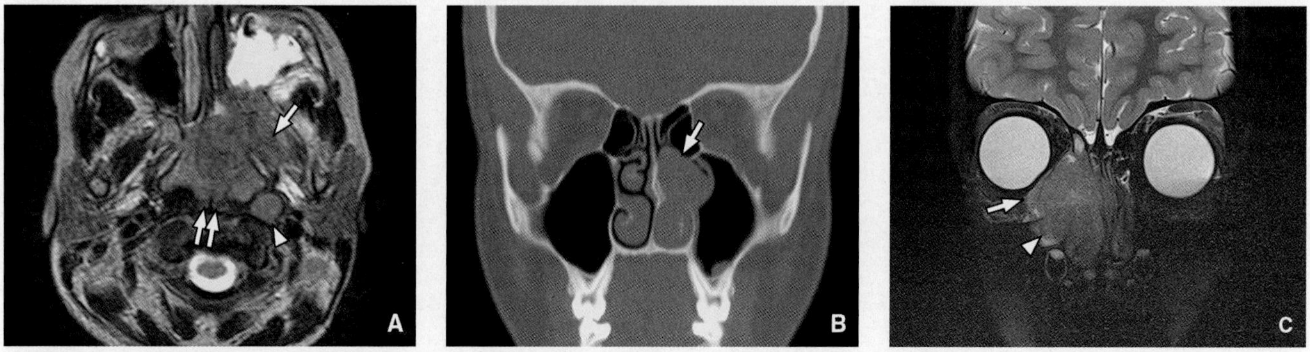

FIGURE 3.76 **Sinonasal malignancies in three different pediatric patients. A:** Nasopharyngeal carcinoma in an 11-year-old girl. Axial T2-weighted MR image shows a large mass in the nasopharynx occluding the lumen. It invades the longus colli muscles, especially on the left (*paired arrows*). It also extends laterally to invade the lateral pterygoid muscle and cranial nerve V3 in foramen ovale (*arrow*). There is a large metastatic left node of Rouviere (*arrowhead*). **B:** Non-Hodgkin lymphoma in a 14-year-old girl. Coronal bone window CT image shows a lobulated mass (*arrow*) in the left nasal cavity. There is erosion of the left middle turbinate. PET revealed avid FDG uptake in this lesion (not shown). **C:** Granulocytic sarcoma (chloroma) in a 3-year-old girl. Coronal T2-weighted fat-suppressed MR image shows a lobulated mass in the right nasal cavity, invading the right orbit (*arrow*) and the maxillary sinus (*arrowhead*). It is relatively hypointense, reflecting high cellularity.

TABLE 3.2 Features of Pediatric Rhabdomyosarcoma (RMS), Nasopharyngeal Carcinoma (NPC), and Lymphoma in the Sinonasal Region

	RMS	NPC	Lymphoma
Average age of presentation	Age 2–5 y; Age 15–19 y	Age >13 y; Adults	Variable
Gender predilection	Slightly more in males	More in males	More in males
Imaging appearance	Heterogeneous; "botryoid sign"	More homogeneous in children than in adults	Homogeneous
Bone destruction	Yes	Yes	Variable
Lymph node involvement	12%–50%	80%–90%	98% Hodgkin lymphoma 50%–60% non-Hodgkin lymphoma
Intracranial extension via skull base	Yes	Yes	Yes

nonendemic areas, accounting for only 10% of all childhood lymphomas. In particular, sinonasal lymphomas are more prevalent in Asian populations.[166]

The major types of lymphomas are Hodgkin lymphoma and NHL, which are more common in male than female children.[167] The two types seen in the sinonasal region are B-cell NHL (more common, typically seen in middle-aged men) and NK/T-cell lymphomas. NK/T-cell lymphomas present at a younger age and are seen mostly in the nasal cavity, with a strong association with EBV infection.[168]

Pediatric patients with low-grade sinonasal NHL present with nasal obstruction (Fig. 3.76B), whereas those with high-grade NHL present with nonhealing ulcer, cranial nerve palsies, epistaxis, or pain, reflecting the destructive nature of these tumors. On imaging, a destructive soft tissue mass is more commonly seen in the nasal cavity than in the sinuses, and may mimic RMS, ENB, squamous cell carcinoma, and granulomatosis with polyangiitis (Wegener granulomatosis). Lymphoma typically appears homogeneous, with intermediate signal intensity on T2-weighted sequence and moderate enhancement. It may remodel or destroy adjacent bone.[168]

Treatment consists of combined radiation and chemotherapy. For localized disease within the sinonasal region, prognosis is generally favorable.

Leukemia

Leukemia rarely involves the sinonasal region as a localized tumor, but may produce diffuse osseous disease. Sinus or nasal issues related to leukemia are more commonly due to infection or hemorrhage. A chloroma (granulocytic sarcoma or extramedullary myeloid tumor/sarcoma) is a solid mass composed of primitive precursors of the granulocytic series of white blood cells that include myeloblasts, promyelocytes, and myelocytes (Fig. 3.77). Occasionally, chloroma occurs as a soft tissue or osseous lesion in the sinonasal region. Sixty percent of affected patients are younger than age 15 years.[169] On imaging, chloromas are bulky masses that appear iso- to hyperdense on CT, with variable signal on T2-weighted MR images and moderate to marked enhancement (Fig. 3.76C).

Osseous and Chondroid Tumors

Osteomas are benign tumors typically seen in the frontal and ethmoid sinuses (Fig. 3.78), but are rare in childhood. They may appear predominantly soft tissue density or

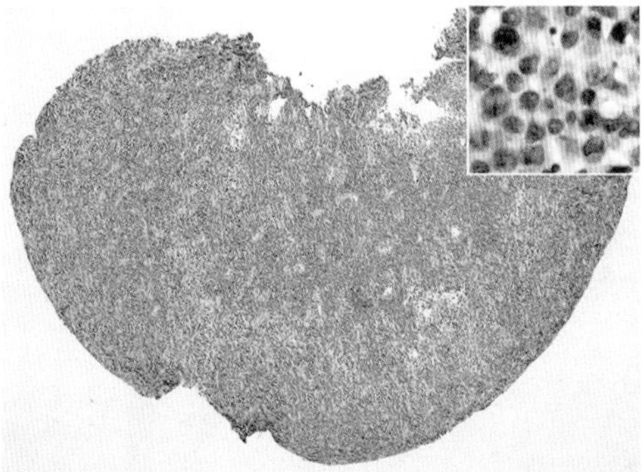

FIGURE 3.77 **Chloroma (extramedullary myeloid tumor) in a 2-year-old girl.** The tumor arose as a polypoid nasal mass following a diagnosis of acute myeloid leukemia. The densely packed cells have a high nucleus-to-cytoplasm ratio (hematoxylin and eosin, original magnification, 40×; **inset**, 600×).

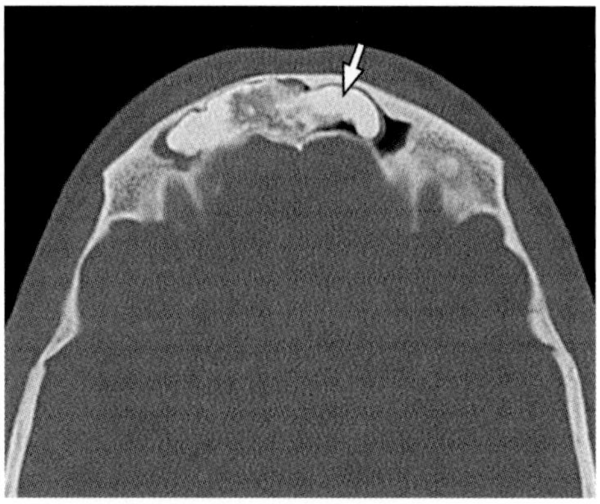

FIGURE 3.78 **Sinus osteoma in an 18-year-old girl.** Axial bone window CT image shows a frontal sinus osteoma (*arrow*) that is predominantly sclerotic, with small areas of soft tissue density.

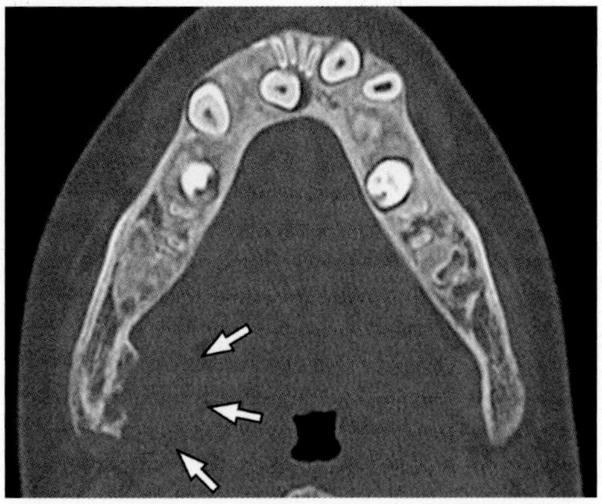

FIGURE 3.79 **Gardner syndrome in a 12-year-old boy.** Axial bone window CT image through the mandible demonstrates the characteristic "cotton wool jaw" appearance. There are multiple osteomas, as well as dental abnormalities such as supernumerary teeth. At the posterior edge of the right mandible, there is irregularity in the contour of the bone due to involvement by an adjacent desmoid tumor (*arrows*) that can be faintly discerned on this bone window CT image.

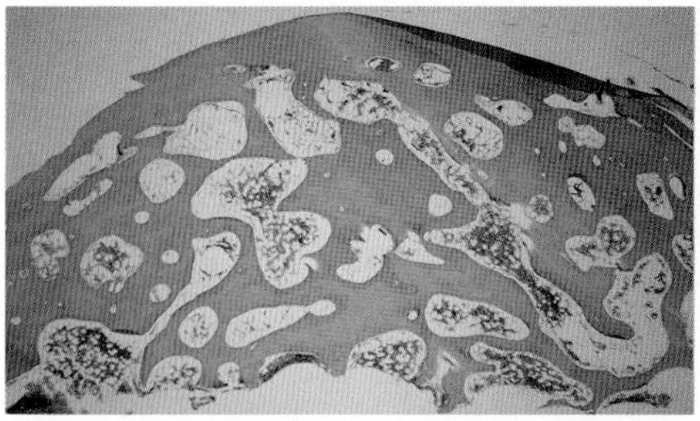

FIGURE 3.80 **Osteoma in a 15-year-old boy.** There is a dome-shaped protrusion of compact bone along the cortical surface of the frontal bone (hematoxylin and eosin, original magnification, 20×).

completely sclerotic. Multiple osteomas, dental abnormalities (e.g., "cotton-wool jaw," supernumerary teeth, odontomas), and desmoid tumors are features of Gardner syndrome (Fig. 3.79).[170] Microscopically, osteomas are typically dome-shaped growths attached to the surface of underlying bone, consisting of predominantly lamellar bone (Fig. 3.80).

Osteochondroma (osteocartilaginous exostosis) is a developmental lesion rather than a true neoplasm, composed of cortical and medullary bone with an overlying hyaline cartilage cap, and is contiguous with the underlying parent bone cortex and medullary canal.[171] They may be solitary or multiple and can arise after radiation or be syndromic, as in autosomal dominant hereditary multiple exostoses (HME). Malignant transformation into osteosarcoma or chondrosarcoma can occur.

Fibrous dysplasia is an idiopathic, benign fibro-osseous disorder that occurs in monostotic and polyostotic forms, sometimes associated with syndromes such as McCune-Albright syndrome. It frequently involves the facial bones, skull, maxilla, and mandible, with potential encroachment upon the skull base foramina (Fig. 3.81A), orbits (Fig. 3.10), nasal cavity (Fig. 3.81B), and sinuses. CT demonstrates the classic ground-glass appearance, sometimes with inhomogeneous soft tissue density or sclerotic foci. On MRI, variably hypointense signal on T2-weighted MR images compared to muscle is characteristic, and there is often enhancement, mimicking an ominous neoplasm.

Melanotic neuroectodermal tumor of infancy (MNTI, retinal anlage tumor) is a benign neoplasm of infancy that most commonly occurs in the maxilla but may also be seen in the mandible and skull (typically anterior fontanelle). Radiographic features have been likened to those of chronic hematoma. Melanin pigment in the tumor may cause high signal intensity on T1-weighted MR images and low signal on T2-weighted MR images. Histologically, two populations of primitive cells form nests in a densely collagenous stroma; the larger primitive cells contain melanin pigment.[172]

Chondrosarcoma may arise de novo, from a preexisting osteochondroma, or following radiation therapy. Chondroid matrix ("rings-and-arcs" calcifications) is not always seen. Chordomas are rare in childhood, typically arising from notochordal remnants in the midline. Osteosarcoma and Ewing sarcoma are highly invasive, with potential for regional and distant metastases. In the head and neck, these sarcomas are most commonly seen in the maxilla and mandible. On imaging of Ewing sarcoma, a bone lesion or a soft tissue mass

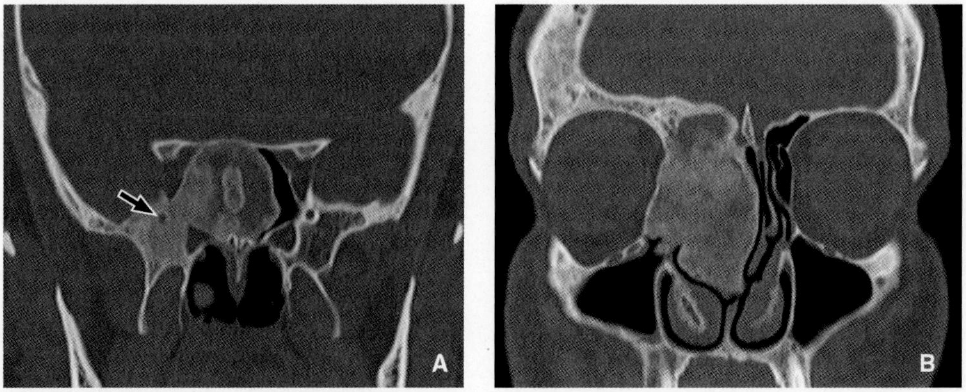

FIGURE 3.81 **Fibrous dysplasia in two different pediatric patients. A:** Coronal bone window CT image shows an area of ground glass density representing fibrous dysplasia, expanding the right sphenoid bone with resultant narrowing of foramen rotundum (*arrow*). **B:** Coronal bone window CT image shows fibrous dysplasia involving the nasal lamella. Osseous expansion causes leftward deviation of the nasal septum and lateral deviation of the lamina papyracea. The latter results in mass effect on the right orbital contents.

with bone destruction and spiculated periosteal reaction is most often seen. Osteosarcoma appears as an aggressive osseous and soft tissue mass with florid new bone formation.

Other Sinonasal Masses

Schneiderian papilloma is comprised of inverted, oncocytic, and exophytic (fungiform) papilloma subtypes. The inverted papilloma is rare in childhood and is so named because of its histologic appearance—there is inversion of the surface epithelium into the underlying stroma (Fig. 3.82). A "convoluted cerebriform pattern" has been described as a characteristic MR imaging feature of inverted papillomas, with alternating bands of hyperintense and hypointense soft tissue on T2-weighted and contrast-enhanced T1-weighted MR images (Fig. 3.83). However, malignant tumors occasionally also exhibit this feature.[173] A focal area within the mass that does not have the cerebriform pattern or has extensive bone erosion may suggest malignant transformation.[173,174] Inverted papillomas are surgically resected.

LCH manifests as tumor-like soft tissue masses with bone destruction and is included in the differential diagnosis for a sinonasal mass with bone involvement. It is histologically characterized by infiltrations consisting of Langerhans-type histiocytes, often admixed with eosinophils.[175] On imaging, LCH usually enhances and produces sharply defined lytic destruction of bone.

Nasal chondromesenchymal hamartoma is a rare but distinctive mass that may involve the sinonasal region and/or nasopharynx unilaterally or bilaterally. It is composed of cystic spaces lined by respiratory epithelium. Its walls contain cartilage nodules as well as stroma. Presentation is typically in the first two decades of life.[176] Although termed a "hamartoma," this entity is best conceptualized as a benign neoplasm and a marker for the pleuropulmonary blastoma family cancer syndrome, often characterized by mutations in the *DICER1* gene. Because of this association, additional radiographic findings such as lung cyst or mass, thyroid nodule, renal cyst, gonadal mass, or other findings typical of pleuropulmonary blastoma family cancer syndrome should prompt the radiologist to consider the diagnosis of nasal chondromesenchymal hamartoma.

Maxillofacial Trauma

Only 5% to 15% of all facial fractures are seen in children,[177] with two peaks in frequency seen, at age 6 to 7 years and age 12 to 14 years.[178,179] The most common cause is motor vehicle accidents, followed by sports-related injury, violence, and accidental causes such as a fall. Facial fractures are also seen in 2.3% of abused children.[178] In all cases, the radiologist should search for potential associated CNS injuries.

CT is the modality of choice for imaging pediatric maxillofacial trauma. Multiplanar reformatting and three-dimensional volume rendering facilitate accurate diagnosis by radiologists and provide precise anatomic depiction useful for surgical planning.

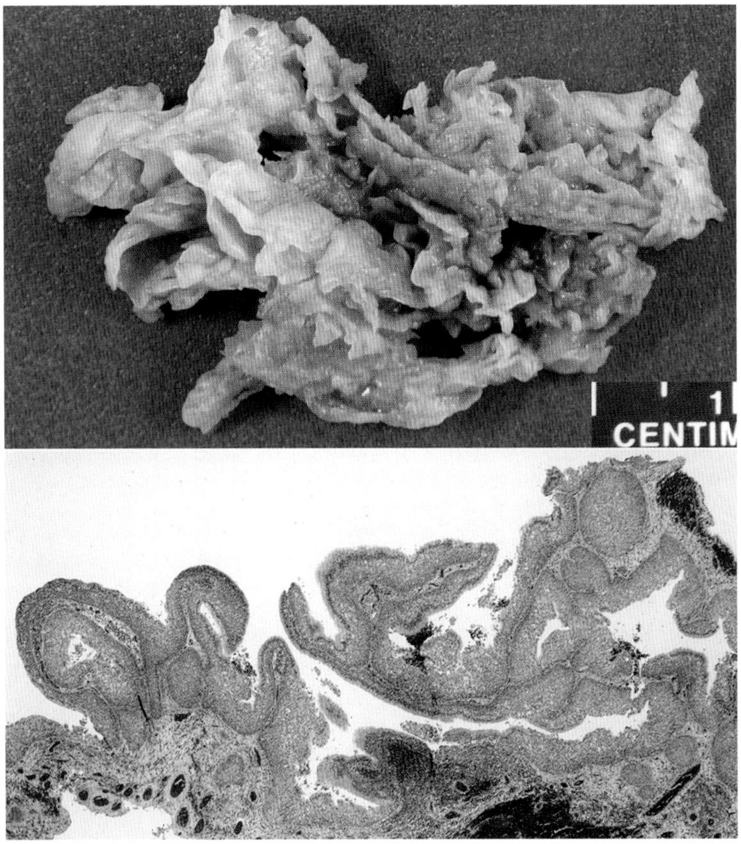

FIGURE 3.82 **Schneiderian papilloma in a 13-year-old boy.** Grossly, numerous exophytic fronds are seen **(top)**. Microscopically, an "inverted" component accompanies the exophytic growth (**bottom**, hematoxylin and eosin, original magnification, 40×).

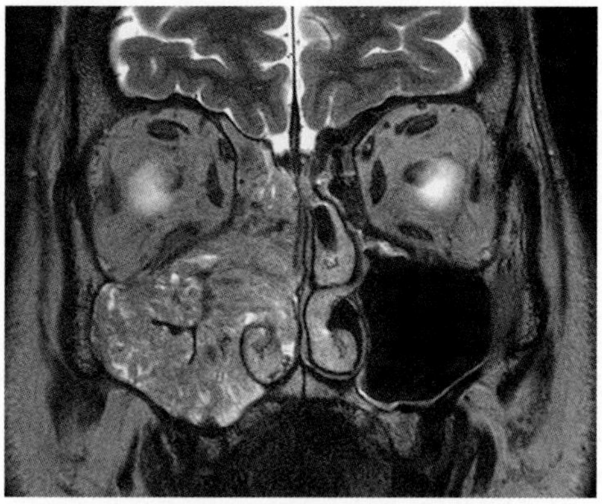

FIGURE 3.83 **Inverted papilloma.** Coronal T2-weighted fat-suppressed MR image demonstrates the "convoluted cerebriform pattern" of an inverted papilloma.

Nasal Fractures

Nasal fractures account for half of all pediatric facial fractures. Fractures are more common in the second decade (Fig. 3.84). The cartilaginous nasal septum may be fractured or displaced (Fig. 3.84). Septal thickening by a subperiosteal hyperdense fluid collection is suggestive of a septal hematoma, which must be promptly drained to prevent complications such as septal avascular necrosis, abscess, perforation, superinfection, and later growth disturbances including saddle nose deformity.[177]

Mandibular Fractures

In children, the most commonly fractured portion of the mandible is the condyle, because of its prominent vascularization and thin cortical rim surrounding a large amount of medullary bone. Condylar fractures are often the result of a blow to the chin. In older children and adolescents, fractures occur more commonly at the condylar neck.[9] One-fifth of condylar fractures are bilateral,[178] and there may be an associated parasymphyseal fracture and/or fracture of the tympanic plate of the temporal bone. CT is used to identify fractures, to assess the temporomandibular joint (TMJ) fossa for dislocation, and to locate fracture fragments.

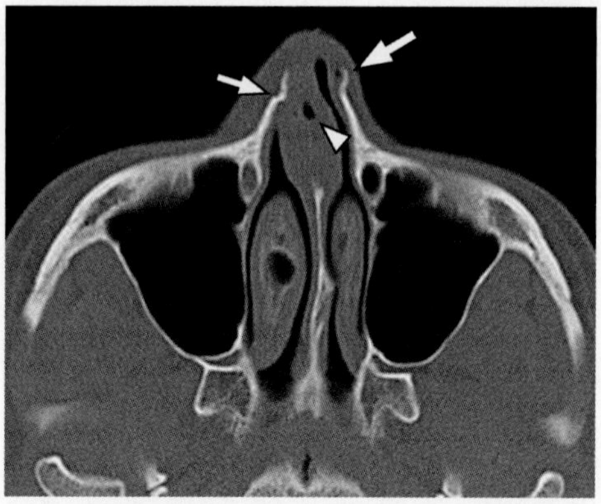

FIGURE 3.84 **Nasal bone fractures, nasal septal fracture, and hematoma.** Axial bone window CT image shows bilateral nasal bone fractures (*small arrow*) and mild lateral splaying of the left fragment (*large arrow*). A small focus of gas (*arrowhead*) in the nasal septum is due to fracture of the septum. There is also thickening of the septum due to a focal hematoma.

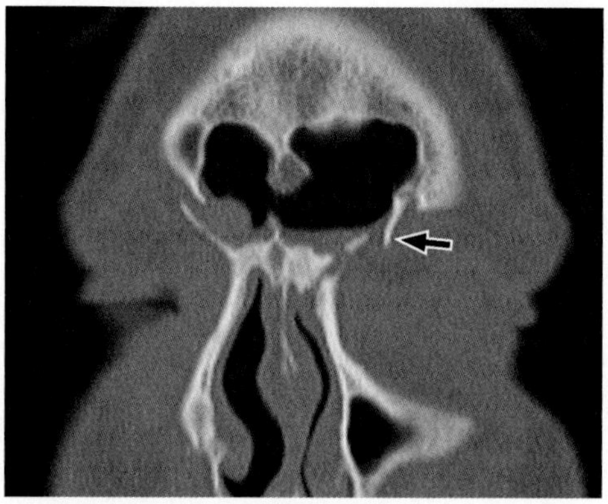

FIGURE 3.85 **Frontal bone fractures.** Coronal bone window CT image demonstrates fractures (*arrow*) involving the margins of the frontal sinuses and orbital roof.

Frontal Bone Fractures

Frontal bone fractures can extend superiorly to the skull vertex or across the orbital roof (Fig. 3.85). Prior to pneumatization of the frontal sinus (younger than age 7 years or so), frontal fractures almost always involve the orbital roof, because of lack of absorption of a frontal impact by a pneumatized sinus. If there is fracture of the posterior wall of the frontal sinus, CSF leak may occur. Frontal bone fracture may be associated with intracranial injuries, orbital fractures, and injuries to orbital contents.

Orbital Fractures

Orbital floor and rim fractures are uncommon in children until the maxillary sinuses are well pneumatized. Orbital roof fractures are more common in young children whose frontal sinuses are not yet pneumatized. When orbital or sinus fractures are seen, it is important to examine the infraorbital canal for injury to the infraorbital nerve, a branch of cranial nerve V2 (Fig. 3.86), as well as the NLD.

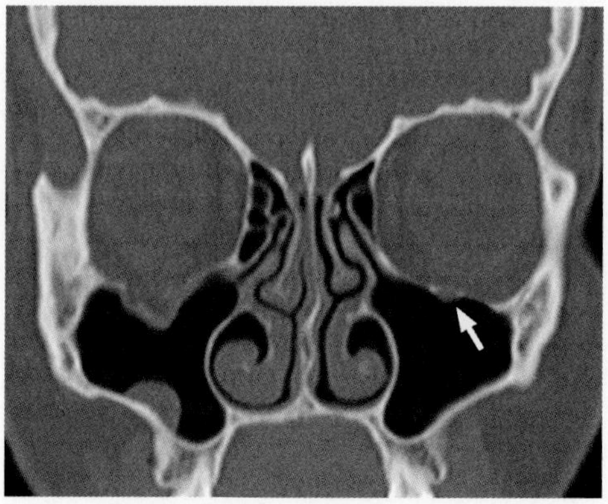

FIGURE 3.86 **Orbital floor fracture.** Coronal bone window CT image shows fracture of the right orbital floor involving the infraorbital canal, through which the infraorbital nerve courses. The normal infraorbital canal (*arrow*) can be seen on the left side.

A blow-out fracture results from a direct frontal blow to the eye causing the floor to fracture and fracture fragments to displace inferiorly to the maxillary sinus (Fig. 3.86). Orbital fat, the inferior rectus muscle, and the inferior oblique muscle may herniate alongside the fragments, with potential entrapment of muscle causing diplopia and enophthalmos. Rarely, a blow-in fracture occurs, with upward displacement of floor fragments that may impinge on adjacent structures. Coronal CT images are useful for assessing these injuries. A "trapdoor fracture" occurs when a floor fracture fragment displaces inferiorly on one edge, but the other edge remains attached to the orbital floor, allowing orbital contents to herniate into the maxillary sinus; subsequently, the fragment spontaneously reduces back to its anatomic location, causing the herniated tissues to be trapped on the maxillary side of the fracture. These fractures are considered surgical emergencies.[180] Orbital emphysema suggests that there is a fracture of a sinus wall, as does high-density fluid in the sinuses. Medial blow-out fractures involve the lamina papyracea, sometimes with herniation of orbital fat with or without a portion of the medial rectus muscle.

Other Midface Injuries

Nonpneumatized sinuses and tooth buds contribute to bone stability. As the maxillary sinuses become pneumatized and deciduous teeth are replaced by permanent teeth, midface fractures occur more frequently. Maxillary fractures may extend bilaterally or to the frontal region, with a high frequency of associated CNS injury and CSF leaks. In older children, adult-type fractures become more common, such as Le Fort fractures and tripod (zygomaticomaxillary complex, trimalar, malar) fractures.[9]

TEMPORAL BONE

Embryology and Development

The inner ear begins to form when the embryo is just 2 mm in crown–rump length. Of all the labyrinthine structures, the cochlea and the endolymphatic sac and duct are the last to differentiate and are more susceptible to developmental malformations. The final otic capsule consists of an endosteal membrane that lines the labyrinth, covered by a thin layer of endosteal bone. Over that is dense enchondral bone. Outside the enchondral layer is periosteal bone. When affected by infection or trauma, the endosteal membrane may proliferate and obliterate the lumen of the labyrinth. The enchondral layer has limited capacity for osteogenic repair, leaving fractures unhealed except for fibrous union. In contrast, the outer periosteal layer reacts readily to infection or trauma with osteogenesis. Over time, the periosteal layer is replaced by haversian bone and then invaded by pneumatic cells.[181]

The middle and outer ears are derived from the branchial apparatus. The first branchial cleft gives rise to the primitive external auditory meatus, and the corresponding first pharyngeal pouch grows up and out toward it, forming the primitive eustachian tube and middle ear cavity. The epithelium of the first branchial cleft and the endoderm of the first pharyngeal pouch then briefly touch at the site of the future tympanic membrane. The auricle develops from the first and second branchial arches. The first branchial arch forms the bodies of the malleus and incus. The second branchial arch forms the manubrium of the malleus, the long and lenticular processes of the incus, and the stapes crura. The stapes footplate arises at least in part from the otic capsule. The tympanic segment of the facial nerve and the styloid process form from the second branchial arch.

The ossicles grow in the first half of fetal life and then ossify. The malleus and incus remain solid and constant in size and shape, whereas the stapes undergoes erosion and thinning soon after it ossifies, such that the adult stapes is less bulky and more delicate than the fetal stapes. As the ossicles develop, the middle ear cavity starts to pneumatize, completing the process at about 30 weeks of fetal life. Pneumatization of the mastoid then begins, progressing through fetal life and childhood. With pneumatization, an epithelium-lined space is created, which becomes aerated subsequently.

Normal Anatomy

The temporal bones are located at either side of the base of the skull. Each temporal bone consists of five parts: squamous portion, mastoid portion, petrous portion, tympanic portion, and the styloid process.

External Ear

The external ear includes the auricle and the external auditory canal (EAC). At the medial end of the EAC is the tympanic membrane, attached to the tympanic annulus. On CT, the tympanic membrane should normally be only faintly seen. The wall of the EAC is fibrocartilaginous in the lateral third and bony in the medial two-thirds (tympanic portion of temporal bone).

Middle Ear

The middle ear, or tympanic cavity, is located within the petrous portion of the temporal bone and is bounded laterally by the tympanic membrane and medially by the cochlear promontory. The upper portion of the tympanic membrane attaches to a sharp bony projection known as the scutum.

The middle ear can be divided into three parts: the mesotympanum is at the level of the tympanic membrane; the epitympanum or attic is superior to the level of the membrane; and the hypotympanum is inferior to the level of the membrane. The eustachian tube opens into the hypotympanum. Immediately above the eustachian tube is the semicanal for the tensor tympani, which is anterior and inferior to the proximal tympanic segment of the facial nerve canal. The tensor tympani tendon attaches to the malleus.

The roof of the middle ear is known as the tegmen tympani. Along the posterior wall of the middle ear are several grooves and protrusions. From lateral to medial, they are the facial recess, pyramidal eminence, sinus tympani, and round window niche. The pyramidal eminence overlies the stapedius muscle, which inserts onto the head of the stapes.

Prussak space is a recess in the superolateral part of the middle ear bordered laterally by the pars flaccida and scutum, superiorly by the lateral malleal ligament, and medially by the neck of the malleus.

Within the middle ear are the ossicles: malleus (head, neck, anterior process, lateral process, and manubrium), incus (body, short process, long process, and lenticular process), and stapes (head/capitellum, anterior crus, posterior crus, and footplate). The manubrium of the malleus attaches to the tympanic membrane at the umbo. The head of the malleus articulates with the body of the incus with the well-known "ice cream cone" configuration seen on axial CT images, forming the incudomalleal joint. The lenticular process comes off of the long process of the incus at a right angle to articulate with the head of the stapes, forming the incudostapedial joint. The stapes footplate attaches to the oval window of the vestibule. The four suspensory ligaments of the ossicles are the superior malleal, lateral malleal, posterior malleal, and posterior incudal ligaments.

Inner Ear

The inner ear is situated in the petrous bone and contains the bony labyrinth, consisting of the vestibule, semicircular canals (SCCs), and cochlea, surrounded by the otic capsule. The bony labyrinth encapsulates the membranous labyrinth, which contains endolymph surrounded by perilymph. The cochlea is part of the hearing apparatus, whereas the vestibule and SCCs have roles in balance and equilibrium.

The vestibule is a perilymphatic space with two main openings: the oval window and the vestibular aqueduct. The vestibular aqueduct houses the endolymphatic sac and duct and courses obliquely from the vestibule to the posterior surface of the petrous bone. The superior, posterior, and lateral SCCs are oriented perpendicular to each other. The dilated ends of the SCCs are known as ampullae.

The cochlea is composed of 2.5 spiral turns (basal, middle, and apical turns, separated by interscalar septae) around a central osseous core known as the modiolus. The osseous spiral lamina projects from the modiolus into the bony canal, which, along with the basilar membrane separates the endolymph-containing cochlear duct from the perilymph-containing scala tympani. Reissner's membrane separates the cochlear duct from the perilymph-containing scala vestibuli on the other side. The lateral aspect of the basal turn bulges into the middle ear, forming the cochlear promontory. The cochlear nerve travels through the anteroinferior IAC through the cochlear nerve canal into the modiolus. From here, it continues onto the organ of Corti, not visible on CT images. The cochlear aqueduct is a bony channel that surrounds the perilymphatic duct and extends from the basal turn of the cochlea to the posteroinferior surface of the petrous temporal bone, leading to subarachnoid space. It is usually filled with arachnoid and fibrous tissue.[181]

The membranous labyrinth consists of interconnecting spaces of the endolymphatic system. It includes the cochlear duct, the vestibular sense organs, the endolymphatic duct and sac, the round window membrane, and the vascular system.

Internal Auditory Canal

The IAC in the petrous bone transmits cranial nerves VII and VIII. Its medial opening is termed the porus acusticus, and its lateral end is termed the fundus. A transverse crest at the fundus called the crista falciformis divides the IAC into superior and inferior compartments. A vertical crest called "Bill's bar" divides the superior compartment into anterior and posterior components.

The facial nerve is situated in the anterosuperior compartment, the cochlear nerve in the anteroinferior compartment, and the superior and inferior vestibular nerves in the superoposterior and inferoposterior compartments. In cross section, the normal cochlear nerve should be the same size or larger in diameter than the normal facial nerve.

Facial Nerve

The facial nerve exits the pons, traverses the cerebellopontine angle (CPA) cistern (cisternal segment), enters the IAC (intracanalicular segment), and travels through the petrous bone (labyrinthine segment), to reach the geniculate ganglion at the anterior genu, giving rise to the greater superficial petrosal nerve. Thereafter, the facial nerve courses posteriorly along the medial aspect of the middle ear (tympanic segment) to reach the posterior genu. On coronal CT images, the tympanic segment can be seen inferior to the lateral SCC and superior to the oval window. After the posterior genu, the facial nerve runs inferiorly within the mastoid bone (mastoid segment), exiting the skull base via the stylomastoid foramen before branching in the parotid gland. The chorda tympani branches off the mastoid segment and travels to the middle ear cavity. On MRI, contrast enhancement can be seen along the facial nerve starting at the anterior genu. The intracanalicular and labyrinthine segments do not normally enhance.

Congenital and Developmental Anomalies

Because the external/middle ear and the inner ear have different embryonic origins, malformations of the external and middle ear often occur in the absence of inner ear anomalies and vice versa, unless there is an underlying syndromic disorder. Malformations of the external ear are invariably associated with anomalies of the middle ear structures because their development is closely linked.

In children, early diagnosis and treatment of hearing loss is crucial in minimizing adverse effects on speech and language development.[182] CT and MR have become important noninvasive tools to help identify pathology.

Anomalies of the External and Middle Ear

A malformed auricle should raise suspicion for anomalies of the first and second branchial arches (Fig. 3.87A).[119] The EAC arises from the first branchial cleft. Partial or complete failure of canalization of the EAC during fetal life results in EAC stenosis or atresia.[183] Malformations of the external ear are associated with malformations of the auricle. A small malformed auricle is known as microtia, and absence of the auricle is termed anotia. Congenital malformations of the external and middle

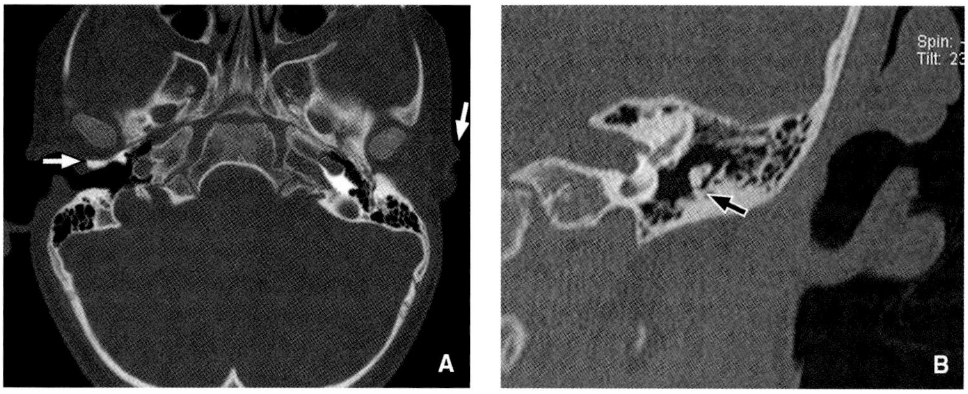

FIGURE 3.87 **External auditory canal (EAC) atresia in a 7-year-old boy. A:** Axial bone window CT image demonstrates left microtia (*long arrow*) and absence of the left EAC and tympanic plate. Note the normal right tympanic plate (*short arrow*). **B:** Coronal CT image through the left ear demonstrates fusion of the malleus to the lateral wall of the middle ear space or "atretic plate" (*arrow*), with deficiency of the manubrium.

ear may occur in isolation, especially when unilateral, or may be related to syndromic/genetic disorders (e.g., BOR syndrome and TCS), chromosomal abnormalities, intrauterine infections, and teratogens (e.g., streptomycin, thalidomide, and salicylates during the first trimester), especially when bilateral.[119] The presence of unilateral or bilateral micrognathia and an abnormally low-set pinna are also indicative of a syndromic etiology.

EAC atresia refers to complete absence of the EAC and is associated with complete absence of the tympanic plate. In the expected location of the tympanic membrane (TM), there is a thick or thin bony plate or membrane or a combination of both. The associated ossicular anomaly typically consists of fusion of the neck of the malleus to the atretic plate (Fig. 3.87B) with deficiency of the manubrium. There is variable abnormality in size, shape, and orientation of the incus and stapes, sometimes with additional sites of ossicular ankylosis. The middle ear space is variably hypoplastic, ranging from severe hypoplasia to mild underdevelopment of the facial recess only. A less severe anomaly is a small blind-ending EAC.

EAC stenosis or narrowing of the cartilaginous and bony EAC is accompanied by hypoplasia of the tympanic plate. Therefore, the presence of even a small tympanic plate distinguishes EAC atresia (absent tympanic plate) from an opacified stenotic EAC. This is relevant as stenotic EACs are at risk for accumulation of debris (keratosis obturans) or EAC cholesteatoma. These erosive processes tend to gradually result

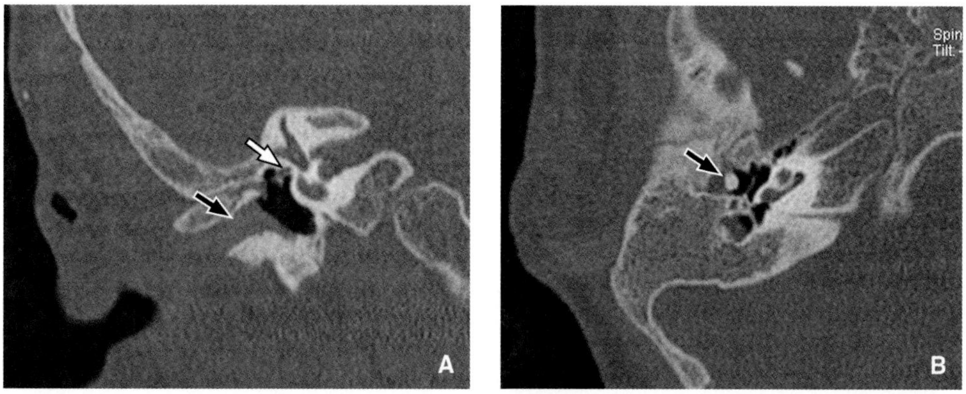

FIGURE 3.88 **External auditory canal (EAC) stenosis in a 5-year-old girl who presented with right ear anomaly and hearing loss. A:** Coronal bone window CT image demonstrates a nonerosive soft tissue plug (*black arrow*) at the site of the EAC. The tympanic plate is present, and the bony diameter of the opacified canal is narrowed. The patient also has oval window atresia and a low-lying tympanic segment of the facial nerve (*white arrow*). **B:** Axial bone window CT image demonstrates the head of the malleus (*arrow*), but the incus is absent. The middle ear cavity is underpneumatized as well. **C:** Axial bone window CT image more caudally shows a laterally displaced internal carotid artery (*arrow*).

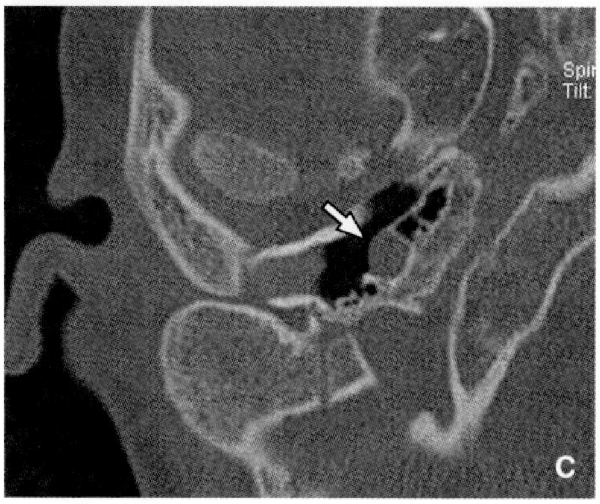

in paradoxical widening of the stenotic canal (Fig. 3.88A).[184] Ossicular anomalies with variation in size, shape, and orientation of the ossicles occur (Fig. 3.88B) but may be subtle.

Other abnormalities seen in association with external ear malformations include hypoplasia or aplasia of the mastoid portion of the temporal bone, TMJ deformity, zygomatic arch defects (e.g., TCS, HFM), and abnormal course and underdevelopment of the internal carotid artery (Fig. 3.88C).[185] The tympanic and mastoid segments of the facial nerve often have aberrancy, with the tympanic segment displaced caudally toward the oval window and the stapes crura (Fig. 3.88A) and the mastoid segment displaced anterolaterally. The oval and round windows may be absent or stenotic (Figs. 3.51B and 3.88A). When there is oval window stenosis or atresia, the tympanic segment of the facial nerve canal is invariably inferiorly located, sometimes running over the expected location of the oval window or lying exposed along the floor of the middle ear space.

TCS, or mandibulofacial dysostosis, is an autosomal dominant heritable disease that is usually caused by a mutation in the treacle gene (*TCOF1*), which is involved in ribosomal gene transcription and plays an important role in craniofacial development.[186] TCS is characterized by symmetric micrognathia with hypoplastic or absent mandibular condyles, hypoplastic/deficient zygomatic arches, and malar flattening. Cleft palate, coloboma, and macrostomia are additional features. Microtia or anotia with low-set auricles is associated with bilateral, relatively symmetric EAC atresia or severe stenosis (Fig. 3.89). There is typically severe hypoplasia or aplasia of the middle ear spaces with rudimentary ossicles or severely malformed, rotated, and fused ossicles (Fig. 3.89). Mastoid pneumatization is usually absent. There is variable inner ear anomaly such as flattening of the cochlear turns and malformation of the vestibules and lateral SCCs.[187]

HFM spectrum comprises a group of disorders characterized by abnormal development of first and second branchial apparatus derivatives. The hallmark of these disorders is unilateral micrognathia with ipsilateral zygomatic arch deficiency and hypoplastic muscles of mastication and parotid gland, sometimes with prominent accessory parotid tissue. Microtia with a low-set auricle is associated with stenosis or atresia of the EAC, with associated middle ear anomalies including stenosis or atresia of the oval window. Although HFM can be bilateral but asymmetric, BOR syndrome should be suspected in bilateral asymmetric micrognathia with branchial cleft anomalies and characteristic inner ear malformations. The presence of epibulbar choristomas (lipodermoids) and vertebral anomalies is characteristic of the Goldenhar phenotype.[188]

Isolated Anomalies of the Middle Ear

Anomalies of the middle ear and ossicles without EAC atresia or stenosis are much less common than middle ear anomalies occurring in conjunction with EAC malformation.

Isolated ossicular anomalies consist of malformation in size, shape, or orientation of one or more ossicles or fusion of the ossicles to each other or to the attic, oval window, cochlear promontory, or bone under the lateral SCC. Fixation of the stapes footplate is the most common form of ossicular fixation but is occult on CT. Additional sites of stapes fixation to surrounding structures can occur. A monopod stapes is characterized by only a single stapes strut. "Malleus bar" is congenital bony fusion of the head of the malleus to the anterior wall of the epitympanum. Additional sites of ankylosis include the tegmen tympani and lateral wall of the attic. The incus may be ankylosed as well.[189,190] In addition to being absent or malformed, ossicular anomaly occasionally manifests as abnormal persistence of bone marrow or mesenchyme. Normally, bone marrow in the head of the malleus and body of the incus is converted to bone and vascular channels; persistence beyond 25 months is considered abnormal.[191]

The course of the facial nerve is often anomalous when there are ossicular chain anomalies, because of their common embryologic origin from the second branchial arch. Most commonly, the tympanic facial nerve is displaced inferiorly and medially and may lie at or inferior to the oval window (Fig. 3.88A), or pass between the two stapes crura. There may

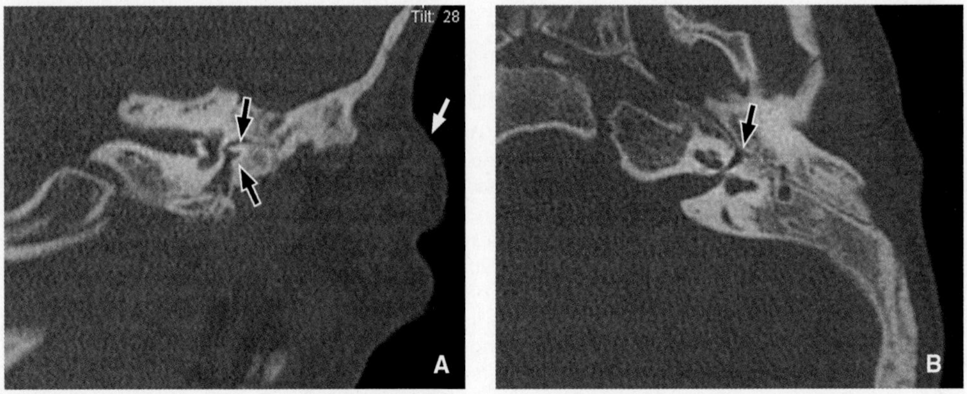

FIGURE 3.89 **Middle and external ear anomalies in a 3-year-old boy with Treacher Collins syndrome. A:** Coronal bone window CT image through the left temporal bone demonstrates microtia (*white arrow*), external auditory canal (EAC) atresia, severe hypoplasia of the middle ear cavity, and fusion of the malleus and incus to the atretic plate (*black arrows*). The facial nerve has an anomalous course (not shown). Inner ear structures, however, are normal. **B:** Axial bone window CT image shows an abnormally wide angle at the anterior genu of the facial nerve (*arrow*). There is underpneumatization of the mastoid bone.

be dehiscence of the bony covering over the tympanic segment, resulting in the nerve protruding into the middle ear cavity. The anterior genu angle may be obtuse (Fig. 3.89B).[192] Facial nerve hypoplasia is associated with some trisomies and a variety of syndromes such as HFM, CHARGE syndrome, and others. Facial nerve aplasia has been described in the Möbius syndrome and with thalidomide exposure.

Oval window stenosis or atresia is often seen with a caudally displaced and dehiscent facial nerve. This is believed to occur because of the abnormally inferior position of the facial nerve mechanically obstructing the stapes, preventing it from making contact with the developing otic capsule, thereby preventing a normal oval window from forming (Fig. 3.88A).

Other abnormalities are absence of the stapedius muscle or tendon, malformation of the pyramidal eminence, and hypoplasia of the tympanic cavity.

Congenital cholesteatoma of the middle ear space is thought to arise from an embryonic rest, and appears as a white mass behind an intact ear drum that is not attributable to prior infection, trauma, or surgery. Imaging is obtained to establish the extent of disease. On CT, congenital cholesteatoma usually appears as a rounded mass located within the mesotympanum, adjacent to the malleus and abutting the cochlear promontory (Fig. 3.90). With increased growth, the cholesteatoma erodes and displaces the ossicles laterally. Extension into the attic, hypotympanum, and mastoid antrum and erosion of surrounding structures is a feature of more advanced disease.

Anomalies of the Inner Ear

Anomalies of the inner ear typically present with SNHL or mixed hearing loss (MHL) and/or with disturbances of balance. Depending on the criteria for imaging, up to 80% of congenital inner ear malformations are not demonstrable at imaging because of microscopic or cellular malformations, where the bony architecture of the inner ear is normal.[193] Imaging is helpful for assessment of congenital inner ear malformations that affect the bony and membranous structures, sometimes suggesting a specific diagnosis. Genetic disorders are increasingly recognized as a cause of SNHL in childhood and are currently thought to cause up to 75% of cases.[194] Approximately 25% to 30% of these are syndromic (e.g., Pendred syndrome, BOR syndrome) and the remainder are nonsyndromic in nature (e.g., *GJB2* mutation). Imaging is particularly helpful for a subset of patients with syndromic hearing loss. Demonstrable inner ear anomalies also result from toxic or teratogenic exposure (e.g., retinoic acid).

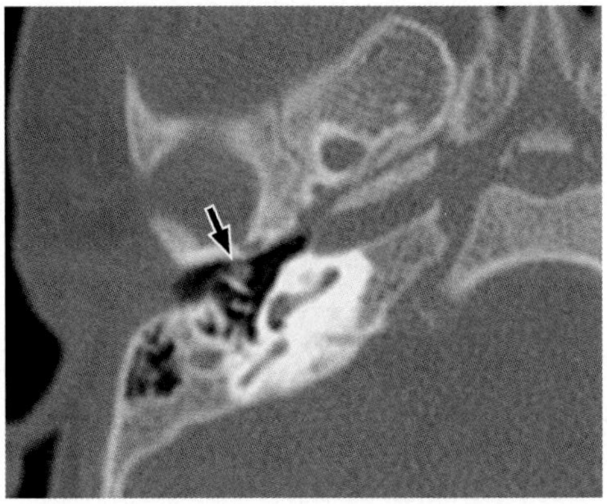

FIGURE 3.90 **Congenital cholesteatoma.** Axial bone window CT image shows a small round nodule (*arrow*) in the anterosuperior middle ear.

In 2002, Sennaroglu and Saatci proposed a descriptive classification system that incorporates some pathologic conditions resulting from insults that occur at different time points during embryologic development and others arising from distinct genetic mutations, with the emphasis that each is anatomically and clinically distinct from the others.[193] However, with increasing recognition of the underlying genetic mechanisms of disease, a proposed single time point for embryonic insult is better replaced with a descriptive classification for inner ear anomalies that incorporates an understanding of the typical features of specific disease entities. These anomalies can be unilateral or bilateral and, when bilateral, are not infrequently asymmetric, even in syndromic disorders. Below is an adapted form of the Sennaroglu classification, in which bony inner ear malformations are grouped as follows:

Cochlear Malformations:

1. Complete labyrinthine aplasia (Michel deformity)
2. Cochlear aplasia
3. Cochlear hypoplasia
4. Common cavity malformation
5. Cystic cochleovestibular malformation (a form of IP-I)
6. Cochlear incomplete partition type I (IP-I)
7. Cochlear incomplete partition type II (IP-II)
8. Cochlear modiolar deficiency
9. Cochlear nerve and cochlear nerve canal aplasia or hypoplasia

Vestibular Malformations:

1. Complete labyrinthine aplasia (Michel deformity)
2. Common cavity malformation
3. Cystic cochleovestibular malformation
4. Vestibular hypoplasia
5. Vestibule–SCC globular anomaly

Superior Semicircular Canal Malformations:

1. SCC aplasia or hypoplasia
2. Vestibule–SCC globular anomaly
3. SCC small bone island

Internal Auditory Canal Malformations:

1. IAC aplasia
2. IAC stenosis
3. IAC enlargement

Vestibular Aqueduct Enlargement:

1. LVA (large vestibular aqueduct)
2. LESA (large endolymphatic sac anomaly)

Complete labyrinthine aplasia is characterized by complete absence of all cochlear and vestibular elements. The cochlear

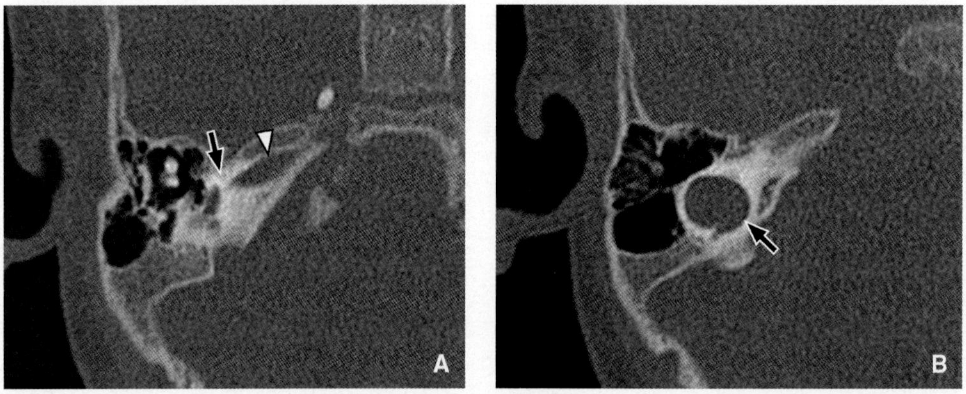

FIGURE 3.91 **Cochlear aplasia in a 9-month-old girl with congenital bilateral sensorineural hearing loss. A:** Axial bone window CT image shows absence of a cochlea in its expected location (*arrow*). The internal auditory canal (IAC) is abnormal in its course, directed posterolaterally (*arrowhead*). **B:** Axial bone window CT image at a more rostral level demonstrates an abnormally dilated vestibule (*arrow*).

promontory is flat. This rare anomaly can be unilateral and sporadic or bilateral and syndromic in nature. It is important to search for anomalies of the ipsilateral internal carotid artery and associated cephaloceles.[195]

Cochlear aplasia is absence of the cochlea in the presence of normal or malformed vestibule and SCC (Fig. 3.91). Patients with cochlear aplasia have no hearing.[193]

Cochlear hypoplasia (CH) refers to a cochlea that is small, usually fewer than two turns, with or without internal structure (Fig. 3.92).

CH type I is a small cochlear bud that lacks internal structure.

CH type II is a small cystic cochlea that lacks internal structure.

CH type III is a small cochlea (<2 turns) with a shortened modiolus and interscalar septa.

Common cavity is a single primitive cystic cavity in place of the cochlea and vestibule, which are not further differentiated beyond this point (Fig. 3.93).

Cystic cochleovestibular anomaly (IP-I) is a globular cochlea that lacks any internal architecture, including the cribriform area. The vestibule is also large and cystic. The cochlea and vestibule thus have a bilobed cystic appearance resembling a "snowman" or "figure of 8." The vestibule and lateral SCC form a single space without an intervening bone island.[193]

IP-I is a cochlea that lacks internal structure (Fig. 3.94). The spectrum of anomaly ranges from mild (cochlea lacks internal structure but the vestibule and SCC are normal or mildly malformed) to severe (cystic cochleovestibular anomaly).

IP-II (previously termed Mondini deformity) is a cochlea with a normal basal turn and deficient interscalar septum between the middle and apical turns, which appear plump (Fig. 3.95A). The modiolus is deficient. The vestibule and lateral SCC are sometimes enlarged (Fig. 3.95B). Associated LVA (Fig. 3.95B) is an important finding with regard to patient management.

Modiolar deficiency, also associated with LVA, is a relatively subtle anomaly where the cochlea demonstrates a normal interscalar septum, but the modiolar struts are asymmetric, resulting in asymmetric scalar chambers.

LVA is the most common inner ear malformation seen in patients with SNHL. LVA typically has a flared morphology (Fig. 3.96) and is usually associated with modiolar deficiency with or without IP-II. MR shows enlargement of the endolymphatic sac and duct lying lateral to the dura and sometimes containing a sediment level (Fig. 3.96). A midpoint

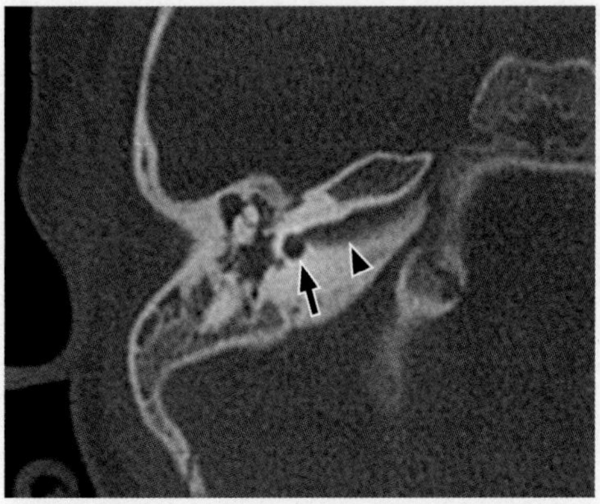

FIGURE 3.92 **Cochlear hypoplasia.** Axial bone window CT image shows a small cochlear bud (*arrow*) off of the internal auditory canal (*arrowhead*). The vestibule is diminutive (not shown).

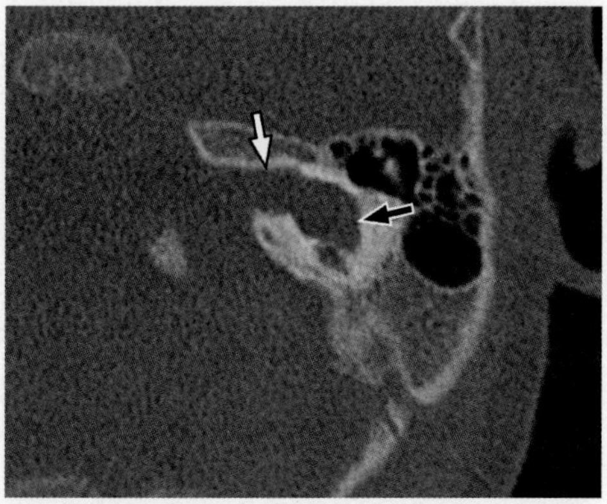

FIGURE 3.93 **Common cavity.** Axial bone window CT image demonstrates a common cavity (*black arrow*) in place of the cochlea and vestibule. An enlarged internal auditory canal (*white arrow*) leads up to it.

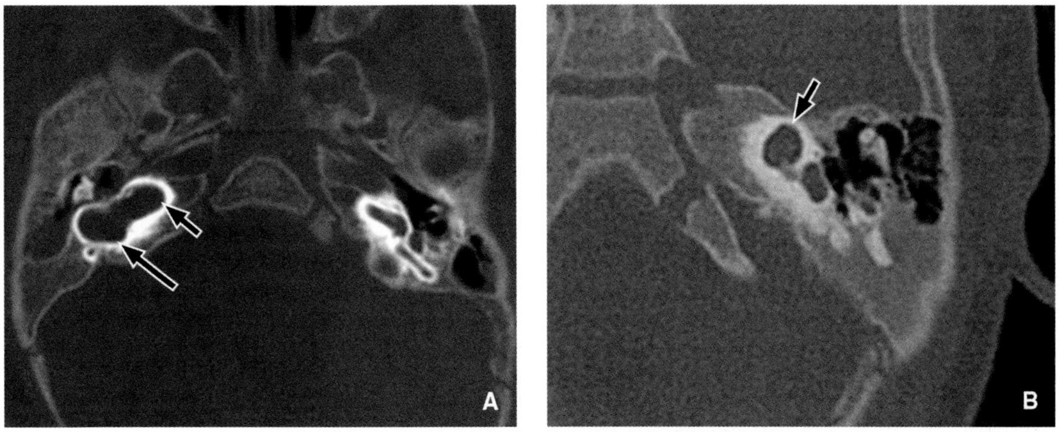

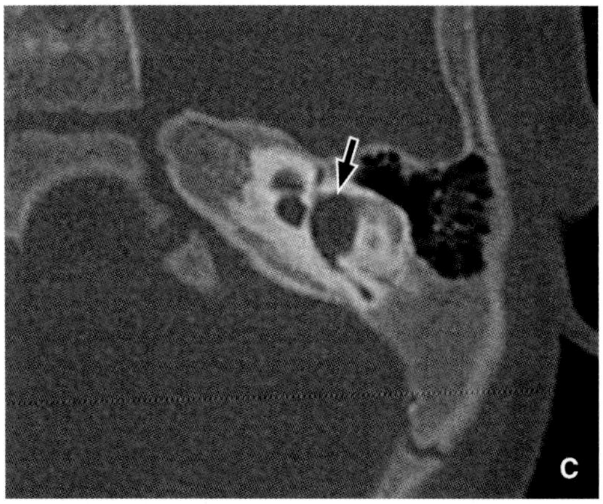

FIGURE 3.94 **Cochlear incomplete partition type I (IP-I). A:** Cystic cochleovestibular anomaly in an infant girl with multiple congenital anomalies. Axial bone window CT image reveals globular dilatation of the right cochlea, which lacks internal structure (*short arrow*). There is wide communication between the cochlea and the globular vestibule-lateral semicircular canal (*long arrow*). The posterior semicircular canal and left inner ear structures appear normal. The cochlear nerve canal appears stenotic and the internal auditory canal appears normal (not shown). **B and C:** Axial bone window CT images in a different pediatric patient demonstrate an empty, cystic cochlea without partitions within (*arrow* in **B**). The vestibule is large and cystic (*arrow* in **C**).

width ≥ 1 mm and an opercular width ≥ 2 mm on CT constitute LVA.[196] More recently, CT images reformatted in the Pöschl plane (parallel to the plane of the superior SCC) have been proposed for more accurate measurements of the vestibular aqueduct, where a width of 1 mm is considered to be the upper limit of normal.[197] The clinical relevance of LVA is the potential for progressive SNHL, sometimes with a sudden decrease in hearing after relatively mild head trauma. Affected children are therefore advised to avoid contact sports. Flared LVA, usually with IP-II or modiolar deficiency, is associated with mutations in the *SLC26A4* gene that encodes for the pendrin protein. *SLC26A4* gene mutations are detected in up to 90% of patients with Pendred syndrome (LVA with thyroid organification defect leading to hypothyroidism and sometimes goiter) and up to 40% of patients with nonsyndromic deafness with LVA (DFNB4).[194] Funnel-shaped LVA is also seen in a variety of other syndromes, for example, BOR syndrome and CHARGE syndrome.[198]

The anatomic description of cochlear anomalies as outlined earlier is helpful in providing a description of cochlear appearance but does not necessarily provide clues as to an underlying syndromic etiology beyond the association of

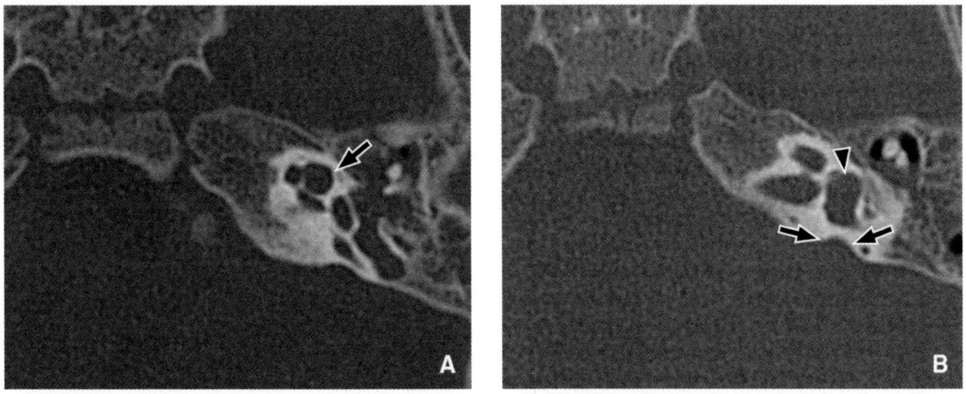

FIGURE 3.95 **Cochlear incomplete partition type II (IP-II). A:** Axial bone window CT image shows coalescence of the middle and apical turns into a cystic apex, without an interscalar septum separating the two (*arrow*). **B:** Axial bone window CT image demonstrates the vestibule which is mildly enlarged (*arrowhead*). The vestibular aqueduct is enlarged as well (*arrows*).

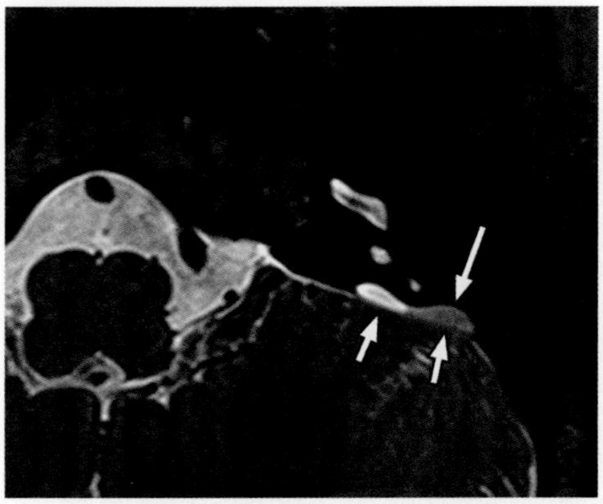

FIGURE 3.96 **Large vestibular aqueduct containing enlarged endolymphatic sac.** Axial T2 SPACE MR image shows an enlarged endolymphatic sac with sedimentation of contents (*long arrow*). Note the location of the endolymphatic sac lateral to the dural reflection (*short arrows*).

IP-II (where the cochlea resembles a baseball cap) and LVA with Pendred syndrome and DFNB4. However, there are some very specific anomalies that do suggest an underlying syndromic diagnosis. In BOR syndrome, the basal turn of the cochlea is tapered and the middle and apical turns are hypoplastic and offset anteriorly, giving the cochlea a characteristic "unwound" appearance. Other typical features include funnel-shaped LVA, SCC malformations including posterior SCC anomaly, middle/external ear and ossicular malformations, and enlarged eustachian tubes. X-linked MHL with stapes gusher (DFNX2) is associated with a malformed corkscrew-shaped cochlea that lacks internal septation, with enlargement of the lateral half of the IAC and sometimes vestibule and SCC enlargement. This is an important diagnosis to make because of the potential for a CSF gusher at attempted stapedectomy or cochleostomy. CHARGE syndrome is associated with absence or flattening of the apical and sometimes middle turn of the cochlea, typically with stenosis or atresia of the cochlear nerve canal. However, the most diagnostic feature of CHARGE syndrome is hypoplasia of the vestibule with aplasia or hypoplasia of the SCC (Fig. 3.51).[199]

SCC malformations are often seen in association with other inner ear anomalies. Malformation most commonly involves the lateral SCC. This can occur as an isolated phenomenon but is also seen in several syndromes such as trisomy 21 and Apert syndrome, in which either there is a small bone island and mildly globular lateral SCC or the lateral SCC forms a common cavity with the vestibule (anlage anomaly).[198] Isolated posterior SCC anomalies are seen in a subtype of Waardenburg syndrome and Alagille syndrome.

Atresia or stenosis of the cochlear nerve canal is associated with aplasia or hypoplasia of the cochlear nerve, often as an isolated finding, particularly in children with congenital unilateral SNHL. However, cochlear nerve aplasia/hypoplasia can occur with aplasia of the vestibular nerve. In infants and children, cochlear nerve aplasia or hypoplasia is usually congenital in nature. Cochlear implants are contraindicated in the setting of cochlear nerve aplasia or severe hypoplasia. MRI is the most sensitive technique for diagnosing cochlear nerve aplasia or hypoplasia.[200] The most helpful sequence is the heavily T2-weighted sequence (e.g., 3D T2 SPACE, DRIVE, FIESTA), which outlines nerves, appearing dark against a background of bright CSF. Oblique sagittal images oriented perpendicular to the long axis of the IAC demonstrates absence or decreased size of the cochlear nerve in the anteroinferior quadrant of the canal reflecting aplasia or hypoplasia (Fig. 3.97). On CT, findings that suggest cochlear nerve aplasia/hypoplasia are absence or stenosis of the cochlear nerve canal or a stenotic IAC.

Infectious and Inflammatory Disorders

Acute Otitis Media

Acute otitis media (AOM) occurs most frequently as a complication of a viral URI.[201,202] Imaging is not necessary in uncomplicated cases. If imaged, one sees opacity in the middle ear with possible fluid levels.[203] There is frequently fluid in the mastoid air cells as well, without bone erosion.

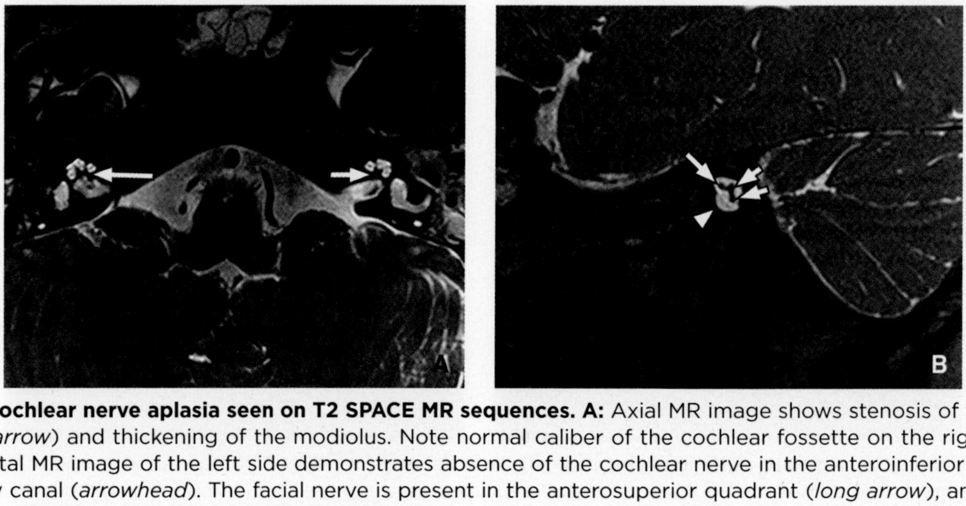

FIGURE 3.97 **Cochlear nerve aplasia seen on T2 SPACE MR sequences. A:** Axial MR image shows stenosis of the left cochlear fossette (*short arrow*) and thickening of the modiolus. Note normal caliber of the cochlear fossette on the right (*long arrow*). **B:** Oblique sagittal MR image of the left side demonstrates absence of the cochlear nerve in the anteroinferior quadrant of the internal auditory canal (*arrowhead*). The facial nerve is present in the anterosuperior quadrant (*long arrow*), and the vestibular nerves are seen posteriorly as an ovoid structure (*double short arrows*) prior to its division into superior and inferior branches.

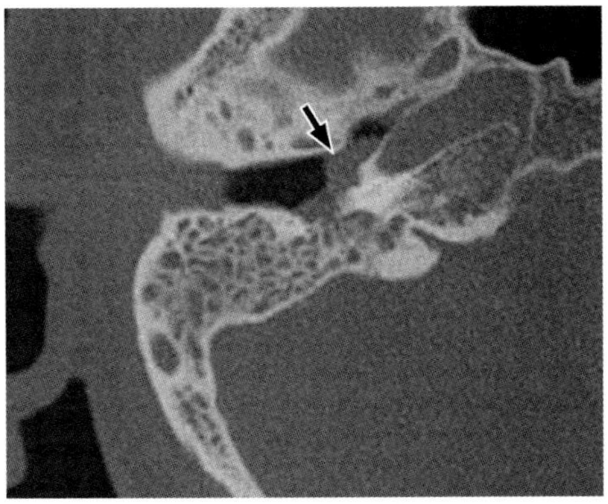

FIGURE 3.98 **Acute mastoiditis.** Axial bone window CT image demonstrates opacification of the mastoid air cells. The mastoid bony septations and cortex remain intact without erosion. The patient also has otitis media, with opacity in the middle ear (*arrow*).

Coalescent Mastoiditis and Petrous Apex Infection

Acute mastoiditis is seen mostly in young children in association with AOM (Fig. 3.98) but can also occur in the setting of obstructive middle ear processes such as cholesteatoma or tumor. Spread of infection to the mastoid trabeculae and cortical bone is known as coalescent mastoiditis, usually heralded by the presence of retroauricular swelling, erythema, or protrusion of the auricle in the setting of recent or coexistent OM and uncontrolled inflammation.[201] Suppurative accumulation under pressure results in acidosis, bony demineralization, ischemia, and osteoclastic resorption of the walls of the mastoid air cells, which then coalesce into larger cavities filled with purulent exudate and granulation tissue.[201]

Imaging is indicated to confirm the diagnosis and detect local and intracranial complications. On CT, the hallmark of coalescent mastoiditis is erosion of mastoid septations, with or without erosion of the retroauricular cortex, sinus plate, and/or tegmen tympani (Fig. 3.99A).

Treatment options depend on clinical course and imaging appearance and range from antibiotics and tympanostomy tube placement to mastoidectomy.

The infection can spread laterally to cause erosion of the external mastoid cortex and a postauricular subperiosteal abscess (Fig. 3.99B).[203] Infection of a pneumatized mastoid tip may extend inferiorly into the soft tissues of the neck deep to the sternocleidomastoid muscle and cause what is known as a Bezold abscess (Fig. 3.99C).[203]

Erosion of the internal mastoid cortex overlying the sigmoid sinus can result in a perisinus epidural abscess. Thrombosis of the sigmoid sinus and/or internal jugular vein (IJV) results from compression due to abscess and/or thrombophlebitis (Figs. 3.99B, C and 3.100) without an abscess. Rarely, venous sinus thrombosis occurs because of acute otomastoiditis without clear-cut evidence of mastoid coalescence, because of thrombophlebitis spreading via emissary veins.

On CT and MR, it can be difficult to distinguish between a perisinus abscess and sigmoid sinus thrombosis. Both lesions appear hypodense with peripheral enhancement on CT; however, a thrombosed sinus appears slightly denser than does an abscess. On MR, loss of normal flow void within the sinus can occur because of compression from a perisinus abscess

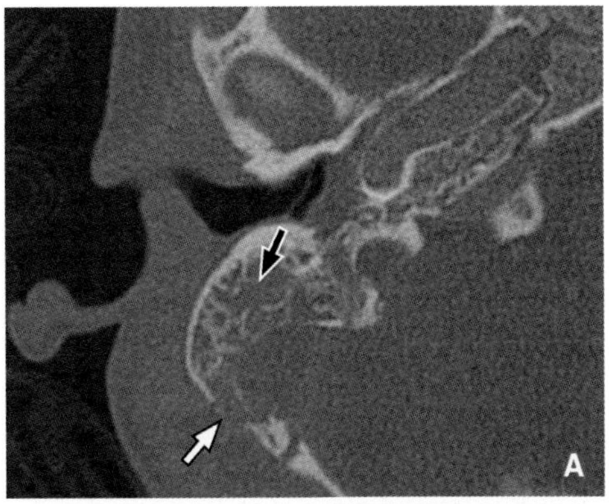

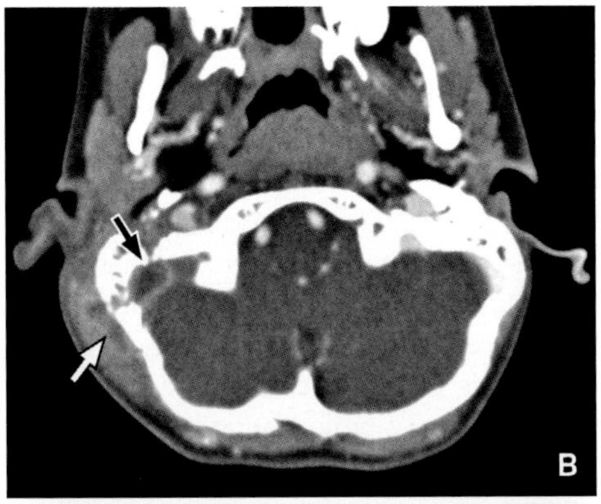

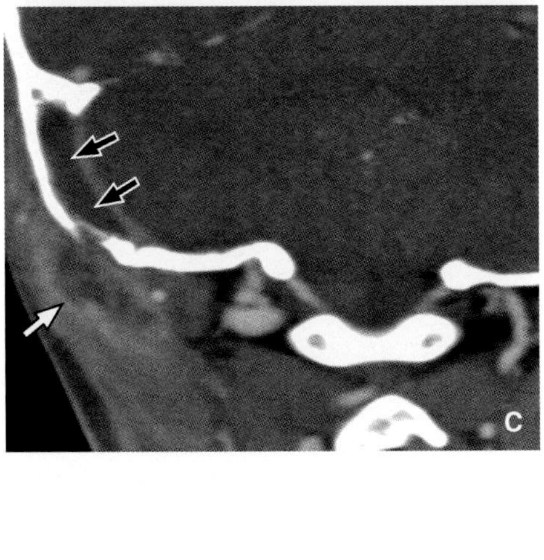

FIGURE 3.99 **Coalescent mastoiditis, Bezold abscess, dural venous sinus thrombosis in a 9-year-old boy who presented with otalgia and hearing loss. A:** Axial bone window CT image demonstrates opacification of the mastoid air cells. In this case, however, there is erosion of the mastoid septations (*black arrow*) and cortex (*white arrow*). **B and C:** Axial and coronal contrast-enhanced CT images show soft tissue swelling and an abscess (*white arrows*). Filling defect in the sigmoid sinus represents thrombus (*black arrows*) as confirmed by the coronal CT image. Note that the axial CT image does not distinguish between an epidural abscess and sigmoid sinus thrombosis.

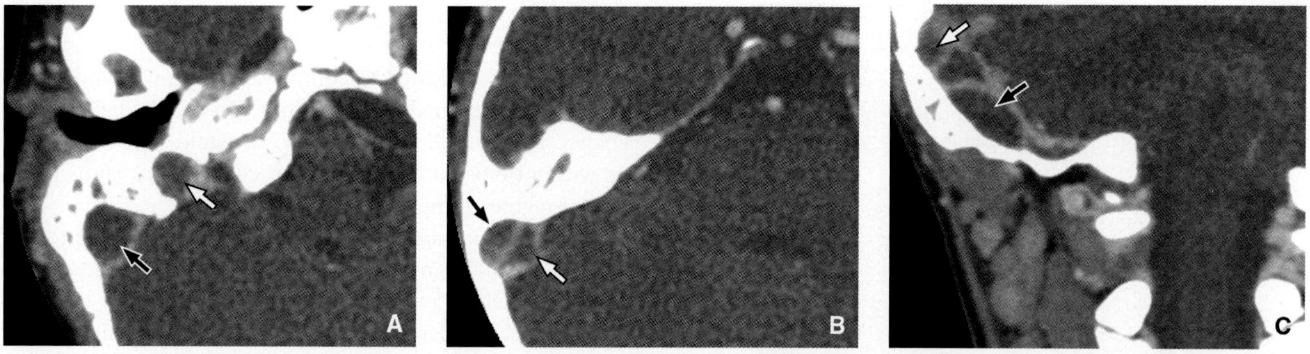

FIGURE 3.100 **Coalescent mastoiditis, epidural abscess, and venous thrombosis. A:** Axial contrast-enhanced CT image demonstrates opacification of right mastoid air cells in this child who had osseous erosion (not shown) consistent with coalescent mastoiditis. There is a rounded hypodensity with peripheral enhancement (*black arrow*) in the expected location of the sigmoid sinus. This could represent either a perisinus epidural abscess compressing the sigmoid sinus or thrombus within the sigmoid sinus. There is thrombus within the internal jugular vein that is of a slightly higher density (*white arrow*). **B:** Axial contrast-enhanced CT image obtained at a more cephalad level than Figure 3.100A reveals epidural abscess (*black arrow*) lateral to thrombus within the sigmoid sinus (*white arrow*). **C:** Coronal reformatted CT image demonstrates the relationship of the epidural abscess (*black arrow*) to thrombus in the sigmoid sinus upstream (*white arrow*) and downstream from the abscess.

or because of thrombus within the sinus, and MR venogram does not always permit distinction between the two. The abscess usually appears hyperintense on T2-weighted MR images, whereas thrombus usually appears somewhat hypointense on T2-weighted MR images. Additional intracranial complications include meningitis, subdural empyema, cerebritis, abscesses, and carotid artery involvement.[201]

If mastoid infection spreads medially to the petrous apex, petrous apex osteomyelitis (in nonpneumatized petrous apex) or petrous apicitis (petrositis; in pneumatized petrous apex) may occur. Gradenigo syndrome refers to a triad of deep retro-orbital pain in the distribution of the trigeminal nerve, diplopia due to sixth nerve palsy, and persistent otorrhea/suppurative otitis media, associated with bacterial otitis media with petrous apicitis.[204] The symptoms are related to local spread of infection from the middle ear and petrous apex to the regional meninges, with involvement of the nearby Gasserian ganglion in Meckel cave and sixth nerve in Dorello canal.

On imaging, petrous apicitis manifests as erosive changes in the petrous apex with fluid in the air cells on CT and abnormal enhancement of the adjacent meninges on MR (Fig. 3.101).[203] Petrous apex osteomyelitis usually occurs in the setting of otomastoiditis and appears as T2 prolongation of the petrous marrow with marrow enhancement on MR. There is typically associated spasm of the petrous segment of the internal carotid artery. Complications are as for mastoiditis but also include cavernous sinus thrombosis and arterial complications. Differential diagnosis includes malignancies such as RMS and metastasis (e.g., from neuroblastoma [Fig. 3.102]).

Chronic Otitis Media

In chronic otitis media, there is long-term damage to the middle ear by infection and inflammation. Common causes include underlying eustachian tube dysfunction and tympanic membrane perforation.[203] On imaging, one may see middle ear effusion, granulation tissue, cholesterol granuloma, and cholesteatoma. There is typically also underpneumatization of the affected mastoid region with sclerosis surrounding the pneumatized portions of the bone.

Acute Labyrinthitis

Labyrinthitis in the pediatric age group typically presents with SNHL and sometimes vertigo. Etiology includes infectious and noninfectious causes (e.g., autoimmune disease, toxins, and trauma). Spread of infection to the inner ear structures can occur via tympanogenic, hematogenic, or meningogenic

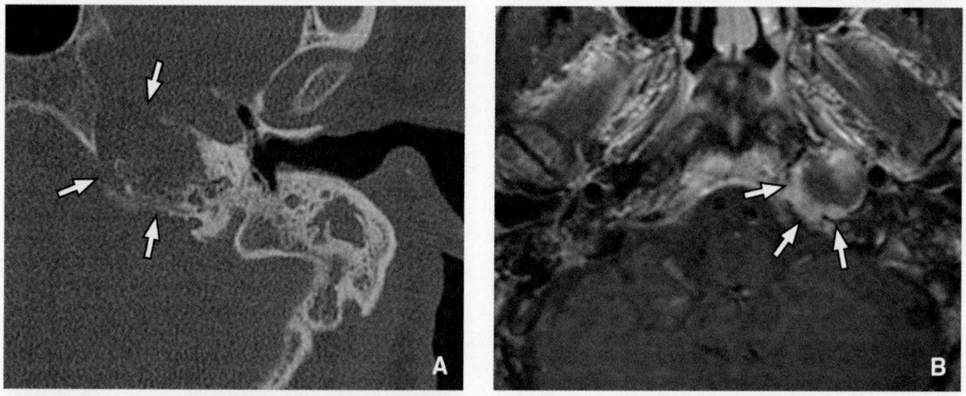

FIGURE 3.101 **Petrous apicitis. A:** Axial bone window CT image demonstrates opacified petrous apex air cells, with bone erosion (*arrows*). **B:** Axial postcontrast T1-weighted MR image shows fluid centrally, with peripheral enhancement (*arrows*).

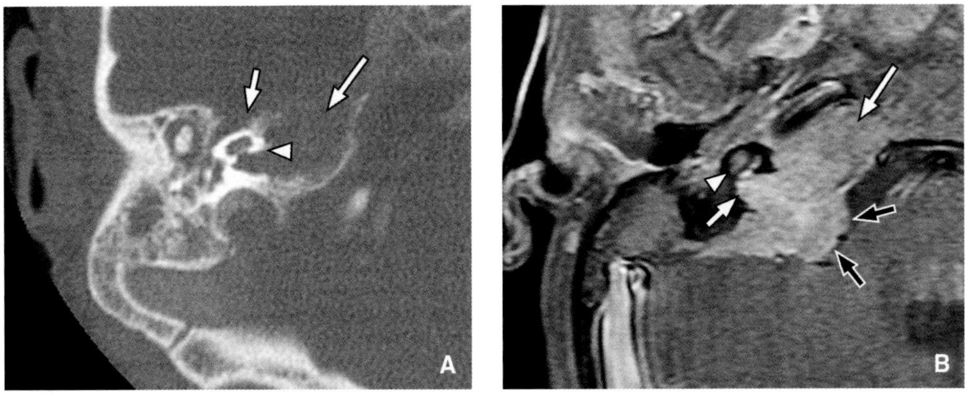

FIGURE 3.102 **Neuroblastoma metastasis in an infant girl who presented with otalgia, otorrhea, and a seventh nerve palsy. A:** Axial contrast-enhanced bone window CT image demonstrates a mass eroding the right petrous apex (*long arrow*), anterior wall of the internal auditory canal (IAC) (*arrowhead*), and the anterior genu of the facial nerve canal (*short arrow*). There is extensive right middle ear space and mastoid opacification. The extent of bony erosion and involvement of the IAC is atypical for petrous apex osteomyelitis. **B:** Axial T1-weighted fat-suppressed MR image shows the extensive enhancing tumor (*long white arrow*) extending into the IAC and into the cochlea (*white arrowhead*), facial nerve canal (*short white arrow*), and middle ear space. The tumor also protrudes into the cerebellopontine angle cistern (*black arrows*). Biopsy of tumor from the middle ear space revealed neuroblastoma. Primary adrenal neuroblastoma was subsequently diagnosed.

routes.[205] An important cause of acute labyrinthitis in children is acute bacterial meningitis due to *H. influenzae* or *S. pneumoniae.* Profound deafness occurs rapidly over weeks, necessitating cochlear implantation.

During the acute stage of infection, MR reveals preservation of fluid signal within the membranous labyrinth, and thin-section, contrast-enhanced, T1-weighted fat-suppressed MR images demonstrate enhancement within the cochlea, vestibule, and SCC. In the subacute phase, there is increasing labyrinthine fibrosis; the enhancement subsides, and there is loss of fluid signal intensity within the membranous labyrinth on thin-section 3D T2-weighted MR images. This phase is followed by progressive labyrinthine ossification within weeks of the initiating event. On CT, ossification commences as hazy increased density within the scala tympani of the cochlea near the round window, and in the SCC. Over weeks, this can progress to florid labyrinthine ossification.

Acquired Cholesteatoma

An acquired cholesteatoma is an accumulation of desquamated keratin epithelium that most frequently occurs in the middle ear, and less commonly in the EAC, mastoid air cells, and petrous apex air cells. It is composed of acellular keratin debris, surrounded by a two-layered lining: the inner layer (matrix) is keratinizing squamous epithelium, and the outer layer (perimatrix) is subepithelial connective tissue (Fig. 3.103). The matrix produces the keratin, whereas the perimatrix produces proteolytic enzymes that are capable of resorbing bone.[203] There are various theories for how acquired middle ear cholesteatomas form. According to the invagination theory, chronic eustachian tube dysfunction leads to a vacuum phenomenon in the middle ear, causing a retraction pocket to form in the TM pars flaccida, and the lining surface epithelium grows over time. According to the epithelial invasion theory, a TM perforation leads to ingrowth of keratinizing stratified squamous epithelium in the middle ear. Most (80%) acquired cholesteatomas are associated with the pars flaccida. Affected pediatric patients can present with chronic otorrhea, TM perforation, and a retraction pocket.

On CT, pars flaccida cholesteatomas are typically seen in Prussak space as a rounded expansile mass with erosion of adjacent bone including the scutum and/or the ossicles, sometimes with medial displacement of the ossicles (Fig. 3.104). The

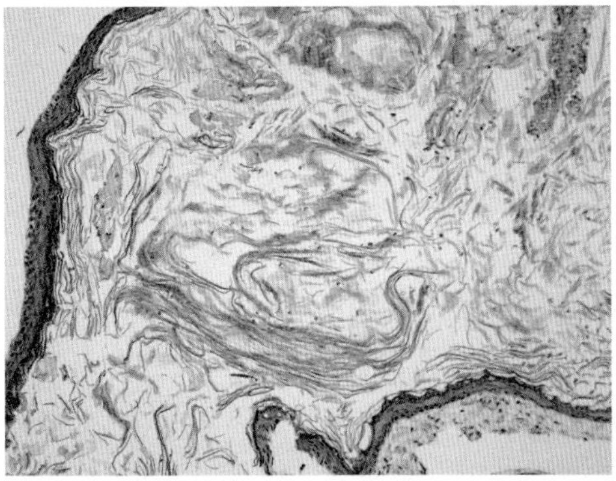

FIGURE 3.103 **Cholesteatoma in a 16-year-old boy.** This middle ear mass shows squamous epithelium with accumulated keratin debris (hematoxylin and eosin, original magnification, 200×).

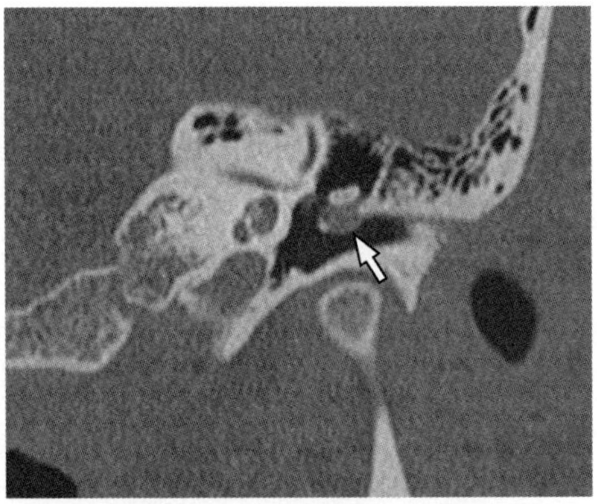

FIGURE 3.104 **Middle ear acquired cholesteatoma.** Coronal bone window CT image demonstrates a rounded soft tissue mass (*arrow*) in the middle ear, displacing the ossicles medially. The long process of the incus is eroded.

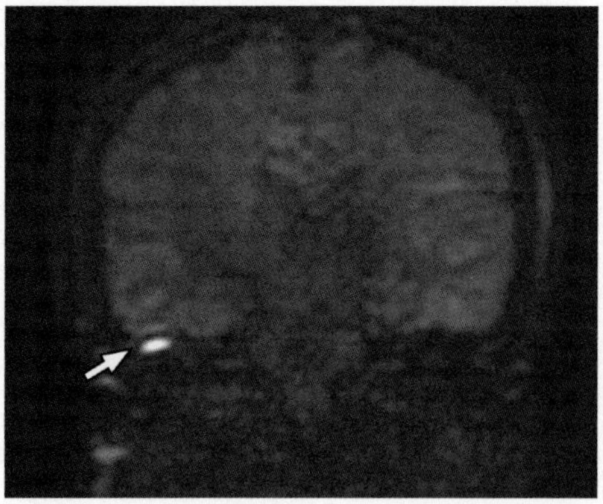

FIGURE 3.105 **Cholesteatoma.** Coronal non-echo-planar diffusion-weighted MR image shows a focus of diffusion reduction on the right, representing a cholesteatoma (*arrow*) in the mastoid region.

lesion may extend into the attic and mastoid air cells. In contradistinction, pars tensa cholesteatomas are usually located medial to the ossicles and displace them laterally. Erosion of the tegmen may result in a meningoencephalocele. Erosion of the otic capsule overlying the lateral SCC results in a labyrinthine fistula. On MRI, cholesteatomas demonstrate characteristic decreased diffusivity. This is best seen on non–echo planar turbo spin echo–based DWI technique (Fig. 3.105). They are hypointense on T1-weighted sequence, mildly hyperintense on T2-weighted sequence, and do not enhance.

Cholesterol Granuloma

Cholesterol granuloma results from rupture of blood vessels in an air space with negative pressure or vacuum phenomenon, as seen in a middle ear cavity where there is eustachian tube dysfunction, in a petrous apex air cell with obstructed drainage, or in a mastoidectomy cavity. With breakdown of red blood cells and tissue elements, cholesterol is released, inciting a foreign body giant cell reaction and formation of a granuloma with cholesterol elements. Cholesterol granuloma can also occur in the setting of a ruptured cholesteatoma, where there is granulomatous response to the cholesterol-rich contents. Because of the presence of blood products and/or cholesterol elements, this lesion is characteristically hyperintense on T1-weighted MR sequences, does not demonstrate fat suppression, and does not enhance, distinguishing it from other entities such as cholesteatoma, fatty tissue, and granulation tissue (Fig. 3.106). In practice, however, features of acquired cholesteatoma and cholesterol granuloma often coexist in the same lesion.

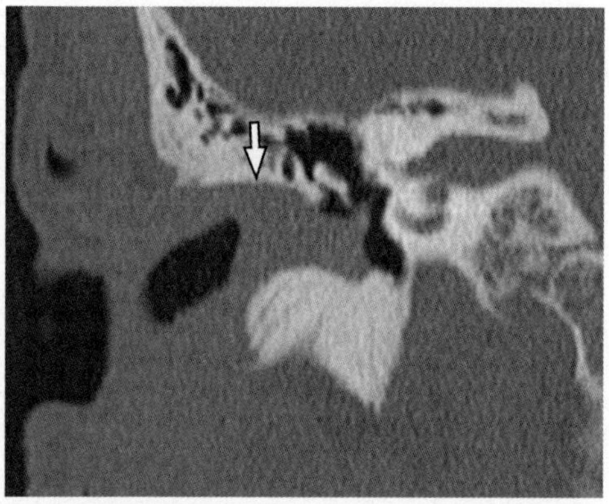

FIGURE 3.107 **Keratosis obturans in a 14-year-old boy with chronic otitis media.** Coronal bone window CT image shows a soft tissue plug in the external auditory canal (EAC) causing expansile scalloping of the roof of the EAC (*arrow*).

Keratosis Obturans

Keratosis obturans represents an accumulation of desquamated keratin debris within the EAC, causing smooth EAC expansion. Affected patients are usually young, presenting with severe pain and conductive hearing loss, and there may be associated sinusitis and bronchiectasis. The presence of EAC stenosis predisposes to the accumulation of keratin debris. CT is important to help confirm smooth expansile scalloping of bone (Fig. 3.107). If there is more extensive bone erosion, diagnoses such as EAC cholesteatoma and malignant neoplasms should be considered.

Malignant Otitis Externa

Malignant otitis externa (MOE) is an aggressive necrotizing infection involving the external ear. There is sometimes associated osteomyelitis of the skull base, typically caused by pseudomonas and seen in immunocompromised patients and diabetics. CT helps to define the extent of bone destruction and abnormal inflammatory soft tissue in air cell spaces

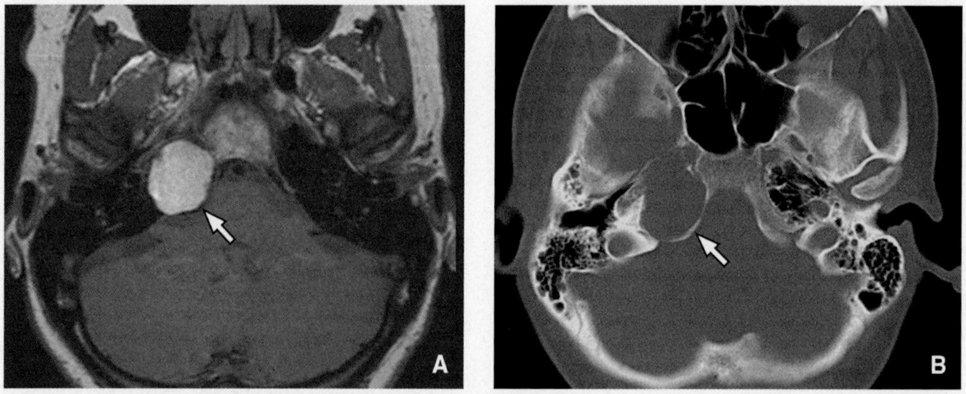

FIGURE 3.106 **Petrous apex cholesterol granuloma. A:** Axial non-contrast-enhanced T1-weighted MR image shows a large, expansile mass (*arrow*) that is intrinsically hyperintense in signal. **B:** Axial bone window CT image shows smooth expansile scalloping of the surrounding bone margins (*arrow*).

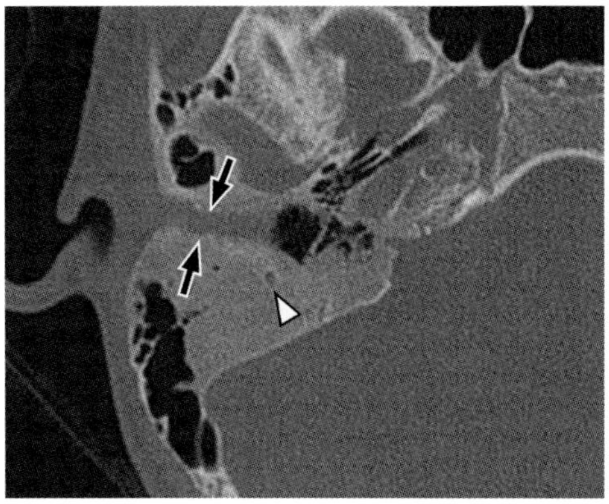

FIGURE 3.108 **Fibrous dysplasia in a 15-year-old boy.** Axial bone window CT image shows homogeneous ground-glass appearance at the tympanic and mastoid portions of the temporal bone. The external auditory canal is narrowed (*arrows*). The mastoid facial nerve canal (*arrowhead*) traverses this region.

(e.g., middle ear, mastoid), whereas MRI is superior for delineating soft tissue involvement in the skull base and neck.

Neoplasms and Tumor-Like Disorders

Temporal bone neoplasms are rare in childhood. Only the more commonly encountered tumors are discussed in this chapter.

Fibrous Dysplasia

CT is the modality of choice for depicting temporal bone fibrous dysplasia, showing expansile bone with a "ground-glass" appearance as well as the effect on skull base foramina and normally air-filled spaces of the temporal bone, which may be narrowed (Fig. 3.108).[206–208] Middle ear encroachment is uncommon.[209] The otic capsule is rarely involved. On MR, fibrous dysplasia appears hypointense on both T1- and T2-weighted sequences, although foci of increased T2 signal may be seen. There is variable enhancement, ranging from moderate to intense.

Exostosis and Osteoma

Exostoses and osteomas involve the EAC and, much less commonly, the IAC.[210] Exostoses are broad-based sessile lesions and are usually multiple and bilaterally symmetrical

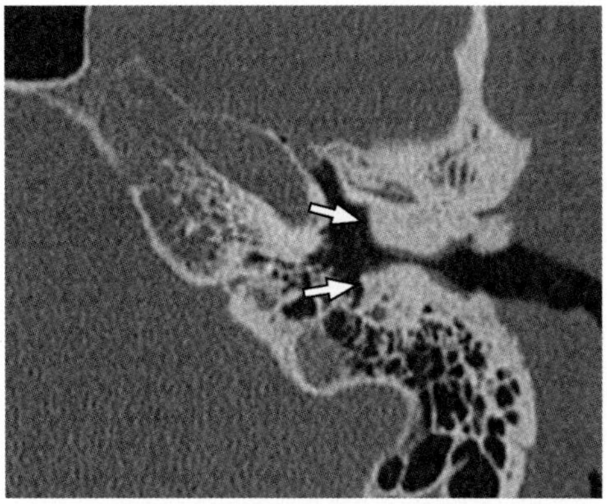

FIGURE 3.109 **External auditory canal (EAC) exostosis.** Axial bone window CT image shows broad-based sessile bony growths (*arrows*) in the medial portion of the EAC.

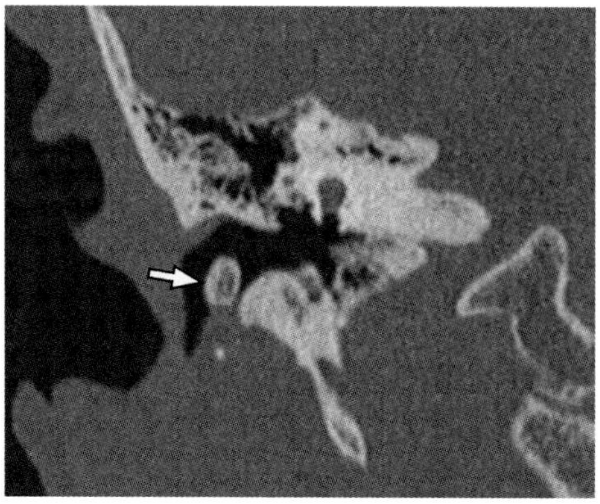

FIGURE 3.110 **External auditory canal (EAC) osteoma.** Coronal bone window CT image shows a solitary, pedunculated bony lesion (*arrow*) in the lateral portion of the EAC near the bony-cartilaginous junction.

(Fig. 3.109).[211] They are thought to be a reactive process related to recurrent cold water exposures or recurrent otitis externa and are therefore common among surfing populations and sometimes referred to as "surfer's ear." Osteomas are pedunculated bony growths, usually solitary with central bone marrow[210] and found more laterally in the EAC near the bony–cartilaginous junction (Fig. 3.110). CT is the optimal modality for diagnosing these entities.

Vestibular Schwannoma

Vestibular schwannomas can be seen anywhere between the CPA cistern and the IAC fundus, frequently causing expansion of the porus acusticus. When seen in a child, even if unilateral, neurofibromatosis type II (NF2) should be considered (Fig. 3.111).[212] It has been recommended that all children with an appropriate family history undergo MRI screening at an early age (age 10 to 12 years) regardless of the auditory brainstem response.[213,214] Patients under the age of 30 years with unilateral vestibular schwannoma should be carefully evaluated for a potential second lesion on the contralateral side, and imaging of the cervical spine is advised.

A vestibular schwannoma has high signal intensity on T2-weighted MR images and enhances (Fig. 3.111A). An unenhanced T1-weighted sequence is important to exclude a lipoma. Heavily T2-weighted MR imaging outlines the dark-appearing tumor well against a background of bright CSF. Tumor growing into the cochlear nerve canal is termed an impacted vestibular schwannoma and is associated with a decreased likelihood of hearing preservation after surgical resection. When large, a vestibular schwannoma may have internal cystic components (Fig. 3.112A), and the ipsilateral labyrinthine fluid often has slightly less intense signal on heavily T2-weighted MR images than does the contralateral normal side, presumably related to higher protein content on the affected side. CT may demonstrate expansile bony scalloping of the IAC walls in bone algorithm (Fig. 3.112B).

Surgical resection is the accepted treatment for removal of schwannoma when feasible. Stereotactic radiation may be considered for high-risk patients or patients with bilateral, recurrent, or residual tumors.[215]

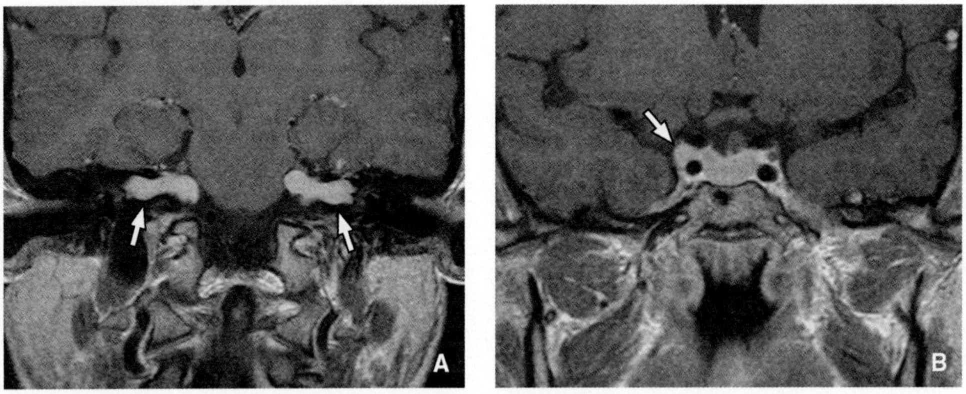

FIGURE 3.111 **Bilateral vestibular schwannomas in neurofibromatosis type 2.** Coronal postcontrast T1-weighted MRI images **(A and B)**. There are homogeneously enhancing masses in bilateral internal auditory canals, representing vestibular schwannomas (*arrows* in **A**). There is also a third nerve schwannoma (*arrow* in **B**) and an ependymoma at the cervicomedullary junction (not shown).

Rhabdomyosarcoma

RMS is the most common primary malignancy of the temporal bone in children, although only 8% to 10% of all head and neck RMS are seen in the middle ear and mastoid region.[216] The embryonal subtype is the most commonly found subtype in the head and neck, although it is not uncommon to see a mixture of subtypes in a lesion.[217]

Affected pediatric patients typically present prior to the age of 5 years. The most common clinical manifestation is chronic otorrhea or chronic otitis media unresponsive to treatment, sometimes with an EAC or retroauricular mass. Cranial nerve palsies indicate advanced disease. Tumors spread by contiguous destruction of soft tissue and bone, extension along nerves, hematogenous spread, and lymphatic spread.

On CT, RMS appears as an enhancing mass with bony destruction of the temporal bone and skull base (Fig. 3.113). Vascular complications include jugular vein compression and invasion. MRI permits soft tissue characterization and detection of intracranial involvement and meningeal invasion. The tumor has intermediate signal on T1- and T2-weighted sequences, decreased diffusivity, and significant enhancement. Differential diagnosis includes metastasis, other malignancies, and LCH. In a young child or infant, a differential diagnosis of an atypical teratoid rhabdoid tumor (ATRT) should be considered.

RMS is highly aggressive with poor survival outcome. With improved treatment, usually combined radiation and chemotherapy, survival has improved significantly with a 5-year disease-free survival rate between 41% (advanced disease) and 81% (nonadvanced disease).[218,219] Radical complete surgical excision is much less commonly performed now because there is no evidence that temporal bone resection adds to survival but has high associated morbidity and physical deformity.[216]

Metastasis

The most common temporal bone metastases are from leukemia and neuroblastoma (Fig. 3.102). CT reveals lytic, permeative bone destruction, and MRI is obtained to detect intracranial involvement. The differential diagnosis includes other malignancies such as RMS. The clinical presentation and imaging appearance can also simulate inflammatory processes such as coalescent mastoiditis or petrous apex infection. By contrast, LCH tends to produce sharply marginated bony destruction.

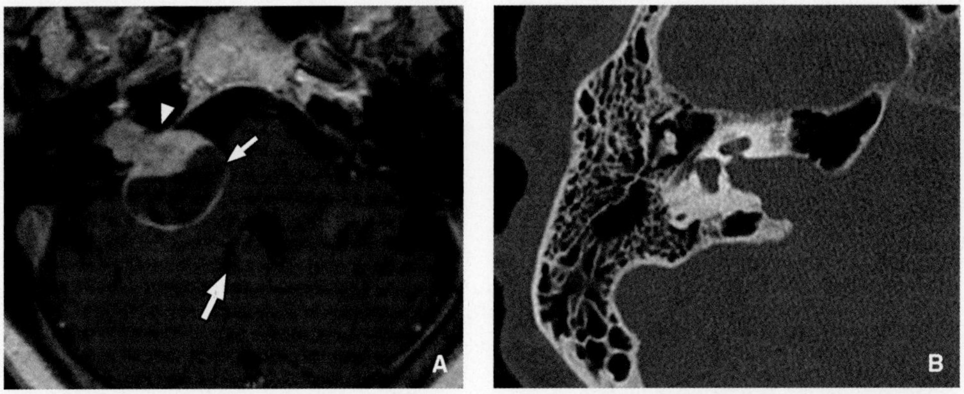

FIGURE 3.112 **Large vestibular schwannoma with cystic change. A:** Axial contrast-enhanced T1-weighted MR image demonstrates an enhancing mass in the internal auditory canal (IAC) and cerebellopontine angle (CPA), expanding the porus acusticus (*arrowhead*). There is cystic change at the periphery (*small arrow*). Note mass effect on the brainstem and cerebellum; the fourth ventricle is compressed (*large arrow*). **B:** Axial bone window CT image shows expansile scalloping of the bony IAC around the mass.

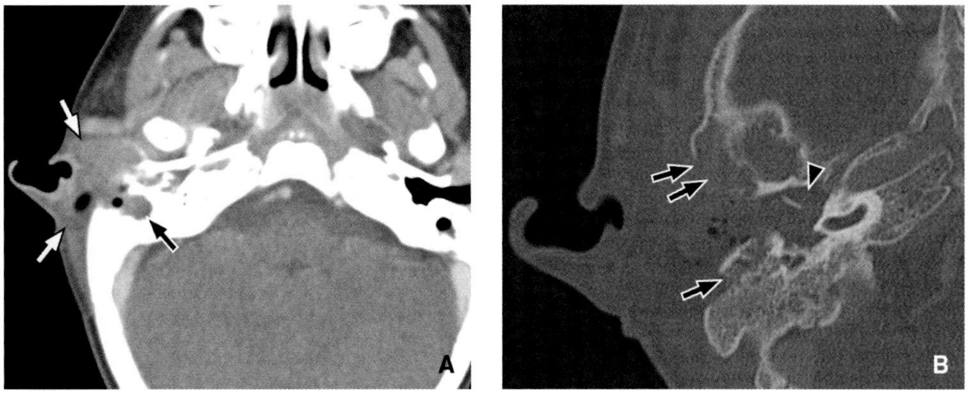

FIGURE 3.113 **Rhabdomyosarcoma in the middle ear and mastoid in a 30-month-old girl. A:** Axial contrast-enhanced CT image in soft tissue algorithm shows enhancing soft tissue (*arrows*) in the periauricular region extending into the middle ear and mastoid. Foci of gas within the mass are related to recent biopsy. **B:** Axial bone window CT image better demonstrates bone erosion (*black arrows*) involving the mastoid and squamosal portions of the temporal bone. Abnormal soft tissue fills the middle ear (*arrowhead*). The patient had an 8-week history of purulent discharge from the right ear. Her parents noticed some gray tissue protruding from the ear. Biopsy from the external and middle ear regions revealed embryonal rhabdomyosarcoma.

Langerhans Cell Histiocytosis

It is estimated that 15% to 61% of patients with LCH have otologic involvement.[220,221] The most frequent symptom is otorrhea resistant to medical therapy. Other signs and symptoms include mastoid swelling, aural polyps, and periauricular eczema.[222] Erosion of the posterior bony EAC with sagging of the canal wall skin, infiltration of the middle ear, involvement of the ossicular chain, and obstruction of the EAC can occur.

CT shows sharply marginated or "punched-out" destruction of the mastoid, squamosal, and/or tympanic portions of the temporal bone (Fig. 3.114A), with occasional petrous apex involvement. The ossicles and the bony labyrinth usually remain relatively preserved despite extensive surrounding bony destruction. Enhancing soft tissue is seen in association with the bone erosion, and there may be intracranial extradural extension. On MR imaging, the abnormal soft tissue has intermediate to high signal on T2-weighted MR images, variable signal on T1-weighted MR images, and enhances markedly (Fig. 3.114B). There is sometimes edema around the lesion.[222]

As mentioned previously, metastasis, RMS, and coalescent mastoiditis can have similar MR appearance, but the sharply marginated bony destruction seen on CT is helpful in suggesting the correct diagnosis. Bilateral temporal bone lesions are suggestive of LCH but can also be seen with metastatic disease.

Historically, treatment included mastoidectomy and radiation therapy; currently, steroid injection is favored. For the multisystemic form of LCH, chemotherapy, steroid injections, and immunotherapy are utilized.[222]

Miscellaneous Tumors

During the first year of life, an avidly enhancing IAC mass is most likely to be an infantile hemangioma (Fig. 3.39B). Associated features include the presence of vascular flow voids within the lesion, the presence of hemangiomas elsewhere, or features of PHACES association such as ipsilateral cerebellar hypoplasia.

In children, paraganglioma is extremely rare, and most cases are familial in nature. Familial tumors constitute 20% of all paragangliomas; these patients have multicentric tumors

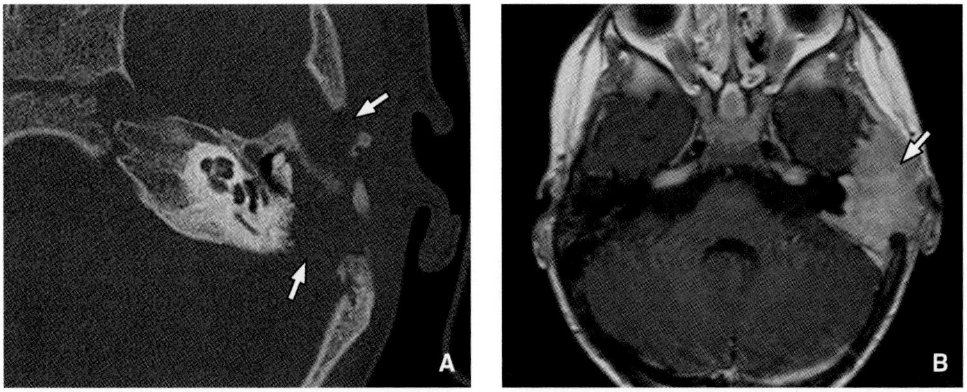

FIGURE 3.114 **Langerhans cell histiocytosis in a 27-month-old boy with a mass in the left temporal bone region. A:** Axial bone window CT image shows sharply marginated destruction of the mastoid and squamosal portions of the temporal bone (*arrows*). The ossicles and the otic capsule remain intact. **B:** Axial contrast-enhanced T1-weighted MR image reveals a soft tissue mass (*arrow*) with marked enhancement.

in 25% to 78% of cases.[223,224] In the head and neck, paragangliomas are historically referred to as "glomus tumors" despite the lack of glomus cells. Those in the middle ear are referred to as glomus tympanicum tumors. Those in the region of the jugular foramen are glomus jugulare tumors. When a glomus jugulare has a component extending into the middle ear, it is called a glomus jugulotympanicum tumor.

Paragangliomas are locally infiltrating but slow growing and are highly vascular. Affected pediatric patients typically present with otologic symptoms or a retrotympanic mass. CT of glomus tympanicum paraganglioma shows a small rounded nodule on or near the cochlear promontory, without bone erosion.[225,226] Glomus jugulare paraganglioma characteristically causes irregular demineralization with a "moth-eaten" appearance of the surrounding bone. MRI reveals avid enhancement of these lesions. A "salt and pepper" appearance on T2-weighted sequences is due to vascular flow voids within the hyperintense tumor. Preoperative angiography and embolization help to reduce intraoperative blood loss during tumor resection.

Traumatic Disorders

Trauma to the temporal bone is usually from blunt head injury. Injury to the tympanic membrane and middle ear without a bony fracture is seen primarily in children, related to instruments such as pencils, hairpins, and cotton tipped applicators (Fig. 3.115).[227]

High-resolution CT with bone algorithm is used to evaluate temporal bone trauma. Submillimeter axial and reformatted coronal images can delineate most fractures, dislocations, and malalignments. Fractures are traditionally classified as longitudinal or transverse, with reference to the long axis of the petrous bone, although in reality most pediatric fractures are oblique. An important consideration is whether the fracture spares or violates the otic capsule.[228]

Most temporal bone fractures are longitudinal, resulting from a moderate to severe temporal or parietal impact. The fracture usually travels through the petrosquamous suture and continues anterior to the otic capsule (otic capsule sparing). Middle ear involvement leads to hemotympanum and ossicular disruption, resulting in conductive hearing loss (Fig. 3.116). The facial nerve is involved in 15% to 20% of these cases.

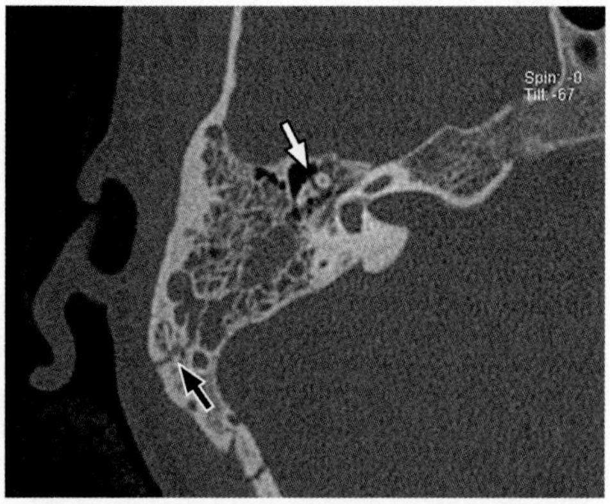

FIGURE 3.116 **Longitudinal temporal bone fracture.** Axial bone window CT image demonstrates a fracture through the temporal bone (*black arrow*), with the fracture line parallel to the long axis of the petrous bone. Increased gap between the head of the malleus and the body of the incus represents incudomalleal distraction (*white arrow*). There is blood in the mastoid air cells and middle ear.

Transverse fractures are less common, resulting from forces along the anteroposterior axis, usually from occipital or frontal impact. Fractures may involve the labyrinth (otic capsule violating) and IAC, causing SNHL and vertigo (Fig. 3.117). The facial nerve is involved in almost 50% of these cases; facial paralysis is often immediate and permanent. Labyrinthine fractures heal slowly and often by fibrous union. Following labyrinthine hemorrhage, labyrinthitis ossificans may result. In the acute stage of labyrinthitis ossificans, enhancement of the inner ear structures may be appreciated on MR images, but CT may appear normal. In the intermediate fibrous stage, heavily T2-weighted MR images demonstrate loss of normal fluid signal in the labyrinth, and the CT may still appear normal. In the

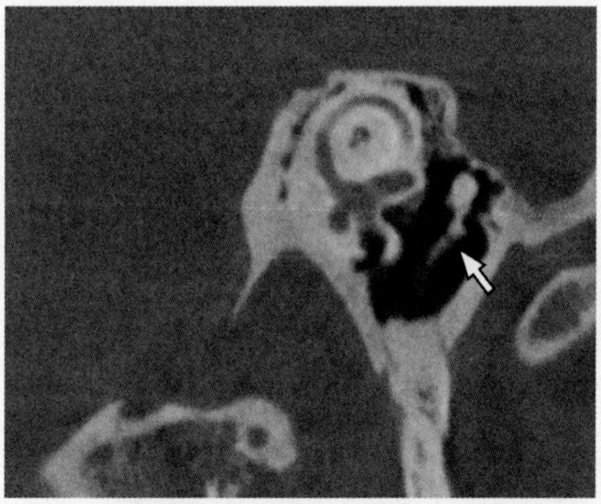

FIGURE 3.115 **Malleus fracture.** Sagittal oblique bone window CT image shows a nondisplaced fracture (*arrow*) through the manubrium of the malleus. The patient thought she felt something in the ear canal and inserted a finger into the canal for digital manipulation. There was subsequent acute onset of pain and conductive hearing loss.

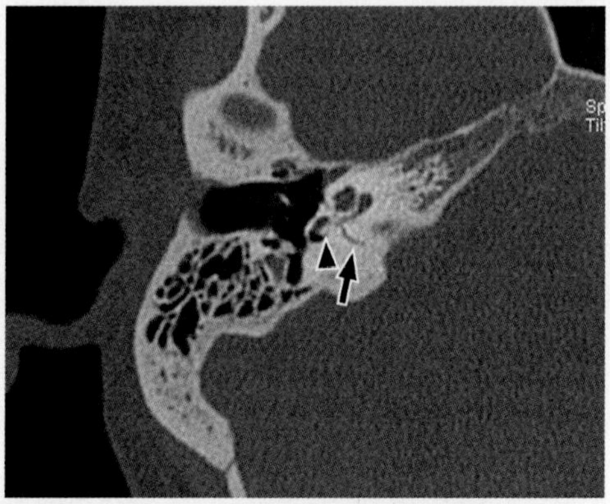

FIGURE 3.117 **Transverse temporal bone fracture.** Axial bone window CT image demonstrates an otic capsule violating fracture through the cochlea (*arrow*) extending to the geniculate and tympanic portions of the facial nerve, with the fracture line perpendicular to the long axis of the petrous bone. Calcific density in the basal turn of the cochlea is due to labyrinthitis ossificans (*arrowhead*).

late ossific stage, CT often reveals abnormal bone attenuation within the cochlea, vestibule, and/or SCCs (Fig. 3.117).[203]

Emergent intervention is warranted when there is herniation of brain into the middle ear, mastoid, or EAC (encephalocele), or injury to the carotid artery. Surgery is also performed when there is hearing loss, facial paralysis, and CSF leak. In general, children recover from temporal bone trauma with fewer complications than do adults, and there is a significantly lower incidence of facial nerve paralysis in children than in adults.[227]

NECK AND UPPER AERODIGESTIVE TRACT

Embryology and Development

Branchial Apparatus

Structures in the head and neck arise from the embryologic branchial apparatus, which consists of branchial arches, branchial (or pharyngeal) pouches, branchial clefts (or grooves), and branchial membranes. In the late somite stage, in the 4th gestational week, the branchial apparatus first becomes identifiable, and development completes by the 6th to 7th week.

The cleft, pouch, and membrane of each arch are caudal to the corresponding arch of the same number. Each arch has a central cartilaginous core that differentiates into bone, cartilage, or ligamentous structures. Each arch also has a muscular component, an aortic arch artery, and a neural element that contains cranial nerve fibers. Some of these muscles may migrate away from their sites of origin, but they still retain their original arch's nerve supply.[229,230] As these muscles migrate, they bring their nerve supply with them, accounting for the oftentimes tortuous routes of cranial nerves. The branchial arch and pouch derivatives are listed in Tables 3.3 and 3.4.

Thymus

In the 6th gestational week, thymic primordia descend from the third pouch and migrate medially along the thymopharyngeal ducts, with the ducts obliterating behind them. By the beginning of the 8th week, the developing thymic masses have approached each other in the midline inferior to the thyroid gland, attached to the pericardium, and begun to descend toward their final position in the superior mediastinum. Finally, mesenchymal cells infiltrate the thymus, and the primitive endodermal cells degenerate into Hassall corpuscles.

TABLE 3.3 Branchial Arch Derivatives

Branchial Arch	Cartilage Derivatives	Muscles	Aortic Arch Vessels	Cranial Nerve
1	Meckel cartilage • Mandible • Sphenomandibular ligament • Anterior malleal ligament • Malleus (head, neck) • Incus (body, short process)	• Muscles of mastication (temporalis, masseter, lateral pterygoid, medial pterygoid) • Mylohyoid • Tensor tympani • Tensor veli palatini • Anterior belly of digastric • Anterior 2/3 of tongue	• Maxillary artery • Common carotid artery	V2 V3
2	Reichert cartilage • Malleus (manubrium) • Incus (long process) • Stapes crura • Styloid process • Stylohyoid ligament • Lesser cornu of hyoid • Upper body of hyoid	• Muscles of facial expression • Stapedius • Stylohyoid • Posterior belly of digastric	• Stapedial artery	VII
3	• Greater cornu of hyoid • Lower body of hyoid	• Stylopharyngeus • Posterior 1/3 of tongue	• Internal carotid artery • Common carotid artery	IX
4	• Thyroid cartilage • Cricoid cartilage • Arytenoid cartilage • Corniculate • Cuneiform	• Most pharyngeal constrictors • Levator veli palatini • Cricothyroid	• Right subclavian artery (right) • Aorta (left)	X (superior laryngeal branch)
5/6		• All intrinsic muscles of the larynx (except cricothyroid)	• Pulmonary arteries • Ductus arteriosus (left)	XI (cranial root) X (recurrent laryngeal branch)

TABLE 3.4 Pharyngeal Pouch Derivatives

Pharyngeal pouch	Derivatives
1	• Middle ear cavity • Eustachian tube • Mastoid air cells
2	• Palatine tonsil • Supratonsillar fossa
3	• Inferior parathyroid glands • Epithelial portion of thymus
4	• Superior parathyroid glands • Parafollicular or C cells of the thyroid gland

Thyroid Gland

The thyroid primordium is a focal endodermal thickening that appears around the 4th gestational week in the ventral midline between the first and second branchial pouches, just caudal to the two median tongue swellings that give rise to the anterior and posterior tongue. This point of origin eventually becomes a small blind pit in the midline at the junction of the anterior two-thirds and posterior one-third of the tongue, known as the foramen cecum.

This primordium elongates downward and bifurcates into the left and right lateral anlagen on either side of the median anlage, eventually becoming the left and right thyroid lobes connected by the isthmus. As the diverticulum descends, it acquires cells from the surrounding endoderm and undergoes cellular proliferation and maturation.[231] At the same time, parafollicular C cells in the ventral portion of the fourth pouch (alternately attributed to the fifth to sixth pouch) localize to a transient embryologic region called the ultimobranchial body on the lateral aspect of each side of the neck. The ultimobranchial bodies then migrate medially, eventually merging with the descending anlagen anterior to the cricoid cartilage forming the definitive thyroid gland.[232] The Zuckerkandl tubercle (ZT) is a protuberance found at the posterolateral border of the thyroid lobes at this point of fusion.[233]

For a period of time, the thyroid gland remains connected to its site of origin (foramen cecum) by the thyroglossal duct. The thyroglossal duct regresses at around the 7th gestational week, when the thyroid gland has reached its final destination at the level of the second and third tracheal cartilages. In almost half the population, the distal half of the thyroglossal duct persists as the pyramidal lobe.

Tongue

The tongue arises from paired lateral lingual swellings in the ventral aspect of the first arches, along with a median swelling known as the tuberculum impar located between the first and second arches, and a second median swelling known as the copula (yoke) spanning the second and third arches. The foramen cecum is seen at the junction of the tuberculum impar and copula in the midline. The oral tongue develops as the lateral lingual swellings expand, with a minor contribution by the tuberculum impar. The root of the tongue develops from the copula along with some tissue from between the third and fourth arches.

For general sensory innervation, the anterior two-thirds of the tongue is innervated by the lingual nerves, branches of the trigeminal nerves, in keeping with the first arch origin of the lateral lingual swellings. The posterior one-third (root) of the tongue is innervated by cranial nerves IX (third arch) and X (fourth arch). For taste, cranial nerves VII (chorda tympani) and IX innervate the taste buds in the anterior two-thirds and posterior one-third of the tongue respectively. For motor function, the intrinsic and extrinsic muscles of the tongue are primarily supplied by cranial nerve XII, apart from the palatoglossus, which is innervated by cranial nerve X.

Normal Anatomy

Compartments of the Neck

The neck is defined superiorly by the lower border of the mandible extending out to the angle of the mandible and mastoid process of the temporal bone. Inferiorly, it is defined by the upper edge of the clavicle and manubrium. Posteriorly, it is defined by the anterior border of the trapezius muscles. On either side, the neck is divided into the anterior and posterior triangles by the sternocleidomastoid muscle, which traverses the neck in an oblique orientation.

The anterior triangle can be further divided by the hyoid bone and the posterior belly of the digastric into suprahyoid and infrahyoid compartments. The suprahyoid compartment contains the midline submental triangle, which is separated from the submandibular triangle on either side by the anterior belly of the digastric muscle and from the oral cavity superiorly by the mylohyoid muscles and their fibrous median raphe. Functionally, the suprahyoid compartment is related to the oral cavity, floor of the mouth, oropharynx, and hypopharynx. The infrahyoid compartment contains the carotid triangle laterally, which is separated from the muscular triangle medially by the superior belly of the omohyoid muscle. The carotid triangle and the lower portion of the muscular triangle are both bordered laterally by the sternocleidomastoid muscle.

The posterior triangle can be further divided by the inferior belly of the omohyoid muscle into the occipital triangle superiorly and the subclavian triangle inferiorly.

The contents of each of these compartments and triangles are listed in Table 3.5.

Fasciae and Spaces of the Neck

There are two main divisions of fasciae: the superficial cervical fascia (SCF) and the deep cervical fascia (DCF). The deep aspect of the thicker SCF contains the platysma, muscles of facial expression, and portions of the anterior and external jugular veins. The thinner, denser DCF surrounds the neck muscles, muscles of mastication, pharyngeal muscles, and the mandible. There are three layers of DCF: the superficial layer of the DCF (SLDCF), the middle layer (MLDCF), and

TABLE 3.5 Contents of the Neck by Compartments

Compartment	Contents
Submental triangle	Lymph nodes Facial artery branches Facial vein branches
Submandibular triangle	Submandibular gland, superficial portion Lymph nodes Retromandibular vein Anterior facial vein
Carotid triangle	Common carotid artery Internal carotid artery External carotid artery Internal jugular vein Cranial nerves IX, X, XI, XII Cervical sympathetic trunk Ansa cervicalis Lymph nodes
Muscular triangle	Infrahyoid "strap" muscles • Superior belly of omohyoid • Sternohyoid • Sternothyroid • Thyrohyoid Larynx Hypopharynx Cervical trachea Cervical esophagus Thyroid gland Parathyroid glands Recurrent laryngeal nerve Lymph nodes (levels IV and VI)
Occipital triangle	Transverse cervical artery and vein Spinal accessory nerve Dorsal scapular nerve Lymph nodes (level V)
Subclavian triangle	Subclavian artery Brachial plexus, trunks Transverse cervical artery and vein Suprascapular artery and vein Lymph nodes

the deep layer (DLDCF). The middle layer itself consists of a pretracheal layer and a visceral layer. The SCF functions in conjunction with the skin and the platysma as a unit, interconnected by connective tissue and muscle fibers that constitute the superficial musculoaponeurotic system (SMAS). SMAS functionally links the superficial muscles to the skin surface, for example, transmitting the effects of muscle contractions to the skin.[234]

The fascial layers create a number of defined spaces in the neck, most of them housing specific anatomic structures, some being potential spaces. Knowledge of these fascial spaces, especially in the suprahyoid neck, greatly simplifies and aids in the interpretation of cross-sectional neck studies. The names and contents of each of these spaces are summarized in Table 3.6.

Cervical Lymph Nodes

Approximately 40% of the lymph nodes in the body are located in the head and neck.[235] Nodes were traditionally named by the location in which they are found. The most recent 2010 modification of the AJCC (American Joint Committee on Cancer) classification is an imaging-based system and has been widely accepted. In this system, there are seven levels. Level IA corresponds to submental nodes. Level IB corresponds to submandibular nodes. Levels II, III, and IV are nodes along the jugular chain from cranial to caudal. Level V nodes are the spinal accessory nodes in the posterior triangle. Level VI nodes are the anterior compartment nodes medial to the carotid arteries. In the original AJCC system, there are level VII nodes that represent nodes inferior to the suprasternal notch. The level system does not include the following nodes, which are named by location: parotid, retropharyngeal (node of Rouvière), facial, and occipital.

The lymphatic system in the head and neck consists of these lymph nodes, along with mucosa-associated lymphoid tissue in Waldeyer ring. The jugulodigastric (level IIA) node is a sentinel node, receiving lymphatic drainage from the tonsils, pharynx, mouth, and facial region. Because these areas are frequently involved by infection or inflammation, especially in children, the jugulodigastric node tends to be larger and more frequently hyperplastic compared to the other nodes. The same is true of Waldeyer ring.

Congenital and Developmental Anomalies

Branchial Anomalies

Branchial anomalies are thought to occur either as vestigial remnants that result from incomplete obliteration of portions of the branchial apparatus or as a result of buried epithelial cell rests.[229,236] Branchial anomalies are therefore classified according to their cleft or pouch of origin, and their provenance can be confirmed surgically by tracing the course of the fistula or sinus tract. There are first, second, third, and fourth branchial anomalies; fifth and sixth branchial anomalies have not been reported.

A pure branchial (cleft) cyst (BCC) has no communication internally to the pharynx or externally to the skin surface. BCCs are lined by stratified squamous epithelium of ectodermal origin, but, rarely, they can arise from pharyngeal pouch endoderm and therefore be lined by columnar epithelium. A branchial fistula forms when there is persistence of a branchial cleft and its corresponding pharyngeal pouch, resulting in an epithelium-lined tract that communicates between the pharyngeal lumen and the skin surface. Because branchial clefts and pouches lie caudal to their corresponding arch, a branchial fistula would lie caudal to the arch, and thus caudal to the arch derivatives after full development. There may be an associated BCC. A branchial sinus is a tract that is only open to the pharyngeal lumen internally or only to the skin surface externally (Fig. 3.118). The latter scenario is more common. There may be an associated BCC.

TABLE 3.6 Contents and Potential Underlying Pathology of the Fascial Spaces

Fascial space	Contents	Pathology
Prestyloid parapharyngeal space	Deep lobe of parotid Minor salivary glands Ascending pharyngeal artery Internal maxillary artery Pterygoid venous plexus Cranial nerve V3 branches Fat Connective tissue	Deep lobe parotid tumor Minor salivary gland tumor Vascular anomaly
Poststyloid parapharyngeal space	Internal carotid artery Internal jugular vein Cranial nerves IX, X, XI, XII Fat	Paraganglioma (rare in children) Schwannoma Neuroblastoma Ganglioneuroblastoma Ganglioneuroma Neurofibroma
Peritonsillar space (potential space)	Fat (Palatine tonsil medial to it) (Parapharyngeal space lateral to it)	Abscess Extension of tonsillar tumor 2nd branchial anomaly Vascular anomaly Neurofibroma
Masticator space	Masseter muscle Lateral pterygoid muscle Medial pterygoid muscle Temporalis muscle Mandibular ramus Cranial nerve V3 branches Internal maxillary artery Fat	Muscle inflammation Rhabdomyosarcoma Other sarcoma Desmoid tumor Mandibular lesion Nerve sheath tumor Vascular anomaly
Submaxillary space (considered lower portion of submandibular space)	Superficial larger portion of submandibular gland Anterior belly of digastric muscle Level I lymph nodes Facial artery Facial vein Fat	Submandibular gland lesions Adenopathy Vascular anomaly Nerve sheath tumor
Sublingual space (considered upper portion of submandibular space)	Deep portion of submandibular gland Wharton duct Sublingual gland and ducts Lingual artery Lingual vein Lingual nerve (sensory V3 and chorda tympani) Cranial nerve XI and XII Fat	Ranula Dermoid Vascular anomaly Nerve sheath tumor
Carotid sheath	Internal carotid artery Common carotid artery Internal jugular vein Cranial nerves IX, X, XI, XII Sympathetic chain Level II, III, IV lymph nodes Fat	Arteritis Aneurysm Carotid dissection Venous thrombosis Nerve sheath tumor Paraganglioma Adenopathy
Retropharyngeal space	Pharynx Medial and lateral (node of Rouvière) retropharyngeal lymph nodes Fat	Adenopathy Edema, phlegmon, abscess Extension of pharyngeal tumor Nerve sheath tumor Vascular anomaly
Danger space (potential space)	Fat (Retropharyngeal space anterior to it) (Prevertebral space posterior to it) (Parapharyngeal space lateral to it)	Phlegmon Abscess

TABLE 3.6 Contents and Potential Underlying Pathology of the Fascial Spaces *(Continued)*

Fascial space	Contents	Pathology
Prevertebral space	Longus colli muscle Longus capitis muscle Phrenic nerve Anterior longitudinal ligament Cervical vertebrae and discs Fat	Calcific tendinitis of the longus colli Sarcoma Nerve sheath tumor Vascular anomaly Phlegmon, abscess Vertebral and disc disease
Perivertebral/paravertebral space	Anterior, middle, posterior scalene muscles Levator scapulae muscle Splenius capitis muscle Splenius cervicis muscle Branchial plexus (roots) Vertebral artery and vein Fat	Muscle disease Brachial plexus nerve sheath tumor Sarcoma
Posterior cervical space	Fat Cranial nerve XI Brachial plexus (trunks, divisions, chords) Lymph nodes Dorsal scapula nerve Long thoracic nerve Cutaneous nerves of cervical plexus	Level V adenopathy Vascular anomaly Lipoma Nerve sheath tumor

Fistulae and sinuses are usually noticed at or soon after birth because of the presence of a pit and/or drainage. Cysts present later and are usually detected as neck masses that may enlarge after an URI. Overall, BCCs are much more common than fistulae or sinuses. Rare bilateral branchial anomalies may be familial and/or syndromic.[237]

On US, BCC usually appears as a rounded anechoic lesion, but it may appear complex with echogenic debris if there is superimposed inflammation (Fig. 3.119A). On CT, an uncomplicated BCC appears cystic with thin smooth walls. Superimposed inflammation causes wall thickening, enhancement, and surrounding edema (Figs. 3.119B and 3.121). BCC contents may be hyperdense from proteinaceous material. On MRI, a noninflamed cyst has low signal on T1-weighted sequence and high signal on T2-weighted sequence (Fig. 3.120). Occasionally, inflammation or proteinaceous content causes T1 shortening with an increase in signal intensity.

The differential diagnosis of BCC depends on location. When suspecting a BCC, it is important to exclude the remote possibility of a cystic or necrotic metastatic node as a mimicker, for example, from a primary thyroid malignancy.

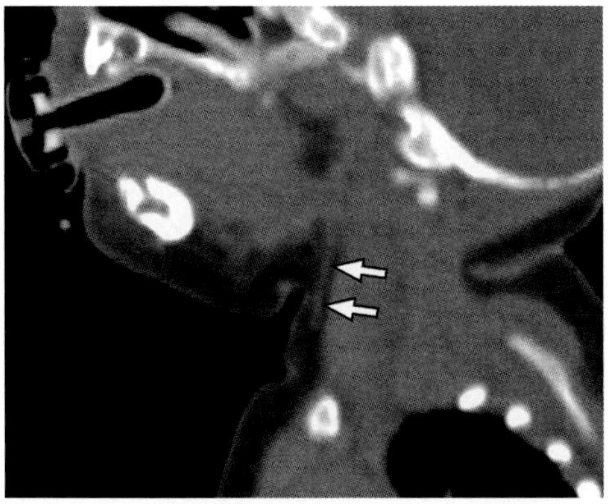

FIGURE 3.118 **Branchial sinus tract in a 5-week-old boy.** This patient presented with a "dimple" in his lower neck which was seen since birth. Physical examination revealed a surface pit at the lower neck adjacent to the sternocleidomastoid muscle. Sagittal CT image shows a thin linear soft tissue tract (*arrows*) traversing the neck, extending from this pit up toward the pharynx at the level of the submandibular gland. There was no obvious opening at the pharyngeal lumen on either physical examination or imaging.

First Branchial Anomalies

Of the first branchial anomalies, two-thirds are cysts, with the remainder evenly split between fistulae and sinuses.[238,239] In 1972, Work classified first branchial anomalies into two types.[240] A Work type I anomaly is considered an EAC duplication, translating to a lesion in the preauricular region with a distal portion anterior or posterior to the pinna. They are generally parallel to the EAC, lateral to the facial nerve, and may be within the parotid gland. If there is a fistulous tract, the tract opens into the EAC. A Work type II anomaly is considered a duplication anomaly of the membranous EAC and pinna, translating to a lesion usually just posterior or inferior to the angle of the mandible that may be lateral to, medial to, or between the branches of the facial nerve within the parotid gland. A Work type II fistulous tracts open into the EAC as well. Although first branchial anomalies most often originate along the EAC, there are rare instances where they originate in the middle ear cavity or nasopharynx. Both Work type I and type II first branchial anomalies relate to the parotid gland and the facial nerve, but their locations relative to these structures vary depending on timing of the embryologic development.

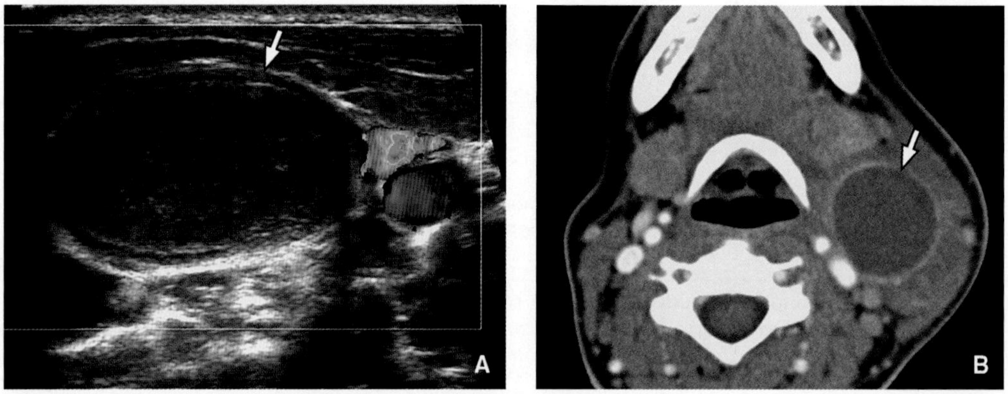

FIGURE 3.119 **Second branchial cyst with inflammatory change. A:** Doppler ultrasound image demonstrates a rounded cystic lesion with internal echogenic debris and wall thickening (*arrow*). **B:** Axial contrast-enhanced CT image shows a large round cystic lesion (*arrow*) with a thick enhancing wall and surrounding edema.

On imaging, first branchial cysts can be seen within or just adjacent to the parotid gland and/or the lower margin of the pinna (Fig. 3.121). If a tract extends toward the EAC, then the diagnosis is unequivocal. If only an intraparotid or periparotid cyst is seen, then differential diagnosis includes LM, dermoid, abscess, necrotic adenopathy from nontuberculous mycobacterial infection (young children), sialocele, and cystic pilomatrixoma.

Second Branchial Anomalies

Second branchial anomalies are the most common, constituting over 92% of all branchial anomalies.[241,242] Cysts are much more common than fistulae or sinuses. For fistulae and sinuses, the external end of the tract usually opens at the anterior border of the sternocleidomastoid muscle at the junction of its middle and lower thirds. It then runs deep to the platysma, ascends lateral to the carotid sheath, passes medially over cranial nerves XII and IX between the external and internal carotid arteries, and opens internally in the region of the palatine tonsillar fossa. A second BCC can occur anywhere along this tract.

Bailey classified second BCCs into four types based on location. Type I BCC is deep to the platysma and the cervical fascia, and anterior to the sternocleidomastoid muscle (Fig. 3.122). Type II is adjacent to the carotid and jugular and may be adherent to them, and is the most common type (Figs. 3.119B and 3.120). Type III extends between the internal and external carotid arteries to the lateral pharyngeal wall. Type IV lies against the lateral pharyngeal wall and is believed to be remnants of the second pharyngeal pouch.

Second BCCs often present following a URI because of stimulation of lymphoid tissue in the cyst wall. As the type II cyst enlarges, it displaces the submandibular gland anteriorly and extends deep to the sternocleidomastoid muscle posteriorly. Histologically, the cysts are lined by squamous to cuboidal or ciliated columnar epithelium, often accompanied by lymphocytic inflammation with follicle formation (Fig. 3.123).

Differential diagnosis of a second BCC includes a lymphatic malformation, metastatic or suppurative lymphadenopathy or abscess, and dermoid/epidermoid. In appropriate locations, a fluid-filled external laryngocele/saccular cyst

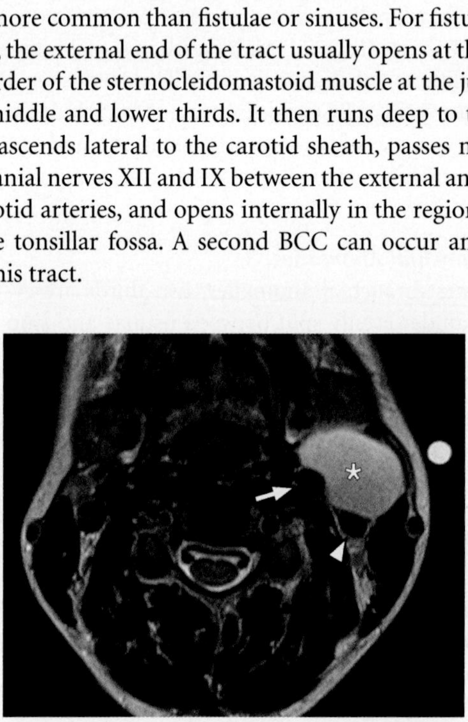

FIGURE 3.120 **Bailey type II second branchial cyst.** Axial T2-weighted MR image shows a homogeneously hyperintense cystic lesion (*asterisk*) posterior to the submandibular gland and anterior to the sternocleidomastoid muscle, adjacent to the common carotid artery (*arrow*) and internal jugular vein (*arrowhead*), compatible with a Bailey type II second branchial cyst.

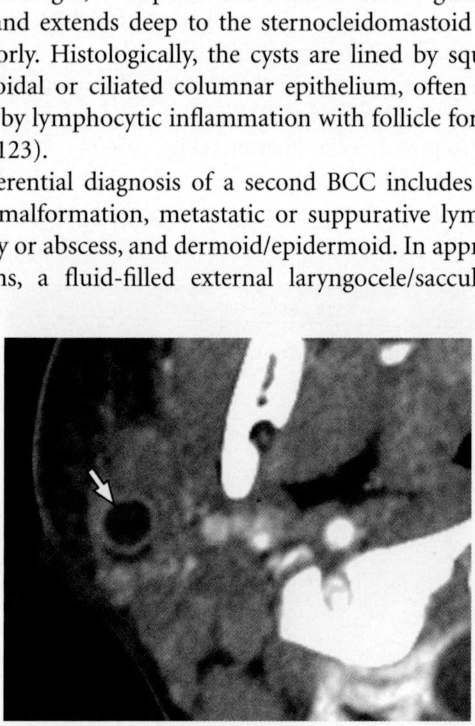

FIGURE 3.121 **First branchial cleft cyst, infected.** Axial contrast-enhanced CT image shows a sharply circumscribed cystic mass (*arrow*) with peripheral enhancement located within the right parotid gland. There is stranding of the subcutaneous fat. After treatment with antibiotics, the lesion was excised and the diagnosis of an infected first branchial cleft cyst was confirmed.

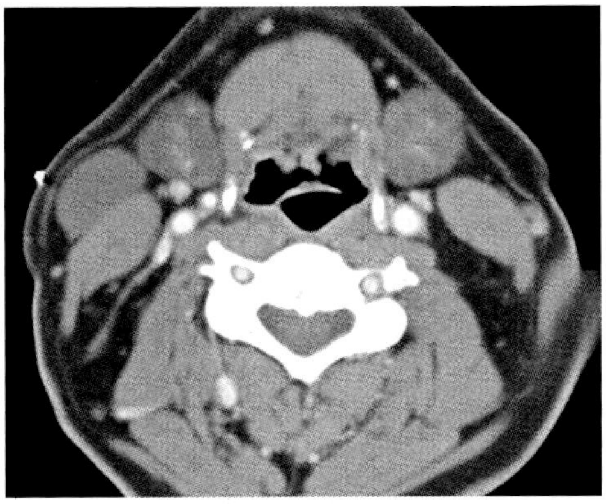

FIGURE 3.122 **Bailey type I second branchial cyst.** Axial contrast-enhanced CT image demonstrates a proteinaceous cystic lesion deep to the platysma, at the anterior aspect of the sternocleidomastoid muscle (marked by a barium dot on the skin surface). The patient subsequently underwent biopsy.

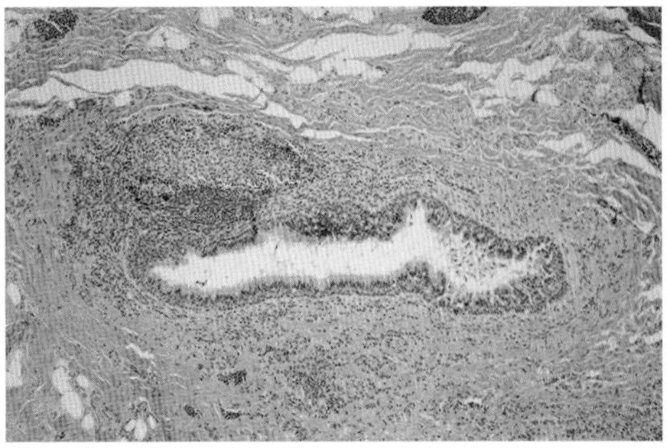

FIGURE 3.123 **Branchial cleft cyst, excised from the right neck of a 1-year-old boy.** The cyst lining contains ciliated columnar epithelium, and it is surrounded by lymphocytic inflammation, including a lymphoid follicle (hematoxylin and eosin, original magnification, 100×).

or a paramedian thyroglossal duct cyst (TGDC) may be considered.

Third and Fourth Branchial Anomalies

Third and fourth branchial anomalies are rare. A third branchial fistulous tract has an external cutaneous opening along the anterior margin of the sternocleidomastoid muscle, inferior to that of a second branchial fistulous tract. It then ascends posterior to the common and internal carotid arteries and passes medially over cranial nerve XII but inferior to cranial nerve IX, continues medially to pierce the thyrohyoid membrane, and opens internally at the superolateral pyriform sinus.

A fourth fistulous tract has a cutaneous opening caudal to those of the second and third fistulae. It ascends the neck, courses medially over cranial nerve XII, continues medially between the external and internal carotid arteries, and then descends again posterior to the common carotid artery. On the left, it then loops under the aortic arch to course posteriorly and then superiorly, lateral to the trachea and the recurrent laryngeal nerve, and opens into the apex of the pyriform sinus. On the right, it loops under the subclavian artery and then superiorly to the apex of the pyriform sinus. On either side, the opening in the pyriform sinus of a fourth branchial fistula/sinus is caudal to that of a third branchial fistula/sinus.

In the literature, third or fourth pharyngeal pouch anomalies have been described to almost always occur on the left side, with patients presenting with recurrent thyroiditis or perithyroidal neck abscess. A third or fourth branchial cyst is rarely seen. On contrast-enhanced CT, there are inflammatory changes and edema around the thyroid gland, usually on the left side (Fig. 3.124A). The thyroid lobe itself may demonstrate inflammatory changes, appearing hypodense with ill-defined margins. There may be an intrathyroidal or perithyroidal abscess. Inflammatory changes and soft tissue thickening can be seen extending cephalad to surround the ipsilateral pyriform sinus.

Recurrent perithyroidal neck infection or recurrent thyroiditis in a child should raise concern for an underlying pyriform sinus tract. Barium pharyngogram may reveal a tract arising from the pyriform sinus, but this must be performed following resolution of inflammatory changes that may compress and efface the tract, resulting in a false-negative study (Fig. 3.124B). Ultimately, direct visualization via pharyngoscopy may be necessary for definitive diagnosis, because

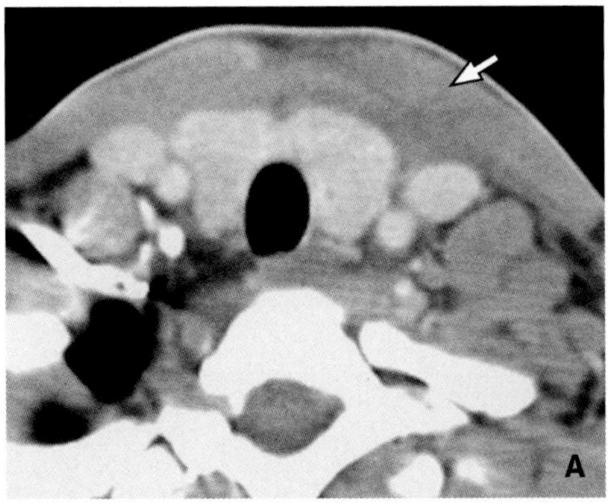

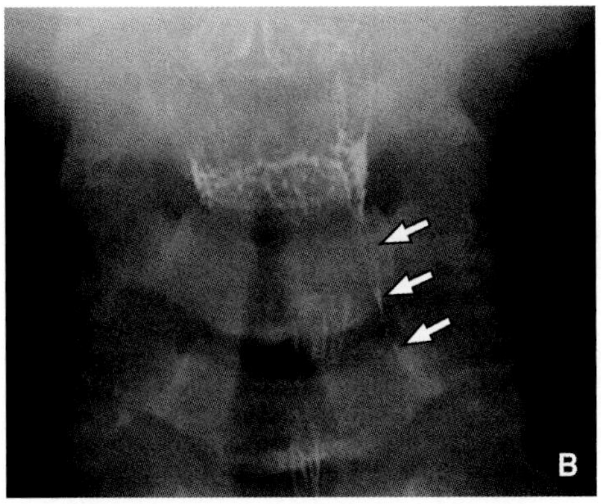

FIGURE 3.124 **Pyriform sinus fistula. A:** Axial contrast-enhanced CT image shows edema and fat infiltration around the left thyroid lobe. The sternocleidomastoid muscle is also inflamed and edematous (*arrow*). **B:** Barium pharyngogram, obtained following resolution of acute infection, shows a fistulous tract (*arrows*) extending inferiorly from the pyriform sinus apex on the left.

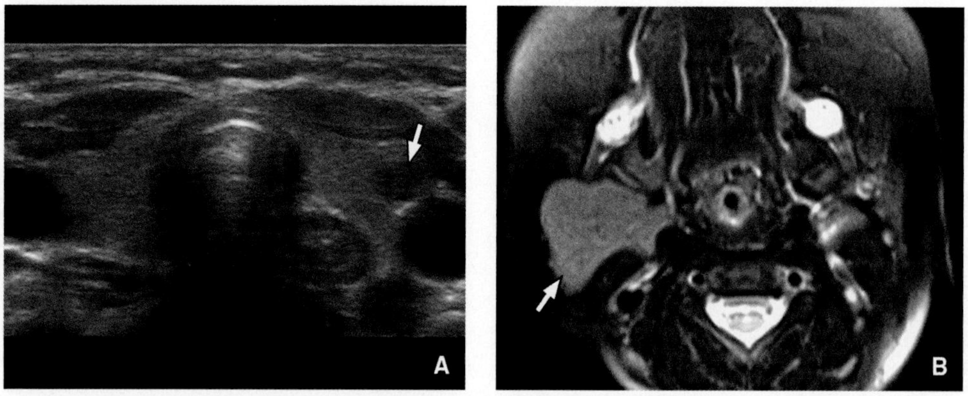

FIGURE 3.125 **Ectopic thymus in two different pediatric patients. A:** Transverse gray-scale ultrasound image demonstrates a hypoechoic focus (*arrow*) within the left thyroid lobe in this 3-year-old girl, incidentally seen during workup of a dermoid in the neck. Biopsy was performed, with pathology revealing thymic tissue. **B:** Axial T2-weighted fat-suppressed MR image shows a characteristic triangular, intermediate signal intensity mass (*arrow*) located posterior to the submandibular gland, lateral to the internal carotid artery, and ventral to the sternocleidomastoid muscle, incidentally detected in this 4-month-old girl.

barium pharyngogram is much less sensitive than direct pharyngoscopy.

Thymic Anomalies

Thymic anomalies result from abnormal descent of thymic primordium into the mediastinum. The descent may be incomplete, thymic tissue may be sequestered along the path of descent, or the thymopharyngeal duct may fail to involute (Fig. 3.125). The ectopic thymic tissue may communicate with the pharynx via an epithelial tract and/or be connected to the orthotopic thymus in the mediastinum. Ectopic thymic cysts occur when portions of the thymopharyngeal duct persist, and are referred to as thymopharyngeal cysts. These are seen more commonly in the left neck.

Thymic cysts can occur anywhere from the angle of the mandible to the sternum, parallel to the sternocleidomastoid muscle (Fig. 3.126) and separate from normal thymus or connected to it by a fibrous band.[243] On imaging, the thymic cyst is off midline, often adjacent to the lower pyriform sinus or just caudal to the thyroid gland. Benign thymic cysts are lined by squamous to columnar epithelium surrounded by variable amounts of thymic lymphoid tissue (Fig. 3.127). Histologic examination may be required to distinguish them from other thymic lesions that may also be cystic, such as a predominantly cystic thymoma, thymic involvement by Hodgkin lymphoma, lymphatic malformation, or teratoma.

Thyroid Anomalies

The thyroid gland or a thyroid lobe may be absent (complete or unilateral agenesis, respectively), thought to result from abnormal migration of thyroid primordium or destruction in utero by maternal antithyroid antibodies.[244,245]

Ectopic thyroid tissue may result from pathologic ascent of thyroid primordium to the tongue, incomplete descent of thyroid primordium to the thyroid bed, or incomplete involution

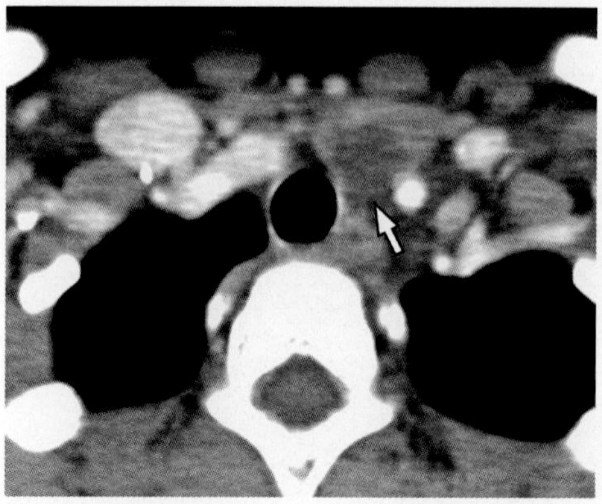

FIGURE 3.126 **Thymic cyst.** Axial contrast-enhanced CT image shows a cystic lesion (*arrow*) at the level of the thoracic inlet, deep to the left sternocleidomastoid muscle. This lesion was biopsied intraoperatively while the patient was undergoing surgical resection of a follicular thyroid carcinoma.

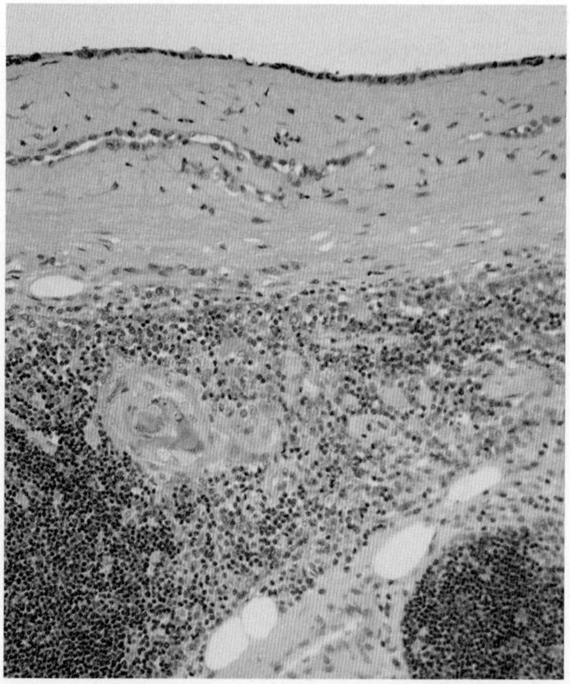

FIGURE 3.127 **Thymic cyst from a 16-year-old boy shows a thin sclerotic fibrous wall lined by epithelium** (hematoxylin and eosin, original magnification, 200x).

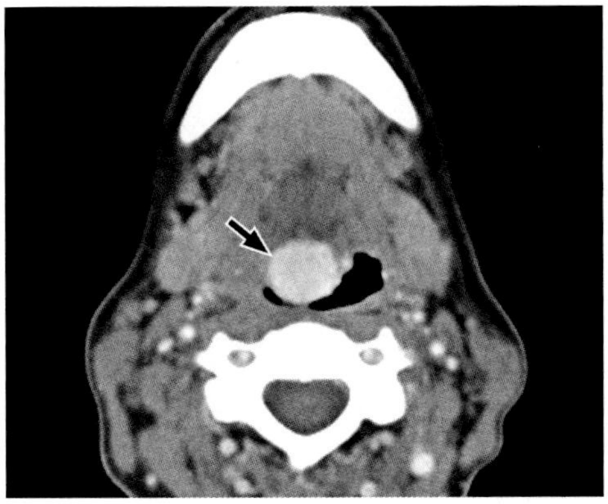

FIGURE 3.128 **Lingual thyroid.** Axial contrast-enhanced CT image demonstrates a hyperdense and enhancing soft tissue mass (*arrow*) at the base of the tongue. Its density is the same as that of the thyroid gland. Images in the lower neck reveal absence of orthotopic thyroid tissue (not shown). These findings are confirmed on a radionuclide I-123 scan (not shown).

of the thyroglossal duct leading to remnants of tissue anywhere along the course of the duct. To be considered true ectopic thyroid, there should be no connection between the ectopic tissue and the normal thyroid bed. Ectopic thyroid is most commonly seen in the midline of the tongue near foramen cecum, where it is referred to as lingual thyroid (Fig. 3.128). Once ectopic thyroid is seen, one should always examine the thyroid bed for normal orthotopic thyroid tissue, absent in 70% to 80% of cases of lingual thyroid.[246] In these cases, if the ectopic tissue is removed, the patient requires lifelong thyroid replacement medication. Ectopic thyroid tissue may be detected by nuclear imaging, usually with technetium-99m pertechnetate, so long as there is no dominant normal thyroid gland present. It is important to bear in mind that, though rare, thyroid gland pathologies, such as goiter, thyroiditis, and thyroid carcinoma, may occur in ectopic thyroid tissue.

Thyroglossal Duct Anomalies

TGDCs account for 70% of congenital neck masses.[247] TGDC is thought to occur when the thyroglossal duct does not involute completely, leaving behind secretory epithelium that may express fluid and result in a cyst. Therefore, TGDCs can occur anywhere along the course of the thyroglossal duct (Figs. 3.129 and 3.130). There is a close relationship between the thyroglossal duct and the body of the hyoid bone embryologically. In rare cases, the duct may even be incorporated into the hyoid bone. Because of this close relationship, TGDCs are often located near the hyoid bone (Figs. 3.129 and 3.131).

Affected pediatric patients usually report a gradually enlarging neck mass in the midline or acute enlargement due to infection. Thyroid tissue may sometimes be found within a TGDC, accounting for instances of associated thyroid pathology such as thyroid malignancy (Fig. 3.132), although this is rare in children.[247] The presence of mineralization and/or necrotic adenopathy is strongly suggestive of the development of carcinoma.

On imaging, suprahyoid TGDCs are almost always found in the midline and usually close to the hyoid bone, at times even causing bony remodeling. In the uncommon off-midline cyst, a "tail" may lead toward the hyoid bone. Infrahyoid TGDCs often lie off midline, closely associated with the strap muscles (Figs. 3.129 and 3.133). As with BCCs, TGDCs can have variable protein content, leading to variable density on CT and intensity on MR imaging. Internal septations may be seen.

The differential diagnosis for midline TGDC is dermoid/epidermoid. An infected TGDC can resemble an infected LM. The differential diagnosis for TGDC arising within the tongue includes vallecular cyst and foregut duplication cyst, although the latter usually involves the anterior third of the tongue.

The definitive treatment of TGDC is the Sistrunk surgical procedure, in which the body of the hyoid bone and TGDC are removed. The recurrence rate with the Sistrunk procedure is only 4%, compared to 50% recurrence when the cyst alone is resected.[248]

Laryngocele

A laryngocele results from obstruction and dilatation of the laryngeal ventricle appendix. When it is air-filled, it is referred to as a laryngocele (Fig. 3.134). When it is fluid-filled, it may be referred to as a saccular cyst. An internal laryngocele is confined within the larynx, delimited by the thyrohyoid membrane. A combined laryngocele protrudes beyond the

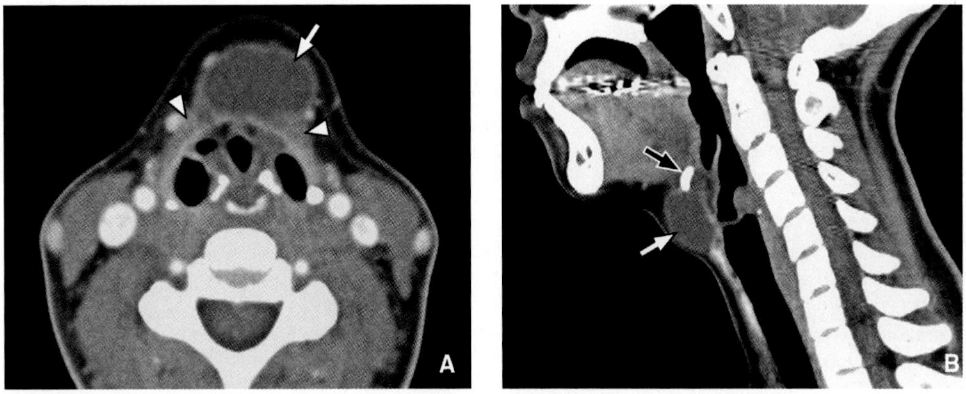

FIGURE 3.129 **Infrahyoid thyroglossal duct cyst.** Axial **(A)** and sagittal reconstructed **(B)** contrast-enhanced CT images demonstrate a well-circumscribed cystic lesion (*white arrow* in **A** and **B**) in the anterior midline of the neck, inferior to the hyoid bone (*black arrow* in **B**), closely associated with the strap muscles (*arrowheads* in **A**). The location is characteristic of a thyroglossal duct cyst.

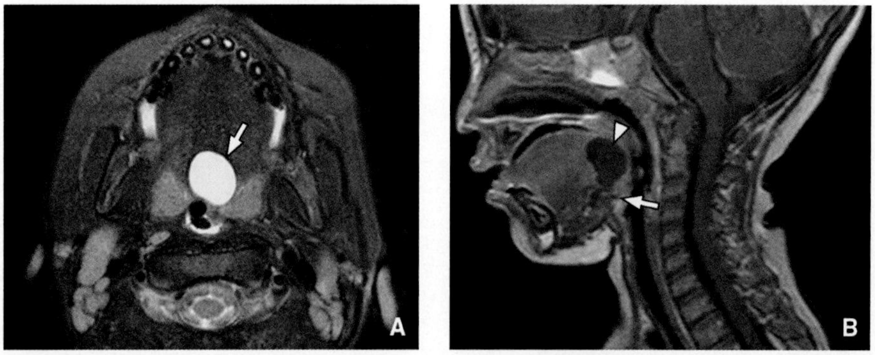

FIGURE 3.130 **Lingual thyroglossal duct cyst. A:** Axial T2-weighted fat-suppressed MR image demonstrates a well-circumscribed, smoothly marginated cystic lesion (*arrow*) at the midline posterior tongue, in the region of the foramen cecum. **B:** Sagittal postcontrast T1-weighted MR image confirms the cystic nature of this lesion (nonenhancing, low signal; *arrowhead*), located at the tongue base just above the hyoid bone (*arrow*). This 28-month-old girl underwent transoral excision of this lesion. Thick mucoid material was seen intraoperatively.

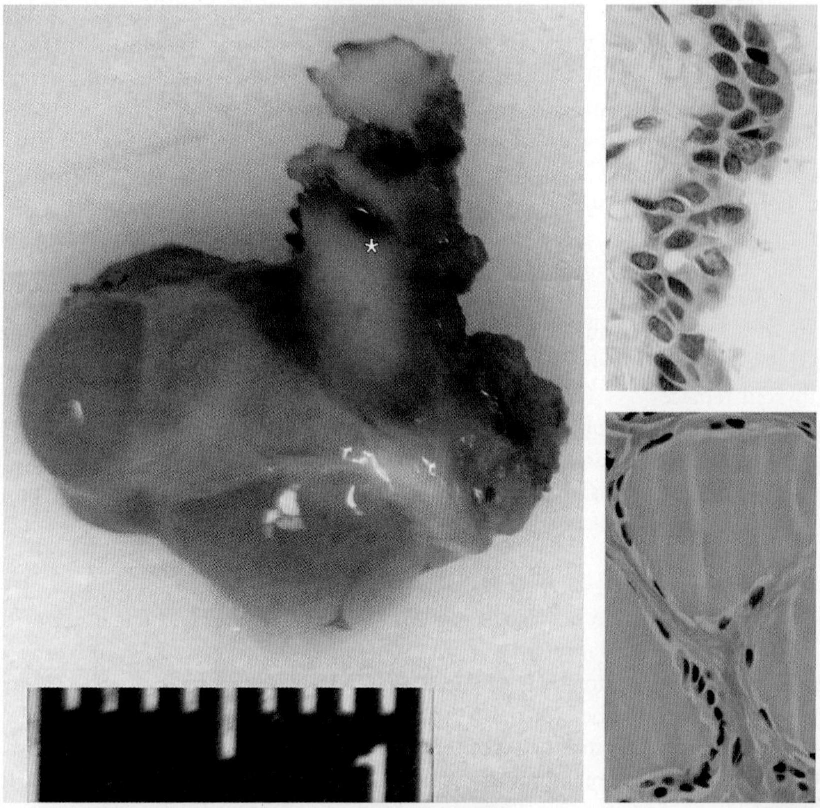

FIGURE 3.131 **Thyroglossal duct cyst in a 2-year-old boy.** This midline neck mass consists grossly **(left)** of a mucus-filled cyst bordering the hyoid bone (*asterisk*). Microscopically, it is lined by respiratory columnar to nonkeratinizing squamous epithelium **(right upper)**, with areas of ectopic thyroid tissue (**right lower**; both hematoxylin and eosin, original magnification, 600×).

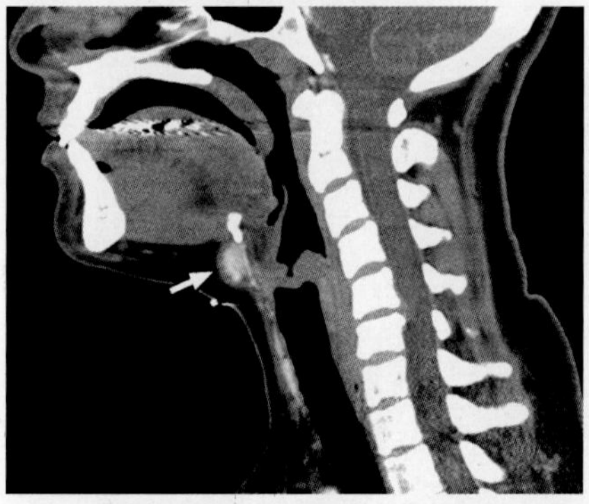

FIGURE 3.132 **Papillary carcinoma within a thyroglossal duct cyst.** Sagittal CT image demonstrates hyperdense and enhancing soft tissue within an infrahyoid cystic lesion (*arrow*). Biopsy revealed papillary carcinoma.

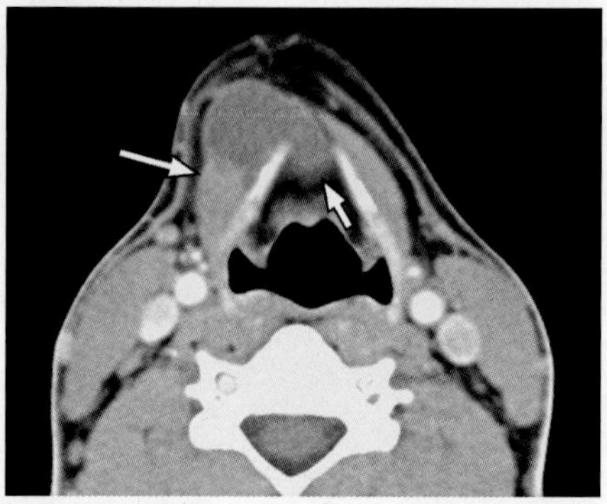

FIGURE 3.133 **Off-midline infrahyoid thyroglossal duct cyst.** Axial contrast-enhanced CT image shows this lesion having a "tail" (*short arrow*) that leads toward the midline larynx between the thyroid cartilage laminae. It is closely related to the right strap muscle (*long arrow*).

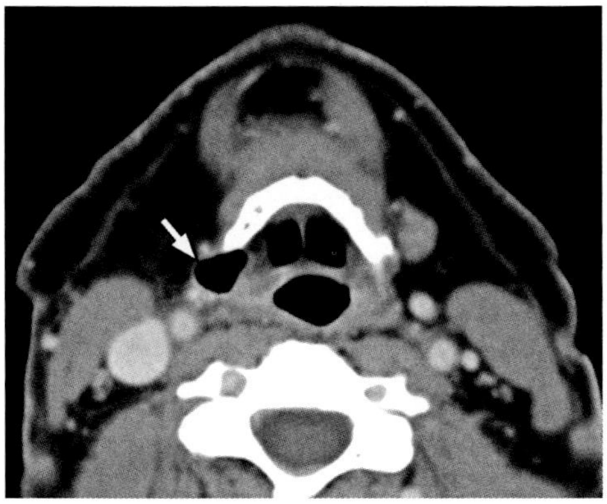

FIGURE 3.134 **Combined laryngocele.** Axial contrast-enhanced CT image demonstrates an air-filled space (*arrow*) with intra- and extralaryngeal components that protrudes laterally beyond the thyrohyoid membrane.

thyrohyoid membrane, such that it has intralaryngeal and extralaryngeal components. On imaging, coronal views are helpful for visualizing the laryngeal ventricle and appendix dilating and extending superiorly.

Salivary Gland Anomalies

The parotid gland begins to form during the 6th gestational week, followed by the submandibular gland in the 7th week and the sublingual gland in the 8th week. The minor salivary glands develop later, between the 9th and 12th weeks.[249]

Salivary gland aplasia is rare. It may involve one or multiple glands, be unilateral or bilateral, occur with other ectodermal defects, and can occur as part of a syndrome, for example, HFM, TCS, and other facial anomalies (Fig. 3.135). Salivary gland aplasia may be seen in lacrimo-auriculo-dento-digital (LADD) syndrome, where patients also have abnormal development of the lacrimal system, deafness or ear anomalies, dental anomalies, and digital anomalies.

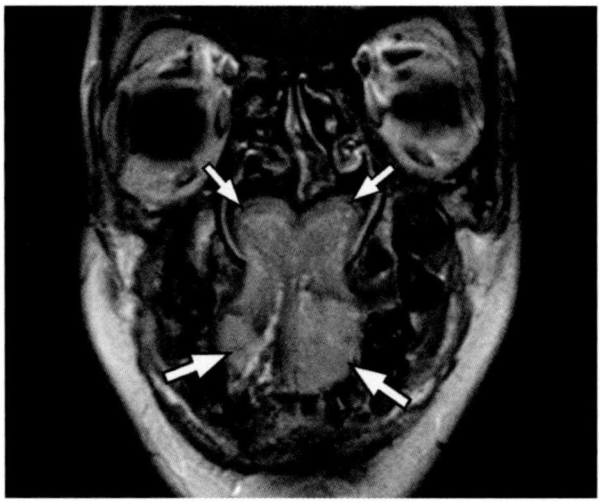

FIGURE 3.135 **Ectopic sublingual/submandibular glands.** Coronal T2-weighted MR image demonstrates lobulated masses (*large arrows*) of salivary gland signal in the anterior superior aspect of the floor of the mouth. No orthotopic sublingual or submandibular gland is present. Note also that the patient has cleft palate, with the tongue (*small arrows*) protruding up toward the nasal cavity. This 10-year-old boy has Treacher Collins syndrome, with temporal bone anomalies shown in Figure 3.89.

Ultrasound, CT, and MRI can all be used to assess the salivary glands.

Other rare developmental abnormalities involving the salivary glands include polycystic disease, congenital sialectasis, ductal agenesis and atresia, imperforate submandibular duct, duplicated gland or duct, and congenital intraglandular cysts. Epidermoid/dermoid cysts (Fig. 3.136), hemangiomas (Fig. 3.137), and vascular malformations can occur in or adjacent to the major salivary glands (Fig. 3.138).

Tongue and Oral Cavity Anomalies

Heterotopic tissues other than lingual thyroid are also occasionally found in the tongue and oral cavity. There have been case reports of neuroglial, respiratory, gastrointestinal,

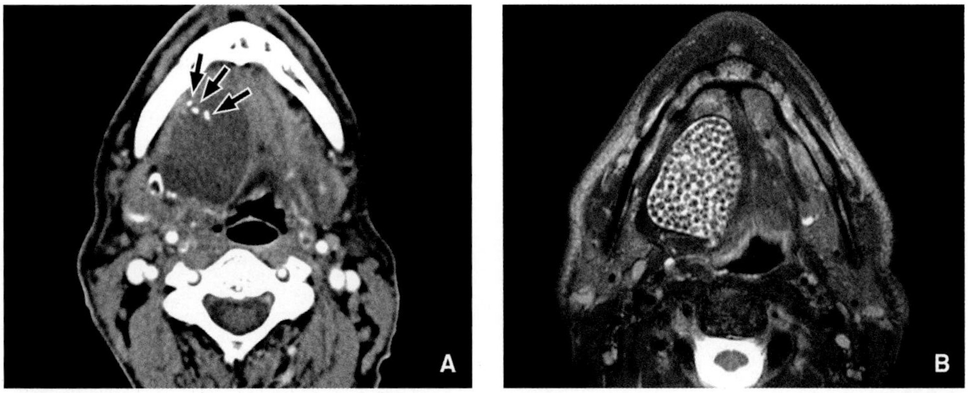

FIGURE 3.136 **Dermoid cyst in the sublingual space. A:** Axial contrast-enhanced CT image shows a smoothly marginated, lobulated mass in the right floor of the mouth. It is generally hypodense, but there are numerous internal foci of low density. A few calcifications (*arrows*) are also present. **B:** Axial T2-weighted fat-suppressed MR image clearly delineates this mass. It is hyperintense, with numerous small round structures within. It displaces the right genioglossus muscle medially and the right mylohyoid muscle laterally. The patient presented with a painless mass in the right floor of the mouth. He was taken to surgery for resection of this lesion, whereupon a well-encapsulated mass surrounded by dense fibrotic tissue was encountered. The cyst was opened up, and "multiple small, greasy, yellow" particles were released. Pathology described a "circumscribed pink-tan mass, which is partially opened to reveal a cystic cavity containing numerous tan, rounded masses of yellow grumous material." Final diagnosis was a dermoid cyst with associated fibrosis, chronic inflammation, and mural histiocytic proliferation consistent with focal rupture.

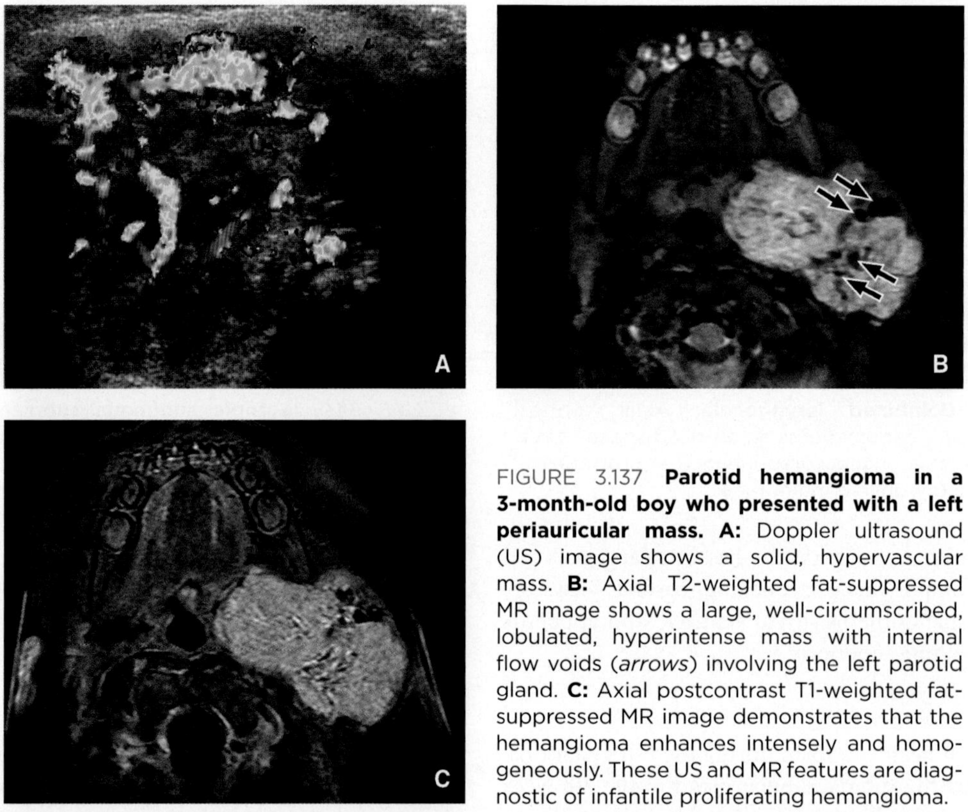

FIGURE 3.137 **Parotid hemangioma in a 3-month-old boy who presented with a left periauricular mass. A:** Doppler ultrasound (US) image shows a solid, hypervascular mass. **B:** Axial T2-weighted fat-suppressed MR image shows a large, well-circumscribed, lobulated, hyperintense mass with internal flow voids (*arrows*) involving the left parotid gland. **C:** Axial postcontrast T1-weighted fat-suppressed MR image demonstrates that the hemangioma enhances intensely and homogeneously. These US and MR features are diagnostic of infantile proliferating hemangioma.

cartilaginous, and osseous tissues found in these regions.[250–254] Hairy polyps can also involve the oral cavity.

Developmental cysts occur in the tongue and floor of the mouth and have been referred to variably as foregut duplication cysts, gastrointestinal mucosal cysts, and choristomas, among other terms. Approximately 55% of patients are asymptomatic with small cysts measuring <3 cm, discovered incidentally on imaging. However, larger cysts present as a mass in the tongue, neck, floor of the mouth, or in the vicinity of the pharynx, sometimes with associated feeding difficulty, snoring, or respiratory distress.[255] The differential diagnosis includes lymphatic malformation, dermoid cyst, and TGDC.

Congenital absence of the tongue is extremely rare and typically occurs in association with other abnormalities such as limb defects or micrognathia. Macroglossia can occur as part of a syndrome such as Beckwith-Wiedemann syndrome or can be related to endocrine disturbance, metabolic disorder, vascular malformation, tumor, or an inflammatory condition.

Tornwaldt Cyst

Tornwaldt cyst is a benign developmental lesion occurring in the midline of the nasopharynx, formed as a result of interaction between the notochord and the pharyngeal endoderm

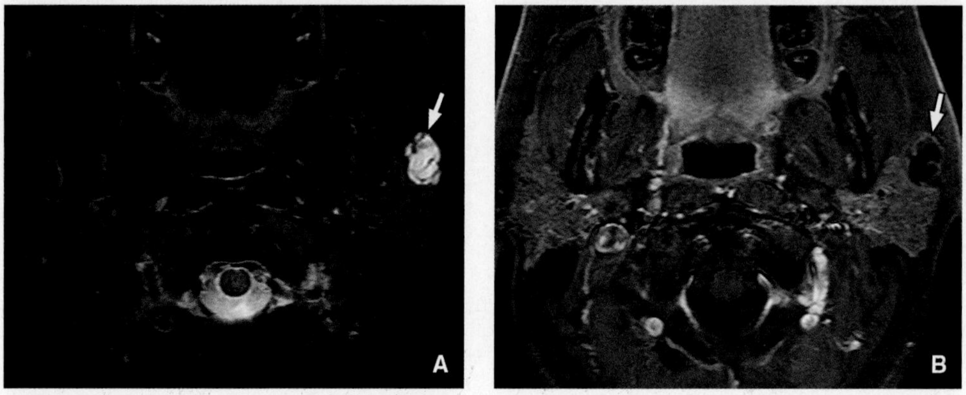

FIGURE 3.138 **Parotid region lymphatic malformation. A:** Axial T1-weighted fat-suppressed MR image shows a well-circumscribed, septated, hyperintense lesion (*arrow*) involving the superficial aspect of the left parotid gland. The differential diagnosis is lymphatic or venous malformation. **B:** Axial postcontrast T1-weighted fat-suppressed MR image shows that the septations enhance (*arrow*), but the lesion is otherwise cystic, confirming that this is a lymphatic malformation.

in utero. The cyst contents are typically proteinaceous.[9] They are seen in 4% of autopsied patients with no sex predilection. Symptoms are uncommon but include ear discomfort and hearing impairment related to eustachian tube obstruction or halitosis and foul taste in the mouth related to leakage or release of cyst contents under pressure.[256]

On MR imaging, Tornwaldt cyst appears as a well-circumscribed, thin-walled, cystic lesion in the midline posterior nasopharyngeal wall, with variable signal on T1-weighted sequence, high signal on T2-weighted sequence, and no enhancement with contrast. On CT, it has mucoid attenuation.

Lymphatic Malformation

Seventy-five percent of all lymphatic malformations (LMs) occur in the head and neck region.[257] LMs are present at birth. Previously occult LMs may present later because of sudden enlargement from intercurrent infection or hemorrhage. Extensive osseous involvement with LM is termed Gorham-Stout syndrome.

LMs may be macrocystic and unilocular or multilocular, or microcystic. On US, macrocystic LMs have echogenic septations, and cyst contents may be variably echogenic depending on proteinaceous or hemorrhagic content. On CT, LMs usually appear hypodense. There may be many (Fig. 3.139), few, or no internal septations. LMs have variable signal intensity on T1- and T2-weighted MR images depending on protein/hemorrhagic content. Hemorrhage occurs not uncommonly in LMs and leads to dependent layering of blood products and characteristic fluid–fluid levels, the signal of which depends on the age and content of the blood products. Dilated veins are sometimes seen in the vicinity of LMs. Hemorrhage and infection can cause sudden enlargement of the LM. Infection causes stranding of the surrounding fat with thickening and irregularity of the margins of the LM.

The differential diagnosis for LM includes VM. However, (1) fluid–fluid levels are not a feature of untreated VMs, (2) VMs enhance gradually because of the presence of venous blood, and (3) phleboliths are characteristic of VMs and are not a feature of pure LMs, although sometimes mixed features of LM and VM may be seen on imaging, particularly in the tongue. Microcystic transpatial LMs sometimes mimic plexiform neurofibroma (Fig. 3.140) or VM. The differential diagnosis for large congenital LMs is primarily congenital teratoma and cystic infantile myofibroma. Fluid–fluid levels are not seen in teratomas, and solid enhancing components, fatty tissue, and mineralized foci that are characteristic of teratomas are not seen in LMs. Depending on location, the differential diagnosis of LM might include ranula, foregut duplication cyst, BCC, TGDC, nodal abscess, and dermoid cyst.

Treatment options include surgery, sclerotherapy, and observation. There is growing utilization of sclerotherapy in patients with macrocystic LM, but there is no consensus on the agent of choice. Sclerosants that have been used include OK-432 (mixture of *S. pyogenes* and benzylpenicillin), bleomycin, doxycycline, acetic acid, alcohol, and hypertonic saline.[257] Rapid diagnosis and treatment is essential for LMs involving critical areas such as the orbit and airway.

Venous Malformation

Venous malformations (VMs) are low-flow vascular malformations that consist of malformed endothelial-lined venous channels. As with LMs, these lesions are present at birth and generally grow commensurate with the growth of the patient, unless complicated by intercurrent thrombophlebitis. VMs present as compressible, cystic masses that enlarge with Valsalva or dependent positioning of the affected body part. Superficial VMs cause bluish discoloration of the skin. Complications of VMs include pain and low-grade coagulopathy. Familial and syndromic forms of VMs occur such as blue rubber bleb nevus syndrome, sometimes with associated intracranial developmental venous anomalies and cavernous malformations.

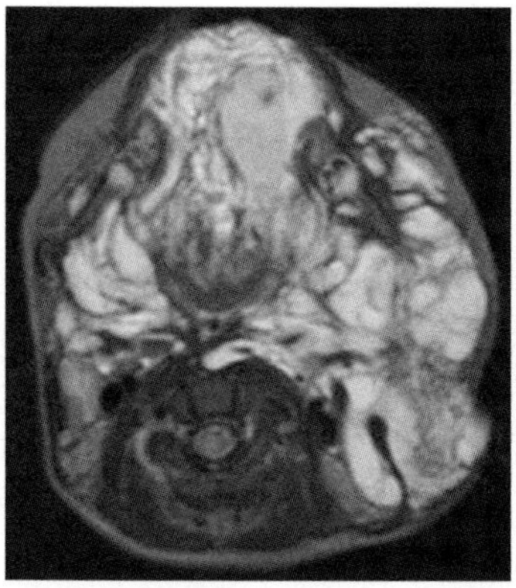

FIGURE 3.139 **Venolymphatic malformation involving multiple spaces of the head and neck.** Axial T2-weighted fat-suppressed MR image demonstrates a multilobulated, transpatial mass infiltrating across multiple spaces including the left parotid region, the left paraspinous region, bilateral masticator spaces, the left retropharyngeal space, the tongue, the oral cavity, and the floor of the mouth. Internal septations are evident. Note mass effect on the airway.

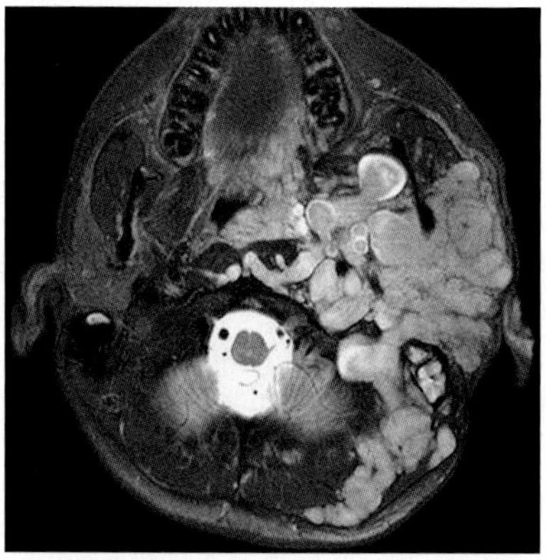

FIGURE 3.140 **Plexiform neurofibroma.** Axial T2-weighted fat-suppressed MR image demonstrates a multilobulated, transpatial mass involving the left parotid, left masticator, left parapharyngeal, bilateral retropharyngeal, and left paraspinous regions. There is also neurofibroma involving the tonsillar tissue. Extension to the floor of the mouth can be seen on images more caudally (not shown).

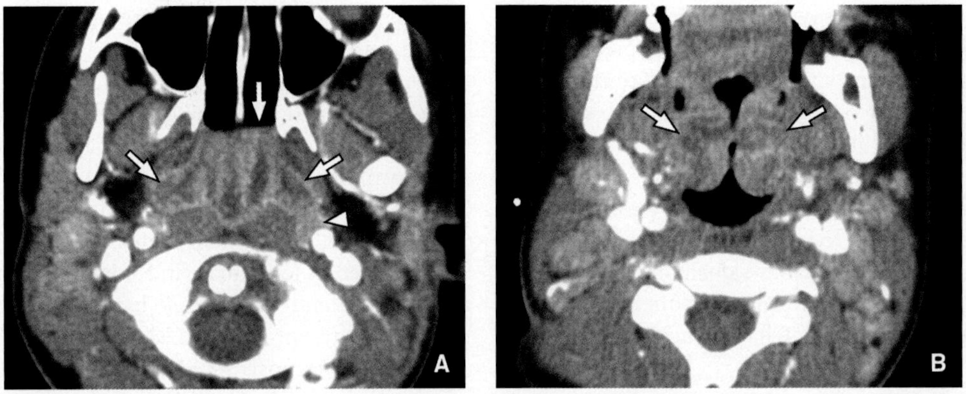

FIGURE 3.141 **Adenotonsillitis. A:** Axial contrast-enhanced CT image shows adenoidal edema and enlargement (*arrows*) resulting in streaky hypodensity with intervening linear enhancement. There is a mildly prominent enhancing node of Rouvière on the left (*arrowhead*). **B:** Axial contrast-enhanced CT image, obtained at a more caudal level than Figure 3.141A, shows that the palatine tonsils are enlarged and edematous (*arrows*), demonstrating similar hypodensity alternating with linear enhancement. These features are diagnostic of adenotonsillitis that occurs because of bacterial (e.g., streptococcal) or viral (e.g., Epstein-Barr virus) infection. There is also mild retropharyngeal edema and cervical lymphadenitis.

On ultrasound, VMs appear as compressible cystic masses with internal echogenicity due to the presence of venous blood. Rounded hyperechoic foci representing phleboliths are characteristic of VM. On contrast-enhanced CT and MR, VMs appear cystic with gradual contrast opacification. Phleboliths are sometimes seen on CT and appear as rounded signal voids on MR. The chief differential diagnosis for VM is LM. Midline facial VMs can be associated with sinus pericranii.

The treatment of choice for VMs is percutaneous sclerotherapy with alcohol. However, VMs tend to recur, necessitating multiple treatments.

Infectious and Inflammatory Disorders

Adenoidal Hypertrophy and Adenotonsillar Inflammation

Adenoidal hypertrophy is extremely common during the first several years of life and then regresses spontaneously from age 8 to 10 through the teenage years (Fig. 3.2). The size of the adenoid relative to the nasopharynx may be more important than actual adenoidal size in terms of symptomatic manifestation.[258] This is particularly true in patients with craniofacial disorders with midface hypoplasia and/or midface retrusion, as seen, for example, in syndromic craniosynostosis and trisomy 21. Adenoidal retention cysts are often seen on MR and are not usually of any clinical significance. These cysts are rounded or ovoid and are often off midline in location, unlike midline Tornwaldt cyst. Adenoidal (adenoidoliths) and tonsillar (tonsilloliths) mineralized concretions are sometimes seen, appearing as small calcific flecks on CT.

Acute adenotonsillitis with lymphadenitis causes marked enlargement and enhancement of the adenoid, tonsils, and lymph nodes on CT, sometimes with marked linear edema of the adenoid and a striated appearance of the edematous tonsils (Fig. 3.141). This appearance is characteristic of streptococcal throat infections and EBV infections. Adenoidal enlargement and intense adenoidal enhancement with retropharyngeal edema and cervical lymphadenopathy may be seen in Kawasaki disease. A peritonsillar or crypt abscess complicating tonsillitis presents as marked unilateral tonsillar enlargement with low attenuation and irregular peripheral enhancement on CT (Fig. 3.142).

Lymphoma and carcinoma are exceedingly rare in the tonsils and adenoid of children. In a patient with a history of organ transplantation, posttransplant lymphoproliferative disease is a consideration. Asymmetric adenoidal enlargement in a teenager can be a feature of EBV-associated NPC.

Retropharyngeal Space Infection

Retropharyngeal nodes drain the nasopharynx, oropharynx, nasal cavity, paranasal sinuses, middle ears, and prevertebral space.[259] These nodes are generally quite large in children because of the high frequency of colds, sinus infections, pharyngitis, and otitis media, but atrophy in teenagers. Bacterial infection (de novo or complicating viral infection) with spread to retropharyngeal nodes causes nodal enlargement

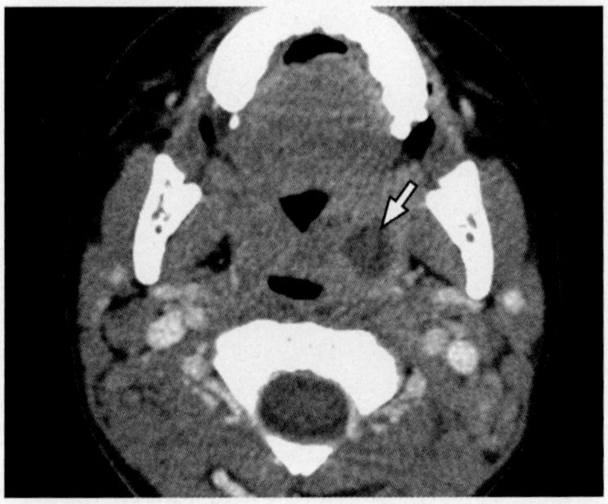

FIGURE 3.142 **Peritonsillar abscess.** Axial contrast-enhanced CT image shows a rounded focus of low density (*arrow*) in the region of the enlarged left tonsil. There is minimal retropharyngeal edema. The patient, who had not responded to IV antibiotics prior to the CT, was taken to the operating room where incision and drainage was performed, with drainage of frank pus from a peritonsillar abscess.

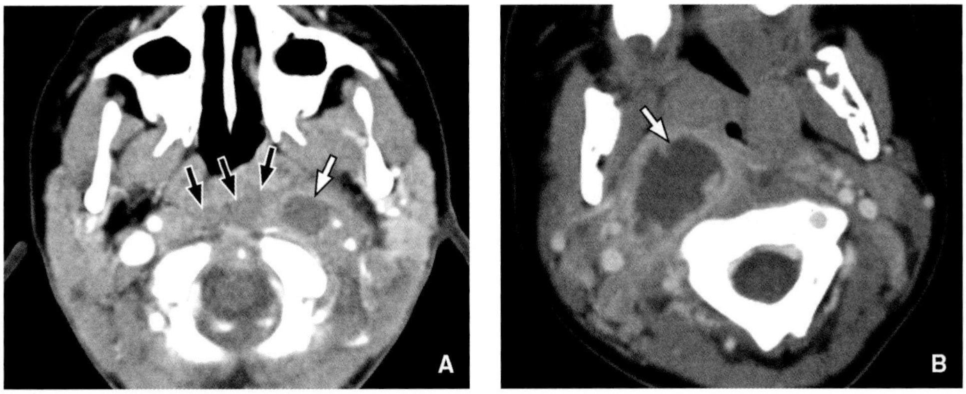

FIGURE 3.143 **Retropharyngeal infection in two different pediatric patients. A:** Suppurative node of Rouviere, retropharyngeal edema in a 6-year-old girl who presented with stiff neck and positive streptococcal throat culture. Axial contrast-enhanced CT image demonstrates enlargement and low attention of a left node of Rouvière (*large arrow*). The appearance could reflect nodal edema or suppuration. There is hypodense fluid infiltrating the retropharyngeal space compatible with retropharyngeal edema (*black arrows*). Note narrowing and displacement of the left internal carotid artery and jugular vein. **B:** Retropharyngeal abscess in a 3-year-old girl who presented with sore throat and drooling. Axial contrast-enhanced CT image shows a large, irregular, peripherally enhancing right retropharyngeal abscess (*arrow*) with associated retropharyngeal edema. Mass effect on the airway is due to a combination of the abscess and enlarged palatine tonsils.

that can progress to nodal edema and suppurative retropharyngeal adenopathy. In this situation, a reactive node has undergone liquefactive necrosis, but the purulent material is still surrounded by an intact nodal capsule, sometimes referred to as an intranodal abscess.[259] This is not uncommonly seen in early childhood and often involves the nodes of Rouvière (lateral retropharyngeal nodes).

On CT, enlarged reactive nodes enhance, whereas suppurative nodes appear hypodense with an intact, thickened, enhancing wall (Fig. 3.143). There may be associated retropharyngeal edema. Treatment usually consists of a trial of intravenous antibiotics. If the patient is clinically unstable, if there is persistent or worsening disease despite antiobiotic therapy, or if the suppurative node is large in size, surgical drainage may be warranted.[260] Progression from suppurative retropharyngeal lymph node to overt retropharyngeal abscess cannot always be predicted on CT. However, marginal irregularity with loss of the typical ovoid nodal configuration is helpful in suggesting progression to a drainable abscess (Fig. 3.143B). On CT and MR imaging, a retropharyngeal abscess has an oval or rounded configuration and a thick enhancing wall. Mass effect on the airway should be reported immediately to the physicians caring for the child. There is also displacement and often narrowing of the ipsilateral internal carotid artery and internal jugular vein. The radiologist should diligently search for a primary source of infection.

Retropharyngeal cellulitis may result when a suppurative retropharyngeal node ruptures, releasing the purulent material and infectious process into the retropharyngeal space. Less commonly, retropharyngeal cellulitis occurs from spread of infection from an adjacent fascial space, or from direct traumatic inoculation.

Not all fluid in the retropharyngeal space is related to infection within the space. Noninfectious retropharyngeal edema may occur, and may be difficult to distinguish from retropharyngeal space cellulitis. Noninfectious edema may be seen in a number of settings including postradiation, calcific tendinitis of the longus colli (Fig. 3.144), IJV thrombosis, and in reaction to an adjacent inflammatory process such as a suppurative retropharyngeal node, as mentioned above.

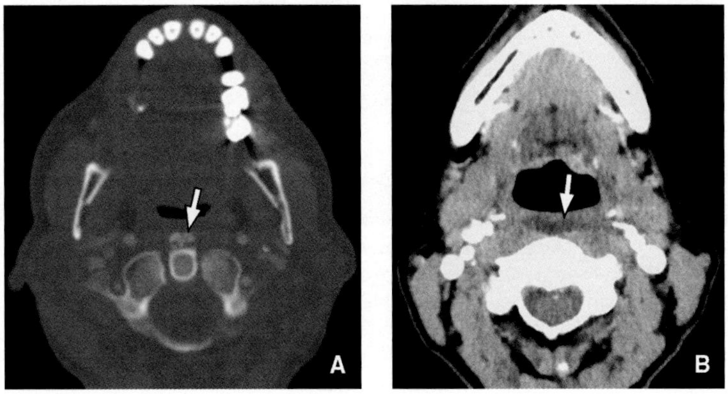

FIGURE 3.144 **Calcific tendinitis of the longus colli.** Axial CT images demonstrate calcific density in the superior oblique fibers of the longus colli muscle (*arrow* in **A**, bone algorithm) due to calcium hydroxyapatite crystal deposition. This incites an inflammatory tendinitis, leading to a retropharyngeal effusion (*arrow* in **B**, soft tissue algorithm).

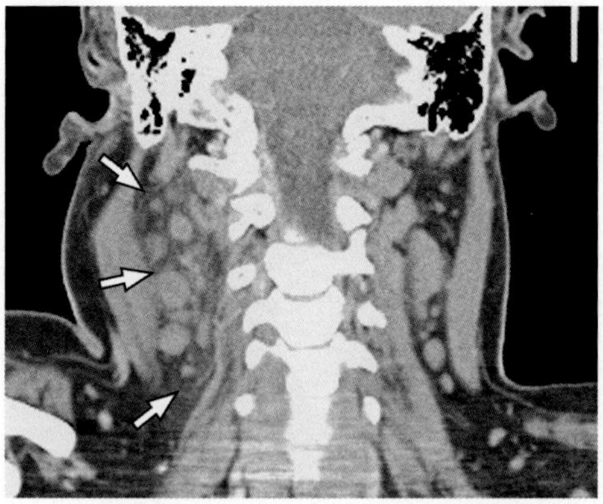

FIGURE 3.145 **Cervical lymphadenitis in an 18-year-old boy with a history of heart transplant who presented with fever and neck tenderness following an upper respiratory tract infection.** Coronal CT image shows enlarged nodes in the neck bilaterally. There is surrounding inflammatory fat stranding (*arrows*) in the right neck.

Findings on plain radiograph include thickening of the retropharyngeal/prevertebral soft tissues that does not vary with the respiratory phase and anterior displacement of the airway. The presence of gas is highly suggestive of an infectious process, provided there has not been a recent history of trauma or surgery. Torticollis may be seen, related to muscle spasm or inflammatory involvement of ligaments.

Complications of a retropharyngeal space infection include airway compromise, IJV thrombosis, carotid artery pseudoaneurysm and rupture, intracranial spread of infection, and mediastinal extension of infection.[261] Cellulitis may be treated with a course of antibiotics,[262] but abscesses often warrant incision and drainage.

Cervical Lymphadenopathy

Cervical lymphadenitis is common in children and typically occurs in the setting of tonsillitis (Fig. 3.145), pharyngitis, or a dental infection. Acute bilateral lymphadenitis is usually associated with systemic or localized viral infection, whereas unilateral lymphadenitis is more suggestive of a local bacterial infection. Bacterial pathogens are commonly *Staphylococcus aureus* and group A streptococcus.[263] If adenitis persists despite antiobiotic treatment, unusual causes should be considered, for example EBV in older children, nontuberculous mycobacteria or Kawasaki disease in young children, and neoplasm such as lymphoma. Other uncommon conditions that cause lymph node enlargement include histiocytoses such as Rosai Dorfman disease (sinus histiocytosis with massive lymphadenopathy) and Kikuchi-Fujimoto disease (histiocytic necrotizing lymphadenitis), and Castleman disease.

Imaging demonstrates the size, number, location, and morphology of the lymph nodes. On US, adenopathy appears as multiple round or oval hypoechoic masses along the jugular chain. On CT and MR imaging, nodal enhancement may be seen. With bacterial infection, the nodes may appear hypoechoic on US and hypodense on CT because of necrosis. In EBV infection, nodes are bilateral, round, and heterogeneous, with loss of normal fatty hila, indistinct margins, and a matted appearance.[264] Nontuberculous mycobacterial (NTM) infection typically presents as a slowly enlarging neck mass in the parotid or submandibular region in an otherwise healthy child aged between 2 and 5 years. There is associated characteristic violaceous discoloration of the overlying skin. Imaging reveals a conglomerate, necrotic nodal mass with extrusion of necrotic material into the subcutaneous fat towards the skin (Fig. 3.146C). Stranding of the surrounding fat is usually minimal to absent.[265] NTM adenitis can affect other cervical lymph nodes, including those in the retropharyngeal space (Fig. 3.146A, B). Affected nodes demonstrate thick enhancing margins, and sometimes calcification.[264] Calcification and nodal necrosis are also seen in fungal infection, cat-scratch disease, tularemia, tuberculosis, treated lymphoma, and metastatic disease (e.g., papillary thyroid carcinoma). In cat-scratch disease, enlarged nodes may become necrotic. Lymphadenopathy, salivary gland enlargement, and multiple parotid cysts are seen in AIDS and autoimmune disorders.

Regional reactive lymphadenitis may be seen with Lemierre syndrome. This condition occurs in otherwise healthy young

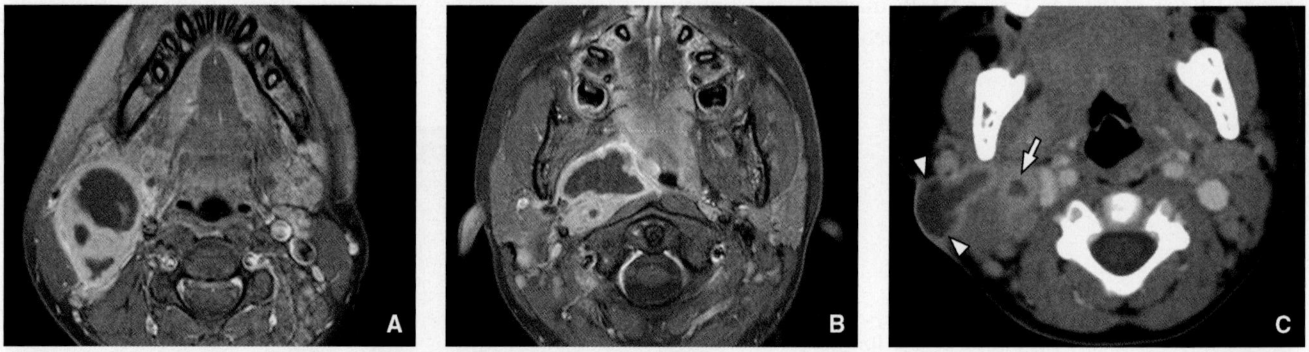

FIGURE 3.146 **Adenopathy from *Mycobacterium avium-intracellulare* (MAI) infection in two different pediatric patients. A and B:** An 11-year-old boy with progressive right cervical lymphadenopathy that did not respond to amoxicillin. Axial postcontrast T1-weighted fat-suppressed MR images demonstrate markedly enlarged necrotic nodes with thick enhancing margins in the right level II jugulodigastric region **(A)** and the right retropharyngeal region (node of Rouvière; **B**). **C:** A 17-month-old girl with a neck mass and violaceous skin discoloration. Axial contrast-enhanced CT image reveals enlarged necrotic level II lymph nodes (*arrow*) with necrotic material extruding into the subcutaneous fat (*arrowheads*) and skin. Note the relative lack of stranding of the surrounding fat.

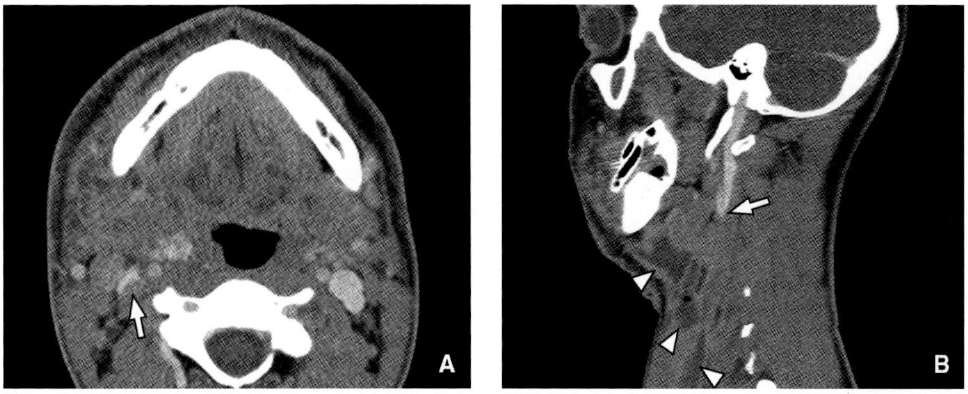

FIGURE 3.147 **Lemierre syndrome complicating neck abscess resulting from dental infection. A:** Axial contrast-enhanced CT image demonstrates partially occlusive thrombus (*arrow*) in the right internal jugular vein (IJV). Note the extensive right facial swelling and edema. **B:** Sagittal contrast-enhanced CT image demonstrates the thrombosed IJV (*arrow*). There are multiple neck abscesses (*arrowheads*) in this patient as a complication of sepsis following dental extraction. The triad of Lemierre syndrome includes neck infection, venous thrombosis, and septic pulmonary emboli (not shown).

patients, in whom an anerobic oropharyngitis leads to septic thrombophlebitis in the ipsilateral IJV (Fig. 3.147). There is frequently associated septicemia, with septic emboli to the lungs and large joints. In some cases, the initiating infection is in the chest rather than in the oropharynx. Pathogens are typically Gram-negative *Fusobacterium*, particularly *F. necrophorum*.[266] On US, echogenic occlusive thrombus is seen in the IJV with loss of compressibility. On CT, the occluded vein is usually enlarged and shows asymmetrically decreased enhancement compared to normal vessels. The vessel wall may enhance because of enhancement of the vasa vasorum. Edema of the surrounding soft tissues is often seen.

Necrotizing Fasciitis

Necrotizing cellulitis or fasciitis is an aggressive infection typically caused by *Streptococcus pyogenes* in otherwise healthy children. Infection is sometimes polymicrobial and *Staphylococcus aureus* (including resistant strains) alone or in combination with streptococcal species and/or other organisms is also commonly isolated. The route of inoculation is typically infected skin lesions such as eczema or varicella.

On contrast-enhanced CT, there is extensive soft tissue thickening of the neck, with stranding of the subcutaneous fat and fat between the fascial compartments, and blurring of the borders of the cervical musculature. Collections of edema are sometimes seen without discrete walled-off abscess. These children are typically toxic. The differential diagnosis includes edema because of a variety of other noninfectious causes including venous thrombosis/obstruction.

Treatment includes appropriate parenteral antibiotics, and prompt and aggressive surgical debridement may be required.[267]

Thyroiditis

In children and adolescents, Hashimoto thyroiditis, also known as chronic lymphocytic thyroiditis, is the most common cause of goiter and accounts for almost all cases of pediatric thyroiditis. Most of these patients are initially euthyroid,[268] but the disease can cause hypothyroidism. In fact, Hashimoto thyroiditis is the most common cause of juvenile hypothyroidism.[269] It is an autoimmune, inflammatory process that is more common in girls, is rare before 5 years of age, and peaks in early to mid puberty. Affected pediatric patients are typically asymptomatic, with a painless neck mass usually incidentally noted.

On CT, the thyroid gland is diffusely enlarged and heterogeneous in appearance. Sonographically, the parenchyma usually appears coarsened, hypoechoic, and hypervascular. A micronodular pattern (hypoechoic nodules 1 to 6 mm, with surrounding echogenic septations) has been found to be highly predictive of Hashimoto thyroiditis (Fig. 3.148).[270,271] Microscopically, the thyroid gland shows diffuse lymphoplasmacytic inflammation, with germinal center formation (Fig. 3.149). Patients with Hashimoto thyroiditis are at an increased risk for thyroid malignancy, including papillary and follicular carcinomas and lymphoma. Therefore, if a discrete nodule or mass is seen on ultrasound, tissue sampling must be performed to exclude a developing malignancy.

Infectious thyroiditis is uncommon[263]; when infection does occur, predisposing conditions such as a pyriform sinus fistula and a thyroglossal duct remnant should be considered.

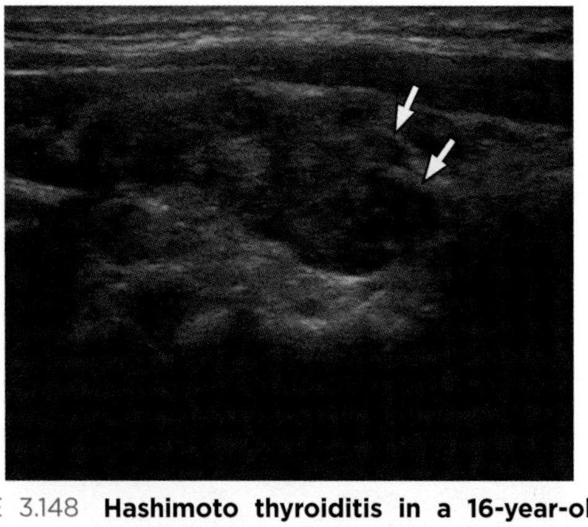

FIGURE 3.148 **Hashimoto thyroiditis in a 16-year-old girl.** Longitudinal gray-scale ultrasound image of the thyroid gland demonstrates multiple hypoechoic nodules in a small gland that appears coarsened and hypoechoic. Some echogenic septations are seen (*arrows*).

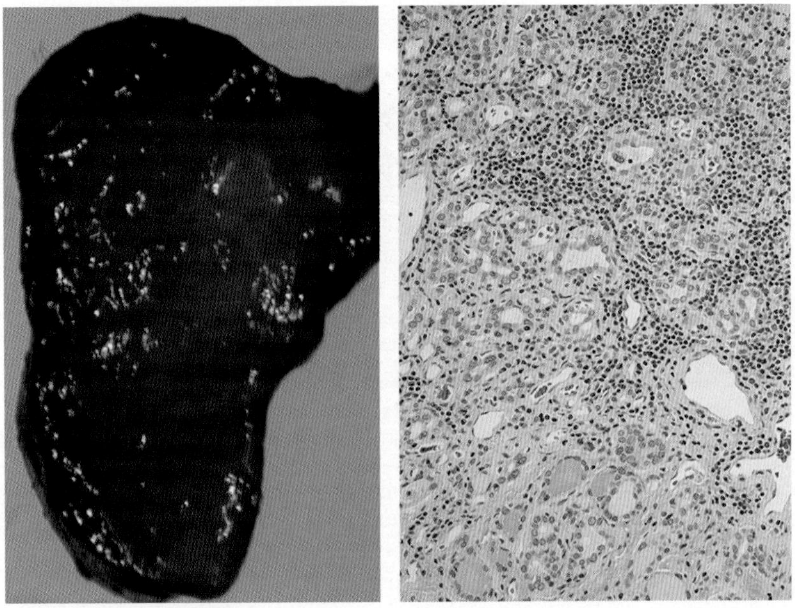

FIGURE 3.149 **Hashimoto thyroiditis in a 16-year-old girl.** Chronic lymphocytic thyroiditis in a thyroidectomy specimen from a patient with antithyroid antibodies (Hashimoto thyroiditis), is characterized by pallor, nodularity, and fine fibrous septa observed grossly **(left)**, and dense lymphocytic inflammation microscopically (**right**, hematoxylin and eosin, original magnification, 200x).

Infectious thyroiditis occurs more commonly in the left lobe than the right, likely related to embryologic anatomy of these predisposing conditions.[272]

The infected thyroid gland appears heterogeneous, with ill-defined areas of decreased echogenicity on ultrasound and hypodensity on CT (Fig. 3.150). A focal rounded hypoechoic/anechoic (US) or hypodense (CT) area suggests an abscess. There is edema and infiltration of the surrounding perithyroidal fat, and enlarged reactive nodes may be seen. Following resolution of an episode of acute suppurative thyroiditis, a barium pharyngogram should be performed to exclude a pyriform sinus fistula (Fig. 3.124B), bearing in mind that this study has a sensitivity of 50% compared to direct pharyngoscopy, and so a false negative result is a possibility.[272]

Salivary Gland Infection and Inflammation

Acute Bacterial and Viral Infections

Most bacterial infections of the salivary glands originate from the oral cavity, with individuals having decreased salivary flow especially at risk. Risk factors include dehydration, sialolithiasis, prior radiation, or a tumor causing ductal obstruction. Immunocompromised states such as HIV infection, malnutrition, and cystic fibrosis also predispose to acute sialoadenitis. In children, foreign bodies and seeds obstructing the duct are additional unusual considerations. Overall, ascending spread of infection is less common in the submandibular gland than in the parotid gland, because the opening of the Wharton duct is smaller and saliva from the submandibular and sublingual glands is thicker and more mucinous, containing antibacterial components such as lysozymes and IgA antibodies. Submandibular sialoadenitis is usually associated with sialolithiasis. Sialodochitis is inflammation of the Stensen or Wharton duct. The duct is often dilated because of downstream obstruction.

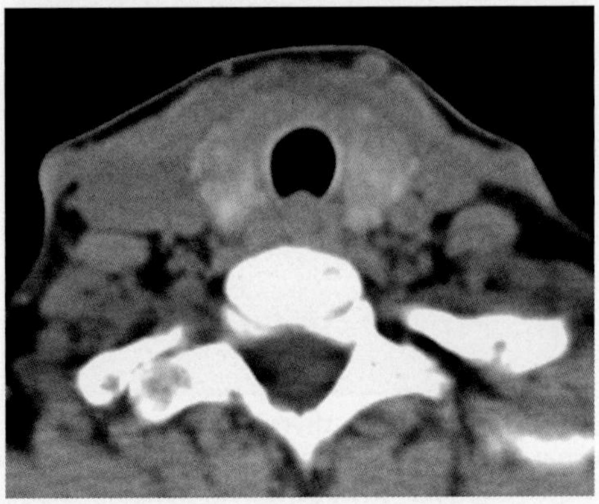

FIGURE 3.150 **Acute thyroiditis on CT.** Axial CT image shows ill-defined hypodense areas within the thyroid gland.

Neonatal suppurative parotitis (NSP) is an uncommon disease.[273] Culture of the purulent exudate from the Stensen duct usually yields *S. aureus*. There is increased risk of NSP in preterm babies, possibly due to their increased risk of dehydration. Ultrasound is useful to assess for potential abscess formation. On CT, the gland appears enlarged, heterogeneously dense, and diffusely enhancing.[274] There is surrounding inflammatory fat stranding, localized facial edema deep to the thickened platysma, regional reactive lymphadenopathy, and occasionally abscess formation (Fig. 3.151). In children, sialoliths most commonly occur within the submandibular gland or in the Wharton duct. Dilated ducts with enhancing walls indicate sialodochitis. On MR, the infected gland may be relatively hyperintense on T2-weighted sequence if there is significant edema, or hypointense if there is primarily inflammatory cell infiltration. Surgical drainage may be necessary in antibiotic resistant cases.

Among viral agents causing sialoadenitis, mumps is most common and is typically associated with parotitis. Other viral agents causing parotitis include coxsackie, parainfluenza, influenza type A, and herpes viruses such as cytomegalovirus (Fig. 3.152).

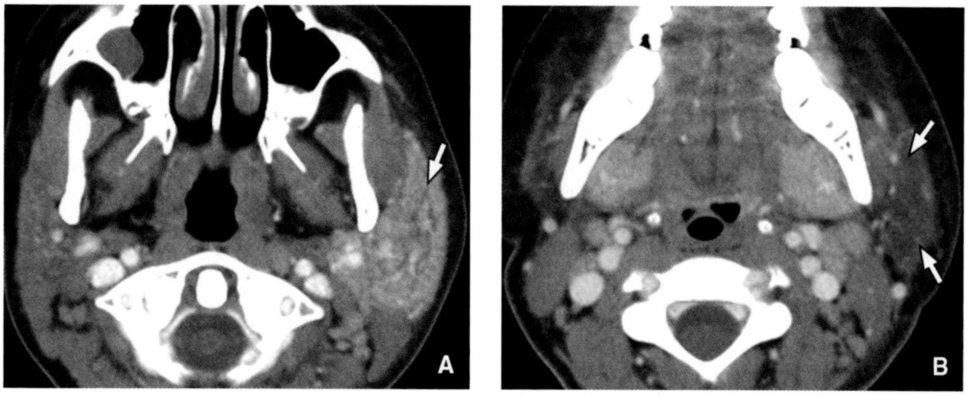

FIGURE 3.151 **Acute parotitis in an 8-year-old girl who presented with acute facial pain and swelling. A:** Axial contrast-enhanced CT image demonstrates the left parotid gland (*arrow*) to be enlarged and avidly enhancing compared to the normal right gland. **B:** A more caudal axial contrast-enhanced CT image shows edema (*arrows*) deep to the platysma muscle and stranding of the subcutaneous fat, consistent with facial cellulitis. This constellation of findings is characteristic of acute parotitis.

Chronic Inflammation

Chronic inflammation of the salivary glands may be seen with recurrent bacterial infections, prior radiation, and autoimmune diseases such as Sjögren syndrome. With chronic sialoadenitis, affected pediatric patients may experience recurrent episodes of acute inflammation separated by periods of quiescence, slow progressive glandular enlargement punctuated by episodes of acute inflammation, or slow progressive painless enlargement of the gland mimicking a neoplastic process. On imaging, the affected gland contains numerous small cysts reflecting ductal ectasia.

Sialolithiasis

Most stones occur in the submandibular gland and along the Wharton duct (80% to 90%) and are solitary (Fig. 3.153). Two-thirds of patients with chronic sialoadenitis have at least one calculus. Not all stones are radiopaque; ~20% of submandibular stones and 40% of parotid stones are not readily detectable on plain films.[275] Ductal stricture can form as a result of a sialolith. Both the stricture and the sialolith can lead to obstructed salivary flow and subsequent bacterial sialoadenitis, glandular atrophy, and/or sialocele formation. CT is the modality of choice for identifying stones. Noncalcified stones may have to be diagnosed by sialography or ultrasound.

Stones in the distal Wharton and Stensen ducts may be removed by opening the duct from a transoral approach, whereas more proximal stones may require surgical excision of the gland and its duct.

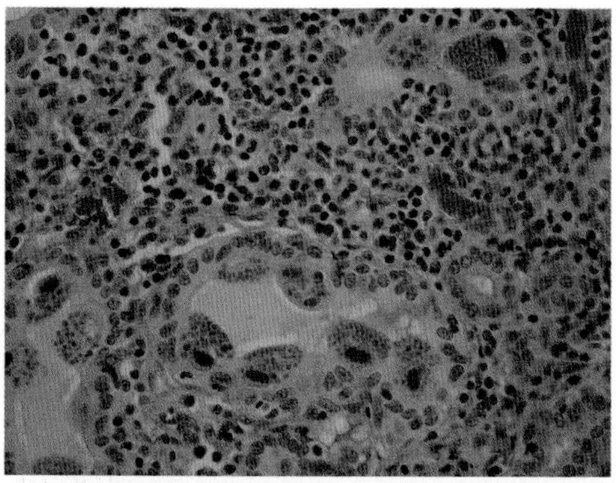

FIGURE 3.152 **Cytomegalovirus (CMV) infection of the parotid in a 5-month-old boy.** Cytomegalovirus sialoadenitis, showing magenta nuclear and cytoplasmic inclusions within ductal epithelial cells and a background of chronic lymphoplasmacytic inflammation (hematoxylin and eosin, original magnification, 600×). The patient presented with seizures, failure to thrive, and increased salivary secretions.

Sjögren Syndrome

In Sjögren syndrome, there is autoimmune lymphocyte-mediated destruction of the exocrine glands. When it affects major salivary glands, usually the parotid, the lymphoid infiltrate produces a localized mass termed a benign lymphoepithelial lesion (BLEL) or Godwin tumor. BLEL is typically a solid mass, but may have a prominent cystic component. Affected patients with Sjögren syndrome are at a much greater risk for developing NHL.[276]

Sjögren syndrome has a characteristic appearance on sialogram termed the "leafless fruit-laden tree": the central ductal system remains relatively normal, while peripherally there are numerous punctate contrast collections throughout the gland. Later in the disease course, the peripheral contrast collections may be larger or more globular, then referred to as the "mulberry tree" (Fig. 3.154). With increasing glandular destruction and ascending infection, the central ducts begin to dilate, and abscesses may develop throughout the gland.

On CT and MR imaging, there is enlargement of the involved gland, which is initially denser on CT, then progressing to a honeycomb appearance where there are small cystic areas, and finally to premature fat deposition. On MR, there is increased fat and sialoectatic foci that are hypointense on T1-weighted sequence and hyperintense on T2-weighted sequence (Fig. 3.155).[277] Rarely, diffuse, bilateral cystic change may be seen within BLEL, with the cysts ranging from a few millimeters to several centimeters. This appearance may then be difficult to distinguish from chronic recurrent parotitis or HIV-associated lymphoepithelial cysts. Any solid masses

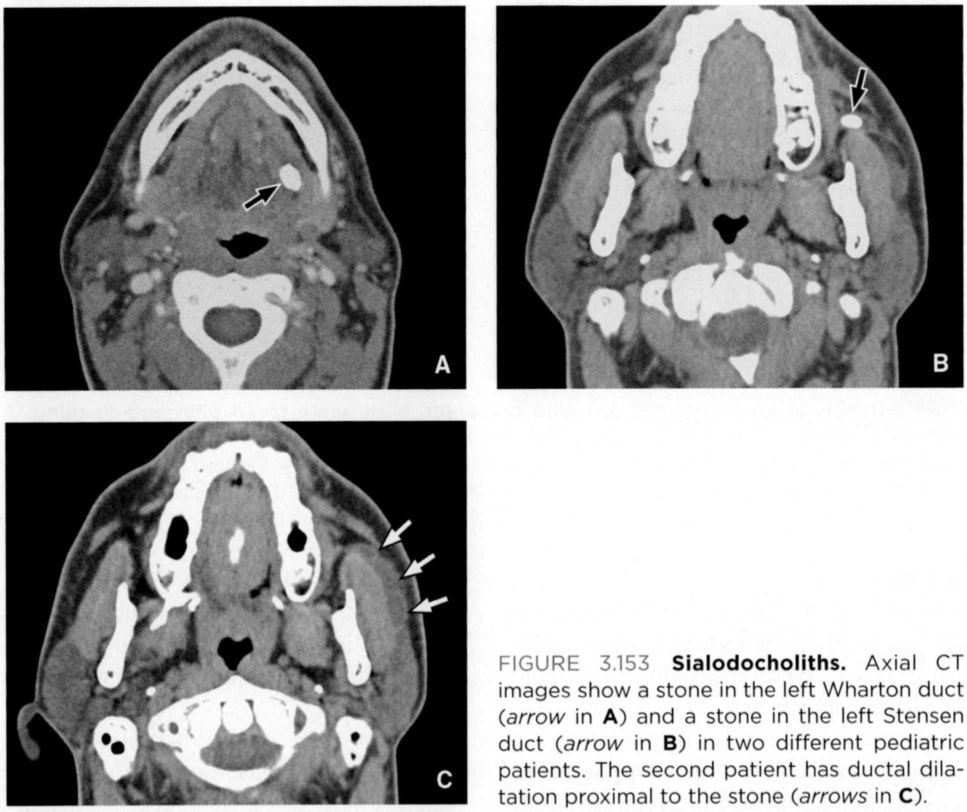

FIGURE 3.153 **Sialodocholiths.** Axial CT images show a stone in the left Wharton duct (*arrow* in **A**) and a stone in the left Stensen duct (*arrow* in **B**) in two different pediatric patients. The second patient has ductal dilatation proximal to the stone (*arrows* in **C**).

within the salivary glands seen in the setting of Sjögren syndrome warrant attention, and should be investigated to exclude the possibility of lymphoma.

Ranula

A ranula is a retention cyst that occurs in association with the sublingual gland, thought to result from obstruction of the gland or its ducts or as a result of trauma, leading to mucus extravasation into the surrounding soft tissues. When it remains within the sublingual space, above the mylohyoid muscle, it is termed a simple ranula. If a simple ranula ruptures and mucinous saliva spills out and extends to the submandibular space, either around the posterior edge of the mylohyoid muscle or through a mylohyoid defect (boutonniere), the resulting pseudocyst is termed a diving or plunging ranula.[278] Definitive treatment includes surgical excision of the sublingual gland.

On CT and MR, a smoothly-marginated, thin-walled, lobulated cystic mass is seen in the sublingual space lateral to the genioglossus muscle (simple ranula) or in the submandibular space lateral to the mylohyoid muscle, sometimes with a visible "tail" leading to the sublingual space or sublingual gland tissue (diving ranula) (Fig. 3.156). If there has been prior infection or hemorrhage, the cyst contents may become quite dense on CT and hyperintense on T1-weighted MR images, and the wall may be thick and enhancing. Differential

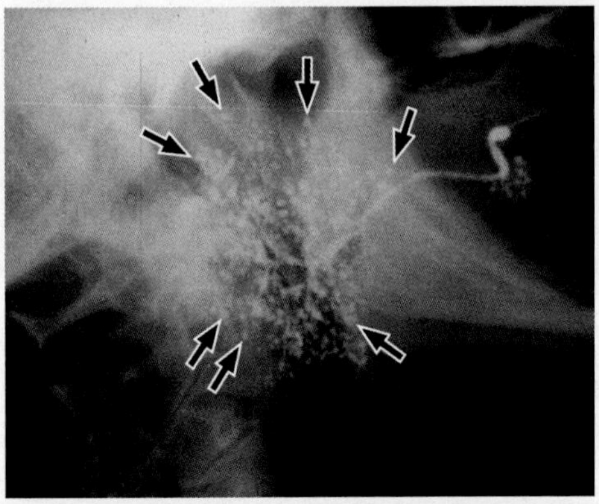

FIGURE 3.154 **Sialogram of Sjögren parotitis.** The central duct is relatively normal in contour and caliber, but peripherally, there are small contrast collections (*arrows*).

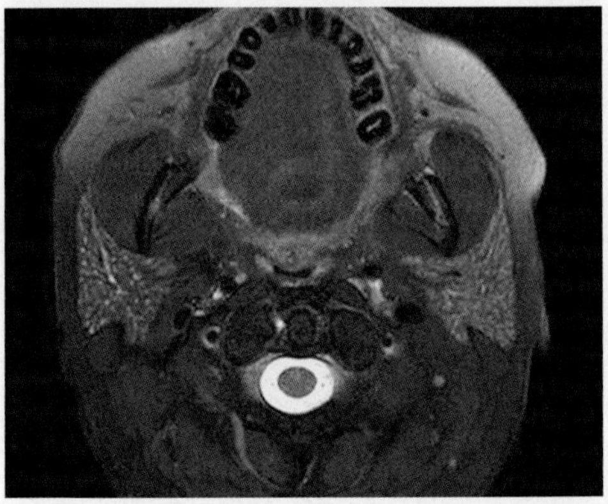

FIGURE 3.155 **Sjögren parotitis.** Axial T2-weighted fat-suppressed MR image shows numerous small cystic areas in the parotid glands. The glands are quite hypointense in signal because of fatty change. This appearance is indistinguishable from chronic recurrent parotitis of childhood.

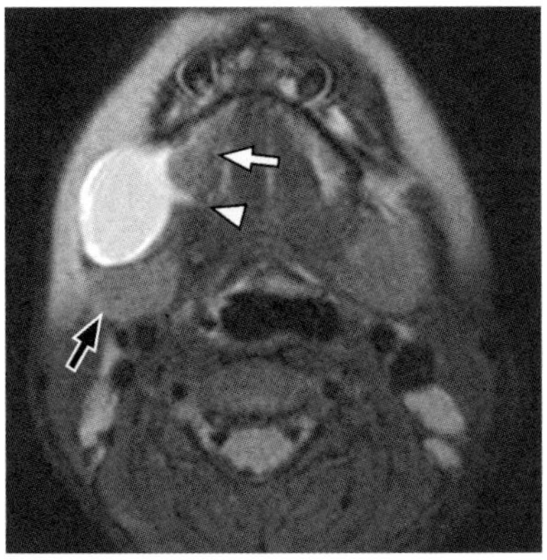

FIGURE 3.156 **Plunging ranula in a 4-year-old girl.** Axial T2-weighted fat-suppressed MR image demonstrates a cystic mass in the right submandibular space lateral to the mylohyoid muscle (*white arrow*), compressing the submandibular gland (*black arrow*). A tail can be seen extending through a mylohyoid defect toward the sublingual space (*white arrowhead*), revealing its origin from the sublingual space.

diagnosis includes dermoid, epidermoid, cystic/necrotic level IB node, and lymphatic malformation, depending on the location.

Neoplasms and Tumor-Like Disorders

Masses in the neck encompass a variety of etiologies, including congenital, vascular, and neoplastic processes. Some of these have already been discussed in previous sections. Other salient ones are discussed below.

Fibromatosis Colli

Fibromatosis colli, sometimes called pseudotumor of infancy or sternocleidomastoid tumor of infancy, is an uncommon, benign, congenital fibrous mass of the sternocleidomastoid muscle occurring in infants. It is the most common neck mass in the newborn. Patients present with torticollis and a firm, nontender mass in the anterior neck, usually in the distal third of the sternocleidomastoid muscle, and more often on the right (75% of cases). Bilaterality is rare.[279] The mass is not present at birth and is usually noted in the first 8 weeks of life. Enlargement over a few weeks may occur.[280] Histopathologically, the mass is composed of benign spindle fibroblasts and collagen around degenerating multinuclear muscle fibers (Fig. 3.157). The exact pathogenesis of fibromatosis colli is unknown. It may be associated with birth trauma, perhaps leading to obstruction of venous outflow in the muscle and subsequent edema, degeneration of muscle fibers, and fibrosis.

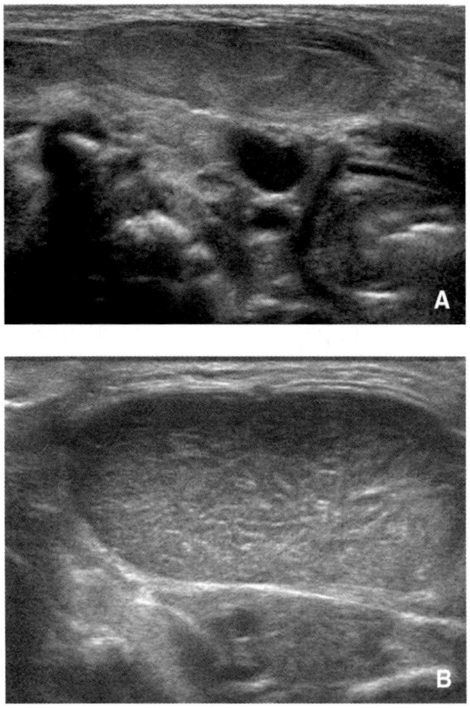

FIGURE 3.158 **Fibromatosis colli in a 29-day-old boy who presented with left sided neck swelling and restriction of movement. A:** Ultrasound image shows the normal sternocleidomastoid muscle on the unaffected *(right)* side. **B:** Ultrasound image demonstrates a thick solid mass at the expected location of the sternocleidomastoid muscle on the affected *(left)* side. It is similar in echogenicity and echotexture to the normal right sternocleidomastoid muscle, except enlarged.

Diagnosis is usually made clinically, based on the presentation, age, and natural history. Imaging can be helpful to distinguish this entity from mimickers such as RMS. Ultrasound reveals a solid mass within the confines of the sternocleidomastoid muscle belly, or diffuse enlargement of the muscle (Fig. 3.158). Echogenicity is variable, and may be increased, decreased, or similar to that of normal muscle. On CT and MR imaging, an isodense/isointense mass is seen within the confines of the sternocleidomastoid muscle, although hemorrhage or mineralization may occur.

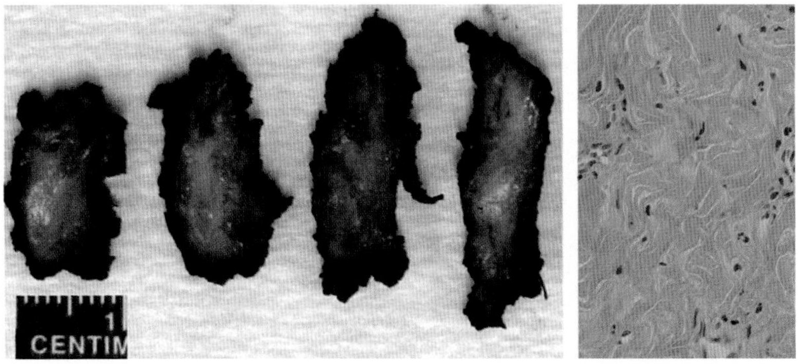

FIGURE 3.157 **Fibromatosis colli (sternocleidomastoid tumor of infancy) in a 1-year-old girl. Left**: the lesion displays a shiny gray-white fibrous cut surface; the black ink was applied by prosector before sectioning, to aid in the evaluation of margin status microscopically. **Right**: histologic examination shows densely collagenized fibrous tissue (hematoxylin and eosin, original magnification, 400x).

Most cases (80%) resolve by the 2nd year with only observation and conservative management such as physical therapy (e.g., massage and stretching), but some progressively worsen and result in facial and skull deformities. Those that persist may need to be treated surgically with tenomyotomy.[281–283]

Dermoid Cyst, Epidermoid Cyst, and Teratoma (Teratoid Cyst)

The spectrum of disorders variably termed dermoid cyst, epidermoid cyst, and teratoma (teratoid cyst) demonstrate overlapping features depending on the definitions used. An epidermoid cyst is a congenital lesion that consists of squamous cell epithelium with a fibrous wall. A dermoid cyst has, in addition to that, skin appendages such as hair follicles and sebaceous glands. A teratoid cyst is an old-fashioned name for a teratoma, composed of multiple types of tissues derived from all three germ cell layers.[284] All three lesions may contain cheesy keratinaceous material, and a teratoma may have variably prominent solid components.

The majority of dermoid and epidermoid cysts in the head and neck are found in the orbit, followed by the oral cavity and the nasal region. The remainder occurs in the neck, scalp, lower lip, and palate, often in the midline. Imaging is important to distinguish dermoid/epidermoid cysts in the sublingual space from those in the submandibular space, as they require different surgical approaches (intraoral versus external cervical).

On ultrasound, dermoid and epidermoid cysts are well-circumscribed, thin-walled echogenic masses (Fig. 3.159A). On CT, they appear as well-circumscribed, unilocular, hypodense masses (Fig. 3.159B). When fat is present, it is usually seen as small internal globules, in contradistinction to a lipoma, which demonstrates homogeneous uniform fat density throughout the lesion. There is usually enhancement of the cyst wall. On MR imaging, epidermoid cysts are hypointense on T1-weighted sequences and hyperintense on T2-weighted sequences, because of fluid within the cyst. Dermoid cysts have variable signal depending on the amount of fat within. Grossly, the resected specimen shows cheesy yellow contents (Fig. 3.19), sometimes with accompanying hair.

Teratoma is the most common congenital head and neck tumor.[285] The detection of a solid and cystic fetal neck mass compressing the airway on US or MR is characteristic. Postnatally, the large mass causes respiratory distress/obstruction and dysphagia. Teratoma most commonly arises in the infrahyoid neck and involves the thyroid gland.

On imaging, teratoma is off midline with the ipsilateral thyroid lobe draped around the tumor, or the ipsilateral thyroid may be difficult to see. On US, CT, and MR, teratoma appears well circumscribed with solid and cystic areas, characteristic foci of calcification, and sometimes fatty tissue. The solid tissue enhances with contrast. Other less common sites include the nasopharynx and paranasal sinuses, oral cavity, and regions adjacent to the skull base. Bony remodeling and erosion are sometimes seen. Grossly, teratomas have areas of soft gelatinous brain tissue, rubbery cartilage nodules, hard calcific areas of bone or tooth, and other elements (Fig. 3.160). Microscopically, the tissue types are intermixed in a disorganized fashion. Malignant teratoma and metastatic disease from teratoma of the head and neck are uncommon in children.

The differential diagnosis for predominantly cystic teratoma is lymphatic malformation. Splaying of thyroid tissue around the periphery and the presence of calcific and fatty foci are characteristic features of teratoma that are not seen in LM. Congenital rhabdomyoma and RMS, congenital hemangioma, and infantile fibrosarcoma are less common congenital solid tumors that lack the cystic changes seen in teratoma. Complete surgical resection of congenital teratoma is usually curative.

Lipoma

Lipomas are soft, mobile fatty masses surrounded by a capsule. They tend to increase in size proportionately with growth of the body. On imaging, the lesion should be of uniform fat density on CT (Fig. 3.161A) and isointense to fat on all MR sequences (Fig. 3.161B). If enhancing soft tissue is seen within the lesion, lipoblastoma should be suspected.

Pilomatrixoma (Calcifying Epithelioma of Malherbe)

Pilomatrixoma (PMX) is a benign tumor of hair follicle matrix cells. Approximately 50% occur in children under the age of 20, and about 50% occur in the head and neck region.[286] The tumor usually presents as a small, hard, slowly growing subcutaneous nodule, sometimes with overlying skin discoloration or ulceration. Rarely, multiple PMXs occur. PMX is typically

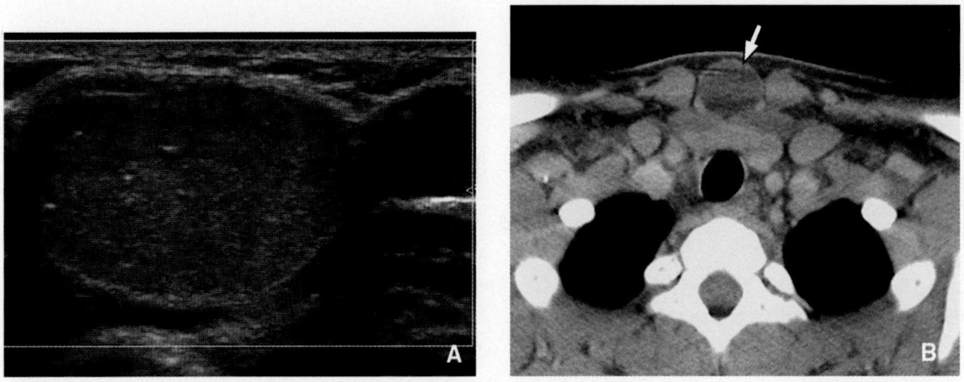

FIGURE 3.159 **Dermoid in a 16-year-old girl who presented with an anterior neck mass. A:** Transverse Doppler ultrasound image of the lower midline neck demonstrates a mass with internal echogenic foci that may represent calcifications. There is no flow within this mass. **B:** Axial contrast-enhanced CT image reveals a well-circumscribed, thin-walled, hypodense mass (*arrow*).

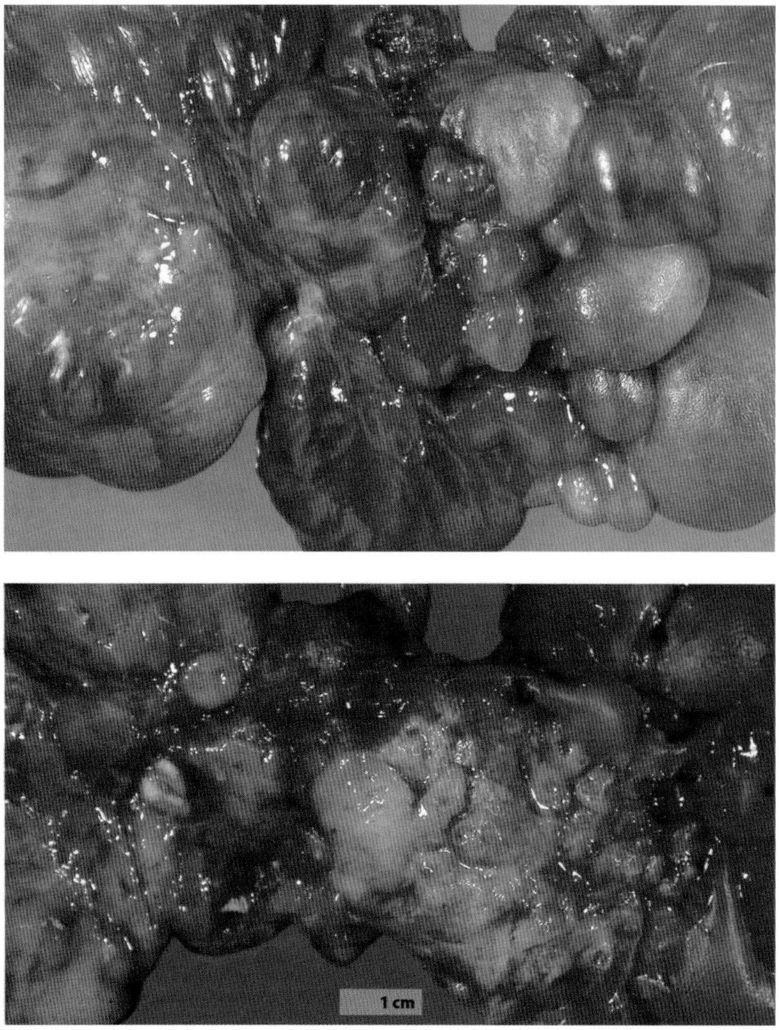

FIGURE 3.160 **Teratoma.** This large congenital teratoma of the naso- and oropharynx was resected on the first day of life. The outer surface is bosselated (**top**), and the cut surface shows marked heterogeneity (**bottom**), which microscopically proved to consist of brain tissue, intestinal tissue, dermal tissue, respiratory tissue, cartilage, liver, and other elements (not shown).

excised without recourse to imaging. Occasionally, imaging is requested, or PMX is seen as an incidental finding on imaging obtained for unrelated reasons.

PMX has a characteristic imaging appearance, typically appearing as a rounded or ovoid, sharply circumscribed subcutaneous mass, <1 cm in size, located in the preauricular region, face, or scalp. Calcification is common, causing the nodule to appear hyperechoic with posterior acoustic shadowing on US, hyperdense on CT (Fig. 3.162), and hypointense on T2-weighted MR images, with minimal peripheral enhancement on fat-suppressed T1-weighted MR images. This appearance is almost pathognomonic of PMX, though the differential diagnosis might include a calcified hematoma or foreign body reaction. The unmineralized and cystic

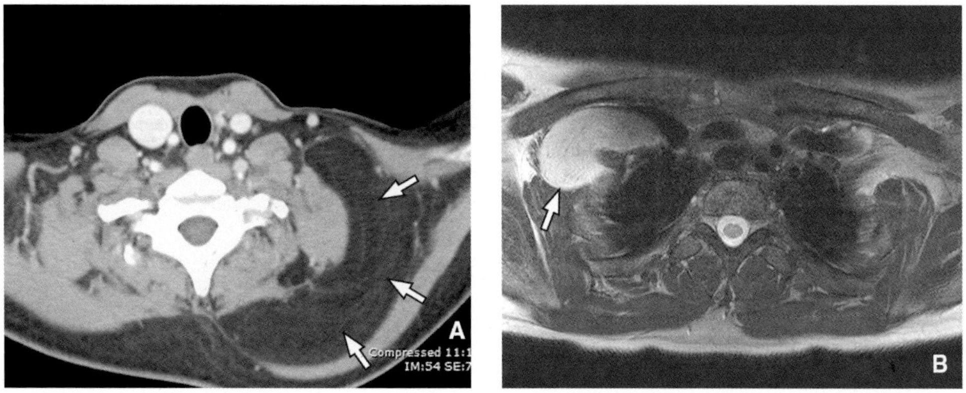

FIGURE 3.161 **Lipoma in two different pediatric patients. A:** Axial contrast-enhanced CT image shows a fat-density mass (*arrows*) in the left paraspinous region. **B:** Axial T2-weighted MR image demonstrates a mass (*arrow*) in the right supraclavicular region that has the same signal as fat on all MRI pulse sequences.

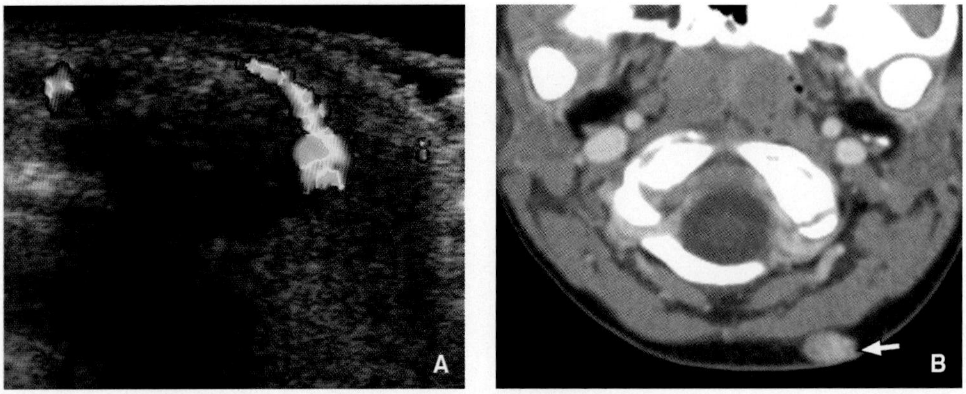

FIGURE 3.162 **Pilomatrixoma. A:** Doppler ultrasound of a posterior scalp nodule shows a heavily calcified, hypovascular lesion with acoustic shadowing. **B:** Axial contrast-enhanced CT shows the sharply defined ovoid hyperdense mass (*arrow*) in the subcutaneous fat extending to the skin.

variants of PMX are uncommon, and for these lesions, differential diagnosis includes neurofibroma (solid lesions) or first branchial cleft cyst (cystic lesions, if periauricular).

The treatment for PMX is complete surgical excision. Rarely, malignant PMX occurs, typically in adults.

Juvenile Xanthogranuloma

Juvenile xanthogranuloma (JXG) is a benign non-LCH that primarily affects children. Although typically presenting as a solitary cutaneous mass that does not require imaging, larger masses or more deep-seated masses do occur in the head and neck region and are then referred for imaging. Sites of predilection include the soft tissues of the pinna and external auditory meatus, and the nasofrontal region and scalp. Disseminated disease occasionally occurs.

On CT, JXG appears sharply circumscribed, enhances, and causes sharply marginated bony destruction. On MR, JXG appears mildly hyperintense relative to gray matter on T1-weighted MR images, hypointense on T2-weighted MR images, and enhances homogeneously.

Rhabdomyoma

Rhabdomyoma is a rare, benign mesenchymal tumor of striated muscle origin that can be divided into cardiac and extracardiac types. Extracardiac rhabdomyomas (fetal and adult subtypes) are extremely rare, but when they occur, they are most commonly found in the head and neck region.[287] The fetal subtype tends to occur in the periauricular soft tissues (Fig. 3.163), and a juvenile variant has a predilection for soft tissues of the face or mucosal sites, including the oropharynx and oral cavity.[288] Fetal rhabdomyoma is sometimes detected during prenatal ultrasound as a solid soft tissue mass in the head and neck region. Differential diagnosis includes RMS, teratoma, hemangioma, and infantile fibrosarcoma. Fetal

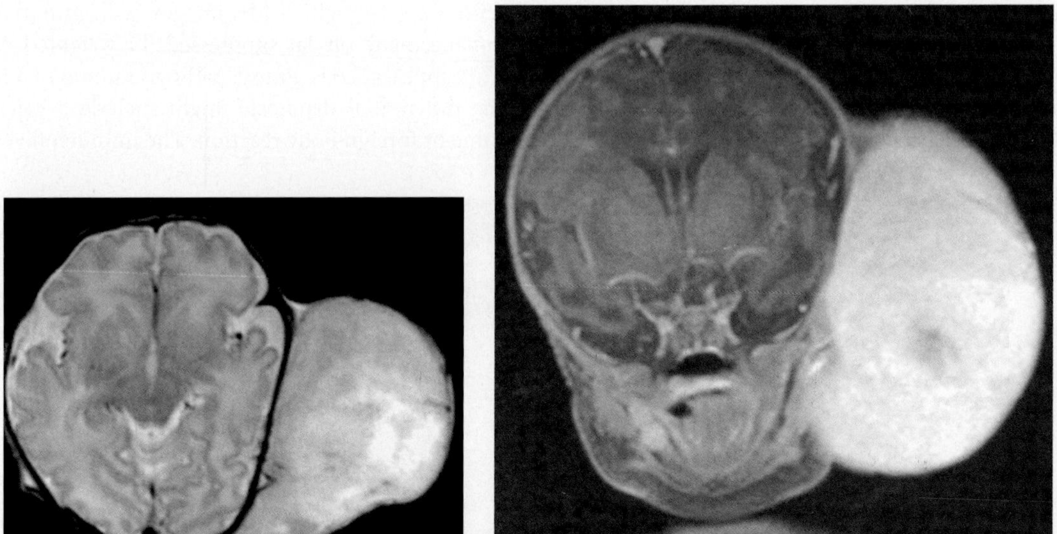

FIGURE 3.163 **Rhabdomyoma in a 1-day-old boy.** Axial T2-weighted and coronal postcontrast T1-weighted MR images reveal a large, well-defined, smoothly marginated mass in the left periauricular region. It has heterogeneous high signal intensity on T2-weighted sequence **(A)** and enhances avidly **(B)**.

MRI is of use to confirm the solid nature of the mass, delineate its margins, and assess for intracranial involvement.[289]

Benign Triton Tumor

Benign triton tumor (neuromuscular hamartoma, neuromuscular choristoma) is a rare neoplasm that manifests as a multinodular expansile mass in or around large nerves,[290] composed of mature peripheral nerve fibers admixed with well-differentiated striated muscle fibers and variable amounts of fibroblastic tissue. Cranial nerve involvement is primarily seen in children, who present with progressive cranial neuropathy and mass effect. The tumor has been variously described as being hyperdense on unenhanced CT, hypointense on T1-weighted MR images, and intermediate to hypointense on T2-weighted MR images. Enhancement ranges from mild to avid (Fig. 3.164).[291]

Nerve Sheath Tumors

Benign nerve sheath tumors include neurofibromas and schwannomas. Plexiform neurofibromas (PNFs) are characteristic of NF1. At least 30% of patients with NF1 will develop at least one PNF.[292] The affected nerves are tortuous, appearing as a "bag of worms." Lesions may be classified as superficial, arising from cutaneous and subcutaneous nerves; displacing, potentially causing pain; and invasive, leading to functional impairment due to their effect on vital structures. All three varieties can lead to significant cosmetic issues. There are two periods of peak growth, the first during early childhood and the second during puberty when there are hormonal changes. Pregnancy may also incite active growth because of hormonal changes.

On CT and MR imaging, they appear as transpatial multilobulated masses with irregular enhancement. They

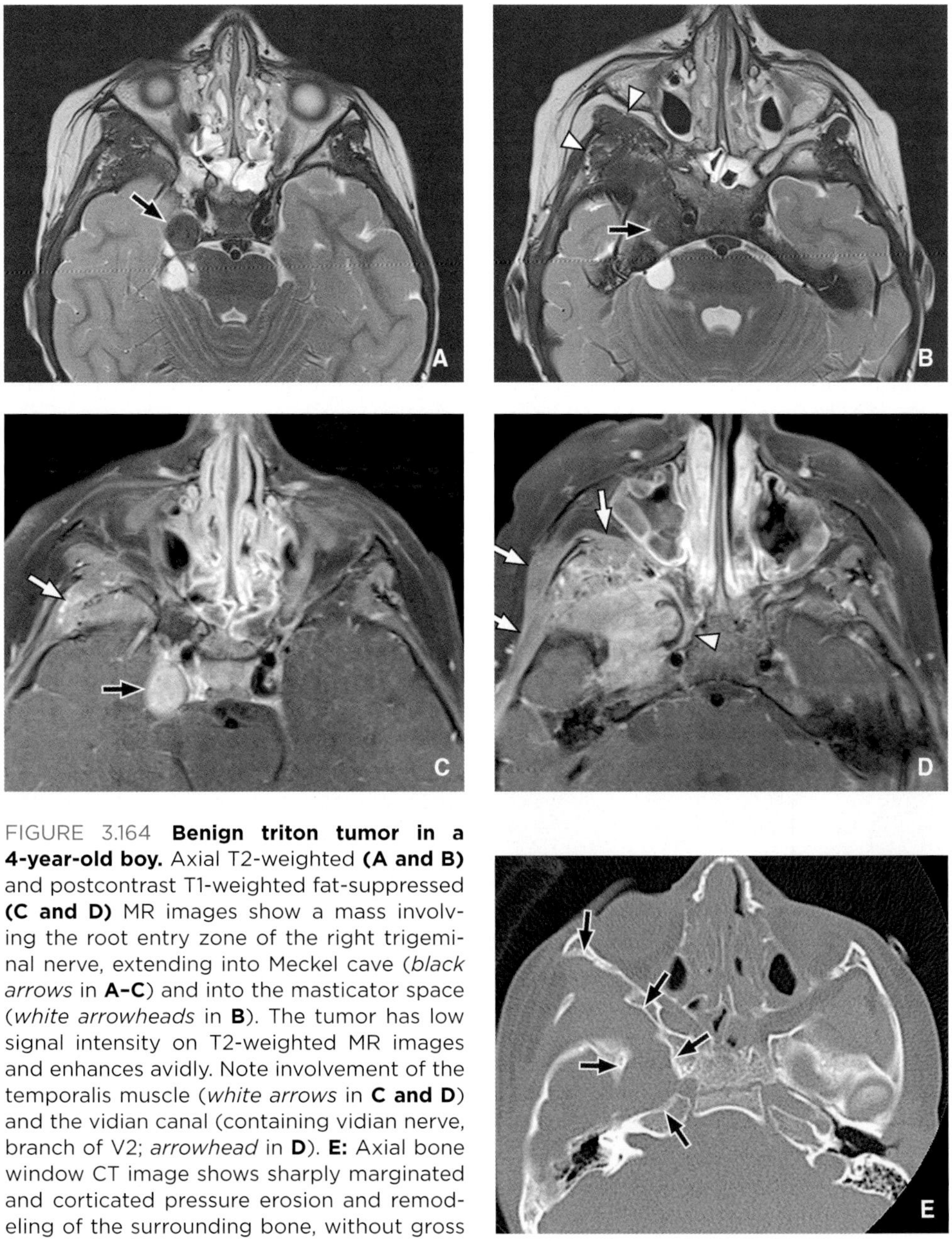

FIGURE 3.164 **Benign triton tumor in a 4-year-old boy.** Axial T2-weighted **(A and B)** and postcontrast T1-weighted fat-suppressed **(C and D)** MR images show a mass involving the root entry zone of the right trigeminal nerve, extending into Meckel cave (*black arrows* in **A–C**) and into the masticator space (*white arrowheads* in **B**). The tumor has low signal intensity on T2-weighted MR images and enhances avidly. Note involvement of the temporalis muscle (*white arrows* in **C and D**) and the vidian canal (containing vidian nerve, branch of V2; *arrowhead* in **D**). **E:** Axial bone window CT image shows sharply marginated and corticated pressure erosion and remodeling of the surrounding bone, without gross destruction (*black arrows*).

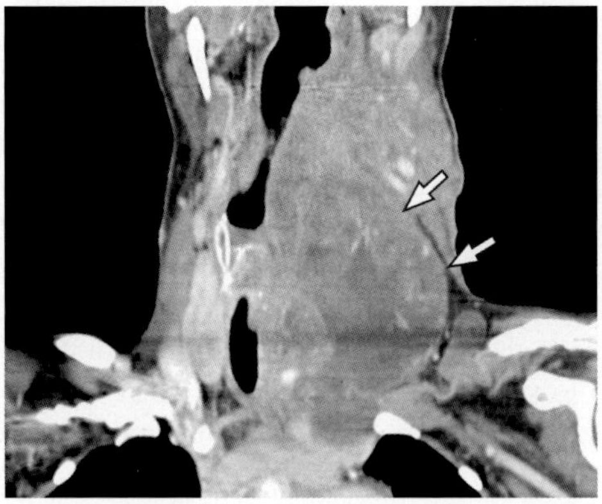

FIGURE 3.165 **Malignant peripheral nerve sheath tumor.** Coronal contrast-enhanced CT image demonstrates a large transpatial mass in the left neck. In the mid to lower neck, there is a focal area that has developed thick soft tissue enhancement (*arrows*). This area has undergone malignant transformation, as confirmed by biopsy.

tend to be isodense to hypodense on CT (Fig. 3.15), hypointense on T1-weighted MR sequence, and of variable signal on T2-weighted sequence depending on fibrous content (Fig. 3.140). There is a risk of degeneration into malignant peripheral nerve sheath tumor (MPNST) (Fig. 3.165). MPNST can also arise de novo.

Schwannomas associated with NF2 are most often bilateral involving the vestibular nerves, but other cranial nerves may also be affected. They are hyperintense on T2-weighted sequence with homogeneous enhancement unless there is internal cystic change. T2 shortening can be seen with more cellular components.

Lymphoma

Hodgkin lymphoma (HL) originates from cells of the monocyte–histiocyte series and accounts for 25% of all malignant lymphomas. The remainder is grouped together as NHLs.[293]

HL is the more common type of lymphoma in the head and neck region and is seen in children and young adults over age 10 years. In children, HL is primarily nodal in location. Extranodal involvement is rare.[168] Patients present with a painless palpable mass that corresponds to an enlarged node or nodal group (Fig. 3.166). The disease spreads from one nodal group to the next contiguous group via lymphatic channels.

On the other hand, extranodal involvement is much more commonly seen with NHL. Up to 30% of patients have an initial presentation of cervical lymphadenopathy with extranodal disease. NHL is more common in older patients and the immunocompromised. The incidence of NHL increases steadily throughout life.[294] After the gastrointestinal tract, the head and neck region is the second most common location for extranodal disease to occur. Areas involved include the Waldeyer ring (accounting for over 50% of cases) (Fig. 3.167), paranasal sinuses, nasal cavity, larynx, oral cavity, salivary glands, thyroid, and orbit.[168] Rapid tumor growth is more suggestive of NHL than HL and results in progressive mass effect and facial asymmetry, swelling, and pain due to extranodal disease. Pediatric NHL is more prone to blood-borne dissemination and is therefore more commonly associated with marrow and intracranial involvement than is HL. Approximately 18% of NHL patients have bone marrow involvement.[295]

Burkitt lymphoma is an aggressive B-cell NHL and is generally seen in children, representing 40% of all childhood NHL.[296] It can be classified into three forms that differ in geographic

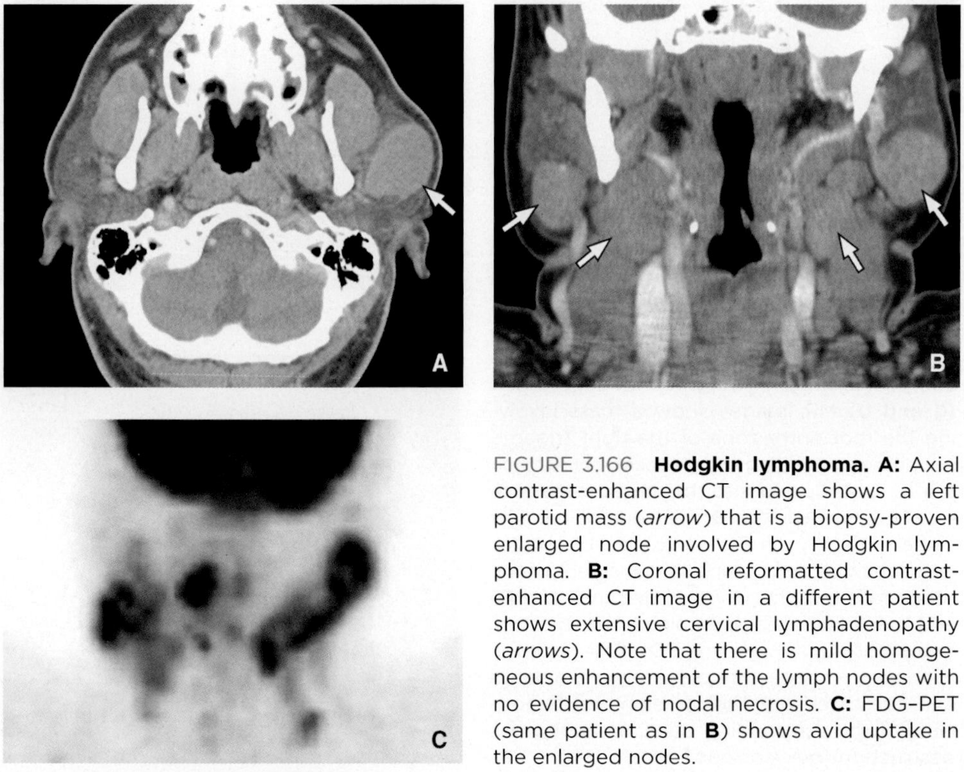

FIGURE 3.166 **Hodgkin lymphoma. A:** Axial contrast-enhanced CT image shows a left parotid mass (*arrow*) that is a biopsy-proven enlarged node involved by Hodgkin lymphoma. **B:** Coronal reformatted contrast-enhanced CT image in a different patient shows extensive cervical lymphadenopathy (*arrows*). Note that there is mild homogeneous enhancement of the lymph nodes with no evidence of nodal necrosis. **C:** FDG-PET (same patient as in **B**) shows avid uptake in the enlarged nodes.

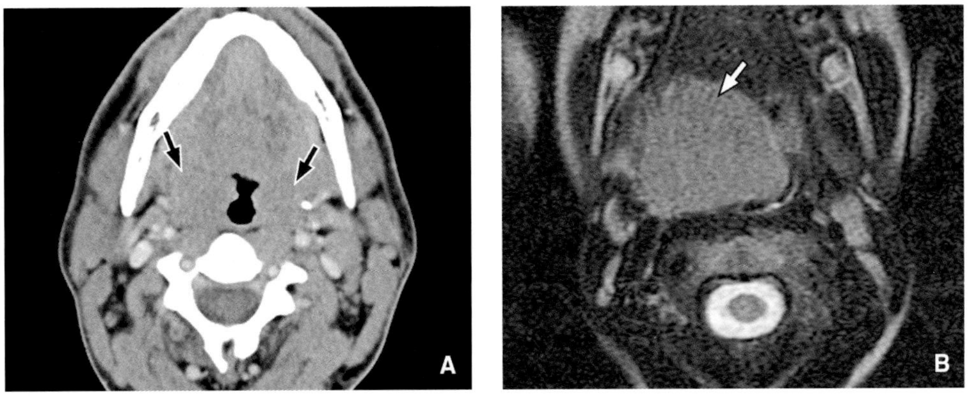

FIGURE 3.167 **Non-Hodgkin lymphoma in two different pediatric patients. A:** Axial contrast-enhanced CT image shows enlargement of the tonsils (*arrows*). **B:** Axial T2-weighted MR image (different patient) reveals a tumor involving the right tonsil (*arrow*) with mass effect on the oropharynx. The mass is very homogeneous and relatively hypointense. Biopsy revealed Burkitt lymphoma.

distribution and EBV association: sporadic, endemic, and immunodeficiency/HIV-associated variants.[165] The incidence of the sporadic form is low, and it is not often associated with EBV (15% to 20% of children). However, the endemic form is associated with EBV in over 95% of cases and is seen mostly in equatorial Africa. In the form associated with immunodeficiency/HIV, ~30% are EBV positive. The mean age of presentation of the endemic African form is 7 years, with the oral cavity, jaw, and kidneys being common sites of involvement. The nonendemic, sporadic form presents later at a mean age of 11 years and more commonly presents as an abdominal mass. Burkitt lymphoma has one of the highest cell proliferation rates of any human neoplasm, with a doubling time of 24 to 48 hours[297] and often has locally aggressive growth patterns.

When there is nodal disease, whether in HL or NHL, multiple nodes are usually involved and involvement may be unilateral or bilateral. Enlargement of the diseased nodes is variable, ranging from a few millimeters to over 10 cm. The middle and lower jugular chain nodes are often enlarged, whereas isolated involvement of the upper jugular chain nodes is unusual. Necrosis is very rarely seen in lymphoma; necrotic nodes in children are usually attributable to acute bacterial infection, subacute granulomatous infection, or Kawasaki disease. However, necrotic nodes with a negative workup for sepsis, persistent fever, and lack of response to adequate antibiotic therapy should prompt biopsy.

Lymphoma in Waldeyer ring often demonstrates multiple foci of disease and may result in airway obstruction. Lymphoma involving the nasopharynx rarely causes adjacent skull base bone erosion. Thyroid lymphoma tends to infiltrate into the adjacent soft tissues, including the aerodigestive tract, and there is often extensive nodal disease as well. Patients with Hashimoto thyroiditis are at an increased risk of acquiring thyroid lymphoma.

CT, MRI, and PET/CT are important tools to aid in staging of lymphomas. CT is useful for assessing bone involvement and for evaluation of cervical lymphadenopathy, whereas MRI is useful for soft tissue delineation in extranodal disease, particularly if there is transpatial disease or if there is intracranial or intraspinal extension. 18F-FDG–PET is utilized for initial staging and follow-up. On CT, the involved structures are isodense to muscle. On MR imaging, they are isointense to muscle on T1-weighted MR images and slightly hyperintense to muscle on T2-weighted MR images, often with very homogeneous signal intensity that is not specific but is quite characteristic of lymphoma. Necrosis and calcification are rare in untreated lymphoma but may be seen in treated lymphoma.

With timely institution of chemotherapy, 5-year survival rate for children with NHL is ~70%. HL, usually diagnosed early, has a cure rate > 90% with chemotherapy. The extent of disease at the time of diagnosis is the key predictor of outcome.[164]

Rhabdomyosarcoma

RMS is a malignant tumor of mesenchymal origin, arising from cells that are destined to differentiate into skeletal muscle. RMS is the most common pediatric soft tissue sarcoma and the second most common head and neck malignancy.[154] The most common sites of origin of RMS in the first decade are the masticator space (Fig. 3.168) and orbit (Fig. 3.34). The sinonasal region is the most common location in the second decade of life (Fig. 3.35). Other sites of involvement include the temporal bone, parotid region, and nasopharynx. The two peak ages of presentation are 2 to 5 years and 15 to 19 years. RMS has association with syndromes such as NF1, Li-Fraumeni, and bilateral or hereditary retinoblastoma, or may be radiation induced, occurring as a second primary malignancy.

Major histologic subtypes are embryonal (75%), alveolar (20%), and pleomorphic (5%). The embryonal subtype is the most common type in the head and neck and is also the most common type to be seen in young children (Fig. 3.168). The alveolar type has the worst prognosis and is seen more commonly in adolescents.

Clinical signs and symptoms depend on tumor location and include a mass, difficulty with chewing, otalgia (eustachian tube obstruction), proptosis, nasal stuffiness, epistaxis, airway obstruction (snoring, obstructive sleep apnea), lymphadenopathy, and cranial nerve palsy.

CT is used to demonstrate bony destruction and reveals an enhancing soft tissue tumor that remodels and erodes bone, with sharply marginated or lytic permeative bony

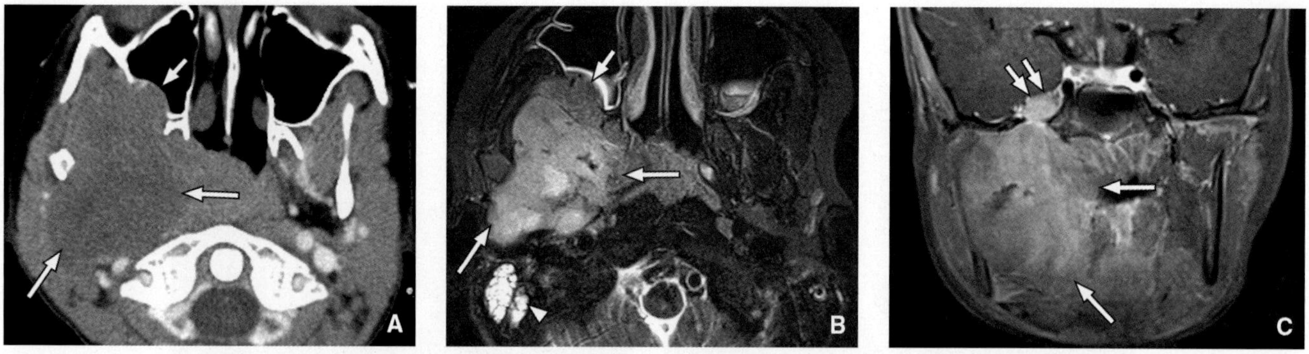

FIGURE 3.168 **Rhabdomyosarcoma (embryonal type) involving the masticator space. A:** Axial contrast-enhanced CT image shows a large mass arising in the right masticator space (*long arrows*) with lateral displacement and erosion of the mandible. There is also erosion of the posterolateral wall of the right maxillary antrum (*short arrow*). **B:** Axial T2-weighted fat-suppressed MR image demonstrates that the tumor (*long arrows*) is of heterogeneous intermediate signal intensity. There is submucosal invasion of the right maxillary antrum (*short arrow*). Note fluid within right mastoid air cells (*arrowhead*) due to eustachian tube obstruction. The right temporomandibular joint is dislocated. **C:** Coronal postcontrast T1-weighted fat-suppressed MR image shows the tumor (*long arrows*), which is extending through foramen ovale (*double arrows*) into the epidural space and into the base of the right cavernous sinus, consistent with parameningeal spread of tumor.

destruction. MR is used to assess soft tissue characteristics. On T2-weighted MR images, RMS typically appears isointense to cortex, though a range of signal intensities can be seen. RMS usually has decreased diffusivity and moderate to marked enhancement on contrast-enhanced images. Tumoral hemorrhage and necrosis are occasionally seen prior to treatment. It is important to detect parameningeal disease on MR. For example, masticator space tumors can extend directly through foramen ovale into the epidural space. Sinonasal, nasopharyngeal, and orbital RMS can erode the sphenoid, ethmoid, or frontal bones or extend through the inferior orbital fissure. Cavernous sinus, epidural, dural, and occasionally intradural spread of tumor results. Metastatic spread of tumor to regional lymph nodes and other parts of the body is best assessed with 18F-FDG–PET and CT.

The differential diagnosis of RMS depends on tumor location and imaging characteristics. Lymphoma can appear indistinguishable from RMS in the orbit, sinonasal region, temporal bone, and nasopharynx. Carcinoma and Ewing sarcoma are also in the differential diagnosis for sinonasal RMS, and NPC for nasopharyngeal RMS. RMS can simulate juvenile nasopharyngeal angiofibroma in the lateral nasal cavity and pterygopalatine fossa; however, RMS is not hypervascular, does not appear fibrous, and tends to cause a more permeative pattern of sphenoid bone destruction than does JNA. LCH, atypical teratoid–rhabdoid tumor, immature teratoma, and metastatic disease simulate RMS in the temporal bone. Ewing sarcoma and desmoid tumor are in the differential diagnosis for masticator space masses.

The prognosis of RMS depends on histologic and molecular subtype, presence of parameningeal disease, and stage of the tumor, and is best for localized disease that is amenable to complete surgical resection. Treatment includes chemotherapy, surgery, and radiation.

The list of other sarcomas that may be seen in the pediatric head and neck is long; it includes but is not limited to congenital fibrosarcoma, Ewing sarcoma, chondrosarcoma, osteosarcoma, epithelioid sarcoma, synovial sarcoma, dermatofibrosarcoma protuberans, alveolar soft part sarcoma, and angiosarcoma.

Thyroid Tumors and Tumor-Like Masses

Thyroid nodules are extremely uncommon in children before puberty.[298–300] Those found in children are more frequently malignant than those in adults.[299,301] US is the modality of choice for morphologic assessment of thyroid nodules. CT is less sensitive and less accurate in terms of evaluation of nodule size, number, and features, for example, degree of vascularity, margin definition, solid or cystic composition, and presence of microcalcifications.

Benign thyroid nodules include hyperplastic (polyclonal and nonneoplastic) and adenomatous nodules (follicular adenomas; monoclonal and neoplastic) (Fig. 3.169), although in practice they are not always distinguishable from each other since, with shifting definitions of the term "neoplasm," it is now well accepted that clonality may in fact be observed in nonneoplastic processes.[302] Thyroid nodules are also a feature of multinodular goiter and autoimmune thyroid disease (e.g., Hashimoto thyroiditis and Graves disease). Multinodular goiter in a child should raise the suspicion for

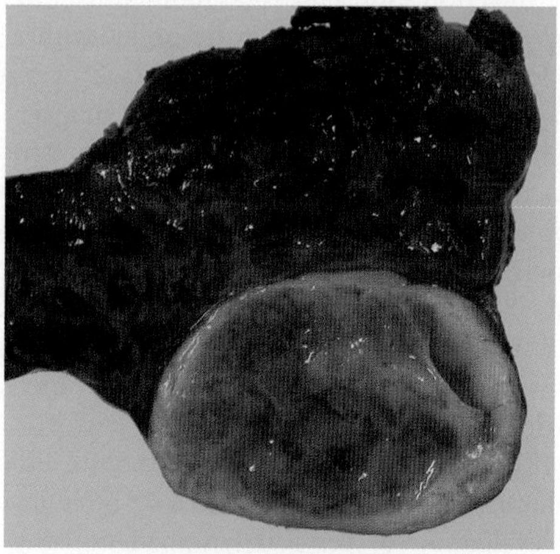

FIGURE 3.169 **Follicular adenoma.** This thyroidectomy specimen from an 11-year-old girl with Cowden syndrome shows a 2 cm well-circumscribed follicular adenoma, standing out as paler than the surrounding normal thyroid tissue.

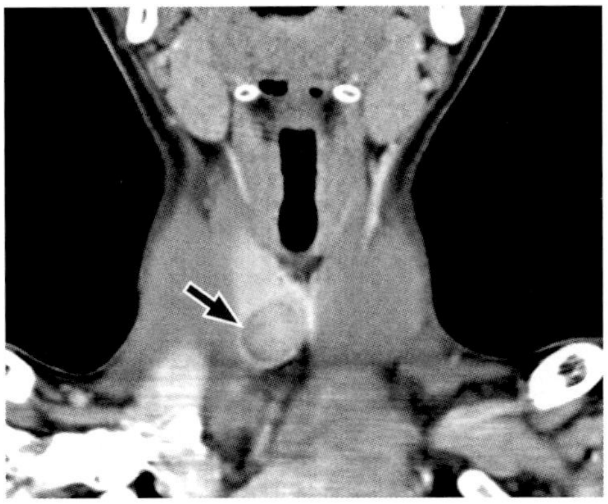

FIGURE 3.170 **Papillary thyroid carcinoma in a 13-year-old girl.** Coronal contrast-enhanced CT image shows a heterogeneous nodule (*arrow*) in the right thyroid lobe. Subsequent biopsy of this nodule confirmed the diagnosis of papillary thyroid carcinoma.

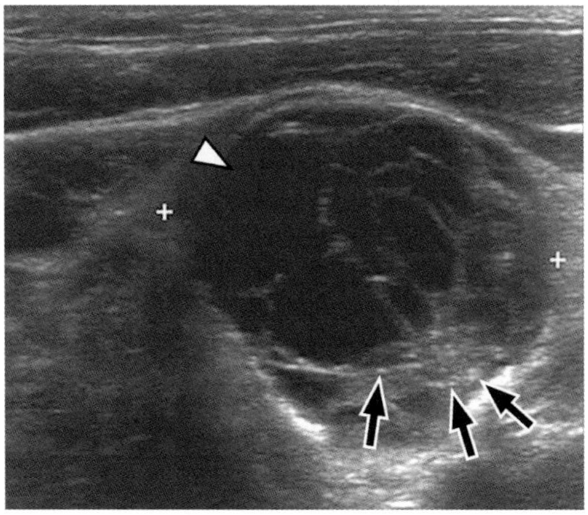

FIGURE 3.172 **Metastatic node from papillary thyroid carcinoma.** Gray-scale ultrasound image shows an enlarged level IV node with cystic components (*arrowhead*) and microcalcifications (*arrows*).

DICER1 syndrome, particularly in the presence of other characteristic lesions such as cystic nephroma and lung cysts.[303]

Most cases of thyroid cancers are sporadic, but some are related to inherited genetic mutations and hereditary cancer syndromes, for example, medullary thyroid carcinoma in the setting of multiple endocrine neoplasia (MEN) type 2, and papillary and follicular cancers in the setting of familial adenomatous polyposis (FAP).[304] Exposure to low to moderate levels of radiation may also increase the risk of papillary and follicular carcinomas.[305,306] It has been suggested that children exposed to increased levels of radiation should be considered for routine periodic thyroid ultrasound.[307,308]

In childhood, differentiated thyroid carcinoma is the most common thyroid malignancy, with ~90% to 95% being papillary thyroid carcinoma and the remainder follicular carcinoma.[309] The medullary subtype is rare in children. Papillary thyroid carcinoma is low grade (Figs. 3.170 and 3.171) and frequently multifocal. On US, the nodule appears hypoechoic and may have microcalcifications and internal vascularity.[310] Cervical nodal metastasis may be seen in up to 50% of cases, mostly in the central compartment and along the lateral cervical chains, and may be calcified, hyperenhancing, or cystic (Fig. 3.172). On T1-weighted MR imaging, metastatic nodes may appear hyperintense, reflecting colloid and thyroglobulin contents.[311] Hematogenous spread to the lungs and bones is uncommon. Prognosis is excellent, with 20-year survival rates >90%. Follicular thyroid carcinoma is uncommon and relatively low grade. Capsular and vascular invasion are common features, and hematogenous spread to the lungs and bones is more common than nodal spread. Prognosis is worse than that of papillary thyroid cancer, with 5-year survival at 90%. Medullary thyroid cancer is rare and has the poorest prognosis of all three subtypes. It may appear as a solitary mass or may invade adjacent soft tissues, metastasize to cervical nodes, or spread hematogenously to the lungs, bones, and liver.[312] Up to 90% secrete calcitonin, which may be used as a marker to track disease progression. Medullary carcinoma does not concentrate iodine and cannot be evaluated by radioactive iodine scintigraphy. However, agents specific to neuroendocrine tissues such as 131-I MIBG and 111-In pentetreotide may be used.

Children with solitary thyroid nodules are usually evaluated by Tc-99m or I-123. Nodules that take up radioactive iodine (hot nodules) are unlikely to be malignant. Biopsy may be warranted, however, for cold nodules. Aspiration may be performed on cystic nodules.

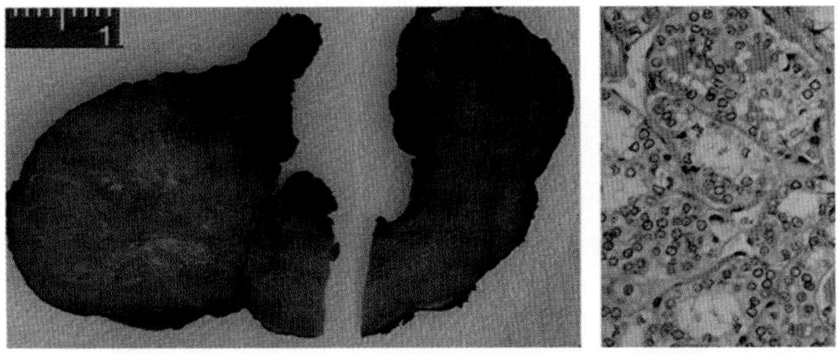

FIGURE 3.171 **Papillary thyroid carcinoma, diffuse sclerosing variant, in a 16-year-old girl.** The right and left lobes and isthmus show diffuse involvement by a tan-white poorly delineated mass with ill-defined white fibrous septa **(left)**. Microscopically, the tumor shows papillary architecture and cells with the characteristic enlarged, clear, and frequently overlapping nuclei (**right;** hematoxylin and eosin, original magnification, 600×).

Salivary Gland Tumors

In childhood, pleomorphic adenoma (benign mixed tumor) and mucoepidermoid carcinoma account for the vast majority of salivary gland epithelial tumors and usually arise in the parotid gland. Sialoblastoma is a rare congenital or infantile primary parotid tumor. Nonepithelial tumors include hemangioma, lymphoma, and neurogenic tumors. In children, nonepithelial tumors predominate, accounting for more than 50% of all lesions. Overall, the most common pediatric salivary gland tumors are hemangiomas, followed by pleomorphic adenomas and mucoepidermoid carcinomas.[313]

Hemangiomas are most commonly seen in the parotid region (Fig. 3.137). On MR, they appear lobulated and sharply defined, with moderately high signal on T2-weighted sequences, flow voids, and intense enhancement. Involuting hemangioma

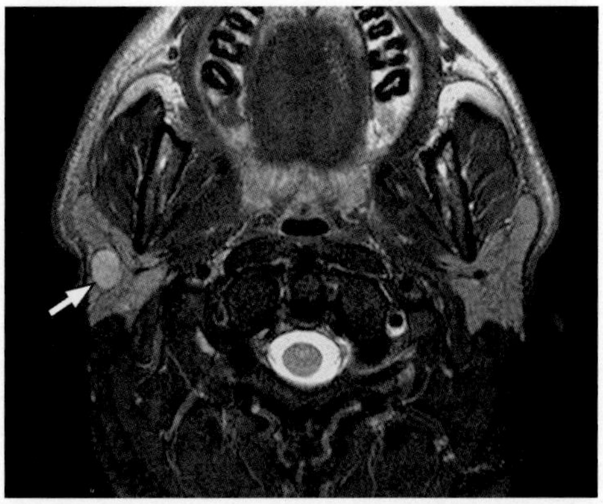

FIGURE 3.173 **Pleomorphic adenoma (benign mixed tumor) of the parotid.** Axial T2-weighted MR image shows a well-marginated rounded mass (*arrow*) in the superficial lobe. It is hypointense on T1-weighted sequence and enhances (not shown).

is characterized by tumor shrinkage, decreased vascularity and enhancement, and increased fibrofatty matrix. Atypical features of an enlarging mass in a young infant such as poorly defined margins, absent flow voids, and moderate or heterogeneous enhancement should prompt a differential diagnosis, which includes kaposiform hemangioendothelioma and sialoblastoma.

Over 80% of pleomorphic adenomas occur in the parotid gland, of which over 90% involve the superficial lobe (Fig. 3.173). These tumors are slow growing and usually appear as solitary, well-circumscribed masses with well-defined bosselated margins (Fig. 3.174). On CT, they are usually hyperdense to the surrounding parenchyma but may be hypodense or cystic appearing. On MR imaging, they usually have high signal intensity on T2-weighted sequences with variable enhancement. Larger tumors may demonstrate necrosis, old hemorrhage, and cystic change. Because of the risk of malignant degeneration, these tumors are usually surgically excised via parotidectomy. Unusual tumor locations include the submandibular glands and minor salivary gland tissue such as within the soft palate.

Although the two most common tumors are both benign, 35% of all salivary gland tumors in children are malignant, seen mostly in older children and adolescents.[314] This is a much higher rate when compared to adults. Mucoepidermoid

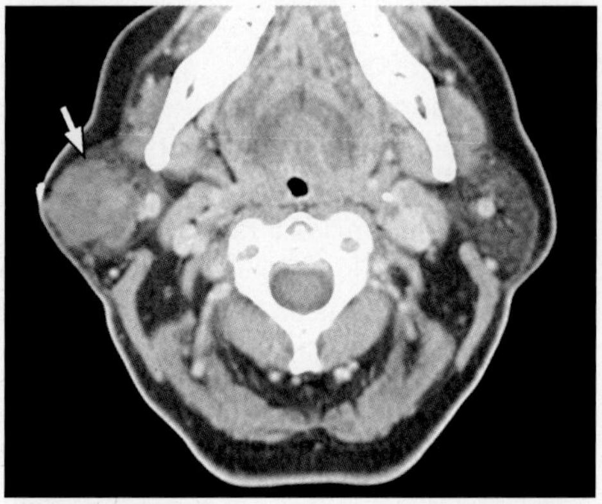

FIGURE 3.174 **Pleomorphic adenoma (benign mixed tumor) of the parotid.** Axial contrast-enhanced CT image shows a mass (*arrow*) with bosselated margins in the superficial lobe on the right.

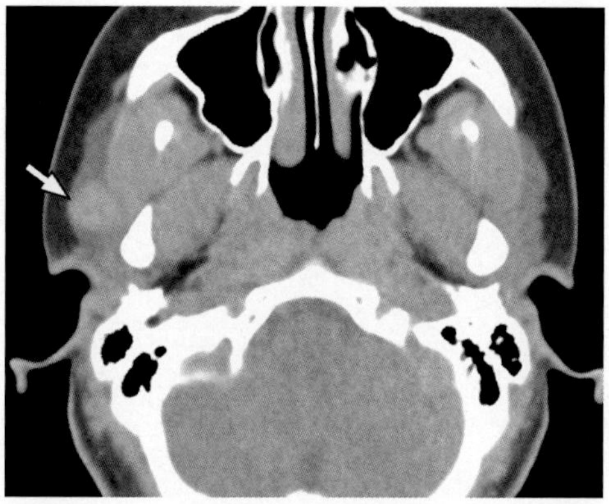

FIGURE 3.175 **Low-grade mucoepidermoid carcinoma in the parotid.** Axial contrast-enhanced CT image demonstrates a rounded and enhancing nodule (*arrow*) in the superficial lobe near the accessory parotid. It has slightly hazy margins but is otherwise not distinctive. Imaging differential includes a benign primary parotid tumor such as pleomorphic adenoma and an enlarged node.

carcinoma is the most common malignant salivary gland tumor in children. Those that are low grade have a similar appearance to a pleomorphic adenoma, with well-defined smooth margins (Fig. 3.175), but higher-grade lesions have poorly defined infiltrative margins and fewer internal cystic areas. On MR, the high-grade tumors have low to intermediate signal on T2-weighted MR images because of high cellularity.

Complete surgical excision with clear margins is the treatment of choice, with the higher-grade varieties receiving adjuvant radiation therapy.

Vascular Variants and Anomalies

Vascular Variants

The dural venous sinuses and IJVs are often asymmetric, with the right side usually appearing larger. The anterior and external jugular veins are also frequently asymmetric or may be absent on one side. The pterygoid plexus of veins may appear asymmetrically prominent on one side as well, mimicking a parapharyngeal mass (Fig. 3.176). The common and internal

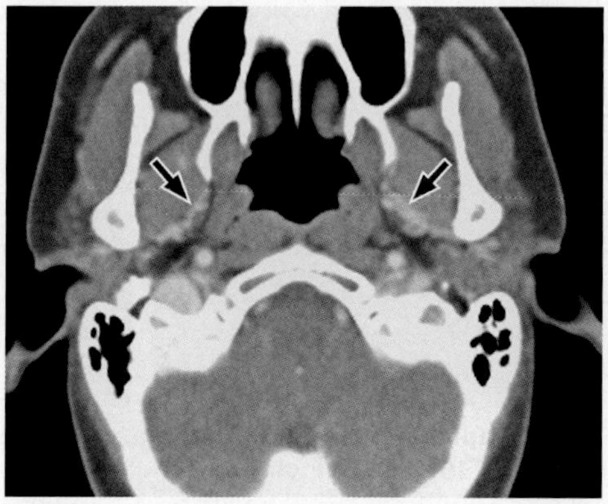

FIGURE 3.176 **Pterygoid venous plexus.** Axial contrast-enhanced CT image shows pterygoid venous plexus bilaterally (*arrows*). It is slightly more prominent on the left. In cases where there is significant asymmetry, the more prominent plexus could be mistaken for enhancing pathology.

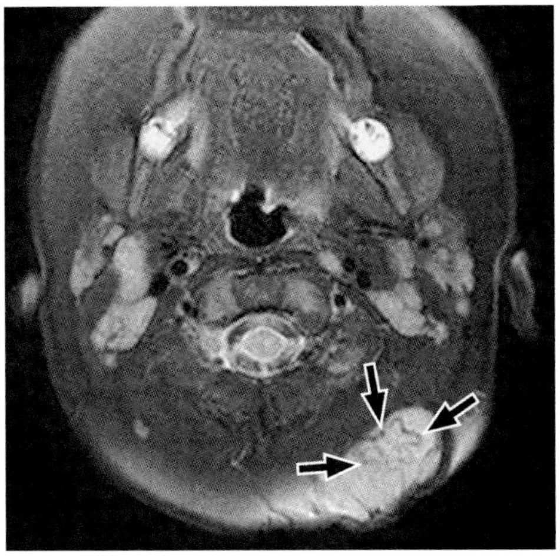

FIGURE 3.177 **Hemangioma in a 4-month-old girl.** The patient's mother noticed a neck mass when she was 3 months old. Axial T2-weighted fat-suppressed MR image shows a mass in the superficial suboccipital region that is hyperintense on T2-weighted sequence, with internal flow voids (*arrows*). It enhances (not shown). Clinical history and imaging characteristics are compatible with an infantile (rather than congenital) hemangioma.

carotid arteries may adopt a medial course in the neck, situated in a retropharyngeal location or abutting the lateral pharyngeal wall, resulting in a pulsatile submucosal retropharyngeal or parapharyngeal mass that may be noted on endoscopy.

Vascular Anomalies

According to the Mulliken and Glowacki classification of vascular lesions, vascular anomalies are divided into tumors—hemangiomas—and vascular malformations, which may be high flow or low flow. High-flow malformations include arteriovenous malformation and arteriovenous fistula; low-flow malformations include venous malformation and lymphatic malformation. In the neck, hemangiomas (Fig. 3.177), venous malformations, and lymphatic malformations are commonly encountered in children. These entities have been discussed in detail earlier in this chapter.

MISCELLANEOUS MASSES AND TUMORS OF THE JAWS

A variety of odontogenic and nonodontogenic lesions affect the maxilla and mandible in children. Fibro-osseous lesions include fibrous dysplasia (as described in earlier sections), ossifying fibroma, giant cell reparative granuloma (giant cell lesion), ABC, and nonossifying fibroma. Fibrous dysplasia and ossifying fibroma (which encompasses cemento-ossifying fibroma and juvenile ossifying fibroma) occur most often in the maxilla as expansile lesions with preservation of bony margins and sometimes with matrix mineralization.

One entity that should not be mistaken for fibrous dysplasia, or for a more aggressive lesion such as osteogenic sarcoma, is chronic nonbacterial osteomyelitis of the mandible. It causes predominantly unilateral but sometimes bilateral mandibular expansion and sclerosis with a lamellated periosteal reaction

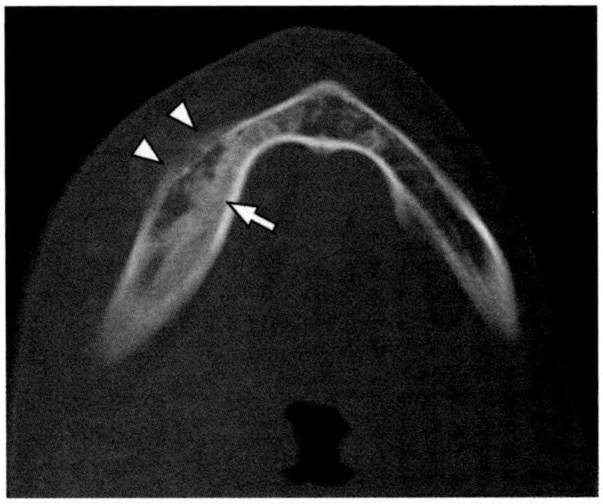

FIGURE 3.178 **Chronic nonbacterial osteomyelitis (chronic sclerosing osteomyelitis) in a 4-year-old girl who presented with slowly progressive right mandibular swelling.** Axial bone window CT image demonstrates expansion and sclerosis of the body of the right mandible (*arrow*). There is periosteal reaction and irregular lucency along the buccal margin of the mandible (*arrowheads*).

(Fig. 3.178) and swelling of the ipsilateral muscles of mastication. A focal expansile lesion with lytic destruction of bone on CT and fluid–fluid levels on CT or MR is characteristic of both giant cell lesion (Fig. 3.179) and ABC. Multiple giant cell lesions are a feature of an allelic variant of Noonan syndrome.[315] Multilocular fibro-osseous radiolucencies of the mandible that are well seen on CT also occur in autosomal dominant cherubism (Fig. 3.180). This condition causes symmetrical expansion of the mandible that develops during early childhood and increases until puberty, then regresses. Histopathologically, the lesions are indistinguishable from giant cell reparative granuloma, solid variant ABC, and brown tumor of hyperparathyroidism. A mutation in the *SH3BP2* gene underlying cherubism has been established.[316] Operative intervention is only required for functional or aesthetic reasons or for aggressive lesions that cause airway obstruction.[317]

Malignant tumors of the maxilla and mandible are as described in the sinonasal section and include primary

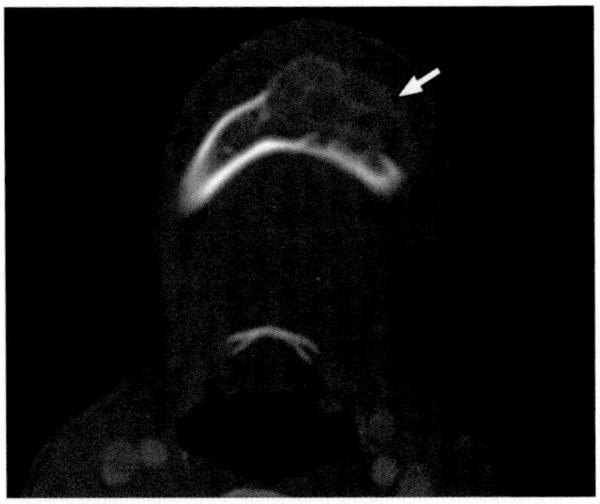

FIGURE 3.179 **Giant cell lesion (giant cell reparative granuloma) in an 11-year-old boy who presented with a mandibular mass.** Axial bone window CT image shows a multilocular, expansile lesion (*arrow*) involving the body of the mandible. Cortical margins are thinned, suggesting a locally aggressive process. The lesion is well away from the teeth, consistent with a nonodontogenic lesion.

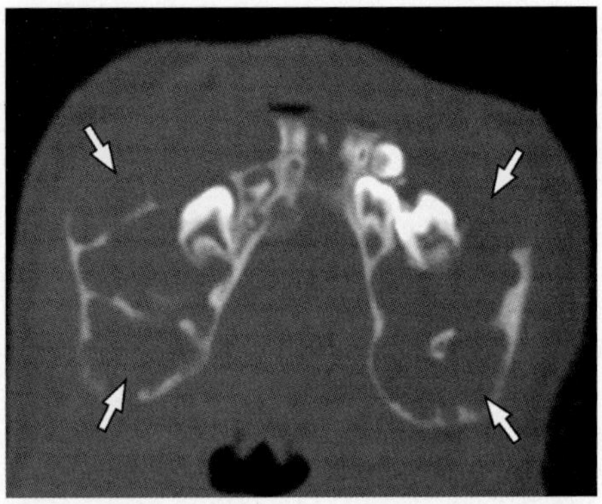

FIGURE 3.180 **Cherubism in a 3-year-old boy who presented with marked facial swelling.** Axial bone window CT image shows extensive bilateral mandibular multilocular expansile lesions (*arrows*) with only strands of intervening bone. The cortex is eroded in areas. There is also diffuse involvement of the maxilla (not shown). This appearance is typical of cherubism, which tends to wane during the teenage years.

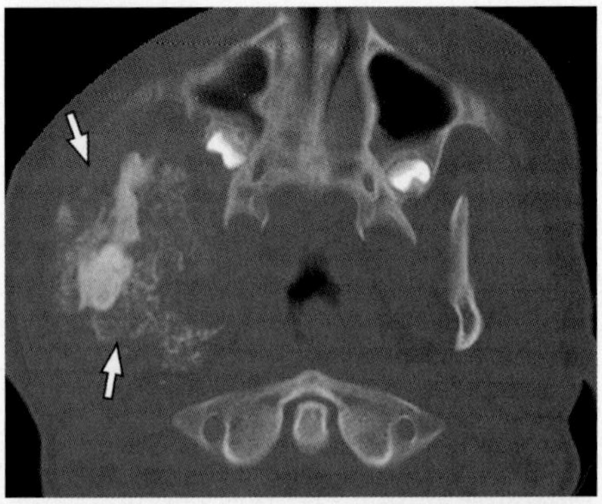

FIGURE 3.181 **Osteogenic sarcoma in a 12-year-old girl who presented with rapid onset of a mandibular mass.** Axial bone window CT image shows a large mass involving the ramus of the right mandible. There is aggressive-appearing periosteal new bone formation with a soft tissue mass involving the muscles of mastication (*arrows*). The appearance is characteristic of osteogenic sarcoma.

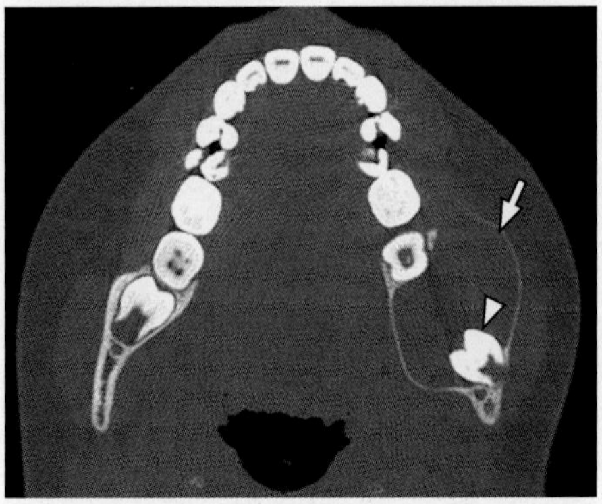

FIGURE 3.182 **Dentigerous cyst in a 14-year-old boy who presented with painless swelling of the mandible.** Axial bone window CT image shows a sharply defined, expansile, lucent lesion (*arrow*) surrounding the crown of an unerupted left third molar tooth (*arrowhead*). Its relationship to a tooth indicates that this is an odontogenic lesion. In this case, the association of the cyst with the crown of an unerupted tooth is characteristic of a dentigerous cyst. Occasionally, however, odontogenic tumors such as ameloblastoma or fibroblastic odontogenic tumor can simulate this appearance on CT.

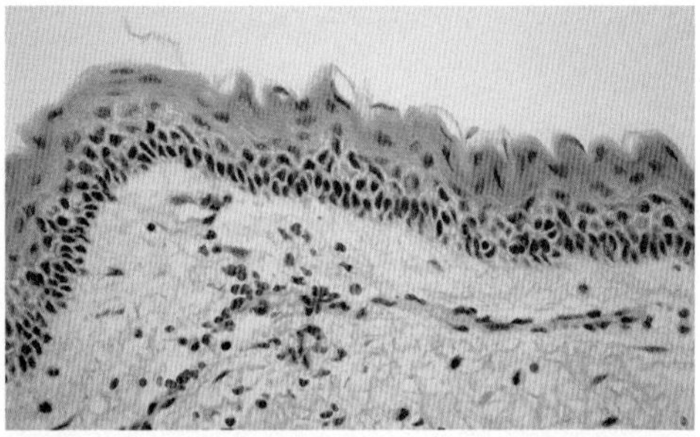

FIGURE 3.183 **Keratocystic odontogenic tumor (odontogenic keratocyst).** This maxillary mass arose in a 10-year-old girl with a previous history of medulloblastoma and extensive calcification of the dura and falx, and therefore was a component of basal cell nevus syndrome. Microscopic examination shows the characteristic wavy appearance of the stratified squamous epithelial lining (hematoxylin and eosin, original magnification, 600×).

tumors, such as osteogenic sarcoma (Fig. 3.181) and Ewing sarcoma, and metastatic tumors, such as neuroblastoma, leukemia, and metastatic Ewing sarcoma.

Odontogenic lesions arise in association with dentition and derive from or recapitulate elements of the tooth apparatus and include benign cysts, tumor-like lesions, and benign and malignant tumors. These lesions present as facial asymmetry, swelling, dental impaction, malocclusion, or facial pain. Odontogenic cysts appear as radiolucent lesions with sharply defined borders on CT. The dentigerous cyst is associated with the crown of an unerupted tooth (Fig. 3.182). Keratocystic odontogenic tumor (KOT) or odontogenic keratocyst is a tumor-like condition of childhood. Single and multiple KOTs are a feature of basal cell nevus syndrome (Gorlin syndrome). On CT, KOT appears as a sharply circumscribed, expansile, lytic lesion that arises in proximity to the molar teeth. Microscopically, it is lined by squamous epithelium with an undulating contour and a thin layer of keratinization (Fig. 3.183). Other odontogenic tumors that occur in childhood include odontoma, cementoblastoma, adenomatoid odontogenic tumor, ameloblastic fibroma, fibroodontoma, and ameloblastoma.

References

1. Rosenberg RA, Cohen NL, Ransohoff J. Long-term hearing preservation after acoustic neuroma surgery. *Otolaryngol Head Neck Surg.* 1987;97(3):270–274.
2. Marsh MA, Xu J, Blamey PJ, et al. Radiologic evaluation of multichannel intracochlear implant insertion depth. *Am J Otol.* 1993;14(4):386–391.
3. Gray RF, Evans RA, Freer CE, et al. Radiology for cochlear implants. *J Laryngol Otol.* 1991;105(2):85–88.
4. Shpizner BA, Holliday RA, Roland JT, et al. Postoperative imaging of the multichannel cochlear implant. *AJNR Am J Neuroradiol.* 1995;16(7):1517–1524.
5. Harwood-Nash DC, Fitz CR. *Neuroradiology in Infants and Children.* St. Louis, MO: Mosby; 1976.
6. Swischuk L. *Imaging of the Newborn, Infant, and Young Child.* 4th ed. Philadelphia, PA: Lippincott Williams & Wilkins; 1997.
7. Swischuk L. *Emergency Imaging of the Acute Ill or Injured Child.* Philadelphia, PA: Lippincott Williams & Wilkins; 2000.

8. Silverman FN, Kuhn JP. *Essentials of Caffey's Pediatric X-Ray Diagnosis*. Chicago, IL: Year Book; 1990.
9. Som PM, Curtin HD. *Head and Neck Imaging*. 5th ed. St. Louis, MO: Elsevier Mosby; 2011.
10. Bluestone CD, Stool SE, Kenna MA. *Pediatric Otolaryngology*. 3rd ed. Philadelphia, PA: WB Saunders; 1996.
11. Teele RL, Share JS. *Ultrasonography of Infants and Children*. Philadelphia, PA: WB Saunders; 1991.
12. Wolpert SM, Barnes PD. *MRI in Pediatric Neuroradiology*. St. Louis, MO: Mosby-Year Book; 1992.
13. Harnsberger HR. *Handbook of Head and Neck Imaging*. 2nd ed. St. Louis, MO: Mosby-Year Book; 1995.
14. Valvassori GE, Mafee MF, Carter BL. *Imaging of the Head and Neck*. New York: Thieme; 1995.
15. Swartz JD, Harnsberger HR. *Imaging of the Temporal Bone*. 2nd ed. New York: Thieme; 1992.
16. Mafee MF, Goldberg MF, Cohen SB, et al. Magnetic resonance imaging versus computed tomography of leukocoric eyes and use of in vitro proton magnetic resonance spectroscopy of retinoblastoma. *Ophthalmology.* 1989;96(7):965–975; discussion 975–966.
17. Beets-Tan RG, Hendriks MJ, Ramos LM, et al. Retinoblastoma: CT and MRI. *Neuroradiology.* 1994;36(1):59–62.
18. Mafee MF, Mafee RF, Malik M, et al. Medical imaging in pediatric ophthalmology. *Pediatr Clin North Am.* 2003;50(1):259–286.
19. Wilms G, Marchal G, Van Fraeyenhoven L, et al. Shortcomings and pitfalls of ocular MRI. *Neuroradiology.* 1991;33(4):320–325.
20. Schueler AO, Hosten N, Bechrakis NE, et al. High resolution magnetic resonance imaging of retinoblastoma. *Br J Ophthalmol.* 2003;87(3):330–335.
21. Galluzzi P, Hadjistilianou T, Cerase A, et al. Is CT still useful in the study protocol of retinoblastoma? *AJNR Am J Neuroradiol.* 2009;30(9):1760–1765.
22. Rauschecker AM, Patel CV, Yeom KW, et al. High-resolution MR imaging of the orbit in patients with retinoblastoma. *Radiographics.* 2012;32(5):1307–1326.
23. Standring S, Berkovitz B, Hackney CM, et al. The orbit and its contents. In: Standring S, ed. *Gray's Anatomy*. 39th ed. Philadelphia, PA: Elsevier; 2005.
24. Snell RS, Lemp M. *Clinical Anatomy of the Eye*. Boston, MA: Blackwell Scientific; 1989.
25. Lustrin ES, Robertson RL, Tilak S. Normal anatomy of the skull base. *Neuroimaging Clin N Am.* 1994;4(3):465–478.
26. Wells RG, Sty JR, Gonnering RS. Imaging of the pediatric eye and orbit. *Radiographics.* 1989;9(6):1023–1044.
27. Mafee MF, Ainbinder D, Afshani E, et al. The eye. *Neuroimaging Clin N Am.* 1996;6(1):29–59.
28. Bilaniuk LT, Farber M. Imaging of developmental anomalies of the eye and the orbit. *AJNR Am J Neuroradiol.* 1992;13(2): 793–803.
29. Hopper KD, Sherman JL, Boal DK. Abnormalities of the orbit and its contents in children: CT and MR imaging findings. *AJR Am J Roentgenol.* 1991;156(6):1219–1224.
30. Hopper KD, Sherman JL, Boal DK, et al. CT and MR imaging of the pediatric orbit. *Radiographics.* 1992;12(3):485–503.
31. American Academy of Ophthalmology. *G C. Section 2. Fundamentals and Principles of Ophthalmology*. San Francisco, CA: American Academy of Ophthalmology; 2008.
32. Mafee MF, Jampol LM, Langer BG, et al. Computed tomography of optic nerve colobomas, morning glory anomaly, and colobomatous cyst. *Radiol Clin North Am.* 1987;25(4): 693–699.
33. Doglietto F, Massimi L, Dickmann A, et al. Microphthalmia and colobomatous cyst of the orbit. *Acta Neurochir.* 2006;148(10): 1123–1125.
34. Lieb W, Rochels R, Gronemeyer U. Microphthalmos with colobomatous orbital cyst: clinical, histological, immunohistological, and electronmicroscopic findings. *Br J Ophthalmol.* 1990;74(1):59–62.
35. Quah BL, Hamilton J, Blaser S, et al. Morning glory disc anomaly, midline cranial defects and abnormal carotid circulation: an association worth looking for. *Pediatr Radiol.* 2005;35(5): 525–528.
36. Auber AE, O'Hara M. Morning Glory syndrome. *MR Imaging Clin Imaging.* 1999;23(3):152–158.
37. Ellika S, Robson CD, Heidary G, et al. Morning glory disc anomaly: characteristic MR imaging findings. *AJNR Am J Neuroradiol.* 2013;34(10):2010–2014.
38. Dollfus H, Verloes A. Dysmorphology and the orbital region: a practical clinical approach. *Surv Ophthalmol.* 2004;49(6):547–561.
39. Howard GM, Ellsworth RM. Differential diagnosis of retinoblastoma. A statistical survey of 500 children. I. Relative frequency of the lesions which simulate retinoblastoma. *Am J Ophthalmol.* 1965;60(4):610–618.
40. Goldberg MF, Mafee M. Computed tomography for diagnosis of persistent hyperplastic primary vitreous (PHPV). *Ophthalmology.* 1983;90(5):442–451.
41. Walsh MK, Drenser KA, Capone A Jr, et al. Early vitrectomy effective for Norrie disease. *Arch Ophthalmol.* 2010;128(4):456–460.
42. Mafee MF, Goldberg MF. Persistent hyperplastic primary vitreous (PHPV): role of computed tomography and magnetic resonance. *Radiol Clin North Am.* 1987;25(4):683–692.
43. Pagon RA, Chandler JW, Collie WR, et al. Hydrocephalus, agyria, retinal dysplasia, encephalocele (HARD +/– E) syndrome: an autosomal recessive condition. *Birth Defects Orig Artic Ser.* 1978;14(6B):233–241.
44. Mandal AK, Chakrabarti D. Update on congenital glaucoma. *Indian J Ophthalmol.* 2011;59(suppl):S148–S157.
45. Barnes PD, Robson CD, Robertson RL, et al. Pediatric orbital and visual pathway lesions. *Neuroimaging Clin N Am.* 1996;6(1): 179–198.
46. Barkovich AJ, Vandermarck P, Edwards MS, et al. Congenital nasal masses: CT and MR imaging features in 16 cases. *AJNR Am J Neuroradiol.* 1991;12(1):105–116.
47. Byrd SE, Naidich TP. Common congenital brain anomalies. *Radiol Clin North Am.* 1988;26(4):755–772.
48. Castillo M. Congenital abnormalities of the nose: CT and MR findings. *AJR Am J Roentgenol.* 1994;162(5):1211–1217.
49. Downey EF Jr, Weinstein ZR. Unusual case of orbital encephalocele. *AJNR Am J Neuroradiol.* 1984;5(2):199–200.
50. Koch BL, Ball WS Jr. Congenital malformations causing skull base changes. *Neuroimaging Clin N Am.* 1994;4(3):479–498.
51. Levy RA, Wald SL, Aitken PA, et al. Bilateral intraorbital meningoencephaloceles and associated midline craniofacial anomalies: MR and three-dimensional CT imaging. *AJNR Am J Neuroradiol.* 1989;10(6):1272–1274.
52. Fitz CR. Holoprosencephaly and septo-optic dysplasia. *Neuroimaging Clin N Am.* 1994;4(2):263–281.
53. Barkovich AJ, Fram EK, Norman D. Septo-optic dysplasia: MR imaging. *Radiology.* 1989;171(1):189–192.
54. Barkovich AJ, Norman D. Anomalies of the corpus callosum: correlation with further anomalies of the brain. *AJR Am J Roentgenol.* 1988;151(1):171–179.

55. Byrd SE, Bohan TP, Osborn RE, et al. The CT and MR evaluation of lissencephaly R. *AJNR Am J Neuroradiol.* 1988;9(5):923–927.
56. Hall-Craggs MA, Harbord MG, Finn JP, et al. Aicardi syndrome: MR assessment of brain structure and myelination. *AJNR Am J Neuroradiol.* 1990;11(3):532–536.
57. Osborn RE, Byrd SE, Naidich TP, et al. MR imaging of neuronal migrational disorders. *AJNR Am J Neuroradiol.* 1988;9(6): 1101–1106.
58. Sobel DF, Kelly W, Kjos BO, et al. MR imaging of orbital and ocular disease. *AJNR Am J Neuroradiol.* 1985;6(2):259–264.
59. Appignani BA, Jones KM, Barnes PD. Primary endodermal sinus tumor of the orbit: MR findings. *AJR Am J Roentgenol.* 1992;159(2):399–401.
60. Rand PK, Ball WS Jr, Kulwin DR. Congenital nasolacrimal mucoceles: CT evaluation. *Radiology.* 1989;173(3):691–694.
61. Castillo M, Merten DF, Weissler MC. Bilateral nasolacrimal duct mucocele, a rare cause of respiratory distress: CT findings in two newborns. *AJNR Am J Neuroradiol.* 1993;14(4): 1011–1013.
62. John PR, Boldt D. Bilateral congenital lacrimal sac mucoceles with nasal extension. *Pediatr Radiol.* 1990;20(4):285–286.
63. Meyer JR, Quint DJ, Holmes JM, et al. Infected congenital mucocele of the nasolacrimal duct. *AJNR Am J Neuroradiol.* 1993;14(4):1008–1010.
64. Guy JR, Quisling RG. Ectopic lacrimal gland presenting as an orbital mass in childhood. *AJNR Am J Neuroradiol.* 1989;10 (5 suppl):S92.
65. Mansour AM, Barber JC, Reinecke RD, et al. Ocular choristomas. *Surv Ophthalmol.* 1989;33(5):339–358.
66. Nugent RA, Lapointe JS, Rootman J, et al. Orbital dermoids: features on CT. *Radiology.* 1987;165(2):475–478.
67. Hesselink JR, Davis KR, Dallow RL, et al. Computed tomography of masses in the lacrimal gland region. *Radiology.* 1979;131(1):143–147.
68. Lallemand DP, Brasch RC, Char DH, et al. Orbital tumors in children. Characterization by computed tomography. *Radiology.* 1984;151(1):85–88.
69. Smirniotopoulos JG, Chiechi MV. Teratomas, dermoids, and epidermoids of the head and neck. *Radiographics.* 1995;15(6): 1437–1455.
70. Kaufman LM, Villablanca JP, Mafee MF. Diagnostic imaging of cystic lesions in the child's orbit. *Radiol Clin North Am.* 1998;36(6):1149–1163, xi.
71. Weber AL, Mikulis DK. Inflammatory disorders of the paraorbital sinuses and their complications. *Radiol Clin North Am.* 1987;25(3):615–630.
72. Hawkins DB, Clark RW. Orbital involvement in acute sinusitis. Lessons from 24 childhood patients. *Clin Pediatr.* 1977;16(5):464–471.
73. Aribandi M, McCoy VA, Bazan C III. Imaging features of invasive and noninvasive fungal sinusitis: a review. *Radiographics.* 2007;27(5):1283–1296.
74. Kitei D, DiMario FJ Jr. Childhood orbital pseudotumor: case report and literature review. *J Child Neurol.* 2008;23(4):425–430.
75. Weber AL, Romo LV, Sabates NR. Pseudotumor of the orbit. Clinical, pathologic, and radiologic evaluation. *Radiol Clin North Am.* 1999;37(1):151–168, xi.
76. Yousem DM, Atlas SW, Grossman RI, et al. MR imaging of Tolosa-Hunt syndrome. *AJR Am J Roentgenol.* 1990;154(1):167–170.
77. Yuen SJ, Rubin PA. Idiopathic orbital inflammation: distribution, clinical features, and treatment outcome. *Arch Ophthalmol.* 2003;121(4):491–499.
78. Yan J, Qiu H, Wu Z, et al. Idiopathic orbital inflammatory pseudotumor in Chinese children. *Orbit.* 2006;25(1):1–4.
79. Bonhomme GR, Waldman AT, Balcer LJ, et al. Pediatric optic neuritis: brain MRI abnormalities and risk of multiple sclerosis. *Neurology.* 2009;72(10):881–885.
80. Goldstein SM, Katowitz WR, Moshang T, et al. Pediatric thyroid-associated orbitopathy: the Children's Hospital of Philadelphia experience and literature review. *Thyroid.* 2008; 18(9):997–999.
81. Maheshwari R, Weis E. Thyroid associated orbitopathy. *Indian J Ophthalmol.* 2012;60(2):87–93.
82. James SH, Halliday WC, Branson HM. Best cases from the AFIP: trilateral retinoblastoma. *Radiographics.* 2010;30(3):833–837.
83. Balmer A, Zografos L, Munier F. Diagnosis and current management of retinoblastoma. *Oncogene.* 2006;25(38): 5341–5349.
84. Cunnane et al. Pathology of the eye and orbit. In: Som PM, Curtin H, eds. *Head and Neck Imaging.* Vol. 1. 5th ed. St. Louis, MO: Elsevier-Mosby; 2011.
85. Balmer A, Munier F, Zografos L. New strategies in the management of retinoblastoma. *J Fr Ophtalmol.* 2002;25(2):187–193.
86. Abramson DH. Second nonocular cancers in retinoblastoma: a unified hypothesis. The Franceschetti Lecture. *Ophthalmic Genet.* 1999;20(3):193–204.
87. Fletcher O, Easton D, Anderson K, et al. Lifetime risks of common cancers among retinoblastoma survivors. *J Natl Cancer Inst.* 2004;96(5):357–363.
88. Abramson DH, Frank CM. Second nonocular tumors in survivors of bilateral retinoblastoma: a possible age effect on radiation-related risk. *Ophthalmology.* 1998;105(4):573–579; discussion 579–580.
89. Mafee MF, Goldberg MF, Greenwald MJ, et al. Retinoblastoma and simulating lesions: role of CT and MR imaging. *Radiol Clin North Am.* 1987;25(4):667–682.
90. Messmer EP, Heinrich T, Hopping W, et al. Risk factors for metastases in patients with retinoblastoma. *Ophthalmology.* 1991;98(2):136–141.
91. Kopelman JE, McLean IW, Rosenberg SH. Multivariate analysis of risk factors for metastasis in retinoblastoma treated by enucleation. *Ophthalmology.* 1987;94(4):371–377.
92. Khelfaoui F, Validire P, Auperin A, et al. Histopathologic risk factors in retinoblastoma: a retrospective study of 172 patients treated in a single institution. *Cancer.* 1996;77(6):1206–1213.
93. Chantada G, Fandino A, Manzitti J, et al. Late diagnosis of retinoblastoma in a developing country. *Arch Dis Child.* 1999;80(2):171–174.
94. Mazzoleni S, Bisogno G, Garaventa A, et al. Outcomes and prognostic factors after recurrence in children and adolescents with nonmetastatic rhabdomyosarcoma. *Cancer.* 2005;104(1):183–190.
95. Mafee MF, Pai E, Philip B. Rhabdomyosarcoma of the orbit. Evaluation with MR imaging and CT. *Radiol Clin North Am.* 1998;36(6):1215–1227, xii.
96. Lewis RA, Gerson LP, Axelson KA, et al. von Recklinghausen neurofibromatosis. II. Incidence of optic gliomata. *Ophthalmology.* 1984;91(8):929–935.
97. Zimmerman RA, Bilaniuk LT, Metzger RA, et al. Computed tomography of orbitalfacial neurofibromatosis. *Radiology.* 1983;146(1):113–116.
98. Reed D, Robertson WD, Rootman J, et al. Plexiform neurofibromatosis of the orbit: CT evaluation. *AJNR Am J Neuroradiol.* 1986;7(2):259–263.

99. Millar WS, Tartaglino LM, Sergott RC, et al. MR of malignant optic glioma of adulthood. *AJNR Am J Neuroradiol.* 1995;16(8):1673–1676.
100. Müller-Forell WS, ed. *Imaging of Orbital and Visual Pathway Pathology*. Berlin, Germany: Springer Verlag; 2005.
101. Kornreich L, Blaser S, Schwarz M, et al. Optic pathway glioma: correlation of imaging findings with the presence of neurofibromatosis. *AJNR Am J Neuroradiol.* 2001;22(10): 1963–1969.
102. Shields JA. *Diagnosis and Management of Orbital Tumors.* Philadelphia, PA: WB Saunders; 1989.
103. Mulliken JB, Glowacki J. Hemangiomas and vascular malformations in infants and children: a classification based on endothelial characteristics. *Plast Reconstr Surg.* 1982;69(3):412–422.
104. Burrows PE, Laor T, Paltiel H, et al. Diagnostic imaging in the evaluation of vascular birthmarks. *Dermatol Clin.* 1998;16(3):455–488.
105. Pascual-Castroviejo I. Vascular and nonvascular intracranial malformation associated with external capillary hemangiomas. *Neuroradiology.* 1978;16:82–84.
106. Frieden IJ, Reese V, Cohen D. PHACE syndrome. The association of posterior fossa brain malformations, hemangiomas, arterial anomalies, coarctation of the aorta and cardiac defects, and eye abnormalities. *Arch Dermatol.* 1996;132(3):307–311.
107. Burrows PE, Robertson RL, Mulliken JB, et al. Cerebral vasculopathy and neurologic sequelae in infants with cervicofacial hemangioma: report of eight patients. *Radiology.* 1998;207(3):601–607.
108. Nozaki T, Nosaka S, Miyazaki O, et al. Syndromes associated with vascular tumors and malformations: a pictorial review. *Radiographics.* 2013;33(1):175–195.
109. Bisdorff A, Mulliken JB, Carrico J, et al. Intracranial vascular anomalies in patients with periorbital lymphatic and lymphaticovenous malformations. *AJNR Am J Neuroradiol.* 2007;28(2):335–341.
110. Kubal WS. Imaging of orbital trauma. *Radiographics.* 2008;28(6):1729–1739.
111. Swallow CE, Tsuruda JS, Digre KB, et al. Terson syndrome: CT evaluation in 12 patients. *AJNR Am J Neuroradiol.* 1998;19(4):743–747.
112. Arevalo JF, Garcia RA, Al-Dhibi HA, et al. Update on sympathetic ophthalmia. *Middle East Afr J Ophthalmol.* 2012;19(1):13–21.
113. Lubin JR, Albert DM, Weinstein M. Sixty-five years of sympathetic ophthalmia. A clinicopathologic review of 105 cases (1913–1978). *Ophthalmology.* 1980;87(2):109–121.
114. Goto H, Rao NA. Sympathetic ophthalmia and Vogt-Koyanagi-Harada syndrome. *Int Ophthalmol Clin.* 1990;30(4):279–285.
115. Weissman JL, Beatty RL, Hirsch WL, et al. Enlarged anterior chamber: CT finding of a ruptured globe. *AJNR Am J Neuroradiol.* 1995;16(4 suppl):936–938.
116. Anand R, Tasman WP. Serous detachment of the neural retina. In: Yanoff M, Duker JS, eds. *Ophthalmology*. St. Louis, MO: Mosby Elsevier; 2009:727–733.
117. Mafee MF, Peyman GA. Retinal and choroidal detachments: role of magnetic resonance imaging and computed tomography. *Radiol Clin North Am.* 1987;25(3):487–507.
118. Gor DM, Kirsch CF, Leen J, et al. Radiologic differentiation of intraocular glass: evaluation of imaging techniques, glass types, size, and effect of intraocular hemorrhage. *AJR Am J Roentgenol.* 2001;177(5):1199–1203.
119. Carlson BM. *Human Embryology and Developmental Biology.* St. Louis, MO: Mosby-Year Book; 1994.
120. Chinwuba C, Wallman J, Strand R. Nasal airway obstruction: CT assessment. *Radiology.* 1986;159(2):503–506.
121. Brown OE, Pownell P, Manning SC. Choanal atresia: a new anatomic classification and clinical management applications. *Laryngoscope.* 1996;106(1 pt 1):97–101.
122. Ramsden JD, Campisi P, Forte V. Choanal atresia and choanal stenosis. *Otolaryngol Clin North Am.* 2009;42(2):339–352, x.
123. Lemmerling M, Dhooge I, Mollet P, et al. CT of the temporal bone in the CHARGE association. *Neuroradiology.* 1998;40(7):462–465.
124. Blake KD, Prasad C. CHARGE syndrome. *Orphanet J Rare Dis.* 2006;1:34.
125. Johnson GF, Weisman PA. Radiological features of dermoid cysts of the nose. *Radiology.* 1964;82:1016–1021.
126. Sessions RB. Nasal dermal sinuses—new concepts and explanations. *Laryngoscope.* 1982;92(8 pt 2 suppl 29):1–28.
127. Chen CY, Huang JH, Choi WM, et al. Parapharyngeal neuroglial heterotopia presenting as a growing single locular cyst: MR imaging findings. *AJNR Am J Neuroradiol.* 2005;26(1):96–99.
128. Klestadt WD. Nasal cysts and the facial cleft cyst theory. *Ann Otol Rhinol Laryngol.* 1953;62(1):84–92.
129. Iida S, Aikawa T, Kishino M, et al. Spheric mass beneath the alar base: MR images of nasolabial cyst and schwannoma. *AJNR Am J Neuroradiol.* 2006;27(9):1826–1829.
130. Cure JK, Osguthorpe JD, Van Tassel P. MR of nasolabial cysts. *AJNR Am J Neuroradiol.* 1996;17(3):585–588.
131. Tanimoto K, Kakimoto N, Nishiyama H, et al. MRI of nasoalveolar cyst: case report. *Oral Surg Oral Med Oral Pathol Oral Radiol Endod.* 2005;99(2):221–224.
132. Verbin R, Barnes L. Cysts and cyst-like lesions of the oral cavity, jaws, and neck. In: Barnes L, ed. *Surgical Pathology of the Head and Neck*. Vol. 2. New York: Marcel Dekker; 1985: 1278–1281.
133. Naidich TP, Blaser SI, Lien RJ, et al. Embryology and congenital lesions of the midface. In: Som PM, Curtin H, eds. *Head and Neck Imaging*. Vol. 1. St. Louis, MO: Elsevier Mosby; 2011.
134. Purandare SM, Ernst L, Medne L, et al. Developmental anomalies with features of disorganization (Ds) and amniotic band sequence (ABS): a report of four cases. *Am J Med Genet A.* 2009;149A(8):1740–1748.
135. Morovic CG, Berwart F, Varas J. Craniofacial anomalies of the amniotic band syndrome in serial clinical cases. *Plast Reconstr Surg.* 2004;113(6):1556–1562.
136. Bromley B, Benacerraf BR. Fetal micrognathia: associated anomalies and outcome. *J Ultrasound Med.* 1994;13(7):529–533.
137. Wald ER. Sinusitis in children. *N Engl J Med.* 1992;326(5): 319–323.
138. Brook I, Foote PA, Hausfeld JN. Frequency of recovery of pathogens causing acute maxillary sinusitis in adults before and after introduction of vaccination of children with the 7-valent pneumococcal vaccine. *J Med Microbiol.* 2006;55 (Pt 7):943–946.
139. Brook I, Gober AE. Frequency of recovery of pathogens from the nasopharynx of children with acute maxillary sinusitis before and after the introduction of vaccination with the 7-valent pneumococcal vaccine. *Int J Pediatr Otorhinolaryngol.* 2007;71(4):575–579.
140. Willing SJ, Faye-Petersen O, Aronin P, et al. Radiologic-pathologic correlation. Capillary hemangioma of the meninges. *AJNR Am J Neuroradiol.* 1993;14(3):529–536.

141. van Alyea OE. *Nasal Sinuses: Anatomic and Clinical Considerations*. 2nd ed. Baltimore, MD: Wiliams & Wilkins; 1951.
142. Som PM, Bradwein MS, Wang BY. Inflammatory diseases of the sinonasal cavities. In: Som PM, Curtin H, eds. *Head and Neck Imaging*. Vol. 1. St. Louis, MO: Elsevier Mosby; 2011.
143. Rak KM, Newell JD II, Yakes WF, et al. Paranasal sinuses on MR images of the brain: significance of mucosal thickening. *AJR Am J Roentgenol.* 1991;156(2):381–384.
144. Yousem DM. Imaging of sinonasal inflammatory disease. *Radiology.* 1993;188(2):303–314.
145. Skomro R, McClean KL. Frontal osteomyelitis (Pott's puffy tumour) associated with Pasteurella multocida: a case report and review of the literature. *Can J Infect Dis.* 1998;9(2):115–121.
146. Moorman CM, Anslow P, Elston JS. Is sphenoid sinus opacity significant in patients with optic neuritis? *Eye.* 1999;13 (pt 1):76–82.
147. Illner A, Davidson HC, Harnsberger HR, et al. The silent sinus syndrome: clinical and radiographic findings. *AJR Am J Roentgenol.* 2002;178(2):503–506.
148. Burduk PK, Dalke K, Mierzwinski J, et al. Silent sinus syndrome in child. *Otolaryngol Pol.* 2007;61(4):458–462.
149. Waitzman AA, Birt BD. Fungal sinusitis. *J Otolaryngol.* 1994;23(4):244–249.
150. Scholtz AW, Appenroth E, Kammen-Jolly K, et al. Juvenile nasopharyngeal angiofibroma: management and therapy. *Laryngoscope.* 2001;111(4 pt 1):681–687.
151. Gullane PJ, Davidson J, O'Dwyer T, et al. Juvenile angiofibroma: a review of the literature and a case series report. *Laryngoscope.* 1992;102(8):928–933.
152. Pryor SG, Moore EJ, Kasperbauer JL. Endoscopic versus traditional approaches for excision of juvenile nasopharyngeal angiofibroma. *Laryngoscope.* 2005;115(7):1201–1207.
153. Curtin HD, Som PM. Pathology of the central skull base. In: Som PM, Curtin HD, eds. *Head and Neck Imaging.* Vol. 1. St. Louis, MO: Elsevier Mosby; 2011.
154. Herrmann BW, Sotelo-Avila C, Eisenbeis JF. Pediatric sinonasal rhabdomyosarcoma: three cases and a review of the literature. *Am J Otolaryngol.* 2003;24(3):174–180.
155. Yousem DM, Lexa FJ, Bilaniuk LT, et al. Rhabdomyosarcomas in the head and neck: MR imaging evaluation. *Radiology.* 1990;177(3):683–686.
156. Robson CD, Rahbar R, Vargas SO, et al. Sinonasal and laryngeal carcinoma in children: correlation of imaging characteristics with clinicopathologic and cytogenetic features. *AJNR Am J Neuroradiol.* 2010;31(2):257–261.
157. Hicks J, Flaitz C. Rhabdomyosarcoma of the head and neck in children. *Oral Oncol.* 2002;38(5):450–459.
158. Kadish S, Goodman M, Wang CC. Olfactory neuroblastoma. A clinical analysis of 17 cases. *Cancer.* 1976;37(3):1571–1576.
159. El Kababri M, Habrand JL, Valteau-Couanet D, et al. Esthesioneuroblastoma in children and adolescent: experience on 11 cases with literature review. *J Pediatr Hematol Oncol.* 2014;36(2):91–95.
160. Som PM, Lidov M, Brandwein M, et al. Sinonasal esthesioneuroblastoma with intracranial extension: marginal tumor cysts as a diagnostic MR finding. *AJNR Am J Neuroradiol.* 1994;15(7):1259–1262.
161. Broski SM, Hunt CH, Johnson GB, et al. The added value of 18F-FDG PET/CT for evaluation of patients with esthesioneuroblastoma. *J Nucl Med.* 2012;53(8):1200–1206.
162. Yabuuchi H, Fukuya T, Murayama S, et al. CT and MR features of nasopharyngeal carcinoma in children and young adults. *Clin Radiol.* 2002;57(3):205–210.
163. Chong VF, Fan YF, Khoo JB. Nasopharyngeal carcinoma with intracranial spread: CT and MR characteristics. *J Comput Assist Tomogr.* 1996;20(4):563–569.
164. Roh JL, Huh J, Moon HN. Lymphomas of the head and neck in the pediatric population. *Int J Pediatr Otorhinolaryngol.* 2007;71(9):1471–1477.
165. Brady G, MacArthur GJ, Farrell PJ. Epstein-Barr virus and Burkitt lymphoma. *J Clin Pathol.* 2007;60(12):1397–1402.
166. Bluestone CD, Alper CM, Stool SE, et al. *Pediatric Otolaryngology*. Vol. 1. Philadelphia, PA: Elsevier Health Sciences; 2002.
167. Friedman ER, Robson CD, Hudgins PA. Pediatric airway disease. In: Som PM, Curtin HD, ed. *Head and Neck Imaging.* Vol. 2. St. Louis, MO: Elsevier Mosby; 2011.
168. Aiken AH, Glastonbury C. Imaging Hodgkin and non-Hodgkin lymphoma in the head and neck. *Radiol Clin North Am.* 2008;46(2):363–378, ix–x.
169. Guermazi A, Feger C, Rousselot P, et al. Granulocytic sarcoma (chloroma): imaging findings in adults and children. *AJR Am J Roentgenol.* 2002;178(2):319–325.
170. Basaran G, Erkan M. One of the rarest syndromes in dentistry: gardner syndrome. *Eur J Dent.* 2008;2(3):208–212.
171. Murphey MD, Choi JJ, Kransdorf MJ, et al. Imaging of osteochondroma: variants and complications with radiologic-pathologic correlation. *Radiographics.* 2000;20(5):1407–1434.
172. Coffin CM, Dehner LP, O'Shea PA. *Pediatric Soft Tissue Tumors: A Clinical, Pathological, and Therapeutic Approach*. Baltimore, MD: Williams & Wilkins; 1997.
173. Jeon TY, Kim HJ, Chung SK, et al. Sinonasal inverted papilloma: value of convoluted cerebriform pattern on MR imaging. *AJNR Am J Neuroradiol.* 2008;29(8):1556–1560.
174. Maroldi R, Farina D, Palvarini L, et al. Magnetic resonance imaging findings of inverted papilloma: differential diagnosis with malignant sinonasal tumors. *Am J Rhinol.* 2004;18(5):305–310.
175. Meyer JS, Harty MP, Mahboubi S, et al. Langerhans cell histiocytosis: presentation and evolution of radiologic findings with clinical correlation. *Radiographics.* 1995;15(5):1135–1146.
176. Priest JR, Williams GM, Mize WA, et al. Nasal chondromesenchymal hamartoma in children with pleuropulmonary blastoma: a report from the International Pleuropulmonary Blastoma Registry registry. *Int J Pediatr Otorhinolaryngol.* 2010;74(11):1240–1244.
177. Alcala-Galiano A, Arribas-Garcia IJ, Martin-Perez MA, et al. Pediatric facial fractures: children are not just small adults. *Radiographics.* 2008;28(2):441–461; quiz 618.
178. Zimmermann CE, Troulis MJ, Kaban LB. Pediatric facial fractures: recent advances in prevention, diagnosis and management. *Int J Oral Maxillofac Surg.* 2006;35(1):2–13.
179. Ferreira PC, Amarante JM, Silva PN, et al. Retrospective study of 1251 maxillofacial fractures in children and adolescents. *Plast Reconstr Surg.* 2005;115(6):1500–1508.
180. Hopper RA, Salemy S, Sze RW. Diagnosis of midface fractures with CT: what the surgeon needs to know. *Radiographics.* 2006;26(3):783–793.
181. Curtin HD, Gupta R, Bergeron RT. Embryology, anatomy, and imaging of the temporal bone. In: Som PM, Curtin HD, eds. *Head and Neck Imaging.* Vol. 1. St. Louis, MO: Elsevier Mosby; 2011.

182. Harrison M, Roush J, Wallace J. Trends in age of identification and intervention in infants with hearing loss. *Ear Hear.* 2003;24(1):89–95.
183. Fisher NA, Curtin HD. Radiology of congenital hearing loss. *Otolaryngol Clin North Am.* 1994;27(3):511–531.
184. Caughey RJ, Jahrsdoerfer RA, Kesser BW. Congenital cholesteatoma in a case of congenital aural atresia. *Otol Neurotol.* 2006;27(7):934–936.
185. Mayer TE, Brueckmann H, Siegert R, et al. High-resolution CT of the temporal bone in dysplasia of the auricle and external auditory canal. *AJNR Am J Neuroradiol.* 1997;18(1):53–65.
186. Valdez BC, Henning D, So RB, et al. The Treacher Collins syndrome (TCOF1) gene product is involved in ribosomal DNA gene transcription by interacting with upstream binding factor. *Proc Natl Acad Sci U S A.* 2004;101(29):10709–10714.
187. Robson CD. Congenital hearing impairment. *Pediatr Radiol.* 2006;36(4):309–324.
188. Lemmerling MM, Vanzieleghem BD, Mortier GR, et al. Unilateral semicircular canal aplasia in Goldenhar's syndrome. *AJNR Am J Neuroradiol.* 2000;21(7):1334–1336.
189. Kurosaki Y, Tanaka YO, Itai Y. Malleus bar as a rare cause of congenital malleus fixation: CT demonstration. *AJNR Am J Neuroradiol.* 1998;19(7):1229–1230.
190. Subotic R, Mladina R, Risavi R. Congenital bony fixation of the malleus. *Acta Otolaryngol.* 1998;118(6):833–836.
191. Yokoyama T, Iino Y, Kakizaki K, et al. Human temporal bone study on the postnatal ossification process of auditory ossicles. *Laryngoscope.* 1999;109(6):927–930.
192. Sando I, Shibahara Y, Takagi A, et al. Frequency and localization of congenital anomalies of the middle and inner ears: a human temporal bone histopathological study. *Int J Pediatr Otorhinolaryngol.* 1988;16(1):1–22.
193. Sennaroglu L, Saatci I. A new classification for cochleovestibular malformations. *Laryngoscope.* 2002;112(12):2230–2241.
194. Albert S, Blons H, Jonard L, et al. SLC26A4 gene is frequently involved in nonsyndromic hearing impairment with enlarged vestibular aqueduct in Caucasian populations. *Eur J Hum Genet.* 2006;14(6):773–779.
195. Ozgen B, Oguz KK, Atas A, et al. Complete labyrinthine aplasia: clinical and radiologic findings with review of the literature. *AJNR Am J Neuroradiol.* 2009;30(4):774–780.
196. Boston M, Halsted M, Meinzen-Derr J, et al. The large vestibular aqueduct: a new definition based on audiologic and computed tomography correlation. *Otolaryngol Head Neck Surg.* 2007;136(6):972–977.
197. Ozgen B, Cunnane ME, Caruso PA, et al. Comparison of 45 degrees oblique reformats with axial reformats in CT evaluation of the vestibular aqueduct. *AJNR Am J Neuroradiol.* 2008;29(1):30–34.
198. Robson CD, Koch BL, Harnsberger HR. *Specialty Imaging: Temporal Bone.* 1st ed: Amirsys Inc. Lippincott Williams & Wilkins; 2013.
199. Morimoto AK, Wiggins RH III, Hudgins PA, et al. Absent semicircular canals in CHARGE syndrome: radiologic spectrum of findings. *AJNR Am J Neuroradiol.* 2006;27(8):1663–1671.
200. Huang BY, Zdanski C, Castillo M. Pediatric sensorineural hearing loss, part 2: syndromic and acquired causes. *AJNR Am J Neuroradiol.* 2012;33(3):399–406.
201. Vazquez E, Castellote A, Piqueras J, et al. Imaging of complications of acute mastoiditis in children. *Radiographics.* 2003;23(2):359–372.
202. Lieberthal AS, Carroll AE, Chonmaitree T, et al. The diagnosis and management of acute otitis media. *Pediatrics.* 2013;131(3):e964–e999.
203. Juliano AF, Ginat DT, Moonis G. Imaging review of the temporal bone: part I. Anatomy and inflammatory and neoplastic processes. *Radiology.* 2013;269(1):17–33.
204. Weissman JL. A pain in the ear: the radiology of otalgia. *AJNR Am J Neuroradiol.* 1997;18(9):1641–1651.
205. Lemmerling MM, De Foer B, Verbist BM, et al. Imaging of inflammatory and infectious diseases in the temporal bone. *Neuroimaging Clin N Am.* 2009;19(3):321–337.
206. Barrionuevo CE, Marcallo FA, Coelho A, et al. Fibrous dysplasia and the temporal bone. *Arch Otolaryngol.* 1980;106(5): 298–301.
207. Lambert PR, Brackmann DE. Fibrous dysplasia of the temporal bone: the use of computerized tomography. *Otolaryngol Head Neck Surg.* 1984;92(4):461–467.
208. Smouha EE, Edelstein DR, Parisier SC. Fibrous dysplasia involving the temporal bone: report of three new cases. *Am J Otol.* 1987;8(2):103–107.
209. Brown EW, Megerian CA, McKenna MJ, et al. Fibrous dysplasia of the temporal bone: imaging findings. *AJR Am J Roentgenol.* 1995;164(3):679–682.
210. Baik FM, Nguyen L, Doherty JK, et al. Comparative case series of exostoses and osteomas of the internal auditory canal. *Ann Otol Rhinol Laryngol.* 2011;120(4):255–260.
211. Kemink JL, Graham MD. Osteomas and exostoses of the external auditory canal: medical and surgical management. *J Otolaryngol.* 1982;11(2):101–106.
212. Martuza RL, Ojemann RG. Bilateral acoustic neuromas: clinical aspects, pathogenesis, and treatment. *Neurosurgery.* 1982;10(1):1–12.
213. Dutcher PO Jr, House WF, Hitselberger WE. Early detection of small bilateral acoustic tumors. *Am J Otol.* 1987;8(1): 35–38.
214. Martuza RL, Eldridge R. Neurofibromatosis 2 (bilateral acoustic neurofibromatosis). *N Engl J Med.* 1988;318(11):684–688.
215. Maya MM, LO, WWM, Kovanlikaya I. Temporal bone tumors and cerebellopontine angle lesions. In: Som PM, Curtin HD, eds. *Head and Neck Imaging.* Vol. 1. St. Louis, MO: Elsevier Mosby; 2011.
216. Sbeity S, Abella A, Arcand P, et al. Temporal bone rhabdomyosarcoma in children. *Int J Pediatr Otorhinolaryngol.* 2007;71(5):807–814.
217. Newton WA Jr, Gehan EA, Webber BL, et al. Classification of rhabdomyosarcomas and related sarcomas. Pathologic aspects and proposal for a new classification: an Intergroup Rhabdomyosarcoma Study. *Cancer.* 1995;76(6):1073–1085.
218. Durve DV, Kanegaonkar RG, Albert D, et al. Paediatric rhabdomyosarcoma of the ear and temporal bone. *Clin Otolaryngol Allied Sci.* 2004;29(1):32–37.
219. Raney RB Jr, Lawrence W Jr, Maurer HM, et al. Rhabdomyosarcoma of the ear in childhood. A report from the Intergroup Rhabdomyosarcoma Study-I. *Cancer.* 1983;51(12): 2356–2361.
220. Cunningham MJ, Curtin HD, Butkiewicz BL. Histiocytosis X of the temporal bone: CT findings. *J Comput Assist Tomogr.* 1988;12(1):70–74.
221. Irving RM, Broadbent V, Jones NS. Langerhans' cell histiocytosis in childhood: management of head and neck manifestations. *Laryngoscope.* 1994;104(1 pt 1):64–70.

222. Fernandez-Latorre F, Menor-Serrano F, Alonso-Charterina S, et al. Langerhans' cell histiocytosis of the temporal bone in pediatric patients: imaging and follow-up. *AJR Am J Roentgenol.* 2000;174(1):217–221.
223. Hodge KM, Byers RM, Peters LJ. Paragangliomas of the head and neck. *Arch Otolaryngol Head Neck Surg.* 1988;114(8):872–877.
224. van der Mey AG, Maaswinkel-Mooy PD, Cornelisse CJ, et al. Genomic imprinting in hereditary glomus tumours: evidence for new genetic theory. *Lancet.* 1989;2(8675):1291–1294.
225. Larson TC III, Reese DF, Baker HL Jr, et al. Glomus tympanicum chemodectomas: radiographic and clinical characteristics. *Radiology.* 1987;163(3):801–806.
226. Som PM, Reede DL, Bergeron RT, et al. Computed tomography of glomus tympanicum tumors. *J Comput Assist Tomogr.* 1983;7(1):14–17.
227. Patel A, Groppo E. Management of temporal bone trauma. *Craniomaxillofac Trauma Reconstr.* 2010;3(2):105–113.
228. Brodie HA, Thompson TC. Management of complications from 820 temporal bone fractures. *Am J Otol.* 1997;18(2):188–197.
229. Maran AG, Buchanan DR. Branchial cysts, sinuses and fistulae. *Clin Otolaryngol Allied Sci.* 1978;3(1):77–92.
230. Smith JF, Kielmovitch I. Branchial cyst anomaly in a newborn. *Otolaryngol Head Neck Surg.* 1989;100(2):163–165.
231. Smuts MS, Hilfer SR, Searls RL. Patterns of cellular proliferation during thyroid organogenesis. *J Embryol Exp Morphol.* 1978;48:269–286.
232. McMullen TPW, Delbridge LW. Thyroid embryology, anatomy, and physiology: a review for the surgeon. In: al HJe, ed. *Endocrine Surgery.* London, UK: Springer-Verlag; 2009.
233. Gil-Carcedo E, Menendez ME, Vallejo LA, et al. The Zuckerkandl tubercle: problematic or helpful in thyroid surgery? *Eur Arch Otorhinolaryngol.* 2013;270(8):2327–2332.
234. Som PM, Curtin HD. Fascia and spaces of the neck. In: Som PM, Curtin HD, eds. *Head and Neck Imaging.* Vol. 2. St. Louis, MO: Elsevier Mosby; 2011.
235. Rouviere H. *Lymphatic System of the Head and Neck.* Ann Arbor, MI: Edwards Brothers; 1938:5–28.
236. Chandler JR, Mitchell B. Branchial cleft cysts, sinuses, and fistulas. *Otolaryngol Clin North Am.* 1981;14(1):175–186.
237. Harnsberger HR, Mancuso AA, Muraki AS, et al. Branchial cleft anomalies and their mimics: computed tomographic evaluation. *Radiology.* 1984;152(3):739–748.
238. Finn DG, Buchalter IH, Sarti E, et al. First branchial cleft cysts: clinical update. *Laryngoscope.* 1987;97(2):136–140.
239. Mukherji SK, Tart RP, Slattery WH, et al. Evaluation of first branchial anomalies by CT and MR. *J Comput Assist Tomogr.* 1993;17(4):576–581.
240. Work WP. Newer concepts of first branchial cleft defects. *Laryngoscope.* 1972;82(9):1581–1593.
241. Liston SL, Siegel LG. Branchial cysts, sinuses, and fistulas. *Ear Nose Throat J.* 1979;58(12):504–509.
242. Cunningham MJ. The management of congenital neck masses. *Am J Otolaryngol.* 1992;13(2):78–92.
243. Som PM, Smoker WR, Curtin HD, et al. Congenital lesions of the neck. In: Som PM, Curtin HD, eds. *Head and Neck Imaging.* Vol. 2. St. Louis, MO: Elsevier Mosby; 2011.
244. Blizzard RM, Chandler RW, Landing BH, et al. Maternal autoimmunization to thyroid as a probable cause of athyrotic cretinism. *N Engl J Med.* 1960;263:327–336.
245. Chandler RW, Blizzard RM, Hung W, et al. Incidence of thyrocytotoxic factor and other antithyroid antibodies in the mothers of cretins. *N Engl J Med.* 1962;267:376–380.
246. Rahbar R, Yoon MJ, Connolly LP, et al. Lingual thyroid in children: a rare clinical entity. *Laryngoscope.* 2008;118(7):1174–1179.
247. Branstetter BF, Weissman JL, Kennedy TL, et al. The CT appearance of thyroglossal duct carcinoma. *AJNR Am J Neuroradiol.* 2000;21(8):1547–1550.
248. Sistrunk WE. The surgical treatment of cysts of the thyroglossal tract. *Ann Surg.* 1920;71(2):121–122.
249. Taji SS, Savage N, Holcombe T, et al. Congenital aplasia of the major salivary glands: literature review and case report. *Pediatr Dent.* 2011;33(2):113–118.
250. Aanaes K, Hasselby JP, Bilde A, et al. Heterotopic neuroglial tissue: two cases involving the tongue and the buccal region. *Oral Surg Oral Med Oral Pathol Oral Radiol Endod.* 2008;105(6):e22–e29.
251. Andressakis DD, Pavlakis AG, Chrysomali E, et al. Infected lingual osseous choristoma. Report of a case and review of the literature. *Med Oral Patol Oral Cir Bucal.* 2008;13(10):E627–E632.
252. Azanero WD, Mazzonetto R, Leon JE, et al. Lingual cyst with respiratory epithelium: a histopathological and immunohistochemical analysis of two cases. *Int J Oral Maxillofac Surg.* 2009;38(4):388–392.
253. Coric M, Seiwerth S, Bumber Z. Congenital oral gastrointestinal cyst: an immunohistochemical analysis. *Eur Arch Otorhinolaryngol.* 2000;257(8):459–461.
254. Rossi-Schneider TR, Salum FG, Cherubini K, et al. Cartilaginous choristoma of the tongue. *Gerodontology.* 2009;26(1):78–80.
255. Kieran SM, Robson CD, Nose V, et al. Foregut duplication cysts in the head and neck: presentation, diagnosis, and management. *Arch Otolaryngol Head Neck Surg.* 2010;136(8):778–782.
256. Baisakhiya N, Deshmukh P, Pawar V. Tornwaldt cyst: a cause of neck pain and stiffness. *Indian J Otolaryngol Head Neck Surg.* 2011;63(suppl 1):147–148.
257. Perkins JA, Manning SC, Tempero RM, et al. Lymphatic malformations: current cellular and clinical investigations. *Otolaryngol Head Neck Surg.* 2010;142(6):789–794.
258. Bahadir O, Caylan R, Bektas D, et al. Effects of adenoidectomy in children with symptoms of adenoidal hypertrophy. *Eur Arch Otorhinolaryngol.* 2006;263(2):156–159.
259. Hoang JK, Branstetter BFT, Eastwood JD, et al. Multiplanar CT and MRI of collections in the retropharyngeal space: is it an abscess? *AJR Am J Roentgenol.* 2011;196(4):W426–W432.
260. Johnston D, Schmidt R, Barth P. Parapharyngeal and retropharyngeal infections in children: argument for a trial of medical therapy and intraoral drainage for medical treatment failures. *Int J Pediatr Otorhinolaryngol.* 2009;73(5):761–765.
261. Nyberg DA, Jeffrey RB, Brant-Zawadzki M, et al. Computed tomography of cervical infections. *J Comput Assist Tomogr.* 1985;9(2):288–296.
262. Glasier CM, Stark JE, Jacobs RF, et al. CT and ultrasound imaging of retropharyngeal abscesses in children. *AJNR Am J Neuroradiol.* 1992;13(4):1191–1195.
263. Dulin MF, Kennard TP, Leach L, et al. Management of cervical lymphadenitis in children. *Am Fam Physician.* 2008;78(9):1097–1098.
264. Fu XS GL, et al. Sonographic appearance of cervical lymphadenopathy due to infectious mononucleosis in children and young adults. *Clin Radiol.* 2014;69(3):239–245.
265. Robson CD, Hazra R, Barnes PD, et al. Nontuberculous mycobacterial infection of the head and neck in immunocompetent children: CT and MR findings. *AJNR Am J Neuroradiol.* 1999;20(10):1829–1835.

266. Screaton NJ, Ravenel JG, Lehner PJ, et al. Lemierre syndrome: forgotten but not extinct: report of four cases. *Radiology.* 1999;213(2):369–374.
267. Brook I, Frazier EH. Clinical and microbiological features of necrotizing fasciitis. *J Clin Microbiol.* 1995;33(9):2382–2387.
268. Bachrach LK, Foley TP Jr. Thyroiditis in children. *Am Acad Pediatr.* 1989;11(6):184–191.
269. Paltiel HJ, Summerville DA, Treves ST. Iodine-123 scintigraphy in the evaluation of pediatric thyroid disorders: a ten year experience. *Pediatr Radiol.* 1992;22(4):251–256.
270. Anderson L, Middleton WD, Teefey SA, et al. Hashimoto thyroiditis: part 1, sonographic analysis of the nodular form of Hashimoto thyroiditis. *AJR Am J Roentgenol.* 2010;195(1): 208–215.
271. Anderson L, Middleton WD, Teefey SA, et al. Hashimoto thyroiditis: part 2, sonographic analysis of benign and malignant nodules in patients with diffuse Hashimoto thyroiditis. *AJR Am J Roentgenol.* 2010;195(1):216–222.
272. Thomas B, Shroff M, Forte V, et al. Revisiting imaging features and the embryologic basis of third and fourth branchial anomalies. *AJNR Am J Neuroradiol.* 2010;31(4):755–760.
273. Spiegel R, Miron D, Sakran W, et al. Acute neonatal suppurative parotitis: case reports and review. *Pediatr Infect Dis J.* 2004;23(1):76–78.
274. Leake D, Leake R. Neonatal suppurative parotitis. *Pediatrics.* 1970;46(2):202–207.
275. Cummings C, Fredrickson J, Harker L, et al, eds. *Otolaryngology-Head and Neck Surgery.* Vol. 2. St. Louis, MO: CV Mosby; 1986.
276. Gadodia A, Bhalla AS, Sharma R, et al. Bilateral parotid swelling: a radiological review. *Dentomaxillofac Radiol.* 2011;40(7):403–414.
277. Takagi Y, Sumi M, Sumi T, et al. MR microscopy of the parotid glands in patients with Sjogren's syndrome: quantitative MR diagnostic criteria. *AJNR Am J Neuroradiol.* 2005;26(5):1207–1214.
278. Macdonald AJ, Salzman KL, Harnsberger HR. Giant ranula of the neck: differentiation from cystic hygroma. *AJNR Am J Neuroradiol.* 2003;24(4):757–761.
279. Crawford SC, Harnsberger HR, Johnson L, et al. Fibromatosis colli of infancy: CT and sonographic findings. *AJR Am J Roentgenol.* 1988;151(6):1183–1184.
280. Lowry KC, Estroff JA, Rahbar R. The presentation and management of fibromatosis colli. *Ear Nose Throat J.* 2010; 89(9):E4–E8.
281. Do TT. Congenital muscular torticollis: current concepts and review of treatment. *Curr Opin Pediatr.* 2006;18(1):26–29.
282. Turkington JR, Paterson A, Sweeney LE, et al. Neck masses in children. *Br J Radiol.* 2005;78(925):75–85.
283. Wei JL, Schwartz KM, Weaver AL, et al. Pseudotumor of infancy and congenital muscular torticollis: 170 cases. *Laryngoscope.* 2001;111(4 pt 1):688–695.
284. Meyer I. Dermoid cysts (dermoids) of the floor of the mouth. *Oral Surg Oral Med Oral Pathol.* 1955;8(11):1149–1164.
285. Robson CD. Imaging of head and neck neoplasms in children. *Pediatr Radiol.* 2010;40(4):499–509.
286. Guinot-Moya R, Valmaseda-Castellon E, Berini-Aytes L, et al. Pilomatrixoma. Review of 205 cases. *Med Oral Patol Oral Cir Bucal.* 2011;16(4):e552–e555.
287. Valdez TA, Desai U, Volk MS. Recurrent fetal rhabdomyoma of the head and neck. *Int J Pediatr Otorhinolaryngol.* 2006;70(6):1115–1118.
288. Sharma SJ, Kreisel M, Kroll T, et al. Extracardiac juvenile rhabdomyoma of the larynx: a rare pathological finding. *Eur Arch Otorhinolaryngol.* 2013;270(2):773–776.
289. O'Callaghan MG, House M, Ebay S, et al. Rhabdomyoma of the head and neck demonstrated by prenatal magnetic resonance imaging. *J Comput Assist Tomogr.* 2005;29(1):130–132.
290. Thakrar R, Robson CD, Vargas SO, et al. Benign triton tumor: multidisciplinary approach to diagnosis and treatment. *Pediatr Dev Pathol.* 2014;17(5):400–405.
291. Castro DE, Raghuram K, Phillips CD. Benign triton tumor of the trigeminal nerve. *AJNR Am J Neuroradiol.* 2005;26(4): 967–969.
292. Mautner VF, Hartmann M, Kluwe L, et al. MRI growth patterns of plexiform neurofibromas in patients with neurofibromatosis type 1. *Neuroradiology.* 2006;48(3):160–165.
293. Lee YY, Van Tassel P, Nauert C, et al. Lymphomas of the head and neck: CT findings at initial presentation. *AJR Am J Roentgenol.* 1987;149(3):575–581.
294. Urquhart A, Berg R. Hodgkin's and non-Hodgkin's lymphoma of the head and neck. *Laryngoscope.* 2001;111(9):1565–1569.
295. Weber AL, Rahemtullah A, Ferry JA. Hodgkin and non-Hodgkin lymphoma of the head and neck: clinical, pathologic, and imaging evaluation. *Neuroimaging Clin N Am.* 2003;13(3): 371–392.
296. Magrath IT. African Burkitt's lymphoma. History, biology, clinical features, and treatment. *Am J Pediatr Hematol Oncol.* 1991;13(2):222–246.
297. Iversen U, Iversen OH, Bluming AZ, et al. Cell kinetics of African cases of Burkitt lymphoma. A preliminary report. *Eur J Cancer.* 1972;8(3):305–308.
298. Millman B, Pellitteri PK. Nodular thyroid disease in children and adolescents. *Otolaryngol Head Neck Surg.* 1997;116 (6 pt 1):604–609.
299. Niedziela M, Korman E, Breborowicz D, et al. A prospective study of thyroid nodular disease in children and adolescents in western Poland from 1996 to 2000 and the incidence of thyroid carcinoma relative to iodine deficiency and the Chernobyl disaster. *Pediatr Blood Cancer.* 2004;42(1):84–92.
300. Niedziela M. Pathogenesis, diagnosis and management of thyroid nodules in children. *Endocr Relat Cancer.* 2006;13(2):427–453.
301. Arda IS, Yildirim S, Demirhan B, et al. Fine needle aspiration biopsy of thyroid nodules. *Arch Dis Child.* 2001;85(4):313–317.
302. Derwahl M, Studer H. Hyperplasia versus adenoma in endocrine tissues: are they different? *Trends Endocrinol Metab.* 2002;13(1):23–28.
303. Rath SR, Bartley A, Charles A, et al. Multinodular Goiter in children: an important pointer to a germline DICER1 mutation. *J Clin Endocrinol Metab.* 2014;99(6): 1947–1948.
304. Harach HR, Williams GT, Williams ED. Familial adenomatous polyposis associated thyroid carcinoma: a distinct type of follicular cell neoplasm. *Histopathology.* 1994;25(6): 549–561.
305. Duffy BJ Jr, Fitzgerald PJ. Cancer of the thyroid in children: a report of 28 cases. *J Clin Endocrinol Metab.* 1950;10(10):1296–1308.
306. Favus MJ, Schneider AB, Stachura ME, et al. Thyroid cancer occurring as a late consequence of head-and-neck irradiation. Evaluation of 1056 patients. *N Engl J Med.* 1976;294(19): 1019–1025.
307. Sklar C, Whitton J, Mertens A, et al. Abnormalities of the thyroid in survivors of Hodgkin's disease: data from the

Childhood Cancer Survivor Study. *J Clin Endocrinol Metab.* 2000;85(9):3227–3232.
308. Wiersinga WM. Thyroid cancer in children and adolescents: consequences in later life. *J Pediatr Endocrinol Metab.* 2001;14(suppl 5):1289–1296; discussion 1297–1288.
309. Bauer AJ. Thyroid nodules and differentiated thyroid cancer. *Endocr Dev.* 2014;26:183–201.
310. Hoang JK, Lee WK, Lee M, et al. US Features of thyroid malignancy: pearls and pitfalls. *Radiographics.* 2007;27(3): 847–860; discussion 861–845.
311. Som PM, Brandwein M, Lidov M, et al. The varied presentations of papillary thyroid carcinoma cervical nodal disease: CT and MR findings. *AJNR Am J Neuroradiol.* 1994;15(6):1123–1128.
312. Gorman B, Charboneau JW, James EM, et al. Medullary thyroid carcinoma: role of high-resolution US. *Radiology.* 1987;162 (1 pt 1):147–150.
313. Lack EE, Upton MP. Histopathologic review of salivary gland tumors in childhood. *Arch Otolaryngol Head Neck Surg.* 1988;114(8):898–906.
314. Ellis GL, Auclair PL. *AFIP Atlas of Tumor Pathology, Tumors of the Salivary Glands.* Fourth Series, Fascicle 9. Washington, DC: American Registry of Pathology; 2008.
315. Bertola DR, Kim CA, Pereira AC, et al. Are Noonan syndrome and Noonan-like/multiple giant cell lesion syndrome distinct entities? *Am J Med Genet.* 2001;98(3):230–234.
316. Prescott T, Redfors M, Rustad CF, et al. Characterization of a Norwegian cherubism cohort; molecular genetic findings, oral manifestations and quality of life. *Eur J Med Genet.* 2013;56(3):131–137.
317. Papadaki ME, Lietman SA, Levine MA, et al. Cherubism: best clinical practice. *Orphanet J Rare Dis.* 2012;7(suppl 1):S6.

CHAPTER 4

Spinal Cord

Benjamin T. Haverkamp • Peter Winningham • Winnie C. Chu • Lisa H. Hutchison • Paul G. Thacker

INTRODUCTION

A variety of disorders affect the pediatric spine. Many present with serious acute symptoms such as paresthesia, paralysis, and loss of sensation or bladder and bowel function. Accurate, prompt diagnosis is essential to prevent development of chronic morbidity and mortality.

In this chapter, we first discuss main imaging modalities and techniques used in the evaluation of spine in infants and children. Next, anatomical and embryologic concepts that are important to understanding congenital and developmental anomalies of the pediatric spine, in addition to normal variants that may simulate disease, are reviewed. A discussion of common infectious disorders, neoplasms, spinal cord trauma, vascular anomalies, and inflammatory processes follows. Emphasis is placed on clinical and imaging findings that are useful in differential diagnosis. Finally, the section on each disorder concludes with a brief discussion of treatment and prognosis.

IMAGING TECHNIQUES

Radiography

Radiographs are insufficient for evaluating the spinal cord and surrounding cerebrospinal fluid. However, radiography is the first imaging modality used to evaluate the spinal column, particularly in pediatric patients with persistent back pain or in posttraumatic patients. Fractures seen on radiography may be better detailed with computed tomography (CT)[1] and magnetic resonance imaging MRI; the latter is useful for evaluating concomitant underlying spinal cord injury.[1] Osteolytic changes and periosteal reaction can be seen with infection and tumors, which need further cross-sectional imaging to assess for mass effect on the cord and/or invasion of the spinal canal. Widening of the spinal canal, a subtle radiographic sign of spinal cord tumors, should be searched for in children with back pain (Fig. 4.1).

Typically, cervical, thoracic, and lumbar spine radiographic series consist of a minimum of two views, a frontal and lateral projection. Specific imaging parameters vary by patient age and size. Although odontoid views are often obtained in children 0 to 8 years of age, their routine utility has been called into question even in posttraumatic patients in this age group.[2] Flexion and extension lateral cervical spine radiographs are often added to evaluate for ligamentous instability in trauma patients. Oblique views of the lumbar spine may be added to identify spondylolysis and, rarely, neuroforaminal expansion.

Ultrasound

Ultrasonography (US) is a well-established and readily available noninvasive technique for newborn and infant spinal cord evaluation.[3–5] Because of the incompletely ossified spinal arches and predominately cartilaginous components, infants have a superb acoustic window allowing sonography to characterize nearly all congenital spinal anomalies.[3] Indeed, the diagnostic value of US in newborns is nearly equal to that of MRI.[3,4] However, as the infant ages and progressive ossification of the posterior elements occurs, the utility of spinal US becomes more limited.[5]

Sonography of the spine is performed with the infant prone using a high-frequency 7- to 12-MHz transducer.

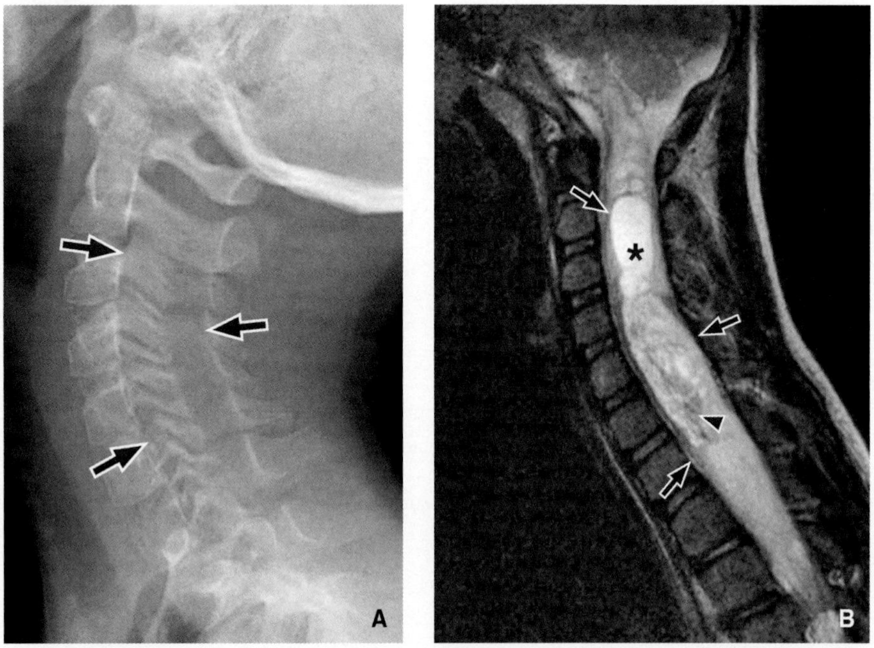

FIGURE 4.1 **Astrocytoma in a 9-year-old girl with a 2-year history of neck pain. A:** Lateral radiograph of the cervical spine demonstrates extensive widening (*arrows*) of the spinal canal. Cervical vertebral bodies show subtle decrease in anteroposterior width. **B:** Sagittal T2-weighted MR image confirms a large intramedullary spinal cord mass (*arrows*) expanding the spinal canal and extending from the foramen magnum to T3. The solid portions of the tumor (*arrowhead*) demonstrate heterogeneous low signal intensity compared to the hyperintense cystic foci (*asterisk*) along the lesion's superior aspect.

Images are obtained in transverse and longitudinal planes. Because of ossification of the posterior elements, paramedian scans may provide the only option for sufficient visualization of the spinal cord beyond 6 months of age.[5] To accurately assess the position of the conus medullaris, vertebral level can be determined by counting inferiorly starting at the twelfth rib and confirmed by counting superiorly from the lumbosacral junction. Indeterminate cases may be further assessed by performing a radiograph after placing a marker on the skin to denote the tip of the conus medullaris. Extended field-of-view (panoramic) US can be used to evaluate the entire lumbosacral spinal canal in a single longitudinal image with up to a 60-cm field of view.[6] In addition, cine images are able to show normal mobility of the cauda equina nerve roots. Color or power Doppler sonography may be added to assess overlying soft tissue or spinal canal masses.[3,4] Lastly, although little literature currently exists to support the clinical value, 3-dimensional (3D) US may be used to eloquently assess the spinal canal.[6]

Computed Tomography

The value of computed tomography (CT) is its ability to assess osseous and paraspinal soft tissue structures. Specifically, it is able to rapidly evaluate acute conditions such as trauma and infection. Fracture patterns can be described with high sensitivity and specificity compared to other imaging modalities. CT is only able to delineate the spinal canal after administration of intrathecal contrast.

CT parameters, particularly mAs, should be adjusted based on patient weight to keep the radiation dose as low as possible. Typical multidetector spine CT technique includes thin collimation and high-resolution bony algorithm in addition to 3-mm standard axial CT images. Reformatted sagittal and coronal CT images are routinely performed as they are particularly advantageous in the posttraumatic patient (Fig. 4.2). Intravenous and intrathecal contrast may rarely be added for specific indications such as assessment of cord pathology in children who cannot undergo MR imaging because of medical devices (such as pacemakers) or orthopedic hardware with artifact obscuring adequate visualization of the area of concern.

Magnetic Resonance Imaging

MR imaging is currently the modality of choice for evaluation of spinal canal contents. It provides superior soft tissue contrast resolution relative to other techniques without exposing the pediatric patient to the harmful effects of ionizing radiation. Furthermore, physiologic information can be garnered by the assessment of cerebrospinal fluid flow characteristics using phase contrast cine imaging and by the evaluation of bone marrow edema patterns on standard T2 and short T1 inversion recovery (STIR) sequences (Fig. 4.2C).

Typical indications for pediatric spinal MRI include neurologic symptoms such as weakness, paresthesia, or loss of bowel or bladder function that may suggest spinal cord mass; posttraumatic spinal cord injury; spinal dysraphism; atypical scoliosis; and leptomeningeal metastatic disease. A complete

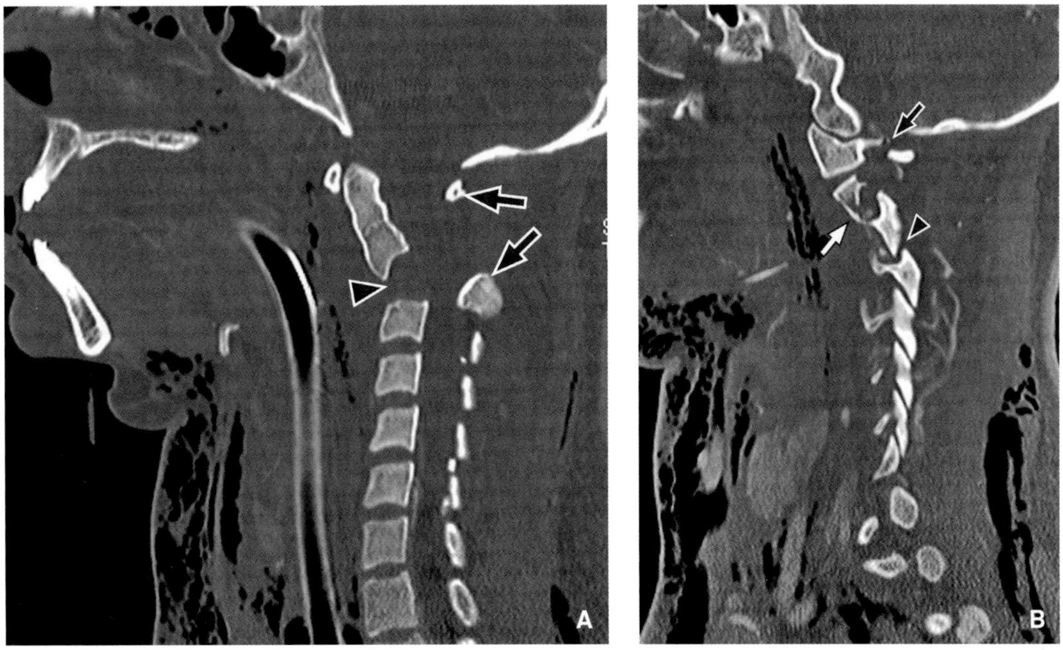

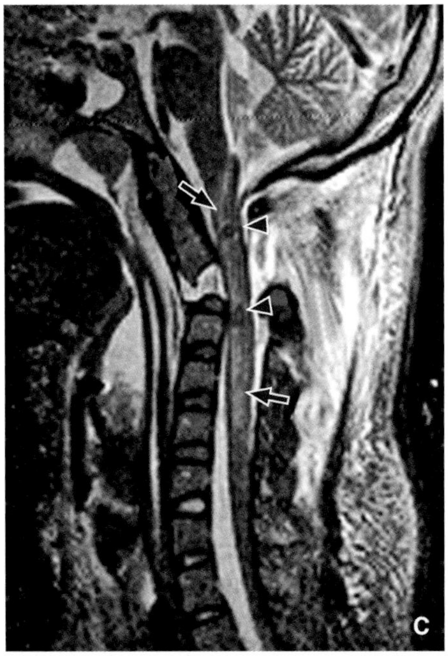

FIGURE 4.2 **Fracture at the C2–C3 disk space in a 5-year-girl after an all-terrain vehicle accident. A:** Sagittal bone window CT image demonstrates widening and severe angulation (*arrowhead*) at the C2–C3 interspace with additional splaying of the C1–C2 posterior elements (*arrows*). Diffuse subcutaneous emphysema is also noted. **B:** Additional sagittal bone window CT image lateral to **A** shows a dislocated, locked facet at C2–C3 (*arrowhead*). Partially visualized fractures of the posterior arch of C1 (*black arrow*) and lateral body of C2 (*white arrow*) are identified. **C:** Sagittal STIR MR image identifies dislocation at the C2–C3 interspace with C2 angulation and severe narrowing of the spinal canal. Full-thickness tears of the anterior and posterior longitudinal ligaments and marked widening of the C1–C2 posterior elements are noted. Diffuse edema (*arrows*) of the brainstem and cervical cord with multiple donut-shaped areas of T2 hypointensity, likely representing focal hemorrhage (*arrowheads*), is present.

discussion of spinal MR imaging protocols is beyond the scope of this chapter. However, a brief discussion of technical factors and common imaging sequences follows.

The small spinal cord volume and relatively increased respiratory and cardiac motion in the pediatric population can make high-quality imaging of the spinal cord challenging. To achieve high-quality MR imaging, smaller fields of view with a larger imaging matrix, thin sections, and no or small interslice gaps are utilized. Because these techniques inherently decrease the signal-to-noise ratio (SNR), an increased number of excitations and longer imaging times are needed. Imaging on a 3 Tesla (T) MRI scanner can increase the SNR to improve image quality or shorten imaging times.[7] A multichannel surface coil should be utilized whenever possible. Only those coils aligned with the region of interest should be employed, with coils outside the imaging field of view turned off as they contribute to image noise.

Conventional spinal MRI protocols consist of sagittal and axial T1- and T2-weighted sequences without fat saturation. However, many institutions also include sagittal, fat-saturated STIR images in order to make edema more conspicuous. For pediatric patients with severe scoliosis, coronal and/or heavily T2-weighted isotropic images with reconstructions in various planes are invaluable. Demyelinating diseases and neoplasms require T1 postgadolinium sequences in at least two planes, typically axial and sagittal.

Newer sequences have recently been reported as advantageous for the evaluation of certain pathologic processes.[8] Specifically, diffusion-weighted MR imaging is able to distinguish epidermoids from arachnoid cysts.[9] Authors demonstrated restricted diffusion in epidermoids compared to arachnoid cysts, which have free diffusivity. More recently, a variant of 3D fast spin echo (FSE) sequences has been introduced. Depending on manufacturer, the acronym for these sequences varies and includes SPACE, FSE-XETA, and VISTA.[8] These imaging sequences are characterized by flip angle modulation during the FSE readout resulting in high-resolution 3D volumetric images, which can be reformatted into multiple imaging planes. Given these capabilities, the utility of these sequences has been described in the evaluation of nerve root avulsions, posttraumatic pseudomeningoceles, scoliosis, and nerve root compression by herniated disk material.[8] Diffusion tensor imaging (DTI) is also a cutting-edge technique that has recently been proposed in the spinal cord. Nerve root avulsion may be characterized by the demonstration of discontinuity between the spinal cord fibers and adjacent nerve roots.[8] DTI has also been utilized in the evaluation of fiber displacement by intramedullary spinal tumors.[10] Nevertheless, DTI's usage in pediatric spinal cord imaging remains largely experimental, and further study is needed before its clinical value can be fully elucidated. Finally, phase contrast images may be added to evaluate cerebrospinal flow characteristics.[11] This sequence is particularly useful to assess motion of the cerebellar tonsils in Chiari I malformations, which may obstruct CSF flow and be associated with progressively enlarging spinal cord syringomyelia.

On T2-weighted MR images, the central canal is occasionally seen as a thin tubular area of hyperintensity.[12] The conus medullaris terminates at or above the L2–L3 disk space, and the thecal sac generally terminates at S2. The filum terminale extends from the conus medullaris as a hypointense cord on T1- and T2-weighted MR imaging, measuring <2 mm.

Other Imaging Modalities

The utility of imaging modalities other than those listed above is limited in the pediatric population. Myelography has been largely supplanted by MRI in children except when MRI is contraindicated. In such cases, CT myelography may be used to assess the spinal cord. Likewise, conventional angiography for diagnostic purposes has been largely replaced by MR and CT angiography for the evaluation of spinal and paraspinal vascular anomalies. However, when MR and CT angiography are inconclusive or if therapeutic intervention is planned, conventional angiography is needed. Currently, nuclear and molecular imaging has a very limited role in the evaluation of the spinal cord. However, with the increased utilization of positron emission tomography with concurrent CT coregistration, CT/PET may take on an increased role in spinal cord disorders, such as evaluation of tumors and treatment response assessment.[13]

NORMAL ANATOMY AND VARIANTS

Spinal Cord Embryology

Knowledge of normal embryology is helpful to understand how congenital spinal lesions develop and their imaging findings. The spinal cord originates from the neural plate, which forms the neural fold and, eventually, the neural tube. Just ventral to the developing neural tube is the notochord, which ultimately forms the vertebral bodies and intervertebral disks. Abnormalities in neural tube development result in open defects occurring in the early embryologic stages of gastrulation (weeks 2 to 3), primary neurulation (weeks 3 to 4), and secondary neurulation (weeks 5 to 6).[14] If mesenchyme migrates into the developing neural tube, a lipomyelocele or lipomyelocystocele can occur.[15] Diastematomyelia develops early during embryogenesis, likely from adhesion between ectoderm and endoderm with splitting of the early notochord.[5]

Synchondrosis Closure

Knowledge of synchondrosis closure is important when evaluating CT studies in the setting of trauma. It can sometimes be challenging to distinguish between a normal developmental process from an acute fracture. Synchondrosis closure in the spine occurs from cranial to caudal. The anterior and posterior atlas arches close around 4 years of age, range 2 to 13 years. The C2 base of dens synchondrosis usually fuses around 9 years of age.[16]

Normal Anatomy

Ultrasound is the screening imaging modality of choice in infants because of its accuracy, relatively low cost compared to MRI, and lack of need for sedation or radiation exposure. In infants, suboccipital US can be used to show the hypoechoic pons, medulla oblongata, and spinal cord.[5] The center of the spinal cord contains two parallel echogenic lines, due to overgrown glial debris, surrounding a hypoechoic center.[5] The conus medullaris, the most caudal portion of the cord, is located at or above the L2–L3 disk level (Fig. 4.3). The filum terminale is a midline echogenic structure that extends from the tip of the conus to the distal thecal sac. It is surrounded by echogenic nerve roots. The spinal cord varies in diameter depending on level, being largest in diameter in the cervical and lumbar regions because of the increased density of efferent and afferent fibers supplying the upper and lower extremities (Fig. 4.4).

Normal Variants

Besides the normal variants previously mentioned, a prominent filum and central echo complex, one must be aware of other variants in order to avoid incorrectly suggesting disease. Common variants are discussed below including filar cysts,

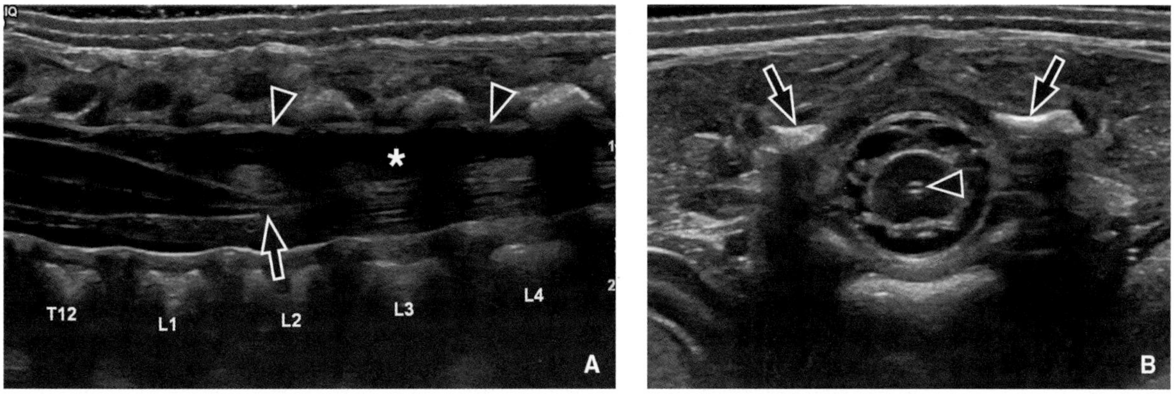

FIGURE 4.3 **Normal lumbar spine ultrasound in a 1-day-old infant with VATER syndrome. A:** Longitudinal ultrasound of the lumbar spine shows the conus medullaris (*arrow*) at the L2 level. Also visible are the dura (*arrowheads*) and cerebrospinal fluid (*asterisk*). Note that the vertebrae are labeled from T12 to L4. **B:** Axial ultrasound of lumbar spine demonstrates the normal central echo complex (*arrowhead*), ventral and dorsal nerve roots, and the transverse processes (*arrows*).

prominent filum terminalis, ventricular terminalis, cauda equina pseudomasses, pseudosinus tracts, and borderline low conus position.

Filar cysts, a common finding on neonatal sonography, are oblong midline cysts located within the filum terminale just below the conus medullaris. They should not be confused with a ventriculus terminalis (discussed below), a different normal variant that is located within the conus medullaris. The frequency in which filar cysts are seen on US is inversely proportional to age up until around 6 months.[17] Seen in isolation, filar cysts are associated with normal developmental milestones. Although common on infant US, no filar cyst has ever been described at autopsy, begging the question as to whether they are merely pseudocysts or related to normal anatomic scaffolding of the neonatal spinal canal (Fig. 4.5).[17]

Prominent filum terminalis is seen as an echogenic linear midline structure extending from the tip of the conus to the distal thecal sac among the cauda equina nerve roots.

Ventriculus terminalis is a cystic structure located within the distal spinal cord just above the conus medullaris. It is thought to be a remnant of the embryologic canalization and retrogressive differentiation processes that form the tip of the conus and coccyx.[18]

Cauda equina pseudomasses occur when infants are scanned while lying on their side and are caused by nerve roots clumping together in the dependent portion of the spinal canal. This can be easily distinguished from a true mass by placing the infant prone and rescanning the region.[4]

Pseudosinus tracts are seen in many infants as a fibrous cord of tissue extending from the coccyx to a skin dimple in the gluteal crease (Fig. 4.6). If the dimple is 2.5 cm above the gluteal crease; if it has skin stigmata such as pigmentation, hair, or a skin tag; or if fluid is draining via this tract, then a true sinus tract requiring surgery is likely present. Without these clinical markers, a pseudosinus tract is most likely, especially if the dimple is within the gluteal crease.

Borderline low conus position between the L2–L3 disk space and the mid L3 vertebral body level is common in infants and has been shown to correlate with normal developmental milestones on clinical follow-up evaluation making

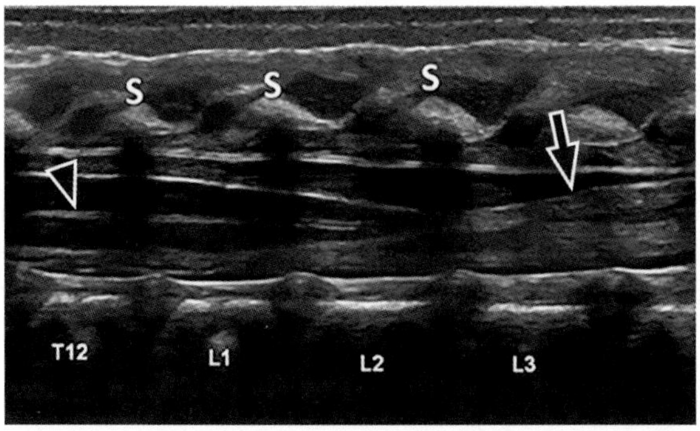

FIGURE 4.4 **Normal sagittal ultrasound in a 3-month old boy with a deep sacral dimple.** Longitudinal ultrasound shows a normal prominent filum terminale (*arrow*) and prominent central echo complex (*arrowhead*). Also note the partially ossified lumbar spinous processes (*S*) beneath which there is acoustic shadowing and decreased visualization of the spinal cord.

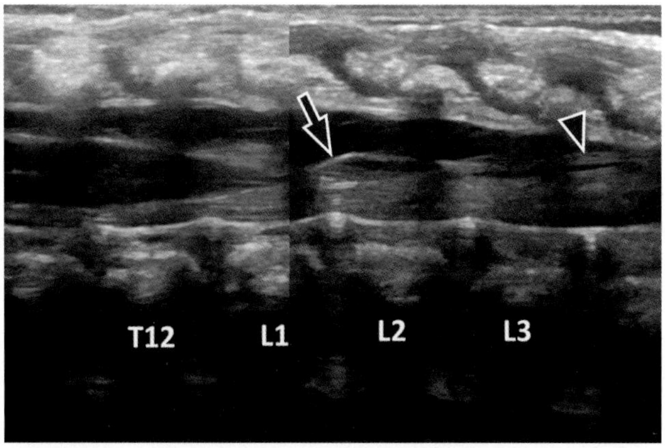

FIGURE 4.5 **Filar cyst in a 1-month-old girl with a dysmorphic gluteal crease.** Longitudinal sonogram shows a well-defined midline hypoechoic oblong cyst (*arrow*) just below the conus medullaris. Also note the normal filum terminale (*arrowhead*).

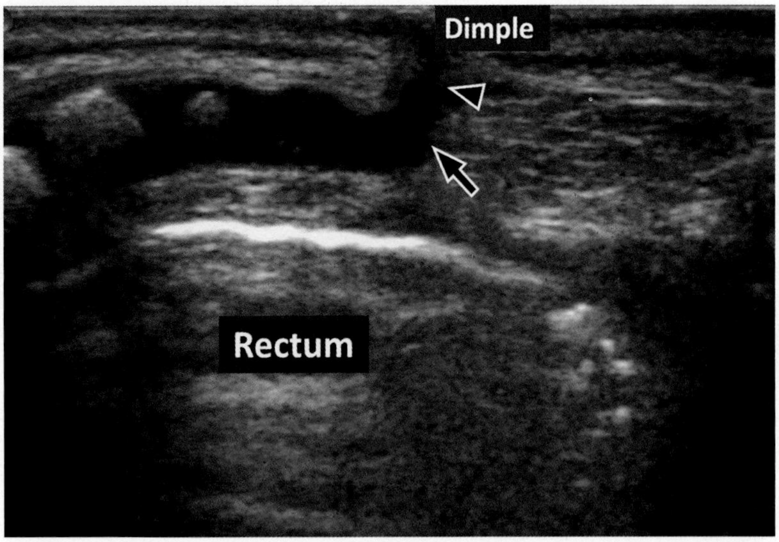

FIGURE 4.6 **Pseudosinus tract and dysmorphic coccyx in a 3-week-old boy with a deep sacral dimple at the top of the gluteal crease.** Longitudinal ultrasound reveals the hypoechoic tip of coccyx (*arrow*) curving toward the skin surface. A pseudosinus tract (*arrowhead*) extends from the dysmorphic coccyx tip to the skin surface.

additional workup and MR imaging unwarranted (Fig. 4.7).[19] However, if clinical concern remains, follow-up sonography may be easily performed up to 6 months of age.

SPECTRUM OF PEDIATRIC SPINAL CORD DISORDERS

Congenital and Developmental Anomalies

Congenital and developmental anomalies of the spine and spinal cord are collectively referred to as spinal dysraphisms, which is a broad term that covers a spectrum of disorders with incomplete or absent fusion of midline mesenchymal and neural structures.

Spinal dysraphisms are approached by first categorizing lesions into open and closed defects.[14] Open spinal dysraphisms (OSDs) have defects in the overlying skin allowing neural tissue with or without its associated subarachnoid space to be exposed to air. Open entities include myelomeningoceles and myeloceles. Hemimyelomeningocele and hemimyelocele are rare entities in the same group, in which the myelo(meningo)cele affects one of two hemicords in the setting of diastematomyelia.[20,21] Closed spinal dysraphisms (CSDs) have components that extend through spinal defects with intact skin overlying neural tissue. Morphologically, CSDs are subcategorized based on the presence or absence of a raised lumbar subcutaneous mass. An approach to classifying spinal dysraphisms is included in Fig. 4.8.

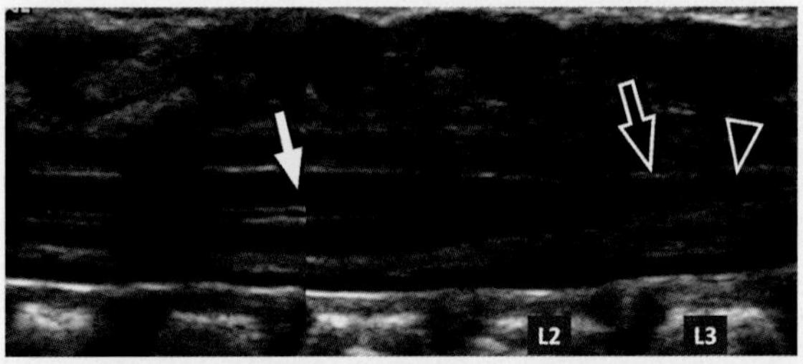

FIGURE 4.7 **Borderline low conus medullaris in a newborn boy with a sacral dimple above the gluteal crease.** Longitudinal ultrasound demonstrates a normal conus (*black arrow*) located just below the L2–L3 disk space posterior to the top of L3. Also noted are a small filar cyst (*arrowhead*) and a ventriculus terminalis (*white arrow*).

Myelomeningocele and Myelocele

Both myelomeningoceles and myeloceles are classified as OSDs having a placode exposed to air. Both are due to defective closure of the primary neural tube[15,22] with persistence of a segment of nonneurulated placode while cutaneous ectoderm does not detach from the neural ectoderm and remains in a lateral position.

Myelomeningoceles are far more common OSDs than myeloceles. The former account for more than 98.8% of OSDs.[23] The previously quoted incidence is 0.6 per 1,000 live births, but the incidence is currently decreasing because of prenatal screening and preventive maternal dietary folic acid supplementation. Myeloceles only account for 1.2% of OSDs and are most common at the lumbar or lumbosacral levels.

On imaging, the main differentiating feature between the two conditions is the relative position of the neural placode with reference to the skin surface.[14] In myelomeningoceles, the neural placode protrudes above the skin surface because of expansion and protrusion of the underlying subarachnoid space (Fig. 4.9). In myeloceles, the ventral subarachnoid space is not protruding; hence, the placode is flush with the skin surface (Fig. 4.10). Although the diagnosis is usually obvious clinically, MRI is useful for surgical planning because it is able to characterize the lesion and assess for associated findings of a Chiari II malformation, including hydrocephalus and hydromyelia.

Chiari II Malformation

There is always consistent association between OSD and the Arnold-Chiari II malformation. The latter is a complex

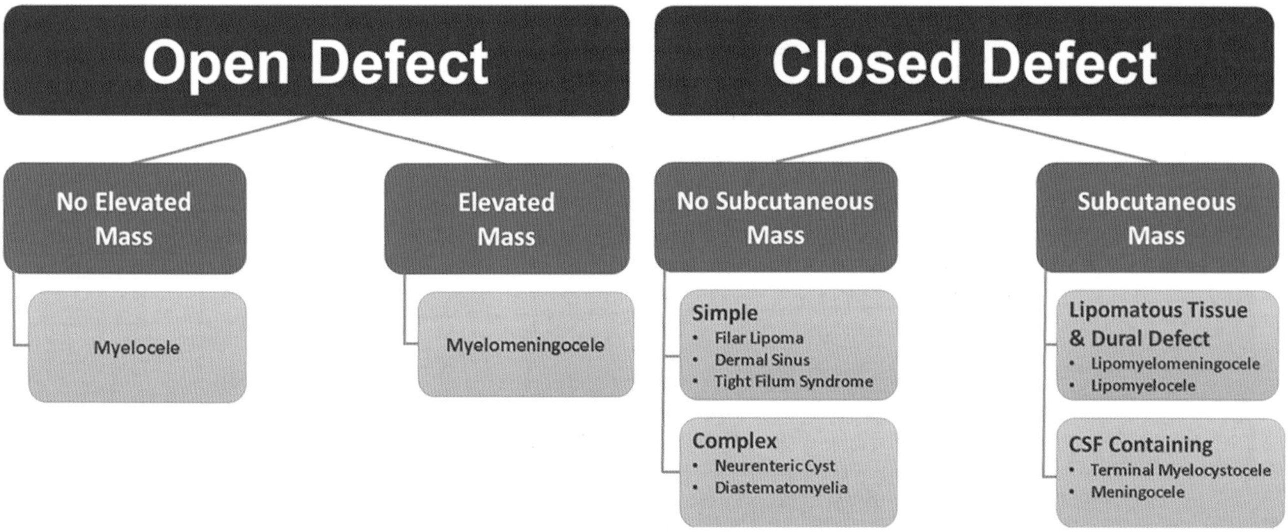

FIGURE 4.8 **Flow chart showing clinical-radiologic classifications of spinal dysraphism.** First division is open versus closed dysraphism. Second division is based on presence or absence of an elevated mass extending through the defect outside the osseous defect.

congenital anomaly of the hindbrain characterized by descent of the cerebellar vermis through the foramen magnum, elongation and kinking of the medulla, caudal displacement of the cervical spinal cord and medulla, and obliteration of the cisterna magna.[24] The pathogenesis is explained by a CSF leak from the OSD, resulting in a lack of appropriate distention of the embryonic ventricular system. The chronic CSF hypotension within the developing neural tube leads to formation of a hypoplastic posterior fossa and subsequent herniation of the cerebellum and brainstem through the foramen magnum.[25] A recent fetal MRI study has suggested that caudal traction by cord tethering also plays a role in a subset of patients with Chiari malformations.[26]

Conventionally, pediatric patients with myelomeningoceles and myeloceles undergo corrective surgery in the postnatal period aimed at covering the exposed placode to prevent ulceration and infection, as well as treating hydrocephalus with a ventricular shunt. Recently, in utero surgery has been performed on selected patients aimed at preventing secondary damage of the spinal cord by a combination of factors such as amniotic fluid exposure, direct trauma, and hydrodynamic pressure[27] based on the "two-hit" hypothesis.[28] The goals of fetal surgery are to reverse hindbrain herniation (Chiari II malformation), reduce the need for ventriculoperitoneal shunting due to hydrocephalus, and prevent later neurologic deficits due to cord tethering.[29]

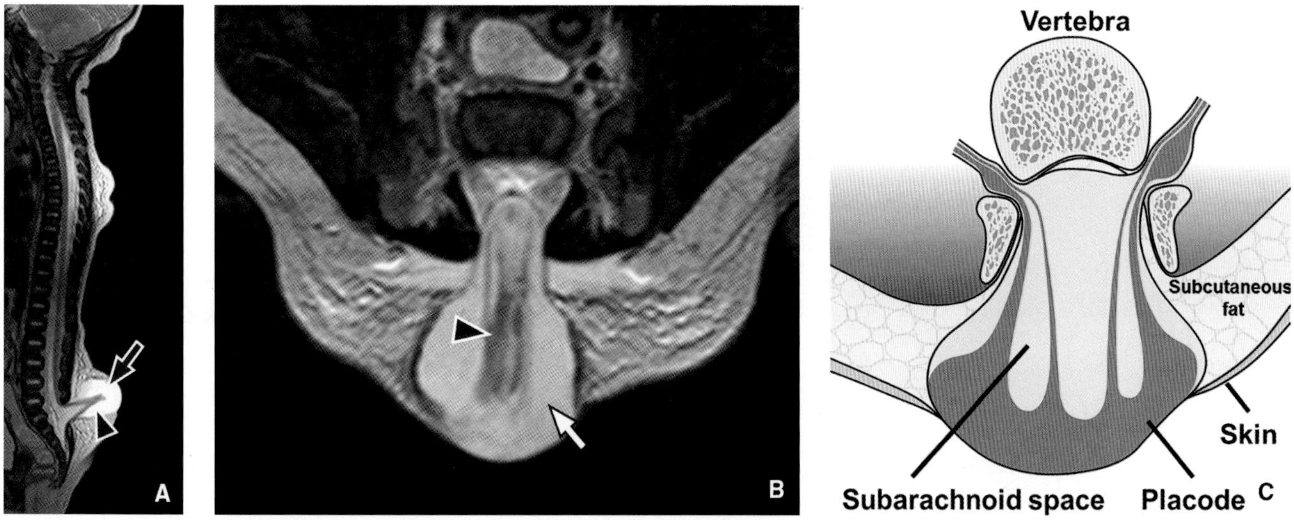

FIGURE 4.9 **Myelomeningocele in a newborn infant girl with open dysraphism.** Sagittal **(A)** and axial **(B)** T2-weighted MR images, as well as axial schematic drawing **(C)** show a tethered spinal cord crossing the meningeal outpouching as a terminal apical placode (*arrowheads*), which is exposed to air. Subarachnoid space is denoted with *black* and *white arrows*.

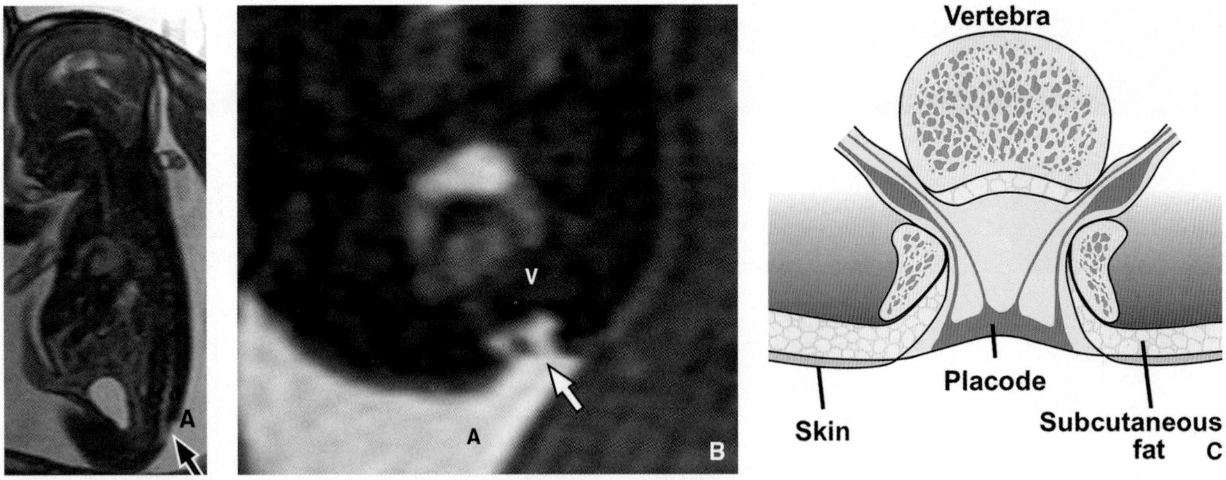

FIGURE 4.10 **Myelocele in a fetus in utero.** Sagittal **(A)** and axial **(B)** T2-weighted MR images demonstrate a skin defect (*arrows*) and sacral spinal dysraphism. The placode is flush with the skin surface and is exposed to the amniotic fluid (*A*) without protrusion of the subarachnoid space through the vertebral (*V*) defect. **C:** Axial schematic representation of myelocele.

Lipomyelocele and Lipomyelomeningocele

Both lipomyeloceles and lipomyelomeningoceles are CSDs that present with a subcutaneous mass at the lumbosacral region beneath the intact skin. Lipomyeloceles are about twice as common as lipomyelomeningoceles.[23] The lipomas are associated with a dural defect. These anomalies account for ~76% of all spinal lipomas and 16.4% of all CSDs. Lipomyeloceles and lipomyelomeningoceles have been attributed to a primary neurulation defect in which there is focal premature disjunction of cutaneous ectoderm from neuroectoderm.[30] The mesenchymal cells enter the neural tube to form fat (lipoma) and prevent further neurulation. The lipoma extends posteriorly through the spinal defect and merges with the subcutaneous fat.

MRI is the imaging modality of choice. The main MR imaging feature that differentiates lipomyeloceles from lipomyelomeningoceles is the position of the placode–lipoma interface relative to the spinal canal. In lipomyeloceles, the placode–lipoma interface is within or at the edge of the spinal canal. The subcutaneous fat extends into the spinal canal and attaches to the spinal cord (Fig. 4.11). In lipomyelomeningoceles, the placode–lipoma interface is outside the spinal canal because of protrusion of the subarachnoid space through the osseous defect. A subcutaneous fatty mass extends through a lumbosacral defect attaching to the open neural placode (Figs. 4.12 and 4.13). The cord is often rotated and asymmetrically tethered by the lipoma, and hydromyelia may be present.[31] There is also unequal development of the nerve roots that may cause cord tethering.

Early surgical treatment is advocated in these pediatric patients to prevent neurologic deficits.[32] The surgical goals include total or subtotal removal of the adipose mass, identification of the lumbosacral fascial defect to release tethering, possible release of the filum terminale, preservation

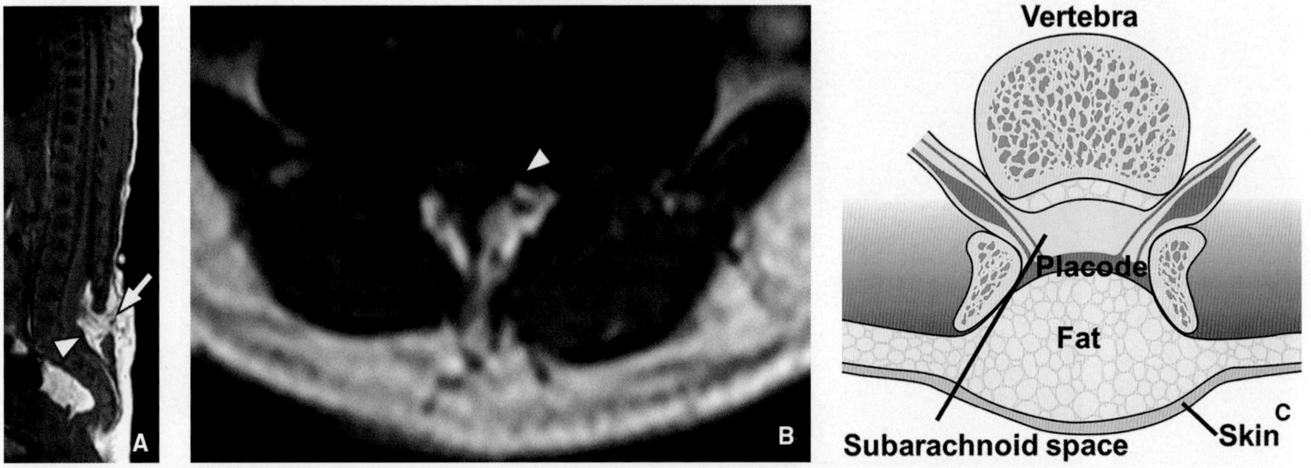

FIGURE 4.11 **Lipomyelocele in a newborn boy.** Sagittal **(A)** and axial **(B)** T1-weighted MR images show the presence of a subcutaneous lipoma (*arrow*) with fatty tissue (*arrowhead*) extending into the spinal canal through a dysraphism and attaching to the neural placode. Note that in **(B)**, the placode–lipoma interface (*arrowhead*) is within the spinal canal, distinguishing it from lipomyelomeningocele. Also note that the overlying skin is intact. **C:** Axial schematic representation of lipomyelocele.

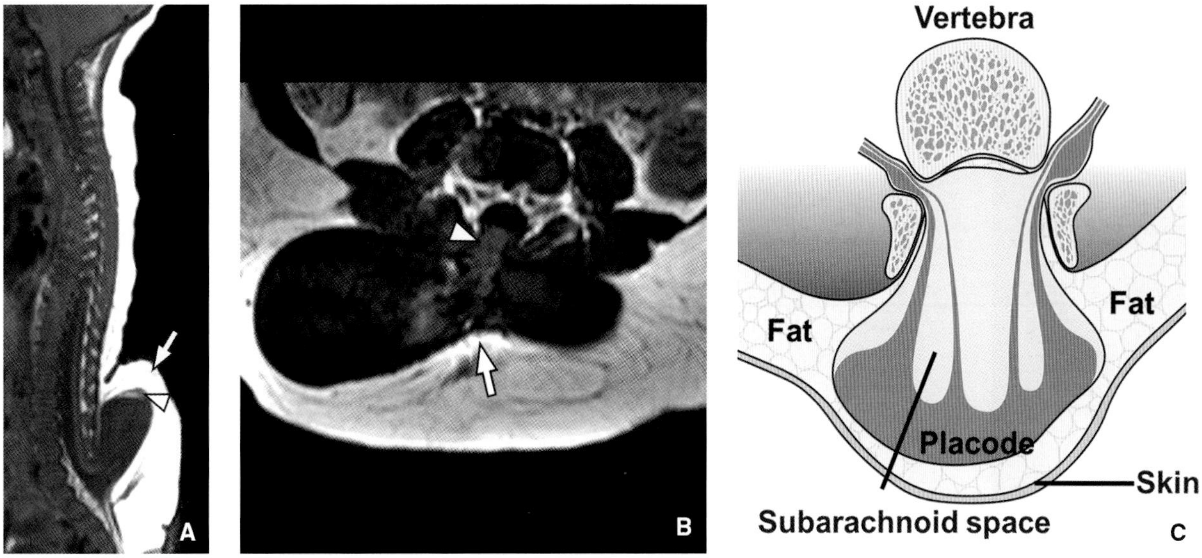

FIGURE 4.12 **Lipomyelomeningocele in a newborn girl.** Sagittal **(A)** and axial **(B)** T1-weighted MR image shows a tethered spinal cord crossing the meningeal outpouching as a terminal placode (*arrowhead*), which is contained within a large subcutaneous lipoma (*arrows*). The placode-lipoma interface and the subarachnoid space extend outside the spinal defect and are covered by skin and subcutaneous tissue, which is also demonstrated in **(C)**, a schematic representation of a lipomyelomeningocele.

of neural elements, and prevention of retethering of the spinal cord.[33]

Meningocele

Posterior meningocele, which is classified under CSD, is uncommon and of unknown etiology. It has been hypothesized that it results from protrusion of meninges through a posterior spinal defect because of subarachnoid space CSF pulsations. Most posterior meningoceles are lumbar or sacral in location, but thoracic and cervical lesions are rarely reported. On imaging, the classic posterior meningocele is characterized by a CSF-filled sac herniating through a posterior spinal defect (Fig. 4.14). By definition, no neural tissue is contained within the sac, although it may be tethered to the neck of the meningocele. Additionally, nerve roots or even the filum terminale may subtly course through the meningocele.[14] Because posterior meningoceles are frequently associated with other occult spinal lesions, MRI of the entire spinal column should be performed for a complete assessment.[34]

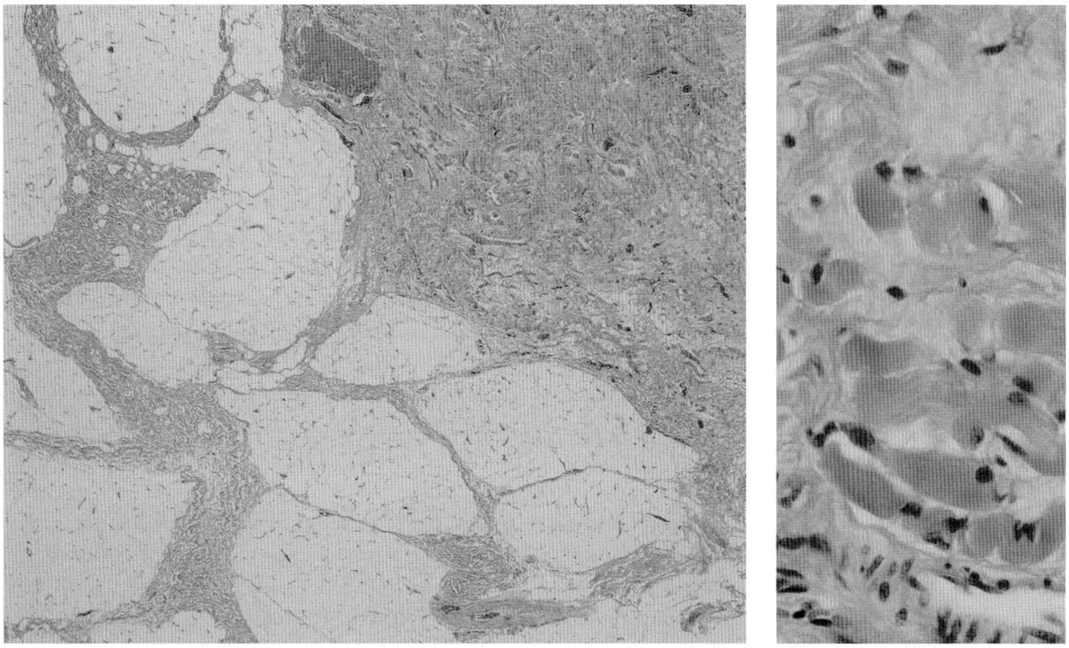

FIGURE 4.13 **Lipomyelomeningocele in a 7-month-old girl with a tethered spinal cord and a lumbar dermal sinus tract.** This complex mass showed abundant fat and a nodular collection of disorganized fibrous tissue and skeletal muscle (hematoxylin and eosin, original magnification; 40×, **right**; 600×, **left**).

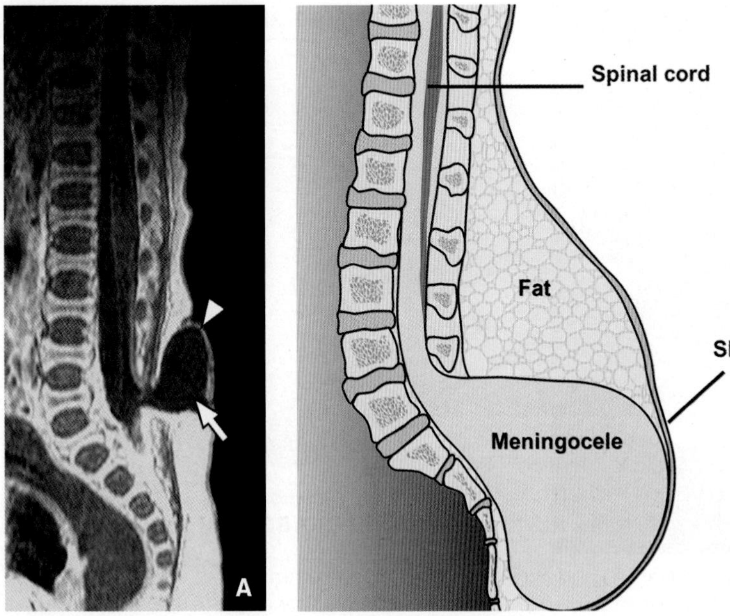

B

FIGURE 4.14 **Meningocele in a newborn girl.** Sagittal T1-weighted MR image **(A)** and corresponding schematic representation **(B)** demonstrate meningeal herniation through a posterior spinal defect forming a CSF-filled sac (*arrow*) without neural contents. The overlying skin (*arrowhead*) is intact. (Case courtesy of In-one Kim, MD, Seoul National University Hospital, South Korea.)

Anterior meningoceles and intrasacral meningoceles are occult spinal dysraphisms without a subcutaneous mass. Anterior meningoceles are presacral in location and found consistently in pediatric patients with caudal agenesis. They may be discovered only in older children or adults complaining of low back pain, urinary incontinence, or constipation.[35] Intrasacral meningocele is an intrasacral extradural cystic lesion caused by arachnoid diverticulum through a small dural defect at the caudal end of the thecal sac. As distinguished from the more common perineural (Tarlov) cysts, intrasacral meningoceles are not associated with any exiting nerve root and, thus, spare the sacral foramina. They may cause sacral pain or sacral nerve root dysfunction by local compression.

Posterior meningoceles generally require surgical repair; anterior and intrasacral meningoceles are surgically treated only when symptomatic. The goal of surgery is to identify the point of herniation through the dura mater and ligate the cyst. After ligation, most affected children have resolution of symptoms.[1]

Terminal Myelocystocele

Terminal myelocystocele (TMC) is a rare form of CSD. The key feature is extrusion of the distal spinal cord into the extraspinal space with its terminal part expanding into a cystic cavity forming the TMC. The functional conus is located in the more rostral part of the TMC. There are a few associated features of TMC that vary from case to case. The intraspinal subarachnoid space may expand and extend into the extraspinal fat space, forming a meningocele surrounding the TMC. Some degree of hydromyelia may occur, usually confined to the lumbosacral region. Rarely, hydromyelia can be enormous and communicate with the TMC. The amount of subcutaneous fat covering the TMC varies, ranging from slightly thicker than normal skin to exuberant lipoma.[36]

The pathogenesis of TMC is not fully understood, but most likely related to an anomaly of secondary neurulation and retrogressive differentiation.[36] It is suggested that TMC may be caused by a time-specific paralysis of apoptosis just before the dehiscence of the cystic distal cord from the future skin, thereby preserving the embryonic components within the cyst.

The key MR imaging feature is that of a “cyst within a cyst” (Fig. 4.15). The inner cyst represents the trumpet-shaped, CSF-filled myelocystocele, which is sometimes in continuity with a hydromyelia cavity (syringocele) within the intraspinal portion of the cord. The outer cyst wall represents the extraspinal extension of the expanded dura, which communicates with the spinal subarachnoid space. The cord is always tethered. Sagittal isotropic 3D reconstructed MR images are particularly able to demonstrate the entire spinal cord in a single plane when scoliosis is present, which can be useful to depict the continuity between the myelocystocele and the spinal cord syringocele.[37]

Early surgical repair is recommended in TMC as it may undergo rapid expansion in infancy, thus causing stretch injury to the conus, which is situated at the proximal part of the cyst. Goals of surgery are to reduce the size of the mass by resection of the nonfunctional caudal cyst wall, untether the placode, and finally, close the syringocele cavity by pia–arachnoid suture.[38,39] The caudal part of the central canal is left open to the subarachnoid space by terminal ventriculostomy to avoid hydrosyringomyelia formation.[40]

Diastematomyelia

Diastematomyelia, or a split cord, is due to failure of midline notochordal integration resulting in two hemicords.[21] Further subtypes of this malformation depend on variable primitive notochordal development.[20] MR imaging features can differentiate subtypes by determining the number of dural sacs containing hemicords and if there is an osteocartilaginous spur or fibrous septum.

Axial MR images are best able to show splitting of the spinal cord as well as associated hydromyelia, low conus position, and intradural lipomas.[41] In type 1 diastematomyelia,

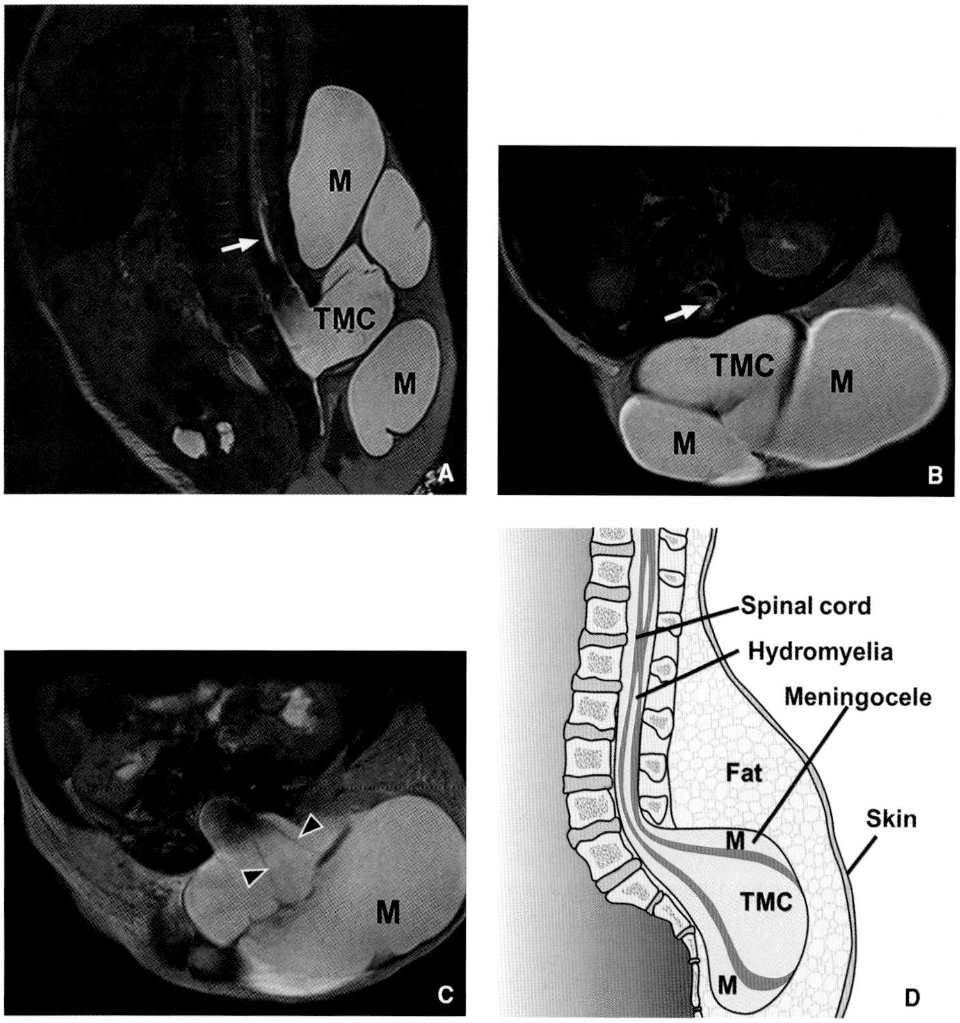

FIGURE 4.15 **Terminal myelocystocele in a newborn girl.** Sagittal T2 **(A)** and axial **(B, C)** T2-weighted MR images show hydromyelia (*arrows*) within the tethered cord, the terminal part of which protrudes through the dorsal spinal defect expanding into a large fluid-filled cyst forming the terminal myelocystocele (*TMC*). Note adjacent extension of the subarachnoid space in the extraspinal fat forming a meningocele (*M*). Multiple cauda equina nerve roots (*arrowheads*) traverse the TMC. Intact skin covers the large cystic mass. (Case courtesy of Sanjay Prabhu, MD, Boston Children's Hospital and Harvard Medical School, Boston, MA.) **D:** Schematic representation of the TMC.

the spinal canal is split into two halves by either an osseous or osteocartilaginous septum (spur), and each dural sac contains a hemicord. The hemicords usually fuse below the spur to form a single cord. Hydromyelia is common in the hemicords and the normal cord above and/or below the splitting. Most cases are also associated with vertebral segmentation anomalies. Osseous anomalies, including the bony septum, may be further evaluated by CT. In type 2 diastematomyelia, a single dural sac contains both hemicords with no osteocartilaginous spur (Fig. 4.16). However, a fibrous septum can occur seen as a thin hypointense band on high-resolution axial and coronal MR images. Again, associated vertebral anomalies are common but generally milder than in type 1 diastematomyelia.

Prophylactic cord untethering and repair of diastematomyelia are advocated for better clinical outcome because residual deficits persist once they are present preoperatively. Associated hydromyelia is always unchanged after surgery, indicating it does not contribute to the neurologic syndrome.[42]

Tethered Cord Syndrome and Filar Lipoma

Tethered cord syndrome is not a single entity but a clinical syndrome that involves progressive neurologic deterioration, in particular, both motor and sensory dysfunction of the lower limbs. Other associated neurologic deficits include spastic gait, muscle atrophy, abnormal reflexes, urinary incontinence, and bony deformities such as scoliosis. The pathogenesis is related to traction of the spinal cord. The cord traction can be directly related to lesions within the spinal canal (in the form of CSD) or secondary to scarring or formation of dermoids after surgical repair of myelomeningocele. When the cord is tethered/stretched, the vascular supply may be compromised, which leads to functional deterioration of nerve cells.[43]

MR imaging shows the classic low conus medullaris position (below the L2–L3 disk space) and variable other associated anomalies of the spine and spinal cord; the most common of which include a tight filum terminale, diastematomyelia,

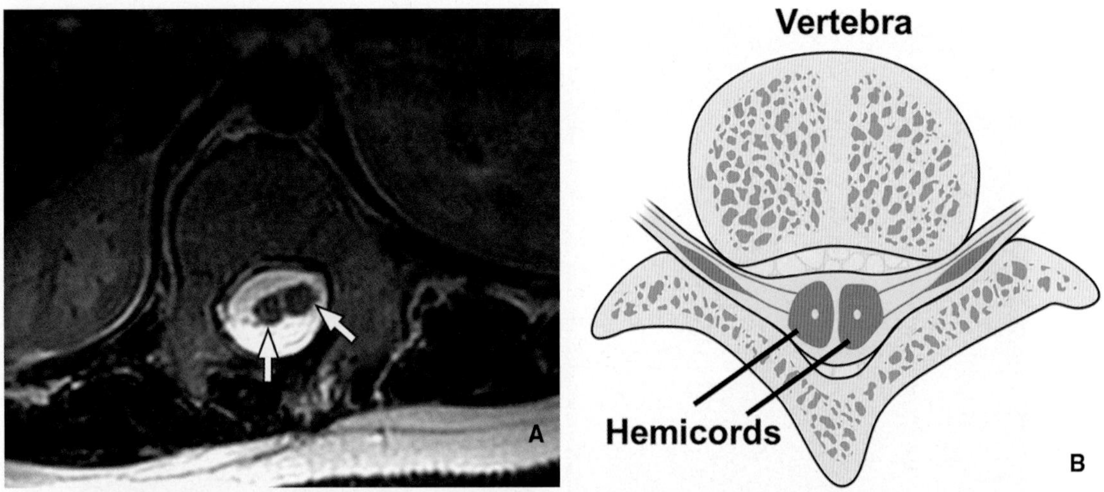

FIGURE 4.16 **Diastematomyelia in an infant boy.** Axial T2-weighted MR image **(A)** and schematic representation **(B)** reveal two hemicords (*arrows*) within a single dural sac. No intervening septum or hydromyelia is seen.

intradural lipomas, and caudal agenesis (Fig. 4.17).[44] The conus may be radiologically "normal" in position in cases of tight filum terminale with or without filar lipomas.[45] The presence of hydromyelia heralds deterioration of neurologic function.

Untethering of the cord is indicated in pediatric patients with progressive or new-onset neurologic symptoms, and the goal of surgery is to improve blood flow within the spinal cord. Surgical success rates vary depending on the nature and severity of anomalies. In general, earlier operative intervention is associated with improved outcome such as pain relief and stabilization of neurologic function. Cord untethering may also halt scoliosis progression.[46]

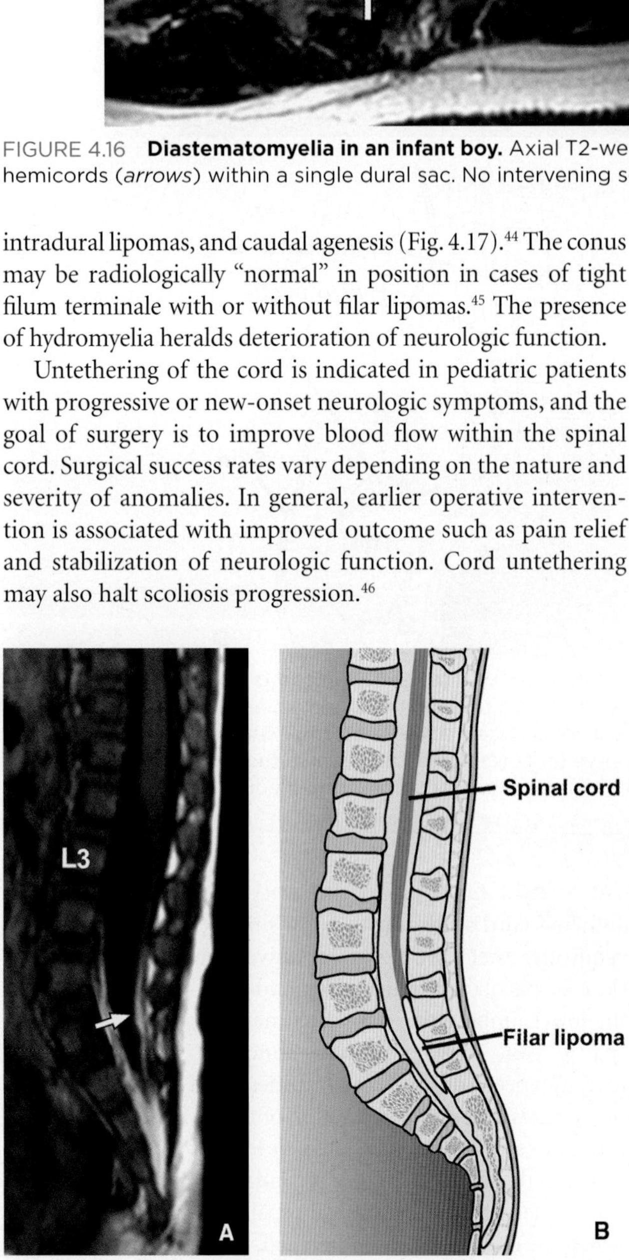

FIGURE 4.17 **Filar lipoma in a 3-month-old boy.** Sagittal T1-weighted MR image **(A)** and schematic representation **(B)** demonstrate hyperintense fat throughout the filum terminale (*arrow*). The spinal cord is low-lying at the L3 level. (Reprinted from Lowe LH, Johanek AJ, Moore CW. Sonography of the neonatal spine: part 2, spinal disorders. *AJR Am J Roentgenol.* 2007;188:739–744, with permission.)

Dermal Sinus

The dermal sinus, a common CSD accounting for ~25% of cases, is an epithelium-lined sinus tract or fistula extending from the skin surface inward where it may connect with the CNS and its meningeal layers.[23] The incidence of dermal sinus is cited as 1 in 2,500 live births, but the exact incidence is unknown.[47] It is most frequently found in the lumbosacral region as a midline dimple or pinpoint ostium above the gluteal crease in the midline, or less commonly, lateral of midline.[48] Associated cutaneous stigmata such as hairy nevi, hyperpigmented patches, or hemangiomas are common. Dermal sinus is believed to be due to incomplete disjunction of cutaneous ectoderm from the neural tube. This leads to the formation of a sinus tract lined by epithelium with dermal elements (Fig. 4.18), all of which may communicate with the CNS.

On MRI, the key feature of a dermal sinus is a hypointense linear focus coursing obliquely and downward in the subcutaneous fat on sagittal images (Fig. 4.19). Associated

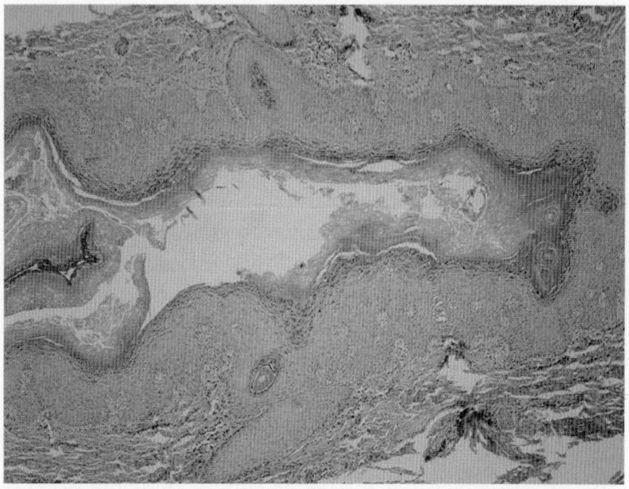

FIGURE 4.18 **Dermal sinus tract in a 1-year-old girl with a sacral dimple.** Note that the tract is lined by keratinizing squamous epithelium with dermal appendages (hematoxylin and eosin, original magnification, 100×).

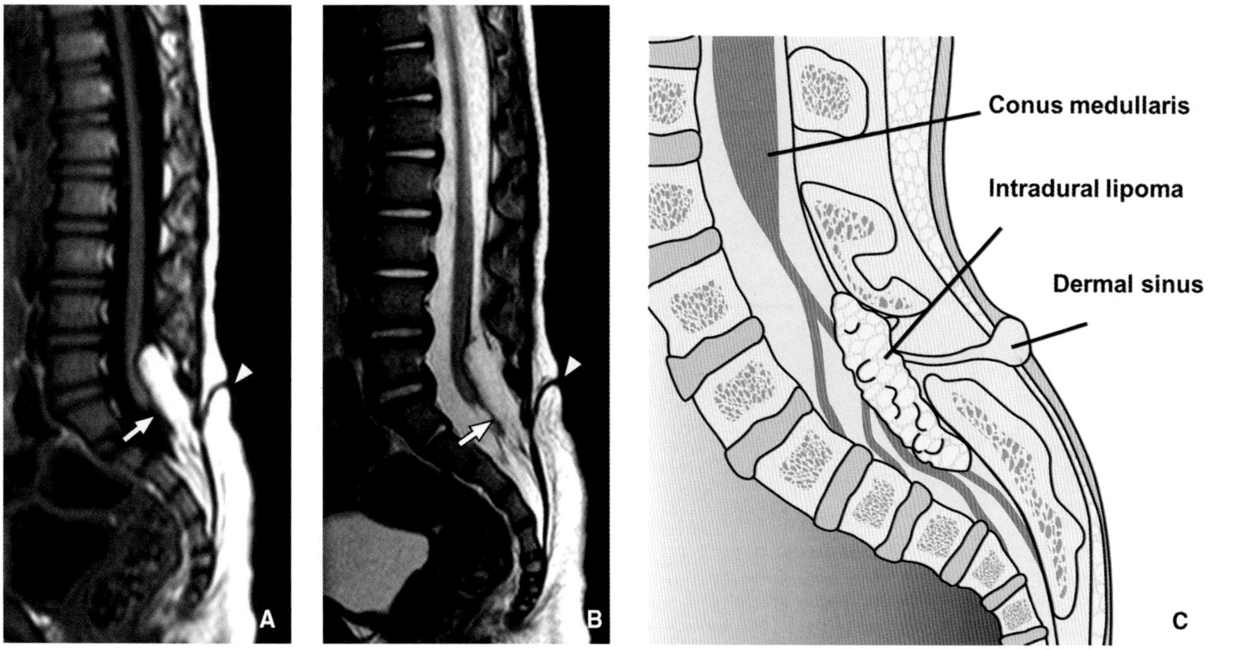

FIGURE 4.19 **Dermal sinus with an intradural lipoma in a 3-year-old boy.** Sagittal T1-weighted MR image **(A)**, sagittal T2-weighted MR image **(B)**, and schematic representation **(C)** show a hypointense subcutaneous sacral dermal sinus (*arrowheads*) within the subcutaneous fat. The spinal cord is tethered and attached to the anterior surface of a T1-hyperintense intradural lipoma (*arrows*) extending from L5 to S2.

intraspinal anomalies are common. Dermal sinuses can be connected to a hypertrophic or fibromatous and/or fatty filum terminale[49] and may have a low conus medullaris and/or an intraspinal lipoma.[50,51] Dermoids at the level of the cauda equina may also be present (inclusion tumor) and are likely due to encystment of part of the dermal sinus tract.[52]

Neonatal lumbar US screening is useful to differentiate a dermal sinus from a coccygeal dimple.[5] US may even be superior to MRI at depicting the relationship of the sinus tract to the conus because of its superior resolution in infants and lack of respiratory artifacts that occur on newborn MRI. However, the utility of US declines in pediatric patients older than 4 months when ossification of the posterior elements of the spine limits the acoustic window.[53]

Untreated dural sinus tracts with subarachnoid connections can serve as a pathway for spread of bacterial infection to the CNS resulting in meningitis and, less frequently, abscess formation. Thus, early surgical sinus tract resection and correction of associated abnormalities are needed.[54]

Intradural Lipoma

Intraspinal lipomas are rare congenital and histologically benign neoplasms that account for <1% of all spinal cord tumors.[55] Of all spinal lipomas, 24% are intradural.[23] Intradural lipomas are most common in the lumbosacral region at the lower thecal sac and present clinically with tethered cord syndrome.[56] They may be solitary or multifocal and may grow to expand the spinal canal. In the cervicothoracic region, they may produce insidious signs of spinal cord compression.

Intradural lipomas are thought to be an anomaly of primary neurulation involving premature disjunction of the neural tube from surrounding ectoderm. The neural plate is left open posteriorly so that mesenchymal cells gain access to the ependymal lining, which induces them to differentiate into fatty tissue.[15,57] The key imaging feature for diagnosis of intradural lipoma is that the mass follows fat signal on all MR sequences including fat suppression sequences (Fig. 4.20). Similarly, it has the same attenuation value as fat on CT and is echogenic on US.

Surgical resection is required in all symptomatic pediatric patients because intradural lipomas may cause mass effect on the conus and nerve roots. The surgical goals are to release tethered neural elements and reduce lesion size. The decision to operate in asymptomatic pediatric patients with intradural lipomas is controversial; however, early decompressive surgery is suggested for patients with large intradural lipomas to prevent clinical worsening if the lesion increases in size as the child grows.[58]

Hydrosyringomyelia

Hydrosyringomyelia is a chronic degenerative process of the spinal cord in which the central canal gradually expands. In children, it is most often developmental, is seen in association with Chiari malformations, and can present at any age.[59] However, it may be idiopathic or acquired because of spinal cord tumors, hemorrhage, infarcts, or trauma. The pathophysiology of hydrosyringomyelia is thought to be related to abnormal cerebrospinal fluid (CSF) flow dynamics. One theory suggests that it may be due to increased pressure in the subarachnoid space, whereas a more recent theory suggests that it is an extracellular accumulation of CSF within the distended spinal cord.[60,61] The clinical presentation of hydrosyringomyelia may include skeletal lesions such as scoliosis or pes cavus and sensory deficits.[62] Other presenting symptoms

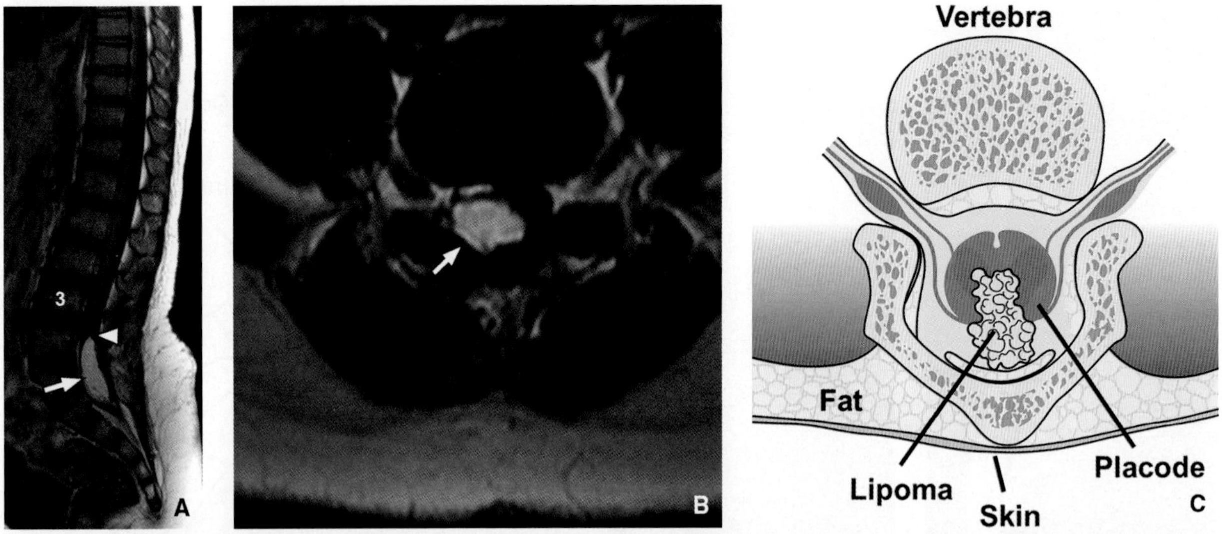

FIGURE 4.20 **Intradural lipoma in a 2-year-old boy.** Sagittal **(A)** and axial **(B)** T1-weighted MR images identify a low-lying conus (*arrowhead*) tethered to a sacral lipoma (*arrow*). Note that the lipoma is intradural and clearly separated from the subcutaneous fat on the axial MR image. Also note slight widening of the spinal canal and "3" indicating the third lumbar vertebra. **C:** Axial schematic representation of intradural lipoma.

may include lower cranial nerve palsy, motor weakness, and muscle atrophy.[62]

Although hydrosyringomyelia may be seen clearly with sonography in infants, MRI with contrast is usually needed for complete assessment of the brain and spinal cord, especially if surgery is planned. The key finding on MRI is T2-hyperintense central cord distention over one or many vertebral segments (Fig. 4.21). When a syrinx is seen, a careful search must be made for an underlying cause, such as a Chiari I malformation, cord tumor, or other cord lesion. Although no contrast enhancement is seen in simple cases of hydrosyringomyelia, contrast is often given during the initial assessment to search for small occult tumors or vascular malformations. MRI allows performance of reconstructed isotropic 3D heavily

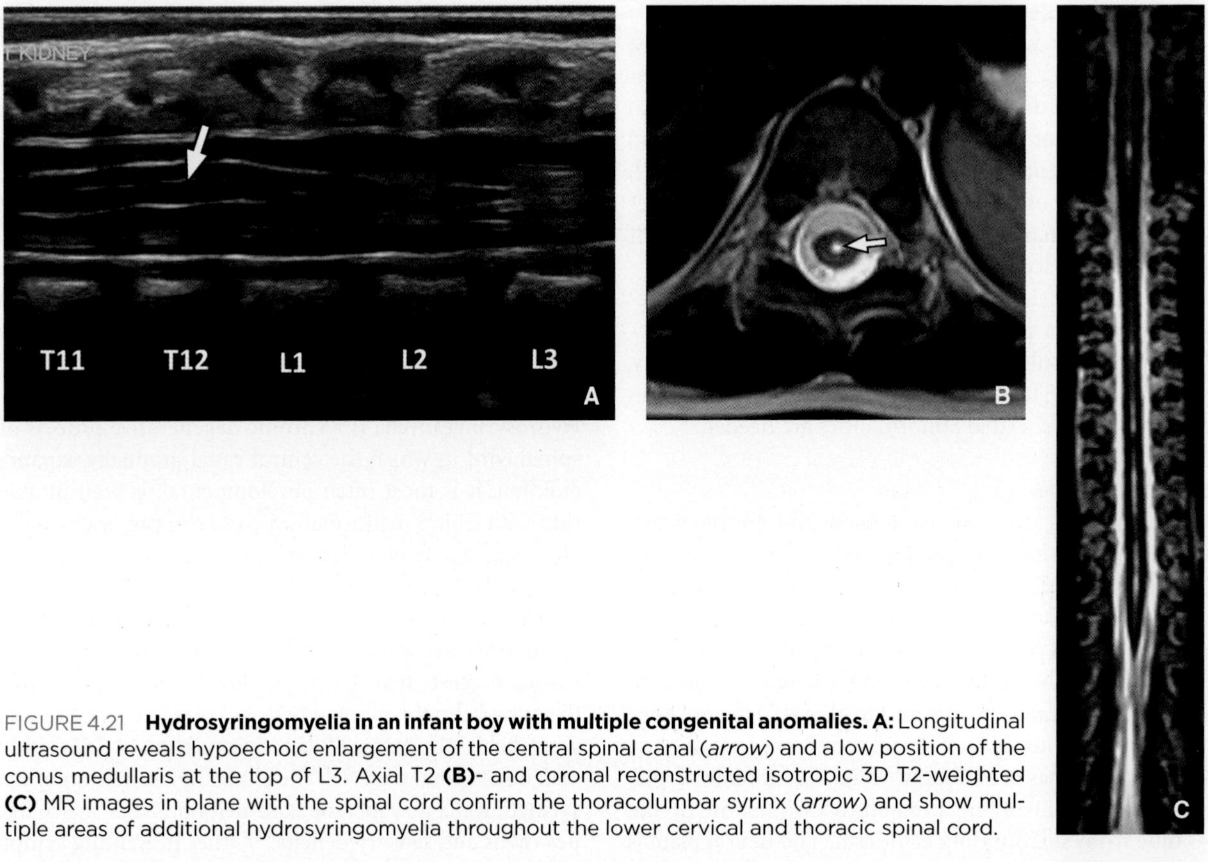

FIGURE 4.21 **Hydrosyringomyelia in an infant boy with multiple congenital anomalies. A:** Longitudinal ultrasound reveals hypoechoic enlargement of the central spinal canal (*arrow*) and a low position of the conus medullaris at the top of L3. Axial T2 **(B)**- and coronal reconstructed isotropic 3D T2-weighted **(C)** MR images in plane with the spinal cord confirm the thoracolumbar syrinx (*arrow*) and show multiple areas of additional hydrosyringomyelia throughout the lower cervical and thoracic spinal cord.

T2-weighted MR images of the entire spinal cord, improving visualization of lesions in the setting of scoliosis and allowing physiologic assessment of CSF flow in Chiari I malformations using phase contrast sequences.[60,63,64]

Treatment of hydrosyringomyelia depends on its cause. Early posterior fossa decompression with or without duraplasty is performed in Chiari I malformations with associated syrinx, leading to symptomatic improvement in 70% to 85% of affected patients.[59,65,66] Spinal cord tumors and vascular lesions may be debulked or resected. Some vascular lesions may undergo catheter embolization, which is discussed in greater detail later in this chapter.

Neurenteric Cysts

Neurenteric cysts are lined by a mucin-secreting epithelium resembling that of the alimentary tract (Fig. 4.22). They can be found anywhere along the spinal canal and are typically located in the cervicothoracic region anterior to the cord. Fewer lesions are found at the lumbar and sacral levels.[67] The pathogenesis is related to endodermal differentiation of primitive streak remnants that remain trapped within a split notochord.

Neurenteric cysts can be viewed as gut duplication within the spinal canal. They include three histologic types. Type 1 is the simplest and most common form, which is thin walled with a layer of stratified or pseudostratified cuboidal or columnar epithelium. The more complex forms are less common, characterized by additional mesodermal elements such as smooth muscle and fat (Type 2) and sometimes ependymal or glial tissue (Type 3). Neurenteric cysts can be isolated or associated with spinal defects or diastematomyelia.[68] The most common pediatric presentation is cord compression,[50] usually in the first decade of life,[69] although meningism (symptoms mimicking meningitis) is the presenting feature in newborns and infants.[70]

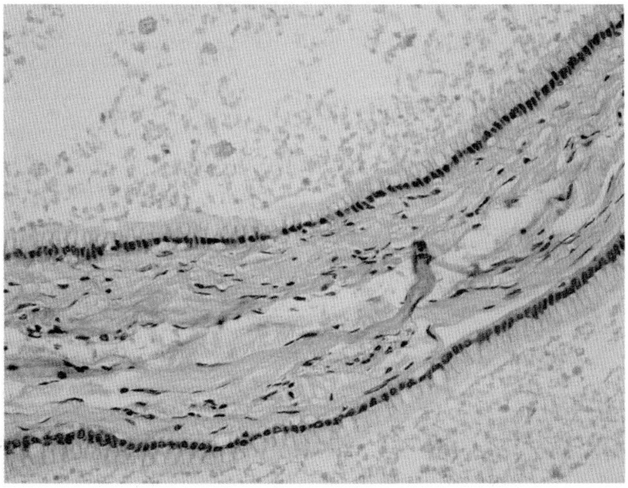

FIGURE 4.22 **Neurenteric cyst in a 9-year-old boy.** This intradural extramedullary mass from the cervical region was cystic, with septa showing a simple enterogenous epithelial lining resembling that of gastric pylorus (hematoxylin and eosin, original magnification, 200×).

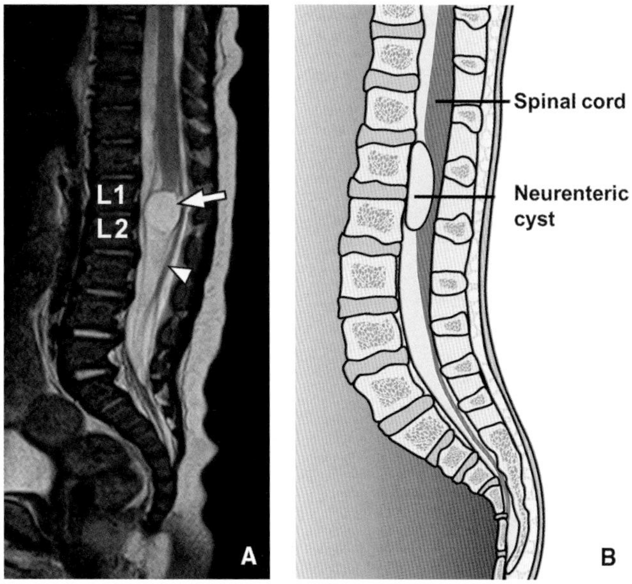

FIGURE 4.23 **Neurenteric cyst in a 2-year-old boy.** Sagittal T1-weighted MR image **(A)** and schematic representation **(B)** show an intradural cyst (*arrow*) ventral to the conus medullaris at L1–L2. Note that the normal filum terminale (*arrowhead*) is displaced by the cyst. (MR image courtesy of In-one Kim, MD, Seoul National University Hospital, South Korea.)

Key imaging features of neurenteric cysts (Fig. 4.23) include a cyst without enhancement that is either T1 isointense or slightly T1 hyperintense on MRI because of variable proteinaceous contents.[71]

The treatment of neurenteric cysts is complete surgical resection.[71] If total excision is not feasible because of adherence of cyst to vital structures, wide fenestration of the cyst wall is performed. The overall prognosis depends on associated anomalies, but usually long-term stability and survival are achieved.[72]

Infectious Disorders

Viral Myelitis

Viral myelitis is rare, but important to consider in children with acute myelopathy. Although many viruses may involve the spinal cord, such as polioviruses, enterovirus 71 (which causes hand-foot-and-mouth disease), arboviruses (e.g., West Nile virus), flaviviruses, coxsackie viruses, human immunodeficiency virus (HIV), Japanese encephalitis virus, and echovirus, isolation of a specific virus is rare.[73–75] The pathophysiology in viral myelitis is not well understood. It may be related to primary viral infection or postinfectious demyelination immune response.[76]

Clinically, affected pediatric patients most often present with sensory loss, bilateral upper and/or lower extremity weakness, aseptic meningitis, rhombencephalitis, myoclonus, tremor, and bladder and bowel dysfunction.[74] Acute flaccid paralysis may occur, indicating spinal cord anterior horn involvement.[76]

Initial workup of these children should include MRI evaluation of the brain and entire spinal cord in order to determine the extent of disease, exclude surgical causes of paralysis, and narrow the differential diagnosis.[76] Spinal cord

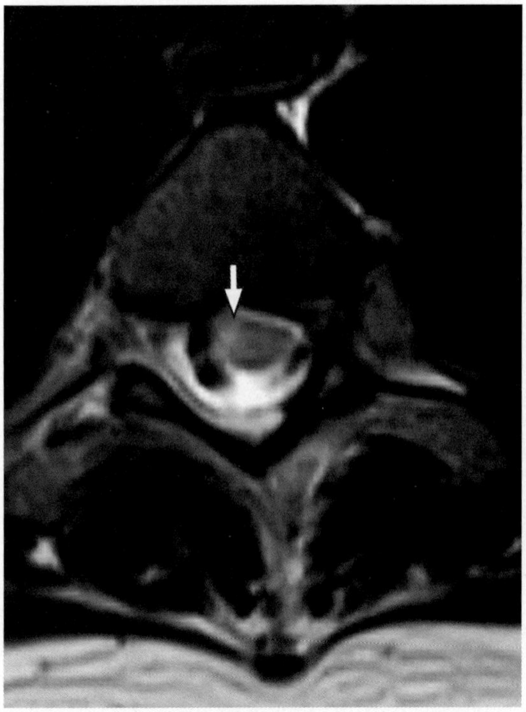

FIGURE 4.24 **Viral myelitis in a 5-year-old girl who presented with arm weakness and pain.** Axial T2-weighted MR image shows a unilateral, mostly anterior lesion (*arrow*) in the thoracic spinal cord.

lesions are T2 hyperintense with variable enhancement. They may be single or multiple, unilateral or bilateral, and classically involve the anterior cord (Fig. 4.24).[75–77] Superficial leptomeningeal enhancement of the spinal cord, nerve roots—especially the ventral roots—and cauda equina may be seen.[75,76] When lesions involve both sides of the cord, the appearance is the same as transverse myelitis.[78] MRI of the brain is useful to look for additional viral lesions and to help exclude other disorders such as multiple sclerosis.

The treatment for viral myelitis is largely supportive. However, it may include methylprednisolone or antiviral medications in cases with PCR sequence identification of a specific virus.[74] The prognosis in viral myelitis varies. In one study of children with enterovirus 71 myelitis, 57% completely recovered and 43% were left with at least a mild deficit.[76,79] Children with bilateral rather than unilateral MRI lesions were more likely to have persistent morbidity such as arm or leg weakness,[76] and those with cardiopulmonary failure associated with brain lesions were more likely to have neurodevelopmental delay and permanent morbidity.[80]

Bacterial Myelitis

Bacterial myelitis is caused by a variety of agents, including *streptococcus*, *staphylococcus*, *Mycoplasma pneumoniae*, *Mycobacterium tuberculosis*, *rickettsia*, and *Borrelia burgdorferi* (Lyme disease/neuroborreliosis).[81] Although intracranial manifestations, such as meningitis, are most common, spinal myelitis and abscess occur occasionally.[82–84] The disease source is hematologic spread of infections from other organ systems, such as skin, lungs, and the gastrointestinal tract.[85]

The pathogenesis of bacterial myelitis may be because of direct bacterial infection and/or a secondary immune-mediated response in which the host produces antibodies that attack the spinal cord.[83,86]

The clinical presentation may be gradual or acute including fever, upper and/or lower extremity weakness, paralysis, and/or paresthesias. Bladder and bowel dysfunction, ataxia, postural instability, back pain, respiratory difficulty, intractable vomiting, and fever may also occur.[83,84,87] Associated septic meningitis, encephalitis, stroke, radiculopathy, and transverse myelitis are seen with Mycoplasma.[86]

MRI is the initial imaging modality of choice in bacterial myelitis. Imaging findings are nonspecific, including T2-hyperintense cord swelling with variable enhancement of the superficial cord and/or nerve roots (Fig. 4.25).[82,85,87] A focal lesion with ring enhancement should raise concern for a bacterial etiology.[85] Lesions of the thoracic cord, enhancing basilar cisterns, and epidural and/or cord abscesses may suggest a diagnosis of tuberculosis (Fig. 4.26).[84] Neuroborreliosis/Lyme disease and tuberculosis may have cranial nerve enhancement as well.[88] The differential diagnosis for spinal cord lesions is lengthy but can be limited by correlating with history, physical findings, and laboratory data.

Treatment depends on the cause of myelitis but typically includes antibacterial medications and methylprednisolone.[85] Bacterial abscesses of the cord usually resolve with antibiotics; however, in cases with associated epidural or soft tissue abscesses, surgical drainage may be required.[83–85] Prognosis varies depending on the severity and extent of infection. Cord atrophy and cavitation portend permanent morbidity.[84]

Neoplastic Disorders

Spinal tumors occur predominantly in young or middle-aged adults and are less common in children. Only 2% of all childhood tumors are spinal in origin. Often symptoms are nonspecific, most commonly manifesting as neck or back pain and clumsiness.[89] More specific symptoms may include motor weakness, changes in gait, spinal curvature, and bowel and bladder dysfunction. In the setting of acute trauma, peritumoral edema may cause paresis or paralysis. This chapter presents an overview of spinal neoplasms, with subsequent detailed discussion of lesions categorized based on anatomic location: intramedullary, intradural extramedullary, and extradural.[90]

The imaging features of spinal neoplasms are often nonspecific with overlapping findings. However, familiarity with age at diagnosis combined with key imaging findings and associations may be helpful in narrowing the differential diagnosis.

Although plain radiographs may show osseous spinal erosions, this is a late finding, making radiography of limited utility for defining and characterizing pediatric spinal cord tumors. Unenhanced CT is helpful to image primary osseous lesions, but it is not the best imaging modality for evaluating the spinal cord. Instead, MRI is the study of choice to define and characterize spinal cord lesions.

Differentiating intramedullary (within the cord) versus extramedullary (outside of the cord) and intradural (within

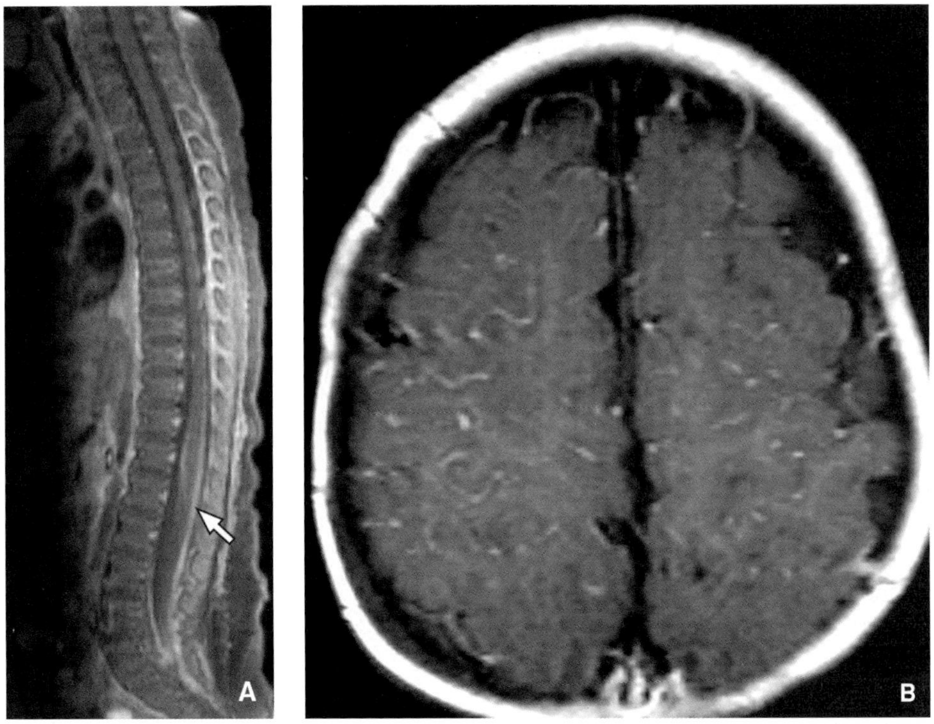

FIGURE 4.25 **Bacterial meningitis (*Streptococcus*) in a 12-month-old girl with decreased arm and leg movement. A:** Sagittal postcontrast T1-weighted MR image of the spine shows enhancement on the surface of the spinal cord and nerve roots (*arrow*) of the cauda equina. **B:** Axial postcontrast T1-weighted MR image of the brain demonstrates leptomeningeal enhancement throughout the brain sulci, right greater than left.

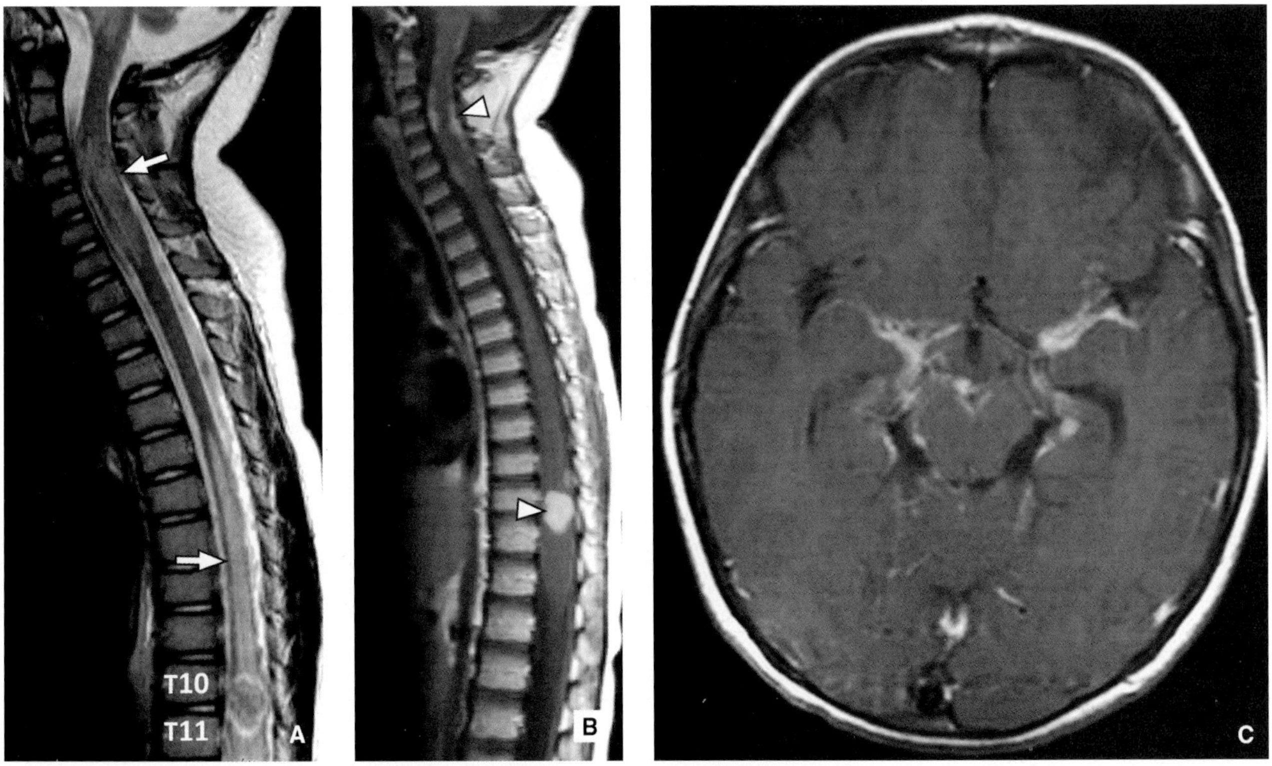

FIGURE 4.26 **Tuberculous myelitis in a 20-month-old boy with seizures and hypotonia.** Sagittal T2-weighted **(A)** and postcontrast T1-weighted **(B)** MR images reveal scattered regions of cord edema (*arrows*) with variable contrast enhancement (*arrowheads*). Note the focal lesion posterior to T10–T11 concerning for developing abscess. **C:** Axial postcontrast T1-weighted MR image of the brain shows extensive enhancement of structures in the basilar cisterns.

the thecal sac) versus extradural (outside the thecal sac, likely osseous) lesions is important and can be accomplished with multiplanar MRI. Intramedullary lesions show cord expansion, whereas extramedullary lesions are separate from the cord in at least one of three planes. Intraoperative ultrasound may be used to determine tumor location and borders during exposure and resection. Baseline postoperative MRI is deferred for at least 12 weeks as surgical changes make early postoperative scans difficult to interpret.[91]

The treatment goal with benign, noninfiltrative spinal neoplasms is complete excision of both the solid tumor and associated syrinx cavities. If any portion of the neoplasm infiltrates the cord, surgical success decreases. Adjuvant radiation therapy and chemotherapy may be used, but the prognosis with an infiltrative, malignant lesion remains dismal.[92]

The surgical approach begins with a laminectomy and myelotomy to access and centrally debulk the tumor. Electrophysiologic monitoring techniques can be helpful when removing the periphery of the tumor, in order to prevent damage to the healthy lateral columns of the spinal cord. The tumor and its associated syrinx cavity are resected to their interface with normal-appearing spinal cord.

In general, preoperative neurologic deficits may persist postoperatively, but most tumors can be removed without new long-term disabilities. Symptomatic recurrences can be managed by reoperation. Residual and recurrent tumor deposits often remain static for years or grow very slowly. If complete tumor excision is not possible with histologically benign pediatric intramedullary gliomas, adjuvant radiation therapy is preferentially avoided because of adverse effects on the immature spinal cord and spinal column.

Surgical management is considered with extradural tumors to establish pathologic diagnosis with biopsy, to decompress the spinal cord in the setting of progressive myelopathy, for reconstruction in cases of spinal instability, and with attempted radical resection for cure. The majority of childhood spinal epidural lesions are responsive to radiation or chemotherapy.[93]

Intramedullary Neoplasms

Pediatric intramedullary tumors occur most commonly in the cervicothoracic cord.[94] These are slow-growing tumors and thus present with nonspecific symptoms. Therefore, diagnosis is often delayed. Up to 67% of affected pediatric patients present with back pain, typically diffuse and worse when lying in a horizontal position, making nighttime pain a common complaint.[95] Younger pediatric patients may present with dull, aching spinal pain, rigidity, muscle spasm, motor regression, and frequent falls.[95,96] Older pediatric patients may present with gait disturbance and/or progressive scoliosis. Extremity weakness and paresthesias are common as well.[96] Symptoms of increased intracranial pressure and hydrocephalus are the presenting complaint in 15% of affected pediatric patients.[95] Imaging findings and associations are summarized in Table 4.1.

Astrocytoma

Approximately 60% of intramedullary tumors in children are astrocytomas, which are most commonly located in the cervical cord.[92,95] Spinal astrocytomas have an equal sex predilection and usually occur in children around 10 years of age; they are rarely seen in neonates and infants.[96] They may present with pain and motor dysfunction, gait disturbance, scoliosis, torticollis (head tilt), and loss or absence of developmental milestones. Symptoms are often protracted.[95,96] Astrocytomas arise from astrocytes and range from benign (grade I) to malignant (grade IV).[97]

Pilocytic astrocytomas are at the benign end of the spectrum (Fig. 4.27), and high-grade astrocytomas and glioblastoma multiforme are at the malignant end of the spectrum.[95]

TABLE 4.1 Pediatric Intramedullary Spinal Neoplasms: Key Imaging Features, Associations, Treatments, and Other Comments

Neoplasm	Key Imaging Features	Associations, Treatments, and Other Comments
Astrocytoma	Cervical region most common	~10 years of age
	Tend to be eccentric within cord +/− syrinx	Treatment—surgical debulking, +/− chemotherapy, and radiation
Ependymoma	Cervical region most common Tend to be central within cord	~13.5 years of age
	Hemosiderin cap on T2-weighted MRI	If multiple lesions, consider NF2
	Drop metastases	Treatment - surgical debulking, +/- chemotherapy, and radiation
Ganglioglioma	Similar appearance to ependymoma	~7 years of age
		Associated with NF2
		Treatment—surgical resection
Hemangioblastoma	Cystic lesion with enhancing mural nodule	Associated with von Hippel-Lindau disease
	Flow voids	Treatment—surgery

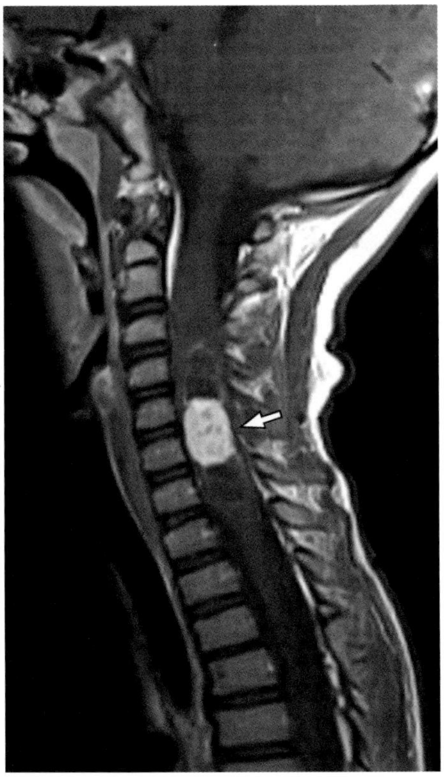

FIGURE 4.27 **Astrocytoma in an 8-year-old boy who presented with upper back pain.** Sagittal postcontrast T1-weighted MR image demonstrates an intramedullary cystic mass with a large central enhancing nodule (*arrow*) and minimal enhancement along cyst margins.

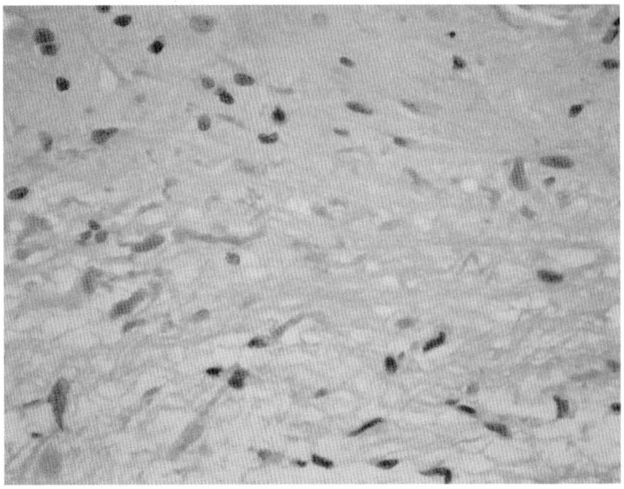

FIGURE 4.29 **Pilocytic astrocytoma in a 4-year-old girl with an intramedullary mass extending from the midthoracic region to the conus medullaris.** Cells have round to elongate nuclei and long hair-like eosinophilic cytoplasmic processes (hematoxylin and eosin, original magnification, 600×).

Grossly, spinal astrocytomas may be cystic, mixed cystic–solid, solid, or variably necrotic. Malignant astrocytomas can mimic spinal vascular malformations because of hypervascularity and variable intratumoral hemorrhage. Lesion size varies from focal to diffuse involvement of the spinal cord. When the disease extends from the cervicomedullary junction to the tip of the conus, it is referred to as holocordal; in astrocytoma, such extensive involvement is usually seen during the first year of life (Figs. 4.28 and 4.29).[98] Astrocytomas can be associated with neurofibromatosis type 1 (NF1).[95]

Contrast-enhanced spinal MRI is critical to identify small tumors with associated syringohydromyelia and to detect subarachnoid seeding. Key imaging features of astrocytomas include cord expansion, eccentric location, T1 hypointensity, heterogeneous T2 hyperintensity, and a cyst with an enhancing mural nodule. Marginal enhancement of the lesion is also common (Fig. 4.30).[94]

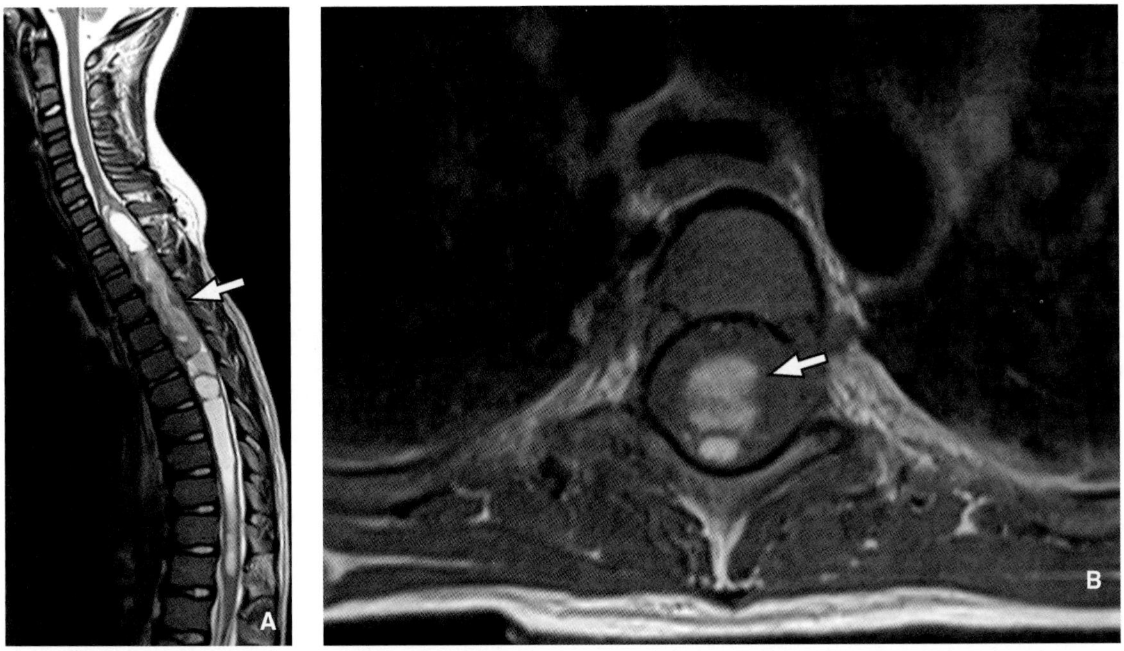

FIGURE 4.28 **Astrocytoma in a 6-year-old boy who presented with pain and decreased right arm use. A:** Sagittal T2-weighted MR image shows an intramedullary cystic cervical cord mass with a mural nodule (*arrow*). Note the small amount of T2 hyperintense cord edema above the mass. **B:** Axial postcontrast T1-weighted MR image shows nodule enhancement (*arrow*).

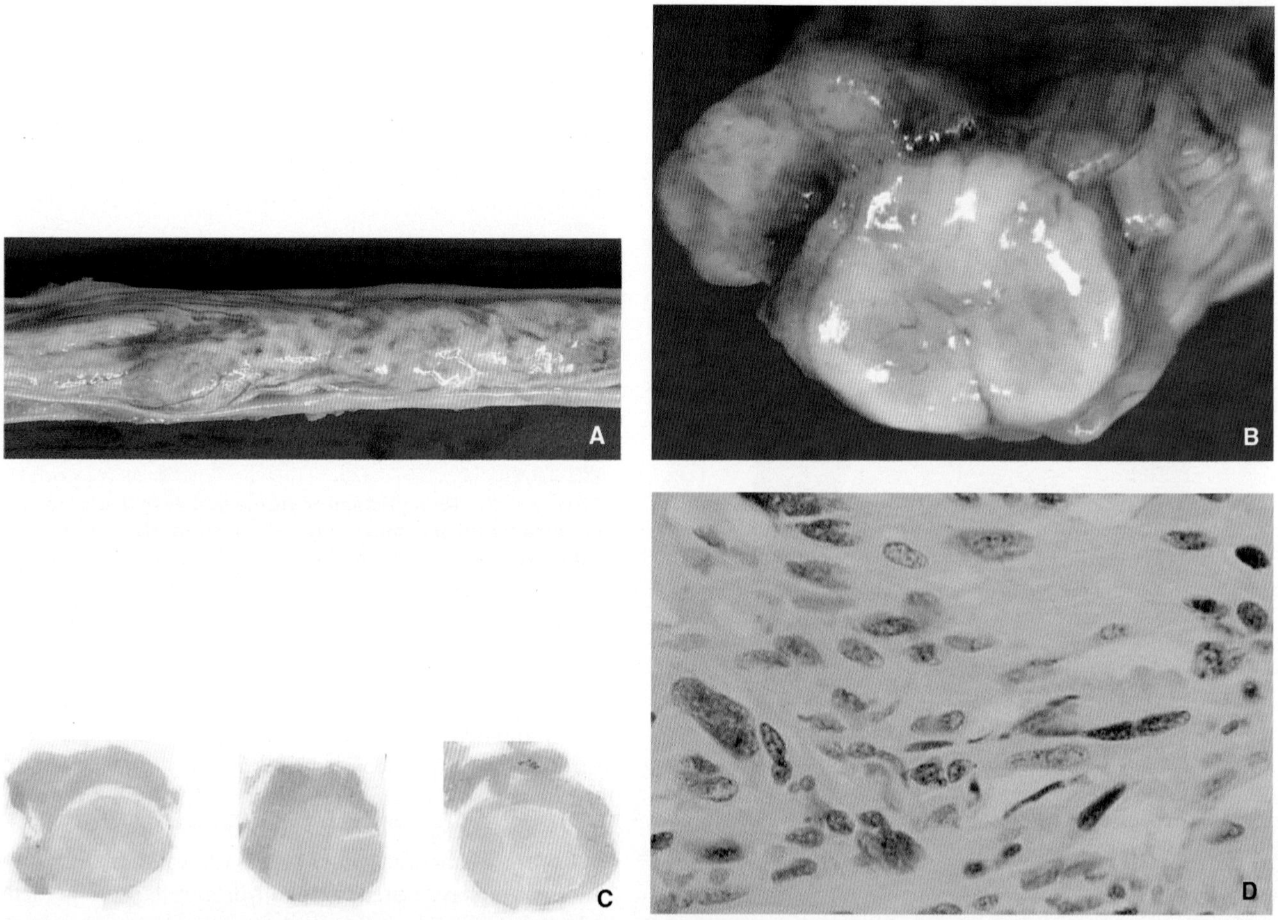

FIGURE 4.30 **Glioblastoma with leptomeningeal spread in a 13-year-old boy (autopsy specimen). A:** On gross inspection, the leptomeninges show areas of opacity and nodularity. **B:** Transverse gross section shows extramedullary intradural tumor. **C:** Microscopic sections confirm leptomeningeal involvement by high-grade glial tumor at multiple levels using hematoxylin and eosin, original magnification, 1x. **D:** Hematoxylin and eosin, original magnification, 400x.

Treatment for intramedullary astrocytoma includes a combination of surgical debulking, maximum safe resection with adjuvant chemotherapy, and, rarely, radiation treatment.[99] Prognosis is most dependent on tumor grade with a 4-year survival rate of 68%.[98,99]

Ependymoma

Up to 30% of intramedullary tumors in children are ependymomas.[95] They present in an older age group, 13 to 14 years, with a slight female predilection.[92] Ependymomas originate from ependymal cells lining the central canal, and as a result, are frequently located centrally within the cord. Ependymomas occur sporadically but may also be associated with neurofibromatosis type 2 (NF2). They may arise within the central spinal cord or filum terminale and frequently span multiple segments. Holocord involvement, as with astrocytomas, is possible.[100] Grossly, ependymomas have well-demarcated borders, typically compressing the adjacent cord as opposed to infiltrating it.[95]

A variety of histologic types of ependymomas exist: cellular, papillary, clear cell, and tanycytic, with cellular ependymoma being the most common. Myxopapillary ependymoma, a separate low-grade type of ependymoma with distinctive histologic features (Fig. 4.31), occurs exclusively in the lower cord and filum terminale.

Surgical management of the myxopapillary subtype is difficult because of varied physical consistency of the lesion and relationship to surrounding nerve roots. When occurring in the cauda equina, this subtype may be associated with subarachnoid hemorrhage, back pain, lower extremity weakness, numbness, and bowel and bladder incontinence.[101]

Ependymomas are identified by their central cord location, cord expansion, well-circumscribed, iso- to hypointense signal on TI-weighted MR images, and iso- to hyperintense signal on T2-weighted MR images. Contrast enhancement varies. A key imaging feature seen in 20% of cases is a rim of T2 hypointense signal along the border of the neoplasm that is referred to as the "cap sign."[95] It represents hemosiderin deposition secondary to intratumoral hemorrhage along the cranial or caudal aspect of the tumor (Figs. 4.32 and 4.33).[102,103] Contrast-enhanced spinal MRI is useful to assess for drop metastasis, a common feature with ependymomas.[102,103] Similarly, cranial MRI is useful in detecting metastatic spread to the brain and resultant hydrocephalus. Multiple ependymomas should prompt consideration of underlying NF2.[104]

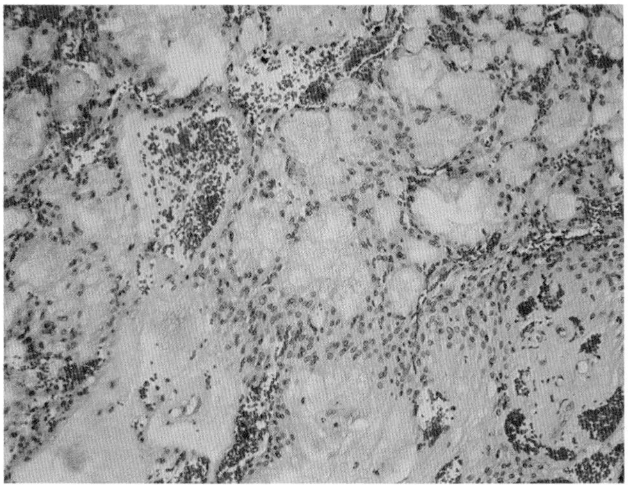

FIGURE 4.31 **Myxopapillary ependymoma in a 16-year-old boy who presented with chronic back pain because of lumbar spinal cord mass.** Microscopic image shows round tumor cells arranged radially around blood vessels and prominent bluish myxoid material between tumor cells and vessels (hematoxylin and eosin, original magnification, 200×).

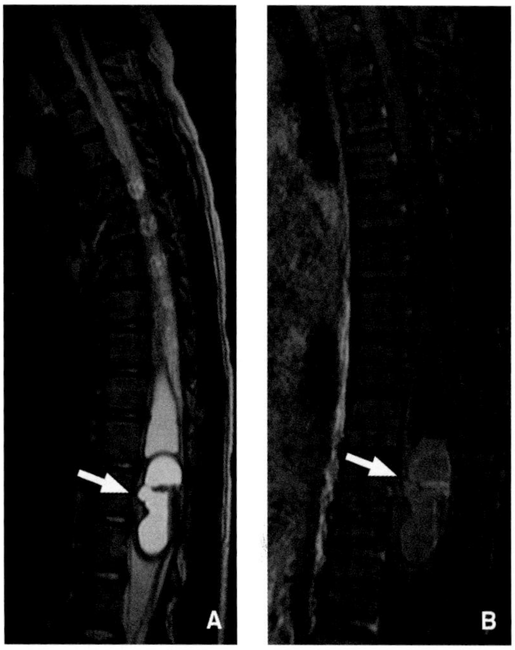

FIGURE 4.33 **Myxopapillary ependymoma in an 11-year-old girl who presented with back pain. A:** Sagittal T2-weighted MR image shows a well-defined hyperintense mass (*arrow*) just below the conus medullaris. An internal fluid–fluid level is seen because of internal hemorrhage. **B:** Axial postcontrast T1-weighted MR image identifies mild heterogeneous enhancement of the mass (*arrow*).

Treatment of ependymomas is strongly dependent on the degree of tumor resection and grade. Myxopapillary ependymomas, tumors with incomplete resections, higher grade lesions, and lesions in the lower spinal cord have been reported to have a higher relapse rate and thus may require additional adjunctive chemotherapy or radiotherapy.[105]

Ganglioglioma

Gangliogliomas account for up to 15% of pediatric intramedullary spinal neoplasms.[95] They present in the first three decades of life with the average age at presentation being around 12 years.[94,106] These neoplasms are composed of ganglion cells and glial elements. Gangliogliomas are typically low grade, slow growing tumors, with a high chance of local recurrence after resection. Histologically, large ganglion-like cells (possibly representing dysplastic neurons) are scattered

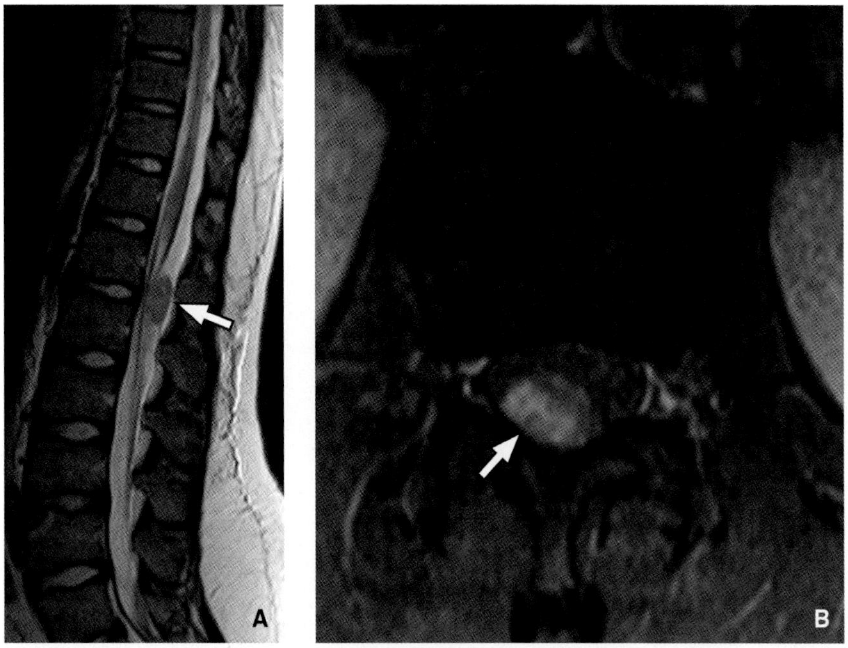

FIGURE 4.32 **Ependymoma in an 11-year-old boy with unexplained altered mental status. A:** Sagittal T2-weighted MR image demonstrates a T2 isointense mass (*arrow*) at T12–L1 displacing the nerve roots ventrally. **B:** Axial postcontrast T1-weighted MR image reveals enhancement of the mass (*arrow*).

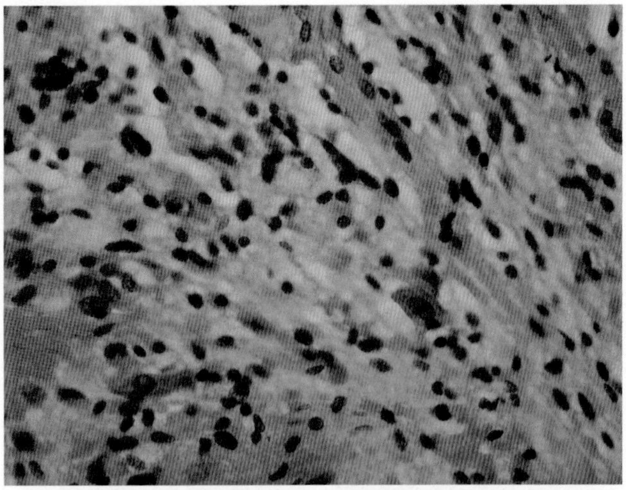

FIGURE 4.34 **Ganglioglioma in a 15-year-old boy with a one year of unilateral leg weakness and atrophy.** This microscopic specimen from the conus medullaris reveals mature ganglion cells admixed with neoplastic glial cells (hematoxylin and eosin, original magnification, 600×).

among proliferating glial cells (Fig. 4.34). Other findings may include eosinophilic granular bodies, stromal desmoplasia, calcification, and lymphoplasmacytic infiltrates.[95]

Gangliogliomas may be solid, cystic, calcified, or hemorrhagic. They demonstrate heterogeneous signal intensity on all sequences.[107] Key imaging features include a heterogeneous mass without peritumoral edema even when large in size, and associated adjacent osseous erosion (Fig. 4.35).[106] Additional helpful imaging characteristics are long tumor length, patchy tumor enhancement, superficial cord enhancement, and mixed signal intensity on T1-weighted MR imaging secondary to dual cellular elements of the tumor.[95] Given this lesion's similar MRI appearance to ependymoma and association with NF2, it should be included in the differential diagnosis whenever ependymoma is considered in the pediatric population.[106]

Gangliogliomas of the spinal cord are surgically resected. The degree of complete surgical resection determines the prognosis. The 5-year survival rate is 83%.[108,109]

Hemangioblastoma

Hemangioblastomas are benign, capillary-rich neoplasms that rarely occur in the pediatric population. Approximately 75% of these neoplasms are intramedullary, but they can be pial, subpial, or combined intramedullary–extramedul lary.[95,110–112] Hemangioblastomas are most common in the cervical and thoracic cord. von Hippel Lindau (VHL) disease should be considered, with screening for VHL gene mutations, when these tumors are diagnosed. Hemangioblastomas are associated with VHL in one-third to one-half of cases.[95]

Key imaging features of hemangioblastomas include a cystic mass with variable T1 signal depending on the proteinaceous content of the cyst fluid, T2 hyperintensity, variable enhancement of mural nodules, and a syrinx in up to 50%. Flow voids are produced by the arterial supply and draining veins of the lesion. Associated hemorrhage and peritumoral edema are common.[113]

Histologically, hemangioblastoma consists of numerous small vascular channels as well as a population of stromal cells that often contain cytoplasmic vacuoles, imparting a clear cell appearance (Fig. 4.36). As with other spinal cord

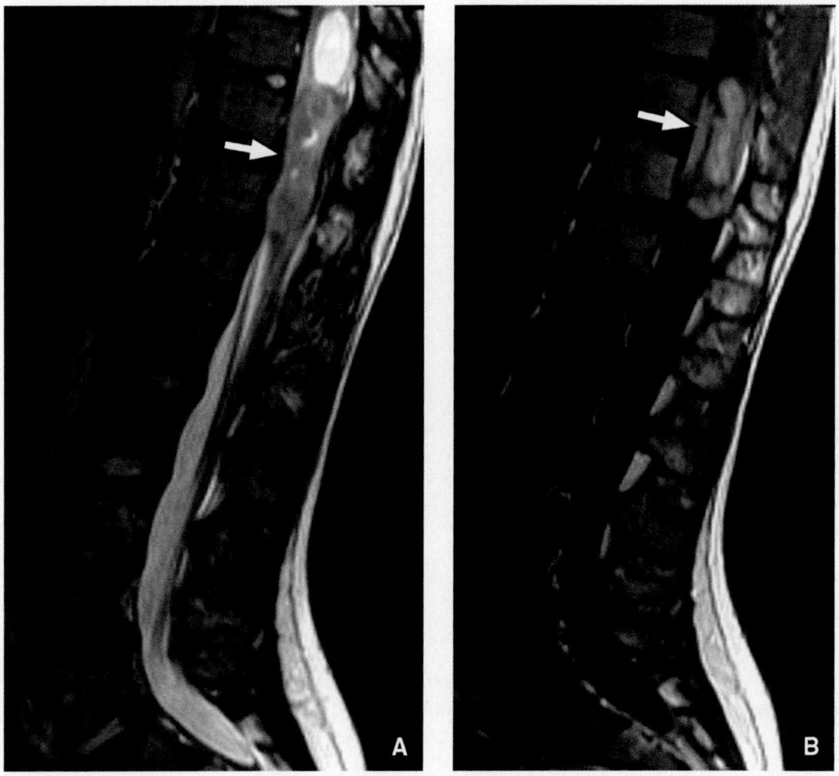

FIGURE 4.35 **Ganglioglioma in an 11-year-old boy with scoliosis and itching. A:** Sagittal T2-weighted MR image demonstrates a heterogeneous lesion (*arrow*) centered at T10–T11. Note the T2 bright cystic component at the superior aspect of the lesion. **B:** Sagittal postcontrast T1-weighted MR image shows lesion enhancement (*arrow*).

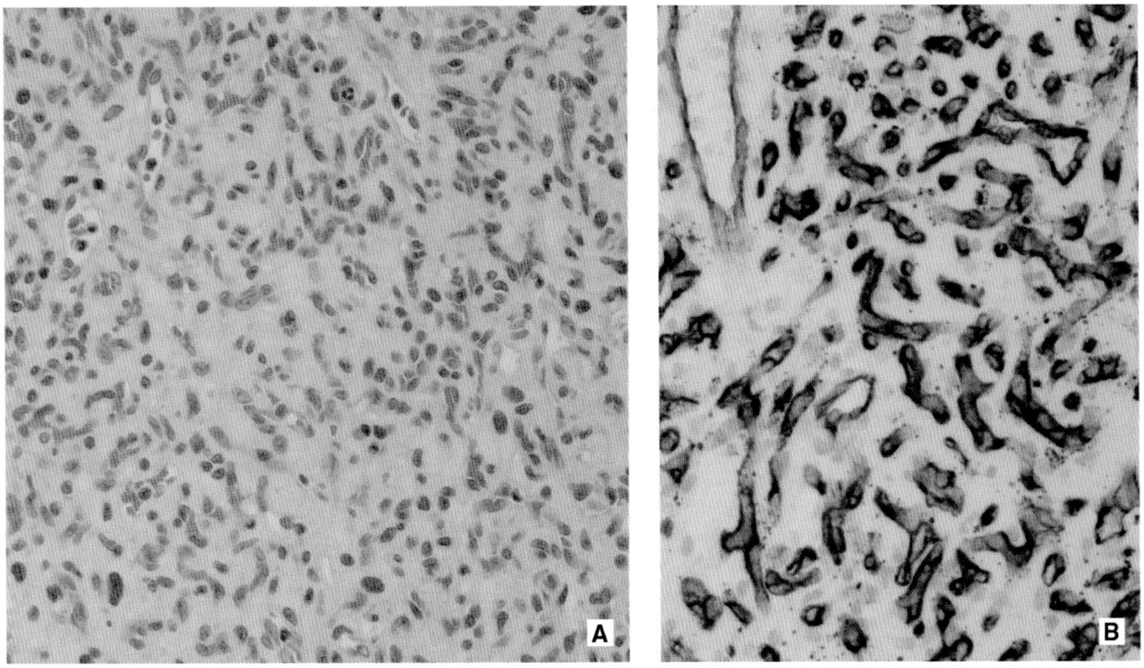

FIGURE 4.36 **Hemangioblastoma in a 13-year-old boy with neck pain. A:** Microscopic material from an intradural mass consists of round uniform tumor cells with abundant cytoplasm and a prominent vascular network (hematoxylin and eosin, original magnification, 400x). **B:** The vascular network is highlighted by an immunostain for CD34 (original magnification, 400x).

tumors, the mainstay of treatment is maximal safe resection. Gamma knife therapy and preoperative embolization may be useful to consider in some cases because of the highly vascular nature of the lesion.[114–116] Recurrence is <25% and is more common in lesions associated with VHL and in the cellular rather than the reticular variant of the tumor.[117]

Treatment of spinal hemangioblastoma includes chemotherapy and surgical resection.[111,112]

Intradural Extramedullary Neoplasms

Intradural extramedullary spinal neoplasms in children include a variety of lesions, the most common being neurofibromas/schwannomas, meningiomas, and leptomeningeal metastases. Imaging findings and associations are summarized in Table 4.2.

Nerve Sheath Tumors (Neurofibroma and Schwannoma)

All types of nerve sheath tumors can occur intradurally. The two main spinal nerve sheath tumors are neurofibroma and schwannoma, with the focus here being on neurofibroma because it is more common in the pediatric population.[118] Neurofibromas may be derived from an intermediate cell or from a combination of Schwann cells and perineural fibroblasts (Fig. 4.37). The majority of spinal neurofibromas are intradural extramedullary. The two morphologic types are fusiform (arising from a single nerve fascicle) and plexiform

TABLE 4.2 Pediatric Intradural Extramedullary Spinal Neoplasms: Key Imaging Features, Associations, Treatments, and Other Comments

Neoplasm	Key Imaging Features	Associations, Treatments, and Other Comments
Nerve sheath tumors (neurofibroma, schwannoma)	Expansion of intervertebral foramina	Associated with NF1 and NF2
	Posterior vertebral body scalloping	Treatment—typically conservative and rarely debulking
	Target sign	
Meningioma	Isointense on noncontrast imaging	Teenagers
	Homogeneous and intense enhancement	Multiple lesions in the setting of NF2
		Treatment—surgical resection
Leptomeningeal metastasis	Lumbosacral region involvement	Common with medulloblastoma, ependymoma, higher grade astrocytoma, and atypical teratoid rhabdoid tumor
	Variable in size and number of lesions	Treatment depends on primary neoplasm

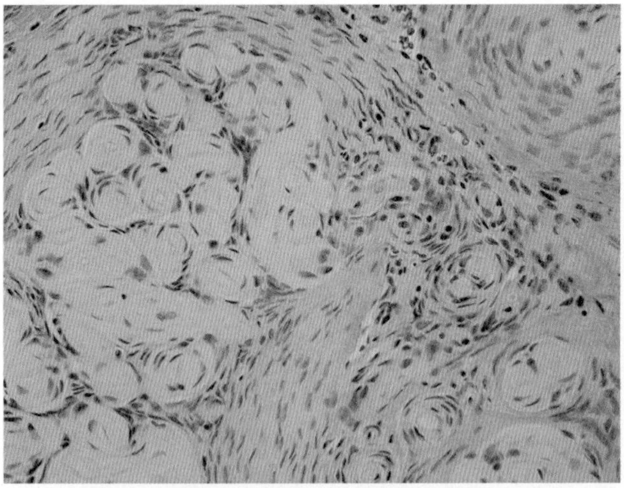

FIGURE 4.37 **Benign nerve sheath tumor in a 3-month-old girl with a hyperpigmented lumbar cutaneous lesion overlying an epidural tract extending to an extramedullary intradural mass.** Benign nerve sheath elements include pacinian and meningothelial differentiation; like many proliferations associated with spinal dysraphism, this lesion occupies an uncertain border zone between hamartoma and neoplasm (hematoxylin and eosin, original magnification, 400×).

(involving multiple nerve branches). The lesions may be single, multiple, or diffuse. Neurofibromas are usually encountered in children with NF1 but may occur as an isolated lesion.[119]

Neurofibromas are of variable T1 signal and T2 hyperintense and enhance after contrast administration. Diffuse neurofibromas may extend along the paraspinal region. Key imaging features of neurofibromas include remodeling and expansion of the intervertebral foramina indicative of slow indolent growth and a target (central low signal with peripheral high signal) sign on T2-weighted MR images (Fig. 4.38). Rib erosion may be seen, and when severe over a long length of a rib, may cause "ribbon ribs." Malignant transformation into malignant peripheral nerve sheath tumor is uncommon but should be considered with large lesions with bone destruction or necrosis.

Neurofibromas that are single are usually resected with a good prognosis. However, in children with neurofibromatosis and plexiform neurofibromas, lesions are only treated when they cause complications such as cord compression. In this situation, debulking is useful to preserve spinal function.[120]

Meningioma

Meningiomas, neoplasms originating from the dural covering of the spinal cord, are rare in childhood.[121] They may occur sporadically, or more often, in association with NF2. When seen in NF2 patients, they may occur intracranially, intraspinally, or both. Typical presenting features include leg pain and weakness. Meningiomas are T1 hypo- to isointense and T2 hyperintense, and they uniformly enhance after contrast administration (Fig. 4.39). Areas of hypointensity may be due to calcification.[122] Microscopically, they typically consist of plump cells with a whorled architectural arrangement (Fig. 4.40). Psammomatous calcifications may be seen.

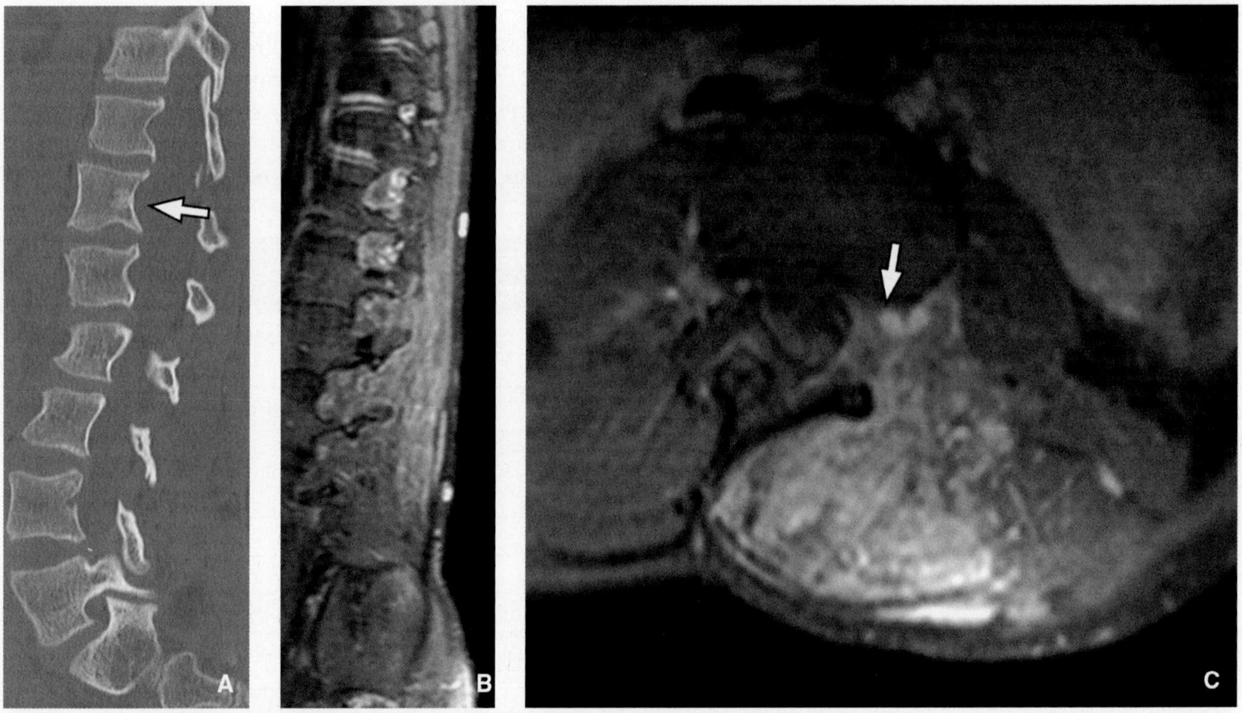

FIGURE 4.38 **Plexiform neurofibroma in 13-year-old girl with neurofibromatosis type 1 and scoliosis. A:** Sagittal reformatted CT image of the spine shows posterior vertebral body scalloping (*arrow*). Sagittal **(B)** and axial **(C)** T1-weighted fat-saturated MR images demonstrate a large, enhancing infiltrative paraspinous mass causing foraminal enlargement (*arrow*, C).

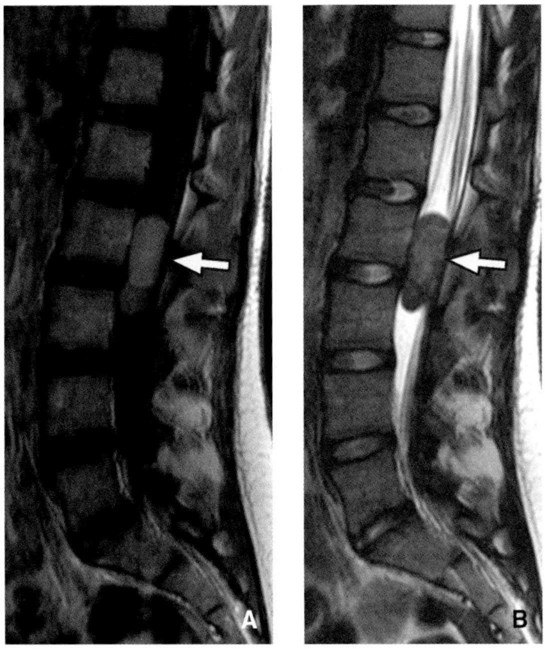

FIGURE 4.39 **Meningioma in a 10-year-old girl with leg pain.** Sagittal T1 **(A)**- and T2 **(B)**-weighted MR images demonstrate a well-defined, intensely enhancing T1- and T2-hyperintense mass (*arrow*) at the L2–L3 level.

Treatment includes surgical resection. However, in subtotally resected lesions, the treatment methods are controversial. The 15-year survival rate has been reported as high as 90%.[123]

Leptomeningeal Metastasis

Metastatic spread to the spinal canal most commonly occurs via the CSF as a result of drop metastases from primary supratentorial and posterior fossa brain neoplasms, such as medulloblastoma, ependymoma, and atypical teratoid rhabdoid tumor.[124]

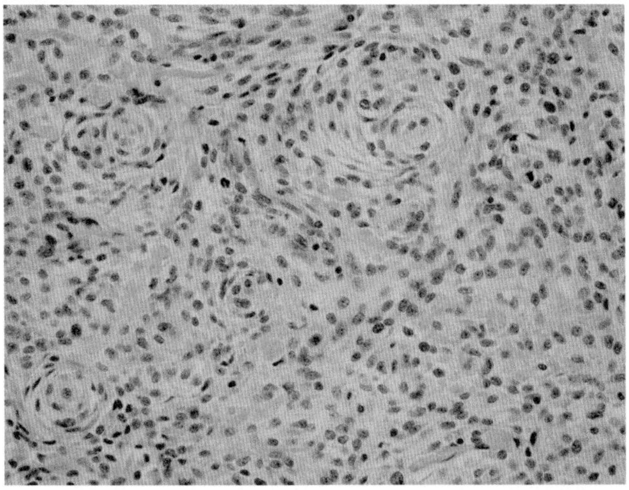

FIGURE 4.40 **Meningioma in a 9-year-old girl with severe back pain because of a T12–S1 intradural mass.** Microscopic examination shows characteristic plump cells in a whorled arrangement (hematoxylin and eosin, original magnification, 400×).

CSF metastases may be solitary, multiple, or diffuse coating the spinal cord and nerve roots. Metastatic nodules may range in size from 1–2 mm to 1–2 cm and may block CSF flow or cause neural compression. The most common site is the distal thecal sac in the lumbosacral area, followed by the thoracic, and finally the cervical spine.[121] To avoid false-positive MRI exams, the spinal cord should be scanned before surgery for newly diagnosed brain tumors with propensity to spread via the CSF. If preoperative MRI is not feasible, MRI should be delayed for 4 to 6 weeks after surgery in order to differentiate from postoperative fluid collections.[125]

The microscopic findings (Fig. 4.41) as well as the treatment and prognosis of leptomeningeal tumor spread depend on the specific primary lesion, a discussion of which is beyond the scope of this chapter.

Extradural Neoplasms

Most childhood extradural neoplasms arise in the paravertebral soft tissues and invade the spinal canal via the intervertebral foramina, including neuroblastoma and sacrococcygeal teratoma (SCT). Primary osseous lesions, such as aneurysmal bone cysts, lymphoma, and Ewing sarcoma, as well as metastatic lesions, may also involve the vertebra and secondarily, the spinal canal. Imaging is utilized to determine the extent of spinal involvement, the degree of neural element compression, and the degree of destabilization of the spinal column by destruction of osseous elements.[103,126]

Neuroblastic Tumors (Neuroblastoma, Ganglioneuroblastoma, and Ganglioneuroma)

Neuroblastic tumors are mainly divided into neuroblastoma, ganglioneuroblastoma, and ganglioneuroma based on the degree of cellular differentiation observed histologically. Neuroblastoma is by far the most common extracranial solid neoplasm, usually presenting between 1 and 5 years of age. Neuroblastomas originate from neuroblasts along the sympathetic chain and arise most commonly in or near the adrenal gland. Spinous metastases can be osseous or involve sympathetic chain ganglia. They may be single or multilevel or extend into the epidural space with spinal cord compression. Larger lesions may have areas of hemorrhage and necrosis. Metastatic involvement of cortical bone, bone marrow, liver, lymph nodes, and skin can occur. Ganglioneuromas are benign tumors at the most mature end of the histologic spectrum; they are generally seen in older children and adults. Ganglioneuroblastomas have intermediate differentiation and generally have a favorable prognosis except for the nodular subtype, which is usually unfavorable. Ganglioneuroblastoma and ganglioneuroma are usually well encapsulated and have imaging findings similar to neuroblastoma, though smaller and better defined. Primary occurrence in the paraspinal region is common.

Key imaging features on US include a solid adrenal or paraspinous mass with vascular encasement and punctate foci of echogenicity indicating calcifications. Both CT and MRI of neuroblastoma show an adrenal or paraspinal soft tissue mass

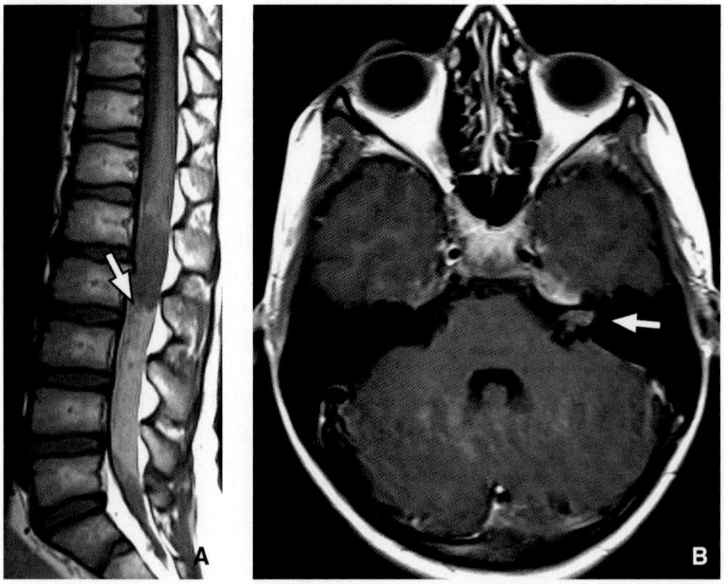

FIGURE 4.41 **Leptomeningeal metastases in a 9-year-old girl with recurrent atypical rhabdoid teratoid tumor after radiation therapy. A:** Sagittal postcontrast T1-weighted MR image demonstrates extensive enhancing solid tissue (*arrow*) filling the distal thecal sac. **B:** Axial postcontrast T1-weighted MR image of the brain shows a metastatic focus (*arrow*) at the left cerebellopontine angle.

with or without intraspinal extension, often encasing, but not invading retroperitoneal vessels. The lesion has variable attenuation and enhancement on CT. It is hypo- to isointense on T1-weighted MR images compared to the spinal cord, demonstrates subtle hyperintensity on T2-weighted MR images, and has variable enhancement after contrast administration (Fig. 4.42). Hypointense areas on T1 and T2 MR sequences may indicate calcifications, which are frequent and punctate. Fat-suppressed T2 MR sequences are useful to determine the extent of osseous disease. Determining if the mass

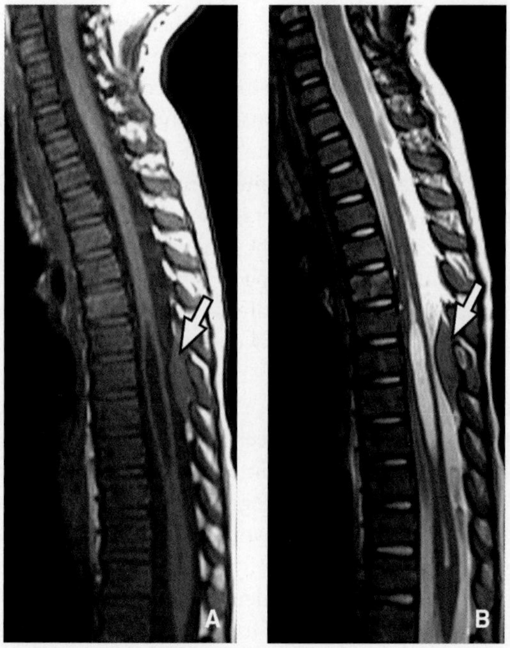

FIGURE 4.42 **Metastatic neuroblastoma in a 2-year-old boy with leg weakness, vomiting, and diarrhea.** Sagittal postscontrast T1- **(A)** and T2- **(B)** weighted MR images show an enhancing epidural mass (*arrows*) at the level of T5 vertebra. Also seen is a syrinx from T5 to L1, and abnormal signal due to marrow metastasis in the T4 vertebra. A primary adrenal neuroblastoma was found (not shown).

extends across the midline is important to stage the lesion. Specifically, stage 2 does not cross the midline, whereas stage 3 does cross the midline.[90]

Spinal neuroblastoma is treated with laminectomy and resection in the setting of cord compression. Otherwise, spinal leptomeningeal neuroblastoma is treated with chemotherapy.[127] Prognosis depends on a number of factors such as stage, grade, age at diagnosis, and various laboratory findings, which are beyond the scope of this chapter.

Sacrococcygeal Teratomas

SCTs are neoplasms derived from all three germ layers. They may contain a wide variety of tissue types, including neural elements, squamous, and intestinal epithelium, skin appendages, cartilage, bone, and teeth (Fig. 4.43). There are four types: 1 (external), 2 (predominantly external with a small intrapelvic portion), 3 (predominantly intrapelvic with small external component), and 4 (intrapelvic). All four types may present in utero or postnatally with an extradural mass and may be associated with sacrococcygeal bony erosions. SCTs can be cystic, mixed cystic–solid, or solid lesions. SCT in infants is benign unless it contains elements of yolk sac tumor or, exceptionally, other admixed histologically malignant elements.

CT is utilized to demonstrate osseous destruction of the sacrum and coccyx, as well as calcification within the lesion. Cystic components of SCT are T1 hypo- and T2 hyperintense. MR signal of hemorrhagic components depends on the age of the hemorrhage. Solid components may enhance after contrast administration (Fig. 4.44). The location of SCT in relationship to the gluteal fold helps to differentiate this lesion from CSDs. Specifically, SCTs typically extend below the gluteal fold and CSDs typically extend above the gluteal fold.[128]

The main treatment of SCTs includes complete surgical resection. Physical and radiologic features suggesting a favorable prognosis are younger age, female sex, mostly cystic composition, the presence of calcifications, and most importantly, completely external location (type 1).[129]

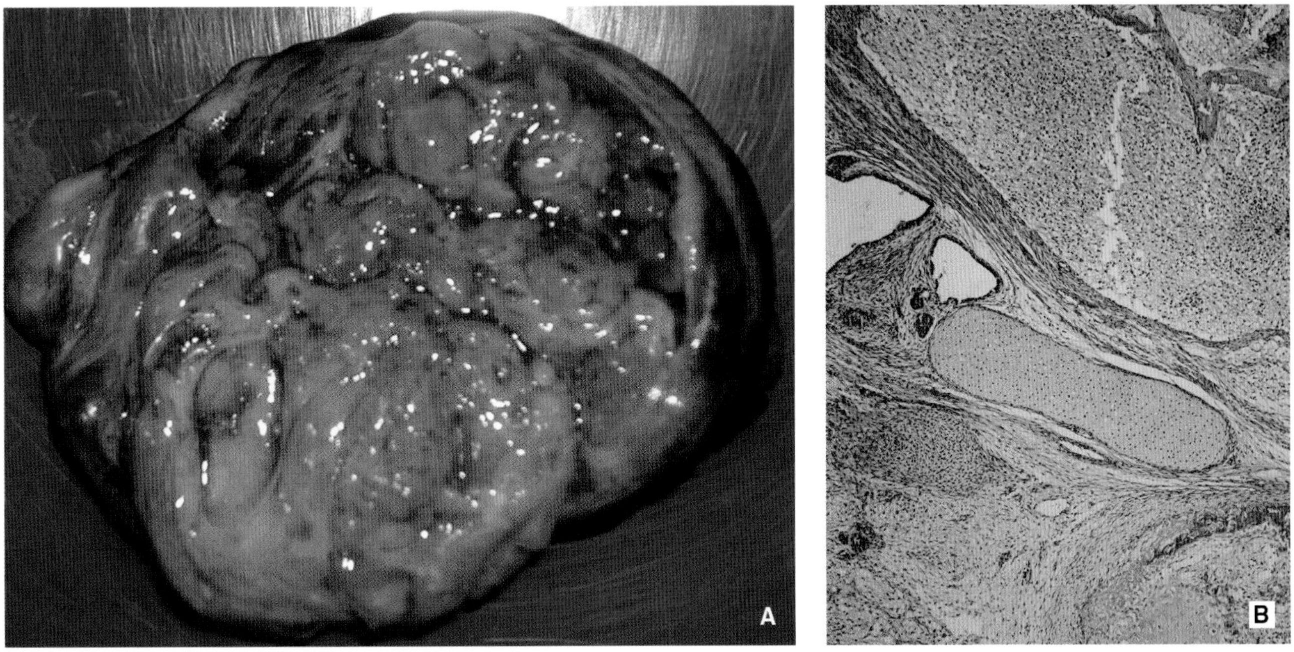

FIGURE 4.43 **Sacrococcygeal teratoma in a 10-day-old girl. A:** Grossly, the mass is partially cystic and shows areas of varying color and consistency. **B:** Microscopically, disorganized tissues and abortive organ structures include cartilage, bone, brain, epithelium, and stromal elements (hematoxylin and eosin, original magnification, 100×).

Lymphoma and Leukemia

Lymphoma involves the spine less commonly than other reticuloendothelial system structures, such as lymph nodes. Single or multiple vertebral bodies may be involved, especially with non-Hodgkin type. There may be diffuse dural infiltration or localized dural-based or spinal cord masses. Epidural deposits from leukemia produce clinical symptoms more often in children than in adults.[130]

Epidural involvement in lymphoma and leukemia is usually isointense on noncontrast T1-weighted MR imaging. Homogeneous postcontrast enhancement is typical. Key imaging features suggesting a lymphomatous or leukemic mass include low sign on T2-weighted MR images, lack of osseous changes, and vascular encasement without occlusion (Fig. 4.45).[131] Involvement of a single vertebra without loss of height is common in lymphoma but may also be seen in Ewing sarcoma. Thus, in children, a vertebral body that has abnormal signal but maintains its height has a differential diagnosis of lymphoma versus Ewing sarcoma.

The treatment of leukemia and lymphoma of the spine is the same as elsewhere in the body. Depending on specific stage, chemotherapy and bone marrow transplant are mainstays of treatment. The prognosis depends on many factors including the specific type of lesion and its stage, a complete discussion of which is beyond the scope of this chapter.[130]

Leptomeningeal Melanosis

Neurocutaneous melanosis is a rare, nonfamilial phakomatosis caused by melanocyte proliferation within the epidermis and leptomeninges. It is characterized by large cutaneous pigmented nevi and melanosis of the leptomeninges. A forme fruste may occur in which only leptomeningeal involvement is present without cutaneous manifestations. In the pediatric population, leptomeningeal involvement may present with signs of raised intracranial pressure and hydrocephalus.

The most common appearance is diffuse leptomeningeal thickening and enhancement after contrast administration, as can be seen with leptomeningeal metastases. Although leptomeningeal metastatic disease is more common than leptomeningeal melanosis, the presence of melanin seen as hyperintense signal on noncontrast T1-weighted MR images should prompt consideration of this disease. The key imaging features of this disorder include T1-hyperintense melanin deposits in the hippocampus and brain stem.[132] Recently, Dandy-Walker Complex has been recognized to occur in up to 10% of children with neurocutaneous melanosis.[133] This association may be a marker for severe melanosis and worse prognosis.[134] Malignant degeneration into melanoma portends a poor prognosis as well because it is nonresponsive to chemotherapy and radiation.[135]

Extradural Bony Lesions

Numerous vertebral osseous abnormalities may extend outside of the spine and produce extradural mass effect. Lesions in the spine tend to either arise from the posterior elements or the vertebral body. Common pediatric posterior element lesions include osteoid osteomas, aneurysmal bone cysts, and osteoblastomas. Common pediatric vertebral body masses include Ewing sarcoma, lymphoma, Langerhans cell histiocytosis, and metastatic disease such as neuroblastoma, leukemia, and primitive neuroectodermal tumor.

The imaging features of extradural bony masses vary depending on the specific type of lesion. Unlike in the majority

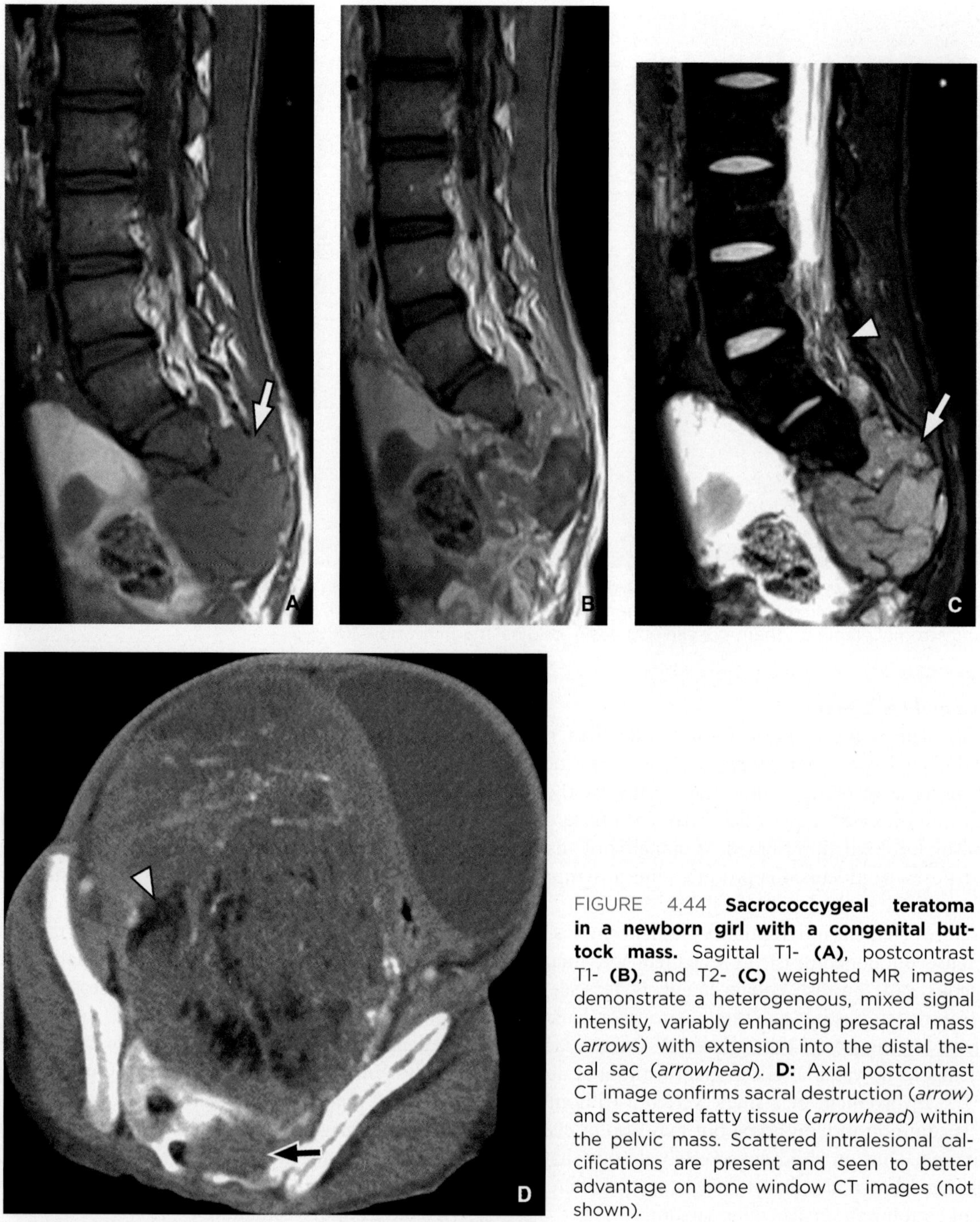

FIGURE 4.44 **Sacrococcygeal teratoma in a newborn girl with a congenital buttock mass.** Sagittal T1- **(A)**, postcontrast T1- **(B)**, and T2- **(C)** weighted MR images demonstrate a heterogeneous, mixed signal intensity, variably enhancing presacral mass (*arrows*) with extension into the distal thecal sac (*arrowhead*). **D:** Axial postcontrast CT image confirms sacral destruction (*arrow*) and scattered fatty tissue (*arrowhead*) within the pelvic mass. Scattered intralesional calcifications are present and seen to better advantage on bone window CT images (not shown).

of spinal tumors, CT plays a greater role in imaging osseous masses and neoplasms and is complimentary to MRI. Vertebral lesions can be grouped into lesions that involve the posterior elements and those that involve the vertebral bodies. Imaging features of posterior element lesions allow a very limited, and often specific, diagnosis.

Osteoid osteomas classically show a focal sclerotic osseous nidus surrounded by a lucent halo on CT and a "double density sign" on nuclear bone scintigraphy. On MRI, the degree of surrounding edema can be impressive and should not be confused with other aggressive lesions. Aneurysmal bone cysts have classic features as well show an expansile, multilocular mass with fluid–fluid levels due to internal hemorrhage and debris (Fig. 4.46). Osteoblastomas demonstrate expansile solid masses of the posterior elements (Fig. 4.47). Compared to osteoid osteoma and aneurysmal bone cysts, osteoblastomas are mostly composed of solid enhancing tissue and rarely contain cystic areas and fluid levels.

The differential diagnosis of vertebral body lesions can be further narrowed by separating single from multilevel lesions. Lesions involving only one vertebral body with no significant loss of vertebral body height are typically either

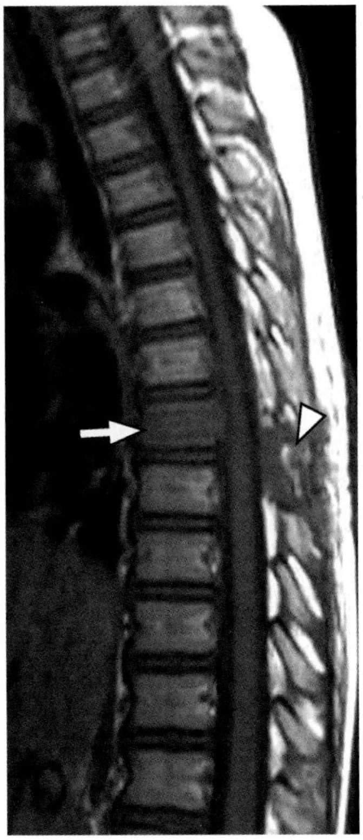

FIGURE 4.45 **Burkitt lymphoma in a 5-year-old boy with back pain, paresthesias, and urinary retention.** Sagittal T1-weighted MR image demonstrates hypointense signal in the T7 vertebral body (*arrow*). Note postbiopsy changes (*arrowhead*) of the posterior elements and soft tissues.

Ewing sarcoma or lymphoma. Both are T1 hypointense and T2 hyperintense and enhance after contrast administration on MRI. Ewing sarcoma tends to have more necrosis (Fig. 4.48). Similar features are seen with multiple vertebral body involvement in lymphoma.[136] Although Langerhans cell histiocytosis may also present with a single vertebra lesion, significant loss of height, or vertebra plana, is the key feature to suggest this diagnosis (Fig. 4.49). Multilevel vertebral disease with moderate loss of height should prompt a differential diagnosis of leukemia versus trauma. Trauma is usually distinguished by appropriate clinical history.

Treatment of this group of lesions depends on the specific mass present. Posterior element osteoid osteomas are treated with radiotherapy ablation, aneurysmal bone cysts with a combination of sclerotherapy and surgery, and osteoblastomas with surgical resection and/or chemotherapy. Vertebral lesions, including leukemia, lymphoma, Langerhans cell histiocytosis, and Ewing sarcoma, are generally treated with chemotherapy. Unifocal Langerhans cell histiocytosis may spontaneously resolve and requires minimal treatment. Prognosis depends on the specific type of lesion present, a full discussion of which is beyond the scope of this chapter.[137–139]

Traumatic Disorders

Delivery Trauma

The majority of trauma related to the process of being born involves various forms of intra- and extracranial hemorrhage. Spinal cord injuries may also occur during the birth process and, rarely, in utero.[140] Thesc injuries present with various neurologic symptoms that are best evaluated with MRI. Besides intracranial hemorrhage, the most common birth-related injuries involve the brachial plexus (Erb palsy) and the spinal cord. Nerve root avulsions can be evaluated with CT myelography,[141] and more often, MRI. It is useful to determine if brachial plexus injuries are preganglionic or postganglionic because there are different implications for each in regard to management. Postganglionic lesions are repaired with nerve grafting or followed conservatively, whereas preganglionic lesions are restored with nerve transfers.[142]

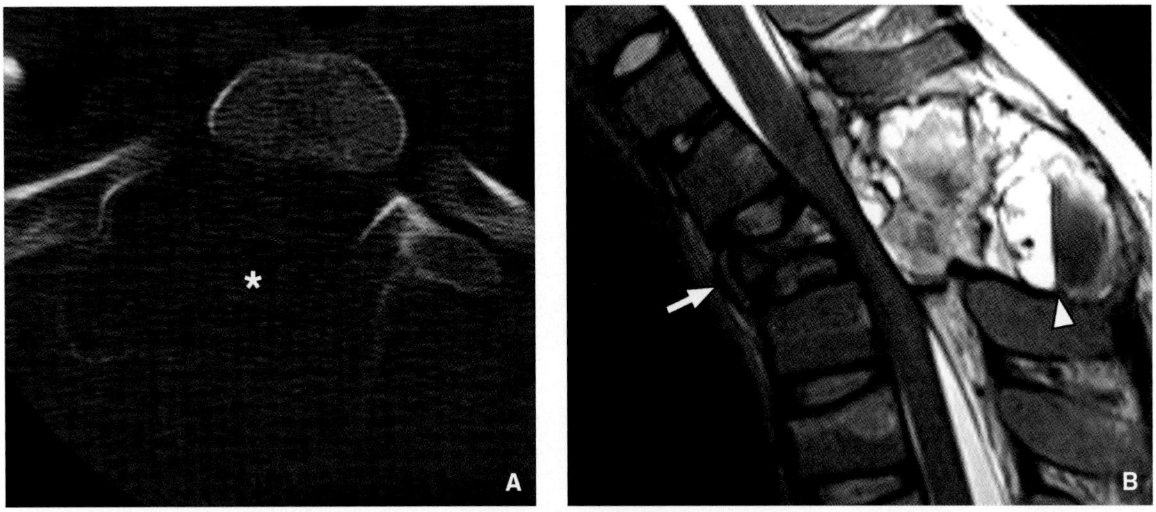

FIGURE 4.46 **Aneurysmal bone cyst in a 10-year-old girl with back pain. A:** Axial bone window CT image shows an expansile lesion (*asterisk*) of the T3 posterior elements. **B:** Sagittal T2-weighted MR image confirms a multiloculated, expansile lesion (*arrowhead*) with fluid levels and mixed signal intensity in the T3 posterior elements. T3 vertebral body compression (*arrow*) causes compression of the adjacent spinal cord.

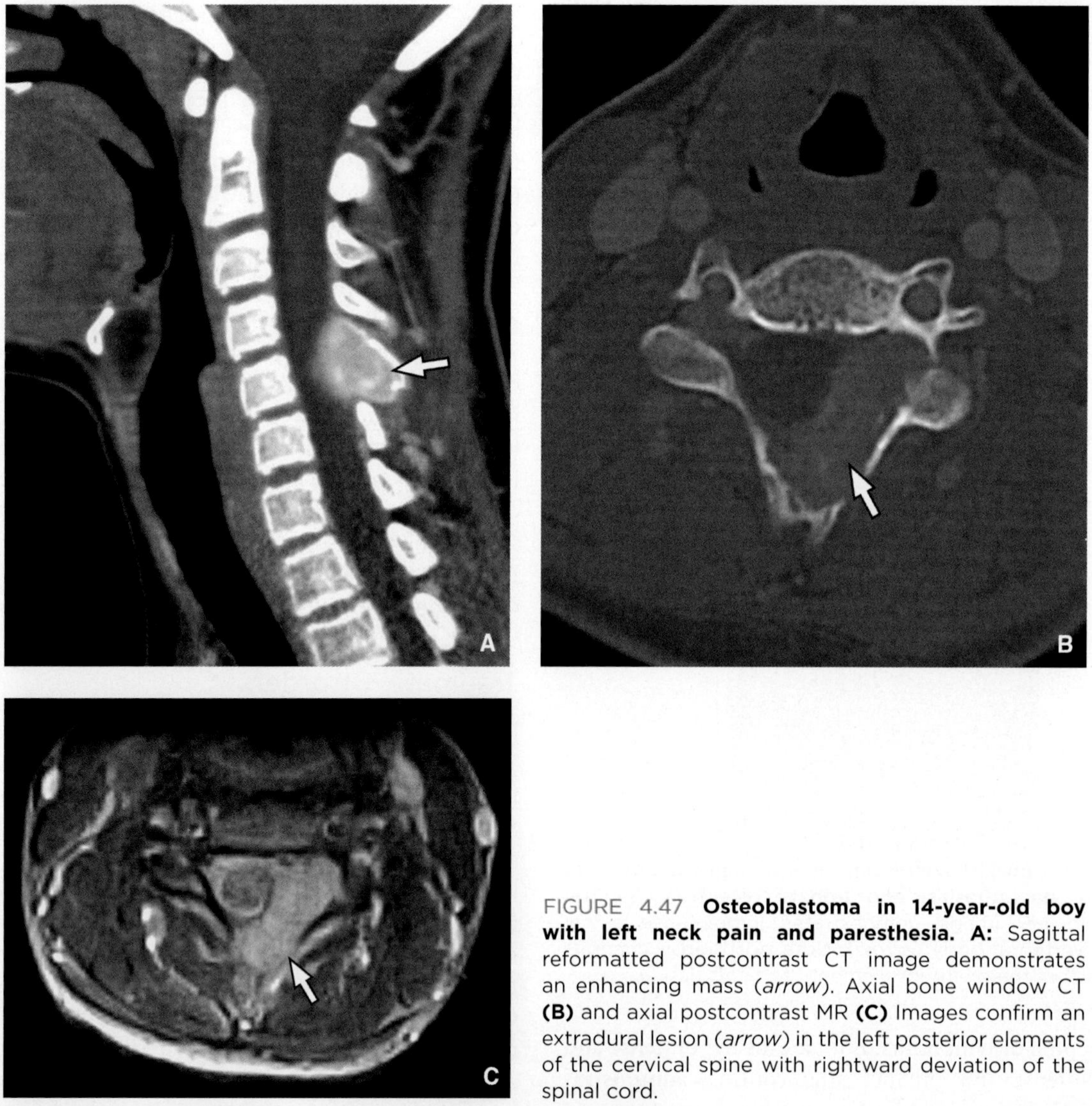

FIGURE 4.47 **Osteoblastoma in 14-year-old boy with left neck pain and paresthesia. A:** Sagittal reformatted postcontrast CT image demonstrates an enhancing mass (*arrow*). Axial bone window CT **(B)** and axial postcontrast MR **(C)** Images confirm an extradural lesion (*arrow*) in the left posterior elements of the cervical spine with rightward deviation of the spinal cord.

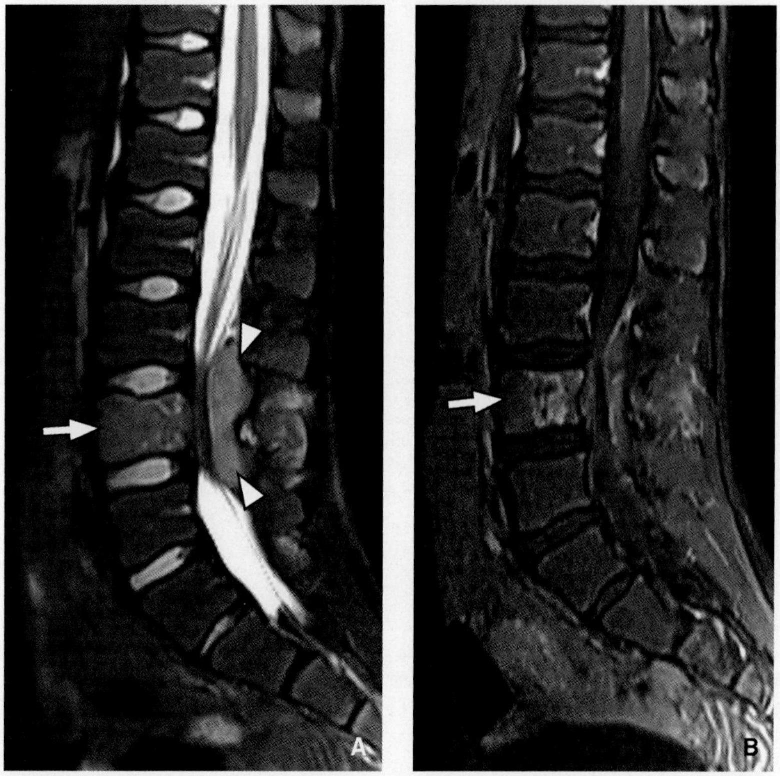

FIGURE 4.48 **Ewing sarcoma in a 6-year-old girl with back pain.** Sagittal T2-weighted **(A)** and sagittal postcontrast fat-saturated T1-weighted **(B)** MR images demonstrate a T2 hyperintense, enhancing L4 vertebral body (*arrow*) with associated posterior epidural soft tissue mass (*arrowheads*) compressing the cauda equina. Note that there is no loss of vertebral height.

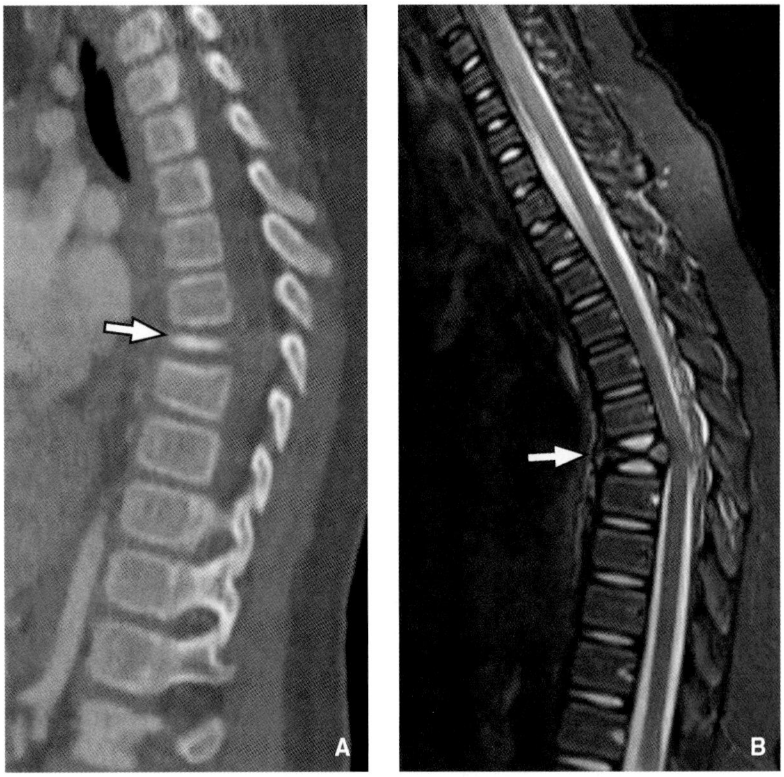

FIGURE 4.49 **Langerhans cell histiocytosis in a 7-year-old girl with back pain. A:** Sagittal reformatted bone window CT image shows focal thoracic kyphosis due to a flattened vertebra, or vertebra plana (*arrow*). **B:** Sagittal T2-weighted MR image confirms kyphosis and vertebra plana (*arrow*). Also noted is projection of the vertebral body posterior cortex into the spinal canal causing some impingement on the spinal cord.

Key imaging findings on MRI in children with Erb palsy include the classic pseudomeningocele and the lesser-known-but-prevalent periscalene soft tissue swelling.[143] Other cord injuries present with cord edema and swelling as well as hemorrhage (Fig. 4.50). High field strength 3 Tesla MRI and new isotropic high-resolution heavily T2-weighted MRI sequences allow 3D postprocessing to make detailed evaluation much easier.[144] Outside the neonatal period, the most common causes for similar nerve root damage are trauma secondary to motor and all-terrain vehicle accidents (Fig. 4.51).

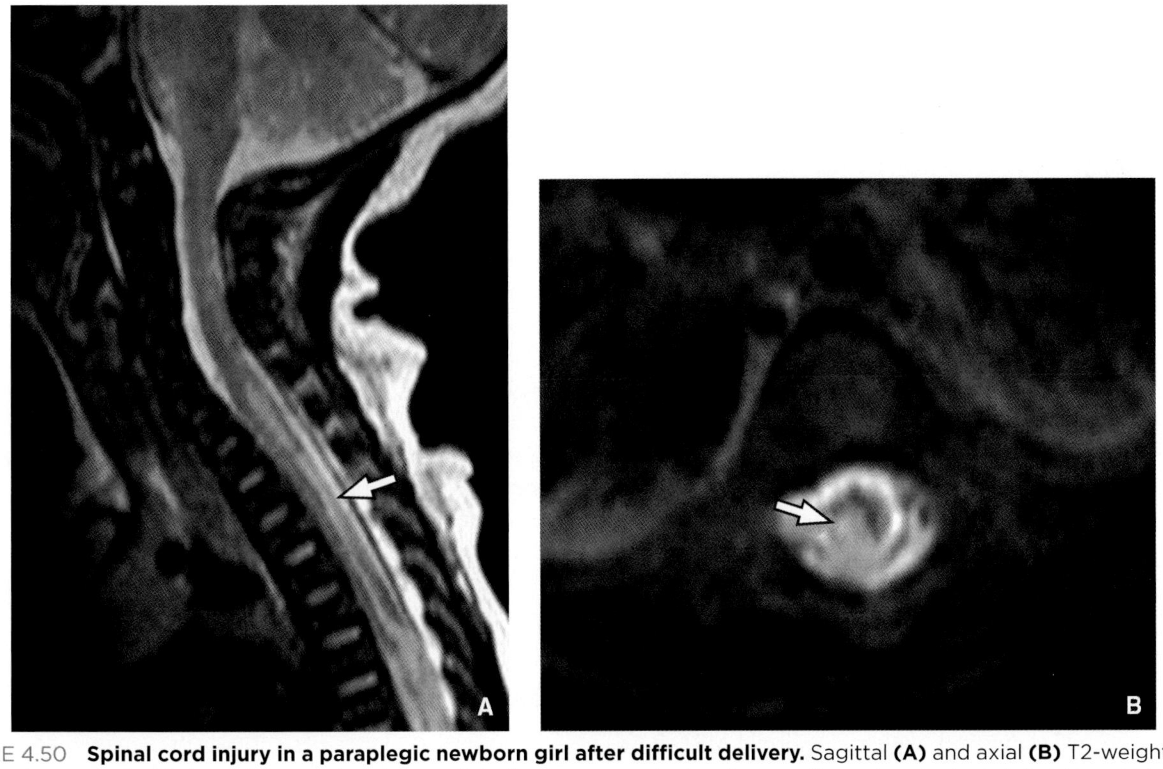

FIGURE 4.50 **Spinal cord injury in a paraplegic newborn girl after difficult delivery.** Sagittal **(A)** and axial **(B)** T2-weighted MR images demonstrate T2-hyperintense signal (*arrow*) in the lower cervical and upper thoracic spinal cord due to cord ischemia and/or infarction.

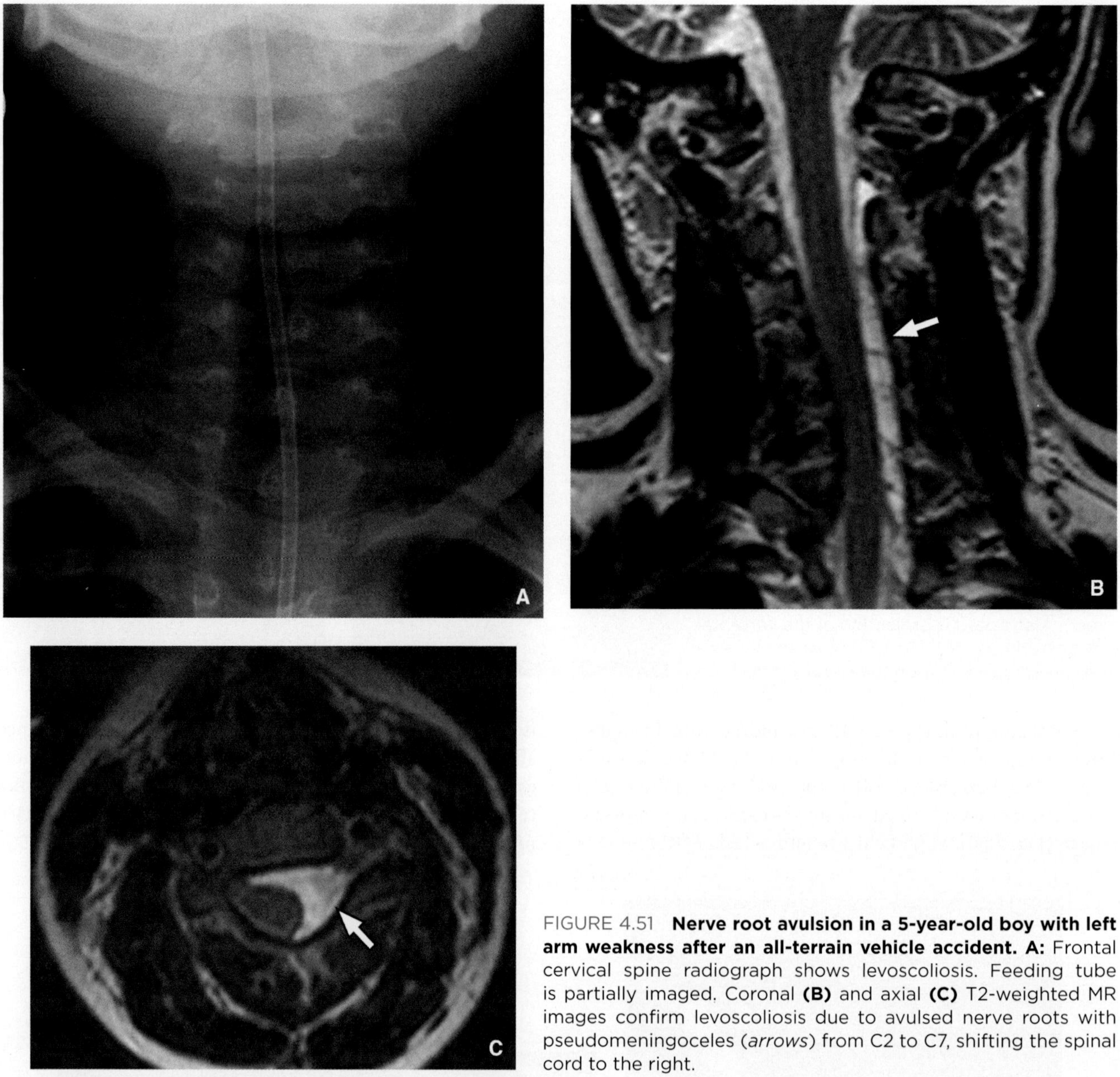

FIGURE 4.51 **Nerve root avulsion in a 5-year-old boy with left arm weakness after an all-terrain vehicle accident. A:** Frontal cervical spine radiograph shows levoscoliosis. Feeding tube is partially imaged. Coronal **(B)** and axial **(C)** T2-weighted MR images confirm levoscoliosis due to avulsed nerve roots with pseudomeningoceles (*arrows*) from C2 to C7, shifting the spinal cord to the right.

Spinal Cord Injury without Radiologic Abnormality

Traumatic injuries in children differ from those in adults because of their disproportionately large heads, weak neck muscles, ligamentous laxity, and incomplete ossification of synchrondroses.[145] Because of these differences, children are more likely to have ligamentous and upper cervical spine injuries compared to adults. Spinal cord injury without radiographic abnormality (SCIWORA), a traumatic injury seen nearly exclusively in children, is diagnosed when no abnormality is found on radiography despite ligamentous and/or spinal cord injury seen on MR imaging (Fig. 4.52).

Although a recent study showed that C-spine CT can be used to clear the cervical spine, it did not detect all soft tissue injuries, which were present on MRI in 17% of patients with normal CTs.[146,147] Key imaging findings in SCIWORA include a normal radiograph with an abnormal MRI showing T2-hyperintense cord edema, which may also have central hypointense hemorrhage in the acute setting or cord transection. Associated soft tissue T2 hyperintensity anterior and/or posterior to the cord is often seen because of ligamentous injury with or without associated hematoma and/or soft tissue swelling. Subtle signal change in the vertebral bodies may be seen with compression fractures.[91,145,146]

Treatment of SCIWORA is supportive in most cases including stabilization of the spine in the setting of trauma. Many injuries require surgical stabilization. Prognosis depends on the severity of the presenting symptoms and the MRI findings. Cord transection and intramedullary blood portend permanent morbidity, and children presenting with complete myelopathy do not fully regain function.[148]

Vascular Disorders

Classification and Terminology

Much has been learned about the histopathophysiology and pathogenesis of vascular malformations in recent years.

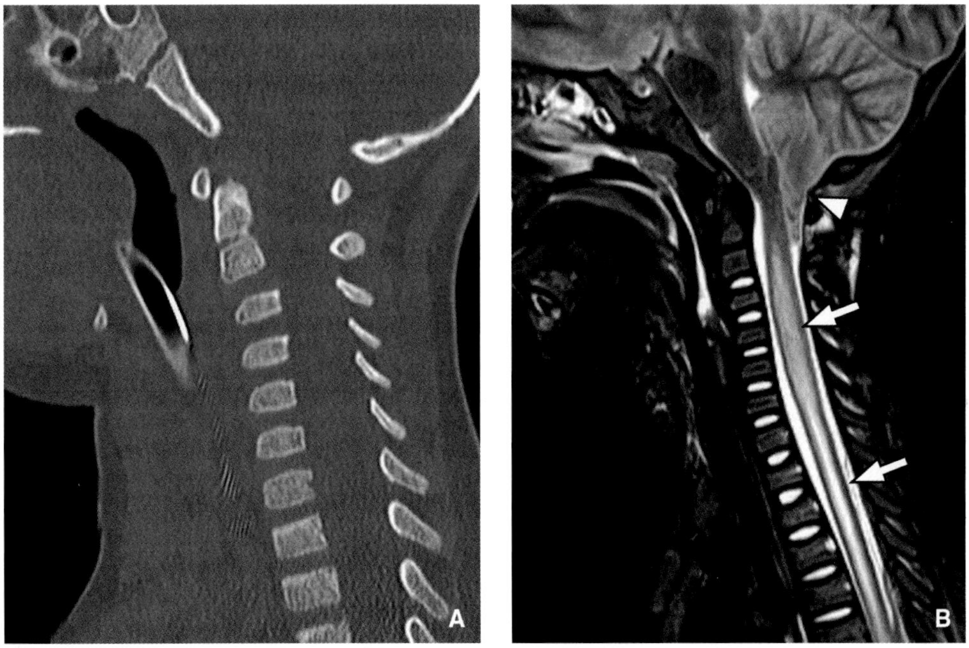

FIGURE 4.52 **Spinal cord injury without radiographic abnormality (SCIWORA) in a 33-month-old boy with severe arm weakness and difficulty breathing after falling from a horse.** The plain radiograph (not shown) was normal. **A:** Sagittal reformatted CT image with bone algorithm is normal. Note presence of endotracheal tube. **B:** Sagittal T2-weighted MR image shows spinal cord edema (*arrows*) throughout the cervical spine. Also noted is cerebellar tonsillar ectopia (*arrowhead*) that was secondary to diffuse cerebral edema in this child who did not survive his injuries.

This new knowledge has caused pediatric subspecialists caring for children with vascular anomalies to adopt a new classification system developed by the International Society for the Study of Vascular Anomalies (ISSVA). This system, which was initially described by Mulliken and Glowacki,[149–151] is useful because of its consistent ability to correlate classification of vascular anomalies in any organ system with histology, presentation, and imaging findings, as well as clinical course and treatment.[152,153] Perhaps of equal importance, use of the new system standardizes nomenclature eliminating past confusing and contradictory terminology that often led to an incorrect diagnosis or delay in treatment.[152,153]

The first step in the ISSVA system is to divide lesions into tumors (neoplasms) and malformations.[150] Tumors grow in size because of disregulated cell proliferation, or mitosis. Conversely, vascular malformations, which are composed of various types of dysmorphic vessels, may enlarge because of internal hemorrhage or inflammation but do not undergo mitosis and are expected to grow proportionately to the child's growth.[152] Herein, we discuss the most common pediatric vascular anomalies found in the spinal cord, including hemangiomas, venous malformations, arteriovenous malformations (AVMs), and arteriovenous fistulas (AVFs). We review current terminology and key imaging features and summarize basic treatment (Table 4.3).

TABLE 4.3 Classification and Treatment of Vascular Anomalies

Tumor Type	Treatment
Infantile hemangioma Congenital hemangioma • RICH (rapidly involuting CH) • NICH (noninvoluting CH)	No treatment unless complicated; antiangiogenic drugs (propranolol, steroids vincristine), rare embolization, or liver transplant for hepatic involvement RICH—same as infantile hemangioma NICH—surgical resection
Vascular Malformation Type	**Treatment**
Slow flow • Venous • Lymphatic	Sclerotherapy, especially mostly cystic lesions Surgery, especially mostly solid lesions and residual masses postsclerotherapy
Fast flow • Arteriovenous malformation • Arteriovenous fistula	Initial catheter embolization and surgical removal in some cases, especially residual disease

CH, congenital hemangioma.

Infantile and Congenital Hemangiomas

Although hemangiomas are neoplasms, they are often discussed under the heading of vascular anomalies, as in this chapter. Hemangiomas are benign neoplasms of blood vessels. Infantile hemangiomas are by far the most common type. Infantile hemangiomas develop between 2 weeks and 2 months of life; this is in contrast to congenital hemangiomas, which are present on day 1 of life. In order to distinguish between infantile and congenital hemangiomas, one must know their time of presentation. Both types of hemangiomas undergo a period of rapid growth, or a proliferative phase, followed by involution where their vessels decrease in size, embedded in variable amounts of residual fibrofatty tissue. Infantile hemangiomas involute gradually, typically resolving completely between 1 year of age and adolescence. Congenital hemangiomas are divided clinically into rapidly involuting (RICH) and noninvoluting (NICH).[154]

Hemangiomas are most common in Caucasian females, are most frequent on the skin or within the liver, and may be single or multiple.[154,155] Infantile hemangiomas have a recently described histopathologic marker, GLUT1 or glucose transporter protein 1.[156] In children, GLUT1 is a marker for infantile hemangiomas. Interestingly, it is also found in placental tissue and perineural cells. The presence of GLUT1 in placental tissue, and the fact that hemangiomas are more common in infants of women who have undergone in utero procedures, has led to the theory that hemangiomas may be at least partially related to in utero placental implants.[157,158] They have also been noted to occur frequently along dermatomal lines in association with regional anomalies of other organs, as well as in the head and neck suggesting a possible neural crest origin.[157,159]

When infantile hemangioma is multifocal and involves the liver, the main differential diagnosis is neuroblastoma because both can cause multiple lesions of the skin and liver. Distinguishing between these two processes is most easily accomplished by checking for urine catecholamines.[160] Although most hemangiomas of the skin and subcutis are diagnosed clinically, imaging is useful in uncertain cases or symptomatic pediatric patients. Symptoms depend on number and location of lesions.[152,157] Cutaneous hemangiomas on the low back may indicate underlying spinal cord pathology, such as tethered cord. They may occur alone or as part of a regional syndrome such as SACRAL (Spinal dysraphism, Anogenital, Cutaneous, Renal, Angioma, Lumbosacral) syndrome.[161]

The imaging features of infantile and congenital hemangiomas (RICH and NICH) overlap, and all may be single or multiple involving one or several organ systems. On US, hemangiomas are solid, usually hypoechoic masses with extensive arterial and venous flow on color and spectral Doppler interrogation[152,162] (Fig. 4.53). On MRI, hemangiomas are T1 hypo- and T2 hyperintense with internal flow voids. Postcontrast CT and MR images show a well-defined, solid, vigorously enhancing mass.[163] Involuting lesions are heterogeneous, containing gradually increasing amounts of fibrofatty tissue. Although a pattern of peripheral enhancement may occur in hemangiomas, it is not specific and cannot be relied upon to make a diagnosis in children.[154] Catheter angiogram findings have been described, although this type of study is rarely performed except as a preamble to treatment.[164]

Microscopic features of infantile hemangiomas, discussed in other chapters, depend on their stage of development. In the spine, they are often one part of a constellation of malformative features of spinal dysraphism (Fig. 4.54). Treatment of infantile hemangiomas and RICHs depends on their symptoms, size, number, and location. Conservative watchful waiting until hemangiomas involute is the initial treatment of choice. However, if lesions become dangerous because of obstruction or compression of vital structures, large amount of shunting, or platelet sequestration. Treatments include chemotherapy (steroids or vincristine), and rarely, embolization or even organ transplant.[164,165] Because NICHs do not involute, surgical resection is required. Although the prognosis of hemangiomas is generally very good, some lesions can cause morbidity and even mortality based on size, number, and location.[166]

Vascular Malformations

Vascular malformations are divided into slow flow (venous malformation and lymphatic malformation) and fast flow (arteriovenous malformation / arteriovenous fistula) malformations depending on the type of dysmorphic vessels present.[151,165]

Slow Flow Malformations

Venous malformations, previously known as cavernous malformations, cavernous angiomas, and cavernomas, are the most common form of slow or low-flow malformation in the spinal cord. They are composed of single layer endothelial venous spaces without neural tissue and are multiple in up to 16% of affected patients.[167] Although they are common in the brain, only 5% of CNS lesions involve the spine.[168] Lymphatic and venous malformations may compress the spinal cord by direct extension from primary masses in the adjacent soft tissues and/or osseous structures.[153] The underlying etiology of venous malformation remains unknown. However, they have been associated with autosomal dominant mutations on chromosomes 3 and 8 with variable penetrance. Other associations include deep venous anomalies in up to 40% of cases and radiation therapy.[168]

On MR imaging, spinal cord venous malformation demonstrates heterogeneous internal T1 and T2 signal due to hemorrhage and blood products of variable age. However, the key imaging feature is a T2 hypointense hemosiderin rim with moderate surrounding edema and mild enhancement (Fig. 4.55). Once a single venous malformation is found, the entire spinal cord and brain should be imaged using susceptibility weighted sequences to search for additional lesions.[169] Spinal venous malformations are not seen on catheter angiography, similar to venous malformations elsewhere in the body.

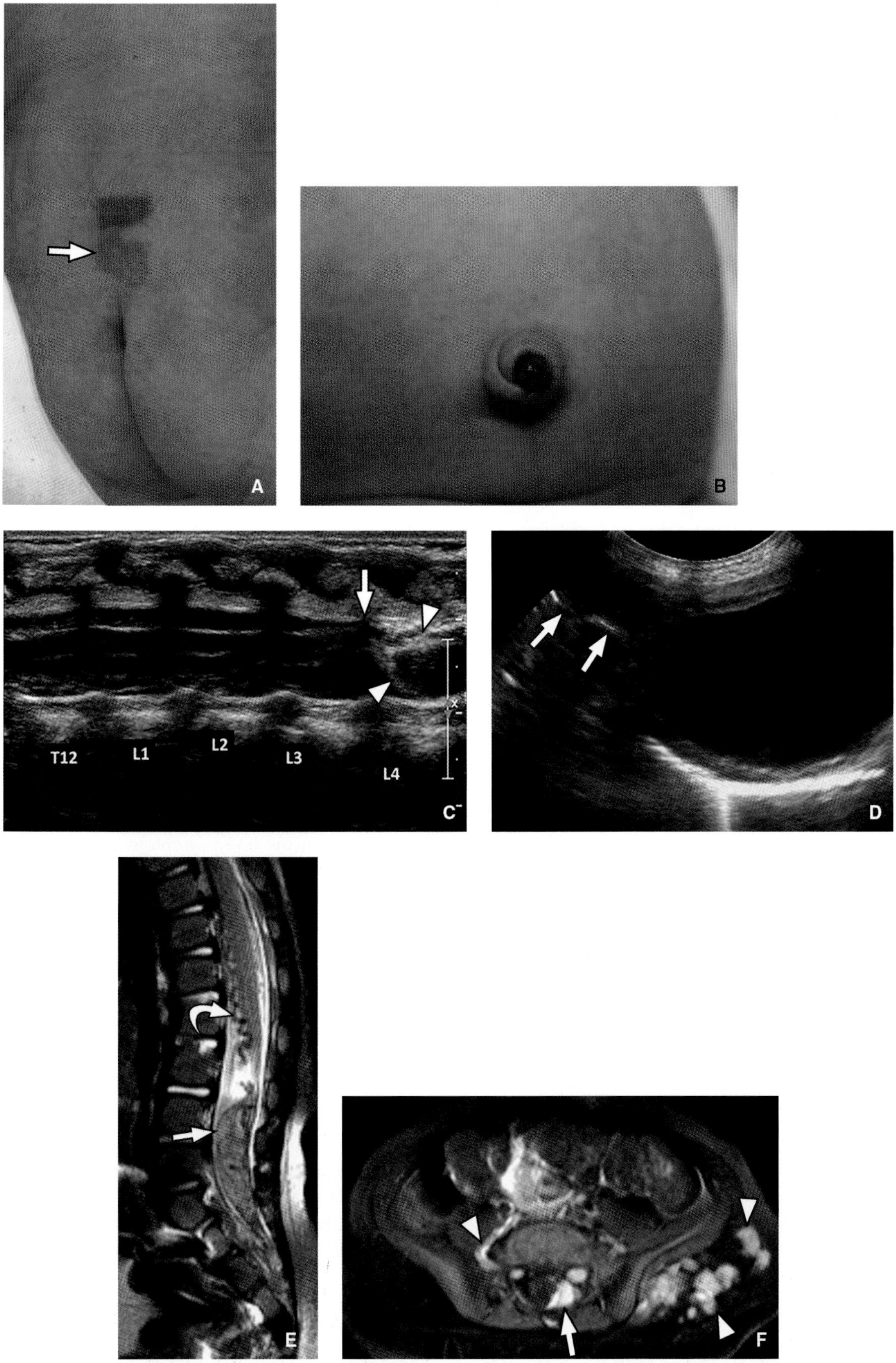

FIGURE 4.53 **Infantile hemangiomas in a 6-month-old boy with spinal segmentation anomalies, imperforate anus, low back hemangiomas, patent urachus, and ambiguous genitalia (SACRAL syndrome). A:** Photographs **(A and B)** show a hemangioma (*arrow*) located just above the gluteal crease and a patent urachus at the umbilicus. **C:** Longitudinal spine ultrasound demonstrates a low conus medullaris (*arrow*) at L4 attached to an echogenic mass (*arrowheads*). **D:** Longitudinal sonogram of the bladder dome confirms the urachus (*arrows*) extending to the skin surface. Sagittal T2-weighted MR image **(E)** of the spine and axial T2-weighted MR image **(F)** of the pelvis demonstrate a slightly T2-hyperintense mass (*straight arrow*) with internal flow voids and vigorous enhancement. Note the presence of several additional hemangiomas (*arrowheads*) in the soft tissues and numerous prominent vessels along the anterior spinal cord surface (*curved arrow*).

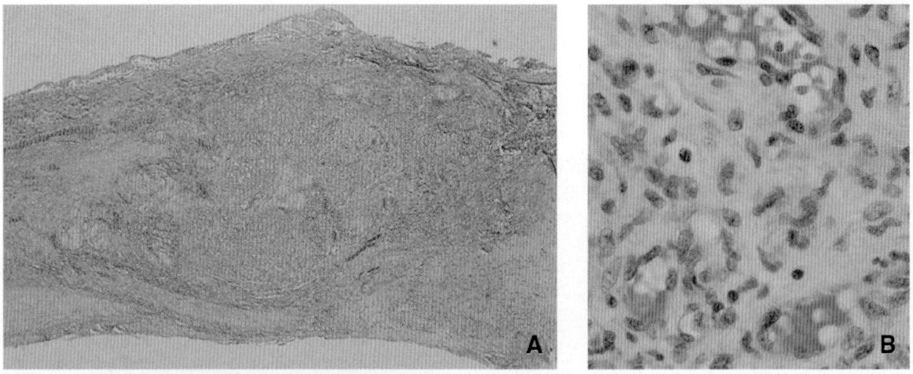

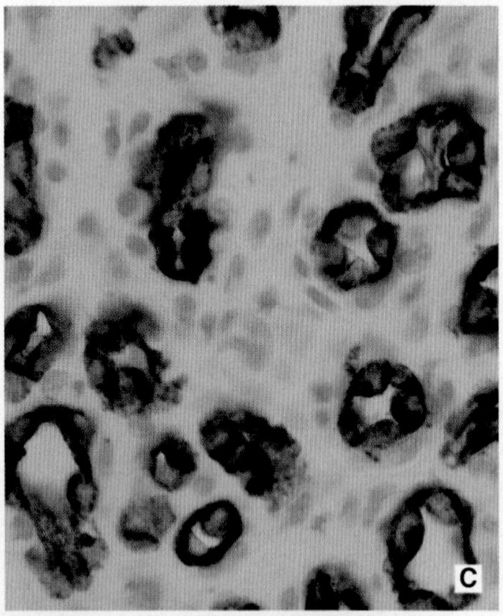

FIGURE 4.54 **Infantile hemangioma in a 4-month-old boy with a midline posterior thoracic cutaneous dermal sinus tract and tethered cord. A:** The hemangioma is admixed with nerve sheath elements including pacinian differentiation and adjacent disorganized brain tissue (hematoxylin and eosin, original magnification, 40×). **B:** The endothelial cells are plump and proliferative (hematoxylin and eosin, original magnification, 400×). **C:** Stain for glut-1 is positive (original magnification, 400×), typical of infantile hemangioma.

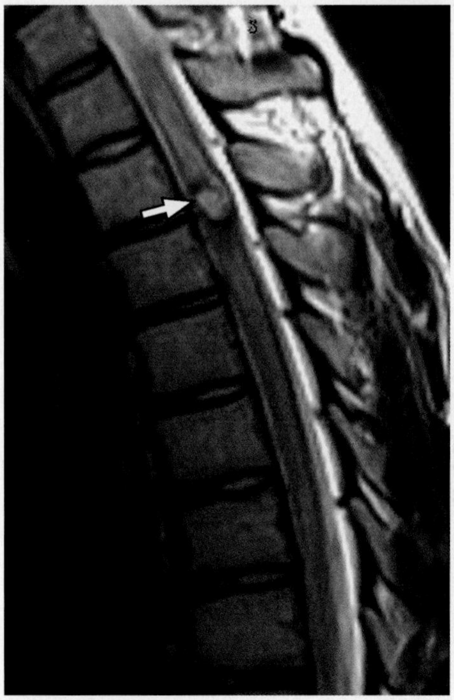

FIGURE 4.55 **Venous malformation in a 16-year-old boy with arm pain and weakness.** Sagittal T2-weighted MR image shows a hyperintense lesion (*arrow*) with a dark hemosiderin rim in the thoracic spinal cord. Note T2 hyperintense edema, in the spinal cord above and below the lesion.

Elsewhere in the body, symptomatic venous malformations are treated with sclerotherapy and/or surgery.[151,163,165] However, those in the spinal cord are usually treated conservatively because of the delicate location.[167,169] Lesions typically do not undergo internal hemorrhage more than once, and outcomes after surgical intervention in spinal cord venous malformations have shown moderate improvement in presenting symptoms in 6% to 23% of cases.[170]

Fast Flow Malformations

Fast, or high-flow vascular malformations are lesions with anomalous communications between arterial and venous structures.[151] They are divided into AVMs, which have a central nidus (cluster of arterioles and venules without an intervening capillary bed), and AVFs, which have a direct arterial to venous connection without a nidus.[163,165,171] AVMs and AVFs are thought to be congenital and acquired, respectively. AVMs are further divided into glomus or metameric types based on the morphology of the nidus.[172] Glomus type AVMs are more common in children and have a tight nidus compared to metameric AVMs, which have a loose nidus.[173] AVMs are twice as common as AVFs in children and can occur throughout the spinal cord. AVFs are subdivided into spinal cord and spinal dural types.[172,173] The former is a far more common type in children than the latter making up nearly all pediatric AVFs.

AVMs and AVFs have a broad range of variable clinical symptoms ranging from acute paralysis to progressive myelopathy including bowel and bladder symptoms, weakness, and sensory loss. Hemorrhage is a common presentation of pediatric AVMs, but not AVFs. Acute presentations of AVMs are due to hemorrhage in more than 50% of cases.[172,174]

Imaging findings of spinal cord AVMs and AVFs are nearly identical. MR imaging and MR angiography are the studies of choice for initial diagnosis because of their lack of radiation exposure and ability to show the spinal cord in multiple planes.[175] Key imaging findings on CT angiography and MRI include tortuous vessels in or on the surface of the spinal cord with or without an associated nidus, cord edema, and/or enhancement (Fig. 4.56).[14,165] A key imaging feature on MR angiography is early venous filling. Ultimately, catheter angiography is required for diagnosis, complete lesion evaluation, and treatment planning.[176,177]

Catheter embolization is the initial treatment of choice for AVMs and AVFs throughout the spinal cord, except for those at the conus, which are surgically removed. However, each lesion requires a specific approach depending on many factors such as size, location, and extent of cord involvement.[172,174] Radiotherapy and microsurgery are other treatment options that may be used alone or in combination with endovascular embolization.[178] The prognosis of AVMs and AVFs depends on the severity of symptoms at the time of diagnosis, with most morbidity persisting partially or completely after treatment.[171,174]

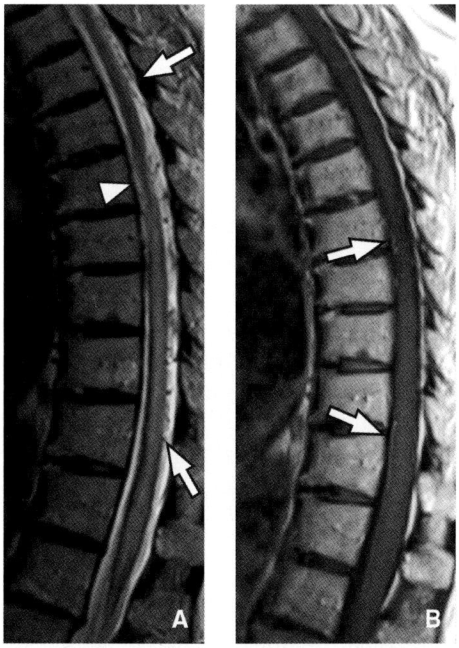

FIGURE 4.56 **Arteriovenous fistula in a 15-year-old boy with back pain and acute leg weakness.** Sagittal T2-weighted **(A)** and postcontrast T1-weighted **(B)** MR images show diffuse increase in T2 signal throughout the spinal cord with tortuous vascular structures (*arrows*) in the surrounding cerebral spinal fluid. Note focal narrowing (*arrowhead*) of the spinal cord suggesting atrophy related to prior ischemia.

Inflammatory Disorders

Transverse Myelitis

Acute transverse myelitis (ATM) is a neurologic disorder characterized by symmetrical abrupt motor, sensory, and autonomic disturbances.[179,180] The term is currently used to describe any cause of the aforementioned clinical symptoms, whereas in the past, transverse myelitis was a term used only for idiopathic cases. ATM is due to a variety of disorders that cause acute spinal cord inflammation, of which viral etiologies are most often blamed, but rarely proven.[180] However, in as many as 60% of affected patients, the etiology is enigmatic. Thus, transverse myelitis is divided into idiopathic and disease-related categories.[180,181]

Across all patient age populations, the incidence of ATM is estimated at between 1.34 and 8 per million per year.[180,181] There are two peaks of incidence for ATM among children, a narrow peak for toddlers under 3 years old, and a larger peak for children between 5 and 17 years old.[181] There is no ethnic, geographic, or familial predisposition, and reports conflict on gender predominance.[181] A recent report regarding children with ATM noted a female predominance of 1.2:1 in children under 10 years of age.[180]

Pediatric ATM is often preceded by a mild prodromal illness ~3 weeks prior to symptom onset.[180] Common presenting symptoms in children include pain, motor deficits, numbness, ataxic gait, priapism, and loss of bowel or bladder function.[180] Nearly all affected pediatric patients have sensory loss in a band-like distribution, reported as numbness or paresthesia. Spinal shock is often present initially because of transient suspension of spinal cord function below the abnormal level.[180] Sympathetic activity below the level of injury is also diminished because of autonomic dysreflexia causing urinary retention and constipation.[180] Deficits are usually abrupt and peak between 4 hours and 21 days of onset.[180]

The Transverse Myelitis Consortium Working Group established inclusion and exclusion criteria for diagnosing idiopathic acute transverse myelitis.[182] Exclusion criteria are as follows: A history of previous spinal radiation, connective tissue disease, ischemia, tumors, CNS infections, and a brain MRI consistent with multiple sclerosis.[182] All of the following inclusion criteria must be met to diagnose idiopathic ATM: Sensory, motor, or autonomic dysfunction, bilateral signs and symptoms, clearly defined sensory level, spinal cord inflammation demonstrated as CSF pleocytosis, enhancing spinal cord lesion on MRI, or elevated IgG, and, finally, progression to nadir between 4 hours and 21 days.[182] Disease-associated ATM requires all inclusion criteria to be met in patients who have one of the conditions listed in the exclusion criteria.[182]

Imaging is beneficial for excluding space-occupying lesions and establishing a diagnosis of ATM or another disorder mimicking ATM.[179,180] Contrast-enhanced MRI is the initial study of choice.[179] Key MRI features include T2-hyperintense and T1-hypointense swelling of the spinal cord over at least three segments with variable enhancement (Fig. 4.57).[179,180] Further imaging with FLAIR and STIR sequences are helpful to suppress CSF and fat signal, respectively.[179] ATM is most

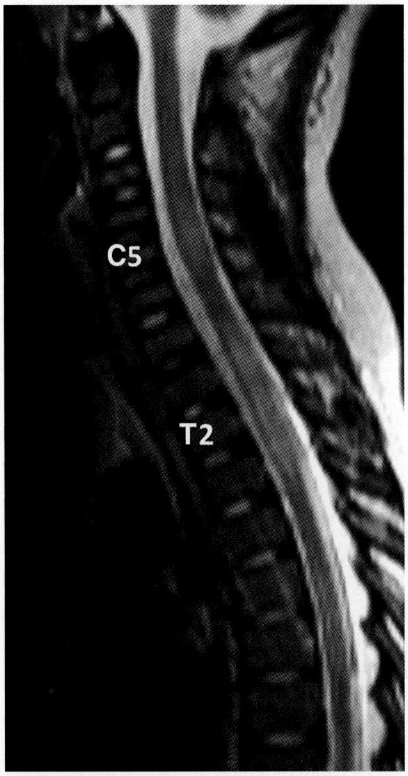

FIGURE 4.57 **Transverse myelitis in a 14-year-old boy with arm pain and weakness.** Sagittal T2-weighted MR image shows patchy signal throughout the spinal cord. Findings are most severe at C5–C6 and T1–T5 levels.

common in the thoracic cord, is generally central, and is more symmetric than cord lesions in multiple sclerosis.[180] Studies have reported that transverse myelitis lesions in pediatric patients average six vertebral segments in length. Cerebral imaging is important to detect disorders mimicking transverse myelitis such as multiple sclerosis.[179]

First-line treatment of ATM is intravenous (IV) methylprednisolone for 1 week, followed by an oral corticosteroid taper.[180] If steroid-resistant exacerbations occur, plasma exchange therapy is initiated.[180] Alternative therapies include IV immunoglobulin and cyclophosphamide.[180] The prognosis of pediatric ATM is based on various factors, including the rapidity of symptom onset, severity of motor weakness at nadir, and need for ventilator support.[180] Complete recovery occurs in 33% to 50% of affected children and outcome is poor in 10% to 20% of cases (lack of ambulation and poor sphincter control).[180] Timely treatment has improved clinical outcomes, including the percentage of children walking independently and the proportion with full recovery at 1 year.[183]

Multiple Sclerosis

Multiple sclerosis (MS) is an autoimmune-mediated disorder that involves inflammatory demyelination in the brain and spinal cord.[184] It is most common in young adults but can occur in children in 3% to 5% of cases.[185,186] Children with MS present in the same manner as adults with relapsing remitting MS, but have episodes of relapse two to three times more frequently.[187] Diagnosis of MS is based on the McDonald criteria, which use clinical and paraclinical assessments (laboratory data and central nervous system MRI findings).[188–190] McDonald criteria revisions made in 2010 allow MRI to play a more important role in the diagnosis of MS by establishing the criteria of dissemination in space (DIS) and time (DIT) more precisely. Specifically, DIS can be demonstrated on MRI by showing at least one T2-hyperintense lesion in two of four locations: Periventricular, juxtacortical, infratentorial, and spinal cord.[188] Revised criteria also allow MRI to establish DIT criteria whenever new T2-hyperintense lesions are found regardless of timing compared to the initial scan.[188] Further, DIT criteria are met when initial MRI identifies enhancing and nonenhancing lesions without requiring a follow-up scan.[191] One author suggests that an additional criterion may be needed in children, stating that an additional 10% of pediatric cases reached the DIS and DIT criteria when enhancing spinal lesions seen on initial MRI were added to the 2010 revised McDonald criteria.[192]

MRI of the brain and spinal cord is critical to the diagnosis of MS. Key brain MRI findings include T2 hyperintense, variably enhancing white matter lesions that are perpendicular to the ventricle margins. These ovoid lesions, known as "Dawson's fingers," are formed by extension of inflammation along perivascular spaces.[193] Lesions at the callososeptal interface are characteristic as well. MS frequently affects the spinal cord with up to 25% of cases presenting with cord lesions only.[194] Key MRI features of spinal cord MS include peripheral T2-hyperintense enhancing lesions with 90% extending over less than two vertebral segments.[195] MS lesions do not respect gray white borders, are most often well defined, are multifocal in 56% of cases, and are mostly located in the dorsolateral cervical spinal cord (Fig. 4.58).[194,196] Silent spinal cord lesions, a unique finding in MS, may allow a diagnosis because they are not seen in other spinal disorders with similar presentations.[197] The differential diagnosis of enhancing spinal MS plaques includes vascular malformations, neoplasms, lupus, and sarcoidosis. These disorders are best distinguished by correlating with clinical history, CSF findings, and brain MRI.

Several treatments are approved for adult MS. Although none are approved in children, the same treatments are used.[198] Treatment options include interferon, steroids, IV immunoglobulins, fingolimod, teriflunomide, mitoxantrone, natalizumab, and cyclophosphamide.[199,200] The prognosis of pediatric MS is highly variable. One third of children have early cognitive impairment with progression within 2 years,[201,202] and progression of motor disabilities takes longer in children than in adults.[203] Cord atrophy may occur and predicts poor prognosis.[204]

Acute Disseminated Encephalomyelitis

Acute disseminated encephalomyelitis (ADEM) is an immune-mediated, monophasic demyelination disorder of the CNS that predominantly involves the white matter of the brain and spinal cord.[205,206] ADEM is rare, with an incidence of eight cases per million people per year.[207] It is often preceded by a viral illness or vaccination and usually occurs in prepubertal children presenting with sensory deficits between 5 and 8 years of age.[208] By comparison, MS is most often

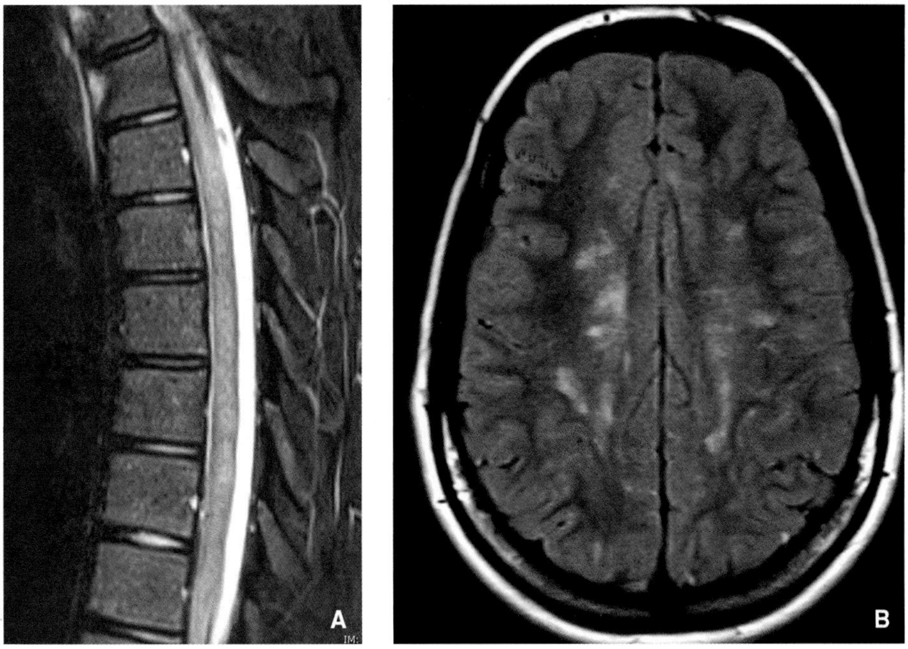

FIGURE 4.58 **Multiple sclerosis in a 15-year-old girl with leg pain and weakness. A:** Sagittal T2-weighted fat-saturated MR image demonstrates diffuse T2-hyperintense signal throughout the thoracic spinal cord. **B:** Axial FLAIR MR image of the brain reveals innumerable hyperintense white matter foci, many of which are oriented perpendicular to the lateral ventricles, typical for multiple sclerosis.

multiphasic occurring in teens and young adults.[209] Other less-common presenting symptoms of spinal cord involvement in ADEM are similar to ATM and MS including extremity pain and weakness, paresthesias, and loss of bowel or bladder function. Up to 10% of cases of ADEM may be eventually reclassified as MS.[210]

Key brain MRI findings that suggest ADEM include bilateral asymmetric confluent T2-hyperintense lesions in the subcortical white matter, thalami, and brain stem. Variable enhancement along the periphery of lesions may be seen along with gray matter involvement of the basal ganglia and less often, spinal cord (Fig. 4.59). Diffusion-weighted MR

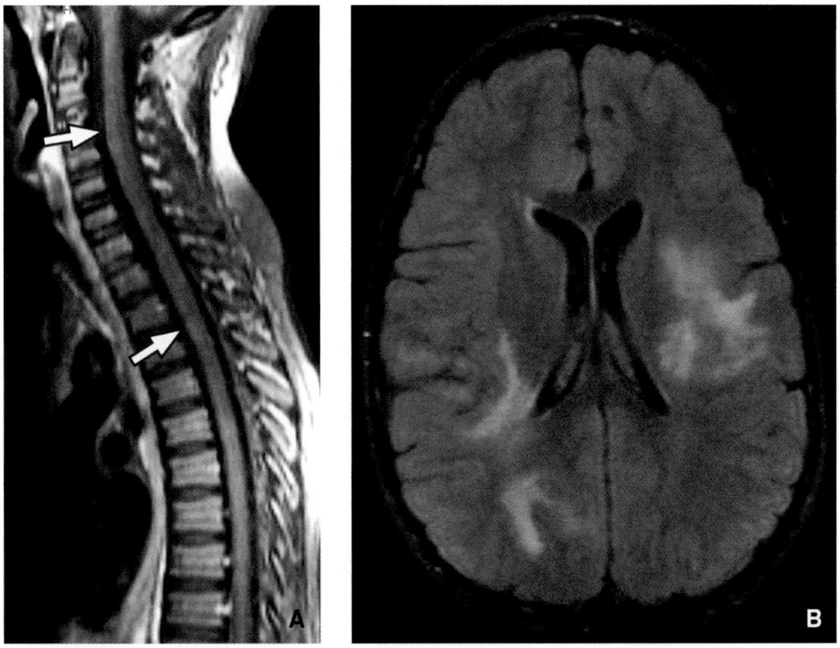

FIGURE 4.59 **Acute disseminated encephalomyelitis in a 13-year-old girl with mental status changes and extremity weakness. A:** Sagittal postcontrast T1-weighted MR image shows subtle ill-defined, patchy enhancement (*arrows*) along the ventral surface of the cervicothoracic spinal cord. **B:** Axial fluid attenuated inversion recovery (FLAIR) MR image demonstrates bilateral confluent regions of white matter hyperintense signal. The regions did not have restricted diffusion or contrast enhancement.

images typically show an increased apparent diffusion coefficient suggesting vasogenic, typically reversible, rather cytotoxic edema. However, in severe cases, restricted diffusion can occur, especially at the lesion margins, and is associated with a worse prognosis.[209,211] Spinal lesions are T2 hyperintense, have occasional enhancement, and are reported in 27% of affected patients.[212]

Treatment of ADEM consists of methylprednisolone, immunoglobulin, and cyclophosphamide.[208] The prognosis of ADEM is generally very good with complete recovery in 1 month in 50% to 60% of cases. Seizures are the most common sequela in up to 30% of children. Death may occur because of respiratory failure in the acute phase in 10% to 30% of children. Some cases may be relapsing, and progression to MS is described in 10% to 35% of cases.[208]

Neuromyelitis Optica or Devic Disease

Neuromyelitis optica (NMO), also known as Devic disease, is a severe demyelinating disorder characterized by optic neuritis and transverse myelitis. Recent evidence has shown that it is humorally mediated and distinct from MS, in spite of similarities in presentation.[213] Disease course may be monophasic or relapsing, the latter being more common in children. The recent discovery of NMO-IgG has helped refine diagnostic criteria, which also require imaging evidence of longitudinally extensive myelitis for diagnosis.

Neuromyelitis optica predominantly affects adults in their late 30s; however, pediatric onset is occasionally seen.[213,214] Among the pediatric population, NMO accounts for ~3% to 4% of demyelinating disease cases.[214] The median age among affected children is 10 to 14 years, although it has been reported in children as young as age 2.[214] Evidence shows a strong female predominance, especially in the relapsing form of the disease, with some reports indicating a three to nine times higher prevalence.[215] NMO is most prevalent among Black North Americans,[214] and affected pediatric patients frequently have other autoimmune disorders such as thyroiditis, lupus, and Sjogren syndrome.[215] The etiology of NMO is not entirely understood, but its coexistence with other autoimmune disorders, and the discovery of the NMO-IgG autoantibody suggests a B-cell mediated process.[213] The antibody targets the aquaporin channels, predominantly found on astrocytes, and it is believed that the proximity to the blood–brain barrier may contribute to injury.[215]

Neuromyelitis optica most often initially presents with ocular pain and/or visual loss due to optic neuritis, or extremity symptoms due to transverse myelitis.[214] These attacks tend to be more severe than optic neuritis associated with multiple sclerosis, with greater visual impairment.[215] Myelitis in NMO presents as complete transverse myelitis involving multiple spinal levels.[214] Depending on the location, this may result in paraparesis, tetraparesis, or sphincter dysfunction, and it is typically more dramatic than myelitis in multiple sclerosis.[214,215] Children with NMO have brain lesions in 68% of cases.[214] In the monophasic course, optic neuritis and myelitis occur within 1 month of each other, and symptoms are generally severe.[213] The relapsing course, which is more common in children, is characterized by relapsing attacks of optic neuritis and transverse myelitis separated by months or years.[214]

Diagnostic criteria for NMO were revised in 2006. Patients must have a history of both optic neuritis and myelitis as absolute criteria, along with at least two out of three of the following supporting criteria: spinal lesions extending over three segments on MRI, a brain MRI that excludes multiple sclerosis, and positive serum NMO-IgG autoantibodies.[214,215]

Key MRI findings include T2-hyperintense lesions that extend over three or more vertebral levels, most frequently involving the central gray matter of the cervical and thoracic cord, cord swelling, and enhancement after contrast.[215] Brain MRI is used to exclude findings typical of multiple sclerosis and is initially normal in 55% to 84% of all patients.[215] Brain lesions are most common in the hypothalamus and brainstem but are nonspecific in 60% of affected patients.[215] Pediatric NMO brain MRIs have occasionally shown white matter, basal ganglia, and hypothalamic lesions.[213]

Treatment of NMO in children is largely the same as in adults.[214] IV corticosteroids are the first-line therapy for acute attacks of optic neuritis and myelitis.[213–215] Most patients respond within 2 weeks, after which they are tapered with oral prednisone.[215] If steroid-resistant exacerbations occur, plasmapheresis is initiated.[213–215] In order to prevent future relapse, affected patients are started on long-term immunosuppressive drugs.[215] Outcomes among NMO patients are overall more severe than those with multiple sclerosis, and patients with monophasic NMO tend to have a better long-term prognosis than patients with a relapsing course.[213] Monocular blindness, ambulatory difficulties, and urinary difficulties are common in relapsing NMO.[213] The 5-year survival rate for monophasic NMO is 90%, and 55% for relapsing NMO within the first year.[213] Affected patients are at risk for mortality because of respiratory failure caused by attacks of ascending cervical myelitis.[213]

Acute Demyelinating Polyradiculoneuritis (Guillain-Barre Syndrome)

Guillain-Barre syndrome (GBS) is a rare autoimmune disorder. The cause of GBS is unknown but believed to be postinfectious because the majority of patients have a history of recent respiratory or GI illness, particularly with *Campylobacter jejuni*.[216] Its incidence is 1 to 2 persons per 100,000 in western countries.[217] Clinically, affected pediatric patients present with symmetric ascending weakness/paralysis, decreased reflexes of deep tendons, and variable sensory symptoms. Urinary retention may occur in cases with rapid onset.[216] Just over half of patients show protein in the CSF without pleocytosis in the first week of illness,[218] which increases to 75% in the second week of illness.[217] Symptoms progress for 10 days on average and then plateau for 1 to 2 weeks, during which time many children cannot walk and 10% require ventilator

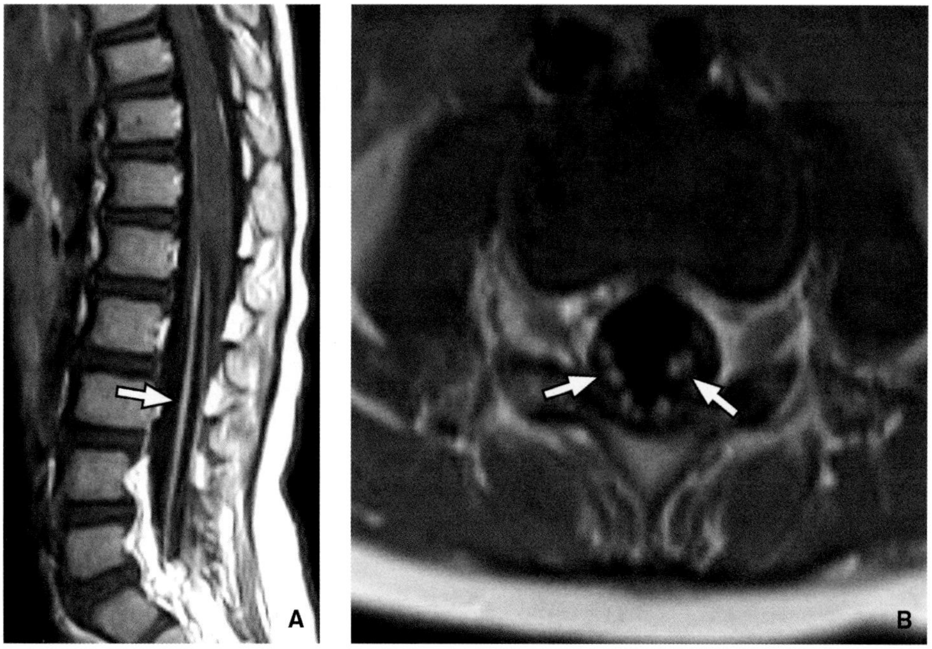

FIGURE 4.60 **Acute demyelinating polyradiculoneuritis (Guillain-Barre syndrome) in a 12-year-old boy with acute leg weakness and loss of bladder function.** Sagittal **(A)** and axial **(B)** postcontrast T1-weighted MR images show enhancement of nerve roots (*arrows*) of the cauda equina.

support.[218] After this time period, symptoms spontaneously regress.

The imaging hallmark of GBS is enhancing cauda equina nerve roots, especially ventral nerve roots, which occurs in 95% of cases (Fig. 4.60).[219] However, recently, authors have also noted enhancing cranial nerves in 83% of affected patients and have advocated for routine brain MRI.[220] Parenchymal brain lesions are rare.

Treatment includes IV immunoglobulins and/or plasmapheresis to remove the offending antibodies.[221] Although full recovery occurs often, 20% of affected patients remain significantly disabled and 5% die because of respiratory failure even with treatment.[217,221]

Hereditary Polyneuropathies (Charcot-Marie-Tooth Disease)

Hereditary sensory and motor neuropathies are often ascribed to Charcot-Marie-Tooth disease (CMT).[222] Although they have been classified into various types based on clinical, electrophysiologic, and genetic characteristics, for the purpose of simplicity, all types will be discussed as CMT in this chapter.[223,224]

CMT, the most common inherited motor sensory neuropathy, affects an estimated 1 in 2,500 individuals.[225,226] The underlying genetic cause is varied, with at least 25 genes currently implicated. These genetic mutations involve proteins with different functions including axonal transport, mitochondrial metabolism, and compaction of myelin.[226] Affected pediatric patients typically present within the first two decades of life with symptoms involving sensory and motor function of the extremities including difficulty running, hindfoot alignment abnormalities (pes cavus), reduced deep-tendon reflexes, and distal extremity sensory loss.[226]

Imaging of CMT relies heavily on MRI, although findings have been described on CT.[227] Radiographs may show neural foraminal enlargement in advanced cases and US has been useful to evaluate peripheral nerve root size. In particular, evaluation of the size of the median nerve has been useful to diagnose some types of CMT.[228] Key imaging findings include enlarged nerves, which are often T2 hyperintense, may enhance, and are most common in the lumbosacral region (Fig. 4.61). Reports have also noted enlarged cranial nerves, peripheral nerves, and nerve roots along the spinal cord.[229] The differential diagnosis of nerve hypertrophy, with or without enhancement, includes chronic inflammatory demyelinating polyneuropathy, or Guillain-Barre syndrome, plexiform neurofibromas in NF1, neurosarcoidosis, and metastatic neoplasms such as leukemia, drop metastasis, and leukemia. The differential can be narrowed based on the degree of nerve root enlargement, enhancement, and smooth versus lobulated nerve morphology.[229]

Currently, there is no effective therapy for CMT. Supportive care is provided in the form of rehabilitative medicine and surgical intervention for soft-tissue abnormalities and skeletal deformities. Experimental models have been valuable for the identification of therapeutic targets, with progesterone antagonists, ascorbic acid, neurotropic factors, and curcumin all currently showing promise as potential therapies.[226] Life expectancy is not altered by CMT, but disability is greater in patients with onset at younger ages.

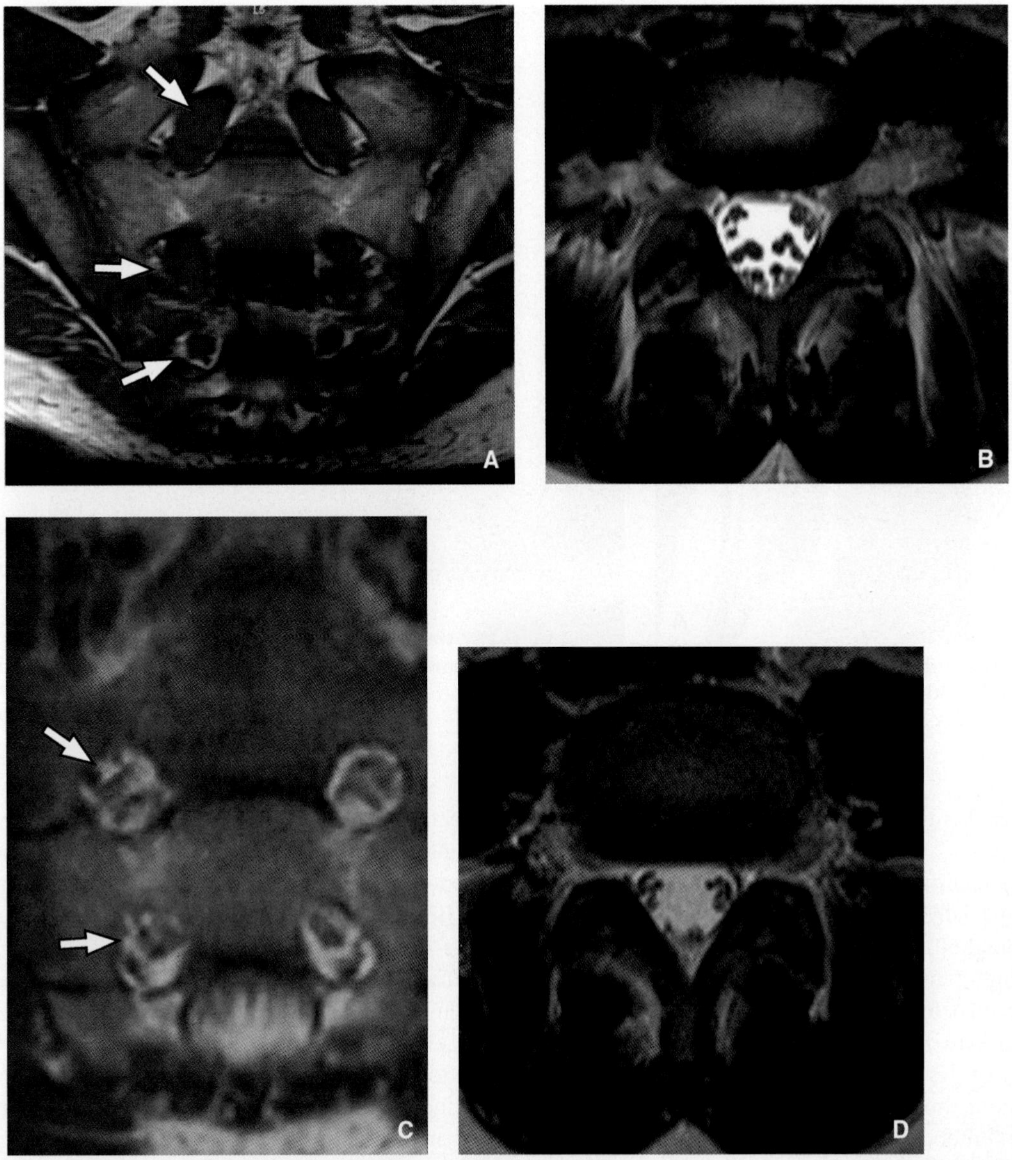

FIGURE 4.61 **Charcot-Marie-Tooth disease in a 13-year-old girl. A and B:** Coronal oblique T1- and axial T2-weighted MR images reveal enlarged exiting sacral nerve roots filling the sacral neural foramina (*arrows*, **A**) and enlarged cauda equina nerve roots in the distal thecal sac **(B)**. **C and D:** Similar images in a normal child demonstrate mostly fat-filled sacral neural foramina (*arrows*, **C**) and normal caliber cauda equina nerve roots **(D)**.

Acknowledgments

The authors wish to thank Maha Jarmakani and Rehan Nizamuddin for their assistance in preparing this manuscript.

References

1. Lohani S, Rodriguez DP, Lidov HG, et al. Intrasacral meningocele in the pediatric population. *J Neurosurg Pediatr.* 2013;11:615–622.
2. Buhs C, Cullen M, Klein M, et al. The pediatric trauma C-spine: is the 'odontoid' view necessary? *J Pediatr Surg.* 2000;35:994–997.
3. Lowe LH, Johanek AJ, Moore CW. Sonography of the neonatal spine: part 2, spinal disorders. *AJR Am J Roentgenol.* 2007;188:739–744.
4. Lowe LH, Johanek AJ, Moore CW. Sonography of the neonatal spine: part 1, normal anatomy, imaging pitfalls, and variations that may simulate disorders. *AJR Am J Roentgenol.* 2007;188:733–738.
5. Unsinn KM, Geley T, Freund MC, et al. US of the spinal cord in newborns: spectrum of normal findings, variants, congenital anomalies, and acquired diseases. *Radiographics.* 2000;20:923–938.
6. Riccabona M, Nelson TR, Weitzer C, et al. Potential of three-dimensional ultrasound in neonatal and paediatric neurosonography. *Eur Radiol.* 2003;13:2082–2093.
7. Phalke VV, Gujar S, Quint DJ. Comparison of 3.0 T versus 1.5 T MR: imaging of the spine. *Neuroimaging Clin N Am.* 2006;16:241–248, ix.
8. Gasparotti R. New techniques in spinal imaging. *Neuroradiology.* 2011;53(suppl 1):S195–S197.

9. Kukreja K, Manzano G, Ragheb J, et al. Differentiation between pediatric spinal arachnoid and epidermoid–dermoid cysts: is diffusion-weighted MRI useful? *Pediatr Radiol.* 2007;37:556–560.
10. Ducreux D, Lepeintre JF, Fillard P, et al. MR diffusion tensor imaging and fiber tracking in 5 spinal cord astrocytomas. *AJNR Am J Neuroradiol.* 2006;27:214–216.
11. Hofmann E, Warmuth-Metz M, Bendszus M, et al. Phase-contrast MR imaging of the cervical CSF and spinal cord: volumetric motion analysis in patients with Chiari I malformation. *AJNR Am J Neuroradiol.* 2000;21:151–158.
12. Walker HS, Dietrich RB, Flannigan BD, et al. Magnetic resonance imaging of the pediatric spine. *Radiographics.* 1987;7:1129–1152.
13. Kamoto Y, Sadato N, Yonekura Y, et al. Visualization of the cervical spinal cord with FDG and high-resolution PET. *J Comput Assist Tomogr.* 1998;22:487–491.
14. Rossi A, Biancheri R, Cama A, et al. Imaging in spine and spinal cord malformations. *Eur J Radiol.* 2004;50:177–200.
15. Naidich TP, McLone DG, Mutluer S. A new understanding of dorsal dysraphism with lipoma (lipomyeloschisis): radiologic evaluation and surgical correction. *AJR Am J Roentgenol.* 1983;140:1065–1078.
16. Karwacki GM, Schneider JF. Normal ossification patterns of atlas and axis: a CT study. *AJNR Am J Neuroradiol.* 2012;33:1882–1887.
17. Irani N, Goud AR, Lowe LH. Isolated filar cyst on lumbar spine sonography in infants: a case-control study. *Pediatr Radiol.* 2006;36:1283–1288.
18. Barkovich AJ, Naidich TP. Congenital anomalies of the spine. In: Norman D, ed. *Contemporary Neuroimaging.* 2nd ed. New York: Raven; 1995:477–540.
19. Thakur NH, Lowe LH. Borderline low conus medullaris on infant lumbar sonography: what is the clinical outcome and the role of neuroimaging follow-up? *Pediatr Radiol.* 2011;41:483–487.
20. Pang D. Split cord malformation: part II: clinical syndrome. *Neurosurgery.* 1992;31:481–500.
21. Pang D, Dias MS, Ahab-Barmada M. Split cord malformation: part I: a unified theory of embryogenesis for double spinal cord malformations. *Neurosurgery.* 1992;31:451–480.
22. Naidich TP, Blaser SI, Delman BD, et al. Congenital anomalies of the spine and spinal cord: embryology and malformations. In: Atlas SW, ed. *Magnetic Resonance Imaging of the Brain and Spine.* Vol. 2. 4th ed. Philadelphia, PA: Lippincott-Raven; 2008.
23. Tortori-Donati P, Rossi A, Cama A. Spinal dysraphism: a review of neuroradiological features with embryological correlations and proposal for a new classification. *Neuroradiology.* 2000;42:471–491.
24. Tortori-Donati P, Rossi A, Biancheri R, et al. Congenital malformations of the spine and spinal cord. In: *Pediatric Neuroradiology.* Berlin Heidelberg: Springer; 2005:1551–1608.
25. McLone DG, Knepper PA. The cause of Chiari II malformation: a unified theory. *Pediatr Neurosci.* 1989;15:1–12.
26. Batty R, Vitta L, Whitby EH, et al. Is there a causal relationship between open spinal dysraphism and Chiari II deformity? A study using in utero magnetic resonance imaging of the fetus. *Neurosurgery.* 2012;70:890–898; discussion 898–899.
27. Adzick NS. Fetal myelomeningocele: natural history, pathophysiology, and in-utero intervention. *Semin Fetal Neonatal Med.* 2010;15:9–14.
28. Meuli M, Meuli-Simmen C, Hutchins GM, et al. The spinal cord lesion in human fetuses with myelomeningocele: implications for fetal surgery. *J Pediatr Surg.* 1997;32:448–452.
29. Danzer E, Johnson MP, Adzick NS. Fetal surgery for myelomeningocele: progress and perspectives. *Dev Med Child Neurol.* 2012;54:8–14.
30. Naidich TP, McLone DG, Fulling KH. The Chiari II malformation: part IV. The hindbrain deformity. *Neuroradiology.* 1983;25:179–197.
31. Tortori-Donati P, Rossi A, Biancheri R, et al. Magnetic resonance imaging of spinal dysraphism. *Top Magn Reson Imaging.* 2001; 12:375–409.
32. Oi S, Nomura S, Nagasaka M, et al. Embryopathogenetic surgicoanatomical classification of dysraphism and surgical outcome of spinal lipoma: a nationwide multicenter cooperative study in Japan. *J Neurosurg Pediatr.* 2009;3:412–419.
33. Sarris CE, Tomei KL, Carmel PW, et al. Lipomyelomeningocele: pathology, treatment, and outcomes. *Neurosurg Focus.* 2012;33:E3.
34. Ersahin Y, Barcin E, Mutluer S. Is meningocele really an isolated lesion? *Childs Nerv Syst.* 2001;17:487–490.
35. Barkovich AJ. Congenital anomalies of the spine. In: *Pediatric Neuroimaging.* Philadelphia, PA: Lippincott Williams & Wilkins; 2000.
36. Pang D, Zovickian J, Lee JY, et al. Terminal myelocystocele: surgical observations and theory of embryogenesis. *Neurosurgery.* 2012;70:1383–1404; discussion 1404–1385.
37. Hashiguchi K, Morioka T, Samura K, et al. Holocord hydrosyringomyelia with terminal myelocystocele revealed by constructive interference in steady-state MR imaging. *Pediatr Neurosurg.* 2008;44:509–512.
38. Choi S, McComb JG. Long-term outcome of terminal myelocystocele patients. *Pediatr Neurosurg.* 2000;32:86–91.
39. Gupta DK, Mahapatra AK. Terminal myelocystoceles: a series of 17 cases. *J Neurosurg.* 2005;103:344–352.
40. Morioka T, Hashiguchi K, Yoshida F, et al. Neurosurgical management of occult spinal dysraphism associated with OEIS complex. *Childs Nerv Syst.* 24:723–729.
41. Emmanouilidou M, Chondromatidou S, Goutsaridou F, et al. MRI evaluation of diastematomyelia and associated abnormalities. *Neuroradiol J.* 2006;19:367–374.
42. Gan YC, Sgouros S, Walsh AR, et al. Diastematomyelia in children: treatment outcome and natural history of associated syringomyelia. *Childs Nerv Syst.* 2007;23:515–519.
43. Yamada S, Knerium DS, Mandybur GM, et al. Pathophysiology of tethered cord syndrome and other complex factors. *Neurol Res.* 2004;26:722–726.
44. Warder DE. Tethered cord syndrome and occult spinal dysraphism. *Neurosurg Focus.* 2001;10:e1.
45. Tubbs RS, Oakes WJ. Urinary incontinence in a patient with Duchenne muscular dystrophy and cord in the normal position with fatty filum terminale. *Childs Nerv Syst.* 2004;20:717–719.
46. Lew SM, Kothbauer KF. Tethered cord syndrome: an updated review. *Pediatr Neurosurg.* 2007;43:236–248.
47. Ramnarayan R, Dominic A, Alapatt J, et al. Congenital spinal dermal sinuses: poor awareness leads to delayed treatment. *Childs Nerv Syst.* 2006;22:1220–1224.
48. Ikwueke I, Bandara S, Fishman SJ, et al. Congenital dermal sinus tract in the lateral buttock: unusual presentation of a typically midline lesion. *J Pediatr Surg.* 2008;43:1200–1202.
49. Jindal A, Mahapatra AK. Spinal congenital dermal sinus: an experience of 23 cases over 7 years. *Neurol India.* 2001;49:243–246.
50. de Oliveira RS, Cinalli G, Roujeau T, et al. Neurenteric cysts in children: 16 consecutive cases and review of the literature. *J Neurosurg.* 2005;103:512–523.

51. Radmanesh F, Nejat F, El Khashab M. Dermal sinus tract of the spine. *Childs Nerv Syst.* 2010;26:349–357.
52. Martinez-Lage JF, Perez-Espejo MA, Tortosa JG, et al. Hydrocephalus in intraspinal dermoids and dermal sinuses: the spectrum of an uncommon association in children. *Childs Nerv Syst.* 2006;22:698–703.
53. Schenk JP, Herweh C, Gunther P, et al. Imaging of congenital anomalies and variations of the caudal spine and back in neonates and small infants. *Eur J Radiol.* 2006;58:3–14.
54. van Aalst J, Beuls EA, Cornips EM, et al. Anatomy and surgery of the infected dermal sinus of the lower spine. *Childs Nerv Syst.* 2006;22:1307–1315.
55. Giuffre R. Intradural spinal lipomas. Review of the literature (99 cases) and report of an additional case. *Acta Neurochir.* 1966;14:69–95.
56. Pierre-Kahn A, Zerah M, Renier D, et al. Congenital lumbosacral lipomas. *Childs Nerv Syst.* 1997;13:298–334; discussion 335.
57. Naidich TP, Zimmerman RA, McLone DG. *Congenital Anomalies of the Spine and Spinal Cord: Embryology and Malformations.* Philadelphia, PA: Lippincott-Raven; 1996.
58. Koyanagi I, Iwasaki Y, Hida K, et al. Factors in neurological deterioration and role of surgical treatment in lumbosacral spinal lipoma. *Childs Nerv Syst.* 2000;16:143–149.
59. Hoffman HJ, Neill J, Crone KR, et al. Hydrosyringomyelia and its management in childhood. *Neurosurgery.* 1987;21:347–351.
60. Vandertop WP. Syringomyelia. *Neuropediatrics.* 2013.
61. Greitz D. Unraveling the riddle of syringomyelia. *Neurosurg Rev.* 2006;29:251–263; discussion 264.
62. Isu T, Iwasaki Y, Akino M, et al. Hydrosyringomyelia associated with a Chiari I malformation in children and adolescents. *Neurosurgery.* 1990;26:591–596; discussion 596–597.
63. Roser F, Ebner FH, Danz S, et al. Three-dimensional constructive interference in steady-state magnetic resonance imaging in syringomyelia: advantages over conventional imaging. *J Neurosurg Spine.* 2008;8:429–435.
64. Bunck AC, Kroeger JR, Juettner A, et al. Magnetic resonance 4D flow analysis of cerebrospinal fluid dynamics in Chiari I malformation with and without syringomyelia. *Eur Radiol.* 2012;22:1860–1870.
65. Hankinson T, Tubbs RS, Wellons JC. Duraplasty or not? An evidence-based review of the pediatric Chiari I malformation. *Childs Nerv Syst.* 2011;27:35–40.
66. Bao C, Yang F, Liu L, et al. Surgical treatment of Chiari I malformation complicated with syringomyelia. *Exp Ther Med.* 2013;5:333–337.
67. Holmes GL, Trader S, Ignatiadis P. Intraspinal enterogenous cysts. A case report and review of pediatric cases in the literature. *Am J Dis Child.* 1978;132:906–908.
68. Mann KS, Khosla VK, Gulati DR, et al. Spinal neurenteric cyst. Association with vertebral anomalies, diastematomyelia, dorsal fistula, and lipoma. *Surg Neurol.* 1984;21:358–362.
69. Rao MB, Rout D, Misra BK, et al. Craniospinal and spinal enterogenous cysts—report of three cases. *Clin Neurol Neurosurg.* 1996;98:32–36.
70. Menezes AH, Ryken TC. Craniocervical intradural neurenteric cysts. *Pediatr Neurosurg.* 1995;22:88–95.
71. Brooks BS, Duvall ER, el Gammal T, et al. Neuroimaging features of neurenteric cysts: analysis of nine cases and review of the literature. *AJNR Am J Neuroradiol.* 1993;14:735–746.
72. Al-Ahmed IH, Boughamoura M, Dirks P, et al. Neurosurgical management of neurenteric cysts in children. *J Neurosurg Pediatr.* 2013;11:511–517.
73. Solomon T, Kneen R, Dung NM, et al. Poliomyelitis-like illness due to Japanese encephalitis virus. *Lancet.* 1998;351:1094–1097.
74. Kincaid O, Lipton HL. Viral myelitis: an update. *Curr Neurol Neurosci Rep.* 2006;6:469–474.
75. Jeha LE, Sila CA, Lederman RJ, et al. West Nile virus infection: a new acute paralytic illness. *Neurology.* 2003;61:55–59.
76. Chen CY, Chang YC, Huang CC, et al. Acute flaccid paralysis in infants and young children with enterovirus 71 infection: MR imaging findings and clinical correlates. *AJNR Am J Neuroradiol.* 2001;22:200–205.
77. Malzberg MS, Rogg JM, Tate CA, et al. Poliomyelitis: hyperintensity of the anterior horn cells on MR images of the spinal cord. *AJR Am J Roentgenol.* 1993;161:863–865.
78. Choudhary A, Sharma S, Sankhyan N, et al. Midbrain and spinal cord magnetic resonance imaging (MRI) changes in poliomyelitis. *J Child Neurol.* 2010;25:497–499.
79. Huang CC, Liu CC, Chang YC, et al. Neurologic complications in children with enterovirus 71 infection. *N Engl J Med.* 1999; 341:936–942.
80. Chang LY, Huang LM, Gau SS, et al. Neurodevelopment and cognition in children after enterovirus 71 infection. *N Engl J Med.* 2007;356:1226–1234.
81. Friess HM, Wasenko JJ. MR of staphylococcal myelitis of the cervical spinal cord. *AJNR Am J Neuroradiol.* 1997;18:455–458.
82. Akgoz A, Mukundan S, Lee TC. Imaging of rickettsial, spirochetal, and parasitic infections. *Neuroimaging Clin N Am.* 2012;22:633–657.
83. Mihai C, Jubelt B. Infectious myelitis. *Curr Neurol Neurosci Rep.* 2012;12:633–641.
84. Wasay M, Arif H, Khealani B, et al. Neuroimaging of tuberculous myelitis: analysis of ten cases and review of literature. *J Neuroimaging.* 2006;16:197–205.
85. Sharif HS. Role of MR imaging in the management of spinal infections. *AJR Am J Roentgenol.* 1992;158:1333–1345.
86. Tsiodras S, Kelesidis I, Kelesidis T, et al. Central nervous system manifestations of Mycoplasma pneumoniae infections. *J Infect.* 2005;51:343–354.
87. DeSanto J, Ross JS. Spine infection/inflammation. *Radiol Clin North Am.* 2011;49:105–127.
88. Baumann M, Birnbacher R, Koch J, et al. Uncommon manifestations of neuroborreliosis in children. *Eur J Paediatr Neurol.* 2010;14:274–277.
89. Wilne S, Walker D. Spine and spinal cord tumours in children: a diagnostic and therapeutic challenge to healthcare systems. *Arch Dis Child Educ Pract Ed.* 2010;95:47–54.
90. Dietrich RB, Kangarloo H. Retroperitoneal mass with intradural extension: value of magnetic resonance imaging in neuroblastoma. *AJR Am J Roentgenol.* 1986;146:251–254.
91. Keiper MD, Zimmerman RA, Bilaniuk LT. MRI in the assessment of the supportive soft tissues of the cervical spine in acute trauma in children. *Neuroradiology.* 1998;40:359–363.
92. Houten JK, Weiner HL. Pediatric intramedullary spinal cord tumors: special considerations. *J Neurooncol.* 2000;47:225–230.
93. Sakai Y, Matsuyama Y, Katayama Y, et al. Spinal myxopapillary ependymoma: neurological deterioration in patients treated with surgery. *Spine.* 2009;34:1619–1624.
94. Huisman TA. Pediatric tumors of the spine. *Cancer Imaging.* 2009;9(Spec No A):S45–S48.
95. Smith AB, Soderlund KA, Rushing EJ, et al. Radiologic–pathologic correlation of pediatric and adolescent spinal neoplasms: part 1, intramedullary spinal neoplasms. *AJR Am J Roentgenol.* 2012;198:34–43.

96. Young Poussaint T, Yousuf N, Barnes PD, et al. Cervicomedullary astrocytomas of childhood: clinical and imaging follow-up. *Pediatr Radiol.* 1999;29:662–668.
97. Roonprapunt C, Houten JK. Spinal cord astrocytomas: presentation, management, and outcome. *Neurosurg Clin N Am.* 2006;17:29–36.
98. Schittenhelm J, Ebner FH, Tatagiba M, et al. Holocord pilocytic astrocytoma—case report and review of the literature. *Clin Neurol Neurosurg.* 2009;111:203–207.
99. Benes V III, Barsa P, Benes V Jr, et al. Prognostic factors in intramedullary astrocytomas: a literature review. *Eur Spine J.* 2009;18:1397–1422.
100. Sarikaya S, Acikgoz B, Tekkok IH, et al. Conus ependymoma with holocord syringohydromyelia and syringobulbia. *J Clin Neurosci.* 2007;14:901–904.
101. Wippold FJ II, Smirniotopoulos JG, Moran CJ, et al. MR imaging of myxopapillary ependymoma: findings and value to determine extent of tumor and its relation to intraspinal structures. *AJR Am J Roentgenol.* 1995;165:1263–1267.
102. Khan SN, Donthineni R. Surgical management of metastatic spine tumors. *Orthop Clin North Am.* 2006;37:99–104.
103. Gebauer GP, Farjoodi P, Sciubba DM, et al. Magnetic resonance imaging of spine tumors: classification, differential diagnosis, and spectrum of disease. *J Bone Joint Surg.* 2008;90(suppl 4): 146–162.
104. Aguilera DG, Mazewski C, Schniederjan MJ, et al. Neurofibromatosis-2 and spinal cord ependymomas: report of two cases and review of the literature. *Childs Nerv Syst.* 2011;27:757–764.
105. Oh MC, Kim JM, Kaur G, et al. Prognosis by tumor location in adults with spinal ependymomas. *J Neurosurg Spine.* 2013;18:226–235.
106. Patel U, Pinto RS, Miller DC, et al. MR of spinal cord ganglioglioma. *AJNR Am J Neuroradiol.* 1998;19:879–887.
107. Jallo GI, Freed D, Epstein FJ. Spinal cord gangliogliomas: a review of 56 patients. *J Neurooncol.* 2004;68:71–77.
108. Lang FF, Epstein FJ, Ransohoff J, et al. Central nervous system gangliogliomas. Part 2: clinical outcome. *J Neurosurg.* 1993;79:867–873.
109. Costa J, Ruivo J, Miguens J, et al. Ganglioglioma of conus medullaris. *Acta Neurochir.* 2006;148:977–980.
110. Bostrom A, Hans FJ, Reinacher PC, et al. Intramedullary hemangioblastomas: timing of surgery, microsurgical technique and follow-up in 23 patients. *Eur Spine J.* 2008;17:882–886.
111. Sardi I, Sanzo M, Giordano F, et al. Monotherapy with thalidomide for treatment of spinal cord hemangioblastomas in a patient with von Hippel–Lindau disease. *Pediatr Blood Cancer.* 2009;53:464–467.
112. Vougioukas VI, Glasker S, Hubbe U, et al. Surgical treatment of hemangioblastomas of the central nervous system in pediatric patients. *Childs Nerv Syst.* 2006;22:1149–1153.
113. Murota T, Symon L. Surgical management of hemangioblastoma of the spinal cord: a report of 18 cases. *Neurosurgery.* 1989;25:699–707; discussion 708.
114. Niemela M, Lim YJ, Soderman M, et al. Gamma knife radiosurgery in 11 hemangioblastomas. *J Neurosurg.* 1996;85:591–596.
115. Eskridge JM, McAuliffe W, Harris B, et al. Preoperative endovascular embolization of craniospinal hemangioblastomas. *AJNR Am J Neuroradiol.* 1996;17:525–531.
116. Zhou LF, Du G, Mao Y, et al. Diagnosis and surgical treatment of brainstem hemangioblastomas. *Surg Neurol.* 2005;63:307–315; discussion 315–306.
117. Hasselblatt M, Jeibmann A, Gerss J, et al. Cellular and reticular variants of haemangioblastoma revisited: a clinicopathologic study of 88 cases. *Neuropathol Appl Neurobiol.* 2005;31: 618–622.
118. Kim NR, Suh YL, Shin HJ. Thoracic pediatric intramedullary schwannoma: report of a case. *Pediatr Neurosurg.* 2009;45:396–401.
119. Jinnai T, Koyama T. Clinical characteristics of spinal nerve sheath tumors: analysis of 149 cases. *Neurosurgery.* 2005;56:510–515; discussion 510–515.
120. Pollack IF, Colak A, Fitz C, et al. Surgical management of spinal cord compression from plexiform neurofibromas in patients with neurofibromatosis 1. *Neurosurgery.* 1998;43:248–255; discussion 255–246.
121. Liu PI, Liu GC, Tsai KB, et al. Intraspinal clear-cell meningioma: case report and review of literature. *Surg Neurol.* 2005;63: 285–288; discussion 288–289.
122. Solero CL, Fornari M, Giombini S, et al. Spinal meningiomas: review of 174 operated cases. *Neurosurgery.* 1989;25:153–160.
123. Cohen-Gadol AA, Zikel OM, Koch CA, et al. Spinal meningiomas in patients younger than 50 years of age: a 21-year experience. *J Neurosurg.* 2003;98:258–263.
124. Parmar H, Hawkins C, Bouffet E, et al. Imaging findings in primary intracranial atypical teratoid/rhabdoid tumors. *Pediatr Radiol.* 2006;36:126–132.
125. Khan ZA, Boscolo E, Picard A, et al. Multipotential stem cells recapitulate human infantile hemangioma in immunodeficient mice. *J Clin Invest.* 2008;118:2592–2599.
126. Sciubba DM, Hsieh P, McLoughlin GS, et al. Pediatric tumors involving the spinal column. *Neurosurg Clin N Am.* 2008;19:81–92.
127. Plantaz D, Rubie H, Michon J, et al. The treatment of neuroblastoma with intraspinal extension with chemotherapy followed by surgical removal of residual disease. A prospective study of 42 patients—results of the NBL 90 Study of the French Society of Pediatric Oncology. *Cancer.* 1996;78:311–319.
128. Fadler KM, Askin DF. Sacrococcygeal teratoma in the newborn: a case study of prenatal management and clinical intervention. *Neonatal Netw.* 2008;27:185–191.
129. Schropp KP, Lobe TE, Rao B, et al. Sacrococcygeal teratoma: the experience of four decades. *J Pediatr Surg.* 1992;27: 1075–1078; discussion 1078–1079.
130. Vazquez E, Lucaya J, Castellote A, et al. Neuroimaging in pediatric leukemia and lymphoma: differential diagnosis. *Radiographics.* 2002;22:1411–1428.
131. Murphey MD, Andrews CL, Flemming DJ, et al. From the archives of the AFIP. Primary tumors of the spine: radiologic pathologic correlation. *Radiographics.* 1996;16:1131–1158.
132. Hayashi M, Maeda M, Maji T, et al. Diffuse leptomeningeal hyperintensity on fluid-attenuated inversion recovery MR images in neurocutaneous melanosis. *AJNR Am J Neuroradiol.* 2004;25:138–141.
133. Kadonaga JN, Barkovich AJ, Edwards MS, et al. Neurocutaneous melanosis in association with the Dandy-Walker complex. *Pediatr Dermatol.* 1992;9:37–43.
134. Chaloupka JC, Wolf RJ, Varma PK. Neurocutaneous melanosis with the Dandy-Walker malformation: a possible rare pathoetiologic association. *Neuroradiology.* 1996;38:486–489.
135. Di Rocco F, Sabatino G, Koutzoglou M, et al. Neurocutaneous melanosis. *Childs Nerv Syst.* 2004;20:23–28.
136. Beltran J, Noto AM, Chakeres DW, et al. Tumors of the osseous spine: staging with MR imaging versus CT. *Radiology.* 1987;162: 565–569.

137. Saccomanni B. Osteoid osteoma and osteoblastoma of the spine: a review of the literature. *Curr Rev Musculoskelet Med.* 2009;2:65–67.
138. Kransdorf MJ, Sweet DE. Aneurysmal bone cyst: concept, controversy, clinical presentation, and imaging. *AJR Am J Roentgenol.* 1995;164:573–580.
139. Kim HJ, McLawhorn AS, Goldstein MJ, et al. Malignant osseous tumors of the pediatric spine. *J Am Acad Orthop Surg.* 2012;20:646–656.
140. Kobayashi S, Kanda K, Yokochi K, et al. A case of spinal cord injury that occurred in utero. *Pediatr Neurol.* 2006;35:367–369.
141. Steens SC, Pondaag W, Malessy MJ, et al. Obstetric brachial plexus lesions: CT myelography. *Radiology.* 2011;259:508–515.
142. Yoshikawa T, Hayashi N, Yamamoto S, et al. Brachial plexus injury: clinical manifestations, conventional imaging findings, and the latest imaging techniques. *Radiographics.* 2006; 26(suppl 1):S133–S143.
143. Wandler E, Lefton D, Babb J, et al. Periscalene soft tissue: the new imaging hallmark in Erb palsy. *AJNR Am J Neuroradiol.* 2010;31:882–885.
144. Chhabra A, Thawait GK, Soldatos T, et al. High-resolution 3T MR neurography of the brachial plexus and its branches, with emphasis on 3D imaging. *AJNR Am J Neuroradiol.* 2013;34:486–497.
145. Roche C, Carty H. Spinal trauma in children. *Pediatr Radiol* 2001;31:677–700.
146. Gargas J, Yaszay B, Kruk P, et al. An analysis of cervical spine magnetic resonance imaging findings after normal computed tomographic imaging findings in pediatric trauma patients: ten-year experience of a level I pediatric trauma center. *J Trauma Acute Care Surg.* 2013;74:1102–1107.
147. Egloff AM, Kadom N, Vezina G, et al. Pediatric cervical spine trauma imaging: a practical approach. *Pediatr Radiol.* 2009;39:447–456.
148. Turgut M, Akpinar G, Akalan N, et al. Spinal injuries in the pediatric age group: a review of 82 cases of spinal cord and vertebral column injuries. *Eur Spine J.* 1996;5:148–152.
149. Mulliken JB, Glowacki J. Classification of pediatric vascular lesions. *Plast Reconstr Surg.* 1982;70:120–121.
150. Mulliken JB, Fishman SJ, Burrows PE. Vascular anomalies. *Curr Probl Surg.* 2000;37:517–584.
151. Mulliken JB. A biologic approach to cutaneous vascular anomalies. *Pediatr Dermatol.* 1992;9:356–357.
152. Kollipara R, Odhav A, Rentas KE, et al. Vascular anomalies in pediatric patients: updated classification, imaging, and therapy. *Radiol Clin North Am.* 2013;51:659–672.
153. Bruder E, Perez-Atayde AR, Jundt G, et al. Vascular lesions of bone in children, adolescents, and young adults. A clinicopathologic reappraisal and application of the ISSVA classification. *Virchows Arch.* 2009;454:161–179.
154. Lowe LH, Marchant TC, Rivard DC, et al. Vascular malformations: classification and terminology the radiologist needs to know. *Semin Roentgenol.* 2012;47:106–117.
155. Mulliken JB, Enjolras O. Congenital hemangiomas and infantile hemangioma: missing links. *J Am Acad Dermatol.* 2004;50:875–882.
156. Leon-Villapalos J, Wolfe K, Kangesu L. GLUT-1: an extra diagnostic tool to differentiate between haemangiomas and vascular malformations. *Br J Plast Surg.* 2005;58:348–352.
157. Restrepo R, Palani R, Cervantes LF, et al. Hemangiomas revisited: the useful, the unusual and the new. Part 1: overview and clinical and imaging characteristics. *Pediatr Radiol.* 2011;41:895–904.
158. North PE, Waner M, Brodsky MC. Are infantile hemangioma of placental origin? *Ophthalmology.* 2002;109:223–224.
159. Berenguer B, Mulliken JB, Enjolras O, et al. Rapidly involuting congenital hemangioma: clinical and histopathologic features. *Pediatr Dev Pathol.* 2003;6:495–510.
160. Rivard DC, Lowe LH. Radiological reasoning: multiple hepatic masses in an infant. *AJR Am J Roentgenol.* 2008;190:S46–S52.
161. Stockman A, Boralevi F, Taieb A, et al. SACRAL syndrome: spinal dysraphism, anogenital, cutaneous, renal and urologic anomalies, associated with an angioma of lumbosacral localization. *Dermatology.* 2007;214:40–45.
162. Paltiel HJ, Burrows PE, Kozakewich HP, et al. Soft-tissue vascular anomalies: utility of US for diagnosis. *Radiology.* 2000;214:747–754.
163. Kollipara R, Dinneen L, Rentas KE, et al. Current classification and terminology of pediatric vascular anomalies. *AJR Am J Roentgenol.* 2013;201:1124–1135.
164. Konez O, Burrows PE, Mulliken JB, et al. Angiographic features of rapidly involuting congenital hemangioma (RICH). *Pediatr Radiol.* 2003;33:15–19.
165. Restrepo R. Multimodality imaging of vascular anomalies. *Pediatr Radiol.* 2013;43(suppl 1):S141–S154.
166. Restrepo R, Palani R, Cervantes LF, et al. Hemangiomas revisited: the useful, the unusual and the new. Part 2: endangering hemangiomas and treatment. *Pediatr Radiol.* 2011;41:905–915.
167. Mottolese C, Hermier M, Stan H, et al. Central nervous system cavernomas in the pediatric age group. *Neurosurg Rev.* 2001;24: 55–71; discussion 72–53.
168. Acciarri N, Galassi E, Giulioni M, et al. Cavernous malformations of the central nervous system in the pediatric age group. *Pediatr Neurosurg.* 2009;45:81–104.
169. Wang M, Dai Y, Han Y, et al. Susceptibility weighted imaging in detecting hemorrhage in acute cervical spinal cord injury. *Magn Reson Imaging.* 2011;29:365–373.
170. Mitha AP, Turner JD, Abla AA, et al. Outcomes following resection of intramedullary spinal cord cavernous malformations: a 25-year experience. *J Neurosurg Spine.* 2011;14:605–611.
171. Song D, Garton HJ, Fahim DK, et al. Spinal cord vascular malformations in children. *Neurosurg Clin N Am.* 2010; 21:503–510.
172. Spetzler RF, Detwiler PW, Riina HA, et al. Modified classification of spinal cord vascular lesions. *J Neurosurg.* 2002;96:145–156.
173. Zozulya YP, Slin'ko EI, Al Q II. Spinal arteriovenous malformations: new classification and surgical treatment. *Neurosurg Focus.* 2006;20:E7.
174. Patsalides A, Knopman J, Santillan A, et al. Endovascular treatment of spinal arteriovenous lesions: beyond the dural fistula. *AJNR Am J Neuroradiol.* 2011;32:798–808.
175. Trop I, Dubois J, Guibaud L, et al. Soft-tissue venous malformations in pediatric and young adult patients: diagnosis with Doppler US. *Radiology.* 1999;212:841–845.
176. Anson JA, Spetzler RF. Interventional neuroradiology for spinal pathology. *Clin Neurosurg.* 1992;39:388–417.
177. Dubois J, Garel L. Imaging and therapeutic approach of hemangiomas and vascular malformations in the pediatric age group. *Pediatr Radiol.* 1999;29:879–893.
178. Juszkat R, Zabicki B, Checinski P, et al. Endovascular treatment of arteriovenous malformation. *Aesthetic Plast Surg.* 2009;33: 639–642.

179. Andronikou S, Albuquerque-Jonathan G, Wilmshurst J, et al. MRI findings in acute idiopathic transverse myelopathy in children. *Pediatr Radiol.* 2003;33:624–629.
180. Wolf VL, Lupo PJ, Lotze TE. Pediatric acute transverse myelitis overview and differential diagnosis. *J Child Neurol.* 2012;27:1426–1436.
181. Bhat A, Naguwa S, Cheema G, et al. The epidemiology of transverse myelitis. *Autoimmun Rev.* 2010;9:A395–A399.
182. Transverse Myelitis Consortium Working Group. Proposed diagnostic criteria and nosology of acute transverse myelitis. *Neurology.* 2002;59:499–505.
183. Defresne P, Meyer L, Tardieu M, et al. Efficacy of high dose steroid therapy in children with severe acute transverse myelitis. *J Neurol Neurosurg Psychiatry.* 2001;71:272–274.
184. Verhey LH, Shroff M, Banwell B. Pediatric multiple sclerosis: pathobiological, clinical, and magnetic resonance imaging features. *Neuroimaging Clin N Am.* 2013;23:227–243.
185. Sindern E, Haas J, Stark E, et al. Early onset MS under the age of 16: clinical and paraclinical features. *Acta Neurol Scand.* 1992;86:280–284.
186. Ghezzi A, Deplano V, Faroni J, et al. Multiple sclerosis in childhood: clinical features of 149 cases. *Mult Scler.* 1997; 3:43–46.
187. Gorman MP, Healy BC, Polgar-Turcsanyi M, et al. Increased relapse rate in pediatric-onset compared with adult-onset multiple sclerosis. *Arch Neurol.* 2009;66:54–59.
188. Swanton JK, Rovira A, Tintore M, et al. MRI criteria for multiple sclerosis in patients presenting with clinically isolated syndromes: a multicentre retrospective study. *Lancet Neurol.* 2007;6:677–686.
189. McDonald WI, Compston A, Edan G, et al. Recommended diagnostic criteria for multiple sclerosis: guidelines from the International Panel on the diagnosis of multiple sclerosis. *Ann Neurol.* 2001;50:121–127.
190. Polman CH, Reingold SC, Banwell B, et al. Diagnostic criteria for multiple sclerosis: 2010 revisions to the McDonald criteria. *Ann Neurol.* 2011;69:292–302.
191. Montalban X, Tintore M, Swanton J, et al. MRI criteria for MS in patients with clinically isolated syndromes. *Neurology.* 2010;74:427–434.
192. Hummel HM, Bruck W, Dreha-Kulaczewski S, et al. Pediatric onset multiple sclerosis: McDonald criteria 2010 and the contribution of spinal cord MRI. *Mult Scler.* 2013;19: 1330–1335.
193. Ge Y. Multiple sclerosis: the role of MR imaging. *AJNR Am J Neuroradiol.* 2006;27:1165–1176.
194. Tartaglino LM, Friedman DP, Flanders AE, et al. Multiple sclerosis in the spinal cord: MR appearance and correlation with clinical parameters. *Radiology.* 1995;195:725–732.
195. Thielen KR, Miller GM. Multiple sclerosis of the spinal cord: magnetic resonance appearance. *J Comput Assist Tomogr.* 1996;20:434–438.
196. Ikuta F, Zimmerman HM. Distribution of plaques in seventy autopsy cases of multiple sclerosis in the United States. *Neurology.* 1976;26:26–28.
197. Lycklama G, Thompson A, Filippi M, et al. Spinal-cord MRI in multiple sclerosis. *Lancet Neurol.* 2003;2:555–562.
198. Chitnis T, Tenembaum S, Banwell B, et al. Consensus statement: evaluation of new and existing therapeutics for pediatric multiple sclerosis. *Mult Scler.* 2012;18:116–127.
199. Kuntz NL, Chabas D, Weinstock-Guttman B, et al. Treatment of multiple sclerosis in children and adolescents. *Expert Opin Pharmacother.* 2010;11:505–520.
200. Banwell B, Reder AT, Krupp L, et al. Safety and tolerability of interferon beta-1b in pediatric multiple sclerosis. *Neurology.* 2006;66:472–476.
201. Amato MP, Zipoli V, Portaccio E. Cognitive changes in multiple sclerosis. *Expert Rev Neurother.* 2008;8:1585–1596.
202. Amato MP, Portaccio E, Goretti B, et al. Cognitive impairment in early stages of multiple sclerosis. *Neurol Sci.* 2010;31:S211–S214.
203. Harding KE, Liang K, Cossburn MD, et al. Long-term outcome of paediatric-onset multiple sclerosis: a population-based study. *J Neurol Neurosurg Psychiatry.* 2013;84:141–147.
204. Losseff NA, Kingsley DP, McDonald WI, et al. Clinical and magnetic resonance imaging predictors of disability in primary and secondary progressive multiple sclerosis. *Mult Scler.* 1996; 1:218–222.
205. Dale RC. Acute disseminated encephalomyelitis. *Semin Pediatr Infect Dis.* 2003;14:90–95.
206. Krupp LB, Banwell B, Tenembaum S, et al. Consensus definitions proposed for pediatric multiple sclerosis and related disorders. *Neurology.* 2007;68:S7–S12.
207. Leake JA, Albani S, Kao AS, et al. Acute disseminated encephalomyelitis in childhood: epidemiologic, clinical and laboratory features. *Pediatr Infect Dis J.* 2004;23:756–764.
208. Hynson JL, Kornberg AJ, Coleman LT, et al. Clinical and neuroradiologic features of acute disseminated encephalomyelitis in children. *Neurology.* 2001;56:1308–1312.
209. Tenembaum S, Chitnis T, Ness J, et al. Acute disseminated encephalomyelitis. *Neurology.* 2007;68:S23–S36.
210. Alper G. Acute disseminated encephalomyelitis. *J Child Neurol.* 2012;27:1408–1425.
211. Honkaniemi J, Dastidar P, Kahara V, et al. Delayed MR imaging changes in acute disseminated encephalomyelitis. *AJNR Am J Neuroradiol.* 2001;22:1117–1124.
212. O'Riordan JI, Losseff NA, Phatouros C, et al. Asymptomatic spinal cord lesions in clinically isolated optic nerve, brain stem, and spinal cord syndromes suggestive of demyelination. *J Neurol Neurosurg Psychiatry.* 1998;64:353–357.
213. Wingerchuk DM. Neuromyelitis optica. *Int MS J.* 2006;13: 42–50.
214. Tillema JM, McKeon A. The spectrum of neuromyelitis optica (NMO) in childhood. *J Child Neurol.* 2012;27:1437–1447.
215. Sahraian MA, Radue EW, Minagar A. Neuromyelitis optica: clinical manifestations and neuroimaging features. *Neurol Clin.* 2013;31:139–152.
216. Rees JH, Soudain SE, Gregson NA, et al. Campylobacter jejuni infection and Guillain–Barre syndrome. *N Engl J Med.* 1995;333:1374–1379.
217. Yuki N, Hartung HP. Guillain–Barre syndrome. *N Engl J Med.* 2012;366:2294–2304.
218. Korinthenberg R. Acute polyradiculoneuritis: Guillain–Barre syndrome. *Handb Clin Neurol.* 2013;112:1157–1162.
219. Baran GA, Sowell MK, Sharp GB, et al. MR findings in a child with Guillain–Barre syndrome. *AJR Am J Roentgenol.* 1993;161: 161–163.
220. Zuccoli G, Panigrahy A, Bailey A, et al. Redefining the Guillain–Barre spectrum in children: neuroimaging findings of cranial nerve involvement. *AJNR Am J Neuroradiol.* 2011;32:639–642.

221. van Doorn PA, Ruts L, Jacobs BC. Clinical features, pathogenesis, and treatment of Guillain–Barre syndrome. *Lancet Neurol.* 2008;7:939–950.
222. Bertorini T, Narayanaswami P, Rashed H. Charcot–Marie–Tooth disease (hereditary motor sensory neuropathies) and hereditary sensory and autonomic neuropathies. *Neurologist.* 2004;10:327–337.
223. Dyck PJ, Lambert EH. Lower motor and primary sensory neuron diseases with peroneal muscular atrophy. I. Neurologic, genetic, and electrophysiologic findings in hereditary polyneuropathies. *Arch Neurol.* 1968;18:603–618.
224. Warner LE, Hilz MJ, Appel SH, et al. Clinical phenotypes of different MPZ (P0) mutations may include Charcot–Marie–Tooth type 1B, Dejerine-Sottas, and congenital hypomyelination. *Neuron.* 1996;17:451–460.
225. Gaeta M, Mileto A, Mazzeo A, et al. MRI findings, patterns of disease distribution, and muscle fat fraction calculation in five patients with Charcot–Marie–Tooth type 2 F disease. *Skeletal Radiol.* 2012;41:515–524.
226. Pareyson D, Marchesi C. Diagnosis, natural history, and management of Charcot–Marie–Tooth disease. *Lancet Neurol.* 2009;8:654–667.
227. Morano JU, Russell WF. Nerve root enlargement in Charcot–Marie–Tooth disease: CT appearance. *Radiology.* 1986;161:784.
228. Martinoli C, Schenone A, Bianchi S, et al. Sonography of the median nerve in Charcot–Marie–Tooth disease. *AJR Am J Roentgenol.* 2002;178:1553–1556.
229. Aho TR, Wallace RC, Pitt AM, et al. Charcot–Marie–Tooth disease: extensive cranial nerve involvement on CT and MR imaging. *AJNR Am J Neuroradiol.* 2004;25:494–497.

CHAPTER 5

Vertebral Column

Esperanza Pacheco-Jacome • Kevin R. Moore • Sara O. Vargas • L. Santiago Medina

INTRODUCTION

Comprehensive imaging evaluation and characterization of vertebral column disorders is essential in the pediatric population. Proper selection of imaging and technique, which can narrow the differential diagnosis, is important for patient outcome. In this chapter, the currently available imaging modalities and important disorders affecting the vertebral column in infants and children are discussed. The characteristic imaging findings and management of congenital and acquired disorders involving the vertebral column in pediatric patients are also reviewed.

IMAGING TECHNIQUES

Radiography

In the evaluation of the vertebral column, radiographs still play an important role. They allow adequate labeling of the vertebrae (i.e., thoracic vs. lumbar) and global evaluation of the bone. Deformity and segmentation abnormalities can be accessed with erect frontal and lateral radiographs of the entire spine with spot images as needed.

In the cervical spine, ideally, a three-view examination including frontal, lateral, and open-mouth views should be obtained. Open-mouth view can be difficult to obtain in patients <5 years or uncooperative pediatric patients. In the thoracic spine, a minimum of a three-view examination including frontal, lateral, and swimmer views should be obtained in order to evaluate the cervicothoracic junction in detail. In the lumbar spine, a minimum of a four-view examination including frontal, lateral, and both oblique views should be obtained. Properly obtained oblique views are important in accurately evaluating the pars interarticularis for spondylolysis. Posteroanterior scoliosis radiographs decrease radiation exposure to the patient. Bending films in the scoliosis survey can be important for surgical planning.

Newer low-dose radiation technology, including low-dose radiation digital stereoradiography system (EOS orthopedic imaging system), allows conventional and 3D reconstructions of the spinal column in a weight-bearing standing or sitting position, allowing assessment in natural posture. This new technology delivers 8 to 10 times less radiation than conventional scoliosis radiographs.[1] 3D reconstruction in the erect position can also be obtained.[2]

Ultrasound

Ultrasound in the newborn period is useful to access the spinal canal contents, which is discussed in Chapter 4 of this book. However, the role of ultrasound in evaluating the osseous spinal column is very limited.

Computed Tomography

In the setting of acute trauma with no neurologic deficit, radiographs followed by computed tomography (CT) are the studies of choice. These allow detailed evaluation of the alignment and integrity of the vertebral column. For craniocervical pathology, such as basilar invagination or complex vertebral column anomalies, the combination of CT (with multiplanar and 3D reconstructions) and magnetic resonance imaging (MRI) allows detailed evaluation not only of the osseous structures but also of the soft tissues and spinal contents including the spinal cord.

Newer multidetector CT (MDCT) with dose reduction technique is ideal because of its ability to cover a long scan range in a few seconds, reducing the need for sedation. The best results are obtained with 3-mm-thick multiplanar reconstructions. 3D reconstructions are always valuable because they allow optimized visualization of all anatomic structures and confirmation of the exact level of pathology. Because of the high complexity of some vertebral anomalies, CT findings should be correlated with radiographic findings. In addition, counting is ideally initiated from C1 or C2, and exact reference levels must be reported in detail in order to avoid unnecessary confusion and risk of error, especially when surgical intervention is being considered.

CT Myelography

In pediatric patients with prior spine instrumentation, a CT myelogram may be required to evaluate the hardware and spinal canal because MRI is often limited by susceptibility artifact. In children with titanium hardware, MRI should be attempted first, because these metallic devices produce less susceptibility artifact than conventional ferrous hardware. Use of titanium instrumentation is currently limited but growing. In pediatric patients with complex meningoceles and vertebral column anomalies, CT myelography can be important in surgical planning to determine the exact relationship of the vertebral column, nerve roots, and cord with respect to the meningocele.

Magnetic Resonance Imaging

MRI plays an important role in the evaluation of the spinal column and its bone marrow. Familiarity with the normal progression of red to fatty marrow according to age is paramount in understanding normal bone marrow patterns and underlying pathology. T1-weighted, T2-weighted, and short tau inversion recovery (STIR) sequences are useful in determining normal bone marrow patterns versus early bone marrow disorders or edema. Pre- and postcontrast T1-weighted MR imaging including fat-saturated sequences allows further characterization of bone marrow–centered lesions. Diffusion-weighted (DW) MR imaging with its appropriate apparent diffusion coefficient (ADC) map is useful in evaluating cystic lesions when the differential diagnosis of dermoid/epidermoid versus arachnoid cyst is being considered. Restricted diffusion is more often seen in dermoid and/or epidermoid cystic lesions.[3]

Nuclear Medicine

18F-FDG-PET plays an important role in the evaluation of metastatic disease to the spine. Familiarity with differences in PET appearance of spinal column bone metastatic disease and pharmacologically induced bone marrow stimulation is of crucial importance. Metastatic disease tends to be more focal and asymmetric, whereas bone marrow–stimulating agents tend to cause more diffuse and symmetric uptake.

Bone scintigraphy with spine 3D SPECT has a special role in evaluating nonfebrile back pain in the older child or adolescent with suspected spondylolysis. Stress changes associated with active pars defects are well-visualized as areas of focally increased radiopharmaceutical uptake.

EMBRYOLOGY OF THE VERTEBRA

The development of the vertebral column passes through three different stages: (1) membranous (precartilaginous) stage, (2) chondrification, and (3) ossification.

Membranous Stage

The intraembryonic mesoderm, (derived from the primitive neuroectoderm) located on each side of the notochord (a mesodermal structure arising from the Hensen node, located between the primitive ectoderm and endoderm) and neural tube, forms a longitudinal column of paraxial mesoderm. By the end of the 3rd week, the paraxial mesoderm divides into somites, located on each side of the developing neural tube and notochord.[4] There are 44 pairs of somites aligned rostrocaudally. The first somite is transient, somites 2 to 4 form the basiocciput, and the others form the axial skeleton, associated musculature, and adjacent dermis of the skin.

During the 4th week, cellular migration occurs. At each somite level, the dermatomes form dorsolaterally, myotomes form medially, and sclerotomes form ventromedially. The sclerotomes (spine) then migrate in three different directions at each level, maintaining their segmental arrangement. Ventromedially, cells migrate and surround the notochord, forming the membranous vertebral column that separates the notochord from the neural tube and gut. Ventrolaterally, cells form two processes: costal (ventral), which later gives origin to the thoracic ribs, and lateral, which gives origin to the transverse processes. Dorsally, cells form the vertebral arches behind the neural tube[4–6] (Fig. 5.1).

On about day 24, the process of resegmentation occurs at the level of the membranous vertebral bodies. Each sclerotomic segment differentiates into a cephalic portion (less condensed) and a caudal portion (more condensed). In the midportion of each sclerotome appears a horizontal sclerotomic cleft (fissure of von Ebner), where each sclerotome divides. The caudal half of each sclerotome then fuses with the cephalic half of the subjacent sclerotome, forming the precartilaginous vertebral centrum. The intervertebral discs form during this time, from the denser caudal portion of the sclerotome. Cells from the caudal portion move cranially to the middle part of each segment, forming the peripheral part of the disc; the annulus fibrosus, which surrounds the notochord, and the enchondral growth plates of the vertebral centra. The intersegmental arteries that were between the somites now enter the center of the forming vertebral bodies.[5–7] The process of resegmentation occurs bilaterally and symmetrically and probably starts at the thoracic region, progressing toward both ends of the embryo (Fig. 5.2).

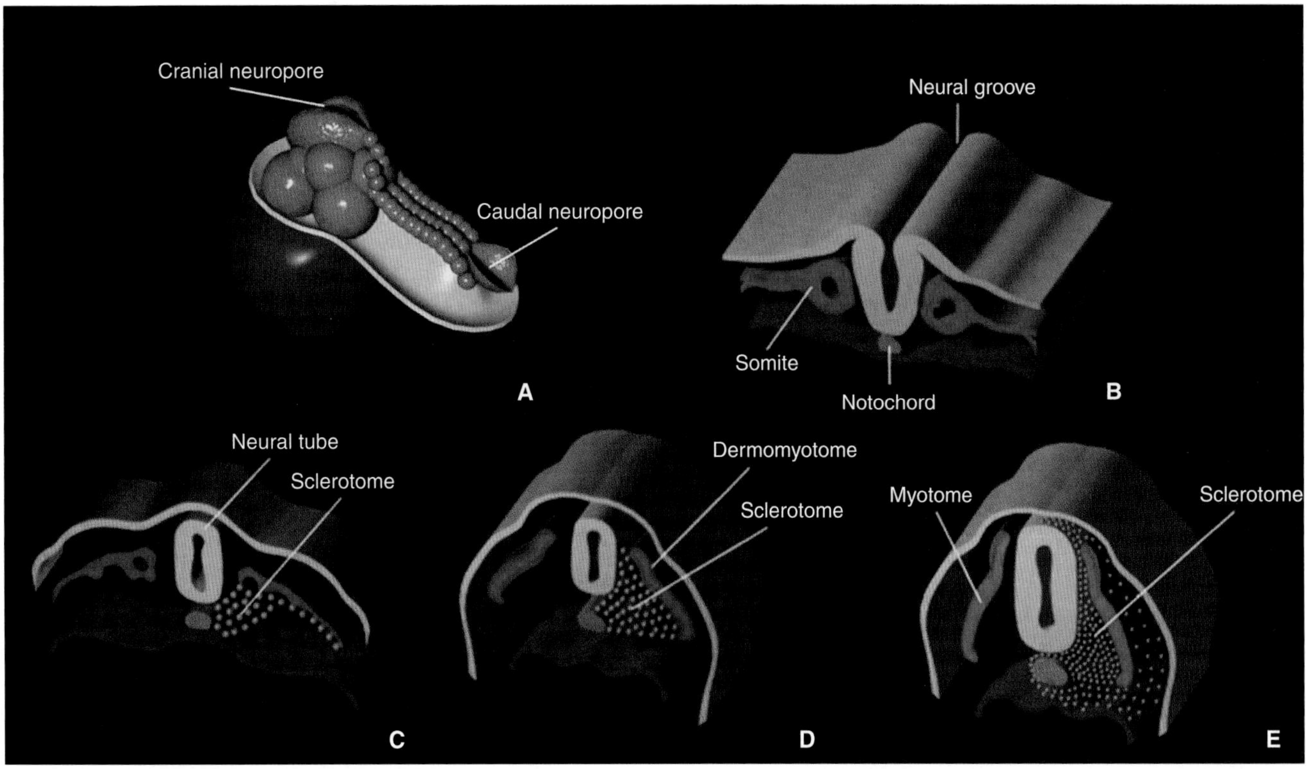

FIGURE 5.1 **Vertebral embryology. A:** Drawing of the embryo during the formation of the somites located to each side of the developing neural tube and notochord. **B:** Coronal depiction of somite formation and closing of the neural tube. **C–E:** Axial drawings of the sclerotome migrating to the neural tube and notochord. **D and E:** Dorsolateral dermatomes and medial myotomes form from the somites.

Chondrification

During the 6th week, chondrification centers appear in the membranous vertebra. The chondrification centers first develop at the cervicothoracic level and then extend downward into the caudal spine. Two chondrification centers appear in each centrum (body) and fuse at the end of the 8th week to form a cartilaginous centrum. The chondrification centers for the neural arches and pars (one on each side of the vertebra) develop later than the centrum, eventually fusing with each other and with the centrum. The transverse and spinous processes develop from extension

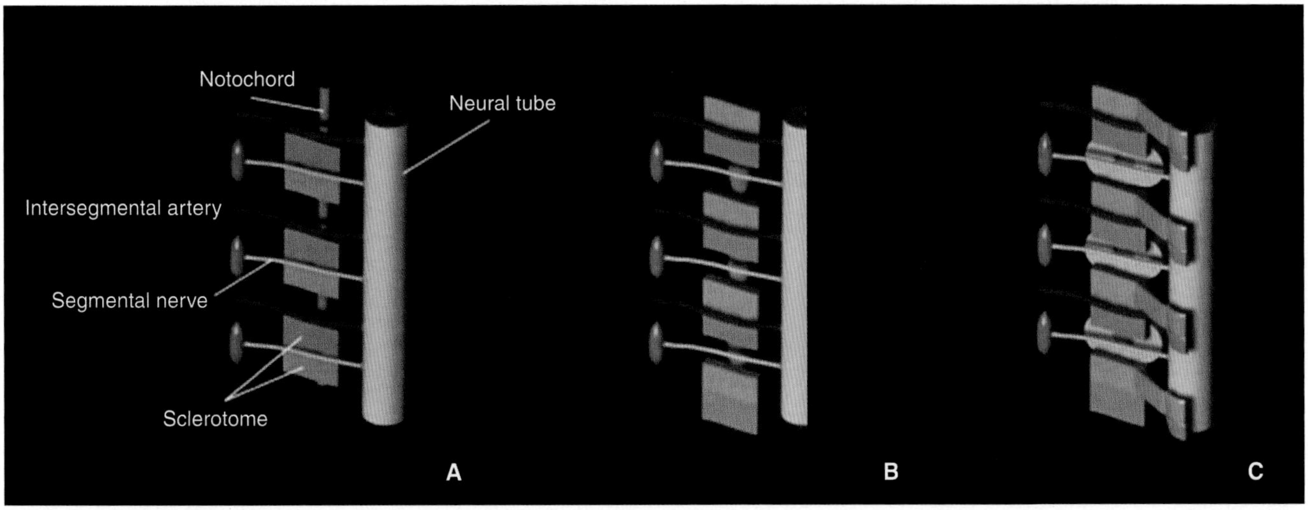

FIGURE 5.2 **Resegmentation of the membranous vertebral bodies. A–C:** The sclerotomic segments differentiate into a cephalic (pink) and a caudal (blue) portion. In the midportion of each sclerotome appears a dividing cleft, the sclerotome cleft. The caudal half of each sclerotome then fuses with the cephalic half of the subjacent sclerotome, forming the precartilaginous vertebral centrum. The intersegmental arteries that were between the somites now enter the center of the forming vertebral bodies. The intervertebral discs form from the rostral surface of the denser caudal portion of the sclerotome. Cells from the caudal sclerotome move cranially to the middle part of each segment, forming the peripheral part of the disc, the annulus fibrosus, which surrounds the notochord.

of chondrification centers in the vertebral arches. With formation and joining of the chondrification centers, there is squeezing of the notochord cells and intervertebral tissue into the disc spaces where the notochord becomes the nucleus pulposus of the disc.[4,7]

Ossification

Ossification begins during the 8th week and ends at about 25 years of age. In the prenatal period, three centers appear by the end of the embryonic period (8 weeks): one for the centrum (body), divided into anterior and posterior components; one ossification center for each pars; and one for each half of the vertebral arch. At birth, each vertebra consists of five bony parts connected by cartilage: the vertebral body, two halves of the neural arch, and two pars ossification centers. The ossification centers do not appear simultaneously at the same level. At 8 weeks, the ossification centers of the posterior arches are first seen in the cervical region, while the vertebral bodies are seen in the lower thoracic and upper lumbar levels, which quickly propagate cranially and caudally[4,7] (Fig. 5.3). During the postnatal period, the halves of each vertebra fuse between years 3 and 5. The arches articulate with the centrum at the cartilaginous neurocentral joints, which grow as the cord enlarges.

Variations from this pattern of ossification occurs at the C1 and C2 level, where the ossification center of the C1 body forms the odontoid process of C2 and the ossification center of the arch of C1 joins anteriorly to form a ring.[4] The C1 vertebra has no vertebral body, and there is no intervertebral disc between C1 and C2.[4]

C1 (atlas) is formed by three ossification centers, which include the anterior arch and two neural arches. The anterior arch is ossified in about 20% of neonates and in 80% by 1 year of age. The posterior neural arches appear by the 7th week of the fetal life, and by age 3, they fuse posteriorly. The posterior and anterior arches fuse around 7 years of age (Fig. 5.4).

At birth, C2 (axis) has four ossification centers: one for each of the two neural arches, one for the body, and one for the odontoid process. In fetal life, the odontoid process forms from two ossification centers that fuse by month 7. The os terminalis is a secondary ossification center at the tip of the odontoid process that fuses by age 12. The odontoid process fuses with the body of C2 by 3 to 6 years of age. The interface of the odontoid with the body is known as the subdental synchondrosis, which may be seen until age 11 and could be mistaken for a fracture. The neural arches fuse posteriorly by age 2 to 3 and anteriorly with the odontoid process between 3 and 6 years of age[8,9] (Fig. 5.5).

After puberty, there are multiple secondary vertebral ossification centers, which include the tip of the spinous process, the tip of each transverse process, and the superior and inferior rims of each vertebral body. By about 25 years, the secondary centers fuse with the rest of the bone[4] (Fig. 5.6).

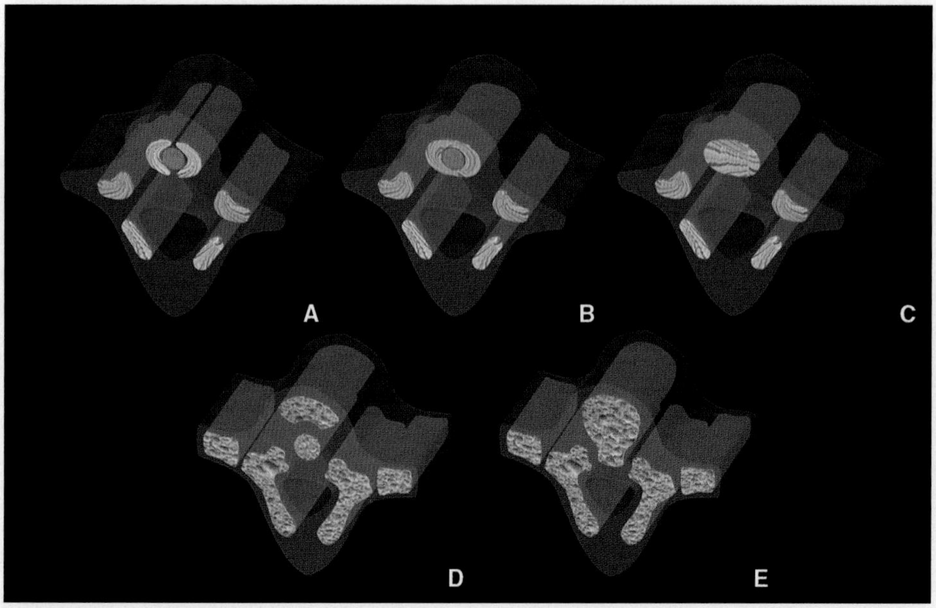

FIGURE 5.3 **Chondrification. A and B:** During the 6th week, two chondrification centers appear in each membranous vertebral centrum and fuse at the end of the 8th week to form a cartilaginous centrum. At the same time, the chondrification centers for the vertebral arches and pars (one on each side) fuse with each other and with the centrum. The transverse and spinous processes develop from extension of vertebral arch chondrification centers. **C:** With the formation and joining of the chondrification centers, there is squeezing of the notochord cells and intervertebral tissue into the disc spaces where the notochord becomes the nucleus pulposus. **Ossification. D:** Three centers appear by the end of the embryonic period (8 weeks): one in the centrum (body), divided into anterior and posterior, and at each half of the developing vertebra, one ossification center for each pars and one for each half of the vertebral arch. **E:** At birth, each vertebra consists of five bony parts connected by cartilage.

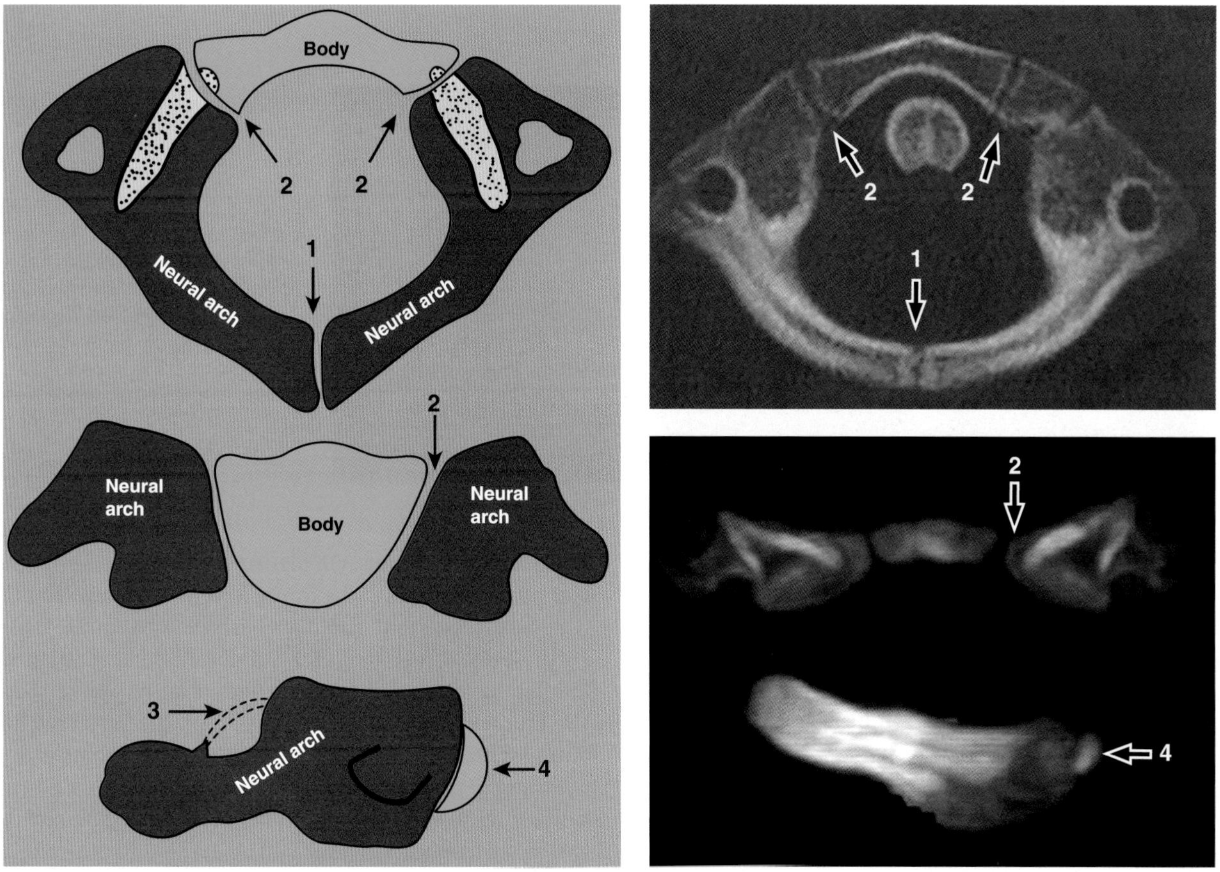

FIGURE 5.4 **C1 vertebra with ossification centers.** In most individuals, the body is not ossified at birth; the ossification center(s) appear during the first year of life. The neural arches appear at about the 7th week of gestation. *1*, The synchondrosis of spinous processes unites by the 3rd year of life. *2*, The neurocentral synchondroses fuse by about the 7th year. *3*, A ligament surrounding the superior neural arch may ossify later in life. *4*, Body of C1. (Drawing modified from Bailey DK. The normal cervical spine in infants and children. *Radiology.* 1952;59:712–719.)

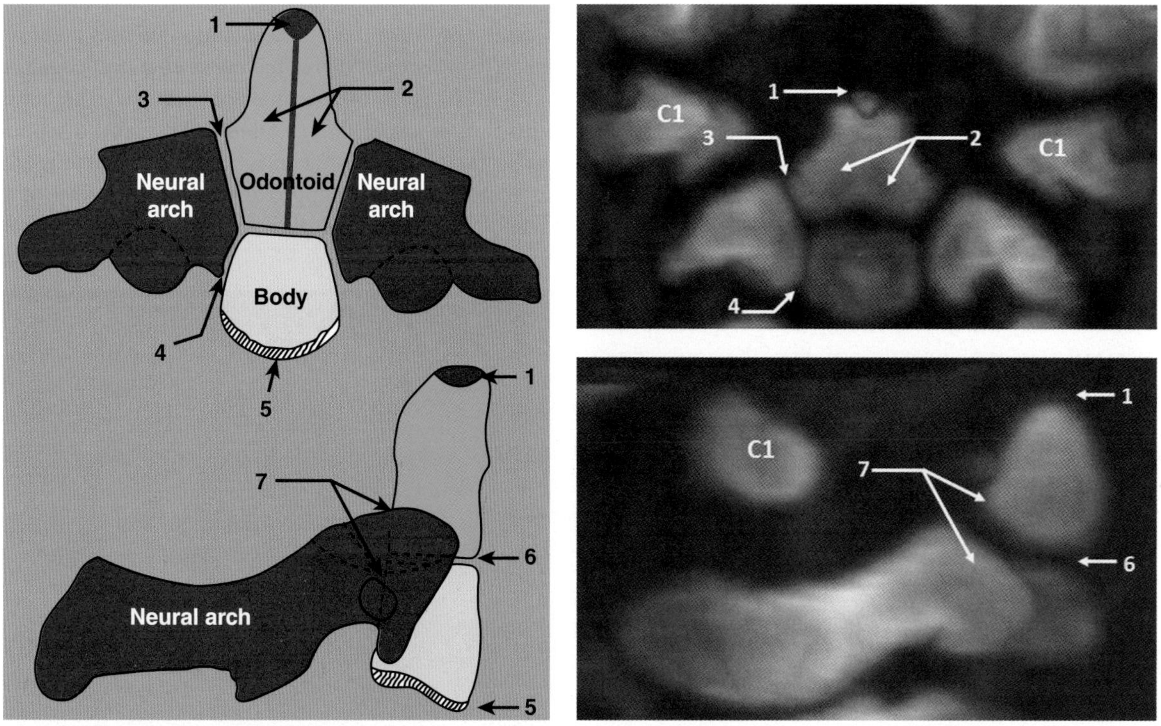

FIGURE 5.5 **C2 vertebra with ossification centers.** *1*, Ossiculum terminale appears by age 3 to 6 and becomes fused by age 12. *2*, Odontoid, two separate ossification centers appear by 5th fetal month and become fused by 7th fetal month. *3*, Synchondrosis between the odontoid and neural arch fuses by 3 to 6 years. *4*, Neurocentral synchondrosis fuses by 3 to 6 years. *5*, Inferior epiphyseal ring appears by puberty and fuses by age 25. *6*, Synchondrosis between the odontoid and body fuses by 3 to 6 years. *7*, Posterior surface of body and odontoid. (Drawing modified from Bailey DK. The normal cervical spine in infants and children. *Radiology.* 1952;59:712–719.)

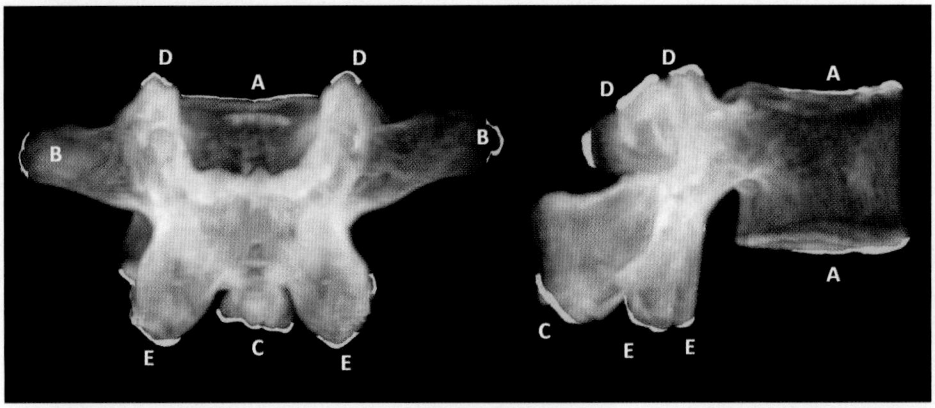

FIGURE 5.6 **Secondary ossification centers.** *A*, The annulus ossification centers (a.k.a, ring apophyses) may appear by age 7 and become fused by approximately age 25. The ossification centers for the transverse processes (*B*), spinous processes (*C*), and superior (*D*) and inferior articular processes (*E*) appear by age 16 and fuse by approximately age 25.

ANATOMY OF THE VERTEBRAE

As described earlier, the bony vertebrae originate from primitive mesoderm, which surrounds the neural tube and notochord. Usually, there are 7 cervical vertebrae, 12 thoracic, 5 lumbar, 5 sacral, and 4 or 5 coccygeal segments. One ossification center appears for each sacral segment in childhood and adolescence. S2 occurs at about 5 to 10 years, S3 occurs from 10 to 15 years, and S3 may occur as late as 20 years.[10] By adulthood, the sacrum has become a single bone.

Transitional anatomy, sometimes with supernumerary or deficient vertebrae, may be seen at the lumbosacral junction ("sacralization" of L5, "lumbarization" of S1), in the cervical, thoracic, or lumbar spine, or in the ribs (cervical rib(s), absent 12th rib(s)).

The morphology of the C1 and C2 vertebrae differs from the other vertebrae and deserves a special discussion. C1 (atlas) is the first spinal vertebra and, in conjunction with C2, connects the skull to the spine. The anterior arch presents a central anterior tubercle for the attachment of the longus colli muscle and anterior longitudinal ligament. Inside the arch is the fovea dentis, a place for the C1 articulation with the odontoid process. The posterior arch is the site of attachment of the posterior atlanto-occipital membrane. It has a groove–foramen for the vertebral artery and ends in a posterior tubercle, which is a rudimentary spinous process. The lateral masses support the weight of the head. They include the superior facets, which articulate with the occipital condyle and allow anterior–posterior movement. The inferior facets articulate with C2 (axis) and allow rotatory movement (Fig. 5.7).

C2 or axis has a special feature, the odontoid process (dens) that articulates with C1. The superior articular facets are mildly convex and oriented upward and laterally. The inferior facets articulate in the same direction as the other cervical vertebrae. The transverse processes are small and perforated, containing the vertebral foramina. The laminae are thick, and the spinous process is large and strong, presenting a bifid end (Figs. 5.8 and 5.9).

The thoracic and lumbar vertebrae are morphologically similar to one another, having an anterior mass or body, a posterior ring or arch, two transverse processes, two superior and inferior articulating facets, and a single posterior spinous process. The thoracic vertebrae have additional costal processes that articulate with the ribs[11] (Fig. 5.10).

In ~50% of neonates, the vertebral bodies have an ovoid configuration on radiography, with a fairly square shape in the thoracic spine. On the lateral view, the vertebrae have a "bone-within-bone" appearance. This configuration is also common in premature infants. There is a single fused ossification center in the vertebral body of a neonate and one ossification center in each neural arch. Anterior and posterior clefts of the vertebral bodies of neonates may be secondary to vascular channels. The anterior cleft may persist for a time in the thoracic spine, and the posterior cleft may be seen in adults. The junction of the neural arches is cartilaginous, which may be mistaken for spina bifida on radiographs. Normal developmental clefts are seen in the neonatal lumbar spine and, to a lesser degree, in the thoracic spine. There is a coronal cleft, which is thought to be related either to a notochord remnant or lack of fusion of the anterior and posterior ossification centers. It is present more often in boys and disappears in a few weeks or months[10](Fig. 5.11). The oval configuration of the vertebrae remains approximately until 2 years of age, and then, the vertebrae become rectangular with rounded cor-

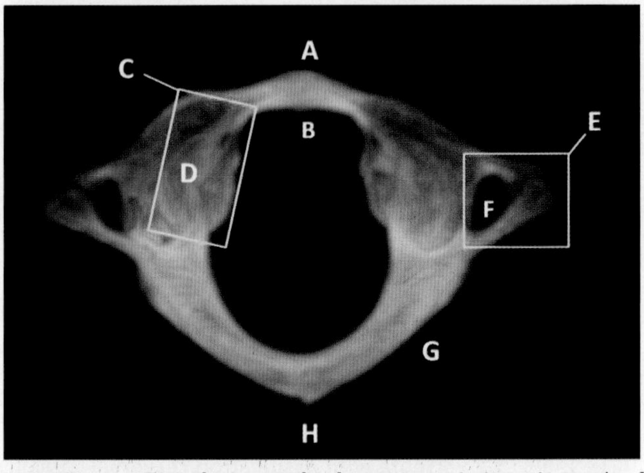

FIGURE 5.7 **C1 (atlas) vertebral anatomy.** *A*, Anterior arch of C1. *B*, Articular facet for the odontoid. *C*, Lateral mass of C1. *D*, Superior articular facet. *E*, Transverse process. *F*, Vertebral foramen. *G*, Lamina. *H*, Posterior arch.

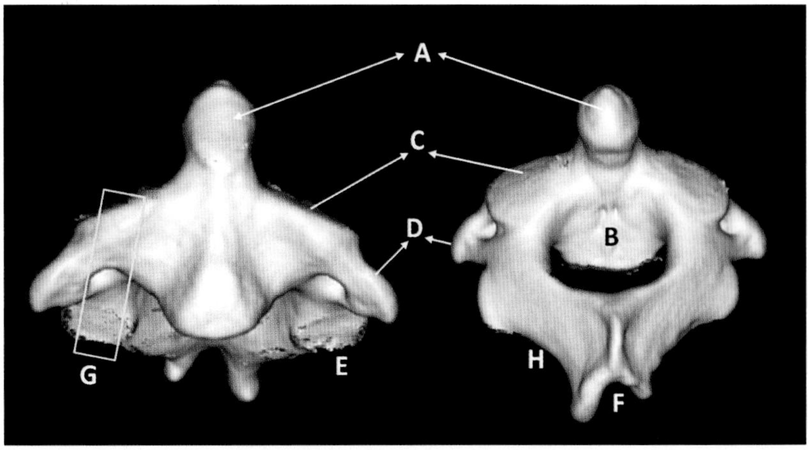

FIGURE 5.8 **C2 vertebral anatomy.** *A*, Odontoid process (dens). *B*, Body. *C*, Superior articular facet. *D*, Transverse process. *E*, Inferior articular facet. *F*, Spinous process. *G*, Lateral mass. *H*, Lamina.

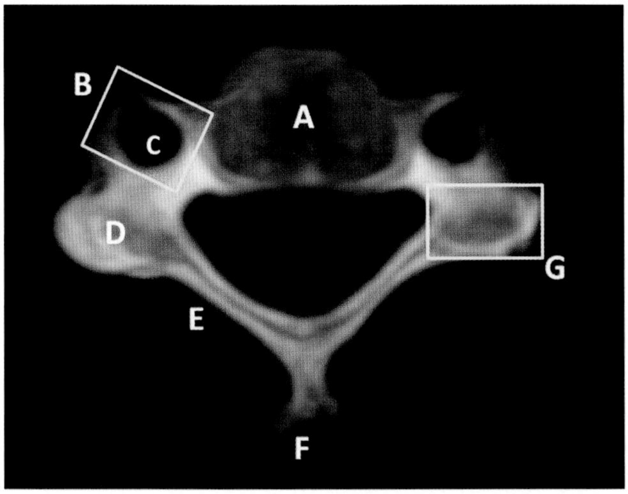

FIGURE 5.9 **Lower cervical vertebral anatomy.** *A*, Body. *B*, Transverse process. *C*, Vertebral foramen. *D*, Superior articular facet. *E*, Lamina. *F*, Spinous process. *G*, Lateral mass.

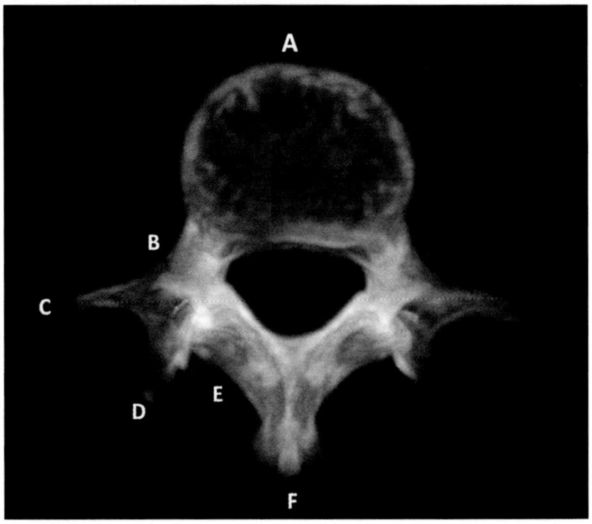

FIGURE 5.10 **Lumbar vertebral anatomy.** *A*, Body. *B*, Pedicle. *C*, Transverse process. *D*, Articulating apophysis. *E*, Lamina. *F*, Spinous process.

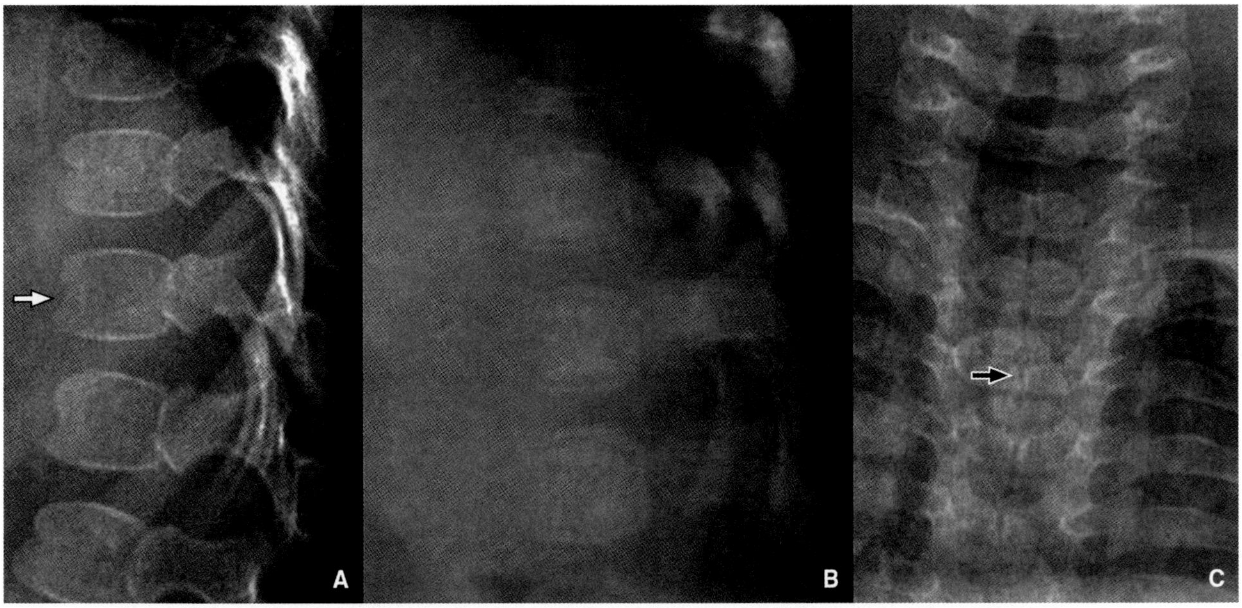

FIGURE 5.11 **Vertebral morphology of the infant. A:** Ovoid configuration and anterior vascular cleft (*white arrow*) in the vertebral body of the newborn. **B:** "Bone-within-bone" vertebral appearance in the newborn or premature infant. **C:** Normal cartilaginous junction (*black arrow*) of the neural arches, which may be mistaken for spina bifida.

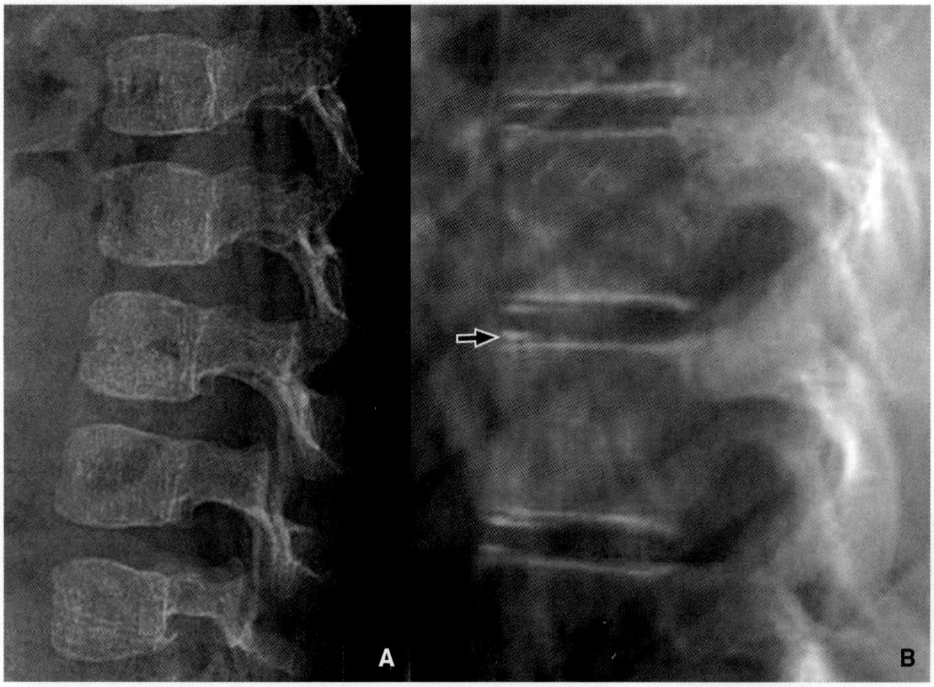

FIGURE 5.12 **Vertebral morphology of the older child. A:** The configuration of the vertebral body is more square in a 2 1/2-year-old child when compared to the ovoid neonatal shape (Fig. 5.11A). **B:** Square vertebral morphology in a 14-year-old boy. Ring apophyses (*arrow*) are demonstrated at the superior and inferior endplates.

ners, which are filled with non-radioopaque cartilage. Later in childhood, further changes in the spine occur, eventually leading to the adult morphology.

The cervical vertebral bodies develop cortical borders superiorly and inferiorly, and the transverse processes enlarge. The lumbar vertebral bodies develop superior and inferior concavity. The ring apophyses begin to appear in the midthoracic and upper lumbar spine at about 6 years of age. They are prominent in later childhood and fused to the vertebral bodies by age 18. These apophyses appear at the corners of the vertebra with a "C"-shaped configuration, and with vertebral growth, a beaked appearance may result[10,12] (Fig. 5.12).

BONE MARROW AND INTERVERTEBRAL DISC

MRI is the modality of choice for evaluating the bone marrow in the developing pediatric spine. In the neonate, the bone marrow is markedly hypointense on the T1-weighted MR images when compared with the intervertebral disc. The vertebrae are hypo- to isointense on the T1-weighted MR images during the first year of life, and then iso- to hyperintense from 1 to 5 years. Subsequently, the vertebrae are hyperintense to the disc on the T1-weighted MR images in older pediatric population. The neonatal anterior vertebral vascular channel disappears in childhood, while the posterior channel may persist into adulthood. Until 6 months of age, the cartilage of the vertebral endplates is hyperintense. Then, it becomes isointense to muscle until 2 years of age, after which time the cartilage is not well seen due to further ossification. The spinous process is initially T1 hypointense and becomes hyperintense after 6 months of age. Bone marrow fatty deposition occurs in stress-related situations that might be seen as a normal variant in the lumbar spine in adolescents[13] (Fig. 5.13).

Two cartilaginous articular plates, the fibrous ring or annulus fibrosus, and the nucleus pulposus compose the intervertebral disc. The annulus fibrosus is made up of connective tissue lamellae that extend from one vertebral surface to the next. The nucleus pulposus is a notochord remnant compressed in the central portion of the disc. In the newborn, the nucleus pulposus is ovoid, and the annulus fibrosus and the cartilaginous endplates are large. By the second decade, an anterior notch forms in the nucleus pulposus, giving it the shape of a thick "C." By this time, the annulus fibrosus bulges convexly into the cartilage, which has thinned significantly.[13]

SPINAL GROWTH

The neonatal spine when viewed laterally has a subtle cervical and lumbosacral lordosis with a gentle thoracic kyphosis. The cervical curvature accentuates with development of head support in the first year of life, and the lumbar lordosis with ambulation by 2 years of age. Then, it becomes more prominent during childhood. The final normal curvatures of the spine typically become fixed after puberty.[10,12]

In the neonate, the cervical spine is 25% of the total spinal length, the thoracic spine 50%, and lumbar spine 25%. By adulthood, the proportions change: the cervical spine comprises one-fifth to one-sixth of the length, and the lumbar segment increases to nearly one-third of the total length.[12] The longitudinal growth of the spine is due to cartilage proliferation in the upper and lower zones of the primary ossification centers of the vertebral bodies, and no growth

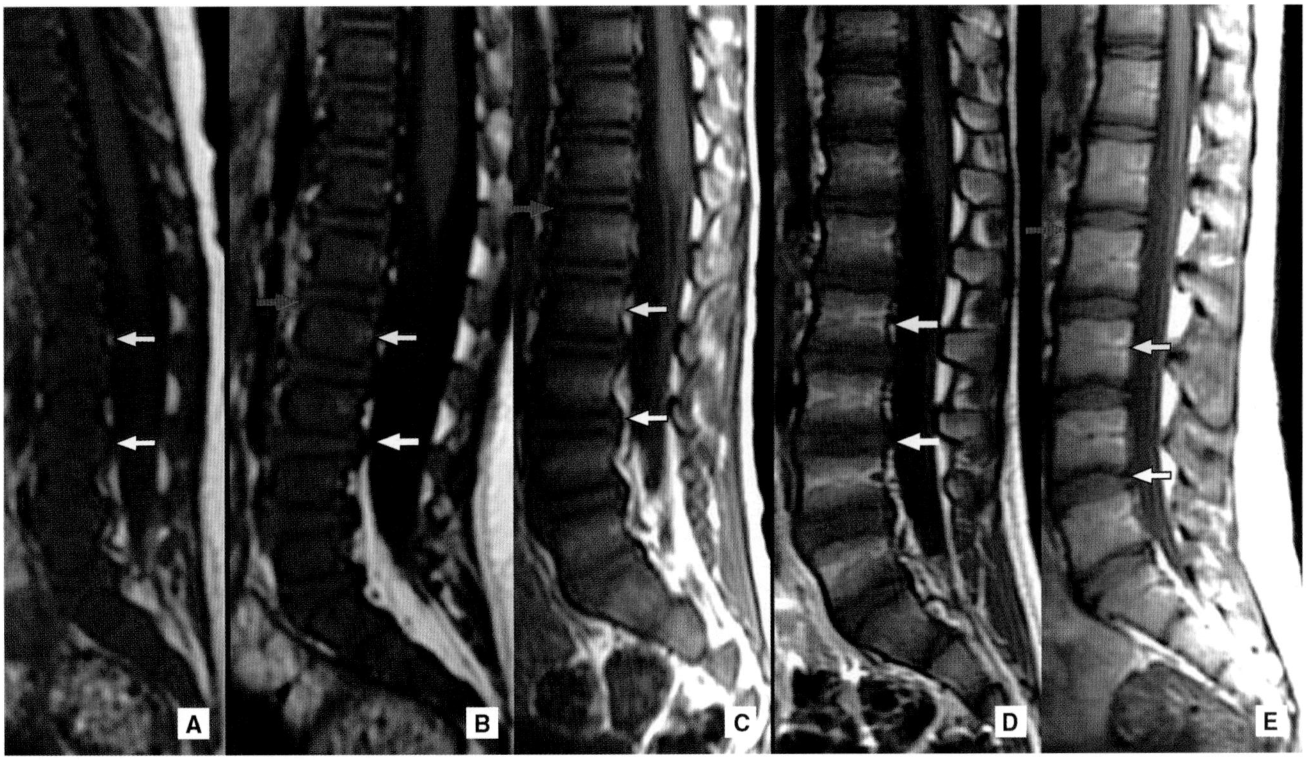

FIGURE 5.13 **Vertebral maturation. A: Neonate:** Oval-shaped vertebra with low signal intensity bone marrow (*yellow arrow*) on T1-weighted MR image. Note the slight hyperintense body center and cartilage. The disc is isointense to muscle (*white arrow*). **B: 8 months old:** More rectangular-shaped vertebral body, asymmetric higher T1 signal intensity, especially in the superior and inferior cartilaginous ossification centers (*red arrow*), early fatty conversion (*yellow arrow*). The disc remains isointense (*white arrow*). **C: 3 years old:** More square-shaped vertebral body, reversal low T1 signal with central fatty deposition (*yellow arrow*). Higher signal of the superior and inferior ossification centers (*red arrow*). The disc remains isointense (*white arrow*). **D: 7 years old:** Homogeneous T1 intermediate signal intensity of the vertebra, with hyperintense center, fatty marrow (*yellow arrow*). Disc is isointense (*white arrow*). **E: 16 years old**: Square-shaped vertebra, higher T1 signal, fatty marrow (*yellow arrow*), lower signal of the ossification centers (*red arrow*), and low signal intensity disc (*white arrow*).

is seen in the annular cartilages.[14] The growth of each vertebra and of the entire spine is modified by the stress of weight bearing. At birth, the average total spine length, not including the sacrum, is 20 cm; at 2 years of age, 45 cm; at puberty, 50 cm; and by adulthood, 75 cm.[10]

ANATOMIC VARIANTS

Anatomic variants of the vertebral column, that can be frequently encountered in the pediatric population, are discussed in this section.

The lateral masses of C1 may be laterally displaced from the odontoid process by as much as 6 mm, which is known as the "pseudo-Jefferson fracture" appearance (Fig. 5.14).

Pseudosubluxation is physiologic anterolisthesis of C2 on C3, and C3 on C4 to a lesser extent. It may resemble a true injury in severe cases. Radiographic evaluation with neutral, flexion, and extension views of the spine with a line from the anterior aspect of the posterior arch of C1 to the anterior aspect of the spinous process of C3 is helpful. The anterior margin of the posterior arch of C1 and the anterior margins of the C2 and C3 spinous processes should align within 1 mm of each other on the flexion and extension view cervical spine radiographs. If a line drawn along the posterior margin of the odontoid intersects or touches the upper posterior corner of C3, no dislocation is present[15] (Fig. 5.15).

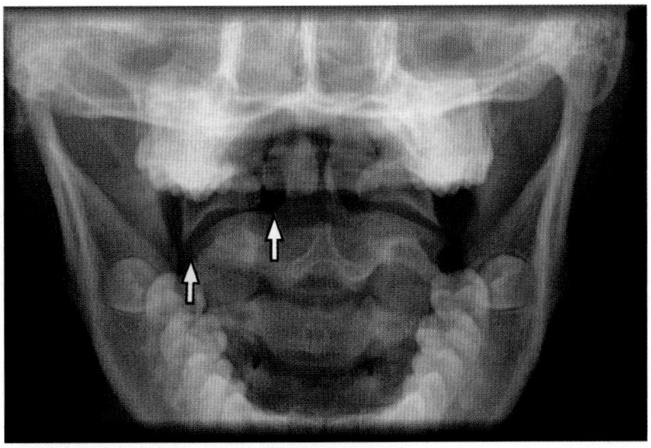

FIGURE 5.14 **Pseudo-Jefferson fracture.** Open-mouth view frontal radiograph demonstrates widening of the C1 lateral mass-odontoid distance (*white arrow*) on the right side and slight offset (*yellow arrow*) of the right lateral mass of C1.

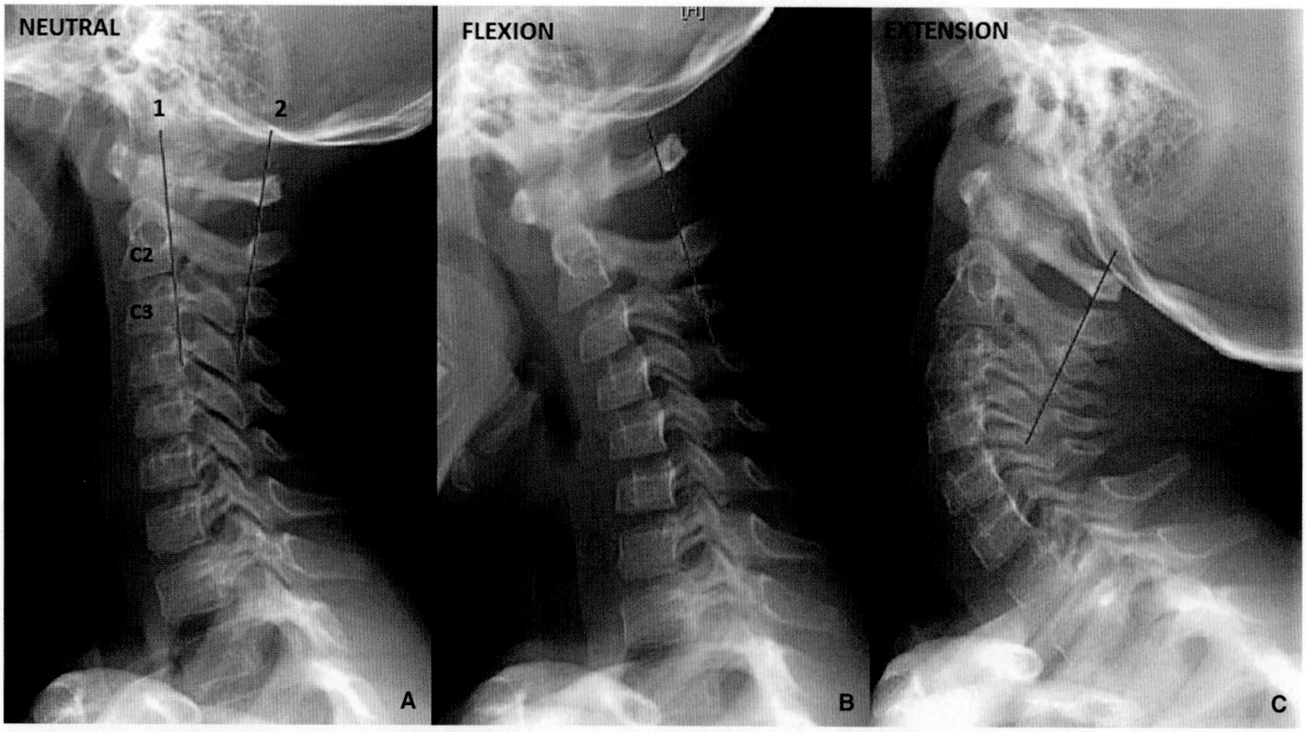

FIGURE 5.15 **Pseudosubluxation, posterior cervical line. A:** Lateral radiograph of the cervical spine in a neutral position demonstrates mild anterior forward position of C2 on C3. *1*, Line along the posterior odontoid touches the superoposterior corner of C3. *2*, The posterior cervical line touches the anterior cortex of the posterior arch of C1 and the C2 and C3 spinous processes. Lateral radiographs of the cervical spine in a flexion position **(B)** and extension position **(C)** illustrate maintenance of the posterior cervical line within a 1 mm distance on the dynamic views.

The variability in the C1–C2 interspinous distance in the younger child is related to ligamentous laxity, which allows spinal hypermobility. However, this distance variability may also be seen in older children. Distances of up to 10 mm or even 12 mm may be normal[15] (Fig. 5.16).

Anterior vertebral wedging may be seen as the vertebral bodies evolve from oval to rectangular shape. It is most evident at C3. The etiology of this wedging may be related to spine hypermobility[15] (Fig. 5.17).

Normal ossification centers, such as the os terminalis of the odontoid, which may be seen normally until 8 years of

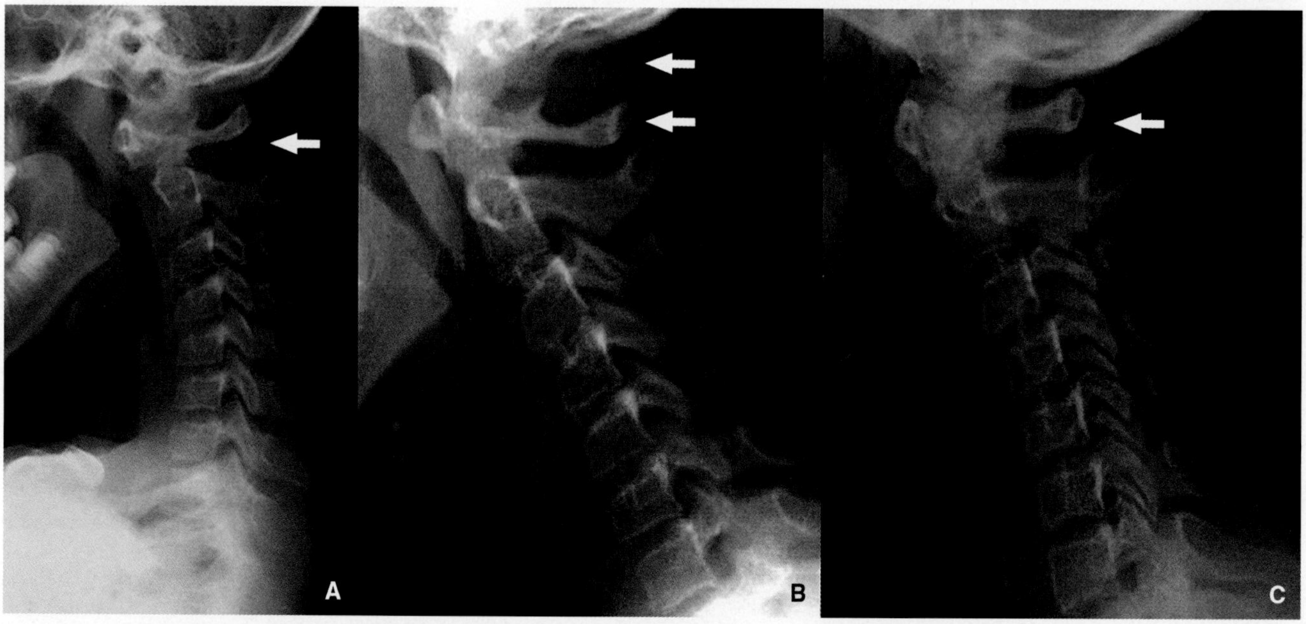

FIGURE 5.16 **C1-C2 interspinous distance.** Lateral views of the cervical spine from three different pediatric patients demonstrate variability in the C1-C2 interspinous distance, due to hypermobility of C1 with flexion. **A:** Increased C1-C2 interspinous distance (*arrow*). **B:** Decreased C1-C2 interspinous distance (*lower arrow*) and increased C1-occiput distance (*upper arrow*). **C:** Average C1-C2 interspinous distance (*arrow*).

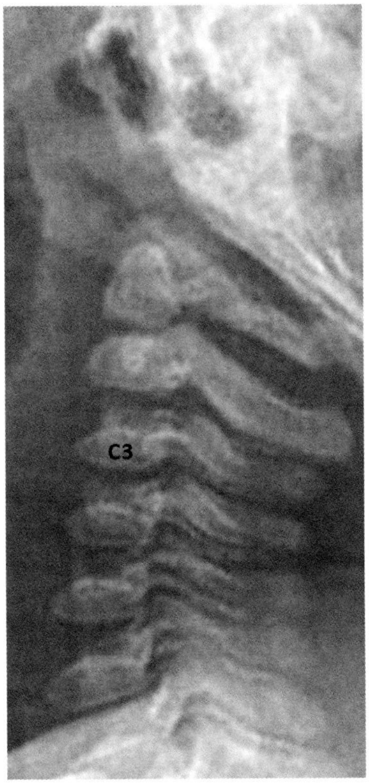

FIGURE 5.17 **Vertebral wedging.** Lateral radiograph in an infant girl shows multiple level anterior vertebral wedging. Vertebral wedging is most prominent at the C3 level.

age, vertebral ring apophyses, and lack of fusion of the arch of C1 may be confused with fractures[15] (Fig. 5.18).

Limbus vertebra is a nontraumatic intraosseous herniation of the nucleus pulposus (Schmorl node), causing fragmentation and corner triangular endplate separation[16] (Fig. 5.19).

Schmorl node is intraosseous herniation of the nucleus pulposus at the center of the vertebral endplate. When multiple, especially in the thoracic spine, Schmorl nodes are associated with Scheuermann disease[16] (Fig. 5.20).

CONGENITAL AND DEVELOPMENTAL ANOMALIES

Absence or Hypoplasia of the Odontoid

Absence or hypoplasia of the odontoid is a rare abnormality with associated underdevelopment of the apical and alar ligaments, which leads to cervical hypermobility[17] (Figs. 5.21 and 5.22).

Os Odontoideum

Os odontoideum is an accessory rounded bony center at the upper dens. The etiology is not clear and may be congenital due to lack of fusion between this center (which originates from the proatlas) and the axis (C2). There is also a traumatic theory about the origin of the os odontoideum, in which interference of the blood supply to the fractured apical segment is implicated. The alar ligament displaces the segment cranially. The os odontoideum should not be confused with the normal ossification center, os terminalis, at the tip of the odontoid, which appears at age 3 and fuses with the dens by age 12[18] (Fig. 5.23).

Vertebral Chondrification or Ossification Developmental Anomalies

These are multiple defects caused by alteration of the normal development of the vertebral cartilage and ossification centers. These defects may be seen in the body or posterior elements of the vertebra[10] (Fig. 5.24).

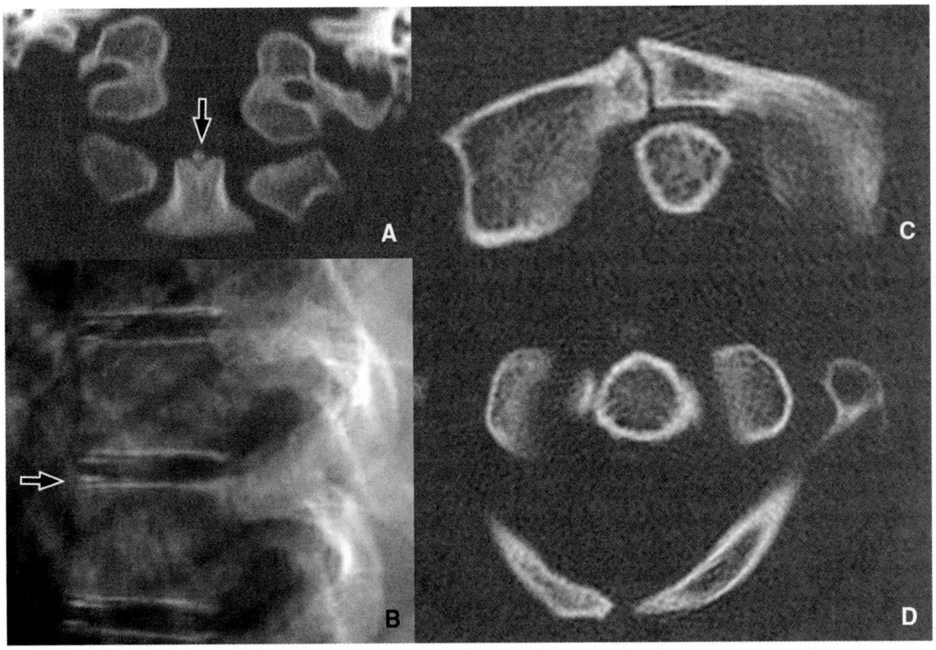

FIGURE 5.18 **Normal variants. A:** Os terminalis (*arrow*) at the tip of the odontoid in a 4-month-old boy. **B:** Superior and inferior ring apophyses (*arrow*), secondary ossification centers, seen in the thoracic vertebrae of a 13-year-old girl. **C and D:** Axial CT images in two pediatric patients show lack of fusion of the anterior and posterior arches of C1, which should not be confused with fractures.

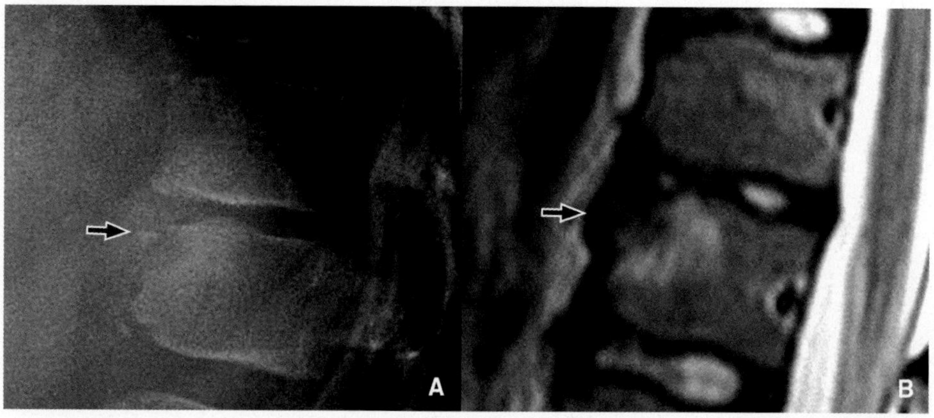

FIGURE 5.19 **Limbus vertebra in a 14-year-old boy. A:** Lateral coned-down radiograph of the lumbar spine shows bony fragmentation (*arrow*) at the anterosuperior margin of the L1 superior endplate. **B:** Sagittal STIR MR image of the L1 vertebra demonstrates bony irregularity (*arrow*) and bone marrow edema.

Anomalies Involving Vertebral Body

Asomia (Agenesis)

Asomia (agenesis) is an uncommon anomaly, which is believed to represent a developmental failure of the vertebral body cartilaginous centers, secondary to vascular insufficiency. Asomia may be a simple abnormality or part of a generalized spinal dysraphism. The posterior elements often remain present.[19]

Hemivertebra

Classical hemivertebra is a relatively common defect where there is absence of half of the vertebral body and neural arch due to developmental failure of the corresponding cartilaginous centers. It is currently believed to be related to ischemic changes. The classical lateral hemivertebrae assume a wedge-shaped configuration with the apex toward the midline. Hemivertebrae may be single or multiple. They may represent an isolated anomaly or present as part of a complex congenital spinal abnormality. Ventral or dorsal hemivertebrae may also occur as a consequence of failure of formation of the right and left cartilaginous centers, respectively.[19,20]

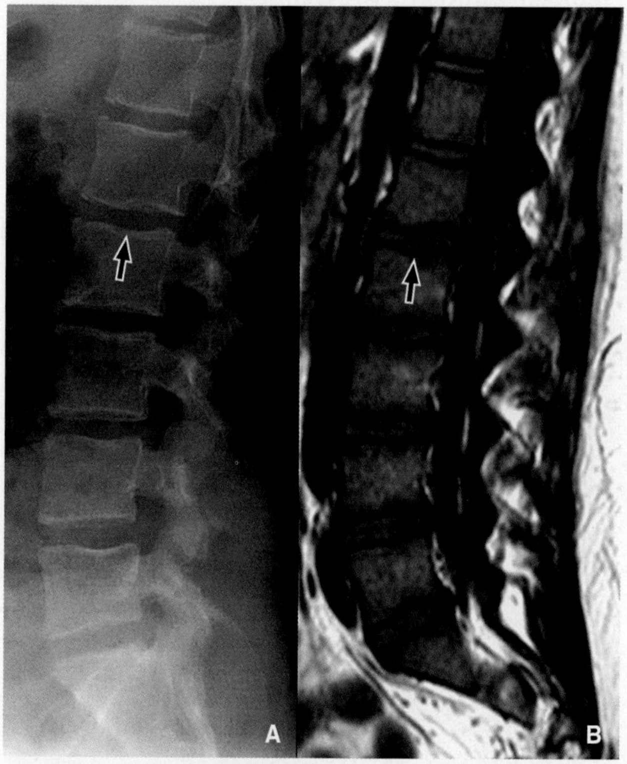

FIGURE 5.20 **Schmorl nodes in an adolescent boy.** Lateral lumbar spine radiograph **(A)** and sagittal T1-weighted MR image of the lumbar spine **(B)** show the central endplate depression (*arrows*) seen in Schmorl nodes.

Sagittal Cleft (Butterfly Vertebra)

Sagittal cleft (butterfly vertebra) is due to the lack of fusion of the two halves of the vertebral body, resulting in two hemivertebrae separated by a sagittal cleft. It is believed to be related to an adhesion between the ectoderm and endoderm that forces the notochord to divide. Sagittal cleft of the vertebral body is relatively common and is usually seen in the thoracic and lumbar spine. It may be associated with abnormality of the intervertebral disc, anterior spina bifida with or without meningocele, diastematomyelia, VACTERL association, and other conditions[19–21] (Fig. 5.25).

Coronal Cleft

Coronal cleft originates from lack of fusion of the ventral and dorsal ossification centers, separated by a cartilaginous cleft. It usually presents in males in the newborn period and is rarely seen after 5 years of age. Coronal cleft may be isolated with no clinical importance or associated with other anomalies such as chondrodysplasia punctata.[19–22]

Anomalies Involving Posterior Elements of the Vertebra

Malformations of the posterior elements result from abnormal development of the neural arch ossification centers and range from mild (spina bifida occulta) to severe (complete absence)[18,19,21] (Fig. 5.26).

Spina Bifida Occulta

Spina bifida occulta is the most common neural arch anomaly, consisting of lack of fusion of the posterior neural arches. The defect may be seen at a single level. The most frequent levels, in descending order, are L5, S1, C1, C7, T1, and the lower thoracic region. Spina bifida occulta is most frequently seen as a solitary defect; however, it may also accompany more complex malformations.[4,20]

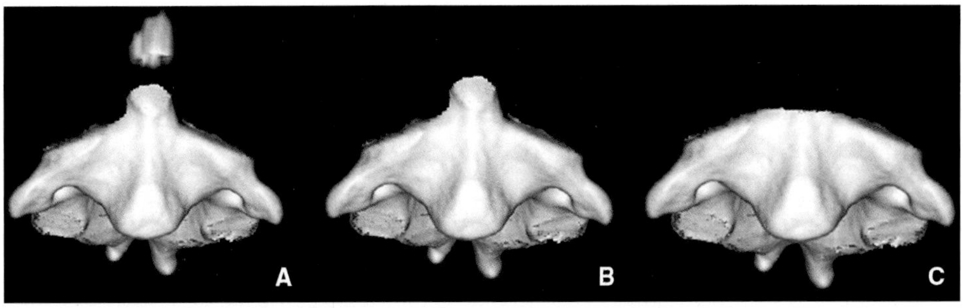

FIGURE 5.21 **Odontoid anomalies.** 3D-reconstructed images of C2 simulate abnormalities of the odontoid process. **A:** Os odontoideum. **B:** Hypoplasia of the odontoid. **C:** Aplasia of the odontoid.

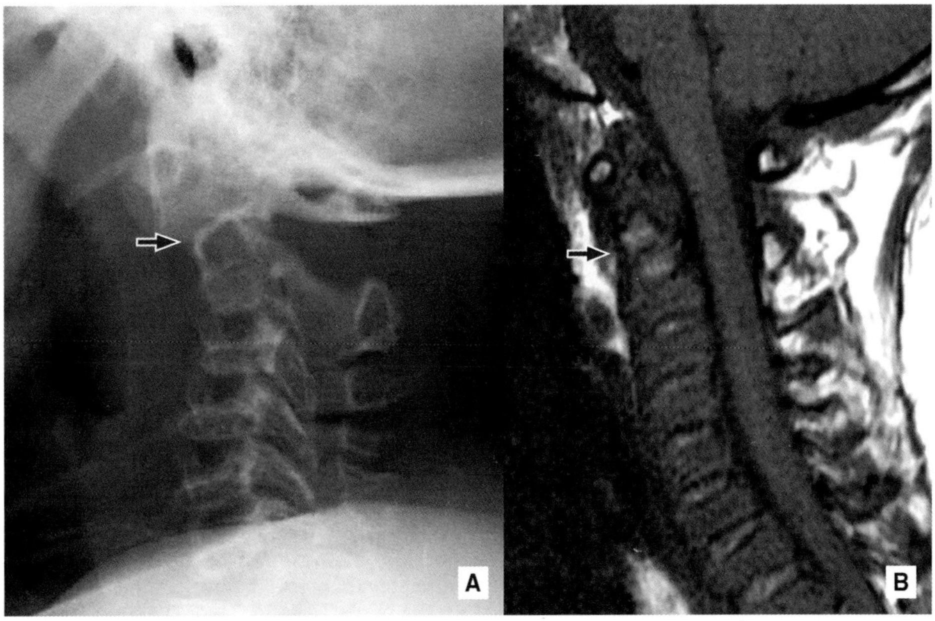

FIGURE 5.22 **Hypoplasia of the odontoid in a 4-year-old boy with Morquio syndrome, dysmorphic features and short stature.** **A:** Lateral cervical spine radiograph shows hypoplasia (*arrow*) of the odontoid. Also noted is platyspondyly of the cervical vertebrae. **B:** Sagittal T1-weighted MR image of the cervical spine demonstrates hypoplasia of the dens (*arrow*), narrowing of the central spinal canal, and cervical platyspondyly.

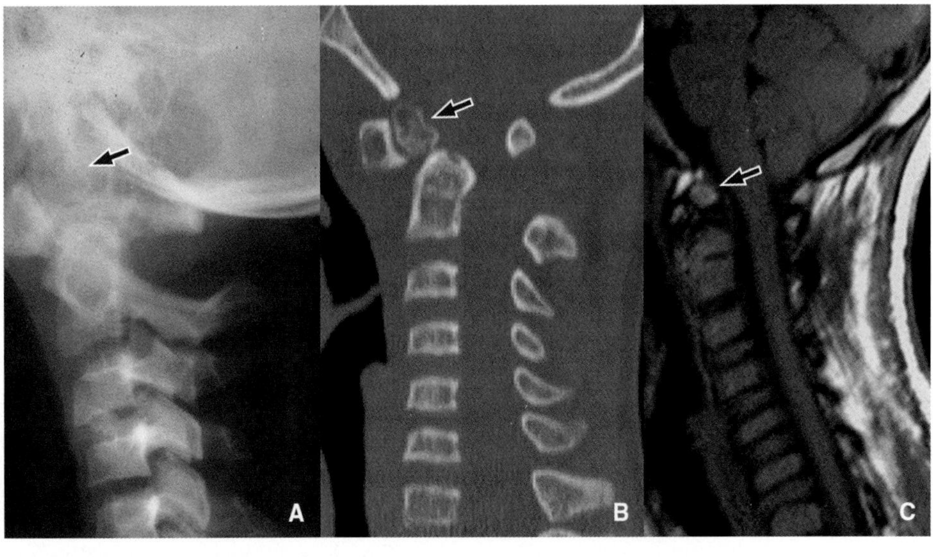

FIGURE 5.23 **Os odontoideum in a 12-year-old girl with osteogenesis imperfecta. (A)** Lateral radiograph, **(B)** sagittal CT image, and **(C)** sagittal T1-weighted MR image of the cervical spine show a bony fragment (*arrows*), above the odontoid, which is an os odontoideum.

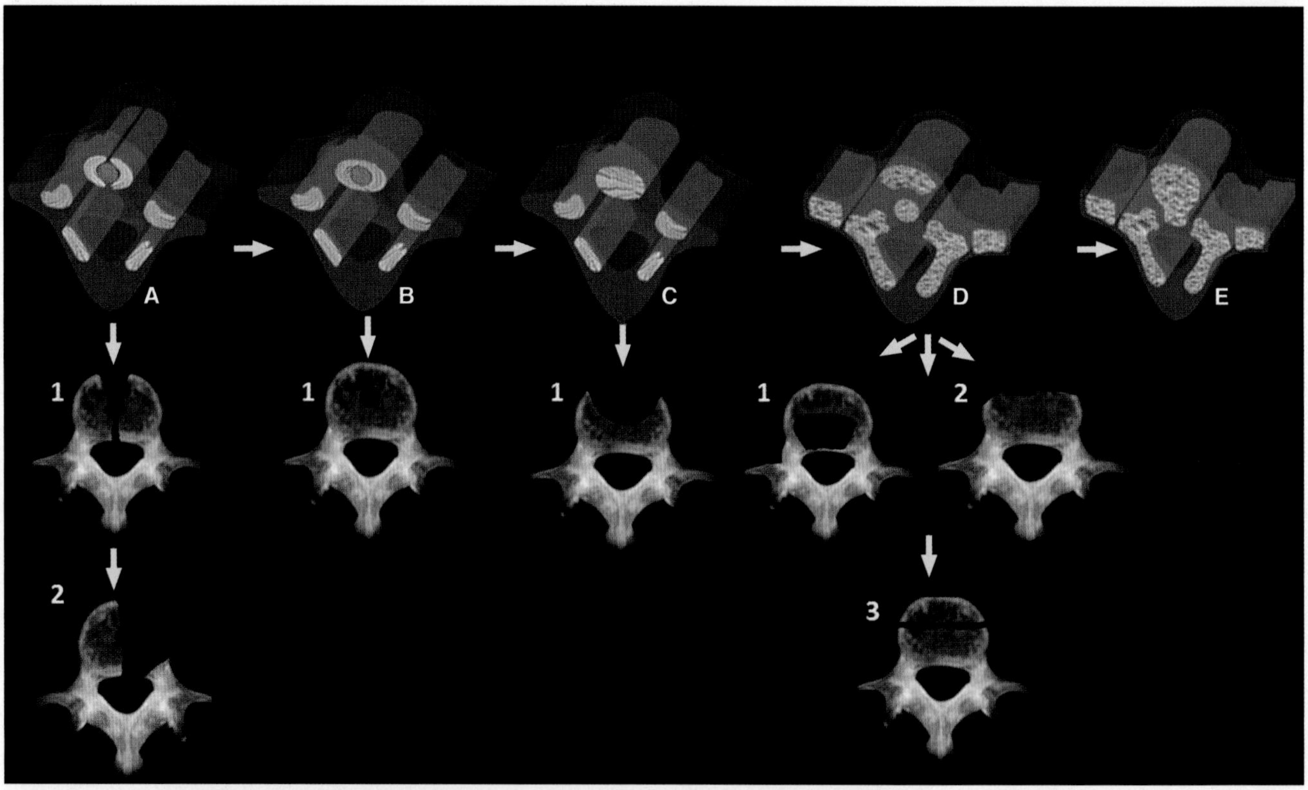

FIGURE 5.24 **Normal development (top line) and abnormalities (lower lines) of the vertebral body.** *A*, Two cartilaginous centers develop into the vertebral body. *A1*, Nonfusion in the midline of these centers gives origin to a sagittal cleft. *A2*, Nonfusion of the cartilaginous centers and lack of development of one of the two ossification centers leads to a **hemivertebra.** *B*, With the formation and joining of the chondrification centers, there is squeezing of the notochord cells and intervertebral tissue into the disc spaces where the notochord becomes the nucleus pulposus of the disc. *B1*, Notochord remnant. *C*, Development of the vertebral body from five ossification centers. *C1*, Nondevelopment of the ossification center: asomia, absent vertebral body. *D*, Developing of an anterior and posterior vertebral body ossification centers. *D1*, Lack of normal development of the anterior body ossification center leads to ventral vertebral hypoplasia. *D2*, Nondevelopment of the posterior ossification center leads to dorsal vertebral hypoplasia. *D3*, Failure of fusion of the anterior and posterior ossification centers leads to coronal cleft. *E*, Fusion of the body ossification centers as a single unit.

Spinal Dysraphism

Spinal dysraphism comprises a group of congenital anomalies of the central nervous system, in which there is maldevelopment of the cutaneous ectoderm (skin), neuroectoderm (neural tube), and bony mesodermal structures. It may involve multiple and consecutive vertebral segments and be associated with other mesenchymal and neural abnormalities. The neural-tissue containing defect may lack skin covering (open dysraphism), with or without protrusion of subarachnoid fluid (myelomeningocele or myelocele, respectively), or be covered by skin and subcutaneous tissue (closed dysraphism), with or without protrusion of the subarachnoid fluid (lipomyelomeningocele or lipomyelocele, respectively). More uncommonly, the externalized meningeal sac contains only subarachnoid fluid without neural elements (e.g., meningocele)[1,20,23] (Fig. 5.27).

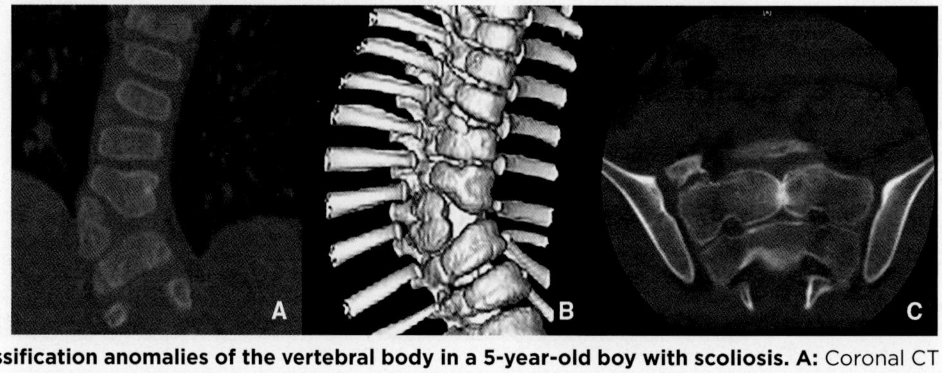

FIGURE 5.25 **Ossification anomalies of the vertebral body in a 5-year-old boy with scoliosis. A:** Coronal CT image of the thoracic spine demonstrates multiple right- and left-sided fused hemivertebrae and dextroscoliosis. **B:** Coronal 3D CT image shows multiple hemivertebrae. **C:** Coronal CT image demonstrates a butterfly S2 vertebra.

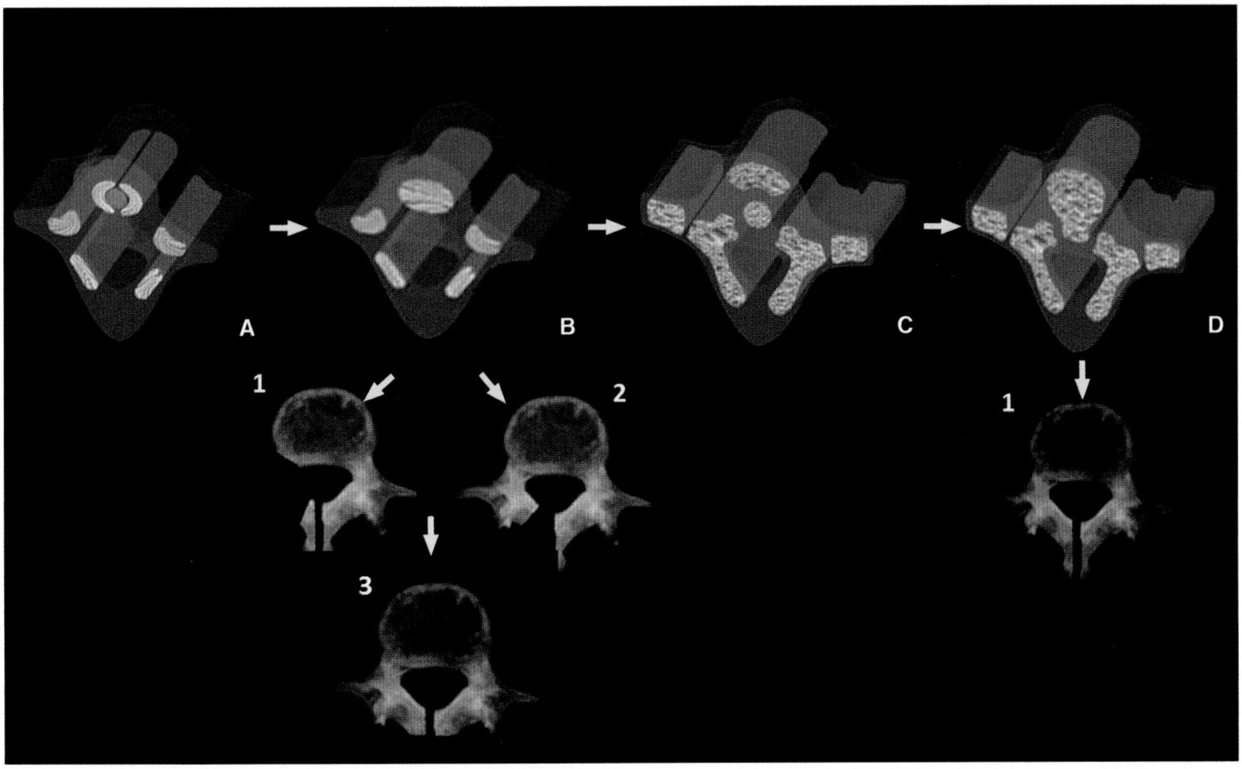

FIGURE 5.26 **Normal development (top line) and abnormalities (lower lines) of the vertebral posterior elements.** *A,* There are three chondrification centers in each side of the developing vertebra: body, pars, and neural arch. *B,* At the same time that the body is forming, the chondrification centers of the vertebral arches and pars (one pair on each side) fuse with each other and with the centrum. *B1,* The chondrification center for the pars fails to develop: pars defect. *B2,* Incomplete development of the cartilaginous centers for the posterior arch: lamina and spinous process defect. *B3,* Absence of both posterior chondrification centers for the neural arch: absence of the posterior arch. *C,* The transverse and spinous processes develop from extension of vertebral arch chondrification centers. *D1,* Incomplete union of the posterior arch: spina bifida.

SEGMENTATION ABNORMALITIES

Complete "Block Vertebra"

This congenital abnormality is secondary to failure in the process of segmentation during fetal life that causes two or more adjacent vertebrae to be partially or completely fused in a single bony block. One or more vertebra(e) may be involved, without or with a rudimentary intervertebral disc. In order of frequency, block vertebra is most common in the lumbar, cervical, and thoracic regions. The morphologic anomalies of the block, such as concave configuration and narrow AP diameter, are due to growth deficiency at the fusion site. There may be associated disorders of embryogenesis in the levels above and below the "block vertebra," such as hemivertebrae or absent vertebra.

The posterior elements of the block may be also malsegmented, and when fused, the spinal curvature is altered, leading to scoliosis and kyphosis. Block vertebra may be associated with dysraphism[21–24] (Fig. 5.28).

Klippel-Feil Syndrome

Klippel-Feil syndrome is a congenital segmentation abnormality, characterized by fusion of two or more cervical vertebrae. The majority of affected pediatric patients have a short neck; limited motion, especially rotation; and a low hairline. There are three types described. In type I, there is extensive fusion of the cervical and upper thoracic vertebrae, usually associated with other anomalies. Type II demonstrates focal

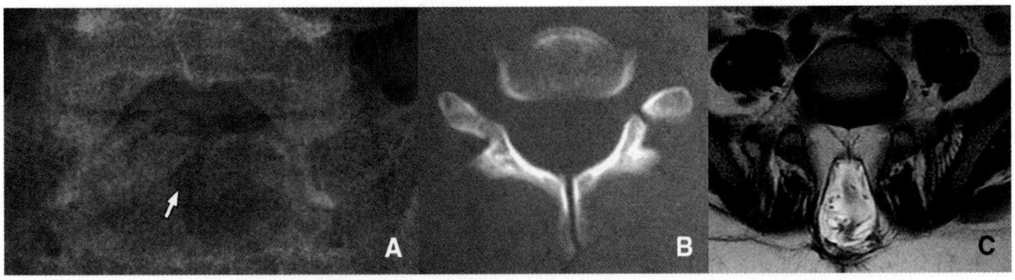

FIGURE 5.27 **Ossification anomalies of the posterior elements in a 4-year-old boy with Chiari II malformation and repaired myelomeningocele. A:** Anteroposterior radiograph of the lumbar spine shows L5 spinal bifida occulta with the "butt-end-twisted" appearance (*arrow*). **B:** Axial CT image demonstrates L5 spinal bifida occulta. **C:** Axial T2-weighted MR image shows a repaired myelomeningocele. Note the lack of posterior elements and vertical orientation of the pedicles.

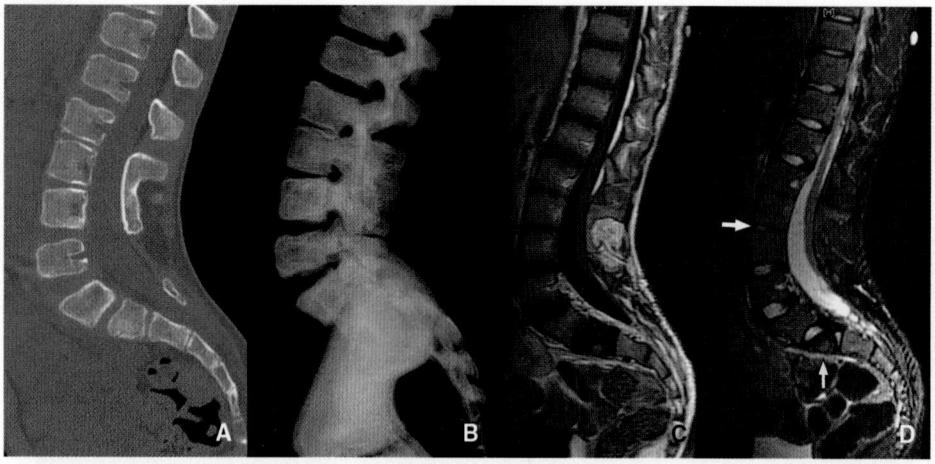

FIGURE 5.28 **Segmentation anomalies in a 14-year-old boy with back pain.** Sagittal CT image **(A)** and sagittal 3D CT image **(B)** of the lumbar spine show "block vertebra" appearance of the L2, L3, L4, and posterior elements. Sagittal T1-weighted MR image **(C)** and sagittal T2-weighted MR image **(D)** of the lumbar spine demonstrate rudimentary intervertebral discs (*white arrow*). Incidentally, a butterfly vertebra of S2 (*yellow arrow*) is also seen.

vertebral fusion of one or two interspaces, usually at the C2-C3 or C5-C6 levels. Type III is associated with thoracic and lumbar spinal anomalies in addition to the findings of type I or type II Klippel-Feil syndrome.

Klippel-Feil syndrome is associated with other bony developmental abnormalities such as vertebral ossification malformations, basilar invagination, and Sprengel deformity. Neural and bony anomalies, in particular Chiari I malformation and diastematomyelia, may occur. Associated renal malformations include renal agenesis, hydronephrosis, horseshoe kidney, duplicated collecting system, renal ectopia, and bilateral tubular ectasia. Congenital heart disease (coarctation of the aorta, atrial septal defect), conductive hearing loss, and rib fusion may also be associated[4,25–27] (Fig. 5.29).

Sprengel Deformity

This congenital abnormality occurs secondary to failure of scapular caudal migration during fetal development because of a fibrous osseous connection. The omovertebral bone articulates with an upper transverse process of the cervical spine. Sprengel deformity is associated with Klippel-Feil syndrome, spina bifida, torticollis, kyphoscoliosis, and atrophy of the regional muscles. The affected scapula is elevated with the inferior angle rotated laterally. Rigault classifies the abnormality in three grades: grade I, superomedial angle lower than the T2 but above the T4 transverse process; grade II, superomedial angle between the C5 and T2 transverse processes; and grade III, superomedial angle above the C5 transverse process[4,20,28] (Fig. 5.30).

Caudal Regression Syndrome

Caudal regression syndrome is a congenital disorder in which the lower spine and/or sacrum is malformed. In addition to vertebral and/or sacral bone, other local tissues derived from the embryonic caudal cell mass may be affected. The caudal cell mass is a conglomerate of totipotential cells responsible for formation of the filum terminale, ventriculus terminalis, conus medullaris, distal lumbosacral vertebra, and urorectal septum, which unites with the cloaca to form the urogenital sinus and the anorectal channel.

Approximately 20% of infants with caudal regression syndrome are born to a mother with diabetes mellitus. There is also an association with OEIS (omphalocele, cloacal exstrophy, imperforate anus, and spinal deformities) complex. VACTERL syndrome (vertebral anomalies, anorectal malformations, cardiac anomalies, tracheoesophageal fistula, renal and limb anomalies) is seen in about 10% of affected patients.

Pang's classification of lumbosacral dysgenesis includes:

Type I: Sacral and partial lumbar agenesis
Type II: Complete sacral agenesis
Type III: Partial sacral agenesis, distal to S2 (most common)

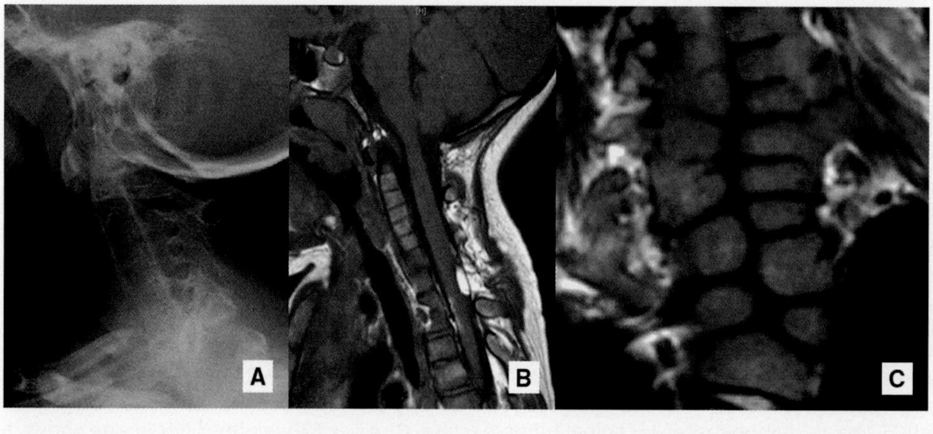

FIGURE 5.29 **Klippel-Feil syndrome in a 6-year-old girl with limited neck mobility. A:** Lateral cervical spine radiograph illustrates the fusion of the cervical vertebra and posterior elements. **B:** Sagittal T1-weighted MR image of the cervical and upper thoracic spine demonstrates the cervical–thoracic-fused vertebrae. **C:** Coronal T1-weighted MR image shows multiples butterfly, hemi-, and block vertebrae.

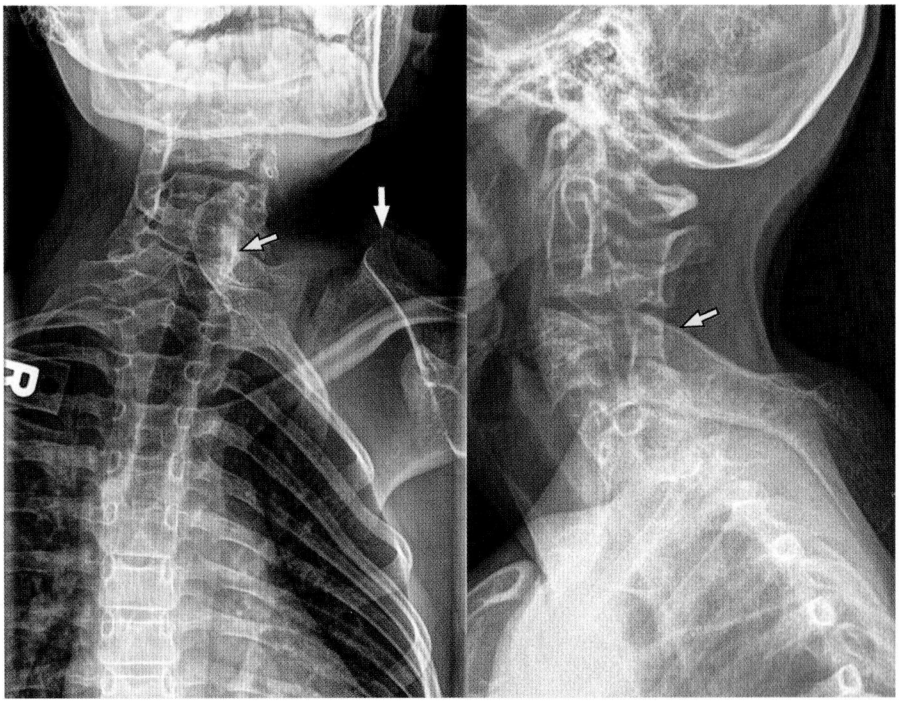

FIGURE 5.30 **Sprengel deformity in a 15-year-old boy who presented with torticollis and limited mobility of the left shoulder.** Frontal and lateral radiographs of the cervical and upper thoracic spine demonstrate elevation of the left scapula (*white arrow*) and fusion of the scapula to the midcervical spine by an omovertebral bone (*yellow arrows*), and multiple segmentation anomalies in the cervical spine.

Type IV: Hemisacrum (second most common)

Type V: Coccygeal agenesis

The MRI findings of caudal regression syndrome include missing distal vertebrae and a "wedge-shaped" configuration of the distal cord when it is located above L1. When the spinal cord ends below L1, there may be other associated findings such as tethered cord, diastematomyelia, fatty or thickened filum, hydromyelia, and mild sacral hypogenesis. Associated abnormalities of the genitourinary and gastrointestinal systems are common[23,29] (Fig. 5.31).

Diastematomyelia

Diastematomyelia is a condition in which all or part of the spinal cord is split. This abnormality originates from aberrant division of the notochord during embryonic life. If the canal of Kovalevsky persists (communication of the yolk sac with the amniotic cavity), or if there is any adhesion between the ectoderm and endoderm, an obstacle to the notochord cells is present. The notochord either deviates to one side or splits to pass around both sides of the obstacle.

The two hemicords may be symmetric or asymmetric, and the length of separation varies. Two types have been described. In type I (40% to 70%), there are two individual sacs separated by an osseous or cartilaginous septum, each containing a hemicord. In type II, there is a single dural sac containing both hemicords, which may be tethered by a nerve root or fibrous bands.

Diastematomyelia is associated with low position of the conus medullaris, thickened filum terminale, segmentation and ossification abnormalities, scoliosis, Sprengel deformity, Klippel-Feil syndrome, Chiari malformation, dermal sinus, lipomyelomeningocele, open dysraphism involving

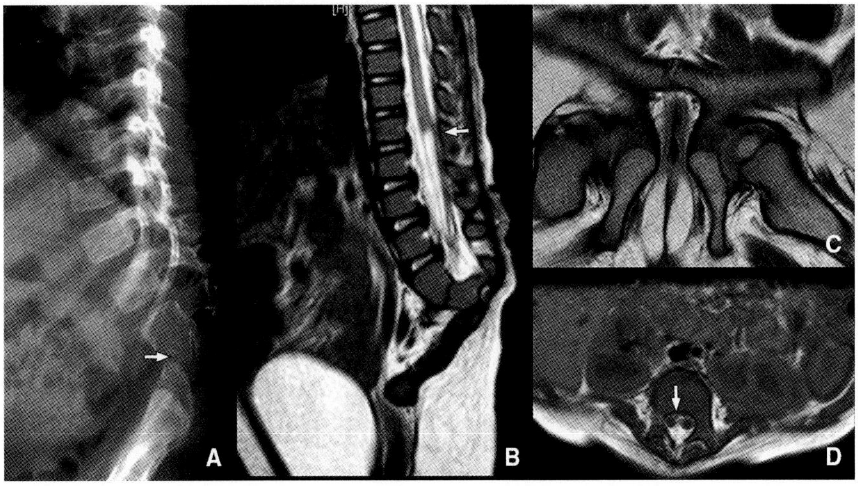

FIGURE 5.31 **Caudal regression syndrome in a 5-year-old girl with history of a diabetic mother and "buttocks deformity." A:** Lateral radiograph of the lumbosacral spine shows absence (*arrow*) of the lumbar segments distal to L2, sacrum, and coccygeal segments. **B:** Sagittal T2-weighted MR image demonstrates the characteristic "wedge-shaped" morphology of the spinal cord (*arrow*). **C:** Coronal T1-weighted MR image of the pelvis shows fusion of the iliac bones due to the missing vertebrae and lack of pubic bone. **D:** Axial T1-weighted MR image demonstrates a divided spinal cord, "diastematomyelia" (*arrow*) associated to caudal regression syndrome. Also, noted is the coronal rotation of the left kidney.

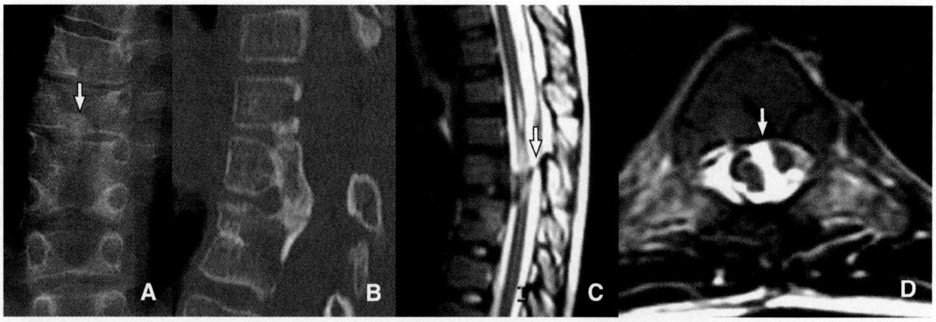

FIGURE 5.32 **Diastematomyelia in a 9-year-old girl who presented with paresthesia. A:** Frontal coned-down radiograph of the lower thoracic spine shows diastematomyelic bony spur (*arrow*). **B:** Sagittal CT image of the lower thoracic spine demonstrates the diastematomyelic bony spur extending into the spinal canal as well as the associated segmentation anomaly of the adjacent vertebra. **C:** Sagittal T2-weighted MR image shows the extension of the diastematomyelic bony spur to the posterior margin of the canal (*arrow*). **D:** Axial T2-weighted MR image demonstrates the divided cord, "diastematomyelia" (*arrow*).

one hemicord (hemimyelocele or hemimyelomeningocele), meningocele manqué, teratoma, and horseshoe kidney[23,24,30,31] (Fig. 5.32).

Currarino Triad

Currarino triad is a rare syndrome first described by Kennedy in 1926 and by Currarino in 1981. It is characterized by anorectal malformation (anal stenosis, anal ectopia, imperforate anus), sacrococcygeal osseous defect (scimitar, comma, or crescent-shaped), and presacral mass, most commonly teratoma or meningocele. In 50% of affected patients, this syndrome is autosomal dominant[32,33] (Fig. 5.33). Mutations in the gene *MNX1* have been reported in almost all familial and many sporadic cases of Currarino triad.

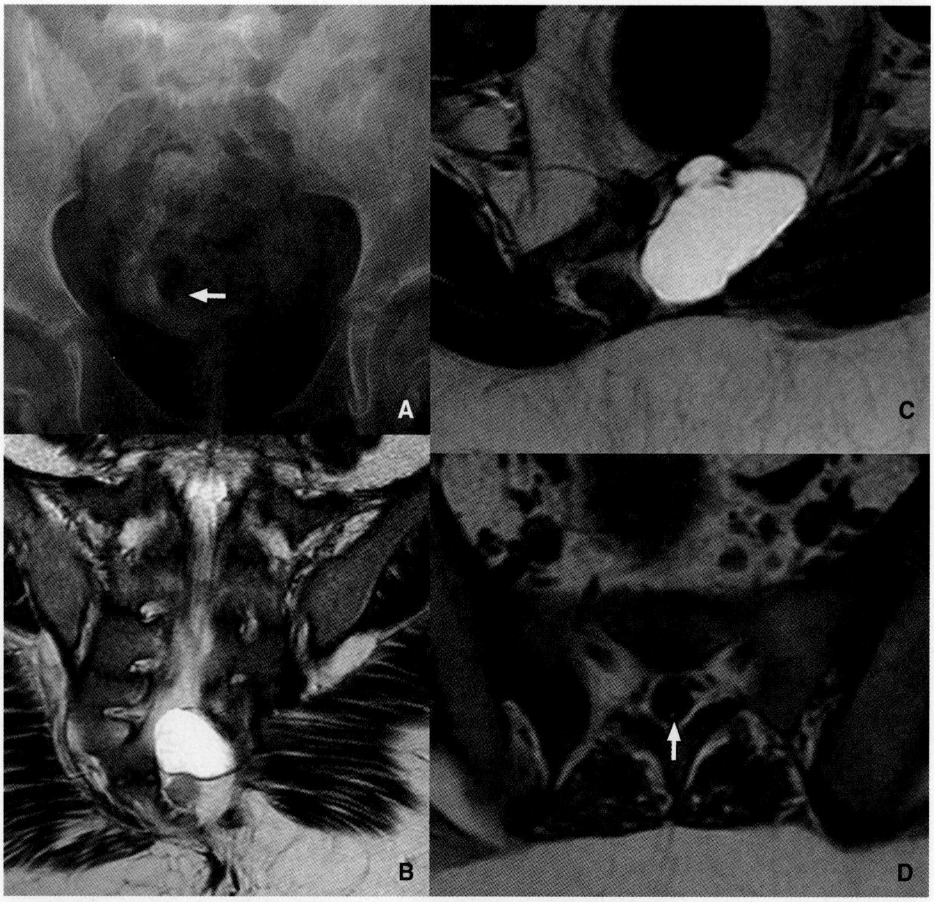

FIGURE 5.33 **Currarino triad and left lateral sacral meningocele in a 16-year-old girl who presented with persistent constipation. A:** Frontal radiograph of the pelvis shows a "scimitar sacrum" (*arrow*). Coronal T2-weighted MR image **(B)** and axial T2-weighted MR image **(C)** demonstrate a lower sacral left lateral meningocele. **D:** Axial T1-weighted MR image shows fatty infiltration (*arrow*) of the filum terminalis.

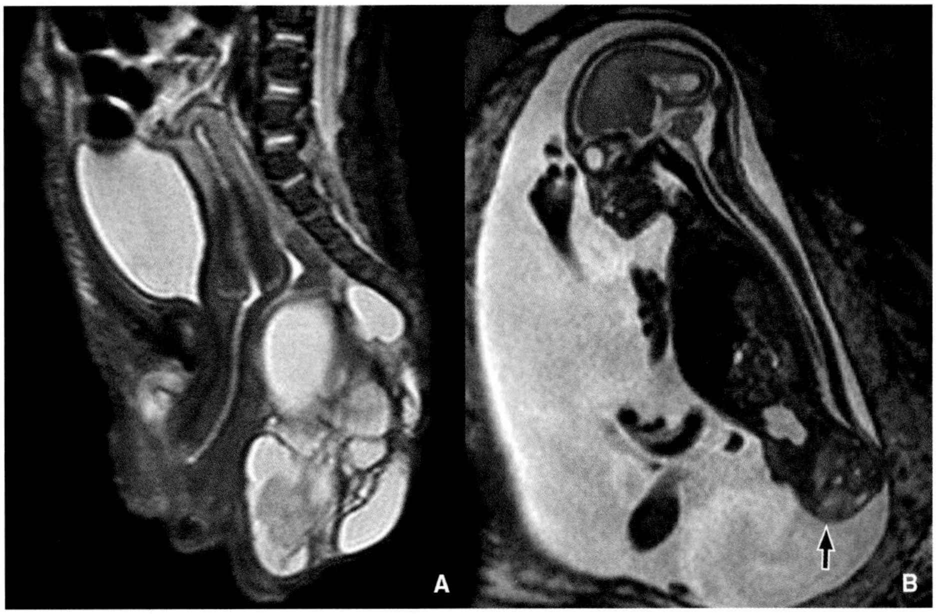

FIGURE 5.34 **Sacrococcygeal teratoma in two different patients. A:** Newborn infant girl with a large cystic and solid, mainly exterior, sacral mass. A small part of the mass extends into the presacral space, consistent with sacrococcygeal teratoma type I. **B:** Fetal MRI obtained in a 20-week-old fetus with a sacral and presacral heterogeneous mass consistent with type I sacrococcygeal teratoma (*arrow*).

Sacrococcygeal Teratoma

Sacrococcygeal teratomas are rare congenital neoplasms presenting in ~1 in 40,000 infants, more commonly in females. They derive from pluripotential cells, are thought to originate from Hensen node, and contain components arising from the three germinal layers. Sacrococcygeal teratomas are classified according to their position in the pelvis. Type I is almost completely external with a minimal portion in the presacral region (47%). Type II is both external and presacral in location (35%). Type III is mainly located in the pelvis and abdomen (8%). Type IV is a presacral mass (10%).[23,32,34]

The majority of sacrococcygeal teratomas are mixed solid and cystic lesions, with only 5% presenting as a cystic neoplasm. Calcifications may be seen in up to 50% of cases. When associated with sacrococcygeal defects, anorectal stenosis, cutaneous stigmata, and genitourinary anomalies, a familial form with dominant inheritance is suggested[23,32,34] (Fig. 5.34).

INFECTIOUS DISORDERS

Terminology and Pathways of Spread

The general term "infectious spondylitis" refers to an infection of the vertebral column and surrounding soft tissues. It does not imply a specific pathologic agent or location. Discitis refers to infection of the intervertebral disc itself. Vertebral osteomyelitis indicates purulence or frank abscess within the osseous vertebral elements. Subdural or epidural abscess (empyema) is purulence within the central spinal canal, whereas paraspinal abscess refers to a suppurative process centered in the paravertebral soft tissues. Practically speaking, multiple compartments are frequently involved concurrently. Because of this, it is important to accurately document all involved areas to facilitate prognostication and treatment planning.

It is crucial to understand the multiple potential pathways for infection spread in the spine. These include direct spread from a contiguous source (e.g., decubitus ulcer to sacrum, disc space to psoas muscle), lymphatic spread, hematogenous spread, and direct CSF spread (e.g., meningitis). Hematogenous spread is the most important pathway for spinal infection. Both arterial (arterioles in the vertebral endplate metaphyseal equivalent) and venous (spinal "Batson" plexus) conduits are important. Spread routes in adults and children differ because of anatomical features related to developmental maturity. In adults, spondylitis frequently commences in the vertebral endplate with secondary involvement of the disc space, paravertebral soft tissues, and epidural space. Conversely, in children, vascular channels extending across the vertebral endplate (not present in adults) permit primary infection of the intervertebral disc space leading to secondary infection of the vertebral endplate.

Pyogenic Spondylodiscitis

Pyogenic spondylodiscitis refers to a pus-forming spinal infection, typically caused by bacteria, and less commonly, by fungus. Age distribution is bimodal, with peaks in both the pediatric age group and the sixth to seventh decades. In children, infection usually commences in the disc space with spread to the adjacent vertebra and paraspinal soft tissues and/or epidural space. On the other hand, in adults, the metaphyseal equivalent of the vertebral body is usually the first site of infection, with secondary spread to the disc and adjacent soft tissues.

Spondylodiscitis can be difficult to clinically diagnose, particularly in young preverbal children; therefore, a heightened index of clinical suspicion is needed. All spinal segments may be affected, although lumbar is more common than thoracic or cervical location. Presenting symptoms can be confusing or misleading,[35] especially in young children, and include refusal to walk (63%), back pain (27%), inability to flex the lower back (50%), and loss of normal lumbar lordosis (40%).[36] Laboratory tests and cultures may be falsely negative or unhelpful.[36]

Staphylococcus aureus is the most common pathogen, although gram-negative bacilli and other less common pathogens may be seen in immunocompetent and immunocompromised patients including intravenous drug abusers.[37,38] In sickle cell disease, one should always consider salmonella. Pathogen identification is made either from blood culture or direct tissue sampling (percutaneous or surgical biopsy).

Characteristic imaging findings of pyogenic vertebral osteomyelitis on radiographs include bone loss and ill definition of the vertebral endplates, sometimes with sclerosis in more chronic indolent infections. The disc space height is reduced, although this can be difficult to appreciate early in the infection. Multiplanar CT imaging can frequently show these findings better than radiographs, but is generally not indicated for initial screening. Spondylodiscitis may be detected when present on thoracic or abdominal CT for imaging evaluation of chest or abdominal pain, and review of the spinal axis should be part of the routine search in all patients presenting with these symptoms. The primary use of CT is for biopsy, localization, and presurgical planning for stabilization procedures. MRI with intravenous contrast is most sensitive for detecting spondylodiscitis. MRI also best evaluates the adjacent soft tissues and spinal cord. Bone marrow edema is seen early; vertebral collapse is usually a later finding. Bone marrow edema shows T1 hypointensity and T2 hyperintensity and is most conspicuous on STIR or fat-saturated T2-weighted MRI sequences (Fig. 5.35A, B).

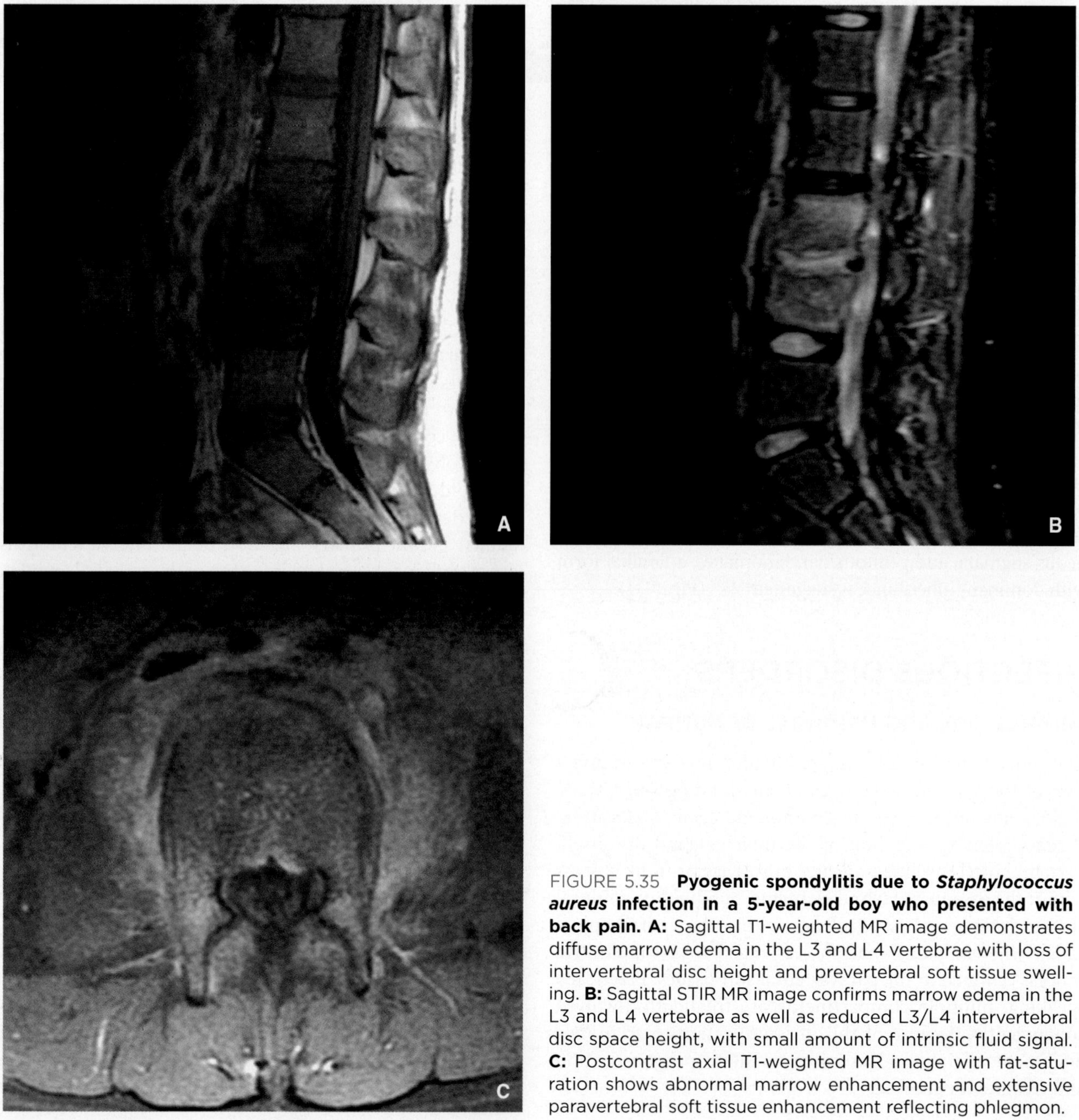

FIGURE 5.35 **Pyogenic spondylitis due to *Staphylococcus aureus* infection in a 5-year-old boy who presented with back pain. A:** Sagittal T1-weighted MR image demonstrates diffuse marrow edema in the L3 and L4 vertebrae with loss of intervertebral disc height and prevertebral soft tissue swelling. **B:** Sagittal STIR MR image confirms marrow edema in the L3 and L4 vertebrae as well as reduced L3/L4 intervertebral disc space height, with small amount of intrinsic fluid signal. **C:** Postcontrast axial T1-weighted MR image with fat-saturation shows abnormal marrow enhancement and extensive paravertebral soft tissue enhancement reflecting phlegmon.

Intravenous contrast-enhanced, fat-saturated T1-weighted MRI is essential to discern phlegmon or cellulitis from frank abscess (Fig. 5.35C) and may also reveal intradural pial enhancement along the spinal cord or cauda equina.

Differential diagnostic considerations include neoplasm and noninfectious spondyloarthropathies, but clinical findings may help distinguish these entities. Therapy is pathogen-specific antibiotic therapy. Surgical decompression and stabilization are reserved for pediatric patients with spinal cord compression and/or instability.

Tuberculous Spondylodiscitis

Tuberculous spondylodiscitis occurs following *Mycobacterium tuberculosis (TB)* infection spread from the lungs to the spinal axis via either hematogenous or lymphatic routes. The initial site of spinal infection occurs in the anterior vertebral body with spread to adjacent vertebral bodies via subligamentous (anterior longitudinal ligament) spread.[39] Relative sparing of the intervertebral disc space (in comparison to pyogenic spondylodiscitis) is attributed to absence of proteolytic enzyme activity.

Clinical presentation usually includes back pain and variable fever. Spinal cord compression producing paraplegia may result from associated epidural abscess or acute angle kyphosis. In fact, tuberculous spondylitis with resulting deformity is the leading cause of paraplegia in developing countries.[40] In general, clinical onset is more insidious than that seen with pyogenic spondylitis. Clinical and imaging findings are similar to other granulomatous spinal infections (e.g., Brucellosis, fungal), with the comment that neurologic deficits are reported more commonly in TB spondylitis. TB spondylitis incidence is increasingly related to association with coinfection in immunocompromised individuals.[41]

Imaging findings in tuberculous vertebral osteomyelitis,[42] in comparison to pyogenic spondylitis, are most often in the midthoracic or thoracolumbar spine. Although radiographs are frequently obtained for initial evaluation, their utility is limited early in the infection process because early vertebral osteomyelitis is often occult on radiographs for several weeks after infection onset. Vertebral body collapse with gibbous kyphotic deformity on radiography is a classic imaging appearance of longer-standing infection. Endplate destruction may not be evident, and in fact, relative lack of disc space involvement strongly suggests the diagnosis of tuberculous spondylitis. In addition, paraspinal calcifications are common and also strongly help suggest the diagnosis.

As with pyogenic spondylitis, the role of multiplanar spine CT is primarily for biopsy guidance and surgical stabilization planning. It can also demonstrate bone complications of infectious spondylitis such as vertebral collapse and spinal deformity. As with pyogenic spondylitis, MRI with intravenous contrast is the best modality to evaluate both vertebral and adjacent soft tissue involvement. Unlike pyogenic infection, large paraspinal and epidural abscesses (frequently with calcification) are common. It is critical to assess for spinal cord compression related to epidural abscess or vertebral collapse and/or subluxation. Nuclear medicine bone scan and gallium scan can both demonstrate increased radiotracer uptake in the infected area, but do not provide high enough spatial resolution to facilitate surgical planning or exclude cord compression. WBC scan may be false negative, particularly in chronic osteomyelitis. Therefore, nuclear scintigraphy has a limited role in the imaging evaluation of tuberculous spondylitis.

Differential diagnostic considerations include pyogenic spondylitis, extradural neoplasms, and (rarely) congenital kyphoscoliosis secondary to vertebral segmentation anomalies. Identification of *M. tuberculosis* species and drug sensitivity testing can be achieved via peripheral blood or direct tissue sampling (percutaneous or surgical biopsy), allowing selection of specific antimycobacterial antibiotic therapy. Surgical decompression and stabilization are reserved for pediatric patients with spinal cord compression and/or instability.

Epidural Empyema

Epidural spinal infection resides within the epidural space and the most commonly isolated pathogens are *Staphylococcus* aureus and *Mycobacterium tuberculosis* (depending on patient population).

Imaging evaluation typically reveals an epidural fluid density/signal mass in the osseous spinal canal with variable dural sac and spinal cord compression (Fig. 5.36A). Although, classically, rim enhancement of the epidural fluid collection is described, many epidural infections demonstrate more homogeneous enhancement with relatively small areas of fluid (Fig. 5.36B). Diffusion-weighted MRI can show restriction within frank empyema. Concurrent discitis and vertebral osteomyelitis are often observed, but are not universally present if the abscess originated from direct inoculation or hematogenous spread to the extradural space.

Differential diagnostic considerations include extradural neoplasm and hematoma. Following percutaneous or surgical aspiration, affected pediatric patients are treated with pathogen-specific antimicrobial therapy. Duration and breadth of therapy are based on pathogen type, severity of infection, and comorbid disease.

Paraspinal Abscess

Paraspinal abscesses reside in either the prevertebral or paravertebral spaces and are often distributed along muscular planes. The most common paravertebral locations are within or adjacent to the iliacus or psoas and the dorsal paraspinal (erector spinae) muscles (Fig. 5.37). Paraspinal abscesses may be single or multiple and either unilocular or multilocular. As with extradural abscess, the most commonly isolated pathogens are *Staphylococcus aureus* and *Mycobacterium tuberculosis* (depending on patient population). Associations

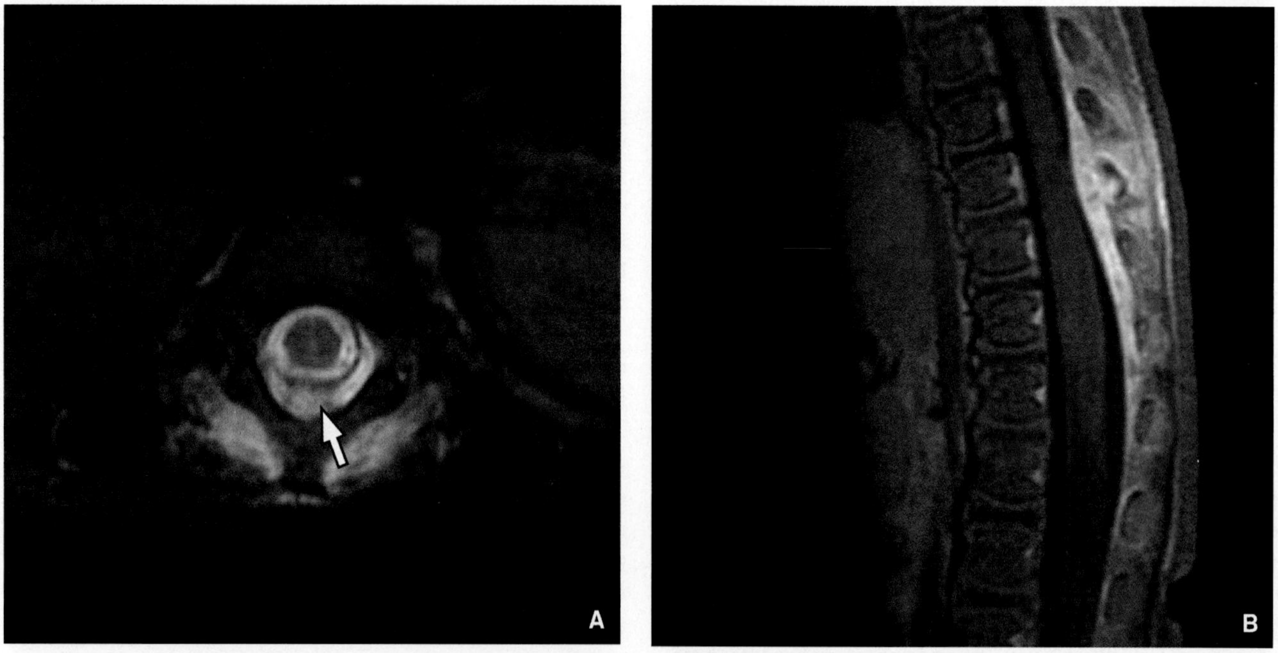

FIGURE 5.36 **Epidural abscess in an infant girl who presented with fever. A:** Axial T2-weighted MR image with fat-saturation shows abnormal epidural T2 hyperintensity (*arrow*) displacing the dural sac and cord anteriorly. There is also abnormal edema extending into the erector spinae muscles. **B:** Postcontrast sagittal T1-weighted MR image with fat-saturation confirms robust epidural thickening and heterogeneous enhancement extending into the dorsal soft tissues.

with intravenous drug abuse, hematogenous spread from other sites, and direct inoculation following trauma are possible, but paravertebral abscesses in pediatric patients frequently arise secondary to concurrent discitis. Imaging characteristics of paravertebral abscess are similar to those of abscesses in other locations.

The primary differential diagnostic considerations include primary or metastatic neoplasm, retroperitoneal hematoma, and extramedullary hematopoiesis, although clinical presentation and associated clinical findings are frequently definitive and specific. Treatment is similar to that previously described for pyogenic and mycobacterial spine infections.

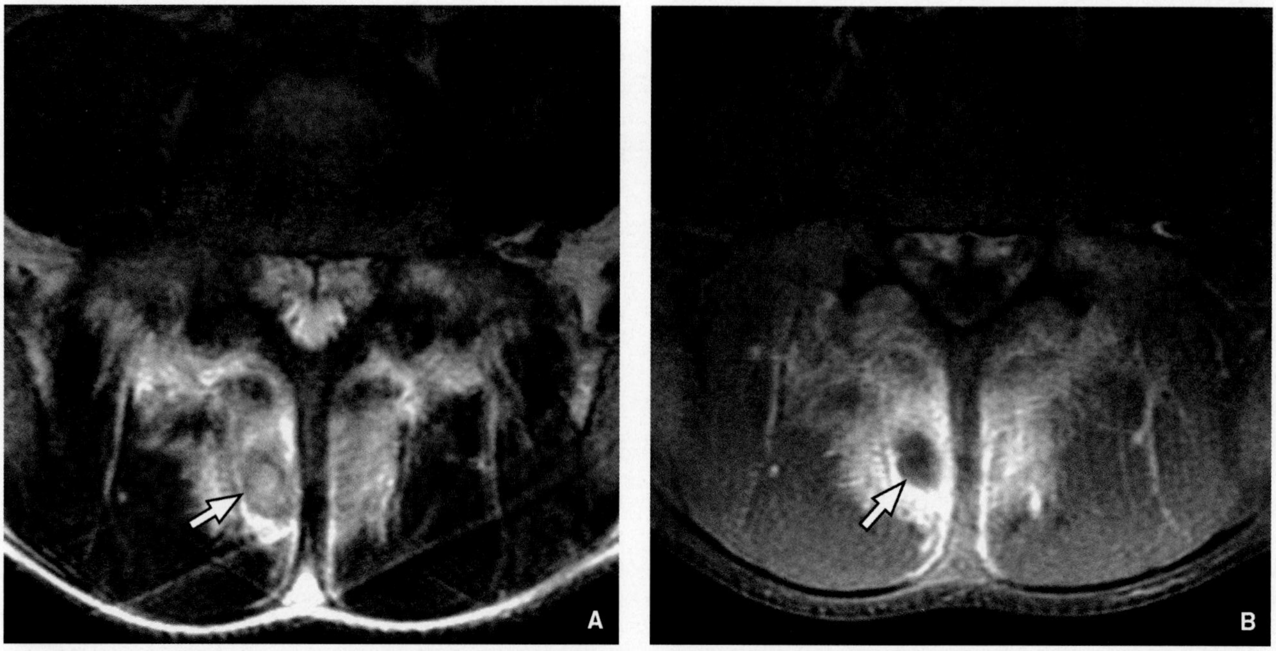

FIGURE 5.37 **Paraspinal abscess in a 14-year-old boy who presented with fever and back pain. A:** Axial T2-weighted MR image shows diffuse edema in the erector spinae muscles. The right muscle complex also demonstrates a rounded hyperintense focus (*arrow*) with a hypointense rim, typical of abscess. **B:** Postcontrast axial T1-weighted MR image with fat-saturation confirms a central hypointense abscess (*arrow*) surrounded by robust inflammatory muscle enhancement.

TRAUMATIC DISORDERS

Cervical Spine Injury

Pediatric spinal injury is relatively infrequent. The majority occurs in the cervical spine, especially in children under 9 years old. The mortality of such injuries is higher because of the vital functions controlled by the injured cervical spinal cord. The anatomy of the cervical spine predisposes children under the age of nine to injury, most frequently at levels C2-C3. The underlying cause of cervical spinal injury varies with age. In infants and children younger than 3 years, obstetrical trauma, motor vehicle accidents, falls, and child abuse are among the most frequent causes. Between 3 and 10 years, falls and auto–pedestrian accidents are more common. Sports and motor vehicle accidents are the most frequent causes of injury in older children. Other predisposing underlying conditions for cervical spinal injury include disorders such as Down syndrome and mucopolysaccharidosis.[43]

In the evaluation of acute cervical spinal injury in the pediatric population, the use of radiographs is controversial due to its low sensitivity.[44] Three-view radiographs (AP, lateral, and odontoid views) have higher sensitivity than the single lateral view in the diagnosis of cervical spine injury. However, multiple views in children should be limited due to the low risk of injuries of the cervical spine and increased amount of overall radiation. The National Emergency X-Radiography Utilization Study (NEXUS) defined low-risk patients for cervical injury as those with no focal point of tenderness along the spine, no altered mental status, and no neurologic deficit, who are not intoxicated and have no distracting injuries.[45] The use of flexion and extension views is controversial in the setting of acute trauma. These views may be useful in assessing ligamentous injury; however, they should only be attempted in an alert cooperative pediatric patient who can follow commands and with close supervision from the trauma team.

MDCT has been shown to have higher sensitivity (98.5%) than radiographs in the diagnosis of fracture and associated injuries.[44] MDCT is faster and provides more anatomic detail, especially with multiplanar and 3D reconstructions. It is readily available in most trauma centers and decreases the study time as well as the use of sedation. Therefore, MDCT is currently the study of choice in the evaluation of acute cervical trauma, especially in pediatric patients with high and moderate risk of injury due to factors including altered mental status and multisystem trauma.[46,47] MDCT has a very high sensitivity (98.5%)[44] in the diagnosis of spine injury, and a negative predictive value as high as 98.9%.[48] However, MRI still has an important role in the evaluation of pediatric patients with acute spinal trauma when there are associated neurologic findings (due to spinal cord or nerve injury); in the obtunded, intubated, or noncooperative pediatric patient; and in those in whom ligamentous injury or spinal cord injury without radiographic abnormality (SCIWORA) is suspected.

Normal Cervical Spine Measurements

A clear knowledge of vertebral bony and ligamentous anatomy as well as normal spine measurements is fundamental to accurate diagnosis of cervical spinal injury. This is especially true in injuries that compromise the craniocervical junction and upper cervical spine.

Prevertebral Soft Tissues

For the evaluation of the prevertebral soft tissues, the head should be fully extended with the airway in inspiration. The measurement at the C3 level from the posterior pharyngeal wall to the vertebra should be no more than 6 mm, and at C4, 14 mm. However, Swischuk has found the morphology of the pharyngeal and tracheal walls more useful in the evaluation of neck soft tissues.[15] If the pharyngeal wall is located posterior to the posterior tracheal wall, the soft tissues are most likely normal. If the posterior pharyngeal wall is straight or curved to the same anterior-posterior position as the posterior tracheal wall, the soft tissues are likely thickened.[15]

Atlanto-Odontoid Distance

Measurement of the distance between the anterior aspect of the odontoid process and posteroinferior margin of the anterior arch of C1 is normally between 2 and 3 mm, and in 5% of children, it may measure up to 5 mm[15] (Fig. 5.38).

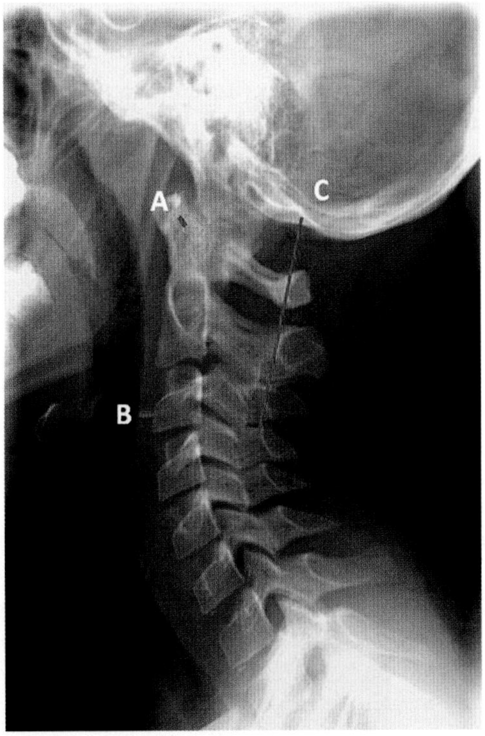

FIGURE 5.38 **Cervical spinal measurements on a lateral radiograph.** *A*, Atlanto-odontoid distance is the measurement between the posterior margin of the anterior arch of C1 and the anterior aspect of the odontoid. In children, up to 5 mm is normal. *B*, Prevertebral soft tissue measurement, from the posterior pharyngeal wall to the C3 vertebra, should be no more than 6 mm. *C*, Posterior cervical line is the line that passes along the anterior margin of the spinous process of C1, C2, and C3. This line may miss the anterior cortex of the C2 spinal process by no more than 1 mm.

Basion–Odontoid Distance

Basion–odontoid distance is a measurement from the tip of the clivus (basion) to the tip of the odontoid (Fig. 5.39). This distance is used in the diagnosis of atlanto-occipital dislocation and should not be >12 mm at any age. Caution must be taken in pediatric patients under 13 years of age, where use of this measurement is limited due to variability in the ossification centers, especially of the dens.[49,50]

Basion–Posterior Axial Line Distance

Basion–posterior axial line distance is a line drawn parallel along the posterior margin of the odontoid process into the cranium (Fig. 5.39). The distance from the basion to this line should be 12 mm or less. In children, the basion is virtually always anterior to this line, however, by no more than 12 mm. This measurement and the basion-odontoid distance are reliable in the diagnosis of atlanto-occipital dislocation.[16,49]

Clivus Line (Wachenheim Line)

Clivus line (Wachenheim line) is a line drawn from the clivus to the odontoid (Fig. 5.39). Normally, the line must intersect or be tangential to the dens.

BC/OA Power Ratio

BC/OA power ratio is defined as the distance between the inferior margin of the clivus (basion) and the posterior arch of C1, divided by the distance from the anterior arch of C1 to the posterior margin of the foramen magnum (opisthion). If the value is >1, atlanto-occipital dislocation should be suspected (Fig. 5.39).

Craniocervical Injuries

Craniocervical injuries are usually fatal and secondary to sudden deceleration, such as in high-speed motor vehicle accidents or falls from great height. The special anatomy of the craniocervical junction in children predisposes them to these injuries compared to the adult population, as the occipital condyles are small, the atlanto-occipital articulation is horizontally oriented, the ligaments are more lax, and the head to body weight ratio is greater.[21,51] Hyperflexion injuries of the upper cervical vertebrae are more frequent in the young because the apex of the flexion curvature is in the upper cervical spine. As the apex is transferred to the midcervical spine when the child matures into adolescence, the injury point is also transferred to the midcervical spine.[49]

The craniocervical junction is formed by the atlantoaxial joint and, laterally, by the atlantoaxial and atlanto-occipital articulations. The atlantoaxial joint is a synovial articulation, which allows rotation of C1 and C2 with respect to each other.[49] The surrounding musculature and several ligaments support these joints. The anterior atlantoaxial-occipital ligament connects the inferior clivus to anterior margin of C2 and joins the anterior aspect of C1. The posterior atlanto-occipital ligament extends from the opisthion to the posterior ring of C1. These ligaments prevent anterior and posterior distraction of the craniocervical junction. The tectorial membrane is a continuation of the periosteum of the clivus that attaches to the posterior aspect of C2. The apical ligament is a fibrous cord from the anterior margin of the foramen magnum to the tip of the odontoid. The paired alar ligaments extend from the lateral aspects of the dens to the medial aspects of the occipital condyles, limiting rotation to the contralateral side and stabilizing the craniocervical junction in the coronal plane. The alar ligament is

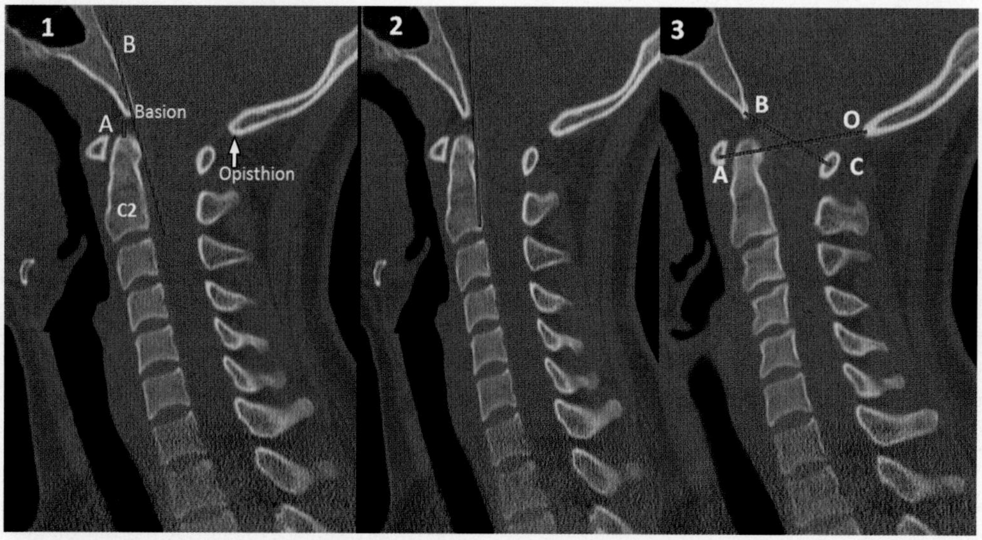

FIGURE 5.39 **Spinal measurements.** *1, A*: Basion–odontoid distance is the measurement from the tip of the clivus to the odontoid. It should not be >12 mm at any age. Its use is limited in patients younger than 13 years due to variable ossification centers. *1, B*: Clivus line (Wachenheim line) is the line drawn along the posterior margin of the clivus, which must intersect or be tangential to the odontoid. *2*, Basion–posterior axial line distance is a line drawn parallel along the posterior margin of the odontoid process into the cranium. The distance from the basion to this line must be 12 mm or less. *3*, BC/OA power ratio is the distance between the basion and posterior arch of C1, divided by the distance from the opisthion to the anterior arch of C1. Normally, this measurement should not be >1.

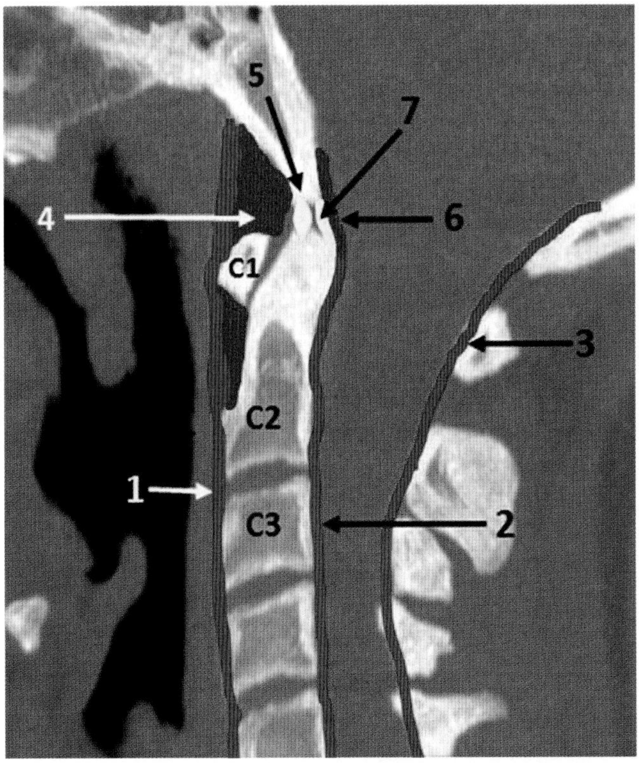

FIGURE 5.40 **Ligaments and membranes of the craniocervical junction.** *1*, Anterior longitudinal ligament. *2*, Posterior longitudinal ligament. *3*, Posterior atlanto-occipital ligament. *4*, Anterior atlanto-occipital membrane. *5*, Apical ligament. *6*, Tectorial membrane. *7*, Cruciate ligament.

comprised of atlantal and occipital components. The transverse ligament is a broad, strong, mainly collagenous band, which extends across the atlas ring behind the odontoid process. The cruciform ligament is part of the atlantoaxial joint and consists of the transverse ligament of the atlas with fibers from the longitudinal band: the strong upper portion of the longitudinal band inserts in the occipital bone, and the inferior weaker portion in the posterior surface of the axis[11,16] (Figs. 5.40 and 5.41).

Atlanto-Occipital Distraction

Ligamentous atlanto-occipital dislocation, displaced occipital condylar fracture with avulsion of the alar ligament, and tectorial membrane disruption comprise most distraction injuries of the craniocervical junction. By definition, these injuries compromise the alar ligament and disrupt the tectorial membrane. They may be associated with condylar fractures. When the ligamentous disruption is associated with a condylar fracture, severe atlanto-occipital discontinuity can occur. These injuries are often fatal due to cardiorespiratory arrest from spinal cord and brainstem injury. Those that survive may become quadriplegic. Associated injury to the nerves and vessels (with subarachnoid hemorrhage), hematomas, and axonal injury have been described.

The imaging findings consist of extensive soft tissue swelling with an abnormal basion–posterior axial line distance (Fig. 5.42). The basion–odontoid distance is useful in pediatric patients older than 13 years of age, when ossification of the odontoid is complete. Occipital condylar fractures are best seen on CT. Evaluation of ligamentous and other soft tissue injuries can be accomplished with MRI[16,49,51–56].

Atlantoaxial Injuries

Atlantoaxial injuries include traumatic ligamentous disruption, odontoid separation, rotatory subluxation, and C1-C2 fractures. These injuries can occur secondary to severe extension and distraction forces, which damage the alar and transverse ligaments, tectorial membrane, and articular capsule. Type I fracture of the odontoid (where the alar ligament inserts) may be associated. Imaging evaluation demonstrates soft tissue swelling, C1-C2 dislocation or subluxation with widening of the C1-C2 facets by more than 5 mm, epidural hematoma, and spinal cord injury[16,49,51,55,56] (Figs. 5.43 and 5.44).

Atlas Fracture (Jefferson Fracture)

Atlas fracture or Jefferson fracture is the result of axial compression forces transmitted through the occipital condyles to the lateral masses of C1. The stability of this fracture depends on integrity of the transverse ligament. When the transverse ligament is disrupted, the fracture becomes unstable. Radiographs show the odontoid displaced more than 6 mm from the lateral masses of C1. CT demonstrates fracture of the C1 ring into at least two parts and a decreased

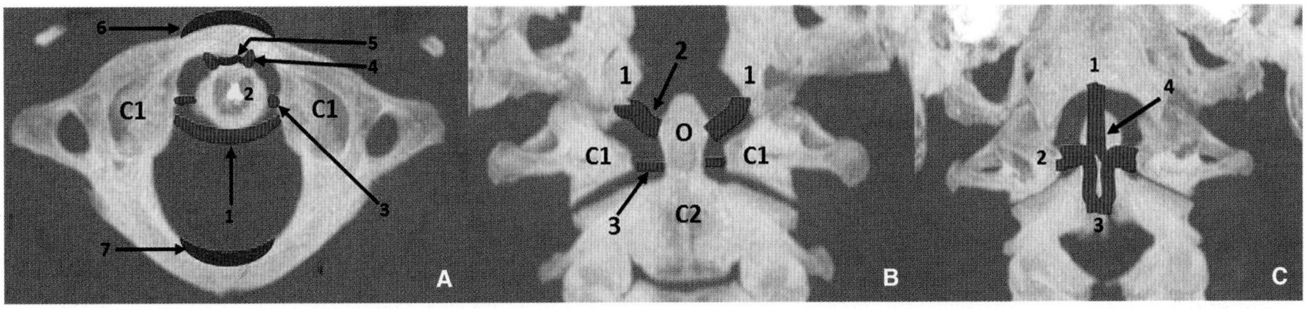

FIGURE 5.41 **Ligaments of the craniocervical junction. A:** *A1*, Transverse ligament. *A2*, Apical ligament. *A3*, Occipital portion of the ligament. *A4*, Atlantal portion of the alar ligament. *A5*, Anterior atlantodental ligament. *A6*, Anterior atlanto-occipital membrane. *A7*, Posterior atlanto-occipital membrane. **B:** *B1*, Occipital condyles. *B2*, Alar ligaments from the occipital condyles to the odontoid process. *B3*, Transverse ligament spanning the lateral masses of C1 behind the odontoid (O). **C:** Cruciate ligament. *C1*, Clivus. *C2*, Lateral masses of C1. *C3*, Odontoid body. *C4*, Attachment point of the cruciate ligament.

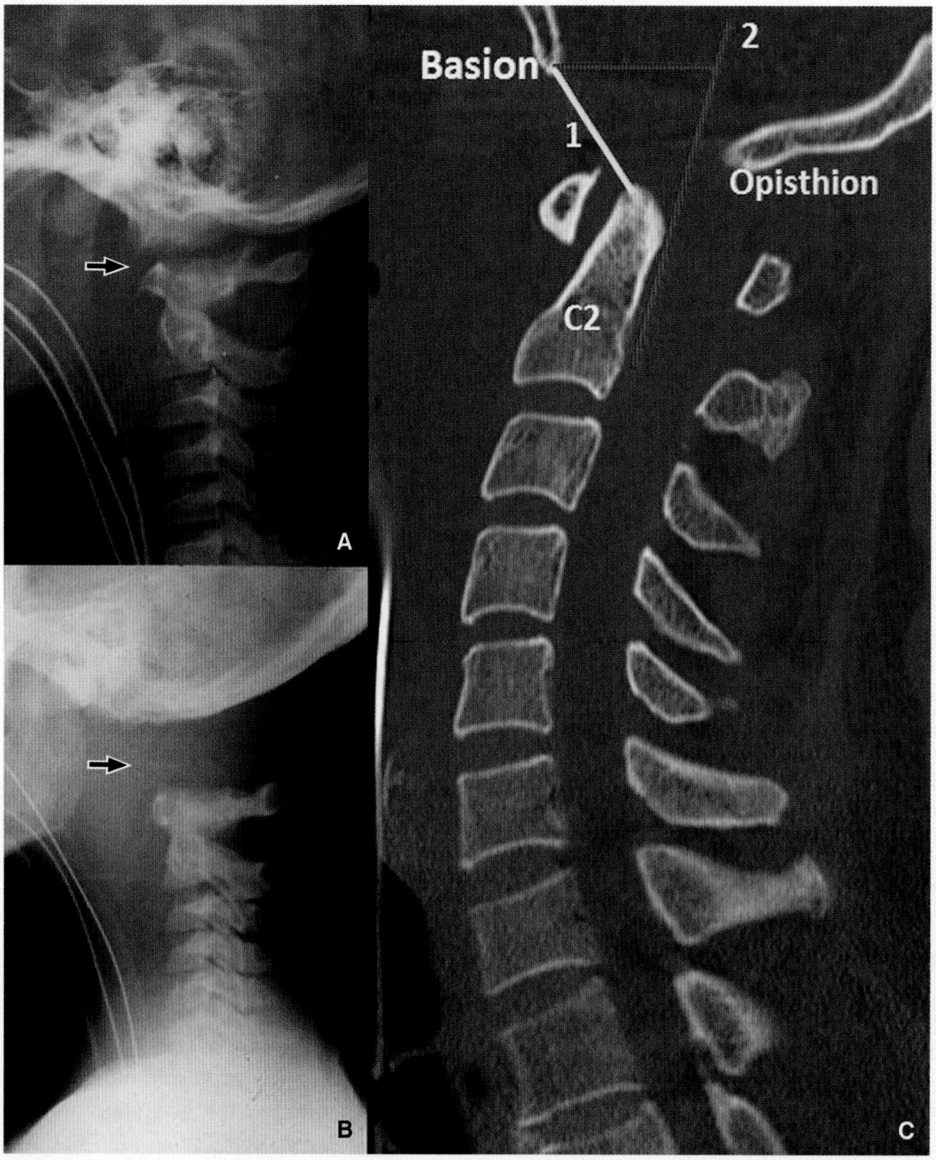

FIGURE 5.42 **Atlanto-occipital dislocation/distraction injuries in three different pediatric patients with history of high speed motor vehicle accident.** **A:** Lateral radiograph of cervical spine shows widening of the atlanto-occipital distance (*arrow*) to more than 12 mm. **B:** Lateral radiograph of cervical spine demonstrates atlanto-occipital distraction injury of the head and neck as well as anterior and superior displacement (*arrow*) of the head in relation to the cervical spine. **C:** Sagittal reformatted CT image of the cervical spine shows abnormal orientation of the base of the skull relative to the upper cervical spine. There is more than 12 mm of displacement of the basion from the basion–posterior axial line (*red lines*) and the basion-odontoid distance (*yellow line*) is greater than 12 mm in a child with atlanto-occipital dislocation. There is also significant pre-vertebral soft tissue edema.

AP diameter of the spinal canal, which is associated with spinal cord injury[16,51,55,56] (Fig. 5.45).

Atlantoaxial Rotatory Fixation

There is variable limitation or fixation of the rotational capability of the C1-C2 articulation, which is responsible for ~50% of cervical rotation. Children are predisposed to atlatoaxial rotatory fixation (AARF) due to such factors as ligamentous laxity and the large synovial folds at the C1-C2 articulation. AARF has been associated with trauma and infection (Grisel syndrome), and in about one-third of the patients, no cause is found. Association with other entities such as craniocervical abnormalities and Down, Marfan, and Morquio syndromes, has been described. The characteristic clinical presentation of these patients is torticollis, neck pain, and no associated neurologic findings.

There are four types of AARF described by Fielding and Hawkins. Type I is the most common, with no displacement of C1. Type II demonstrates from 3 to 5 mm anterior displacement of C1 on C2, with implied abnormality of the transverse ligament. In type III, there is more than 5 mm displacement, and the alar and transverse ligaments are deficient. Type IV demonstrates posterior displacement of C1 over C2.

Diagnosing AARF with radiographs is often difficult. The lateral view of the spine demonstrates lack of superimposition of the posterior arch and lateral masses of C1. The AP view shows the odontoid displaced toward the one of lateral masses of C1. The diagnoses of fixation and subluxation can be more accurately achieved with dynamic CT. Initially, CT is performed at rest and then is repeated with voluntary rotation to both sides. Normally, there is anterior displacement of the lateral masses of C1 relative to C2, when the head is turned to either side[57] (Fig. 5.46).

Odontoid Fracture

Fracture of the odontoid (dens) results from diverse mechanisms and is the most common injury of C2. In children

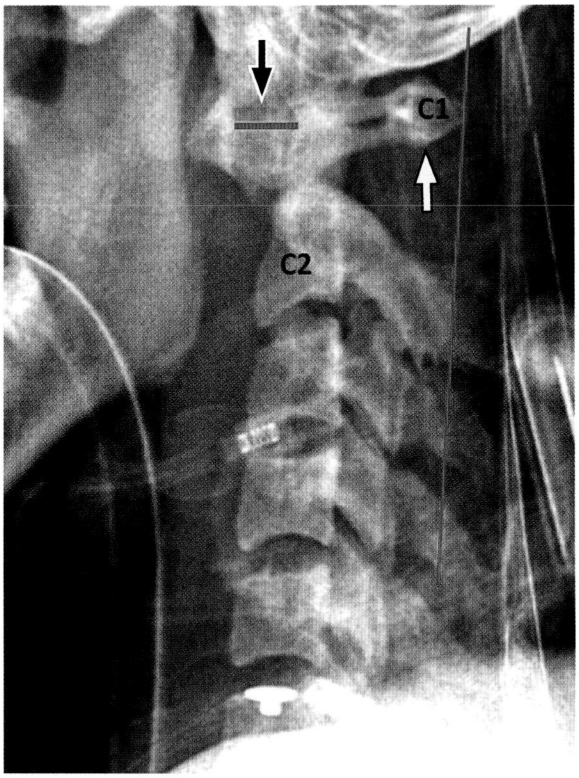

FIGURE 5.43 **Atlantoaxial injury in a 14-year-old boy involved in a motor vehicle accident.** Cross-table lateral radiograph of the cervical spine shows marked increase of the atlantoaxial distance (*black arrow, horizontal red line*). Malalignment of the posterior spinolaminar line (*vertical red line*) is also seen. C1 is anteriorly displaced (*white arrow*). Prevertebral soft tissue swelling is also present.

<7 years, odontoid fractures usually occur through the dens–body synchondrosis (Fig. 5.47). In older children, in whom the synchondrosis is fused, the fracture pattern is similar to the adult population. Type I involves the tip of the odontoid from the attachment site of the alar ligament. Type II is a transverse fracture of the base of the dens that may be associated with nonunion. It is the most common type. Type III involves a horizontal fracture through the body of C2 (Fig. 5.48).

On the lateral cervical spine radiograph, prevertebral soft tissue edema, mild anterior tilt of the odontoid, and widening of the synchondrosis may indicate odontoid fracture. CT with multiplanar and 3D reformatted images and MRI can improve the diagnosis and characterization of odontoid fractures[16,51,55,56] (Figs. 5.49 and 5.50).

Traumatic Spondylolisthesis (Hangman Fracture)

Traumatic spondylolisthesis is a hyperextension force–induced injury typically producing vertical fractures through both pars interarticularis of C2, with anterior subluxation of C2 on C3. The atypical form of this injury compromises the body of C2 posteriorly and in the coronal plane. Radiography shows the fracture line along the pars interarticularis and posterior C2 body, and widening of the C2-C3 disc space. CT is recommended for accurate characterization of this injury (Fig. 5.51).

Differentiating between Hangman fracture and congenital pars defects of C2 is sometimes challenging in the pediatric population. The congenital pars defect presents with smooth and sclerotic bony margins, and there is hypoplasia of the posterior arch of C2 and adjacent arches. Also, a history of trauma is absent in the congenital pars defects of C2[16,51,55,56] (Fig. 5.52).

Lower Cervical Spine Hyperflexion Injuries

Hyperflexion injuries present with anterior compression forces and posterior distraction forces, characteristically in the midcervical spine of older children. Associated vertebral body fractures with secondary compression or "teardrop" fractures can be seen. The "teardrop" fragment results from avulsion of the inferior corner of the vertebra (usually the ring apophysis), which is attached to the anterior longitudinal ligament. Distraction and pulling forces injure the posterior elements, damaging the posterior longitudinal and spinous ligaments, with secondary widening of the posterior elements, and occasionally, the posterior disc space. Injury of the spinal cord may be seen in severe, comminuted fractures of the vertebral body, which may narrow the canal and compress or transect the spinal cord.

Disruption of the facet joint with or without facet fracture may occur in hyperflexion injury. The radiographic findings may be subtle, with facet separation taking on a V-shaped configuration. In severe cases, the posterior corner of the superior facet becomes perched on the anterior corner of the inferior facet, which is referred as the "perched

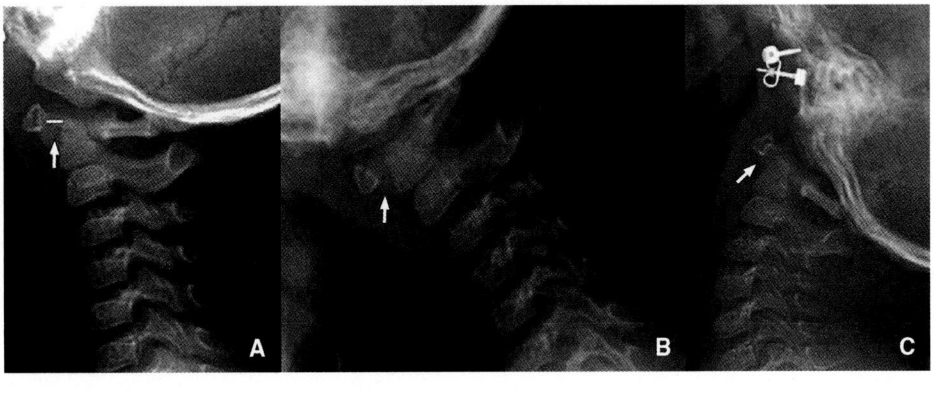

FIGURE 5.44 **Atlantoaxial subluxation in a 3-year-old boy with Down syndrome. A:** Lateral radiograph of the cervical spine shows C1-C2 atlantoaxial subluxation. Widening of the C1-C2 distance (*arrow*) and pyramidal shape of the odontoid are also seen. **B and C:** Lateral radiographs of cervical spine obtained during flexion **(B)** and extension **(C)** show motion (*arrow*) of the C1-C2 articulation, with increased widening during flexion and relative narrowing in extension.

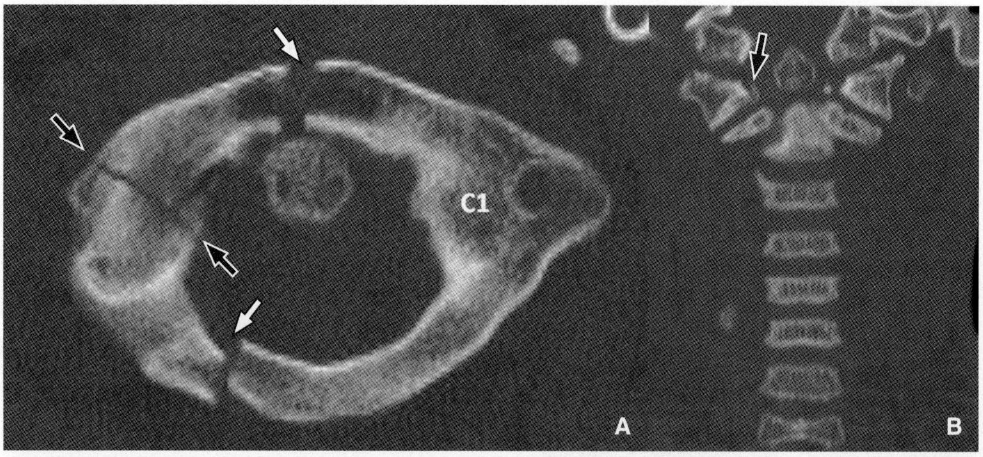

FIGURE 5.45 **Jefferson fracture in a 7-year-old boy who presented with multiple osseous injuries after falling off a third-floor apartment balcony. A:** Axial CT image shows fractures (*white arrows*) of the anterior and posterior arches of the C1 vertebra and fracture–avulsion fracture (*black arrows*) of the right lateral mass. **B:** Coronal CT image shows the avulsion fracture (*arrow*) of the right lateral mass of C1 as well as multiple compression fractures of more inferior cervical vertebrae.

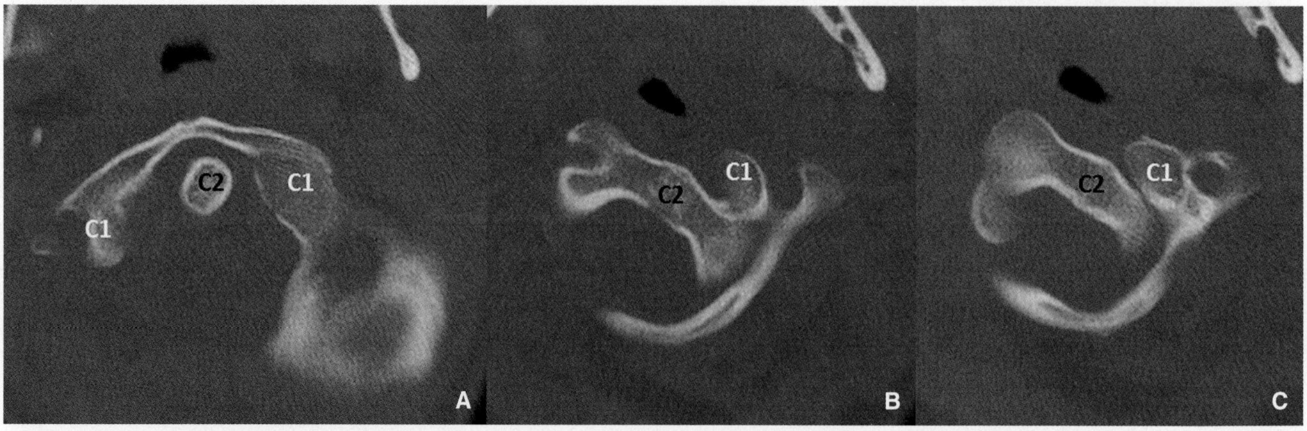

FIGURE 5.46 **A–C: Type 3 rotatory fixation in an 8-year-old girl who presented with torticollis.** Three axial CT images (with right and left head rotation) show that there is no change of anterior positioning of the left lateral mass of C1 in relationship with the posteriorly fixed C2 vertebra.

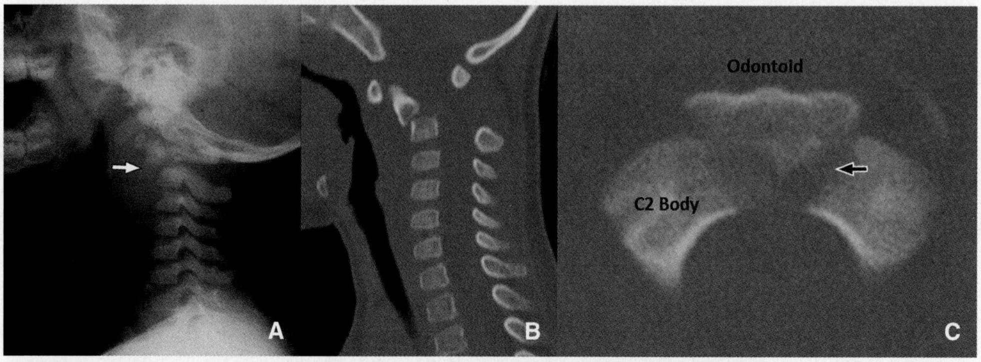

FIGURE 5.47 **Fracture of the C2 synchondrosis in a 3-year-old boy with a history of closed head injury. A:** Lateral radiograph of the cervical spine shows anterior displacement (*arrow*) of the odontoid from the body of C2 and soft tissue swelling. **B:** Sagittal CT image demonstrates angulation of the odontoid process and prevertebral soft tissue swelling. **C:** Axial CT image shows an anteriorly displaced fracture (*arrow*) at the synchondrosis.

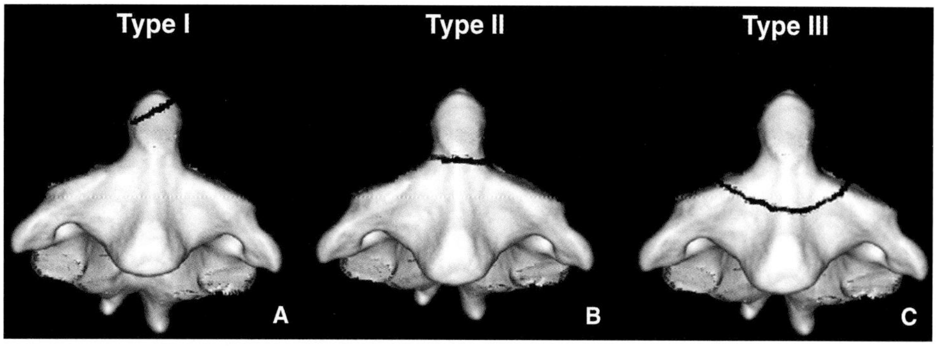

FIGURE 5.48 **Types of odontoid fractures.** 3D reformatted models of C2 recreate the three types of odontoid fractures as described by Anderson and D'Alonzo, according to the localization of the fracture plane. **A:** Type I odontoid fracture, which involves the odontoid tip. **B:** Type II odontoid fracture, which involves the base of the dens. **C:** Type III odontoid fracture, which involves the body of C2.

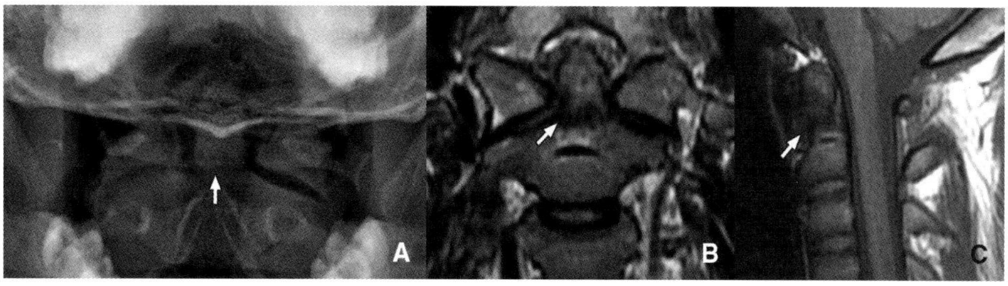

FIGURE 5.49 **Type II odontoid fracture in a 14-year-old boy with history of trauma. A:** Frontal radiograph of odontoid shows a transverse fracture (*arrow*) at the base of the odontoid. Coronal STIR **(B)** and sagittal T1-weighted **(C)** MR images demonstrate a low signal intensity line (*arrows*) representing a fracture at the odontoid base, as well as adjacent bone marrow edema.

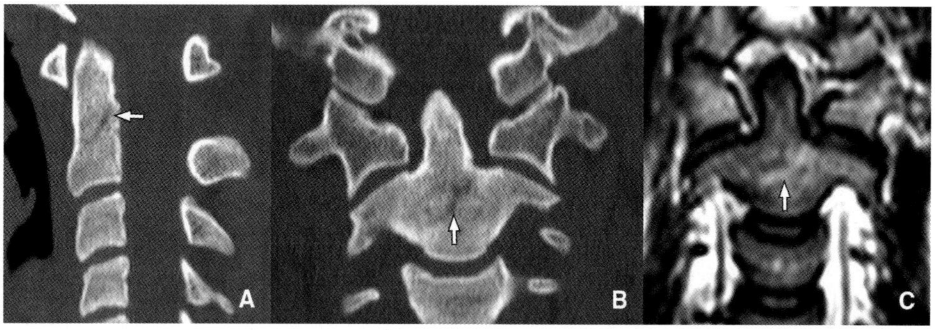

FIGURE 5.50 **Type III odontoid fracture in a 16-year-old girl involved in a motor vehicle accident.** Sagittal CT image **(A)** and coronal CT image **(B)** of the odontoid show a fracture line (*arrows*) extending into the odontoid body. **C:** Coronal fast spin-echo T2-weighted MR image demonstrates bone marrow edema (*arrow*) along the fracture.

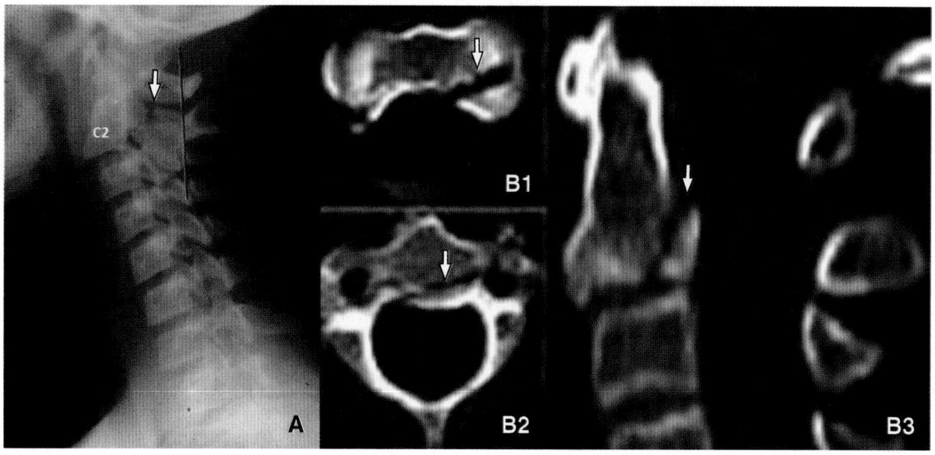

FIGURE 5.51 **Hangman fracture in a 17-year-old girl with hyperextension injury after hitting the dashboard in a car accident. A:** Lateral radiograph of the cervical spine shows fractures (*arrow*) of both C2 pars interarticularis with mild anterior anterolisthesis of C2 on C3 and deviation of the posterior arch of C2 from the posterior spinal cervical line (*red line*). **B:** Axial and sagittal CT images of an atypical hangman fracture demonstrate fractures (*arrows*) of the C2 lateral mass (*B1*), body and vertebral foramen (*B2*), and the body (*B3*).

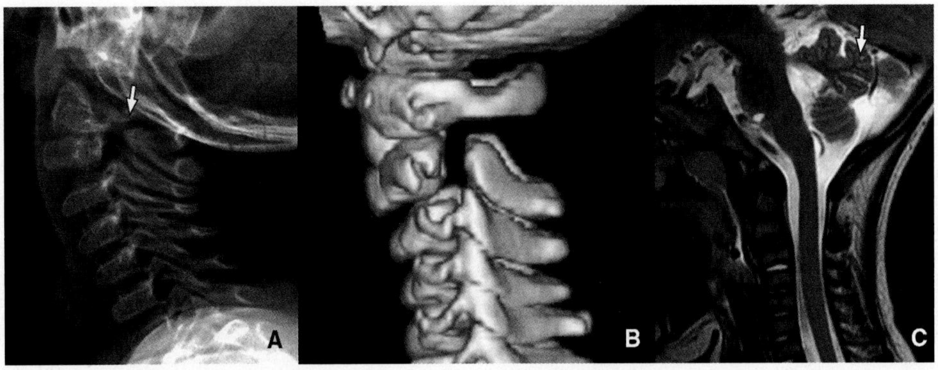

FIGURE 5.52 **Congenital C2 spondylolysis detected as an incidental finding in a 2-year-old girl with the diagnosis of "cobblestone lissencephaly." A:** Lateral radiograph of the cervical spine shows a congenital defect (*arrow*) involving the C2 pars interarticularis. Also noted are anterolisthesis of C2 on C3, a pyramid-shaped odontoid, and lack of prevertebral soft tissue edema. **B:** 3D CT image demonstrates the C2 spondylolysis. **C:** Sagittal T2-weighted MR image shows the small cerebellum with cystic changes (*arrow*) in a different child with lissencephaly.

facet" sign. Facet injury is often associated with spinal cord syndromes[16,51,55,56] (Figs. 5.53, 5.54, and 5.55).

Lower Cervical Spine Hyperextension Injuries

These injuries are rare in children, representing about 3% of spinal injuries.[51] In hyperextension injuries, compression forces are posterior and distraction forces are anterior, leading to anterior superior endplate avulsion fractures, widening of the anterior disc space, and ligamentous injury.

The initial imaging evaluation of hyperflexion and hyperextension injuries must include CT with multiplanar and 3D reformatted images and, in some cases, MRI for better evaluation of the cord, ligament, disc space, soft tissues, and other involved anatomic structures[16,51,54–56] (Fig. 5.56).

Spinal Cord Injury Without Radiographic Abnormality (SCIWORA)

Spinal cord injury without radiographic abnormality (SCIWORA) is related to ligamentous laxity and hypermobility of the pediatric spine, which predisposes to stretching or direct impact on the cord with hyperextension. Others suggest that this cord lesion is the result of cord ischemia, as a result of hypoperfusion on vessel injury. SCIWORA is more frequently observed in younger children.

No abnormality is seen on radiography or CT in pediatric patients with SCIWORA. MRI shows areas of cord edema or hemorrhage, ligamentous injury, disc abnormalities, and extra-axial hemorrhage. The outcome of this injury depends on the severity of the findings, ranging from no or minimal deficits in children with isolated cord edema to complete paralysis in those with cord disruption or severe hemorrhage[8,55] (Fig. 5.57).

Thoracolumbar Spine Injuries

The injury pattern of thoracolumbar spine injury varies according to the applied forces: flexion, extension, rotation, and/or shearing forces. The site of injury is more frequently seen at the transitional points in the cervicothoracic and thoracolumbar regions.

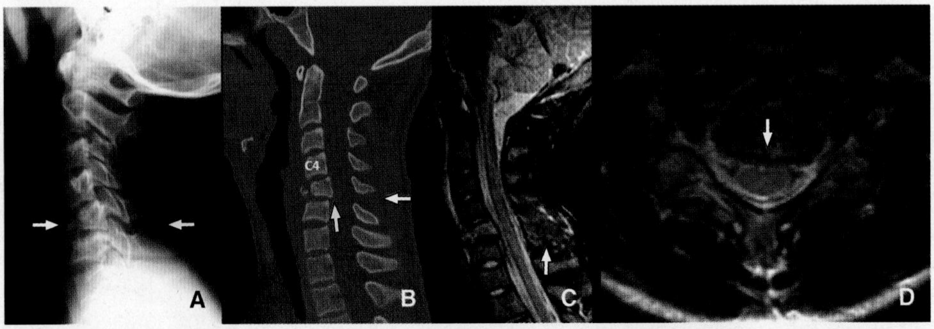

FIGURE 5.53 **Hyperflexion injury of the mid- and lower cervical spine in a 15-year-old boy who presented with numbness of the arms after a motor vehicle accident. A:** Lateral cervical spine radiograph shows a "teardrop" fracture (*white arrow*) of C5 with mild posterior displacement of the C5 body into the canal. Widening (*yellow arrow*) of the C5-C6 interspace implies ligamentous injury. **B:** Sagittal CT image demonstrates the C5 fracture, posterior displacement (*yellow arrow*) of C5, and widening (*white arrow*) of the interspinous distance ("fanning") at C5-C6. **C:** Sagittal STIR MR image demonstrates mass effect upon the cord and posterior ligamentous injury (*arrow*). **D:** Axial T2-weighted MR image demonstrates mass effect upon the cord secondary to C5 posterior displacement (*arrow*).

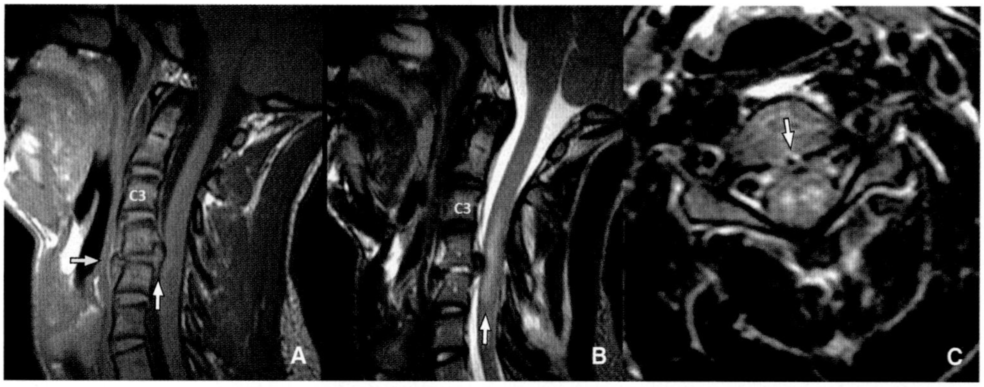

FIGURE 5.54 **Hyperflexion injury of the mid- and lower cervical spine in a 16-year-old boy involved in a motor vehicle accident. A:** Sagittal T1-weighted MR image of the cervical spine shows anterior narrowing (*yellow arrow*) and posterior widening (*white arrow*) of the C4-C5 disc space with an acutely herniated disc. **B:** Sagittal T2-weighted MR image of the cervical spine demonstrates a cord contusion (*arrow*). **C:** Axial T2-weighted MR image shows narrowing of the spinal canal and the herniated disc impinging upon the edematous cord (*arrow*).

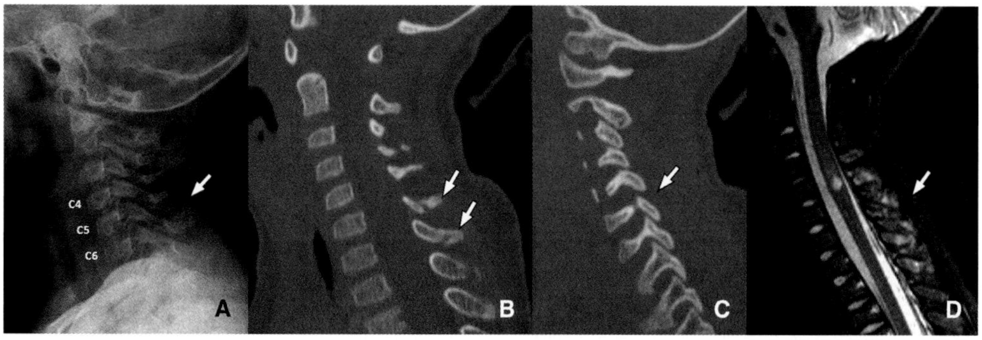

FIGURE 5.55 **Hyperflexion injury of the mid- and lower cervical spine in a 3-year-old boy involved in a motor vehicle accident. A:** Lateral radiograph of the cervical spine shows widening of the interspinous distance (*arrow*) between C4 and C5. **B:** Sagittal CT image demonstrates multilevel spinous process fractures (*arrows*). **C:** Parasagittal reformatted CT image shows widening (*arrow*) of the C5-C6 facet joint. **D:** Sagittal STIR MR image demonstrates signal abnormality (*arrow*) in the ligaments and spinous processes as well as cord injury.

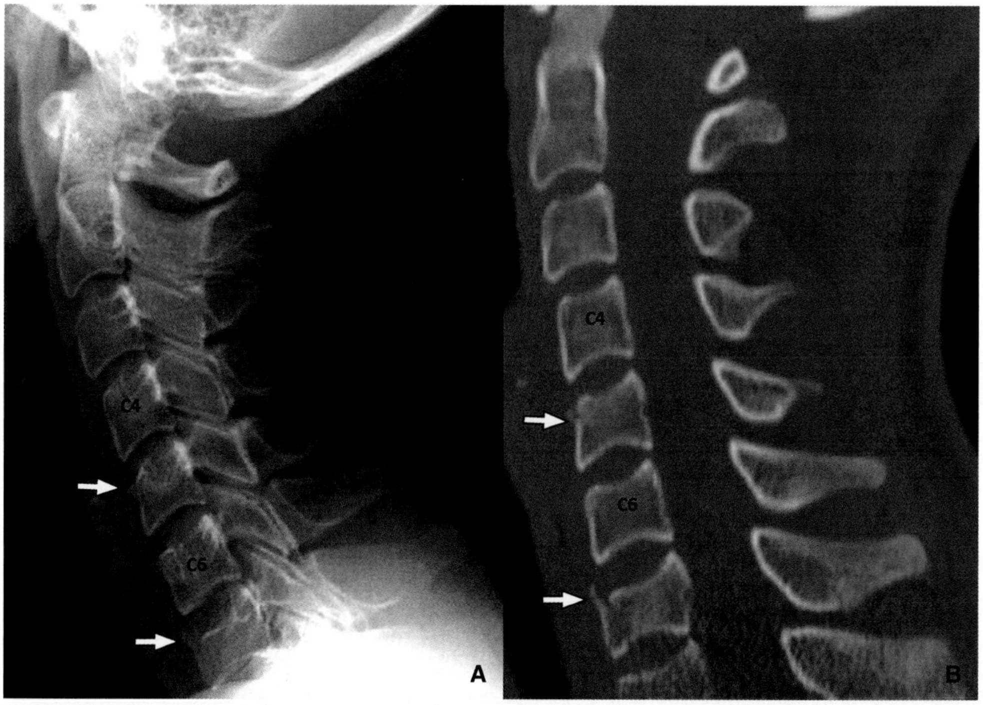

FIGURE 5.56 **Hyperextension injury of the mid- and lower cervical spine in a 2-year-old girl who was an unrestrained passenger in a motor vehicle accident. A and B:** Lateral radiograph **(A)** and sagittal CT image **(B)** show compression of the superior end plates and avulsion fractures (*arrows*) at C5 and C7. Also noted are widening of the C6-C7 anterior intervertebral disc space and prevertebral soft tissues swelling.

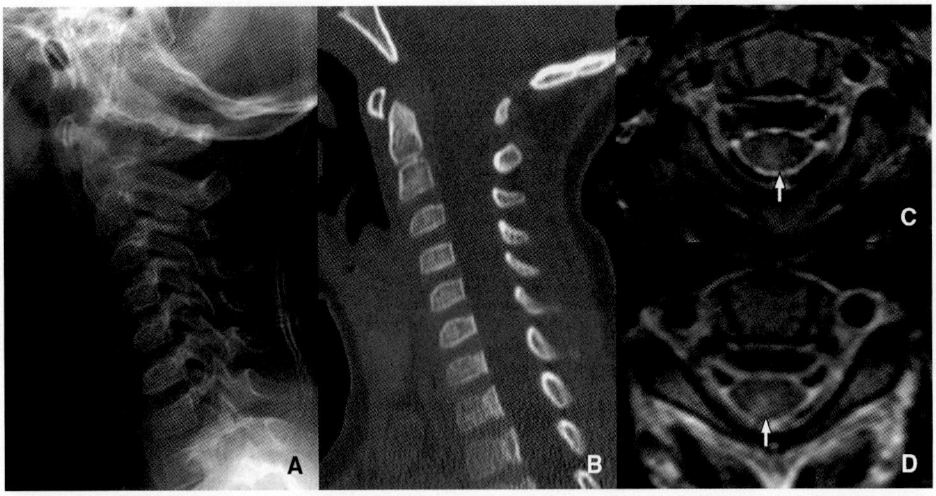

FIGURE 5.57 **Spinal cord injury without radiographic abnormality (SCIWORA) in a 2-year-old boy who presented with decreased motor function in the upper extremities after a fall onto his back. A and B:** Lateral radiograph and sagittal CT image of the cervical spine show no appreciable abnormality. **C and D:** Axial T2-weighted MR images demonstrate abnormal high signal intensity (*arrows*) in the spinal cord, consistent with cord edema and/or contusion.

There are four major types of fracture in the thoracolumbar region: compression fracture, burst fracture, seat-belt injury (Chance fracture), and fracture-dislocation, which are discussed in the following sections.

Compression Fracture

Compression fractures are defined by failure of the anterior column under compression; the middle column is intact and acts as a fulcrum; in severe injuries, the posterior column may be partially compromised.[52] Compression fractures are classified as simple or severe, depending on the percentage of vertebral body compression: compression fracture of the thoracolumbar spine is termed simple and stable when <50% of the vertebral body is compromised or collapsed. When more than 50% of the vertebral body is involved, it is considered severe and unstable (Fig. 5.58).

Burst Fracture

Burst fractures are the result of failure of the anterior and middle vertebral columns because of axial loading or hyperflexion forces applied to one or both endplates of the same vertebra.[52] These fractures are unstable in the lumbar spine and thoracolumbar region. Because of support from the rib cage, they are stable in the thoracic spine. The association

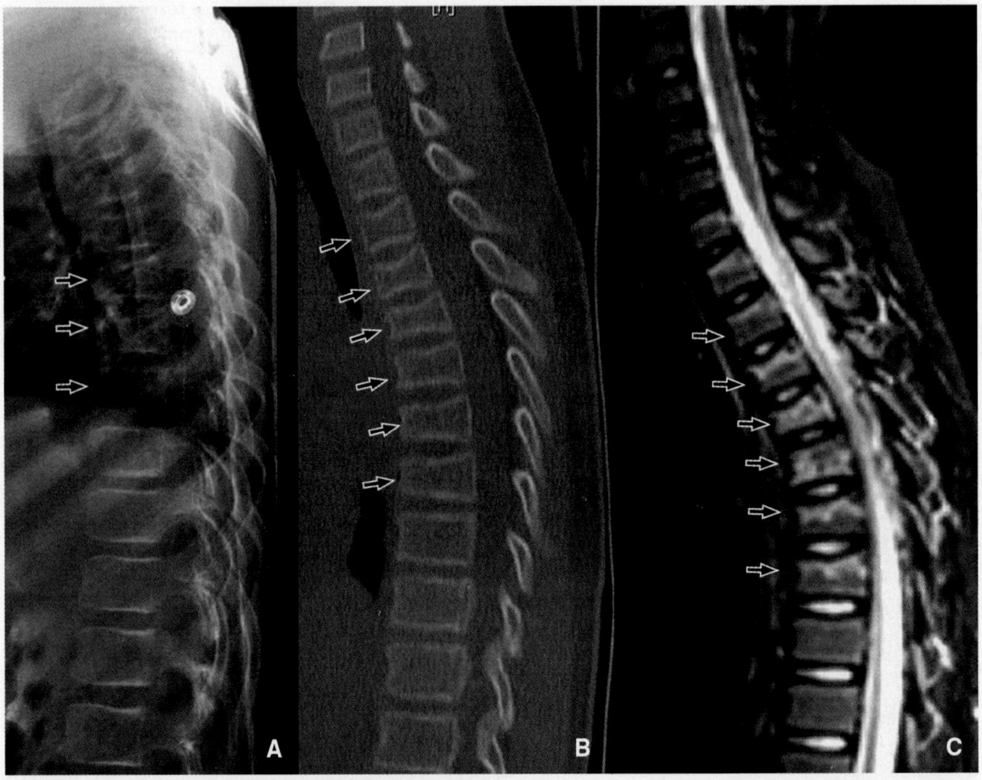

FIGURE 5.58 **Thoracic spine compression fractures in a 14-year-old girl who fell off a horse. A–C:** Lateral radiograph **(A)**, sagittal CT image **(B)**, and sagittal T2-weighted MR image **(C)** of the thoracic spine show multilevel compression fractures (*arrows*) with no fragmentation or compromise of the spinal canal. MRI shows bone marrow edema at the affected levels.

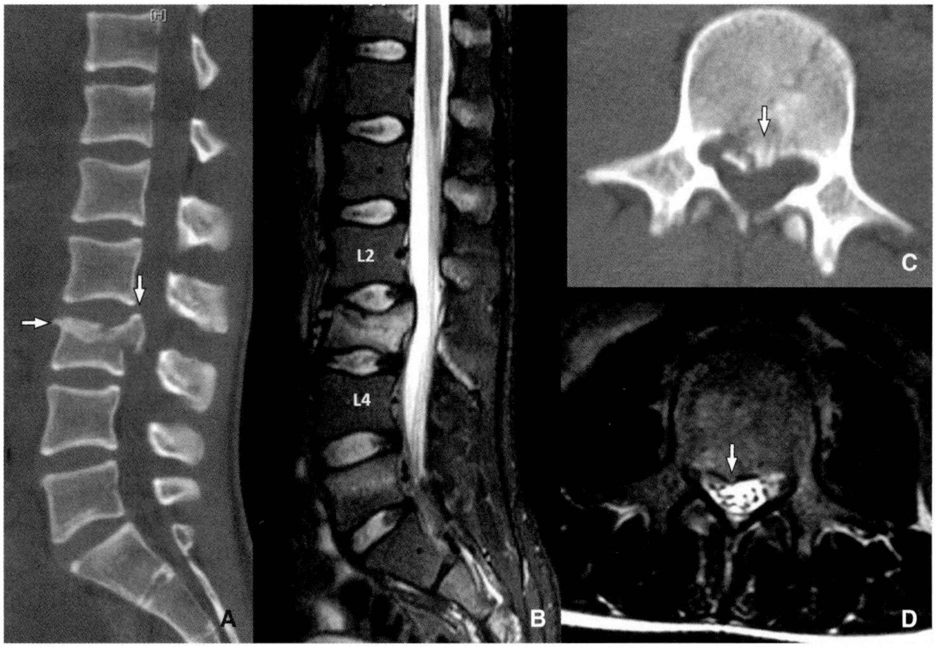

FIGURE 5.59 **Lumbar spine burst fracture in a 13-year-old boy injured in a motor vehicle accident. A:** Sagittal CT image of the lumbar spine shows a comminuted fracture (*horizontal arrow*) of L3 with a retropulsed fragment (*vertical arrow*) projecting into the spinal canal. **B:** Sagittal STIR MR image demonstrates the bone marrow edema and deformity of L3, posterior displacement of a fragment into the canal, elevation of the posterior longitudinal ligament, and narrowing of the canal. Also noted is bone marrow edema at L5. **C:** Axial CT image at L3 level shows the bony fragment (*arrow*) displaced into the spinal canal. **D:** Axial T2-weighted MR image demonstrates the displaced bony fragment (*arrow*) exerting mass effect on the thecal sac.

with neurologic injury from this type of spinal injury is strong due to spinal cord vascular compromise (Fig. 5.59).

Seat-Belt Injury (Chance Fracture)

Seat-belt injuries are the result of posterior and middle column failure, secondary to tension forces generated by flexion-distraction with its axis in the anterior column.[52] Characteristically, there is horizontal separation of the transverse processes and pedicles. In addition, fracture separation of the spinous process; fracture of the pedicle, lamina, and part of the vertebral body; distraction injury of the facets and intervertebral disc; and ligamentous disruption may be associated with seat-belt injuries. These fractures are often unstable and associated with other bony and soft tissue injuries, such as muscular, vascular, and visceral injuries[58] (Fig. 5.60).

Fracture–Dislocation

Fracture–dislocations are unstable thoracolumbar injuries, where the anterior, middle, and posterior columns

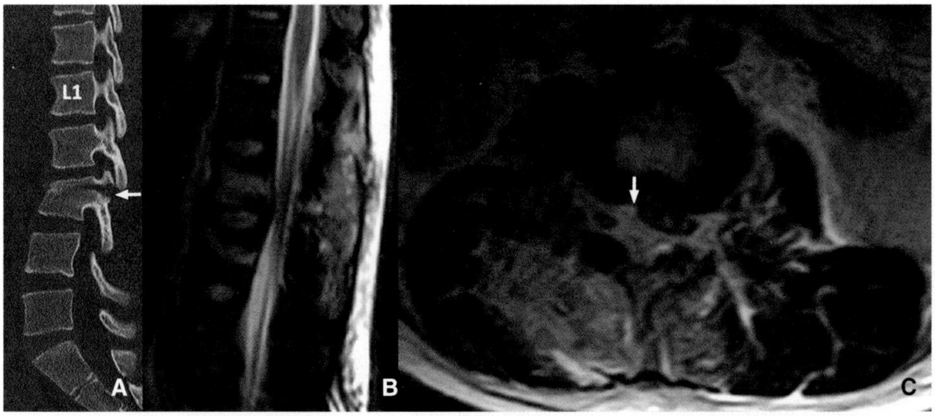

FIGURE 5.60 **Seat-belt injury, "chance fracture," in a 9-year-old girl involved in a motor vehicle accident. A:** Sagittal CT image of the lumbar spine shows a transverse fracture (*arrow*) through the pars interarticularis and body of the L3 vertebra. **B:** Sagittal T2-weighted MR image of the lumbar spine demonstrates bone marrow edema and extensive soft tissue injury in the paraspinal muscles. **C:** Axial T2-weighted MR image at the L2-L3 level shows the extensive paraspinal muscle injury and epidural edema/hematoma with mass effect and displacement of the thecal sac/cauda equina (*arrow*).

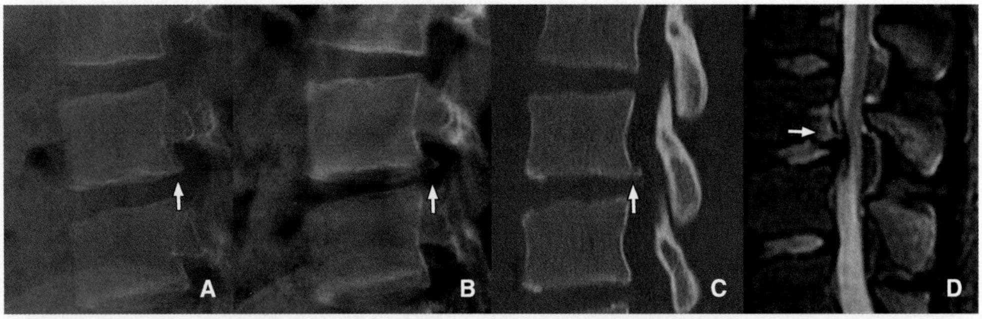

FIGURE 5.61 **Fracture of the ring apophyses in a 5-year-old male athlete who presented with progressively worsening back pain. A:** Lateral coned-down radiograph of L3 shows minimal irregularity (*arrow*) of the L3 posterior and inferior margin. **B:** Three months later, a lateral coned-down radiographs shows obvious bony irregularity (*arrow*). **C:** Sagittal CT image demonstrates the fracture (*arrow*) of the ring apophysis. **D:** Sagittal STIR MR image shows bone marrow edema (*arrow*), corner irregularity, bulging of the L3-L4 disc, and elevation of the posterior longitudinal ligament.

are compromised under compression, tension, and rotation or shear forces.[52] There are three major subtypes according to mechanism of injury: flexion–rotation, shear, and flexion-distraction. Characteristic imaging findings of fracture–dislocation injuries are subluxation and dislocation of the spinal column. Narrowing of the spinal canal, retropulsed fragments, jumped facets, and compromise of the intervertebral disc, rib and transverse processes may be associated.

Ring Apophysis Fracture

Ring apophysis fractures may occur at any spinal level, usually in adolescents (Fig. 5.61). Clear understanding of the imaging findings of ring apophysis fracture is important because the imaging appearance may simulate a herniated disc. When ring apophysis fracture is isolated, it is typically located at the L4 level[16].

Spondylolysis

Spondylolysis is characterized by a defect of the pars interarticularis between the superior and inferior articulating processes. This usually occurs in the lumbar spine at L4 and L5 and may or may not be associated with spondylolisthesis. Spondylolysis is usually due to trauma in the pediatric population. However, other etiologies are congenital malformations including pars hypoplasia, neoplasms, infections, and osteogenesis imperfecta[16,19] (Fig. 5.62).

NEOPLASTIC DISORDERS

Benign Tumors of the Spine

Osteoid Osteoma

Osteoid osteoma is a small benign osteoid–producing lesion of the bone. When it involves the vertebrae, it most frequently occurs in the posterior elements and usually presents between 10 and 20 years of age. Affected pediatric patients may present with either painful or painless scoliosis.

On radiographs, osteoid osteoma typically demonstrates a radiolucent area called the nidus, which is surrounded by a rim or halo of radiodense cortical hypertrophy or hyperostosis. Bone scan is highly sensitive for the detection of osteoid osteoma. CT demonstrates a lucent nidus with surrounding reactive bony sclerosis, sometimes with a central sclerotic dot of osteoid. The evaluation of osteoid osteoma by MRI is sometimes limited due to small size of the lesion; however, there is usually heterogeneous bone marrow signal intensity and substantial signal abnormality and enhancement of the surrounding soft tissues[59–61] (Fig. 5.63).

The most significant symptom of osteoid osteoma is nighttime pain (due to prostaglandin release), which is treated with aspirin, ibuprofen, or other anti-inflammatory medications. Alternative treatment for pediatric patients who do not respond to medications is local radiofrequency ablation or surgical resection.

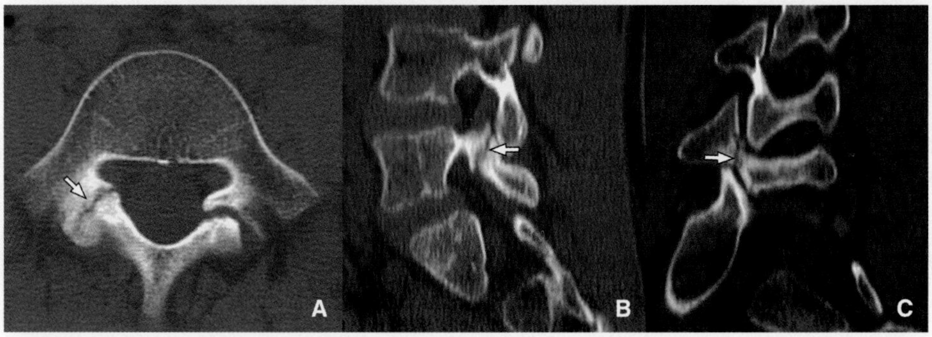

FIGURE 5.62 **Spondylolysis in a 6-year-old boy who presented with recurrent back pain. A:** Axial CT image shows a right L5 pars interarticularis defect (*arrow*) with sclerotic changes along the margins. **B and C:** Sagittal **(B)** and parasagittal **(C)** reformatted CT images also demonstrate the defect (*arrows*).

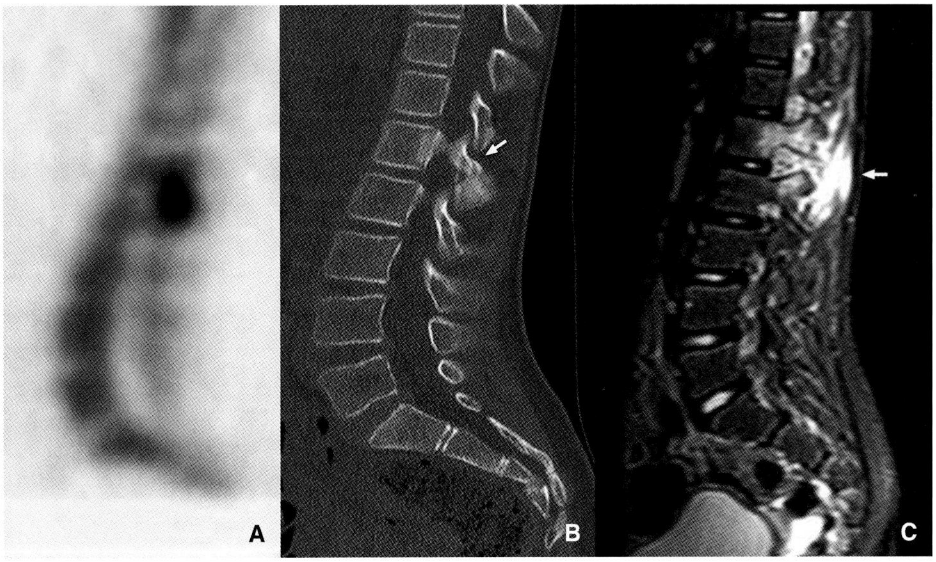

FIGURE 5.63 **Osteoid osteoma in a 5-year-old boy who presented with back pain that comes and goes during the day. A:** Sagittal SPECT bone scan image shows focal increased perfusion in the posterior elements of the upper lumbar spine. **B:** Sagittal CT image demonstrates a focal lucency (*arrow*) with a sclerotic center in the posterior elements of L1. Associated reactive sclerosis of the adjacent bone is also seen. **C:** Sagittal STIR MR image shows substantial soft tissue and bone marrow edema (*arrow*) associated with the osteoid osteoma.

Osteoblastoma

Osteoblastoma is a benign bone tumor, histologically indistinguishable from but larger than osteoid osteoma (Fig. 5.64). Size definitions vary, but typically, >2 cm is the arbitrary measurement used to distinguish osteoblastoma from osteoid osteoma. Osteoblastoma of the spine typically occurs in the second and third decades of life and may present with painful scoliosis or fracture. This lesion is localized in the posterior elements and may extend to the vertebral body.

There are two imaging appearances of osteoblastoma: (1) a localized osteoid nidus similar to an osteoid osteoma or (2) a cystic, expansile, more aggressive lesion, perhaps with hemorrhage, similar in appearance to an aneurysmal bone cyst[59–61] (Fig. 5.65).

Surgical excision is currently recommended for surgically accessible osteoblastomas. The use of radiation or chemotherapy is controversial because their effectiveness is questionable and they may raise risk of malignant degeneration.

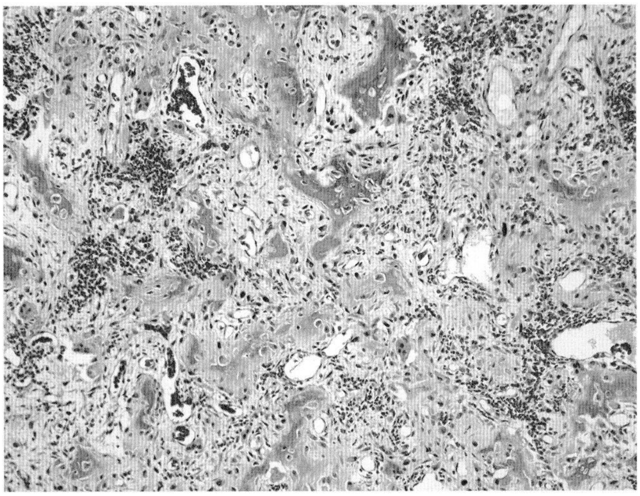

FIGURE 5.64 **Osteoblastoma involving the T10 vertebra in a 16-year-old boy.** Spicules of woven bone are embedded within a richly vascularized stroma (hematoxylin and eosin, original magnification, 200x).

Aneurysmal Bone Cyst

Aneurysmal bone cyst is a benign neoplasm of bone, characterized genetically by a rearrangement of the *USP6* gene on chromosome 17p. Approximately 75% of aneurysmal bone cysts are localized in the posterior elements of the lower

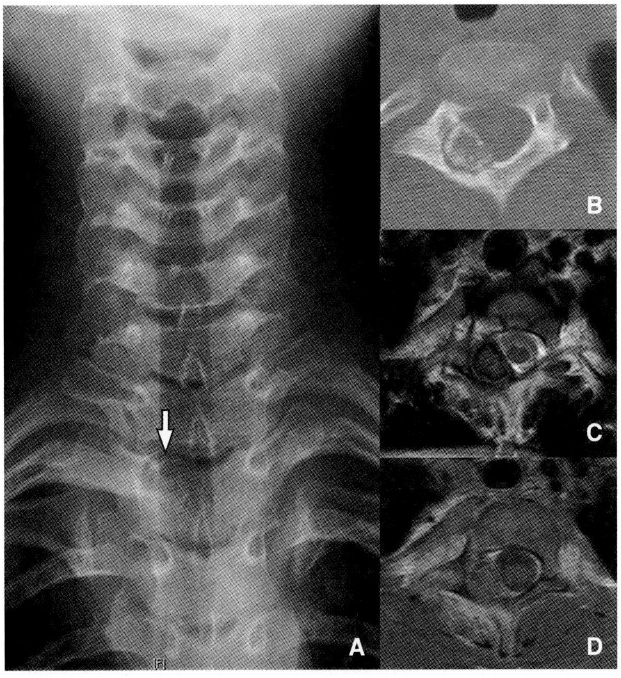

FIGURE 5.65 **Osteoblastoma in a 14-year-old girl who presented with neck pain. A:** Frontal view of the cervical spine shows asymmetric lucency (*arrow*) of the right T2 pedicle. **B:** Axial CT image at T2 demonstrates a mainly sclerotic right laminar lesion protruding into the spinal canal. Associated reactive sclerosis of the adjacent bone is also seen. **C:** Axial T2-weighted MR image shows mass effect upon the spinal cord secondary to the osteoblastoma, as well as soft tissue edema. **D:** Postcontrast axial T1-weighted MR image with fat-saturation demonstrates diffuse enhancement of the soft tissues, bone, and osteoblastoma.

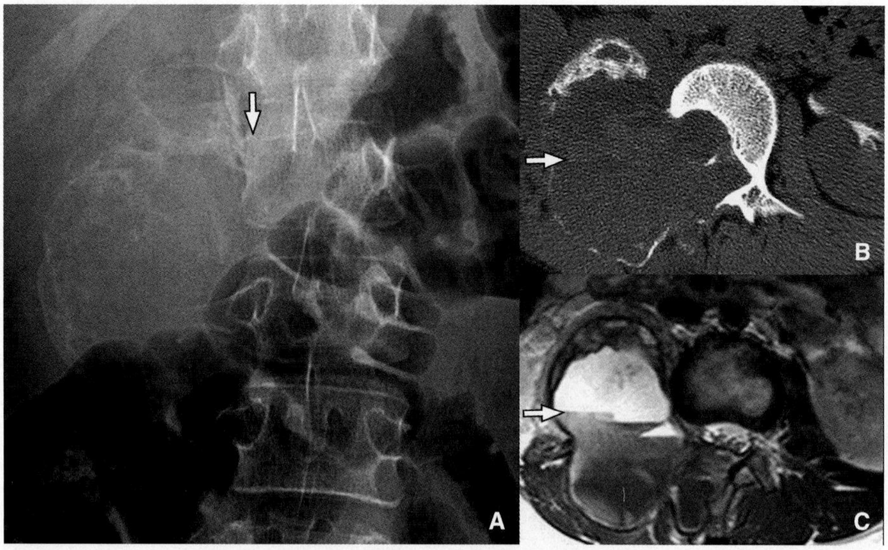

FIGURE 5.66 **Aneurysmal bone cyst in a 16-year-old boy who presented with low back pain associated with scoliosis. A:** Frontal coned-down radiograph of the upper lumbar spine shows an "eggshell" bony density in the right paraspinal region and absence of the right L2 pedicle (*arrow*). **B and C:** Axial CT image **(B)** and axial T2-weighted MR image **(C)** demonstrate blood-fluid levels (*arrows*) within the bony mass, epidural extension, and mass effect upon the thecal sac. Extra-axial extension of the aneurysmal bone cyst displaces the paraspinal muscles and inferior vena cava.

thoracic and lumbosacral spine and 25% in the cervical spine. Lesions may extend to the vertebral body. They usually present in the first two decades of life with painful scoliosis, vertebral expansion and/or compression, radicular pain, or spinal cord compression because of vertebral expansion and hemorrhage.

On radiographs, aneurysmal bone cysts of the spine typically present as sharply defined, expansile osteolytic lesions, with thin sclerotic margins. An absent pedicle is the characteristic finding of vertebral body involvement by large aneurysmal bone cysts on radiographs. CT, which can provide better assessment of the internal fluid–fluid levels as well as cortical breach and extension into adjacent soft tissues, is useful. MRI can also clearly demonstrate the fluid–fluid levels and may provide additional information by demonstrating nerve root or cord compression[59–61] (Fig. 5.66). It is important to recognize that fluid–fluid levels within osseous lesions are not unique to aneurysmal bone cysts. They can be also seen in benign and malignant bone lesions including simple bone cysts, chondroblastomas, giant cell tumors, and telangiectatic osteosarcomas.

Selective arterial embolization has been used in the primary medical treatment of aneurysmal bone cysts, when it is technically possible and there is no evidence of fracture or neurologic compromise. Selective arterial embolization can be performed a few days before surgery in order to reduce the amount of hemorrhage. In pediatric patients for whom surgical management is necessary, an intralesional curettage or excision is the currently recommended procedure.

Vertebral Venous Malformation ("Hemangioma" of Bone)

So-called hemangioma of bone is an intraosseous mass of benign thin-walled blood vessels (Fig. 5.67). It is best conceptualized as a venous malformation, distinct from true hemangiomas such as epithelioid hemangioma. It usually occurs in the vertebral bodies of the thoracic and lumbar spine and, less frequently, in the cervical spine and sacrum. It most commonly occurs in middle age but may be seen in the pediatric population.

The radiographic and CT appearance of spinal "hemangioma" has a "corduroy" or "accordion" appearance of vertically-oriented coarse and thickened trabeculae. The characteristics of these lesions on MRI include high signal on both T1- and T2-weighted MR images without bone destruction. Some "hemangiomas" of bone present as enhancing masses with abnormal soft tissue, distortion of the vertebra, and epidural extension in the spine[59–61] (Fig. 5.68).

The management of vertebral "hemangiomas" depends on the symptoms. No treatment is required for asymptomatic, incidentally found "hemangiomas." In children with painful "hemangiomas" associated with spinal cord compression, arterial embolization followed by laminectomy is currently recommended. In children with pain but no spinal cord

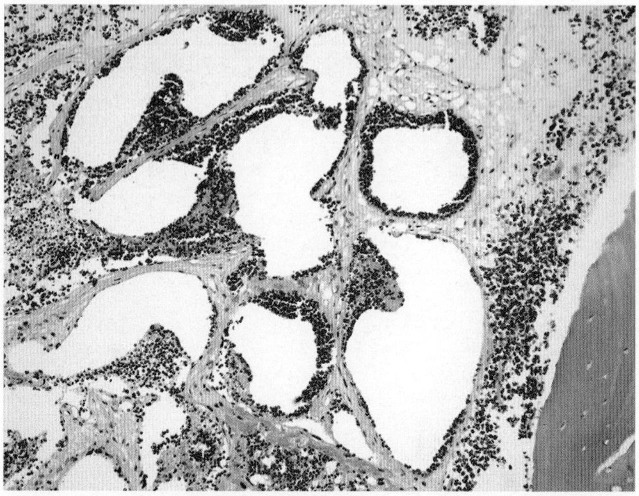

FIGURE 5.67 **Venous malformation, or "hemangioma" of bone, involving the T8 vertebra in an 11-year-old boy with symptoms of spinal cord compression.** Numerous thin-walled blood-filled channels resembling veins are present within the bone, constituting a lesion that is best considered a venous malformation (hematoxylin and eosin, original magnification, 200x).

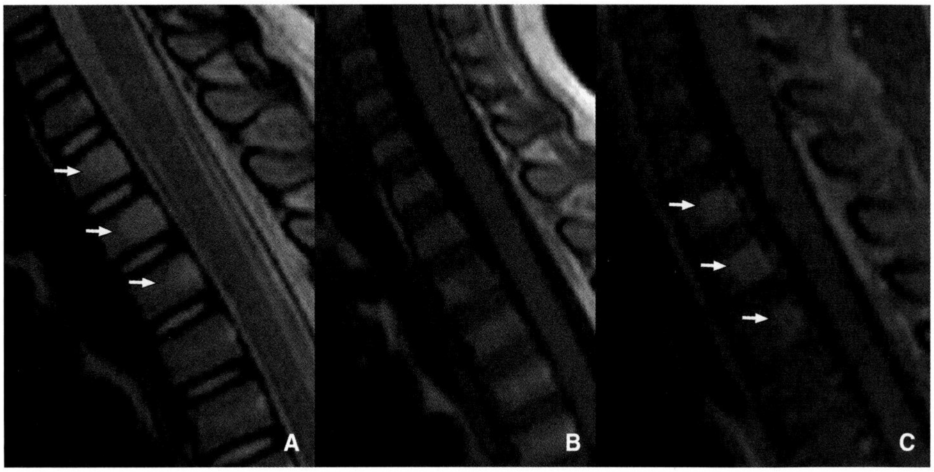

FIGURE 5.68 **Venous malformation, ("hemangioma" of bone) in a 3-year-old girl who presented with back pain. A:** Sagittal T2-weighted MR image shows multilevel focal, rounded areas of high signal intensity (*arrows*) in the vertebral bodies of the lower cervical and upper thoracic spine. **B:** Sagittal T1-weighted MR image demonstrates low signal intensity of these lesions **(A)**. **C:** Postcontrast sagittal T1-weighted MR image with fat-saturation shows homogeneous enhancement of these lesions (*arrows*).

compression, arterial embolization is the management of choice. Vertebroplasty is used to improve pain, especially in pediatric patients with compression fractures without neurologic deficits.

Aggressive and Malignant Tumors of the Spine

Langerhans Cell Histiocytosis

Formerly known by the terms histiocytosis X and eosinophilic granuloma, Langerhans cell histiocytosis (LCH) is now the preferred term for disorders characterized by abnormal proliferation and accumulation of Langerhans cells that produce mass lesions in affected tissues.[62] Although LCH of bone is not malignant, it is included in this section because its aggressive and destructive radiographic features place it in the differential diagnosis with Ewing sarcoma, neuroblastoma, hematopoietic neoplasms, and hematogenous metastases. Osteomyelitis and giant cell tumor are also in the radiographic differential diagnosis. LCH can involve any bone, but most lesions occur in the skull (especially calvarium and temporal bone), pelvis, spine, mandible, ribs, and tubular bones.[62] LCH lesions may be solitary or multiple.[63]

In the spine, these lesions occur primarily within the osseous vertebral elements, particularly the vertebral body. Although the thoracic spine is involved most frequently, lumbar and cervical spine lesions are also seen. Associated abnormalities may include infiltration of the hypothalamic/pituitary axis (producing diabetes insipidus), hearing loss related to temporal bone destruction, orbital lesions producing proptosis, cutaneous nodules, lymph node enlargement, and lung involvement. The natural history of LCH is variable, but bone lesions (particularly solitary skull and spine lesions) generally have a good prognosis. Some patients with aggressive or multiple lesions may have a more fulminant clinical course.[63]

The classic imaging appearance of spinal LCH on plain radiography is a lytic lesion producing substantial (often asymmetric) vertebral body collapse ("vertebra plana")[62] (Fig. 5.68A) or a nonspecific aggressive-appearing destructive lesion. Radiographic skeletal surveys are utilized to screen for additional lesions and to evaluate response to therapy. CT can confirm a lytic lesion, which is frequently associated with substantial loss of vertebral height. MRI can demonstrate a destructive lesion with T1 hypointensity and T2 hyperintensity (Fig. 5.69B). These MR signal characteristics are typical of a cellular ("small round blue cell") lesion. Contrast enhancement is frequently heterogeneous in active LCH lesions and may be absent in chronic lesions. The disc space is characteristically spared in most cases. On both CT and MRI, the soft tissue component is frequently small (Fig. 5.69C), which helps distinguish LCH from primary malignant spine neoplasms. Nuclear scintigraphy does not have a routine role in the imaging assessment of LCH. Uptake on bone scintigraphy is variable and false-negative results are common.

In the absence of systemic disease or spinal deformity, conservative management with observation or nonsteroidal anti-inflammatory medications only may be indicated for spinal LCH in the pediatric population. Extensive or severe disease may require aggressive medical management with chemotherapy or surgical intervention.[11] Vertebra plana deformity, in contrast to neoplastic destructive lesions, often shows striking restoration of vertebral height with lesion healing.[64]

Ewing Sarcoma

Ewing sarcoma (primitive neuroectodermal tumor) is a "small round blue cell" neoplasm of neuroectodermal origin. Ewing sarcoma arises principally in children and young adults and comprises roughly 3% of all pediatric malignancies. Ninety percent present in the first and second decades of life, with a peak incidence between 5 and 13 years of age.[65] Ewing sarcoma is the most common malignant spinal bone tumor in children.[65] Genetic analysis reveals a characteristic translocation, typically between the *EWS* gene on chromosome 22 and *FLI1* on chromosome 11. Approximately 5% of all Ewing sarcomas involve the spine, with the sacrum being the most common location, followed by the lumbar, thoracic, and cervical spine (rare).[66,67] In most pediatric patients, the vertebral body is affected before the neural arch, although some lesions arise within the epidural or paraspinal soft tissues. Tumor

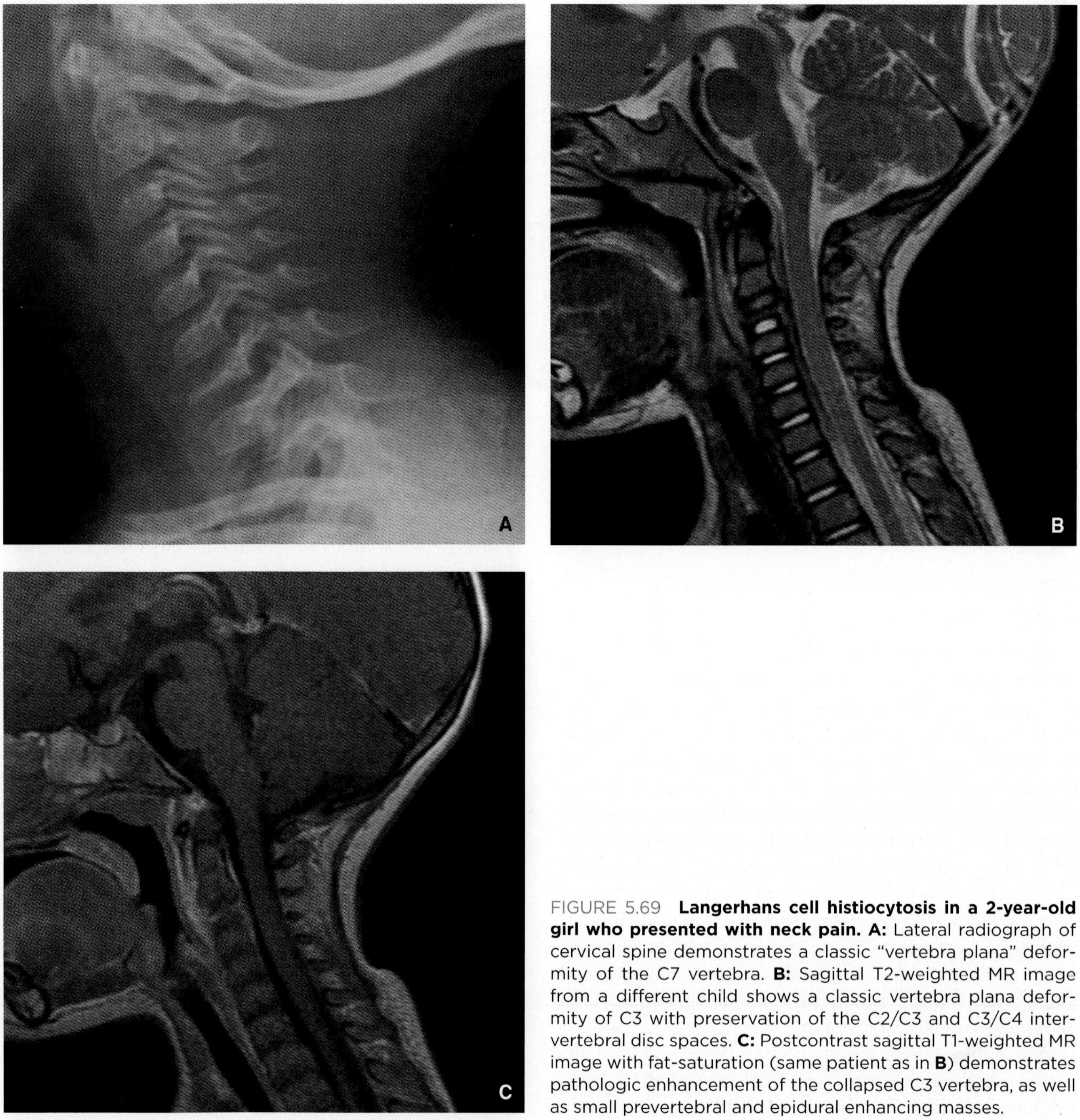

FIGURE 5.69 **Langerhans cell histiocytosis in a 2-year-old girl who presented with neck pain. A:** Lateral radiograph of cervical spine demonstrates a classic "vertebra plana" deformity of the C7 vertebra. **B:** Sagittal T2-weighted MR image from a different child shows a classic vertebra plana deformity of C3 with preservation of the C2/C3 and C3/C4 intervertebral disc spaces. **C:** Postcontrast sagittal T1-weighted MR image with fat-saturation (same patient as in **B**) demonstrates pathologic enhancement of the collapsed C3 vertebra, as well as small prevertebral and epidural enhancing masses.

"percolates" through tiny perforations in the cortex rather than through large areas of frank cortical destruction, and peripheral nerve spread has been described. Ewing sarcoma metastases to other bones, regional soft tissues, lymph nodes, and lung are frequently present at initial diagnosis. Neurologic deficits result from spinal cord or peripheral nerve compression/neoplastic infiltration in affected patients. Some pediatric patients present with fever, leukocytosis, and elevated erythrocyte sedimentation rate, clinically mimicking osteomyelitis.

Radiographs typically demonstrate a permeative lytic lesion of the vertebral body or sacrum (Fig. 5.70A), often with a large associated soft tissue mass. The lesion is usually centered in the vertebral body (as opposed to the posterior elements), although spread into the posterior elements is relatively common.[67] Bone changes are permeative without large areas of cortical destruction, recapitulating the previously described gross findings of tumor permeating through tiny perforations to form a soft tissue mass. The zone of transition is wide and tumor margins are typically difficult to determine. Vertebra plana is occasionally seen, simulating LCH in the pediatric population, although a large soft tissue mass at presentation should lead the radiologist to favor Ewing sarcoma over LCH. CT can confirm a permeative, moth-eaten bone destruction pattern (Fig. 5.70B). Some lesions show bony sclerosis, representing host reaction rather than tumor matrix. Absence of calcification in the soft tissue mass helps distinguish Ewing sarcoma from osteosarcoma. The disc space is usually spared, helping to distinguish Ewing sarcoma

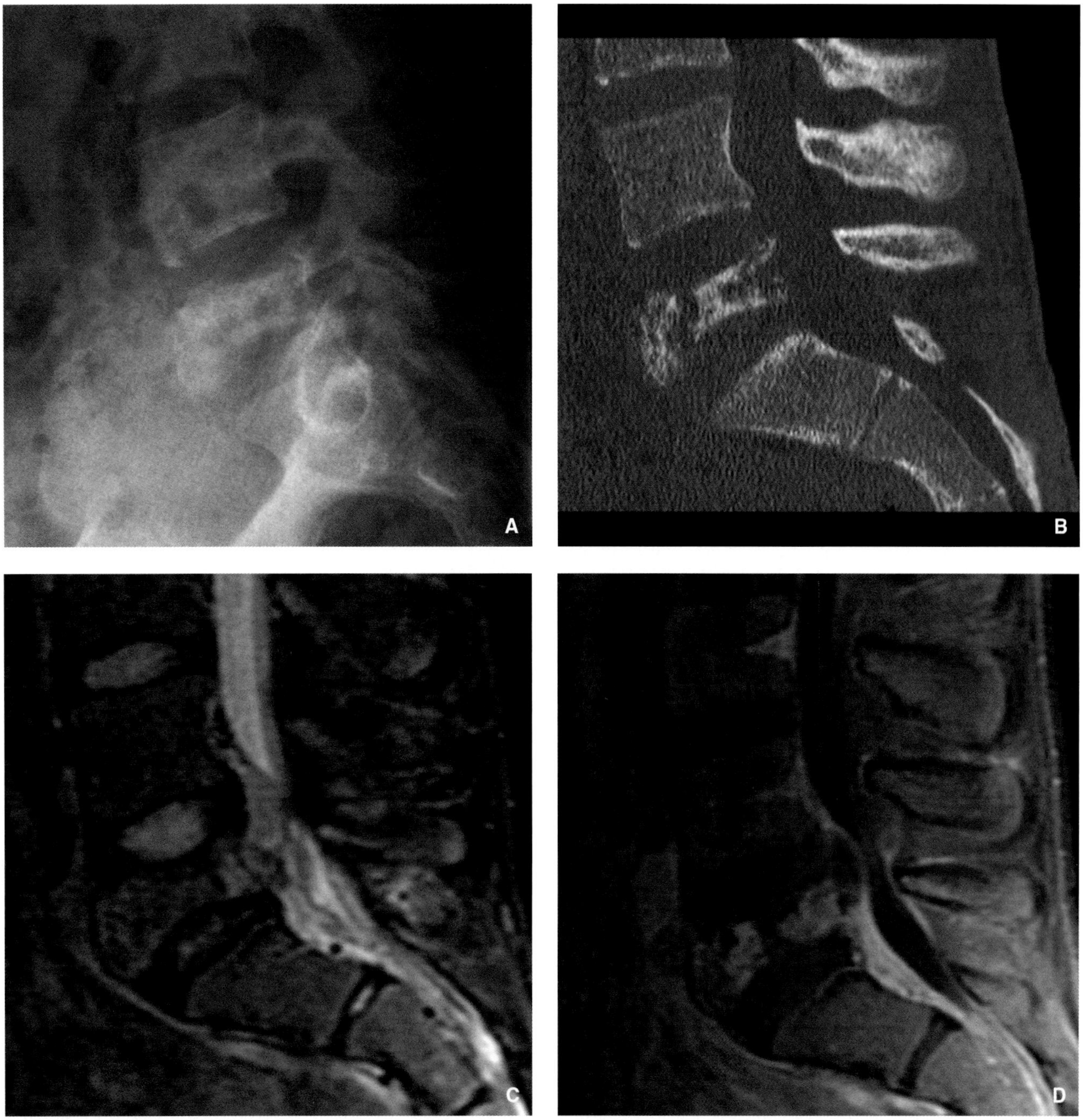

FIGURE 5.70 **Ewing sarcoma in a 15-year-old girl who presented with progressively worsening back pain. A:** Lateral radiograph of the lumbosacral junction shows a permeative L5 vertebral body lesion with substantial vertebral height loss. **B:** Sagittal CT image confirms permeative bone destruction and pathologic compression fracture involving L5 vertebral body. **C:** Sagittal STIR MR image shows relatively mild T2 hyperintensity of the L5 vertebral body bone marrow, which is typical of cellular neoplasms, and an epidural soft tissue mass extending into the spinal canal. **D:** Postcontrast sagittal T1-weighted MR image with fat-saturation demonstrates robust heterogeneous enhancement of the pathologic vertebra and epidural soft tissue mass.

from spondylodiscitis. MRI typically shows a poorly defined soft tissue or bone mass with signal intensity lower than muscle and disc on T1-weighted MR images and intermediate to high signal intensity on T2-weighted and STIR MR images (Fig. 5.70C). Unfortunately, it is frequently difficult to distinguish between tumor and peritumoral edema on MRI. Central necrosis and heterogeneous enhancement following intravenous contrast are typical (Fig. 5.70D). PET imaging usually shows increased FDG uptake in the primary tumor and metastases. In general, MRI is currently the most useful imaging modality for tumor characterization and treatment planning. The role of CT is relatively limited to determining the extent of bone destruction and evaluating chondroid or osteoid (to help discern from chondrosarcoma and osteosarcoma). Chest CT is used to screen for and follow lung metastases.

The differential diagnostic considerations include LCH, osteosarcoma, neuroblastoma, and osteomyelitis in the pediatric population. Other possible, but much less likely, considerations include chordoma, giant cell tumor, and chondrosarcoma, although their typical imaging appearances are different from Ewing sarcoma in children. The current management strategy of choice for Ewing sarcoma is a multimodality approach including surgery, chemotherapy, and radiation therapy. Specifics depend on the size, extent, and grade of tumor, as well as the presence of distant metastasis.[65,68–70]

Chondrosarcoma

Chondrosarcoma is the second most common nonlymphoproliferative primary malignant spinal neoplasm (after chordoma) in adults with the peak age of presentation in the fifth decade.[67] It is rare in the pediatric population, accounting for <10% of primary malignant bone tumors in children.[71] Most spinal chondrosarcomas are primary, although secondary tumors arising in preexisting lesions (e.g., osteochondroma) may occur.

On radiographs, chondrosarcoma may be centered in the vertebral body, posterior elements, or both. The accompanying soft tissue mass is usually large. Characteristic chondroid matrix (C-shaped arcs and rings) is seen in most tumors on radiography and CT, which can permit a specific diagnosis of chondrosarcoma. Apart from the presence of chondroid matrix, chondrosarcoma and chordoma may have a similar imaging appearance. MRI can best characterize soft tissue extent and involvement of regional structures. High lesional signal intensity on T2-weighted MR images is common and helps distinguish chondrosarcoma from more cellular neoplasms such as Ewing sarcoma. Chest CT is utilized to screen for and follow lung metastases in affected pediatric patients.

Chondrosarcoma is frequently low grade, resulting in substantially better long-term survival than osteosarcoma in the pediatric population. Treatment often includes chemotherapy or surgery depending on tumor extent and grade as well as the presence of metastasis.

Osteosarcoma

Spinal osteosarcoma is rare (5% of spinal sarcomas) and generally presents in adult patients during the fourth decade.[67] Pediatric presentations of spinal osteosarcoma are rare. The most common locations for primary spinal osteosarcoma are the thoracic and lumbar spine.[72] Bone destruction and large soft tissue mass are typically present.

Radiographs and CT demonstrate osteoid matrix in the majority of osteosarcomas, permitting distinction from other spinal sarcomas such as Ewing sarcoma. However, it is important to recognize that telangiectatic osteosarcomas may present as lytic lesions without osteoid matrix. MRI can best demonstrate soft tissue mass extent and relationship to important adjacent structures. MR signal intensity of spinal osteosarcoma is relatively nonspecific, although matrix may be visible as relatively hypointense foci within the tumor mass. Contrast enhancement is usually conspicuous. Telangiectatic osteosarcoma may demonstrate fluid–fluid levels in the cystic portions, mimicking aneurysmal bone cyst. Chest CT is used to screen for and follow lung metastases.

Both surgery and chemotherapy are used for local disease and metastatic control in children with spinal osteosarcoma. Unfortunately, overall prognosis is very poor,[73,74] and long-term survivors are at increased risk for developing a second malignancy.

Chordoma

Chordoma is a malignant neoplasm arising from notochord remnants (Fig. 5.71). As a result, the tumor center is frequently within the posterior vertebral body. Chordoma arises in the sacrum most commonly (50%), followed by the clivus (35%), and non-sacral vertebrae (15%). Chordoma most commonly presents in the fifth to sixth decades, with <5% of presentations occurring in pediatric patients.[65,75] The soft tissue mass is frequently large in comparison to the extent of osseous destruction. Slow tumor growth correlates with slow onset of symptoms in the majority of affected patients.

Chordoma's imaging appearance is characteristic (although overlap exists with chondrosarcoma) in comparison to other malignant spinal neoplasms. Radiographs show a heterogeneous destructive lesion, often associated with some sclerosis or intratumoral calcifications. The size of the soft tissue component of tumor is frequently underappreciated on radiographs. CT can better demonstrate a lytic destructive lesion with a soft tissue mass disproportionately larger than the bone defect. The osseous margins of chordoma are usually fairly well-circumscribed. Amorphous intratumoral calcification is inconsistently seen and must be distinguished from chondroid or osteoid matrix. In general, intratumoral calcification is much less conspicuous on radiographs than CT. MRI is the best imaging modality for demonstrating tumor relationship to the spinal cord and regional soft tissue structures. MRI often shows a large soft tissue mass with markedly high T2 signal intensity (Fig. 5.72) and relatively low T1 signal intensity. Heterogeneous contrast enhancement of tumor is typically seen. The tumor may span two or more vertebral levels and extend into the intervertebral disc space(s). Intratumoral calcifications are not well seen on MRI. Therefore, correlation with CT or radiography is helpful when trying to distinguish chordoma from chondrosarcoma. Differential diagnostic considerations primarily include chondrosarcoma and ecchordosis physaliphora (because of marked T2 prolongation), although giant cell tumor, metastasis, and plasmacytoma should also be considered.

Despite slow tumor growth, prognosis of pediatric patients with chordoma is poor, mainly because of difficulty in achieving a total and complete surgical resection due to involvement of locoregional structures.

Lymphoma

Lymphoma represents a relatively large group of lymphoreticular neoplasms that may arise in bone (osseous lymphoma), epidural soft tissues (epidural lymphoma), meninges (lymphomatous leptomeningitis), spinal cord (intramedullary lymphoma), or peripheral nerves (peripheral neurolymphomatosis)

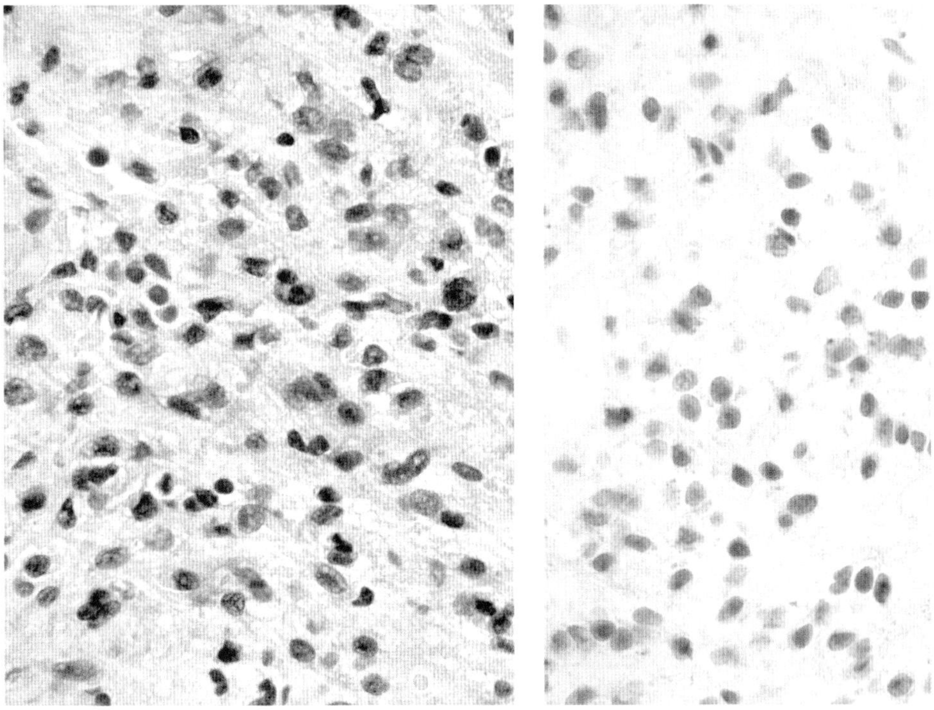

FIGURE 5.71 **Chordoma of the cervical spine in a 16-year-old boy.** The cells are round with occasionally bubbly ("physaliferous") pink cytoplasm (**left**, hematoxylin and eosin, original magnification, 600x). Immunostaining for brachyury, a marker of notochordal differentiation, highlights tumor nuclei (**right**, original magnification, 600x) and has afforded recognition of an expanded histologic spectrum of disease including poorly differentiated chordomas resembling small round blue cell tumors.

in addition to more typical locations such as lymph nodes.[76] Epidural lymphoma is most common in the thoracic spine, whereas intramedullary lymphoma favors the cervical spine. Spinal involvement by non-Hodgkin lymphoma is more common than Hodgkin lymphoma. Most spinal lymphomas are of B-cell origin. Secondary spinal involvement is more common than primary spinal lymphoma. Back pain is the most common clinical presentation in pediatric patients with lymphomatous spinal involvement, although some affected children may present with neural compressive or systemic symptoms.

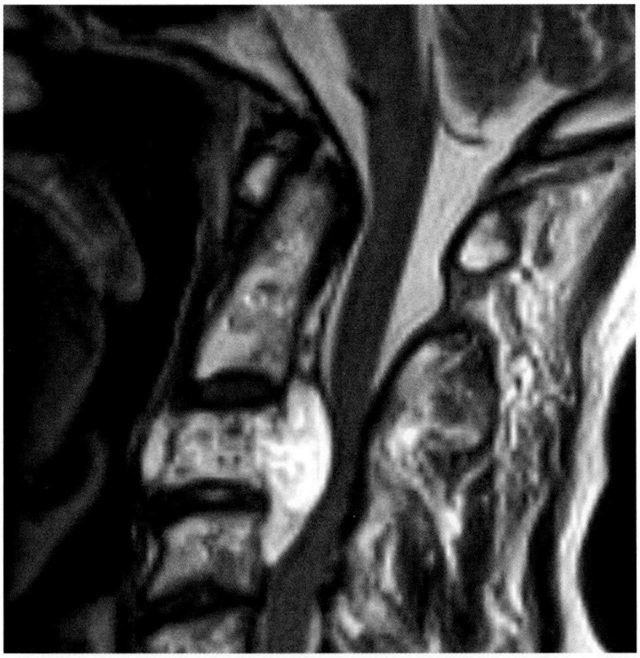

FIGURE 5.72 **Chordoma involving the C3 vertebral body in a 17-year-old boy who presented with neck pain and myelopathy.** Sagittal T2-weighted MR image shows a destructive C3 vertebral body lesion with a soft tissue mass and marked ("lightbulb") T2 hyperintensity characteristic of chordoma. Note that the lesion center is in the posterior vertebral body.

Imaging manifestations of spinal lymphoma are myriad and reflect site of origin as well as growth pattern. The role of radiography is limited to initial evaluation of back pain in affected children and, if abnormal, usually shows nonspecific neoplastic bone destruction. Rarely, affected patients' radiographs may show sclerosis ("ivory vertebra") or vertebra plana, mimicking LCH. CT with multiplanar and 3D reformatted images is useful to characterize the extent of bone destruction and may show tumor spread across the disc spaces. MRI is the most useful imaging tool for spinal lymphoma because it best demonstrates bone marrow involvement and soft tissue extent relative to regional structures. Signal intensity is relatively isointense on T1-weighted MR images and hyperintense on T2-weighted MR image compared to muscle. MRI characteristics are nonspecific for distinguishing lymphoma from other cellular spinal neoplasms and mimics such as Ewing sarcoma, primitive neuroectodermal tumor, and LCH. 18F-FDG PET is used for staging, monitoring response to treatment, and risk stratification.

The prognosis for pediatric patients with spinal lymphoma is poor. Radiotherapy is currently the treatment of choice, sometimes conferring preserved neurologic function and extended survival. Unfortunately, there is currently a paucity of information regarding the role of chemotherapy.

Metastasis

Spine metastases are much less common in children than adults, with metastatic spread of neuroblastoma, hematopoietic neoplasms, or primary bone tumors most commonly encountered. Metastatic neoplasms reach the spinal axis by direct spread from contiguous structures, lymphatic dissemination, hematogenous dissemination, circulation through the CSF, or a combination of these mechanisms. Hematogenous dissemination is the most common pathway for metastatic tumor spread to the vertebral elements. Imaging characteristics of spinal metastasis may reflect features of the primary tumor, although the most frequent appearance is a nonspecific destructive mass lesion. Diagnosis is facilitated by knowledge of primary tumor type, location, and stage. Treatment is variable and based on primary tumor type as well as location and extent of metastasis.

Neuroblastic Tumors

Neuroblastic tumors are embryonal neoplasms derived from the primordial neural crest cells that form the sympathetic nervous system.[77–79] In order of increasing aggressiveness, they are ganglioneuroma (benign), ganglioneuroblastoma (usually benign) (Fig. 5.73A), and neuroblastoma (malignant) (Fig. 5.73B). Neuroblastoma is primarily a neoplasm of infants and young children (75% <2 years of age). Ganglioneuroma and ganglioneuroblastoma are more common in older age groups. Approximately 40% of neuroblastomas arise in the adrenal gland. Primary extra-adrenal neuroblastomas most commonly involve the paraspinal ganglia, resulting in an anterior paraspinal soft tissue mass.

On radiographs, a paraspinal mass (sometimes associated with scoliosis) is characteristic, although findings can be subtle even with large masses. Detection of tumor calcification is helpful because the majority of neuroblastomas show calcification. CT can better demonstrate the presence of an enhancing paraspinal mass and its extent, as well as detect pulmonary and osseous metastasis. Neuroblastoma frequently engulfs rather than displaces adjacent vessels, in contrast to Wilms tumor. Ganglioneuroma and ganglioneuroblastoma usually show adjacent bone erosion rather than frank destruction. They may also erode or remodel the ribs, producing rib splaying as well as enlargement of involved neural foramina. Conversely, neuroblastoma more often produces local bone destruction (although foraminal extension may occur through otherwise normal-appearing neural foramina). MRI is the most helpful imaging modality for evaluating neuroblastic tumors because it best demonstrates soft tissue mass size, relationship to regional structures, and involvement of bone marrow and neural foraminal spread at one or more levels. On MRI, neuroblastoma often shows mild T2 hyperintensity relative to muscle, reflecting cellular tumor histology with a relatively high nuclear-to-cytoplasmic ratio ("small round blue cell tumor") and heterogeneous contrast enhancement.

Unlike for most spinal neoplasms, there is a well-defined role for nuclear scintigraphy for neuroblastoma both in initial characterization and treatment surveillance. I-123 MIBG, a radiotracer taken up by sympathetic catecholaminergic cells, is useful for staging and posttherapy surveillance with the caveat that up to 10% of neuroblastomas do not accumulate MIBG.[80] Differential diagnostic considerations include Ewing sarcoma, nerve sheath tumor, and lymphoma in the pediatric population. Adrenal primary lesions may mimic Wilms tumor, although the latter typically shows a tumor center within the kidney, "claw sign" reflecting normal renal tissue around the tumor margin, and lack of tumoral calcification.

Prognosis of neuroblastic tumors depends on age at presentation, staging, tumor histology, and genetic factors.[78,79]

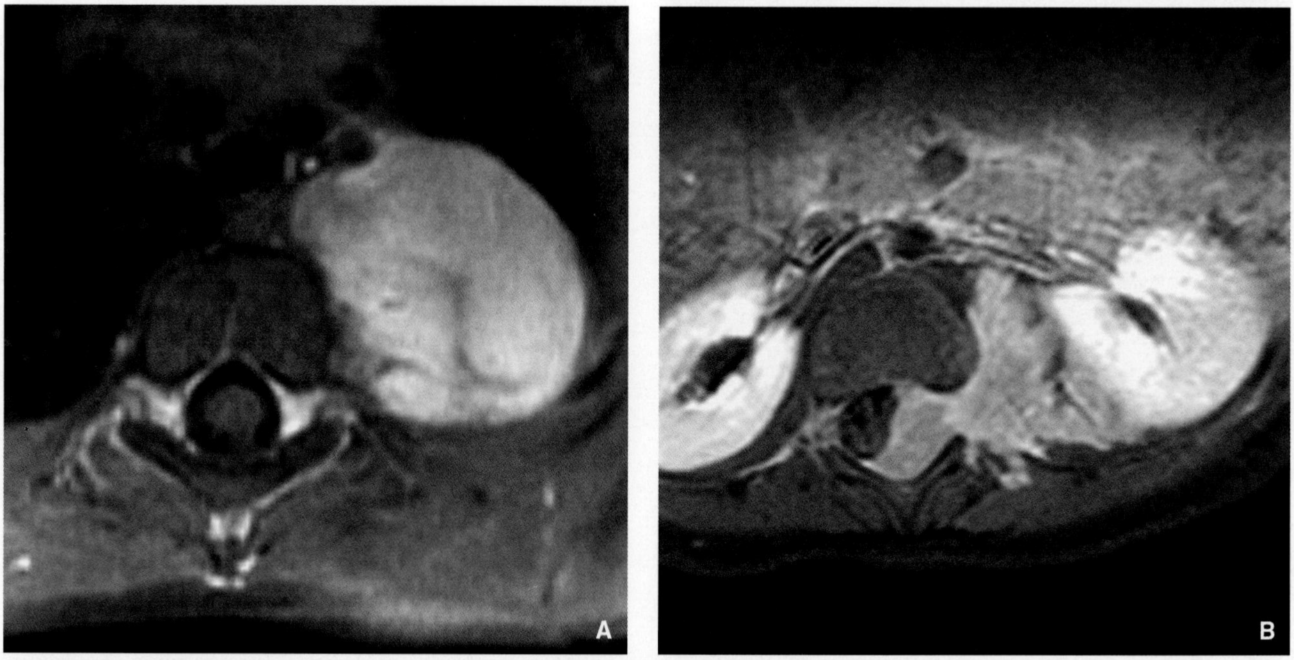

FIGURE 5.73 **Neuroblastic tumors in a six-year-old boy (A) and a 7-month-old girl (B). A:** Ganglioneuroblastoma. Postcontrast axial T1-weighted MR image with fat-saturation demonstrates an enhancing thoracic paraspinal mass without foraminal extension. **B:** Neuroblastoma. Postcontrast axial T1-weighted MR image with fat-saturation shows an enhancing paraspinal tumor with foraminal extension and dural sac displacement.

Patients diagnosed at less than 1 year of age frequently have a better prognosis than older children. This is particularly true in those with liver, bone marrow, and skin metastases only (stage 4S) whose tumor may spontaneously regress. Surgical resection is current management of choice for ganglioneuroma. A combination of surgery and chemotherapy is usually used for ganglioneuroblastoma and neuroblastoma.

Peripheral Nerve Sheath Tumors

Peripheral nerve sheath tumors include neurofibroma (localized, diffuse, and plexiform), schwannoma, and malignant peripheral nerve sheath tumor (MPNST). All may be solitary or multiple, with syndromic associations (neurofibromatosis types 1 and 2) that are well known in clinical practice.

Neurofibroma

Neurofibroma (NF) is a benign neoplasm containing a combination of fibroblasts, Schwann cells, myxoid material, and peripheral nerve fibers. Although the Schwann cells are neoplastic, nerve fibers are characteristically intermixed within the tumor, facilitating pathologic distinction from schwannoma. Approximately 90% of NFs are sporadic. NF may be localized, diffuse, or plexiform. Plexiform NFs are virtually pathognomonic for neurofibromatosis type 1. Malignant transformation (to MPNST) is rare with solitary NF, but occurs in up to 10% of plexiform NF in neurofibromatosis type 1 patients. Deep-seated NFs are at particular risk for malignant transformation. NFs occur all over the body. In the spinal region, they may be extradural paraspinal, intradural/extramedullary, or transpatial. The nerve of origin may be very small in some localized NFs resulting in the tumor not having an obvious relationship to spinal or major peripheral nerves.

In the assessment of spinal manifestations of neurofibromatosis type 1, the primary role of radiography is to assess for scoliosis, kyphosis, and bone remodeling. Radiography has a limited role for imaging of NF directly. CT can demonstrate a rounded or fusiform (localized NF) or ill-defined infiltrating (plexiform NF) soft tissue mass with variable but generally mild enhancement. It is frequently difficult to accurately define plexiform NF margins using CT. MRI is most useful for characterization and treatment planning, particularly for plexiform tumors. Signal intensity of NF on T1-weighted MR images is similar to spinal cord and nerve roots. T2-weighted MRI findings classically show a characteristic "target sign" appearance with peripheral hyperintensity and central hypo- to isointensity (Fig. 5.74). STIR MR imaging is optimal for demonstrating the neoplasm on a background of relatively dark fat and muscle. After contrast administration, NFs typically enhance although usually mildly compared to schwannoma and solid musculoskeletal tumors. Differential diagnostic considerations in the pediatric population include schwannoma, MPNST, perineural root sleeve cyst, and chronic immune demyelinating polyneuropathy.

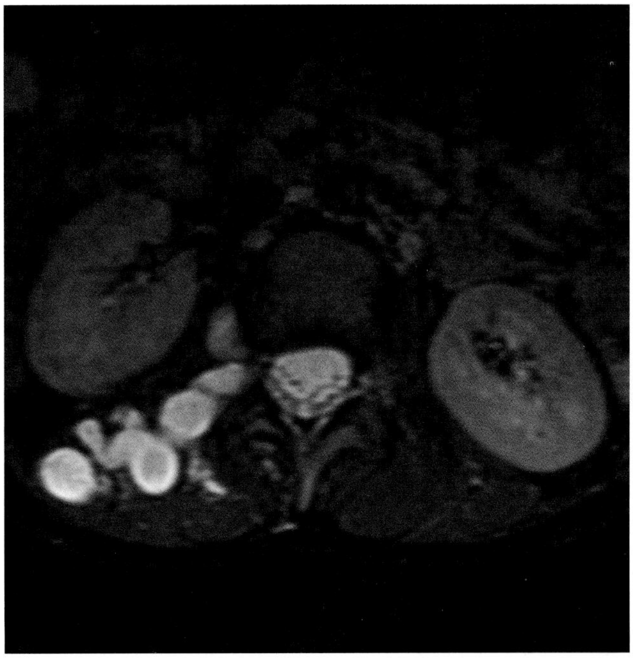

FIGURE 5.74 **Plexiform neurofibroma in a 5-year-old girl.** Axial STIR MR image demonstrates a paraspinal plexiform neurofibroma (NF1) arising from the lumbar plexus with classic "target signs."

The majority of NFs are managed with observation. However, some may need to be surgically removed for cosmetic purposes or in order to alleviate functional impairments. In addition, some NFs may require surgical biopsy to investigate for malignant degeneration.

Schwannoma

Schwannoma is a nerve sheath neoplasm arising from Schwann cells. The majority of tumors are intradural/extramedullary in location with a smaller number being entirely extradural or both intra- and extradural in location ("dumbbell" neoplasm). Multiple schwannomas are a feature of neurofibromatosis type 2 (NF2), although sporadic schwannomas are substantially more common.

Radiography has a limited role in the assessment of schwannoma, but may show local bone remodeling. CT usually demonstrates a well-circumscribed mass that robustly enhances after administration of contrast. Enhancement is typically more robust than that seen with NF. Intrinsic cystic changes are common, compared to NF, where cystic changes are not characteristic. Larger schwannomas frequently remodel adjacent bone, typically with well-circumscribed, sharp margins. MRI is most useful for detecting and characterizing the tumor and its relationship to regional bones and soft tissues. Schwannoma is iso- to hypointense on T1-weighted and hyperintense on T2-weighted MR images. Intrinsic cystic changes show fluid signal characteristics. Rarely, schwannoma demonstrates imaging findings resembling a "target sign." Differential diagnostic considerations include NF, MPNST, myxopapillary ependymoma, perineural root sleeve cyst, and leptomeningeal carcinomatosis.

The current preferred management approach for schwannoma is total surgical resection where possible.

Malignant Peripheral Nerve Sheath Tumor

MPNST is a soft tissue sarcoma arising either spontaneously or from malignant degeneration of a NF (especially plexiform NF). MPNST may be sporadic or associated with neurofibromatosis type 1 (NF1). Clinical presentation of MPNST is earlier in NF1 patients than in the general population. MPNST most commonly arises in the brachial plexus, lumbosacral plexus, or sciatic nerve.

Radiography has a limited role in MPNST evaluation. CT and MRI typically show a large infiltrating mass with a propensity for intrinsic hemorrhage. Margins of the tumor are commonly ill-defined (compared to benign NF) with avid contrast enhancement. Detection of local soft tissue invasion or bone destruction helps in the identification of malignant lesion, although it is important to recognize that MPNST may present as relatively small, rounded, noninvasive lesion that is indistinguishable from benign NF on imaging. In those cases, biopsy is the only definitive way to confirm the correct diagnosis. As a metabolically active tumor, MPNST typically displays FDG avidity, helping to distinguish it from benign NF. Differential considerations include schwannoma, NF, and other soft tissue sarcomas in the pediatric population.

Both surgery and chemotherapy play important roles in the treatment of MPNST.

Other Paraspinal Tumors

Other malignant pediatric tumors that demonstrate a predilection for the paraspinal soft tissues include extrarenal malignant rhabdoid tumor, soft tissue myoepithelioma, and extrarenal Wilms tumor. They typically present as solid masses with nonspecific radiologic features, and tissue sampling is required for a definitive diagnosis.

SPINAL DYSPLASIA SYNDROMES

Three bone dysplasia syndromes that mainly affect the vertebral column in the pediatric population include spondyloepiphyseal dysplasia, achondroplasia, and trisomy 21. Achondroplasia and trisomy 21 are discussed in Chapter 21 (Musculoskeletal Normal Growth, Normal Development, and Congenital Disorders) of this book. This chapter discusses spondyloepiphyseal dysplasia in the following section.

Spondyloepiphyseal Dysplasia

Spondyloepiphyseal dysplasia (SED) dwarfism is characterized by a disproportionately short trunk relative to the extremities. Epiphyseal deformities are characteristic and permit a specific diagnosis. SED results from type II collagenopathy,[81] with both congenital (congenital, autosomal dominant) and later onset (tarda, X-linked recessive) forms described. Life expectancy is normal, although orthopedic deformities may produce substantial morbidity.[82]

Radiographs are useful for establishing the correct diagnosis, showing absent or abnormal epiphyses that may be poorly ossified or flat and irregular. Epiphyseal equivalent involvement in the spine results in platyspondyly or flattened vertebra. The chest is frequently bell-shaped, with flared ribs. Spine imaging is characteristic of a dysplasia but may not be specific for SED. It is important to evaluate the cervical spine in SED patients, because odontoid process hypoplasia with associated atlantoaxial instability may produce spinal cord compression. CT is helpful to better define osseous anomalies, particularly at the craniovertebral junction, which is particularly difficult to evaluate with radiographs in affected young children. MRI can also demonstrate non-osseous findings of SED. In addition, MRI can provide evaluation of the spinal cord for compressive myelopathy or syringohydromyelia. MR also best demonstrates underossified portions of the spine that may be difficult to visualize on radiographs or CT. Differential considerations include mucopolysaccharidoses (particularly MPS 4, Morquio syndrome), achondroplasia, and thanatophoric dysplasia.

MISCELLANEOUS CONDITIONS

Scoliosis

Adolescent idiopathic scoliosis accounts for 89% of all idiopathic scoliosis, making it the most common form of scoliosis in children.[83] Severe curves >40 degrees have a prevalence of 1 in 1,000.[84] Less severe scoliosis with curves >10 degrees but <40 degrees has a prevalence of 2% to 3%.[84] Juvenile idiopathic scoliosis with age of onset usually between 4 and 10 years is more common than infantile scoliosis with age of onset between 0 and 3 years.[85]

Failure of vertebral segmentation causes congenital scoliosis.[86] The most common type of vertebral anomaly is a hemivertebra. However, the most severe scoliosis is associated with a unilateral unsegmented bar with a contralateral hemivertebra.[86] In neuromuscular diseases, scoliosis is seen in 25% to 100% of affected children depending on the underlying disorder.[87]

Imaging evaluation of scoliosis should always start with excellent quality posteroanterior (PA) projection radiographs with the patient standing or in the most upright position possible, with coverage from the cervicothoracic junction to the inferior sacrococcygeal region (Fig. 5.75). Ionizing radiation exposure from excessive follow-up radiography in pediatric patients with scoliosis and other chronic spine disorders has been associated with increased breast cancer incidence and mortality.[88] Studies have also shown that replacing the anteroposterior view with the PA view results in a three- to sevenfold dose reduction to the breast and thyroid tissue.[89,90] Newer low-dose radiation digital stereoradiography systems (EOS imaging) can further reduce overall radiation exposure.

Several previous studies have shown an increased prevalence of neural axis abnormalities in patients with infantile or juvenile scoliosis: 22% in patients with the infantile type and 26% in patients with the juvenile type.[91,92] Abnormalities reported include Chiari I malformation, syrinx, tethered

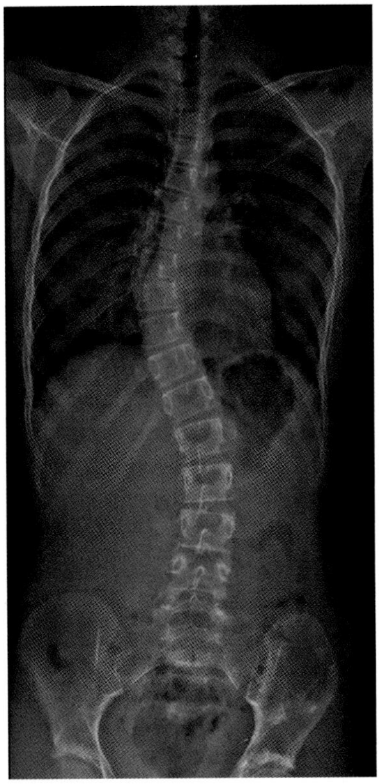

FIGURE 5.75 **Scoliosis in a 14-year-old girl who presented with progressively worsening spine deformity and pain.** Frontal radiograph of thoracic and lumbar spine shows "S"-shaped thoracolumbar scoliosis. Thoracic dextroscoliosis is centered at the T7 vertebral body level, and compensatory levoscoliosis is centered at the L2 vertebral body level.

cord, osteoid osteoma, and brainstem neoplasm. Detecting underlying neural axis lesions is important for optimizing clinical outcomes. For example, decompression of Chiari I malformation in patients with scoliosis and syringomyelia has been shown to result in stabilization or improvement in the degree of scoliosis.[93] Spinal instrumentation for scoliosis with an underlying untreated syrinx can cause progressive neurologic deterioration.[94,95]

Currently, MRI is recommended in all cases of infantile and juvenile scoliosis, particularly in cases with underlying vertebral segmentation anomalies. MRI of the entire spine can exclude underlying spinal canal or cord lesions. Imaging of the entire spine is important to avoid missing lesions including hydrosyringomyelia, diastematomyelia, and neoplasms. Multiplanar T1- and T2-weighted MR images, ideally in all three planes but with a minimum of the axial and sagittal planes, must be obtained. If a syrinx or hydrosyringomyelia is found, administration of contrast is mandatory to exclude an underlying neoplasm.

Additional indications for MRI include abnormal neurologic examination, focal or disabling back pain, and a severe or rapidly progressive spinal curve.[96,97] The presence of levoconvex scoliosis as a risk factor for an underlying lesion is currently controversial. A large study has shown that this parameter alone is not an important indicator of underlying neural axis abnormalities.[98]

The most accurate measurement parameter for spinal scoliosis is the Cobb angle. This angle is evaluated by measuring the difference in angulation between the superior endplate of the upper end vertebra and the inferior endplate of the lower end vertebra of the scoliosis on the frontal view. The end vertebral bodies are the ones most tilted with respect to a horizonal line on a standing or upright radiograph. Most studies demonstrate that an increase in the Cobb angle by 5 or more degrees is consistent with idiopathic scoliosis curve progression.[99–102] The presence of segmentation anomalies as part of the scoliosis pattern makes the estimation of the Cobb angle more difficult. Determining skeletal maturity using the Risser staging is important in predicting the risk of curve progression. In Risser stage 0 (iliac crest apophysis not present) and stage 1 (25% present), the risk of curve progression in idiopathic scoliosis is 60% to 70%.[103] However, if the patient is Risser stage 3, (75% of apophysis present) or greater, the risk of curve progression falls to <10%.[103]

Treatment of scoliosis addresses the underlying etiology, such as craniocervical decompression surgery for Chiari I malformation. For idiopathic scoliosis, brace placement and surgical correction are options chosen on the basis of severity.

Scheuermann Disease

Scheuermann disease, also discussed in Chapter 25 (Musculoskeletal Disorders Due to Endocrinopathy, Metabolic Derangement, and Arthropahy) is the most common cause of hyperkyphosis in children. A diagnosis of Scheuermann disease is made following identification of abnormal kyphosis (generally >40 degrees) accompanied by vertebral endplate irregularity, more than three consecutive anteriorly wedged vertebra, and multiple Schmorl nodes (Fig. 5.76).

Scheuermann disease is most frequently identified in the thoracic spine, but many patients also show some thoracolumbar involvement. The lumbar spine is less commonly involved and cervical involvement is rare. A minority of affected pediatric patients have concurrent scoliosis. Scheuermann disease usually presents in adolescence, but may not be recognized until adulthood. Etiology and inheritance are unclear, but there appears to be a heritable component in some patients.[104] Some affected pediatric patients may present after participating in sports that have exposed them to substantial spinal loading, such as gymnastics, rodeo riding, or weight-lifting.[105] Typical presenting signs and symptoms include kyphosis and back pain worsened by activity.

Although the classic late findings of Scheuermann disease can be easily recognized, it can be challenging to make the diagnosis early in the disease course. Plain radiography is used for initial diagnosis in most patients. The role of CT is primarily for presurgical planning, although endplate irregularities are frequently more conspicuous on CT than radiography. MRI is reserved for detecting complications of Scheuermann disease including pedicular and pars stress fractures or intervertebral disc herniation. Primary differential considerations include postural kyphosis, traumatic anterior wedge compression fractures, congenital kyphosis with

FIGURE 5.76 **Scheuermann disease in a 17-year-old rodeo rider who presented with back pain.** Sagittal STIR MR image shows kyphosis, multiple anteriorly wedged vertebra, and numerous endplate undulations with Schmorl nodes.

segmentation anomalies, neuromuscular disease, spondylodysplasias, and infectious spondylitis.

Physical therapy and pain control are the primary therapeutic interventions in children with Scheuermann disease, with bracing and surgery reserved for severe or worsening orthopedic deformity.

Acknowledgment

We want to thank Nolan Altman, MD; Cynthia Cristoph, MD; Donald Morel; and Sury Alvarado for their excellent assistance.

References

1. Dubousset J, Charpak G, Dorion I, et al. A new 2D and 3D imaging approach to musculoskeletal physiology and pathology with low-dose radiation and the standing position: the EOS system. *Bull Acad Natl Med.* 2005;189(2):287–297.
2. Glaser DA, Doan J, Newton PO. Comparison of 3-dimensional spinal reconstruction accuracy: biplanar radiographs with EOS versus computed tomography. *Spine.* 2012;37(16):1391–1397.
3. Kukreja K, Manzano G, Ragheb J, et al. Differentiation between pediatric spinal arachnoid and epidermoid-dermoid cysts: is diffusion-weighted MRI useful? *Pediatr Radiol.* 2007;37:556–560.
4. Moore P. The skeletal system. In: *The Developing Human Clinically Oriented Embryology*. 6th ed. Philadelphia, PA: W.B. Saunders; 1998:405–424.
5. Sadler TW. Central nervous system. In: *Langman's Medical Embryology*. 9th ed. Baltimore, MD: Lippincott Williams & Wilkins; 2004:433–448.
6. Moore P. Organogenesis period: fourth to eight weeks. In: *The Developing Human Clinically Oriented Embryology*. 6th ed. Philadelphia, PA: W.B. Saunders; 1998:83–105.
7. Sadler TW. Skeletal system. In: *Langman's Medical Embryology*. 9th ed. Baltimore, MD: Lippincott Williams & Wilkins; 2004:171–197.
8. Lustrin ES, Karakas S, Ortiz O, et al. Pediatric cervical spine: normal anatomy, variants, and trauma. *Radiographics.* 2003;23:539–560.
9. Bailey DK. The normal cervical spine in infants and children. *Radiology.* 1952;59:712–719.
10. Harwood-Nash DC, Fitz CR. The normal spine. In: Harwood-Nash DC, Fitz CR, eds. *Neuroradiology in Infants and Children, Vol. III*. 1st ed. St. Louis, MO: CV Mosby Company; 1976:1054–1071.
11. Williams A, Newell RLM, Collins P. Back and macroscopic anatomy of spinal cord. In: Standring S, ed. *Gray's Anatomy*. 39th ed. London, UK: Elsevier Churchill Livingstone; 2005:725–798.
12. Slovis TL. The normal vertebra. In: Slovis T, ed. *Caffey's Pediatric Diagnostic Imaging*. Vol. 1. 11th ed. Philadelphia, PA: Mosby Elsevier; 2008:871–885.
13. Babyn SP, Ranson M, McCarville E. Normal bone marrow. Signal characteristics and fatty conversion. *Magn Reson Imaging Clin N Am.* 1998;6(3):473–495.
14. Beadle OA. *The Intervertebral Discs*. Special report Series No.161, Medical Research Council London, His Majesty's Stationery Office; 1931.
15. Swischuk L. Normal variations. In: Swischuk L, ed. *Imaging of the Cervical Spine in Children*. 1st ed. Springer-Verlag; 2002:13–38.
16. Harris J Jr, Harris W, Novelline R. Spine including soft tissues of the pharynx and neck. In: Harris J Jr, Harris W, Novelline R, eds. *The Radiology of Emergency Medicine*. 3rd ed. Baltimore, MD: Lippincott Williams & Wilkins; 1993:128–282.
17. Von Torlkus D, Gehle W. *The Upper Cervical Spine Morphology, Pathology, and Traumatology, An X Ray Atlas*. New York, NY: Grune & Stratton; 1972.
18. Swischuk L. Anomalies and normal variations of the dens. In: Swischuk L, ed. *Imaging of the Cervical Spine in Children*, 1st ed. Springer-Verlag; 2002:57–73.
19. Macpherson RI, Genez B. Spine. In: Reed MH, ed. *Pediatric Skeletal Radiology*. 1st ed. Baltimore, MD: Lippincott Williams & Wilkins; 1992:209–296.
20. Harwood-Nash DC, Fitz CR. Abnormal Spine. In: Harwood-Nash D, Fitz CR, eds. *Neuroradiology in Infants and Children. Vol. III*, 1st ed. St. Louis, MO: CV Mosby Company; 1976:1072–1124.
21. Kumar R, Guinto FC, Madewell JE, et al. The vertebral body: radiographic configuration in various congenital and acquired disorders. *Radiographics.* 1988:455–485.
22. Mooney III J, Slovis TL. Congenital malformations. In: Slovis TL, ed. *Caffey's Pediatric Diagnostic Imaging*, Vol. 1. 11th ed. Philadelphia, PA: Mosby Elsevier; 2008:886–898.
23. Barkovich J, Raybaund C. Congenital anomalies of the spine. In: Barkovich J, Raybaund C, eds. *Pediatric Neuroimaging*. 5th ed. Baltimore, MD: Lippincott Williams & Wilkins; 2012:857–922.
24. Naidich TP, Zimmerman RA, Mclone DG, et al. Congenital anomalies of the spine and spinal cord, embryology and malformations. In: Atlas SY, ed. *Magnetic Resonance imaging of the Brain and Spine*. 2nd ed. Lippincott-Raven; 1996:1265–1335.
25. Swischuk L. Anomalies. In: Swischuk L, ed. *Imaging of the Cervical Spine in Children*. 1st ed. Springer-Verlag; 2002:39–56.
26. Sullivan JA, Keenan MAE, et al. Klippel-Fail syndrome. *Medscape*, February 7; 2012.
27. Ulmer JL, Elser AE, Williams DW III. Klippel-Feil syndrome: CT and MR of the acquired and congenital abnormalities of the cervical spine and cord. *J Comput Assit Tomogr.* 1993;17:215–224.

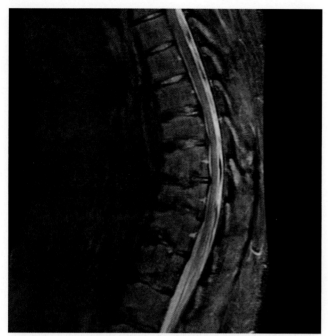

28. Rigault P, Pouliquen JC, et al. Congenital elevation of the scapula in children, Anatomo-pathological and therapeutic study apropos of 27 cases. *Rev Chir Orthop Repatrice Appar Mot.* 1976;62(1):5–26.
29. Pang D. Sacral agenesis and caudal spinal cord malformations. *Neurosurgery.* 1993;32:755–779.
30. Dias MS, McLone D. Normal and abnormal early development of the nervous system. In: McLone D, ed. *Pediatric Neurosurgery: Surgery of the Developing Nervous System.* Philadelphia, PA: Saunders; 2001:31–71 [Chapter 4].
31. Rufner S, et al. Imaging of congenital spine and spinal cord malformations. *Neuroimaging Clin N Am.* 2011;21(3):659–676.
32. Kocaoglu M, Frush D. Pediatric presacral masses. *Radiographics.* 2006;26:833–857.
33. Fernbach SK, Poznanski AK. Pediatric case of the day. *Radiographics.* 1989;9(5):968–971.
34. Avni FE, Guibaud L, Robert Y, et al. MRI imaging of fetal sacrococcygeal teratoma: diagnosis and assessment. *Am J Roentgenol.* 2002;178:179–183.
35. Kowalski TJ, Layton KF, Berbari EF, et al. Follow-up MR imaging in patients with pyogenic spine infections: lack of correlation with clinical features. *Am J Neuroradiol.* 2007;28(4):693–699.
36. Brown R, Hussain M, McHugh K, et al. Discitis in young children. *J Bone Joint Surg Br.* 2001;83-B(1):106–111. doi:10.1302/0301-620X.83B1.10865.
37. Garron E, Viehweger E, Launay F, et al. Nontuberculous spondylodiscitis in children. *J Pediatr Orthop.* 2002;22(3):321–328.
38. Hadjipavlou AG, Mader JT, Necessary JT, et al. Hematogenous pyogenic spinal infections and their surgical management. *Spine.* 2000;25(13):1668–1679.
39. Teo HEL, Peh WCG. Skeletal tuberculosis in children. *Pediatr Radiol.* 2004;34(11):853–860. doi:10.1007/s00247-004-1223-7.
40. Vadivelu S, Effendi S, Starke JR, et al. A review of the neurological and neurosurgical implications of tuberculosis in children. *Clin Pediatr.* 2013;52(12):1135–1143. doi:10.1177/0009922813493833.
41. Prasad A, Manchanda S, Sachdev N, et al. Imaging features of pediatric musculoskeletal tuberculosis. *Pediatr Radiol.* 2012;42(10):1235–1249. doi:10.1007/s00247-012-2439-6.
42. Andronikou S, Jadwat S, Douis H. Patterns of disease on MRI in 53 children with tuberculous spondylitis and the role of gadolinium. *Pediatr Radiol.* 2002;32(11):798–805. doi:10.1007/s00247-002-0766-8.
43. Grimme J, Castillo M. Congenital anomalies of the spine. *Neuroimag Clin N Am.* 2007;17(1):1–16.
44. Nunez D Jr, Amhad AA, et al. Clearing the cervical spine in multiple trauma victims: a time-effective protocol using helical computed tomography. *Emerg Radiol.* 1994;1:273–278.
45. Munera F, Rivas L, Nunez D, et al. Imaging evaluation of adult spinal injuries: emphasis on multidetector CT in cervical spine trauma. *Radiology.* 2012;263(3):645–659.
46. Bailitz J, Starr F, et al. CT should replace three-view radiographs as initial screening test in patients at high, moderate and low risk for blunt cervical spinal injury: a prospective comparison. *J Trauma.* 2009;66(6):1605–1609.
47. Nunez D, Zuluaga A, et al. Cervical spine trauma: how much more do we learn by routinely using helical CT? *Radiographics.* 1996;16:1307–1318.
48. Hogan GJ, Mirvis SE, Shanmuganat K, Scalea TM. Exclusion of unstable cervical injury in obtunded patients with blunt trauma: Is MR imaging needed when multidetector row CT findings are normal? *Radiology.* 2005;237(1):106–113.
49. Deleganis AV, Baxter AB. et al. Radiologic spectrum of craniocervical distraction injuries. *Radiographics.* 2000;20:S237–S250.
50. Harris JH, Mirvis SE. *The Radiology of Acute Cervical Spine Trauma.* 3rd ed. Baltimore, MD: Lippincott Williams & Wilkins; 1996:20–25.
51. Backstrom JW, Junewick JJ. Vertebral trauma. In: Slovis T, ed. *Caffey's Pediatric Diagnostic Imaging.* Vol. 1. 11th ed. Philadelphia, PA: Mosby Elsevier; 2008:899–924.
52. Denis F. Spinal instability as defined by the three-column spine concept in acute spinal trauma. *Clin Orthop Relat Res.* 1984:189: 65–76.
53. Daffner R, Deeb Z, Rothfus W. Fingerprints of vertebral trauma-a unifying concept based in mechanisms. *Skeletal Radiol.* 1986;15:518–525.
54. Rao S, Waysliw C, Nunez D. Spectrum of imaging findings in hyperextension injuries of the neck. *Radiographics.* 2005;25: 1239–1254.
55. Swischuk L. Trauma. In: Swischuk L, ed. *Imaging of the Cervical Spine in Children.* 1st ed. Springer-Verlag; 2002:75–121.
56. Zuluaga A, Nunez D. Plain film radiography and computed tomography of the cervical spine: part II. Classification and subtypes of spinal injury. In: *Spinal Trauma Imaging, Diagnosis and Management.* Baltimore, MD: Lippincott Williams & Wilkins; 2007:73–155.
57. Haque S, Bilal Shafi B, Kaleen M. Imaging of torticollis in children. *Radiographics.* 2012;32:557–571.
58. Groves C, Cassar-Pullicino V, et al. Chance-type flexion-distraction injuries in the thoracolumbar spine: MR imaging characteristics. *Radiology.* 2005;236:601–608.
59. Sze G. Neoplastic disease of the spine and spinal cord. In: Atlas SW, ed. *Magnetic Resonance Imaging of the Brain and Spine.* 2nd ed. Lippincott-Raven; 2007:1339–1360.
60. Strain J, Kuhn JP. Neoplasms of the vertebrae. In: Slovis T, ed. *Caffey's Pediatric Diagnostic Imaging,* Vol. 1. 11th ed. Philadelphia, PA: Mosby Elsevier; 2008:934–940. [Chapter 60].
61. Rossi A, Gandolfo C, Morana G. et al. Tumors of the spine in children. *Neuroimag Clin N Am.* 2007;17(1):25–29.
62. Azouz EM, Saigal G, Rodriguez MM, et al. Langerhans? Cell histiocytosis: pathology, imaging and treatment of skeletal involvement. *Pediatr Radiol.* 2004;35(2):103–115. doi:10.1007/s00247-004-1262-0.
63. Lee S-K, Jung T-Y, Jung S, et al. Solitary Langerhans cell histocytosis of skull and spine in pediatric and adult patients. *Childs Nerv Syst.* 2014;30(2):271–275. doi:10.1007/s00381-013-2198-1.
64. Garg S, Mehta S, Dormans JP. Langerhans cell histiocytosis of the spine in children long-term follow-up. *J Bone Joint Surg Am.* 2004;86-A(8):1740–1750. doi:10.2106/JBJS.L.01386.
65. Klimo P, Codd PJ, Grier H, et al. Primary pediatric intraspinal sarcomas. Report of 3 cases. *J Neurosurg Pediatr.* 2009;4(3):222–229. doi:10.3171/2009.3.PEDS08272.
66. Menezes AH. Craniovertebral junction neoplasms in the pediatric population. *Childs Nerv Syst.* 2008;24(10):1173–1186. doi:10.1007/s00381-008-0598-4.
67. Murphey MD, Andrews CL, Flemming DJ. From the archives of the AFIP. Primary tumors of the spine: radiologic pathologic correlation. *Radiographics.* 1996;16(5):1131–1158. doi:10.1148/radiographics.16.5.8888395;issue:issue:10.1148/radiographics.1996.16.issue-5;page:string:Article/Chapter.
68. Kumar R, Giri PJ. Pediatric extradural spinal tumors. *Pediatr Neurosurg.* 2008;44(3):181–189. doi:10.1159/000120147.

69. Kim HJ, McLawhorn AS, Goldstein MJ, et al. Malignant osseous tumors of the pediatric spine. *J Am Acad Orthop Surg.* 2012;20(10):646–656. doi:10.5435/JAAOS-20-10-646.
70. Ellis JA, Rothrock RJ, Moise G, et al. Primitive neuroectodermal tumors of the spine: a comprehensive review with illustrative clinical cases. *Neurosurg Focus.* 2011;30(1):E1. doi:10.3171/2010.10.FOCUS10217.
71. Mosier SM, Patel T, Strenge K, et al. Chondrosarcoma in childhood: the radiologic and clinical conundrum. *J Radiol Case Rep.* 2012; 6(12):32–42. doi:10.3941/jrcr.v6i12.1241.
72. Zils K, Bielack S, Wilhelm M, et al. Osteosarcoma of the mobile spine. *Ann Oncol.* 2013;24(8):2190–2195. doi:10.1093/annonc/mdt154.
73. Ozaki T, Flege S, Liljenqvist U, et al., Osteosarcoma of the spine. *Cancer.* 2002;94(4):1069–1077.
74. Longhi A, Errani C, De Paolis M, et al. Primary bone osteosarcoma in the pediatric age: state of the art. *Cancer Treat Rev.* 2006;32(6):423–436. doi:10.1016/j.ctrv.2006.05.005.
75. Choi GH, Yang M-S, Yoon DH, et al. Pediatric cervical chordoma: report of two cases and a review of the current literature. *Childs Nerv Syst.* 2010;26(6):835–840. doi:10.1007/s00381-009-1076-3.
76. Moore KR, Blumenthal DT, Smith AG, et al. Neurolymphomatosis of the lumbar plexus: high-resolution MR neurography findings. *Neurology.* 2001;57(4):740–742.
77. Kornreich L, Horev G, Kaplinsky C, et al. Neuroblastoma: evaluation with contrast enhanced MR imaging. *Pediatr Radiol.* 1991;21(8):566–569.
78. Monclair T, Brodeur GM, Ambros PF, et al. The International Neuroblastoma Risk Group (INRG) staging system: an INRG Task Force report. *J Clin Oncol.* 2009;27(2):298–303. doi:10.1200/JCO.2008.16.6876.
79. Brisse HJ, McCarville MB, Granata C, et al. Guidelines for imaging and staging of neuroblastic tumors: consensus report from the International Neuroblastoma Risk Group Project. *Radiology.* 2011;261(1):243–257. doi:10.1148/radiol.11101352.
80. DuBois SG, Matthay KK. Radiolabeled metaiodobenzylguanidine for the treatment of neuroblastoma. *Nucl Med Biol.* 2008;35:S35–S48. doi:10.1016/j.nucmedbio.2008.05.002.
81. Anderson IJ, Goldberg RB, Marion RW, et al. Spondyloepiphyseal dysplasia congenita: genetic linkage to type II collagen (COL2AI). *Am J Hum Genet.* 1990;46(5):896–901.
82. Kocyigit H, Arkun R, Ozkinay F, et al. Spondyloepiphyseal dysplasia tarda with progressive arthropathy. *Clin Rheumatol.* 2000;19(3):238–241. doi:10.1007/s100670050166.
83. Riseborough EJ, Wynne-Davies R. A genetic survey of idiopathic scoliosis in Boston, Massachusetts. *J Bone Joint Surg Am.* 1973;55(5):974–982.
84. Miller NH. Cause and natural history of adolescent idiopathic scoliosis. *Orthop Clin North Am.* 1999;30(3):343–352, vii.
85. Al-Arjani AM, Al-Sebai MW, Al-Khawashki HM, et al. Epidemiological patterns of scoliosis in a spinal center in Saudi Arabia. *Saudi Med J.* 2000;21(6):554–557.
86. Shahcheraghi GH, Hobbi MH. Patterns and progression in congenital scoliosis. *J Pediatr Orthop.* 1999;19(6):766–775.
87. Campos MA, Weinstein SL. Pediatric scoliosis and kyphosis. *Neurosurg Clin N Am.* 2007;18(3):515–529.
88. Doody MM, Lonstein JE, Stovall M, et al. Breast cancer mortality after diagnostic radiography: findings from the U.S. Scoliosis Cohort Study. *Spine.* 2000;25(16):2052–2063.
89. Levy AR, Goldberg MS, Mayo NE, et al. Reducing the lifetime risk of cancer from spinal radiographs among people with adolescent idiopathic scoliosis. *Spine.* 1996;21(13):1540–1547; discussion 8.
90. Levy AR, Goldberg MS, Hanley JA, et al. Projecting the lifetime risk of cancer from exposure to diagnostic ionizing radiation for adolescent idiopathic scoliosis. *Health Phys.* 1994;66(6):621–633.
91. Evans SC, Edgar MA, Hall-Craggs MA, et al. MRI of 'idiopathic' juvenile scoliosis. A prospective study. *J Bone Joint Surg Br.* 1996; 78(2):314–317.
92. Dobbs MB, Lenke LG, Szymanski DA, et al. Prevalence of neural axis abnormalities in patients with infantile idiopathic scoliosis. *J Bone Joint Surg Am.* 2002;84-A(12):2230–2234.
93. Eule JM, Erickson MA, O'Brien MF, et al. Chiari I malformation associated with syringomyelia and scoliosis: a twenty-year review of surgical and nonsurgical treatment in a pediatric population. *Spine.* 2002;27(13):1451–1455.
94. Davids JR, Chamberlin E, Blackhurst DW. Indications for magnetic resonance imaging in presumed adolescent idiopathic scoliosis. *J Bone Joint Surg Am.* 2004;86-A(10):2187–2195.
95. Ozerdemoglu RA, Transfeldt EE, Denis F. Value of treating primary causes of syrinx in scoliosis associated with syringomyelia. *Spine.* 2003;28(8):806–814.
96. Ramirez N, Johnston CE, Browne RH. The prevalence of back pain in children who have idiopathic scoliosis. *J Bone Joint Surg Am.* 1997;79(3):364–368.
97. Sato T, Hirano T, Ito T, et al. Back pain in adolescents with idiopathic scoliosis: epidemiological study for 43,630 pupils in Niigata City, Japan. *Eur Spine J.* 2011;20(2):274–279.
98. Morcuende JA, Dolan LA, Vazquez JD, et al. A prognostic model for the presence of neurogenic lesions in atypical idiopathic scoliosis. *Spine.* 2004;29(1):51–58.
99. Morrissy RT, Goldsmith GS, Hall EC, et al. Measurement of the Cobb angle on radiographs of patients who have scoliosis. Evaluation of intrinsic error. *J Bone Joint Surg Am.* 1990;72(3):320–327.
100. Carman DL, Browne RH, Birch JG. Measurement of scoliosis and kyphosis radiographs. Intraobserver and interobserver variation. *J Bone Joint Surg Am.* 1990;72(3):328–333.
101. Shea KG, Stevens PM, Nelson M, et al. A comparison of manual versus computer-assisted radiographic measurement. Intraobserver measurement variability for Cobb angles. *Spine.* 1998;23(5):551–555.
102. Pruijs JE, Hageman MA, Keessen W, et al. Variation in Cobb angle measurements in scoliosis. *Skeletal Radiol.* 1994;23(7):517–520.
103. Lonstein JE, Carlson JM. The prediction of curve progression in untreated idiopathic scoliosis during growth. *J Bone Joint Surg Am.* 1984;66(7):1061–1071.
104. Damborg F, Engell V, Nielsen J, et al. Genetic epidemiology of Scheuermann's disease. *Acta Orthop.* 2011;82(5):602–605. doi:10.3109/17453674.2011.618919.
105. Lowe TG, Line BG. Evidence based medicine: analysis of Scheuermann kyphosis. *Spine.* 2007;32(19 Suppl):S115–S119. doi:10.1097/BRS.0b013e3181354501.

PART II
PEDIATRIC THORACIC RADIOLOGY

Edward Y. Lee

CHAPTER 6

Lung

Bernard F. Laya • Behrang Amini • Evan J. Zucker • Tracy Kilborn • Sara O. Vargas • Edward Y. Lee

INTRODUCTION

As the main organ of respiration, the lungs perform the important function of oxygen transport from the atmosphere into the bloodstream as well as the release of carbon dioxide from the bloodstream into the atmosphere. This process is made possible through the lungs' intricate tissue framework, which allows gas exchange at the alveolar level. Lung development start as early as the 4th week of life, but maturation and development continue up to early adolescence. Any insult or interruption during normal development could lead to various forms of congenital and developmental malformations. Injury to a fully developed lung could lead to either transient or long-term sequelae. These injuries could be infectious, inflammatory, neoplastic, traumatic, and idiopathic in etiology.

Medical imaging not only has allowed visualization of anatomy and function of the lungs but also has led to increased detection and diagnosis of various congenital and acquired lung disorders in the pediatric population. Along the way, imaging has helped improve our knowledge and understanding on the etiology, onset, timing, and course of these abnormalities and has made an impact in the treatment and management of lung disease. In this chapter, imaging techniques for evaluating lungs and normal anatomy in pediatric patients are discussed. In addition, various congenital and acquired disorders commonly affecting infants and children are reviewed including clinical features, characteristic imaging findings, relevant pathologic findings, and current treatment approaches.

IMAGING TECHNIQUES

Radiography

The chest radiograph is the most frequently performed radiographic examination in pediatric patients. Assessment of the technical quality of a chest radiograph is important prior to interpretation. Special attention should be given to proper patient positioning, inspiratory effort, and x-ray exposure during the procedure. In most clinical indications, a single frontal projection of the chest is sufficient, but a lateral view may be helpful to demonstrate an abnormality in the mediastinum and at the lung base in the pediatric population (Fig. 6.1). Additional views such as cross-table lateral or lateral decubitus views may be obtained in assessing pleural effusion, pneumothorax, and foreign body.

In neonates and children under 2 years of age, the frontal chest radiographs are obtained supine, anteroposterior (AP). For toddlers, an erect (AP) view is obtained unless the patient is old enough to cooperate for an upright posteroanterior (PA) view. The cardiomediastinal width appears exaggerated on both the supine position and the AP projection. Attention to the degree of rotation in the frontal radiograph is important because it can cause unequal lucency of the two lungs, which can mimic pathologic lung hyperlucency (Fig. 6.2). Chest radiographs obtained in expiratory phase result in crowding of pulmonary vessels, which can be mistaken for pulmonary edema, atelectasis, consolidation, or even lymphadenopathy (Fig. 6.2). Inspiratory effort is adequate if the eighth or ninth posterior ribs are visible above the diaphragm. Exposure is

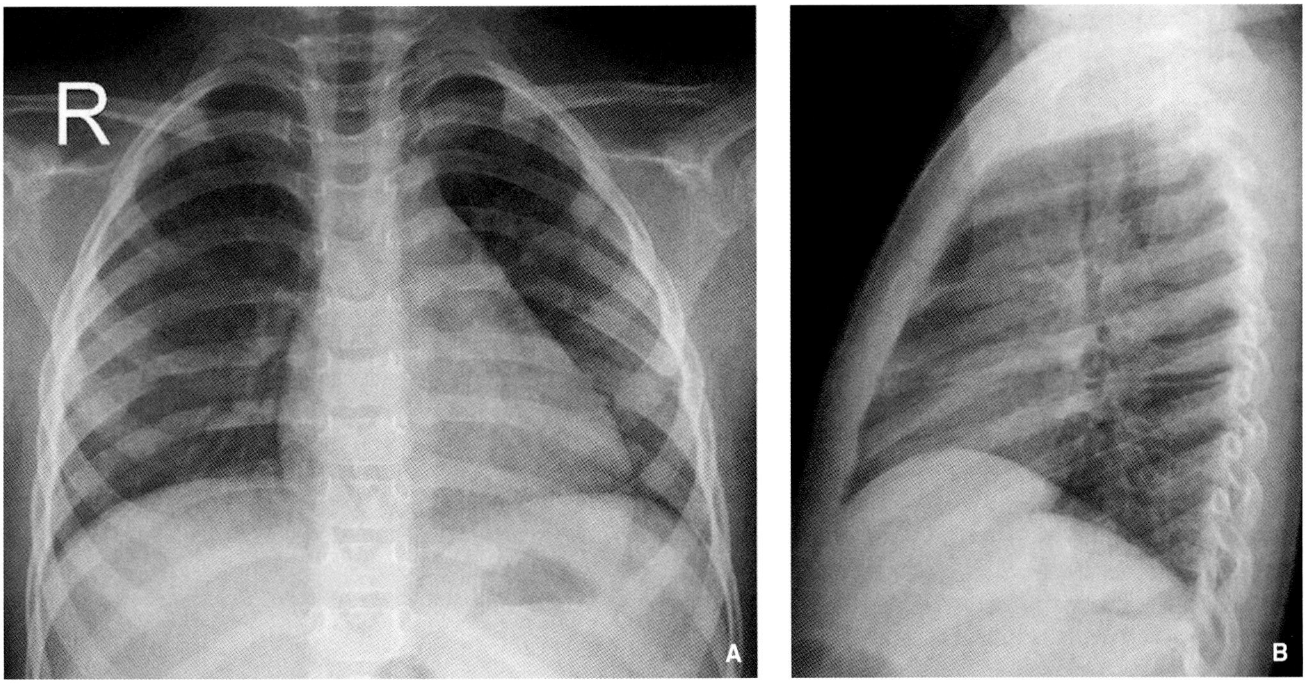

FIGURE 6.1 **Standard chest radiographic views in a 2-year-old boy.** Frontal **(A)** and lateral **(B)** views demonstrate adequate radiographic technique. On the frontal view, the clavicles are equidistant. There is faint visualization of the thoracic vertebral bodies and major vessels through the heart indicative of adequate exposure. At least, eight or nine posterior ribs are noted above the diaphragm indicative of adequate inspiration.

adequate if the thoracic spine, intervertebral discs, and the pulmonary vessels are just faintly visible through the heart shadow. Finally, particular attention should be given to artifacts (e.g., incubator holes, skin folds, bandages and dressing), which could be mistaken for abnormalities.

Changes in the normal appearance of the chest radiograph from neonatal, childhood, and teenage years must be clearly understood. In a neonate, there is a more triangular configuration of the chest with wider AP diameter. Air bronchograms are frequently seen projecting through the cardiac shadow but should be considered pathologic when seen more peripherally. The thymus gland, which is variable in size, gives rise to a prominent anterior mediastinal shadow in infancy, with its characteristic "sail" shape or wavy margins interdigitating with the intercostal spaces.[1] It is important to identify abnormal radiologic signs by systematically reviewing all thoracic organs and systems. Although some chest radiographic findings are pathognomonic for specific conditions, in most cases, the diagnostic process depends upon correlating the chest radiographic findings with the clinical scenario. In some situations, the

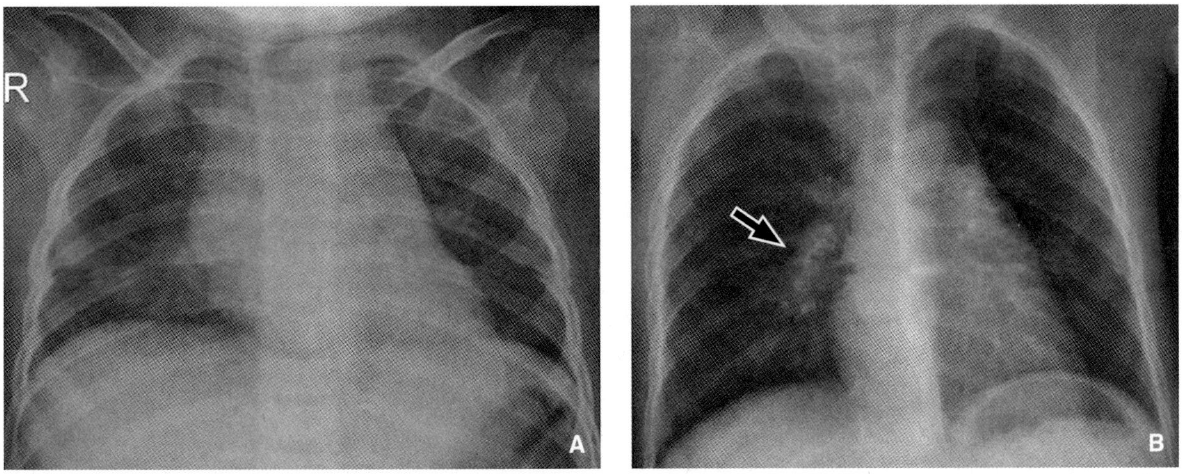

FIGURE 6.2 **Effect of respiratory effort and technique on the chest radiographs. A:** Frontal chest radiograph obtained in expiratory phase demonstrates vascular crowding, often mistaken for airspace disease or pulmonary edema. **B:** Frontal radiograph with patient rotated to the right shows asymmetric lung density with the left side being more lucent. The hilum (*arrow*) becomes more prominent on the side of rotation, which can be mistaken for enlarged hilar lymph nodes.

diagnosis may only be confirmed on follow-up study, based on the observed radiologic signs and clinical features.

Ultrasound

In evaluation of pediatric chest, ultrasound (US) is mainly used for assessing pleural fluid, differentiating simple from complex pleural effusion. Substantial improvements in US have included the use of higher-resolution transducers, tissue-harmonic imaging, color flow technique, and panoramic views, all improving spatial resolution as well as tissue penetration and characterization. In addition, the chest in young children has immature costal and sternal cartilage and thin subcutaneous adipose tissue, which enable increased applicability of US in the evaluation of the pediatric chest. US has various advantages including real-time scanning, no sedation, no specific preparation, and no exposure to radiation. It can be used for planning thoracentesis, thoracotomy, and image-guided drainage.[2] Because of its portability, US can be performed at the bedside, and small children can even be scanned in their parents' arms, reducing anxiety and improving cooperation, which is necessary for optimal imaging.

Optimal frequency of the transducer for chest US varies with age of the patient, anatomic location, and planned approach. Neonates and small infants are easily examined with high-frequency linear transducers, but older children and adolescents require lower-frequency transducers. Smaller sector, vector, or tightly curved array transducers are required in order to insonate between ribs, below the diaphragm, or from the suprasternal notch.[3–5] Real-time focused US is useful in assessing a variety of chest pathologies including superficial lesions when the chest radiograph is negative, diaphragmatic pathologies, characterization and quantification of pleural effusions, and evaluation of the mediastinum.

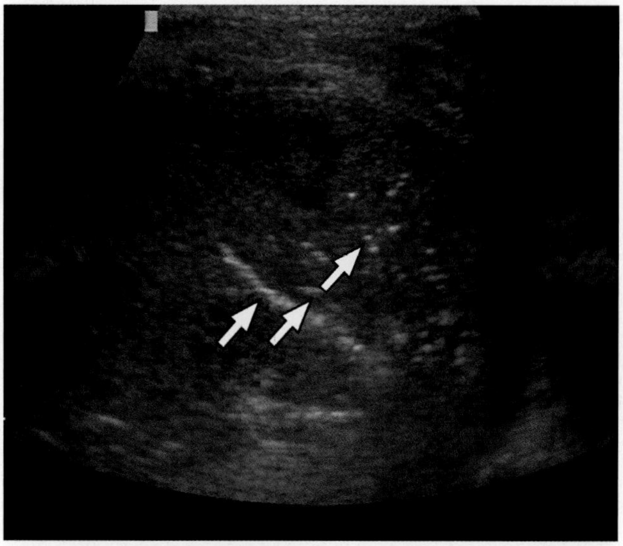

FIGURE 6.3 **Left lower lobe pneumonia in a 4-year-old boy.** Gray scale ultrasound image shows consolidated lung which has similar appearance and echogenicity to those of the normal hepatic parenchyma, a sign termed "hepatization." Linear and branching echogenic densities (*arrows*) correspond to sonographic air bronchograms.

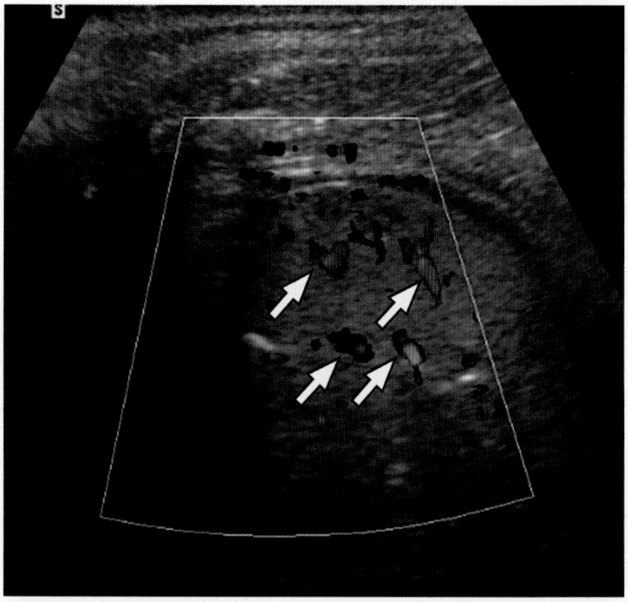

FIGURE 6.4 **Right lower lobe pneumonia in a 3-year-old girl.** Color Doppler ultrasound image shows presence of pulmonary vessels (*arrows*) within an area of pulmonary consolidation.

The lung, which is mostly air, normally absorbs most of the sound waves and causes reverberations. In atelectasis or consolidated lung, the US beam can be transmitted, and imaging shows heterogeneous, low echogenicity similar to the liver (known as lung hepatization). Within the solid-appearing lung, multiple linear-branching bright dots represent air in the bronchi, which are referred to as *sonographic air bronchograms* (Fig. 6.3). Entrapped fluid or mucoid material within bronchi in necrotizing or postobstructive pneumonias produces hypoechoic branching structures, *sonographic fluid bronchograms*. Development of lung abscess from pneumonic consolidation can be readily assessed in US.

Although CT is currently an imaging modality of choice, US can also be utilized in the evaluation of neoplastic masses and various nonneoplastic lung malformations including congenital pulmonary airway malformation (CPAM) and pulmonary sequestration (PS).[3–6] Color flow is helpful in characterization of vascularity and flow pattern within the lesion and adjacent vessels (Fig. 6.4). B lines or comet tail artifacts at the surface of aerated lung in US are believed to represent thickened interlobular septa in interstitial lung disease. These correlate with CT findings of pulmonary fibrosis in children.[7–9]

Computed Tomography

Computed tomography (CT) is a valuable imaging modality in the evaluation of various congenital and acquired lung disorders in infants and children. CT is currently indicated for evaluation of interstitial lung disease, congenital lung malformations, primary and secondary neoplasms, and traumatic injuries. In addition, CT is often used in evaluation of extensive pulmonary infection as well as its complications. CT,

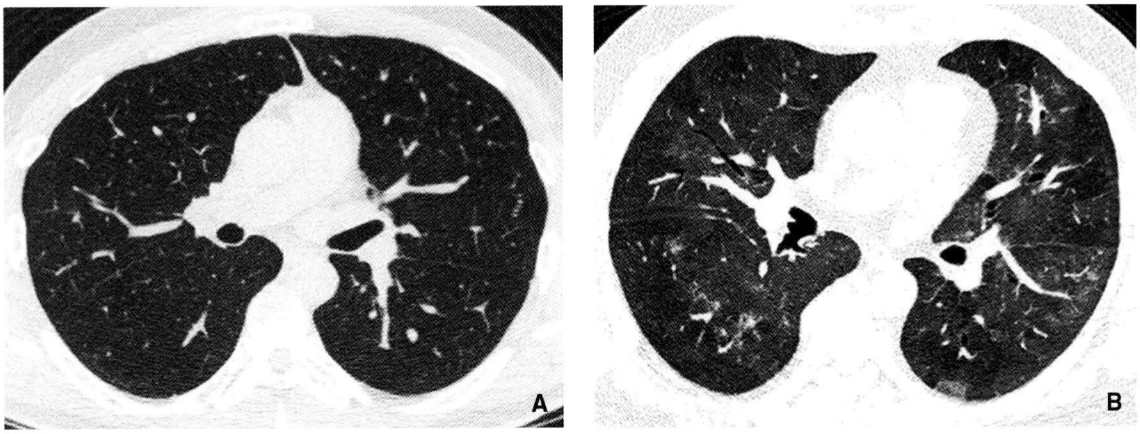

FIGURE 6.5 **CT of normal lung parenchyma and diffuse ground-glass opacification. A:** Axial CT image of lungs shows well-aerated normal lung parenchyma. Patent normal bilateral mainstem bronchi are also seen. **B:** Axial CT image of lungs demonstrates diffuse ground-glass opacities, which were not seen on chest radiographs.

particularly currently available, multidetector CT (MDCT), has the advantage of faster scanning and decreased motion artifact yielding a highly detailed evaluation of the chest in a short period of time resulting in lower rate of sedation, greater optimization of intravascular contrast, and better image quality (Fig. 6.5). This is further enhanced by multiplanar reformats and various 3D rendering techniques[10,11] (Fig. 6.6).

In recent years, the faster MDCT scanners have substantially reduced the rate of sedations, but many children below the age of 5 still may need to be sedated. Neonates and small infants can be scanned during normal sleep or after feeding with proper immobilization.[12] Intravenous administration of nonionic contrast is advisable for most congenital malformations with anomalous vascular component and tumors with a usual dose of 1 to 2 mL/kg with a maximum of 100 mL.[10] Contrast material can be administered by manual or mechanical injection depending on the size, location, and stability of the angiocatheter. Mechanical injection of contrast material is preferred because it provides a reproducible and more homogeneous contrast enhancement.[11]

A thoracic MDCT study with narrower collimation (<1 mm) provides data with isotropic resolution, which results in more detailed images of the lung, airway, mediastinum, and vasculature.[10,13] High-resolution CT (HRCT) is a type of thoracic CT technique where 1-mm noncontiguous scans of the entire chest are obtained every 10- or 20-mm interval. Intravenous contrast is usually not administered, but the images are displayed in high-resolution algorithm for optimal

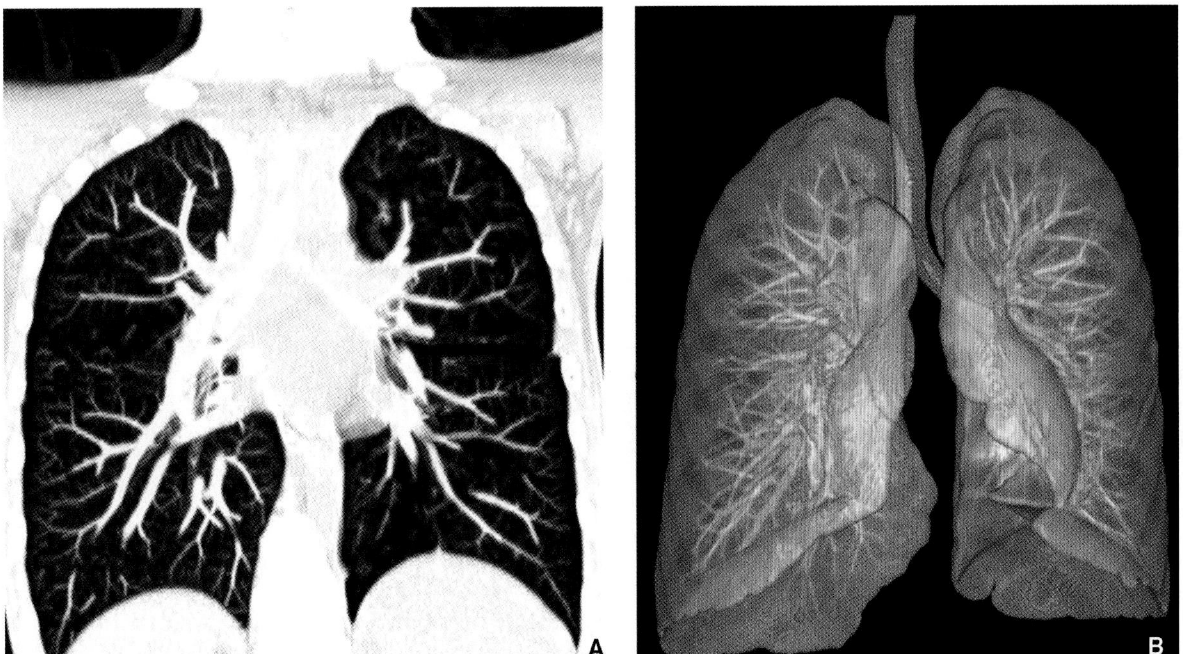

FIGURE 6.6 **Reformatted CT images. A:** Maximal intensity projection reconstruction CT image in coronal view and lung window setting highlights the lung parenchyma in relation to the pulmonary arterial vasculature. **B:** External surface rendered 3D reconstruction CT image of the airways and both lungs.

lung parenchymal detail. HRCT is valuable for the detection and characterization of diffuse lung disorders and chronic lung diseases requiring repeated CT follow-up examinations, for patients with conditions such as interstitial lung disease, chronic infiltrative lung disease, and pulmonary involvement from systemic diseases.[12–14] Chest CT obtained in full inspiration and expiration can be helpful in the evaluation of air trapping often seen in children with underlying small airway diseases; however, it should be used with caution because of the increased overall radiation dose.[12]

Current computer software allows characterization and assessment of pulmonary nodules and masses, which can be performed automatically or semiautomatically by computer-aided diagnosis based on CT densitometry.[15] Advanced imaging applications obtaining quantitative measurement parameters used for functional thoracic imaging are now being performed. These measures, achieved by spirometric monitoring, include lung density, lung volume, airway luminal area, airway wall thickness, and airway wall area.[16] Dual-energy CT lung perfusion and ventilation at a single scanning is another advanced functionality performed on CT scan for the diagnosis of pulmonary embolism and various airway diseases.[17]

Although CT is a valuable imaging modality for assessing various lung disorders in pediatric patients, CT is the main source for the increasing radiation exposure from medical diagnostic imaging, a problem that is particularly pertinent in children, who are more sensitive than adults to radiation.[18] Therefore, it is important to ensure that each CT study performed is clinically justified and that conscious efforts to reduce unnecessary high-dose radiation exposure shall be done according to principle of ALARA (as low as reasonably achievable). Body size-adapted protocols, considering the patient's weight or dimensions, should be taken to account when assigning tube potential (kV) and the product of tube current and time (mAs).[14,19] Recommended kV and mAs for both routine volumetric chest CT examination and HRCT of the lungs are shown in Tables 6.1 and 6.2; it remains the responsibility of the radiologist to further optimize the scanning parameters and ensure that the protocol is customized for the need of each individual pediatric patient. Other CT parameters including collimation, field of view, pitch, reconstruction intervals, scanning time, and exposure factors should be optimized. Furthermore, special filters (present in more advanced CT scanners), automated current modulation options, iterative dose reconstruction, and avoidance of multiphasic CT studies are all helpful in reducing the radiation burden to the pediatric patient.[12]

TABLE 6.1 Recommended Imaging Protocol Guideline for Routine Volumetric Chest CT in Children

Weight	kV	Effective mAs	Rotation Time (s)
<9 kg	80	100	0.5
10–15 kg	100	70	0.5
16–25 kg	100	80	0.5
26–35 kg	100	95	0.5
36–45 kg	100	110	0.5

TABLE 6.2 Recommended Imaging Protocol Guideline for Sequential Chest HRCT in Children

Weight	kV	mAs	Rotation Time (s)
<15 kg	100	50	0.5
16–25 kg	100	60	0.5
26–35 kg	100	70	0.5
36–45 kg	100	80	0.5

Magnetic Resonance Imaging

Magnetic resonance imaging (MRI) has become an established noninvasive modality as a reliable cross-sectional imaging of various organ systems. However, MRI of the lung differs profoundly from imaging other organs because of the lung's inherent low proton density, high loss of signal due to susceptibility, and substantial motion artifacts. Because there is virtually no signal in the lung, a pathologic process with high liquid or proton content is clearly visible on the MRI (Figs. 6.7 and 6.8). This quality is less helpful in pathologic processes also lacking signal, such as air-filled bullae, emphysema, and other cystic structures.[20] Artifacts from cardiac and respiratory motion have been the main reason for difficulty in obtaining reproducible and diagnostic MR images of the lung, but with the help of currently available fast imaging techniques combined with electrocardiograph gating and respiratory gating, pathologic lung lesions have been increasingly thoroughly examined in recent years.[20,21]

Pulmonary diseases involving alveolar infiltration or exudation patterns including pneumonia and pulmonary edema are reliably depicted on MRI[22,23] (Fig. 6.8). Unfortunately, early and subtle interstitial lung diseases are not easily visualized on MRI, and CT remains the superior tool for this indication. Congenital malformations such as PS with an anomalous feeding vessel can be readily imaged by MR angiography, but diagnostic difficulties occur in hybrid lesions with pulmonary malformations that do not have anomalous vessels. There has been a paucity of literature regarding evaluation of primary lung tumors on MRI, but pulmonary metastasis measuring 5 mm and larger has been reliably diagnosed with MRI in the pediatric population.[20,24]

Combining functional studies with morphologic assessment at high spatial and temporal resolution but without the risk of ionizing radiation is a major advantage of MRI. These functional MRI studies of the lungs include measurements of perfusion, blood flow, ventilation, gas exchange, as well as

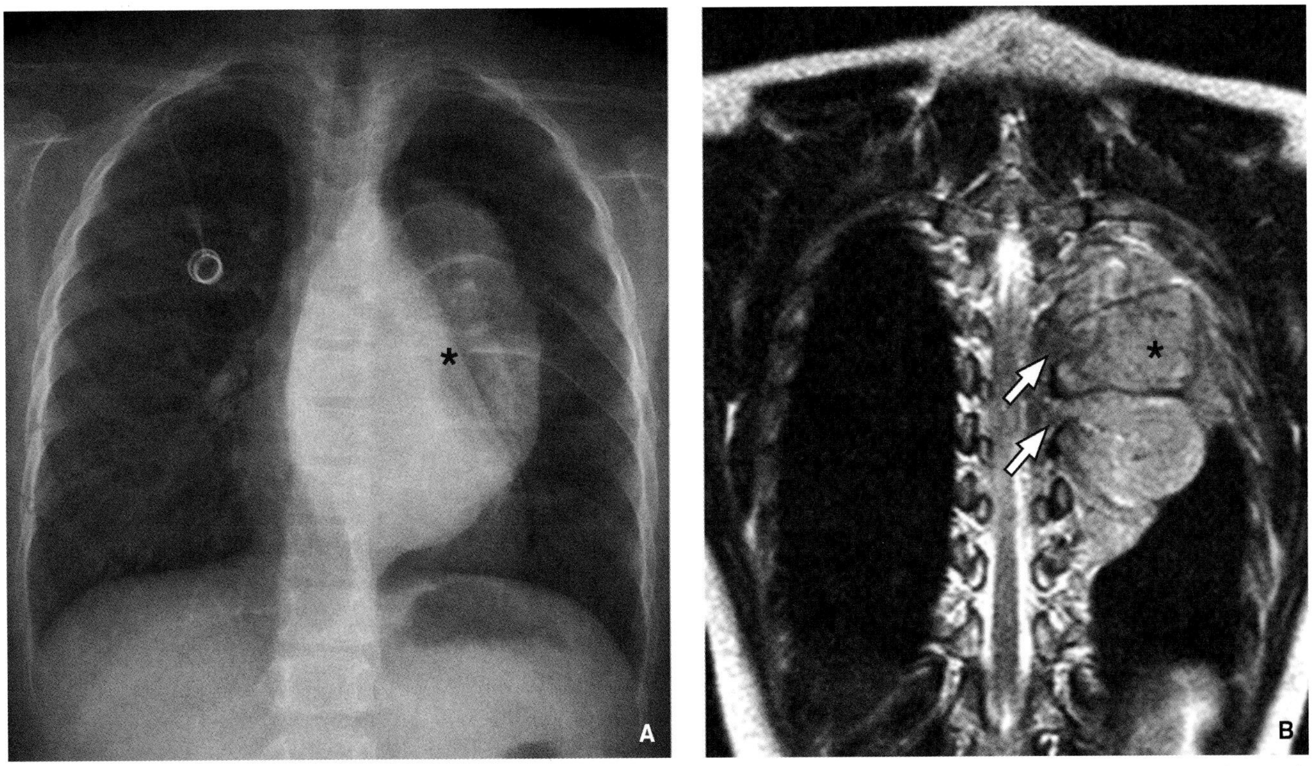

FIGURE 6.7 **Neurogenic tumor on chest MRI in a 5-year-old boy who presented with chest pain. A:** Frontal chest radiograph shows a large left paraspinal region mass (*asterisk*), likely mediastinal in location. **B:** Coronal T2-weighted MR image confirms the neurogenic, posterior mediastinal mass (*asterisk*) that communicates with the exiting thoracic nerve roots on the left (*arrows*).

respiratory motion and mechanics. MRI perfusion imaging, which can be either with or without contrast enhancement, can be performed alone or along with ventilation imaging to create ventilation/perfusion MR imaging.[16,24,25] Oxygen-enhanced imaging evaluates oxygen delivery at the alveolar level, useful in the assessment of a large number of pulmonary diseases.[24] MRI with inhaled hyperpolarized noble gases helium-3 (^{3}He) and xenon-129 (^{129}Xe), which provides both structural and functional pulmonary measurements, is currently being performed in some imaging centers with polarizer availability.[16,24,25]

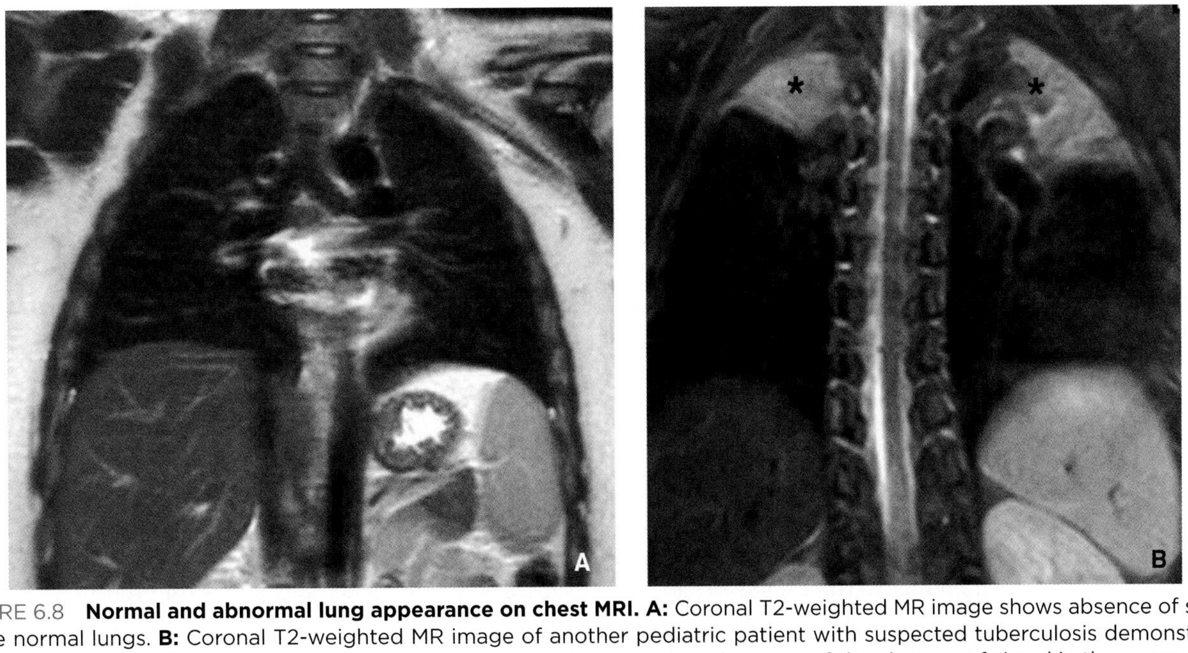

FIGURE 6.8 **Normal and abnormal lung appearance on chest MRI. A:** Coronal T2-weighted MR image shows absence of signal in the normal lungs. **B:** Coronal T2-weighted MR image of another pediatric patient with suspected tuberculosis demonstrates pulmonary consolidations (*asterisks*) on both upper lobes, which stand out because of the absence of signal in the surrounding normal lung parenchyma.

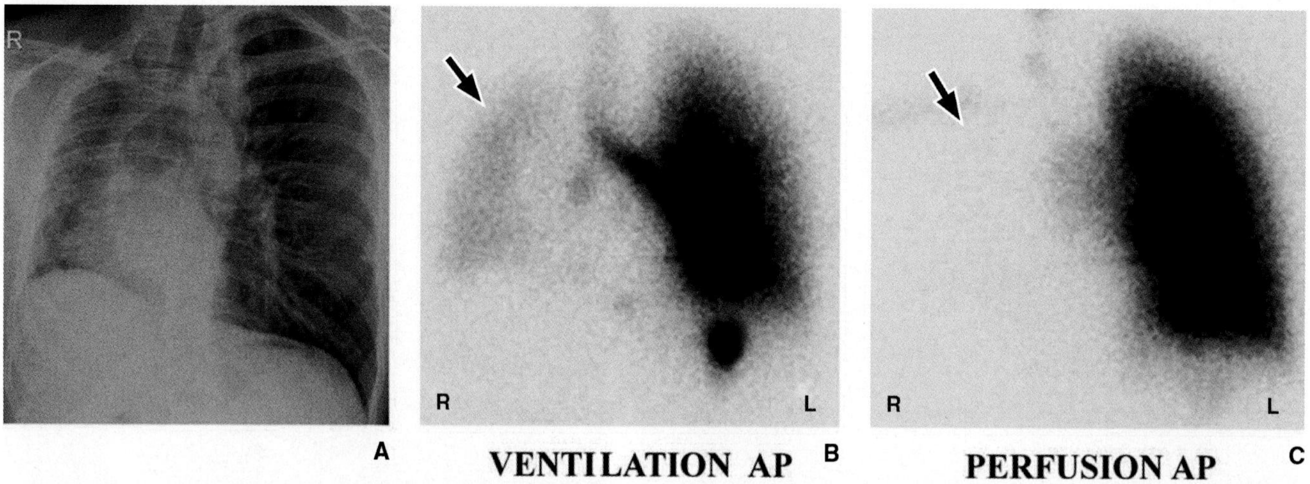

FIGURE 6.9 **Ventilation and perfusion nuclear medicine scan in a 7-year-old girl with congenital venolobar syndrome.** **A:** Frontal chest radiograph shows diminished right lung volume. **B:** Ventilation scan with technetium 99m DTPA aerosol shows normal ventilation on the left lung, but ventilation to the right lung is diminutive (*arrow*). **C:** Perfusion scan with technetium 99m MAA shows normal perfusion to the left lung, but there is complete absence of perfusion on the right lung (*arrow*).

Nuclear Medicine

Nuclear medicine studies such as scintigraphy as well as positron emission tomography (PET) and PET/CT are currently widely used in the pediatric patients. Scintigraphic methods are available for imaging and quantifying both lung ventilation (V) and perfusion (Q), and pulmonary embolism remains an important indication for this study. Other indications of V/Q scintigraphy in children include quantitative evaluation of differential and regional lung perfusion in children with congenital heart disease, evaluation of lung volumes and ventilation in pediatric patients with bronchial or parenchymal lung diseases, and identification of ventilation/perfusion mismatches in pediatric patients with developmental or acquired lung disease.[26,27]

The radiopharmaceutical for lung perfusion scans is technetium 99m labeled macroaggregated albumin (^{99m}Tc-MAA) with particle size of 20 to 100 μm. The distribution of ^{99m}Tc-MAA within the lungs reflects differential and regional blood flow, and quantitative assessment of lung perfusion can be performed. The particles have a biologic half-life of a few hours and have essentially no physiologic effect on normal lung function. The average number of injected particles is 500,000 in adult dose, but in children, the number of particles should be adjusted to the age or weight to keep the number of particles as low as possible.[28] For the ventilation part of the test, the use of radiolabeled aerosolized particles such as ^{99m}Tc-labeled diethylenetriamine pentaacetic acid (DTPA) is the most commonly used radiopharmaceutical because of the fast renal clearance, which lowers the radiation burden.[29] Because aerosolized DTPA persists in the lung airways, images can be acquired in multiple projections, but dynamic ventilation studies cannot be performed[30] (Fig. 6.9). Xenon (^{133}Xe) is an inert gas that is also used for imaging lung ventilation. ^{133}Xe gas can be administered successfully to patients with limited cooperation, such as infants, and to patients intubated with an endotracheal tube (ETT). The ^{33}Xe ventilation scan is generally performed prior to the perfusion exam, as downscatter from the Tc-99m would severely degrade image quality. The advantage of xenon exam is the ability to obtain single breath, equilibrium, and washout images providing a better evaluation of ventilation and better sensitivity for obstructive lung disease.[27,29]

The clinical introduction of PET and PET/CT has transformed the clinical practice of nuclear medicine and molecular oncologic imaging, where ^{18}F-FDG has been widely used for diagnoses, staging, follow-up, and assessing the response to therapy for nearly all forms of malignancy. FDG PET is usually not able to detect small (<1 cm) pulmonary tumors or lung metastases, but many of the primary malignant lung tumors of children have been demonstrated to be FDG avid. For most lung lesions in children, FDG PET usually is not the primary diagnostic tool, but can be useful for staging and posttreatment follow-up.[26]

NORMAL ANATOMY AND NORMAL VARIANTS

Normal Lung Development

Development of lung starts as early as 3 weeks of embryonic life and continues into postnatal life up to early adulthood. The events of antenatal growth and development of human lung have traditionally been divided into five stages, namely, embryonic (0 to 6 weeks in utero), pseudoglandular (6 to 16 weeks in utero), canalicular (16 to 28 weeks in utero), saccular (28 to 34 weeks in utero), and alveolar stages (36 weeks in utero to 2 years).

At around 3 to 4 weeks of embryonic life, the lung develops as an outgrowth of the ventral wall of the primitive foregut, the laryngotracheal groove. At around the 5th week, the trachea branches into the right and left main bronchi and subsequently into lobar and segmental bronchi. During the pseudoglandular stage, there is further branching of the airway, and by the end of this stage, there is already formation of all nonrespiratory components of the bronchial tree

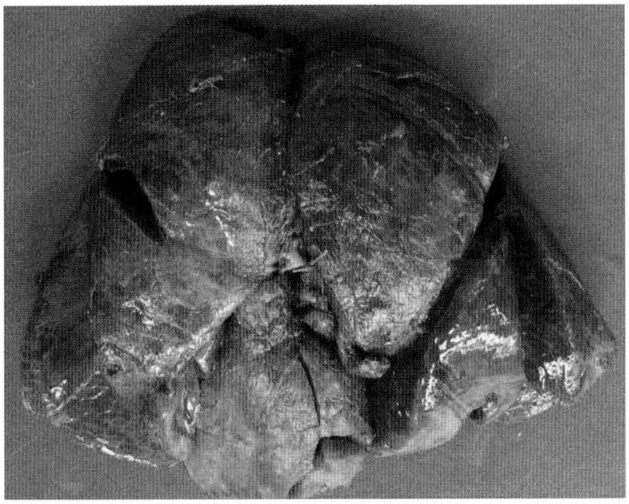

FIGURE 6.10 **Abnormal lobation, trilobed left lung, in a 3-month-old boy with heterotaxy syndrome (asplenia complex).** In this image, the heart and lungs show fibrous adhesions due to previous surgery for complex congenital heart disease.

including conducting airways and terminal bronchioles. The formation of early pulmonary parenchyma and the respiratory bronchioles, alveolar ducts, and primitive alveoli characterize the canalicular or acinar stage. It is also during this stage that type I and II pneumocytes are differentiated, and by the end of 24 weeks, surfactant is already detectable. Between 28 and 36 weeks of gestation, division of the airways is almost complete with further dilatation of the acinar tubules and early development of true alveoli. The alveolar phase of lung development extends from ~36 weeks' gestation until ~2 years postnatal, but most alveolarization occurs within 5 to 6 months following delivery at term. The alveolar multiplication continues in the postnatal period at least up to the age of 2 to 3 years, and alveolar size and surface area increase until after adolescence.[31–33]

Lobes, Fissures, and Variations

The lungs have the general shape of a half cone. Both are contained within their own pleural sac and separated from each other by the mediastinal pleura and structures of the mediastinum. Each lung is attached by its root and pulmonary ligament to the heart and trachea but is otherwise free in the thoracic cavity. Each lung extends from the apical portion in the base of the neck, above the clavicles, to the most inferior basal portion resting on the corresponding hemidiaphragm. They are bordered by the mediastinal surface anteriorly where the two lobes almost meet and at the costovertebral gutter posteriorly. The right lung is usually wider than the left, but has less vertical extent because the dome of the right hemidiaphragm is higher. The right lung has three lobes, and the left has two, with occasional exceptions to this rule (Fig. 6.10).

Interlobar fissures are depressions that extend from the outer surface of the lung to its inner and hilar regions. The lung is covered by the visceral pleura, extending deep into the fissures, which separates the adjacent lobes. The right major fissure originates posteriorly from the lower margin of T4 posteriorly to the sixth costochondral junction anteriorly. A minor or horizontal fissure is seen only on the right that begins at the midaxillary line of the major fissure and runs horizontally to the level of the fourth costal cartilage. The right major fissure separates the right upper and middle lobes from the right lower lobe, whereas the right minor fissure separates the right upper and middle lobes (Fig. 6.11).

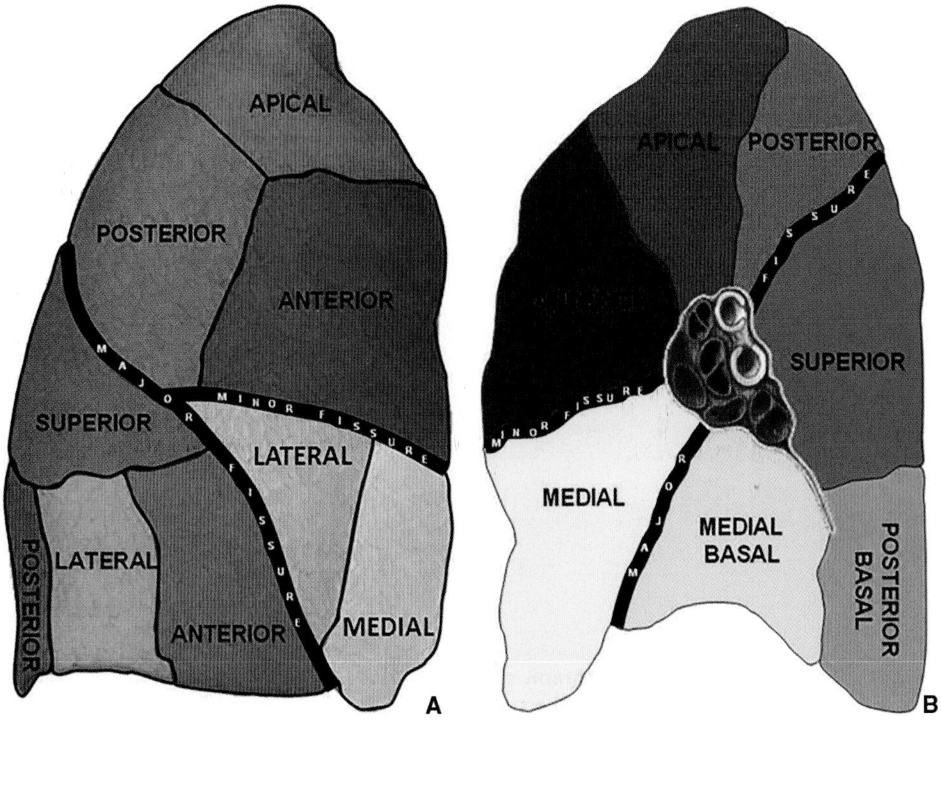

FIGURE 6.11 **Schematic representation of the (A) lateral and (B) medial surfaces of the right lung shows the major and minor fissures, lobes, and bronchopulmonary segments.**

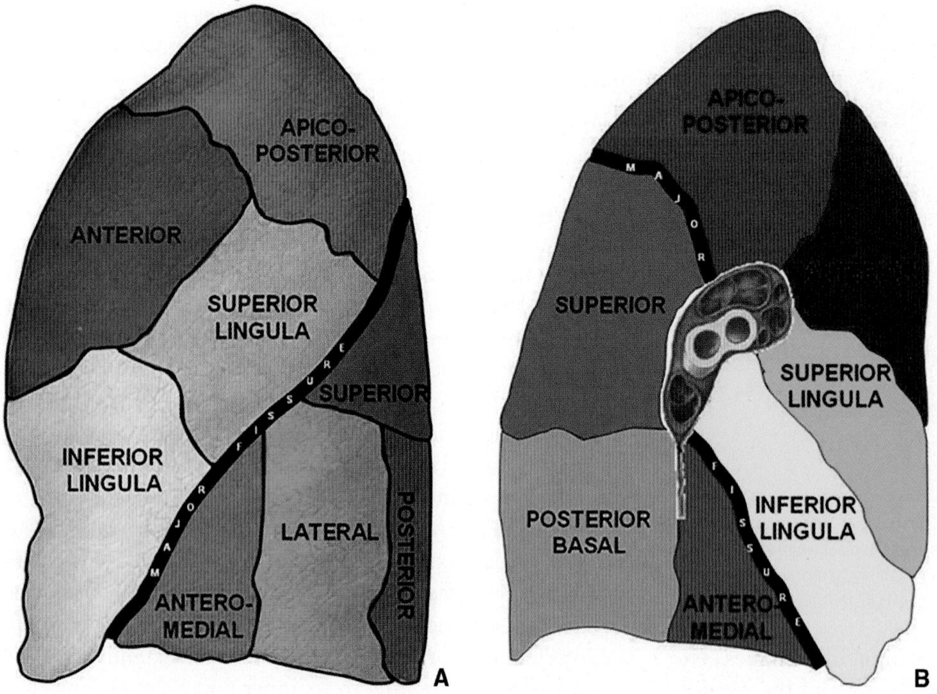

FIGURE 6.12 **Schematic representation of the (A) lateral and (B) medial surfaces of the left lung shows the major fissure, lobes, and bronchopulmonary segments.**

The left major or oblique fissure originates at the T3 level posteriorly and follows the path of the sixth rib extending anteriorly. The left major fissure separates the left lung into upper and lower lobes (Fig. 6.12).

Variations of the interlobar fissural anatomy occur even in healthy individuals. Incomplete or interrupted fissures are often seen with areas of parenchymal fusion between the lobes. There is significant proportion of the population with fissural variations and degrees of adjacent lobar fusion.[34,35] Accessory fissures are occasionally seen, which form the accessory lobes or segments. On occasion, such fissures are visible as linear shadows on the chest radiograph. Examples are the cardiac lobes formed by accessory intersegmental fissure in the medial basal segments (Fig. 6.13), the azygos lobe caused by the arch of azygos vein creating a depression in the right upper lobe (Fig. 6.14), and the left minor fissure.[36–38]

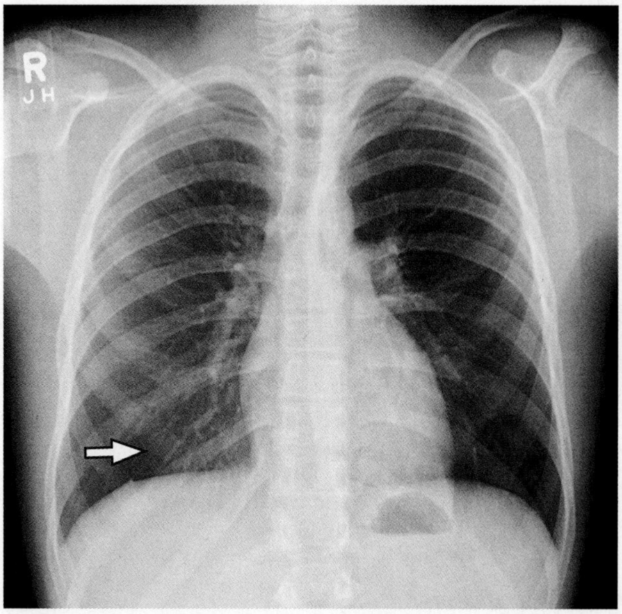

FIGURE 6.13 **Frontal chest radiograph shows an intersegmental accessory fissure (*arrow*) in the right lower lobe.**

Bronchopulmonary Segment (Anatomic Unit of the Lung)

The bronchopulmonary segment is the anatomic unit of the lung. This unit possesses its own bronchus (third-order bronchus), pulmonary arterial, venous, and lymphatic systems. Bronchopulmonary segments can be removed individually without disturbing the function of adjacent segments. It was Jackson and Huber in 1943[39] that initially proposed a simple and consistent system of nomenclature on bronchopulmonary segments. In 1949, the Thoracic Society of Great Britain formed a committee with the task of defining the anatomy and establishing a standard nomenclature on bronchopulmonary segments.[40] Subsequently, in 1989, the latest Nomina Anatomica nomenclature for the lung segments was published that is essentially similar to Jackson and Huber's but the numerical designation for the upper lobes slightly vary.

The right upper lobe bronchus divides into three segmental bronchi supplying the apical, the anterior, and the posterior segments, respectively. The middle lobe bronchus gives rise to two segmental bronchi and corresponding lateral and medial segments. The first bronchial branch of the right lower lobe is the superior segmental branch supplying the superior segment. The rest of the right lower lobe bronchus terminates into four basal bronchi to supply four

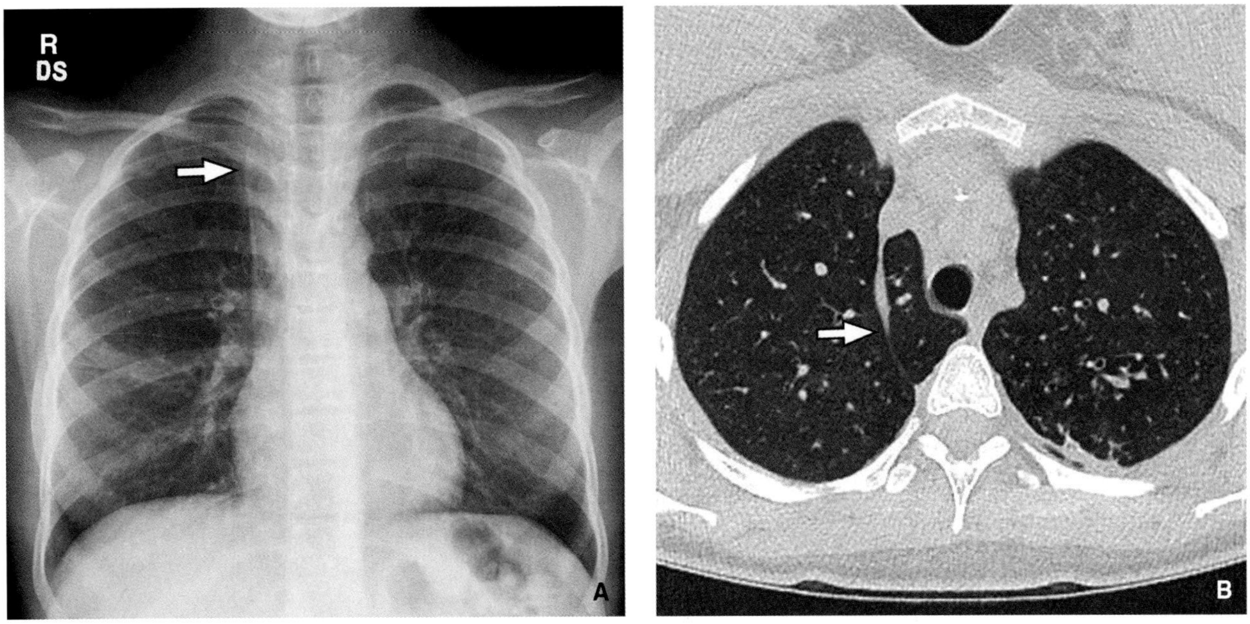

FIGURE 6.14 **Azygous fissure.** Frontal chest radiograph **(A)** and axial CT image **(B)** show an azygous fissure (*arrow*), a developmental variant.

basal segments: medial basal, anterior basal, lateral basal, and posterior basal segments (Fig. 6.11).

The left upper lobe bronchus bifurcates into superior and inferior trunks. The superior trunk supplies the anterior and apicoposterior segments whereas the inferior trunk supplies the lingula, and gives rise to the superior and inferior lingular segments. The lingula is the anteroinferior projection of the left upper lobe and is considered the middle lobe equivalent. The first branch of the left lower bronchus supplies the superior segment whereas the remaining trunk of the left lower lobe bronchus gives rise to the common anteromedial basal, lateral basal, and posterior basal bronchus and corresponding segments. Because of the common segmental branching by subsegmental bronchopulmonary units (apicoposterior segment of the left upper lobe and anteromedial basal segment of the left lower lobe), the left lung has a total of 8 segments (compared to 10 on the right lung) (Fig. 6.12).

Each bronchopulmonary segment is pyramidal in shape with its base at the pleural surface and the apex pointing toward the center of the lung. Each segment is surrounded by a connective tissue covering that is an extension of the pleural surface. A segmental bronchus is located in the middle of each segment and gives two to three subsegmental bronchial branches. There is further branching of the subsegmental bronchi until it reaches the pulmonary lobule, which is the physiologic unit of the lung. Segmental pulmonary arterial branches are also seen in the middle of a lung segment just posterior to its accompanying segmental bronchi. The pulmonary lymphatic drainage pathway courses alongside the segmental arteries and bronchi and into the subsegmental and segmental nodal stations. One main segmental vein drains each bronchopulmonary segment, which courses along the intersegmental planes, and provides delineation from each individual segment.[36]

Pulmonary Lobule (Physiologic Unit of the Lung)

The secondary pulmonary lobule refers to the smallest fundamental unit of lung structure. It is demarcated by connective tissue septa, and it can be conceptualized as a miniature lung complete with airways, pulmonary arteries, veins, lymphatics, and interstitium. It is variable in size, ranging from 1 to 2.5 cm in diameter, and has an irregular polyhedral shape.[41,42] The main components of the secondary pulmonary lobule are the interlobular septa and septal structures, the centrilobular region, and the lobular parenchyma. The interlobular septa are bands of fibrous connective tissue that extend inward from the pleural surface.[42,43] Branches of the pulmonary veins and lymphatics lie within the interlobular septa. When the septa are not clearly visible, their locations can be inferred by identifying septal pulmonary vein branches. The centrilobular region contains the lobular bronchiole or preterminal bronchiole, which supplies the pulmonary lobule. It gives rise to smaller terminal bronchioles, and respiratory bronchioles. The central portion of the lobule also contains the intralobular artery and bronchiolar branches that supply the lobule, as well as lymphatics and supporting connective tissue (Fig. 6.15).

Thin-section HRCT shows a linear, branching, or dot-like opacity in the center of a lobule that represents the intralobular artery branch or its divisions. The intralobular bronchioles are not readily seen on CT, and their visibility depends on their wall thickness rather than diameter. The vasculature within the interlobular septa is supported by a fine network of connective tissue stroma[42,43] (Fig. 6.16). Each secondary pulmonary lobule is usually made up of 3 to 24 variably sized pulmonary acini.[44] Each acinus ranges 6 to 10 mm in size and is where most of the gas exchange occurs in the lungs. The acinus includes the

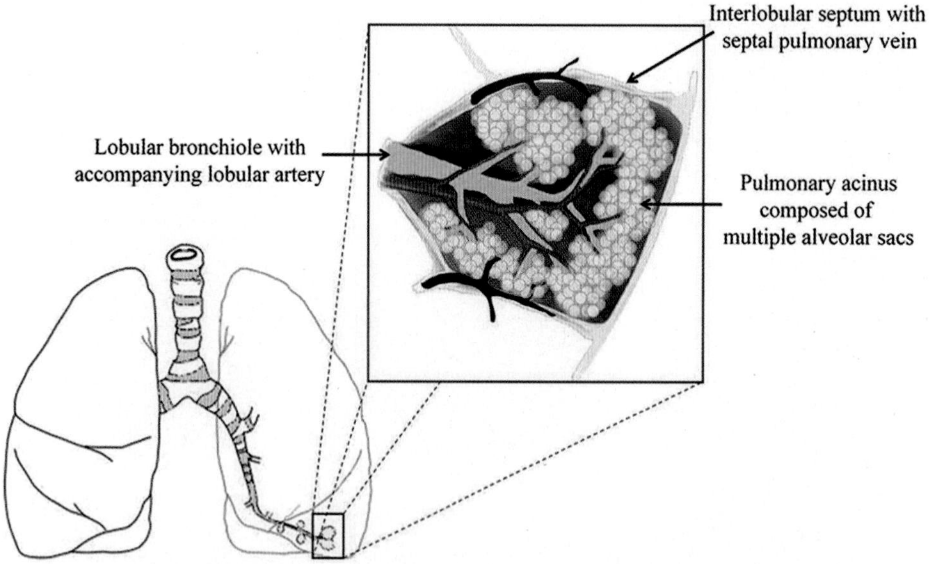

FIGURE 6.15 **Diagrammatic depiction of the lung and the secondary pulmonary lobule (inset) with its components.**

respiratory bronchioles (primary and secondary), the alveolar ducts, and the alveolar sacs. Respiratory bronchioles, distal continuations of the terminal bronchioles, have progressively more alveoli in their walls with successive distal generations. The last conducting structure, the alveolar duct, is entirely lined by alveoli. The alveolar ducts terminate in alveolar sacs, which are globular aggregations of adjacent alveoli.[45–47]

SPECTRUM OF LUNG DISORDERS

Congenital and Developmental Anomalies

Congenital lung malformations consist of a spectrum of vascular, parenchymal, and/or bronchial developmental abnormalities with an estimated annual incidence ranging from 30 to 42 cases per 100,000 population.[11] They can be detected prenatally, in infancy or later in childhood, or even in adult life.[11,12] With recent advances in prenatal imaging evaluation, detection of asymptomatic congenital lung malformations has been increasing in frequency, but many also present with acute respiratory distress or recurrent infections in older children.

There are currently four main postulated theories regarding the development of congenital pulmonary malformations: (1) defective foregut budding, differentiation, and separation; (2) airway obstruction; (3) vascular abnormality; and (4) genetic cause. These proposed mechanisms may act alone or in combination.[11] Defective budding, differentiation, and separation of the primitive foregut, which occur early in the tracheobronchial tree development between 24 and 36 days of gestation, are believed to be the most frequent causes of the congenital pulmonary malformations.[48–50] Another proposed etiology is airway obstruction with development of pulmonary dysplastic changes,[51] where the spectrum of pathologic manifestations depends on the degree, variability in the timing, location, and extent of airway obstruction.[52] Vascular abnormality has also been frequently suggested as an underlying cause of congenital pulmonary anomalies, including absent pulmonary artery associated with pulmonary agenesis.[50] More recently, underlying genetic mechanisms have been implicated, specifically those related to impairment in the signaling pathways responsible for airway development.[53,54] Given the diversity of congenital pulmonary malformations, it is likely that the etiology

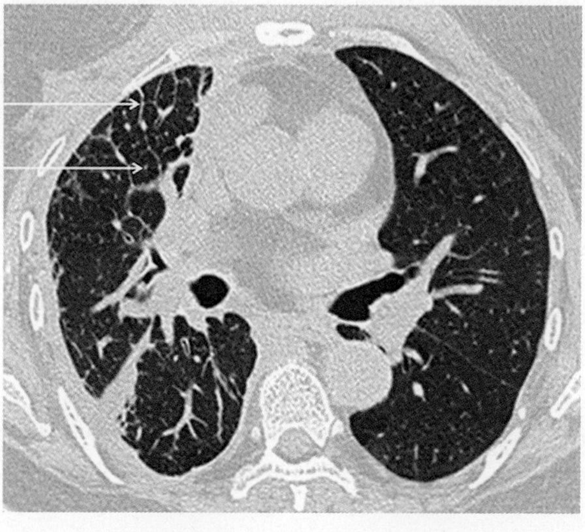

FIGURE 6.16 **HRCT image shows an abnormal right lung depicting individual pulmonary lobules bordered by the thickened interlobular septa.** Within the central portion of the lobule is a dot-like structure representing the lobular artery. Notice that the interlobular septa are difficult to visualize on a normal CT image, as seen on the left lung for comparison.

is multifactorial, representing a combination of the four postulated theories.[55]

There have been several ways of classifying congenital pulmonary malformations depending on embryology, morphologic appearance, or radiologic manifestations. Some malformations represent abnormalities or anomalies with primarily single component such as congenital lobar emphysema (CLE) (parenchymal abnormality), arteriovenous malformation (AVM) (vascular abnormality), foregut duplication cyst (foregut anomaly), and bronchial atresia (airway anomaly), but they can also involve two or more components with various degrees of involvement[56] (Fig. 6.17). PS is an example of a complex malformation that can have both pulmonary and vascular anomalies.

Imaging evaluation plays a crucial role in prompt and accurate diagnosis of these congenital lung malformations. Advances in both prenatal and postnatal imaging have also improved our knowledge of the etiology, onset, timing, and course of these congenital pulmonary malformations.[11] Congenital pulmonary malformations are increasingly detected with prenatal US because of its routine use in prenatal care. Advances in fetal MRI in recent years also played a role in detecting and understanding these malformations in utero.[57] Postnatally, chest radiograph remains very helpful for screening of symptomatic or asymptomatic patients, but advanced imaging modalities such as CT and MR imaging are used for confirmation and further characterization of congenital pulmonary malformations.

Bronchial Atresia

Bronchial atresia, also known as bronchial mucocele, is a congenital lung lesion typically characterized by stenosis or obliteration of subsegmental, segmental, or lobar bronchus, with peribronchial emphysema. As a result, there is accumulation of mucus distal to the bronchial narrowing, accounting for the term "mucocele."[58,59] The upper lobe bronchi are more frequently affected, and the middle and lower lobe bronchi are rarely affected.[60,61] The exact cause of bronchial atresia is unknown, but it is hypothesized to be due to intrauterine ischemia leading to focal bronchial interruption.[62,63] Bronchial atresia has been seen in patients with concomitant intralobar PS, CPAM, and CLE (also known as congenital lobar overinflation [CLO]), which reaffirms the possible etiologic association of this group of congenital lung malformations.[52,63,64] Bronchial atresia is often discovered incidentally on postnatal imaging because it is typically asymptomatic. However, affected pediatric patients may present with recurrent infections or respiratory compromise.[51,52,63,64]

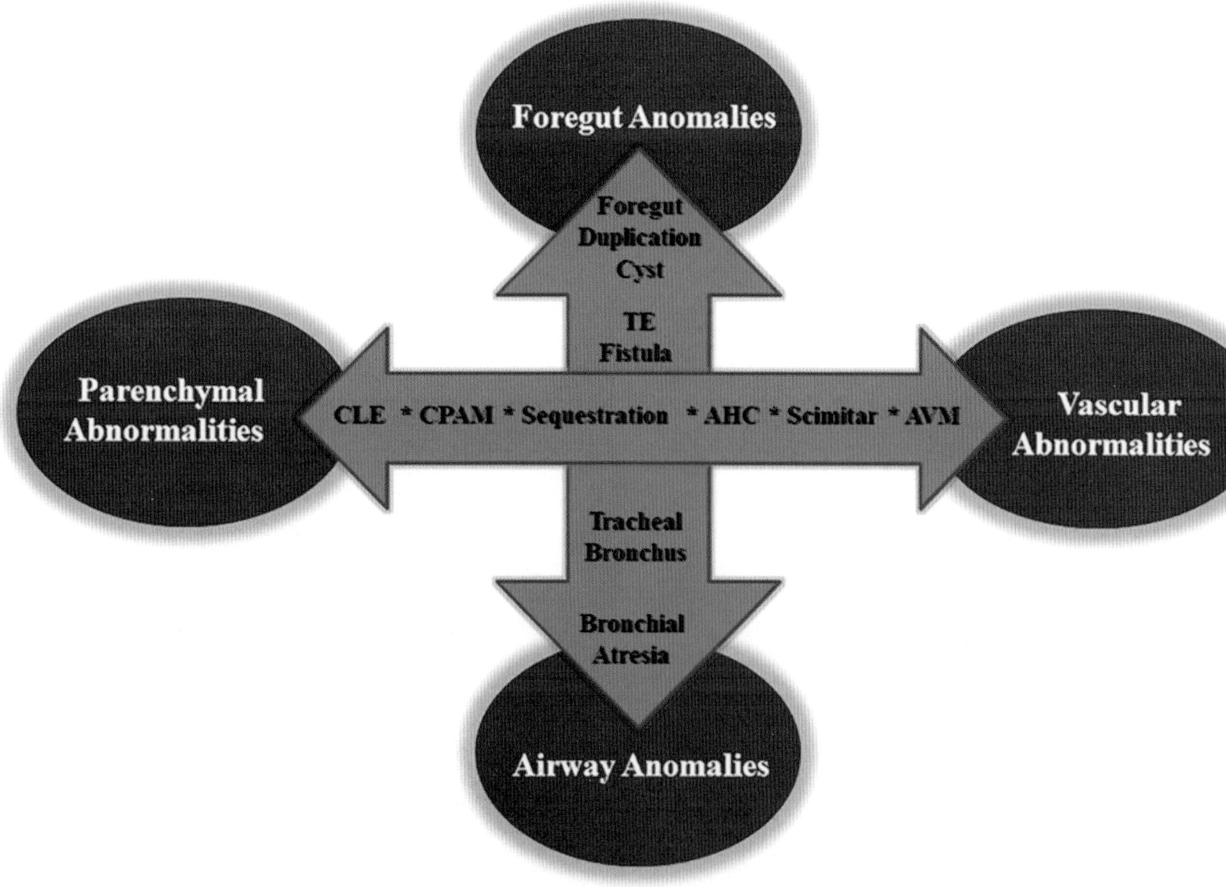

FIGURE 6.17 **Diagram depicting the spectrum of congenital pulmonary malformations.** These malformations represent a continuum of four principal components including pulmonary, foregut, vascular, and airway anomalies (*red circle*). Malformations can contain only one major component such as CLE, congenital lobar emphysema; CPAM, congenital pulmonary airway malformation; AHC, aplasia-hypoplasia complex; or AVM, arteriovenous malformation. TE, tracheoesophageal.

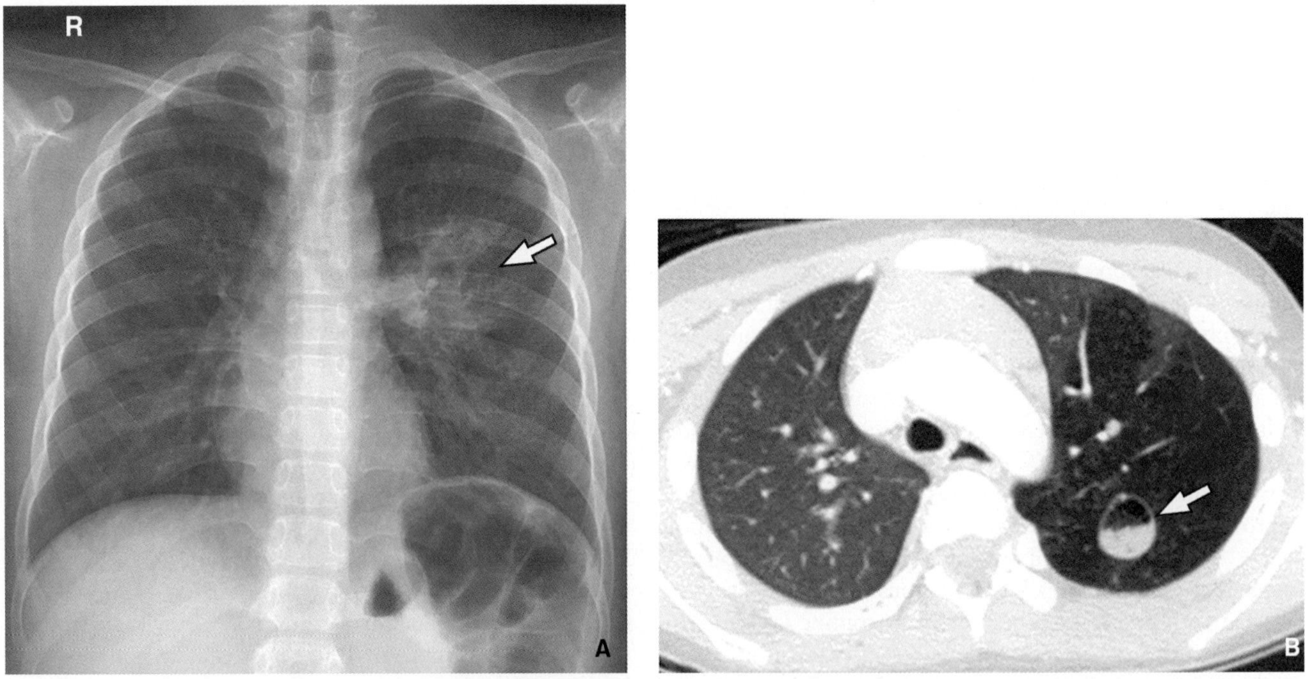

FIGURE 6.18 **Bronchial atresia in a 7-year-old boy who presented with recurrent pneumonia. A:** Frontal radiograph demonstrates a hazy opacity (*arrow*) in the left upper lobe. **B:** Axial lung window CT image obtained after a course of antibiotic therapy shows a rounded lesion (*arrow*) with air–fluid levels and surrounding hyperlucency in the left upper lobe.

Bronchial atresia typically appears as an oval, tubular, or branching structure that is of increased echogenicity on prenatal US and homogenously high signal intensity on T2-weighted images on MR. On chest radiograph, it appears as a round or oval-shaped opacity typically located in the apical or apicoposterior segment of the upper lobes, which represents impacted mucus within the dilated bronchus ("mucocele"). MDCT with both 2D and 3D reconstructions can accurately demonstrate the dilated round, oval, or tubular-shaped bronchial mucocele, typically seen at the hilar aspect of an adjacent area of hyperlucency with decreased vascularity (Fig. 6.18). The associated surrounding hyperlucency is attributable to collateral ventilation through intra-alveolar pores of Kohn, bronchoalveolar channels of Lambert, and interbronchiolar channels, with "air trapping" as well as a component of maldevelopment.[11,65,66]

There is currently substantial debate regarding the treatment of bronchial atresia. For some, the management of choice is usually surgical resection, even in asymptomatic patients, because of the increased risk of infection.[67] Others believe that treatment should be conservative, with regular chest radiograph follow-up, with surgery reserved for patients with severe or recurrent infection or ineffective medical treatment. If surgery is required, minimally invasive thoracoscopic surgery and, if possible, local resection should be performed as a first option.[63]

Bronchogenic Cyst

Bronchogenic cysts are developmental anomalies, thought to arise from abnormal budding of the tracheobronchial tree during airway development between the 26th and 40th days of fetal life. This ectopic or supernumerary bud subsequently differentiates into a blind-ending pouch, typically filled with mucus[68] (Fig. 6.19). These cysts are a part of the spectrum of foregut duplication cysts that include bronchogenic cysts, enteric cysts, and neurenteric cysts. Around 70% of bronchogenic cysts are located in the mediastinum at the subcarinal, hilar, or right paratracheal locations, but they can also be intraparenchymal in location, particularly in the lower lobes (14%). When intraparenchymal, they may be better conceived of as a congenital or acquired mucocele/sequestration than as a type of foregut duplication cyst. Rarely, bronchogenic cyst can be seen in the neck, pericardium, or abdominal cavity.[61,69–71] These cysts may contain fluid, air, or both. Most bronchogenic cysts are found incidentally. Symptomatic pediatric patients usually present with chest pain, dysphagia, and respiratory distress, if

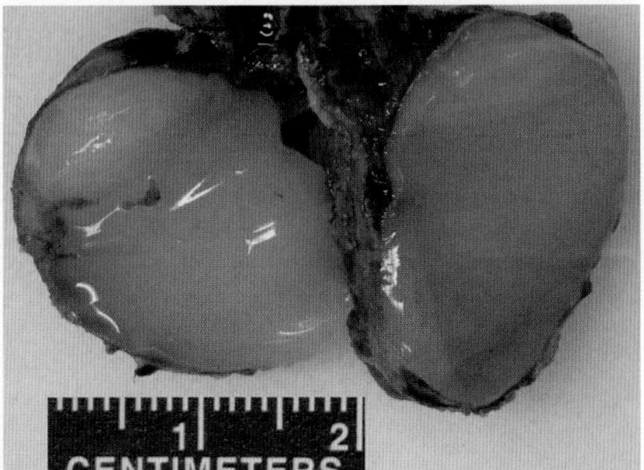

FIGURE 6.19 **Bronchogenic cyst from a 12-year-old boy.** The cut surface shows accumulated pale mucus. Microscopic examination (not shown) confirmed the presence of respiratory mucosa and occasional mural cartilage plates.

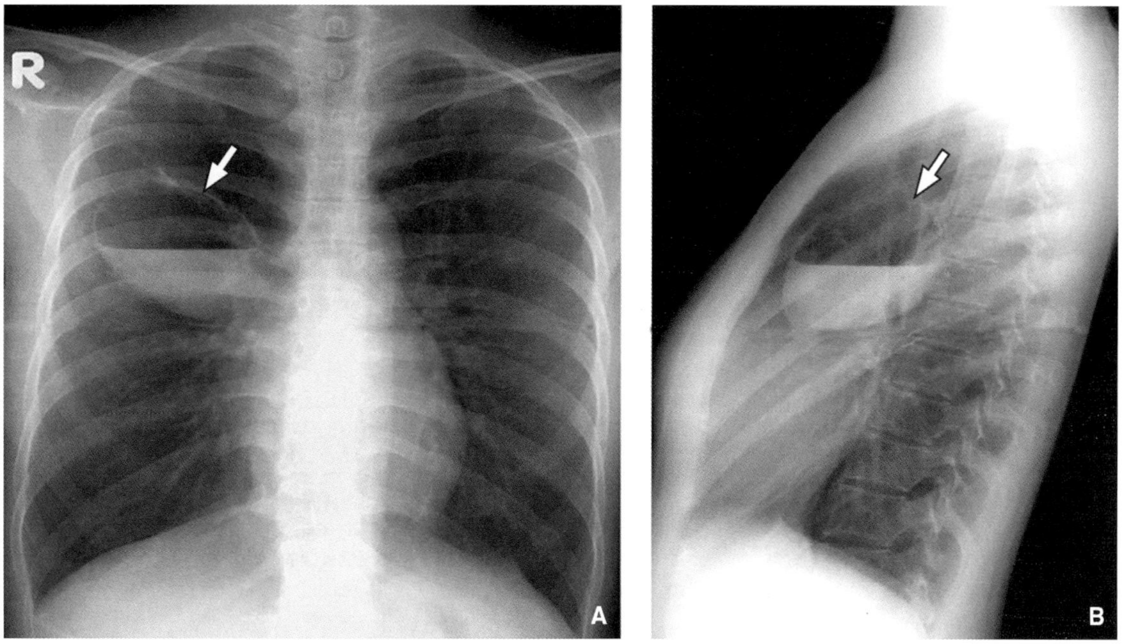

FIGURE 6.20 **Bronchogenic cyst in an 8-year-old boy who presented with persistent cough and chest pain.** Frontal **(A)** and lateral **(B)** chest radiographs demonstrate an oval-shaped, well-circumscribed, thinly marginated lesion (*arrow*) in the right upper lobe with air–fluid level.

the lesion causes a mass effect on the adjacent esophagus and airway. Mediastinal bronchogenic cysts usually do not communicate with the bronchial tree, but intrapulmonary bronchogenic cysts often have a bronchial communication, which may be responsible for recurrent infections. Infected bronchogenic cysts are more often seen in older children.[11,72]

The typical radiographic appearance of a bronchogenic cyst is a round or oval, well-circumscribed, noncalcified mass located within the middle mediastinal compartment. It can be lucent if air filled or there can be air–fluid levels[61,70,71] (Fig. 6.20). The lesion is hypoechoic on US, indicating internal fluid content. On CT, bronchogenic cysts usually appear as well-defined fluid density lesions, although they can have higher attenuation than water density due to proteinaceous debris from mucoid material or previous hemorrhage[60] (Fig. 6.21). On MRI, bronchogenic cysts demonstrate high

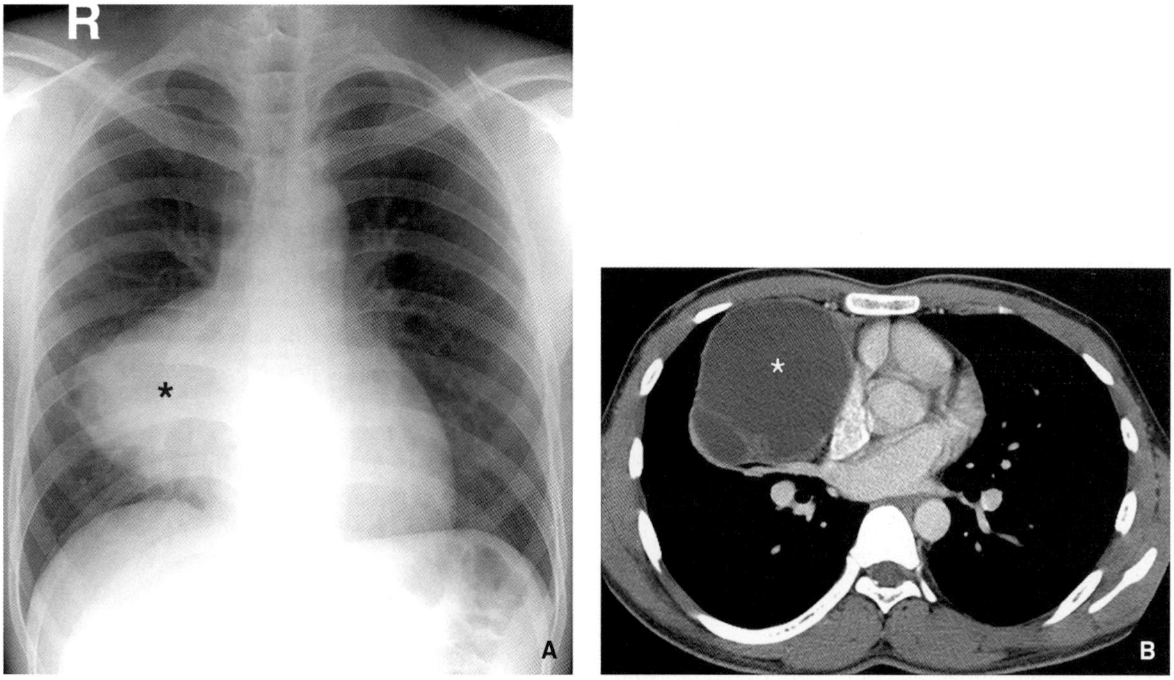

FIGURE 6.21 **Bronchogenic cyst in a 9-year-old boy who presented with chest pain and shortness of breath. A:** Frontal chest radiograph shows a large, rounded soft tissue mass (*asterisk*) adjacent to the right cardiac border. **B:** Axial enhanced CT image demonstrates a large, rounded, well-circumscribed, and fluid-filled mass (*asterisk*) with minimal peripheral septations, proven to be a bronchogenic cyst.

signal intensity on T2-weighted MR images, but signal is variable on T1-weighted MR images depending on the internal contents of the cyst.[73] Normally, no intracystic enhancement is seen on CT or MR images following contrast administration, although minimal enhancement of the wall may be present.[55] Associated septations are occasionally seen.[55,71] The presence of air–fluid level, thick enhancing wall, and surrounding inflammatory changes are clues to infected bronchogenic cysts.[71,74]

The current appropriate management for bronchogenic cyst is complete or partial surgical resection, especially in pediatric patients with repeated infections. Percutaneous or transbronchial needle aspiration, although not a definitive treatment, may reduce mass effect and may help minimize the incision size during subsequent resection.[11,61,75]

Congenital Pulmonary Airway Malformation

CPAM is the most common congenital lung malformation, with an incidence of 1:25,000 to 1:35,000 live births, and representing 30% to 47% of fetal thoracic lung lesions.[51,57,76,77] Also known as congenital cystic adenomatoid malformations (CCAMs), CPAMs are a group of congenital cystic and noncystic lung masses characterized by proliferation of distal airway-like structures and suppression of normal alveolar formation resulting in a cystic gross appearance[78,79] (Fig. 6.22). They are usually unilateral and confined to a single lobe (95%) but can rarely be seen bilaterally.[80] In the majority of CPAMs, blood supply is from the pulmonary artery and venous drainage is into the pulmonary vein. The lesion may communicate with the proximal airways, although this communication is abnormal.[59,61]

Affected pediatric patients usually present with respiratory difficulty or superimposed infection between the neonatal period and 2 years of age unless previously detected by prenatal imaging studies. Given the strong association of CPAM-like changes with bronchial atresia, the postulated etiology of intrauterine obstruction of the airway has become increasingly well accepted.[53,64,81] CPAM's atretic bronchi are continuous with the proximal tracheobronchial tree, and CPAMs do not have a systemic arterial supply; however, CPAM-like parenchymal changes may be seen in PS, which is distinguished from CPAM by the presence of its systemic arterial supply.[59] "Hybrid lesions" are further discussed under the Pulmonary Sequestration section of this chapter.

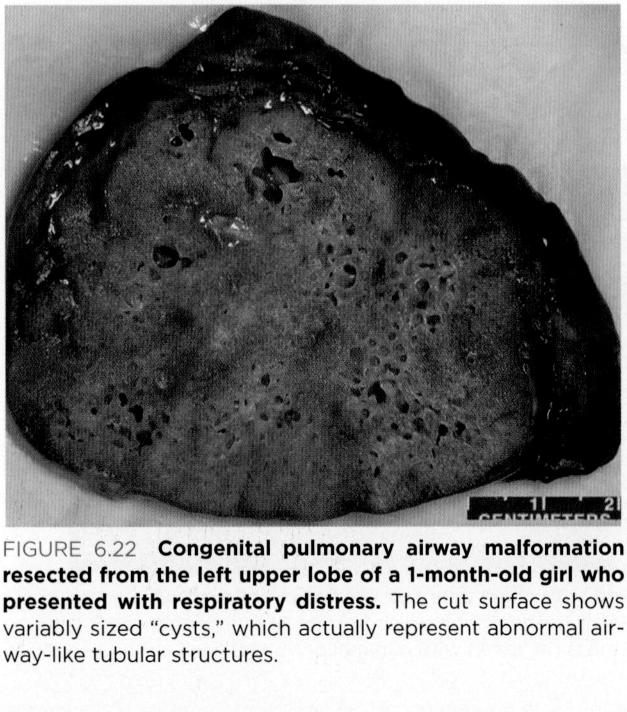

FIGURE 6.22 **Congenital pulmonary airway malformation resected from the left upper lobe of a 1-month-old girl who presented with respiratory distress.** The cut surface shows variably sized "cysts," which actually represent abnormal airway-like tubular structures.

The most recent CPAM classification by Stocker, which consists of five types,[78] is an expansion of his original CCAM classification and is mainly based on the cyst size and histologic resemblance to segments of the developing bronchial tree and airspaces. Type CPAM 0 is characterized by acinar dysgenesis or dysplasia of the trachea or bronchus involving all lung lobes, and therefore is not compatible with life. Type 1 CPAM is characterized by single or multiple cysts (>2 cm) resembling bronchi or bronchioles. Type 2 CPAM is characterized by single or multiple cysts (≤2 cm) resembling bronchioles. Type 3 CPAM is predominantly solid "adenomatoid" tissue with small cysts (<0.5 cm) resembling bronchioles and alveolar ducts. Type 4 CPAM is characterized by large air-filled cysts resembling distal acini.[11,55,78,82] Type 0 CPAM (acinar dysplasia) is histologically and biologically quite distinct from the other types. In practice, types 1 to 4 CPAM may be difficult to distinguish from each other grossly and histologically.

The radiologic features of CPAM types 1 to 4 depend on the content, size, and number of "cysts", which actually consist of malformed thin-walled airway-like tubular structures. Chest radiograph typically shows multiple air-filled thin-walled cysts of varying sizes. At birth, these cysts are fluid filled, but later as the cysts aerate, air–fluid levels may appear.[33,75] Some lesions are not readily apparent on radiographs, and either CT or MRI would more accurately identify and characterize the lung malformation. A solid component of the lesion may also be seen. Type 0 CPAM, which is incompatible with life, is not usually imaged. Type 1 CPAM presents with either one or two dominant cysts larger than 2 cm, amidst a few smaller cysts. Type 2 CPAM usually presents with multicystic mass, with cysts ≤2 cm in diameter. Type 3 CPAM appears solid at imaging because the cysts are microscopic and can only be identified through histologic evaluation (Fig. 6.23). Type 4 CPAM usually presents as very large cysts with lobar expansion or sometimes with pneumothorax, causing mass effect and mediastinal shift. A predominantly cystic pleuropulmonary blastoma (PPB) can mimic in particular types 1 and 4 CPAM.[83,84] In pediatric patients with infected CPAM, fluid-filled cysts with air–fluid levels along with thick contrast enhancement of the cystic walls can be seen[4,11,55] (Fig. 6.24).

In infected CPAM, US-guided percutaneous drainage can alleviate mass effect or enhance the treatment of infection, with delay of surgical resection until after resolution of a pneumonia.[4] Surgical resection by either lobectomy or segmentectomy is the current management of choice for CPAM in symptomatic patients.[75,85,86] For asymptomatic infants and children, there is no consensus on when surgery is indicated.[4] Important justifications for resection include recurrent infections and complications as well as difficulty in distinguishing between CPAM and PPB.[84] Because PPB is often familial and is known to be

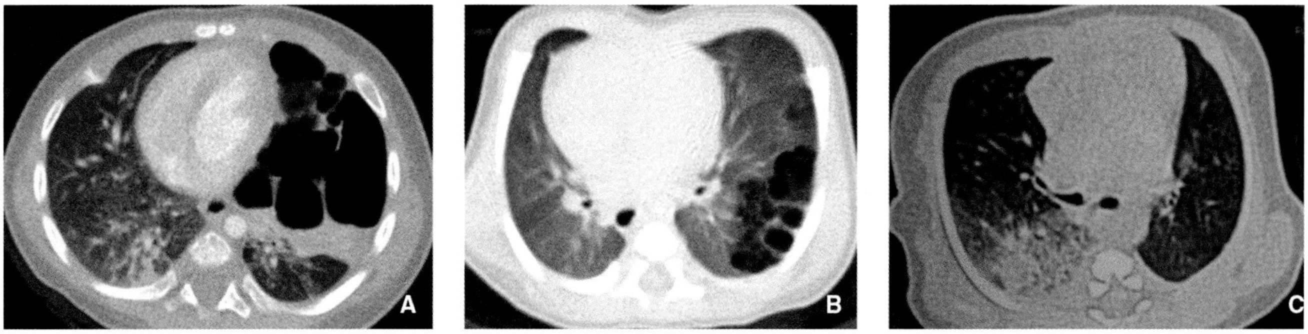

FIGURE 6.23 **Spectrum of congenital pulmonary airway malformation (CPAM) lesions on CT. A:** Axial lung window CT image demonstrates multiple, large (>2 cm) cystic lesions in the left lower lobe compatible with type 1 CPAM. **B:** Axial lung window CT image shows multiple small (≤2 cm), air-filled, cystic lesions are seen in the posterior basal segment of the left lower lobe consistent with type 2 CPAM. **C:** Axial lung window CT image demonstrates an opacity on the right lower lobe with some areas showing tiny cystic changes. This finding had been persistent on successive follow-up studies and was later proven to be type 3 CPAM.

associated with mutations in the *DICER1* gene, family history and/or genetic testing may help with surgical decision-making.

Congenital Lobar Emphysema

CLE, also called as congenital lobar overinflation (CLO) or infantile lobar emphysema, is a progressive lobar hyperinflation anomaly due to overdistension of the alveoli[14,61,87,88] (Fig. 6.25). It can be associated with either intrinsic and/or extrinsic bronchial obstruction or inherent defect in bronchial wall anatomy and structure.[14,61,87,88] The incidence of CLE is 1 in 20,000 to 1 in 30,000 births.[33,89]

There are two types of CLE distinguished histologically based on the number of alveoli: the hypoalveolar and polyalveolar types. Hypoalveolar type has fewer than expected number but markedly overdistended alveoli, whereas there is threefold to fivefold greater than expected number of alveoli in the polyalveolar type. In polyalveolar CLE, the hyperinflation of the lobe is due to the increase in number of normally inflated air spaces.[90] Pediatric patients affected with hypoalveolar type CLE typically present in the first 6 months of life with respiratory distress due to mass effect and compression of the affected hyperinflated lobe upon the adjacent lung and mediastinal structures.[14,61,72]

Chest radiograph in CLE initially shows opacity from fetal lung fluid retention. As the fluid is reabsorbed and replaced by air, lobar hyperinflation results causing a mass effect on the adjacent lung and mediastinal structures (Fig. 6.26). On CT, there is visualization of attenuated vessels indicative of reduced vascularity within the overinflated lung segment, along with effacement of adjacent structures and mediastinal shift[14,61,72] (Fig. 6.27). The left upper lobe is the most frequently affected (42%), followed by the right middle (35%) and right upper lobe (21%).[51,56,76,80,91] Rarely, CLE may show bilateral or multifocal involvement.[92] It is important to have a clear understanding of the imaging features of CLE because it may be confused with pneumothorax or a congenital or acquired lung cyst.

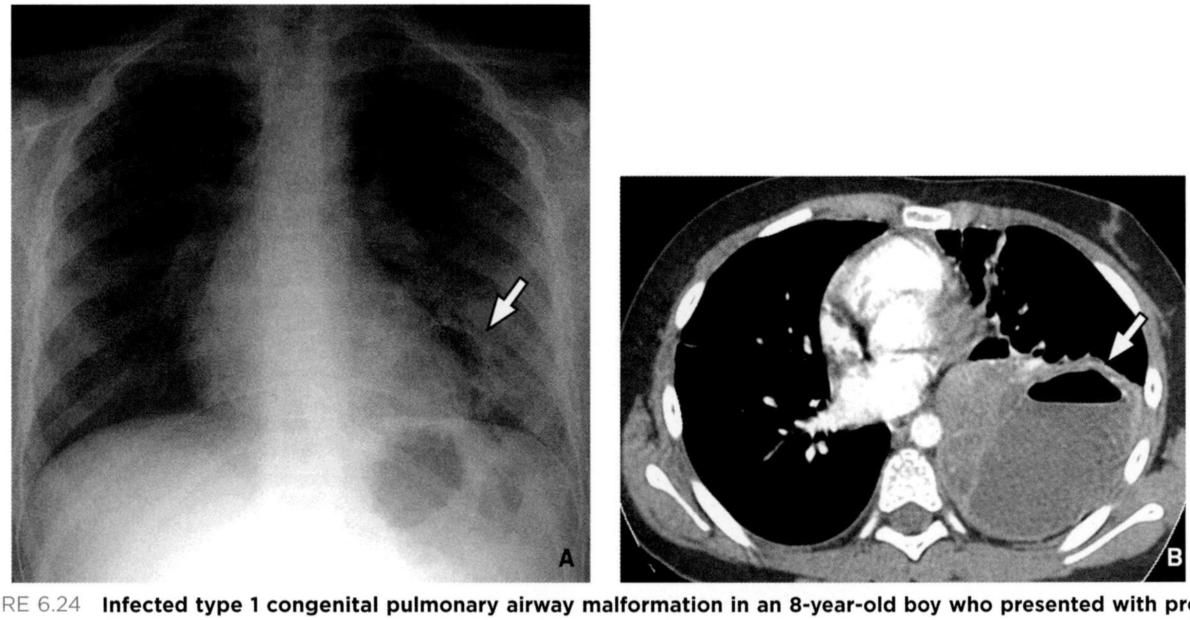

FIGURE 6.24 **Infected type 1 congenital pulmonary airway malformation in an 8-year-old boy who presented with productive cough, high fever, and recurrent pulmonary infections. A:** Frontal chest radiograph shows a cystic structure (*arrow*) in the left lower lobe with hazy opacity of the adjacent lung parenchyma. **B:** Axial enhanced CT image obtained a few days after chest radiograph **(A)** shows a large cystic lesion (*arrow*) in the left lower lobe with air-fluid levels, thick margins, and septations.

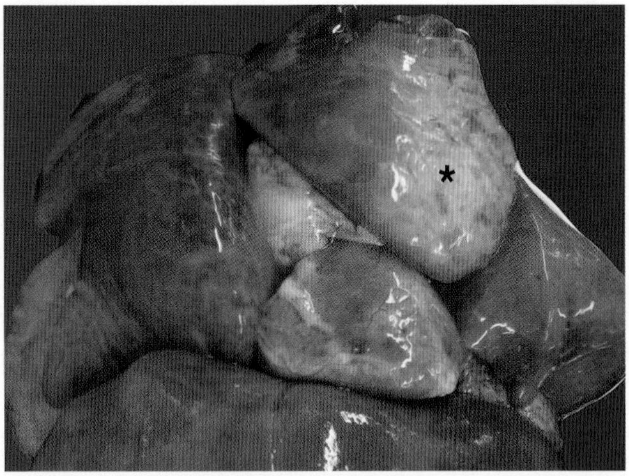

FIGURE 6.25 **Congenital lobar emphysema identified at autopsy in a 12-month-old boy with multiple congenital anomalies.** The affected left upper lobe is pale and hyperexpanded (*asterisk*).

Treatment options for CLE depend on the clinical presentation of patients. Asymptomatic children or those with only mild symptoms may be managed conservatively with continuous follow-up as some studies showed gradual reduction in size of the lesion. For symptomatic children, lobectomy by open or thoracoscopic approach is the current management of choice.[86,88,93,94]

Pulmonary Sequestration (Including "Hybrid Lesion")

PS is characterized by nonfunctioning lung parenchyma, which does not communicate with the tracheobronchial tree and receives blood supply from systemic artery. PS is believed to be due to abnormal budding of the primitive foregut and is often associated with bronchial atresia.[52] Anatomically, it can be classified as intralobar (75%) and extralobar (25%) PS.[33,56,59,61,95]

Intralobar PS lies within visceral pleura, intimately connected to the adjacent lung, and usually occurs in the posterobasal segment of the lower lobe. The arterial supply is from the abdominal or thoracic aorta, and venous drainage is usually through the ipsilateral inferior pulmonary veins, into the left atrium (Figs. 6.28 and 6.29). Intralobar sequestrations communicate with adjacent lung parenchyma through the pores of Kohn, which allow infection to occur; resolution is incomplete or slow because of inadequate bronchial drainage.[33,56,59,61,95] Clinically, intralobar sequestration often presents as recurrent pneumonia in adolescents and adults.[75]

Extralobar PS is most commonly seen in infants. It is surrounded by its own pleura and is usually located near the left lower lobe. The arterial supply is via the thoracic or abdominal aorta, and the venous drainage is usually via the systemic veins (Figs. 6.28, 6.30, and 6.31). The sequestered lobe may cause substantial arteriovenous shunting, leading to high-output cardiac failure.[33] The location of 77.4% of these lesions is between the diaphragm and the lower lobe, whereas 9.7% are in an infradiaphragmatic location.[33,96,97] Extralobar sequestration is commonly associated with other congenital anomalies including congenital diaphragmatic defect, chest wall and vertebral deformities, hindgut duplications, and congenital heart disease.[33,72] Extralobar PS usually manifests early in infancy with chronic cough and respiratory distress.[75]

Most intralobar and extralobar PSs show the same parenchymal maldevelopment that is typical of CPAM. The term "hybrid lesion" has been applied to this phenomenon, which has been attributed to the bronchial atresia common to both CPAM and PSs[33,54,97–99] (Fig. 6.32). Typically, these PSs with CPAM-like parenchymal maldevelopment have a better prognosis compared with a true CPAM, which lacks systemic feeding vessels.[100,101]

Radiologic findings of PS vary depending on the type, presence of other congenital malformations such

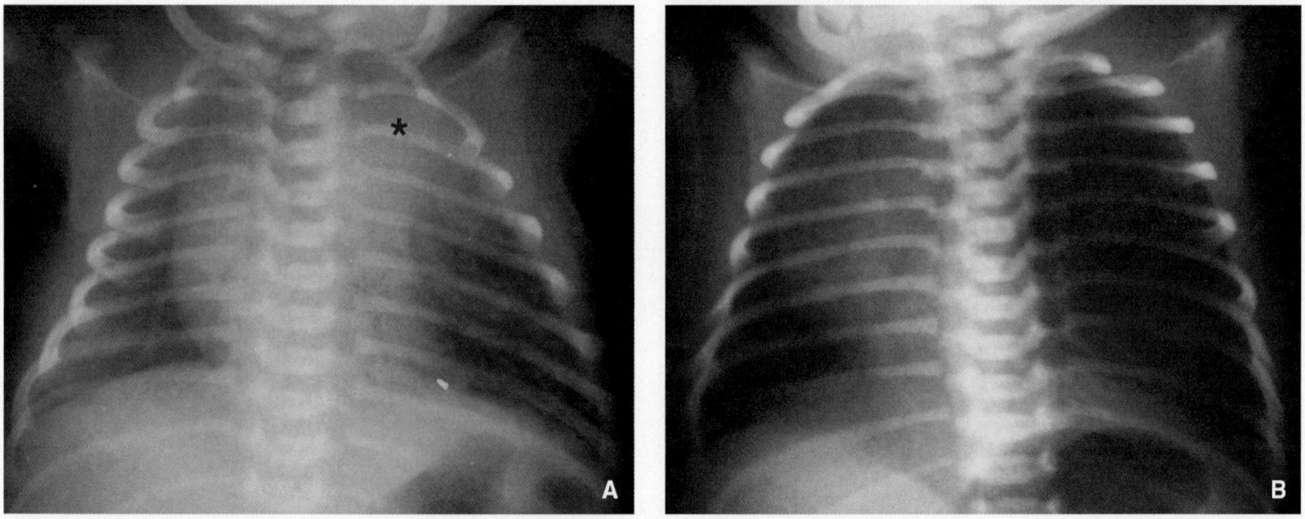

FIGURE 6.26 **Congenital lobar emphysema in an afebrile neonate who presented with tachypnea. A:** Frontal chest radiograph shows a nonspecific opacity (*asterisk*) in the left upper lobe. **B:** Follow-up frontal chest radiograph obtained 5 days later shows that the opacity was replaced by hyperlucency with cardiomediastinal shift to the right.

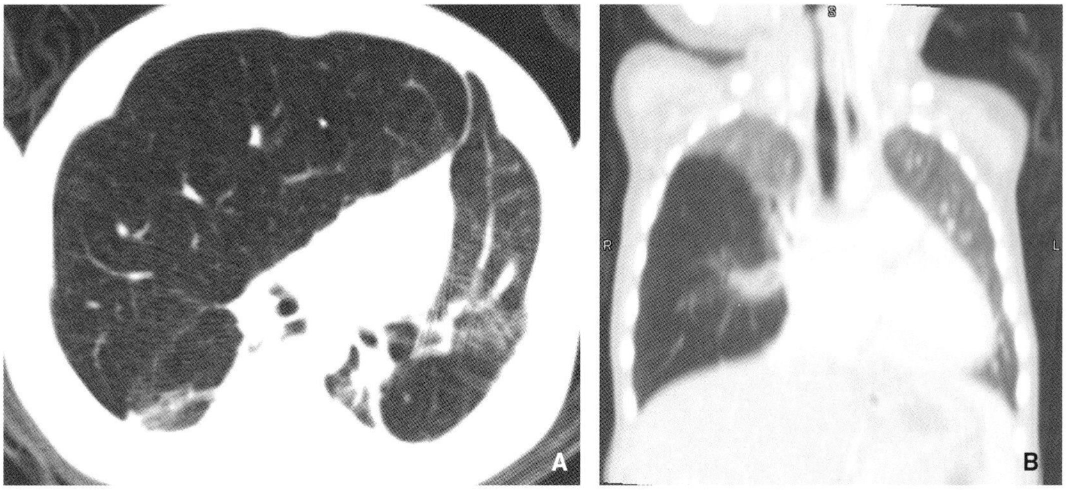

FIGURE 6.27 **Congenital lobar emphysema in a neonate who presented with respiratory distress. A:** Axial lung window CT image shows hyperaeration of the right middle lobe with cardiomediastinal shift to the left. There are attenuated pulmonary vessels in the hyperaerated lungs. **B:** Coronal reformatted CT image of another neonate shows substantial hyperaeration of the right middle lobe with attenuation of the pulmonary vessels.

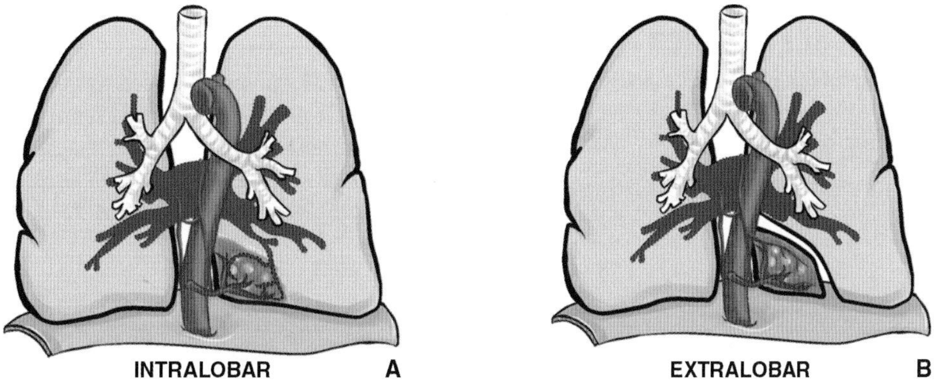

FIGURE 6.28 **Diagrammatic representation of two types of pulmonary sequestration. A:** Intralobar pulmonary sequestrations are lesions mostly confined to the lower lobes, intimately connected with the adjacent lung, usually have venous drainage through the pulmonary veins and have no separate pleural covering. **B:** Extralobar pulmonary sequestrations are accessory lobes with separate pleural covering and have an anomalous venous drainage through a systemic vein.

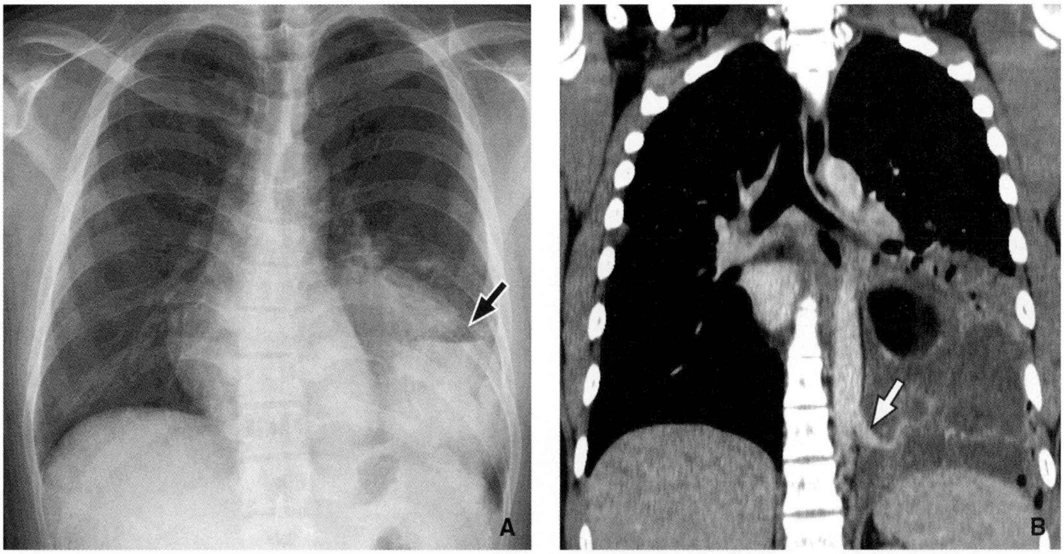

FIGURE 6.29 **Intralobar pulmonary sequestration in a 5-year-old girl with fever and productive cough. A:** Frontal chest radiograph reveals an opacity (*arrow*) in the left lower lobe with associated air–fluid level. **B:** Coronal reformatted CT image shows a complex lesion with solid and cystic component. An anomalous arterial supply (*arrow*) to the lesion originates from the descending thoracic aorta.

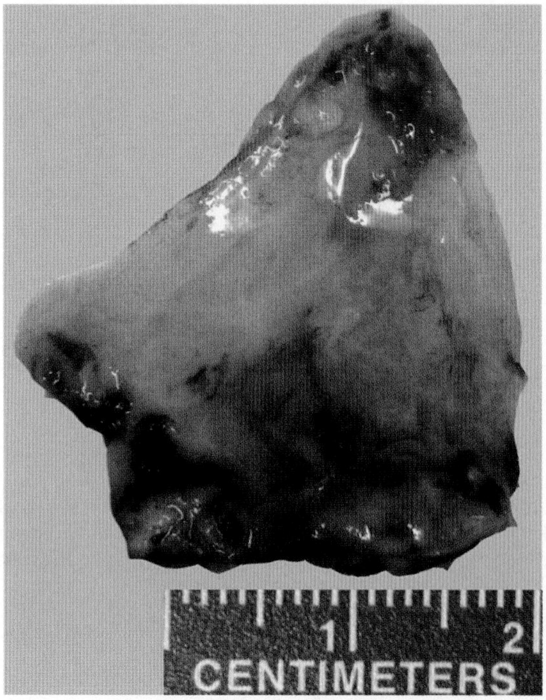

FIGURE 6.30 **Extralobar pulmonary sequestration from an 11-month-old boy.** The resected lung lesion is invested by its own shiny pleura. The accumulation of "hilar" mucus, seen as a large area of pallor, had led to a clinical diagnosis of bronchogenic cyst, but pathologic examination showed peripheral lung tissue with CPAM-like changes, confirming the diagnosis of extralobar pulmonary sequestration.

as CPAM-like maldevelopment (hybrid lesions), and superimposed infection. Chest radiograph usually shows a soft tissue opacity, particularly at the lung base. Cystic areas, either air filled or fluid filled with air–fluid levels, can be seen (Figs. 6.29 and 6.32). On US, PS is usually a homogeneous round, oval or triangular echogenic mass most commonly located at the lung base, adjacent to the diaphragm. It has a systemic feeding vessel, which is better appreciated on Doppler US examination.[57,100,101] MDCT with 3D reconstruction shows a heterogeneously enhancing solid lung parenchymal mass or a complex cystic lesion sometimes with internal air–fluid levels usually at the region of the lower lobes, although infradiaphragmatic and abdominal lesions had been reported. CT can accurately detect the anomalous arterial supply coming from either the thoracic or abdominal aorta as well as its venous drainage. Assessment of concomitant congenital lesions can also be obtained with CT[14,54,61] (Figs. 6.29, 6.31, and 6.32). MRI characterizes the lesion by differentiating the content as solid, cystic, hemorrhagic, or containing mucus components. PS appears as a T2 hyperintense lesion in the lower lobe although cysts of varying size can be seen in hybrid lesions.[57,77,80] Three major radiologic differential diagnoses that need to be considered with PS are CPAM, CLE, and diaphragmatic hernia.

The current management of PS, especially for those presenting with recurrent infection, is surgical excision. Because of the presence of a dominant feeding artery supplying

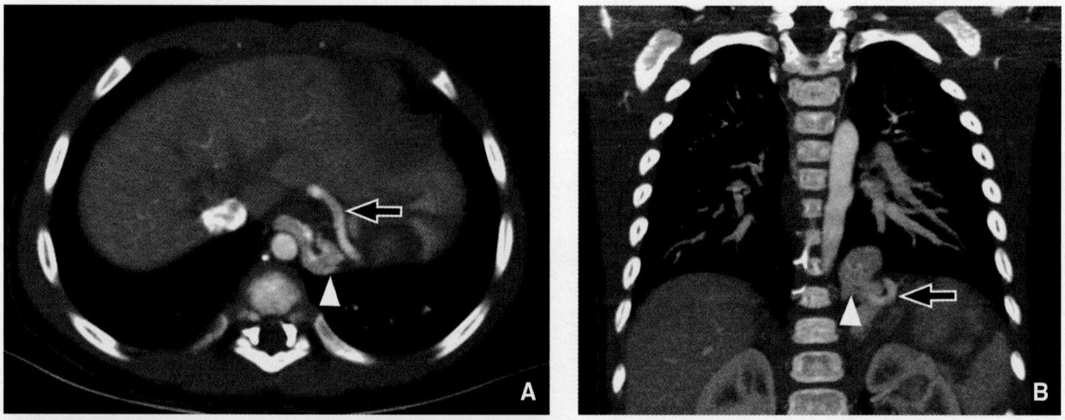

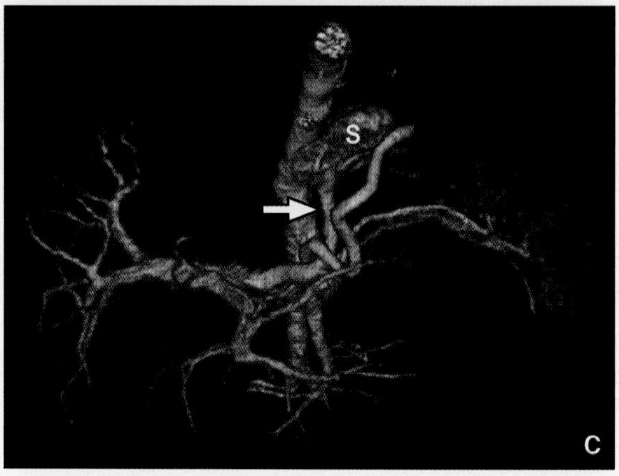

FIGURE 6.31 **Extralobar pulmonary sequestration in a neonate.** Axial **(A)** and coronal reformatted **(B)** CT images following administration of intravenous contrast reveal a well-defined, contrast-enhancing lesion (*white arrowheads*) with a prominent arterial supply (*black arrows*) at the medial basal region of the left lower lobe above the left hemidiaphragm. 3D reconstruction CT image **(C)** shows the arterial supply (*arrow*) of the extralobar pulmonary sequestration (*S*) originating from a branch of the abdominal aorta.

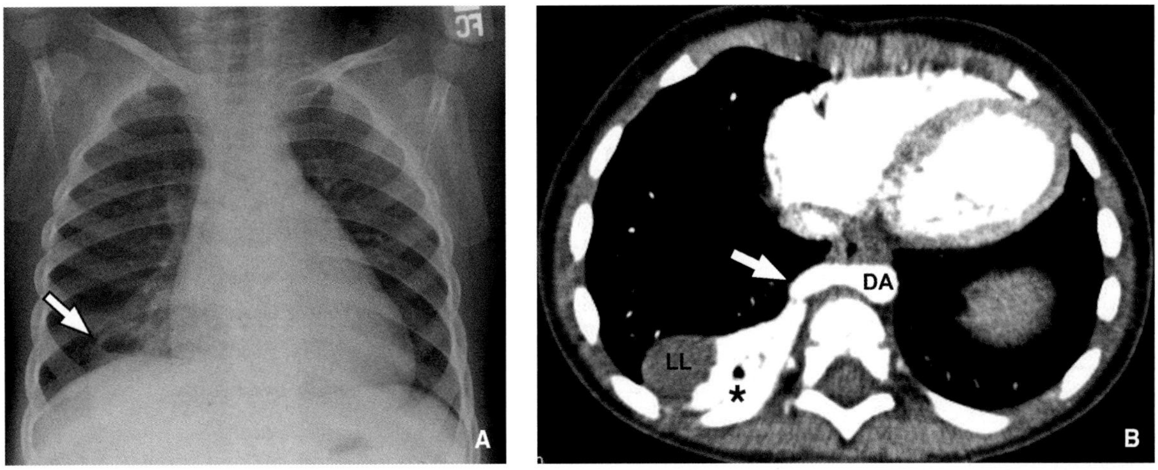

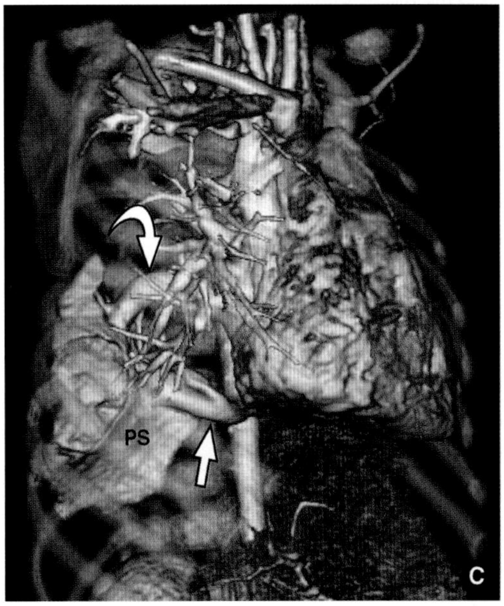

FIGURE 6.32 **Hybrid congenital lung lesion consists of pulmonary sequestration and bronchogenic cyst in a 22-month-old girl who presented with prenatal diagnosis of a focal lung lesion. A:** Frontal chest radiograph shows a focal lung lesion (*arrow*) with areas of lucency and opacity projecting over the right lower lobe and hemidiaphragm. **B:** Axial enhanced CT image demonstrates an enhancing focal lesion (*asterisk*) with an anomalous arterial supply (*arrow*) arising from descending aorta (*DA*). Adjacent to this enhancing focal lesion, an oval-shaped low attenuation lesion (*LL*) is also seen, which was later found to be a bronchogenic cyst on pathology. **C:** 3D volume rendered CT image shows a pulmonary sequestration (*PS*) with an anomalous arterial supply (*straight arrow*) arising from the descending aorta and an anomalous drainaging vein (*curved arrow*) into the right inferior pulmonary vein.

the lesion, some PSs in children have been managed with embolization of the feeding arteries, reportedly with a high success rate.[11,55,102,103]

Infectious Disorders

Pneumonia or lower respiratory tract infection is the most common cause of illness in children resulting in a significant cause of morbidity and mortality. There are over 156 million cases of pneumonia in children <5 years of age worldwide annually[104] and approximately one-third of children develop pneumonia within the first year of life.[105] Childhood mortality from lower respiratory infections is low in developed countries but is a main cause of mortality in developing countries.[106] Pulmonary infections can be severe in young children and account for one-fifth of all deaths under 5 years of age. Of these mortalities, 70% occur in Africa and Southeast Asia.[107]

Determining the underlying etiology of pneumonia in a child is often difficult, but the patient's age can be helpful. Viral pneumonia is rare in neonates because of conferred maternal antibody protection. Group B *Streptococcus* and Gram-negative enteric bacteria obtained via vertical transmission during childbirth are the most common cause of pneumonia in neonates (birth to 20 days). From age 3 weeks to 3 months, *Streptococcus pneumoniae* is the most common bacterial pathogen, but in infants older than 4 months and in preschool-aged children, viruses are the most frequent cause of community-acquired pneumonia. For school-aged children, bacterial infection from *Streptococcus* increases, but viral infection remains the most common cause.[108,109] Bacterial pneumonia can occur at any time of the year in preschool- and school-aged children and adolescents[110] (Table 6.3). Other infectious agents causing pneumonia include *Mycoplasma*, *Mycobacteria*, fungi, protozoa, and parasites. Coinfection with two or more microbial agents can also occur.

Unfortunately, clinical signs and symptoms are nonspecific, and some children can present with nonrespiratory symptoms. Physical examination is also less reliable in children than adults.[111] Sputum cultures are unreliable in children and nearly impossible to obtain in infants.[108] Nasopharyngeal and throat cultures correlate poorly with lower respiratory tract agents.[112]

TABLE 6.3 Frequently Encountered Causes of Community-Acquired Pneumonia in the Pediatric Population

Newborn to 3 weeks *Escherichia coli* Group B *Streptococcus* *Listeria monocytogenes*
3 weeks to 3 months Respiratory viruses *Chlamydia trachomatis* *Bordetella pertussis* *Streptococcus pneumoniae*
4 months to 5 years Respiratory viruses *Chlamydia pneumoniae* *Mycoplasma pneumoniae* *Staphylococcus aureus* *Streptococcus pneumoniae*
5 to 15 years Respiratory viruses *Chlamydia pneumoniae* *Mycoplasma pneumoniae* *Streptococcus pneumoniae* *Staphylococcus aureus*

Viral Infection

Viruses are a common cause of lower respiratory tract infections among children. Different sampling techniques, detection methodologies, and geographical areas can greatly influence the observed burden from each virus.[113,114] In developed countries, infants and preschool-aged children experience a mean of 6 to 10 viral infections annually, and school-aged children and adolescents experience 3 to 5 illnesses annually.[115]

Peripheral airways disease and bronchiolitis are common terms ascribed to viral lower respiratory infection. Following inhalation of infected aerosols in the nasopharynx and upper respiratory tract, it migrates to small airways and alveoli. There is resultant inflammation and necrosis of the ciliated epithelial cells, goblet cells, and bronchial mucous glands, which leads to bronchial and bronchiolar edema, often with involvement of the peribronchial tissue and interlobular lung septa. These gross and microscopic findings are seen in all viral lower respiratory tract diseases.[116,117] The airway reacts with bronchoconstriction and increased mucous secretion, which narrows the small airways causing peripheral atelectasis.[118] Affected pediatric patients typically present with cough, coryza, and wheezing, although severe respiratory distress that requires hospitalization also occurs.

RNA Viruses

Respiratory Syncytial Virus

Respiratory syncytial virus (RSV) is an enveloped, nonsegmented, negative-stranded RNA virus, member of the Paramyxoviridae family. It is the most common viral cause of lower respiratory tract infection in infants.[119] An RSV infection can occur and recur at any age, and by age two, most children would have had an RSV infection manifesting as bronchiolitis. The infection begins with replication of the virus in the nasopharynx and spreads to the small bronchiolar epithelium causing edema, increased mucus production, and eventual necrosis and regeneration of these epithelial cells. This leads to small airway obstruction, air trapping, and increased airway resistance. It is diagnosed based on patient history and physical examination, and children typically present with cough, coryza, and wheezing.[120] Children <3 months, those born prematurely (<35 weeks of gestation), and those with unrepaired cardiac disease or chronic lung disease are at increased risk of severe RSV infection.[120,121] Children with more severe disease usually display grunting, nasal flaring, and intercostal retractions.

Human Metapneumovirus

Human metapneumovirus (hMPV), a recently discovered member of family Paramyxoviridae, is a pleomorphic, enveloped virion, containing single-stranded RNA.[122,123] Early reports indicate that hMPV was found in ~10% of children, and most children have serologic evidence of infection by 5 years of age.[122,124] The mean age of patients with hMPV was greater (12 to 36 months) compared to RSV patients predominantly in infants (<12 months).[125] Clinical disease associated with hMPV appears to be similar to that associated with RSV and other viral infections, ranging from mild upper respiratory tract infection to bronchiolitis and bronchopneumonia.[122–124,126] Occasionally, hMPV may also cause severe illness that requires treatment at intensive care units (ICUs). Frequent coinfection of hMPV with other pathogens has been described. Like other respiratory viruses, hMPV may predispose to secondary bacterial infection.[122–124,126]

Parainfluenza Virus

Human parainfluenza viruses (HPIVs) are enveloped, medium-sized, RNA viruses. HPIV are divided into types 1 to 4. Subgroups or genotypes of HPIV-1 to HPIV-3 have been described as major causes of lower respiratory infections in infants and young children, the immunocompromised, the chronically ill, and the elderly. Each subtype can cause somewhat unique clinical diseases in different hosts. It is associated with all kinds of upper and lower respiratory tract illness from croup, bronchiolitis, and pneumonia. Immunocompromised children appear to be susceptible to developing severe and even fatal lower respiratory tract infection.[127] Many factors have been found that predispose to these infections, including malnutrition, overcrowding, vitamin A deficiency, lack of breast-feeding, and environmental causes.[127,128]

Measles

Measles (rubeola) is a single-stranded RNA-enveloped virus causing an acute disease characterized by fever, cough, conjunctivitis, runny nose, and an erythematous maculopapular rash in affected children. Other manifestations are neurologic complications, otitis media, croup, and bronchopneumonia (5% to 15%). Severe respiratory failure or neurologic complications occur in younger (<5 years old) and immunocompromised patients. Incidence of this disease has significantly diminished through the years because of vaccination, but outbreaks still occur. Although serologic tests are available, diagnosis can be challenging outside of an outbreak situation because physicians have not seen measles during their training, and it is not readily included in the differential diagnosis.[129,130]

DNA Viruses

Adenovirus

Adenovirus is less frequent but an important cause of acute respiratory illness in children. Most infections are mild and indistinguishable from other viral infections, but some diseases result in considerable residual sequelae and even fatal outcome.[131,132] Adenovirus infections can occur endemically or in epidemics. The incidence of infection peaks in pediatric patients who are 6 months to 5 years of age. Several serotypes have been identified in humans, but types 1, 2, 3, 5, 7, and 21 are usually seen in lower respiratory infections.[132] It can spread in other organs other than the respiratory system in previously healthy and immunocompromised.[133] When adenovirus involves the lower respiratory tract, it can cause necrotizing bronchitis, bronchiolitis, and bronchopneumonia. Widespread bronchiolar obliteration as well as bronchiectasis have been noted as sequelae. Adenovirus accounts for 2% to 7% of lower respiratory tract illness in young children admitted to the hospital.[134]

Cytomegalovirus

Cytomegalovirus (CMV) is the largest and most complex member of the herpesvirus family that infects humans. Infants and children are an important source of infection through close contact allowing for direct and indirect person-to-person contact.[135] Infection is less severe in the immunocompetent individual than in the immunocompromised. CMV pneumonia is one of the most common pulmonary complications after organ and bone marrow transplantation (BMT). Approximately one-third of infected patients subsequently develop CMV pneumonia with a median onset time of 50 to 60 days posttransplantation[136,137] (Fig. 6.33).

Varicella Zoster Virus

Varicella zoster, the virus that causes chickenpox, also belongs to the herpesvirus family. Varicella virus infection is a highly contagious but a benign, self-limited disease. The same virus also causes herpes zoster upon reactivation. Infection is generally mild, but there is an increased risk of complications in immunocompromised individuals and neonates. Serious complications include secondary bacterial skin and soft tissue infections, encephalitis, coagulopathy, and pneumonia. Hospitalization rates because of chickenpox are considerably high in developed countries, especially among children.[138] Varicella involving the lower respiratory tract is a more severe complication in adults, but immunocompromised children are also at high risk, presenting with cough, fever, dyspnea, and chest pain, in addition to the vesicular rash.[139]

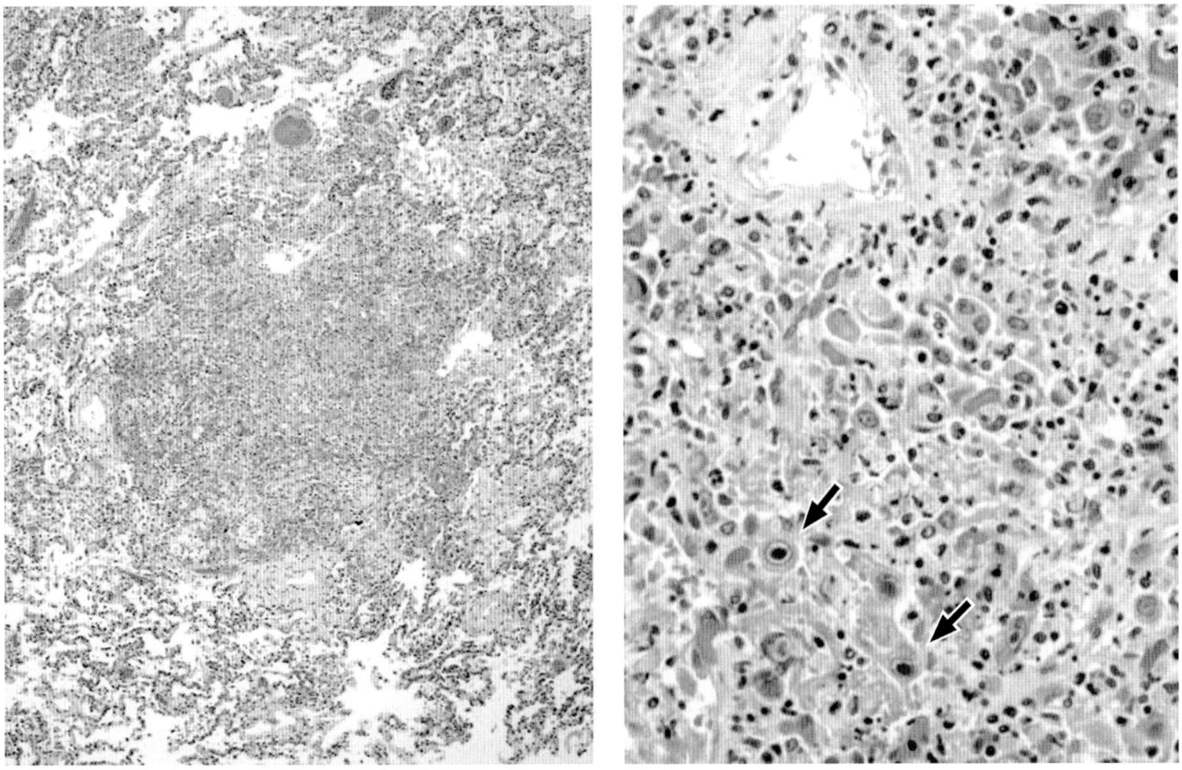

FIGURE 6.33 **Cytomegalovirus (CMV) pneumonia.** CMV often affects alveolated lung tissue by forming discrete nodules of fibrin-rich consolidation (**left**, hematoxylin and eosin, original magnification, 200×). The characteristic viral inclusions (*arrows*) are diagnostic (**right**, hematoxylin and eosin, original magnification, 600×).

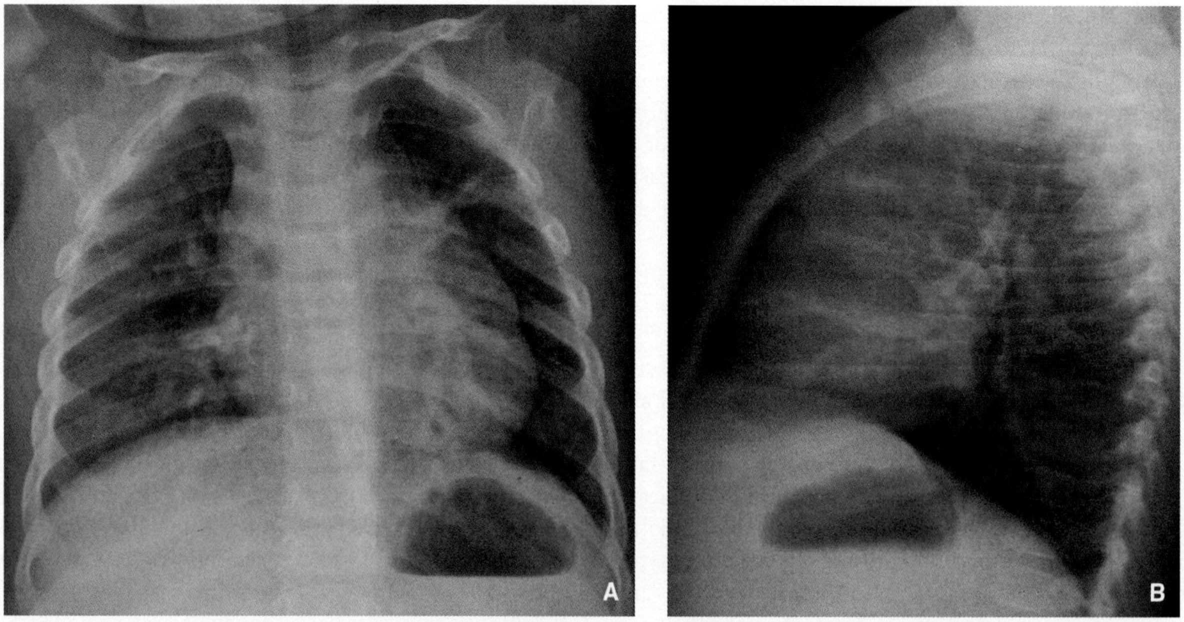

FIGURE 6.34 **Typical radiographic appearance of viral pulmonary infection in a 6-month-old girl who presented with cough, runny nose, and low-grade fever.** Frontal **(A)** and lateral **(B)** views of chest radiograph show hyperaeration, increased peribronchial interstitial markings particularly in the parahilar regions, and areas of subsegmental atelectasis.

Human Immunodeficiency Virus

Human immunodeficiency virus (HIV) is a slowly replicating retrovirus that causes acquired immunodeficiency syndrome (AIDS). HIV damages or destroys vital cells in the human immune system such as helper T cells, macrophages, and dendritic cells, leaving them unable to fight infections and certain cancers. Children represent 2% of the reported cases of HIV infection. Most children are infected after vertical transmission from their mothers, and the majority develop AIDS early in life.[140] Other causes of childhood HIV include sexual transmission, illicit drug use, and blood transfusions, particularly in underdeveloped countries. Respiratory illnesses are important cause of morbidity in these children and are the primary cause of death in 50% of cases.[141,142] HIV-infected individuals who have a CD4 cell count of ≥200 are predisposed to bronchial infections and bacterial pneumonia, whereas patients with CD4 cell count of <200 are predisposed to opportunistic infections such as *Pneumocystis jiroveci*.[143] There is also increased susceptibility to *Mycobacterium tuberculosis* and *M. avium-intracellulare* in children with HIV/AIDS.[144] These specific infections are discussed separately in this chapter.

Other Viruses

Other viral groups have been reported to cause severe infection causing respiratory failure and even death. The severe acute respiratory syndrome (SARS) outbreak in 2003, caused by Coronavirus A (SARS-CoV), was reported in 29 different countries with over 8,000 cases. SARS presents with a prodrome of flu-like illness, followed by cough, dyspnea, and possibly acute respiratory distress.[145] Pandemic influenza viruses including A H5N1 (avian influenza virus), originating from Asia,[146] and influenza A H1N1, an influenza virus of swine origin, first reported in Mexico in 2009,[147] have spread over many parts of the world. Recently, the Middle East Respiratory Syndrome Coronavirus (MERS-CoV), a SARS-like virus, which was first detected in Saudi Arabia in 2012, has spread to other countries in the Middle East and Europe.[148]

Imaging of Viral Lung Infection

Chest radiographs can be normal especially in mild viral infections. The most typical chest radiographic appearances of commonly encountered viral disease are peribronchial thickening or cuffing, hyperaeration, and subsegmental atelectasis (Fig. 6.34). Bilateral peribronchial thickening or cuffing of the bronchial walls radiate from the hila into the lung. Narrowing of the distal airway lumens due to bronchiolar wall edema and mucous plugging results in air trapping and subsequent hyperinflation with areas of segmental and subsegmental atelectasis.[108,110,115,117] However, these patterns have been found to be nonspecific because they can also be seen in nonviral lower respiratory tract infections including bacterial pneumonia as well as reactive small airway disease such as asthma.[149,150]

Other studies support the notion that viral infection can often mimic the radiographic findings of bacterial pneumonia.[111,117] In a more recent study, the predominant radiologic finding of viral pneumonia was bilateral patchy areas of consolidation, with interstitial prominence, diffuse areas of consolidation, and lobar consolidation, less observed[151] (Fig. 6.35). This is also true for pandemic and outbreak viruses including influenza A H5N1 and A H1N1, where the initial radiographic manifestation is the presence of focal or diffuse interstitial opacities but rapidly progress to bilateral areas of consolidation.[147,152] In varicella and CMV, ground-glass or diffuse nodular opacities that may progress to large segmental areas of patchy airspace disease in the bases and perihilar regions can be seen (Fig. 6.36). Complete clearing is expected, but punctate calcifications may be seen

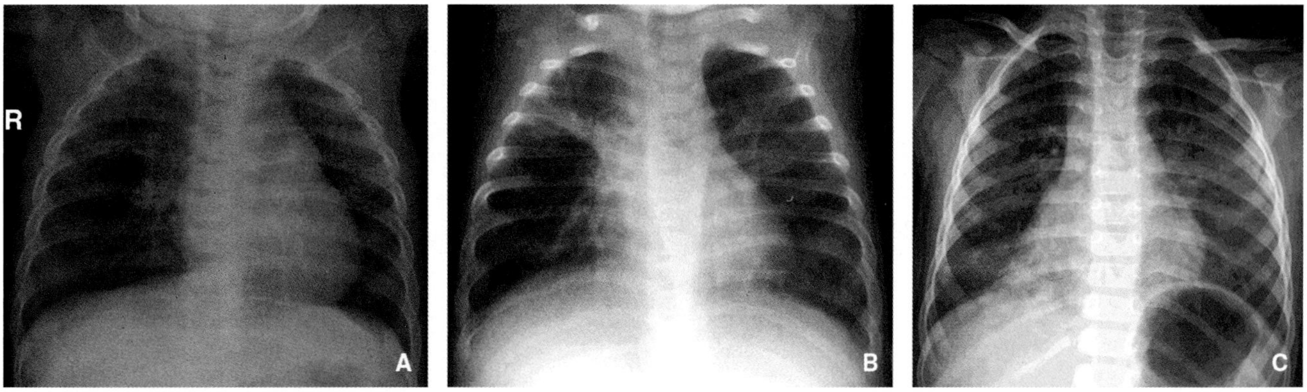

FIGURE 6.35 **Spectrum of radiographic findings in viral pulmonary infection. A:** Frontal chest radiograph in a 10-month-old boy with respiratory syncytial virus infection shows bilateral hyperaeration without focal consolidations. **B:** Frontal chest radiograph in a 7-month-old girl with measles infection shows hyperaeration and multiple areas of subsegmental atelectasis. **C:** Frontal chest radiograph in a 2-year-old boy with parainfluenza virus infection demonstrates the typical peribronchial thickening with multifocal patchy airspace opacities particularly in both lower and right middle lobes.

after acute illness in children with varicella pneumonia.[153] CT is rarely required in the investigation of viral pneumonia, but the findings reflect the underlying pathologic process depending on the virulence of the virus. The spectrum of CT findings includes interlobular septal thickening, bronchial/bronchiolar thickening, ground-glass opacity, nodules, and consolidation.[119]

Lung disease is common among HIV-infected children, and changes reflective of chronic lung disease are commonly seen on radiographs.[154] Children with HIV/AIDS have increased susceptibility to other viral, bacterial, fungal, protozoal, and opportunistic infections, with lobar or segmental consolidations as the most common radiographic patterns.[140] Abnormal chest radiographs have been reported in up to 90% of patients with HIV/AIDS showing the typical findings of diffuse bilateral interstitial prominence without a pleural effusion. As the disease progresses, alveolar opacification may also develop. HRCT is the modality of choice to evaluate those symptomatic pediatric patients with an otherwise normal chest radiograph.[155] *M. tuberculosis* and *M. avium-intracellulare* infection can be seen in AIDS patients, and the radiographic appearance mimics that seen in immunocompetent children with the same infection.[142] The imaging appearance of *M. tuberculosis* and nontuberculous mycobacterial infections, as well as *Pneumocystis jiroveci*, the most common opportunistic pulmonary infection in children with HIV/AIDS, is discussed separately in this chapter.

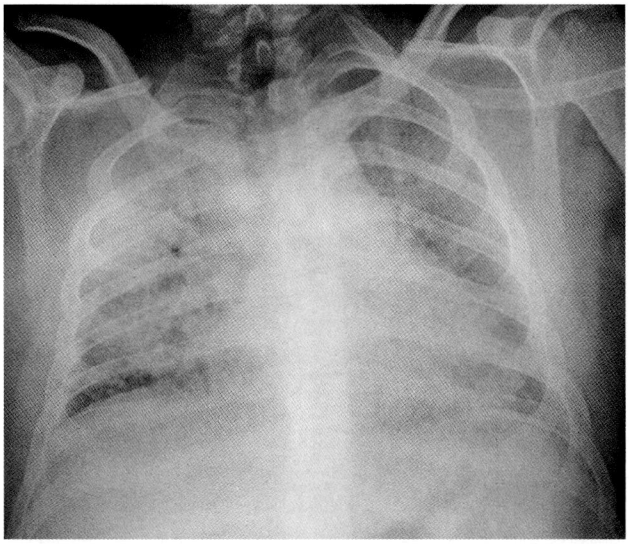

FIGURE 6.36 **Varicella pneumonia in a 5-year-old girl.** Frontal chest radiograph shows diffuse nodular opacities with segmental areas of patchy airspace disease in the right upper lobe and right perihilar region.

Treatment of Viral Lung Infection

For the most part, management of bronchiolitis or lower respiratory infections from a viral cause has been mainly supportive, with particular attention to maintaining hydration, oxygenation, and management of secretions. Most affected children recover uneventfully with supportive care. In some children younger than 60 days and those with severe symptoms, hospitalization would be beneficial.[120] An antiviral therapy for bronchiolitis has not been fully established although antibiotic treatment for confirmed superimposed bacterial infection should be initiated. There have been reports on the role of inhaled bronchodilators, epinephrine, and steroids, but their use remains controversial.[156–159] With regard to HIV/AIDS, the incidence of related deaths among children has been declining. Available vaccines have lower efficacy in children infected with HIV, but are still protective. The use of co-trimoxazole prophylaxis and treatment with antiretroviral agents has reduced the incidence and severity of HIV-associated pneumonia and has substantially improved the outcome for children with HIV infection.[107,160,161]

Bacterial Infection

Bacterial pneumonia is most often a descending process, acquired via travel of bacteria from the oropharynx to the airways then alveoli. Much less commonly, it arises from a hematogenous route and rarely by direct extension from the chest wall or an extrathoracic site. The bacteria incite an intra-alveolar inflammatory exudate, with hyperemia and engorgement of the arterial blood vessels[152,162] (Fig. 6.37). The typical distribution

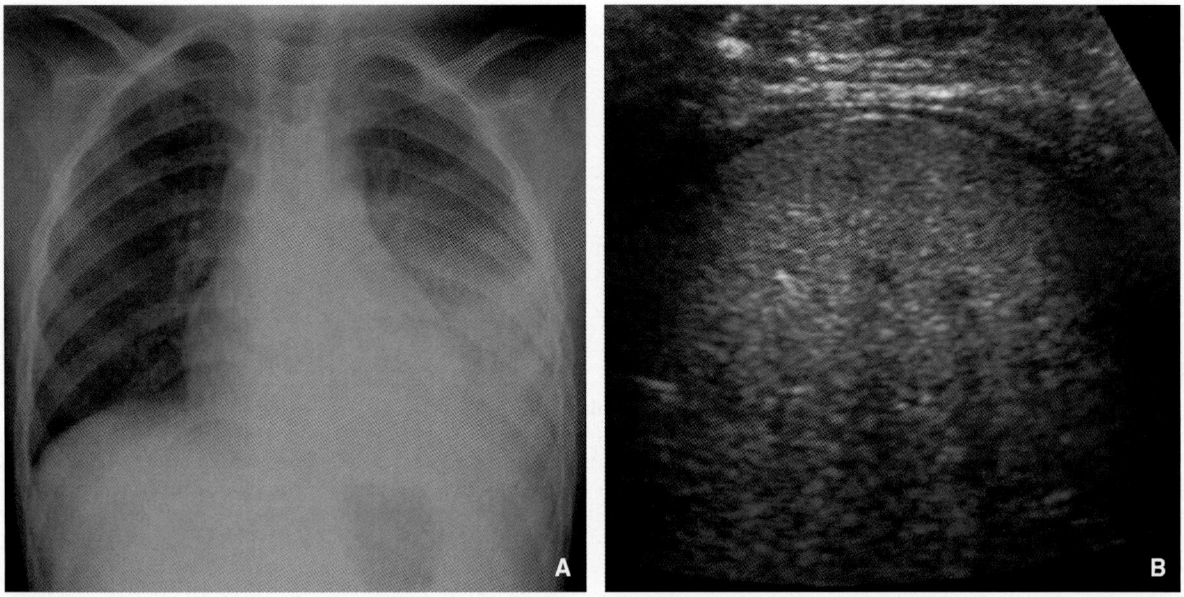

FIGURE 6.37 **Lobar bacterial pneumonia in a 3-year-old boy. A:** Frontal chest radiograph shows dense pulmonary consolidation involving the left lower lobe. **B:** Focused ultrasound of the left lower lobe confirms the consolidation with homogenous echogenic pattern similar to liver, thus called "hepatization" of the lung.

is lobar or segmental, depending on the stage of progression at the time the radiograph is obtained.[108,112,163] Bacterial infection is highly probable in children with alveolar opacification on the chest radiograph, but interstitial prominence is seen in both viral and bacterial pneumonias.[150,164] If the process extends to the pleural space, associated pleural effusion is present. Bronchopneumonia, the typical pattern of a descending pneumonia, is characterized by peribronchiolar inflammation that spreads to the adjacent parenchyma, causing patchy nodules and consolidation (Fig. 6.38).[152]

The pattern of lung response to infection is more influenced by age rather than the offending organism. Lobar and alveolar lung opacities are more common in older children and are more frequently due to bacterial infections, whereas interstitial opacities are seen in all age groups, and are therefore nonspecific as to the type of causative organism.[149] *Staphylococcus* occurs commonly in early infancy, *Haemophilus* most often between 6 and 12 months, and *S. pneumoniae* more commonly between 1 and 3 years old.[153]

Streptococcus pneumoniae

The most common cause of bacterial pneumonia is *S. pneumoniae* or pneumococcus, a Gram-positive, anaerobic, extracellular pathogen characterized by a thick polysaccharide capsule.[163,165] This immunogenic capsule is the major virulence factor in pneumococcus.[166] Children, especially under 2 years of age, lack specific functions for immune responses to polysaccharide antigens making them susceptible to pneumococcal infection and colonization.[167,168] Pneumococcal pneumonia is a major cause of pediatric morbidity and mortality worldwide, annually resulting in ~800,000 deaths in children <5 years of age. In addition to pneumonia, it can also cause meningitis and sepsis.[169] Infection usually begins with prodromal symptoms, such as cough, rhinitis, or vomiting, which develop during one to several days and are later followed by high fever.[163]

The typical chest radiographic presentation is a lung alveolar opacification producing a homogenous pattern involving partial or complete segments of the lung and occasionally the entire lobe (Fig. 6.39). Airways are not primarily involved

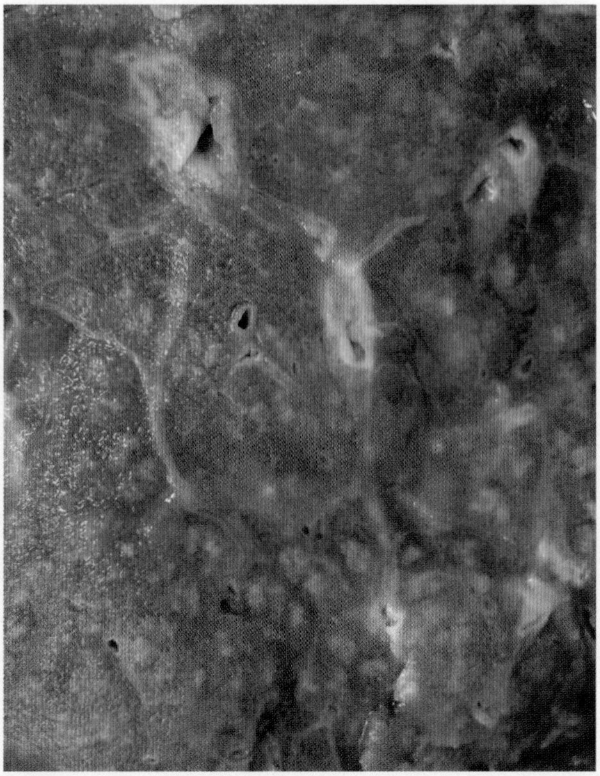

FIGURE 6.38 **Bronchopneumonia pattern of bacterial pneumonia in a 16-year-old lung transplant patient who was found dead in bed.** Multifocal florette-shaped areas of pallor reflect neutrophilic inflammation and highlight the anatomy of the disease, which involves terminal airways and variable amounts of surrounding alveoli.

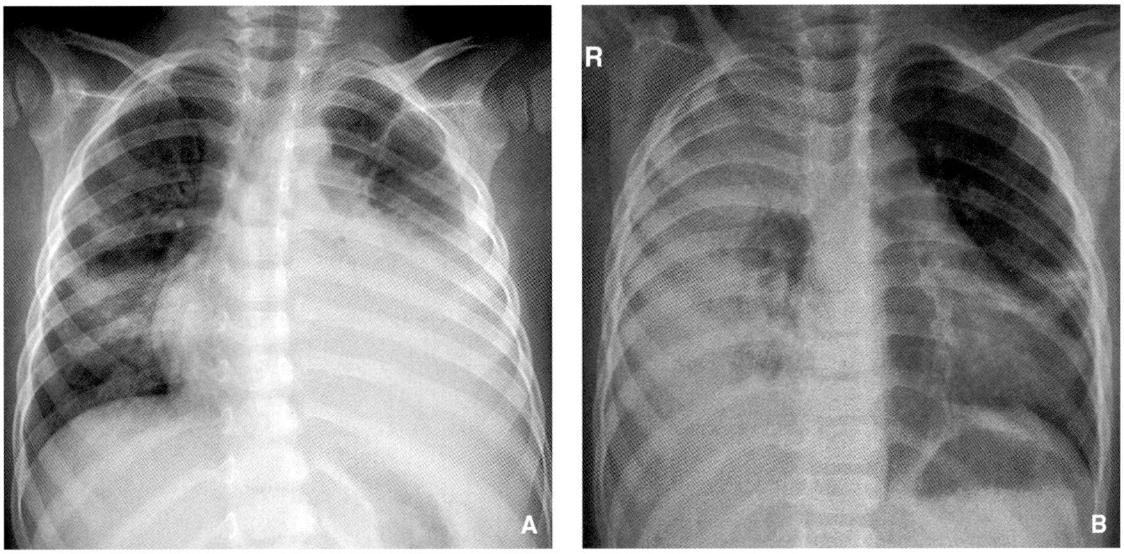

FIGURE 6.39 ***Streptococcus pneumoniae* pneumonia in two children. A:** Frontal chest radiograph reveals a dense consolidation of the left lower lobe and lingula as well as a focal region on the right lower lobe. Presence of left pleural effusion is also seen. **B:** Frontal chest radiograph shows a near-complete opacification of the right hemithorax with consolidation and effusion. Also noted are patchy airspace opacities in the left mid- to lower lung zones.

and remain patent; therefore, lobar volume tends to be preserved and air bronchograms may be seen.[163,166,170] This finding is believed to be present in about 85% of all cases.[170] Parapneumonic effusions are fairly common in pneumococcal pneumonia. Interstitial prominence without focal lung consolidation can sometimes present at the time of diagnosis.[163]

Round pneumonia is an imaging manifestation of community-acquired pneumonia in children. *S. pneumoniae* is the most common etiologic agent, seen in 90% of cases, but *Klebsiella pneumoniae* and *Haemophilus influenza* have also been implicated.[171,172] In the immunocompromised patients, it can be due to fungi and mycobacterium. Ninety percent of round pneumonia is seen in children <12 years owing to smaller alveoli, closely apposed septa, and underdeveloped airway collaterals (pores of Kohn and channels of Lambert).[171,172] Older children are less susceptible to round pneumonia because they have more developed pathways of collateral ventilation and larger alveoli. When a round opacity is seen in older age groups, atypical microorganisms, immunodeficiencies, underlying lesions, and other rare etiologies, such as a primary malignancy, must be considered.[171]

Round pneumonia typically presents radiographically as a solitary, well-circumscribed, homogeneous spherical lesion >3 cm (range 1 to 12 cm).[171,172] The lesion has a predilection for the posterior segment of the lower lobe and is commonly in contact with the pleura, hilum, or pulmonary fissure (Fig. 6.40). Satellite lesions are sometimes present, and air bronchograms can be seen in up to 20% of cases.[171,172]

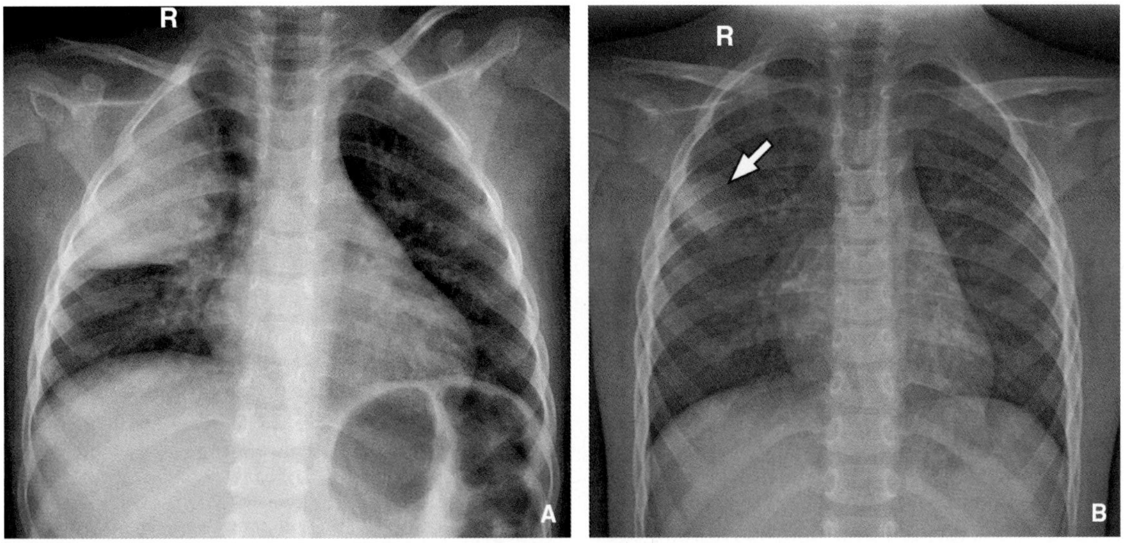

FIGURE 6.40 **Round pneumonia in two pediatric patients. A:** Frontal chest radiograph of a 4-year-old girl who presented with cough, fever, and right-sided chest pain shows a dense spherical opacity in the right upper lobe adjacent to the pleural surface. **B:** Frontal chest radiograph of a 5-year-old boy who presented with fever and cough demonstrates a rounded opacity (*arrow*) in the right upper lobe compatible with a round pneumonia.

Calcifications, cavitations, lymphadenopathy, or pleural effusions are uncommon.[171,172]

Streptococcus pyogenes

Streptococcus pyogenes (group A *Streptococcus*) is a spherical Gram-positive bacterium that causes a wide range of syndromes ranging from localized illness, such as pharyngitis, to invasive disease, such as bacteremia, pneumonia, necrotizing fasciitis, and streptococcal toxic shock syndrome.[173] In the neonatal age group, group B *Streptococcus* is a leading cause of sepsis, which includes pneumonia and meningitis. Inadequate treatment of *S. pyogenes* infections, predominantly throat infections, can result in the serious postinfectious sequela such as acute rheumatic fever, which may lead to rheumatic heart disease. The burden of poststreptococcal sequelae is great in developing countries but relatively rare in developed countries.[174]

S. pyogenes pneumonia presents radiographically as an alveolar patchy or dense consolidation. It can be segmental or lobar, with lower lobe predisposition. Although it is typically unilateral, it can also affect both lungs. Complicated pneumonia with development of necrotizing pneumonia and abscess can be seen (Fig. 6.41). Presence of parapneumonic effusions and empyema is common especially in neonates and young children. Presence of empyema in these neonates is potentially fatal.[175,176] It can have radiographic appearance similar to *S. pneumoniae* and staphylococcal pneumonia although pneumatoceles are less commonly observed.

Staphylococcus aureus

Staphylococcus aureus is a Gram-positive, catalase-positive coccus. It is an infrequent, but recognized cause of community-acquired pneumonia that primarily affects infants under the age of 1 year. It can occur as a superimposed infection especially in the immunocompromised patients. *S. aureus* can invade the lung directly through the tracheobronchial tree (primary disease) or via hematogenous seeding (secondary disease). Most of the community-acquired (CA) staphylococcal infections are caused by methicillin-resistant *S. aureus* (MRSA).[177] A virulent form of staphylococcal pneumonia has been recognized, associated with the Panton-Valentine leukocidin (PVL) toxin that causes alveolar hemorrhage and necrosis of the interlobular septa. This form of pneumonia rapidly progresses within a few days from a flu-like illness to a severe pneumonia, with high fever, hypotension, tachycardia, cyanosis, hemoptysis, and leucopenia, and carries a high mortality rate (Fig. 6.42).[177,178] Staphylococcal pneumonia secondary to septicemia or hematogenous seeding is sometimes referred to as septic embolism. In these pediatric patients, there is usually a distant source infection in the skin, soft tissue, and bones.[179,180]

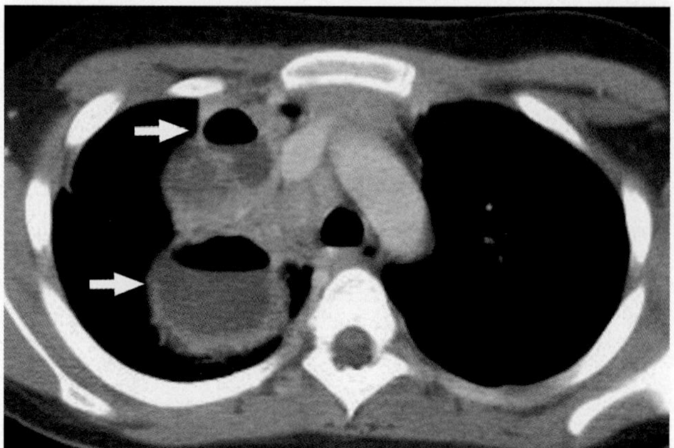

FIGURE 6.41 ***Streptococcus pyogenes* abscesses in a 12-year-old boy who presented with cough, fever, and chest pain.** Axial enhanced CT image demonstrates low-attenuation cystic masses (*arrows*) with air-fluid levels in the right upper lobe compatible with abscesses.

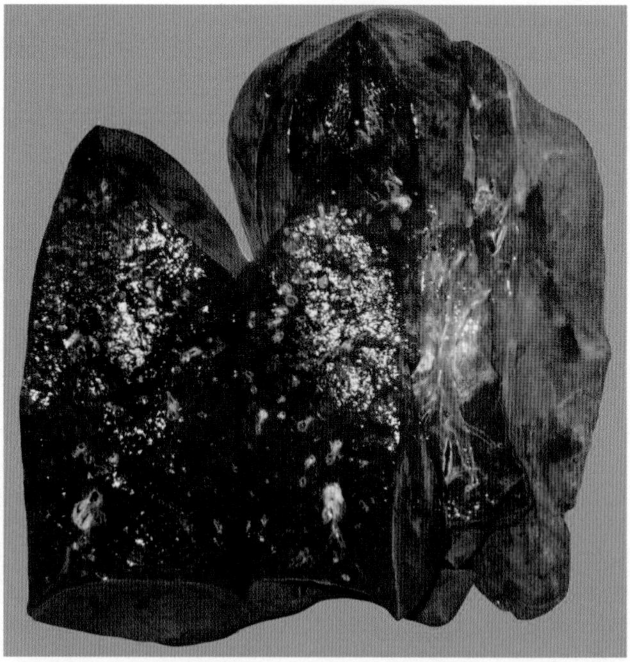

FIGURE 6.42 **Staphylococcal pneumonia due to methicillin-resistant Staphylococcus aureus in a previously healthy 15-year-old boy.** At autopsy, the lungs showed widespread areas of pallor corresponding to advanced necrotizing bronchopneumonia. Dark maroon hemorrhage is also seen.

S. aureus pneumonia in children typically has a bronchopneumonia pattern. It can initially have segmental distribution but could affect the entire lobe. It is unilateral in a majority of cases and associated with high rates of complications,[181] particularly pleural effusion and empyema, which occur in more than 90% of children[182,183] (Fig. 6.43). Pneumatoceles are a late complication without prognostic significance except that they can rupture causing pneumothorax. *S. aureus* can also present as a round pneumonia in younger children. When the route of acquisition is hematogenous, then multiple bilateral pulmonary nodular masses and/or cavities are characteristic.

Haemophilus influenzae

Haemophilus influenzae is a Gram-negative, rod-shaped bacterium. In infants and young children, it causes bacteremia,

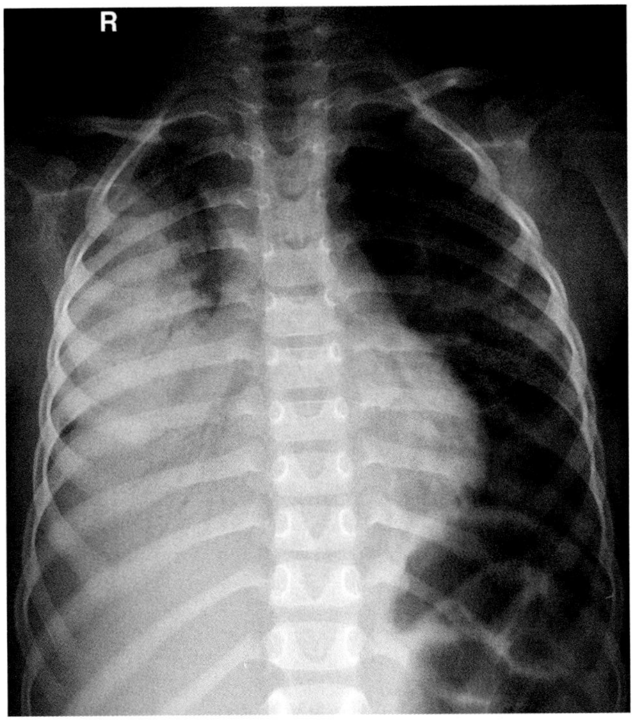

FIGURE 6.43 **Methicillin-resistant *Staphylococcus aureus* pneumonia in a 3-year-old boy.** Frontal chest radiograph shows dense consolidation on the right lung with air bronchograms.

pneumonia, cellulitis, epiglottitis, and meningitis. Childhood *Haemophilus* infection is now markedly decreased because of the widespread vaccination for this organism.

The radiographic appearance of *H. influenza* pneumonia is nonspecific. It can present as bronchopneumonia, consolidation, and reticulonodular pattern in combination with airspace consolidation or can display a combination of patterns[168] (Fig. 6.44). The segmental or lobar opacification is mostly unilateral and can be complicated by empyema.[184]

Bordetella pertussis

Pertussis (whooping cough) is a highly contagious respiratory bacterial infection caused by a Gram-negative, aerobic, capsulated coccobacillus *Bordetella pertussis* and related species. It infects mainly the upper respiratory tract in infants and young children, usually starting as a mild upper airway disease (catarrhal stage), progressing to coughing spells characterized by an inspiratory whoop commonly followed by vomiting (paroxysmal stage), and ending over several weeks (convalescent stage).[185] Pneumonia (due to *B. pertussis* or to a secondary bacterial pathogen) is a common complication. Untreated patients may be contagious for 3 weeks or more following onset of the cough. The spread of pertussis can be prevented by immunization.

Typical radiographic manifestations include streaky perihilar interstitial prominence with most often unilateral hilar adenopathy, a pattern sometimes called the "shaggy heart" appearance[153] (Fig. 6.45). Because this is primarily an airway disease, the radiographic appearance may mimic a viral airway disease pattern.

Pseudomonas aeruginosa

Pseudomonas aeruginosa, a Gram-negative, aerobic, rod-shaped bacterium, is a common cause of severe nosocomial pulmonary infection especially in the ICU.[168] In addition to the lungs, it can also affect other systems including the kidneys and the urinary tract, central nervous system, skin, bone and joints, eyes, and ears; it can also cause bacteremia and sepsis, especially in immunocompromised pediatric patients. Children with cystic fibrosis (CF) are highly susceptible to *Pseudomonas* colonization and infection even as early as preschool years.[186]

The common radiographic manifestation is usually that of bronchopneumonia consisting of bilateral multifocal areas of consolidation.[168] Small pulmonary abscesses and cavitary necrosis may occur. On CT, *Pseudomonas* infection

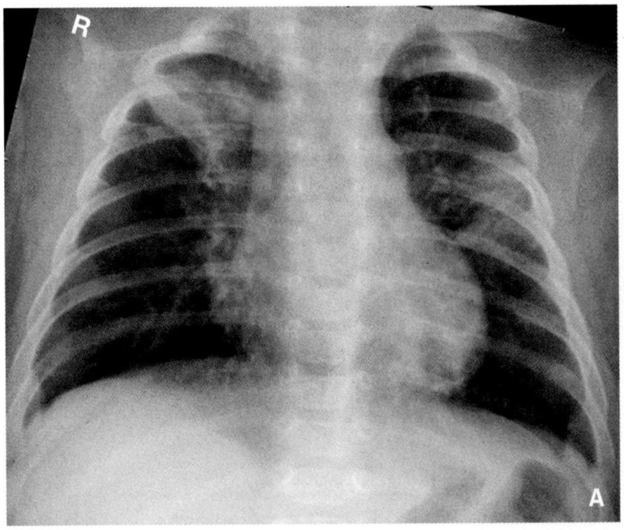

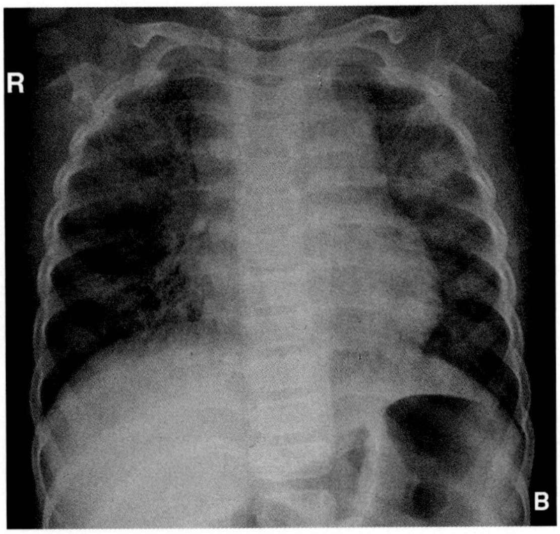

FIGURE 6.44 ***Haemophilus influenzae* pneumonia in two pediatric patients.** Frontal radiographs of an 8-month-old boy **(A)** and a 15-month-old girl **(B)** show a nonspecific radiographic pattern with a combination of interstitial thickening and multifocal airspace consolidation.

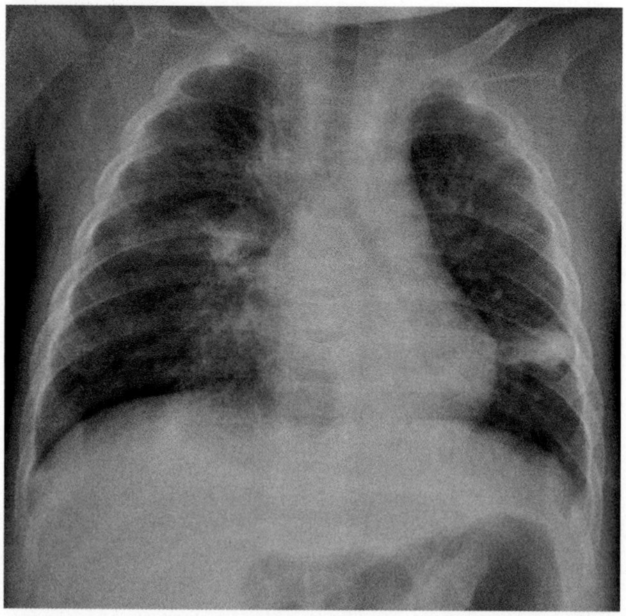

FIGURE 6.45 ***Pertussis* pneumonia in an 18-month-old boy who presented with whooping cough.** Frontal chest radiograph shows dense streaky perihilar opacities, a pattern sometimes called the "shaggy heart" appearance.

commonly presents with multifocal airspace consolidation with nodular features, with some patients demonstrating tree-in-bud opacities[187] (Fig. 6.46).

Legionella pneumophila

Legionella pneumophila, an aerobic, pleomorphic, and flagellated, Gram-negative bacterium, is the causative agent for two clinical syndromes: Pontiac fever and Legionnaires disease, both are collectively known as legionellosis. Pontiac fever is generally a self-limited, influenza-like illness, whereas Legionnaires disease is a common cause of serious bacterial pneumonia. Risk factors for Legionnaires disease include older age group, those with underlying chronic illness, and immunosuppression. Lung infection from *Legionella pneumophila* is relatively uncommon in children.[188]

Initial radiographs can be normal but rapidly progresses into poorly demarcated focal opacifications. It could be unilateral and unifocal but could become multifocal and become confluent, with or without pleural effusions[168] (Fig. 6.47). It could also present as multiple cavitating pulmonary nodules, but this is less commonly observed.[189]

Bacteria-like Organism Infection

Chlamydia pneumoniae

Chlamydia trachomatis is an obligate intracellular human bacterium.[190] Genital chlamydial infection is recognized as the world's most common sexually transmitted disease and the high prevalence in women of childbearing age results in exposure of neonates during childbirth. Neonatal infection is acquired after passage of the fetus through the birth canal. The infant typically presents at 3 to 6 weeks of age with respiratory symptoms and occasional pulmonary hemorrhage. *C. trachomatis* should be suspected in infants who are afebrile or nontoxic and have a dry cough. These pediatric patients often have concomitant conjunctivitis and peripheral eosinophilia.[109] *Chlamydia pneumoniae* was reported as a pathogen for human pneumonia in 1989 and is now the third most common pathogen after *S. pneumoniae* and *Mycoplasma pneumoniae* in community-acquired pneumonia. It is seen in school-aged children, teenagers, and adults. This atypical pneumonia is clinically characterized by a nonproductive cough or a mildly elevated or normal white blood cell count, but severe disease can occur.[191]

The radiographic appearance of infants with *Chlamydia* pneumonia is not distinctive and shares findings similar to

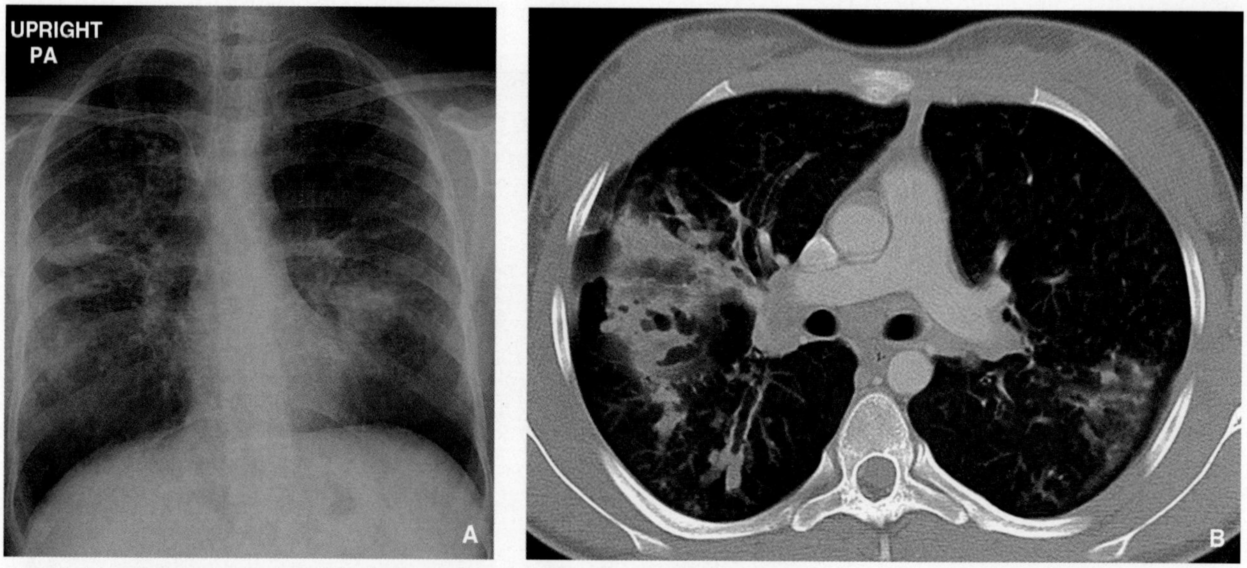

FIGURE 6.46 ***Pseudomonas* infection in a 7-year-old boy with cystic fibrosis. A:** Frontal chest radiograph shows diffuse underlying bronchiectatic lung changes in keeping with the patient's known history of underlying cystic fibrosis. In addition, bilateral multifocal areas of lung consolidation are also seen. **B:** Axial CT image shows multifocal airspace consolidations along with chronic lung changes including tubular bronchiectasis due to underlying cystic fibrosis.

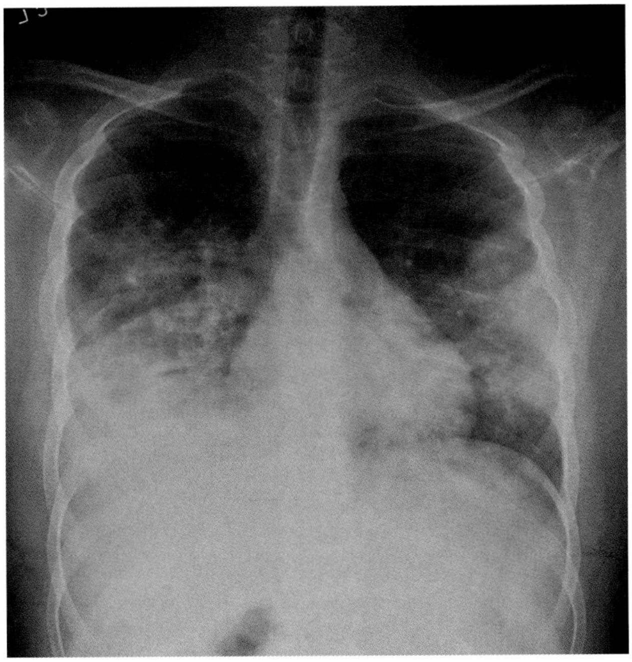

FIGURE 6.47 ***Legionella* pneumonia in a 15-year-old girl who presented with cough and fever.** Frontal chest radiograph demonstrates multifocal confluent airspace opacifications with right-sided effusion.

viral disease. Most chest radiographs show bilateral hyperaeration and diffuse interstitial prominence with a variety of radiographic patterns including interstitial and reticulonodular opacities as well as atelectasis and bronchopneumonia. Lobar consolidation and pleural effusion are not usually seen[192] (Fig. 6.48).

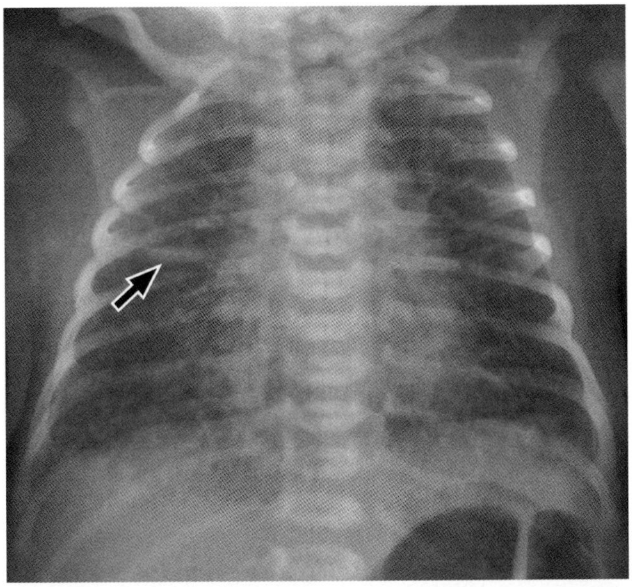

FIGURE 6.48 ***Chlamydia* infection in a 1-week-old infant boy who presented with conjunctivitis.** Frontal chest radiograph shows bilateral diffuse coarse interstitial opacities as well as hyperaeration. Small amount of pleural effusion is seen along the minor fissure (*arrow*). (Case courtesy of Louis Allan B. Serrano, MD, De La Salle University Medical Center, Manila, Philippines.)

Mycoplasma pneumoniae

M. pneumoniae is a common ubiquitous organism and treatable cause of community-acquired pneumonia. After infection, damage is directed toward the bronchiolar mucosa, and later, the peribronchial tissue and interlobular septa become edematous and infiltrated with inflammatory cells.[155] Clinical manifestations include tracheobronchitis, pneumonia, pharyngitis, and otitis media. The symptoms of mycoplasma pneumonia are less severe compared to typical bacterial pneumonia.[153] Mycoplasma infection, referred to as "atypical pneumonia," accounts for up to 30% of all pneumonia in the general population, with the highest incidence in children between 3 and 14 years of age. It causes up to 35% of all cases of outpatient pneumonia and 3% to 18% of pneumonia cases necessitating hospitalization.[193]

There is a broad spectrum of radiographic findings in mycoplasma pneumonia, with patterns typically intermediate between the typical viral and bacterial pneumonia.[112,193,194] Findings can be focal, segmental, or widespread with a reticulonodular pattern or nodular opacities[162] or confluent and patchy consolidation.[168,195] In a study by Hsieh and colleagues, bilateral peribronchial and perivascular interstitial opacities were most frequently seen[193] (Fig. 6.49). Clinical and laboratory findings are essential for the diagnosis of mycoplasma pneumonia because radiographic findings alone are not sufficiently distinctive.[112,161,194,195] Children who require hospitalization for mycoplasma pneumonia are reported to demonstrate an increased incidence of follow-up HRCT showing features of obliterative bronchiolitis, which include air trapping, mosaic perfusion pattern, bronchial wall thickening, and bronchiectasis.[196]

Treatment of Bacteria and Bacteria-like Lung Infection

Treatment decisions of bacterial and bacteria-like lung infections should be based on diagnostic algorithms that begin with the age of the child, then consider clinical and epidemiologic factors, and finally take into account the results of imaging if there are any pneumonic complications. Antibiotic therapy should be initiated promptly focused on the causative agent, either presumed (empirical treatment) or preferably directed by the results of culture or other laboratory assays. In very young children who appear toxic, hospitalization and intravenous antibiotics are needed. The symptoms in outpatients who present with community-acquired pneumonia can help determine the treatment.[109]

Mycobacterial Infection

Tuberculosis (TB), caused by *Mycobacterium tuberculosis,* is a major global health problem, and the burden remains enormous. In 2013, an estimated 9 million people developed TB (13% with HIV coinfection), and 1.5 million died from the disease.[197] Majority of cases were in the Southeast Asia, Africa, and Western Pacific regions. Around 3.5% of newly diagnosed TB cases and 20.5% of those previously treated for TB have multidrug-resistant TB.[197] Among children under 15 years, there were an estimated 550,000 new TB cases and 80,000 TB deaths in 2013.[197]

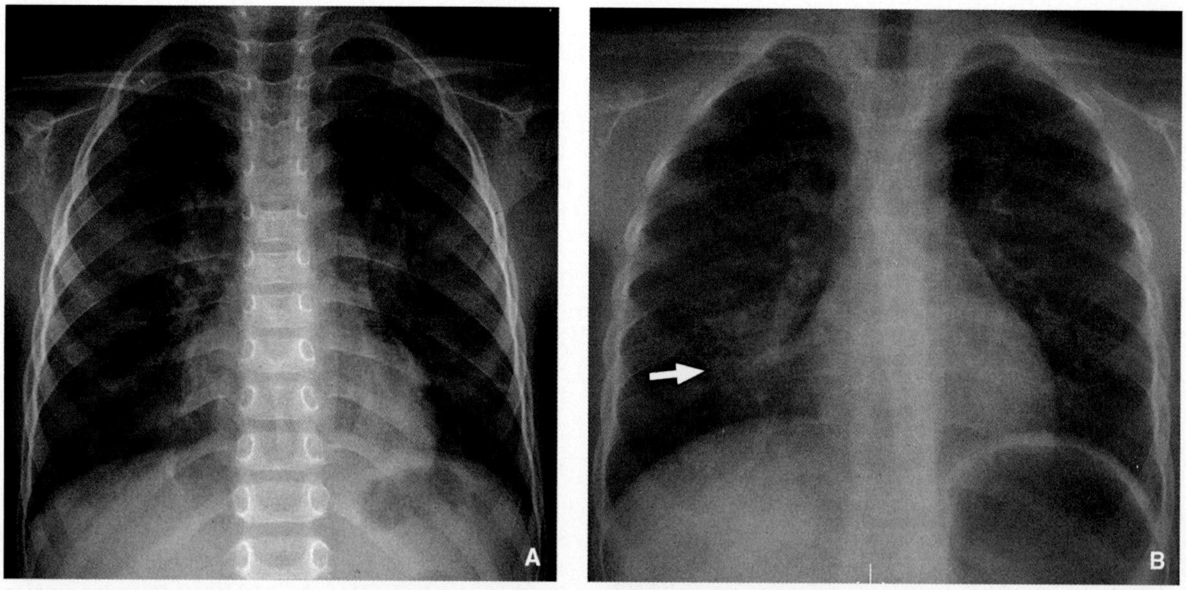

FIGURE 6.49 **Variable radiographic appearance of *Mycoplasma pneumonia* infection in two different children. A:** Frontal chest radiograph of a 7-year-old girl shows generalized interstitial thickening in the perihilar regions along with areas of subsegmental atelectasis and hyperaeration. **B:** Frontal chest radiograph of a 9-year-old boy demonstrates patchy subtle area of airspace opacification (*arrow*) in the right lower lung zone.

After being inhaled, mycobacteria settle in the alveoli inciting an inflammatory reaction. The bacilli also spread to nearby mediastinal and hilar lymph nodes. In an otherwise healthy child, the infection is contained by an intact immune system, the bacilli become dormant, and the infection goes into latency, where children are reactive to tuberculin skin test (TST) or Quantiferon test, but have no clinical evidence of TB disease.[198] The contained alveolar site of infection (Ghon focus), the infected lymph nodes, and associated lymphangitis form the "primary (Ranke) complex." Primary progressive TB disease occurs if the host is unable to contain the infection and disease progression occurs. Risk factors for disease progression include malnutrition, immune suppression including HIV infection, and young age (<5 years old).

Progression of primary pulmonary tuberculosis manifests in the lungs, the lymph nodes, pleural space, or adjacent structures in the thorax; there can also be involvement of distant body parts through hematogenous dissemination.[199] Samples from sputum, or less commonly bronchoalveolar lavage, fine needle aspiration, or biopsy, are used for laboratory confirmation of disease. Acid-fast bacilli stains, microbiologic cultures, and molecular assays can all contribute to diagnosis. Xpert MTB/RIF, a rapid molecular diagnostic test, has been endorsed by the World Health Organization (WHO) for TB detection and identification of rifampicin resistance.[200]

Lymphadenopathy in the hilar, paratracheal, subcarinal, or mediastinal regions, with or without accompanying lung parenchymal disease (Ghon focus), is regarded as the radiographic hallmark of primary TB infection. The Ghon foci typically calcify over time (Fig. 6.50). They may be too small to see radiographically. A right-sided predominant distribution of the lymph nodes has been well recognized although it could be on the left or bilateral.[201] In primary progressive TB disease, the lymph nodes are enlarged and edematous and may cause compression of the adjacent bronchus and can lead to hyperinflation or atelectasis of the affected lung segment. Both anterior and lateral views are required for optimal lymph node visualization, although it may remain difficult to visualize enlarged lymph nodes with certainty (Fig. 6.51). CT has a higher sensitivity for lymphadenopathy detection, which may show a characteristic appearance consisting of central areas of low attenuation with peripheral rim enhancement and

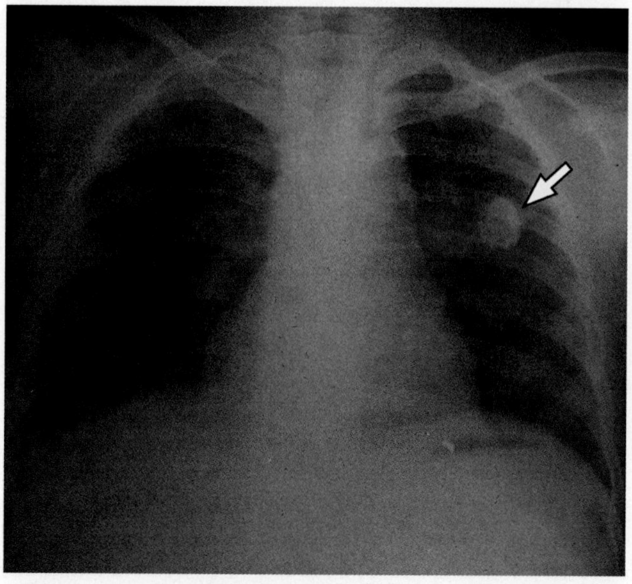

FIGURE 6.50 **A calcified Ghon focus of tuberculous (TB) infection in an 8-year-old girl.** Frontal chest radiograph obtained as a school requirement shows a calcified Ghon focus (*arrow*) of TB on the left upper lobe. Patient had a positive tuberculin skin test.

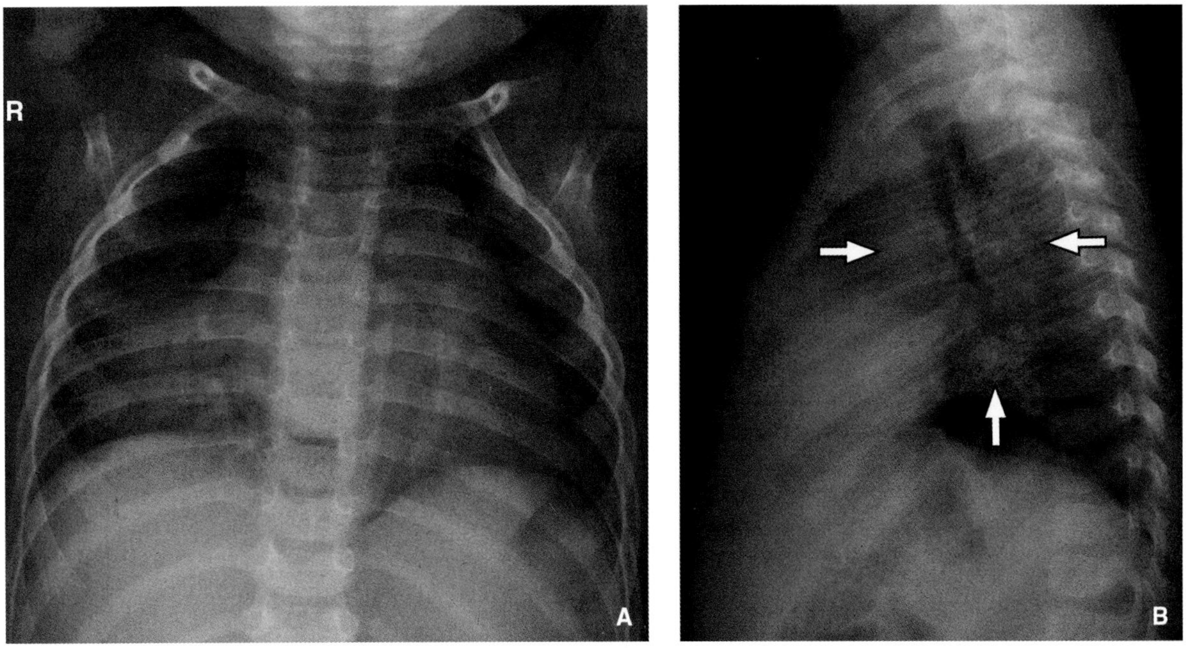

FIGURE 6.51 **Primary tuberculous (TB) infection in a 2-year-old girl whose mother has active TB.** Frontal **(A)** and lateral **(B)** views of chest radiograph reveal a right middle lobe consolidation along with significant lymphadenopathy (*arrows*) best seen on the lateral view.

obliteration of perinodal fat. Calcification within the nodes is seen in 15%.[202] It could also present with ghost-like pattern of enhancement of enlarged lymph nodes[203] (Fig. 6.52).

Parenchymal involvement in primary progressive pulmonary TB disease most commonly appears as homogeneous consolidation, although it can appear patchy, linear, nodular, and mass-like. Caseating necrosis, liquefaction, or calcifications can be seen within the consolidation and can progress into extensive lung damage[204] (Fig. 6.53). Bronchopneumonic

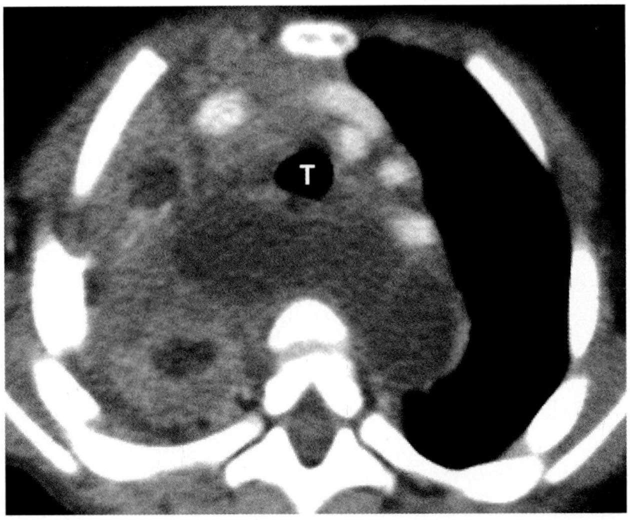

FIGURE 6.52 **Progressive tuberculous lymphadenopathy in a 4-year-old boy who presented with fever and respiratory distress.** Axial enhanced CT image shows an extensive lymphadenopathy with caseated necrosis along the paratracheal region and upper mediastinum. Trachea (*T*) is shifted to the left side and superiorly because of underlying lymphadenopathy.

consolidation could result from intrabronchial spread of a parenchymal cavity or after eruption of a caseated lymph node into the bronchial tree. The radiographic pattern shows large irregular patchy infiltration usually involving more than one lobe of a single lung. CT may show poorly defined nodules or rosettes of nodules, 2 to 10 mm in diameter that can be identified as centrilobular or branching centrilobular opacities mimicking the "tree-in-bud" appearance[203–206] (Fig. 6.54).

Hematogenous (miliary) dissemination, usually seen in very young and immunocompromised patients, can affect virtually any organ in the body. Miliary tuberculosis manifests radiographically in the lung as nodular interstitial granulomas, usually 1 to 2 mm in size, throughout both lungs. CT is more sensitive than chest radiograph for the detection of miliary TB[202] (Fig. 6.55). Congenital tuberculosis, defined as an infection transmitted from the mother to the fetus via transplacental route or via the birth canal, usually presents as a miliary pattern on imaging.

Tuberculous pleural effusion and chronic TB empyema can be seen as complications with or without pleural calcification.[207] Pericarditis and pericardial effusion can also be seen as complications. Cross-sectional imaging such CT is a sensitive imaging tool to confirm the diagnosis and assess sequelae including constrictive pericarditis.[208]

Postprimary TB, reactivation TB disease, or adult-type TB disease is often seen in children over 10 years of age and adults. The typical radiographic pattern is bilateral ill-defined parenchymal densities mainly involving the apical segments of the upper lobes (Fig. 6.56). It is usually associated with nodular and linear fibrosis. There could be associated distortion of the adjacent mediastinal and bronchovascular structures. Cavitation with air–fluid levels, pleural effusions,

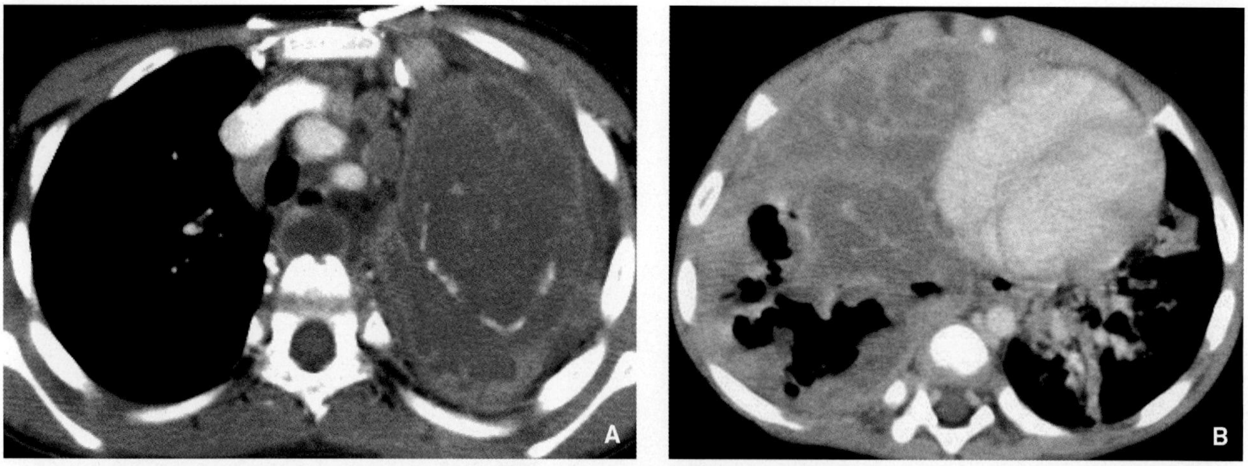

FIGURE 6.53 **Primary progressive pulmonary tuberculosis in two different pediatric patients. A:** Axial enhanced CT image reveals necrotic lung consolidation with calcifications in the left upper lobe. **B:** Axial enhanced CT image of another pediatric patient with extensive right lung disease with necrosis and cavitation.

bronchiectasis, and even colonization of the cavities with *Aspergillus* species can be seen.[207] Rarely, Rasmussen aneurysm, a pseudoaneurysm caused by erosion of a peripheral pulmonary artery branch by an adjacent tuberculous cavity lesion, occurs.[208]

Antimycobacterial therapy is the cornerstone of TB treatment. Most common medications include isoniazid, rifampin, ethambutol, and pyrazinamide. These are taken for at least 6 to 9 months depending on age, overall health, possible drug resistance, organ involvement, and form of disease. Hematogenous dissemination in various body parts would entail longer and more aggressive treatment. Completing the treatment course is essential to avoid development of drug-resistant strains, which are much more dangerous and difficult to treat. Directly observed therapy (DOT) program, where a health care worker helps in administration of medication, has helped increase compliance.

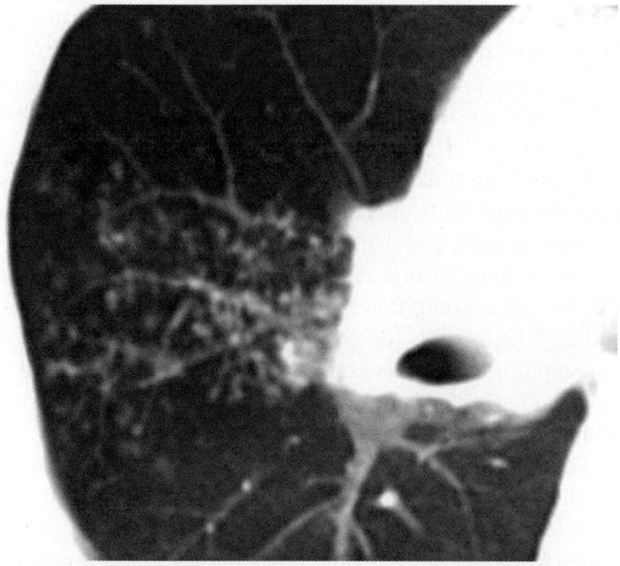

FIGURE 6.54 **Tree-in-bud pattern of tuberculous (TB) infection.** Axial lung window CT image shows variable-sized pulmonary nodules in a branching pattern mimicking the "tree-in-bud" appearance. This represents bronchopneumonic pattern of disease spread in TB.

Nontuberculous Mycobacterial Infection

Nontuberculous mycobacteria (NTM) are species of the genus *Mycobacterium* that do not belong to the *Mycobacterium tuberculosis* complex. These human opportunistic pathogens are widespread in the environment and have been isolated from water, soil, food products, as well as domestic and wild animals. Transmission is through ingestion or inhalation of water, particulate matter or aerosols, or through trauma.[209] *M. avium, M. intracellulare, and M. abscessus* are the species most frequently isolated from children.[210] NTM may produce infection in pediatric patients with normal immunity, but infection is more significant in immunocompromised children and those with CF. NTM most commonly manifests as one of four clinical syndromes: (1) lymphadenopathy, (2) skin and soft tissue infection, (3) pulmonary disease (particularly with underlying pulmonary conditions), (4) disseminated disease in immunocompromised children.

The clinical features of pulmonary disease are variable and include chronic or recurrent cough, increased sputum production, dyspnea, hemoptysis, chest pain, rhonchi, crackles, wheezing, and stridor. Constitutional findings, which are more prevalent in the immunocompromised, may include fever, fatigue, malaise, and weight loss.[211] Diagnosis of NTM is based on a combination of clinical, radiographic, and laboratory criteria.

Mediastinal and hilar lymph node enlargement is the most common radiographic manifestation of NTM in children, similar to *M. tuberculosis* infection (Fig. 6.57). With advanced disease, signaled by generalized complaints, there is increased development of pulmonary abnormality.[212,213] Pulmonary abnormalities include multiple nodules and consolidations, which may show cavitation. Multifocal bronchiectasis could also be seen and better visualized in HRCT. In NTM hypersensitivity-like pneumonitis ("hot tub lung"), radiographic

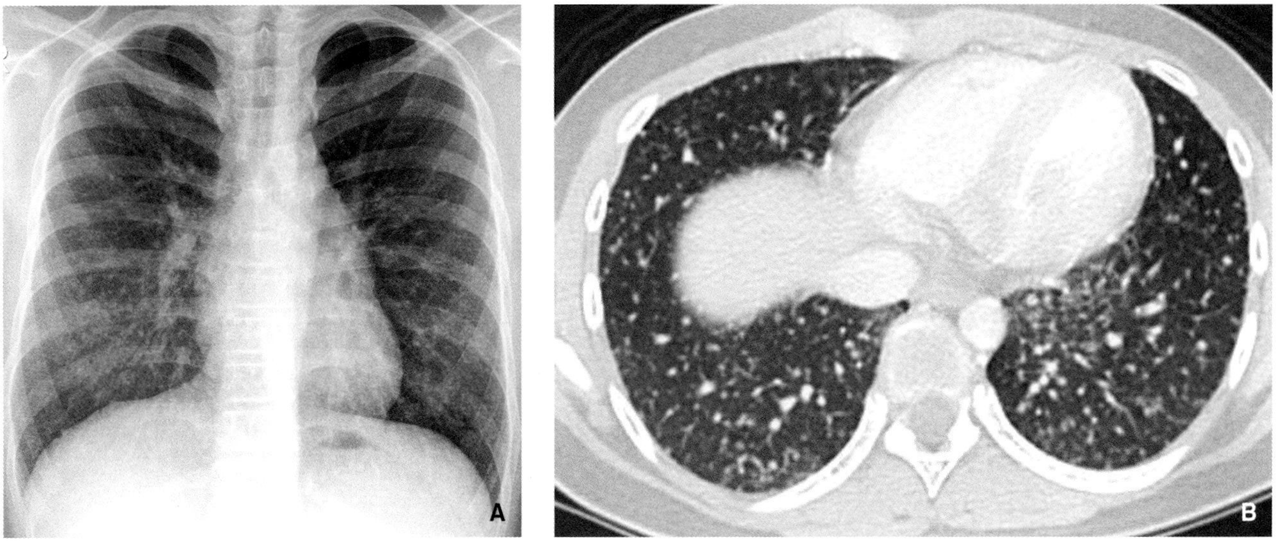

FIGURE 6.55 **Miliary pattern of tuberculous (TB) infection.** Frontal chest radiograph **(A)** and axial lung window CT image **(B)** show small (1 to 2 mm), uniform nodular densities scattered throughout both lungs compatible with disseminated TB infection.

features may resemble those seen in variably florid hypersensitivity pneumonitis.[214]

Antimycobacterial treatment is generally warranted for children who meet clinical and microbiologic criteria for NTM pulmonary disease. However, the potential risks and benefits of antimycobacterial therapy must be considered before initiating treatment. Speciation and drug susceptibility testing are recommended for clinically significant NTM pulmonary isolates. However, it may be necessary to initiate empiric therapy before speciation is complete, particularly when *M. tuberculosis* cannot be excluded.

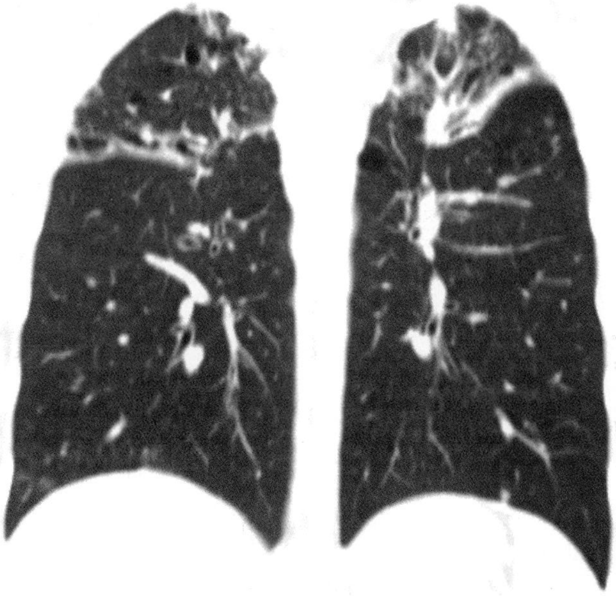

FIGURE 6.56 **Reactivation tuberculous (TB) or adult-type TB infection pattern in a 13-year-old girl who presented with chronic cough.** Coronal reformatted CT image in the lung window setting shows bilateral apical fibrosis with nodules and cavities.

Fungal Infection

Aspergillosis

Aspergillus species are ubiquitous saprophytic molds commonly found in decaying materials. Although there are more than 900 species, the agent responsible for more than 90% of human infections is *Aspergillus fumigatus*. The respiratory tract is the usual entry site of infection, although other routes of entry include the skin, GI tract, and nasopharynx. Involvement of the respiratory tract can manifest as (1) allergic disease (sinusitis, asthma, alveolitis) following repeated exposure to *Aspergillus* antigens; (2) saprophytic infestation involving mycelial growth in the body of the host, resulting in allergic bronchopulmonary aspergillosis (ABPA); (3) colonization of necrotic tissue and airway cavities (aspergilloma); and (4) invasive disease, which is usually acute and rapidly progressive severe disease.[215] These four types of involvement by aspergillus are an idealized schema of disease but may not always be so distinct.

ABPA occurs in patients with chronic respiratory disease (e.g., asthma and CF) where the fungi are trapped in tenacious secretions, leading to an immune response that exacerbates their respiratory symptoms. Chronic mucosal colonization causes elevated immunoglobulin G (IgG) and immunoglobulin E (IgE) levels, which lead to recurrent bronchospasm. On imaging studies, ABPA is characterized by mucoid impaction of the proximal bronchi, seen as finger-like shadows involving the upper lobes on the chest radiograph. This radiographic pattern is referred to as "finger-in-glove" sign (Fig. 6.58). CT demonstrates the mucoid impaction of the central airways and the bronchiectasis of the segmental or subsegmental airways.[215]

Aspergilloma or mycetoma (fungus ball) is a colonization of intertwined fungal hyphae growing in a preformed space such as an ectatic bronchus or a postpneumonic cavity. Aspergillomas typically demonstrate a rounded soft tissue mass within a cavity forming an "air-crescent" sign. The fungal ball may move within the cavity according to the patient's position[215] (Fig. 6.59).

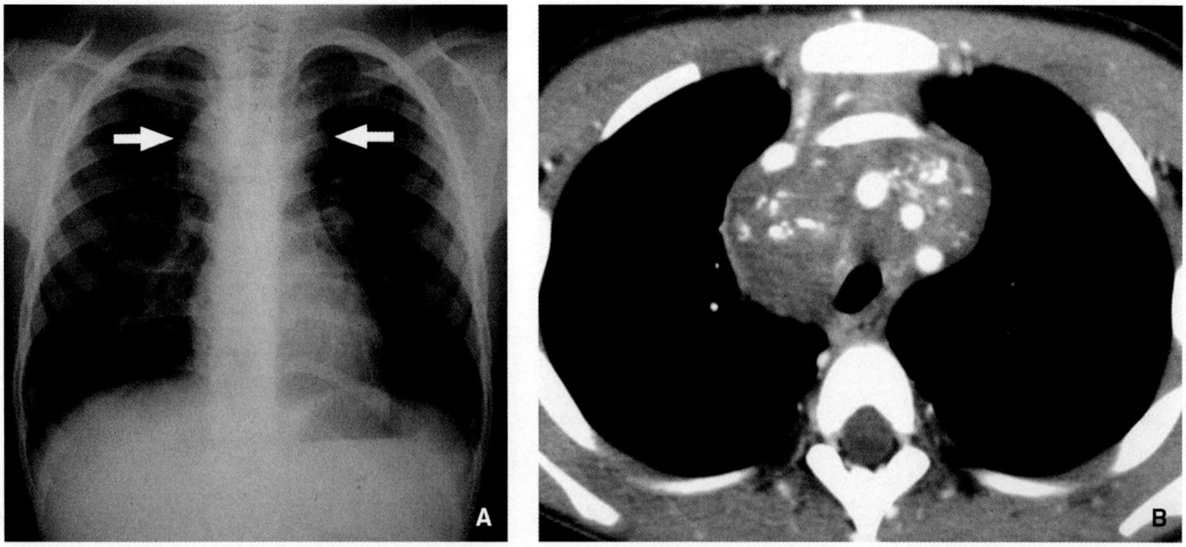

FIGURE 6.57 **Nontuberculous *Mycobacterium* infection in a 10-year-old boy who presented with palpable cervical lymphadenopathy. A:** Frontal chest radiograph shows mediastinal widening (*arrows*) with mild buckling of the trachea to the left. **B:** Axial enhanced CT image confirms the mass as matted lymph nodes with mottled calcifications.

Invasive disease occurs in the immunocompromised, commonly in the setting of neutropenia and AIDS. It ranges from localized abscess formation (Fig. 6.60) to an aggressive, rapidly disseminating and destructive disease with high mortality.[216] The former can lead to widespread organ involvement, including pulmonary, cerebral, ocular, and cutaneous disease. In the lungs, it is characterized by the occlusion of large or medium-sized arteries by plugs of hyphae causing pulmonary hemorrhage, arterial thrombosis, and infarction.[217] For invasive pulmonary aspergillosis, radiographic findings are mostly nonspecific, with multiple nodules or areas of consolidation[218]; however, pleural-based wedge-shaped lesions and cavitations can suggest aspergillus pneumonia. The typical CT finding is the "halo sign", which consists of a pulmonary nodule or mass surrounded by ground-glass attenuation representing hemorrhage[144,215,218] (Fig. 6.61).

Aspergillosis treatment is based on the disease manifestation. When invasive aspergillosis is strongly suspected in an immunocompromised patient, antifungal medications are empirically administered. ABPA exacerbations are treated with corticosteroids to reduce serum IgE levels. Surgical care

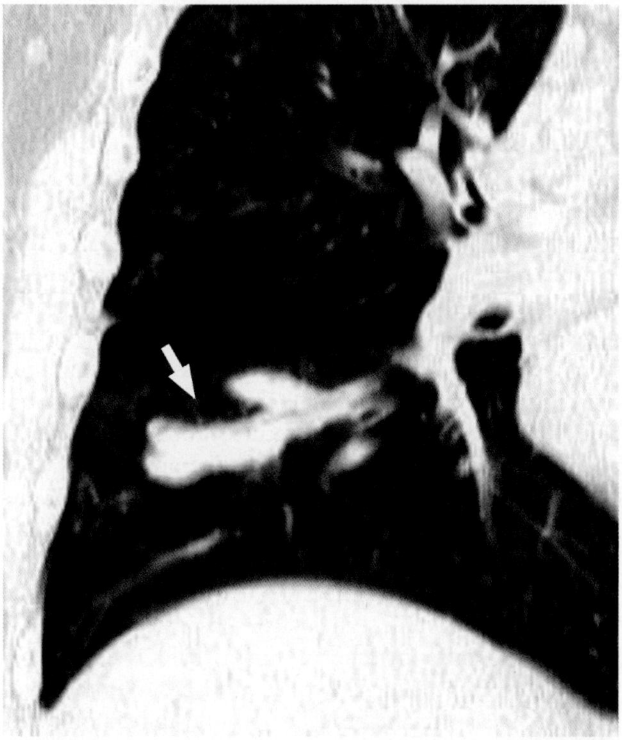

FIGURE 6.58 **ABPA in a 12-year-old boy with asthma.** Coronal reformatted CT image in the lung window setting shows mucoid impaction (*arrow*), which results in a bronchocoele, "finger-in-glove" sign.

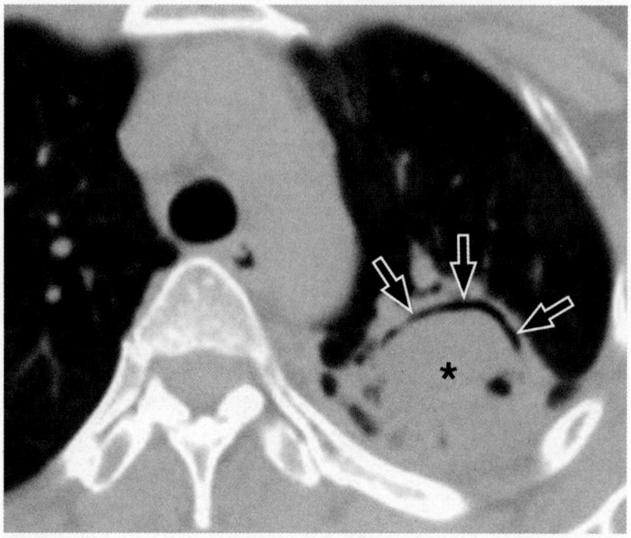

FIGURE 6.59 **Aspergilloma (fungal ball) in a 10-year-old boy.** Axial CT image in the lung window setting shows a round soft tissue mass (*asterisk*) within a cavity forming an "air-crescent" sign (*arrows*), which is typical of aspergilloma.

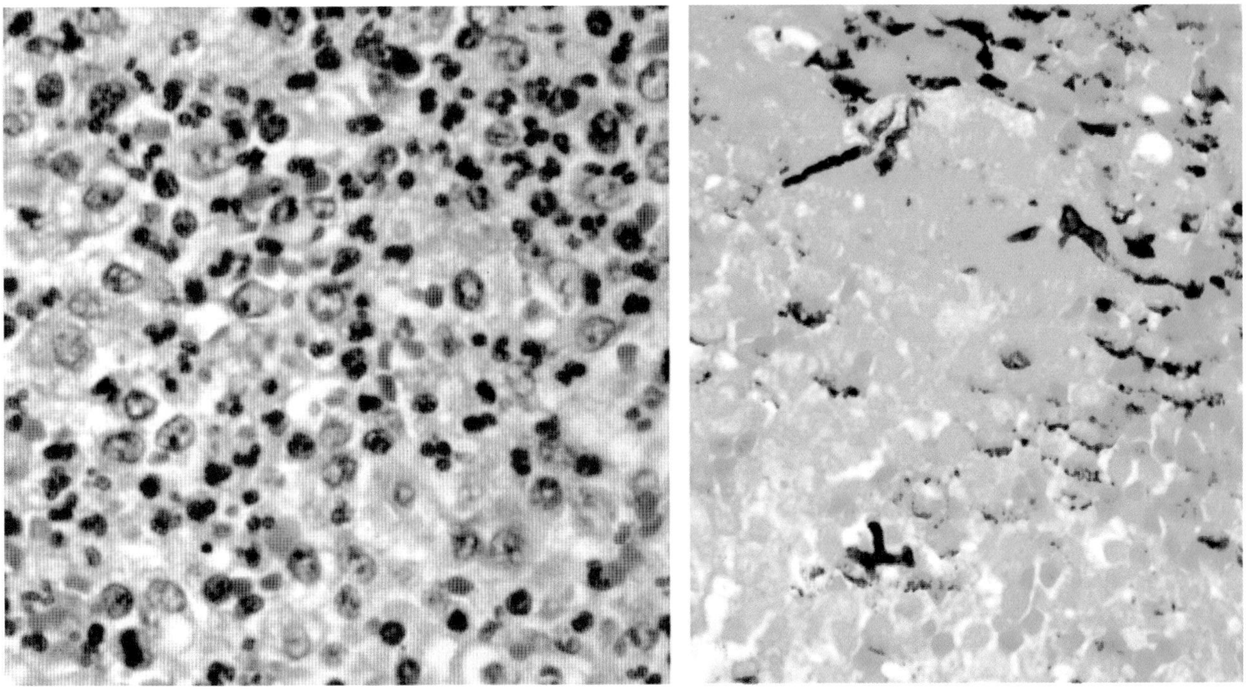

FIGURE 6.60 ***Aspergillus* causing lung abscesses in a 12-year-old girl with acute myelogenous leukemia.** The abscess cavity contains predominantly neutrophils and macrophages (**left**; hematoxylin and eosin stain, original magnification, 600×) and branching septate hyphal fungal forms (**right**; Grocott methenamine silver stain, original magnification, 600×).

for aspergilloma is typically reserved for patients with severe hemoptysis.

Histoplasmosis

Histoplasma capsulatum is a dimorphic fungus that causes histoplasmosis. It is found in the soil of endemic areas including Central United States particularly the Ohio and Mississippi river valleys, Central America, Northern South America, and some parts of Asia.[219] After inhalation, the spores germinate within the alveoli, inciting an intense tissue reaction characterized by granulomas, which may calcify. The infection also spreads into the hilar or mediastinal lymph nodes.[220] Histoplasmosis is generally an asymptomatic and self-limited disease that rarely requires therapy in children other than the very young or immunocompromised.

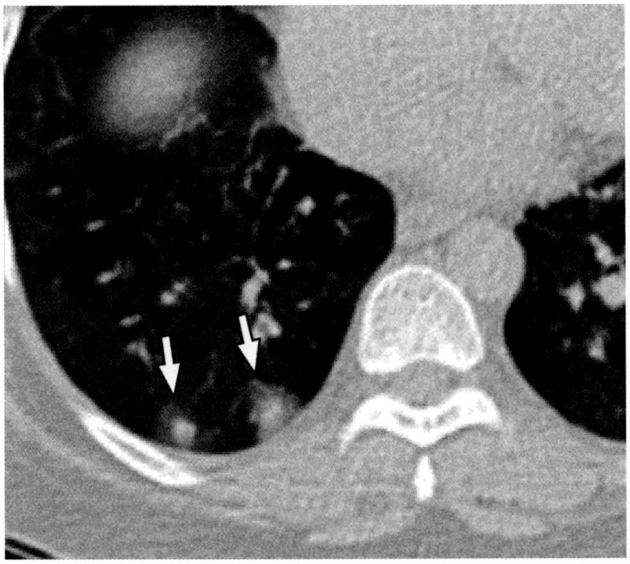

FIGURE 6.61 **Invasive pulmonary aspergillosis infection in a 7-year-old girl with leukemia.** Axial lung window CT image shows pulmonary nodules (*arrows*) with the typical "halo sign", which consists of a pulmonary nodule surrounded by ground-glass attenuation representing adjacent hemorrhage.

Disease falls in one of three phases: acute, chronic, and disseminated disease. Acute pulmonary histoplasmosis, a self-limited illness, usually develops 12 to 14 days after exposure. It is characterized by nonspecific symptoms including fever, headache, cough, chest pain, and sometimes erythema nodosum/multiforme. Chronic pulmonary histoplasmosis occurs in patients with chronic lung disease and presents similar to TB. Disseminated disease occurs in pediatric patients with impaired immunity. It is characteristically a fulminant illness involving multiple organs, which may or may not involve the lungs.[219] Organisms seen on biopsy appear as small round forms with narrow-based budding. For definitive speciation, laboratory testing for antigen, *Histoplasma*-specific antibodies, and/or molecular signature is required; characteristic radiologic features are also helpful in the diagnosis.

Radiologic manifestations are similar to TB and parallel the clinical phase of the disease. Acute histoplasmosis usually manifests as focal parenchymal consolidation with or without ipsilateral hilar adenopathy. Pulmonary nodule representing a histoplasmoma may result after healing but with large inoculum exposures, widespread consolidation or diffuse nodular opacifications with calcifications may occur. Calcified mediastinal and hilar lymph nodes are often seen in patients with

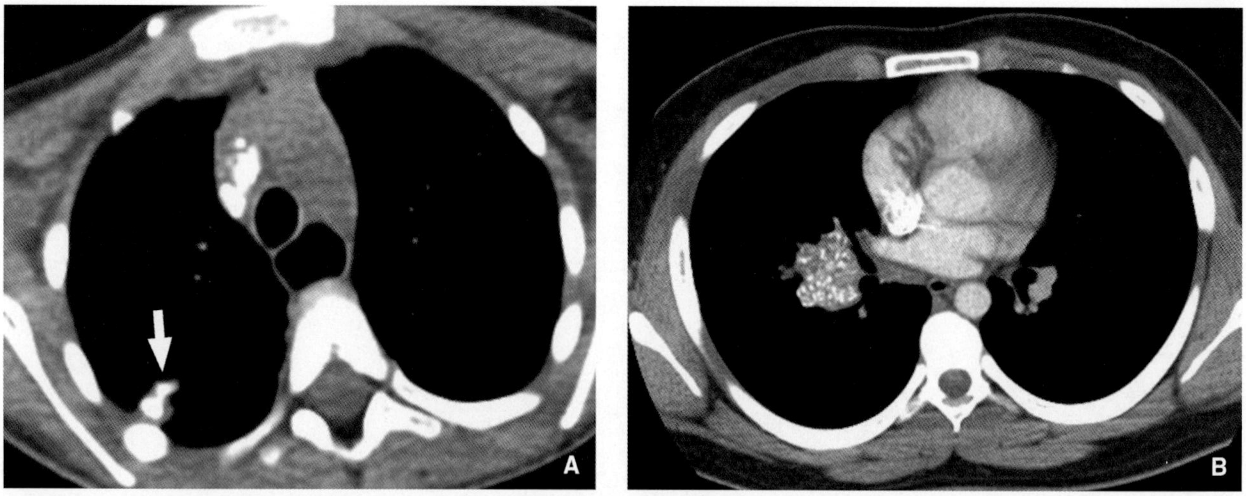

FIGURE 6.62 **Histoplasmosis infection in a 4-year-old boy.** Axial enhanced CT images **(A)** and **(B)** show a calcified pulmonary nodule in the right upper lobe (*arrow*) along with calcified lymph nodes in the pretracheal region and right hilar area. (Case courtesy of Beth Kline-Fath, MD, Cincinnati Children's Hospital Medical Center, Cincinnati, OH.)

calcified pulmonary nodules (Fig. 6.62). Chronic histoplasmosis radiographically manifests as an upper lobe fibrocavitary disease indistinguishable from postprimary tuberculosis. Disseminated disease may show miliary or diffuse reticulonodular pattern that could progress to diffuse airspace opacification[220] (Fig. 6.63).

Mediastinal histoplasmosis may complicate the pulmonary disease. It can be in the form of enlarged and lobulated mediastinal lymph nodes forming granulomas, which may cause symptoms related to mass effect on adjacent structures, or it could be from mediastinal fibrosis, which occurs less frequently but can gradually compress adjacent structures.[221]

For immunocompetent hosts, most acute forms of histoplasmosis resolve without specific treatment. Systemic antifungal treatment (amphotericin B, itraconazole, ketoconazole, or fluconazole) is indicated for more severe disease especially in chronic pulmonary histoplasmosis, disseminated histoplasmosis, or any disease manifestation in an immunocompromised pediatric patient. The specific antifungal agent, dose, and length of administration vary with the form and disease manifestation.

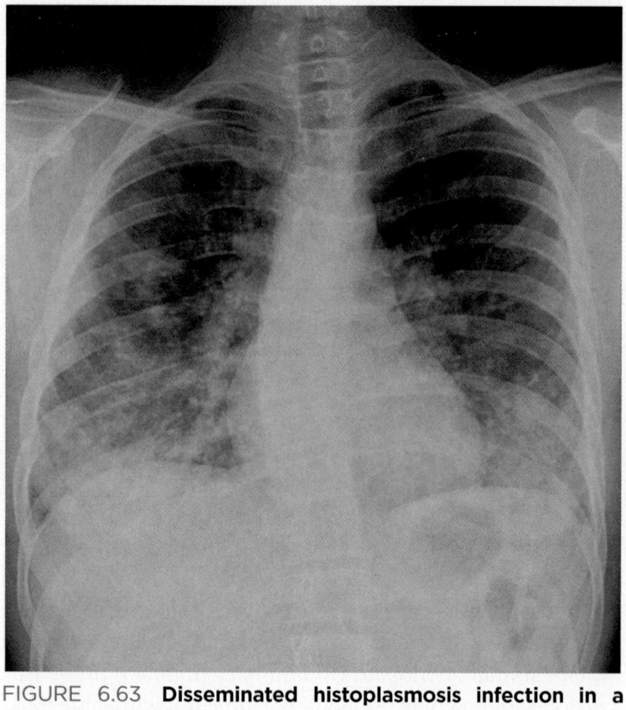

FIGURE 6.63 **Disseminated histoplasmosis infection in a 15-year-old girl.** Frontal chest radiograph shows multiple nodular opacities throughout both lungs. Following therapy, the patient did well without sequelae. (Case courtesy of Elizabeth H. Ey, MD, Dayton Children's Hospital Medical Center, Dayton, OH.)

Coccidioidomycosis

Coccidioidomycosis is caused by *Coccidioides immitis* and *Coccidioides posadasii*, two distinct but morphologically identical species of a soil fungus with identical manifestations of infection. It is endemic to certain regions in the United States including California (San Joaquin Valley), Arizona, Nevada, New Mexico, Utah, and Texas, as well as regions of Mexico, and Central and South America.

Inhalation of spores is the route of infection, and the most common clinical manifestation is self-limited or subacute community-acquired pneumonia.[222] Some affected pediatric patients develop symptomatic disease, ranging from a mild influenza-like illness, pneumonia, and rarely respiratory failure. A more involved presentation, with the constellation of fever, arthralgias, erythema nodosum or erythema multiforme, and chest pain, is commonly referred to as San Joaquin Valley fever or desert rheumatism. In addition to pneumonia, mediastinitis is also a common presentation in the pediatric population, which requires longer hospitalization.[223] Disseminated infection, virtually involving any organ of the body, is seen in minority of affected children especially those with impaired immune status.

Radiographs of affected pediatric patients may show pulmonary nodules or consolidation with associated enlargement of mediastinal or hilar lymph nodes. In immunocompetent children, most of these lesions resolve spontaneously. However, persistent pulmonary lesions can eventually

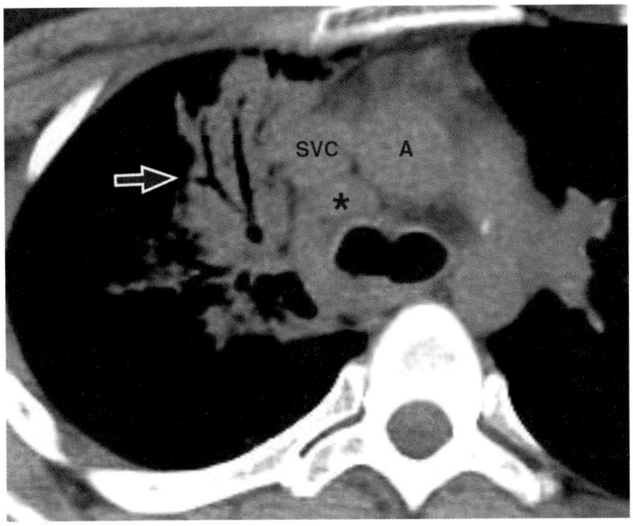

FIGURE 6.64 **Cocidioidomycosis infection in a 17-year-old boy who presented with cough and chest pain after traveling to northern Mexico.** Axial CT image shows consolidation with air bronchograms in the right upper lobe (*arrow*) and mediastinal lymphadenopathy (*asterisk*). *A*, aorta; *SVC*, superior vena cava.

degenerate into thin-walled cavities. The regional nodes may also erode into an adjacent bronchus with endobronchial spread of the infection and the development of bilateral diffuse pneumonia. In younger children, diffuse nodular opacities throughout both lungs along with areas of more severe focal consolidation are seen[224] (Fig. 6.64). Similar imaging manifestations are also seen in TB and histoplasmosis.

Management of coccidioidomycosis involves defining the extent of infection and identifying host factors that affect severity of disease. Most infected pediatric patients are asymptomatic or have self-limited symptoms and require only supportive care. Symptomatic children with no risk factors for complications often require only periodic reassessment to demonstrate resolution of their self-limited process. Pediatric patients with extensive spread of infection or those at high risk of complications because of immunosuppression or other preexisting factors require a variety of treatment strategies that may include antifungal drug therapy, surgical debridement, or a combination of both. Azoles, primarily fluconazole and itraconazole, are the antifungals of choice for most chronic pulmonary or disseminated cocidioidomycosis infections.[220]

Pneumocystis jiroveci

Pneumocystis jiroveci (previously classified as *Pneumocystis carinii*) is considered a fungus based on nucleic acid and biochemical analysis. These organisms are commonly found in the lungs of healthy individuals and most children who have been exposed to the organism.[225] It is an important opportunistic human pathogen in the immunocompromised host and the most common cause of death among children receiving chemotherapy for leukemia prior to the inclusion of *Pneumocystis jiroveci* prophylaxis.[226] It is also the most common opportunistic pulmonary infection in children with HIV/AIDS, occurring in up to 50%.[144]

Once inhaled, the trophic form of *Pneumocystis jiroveci* organisms attach to the alveoli inciting the infectious process. Multiple host immune defects allow for uncontrolled replication of the organisms and development of illness. *Pneumocystis jiroveci* pneumonia typically follows a subacute indolent time course, with symptoms that include exertional dyspnea, fever, nonproductive cough, chest discomfort, and weight loss. Children with severe disease may have cyanosis, nasal flaring, and intercostal retractions.

The chest radiographic findings may be normal in pediatric patients with early or mild disease,[227] but the majority of children with *Pneumocystis jiroveci* pneumonia have abnormal chest radiographs.[228] Imaging appearance is variable, but the typical radiographic findings include diffuse bilateral interstitial or nodular opacification extending from the perihilar region with hyperinflation (Fig. 6.65). There is often progres-

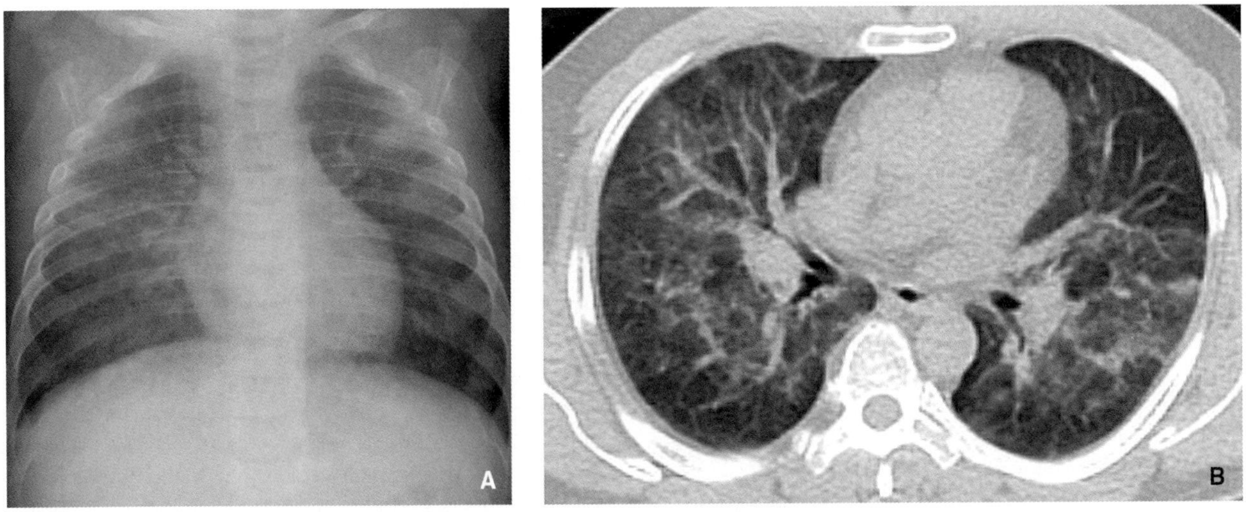

FIGURE 6.65 ***Pneumocystis jiroveci* infection in a 2-year-old boy with primary immune deficiency. A:** Frontal chest radiograph shows bilateral diffuse interstitial nodular opacities extending from the perihilar regions and hyperinflation. **B:** Axial CT image reveals patchy ground-glass attenuation with a background of interlobular septal thickening.

sion to widespread alveolar opacities with air bronchogram.[228] Cavitary nodules and cysts can also be seen, with pneumothorax and/or pneumomediastinum as common complications. Pleural effusions and intrathoracic adenopathy are rare.

Typical HRCT findings include patchy or diffuse ground-glass attenuation with a background of interlobular septal thickening known as "crazy-paving" pattern. Consolidations, cavities, centrilobular opacities, and nodules are best appreciated on the CT compared to the chest radiograph.[142,144] Cystic changes can be seen related to aerosolized pentamidine and trimethoprim prophylaxis.[228] A normal CT alone does not exclude *Pneumocystis jiroveci* infection. Gallium scanning is highly sensitive for detecting *Pneumocystis jiroveci* infection but with low and variable specificity.

The typical appearance of *Pneumocystis jiroveci* pneumonia is that of an eosinophilic intra-alveolar exudate resembling alveolar proteinosis; special stains reveal round yeast-like forms within the material (Fig. 6.66). The exudate and diagnostic organisms may be recovered via bronchoalveolar lavage or biopsy. A minority of affected pediatric patients (5%) show granulomatous inflammation rather than the characteristic exudative pattern.

Although it is classified as a fungal pneumonia, *Pneumocystis jiroveci* does not respond to antifungal treatment. Trimethoprim-sulfamethoxazole (TMP-SMX) is the recommended drug for treatment. Corticosteroids are used as adjunctive initial therapy in patients with HIV infection who have severe *Pneumocystis jiroveci* pneumonia.[226] The incidence of *Pneumocystis jiroveci* pneumonia has decreased significantly since initiation of prophylaxis; however, breakthrough cases occur. Myelosuppression is the most important adverse effect of TMP-SMZ and the most frequent cause for choosing alternative prophylactic agents in children undergoing chemotherapy. Aerosolized pentamidine and atovaquone are alternative prophylactic agents that must be used in pediatric patients with developing myelosuppression secondary to TMP-SMZ or dapsone.[229]

Candidiasis

Candida is the most common cause of fungal infections worldwide. Many species are harmless to hosts including humans; however, they can act as opportunistic pathogens when the immune system is compromised. *Candida albicans* is the most commonly isolated species, but other species such as *C. tropicalis, C. parapsilosis,* and *C. lusitaniae* have also been implicated.[230] *Candida* pneumonia may be due to aspiration from oral or upper airway flora (descending pneumonia) or via disseminated infection from a distant site (hematogenous pneumonia). *Candida* pneumonia from a hematogenous source can be seen in patients with chronic debilitating disease and the immunocompromised.[218,231]

The most common symptoms of *Candida* pneumonia from a descending source are fever, tachypnea, dyspnea, and chest pain. Hematogenously acquired *Candida* pneumonia usually presents as part of the complex of symptoms depending on other organs involved. Diagnosis is difficult because there is no specific clinical or radiologic presentation. In addition, the presence of *Candida* in sputum or respiratory specimens sometimes represents contamination. A definitive diagnosis of *Candida* pneumonia requires histopathologic proof of lung invasion.[231]

There is no clear radiologic pattern that indicates either descending or hematogenous *Candida* pneumonia. Many of the affected pediatric patients have normal chest radiographs, but when abnormal, most common findings are bilateral interstitial or multifocal alveolar patchy opacifications. A miliary pattern is common in hematogenous *Candida* pneumonia.[232] Cavitary masses and exudative pleural effusions have also been described. CT features are nonspecific and vary with pathologic pattern and stage of the disease. A common finding is a miliary pattern with multiple nodules usually ranging from 3 to 30 mm in diameter, either well defined or associated with other parenchymal findings such as airspace consolidation, tree-in-bud changes, or ground-glass opacities[233] (Fig. 6.67). Sometimes, a CT halo sign may be seen around the nodular lesions.[218]

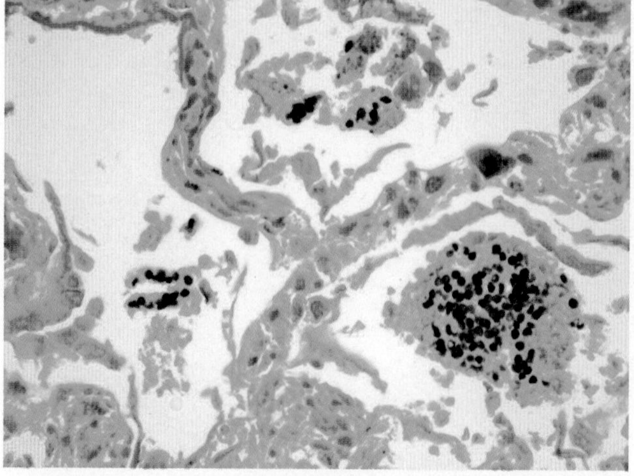

FIGURE 6.66 ***Pneumocystis jiroveci* infection involving the lung.** Grocott methenamine stain highlights round yeast-like forms with a frequent collapsed or deflated appearance. The organisms are located within a fluffy intra-alveolar proteinaceous exudate (original magnification, 600×).

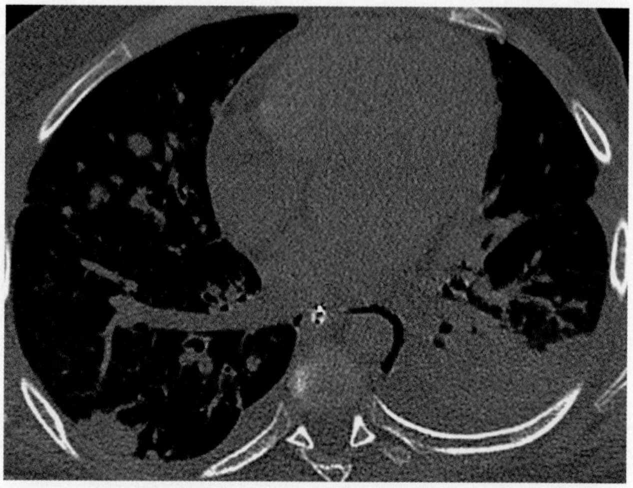

FIGURE 6.67 **Disseminated candidiasis infection in a 4-year-old girl who is immunosuppressed.** Axial CT image shows multiple small pulmonary nodules of variable size in both lungs compatible with disseminated *Candida* infection. Also noted is left lower lobe consolidation. (Case courtesy of Elizabeth H. Ey, MD, Dayton Children's Hospital Medical Center, Dayton, OH.)

Antifungal therapy with amphotericin B or fluconazole is given for *Candida* pneumonia. However, because many *Candida* infections involving the lungs are secondary to hematogenous dissemination, treatment of distant disease or fungemia should be considered.[233]

Parasitic Infection

Pulmonary Paragonimiasis

Paragonimiasis is a parasitic infection, also known as lung fluke disease, caused by a trematode, *Paragonimus westermani,* or other species. It is endemic in East Asia, Southeast Asia, Latin America, and Africa. Infection often occurs by ingestion of *Paragonimus* metacercariae through raw or partially cooked freshwater crab or crayfishes. The metacercariae lodge in the small intestine and penetrate the peritoneal cavity, diaphragm, pleural cavity, and eventually enter the lung parenchyma where they mature and can cause disease. Infrequently, the metacercariae migrate to other tissues, which is termed extrapulmonary paragonimiasis. Pediatric patients with pulmonary paragonimiasis may be asymptomatic, but typical presenting symptoms include chronic cough with rusty-brown sputum, hemoptysis, pleurisy, and fever.[234–236]

Radiologic findings often correlate well with the stage of the disease. Pleural effusion or pneumothorax can be seen because of penetration of the juvenile worms through the pleural cavity. Once the parasites get to the lung, patchy airspace consolidation or nodules with surrounding ground-glass opacity are seen, which reflects exudative or hemorrhagic pneumonia. These nodules and opacities can cavitate. Many nodules have linear track to the peripheral surface that may correspond to the worm migration track. During the late stage, worm cysts, measuring 0.5 to 1.5 cm, are better visualized after the consolidation resolves and manifest as either solitary or multiple nodules or gas-filled cysts depending on their content and their communication with the airway. A crescent-shaped area of increased opacity within the cyst represents worms attached to the wall[235–237] (Fig. 6.68).

The anthelmintic drugs recommended by the World Health Organization for the treatment of paragonimiasis are praziquantel and triclabendazole. Promotion and education on healthy eating habits are also very important in the prevention and spread of the disease.[234]

Echinococcus Infection

Echinococcosis is a parasitic infection in humans caused by dog tapeworm *Echinococcus granulosus* in its larval stage. Also known as hydatid disease or hydatidosis, it is endemic in many sheep- and cattle-raising countries throughout the world.[238] Definitive hosts are canines (usually dogs), and the intermediate hosts are usually grazing animals (sheep and cattle). Humans acting as intermediate hosts become infected through ingestion of contaminated water or vegetables. When eggs of adult tapeworm are ingested, embryos are freed and migrate through the host's gastrointestinal mucosa, enter the portal vein and lymphatic system, to various parts of the body where the embryo develops into a cyst, which increases 2 to 3 cm in size every year.[239] The wall of the cysts contains three layers: the outermost pericyst, the middle laminated membrane layer, ectocyst, and innermost germinal layer, endocyst.[238,239] The lungs are the most common site of infection in children and the second most common site of infection in adults. The majority of infected pediatric patients remain asymptomatic, but common symptoms include cough, chest pain, hemoptysis, and vomica.[239,240]

Abnormalities that are incidentally seen on routine chest radiographs are helpful in the diagnosis. The most common radiographic manifestation is a dense, well-demarcated rounded opacity that could mimic a bronchogenic cyst or a

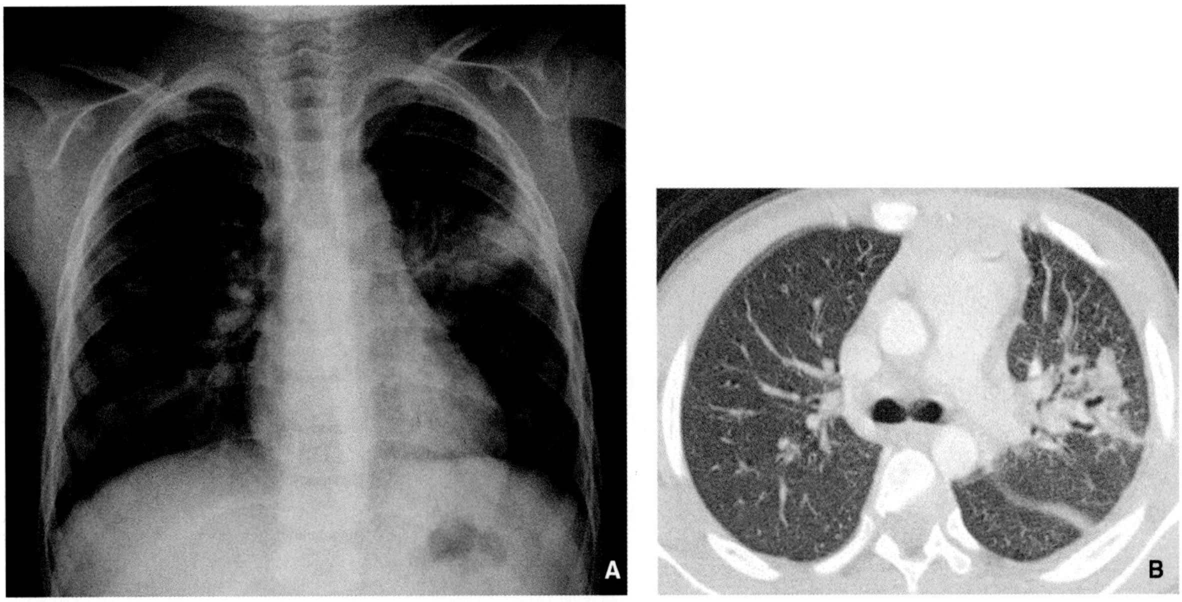

FIGURE 6.68 **Pulmonary paragonimiasis infection in a 4-year-old boy. A:** Frontal chest radiograph shows a nonspecific patchy airspace opacification in the left upper lobe. **B:** Axial lung window CT image confirms this consolidation with associated mild bronchiectasis. (Case courtesy of Kay Pacharn, MD, Siriraj Hospital, Bangkok, Thailand.)

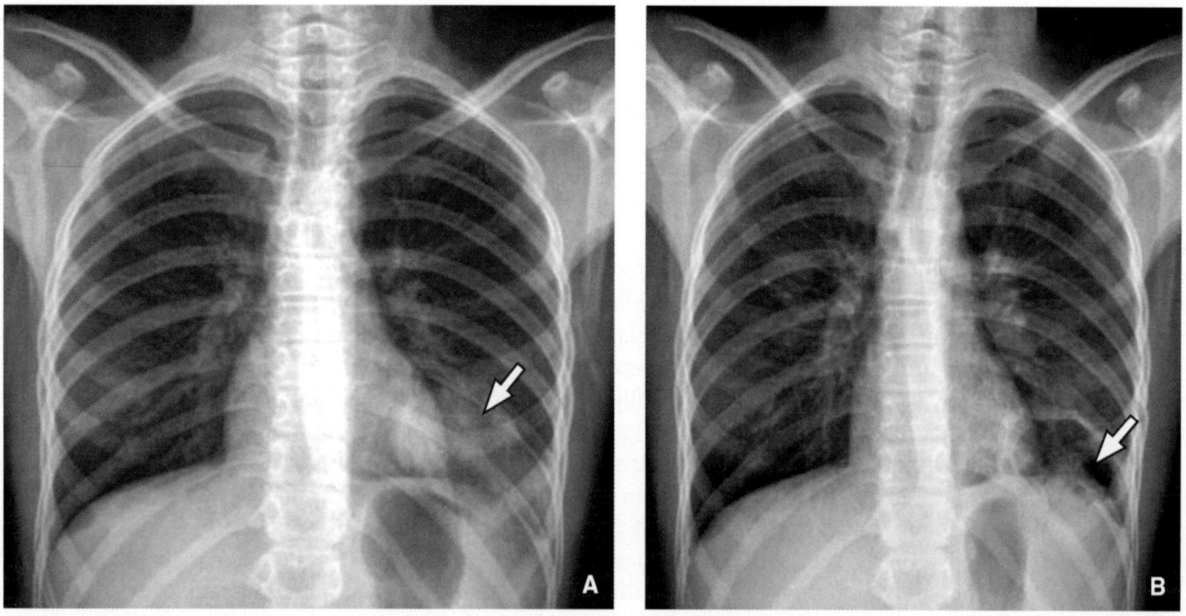

FIGURE 6.69 **Hydatid disease from Echinococcus infection in a 12-year-old girl who presented with fever and left-sided chest pain. A:** Frontal chest radiograph shows a rounded opacity (*arrow*) at the base of the left lung. **B:** Follow-up chest radiograph obtained a week later shows a membrane (*arrow*) within the cystic lesion, compatible with the "water lily sign." (Case courtesy of Ali Yikilmaz, MD, Istanbul Medeniyet University Medical School, Goztepe Research and Training Hospital, Istanbul, Turkey.)

neoplasm. As the cyst grows and erodes the adjacent bronchioles, air between the endocyst and pericyst can produce a "crescent" or "inverse crescent" sign. If air continues to enter the cyst cavity, the endocyst membrane can be seen floating in the most dependent part of the pericyst cavity producing the typical "water-lily" sign appearance[240,241] (Fig. 6.69). An infected cyst has higher attenuation/density, thick walls, with air–fluid level and surrounding pneumonia, similar to typical lung abscess.[240]

A pathology-based classification for this disease has been described: Type I hydatid cysts have a well-defined round or oval cystic mass, which has an anechoic appearance on US and are near water density on CT. Type II hydatid cysts have many daughter cysts and/or matrix within the parent cyst with or without cyst wall calcification. Type III hydatid cysts are calcified, nonviable degenerated cysts.[238,242]

The fundamental medical management of *Echinococcus* infection is administration of antiparasitic drugs such as benzimidazoles (mebendazole and albendazole) at high doses. Intravenous amphotericin B may be used as a rescue drug in pediatric patients resistant or intolerant to benzimidazoles.

Complications of Lung Infections

Lung parenchymal complications from pulmonary infections represent a spectrum of abnormalities including necrotizing pneumonia, lung abscess, pneumatocele, pulmonary gangrene, and bronchiectasis. Imaging, particularly CT, has been shown to be highly accurate in the identification of the presence and extent of these lung parenchymal complications.

Necrotizing Pneumonia

Necrotizing pneumonia, or cavitary necrosis, is a complication of severe lobar pneumonia characterized by underlying necrosis and liquefaction of lung tissues leading to multiple cavities. It is most commonly caused by *S. pneumoniae*[243] although *Aspergillus* and *Legionella* have also been implicated in the pediatric population.[244] Inflammation from infection causes thrombotic occlusion of alveolar capillaries that results in ischemia or infarction. There is necrosis and liquefaction of the affected lung tissue forming fluid-filled or air-filled cavities. The adjacent visceral pleura is particularly fragile and tends to rupture, causing bronchopleural fistula.[245] CT is more sensitive than radiographs for the diagnosis of necrotizing pneumonia. CT shows lung consolidation with decreased parenchymal enhancement, loss of lung–pleura margin, and multiple thin-walled cavities lacking an enhancing border (Fig. 6.70). US may also show similar findings of necrotizing pneumonia within the consolidation.[244–246] Necrotizing pneumonia indicates an intense, usually prolonged illness, but it usually resolves without surgical intervention in the pediatric population.[243,245]

Lung Abscess

Lung abscesses are cavities containing purulent material that occur within an area of pre-existing lung infection, aspiration, or from hematogenous spread.[247] Imaging studies such as chest radiograph and CT show a thick-walled, circumscribed area of necrosis often associated with air–fluid level, usually 2 cm or greater within an area of lung infection (Fig. 6.71). Systemic antibiotics and physiotherapy with postural drainage are the initial treatment of choice. Lung abscesses in children under 7 years often do not drain spontaneously and are less likely to respond to medical treatment. In these pediatric patients, surgical or percutaneous drainage is likely to be required.[248]

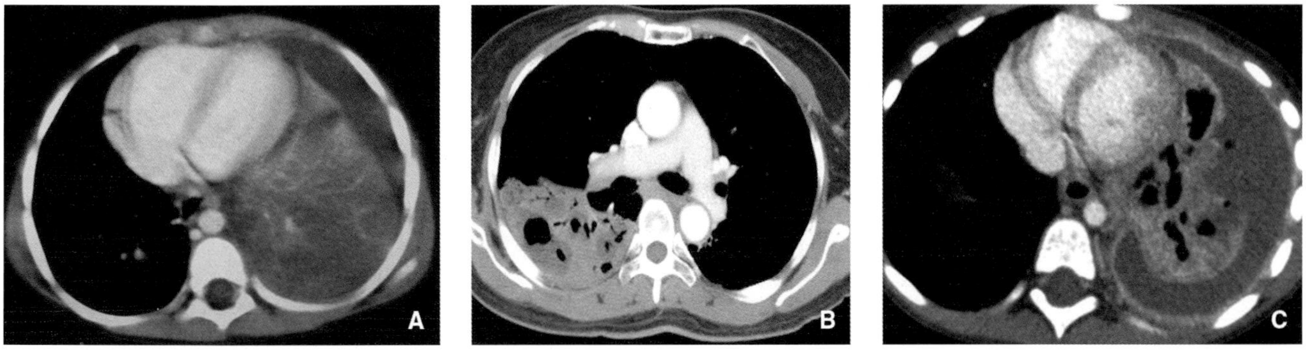

FIGURE 6.70 **Spectrum of necrotizing pneumonia appearance on CT in three pediatric patients. A:** Axial enhanced CT image shows left lower lobe consolidation with diminished perfusion at the posterior region. Moderate-sized pleural effusion is also seen. **B:** Axial enhanced CT image demonstrates an evolution of lung ischemia with development of multiple fluid-filled and air-filled cavities. **C:** Axial enhanced CT image shows cavitary necrosis of the consolidated left lung with bronchopleural fistula. The associated pleural fluid has an enhancing pleural surface, also known as the "split pleura" sign suggesting underlying pleural empyema.

Pneumatocele

Pneumatoceles are thin-walled cysts without septations that develop within the lung after an acute pneumonia, infarction, or other lung injury resulting in resorption of necrotic tissue. They are most often a sequelae of *S. aureus* infection[152] (Fig. 6.72).

Pulmonary Gangrene

Pulmonary gangrene is a rare complication of severe lung infection with devitalization of lung parenchyma (Fig. 6.73). It has been given various names including spontaneous amputation, massive sequestration of the lung, and spontaneous lobectomy. Most cases are due to *Klebsiella*, *S. aureus*, *Haemophilus influenzae*, pneumococci, and *Pseudomonas*. It is also described in TB, aspergillosis, and mucormycosis. When the entire lobe becomes involved, empyema results. However, when an intrapulmonary portion of the pulmonary parenchyma undergoes necrosis, it forms a cavity with gangrenous lung tissue floating inside the cavity. A "crescent sign" may be seen when the devitalized lung separates from the viable lung.[249]

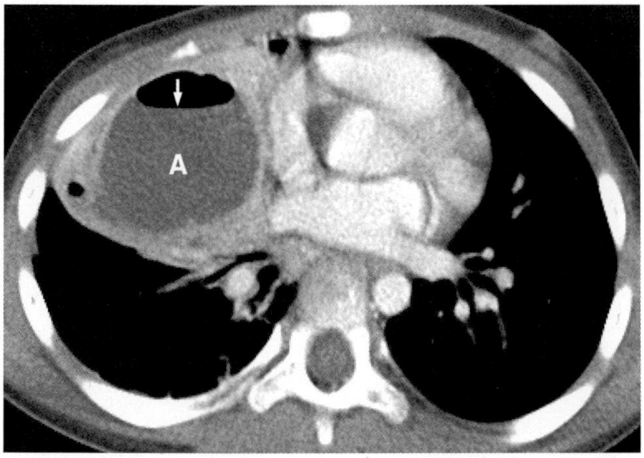

FIGURE 6.71 **Lung abscess in a 5-year-old boy who presented with cough and high fever.** Axial enhanced CT image shows a large abscess (A) in the right lung with air-fluid level (*arrow*) and thick irregular border.

Bronchiectasis

Bronchiectasis is the most common long-term sequelae of lung parenchymal damage from pneumonia.[218,247] It is the permanent abnormal enlargement of the diameter of the bronchus related to damage of the bronchial walls (Fig. 6.74). It is best demonstrated on HRCT, and the main diagnostic features include the internal diameter of the bronchus being wider than its adjacent pulmonary artery, failure of the bronchus to taper peripherally, and visualization of bronchi in the outer 1 to 2 cm of the lung zones[115,250] (Fig. 6.75).

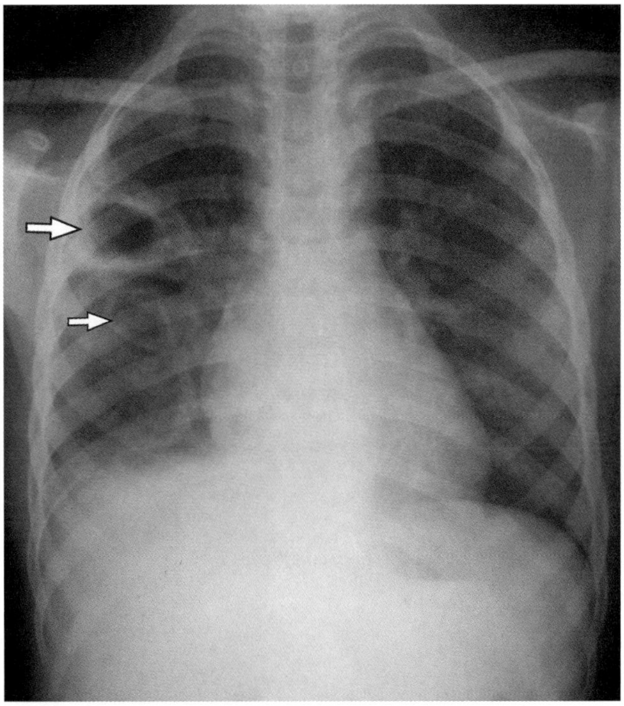

FIGURE 6.72 **Postinfectious pneumatocele from prior *Staphylococcus aureus* infection in a 7-year-old girl.** Frontal chest radiograph shows two air-filled cavities (*arrows*) without septations. The more superior cavity has a slightly thicker border, but the inferior cavity has an almost imperceptible border.

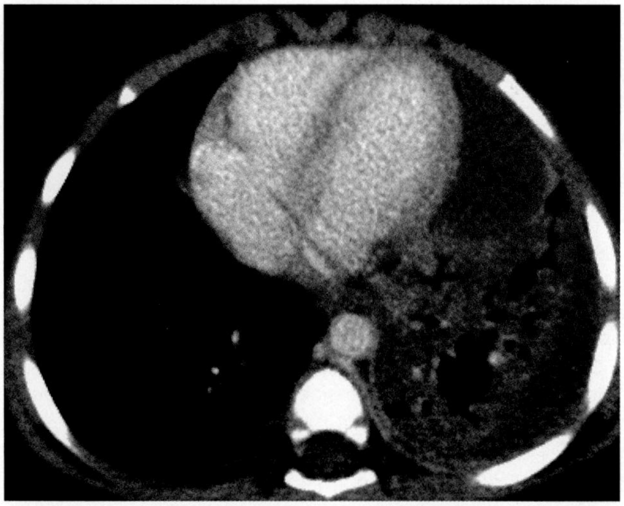

FIGURE 6.73 **Pulmonary gangrene in a 2-year-old boy.** Axial enhanced CT image shows a left lung consolidation with an absence of contrast enhancement, replaced with air and fluid. The integrity of the visceral pleura is no longer maintained.

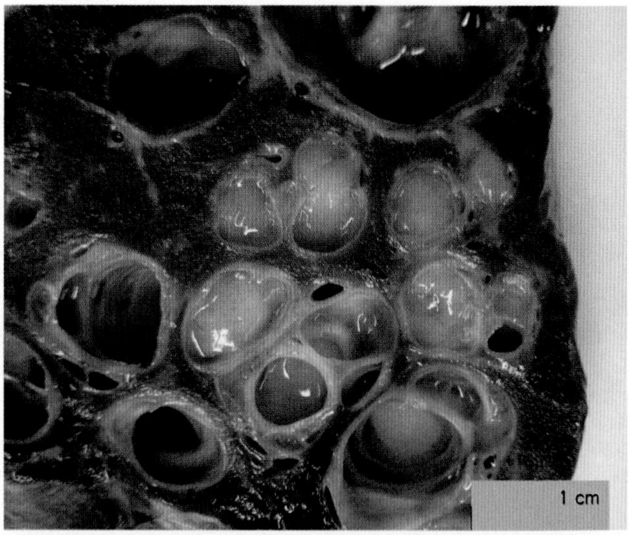

FIGURE 6.74 **Severe bronchiectasis in a 10-year-old girl.** Resection of a portion of the right lung showed markedly dilated airways.

Neoplastic Disorders

Primary pulmonary neoplasms are relatively rare in the pediatric population with inflammatory or reactive masses that occur more frequently than malignancies by a factor of 10.[251] Among the neoplastic conditions affecting the lung in the pediatric population, metastases outnumber primary lung neoplasm by a ratio of 5–11:1.[251,252] When primary lung neoplasms are encountered, they are more likely malignant than benign neoplasms by a ratio of ~3:1.[253]

The low incidence of pulmonary malignancy often results in a low index of suspicion for underlying neoplasm in infants and children. This may result in delays in achieving a correct diagnosis as well as initiating appropriate treatment. In the pediatric population, pulmonary neoplasm should be considered when a patient's clinical presentation and chest radiographic findings are incongruent and/or when unusual chest radiographic findings are encountered, as in the case of a child with a clinical presentation of pneumonia who does not respond to antibiotic therapy as expected.[252] In addition, certain genetic syndromes and familial disease can predispose pediatric patients to pulmonary neoplasia.

Benign Primary Neoplasms

Benign primary neoplasms of the lung account for ~1% to 5% of lung tumors[254]; however, they can mimic more aggressive processes on imaging studies. Familiarity with these lesions is important for optimal management of a child who presents with a suspected primary lung neoplasm. The two most common benign primary neoplasms of the lung in the pediatric population are sclerosing pneumocytoma and pulmonary hamartoma.

Sclerosing Pneumocytoma

Sclerosing pneumocytoma, also known as sclerosing hemangioma, is a rare benign pulmonary neoplasm of pneumocyte

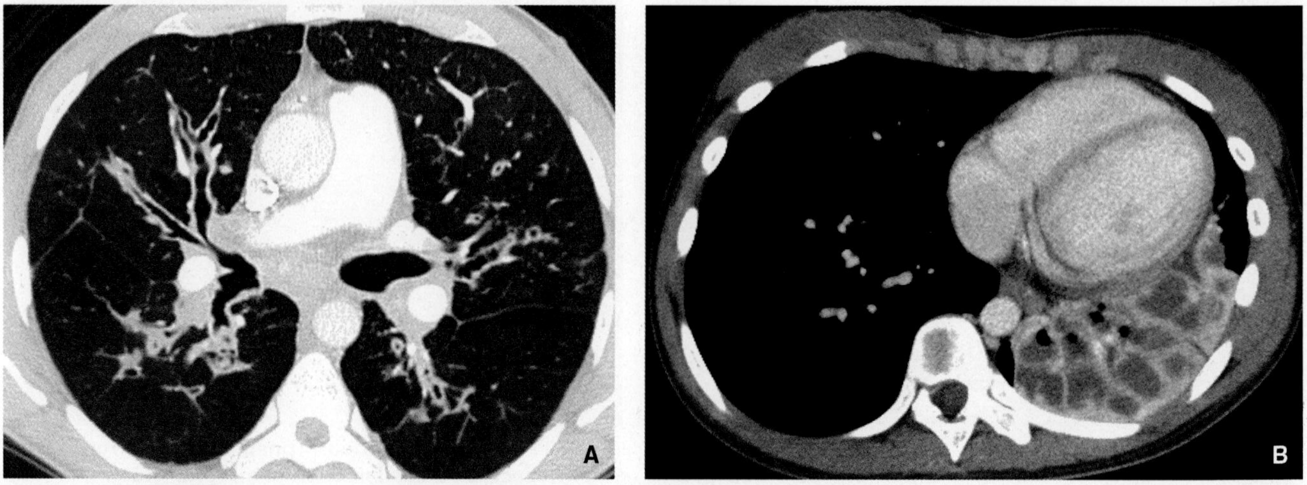

FIGURE 6.75 **Bronchiectasis in two pediatric patients. A:** Axial lung window CT image shows thick-walled, dilated bronchi with diameters wider than the adjacent pulmonary arteries compatible with tubular bronchiectasis. **B:** Axial enhanced CT image of another pediatric patient with dilated distal bronchi in the left lower lobe. The bronchi have a cystic configuration with thick walls and are filled with secretions.

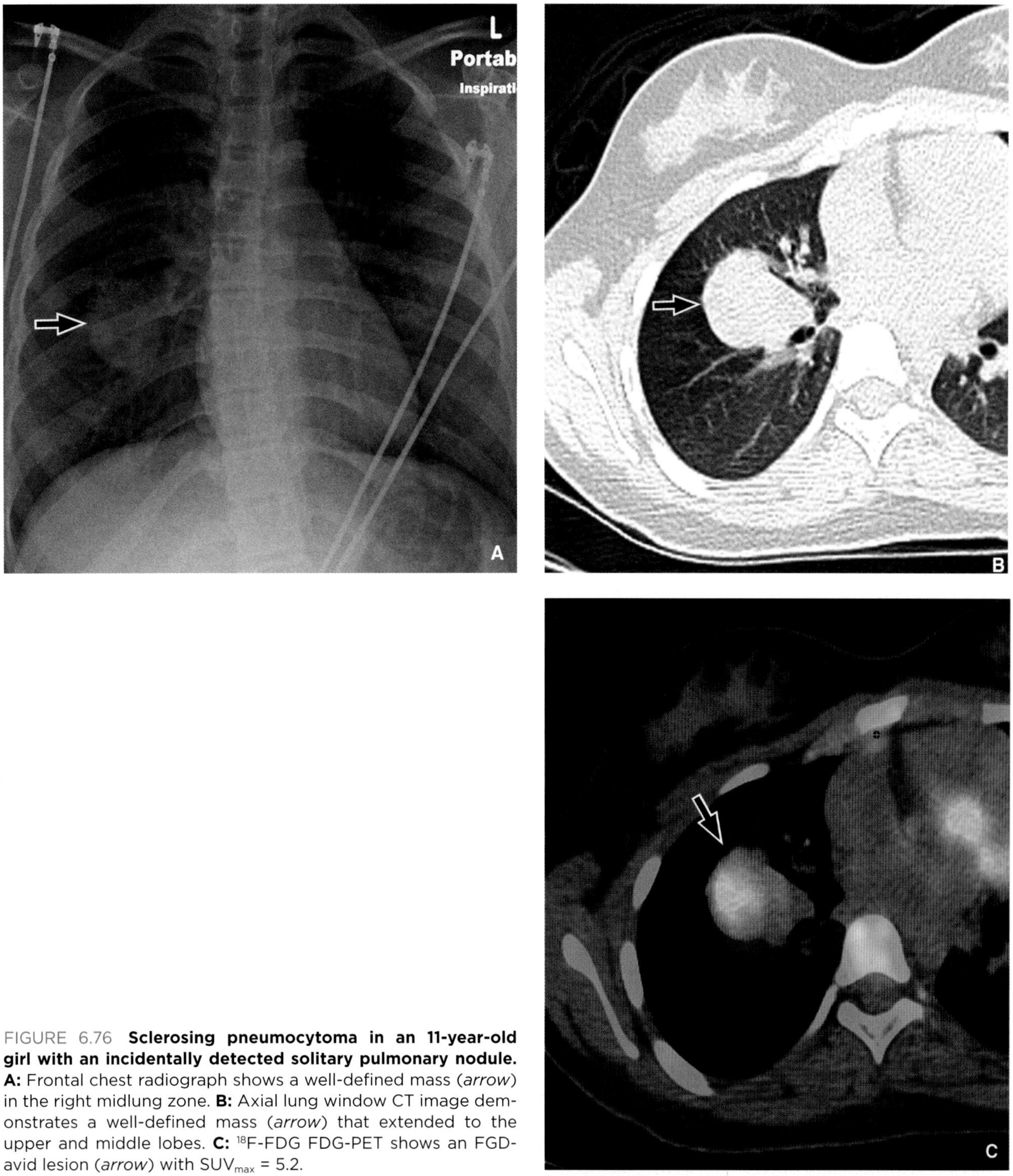

FIGURE 6.76 **Sclerosing pneumocytoma in an 11-year-old girl with an incidentally detected solitary pulmonary nodule. A:** Frontal chest radiograph shows a well-defined mass (*arrow*) in the right midlung zone. **B:** Axial lung window CT image demonstrates a well-defined mass (*arrow*) that extended to the upper and middle lobes. **C:** ^{18}F-FDG FDG-PET shows an FGD-avid lesion (*arrow*) with SUV_{max} = 5.2.

origin. It is currently categorized as an adenoma because it behaves as a benign lesion with rare lymph node metastasis that does not appear to affect the benign course.[255] There is a 5:1 female-to-male ratio. Although sclerosing pneumocytoma predominantly affects middle-aged adults, it can also occur in adolescents.[256] The majority of affected pediatric patients are asymptomatic, and the lesions are typically incidentally detected. The typical clinical presentation of symptomatic patients include hemoptysis, cough, and chest pain.[257]

Typical findings of sclerosing pneumocytoma on chest radiograph include a small solitary nodule with well-defined margins (Fig. 6.76A).[258] Approximately 4% of cases present as multiple pulmonary nodules.[257] An air meniscus sign (crescent-shaped lucency) can be present in some cases and is similar to that seen with invasive pulmonary aspergillosis in immunocompromised pediatric patients. The crescent of lucency is thought to represent trapped air following peritumoral hemorrhage and clearance through the airway.[259] CT findings mir-

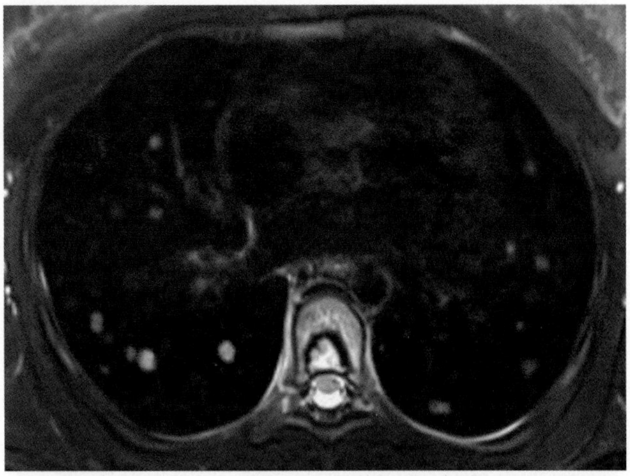

FIGURE 6.77 **Sclerosing pneumocytoma in a 17-year-old girl who presented with shortness of breath.** Axial T2-weighted MR image shows well-defined multiple small pulmonary nodules in both lungs with increased signal intensity.

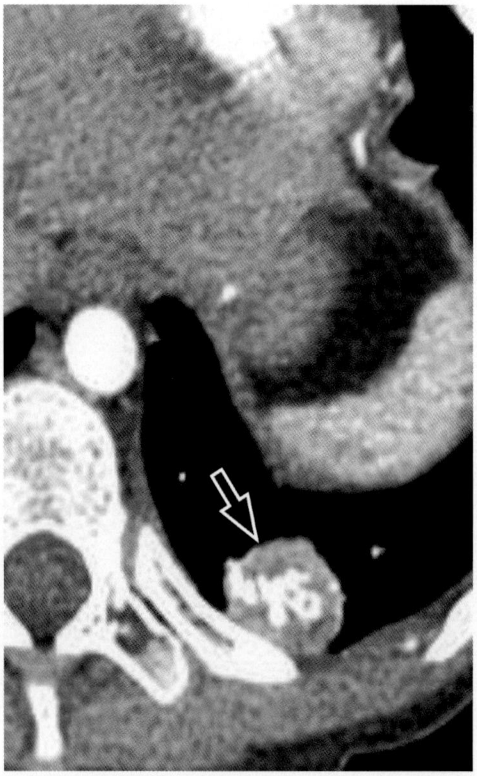

FIGURE 6.78 **Pulmonary hamartoma in a 3-year-old boy with an incidentally detected pulmonary nodule.** Axial enhanced CT image shows a round lung lesion (*arrow*) in the left lower lobe with characteristic popcorn calcification.

ror the radiographic appearance of a well-defined pulmonary lesion (Fig. 6.76B). Cystic areas of low attenuation and foci of calcification within the lesion may be present. After contrast administration, avid enhancement is typically seen.[258] Local invasion or lymph node metastases from pulmonary sclerosing hemangioma are rare particularly in the pediatric population.[257] MRI findings of sclerosing pneumocytoma are variable. Lesions can be hyperintense on both T1- and T2-weighted MR images and show intense contrast enhancement or appear heterogeneous because of underlying hemorrhage and cystic change (Fig. 6.77).[260] The majority of lesions are hypermetabolic on ^{18}F-FDG PET (Fig. 6.76C) and can be falsely interpreted as malignancy because of their high FDG avidity.[261]

Surgical resection is the current management of choice which usually results in excellent prognosis.

Pulmonary Hamartoma

Pulmonary hamartomas are benign neoplasms composed of variable amounts of cartilage, fat, connective tissue, and smooth muscle.[262] They are the most common benign lung tumor in adults, but can also occur in pediatric patients.[263] These lesions typically grow slowly, usually do not result in symptoms, and are often detected incidentally on imaging studies.

The typical chest radiographic appearance of pulmonary hamartoma is that of a well-circumscribed, round or oval nodule, usually with lobulated contours and located in the periphery of the lung. Larger lesions are more likely to have the characteristic popcorn calcification.[263] CT typically reveals a well-circumscribed lesion with lobulated contours and can better demonstrate fatty and calcific components of the lesion (Fig. 6.78). The presence of fat and "popcorn" calcifications (seen on CT in 50% and 5% to 15% of cases, respectively) is highly predictive for pulmonary hamartomas[264]; however, accurate diagnosis becomes challenging when neither of these elements are present.[265] On MRI, pulmonary hamartomas tend to have intermediate signal intensity on T1-weighted MR images and high signal intensity on T2-weighted MR images. After contrast administration, pulmonary hamartoma may have avidly enhancing internal septations. Calcifications, when present, can appear as low signal foci on all MRI sequences; however, fat may not be easily seen on MRI.[266] Although the majority of pulmonary hamartomas are not FDG avid, false-positive cases have been reported.[267]

The definitive diagnosis of pulmonary hamartoma can be made based on either transthoracic needle aspiration or core needle biopsy with pathologic evaluation in cases that do not show characteristic imaging features.

Malignant Primary Neoplasms

The majority of malignant neoplasms of the lung in the pediatric population are metastases, with primary neoplasms of the lung and large airway representing a small minority of all malignancies in this age group.[251–253] Early and accurate diagnosis is important to avoid progression to advanced stages.

Pleuropulmonary Blastoma

Pleuropulmonary blastoma (PPB) is a potentially aggressive primary malignant lung neoplasm. PPB encompasses a spectrum of pulmonary neoplastic lesions ranging from cystic (type I) to cystic and solid (type II) to solid (type III). Increasing solid growth corresponds to increasing aggressiveness and poor prognosis. PPB is part of the inherited syndrome of *DICER1* mutation, in which affected pediatric patients and their family members are prone to PPB, cystic

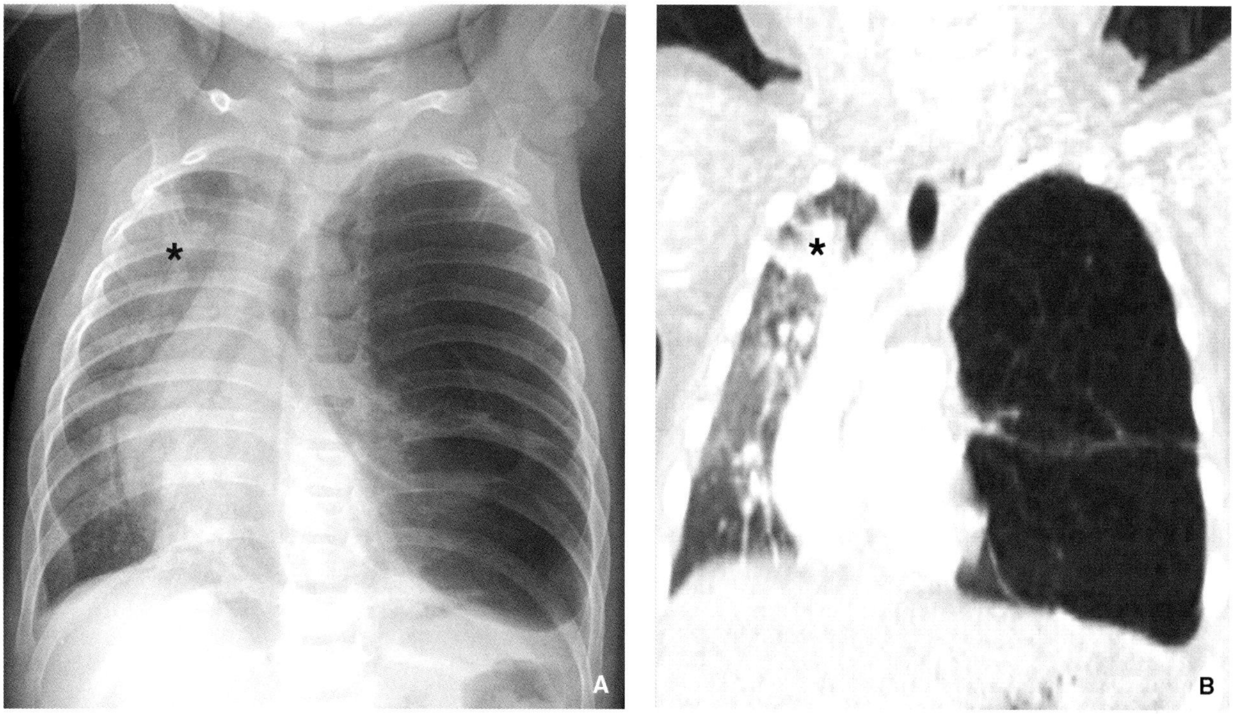

FIGURE 6.79 **Type I pleuropulmonary blastoma in a 9-month-old boy. A:** Frontal chest radiograph shows a large cystic lesion in the left chest, associated with a small left pleural effusion, rightward mediastinal shift, and compressive atelectasis in the right lung (*asterisk*). **B:** Coronal reformatted lung window CT image confirms a large cystic lesion in the left chest, rightward mediastinal shift, and compressive atelectasis (*asterisk*) in the right lung.

nephroma, multinodular thyroid, Sertoli-Leydig cell tumor, embryonal rhabdomyosarcoma, and nasal chondromesenchymal hamartoma.[268] It is postulated that benign epithelial cells within PPB induce tumor growth via dysregulated stromal–epithelial interaction due to loss of *DICER1*, a regulator of microRNA.[268]

Pediatric patients with type I PPB may be asymptomatic or present with respiratory distress with or without pneumothorax.[62] Infants and children with type II and III PPBs often present with dyspnea, fever, cough, and chest or abdominal pain. The median age of diagnosis for PPBs is 3 years and varies among the three types.[269] Pediatric patients with type I PPB present at a median age of 10 months, whereas those with type III PPB present at a median age of 44 months.[269] Approximately 25% of affected pediatric patients have features in keeping with a familial cancer syndrome.[270]

The typical radiographic appearance of a PPB is that of a lung mass with or without visible cysts (Fig. 6.79A). For unknown reasons, the tumor has a predilection for the right lung (20). The cystic type PPB may bear a radiographic resemblance to CPAM on imaging studies. Large solid lesions without visible cysts can result in complete opacification of the hemithorax with contralateral mediastinal shift on chest radiograph. Pleural effusion and pneumothorax in type II PPB can also be present.[268] On CT, type I PPBs appear as cystic lung lesions with variable numbers of cysts (Fig. 6.79B) typically ranging in size from 2 to 9 cm in diameter.[268] Mass effect on adjacent structures can result in lobar expansion, sometimes with contralateral mediastinal shift. Type II PPBs have solid components together with air-filled cysts with or without air–fluid levels.[271] Intralesional hemorrhage or infection can occupy the cysts and result in a more solid appearance.[272] Large lesions can be accompanied by pleural effusion and contralateral mediastinal shift.[271] Type III PPBs are solid lesions with heterogeneous contrast enhancement with or without pleural effusion, atelectasis, and mediastinal shift.[271,273] The MRI appearance of PPBs depends on the mixture of cystic and solid components, with the latter appearing as areas of heterogeneous contrast enhancement.[273] ^{18}F-FDG-PET appearance of a type III PPB is heterogeneous, predominantly peripheral, FDG avidity (Fig. 6.80).[273] Multiple

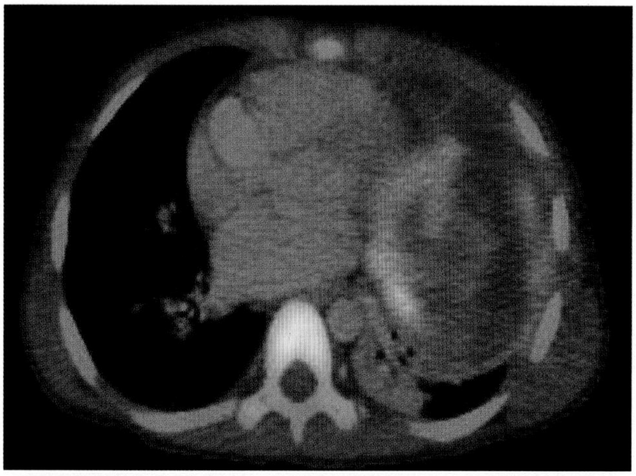

FIGURE 6.80 **Type III pleuropulmonary blastoma in a 3-year-old girl.** ^{18}F-FDG FDG-PET image shows a predominantly peripheral FGD-avid lesion in the left hemithorax.

primary PPBs can occur in the same patient and may be difficult to distinguish from metastasis or recurrence.

The current management depends on the type of PPBs. Surgical excision may be adequate for pediatric patients with small type I PPB. Neoadjuvant chemotherapy can help decrease the tumor size and increase the chance of complete resection in large PPBs with a solid component. Metastatic disease, most usually located in the brain, can be sometimes seen in pediatric patients with type II and III PPBs, which is treated with chemotherapy. On pathology, type I PPB is a multicystic mass with thin fibrous septa lined by benign frequently cuboidal epithelium. The septa may contain hypercellular stroma as well as benign cartilage nodules underlying the epithelium, resembling a "cambium layer." In type II and III PPBs, malignant components commonly include areas resembling embryonal rhabdomyosarcoma with anaplasia. Other components may also include areas resembling fibrosarcoma and chondrosarcoma. In addition, rarer bizarre components such as neuroblastoma may be seen.

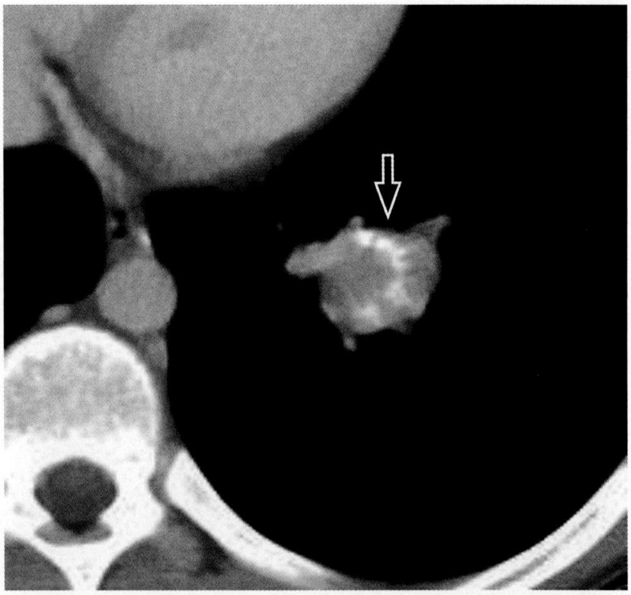

FIGURE 6.81 **Carcinoid tumor in a 14-year-old boy who presented with fever and cough.** Axial unenhanced CT image shows a round mass (*arrow*) with internal calcification located in the left lower lobe. The diagnosis of typical carcinoid tumor was confirmed on surgical pathology.

Carcinoid Tumor

Primary neuroendocrine tumors of the lung include typical and atypical carcinoid tumors, large cell neuroendocrine carcinoma, and small cell carcinoma. Typical and atypical lung carcinoid tumors represent low- and intermediate-risk types of neuroendocrine tumors. Typical carcinoid tumors are characterized by fewer than 2 mitoses per 2 mm^2 (10 high-power fields) and no necrosis, whereas atypical carcinoid tumors have 2 to 10 mitoses per 2 mm^2 and/or foci of necrosis.[274]

The majority of lung carcinoid tumors arise in the large intrapulmonary airways.[275] In children, the mean age of presentation is 12 years with a male-to-female ratio of 1.4:1.[276] Peripheral lung lesions are less likely to cause symptoms compared to central endobronchial lesions. Carcinoid syndrome, which includes flushing, diarrhea, heart failure, and bronchoconstriction, is rare in pediatric patients with lung carcinoid tumors.[276]

Radiographs typically reveal round or ovoid opacities with well-circumscribed margins.[275] The parallel sign describes the orientation of nonspherical lung carcinoid tumors along the axis of the nearest major bronchus or pulmonary arterial branch.[275] On CT, lung carcinoid tumors present as soft tissue attenuation masses with well-defined or lobulated margins (Fig. 6.81). Internal calcification is more likely to be seen with centrally located carcinoid tumors than with those located in the periphery. Administration of intravenous contrast typically shows intense enhancement in carcinoid tumors.[275]

The current management of choice for lung carcinoid tumors is complete surgical resection, which results in >90% 10-year survival in pediatric patients.[274]

Inflammatory Myofibroblastic Tumor

Inflammatory myofibroblastic tumor (IMT) is recognized as a clonal neoplasm, now nosologically separate from primary inflammatory processes ("inflammatory pseudotumor" and "plasma cell granuloma"). It is an indolent tumor with a capacity for recurrence and occasional metastasis.[277] It has a predilection for children, adolescents, and young adults. In the pediatric age group, the median age at diagnosis is 9 years. IMT was first described in the lung but soon was recognized to occur in other sites, particularly the head and neck, mediastinum, and abdomen and pelvis (mesentery, omentum, and soft tissue).[278] Within the lung, the tumors are typically solitary but occasionally multiple.[279,280] Approximately 12% of IMT present as endobronchial lesions.[281] Approximately 50% of affected patients are asymptomatic.[279–282] Symptoms are more likely with endobronchial than with parenchymal lesions and can include fever, cough, chest pain, hemoptysis, and pneumonitis.[279–282] Elevated erythrocyte sedimentation rate, thrombocytosis, anemia, and hyperglobulinemia, attributed to tumor cytokines, may also occur.[278]

Chest radiograph typically reveals a solitary, well-circumscribed lesion, usually located in the lower lobes[279] (Fig. 6.82A). The typical CT appearance is that of a well-marginated lesion with lobulated contours and heterogeneous attenuation (Fig. 6.82B). The amount of calcification and degree of contrast enhancement are variable. Amorphous, mixed, fine fleck-like or dense calcification patterns have been reported.[279,283] On MRI (Fig. 6.82C–E), IMTs typically have low to intermediate signal intensity on T1-weighted MR images and high signal intensity on T2-weighted weighted MR images.[279,284] One case report has shown homogeneous delayed enhancement in IMTs.[284] Because of the presence of inflammatory cells, ^{18}F-FDG PET can reveal areas of increased avidity in these lesions.[285]

Surgical resection is the current management of choice, which often results in cure if clear surgical margin can be

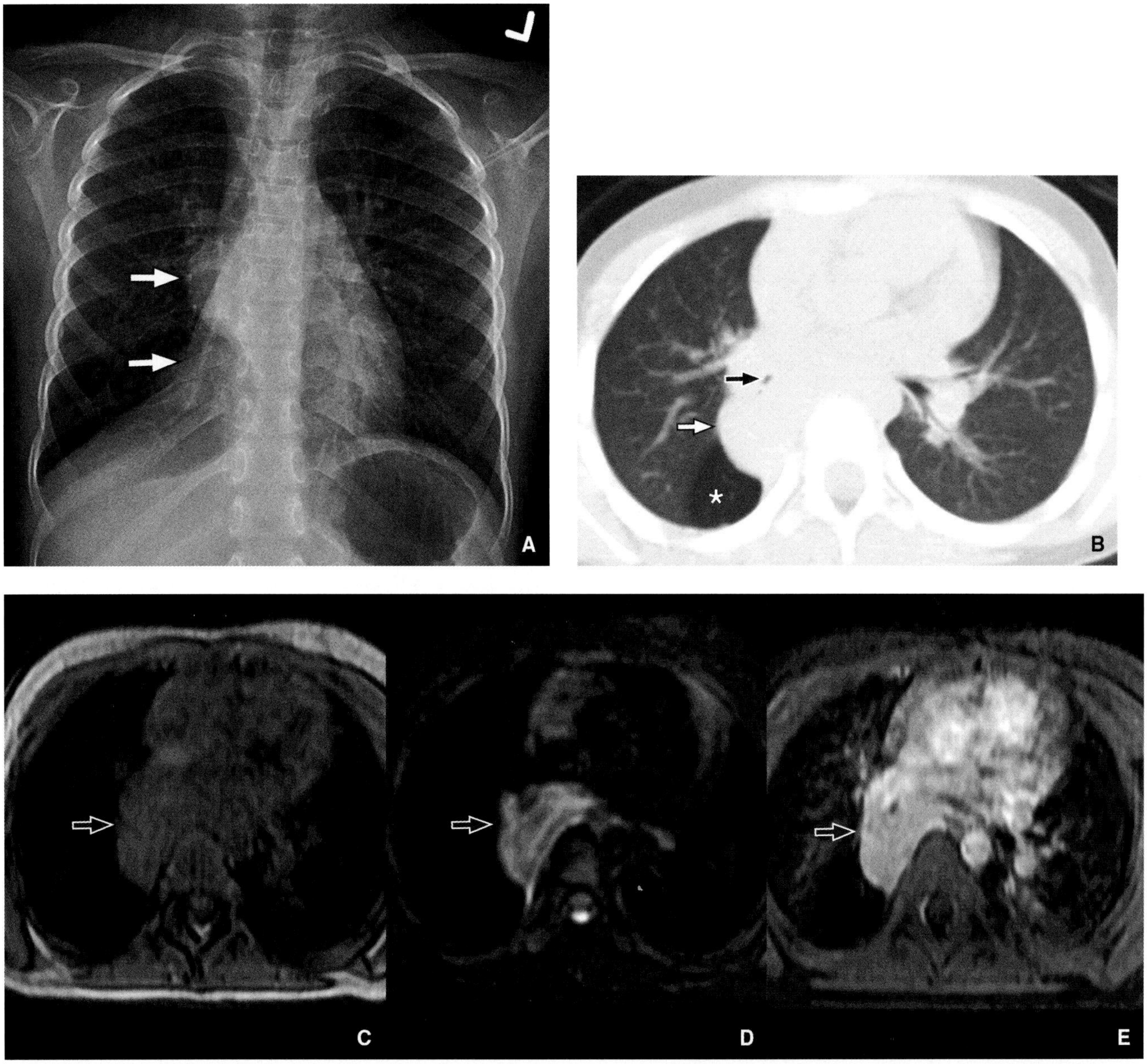

FIGURE 6.82 **Inflammatory myofibroblastic tumor (IMT) in a 5-year-old girl who presented with cough unresponsive to antibiotics. A:** Frontal chest radiograph shows two lung masses (*arrows*) in the right lower lobe abutting the mediastinum. **B:** Axial lung window CT image shows the more superior of the two masses (*white arrow*), which results in narrowing of the right lower lobe bronchus (*black arrow*) and air trapping (*asterisk*) in the right lower lobe. **C–E:** Three axial MRI images show a mass (*arrows*) with intermediate signal intensity on T1-weighted MR image **(C)**, high signal intensity on T2-weighted MR image **(D)**, and contrast enhancement on T1-weighted MR image **(E)**.

achieved. Microscopic examination reveals a proliferation of myofibroblastic spindle-shaped tumor cells with admixed inflammation typically rich in plasma cells and lymphocytes (Fig. 6.83).[277] Genetically, the tumors can harbor a rearrangement of the *ALK* gene (with any of a variety of partners) or less often a *ROS1* or *PDGFRβ* gene rearrangement.[277]

Lymphoma (Including Posttransplant Lymphoproliferative Disorder)

Primary lymphoma of the lung without mediastinal involvement is exceedingly rare and has been reported in three patients.[286–290] The more common presentation of pulmonary lymphoma is in the setting of extrapulmonary Hodgkin and non-Hodgkin lymphoma (HL and NHL, respectively) and posttransplant lymphoproliferative disorder (PTLD). PTLD is the most common malignant complication of solid organ transplantation in children and can be seen in 2% of pediatric renal transplant recipients and up to 20% of pediatric lung or intestinal transplant recipients.[291–293] Currently, the pathophysiology and etiology are not completely understood. However, Epstein-Barr virus infection and transplant-related immunosuppression have been clearly linked.[291] Thoracic involvement in PTLD is most common after lung or heart–lung transplantation.[294]

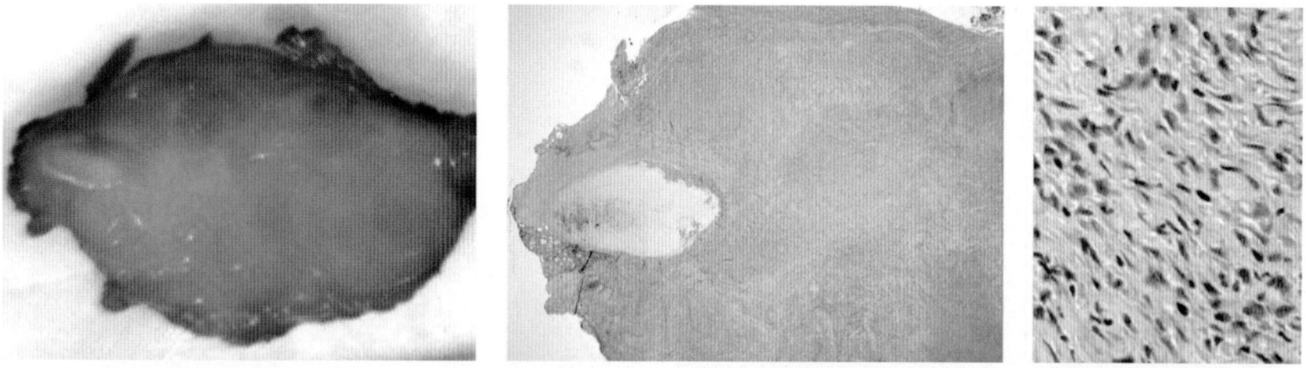

FIGURE 6.83 **Inflammatory myofibroblastic tumor resected from the bronchus intermedius of a 10-year-old boy.** Grossly **(left)** and microscopically (**middle**; hematoxylin and eosin, original magnification, 20×), the tumor is seen in the bronchial wall, surrounding and destroying bronchial cartilage. High-power magnification shows spindle-shaped (myo)fibroblastic cells (**right**; hematoxylin and eosin, original magnification, 600×).

In pediatric patients with HL, NHL, and PTLD, pulmonary parenchymal disease is seen in 13% at some point during the course of the disease without a significant difference in incidence among the three groups.[295] Three main radiologic patterns of pulmonary lymphoma from HD and NHL are nodular, bronchovascular–lymphangitic, and pneumonic–alveolar appearances.[296] The typical imaging manifestations of pediatric patients with lymphoproliferative disorders (HL, NHL, and PTLD) in the lung are solitary or multiple pulmonary nodules, seen in 90% of cases (Fig. 6.84) and pulmonary mass in 39%.[295] Other thoracic manifestations of pediatric lymphoproliferative disorders are interstitial disease (9%), alveolar disease (9%), cavitation (9%), and pleurally based masses (9%).[295] Pleural effusion can be seen in addition to the above features in 9% of cases, and the majority of affected patients have at least two of the above lung findings.[295]

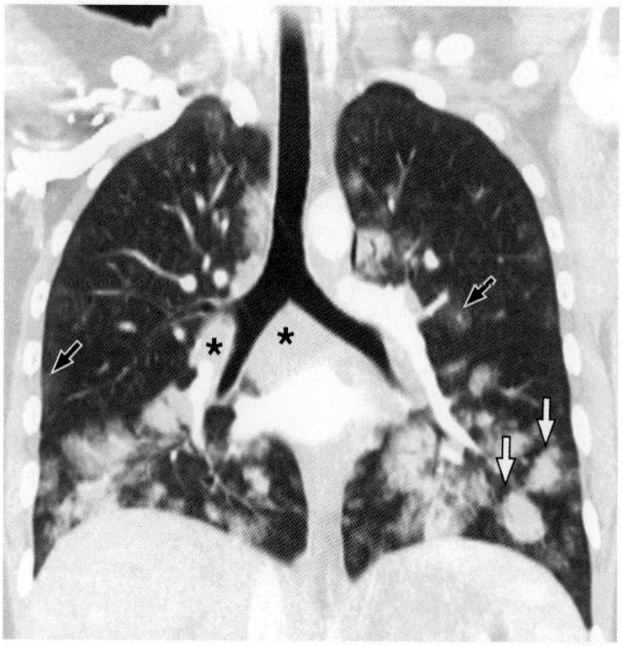

FIGURE 6.84 **Immunodeficiency and Epstein-Barr virus-related lymphoproliferative disorder in a 14-year-old girl.** Coronal reformatted lung window CT image shows multiple ground-glass (*black arrows*) and confluent (*white arrows*) pulmonary nodules and mediastinal and hilar adenopathy (*asterisks*).

In recent years, chemotherapy alone or combined-modality treatment with chemotherapy and radiation therapy has made HL one of the most curable cancers.[289] In contrast to NHL in adults, almost all childhood NHL cases are high grade; however, outcomes are better for children.[290] Because NHL in children is considered a disseminated disease, local control of discrete sites of involvement with surgery or radiotherapy is not commonly attempted.[290]

Secondary Neoplasms (Metastatic Disease)

Pulmonary metastases are 5 to 11 times more common than primary lung malignancies and represent ~80% of parenchymal tumors in the pediatric population.[251,252] The most common sources of pediatric lung metastases include Wilms tumor (31%), osteosarcoma (20%), and Ewing sarcoma (9%). Sarcomas as a group account for 47% of lung metastases in the pediatric population.[252]

On chest radiographs or CT, pulmonary metastases present as single (Fig. 6.85) or multiple well-defined nodules (Fig. 6.86) that are often peripherally located and tend to involve the lower lobes.[297] A reticular or miliary pattern is rare but can also be seen in patients with lymphangitic spread.[297] Cavitation and pneumothorax are rare but are more commonly seen in association with Wilms tumor, Hodgkin lymphoma, and osteosarcoma.[297] Metastases from osteosarcoma (Fig. 6.86A) or synovial sarcoma can present with internal mineralization (calcification), similar to that seen with the primary lesion.

In addition to controlling the primary neoplasms, surgical resection of pulmonary metastases (metastasectomy) may improve survival in pediatric patients with a wide range of solid tumors.[298]

Traumatic Disorders

Trauma is the leading cause of death in pediatric patients older than 1 year.[299] More than 45% of all deaths in children from 1 to 14 years are the result of trauma.[300-302]

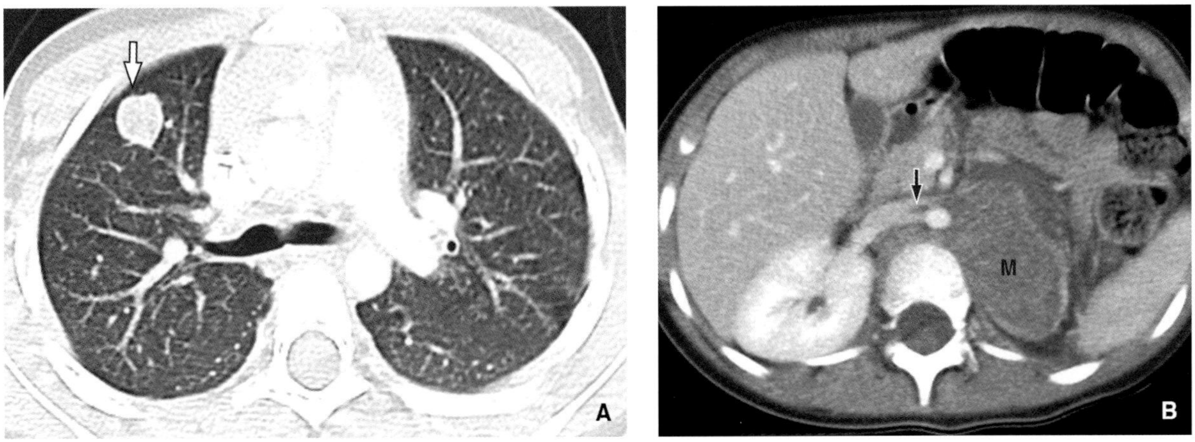

FIGURE 6.85 **Solitary pulmonary metastasis in a 3-year-old girl with Wilms tumor. A:** Axial lung window CT image shows a solitary nodule (*arrow*) in the right upper lobe. **B:** Axial enhanced CT image of the abdomen shows the primary left renal mass (*M*) with extension into the left renal vein (*arrow*).

Thoracic injuries in children occur less frequently than adults, but remain a significant cause of morbidity and mortality in pediatric trauma patients. The presence of chest trauma in an injured child is usually indicative of a significant trauma.[12] Blunt force injuries to the thorax are 6 times more common than penetrating injuries in pediatric patients.[303]

Commonly encountered causes of thoracic injury in children include motor vehicle crashes, falls, pedestrian versus motor vehicle accidents, bicycle accidents, playground mishaps, child abuse, and gun-related injuries.[299,304–308] The mechanism of the trauma generally determines the types of injuries, but pediatric chest trauma injury patterns usually differ from those observed in adults. The increased compliance of the pediatric chest wall has been suggested as a reason for unique pediatric injury patterns and outcomes.[309] Lung injury, hemothorax, pneumothorax, mediastinal injuries, and rib fractures may present in isolation or in combination.[302] They are also seen in association with head, abdominal, and other organ injuries.

Imaging evaluation plays an important role in the initial management of chest trauma in children, allowing for prompt diagnoses and expedited patient care. Chest radiograph remains the most important imaging modality for

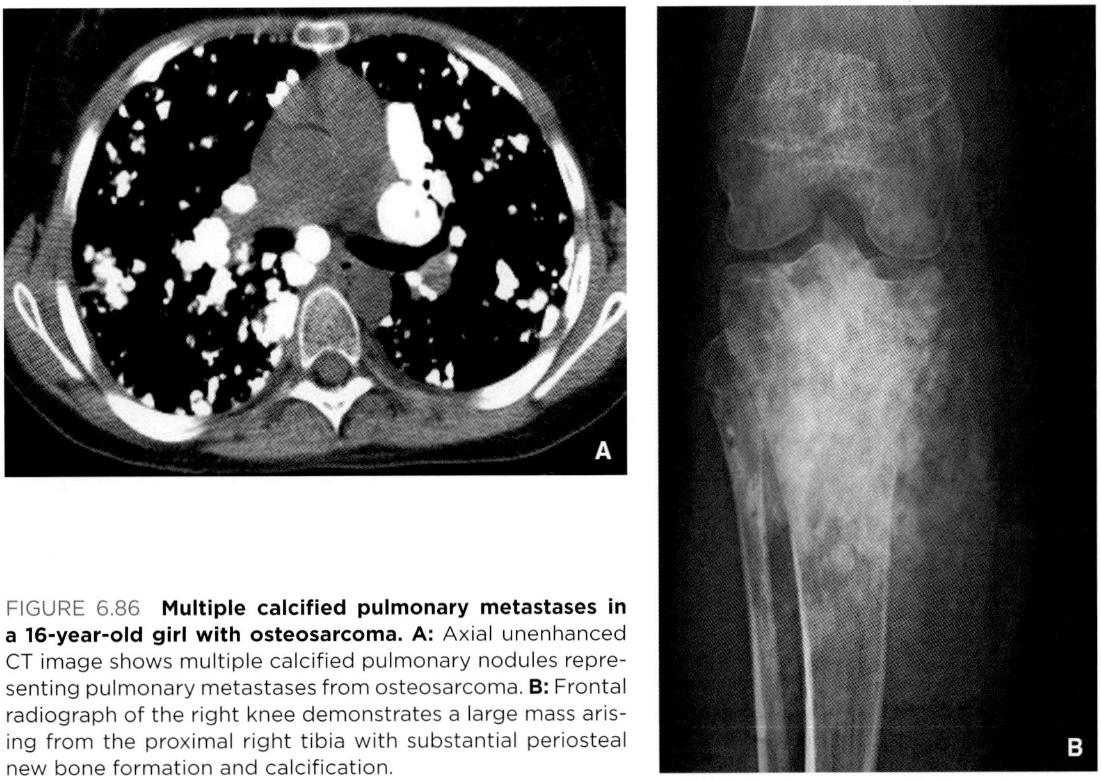

FIGURE 6.86 **Multiple calcified pulmonary metastases in a 16-year-old girl with osteosarcoma. A:** Axial unenhanced CT image shows multiple calcified pulmonary nodules representing pulmonary metastases from osteosarcoma. **B:** Frontal radiograph of the right knee demonstrates a large mass arising from the proximal right tibia with substantial periosteal new bone formation and calcification.

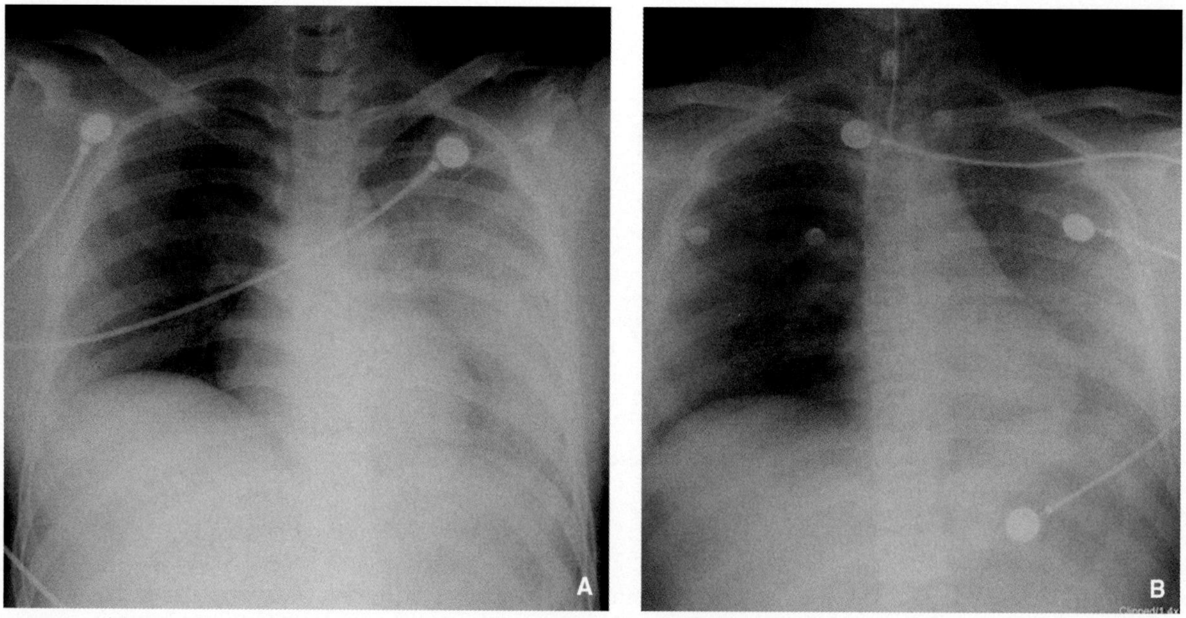

FIGURE 6.87 **Pulmonary contusion in a 12-year-old boy injured in a motor vehicular accident. A:** Frontal chest radiograph obtained upon admission to the hospital shows an opacity in the left hemithorax. There is no fracture of the adjacent ribs. **B:** Follow-up chest radiograph obtained at 48 hours demonstrates substantial resolution of the pulmonary contusion.

initial triage; however, subtle changes may be difficult to visualize on radiographs. In addition, suboptimal radiographic techniques and artifacts, which are related to the complex nature of pediatric trauma, can limit the ability to detect underling true pathology.[303] CT is currently the imaging modality of choice in the evaluation of symptomatic pediatric patients with chest trauma or polytrauma because CT provides a more detailed evaluation of thoracic structures, and, therefore, it is more sensitive in detecting injury than chest radiograph.[12,307]

Pulmonary Contusion

Pulmonary contusion is the most common traumatic thoracic injury in children and commonly associated with motor vehicle crashes, blast injuries, or blunt-instrument trauma.[302,309] It is associated with a 15% to 20% mortality rate.[310,311] There is greater flexibility of the thoracic cage in young children allowing rib compression during trauma, translating the energy to the lung parenchyma. Such traumatic impact on the lung causes alveolar hemorrhage, interstitial edema, and consolidation. This occurs with less rib fractures in children compared to adults.[302,308,312–314]

Clinical course of pulmonary contusions varies with the degree and volume of injury. Approximately 20% of affected children develop pneumonia as a complication, which may progress to respiratory failure. Respiratory insufficiency, acute respiratory distress syndrome, and long-term changes in respiratory function and radiographic abnormalities have also been noted.[302,315–317]

The radiologic findings in pulmonary contusion can vary considerably. Chest radiographs usually manifest as ill-defined areas of peripherally located nonanatomic consolidation, often in the absence of rib fractures or chest wall bruising[308] (Fig. 6.87). Contusions can be confluent or extensive, solitary or multifocal, and unilateral or bilateral.[302] Contusions may occur directly at the site of impact or in the contralateral hemithorax in a contrecoup fashion.[308] They usually become apparent within 6 hours of the injury, but may not be visualized on initial chest radiographs.[308,311] On chest CT, they manifest as ill-defined focal or diffuse ground-glass or consolidative airspace opacities without air bronchograms[12,299,318,319] (Fig. 6.88). These nonsegmental opacities often spare the subpleural lung, so-called "subpleural sparing" sign.[12,319] In most cases, contusions typically resolve within 7 days.[308,320] Occasionally, they are difficult to differentiate from aspiration-related lung abnormality, which may

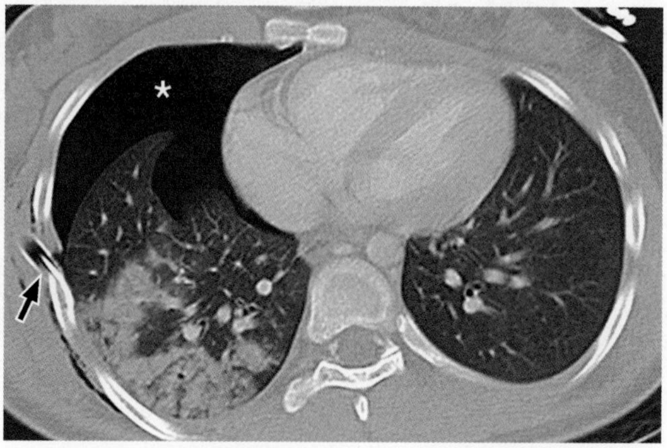

FIGURE 6.88 **Pulmonary contusion with pneumothorax in a 16-year-old girl involved in a motor vehicle accident.** Axial lung window CT image shows patchy consolidative densities in the right lower lobe compatible with pulmonary contusion. A chest tube (*arrow*) is noted to decompress the associated pneumothorax (*asterisk*). (Case courtesy of Elizabeth H. Ey, MD, Dayton Children's Hospital Medical Center, Dayton, OH.)

occur at the time of injury, during intubation, or during the evaluation phase.[302] Aspiration-related lung abnormality is typically segmental and located in the dependent portions of the lungs, whereas contusions are nonsegmental and variably distributed.[308]

The current management of pulmonary contusion is mainly supportive, with supplemental oxygen and analgesia for the chest wall injury.

Pulmonary Laceration

Pulmonary lacerations are tears in the lung parenchyma that result from the compressive rupture, compressive shear, rib penetration, or adhesive shearing of the lung in the setting of thoracic injury.[299,321] They are uncommon following chest trauma in children and are associated with high degree of mortality (>40%).[308,311,322] When lacerations occur deeper within the lung parenchyma, cavities containing blood (hematoma) or with air (pneumatocele) may form. Peripheral lacerations, depending on the size and extent, could result to pneumothorax or even bronchopleural fistula.[311]

Pulmonary lacerations are frequently occult and may not be evident on initial radiographs especially in the background of pulmonary contusions[299,308,321] (Fig. 6.89A). On CT, lacerations commonly appear as linear areas of lucency containing air attenuation within the lung parenchyma (Fig. 6.89B). They may be better appreciated on reformatted CT images.[299,321] Pulmonary hematomas that developed from the laceration appear as rounded opacities of soft tissue density on chest radiograph. Fluid levels can be seen on erect views.[14]

The pulmonary laceration itself has little associated morbidity and typically heals without intervention, although secondary complications, such as hemorrhage, pneumothorax, or bronchopleural fistula, require specific management.[299]

Posttraumatic Pneumatocele

Posttraumatic pneumatoceles are cavitary lesions in the lung parenchyma associated with blunt thoracic trauma.[323] It has been suggested that they result from forces applied to the compliant pediatric chest that result in distention and rupture of the most distal airways and interstitium.[324] Pneumatoceles usually represent more extensive lung tissue disruption and injury than pulmonary contusion. Affected pediatric patients may be asymptomatic or could present with nonspecific symptoms, including hemoptysis, chest pain, dyspnea, cough, mild fever, after trauma.[325,326]

Pneumatoceles typically present as round or oval-shaped, discrete air pockets within the lung parenchyma without discernible walls[323] (Fig. 6.90). They are variable in size, either solitary or multiple, and can be seen anywhere throughout the lungs, although they have the tendency to be central in location. Pneumatoceles are often associated with surrounding pulmonary contusion, which make them more difficult to detect. Small pneumatoceles often remain radiographically occult.[299] CT is superior to chest radiograph for demonstrating pneumatoceles with a reported sensitivity of 96%.[323]

Pneumatoceles generally resolve over several weeks to months.[311,325,326] Secondary infection is unusual and routine use of prophylactic antibiotic treatment is not recommended. If a nonresolving pneumothorax is seen along with a pneumatocele, the diagnosis of bronchopleural fistula should be considered.[311]

Vasculitic, Inflammatory, Vascular, and Other Disorders

Granulomatosis with Polyangiitis

Granulomatosis with polyangiitis (GPA), formerly known as Wegener granulomatosis, is a systemic vasculitis that manifests as the classic triad of upper airway, lower respiratory tract,

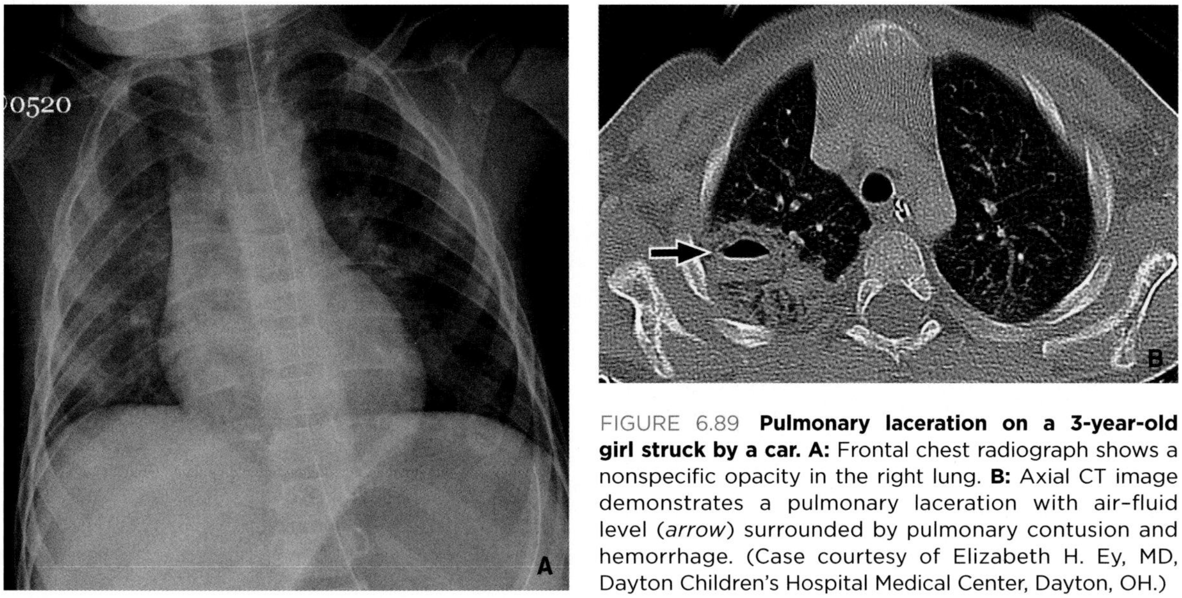

FIGURE 6.89 **Pulmonary laceration on a 3-year-old girl struck by a car. A:** Frontal chest radiograph shows a nonspecific opacity in the right lung. **B:** Axial CT image demonstrates a pulmonary laceration with air–fluid level (*arrow*) surrounded by pulmonary contusion and hemorrhage. (Case courtesy of Elizabeth H. Ey, MD, Dayton Children's Hospital Medical Center, Dayton, OH.)

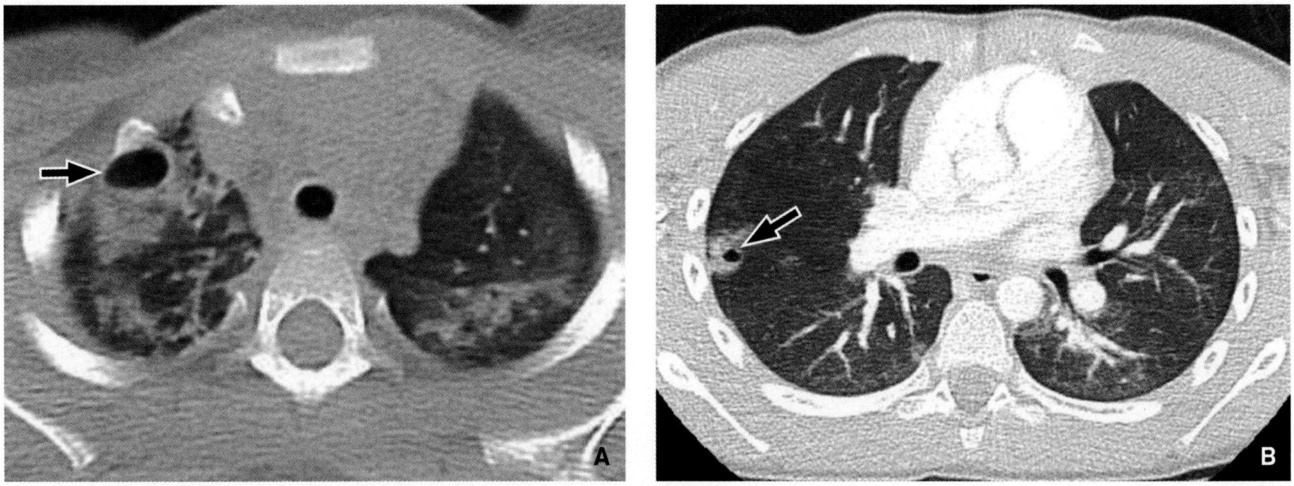

FIGURE 6.90 **Posttraumatic pneumatocele in two pediatric patients. A:** Axial lung window CT image of a 3-year-old girl who fell from a tractor shows an air-filled cyst (arrow) with a thin wall, surrounded by pulmonary contusion. (Case courtesy of Bradley Maxfield, MD, Children's Hospital of Wisconsin, Milwaukee, WI.) **B:** Axial lung window CT image of a 12-year-old boy also shows similar findings compatible with posttraumatic pneumatocele (*arrow*). (Case courtesy of Aaron Betts, MD, Cincinnati, OH.)

and renal disease with various degrees of involvement.[327,328] In the lung, GPA is characterized by necrotizing granulomatous inflammation often accompanied by a necrotizing vasculitis.[329–334] It is relatively rare in children, with an incidence of one in 1 million.[330,331] GPA involves the lung in most clinically recognized cases (74% to 87% of affected children),[331,335] with symptoms including cough, dyspnea, and/or hemoptysis with pleuritic chest pain, fever, arthralgias, and skin rashes, or ulceration.[333] A positive serum antineutrophilic cytoplasmic antibodies (ANCA) has a positive predictive value approaching 99% in the appropriate clinical setting.[330,331,333]

The precise radiographic findings of pediatric GPA are difficult to state because there are no large studies in the pediatric population. Diffuse interstitial and alveolar opacifications were the most frequent chest radiographic findings reported in small group of affected children.[336] Pulmonary nodules or masses are the most common abnormality seen at HRCT (90%) and usually occur bilaterally. The nodules usually have a diameter of more than 5 mm, have no zonal predilection, show occasional cavitation (17% of cases), and tend to resolve and reappear in the same or other sites at follow-up examinations.[331,333,336,337] Some of the consolidated nodules may have a surrounding ground-glass opacity representing hemorrhage (Fig. 6.91). This pattern, described as "halo sign", is also seen in hypervascular metastases, lymphoproliferative disorders, and angioinvasive *Aspergillosis* infection. The "reverse halo sign", where the central area of ground-glass opacity (hemorrhage) is surrounded by a ring of consolidation representing the organizing pneumonia, can also be seen in patients with GPA.[337] Patchy areas of ground-glass opacities (52%) and airspace consolidation (45%) constitute other common CT findings. Furthermore, bronchial stenosis due to granulomatous

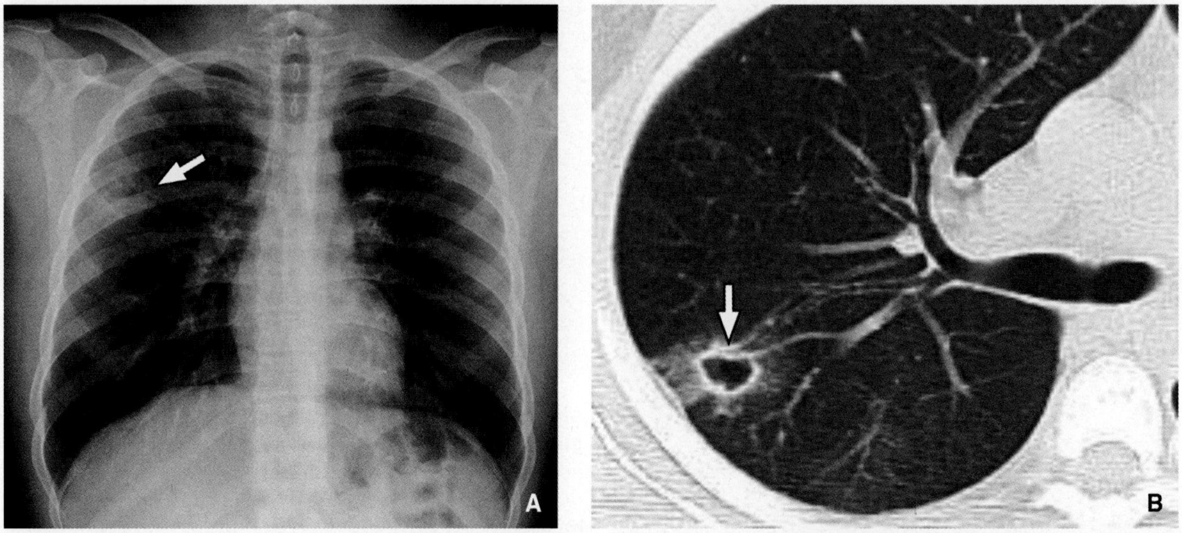

FIGURE 6.91 **Granulomatosis with polyangiitis in a 7-year-old girl who presented with chronic cough, shortness of breath, and chest pain. A:** Frontal chest radiograph demonstrates a small cavitary lesion (*arrow*) in the right upper lobe. **B:** Axial lung window CT image of the same patient shows a cavitary nodule (*arrow*) surrounded by ground-glass opacity representing hemorrhage (halo sign).

inflammation of the respiratory tract is found in about 3% of affected patients.[331,333,336]

Cyclophosphamide and corticosteroids comprise the mainstay of therapy for GPA in the pediatric population. In refractory cases, biologic therapy such as rituximab and anti–tumor necrosis factor inhibitors is increasingly being used.[330,338]

Churg-Strauss Syndrome

Churg-Strauss syndrome (CSS), also known as allergic granulomatosis and angiitis, is a primary systemic vasculitis of unknown etiology affecting small and medium-sized vessels.[339,340] Affected pediatric patients usually present with a history of asthma, allergic rhinitis, and blood eosinophilia.[328,332,339,340] In children, cardiorespiratory manifestations are seen more frequently than in adults.[340,341]

Chest radiographs are abnormal in 70% of patients with CSS.[328] The most common radiographic findings are bilateral patchy pulmonary opacification or consolidation without a clear lobar distribution as well as lung nodules. The areas of consolidation can be predominantly peripheral and transient.[332,334,342] Bilateral multifocal migratory consolidation or ground-glass opacities are typical findings on HRCT[328,332] (Fig. 6.92). CT may also show interlobular septal thickening, bronchial wall thickening, nodules, and hyperinflation.[328,332,337,343] In addition, unilateral or bilateral pleural effusions are seen in 10% to 50% of affected patients and may be caused by heart failure from associated cardiomyopathy or eosinophilic pleuritis.[342] Rarely, diffuse pulmonary hemorrhage may also present.[337]

The mainstay of treatment of CSS is corticosteroids, although cytotoxic agents including cyclophosphamide and plasma exchange are added in the therapy for affected patients with poor prognostic factors.[40,334,344]

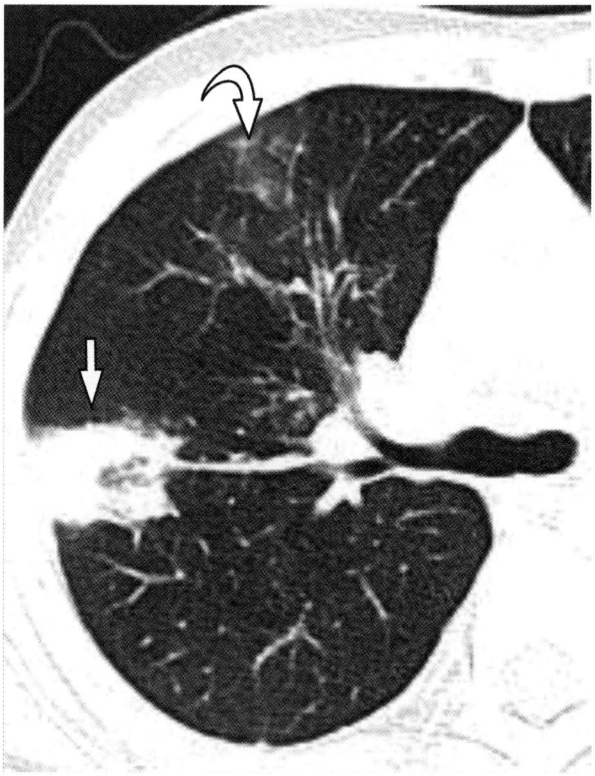

FIGURE 6.92 **Churg-Strauss syndrome in a 6-year-old girl with asthma and sinusitis who presented with malaise, urticarial rash, and eosinophilia.** Axial lung window CT image shows predominantly peripheral patchy areas of consolidation (*straight arrow*) and ground-glass opacity (*curved arrow*) without cavitation.

Goodpasture Syndrome

Goodpasture syndrome is a rare pulmonary–renal syndrome in childhood with substantial morbidity and mortality.[345,346] The syndrome consists of a triad of pulmonary hemorrhage, rapidly progressive glomerulonephritis, and anti–glomerular basement membrane (anti-GBM) antibodies, either in circulation or fixed to the kidney.[345]

Chest radiographs of pediatric patients with acute presentation of the disease demonstrate diffuse, bilateral alveolar opacification compatible with pulmonary hemorrhage[345,347] (Fig. 6.93). CT often shows bilateral ground-glass opacities and consolidation.[337,348] As a result of repeated lung hemorrhages, a reticulonodular pattern may be seen on follow-up CT.[349]

Corticosteroids, immunosuppressant agents such as cyclophosphamide, and plasmapheresis are standard therapeutic regimen in pediatric patients with Goodpasture syndrome.[345,350] Renal transplantation can be performed in patients requiring chronic hemodialysis after the disappearance of the circulating anti-GBM antibodies.[345]

Sickle Cell Disease

Sickle cell disease (SCD) is an inherited abnormality of the β-globin chain of hemoglobin (Hb) resulting in a spectrum of hemolytic anemia. The most common type of SCD is sickle cell anemia. Other types of SCD are caused by combinations of Hb S with Hb C or β-thalassemia. This disease is prevalent in Africa,

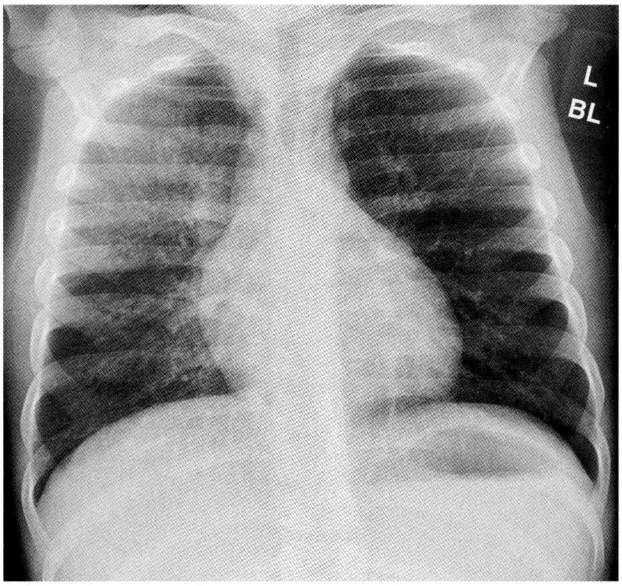

FIGURE 6.93 **Goodpasture syndrome in a 4-year-old boy who presented with hemoptysis and glomerulonephritis.** Frontal chest radiograph shows hazy airspace opacification seen on the right lung compatible with pulmonary hemorrhage.

the Middle East, Mediterranean countries, and India. Due to migration, it is now seen in America, Caribbean, and Europe.

The fundamental abnormality of SCD is the nucleotide substitution in the sixth codon of the β-globin chain, with hydrophobic valine residue replacing a normal hydrophilic glutamic acid, which is prone to polymerization under low oxygen conditions. The resultant abnormal Hb S damages the red blood cell (RBC) membrane, drastically shortening the RBC life span to as short as 12 days instead of 120 days. The RBCs also become dehydrated, relatively inflexible, abnormally adhesive, and form "sickle cells." These deformed cells are prone to adhere to the endothelial lining of blood vessels impeding blood flow, causing vaso-occlusion, leading to ischemia, infarction, and ischemia reperfusion injury of organs and tissues. Although it is fundamentally a blood disease, SCD affects the entire body, from infancy to adulthood.[351–353] Diagnosis is made by evaluation of the complete blood count, peripheral blood morphology, and a combination of Hb separation techniques, family studies, and genetic testing.

Affected patients in the first few months of life are asymptomatic, because they still have fetal Hb, which prevents polymerization of Hb S, and usually lasts for about 3 months. The common clinical manifestations of SCD in children are anemia, jaundice, recurrent vaso-occlusive crises, and infections by encapsulated bacteria, such as *Streptococcus pneumoniae*, due to functional asplenia.[351,352] Pulmonary complications such as pneumonia and acute chest syndrome (ACS) are the most common causes of death and hospital admission in SCD.

ACS is defined as a pulmonary illness with fever, chest pain, leukocytosis, and a new pulmonary opacity on a chest radiograph in a pediatric patient with SCD.[354] Several etiologies for ACS have been proposed, which are both clinically and radiographically difficult to differentiate. Infection has been initially proposed as an etiology,[351,354] but other reported underlying causes include infarction (due to microvascular occlusion), hypoperfusion, and fat embolism.[351,352,355] With current multidisciplinary care and substantial advances in intervention, almost all children (>95%) born with SCD in developed nations now survive to adulthood.[353,356]

The chest radiographic features of ACS are new foci of segmental, lobar, or multilobar consolidation with or without a pleural effusion (Fig. 6.94). Lower lobe airspace disease with rapid onset and rapid resolution following therapy was seen in children with no identifiable cause for their symptoms. In patients with an identifiable etiology (usually pneumonia), patients had a prolonged radiographic course with improvement not seen until 4 days posttherapy.[355,357] It is also important to note that a normal chest radiograph does not exclude incipient ACS.[351,355] HRCT often reveals ground-glass opacification without lobar distribution and may have a scattered or mosaic pattern. In addition, there may be diminished vascular markings and areas of scarring from the vaso-occlusion. In older SCD children, chronic interstitial lung changes manifested by interlobular septal thickening, parenchymal bands, pleural tags, dilated secondary pulmonary lobules, traction bronchiectasis, and architectural distortion can be also present. Despite this, it is important to note that there is no significant correlation between the severity of ACS and the extent of radiologic findings.[351,358,359]

Other extrapulmonary intrathoracic findings in patients with SCD include cardiomegaly and H-shaped thoracic vertebral bodies. In the spine, marrow hyperplasia and sickling result in ischemia, repeated microinfarctions, and occasional infections. This leads to weakening of the bone and intrusion of the disk into the vertebral endplate. On imaging, there is osteoporosis, vertebral cortical thinning, and smooth biconcave deformity of the vertebral bodies, referred to as "fish-mouth" or

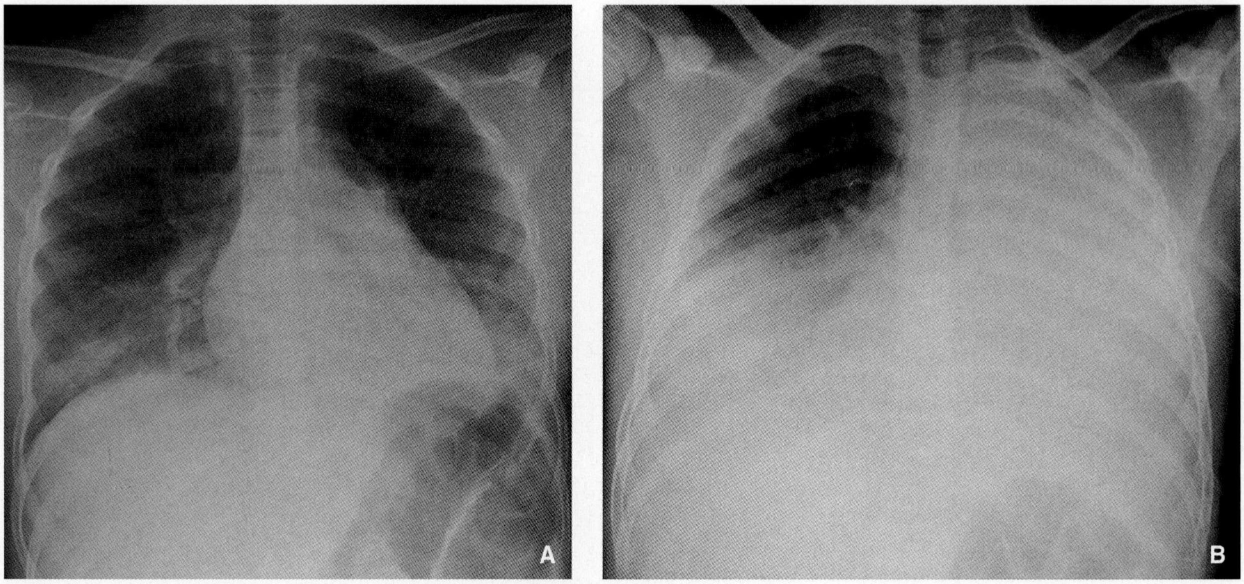

FIGURE 6.94 **Sickle cell disease (SCD) and acute chest syndrome (ACS). A:** Frontal chest radiograph of a 6-year SCD patient shows bibasilar lung opacities. Also noted is cardiomegaly. **B:** Frontal radiograph of another SCD pediatric patient who presented with ACS demonstrates opacities in the right middle and lower lobes and complete opacification of the left hemithorax likely related to underlying airspace consolidation and effusion. (Case courtesy of Elizabeth H. Ey, MD, Dayton Children's Hospital Medical Center, Dayton, OH.)

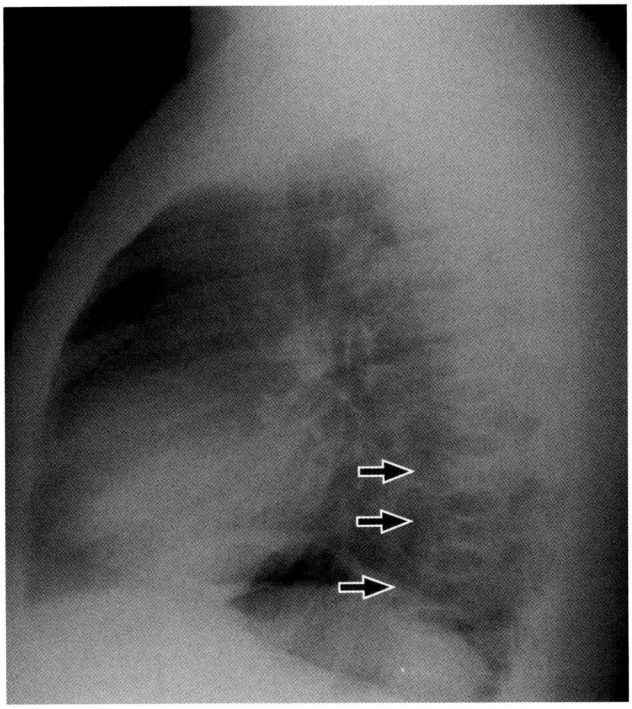

FIGURE 6.95 **A 17-year-old girl with sickle cell disease.** Lateral radiograph shows "H"-shaped thoracic vertebral bodies (*arrows*).

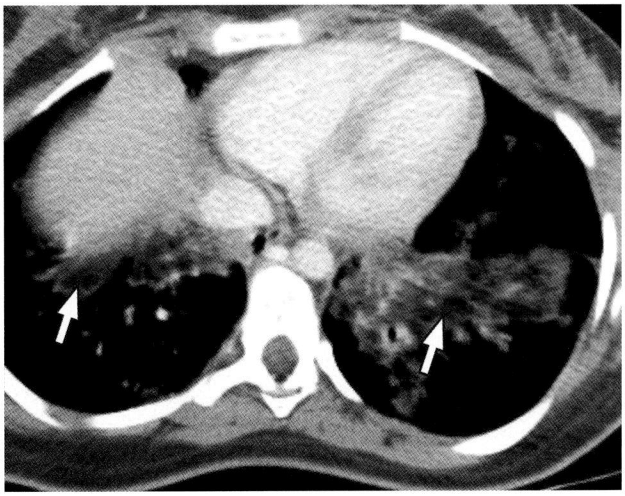

FIGURE 6.96 **Lipid pneumonia in a 15-year-old girl with a history of taking mineral-based laxatives for treatment of constipation.** Axial enhanced CT image shows bilateral lower lobe consolidations with areas of fatty attenuation (*arrows*). Given the history and CT findings, diagnosis of lipid pneumonia was made.

"H-shaped" vertebrae (Fig. 6.95). Vertebral collapse or wedging with resultant kyphosis can also occur.[360,361]

The substantial improvement in survival of SCD patients over the past four decades is the result of a variety of interventions, including newborn screening, prophylactic penicillin, immunizations against *H. influenzae* type b and *S. pneumoniae*, advances in diagnostic and supportive care, and the increased use of disease-modifying treatments such as hydroxyurea, chronic transfusions, and stem cell transplantation.[352,353]

Lipid Pneumonia

Lipid pneumonia (exogenous lipid pneumonia) in children results from the aspiration of mineral, vegetable, or animal oils. Exposure to fat or oil depends upon various customs in feeding, bathing, mouth or nose cleaning, and therapeutic intervention.[362] Oily substances inhibit the cough reflex and ciliary motion, and as a result, they easily progress down to dependent portions of the lung. Pre-existing conditions such as cleft palate, gastroesophageal reflux, achalasia, anesthesia, coma, and forced ingestion of medication enhance this complication.[362,363] Mineral oils trigger only mild inflammatory response, but animal oils tend to provoke a more severe inflammatory reaction in the lungs.[364] In adults, the symptoms are usually mild and rarely progress to respiratory failure, but children usually suffer an acute, more severe, and widespread aspiration pneumonia.[363]

Diagnosis can be difficult because affected pediatric patients usually present with nonspecific symptoms such as cough, fever, sputum production, and progressive dyspnea. Diagnosis is often delayed because lipid pneumonia is not initially considered until after there is poor response to antimicrobials and the history of oil inhalation or ingestion is elicited much later. Increased lipid-laden macrophages in bronchoalveolar lavage fluid may suggest the lipid pneumonia, but they are also seen in many other conditions.[365]

Lipid pneumonia can radiographically manifest within 30 minutes of aspiration or inhalation, and pulmonary opacities can be seen in most patients within 24 hours. Typical appearance is a bilateral ground-glass opacity or consolidation with segmental or lobar distribution and predominantly involves the middle and lower lobes.[366] A diffuse bilateral, parahilar opacification has also been previously described.[363,367] The CT is considered the imaging modality of choice for the diagnosis of lipid pneumonia.[368] The main CT findings are bilateral airspace consolidations in the posterior lung bases, usually with areas of fatty attenuation ranging from −30 to −150 Hounsfield units (HU) (Fig. 6.96). Areas of ground-glass attenuation and a crazy-paving pattern are also common findings on CT in affected children.[364,366–369] Interstitial thickening, with or without volume loss of the affected lung, nodular or irregular mass-like lesions, cavitation, and pleural effusion have also been reported.[362,363] In some affected pediatric patients, fat attenuation is less conspicuous in the presence of superimposed inflammation.[366]

The mainstay of management of lipid pneumonia includes avoiding ongoing exposure to the offending agent, treating any underlying infection, and providing supportive care. There have been reports of systemic corticosteroids used to slow the inflammatory response, but it is not routinely used.[370,371]

Unique Lung Disorders in Neonates

Respiratory distress from pulmonary disease is common in the early neonatal period and occurs in up to 7% of newborn infants.[93,372] Generally, pulmonary abnormalities in neonates can be mainly categorized into medical diseases and surgical diseases. This chapter focuses on five most commonly encountered medical diseases of the neonatal lung including hyaline membrane disease (HMD), transient tachypnea of the newborn (TTN), meconium aspiration syndrome (MAS), neonatal pneumonia, and pulmonary interstitial emphysema (PIE). Table 6.4 summarizes the typical radiographic imaging features of these neonatal lung conditions, but because of significant overlap, clinical correlation including the prenatal and perinatal history, gestational age, and current clinical condition is important in providing an accurate diagnosis.

TABLE 6.4 Summary of Clinical and Radiologic Features of Unique Lung Disorders in Neonates

Disorder	Clinical Findings	Risk Factors	Radiographic Findings
Hyaline membrane disease (HMD) Also referred to as surfactant deficiency disorder (SDD) or respiratory distress syndrome (RDS)	• Grunting, nasal flaring, retractions, tachypnea, and cyanosis within minutes of birth	• Prematurity • Maternal diabetes mellitus (DM) • Multiple gestations • Cesarian section delivery • Perinatal asphyxia	• Low lung volume • Symmetric diffuse reticulogranular lung opacities with air bronchograms • Findings usually noted shortly after birth but with maximum severity at 12–24 h of life • May mimic neonatal pneumonia, meconium aspiration, and pulmonary interstitial emphysema (PIE).
Transient tachypnea of the newborn (TTN) Also referred to as wet lung disease or retained fetal lung fluid	• Infant initially normal, then becomes tachypneic • Rapid clinical improvement usually within 1 or 2 d	• Cesarian section delivery • Precipitous delivery • Hypotonic and sedated infants • Delivery prior to 38 weeks of gestation • Low birth weight • Macrosomia • Maternal DM or asthma	• Hyperinflated lungs with diffuse prominent parahilar and interstitial markings • Minimal pleural or fissural fluid • Transient minimal cardiac enlargement • Rapid radiographic improvement usually within 1 or 2 d
Meconium aspiration syndrome (MAS)	• Meconium-stained amniotic fluid	• Postmaturity • Small for gestational age • Intrauterine stress and/or hypoxemia • Maternal hypertension, DM, respiratory disease, and cardiovascular disease	• Hyperinflated lungs with bilateral diffuse and asymmetric patchy opacities • Pattern may be varied and often cannot be distinguished from neonatal pneumonia • May develop PIE, pneumomediastinum, and pneumothorax as complication of ventilator support • Pulmonary hemorrhage and pleural effusion can also develop
Neonatal pneumonia	• Early onset: first 48 h up to first week of life • Late onset: next 3 wk	• Prematurity • Prolonged rupture of membranes • Maternal infection, especially chorioamnionitis • Invasive mechanical ventilation	• Typically bilateral, multifocal patchy opacities with or without pleural effusion • Pattern may mimic TTN, MAS, or HMD
Pulmonary interstitial emphysema (PIE)	• Associated with administration of positive pressure ventilation and resuscitation • May occur spontaneously	Premature infants are more prone than term infants	• Coarse, nonbranching linear or cystic lucencies tracking along the bronchovascular sheaths from the hilum to periphery • Usually diffuse and bilateral but may be unilateral or unilobar • CT: linear and dot-like structures within cysts • May appear similar to bronchopulmonary dysplasia, congenital lobar emphysema, or congenital pulmonary airway malformation • Can occur with pneumomediastinum, pneumothorax, and subcutaneous emphysema

Hyaline Membrane Disease

HMD, also called respiratory distress syndrome or surfactant deficiency disorder, remains one of the most important causes of neonatal respiratory distress. HMD is a disease resulting from pulmonary immaturity and deficiency of surfactant, a lipoprotein complex produced by type II pneumocytes, which decreases surface tension and prevents collapse of the alveoli. Surfactant deficiency leads to a cascade of events, which includes development of hyaline membranes containing fibrin and cellular debris; abnormal pulmonary compliance and atelectasis, leading to poor gas exchange, also develop.[373] It is important to note that hyaline membranes are not specific to surfactant deficiency and may occur because of any of the numerous insults associated with acute respiratory distress syndrome.

Prematurity is the most significant risk factor for developing HMD, and the incidence is inversely related to gestational age and weight. HMD occurs in 60% to 80% of babies born <28 weeks and 15% to 30% of babies born between 32 and 36 weeks.[31,373–375] Although it may be present beyond 36 weeks or at term, it is uncommon, and other diagnoses should be considered.[374] Males are affected almost twice as often as females, and HMD is more common in whites than in blacks. Other risk factors include maternal diabetes, multiple gestations, cesarean section, and infants exposed to perinatal asphyxia.[31,373–375]

Affected infants are usually symptomatic within minutes of birth with grunting, nasal flaring, retractions, tachypnea, and cyanosis. The rigid, noncompliant lungs and the associated hypoxia and acidosis may lead to persistent pulmonary hypertension and left-to-right shunting across a patent ductus arteriosus.[31,373,376] Advances in neonatal care have markedly improved the outlook for premature infants with HMD. Prematurity with HMD requiring continued ventilation is a significant risk factor for development of bronchopulmonary dysplasia (BPD).[31,377] BPD, congenital surfactant dysfunction in full-term infants, as well as other diffuse lung disease as a result of gene mutations are discussed in the section on diffuse lung disorders in this chapter.

The typical radiographic findings of HMD are small lung volume, symmetric diffuse reticulogranular lung opacities, and air bronchograms (Fig. 6.97). However, the radiographic findings depend on the severity of the disorder that results from surfactant deficiency (Fig. 6.98). These radiographic findings are usually noted shortly after birth, but occasionally do not reach maximum severity until 12 to 24 hours of life.[373] In mild disease, the lungs show fine ground-glass shadowing, but more severe disease could show more widespread lung opacity with air bronchograms or even a complete white-out with obscuration of the cardiac border.[375]

The underaeration of the lungs may no longer be seen in neonates who have already been intubated and whose lungs have been ventilated. The use of artificial surfactant has also produced several significant changes in radiographic appearance of HMD. Usually, the surfactant given via the ETT is not evenly distributed throughout the lungs. Therefore, it is common to see some areas of lungs that have improved aeration and other areas maintaining the hazy reticulogranular opacities. This may mimic and should not be confused with other neonatal lung conditions such as neonatal pneumonia or meconium aspiration. Because of surfactant's effective distention of multiple alveolar units, it may also produce a radiographic appearance similar to PIE or even pneumothorax, but it has no

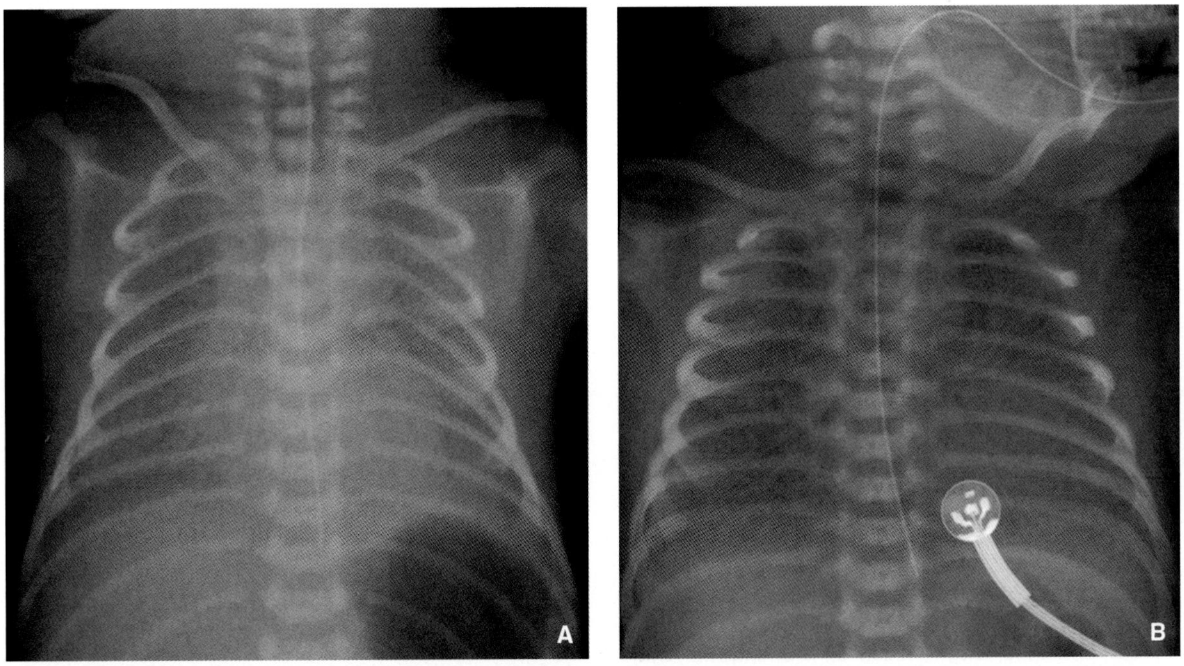

FIGURE 6.97 **Hyaline membrane disease (HMD) or surfactant deficiency disorder (SDD) in two premature neonates.** Frontal chest radiographs of a 31-week premature infant **(A)** and a 35-week premature neonate **(B)** both show the typical radiographic pattern of HMD or SDD which includes hypoaeration, reticulogranular opacity, and presence of air bronchograms. The degree of lung opacification is more substantial in the 31-week premature infant **(A)**.

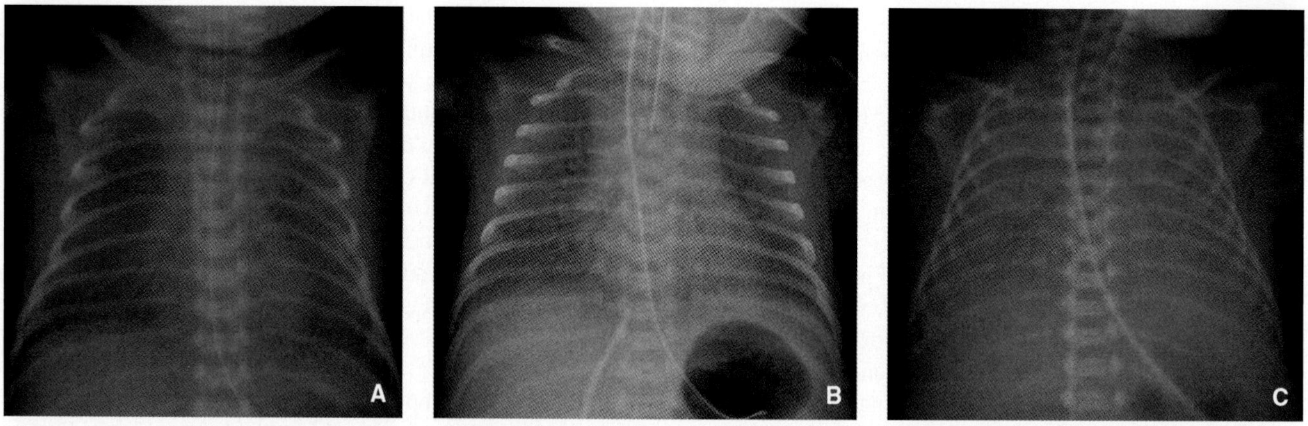

FIGURE 6.98 **Hyaline membrane disease or surfactant deficiency disorder following intubation and surfactant therapy in three premature neonates. A:** Frontal chest radiograph shows improved lung aeration pattern due to surfactant therapy, but subsegmental lung collapse remain in the left upper lobe. **B:** Frontal chest radiograph demonstrates that there is effective distention of the multiple alveolar units further accentuating the air bronchogram. **C:** Frontal chest radiograph shows the presence of lung opacity despite surfactant therapy that may suggest underlying pulmonary edema, presence of patent ductus arteriosus, superimposed infection, or even hemorrhage.

influence on the clinical outcome.[31,373,378] Left-to-right shunting through a patent ductus arteriosus compounding HMD may be recognized radiographically before clinical symptoms or a murmur develops. It is heralded by the development of pulmonary edema, which manifests radiographically as diffuse pulmonary opacification with an enlarging heart. Other considerations for diffuse lung opacity in HMD include hypoventilation due to decreasing ventilator support, superimposed infection, and less commonly, diffuse pulmonary hemorrhage. Most premature infants that survive HMD but require continued ventilation support eventually develop chronic BPD (or also known as chronic lung disease) (Fig. 6.99).

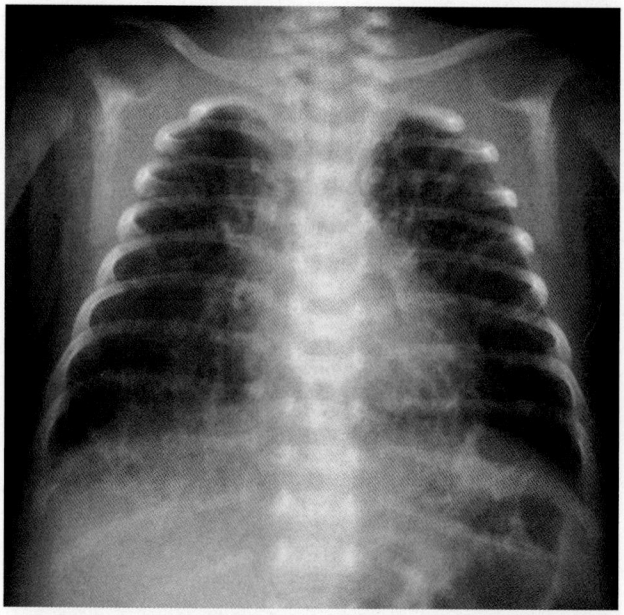

FIGURE 6.99 **Chronic lung disease or bronchopulmonary dysplasia in a 2-month-old, former 28 weeks' gestation infant boy.** Frontal chest radiograph shows hyperaerated lungs with bilateral coarse reticular opacities giving an almost diffuse cystic or "bubbly" appearance.

In recent years, strategies to delay labor and antenatal administration of glucocorticoids to mothers with expectant premature delivery have substantially reduced the incidence of HMD. Surfactant replacement therapy and more advanced ventilatory strategies have also improved the early management and survival of these neonates and infants.[31,373,378]

Transient Tachypnea of the Newborn

TTN is also referred to as retained fetal lung fluid or wet lung disease. It is a benign transient condition caused by delayed clearance of fetal lung fluid. Under normal circumstances, the fetal lung fluid is cleared from the lungs at or shortly after birth via the tracheobronchial system, the interstitial lymphatics, and the capillaries.[373] TTN is now recognized as the most common cause of respiratory distress in newborn term infants.[372] The primary risk factor for TTN is delivery via cesarean section where the usual mechanisms to clear the neonatal lung fluid during labor do not occur. Other risk factors include infants with precipitous delivery, hypotonic and sedated infants,[373,379] delivery prior to 38 weeks of gestation, male gender, low birth weight, macrosomia, and maternal diseases such as gestational diabetes and asthma.[372] Typically, affected infant is normal immediately after birth but becomes tachypneic over the next few hours. Despite mild to moderate signs of respiratory distress, there is usually normal oxygenation. Some infants develop an oxygen requirement that necessitates admission to the neonatal unit for a few days.[380] There have been reports that TTN may be associated with development of asthma later in childhood, especially among males.[381,382]

Typically radiographic features of TTN are diffusely prominent parahilar interstitial markings along with hyperinflation (Fig. 6.100). However, there is variability of radiographic manifestations, which may appear similar to HMD, pulmonary edema, meconium aspiration, or neonatal pneumonia.[373,375] In such cases, clinical history would play an important role. A small amount of pleural effusion and fluid

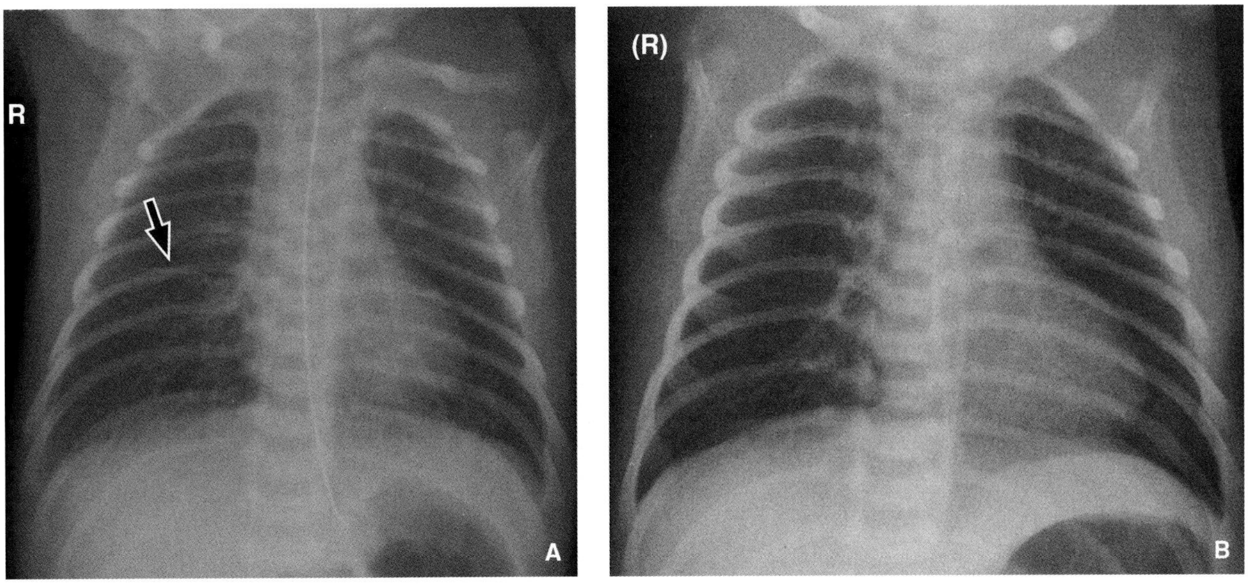

FIGURE 6.100 **Transient tachypnea of the newborn (TTN) in a term neonate delivered via cesarian section. A:** Frontal chest radiograph obtained at the date of delivery shows hyperaeration and prominent parahilar interstitial markings along with small amount of minor fissural fluid (*arrow*). **B:** Frontal chest radiograph obtained 3 days later shows clear lungs.

in the fissures is also frequently seen, and in some cases, there is transient minimal cardiac enlargement. An important hallmark of TTN is the rapid clinical and radiologic improvement, usually within 1 or 2 days.[372,375]

TTN is a benign, self-limited condition and affected infants almost always recover fully. Some affected infants may require oxygen therapy or other forms of respiratory support for a couple of hours after birth to aid recovery.

Meconium Aspiration Syndrome

MAS is a result of perinatal inhalation and aspiration of the meconium leading to hypoxia and fetal distress. Meconium is the fetal colonic material that is usually passed during the first 24 hour after birth and is rarely found in the amniotic fluid prior to 34 weeks. MAS usually occurs in babies who are postmature (mean gestational age has been reported as 290 or 10 days past the expected day of delivery) or small for gestational age or where there has been intrauterine stress causing hypoxemia. Other risk factors include maternal hypertension, diabetes mellitus, and cardiovascular disease.[373,383]

MAS is diagnosed by the presence of meconium in the airway below the vocal cords (Fig. 6.101). There is meconium staining of the amniotic fluid in ~5% to 30% of live births, and MAS develops in 2% to 10% of newborns born with meconium staining.[372] The aspirated meconium causes lung injury both by plugging the small- and medium-sized airways and causing obstruction and by inciting chemical inflammatory response, pulmonary vasoconstriction, and secondary surfactant deficiency.[375,383,384] Meconium also increases the risk for developing superimposed bacterial infection and persistent pulmonary hypertension of the newborn (PPHN). As a consequence of prolonged ventilation in some severely affected patients, air leak phenomenon and eventually BPD may develop.[372,373]

The radiographic findings in MAS vary depending on the severity of aspiration. Typical radiographic findings include hyperinflated lungs with bilateral diffuse and asymmetric patchy parahilar opacities (Figs. 6.102 and 6.103). These opacities can have various patterns due to diversity in the disease presentation, and often, it cannot be distinguished from neonatal pneumonia. Air leak complications including PIE, pneumomediastinum, and pneumothorax are frequently but not always a result of positive-pressure ventilatory support. Pleural effusion and pulmonary hemorrhage may also develop.[373,375,383]

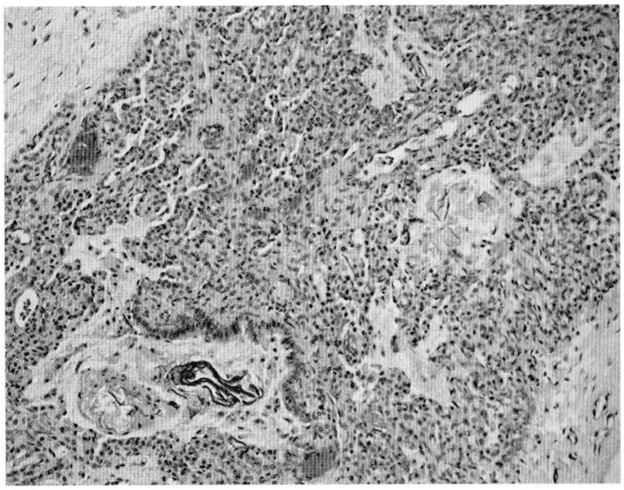

FIGURE 6.101 **Meconium aspiration in a 12-day-old infant boy with respiratory distress and a history of meconium-stained amniotic fluid.** Lung biopsy shows abundant anucleate squames and other amnionic debris in the distal airways and airspaces (hematoxylin and eosin, original magnification, 400×).

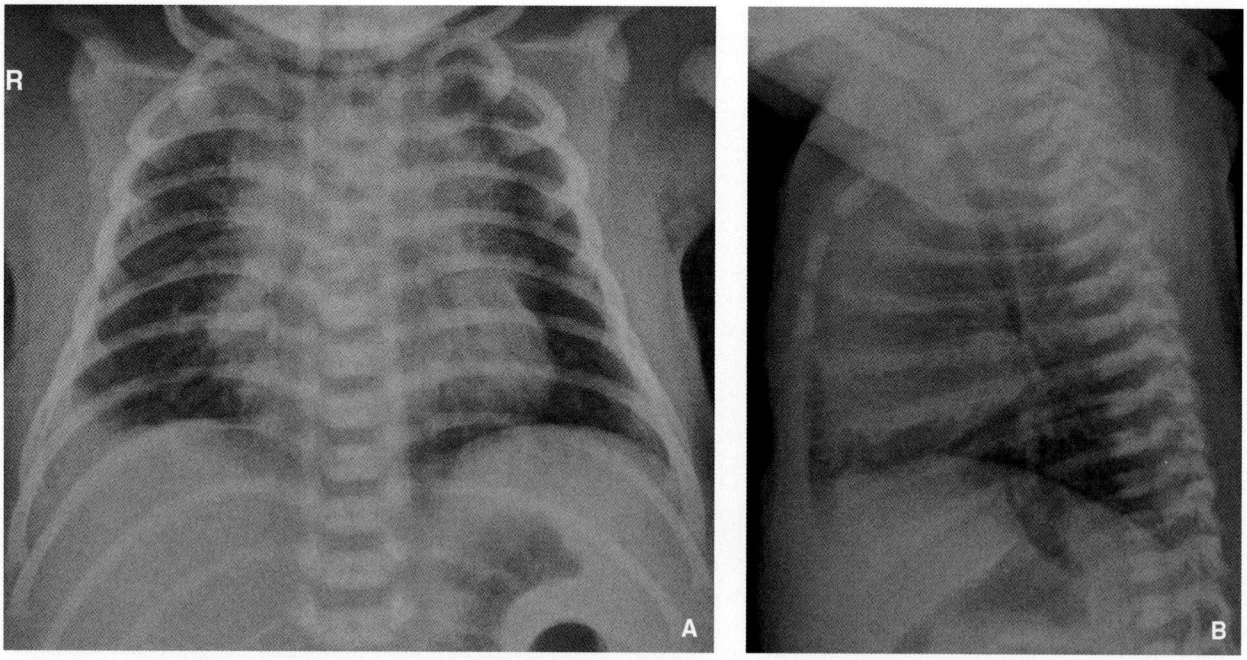

FIGURE 6.102 **Meconium aspiration in a 42-week-old (post-term) neonate.** Frontal **(A)** and lateral **(B)** views of chest radiograph show hyperaerated lungs with diffuse parahilar opacities. There is also small amount of right pleural effusion.

The incidence of MAS continues to decline because of improving obstetric practice in post-term mothers along with closer fetal monitoring.[383,385] Most infants with MAS recover within 2 to 3 days and only require supportive therapy. Treatment for more severe MAS include high-frequency ventilation, exogenous surfactant, inhaled nitrous oxide, liquid ventilation, and medications to reduce pulmonary hypertension. Because the development of neonatal pneumonia is always a consideration, antibiotics are often administered.[372,373,383] In some cases where the neonate fails to respond to conventional therapy, extracorporeal membrane oxygenation (ECMO) therapy is used.[372,386]

Neonatal Pneumonia

Neonatal pneumonia refers to lower respiratory infection that occurs during the first 28 days of life causing respiratory distress. Early-onset neonatal pneumonia presents in the first 48 hours up to the first week of life, whereas late-onset neonatal

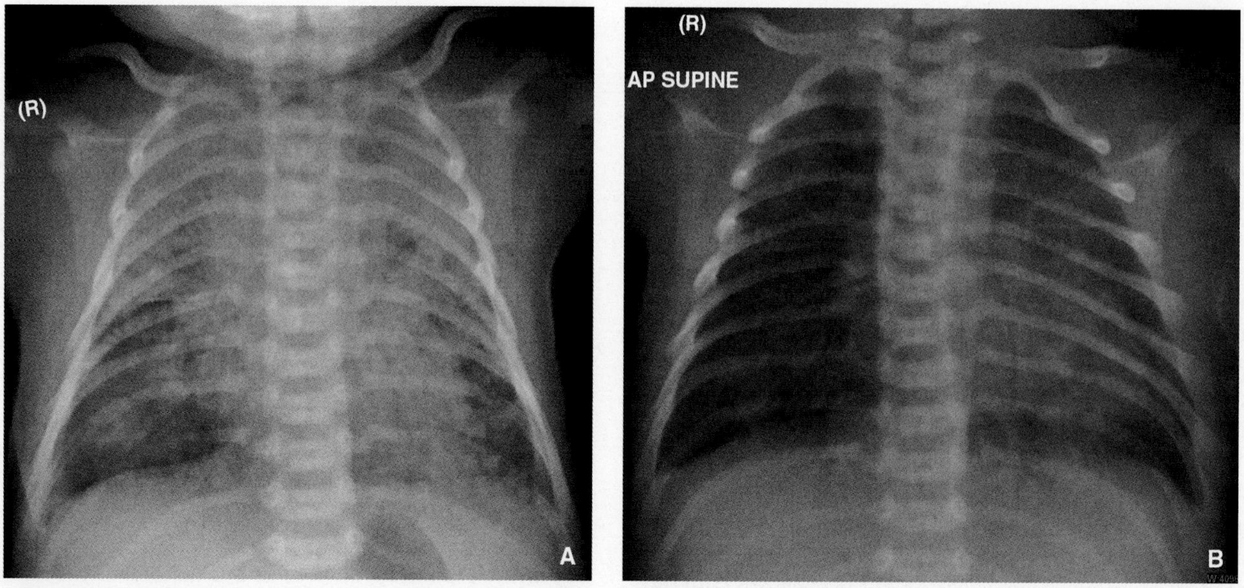

FIGURE 6.103 **Meconium aspiration in a 41 weeks' gestation infant before and after therapy. A:** Frontal chest radiograph shows hyperaeration and coarse multifocal opacities in both lungs. **B:** Frontal chest radiograph obtained 10 days following appropriate management and therapy demonstrates substantial clearing of the lung opacities but with residual hyperaeration and interstitial thickening.

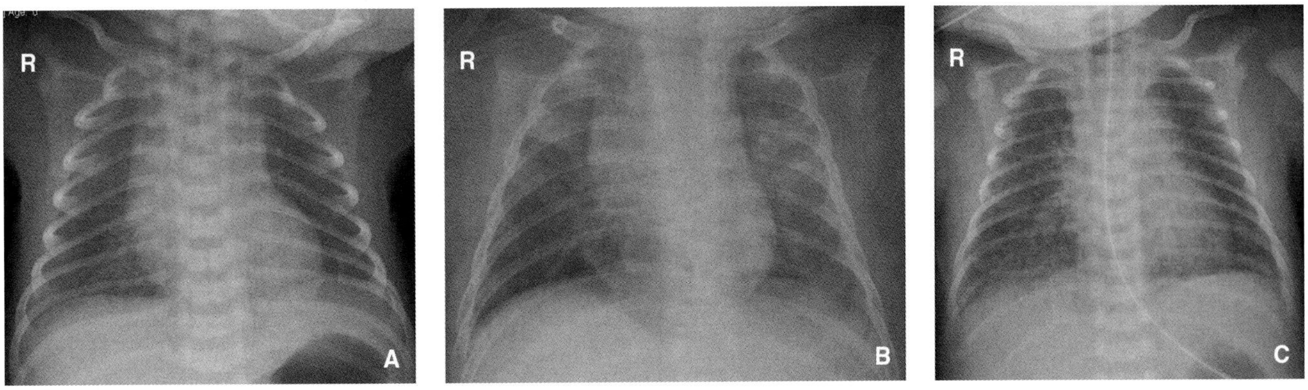

FIGURE 6.104 **Spectrum of chest radiographic findings of neonatal pneumonia in three neonates.** Frontal chest radiographs show mild focal opacity in the right lower lobe **(A)**, multifocal opacities involving both lungs **(B)**, and diffuse interstitial opacities **(C)**.

pneumonia occurs in the next 3 weeks.[387] It is the most common cause of neonatal sepsis, causing substantial morbidity and mortality. Neonatal pneumonia can be acquired in utero, during passage, or just after birth. The major risk factors are prematurity, prolonged rupture of the membranes, maternal infection, and invasive mechanical ventilation.[2,3] Birth weight and age of onset are both strongly associated with the mortality risk from pneumonia.[388,389] Bacterial etiology is the most common cause and includes group B *Streptococcus*, *S. pneumoniae*, *S. aureus*, *Listeria*, and *Escherichia coli*. Some viruses, including *Herpes* and atypical organisms such as *Chlamydia*, are also associated with neonatal pneumonia. Diagnosis depends on a high index of suspicion from the clinical and radiologic findings.[372–387]

Neonatal pneumonia is frequently a systemic disease, and the typical radiographic manifestation is bilateral, multifocal patchy opacifications with or without pleural effusion (Fig. 6.104). This radiographic pattern is nonspecific and overlaps with other neonatal lung diseases. It may mimic the parahilar interstitial thickening of TTN or the patchy parahilar opacifications of MAS. Neonatal pneumonia may also present with reticulogranular opacifications throughout the lungs similar to HMD. However, the presence of pleural effusion is more commonly associated with pneumonia rather than HMD.[372,373,375]

Antibiotic therapy is the mainstay of therapy in neonatal pneumonia. Supportive care such as oxygen, thermoregulation, prevention of hypoglycemia, and parenteral nutrition or nasogastric tube feeding is often required.[387,388] Screening for group B *Streptococcus* infection in the third trimester of pregnancy and treatment of those infected have reduced the incidence of associated pneumonia.[390]

Pulmonary Interstitial Emphysema

PIE is a form of air leak with air dissecting along the interstitial spaces of the lung. Although this condition is associated with administration of positive pressure ventilation and resuscitation, it can also occur spontaneously. PIE can be subclassified as an acute transient process lasting for a few days or it can be persistent. The pattern of involvement could be diffuse and bilateral or it could be localized in one lobe or lung.[391] PIE is more common in premature than term infants because there is looser texture of the interstitial tissue in premature infants allowing gas to accumulate at lower pressures than in term infants. Unilateral PIE may occur if the tip of an ETT is misplaced and directed into only one of the main bronchi.[392] Although it can occur alone, PIE can coexist with other air leak complications including pneumothorax, pneumomediastinum, pneumopericardium, subcutaneous emphysema, and even pneumoperitoneum.[375]

On radiographs, PIE appears as coarse nonbranching linear or cystic lucencies tracking along the bronchovascular sheaths, from the hilum to the periphery of the lungs.[375] These lucencies vary from the typical branching pattern of air bronchograms and sometimes get wider in the periphery of the lungs. Although it can be unilateral or unilobar, it is generally a diffuse bilateral process (Fig. 6.105). PIE can sometimes be confused with lung changes seen in BPD, but the two can be distinguished through history and comparison with old studies. PIE may

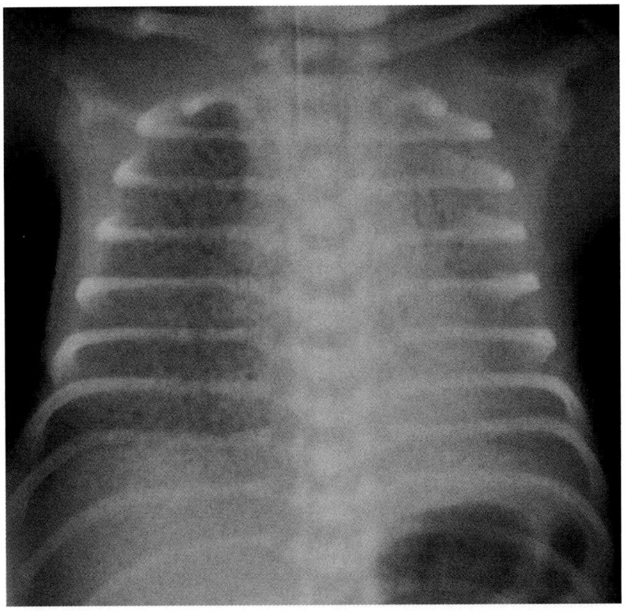

FIGURE 6.105 **Unilateral pulmonary interstitial emphysema (PIE) in a 2-week-old ventilated neonate with history of prematurity.** Frontal chest radiograph shows nonbranching linear lucencies in the right lung consistent with PIE.

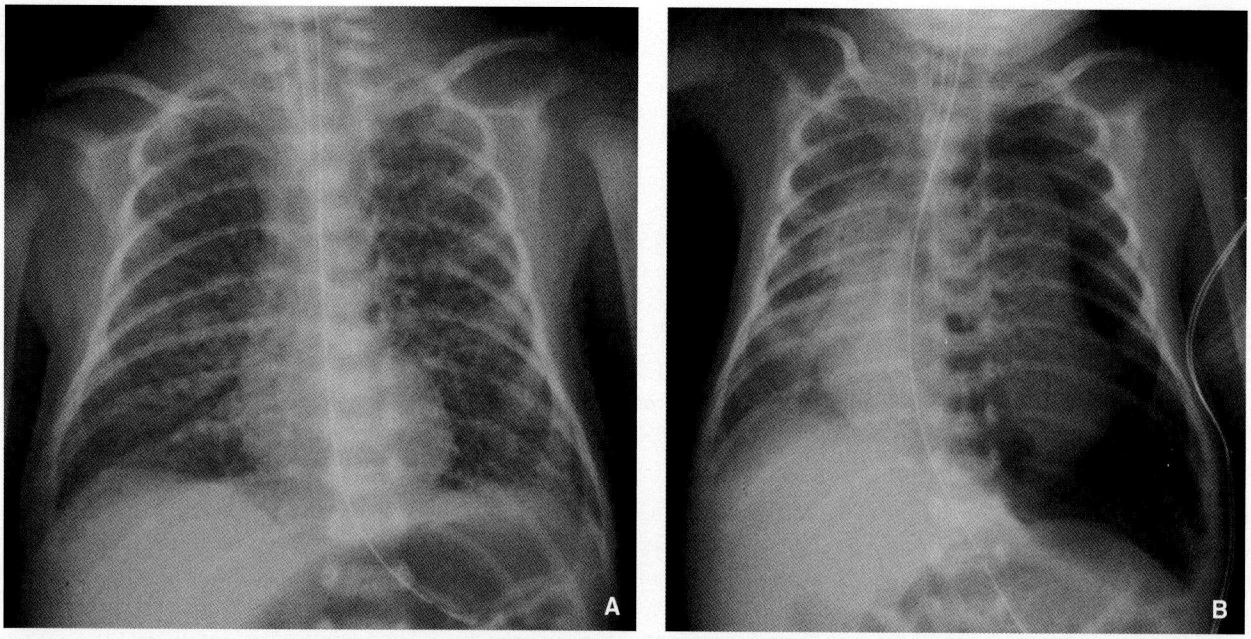

FIGURE 6.106 **Pulmonary interstitial emphysema (PIE) and sequelae in a premature infant boy in mechanical ventilation. A:** Frontal chest radiograph shows coarse nonbranching linear and cystic lucencies in both lungs compatible with PIE. **B:** Follow-up frontal radiograph obtained 24 hours later demonstrates large pneumothorax on the left with cardiomediastinal shift to the right.

persist and form localized thin-walled cysts, which can cause mass effect on adjacent structures. In some cases, the imaging appearance of PIE may mimic CLE or CPAM.[31,375,391,393] On CT, the linear and dot-like structures of soft tissue attenuation are seen within the cysts, which have been attributed to bronchovascular bundles surrounded by interstitial gas.[31,394] PIE can occur with pneumomediastinum, pneumothorax, subcutaneous emphysema, and other forms of air leak (Fig. 6.106). Pathologic examination shows dissected spaces predominately along bronchovascular bundles interlobular septa and pleura (Fig. 6.107).

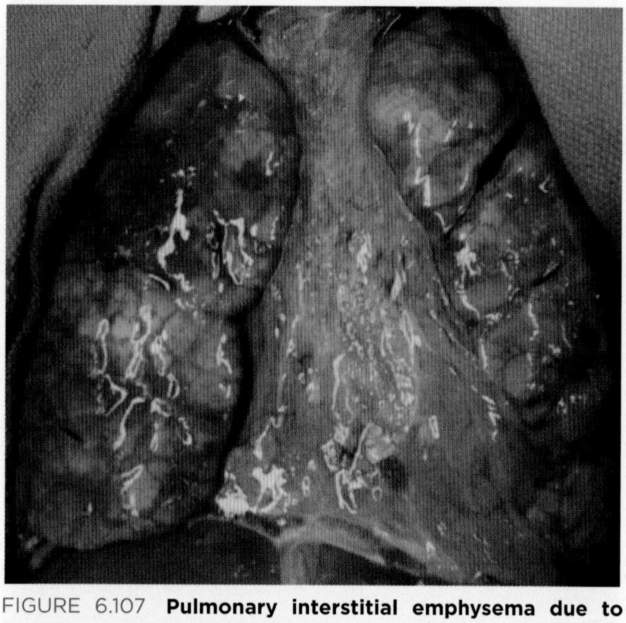

FIGURE 6.107 **Pulmonary interstitial emphysema due to positive-pressure ventilation in the setting of necrotizing bacterial pneumonia in a 15-year-old boy.** From the pleural surface, the lobular architecture of the lung is accentuated because of widening of the interlobular septa by air. Small crepitant air bubbles also fill the mediastinal soft tissue.

Management of PIE is guided by the severity of the disease. More benign clinical presentations have been managed conservatively through lateral decubitus positioning, selective bronchial intubation, selective bronchial occlusion, steroids, surfactant, and tube thoracostomy. Management of more severely affected neonates includes high-frequency ventilation, ECMO, pleurotomy, and lobectomy in selected patients.[391]

Diffuse Lung Disorders

The pediatric diffuse lung disorders are a rare and heterogeneous group of diseases associated with significant chronic illness and even death. Clinically, they present with dyspnea, tachypnea, crackles and hypoxemia. The diffuse lung disorders are commonly referred to as the childhood interstitial lung diseases (chILD). However, the former term is considered more appropriate because the disorders may in fact affect the alveoli, blood vessels, lymphatics, and pleural spaces in addition to the pulmonary interstitium. Some diffuse lung disorders occur predominantly or exclusively in infancy, as defined by the revised chILD classification scheme (Table 6.5), whereas others may occur at any age.[395–401]

Diffuse Lung Disorders in Infants

Diffuse Developmental Disorders

The three main disorders within this category are acinar dysplasia, congenital alveolar dysplasia (CAD), and alveolar capillary dysplasia with malalignment of pulmonary veins (ACD/MPV).[395–401] They are thought to be caused by aberrations of early prenatal lung development and characterized by severe dysfunction in alveolar gas exchange.

TABLE 6.5 Classification System of Interstitial Lung Diseases in Infants

Diffuse Developmental Disorders Acinar dysplasia Congenital alveolar dysplasia Alveolar capillary dysplasia with malalignment of pulmonary veins
Alveolar Growth Disorders Prenatal: secondary pulmonary hypoplasia Postnatal: chronic lung disease • Prematurity-related chronic lung disease (bronchopulmonary dysplasia) • Chronic lung disease in term infant Associated chromosomal or genetic abnormalities • Trisomy 21 • Other (e.g., filamin A mutation) Associated congenital heart disease
Surfactant Dysfunction/Related Abnormalities Surfactant dysfunction disorders • *SpB* genetic mutations (pulmonary alveolar proteinosis and variants) • *SpC* genetic mutations (chronic pneumonitis of infancy; also pulmonary alveolar proteinosis, diffuse interstitial pneumonitis, and nonspecific interstitial pneumonia) • Adenosine triphosphate–binding cassette transporter protein A3 genetic mutation (pulmonary alveolar proteinosis; also chronic pneumonitis of infancy, diffuse interstitial pneumonitis, and nonspecific interstitial pneumonia) • Congenital granulocyte macrophage colony-stimulating factor receptor deficiency (pulmonary alveolar proteinosis histologic pattern) • Thyroid transcription factor-1 genetic mutations • Others: histology consistent with surfactant dysfunction, unrecognized genetic disorder Lysinuric protein intolerance (pulmonary alveolar proteinosis histologic pattern)
Specific Conditions of Unknown or Poorly Understood Etiology Neuroendocrine cell hyperplasia of infancy Pulmonary interstitial glycogenosis • Primary • Associated with other pulmonary conditions, especially alveolar growth disorders

Modified from Lee EY, Cleveland RH, Langston C. Interstitial lung disease in infants and children: new classification system with emphasis on clinical, imaging, and pathologic correlation. In: Cleveland RH, ed. Imaging in Pediatric Pulmonology. New York: Springer; 2011, with permission.

Lungs with acinar dysplasia are small and contain only airway structures, lacking alveoli and incompatible with life (Fig. 6.108). CAD is a poorly described entity in which alveolar septa are diffusely widened, somewhat resembling "pulmonary interstitial glycogenosis" (PIG) and reminiscent of alveolar capillary dysplasia without malalignment of pulmonary veins. ACD/MPV is characterized clinically by severe pulmonary hypertension with respiratory failure in the newborn period. Histologically, large veins course in an abnormal location adjacent to pulmonary arteries and airways (Fig. 6.109). Alveolar septa are thickened, and capillaries lack apposition to alveolar epithelium. Additional lung abnormalities may include medial hypertrophy of pulmonary arteries, underdevelopment of pulmonary lobules sometimes with alveolar enlargement and reduced capillary density, and prominent regional or diffuse lymphangiectasis. *FOXF1* gene mutations and 16q24.1 microdeletions are implicated in some cases of ACD/MPV, whereas no known genetic basis exists for acinar dysplasia or CAD.[395–400,402–406] Associated extrapulmonary congenital anomalies (cardiovascular, gastrointestinal, genitourinary) are present in more than 80% of ACD/MPV patients and can aid in diagnosis. Pediatric patients with diffuse developmental disorders typically present at term with progressive respiratory distress and cyanosis.[399]

Because of the rarity and severity of these diseases, in general, only portable chest radiographs are available with nonspecific and even normal findings. As disease progresses, radiographs show progressive diffuse hazy bilateral pulmonary

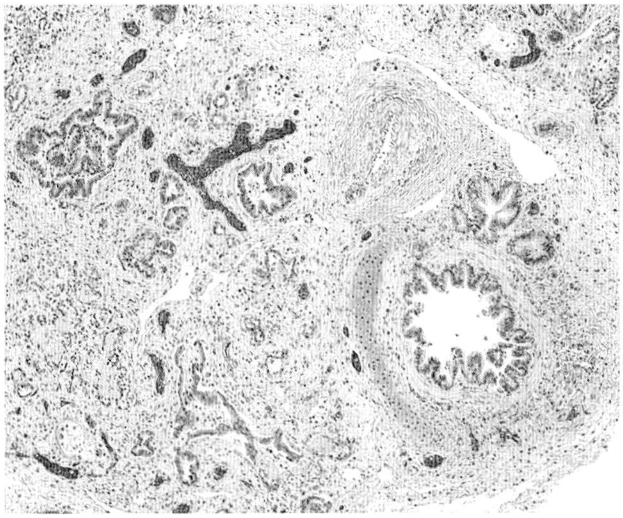

FIGURE 6.108 **Acinar dysplasia.** Histologic examination from the autopsy of a 2-day-old term infant boy with small lungs and respiratory failure at birth shows the characteristic lack of alveoli (hematoxylin and eosin, original magnification, 100×).

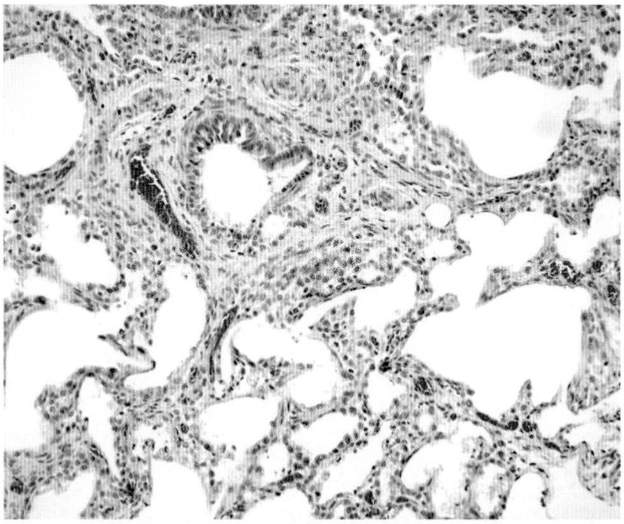

FIGURE 6.109 **Alveolar capillary dysplasia with malalignment of pulmonary veins (ACD/MPV).** Lung biopsy specimen from a 2-week-old girl with respiratory failure shows a large vein running with the bronchovascular bundle, marked pulmonary arterial hypertensive changes, and widened alveolar septa (hematoxylin and eosin, original magnification, 200×).

opacities and hypoinflation, mimicking findings of surfactant deficiency syndrome or congenital surfactant metabolism disorders. Lung volumes may be increased with ventilator support. About 50% of affected pediatric patients develop air leaks such as pneumomediastinum or pneumothorax, likely related to barotrauma.[395–400,407–410]

Diffuse developmental disorders usually result in death within the first 2 months of life due to rapidly worsening respiratory failure, despite aggressive supportive care. Affected pediatric patients usually do not survive long enough to receive a lung transplant, the only viable treatment. Because 10% of ACD/MPV cases are heritable, genetic counseling may be offered to family members of afflicted infants.[395–400,402–411]

Alveolar Growth Disorders

Alveolar growth disorders are characterized by alveolar formation defects with enlargement of airspaces, lack of alveolar septation, and lobular simplification. Although caused by abnormal lung development, they are not preprogrammed to occur as in the case of diffuse developmental disorders but rather arise because of a superimposed prenatal or postnatal event or in

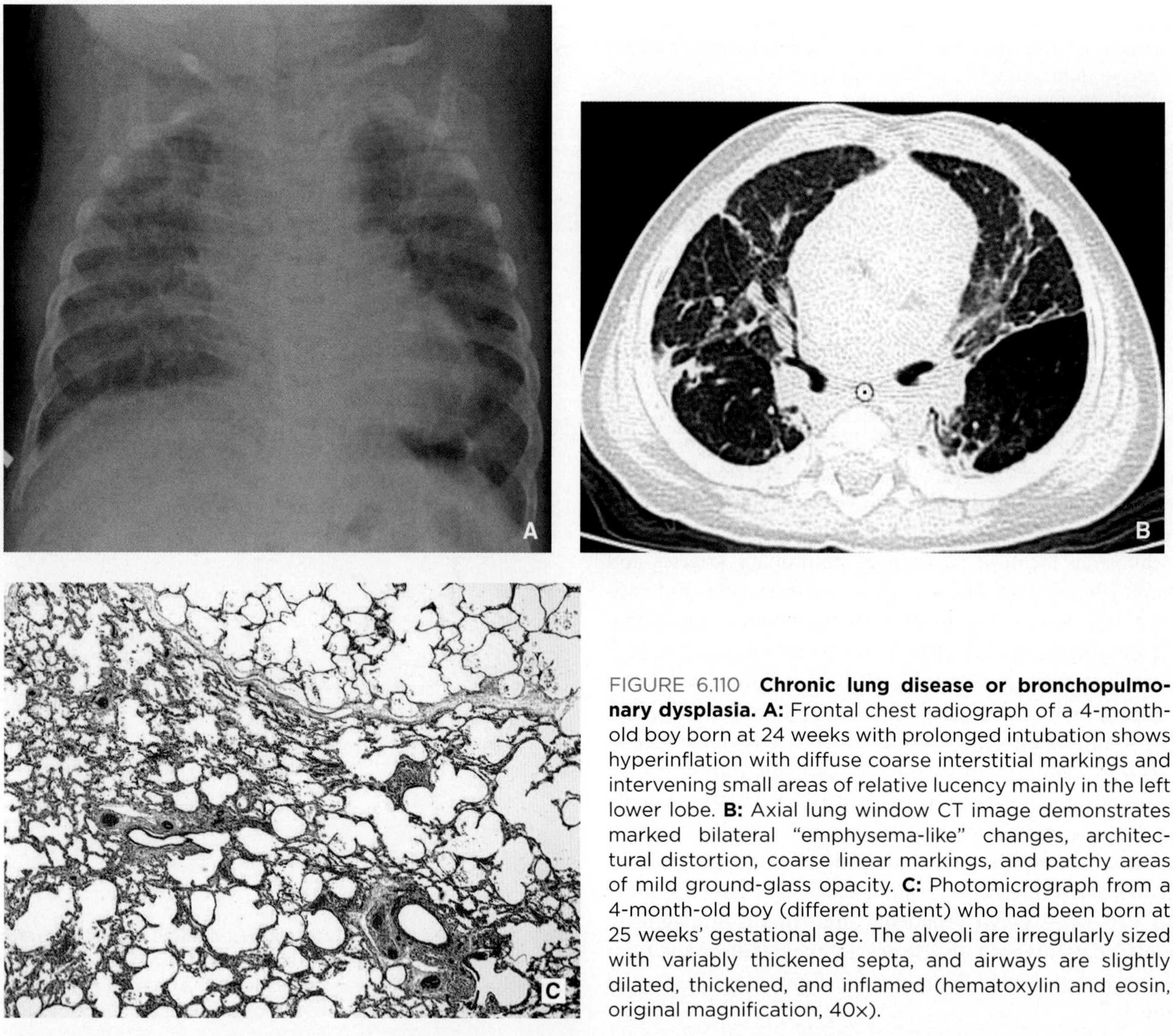

FIGURE 6.110 **Chronic lung disease or bronchopulmonary dysplasia. A:** Frontal chest radiograph of a 4-month-old boy born at 24 weeks with prolonged intubation shows hyperinflation with diffuse coarse interstitial markings and intervening small areas of relative lucency mainly in the left lower lobe. **B:** Axial lung window CT image demonstrates marked bilateral "emphysema-like" changes, architectural distortion, coarse linear markings, and patchy areas of mild ground-glass opacity. **C:** Photomicrograph from a 4-month-old boy (different patient) who had been born at 25 weeks' gestational age. The alveoli are irregularly sized with variably thickened septa, and airways are slightly dilated, thickened, and inflamed (hematoxylin and eosin, original magnification, 40×).

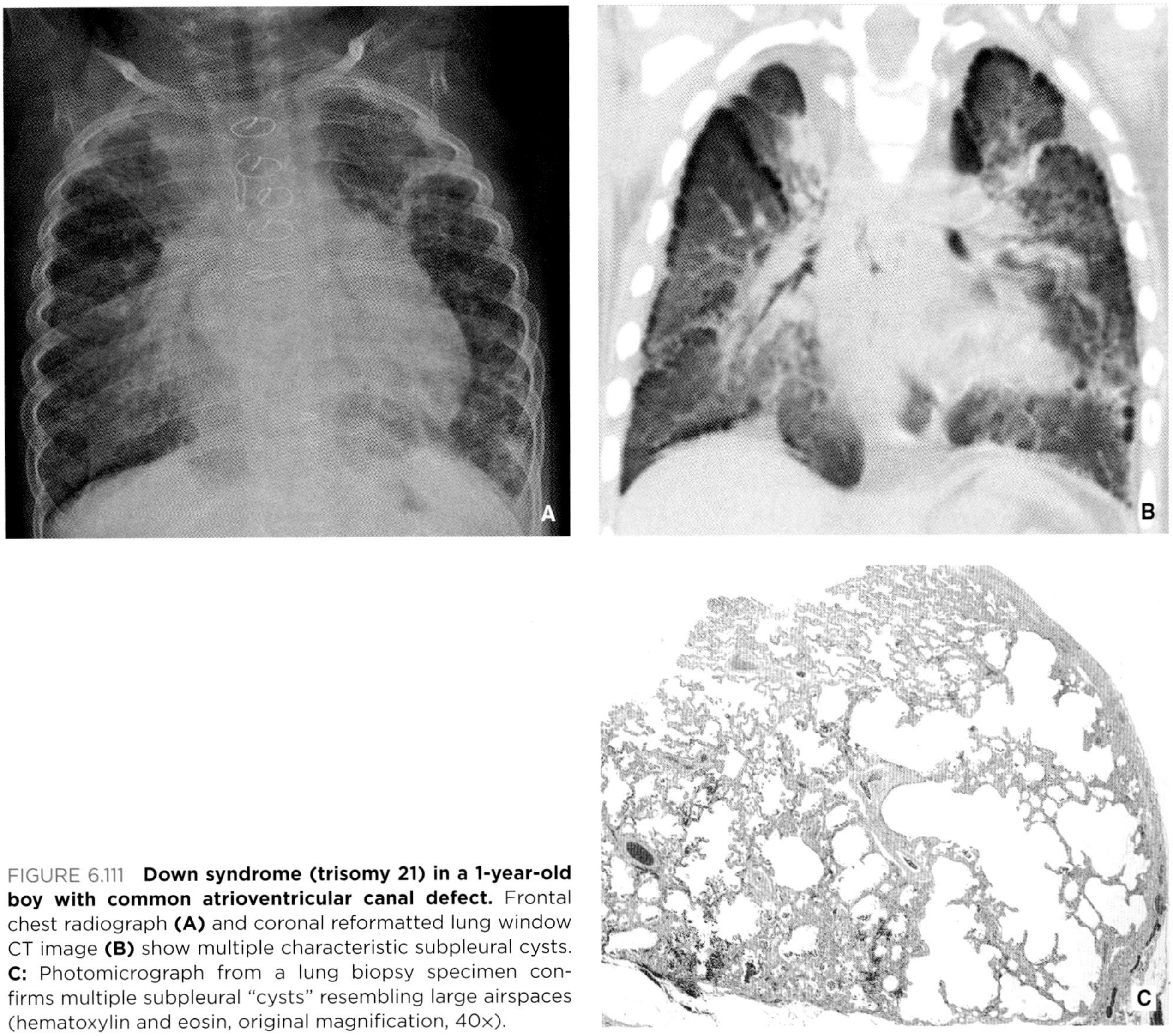

FIGURE 6.111 **Down syndrome (trisomy 21) in a 1-year-old boy with common atrioventricular canal defect.** Frontal chest radiograph **(A)** and coronal reformatted lung window CT image **(B)** show multiple characteristic subpleural cysts. **C:** Photomicrograph from a lung biopsy specimen confirms multiple subpleural "cysts" resembling large airspaces (hematoxylin and eosin, original magnification, 40×).

association with chromosomal abnormalities or congenital heart disease. Prematurity-related chronic lung disease (also known as BPD) may be the most familiar version encountered in daily practice (Fig. 6.110). Alveolar growth disorders are the most common form of infant diffuse lung disease, comprising ~43% of cases.[395–401] Affected infants and children present with variably progressive respiratory distress.[399]

Although both radiographic and CT findings are in general variable, some specific alveolar growth disorders demonstrate distinct imaging patterns. For example, chest radiographs in chronic neonatal lung disease of prematurity characteristically show coarse reticular opacities, cystic lucencies, and disordered lung aeration due to alveolar septal fibrosis and hyperinflation. Small subpleural cysts are typical of infants with Down or Turner syndrome (Fig. 6.111). In patients with X-linked filamin A (*FLNA*) genetic mutations, chest imaging demonstrates severe hyperinflation with hyperlucent lung parenchyma and peripheral pulmonary vascular attenuation affecting all lobes as well as central pulmonary artery enlargement and atelectasis[31,395–400,402,412–416] (Fig. 6.112).

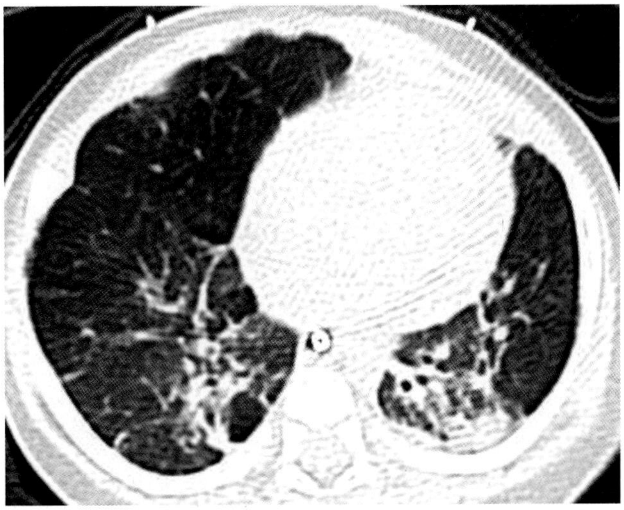

FIGURE 6.112 **Filamin A (FLNA) mutation in a 7-month-old boy.** Axial lung window CT image shows marked multilobar hyperlucency with vascular attenuation resembling panlobar emphysema. Also noted is atelectasis in the posterior lungs bilaterally.

Extrapulmonary findings may also be encountered such as periventricular gray matter heterotopia, skeletal dysplasia, joint laxity, patent ductus arteriosus, and progressive aortic root dilation.[399]

In pediatric patients with alveolar growth disorders, lung biopsy may be useful to establish a definitive diagnosis because many also have patchy PIG (detailed below), which is potentially steroid responsive. Minimizing injurious respiratory support is the primary method of reducing prematurity-related chronic lung disease severity and incidence. Pediatric patients with *FLNA* mutations may require lung transplantation because of particularly severe respiratory decline.[31,395–400,402,411–418]

Surfactant Dysfunction Disorders

The genetic surfactant disorders are characterized by mutations in genes necessary for normal surfactant metabolism. Such genes include *SFTPB* for surfactant protein B (SpB), *SFTPC* for surfactant protein C (SpC), and the ATP-binding cassette subfamily A member 3 (*ABCA3*) for the ABCA3 protein involved in surfactant processing. Additionally, rare genetic disorders such as thyroid transcription factor-1 (TTF-1) gene (NKX2-1) mutations ("brain–lung–thyroid syndrome"), lysinuric protein intolerance, and GM-CSF receptor mutations resulting in impaired surfactant metabolism are included in this category.[395–400,419–438]

Although rare, genetic surfactant metabolism disorders are a frequent cause of unexplained respiratory distress syndrome in term newborns. Clinical presentations include respiratory failure, persistent tachypnea, and hypoxemia.[399] By contrast, acquired surfactant metabolism disorders, such as the development of anti-GM-CSF autoantibodies leading to pulmonary alveolar proteinosis (PAP), occur in older children and adults.

Chest radiographs in pediatric patients with surfactant disorders show diffuse or patchy hazy granular opacities, similar to those seen in respiratory distress syndrome of prematurity (Figs. 6.113A and 6.114A). CT demonstrates diffuse ground-glass or consolidative opacity and interlobular septal thickening (Figs. 6.113B and 6.114B). A geometric crazy-paving pattern typical of PAP (detailed separately below) may be present. As patients age, ground-glass opacities often recede and thin-walled parenchymal cysts develop, increasing in size and number over time (Fig. 6.115). Skeletal abnormalities such as pectus excavatum are commonly observed in patients surviving beyond infancy; this association is thought to be related to the effects of chronic, restrictive lung disease on the growing chest wall.[395–400,419–438]

Histologically, genetic surfactant disorders show varying proportions of alveolar proteinosis, type 2 pneumocyte hyperplasia, intra-alveolar macrophages, and fibrosis, often accompanied by alveolar growth disturbance (Fig. 6.114C). Genetic testing for surfactant mutations can help to confirm diagnosis, but is rarely considered definitive without supporting histology, because many mutations are of unknown clinical significance. Chronic ventilator support is the mainstay of treatment, possibly supplemented by corticosteroids and prophylaxis for pulmonary infection. Lung transplantation is an option for severe disease. Development of targeted genetic therapies for specific surfactant mutations is an area of active investigation.[395–400,411,419–438]

Specific Conditions of Unknown or Poorly Understood Etiology

Neuroendocrine Cell Hyperplasia of Infancy

Neuroendocrine cell hyperplasia of infancy (NEHI) is a recently discovered disease pattern with an unclear etiology. On a pathologic level, the disorder is characterized by abnormally increased numbers of pulmonary neuroendocrine cells (PNECs) in the epithelium of peripheral airways. PNECs are involved in fetal lung development and oxygen sensing but normally significantly dissipate after the neonatal period.[395–400,402,411,439–446] NEHI patients are usually term newborns who present with persistent tachypnea, retractions, hypoxemia, and crackles by 3 months of age, notably with lack of significant cough or wheeze.[399]

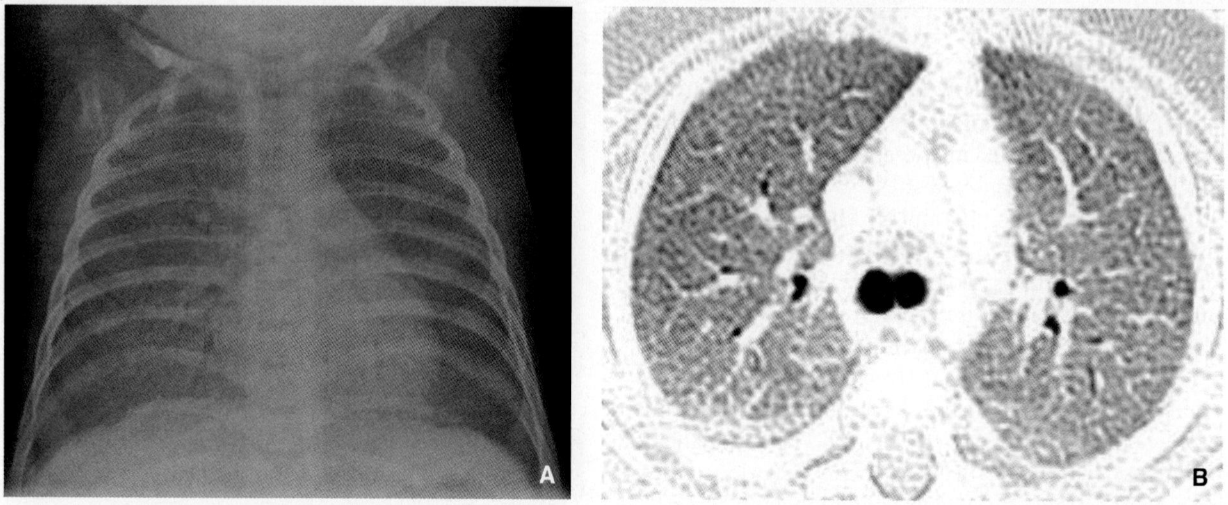

FIGURE 6.113 **Surfactant protein B (SpB) deficiency in a term infant boy who presented with respiratory distress after birth. A:** Frontal chest radiograph shows diffuse granular opacities in both lungs resembling respiratory distress syndrome of prematurity. **B:** Axial lung window CT image demonstrates symmetric diffuse ground-glass opacity and interlobular septal thickening in both lungs.

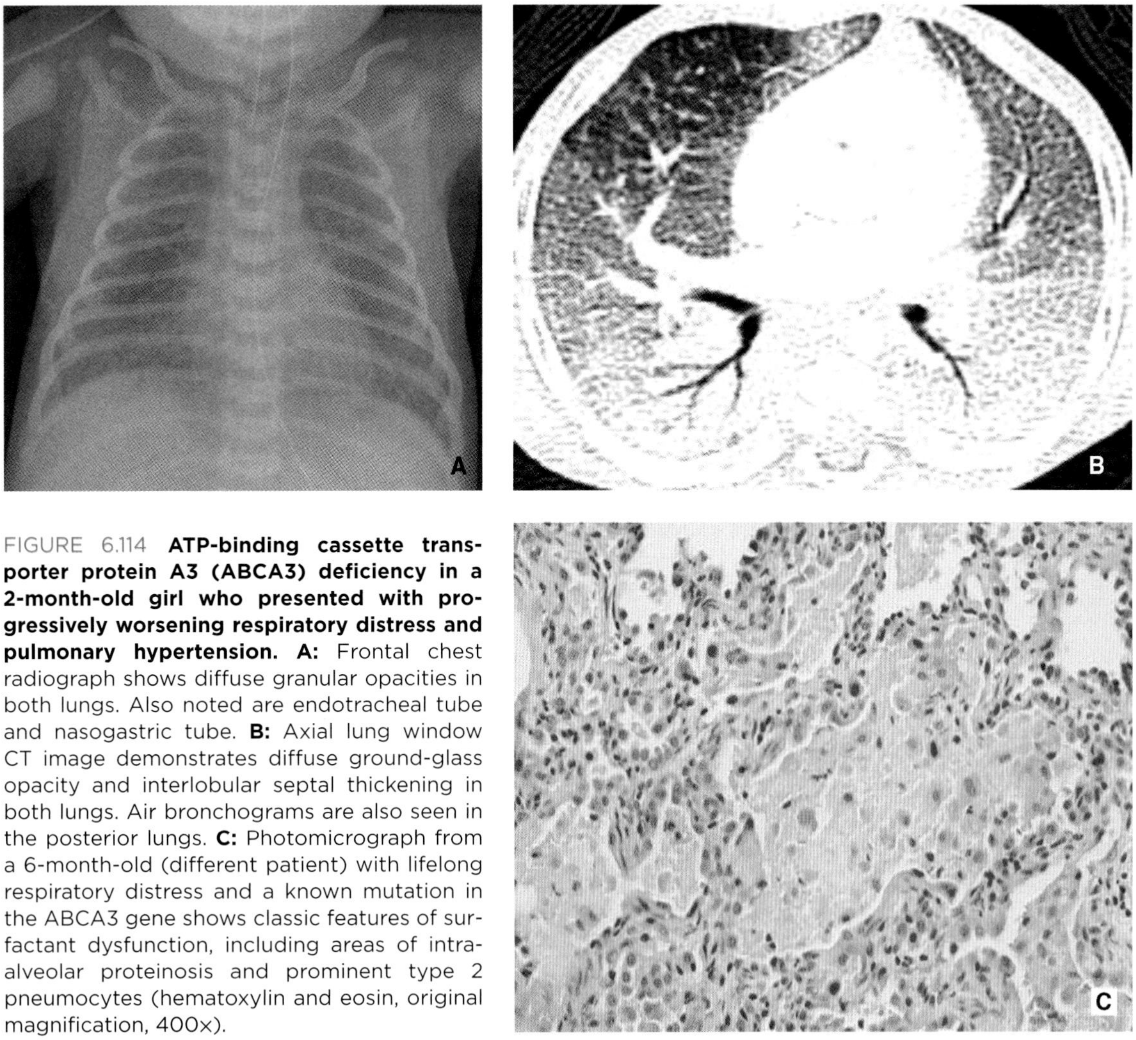

FIGURE 6.114 **ATP-binding cassette transporter protein A3 (ABCA3) deficiency in a 2-month-old girl who presented with progressively worsening respiratory distress and pulmonary hypertension. A:** Frontal chest radiograph shows diffuse granular opacities in both lungs. Also noted are endotracheal tube and nasogastric tube. **B:** Axial lung window CT image demonstrates diffuse ground-glass opacity and interlobular septal thickening in both lungs. Air bronchograms are also seen in the posterior lungs. **C:** Photomicrograph from a 6-month-old (different patient) with lifelong respiratory distress and a known mutation in the ABCA3 gene shows classic features of surfactant dysfunction, including areas of intra-alveolar proteinosis and prominent type 2 pneumocytes (hematoxylin and eosin, original magnification, 400×).

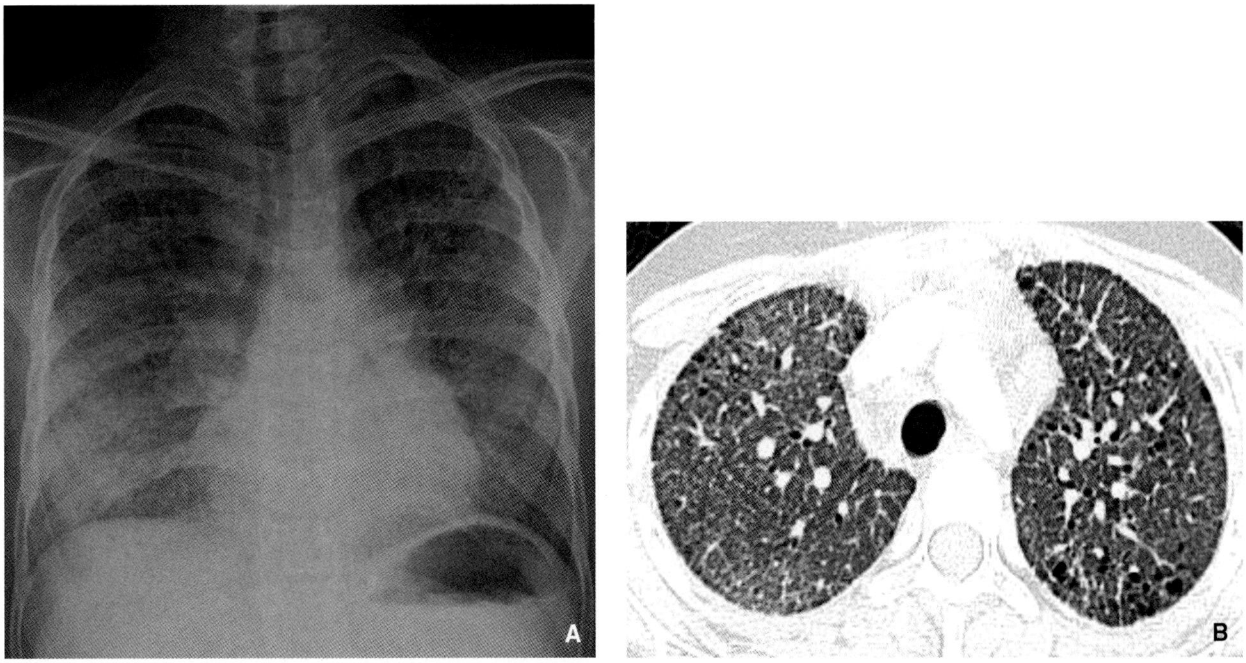

FIGURE 6.115 **ATP-binding cassette transporter protein A3 (ABCA3) deficiency in a 12-year-old girl. A:** Frontal chest radiograph shows interstitial thickening and multiple small cystic changes in both lungs. **B:** Axial lung window CT image better demonstrates multiple small cystic changes along with mild septal thickening in both lungs.

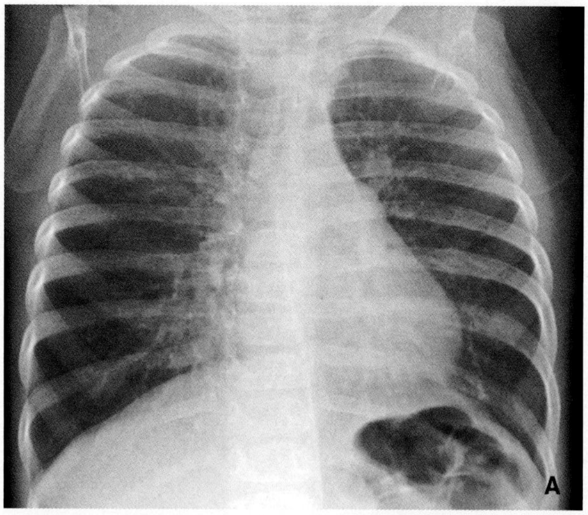

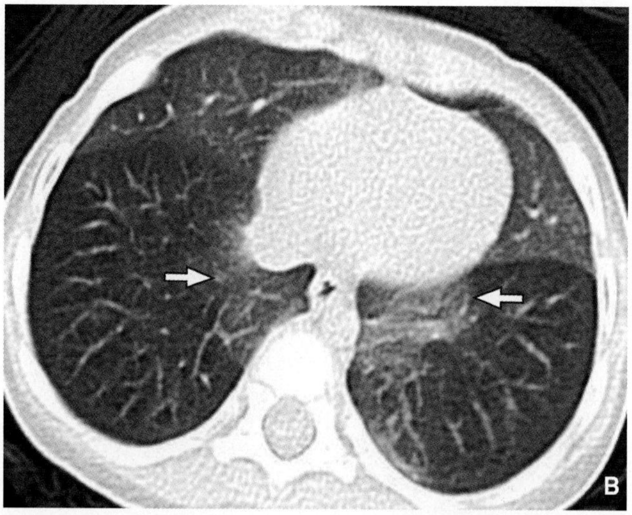

FIGURE 6.116 **Neuroendocrine cell hyperplasia of infancy (NEHI) in a 5-month-old girl who presented with persistent tachypnea and hypoxemia. A:** Frontal chest radiograph shows opacity along the bilateral paramediastinal regions and hyperinflation. **B:** Axial lung window CT image shows geographic ground-glass opacities of the right middle lobe, lingula, and bilateral paramediastinal lung regions (*arrows*).

Chest radiographs show variable increased perihilar opacity and hyperinflation, mimicking bronchiolitis or reactive airways disease (Fig. 6.116A). CT findings are characteristics with air trapping and a mosaic attenuation pattern involving at least four lobes and geographic, paramediastinal ground-glass opacities particularly in the right middle lobe and lingua (Fig. 6.116B). In fact, the sensitivity and specificity of HRCT for the diagnosis is reported to be 78% to 83% and 100% when exams are evaluated by experienced pediatric chest radiologists.[396,397,399] Thus, characteristic CT features in combination with an appropriate clinical history may eliminate the need for lung biopsy to establish a confident diagnosis.[395–400,402,411,439–446] When procured, biopsy shows nearly-normal lung tissue with variably subtle chronic airway changes resembling those seen in postviral injury. Immunostaining for bombesin highlights increased numbers of neuroendocrine cells.

Treatment for NEHI is supportive, aimed at ensuring adequate oxygenation, preventing infection, and sustaining nutritional intake. Affected pediatric patient may have persistent symptoms necessitating prolonged oxygen therapy. However, the prognosis is favorable, with no reported deaths or progression to respiratory failure attributable directly to the disorder.[395–400,402,411,439–446]

Pulmonary Interstitial Glycogenosis

PIG is a disorder of unknown etiology that may result from disordered lung growth and development. It is characterized histopathologically by accumulation of immature alveolar septal mesenchymal cells that contain copious cytoplasmic glycogen (Fig. 6.117). There are two subtypes: the more common "patchy" type, which often coexists with alveolar growth disorders, and the rare "diffuse" type, which is not associated with growth disorders.[395–400,402,411,412,447–452] Affected pediatric patients present with tachypnea and hypoxemia usually by several hours and never later than 6 months after birth.[399]

Chest radiographs in pediatric patients with PIG show worsening hyperinflation over time. Diffuse fine interstitial markings progress to coarse interstitial or alveolar opacities. CT findings may include hyperinflated/hyperlucent areas, pulmonary architectural distortion, ground-glass opacities (diffuse, segmental, or subsegmental), interlobular septal thickening, and reticular changes, often subpleural in location. In patchy PIG, unlike the diffuse type, CT may show multiple, small, scattered cystic changes (Fig. 6.118). These cysts may in fact be attributable to a concomitant alveolar growth abnormality rather than to PIG itself.[395–400,402,411,412,447–452]

Pediatric patients with PIG usually require supplemental oxygen and tend to benefit from steroid therapy, which is thought to accelerate lung maturation. Although

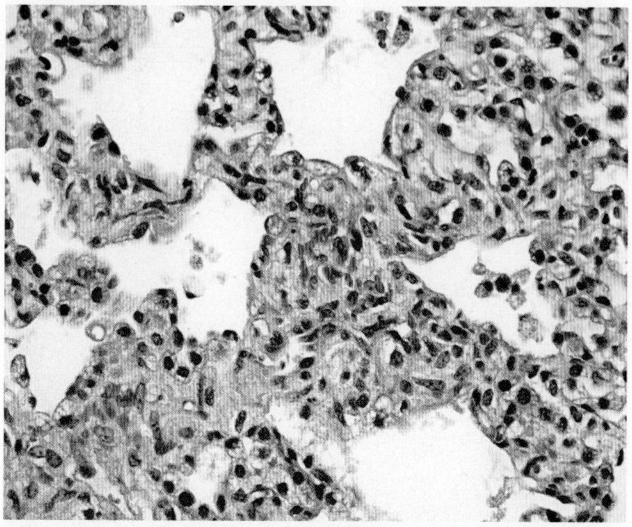

FIGURE 6.117 **Pulmonary interstitial glycogenosis (PIG).** Photomicrograph shows the expansion of alveolar septa containing glycogen-rich interstitial cells typical of this disorder (hematoxylin and eosin, original magnification, 600×).

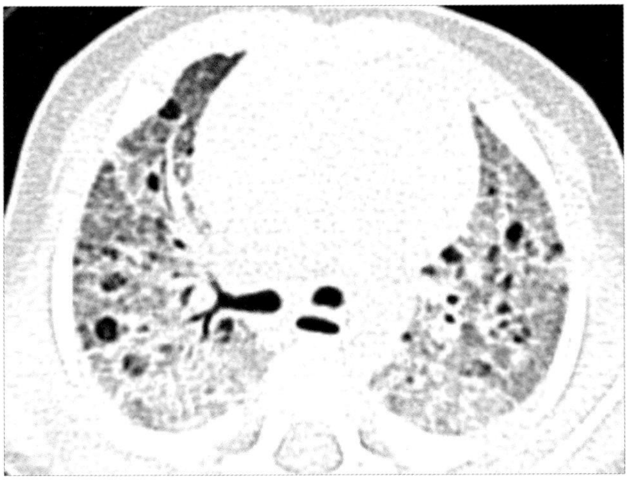

FIGURE 6.118 **Pulmonary interstitial glycogenosis (PIG) in a full-term 5-week-old girl who presented with tachypnea and hypoxemia.** Axial lung window CT image shows diffuse ground-glass opacification, interstitial thickening as well as small and multiple cyst-like hyperlucent disordered pulmonary lobules in both lungs.

hyperinflation may persist for years, the prognosis is favorable with no reported deaths attributable to PIG. The prognosis worsens when there is a coexisting growth disorder or pulmonary arterial hypertension.[395–400,402,411,412,447–452]

Other Childhood Diffuse Lung Disorders

Pulmonary Alveolar Proteinosis

PAP is a rare disorder that is characterized by an abnormal accumulation of lipoproteinaceous surfactant within the alveoli, hindering normal gas exchange. The congenital form is usually more severe and can be seen in the setting of a genetic surfactant deficiency, as discussed above. The acquired form of PAP tends to occur in older children and adults. It is most commonly caused by autoantibodies against granulocyte macrophage colony-stimulating factor (GM-CSF) but can arise in many processes that impair alveolar macrophage-dependent surfactant clearance.[395–398,402,453–459] A recently discovered pediatric etiology is MonoMAC syndrome (*GATA2* mutation).[460] It is also associated with monocytopenia, lymphopenia, mycobacterial/fungal infection, myelodysplasia, and myeloid leukemias.[460] Pediatric patients with PAP typically present with slowly progressive dyspnea and nonproductive cough. Because symptoms are often indolent, and even absent in 30% of cases, the diagnosis of PAP may be delayed or missed.[395,461,462]

The various causes of PAP share similar imaging appearances. Chest radiographs usually show symmetric perihilar opacities extending to the lung periphery (Fig. 6.119A). The opacities are usually less consolidative and dense than would be typical of bacterial pneumonia. CT characteristically demonstrates a crazy-paving pattern (Fig. 6.119B), with bilateral ground-glass opacities superimposed on smooth intra- and interlobular septal thickening in polygonal shapes.[395–398,402,453–459]

A definitive diagnosis of PAP can be made by bronchoscopy with bronchoalveolar lavage or transbronchial (or if necessary surgical) biopsy. Repeated whole-lung lavage is the treatment for acquired PAP. Aerosolized GM-CSF therapy may also be useful in autoimmune cases. Acquired PAP generally has a favorable prognosis, whereas congenital PAP is often fatal without lung transplantation.[395–398,402,453–459,461,462]

Langerhans Cell Histiocytosis

Langerhans cell histiocytosis (LCH) is characterized by a clonal proliferation of large dendritic cells (Langerhans cells). Pulmonary LCH in children is rarely isolated without multisystem involvement. In contrast to the adult form, it is

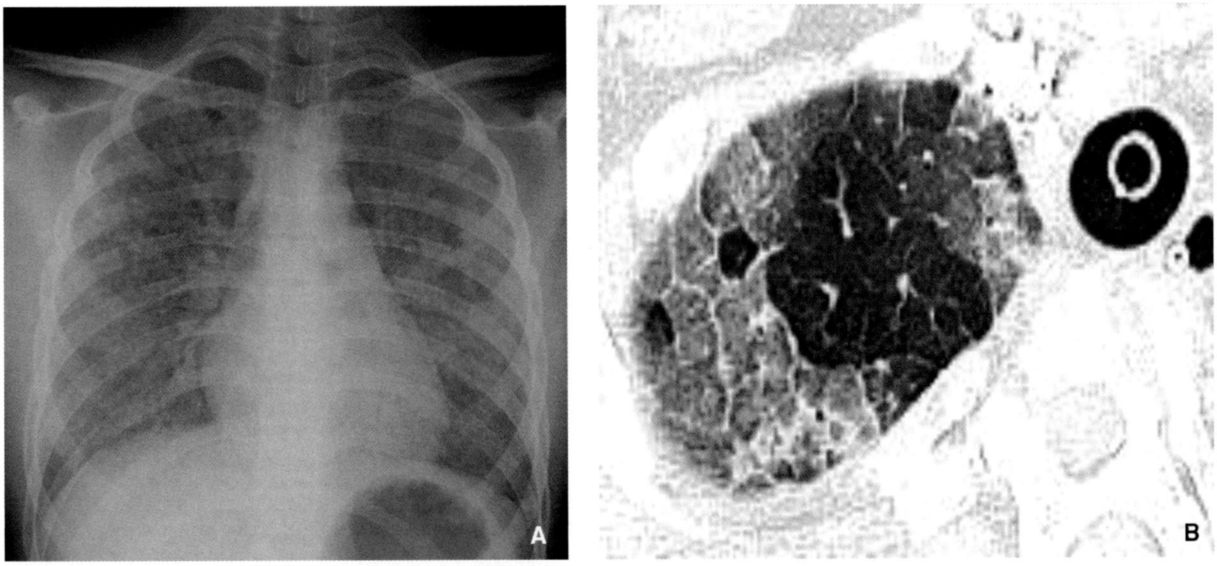

FIGURE 6.119 **Pulmonary alveolar proteinosis (PAP) in a 17-year-old boy who presented with respiratory failure. A:** Frontal chest radiograph shows symmetric and diffuse lung opacification and interstitial thickening in both lungs. **B:** Axial lung window CT image demonstrates a crazy-paving pattern of lungs characterized by a combination of ground-glass opacities with smooth intra- and interlobular septal thickening in polygonal shapes. Also noted are endotracheal tube and nasogastric tube.

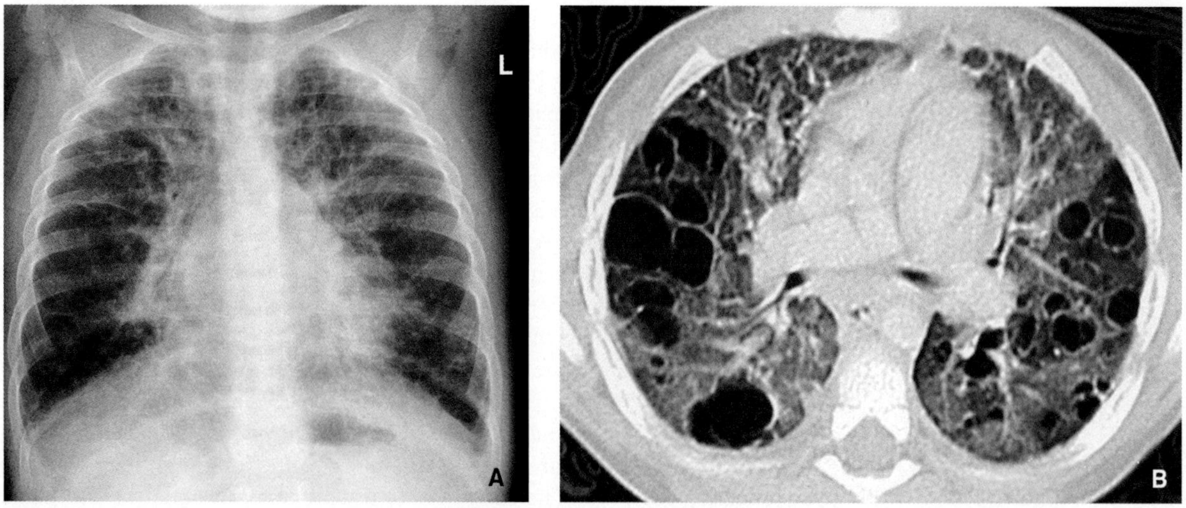

FIGURE 6.120 **Langerhans cell histiocystosis (LCH) in a 3-year-old boy. A:** Frontal chest radiograph shows pulmonary fibrosis characterized by architectural distortion and honeycombing as well as areas of cystic lung changes and small pulmonary nodules. Hyperinflation is also seen. **B:** Axial lung window CT image demonstrates multiple thin-walled cysts in varying size and several small pulmonary nodules.

not associated with smoking. LCH typically affects children between the ages of 1 and 15 with an annual incidence of 1 in 200,000.[395,397,398] Presenting pulmonary complaints are nonspecific such as cough and dyspnea.[395,397,398]

Chest radiographs early in the disease course show indistinct reticulonodular opacities located primarily in the upper lungs. Late-stage findings include architectural distortion and honeycombing characteristic of pulmonary fibrosis (Fig. 6.120A). HRCT is the preferred imaging modality demonstrating characteristic small (<5 mm) nodules in a centrilobular or peribronchiolar distribution involving both lungs. In about a third of patients, the nodules undergo cavitation to form bizarrely shaped thin-walled cysts (Fig. 6.120B), which can rupture and cause spontaneous pneumothorax.[337,395,397,398] Childhood pulmonary LCH, unlike the adult form, does not spare the lung bases near the costophrenic angles.[463,464] Thymic enlargement and intrathymic calcification, cavitation, and cyst formation are additional chest imaging clues to an LCH diagnosis[398] (Fig. 6.121).

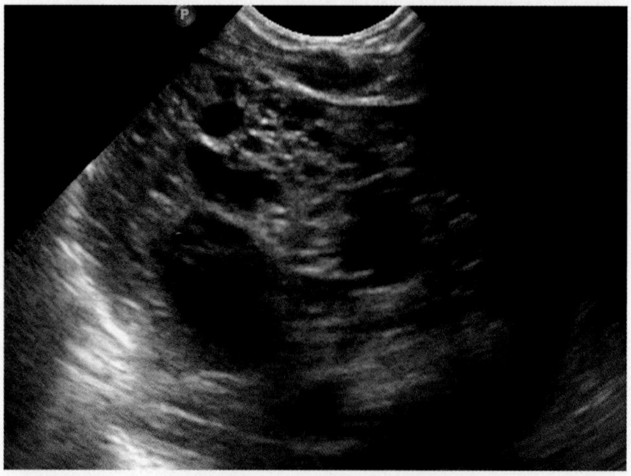

FIGURE 6.121 **Langerhans cell histiocytosis in a 1-week-old girl.** Ultrasound of thymus shows multiple cysts in varying size.

LCH is treated using a variety of combination chemotherapy regimens. Even with successful treatment, pulmonary fibrosis may still ensue because of the effects of cytokines.[397,398,465]

Pulmonary Lymphangiectasia and Lymphangiomatosis

Pulmonary lymphangiectasia and lymphangiomatosis are rare disorders of the pulmonary lymphatics, which normally function to remove lung fluid and protein. In pulmonary lymphangiectasia, there is abnormal dilatation of the lymphatics in pulmonary interstitial and subpleural spaces. It may be congenital (with some associated genetic syndromes) or acquired (because of pulmonary lymphatic or venous obstruction). In pulmonary lymphangiomatosis, there is proliferation of complex lymphatic channels with subsequent lymphatic dilatation. Both disorders may be isolated to the lung or involve other thoracic and/or extrathoracic sites.[395–398,412,466–472] Pediatric patients with congenital lymphangiectasia usually present at birth with marked respiratory distress, tachypnea, and cyanosis. Older surviving children often present with recurrent cough, wheeze, increased respiratory effort, crackles, and sometimes congestive heart failure.[395]

Chest radiographs in affected pediatric patients presenting with classic symptoms of respiratory distress show diffuse hazy bilateral lung opacities similar to those seen in surfactant deficiency disorders. CT demonstrates patchy ground-glass opacities; diffuse, smooth thickening of the interlobular septa and peribronchovascular interstitium; and pleural effusions (often chylous) (Fig. 6.122). In surviving neonates or children presenting later in infancy, greater hyperinflation, less diffuse opacity, and less severe septal thickening are typical. MRI shows T2 hyperintensity of the pulmonary interstitium and pleural effusions. Pulmonary findings are similar in pulmonary lymphangiectasia and lymphangiomatosis. However, lymphangiomatosis presents in late childhood and is more

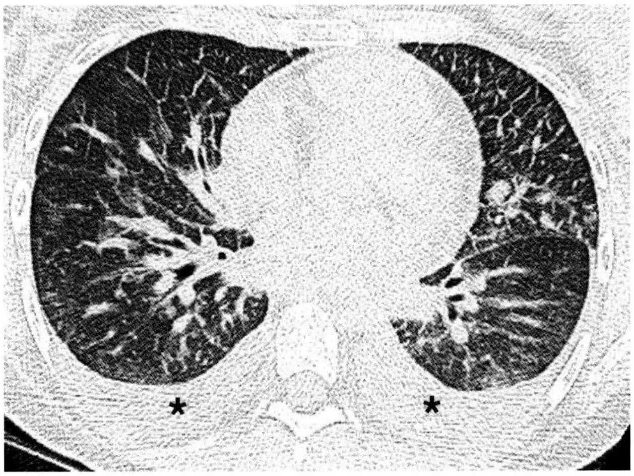

FIGURE 6.122 **Pulmonary lymphangiectasia in a 16-year-old girl.** Axial lung window CT image shows patchy ground-glass opacities, diffuse smooth thickening of the interlobular septa, and peribronchovascular interstitium. Also noted are bilateral pleural effusions (*asterisks*).

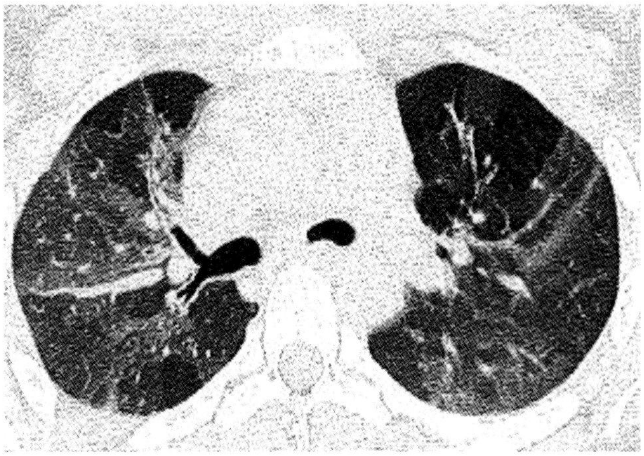

FIGURE 6.123 **Bronchiolitis obliterans (BO) in a 17-year-old girl with graft-versus-host disease.** Axial lung window CT image shows patchy bilateral ground-glass opacities with mosaic attenuation pattern suggesting underlying air trapping.

likely to involve extrapulmonary sites, with mediastinal soft tissue edema and lytic bone lesion.[395–398,412,466–472]

Pediatric patients with congenital lymphangiectasia may be stillborn or die within several hours after birth because of severe lung hypoplasia associated with pleural effusions. Short-term survivors inevitably require pleural drainage and mechanical ventilation. Long-term survivors experience variable respiratory compromise managed with home supplemental oxygen, fluid restriction, dietary measures, and symptomatic support.[395–398,412,466–473]

Bronchiolitis Obliterans

Bronchiolitis obliterans (BO) is characterized by small airway luminal narrowing caused by a fibroblastic reparative response to injury, usually due to a viral infection such as adenovirus or influenza. Other inciting conditions include chronic allograft rejection in lung transplant patients, graft-versus-host disease, and Stevens-Johnson syndrome. Swyer-James-Macleod syndrome is a form of BO affecting predominantly one lung, becoming symptomatic months to years after an initial infection. Unfortunately, there is inconsistent terminology for BO in the literature, often leading to confusion. The clinical manifestation of BO may be termed BO syndrome.[395–398,412,474–479] Pediatric patients with the postinfectious form present acutely with fever and cough similar to an episode of viral bronchiolitis and subsequently develop dyspnea, tachypnea, wheezing, and hypoxemia lasting at least 2 months after the initial lung injury.[395–398,412,474–479]

Chest radiographs in BO most commonly demonstrate hyperinflation but are overall nonspecific and may be normal. Findings on CT include air trapping (more pronounced with expiration), parenchymal hyperlucency, mosaic attenuation, bronchiectasis, bronchial wall thickening, and pulmonary vascular attenuation (Fig. 6.123). The Swyer-James-Macleod variant of BO is characterized radiographically by a hyperlucent lung on the affected side with relatively diminished perfusion and normal or decreased volume; however, CT may show bilateral abnormalities in half of the cases. Hyperlucency combined with pulmonary vascular attenuation is highly specific for moderate/severe nontransplant BO and considered diagnostic when correlating clinical history, and a fixed obstructive pattern on pulmonary function testing (PFT) is present.[395–398,412,474–479]

Follow-up imaging is useful to distinguish normally healing viral bronchiolitis from BO; by several months, imaging findings normalize in typical viral bronchiolitis but persists or worsens in BO. Corticosteroids and azithromycin have shown benefit in treating BO associated with lung transplantation.[395–398,412,474–481]

Hypersensitivity Pneumonitis

Hypersensitivity pneumonitis (also known as extrinsic allergic alveolitis) results from an abnormal pulmonary inflammatory response to an inhalational antigen, such as birds, fungi, or dusts. The acute form presents with flu-like symptoms such as high fever, nonproductive cough, and dyspnea. The subacute and chronic forms lack fever and present with more indolent cough, dyspnea on exertion, and variable anorexia, fatigue, and malaise depending on the duration of exposure.[395–398,402,466,482–486]

Abnormal chest radiographic findings shared by both acute and subacute hypersensitivity include diffuse micronodular interstitial prominence and mid- to lower lung opacities that may resemble pulmonary edema or pneumonia (Fig. 6.124A). However, 40% of radiographs are normal, with underlying abnormalities visible only on CT. HRCT shows small (1 to 3 mm) ill-defined centrilobular nodules (reflecting bronchiolitis), ground-glass opacities (reflecting alveolitis), and air trapping (Fig. 6.124B). The upper lungs are relatively spared. The chronic form is characterized by volume loss and fibrotic changes with irregular reticular opacities, honeycombing, and architectural distortion; findings may be visible by radiography or CT[395–398,402,466,482–486] (Fig. 6.125). The subacute/chronic

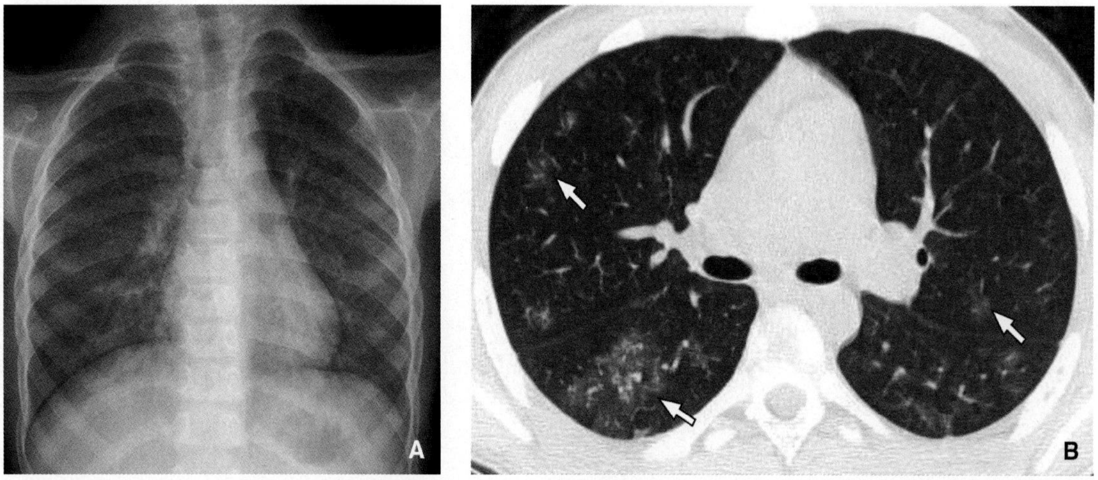

FIGURE 6.124 **Acute hypersensitivity pneumonitis in a 4-year-old boy. A:** Frontal chest radiograph shows diffuse and patchy opacities mainly in the mid- to lower lung zones. **B:** Axial lung window CT image demonstrates small ill-defined centriloblar nodules and patchy ground-glass opacities in both lungs (*arrows*).

form may undergo biopsy, typically showing a mild alveolar septal lymphocytic infiltrate as well as mild chronic airway inflammation, often accompanied by small poorly formed interstitial granulomas and sometimes by fibrosis (Fig. 6.126).

Eliminating exposure to the underlying inciting antigen is the current treatment of choice. Children with the acute form of the disease usually are completely well 24 hours after antigen cessation, and imaging findings in both the acute and subacute forms of the disease eventually regress. In contrast, the fibrotic changes typical of the chronic form persist and may even progress. In these cases, corticosteroids are useful in symptom relief but do not affect long-term outcomes.[395–398,402,466,482–486]

Diffuse Pulmonary Hemorrhage Disorders

The diffuse pulmonary hemorrhage disorders are subdivided according to the presence or absence of capillaritis, an inflammatory disruption of the interstitial capillary network. Disorders with capillaritis include idiopathic pulmonary capillaritis, GPA (formerly known as Wegener granulomatosis), microscopic polyangiitis, Goodpasture syndrome, idiopathic pulmonary–renal syndrome, lupus, and drug-induced capillaritis. Disorders without capillaritis include idiopathic pulmonary hemosiderosis, acute idiopathic pulmonary hemorrhage of infancy, Heiner syndrome (pulmonary disease caused by food sensitivity, usually to cow milk), coagulation disorders, and pulmonary vascular disease such as pulmonary AVMs and pulmonary veno-occlusive disease (PVOD). Many pediatric patients with pulmonary hemorrhage disorders present with iron deficiency anemia rather than frank hemoptysis, which can range from severe and life-threatening

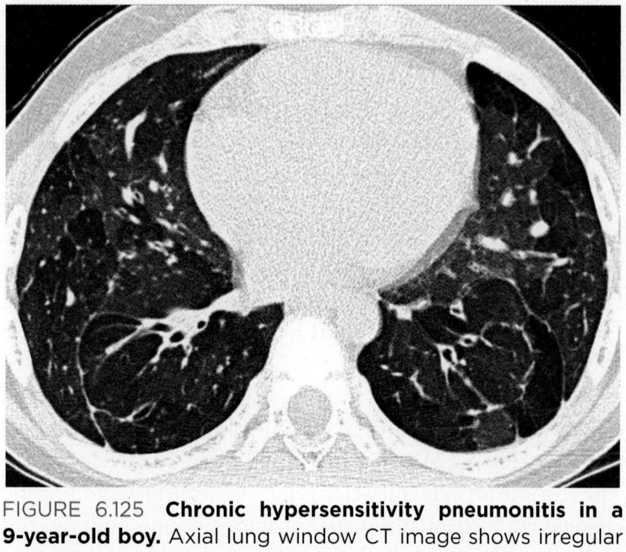

FIGURE 6.125 **Chronic hypersensitivity pneumonitis in a 9-year-old boy.** Axial lung window CT image shows irregular reticular opacities and architectural distortion as well as areas of hyperinflation in both lungs.

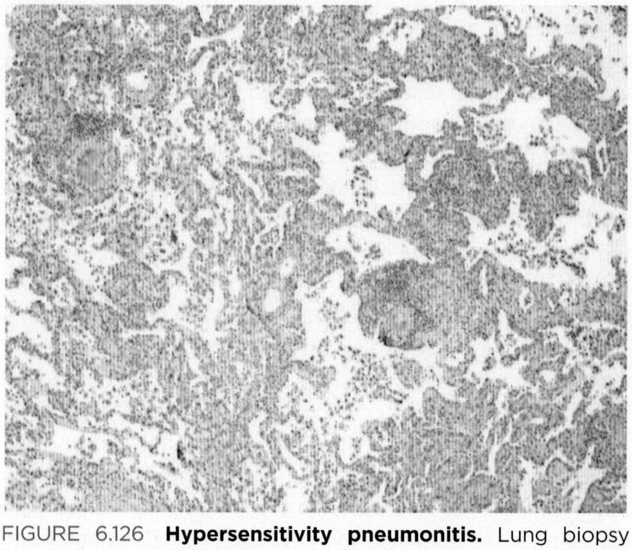

FIGURE 6.126 **Hypersensitivity pneumonitis.** Lung biopsy from a 3-year-old girl with mycobacterium-avium-intracelluare-related hypersensitivity ("hot tub lung") shows areas of hypersensitivity pneumonitis, characterized by a sparse lymphocytic pneumonitis and airway-centered poorly formed granulomas (hematoxylin and eosin, original magnification, 100×).

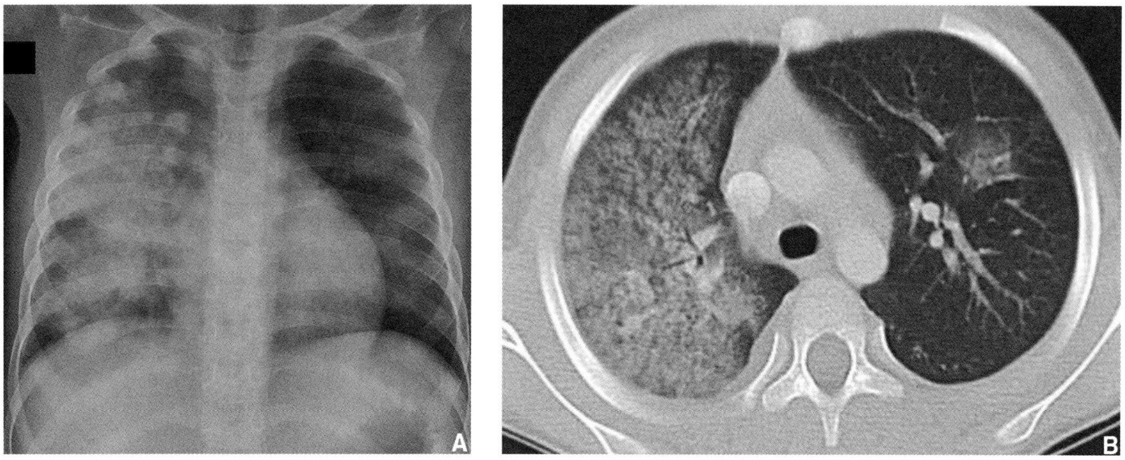

FIGURE 6.127 **Pulmonary hemorrhage in a 4-year-old boy with granulomatosis with polyangiitis. A:** Frontal chest radiograph shows diffuse opacity in the right greater than left lung. **B:** Axial lung window CT image confirms diffuse ground-glass opacity in the right more than left lung.

to minor blood-streaked sputum. Disorders with capillaritis are often accompanied by serologic positivity to ANCA and renal disease.[393,395–398]

Bilateral symmetric airspace opacities in a "butterfly" or "batwing" configuration are the classic radiographic findings in acute diffuse pulmonary hemorrhage. However, the airspace disease may be asymmetric or unilateral (Fig. 6.127A). HRCT, with greater sensitivity, shows patchy ground-glass and/or consolidative opacities in the acute setting (Fig. 6.127B). Repetitive or organizing hemorrhage may lead to interlobular septal thickening, nodular opacities, and even a crazy-paving pattern. Additionally, tiny juxtapleural or parenchymal cysts may be present. Fluffy centrilobular opacities are suggestive of, but not specific for, disorders with capillaritis.[395–398,487–491]

Ultimately, imaging cannot reliably distinguish the various causes of pulmonary hemorrhage. Lung biopsy can contribute to diagnosis; however, the absence of capillaritis in a biopsy sample does not exclude the possibility of healed or unsampled capillaritis. Therefore, careful correlation with serologic and other findings can be helpful to determine whether intensive immunosuppressive therapy may be required. Imaging abnormalities usually recede with proper treatment.[395–398,487–492]

Nonspecific Interstitial Pneumonia

Nonspecific interstitial pneumonia (NSIP) is characterized by a distinct histopathologic appearance consisting of spatially and temporally uniform interstitial lymphoplasmacytic inflammation with variable fibrosis. It may be idiopathic, familial, or secondary to a variety of conditions such as autoimmune connective tissue and collagen vascular diseases, genetic surfactant disorders, and hypersensitivity pneumonitis.[395–398,402,490–496] Common clinical findings include dyspnea and cough and restrictive PFTs.[497]

NSIP is best characterized by HRCT. Typical imaging findings consist of ground-glass and fine linear opacities predominantly at the lung periphery. Over time, volume loss (especially lower lobe), traction bronchiectasis, and honeycombing may develop[395–398,402,493–497] (Fig. 6.128).

Immunosuppressant therapy is often helpful for disorders associated with NSIP. CT findings may persist if there is underlying fibrosis. Lung transplantation may be required in pediatric patients with progressive disease.[395–398,402,493–497]

Connective Tissue and Collagen Vascular Diseases

These heterogeneous rheumatologic diseases, such as systemic lupus erythematosus (SLE) and rheumatoid arthritis (RA), are characterized by chronic inflammation and thought to have an autoimmune basis. Although these entities present with different clinical symptoms, physical exam findings, and serologic results, they share an NSIP (most commonly) on histopathologic analysis. Vasculopathy/vasculitis, pleuritis, pulmonary lymphoid hyperplasia, and chronic and organizing pneumonia (detailed below) may also be present.[395–398,402,493–496,498–500] Complications of immunosuppressive therapy can represent another important category of pulmonary findings in these pediatric patients.

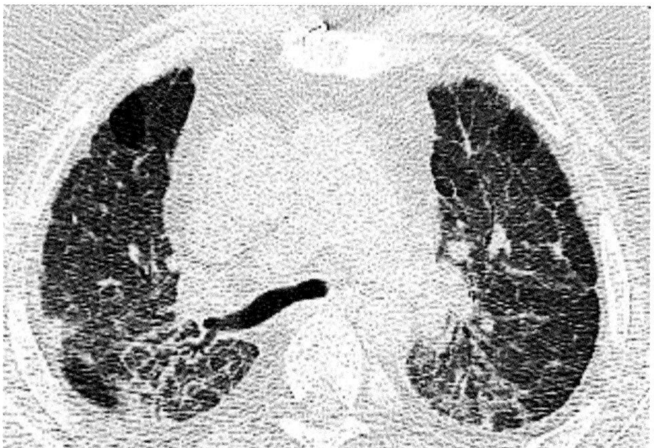

FIGURE 6.128 **Nonspecific interstitial pneumonia (NSIP) in a 17-year-old boy.** Axial lung window CT image shows areas of ground-glass and linear opacities with mild bronchiectasis.

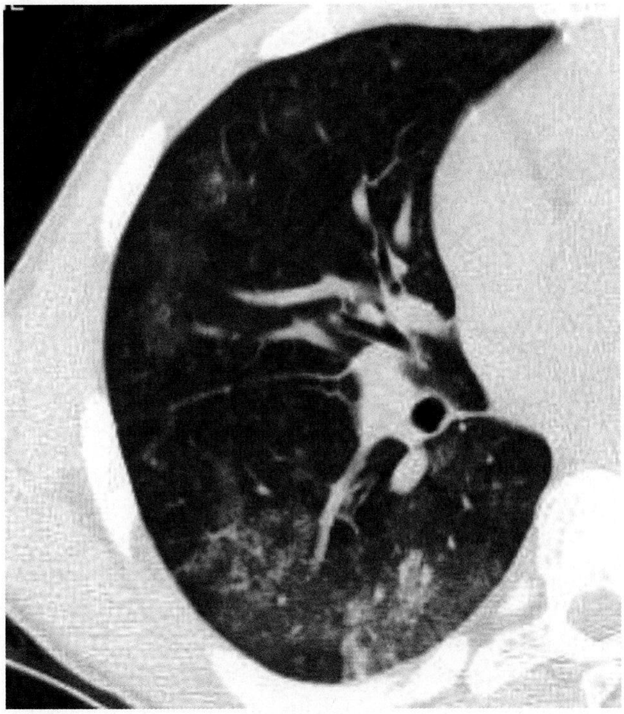

FIGURE 6.129 **Pulmonary hemorrhage in a 16-year-old girl with scleroderma.** Axial lung window CT image shows patchy areas of airspace opacification representing blood products.

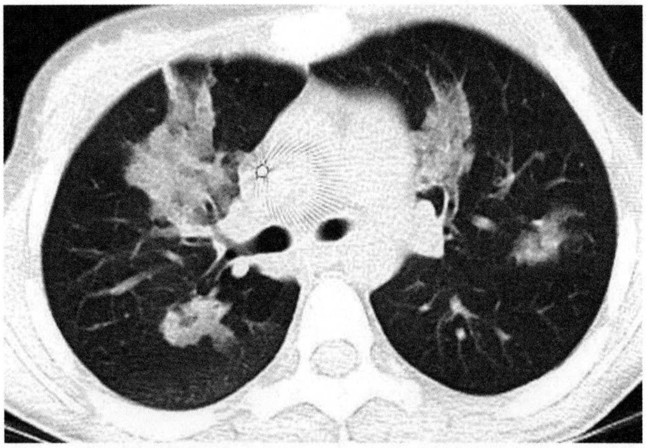

FIGURE 6.130 **Cryptogenic organizing pneumonia (COP) in a 7-year-old boy.** Axial lung window CT image demonstrates multifocal areas of ground-glass and consolidative opacities, some with subtle air bronchograms in both lungs.

Imaging cannot reliably differentiate the various connective tissue diseases, as they share an NSIP imaging pattern (as previously described). Ancillary findings such as a dilated esophagus in scleroderma may allow a definitive diagnosis. Unlike adult SLE, the childhood form tends to present with pulmonary hemorrhage and vasculitis rather than interstitial lung disease[395–398,402,493–496,498–500] (Fig. 6.129).

For most disorders, immunosuppressive therapy is the treatment of choice. Imaging findings may recede with clinical improvement; however, fibrosis is irreversible. Ongoing research focuses on targeting specific genes involved in inflammatory pathways.[395–398,402,493–496,498–500]

Organizing Pneumonia

On a histologic level, organizing pneumonia is characterized by organizing fibrosis in the alveoli and distal airways, including the bronchioles and alveolar ducts. When idiopathic, it is termed cryptogenic organizing pneumonia (COP). Organizing pneumonia may be secondary to conditions that stimulate a lung reparative response, such as healing infectious pneumonia, drug reaction, aspiration injury, autoimmune disease, and BMT. Currently, use of the term bronchiolitis obliterans organizing pneumonia (BOOP) has fallen out of favor because of potential confusion with BO, a distinct disorder (described previously).[395–398,501–503] Children with organizing pneumonia generally present with subacute dyspnea, cough, and fever, however, symptoms are variable.[504]

Although organizing pneumonia does not have a pathognomonic imaging appearance, CT usually shows peripheral patchy consolidation, often with internal air bronchograms and areas of mild bronchial dilatation (Fig. 6.130). Ground-glass opacity may surround the consolidated areas. Other findings may include the atoll or reverse halo sign (central ground-glass opacity surrounded by consolidation), small pulmonary nodules in a bronchovascular distribution, perilobular thickening, linear and band-like subpleural opacities, and progressive fibrosis.[395–398,501–503]

Corticosteroids are the current treatment of choice for most cases of organizing pneumonia, regardless of the underlying cause. Up to 80% cure rate is reported. Imaging findings reflecting inflammation recede with treatment, whereas fibrotic changes remain or even progress.[395–398,477,501–503]

Pulmonary Infiltrate with Eosinophilia

A variety of eosinophilic lung diseases exist, all characterized by peripheral or tissue eosinophilia and interstitial and intra-alveolar eosinophils on pathology. There are three main subtypes: eosinophilic disease of known cause, eosinophilic disease of unknown cause, and eosinophilic vasculitis. Diseases of known cause include ABPA (Fig. 6.131), bronchocentric granulomatosis (BG), drug reactions, and fungal and parasitic infections. Diseases of unknown cause include acute eosinophilic pneumonia (AEP) (Fig. 6.132), chronic eosinophilic pneumonia (CEP) (Figs. 6.133 and 6.134), simple pulmonary eosinophilia (SPE or Loffler syndrome), and idiopathic hypereosinophilic syndrome (IHS). The primary eosinophilic vasculitis is allergic angiitis and granulomatosis (CSS).[395–398,505–508] AEP presents with acute febrile illness and hypoxemia and is more common in adolescents than in young children. CEP presents with chronic, progressive respiratory and systemic symptoms and is more often seen in older children or adult patients with asthma than in pediatric patients.[395]

Imaging features of the eosinophilic lung diseases are usually nondiagnostic, consisting of nonspecific interstitial and/or alveolar opacities. However, certain imaging appearances are characteristic of specific disorders. For example, radiographs in AEP show bilateral reticular opacities that may be accompanied by consolidation and pleural effusion.

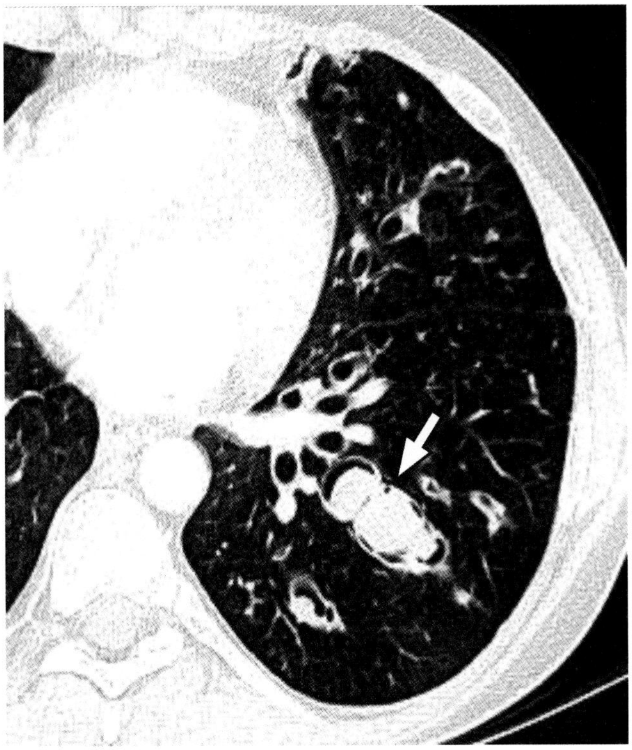

FIGURE 6.131 **ABPA in a 13-year-old boy with known cystic fibrosis.** Axial lung window CT image shows mucoid impaction of the dilated bronchus known as the "finger-in-glove" sign (*arrow*). Also seen are bronchiectatic lung changes in other areas of left lung.

CT demonstrates bilateral patchy ground-glass opacities, commonly with areas of consolidation, interlobular septal thickening, and/or ill-defined nodules (Fig. 6.132). These features overlap with more common diseases such as pulmonary edema and acute respiratory distress syndrome (ARDS), potentially leading to delayed diagnosis. Peripheral consolidation with sparing of the central lung zones ("photographic negative" or "reversed" pulmonary edema pattern) is highly specific for the diagnosis of CEP or drug-induced PIE when peripheral eosinophilia is also present (Figs. 6.133 and 6.134). SPE and IHS characteristically show pulmonary nodules with ground-glass halos. ABPA demonstrates central bronchiectasis; concurrent mucoid impaction of the large airways may be present, creating an appearance known as the "finger-in-glove" sign (Fig. 6.131). BG shows focal nodules and masses or lobar atelectasis and consolidation. Findings in

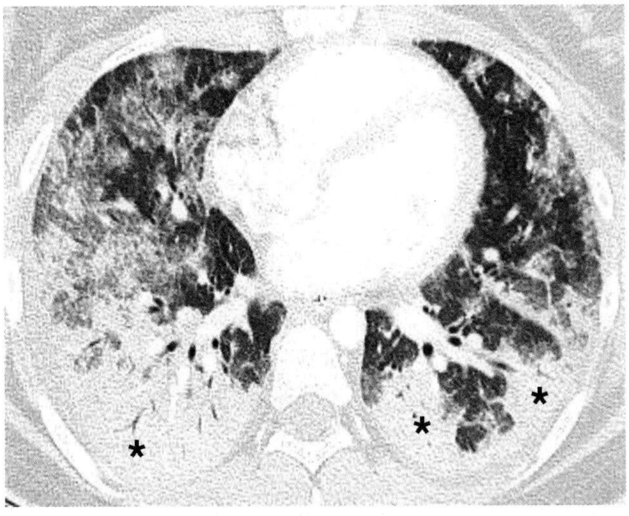

FIGURE 6.132 **Acute eosinophilic pneumonia in a 15-year-old girl who presented with fever and hypoxemic respiratory failure.** Markedly elevated numbers of eosinophils in bronchoalveolar lavage fluid were identified. Axial lung window CT image shows bilateral patchy ground-glass opacities with areas of consolidation (*asterisks*) and several small nodules.

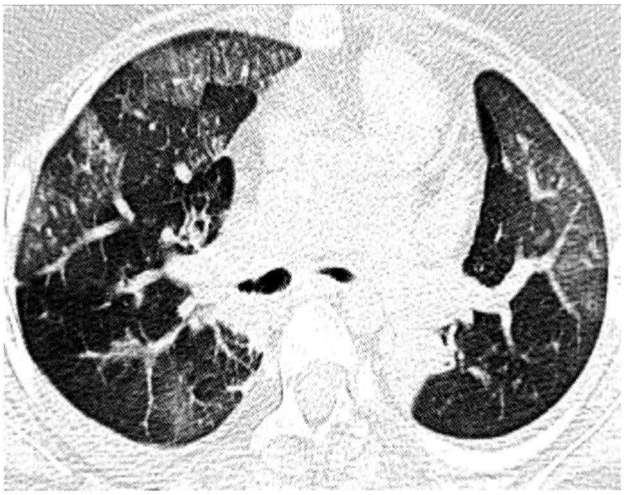

FIGURE 6.133 **Chronic eosinophilic pneumonia in a 10-year-old boy with asthma who presented with dry cough, shortness of breath, and malaise.** Elevated numbers of eosinophils in bronchoalveolar lavage fluid and in peripheral blood were identified. Axial lung window CT image shows peripheral ground-glass opacification and consolidation known as "photographic negative" or "reversed" pulmonary edema pattern.

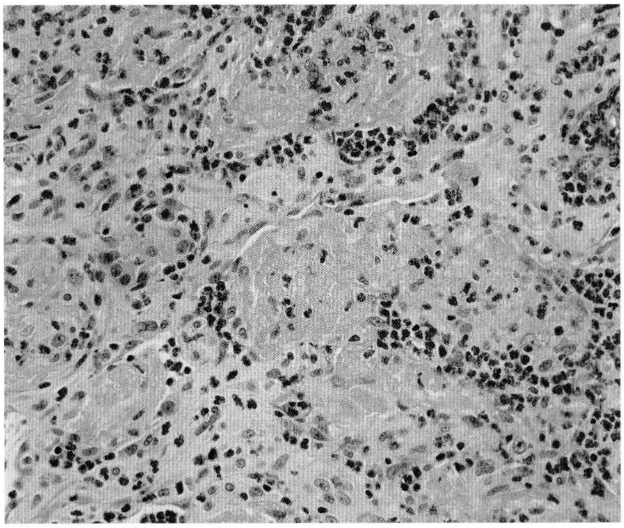

FIGURE 6.134 **Eosinophilic pneumonia.** Photomicrograph demonstrates numerous eosinophils within alveolar septa and organizing fibrin-rich airspace exudate (hematoxylin and eosin, original magnification, 400×).

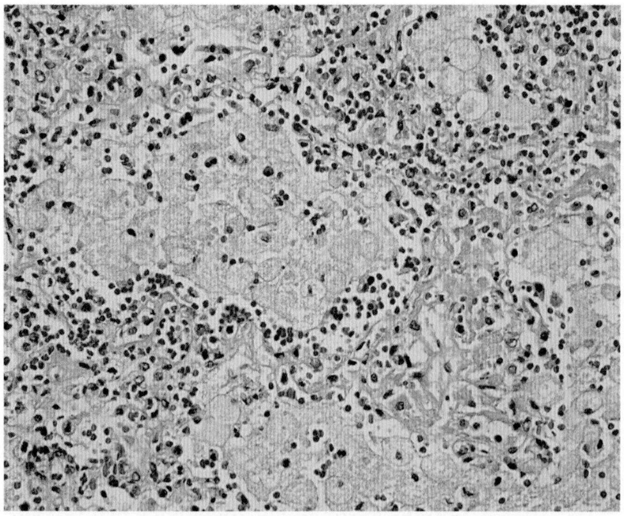

FIGURE 6.135 **Niemann-Pick disease.** Photomicrograph demonstrates macrophages filling the alveolar spaces (hematoxylin and eosin, original magnification, 400×).

Churg-Strauss include interlobular septal thickening, centrilobular nodules, subpleural consolidation, and bronchial wall thickening.[395–398,505–508]

Although imaging may not allow for specific diagnosis, it can still help localize targets for potential lung biopsy. Corticosteroids are the most effective treatment and generally result in rapid and complete clinical response. CEP, unlike AEP, may recur once steroids are discontinued. Treatments for specific eosinophilic diseases should be tailored to the underlying etiology, such as antiparasitic medication for parasite-induced eosinophilic lung disease.[395–398,505–508]

Storage Diseases

The lysosomal storage diseases are genetic metabolic disorders that result in impaired lysosomal function. In Gaucher disease and Niemann-Pick disease, lipid-laden "foamy" macrophages (Gaucher cells or Niemann-Pick cells, respectively) build up in tissues and may infiltrate the lung, causing respiratory symptoms (Fig. 6.135). Gaucher disease is the most common lysosomal storage disorder. Symptomatic pulmonary involvement in Gaucher disease is rare and if it occurs tends to be late in the disease course; it is more common in the type III neuronopathic form.[396–398,509–512]

Imaging findings indicating pulmonary involvement of Gaucher disease are nonspecific. Chest radiographs may demonstrate reticulonodular opacities. CT may show ground-glass opacities, consolidation, bronchial wall thickening, interstitial thickening, lymphadenopathy, and thymic enlargement. Pulmonary involvement in Niemann-Pick disease tends to progress from caudal to cranial. Diffuse interstitial thickening is typical of the type B form (Fig. 6.136), whereas a crazy-paving pattern is characteristic of the type C2 form.[396–398,509–512]

Targeted enzyme replacement therapy, approved by the U.S. Food and Drug Administration (FDA), is available for several of the lysosomal storage diseases. The imaging findings in pulmonary Gaucher disease gradually improve with treatment, although complete normalization is generally not achieved. Chest radiographs are currently recommended every 2 years in Gaucher disease to monitor for lung involvement.[396–398,509–512]

Chronic Granulomatous Disease

Chronic granulomatous disease (CGD) is a rare hereditary immunodeficiency disorder due to a mutation in one of the four genes encoding subunits of the phagocyte nicotinamide adenine dinucleotide phosphate (NADPH). The mutation results in dysfunctional phagocyte NADPH oxidase activity, leading to impaired mechanisms for fighting intracellular catalase-positive bacteria as well as fungi. The disease occurs in ~1 in 200,000 to 250,000 children born in the United States, with a male to female ratio that is 3:1.[395–397,513–515] CGD

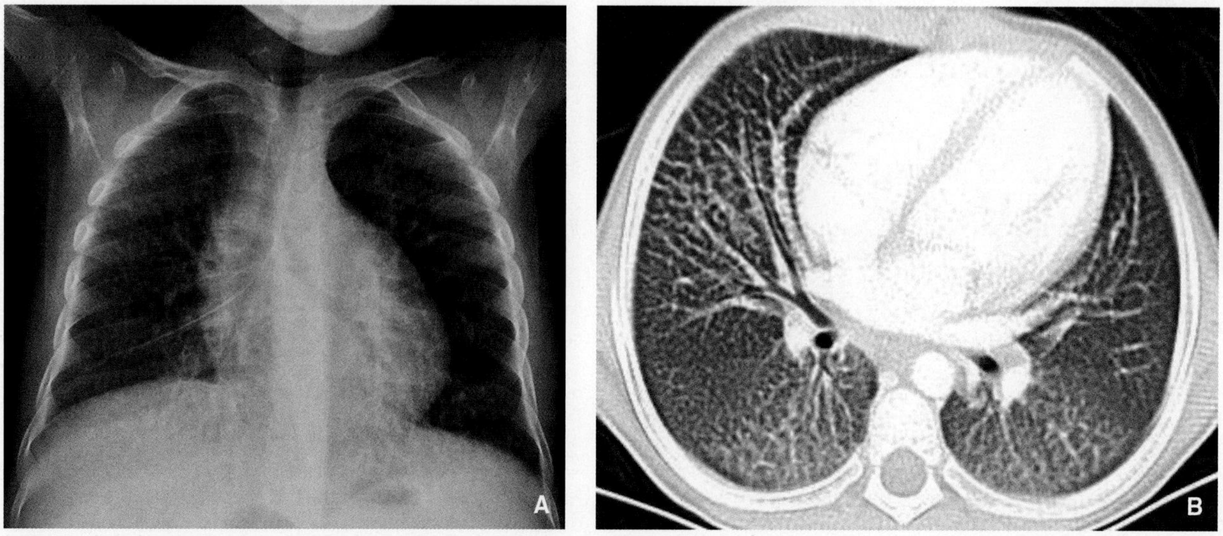

FIGURE 6.136 **Niemann-Pick disease in a 14-year-old boy.** Frontal chest radiograph **(A)** and axial lung window CT image **(B)** show diffuse bilateral interstitial thickening.

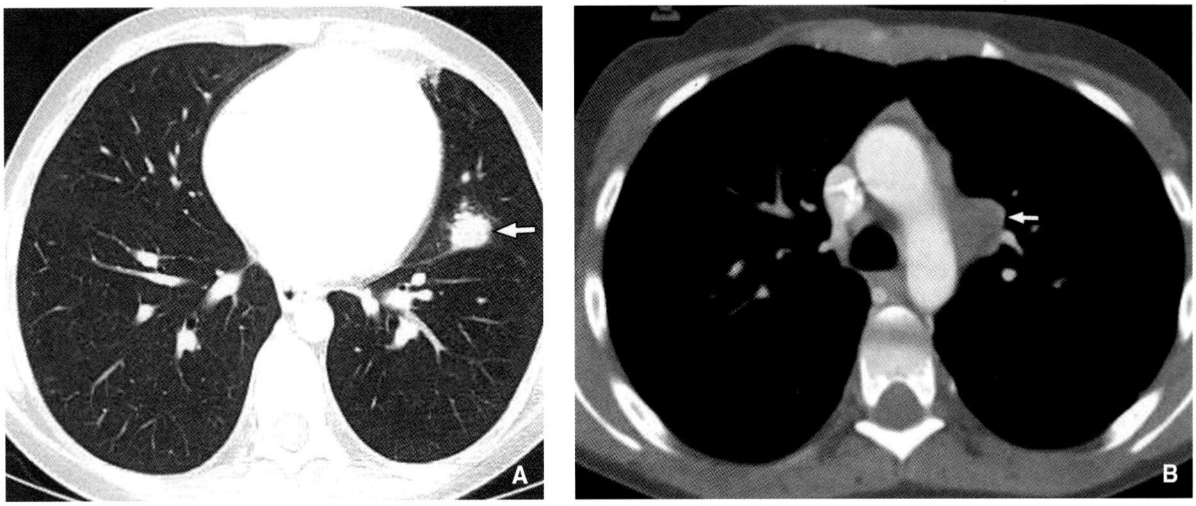

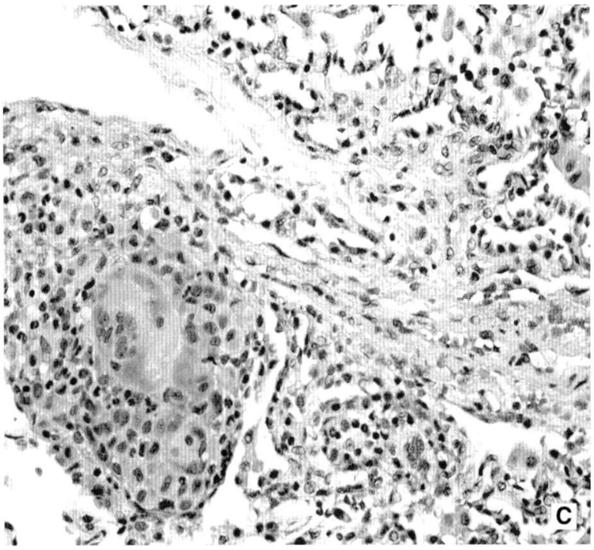

FIGURE 6.137 **Chronic granulomatous disease (CGD) in a 17-year-old boy. A:** Axial lung window CT image shows an irregular area of lingular consolidation (*arrow*) abutting the left major fissure with hazy surrounding ground-glass attenuation. **B:** Axial enhanced CT image demonstrates prevascular mediastinal lymphadenopathy (*arrow*). **C:** Photomicrograph in a 3-year-old boy (different patient) with CGD and a history of various fungal infections shows a small granuloma (hematoxylin and eosin, original magnification, 400×).

is typically inherited in an X-linked fashion in boys, whereas it may be autosomal recessive or X-linked (skewed lyonization) in girls. Affected children typically present by age 2 with recurrent infections; pulmonary involvement is most common, followed by skin and gastrointestinal tract and then liver and bone.[395–397,513–515]

Imaging findings in pediatric patients with CGD are variable. Acute findings may include ground-glass opacities, consolidation, tree-in-bud opacities, and centrilobular, random, and/or miliary nodules (Figs. 6.137 and 6.138). Chronic findings may include air trapping, septal thickening, bronchiectasis, abscess formation, cysts, fibrosis, and honeycombing. Mediastinal and/or hilar lymphadenopathy, pleural thickening, empyema, rib or vertebral osteomyelitis, and chest wall invasion are also common[395–397,513–515] (Fig. 6.137B).

A variety of methods are used to treat CGD, including lipophilic antibiotics, antifungals, interferon-γ, abscess drainage, surgical resection, and stem cell transplantation. Prophylactic antibiotics are efficacious. With improved treatments, children with CGD now may survive into adulthood.[395–397,513–515]

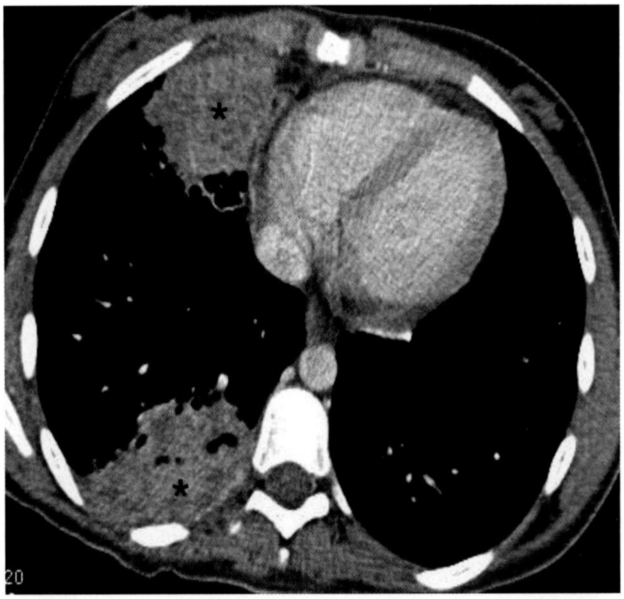

FIGURE 6.138 **Chronic granulomatous disease in a 16-year-old girl.** Axial enhanced CT image shows areas of consolidations (*asterisks*).

Cystic Fibrosis

Inherited in an autosomal recessive fashion, CF is the most common genetic disorder causing chronic pulmonary disease in children, occurring in 1 in 2,500 white live births.[395,507,516–518] It results from mutations in the cystic fibrosis transmembrane regulator (CFTR) gene. Affected children are more commonly of European descent and tend to present at infancy with chronic recurrent pulmonary infections or with nonpulmonary manifestations such as meconium ileus, failure to thrive, or malabsorption. Definitive diagnosis may be made via a sweat test and/or direct genetic panel.[395,507,516–518]

Chest imaging early in the course of CF may be normal or demonstrate mild-to-moderate air trapping and/or bronchiectasis. Later-stage findings include upper lobe predominant bronchiectasis, bronchial wall thickening, centrilobular and tree-in-bud opacities, and mucus plugging with air trapping. Mucoid impaction may produce a finger-in-glove pattern similar to that observed in ABPA. Mediastinal and hilar lymphadenopathy may develop because of chronic/recurrent infections. CT is more sensitive than PFTs for detecting mild or localized lung disease (Fig. 6.139). Although primarily limited to research settings, radiographic and CT scoring systems are available for assessing the extent and severity of CF and can be used as surrogate endpoints in clinical studies.[395,516–518] MRI is currently now fully proven to be useful for evaluating pediatric patients with CF. However, with recently developed high-resolution and fast imaging sequences, MRI, which is not associated with ionizing radiation exposure, may play an important role in evaluation of pediatric patients with CF who often require repetitive imaging assessment.

CF treatment to date has focused on managing and preventing the sequelae of the disease in the pediatric population. Standard therapies include oral azithromycin, inhaled tobramycin, and additional antibiotics as needed depending on the type of infections present and resistance pattern. Hypertonic saline and dornase alfa (Pulmozyme), which

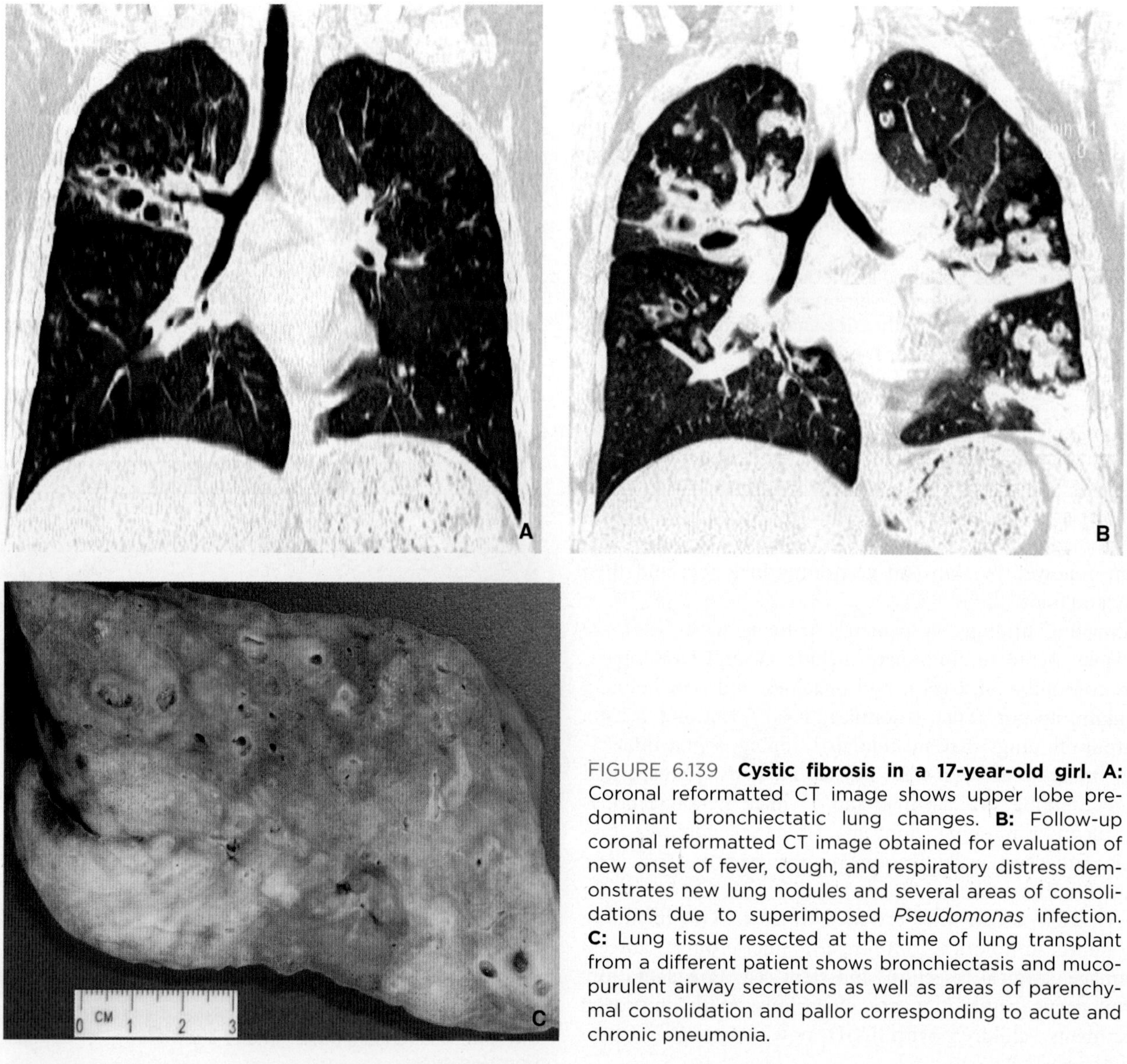

FIGURE 6.139 **Cystic fibrosis in a 17-year-old girl. A:** Coronal reformatted CT image shows upper lobe predominant bronchiectatic lung changes. **B:** Follow-up coronal reformatted CT image obtained for evaluation of new onset of fever, cough, and respiratory distress demonstrates new lung nodules and several areas of consolidations due to superimposed *Pseudomonas* infection. **C:** Lung tissue resected at the time of lung transplant from a different patient shows bronchiectasis and mucopurulent airway secretions as well as areas of parenchymal consolidation and pallor corresponding to acute and chronic pneumonia.

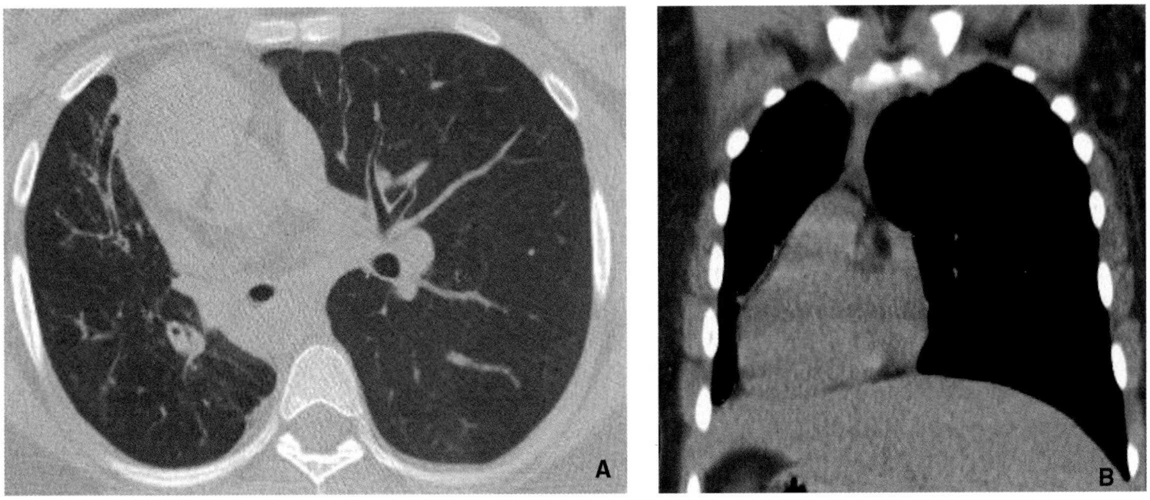

FIGURE 6.140 **Immotile cilia syndrome in a 7-year-old boy. A:** Axial lung window CT image shows bronchiectasis, peribronchial thickening, and mucus plugging in the small right lung. The left lung is hyperinflated with areas of mild mosaic ground-glass attenuation suggestive of air-trapping. **B:** Coronal reformatted CT image demonstrates situs inversus with a left-sided liver, right-sided stomach, and right-sided cardiac apex.

functions to break down thick secretions, are also efficacious and routinely used. Additionally, in 2012, the novel small molecule ivacaftor (Kalydeco) received FDA approval for CF in patients with at least one *G551D* mutation.[519] Despite these advances, lung transplantation is a common end resort.

Immotile Cilia Syndrome

Also known as primary ciliary dyskinesia (PCD), immotile cilia syndrome is an autosomal recessive genetic disorder characterized by impaired ciliary function, leading to chronic lung, sinus, and middle ear disease. The prevalence is ~1/12,000 to 1/60,000. Situs inversus occurs in 50% of cases on a random basis.[337,520–523] Affected pediatric patients usually present with chronic respiratory tract infections in early childhood and eventual chronic bronchitis, rhinosinusitis, otitis, and male infertility. The triad of situs inversus, bronchiectasis, and sinusitis is known as Kartagener syndrome, seen in half of PCD cases.[337,520–523] Polysplenia and pectus exacavtum occur in 8% of affected patients.[337]

Chest radiographs and CT show regional consolidation corresponding to areas of acute infection. Other common findings include peribronchial thickening, mucus plugging, bronchiectasis, ground-glass opacity, and air trapping. Small pulmonary nodules in a tree-in-bud pattern may also present. Unlike CF, which demonstrates upper lobe predominance, PCD tends to affect the middle lobe, lingula, and lower lobes. In fact, middle lobe bronchiectasis in a child is very suggestive of ciliary dyskinesia[337,520–522] (Fig. 6.140).

The subset of PCD patients with evident structural ciliary abnormalities can be diagnosed by electron microscopic examination of ciliated tissue from the nasopharynx or airways. Genetic testing for known gene abnormalities in ciliary dysfunction is an emerging field. No specific treatment currently exists for PCD. Management is currently focused on treating infections, improving or maintaining lung function, promoting mucus clearance, and preventing chronic damage to the lung.[523]

Disorders Masquerading as Diffuse Lung Disease

These disorders have similar clinical presentations to the diffuse lung diseases but are conceptually distinct with substantial differences in management. They are primarily vascular in nature and often best assessed with CT angiography.[395] Pulmonary edema and pulmonary arterial hypertensive (PAH) vasculopathy are key entities included in this category.

Cardiogenic and Noncardiogenic Pulmonary Edema

Pulmonary edema is caused by an excess of fluid within lung tissues, due to either cardiogenic or noncardiogenic causes (Fig. 6.141). Affected pediatric patients present with variable dyspnea, hypoxia, and hyperhidrosis depending on the severity of pulmonary edema.[395]

Imaging findings reflect the severity of disease, beginning with pulmonary vascular redistribution (only with upright positioning), followed by interstitial, and then alveolar edema. Radiographs in milder disease show vascular redistribution, haziness of the vascular and bronchial walls, thickening of the pleural fissures, and Kerley B lines (thickening of the interlobular septa with thin, nonbranching lines abutting the pleura) (Fig. 6.141). Radiographs in severe disease demonstrate alveolar opacities and air bronchograms with poorly defined borders. CT shows ground-glass opacities, fissural thickening, smooth interlobular septal thickening, and often pleural effusions (Fig. 6.142). Cardiogenic pulmonary edema is often accompanied by left atrial and ventricular enlargement.[395]

Definitive treatment of pulmonary edema depends on the underlying cause. Supportive measures such as diuretics, supplemental oxygen, and if needed mechanical ventilation are often utilized. In neurogenic pulmonary edema, treating the underlying brain insult helps prevent secondary insults but has not been proven to improve pulmonary function.[524]

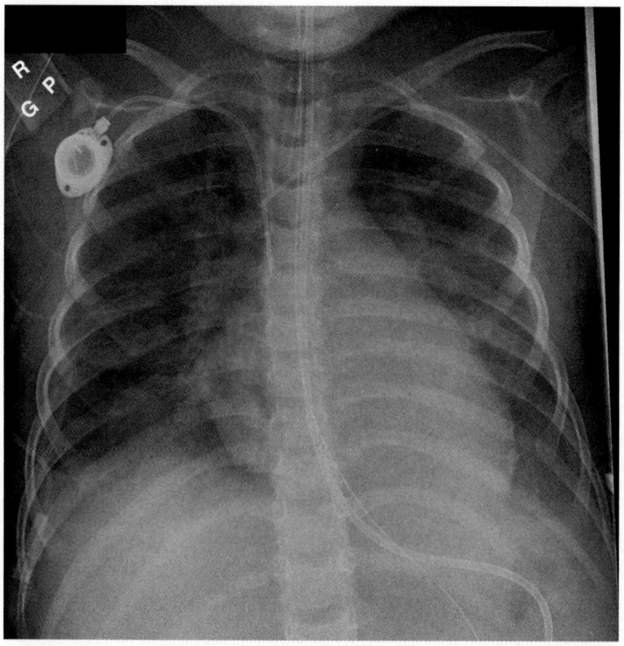

FIGURE 6.141 **Pulmonary edema in a 6-year-old boy with renal failure.** Frontal chest radiograph shows cardiomegaly, bilateral pleural effusions, and indistinctness of the pulmonary vasculature consistent with interstitial edema. Retrocardiac opacity, left greater than right, is compatible with superimposed atelectasis or consolidation. Also noted are supporting lines and tubes.

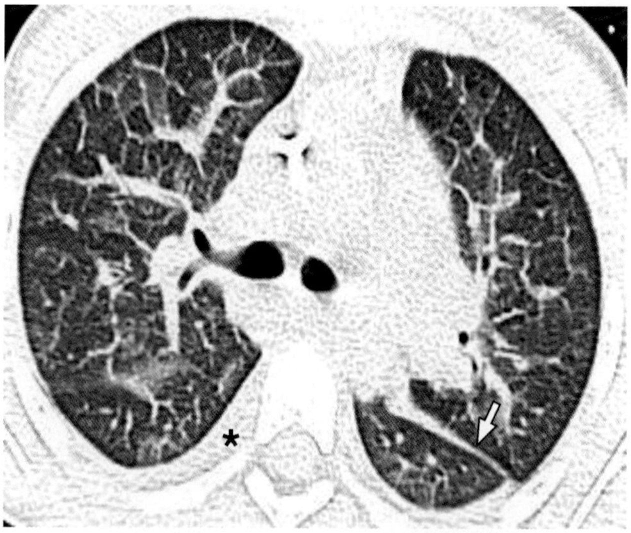

FIGURE 6.142 **Pulmonary edema in a 6-year-old girl with head injury after motor vehicle accident.** Axial lung window CT image shows bilateral ground-glass opacities, smooth interlobular septal thickening, fissural thickening (*arrow*), and pleural effusion (*asterisk*).

Pulmonary Arterial Hypertensive Vasculopathy

PAH is defined as a mean pulmonary artery pressure >25 mm Hg at rest or >30 mm Hg during exertion with increased pulmonary vascular resistance. It may be idiopathic or occur in association with parenchymal lung disease, thromboembolic disease, liver disease, pulmonary venous disease, and/or cardiac disease such as left-to-right shunts.[395] Only 10% of PAH cases occur in children, with a 2:1 female predominance. If not idiopathic or familial, it usually is secondary to congenital heart disease. Affected pediatric patients present with dyspnea, chest pain, fatigue, and syncope. Symptoms are often exacerbated by exertion.[525]

Imaging findings in PAH include enlargement of the central pulmonary arteries, abrupt tapering or narrowing of peripheral pulmonary arteries, dilated bronchial arteries (Fig. 6.143A). A mosaic attenuation of the lungs reflecting variable lung perfusion may be present (Fig. 6.143B). This pattern may be confused with interstitial lung disease; however, additional features such as right ventricular and atrial enlargement and right ventricular hypertrophy, along with correlating clinical history, help solidify the diagnosis of PAH.[395]

Treatment for PAH is tailored to the severity of functional impairment. Conventional agents include calcium channel blockers and prostanoid analogs. Newer endothelin

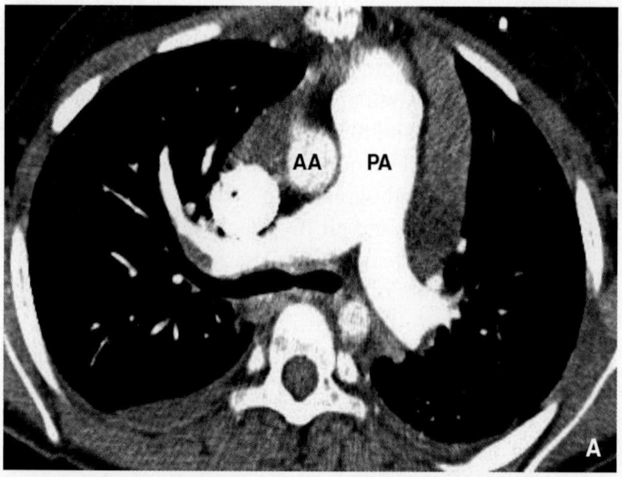

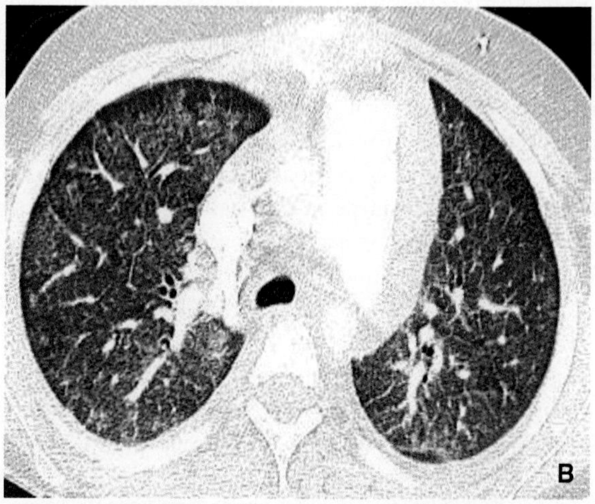

FIGURE 6.143 **Pulmonary artery hypertension in a 12-year-old girl who presented with dyspnea and chest pain. A:** Axial enhanced CT image shows dilation of the central pulmonary arteries (*PA*), which are larger than adjacent ascending aorta (*AA*). **B:** Axial lung window CT image demonstrates a mosaic attenuation of the lungs due to variable underlying lung perfusion.

antagonists and phosphodiesterase-V inhibitors such as sildenafil appear beneficial and are increasingly being used.[525]

Catheters and Tubes

A hospitalized child, particularly those in the neonatal intensive care unit (NICU) and the pediatric intensive care unit (PICU), often undergoes several medical interventions and therapies requiring various catheter or tube placement. Such catheters include venous catheters necessary for hydration, nutrition, and intravenous drug therapy, as well as arterial catheters used for laboratory sampling and arterial oxygen or blood pressure monitoring. Other nonvascular tubes including ETT for ventilation and enteric tubes for either nutritional support or decompression are also frequently encountered.

One of the important purposes of obtaining a chest and/or abdomen radiograph is to confirm the location of these tubes and catheters. Proper attention to technique should be given to accurately identify these catheters and tubes in their entirety. Early recognition of malposition is crucial for avoiding serious complications. Therefore, it is important to understand the indication, correct position, as well as the potential complications that may arise from the placement of theses catheters and tubes.

Umbilical Arterial Catheter

Placement of the umbilical arterial catheter is indicated for blood gas or laboratory sample analysis, arterial oxygen level or continuous blood pressure monitoring, exchange transfusions, cardiac catheterization, and infusion of medications.[526]

The catheter pathway is through either one of the two umbilical arteries, into the internal iliac artery, to the common iliac artery and into the abdominal aorta[526,527] (Fig. 6.144). The optimal position could be either a "*high*" or "*low*" line depending on the exact location of the catheter tip in relation to the visceral arteries. The high line has its final tip position between T7–T9 vertebral bodies (Fig. 6.145A), above the celiac axis, whereas the low line has its tip between L3–L5 vertebral bodies, below the renal arteries[375,526] (Fig. 6.145B). On the frontal radiograph, a characteristic inferior curve is seen as the catheter enters the umbilical artery and into the internal iliac artery, then it takes a superior curve as it enters and ascends into the aorta. On the lateral radiograph, the catheter demonstrates the typical downward curve in the pelvic region before it ascends superiorly into the aorta, just anterior to the vertebral bodies (Fig. 6.145C). Most neonatologists prefer high lines because of decreased incidence of complications.[526,528]

An umbilical artery catheter may be malpositioned in the subclavian artery, celiac axis, inferior gluteal artery, and renal artery. Complications from UAC may include intracranial hemorrhage, vasospasm, or arterial thrombosis leading to ischemia and other perfusion abnormalities, arterial damage, and infections. The catheter can also fragment or break causing leaks and extravasations. The reported incidence of necrotizing enterocolitis associated with UAC placement is 3.9% with high catheter position and 2.9% with low catheter position.[528]

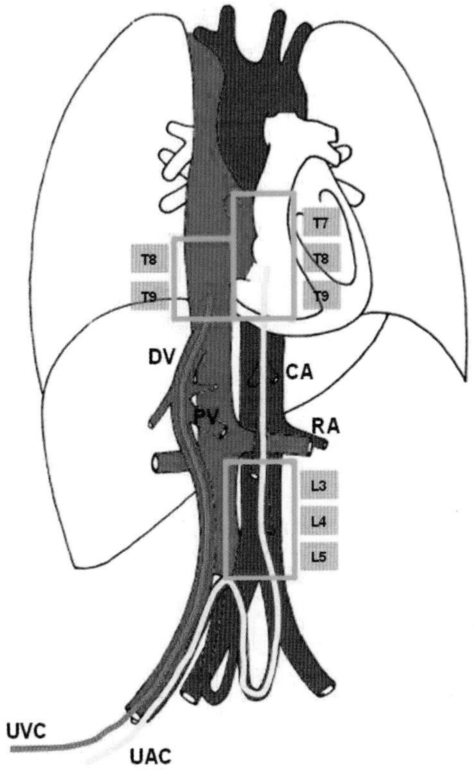

FIGURE 6.144 **Diagram showing the normal course and optimal termination (green boxes) of the umbilical arterial catheter (*UAC*) and umbilical venous catheter (*UVC*).** *CA*, celiac artery; *DV*, ductus venosus; *PV*, portal vein; *RA*, renal artery.

Umbilical Venous Catheter

The common indications for umbilical venous catheter (UVC) placement includes infusion of hypertonic fluid solutions and fluid resuscitation, access for medication or nutrition, central venous pressure monitoring, and exchange transfusion. Its use has been increasing because of low birth weight infants, more aggressive therapy, and increasing heparin use.

The path of the catheter is from the umbilical vein to the left portal vein, then to the middle or left hepatic vein via the ductus venosus, and into the inferior vena cava (IVC).[526,527] The optimum tip position for the UVC is at the junction of the IVC and right atrium, at T8–T9 vertebral level[526,529] (Fig. 6.144). On the frontal radiograph, the catheter runs cephalad within the umbilical vein and slightly curves to the right as it enters the liver via the portal vein and then makes a subtle curve to the left as it enters the ductus venosus and into the hepatic vein, before it enters the IVC (Fig. 6.146A). On the lateral view, the venous catheter ascends anteriorly into the umbilical vein and then takes a posterior curve, traversing the liver and ascends into the IVC (Fig. 6.146B).

Mechanical complications or occlusions are common complication of UVC placement, with an incidence of 41%.[530] The catheter could be malpositioned within the liver parenchyma (Fig. 6.147A), which may lead to portal vein thrombosis and potential portal hypertension,[526] hepatic hematoma,[529] or even erosion of the catheter into the liver parenchyma.[531] The catheter can also be malpositioned in the superior

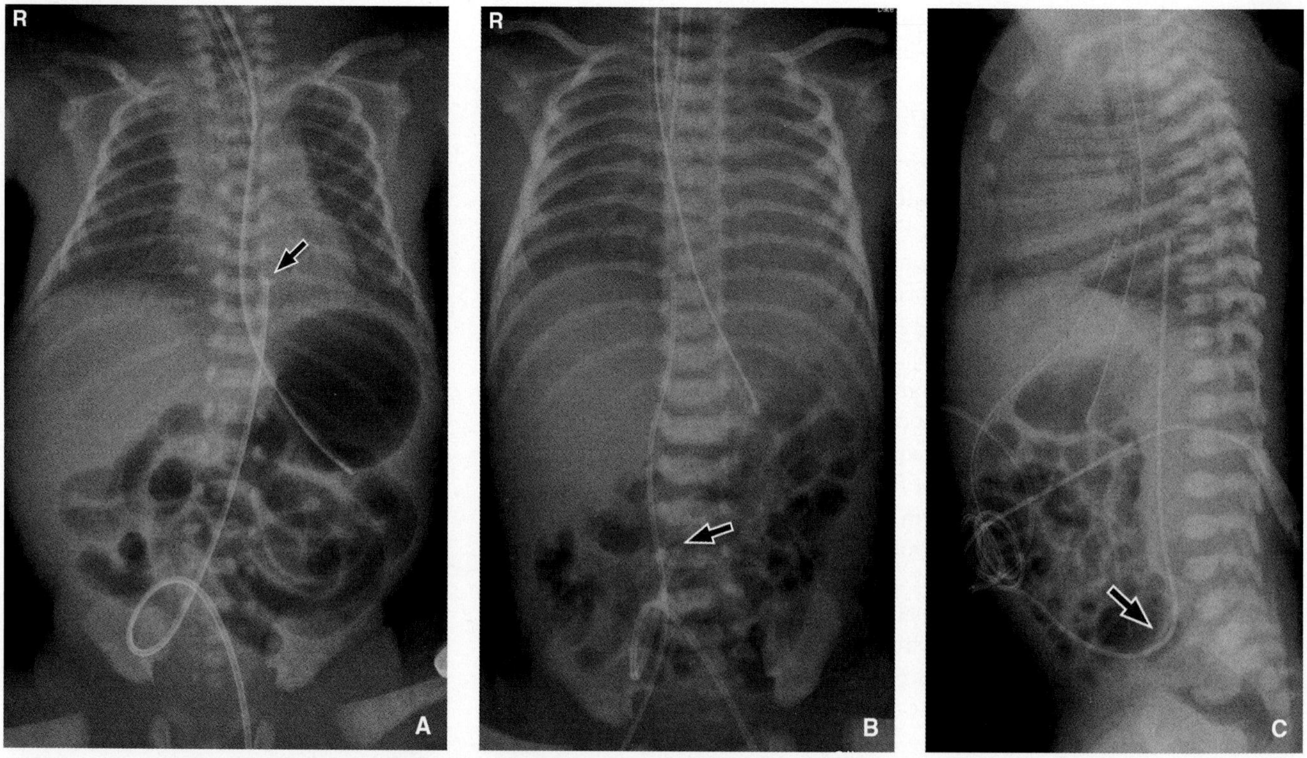

FIGURE 6.145 **Radiographic appearance of umbilical artery catheter (UAC). A:** Frontal radiograph demonstrate a "high" -position UAC with its tip (*arrow*) at T9 vertebral level. **B:** Frontal radiograph of another neonate with a "low"-position UAC with its tip (*arrow*) at the level of L4. Notice that the patient also has an umbilical vein catheter. **C:** Lateral radiograph demonstrates the characteristic pelvic loop of the UAC before it ascends into the aorta.

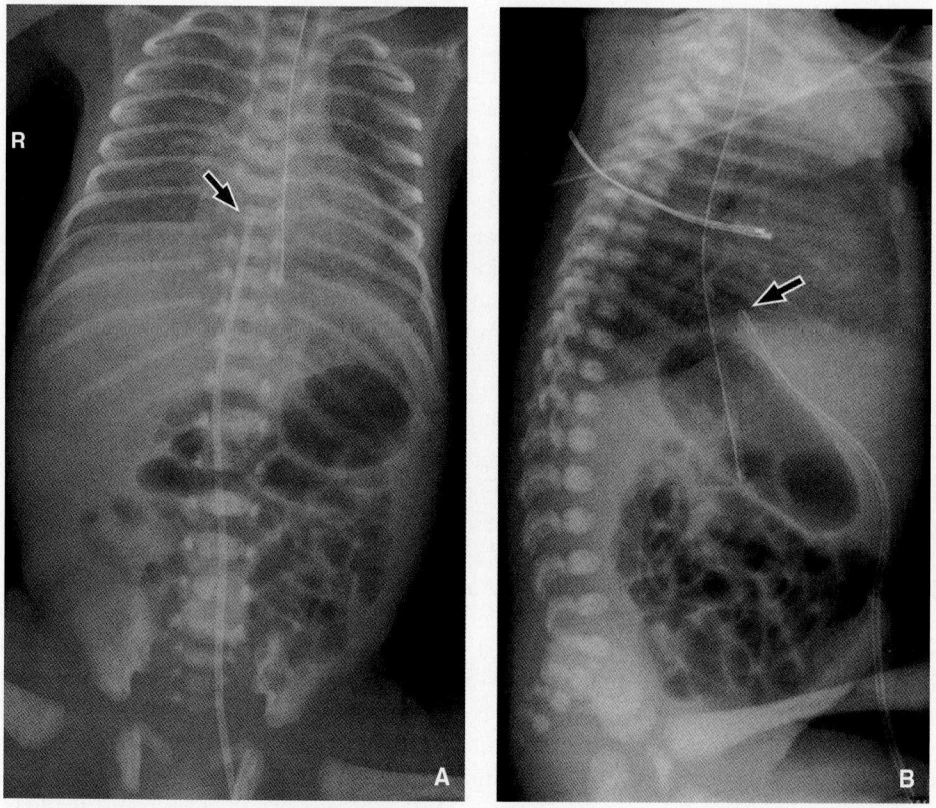

FIGURE 6.146 **Radiographic appearance of umbilical venous catheter (UVC). A:** Frontal radiograph demonstrates the UVC ascending into the inferior vena cava (IVC) with its tip (*arrow*) at the IVC and right atrium junction, at T7 vertebral level. **B:** On lateral radiograph, the UVC ascends anteriorly in the umbilical vein and courses posteriorly as it ascends into the IVC (*arrow*).

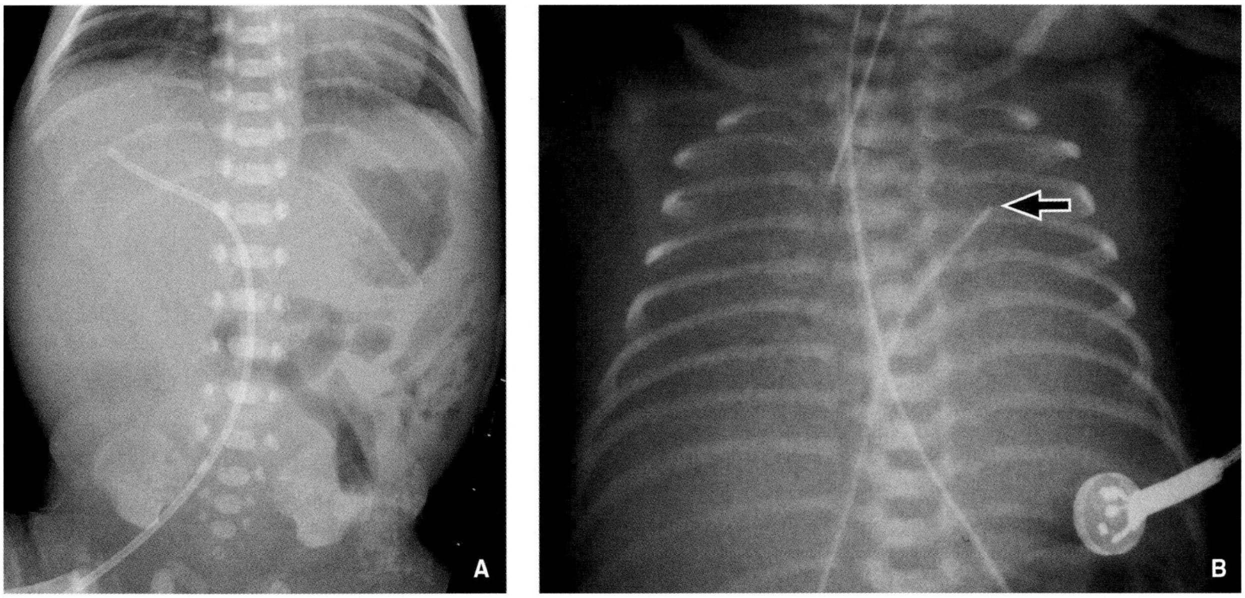

FIGURE 6.147 **Malpositioned umbilical vein catheter (UVC). A:** On frontal radiograph, UVC is seen coursing along the right hepatic lobe with tip likely within the right portal vein. **B:** On frontal radiograph, UVC placement in a neonate with surfactant deficiency disorder or hyaline membrane disease is very high in the left chest. The tip (*arrow*) is likely in the left pulmonary artery.

mesenteric vein, splenic vein, and occasionally, the catheter can be malpositioned in the heart or lungs (Fig. 6.147B), which can lead to pulmonary leak, hemorrhage, edema, and even infarction.[532,533] UVC-related infection is not uncommon, with *Staphylococcus* as the most common pathogen.

Central Venous Catheter

Central venous catheters are indicated when a continuous intravenous access is necessary, but there is no available peripheral venous access or when the UVC can no longer be used. These catheters can be used for hydration, nutrition, and drug administration.

Although surgeons have previously been placing these catheters by way of either percutaneous technique or cutdown, radiologists have been inserting these catheters with increasing frequency under US and even fluoroscopic guidance. The most common sites are the internal jugular, subclavian, femoral, facial, and external jugular veins. Optimal placement of the catheter tip for lines placed above the heart is at the junction of the superior vena cava (SVC) and the right atrium[526,534] (Fig. 6.148), and for femoral venous catheters, the ideal position of the tip is at the IVC and right atrium junction.[526] Pneumothorax should be carefully evaluated for, particularly with multiple unsuccessful attempts. For catheters placed under fluoroscopic guidance, postoperative chest radiographs in asymptomatic patients may not be necessary.[535]

Bleeding at the placement site with hematoma formation can occur during the process of insertion and even after the procedure. Pneumothorax could be a complication particularly with subclavian vein insertions. Other complications include malpositioned lines[536] (Fig. 6.149), dislodgement, leaking, and catheter occlusion.[537] Venous thrombosis occurs, which is higher in the saphenous veins compared to the internal jugular or subclavian lines. The risk of thrombosis is higher in smaller children, patients with inherent hypercoagulable state such as dehydration and sepsis, as well as malpositioned lines. Catheter-related infections occur with *Staphylococcus* and fungal infections as most common pathogens.[526] However, there is no significant association between the rate of infection and the site of catheter insertion, and the femoral vein catheterization carries a risk of infection similar to internal jugular catheterization.[538,539]

Peripherally Inserted Central Venous Catheter

Peripherally inserted central venous catheters (PICCs) have been increasingly placed if an intravenous access site is needed for an extended period of time (longer than the conventional peripheral intravenous line). The preferred veins for access in the upper extremity are the basilic and cephalic veins. The catheter is introduced by way of a peripheral vein and advanced to its final position, which is at SVC and right atrium junction if placed from the upper extremities (Fig. 6.150) and the IVC and right atrium junction when placed from the lower extremities.

Changes in the arm position influence the tip location of the PICC, moving it an average of 2.2 rib spaces. Elbow bending and arm adduction cause the tip to move deeper into the chest, compared to when the arm was straight and abducted 90 degrees. The side, site, and vein selected for access do not significantly influence the range of movement.[540]

Guidance for the initial puncture of the peripheral vein can be done by direct visualization or by US, but fluoroscopy is sometimes used as the catheter is advanced into its final position. Nurses with advanced intravenous access skills can insert these catheters with good safety profile and success rate, with low postprocedural complications.[541] However, pediatric PICC placement without fluoroscopic guidance required

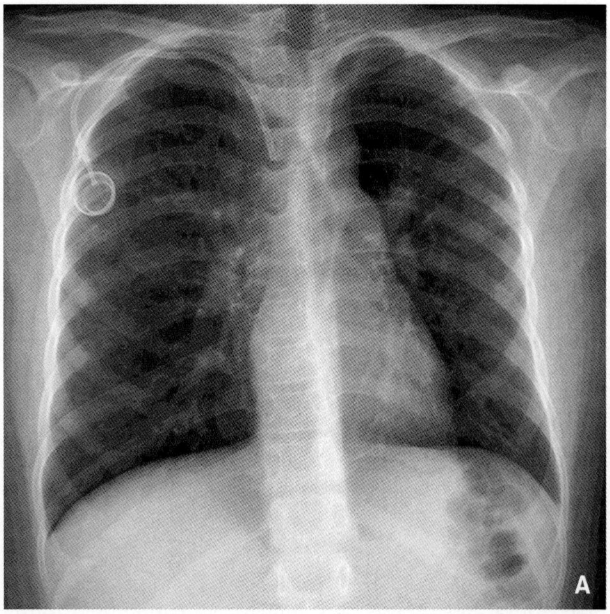

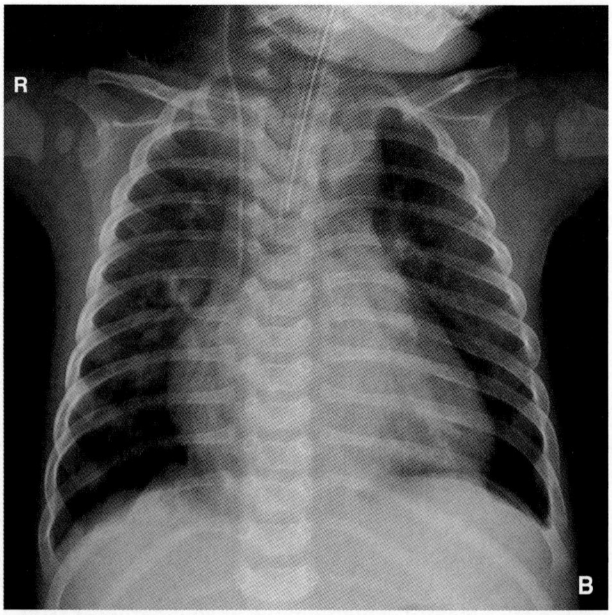

FIGURE 6.148 **Appropriate central venous catheter placement. A:** Frontal chest radiograph of a 10-year-old boy with leukemia, which shows a venous catheter in the right subclavian vein, with its tip within the superior vena cava (SVC). **B:** Frontal chest radiograph of a 7-year-old girl with congenital heart disease shows a right internal jugular vein catheter with its tip at the SVC and right atrium junction. Note that the child also has an ETT.

further catheter manipulation in 86% and needed repeated chest radiographs for confirmation.[542] Radiologists, with their imaging skills, have been inserting PICC lines under fluoroscopic guidance. Complications are mostly associated with local trauma during insertion. Mechanical problems including leaks and tears, as well as thrombosis and infection seen in regular central venous catheters, are also associated with PICC lines.[526,543]

Extracorporeal Membrane Oxygenation

ECMO is a well-established mode of treating acute, severe but reversible respiratory and cardiac failure with no response to optimal ventilator or pharmacologic treatment. The desaturated blood is usually removed through a venous cannula placed

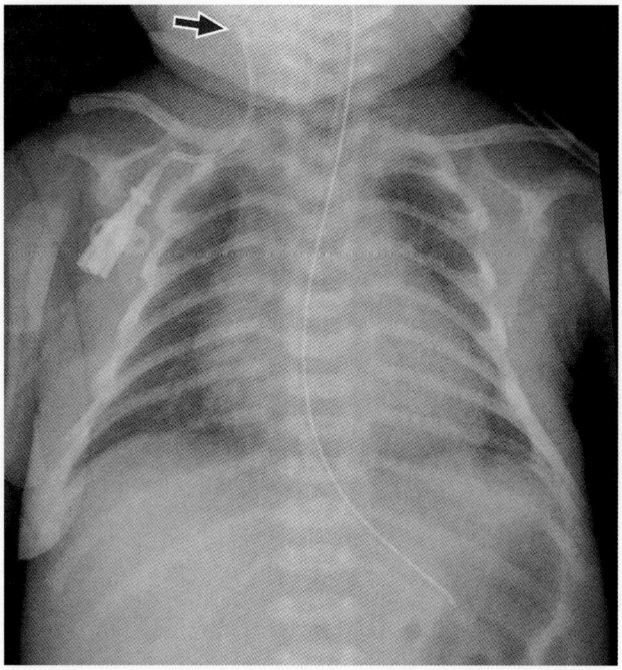

FIGURE 6.149 **Misplaced central venous catheter.** Frontal chest radiograph shows a right subclavian vein catheter placed with its tip (*arrow*) directed superiorly toward the right internal jugular vein.

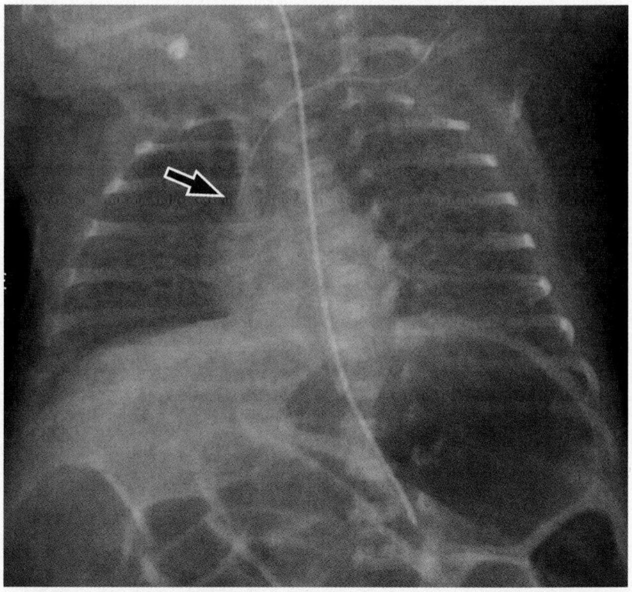

FIGURE 6.150 **Appropriate placement of peripherally inserted central venous catheter (PICC).** Frontal chest radiograph of a premature infant with a PICC line inserted through the left upper extremity shows the tip (*arrow*) of the catheter to be at the junction of superior vena cava and the right atrium.

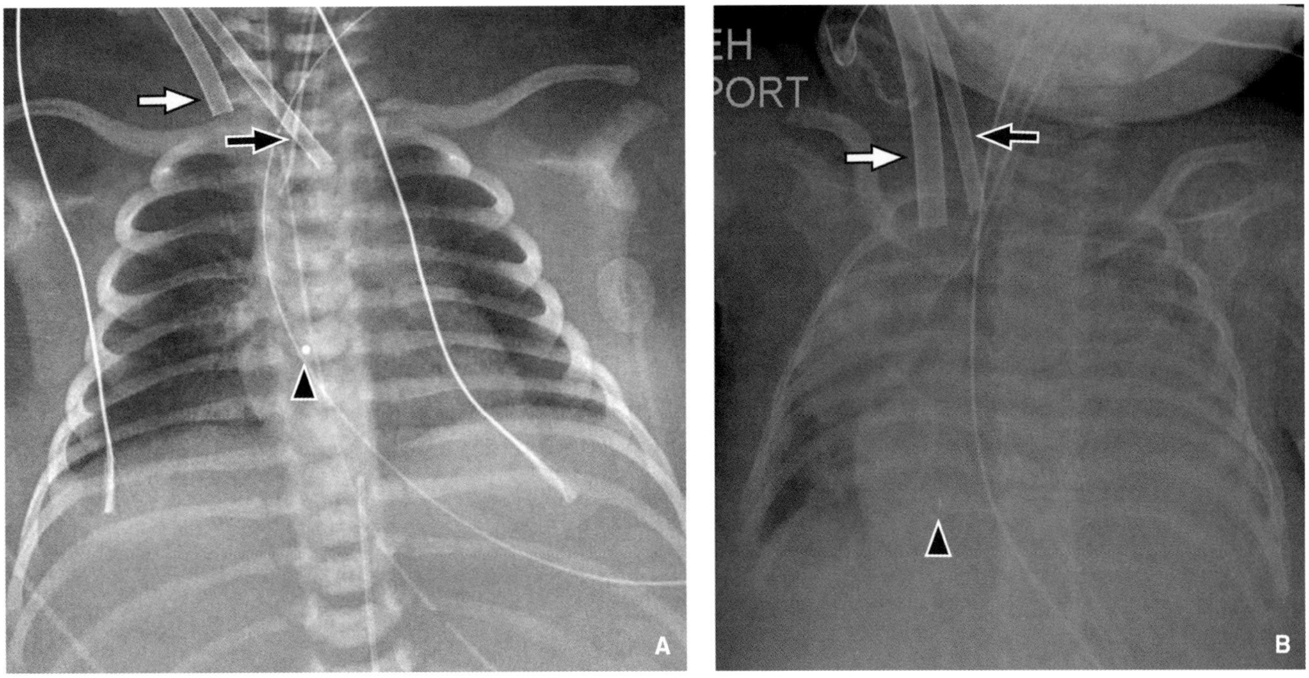

FIGURE 6.151 **Venoarterial extracorporeal membrane oxygenation (ECMO).** Frontal chest radiographs from two different pediatric patients on ECMO **(A and B)** show the right internal jugular vein (*white arrows*) and the right common carotid artery (*black arrows*) cannulas on the right neck region. The small radiopaque bead in the right atrium (*arrowheads*) signifies the tip of the venous catheter. (Case courtesy of Beth Kline-Fath, MD, Cincinnati Children's Hospital Medical Center, Cincinnati, OH.)

via the right internal jugular vein and extending into the right atrium. This blood passes through a membrane oxygenator and the reoxygenated blood is returned through an arterial cannula placed via the right common carotid artery and extending to the level of the aortic arch (venoarterial). A dual-lumen, single-cannula venovenous system that obviates the need to cannulate the right common carotid artery has also been developed.[544]

The most common neonatal diagnoses in neonates treated with ECMO are MAS, congenital diaphragmatic hernia, PPHN, respiratory distress syndrome, sepsis, pneumonia, and air leak syndrome. MAS carries the highest survival (94%), whereas congenital diaphragmatic hernia on ECMO only has a survival of 52%. In older children, the most common diagnoses for bypass support are viral pneumonia, bacterial pneumonia, ARDS, and aspiration pneumonia, which carry a high survival rate.[545]

For the more commonly used venoarterial ECMO bypass, chest radiograph usually reveals two large catheters in the right side of the neck. The laterally located venous catheter is within the right internal jugular vein, but its more distal tip is within the right atrium, recognized by a radiopaque bead (Fig. 6.151). The more medially located cannula is within the right common carotid artery. It is important to note that various degrees of pulmonary opacification can be seen in chest radiographs of patients undergoing ECMO, which may not be an accurate predictor of the patient's clinical status.[546]

The most common complication of ECMO is intracranial, pulmonary, or gastrointestinal hemorrhage. This is mostly due to the anticoagulation medications administered while the patient is on bypass. Other complications are related to the catheter-induced vascular trauma such as aortic dissection and pseudoaneurysm formation, as well as thromboemboli, infarction, and SVC syndrome.[526,547]

Endotracheal Tube

ETTs are frequently placed in hospitalized pediatric patients who need ventilator support, particularly in the NICU and PICU. The diameter and depth of insertion of the ETT are determined by the patient's size and age.

Radiographic confirmation is made possible by a radiopaque stripe that terminates at the most distal point of the tube's beveled tip. Chest radiographs obtained for the purposed of ETT evaluation should include the mandible in order to accurately assess tube position. In the vast majority of patients, ideal placement of the tip is in the midtrachea, approximately halfway between the inferior margin of the clavicles and the carina.[534] In neonates, the optimal placement has been reported from 0.2 to 2 cm above the carina[527,548] (Fig. 6.152A). The ETT changes in position with the neonate's head movement, the tip of ETT moving inferiorly with flexion of the head and superiorly with extension and lateral rotation of the head.[527]

Common complications of endotracheal intubation include malposition, most often in the right main bronchus (Fig. 6.152B) because of its more obtuse course compared to the left main bronchus. Malpositioned tubes are potentially dangerous because they may result in atelectasis and selective pulmonary distention. Malposition is much more common in children than adults and is seen in 15.5% of PICU patients.[536] Furthermore, 25% of the radiographically confirmed incorrectly placed ETTs continued to be malpositioned after repositioning.[549] Prolonged endotracheal intubation can also lead to subglottic stenosis and granuloma formation.[527]

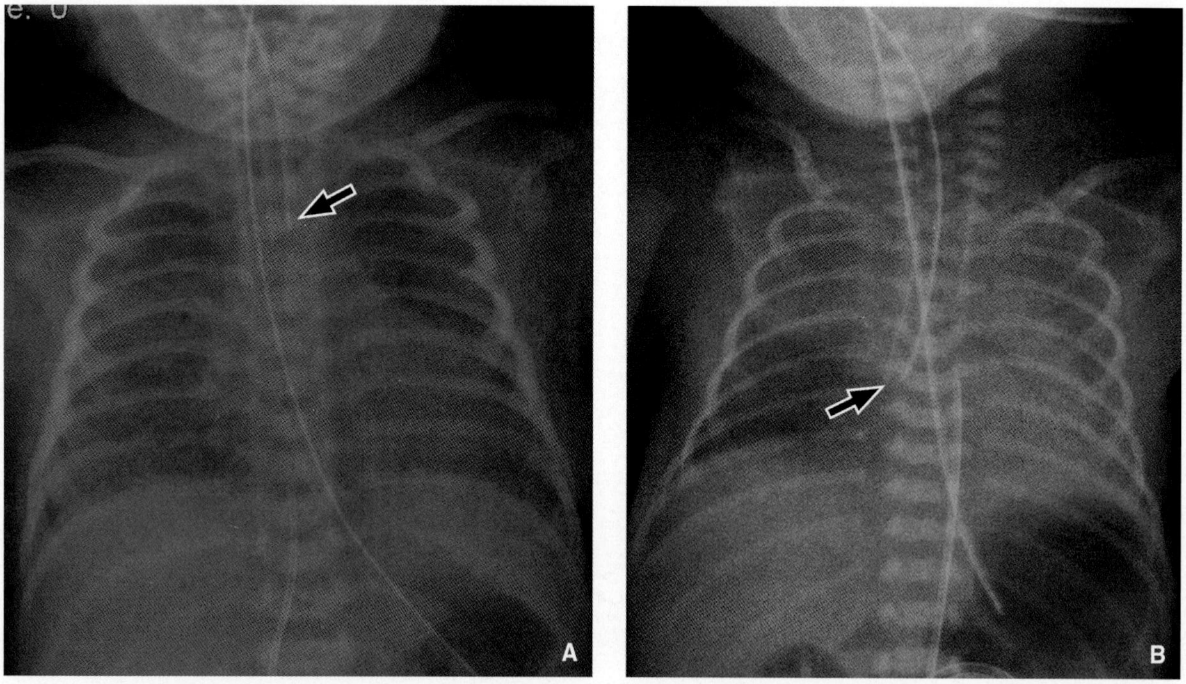

FIGURE 6.152 **Endotracheal tube (ETT) in two neonates. A:** Frontal chest radiograph of a neonate with surfactant deficiency disorder or hyaline membrane disease demonstrates the ETT with characteristic radiopaque stripe, appropriately placed with its tip (*arrow*) in the thoracic mid-trachea. **B:** Frontal chest radiograph of another neonate shows a malpositioned ETT with its tip (*arrow*) in the bronchus intermedius, causing atelectasis of the right upper lobe. Also noted is decreased left lung volume with atelectasis.

Enteric Tube

Nasogastric or orogastric tubes are placed in children mainly to decompress a distended stomach and sometimes for feeding. Duodenal tubes are placed primarily to infuse nutritional support particularly in chronically ill patients.

Radiographs are often obtained to confirm placement of enteric tubes. The ideal position for duodenal tube is ~1 cm proximal to the duodenojejunal junction or ligament of Trietz.[527] Nasogastric or orogastric tube tips are sometimes confirmed by auscultation if it is within the stomach. However, checking the placement of enteral tubes with traditional methods does not prevent misplacement in the respiratory tree,[550] thus validating the need for imaging in confirming the location of these tubes.

Malposition of enteric tubes is fairly common particularly in PICU[536] and is often seen in radiographs. Enteric tubes are sometimes noted within the esophagus and the gastroesophageal junction, which promotes gastroesophageal reflux. It can be looped within the oropharyngeal area and even within the esophagus (Fig. 6.153). Inadvertent cannulation of the

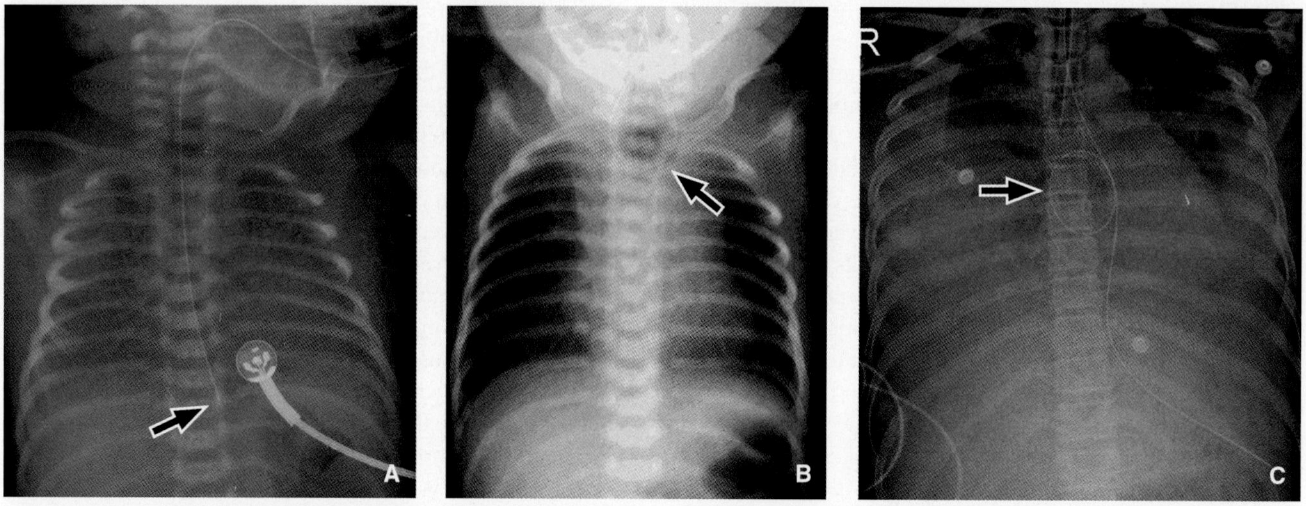

FIGURE 6.153 **Malpositioned orogastric tubes (OGT) on chest radiographs. A:** Frontal chest radiograph shows the OGT tip (*arrow*) to be in the distal esophagus, which defeats the purpose of gastric decompression. **B:** Frontal chest radiograph demonstrates the enteric tube (*arrow*) coiled back in the upper esophagus, initially mistaken for esophageal atresia. **C:** Frontal chest radiograph of a 12-year-old boy with severe pneumonia shows the enteric tube looped (*arrow*) within the midesophagus.

trachea, bronchus, or even the lung is occasionally encountered, which carries a degree of morbidity and possibly mortality. Malpositioned tubes can also lead to perforations with substantial complications. Therefore, timely recognition and immediate reposition of malpositioned enteric tubes are essential for optimal pediatric patient care.

References

1. Arthur R. Interpretation of pediatric chest x-ray. *Curr Paediatr.* 2003;13:438–447.
2. Supakul N, Karmazyn B. Ultrasound of the pediatric chest-the ins and outs. *Semin Ultrasound CT MRI.* 2013;34(3):274–285.
3. Kim OH, Kim WS, Kim MJ, et al. US in the diagnosis of pediatric chest diseases. *Radiographics.* 2000;20:653–671.
4. Coley BD. Chest sonography in children: current indications, techniques, and imaging findings. *Radiol Clin North Am.* 2011; 49:825–846.
5. Mong A, Epelman M, Darge K. Ultrasound of the pediatric chest. *Pediatr Radiol.* 2012;42:1287–1297.
6. Baez JC, Sodhi KS, Restrepo R, et al. Sonographic evaluation of congenital and acquired thoracic disorders in pediatric patients. *Ultrasound Clin.* 2013;8(3):265–284.
7. Pieper CH, Smith J, Brand EJ. The value of ultrasound examination of the lungs in predicting bronchopulmonary dysplasia. *Pediatr Radiol.* 2004;34:227–231.
8. Tardella M. Ultrasound in the assessment of pulmonary fibrosis in connective tissue disorders: correlation with high-resolution computed tomography. *J Rheumatol.* 2012;39:1641–1647.
9. Toma P, Owens CM. Chest ultrasound in children: critical appraisal. *Pediatr Radiol.* 2013;43:1427–1434.
10. Watson T, Owens CM. Computed tomography in children with lung disease. How, when and why? Myths and mystery unraveled. *Paediatr Child Health.* 2013;23(3):125–132.
11. Lee EY, Dorkin H, Vargas SO. Advances in pediatric thoracic imaging of congenital pulmonary malformations in pediatric patients: review and update on etiology, classification, and imaging findings. *Radiol Clin North Am.* 2011;49(5):921–948.
12. Lobo L, Antunes D. Chest CT in infants and children. *Eur J Radiol.* 2013;82(7):1108–1117.
13. Park KM, Owens CM. When should CT be performed in children with lung disease? *Paediatr Child Health.* 2009;19(6):282–290.
14. Young C, Xie C, Owens CM. Paediatric multi-detector row chest CT: what you really need to know. *Insights Imaging.* 2012;3: 229–246.
15. Goo JM. A computer-aided diagnosis for evaluating lung nodules on chest CT: the current status and perspective. *Korean J Radiol.* 2011;12:145–155.
16. Goo HW. Advanced functional thoracic imaging in children: from basic concepts to clinical applications. *Pediatr Radiol.* 2013;43:262–268.
17. Goo HW. Initial experience of dual-energy lung perfusion CT using a dual-source CT system in children. *Pediatr Radiol.* 2010;40:1536–1544.
18. Brenner D, Elliston C, Hall E, et al. Estimated risks of radiation-induced fatal cancer from pediatric CT. *AJR Am J Roentgenol.* 2001;176(2):289–296.
19. Goo HW. CT radiation dose optimization and estimation: an update for radiologists. *Korean J Radiol.* 2012;13(1):1–11.
20. Hirsch W, Sorgea I, Krohmera S, et al. MRI of the lungs in children. *Eur J Radiol.* 2008;68:278–288.
21. Wielpütz M, Kauczor HU. MRI of the lung: state of the art. *Diagn Interv Radiol.* 2012;18:344–353.
22. Yikilmaz A, Koc A, Coskun A, et al. Evaluation of pneumonia in children: comparison of MRI with fast imaging sequences at 1.5 T with chest radiographs. *Acta Radiol.* 2011;52(8):914–919.
23. Sodhi KS, Khandelwal N, Saxena AK, et al. Rapid lung MRI: paradigm shift of febrile neutropenia in children with leukemia: a pilot study. *Leuk Lymphoma.* 2015;57(1):70–75.
24. Liszewski MC, Hersman FW, Altes TA, et al. Pediatric body imaging with advanced MDCT and MRI magnetic resonance imaging of pediatric lung parenchyma, airways, vasculature, ventilation, and perfusion. *Radiol Clin North Am.* 2013;51(4): 555–582.
25. Kirby M, Coxson HO, Parraga G. Pulmonary functional magnetic resonance imaging for paediatric lung disease. *Paediatr Respir Rev.* 2013;14(3):180–189.
26. Grant FD, Treves ST. Advances in pediatric thoracic imaging nuclear medicine and molecular imaging of the pediatric chest: current practical imaging assessment. *Radiol Clin North Am.* 2011;49(5):1025–1051.
27. Shammas A, Vali R, Charron M. Pediatric nuclear medicine in acute care. *Semin Nucl Med.* 2013;43:139–156.
28. Parker JA, Coleman RE, Grady E, et al: SNM practice guideline for lung scintigraphy 4.0. *J Nucl Med Technol.* 2012;40(1):57–65.
29. Ciofetta G, Piepsz A, Roca I, et al. Guidelines for lung scintigraphy in children. *Eur J Nucl Med Mol Imaging.* 2007;34(9): 1518–1526.
30. Trujillo NP, Pratt JP, Talusani S,et al. DTPA aerosol in ventilation/perfusion scintigraphy for diagnosing pulmonary embolism. *J Nucl Med.* 1997;38:1781–1783.
31. Agrons GA, Courtney SE, Stocker JT, et al. From the archives of AFIP: lung disease in premature neonates: radiologic-pathologic correlation. *Radiographics.* 2005;25(4):1047–1073.
32. Joshi S, Kotecha S. Lung growth and development. *Early Hum Dev.* 2007;83:789–794.
33. Correia-Pinto J, Gonzaga S, Huang Y, et al. Congenital lung lesions—underlying molecular mechanisms. *Semin Pediatr Surg.* 2010;19:171–179.
34. Medlar EM. Variations in interlobar fissures. *AJR Am J Roentgenol.* 1947;57:723–725.
35. Aziz A, Ashizawa K, Nagaoki K, et al. High resolution CT anatomy of the pulmonary fissures. *J Thorac Imaging.* 2004;19(3): 186–191.
36. Ugalde P, Camargo JDJ, Deslauriers J. Lobes, fissures, and bronchopulmonary segments. *Thorac Surg Clin.* 2007;17: 587–599.
37. Ariyurek OM, Gulsun M, Demirkazik FB. Accessory fissures of the lung: evaluation by high-resolution computed tomography. *Eur Radiol.* 2001;11(12):2449–2453.
38. Murlimanju BV, Prabhu LV, Shilpa K, et al. Pulmonary fissures and lobes: a cadaveric study with emphasis on surgical and radiological implications. *Clin Ter.* 2012;163(1):9–13.
39. Jackson CL, Huber JF. Correlated anatomy of the bronchial tree and lung with a system of nomenclature. *Dis Chest.* 1943; 9:319–326.
40. Brock RC. The nomenclature of broncho-pulmonamy anatomy: an international nomenclature accepted by the Thoracic Society. *Thorax.* 1950;5:222–228.
41. Osborne DR, Effmann EL, Hedlund LW. Postnatal growth and size of the pulmonary acinus and secondary lobule in man. *AJR Am J Roentgenol.* 1983;140:449–454.

42. Webb WR. Thin-section CT of secondary pulmonary lobule. *Radiology.* 2006;239:322–338.
43. Weibel ER. Looking into the lung: what can it tell us? *AJR Am J Roentgenol.* 1979;133:1021–1031.
44. Itoh H, Murata K, Konishi J, et al. Diffuse lung disease: pathologic basis for the high-resolution computed tomography findings. *J Thorac Imaging.* 1993;8:176–188.
45. Hansen J, Ampaya E, Bryant G, et al. Branching patterns of airways and air spaces of a single human terminal bronchiole. *J Appl Physiol.* 1975;38:983–989.
46. Schreider JP, Raabe OG. Structure of the human respiratory acinus. *Am J Anat.* 1981;162:221–223.
47. Smith LJ, McKay KO, Van Asperen PP, et al. Normal development of the lung and premature birth. *Paediatr Respir Rev.* 2010;11(3):135–142.
48. Heithoff KB, Sane SM, Williams HJ, et al. Bronchopulmonary foregut malformations. A unifying etiological concept. *AJR Am J Roentgenol.* 1976;126:46–55.
49. Johnson AM, Hubbard AM. Congenital anomalies of the fetal/neonatal chest. *Semin Roentgenol.* 2004;39:197–214.
50. Panicek DM, Heitzman ER, Randall PA, et al. The continuum of pulmonary developmental anomalies. *Radiographics.* 1987;7:747–772.
51. Langston C. New concepts in the pathology of congenital lung malformations. *Semin Pediatr Surg.* 2003;12:17–37.
52. Riedlinger WF, Vargas SO, Jennings RW, et al. Bronchial atresia is common to extralobar sequestration, intralobar sequestration, congenital cystic adenomatoid malformation, and lobar emphysema. *Pediatr Dev Pathol.* 2006;9:361–373.
53. Wagner AJ, Stumbaugh A, Tigue Z, et al. Genetic analysis of congenital cystic adenomatoid malformation reveals a novel pulmonary gene: fatty acid binding protein-7 (brain type). *Pediatr Res.* 2008;64:11–16.
54. Klein JD, Turner CG, Dobson LJ, et al. Familial case of prenatally diagnosed intralobar and extralobar sequestrations with cystadenomatoid change. *J Pediatr Surg.* 2011;46:E27–E31.
55. Thacker PG, Rao AG, Hill JG, et al. Congenital lung anomalies in children and adults: current concepts and imaging findings. *Radiol Clin North Am.* 2014;52:155–181.
56. Newman B. Congenital bronchopulmonary foregut malformation: concepts and controversies. *Pediatr Radiol.* 2006;36:773–791.
57. Bulas D, Egloff AM. Fetal chest ultrasound and magnetic resonance imaging: recent advances and current clinical applications. *Radiol Clin North Am.* 2011;49(5)805–823.
58. Ramsay BH, Byron FX. Mucocele, congenital bronchiectasis, and bronchogenic cyst. *J Thorac Surg.* 1953;26(1):21–30.
59. Biyyam DR, Chapman T, Ferguson MR, et al. Congenital lung abnormalities: embryologic features, prenatal diagnosis, and postnatal radiologic-pathologic correlation. *Radiographics.* 2010;30:1721–1738.
60. Williams AJ, Schuster SR. Bronchial atresia associated with a bronchogenic cyst: evidence of early appearance of atretic segments. *Chest.* 1985;87:396–398.
61. Berrocal T, Madrid C, Novo S, et al. Congenital anomalies of the tracheobronchial tree, lung, and mediastinum: embryology, radiology, and pathology. *Radiographics.* 2004;24(1):e17.
62. Griffin N, Devaraj A, Goldstraw P, et al. CT and histopathological correlation of congenital cystic pulmonary lesions: a common pathogenesis? *Clin Radiol.* 2008;63(9):995–1005.
63. Wang Y, Dai W, Sun Y, et al. Congenital bronchial atresia: diagnosis and treatment. *Int J Med Sci.* 2012;9(3):207–212.
64. Discioscio V, Feraco P, Bazzocchi A, et al. Congenital cystic adenomatoid malformation of the lung associated with bronchial atresia involving a different lobe in an adult patient: a case report. *J Med Case Reports.* 2010;4:164–166.
65. Kawamoto S, Yuasa M, Tsukuda S, et al. Bronchial atresia: three-dimensional CT bronchography using volume rendering technique. *Radiat Med.* 2001;19(2):107–110.
66. Matsushima H, Takayanagi N, Satoh M, et al. Congenital bronchial atresia: radiologic findings in nine patients. *J Comput Assist Tomogr.* 2002;26(5):860–864.
67. Cappeliez S, Lenoir S, Validire P, et al. Totally endoscopic lobectomy and segmentectomy for congenital bronchial atresia. *Eur J Cardiothorac Surg.* 2009;36(1):222–224.
68. Aktgu S, Yuncu G, Halilocolar H, et al. Bronchogenic cysts: clinico-pathological presentation and treatment. *Eur Respir J.* 1996;9:2017–2021.
69. Nuchtern JG, Harberg FJ. Congenital lung cysts. *Semin Pediatr Surg.* 1994;3:233–243.
70. Winters WD, Effman EL. Congenital masses of the lung: prenatal and postnatal imaging evaluation. *J Thorac Imaging.* 2001;16:196–206.
71. McAdams HP, Kirejczyk WM, Rosado-de-Christenson ML, et al. Bronchogenic cyst: imaging features with clinical and histopathologic correlation. *Radiology.* 2000;217:441–446.
72. Paterson A. Imaging evaluation of congenital lung abnormalities in infants and children. *Radiol Clin North Am.* 2005;43:303–323.
73. Lee EY. Evaluation of non-vascular mediastinal masses in infants and children: an evidence-based practical approach. *Pediatr Radiol.* 2009;39:S184–S190.
74. Suen HC, Mathisen DJ, Grillo HC, et al. Surgical management and radiological characteristics of bronchogenic cysts. *Ann Thorac Surg.* 1993;55:476–481.
75. Jain A, Anand K, Kumar A. Congenital cystic lung diseases. *J Clin Imaging Sci.* 2013;3:5. doi: 10.4103/2156-7514.106620.
76. Laberge JM, Flageole H, Pugash D, et al. Outcome of the prenatally diagnosed congenital cystic adenomatoid lung malformation: a Canadian experience. *Fetal Diagn Ther.* 2001;16:178–186.
77. Epelman M, Kreiger PA, Servas S, et al. Current imaging of prenatally diagnosed congenital lung lesions. *Semin Ultrasound CT MR.* 2010;31:141–157.
78. Stocker JT. Congenital pulmonary airway malformation—a new name for an expanded classification of congenital cystic adenomatoid malformation of the lung. *Histopathology.* 2002;41:424–431.
79. Wilson RD, Hedrick HL, Liechty KW, et al. Cystic adenomatoid malformation of the lung: review of genetics, prenatal diagnosis, and in utero treatment. *Am J Med Genet A.* 2006;140:151–155.
80. Daltro P, Werner H, Gasparetto T, et al. Congenital chest malformations: a multimodality approach with emphasis on fetal MR imaging. *Radiographics.* 2010;30:385–395.
81. Imai Y, Mark EJ. Cystic adenomatoid change is common to various forms of cystic lung diseases of children: a clinicopathologic analysis of 10 cases with emphasis on tracing the bronchial tree. *Arch Pathol Lab Med.* 2002;126:934–940.
82. Yikilmaz A, Lee EY. CT imaging of mass-like nonvascular pulmonary lesions in children. *Pediatr Radiol.* 2007;37(12):1253–1263.
83. Hill DA. USCAP Specialty Conference: case 1-type I pleuropulmonary blastoma. *Pediatr Dev Pathol.* 2005;8(1):77–84.
84. Hill DA, Jarzembowski JA, Priest JR, et al. Type 1 pleuropulmonary blastoma: pathology and biology study of 51 cases from the international pleuropulmonary blastoma registry. *Am J Surg Pathol.* 2008;32:282–295.

85. Vu LT, Farmer DL, Nobuhara KK, et al. Thoracoscopic versus open resection for congenital cystic adenomatoid malformations of the lung. *J Pediatr Surg.* 2008;43(1):35–39.
86. Masters IB. Congenital airway lesions and lung disease. *Pediatr Clin North Am.* 2009;56:227–242.
87. Olutoye OO, Coleman BG, Hubbard AM, et al. Prenatal diagnosis and management of congenital lobar emphysema. *J Pediatr Surg.* 2000;35(5):792–795.
88. Ozcelik U, Gocmen A, Kiper N, et al. Congenital lobar emphysema: evaluation and long-term follow up of thirty cases at a single center. *Pediatr Pulmonol.* 2003;35:384–391.
89. Thakral CL, Maji DC, Sajwani MJ. Congenital lobar emphysema: experience with 21 cases. *Pediatr Surg Int.* 2001;17: 88–91.
90. Cleveland RH, Weber B. Retained fetal lung liquid in congenital lobar emphysema: a possible predictor of polyalveolar lobe. *Pediatr Radiol.* 1993;23:291–295.
91. Kumar A, Bhatnagar V. Respiratory distress in neonates. *Indian J Pediatr.* 2005;72:425–428.
92. Hugosson C, Rabeeach A, Al-Rawaf A, et al. Congenital lobar emphysema. *Pediatr Radiol.* 1995;25:649–651.
93. Eber E. Antenatal diagnosis of congenital thoracic malformations: early surgery, late surgery, or no surgery? *Semin Respir Crit Care Med.* 2007;28(3):355–366.
94. Nazem M, Hosseinpour M. Evaluation of early and late complications in patients with congenital lobar emphysema: a 12 year experience. *Afr J Paediatr Surg.* 2010;7:144–146.
95. Stocker JT. Cystic lung disease in infants and children. *Fetal Pediatr Pathol.* 2009;28:155–184.
96. Savic B, Birtel FJ, Tholen W, et al. Lung sequestration: report of seven cases and review of 540 published cases. *Thorax.* 1979;34:96–101.
97. Olivieri C, Nanni L, Busatoa G, et al. Intradiaphragmatic hybrid lesion in an infant: case report. *J Pediatr Surg.* 2012;47:E25–E28.
98. Cass DL, Crombleholme TM, Howell LJ, et al. Cystic lung lesions with systemic arterial blood supply: a hybrid of congenital cystic adenomatoid malformation and bronchopulmonary sequestration. *J Pediatr Surg.* 1997;32:986–990.
99. Conran RM, Stocker JT. Extralobar sequestration with frequently associated congenital cystic adenomatoid malformation, type 2: report of 50 cases. *Pediatr Dev Pathol.* 1999;2:454–463.
100. Vijayaraghavan SB, Rao PS, Selvarasu CD, et al. Prenatal sonographic features of intralobar bronchopulmonary sequestration. *J Ultrasound Med.* 2003;22:541–544.
101. Sepulveda W. Perinatal imaging in bronchopulmonary sequestration. *J Ultrasound Med.* 2009;28:89–94.
102. Lee BS, Kim JT, Kim EA, et al. Neonatal pulmonary sequestration: clinical experience with transumbilical arterial embolization. *Pediatr Pulmonol.* 2008;43:404–413.
103. Lee KH, Sung KB, Yoon HK, et al. Transcatheter arterial embolization of pulmonary sequestration in neonates: long term follow-up results. *J Vasc Interv Radiol.* 2003;14:363–367.
104. Rudan I, Boschi-Pinto C, Biloglav Z, et al. Epidemiology and etiology of childhood pneumonia. *Bull World Health Organ.* 2008;86(5):408–418.
105. Kusel MM, de Klerk NH, Holt PG, et al. Role of respiratory viruses in acute upper and lower respiratory tract illness in the first year of life: a birth cohort study. *Pediatr Infect Dis J.* 2006; 25(8):680–686.
106. Nair H, Simooes EA, Rudan I, et al. Global and regional burden of hospital admissions for severe acute lower respiratory infections in young children in 2010: a systematic analysis. *Lancet.* 2013;381(9875):1380–1390.
107. Williams BG, Gouws E, Boschi-Pinto C, et al. Estimates of worldwide distribution of child deaths from acute respiratory infections. *Lancet Infect Dis.* 2002;2(1):25–32.
108. Condon VR. Pneumonia in children. *J Thorac Imaging.* 1991; 6:31–44.
109. Ostapchuk M, Roberts DM, Haddy R, et al. Community acquired pneumonia in infants and children. *Am Fam Physician.* 2004;70(5):899–908.
110. Alter SJ. Vidwan NK, Sobande PO, et al. Common childhood bacterial infections. *Curr Probl Pediatr Adolesc Health Care.* 2011;41:256–283.
111. Donnelly LF. Practical issues concerning imaging of pulmonary infection in children. *J Thorac Imaging.* 2001;16:238–250,
112. Donnelly LF. Maximizing the usefulness of imaging in children with community-acquired pneumonia. *AJR Am J Roentgenol.* 1999;172:505–512.
113. Korppi M, Heiskanen-Kosma T, Jalonen E, et al. Aetiology of community-acquired pneumonia in children treated in hospital. *Eur J Pediatr.* 1993;152(1):24–30.
114. Shafik CF, Mohareb EW, Yassin AS. Viral etiologies of lower respiratory tract infections among egyptian children under five years of age. *BMC Infect Dis.* 2012;12:350. doi: 10.1186/1471-2334-12-350.
115. Glezen P, Denny FW. Epidemiology of acute lower respiratory disease in children. *N Engl J Med.* 1973;288:498–505.
116. Osborne D. Radiologic appearance of viral disease of the lower respiratory tract in infants and children. *AJR Am J Roentgenol.* 1978;130:29–33.
117. Aherne W, Bird T, Court DS, et al. Pathological changes in virus infection of the lower respiratory tract in children. *J Clin Pathol.* 1970;23:7–18.
118. Swischuk LE, Hayden CK. Viral versus bacterial infections in children: is roentgenographic differentiation possible? *Pediatr Radiol.* 1986;16:278–284.
119. Franquet T. Imaging of pulmonary viral pneumonia. *Radiology.* 2011;260(1):18–39.
120. Dawson-Caswell M, Muncie HL. Respiratory syncytial virus in children. *Am Fam Physician.* 2011;83(2):141–146.
121. Weisman LE. Populations at risk for developing respiratory syncytial virus and risk factors for respiratory syncytial virus severity: infants with predisposing conditions. *Pediatr Infect Dis J.* 2003;22(2 suppl):S33–S37.
122. Peret TC, Boivin G, Li Y, et al. Characterization of human metapneuomovirus isolated from patients in North America. *J Infect Dis.* 2002;185:1660–1663.
123. Maggi F, Pifferi M, Vatteroni M, et al. Human metapneumovirus associated with respiratory tract infections in a 3-year study of nasal swabs from infants in Italy. *J Clin Microbiol.* 2003; 41(7):2987–2991.
124. Lin PY, Lin Ty, Huang YC, et al. Human metapneumovirus and community-acquired pneumonia in children. *Chang Gung Med J.* 2005;28:638–638.
125. Kim CK, Choi J, Callaway Z, et al. Clinical and epidemiological comparison of human metapneumovirus and respiratory syncytial virus in Seoul, Korea, 2003–2008. *J Korean Med Sci.* 2010;25:324–327.
126. Heikkinen T, Osterback R, Peltola V, et al. Human metapneumovirus infections in children. *Emerg Infect Dis.* 2008; 14(1):101–106.

127. Henrickson KJ. Parainfluenza viruses. *Clin Microbiol Rev.* 2003;16(2):242–264.
128. McIntosh K. Pathogenesis of severe acute respiratory infections in the developing world: respiratory syncytial virus and parainfluenza viruses. *Rev Infect Dis.* 1991;13:S492–S500.
129. Peltola H, Heinonen OP, Valle M, et al. The elimination of indigenous measles, mumps, and rubella from Finland by a 12-year, two-dose vaccination program. *N Engl J Med.* 1994; 331(21):1397–1402.
130. Posfay-Barbe KM. Infections in pediatrics: old and new diseases. *Swiss Med Wkly.* 2012;142:w13654. doi: 10.4414/smw.2012.13654.
131. Becroft DMO. Bronchiolitis obliterans, bronchiectasis, and other sequelae of adenovirus type 21 infection in younger children. *J Clin Pathol.* 1971;24:72–82.
132. Hong JY, Lee HJ, Piedra PA, et al. Lower respiratory tract infections due to adenovirus in hospitalized Korean children: epidemiology, clinical features, and prognosis. *Clin Infect Dis.* 2001;32(10):1423–1429.
133. Munoz FP, Piedra PA, Demmler GJ. Disseminated adenovirus disease in immunocompromised and immunocompetent children. *Clin Infect Dis.* 1998;27:1194–1200.
134. Osborne D, White P. Radiology of epidemic adenovirus 21 infection of the lower respiratory tract in infants and young children. *AJR Am J Roentgenol.* 1979;133:397–400.
135. Nasetta L, Kimberin D, Whitley R. Treatment of congenital cytomegalovirus infection: implications for future therapeutic strategies. *J Antimicrob Chemother.* 2009;63:862–867. doi:10.1093/jac/dkp083.
136. Gasparetto EL, Ono SE, Escuissato D, et al. Cytomegalovirus pneumonia after bone marrow transplantation: high resolution CT findings. *Br J Radiol.* 2004;77(921):724–727.
137. Cunningham I. Pulmonary infections after bone marrow transplant. *Semin Respir Infect.* 1992;7:132–138.
138. Chan JY, Tian L, Kwan Y, et al. Hospitalizations for varicella in children and adolescents in a referral hospital in Hong King, 2004 to 2008: a time series study. *BMC Public Health.* 2011;11:366. doi: 10.1186/1471-2458-11-366.
139. Kim JS, Ryu CW, Lee SI, et al. High resolution CT findings of varicella zoster pneumonia. *AJR Am J Roentgenol.* 1999; 172:113–116.
140. Marks MJ, Haney PJ, McDermott MP, et al. Thoracic diseases in children with AIDS. *Radiographics.* 1996;16:139–1362.
141. Marolda J, Paca B, Bonforte J, et al. Pulmonary manifestations of HIV infection in children. *Pediatr Pulmonol.* 1991;10:231–235.
142. Collingsworth CL. Thoracic disorders in the immunocompromised. *Radiol Clin North Am.* 2005;43:435–447.
143. Franquet T, Müller NL, Lee KS, et al. Pulmonary candidiasis after hematopoietic stem cell transplantation: thin-section CT findings. *Radiology.* 2005;236(1):332–337.
144. Jeanes AC, Owens CM. Chest imaging in the immunocompromised child. *Pediatr Respir Rev.* 2002;3:59–69.
145. Thibodeau KP, Viera AJ. Atypical pathogens and challenges in community acquired pneumonia. *Am Fam Physician.* 2004; 69(7):1699–1706.
146. Brodzinski H, Ruddy RM. Review of new and newly discovered respiratory tract viruses in children. *Pediatr Emerg Care.* 2009;25:352–360.
147. Lee EY, McAdam A, Chaudry G, et al. Swine-origin influenza A (H1N1) viral infection in children: initial chest radiographic findings. *Radiology.* 2010;254(3):934–941. doi: 10.1148/radiol.09092083.
148. Assiri A, McGeer A, Perl TM. Hospital outbreak of Middle East respiratory syndrome coronavirus. *N Engl J Med.* 2013; 369(5):407–416. doi: 10.1056/NEJMoa1306742.
149. Westra SJ, Choy G. What imaging should we perform for the diagnosis and management of pulmonary infections? *Pediatr Radiol.* 2009;39(suppl 2):S178–S183.
150. Virkki R, Juven T, Rikalainen H, et al. Differentiation of bacterial and viral pneumonia in children. *Thorax.* 2002;57: 438–441.
151. Guo W, Wang J, Sheng M, et al. Radiological findings in 210 pediatric patients with viral pneumonia: a retrospective case study. *Br J Radiol.* 2012;85(1018):1385–1389.
152. Daltro P, Santos EN, Gasparetto TD, et al. Pulmonary infections. *Pediatr Radiol.* 2011;41(suppl 1):S69–S82.
153. Blickman H. Inflammatory lung disease, Chapter 2. In: *Pediatric Radiology, The Requisites.* 2nd ed. Baltimore, MD: Mosby; 1998.
154. Desai SR, Copley SJ, Barker RD, et al. Chest radiography in 75 adolescents with vertically-acquired human immunodeficiency virus (HIV) infection. *Clin Radiol.* 2011;66(3): 257–263.
155. Franquet T. Imaging of pneumonia: trends and algorithms. *Eur Respir J.* 2001;18:196–208.
156. Langley JM, Smith MB, LeBlanc JC, et al. Racemic epinephrine compared to salbutamol in hospitalized young children with bronchiolitis: a randomized control trial. *BMC Pediatr.* 2005;5(1):1–7.
157. Plint AC, Johnson DW, Patel H, et al. Epinephrine and dexamethasone in children with bronchiolitis. *N Engl J Med.* 2009;360(20):2079–2089.
158. Wainwright MB, Altamirano L, Medico-Cirujano MC, et al. A multicenter randomized, double blind, controlled trial of nebulized epinephrine in infants with acute bronchiolitis. *N Engl J Med.* 2003;349:27–35.
159. Blickman JG. Comparison of nebulized epinephrine to albuterol in bronchiolitis. *Acad Emerg Med.* 2008;15(4):305–313.
160. Johnson LF, Davies MA, Moultirie H. The effect of early initiation of antiretroviral treatment in infants on pediatric AIDS mortality in South Africa: a model-based analysis. *Pediatr Infect Dis.* 2012;31(5):474–480.
161. Van Dyke RB, Patel K, Siberry GK, et al. Antiretroviral treatment of US children with perinatally acquired HIV infection: temporal changes in therapy between 1999 and 2009 and predictors of immunologic and virologic outcomes. *J Acquir Immune Defic Syndr.* 2011;57(2):165–173.
162. John SD, Ramanathan J, Swischuk LE. Spectrum of clinical and radiographic findings in pediatric mycoplasma pneumonia. *Radiographics.* 2001;21:121–131.
163. Toikka P, Virkki R, Mertsola J, et al. Bacterimic pneumococcal pneumonia in children. *Clin Infect Dis.* 1999;29(3):568–572.
164. Korppi M, Kiekara O, Heiskanen-Kosma T, et al. Comparison of radiological findings and microbial aetiology of childhood pneumonia. *Acta Paediatr.* 1993;82(4):360–363.
165. Tomanen E, Austrian R, Masure HR. Pathogenesis of Pneumococcal infection. *N Engl J Med.* 2009;332:1280–1284.
166. Hausdorff WP, Bryant J, Paradiso PR, et al. Which pneumococcal serogroups cause the most invasive disease: implications for conjugate vaccine formulation and use, part I. *Clin Infect Dis.* 2000;30:100–121.

167. Kin N, Crawford D, Liu J, et al. DNA microarray gene expression profile of marginal zone versus follicular B cells and idiotype marginal zone B cells before and after immunization with *Streptococcus pneumonia*. *J Immunol.* 2008;180:6663–6674.
168. Reynolds JH, McDonald G, Alton H, et al. Pneumonia in the immunocompetent patient. *Br J Radiol.* 2010;83(996): 998–1009. doi: 1259/bjr/31200593.
169. O'Brien KL, Wolfson LJ, Watt JP, et al. Burden of disease caused by *Streptococcus pneumoniae* in children younger than 5 years: global estimates. *Lancet.* 2009;374:893–902.
170. Ort S, Ryan JL, Barden G, et al. Pneumococcal pneumonia in hospitalized patients. Clinical and radiological presentations. *J Am Med Assoc.* 1983;249:214–218.
171. Kim Y, Donnelly LF. Round pneumonia: imaging findings in a large series of children. *Pediatr Radiol.* 2007;37:1235–1240.
172. Restrepo R, Palani R, Matapathi U, et al. Imaging of round pneumonia and mimics in children. *Pediatr Radiol.* 2010;40(12): 1931–1940.
173. O'Loughlin RE, Roberson A, Cieslak PR, et al. The epidemiology of invasive group A streptococcal infection and potential vaccine implications: United States, 2000–2004. *Clin Infect Dis.* 2007;45:853–862.
174. Carapetis J, Steer AC, Mulholland EK, et al. The global burden of group A streptococcal diseases. *Lancet Infect Dis.* 2005; 5:685–694.
175. Gupta R, Faridi MM, Gupta P. Neonatal empyema thoracis. *Indian J Pediatr.* 1996;63:704–706.
176. Thaarup J, Ellermann-Eriksen S, Stjernholm J. Neonatal pleural empyema with group A *Streptococcus*. *Acta Paediatr.* 1997; 86(7):769–791.
177. Gillet Y, Vanhems P, Lina G, et al. Factors predicting mortality in necrotizing community-acquired pneumonia caused by Staphylococcus aureus containing panton-valentine leukocidin. *Clin Infect Dis.* 2007;45:315–321.
178. Thomas B, Pugalenthi A, Chivers M. Pleuropulmonary complications of PVL-positive *Staphylococcus aureus* infection in children. *Acta Paediatr.* 2009;98:1372–1375.
179. Wong KS, Lin TY, Huang YC, et al. Clinical and radiographic spectrum of septic pulmonary embolism. *Arch Dis Child.* 2002; 87(4):312–315.
180. Celebi S, Hacimustafaoglu M, Demirkaya M. Septic pulmonary embolism in a child. *Indian Pediatr.* 2008;45(5):415–417.
181. Erdem G, Bergert L, Len K, et al. Radiological findings of community-acquired methicillin-resistant and methicillin-susceptible *Staphylococcus aureus* pediatric pneumonia in Hawaii. *Pediatr Radiol.* 2010;40(11):1768–1773.
182. Macfarlane J, Rose D. Radiographic features of staphylococcal pneumonia in adults and children. *Thorax.* 1996;51:539–540.
183. Gonzalez BE, Hulten KG, Dishop MK, et al. Pulmonary manifestations in children with invasive community-acquired *Staphylococcus aureus* infection. *Clin Infect Dis.* 2005;41(5): 583–590.
184. Asmar BI, Slovis TL, Reed JO, et al. Hemophilus influenzae type B pneumonia in 43 children. *J Pediatr.* 1978;93:389–393.
185. Mastrantonio P, Stefanelli P, Giuliano M, et al. Bordetella parapertussis infection in children: epidemiology, clinical symptoms, and molecular characteristics of isolates. *J Clin Microbiol.* 1998;36(4):999–1002.
186. Burns JL, Gibson RL, McNamara S, et al. Longitudinal assessment of *Pseudomonas aeruginosa* in young children with cystic fibrosis. *J Infect Dis.* 2001;183:444–452.
187. Shah RM, Wechsler R, Salazar AM, et al. Spectrum of CT findings in nosocomial *Pseudomonas aeroginosa* pneumonia. *J Thorac Imaging.* 2002;17(1):53–57.
188. Neil K, Berkelman R. Increasing incidence of legionellosis in the united states, 1990–2005: changing epidemiologic trends. *Clin Infect Dis.* 2008;47(5):591–599.
189. Quagliano PV, Das NL. Legionella pneumonia causing multiple cavitating pulmonary nodules in a 7-month-old infant. *AJR Am J Roentgenol.* 1993;161:367–368.
190. Zaleznik DF. Pneumina caused by *Chlamydia pneumoniae* in adults. In: Bartlett JG, ed. *UpToDate.* Waltham, MA. Accessed December 2, 2016.
191. Lieberman D, Ben-Yaakov M, Lazarovich Z, et al. *Chlamydia pneumonia* community-acquired pneumonia: a review of 62 hospitalized adult patients. *Infection.* 1996;24:109–114.
192. Radkowski MA, Kranzler JK, Baem MO, et al. *Chlamydia trachomatis* in infants: radiography in 125 cases. *AJR Am J Roentgenol.* 1981;137(4):703–706.
193. Hsieh SC, Kuo YT, Chern MS, et al. Mycoplasma pneumonia: clinical and radiographic features in 39 children. *Pediatr Int.* 2007;49(3):363–367.
194. Reittner P, Muller NL, Heyneman L, et al. Mycoplasma pneumonia pneumonia: radiographic and HRCT features in 28 patients. *AJR Am J Roentgenol.* 2000;174:37–41.
195. Guckel C, Benz-Bohm G, Widemann B. Mycoplama pneumonias in childhood. Roentgen features, differential diagnosis and review of literature. *Pediatr Radiol.* 1989;9(8):499–503.
196. Kim CK, Chung CY, Kim JS, et al. Late abnormal findings on high resolution computed tomography after mycoplasma pneumonia. *Pediatrics.* 2000;105:372–378.
197. World Health Organization (WHO). The burden of disease caused by TB. World Health Organization Tuberculosis Report 2014. Geneva. 2014:7–31.
198. Inselman LS. Tuberculosis in children: an update. *Pediatr Pulmonol.* 1996;21:101–120.
199. Nelson LJ, Wells CD. Global epidemiology of childhood TB. *Int J Tuberc Lung Dis.* 2004;8(5):536–647.
200. Nicol MP, Workman L, Isaacs W, et al. Accuracy of the Xpert MTB/RIF test for the diagnosis of pulmonary tuberculosis in children admitted to hospital in cape town, south africa: a descriptive study. *Lancet Infect Dis.* 2011;11(11): 819–824.
201. Leung AN, Muller NL, Pineda PR, et al. Primary tuberculosis in childhood: radiographic manifestations. *Radiology.* 1992; 182:87–91.
202. Kim WS, Moon WK, Kim IO, et al. Pulmonary tuberculosis in children: evaluation with CT. *AJR Am J Roentgenol.* 1997; 168:1005–1009.
203. Andronikou S, Joseph E, Lucas S, et al. CT scanning for the detection of tuberculous mediastinal and hilar lymphadenopathy in children. *Pediatr Radiol.* 2004;34:232–236.
204. Marais BJ, Gie RP, Schaaf HS, et al. The natural history of childhood intrathoracic tuberculosis: a critical review of prechemotherapy literature. *Int J Tuberc Lung Dis.* 2004; 8:392–402.
205. Moon WK, Kim WS, Kim, IO. Complicated pleural tuberculosis in children: CT evaluation. *Pediatr Radiol.* 1999;29: 153–157.
206. Marais BJ. State of the Art series: global pediatric pulmonary issues-tuberculosis in children. *Pediatr Pulmonol.* 2008;43: 322–329.

207. Leung AN. Pulmonary tuberculosis: the essentials. *Radiographics.* 1999;210:307–322.
208. Kim HY, Song KS, Goo JM, et al. Thoracic sequelae and complications of tuberculosis. *Radiographics.* 2001;21(4):839–858.
209. Falkinham JO. The changing pattern of nontuberculous mycobacterial disease. *Can J Infect Dis.* 2003;14(5):281–286.
210. Esther CR, Henry MM, Molina PL, et al. Nontuberculous mycobacterial infection in young children with cystic fibrosis. *Pediatr Pulmonol.* 2005;40(1):39–44.
211. Griffith DE, Girard WM, Wallace RJ. Clinical features of pulmonary disease caused by rapidly growing mycobacteria. An analysis of 154 patients. *Am Rev Respir Dis.* 1993;147:1271–1278.
212. Nolt D, Michaels MG, Wald ER. Intrathoracic disease from nontuberculous mycobacteria in children: two cases and a review of the literature. *Pediatrics.* 2003;112;e434–e439.
213. Freeman AF, Olivier KN, Rubio TT, et al. Intrathoracic nontuberculous mycobacterial infections in otherwise healthy children. *Pediatr Pulmonol.* 2009;44:1051–1056.
214. Johnson MM, Odell JA. Nontuberculous mycobacterial pulmonary infections. *J Thorac Dis.* 2014;6(3):210–220.
215. Foster K, Alton H. Chronic lung infection in children. *Paediatr Respir Rev.* 2003;4:225–229.
216. Thomas KE, Owens CM, Veys PA, et al. The radiological spectrum of invasive aspergillosis in children: a 10-year review. *Pediatr Radiol.* 2003;33:453–460.
217. Copley SJ. Application of computed tomography in childhood respiratory infections. *Br Med Bull.* 2002;61:263–279.
218. Eslamy HK, Newman B. Pneumonia in normal and immunocompromised children: an overview and update. *Radiol Clin North Am.* 2011;49:895–920.
219. Houston S. Histoplasmosis and pulmonary involvement in the tropics. *Thorax.* 1994;49:598–601.
220. McAdams HP, Rosado-de-Christenson ML, Lesar M. Thoracic mycoses from endemic fungi: radiologic-pathologic correlation. *Radiographics.* 1995;15:255–270.
221. Kirchner SG, Hernanz-Schulman M, Stein SM, et al. Imaging of Pediatric mediastinal histoplasmosis. *Radiographics.* 1991;11:365–381.
222. Galgiani JN, Ampel NM, Blair JE, et al. Coccidioidomycosis. *Clin Infect Dis.* 2005;41:1217–1223.
223. McCarty JM, Demetral LC, Dabrawski L, et al. Pediatric coccidioidomycosis in central California: a retrospective case series. *Clin Infect Dis.* 2013;56(11):1579–1585.
224. Child DD, Newell JD, Bjelland JC, et al. Radiographic findings of pulmonary coccidioidomycosis in neonates and infants. *AJR Am J Roentgenol.* 1985;145:261–263.
225. Slogrove AL, Cotton MF, Esser MM. Severe infections in HIV-exposed uninfected infants: clinical evidence of immunodeficiency. *J Trop Pediatr.* 2010;56(2):75–81.
226. Shankar SM, Nania JJ. Management of *Pneumocystis jiroveci* pneumonia in children receiving chemotherapy. *Pediatr Drugs.* 2007;9(5):301–309.
227. De Lorenzo LJ, Huang CT, Maguire GP, et al. Roentgenographic patterns of pneumocystis carinii pneumonia in 104 patients with AIDS. *Chest.* 1987;91(3):323–327.
228. George R, Andronikou S, Theron S, et al. Pulmonary infections in HIV-positive children. *Pediatr Radiol.* 2009;39:545–554.
229. Mofenson LM, Brady MT, Danner SP, et al. Guidelines for the prevention and treatment of opportunistic infections among HIV-exposed and HIV-infected children: recommendations from CDC, the National Institutes of Health, the HIV Medicine Association of the Infectious Diseases Society of America, the Pediatric Infectious Diseases Society, and the American Academy of Pediatrics. *MMWR Recomm Rep.* 2009;58:1–166.
230. El-Mahallawy HA, Attia I, Ali-El-Din NH, et al. A prospective study on fungal infection in children with cancer. *J Med Microbiol.* 2002;51:601–605.
231. Pasqualotto AC. Candida and the paediatric lung. *Paediatr Respir Rev.* 2009;10(4):186–191.
232. Buff SJ, McLelland R, Gallis HA, et al. *Candida albicans* pneumonia: radiographic appearance. *AJR Am J Roentgenol.* 1982;138:645–648.
233. Pappas PG, Rex JH, Sobel JD, et al. Guidelines for treatment of candidiasis. *Clin Infect Dis.* 2004;38(2):161–189.
234. Xu HZ, Tang LF, Zheng XP, et al. Paragonimiasis in chinese children: 58 cases analysis. *Iran J Pediatr.* 2012;22(4):505–511.
235. Martinez S, Restrepo CS, Carillo JA, et al. Thoracic manifestations of tropical parasitic infections: a pictorial review. *Radiographics.* 2005;25:135–155.
236. Henry TS, Lane MA, Weil GJ, et al. Chest CT features of North American paragonimiasis. *AJR Am J Roentgenol.* 2012;198(5):1076–1083.
237. Procop GW. North American paragonimiasis (caused by Paragonimus kellicotti) in the context of global paragonimiasis. *Clin Microbiol Rev.* 2009;22:415–446.
238. Yuksel M, Dermirpolat G, Sever A, et al. Hydatid disease involving some rare locations in the body: a pictorial assay. *Korean J Radiol.* 2007;8:531–540.
239. Czermak BV, Unsinn KM, Gotwald T, et al. Echinococcus granulosus revisited: radiologic patterns seen in pediatric and adult patients. *AJR Am J Roentgenol.* 2001;177:1051–1056.
240. Santivanez S, Garcia HH. Pulmonary cystic echinococcosis. *Curr Pin Pulm Med.* 2010;16(3):257–261.
241. Pinch LW, Wilson JF. Non-surgical management of cystic hydatid disease in alaska. *Ann Surg.* 1973;178(1):45–48.
242. Lewall DB. Hydatid disease: biology, pathology, imaging, and classification. *Clin Radiol.* 1998;53:863–874.
243. Chen KC, Su YT, Chiu KC, et al. Clinical analysis of necrotizing pneumonia in children: three year experience in a single medical center. *Acta Paediatr Taiwan.* 2003;44(6):343–348.
244. Hodina M, Hanquinet S, Scnyder P, et al. Imaging of cavitary necrosis in complicated pneumonia. *Eur Radiol.* 2002;12(2):391–396.
245. Hoffer FA, Bloom DA, Colin AA, et al. Lung abscess versus necrotizing pneumonia: implications for interventional therapy. *Pediatr Radiol.* 1999;29:87–91.
246. Kurian J, Levin TL, Han BK, et al. Comparison of ultrasound and CT in the evaluation of pneumonia complicated by parapneumonic effusion in children. *AJR Am J Roentgenol.* 2009;193:1648–1654.
247. Lynch DA, Brasch RC, Hardy KA, et al. Pediatric pulmonary disease: assessment with high-resolution ultrafast CT. *Radiology.* 1990;176:243–248.
248. Erasmus J, Page McAdams H, Rossi S, et al. Percutaneous management of intrapulmonary air and fluid collections. *Radiol Clin North Am.* 2000;38:385–393.
249. Kothari PR, Jiwane A, Kulkarni B. Pulmonary gangrene complicating bacterial pneumonia. *Indian Pediatr.* 2003;40(8):784–785.
250. Kornreich L, Horev G, Ziv N, et al. Bronchiectasis in children: assessment by CT. *Pediatr Radiol.* 1993;23:12–123.

251. Cohen MC, Kaschula RO. Primary pulmonary tumors in childhood: a review of 31 years' experience and the literature. *Pediatr Pulmonol.* 1992;14(4):222–232.
252. Dishop MK, Kuruvilla S. Primary and metastatic lung tumors in the pediatric population: a review and 25-year experience at a large children's hospital. *Arch Pathol Lab Med.* 2008;132(7): 1079–1103.
253. Hancock BJ, Di Lorenzo M, Youssef S, et al. Childhood primary pulmonary neoplasms. *J Pediatr Surg.* 1993;28(9):1133–1136.
254. Arrigoni MG, Woolner LB, Bernatz PE, et al. Benign tumors of the lung. A ten-year surgical experience. *J Thorac Cardiovasc Surg.* 1970;60(4):589–599.
255. Beasley MB, Travis WD. Sclerosing Pneumocytoma. In: Travis WD, Brambilla E, Burke AP, et al., eds. *World Health Organization Classification of Tumours Pathology and Genetics of Tumours of the Lung, Pleura, Thymus and Heart.* Lyon, France: IARC Press; 2015:110–111.
256. Liebow AA, Hubbell DS. Sclerosing hemangioma (histiocytoma, xanthoma) of the lung. *Cancer.* 1956;9(1):53–75.
257. Devouassoux-Shisheboran M, Hayashi T, Linnoila RI, et al. A clinicopathologic study of 100 cases of pulmonary sclerosing hemangioma with immunohistochemical studies: TTF-1 is expressed in both round and surface cells, suggesting an origin from primitive respiratory epithelium. *Am J Surg Pathol.* 2000;24(7):906–916.
258. Im JG, Kim WH, Han MC, et al. Sclerosing hemangiomas of the lung and interlobar fissures: CT findings. *J Comput Assist Tomogr.* 1994;18(1):34–38.
259. Nam JE, Ryu YH, Cho SH, et al. Air-trapping zone surrounding sclerosing hemangioma of the lung. *J Comput Assist Tomogr.* 2002;26(3):358–361.
260. Fujiyoshi F, Ichinari N, Fukukura Y, et al. Sclerosing hemangioma of the lung: MR findings and correlation with pathological features. *J Comput Assist Tomogr.* 1998;22(6):1006–1008.
261. Lee E, Park CM, Kang KW, et al. 18F-FDG PET/CT features of pulmonary sclerosing hemangioma. *Acta Radiol.* 2013; 54(1):24–29.
262. Johansson M, Dietrich C, Mandahl N, et al. Recombinations of chromosomal bands 6p21 and 14q24 characterise pulmonary hamartomas. *Br J Cancer.* 1993;67(6):1236–1241.
263. Bateson EM, Abbott EK. Mixed tumors of the lung, or hamarto-chondromas. A review of the radiological appearances of cases published in the literature and a report of fifteen new cases. *Clin Radiol.* 1960;11:232–247.
264. Potente G, Macori F, Caimi M, et al. Noncalcified pulmonary hamartomas: computed tomography enhancement patterns with histologic correlation. *J Thorac Imaging.* 1999;14(2): 101–104.
265. Guo W, Zhao YP, Jiang YG, et al. Surgical treatment and outcome of pulmonary hamartoma: a retrospective study of 20-year experience. *J Exp Clin Cancer Res.* 2008;27:8.
266. Alexopoulou E, Economopoulos N, Priftis KN, et al. MR imaging findings of an atypical pulmonary hamartoma in a 12-year-old child. *Pediatr Radiol.* 2008;38(10):1134–1137.
267. Sminohara S, Hanagiri T, Kuwata T, et al. Clinical characteristics of pulmonary hamartoma resected surgically as undiagnosed pulmonary nodule. *J UOEH.* 2012;34(1):41–46.
268. Messinger YH, Stewart DR, Priest JR, et al. Pleuropulmonary blastoma: a report on 350 central pathology-confirmed pleuropulmonary blastoma cases by the International Pleuropulmonary Blastoma Registry. *Cancer.* 2015;121(2): 276–285.
269. Priest JR, McDermott MB, Bhatia S, et al. Pleuropulmonary blastoma: a clinicopathologic study of 50 cases. *Cancer.* 1997; 80(1):147–161.
270. Priest JR, Watterson J, Strong L, et al. Pleuropulmonary blastoma: a marker for familial disease. *J Pediatr.* 1996; 128(2):220–224.
271. Orazi C, Inserra A, Schingo PM, et al. Pleuropulmonary blastoma, a distinctive neoplasm of childhood: report of three cases. *Pediatr Radiol.* 2007;37(4):337–344.
272. Amini B, Huang SY, Tsai J, et al. Primary lung and large airway neoplasms in children: current imaging evaluation with multidetector computed tomography. *Radiol Clin North Am.* 2013;51(4):637–657.
273. Geiger J, Walter K, Uhl M, et al. Imaging findings in a 3-year-old girl with type III pleuropulmonary blastoma. *In Vivo.* 2007;21(6):1119–1122.
274. Travis WD, Rush W, Flieder DB, et al. Survival analysis of 200 pulmonary neuroendocrine tumors with clarification of criteria for atypical carcinoid and its separation from typical carcinoid. *Am J Surg Pathol.* 1998;22(8):934–944.
275. Chong S, Lee KS, Chung MJ, et al. Neuroendocrine tumors of the lung: clinical, pathologic, and imaging findings. *Radiographics.* 2006;26(1):41–57; discussion 57–48.
276. Yu DC, Grabowski MJ, Kozakewich HP, et al. Primary lung tumors in children and adolescents: a 90-year experience. *J Pediatr Surg.* 2010;45(6):1090–1095.
277. Borczuk A, Coffin C, Fletcher CDM. Inflammatory myofibroblastic tumor. In: Travis WD, Brambilla E, Burke AP, et al., eds. *World Health Organization Classification of Tumours Pathology and Genetics of Tumours of the Lung, Pleura, Thymus and Heart.* Lyon, France: IARC Press; 2015:121–122.
278. Coffin CM, Alaggio R. Fibroblastic and myofibroblastic tumors in children and adolescents. *Pediatr Dev Pathol.* 2012;15 (1 suppl):127–180.
279. Agrons GA, Rosado-de-Christenson ML, Kirejczyk WM, et al. Pulmonary inflammatory pseudotumor: radiologic features. *Radiology.* 1998;206(2):511–518.
280. Pettinato G, Manivel JC, De Rosa N, et al. Inflammatory myofibroblastic tumor (plasma cell granuloma). Clinicopathologic study of 20 cases with immunohistochemical and ultrastructural observations. *Am J Clin Pathol.* 1990;94(5):538–546.
281. Matsubara O, Tan-Liu NS, Kenney RM, et al. Inflammatory pseudotumors of the lung: progression from organizing pneumonia to fibrous histiocytoma or to plasma cell granuloma in 32 cases. *Hum Pathol.* 1988;19(7):807–814.
282. Hartman GE, Shochat SJ. Primary pulmonary neoplasms of childhood: a review. *Ann Thorac Surg.* 1983;36(1):108–119.
283. Kim TS, Han J, Kim GY, et al. Pulmonary inflammatory pseudotumor (inflammatory myofibroblastic tumor): CT features with pathologic correlation. *J Comput Assist Tomogr.* 2005;29(5):633–639.
284. Takayama Y, Yabuuchi H, Matsuo Y, et al. Computed tomographic and magnetic resonance features of inflammatory myofibroblastic tumor of the lung in children. *Radiat Med.* 2008;26(10):613–617.
285. Huellner MW, Schwizer B, Burger I, et al. Inflammatory pseudotumor of the lung with high FDG uptake. *Clin Nucl Med.* 2010;35(9):722–723.
286. Veliath AJ, Khanna KK, Subhas BS, et al. Primary lymphosarcoma of the lung with unusual features. *Thorax.* 1977;32(5):632–636.
287. Sery Z. Pulmonary resection in children. *Surgery.* 1963;54: 810–814.

288. National Cancer Institute (U.S.), Surveillance Program, SEER Program (National Cancer Institute (U.S.)), National Center for Health Statistics (U.S.), National Institutes of Health (U.S.). *SEER Cancer Statistics Review, 1975-2008. NIH Publication.* Bethesda, MD: U.S. Dept. of Health and Human Services, Public Health Institute, National Institutes of Health, National Cancer Institute; 2011.
289. Freed J, Kelly KM. Current approaches to the management of pediatric Hodgkin lymphoma. *Paediatr Drugs.* 2010;12(2):85–98.
290. Gross TG, Termuhlen AM. Pediatric non-Hodgkin lymphoma. *Curr Hematol Malig Rep.* 2008;3(3):167–173.
291. Mynarek M, Schober T, Behrends U, et al. Posttransplant lymphoproliferative disease after pediatric solid organ transplantation. *Clin Dev Immunol.* 2013;2013:814973.
292. Wilde GE, Moore DJ, Bellah RD. Posttransplantation lymphoproliferative disorder in pediatric recipients of solid organ transplants: timing and location of disease. *AJR Am J Roentgenol.* 2005;185(5):1335–1341.
293. Siegel MJ, Lee EY, Sweet SC, et al. CT of posttransplantation lymphoproliferative disorder in pediatric patients of lung allograft. *AJR Am J Roentgenol.* 2003;181(4):1125–1131.
294. Hryhorczuk AL, Kim HB, Harris MH, et al. Imaging findings of children with proliferative disorders following multivisceral transplantation. *Pediatr Radiol.* 2015;45(8):1138–1145.
295. Maturen KE, Blane CE, Strouse PJ, et al. Pulmonary involvement in pediatric lymphoma. *Pediatr Radiol.* 2004;34(2):120–124.
296. Berkman N, Breuer R, Kramer MR, et al. Pulmonary involvement in lymphoma. *Leuk Lymphoma.* 1996;20(3–4):229–237.
297. McCahon E. Lung tumours in children. *Paediatr Respir Rev.* 2006;7(3):191–196.
298. Tronc F, Conter C, Marec-Berard P, et al. Prognostic factors and long-term results of pulmonary metastasectomy for pediatric histologies. *Eur J Cardiothor Surg.* 2008;34(6):1240–1246.
299. Hammer MR, Dillman JR, Chong ST, et al. Imaging of pediatric thoracic trauma. *Semin Roentgenol.* 2012;47(2):135–146.
300. Avarello JT, Cantor RM. Pediatric major trauma: an approach to evaluation and management. *Emerg Med Clin North Am.* 2007;25:803–836.
301. Jaffe D. Emergency management of blunt trauma in children. *N Engl J Med.* 1991;324:1477–1482.
302. Bliss D, Silen M. Pediatric thoracic trauma. *Crit Care Med.* 2002;30(11 suppl):S409–S415.
303. Westra SJ, Wallace EC. Imaging evaluation of pediatric chest trauma. *Radiol Clin North Am.* 2005;43:267–281.
304. Haider AH, Risucci D, Omer S, et al. Determination of national pediatric injury prevention priorities using the injury prevention priority score. *J Pediatr Surg.* 2004;39:976–978.
305. Cyr C, Xhignesse M, Lacroix J, et al. Severe injury mechanisms in two paediatric trauma centres. Determination of prevention priorities. *Paediatr Child Health.* 2008;13:165–170.
306. Manson D, Babyn PS, Palder S, et al. CT of blunt chest trauma in children. *Pediatr Radiol.* 1993;23:1–5.
307. Markel TA, Kumar R, Koontz NA, et al. The utility of computed tomography as a screening tool for the evaluation of pediatric blunt chest trauma. *J Trauma.* 2009;67:23–28.
308. Moore MA, Wallace EC, Westra SJ. Advances in pediatric thoracic imaging chest trauma in children: current imaging guidelines and techniques. *Radiol Clin North Am.* 2011 49(5):949–968.
309. Cohn SM. Pulmonary contusion: review of the clinical entity. *J Trauma.* 1997;42:973–979.
310. Sartorelli KH, Vane DW. The diagnosis and management of children with blunt injury of the chest. *Semin Pediatr Surg.* 2004;13:98–105.
311. Moore MA, Wallace EC, Westra SJ, et al. The imaging of paediatric thoracic trauma. *Pediatr Radiol.* 2009;39:485–496.
312. Nakayama DK, Ramenofsky ML, Rowe MI. Chest injuries in children. *Ann Surg.* 1989;210:770–775.
313. Hamrick MC, Duhn RD, Carney DE, et al. Pulmonary contusion in the pediatric population. *Am Surg.* 2010;76:721–724.
314. Patel RP, Hernanz-Schulman M, Hilmes MA, et al. Pediatric chest CT after trauma. Impact on surgical and clinical management. *Pediatr Radiol.* 2010;40:1246–1253.
315. Allen GS, Cox CS, Moore FA, et al. Pulmonary contusion: are children different? *J Am Coll Surg.* 1997;185:229–233.
316. Allen GS, Cox CS. Pulmonary contusion in children: diagnosis and management. *South Med J.* 1998;91:1099–1106.
317. Davis SL, Furman DP, Costarino AT. Adult respiratory distress syndrome in children: associated disease, clinical course and predictors of death. *J Pediatr.* 1993;123:35–45.
318. Kwon A, Sorrells DL, Kurkchubasche AG, et al. Isolated computed tomography diagnosis of pulmonary contusion does not correlate with increased morbidity. *J Pediatr Surg.* 2006;41:78–82.
319. Donnelly LF, Klosterman LA. Subpleural sparing: a CT finding of lung contusion in children. *Radiology.* 1997;204(2):385–387.
320. Deunk J, Poels TC, Brink M, et al. The clinical outcome of occult pulmonary contusion on multidetector-row computed tomography in blunt trauma patients. *J Trauma.* 2010;68(2):387–394.
321. Wagner RB, Crawford WO, Schimpf PP, et al. Classification of parenchymal injuries of the lung. *Radiology.* 1988;167(1):77–82.
322. Cooper A, Barlow B, DiScala C, et al. Mortality and truncal injury: the pediatric perspective. *J Pediatr Surg.* 1994;29(1):33–38.
323. Tsitouridis I, Tsinoglou K, Tsandiridis C, et al. Traumatic pulmonary pseudocysts: CT findings. *J Thorac Imaging.* 2007;22:247–251.
324. Galea MH, Williams N, Mayell MJ, et al. Traumatic pneumatocele. *J Pediatr Surg.* 1992;27:1523–1524.
325. Chon SH, Lee CB, Kim H, et al. Diagnosis and prognosis of traumatic pulmonary psuedocysts: a review of 12 cases. *Eur J Cardiothorac Surg.* 2006;29(5):819–823.
326. Cheung NK, James A, Kumar R. Large Traumatic pneumatocele in a 2-year-old child. *Case Rep Pediatr.* 2013;2013:940189. doi: 10.1155/2013/940189.
327. Chung MP, Yi CA, Lee HY, et al. Imaging of pulmonary vasculitis. *Radiology.* 2010;255(2):322–341. doi: 10.1148/radiol.10090105.
328. Frankel SK, Jayne D. The pulmonary vasculitides. *Clin Chest Med.* 2010;31:519–536.
329. Jennette JC, Falk RJ, Andrassy K, et al. Nomenclature of systemic vasculitides. Proposal of an international consensus conference. *Arthritis Rheum.* 1994;37(2):187–192.
330. Dedeoglu F, Sundel RP. Vasculitis in children. *Rheum Dis Clin North Am.* 2007;33:555–583.
331. Levine D, Akikusa J, Manson D, et al. Chest CT findings in pediatric Wegener's granulomatosis. *Pediatr Radiol.* 2007;37(1):57–62.
332. Castañer E, Alguersuari A, Gallardo X, et al. When to suspect pulmonary vasculitis: radiologic and clinical clues. *Radiographics.* 2010;30:33–53.

333. O'Sullivan BP. Pulmonary complications of systemic vasculitides. *Paediatr Respir Rev.* 2012;13(1):37–43.
334. Martín-Suné N, Ríos-Blanco JJ. Pulmonary affectation of vasculitis. *Arch Bronconeumol.* 2012;48(11):410–418.
335. Rottem M, Fauci AS, et al. Wegener granulomatosis in children and adolescents: clinical presentation and outcome. *J Pediatr.* 1993;122:26–31.
336. Wadsworth D, Siegel M, Day D. Wegener's granulomatosis in children: chest radiographic manifestations. *AJR Am J Roentgenol.* 1994;163:901–904.
337. García-Peña P, Boixadera H, Barber I, et al. Thoracic findings of systemic diseases at high-resolution CT in children. *Radiographics.* 2011;31:465–482.
338. Eleftheriou D, Brogan PA. Vasculitis in children. *Paediatr Child Health.* 2014;24(2):58–63. http://dx.doi.org/10.1016/j.paed.2013.07.006
339. Kelly A, Tizard JE. Vasculitis in children. *Paediatr Child Health.* 2009;20:2.
340. Zwerina J, Eger G, Englbrecht M, et al. Churg-Strauss syndrome in childhood: a systematic literature review and clinical comparison with adult patients. *Semin Arthritis Rheum.* 2009; 39:108–115.
341. Boyer D, Vargas SO, Slattery D, et al. Churg-Strauss syndrome in children: a clinical and pathologic review. *Pediatrics.* 2006; 118(3):e914–e920.
342. Silva CI, Müller NL, Fujimoto K, et al. Churg-Strauss syndrome: high resolution CT and pathologic findings. *J Thorac Imaging.* 2005;20(2):74–80.
343. Lynch DA, Hay T, Newell JD, et al. Pediatric diffuse lung disease: diagnosis and classification using high-resolution CT. *AJR Am J Roentgenol.* 1999;173(3):713–718.
344. Guillevin L, Lhote F, Gayraud M, et al. Prognostic factors in polyarteritis nodosa and Churg-Strauss syndrome. A prospective study in 342 patients. *Medicine.* 1996;75:17–28.
345. Poddar B, Singhal S, Azim A, et al. Goodpasture's syndrome in children. *Saudi J Kidney Dis Transpl.* 2010;21(5):935–939.
346. Koscielska-Kasprzak K, Bartoszek D, Myszka M, et al. The complement cascade and renal disease. *Arch Immunol Ther Exp (Warsz).* 2014;62(1):47–57.
347. Kim YO, Choi JY, Park JI, et al. A case of Goodpasture's syndrome with massive pulmonary hemorrhage. *J Korean Med Sci.* 2000;15:99–102.
348. Mayberry JP, Primack SL, Müller NL. Thoracic manifestations of systemic autoimmune diseases: radiographic and high-resolution CT findings. *Radiographics.* 2000;20(6):1623–1635.
349. Lucaya J, Garel L, Piqueras J. Clinical quiz: Goodpasture's syndrome along with Wegner's granulomatosis with pulmonary hemorrhage. *Pediatr Radiol.* 2003;33(8):591–592.
350. Bogdanović R, Minić P, Marković-Lipkovski J, et al. Pulmonary renal syndrome in a child with coexistence of anti-neutrophil cytoplasmic antibodies and anti-glomerular basement membrane disease: case report and literature review. *BMC Nephrol.* 2013;14:66. doi: 10.1186/1471-2369-14-66.
351. Madani G, Papadopoulou AM, Holloway B, et al. The radiological manifestations of sickle cell disease. *Clin Radiol.* 2007; 62:528–538.
352. Kanter J, Kruse-Jarres R. Management of sickle cell disease from childhood through adulthood. *Blood Rev.* 2013;27:279–287.
353. Quinn CT. Sickle cell disease in childhood from newborn screening through transition to adult medical care. *Pediatr Clin North Am.* 2013;60:1363–1381.
354. Charache S, Scott JC, Charache P. "Acute chest syndrome" in adults with sickle cell anemia. Microbiology, treatment, and prevention. *Arch Intern Med.* 1979;139:67–69.
355. Martin L, Buonomo C. Acute chest syndrome of sickle cell disease: radiographic and clinical analysis of 70 cases. *Pediatr Radiol.* 1997;27:637–641.
356. Telfer P, Coen P, Chakravorty S, et al. Clinical outcomes in children with sickle cell disease living in England: a neonatal cohort in East London. *Haematologica.* 2007;92(7):905–912.
357. Crowley JJ, Sarnaik S. Imaging of sickle cell disease. *Pediatr Radiol.* 1999;29:646–661.
358. Bhalla M, Abboud MR, McLoud TC, et al. Acute chest syndrome in sickle cell disease: CT evidence of microvascular occlusion. *Radiology.* 1993;187:45–49.
359. Aquino SL, Gamsu G, Fahy JV. Chronic pulmonary disorders in sickle cell disease: findings at thin section CT. *Radiology.* 1994;193:807–811.
360. Roger E, Letts M. Sickle cell disease of the spine in children. *Can J Surg.* 1999;42(4):289–292.
361. Ejundu VC, Hine AL, Mashayeshi M, et al. Musculoskeletal manifestations of sickle cell disease. *Radiographics.* 2007; 27(4):1005–1021.
362. Hugosson CO, Riff EJ, Moore CCM, et al. Lipoid pneumonia in infants: a radiological-pathological study. *Pediatr Radiol.* 1991;21:193–197.
363. De Oliveira GA, Del Caro SR, Bender Lamego CM, et al. Radiographic plain film and CT findings in lipoid pneumonia in infants following aspiration of mineral oil used in the treatment of partial small bowel obstruction by Ascaris lumbricoides. *Pediatr Radiol.* 1985;15:157–160.
364. Baron SE, Haramati LB, Rivera VT. Radiological and clinical findings in acute and chronic exogenous lipoid pneumonia. *J Thorac Imaging.* 2003;18:217–224.
365. Kazachkov MY, Muhlebach MS, Livasy CA, et al. Lipid-laden macrophage index and inflammation in bronchoalveolar lavage fluids in children. *Eur Respir J.* 2001;18(5):790–795.
366. Betancourt SL, Martinez-Jimenez S, Rossi SE, et al. Lipoid pneumonia: spectrum of clinical and radiologic manifestations. *AJR Am J Roentgenol.* 2010;194:103–109.
367. Lee KH, Kim WS, Cheon JE, et al. Squalene aspiration pneumonia in children: radiographic and CT findings as the first clue to diagnosis. *Pediatr Radiol.* 2005;35:619–623.
368. Agarwal R. Low-attenuation consolidation: the most characteristic finding in lipoid pneumonia. *Eur J Intern Med.* 2006; 17(4):307.
369. Zanetti G, Marchiori E, Gasparetto TD, et al. Lipoid pneumonia in children following aspiration of mineral oil used in the treatment of constipation: high-resolution CT findings in 17 patients. *Pediatr Radiol.* 2007;37:1135–1139.
370. Hadda V, Khilnani GC, Bhalla AS, et al. Lipoid pneumonia presenting as non resolving community acquired pneumonia: a case report. *Cases J.* 2009;2:9332. doi: 10.1186/1757-1626-2-9332.
371. Banjar H. Lipoid Pneumonia: a review. *Bahrain Med Bull.* 2003;25(1):36–39.
372. Edwards MO, Kotecha SJ, Kotecha S. Respiratory distress of the term newborn infant. *Paediatr Respir Rev.* 2013;14:29–37.
373. Cleveland RH. A radiologic update on medical diseases of the newborn chest. *Pediatr Radiol.* 1995;25:631–637.
374. Holme N, Chetcuti P. The pathophysiology of respiratory distress syndrome in neonates. *Paediatr Child Health.* 2012; 22(12):507–512.

375. Arthur R. The neonatal chest x-ray. *Paediatr Respir Rev.* 2001;2(4):311–323.
376. Mahoney AD, Jain L. Respiratory disorders in moderately preterm, late preterm, and early term infants. *Clin Perinatol.* 2013;40:665–678.
377. Bancalari E, Claure N. Definitions and diagnostic criteria for bronchopulmonary dysplasia. *Semin Perinatol.* 2006;30(4): 164–170.
378. Slama M, Andre C, Huon C, et al. Radiological analysis of hyaline membrane disease after exogenous surfactant treatment. *Pediatr Radiol.* 1999;29:56–60.
379. Jain L, Eaton DC. Physiology of fetal lung fluid clearance and the effect of labor. *Semin Perinatol.* 2006;30(1):34–43.
380. Tutdibi E, Gries K, Bucheler M, et al. Impact of labor on outcomes in transient tachypnea of the newborn: population-based study. *Pediatrics.* 2010;125:e577–e583.
381. Liem JJ, Huq SI, Ekuma O, et al. Transient tachypnea of the newborn may be an early clinical manifestation of wheezing symptoms. *J Pediatr.* 2007;151:29–33.
382. Thavagnanam S, Fleming J, Bromley A, et al. A metaanalysis of the association between Caesarean section and childhood asthma. *Clin Exp Allergy.* 2008;38:629–633.
383. Walsh MC, Fanaroff JM. Meconium stained fluid: approach to the mother and the baby. *Clin Perinatol.* 2007;(34) 653–665.
384. Ross MG. Meconium aspiration syndrome—more than intrapartum meconium. *N Engl J Med.* 2005;353:946–948.
385. Dargaville PA, Copnell B. The epidemiology of meconium aspiration syndrome: incidence, risk factors, therapies, and outcome. *Pediatrics.* 2006;117:1712–1721.
386. Ford JW. Neonatal ECMO: current controversies and trends. *Neonatal Netw.* 2006;25(4):229–238.
387. Nissen MD. Congenital and neonatal pneumonia. *Paediatr Respir Rev.* 2007;8:195–203.
388. Duke T. Neonatal pneumonia in developing countries. *Arch Dis Child Fetal Neonatal Ed.* 2005;90:F211–F219.
389. Beeton ML, Maxwell NC, Davies PL, et al. Role of pulmonary infection in the development of chronic lung disease of prematurity. *Eur Respir J.* 2011;37:1424–1430.
390. Schrag SJ, Zell ER, Lynfield R, et al. A population based comparison of strategies to prevent early-onset group B streptococcal disease in neonates. *N Engl J Med.* 2002;347:233–239.
391. Berk DR, Varich LJ. Localized persistent pulmonary interstitial emphysema in a preterm infant in the absence of mechanical ventilation. *Pediatr Radiol.* 2005;35:1243–1245.
392. Boothroyd AE, Barson AJ. Pulmonary interstitial emphysema—a radiological and pathological correlation. *Pediatr Radiol.* 1988;18:194–199.
393. Miller JD, Carlo WA. Pulmonary complications of mechanical ventilation in neonates. *Clin Perinatol.* 2008;(35):273–281.
394. Donnelly LF, Lucaya J, Ozelame V, et al. CT findings and temporal course of persistent pulmonary interstitial emphysema in neonates: a multi-institutional study. *AJR Am J Roentgenol.* 2003;180:1129–1132.
395. Lee EY, Cleveland RH, Langston C. Interstitial lung disease in infants and children: new classification system with emphasis on clinical, imaging, and pathologic correlation. In: Cleveland RH, ed. *Imaging in Pediatric Pulmonology*. New York: Springer; 2011.
396. Zucker EJ, Guillerman RP, Fishman MP, et al. Diffuse lung disease. In: Coley BD, ed. *Caffey's Pediatric Diagnostic Imaging.* 12th ed. Philadelphia, PA: Elsevier/Saunders; 2013.
397. Guillerman RP, Brody AS. Contemporary perspectives on pediatric diffuse lung disease. *Radiol Clin North Am.* 2011;49: 847–868.
398. Guillerman RP. Imaging of childhood interstitial lung disease. *Pediatr Allergy Immunol Pulmonol.* 2010;23:43–68.
399. Lee EY. Interstitial lung disease in infants: new classification system, imaging technique, clinical presentation and imaging findings. *Pediatr Radiol.* 2013;43:3–13.
400. Kurland G, Deterding RR, Hagood JS, et al. An official american thoracic society clinical practice guideline: classification, evaluation, and management of childhood interstitial lung disease in infancy. *Am J Respir Crit Care Med.* 2013;188:376–394.
401. Langston C, Dishop MK. Infant lung biopsy: clarifying the pathologic spectrum. *Pathol Int.* 2004;54:s419–s421.
402. Dishop MK. Diagnostic pathology of diffuse lung disease in children. *Pediatr Allergy Immunol Pulmonol.* 2010;23: 69–85.
403. Sen P, Thakur N, Stockton DW, et al. Expanding the phenotype of alveolar capillary dysplasia (ACD). *J Pediatr.* 2004;145:646–651.
404. Licht C, Schickendantz S, Sreeram N, et al. Prolonged survival in alveolar capillary dysplasia syndrome. *Eur J Pediatr.* 2004; 163:181–182.
405. Stankiewicz P, Sen P, Bhatt SS, et al. Genomic and genic deletions of the FOX gene cluster on 16q24.1 and inactivating mutations of FOXF1 cause alveolar capillary dysplasia and other malformations. *Am J Hum Genet.* 2009;84:780–791.
406. Eulmesekian P, Cutz E, Parvez B, et al. Alveolar capillary dysplasia: a six-year single center experience. *J Perinat Med.* 2005;33:347–352.
407. Michalsky MP, Arca MJ, Groenman F, et al. Alveolar capillary dysplasia: a logical approach to a fatal disease. *J Pediatr Surg.* 2005;40:1100–1105.
408. Hugosson CO, Salama HM, Al-Dayel F, et al. Primary alveolar capillary dysplasia (acinar dysplasia) and surfactant protein B deficiency: a clinical, radiological and pathological study. *Pediatr Radiol.* 2005;35:311–316.
409. Gillespie LM, Fenton AC, Wright C. Acinar dysplasia: a rare cause of neonatal respiratory failure. *Acta Paediatr.* 2004;93: 712–713.
410. Newman B, Yunis E. Primary alveolar capillary dysplasia. *Pediatr Radiol.* 1990;21:20–22.
411. Deterding RR. Infants and young children with children's interstitial lung disease. *Pediatr Allergy Immunol Pulmonol.* 2010;23:25–31.
412. Deutsch GH, Young LR, Deterding RR, et al. Diffuse lung disease in young children: application of a novel classification scheme. *Am J Respir Crit Care Med.* 2007;176:1120–1128.
413. Owens C. Radiology of diffuse interstitial pulmonary disease in children. *Eur Radiol.* 2004;14:L2–L12.
414. Mahut B, De Blic J, Emond S, et al. Chest computed tomography findings in bronchopulmonary dysplasia and correlation with lung function. *Arch Dis Child Fetal Neonatal Ed.* 2007;92:F459–F464.
415. Biko DM, Schwartz M, Anupindi SA, et al. Subpleural lung cysts in Down syndrome: prevalence and association with coexisting diagnoses. *Pediatr Radiol.* 2008;38:280–284.
416. Taylor PA, Dishop MK, Lotze TE, et al. Congenital multilobar emphysema: a characteristic lung growth disorder attributable to Filamin A gene mutations. *Pediatr Radiol.* 2009;39(suppl 3): S516.

417. Mosca F, Colnaghi M, Fumagalli M. BPD: old and new problems. *J Matern Fetal Neonatal Med.* 2011;24(suppl 1): 80–82.
418. Kugelman A, Durand M. A comprehensive approach to the prevention of bronchopulmonary dysplasia. *Pediatr Pulmonol.* 2011;46(12):1153–1165.
419. Garmany TH, Wambach JA, Heins HB, et al. Population and disease-based prevalence of the common mutations associated with surfactant deficiency. *Pediatr Res.* 2008;63:645–649.
420. Cole FS, Hamvas A, Rubinstein P, et al. Population-based estimates of surfactant protein B deficiency. *Pediatrics.* 2000; 105:538–541.
421. Gower WA, Popler J, Hamvas A, et al. Clinical improvement in infants with ILD due to mutations in the surfactant protein C gene (SFTPC). *Am J Respir Crit Care Med.* 2010;181:A6733.
422. Rosen DM, Waltz DA. Hydroxychloroquine and surfactant protein C deficiency. *N Engl J Med.* 2005;352:207–208.
423. Karjalainen MK, Haataja R, Hallman M. Haplotype analysis of ABCA3: association with respiratory distress in very premature infants. *Ann Med.* 2008;40:56–65.
424. Clement A, Corvol H, Epaud R, et al. Dramatic improvement by macrolides in surfactant deficiency with ABCA3 mutation. *Am J Respir Crit Care Med.* 2009;179:A3011.
425. Doan ML, Guillerman RP, Dishop MK, et al. Clinical, radiological, and pathological features of ABCA3 mutations in children. *Thorax.* 2008;63:366–373.
426. Guillot L, Carre A, Szinnai G, et al. NKX2-1 mutations leading to surfactant protein promoter dysregulation cause interstitial lung disease in "Brain-Lung-Thyroid Syndrome." *Hum Mutat.* 2010;31:E1146–E1162.
427. Iwatani N, Mabe H, Devriendt K, et al. Deletion of NKX2.1 gene encoding thyroid transcription factor-1 in two siblings with hypothyroidism and respiratory failure. *J Pediatr.* 2000; 137:272–276.
428. Deterding R, Dishop MK, Uchida DA, et al. Thyroid transcription factor 1 gene abnormalities;an under recognized cause of children's interstitial lung disease. *Am J Respir Crit Care Med.* 2010;181:A6725.
429. Galambos C, Levy H, Cannon CL, et al. Pulmonary pathology in thyroid transcription factor-1 deficiency syndrome. *Am J Respir Crit Care Med.* 2010;182:549–554.
430. Willemsen MA, Breedveld GJ, Wouda S, et al. Brain-thyroid-lung syndrome: a patient with severe multi-system disorder due to a de novo mutation in the thyroid transcription factor 1 gene. *Eur J Pediatr.* 2005;164:28–30.
431. Bush A. Paediatric interstitial lung disease: not just kid's stuff. *Eur Respir J.* 2004;24:521–523.
432. Olsen E ØE, Sebire NJ, Jaffe A, et al. Chronic pneumonitis of infancy: high-resolution CT findings. *Pediatr Radiol.* 2004; 34:86–88.
433. Hamvas A. Inherited surfactant protein-B deficiency and surfactant protein-C associated disease: clinical features and evaluation. *Semin Perinatol.* 2006;30:316–326.
434. Soraisham AS, Tierney AJ, Amin HJ. Neonatal respiratory failure associated with mutation in the surfactant protein C gene. *J Perinatol.* 2006;26:67–70.
435. Prestridge A, Woodridge J, Deutsch G, et al. Persistent tachypnea and hypoxia in a 3-month-old term infant. *J Pediatr.* 2006;149:702–706.
436. Stevens PA, Pettenazzo A, Brasch F, et al. Nonspecific interstitial pneumonia, alveolar proteinosis, and abnormal proprotein trafficking resulting from a spontaneous mutation in the surfactant protein C gene. *Pediatr Res.* 2005;57:89–98.
437. Thouvenin G, Taam RA, Flamein F, et al. Characteristics of disorders associated with genetic mutations of surfactant protein C. *Arch Dis Child.* 2010;95:449–454.
438. Mechri M, Epaud R, Emond S, et al. Surfactant protein C gene (SFTPC) mutation-associated lung disease: high-resolution computed tomography (HRCT) findings and its relation to histological analysis. *Pediatr Pulmonol.* 2010;45:1021–1029.
439. Kerby GS, Wilcox SL, Hay TC, et al. Infant pulmonary function testing in children with neuroendocrine cell hyperplasia with and without lung biopsy. *Am J Respir Crit Care Med.* 2009;179:A3671.
440. Deterding RR, Pye C, Fan LL, et al. Persistent tachypnea of infancy is associated with neuroendocrine cell hyperplasia. *Pediatr Pulmonol.* 2005;40:157–165.
441. Popler J, Young LR, Deterding RR. Beyond infancy: persistence of chronic lung disease in neuroendocrine cell hyperplasia of infancy (NEHI). *Am J Respir Crit Care Med.* 2010;181:A6721.
442. Brody AS, Guillerman RP, Hay TC, et al. Neuroendocrine cell hyperplasia of infancy: diagnosis with high-resolution CT. *AJR Am J Roentgenol.* 2010;194:238–244.
443. Popler J, Gower WA, Mogayzel PJ Jr, et al. Familial neuroendocrine cell hyperplasia of infancy. *Pediatr Pulmonol.* 2010;45:749–755.
444. Bramson RT, Cleveland R, Blickman JG, et al. Radiographic appearance of follicular bronchitis in children. *AJR Am J Roentgenol.* 1996;166:1447–1450.
445. Young LR, Brody AS, Inge TH, et al. Neuroendocrine cell distribution and frequency distinguish neuroendocrine cell hyperplasia of infancy from other pulmonary disorders. *Chest.* 2011;139:1060–1071.
446. Deterding R. Evaluating infants and children with interstitial lung disease. *Semin Respir Crit Care Med.* 2007;28: 333–341.
447. Canakis AM, Cutz E, Manson D, et al. Pulmonary interstitial glycogenosis: a new variant of neonatal interstitial lung disease. *Am J Respir Crit Care Med.* 2002;165:1557–1565.
448. Onland W, Molenaar JJ, Leguit RJ, et al. Pulmonary interstitial glycogenosis in identical twins. *Pediatr Pulmonol.* 2005;40:362–366.
449. Castillo M, Vade A, Lim-Dunham JE, et al. Pulmonary interstitial glycogenosis in the setting of lung growth abnormality: radiographs and pathologic correlation. *Pediatr Radiol.* 2010;40:1562–1565.
450. Smets K, Dhaene K, Schelstraete P, et al. Neonatal pulmonary interstitial glycogen accumulation disorder. *Eur J Pediatr.* 2004;163:408–409.
451. Deutsch GH, Young LR. Pulmonary interstitial glycogenosis: words of caution. *Pediatr Radiol.* 2010;40:1471–1475.
452. Lanfranchi M, Allbery SM, Wheelock L. Pulmonary interstitial glycogenosis. *Pediatr Radiol.* 2010;40:361–365.
453. Albafouille V, Sayegh N, De Coudenhove S, et al. CT scan patterns of pulmonary alveolar proteinosis in children. *Pediatr Radiol.* 1999;29:147–152.
454. Vrielynck S, Mamou-Mani T, Emond S, et al. Diagnostic value of high-resolution CT in the evaluation of chronic infiltrative lung disease in children. *AJR Am J Roentgenol.* 2008;191:914–920.
455. Copley SJ, Padley SP. High-resolution CT of paediatric lung disease. *Eur Radiol.* 2011;11:2564–2575.

456. Suzuki T, Sakagami T, Rubin BK, et al. Familial pulmonary alveolar proteinosis caused by mutations in CSF2RA. *J Exp Med.* 2008;205:2703–2710.
457. Martinez-Moczygemba M, Doan ML, Elidemir O, et al. Pulmonary alveolar proteinosis caused by deletion of the GM-CSFRalpha gene in the X chromosome pseudoautosomal region 1. *J Exp Med.* 2008;205:2711–2716.
458. Robinson TE, Trapnell BC, Goris ML, et al. Quantitative analysis of longitudinal response to aerosolized granulocyte-macrophage colony-stimulating factor in two adolescents with autoimmune pulmonary alveolar proteinosis. *Chest.* 2009;135:842–848.
459. Miller AL, Schissel S, Levy BD, et al. Clinical problem-solving. A crazy cause of dyspnea. *N Engl J Med.* 2011;364:72–77.
460. Hsu AP, Sampaio EP, Khan J, et al. Mutations in GATA2 are associated with the autosomal dominant and sporadic monocytopenia and mycobacterial infection (MonoMAC) syndrome. *Blood.* 2011;118:2653–2655.
461. Tabatabaei SA, Karimi A, Tabatabaei SR, et al. Pulmonary alveolar proteinosis in children: a case series. *J Res Med Sci.* 2010;15:120–124.
462. Leth S, Bendstrup E, Vestergaard H, et al. Autoimmune pulmonary alveolar proteinosis: treatment options in year 2013. *Respirology.* 2013;18:82–91.
463. Seely JM, Salahudeen S Sr, Cadaval-Goncalves AT, et al. Pulmonary Langerhans cell histiocytosis: a comparative study of computed tomography in children and adults. *J Thorac Imaging.* 2012;27:65–70.
464. Bano S, Chaudhary V, Narula MK, et al. Pulmonary Langerhans cell histiocytosis in children: a spectrum of radiologic findings. *Eur J Radiol.* 2014;83(1):47–56.
465. Minkov M. Multisystem Langerhans cell histiocytosis in children: current treatment and future directions. *Paediatr Drugs.* 2011;13:75–86.
466. Clement A, Nathan N, Epaud R, et al. Interstitial lung disease in children. *Orphanet J Rare Dis.* 2010;5:22.
467. Esther CR Jr, Barker PM. Pulmonary lymphangiectasia: diagnosis and clinical course. *Pediatr Pulmonol.* 2004;38:308–313.
468. Barker PM, Esther CR Jr, Fordham LA, et al. Primary pulmonary lymphangiectasia in infancy and childhood. *Eur Respir J.* 2004;24:413–419.
469. Copley SJ, Coren M, Nicholson AG, et al. Diagnostic accuracy of thin-section CT and chest radiography of pediatric interstitial lung disease. *AJR Am J Roentgenol.* 2000;174:549–554.
470. Faul JL, Berry GJ, Colby TV, et al. Thoracic lymphangiomas, lymphangiectasias, lymphangiomatosis, and lymphatic dysplasia syndrome. *Am J Respir Crit Care Med.* 2000;161: 1037–1046.
471. Swenson SJ, Hartman TE, Mayor JR, et al. Diffuse pulmonary lymphangiomatosis: CT findings. *J Comput Assist Tomogr.* 1995; 19:348–352.
472. Chung CJ, Fordham LA, Barker P, et al. Children with congenital pulmonary lymphangiectasia: after infancy. *AJR Am J Roentgenol.* 1999;173:1583–1588.
473. Bellini C, Boccardo F, Campisi C, et al. Pulmonary lymphangiectasia. *Lymphology.* 2005;38:111–121.
474. Yalçin E, Dog D, Halilog M, et al. Postinfectious bronchiolitis obliterans in children: clinical and radiological profile and prognostic factors. *Respiration.* 2003;70:371–375.
475. Zhang L, Irion K, da Silva Porto N, et al. High-resolution computed tomography in pediatric patients with postinfectious bronchiolitis obliterans. *J Thorac Imaging.* 1999;14:85–89.
476. Smith KJ, Dishop MK, Fan LL, et al. Diagnosis of bronchiolitis obliterans with computed tomography in children. *Pediatr Allergy Immunol Pulmonol.* 2011;23:253–259.
477. Moonnumakal SP, Fan LL. Bronchiolitis obliterans in children. *Curr Opin Pediatr.* 2008;20:272–278.
478. Mattiello R, Sarria EE, Mallol J, et al. Post-infectious bronchiolitis obliterans: can CT scan findings in early age anticipate lung function? *Pediatr Pulmonol.* 2010;45:315–319.
479. Lucaya J, Gartner S, García-Peña P, et al. Spectrum of manifestations of Swyer-James-Macleod syndrome. *J Comput Assist Tomogr.* 1998;22:592–597.
480. Kim TO, Oh IJ, Kang HW, et al. Temozolomide-associated bronchiolitis obliterans organizing pneumonia successfully treated with high-dose corticosteroid. *J Korean Med Sci.* 2012;27:450–453.
481. Vos R, Vanaudenaerde BM, Verleden SE, et al. Antiinflammatory and immunomodulatory properties of azithromycin involved in treatment and prevention of chronic lung allograft rejection. *Transplantation.* 2012;94(2):101–109.
482. MacDonald S, Müller NL. Insights from HRCT: how they affect the management of diffuse parenchymal lung disease. *Semin Respir Crit Care Med.* 2003;24:357–364.
483. Fan LL. Hypersensitivity pneumonitis in children. *Curr Opin Pediatr.* 2002;14:323–326.
484. Hartman TE. The HRCT features of extrinsic allergic alveolitis. *Semin Respir Crit Care Med.* 2003;24:419–426.
485. Vece TJ, Fan LL. Interstitial lung disease in children older than 2 years. *Pediatr Allergy Immunol Pulmonol.* 2010;23:33–41.
486. Zacharisen MC, Fink JN. Hypersensitivity pneumonitis and related conditions in the work environment. *Immunol Allergy Clin North Am.* 2011;31:769–786.
487. Fullmer JJ, Langston C, Dishop MK, et al. Pulmonary capillaritis in children: a review of eight cases with comparison to other alveolar hemorrhage syndromes. *J Pediatr.* 2005;146: 376–381.
488. Susarla SC, Fan LL. Diffuse alveolar hemorrhage syndromes in children. *Curr Opin Pediatr.* 2007;19:314–320.
489. Nuesslein TG, Teig N, Rieger CH. Pulmonary haemosiderosis in infants and children. *Paediatr Respir Rev.* 2006;7:45–48.
490. Ravenel JG, McAdams HP. Pulmonary vasculitis: CT features. *Semin Respir Crit Care Med.* 2003;24:427–436.
491. Connolly B, Manson D, Eberhard A, et al. CT appearance of pulmonary vasculitis in children. *AJR Am J Roentgenol.* 1996; 167:901–904.
492. Godfrey S. Pulmonary hemorrhage/hemoptysis in children. *Pediatr Pulmonol.* 2004;37:476–484.
493. Brody AS. Imaging considerations: interstitial lung disease in children. *Radiol Clin North Am.* 2005;43:391–403.
494. Gordon IO, Cipriani N, Arif Q, et al. Update in nonneoplastic lung diseases. *Arch Pathol Lab Med.* 2009;63:366–373.
495. Kligerman SJ, Groshong S, Brown KK, et al. Nonspecific interstitial pneumonia: radiologic, clinical, and pathologic considerations. *Radiographics.* 2009;29:73–87.
496. Flaherty KR, Martinez FJ. Nonspecific interstitial pneumonia. *Semin Respir Crit Care Med.* 2006;27:652–658.
497. Travis WD, Hunninghake G, King TE Jr, et al. Idiopathic nonspecific interstitial pneumonia: report of an American Thoracic Society project. *Am J Respir Crit Care Med.* 2008; 177:1338–1347.
498. Lilleby C, Aalokeen TM, Johansen B, et al. Pulmonary involvement with childhood-onset systemic lupus erythematosus. *Clin Exp Rheumatol.* 2006;24:203–208.

499. Schirmer M, Dejaco C, Duftner C. Advances in the evaluation and classification of chronic inflammatory rheumatic diseases. *Discov Med.* 2012;13:299–304.
500. Leask A. Emerging targets for the treatment of scleroderma. *Expert Opin Emerg Drugs.* 2012;17:173–179.
501. Fan LL, Deterding RR, Langston C. Pediatric interstitial lung diseases revisited. *Pediatr Pulmonol.* 2004;38:369–378.
502. Polverosi R, Maffesanti M, Dalpiaz G. Organizing pneumonia: typical and atypical HRCT patterns. *Radiol Med.* 2006;111:202–212.
503. Epler GR. Bronchiolitis obliterans organizing pneumonia, 25 years: a variety of causes, but what are the treatment options? *Expert Rev Respir Med.* 2011;5:353–361.
504. Masetti R, Cazzato S, Prete A, et al. Organizing pneumonia primed by high-dose chemotherapy and lung irradiation: two pediatric cases. *J Pediatr Hematol Oncol.* 2011;33:e202–e204.
505. Jeong YJ, Kim KI, Seo IJ, et al. Eosinophilic lung diseases: a clinical, radiologic, and pathologic overview. *Radiographics.* 2007;27:617–637.
506. Oermann CM, Panesar KS, Langston C, et al. Pulmonary infiltrates with eosinophilia syndromes in children. *J Pediatr.* 2000;136:351–358.
507. Martinez S, Heyneman LE, McAdams HP, et al. Mucoid impactions: finger-in-glove sign and other CT and radiographic features. *Radiographics.* 2008;28:1369–1382.
508. Fernández Pérez ER, Olson AL, Frankel SK. Eosinophilic lung diseases. *Med Clin North Am.* 2011;95:1163–1187.
509. McHugh K, Olsen E ØE, Vellodi A. Gaucher disease in children: radiology of non-central nervous system manifestations. *Clin Radiol.* 2004;59:117–123.
510. Goiten O, Elstein D, Abrahamov A, et al. Lung involvement and enzyme replacement therapy in Gaucher's disease. *QJM.* 2001;94:407–415.
511. Guillemot N, Troadec C, de Villemeur TB, et al. Lung disease in Niemann-Pick disease. *Pediatr Pulmonol.* 2007;42:1207–1214.
512. Griese M, Brasch F, Aldana VR, et al. Respiratory disease in Niemann-Pick type C2 is caused by pulmonary alveolar proteinosis. *Clin Genet.* 2010;77:119–130.
513. Towbin AJ, Chaves I. Chronic granulomatous disease. *Pediatr Radiol.* 2010;40:657–668.
514. Khanna G, Kao SC, Kirby P, et al. Imaging of chronic granulomatous disease in children. *Radiographics.* 2005;25:1183–1195.
515. Gungor T, Engel-Bicik I, Eich G, et al. Diagnostic and therapeutic impact of whole body positron emission tomography using fluorine-18-fluoro-2-deoxy-D-glucose in children with chronic granulomatous disease. *Arch Dis Child.* 2001 85:341–345.
516. Cleveland RH, Neish AS, Zurakowski D, et al. Cystic fibrosis: predictors of accelerated decline and distribution of disease in 230 patients. *AJR Am J Roentgenol.* 1998;171:1311–1315.
517. Ramsey BW. Use of lung imaging studies as outcome measures for development of new therapies in cystic fibrosis. *Proc Am Thorac Soc.* 2007;4:359–363.
518. Brody AS, Sucharew H, Campbell JD, et al. Computed tomography correlates with pulmonary exacerbations in children with cystic fibrosis. *Am J Respir Crit Care Med.* 2005;172:1128–1132.
519. Ramsey BW, Davies J, McElvaney NG, et al. A CFTR potentiator in patients with cystic fibrosis and the G551D mutation. *N Engl J Med.* 2011;365:1663–1672.
520. Noone PG, Leigh MW, Sannuti A, et al. Primary ciliary dyskinesia: diagnostic and phenotypic features. *Am J Respir Crit Care Med.* 2004;169:459–467.
521. Brown DE, Pittman JE, Leigh MW, et al. Early lung disease in young children with primary ciliary dyskinesia. *Pediatr Pulmonol.* 2008;43:514–516.
522. Kennedy MP, Noone PG, Leigh MW, et al. High-resolution CT of patients with primary ciliary dyskinesia. *AJR Am J Roentgenol.* 2007;188:1232–1238.
523. Pifferi M, Di Cicco M, Piras M, et al. Up to date on primary ciliary dyskinesia in children. *Early Hum Dev.* 2013;89(suppl 3):S45–S48.
524. Nguyen TT, Hussain E, Grimason M, et al. Neurogenic pulmonary edema and acute respiratory distress syndrome in a healthy child with febrile status epilepticus. *J Child Neurol.* 2012;28(10):1287–1291.
525. Wardle AJ, Tulloh RM. Evolving management of pediatric pulmonary arterial hypertension: impact of phosphodiesterase inhibitors. *Pediatr Cardiol.* 2013;34:213–219.
526. Hogan MJ. Neonatal vascular catheters and their complications. *Radiol Clin North Am.* 1999;37(6):1109–1125.
527. Das Narla L, Hom M, Lofland GK, et al. Evaluation of umbilical catheter and tube placement in premature infants. *Radiographics.* 1991;11:849–863.
528. Barrington J. Umbilical artery catheters in the newborn: effects of position of the catheter tip. *Cochrane Database Syst Rev.* 2000;2:CD000505.
529. Schlesinger AE, Braverman RM, DiPietro MA, et al. Neonates and umbilical venous catheters: normal appearance, anomalous positions, complications, and potential aid to diagnosis. *AJR Am J Roentgenol.* 2003;180:1147–1153.
530. Seguin J, Fletcher MA, Landers S, et al. Umbilical venous catheterizations: audit by the study group for complications of perinatal care. *Am J Perinatol.* 1994;11(1):67.
531. Coley BD, Seguin J, Cordero L, et al. Neonatal total parenteral nutrition ascites from liver erosion by umbilical vein catheters. *Pediatr Radiol.* 1998;28(12):923–927.
532. Bjorklund LJ, Malmgren M, Lindroth M. Pulmonary complications of umbilical venous catheters. *Pediatr Radiol.* 1995;25:149–152.
533. Green JS, Lamont AC. Pulmonary complications of umbilical venous catheters. *Pediatr Radiol.* 1996;26:239.
534. Teele SA, Emani SM, Thiagarajan RR, et al. Catheters, wires, tubes and drains on postoperative radiographs of pediatric cardiac patients: the whys and wherefores. *Pediatr Radiol.* 2008;38:1041–1053.
535. Keckler SJ, Spilde TL, Ho B, et al. Chest radiograph after central line placement under fluoroscopy: utility or futility? *J Pediatr Surg.* 2008;43(4):854–856.
536. Valk JW, Plotz FB, Schuerman F, et al. The value of routine chest radiographs in a paediatric intensive care unit: a prospective study. *Pediatr Radiol.* 2001;31:343–347.
537. Hruszkewycz V, Holtrop PC, Batton DG, et al. Complications associated with central venous catheters inserted in critically ill neonates. *Infect Control Hosp Epidemiol.* 1991;129:544–548.
538. Vilela R, Jácomo A, Tresoldi AT. Risk factors for central venous catheter related infections in pediatric intensive care. *Clinics.* 2007;62(5):537–544.
539. Reyes JA, Habash ML, Taylor RP. Femoral central venous catheters are not associated with higher rates of infection in the pediatric critical care population. *Am J Infect Control.* 2012;40(1):43–47.

540. Connolly B, Amaral A, Walsh S, et al. Influence of arm movement on central tip location of peripherally inserted central catheters (PICCs). *Pediatr Radiol.* 2006;36(8):854–850.
541. Gamulka B, Mendoza C, Connolly B. Evaluation of a unique, nurse-inserted, peripherally inserted central catheter program. *Pediatrics.* 2005;115:1602–1606.
542. Fricke BL, Racadio JM, Duckworth T. Placement of peripherally inserted central catheters without fluoroscopy in children: initial catheter tip position. *Radiology.* 2005;253:887–892.
543. Braswell LE. Peripherally inserted central catheter placement in infants and children. *Tech Vasc Interv Radiol.* 2011;14(4):204–211.
544. Gross GW, McElwee DL, Baumgart S, et al. Bypass cannulas utilized in extracorporeal membrane oxygenation in neonates: radiographic findings. *Pediatr Radiol.* 1995;25:337–340.
545. Frenckner B, Radell P. Respiratory failure and extracorporeal membrane oxygenation. *Semin Pediatr Surg.* 2008;17(1):34–41.
546. Schlesinger AE, Cornish JD, Null DM. Dense pulmonary opacification in neonates treated with extracorporeal membrane oxygenation. *Pediatr Radiol.* 1986;16:448–451.
547. Zreik H, Bengur AR, Meliones JN, et al. Superior vena cava obstruction after extracorporeal membrane oxygenation. *J Pediatr.* 1995;127:314–316.
548. Schmolzer GM, O'Reilly M, Davis PG, et al. Confirmation of correct tracheal tube placement in newborn infants. *Resuscitation.* 2013;84(6):731–737.
549. Levy FH, Bratton SL, Jardine DS. Routine chest radiographs following repositioning of endotracheal tubes are necessary to assess correct position in pediatric patients. *Chest.* 1994;106:1508–1510.
550. Creel AM, Winkler MK. Oral and nasal enteral tube placement errors and complications in a pediatric intensive care unit. *Pediatr Crit Care Med.* 2007;8(2):161–164.

CHAPTER 7

Pleura

Rama S. Ayyala • Shunsuke Nosaka • Khalid Khashoggi • Janina M. Patsch • Zaleha Abdul Manaf • Edward Y. Lee

INTRODUCTION

In children, various pathologic disorders can affect the pleura and the pleural space with imaging playing a vital role in determining the underlying etiology, location, and extension. Pleural abnormalities can be subtle and often require careful investigation with multiple imaging modalities in the pediatric population. This chapter provides an overview of the currently available imaging modalities to evaluate pleural abnormalities and the normal pleural anatomy in the pediatric population (Table 7.1). In addition, pleural pathology commonly encountered in infants and children is reviewed, with correlative imaging findings and pathology in selected cases.

IMAGING TECHNIQUES

Radiography

Standard radiographs of the chest are usually the first-line imaging modality to assess for pleural abnormalities in children, given their wide availability, relative inexpensiveness, and easy acquisition. Typical examination includes anteroposterior (AP) radiograph of the chest in infants and young children or posteroanterior (PA) radiograph of the chest in older children. Radiographs optimally should be obtained with the patient in the standing position, with an appropriate inspiratory effort. However, depending on the age and condition of the patient, radiographs may only be able to be obtained in the supine position. Lateral decubitus radiographs can be added for further characterization of a questionable abnormality seen on an AP or PA radiograph, such as an opacity, which may represent a pleural effusion, or to evaluate for a pneumothorax (Fig. 7.1). Although radiographs are an excellent first-line imaging modality to assess pleural abnormalities, additional imaging studies may be necessary for confirmation and further characterization of radiographic findings.

Ultrasound

Ultrasound (US) is a frequently used noninvasive modality for evaluation of the pleura in the pediatric population. It is relatively accessible and easy to perform, with the additional advantage of allowing for real-time imaging. In addition, US can be performed portably, does not require sedation or intravenous access for contrast administration, and is unique in that children are not exposed to the potentially harmful effects of ionizing radiation. However, proper technique is essential for obtaining diagnostic quality US information in the pediatric population.

Three major technical factors that affect the quality of US imaging include proper US transducer selection, appropriate patient positioning, and optimal imaging approach.[1] For optimal evaluation of pleural abnormalities in pediatric patients, curved or linear array transducers (7.5 to 15.0 MHz) should be used. Real-time gray-scale US is the standard imaging used to visualize most pleural abnormalities. However, color Doppler imaging can provide added value, particularly in order to differentiate vascular and nonvascular pleural lesions.

Chest US for evaluation of pleural disorders is usually performed with the patient in the supine position, with imaging typically performed via either frontal or lateral approach. Imaging can also be performed with the patient in upright position via a posterior approach, which permits optimal visualization of the posterior pleural lesions and small layering effusions.

TABLE 7.1 Advantages and Disadvantages of Imaging Modalities for Evaluating Pleura

	Advantages	Disadvantages
Radiography	• Easily accessible • Easy to acquire • Inexpensive	• Patient position dependent • Difficult to differentiate pleural vs. parenchymal abnormality
Ultrasound	• Lack of ionizing radiation • No need for intravenous contrast • Easily accessible • Best to characterize simple vs. complex effusion	• Operator dependent
CT	• Delineate extension of a pleural abnormality into adjacent structures • Intravenous contrast helps differentiate pleural and parenchymal process	• Ionizing radiation • Intravenous access for contrast may be needed • Sedation in young patients for optimal study
MRI	• Lack of ionizing radiation • Characterize pleural abnormality and its relation to adjacent structures	• Intravenous access for contrast may be needed • Sedation in young patients for optimal study • Longer examination time

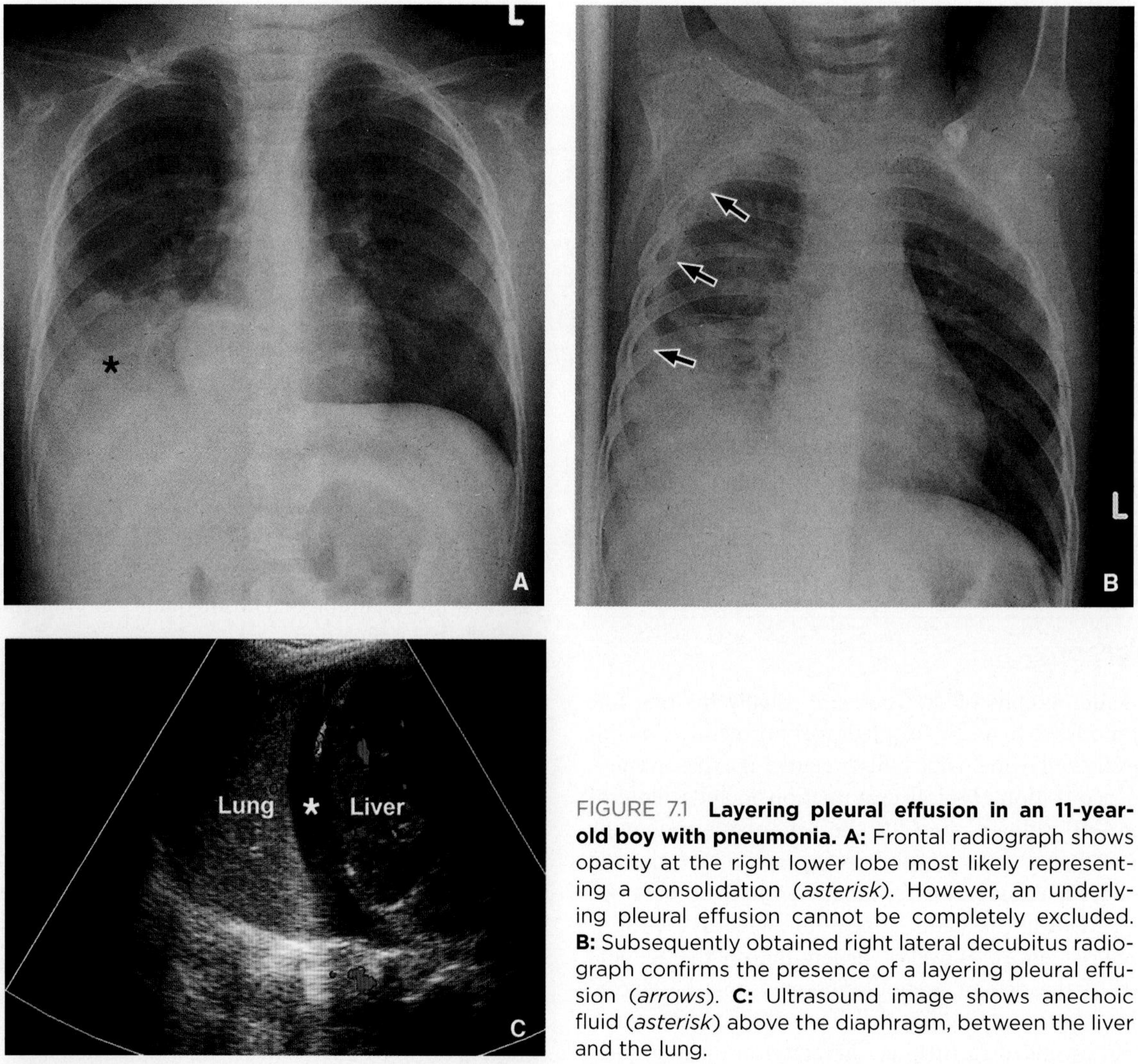

FIGURE 7.1 **Layering pleural effusion in an 11-year-old boy with pneumonia. A:** Frontal radiograph shows opacity at the right lower lobe most likely representing a consolidation (*asterisk*). However, an underlying pleural effusion cannot be completely excluded. **B:** Subsequently obtained right lateral decubitus radiograph confirms the presence of a layering pleural effusion (*arrows*). **C:** Ultrasound image shows anechoic fluid (*asterisk*) above the diaphragm, between the liver and the lung.

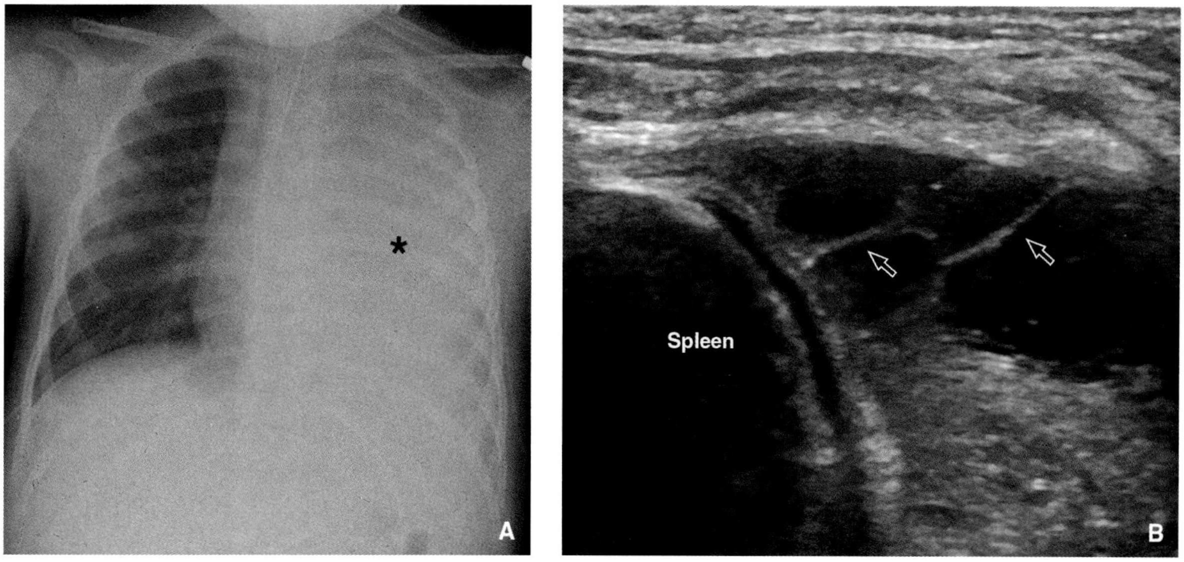

FIGURE 7.2 **Pleural effusion in a 20-month-old girl. A:** Frontal radiograph shows complete opacification of the left hemithorax (*asterisk*) with mediastinal shift to the contralateral side **(right side)**. **B:** Ultrasound image demonstrates a complex pleural effusion with multiple internal septations (*arrows*).

Currently, US is often used in evaluation of pediatric patients with an opaque hemithorax on chest radiograph in order to delineate pleural effusion from underlying parenchymal pathology.[2] When a pleural effusion is present, it can also aid in estimating the size of a pleural effusion and characterize a pleural effusion as simple or complex (Fig. 7.2).[3] Finally, US can aid in therapy by serving as a guidance tool in chest drain insertion or thoracentesis.[2]

Computed Tomography

In conjunction with radiographs and US, computed tomography (CT) is an effective imaging modality to help further evaluate abnormal pleural findings, which may be difficult to be characterized on radiographs and US alone. CT is a superior imaging modality to delineate complex anatomy, allowing for evaluation of the pleural space in addition to lung parenchyma, mediastinum, and chest wall. However, CT should be reserved for indeterminate or challenging cases that need additional information for proper pediatric patient management in order to limit exposure of children to ionizing radiation. Another advantage of CT is the ability to use intravenous contrast for characterization of pleural fluid or lesion. For instance, contrast-enhanced CT can show pleural thickening and enhancement, which suggests empyema, and help differentiate a lung abscess (Fig. 7.3). CT can optimally show the presence of a pleural effusion or pneumothorax, especially if small in volume. However, unlike US, CT is not optimal to visualize internal septations and debris within complex pleural effusions. Lastly, CT is the preferred modality for imaging of primary and metastatic pleural neoplasms allowing prompt diagnosis and guidance of treatment (Fig. 7.4). Not only the primary mass can be characterized with CT but also disease extent and additional lesions can be identified.

Magnetic Resonance Imaging

Magnetic resonance imaging (MRI) is an excellent imaging modality for evaluating pleural abnormalities, particularly in pediatric patients, because of its superior ability to characterize soft tissues without ionizing radiation exposure. However, MRI may not be as widely available as CT, making it more challenging to obtain in all cases. In addition, MRI is a longer examination given the multiple sequences performed; therefore, it may require sedation in the young pediatric population to obtain optimal and diagnostic images. Currently, the role of MRI in the evaluation of pleura is reserved for

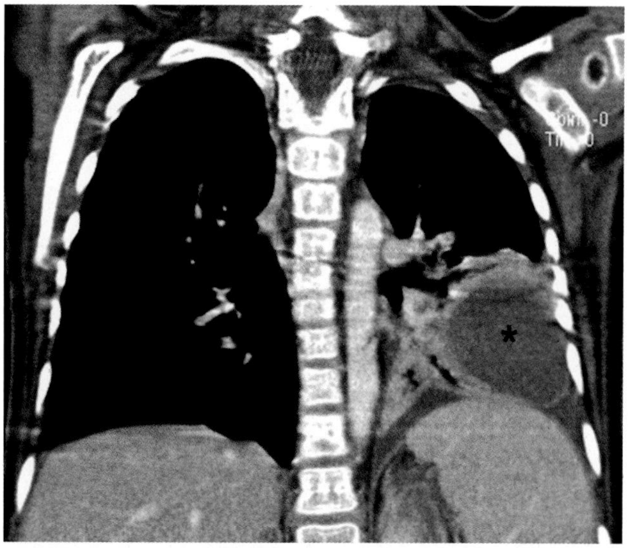

FIGURE 7.3 **Lung abscess in a 33-month-old boy with pneumonia.** Contrast-enhanced coronal reformatted CT image shows a round low-attenuation fluid collection (*asterisk*) centered within the left lower lobe with peripheral contrast enhancement most consistent with a lung abscess.

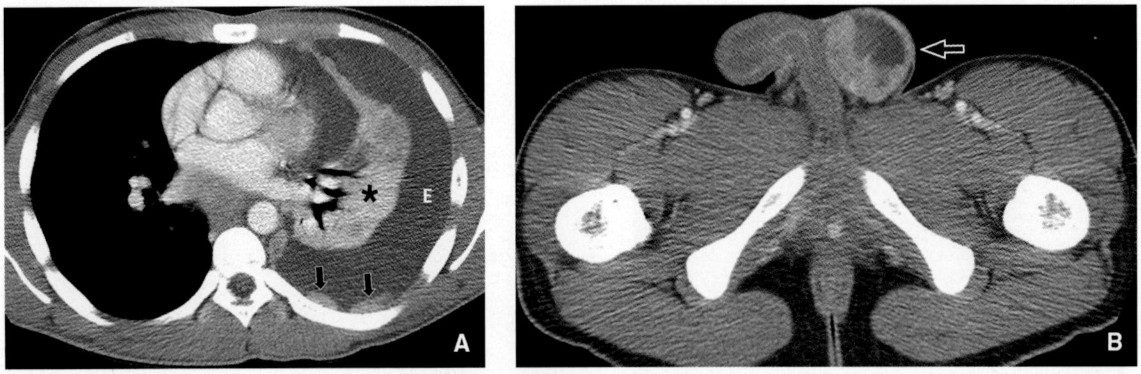

FIGURE 7.4 **Pleural metastasis in a 16-year-old boy with testicular cancer. A:** Contrast-enhanced axial CT image shows multiple enhancing pleural-based masses (*arrows*) with adjacent pleural effusion (*E*) and consolidation of the left lower lobe (*asterisk*). **B:** Contrast-enhanced axial CT image of the lower pelvis demonstrates a heterogeneously enhancing left testicular mass (*arrow*).

problem-solving in specific situations when further characterization of the pleural lesions is necessary after other imaging studies. Various signal characteristics on MRI can help diagnose pleural disease and help differentiate benign from malignant pleural processes. However, histologic evaluation is often ultimately necessary for a definitive diagnosis (Fig. 7.5). MRI examinations for evaluation of the pleura mainly consist of T1- and T2-weighted MR images, as well as postcontrast T1-weighted MR images in axial and coronal planes. MR images in sagittal plane can be useful for assessing pleural abnormalities adjacent to the sternum or spine.

NORMAL ANATOMY

Pleura is a continuous surface epithelium that lines the thoracic cavity and the lungs. The visceral pleura adheres to the lungs and is in continuity with the parietal pleura, which covers the inner thoracic wall, diaphragm, and medial mediastinum. The visceral pleura invaginates into the interlobar fissures of the lung, as well as into accessory fissures if present (Fig. 7.6). In healthy children, the pleural membranes are typically 0.2 to 0.4 mm thick with ~4 to 18 mL of physiologic fluid in the space, forming a layer 5 to 10 μm thick.[3] Parietal and visceral pleura contain blood vessels and lymphatics. Visceral pleura is supplied by bronchial arteries, whereas parietal pleura is supplied by systemic arteries, including the phrenic artery and intercostal arteries. Venous drainage for the visceral pleura is to the pulmonary veins, whereas the venous drainage for the parietal pleura is to the intercostal and phrenic veins.

The pleural space is a potential space that normally contains a small amount of physiologic pleural fluid. Only the lymphatics of the parietal pleura communicate with the pleural space via 8- to 10-μm holes, which exude fluid into the pleural space (Fig. 7.7). This fluid is typically taken up by mediastinal lymph nodes, which drains into the thoracic duct and ultimately into the systemic venous system. Normal physiologic fluid is evenly distributed in the pleural space, decreasing friction between the visceral and parietal pleura during movement of the lungs against the chest wall with normal respiration.[4] Pleura and the pleural space only become visible on imaging studies when an abnormality is present.

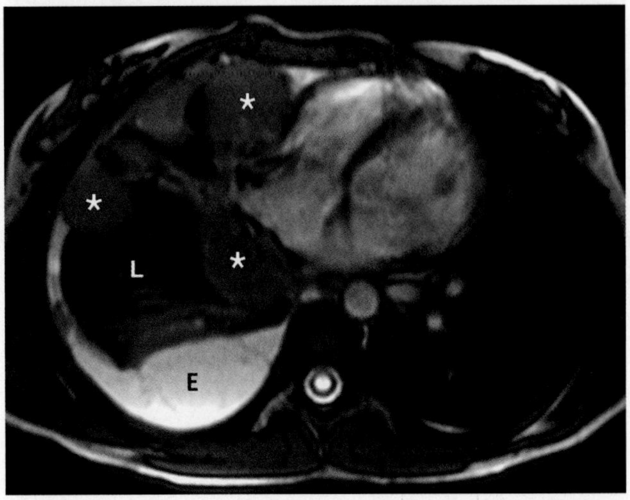

FIGURE 7.5 **Pleural metastasis in a 15-year-old boy with synovial cell sarcoma.** Axial T2-weighted MR image shows multiple low-signal pleural-based masses (*asterisk*) in the right hemithorax. (*L*, lung; *E*, pleural effusion.)

SPECTRUM OF PLEURAL DISORDERS

Pneumothorax

Pneumothorax is defined as air within the potential pleural space. Although there are various underlying etiologies of pneumothorax, they can be broadly categorized into either spontaneous (i.e., primary) or iatrogenic (i.e., secondary) pneumothorax. Spontaneous pneumothorax can occur in a previously healthy child resulting from spontaneous rupture of a preexisting bleb, usually located in the apex of the lung (Fig. 7.8), or may be a consequence of an underlying pulmonary disorder, such as asthma or cystic fibrosis. Secondary or iatrogenic pneumothorax can occur in the setting of a

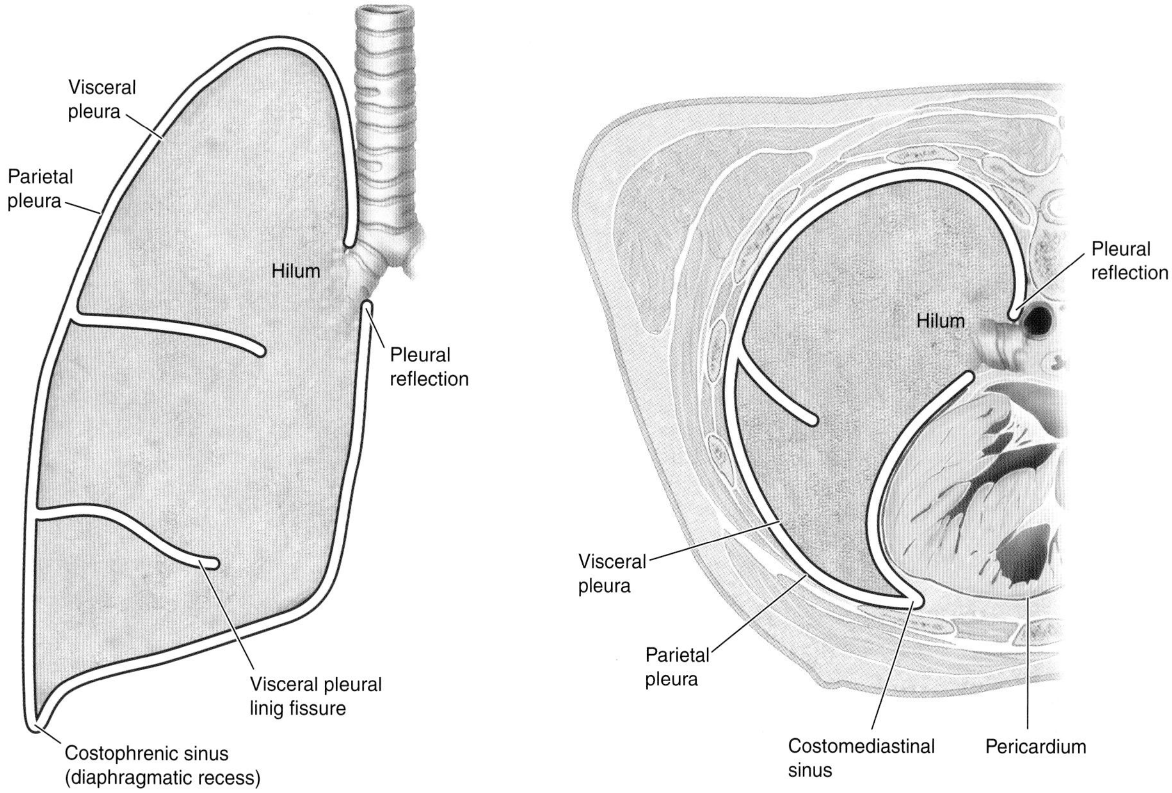

FIGURE 7.6 **Normal pleural anatomy.** Schematic diagram of the lungs shows the parietal pleura outlining the chest wall and the visceral pleura overlying the lung as well as invaginating into the different fissures. The parietal and visceral pleural are continuous (pleural reflections) creating the potential pleural space.

recent intervention, such as a lung biopsy, thoracentesis, or mechanical ventilation.[5] Iatrogenic pneumothorax can be also secondary to blunt or penetrating trauma, with or without an associated rib fracture (Fig. 7.9). Air can be introduced into the pleural space not only from an external wound but also secondary to pulmonary, esophageal, or tracheobronchial injuries.

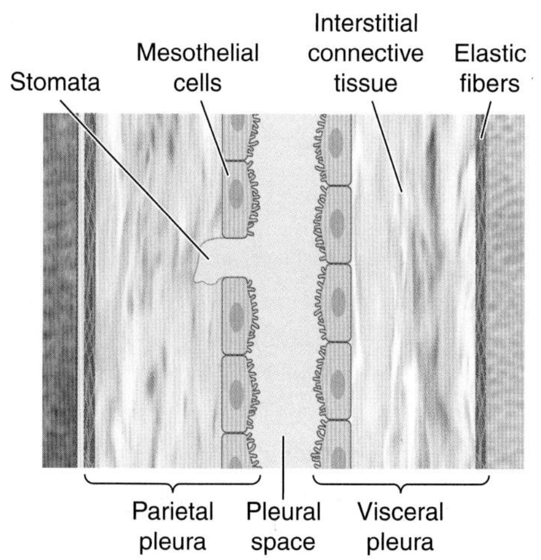

FIGURE 7.7 **Normal pleural anatomy.** The lymphatics of the parietal pleura produce the majority of the pleural fluid, which is exuded into the pleural space via stomata. The mesothelial cells secrete a surfactant-like substance that lubricates the pleural cavity.

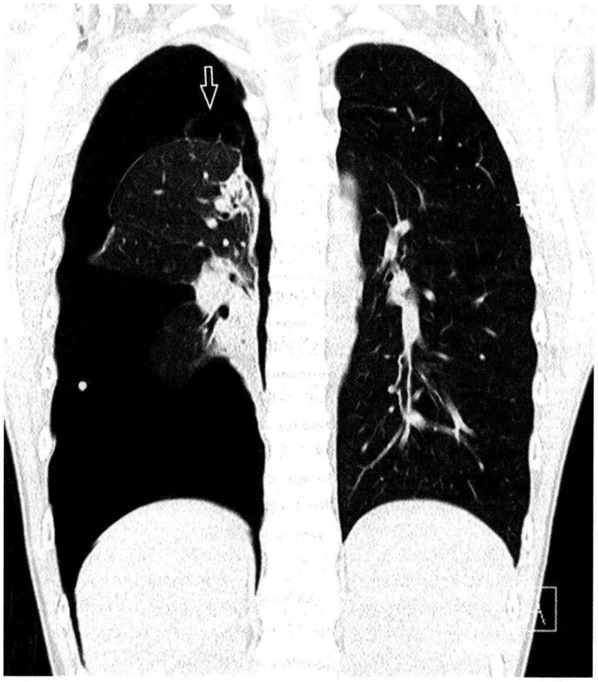

FIGURE 7.8 **Spontaneous pneumothorax in a 15-year-old boy who presented with acute shortness of breath and right-sided chest pain.** Coronal reformatted lung window CT image shows a large right pneumothorax with collapse of the right lung. Also noted are small blebs (*arrow*) at the right lung apex most likely the cause of this patient's spontaneous pneumothorax.

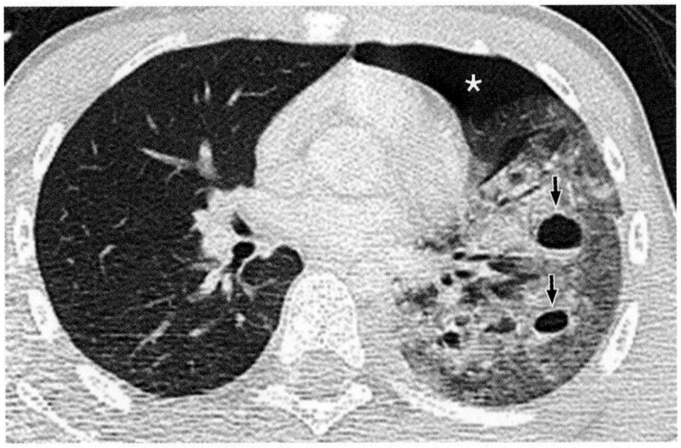

FIGURE 7.9 **Traumatic pneumothorax in an 8-year-old boy status post motor vehicle accident.** Axial lung window CT image shows a left pneumothorax (*asterisk*). Opacities in the left lung are consistent with lung contusions with pneumatoceles (*arrows*) containing fluid (hemorrhage).

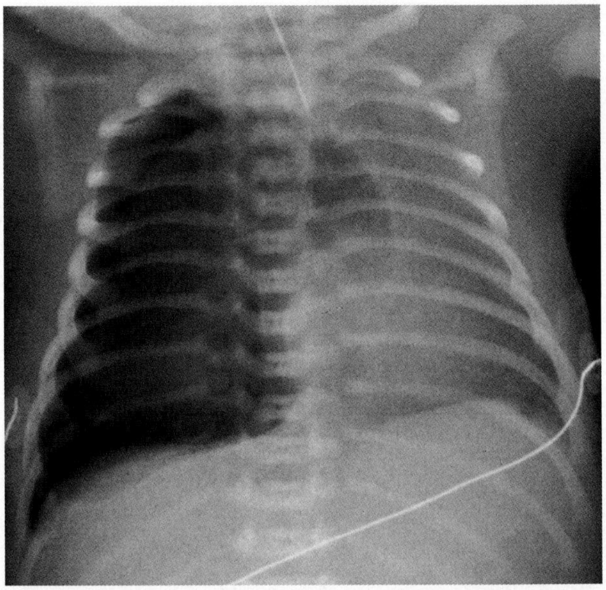

FIGURE 7.10 **Tension pneumothorax in a newborn boy who presented with desaturation and absent breath sound in the right hemithorax.** Frontal chest radiograph shows a large right pneumothorax with associated mediastinal shift to the contralateral side and flattening of the right hemidiaphragm, characteristic radiographic findings suggesting underlying tension pneumothorax.

The incidence of spontaneous pneumothorax is ~1.2 to 6 cases per 100,000 girls and 7.4 to 18 cases per 100,000 boys, with a mean age at presentation being 14 to 15.9 years in the pediatric population.[5] The common demographic of pediatric patients with a spontaneous primary pneumothorax is tall, thin boys with low body mass index.[6] Affected pediatric patients typically present with sudden-onset shortness of breath and unilateral chest pain. In the setting of thoracic trauma, one-third of thoracic injuries are associated with pneumothorax. A concerning adverse outcome of a traumatic pneumothorax is a tension pneumothorax, which occurs when the pleural defect acts as a one-way valve, allowing air to flow into the pleural cavity without escape. The increasing volume and accumulation of air in the pleural space cause mass effect on the adjacent structures, resulting in mediastinal shift to the contralateral side and possible vascular compromise of the heart and the great vessels (Fig. 7.10).[5] Physical examination findings specific to tension pneumothorax include engorged neck veins and deviation of the airway to the contralateral side.

Standing AP or PA radiographs are an initial imaging method for evaluating pediatric patients clinically suspected of having pneumothorax. On frontal chest radiographs, pneumothorax typically presents as lucency and collapsed lung with visible pleural surface (Fig. 7.11). When the pneumothorax is localized in the subpulmonic region, lucency can be localized and projects over the lower lung zone, just above the diaphragm (Fig. 7.12). In the setting of both air and fluid in the pleural space, which is known as hydropneumothorax, the interface between the air and fluid can be seen on an erect radiograph as a horizontal line extending across the entire length of the hemithorax (Fig. 7.13). In critically ill pediatric patients who cannot tolerate standing, chest radiographs can be obtained in the supine position, which unfortunately decreases sensitivity for evaluation of pneumothorax. However, given air rises to the nondependent position, pneumothorax can be seen on a supine radiograph as global lucency in the chest without clear visualization of pleural line, especially in neonates and infants (Fig. 7.14). Lateral radiographs are not necessary as the initial evaluation; however, lateral decubitus radiographs can be useful in challenging cases particularly when the amount of intrathoracic free air is small. In severely ill

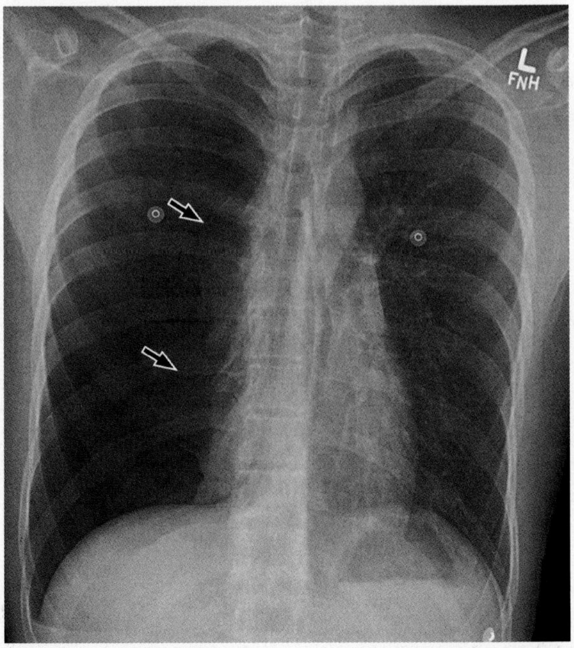

FIGURE 7.11 **Pneumothorax in a 16-year-old boy who presented with acute shortness of breath and right-sided chest pain.** Frontal chest radiograph shows a large right pneumothorax with collapse of the right lung. The pleural line (*arrows*) is well visualized given the large amount of air in the pleural space.

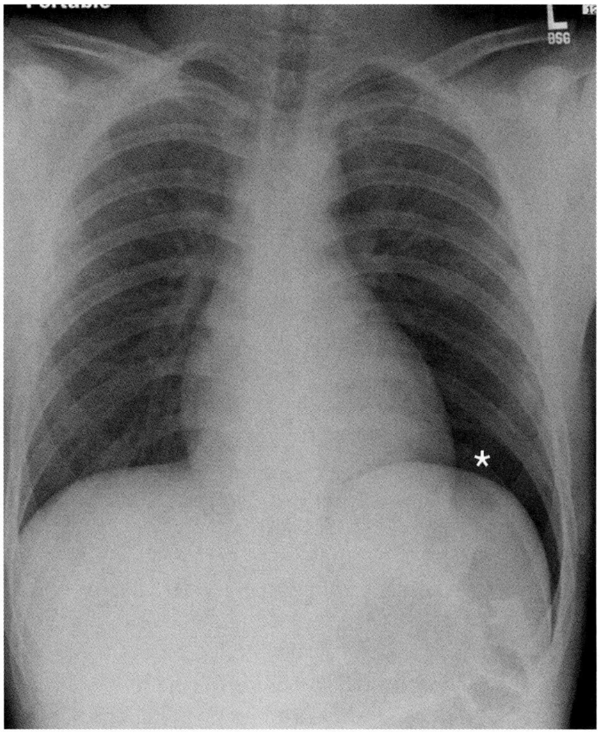

FIGURE 7.12 **Subpulmonic pneumothorax in a 14-year-old boy with left-sided chest pain.** Frontal chest radiograph shows lucency at the left lung base (*asterisk*), consistent with air tracking in the subpulmonic space (pleural space between the lung and diaphragm).

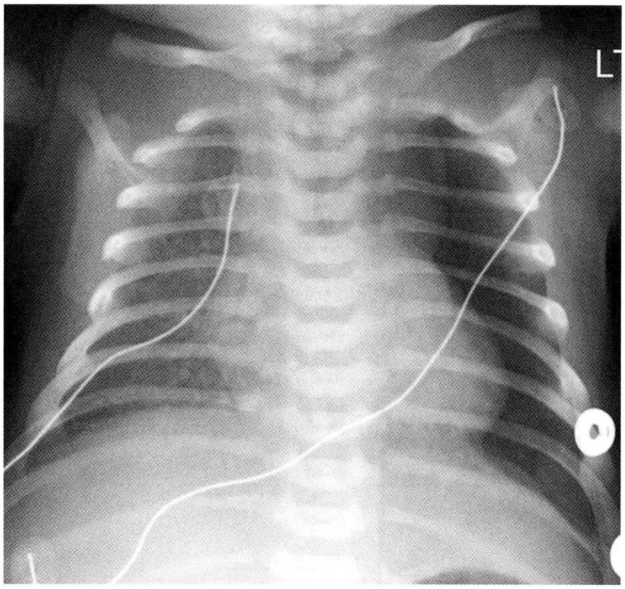

FIGURE 7.14 **Anterior pneumothorax in a newborn girl with respiratory distress.** Frontal chest radiograph obtained in a supine position shows lucency in the left hemithorax because of an anteriorly placed pneumothorax. Mildly coarse diffuse opacity is seen in the right hemithorax secondary to meconium aspiration.

patients, a cross-table lateral radiograph or decubitus radiograph can be performed.

US is not typically performed for evaluation of pneumothorax. However, it can be an incidental finding; therefore, it is important to recognize the sonographic findings of pneumothorax. In a healthy pediatric patient, sliding of the echogenic surface of the visceral pleura on the parietal pleura during normal respiration is noted, known as the "lung sliding sign." When air is introduced into the pleural space, the interface is obscured; therefore, the normal sliding motion is not visualized (Fig. 7.15). This can be further investigated using M-mode or power Doppler, which can increase the sensitivity for detecting pneumothorax.[7] Overall, US has a sensitivity of 86% to 98% and specificity of 97% to 100% in detection of pneumothorax.[8]

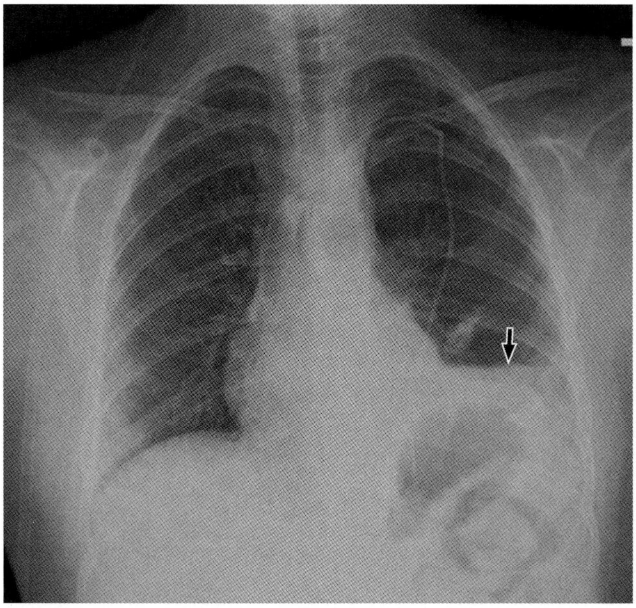

FIGURE 7.13 **Hydropneumothorax in a 9-year-old girl.** Frontal chest radiograph shows the horizontal line (*arrow*) delineating fluid layering within the pleural space of the left hemithorax. Also noted is a moderate size left pneumothorax.

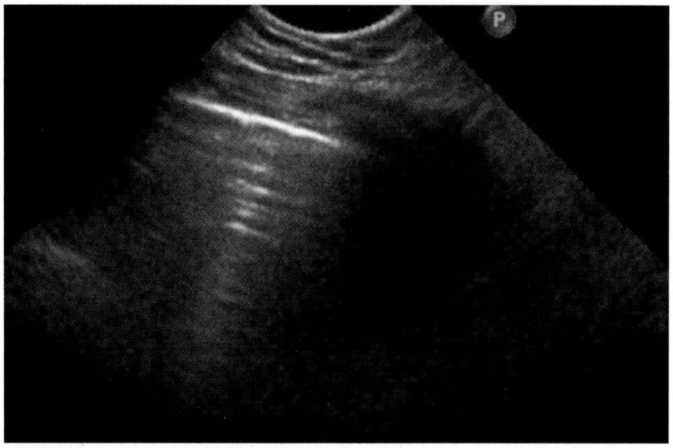

FIGURE 7.15 **Pneumothorax detected on ultrasound.** Transverse ultrasound image of the right lower hemithorax demonstrates an iatrogenic pneumothorax in a critical care pediatric patient because of barotrauma. (Reprinted with permission from Baez JC, Sodhi KS, Restrepo R, et al. Sonographic evaluation of congenital and acquired thoracic disorders in pediatric patients. *Ultrasound Clin.* 20138(3):265–284, with permission, editor Harriet J. Paltiel.)

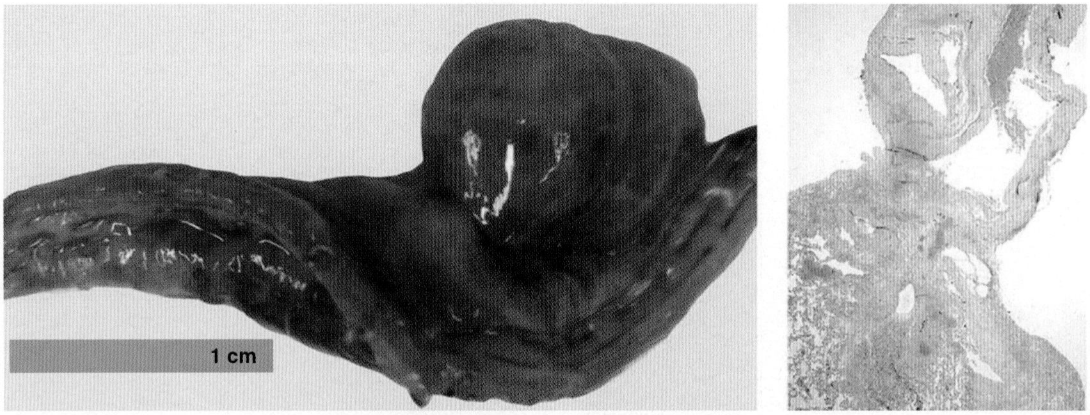

FIGURE 7.16 **Apical bleb in a 16-year-old boy with recurrent spontaneous pneumothorax.** The resected specimen shows a cystic protrusion from the pleural surface **(left)**. Microscopically, large pleural and subpleural air-filled spaces are seen (**right**, hematoxylin and eosin, original magnification, 40×).

CT is currently the gold standard imaging study for diagnosis of pneumothorax. In pediatric patients with spontaneous primary pneumothorax or recurrent pneumothoraces, CT is performed to evaluate for underlying etiology, such as subpleural blebs or bullae.[9–11] These are typically located at the lung apices (Figs. 7.8 and 7.16); therefore, in cases of suspected blebs or bullae, a limited CT of the apices can be performed in order to limit radiation exposure.[9] Additionally, in the setting of persistent pneumothorax despite treatment, an underlying bronchopleural fistula should be suspected and can be optimally evaluated with CT (Fig. 7.17). Lastly, CT can also help assess for additional injuries in the setting of a traumatic pneumothorax.

Currently, no specific management guidelines have been established for treatment of pneumothorax in the pediatric population. However, in asymptomatic pediatric patients, observation is the first-line management, which is typically reserved for cases of small pneumothorax. In symptomatic pediatric patients with moderate to large pneumothorax, more aggressive and immediate intervention is needed. Administration of oxygen can be implemented to increase resorption of the pneumothorax. Direct interventions such as simple aspiration or placement of a thoracostomy tube allow for prompt decompression of the pneumothorax. In cases of tension pneumothorax, immediate needle decompression with a large-bore needle or angiocatheter at the second intercostal space along the midclavicular line is indicated. In any situation, follow-up chest radiographs for confirmation of interval resolution of pneumothorax before discharge are recommended, especially in children who underwent thoracostomy tube or needle decompression of pneumothorax.

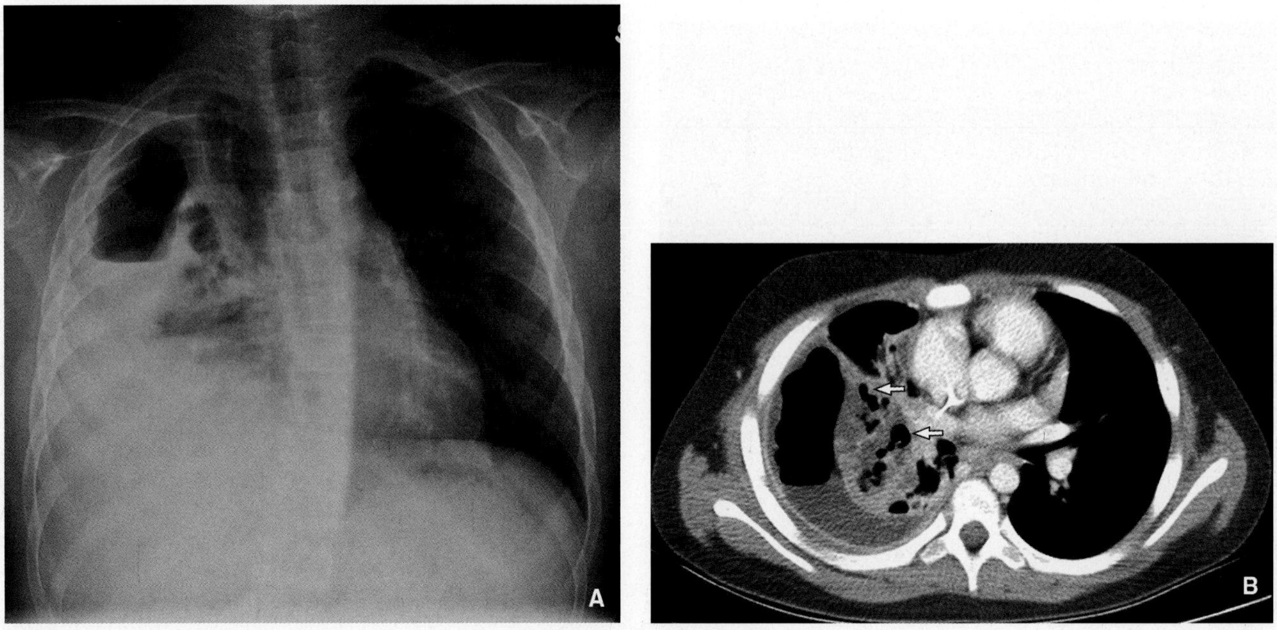

FIGURE 7.17 **Bronchopleural fistula in a 12-year-old girl with pneumonia. A:** Frontal chest radiograph shows a large right hydropneumothorax with adjacent consolidation. **B:** Contrast-enhanced axial CT image demonstrates the right hydropneumothorax with multiple cavitations (*arrows*) within the consolidated lung consistent with underlying necrosis. Given the accumulation of air within the pleural space in the setting of the necrosis, an underlying bronchopleural fistula was presumed present.

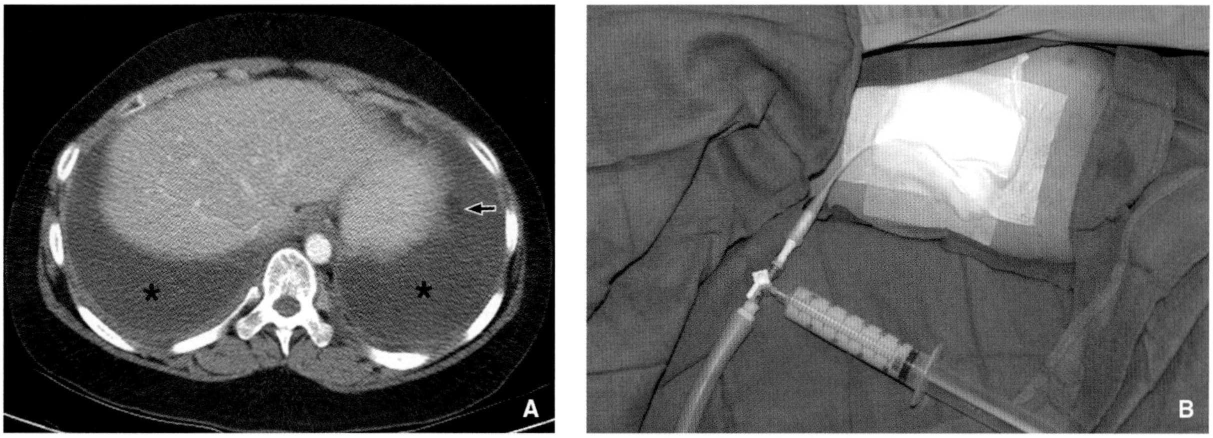

FIGURE 7.18 **Chylous pleural effusion in a 16-year-old girl with underlying systemic lupus erythematosus. A:** Contrast-enhanced axial CT image shows bilateral pleural effusions (*asterisks*). A focal hypodensity (*arrow*) was present with Hounsfield units consistent with fat. **B:** Analysis of the drained pleural fluid confirmed bilateral chylothoraces.

Pleural Effusions

Fluid can accumulate in the potential space between the visceral and parietal pleura, as a result of dysfunction of the normal lymphatic system of the pleura. Pleural effusions result from either overproduction of lymphatic fluid or decreased resorption of lymphatic fluid (Fig. 7.18). Three main underlying etiologies of pleural effusions include infectious, inflammatory, and neoplastic processes. Pleural effusions can be mainly categorized as transudative or exudative. Transudates are usually seen in systemic disorders affecting the normal function of the lymphatic system in the pediatric population. Typical etiologies include heart failure, nephrotic syndrome, and cirrhosis. Exudates are caused by increased formation of pleural fluid by localized infections or pathologic processes. Exudative pleural effusion can be seen in the setting of pneumonia, pulmonary inflammatory disorders, or neoplasms. The most common etiology of pleural effusion in children is pleuropulmonary infection.[12] Children with small pleural effusions can be asymptomatic; however, larger pleural effusions can cause chest pain and respiratory compromise.

Radiographs are usually the first-line imaging modality for evaluation of pleural effusion in the pediatric population. Radiographic appearance can vary based on the patient positioning, volume of the effusion, and the presence of septations. Standing AP or PA lateral radiographs usually show blunting of the costophrenic angles, which changes in position on lateral decubitus radiographs with free-flowing fluid (Fig. 7.19). On supine radiographs, a free-flowing pleural

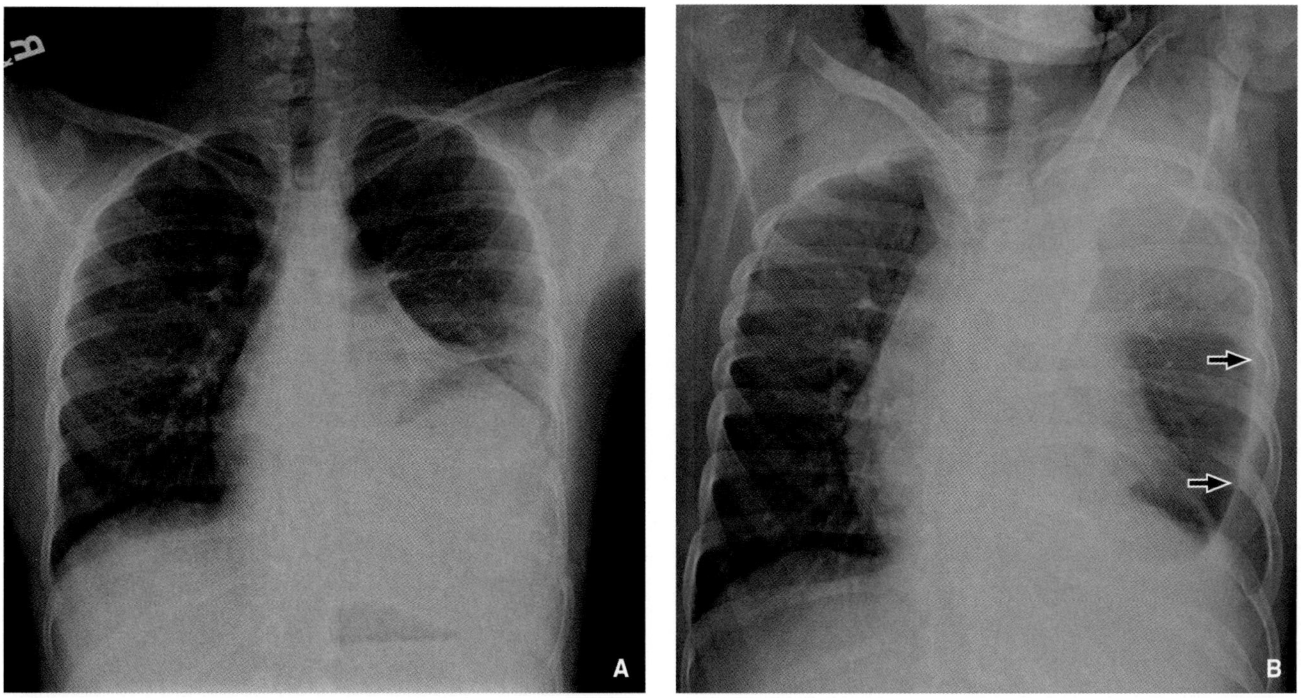

FIGURE 7.19 **Pleural effusion in a 10-year-old boy with pneumonia. A:** Frontal chest radiograph obtained in standing position shows opacity at the left lung base with nonvisualization of the left costophrenic angle suggesting an underlying pleural effusion. **B:** Left lateral decubitus radiograph confirms a layering pleural effusion (*arrows*).

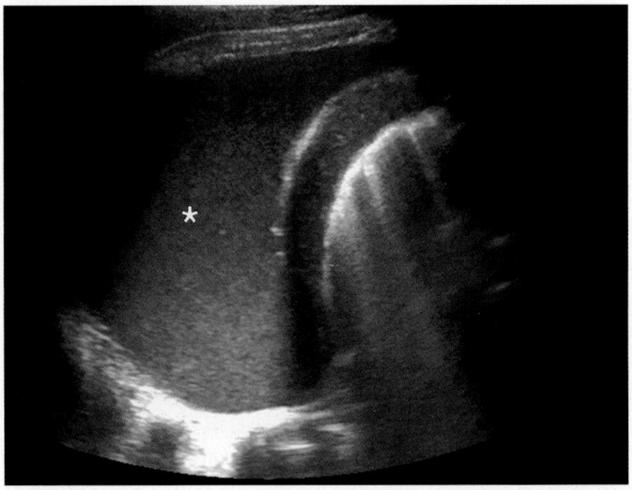

FIGURE 7.20 **Complex pleural effusion in a 5-year-old girl with pneumonia.** Gray-scale ultrasound image shows low-level echoes within a left pleural effusion (*asterisk*).

effusion layers posteriorly, causing diffuse hazy appearance of the hemithorax. A lentiform pleural-based opacity with no change in appearance with change in patient positioning suggests a loculated effusion.

US is currently the best imaging modality in detection and characterizing pleural fluid. Pleural effusions on US can be categorized as simple or complex. Simple pleural effusion is characterized by free-flowing, homogenously anechoic fluid (Fig. 7.1). Varying sonographic appearances can be seen with complex effusions, including low-level echoes with or without septations (Figs. 7.20 and 7.21). CT or MRI can detect small pleural effusions, as well as evaluate the remainder of the intrathoracic cavity for additional associated abnormalities (Figs. 7.4 and 7.5).

Small pleural effusions in asymptomatic pediatric patients can be treated conservatively. The treatment of choice for moderate or large pleural effusions particularly in symptomatic pediatric patients is thoracentesis, which can be both therapeutic and diagnostic. Indications for thoracentesis in children include respiratory compromise, mediastinal shift, pleuritic chest pain, and underlying lung disease. Management of parapneumonic effusions and loculated fluid collections are discussed later in this chapter.[12]

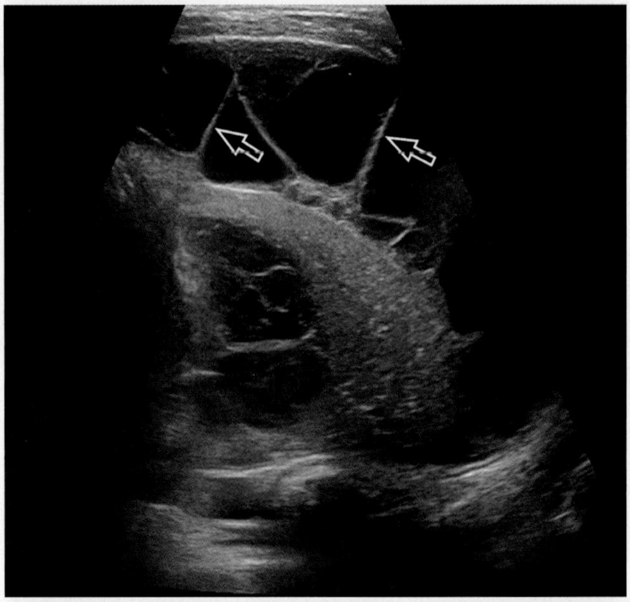

FIGURE 7.21 **Complex pleural effusion in a 6-year-old boy with pneumonia.** Gray-scale ultrasound image shows multiple septations (*arrows*) interspersed with anechoic fluid within the pleural effusion.

Parapneumonic Effusion and Empyema

Parapneumonic effusion is accumulation of mobile fluid in the pleural space secondary to underlying lung infection. These effusions may be free flowing or can become loculated, otherwise known as an empyema. Bacterial pneumonia is a common cause of parapneumonic effusions in children, specifically with *Streptococcus pneumoniae* and *Staphylococcus aureus* as the most common causative organisms.

There are three main stages of progression of a parapneumonic effusion: exudative, fibrinopurulent, and organizing. Free-flowing fluid secreted into the pleural space secondary to the inflammatory process defines an exudative effusion. As the infection progresses, fibrin begins to accumulate in the pleural fluid. In the early fibrinopurulent phase, fibrin causes the pleural fluid to thicken, leading to septations and loculations. In the late fibrinopurulent stage, pus accumulates in the pleural space. In the organizing phase, a thick rind of pleura forms around the fluid, which can impair respiratory function by limiting lung re-expansion, as well as render the pleural space vulnerable to recurrent infections.

On chest radiographs in pediatric patients with parapneumonic effusion, lack of mobility of the effusion with changing patient positioning suggests a complex effusion. US is the best imaging modality to characterize a parapneumonic effusion with typical findings including low-level echoes, layering debris, and internal septations. Empyema is characterized by a fibrous capsule surrounding the complex pleural fluid (Fig. 7.22). CT is not routinely performed in evaluation of

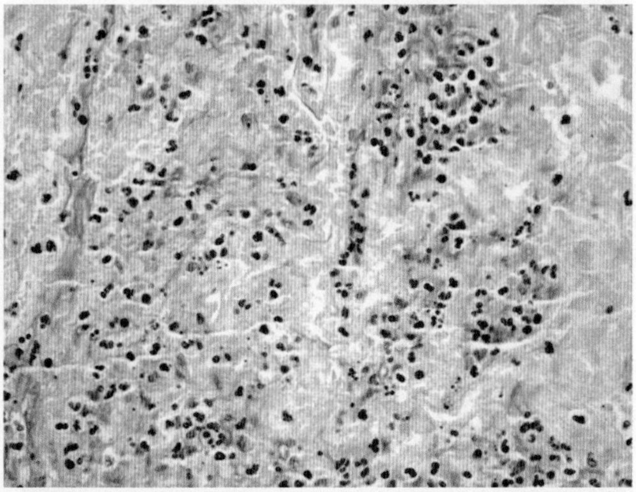

FIGURE 7.22 **Empyema from a 3-year-old girl with a complicated pneumonia.** The pleural decortication specimen shows fibrinopurulent material, including neutrophils, cellular debris, and fibrin (hematoxylin and eosin, original magnification, 600×).

parapneumonic effusions and it has been reported that CT characteristics of parapneumonic effusions do not allow radiologists to accurately predict empyema.[13] However, CT can be valuable for evaluating other abnormalities such as lung abscess or bronchopleural fistula (Figs. 7.3 and 7.17). On CT, an empyema is a loculated pleural-based collection with contrast enhancement of the thickened pleural walls, known as the "split pleura sign" (Fig. 7.23). This can be differentiated from lung abscesses, which are intraparenchymal and can have an internal air–fluid level (Fig. 7.3). Although less sensitive than US, CT may also show underlying septations within a parapneumonic effusion. Air within a parapneumonic effusion or empyema without recent history of an intervention suggests the presence of a bronchopleural fistula (Fig. 7.17).

Treatment of a parapneumonic effusion is different for simple versus complex effusions. A simple effusion can be treated with thoracentesis or percutaneous placement of a chest tube. Treatment of complex parapneumonic effusions and empyema in pediatric patients is currently controversial. Treatment options include drainage via chest tube, with or without instillation of a fibrinolytic agent into the pleural space. More invasive treatment options include video-assisted thoracoscopy (VATS) or open thoracotomy. Complication such as bronchopleural fistula can be managed initially with percutaneous decompression via thoracostomy tube. If conservative management fails, VATS or open thoracotomy may be performed to surgically repair the fistula.

Follow-up imaging involves radiographs, which can be obtained 4 to 6 weeks posttreatment to assess interval decrease or resolution of the parapneumonic effusion or empyema. If treatment is successful, radiographs typically return to baseline after ~3 to 6 months in the pediatric population. However, if affected pediatric patients continue to be symptomatic after treatment, additional follow-up imaging with US or CT may be beneficial to assess for underlying complications.

Pleural Neoplasms

In general, primary pleural neoplasms are rare in children, whereas secondary tumors, either metastatic or via direct invasion, are more common (Table 7.2). Benign primary pediatric pleural tumors that have been reported include lipoma, myofibroma, and calcifying fibrous tumor. Malignant primary pleural tumors include desmoplastic round cell tumor, solitary fibrous tumor, and mesothelioma. The most common tumors that metastasize to the pleura in children are neuroblastoma (Fig. 7.24), lymphoma, Wilms tumor, rhabdomyosarcoma, and other sarcomas.

Treatment of pleural neoplasms differs for primary versus secondary (metastatic) tumors. Primary tumors are typically treated by surgical resection, often combined with chemotherapy. The mainstay of treatment for secondary pleural tumors is directed to the underlying primary neoplasm; however, debulking or complete surgical resection of metastatic pleural tumor may be indicated in symptomatic pediatric patients.

Primary Pleural Neoplasms

Benign Primary Pleural Neoplasms

Lipoma is a rare benign pleural neoplasm in children, commonly incidentally found by imaging. Chest wall lipoma often protrudes into the pleural cavity, which is rarely symptomatic.[14] On US, pleural lipoma is a typically hyperechoic lesion with well-circumscribed borders. CT demonstrates a lesion with low attenuation similar to that of the adjacent subcutaneous fat, which can confirm the diagnosis (Fig. 7.25). It is usually intimately associated with the chest wall and extends into the pleural space. MRI with fat saturation technique may be useful in characterizing and confirming a pleural lipoma (Table 7.2).

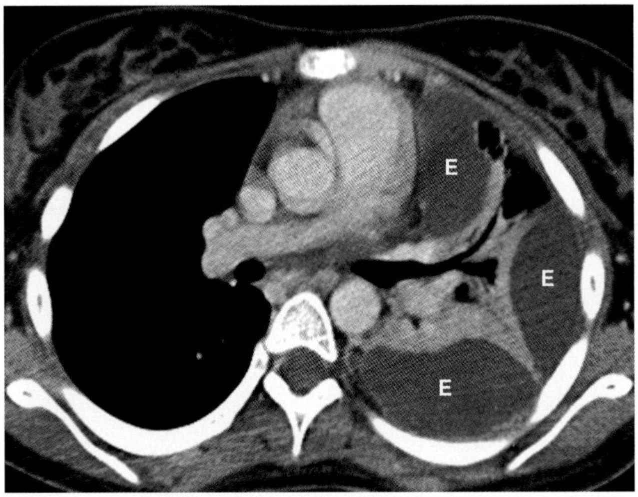

FIGURE 7.23 **Empyema in a 14-year-old girl.** Contrast-enhanced axial CT image shows loculated empyema (E) in the left hemithorax with enhancement of the pleura demonstrating the *split pleura* sign.

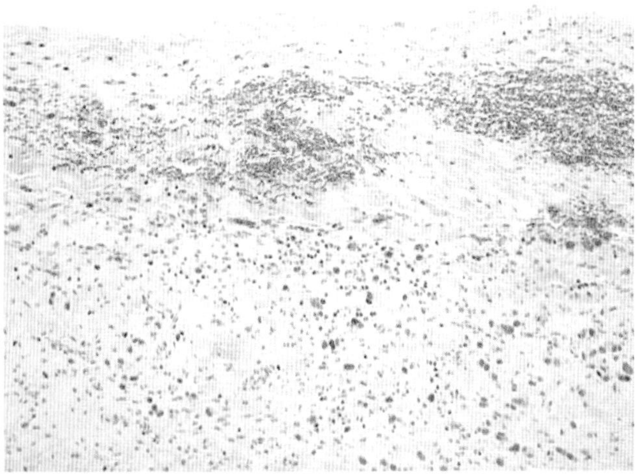

FIGURE 7.24 **Pleural involvement by neuroblastoma in a 7-year-old girl.** Tumor infiltrates the pleura, associated with hemosiderosis and fibrosis (hematoxylin and eosin, original magnification, 200×).

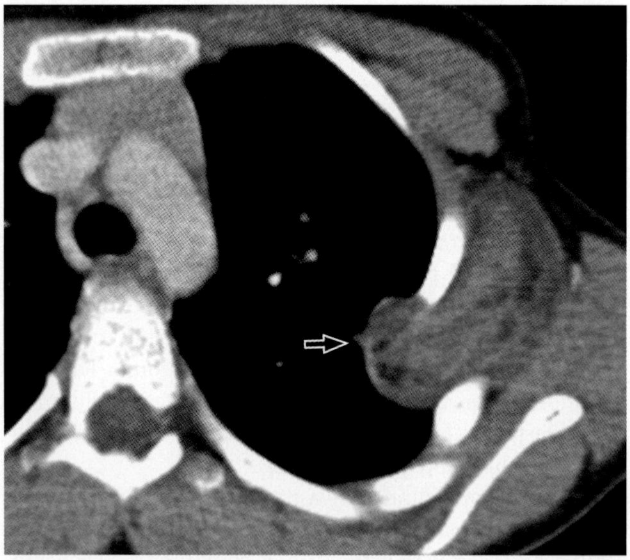

FIGURE 7.25 **Lipoma in a 7-year-old boy.** Contrast-enhanced axial CT image shows a mass (*arrow*) in the left chest wall extending into the pleural space. Areas of low attenuation within the mass demonstrate Hounsfield units confirming fat.

Infantile myofibroma/myofibromatosis is a benign tumor composed of mature and immature myofibroblastic cells with hemangiopericytoma-like vessels. It is an unusual condition, which can be solitary or multicentric. Infantile myofibromatosis may involve various sites such as skin, muscle, bones, and viscera. Pulmonary and pleural involvement is rare. The US appearance of infantile myofibromatosis can be variable; therefore, there are no specific characteristic imaging findings described. On CT, the lesion often demonstrates isointense attenuation to adjacent muscle with some peripheral enhancement. Like US, the MR appearance of the lesions can be variable; however, they typically have a T1 hypointense and T2 hyperintense center with peripheral enhancement on postcontrast images.[15]

TABLE 7.2 Pleural Neoplasms in Children

Primary Pleural Neoplasms
- Benign primary pleural neoplasms
  - Lipoma
  - Hemangioma/lymphatic malformation
  - Infantile myofibromatosis
  - Solitary fibrous tumor
- Malignant primary pleural neoplasms
  - Desmoplastic small round cell tumor
  - Mesothelioma
  - Ewing sarcoma (Askin tumor)
  - Pleuropulmonary blastoma

Secondary Malignant Pleural Neoplasms
- Metastases
  - Neuroblastoma
  - Lymphoma
  - Wilms tumor
  - Sarcomas

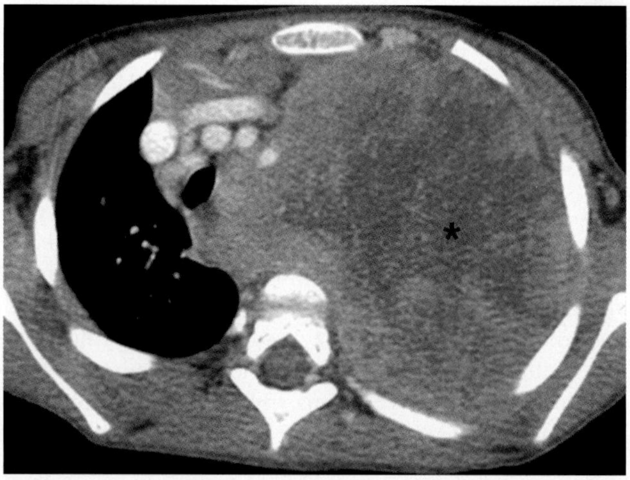

FIGURE 7.26 **Desmoplastic small round cell tumor in a 5-year-old boy who presented with chest pain and weight loss.** Contrast-enhanced axial CT image shows large heterogeneously enhancing mass (*asterisk*) in the left hemithorax, causing contralateral mediastinal shift and crossing midline.

Malignant Primary Pleural Neoplasms

Desmoplastic small round cell tumor is a rare malignancy that most commonly presents as single or multiple masses in the abdominal cavity. However, it rarely can present as primary neoplasm of the pleura in the second or third decade of life with a male predilection. With pleural involvement, affected pediatric patients can be symptomatic with chest pain and respiratory symptoms. If the disease is located in a paraspinal pleural location, it can also present with scoliosis. On imaging studies, desmoplastic small round cell tumor often presents as a large, heterogeneous enhancing mass with associated pleural effusions or destruction of adjacent osseous structures (Fig. 7.26).

Mesothelioma is substantially more common in the adult population. However, it rarely occurs in children in the second decade. There is a predilection for pleura with a male predominance and poor prognosis.[16]

Secondary Malignant Pleural Neoplasms

Malignant neoplasms can affect the pleura primarily by direct invasion from adjacent intrapulmonary, mediastinal, or chest wall lesions (Fig. 7.27) or hematogenously. In pediatric patients, metastatic pleural neoplasms usually arise from neuroblastoma, lymphoma (Fig. 7.28), Wilms tumor, synovial sarcoma, and other sarcomas. Tumors that may reach the pleura by direct extension from the chest wall include Ewing

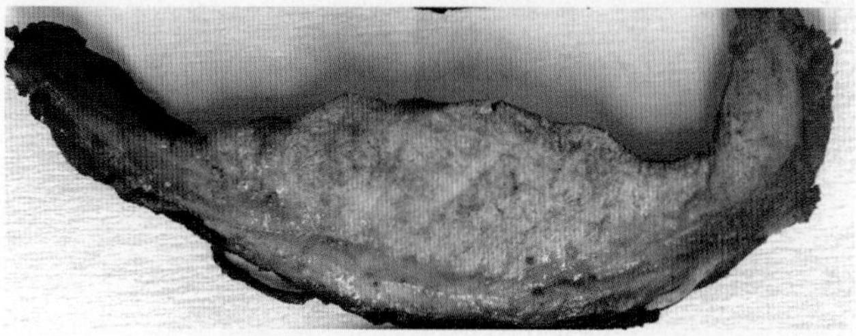

FIGURE 7.27 **Ewing sarcoma in a 4-year-old girl, involving the rib and surrounding soft tissue, with extension to the pleura (upper aspect).**

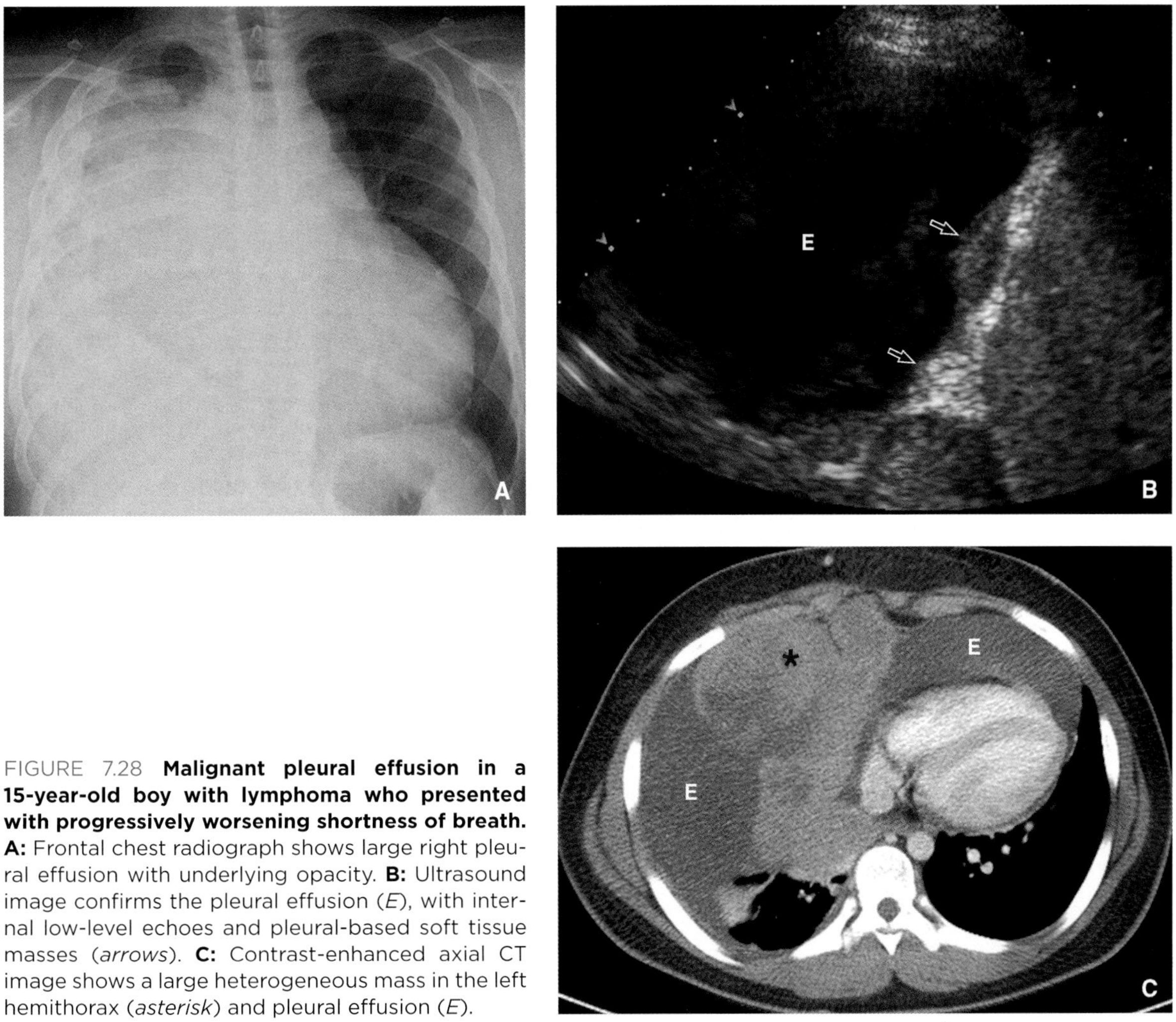

FIGURE 7.28 **Malignant pleural effusion in a 15-year-old boy with lymphoma who presented with progressively worsening shortness of breath.** **A:** Frontal chest radiograph shows large right pleural effusion with underlying opacity. **B:** Ultrasound image confirms the pleural effusion (*E*), with internal low-level echoes and pleural-based soft tissue masses (*arrows*). **C:** Contrast-enhanced axial CT image shows a large heterogeneous mass in the left hemithorax (*asterisk*) and pleural effusion (*E*).

sarcoma (Askin tumor) (Fig. 7.29), malignant peripheral nerve sheath tumor, and other sarcomas.

On chest radiograph, the most common finding of metastatic pleural neoplasm is pleural effusion. Sometimes, it can be difficult to differentiate the pleural tumor from the underlying pleural fluid (Fig. 7.28A). US can be a helpful tool to characterize the pleural effusion as well as to evaluate the underlying mass (Fig. 7.28B). Although both CT and MRI can be used to characterize malignant pleural neoplasms as well as evaluate the extent and involvement of adjacent structures, contrast-enhanced MRI has superior ability to CT for evaluation of diaphragm or chest wall involvement from malignant pleural neoplasms.[17] In one study, high signal intensity of pleural-based masses in relation to the intercostal muscles on T2-weighted MR images had a sensitivity of 91% and specificity of 80% for diagnosing pleural malignancy.[16] In addition, enhancement on the postcontrast T1-weighted MR images had a sensitivity of 93% and specificity of 73% for detecting pleural malignancy.[16] MRI findings that suggest pleural malignancy include pleural nodularity, pleural thickness >10 mm, mediastinal or circumferential pleural involvement, or invasion of the chest wall and/or diaphragm.[16] The combination of these MRI findings has an overall sensitivity of 96% and specificity of 80% for detecting pleural malignancy.[17] However, although these MRI findings are helpful, given the overlap of imaging appearance of primary and metastatic pleural neoplasms, definitive diagnosis relies on pathological examination of biopsy samples, which can be obtained with image guidance.

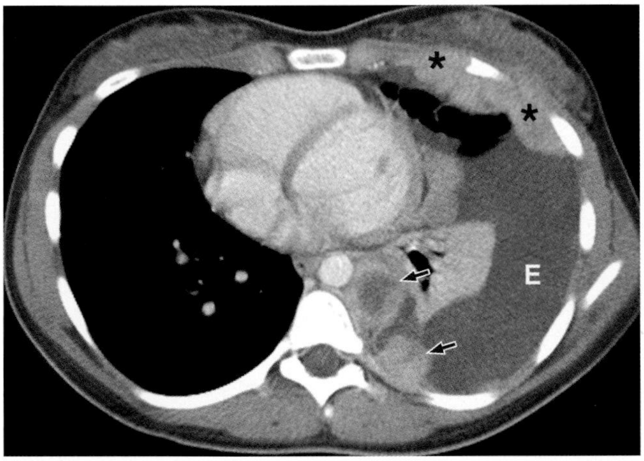

FIGURE 7.29 **Pleural spread of Ewing sarcoma (Askin tumor) in a 14-year-old girl.** Contrast-enhanced axial CT image shows heterogeneously enhancing pleural-based masses (*arrows*) and large left pleural effusion (*E*). The anteriorly located pleural-based masses (*asterisk*) extending into the anterior chest wall are also seen.

References

1. Baez JC, Sodhi KS, Restrepo R, et al. Sonographic evaluation of congenital and acquired thoracic disorders in pediatric patients. *Ultrasound Clin.* 2013:8(3)265–284.
2. Balfour-Lynn IM, et al. BTS guidelines for the management of pleural infection in children. *Thorax.* 2005;60 (suppl 1):i1–i21.
3. Heffner JE, Klein JS, Hampson C. Diagnostic utility and clinical application of imaging for pleural space infections. *Chest.* 2010;137(2):467–479.
4. Sevin CM, Light RW. Microscopic anatomy of the pleura. *Thorac Surg Clin.* 2011;21(2):173–175, vii.
5. Johnson NN, Toledo A, Endom EE. Pneumothorax, pneumomediastinum, and pulmonary embolism. *Pediatr Clin North Am.* 2010;57(6):1357–1383.
6. Robinson PD, Cooper P, Ranganathan SC. Evidence-based management of paediatric primary spontaneous pneumothorax. *Paediatr Respir Rev.* 2009;10(3):110–117; quiz 117.
7. Coley BD. Pediatric chest ultrasound. *Radiol Clin North Am.* 2005;43(2):405–418.
8. Wilkerson RG, Stone MB. Sensitivity of bedside ultrasound and supine anteroposterior chest radiographs for the identification of pneumothorax after blunt trauma. *Acad Emerg Med.* 2010;17(1):11–17.
9. Guimaraes CV, Donnelly LF, Warner BW. CT findings for blebs and bullae in children with spontaneous pneumothorax and comparison with findings in normal age-matched controls. *Pediatr Radiol.* 2007;37(9):879–884.
10. Warner BW, Bailey WW, Shipley RT. Value of computed tomography of the lung in the management of primary spontaneous pneumothorax. *Am J Surg.* 1991;162(1):39–42.
11. Choudhary AK, et al. Primary spontaneous pneumothorax in children: the role of CT in guiding management. *Clin Radiol.* 2005;60(4):508–511.
12. Efrati O, Barak A. Pleural effusions in the pediatric population. *Pediatr Rev.* 2002;23(12):417–426.
13. Donnelly LF, Klosterman LA. CT appearance of parapneumonic effusions in children: findings are not specific for empyema. *AJR Am J Roentgenol.* 1997;169(1):179–182.
14. Granville L, et al. Review and update of uncommon primary pleural tumors: a practical approach to diagnosis. *Arch Pathol Lab Med.* 2005;129(11):1428–1443.
15. Koujok K, Ruiz RE, Hernandez RJ. Myofibromatosis: imaging characteristics. *Pediatr Radiol.* 2005;35(4):374–380.
16. Coffin CM, Dehner LP. Mesothelial and related neoplasms in children and adolescents: a clinicopathologic and immunohistochemical analysis of eight cases. *Pediatr Pathol.* 1992;12(3):333–347.
17. Hierholzer J, et al. MRI and CT in the differential diagnosis of pleural disease. *Chest.* 2000;118(3):604–609.

CHAPTER 8

Airway

Evan J. Zucker • Supika Kritsaneepaiboon • Omolola M. Atalabi • Ricardo Restrepo • Yumin Zhong • Sally A. Vogel • Edward Y. Lee

INTRODUCTION

Airway disease is common in the pediatric population, and imaging is an essential component of the diagnostic evaluation. Prompt recognition and accurate diagnosis are crucial, as many disorders can be potentially life threatening. Affected pediatric patients often present with stridor, wheezing, and respiratory distress because of acute airway obstruction. With smaller and more collapsible airways, infants and children tend to develop symptoms earlier than do their adult counterparts.[1] Chronic airway obstruction may manifest as recurrent pulmonary infections or obstructive sleep apnea (OSA).[2]

In this chapter, an overview of pediatric airway disease is provided. First, the variety of imaging techniques currently available for evaluating the pediatric airway is discussed. The normal anatomy of the pediatric airways is reviewed. Finally, selected pediatric airway disorders important for everyday practice, focusing on pathophysiology, clinical features, imaging assessment, and treatment approaches, are presented.

IMAGING TECHNIQUES

Radiography

In pediatric patients, who present with potential airway disorder, imaging assessment typically begins with frontal and lateral views of the neck and/or chest (Figs. 8.1 to 8.5). Relatively inexpensive and widely available radiographs are the first-line modality for helping to exclude foreign body aspiration and other causes of respiratory distress.[1,2]

The airway is best evaluated with a magnification high-kilovoltage (kV) technique with the anteroposterior (AP) view tightly coned to the neck and selectively filtered to eliminate overlying bony shadows from the cervical spine[3] (Table 8.1). Proper positioning is essential for the lateral neck view, which should be performed in inspiration with moderate neck extension. Rotation, flexion, or expiration may lead to inaccurate interpretation[1,2] (Fig. 8.4). However, an optimal exam may be difficult to achieve in

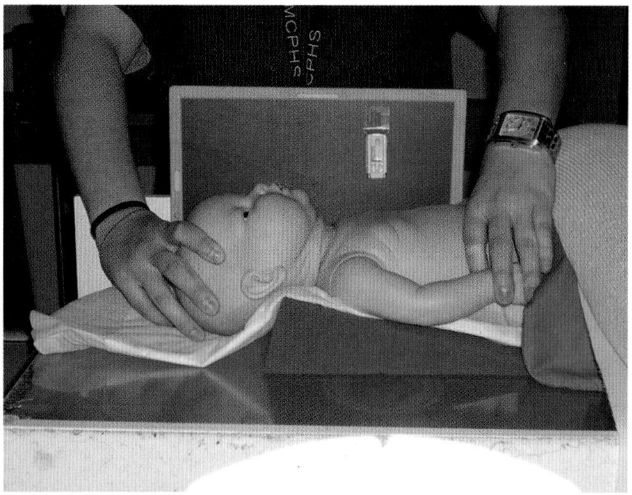

FIGURE 8.1 **Position for lateral airway radiography in an infant.** The lateral radiograph is obtained in deep inspiration with the neck extended. Radiographer can stabilize the optimal neck position of the patient while obtaining the neck radiograph.

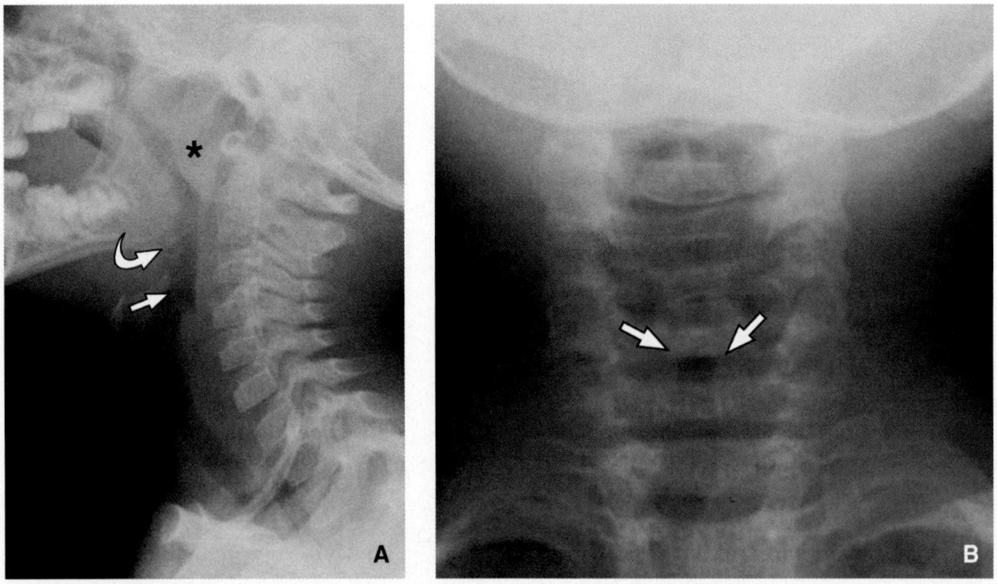

FIGURE 8.2 **Lateral and anteroposterior airway radiographs. A:** Lateral radiograph shows normal degree of oropharyngeal distension, "small finger-sized" epiglottis (*curved arrow*) and thin aryepiglottic folds (*straight arrow*). Moderate enlargement of adenoids (*asterisk*) is also seen. **B:** Anteroposterior airway radiograph demonstrates normal symmetric subglottic "shoulders" (*arrows*).

actual practice in the moving, crying infant. To help solve this problem, a variety of immobilization devices are available for children <4 years old. Pacifiers are also useful. An important caveat is that pediatric patients with suspected airway obstruction should never be forced into a position they do not wish to assume, because this may lead to acute respiratory decompensation, which is potentially life threatening.

Chest radiographs should be obtained near the end of quiet inspiration. In infants, supine AP views of the chest are more easily obtained and adequate because the degree of magnification is similar compared to AP or posteroanterior (PA) erect radiographs. Lateral radiographs are rarely needed. In cooperative children (generally >4 years of age), PA and lateral erect views should be obtained, either standing or sitting (Figs. 8.5 and 8.6). Evaluation for air trapping, an indirect sign of tracheobronchial foreign body obstruction, can be further evaluated with expiratory views in cooperative older children (Fig. 8.7) or the less technically challenging lateral decubitus views in younger uncooperative patients[1] (Fig. 8.8). Gonadal shielding is used to help limit radiation exposure.

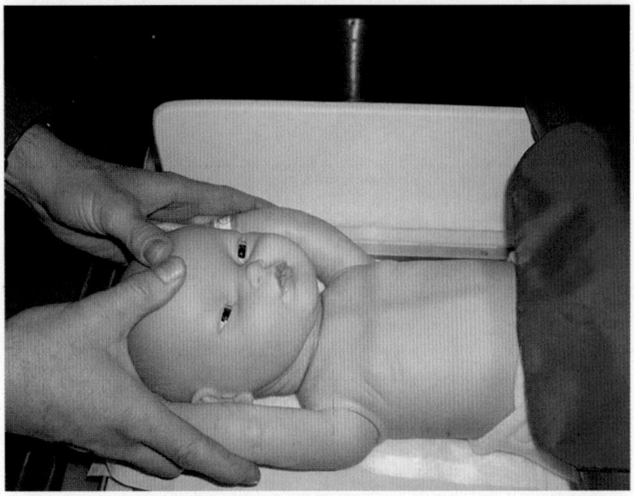

FIGURE 8.3 **Well-coned anteroposterior chest radiograph.** Radiographer can stabilize the child for the optimal chest position while obtaining chest radiograph. Note the lead drape over the lower abdomen.

Ultrasound

Although in general an ideal pediatric imaging modality due to the lack of ionizing radiation, no need for sedation, and ability for real-time assessment in multiple planes, ultrasound (US) has traditionally played a limited role in evaluating the airway. Ultrasound is useful for assessing neck masses, helping to distinguish cystic from solid masses. Lesion vascularity and the patency of vessels and vascular catheters can be readily assessed with Doppler ultrasound.

Although not widely used, techniques for sonographic airway assessment have been described. Patients are imaged supine with a pillow under the shoulders, the head extended, and the neck flexed ("sniffing" position). A linear high-frequency transducer is best for superficial airway structures (within 2 to 3 cm from the skin), with images obtained in the transverse plane (Fig. 8.9). A curved low-frequency transducer is most useful for sagittal and parasagittal views of structures in the submandibular and supraglottic regions. Sonography complements the physical examination and direct visualization methods such as laryngoscopy. Ultrasound may also provide imaging guidance for procedures such as percutaneous tracheostomy.[4,5]

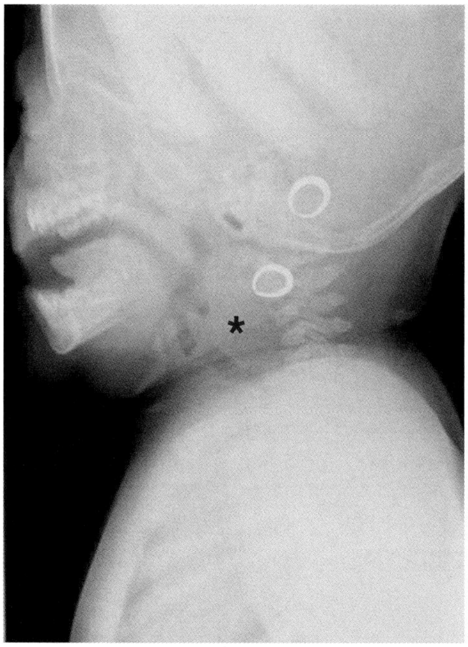

FIGURE 8.4 **Suboptimal quality lateral airway radiograph due to overlying earrings and fingers with suboptimal neck extension obtained in expiration.** Widening (*asterisk*) of the retropharyngeal soft tissues during expiration may mimic a retropharyngeal abscess.

Airway Fluoroscopy

Airway fluoroscopy is useful for evaluating dynamic abnormalities such as laryngomalacia and tracheomalacia (Fig. 8.10). It may be combined with a barium swallow study.[2] The entire airway from nasopharynx to main bronchi can be evaluated safely, rapidly, and noninvasively in frontal, lateral, and oblique projections. In accordance with the As Low As Reasonably Achievable (ALARA) principle, radiation dose reduction techniques should be implemented whenever possible such as pulsed fluoroscopy and restricting time spent using the fluoroscopic pedal. Evaluation may be limited in uncooperative infants and young children and older children with larger body habitus.[1,2]

Dynamic sleep airway fluoroscopy is useful for assessing such conditions as OSA. The patient is sedated with continuous vital sign and pulse oximetry monitoring. When signs of airway occlusion occur, fluoroscopic evaluation for 10 to 20 seconds is performed at selected anatomical sites in the lateral supine position and correlated with clinical findings. The oropharynx at the level of the base of the tongue, hypopharynx, and intrathoracic trachea is typically assessed. Downward pulling of the arms improves neck visualization, whereas an arms-above-head position maximizes assessment of the intrathoracic trachea. A maximum of 2-minute fluoroscopy is used to limit radiation exposure.[6]

Computed Tomography

Multidetector computed tomography (MDCT) with multiplanar two-dimensional (2D) and three-dimensional (3D) reformation is now the noninvasive gold standard for evaluation of the pediatric airway (Fig. 8.11). Combining precise anatomical detail with rapid scan times, MDCT often eliminates the need for sedation and intubation to achieve diagnostic imaging. Newer techniques including paired inspiratory–expiratory MDCT, cine MDCT, and four-dimensional (4D) MDCT permit dynamic airway assessment.[7–9] Nevertheless, use of CT is tempered by growing concerns about risks of radiation exposure particularly in children.[10]

TABLE 8.1 Radiography Technique for Soft Tissue Neck

Age	View	KVP	MAS	AEC	Grid	SID	FSS
0–3 mo	AP	60	1.5	Off	No	40"	Small
3–12 mo	AP	60	2	Off	No	40"	Small
1–3 y	AP	65	2	Off	No	40"	Small
3–6 y	AP	65	5	Active	Grid	40"	Small
6–10 y	AP	70	5	Active	Grid	40"	Small
>10 y	AP	75	8	Active	Grid	40"	Small
Age	**View**	**KVP**	**MAS**	**AEC**	**Grid**	**SID**	**FSS**
0–3 mo	Lateral	60	4	Off	No	72"	Small
3–12 mo	Lateral	60	5	Off	No	72"	Small
1–3 y	Lateral	65	6	Off	No	72"	Small
3–6 y	Lateral	65	6.5	Off	No	72"	Small
6–10 y	Lateral	70	7	Off	No	72"	Small
>10 y	Lateral	75	15	Off	Grid	72"	Large

KVP, kilovoltage; MAS, current; AEC, automatic exposure control; SID, source to image-receptor distance; FSS, focal spot size.

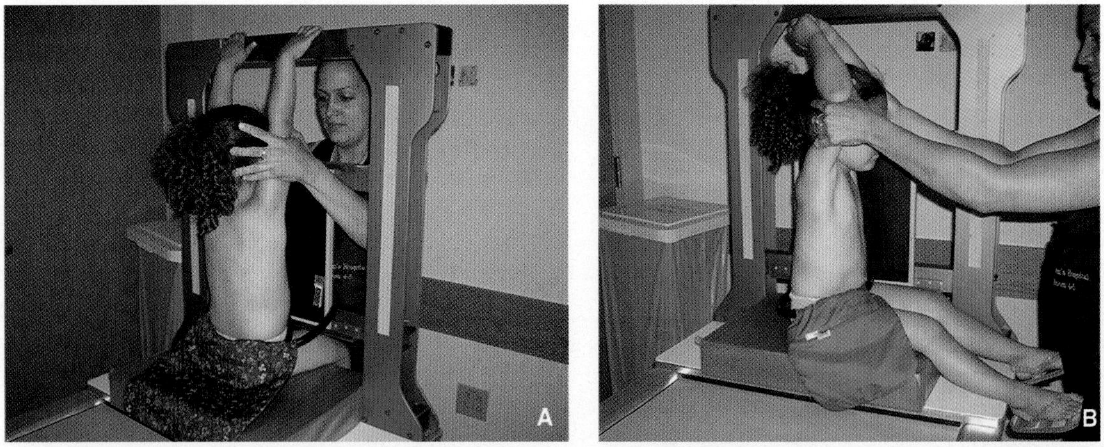

FIGURE 8.5 **Positioning for upright chest radiograph in cooperative older children.** Posteroanterior **(A)** and lateral **(B)** radiograph in an upright position can be obtained in sitting position and with the arm elevated.

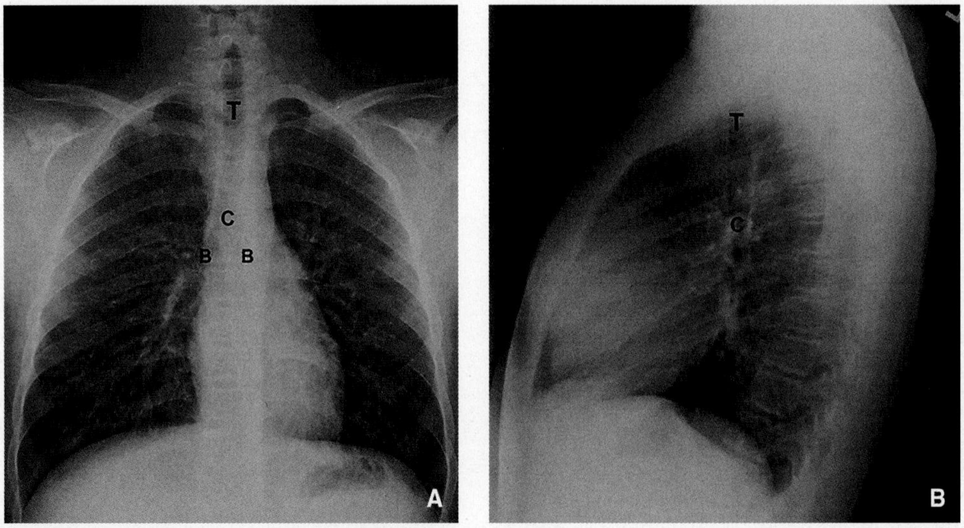

FIGURE 8.6 **Normal chest radiograph in an older child. A:** Posteroanterior chest radiograph shows trachea (*T*), carina (*C*), and bilateral mainstem bronchi (*B*). **B:** Lateral chest radiograph demonstrates trachea (*T*) and carina (*C*).

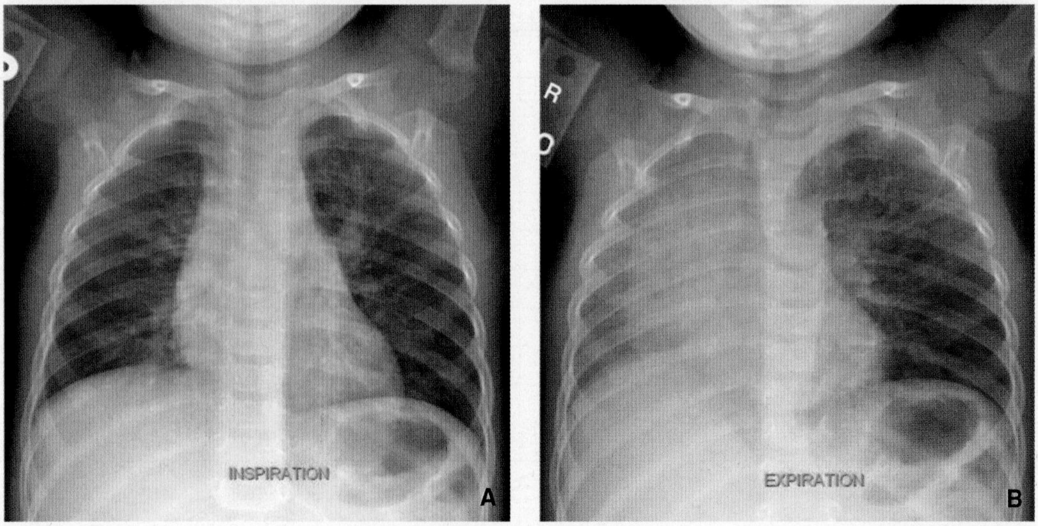

FIGURE 8.7 **Chest radiographs obtained at end inspiration and end expiration in a 5-year-old girl.** This patient was subsequently diagnosed a nonradiopaque foreign body lodged in the left mainstem bronchus by bronchoscopy. **A:** Frontal chest radiograph obtained at end inspiration shows fairly symmetric lung aeration. **B:** Frontal chest radiograph obtained at end expiration demonstrates expected decreased right lung volume but substantial hyperinflation of the left lung indicating underling air trapping due to left mainstem bronchial obstruction.

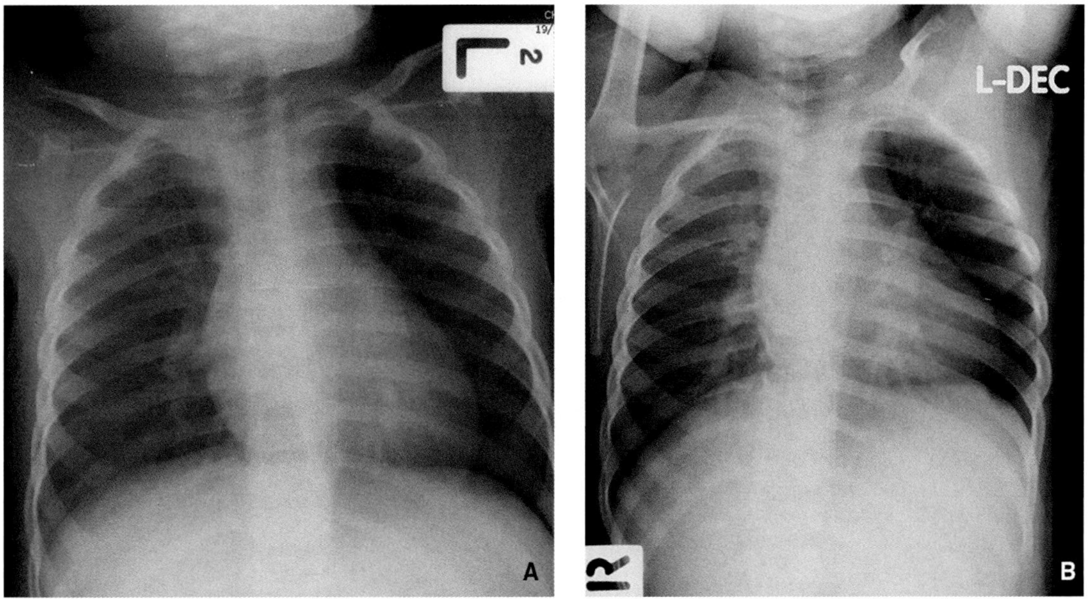

FIGURE 8.8 **Value of lateral decubitus view.** A 2-year-old girl who presented with acute wheezing and coughing after playing with her brother's plastic building toys. The patient was subsequently diagnosed with a nonradiopaque foreign body lodged in the left mainstem bronchus by bronchoscopy. **A:** Frontal radiograph shows mildly hyperinflated left lung compared to the right lung. **B:** Left-sided lateral decubitus view demonstrates persistent hyperinflation of the left lung.

Specific parameters for large airway imaging are dependent on the type of CT scanner. However, in general, optimal imaging can be achieved with ≥16-row MDCT and the following parameters: 0.75-mm collimation for 16-MDCT scanner, 0.625-mm collimation for 32-MDCT scanner, and 0.6-mm collimation for 64-MDCT scanner; high-speed mode; and a pitch equivalent of 1.0 to 1.5. Use of age- or weight-adjusted milliamperage (mA), lowest possible kV, and anatomically based real-time automated exposure control helps reduce radiation exposure. The intrinsic contrast between the air-filled large airways and adjacent mediastinal soft tissues also allows for lower-dose technique. Suggested parameters for tube current and kV from Boston Children's Hospital are shown in Table 8.2. In addition to traditional coronal and sagittal reconstructions, curved planar reformats along the long axis of the trachea and bronchi can be routinely obtained to allow more accurate measurements of the trachea and bronchi[1,2,7,11] (Fig. 8.11D).

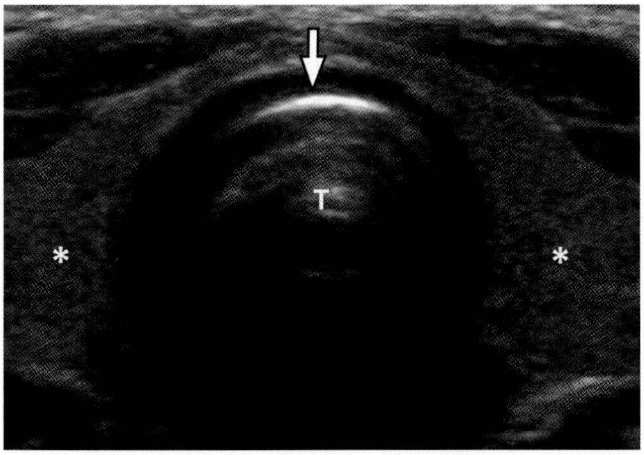

FIGURE 8.9 **Normal trachea seen on ultrasound.** Air within the nondependent portion of the trachea (*T*) in supine position of the patient shows increased echogenicity (*arrow*) with posterior shadowing. Also seen is normal thyroid gland (*asterisks*) on both sides of the trachea.

Magnetic Resonance Imaging

Magnetic resonance imaging (MRI) offers excellent contrast resolution without ionizing radiation. However, long scan times may require sedation to prevent patient motion. MRI of the neck and upper airway generally takes 30 to 60 minutes with current techniques (Fig. 8.12). Intravenous gadolinium contrast is useful for assessing suspected neoplastic or infectious causes of upper airway obstruction.[2]

Beyond static MRI for anatomical evaluation, cine MRI utilizing fast gradient-echo sequences is an emerging modality allowing dynamic airway assessment for such conditions as OSA and velopharyngeal insufficiency.[2,12–17] Studies can be performed on either a 1.5 or 3.0 Tesla (T) MRI unit. The patient is sedated and placed in the head-and-neck vascular coil. In small pediatric patients, the airway from the superior nasal passages to the carina can be visualized in its entirety. In larger pediatric patients, the inferior aspect of the trachea may be outside the field of view. After a 3D localizer image is obtained, sagittal and axial T1-weighted spin-echo (SE) (representative parameters: repetition time [msec]/echo time [msec] of 400/minimal, 22-cm field of view, 4-mm section thickness with 1-mm gap, 256 × 192 matrix, two signals acquired) and sagittal and axial fast SE inversion recovery (IR)

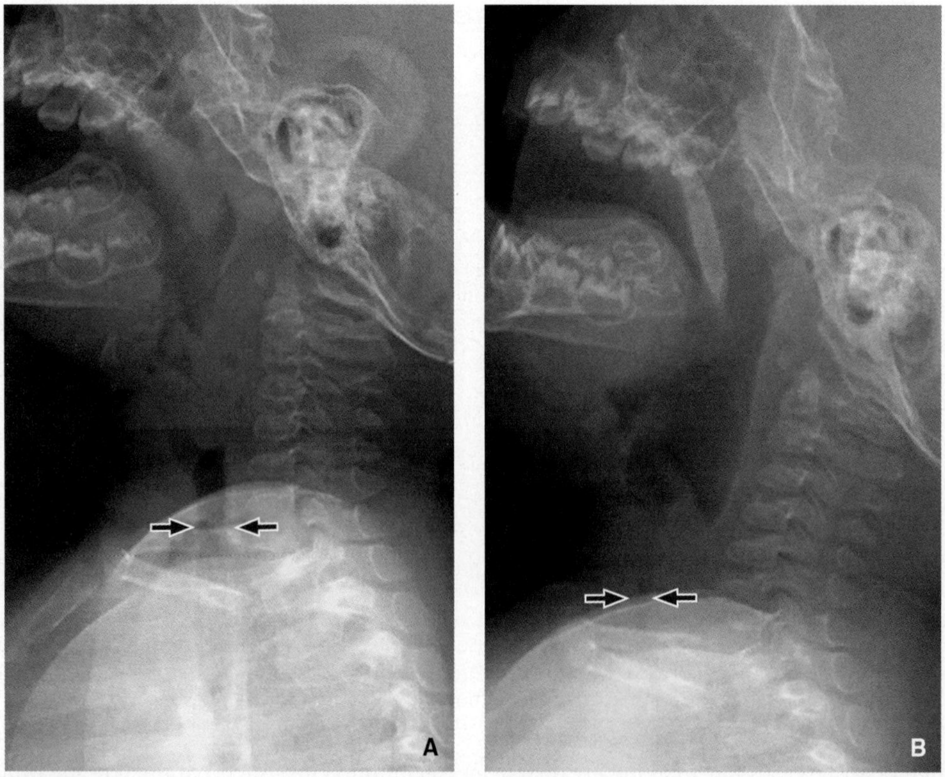

FIGURE 8.10 **Tracheomalacia in a 4-year-old girl who presented with chronic cough and recurrent pulmonary infection.** Subsequently performed bronchoscopy confirmed the diagnosis of marked tracheomalacia. **A:** Lateral radiograph obtained at end inspiration during airway fluoroscopy study of airway shows patent trachea (*arrows*). **B:** Lateral radiograph obtained at end expiration during airway fluoroscopy study demonstrates marked (>75%) collapse of the trachea (*arrows*), consistent with tracheomalacia.

(representative parameters: 5,000/34, echo train length of 12, 22-cm field of view, 6-mm section thickness with 2-mm gap, 256 × 192 matrix, two signals acquired) sequences are obtained. Cine MR is performed in midline sagittal and axial planes at the midportion of the tongue using a fast gradient-echo sequence (representative parameters: 8,200/3,600, 80-degree flip angle, 12-mm section thickness) with 128 consecutive images captured in ~2 minutes and viewed on cine mode.[2,16]

NORMAL ANATOMY AND VARIANTS

The airway includes the nose, paranasal sinuses, pharynx (nasopharynx, oropharynx, and hypopharynx), larynx, trachea, main bronchi, peripheral bronchi, and bronchioles. The nasopharynx is located posterior to the nasal cavity and superior to the soft palate (Fig. 8.12). The oropharynx is situated between the soft palate and tip of the epiglottis. The hypopharynx (laryngopharynx) is bounded by the tip of the epiglottis and the cricoid cartilage. The larynx, bounded by the cricoid cartilage and the tongue base, includes the thyroid and cricoid cartilage, paired arytenoids, and epiglottis.[18] The supraglottic larynx includes the epiglottis, aryepiglottic folds, and false vocal cords, extending to the laryngeal ventricle. The glottic larynx extends from the laryngeal ventricle to the inferior margin of the true vocal cords. Finally, the subglottic larynx then extends to the level of the inferior margin of the cricoid cartilage, subglottic larynx, and upper trachea.

The trachea, a cartilaginous and membranous tube, extends from the larynx at approximately the level of C6 to the upper border of T5 (Fig. 8.13). There it divides into the right and left main bronchi. The right main bronchus divides into the right upper lobe bronchus and bronchus intermedius, which further branches into the right middle and lower lobe bronchi (Figs. 8.13 and 8.14). The left main bronchus divides into the left upper and lower lobe bronchi. There are three right upper lobe segmental bronchi (apical, anterior, and posterior), two right middle lobe segmental bronchi (lateral and medial), and five right lower lobe segmental bronchi (superior, medial basal, anterior basal, lateral basal, and posterior basal). There are four left upper lobe segmental bronchi (apicoposterior, anterior, superior lingular, and inferior lingular) and four left lower lobe segmental bronchi (superior, anteromedial, lateral basal, and posterior basal) (Figs. 8.13 and 8.14). Many normal variations in airway branching anatomy exist.

In initially assessing the upper airway, the lateral neck radiograph is most useful. On a normal exam, the following structures can be identified: nasopharynx, adenoids, hard

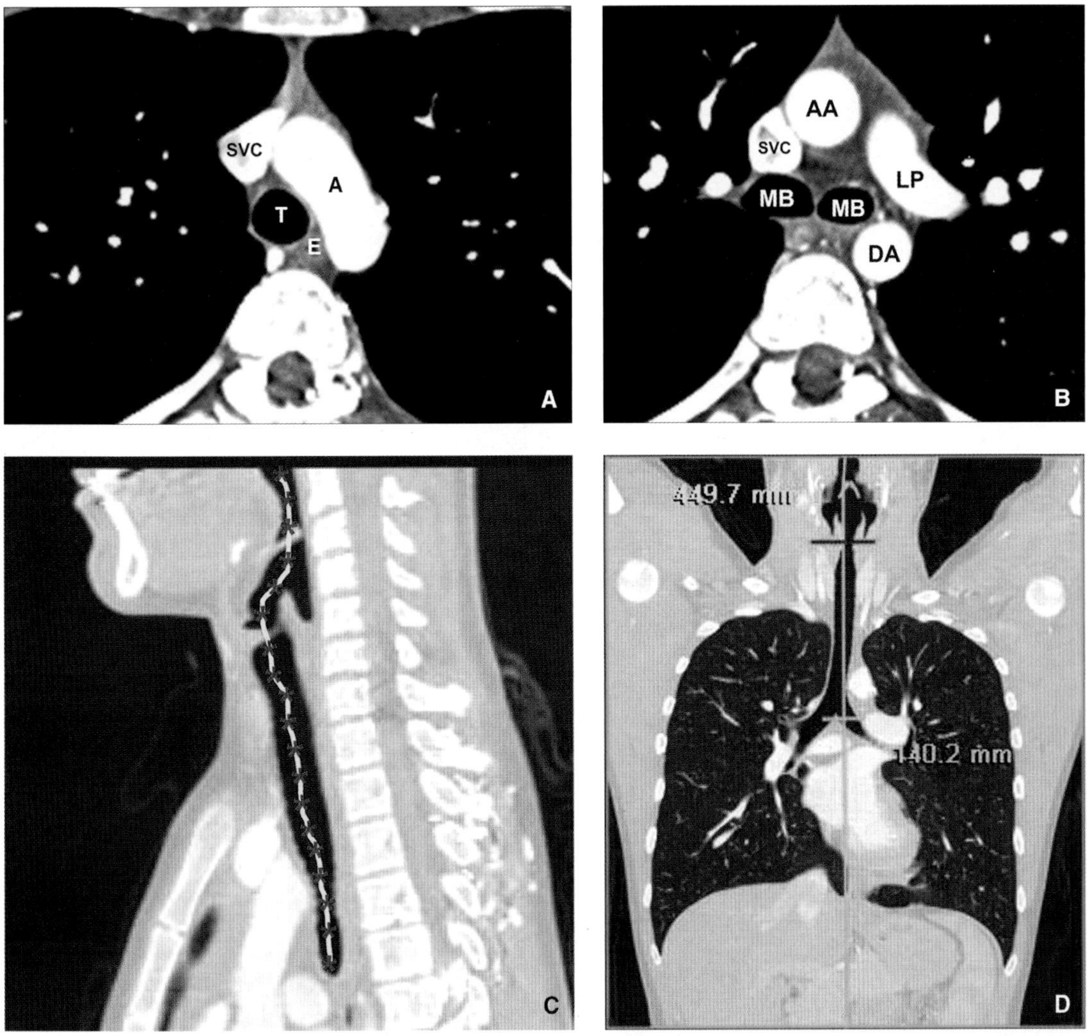

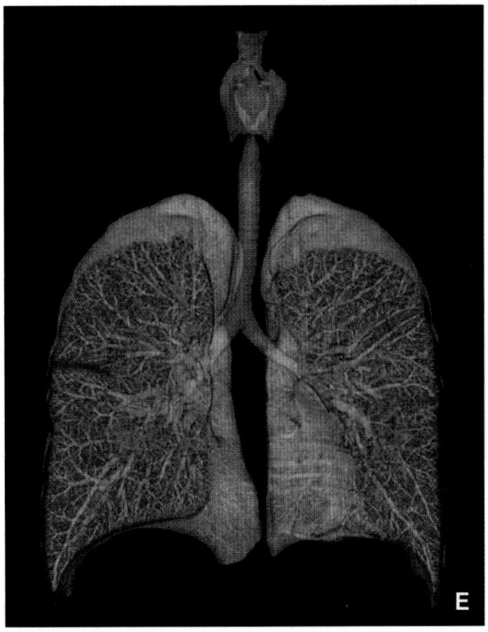

FIGURE 8.11 **Normal large airway in a 6-year-old girl. A:** Enhanced axial CT image at the aortic arch level shows normal round and patent trachea (*T*) obtained at end inspiration. (*A*, aortic arch; *SVC*, superior vena cava; *E*, esophagus.) **B:** Enhanced axial CT image shows normal and patent bilateral mainstem bronchi (*MB*). (*AA*, ascending aorta; *DA*, descending aorta; *SVC*, superior vena cava; *LP*, left main pulmonary artery.) **C:** Sagittal reformatted lung window CT image of the large airway. A reference line (*yellow line* and *red asterisks*) through the center of the airway for reconstruction of a curved coronal reformatted CT image. **D:** Curved coronal reformatted CT image shows a straightened view of the entire trachea. **E:** 3D external volume-rendered CT image (i.e., virtual bronchography) of normal airway.

(Continued)

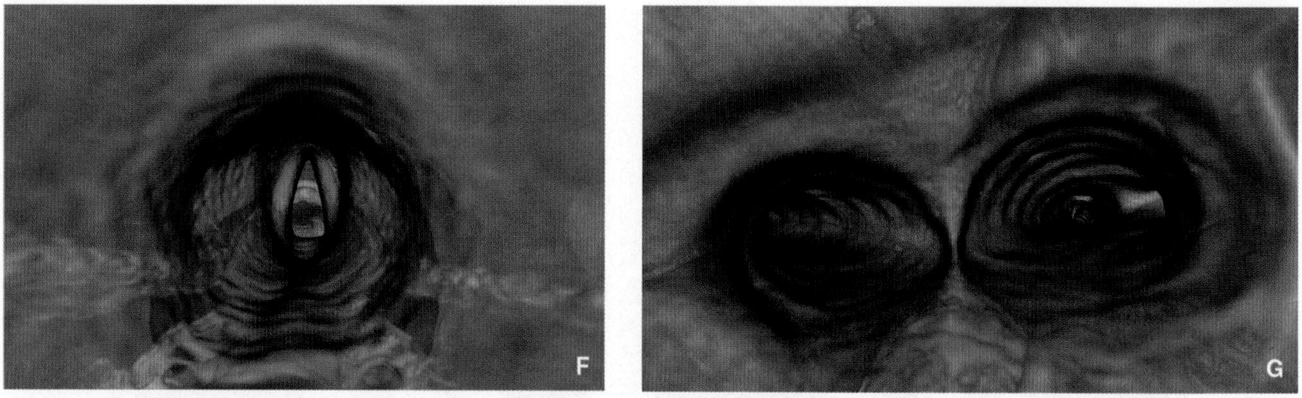

FIGURE 8.11 *(Continued)* **F:** 3D internal volume-rendered CT image (i.e., virtual bronchoscopy) of airway obtained at glottis level. Mildly opened glottis is seen. **G:** 3D internal volume-rendered CT image of airway obtained at the level of carina. Bilateral mainstem bronchi are patent.

and soft palate, uvula, oropharynx, tongue, mandible, base of the tongue, vallecula, epiglottis, aryepiglottic folds, pyriform sinuses, laryngeal ventricle, true and false vocal cords, subglottic larynx, and upper trachea (Fig. 8.2).

In children 5 years old or less, lateral deviation of the trachea is normal and should not be mistaken for pathology (Fig. 8.15). This phenomenon, which tends occur at or just above the thoracic inlet opposite the side of the aortic arch, is felt possibly because of the relatively long tracheal length with respect to the child's short neck and rib cage.[1,19] Other common normal variants are anterior buckling of the trachea and widening of the retropharyngeal soft tissues during expiration and neck flexion, features that may mimic a retropharyngeal abscess[20] (Fig. 8.4).

TABLE 8.2 Tube Current and kV by Patient Weight for Central Airway MDCT

Weight (kg)	Tube Current (mAs) Insp./Exp.	kV
<10	40/20	80
10–14	50/25	80
15–24	60/30	80
25–34	70/35	80
35–44	80/40	80
45–54	90/40	90
55–70	100–120/40	100–120

For tube current and kilovoltage by patient weight for end-expiratory MDCT examination, mAs should be reduced by 50% to a maximum of 40 mA while maintaining the same level of kV for end-inspiratory MDCT examination.

Insp, inspiratory; Exp, expiratory; mA, milliamperage; kV, kilovoltage; MDCT, multidetector computed tomography.

Reprinted from Lee EY, Boiselle PM. Tracheobronchomalacia in infants and children: multidetector CT evaluation. Radiology. 2009;252:7–22, with permission.

SPECTRUM OF PEDIATRIC AIRWAY DISORDERS

Congenital and Developmental Anomalies

Choanal Atresia/Stenosis

Choanal atresia is a congenital obstruction of the nasopharynx characterized by narrowing and closure of the posterior choanae and medialization of the pterygoid plates and lateral wall of the nose.[2,21] It is the most common etiology of neonatal nasal obstruction with an estimated incidence of 1 in 5,000 to 1 in 9,000 births, occurring twice as often in females as in males, more often unilateral than bilateral.[2,21,22] Although osseous obstruction of the choanae was previously thought most common (90%) (Fig. 8.16), with membranous obstruction in the remaining 10% (Fig. 8.17), more recent data suggest a mixed bony/membranous cause in 70% of cases and a pure bony abnormality in 30%.[21] Unilateral choanal atresia may be asymptomatic until the patient develops nasal stuffiness, rhinorrhea, or infection later in life. Failure to pass a nasal enteric tube is a suspicious clinical history. Bilateral choanal atresia can cause severe respiratory distress, as neonates are obligate nose

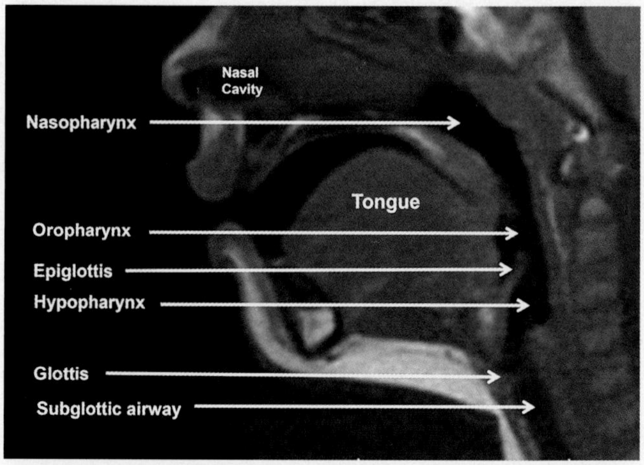

FIGURE 8.12 **Normal anatomy of the upper airway.** T1-weighted sagittal MR image shows normal anatomy of the upper airway.

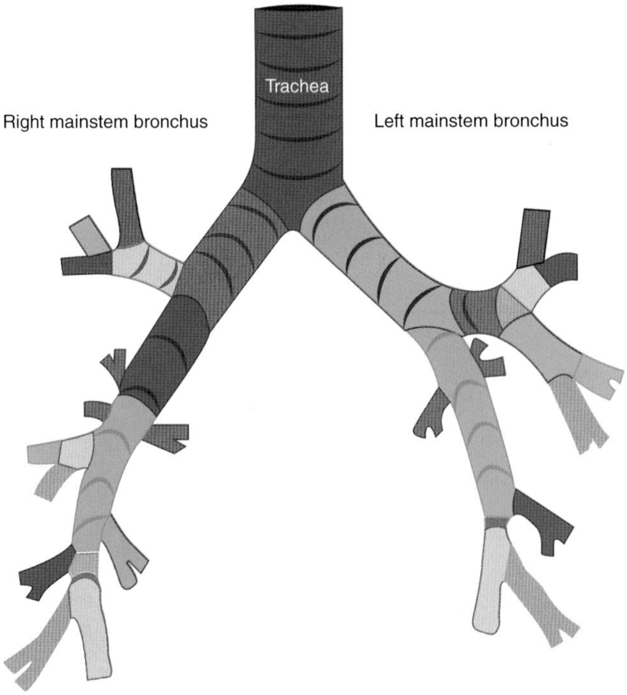

FIGURE 8.13 **Normal bronchial anatomy.**

breathers.[2] Associated anomalies such as coloboma, heart defects, and mental retardation and syndromes including CHARGE (coloboma, heart disease, choanal atresia, growth and mental retardation, genital hypoplasia, ear anomalies with deafness), Crouzon, Pfeiffer, Antley-Bixler, Marshall-Smith, Schinzel-Giedion, and Treacher Collins occur in ~50% of affected patients.[2,21,23]

CT best demonstrates the underlying anatomic abnormalities[2,24] (Fig. 8.16). Characteristic findings are narrowing of the posterior choanae to a width <0.34 cm in children <2 years old, inward bowing of the posterior maxilla, fusion or thickening of the vomer, and a bone or soft tissue septum across the posterior choanae.[2,25] Choanal stenosis may mimic atresia depending on the degree of narrowing and is also best characterized by CT.[2] CT virtual endoscopy, a 3D postprocessing technique requiring ~10 additional minutes per examination but no additional radiation, can be useful in diagnosis and preoperative planning.[26] Instillation of 1 to 3 drops diluted nonionic contrast material through the nostril has also been used to better characterize the communication of the posterior choanae with the nasopharynx.[27]

Surgery is the management of choice for choanal atresia/stenosis involving perforation of the obstructing septum to create a permanently patent airway.[2] A variety of surgical techniques have been used including transnasal puncture, transpalatal resection, stent placement, endoscopic resection, and choanal resection.[2,21] However, there is currently no definitively preferred evidence-based strategy.[22] Correction of unilateral choanal atresia can be delayed until 6 to 9 years of age when the midface reaches almost adult size. In contrast, bilateral choanal atresia requires immediate intervention to reestablish airway patency.[2] CT navigation systems may be helpful in complex cases. Adjuncts such as mitomycin C and laser demonstrate no clear benefit.[21] Surgical success ultimately depends on the type of atresia, approach used, type of stent and duration of placement, and the presence of other anomalies.[2]

Congenital Nasal Pyriform Aperture Stenosis

Congenital nasal pyriform aperture stenosis (CNPAS) is a rare cause of upper airway obstruction in the newborn caused by excessive growth of the medial nasal process of the maxilla.[2] Affected pediatric patients may present with respiratory distress, episodic apnea, cyclical cyanosis, or sudden total airway obstruction.[28,29] Inability to pass a 5-French (F) catheter or endoscope through the nasal cavity is characteristic.[28] Clinically, CNPAS is indistinguishable from bilateral choanal atresia.[2] The disorder may be part of the holoprosencephaly spectrum with a single central maxillary incisor reported in up to 75% of cases as well as other central nervous system (CNS) anomalies.[2,25,28,29] Other associations include chromosomal abnormalities and pituitary hormonal deficiencies.[2,28,29]

CT is the imaging modality of choice, with thin (1.5 to 2 mm) contiguous axial images acquired parallel to the hard palate and roof of the orbit. Multiplanar 2D reformats are helpful but generally not required for diagnosis. Characteristic findings are soft tissue density extending across the nostrils just inside the nares, overgrowth and medial displacement of the nasal processes of the maxilla, and narrowing of the pyriform aperture (Fig. 8.18). Narrowing of the pyriform aperture, bounded by the nasal bone superiorly, the nasal process of the maxilla laterally, and the horizontal process inferiorly, to a width <11 mm in a term infant is considered diagnostic.[2,28,30,31] MR is useful for assessing associated intracranial abnormalities in affected pediatric patients.[32]

Affected children with mild symptoms can be treated conservatively with humidification, topical nasal decongestants, nasal stenting, and placement of an oropharyngeal airway. More severe disease may require surgical intervention.[2,28,29,32] In general, the prognosis is excellent after treatment.[28]

Adenoid and Palatine Tonsil Enlargement

Pathologic enlargement of the normally immunoprotective adenoids and palatine tonsils is a common cause of upper airway obstruction in pediatric patients. Located in the nasopharynx roof just beneath the sphenoid sinus and anterior to the basiocciput, the adenoids are an aggregation of lymphoid tissue absent at birth that rapidly grows during infancy. They reach a maximum size of 7 to 12 mm between 2 years of age and progressively decrease in size during puberty. Similarly, the palatine (faucial) tonsils are masses of lymphoid tissue located between the glossopalatine and pharyngopalatine arches. Hypertrophy of the adenoids and palatine tonsils caused, for example, by chronic inflammation or prior infection may result in

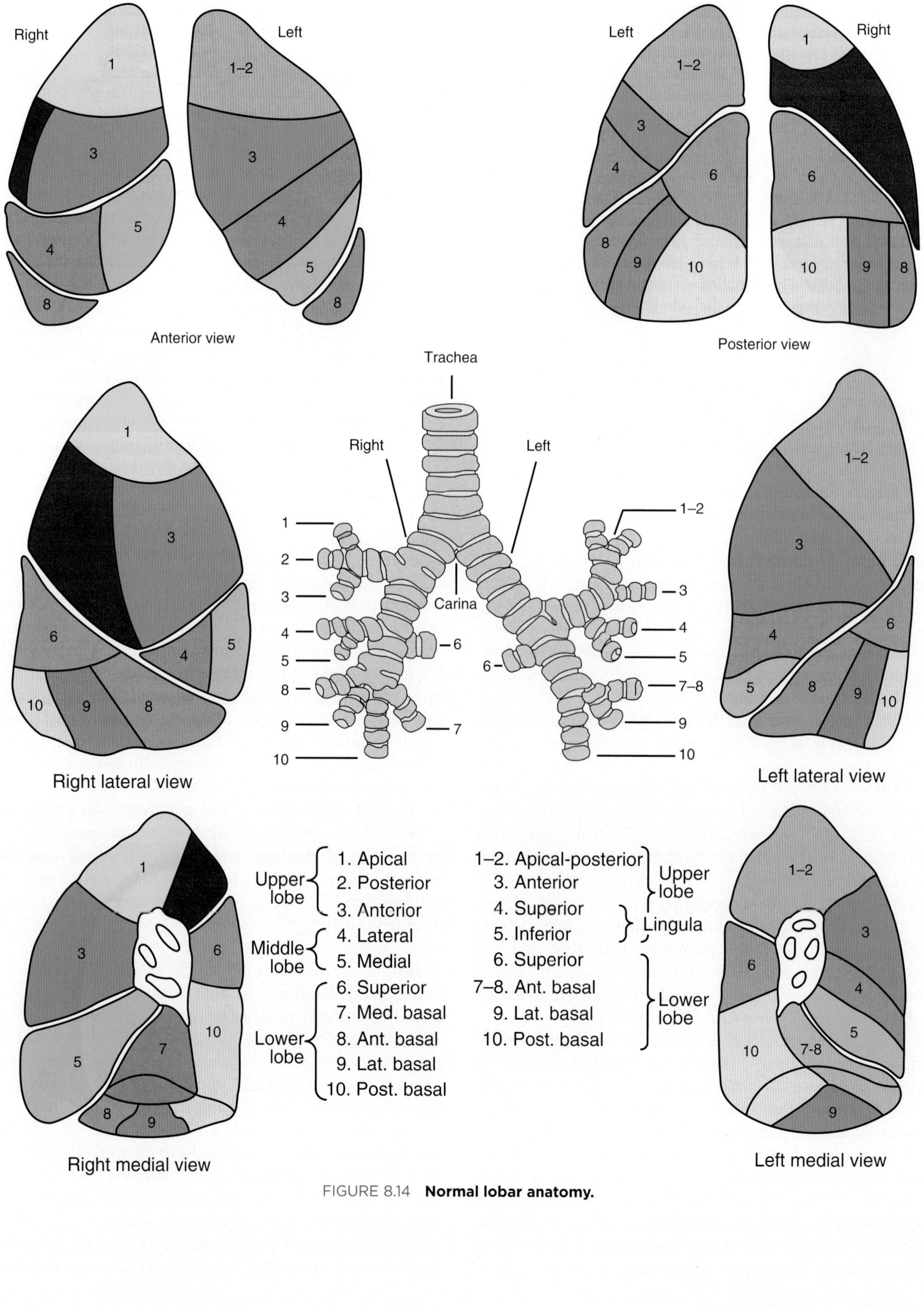

FIGURE 8.14 **Normal lobar anatomy.**

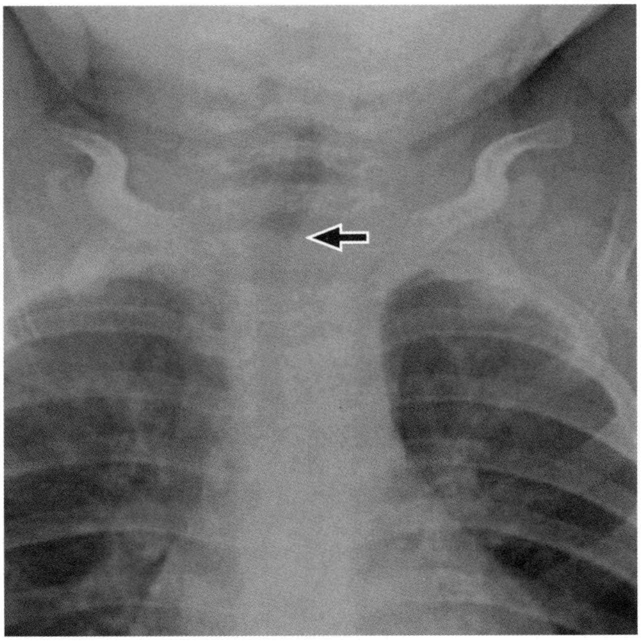

FIGURE 8.15 **Normal trachea deviation (also known as buckling) in an 11-month-old boy who underwent chest radiograph for fever and cough.** Coned radiograph shows normal deviation (*arrow*) of the trachea to the right of midline at the thoracic inlet level.

nasopharyngeal and oropharyngeal obstruction. Potential sequelae include chronic hypoxemia and hypercarbia from hypoventilation and OSA.[2,14,33–37]

Imaging evaluation begins with radiography. The adenoids are considered enlarged if they appear to touch the hard palate on a lateral view of the upper airway (Fig. 8.19). A more objective method is to calculate the adenoidal–nasopharyngeal ratio or adenoidal divided by nasopharyngeal size. A value >0.8 suggests enlarged

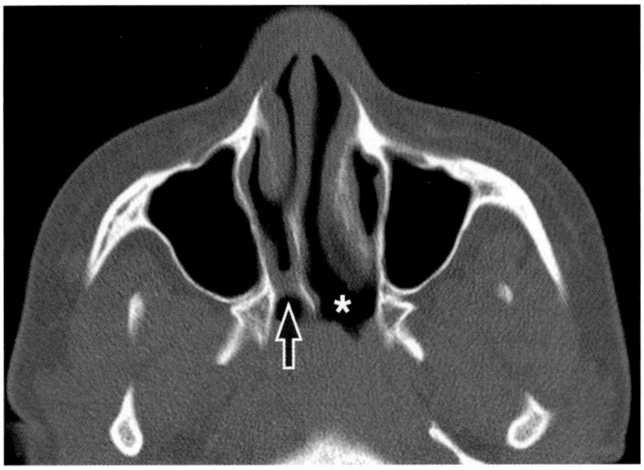

FIGURE 8.17 **Membranous type of choanal atresia.** Axial bone window CT image of the facial bones in a newborn girl who presented with respiratory distress shows narrowed posterior choanae on the right side with soft tissue density (*arrow*) compatible with right-sided membranous type of choanal atresia. Left-sided posterior choanae (*asterisk*) is normal and patent.

adenoids.[2,38,39] The palatine tonsils are considered enlarged when the tonsillar shadow is sufficiently prominent to extend into the hypopharynx. The tonsillar–pharyngeal (T/P) ratio, or width of the tonsil divided by depth of the pharyngeal space on a lateral neck radiograph, has been used to screen children with suspected OSA.[2,40] Sedated video fluoroscopy has traditionally been obtained for dynamic airway evaluation.[2,41] More recently, cine MRI has been used, able to provide volumetric measurements of the tonsils and adenoids as well as dynamic airway assessment.[2,14,42]

Active adenoid and tonsillar infection (with associated enlargement) is treated with antibiotics. For chronic

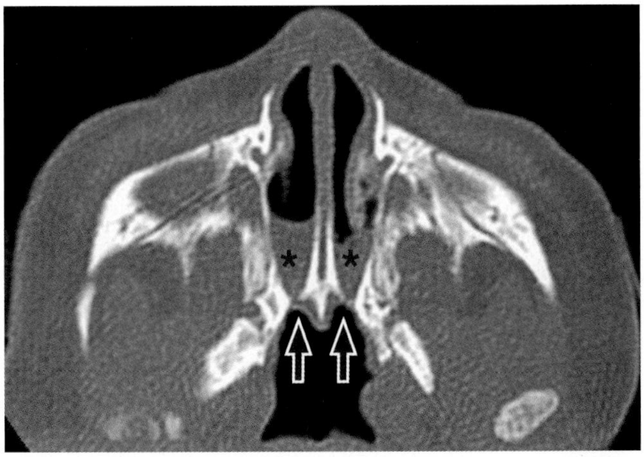

FIGURE 8.16 **Osseous type choanal atresia in a newborn boy who presented with respiratory distress and inability to pass a nasogastric tube.** Axial bone window CT image of the facial bones shows bony obliteration of both choanae with diamond-shaped vomers (*arrows*). Accumulated secretions (*asterisks*) are also present in the dependent potions of the nasal passages.

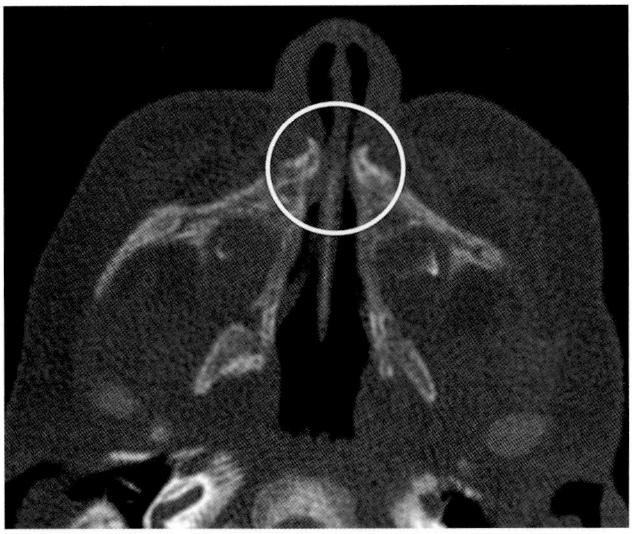

FIGURE 8.18 **Congenital pyriform aperture stenosis in a newborn girl who presented with dyspnea while feeding.** Axial bone window CT image of the facial bone shows marked narrowing (*circled area*) of the nasal passages anteriorly due to closed apposition of the maxilla anteriorly.

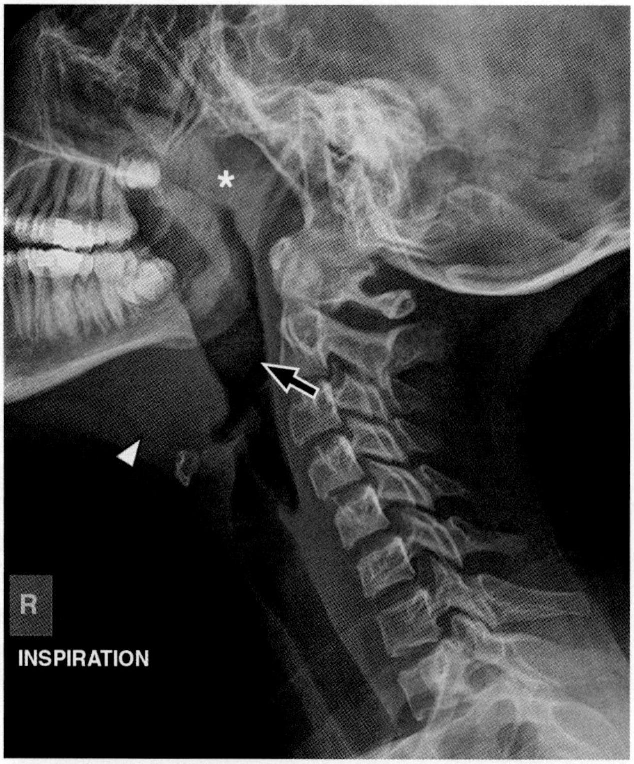

FIGURE 8.19 **Adenoid, palatine, and lingual tonsillar hypertrophy in a 12-year-old girl who presented with progressively worsening oral breathing and snoring.** Lateral radiograph of the upper airway shows moderate prominence of the adenoids (*asterisk*) causing narrowing of the nasopharynx. There is also substantial enlargement of the lingual tonsils (*arrowhead*) and palatine tonsils (*arrow*).

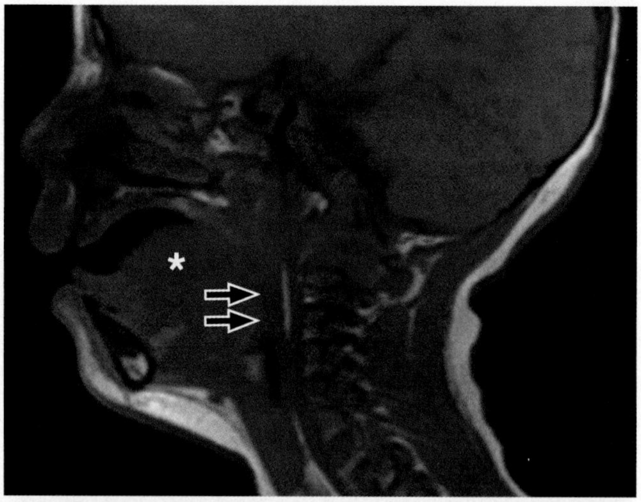

FIGURE 8.20 **Macroglossia in a 4-year-old boy with Down syndrome and respiratory distress.** A sagittal T2-weighted MR image shows a large tongue (*asterisk*) without abnormal internal signal. Glossoptosis or posterior displacement of the tongue is also seen (*arrows*).

enlargement, particularly when associated with airway compromise or OSA, adenoidectomy and/or tonsillectomy may be required. Surgery may also help relieve associated recurrent sinus or ear infections.[2]

Macroglossia

Macroglossia refers to a chronic and painless enlargement of the tongue, which protrudes beyond the teeth or alveolar ridge at rest. It should be differentiated from acute glossitis, characterized by painful and rapid tongue enlargement.[2,43] Causes include hypothyroidism, idiopathic hyperplasia, and various syndromes including the mucopolysaccharidoses, Down, and Beckwith-Wiedeman.[2,44,45] A variant termed relative macroglossia refers to a proportionately large tongue in relation to a small mandible (micrognathia). Presenting symptoms include noisy breathing, drooling, dysphagia, and speech difficulty. Most concerning is the potential for upper airway obstruction.[2,45,46]

Sleep fluoroscopy can be used to assess progressive respiratory distress in affected pediatric patients. The enlarged tongue may be seen falling posteriorly during sleep and obstructing the posterior pharynx.[2,41] Cross-sectional imaging with CT and MRI is also useful in assessing the tongue and helping to exclude underlying masses[2,47] (Fig. 8.20).

In macroglossia related to an underlying systemic process, medical management may be sufficient. Otherwise, surgery with reduction glossectomy is the treatment of choice in symptomatic patients, helping to prevent future airway, speech, and orthodontic problems. Acute upper airway obstruction requires immediate attention and intervention such as tracheostomy.[2,47]

Laryngomalacia

Laryngomalacia is a benign, often transient, condition characterized by abnormal laxity of the pharyngeal soft tissues due to immaturity of the laryngeal cartilages and muscles. These abnormalities cause inspiratory collapse of the epiglottis, arytenoids, and aryepiglottic folds resulting in partial upper airway obstruction. Laryngomalacia is the most common congenital laryngeal anomaly. It is also the most common cause of symptomatic airway obstruction in infants presenting with stridor, which worsens with rest and improves with activity.[2,48–50]

Airway fluoroscopy characteristically demonstrates downward and posterior bending of the epiglottis and anterior buckling of the aryepiglottic folds, narrowing and eventually occluding the upper airway (Fig. 8.21). However, airway fluoroscopy, while relatively specific for the diagnosis, has poor sensitivity. Thus, even when normal, further evaluation with laryngoscopy should be performed if there is persistent clinical suspicion.[2,48,51,52]

Most cases of laryngomalacia are self-limited and resolve without intervention by the first year of life.[2] Acid-suppressing medication should be given in patients with concurrent laryngomalacia and feeding symptoms.[53] Persisting symptoms require surgical intervention to prevent complications such as airway obstruction and even sudden death. Current management techniques include supraglottoplasty, aryepiglottic fold incision, epiglottopexy, and tracheostomy.[2,54]

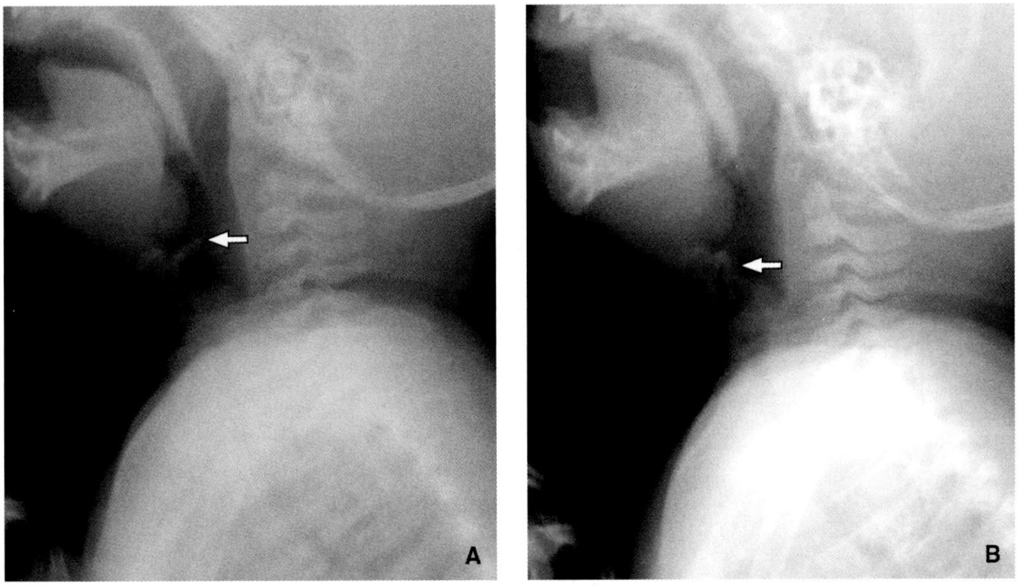

FIGURE 8.21 **Laryngomalacia in a 2-month-old infant with stridor. A:** Lateral radiograph of the upper airway demonstrates the normal position of the epiglottis (*arrow*). **B:** Lateral radiograph of the upper airway shows laxity of the epiglottis (*arrow*) with posterior and downward movement obstructing the airway. (Reprinted from Laya BF, Lee EY. Congenital causes of upper airway obstruction in pediatric patients: updated imaging techniques and review of imaging findings. *Sem Roentgenol.* 2012;47(2):147–158, with permission. Case courtesy of Khristine Grace C. Pulido, MD, Manila, Philippines.)

Tracheal Agenesis

Congenital tracheal agenesis is a rare and generally fatal anomaly. Although the pathogenesis is uncertain, it is postulated to result from failed embryologic separation of the trachea and esophagus during anterior budding of the proximal foregut.[55] The estimated incidence is 1 in 50,000 newborns with a male/female ratio of 2:1.[56] Over 150 cases have been reported since its initial description by Payne in 1900.[56,57] More than 50% of affected patients are premature, and over half of pregnancies are associated with polyhydramnios.[56,58] Associated congenital anomalies are present in 50% to 94% of cases. Affected pediatric patients typically present emergently with cyanosis, severe respiratory distress, inadequate gas exchange, lack of audible crying, and failed endotracheal intubation.[56]

Anatomically, the trachea is typically blind-ending below the level of the larynx, with gas exchange occurring through a distal esophageal fistula.[59] As originally described by Floyd et al.,[60] there are three recognized subtypes (Fig. 8.22). In type I, the proximal trachea is atretic. The preserved short distal trachea communicates with the esophagus via a tracheoesophageal fistula (TEF). Type II is most common, occurring in 60% of cases. The trachea is nearly or entirely absent. Two main bronchi join to form a midline carina, which most often fistulizes with the esophagus. In type III, the trachea and carina are absent. The main bronchi arise directly from the distal esophagus at separate origins.[55,56,59,60]

Chest radiographs are generally nondiagnostic but may demonstrate a missing tracheal air column, an abnormally low position of the tracheal bifurcation, an abnormally posterior "endotracheal" tube/esophageal intubation, or gaseous distention of the distal esophagus, stomach, and proximal small bowel (Fig. 8.23). Historically, barium studies were performed to assess for bronchoesophageal fistulas but are now generally avoided due to potential airway compromise.[55,59,61] CT with multiplanar reformations (MPRs) is the test of choice, which can show the entire length of atresia and precise location of esophageal fistula.[55,59]

Few treatment options currently exist. If diagnosed prenatally by fetal ultrasound and MRI, the ex utero intrapartum tracheotomy (EXIT) procedure may be successful if the distal trachea is patent. Surgical attempts to reconstruct the upper airway using the esophagus or synthetic material thus far have been ineffective in allowing long-term survival.[62]

Tracheal Bronchus

Historically, tracheal bronchus was strictly defined as a right upper lobe bronchus arising from the trachea (also known as "bronchus suis" or pig bronchus due to similar morphology in pigs). The entity now encompasses a variety of bronchial anomalies originating from the trachea or main bronchi directed toward the upper lobes. Based on bronchographic and bronchoscopic series, the prevalence of right and left tracheal bronchus is 0.1% to 0.2% and 0.3% to 1%, respectively.[1,7,63,64] Although generally isolated and incidental, reported associations include Down syndrome, rib anomalies, TEF, VATER (vertebral defects, anal atresia, tracheoesophageal fistula, esophageal atresia, renal defects, radial dysplasia) syndrome, partial anomalous pulmonary venous return, congenital lobar emphysema, and cystic lung malformations.[63–65] Affected infants and children are usually asymptomatic but may present with recurrent pneumonia, atelectasis, or air

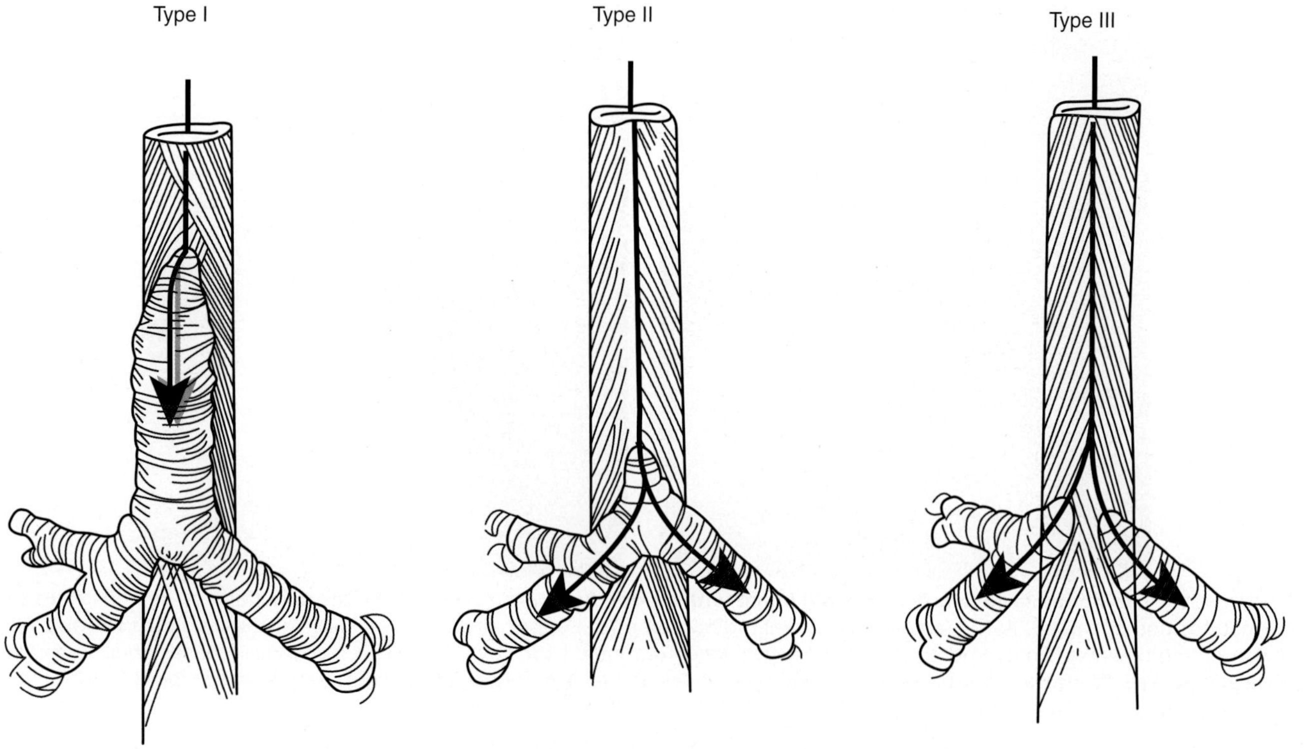

FIGURE 8.22 **Diagram of three types of congenital tracheal agenesis.** In congenital tracheal agenesis type I, the proximal trachea is atretic. The preserved short distal trachea communicates with the esophagus via a tracheoesophageal fistula. In congenital tracheal agenesis type II, the trachea is nearly or entirely absent. Two main bronchi join to form a midline carina, which most often fistulizes with the esophagus. In congenital tracheal agenesis type III, the trachea and carina are absent. The main bronchi arise directly from the distal esophagus at separate origins.

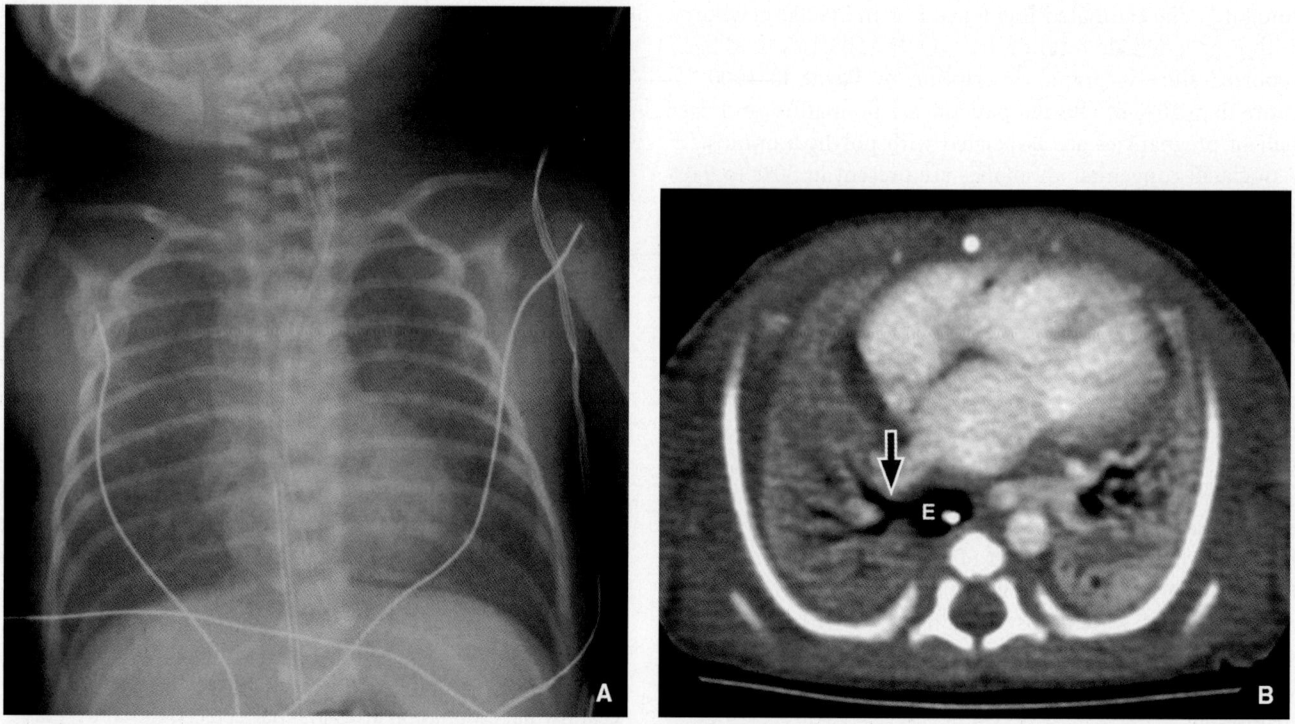

FIGURE 8.23 **Tracheal agenesis in a 3-day-old boy with multiple congenital malformations including DiGeorge syndrome, tetralogy of Fallot, right aortic arch, and discontinuous pulmonary artery who presented with severe respiratory distress.** **A:** Frontal chest radiograph shows a missing tracheal air column. **B:** Enhanced axial CT image shows an absent trachea and right mainstem bronchus (*arrow*) directly arising from the distended esophagus (*E*). Also noted is a nasogastric tube within the esophagus. (Case courtesy of Jonathan R. Dillman, MD, MSc, Cincinnati Children's Hospital Medical Center, Cincinnati, OH.)

trapping, persistent cough, stridor, acute respiratory distress, or hemoptysis.[63,64] A classic history is persistent right upper lobe atelectasis following endotracheal intubation because of obstruction of the unsuspected aberrant bronchus by the endotracheal tube.[25,26]

A "true tracheal bronchus" arises from the trachea generally <2 cm and no more than 6 cm from the carina, typically at the right lateral aspect.[1,7,63,64] If the segmental bronchi of the parent anatomic bronchus supplying the same (upper) lobe as the tracheal bronchus are preserved, the tracheal bronchus is termed supernumerary. Otherwise, the tracheal bronchus is termed displaced. Blind-ending supernumerary bronchi are called tracheal diverticula. Supernumerary bronchi ending in aerated or bronchiectatic lung are called apical accessory lungs or tracheal lobes.[64]

Chest radiography may demonstrate the anomalous air-filled bronchus. However, CT is the preferred imaging modality for diagnosis. Newer postprocessing techniques such as 3D airway reconstruction and CT virtual bronchoscopy (CTVB) can help facilitate assessment[1,66,67] (Fig. 8.24).

Asymptomatic patients require no treatment. However, surgical resection of the tracheal bronchus is recommended in those symptomatic.[7] Additionally, preoperative recognition of tracheal bronchus helps optimize airway management; this is especially important in critically ill patients undergoing complex surgeries.[66,68]

Tracheal Diverticulum

Tracheal diverticulum is a rare abnormality characterized by an outpouching of the posterolateral tracheal wall because of focal weakness of the trachealis muscle. The congenital form results from malformed supernumerary tracheal branches. The acquired form is caused by increased transluminal pressure within the trachea in patients with chronic cough or obstructive lung disease. Most affected pediatric patients are asymptomatic. However, large diverticula may harbor debris and cause recurrent pulmonary infections. Presenting symptoms also include foreign body sensation, neck or cervical swelling, and dysphagia.[1,69–73] The Mounier-Kuhn syndrome (tracheobronchomegaly) is associated with multiple tracheal diverticula.[74]

CT with multiplanar 2D and 3D reformats accurately demonstrates a direct connection between the trachea and diverticulum, which can be difficult to visualize with bronchoscopy[1,69–73] (Fig. 8.25). Diverticula more commonly occur on the right side; this may be related to the supporting esophagus and aortic arch on the left preventing diverticulum formation.[72,73] Congenital diverticula are typically small and narrow mouthed, arising 4 to 5 cm below the true vocal cords, whereas acquired diverticula are larger and wide mouthed.[1,69–73]

Asymptomatic tracheal diverticula merit only conservative management with antibiotics, mucolytics, and physiotherapy

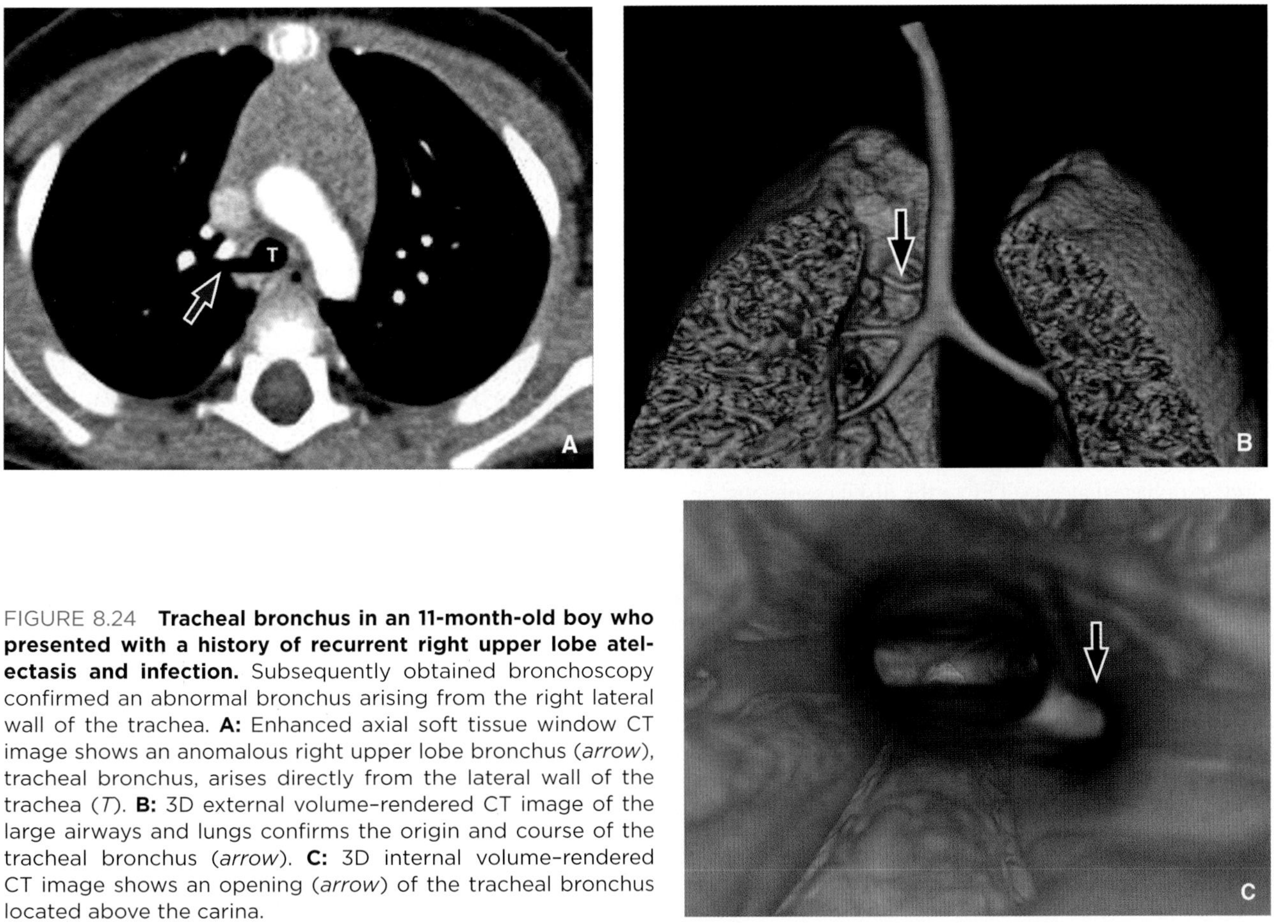

FIGURE 8.24 **Tracheal bronchus in an 11-month-old boy who presented with a history of recurrent right upper lobe atelectasis and infection.** Subsequently obtained bronchoscopy confirmed an abnormal bronchus arising from the right lateral wall of the trachea. **A:** Enhanced axial soft tissue window CT image shows an anomalous right upper lobe bronchus (*arrow*), tracheal bronchus, arises directly from the lateral wall of the trachea (*T*). **B:** 3D external volume-rendered CT image of the large airways and lungs confirms the origin and course of the tracheal bronchus (*arrow*). **C:** 3D internal volume-rendered CT image shows an opening (*arrow*) of the tracheal bronchus located above the carina.

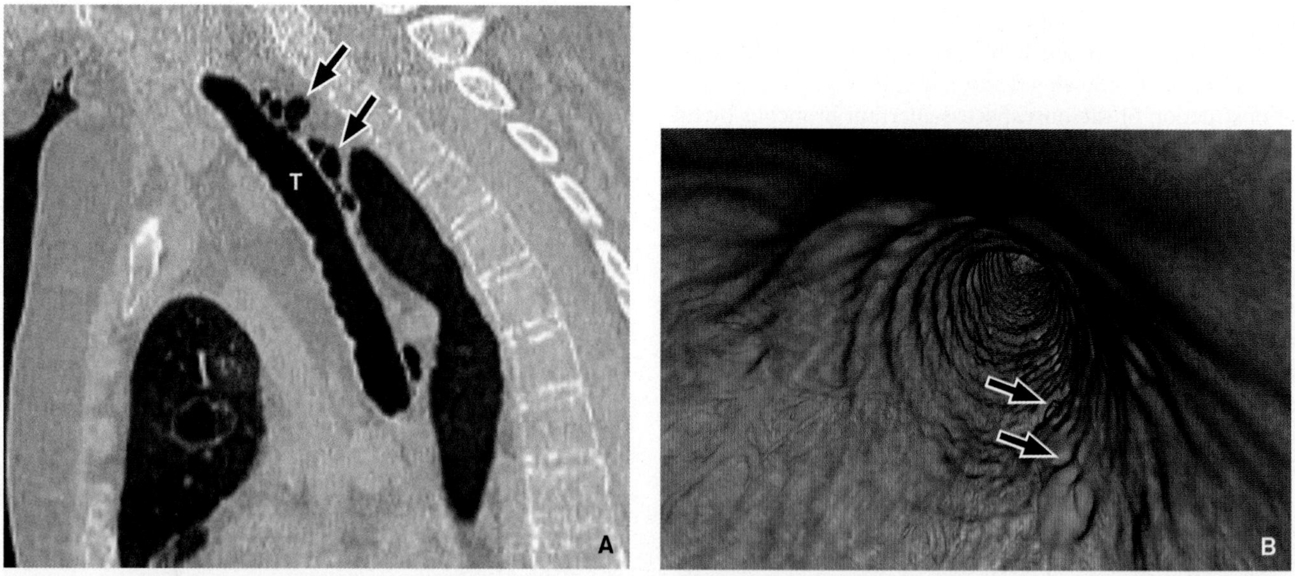

FIGURE 8.25 **Tracheal diverticulum in a 13-year-old boy who presented with chronic cough and recurrent pulmonary infection. A:** Sagittal minimum intensity projection CT image shows multiple outpouchings (*arrows*) of the posterolateral tracheal wall, consistent with tracheal diverticuli. (*T*, trachea.) **B:** A 3D internal volume-rendered CT image confirms openings (*arrows*) of the multiple tracheal diverticuli.

as needed.[72] Surgical resection is the treatment of choice in symptomatic pediatric patients. Outcomes are usually excellent.[1]

Esophageal Bronchus or Lung

Esophageal bronchus and esophageal lung are rare congenital bronchopulmonary foregut malformations (BPFM) in which a bronchus arises directly from the esophagus.[1,75] They are part of a spectrum of anomalies referred to as communicating bronchopulmonary foregut malformations (CBPFM) in which the respiratory and gastrointestinal tracts communicate.[76] In esophageal bronchus, a lobar bronchus arises from the esophagus, typically supplying the right lower lobe medial basal segment. In esophageal lung, a main bronchus arises from the esophagus, supplying an entire lung. Both anomalies occur more commonly on the right side.[1,75–77]

Esophageal lung, with only 20 known cases in the literature, shows no sex predilection, whereas esophageal bronchus has a female/male ratio of 1.5:1. Reported associations include esophageal atresia, TEF to the distal esophagus, duodenal stenosis with annular pancreas, imperforate anus, vertebral anomalies, ambiguous genitalia, and congenital heart disease.[75–77] Affected pediatric patients typically present with recurrent pulmonary infections by the first 8 months of age if the diagnosis is not made incidentally during the neonatal period.[76,77] However, symptoms can range from none at all to fulminant respiratory failure depending on the severity of malformation. The latest reported age at diagnosis of esophageal bronchus is 27.[76]

The imaging evaluation begins with chest radiography, which may demonstrate consolidation or collapse in the lung or portion of the lung supplied by the anomalous bronchus. Barium esophagogram establishes a direct communication between the bronchus and esophagus (Fig. 8.26A). CT with mutliplanar 2D as well as 3D reformats confirms the diagnosis and provides a precise anatomical and vascular roadmap for surgical planning (Fig. 8.26B). Esophageal bronchus and lung must be differentiated from extralobar pulmonary sequestration, a potential mimic. Distinguishing features include arterial blood supply from the pulmonary circulation (vs. systemic circulation in extralobar sequestration), esophageal origin of the bronchus, and whole lung involvement in esophageal lung (vs. segmental distribution in extralobar sequestration).[1,75–77]

Resection of the lung or lobe destroyed by recurrent infection followed by repair of the esophageal communication is the treatment of choice. However, if the diagnosis is made in the neonatal period before lung damage occurs, bronchial reimplantation may be successful.[75] Selective ventilation of the aberrant pulmonary tissue helps determine if viable functional oxygenation capacity remains prior to attempts at bronchial reconstruction.[78]

Congenital Tracheal Stenosis

Congenital tracheal stenosis (CTS) is a rare disorder characterized by focal or diffuse complete tracheal cartilage rings that cause absent or deficient tracheal membranes. These findings result in fixed tracheal narrowing.[1,7,9] Associated cardiovascular anomalies are present in the majority of patients, most commonly left pulmonary artery sling.[1,79] Isolated CTS is unusual, occurring in 10% to 25% of patients.[80] Affected pediatric patients usually present in the first year of life with biphasic stridor, wheezing, and recurrent pneumonia.[7]

As originally classified by Cantrell and Guild, there are three anatomic subtypes (Fig. 8.27). Type I is generalized hypoplasia with total tracheal involvement and normal

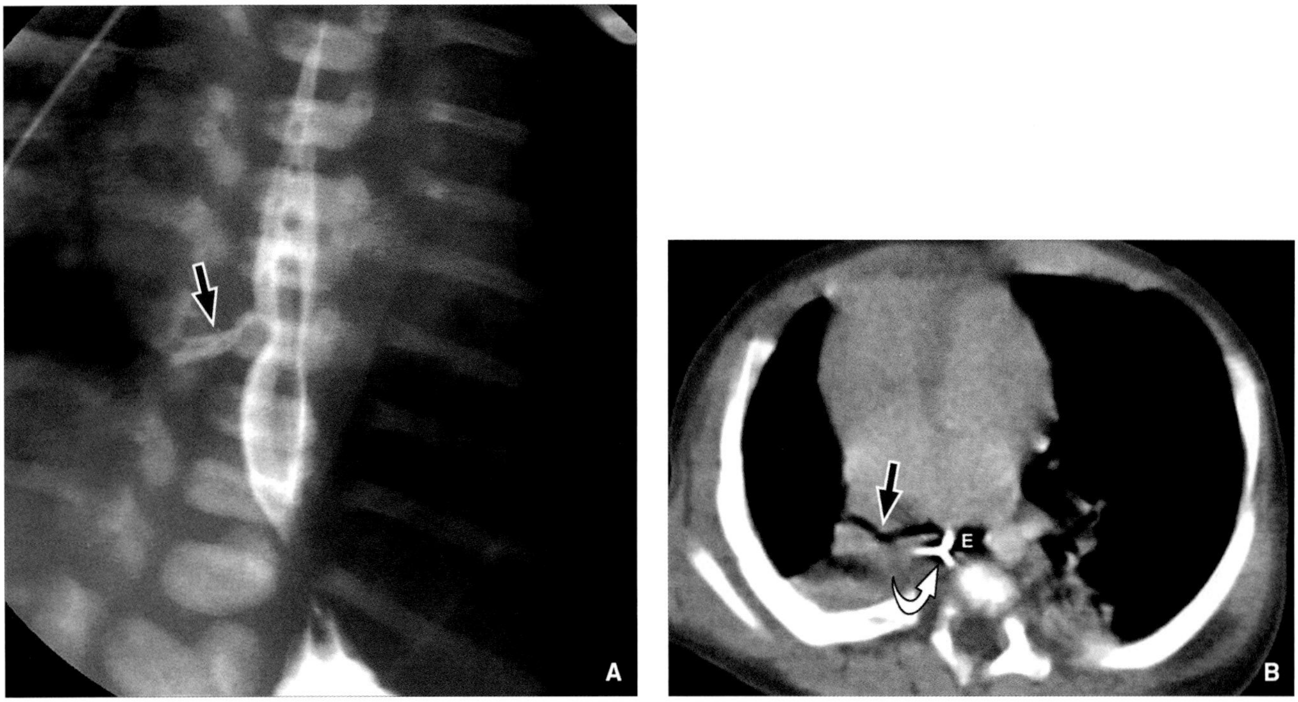

FIGURE 8.26 **Esophageal bronchus in a 1-month-old boy with respiratory distress and feeding difficulty. A:** Esophagogram shows a barium-filled medial right lower lobe bronchus (*arrow*) directly arising from the distal esophagus, consistent with esophageal bronchus. **B:** Enhanced axial CT image demonstrates right lower lobe bronchus (*straight arrow*) arising from the esophagus (*E*). Also noted is a nasogastric tube (*curved arrow*) with streaky metallic artifact in the esophagus. Consolidation in the posterior right lower lobe related to aspiration is also seen.

bronchi and distal airway. Type II is a funnel-like stenosis with gradual tapering of the airway and a normal subglottic and stenotic carinal end of the trachea. Type III is a segmental stenosis involving a short segment of airway, ~2 to 5 cm in length.[80,81] The estimated proportions of each type are 30%, 20%, and 50%, respectively.[7] More recently, Antón-Pacheco et al. proposed an alternative functional classification depending on whether symptoms are mild, moderate, or severe and whether associated anomalies are present or absent.[80,82]

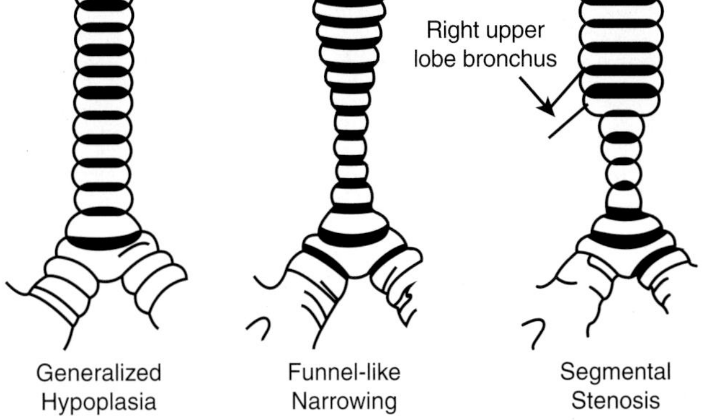

FIGURE 8.27 **Diagram of three types of congenital tracheal stenosis.**

Initial imaging evaluation with chest radiography and fluoroscopy may demonstrate tracheal narrowing. However, MDCT with 2D and 3D reformations, which is the current imaging modality and postprocessing technique of choice, can demonstrate the exact location and extent of stenosis as well as other associated congenital anomalies[1,7,9] (Figs. 8.28 and 8.29). CTVB can provide images on par with actual rigid bronchoscopy, although direct head-to-head comparison studies are still needed in pediatric patients. MRI is generally more challenging in tracheal imaging but is useful in demonstrating associated anomalies such as vascular malformations.[80]

Historically, CTS was mostly managed conservatively. Surgical correction is now preferred whenever possible in symptomatic pediatric patients, associated with significant gains in patient survival. For short-segment tracheal stenosis (≤5 cm), segmental resection with end-to-end anastomosis is the treatment of choice. For long-segment stenosis (>5 cm), patch or tracheal autograft repair was traditionally performed.[1,80,82] However, a newer procedure known as slide tracheoplasty is now felt to be superior, limiting risks of stricture and granulation tissue formation by avoiding extensive mobilization and tension at the suture line.[80,82]

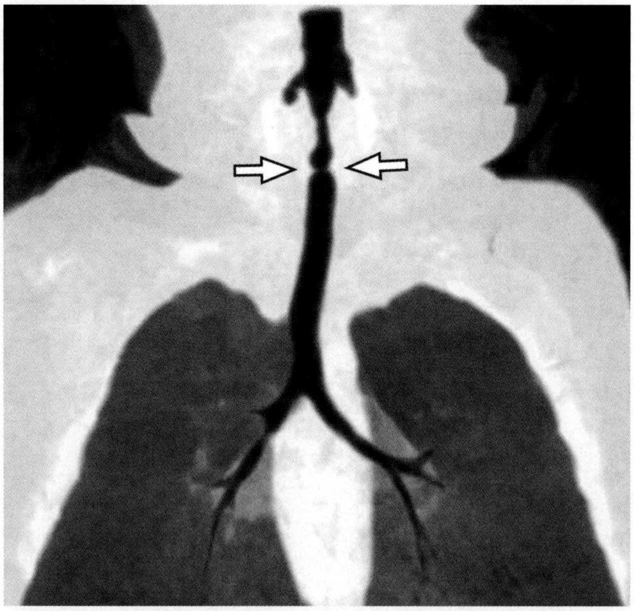

FIGURE 8.28 **Congenital proximal tracheal stenosis in a newborn baby girl with severe respiratory distress.** Coronal minimum intensity projection CT image shows a high-grade congenital stenosis (*arrows*) in the subglottic region. Subsequently obtained bronchoscopy confirmed the congenital tracheal stenosis.

Infectious Disorders

Croup

Croup is a very common acute pediatric airway disorder characterized by diffuse laryngeal and tracheal inflammation and marked subglottic laryngeal swelling and narrowing.[83] Viral croup (laryngotracheitis), in which a virus directly incites the inflammation, should be distinguished from spasmodic croup, an allergic inflammatory reaction to a viral infection.[84] However, these subtypes are functionally very similar, occurring in children <6 years old (peak incidence at 7 to 36 months old) with similar underlying pathogens (typically parainfluenza virus 1) and presenting symptoms (inspiratory stridor, barking cough, and hoarseness). There is a male/female predilection of 1.5/1. Croup is most prevalent in mid-autumn and least common in the summer.[85]

Imaging is generally not required for a clinical diagnosis of croup. However, radiography may be obtained if more complex pathology is anticipated. Half of neck radiographs in pediatric patients with (isolated) croup are normal.[84] The classic appearance on the AP neck radiograph is known as the "steeple sign" with absence of the normal shouldering edges of the subglottic airway and tapered narrowing up to the glottis[84,86,87] (Fig. 8.30). The lateral neck radiograph is characterized by loss of the normally sharp margins of the subglottic airway.[84] Additionally, during inspiration (against a fixed obstruction), there is distention of the hypopharynx and larynx with cervical tracheal narrowing; these changes may be diminished or even absent in expiration.[83,84] Advanced imaging is generally not indicated but may be pursued in the workup of recurrent croup to exclude an underlying lesion.[88]

Therapy is tailored according to clinical severity, as may be classified by the Westley croup score.[85,89,90] The first-line treatment for croup is a single dose of corticosteroids, resulting in fewer hospital admissions and shorter emergency department (ED) visits. Nebulized or L-epinephrine reduces symptom severity in pediatric patients with moderate to severe croup.

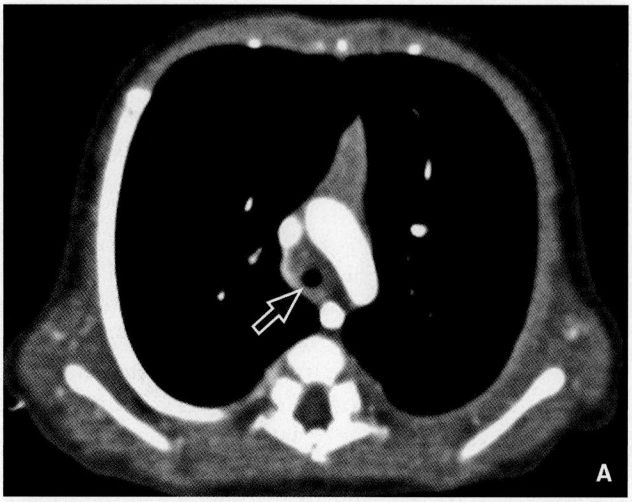

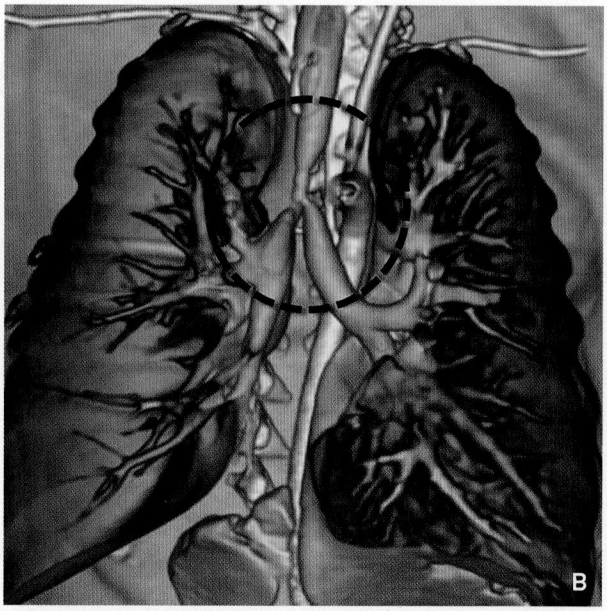

FIGURE 8.29 **Congenital distal tracheal stenosis in a newborn boy who presented with stridor and desaturation.** Bronchoscopy and surgery confirmed the diagnosis of congenital stenosis involving the distal trachea, carina, and proximal mainstem bronchi. **A:** Enhanced axial CT image shows a narrowed trachea (*arrow*) at the level of aortic arch. There is no extrinsic compression upon the trachea. **B:** 3D external volume-rendered CT image demonstrates congenital stenosis (*circle*) involving the distal trachea as well as carina and bilateral mainstem bronchi.

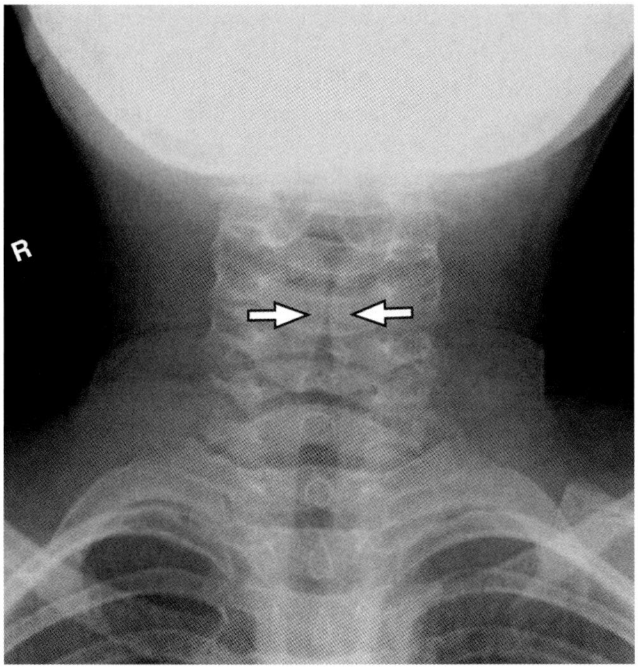

FIGURE 8.30 **Croup in a 5-year-old boy who presented with "barking cough."** Frontal radiograph shows symmetric subglottic narrowing (*arrows*), with loss of normal shouldering.

Heliox has an uncertain benefit, and humidified air has no clear evidence-based use.[90]

Bacterial Tracheitis

Bacterial tracheitis, also referred to as membranous laryngotracheobronchitis, membranous croup, and exudative tracheitis, is a rare, life-threatening infectious cause of acute airway obstruction caused by thick, adherent tracheal membranes. The condition occurs in children 6 months to 14 years old with a peak incidence at 3 to 8 years old. It is usually preceded by an acute upper respiratory viral infection and is most common in the fall and winter.[91] In the past, *Staphylococcus aureus* was the most prevalent underlying pathogen, although a variety of bacteria are now recognized including *Haemophilus influenzae*, *Streptococcus pyogenes*, *Streptococcus pneumoniae*, *Moraxella catarrhalis*, and *Branhamella catarrhalis*.[92] Typical presenting symptoms are cough and stridor followed by hoarseness, fever, and tachypnea. Odynophagia and drooling are unusual. Rapid decline or lack of response to medical therapy for suspected croup should raise clinical suspicion for bacterial tracheitis.[91]

Findings on neck and chest radiography include subglottic tracheal narrowing, proximal tracheal contour irregularity, and tracheal membranes (characteristically linear)[93,94] (Fig. 8.31). The membranes may partially or completely detach and mimic tracheal foreign bodies.[93] Irregularities over the anterior tracheal wall on the lateral view have been called the "candle dripping" sign.[91] Rarely, membranous croup may present with pneumomediastinum.[94,95]

Endotracheal intubation or a surgical airway is often necessary due to concern for impending airway compromise.[91,92]

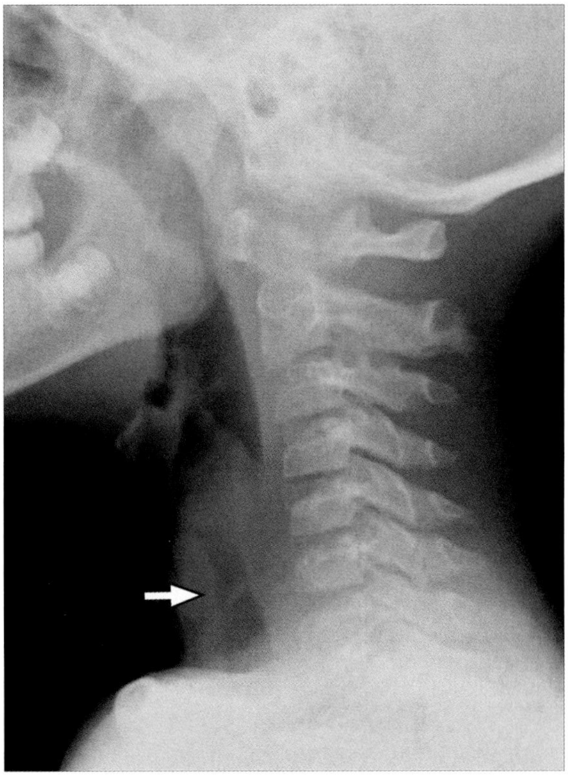

FIGURE 8.31 **Bacterial tracheitis in a 7-year-old boy who presented with fever, coughing, and respiratory distress.** Lateral radiograph shows irregular narrowing (*arrow*) of the trachea and internal linear opacity, which was confirmed to be tracheal membranes on bronchoscopy.

After initial nasolaryngoscopy when possible, rigid laryngoscopy and bronchoscopy are performed, not only confirming the diagnosis but also enabling treatment through direct debridement of mucopurulent debris and sampling for culture. Broad-spectrum intravenous (IV) antibiotics are also administered, later tailored to culture data.[92] Corticosteroids are a useful adjunct to decrease airway edema.[91]

Epiglottitis

Epiglottitis, also known as bacterial croup and supraglottitis, is an uncommon potentially life-threatening bacterial infection of the epiglottis and surrounding structures, including the aryepiglottic folds, arytenoids, and supraglottic larynx, causing acute airway obstruction. In the past, *Haemophilus influenzae* type b (Hib) was the most common underlying pathogen. With the advent of Hib vaccination, the incidence dropped from 41 cases per 100,000 children in 1987 to 1.3 cases per 100,000 children in 1997.[96] Accordingly, a variety of inciting organisms are now recognized including streptococci, staphylococci, pseudomonas, viruses, and candida as well as noninfectious causes such as angioneurotic edema and corrosive ingestion.[49,84] Historically occurring in children 2 to 5 years old, epiglottitis now appears to affect older children, with a mean age of 11.6 years old during the period 1998–2002. Characteristic presenting symptoms are the "4 Ds" (drooling, dysphagia, dyspnea, and dysphonia), high fever, and irritability. Symptoms in the post–Hib era

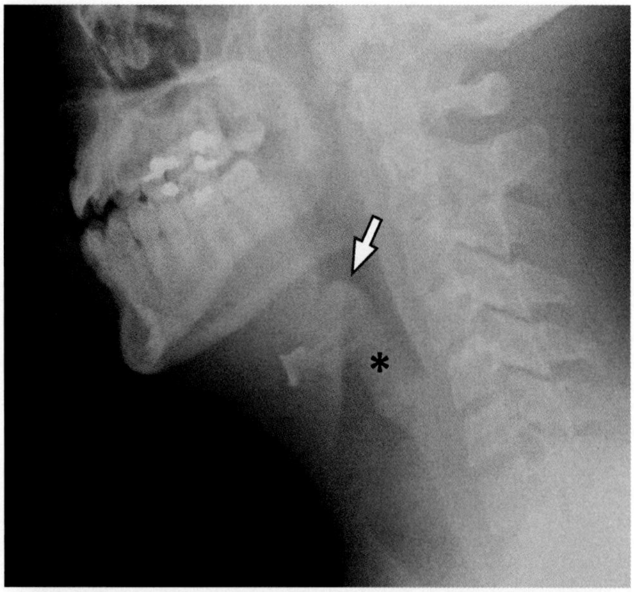

FIGURE 8.32 **Epiglottitis in a 6-year-old girl who presented with respiratory distress, stiff neck, and fever.** Lateral radiograph shows a markedly enlarged epiglottis (*arrow*) and marked thickening of aryepiglottic folds (*asterisk*).

may differ, with low-grade fever, viral prodrome, and croup-like cough.[49,96]

Radiography (without fluoroscopy) is generally sufficient for diagnosis.[52] Typical findings on the lateral neck radiograph are marked thickening of the epiglottis and aryepiglottic folds[49,84] (Fig. 8.32). The imprint of the swollen epiglottis on the airway is termed the "thumb sign"[97,98] (Fig. 8.33). To best differentiate between epiglottitis and other clinical mimics, the aryepiglottic folds should be measured just behind the epiglottis, with a mean thickness of 5.1 mm in this location

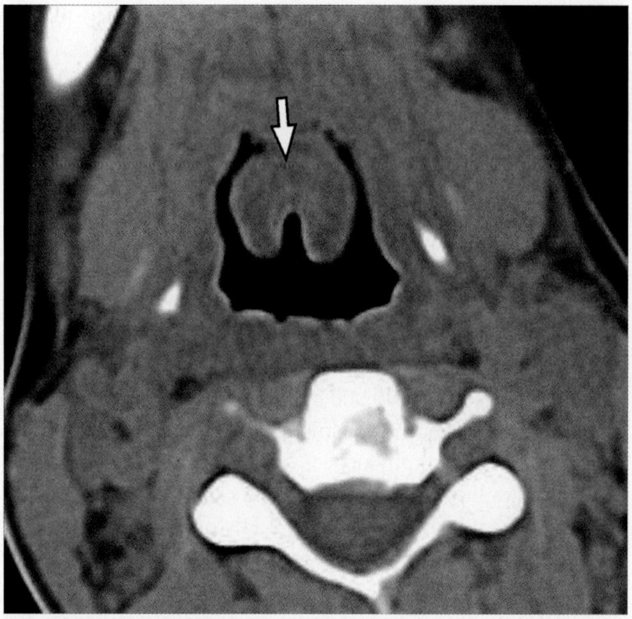

FIGURE 8.33 **Epiglottitis in a 5-year-old boy who presented with fever, drooling, and neck pain.** Axial CT image shows a markedly enlarged epiglottis (*arrow*).

compared to 1.5 mm in pediatric patients with croup and 1.7 mm in normal controls.[99] On the frontal neck radiograph, a steeple or funnel configuration of the glottic and subglottic airway may sometimes be seen secondary to inflammation.[49] An important caveat is the normal variant known as the omega epiglottis, a uniformly thickened epiglottis with a horseshoe configuration associated with tracheomalacia. However, in contrast to epiglottitis, the aryepiglottic folds are normal thickness.[84]

More recent research in adult patients suggests additional diagnostic tools in the imaging evaluation of epiglottitis. Absent visualization of the valleculae on the lateral neck radiograph ("vallecula sign") was associated with accurate diagnosis.[100] In patients too unstable for radiography, bedside ultrasonography has been used, showing the "alphabet P sign" formed by the hyoid bone and its acoustic shadow, preepiglottic space, and swollen epiglottis at the level of the thyrohyoid membrane.[101] Sonographic AP diameter measurements of the epiglottis also can help separate epiglottitis patients from normal controls.[102]

At all times during the assessment for suspected epiglottitis, care should be taken to minimize patient anxiety and excessive manipulation of the airway, allowing the child to remain in a "position of comfort," to help prevent acute airway compromise. Laryngoscopy under anesthesia should be performed, with supraglottic culture and endotracheal intubation. Broad-spectrum antibiotics effective against β-lactamase–producing organisms should be administered, later tailored to culture data. The duration of antibiotics is dependent on clinical status, but symptoms often improve in 1 to 2 days.[96]

Tuberculosis

Tuberculosis (TB), caused by *Mycobacterium tuberculosis*, is a communicable and often persistent infection.[1] Although rates have declined with better diagnostic and therapeutic methods, TB remains the leading infectious cause of death worldwide, with children comprising 10% to 20% of affected patients. Human immunodeficiency virus (HIV) is a major risk factor.[103] TB usually affects the airways via extrinsic tracheobronchial compression by infectious mediastinal and/or hilar lymphadenopathy and uncommonly extension of paraspinal (Pott) disease.[1,104] However, direct airway involvement is possible and found in up to 43% of children with active TB. Airway obstruction may result from caseation, mucus plugging, and rarely large granuloma formation. Mucosal inflammation and edema may cause tracheobronchial narrowing. In late stages, bronchial fibrostenosis may occur.[105] The distal trachea and proximal main bronchi are most commonly involved.[7] Fistula formation can also occur with advanced airway disease.[1]

The characteristic radiographic presentation of primary TB in children is lymphadenopathy possibly accompanied by lung parenchymal abnormalities.[106,107] Radiographs may demonstrate extrinsic airway compression or intrinsic airway involvement. However, MDCT with 2D and 3D reconstructions is superior for this purpose (Figs. 8.34 and 8.35A). Additionally, it can demonstrate typical parenchymal findings such as "tree-in-bud" nodular opacities and air-space consolidation as well as extrapulmonary manifestations of TB[1] (Fig. 8.35B). Classically, TB lymph nodes by CT are low attenuation centrally with rim enhancement or calcification.[108] Airway involvement is characterized by tracheobronchial thickening and narrowing.[7]

Early anti-TB therapy to prevent airway involvement and resultant bronchial fibrostenosis is paramount.[7] In pediatric patients already with endobronchial involvement, a variety of treatment strategies have been tried including steroids, bronchoscopic dilatation, and endobronchial stenting with variable success, frequent recurrence, and potential morbidity. For advanced fibrostenosis, surgical management is necessary with excision and primary bronchial anastomosis for simple

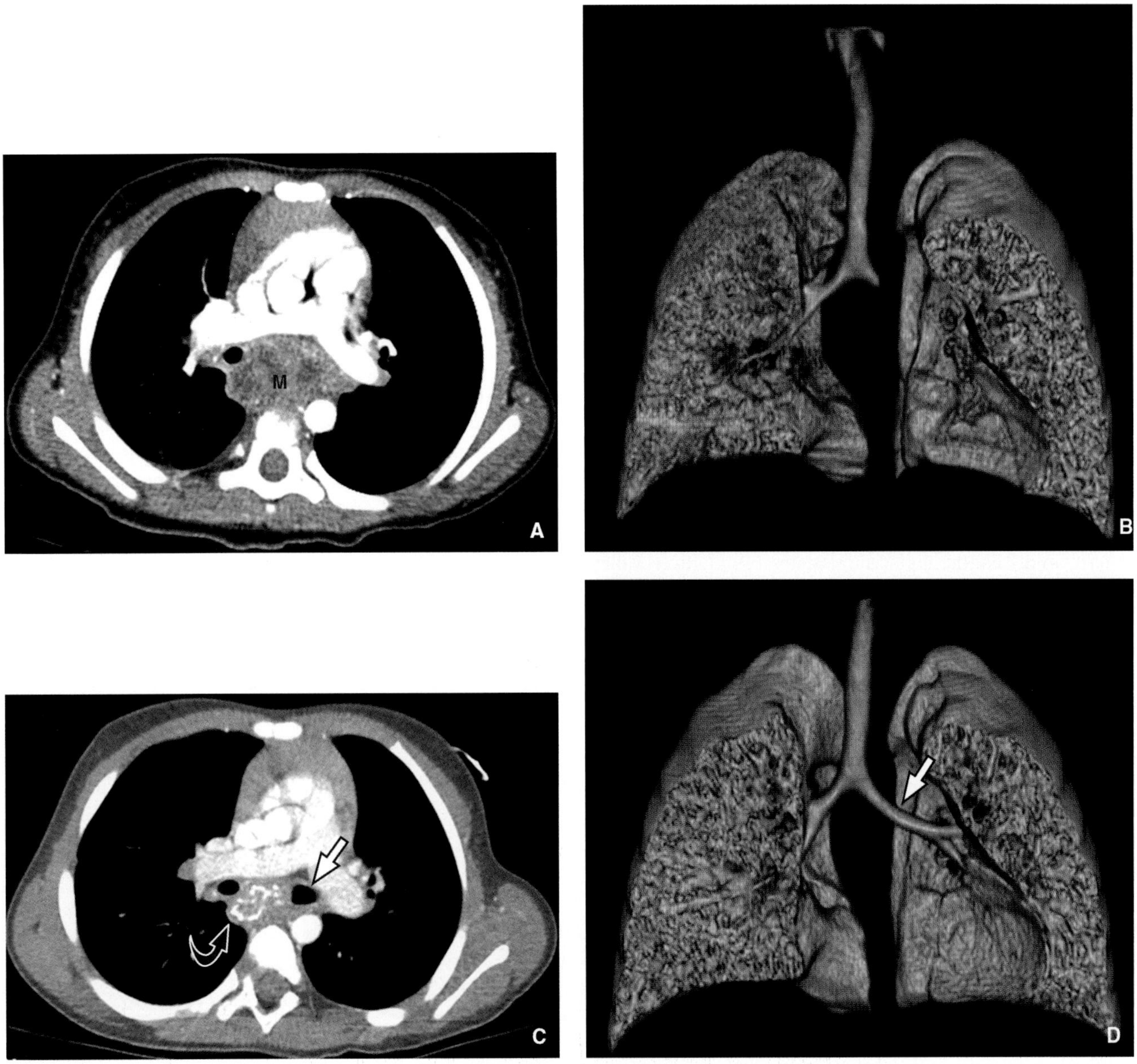

FIGURE 8.34 **TB infection with an obstruction of left mainstem bronchus in a 1-year-old boy who presented with respiratory distress, cough, fever, and abnormal chest radiographs. A:** Enhanced axial CT image shows a complete obstruction of the left mainstem bronchus by the heterogeneously enhancing subcarinal mass (*M*). **B:** 3D external volume-rendered CT image demonstrates an obstruction of the left mainstem bronchus. **C:** Enhanced axial CT image obtained 1 year after treatment shows an interval resolution of the previously noted obstruction of the left mainstem bronchus (*straight arrow*). Previously noted subcarinal lymphadenopathy (*curved arrow*) has been decreased in size and now partially calcified. **D:** 3D external volume-rendered CT image obtained 1 year after treatment shows a patent left mainstem bronchus (*arrow*). (Reprinted from Lee EY, Greenberg SB, Boiselle PM. Multidetector computed tomography of pediatric large airway diseases: state-of-the-art. *Radiol Clin North Am.* 869–894, with permission.)

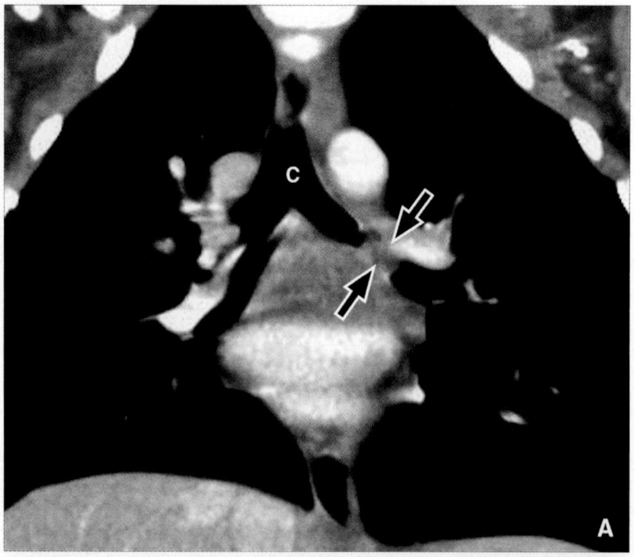

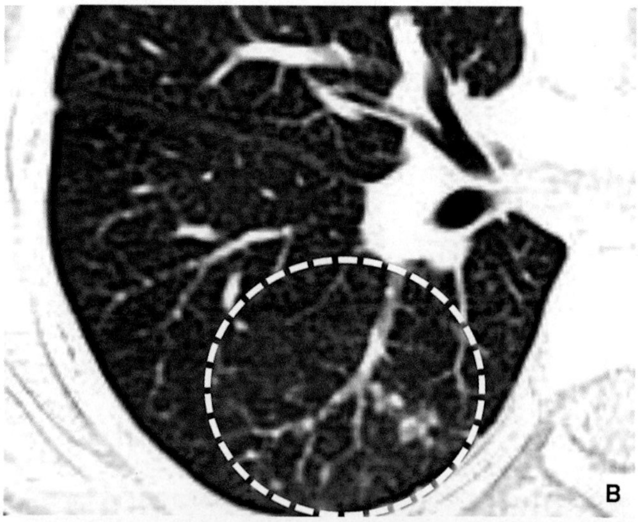

FIGURE 8.35 **Endobronchial tuberculosis infection in a 4-year-old girl with known tuberculosis infection who presented with respiratory distress.** Microbacterial culture obtained during bronchoscopy confirmed the diagnosis of endobronchial tuberculosis infection. **A:** Enhanced coronal reformatted CT image shows a heterogeneously enhancing endobronchial lesion (*arrows*) located in the left mainstem bronchus. (*C*, carina.) **B:** Axial lung window CT image demonstrates "tree-in-bud" nodular opacities (*circle*), which are typical for tuberculosis lung infection.

strictures and bronchoplasty with removal of damaged lung parenchyma in more complex cases.[104]

Histoplasmosis (Fibrosing Mediastinitis)

Histoplasmosis is an infection caused by the fungus *Histoplasma capsulatum*. Inoculation is generally through the respiratory tract.[109] In the United States, it is most common in the southeastern, mid-Atlantic, and central states (Ohio River Valley region).[1] Histoplasmosis is more common among pigeon or chicken breeders, in locations where bats are common (caves), and in old demolition sites.[65] Most cases are self-limited with no symptoms. If symptoms do occur, they are generally mild and nonspecific, such as fever, cough, and malaise.[109,110] Advanced pulmonary and disseminated disease is more common in infants and in pediatric patients with HIV.[109,111] An uncommon manifestation of histoplasmosis is fibrosing mediastinitis (also known as sclerosing mediastinitis or mediastinal fibrosis), characterized by abnormal proliferation of dense acellular collagen and fibrous tissue in the mediastinum.[7,112–114]

Radiographs may demonstrate such findings as hilar or mediastinal lymphadenopathy and lobar consolidation in acute pulmonary histoplasmosis.[109] However, CT is preferable for more definitive characterization and assessment of airway and vascular compromise. MRI may be a useful adjunct. Pulmonary nodules (1 to 3 cm) and enlarged mediastinal and/or hilar lymph nodes with calcification are typical[1] (Fig. 8.36). Rarely, there may be a mediastinal granuloma characterized by a lobulated mass of lymph nodes several centimeters in thickness surrounded by a thin capsule sometimes with calcification.[109,110]

In patients with histoplasmosis, fibrosing mediastinitis most commonly presents as a focal soft tissue mass typically in the right paratracheal, subcarinal, or hilar regions; calcification is present in 63% of cases. A diffuse form of mediastinal fibrosis lacking calcification with infiltration potentially of all mediastinal compartments is less commonly infectious in origin and more typical of idiopathic fibrosing disorders such as mediastinal fibrosis.[7] On MRI, the infiltrating tissue of fibrosing mediastinitis typically demonstrates heterogeneous T1 signal and enhancement. T2 signal is variable. However, the presence of low T2 signal is a helpful differentiating factor, as malignancy is more typically associated with

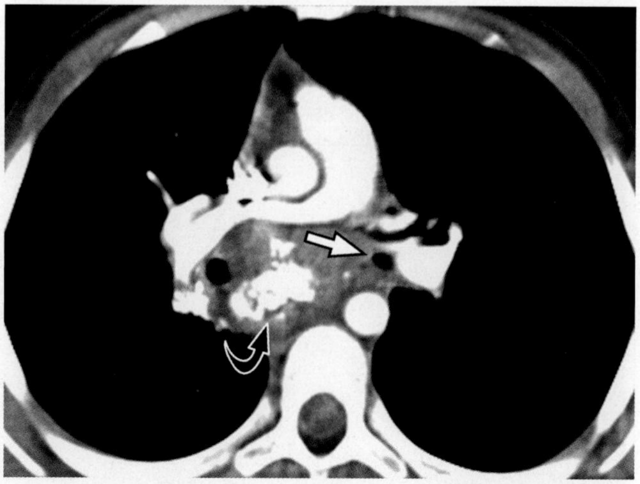

FIGURE 8.36 **Fibrosing mediastinitis caused by *Histoplasma capsulatum* infection in a 9-year-old girl who presented with 1-month history of cough and dyspnea.** Enhanced axial CT image shows narrowing of the left mainstem bronchus (*straight arrow*) from heterogeneously enhancing and partially calcified subcarinal soft tissue mass (*curved arrow*) (Reprinted from Lee EY, Greenberg SB, Boiselle PM. Multidetector computed tomography of pediatric large airway diseases: state-of-the-art. *Radiol Clin North Am.* 2011;49[5]:869–893, with permission.).

T2 hyperintensity.[113] Imaging can also be used to demonstrate extrapulmonary manifestations of histoplasmosis both within the chest (e.g., cardiomegaly in pericarditis) and outside the chest (e.g., organomegaly, CNS involvement).[65]

Antifungal agents are the mainstay of treatment. Amphotericin B deoxycholate is well tolerated and preferred in children. Therapy may not be required in pediatric patients with acute, uncomplicated disease, whereas children with disseminated disease require at least 4 to 6 weeks of treatment.[109] For fibrosing mediastinitis, corticosteroids are also used. Surgical correction for airway and/or vascular involvement may ultimately be required.[7] In adult patients with mediastinal fibrosis, less invasive methods such as balloon angioplasty and stenting have been used successfully to treat vascular complications.[115,116]

Neoplastic Disorders

Benign Neoplasm

Subglottic Hemangioma

Subglottic hemangioma is one of the most common benign large airway neoplasms in pediatric patients, the other being recurrent laryngotracheal papillomatosis.[1,7] Overall, it is a rare disease, comprising 1.5% of congenital laryngeal anomalies. However, prompt recognition is essential, as subglottic hemangioma can cause acute airway compromise, with a 50% mortality rate if left untreated.[117,118] Affected pediatric patients are more likely Caucasian and female with a history of low birth weight, prematurity, and multiple gestations. The diseases typically manifests clinically at ages 6 to 12 weeks, as the lesion grows.[117] Presenting symptoms include inspiratory or biphasic stridor, respiratory distress, and feeding difficulties and may be mistaken for more benign etiologies such as croup.[1,118] Hemoptysis can also occur.[7]

The classic radiographic appearance is asymmetric narrowing of the subglottic airway on the frontal neck view[119] (Fig. 8.37A). However, this asymmetric narrowing is not specific and can be seen with other entities such as cysts, granulomas, and papillomas. Moreover, many cases of subglottic hemangioma present with symmetric subglottic airway narrowing. The lateral neck radiograph is generally less useful.[120] CT shows a round, well-circumscribed, avidly enhancing soft tissue mass generally arising from the posterolateral aspect of the subglottic trachea[1,7,121] (Fig. 8.37B). On MRI, the lesion is T1 isointense to muscle, T2 hyperintense, and enhances intensely.[122] Ultrasound has more recently been used, showing a hypoechoic solid mass at the posterolateral aspect of the subglottic airway with marked vascularity on color Doppler.[123]

Many therapeutic strategies have been tried for treating subglottic hemangioma, including external radiation, tracheotomy, surgical excision, sclerotherapy, systemic steroids, cryotherapy, radium implantation, laser ablation, and interferon therapy.[118] Laser therapy is currently the treatment of choice (best with smaller lesions).[1,7,118] Emerging research suggests propranolol may be an effective treatment adjunct or even monotherapy in some cases of subglottic hemangioma, although the evidence is currently better established for cutaneous hemangioma.[117,118]

Recurrent Respiratory Papillomatosis

Juvenile or recurrent respiratory papillomatosis (RRP) is a rare disorder typified by multiple laryngeal or tracheal lesions in children typically <4 years old.[7] It is caused by human papillomavirus (HPV) types 6 and 11, acquired either in utero or during delivery via the birth canal.[1,7,124] The estimated incidence is 4.3 per 100,000 people in the United States. An adult-onset form also exists, but the childhood type is generally more aggressive.[124] Affected pediatric patients present with stridor and voice changes.[7]

CT is preferred over radiographs for evaluation, showing multiple intraluminal lesions that represent papillomas[1,7,125] (Fig. 8.38). The larynx is almost always involved[1] (Fig. 8.39). In 5% of children with the disease, there is lung involvement consisting of multiple solid and/or cystic nodules.[1,7,125,126] Rarely, lesions may undergo malignant degeneration into

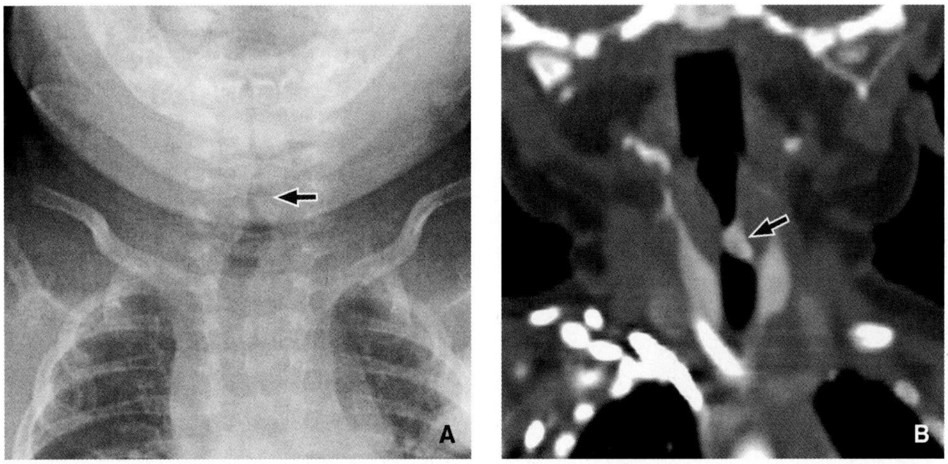

FIGURE 8.37 **Subglottic hemangioma in a 1-month-old girl who presented with worsening biphasic stridor. A:** Frontal radiograph shows an asymmetric narrowing (*arrow*) of the subglottic airway. **B:** Enhanced coronal CT image demonstrates the location and extent of the subglottic hemangioma (*arrow*) and degree of airway narrowing.

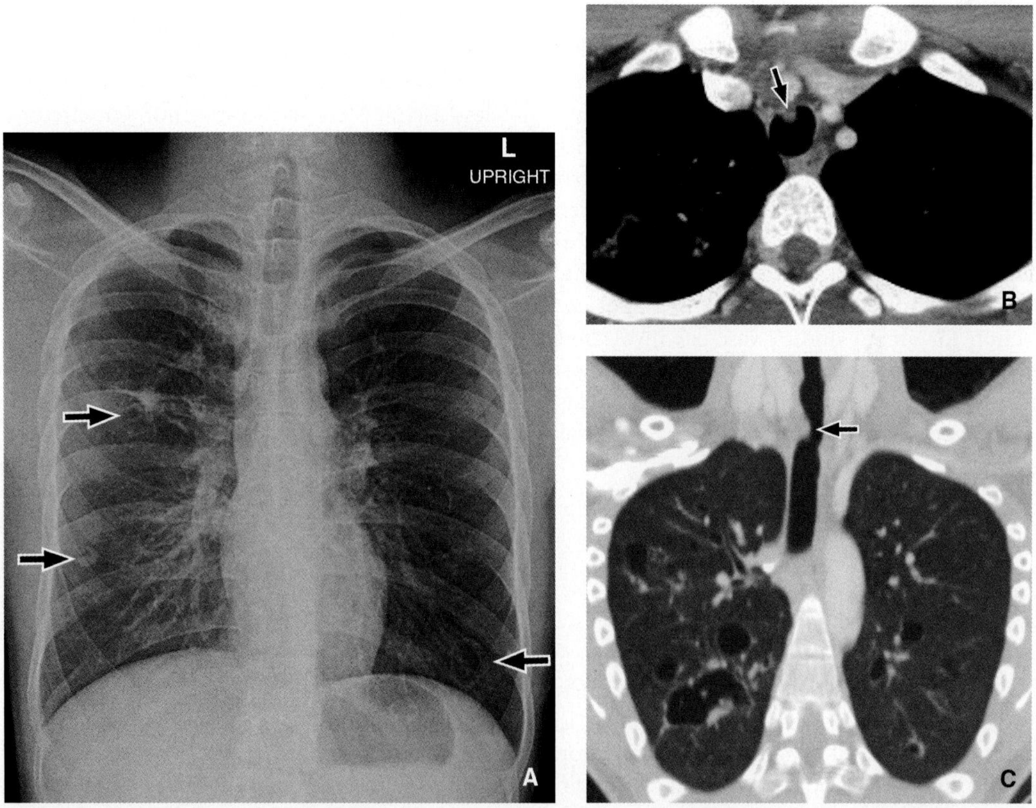

FIGURE 8.38 **Recurrent respiratory papillomatosis in a 16-year-old boy with known diagnosis who presented with hoarseness. A:** Frontal chest radiograph shows multiple cavitary lesions (*arrows*) in both lungs. **B:** Enhanced axial CT image demonstrates an intratracheal lesion, tracheal papilloma (*arrow*) located in the non-dependent portion of the trachea. **C:** Coronal reformatted lung window CT image shows an intratracheal lesion (*arrow*). Multiple cavitary lesions in both lungs are also seen.

squamous cell carcinoma, more common in patients with history of smoking or radiation treatment. There should be heightened concern if significant or rapid change is detected on follow-up imaging.[127] RRP lesions with increased uptake on 2-[^{18}F]-fluoro-2-deoxy-D-glucose (F-18 FDG)–positron emission tomography (PET) are more likely to be malignant.[128]

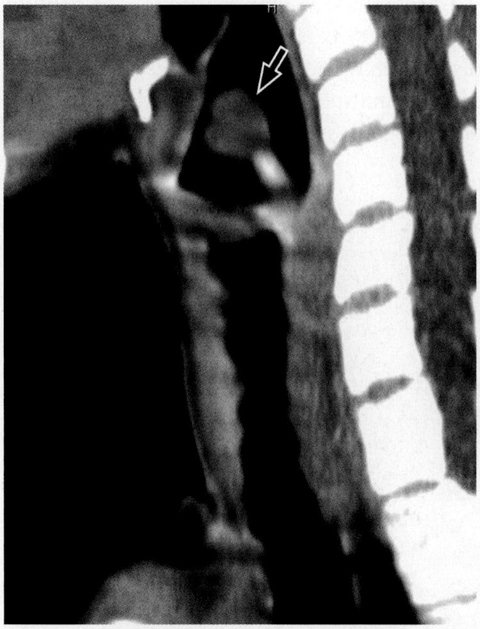

FIGURE 8.39 **Laryngeal papillomatosis in a 7-year-old girl with respiratory distress.** Sagittal reformatted CT image shows a large laryngeal papilloma (*arrow*). (Case courtesy of Hector Hugo Robledo, MD, Hospital de Niños de la Santísima Trinidad de Córdoba, Córdoba, Argentina.)

In pediatric patients with RRP, medical treatment strategies are used to prevent disease progression, whereas more invasive means are used to eliminate lesions as they occur. Antiviral and cytotoxic agents are used to slow papilloma growth.[1,7] In some series, antireflux medications helped promote remission. Mechanistically, it is thought that laryngopharyngeal reflux disease may trigger RRP through acidic mucosal damage or inflammation.[124] Techniques for excising endoluminal lesions include electrocautery, cryotherapy, and carbon dioxide (CO_2) laser.[1,7] Photodynamic therapy is also potentially beneficial. It is hypothesized that the HPV vaccine may result in a decreased incidence of RRP, but further epidemiologic study is needed.[124]

Malignant Neoplasm

Carcinoid Tumor

While overall rare, carcinoid is the most common malignant large airway neoplasm in the pediatric population.[7] The incidence of bronchial carcinoid in the general population is 3 to 5 cases per 1,000,000 people per year, accounting for 1% to 2% of lung cancers.[129] Neuroendocrine in origin, the tumor can produce hormones and neuroamines such as corticotrophin (adrenocorticotropic hormone), gastrin, insulin, vasoactive intestinal peptide, somatostatin, bradykinin, serotonin, and histamine.[1,7,130] Affected pediatric patients present with cough, wheeze, airway obstructive symptoms (atelectasis, obstructive pneumonitis, pleuritic pain, and dyspnea), and sometimes hemoptysis because of carcinoids vascularity[7,130] (Fig. 8.40A). The classic "carcinoid syndrome" with symptoms of flushing and diarrhea because of serotonin production by the tumor is rare in bronchial carcinoid and even less common in children.[129,130]

Carcinoid within the airway is best visualized on CT particularly with multiplanar 2D and 3D reformations[7] (Fig. 8.40). The tumor is characterized by a round, oval, or polypoid endobronchial nodule or mass.[1] Distal hyperinflation may be seen secondary to the "ball-valve" effect of the tumor.[131] Contrast enhancement is variable, ranging from mild to marked. Diffuse or punctuate calcification is seen in 30% of bronchial carcinoid tumor cases.[1] The tumor is most commonly located within the mainstem or lobar bronchi. However, 15% occur in segmental bronchi or the lung periphery.[1,7] As somatostatin receptors are present on most bronchial carcinoids, somatostatin receptor scintigraphy utilizing [^{111}In-DTPA-D-Phe^{1}]-octreotide is helpful in tumor detection and disease monitoring.[130,132]

Surgical resection is the most commonly accepted treatment for bronchial carcinoid, taking care to conserve as much lung parenchyma as possible. Endoscopic and laser ablation are often inadequate even for small lesions because of unsuspected bronchial wall infiltration ("iceberg phenomenon") and lack of lymph node evaluation.[129] Octreotide also has a potential therapeutic benefit.[130]

Mucoepidermoid Tumor

Mucoepidermoid is the second most common primary malignant airway tumor in the pediatric population.[1,7] It comprises 10% of malignant primary pediatric pulmonary neoplasms and 0.1% to 0.2% of all primary lung cancers.[133,134] Mucoepidermoid arises from the minor salivary glands of the large airways and most frequently involves the mainstem or proximal lobar bronchi with no side predilection.[1,7,133] The tumor generally presents as an exophytic luminal mass (sessile, polypoid with a broad-based connection

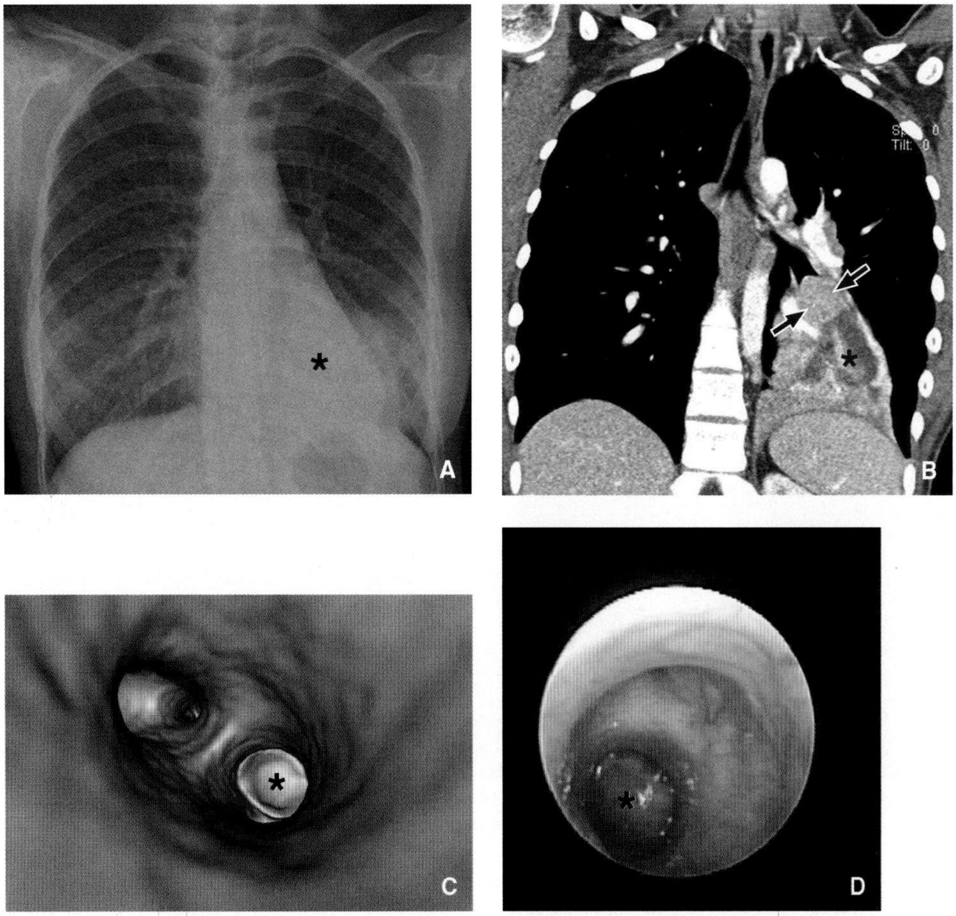

FIGURE 8.40 **Endobronchial carcinoid tumor in a 16-year-old girl who presented with recurrent left lower lobe pneumonia for the last 3 years.** Surgical pathology confirmed the diagnosis of endobronchial carcinoid tumor. **A:** Frontal chest radiograph shows an opacity (*asterisk*) in the left lower lobe. **B:** Enhanced coronal reformatted CT image demonstrates an enhancing endobronchial mass (*arrows*) located in the left lower lobe bronchus with postobstructive bronchiectasis and mucus plugging (*asterisk*). **C:** 3D internal volume-rendered CT image shows obstruction (*asterisk*) of the left lower lobe bronchus due to an endobronchial mass. **D:** Conventional bronchoscopy finding (*asterisk*) is similar to finding seen on 3D virtual bronchoscopy (40C). (Bronchoscopy image courtesy of Robert Shamberger, MD, Boston Children's Hospital and Harvard Medical School, Boston, MA.)

to the bronchial wall, or pedunculated with a stalk) covered by intact respiratory epithelium.[7,135] There are two histologic subtypes (low and high grades) based on cellular differentiation and mitotic activity; in children, the low-grade form is most common[1,7,136] (Fig. 8.41A, B). Presenting symptoms include cough, hemoptysis, bronchitis, wheezing, fever, chest pain, and rarely clubbing.[135]

Radiographs may demonstrate an endotracheal or endobronchial nodule, a solitary pulmonary nodule or mass, a mass with postobstructive pneumonia or atelectasis, or mass with distal cavitary lesion[137] (Fig. 8.41C). CT is more sensitive than radiographs for detection and typically demonstrates a sharply marginated, oval or lobulated intraluminal mass, 1 to 4 cm in size, which follows the contours of the airways[7,137,138] (Fig. 8.41D). Aggressive features such as large size (>5 cm), irregular borders, and infiltration of the adjacent mediastinal or pulmonary structures are more typical of high-grade mucoepidermoid.[1] Mucoepidermoid typically mildly and diffusely enhances and contains punctuate calcifications in approximately half of cases.[1,137] A crescent of air may be found at the periphery of the primary mass corresponding to the residual ectatic bronchus occupied by the lesion.[137] CT can also demonstrate postobstructive pneumonia, subsegmental atelectasis, air trapping, and distal bronchial dilatation and mucoid impaction associated with the tumor.[93,94] Although the appearance on ^{18}F-FDG–PET is variable, higher uptake is

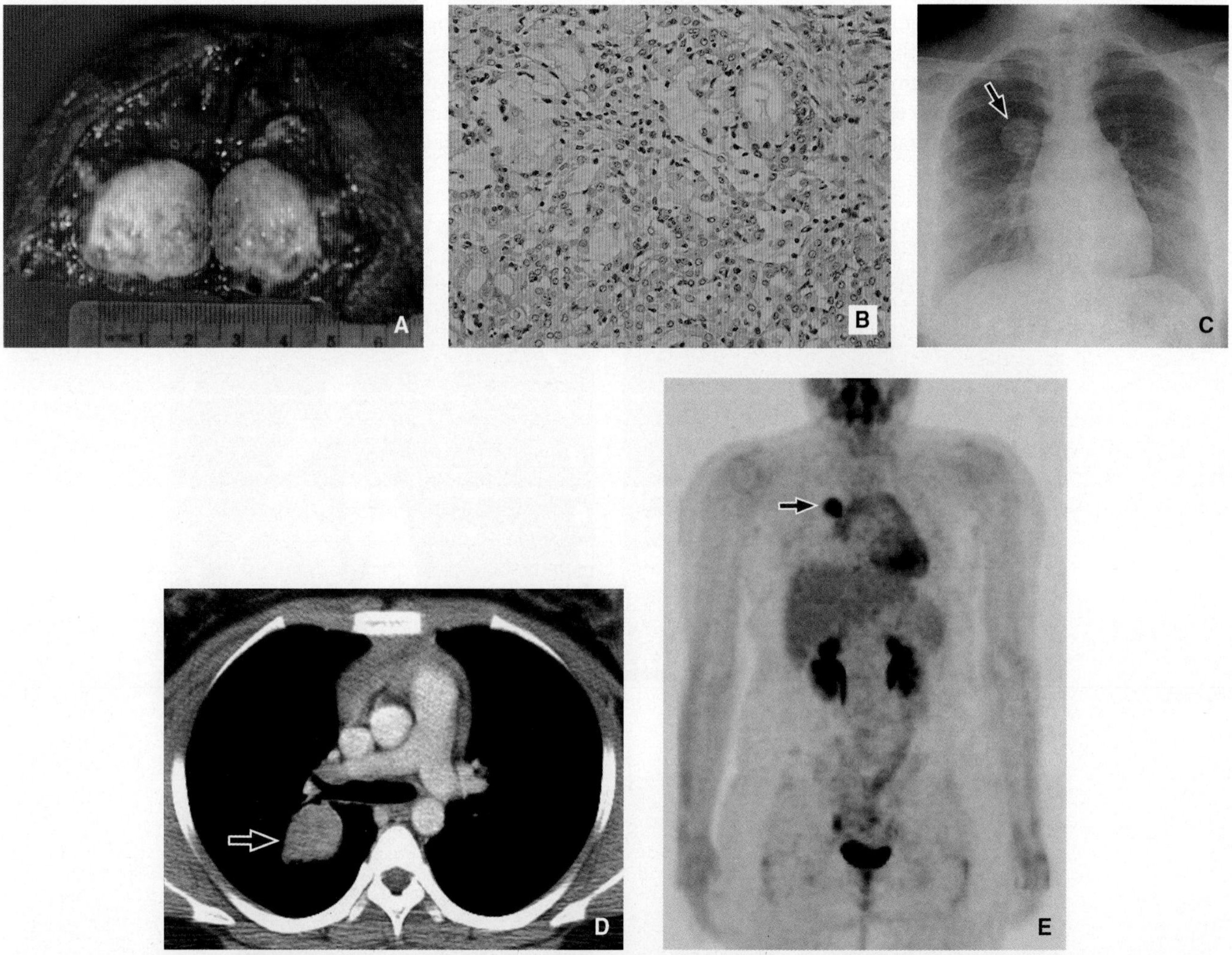

FIGURE 8.41 **Mucoepidermoid carcinoma of bronchus in a 15-year-old girl who presented with fever, cough, a single episode of minor hemoptysis, and flu-like symptoms, which persisted for several days. A:** The tumor nodule (bisected here) is sharply circumscribed with a yellow-tan glistening mucoid cut surface, which demonstrates numerous nearly microscopic cysts. **B:** Low-grade mucoepidermoid carcinoma of the bronchus shows a mixture of squamoid, intermediate, and mucus-producing epithelium (H&E, original magnification × 40). **C:** Posteroanterior chest radiograph demonstrates a well-circumscribed and round opacity (*arrow*) located in the medial right upper lobe, suprahilar region, without associated calcification or mediastinal lymphadenopathy. **D:** Enhanced axial CT image shows a smooth well-circumscribed soft tissue mass (*arrow*) without significant contrast enhancement located within the posterior segment of the right upper lobe at its origin. **E:** A maximum intensity projection of the ^{18}F-FDG–PET study demonstrates markedly increased ^{18}F-FDG uptake within the pulmonary mass (*arrow*), without evidence of metastatic disease. There is expected intense physiologic ^{18}F-FDG uptake in the brain, myocardium, and genitourinary system. (Reprinted from Lee EY, et al. Mucoepidermoid carcinoma of bronchus in a pediatric patients: 18F-FDG PET findings. *Pediatr Radiol.* 2007;37:1278–1282, with permission.)

associated with higher-grade tumors[136] (Fig. 8.41E). PET may be useful in metastatic workup and staging.[133]

Complete surgical resection with primary reanastomosis or sleeve resection is currently the treatment of choice.[1] As in the case of carcinoid, endoscopic resection is discouraged because of the iceberg-like appearance of the tumor.[134] Recent research suggests specific reciprocal chromosomal translocations are implicated in the tumorigenesis of mucoepidermoid, which may ultimately allow for targeted chemotherapeutic agents.[135]

Traumatic Disorders

Acquired Tracheobronchial Stenosis

Acquired tracheobronchial stenoses typically occur in children with prior airway instrumentation or surgery, most commonly in the setting of long-term endotracheal or tracheostomy tube placement.[1,7] Benign tracheal strictures occur in up to 10% to 15% of patients with prolonged intubation.[9] The tube causes pressure ischemia, which results in tracheal necrosis, subsequent fibrosis, and eventual stenosis.[1,7] Most strictures occur at the level of the endotracheal tube balloon or tracheostomy stoma.[1,7,9] Acquired bronchial stenoses often occur in pediatric patients with prior lung transplantation, generally at the site of surgical anastomosis.[1,7,139,140]

MDCT with multiplanar 2D and 3D reconstructions can precisely locate and characterize acquired strictures and is the imaging test of choice for evaluation[1,7] (Fig. 8.42). Curved coronal and virtual bronchoscopic reformats improve visualization and diagnostic accuracy compared to axial images alone.[7,140] Typical CT findings are focal proximal tracheal narrowing with eccentric or concentric soft tissue thickening because of intimal hyperplasia.[7] With bronchoscopy as the gold standard, MDCT demonstrates a sensitivity and specificity of 92% and 100%, respectively, for detecting postintubation stenosis.[7,141]

Currently, various methods are available for treating acquired tracheobronchial stenoses. Less invasive approaches such as balloon angioplasty are preferred when possible particularly in pediatric patients. Alternatives include use of dilators, laser, surgery, and/or insertion of prosthetic material.[142,143] In patients who underwent poststenting for airway strictures, MDCT is useful in detecting complications such as stent fracture or migration.[144]

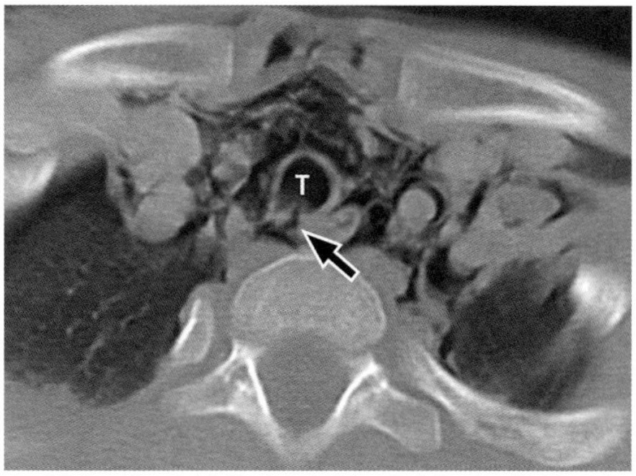

FIGURE 8.43 **Traumatic tracheal laceration in a 13-year-old girl who developed acute chest pain and severe dyspnea after a motor vehicle accident.** Axial lung window CT image at the thoracic inlet level shows a focal disruption (*arrow*) of the posterior wall of the trachea. Extensive pneumomediastinum is also seen. (*T*, trachea.)

Tracheobronchial Injury

Tracheobronchial injury is unusual in children, occurring in <1% of patients with penetrating or blunt thoracic trauma.[1,145,146] However, it should not be overlooked, as the mortality rate approaches 30% because of delayed diagnosis in 25% of cases.[1,145,147] Tracheal disruption usually occurs just superior to the carina (Fig. 8.43). Bronchial injury generally occurs within 2.5 cm of the carina, most commonly affecting the proximal right mainstem bronchus.[1,145–156]

On radiographs, there may be persistent, extensive pneumothorax and/or pneumomediastinum with air extending into the subcutaneous tissues of the neck and chest wall

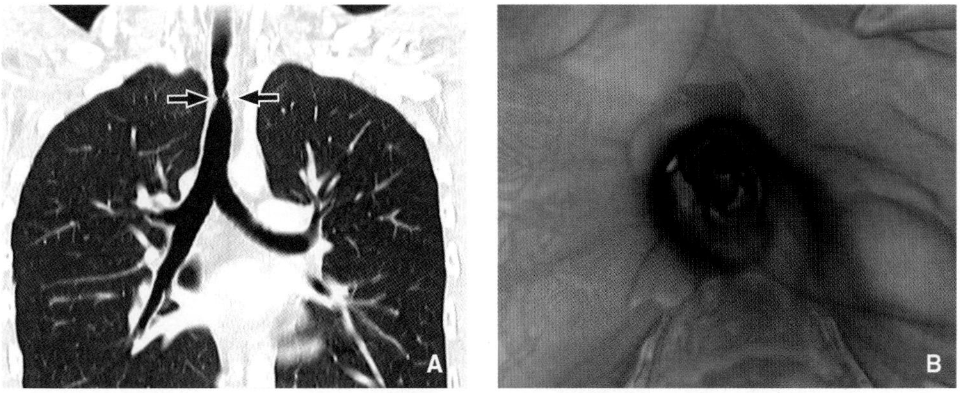

FIGURE 8.42 **Acquired tracheal stenosis caused by previous long-term placement of endotracheal tube in a 15-year-old boy.** The patient subsequently underwent bronchoscopy, which confirmed the tracheal stenosis. **A:** Coronal reformatted lung window CT image shows an irregular thickening and narrowing (*arrows*) of the trachea at the thoracic inlet level where the endotracheal tube balloon was previously placed. **B:** 3D internal volume-rendered CT image of the airways shows an irregular narrowing of the trachea.

even with a normally functioning chest and/or mediastinal tube.[1,145–156] The injured bronchus may be distended.[145] If completely avulsed, the affected lung collapses in a dependent position, attached to the hilum only by vascular structures. This finding is known as the "fallen lung sign."[1,145–156] Other suspicious appearances include an abnormal endotracheal tube position and rib fractures, especially involving the anterior portion of the first through third ribs.[1,145,149] MDCT with multiplanar 2D and 3D reformats is far superior to radiography in accurately locating the site of airway disruption, which is particularly useful in presurgical planning.[1,145,155]

Management is tailored to the severity and location of injury.[1] Conservative measures may be adequate if the disruption involves <33% of the circumference of tracheobronchial tree, and there is full lung expansion and early air leak cessation on chest tube insertion. Intubation across or tracheostomy though tracheal tears located anteriorly may also be sufficient.[156] In other cases, surgical repair is indicated, also helping to prevent scarring and infection.[1,156] Techniques include primary anastomosis or reimplantation coupled with temporary tracheostomy or intubation.[1,147,148,150,153] Pulmonary resection or pneumonectomy should not be performed unless there is also severe pulmonary contusion.[156]

Reactive Airway Disease (Asthma)

Asthma, or reactive airway disease, is characterized by small airway narrowing and abnormally elevated airflow resistance. These findings result from bronchial smooth muscle contraction and wall inflammation, bronchospasm, and increased mucus production in response to internal or external triggers.[157] Asthma is the most common chronic illness in children and a major cause of hospitalization. Racial minority, lower socioeconomic status, and abnormal glucose and lipid metabolism appear to be risk factors, but multiple confounding variables prevent definitive analysis.[158,159] Acute-onset wheeze, cough, and dyspnea are typical presenting symptoms.[157]

Radiographic findings vary depending on the degree of airway obstruction. Hyperinflation with flattening of the diaphragms, increased retrosternal clear space, and peripheral arterial attenuation is characteristic because of expiratory air trapping. Other potential findings include bronchial wall thickening and peribronchial cuffing, usually perihilar in location, and bronchiectasis (Fig. 8.44A). Focal atelectasis may be present if there is severe airway narrowing or mucus plugging.[157] High-resolution computed tomography (HRCT) provides more detailed anatomical assessment and effectively demonstrates air trapping (Fig. 8.44B, C). However, CT correlation with asthma severity is variable. Nuclear medicine ventilation scintigraphy provides more pertinent data on regional airflow dynamics but is rarely used in clinical practice.[160] Investigational studies into the use of hyperpolarized helium-3 (HP ^{3}He) MRI appear promising in detecting ventilation defects in asthma while preserving spatial resolution.[160,161]

A variety of medications are available for asthma including short- and long-acting β-agonists, inhaled corticosteroids, leukotriene receptor antagonists, and anti-IgE therapy, often used in combination to decrease bronchial constriction and inflammation. The exact regimen is tailored to the severity of symptoms. Treatment adherence is paramount to help prevent acute exacerbations potentially leading to ED visits, inpatient hospitalization, and/or endotracheal intubation.[159]

Obstructive Sleep Apnea

Obstructive sleep apnea (OSA) refers to transient upper airway obstruction during sleep despite attempts to breathe. OSA is common, affecting up to 3% of all children or 2 million in the United States alone, most often because of enlarged adenoids and palatine tonsils. However, any underlying factors increasing airway resistance elevate risk for OSA, including obesity, craniofacial anomalies, congenital syndromes (Down, achondroplasia, mucopolysaccharidoses), and prior surgery.[6,162] Lingual tonsil enlargement is a recognized cause of sleep apnea in children with obesity and/or Down syndrome, occurring more frequently in patients with prior palatine tonsillectomy and

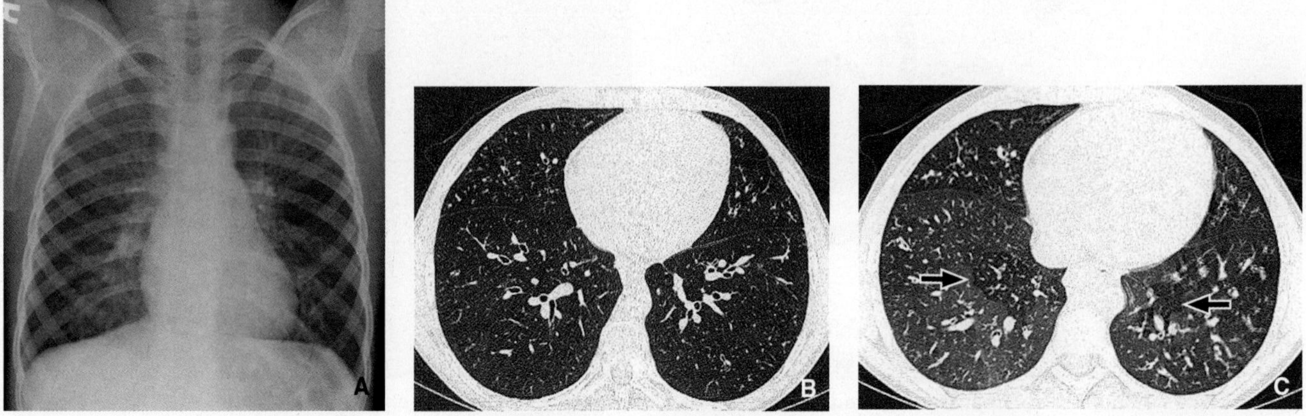

FIGURE 8.44 **Acute asthma attack in a 5-year-old boy who presented with wheezing, cough, and dyspnea. A:** Frontal chest radiograph shows hyperinflation with flattening of the diaphragms. Peribronchial wall thickening and cuffing are also seen. **B:** Axial lung window CT image obtained at end inspiration shows mild bronchial wall thickening. **C:** Axial lung window CT image obtained at end expiration demonstrates geographic air trapping (*arrows*) in both lungs .

adenoidectomy.[163] Presenting symptoms may include snoring, excessive daytime sleepiness (more common in adults), hyperactivity, attention deficit disorder, diminished hearing, physical debilitation, and failure to thrive.[14,162] Although prone to technical variation, overnight polysomnography is the gold standard for diagnosis, with obstructive apnea defined as >90% reduction in airflow despite continuing respiratory efforts when the event lasts at least two missed breaths.[162]

Radiography, CT, and MRI can used to exclude other potential causes of extrinsic airway compression or intrinsic narrowing. Thereafter, dynamic techniques may be used to accurately evaluate OSA. Dynamic sleep fluoroscopy can help detect the location of airway obstruction during desaturation episodes.[6,164] Cine MRI has more recently been used[12–16] (Fig. 8.45). Patients with OSA have a greater mean change in airway diameter including the nasopharynx, oropharynx, and hypopharynx compared to normal controls.[14]

Adenotonsillectomy is generally effective in patients with OSA because of enlarged tonsils and adenoids. Various surgical methods are used in children with underlying craniofacial anomalies. Less invasive approaches include continuous positive airway pressure (CPAP), bi-level positive airway pressure (BiPAP), nocturnal oxygen supplementation (temporary measure), and orthodontic maxillary expansion which increases the width of the maxilla and reduces nasal resistance.[162]

Tracheobronchomalacia

In tracheobronchomalacia (TBM), there is disproportionate expiratory collapse of the trachea or bronchi caused by softening of the airway walls, weakening of the supporting cartilage, and/or hypotonia of the supporting muscles.[1,2,7,11,165–170] There are two types: primary (congenital) and secondary (acquired). Primary TBM is commonly attributed to prematurity, congenital TEF, and congenital cartilage disorders. Secondary TBM may occur as a result of prior intubation, infection, surgery, and extrinsic compression from mediastinal vascular abnormalities.[1,7,11,165] Anomalies associated with TBM include cardiovascular defects, bronchopulmonary dysplasia, gastroesophageal reflux, and neurologic impairment.[165] Symptoms, worse during crying or forced expiration, include wheeze, cough, stridor, dyspnea, cyanosis, and recurrent respiratory infections.[2] Because of the nonspecific clinical presentation, TBM may be overlooked.[1,7,11,165]

The diagnosis of TBM is made when there is >50% airway collapse on expiration. This criterion, originally based on rigid bronchoscopy, is now also used for imaging studies. In the past, TBM was primarily assessed with chest radiography and airway fluoroscopy (Fig. 8.10). However, MDCT with multiplanar 2D and 3D reformats is now preferred. Providing precise anatomical detail, CT accurately localizes the malacia and characterizes its severity and extent, also allowing quantitative measurements (Fig. 8.46). CT is also useful for assessing underlying causes and associated anomalies. Further, air trapping, common among children with TBM, is readily detected by CT.[170] Paired inspiratory–expiratory MDCT is most often performed to evaluate for suspected TBM. To help reduce radiation exposure, the tube current may be reduced by 50% during expiration while maintaining diagnostic ability. Newer techniques include cine imaging with the 64-MDCT scanner and four-dimensional imaging with the 320-MDCT scanner, allowing real-time dynamic 4D airway assessment.[1,2,7,11,165–170]

Because the tracheal cartilage stiffens and strengthens with age, primary TBM often gradually improves with age, even resolving by 1 to 2 years in mild-to-moderate cases.[2,11,165] Supportive therapies include antibiotics for associated respiratory infections, humidified oxygen therapy, and pulmonary physiotherapy. For pediatric patients not responsive to conservative measures, more aggressive options are available, including CPAP, tracheostomy, airway stenting, and surgery such as tracheoplasty or aortopexy.[1,2,11,165]

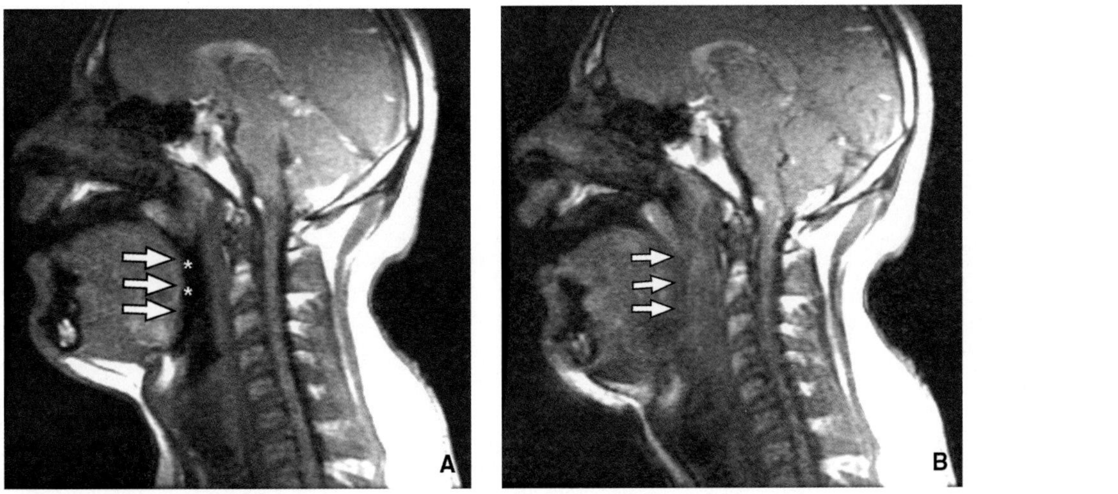

FIGURE 8.45 **Obstructive sleep apnea in a child with glossoptosis. A:** Sagittal cine MRI sleep study image shows the posterior edge of the tongue (*arrows*) in relation to the patent pharyngeal space (*asterisks*). **B:** Sagittal cine MRI sleep study image coinciding with an episode of oxygen desaturation shows the posterior displacement of the tongue (*arrows*) and resultant obliteration of the pharyngeal space. (Reprinted from Laya BF, Lee EY. Congenital causes of upper airway obstruction in pediatric patients: updated imaging techniques and review of imaging findings. *Sem Roentgenol.* 2012;47(2):147–158, with permission. Case courtesy of Lane F. Donnelly, MD, Orlando, FL.)

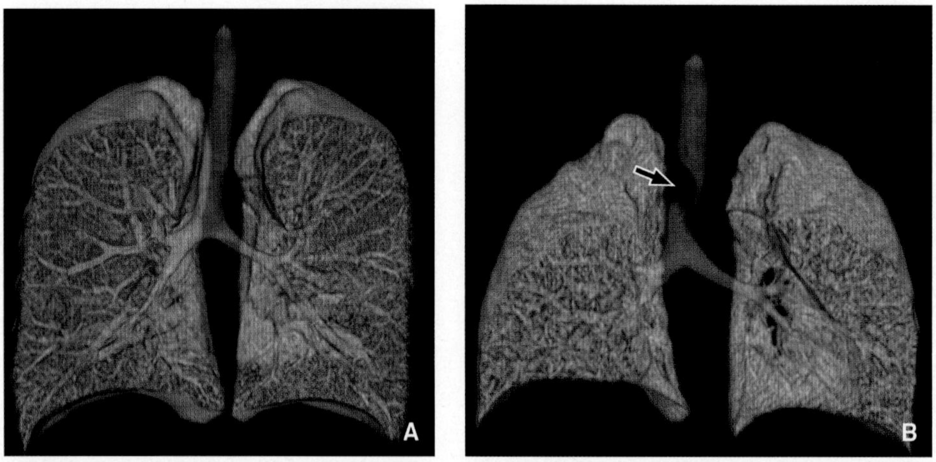

FIGURE 8.46 **Tracheomalacia in an 11-year-old boy with history of recurrent respiratory distress and pneumonia.** Subsequently obtained bronchoscopy confirmed the diagnosis of focal severe tracheomalacia. **A:** 3D external volume-rendered CT image obtained at end inspiration shows patent trachea and bilateral mainstem bronchi. Lungs are well aerated. **B:** 3D external volume-rendered CT image obtained at end expiration demonstrates almost complete focal collapse (*arrow*) of the mid- to distal trachea, which is diagnostic of focal tracheomalacia. Also noted is decreased overall lung volume in comparison to end inspiration **(A)**.

Foreign Body Aspiration

Foreign body aspiration is a common and potentially life-threatening etiology of acute respiratory distress in pediatric patients. Children ages 6 months to 3 years are usually affected, due to their tendency to place objects into their mouths, their lack of ability to chew certain foods due to missing molars, and their uncoordinated swallowing mechanism.[1,7,171] Edible and inedible food items are most likely to be aspirated, peanuts being the leading offender.[172] Foreign bodies usually lodge in the right main bronchus because it is larger than the left main bronchus and directly aligned with trachea in upright patients. Classically, affected children present with coughing, wheezing, and potentially stridor after an acute choking episode, but they may be asymptomatic.[1,7]

Chest radiography is the first-line imaging modality. Findings may include an identifiable, radiopaque foreign body; unilateral emphysema, hyperinflation, or localized air trapping on the affected side; bilateral emphysema or hyperinflation; focal air-space disease such as pneumonia and/or atelectasis;

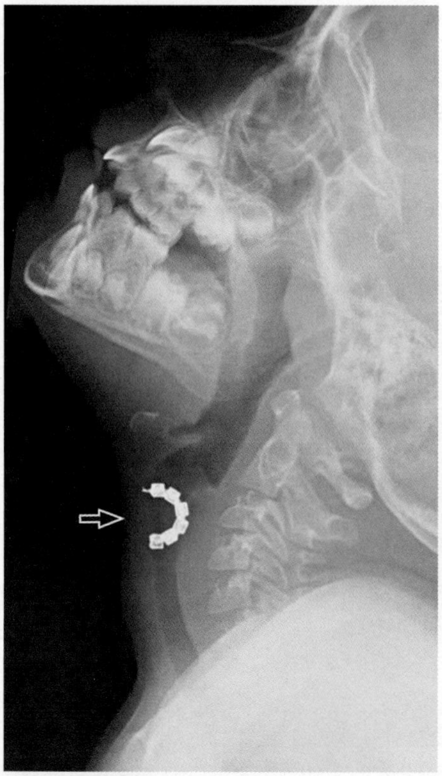

FIGURE 8.47 **Radiopaque foreign body aspiration lodged in a 4-year-old girl who presented with acute respiratory distress after swallowing an earring.** Lateral radiograph of the airway shows the radiopaque earring (*arrow*) lodged in the proximal trachea, just below glottis level.

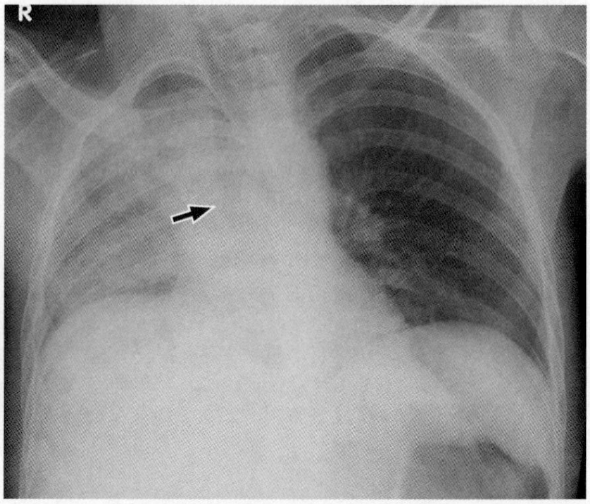

FIGURE 8.48 **Nonradiopaque foreign body aspiration in a 3-year-old boy who presented with acute respiratory distress after eating a hot dog.** Frontal chest radiograph shows an acute cutoff (*arrow*) of the proximal right mainstem air column and decreased right lung volume with atelectasis. The patient subsequently underwent bronchoscopy, which confirmed the aspirated hot dog fragment lodged in the proximal right mainstem bronchus.

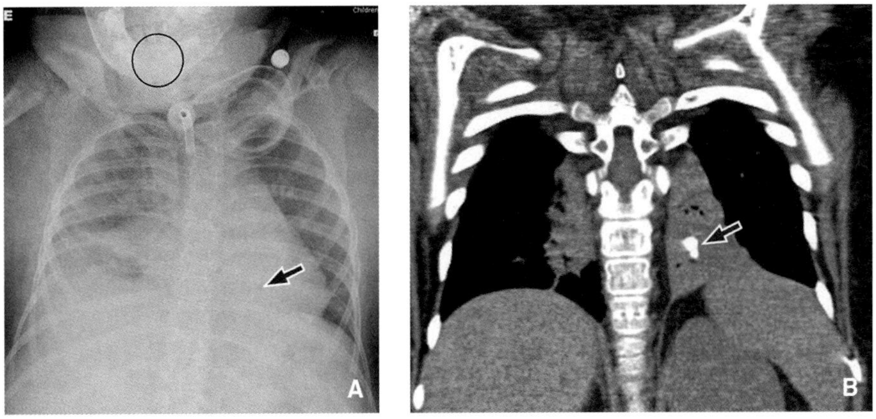

FIGURE 8.49 **Teeth aspiration in a 6-year-old boy with known cerebral palsy and tracheostomy who presented with acute respiratory distress and desaturation.** The patient subsequently underwent bronchoscopy, which retrieved the aspirated teeth. **A:** Frontal chest radiograph shows two square-shaped opacities (*arrow*) projecting over the left lower lobe. Also noted are missing two lower teeth (*circle*). **B:** Nonenhanced coronal reformatted CT image demonstrates aspiration teeth (*arrow*) with surrounding consolidation.

pleural effusion; subcutaneous emphysema; pneumothorax; or mediastinal shift[171,173–175] (Figs. 8.47 to 8.49). In addition to the standard frontal and lateral views, forced expiratory or bilateral decubitus views have traditionally been obtained to better assess for air trapping, a useful indirect sign of foreign body aspiration (Figs. 8.7 and 8.8). However, a recent study demonstrated that obtaining bilateral decubitus views increased the rate of false-positive diagnoses without increasing true-positive diagnoses. Expiratory views modestly increased the rate of true-positive diagnoses without increasing false-positive diagnoses; however, routine use must be weighed against potential excess radiation exposure due to the technically challenging nature of the exam and frequent need for repeat radiographs.[84,173]

It should be cautioned that only 10% of airway foreign bodies are radiopaque and can be detected on chest radiographs[1,7,128,173] (Fig. 8.49A). Further, the sensitivity and specificity for detection of foreign body aspiration with chest radiography are in the range of 68% to 74% and 45% to 67%, respectively.[1,7,126,176] Therefore, if there is high clinical concern in the setting of negative or equivocal radiographs, further evaluation should include conventional bronchoscopy or CT.[1,7,177,178] Although CT has an accuracy of close to 100%, its use should be weighed against radiation concerns.[1,7] The foreign body may be visible as an endoluminal mass of variable attenuation depending on the composition of the aspirated material. Secondary signs (as for chest radiography) include postobstructive air trapping, atelectasis, and consolidation.[1,7,9] CT is also helpful in cases of suspected residual foreign body postbronchoscopy.[7,176] 3D CT with virtual bronchoscopic reconstruction is useful in determining the need for bronchoscopy and the precise location of the foreign body.[179]

Rigid bronchoscopy with removal of the aspirated foreign body is, in general, the treatment of choice.[171,175] As residual foreign body after initial bronchoscopy is common, there should be a low threshold to repeat bronchoscopy given the appropriate clinical suspicion. For peripheral foreign bodies that cannot be removed bronchoscopically, alternative treatments include corticosteroids, bronchodilators, postural drainage, and tapotement (rhythmic percussion) to facilitate noninvasive removal.[175,180]

References

1. Lee EY, Restrepo R, Dillman JR, et al. Imaging evaluation of pediatric trachea and bronchi: systematic review and updates. *Semin Roentgenol.* 2012;47:182–196.
2. Laya BF, Lee EY. Congenital causes of upper airway obstruction in pediatric patients: updated imaging techniques and review of imaging findings. *Semin Roentgenol.* 2012;47:147–158.
3. Slovis TL. Noninvasive evaluation of the pediatric airway: a recent advance. *Pediatrics.* 1977;59:872–880.
4. Vats A, Worley GA, de Bruyn R, et al. Laryngeal ultrasound to assess vocal fold paralysis in children. *J Laryngol Otol.* 2004;118:429–431.
5. Singh M, Chin KJ, Chan VW, et al. Use of sonography for airway assessment: an observational study. *J Ultrasound Med.* 2010;29: 79–85.
6. Donnelly LF, Strife JL, Myer CM. Dynamic sleep fluoroscopy in children with obstructive sleep apnea. *Appl Radiol.* 2001; 30–34.
7. Lee EY, Greenberg SB, Boiselle PM. Multidetector computed tomography of pediatric large airway diseases: state-of-the-art. *Radiol Clin North Am.* 2011;49:869–893.
8. Lee EY. Advancing CT and MR imaging of the lungs and airways in children: imaging into practice. *Pediatr Radiol.* 2008;38 (suppl 2):S208.
9. Lee EY, Siegel MJ. MDCT of tracheobronchial narrowing in pediatric patients. *J Thorac Imaging.* 2007;22:300–309.
10. Pearce MS, Salotti JA, Little MP, et al. Radiation exposure from CT scans in childhood and subsequent risk of leukaemia and brain tumours: a retrospective cohort. *Lancet.* 2012;380: 499–505.
11. Lee EY, Boiselle PM. Tracheobronchomalacia in infants and children: multidetector CT evaluation. *Radiology.* 2009;252: 7–22.
12. Shenoy-Bhangle A, Nimkin K, Gee MS. Pediatric imaging: current and emerging techniques. *J Postgrad Med.* 2010;56:98–102.
13. Donnelly LF, Casper KA, Chen B, et al. Defining normal upper airway motion in asymptomatic children during sleep by means of cine MR techniques. *Radiology.* 2002;223:176–180.
14. Donnelly LF, Surdulescu V, Chini BA, et al. Upper airway motion depicted at cine MR imaging performed during sleep: comparison between young patients with and those without obstructive sleep apnea. *Radiology.* 2003;227:239–245.

15. Abbott MB, Donnelly LF, Dardzinski BJ, et al. Obstructive sleep apnea: MR imaging volume segmentation analysis. *Radiology.* 2004;232:889–895.
16. Donnelly LF. Obstructive sleep apnea in pediatric patients: evaluation with cine MR sleep studies. *Radiology.* 2005;236: 768–778.
17. Atik B, Bekerecioglu M, Tan O, et al. Evaluation of dynamic magnetic resonance imaging in assessing velopharyngeal insufficiency during phonation. *J Craniofac Surg.* 2008;19: 566–572.
18. Adewale L. Anatomy and assessment of the pediatric airway. *Paediatr Anaesth.* 2009;19(suppl 1):1–8.
19. Chang LW, Lee FA, Gwinn JL. Normal lateral deviation of the trachea in infants and children. *Am J Roentgenol Radium Ther Nucl Med.* 1970;247–251.
20. Eslamy HK, Newman B. Imaging of the pediatric airway. *Paediatr Anaesth.* 2009;(suppl 1):9–23.
21. Ramsden JD, Campisi P, Forte V. Choanal atresia and choanal stenosis. *Otolaryngol Clin North Am.* 2009;42:339–352.
22. Cedin AC, Atallah AN, Andriolo RB, et al. *Cochrane Database Syst Rev.* 2012;2:CD008993.
23. Castillo M. Congenital abnormalities of the nose: CT and MR findings. *AJR Am J Roentgenol.* 1994;162:1211–1217.
24. Slovis TL, Renfro B, Watts FB, et al. Choanal atresia: precise CT evaluation. *Radiology.* 1985;155:345–348.
25. Lowe LH, Booth TN, Joglar JM, et al. Midface anomalies in children. *Radiographics.* 2000;20:907–922.
26. Thomas BP, Strother MK, Donnelly EF, et al. CT virtual endoscopy in the evaluation of large airway disease: review. *AJR Am J Roentgenol.* 2009;192(3 suppl):S20–S30.
27. Al-Noury K, Lotfy A. Role of multislice computed tomography and local contrast in the diagnosis and characterization of choanal atresia. *Int J Pediatr.* 2011;2011:280763.
28. Sanal B, Demirhan N, Koplay M, et al. Congenital nasal pyriform aperture stenosis: clinical and radiologic findings and treatment. *Jpn J Radiol.* 2009;27:389–391.
29. Osovsky M, Aizer-Danon A, Horev G, et al. Congenital pyriform aperture stenosis. *Pediatr Radiol.* 2007;37:97–99.
30. Belden CJ, Mancuso AA, Schmalfuss IM. CT features of congenital nasal piriform aperture stenosis: initial experience. *Radiology.* 1999;213:495–501.
31. Rollins N, Booth T, Biavati M. Case 40: congenital pyriform aperture stenosis. *Radiology.* 2001;221:392–394.
32. Baxter DJ, Shroff M. Congenital midface abnormalities. *Neuroimaging Clin N Am.* 2011;21:563–584.
33. Vogler RC, Ii FJ, Pilgram TK. Age-specific size of the normal adenoid pad on magnetic resonance imaging. *Clin Otolaryngol Allied Sci.* 2000;25:392–395.
34. Capitanio MA, Kirkpatrick JA. Nasopharyngeal lymphoid tissue. Roentgen observations in 257 children 2 years of age or less. *Radiology.* 1970;96:389–391.
35. Donnelly LF, Shott SR, LaRose CR, et al. Causes of persistent obstructive sleep apnea despite previous tonsillectomy and adenoidectomy in children with Down syndrome as depicted on static and dynamic cine MRI. *AJR Am J Roentgenol.* 2004; 183:175–181.
36. Fernbach SK, Brouillette RT, Riggs TW, et al. Radiologic evaluation of adenoids and tonsils in children with obstructive sleep apnea: plain films and fluoroscopy. *Pediatr Radiol.* 1983; 13:258–265.
37. Chan J, Edman JC, Koltai PJ. Obstructive sleep apnea in children. *Am Fam Physician.* 2004;69:1147–1154.
38. Fujioka M, Young LW, Girdany BR. Radiographic evaluation of adenoidal size in children: adenoidal-nasopharyngeal ratio. *AJR Am J Roentgenol.* 1979;133:401–404.
39. Brooks LJ, Stephens BM, Bacevice AM. Adenoid size is related to severity but not the number of episodes of obstructive apnea in children. *J Pediatr.* 1998;132:682–686.
40. Li AM, Wong E, Kew J, et al. Use of tonsil size in the evaluation of obstructive sleep apnoea. *Arch Dis Child.* 2002;87:156–159.
41. Gibson SE, Myer CM III, Strife JL, et al. Sleep fluoroscopy for localization of upper airway obstruction in children. *Ann Otol Rhinol Laryngol.* 1996;105:678–683.
42. Donnelly LF, Casper KA, Chen B. Correlation on cine MR imaging of size of adenoid and palatine tonsils with degree of upper airway motion in asymptomatic sedated children. *AJR Am J Roentgenol.* 2002;179:503–508.
43. Gupta OP. Congenital macroglossia. *Arch Otolaryngol.* 1971;93: 378–383.
44. Rizer FM, Schechter GL, Richardson MA. Macroglossia: etiologic considerations and management techniques. *Int J Pediatr Otorhinolaryngol.* 1985;8:225–236.
45. Morgan WE, Friedman EM, Duncan NO, et al. Surgical management of macroglossia in children. *Arch Otolaryngol Head Neck Surg.* 1996;122:326–329.
46. Myer CM, Hotaling AJ, Reilly JS. The diagnosis and treatment of macroglossia in children. *Ear Nose Throat J.* 1986;65:444–448.
47. Murthy P, Laing MR. Macroglossia. *BMJ.* 1994;309:1386–1387.
48. Nussbaum E, Maggi JC. Laryngomalacia in children. *Chest.* 1990;98:942–944.
49. John SD, Swischuk LE. Stridor and upper airway obstruction in infants and children. *Radiographics.* 1992;12:625–643.
50. Tucker GF. Laryngeal development and congenital lesions. *Ann Otol Rhinol Laryngol.* 1980;74:142–145.
51. Sivan Y, Ben-Ari J, Soferman R, et al. Diagnosis of laryngomalacia by fiberoptic endoscopy: awake compared with anesthesia-aided technique. *Chest.* 2006;130:1412–1418.
52. Berg E, Naseri I, Sobol SE. The role of airway fluoroscopy in the evaluation of children with stridor. *Arch Otolaryngol Head Neck.* 2008;134:415–418.
53. Landry AM, Thompson DM. Laryngomalacia: disease presentation, spectrum, and management. *Int J Pediatr.* 2012; 2012:753526.
54. Ahmad SM, Soliman AM. Congenital anomalies of the larynx. *Otolaryngol Clin North Am.* 2007;40:177–191.
55. Strouse PJ, Newman B, Hernandez RJ, et al. CT of tracheal agenesis. *Pediatr Radiol.* 2006;36:920–926.
56. Heimann K, Bartz C, Naami A, et al. Three new cases of congenital agenesis of the trachea. *Eur J Pediatr.* 2007;166:79–82.
57. Payne W. Congenital absence of the trachea. *Brooklyn Med J.* 1900; 14:568.
58. Ergun S, Tewfik T, Daniel S. Tracheal agenesis: A rare but fatal congenital anomaly. *Mcgill J Med.* 2011;13:10.
59. Pumberger W, Metz V, Birnbacher R, et al. Tracheal agenesis: evaluation by helical computed tomography. *Pediatr Radiol.* 2000; 30:200–203.
60. Floyd J, Campbell DC Jr, Dominy DE. Agenesis of the trachea. *Am Rev Respir Dis.* 1962;86:557–560.
61. Effmann EL, Spackman TJ, Berdon WE, et al. Tracheal agenesis. *Am J Roentgenol Radium Ther Nucl Med.* 1975;125:767–781.
62. Krause U, Rödel RM, Paul T. Isolated congenital tracheal stenosis in a preterm newborn. *Eur J Pediatr.* 2011;170:1217–1221.
63. Ghaye B, Szapiro D, Fanchamps JM, et al. Congenital bronchial abnormalities revisited. *Radiographics.* 2001;21:105–119.

64. Berrocal T, Madrid C, Novo S, et al. Congenital anomalies of the tracheobronchial tree, lung, and mediastinum: embryology, radiology, and pathology. *Radiographics.* 2004;24:e17.
65. O'Sullivan BP, Frassica JJ, Rayder SM. Tracheal bronchus: a cause of prolonged atelectasis in intubated children. *Chest.* 1998;113:537–540.
66. Manjunatha YC, Gupta AK. Tracheal bronchus (pig bronchus). *Indian J Pediatr.* 2010;77:1037–1038.
67. Gower WA, McGrath-Morrow SA, MacDonald KD, et al. Tracheal bronchus in a 6-month-old infant identified by CT with three-dimensional airway reconstruction. *Thorax.* 2008;63:93–94.
68. Iwamoto T, Takasugi Y, Hiramatsu K, et al. Three-dimensional CT image analysis of a tracheal bronchus in a patient undergoing cardiac surgery with one-lung ventilation. *J Anesth.* 2009;23:260–265.
69. Teh BM, Hall C, Kleid S. Infected tracheocoele (acquired tracheal diverticulum): case report and literature review. *J Laryngol Otol.* 2011;125:540–545.
70. Sharma BG. Tracheal diverticulum: a report of 4 cases. *Ear Nose Throat J.* 2009;88:E11.
71. Soto-Hurtado EJ, Peñuela-Ruíz L, Rivera-Sánchez I, et al. Tracheal diverticulum: a review of the literature. *Lung.* 2006;184:303–307.
72. Shah M, Joshi JM. Tracheal diverticulum. *Indian J Chest Dis Allied Sci.* 2012;54:39–40.
73. Goo JM, Im JG, Ahn JM, et al. Right paratracheal air cysts in the thoracic inlet: clinical and radiologic significance. *AJR Am J Roentgenol.* 1999;173:65–70.
74. Celik B, Bilgin S, Yuksel C. Mounier-Kuhn syndrome: a rare cause of bronchial dilation. *Tex Heart Inst J.* 2011;38:194–196.
75. Pimpalwar AP, Hassan SF. Esophageal bronchus in an infant—a rare cause of recurrent pneumonia. *J Pediatr Surg.* 2012;47:e5–e8.
76. Verma A, Mohan S, Kathuria M, et al. Esophageal bronchus: case report and review of the literature. *Acta Radiol.* 2008;49:138–141.
77. Sugandhi N, Sharma P, Agarwala S, et al. Esophageal lung: presentation, management, and review of literature. *J Pediatr Surg.* 2011;46:1634–1637.
78. Michel JL, Revillon Y, Salakos C, et al. Successful bronchotracheal reconstruction in esophageal bronchus: two case reports. *J Pediatr Surg.* 1997;32:739–742.
79. Antón-Pacheco JL, Kalicinski P, Kansy A, et al. Slide tracheoplasty in an infant with congenital tracheal stenosis and oesophageal atresia with tracheoesophageal fistula. *Eur J Cardiothorac Surg.* 2012;42(5):892–893.
80. Herrera P, Caldarone C, Forte V, et al. The current state of congenital tracheal stenosis. *Pediatr Surg Int.* 2007;23:1033–1044.
81. Cantrell JR, Guild HG. Congenital stenosis of the trachea. *Am J Surg.* 1964;108:297–305.
82. Antón-Pacheco JL, Cano I, García A, et al. Patterns of management of congenital tracheal stenosis. *J Pediatr Surg.* 2003;38:1452–1458.
83. Currarino G, Williams B. Lateral inspiration and expiration radiographs of the neck in children with laryngotracheitis (croup). *Radiology.* 1982;145:365–366.
84. Chapman T, Sandstrom CK, Parnell SE. Pediatric emergencies of the upper and lower airway. *Appl Radiol.* 2012;10–17.
85. Cherry JD. Clinical practice. Croup. *N Engl J Med.* 2008;358:384–391.
86. Salour M. The steeple sign. *Radiology.* 2000;216:428–429.
87. Huang CC, Shih SL. Images in clinical medicine. Steeple sign of croup. *N Engl J Med.* 2012;367:66.
88. Lin CY, Chi H, Shih SL, et al. A 4-year-old boy presenting with recurrent croup. *Eur J Pediatr.* 2010;169:249–251.
89. Westley CR, Cotton EK, Brooks JG. Nebulized racemic epinephrine by IPPB for the treatment of croup: a double-blind study. *Am J Dis Child.* 1978;132:484–487.
90. Pitluk JD, Uman H, Safranek S. Clinical inquiries. What's best for croup? *J Fam Pract.* 2011;60:680–681.
91. Miranda AD, Valdez TA, Pereira KD. Bacterial tracheitis: a varied entity. *Pediatr Emerg Care.* 2011;27:950–953.
92. Shargorodsky J, Lee GS, Whittemore KR. Bacterial tracheitis: a therapeutic approach. *Laryngoscope.* 2010;120:2498–2501.
93. Han BK, Dunbar JS, Striker TW. Membranous laryngotracheobronchitis (membranous croup). *AJR Am J Roentgenol.* 1979;133:53–58.
94. Sammer M, Pruthi S. Membranous croup (exudative tracheitis or membranous laryngotracheobronchitis). *Pediatr Radiol.* 2010;40:781.
95. Hedlund GL, Wiatrak BJ, Pranikoff T. Pneumomediastinum as an early radiographic sign in membranous croup. *AJR Am J Roentgenol.* 1998;170:55–56.
96. Wheeler DS, Dauplaise DJ, Giuliano JS Jr. An infant with fever and stridor. *Pediatr Emerg Care.* 2008;24:46–49.
97. Podgore JK, Bass JW. Letter: The "thumb sign" and "little finger sign" in acute epiglottitis. *J Pediatr.* 1976;88:154–155.
98. Grover C. Images in clinical medicine. "Thumb sign" of epiglottitis. *N Engl J Med.* 2011;365:447.
99. John SD, Swischuk LE, Hayden CK Jr, et al. Aryepiglottic fold width in patients with epiglottitis: where should measurements be obtained? *Radiology.* 1994;190:123–125.
100. Ducic Y, Hébert PC, MacLachlan L, et al. Description and evaluation of the vallecula sign: a new radiologic sign in the diagnosis of adult epiglottitis. *Ann Emerg Med.* 1997;30:1–6.
101. Hung TY, Li S, Chen PS, et al. Bedside ultrasonography as a safe and effective tool to diagnose acute epiglottitis. *Am J Emerg Med.* 2011;29:359.e1–359.e3.
102. Ko DR, Chung YE, Park I, et al. Use of bedside sonography for diagnosing acute epiglottitis in the emergency department: a preliminary study. *J Ultrasound Med.* 2012;31:19–22.
103. Perez-Velez CM. Pediatric tuberculosis: new guidelines and recommendations. *Curr Opin Pediatr.* 2012;24:319–328.
104. Ochoa TJ, Rojas R, Gutierrez M, et al. Severe airway obstruction in a child with Pott's disease. *Pediatr Infect Dis J.* 2006;25:649–651.
105. Wong JS, Ng CS, Lee TW, et al. Bronchoscopic management of airway obstruction in pediatric endobronchial tuberculosis. *Can Respir J.* 2006;13:219–221.
106. Leung AN, Müller NL, Pineda PR, et al. Primary tuberculosis in childhood: radiographic manifestations. *Radiology.* 1992;182:87–91.
107. Weber AL, Bird KT, Janower ML. Primary tuberculosis in childhood with particular emphasis on changes affecting the tracheobronchial tree. *Am J Roentgenol Radium Ther Nucl Med.* 1968;103:123–132.
108. Kim WS, Moon WK, Kim IO, et al. Pulmonary tuberculosis in children: evaluation with CT. *AJR Am J Roentgenol.* 1997;168:1005–1009.
109. Fischer GB, Mocelin H, Severo CB, et al. Histoplasmosis in children. *Paediatr Respir Rev.* 2009;10:172–177.
110. Kirchner SG, Hernanz-Schulman M, Stein SM, et al. Imaging of pediatric mediastinal histoplasmosis. *Radiographics.* 1991;11:365–381.

111. Weinberg GA, Kleiman MB, Grosfeld JL, et al. Unusual manifestations of histoplasmosis in childhood. *Pediatrics.* 1983;72:99–105.
112. Sherrick AD, Brown LR, Harms GF, et al. The radiographic findings of fibrosing mediastinitis. *Chest.* 1994;106:484–489.
113. Rossi SE, McAdams HP, Rosado-de-Christenson ML, et al. Fibrosing mediastinitis. *Radiographics.* 2001;21:737–757.
114. Devaraj A, Griffin N, Nicholson AG, et al. Computed tomography findings in fibrosing mediastinitis. *Clin Radiol.* 2007;62:781–786.
115. Smith JS, Kadiev S, Diaz P, et al. Pulmonary artery stenosis secondary to fibrosing mediastinitis: management with cutting balloon angioplasty and endovascular stenting. *Vasc Endovascular Surg.* 2011;45:170–173.
116. Ferguson ME, Cabalka AK, Cetta F, et al. Results of intravascular stent placement for fibrosing mediastinitis. *Congenit Heart Dis.* 2010;5:124–133.
117. Raol N, Metry D, Edmonds J, et al. Propranolol for the treatment of subglottic hemangiomas. *Int J Pediatr Otorhinolaryngol.* 2011;75:1510–1514.
118. Javia LR, Zur KB, Jacobs IN. Evolving treatments in the management of laryngotracheal hemangiomas: will propranolol supplant steroids and surgery? *Int J Pediatr Otorhinolaryngol.* 2011;75:1450–1454.
119. Sutton TJ, Nogrady MB. Radiologic diagnosis of subglottic hemangioma in infants. *Pediatr Radiol.* 1973;1:211–216.
120. Cooper M, Slovis TL, Madgy DN, et al. Congenital subglottic hemangioma: frequency of symmetric subglottic narrowing on frontal radiographs of the neck. *AJR Am J Roentgenol.* 1992; 159:1269–1271.
121. Koplewitz BZ, Springer C, Slasky BS, et al. CT of hemangiomas of the upper airways in children. *AJR Am J Roentgenol.* 2005;184:663–670.
122. Nozawa K, Aihara T, Takano H. MR imaging of a subglottic hemangioma. *Pediatr Radiol.* 1995;25:235–236.
123. Rossler L, Rothoeft T, Teig N, et al. Ultrasound and colour Doppler in infantile subglottic haemangioma. *Pediatr Radiol.* 2011;41:1421–1428.
124. Venkatesan NN, Pine HS, Underbrink MP. Recurrent respiratory papillomatosis. *Otolaryngol Clin North Am.* 2012;45:671–694.
125. Williams SD, Jamieson DH, Prescott CA. Clinical and radiological features in three cases of pulmonary involvement from recurrent respiratory papillomatosis. *Int J Pediatr Otorhinolaryngol.* 1994; 30:71–77.
126. Glikman D, Baroody FM. Images in clinical medicine. Recurrent respiratory papillomatosis with lung involvement. *N Engl J Med.* 2005;352:e22.
127. Lui D, Kumar A, Aggarwal S, et al. CT findings of malignant change in recurrent respiratory papillomatosis. *J Comput Assist Tomogr.* 1995;19:804–807.
128. Szyszko T, Gnanasegaran G, Barwick T, et al. Respiratory papillomatosis of lung and F-18 FDG PET-CT. *Clin Nucl Med.* 2009;34:521–522.
129. Avanzini S, Pio L, Buffa P, et al. Intraoperative bronchoscopy for bronchial carcinoid parenchymal-sparing resection: a pediatric case report. *Pediatr Surg Int.* 2012;28:75–78.
130. Moraes TJ, Langer JC, Forte V, et al. Pediatric pulmonary carcinoid: a case report and review of the literature. *Pediatr Pulmonol.* 2003;35:318–322.
131. Curtis JM, Lacey D, Smyth R, et al. Endobronchial tumours in childhood. *Eur J Radiol.* 1998;29:11–20.
132. Hervás Benito I, Bello Arques P, Loaiza JL, et al. Somatostatin receptor scintigraphy in pediatric bronchial carcinoid tumor. [Article in Spanish]. *Rev Esp Med Nucl.* 2010;29:25–28.
133. Lee EY, Vargas SO, Sawicki GS, et al. Mucoepidermoid carcinoma of bronchus in a pediatric patient: (18)F-FDG PET findings. *Pediatr Radiol.* 2007;37:1278–1282.
134. Granata C, Battistini E, Toma P, et al. Mucoepidermoid carcinoma of the bronchus: a case report and review of the literature. *Pediatr Pulmonol.* 1997;23:226–232.
135. Liu X, Adams AL. Mucoepidermoid carcinoma of the bronchus: a review. *Arch Pathol Lab Med.* 2007;131:1400–1404.
136. Park CM, Goo JM, Lee HJ, et al. Tumors in the tracheobronchial tree: CT and FDG PET features. *Radiographics.* 2009;29:55–71.
137. Kim TS, Lee KS, Han J, et al. Mucoepidermoid carcinoma of the tracheobronchial tree: radiographic and CT findings in 12 patients. *Radiology.* 1999;212:643–648.
138. Yikilmaz A, Lee EY. CT imaging of mass-like nonvascular pulmonary lesions in children. *Pediatr Radiol.* 2007;37:1253–1263.
139. Medina LS, Siegel MJ, Glazer HS, et al. Diagnosis of pulmonary complications associated with lung transplantation in children: value of CT vs. histopathologic studies. *AJR Am J Roentgenol.* 1994;162:969–974.
140. McAdams HP, Palmer SM, Erasmus JJ, et al. Bronchial anastomotic complications in lung transplant recipients: virtual bronchoscopy for noninvasive assessment. *Radiology.* 1998;209:689–695.
141. Sun M, Ernst A, Boiselle PM. MDCT of the central airways: comparison with bronchoscopy in the evaluation of complications of endotracheal and tracheostomy tubes. *J Thorac Imaging.* 2007;22:136–142.
142. Brown SB, Hedlund GL, Glasier CM, et al. Tracheobronchial stenosis in infants: successful balloon dilation therapy. *Radiology.* 1987;164:475–478.
143. Polonovski JM, Hertz Panier L, Francois M, et al. Balloon dilatation of tracheobronchial stenoses in children. Apropos of 4 cases. [Article in French]. *Ann Otolaryngol Chir Cervicofac.* 1991;108:411–416.
144. Dialani V, Ernst A, Sun M, et al. MDCT detection of airway stent complications: comparison with bronchoscopy. *AJR Am J Roentgenol.* 2008;191:1576–1580.
145. Hammer MR, Dillman JR, Chong ST, et al. Imaging of pediatric thoracic trauma. *Semin Roentgenol.* 2012;47:135–146.
146. Ozdulger A, Cetin G, Erkmen Gulhan S, et al. A review of 24 patients with bronchial ruptures: is delay in diagnosis more common in children? *Eur J Cardiothorac Surg.* 2003;23:379–383.
147. Nakayama DK, Ramenofsky ML, Rowe MI. Chest injuries in childhood. *Ann Surg.* 1989;210:770–775.
148. Jackimczyk K. Blunt chest trauma. *Emerg Med Clin North Am.* 1993;11:81–96.
149. Harvey-Smith W, Bush W, Northrop C. Traumatic bronchial rupture. *AJR Am J Roentgenol.* 1980;134:1189–1193.
150. Ein SH, Friedberg J, Shandling B, et al. Traumatic bronchial injuries in children. *Pediatr Pulmonol.* 1986;2:60–64.
151. Mahboubi S, O'Hara AE. Bronchial rupture in children following blunt chest trauma. Report of five cases with emphasis on radiologic findings. *Pediatr Radiol.* 1981;10:133–138.
152. Hrkac Pustahija A, Vukelic Markovic M, Ivanac G, et al. An unusual case of bronchial rupture—pneumomediastinum appearing 7 days after blunt chest trauma. *Emerg Radiol.* 2009;16:163–165.
153. Scaglione M, Romano S, Pinto A, et al. Acute tracheobronchial injuries: impact of imaging on diagnosis and management implications. *Eur J Radiol.* 2006;59:336–343.

154. Le Guen M, Beigelman C, Bouhemad B, et al. Chest computed tomography with multiplanar reformatted images for diagnosing traumatic bronchial rupture: a case report. *Crit Care.* 2007;11:R94.
155. Wan YL, Tsai KT, Yeow KM, et al. CT findings of bronchial transection. *Am J Emerg Med.* 1997;15:176–177.
156. Bingol-Kologlu M, Fedakar M, Yagmurlu A, et al. Tracheobronchial rupture due to blunt chest trauma: report of a case. *Surg Today.* 2006;36:823–826.
157. Rencken I, Patton WL, Brasch RC. Airway obstruction in pediatric patients. From croup to BOOP. *Radiol Clin North Am.* 1998;36:175–187.
158. McColley SA, Morty RE. Update in pediatric lung disease 2011. *Am J Respir Crit Care Med.* 2012;186:30–34.
159. Kazani S, Israel E. Update in asthma 2011. *Am J Respir Crit Care Med* 2012;186:35–40.
160. Ley-Zaporozhan J, Puderbach M, Kauczor HU. MR for the evaluation of obstructive pulmonary disease. *Magn Reson Imaging Clin N Am.* 2008;16:291–308.
161. Fain S, Schiebler ML, McCormack DG, et al. Imaging of lung function using hyperpolarized helium-3 magnetic resonance imaging: review of current and emerging translational methods and applications. *J Magn Reson Imaging.* 2010;32:1398–1408.
162. Schwengel DA, Sterni LM, Tunkel DE, et al. Perioperative management of children with obstructive sleep apnea. *Anesth Analg.* 2009;109:60–75.
163. Guimaraes CV, Kalra M, Donnelly LF, et al. The frequency of lingual tonsil enlargement in obese children. *AJR Am J Roentgenol.* 2008;190:973–975.
164. Felman AH, Loughlin GM, Leftridge CA Jr, et al. Upper airway obstruction during sleep in children. *AJR Am J Roentgenol.* 1979;133:213–216.
165. Carden KA, Boiselle PM, Waltz DA, et al. Tracheomalacia and tracheobronchomalacia in children and adults: an in-depth review. *Chest.* 2005;127:984–1005.
166. Lee EY, Mason KP, Zurakowski D, et al. MDCT assessment of tracheomalacia in symptomatic infants with mediastinal aortic vascular anomalies: preliminary technical experience. *Pediatr Radiol.* 2008;38:82–88.
167. Lee EY, Zurakowski D, Waltz DA, et al. MDCT evaluation of the prevalence of tracheomalacia in children with mediastinal aortic vascular anomalies. *J Thorac Imaging.* 2008;23: 258–265.
168. Lee EY, Litmanovich D, Boiselle PM. Multidetector CT evaluation of tracheobronchomalacia. *Radiol Clin North Am.* 2009; 47:261–269.
169. Lee EY, Strauss KJ, Tracy DA, et al. Comparison of standard-dose and reduced-dose expiratory MDCT techniques for assessment of tracheomalacia in children. *Acad Radiol.* 2010;17:504–510.
170. Lee EY, Tracy DA, Bastos M, et al. Expiratory volumetric MDCT evaluation of air trapping in pediatric patients with and without tracheomalacia. *AJR Am J Roentgenol.* 2010;194: 1210–1215.
171. Grover S, Bansal A, Singhi SC. Airway foreign body aspiration. *Indian J Pediatr.* 2011;78:1401–1403.
172. Kaushal P, Brown DJ, Lander L, et al. Aspirated foreign bodies in pediatric patients, 1968–2010: a comparison between the United States and other countries. *Int J Pediatr Otorhinolaryngol.* 2011;75:1322–1326.
173. Brown JC, Chapman T, Klein EJ, et al. The utility of adding expiratory or decubitus chest radiographs to the radiographic evaluation of suspected pediatric airway foreign bodies. *Ann Emerg Med.* 2013;61(1):19–26.
174. Svedström E, Puhakka H, Kero P. How accurate is chest radiography in the diagnosis of tracheobronchial foreign bodies in children? *Pediatr Radiol.* 1989;19:520–522.
175. Paksu S, Paksu MS, Kilic M, et al. Foreign body aspiration in childhood: evaluation of diagnostic parameters. *Pediatr Emerg Care.* 2012;28:259–264.
176. Shin SM, Kim WS, Cheon JE, et al. CT in children with suspected residual foreign body in airway after bronchoscopy. *AJR Am J Roentgenol.* 2009;192:1744–1751.
177. Bai W, Zhou X, Gao X, et al. Value of chest CT in the diagnosis and management of tracheobronchial foreign bodies. *Pediatr Int.* 2011;53:515–518.
178. Koşucu P, Ahmetoğlu A, Koramaz I, et al. Low-dose MDCT and virtual bronchoscopy in pediatric patients with foreign body aspiration. *AJR Am J Roentgenol.* 2004; 183:1771–1777.
179. Jung SY, Pae SY, Chung SM, et al. Three-dimensional CT with virtual bronchoscopy: a useful modality for bronchial foreign bodies in pediatric patients. *Eur Arch Otorhinolaryngol.* 2012;223–228.
180. Cataneo AJ, Cataneo DC, Ruiz RL Jr. Management of tracheobronchial foreign body in children. *Pediatr Surg Int.* 2008;24:151–156.

CHAPTER 9

Heart

Lorna P. Browne • Edward Y. Lee • Oleksandr Kondrachuk • Marielle V. Fortier • Zhu Ming • Cynthia K. Rigsby

INTRODUCTION

In recent years, congenital and acquired forms of cardiac disease have been encountered with increasing frequency in the pediatric population. This is because more children with congenital heart disease survive longer mainly due to the substantial advances in surgical techniques and management. Radiologic imaging remains at the forefront of the diagnostic evaluation in children with clinically suspected or known congenital heart disease. However, the inherent complexity of these conditions continues to be a challenge for many radiologists.

The objective of this chapter is to enhance the understanding of congenital and acquired forms of cardiac disease occurring in the pediatric population by using a stepwise approach to cardiac anatomy and diagnosis that can be applied by the novice resident or expert radiologist. First, the various imaging techniques currently available for evaluating pediatric cardiac disease are discussed. The normal anatomy of the heart including the systemic and pulmonary arterial and venous vessels is reviewed. The beneficial use of the segmental approach to diagnosis is presented. Finally, a variety of the commonly encountered pediatric cardiac diseases focusing on pathophysiology, clinical features, imaging assessment, and treatment options are discussed.

IMAGING TECHNIQUES

Several imaging modalities are currently utilized in the evaluation of infants and children with suspected congenital or acquired cardiac disease, including radiography, echocardiography, computed tomography (CT), and magnetic resonance imaging (MRI), each of which has its own distinct advantages and disadvantages.

Radiography

Chest radiography is a useful initial evaluation in the infant or child with suspected cardiac disease, but its role in diagnosis has been supplanted by other imaging modalities. Still, many congenital cardiac conditions, such as tetralogy of Fallot (TOF), transposition of great arteries (TGA), supracardiac total anomalous pulmonary venous return (TAPVR), and Ebstein anomaly, have classical radiographic appearances.[1] Currently, chest radiography is frequently used to screen pediatric patients with suspected underlying cardiac disease for assessment of cardiac size and evaluation of pulmonary vasculature. In addition, it is also used in pediatric patients with known cardiac disease in order to evaluate the pulmonary circulation for evidence of pulmonary venous congestion and response to intervention.

Echocardiography

Echocardiography (echo) is unrivaled in its ability to evaluate the intracardiac structures with excellent temporal and spatial resolution. It is commonly the first test performed in a neonate with suspected cardiac disease, usually before chest radiography. Limitations of echo include poor echo windows in older children or those with skeletal malformations and its inability to adequately visualize the extracardiac arterial and venous vasculature.[2] In general, echo falls more within the purview of a pediatric cardiologist than a pediatric radiologist. Therefore, for the most part, this chapter is dedicated to the other (nonecho) imaging modalities that are currently used for evaluation of congenital and acquired forms of cardiac disease in the pediatric population.

Computed Tomography

Previously, pediatric cardiac computed tomography angiography (CTA) was associated with relatively long acquisition times and high radiation doses, limiting its utility in pediatric cardiac imaging. However, the advent of prospective ECG gating, ultrafast gantry rotation times, dual-source technology/volume acquisition, variable pitch (higher pitch with fast heart rate), and radiation dose modulation has enabled successful pediatric cardiac CTA with low radiation doses (~1 to 3 mSv or less), frequently not requiring sedation or breath-holding.[2] Although high heart rates (>100 bpm) are typical in infants and young children, beta blockade and vasodilation agents are not used routinely. Common applications of pediatric cardiac CTA include evaluation for anomalous coronary arteries, anomalous pulmonary veins, pulmonary artery stenosis/atresia, major arteriopulmonary collateral arteries (MAPCAs), and aortic root dilatation/dissection.[2]

Magnetic Resonance Imaging

The cardiac MRI evaluation of pediatric congenital heart anomalies can be subdivided into an assessment of cardiovascular morphology, quantification of ventricular function, and quantification of flow. Each of these assessments involves dedicated MRI sequences optimized for their individual role.[3]

Evaluation of cardiovascular morphology is performed using static spin-echo "black blood" sequences (T1/T2) or cine gradient-echo "bright blood" sequences (2D steady-state free precession [SSFP]). Spin-echo black blood techniques allow a static overview of the extracardiac thoracic vasculature. Cine gradient-echo imaging allows a dynamic assessment of the thoracic vessels with multiple frames acquired throughout the cardiac cycle. This provides a more accurate depiction of stenosis/aneurysms in vessels whose diameters are changing throughout the cardiac cycle.[3,4] Coronary artery evaluation involves a specific sequence (3D SSFP), which yields high-resolution images only during a short period of each cardiac cycle when the heart is relatively motionless (usually end diastole for lower heart rates and end systole for higher heart rates). As this is a long sequence, typically taking 5 minutes or longer, respiratory motion is minimized by using a respiratory navigator during image acquisition. This technique is timed to have imaging occur during a small length of diaphragmatic excursion. Finally, contrast-enhanced 3D magnetic resonance angiography (MRA) also provides excellent morphologic assessment of the thoracic and abdominal vasculature with time-resolved techniques. Such techniques enable a fast acquisition that can be used to isolate the pulmonary and systemic arterial phases of contrast enhancement.[5]

Evaluation of ventricular function is performed with cine 2D SSFP sequences that are optimized to provide excellent myocardial blood pool differentiation.[3,4] Images are obtained in various planes that are similar to those acquired on echo and include a two-chamber plane (coronal oblique view demonstrating the right/left atrium and accompanying ventricle), a four-chamber plane (transverse oblique covering both atria and ventricles), and a short-axis plane (sagittal oblique across the right ventricle [RV] and left ventricle [LV]) (Fig. 9.1). Additional views, such as left and right outflow tract planes as well as aortic root planes (Fig. 9.2), may also be acquired depending on the pathology being evaluated.

Ventricular volume is calculated by summing the individual volumes of the ventricles on each of the short-axis or four-chamber slices acquired in end diastole and end systole, using specialized postprocessing software. Wall motion abnormalities are demonstrated by visualization of the images in a dynamic mode throughout the cardiac cycle. Immediately following the intravenous administration of gadolinium, first-pass perfusion sequences may show areas of delayed or absent myocardial perfusion related to ischemia or infarction, respectively.[4,5] Administration of a pharmacologic stress agent such as adenosine or dobutamine (stress perfusion) can be utilized to elicit decreased first-pass perfusion that is not

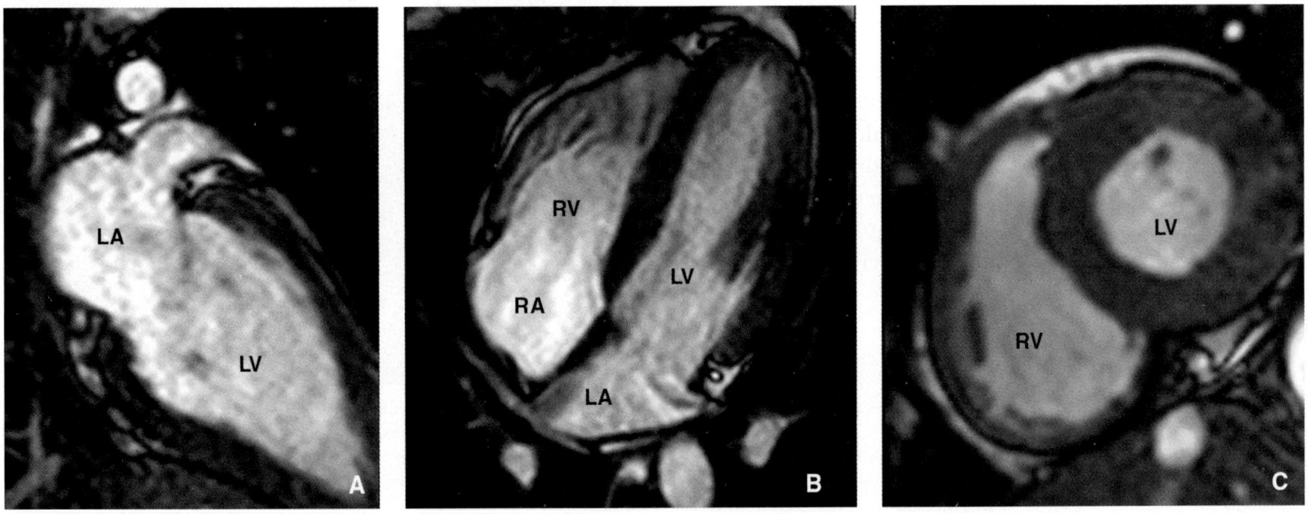

FIGURE 9.1 **Standard cardiac magnetic resonance imaging planes.** Bright blood magnetic resonance images in **(A)** two-chamber, **(B)** four-chamber, and **(C)** short-axis geometries. *LA*, left atrium; *LV*, left ventricle; *RA*, right atrium; *RV*, right ventricle.

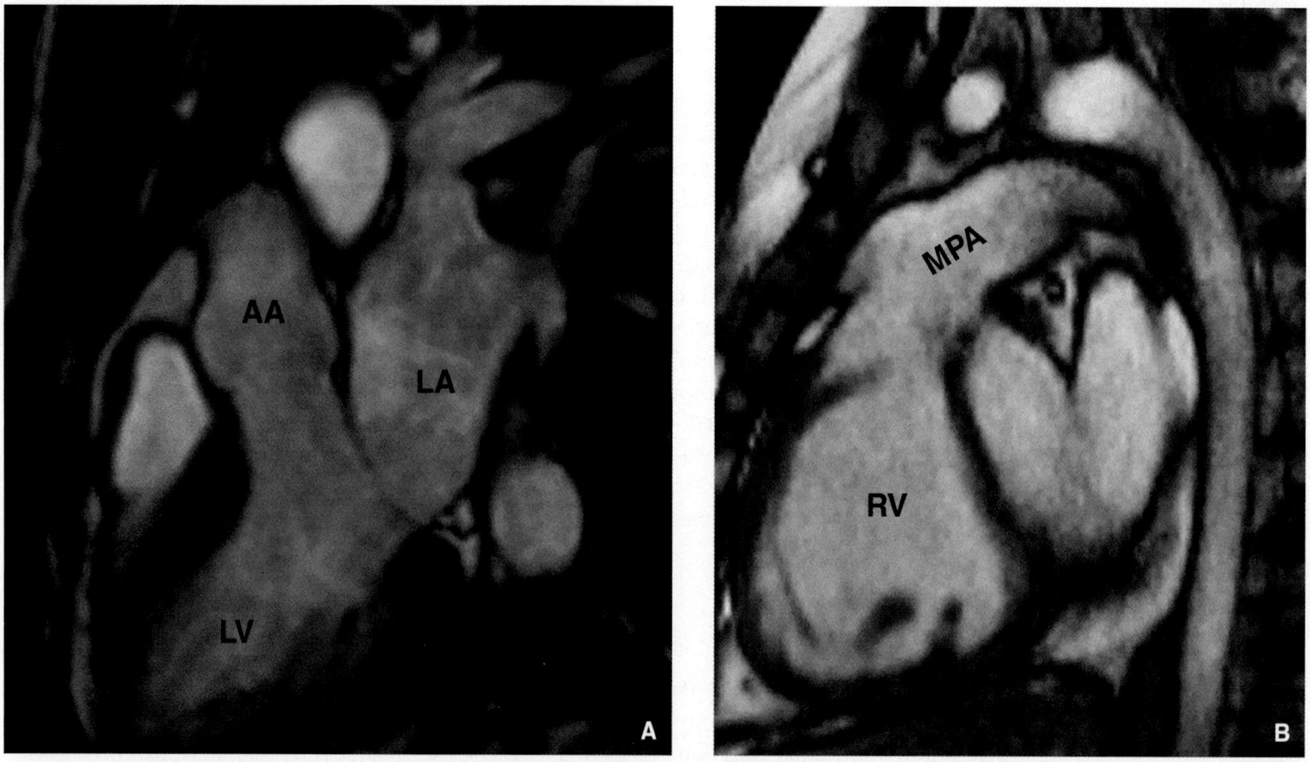

FIGURE 9.2 **Outflow tract cardiac magnetic resonance imaging planes.** Bright blood magnetic resonance images in **(A)** left ventricular outflow tract/three-chamber view **(B)** right ventricular outflow tract. *AA*, ascending aorta; *LA*, left atrium; *LV*, left ventricle; *MPA*, main pulmonary artery; *RV*, right ventricle.

visible under resting conditions. In general, adenosine is preferred because of its ease of administration, fast action, and short half-life. However, unlike in adults, stress perfusion in pediatrics is usually reserved for those patients clinically felt to be high risk for myocardial ischemia, such as those with coronary artery involvement in Kawasaki disease or in heart transplant patients with suspected coronary artery vasculopathy. Approximately 10 minutes after administration of gadolinium, myocardial viability sequences can be performed to demonstrate retained gadolinium in regions of myocardial fibrosis (Fig. 9.3).

Flow evaluation is performed with cine phase-contrast sequences (Fig. 9.4). Flow sequences are used to assess stroke volumes and regurgitant fractions across the aortic and pulmonary valves. In addition, flow sequences can be used to measure the volume of systemic to pulmonary shunting, known as the Qp:Qs ratio where Qp is the volume of pulmonary blood flow and Qs is the volume of systemic blood flow.[4,5] The Qp:Qs ratio is an important quantification in the evaluation of septal defects and other left-to-right shunts. Pressure gradients across stenoses may be derived using the modified Bernoulli equation ($4 \times V^2 = \Delta P$, where ΔP is the pressure gradient in mm Hg and V is the measured peak velocity by cine phase contrast in m/s).

The entire cardiac MRI examination, including a morphologic assessment, ventricular function, and flow analysis, is expected to take between 60 and 90 minutes; therefore,

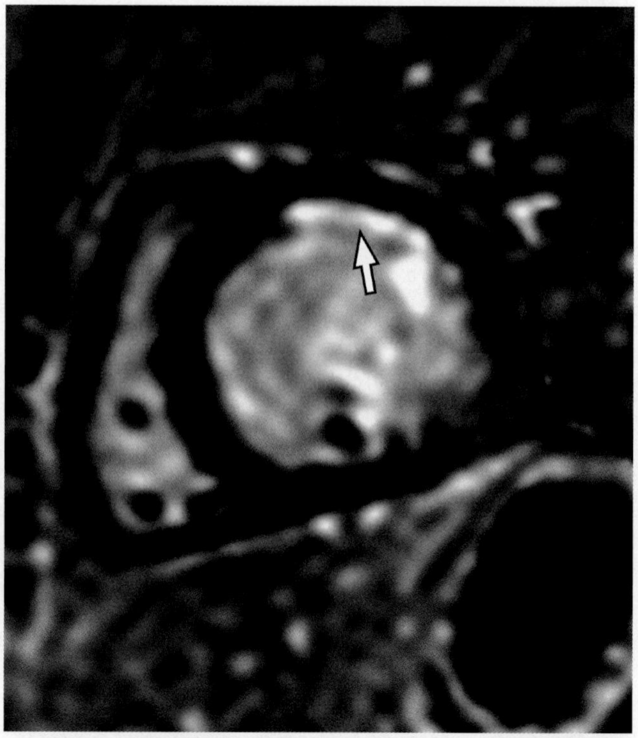

FIGURE 9.3 **Delayed cardiac wall enhancement.** Short-axis plane phase-sensitive inversion recovery magnetic resonance image shows an area of subendocardial enhancement (*arrow*) in the anterolateral wall of the left ventricle.

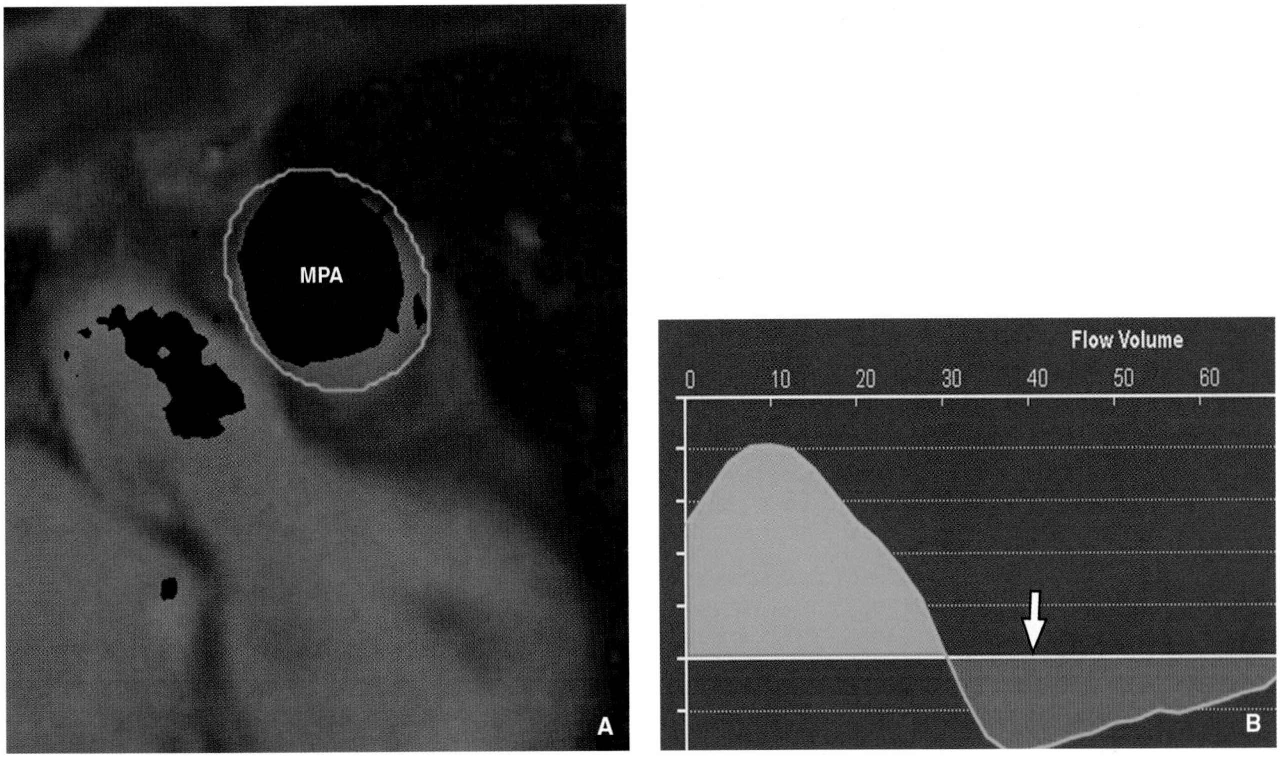

FIGURE 9.4 **Flow quantification using phase-contrast angiography.** Phase contrast across the main pulmonary artery (*MPA*) demonstrates an approximately 40% pulmonary regurgitant fraction (green circle on **A** and arrow on **B**).

frequently, general anesthesia or conscious sedation is necessary in the pediatric population.

NORMAL ANATOMY

A clear understanding of normal cardiac anatomy is fundamental to the imaging interpretation of congenital heart anomalies and abnormalities.

The normal pediatric heart occupies ~60% of the cardiothoracic diameter on chest radiography in the neonatal period and early infancy, decreasing to about 50% in later childhood life and adolescence. When evaluating both normal and complex cardiovascular anatomy on cross-sectional imaging techniques such as CT or MRI, a segmental approach, which can enhance interpretation, is recommended.[6] This approach broadly encompasses a series of steps that assess the positions of the cardiac chambers and great vessels and their relationships in a sequential fashion, as if the interpreter were a red blood cell traveling from the systemic veins into the heart and ultimately terminating in the systemic arteries.

The first step is the evaluation of visceral situs. This involves confirmation of rightward location of the liver and inferior vena cava (IVC) and leftward location of the spleen and stomach. The cardiac position (referred to as cardiac situs) is determined by the position of the cardiac apex, which is normally inferior and leftward and termed levocardia. Mesocardia refers to a heart in a more midline location. Dextrocardia indicates that the heart is located in the right chest with the apex pointing rightward. In dextroversion, the heart is shifted rightward, either through mass effect or pulmonary volume loss, but the cardiac apex still points to the left.

The next step involves evaluation of the systemic venous anatomy, including confirmation of a single right-sided superior vena cava (SVC), normal position of the right and left innominate veins, and the presence of a normal suprarenal IVC. Commonly encountered systemic venous anomalies include bilateral SVCs (usually without a left innominate vein) and an interrupted IVC with azygos continuation.

The atrial situs evaluation comes next. It is the morphology of the atria and their venous inflow, rather than their location in the chest, which determines whether the atria are termed right or left. The atrium that receives the suprahepatic IVC and has a broad-based atrial appendage is considered to be the right atrium. The SVC is more variable in its drainage than the suprahepatic IVC. Therefore, it is not used in determination of atrial morphology. The atrium that has a long and narrow atrial appendage is termed the left atrium and normally should receive the four pulmonary veins.

The determination of ventricular morphology can establish what type of ventricular looping took place during embryonic cardiac development and also the type of atrioventricular valve (AVV) supplies the ventricles. The RV has a number of prominent trabeculations along the septum and ventricular free wall. One of these trabeculations is particularly prominent and is known as the moderator band (Fig. 9.5). The moderator band runs from the ventricular free wall to the interventricular septum and is relatively closely located to the cardiac apex. The moderator band can be easily identified on an axial CT view of the chest and a four-chamber view

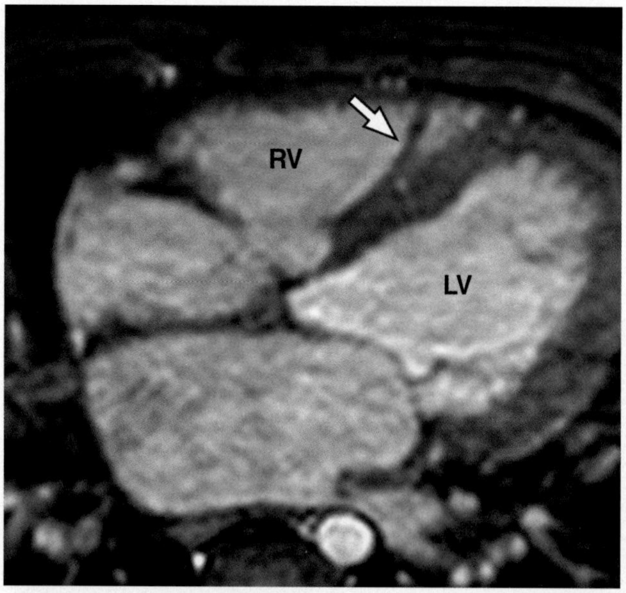

FIGURE 9.5 **Moderator band.** Bright blood magnetic resonance image in four-chamber plane shows the moderator band (*arrow*) in the right ventricle extending from the free wall to the ventricular septum. *LV*, left ventricle; *RV*, right ventricle.

on cardiac MRI and is a reliable determinant of ventricular morphology. The tricuspid valve follows the RV. Typically, the tricuspid valve is located very slightly closer to the cardiac apex than the mitral valve. The tricuspid valve has three leaflets, including the septal leaflet (attached to the interventricular septum) and anterior and posterior leaflets. The LV is supplied by the mitral valve and typically has two papillary muscles along its free wall (anterolateral and posteromedial). However, these papillary muscles are more variable in appearance than moderator band in terms of correctly identifying ventricular morphology. If the RV is located anteriorly and rightward relative to the LV, then normal ventricular "D" looping is deemed to have occurred. If the ventricle containing the moderator band is located posteriorly and leftward, then ventricular inversion or "L" looping has occurred. This is discussed in more detail later in the chapter in TGA.

Evaluation of the great arteries starts with evaluation of the conus (infundibulum). The conus is the muscular sleeve that is normally located under the pulmonary valve around the infundibulum of the heart. It forms the superior portion of the interventricular septum. In addition, it separates the pulmonary valve from the AV and the aortic valves. Its presence, absence, or variation in appearance forms a central role in the development of complex malformations such as TOF, interrupted arch, TGA, and double outlet right ventricle (DORV).

The next step is the assessment of great vessel arrangement and ventriculoarterial connections. Normally, the LV is attached to the aorta, and the RV is attached to the main pulmonary artery (MPA). If this normal arrangement is present, the ventriculoarterial connection is described as concordant. If the LV is connected to the pulmonary artery and the RV is connected to the aorta, the arrangement is described as discordant. The normal relationship of the great arteries results in the aortic valve annulus located rightward and posterior to the pulmonary valve annulus (termed situs solitus of the great vessels). Situs inversus of the great vessels is the term used when the aortic annulus is located leftward and posterior of the pulmonary valve yet normal ventriculoarterial concordance is maintained (i.e., LV → Aorta and RV → MPA). In discordant ventriculoarterial connections (i.e., LV → MPA and RV → Aorta), the great vessels are described as being transposed. In this case, the aortic valve annulus may be either rightward and anterior to the pulmonary valve (D-transposed) or leftward and anterior to the pulmonary valve (L-transposed).

Once the cardiac segmental anatomy is established, the interatrial and interventricular septa are assessed for defects, and the great vessels are interrogated for stenoses or other abnormalities.

Approaching the cardiac anatomy using the above segmental approach greatly assists in correctly identifying and classifying cardiac malformations.[6]

Atria

The atria are the cardiac chambers that receive the systemic and pulmonary venous drainage. The right atrium forms the right heart border of the cardiac silhouette on frontal chest radiographs. It receives systemic venous blood from the two venae cavae and from the coronary veins via the coronary sinus. Then the right atrium expels blood through the tricuspid valve into the RV. The interior of the right atrium has a smooth posterior wall and a muscular anterior wall that is separated by a crescent-shaped muscular ridge, the crista terminalis. The inferior vena caval orifice is guarded by the Eustachian valve and the coronary sinus by the Thebesian valve. Both the inferior vena caval orifice and the coronary sinus orifice are located along the inferior border of the atrium. The superior vena caval orifice is valveless, but the pacemaker of the heart, the sinoatrial (SA) node, is located just posterior to the superior vena caval orifice.

The left atrium forms the posterior border of the heart on lateral chest radiographs. The left atrium is located just below the carina and left main bronchus. Such location of the left atrium with respect to the carina and left main bronchus explains why the carina appears splayed and left main bronchus appears elevated on frontal chest radiographs in cases of severe left atrial enlargement. The left atrium typically receives at least four pulmonary veins and expels blood through the mitral valve into the LV. There is a normal ridge of tissue known as the Coumadin ridge, which separates the left upper pulmonary vein from the left atrium that is confluent with the wall of the left atrial appendage. This should not be confused with cor triatriatum.[7]

Atrial Septum

The interatrial septum not only separates the left and right atria but also has a small portion that separates the right atrium from the LV, known as the AV septum. The importance of the AV portion is that it represents one of the boundaries of the triangle of Koch that is the anatomic landmark for the AV node. In addition to the SA node, the AV node forms part of the conduction system of the heart. Along the midportion of the interatrial septum lies a small depression known as the fossa ovalis/foramen ovale that represents the remnant of the ostium secundum and should close shortly after birth.[7]

Ventricles

The RV forms most of the inferior border of the cardiac silhouette on frontal chest radiographs. Normally, the RV is anterior and rightward with respect to the LV. The RV can be divided into inlet, trabecular, and outlet portions. The inlet portion is derived in association with the tricuspid valve and contains the chordal attachments. The trabecular portion contains prominent muscle bundles that traverse the chamber from the free wall to the interventricular septum and include the moderator band. Other important named muscle bundles include the parietal band and the septal band. The parietal band separates the tricuspid and pulmonary valves. The septal band, which is Y-shaped, merges with apical trabeculations, gives rise to the moderator band (Fig. 9.5), and ends in the tricuspid papillary muscle. These three muscle bands form a circular ring known as the crista supraventricularis, which separates the trabecular portion of the ventricle from the outlet portion. The outlet portion of the RV is contained within a collar of muscle known as the conus arteriosus ("conus," or infundibulum), and it separates the pulmonary and tricuspid valves.

The LV forms the left border of the heart on frontal chest radiographs. The muscle bundles of the septal and free walls of the LV are arranged in a spiral fashion and also crisscross one another. As a consequence, systole results in twisting contractions, which "wring" the blood out of the LV. The LV is also divided into inlet, trabecular, and outlet portions. The inlet portion of the LV is short and contains the mitral chordal attachments. The trabecular portion contains the anterolateral and posteromedial papillary muscles and fine apical trabeculations. The outlet portion is quite long and does not have a conus infundibulum muscular ring (as is seen in the right ventricular outlet), so the aortic and mitral valves normally are in fibrous continuity.

Division of the LV into four segments is used in imaging when assessing myocardial function and evaluating for perfusion defects. In this segmentation scheme, the LV is considered to be a circular structure, and the four segments are septal (interventricular septum), anterior (superior wall), inferior (inferior wall), and lateral (mid free wall). The locations where these quadrants overlap are termed anteroseptal, anterolateral, inferoseptal, and inferolateral.[7]

Interventricular Septum

The ventricular septum is divided in a similar way to the ventricular chambers. The inlet septum is bordered by tricuspid valve attachments, the outlet septum lies superior to the crista supraventricularis, and the trabecular septum is located between the inlet and outlet portions. Such division is useful when trying to localize ventricular septal defects (VSDs). One additional portion of the outlet septum is termed the membranous septum, which is a very small portion of the septum that lies between the pulmonary valve annulus and

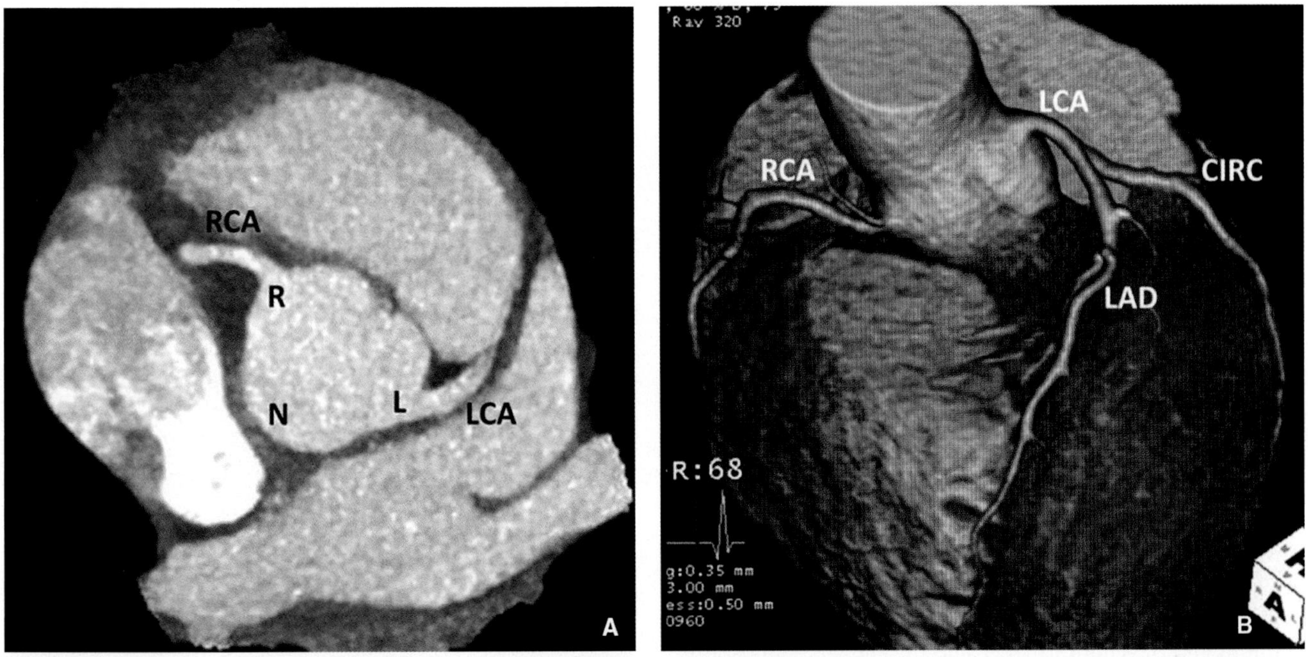

FIGURE 9.6 **Normal coronary arteries. A:** Axial maximum intensity projection (MIP) CT image demonstrates normal origin of the right coronary artery (*RCA*) and left coronary artery (*LCA*) from the right (*R*) and left (*L*) sinuses of Valsalva. (*N*, noncoronary sinus.) **B:** Three-dimensional volume-rendered CT image shows normal courses of the *RCA*, *LCA*, left anterior descending coronary artery (*LAD*), and left circumflex coronary artery (*CIRC*).

inferior aspect of the tricuspid valve annulus. The AV bundle (of HIS) runs through the membranous septum and is the only normal route for connection between the AV node and the ventricular myocardial conduction system.[7]

Coronary Arteries

The right and left main coronary arteries (RCA and LCA) originate from the center of the right and left aortic sinuses of Valsalva, which are located on either side of the aortic root, facing the pulmonary valve[8] (Fig. 9.6). The third aortic sinus, known as the noncoronary sinus, is located posterior to the other two aortic sinuses. The right and left coronary arteries arise from their respective aortic sinuses about halfway between the aortic valve annulus and the sinotubular junction. The right coronary artery (RCA) travels in the right AV groove and supplies the right ventricular free wall via a conal branch and multiple marginal branches. The left coronary artery rapidly divides into left anterior descending (LAD) and circumflex branches. The LAD artery travels in the anterior interventricular groove. It usually supplies the myocardium of the left ventricular free wall via diagonal branches and the anterior interventricular septum via septal branches. The circumflex artery travels within the left AV groove. It terminates in obtuse marginal branches that supply the lateral wall of the LV and part of the anterolateral papillary muscle.[8]

The artery that gives rise to the posterior descending artery (PDA), which supplies the inferior interventricular septum, inferior left ventricular free wall, and the AV node, is considered to be the dominant coronary artery. In ~70% of individuals, the RCA gives rise to the PDA (right coronary dominant); in 10%, the circumflex artery gives rise to branches to the posterior right ventricular surface (left circumflex [LCX] dominant); and in the remaining 20%, the PDA is supplied by branches from both right coronary and LCX arteries (codominant).[8]

CONGENITAL CARDIAC MALFORMATIONS

Septal Defects

Atrial Septal Defects

Atrial septal defect (ASD) arises from failure of closure of portions of the interatrial septum (ostium primum and ostium secundum) or maldevelopment of the portion of the atrium that receives the vena cava (sinus venosus defects). There are three major types of ASDs: ostium primum, ostium secundum, and sinus venous defects[9] (Fig. 9.7).

The atrial septum is formed from the septum primum. This starts in the roof of the primitive common atrium and grows toward the endocardial cushions, located between the primitive atria and ventricles. The gap between the septum primum and the endocardial cushion is known as an ostium primum. The gap gradually decreases as the septum primum and the endocardial cushions fuse to form the interatrial septum and atrioventricular valves, respectively. If the septum

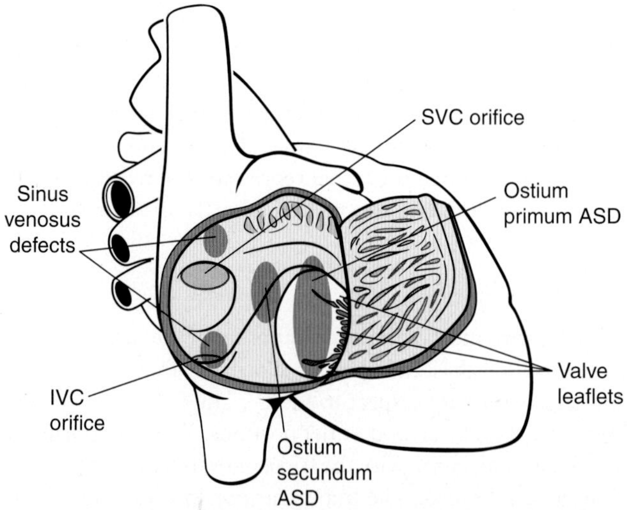

FIGURE 9.7 **Diagram of the location of the three types of atrial septal defects.** ASD 1: primum atrial septal defects. ASD 2: secondum atrial septal defects. ASD 3: sinus venosus superior/inferior atrial septal defects.

primum and endocardial cushions fail to fuse completely, an ostium primum ASD results (10% to 15% of ASDs), which is an ASD that is located close to the AV (mitral and tricuspid) valves. It is usually associated with maldevelopment of the atrioventricular valves (AVVs).[9]

The ostium secundum results from small perforations, which form in the septum primum and which gradually coalesce. The ostium secundum is usually partially covered by a valve of tissue formed by a fold in the septum primum. This fold (septum secundum) usually fuses completely with the rest of the interatrial septum shortly after birth closing the ostium secundum. Persistence is known as a patent foramen ovale or ostium secundum ASD comprising of 80% of all ASDs (Fig. 9.8).[9]

The sinus venosus is the posterior portion of the right atrium formed by the incorporation of primitive cardinal veins into the primitive atrium.[10] Sinus venosus defects (5% to

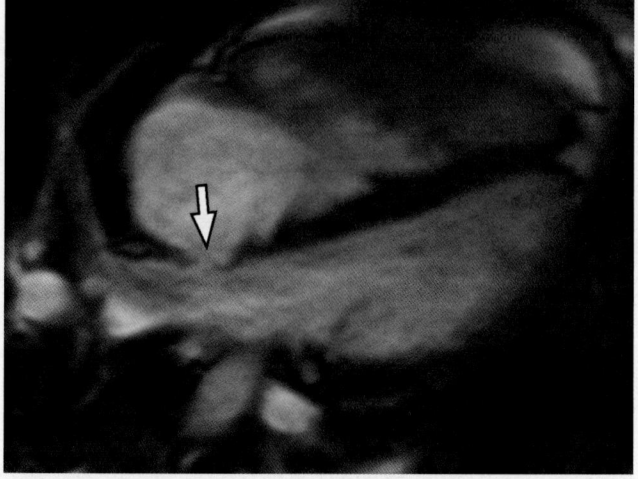

FIGURE 9.8 **Ostium secundum atrial septal defect.** Bright blood magnetic resonance image in four-chamber plane shows ostium secundum atrial septal defect (*arrow*).

10% of all ASDs) occur as a result of either malposition of the interatrial septum or malposition of the SVC/IVC resulting in a vena cava that overrides the atrial septum. Therefore, a sinus venous defect is actually a defect above or below the interatrial septum and not truly within the septum like ostium primum and secundum defects. A superior sinus venous defect where the SVC meets the interatrial septum is much more common than the inferior sinus venosus type. The resulting gap between the interatrial septum and the vena cava causes pulmonary venous blood in the left atrium to be drawn into the lower pressure right atrium. In addition, at least 85% patients with superior type sinus venosus defects have concomitant anomalous partial anomalous pulmonary venous drainage from the right upper lobe into the SVC (Fig. 9.9).

All ASDs result in a left-to-right shunt, which may lead to complications. A small ostium secundum defect may close spontaneously in the first 2 years of life. The remaining ASDs or ostium secundum ASDs in patients older than 2 years of age are unlikely to close. An untreated large ASD leads to increased pulmonary blood flow, right atrial and right ventricular enlargement, and pulmonary hypertension.[9]

On chest radiographs, cardiomegaly and pulmonary vascular congestion with an enlarged central pulmonary vessels and variable amounts of pulmonary edema depending on the size of the shunt are seen. Currently, cardiac gated CTA is occasionally used to assess ostium secundum ASDs for possible percutaneous septal device closure. A 5 mm rim of tissue separating the ASD from each of the following structures: aortic annulus, SVC orifice, IVC orifice, right upper pulmonary venous orifice and the atrioventricular valve is needed for successful device placement. Cardiac MRI can evaluate the presence and location of the ASD, which is close to the tricuspid and mitral valves in ostium primum defects, midinteratrial septum in ostium secundum defects, and posterior aspect of cavoatrial junction in sinus venous defects. It also provides information regarding the size of the rim of septal tissue that surrounds an ostium secundum ASD, which helps determine candidacy for percutaneous closure. In addition to the assessment of right ventricular function, cardiac MRI can also quantify the shunt volume or Qp:Qs (ratio of volume of blood in the pulmonary circulation: volume of blood in the systemic circulation) by comparing stroke volumes in the RV and MPA to stroke volumes in the LV and aorta. Furthermore, cardiac MRI provides excellent evaluation of the pulmonary veins given the association of anomalous pulmonary venous drainage in sinus venosus type defects.

Ostium secundum defect closure can be achieved either surgically using a pericardial/Gore-Tex patch or percutaneously using a septal closure device in select cases.[11] Surgical ostium primum defect closure involves placing a patch. The type of surgical repair undertaken for repairing sinus venosus defects is dependent upon the location of the drainage of the anomalous pulmonary veins. The Warden procedure is generally performed when the anomalous pulmonary veins return to the SVC. This procedure involves oversewing the SVC above the anomalous pulmonary venous connection and anastomosing the proximal end of the SVC to the right atrial appendage.[10] The anomalous pulmonary vein(s) and caudal end of the SVC are baffled to the left atrium through the sinus venosus defect thus closing the defect. A single patch closure of the sinus venosus defect is performed if the anomalous pulmonary veins drain to the right atrium or SVC/right atrial junction.[12]

Atrioventricular Septal Defects

The two endocardial cushions are located between the primitive atria and ventricles. They normally fuse to form the mitral and tricuspid valves and the crux of the heart, at the junction of the interatrial and interventricular septa.[13] Atrioventricular

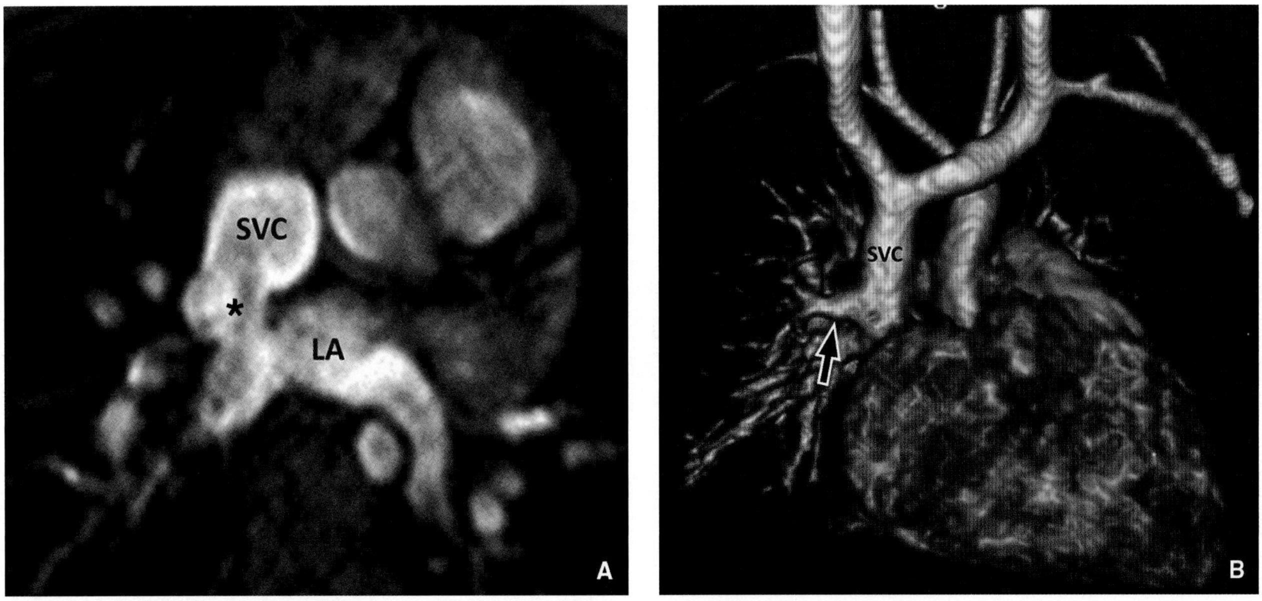

FIGURE 9.9 **Sinus venous defect. A:** Axial bright blood magnetic resonance (MR) image demonstrates a superior sinus venous defect (*asterisk*) between the posterior wall of superior vena cava (*SVC*) and anterior left atrium (*LA*). **B:** Three-dimensional volume-rendered MR image shows partial anomalous pulmonary venous return (*arrow*) from right upper lobe to SVC.

septal defects (AVSDs) are malformations caused by failure of fusion of the endocardial cushions that result in a deficient AV septum with a common atrioventricular valve (AVV) rather than separate mitral and tricuspid valve openings.[14] This common AVV often has five to six leaflets and a complex arrangement of chordal attachments. Normally, the aortic valve is situated between the tricuspid and mitral valves. However, when there is common AVV, the aortic valve becomes displaced superiorly, resulting in an elongated and potentially narrowed left ventricular outflow tract.

If the AVV is positioned centrally over the ventricles, it is termed a balanced AV septal defect and results in a large left-to-right shunt. An unbalanced AV septal defect results when the common AVV is located more over one ventricle than the other. This affects ventricular development and a single ventricle physiology usually results. For instance, if the AVV is situated more over the RV, then LV becomes underdeveloped and a hypoplastic left heart physiology results. Such location of the AVV may be exacerbated by coexistent left ventricular outflow tract stenosis resulting from the displaced aortic valve. This is discussed more fully in the single ventricle portion of the chapter.

AVSDs result in significant left-to-right shunting. Therefore, clinical presentation is in the early neonatal period with respiratory distress, murmur, and congestive cardiac failure. AVSDs are commonly associated with Down syndrome and anomalies of atrial and visceral situs.[15]

Chest radiography demonstrates global cardiomegaly (Fig. 9.10), sometimes with a horizontal superior right atrial border, severe pulmonary vascular engorgement, and pulmonary edema.[1] CT usually has no role in the evaluation of AVSDs. Cardiac MRI is usually reserved for complex cases not completely assessed on echo. In these cases, cardiac MRI can quantify shunt volume and AVV regurgitation, depict complex intracardiac anatomy, and determine ventricular size and function, which may facilitate presurgical planning (Fig. 9.11).

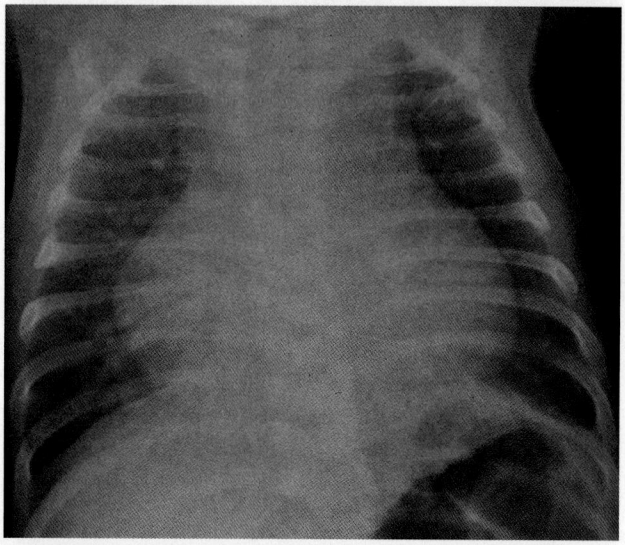

FIGURE 9.10 **Balanced atrioventricular septal defect.** Frontal chest radiograph shows increased pulmonary vascularity and global cardiomegaly.

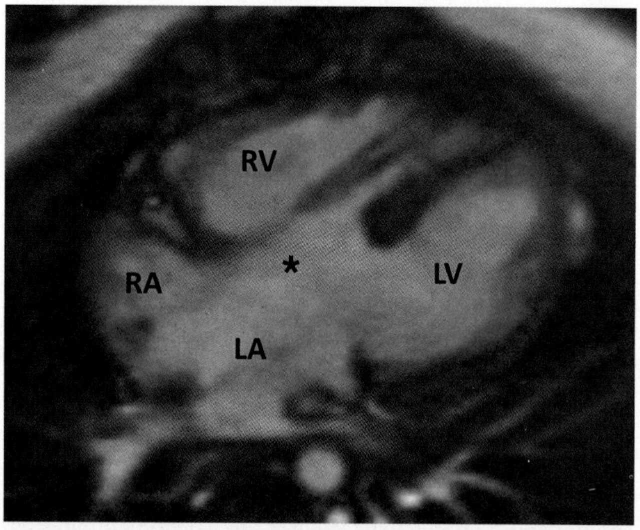

FIGURE 9.11 **Balanced atrioventricular septal defect.** Bright blood magnetic resonance image in four-chamber plane demonstrates large atrioventricular septal defect (*asterisk*). *LA*, left atrium; *LV*, left ventricle; *RA*, right atrium; *RV*, right ventricle.

Surgical correction of balanced AVSDs can be achieved by closure of the ostium primum ASD and inlet VSD using one or two patches, which are then used to recreate separated atrioventricular valves.[15,16] Surgical correction of unbalanced defects depends on the type of physiology and is discussed in the single ventricle portion of the chapter.

Ventricular Septal Defects

VSDs are holes in the interventricular septum. They can occur as an isolated defect or be part of more complex congenital heart anomalies such as conotruncal anomalies (TOF, TGA, DORV) or AVSDs. VSDs are the second most commonly encountered congenital heart defects after bicuspid aortic valves.[17]

The interventricular septum first appears as a muscular ridge close to the cardiac apex at the end of the 4th week. Then, it grows cephalad as the RV and LV enlarge, eventually fusing with bulbus cordis (primitive ventricular outflow tract). The inlet portion of the ventricular septum is thought to arise from the endocardial cushions. The membranous portion of the ventricular septum forms last and results from the formation of fibrous valvar leaflets arising from the endocardial cushions. The union of the endocardial cushions with the muscular interventricular septum is still not completely understood with differing hypotheses. However, final fusion between the muscular septum, membranous septum, and inlet septum occurs at approximately the 8th gestational week.

There are four types of VSDs that reflect the embryologic development of the interventricular septum: inlet, muscular, perimembranous, and subarterial[17] (Fig. 9.12). The inlet type of VSD extends from the fibrous annulus of the AVV and is often associated with an endocardial cushion defect. Muscular defects may appear anywhere throughout the muscular portion of the ventricular septum. Small muscular VSDs

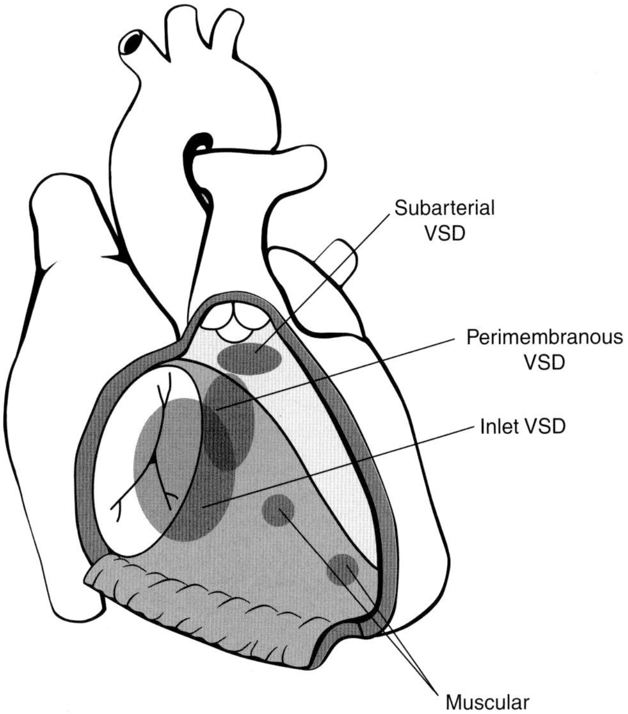

FIGURE 9.12 Diagram of the location of the four types of ventricular septal defects (VSDs) including subpulmonary VSD (subarterial), membranous VSD (perimembranous), atrioventricular canal defect (inlet type), and muscular VSD (muscular).

usually close spontaneously, and larger VSDs generally require surgical intervention. Occasionally, the muscular part of the septum can have innumerable VSDs, resulting in the so-called Swiss cheese interventricular septum. Perimembranous VSDs are the most common type to require surgical intervention and are characterized by a defect in the membranous portion of the ventricular septum. The subarterial or malalignment type of VSD appears just below the aortic valve cusps. Perimembranous and subarterial VSDs are often referred to as outlet VSDs and are associated with conotruncal anomalies such as TOF and TGA.[17]

Clinical presentation depends on the size of the defect and whether other cardiac anomalies are present. Small isolated VSDs often require no treatment and usually spontaneously close during childhood, whereas larger defects may manifest with failure to thrive and signs of congestive heart failure. Chronic left-to-right shunting may result in pulmonary hypertension leading to reversal of shunting known as Eisenmenger syndrome.[18]

Chest radiography appearances of VSDs depend of the size of the VSD and vary from normal cardiac size to severe cardiomegaly with normal pulmonary vascularity to severe pulmonary vascular engorgement and pulmonary edema (Fig. 9.13). CT has no role in the evaluation of VSDs although they are sometimes found incidentally (Fig. 9.14). Cardiac MRI is used usually reserved for evaluation of complex cases, which are not completely assessed on echo (Fig. 9.15). In these cases, cardiac MRI can quantify shunt volume, depict associated

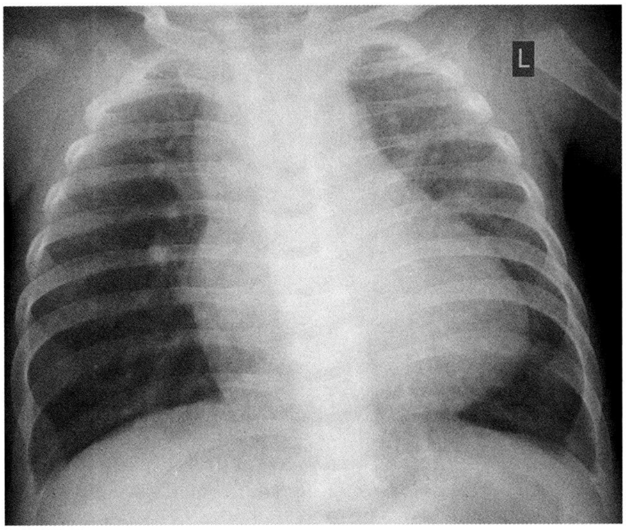

FIGURE 9.13 **Ventricular septal defect.** Frontal chest radiograph shows increased pulmonary vascularity and cardiac enlargement.

intracardiac or valvar anomalies, and determine ventricular size and function, which may facilitate presurgical planning.

Surgical closure is favored for treatment of VSDs that are unlikely to close spontaneously or are associated with a significant left-to-right shunt. This is usually performed using a patch of synthetic material.[18] Percutaneous device closure of these defects is rarely performed because of the reported incidence of both early- and late-onset complete heart block after device closure of perimembranous VSDs, which occurs presumably secondary to device trauma to the adjacent AV node. Occasionally, percutaneous closure of muscular VSDs is performed using a septal occluder device.[19]

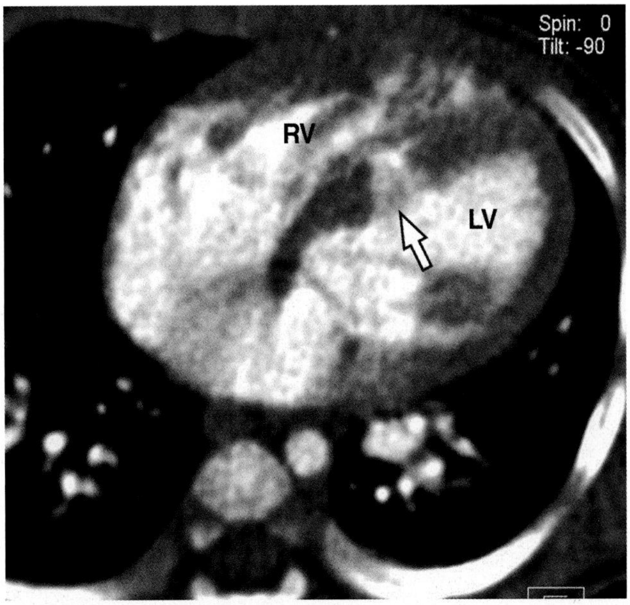

FIGURE 9.14 **Ventricular septal defect.** Axial enhanced CT image shows a large muscular VSD (*arrow*), partially covered by right ventricular muscle bundles. *LV*, left ventricle; *RV*, right ventricle.

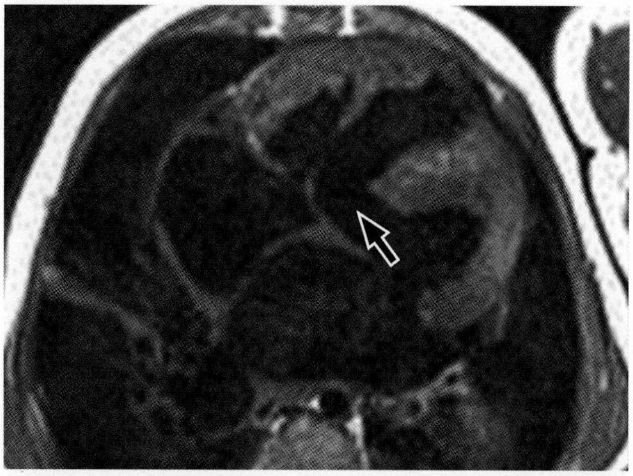

FIGURE 9.15 **Perimembranous ventricular septal defect.** Black blood magnetic resonance image shows a perimembranous ventricular septal defect (*arrow*) with muscular extension in a 2-month-old girl with double outlet right ventricle.

Atrioventricular Valve Stenosis and Regurgitation

Mitral Stenosis

Congenital mitral stenosis is very rare and usually occurs in association with other left heart lesions including hypoplastic left heart syndrome (HLHS) and aortic stenosis/atresia. Asymmetric congenital mitral stenosis is termed parachute mitral valve, which may be associated with a single papillary muscle with fused chordal attachments, giving the mitral valve an unbalanced appearance.[7] The most common cause of acquired mitral stenosis in young patients is rheumatic heart disease (Fig. 9.16). Patients with mild stenosis are usually asymptomatic, whereas patients with more severe disease develop pulmonary venous congestion.

Chest radiography may be normal or demonstrate pulmonary vascular congestion and interstitial edema depending on the degree of underlying obstruction. Cardiac MRI and CTA currently do not usually have a role in evaluating mitral stenosis.

Surgical repair of congenital mitral stenosis involves valvuloplasty and often later valve replacement surgery.

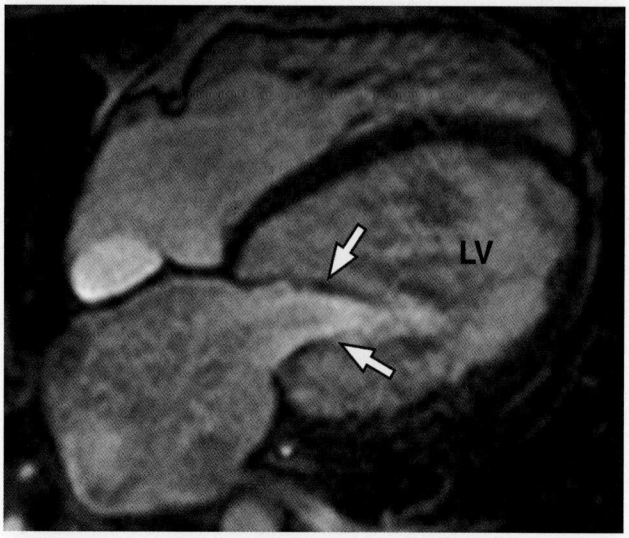

FIGURE 9.16 **Mitral stenosis.** Axial bright blood magnetic resonance image shows turbulent jets arising from the tips of stenosed mitral valve leaflets (*arrows*). *LV*, left ventricle.

Mitral Regurgitation

Congenital mitral regurgitation is very rare. It is usually seen in association with a cleft in the mitral valve, connective tissue disorders such as Marfan syndrome, or secondary to ventricular dysfunction, trauma, or myocardial infarction.[7] Mitral valve prolapse is thought to be related to an inherent abnormality in the myxomatous matrix/collagenous structure of the mitral valve.[20] Clinically, symptoms depend on severity of disease. Infants and children with severe disease usually demonstrate symptoms of pulmonary vascular congestion at <3 years of age.

Chest radiography may reveal elevation of the left main bronchus, splaying of the carina, and an enlarged posterior cardiac shadow on the lateral projection related to left atrial enlargement. Although echo is the primary diagnostic test for evaluating mitral regurgitation, cardiac MRI is frequently used in the overall cardiovascular assessment in patients with connective tissue disorders such as Marfan syndrome. Mitral regurgitation can be seen as a regurgitant jet arising from the valve leaflets during ventricular systole, usually resulting in left atrial dilatation (Fig. 9.17). Mitral valve prolapse is best appreciated on the left ventricular outflow tract/three-chamber view. This view shows the anterior mitral valve leaflet prolapsing into the atrium during systole with an accompanying regurgitant jet into the left atrium (Fig. 9.18).

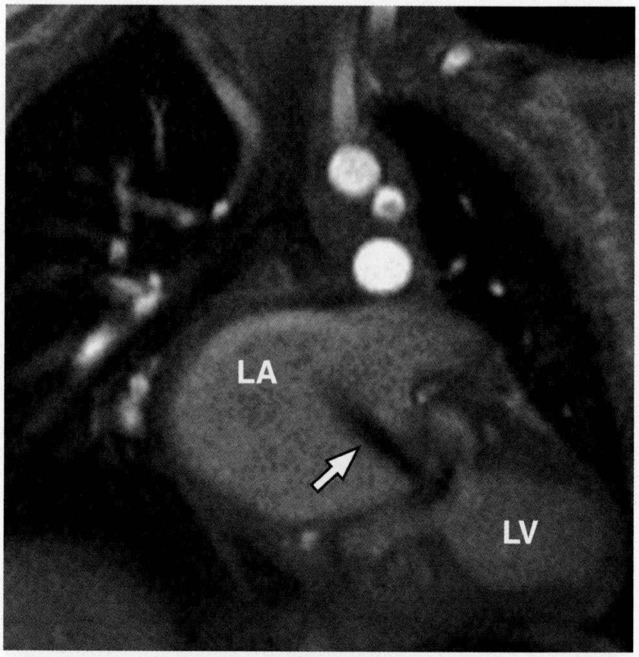

FIGURE 9.17 **Mitral regurgitation.** Two-chamber plane magnitude phase-contrast magnetic resonance image demonstrates mitral valve regurgitation jet (*arrow*) into an enlarged left atrium (*LA*). *LV*, left ventricle.

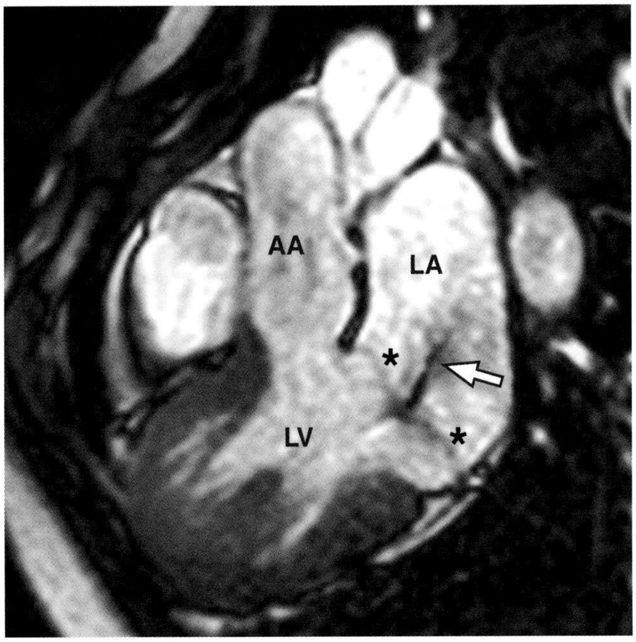

FIGURE 9.18 **Mitral valve prolapse.** Bright blood magnetic resonance image in left ventricular outflow tract plane shows mitral valve leaflets (*asterisks*) prolapsing into the left atrium (*LA*) with a prominent regurgitant jet (*arrow*). *AA*, ascending aorta; *LV*, left ventricle.

A cleft in the mitral valve can usually be surgically repaired either primarily or with a patch. Occasionally, annular plication is used in severe mitral valve prolapse with redundant leaflets. Mitral valve replacement is occasionally necessary in pediatric patients with severe mitral regurgitation or those who have failed more conservative surgical measures.

Tricuspid Stenosis

Congenital tricuspid stenosis is usually associated with other anomalies of the right heart including right ventricular hypoplasia and right ventricular outflow tract (RVOT) obstruction/pulmonary atresia (Fig. 9.19). Isolated tricuspid stenosis is extremely rare. Tricuspid stenosis is similar to tricuspid atresia clinically, on imaging, and surgically.[7]

Tricuspid Regurgitation

Primary tricuspid valve dysplasia resulting in tricuspid regurgitation is most common in the setting of Ebstein anomaly and TGA. However, secondary tricuspid regurgitation may be seen in any congenital or acquired cardiac disease that leads to right ventricular volume overload, arising from secondary tricuspid annular distortion, and dilatation.[7] Clinically, affected pediatric patients present with variable signs of right heart failure depending on the degree of underlying regurgitation.

Chest radiography may show right heart prominence related to right atrial enlargement. Cardiac MRI and CT are primarily used to identify the secondary causes of tricuspid regurgitation leading to right ventricular dysfunction (Fig. 9.20).

Ebstein Anomaly

Ebstein anomaly is a relatively rare and isolated anomaly of the tricuspid valve in which there is displacement of the septal and posterior tricuspid valve leaflets beyond the tricuspid annulus into the RV[21,22] (Fig. 9.21). The portion of the RV between the tricuspid valve annulus and the displaced leaflets forms an "atrialized" portion of the right ventricular chamber (Fig. 9.22). The tricuspid valve is usually markedly dysplastic and regurgitant. In most cases, there is also an ASD or patent foramen ovale.[21,22]

The majority of affected pediatric patients present with cyanosis. Cyanosis is worst in the neonatal period where the functionally small RV may not be able to generate sufficient pressures to overcome the high pulmonary vascular resistance present after birth. After the pulmonary vascular resistance drops, typically around the 6th week, the cyanosis typically resolves only to reappear in the adolescent period, thought to be due to worsening tricuspid regurgitation.[21]

Chest radiography classically demonstrates a moderately to severely enlarged right heart with diminished pulmonary

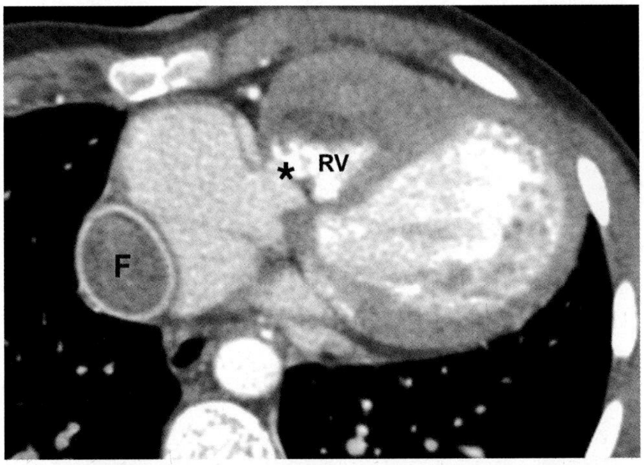

FIGURE 9.19 **Tricuspid stenosis.** Axial enhanced CT image shows thickened tricuspid valve with narrowed valve annulus (*asterisk*) and hypoplastic right ventricle (*RV*). Also noted is an extracardiac Fontan (*F*) shunt.

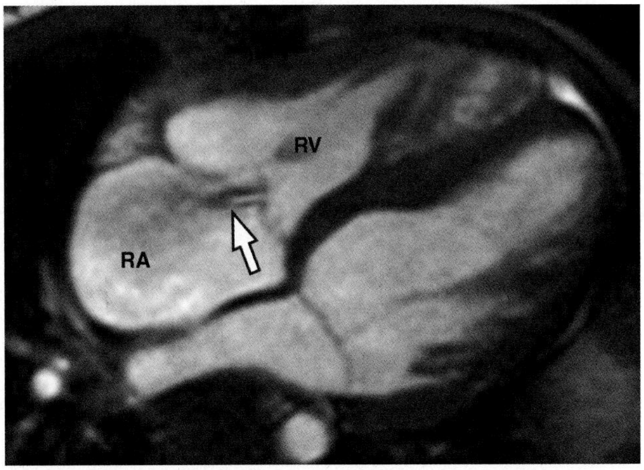

FIGURE 9.20 **Tricuspid regurgitation.** Axial bright blood magnetic resonance image in four-chamber plane shows tricuspid regurgitant jet (*arrow*) and enlarged right atrium (*RA*). *RV*, right ventricle.

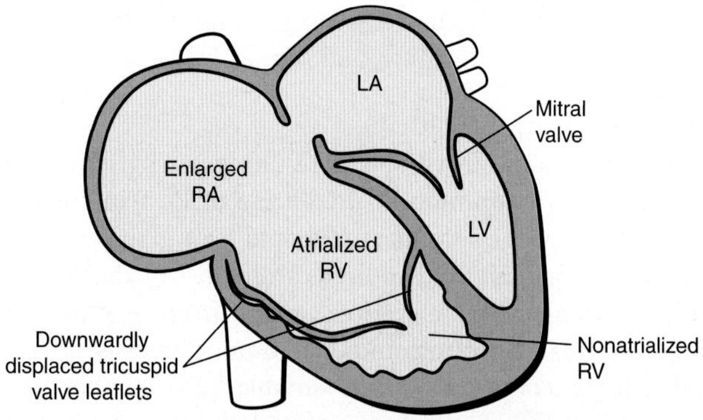

FIGURE 9.21 **Diagram of the anatomy of Ebstein anomaly.** The tricuspid valve is downwardly displaced and adherent to the interventricular septum. Part of the right ventricle is "atrialized," being located superior to the tricuspid valve. *LA*, left atrium; *LV*, left ventricle; *RA*, right atrium; *RV*, right ventricle.

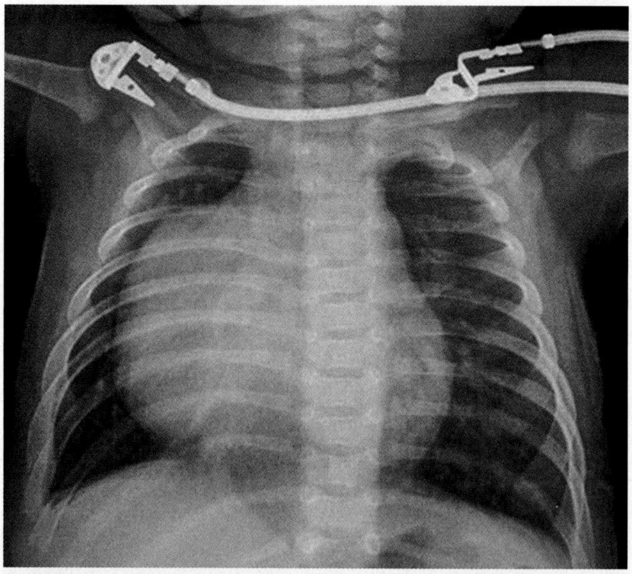

FIGURE 9.23 **Ebstein anomaly.** Frontal chest radiograph demonstrates enlarged right cardiac margin.

vascularity[1,22] (Fig. 9.23). Echo is used for initial diagnosis. However, MRI is playing an increasing role in the presurgical and postrepair assessment of right ventricular volumes, tricuspid valve morphology/regurgitation, and associated atrial or ventricular shunts.

Surgical repair involves tricuspid valve plication, annuloplasty, or tricuspid valve replacement. In the neonatal stage, if cyanosis is severe, a palliative modified Blalock-Taussig (BT) shunt maybe required to supplement pulmonary arterial blood supply.[22]

Complex Univentricular Connections

Complex univentricular connections are congenital malformations that result in the atrioventricular valvar unit emptying into one ventricular chamber. These entities include HLHS, tricuspid atresia, double inlet LV, and unbalanced AVSDs. In these cases, the second ventricular chamber that is not supplied by an AVV is hypoplastic or atretic. The AVV unit may be composed of one common AVV, a normal-appearing mitral and tricuspid valve, or either a mitral or tricuspid valve. If present, the hypoplastic second ventricular chamber that is not supplied by an AVV is connected to the main ventricle by a VSD.

Hypoplastic Left Heart Syndrome

HLHS is the most common single ventricle anomaly. HLHS has a series of congenitally small left-sided structures including a stenosed/atretic mitral valve, small LV, stenosed/

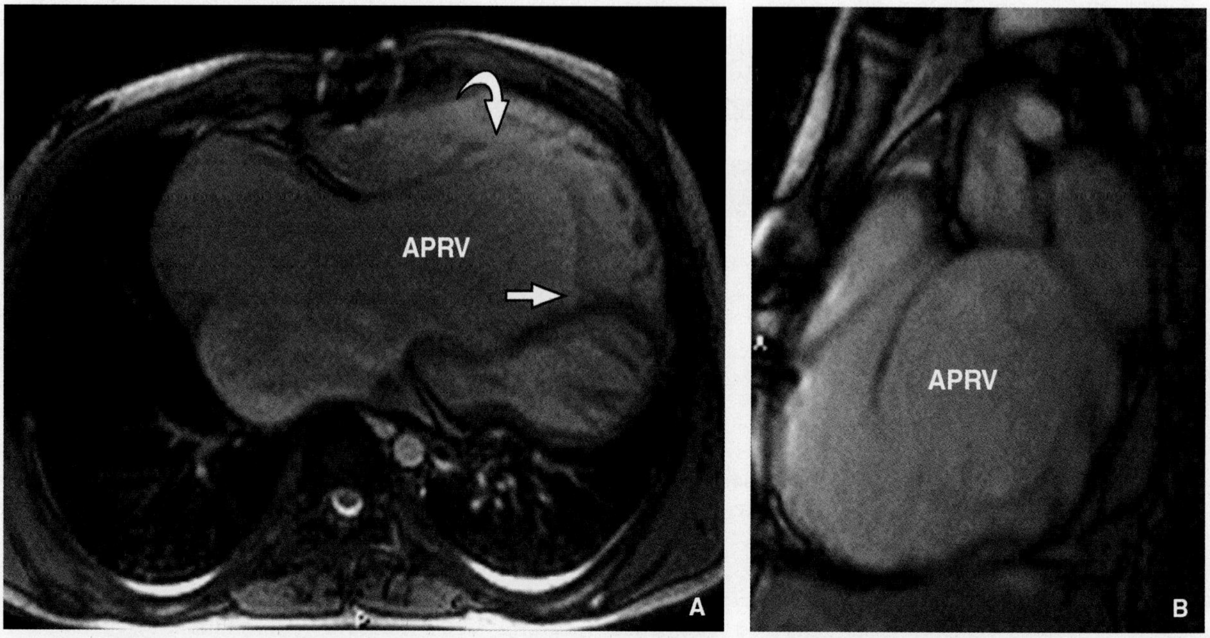

FIGURE 9.22 **Ebstein anomaly.** Bright blood magnetic resonance images in a four-chamber plane **(A)** and left ventricular outflow tract plane **(B)** show downward displacement of the attachment of the septal leaflet (*straight arrow*). The anterior leaflet (*curved arrow*) is large and "sail-like" resulting in an atrialized portion of the right ventricle (*APRV*).

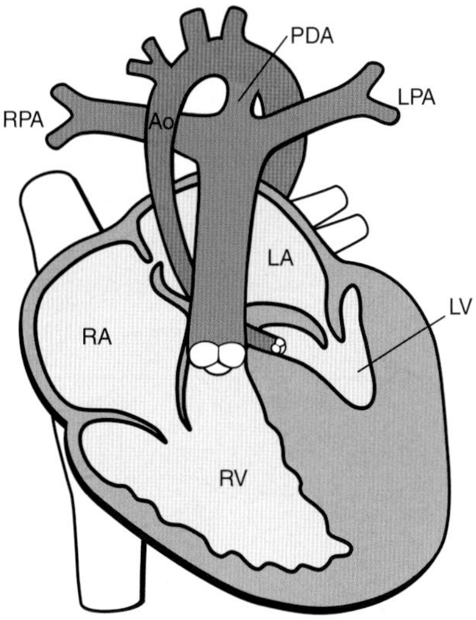

FIGURE 9.24 **Diagram of hypoplastic left heart associated with aortic atresia.** The left ventricle (*LV*) is hypoplastic and hypertrophied. The ascending aorta (*Ao*) is very hypoplastic. *LA*, left atrium; *LPA*, left pulmonary artery; *RA*, right atrium; *RPA*, right pulmonary artery; *RV*, right ventricle.

atretic aortic valve, small ascending aorta, and tubular hypoplasia of the aortic arch and aortic coarctation (Figs. 9.24 and 9.25).[23] If there is severe aortic valve stenosis/atresia, then the ascending aorta and aortic arch may demonstrate retrograde filling from the ductus arteriosus, rather than anterograde flow through the aortic valve. In this situation, the coronary arteries also rely on retrograde flow leading to chronic myocardial hypoperfusion. Most of the oxygenated pulmonary venous blood crosses through an ASD into the pulmonary artery via the right heart and reaches the systemic arterial circulation through the ductus arteriosus.[23,24] The descending aorta is usually normal caliber because of the presence of an enlarged ductus arteriosus. Clinical presentation is during the first few weeks of life coinciding with the closure of the ductus arteriosus. Manifestations vary depending on the degree of left-sided obstruction and include failure to thrive, hypoperfused extremities, cardiac failure, and metabolic acidosis.[7,23]

On chest radiography, the cardiac size can be normal or increased and there is reduced size of the aortic knuckle (Fig. 9.26). Additionally, there is usually pulmonary vascular congestion that is increased in the presence of a restrictive ASD. Echo is used to clearly delineate the intracardiac anatomy in the prerepair setting of HLHS. Once diagnosed, affected infants usually undergo immediate palliative surgery without additional imaging.

Cardiac MRI has a limited role in the preoperative assessment of HLHS. However, it can provide useful information in pediatric patients with less severe forms of left-sided obstruction and larger LVs who may benefit from a biventricular type of cardiac repair rather than a univentricular type of palliation.[25] In these instances, cardiac MRI may be used to estimate the left ventricular end diastolic volume (LVEDV) and screen for the presence of endocardial fibroelastosis, which is used as a predictor of potential outcome. Predictors of a failed biventricular repair include a small LV (LVEDVs indexed to body surface area of <15 to 20 mL/m^2), large VSD with right-to-left systolic shunting, severe mitral annular hypoplasia, and a dysplastic aortic valve.[25] Other indications for CTA or MRA in pediatric patients with HLHS include aortic arch assessment, in order to assess for aortic coarctation and tubular arch hypoplasia.

Biventricular repair is reserved for a subset of children with the mildest forms of HLHS and least aortic and mitral valvar stenosis.[25] Biventricular repair involves reconstruction of the ascending aorta with the MPA, a RV-PA conduit, and closure of the atrial and ventricular septal defects.

In the majority of patients with HLHS, the LV is too small to function as the systemic ventricle. Therefore, a staged single

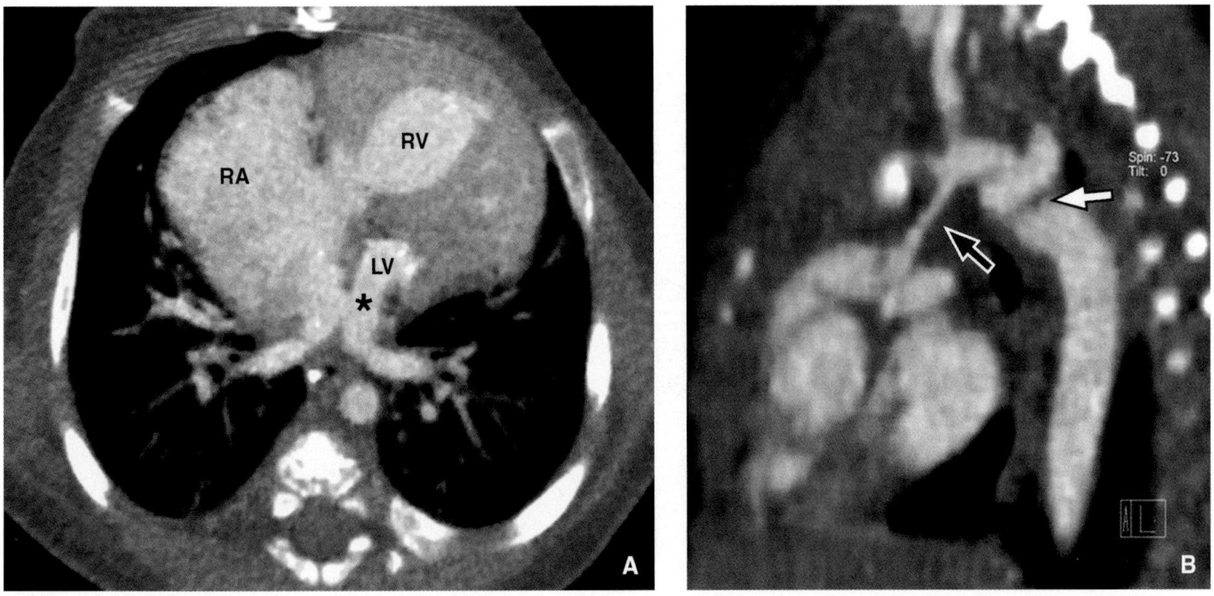

FIGURE 9.25 **Hypoplastic left heart syndrome. A:** Axial enhanced CT image shows mitral valve annular stenosis (*asterisk*) and hypoplastic left ventricle (*LV*). *RA*, right atrium; *RV*, right ventricle. **B:** Sagittal reformatted enhanced CT image demonstrates tubular hypoplasia of ascending aorta (*black arrow*) and coarctation (*white arrow*) at aortic isthmus.

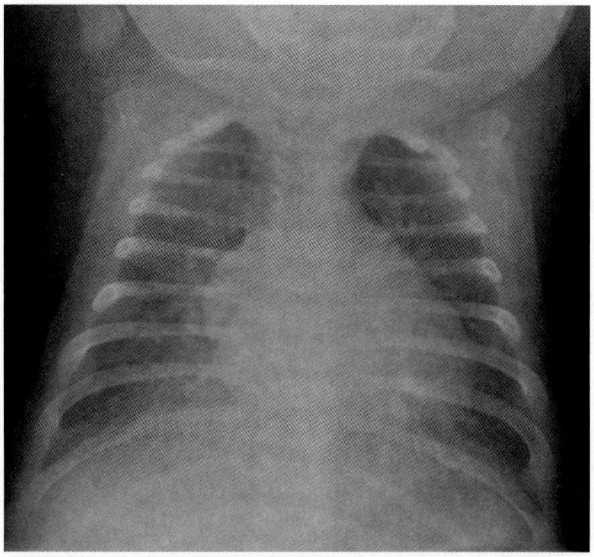

FIGURE 9.26 **Hypoplastic left heart syndrome.** Frontal chest radiograph in a 1-day-old girl shows increased pulmonary vascularity and cardiomegaly. Aortic knuckle is not clearly visualized.

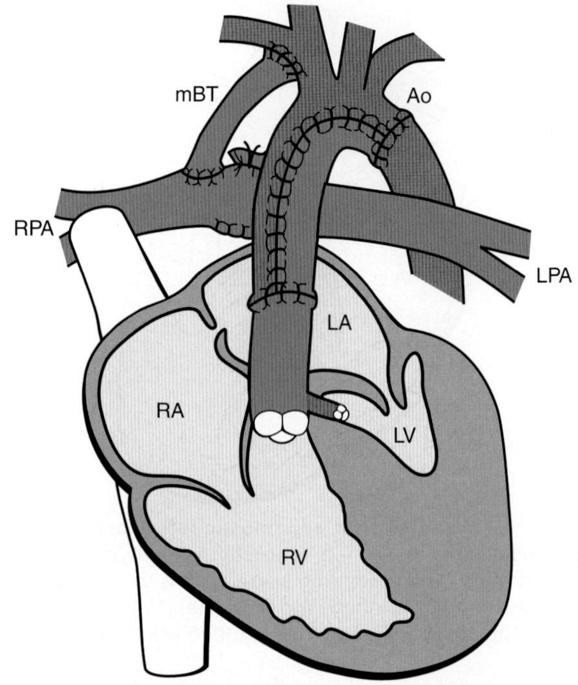

FIGURE 9.27 **Diagram of the Norwood stage 1 operation.** The pulmonary artery has been transected at its bifurcation and the distal end oversewn. Pulmonary blood flow is provided by a modified Blalock-Taussig shunt (mBT shunt). The aortic arch is augmented with a patch and connected to the proximal main pulmonary artery. An atrial septectomy is also performed so that pulmonary venous blood can reach the right atrium and then right ventricle without obstruction. *LA*, left atrium; *LPA*, left pulmonary artery; *LV*, left ventricle; *RA*, right atrium; *RPA*, right pulmonary artery; *RV*, right ventricle.

ventricle palliation is performed,[23,24] which results in the RV functioning as the systemic ventricle. This staged complex surgical procedure is performed in three stages, known as the Norwood I, the Glenn shunt (occasionally referred to as superior cavopulmonary anastomosis/Norwood II), and the Fontan shunt (occasionally referred to as Norwood III/total cavopulmonary anastomosis) procedure.[23,24]

The first stage, known as the Norwood I procedure, is performed immediately after birth (Figs. 9.27 and 9.28; Table 9.1).

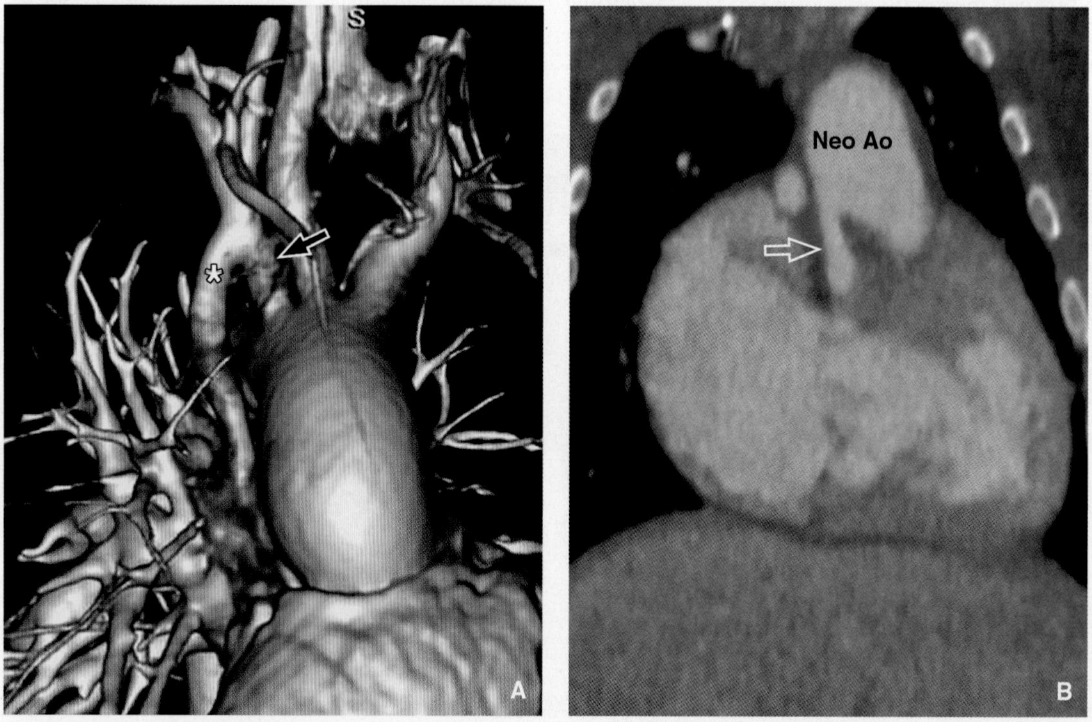

FIGURE 9.28 **Norwood procedure. A:** Three-dimensional volume-rendered CT image **(A)** shows stage 1/modified Blalock-Taussig shunt (*asterisk*) connecting right subclavian artery (*arrow*) to right pulmonary artery. **B:** Coronal reformatted enhanced CT image demonstrates the hypoplastic ascending aorta (*arrow*), which has been anastomosed to the main pulmonary artery using a Damus Kaye Stansel anastomosis creating the neoaorta (*Neo Ao*).

TABLE 9.1 Simplified Description of Selected Named Surgical Procedures for Treatment of Congenital Cardiovascular Anomalies

Surgical procedure	Congenital heart anomalies	Description
Norwood I procedure	Hypoplastic left heart syndrome	First stage of three-stage palliation. Performed shortly after birth. Utilizes main pulmonary artery (MPA) to augment the hypoplastic ascending aorta. Modified Blalock-Taussig (BT) shunt or Sano shunt to augment pulmonary blood flow
Modified BT shunt **Sano shunt**	• Pulmonary atresia/severe pulmonary stenosis including tetralogy of Fallot • Hypoplastic left heart syndrome • Tricuspid atresia	• Modified BT shunt: shunt connecting the subclavian artery (generally right subclavian) to the pulmonary artery (generally right pulmonary artery [RPA]) • Sano shunt: shunt from right ventricle (RV) to branch pulmonary arteries
Glenn shunt	Single ventricle morphologies including hypoplastic left heart syndrome, tricuspid atresia, unbalanced atrioventricular (AV) canal defects	Second stage of single ventricle palliation performed at ~3–6 mo of age. Distal superior vena cava (SVC) resected from the right atrium and connected to the RPA (at same time, modified BT or Sano shunt is taken down)
Fontan shunt	Single ventricle morphologies including hypoplastic left heart syndrome, tricuspid atresia, unbalanced AV canal defects	Final stage of single ventricle palliation performed at 18 mo to 4 years of age. Inferior vena cava (IVC) resected from the right atrium and connected to the RPA (Glenn shunt remains in place) resulting in total cavopulmonary anastomosis
Tetralogy of Fallot repair	Tetralogy of Fallot	Closure of ventricular septal defect (VSD) and right ventricular outflow tract (RVOT) and pulmonary valve obstruction
Unifocalization procedure	Pulmonary atresia with major arteriopulmonary collateral arteries (MAPCAs)	MAPCAs are isolated from the aorta/systemic arterial supply and anastomosed to central branch pulmonary arteries
Jatene "arterial switch" procedure	D-transposition of the great arteries (D-TGA)	The aorta and MPA resected above the level of their valves and translocated to their correct anatomical location with coronary artery reimplantation. Performed shortly after birth
Mustard or Senning atrial switch	D-transposition of the great arteries (D-TGA)	Systemic venous return and pulmonary venous return baffled to the left and right atrium, respectively. Now replaced by the arterial switch procedure
Coronary artery unroofing	Anomalous origin of left coronary artery/right coronary artery from contralateral coronary sinus with intramural interarterial course	Anomalous ostium is elongated and the neo-ostium placed into the proper sinus by resecting the intervening aortic wall
Warden procedure	• Superior sinus venosus defect • Right upper lobe partial anomalous pulmonary venous return to SVC	The SVC is divided below the right upper lobe pulmonary vein (RULPV). The RULPV and inferior SVC are baffled to the left atrium with closure of the sinus venous defect, and the superior SVC is anastomosed to right atrial appendage
Ross procedure	Aortic stenosis	Aortic valve replacement using patients own pulmonary valve (autograft) and placement of a pulmonary valve homograft
Konno procedure	Aortic stenosis with left ventricular outflow tract obstruction	Aortic valve replacement and widening of left ventricular outflow tract using a patch
David procedure	Aortic root aneurysmal dilatation	Aortic valve sparing aortic root replacement
Rastelli procedure	• D-TGA/double outlet right ventricle with pulmonary atresia/stenosis and VSD	Routing of LV blood flow to the aorta through the VSD and placement of a valved conduit from RV to the pulmonary artery

Note: Intracardiac surgical shunts are referred to as baffles; extracardiac shunts are referred to as conduits.

This procedure sacrifices the MPA in order to refashion an ascending aorta capable of sustaining the systemic arterial supply. The MPA is resected and separated from the right and left pulmonary arteries. The MPA is then used to augment the hypoplastic ascending aorta and proximal arch (the Damus-Kaye-Stansel maneuver). As the MPA has been resected, pulmonary arterial supply has to be reestablished. This can be accomplished using either a modified BT shunt from the right subclavian artery to the right pulmonary artery (RPA) (Fig. 9.28) or modified Sano shunt (RV) to confluence of branch pulmonary arteries (Fig. 9.29).[23,24]

The second stage of repair is the bidirectional Glenn shunt, which is usually performed at 6 to 9 months of life. It involves anastomosing the SVC to the pulmonary artery and taking down the modified BT/Sano shunt (Figs. 9.30 and 9.31). Following the Glenn shunt, all the venous blood from the head and arms returns directly to the branch pulmonary arteries without going into the heart.

The Fontan shunt is the final surgical stage in a single ventricle palliation. It is usually performed between 18 months and 4 years of age and involves connecting the IVC to the undersurface of the RPA. The Glenn shunt is left in place, so that after the Fontan procedure, all the SVC and IVC blood

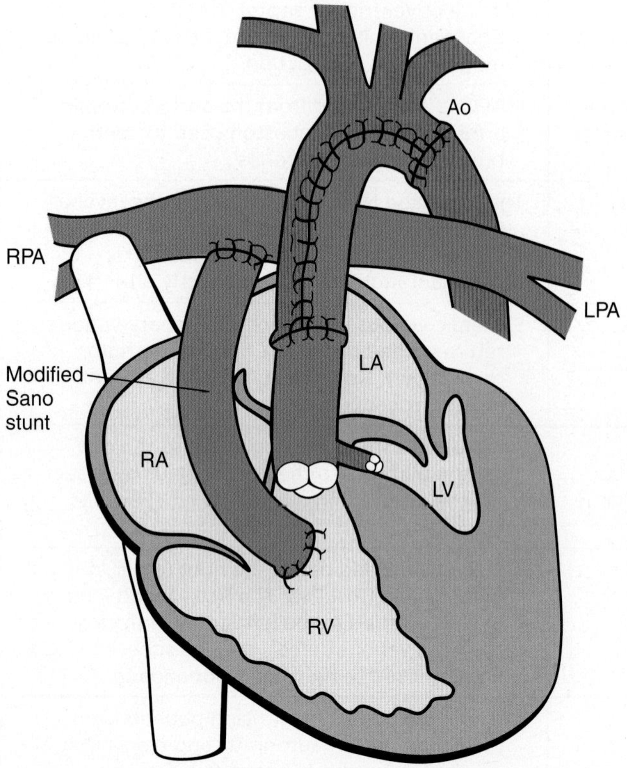

FIGURE 9.29 **Diagram of the Sano modification for stage 1 palliation of hypoplastic left heart syndrome.** A Gore-Tex tube graft connects the right ventricle and pulmonary arteries, provides pulmonary blood flow, and replaces the modified Blalock-Taussig shunt used in the Norwood stage 1 procedure. The Sano modification provides higher systemic diastolic pressures and presumably better coronary perfusion than the Norwood stage 1 procedure. *Ao*, aorta; *LA*, left atrium; *LPA*, left pulmonary artery; *LV*, left ventricle; *RA*, right atrium; *RPA*, right pulmonary artery; *RV*, right ventricle.

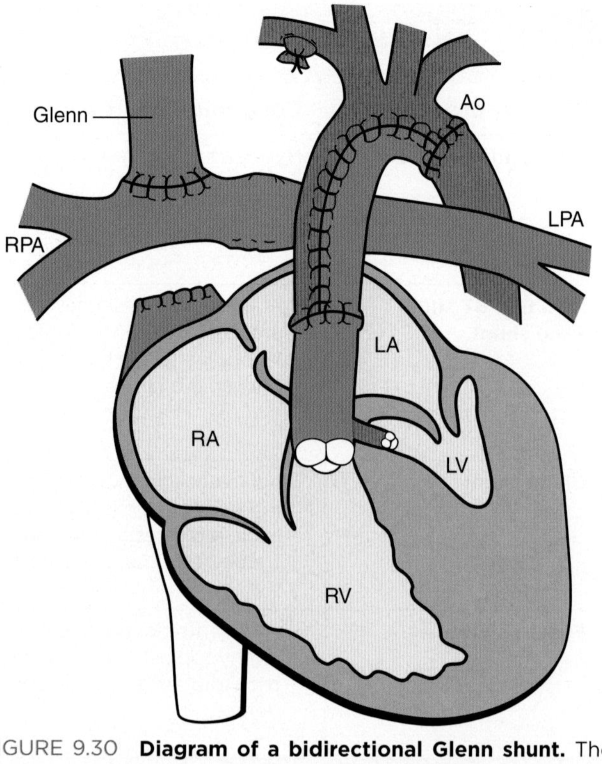

FIGURE 9.30 **Diagram of a bidirectional Glenn shunt.** The SVC is removed from the heart and connected end to side to the right pulmonary artery (*RPA*), which is in continuity with the left pulmonary artery (*LPA*). The main pulmonary artery has been separated from the heart and oversewn. *Ao*, aorta; *Glenn*, Glenn shunt; *LA*, left atrium; *LV*, left ventricle; *RA*, right atrium; *RV*, right ventricle.

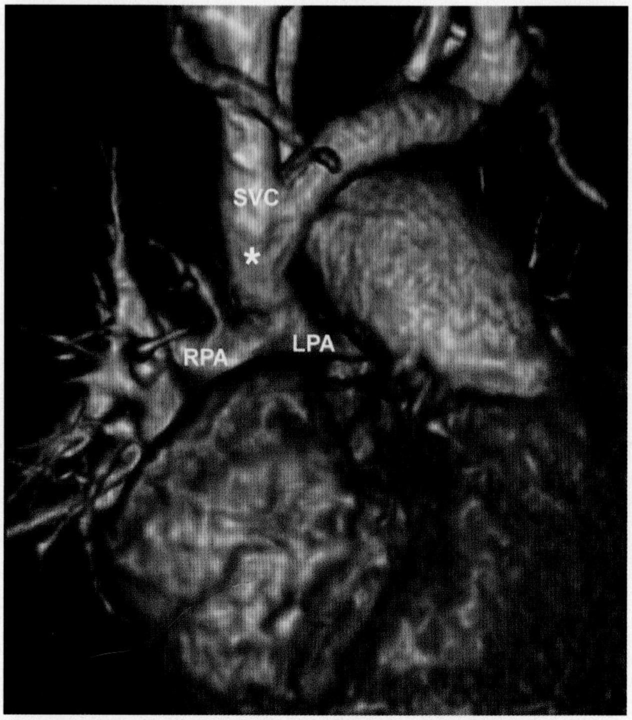

FIGURE 9.31 **Bidirectional Glenn procedure.** Three-dimensional volume-rendered CT image shows stage II/Glenn shunt. Glenn shunt (*asterisk*) is located between superior vena cava (*SVC*) and right pulmonary artery (*RPA*). *LPA*, left pulmonary artery.

flow returns directly to the pulmonary arteries without going through the heart (total cavopulmonary anastomosis) (Fig. 9.32). There are two types of Fontan shunts currently performed: the lateral tunnel and the extracardiac conduit (Fig. 9.33). In the lateral tunnel Fontan conduit, an intra-atrial baffle is placed in the lateral part of the right atrium connecting the IVC with the undersurface of the RPA. In the extracardiac Fontan conduit, the IVC is transected at the inferior cavoatrial junction. Then, a conduit lying outside the heart is interposed between the IVC and the inferior surface of the RPA.[23,24]

Previously, cardiac catheterization was considered the standard of care to assess suitability of the pulmonary circulation, systemic vessels, and single ventricle for subsequent Glenn and Fontan surgeries. However, in recent years, cardiac MRI has assumed a central role in pre-Glenn and pre-Fontan assessment. Cardiac MRI has been shown to noninvasively and successfully evaluate function of the single ventricle, the presence of ventricular myocardial and endocardial fibrosis, the size of pulmonary arteries, and the suitability of systemic vasculature. Such information is valuable when attempting to select pediatric patients who are unlikely to require percutaneous interventions or to need hemodynamic measurements prior to palliation.[26,27]

After the Fontan procedure, there is usually systemic venous stasis, which is associated with an increased risk of thromboembolism and predisposes to the formation of extensive venous collateral vessels. Aortopulmonary

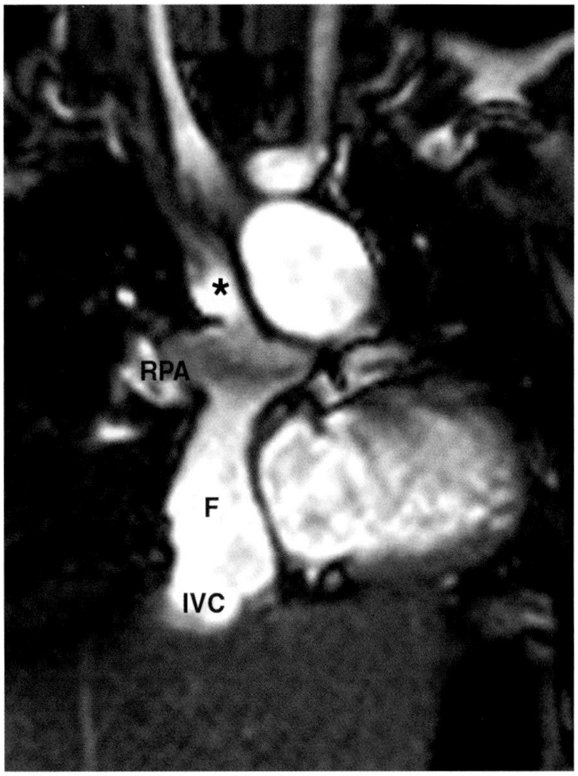

FIGURE 9.32 **Fontan procedure.** Coronal oblique bright blood magnetic resonance image demonstrates Fontan (*F*) shunt between inferior vena cava (*IVC*) and right pulmonary artery (*RPA*) with Glenn shunt (*asterisk*) as previously placed.

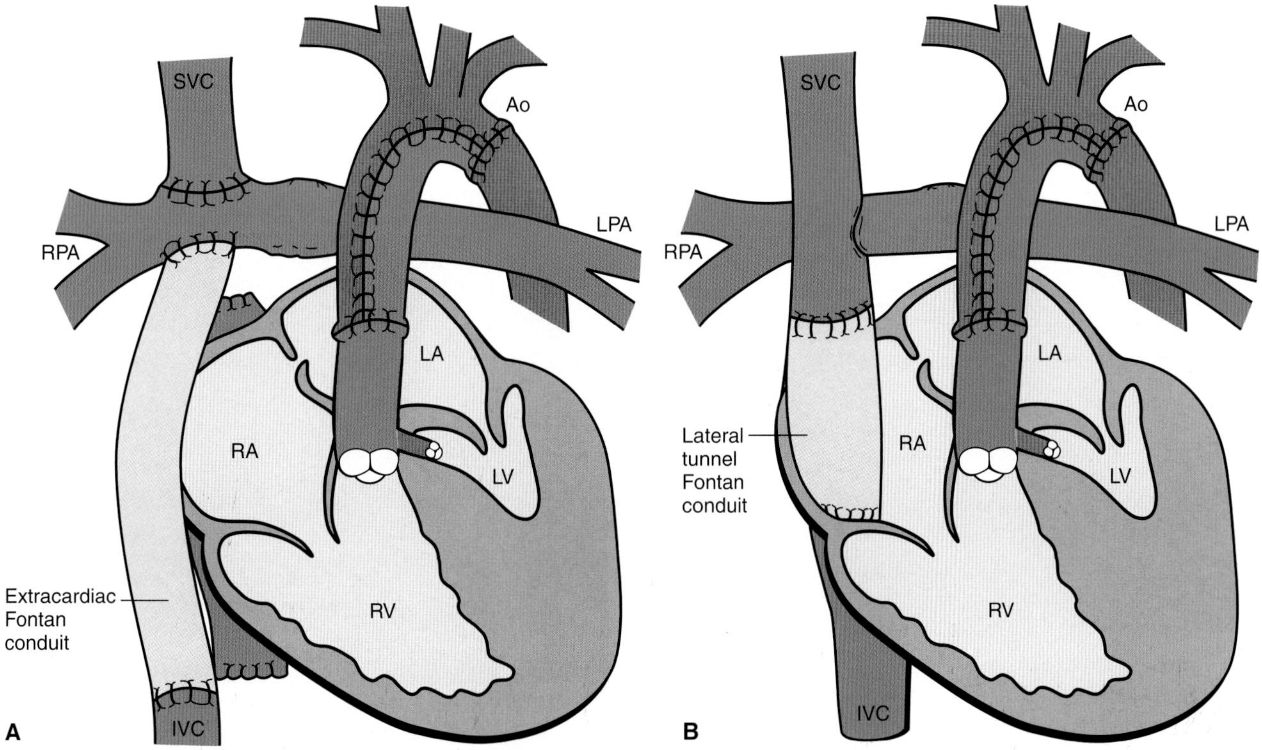

FIGURE 9.33 **Diagram of an extracardiac Fontan (left) and a lateral tunnel Fontan (right) procedure.** The inferior vena cava (*IVC*) and right pulmonary artery (*RPA*) are connected by placement of **(A)** an extracardiac conduit, and **(B)** a lateral tunnel conduit within the right atrium. In each, a previous bidirectional Glenn shunt (Figure 9.30) has been performed (end-to-side anastomosis of the superior vena vena [*SVC*] with the RPA). *Ao*, aorta; *LA*, left atrium; *LPA*, left pulmonary artery; *LV*, left ventricle; *RA*, right atrium; *RV*, right ventricle.

collateral vessels may also form, which in addition to the venous collaterals, increase preload and risk of dysfunction on the single ventricle. The post-Fontan cardiac MRI assessment involves evaluation of ventricular function as well as systemic veins, pulmonary veins, and pulmonary arteries for evidence of obstruction or thrombosis. In addition, screening for venovenous or aortopulmonary collateral vessels should be performed.[28]

Tricuspid Atresia

Diseases of the tricuspid valve are relatively rare. Tricuspid atresia is complete absence of the normal communication between the right atrium and RV. There is always a patent foramen ovale or ASD that allows for necessary right-to-left shunting at the atrial level. The RV is often hypoplastic, and there is usually a VSD to allow communication between the systemic and pulmonary circulations. There is often associated pulmonary stenosis or atresia, and the great arteries may be transposed or malposed.[29,30]

Clinically, the majority of affected pediatric patients present with cyanosis, heart failure, and a loud murmur shortly after birth.[30] Chest radiography may be normal without pulmonary obstruction, but in the setting of obstruction to pulmonary artery blood flow, cardiomegaly with an enlarged right heart border (indicating right atrial enlargement) usually develops and the pulmonary vascularity is reduced.

Echo is usually the primary method of diagnosis. On chest radiography (Fig. 9.34), a normal heart size, decreased pulmonary vascularity, and a concave MPA segment are usually seen. However, cardiomegaly with either normal or increased pulmonary vascularity may be seen in the setting of a concomitant large VSD. On CTA or cardiac MRI, a thickened atretic tricuspid valve or increased fat deposition in the right AV groove with severe right ventricular hypoplasia is usually present. CTA and cardiac MRI are usually reserved for evaluation of patients before and after surgical palliation.

Surgical treatment involves the establishment of pulmonary artery blood supply, which in the neonatal period is achieved by a modified BT shunt (right subclavian artery to RPA). Subsequently, during infancy after the pulmonary vascular resistance drops, the BT shunt is taken down, and a Glenn shunt/superior cavopulmonary anastomosis (SVC to RPA) is performed. Similar to HLHS, the Fontan shunt/total cavopulmonary anastomosis is performed at 18 months to 4 years of age, after which all the SVC and IVC blood returns directly to the pulmonary arteries rather than to the heart.[30]

Double Inlet Left Ventricle

Double inlet LV is a type of complex single ventricular connection in which there is a dominant LV, two AVVs, and a rudimentary right ventricular remnant that communicates with the LV via a small VSD (known as a bulboventricular foramen).[31] Patients with this condition usually have atrial and visceral situs solitus but the ventricular looping may be anomalous. Both AVVs empty into the LV (Fig. 9.35). The great arteries are usually malposed so the left ventricular chamber gives rise to the pulmonary artery and the right ventricular chamber gives rise to the aorta, thereby placing these patients at risk of subaortic stenosis, HLHS, interrupted

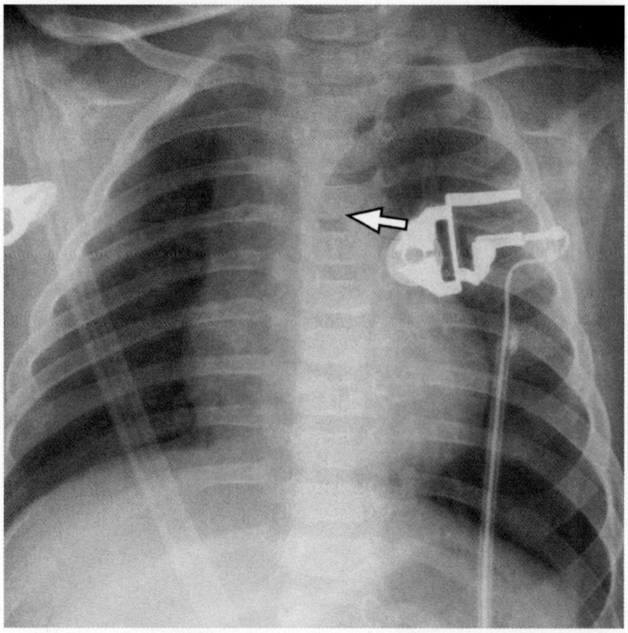

FIGURE 9.34 **Tricuspid atresia.** Frontal chest radiograph in cyanotic infant shows mildly decreased pulmonary vascularity, normal heart size, and concavity (*arrow*) in the region of main pulmonary artery.

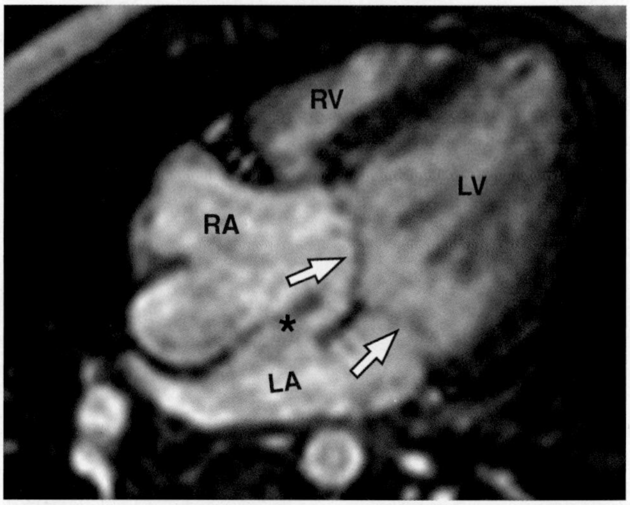

FIGURE 9.35 **Double inlet left ventricle.** Axial bright blood magnetic resonance image in four-chamber plane shows both atrioventricular valves (*arrows*) emptying into the left ventricular chamber (*LV*) with atretic right ventricle (*RV*). The right atrium (*RA*) and left atrium (*LA*) are also connected with ostium secundum atrial septal defect (*).

aortic arch (IAA), and aortic coarctation. Pulmonary outflow tract obstruction may also occur with either concordant or discordant ventriculoarterial connections.[31] Presentation is usually in the neonatal period with cyanosis and congestive heart failure.

Chest radiography usually demonstrates cardiomegaly, and in patients with subaortic stenosis, the pulmonary vascularity is increased. The intracardiac anatomy is usually adequately depicted with echo. If required, cardiac MRI can demonstrate both AVVs emptying into a dominant ventricular chamber with a left ventricular morphology. The rudimentary chamber may be identified as a morphologic RV by the presence of the moderator band. Cardiac MRI can also demonstrate the outflow tract relationships, the presence of outflow tract stenosis, the size of the bulboventricular foramen, and great artery anatomy. CTA may be indicated to better delineate the aortic arch anomalies in patients with aortic coarctation/interruption.

Patients with double inlet LV usually undergo a single ventricle staged surgical palliation. In patients with severe subaortic stenosis and hypoplastic aorta, a Norwood type operation is performed shortly after birth (similar to HLHS), followed by the Glenn and Fontan shunts.[31]

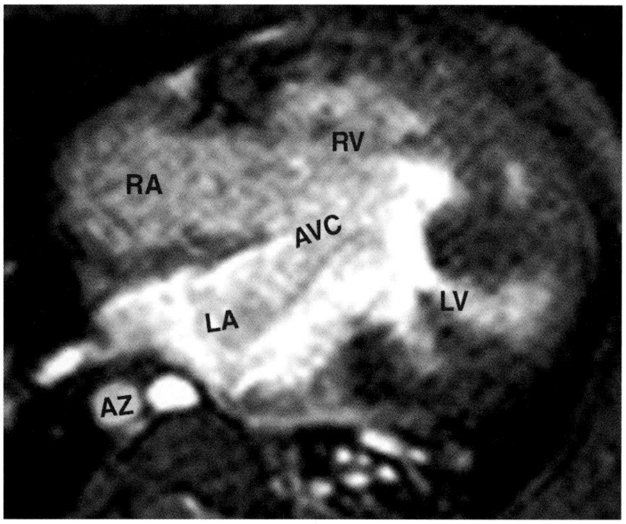

FIGURE 9.36 **Unbalanced atrioventricular canal defect in a 2-month-old girl with heterotaxy.** Bright blood magnetic resonance image in four-chamber plane shows large atrioventricular canal defect (*AVC*) positioned over the right ventricle (*RV*) (i.e., right-sided dominance) resulting in hypoplastic left ventricle (*LV*). Also noted is azygos continuation (*AZ*) of IVC. *LA*, left atrium; *RA*, right atrium.

Unbalanced Atrioventricular Septal Defects

AVSDs result from failure of fusion of the endocardial cushions leading to a deficient AV septum and a common AVV rather than separate openings and attachments for the mitral and tricuspid valves.[32] If this common AVV is positioned so that one ventricle receives the larger proportion of AV inflow and the other ventricle is hypoplastic, an unbalanced AVSD results. Most commonly, there is a dominant RV and hypoplastic LV with similar physiology to HLHS (Fig. 9.36).[32,33] The corollary anomaly with a dominant LV and right ventricular hypoplasia results in a physiology similar to tricuspid atresia. Unbalanced AV canal defects are seen in association with Down syndrome and heterotaxy as well as isolated anomalies.[32,33] Clinically affected pediatric patients usually present with cyanosis, murmur, and cardiac failure. Metabolic acidosis and peripheral ischemia may be present in the setting of HLHS-like morphology.[33,34]

Chest radiography demonstrates cardiomegaly, pulmonary edema, and situs anomalies in the setting of heterotaxy. Echo is used for the initial diagnosis with MRI reserved for borderline cases with less severe forms of left-sided obstruction and larger LVs that potentially could support a biventricular type cardiac repair. In these instances, cardiac MRI can accurately measure the LVEDV, screen for the presence of endocardial fibroelastosis, and assess for left ventricular outflow tract obstruction, which may help predict suitability for a biventricular repair.[25] In cases of heterotaxy, CTA or MRA can accurately depict the complex systemic and pulmonary venous anomalies. Additionally, CTA or MRI can also assess the upper abdomen for concomitant splenic and GI rotation anomalies.

The surgical approach depends on the morphology of the unbalanced defect. It may involve a biventricular repair in patients with milder forms and appropriate biventricular sizes, a three-stage palliation (Norwood, Glenn, Fontan) in patients with a HLHS-like morphology, or a modified BT shunt followed by Glenn and Fontan shunts in patients with a tricuspid atresia-like morphology.[34]

Conotruncal Anomalies

The conotruncal region of the heart comprises of the ventricular outflow tracts, the aortic and pulmonary valves, and the outlet (conal and membranous) portions of the interventricular septum. The embryologic precursors of this region are the distal bulbus cordis and truncus arteriosus. The term conotruncal anomalies encompasses TOF, pulmonary atresia with intact ventricular septum, transposition of great vessels, DORV, truncus arteriosus, and even IAA (IAA is discussed with the arch anomalies portion of this chapter). There is a high incidence of DiGeorge syndrome (chromosome 22q11.2 deletion) in patients with conotruncal anomalies.[35]

Tetralogy of Fallot

TOF arises from a single pathologic defect in the formation of the conus (infundibulum).[36,37] In TOF, the conus is abnormally superiorly and anteriorly displaced, narrowing the RVOT, which leads to right ventricular hypertrophy. An outlet type VSD results where the conus would have formed the superior part of the VSD, and the aorta overrides the VSD (Figs. 9.37 and 9.38). The RVOT narrowing results in a spectrum of pulmonary valve pathology ranging from mild dysplasia to

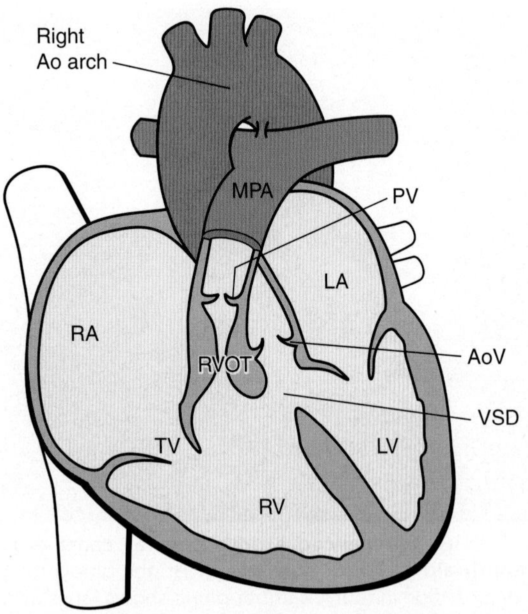

FIGURE 9.37 **Diagram of anatomy of tetralogy of Fallot with right ventricular outflow tract (*RVOT*) and pulmonary valvar stenosis.** The aortic valve (*AoV*) can be seen through the ventricular septal defect (*VSD*). There is RVOT stenosis in the subpulmonary valve region, hypoplastic pulmonary valve (*PV*), hypoplastic pulmonary arteries. A right aortic (*Ao*) arch is present in ~25% of patients. *LA*, left atrium; *LV*, left ventricle; *MPA*, main pulmonary artery; *RA*, right atrium; *RV*, right ventricle.

pulmonary atresia. Absence of the pulmonary valve may also occur in TOF, and this entity is discussed separately later in this chapter. The variable degree of RVOT/pulmonary valve stenosis results in variations in branch pulmonary artery anatomy. In most cases, the pulmonary arteries are normal or mildly diminished in size. However, with pulmonary valve atresia, the branch pulmonary artery anatomy may be very complex. The branch pulmonary arteries may be connected to each other (confluent) and solely supplied either by the ductus arteriosus or by major arteriopulmonary collaterals (MAPCAs).[38,39] Nonconfluent branch pulmonary arteries may be solely supplied by multiple MAPCAs. MAPCAs may also supply individual segments of the lung directly without going through the pulmonary arterial branches.

Clinical presentation depends on the degree of pulmonary stenosis. Patients with severe pulmonary stenosis present in the early neonatal period with cyanosis and failure to thrive. Those with less severe stenosis may develop cyanotic "spells" after periods of exertion. During these spells, children may squat, instinctively attempting to increase systemic vascular resistance in order to decrease right-to-left shunting across the VSD and increase pulmonary blood supply.[37] Eight to twenty-three percent of patients with TOF have DiGeorge syndrome.[35]

Common chest radiographic appearances of TOF (Fig. 9.39) include enlargement of the cardiac silhouette with elevation of the cardiac apex, resulting in a boot-shaped appearance (known as "coeur en sabot"), a right-sided aortic arch (20%), and diminished pulmonary vascularity (usually only presurgical repair).[36,37] In patients with pulmonary atresia, the MPA silhouette is absent and the peripheral pulmonary vascular markings may be increased in the presence of multiple large MAPCAs (Figs. 9.40 and 9.41).[38,39] The prerepair intracardiac anatomy of TOF is usually well established by echo. Prerepair CTA and MRA are reserved for those cases with pulmonary atresia when the complex branch pulmonary artery anatomy cannot be completely evaluated on echo. Depiction of the branch pulmonary artery anatomy, origin, and course of any MAPCAs is vital for preoperative planning of possible surgical repairs. CTA has the ability to evaluate the lung parenchyma, enabling visualization of the individual pulmonary segments and determining areas of over circulation (ground-glass attenuation) compared to regions of relative hypoperfusion (attenuated vessels, relative lucency). For assessing MAPCAs, MRA is somewhat limited by spatial resolution as only vessels that are larger than 0.5 mm are reliably seen. Other anomalies encountered less frequently in the preoperative CTA/cardiac MRI evaluation of TOF include

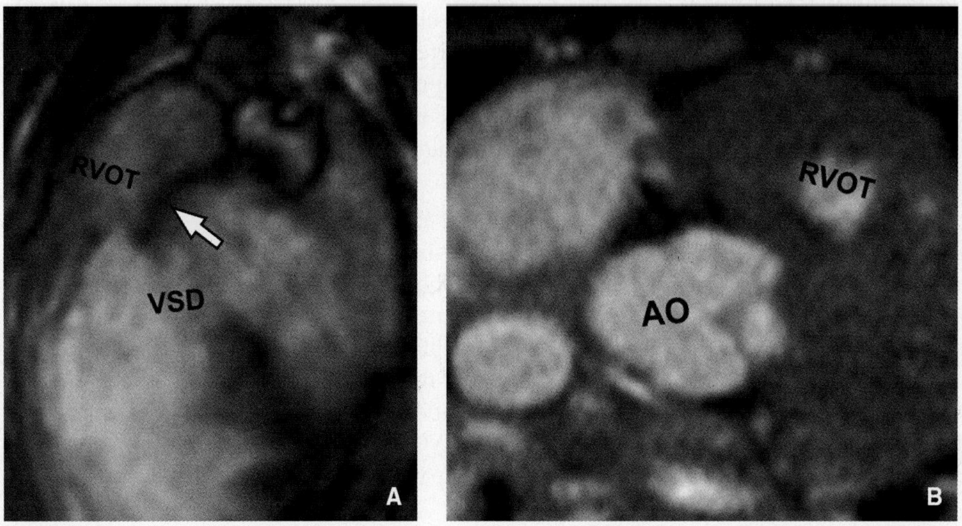

FIGURE 9.38 **Tetralogy of Fallot.** Bright blood magnetic resonance (MR) image **(A)** in right ventricular outflow tract (*RVOT*) plane demonstrates anterior malalignment of conus (*arrow*) resulting in narrowing of RVOT, outlet ventricular septal defect (*VSD*). Axial bright blood MR image **(B)** shows narrowed RVOT and overriding aorta (*AO*).

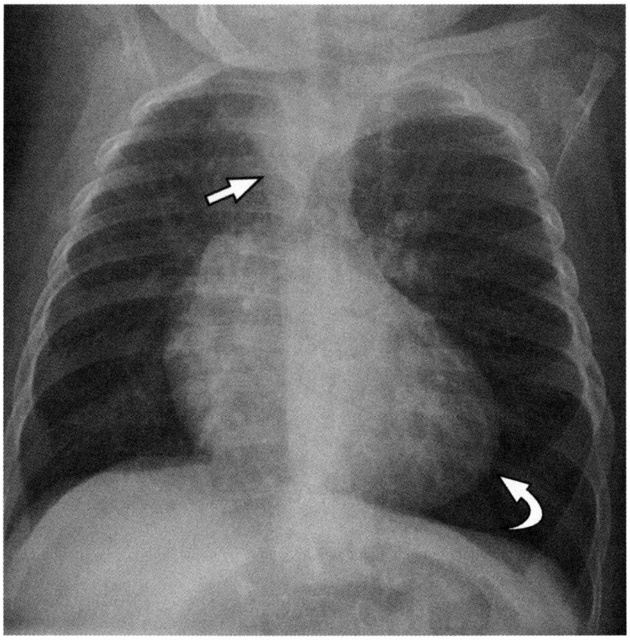

FIGURE 9.39 **Tetralogy of Fallot in a 2-day-old girl.** Frontal chest radiograph demonstrates cardiomegaly with elevated cardiac apex (*curved arrow*). Also noted is a right-sided aortic arch (*straight arrow*).

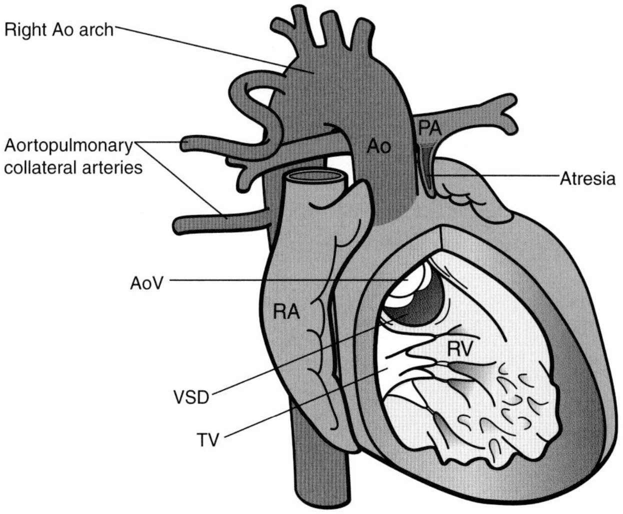

FIGURE 9.40 **Diagram of tetralogy of Fallot associated with pulmonary atresia in right ventricular view.** There is atresia of the right ventricular outflow tract (RVOT)/pulmonary valve and hypoplasia of the confluent branch pulmonary arteries (*PA*). The aortic valve (*AoV*) is visible through the ventricular septal defect (*VSD*). The tricuspid valve (*TV*) is normal. The proximal segments of two arteriopulmonary collateral arteries are shown. A right aortic (*Ao*) arch is present in ~25% of patients. *RA*, right atrium; *RV*, right ventricle.

anomalous coronary arteries, anomalous pulmonary venous return, and ASDs. However, in the majority of TOF cases, MRI is mainly a postrepair surveillance tool (see below).

Lillehei introduced the complete repair of TOF in 1954 and little has changed since its inception.[40] The VSD is closed with a patch. The hypertrophied muscles in the RVOT and variable portions of the stenotic pulmonary valve are resected, and the RVOT may be reconstructed by incorporating a transannular patch of pericardium or synthetic material. In severe forms of pulmonary stenosis, a homograft pulmonary valve, or a conduit containing a prosthetic valve, may be inserted between the RV and the pulmonary artery. The full repair of TOF is usually performed as a primary procedure in the first few months of life.[41]

However, in the setting of small branch pulmonary arteries, an initial modified BT shunt (graft from the right subclavian artery to the RPA) may be performed to allow pulmonary arterial growth in newborn patients prior to a full TOF repair. In TOF patients with pulmonary atresia, nonconfluent branch pulmonary arteries and MAPCAs, a unifocalization procedure may be performed in addition to reconstruction of the RVOT. In the unifocalization procedure, the MAPCAs are isolated from their systemic arterial supply and anastomosed with the branch pulmonary arteries.[39,42] Redundant MAPCAs may be ligated or occluded. Stenotic MAPCAs may need dilatation.[42]

Long-term results after TOF repair are good but almost all patients have some degree of pulmonary regurgitation postrepair. The long-term effects of pulmonary regurgitation

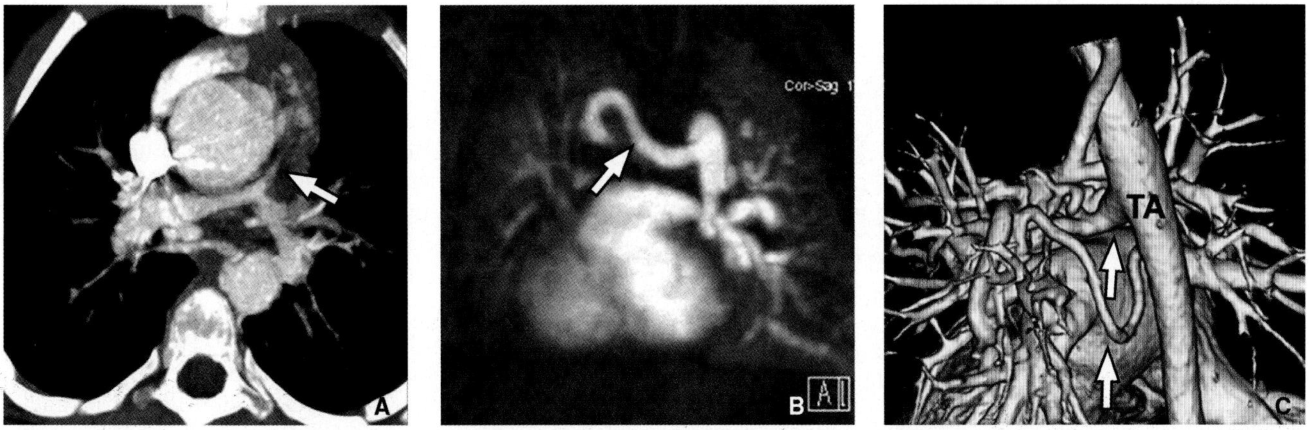

FIGURE 9.41 **Tetralogy of Fallot with pulmonary atresia and multiple large arteriopulmonary collateral arteries (MAPCAs).** Axial enhanced CT image **(A)** shows pulmonary atresia (*arrow*). Coronal magnetic resonance angiography image **(B)** demonstrates large aortopulmonary collateral artery (*arrow*) to right lung from descending thoracic aorta. Three-dimensional volume-rendered CT image **(C)** shows MAPCAs (*arrows*) arising from thoracic aorta (*TA*).

include right ventricular volume overload and decreased RV function.[36,41] Most patients eventually require a pulmonary valve repair or replacement at some point in order to decrease the volume overload on the RV. Cardiac MRI has been accepted as the gold standard for right ventricular volume and function evaluation and for assessment of pulmonary valvar regurgitant fraction providing an important data for the timing of pulmonary valve replacement.[38,43]

Tetralogy of Fallot with Absent Pulmonary Valve

TOF with absent pulmonary valve is a rare subtype of tetralogy. In this condition, an absence of mature pulmonary valvar tissue results in severe pulmonary regurgitation and aneurysmal enlargement of the branch pulmonary arteries (Fig. 9.42).[44] In addition to the right ventricular dilatation typically encountered in conventional TOF, the aneurysmally enlarged branch pulmonary arteries often cause severe narrowing of the left and right mainstem bronchi, resulting in severe respiratory symptoms.

Chest radiography demonstrates bilaterally markedly dilated proximal branch pulmonary arteries, relatively normally appearing peripheral pulmonary vascularity, and

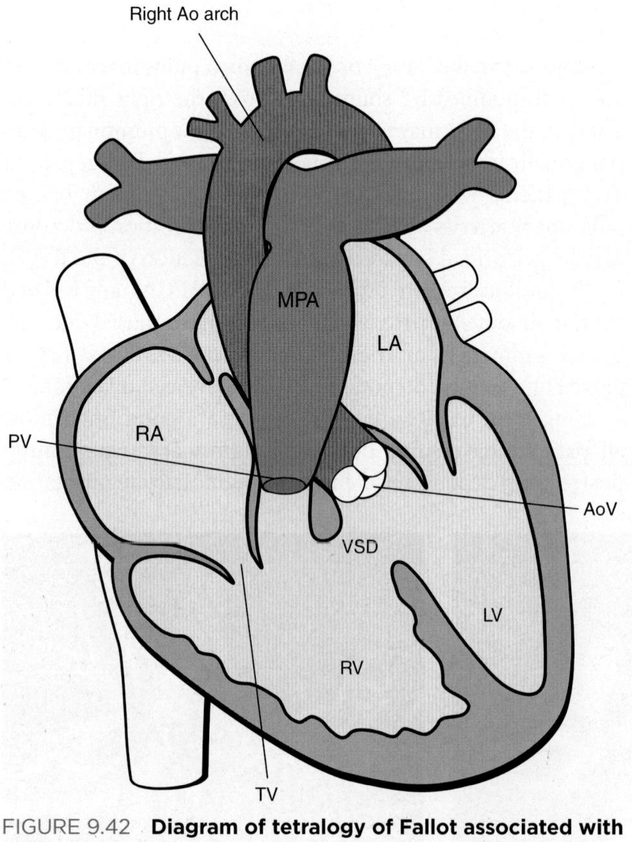

FIGURE 9.42 **Diagram of tetralogy of Fallot associated with absent pulmonary valve.** There is right ventricular outflow tract (RVOT) stenosis and severe pulmonary valve dysplasia/absence. The absent or markedly deficient pulmonary valve leaflets produce pulmonary regurgitation, which leads to the development of markedly dilated pulmonary arteries. The aortic valve (*AoV*) is visible through the ventricular septal defect (*VSD*). The tricuspid valve (*TV*) is normal. A right aortic (*Ao*) arch is present in ~25% of patients. *LA*, left atrium; *LV*, left ventricle; *MPA*, main pulmonary artery; *PV*, pulmonary valve; *RA*, right atrium; *RV*, right ventricle.

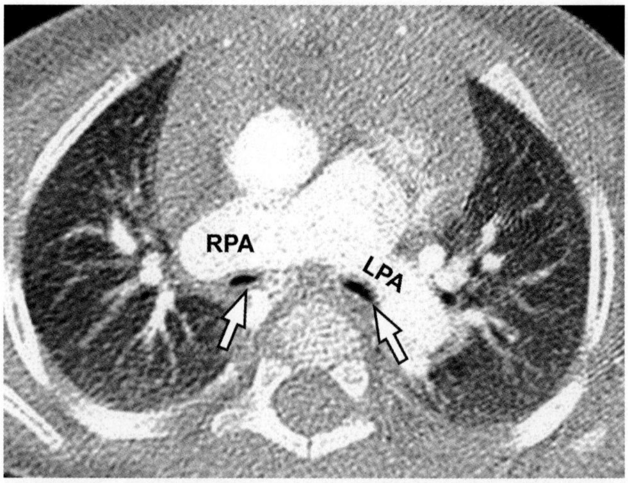

FIGURE 9.43 **Tetralogy of Fallot with absent pulmonary valve.** Axial lung window CT image shows compression (*arrows*) of the right and left main stem bronchi by dilated right pulmonary artery (*RPA*) and left pulmonary artery (*LPA*).

cardiomegaly with apical elevation resulting in the typical boot-shaped cardiac silhouette of TOF. A right aortic arch may be present. CTA can be used to evaluate the branch pulmonary artery size and assess the tracheobronchial tree for bronchial narrowing and associated air-trapping or lung collapse (Fig. 9.43). Cardiac MRI provides information regarding RV function and size, the degree of pulmonary regurgitation, and size of the branch pulmonary arteries. However, cardiac MRI is more limited in its ability to visualize narrowing of the bronchi, which is better appreciated with CT.

Surgical repair of TOF with absent pulmonary valve often involves pulmonary arterial plication or reduction in addition to RVOT reconstruction. However, affected pediatric patients often have intractable respiratory compromise.[44]

Pulmonary Atresia with Intact Ventricular Septum

Pulmonary atresia with intact ventricular septum results from complete obstruction to right ventricular outflow with varying degrees of underlying right ventricular and tricuspid valve hypoplasia. It has Ebstein-like features and there is often significant tricuspid regurgitation.[45] Because of underlying pulmonary atresia, there is an obligatory right-to-left shunt at the atrial level. Blood to the pulmonary arteries is completely dependent on the ductus arteriosus, and prostaglandin must be administered in order to prevent ductal closure.

In pediatric patients with pulmonary atresia and intact ventricular septum, there may be complex branch pulmonary artery anatomy. The branch pulmonary arteries are usually connected to each other (confluent) and supplied by a left-sided ductus arteriosus.[46] Nonconfluent branch pulmonary arteries are either supplied by bilateral ductus arteriosus or by major arteriopulmonary collateral vessels.

On chest radiography, the cardiac silhouette may be mildly enlarged and the pulmonary vascularity is reduced. Echo usually adequately delineates the intracardiac anatomy and presence of a ductal dependent pulmonary arterial circulation, with CTA and MRA reserved for those cases with unusual branch pulmonary artery anatomy, tortuous ductus arteriosus, or rarely MAPCAs.

Transposition of the Great Arteries

TGA by definition infers discordant ventriculoarterial connections such that the ascending aorta arises from the RV and the MPA arises from the LV. There are two types of TGA, D-TGA and L-TGA (Figs. 9.44 and 9.45). In both types of TGA, the RV is connected to the aorta and LV is connected to the pulmonary artery.[30] The difference in these two types of TGA lies in the ventricular arrangement. In D-TGA, there is normal ventricular D-looping (i.e., the right ventricle is anterior and to the right and the left ventricle is posterior and to the left). As a result the flow is right atrium to RV to aorta and left atrium to LV to MPA. In L-TGA, there is L-looping of the ventricles which results in a switch of the ventricular positions. The atria and venous system remain normally positioned. As a result in L-TGA, the right atrium connects to the LV which connects to the MPA, and the left atrium connects to the RV and to the aorta.

The ventriculoarterial connections in D-TGA result in complete separation of systemic and pulmonary circulations. If there is not an associated atrial or ventricular level shunt, an intervention, generally an atrial septostomy, within the first few hours of life is needed to sustain life.[30] In L-TGA, the switching of the ventricular positions in addition to the swapped great artery positions actually restores the normal flow of blood through both systemic-pulmonary circulations and is compatible with life and usually does not require surgical correction. Therefore, L-TGA is described as being "physiologically corrected" as pulmonary blood flow reaches the systemic arteries via the RV. However, as the RV is the systemic ventricle, most patients ultimately develop systemic RV dysfunction in adulthood.[47]

Radiographic features of TGA in the neonatal period include cardiac enlargement and a relatively narrow appearance to the great vessels on the AP projection because of their anterior posterior arrangement (Fig. 9.46). Both CT

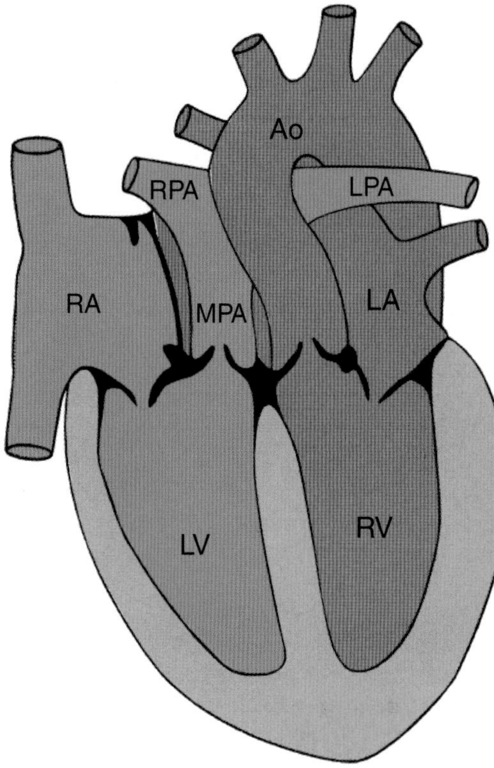

FIGURE 9.45 **Diagram of L-transposition of the great arteries (L-TGA).** The aorta and the pulmonary artery are transpositioned with the aorta anterior and to the left of the pulmonary artery. The position of the right ventricle (*RV*) and left ventricle (*LV*) are also switched (transposed). The aorta (*Ao*) arises from the RV and the pulmonary artery (*MPA*) from the LV. In L-TGA, the circulation through the heart is physiologic or "congenitally corrected" because there is both ventriculoarterial and atrioventricular discordance. *LA*, left atrium; *LPA*, left pulmonary artery; *RA*, right atrium; *RPA*, right pulmonary artery.

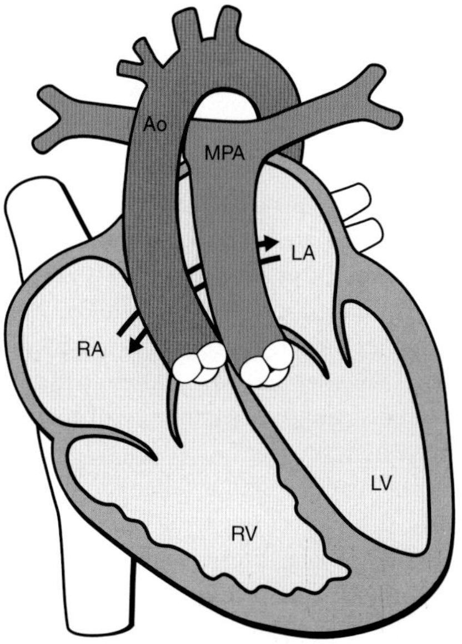

FIGURE 9.44 **Diagram of D-transposition of the great arteries.** The aorta (*Ao*) arises from the right ventricle (*RV*) and the pulmonary artery (*MPA*) from the left ventricle (*LV*). The aorta (*Ao*) is to the right and anterior (not shown) relative to the pulmonary artery. The ventricles are in their normal positions. *LA*, left atrium; *RA*, right atrium.

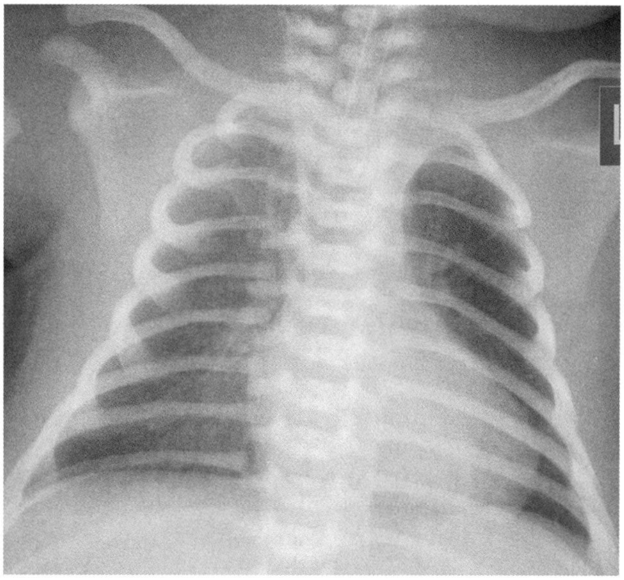

FIGURE 9.46 **D-Transposition of the great arteries.** Frontal chest radiograph shows egg-shaped cardiac silhouette with narrow superior mediastinum, increased pulmonary vascularity, and mild cardiomegaly.

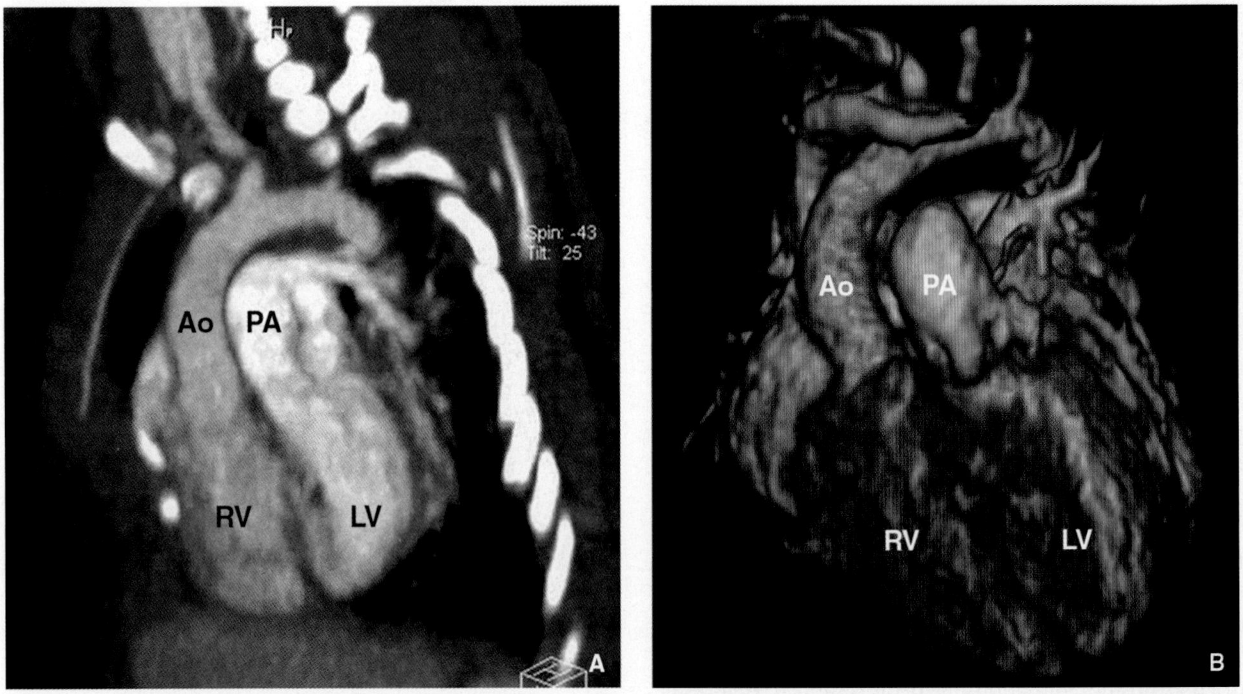

FIGURE 9.47 **D-Transposition of the great arteries.** Sagittal oblique maximum intensity projection image (MIP) **(A)** and three-dimensional volume-rendered CT image **(B)** shows the aorta (*Ao*) arising from the right ventricle (*RV*) and pulmonary artery (*PA*) originating from the left ventricle (*LV*). The aorta (*Ao*) is located anterior to the pulmonary artery (*PA*). The ventricles are in their normal positions.

and MRI are rarely used in the preoperative setting as the cardiac anatomy can be clearly delineated with echo in most cases. Occasionally, cardiac-gated CTA or cardiac MRI may be required to evaluate complex coronary artery anatomy not fully assessed on echo (Fig. 9.47).

D-TGA requires corrective surgery in the first few days of life.[47] The preferred procedure is the Jatene "arterial switch" (Fig. 9.48). For this surgical procedure, the ascending aorta and the MPA are transected above their valves and moved to their anatomically correct positions with the pulmonary bifurcation placed anterior to the ascending aorta (LeCompte maneuver). The coronary arteries are transplanted from the native aortic root to the neoaortic root. Septal defects, if present, are surgically closed. After the arterial switch procedure, many patients develop anastomotic narrowing at the RV to neo-MPA anastomosis, branch pulmonary artery narrowing, and dilatation of the neoaortic root. Late coronary occlusion can develop in 8% to 10% individuals after the arterial switch and although uncommon can cause sudden death. Cardiac MRI is routinely used to evaluate the postarterial switch patient for these complications.[43]

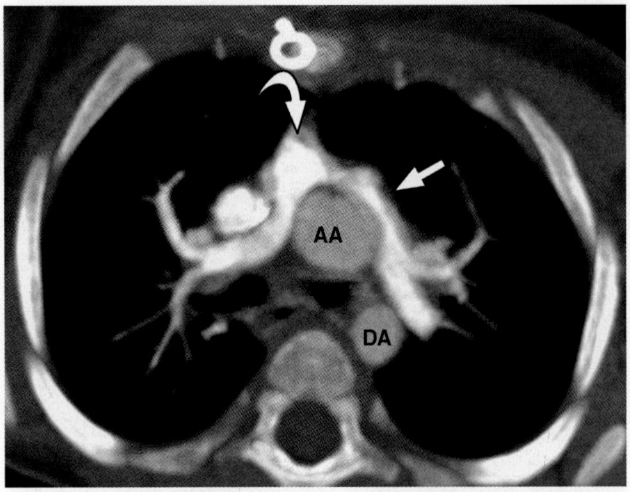

FIGURE 9.48 **D-Transposition of the great arteries after arterial switch operation.** Axial enhanced maximum intensity projection CT image shows main pulmonary artery (*curved arrow*) which is located anterior to the ascending aorta as the result of LeCompte maneuver. Also noted is stenosis (*straight arrow*) of the left pulmonary artery and a dilated ascending aorta (*AA*). *DA*, descending aorta.

Double Outlet Right Ventricle

DORV is a disorder where both the pulmonary artery and the aorta arise from the RV associated with a VSD (Fig. 9.49). In this disorder, there is a great deal of morphologic variability that depends on whether the relationship of the great arteries is normal or abnormal, whether the VSD is closest to the MPA or aorta, and whether or not there is subpulmonic/subaortic stenosis.[48,49]

The most frequent form of DORV is a side-to-side arrangement of the great arteries with a subaortic VSD and subpulmonic stenosis. In this form of DORV, blood flow favors the aorta over the pulmonary artery resulting in TOF-like physiology. Other forms include side-to-side arrangement of the great vessels with a subpulmonic VSD, in which shunted blood flow favors the MPA. This is known as Taussig-Bing anomaly and results similar to physiology to D-TGA, with blood from the LV favoring the MPA and blood from the RV favoring the aorta. In patients with subpulmonary stenosis,

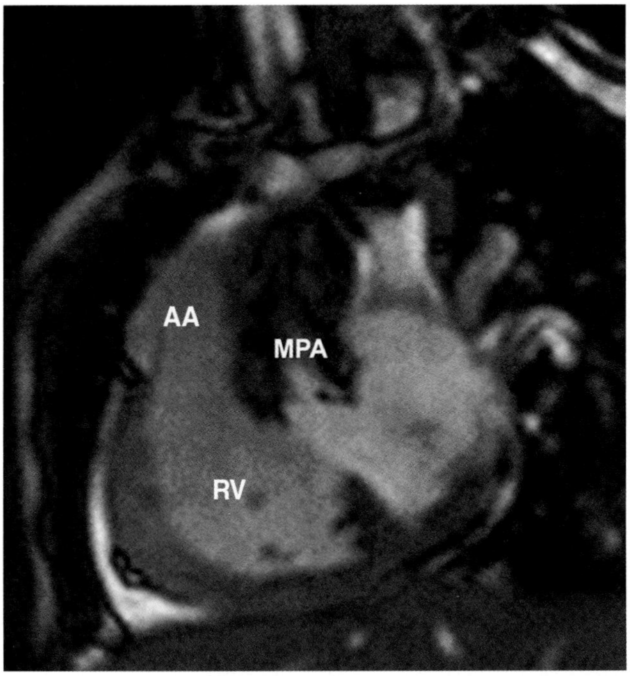

FIGURE 9.49 **Double outlet right ventricle and situs inversus.** Oblique bright blood magnetic resonance image shows both the main pulmonary artery (*MPA*) and the ascending aorta (*AA*) arising from the right ventricle (*RV*).

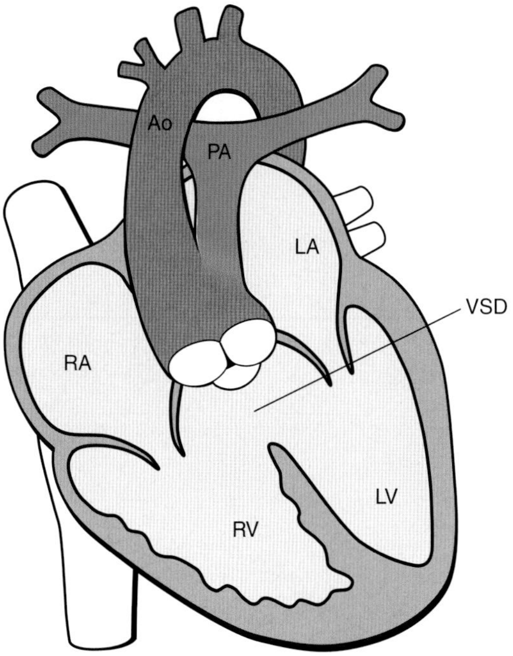

FIGURE 9.50 **Diagram of truncus arteriosus (type 1).** There is one artery exiting the heart, the ascending portion of which supplies the aorta, coronary arteries, and pulmonary arteries. *Ao*, aorta; *LA*, left atrium; *LV*, left ventricle; *PA*, pulmonary artery; *RA*, right atrium; *RV*, right ventricle; *VSD*, ventricular septal defect.

ventricular outflow also favors the aorta, and the RV becomes hypertrophied in a physiology similar to TOF.

Chest radiography usually shows cardiomegaly and may have apical elevation similar to TOF because of right ventricular hypertrophy. The mediastinal contour may be widened due to the side-to-side great vessel alignment. The aortic arch may be right sided. If there is pulmonary stenosis, there will be diminished pulmonary vascularity. DORV with a subpulmonic VSD usually leads to pulmonary vascular congestion. The cardiac anatomy is usually adequately depicted by echo in the neonatal stage, with CT and MRI reserved for cases where it is unclear whether the VSD is too remote from the aorta to enable a baffle type closure. In these cases, MRI may help preoperative planning of potentially complex repairs. In most cases, MRI is mainly used as postoperative surveillance, similar to TGA and TOF.[43] CTA may be of use in assessment of pulmonary artery size, but is not primarily used for an intracardiac assessment.

Surgical repair depends on the type of DORV, but usually involves redirecting left ventricular outflow to the aorta through the VSD by creation of an intraventricular tunnel/baffle using synthetic material. If severe pulmonary stenosis is present, then an RV-PA conduit is placed.[50]

Truncus Arteriosus

Truncus arteriosus is an uncommon conotruncal anomaly resulting in a single arterial trunk arising from normally formed ventricles (Fig. 9.50). Embryologically, the anomaly is thought to be a result of failed septation of the truncus arteriosus. As the outlet portion of the ventricular septum arises from the truncus arteriosus, this too is affected resulting in an outlet VSD.[51] The common trunk straddles a VSD (similar to TOF, TGA, and DORV). The truncal valve is usually dysplastic resulting in truncal stenosis or regurgitation. The coronary arteries are frequently anomalous with single coronary arteries and intramural courses commonly encountered. The pulmonary arteries arise from the common trunk distal to the coronary arteries. Affected pediatric patients typically present in infancy with cyanosis, failure to thrive, and heart failure.

There are four variations of truncus arteriosus described depending on the branch pattern of the pulmonary arteries[30,51,52] (Fig. 9.51) and classified by the Collett and Edwards or Van Praagh classifications. Based on the Collett and Edwards classification, type 1 is characterized by a single pulmonary trunk arising from the common trunk that bifurcates into left and right branch pulmonary arteries. This corresponds to type A1 in the Van Praagh classification. Type II has separate origins of the pulmonary arteries from the posterolateral aspects of the common trunk. Type III is similar to type II except the branch pulmonary arteries arise from the anterolateral aspects of the common trunk. Types I and II correspond to type A2 in the Van Praagh classification. In type IV, the branch pulmonary arteries arise from the descending aorta. However, type IV is a controversial type because many people believe this to be a form of pulmonary atresia with MAPCAs.[51,52]

Chest radiography usually demonstrates cardiomegaly, a right-sided aortic arch (50%) and pulmonary vascular congestion (Fig. 9.52). Echo is usually the primary modality for initial diagnosis. Cardiac MRI or CT usually reserved for complex cases where the pulmonary artery anatomy cannot be delineated on echo or where pulmonary stenosis is suspected

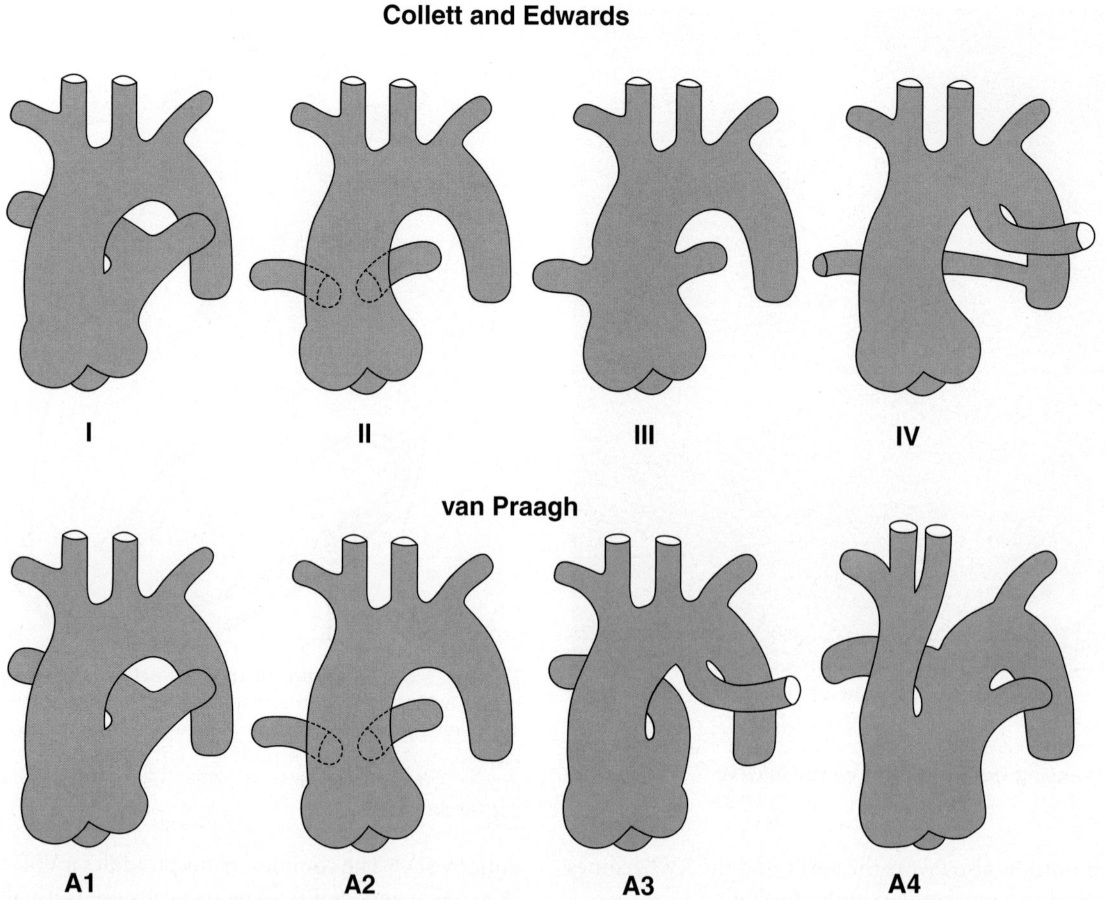

FIGURE 9.51 **Diagrams of Collett and Edwards and van Praagh classifications of truncus arteriosus.** Type I and type A1 are the same. Type II (pulmonary arteries arising separately from the posterior portion of the truncus) and type III (pulmonary arteries arising separately from the lateral walls of the truncus) are grouped as a single A2. Type A3 represents atresia of one of the pulmonary arteries with collateral flow to that lung. Type A4 is truncus associated with interrupted aortic arch.

(Fig. 9.53). CTA can be very useful in delineating anomalous coronary artery courses.

Surgical treatment involves patching the VSD, resecting the pulmonary arteries from the common trunk, and reconstructing the RVOT using an RV-PA conduit.[53] Postoperatively, the truncal valve (which is now the neo-aortic valve) may remain regurgitant and left ventricular dilatation results. The RV-PA conduit eventually undergoes calcification and stenosis leading to right ventricular hypertrophy; ultimately, it results in the need for pulmonary valve replacement in adolescence or adulthood. Cardiac MRI is used as regular surveillance following repair of truncus arteriosus to assess aortic regurgitation, RV-PA stenosis and biventricular size and function, and coronary artery anatomy.

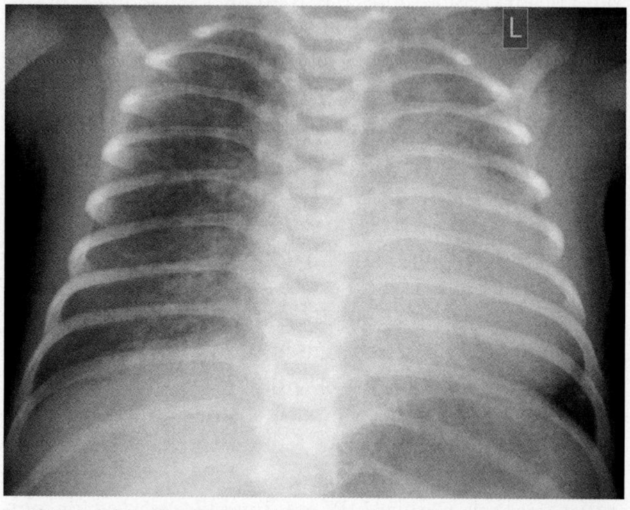

FIGURE 9.52 **Truncus arteriosus.** Frontal chest radiograph shows increased pulmonary vascularity, marked cardiomegaly, and right-sided aortic arch.

Aortic Anomalies

Aortic Stenosis

Aortic stenosis is characterized by the narrowing of the opening of the aortic valve. It is classified into three types, valvar, supravalvar, and subvalvar. The most common type of aortic stenosis in children is valvar type because of underlying bicuspid aortic valve.[54] Normally, the aortic valve is composed of three leaflets that arise from the three sinuses of Valsalva. When two of these leaflets are congenitally fused, the aortic valve is described as being bicuspid. Bicuspid aortic valves are commonly associated with aortic coarctation and Turner

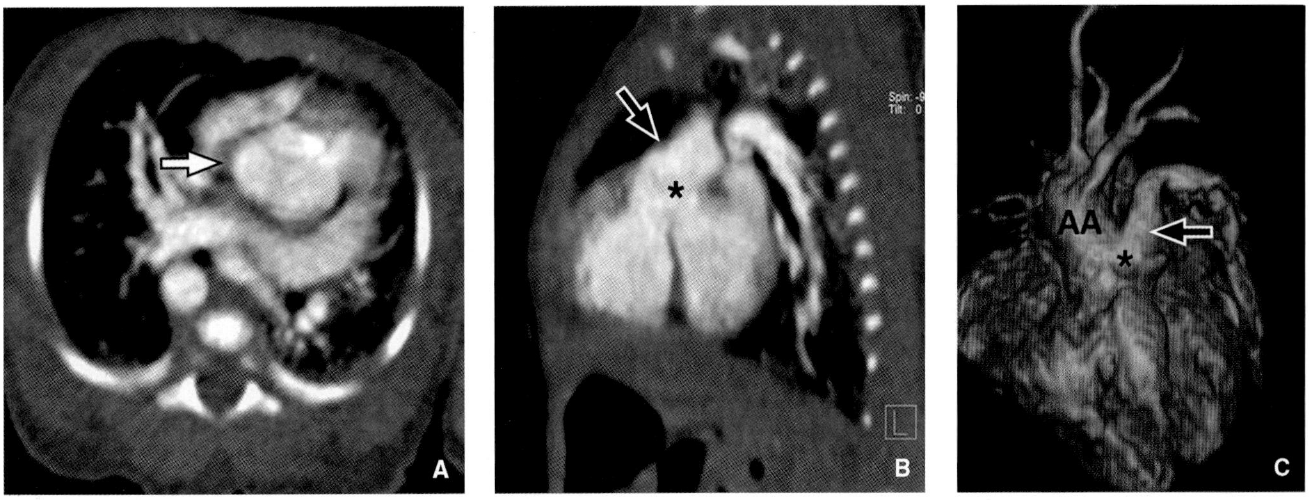

FIGURE 9.53 **Truncus arteriosus type I/A1.** Axial enhanced CT image **(A)** shows the truncal valve (*arrow*). Sagittal reformatted enhanced CT image **(B)** demonstrates ventricular septal defect (*asterisk*) under truncal valve (*arrow*). Three-dimensional volume-rendered CT image **(C)** shows main pulmonary artery (*arrow*) arising from truncal root (*asterisk*). *AA*, ascending aorta.

syndrome. A less common secondary cause of aortic valvar stenosis in the pediatric age group is rheumatic heart disease affecting the aortic valve.[55]

Supravalvar aortic stenosis occurs above the level of the aortic valve at the sinotubular junction. This is seen in patients with Williams syndrome (caused by deletion of chromosomal material from 17q11.23), which is associated with elfin facies, pulmonary stenosis, and midaortic narrowing (Fig. 9.54).[55] Subvalvar aortic stenosis can be seen in conotruncal anomalies and conditions resulting in left ventricular hypertrophy.[55]

Clinical presentation of aortic stenosis varies with its degree and the presence of any associated conditions. Critical aortic stenosis presents in the neonatal period with signs of peripheral ischemia, metabolic acidosis, and pulmonary overload. However, the majority of pediatric patients with isolated aortic stenosis are discovered incidentally because of the presence of a murmur on physical examination. These patients may not develop symptoms until adolescence or adulthood. Patients with rheumatic aortic stenosis acquired during childhood typically do not develop symptoms until after the sixth decade of life.[54]

Chest radiographic features that may be present in more severe forms of aortic stenosis include cardiomegaly and a dilated ascending aorta. Pulmonary vascular congestion may be seen in neonates with critical aortic stenosis. The diagnosis of aortic stenosis is primarily made by echo with additional imaging reserved for those cases with poor echo windows or when there is a concern for aortic coarctation. On cardiac MRI, the three leaflets of the aortic valve have an appearance when viewed en face that is sometimes described as the "Mercedes" sign because it resembles the emblem for Mercedes-Benz cars. In patients with a bicuspid aortic valve,

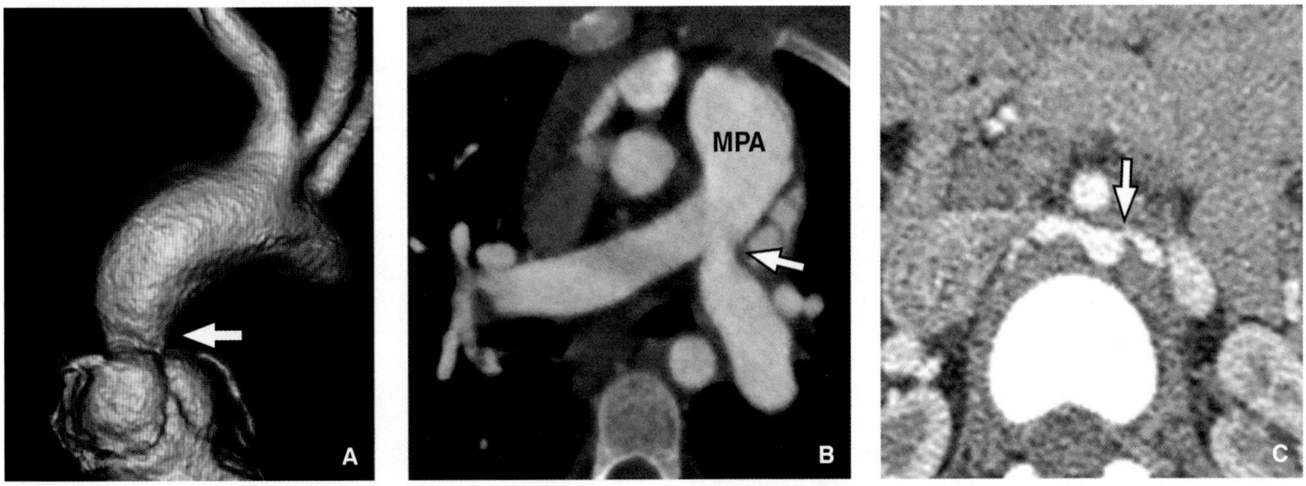

FIGURE 9.54 **Williams syndrome.** Three-dimensional volume-rendered CT image **(A)** shows supravalvar aortic stenosis at the sinotubular junction (*arrow*). Axial enhanced CT image **(B)** demonstrates mild left pulmonary artery stenosis (*arrow*). *MPA*, main pulmonary artery. Axial enhanced CT image **(C)** at level of renal arteries shows midaortic narrowing and left renal artery stenosis (*arrow*).

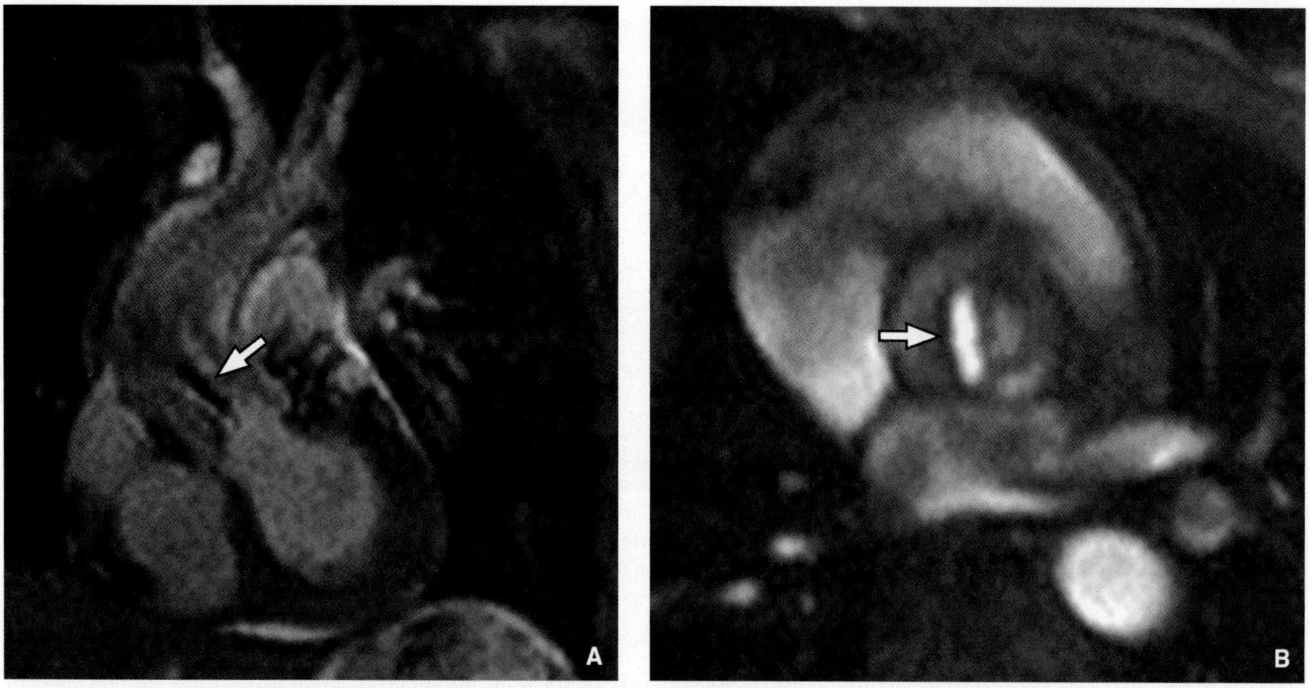

FIGURE 9.55 **Aortic stenosis with bicuspid aortic valve. A:** Oblique cine magnetic resonance (MR) image in coronal plane through left ventricular outflow tract demonstrates turbulent flow (*arrow*) that extends from the aortic valve leaflets into the ascending aorta during systole. **B:** Oblique axial phase-contrast magnitude MR image shows the reduced aortic valve opening (*arrow*).

there is instead a more oval opening in the valve, resembling the mouth of a fish (Fig. 9.55). The hemodynamic effects of turbulent high-velocity jets passing through stenotic valves are felt to be at least partially responsible for the ascending aortic dilatation that develops in patients with aortic stenosis (Fig. 9.56). Significant dilatation may predispose the patient to aortic dissection. CTA and MRA can be used to screen for associated aortic coarctation (see below). Cardiac MRI can quantify the degree of aortic stenosis and aortic insufficiency, which may result from inadequate coaptation of the stenosed valvar leaflets, and also evaluate for secondary left ventricular dilatation and hypertrophy.

The current treatment options include percutaneous balloon dilatation, aortic valvotomy, prosthetic valve replacement, or Ross procedure in which the native pulmonary valve is replaced with the stenosed aortic valve.

Aortic Insufficiency

Aortic valve insufficiency results from backflow of blood through the aortic valve arising from incomplete coaptation of the aortic valvar leaflets. A number of conditions predispose to aortic insufficiency in children including bicuspid aortic valve, disorders resulting in aortic root dilatation such as connective tissue disorders (Ehlers-Danlos, Marfan, and Loeys-Dietz syndromes), inflammatory conditions such as Takayasu arteritis, and conotruncal anomalies including TGA.[54,55] Clinically, most aortic insufficiency is silent apart from a murmur on physical exam and abnormal pulse pattern (known as a water-hammer pulse).

Chest radiography may reveal cardiomegaly in the setting of left ventricular dilatation. There may be a dilated ascending aorta. CT is generally not helpful for the diagnosis of aortic insufficiency alone. MRI is useful to assess for the aortic regurgitant fraction (fractional amount of blood that returns through the aortic valve relative to the amount of blood ejected

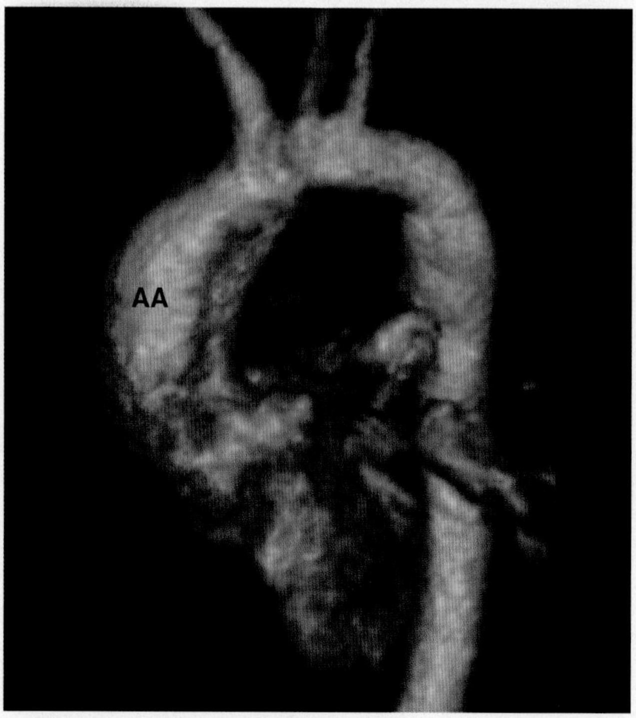

FIGURE 9.56 **Aortic stenosis.** Three-dimensional volume-rendered image from gadolinium-enhanced 3-dimensional magnetic resonance angiography shows dilatation of the ascending aorta (*AA*).

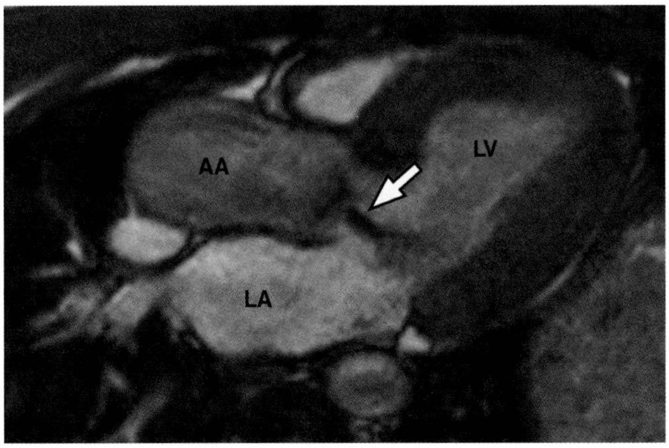

FIGURE 9.57 **Aortic regurgitation.** Bright blood magnetic resonance image in left ventricular outflow tract plane demonstrates aortic regurgitation jet (*arrow*) in a pediatric patient with aortic root and ascending aortic dilatation (*AA*) and mild left ventricular hypertrophy. *LA*, left atrium; *LV*, left ventricle.

through the valve). MRI is also helpful for complete assessment of a dilated aorta and ventricular size and function (Fig. 9.57).

Current management of aortic insufficiency includes the use of vasodilators in stable and asymptomatic children and aortic valve replacement in symptomatic children, particularly those with a left ventricular ejection fraction of <50%.

Aortic Coarctation

Coarctation of the aorta represents 5% to 10% of congenital heart disease (Fig. 9.58). It can be classified into preductal, juxtaductal, and postductal forms according to its location relative to the isthmus, which represents the aortic attachment of the ductus arteriosus.[56,57] Juxtaductal is the most common form and occurs at the isthmus just distal to the takeoff of the left subclavian artery. Two main theories regarding the embryologic development of aortic coarctation that have been proposed include the ductal theory and the hemodynamic theory. The ductal theory hypothesizes that aortic coarctation results from migration of smooth muscle ductal cells that constrict and narrow the aortic lumen. The hemodynamic theory hypothesizes that aortic coarctation results from decreased fetal arch flow secondary to increased ductal flow leading to arch hypoplasia and coarctation.[56,57]

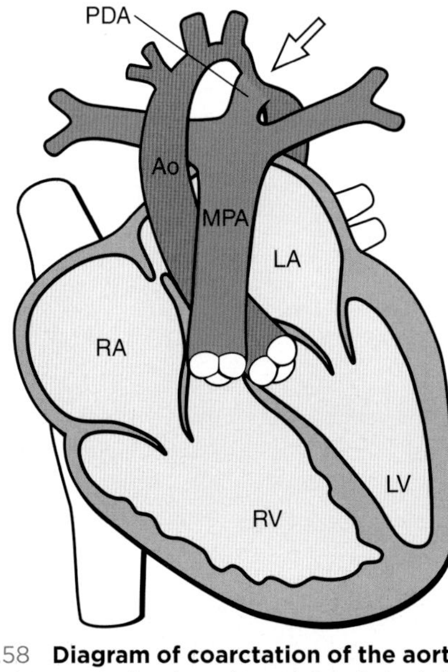

FIGURE 9.58 **Diagram of coarctation of the aorta.** The aorta is narrowed (*arrow*) distal to the origin of the left subclavian artery. The ductus arteriosus or ligamentum arteriosum (neither shown in the figure) typically is located just distal to the coarctation region. *Ao*, aorta; *LA*, left atrium; *LV*, left ventricle; *MPA*, main pulmonary artery; *PDA*, patent ductus arteriosus; *RA*, right atrium; *RV*, right ventricle.

On chest radiography, normal or increased pulmonary vascularity because of passive vascular congestion is seen. In more severe forms of coarctation, there may be associated left ventricular hypertrophy and dilatation. The aortic knob may be small if the distal aortic arch is hypoplastic. The "figure-of-3" sign may be present in patients with a discrete coarctation at the aortic isthmus (Fig. 9.59). This sign is formed by prestenotic dilatation of the aortic arch and left subclavian artery, indentation at the coarctation site, and poststenotic dilatation of the descending aorta. Rib notching under the posterolateral aspects of the fourth to eighth ribs may be seen when the coarctation results in chronic enlargement of the intercostal arteries, which fill the descending aorta via retrograde flow from connections with the internal mammary arteries. Rib notching is usually bilateral, but maybe unilateral in rare case of an aberrant subclavian artery arising after the coarcted segment. In this case, the collateral vessels occur on the contralateral side to the aberrant subclavian artery.

Echo provides adequate data to allow operative planning in the majority of cases of infants and young children who have adequate sonographic acoustic windows. CTA and cardiac MRI provide further information in cases where the coarctation is incompletely defined due to poor acoustic windows or where the coarctation is atypical or complex. CTA and MRA provide morphologic assessment of the entire aorta and

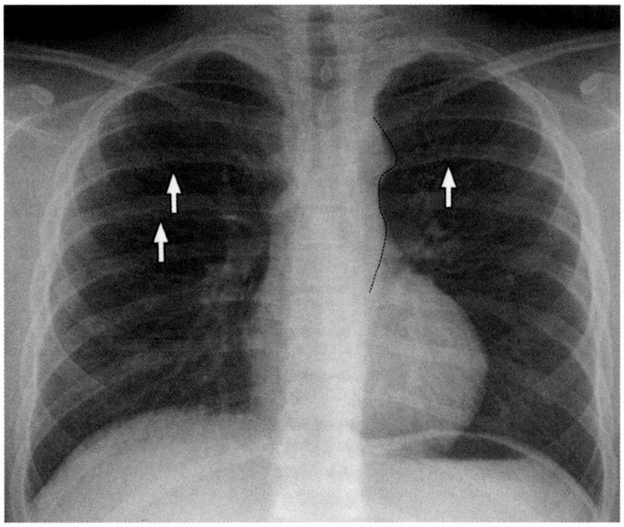

FIGURE 9.59 **Coarctation of the aorta.** Frontal chest radiograph shows "figure-of-3" sign (*dotted line*) and enlarged left cardiac margin representing left ventricular dilatation with rib notching bilaterally (*arrows*).

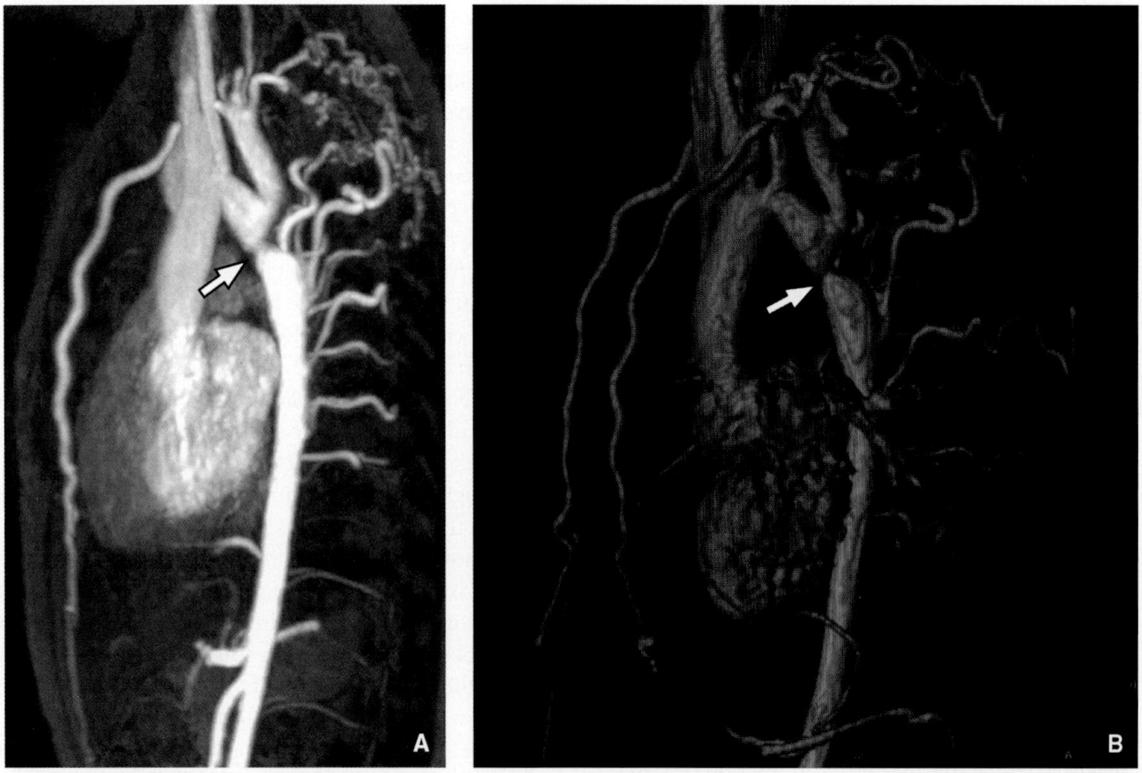

FIGURE 9.60 **Coarctation of the aorta.** Sagittal reformatted enhanced maximum intensity projection CT image **(A)** and 3-dimensional volume-rendered CT image **(B)** show juxtaductal coarctation (*arrows*) and enlarged intercostal collateral vessels.

demonstrate collateral vessels (Fig. 9.60).[56] Phase-contrast MR sequences may quantify collateral flow to the descending aorta and estimate the pressure gradient across the stenotic region. A coarctation is deemed to be significant when the pressure gradient across the coarctation exceeds 20 mm Hg. In contrast, pseudocoarctation, which is characterized by tortuosity of the aortic arch results in turbulent blood flow, but is without a hemodynamically significant pressure gradient or collateral flow (Fig. 9.61).

Surgical procedures for aortic coarctation include surgical resection of the stenotic segment with an extended end-to-end anastomosis in neonates, infants, and young children. In patients who cannot be repaired in this fashion, resection of the coarctation with placement of an interposition graft can be performed. Percutaneous corrective procedures include balloon angioplasty alone or balloon angioplasty and stent placement. In general, infants with complex arch anatomy or long segment arch hypoplasia are considered candidates for surgical repair, with percutaneous therapies favored in adults, short-segment stenoses, and restenoses.[58]

Complications that occur after surgical repair and balloon angioplasty/stenting include recoarctation, dissection, and aneurysm formation. Recurrent coarctation is more common with surgical repairs in infancy. Aneurysm formation is most common following a subclavian flap repair, having a reported incidence of 27% and typically occurring on the side opposite the flap.[58]

Although echo is typically used for routine follow-up of patients after coarctation repair or stenting, CT, and cardiac MRI can both be used to evaluate for complications such as restenosis or pseudoaneurysm formation in patients with suspicious features on echo.

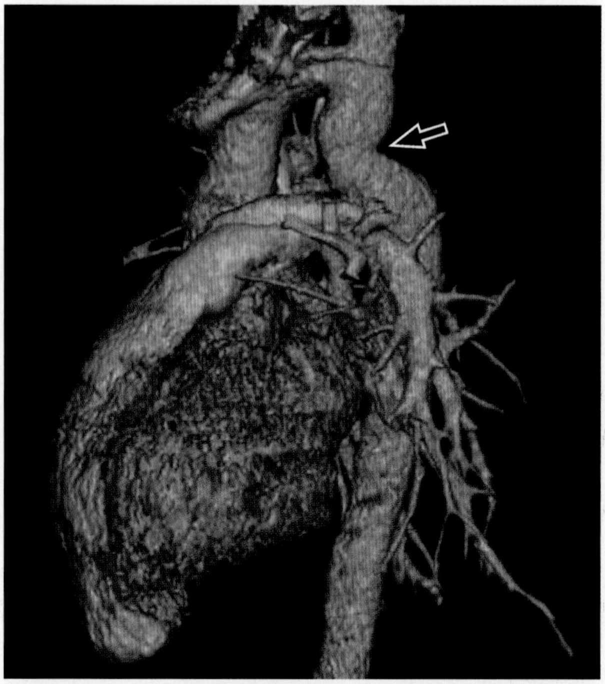

FIGURE 9.61 **Pseudocoarctation of the aorta.** Three-dimensional volume-rendered CT image shows kinking (*arrow*) of the aortic arch without obstruction.

Interrupted Aortic Arch

IAA is a relatively rare disorder that results in lack of continuity between the ascending aorta and descending aorta. There are three types depending on where in the thoracic aorta the interruption occurs.[59] In type A, the interruption is located distal to the left subclavian artery. In type B, the most common type, the interruption occurs between the left common carotid artery and left subclavian artery. Type C is the least common type, and the interruption occurs between the right brachiocephalic and left common carotid arteries. In any of the three types of IAA, there may be an aberrant right/left subclavian artery. Aortic interruption is usually seen in association with a large VSD and a large ductus arteriosus (known as a "ductal arch"). The ductus arteriosus is the major arterial supply of the descending aorta. The subvalvar area of the LV can be hypoplastic in 50% to 80% of patients.

Typical clinical presentation of IAA is in the neonatal period with lethargy, poor feeding, mottled appearing lower extremities, and reduced pulses in the lower extremities. Approximately 50% of patients with IAA have DiGeorge syndrome.[35]

Chest radiography in IAA may demonstrate cardiomegaly and increased pulmonary vascularity (Fig. 9.62). In DiGeorge syndrome, the thymus is typically absent. Echo usually makes the primary diagnosis, but CTA and MRA are increasingly used to characterize the aortic anatomy, ductal arch, and any collaterals that may be present (Fig. 9.63). Cardiac MRI may be used to evaluate the subaortic anatomy.[59]

Surgical reconstruction of the arch is usually performed with side-to-side anastomosis with arch augmentation as needed. If the subaortic region is of appropriate size, the VSD is usually closed with a patch during the primary repair. If there is subaortic narrowing, repair becomes more complex and may include a Ross-Konno procedure or in severe subaortic obstruction a Norwood I procedure with closure of VSD and RV-PA conduit (Rastelli procedure).[59,60]

Cardiac MRI is used routinely in the postoperative surveillance of patients following a Ross-Konno procedure or a Norwood-Rastelli procedure, with evaluation for neoaortic root dilatation, neoaortic valve regurgitation, RV-PA conduit stenosis, biventricular size and function, and coronary ischemia (after the Ross-Konno).

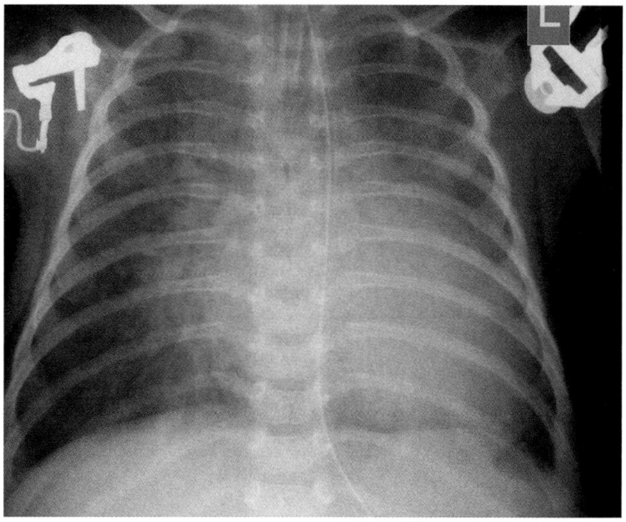

FIGURE 9.62 **Interrupted aortic arch.** Frontal chest radiograph in a newborn demonstrates increased pulmonary vascularity and marked cardiomegaly. Also noted are endotracheal tube and nasogastric tube.

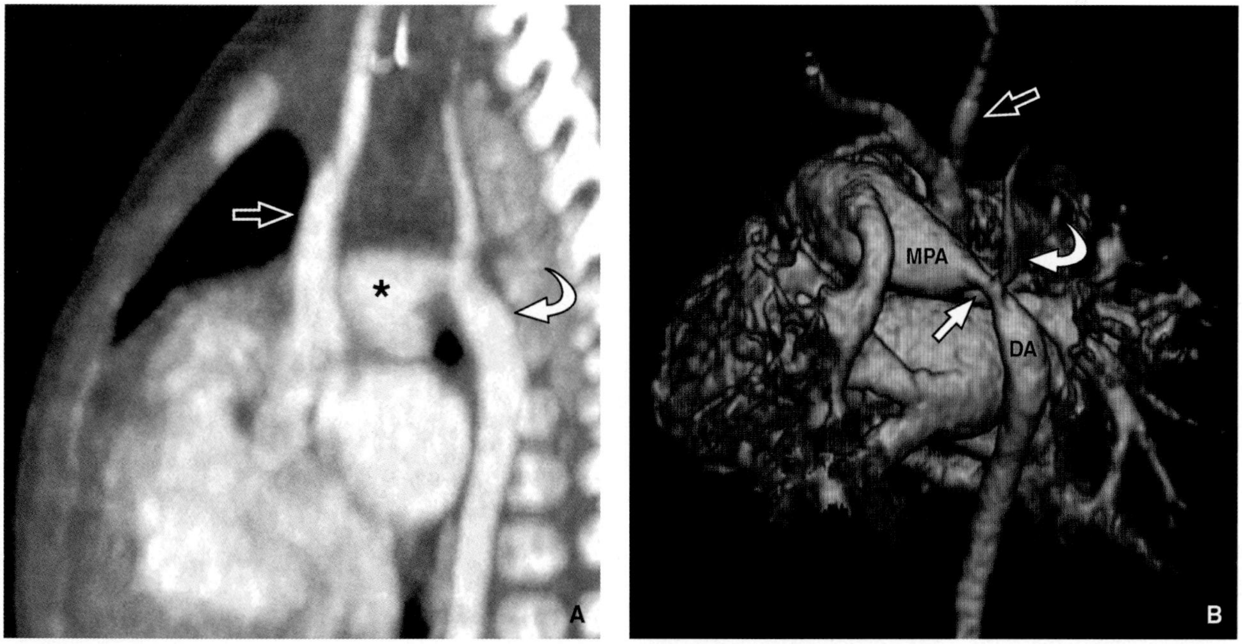

FIGURE 9.63 **Interrupted aortic arch.** Sagittal oblique enhanced CT image **(A)** shows discontinuity between the ascending (*straight arrow*) and descending aorta (*curved arrow*). Blood to the descending aorta is supplied by enlarged patent ductus arteriosus (*asterisk*). Three-dimensional volume-rendered CT image **(B)** demonstrates interruption of the aortic arch between the right common carotid (*black arrow*) and right subclavian (*curved arrow*) arteries. Blood to the descending aorta is supplied by the patent ductus arteriosus (*white arrow*). *DA*, descending aorta; *MPA*, main pulmonary artery.

Coronary Artery Anomalies

Anomalies of the coronary arteries comprise of anomalies of origin, anomalies of course, and anomalous fistulous connections.

Anomalous Origin or Course of Coronary Artery

The left and right main coronary arteries usually arise from the center of the left and right sinuses of Valsalva, respectively. Anomalies of coronary artery origin include (1) individual origins of the LAD and LCX from the left sinus of Valsalva with absence of left main coronary artery (LMCA); (2) anomalously high/low takeoff of the RCA or LMCA from above or below the left sinus of Valsalva; (3) LMCA origin from the right sinus of Valsalva; (4) RCA origin from the left sinus of Valsalva; (5) a single coronary ostium from left or right sinus of Valsalva resulting in a single coronary artery, which then divides into LMCA and RCA; and (6) LMCA origin from the MPA (anomalous origin of the LCA from the pulmonary artery [ALCAPA]).[61,62]

Separate origins of the LAD and LCX with absence of the LMCA occur in ~1% of the population and are associated with a bicuspid aortic valve. Anomalies of high or low takeoff of the RCA or LMCA from above or below the appropriate sinus may occasionally have clinical consequence.[63] Anomalous origin of the LMCA from the right sinus of Valsalva and RCA from the left sinus of Valsalva are believed to be relatively common with a prevalence in the range of 0.1% to 0.3% of the population.[64]

When the RCA arises from the left sinus of Valsalva as either a separate ostium or the same ostium as the LMCA (single coronary ostium), the RCA has different possible routes to reach its normal location in the right AV groove. It can course through the interventricular septum (transseptal), anterior to the pulmonary artery (prepulmonic), dorsal to the aorta (retroaortic), or between the aorta and pulmonary trunk (interarterial) to reach the right AV groove.[61]

The transseptal, prepulmonic, and retroaortic courses are generally considered clinically insignificant. An interarterial RCA may have a proximal course that travels within the wall of the aortic root (interarterial and intramural). This type of anomalous course is occasionally associated with syncope, chest pain, or sudden death in adolescents and young adults.[61,64]

Surgical repair of an anomalous RCA from the left sinus of Valsalva is controversial due the relative frequency of the anomaly in asymptomatic patients and relative low incidence of associated sudden death in postmortem studies.[62,64] However, surgical correction is usually indicated in symptomatic pediatric patients.

Similar to the anomalous RCA, when the LMCA arises from the right sinus of Valsalva as either a separate ostium or the same ostium (single coronary ostium), the LMCA has different possible routes to its normal anterior interventricular groove location. It can course through the interventricular septum (transseptal), anterior to the pulmonary artery (prepulmonic), behind the aorta (retroaortic), or between the aorta and pulmonary trunk (interarterial) to reach its myocardial territory.[61] Similar to anomalous RCA, the transseptal, prepulmonic, and retroaortic courses are usually clinically insignificant, although occasionally a transseptal course may become narrowed as it travels through a tunnel of ventricular septum. However, an anomalous origin of the LMCA from the right sinus of Valsalva with an interarterial and intramural course is strongly associated with risk of ischemia and sudden death, so surgical correction with an unroofing procedure or translocation is recommended in all cases.[61,62,64]

The chest radiography of pediatric patients with anomalous origin or course of coronary artery is generally normal. Cardiac CTA or MRI may be required for presurgical confirmation of coronary anomalies (Figs. 9.64 and 9.65). In

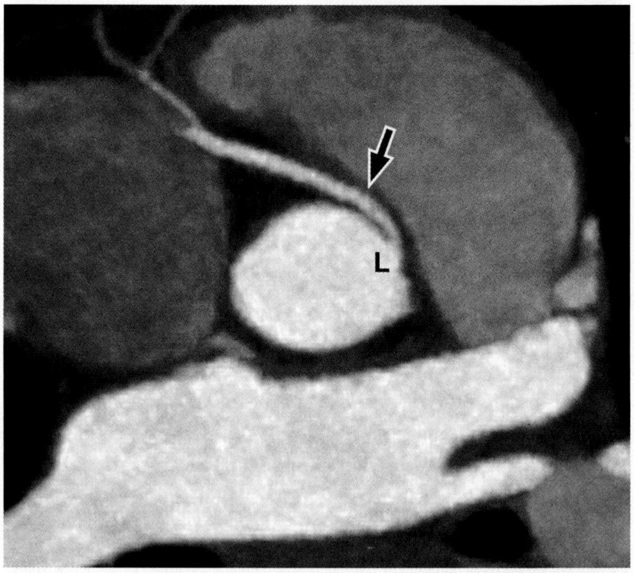

FIGURE 9.64 **Anomalous right coronary artery from the left sinus of Valsalva.** Axial enhanced maximum intensity projection CT image shows an anomalous origin of the right coronary artery (*arrow*) from the left sinus of Valsalva (*L*) with an interarterial and proximal intramural course.

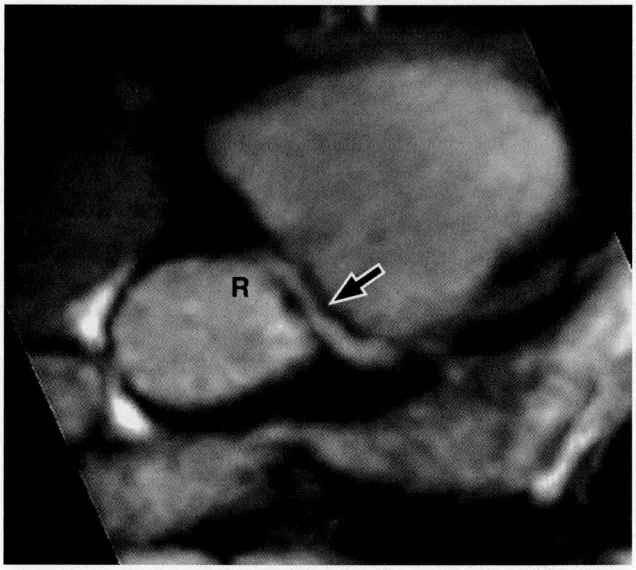

FIGURE 9.65 **Anomalous left coronary artery from the right sinus of Valsalva.** Axial bright blood magnetic resonance image shows an anomalous origin of the left coronary artery (*arrow*) from the right sinus of Valsalva (*R*) with an interarterial and proximal intramural course.

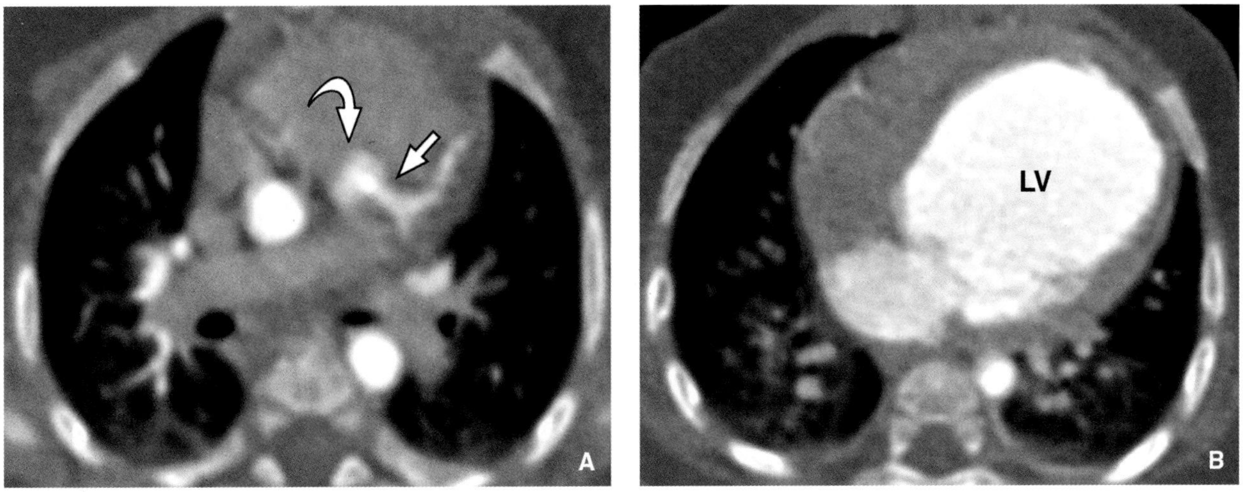

FIGURE 9.66 **Anomalous left coronary artery from the pulmonary artery.** Axial enhanced CT images **(A, B)** show an anomalous origin of the left coronary artery (*straight arrow*) from the pulmonary artery. The main pulmonary artery (*curved arrow*) is filled with contrast medium from the left coronary artery (coronary steal phenomenon), and there is a marked global left ventricular dilatation (*LV*).

addition to demonstrating the coronary artery anatomy, cardiac MRI with stress perfusion and delayed gadolinium enhancement imaging may be used to demonstrate changes of ischemia or infarction, respectively, in the myocardial territory supplied by the LMCA.

The preferred surgical repair of anomalous RCA or LMCA from the opposite sinus of Valsalva is coronary artery unroofing.[65] The unroofing procedure involves resection of the aortic wall between the aortic lumen and the intramural portion of the coronary artery with placement of the ostium in the appropriate sinus. If the intercoronary commissure would be at risk from unroofing, a reimplantation procedure between the anomalous coronary and the appropriate sinus of Valsalva is performed.

Anomalous Left Coronary Artery from the Pulmonary Artery

ALCAPA is a rare congenital cardiovascular abnormality. Most cases of ALCAPA present with heart failure at ~6 to 8 weeks of age, coinciding with a decrease in pulmonary vascular resistance.[66] In the first 6 weeks of life, the pulmonary vascular resistance remains high; therefore, blood from the MPA favors the lower pressure LCA over the higher pressure pulmonary circulation. However, when the pulmonary vascular resistance drops, a coronary steal phenomenon results with reversal of left coronary artery circulation with flow of blood to the now lower pressure pulmonary circulation. Collateral vessels from the normal RCA to the left coronary circulation develop, and ~15% of patients develop such extensive collateral circulations that presentation occurs much later, with rare cases of presentation during adulthood described.[66]

Chest radiography usually demonstrates cardiomegaly and pulmonary edema resulting from myocardial ischemia. Echo is most frequently used to make this diagnosis, with other modalities (CT/MRI/cardiac catheterization) reserved for challenging cases. Because of the small size and frequently tenuous medical condition of these children, CT is preferred over MRI, because of the speed of acquisition and better spatial resolution. The anomalous LMCA usually arises from the posterior facing sinus of the pulmonary trunk close to the left sinus of Valsalva (Figs. 9.66 and 9.67). The LV is usually enlarged and decreased left ventricular systolic function may be demonstrated (Fig. 9.66B).

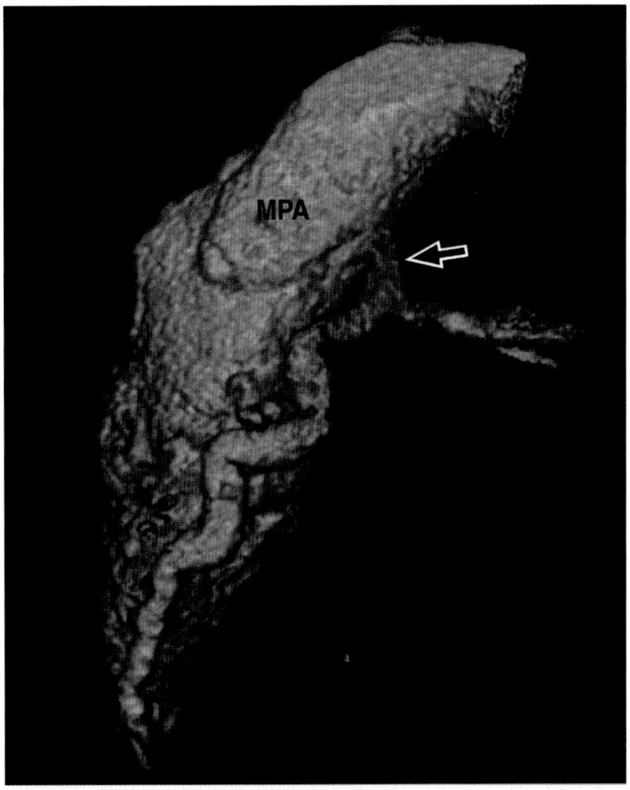

FIGURE 9.67 **Anomalous left coronary artery from the pulmonary artery (late presentation).** Three-dimensional volume-rendered CT image shows an anomalous origin of the left coronary artery (*arrow*) from the main pulmonary artery (*MPA*).

Currently, there are two main surgical management options available for treating ALCAPA in symptomatic children. Most commonly, the LMCA can be surgically detached from the pulmonary artery and reimplanted into the ascending aorta.[67] Less commonly, a tunnel from the aorta to the anomalous LMCA can be created, and then the connection between the LMCA and the pulmonary artery is closed.[68]

Coronary Artery Fistula

Coronary artery fistulas are anomalous connections between one of the major coronary artery branches and the ventricle (known as a coronary-cameral fistula) or between a coronary artery and any portion of the systemic/pulmonary circulations (e.g., a coronary artery to pulmonary artery fistula).[61,69] A coronary artery fistula results in bypassing of the normal myocardial vascular bed by the fistulous connection. The majority of coronary artery fistulae are small and clinically insignificant. However, large fistulae (>3 × size of the normal coronary artery) may cause murmurs on physical exam, arrhythmias, or myocardial ischemia.[69]

Chest radiography is usually normal except in cases of a large left-to-right shunt, when cardiomegaly and pulmonary edema may result. CTA and cardiac MRI both provide excellent delineation of large fistulous connections, with MRI preferred for larger lesions when an estimate of shunt fraction may help determine whether closure is required. CTA provides high spatial resolution and so is preferred for small lesions.

Small incidental coronary artery fistulas may be left untreated with intervention reserved for those cases with a large left-to-right shunt. The shunt may be closed percutaneously at the time of cardiac catheterization with occlusive devices/coils or surgically via direct ligation.[69]

Anomalous Venous Connections

Anomalous venous connections can be classified as anomalous connections of systemic or pulmonary venous drainage. These anomalous drainage patterns result from an abnormal embryologic venous development.

Systemic Venous Anomalies

The systemic venous system arises from the development and subsequent regression of portions of a complex cardinal venous system, which is present from approximately the end of the 4th embryologic week[70] (Fig. 9.68). At the end of the 4th week of gestation, there are two sinus venosus horns in the early fetal heart. These sinus venous horns receive the paired common cardinal veins, which in turn drain the bilateral anterior and posterior cardinal veins. The distal left common cardinal vein and left posterior cardinal vein degenerate, leaving the left sinus venous to form the coronary sinus. The left anterior cardinal vein anastomoses with the right anterior cardinal vein, and both become known as the innominate veins, with the right common cardinal vein forming the SVC.[70]

Blood caudal to the heart initially returns via the paired posterior cardinal veins. However, additional plexuses known as the subcardinal and supracardinal veins develop, which anastomose with the posterior cardinal veins. The intrahepatic portion of the IVC forms from the vitelline veins within the liver. The renal veins and renal and suprarenal portions of the IVC form from anastomoses between supracardinal, subcardinal veins, and posterior cardinal veins. The infrarenal portion of the IVC forms from the right supracardinal vein. The posterior cardinal veins and left supracardinal vein regress. The right subcardinal vein becomes the azygos vein, and the left subcardinal vein becomes the hemiazygos vein[70] (Fig. 9.69).

Common systemic venous anomalies arise from the inappropriate persistence or regression of one or more of the cardinal, subcardinal, or supracardinal veins. Although most systemic venous anomalies are isolated, anomalies of systemic venous drainage are commonly seen as part of the heterotaxy spectrum.

A left-sided SVC results when the left common cardinal vein fails to regress, with the left SVC draining into the right atrium via the coronary sinus (Fig. 9.69). This is usually associated with a left innominate vein emptying directly into the left SVC rather than bridging the mediastinum into the right SVC. In most cases of a left SVC, a normal or small right SVC is also present.[70]

A left-sided IVC results from persistence of the left supracardinal vein. In most cases, the right supracardinal vein regresses, resulting in a left IVC that crosses the midline at the renal vein level and then continues normally into the liver. A duplicated IVC results when neither right nor left supracardinal veins regress.[70]

Interruption of the suprarenal IVC results from failure of the supracardinal veins to form appropriate anastomoses with the vitelline veins in the liver. In this case, blood is shunted through the right supracardinal and subcardinal venous systems into the azygos vein. The azygos vein drains the intra-abdominal venous return into the SVC via the azygos arch. The suprahepatic IVC formed by the confluence of the hepatic veins returns normally to the right atrium.[70]

Clinically, systemic venous anomalies are usually silent and found incidentally on cross-sectional imaging. Chest radiography is normal unless there are coexistent cardiac or situs anomalies. CTA and MRA with 2D and 3D reformations can best demonstrate the venous anomalies and subsequent collateral venous pathways that have developed.

Surgical correction of systemic venous anomalies is not performed unless obstruction or anomalous drainage is present, but awareness of the systemic venous pathway may be relevant for other procedures such as a vena cava filter placement or cardiac catheterization.[70]

Pulmonary Venous Anomalies

The embryologic development of normal pulmonary venous drainage is simpler than the systemic veins. Between the 5th and 7th gestational weeks, the pulmonary veins develop as outgrowths from the left atrium and anastomose with the developing vascular plexus in each lung bud.[71]

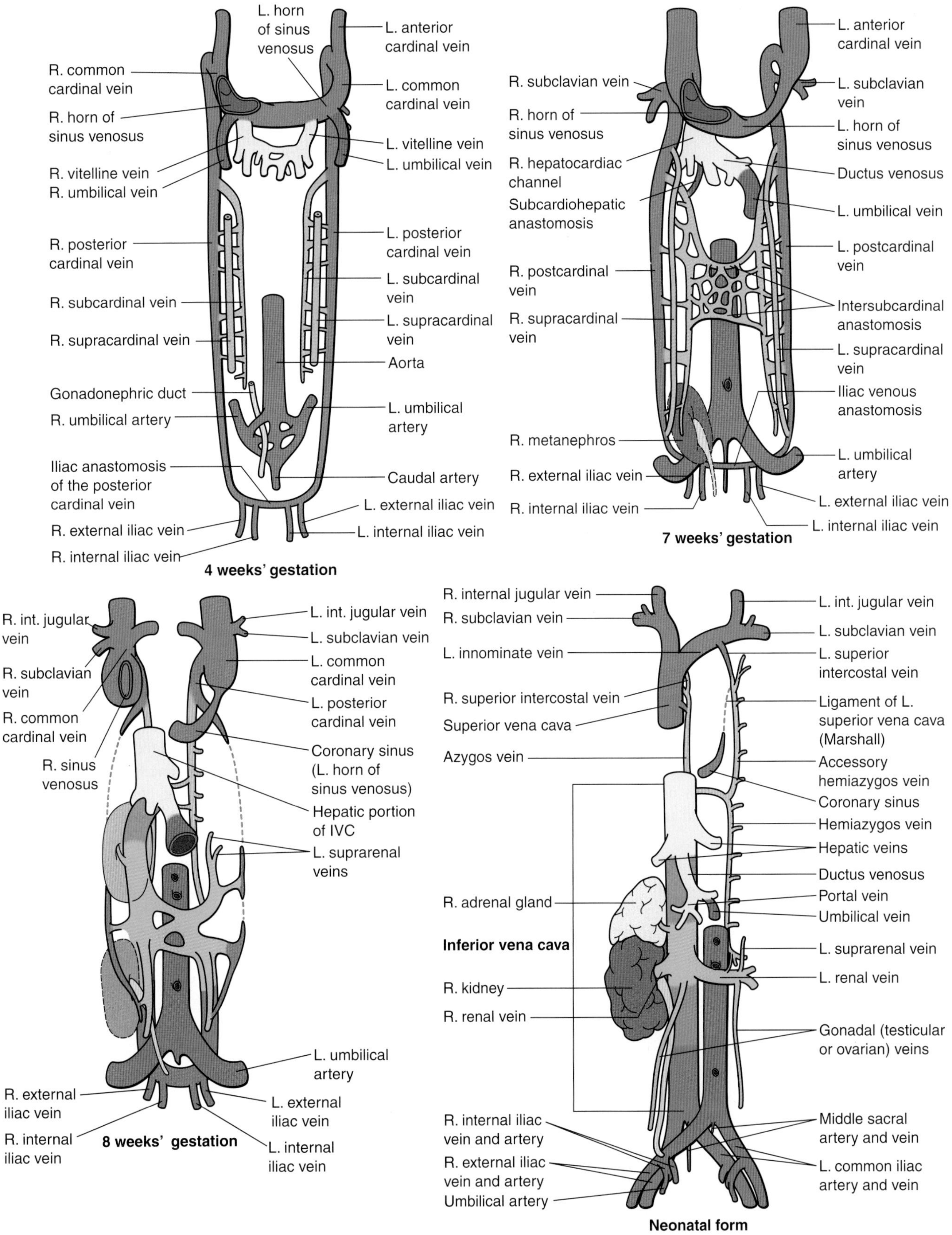

FIGURE 9.68 **Embryology of systemic veins.**

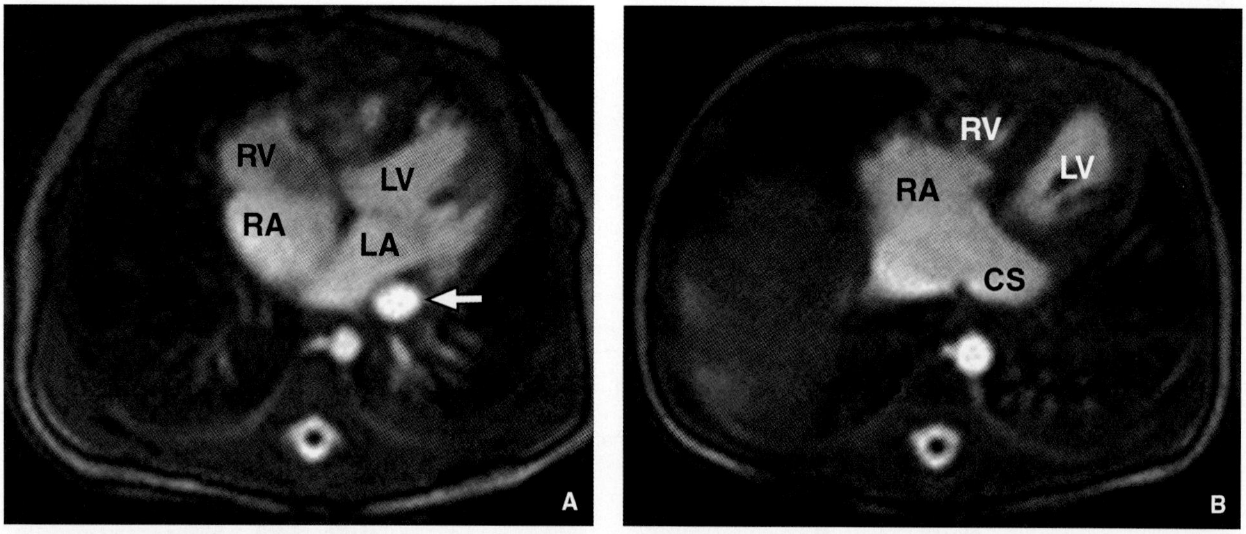

FIGURE 9.69 **Persistent left superior vena cava.** Axial bright blood magnetic resonance images **(A, B)** show persistent left superior vena cava (*arrow*) draining into the right atrium (*RA*) via a dilated coronary sinus (*CS*). *LA*, left atrium; *LV*, left ventricle; *RV*, right ventricle.

Partial Anomalous Pulmonary Veins

In partial anomalous pulmonary venous return (PAPVR), one or more pulmonary veins return to the systemic veins rather than the left atrium (Fig. 9.70). The most common type of PAPVR is anomalous drainage of the right upper lobe pulmonary vein to the SVC (Fig. 9.71). This type of anomalous drainage is associated with a sinus venosus septal defect in a high percentage of cases. Left upper lobe pulmonary venous connection to the left innominate vein is also a relatively common type of PAPVR. It is frequently an incidental finding in pediatric patients investigated for other reasons.[71] Left upper lobe pulmonary venous connection to the left innominate vein typically does not result in a large left-to-right shunt. Scimitar syndrome is associated with PAPVR from the right lung to the IVC and is discussed in the great vessel chapter (Chapter 10).

Chest radiography in PAPVR is typically normal if there is not a large left-to-right shunt. If there is an associated sinus venosus septal defect, there may be cardiomegaly and prominent pulmonary vascularity. CTA and MRA with 2D and 3D reformations can easily demonstrate the anatomy of anomalous pulmonary veins. Cardiac MRI can also quantify the shunt fraction, which helps determine whether surgical correction is necessary.

Surgery may be performed when >1 pulmonary vein is anomalous or there is a large left-to-right shunt (>1.5:1). The anomalous pulmonary vein is typically resected from its systemic venous connection and redirected into the left atrium via a baffle or direct anastomosis.[71]

Total Anomalous Pulmonary Veins

In total anomalous pulmonary venous return (TAPVR), all of the pulmonary venous return is anomalously connected to the systemic or portal venous systems. An ASD is obligatory in order for this defect to be compatible with life. TAPVR is commonly seen as part of the heterotaxy malformation. There are four types of TAPVR, which include supracardiac, cardiac, infracardiac, and mixed types[71] (Fig. 9.72).

In supracardiac type of TAPVR, the right pulmonary veins (RPVs) join the left pulmonary veins (LPVs) close to the left atrial appendage. This venous confluence forms an ascending vertical vein, which ascends on the left side of the mediastinum and drains into the left innominate vein, and the blood returns to the right heart via the SVC. There is an obligatory ASD in order for this to be compatible with life. The anomalous pulmonary veins often drain without stenosis (unobstructed) into the left innominate vein. However, obstruction can occur at the level of the left mainstem bronchus. Affected pediatric patients usually present with cyanosis and cardiac failure shortly after birth if there is obstruction. If there is no obstruction, affected patients may present later in childhood or adolescence.

On chest radiography in older children, the enlarged left innominate vein and SVC can be seen as a widened prominent superior mediastinal silhouette and together with an enlarged cardiac silhouette results in an appearance of a snowman (Fig. 9.73).[71] In younger children who present with cyanosis and cardiac failure because of obstruction, there may be pulmonary venous congestion seen. CTA and MRA can easily depict the course of the obstructed or non-obstructed anomalous pulmonary veins and the enlarged right heart chambers from the large left-to-right shunt if there is no obstruction to venous flow.

In the infracardiac type of TAPVR, the LPVs and RPVs typically join posterior to the left atrium very close to their normal drainage position. However, rather than emptying into the left atrium, they form a descending vertical vein, which crosses the diaphragm and empties into an abdominal vein, usually the portal vein or a hepatic vein. The descending vertical vein typically is obstructed at its diaphragmatic hiatus and marked pulmonary venous congestion results.[71] Children with infracardiac TAPVR also present with cyanosis and respiratory distress.

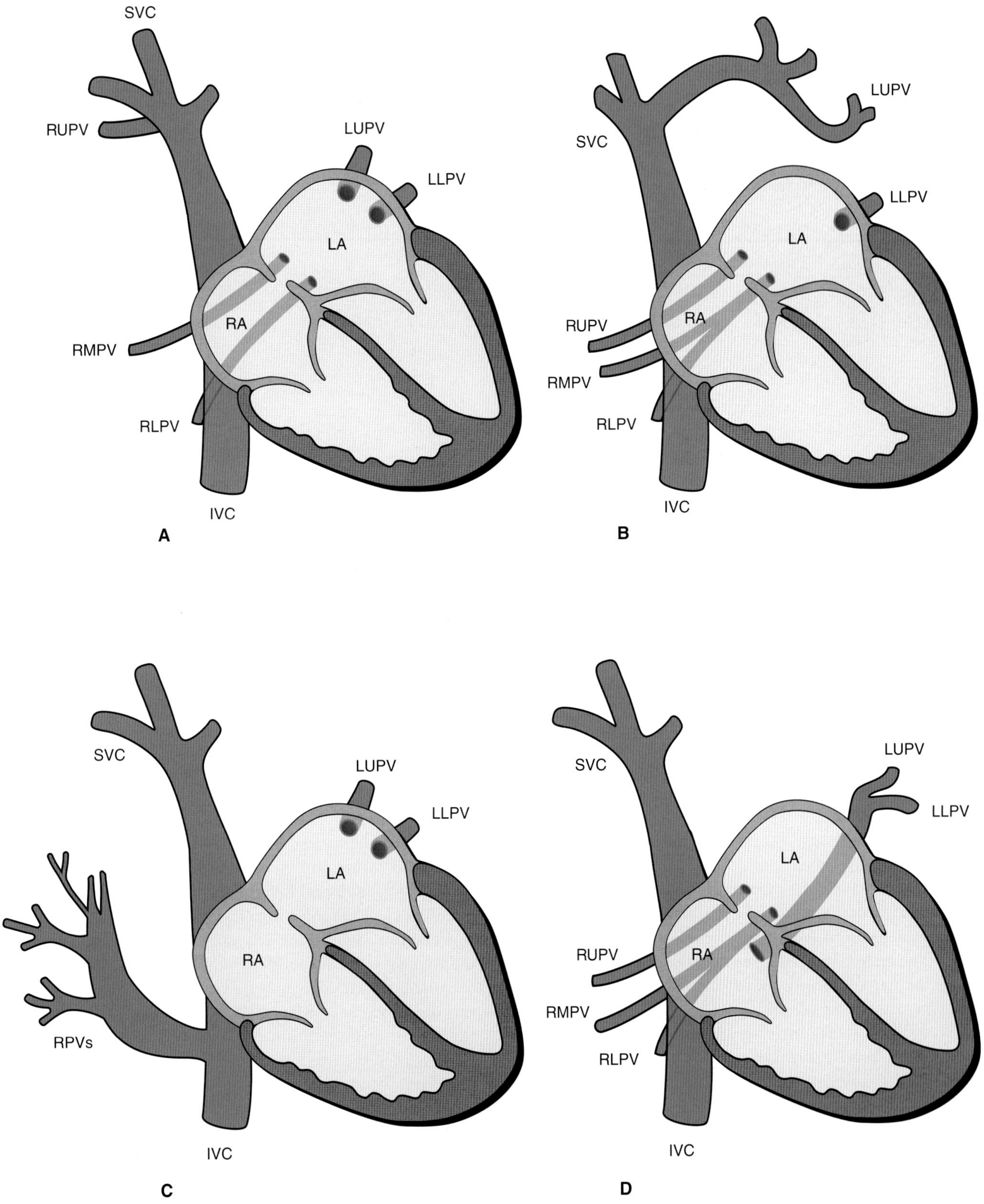

FIGURE 9.70 **Diagram of several different types of partial anomalous pulmonary venous return. A:** Drainage of the right upper pulmonary vein (*RUPV*) to the superior vena cava (*SVC*). **B:** Drainage of the left upper pulmonary vein (*LUPV*) via a vertical vein to the innominate vein. **C:** Drainage of the right pulmonary veins (*RPVs*) to the inferior vena cava (*IVC*). This is the scimitar syndrome. **D:** Drainage of the left upper pulmonary vein (*LUPV*) and left lower pulmonary vein (*LLPV*) into the coronary sinus. *IVC*, inferior vena cava; *LA*, left atrium; *LPV*, left pulmonary vein; *RA*, right atrium; *RLPV*, right lower pulmonary vein; *RMPV*, right middle pulmonary vein.

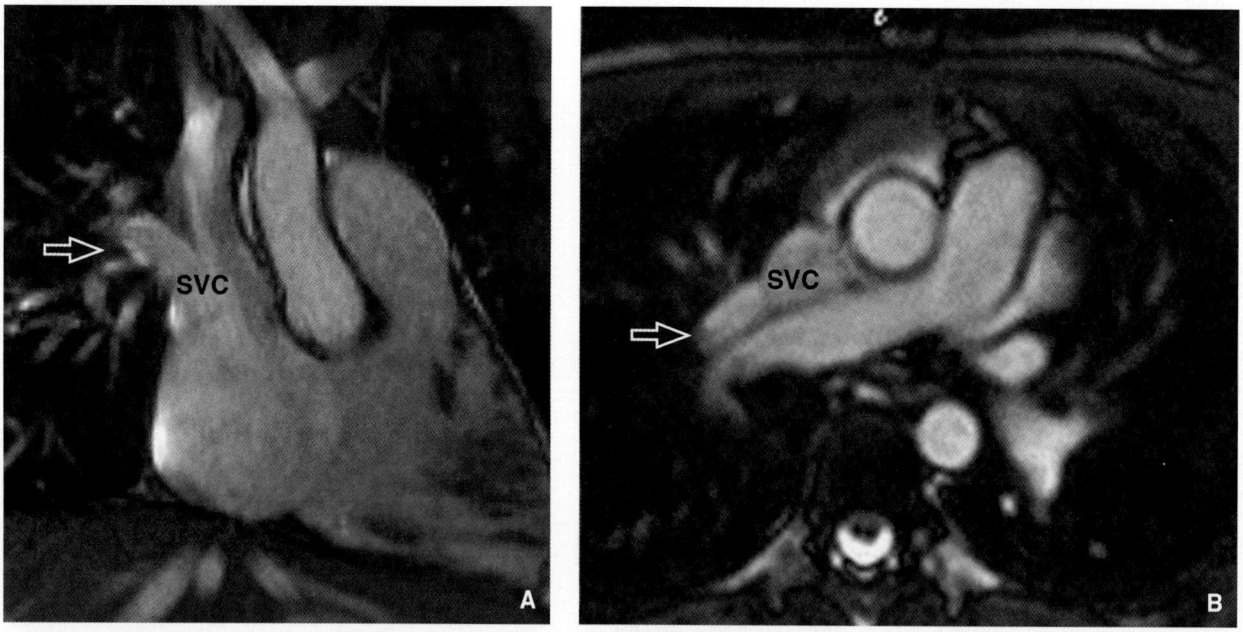

FIGURE 9.71 **Right upper lobe partial anomalous pulmonary venous return.** Coronal oblique **(A)** and axial **(B)** bright blood magnetic resonance images show an anomalous right upper lobe pulmonary vein (*arrows*) draining into superior vena cava (*SVC*).

Chest radiography demonstrates marked septal thickening without cardiac enlargement, which may erroneously result in a diagnosis of pulmonary parenchymal disease (Fig. 9.74A). CTA and MRA demonstrate the infracardiac course of the vertical vein and the degree of obstruction and upstream pulmonary venous distention (Fig. 9.74B). When performing a CTA or MRA in an infant with a potential infracardiac type of TAPVR, it is important to include the liver in order to adequately evaluate the intra-abdominal venous course.

The cardiac-type TAPVR occurs when the pulmonary veins drain anomalously directly into the right atrium via the coronary sinus.[71] This type of anomalous pulmonary venous drainage is usually well assessed on echo and rarely requires CTA or MRA assessment.

In mixed TAPVR, the pulmonary venous return is a combination of cardiac, supracardiac, or infracardiac connections.

Surgical repair of TAPVR involves closure of the ASD, ligation of the vertical vein, and creating a wide neoanastomosis of the pulmonary veins with the left atrium or left atrial appendage. The most common postsurgical complication is pulmonary venous obstruction at the anastomosis.[72] The sutureless repair, introduced in 1998, allows for minimal suturing of the anomalous pulmonary vein insertion and is associated with decreased postoperative pulmonary venous stenosis.[72]

Cor Triatriatum

Cor triatriatum is a congenital anomaly resulting in a heart with three atria (tri atria). Classically, this occurs in the left atrium (cor triatriatum sinister) as a result of failure to incorporate the common pulmonary vein.[73] This leads to an accessory left atrial chamber that receives all the pulmonary veins and lies posterior to the main left atrial chamber. These two chambers communicate through several small septations in the thin membrane separating the two chambers. There are varying degrees of obstruction/communication between the two chambers. Occasionally, there is no communication between the two left atria. Instead, the accessory left atrium receives all the pulmonary veins and connects with the right atrium either directly or indirectly via a vertical vein into the left innominate vein similar to supracardiac TAPVR.[73,74] The majority of affected pediatric patients present in the first few years of life with failure to thrive or respiratory symptoms frequently attributed to underlying pulmonary disease.

Chest radiography reveals pulmonary venous congestion and signs of left atrial enlargement, which is characterized by splayed carina and elevated left main stem bronchus on frontal projection and bulging of the posterior cardiac margin on the lateral projection (Fig. 9.75).[73,74]

Echo can identify the accessory left atrium receiving the pulmonary veins and obstructing membrane in most cases. CTA and cardiac MRI may be performed in cases in which the diagnosis is unclear. CTA and cardiac MRI can show the course of the pulmonary veins and degree of obstruction between the two left atrial chambers (Fig. 9.76). CT can also demonstrate the pulmonary parenchymal ground-glass opacity resulting from venous congestion and edema.

The current management of cor triatriatum involves surgical resection of the obstructing membrane between the two left atrial chambers.

Cardiac Malpositions and Anomalies of Atrial and Visceral Situs

The term situs refers to the position of the organs within the body. Normal position is termed situs solitus. A direct mirror image appearance to the organ arrangement about the left/right

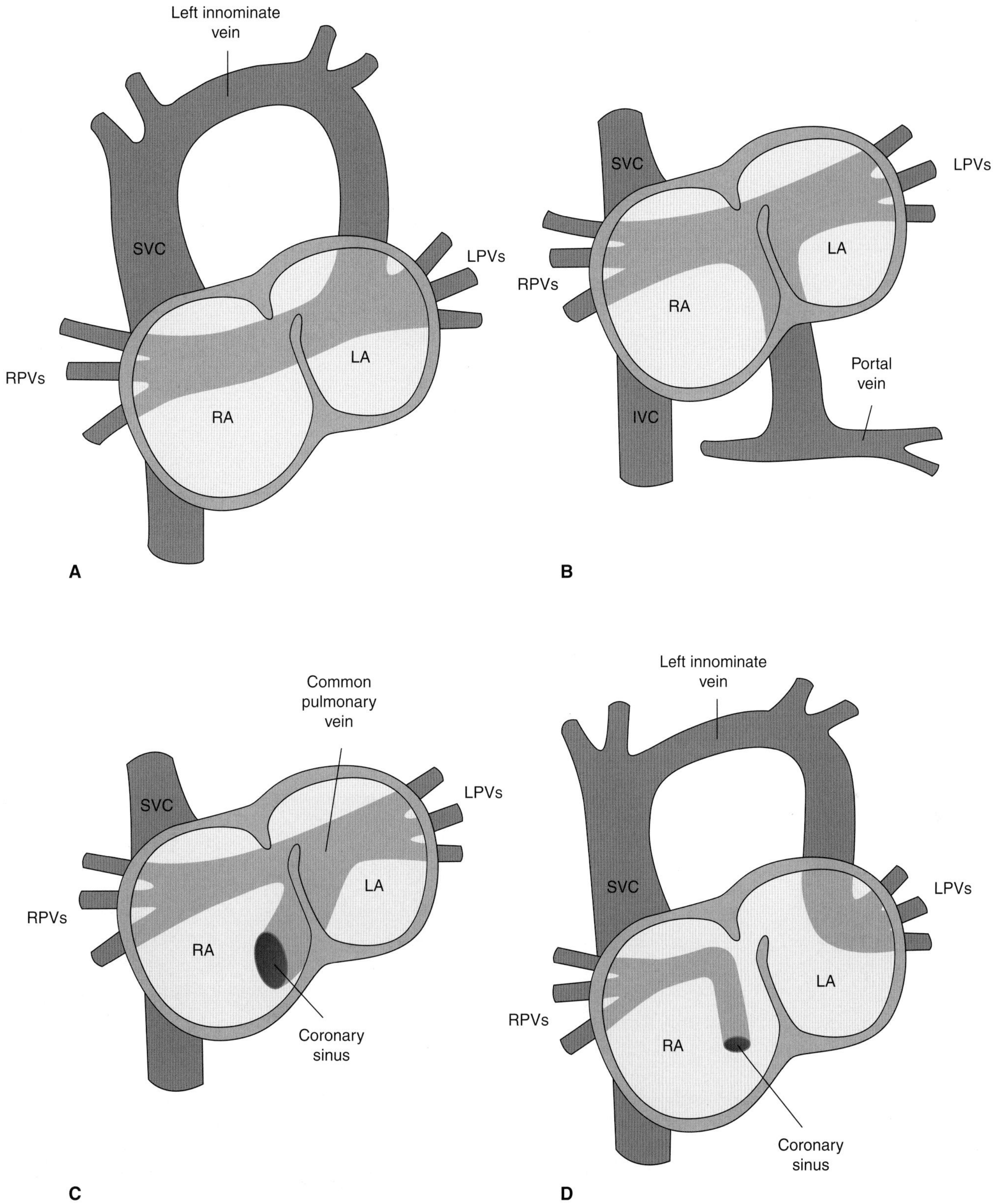

FIGURE 9.72 **Diagram depicting the various types of total anomalous pulmonary venous return.** For each type, there is an atrial communication enabling blood to reach the left side of the heart. **A:** Supracardiac—the RPVs and LPVs join in a confluence posterior to the left atrium and are connected via an ascending vertical vein to the innominate vein, which drains to the superior vena cava (*SVC*). **B:** Infracardiac: the confluence of pulmonary veins drains via a descending vertical vein to the portal venous system. **C:** Cardiac: the right and LPVs drain into the coronary sinus. **D:** Mixed pattern: the diagram depicts anomalous supracardiac pulmonary venous return of the LPVs via an ascending vertical vein to the innominate vein, and anomalous cardiac pulmonary venous return of the RPVs to the coronary sinus. *LA*, left atrium; *LPVs*, left pulmonary veins; *RA*, right atrium; *RPVs*, right pulmonary veins.

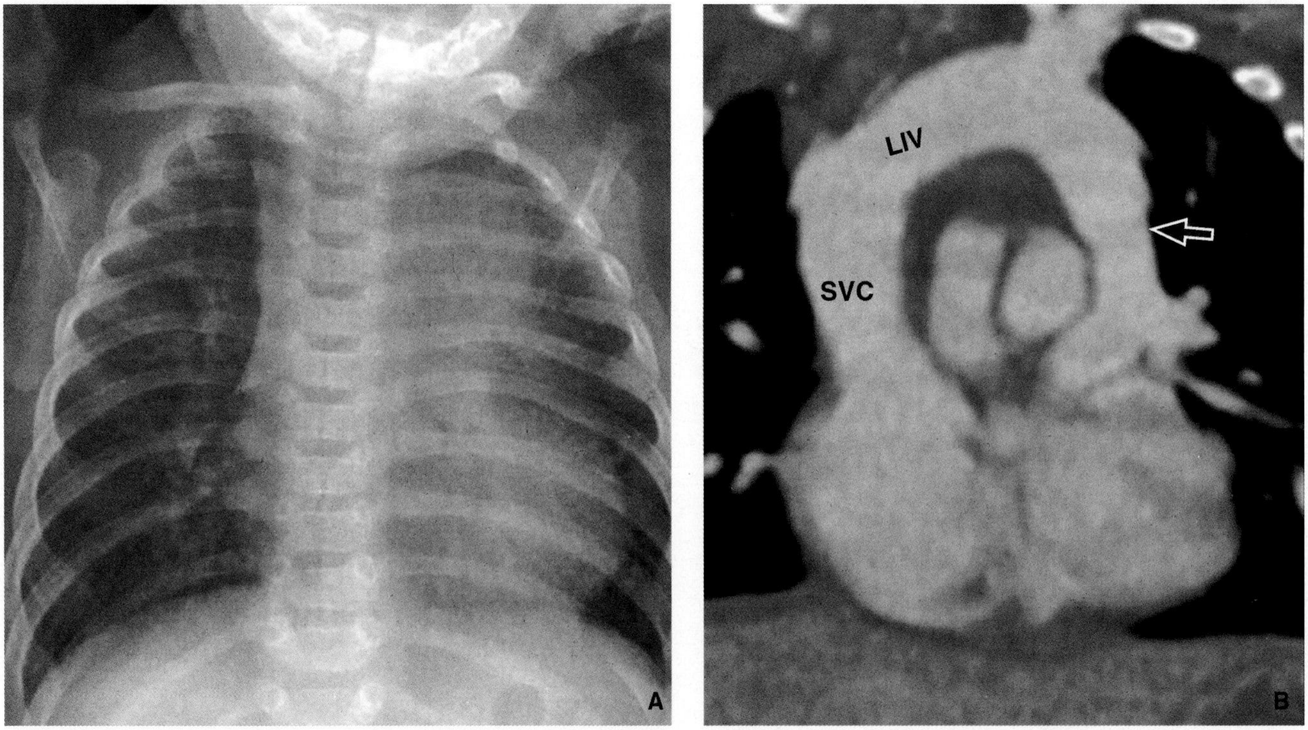

FIGURE 9.73 **Supracardiac type total anomalous pulmonary venous return.** Frontal chest radiograph **(A)** shows cardiomegaly and enlarged superior mediastinal silhouette. These radiographic findings are known as snowman sign which refers to the configuration of the heart and superior mediastinal borders resembling a snowman. **B:** Coronal reformatted enhanced CT image demonstrates total anomalous pulmonary venous return (*arrow*) into the left innominate vein (*LIV*). *SVC*, superior vena cava.

axis is termed situs inversus. Disorders of situs with arrangements, which are neither solitus nor inversus, are termed heterotaxy.[75] The terms situs ambiguous, left-sided isomerism and polysplenia syndrome, or right-sided isomerism and asplenia are synonymous with heterotaxy and are frequently used interchangeably. Unlike situs solitus and situs inversus totalis, heterotaxy disorders are associated with complex and sometimes quite unusual cardiovascular arrangements.[76,77]

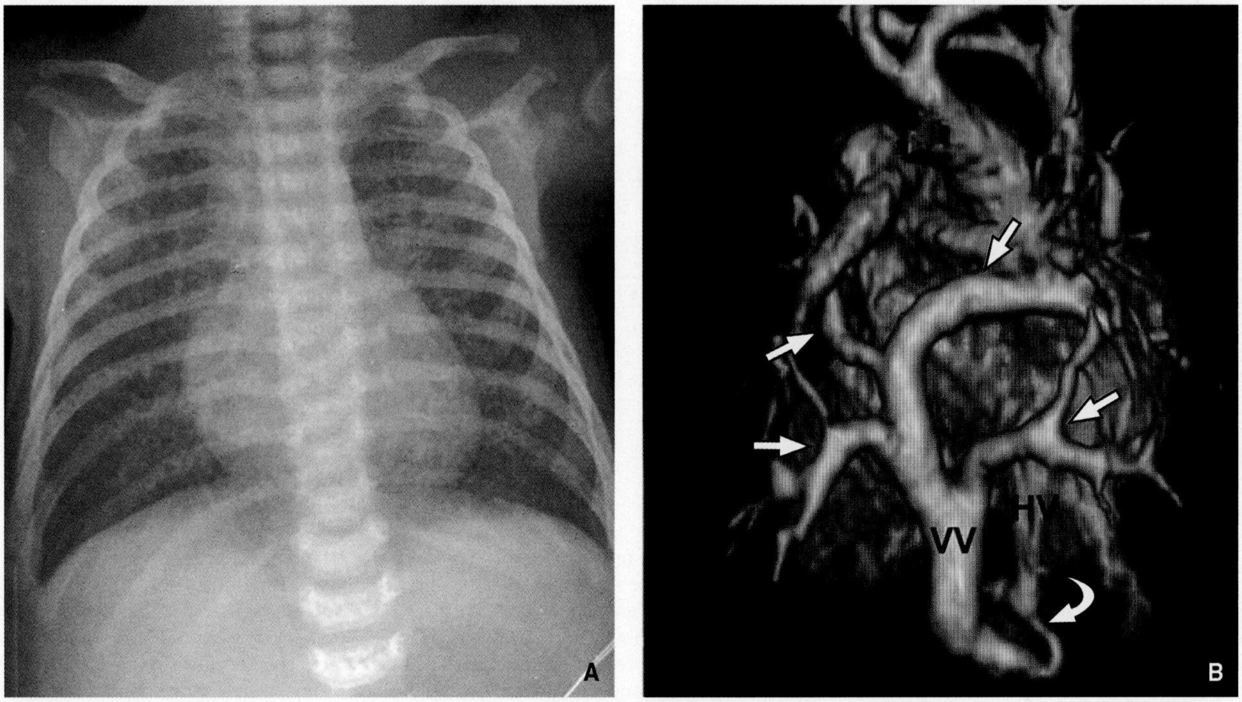

FIGURE 9.74 **Infracardiac total anomalous pulmonary venous return.** Frontal chest radiograph **(A)** shows interstitial edema with normal-sized heart. **B:** Three-dimensional volume-rendered enhanced CT image demonstrates infracardiac type of total anomalous pulmonary venous return. All pulmonary veins (*arrows*) are joined in a pulmonary venous confluence. Descending vertical vein (*VV*) drains into the left hepatic vein (*HV*). Also noted is marked narrowing (*curved arrow*) at the insertion of the VV into the left HV.

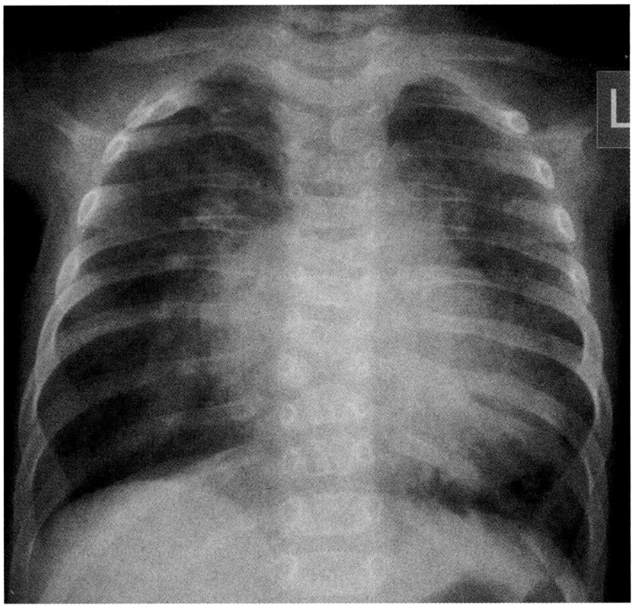

FIGURE 9.75 **Cor triatriatum.** Frontal chest radiograph demonstrates pulmonary venous congestion and cardiomegaly.

Situs is determined very early in embryologic life between the 4th and 7th weeks of embryologic development and is dependent on normal function of the cilia. Interference with normal cilial motion during this embryologic period may result in situs anomalies.[77]

Situs Inversus

In situs inversus totalis, the position of all the organ systems is completely reversed about the left–right axis of the body. In this condition, the apex of the heart, stomach, and spleen are located on the right, and the liver and IVC are located on the left. The constellation of findings of situs inversus, nasal polyposis with chronic sinusitis, and bronchiectasis is termed Kartagener syndrome, which is caused by immotile cilia.[76,77] The classic presentation of Kartagener syndrome is with recurrent infections and purulent cough related to bronchiectasis.

Chest radiography demonstrates the cardiac apex pointing to the right (dextrocardia) and a right-sided stomach bubble. In the setting of Kartagener syndrome, lower lobe bronchiectasis and peribronchial thickening may also be visible. CT typically shows the presence of right-sided branching of left bronchial tree, left-sided branching of right bronchial tree, bronchiectasis, peribronchial thickening, and peripheral mucus plugging (Fig. 9.77). MRI does not usually have a role to play in the evaluation of situs inversus but may detect it incidentally when performed for other reasons.

Pediatric patients with situs inversus without Kartagener disease have a normal life expectancy without medical or surgical treatment necessary.[76,77] The majority of children with Kartagener syndrome are managed medically for their recurrent infections.

Left-Sided Isomerism

Isomerism means mirror image arrangement. In left-sided isomerism, the tracheobronchial tree, segmental anatomy of the lungs, and atrial appendages all demonstrate a bilateral left-sided arrangement. Affected patients generally have a liver in a midline position and multiple small spleens in the right upper quadrant (polysplenia) (Fig. 9.78). For this reason, left-sided isomerism is often referred to as polysplenia syndrome.[78,79] Intracardiac anomalies are common and include atrial and ventricular septal defects and balanced AVSDs. Systemic and pulmonary venous anomalies are also common in left-sided isomerism, including left-sided SVC, interrupted IVC with azygos continuation and TAPVR or PAPVR.[8,79] In addition, GI anomalies including anomalies of rotation (in 40% to 90%) and biliary atresia (10% to 20%) are

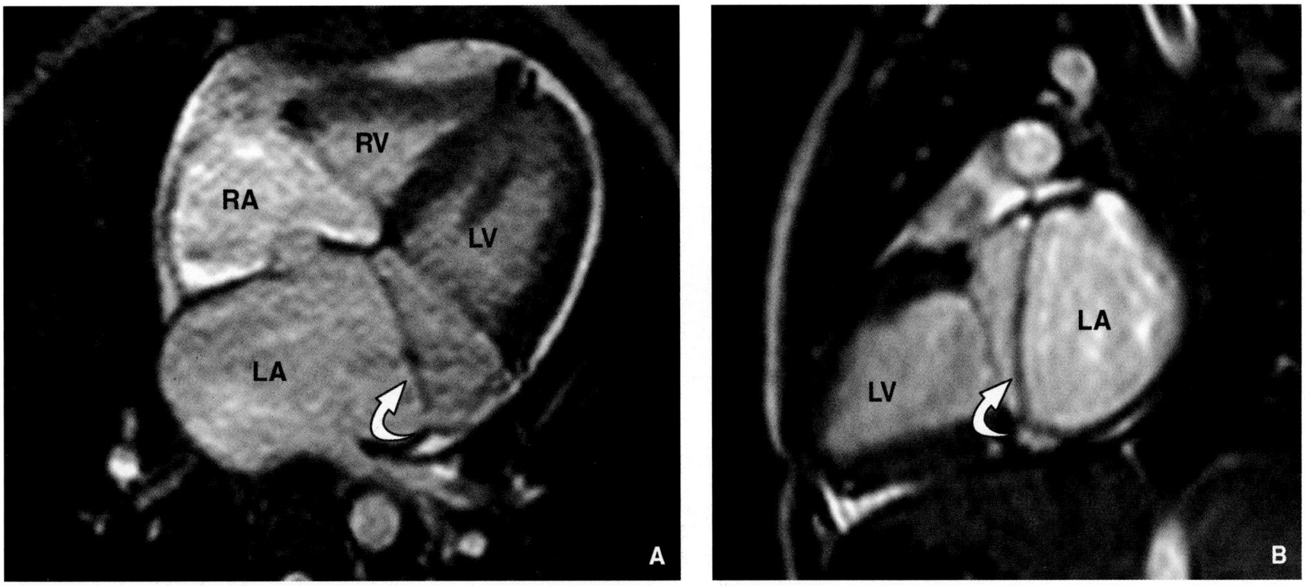

FIGURE 9.76 **Cor triatriatum.** Bright blood magnetic resonance images in four-chamber plane **(A)** and two-chamber plane **(B)** show obstructing septum (*curved arrows*) in the left atrium with enlarged proximal left atrial (*LA*) chamber. *LV*, left ventricle; *RA*, right atrium; *RV*, right ventricle.

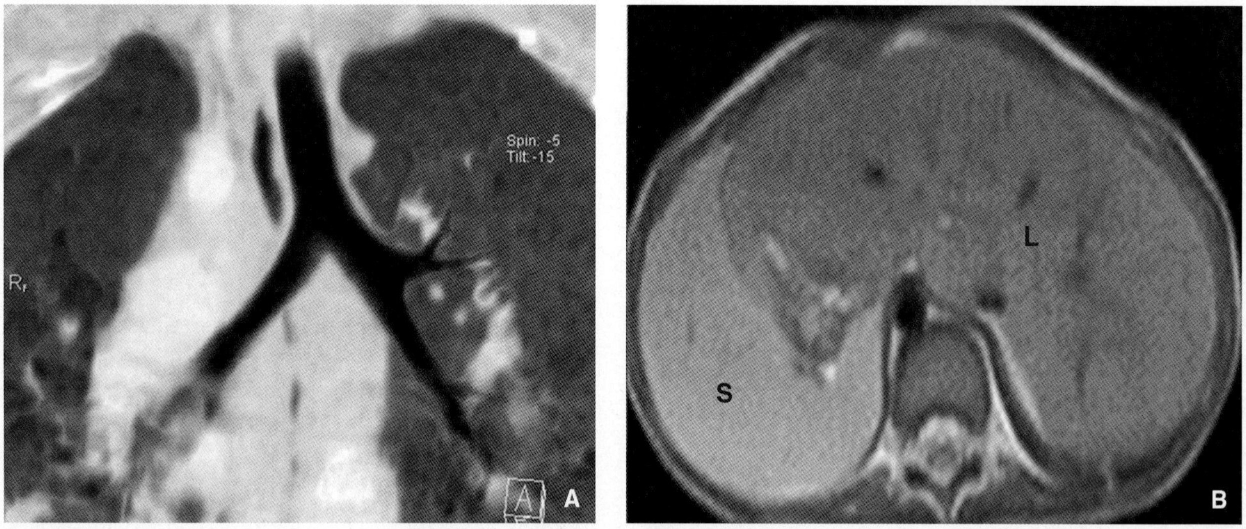

FIGURE 9.77 **Situs inversus. A:** Coronal minimum intensity projection (MinIP) CT image shows right-sided branching of the bronchial tree in the left lung and left-sided branching of the bronchial tree in the right lung. **B:** Axial MR image demonstrates the liver (*L*) on the left side and the spleen (*S*) in the right side of the abdomen.

also present.[80,81] Clinical presentation is usually with cyanosis or cardiac failure at or shortly after birth related to the severity of anomalous pulmonary venous return or intracardiac anomalies.

Chest radiography may demonstrate cardiomegaly and pulmonary vascular congestion depending on the cardiovascular anomalies. CTA provides excellent definition of the anatomy of anomalous pulmonary venous return and systemic venous anomalies. Cardiac MRI can evaluate ventricular function and size in the evaluation for candidacy for biventricular repair as well as delineating the course of the extracardiac systemic and pulmonary vascularity. Cardiac CTA and MRI both can demonstrate the isomerism of the tracheobronchial tree, with bilateral left-sided bronchi, which course under the accompanying pulmonary artery (hyparterial bronchi) and the abnormal morphology of the atrial appendages with both demonstrating a left appendage (long finger-like projection). Upper GI may demonstrate malrotation, and ultrasound of the abdomen may be performed in cases of suspected biliary atresia where a normal gallbladder is absent.

Complex surgical repairs involving establishing normal pulmonary venous drainage and either a biventricular repair or single ventricle repair of the complex cardiac anomalies. In addition, despite the presence of multiple small spleens, affected pediatric patients may be immunocompromised and require antibiotic prophylaxis.

Right-Sided Isomerism

In right-sided isomerism, there is a mirror image appearance with bilateral right-sided branching of the tracheobronchial tree, trilobed lungs (both right and left lungs have middle lobes), and bilateral right atrial appendage morphology.[78,79] Affected pediatric patients usually have no identifiable splenic tissue ("asplenia") and a midline liver (Fig. 9.79). Complex intracardiac anomalies are usually present and include AVSDs and DORV. Systemic and pulmonary venous anomalies are

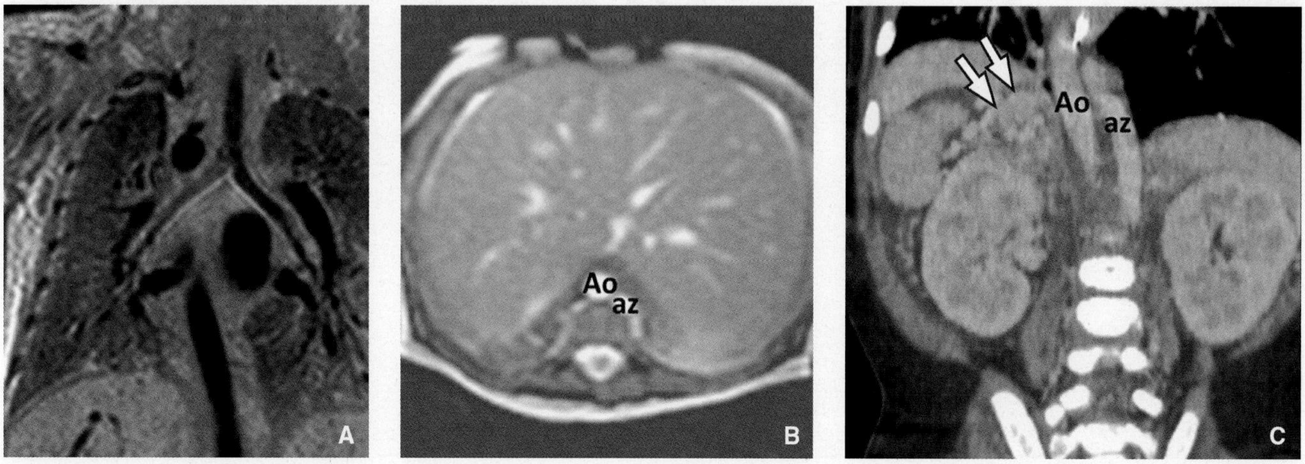

FIGURE 9.78 **Left-sided isomerism.** Coronal oblique black blood magnetic resonance (MR) image **(A)** shows bilateral left-sided bronchial branching in both lungs. Axial bright blood MR image **(B)** demonstrates azygos continuation (*az*) of inferior vena cava (IVC) and a midline liver. Coronal reformatted enhanced CT image **(C)** shows right-sided polysplenia (*arrows*) and azygos continuation of IVC. *Ao*, aorta.

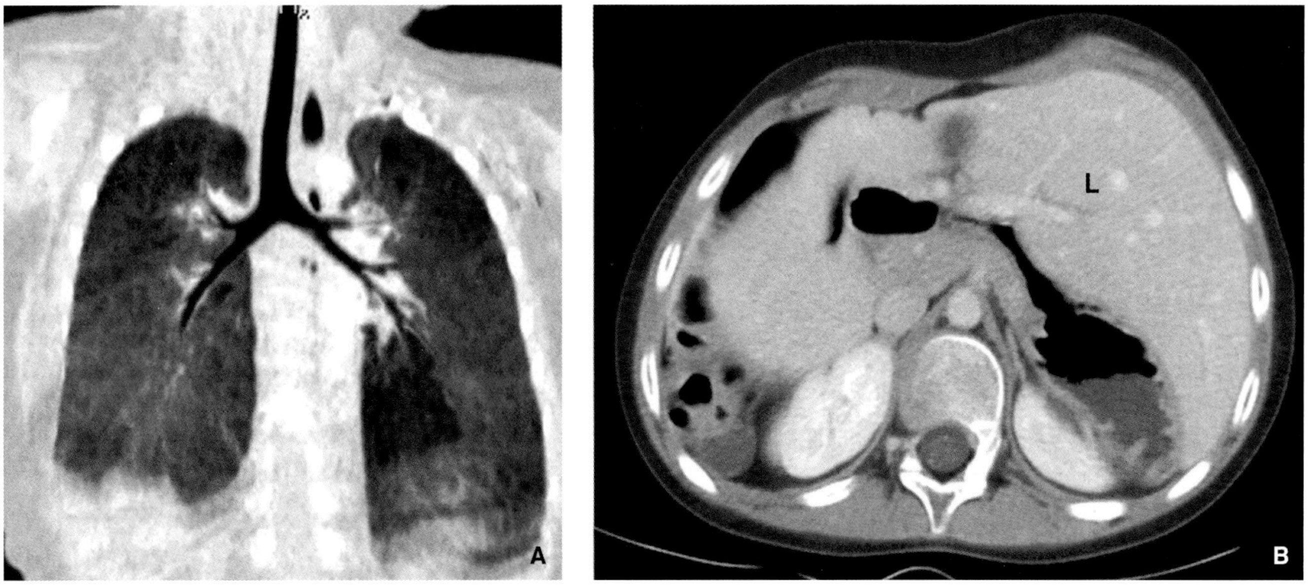

FIGURE 9.79 **Right-sided isomerism.** Oblique coronal minimum intensity projection (MinIP) CT image **(A)** shows bilateral right-sided branching of the tracheobronchial tree. Axial enhanced CT image **(B)** demonstrates left sided liver (*L*) and asplenia.

more commonly encountered in left-sided isomerism. GI malrotation is present in 40% to 90%. Affected pediatric patients usually present with cyanosis or cardiac failure, which develops shortly after birth.

Chest radiography may demonstrate cardiomegaly and pulmonary vascular congestion related to the underlying complex congenital cardiac anomalies. The stomach bubble may either be left- or right-sided. The liver silhouette appears midline. CTA may be helpful in the evaluation of associated cardiovascular anomalies including aortic hypoplasia/atresia, pulmonary atresia, or MAPCAs. Cardiac MRI is used to delineate the size of ventricles for possible biventricular repair.[25] Both CTA and cardiac MRI demonstrate the isomerism of the tracheobronchial tree, with bilateral right-sided bronchi, which course over both branch pulmonary arteries (epiarterial bronchi) and bilateral right-sided atrial appendages (short broad-based origins). Upper GI examination is usually required to evaluate for possible concomitant malrotation. A biventricular repair or staged single ventricle palliation are usually required to correct the cardiac anomalies.

Situs Ambiguus

Occasionally, pediatric patients demonstrate mixed features and therefore do not fit perfectly into a distinct category of solitus, inversus, or right- or left-sided isomerism, and these are simply termed situs ambiguus.[75,79]

Congenital Pericardial Malformation

Congenital Absence of the Pericardium

Congenital absence of the pericardium is an extremely rare entity, which can vary from partial pericardial absence to complete absence. Partial absence of the left-sided pericardium is the most common form.[82] Affected pediatric patients are usually asymptomatic; however, occasional chest pain may occur.

Chest radiography is commonly normal in patients with partial pericardial absence, but in patients with complete absence, the cardiac silhouette is commonly rotated to the right, the convexities for the aortic knuckle and MPA convexities are unusually prominent and lung interposed between the inferior cardiac border, and the left hemidiaphragm may be visible.[82] On CTA and MRI, the absence of the pericardium and pericardial fat may be directly visualized, and lung tissue may invaginate between the spaces usually occupied by pericardial fat.[82]

Most pediatric patients with congenital absence of the pericardium require no treatment. However, surgical treatment may be required for complications such as herniation and strangulation of the left atrial appendage or part of the left ventricular myocardium.[82]

ACQUIRED CARDIAC DISORDERS

Cardiomyopathies

Cardiomyopathies are primary diseases of the myocardium. They are a diverse group of diseases that vary considerably in their underlying etiology, presentation, and natural history. Hypertrophic cardiomyopathy, dilated cardiomyopathy, restrictive cardiomyopathy and arrhythmogenic right ventricular dysplasia (ARVD), and left ventricular noncompaction are five main cardiomyopathies encountered in the pediatric population and discussed in this section.[83]

Hypertrophic Cardiomyopathy

Hypertrophic cardiomyopathy (idiopathic hypertrophic cardiomyopathy) is characterized by a thickened left ventricular wall in the absence of other cardiac or systemic processes that may result in left ventricular hypertrophy such as aortic stenosis, coarctation of the aorta, or systemic hypertension.[83,84] The left ventricular wall is thickened, characteristically asymmetrically, with predominant involvement of a left ventricular segment such as the left ventricular apex, left ventricular free wall, or basal portion of the interventricular septum (Fig. 9.80). Histologic changes may include disorganized myocytes, patchy fibrosis, and expanded extracellular matrix.[83] There are a number of genetic mutations associated with hypertrophic cardiomyopathy (including beta-myosin heavy chain and myosin-binding protein C) with an autosomal dominant inheritance pattern.[83,84]

Clinically, affected pediatric patients with hypertrophic cardiomyopathy may present with myocardial ischemia or ventricular tachyarrhythmias during exercise. The severity of symptoms shows good agreement with the degree of left ventricular obstruction and extent of fibrosis.

The majority of pediatric patients with hypertrophic cardiomyopathy may have a normal heart appearance on chest radiographs initially, although cardiomegaly may become evident with increasing age. Echo is the primary imaging modality used in identifying hypertrophic cardiomyopathy. CTA usually has no diagnostic role in hypertrophic cardiomyopathy. Pediatric patients with suspected or genotype-positive hypertrophic cardiomyopathy are usually referred for further evaluation with cardiac MRI. Cardiac MRI has a number of useful applications in evaluating hypertrophic cardiomyopathy; including assessment of left ventricular myocardial morphology; left ventricular size and function; left ventricular myocardial mass; quantification of the severity of left ventricular obstruction; evaluation for systolic anterior motion of the mitral valve, which may increase left ventricular outflow obstruction; and evaluate for fibrosis with myocardial delayed enhancement (Fig. 9.80C).[83] Affected pediatric patients often undergo serial MRIs in order to assess progression or response to therapy. In addition, MRI may be used to screen family members for features of hypertrophic cardiomyopathy and screen for other causes of left ventricular hypertrophy including aortic stenosis and coarctation in borderline cases.

Medical management with multiple drugs used for heart failure treatment including beta-blockers, ace inhibitors, and angiotensin receptor blockers are often used initially. Prophylactic

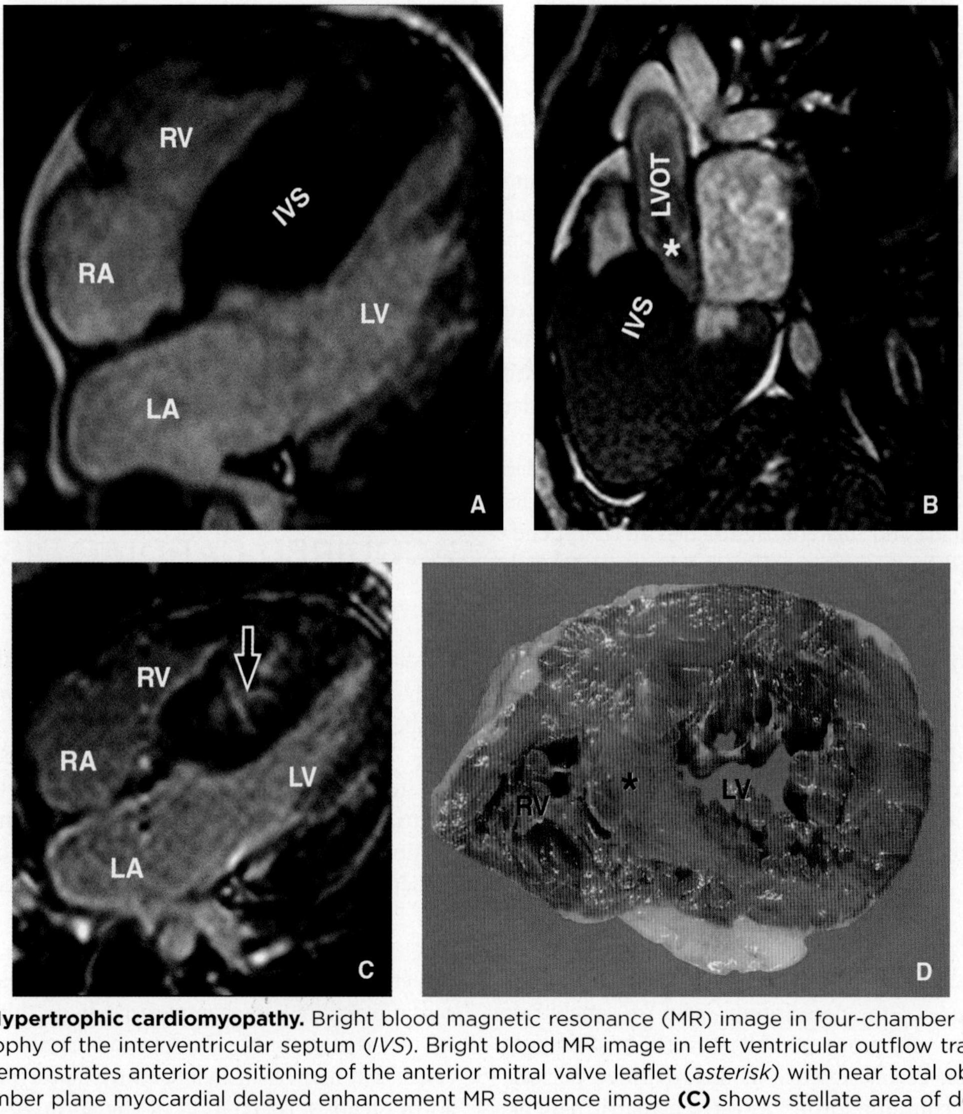

FIGURE 9.80 **Hypertrophic cardiomyopathy.** Bright blood magnetic resonance (MR) image in four-chamber plane **(A)** shows marked hypertrophy of the interventricular septum (*IVS*). Bright blood MR image in left ventricular outflow tract (*LVOT*) plane **(B)** in systole demonstrates anterior positioning of the anterior mitral valve leaflet (*asterisk*) with near total obstruction of the LVOT. Four-chamber plane myocardial delayed enhancement MR sequence image **(C)** shows stellate area of delayed enhancement in the midmyocardium (*arrow*). Explant specimen of a 12-year-old boy with hypertrophic cardiomyopathy image **(D)** demonstrates severe left ventricular hypertrophy, most pronounced in the interventricular septum (*asterisk*). *LA*, left atrium; *LV*, left ventricle; *RA*, right atrium; *RV*, right ventricle.

implantable cardioverter defibrillators may be placed in high-risk pediatric patients to avoid life-threatening ventricular arrhythmias and restore sinus rhythm by delivering a defibrillating shock.[83,84] Septal myomectomy may be used to resect the obstructing tissues in the left ventricular outflow tract.[84]

Dilated Cardiomyopathy

Dilated cardiomyopathy is characterized by a poorly functioning and dilated LV. Infectious, inflammatory, ischemic, toxic, and hereditary factors have been associated with the development of dilated cardiomyopathy in pediatric population, although in the majority of cases, the cause remains unidentified.[83] Familial dilated cardiomyopathy is inherited as an autosomal dominant trait or occasionally as an X-linked trait in males, although a common gene has not been found. At the cellular level, it is characterized by a loss and decreased regenerative capacity of myocytes with an increased extracellular matrix composed of poorly cross-linked collagen.[83] These processes result in wall thinning, ventricular dilatation, and fibrosis.

Clinically, affected pediatric patients present with symptoms and signs of heart failure, which often correlates well with underlying deteriorating myocardial dysfunction. Occasionally, an inflammatory etiology such as a previous viral infection resulting in myocarditis may be elicited.

On chest radiography, there is usually moderate to severe cardiac enlargement with a variable degree of pulmonary edema. Cardiac MRI can provide accurate quantification of left ventricular size and function (Fig. 9.81) and assess the volume of fibrosis using late gadolinium enhancement techniques. The left ventricular myocardium usually appears thinned, and left ventricular aneurysms may be present. Serial cardiac MRIs can be used to monitor response to medical management and guide prognosis. There is currently no diagnostic role for CTA in evaluating dilated cardiomyopathy in the pediatric population.

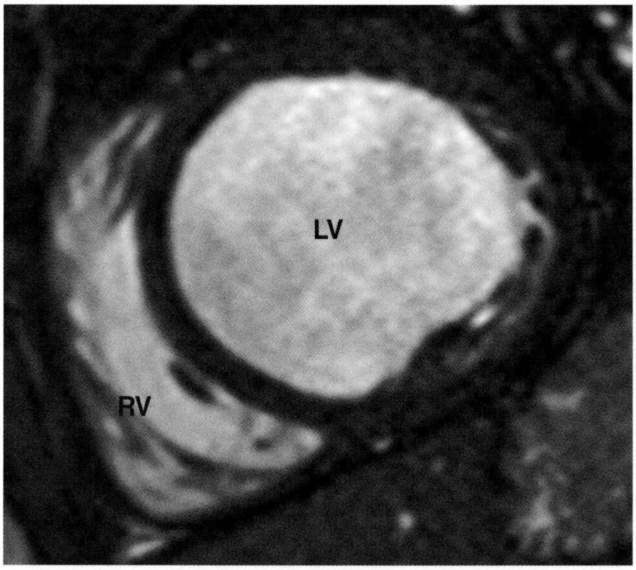

FIGURE 9.81 **Dilated cardiomyopathy.** Bright blood magnetic resonance image in short-axis plane shows severely dilated left ventricular (*LV*) chamber. *RV*, right ventricle.

Medical treatments to improve myocardial function and decrease left ventricular afterload are the mainstay of treatment. Cardiac transplantation is considered if short-term survival is considered unlikely or in patients unresponsive to medical management. Left ventricular assist devices are frequently used as a bridge to cardiac transplantation in pediatric patients with severely impaired cardiac function.[83]

Restrictive Cardiomyopathy

Restrictive cardiomyopathy is the most infrequently encountered cardiomyopathy in the pediatric population and is characterized by restricted left and right ventricular filling and resultant reduced ventricular diastolic volumes.[83,85] There is usually normal ventricular systolic function (i.e., ejection fraction) and normal or mildly hypertrophied myocardial wall. The etiologies include idiopathic (most common), infiltrative myocardial, and endomyocardial conditions including endocardial fibroelastosis (Fig. 9.82), endomyocardial fibrosis (common in tropics), storage disorders, hemochromatosis, and hypereosinophilia syndrome.[85] Pathophysiologically, the cardinal features are hypothesized to be due to either an increased myocardial stiffness with decreased compliance or decreased myocardial relaxation with an end result of increased ventricular pressures.[85] Clinically, the majority of affected pediatric patients have dyspnea with exertion, frequently resulting in an initial misdiagnosis of reactive airway disease.

Chest radiography usually demonstrates cardiomegaly and variable degrees of pulmonary edema. Echo, usually the primary diagnostic test, can demonstrate altered hemodynamics and ventricular appearances. However, cardiac

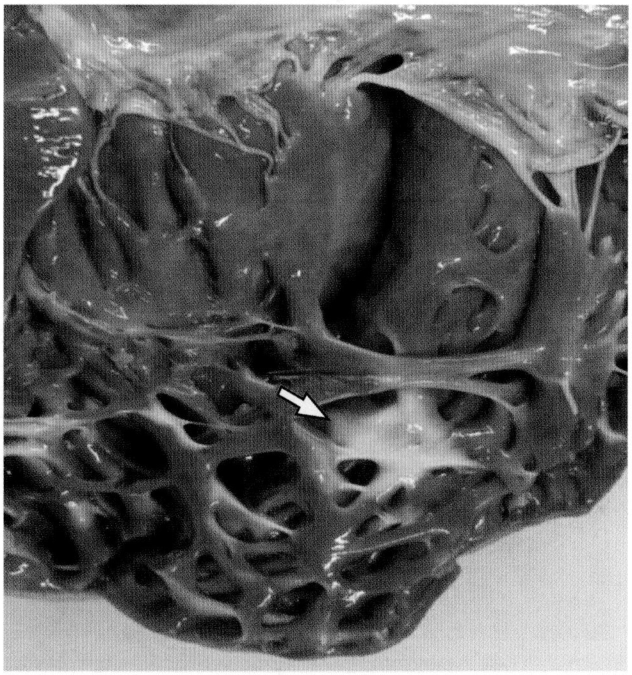

FIGURE 9.82 **Endocardial fibroelastosis.** Gross specimen of cardiac explant demonstrates localized endocardial fibroelastosis appearing as a patch of white fibrous thickening (*arrow*) of the left ventricular endocardium.

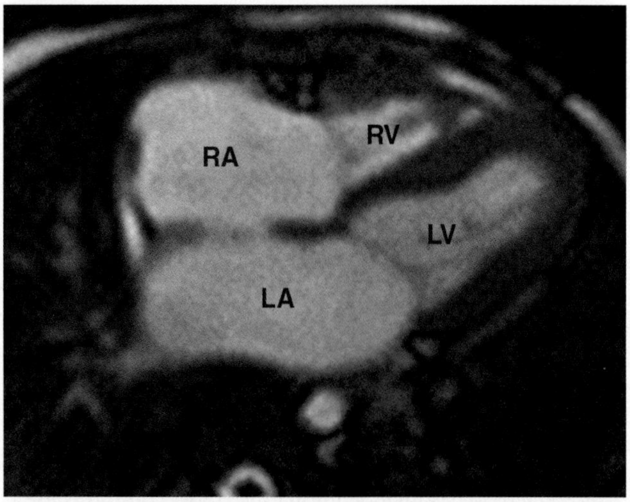

FIGURE 9.83 **Restrictive cardiomyopathy.** Axial bright blood magnetic resonance image shows the relatively small size of the right ventricle (*RV*) and left ventricle (*LV*), with dilatation of the right atrium (*RA*) and left atrium (*LA*).

MRI is frequently requested for differentiating restrictive cardiomyopathy from constrictive pericardial disease. In both restrictive cardiomyopathy and constrictive pericardial disease, the ventricles demonstrate an elongated narrowed appearance with atrial dilatation (Fig. 9.83). In restrictive cardiomyopathy, myopathic changes may be evident, including hypertrophied myocardium, T2 changes in the myocardium representing edema, myocardial or endomyocardial delayed enhancement from infiltrative conditions, and normal septal motion.[86] In restrictive cardiomyopathy, the pericardium is usually normal. In constrictive pericarditis, there is usually pericardial thickening or effusion and paradoxical motion of the interventricular septum in inspiration.[86]

Management of restrictive cardiomyopathy is usually difficult and involves treatments directed at the underlying etiologies such as phlebotomy for iron overload or procedures such as endocardial stripping for endocardial fibroelastosis, in addition to standard heart failure treatments.[83–85] In severe cases, cardiac pacing, left ventricular assist devices, or cardiac transplantation may be considered.[87]

Arrhythmogenic Right Ventricular Dysplasia

ARVD is a genetically inherited cardiomyopathy resulting in structural abnormalities in the RV, including progressive fibrofatty deposition in the right ventricular myocardium. Several genes have been identified that are associated with autosomal dominant inheritance of ARVD. The diagnosis of ARVD is based on a combination of major and minor criteria, using family history in conjunction with ECG, echo, and MRI findings.[88] Clinically, affected children present with ventricular tachycardias, which may be life-threatening. ARVD is reported to be associated with up to 10% of cases of unexpected sudden cardiac death in adolescents and young adults.[88]

Radiographically, ARVD is often occult until it presents as cardiomegaly because of the development of left and right ventricular dilatation in advanced cases. Cardiac MRI is used to screen patients for changes of ARVD, including right ventricular dysfunction, elevated right ventricular indexed volume, right ventricular wall motion abnormalities, fatty deposition, and delayed enhancement (representing fibrosis) in the right ventricular myocardium.[88,89] The evaluation for macroscopic right ventricular fibrofatty change in adolescents and young adults is impaired by the normally very thin right ventricular myocardial free wall[90] (Fig. 9.84). In addition, as it is a progressive condition, macroscopic disease may not be evident in the early stages, and frequently serial MRIs are required.[89] CT currently has no role in the diagnosis of ARVD.

Pediatric patients with a history of ARVD who have had a sustained ventricular tachycardia or near sudden cardiac death event may need placement of an automatic implantable defibrillator. Antiarrhythmogenic agents and ablative therapies aimed at limiting the arrhythmias are usually required.

Left Ventricular Noncompaction

Left ventricular noncompaction is a relatively rare cardiomyopathy that can be diagnosed at any age. It is characterized by deep trabeculations ("noncompaction") in the subendocardial

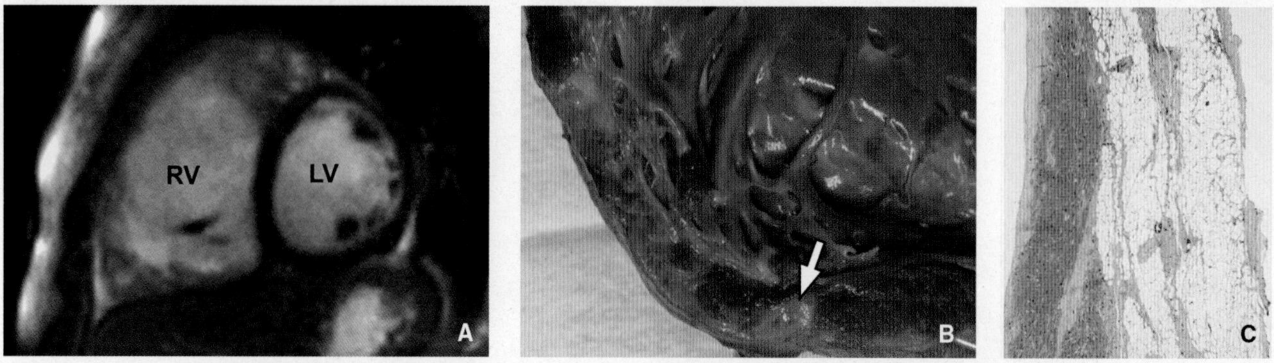

FIGURE 9.84 **Arrhythmogenic right ventricular dysplasia (ARVD) in early adolescence.** Bright blood magnetic resonance image **(A)** in short axial axis plane shows dilated right ventricular (*RV*) chamber. Of note, no fat or fibrous tissue could be demonstrated on MR image. *LV*, left ventricle. ARVD in the explanted heart of a 15-year-old boy **(B, C)**. The right ventricular wall is thin and consists largely of yellow fat (*arrow*), with only scant admixed myocytes seen microscopically (**right**, hematoxylin and eosin; original magnification, 40×).

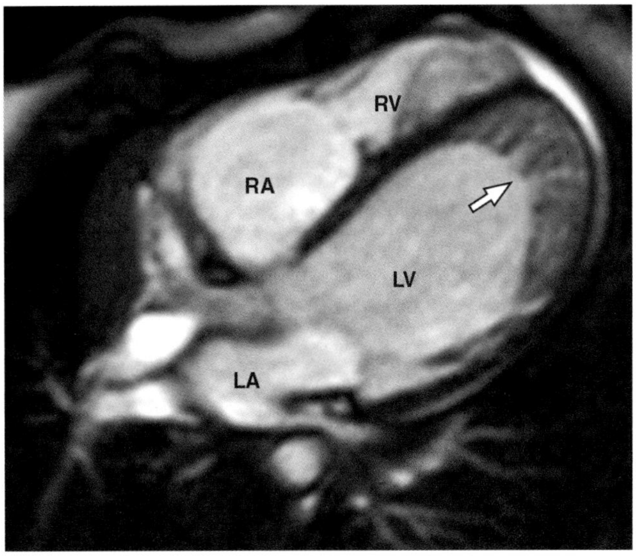

FIGURE 9.85 **Left ventricular noncompaction in a 3-year-old boy.** Bright blood magnetic resonance image in four-chamber plane shows abnormally thick layer of noncompacted myocardium (*arrow*) in the apex of a dilated left ventricular chamber. *LA*, left atrium; *LV*, left ventricle; *RA*, right atrium; *RV*, right ventricle.

layer of the left ventricular myocardium. The subepicardial layer is compacted normally. It is a congenital condition thought to result from an intrauterine arrest in myocardial compaction.[91,92] Pediatric patients with left ventricular noncompaction typically come to medical attention in adolescence or early adulthood with ventricular arrhythmias or heart failure, although neonatal and infantile presentations may also occur.

Echo provides initial diagnostic assessment, based on a ratio of compacted to noncompacted myocardial layers. Cardiac MRI diagnostic criteria include a ratio of noncompacted to compacted myocardium of >2.3 during diastole[91] or a trabeculated myocardial mass of >20% the total myocardial mass. Cardiac MRI is the preferred diagnostic tool as it provides good diagnostic sensitivity and specificity and may localize the involved segments (Fig. 9.85). The degree of delayed myocardial hyperenhancement of the trabeculated noncompacted myocardium correlates well with disease severity and can help stratify risk.[92]

Treatment options depend on the disease severity and include heart failure therapies, antiarrhythmic agents, implantable automated defibrillators, and cardiac transplant.

Arteriopathies

Marfan Syndrome

Marfan syndrome is an inherited connective tissue disorder caused by a defect in the gene that codes for fibrillin 1 (*FBN1*, at 15q21.1).[55] The prevalence of Marfan syndrome is ~1 in 4,000 individuals.[55] Musculoskeletal manifestations include above average height, pectus excavatum or pectus carinatum, scoliosis, and arachnodactyly (long spidery fingers). Cardiac manifestations include mitral valve prolapse and regurgitation, aortic root dilatation, arterial aneurysms, and risk of arterial dissection and rupture. Other manifestations include spontaneous pneumothoraces, dislocation of lens of the eye, and dural ectasia in the spinal canal.[55]

Chest radiography usually shows a pectus deformity and scoliosis. It may also demonstrate aortic root or thoracic aortic enlargement. Cardiac MRI is used to screen for cardiovascular complications including mitral and aortic valvar regurgitation and aortic dilatation. Classically, the ascending aorta is most dilated at the sinotubular junction, losing the normal indentation above the level of the sinuses of Valsalva.[55] CTA can be used to assess aortic root dilatation in patients with Marfan syndrome (Fig. 9.86) in addition to MRI, but is mostly used in the acute setting when aortic dissection is suspected.

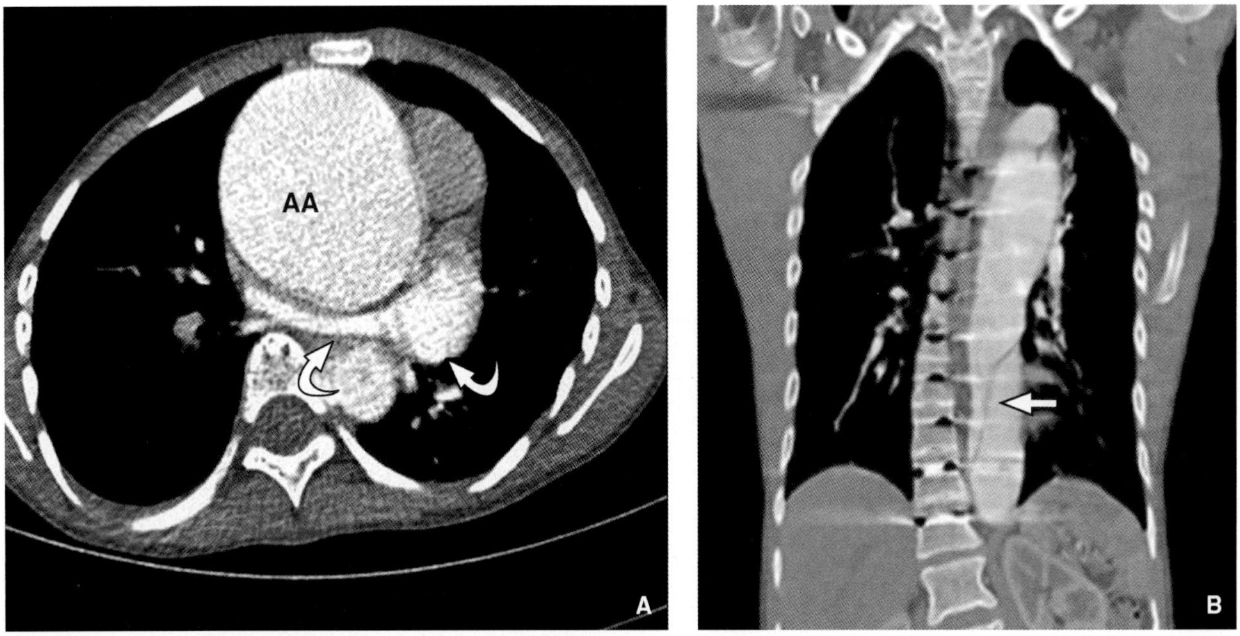

FIGURE 9.86 **Marfan syndrome.** Axial enhanced CT image **(A)** shows marked dilatation of the proximal ascending aorta (*AA*) compressing adjacent pulmonary artery (*curved arrows*). Coronal reformatted enhanced CT image **(B)** obtained from a different pediatric patient with Marfan syndrome demonstrates dissection (*arrow*) in the dilated descending thoracic aorta.

Medical treatments include losartan, a drug that blocks angiotensin receptors in vascular smooth muscle, preventing vasoconstriction and decreasing aortic root dilatation in patients with Marfan syndrome. Surgical repair of the aortic root is recommended when the aortic diameter reaches 5.0 cm. Rapid growth >0.5 cm/year, family history of dissection at a diameter <5.0 cm, or the presence of significant aortic regurgitation may also be indications for surgery. Once the aortic diameter reaches 6.0 cm, there is a fourfold increased risk of dissection and rupture.[93,94]

Loeys-Dietz Syndrome

Loeys-Dietz syndrome is a recently characterized connective tissue disorder, which may arise from a de novo mutation or be inherited in an autosomal dominant fashion. It is caused by mutations in the genes encoding transforming growth factor beta-receptor type 1 or type 2 (*TGFBR1* or *TGFBR2*).[55,95] This arteriopathy has cardiovascular, musculoskeletal, and ocular manifestations similar to Marfan syndrome. However, it is more aggressive, with more severe aneurysm formation at an earlier age than Marfan syndrome and increased risk of arterial dissection and rupture.[95] The musculoskeletal manifestations also are more severe, and in addition to scoliosis and pectus deformity, patients demonstrate vertebral instability leading to subluxation and craniosynostosis. Bifid uvula and hypertelorism are other characteristic features.[95]

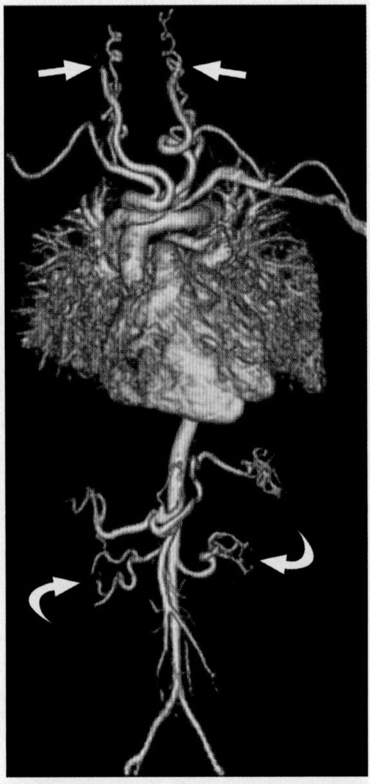

FIGURE 9.87 **Loeys-Dietz syndrome.** Three-dimensional volume-rendered image from magnetic resonance angiography shows corkscrew-shaped extracranial vertebral arteries (*straight arrows*) and marked tortuosity of subclavian arteries, hepatic artery, splenic artery, and bilateral renal arteries (*curved arrows*).

Chest radiography in Loeys-Dietz syndrome may show aortic dilatation, scoliosis, and pectus deformity. Cardiac MRI is used to serially evaluate patients for mitral valve prolapse and regurgitation, aortic dilatation and regurgitation, and arterial aneurysms. Pediatric patients with Loeys-Dietz syndrome demonstrate marked tortuosity of the extracranial vertebral arteries, and the degree of tortuosity appears to correlate with the severity of the arterial complications (Fig. 9.87). Excessive vertebral artery tortuosity was initially thought to be pathognomic of Loeys-Dietz syndrome. However, now, it is known to occur in patients with other arteriopathies including Marfan syndrome, although in general tortuosity is most pronounced in patients with Loeys-Dietz syndrome. Tortuosity of other arteries is also frequently present (Fig. 9.87).

Medical management with beta-blockers and losartan therapy has been shown to decrease the rate of aortic dilatation in patients with Loeys-Dietz syndrome.[55] Early surgical or interventional treatment of aneurysms is recommended for young children with severe systemic manifestations and prominent craniofacial features, which are associated with more severe aortic disease. Once the aortic diameter exceeds the 99th percentile for age and the aortic valve annulus reaches 1.8 to 2.0 cm, surgical treatment is recommended in order to decrease risk of rupture.[94] Despite the interventions, the natural history of Loeys-Dietz syndrome is death from complications at a mean of 26.1 years.[95]

Ehlers-Danlos Syndrome

Ehlers-Danlos syndrome encompasses a group of several inherited disorders with autosomal recessive trait resulting from a genetic defect in collagen synthesis.[55] This syndrome is clinically heterogeneous as the underlying collagen abnormality is different for each type. Joint laxity, easy bruising, and skin hyperelasticity are hallmarks of the condition. Among different types of Ehlers-Danlos syndrome, type IV Ehlers-Danlos syndrome is associated with severe arteriopathy with aneurysms, arterial dissection, and rupture with possible catastrophic consequences. The majority of patients with type IV Ehlers-Danlos syndrome have a characteristic facial appearance with thin lips and philtrum and large eyes.[55] Musculoskeletal manifestations include congenital hip dysplasia, joint dislocation, and clubfeet.

Chest radiography often shows aortic root or thoracic aortic enlargement and scoliosis. Cardiac MRI is used to serially evaluate the size of the aortic root and or ascending aortic dilatation. CTA is most frequently used in the setting of acute chest pain to evaluate for aortic dissection.

Surgical repair of the aortic root at 5 cm is suggested in order to decrease risk of dissection and rupture in pediatric patients with Ehlers-Danlos syndrome.[55]

Filamin A Mutation

Filamin A mutation is an X-linked disorder arising from mutations in the FLNA (encoding filamin A) gene. Affected individuals have a phenotype similar to Ehlers-Danlos syndrome with aortic dilatation, cardiac valvar dysplasia, and joint hypermobility.[96] Distinguishing features of filamin

A mutation include periventricular heterotopia and diffuse lung disease, which are not seen in other arteriopathies.[97]

Cardiac Tumors

Cardiac tumors in the pediatric population are exceedingly rare with a reported incidence of ~0.002%.[98] The vast majority (>90%) of cardiac tumors encountered in children are benign. However, they retain the potential for serious complications, including obstruction, arrhythmias, and embolic phenomena because of their potentially critical location.[99] Additionally, they may be a marker of syndromic disease.

For evaluation of cardiac tumors, MRI is the current imaging modality of choice after initial evaluation with echo. MRI can be used to identify the size, number, and location of cardiac tumors. Although MRI can be also used to characterize the cardiac tumors based on T1, T2, perfusion, and delayed enhancement MR imaging findings, it typically lacks sufficient sensitivity and specificity to obviate a tissue diagnosis.[98] CTA usually has no role in detection and characterization of pediatric cardiac tumors.

Benign Cardiac Tumors

Cardiac Rhabdomyoma

Cardiac rhabdomyoma is the most common primary pediatric cardiac tumor. It accounts for ~45% to 75% of all pediatric cardiac tumors and is typically diagnosed in utero or during neonatal period.[98] Cardiac rhabdomyomas are composed of large vacuolated myocytes (Fig. 9.88). They are distinct from soft tissue rhabdomyomas, which recapitulate skeletal muscle.

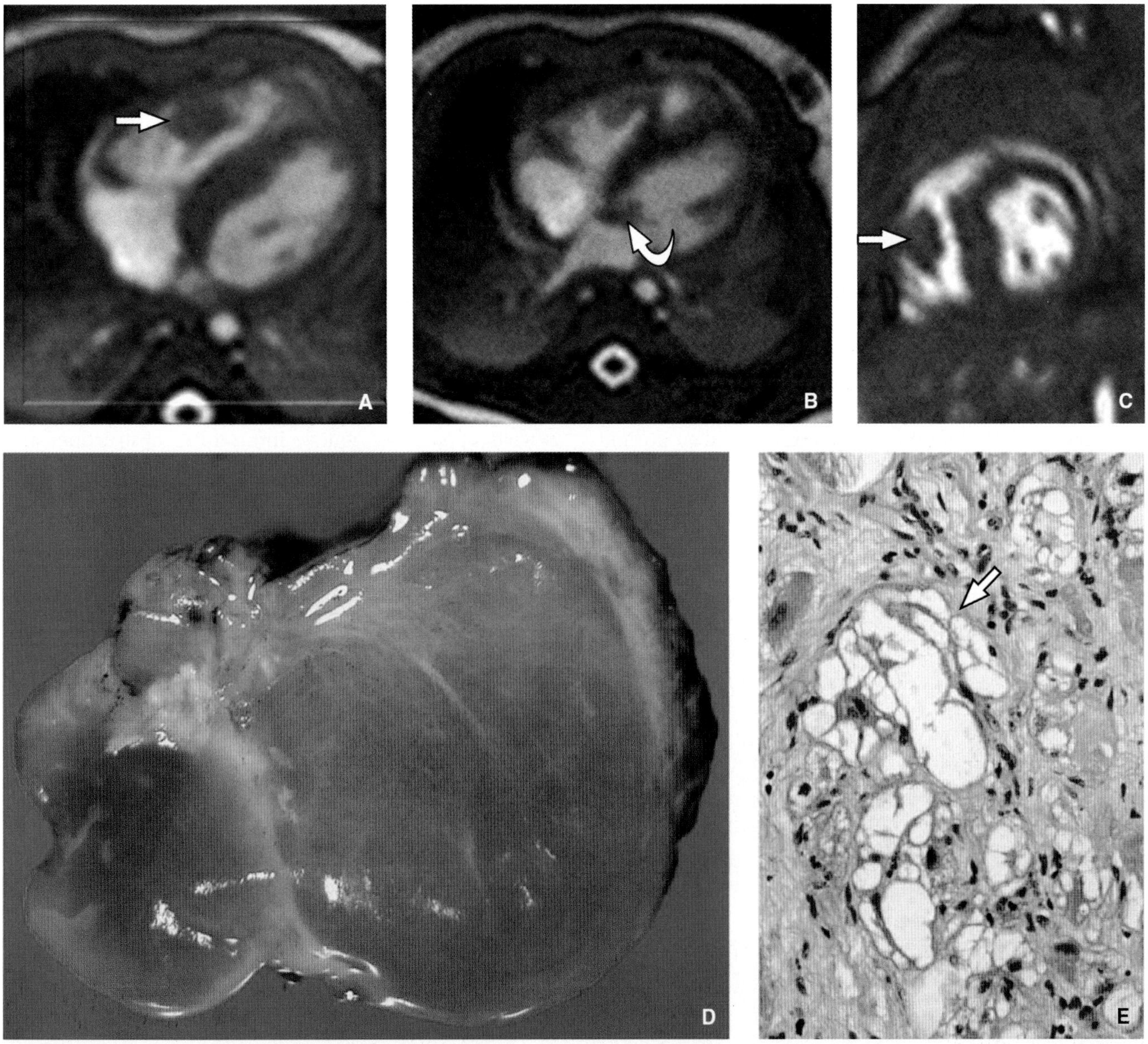

FIGURE 9.88 **A–C: Cardiac rhabdomyoma.** Bright blood magnetic resonance images in four-chamber plane **(A,B)** and short-axis plane **(C)** show rhabdomyomas in the right ventricle (*RV*) (*straight arrows*) and at the base of the anterior leaflet of mitral valve (*curved arrow*). **D, E:** Cardiac rhabdomyoma, excised from the right ventricle of a newborn, shows a homogeneous pale cut surface **(D)**. Microscopic examination shows vacuolated cytoplasm (*arrow*) (hematoxylin and eosin **(E)**; original magnification, 400×).

They have been variously classified as hamartomas or benign neoplasms. Fifty to seventy percent of patients with cardiac rhabdomyomas have tuberous sclerosis.[98]

The clinical presentation of a child with cardiac rhabdomyomas is related to the size, number, and position of the masses. Large exophytic rhabdomyomas attached to the myocardium may obstruct the intraventricular lumen (intracavitary rhabdomyomas) or obstruct the orifice for the AV or pulmonary or aortic valves. Extensive myocardial involvement with multiple small rhabdomyomas may be associated with diminished myocardial function.[98]

Chest radiography may demonstrate cardiomegaly and pulmonary vascular congestion in large obstructing cardiac rhabdomyomas. On echo, cardiac rhabdomyomas are characteristically markedly echogenic. On cardiac MRI, these lesions are homogeneous and show mildly high T2 signal with respect to the surrounding normal myocardium. The masses are typically well-circumscribed and have a predilection for the ventricular myocardium (Fig. 9.88).[99]

Most rhabdomyomas regress spontaneously over the first year of life. Therefore, surgical resection is reserved for those patients with cardiac rhabdomyomas causing hemodynamic compromise or life-threatening arrhythmias.[98]

Cardiac Fibroma

Cardiac fibroma is the second most common pediatric primary cardiac tumor. It is most frequently found in the free wall of the LV, interventricular septum or left ventricular apex. These tumors are intramural masses composed of fibroblasts and extracellular matrix rich in collagen and elastic fibers. Cardiac fibromas are typically detected during the neonatal period.[98] Clinical manifestations depend on size and number, and similar to rhabdomyomas, large lesions may obstruct the ventricular inflow, outflow, or valvar function.[98] Patients with Gorlin syndrome have an increased incidence of cardiac fibromas.

Chest radiography in cardiac fibroma may show mild to severe cardiomegaly and pulmonary edema depending on the size of the lesion and degree of ventricular dysfunction. On cardiac MRI, fibromas are one of the few cardiac tumors that have a relatively specific enhancement pattern. They typically demonstrate decreased first-pass perfusion and intense delayed enhancement because of the presence of underlying fibrous tissue.[99] On other MR sequences, fibromas are similar in signal to the surrounding myocardium (Fig. 9.89).

Unlike rhabdomyomas, cardiac fibromas do not typically regress.[98] Total or subtotal surgical resection can be performed in most fibromas, whereas cardiac transplantation may be required for pediatric patients with extensive tumor involvement causing severely diminished cardiac function.[98]

Cardiac Myxoma

Cardiac myxoma is most frequently seen in adults but occasionally occurs in children. It is the third most common primary pediatric cardiac tumor.[98] Cardiac myxoma is usually solitary with a predilection for the atria (left > right). It is frequently pedunculated and usually attached to the interatrial septum at the foramen ovale. It is often quite mobile and potentially may impair normal AVV function resulting in regurgitation or stenosis. Histologically, cardiac myxomas are composed of strands/cords of cells in a myxoid matrix (Fig. 9.90). Cardiac myxomas have been associated with multiple syndromes and endocrine abnormalities including the Carney complex, characterized by myxomas of the heart and other sites, skin hyperpigmentation, and endocrine overactivity.[98]

Older patients with cardiac myxoma classically have a triad of systemic illness, intracardiac obstruction, and emboli. However, clinical presentation of pediatric patients with cardiac myxoma is usually nonspecific which may delay diagnosis. Peripheral embolization of tumor material is common, potentially to the coronaries, carotids, and pulmonary

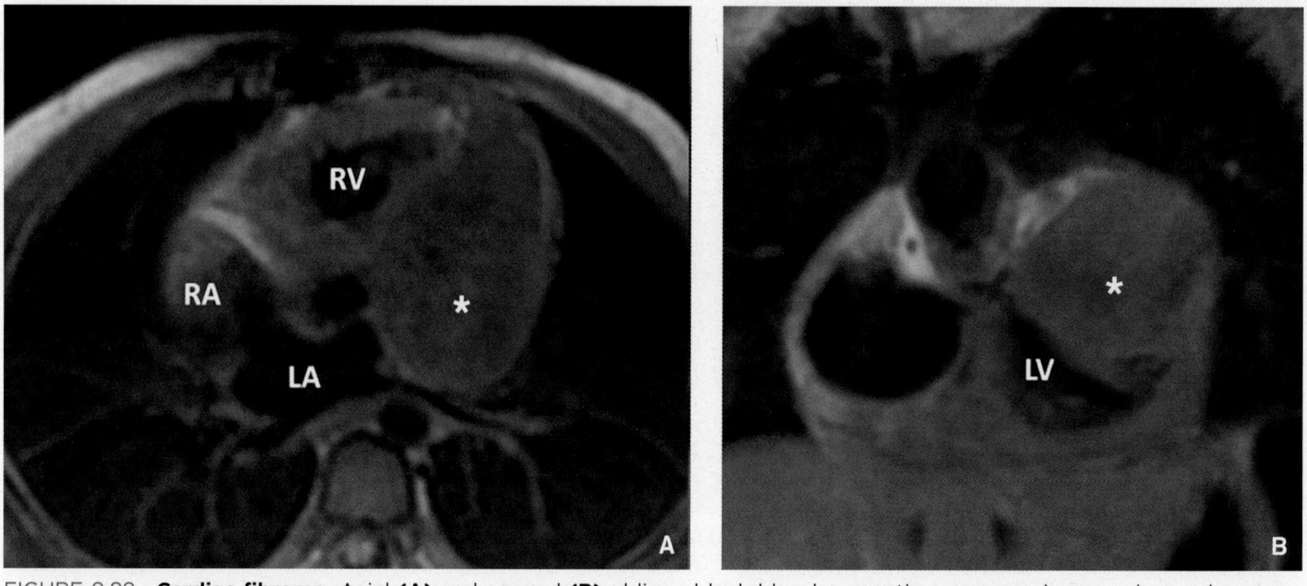

FIGURE 9.89 **Cardiac fibroma.** Axial **(A)** and coronal **(B)** oblique black blood magnetic resonance images show a homogeneous left ventricular mass (*asterisk*) with similar signal intensity to myocardium compressing the left ventricular (*LV*) chamber. *RA*, right atrium; *RV*, right ventricle.

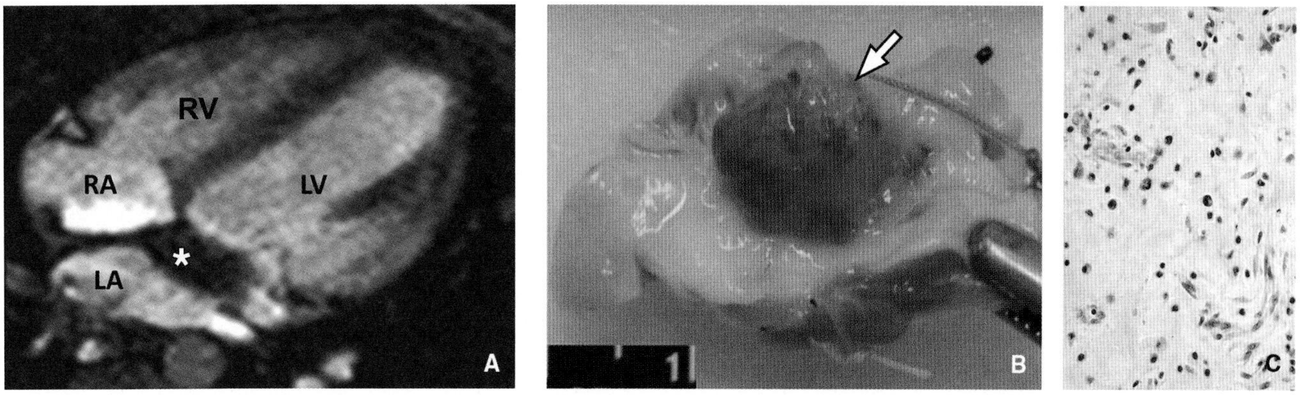

FIGURE 9.90 **A: Cardiac myxoma.** Axial bright blood magnetic resonance image **(A)** shows hypointense mass in the left atrium (*asterisk*) arising from interatrial septum in the region of the foramen ovale. *LA*, left atrium; *LV*, left ventricle; *RA*, right atrium; *RV*, right ventricle. **B, C:** Gross specimen **(B)** of cardiac myxoma (*arrow*), which projects from the left atrial endocardial surface. Microscopic image **(C)** shows a pale blue myxoid matrix containing scattered inflammatory cells, myxoma cells, hemosiderin-laden macrophages, and small blood vessels (hematoxylin and eosin; original magnification, 400x).

arteries, and can result in thrombosis, infarction, and stroke. Delayed development of peripheral arterial aneurysms years after previous myxoma resection has been attributed to earlier embolic phenomena.[7,98]

Chest radiography may be normal or demonstrate atrial enlargement and pulmonary edema. Cardiac MRI can show the classical appearance of a pedunculated mass attached to the interatrial septum (Fig. 9.90). Cardiac myxomas are often hyperintense on T2-weighted MR sequences and demonstrate heterogeneous enhancement after gadolinium administration.[98]

The current management of cardiac myxomas is surgical resection, which also may involve the resection of portions of the interatrial septum. After surgical resection, patients require surveillance for disease recurrence and for the presence of peripheral arterial aneurysms. The incidence of recurrence is ~5%.[98]

Cardiac Teratoma

Cardiac teratoma is a rare primary cardiac tumor, which is typically located within the pericardium (intrapericardial). It is usually a large tumor that may cause severe obstruction of the SVC[7] (Fig. 9.91). Histologically, cardiac teratomas are composed of the three germ layers (mesoderm, endoderm, and ectoderm), resulting in a characteristically heterogeneous tumor, which often contains fatty or calcified tissue.

Chest radiography usually demonstrates cardiomegaly with or without calcifications. Vascular congestion because of obstruction may also present. Cardiac CTA or MRI can show the presence of fat and calcification in addition to other solid/cystic component of tumor, which usually indicates the diagnosis.[99] Concomitant pericardial effusion is also often present.

Cardiac teratomas are treated with surgical resection and decompression of the pericardial effusion with excellent long-term success rates.[7,98]

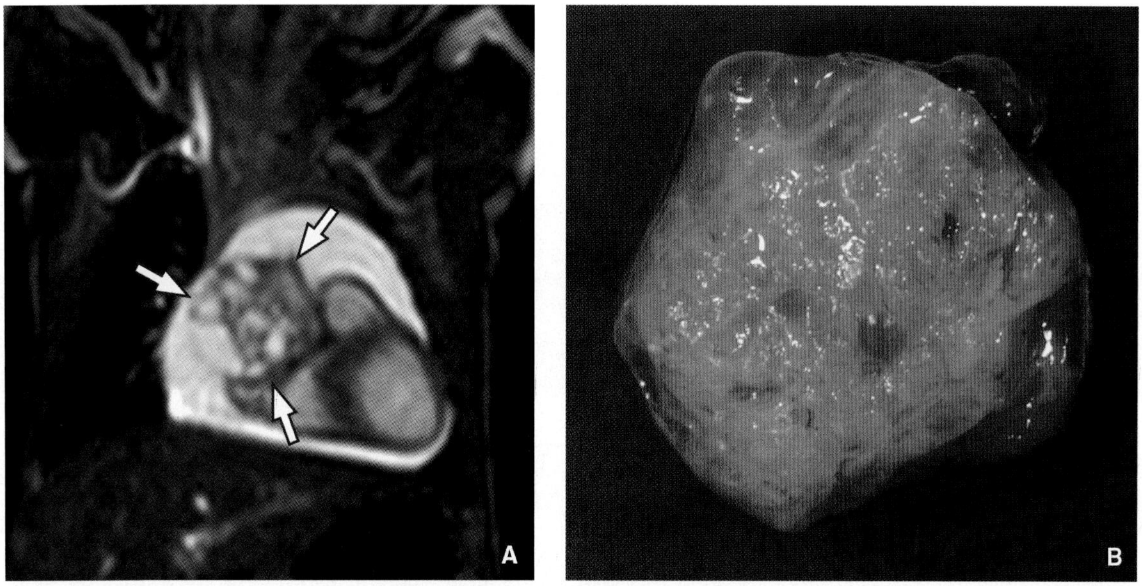

FIGURE 9.91 **Pericardial teratoma in a 4-week-old girl.** Coronal T2-weighted magnetic resonance image **(A)** shows a large heterogeneous mass arising from the pericardium near the right atrium (*arrows*). Also noted is a large pericardial effusion. Gross specimen **(B)** of pericardial teratoma, which is partially cystic and measures ~4 cm.

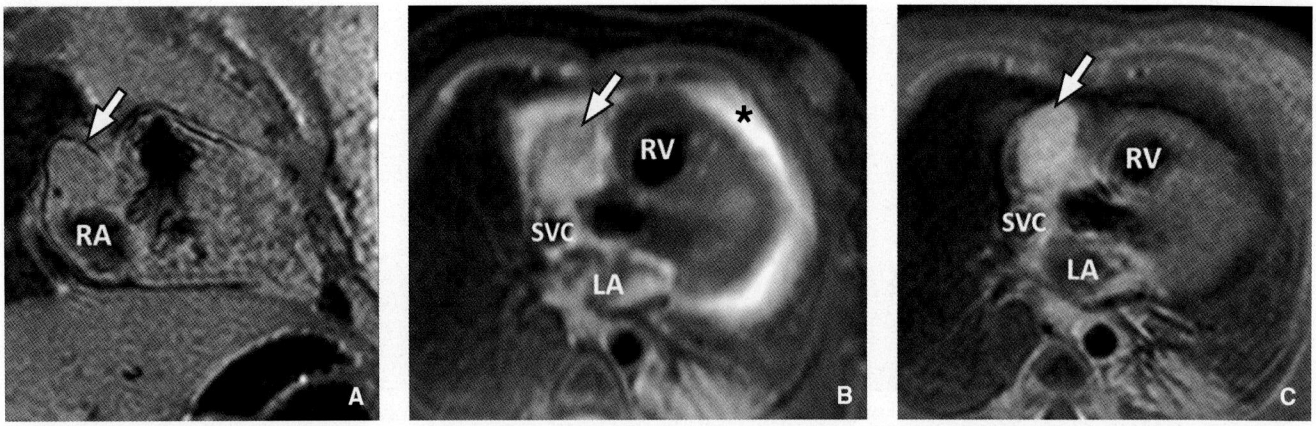

FIGURE 9.92 **Cardiac hemangioma.** Coronal oblique black blood T1-weighted magnetic resonance (MR) image **(A)** shows a mass (*arrow*) adjacent to right atrial appendage. Axial fat-saturated black blood T2-weighted MR image **(B)** demonstrates a T2 hyperintense mass (*arrow*) and moderate pericardial effusion (*asterisk*). Axial postcontrast T1-weighted MR image **(C)** shows moderate homogeneous contrast enhancement of the mass (*arrow*). *LA*, left atrium; *RA*, right atrium; *RV*, right ventricle; *SVC*, superior vena cava.

Cardiac Hemangioma

Cardiac hemangioma is almost always a single tumor and can occur anywhere within the heart. Histologically, there are many types of hemangiomas that can involve the heart. The clinical course of cardiac hemangioma depends on the size of the lesion and the histologic variation.[98]

Chest radiography may be normal or show cardiomegaly. On cardiac MRI, cardiac hemangiomas typically demonstrate intense enhancement on first-pass perfusion sequences similar to angiosarcoma.[99] Affected pediatric patients may have a nonhemorrhagic pericardial effusion (Fig. 9.92).

Congenital cardiac hemangiomas may regress in size with beta-blocker therapy, whereas noninvoluting tumors may require surgical intervention.[98]

Malignant Cardiac Tumors

Primary Malignant Cardiac Tumors

Primary malignant cardiac tumors comprise <7% of primary pediatric cardiac tumors. They include, among others, angiosarcoma, fibrosarcoma, and rhabdomyosarcoma. Among these, angiosarcoma is the most frequent primary malignant cardiac tumor and most often involves the right atrium and pericardium.[7] Typical, clinical presentation of primary malignant cardiac tumors include right heart failure, cardiac tamponade, and SVC obstruction.

Chest radiography usually demonstrates cardiac enlargement and pulmonary edema, but may also show pulmonary metastatic disease. On cardiac MRI and CT, primary malignant cardiac tumors are intensely vascular with hyperenhancement on first-pass perfusion sequences similar to hemangiomas (Fig. 9.93). Concomitant hemorrhagic and pericardial effusions may be also present.[99]

Affected pediatric patients have poor prognosis because surgical resection is often challenging because of tumor extension into the myocardium. Additionally, the majority of affected patients already have metastatic disease to the lungs, liver, or central nervous system when the diagnosis is made.[7]

Secondary Malignant Cardiac Tumors

Secondary malignant cardiac tumors in children most frequently arise via direct inferior venocaval extension of Wilms tumor, neuroblastoma, or adrenocortical carcinoma.

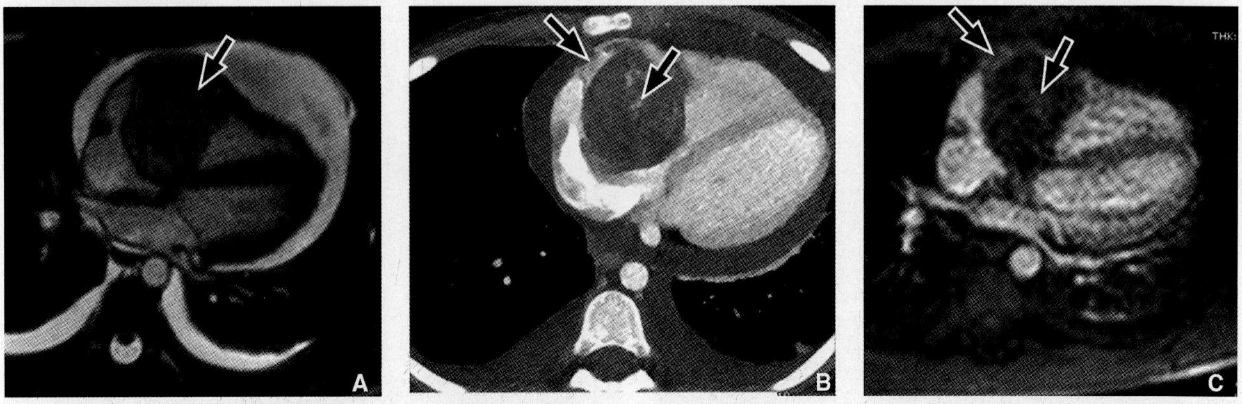

FIGURE 9.93 **Primary cardiac angiosarcoma.** Axial oblique bright blood magnetic resonance (MR) image **(A)** shows mass (*arrow*) at right atrioventricular junction obliterating tricuspid valve inflow. There is also a large pericardial effusion (hemorrhagic) and bilateral pleural effusions. Axial enhanced CT image **(B)** demonstrates areas of hyperattenuation (*arrows*) within the mass. Axial perfusion MR image **(C)** shows early hyperenhancement of the periphery and central portions (*arrows*) of the mass, which corresponds to the areas of hyperattenuation on CT (Figure 9.93B).

Non-Hodgkin lymphoma is also one of the common pediatric malignancies that may result in intracardiac metastases. Secondary cardiac malignancies may result in pericardial effusions, congestive cardiac failure, emboli, and arrhythmias. Treatment and prognosis depend on histology and extent of cardiac involvement.[7]

Kawasaki Disease

Kawasaki disease is a systemic inflammatory condition resulting in a small- and medium-sized arteritis. It causes vessel aneurysm and stricture formation. Kawasaki disease has a predilection for causing coronary artery aneurysms but also frequently involves the axillary, subclavian, and iliac arteries.[100] Kawasaki disease is sometimes referred to as mucocutaneous lymph node syndrome because it also causes lymph node enlargement and inflammatory changes of the tongue and skin. The etiology of Kawasaki syndrome is currently unknown. There is an increased prevalence in patients of Asian descent, boys, and young children.[100] Age at presentation is usually <5 years old, typically with high fever and lymph node enlargement. Physical examination may reveal a strawberry tongue (red and inflamed appearance) and a desquamative rash on the palms of the hands and soles of the feet.

Echo is performed to screen pediatric patients with Kawasaki disease for the presence coronary artery involvement. Coronary dilatation may be seen in the first 7 days of symptoms, but peak involvement is usually at 4 weeks. If coronary abnormalities are seen on echo, cardiac CTA or MRI may be obtained for further evaluation. Both cardiac CTA and MRI can evaluate the coronary arteries for aneurysms, stenoses, and thrombus formation (Fig. 9.94). In addition, cardiac CTA and MRA can assess other thoracic or abdominal arterial involvement. Cardiac MRI may also be used to assess disease activity and response to therapy. Persistent mural edema and enhancement on MRI suggest active inflammation, whereas ischemic sequelae (diminished perfusion and scar) may be assessed with stress myocardial first-pass perfusion and delayed enhancement sequences.[101]

Medical management consists of anti-inflammatory agents, immune modulating agents, and gamma globulins.[100,102] Response to treatment is variable, with best outcomes reported in children who receive treatment within the first 10 days and those without coronary artery involvement.[102] Occasionally, coronary artery bypass grafting (CABG) is required in cases of severe coronary stenoses, and rarely, cardiac transplantation may be needed in the setting of ventricular failure.[100,102]

Myocarditis

Myocarditis is inflammation of the myocardium, excluding the ones due to infarction. The majority of cases are related to viral disease including adenovirus, enterovirus, parvovirus, and coxsackievirus. However, frequently, no viral agent is identified and the cause remains idiopathic.[103–105] Clinical presentation of myocarditis depends on the age of the child and severity of myocardial dysfunction. Usual symptoms include an upper respiratory tract infection and gastroenteritis preceding the onset of chest pain, arrhythmia, or congestive cardiac failure.

Chest radiography may show cardiomegaly and pulmonary vascular congestion. Troponin levels, ECG, and echo evaluation are used as the primary diagnostic tests. Myocardial biopsy remains the gold standard for diagnosis, but cardiac MRI is playing an increasingly important role in the diagnosis of myocarditis and in predicting prognosis (Fig. 9.95). The presence of edema on T2-weighted sequence represents areas of myocardial inflammation that may be reversible. In contrast, large areas of fibrosis/scar on delayed enhancement may reflect irreversible myocardial injury and may precede the development of dilated cardiomyopathy.[103,104]

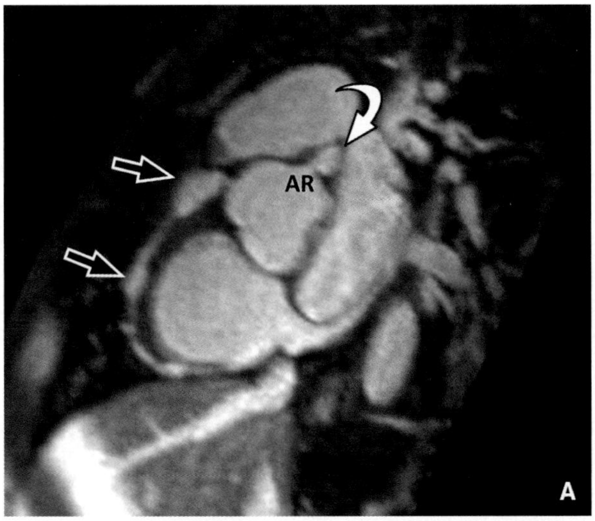

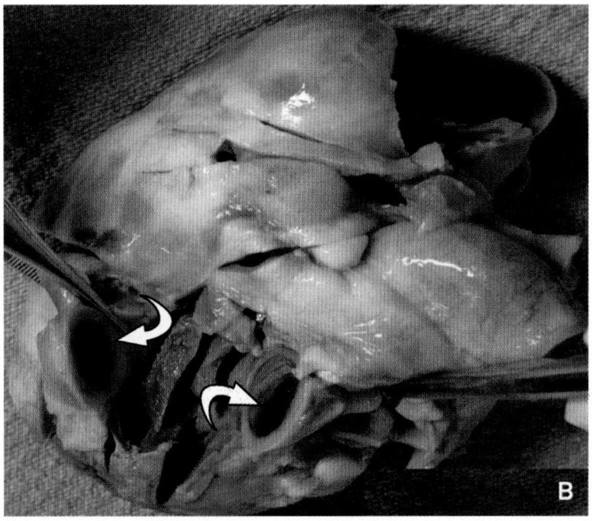

FIGURE 9.94 **Kawasaki disease. A:** Sagittal oblique 3D steady-state free precession (coronary artery sequence) MR image shows beaded appearance (*arrows*) to the right coronary artery and an aneurysm (*curved arrow*) at left coronary artery origin from aortic root (*AR*). Gross specimen **(B)** shows large thrombosed coronary artery aneurysms (*curved arrows*) because of Kawasaki disease in a 15-month-old boy.

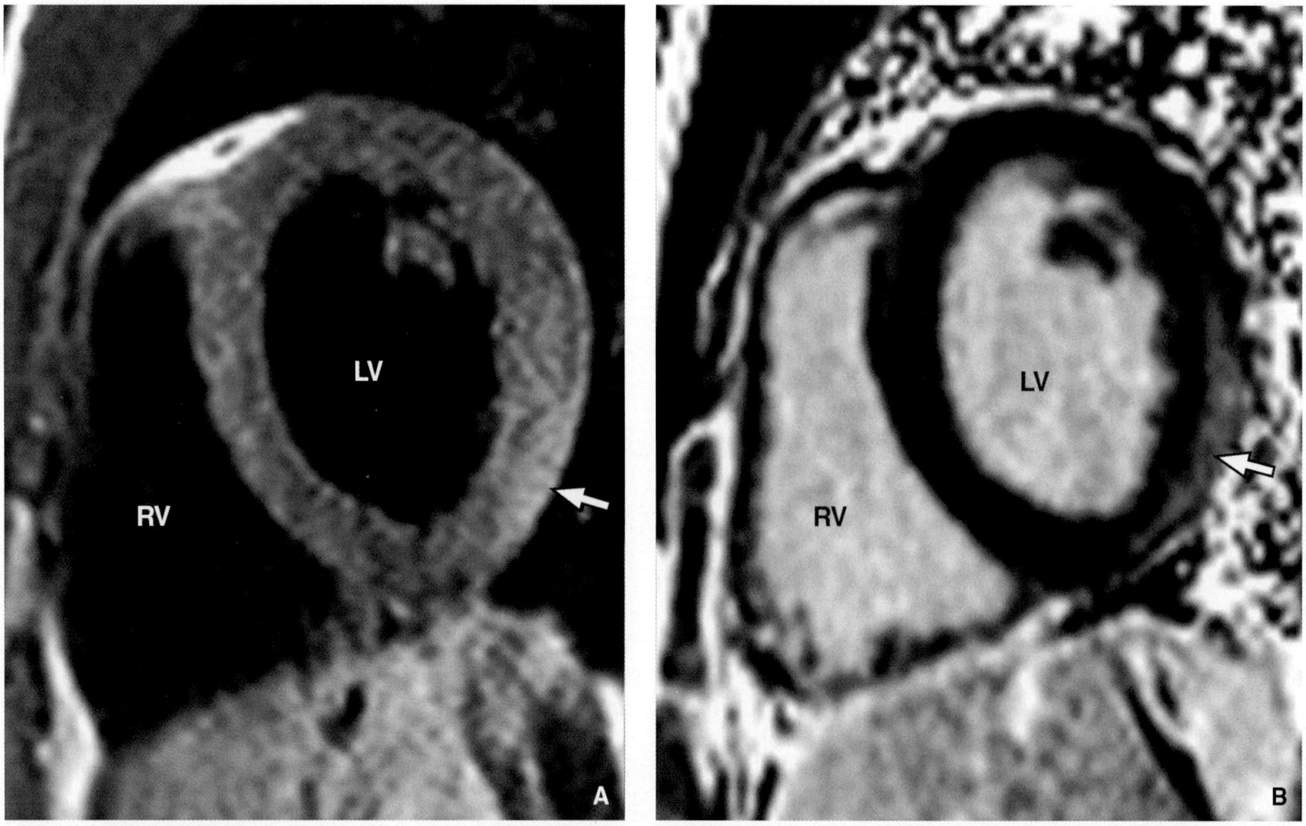

FIGURE 9.95 **Myocarditis.** Black blood T2-weighted magnetic resonance (MR) image **(A)** in short-axis plane shows subepicardial increased T2 signal (*arrow*) in free wall of the left ventricle (*LV*). Myocardial delayed enhancement sequence MR image **(B)** shows subepicardial delayed enhancement in same area (*arrow*) as Figure 9.95A. *RV*, right ventricle.

Medical management of myocarditis is usually supportive with antiarrhythmogenic agents or heart failure therapies. Antiviral and immunosuppressant agents have not been shown to affect prognosis and are not used routinely.[103] Cardiac pacing, ventricular assist devices, and heart transplantation are occasionally used in severe cases or when dilated cardiomyopathy results.

Pericardial Disorder

Pericarditis

The visceral and parietal membranes of the pericardium enclose the heart, pulmonary artery, and proximal ascending aorta. Acute pericarditis is an inflammatory condition of the pericardium caused by a variety of etiologies including infectious, autoimmune (juvenile idiopathic arthritis and systemic lupus erythematosus), metabolic (uremia), malignant, and iatrogenic (secondary to drugs and cardiac surgery) conditions.[106] Viral infections, including coxsackievirus, adenovirus, and echovirus, are the most common cause of pericarditis in the pediatric population. In the past, tuberculosis (TB) was a common cause of pericarditis. However, it is now rarely seen except in immunosuppressed pediatric patients and TB endemic regions.[107]

Acute pericarditis can be complicated by cardiac tamponade if the pericardial effusion rapidly accumulates and obstructs cardiac filling.[108] Constrictive pericarditis arises from chronic pericardial inflammation resulting in a thickened adherent pericardium that impedes filling of the ventricles.[108]

Clinically, the majority of children with pericarditis present with acute inspiratory chest pain. Affected pediatric patients often have a history of a viral prodrome or recent gastroenteritis. On auscultation, a scratchy sound may be heard over the anterior chest wall (Hammond crunch), and the heart sounds may be muffled by a pericardial effusion. The ECG can demonstrate ST segment elevation or inverted T waves.[106]

Chest radiography may be normal or demonstrate global cardiac enlargement, resulting in a triangular appearance sometimes referred to as a "water-bottle" heart (Fig. 9.96).[106,108,109] Echo is usually used to make the diagnosis. In some cases, if the diagnosis is unclear on echo, cardiac MRI may be performed. Cardiac MRI is also used to distinguish between restrictive cardiomyopathy and constrictive pericarditis, both of which result in a narrowed ventricular morphology and severe atrial dilatation and dilated systemic veins. Distinguishing features of constrictive pericarditis on MRI include pericardial thickening (pericardial thickness of >5 mm), pericardial effusion, myocardial tethering to the inflamed pericardium (which may be evident on functional sequences or following myocardial tagging), and paradoxical motion of the interventricular septum.[86,108]

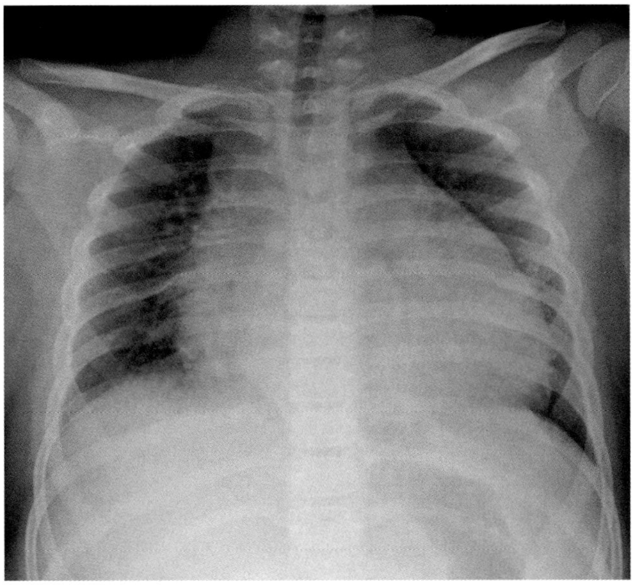

FIGURE 9.96 **Pericarditis.** Frontal chest radiograph shows global cardiomegaly in an adolescent boy with a large pericardial effusion because of underlying pericarditis. The shape of the cardiac silhouette on this erect frontal chest radiograph is "water-bottle" appearance. The water-bottle sign or configuration refers to the shape of the cardiac silhouette on erect frontal chest radiograph in patients who have a very large pericardial effusion.

Management of pericarditis is directed at identifying and treating the underlying cause. For children with viral etiology, NSAIDs are the mainstay of treatment.[104] Use of steroids is controversial because of the potential risk of reactivation of infection because of immunocompromised status. Colchicine may provide some therapeutic benefit in patients not responding to NSAID therapy.[106] Pericardiocentesis is usually reserved for pediatric patients with a severe pericardial effusion at risk for cardiac tamponade. In severe cases unresponsive to other therapies, a pericardial window or pericardial stripping may be necessary.[106]

References

1. Schweigmann G, Gassner I, Maurer K. Imaging the neonatal heart—essentials for the radiologist. *Eur J Radiol.* 2006;60:159–170.
2. Watts JR Jr, Sonavane SK, Singh SP, et al. Pictorial review of multidetector CT imaging of the preoperative evaluation of congenital heart disease. *Curr Probl Diagn Radiol.* 2013;42(2):40–56.
3. Bonello B, Kilner PJ. Review of the role of cardiovascular magnetic resonance in congenital heart disease, with a focus on right ventricle assessment. *Arch Cardiovasc Dis.* 2012;105:605–613.
4. Burchill LJ, Mertens L, Broberg CS. Imaging for the assessment of heart failure in congenital heart disease: ventricular function and beyond. *Heart Fail Clin.* 2014;10:9–22.
5. Chung T. Magnetic resonance angiography of the body in pediatric patients: experience with a contrast-enhanced time-resolved technique. *Pediatr Radiol.* 2005;35:3–10.
6. Lapierre C, Déry J, Guérin R, et al. Segmental approach to imaging of congenital heart disease. *Radiographics.* 2010;30:397–411.
7. Allen HD. *Moss and Adams' Heart Disease in Infants, Children, and Adolescents: Including the Fetus and Young Adult.* 4th ed. Philadelphia, PA: Lippincott Williams & Wilkins; 2008.
8. Attili A, Hensley AK, Jones FD, et al. Echocardiography and coronary CT angiography imaging of variations in coronary anatomy and coronary abnormalities in athletic children: detection of coronary abnormalities that create a risk for sudden death. *Echocardiography.* 2013;30(2):225–233.
9. Braunwald E. Atrial septal defect. In: Braunwald E, ed. *Heart Disease: A Text of Cardiovascular Medicine.* 4th ed. Philadelphia, PA: WB Saunders; 1992:906–908.
10. Davia J, Cheitlin M, Bedynek J. Sinus venosus atrial septal defect: analysis of fifty cases. *Am Heart J.* 1973;2:177–185.
11. Bialkowski J, Karwot B, Szkutnik M, et al. Closure of atrial septal defects in children: surgery versus Amplatzer device implantation. *Tex Heart Inst J.* 2004;31:220–223.
12. Stewart RD, Bailliard F, Kelle AM, et al. Evolving surgical strategy for sinus venosus atrial septal defect: effect on sinus node function and late venous obstruction. *Ann Thorac Surg.* 2007;84:1651–1655.
13. Wenink AC, Zevallos JC. Developmental aspects of atrioventricular septal defects. *Int J Cardiol.* 1988;18:65–78.
14. Rastelli GC, Kirklin JW, Titus JL. Anatomic observations on complete form of persistent common atrioventricular canal with special reference to atrioventricular valves. *Mayo Clin Proc.* 1966;41:296–308.
15. Miller A, Siffel C, Lu C, et al. Long-term survival of infants with atrioventricular septal defects. *J Pediatr.* 2010;156:994–1000.
16. Bando K, Turrentine MW, Sun K, et al. Surgical management of complete atrioventricular septal defects. A twenty-year experience. *J Thorac Cardiovasc Surg.* 1995;110:1543–1552.
17. Van Praagh R, Geva T, Kreutzer J. Ventricular septal defects: how shall we describe, name and classify them? *J Am Coll Cardiol.* 1989;14:1298–1299.
18. Kidd L, Driscoll DJ, Gersony WM, et al. Second natural history study of congenital heart defects. Results of treatment of patients with ventricular septal defects. *Circulation.* 1993;87:I38–I51.
19. Fu YC, Bass J, Amin Z, et al. Transcatheter closure of perimembranous ventricular septal defects using the new Amplatzer membranous VSD occluder: results of the U.S. phase I trial. *J Am Coll Cardiol.* 2006;47:319–325.
20. Guy TS, Hill AC. Mitral valve prolapse. *Annu Rev Med.* 2012;63:277–292.
21. Attie F, Casanova JM, Zabal C, et al. Ebstein's anomaly. Clinical profile in 174 patients. *Arch Inst Cardiol Mex.* 1999;69:17–25.
22. Boston US, Goldberg SP, Ward KE, et al. Complete repair of Ebstein anomaly in neonates and young infants: A 16-year follow-up. *J Thorac Cardiovasc Surg.* 2011;141:1163–1169.
23. Norwood WI, Kirklin JK, Sanders SP. Hypoplastic left heart syndrome: experience with palliative surgery. *Am J Cardiol.* 1980;45:87–91.
24. Carlo WF, Carberry KE, Heinle JS, et al. Interstage attrition between bidirectional Glenn and Fontan palliation in children with hypoplastic left heart syndrome. *J Thorac Cardiovasc Surg.* 2011;142:511–516.
25. Schwartz ML, Gauvreau K, Geva T. Predictors of outcome of biventricular repair in infants with multiple left heart obstructive lesions. *Circulation.* 2001;104:682–687.
26. Brown DW, Gauvreau K, Powell AJ, et al. Cardiac magnetic resonance versus routine cardiac catheterization before bidirectional glenn anastomosis in infants with functional single ventricle: a prospective randomized trial. *Circulation.* 2007;116:2718–2725.

27. Fogel MA, Pawlowski TW, Whitehead KK, et al. Cardiac magnetic resonance and the need for routine cardiac catheterization in single ventricle patients prior to Fontan: a comparison of 3 groups: pre-Fontan CMR versus cath evaluation. *J Am Coll Cardiol.* 2012;60:1094–1102.
28. Glatz AC, Rome JJ, Small AJ, et al. Systemic-to-pulmonary collateral flow, as measured by cardiac magnetic resonance imaging, is associated with acute post-Fontan clinical outcomes. *Circ Cardiovasc Imaging.* 2012;5:218–225.
29. Rao PS. Tricuspid atresia: anatomy, imaging, and natural history. In: Braunwald E, Freedom R, eds. *Atlas of Heart Disease: Congenital Heart Disease.* Vol. 12. Philadelphia, PA: Current Medicine; 1997:14.1.
30. Waldman JD, Wernly JA. Cyanotic congenital heart disease with decreased pulmonary blood flow in children. *Pediatr Clin North Am.* 1999;46:385–404.
31. Himeshkumar V, Hagler DJ. Double inlet left ventricle. *Curr Treat Options Cardiovasc Med.* 2007:9:391–398.
32. Nadas AS. Endocardial cushion defects. In: Flyer DC, ed. *Nadas' Pediatric Cardiology.* Hanley & Belfus, Inc.; 1992:577–586.
33. Drinkwater DC, Laks H. Unbalanced atrioventricular septal defects. *Semin Thorac Cardiovasc Surg.* 1997;9(1):21–25.
34. Apfel HD, Gersony WM. Clinical evaluation, medical management and outcome of atrioventricular canal defects. *Prog Pediatr Cardiol.* 1999;10:129–136.
35. Amati F, Mari A, Digilio MC, et al. 22q11 deletion in patients with conotruncal anomalies cardiac malformations: A prospective study. *Eur J Pediatr.* 1995:154:878–881.
36. Boechat MI, Ratib O, Williams PL, et al. Cardiac MR imaging and MR angiography for assessment of complex tetralogy of Fallot and pulmonary atresia. *Radiographics.* 2005;25:1535–1546.
37. Hill G. Repair and follow-up of Tetralogy of Fallot with pulmonary stenosis. *Congenit Heart Dis.* 2013;8:174–177.
38. Holmqvist C, Hochbergs P, Björkhem G, et al. Pre-operative evaluation with MR in tetralogy of fallot and pulmonary atresia with ventricular septal defect. *Acta Radiol.* 2001;42:63–69.
39. McElhinney DB, Reddy VM, Hanley FL. Tetralogy of Fallot with major aortopulmonary collaterals: early total repair. *Pediatr Cardiol.* 1998;19:289–296.
40. Lillehei CW, Cohen M, Warden HE, et al. Direct vision intracardiac surgical correction of the tetralogy of fallot, pentalogy of fallot, and pulmonary atresia defects report of first ten cases. *Ann Surg.* 1955;142(3):418 442.
41. Park CS, Lee JR, Lim HG, et al. The long-term result of total repair for tetralogy of Fallot. *Eur J Cardiothorac Surg.* 2010;38:311–317.
42. Puga FJ, Leoni FE, Julsrud PR, et al. Complete repair of pulmonary atresia, ventricular septal defect, and severe peripheral arborization abnormalities of the central pulmonary arteries. Experience with preliminary unifocalization procedures in 38 patients. *J Thorac Cardiovasc Surg.* 1989;98(6):1018–1028.
43. Dorfman AL, Geva T. Magnetic resonance imaging evaluation of congenital heart disease: conotruncal anomalies. *J Cardiovasc Magn Reson.* 2006;8:645–659.
44. Zucker N, Rozin I, Levitas A, et al. Clinical presentation, natural history, and outcome of patients with the absent pulmonary valve syndrome. *Cardiol Young.* 2004;14(4):402–408.
45. Choi YH, Seo JW, Choi JY, et al. Morphology of the tricuspid valve in pulmonary atresia with intact ventricular septum. *Pediatr Cardiol.* 1998;19:381–389.
46. Freedom RM. *Pulmonary Atresia with Intact Ventricular Septum.* Mount Kisco, NY: Futura Publishing; 1989.
47. Warnes CA. Transposition of the great arteries. *Circulation.* 2006;114:2699–2709.
48. Walters HL III, Mavroudis C, Tchervenkov CI, et al. Congenital heart surgery nomenclature and database project: double outlet right ventricle. *Ann Thorac Surg.* 2000;69(4 suppl):S249–S263.
49. Demir MT, Amasyall Y, Kopuz C, et al. The double outlet right ventricle with additional cardiac malformations: an anatomic and echocardiographic study. *Folia Morphol (Warsz).* 2009;68:104–108.
50. Brown JW, Ruzmetov M, Okada Y, et al. Surgical results in patients with double outlet right ventricle: a 20-year experience. *Ann Thorac Surg.* 2001;72:1630–1635.
51. Collett RW, Edwards JE. Persistent truncus arteriosus: a classification according to anatomic types. *Surg Clin North Am.* 1949;29:1245–1270.
52. Van Praagh R, Van Praagh S. The anatomy of common aorticopulmonary trunk (truncus arteriosus communis) and its embryologic implications. A study of 57 necropsy cases. *Am J Cardiol.* 1965;16(3):406–425.
53. Sojak V, Lugo J, Koolbergen D, et al. Surgery for truncus arteriosus. *Multimed Man Cardiothorac Surg.* 2012;2012.
54. Helms AS, Bach DS. Heart valve disease. *Prim Care.* 2013;40:91–108.
55. Cury M, Zeidan F, Lobato AC. Aortic disease in the young: genetic aneurysm syndromes, connective tissue disorders, and familial aortic aneurysms and dissections. *Int J Vasc Med.* 2013;2013:267215.
56. Predey TA, McDonald V, Demos TC, et al. CT of congenital anomalies of the aortic arch. *Semin Roentgenol.* 1989;24:96–113.
57. Frigerio A, Stevenson DA, Grimmer JF. The genetics of vascular anomalies. *Curr Opin Otolaryngol Head Neck Surg.* 2012;20(6):527–532.
58. Dodge-Khatami A, Backer CL, Mavroudis C. Risk factors for recoarctation and results of reoperation: a 40-year review. *J Card Surg.* 2000;15:369.
59. Jacobs ML, Chin AJ, Rychik J. Interrupted aortic arch. Impact of subaortic stenosis on management and outcome. *Circulation.* 1995;92(9 suppl):II128–II131.
60. Serraf A, Lacour-Gayet F, Robotin M, et al. Repair of interrupted aortic arch: a ten-year experience. *J Thorac Cardiovasc Surg.* 1996;112(5):1150–1160.
61. Shriki JE, Shinbane JS, Rashid MA, et al. Identifying, characterizing, and classifying congenital anomalies of the coronary arteries. *Radiographics.* 2012;32:453–468.
62. Cheitlin MD, MacGregor J. Congenital anomalies of coronary arteries: role in the pathogenesis of sudden cardiac death. *Herz.* 2009;34(4):268–279.
63. Rosenthal RL, Carrothers IA, Schussler JM. Benign or malignant anomaly? Very high takeoff of the left main coronary artery above the left coronary sinus. *Tex Heart Inst J.* 2012;39(4):538–541.
64. Peñalver JM, Mosca RS, Weitz D, et al. Anomalous aortic origin of coronary arteries from the opposite sinus: a critical appraisal of risk. *BMC Cardiovasc Disord.* 2012;12:83.
65. Van der Mieren G, Van Kerrebroeck C, Gutermann H, et al. Surgical angioplasty and unroofing technique for intramural coronary anomaly. *Interact Cardiovasc Thorac Surg.* 2011;13:424–426.

66. Zheng J, Ding W, Xiao Y, et al. Anomalous origin of the left coronary artery from the pulmonary artery in children: 15 years experience. *Pediatr Cardiol.* 2011;32:24–31.
67. Jin Z, Berger F, Uhlemann F. Improvement in left ventricular function in 11 consecutive pediatric patients with anomalous origin of the left coronary artery from the pulmonary artery. Early results of a serial ehcocardiographc follow up. *Eur Heart J.* 1994;15:1044–1049.
68. Takeuchi S, Imamura H, Katsumoto K. New surgical method for repair of anomalous origin of the left coronary artery from the pulmonary artery utilizing the trap door flap method. *J Thorac Cardiovasc Surg.* 1979;78:7–11.
69. Zenooz NA, Habibi R, Mammen L, et al. Coronary artery fistulas: CT findings. *Radiographics.* 2009;29:781–789.
70. Mazzucco A, Bortolotti U, Stellin G, et al. Anomalies of the systemic venous return: a review. *J Card Surg.* 1990;5(2):122–133.
71. Katre R, Burns SK, Murillo H, et al. Anomalous pulmonary venous connections. *Semin Ultrasound CT MR.* 2012;33:485–499.
72. Azakie A, Lavrsen MJ, Johnson NC, et al. Early outcomes of primary sutureless repair of the pulmonary veins. *Ann Thorac Surg.* 2011;92:666–671.
73. Gheissari A, Malm JR, Bowman FO Jr, et al. Cor triatriatum sinistrum: one institution's 28-year experience. *Pediatr Cardiol.* 1992;13:85–88.
74. Ibrahim T, Schreiber K, Dennig K, et al. Images in cardiovascular medicine. Assessment of cor triatriatum sinistrum by magnetic resonance imaging. *Circulation.* 2003;108(15):e107.
75. Jacobs JP, Anderson RH, Weinberg PM, et al. The nomenclature, definition and classification of cardiac structures in the setting of heterotaxy. *Cardiol Young.* 2007;17(suppl 2):1–28.
76. Garg N, Agarwal BL, Modi N, et al. Dextrocardia: an analysis of cardiac structures in 125 patients. *Int J Cardiol.* 2003;88:143–155.
77. Nonaka S, Shiratori Y, Saijoh Y, et al. Determination of left-right patterning of the mouse embryo by artificial nodal flow. *Nature.* 2002;418:96–99.
78. Ticho BS, Goldstein AM, Van Praagh R. Extracardiac anomalies in the heterotaxy syndromes with focus on anomalies of midline-associated structures. *Am J Cardiol.* 2000;85:729–734.
79. Applegate KE, Goske MJ, Pierce G, et al. Situs revisited: imaging of the heterotaxy syndrome. *Radiographics.* 1999;19:837–852.
80. Strouse PJ. Disorders of intestinal rotation and fixation ("malrotation"). *Pediatr Radiol.* 2004;34(11):837–851.
81. Tashjian DB, Weeks B, Brueckner M, et al. Outcomes after a Ladd procedure for intestinal malrotation with heterotaxia. *J Pediatr Surg.* 2007;42(3):528–531.
82. Murat A, Artas H, Yilmaz E, et al. Isolated congenital absence of the pericardium. *Pediatr Cardiol.* 2008;29:862–864.
83. Hong YM. Cardiomyopathies in children. *Korean J Pediatr.* 2013;56:52–59.
84. Maron BJ, Maron MS. Hypertrophic cardiomyopathy. *Lancet.* 2013;381:242–255.
85. Kushwaha SS, Fallon JT, Fuster V. Restrictive cardiomyopathy. *N Engl J Med.* 1997;336:267–276.
86. Goldstein JA. Differentiation of constrictive pericarditis and restrictive cardiomyopathy. *ACC Ed Highlights.* 1998;14–22.
87. Topilsky Y, Pereira NL, Shah DK, et al. Left ventricular assist device therapy in patients with restrictive and hypertrophic cardiomyopathy. *Circ Heart Fail.* 2011;4:266–275.
88. Tandri H, Saranathan M, Rodriguez ER, et al. Noninvasive detection of myocardial fibrosis in arrhythmogenic right ventricular cardiomyopathy using delayed-enhancement magnetic resonance imaging. *J Am Coll Cardiol.* 2005;45:98–103.
89. Fogel MA, Weinberg PM, Harris M, et al. Usefulness of magnetic resonance imaging for the diagnosis of right ventricular dysplasia in children. *Am J Cardiol.* 2006;97(8):1232–1237.
90. Marcus FI, McKenna WJ, Sherrill D, et al. Diagnosis of arrhythmogenic right ventricular cardiomyopathy/dysplasia: proposed modification of the task force criteria. *Circulation.* 2010;121(13):1533–1541.
91. Petersen SE, Selvanayagam JB, Wiesmann F, et al. Left ventricular non-compaction: insights from cardiovascular magnetic resonance imaging. *J Am Coll Cardiol.* 2005;46(1):101–105.
92. Dodd JD, Holmvang G, Hoffmann U, et al. Quantification of left ventricular noncompaction and trabecular delayed hyperenhancement with cardiac MRI: correlation with clinical severity. *AJR Am J Roentgenol.* 2007;189(4):974–980.
93. Milewicz DM, Dietz HC, Miller DC. Treatment of aortic disease in patients with Marfan syndrome. *Circulation.* 2005;111:e150–e157.
94. Hiratzka LF, Bakris GL, Beckman JA, et al. 2010 ACCF/AHA/AATS/ACR/ASA/SCA/SCAI/SIR/STS/SVM Guidelines for the diagnosis and management of patients with thoracic aortic disease. A Report of the American College of Cardiology Foundation/American Heart Association Task Force on Practice Guidelines, American Association for Thoracic Surgery, American College of Radiology, American Stroke Association, Society of Cardiovascular Anesthesiologists, Society for Cardiovascular Angiography and Interventions, Society of Interventional Radiology, Society of Thoracic Surgeons, and Society for Vascular Medicine. *J Am Coll Cardiol.* 2010;55(14).
95. Loeys BL, Dietz HC. Loeys-Dietz syndrome. In: Pagon RA, Adam MP, Bird TD, et al., eds. *GeneReviews.* Seattle, WA: University of Washington; 2008:1993–2013.
96. Reinstein E, Frentz S, Morgan T, et al. Vascular and connective tissue anomalies associated with X-linked periventricular heterotopia due to mutations in Filamin A. *Eur J Hum Genet.* 2013;21(5):494–502.
97. Masurel-Paulet A, Haan E, Thompson EM, et al. Lung disease associated with periventricular nodular heterotopia and an FLNA mutation. *Eur J Med Genet.* 2011;54(1):25–28.
98. Beghetti M, Gow RM, Haney I, et al. Pediatric primary benign cardiac tumors: a 15-year review. *Am Heart J.* 1997;134:1107–1114.
99. Beroukhim RS, Prakash A, Buechel ER, et al. Characterization of cardiac tumors in children by cardiovascular magnetic resonance imaging: a multicenter experience. *J Am Coll Cardiol.* 2011;58:1044–1054.
100. Barron K. Kawasaki disease: etiology, pathogenesis and treatment. *Cleve Clin J Med.* 2002;69:SII69–SII78.
101. Greil GF, Stuber M, Botnar RM, et al. Coronary magnetic resonance angiography in adolescents and young adults with Kawasaki disease. *Circulation.* 2002;105:908–911.
102. Newburger J, Takahashi M, Gerber M, et al. Diagnosis, treatment, and long term management of Kawasaki disease: a statement for health professionals from the committee on rheumatic fever, endocarditis and Kawasaki disease, Council on cardiovascular disease in young American Heart Association. *Circulation.* 2004;110:2747–2771.
103. Karatolios K, Pankuweit S, Maisch B. Diagnosis and treatment of myocarditis: the role of endomyocardial biopsy. *Curr Treat Options Cardiovasc Med.* 2007;9:473–481.

104. Klugman D, Berger JT, Sable CA, et al. Pediatric patients hospitalized with myocarditis: a multi-institutional analysis. *Pediatr Cardiol.* 2009;31(2):222–228.
105. Durani Y, Egan M, Baffa J, et al. Pediatric myocarditis: presenting clinical characteristics. *Am J Emerg Med.* 2009;27: 942–947.
106. Dudzinski DM, Mak GS, Hung JW. Pericardial diseases. *Curr Probl Cardiol.* 2012;37(3):75–118.
107. Mastroianni A, Coronado O, Chiodo F. Tuberculous pericarditis and AIDS: case reports and review. *Eur J Epidemiol.* 1997;13:755–759.
108. Imazio M, Brucato A, Maestroni S, et al. Risk of constrictive pericarditis after acute pericarditis. *Circulation.* 2007;1006: 1026–1028.
109. Yared K, Baggish AL, Picard MH, et al. Multimodality imaging of pericardial diseases. *JACC Cardiovasc Imaging.* 2010;3:650–660.

CHAPTER 10

Great Vessels

Monica Epelman • Pilar Garcia-Pena • Eric J. Chong Barboza • Magdalena Gormsen • Fatma Hamza Makame • Edward Y. Lee

INTRODUCTION

Congenital and acquired thoracic vascular abnormalities involve the thoracic aorta and branch arteries, pulmonary arteries, thoracic systemic veins, and pulmonary veins. Imaging evaluation of these vascular abnormalities typically requires a combination of radiographs, ultrasound (echocardiography), computed tomography angiography (CTA), magnetic resonance imaging (MRI), magnetic resonance angiography (MRA), and catheter angiography (CA). In recent years, technological advances in multidetector-row computed tomography (MDCT) and MRI have greatly advanced the noninvasive diagnosis of these vascular anomalies in the pediatric population. The use of multiplanar (2D) and 3D visualization techniques in both aforementioned modalities provides comprehensive multiprojectional anatomical displays for interactive interpretation, treatment planning, and postoperative and postendovascular evaluation.[1–6]

Clear knowledge and understanding of a cost-effective approach and the appropriate utilization of the available imaging modalities are required in today's clinical environment. The approach should be based on the type of underlying vascular abnormality, the inherent advantages and limitations of each imaging modality, and the overall performance of each imaging modality. In this chapter, up-to-date imaging techniques for evaluating the great vessels in infants and children are presented, and normal anatomy is reviewed. In addition, commonly encountered congenital and acquired thoracic vascular abnormalities are discussed with reference to clinical features, characteristic imaging findings, and treatment approaches.

IMAGING TECHNIQUES

Radiography

Chest radiography is readily available and provides a rapid and inexpensive means of obtaining initial diagnostic information in infants and children with clinically suspected thoracic vascular abnormalities. The chest radiograph provides valuable information concerning the structure and function of the cardiovascular system by permitting assessment of the size and extent of pulmonary vascularization as well as the size of the cardiac chambers. Although a chest radiograph is rarely sufficient to make a specific underlying cardiovascular diagnosis, for a small amount of radiation exposure (0.02 to 0.04 mSv), it may guide early treatment and subsequent advanced imaging and also serve as a baseline in certain conditions.

Chest radiographic examination usually consists of frontal and lateral views of the chest. In the case of neonates, chest radiographs are typically combined with an abdominal–pelvic radiograph, a so-called babygram, in order to facilitate the confirmation of appropriate positioning for all support devices including lines and tubes placed during initial evaluation. Subsequent chest radiographs should extend to at least the midabdomen, with or without the pelvis, depending upon the type of device, to account for variable degrees of inspiration. Such radiographs are obtained at the discretion of the medical team not only to permit the assessment of cardiovascular status but also especially to allow the evaluation of support devices, as malpositioned devices can lead to iatrogenic complications. In addition, the course of the support devices can offer clues to the individual patient's underlying vascular

TABLE 10.1 Abnormal Course of Support Devices Suggesting Vascular Anomalies or Congenital Heart Disease

Device	Abnormal Course
Endotracheal tube	If deviated leftward, may suggest a right aortic arch
Umbilical venous line	If ascends to the left of the spine, may suggest a left-sided or a double IVC May be seen in heterotaxy
Umbilical arterial line	If ascends to the chest on the right, may suggest a right aortic arch If ascends to the chest on the left, but crosses to the right of the spine, may suggest a right aortic arch with a circumflex aorta
PICC line	If descends along the left mediastinum → left-sided SVC to coronary sinus If ascends to the left of the spine → left-sided or a double IVC
Enteric tube	If terminates in the right upper quadrant → right-sided stomach → heterotaxy

PICC, peripherally inserted central catheter; IVC, inferior vena cava; SVC, superior vena cava.

anatomy and provide a basis for the evaluation of congenital vascular abnormalities (Table 10.1).

Ultrasound and Echocardiography

Ultrasound (US) and transthoracic echocardiography (ECHO) are usually the next diagnostic modalities employed in the assessment of infants and children with clinically suspected of having thoracic vascular abnormalities. Vascular US is used to visualize the peripheral vascular system, and ECHO is used for the heart, coronary arteries, pulmonary vasculature, thoracic aorta, and intrathoracic systemic veins. US and ECHO have advantages over other imaging modalities because they permit the noninvasive evaluation of morphology, function, and flow without exposure to radiation or potentially nephrotoxic contrast medium. Real-time gray-scale US images and cine loops are acquired in multiple projections to the heart, aorta, central pulmonary arteries and veins, and central intrathoracic systemic veins to depict various segments of the cardiac anatomy and vascular branches. In addition, flow characteristics such as direction and velocity can be determined by Doppler. However, US and ECHO are limited by acoustic impedance, operator skill, and ability to visualize peripheral vascular segments, including those of the pulmonary arteries, pulmonary veins, and supra-aortic branch arteries.[3–5]

Computed Tomography

Nowadays, the evaluation of great vessel abnormalities can usually be performed with MDCT using CTA protocol without sedation and electrocardiographic gating. Because of the inherent radiation risk, CT should be judiciously used in pediatric patients. CT is typically indicated for evaluation of mediastinal vascular abnormality in infants and children when (1) there is a high sedation or general anesthesia risk; (2) coassessment of noncardiovascular structures, especially the airway and lungs, is required; (3) emergent imaging is necessary; and (4) higher spatial resolution is needed. Other advantages of CT include wide clinical availability and short examination times.

With the latest generation CT scanners, acquisition time <2 seconds is feasible for mediastinal vascular imaging in pediatric patients. On the other hand, a typical MRI examination is currently acquired over 30 to 45 minutes. Obtaining selected MRI sequences may potentially decrease the total examination time to 10 to 15 minutes, but in most instances, this does not entirely obviate the need for sedation or general anesthesia in infants and young children who cannot follow breathing instruction.

Thoughtful patient preparation before CT imaging can lead to high-quality CT data set for accurately assessing great vessels, which in turn can result in optimal patient care. In order to optimize photon delivery and minimize the adverse effect of noise, the targeted region needs to be isocentered in the gantry. All external metallic objects and support devices with metallic components (e.g., weighted feeding tubes) should be removed, if possible, from the region to be scanned. This is because the presence of radiodense material may result in streak artifacts and can aggravate the effects of noise when low-dose parameters are used.[4] Similarly, the upper extremities are raised above the head and out of the field of view when performing chest CT, whereas they are placed at the patient's side for head and neck CT studies.

Because of their inherent dependence upon radiation, CT protocols in pediatric patients should strive for only one core series (i.e., a single-phase angiographic scan). Such CT examination is typically obtained using the lowest possible voltage (80 kVp is usually sufficient for most pediatric patients under 60 kg) and with weight-based low-dose milliamperage following as low as reasonably achievable (ALARA) principle. In addition, at lower tube voltages (80 kVp), the use of iodinated contrast material is more efficient and yields higher attenuation of the vascular structures scanned because 80 kVp is closer to the k-edge of iodine (33.2 keV).[7,8]

For mediastinal vascular imaging with CTA, highly concentrated iodine contrast medium (300 to 370 mg I/mL) is administered according to weight (2 mL/kg, not to exceed 5 mL/kg or a total of 100 mL), at the highest weight-based injection rate possible via a pressure-limiting power injector (e.g., a pressure limit set to 200 to 250 psi).[3–5] The injection rate currently used varies according to the patient's weight

TABLE 10.2 Recommended Intravenous Catheter Sites in Relation to Anatomy

Type of Study	Preferred IV Catheter Site	Second Choice	Other Possible Location
Chest CTA/MRA with left aortic arch	Right AC	Foot	Last resource: left AC
Chest CTA/MRA with right aortic arch	Left AC	Foot	Last resource: right AC
Abdomen/pelvis CTA/MRA	Right or left AC	Last resource: foot	
Right upper extremity CTA/MRA	Left AC	Foot	Last resource: right AC
Left upper extremity CTA/MRA	Right AC	Foot	Last resource: left AC
Both upper extremities CTA/MRA	Foot		
Bilateral lower extremities CTA/MRA	Right or left AC		

AC, antecubital; IV, intravenous.

and IV access. For example, the injection rate of ~1.0 mL/s can be used in infants. For adult-sized older children, the contrast can be injected at 3 to 5 mL/s. The antecubital location is the preferred access site for the larger vein size needed to accommodate high flow rates of IV contrast administration for CTA. In neonates and young infants, a forearm, hand, or foot vein may also be considered. In such cases, the use of a power injectable, peripherally inserted central catheter is a more desirable and safer option.[4] On the basis of hemodynamic and anatomic data, the injection of IV contrast medium should be performed into the right upper extremity vein in order to limit streak artifacts from the dense contrast across the aortic arch, which can occur when the left upper extremity vein is used[9] (Table 10.2). Initially, the test injection should be performed using peripheral IV access with saline with a flow rate similar to that planned for the contrast medium for CTA. If the test injection is uneventful, the contrast injection, followed by a saline chase to clear the venous inflow and optimize the volume of contrast medium that reaches the target region, can be subsequently obtained.

CT imaging using automated bolus tracking should be considered because this method permits the use of a lower total amount of contrast agent and optimizes the accurate timing of the CT scanning.[3,10,11] A region of interest (ROI) is placed in the vessel to be evaluated, and the CT imaging is triggered automatically when a predefined enhancement threshold (e.g., 90 to 150 HU) is achieved. In general, the minimum amount of coverage and the shortest possible scan times (fast gantry rotation times, high pitch, and volumetric CT techniques) should be used. If possible, coverage should be tailored to the specific clinical question, and radiosensitive organs such as the thyroid should be avoided or limited. CTA for the evaluation of mediastinal vascular abnormality is typically obtained under suspended respiration or during quiet breathing.

Once axial CT data set is obtained, they can be reconstructed into 3- or 5-mm-thick axial CT images for routine viewing and into at least 1.5 mm axial CT images with 50% overlap for reconstructions and to maximize 3D displays[3–5,11] (Table 10.3). The use of 3D visualization techniques provides comprehensive multiprojectional anatomical displays of often complex mediastinal vascular abnormalities for interactive interpretation, treatment planning, and postoperative and postendovascular evaluation.[1–5] Volume-rendered (VR) and maximum intensity projection (MIP) images are currently available and clinically helpful for (1) depiction of the spatial relationship between the vessels in question and the adjacent structures, (2) grading of vascular stenosis and extent, and (3) improved delivery of the findings obtained by imaging to the referring clinicians and families.[1] The use of interactive 3D workstations not only facilitates the evaluation of the vascular structures, which are better depicted in the z-axis, but also assists in overcoming the noise that may occur with the use of low-dose protocols.[4–6]

Magnetic Resonance Imaging

MRI is an increasingly utilized imaging modality for evaluating the great vessels, particularly in the pediatric population. However, it is rarely used as a first-line imaging modality. MRI typically complements US or ECHO as a noninvasive alternative to conventional CA. When used to evaluate more central vascular structures such as great vessels, three main types of MRI techniques are currently available that include (1) ECG-gated "black-blood" MR imaging, (2) static and cine "white-blood" MR imaging, and (3) a 3D contrast-enhanced angiographic MR imaging.

Black-blood MR imaging refers to the low signal exhibited by cardiovascular structures. It is used primarily to delineate anatomy and morphology and to visualize spatial relationships, particularly those of vascular structures and the adjacent central airway.[5,12,13] In the past, spin-echo sequences were used for black-blood imaging; today, these techniques have been largely supplanted by fast spin-echo (FSE) and turbo spin-echo (TSE) techniques.[14] These MRI sequences are ECG gated at end diastole and may be obtained with or without double inversion recovery techniques in order to null the signal from blood. They also may be obtained in any desired plane, including the sagittal oblique or "candy cane" view. Care should be taken with slow-flowing blood and when gadolinium is present because these conditions may interfere

TABLE 10.3 Cardiovascular Advanced Visualization Techniques

	Display	Principle Use	Advantages	Disadvantages
MPR	2D	• Structural detail • Quantitative analysis	• "Slice" through data set in coronal, sagittal, and oblique projections • Real-time multiplanar interrogation • Simplify image interpretation	• Limited spatial perception
CPR	2D	• Structural detail • Centerline display • Simplify MPR	• Single anatomical display • Longitudinal cross-sectional anatomical display	• Operator dependent
Ray-Sum	2D	• Structural overview	• "Slice" through data set in axial, coronal, sagittal, and oblique projections • Real-time multiplanar interrogation • Radiograph-like display	• Loss of structural detail with increased slab thickness

MIP	2D	• Structural overview
		• Angiographic display
			• "Slice" through data set in axial, coronal, sagittal, and oblique projections
			• Real-time multiplanar interrogation
			• Improved depiction
			  • Small caliber vessels
			  • Poorly enhanced vessels
			• Communicate findings
				• Anatomical overlap (vessels, bone, viscera) with increased slab thickness
				• Visualization degraded by high-density structures (i.e., bone, calcium, stents, coils)
				• Loss of structural detail with increased slab thickness
				• Limited grading of stent lumens

MinIP	2D	• Structural Overview • Airway • Air trapping in the lung • Soft tissue air	• "Slice" through data set in axial, coronal, sagittal, and oblique projections • Real-time multiplanar interrogation • Depict low-density structures • Communicate findings	• Anatomical overlap • Loss of structural detail with increased slab thickness
VR	3D	• Structural overview • Angiographic display	• "Slice" through data set in axial, coronal, sagittal, and oblique projections • Real-time multiplanar interrogation • Depict structural relationships • Accurate spatial perception • Communicate findings	• Dependent upon opacity-transfer function • Anatomical overlap • Loss of structural detail with increased slab thickness

2D, two dimensional; 3D, three dimensional; MPR, multiplanar reformation; CPR, curved planar reformation; MIP, maximum intensity projection; MinIP, minimum intensity projection; VR, volume rendered.

Reprinted from Hellinger JC, Pena A, Poon M, et al. Pediatric computed tomographic angiography: imaging the cardiovascular system gently. Radiol Clin North Am. 2010;48(2):439–467, with permission. Ref. 4.

with the nulling of flowing blood and may appear bright on the sequence, potentially resulting in artifacts that may lead to misinterpretation. For this reason, gadolinium should be administered only after black-blood imaging has been performed.[14] T1-weighted gradient echo sequences performed before and after contrast administration are usually used instead of black-blood MR images for the assessment of vessel wall thickening in cases of vasculitis.[15]

Bright-blood or white-blood MR imaging may consist of static and/or cine images. Static white-blood images are generally obtained with the steady-state free precession (SSFP) technique; a full stack of the entire chest can be acquired in <30 seconds, providing a useful adjunct to the more time-consuming acquisition of a black-blood MR imaging sequence for anatomic depiction. Cine white-blood MR imaging is typically used to evaluate cardiac function and is usually obtained either with gradient-echo sequences or with a balanced-SSFP pulse sequence. These MRI sequences provide cine images that permit visualization of cardiac or valvular motion in multiple frames over the entire cardiac cycle, allowing assessment of cardiac function and calculation of ventricular volumes. The SSFP pulse sequence demonstrates high signal-to-noise and high contrast-to-noise ratios between the blood pool and myocardial interface.[11–14,16]

Angiographic techniques include time-of-flight MRA, multiphase (arterial and venous) 3D T1-weighted contrast-enhanced MRA, and time-resolved MRA. Contrast-enhanced acquisitions are often conducted in the coronal plane, depending on the required anatomical coverage and breath-hold duration. The use of time-resolved MRA permits the depiction of reliable first-pass imaging that is independent of the timing of contrast injection and acquisition, resulting in clear depiction of dextro and levo phases and providing insight into the hemodynamics of the disease process and the assessment of collateral circulation. Multiplanar reformatting, maximum-intensity projection, volume rendering, and virtual endoscopy are useful adjuncts for enhancing interpretation[5,6,12,13,16–18] (Table 10.3).

Phase-contrast imaging with velocity-encoded imaging is a useful adjunct to the acquisition of angiographic MR images. It is primarily used as a noninvasive method to accurately quantify velocity, flow, and related pressure gradients. Pulmonary blood flow (Qp) and systemic blood flow (Qs) may be assessed with this technique and used to calculate the pulmonary-to-systemic flow ratio (Qp:Qs) and to determine the shunt fraction. A Qp:Qs >1.5 usually indicates a significant left-to-right shunt that may require intervention.[5,19]

Nuclear Medicine

Nuclear medicine studies involving the pediatric thorax are primarily used to evaluate myocardial perfusion and viability in adult patients. Lung ventilation/perfusion imaging, which is at times used for the diagnosis of pulmonary embolism in adult, is mainly employed for quantification of differential and regional lung perfusion in congenital heart disease in pediatric patients. Right-to-left shunts may be demonstrated during the course of a perfusion scan by showing accumulation of the radiotracer within capillary beds of other organs, typically the brain and kidneys.[20]

Catheter Angiography

Catheter angiography remains the reference standard for vascular imaging in both pediatric and adult patients. However, it is invasive and exposes the pediatric patient to radiation and to the nephrotoxic effects of iodinated contrast media. Catheter angiography also typically requires the use of sedation or general anesthesia. In today's clinical practice, Catheter angiography is primarily used for interventions. In rare instances, it is used as a problem-solving tool for issues related to morphology, flow, or function that cannot be fully answered by the other noninvasive imaging modalities.[4,5]

NORMAL ANATOMY

Aorta

The normal thoracic aorta can be divided into four major segments: the aortic root, the ascending aorta, the aortic arch, and the descending aorta. The aortic root is the segment of the aorta that originates from the left ventricle. The aortic root includes the aortic valve annulus, the aortic valve cusps, and the sinuses of Valsalva, including the right, left, and noncoronary sinuses, which serve as attachments for the valve leaflets and house the coronary arteries ostia. The ascending aorta extends from the sinotubular junction to the first branch of the aortic arch, typically the brachiocephalic or innominate artery. In normal individuals, the sinotubular junction is characteristically distinguished by a sharp waist to which the aortic leaflets attach. The aortic arch extends from the origin of the brachiocephalic artery to the insertion of the ductus or ligamentum arteriosum. The aortic arch gives origin to the major head and neck arteries. From anterior to posterior, these typically consist of the brachiocephalic, left common carotid, and left subclavian arteries. Common normal variants include a bovine arch consisting of a common origin of the brachiocephalic artery and the left common carotid artery and a direct origin of the left vertebral artery off the aortic arch between the origins of the left common carotid and left subclavian arteries. The descending aorta begins at the aortic isthmus, which is marked by the location of the ductus or ligamentum arteriosum.[21] The descending aorta is further subdivided into thoracic and abdominal portions at the aortic hiatus.[15,22,23]

Standardized, reproducible aortic landmarks for measurement were published in 2010 in an ACCF/AHA guideline.[15] The published guideline notes that external diameter measurements should be made perpendicular to the longitudinal or flow axis of the vessel (Fig. 10.1). It should be noted that, in the cardiology literature, the aortic isthmus is considered only the point at which the ligamentum arteriosum inserts.[15,21]; however, several authors in the radiologic literature consider the aortic isthmus to represent the portion of the distal aortic arch that extends from the left subclavian artery to the insertion of the ligamentum arteriosum.[22,24–26] In 2008, Kaiser et al.[27] established normal values for thoracic aortic dimensions related to body growth in children and adolescents aged 2 to 20 years using images obtained by contrast-enhanced MR angiography. These authors provided an Excel file that permits the calculation of percentiles and z-scores and graphical display of the calculated values on the normative curves. These data are especially suitable for pediatric patients and may be utilized for the diagnosis, treatment planning, and follow-up of aortic abnormalities in the pediatric population. Given the lack of normative data obtained with contrast-enhanced MR angiography in neonates and young infants with body surface areas <0.5 m^2, Madan and colleagues[28] recommend the use of ECHO-based z-scores for this subset of patients.

Pulmonary Artery

The main pulmonary artery (MPA) originates during the 4th week of embryogenesis after the conotruncal division is formed. Originating from the right ventricular outflow tract, it transports deoxygenated blood to the lungs for oxygenation, a distinctive function of the pulmonary arteries. The MPA follows an intrapericardial direction coursing superiorly and posteriorly. The MPA then passes anteriorly and to the left of the

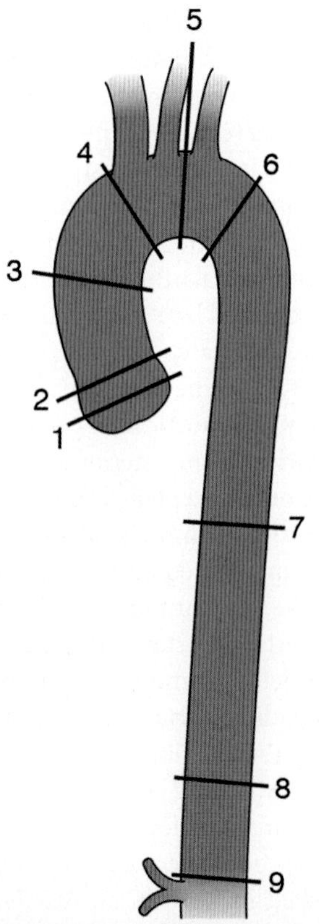

FIGURE 10.1 **Normal aortic segments with standard landmarks for reporting aortic diameter.** Locations: (*1*) sinuses of Valsalva; (*2*) sinotubular junction; (*3*) midascending aorta; (*4*) proximal aortic arch; (*5*) midaortic arch; (*6*) proximal descending thoracic aorta (begins at the isthmus); (*7*) middescending aorta; (*8*) aorta at diaphragmatic hiatus; (*9*) abdominal aorta at the celiac axis origin. (Based on Hiratzka LF, Bakris GL, Beckman JA, et al. 2010 ACCF/AHA/AATS/ACR/ASA/SCA/SCAI/SIR/STS/SVM guidelines for the diagnosis and management of patients with thoracic aortic disease: executive summary. A report of the American College of Cardiology Foundation/American Heart Association Task Force on Practice Guidelines, American Association for Thoracic Surgery, American College of Radiology, American Stroke Association, Society of Cardiovascular Anesthesiologists, Society for Cardiovascular Angiography and Interventions, Society of Interventional Radiology, Society of Thoracic Surgeons, and Society for Vascular Medicine. *Catheter Cardiovasc Interv.* 2010;76[2]:E43–E86. *Ref. 15.*)

ascending aorta before giving origin to the right and left pulmonary arteries, which are derived from the sixth pharyngeal arch. The left pulmonary artery (LPA) is shorter and slightly smaller than the right pulmonary artery (RPA). The ductus or its remnant, the ligamentum arteriosum, courses posteriorly and superiorly to the undersurface of the aortic arch just distal to the origin of the left subclavian artery. The RPA and LPA travel along the bronchi down to the subsegmental level matching the adjacent bronchi in course and caliber.[22,29–31]

The relationship of the pulmonary arteries to the central airway is important for the assessment of thoracic situs because there is good agreement between this relationship and atrial laterality, one of the most important factors in determining situs. The relationship between the pulmonary arteries and the central bronchi can be easily demonstrated on multiplanar (2D) and 3D reconstructions. Identification of the right eparterial bronchus, meaning that the first branch of the right mainstem bronchus is above the level of the RPA, and the left hyparterial bronchus, meaning that the first branch of the left mainstem bronchus is below the level of the LPA, is considered predictive of thoracic situs solitus.[29]

Pulmonary Veins

In most instances, there are four individual pulmonary veins, two for each lung. However, there is substantial variation in the number and branching pattern of the pulmonary venous drainage, with variation on the right considerably greater than that on the left. The most common variation, which is seen in ~25% of cases, is the presence of an additional third pulmonary vein on the right side that independently drains the right middle lobe.[32–34]

Superior Vena Cava

The superior vena cava (SVC) serves as the major draining route for the veins of the head and neck and the bilateral upper extremities. The SVC is formed by the confluence of the right and left brachiocephalic veins. The SVC courses caudally and drains into the morphologic right atrium.[33–36]

Inferior Vena Cava

The suprahepatic inferior vena cava (IVC) is a short intrathoracic portion of the IVC that drains the lower half of the body into the right atrium. It crosses the diaphragm at the level of T8 after receiving the hepatic veins. Imaging confirmation of IVC drainage into the right atrium is an important clue in the determination of atrial situs solitus because it is unusual for the IVC to drain elsewhere.[33,34]

SPECTRUM OF GREAT VESSEL ABNORMALITIES

Congenital Great Vascular Anomalies

Aorta

Cervical Aortic Arch

Cervical aortic arch (CAA) is a rare vascular anomaly in which the aortic arch is in a supraclavicular location (Fig. 10.2). Clinically, it may present as a pulsatile lesion in the ipsilateral supraclavicular fossa. This vascular anomaly is believed to be the result of persistence of the embryonic third arch with regression of the expected fourth arch. CAA has been described in association with chromosome 22q 11 deletion.[5,22,37]

Left Aortic Arch with an Aberrant Right Subclavian Artery

A left aortic arch with an aberrant right subclavian artery is the most common type of aortic arch anomaly. In this vascular anomaly, the aortic arch gives rise, in sequence, to the

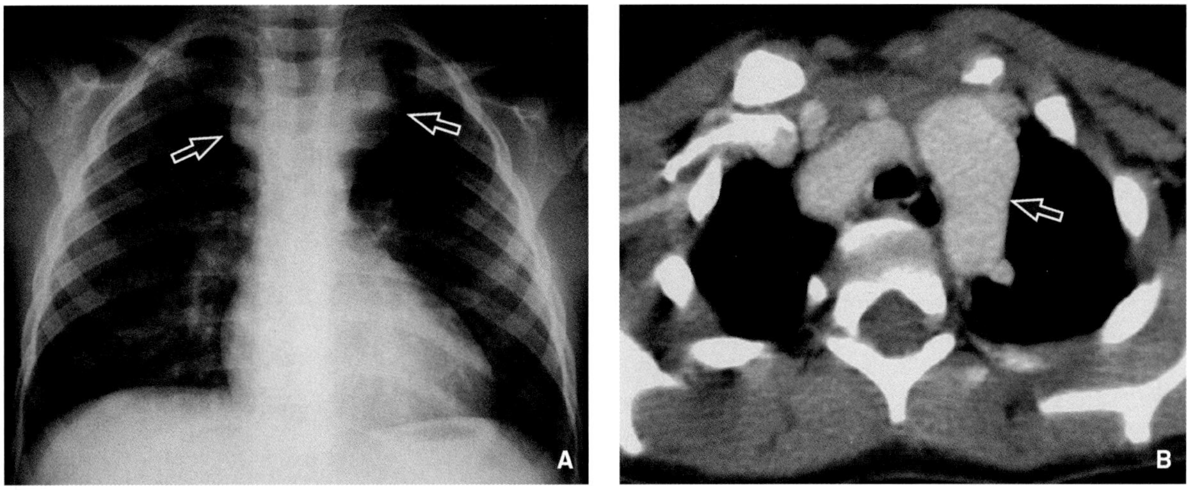

FIGURE 10.2 **Cervical aortic arch in a 3-year-old girl who presented with a pulsatile left upper chest mass. A:** Frontal chest radiograph shows a superior mediastinal lesion (*arrows*). **B:** Axial enhanced CT image demonstrates a left aortic arch (*arrow*) which is located in a supraclavicular region.

right common carotid artery, the left common carotid artery, the left subclavian artery, and the aberrant right subclavian artery, which takes a retroesophageal course. This vascular anomaly does not form a vascular ring because the trachea and esophagus are not entirely surrounded by vessels and/or ligaments. In the older literature, the presence of this variant was reported to result in so-called dysphagia lusoria in elderly patients. In these cases, the aberrant right subclavian artery is smooth in its contours, nearly equal in caliber throughout its intrathoracic course and tapers gradually[37–39] (Fig. 10.3).

Vascular Rings

Vascular rings are a spectrum of congenital mediastinal vascular anomalies resulting from abnormal development of the embryonic aortic arches. As a result of these vascular anomalies, the trachea and esophagus are completely surrounded by vessels or their atretic portions, potentially resulting in airway or esophageal compression.[5,38–43] The vessels conforming the vascular ring may include the aortic arch or arches, aortic arch branch vessels, pulmonary branch arteries, and the ductus arteriosus or the ligamentum arteriosum.[38,39]

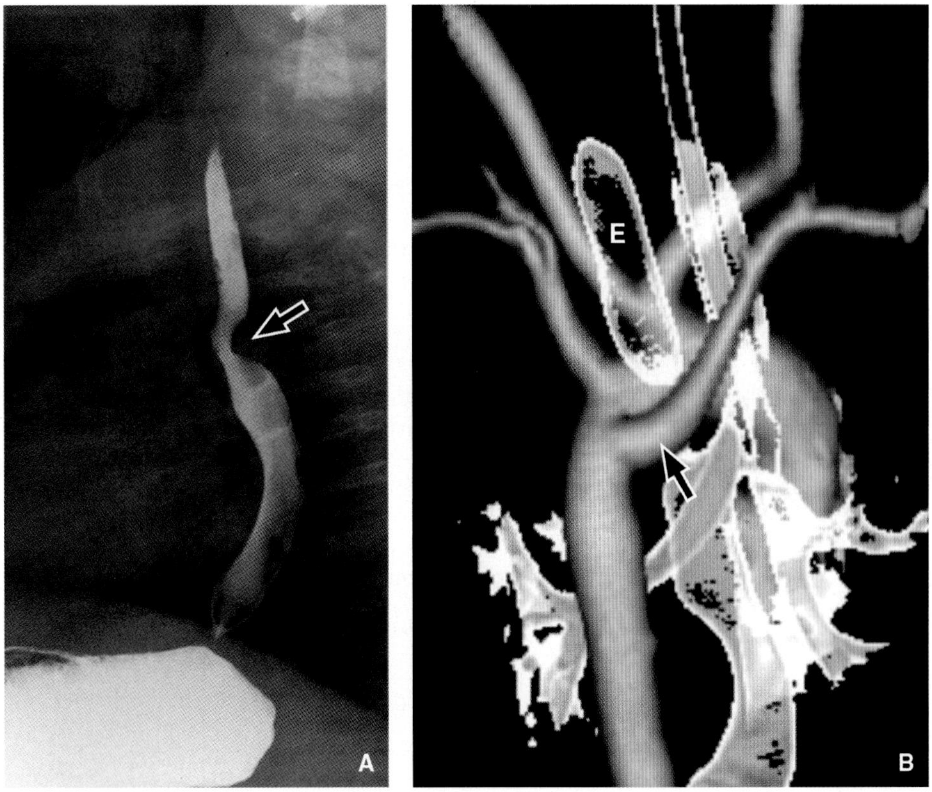

FIGURE 10.3 **Left aortic arch with an aberrant right subclavian artery in a 2-month-old boy who presented with intermittent stridor. A:** Lateral view of esophagogram shows mass effect (*arrow*) upon the posterior aspect of the barium containing esophagus. **B:** 3D volume-rendered CT image demonstrates an aberrant right subclavian artery (*arrow*), which is smooth in caliber and without evidence of a Kommerell diverticulum or airway compression. However, the compression on the esophagus (*E*) is again seen.

Affected pediatric patients may be asymptomatic, and the anomaly may be incidentally discovered in adulthood. Alternatively, the resulting airway compression may produce substantial respiratory symptoms such as a distinctive stridor worsening with feedings, cyanotic episodes, and even respiratory arrest, particularly in neonates and young infants.[38,40,41,43–46] Aortic arch anomalies have been reported in association with chromosome 22q11 deletion.[5,37] Moreover, chromosome 22q11 deletion is found in ~25% of patients with aortic arch anomalies who lack associated intracardiac defects.[44]

In the past, barium esophagography used to be the primary imaging modality for the evaluation of vascular rings during the early 1930s. However, CA became the reference standard in the 1960s. Currently, CT and MRI have largely replaced the aforementioned modalities given their higher sensitivity (approaching 100%) for the diagnosis of vascular rings in noninvasive manner.[43]

Symptomatic vascular rings are currently surgically managed to reduce compression of the airway and esophagus in the pediatric population (Table 10.4).

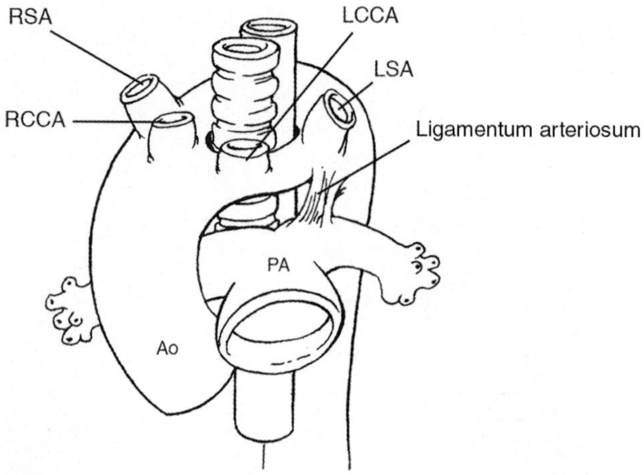

FIGURE 10.4 **Double aortic arch.** *Ao*, ascending aorta; *LCCA*, left common carotid artery; *LSA*, left subclavian artery; *PA*, pulmonary artery; *RCCA*, right common carotid artery; *RSA*, right subclavian artery.

Double Aortic Arch with Variants

Double aortic arch (DAA) is the result of persistence of both the right and left embryonic fourth arches (Fig. 10.4). It is the most common form of symptomatic vascular ring. DAA is seldom associated with congenital heart disease; if present, the congenital disease is usually tetralogy of Fallot.

In the majority of DAA, both arches remain patent; however, in some cases, an atretic segment may be present in either arch. The atretic segment is more typically seen in the left arch and is characteristically located following the take-off of the left subclavian artery.[1,5,38,39] Therefore, in the majority of cases, the right arch is dominant. Typically, the right arch is more superiorly located than the left arch, as is best seen on coronal cross-sectional images. In these instances, the descending aorta is more frequently seen on the left side.[38] Less frequently, the two arches are codominant and equivalent in size or the right arch is atretic and the left arch is dominant. When both arches are patent and similar in size, each arch shows relatively symmetric origins of each of the four major supraaortic vessels (right and left carotid and subclavian arteries) from the respective arch, constituting an important imaging clue (four-vessel sign) in the diagnosis of this mediastinal vascular anomaly. However, in instances in which the right arch is dominant, the branching pattern may be indistinguishable from those of the right aortic arch with mirror image branching. In this situation, the only clue for diagnosis would be a left-sided descending aorta on the side opposite that of the arch[5,38,39] (Figs. 10.5 and 10.6).

TABLE 10.4 Surgical Management of Symptomatic Vascular Rings

Right aortic arch with an aberrant left subclavian artery	Surgical division of left ligamentum arteriosum Left thoracotomy approach
Double aortic arch	Surgical division of the smaller arch and the ligamentum (if present) Thoracotomy ipsilateral to the smaller arch
Circumflex left aortic arch	Surgical division of right ligamentum arteriosum Right or midline thoracotomy approach

Surgical division of the underlying vascular ring is current management of choice for symptomatic pediatric patients with DAA. When considering surgical division, it should be recognized that a ligamentum arteriosum or, in some cases, a patent ductus arteriosus may be present, which should be also divided in addition to one of the arches. If not, the ligamentum may still form a vascular ring once the arches are divided, without amelioration of the symptoms.[38,39]

Circumflex Left Aortic Arch

In this rare aortic vascular anomaly, the aortic arch is left sided and the aorta loops around the trachea, coursing posterior to the esophagus to the right side of the spine and resulting in a proximal right descending aorta opposite the side of the arch. A right-sided ligamentum or a right-sided ductus typically completes the vascular ring. Therefore, unlike most instances, a right thoracotomy approach is needed in order to divide the vascular ring although a midline approach may also be utilized. This aortic vascular anomaly may occur in association with an aberrant right subclavian artery. In this situation, the aberrant subclavian artery is not retroesophageal in its course despite the fact that it arises from the descending aorta as the last arch vessel as it passes from its horizontal to its more nearly vertical course.[5,37]

Right Aortic Arch with Variants

Three main types of right aortic arch anomalies may be seen in association with vascular rings:

1. Right aortic arch with an aberrant left subclavian artery off a Kommerell diverticulum
2. Right aortic arch with left descending aorta (right circumflex aortic arch) (Fig. 10.7)

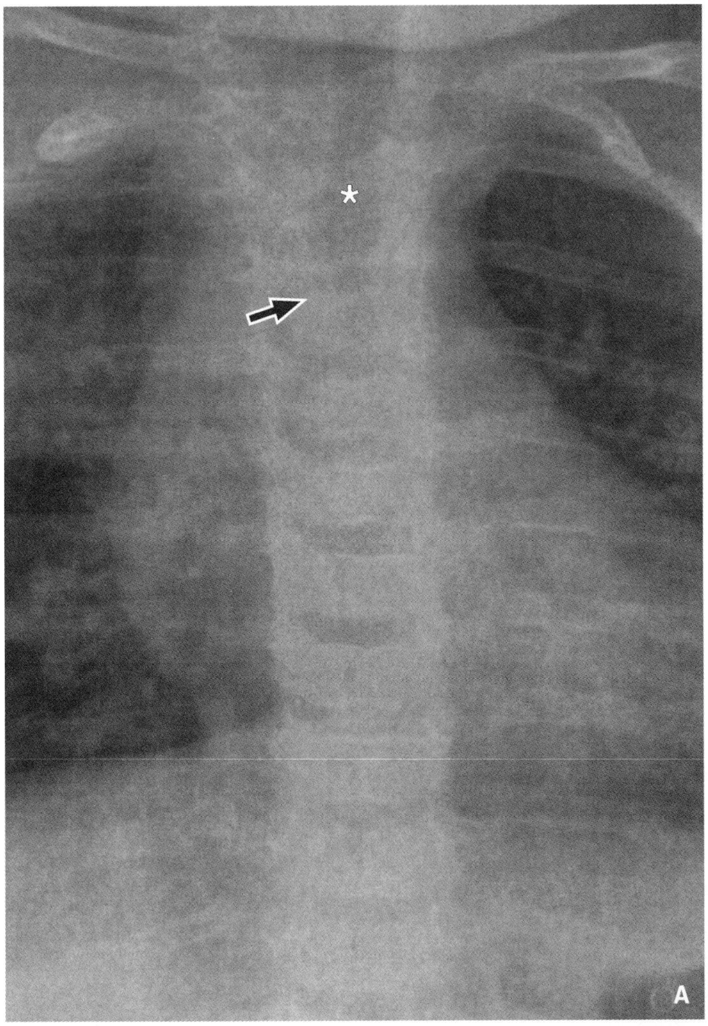

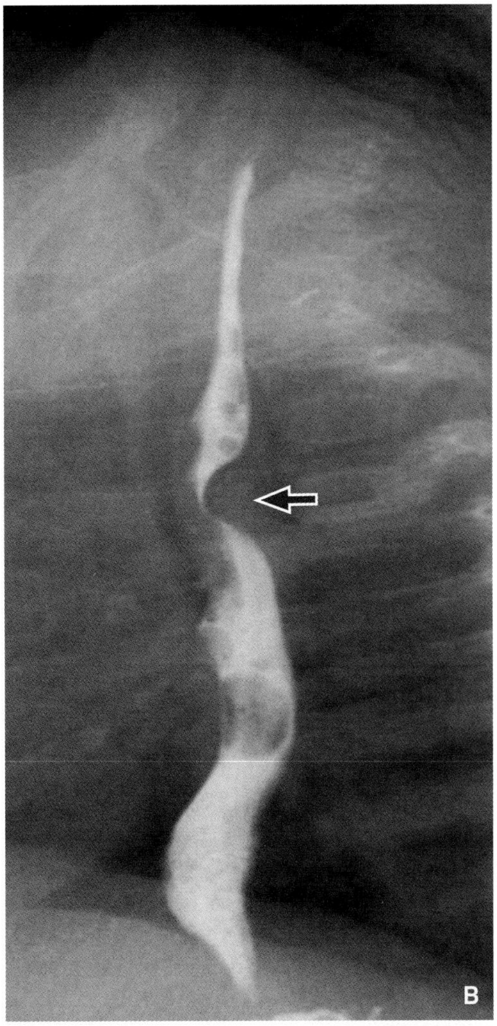

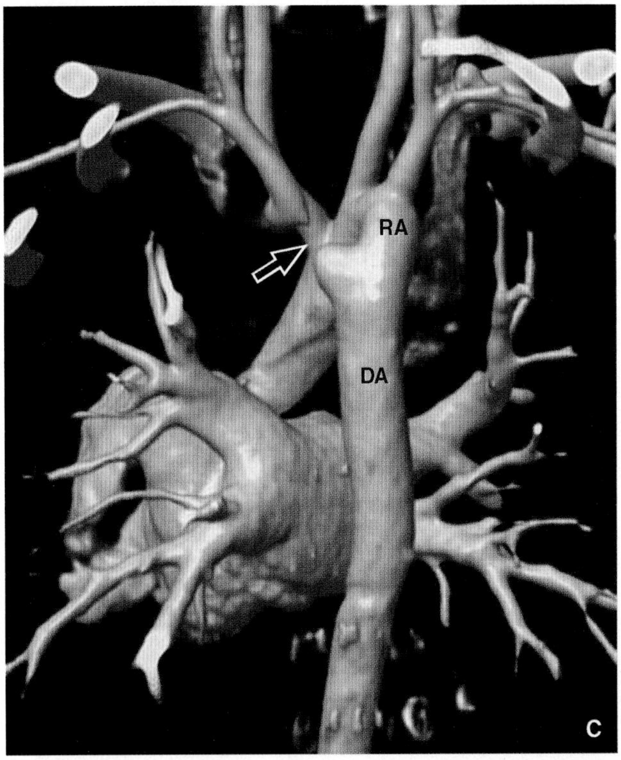

FIGURE 10.5 **Double aortic arch with a dominant right arch and a smaller left arch with an atretic segment in a 2-year-old girl who presented with a history of recurrent pulmonary infections and an abnormality on chest radiograph. A:** Frontal chest radiograph shows mild deviation of the trachea (*asterisk*) to the left with an indentation (*arrow*) on the right lateral wall of the trachea suggesting a right sided aortic arch. **B:** Lateral esophagogram image demonstrates a posterior indentation (*arrow*) with narrowing of the esophagus. **C:** Posterior view of 3D volume-rendered CT image shows a double aortic arch with a dominant right arch (*RA*) and a smaller left arch with an atretic segment (*arrow*). (*DA*, descending aorta.) 3D volume-rendered CT images facilitate evaluation of arch dominance and location.

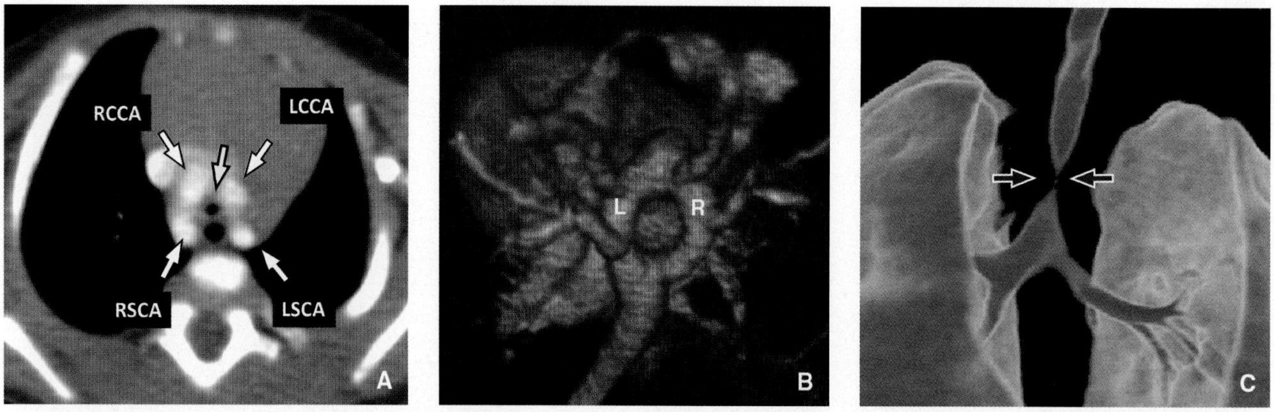

FIGURE 10.6 **Double aortic arch in an 18-month-old boy who presented with progressively worsening stridor. A:** Axial enhanced CT image shows symmetric origins of the four arch vessels (*white arrows*), also known as "four-vessel" sign, arising separately from the two aortic arches. (*RCCA*, right common carotid artery; *RSCA*, right subclavian artery; *LCCA*, left common carotid artery; *LSCA*, left subclavian artery). Both aortic arches are nearly equal in size and encircle the narrowed trachea (*yellow arrow*). **B:** Superior view of 3D volume-rendered CT image demonstrates the characteristic vascular anatomy of a double aortic arch to better advantage. In this instance, the right (*R*) and left (*L*) aortic arches have relative codominance, forming a complete vascular ring. **C:** 3D volume-rendered CT image shows the marked tracheal compression (*arrows*) at the level of the double aortic arch.

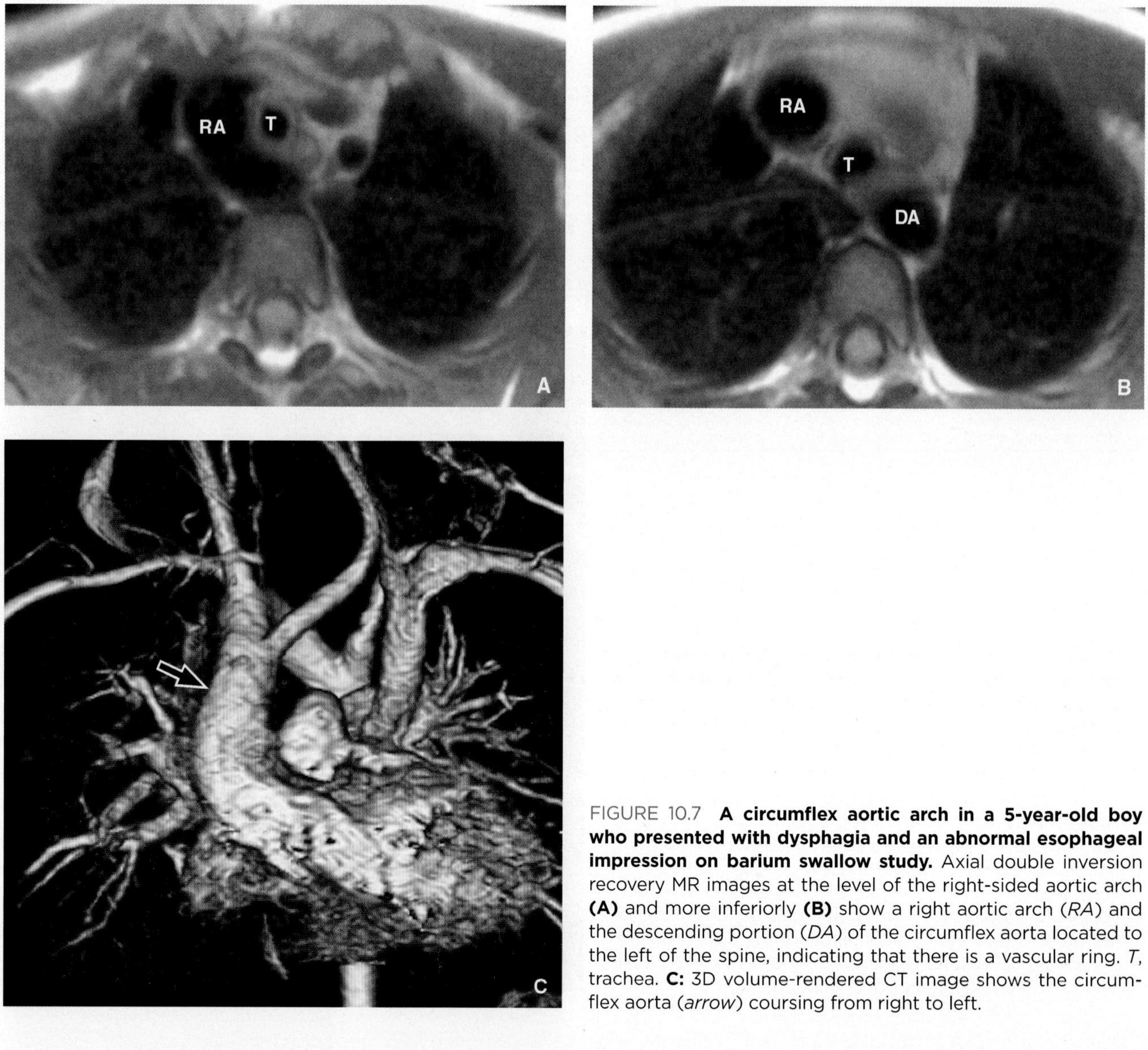

FIGURE 10.7 **A circumflex aortic arch in a 5-year-old boy who presented with dysphagia and an abnormal esophageal impression on barium swallow study.** Axial double inversion recovery MR images at the level of the right-sided aortic arch **(A)** and more inferiorly **(B)** show a right aortic arch (*RA*) and the descending portion (*DA*) of the circumflex aorta located to the left of the spine, indicating that there is a vascular ring. *T*, trachea. **C:** 3D volume-rendered CT image shows the circumflex aorta (*arrow*) coursing from right to left.

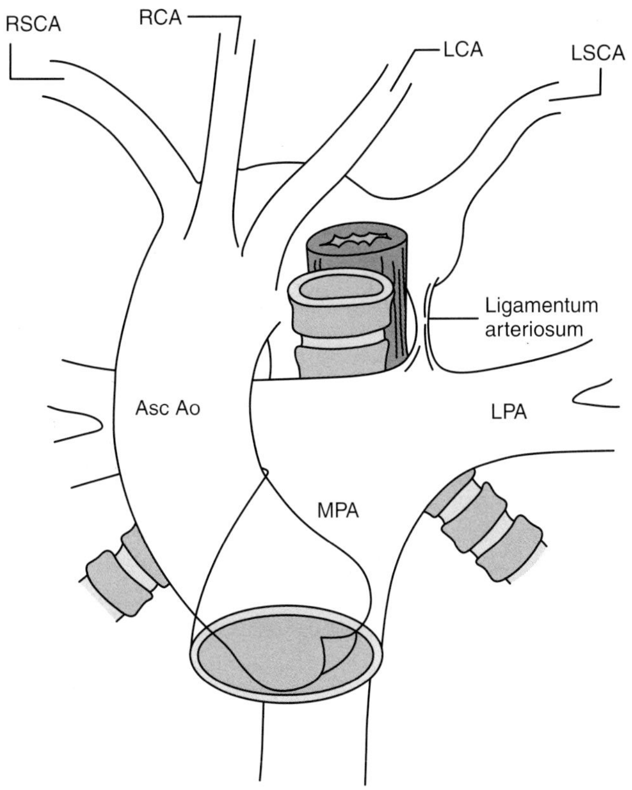

FIGURE 10.8 **Right aortic arch with an aberrant left subclavian artery.** *Asc AO*, ascending aorta; *LCA*, left common carotid artery; *LPA*, left pulmonary artery; *LSCA*, left subclavian artery; *MPA*, main pulmonary artery; *RCA*, right common carotid artery; *RSCA*, right subclavian artery.

3. Right aortic arch with mirror-image branching and a left retroesophageal ductus arteriosus or ligamentum arteriosum (Fig. 10.8)

Right Aortic Arch with an Aberrant Left Subclavian Artery Off a Kommerell Diverticulum

This is the second most common type of symptomatic vascular ring after the DAA in the pediatric population (Fig. 10.9). However, it is often asymptomatic and incidentally discovered. In sequential order, the branching pattern of this aortic arch anomaly consists of the left common carotid artery, the right common carotid artery, the right subclavian artery, and the aberrant left subclavian artery. The latter originates from a diverticulum of Kommerell, which is the result of the embryonic origin of the left aberrant subclavian artery off the patent ductus arteriosus. Therefore, as a rule of thumb, it is important to recognize that a diverticulum of Kommerell is typically associated with the presence of an ipsilateral ligamentum arteriosum that is not visible with contemporary imaging techniques. Such ligamentum arteriosum connects the pulmonary artery to the aortic diverticulum, thereby constituting a vascular ring.

Right Aortic Arch with Left Descending Aorta (Right Circumflex Aortic Arch)

In this aortic vascular anomaly, the aortic arch is right sided, whereas the descending aorta is left sided (Figs 10.7 and 10.10). A left ductus or ligamentum arteriosum completes the vascular ring. This is the third most common type of vascular ring.[37–39] The right-sided aortic arch courses posterior to the trachea and esophagus in a so-called right circumflex aortic arch configuration and then makes an acute turn. Inferiorly, the descending aorta courses along the left side of the spine. This is unlike cases of right aortic arch in which the descending aorta, after coursing over the right mainstem bronchus, gradually descends for some distance on the right and then

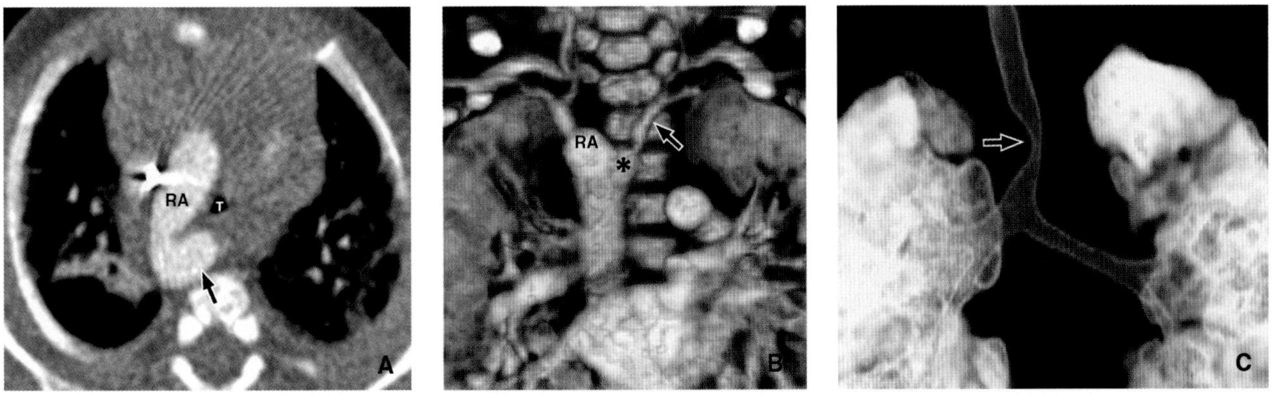

FIGURE 10.9 **Right aortic arch with an aberrant left subclavian artery off a Kommerell diverticulum in a 5-month-old girl who presented with worsening stridor. A:** Axial enhanced CT image shows a right aortic arch (*RA*) with a Kommerell diverticulum (*arrow*). Trachea (*T*) compression is also seen. **B:** 3D volume-rendered CT image demonstrates an aberrant origin of the left subclavian artery (*arrow*) off a Kommerell diverticulum (*asterisk*). The Kommerell diverticulum (*asterisk*) is larger in caliber than the subclavian artery (*arrow*) because it represents a remnant of the ductus arteriosus that once carried much of the systemic blood flow during fetal life. The atretic portion of the ligamentum arteriosum completes the ring, but is not visible with current CT techniques. *RA*, right aortic arch. **C:** Coronal external volume-rendered CT image of the airways and lungs shows the narrowing (*arrow*) of the trachea because of underlying vascular ring.

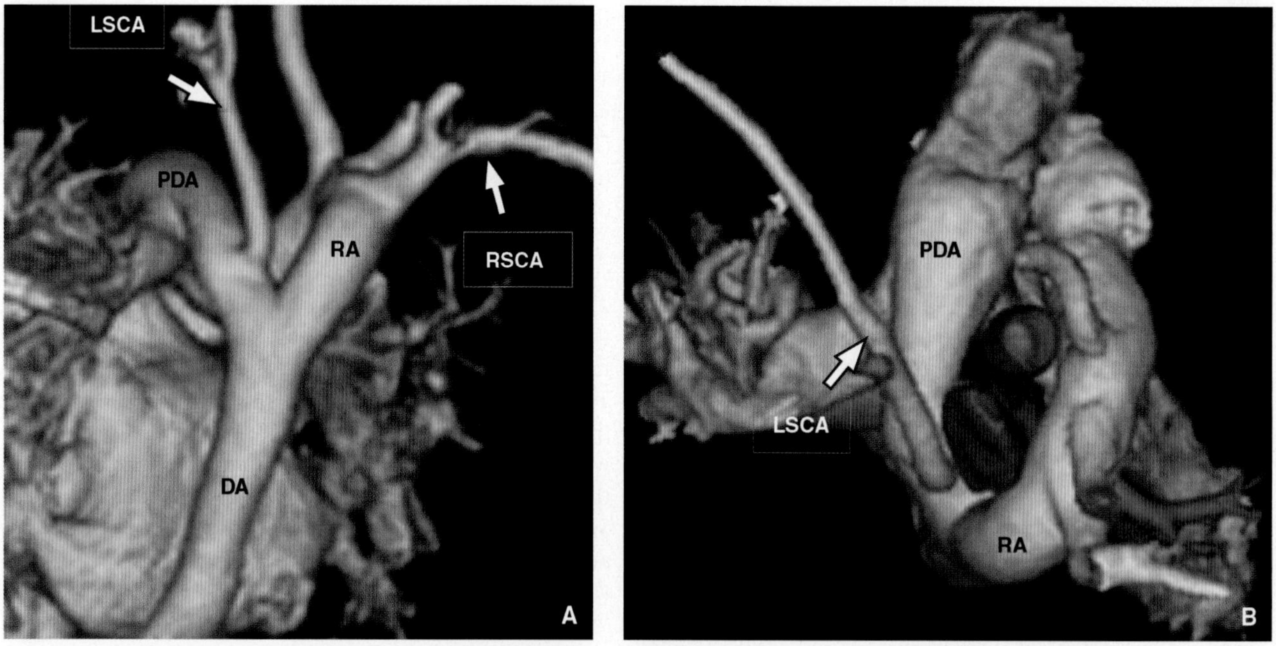

FIGURE 10.10 **Right aortic arch with left descending aorta (right circumflex aortic arch) in a 3-month-old boy who presented with increasing respiratory distress.** Posterior view **(A)** and cranial view **(B)** of 3D volume-rendered CT images show a right-sided aortic arch (*RA*). There is also a prominent, patent ductus arteriosus (*PDA*) completing the vascular ring. Note that the aberrant left subclavian artery (*LSCA*) originates from the PDA. (*RSCA*, right subclavian artery.)

progressively courses into the left before reaching the aortic hiatus.

Right Aortic Arch with Mirror-Image Branching and A Left Retroesophageal Ductus Arteriosus or Ligamentum Arteriosum

A right aortic arch with mirror image branching and a left retroesophageal ductus arteriosus or ligamentum arteriosum is a rare aortic vascular anomaly. It is the only type of right aortic arch with mirror-image branching that constitutes a vascular ring (Fig. 10.11). The branching sequence is as follows: brachiocephalic artery (left common carotid and left subclavian arteries) form the first branch, followed by the right common carotid and the right subclavian arteries. A left-sided patent ductus arteriosus or a ligamentum arteriosum off a prominent aortic diverticulum completes the vascular ring. This aortic vascular anomaly should not be confused with right aortic arch with mirror image branching (Fig. 10.11), a condition that is characteristically associated with patients with tetralogy of Fallot. In these instances, the ductus or ligamentum is usually right sided and does not form a complete vascular ring.

Pulmonary Artery

Pulmonary Agenesis, Aplasia, and Hypoplasia

Pulmonary underdevelopment may be classified into three major categories: (1) pulmonary agenesis characterized by absence of the lung, bronchus, and pulmonary artery (Fig. 10.12); (2) pulmonary aplasia defined by the presence of a rudimentary bronchus as well as absent lung and pulmonary artery; and (3) pulmonary hypoplasia consisting of a rudimentary bronchial tree and pulmonary artery with a variable amount of lung parenchyma.[47–50] Pulmonary agenesis may be isolated or may be part of a syndrome such as chromosome 22q11 deletion and Goldenhar. It also may be part of a syndrome such as VACTERL (vertebral defects, anal atresia, cardiac defects, tracheo-esophageal fistula, renal anomalies, and limb abnormalities) association.[49,51]

The underlying etiology of pulmonary agenesis or aplasia remains uncertain, and genetic, teratogenic, and mechanical factors may all contribute. Given the common association between lung agenesis and ipsilateral radial ray defects or hemifacial microsomia, it has been postulated that in some cases, it may result from maldevelopment of or abnormal blood supply to the first and second embryonic arches.[52] On the other end of the spectrum, often no identifiable cause can be found for lung hypoplasia.[47]

On frontal chest radiographs, the affected hemithorax is usually small and radiopaque, with ipsilateral mediastinal shift and hemidiaphragmatic elevation related to volume loss (Fig. 10.12A). The normal contralateral lung exhibits compensatory hyperinflation and herniation across the midline, manifested by a band of increased retrosternal lucency on lateral projections. Not infrequently, vertebral segmentation and rib anomalies may be observed.[47,50] CT is useful in delineating the anatomy and spatial relationship between the

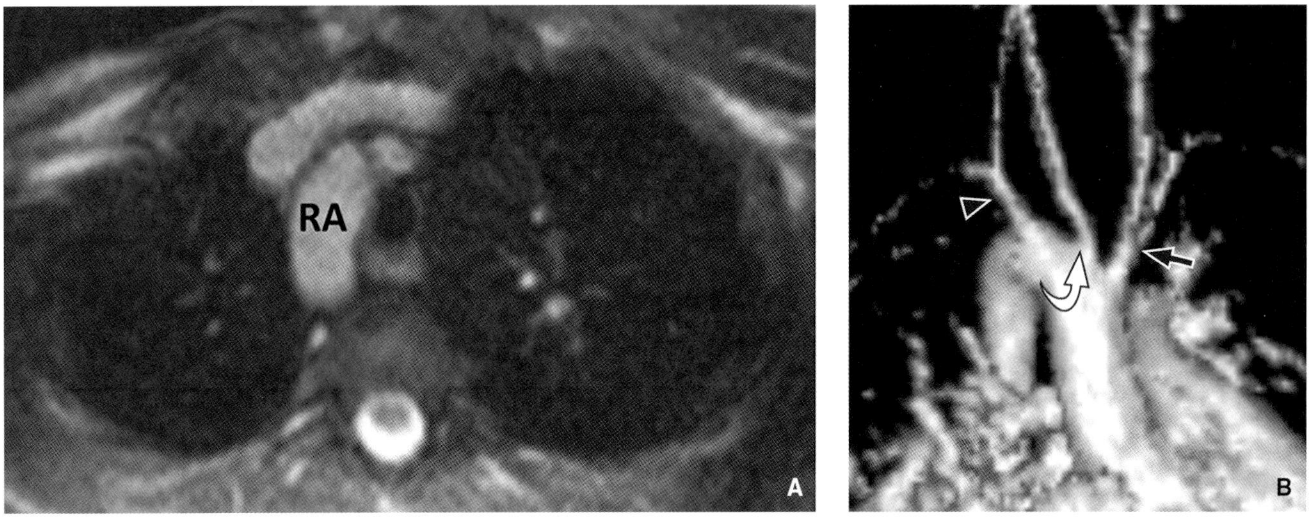

FIGURE 10.11 **Right aortic arch with mirror image branching in a 5-year-old boy who presented with abnormal chest radiograph obtained for evaluation of pneumonia.** Axial white-blood **(A)** and coronal 3D volume-rendered **(B)** MR images show a right aortic arch (*RA*) with mirror image branching. First branch, innominate equivalent with a common trunk (*straight arrow*) for the left common carotid and left subclavian artery, followed by the right common carotid artery (*curved arrow*) and right subclavian artery (*arrowhead*) are seen.

abnormal vasculature and adjacent airway. Furthermore, the multiplanar and 3D reformatted CT images may aid in differentiation between pulmonary agenesis, pulmonary aplasia, and severe pulmonary hypoplasia by better depicting the bronchial stump and/or rudimentary bronchial tree[47,50,53] (Fig. 10.12).

The prognosis for pediatric patients with pulmonary agenesis, aplasia, or hypoplasia depends on the extent of lung underdevelopment and the type of coexisting malformation(s) present.[47] The prognosis for pediatric patients with right-sided lung agenesis is poorer than that of patients with left-sided agenesis; this is attributable to the greater distortion of the airway and cardiovascular structures as well as a reported increased incidence of coexistent cardiovascular anomalies in the former.[49] The most commonly reported associated anomalies involve the heart and the gastrointestinal system, followed in order of frequency by skeletal, vascular, craniofacial, and genitourinary anomalies.[47,49,53,54]

Management is currently aimed at improving respiratory status and symptoms related to the coexisting congenital malformations. It is recommended that regular immunizations

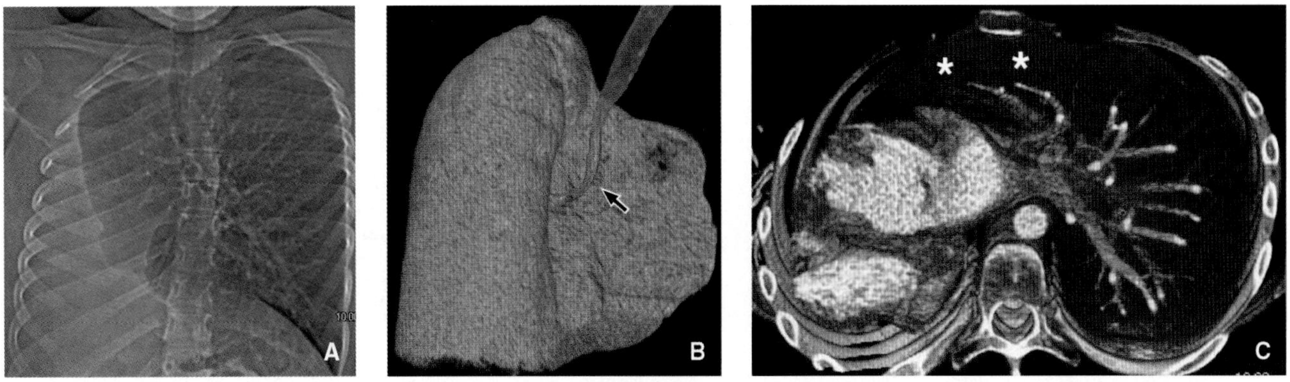

FIGURE 10.12 **Pulmonary agenesis in a 15-year-old girl who presented with worsening asthma. A:** Frontal scout CT image shows marked hyperinflation of the left lung that extends across the midline anteriorly and herniates toward the right. There is dextroposition of the heart into the right hemithorax. **B:** Coronal posterior view 3D volume-rendered CT image of the central airways and lungs demonstrates complete agenesis of the right bronchus and lung. A normal left mainstem bronchus (*arrow*) is seen. **C:** Axial 3D volume-rendered CT image also shows dextroposition of the heart and compensatory hyperexpansion of the left lung, particularly of the left upper lobe (*asterisks*), which herniates into the right hemithorax.

and flu vaccinations during the winter months should be given to affected children with substantial underlying lung deficiency. In infants under the age of 2, some authors advocate preventive care with palivizumab during the respiratory syncytial virus season.[49] In rare instances, when the associated cardiovascular anomalies result in substantial airway compromise, surgery may be required.[49,50]

Pulmonary Artery Sling (Aberrant Left Pulmonary Artery)

Pulmonary artery sling (PAS) occurs as a result of an anomalous origin of the LPA from the posterior aspect of the RPA (Fig. 10.13). The anomalous LPA courses over the right mainstem bronchus and then from right to left between the trachea and the esophagus, reaching the left lung hilum. When it does, it forms a sling around the distal trachea[5,43,47,50,55,56] (Figs. 10.14 and 10.15). This type of vascular ring is completed by a left ligamentum arteriosum connecting the MPA or RPA to the left descending aorta, resulting in a complete vascular ring that enfolds the trachea but spares the esophagus.[5,47] It is postulated that PAS develops as a result of abnormal proximal left sixth arch involution and that a secondary connection to the right sixth branchial arch is acquired through the embryonic peritracheal vessels.[5,50,55,56] PAS most commonly presents in infancy with respiratory symptoms such as stridor, apneic spells, wheezing, recurrent pneumonia, and/or hypoxia. The timing and severity of the symptoms mainly depend on the severity of the accompanying airway abnormalities, which may be disproportionally exacerbated by a superimposed acute upper respiratory infection.[43,50,56–58] Cardiovascular, gastrointestinal, and right-lung anomalies including lung hypoplasia, aplasia, agenesis, and scimitar syndrome may coexist with PAS.[47,56,57]

Two major types of PAS are current recognized. In type I PAS, the carina is normally positioned at the T4-5 level. In the vast majority of type I cases, the airway is intrinsically normal and may or may not have an associated tracheal bronchus. In these instances, the anomalous LPA may extrinsically compress the posterior wall of the distal trachea and the lateral aspect of the right mainstem bronchus. Tracheobronchomalacia may develop in these areas adjacent to pulsating vessels, and right lung atelectasis or air trapping may subsequently ensue.[47,56,57] Type

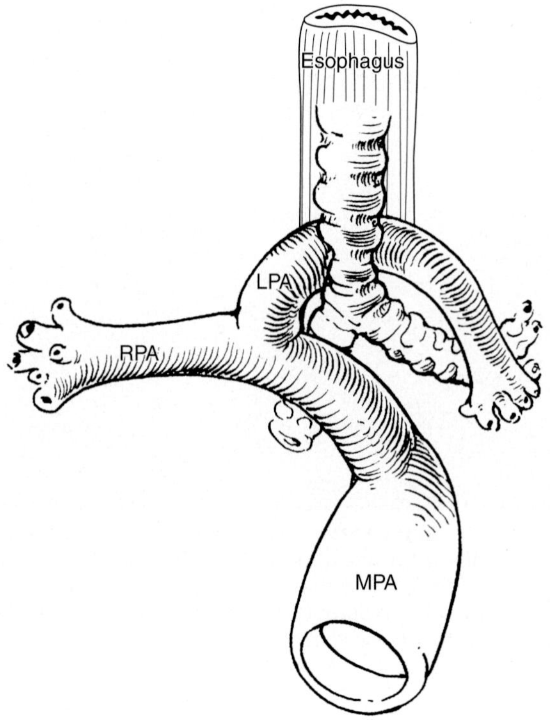

FIGURE 10.13 **Pulmonary artery sling.** The left pulmonary artery (*LPA*) arises from the right pulmonary artery (*RPA*) and courses between the trachea and the esophagus while entering the left hilum. *MPA*, main pulmonary artery.

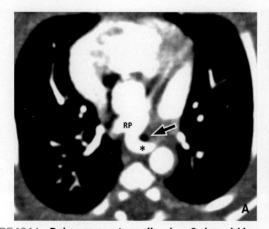

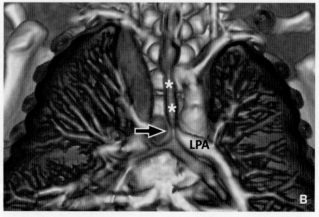

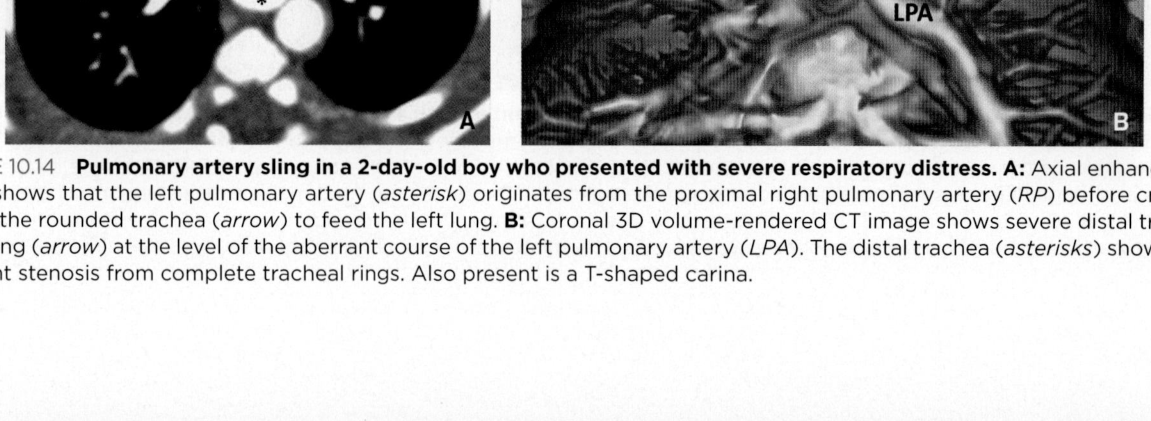

FIGURE 10.14 **Pulmonary artery sling in a 2-day-old boy who presented with severe respiratory distress. A:** Axial enhanced CT image shows that the left pulmonary artery (*asterisk*) originates from the proximal right pulmonary artery (*RP*) before crossing behind the rounded trachea (*arrow*) to feed the left lung. **B:** Coronal 3D volume-rendered CT image shows severe distal tracheal narrowing (*arrow*) at the level of the aberrant course of the left pulmonary artery (*LPA*). The distal trachea (*asterisks*) shows long segment stenosis from complete tracheal rings. Also present is a T-shaped carina.

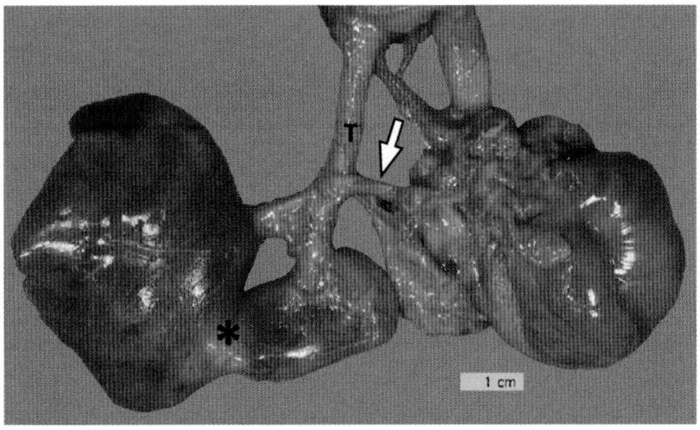

FIGURE 10.15 **Pulmonary artery sling in a 3-day-old girl who died of complications of tracheal atresia (with complete distal rings) and pulmonary hypoplasia.** The left pulmonary artery (*arrow*) branches off a dilated pulmonary trunk and courses posterior to the narrowed trachea (*T*). In this example, the right lung is attached to the left lower lobe ("horseshoe lung") (*asterisk*).

II PAS is characterized by a more inferiorly positioned carina at the level of T6. Type II PAS is usually associated with long-segment tracheal stenosis with complete cartilaginous rings and abnormal bronchial branching, including an inverted T-shaped carina and a right-bridging bronchus.[50,56,58]

PAS imaging findings mainly depend on the type of PAS and presence of coexisting anomalies. In type I PAS, substantial right-sided hyperinflation or atelectasis because of partial obstruction and right mainstem bronchomalacia may be appreciated on frontal chest radiograph. A right-sided tracheal bronchus may be observed in some instances. In type II PAS, bilateral hyperinflation may be present, particularly in cases associated with long-segment tracheal stenosis. In this situation, the trachea may appear narrow or difficult to resolve on a frontal chest radiograph, and the carina may appear low and horizontal in position. This constellation of radiographic findings should raise suspicion for underlying type II PAS.[57,59] Occasionally, on lateral chest radiographs and on lateral esophagograms, a small, rounded, soft tissue density may be present between the midtrachea and the esophagus, consistent with the presence of an anomalous LPA coursing between these two structures. This may be seen in both types of PAS.[50,57,59]

Currently, CTA and MRI with 3D reformatted CT images are two main noninvasive imaging modalities for the assessment of PAS because the presence, origin, size, and entire course of the anomalous LPA can be accurately depicted on the 3D reformatted images obtained with both imaging modalities. However, CT has an advantage over MRI because it can better demonstrate the large airway and lung abnormalities often associated with PAS. Paired inspiratory/expiratory or dynamic 4D airway CT imaging techniques can accurately demonstrate the presence, degree, and extent of the large airway abnormalities such as stenosis or malacia as well as air trapping in the lungs often seen in pediatric patients with PAS.[2,5,50]

Asymptomatic pediatric patients with PAS may be followed clinically. In some very mild cases, there are some anecdotal reports of spontaneous improvement. Symptomatic type I PAS pediatric patients may benefit from LPA reimplantation and excision of the patent ductus arteriosus or ductal ligament. In symptomatic type II PAS patients, LPA reimplantation or anterior translocation alone may not result in improvement of respiratory symptoms if the long-segment large airway stenosis is not properly addressed, usually by slide tracheoplasty.[50,56,57]

Proximal Interruption of the Pulmonary Artery

Proximal interruption of the pulmonary artery is characterized by discontinuous pulmonary arteries in which the site of interruption involves the proximal portion of the RPA or LPA.[47,57,60,61] The more distal, hilar portion of the pulmonary artery and the intrapulmonary vascular network remain patent. The interrupted proximal pulmonary artery is characteristically located on the contralateral side of the aortic arch. It is more commonly seen on the right side. Interruption of the proximal LPA is less common and is frequently associated with congenital heart disease, typically tetralogy of Fallot and heterotaxy. This vascular anomaly occurs in isolation in ~40% of the reported cases.[61] Although asymptomatic children with this condition may be detected incidentally, some affected pediatric patients may present with symptoms related to recurrent pulmonary infections, hemoptysis, and pulmonary hypertension.[47,57,58]

Some authors prefer to use the term "ductal origin of the pulmonary artery" to describe this vascular anomaly because that term provides more insight into the embryology of this lesion and better illustrates its physiopathology.[62,63] This malformation is due to the abnormal involution of the proximal sixth aortic arch. This results in "absence" of the proximal pulmonary artery and persistent connection of the hilar pulmonary artery to the distal sixth arch, which ultimately becomes the ductus arteriosus. In the case of proximal interruption of the proximal pulmonary artery, the affected hilar pulmonary artery supplying the ipsilateral lung continues to develop via the blood supply from the ductus arteriosus, which originates either from the base of the right innominate artery, or occasionally from an aberrant right subclavian artery.[47,57,61] Progressive closure of the ductus results in loss of blood supply to the hilar pulmonary artery and lung. Perfusion of the affected lung becomes dependent on collateral systemic vessels, primarily the aortopulmonary and bronchial arteries, but also the transpleural branches of the intercostal, internal mammary, subclavian, and innominate arteries.[47,55,62–64]

On chest radiographs, the affected lung and hilum are usually smaller in size than those on the unaffected side. Additional chest radiographic findings may include ipsilateral mediastinal shift, ipsilateral narrowed intercostal spaces, and rarely, rib notching in the case of prominent intercostal collaterals.[47,58,64] On CT, the interrupted pulmonary artery characteristically terminates within 1 cm of its origin from the MPA (Fig. 10.16). Serrated pleural thickening and subpleural parenchymal bands may be also observed. Such findings result from the direct anastomosis of transpleural systemic collaterals with peripheral branches of the pulmonary arteries. On high-resolution CT, reticular opacities, septal thickening, subpleural consolidation, tiny cystic lung changes, and pleural thickening may be present.[65] Airway branching and anomalies in pulmonary lobation are not uncommon in affected children. Additional osseous findings may include an asymmetric thoracic cage and scoliosis.[47,50,55,57,58,60,61,64]

Early and accurate diagnosis of this vascular anomaly is important because early surgical intervention may provide adequate blood supply to the affected lung, allowing improved lung and pulmonary arterial growth. Flow reconstitution may be achieved either by using an interposition graft or with a direct anastomosis when possible.[61] Surveillance is indicated for the late-presenting older children who are considered unsuitable for intervention. Affected pediatric patients who present with recurrent hemoptysis or pulmonary hypertension may benefit from coil embolization of large systemic collaterals.[47,59,66]

Pulmonary Arteriovenous Malformation

Pulmonary arteriovenous malformation (AVM) is a low-resistance, high-flow vascular malformation consisting of a direct

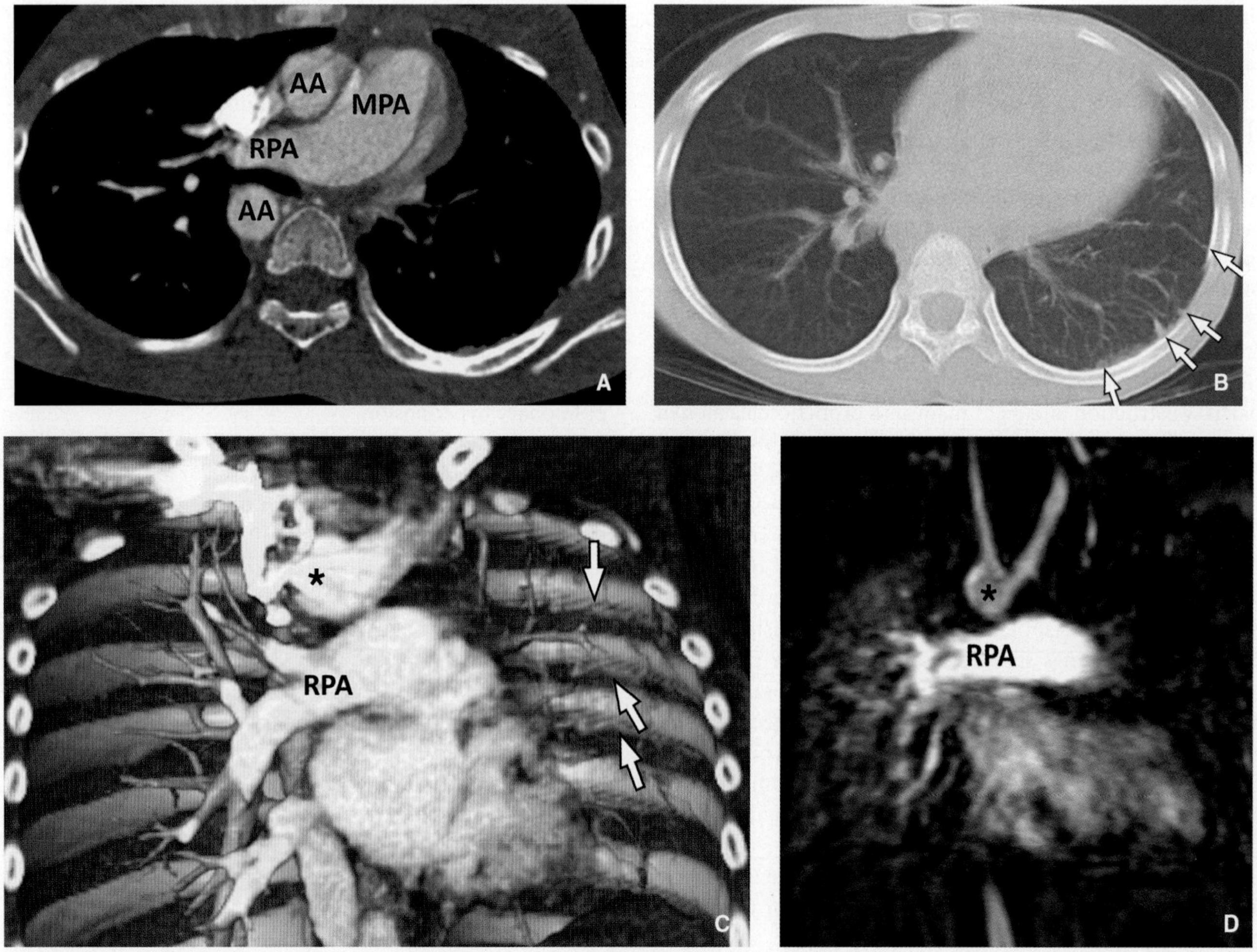

FIGURE 10.16 **Proximal interruption of the left pulmonary artery in a 10-year-old girl who presented with recurrent cough and shortness of breath. A:** Axial enhanced CT image shows absence of the left pulmonary artery. Pulmonary blood flow is from the main pulmonary artery (*MPA*) to the right pulmonary artery (*RPA*). The aortic arch (*AA*) is right sided. **B:** Axial lung window CT image demonstrates a smaller left lung with very mild mediastinal shift and serrated pleural thickening (*arrows*), reflective of transpleural systemic collaterals in direct anastomosis with peripheral branches of the pulmonary arteries. **C:** 3D volume-rendered CT image shows normal right pulmonary artery (*RPA*) arborization and poor vascularity in the left lung. Prominent left intercostal arteries (*arrows*) provide collateral flow to the left lung. Note the right-sided aortic arch (*asterisk*). **D:** Coronal MRA image in the pulmonary arterial phase shows nearly no enhancement of the left lung. *RPA*, right pulmonary artery. Right-sided aortic arch (*asterisk*).

connection between pulmonary arteries and veins without an intervening capillary network. This vascular anomaly with bypassing of the capillary network has two important physiologic consequences. First, the direct communication acts a right-to-left shunt and may result in hypoxemia. Second, blood flowing through a pulmonary AVM circumvents the filter function of the normal pulmonary capillary bed, thereby predisposing affected pediatric patients to paradoxical embolism and ultimately causing strokes or cerebral absc esses.[47,50,58,67]

Pulmonary AVMs can be congenital or acquired. The acquired form of pulmonary AVM is usually seen in pediatric patients with prior history of bidirectional cavopulmonary shunts, hepatopulmonary syndrome, trauma, or infections such as schistosomiasis, tuberculosis, or actinomycosis.[47,58,67] In its congenital forms, pulmonary AVM may occur sporadically, although it is characteristically seen in 30% to 50% of family members with hereditary hemorrhagic telangiectasia (HHT), also known as Rendu-Osler-Weber syndrome. HHT is an autosomal dominant vascular disorder that is diagnosed clinically by applying the so-called Curaçao criteria.[68] A definite diagnosis of HHT is accepted if at least three of the following are present: (1) spontaneous, recurrent epistaxis; (2) multiple mucocutaneous telangiectases at characteristic sites (i.e., lips, oral cavity, fingers, nose); (3) visceral involvement, including but not limited to gastrointestinal telangiectasia and pulmonary, hepatic, cerebral, and spinal AVMs; and (4) family history of a first-degree relative with HHT according to these criteria. The disease is considered possible if only two criteria are present and unlikely if one or no criteria are present.[67–70] Given that each offspring of an affected person has a 50% risk of inheriting the condition, family members of HHT patients should be screened for pulmonary AVMs.[47,71]

Small pulmonary AVMs may be asymptomatic, particularly in children. However, larger or multiple pulmonary AVMs may act as a direct right-to-left shunt, bypassing the pulmonary capillary bed, and resulting in paradoxical emboli to the brain that may present as transient ischemic attack, stroke, or classically, brain abscess. In addition, these larger pulmonary AVMs may result in desaturation with resulting exercise intolerance and, in severe cases, cyanosis and clubbing.[72] Clinically, these affected pediatric patients may present with dyspnea on exertion, cyanosis, chest pain, palpitations, and hemoptysis.

On chest radiographs, pulmonary AVM may appear as a well-circumscribed serpiginous or lobulated opacity. Occasionally, curvilinear opacities directed toward the hilum and representing the feeding artery or draining vein may be seen. Most pulmonary AVMs are situated within the lower lobes. Unfortunately, small pulmonary AVMs located in areas obscured by normal structures, such as those in the retrocardiac area or the pulmonary hila, may be easily overlooked on chest radiographs. For these small pulmonary AVMs, further evaluation with cross-sectional imaging studies such as CTA or MRA is often needed for a complete assessment.

Traditionally, pulmonary AVMs have been evaluated with conventional pulmonary angiography. However, in recent years, MDCT with CTA technique has become the preferred imaging modality and technique for a complete assessment of pulmonary AVMs (Figs. 10.17 and 10.18). On CTA, pulmonary AVMs may be single or multiple, unilateral or bilateral, and simple or complex. Simple pulmonary AVMs

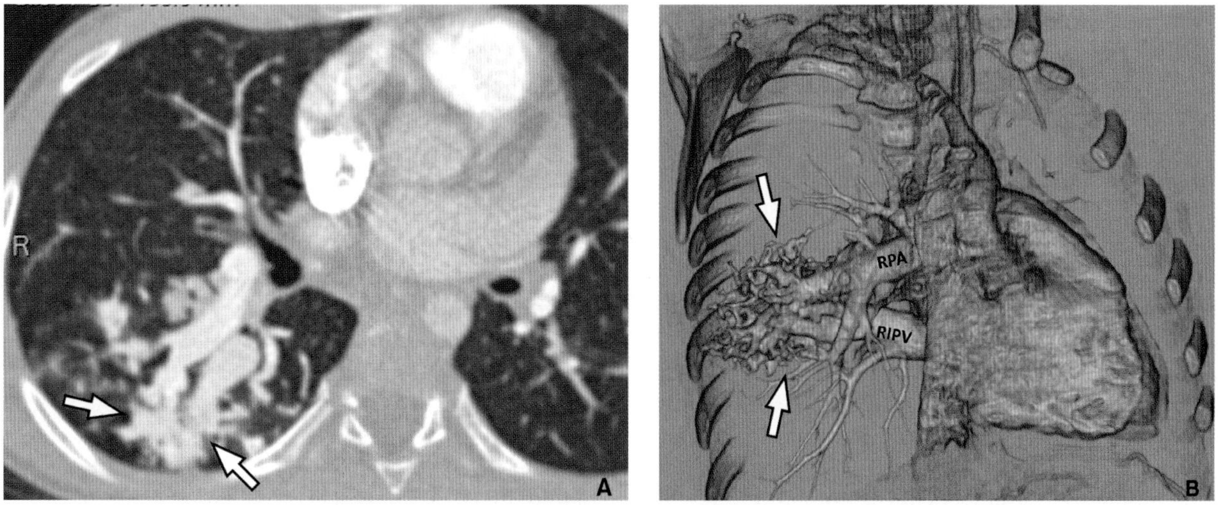

FIGURE 10.17 **Pulmonary arteriovenous malformation (AVM) in an 8-year-old girl with a family history of hereditary hemorrhagic telangiectasia and an abnormal bubble echocardiogram with findings concerning for intrapulmonary shunting. A:** Axial CT image shows a large pulmonary AVM (*arrows*) in the superior segment of the right lower lobe. **B:** Coronal-oblique 3D volume-rendered CT image demonstrates a large pulmonary AVM (*arrows*) with a feeding artery from the right main pulmonary artery (*RPA*) and a draining vein into an enlarged right inferior pulmonary vein (*RIPV*).

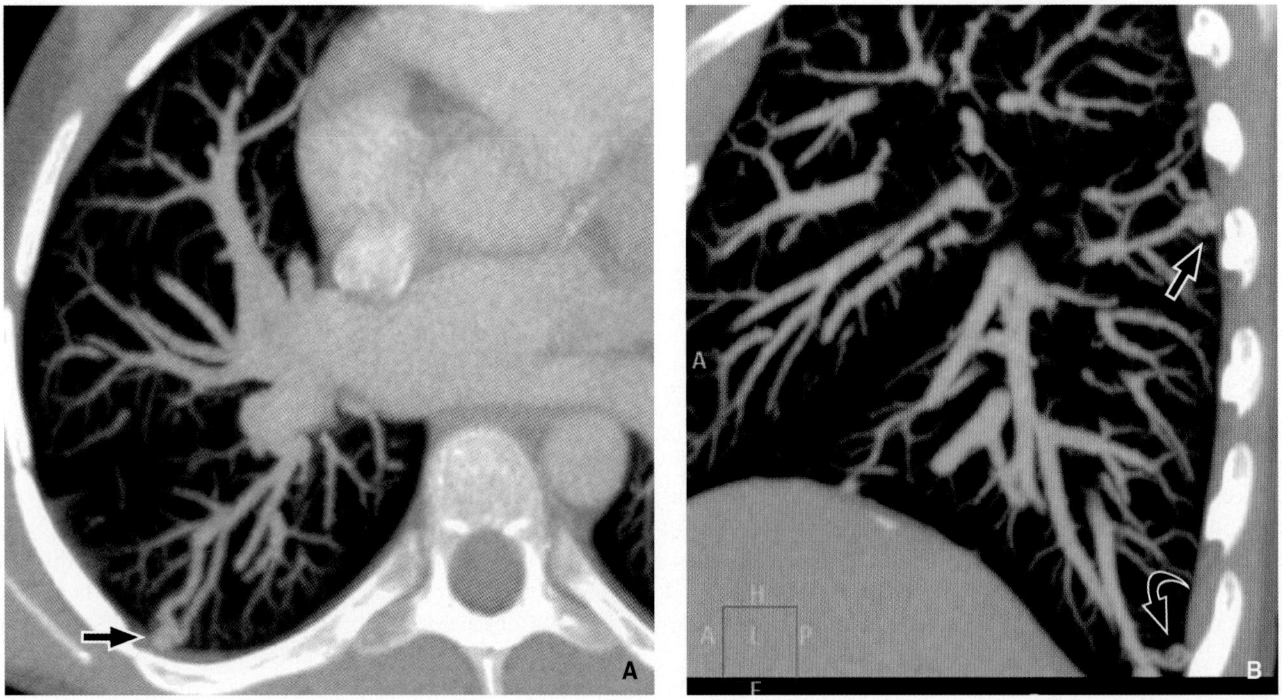

FIGURE 10.18 **Multiple pulmonary arteriovenous malformations in a 14-year-old girl with hereditary hemorrhagic telangiectasia.** Axial **(A)** and sagittal **(B)** maximum intensity projection CT images show a small pulmonary arteriovenous malformation (AVM) (*straight arrow*) in the superior segment of the right upper lobe. An additional pulmonary AVM (*curved arrow*) is noted at the costophrenic sulcus area.

receive their blood supply through a single feeding artery, whereas complex AVMs receive their blood supply through two or more arteries that arise from at least two different segmental pulmonary arteries and connect with at least two draining veins. CTA with 3D reformatted CT images plays an important role in the preinterventional and posttreatment evaluation of pediatric patients with pulmonary AVM. Such CT images can clearly depict the number, size, extent, and angioarchitecture of the pulmonary AVMs in exquisite detail. This permits optimal planning for the embolization procedure, a factor that is of utmost importance when managing complex lesions.[47,72] Recently, the use of MRA is also found to be useful for the assessment of pulmonary AVMs.[70,73] Given the risk of paradoxical emboli in affected patients, great care should be taken with the IV placement and connection to the power injector to ensure an air-bubble-free contrast administration during CTA and MRA imaging.[72]

In regard to the management of pulmonary AVMs in children, there is currently no specific standard of care as to which patients should be treated, particularly if patients are asymptomatic and under 12 years of age.[74,75] This is because immature, developing lungs in this setting may be at increased risk for reperfusion via pulmonary collaterals, which are even more difficult to treat. Nevertheless, a few studies have shown the efficacy and safety of pulmonary AVM treatment in children,[67] and there is general agreement that symptomatic pulmonary AVMs with feeding arteries equal or larger than 3 mm detected by CT should be treated.[50,72] However, symptomatic paradoxical emboli have been reported in patients with sub-3 mm feeding arteries. Consequently, many HHT centers are currently treating pulmonary AVMs with <3 mm feeding arteries.[67,76] The current management choice for pulmonary AVMs is transvenous transcatheter embolotherapy, which can be performed with a variety of devices including fibered steel coils, fibered platinum Nester coils, fibered microcoils, hydrophilic coils, and self-expandable nitinol plugs.[70] In addition, antibiotic prophylaxis prior to dental and surgical interventions is recommended in children with pulmonary AVMs in order to reduce the risk of paradoxical embolic episodes and abscess.[67,70]

Pulmonary Arterial Hypertension

Pulmonary arterial hypertension (PAH) occurs across a wide spectrum of clinical conditions (Fig. 10.19). The most current clinical classification, which supersedes the Dana Point classification, was established at the fifth World Symposium held in 2013 in Nice, France[77] (Table 10.5). Unlike PAH in adults, PAH in children is usually idiopathic or associated with congenital heart disease (CHD), chronic lung disease, or hematologic disorders, including sickle cell disease. Underlying pathologic features of PAH include dilation and atherosis of the large hilar pulmonary arteries. Smaller

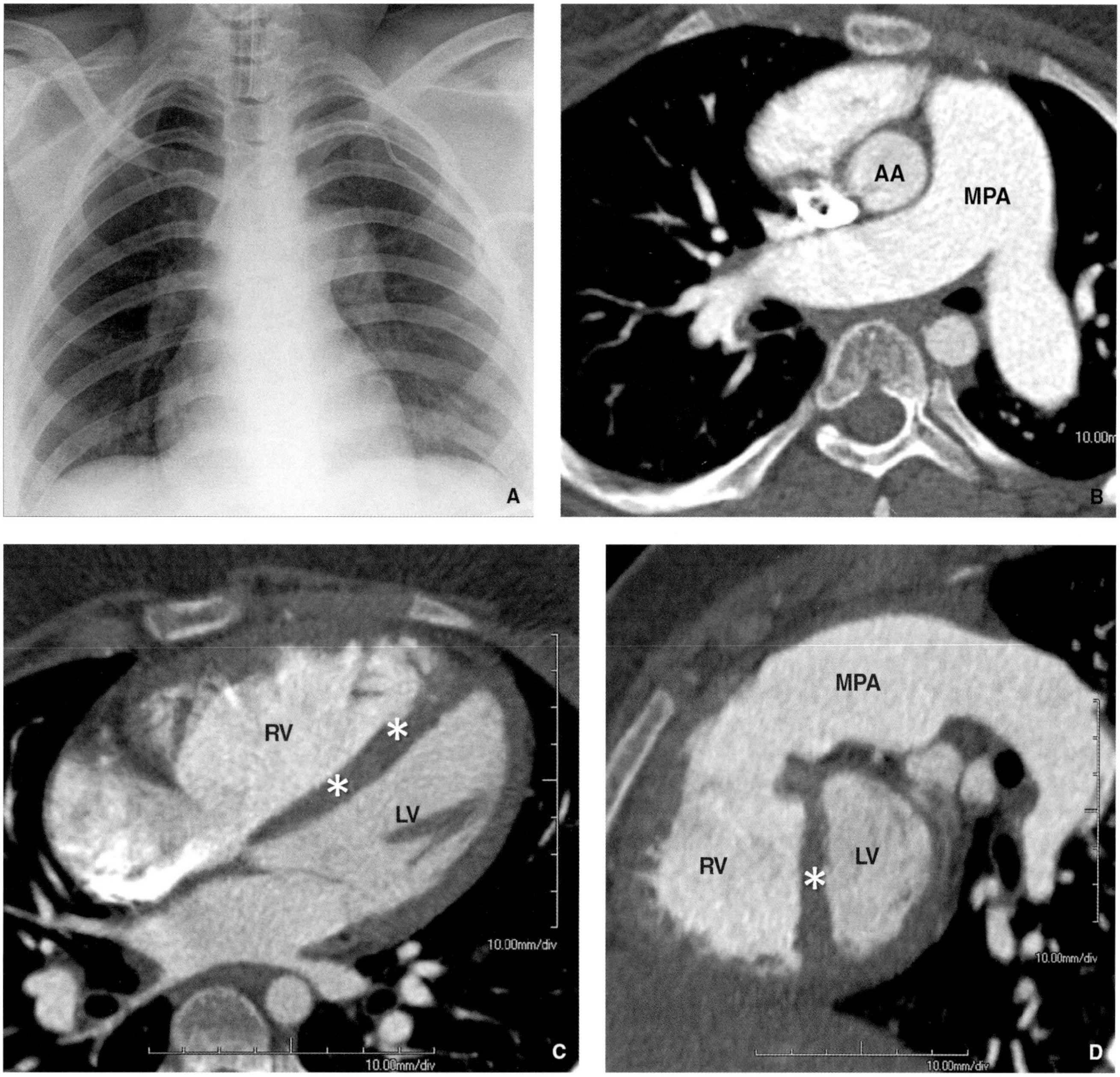

FIGURE 10.19 **Pulmonary arterial hypertension in a 15-year-old girl who presented with worsening fatigue. A:** Frontal chest radiograph shows characteristic imaging findings of pulmonary arterial hypertension with enlarged main, right and left pulmonary arteries tapering in the lung periphery. **B:** Axial enhanced CT image demonstrates central pulmonary arterial enlargement with abrupt tapering toward the periphery. Note that the transverse dimension of the main pulmonary artery (*MPA*) exceeds the transverse dimension of the ascending aorta (*AA*) at the same level, a finding consistent with pulmonary arterial hypertension. **C, D:** Axial enhanced **(C)** and short-axis reformatted enhanced **(D)** CT images show an enlarged right ventricle (*RV*) with right ventricular hypertrophy. There is flattening of the interventricular septum (*asterisks*), which results in a D-shaped configuration of the left ventricle (*LV*) on the short-axis reformatted CT image, a finding that may indicate elevated pulmonary arterial pressures. Note right ventricular hypertrophy as a result of long-standing pulmonary arterial pressure elevation. **E:** Axial lung window CT image shows a pattern of mosaic perfusion.

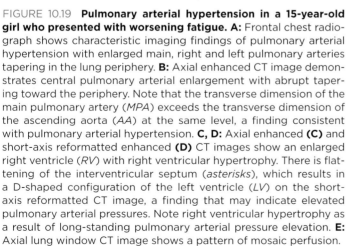

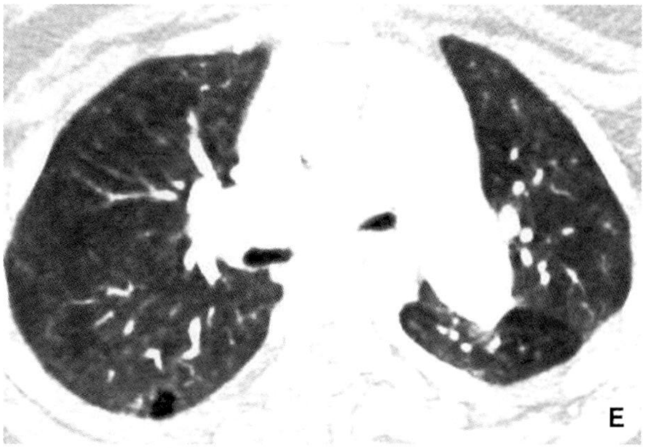

TABLE 10.5 Classification of Pulmonary Arterial Hypertension*

1. Pulmonary arterial hypertension	1.1 Idiopathic PAH	
	1.2 Heritable PAH	1.2.1 BMPR2 1.2.2 ALK-1, ENG, ***SMAD9***, ***CAV1***, ***KCNK3*** 1.2.3 Unknown
	1.3 Drug and toxin induced	
	1.4 Associated with:	1.4.1 Connective tissue disease 1.4.2 HIV infection 1.4.3 Portal hypertension 1.4.4 Congenital heart diseases 1.4.5 Schistosomiasis
	1′ Pulmonary venoocclusive disease and/or pulmonary capillary hemangiomatosis	
	1″ Persistent pulmonary hypertension of the newborn (PPHN)	
2. Pulmonary hypertension due to left heart disease	2.1 Left ventricular systolic dysfunction	
	2.2 Left ventricular diastolic dysfunction	
	2.3 Valvular disease	
	2.4 Congenital/acquired left heart inflow/outflow tract obstruction and congenital cardiomyopathies	
3. Pulmonary hypertension due to lung diseases and/or hypoxia	3.1 Chronic obstructive pulmonary disease	
	3.2 Interstitial lung disease	
	3.3 Other pulmonary diseases with mixed restrictive and obstructive pattern	
	3.4 Sleep-disordered breathing	
	3.5 Alveolar hypoventilation disorders	
	3.6 Chronic exposure to high altitude	
	3.7 Developmental lung diseases	
4. Chronic thromboembolic pulmonary hypertension		
5. Pulmonary hypertension with unclear multifactorial mechanisms	5.1 Hematologic disorders: ***chronic hemolytic anemia***, myeloproliferative disorders, splenectomy	
	5.2 Systemic disorders: sarcoidosis, pulmonary histiocytosis, lymphangioleiomyomatosis	
	5.3 Metabolic disorders: glycogen storage disease, Gaucher disease, thyroid disorders	
	5.4 Others: tumoral obstruction, fibrosing mediastinitis, chronic renal failure, ***segmental PH***	

BMPR, bone morphogenetic protein receptor type II; CAV1, caveolin-1; ENG, endoglin; HIV, human immunodeficiency virus; PAH, pulmonary arterial hypertension.

** The 5th World Symposium on Pulmonary Hypertension, held February 2013 in Nice, France.*

Main modifications to the previous Dana Point classification are in ***italics***.

Reproduced from Simonneau G, Gatzoulis MA, Adatia I, et al. Updated clinical classification of pulmonary hypertension. J Am Coll Cardiol. 2013;62(25 suppl):D34–D41, with permission. Ref. 77.

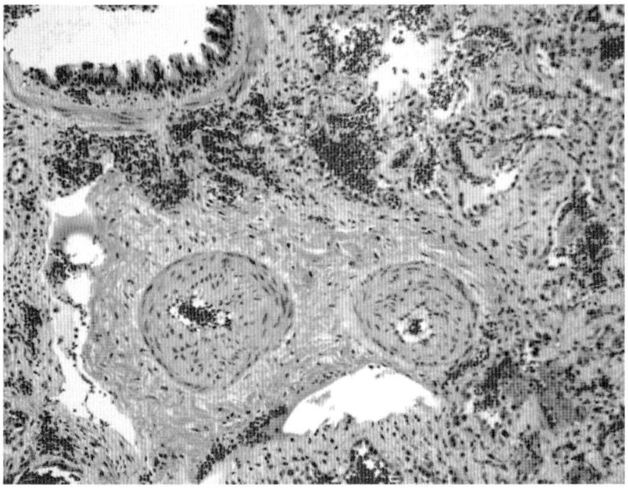

FIGURE 10.20 **Pulmonary arterial hypertension in an 11-year-old girl who presented with fatigue rapidly progressing to cardiac failure.** Biopsy shows markedly thickened arterial media (hematoxylin and eosin, original magnification, 200x). Ultimately, an *EIF2AK4* gene mutation was identified, providing an explanation for an otherwise idiopathic condition.

intrapulmonary arteries typically show varying degrees of concentric medial hypertrophy (Fig. 10.20). Occasionally, concomitant venous hypertensive changes are seen, usually an indication that the PAH is due to venous obstructive disease. Although the symptoms of PAH are often insidious in onset and nonspecific, affected children may present with decreased energy, growth retardation, avoidance of strenuous activity, or cyanosis.

PAH is defined by a mean pulmonary pressure exceeding 25 mm Hg at right heart catheterization after 3 months of age if blood flow to all lung segments is equal and there is increased pulmonary vascular resistance.[77–83] ECHO is a widely available, noninvasive, reproducible, and relatively inexpensive modality for screening for PAH by measurement of systolic pulmonary arterial pressure using peak tricuspid regurgitant jet velocity. For the detection of moderate PAH, the sensitivity of ECHO ranges from 79% to 100%, and its specificity ranges from 68% to 98%.[82] ECHO is also useful for the evaluation of cardiac anatomy, left ventricular systolic and diastolic dysfunction, abnormal ejection fraction, valvular abnormalities, and intracardiac shunts.[82,84]

Regardless of the underlying etiology, the imaging findings of PAH on CT include (1) enlarged central pulmonary arteries with dilatation of the MPA to a diameter exceeding that of the ascending aorta at the same level, (2) peripheral tapering with pruning of the distal pulmonary arterial vasculature, (3) right ventricular hypertrophy and (4) right ventricular and atrial dilatation with flattening of the interventricular septum and posterior displacement of the left ventricle by the enlarged right cardiac chambers[82,85] (Fig. 10.19). In addition, CT can also show diffuse lung disease often associated with PAH. Such lung disease frequently present as a pattern of mosaic attenuation characterized by increased arterial vessel caliber in the geographic areas with increased attenuation and diminutive vessel caliber in the geographic areas with decreased attenuation (oligemia).[82]

In addition to CT, MRI can be also valuable because it can provide additional functional information and quantification of shunts in children with PAH.[84] MRI permits direct assessment of right ventricular volumes and morphology, septal and tricuspid valve motion, and ejection fraction, all of which have prognostic significance in pediatric patients with PAH.[82,84]

In infants and children in whom PAH is suspected, the level of brain-type natriuretic peptide (BNP) should be checked. BNP is a serum marker of ventricular dysfunction and a useful marker for monitoring disease severity and progression in pediatric PAH.[79,86] The current mainstay of pediatric PAH therapy includes ventilation strategies aimed at recruiting lung volume and monotherapy or combination therapy with pulmonary vasodilators, which may include calcium channel antagonists, prostacyclin analogs, endothelin receptor antagonists, and the phosphodiesterase type 5 inhibitors such as sildenafil and tadalafil. Atrial septostomy may be considered in children with worsening PAH as an initial procedure or before consideration of lung transplantation.[78] It should be noted that the FDA recently released a strong warning against the chronic use of sildenafil for PAH in pediatric patients.[83,87] Care should be taken in cases of PAH because of downstream obstructions, such as pulmonary vein stenosis, because the use of vasodilators in these conditions may result in fatal pulmonary edema if used before the obstruction is relieved.[79,82,85,88] Noninvasive and highly sensitive imaging study such as CTA with 3D reformatted CT images can be useful for evaluating the patency of the pulmonary veins in this patient population.[89]

Pulmonary Vein

Pulmonary Vein Stenosis

Pulmonary vein stenosis (PVS) refers to stenosis of the large (extrapulmonary) pulmonary veins (Fig. 10.21). It may occur as an isolated lesion (Fig. 10.22) or may be secondary to interventional therapy or to cardiovascular surgery (Fig. 10.23). In pediatric patients, secondary PVS is seen most commonly following anomalous pulmonary vein reimplantation surgery, whereas it is most frequently seen following radiofrequency ablation for atrial fibrillation in adults. The congenital form of PVS is thought to result from the uninhibited proliferation of myofibroblast-like cells and matrix deposition, resulting in luminal narrowing of the pulmonary veins.[50,58,90–92] In this case, the term "primary" pulmonary vein stenosis would be more appropriate because there is increasing evidence that the disease is not static with progressive worsening and that it may not even be present at the time of birth.

PVS is strongly associated with prematurity and other forms of CHD, with a range of co-occurrence of 30% to

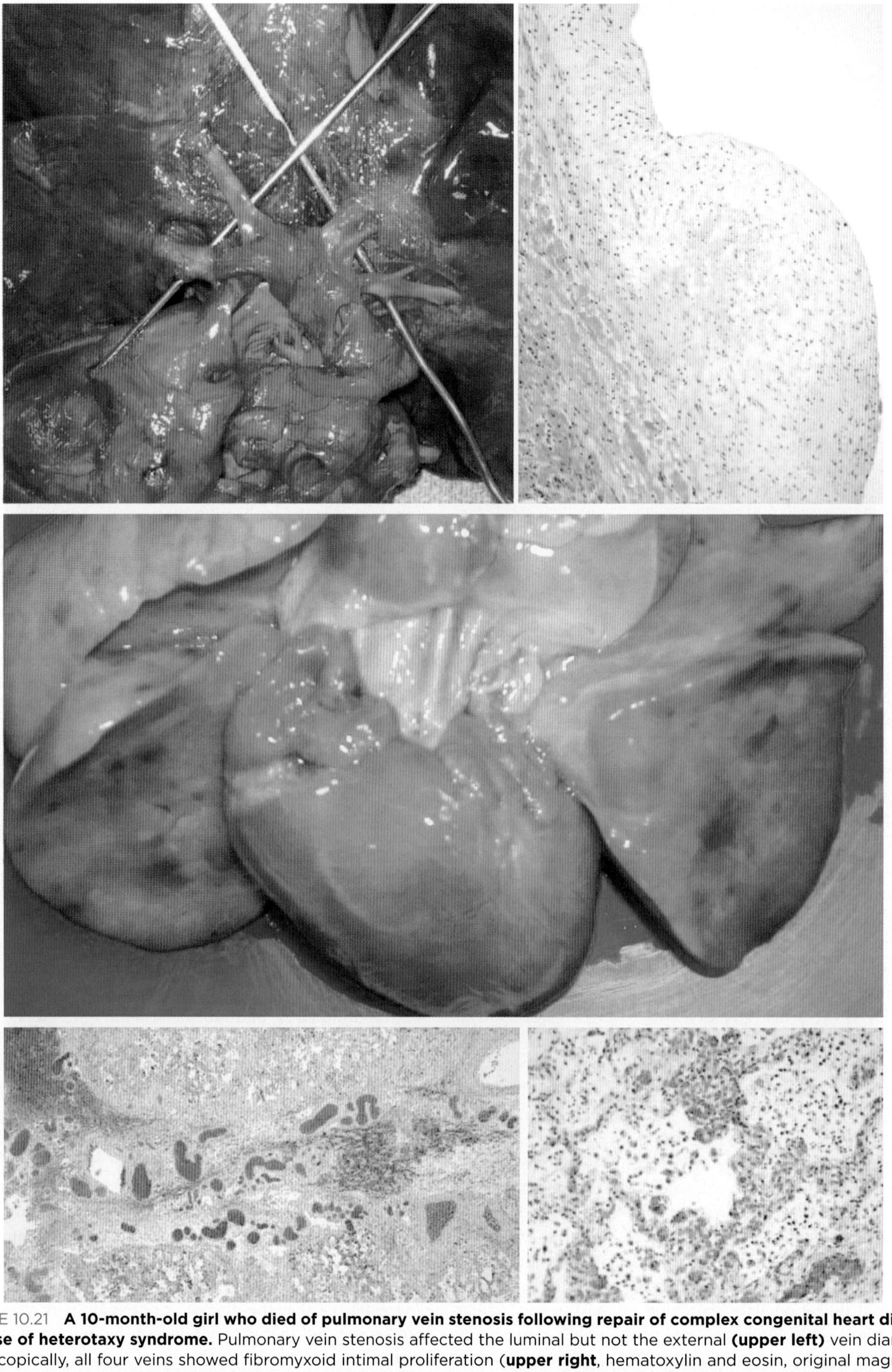

FIGURE 10.21 **A 10-month-old girl who died of pulmonary vein stenosis following repair of complex congenital heart disease because of heterotaxy syndrome.** Pulmonary vein stenosis affected the luminal but not the external **(upper left)** vein diameter. Microscopically, all four veins showed fibromyxoid intimal proliferation (**upper right**, hematoxylin and eosin, original magnification, 200x). On the external surface of the lungs, there are leopard-like spots **(middle)** reflecting pulmonary capillary hemangiomatosis-like foci because of chronic venous obstruction. Venous hypertensive changes dominate the microscopic findings. There is interlobular septal expansion with thick-walled and reduplicated venous channels (**lower left**, hematoxylin and eosin, original magnification, 40x) as well as patchy alveolar septal thickening by pulmonary capillary hemangiomatosis-like foci (**lower right**, hematoxylin and eosin, original magnification, 200x).

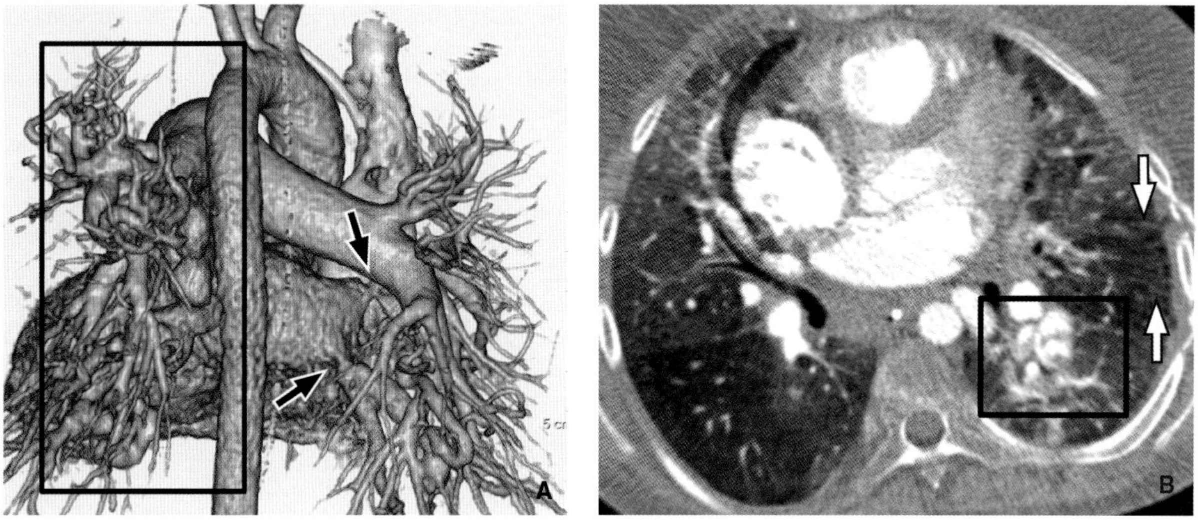

FIGURE 10.22 **Pulmonary vein stenosis in a 10-year-old girl. A:** Posterior oblique 3D volume-rendered CT image demonstrates at least moderate degree right superior and inferior pulmonary vein stenosis (*arrows*). The left superior pulmonary vein was completely occluded at the atrial insertion. There is compensatory varicose enlargement of left superior and left inferior pulmonary veins (*box*), which drain jointly, likely because of the redirection of flow. **B:** Axial enhanced CT image shows smooth interlobular septal thickening (*arrows*) and a pattern of mosaic perfusion related to pulmonary hypertension. Again noted is compensatory varicose enlargement of left inferior pulmonary veins (*box*).

80%.[58,91] Therefore, echocardiographic evaluation of the pulmonary veins should be performed in all patients with CHD, especially because some studies have established that worsening PVS can occur in patients with prior normal pulmonary venous flow patterns.[93,94] PVS may also occur in isolation; in those cases, it generally follows a rapid course.

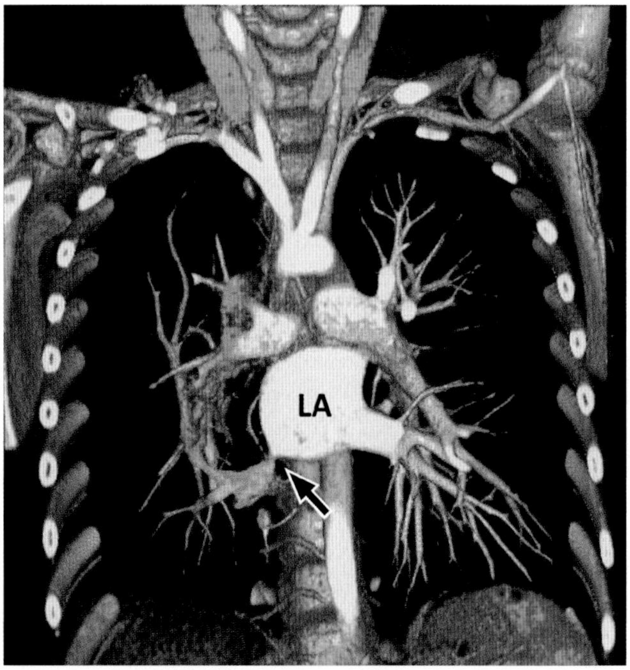

FIGURE 10.23 **Pulmonary vein stenosis in a 6-year-old girl status post scimitar vein reimplantation.** Coronal 3D volume-rendered CT image shows severe stenosis (*arrow*) of the reimplanted scimitar vein at the atrial insertion. *LA*, left atrium.

Most cases of PVS present in infancy with a history of worsening respiratory difficulties and recurrent pneumonia. With disease progression, pulmonary hypertension develops and becomes increasingly prominent. Hemoptysis may become a key concern, particularly in older patients.[91] Therefore, all pulmonary veins in young patients with unexplained pulmonary hypertension should be thoroughly assessed for signs of PVS. Usually, the age at diagnosis and the severity of symptoms are contingent on the number of pulmonary veins involved and the severity of pulmonary venous obstruction of individual veins.[91,95] Breinholt et al. found that the mortality rate approaches 85% in patients with PVS involving three or four veins versus 0% if the condition involves only one or two veins.[93]

In infants and young children with PVS, ECHO is usually the first line of imaging, and all pulmonary veins can usually be seen in most patients. Turbulent flow on color Doppler with flow velocities >1.6 m/s may potentially indicate hemodynamically significant obstruction.[96] On chest radiographs, findings of PVS include patchy reticular opacities and thickened septa, reflecting the impaired venous drainage in the diseased lung. In severe cases, the imaging findings may be indiscernible from pulmonary venous atresia, with smooth septal thickening, reticular opacities, patchy ground-glass centrilobular opacities, and smooth or nodular pleural thickening.[97]

On CT, PVS manifests with pulmonary vein thickening and narrowing that commonly affects the pulmonary venous-left atrial junction. However, the abnormality may progressively extend to involve more central and peripheral segments, resulting in long-segment narrowing, particularly in advanced cases.[47,58,98] For evaluation of PVS on CT, the routine acquisition of 3D volume-rendered CT images is recommended for the accurate assessment of central PVS because 3D volume-rendered CT images can significantly enhance depiction of the stenotic abnormalities seen in PVS, improving diagnostic accuracy and reader confidence in this setting.[89] In addition, prominent soft tissue located adjacent to the affected pulmonary veins and left atrium, which represent proliferative myofibroblastic cells, may be also seen. On lung window CT images, a pattern of diffuse, multifocal regions of mosaic attenuation may be present. Typically, oligemia is observed in the hypoattenuating regions, as expected given the underlying vascular etiology of this mosaic pattern.[99] This differs from the pattern observed in small airways disease, in which the vascular structures are unaffected.[99] Enlarged mediastinal lymph nodes related to vascular congestion may be also present.[100]

MRI may show similar findings in pediatric patients with PVS although to a lesser extent given that CT offers better spatial resolution. However, MRI may provide additional physiologic information, and the clinical significance of the stenosis may be readily assessed by quantifying pulmonary venous and arterial flow in the involved and uninvolved lung portions.[92] Although it is currently not routinely used for evaluation of PVS, on V/Q scans, PVS may show a mottled appearance with patchy distribution of the radiotracer but without discrete segmental or subsegmental defects that can be demonstrated on CT. This is presumably related to increased downstream resistance to the flow of the macroaggregated albumin particles but not to the power injection of the contrast in CTA or pulmonary angiograms.[97,100]

PVS may be amenable to balloon angioplasty, with stent placement usually considered only as a last mode of therapy before lung transplantation.[91] Special care should be taken in pediatric patients with PVS because stent implantation before surgery may complicate and limit the later surgical approach. Despite the introduction of new surgical venoplastic techniques based on the premise of reducing trauma to the veins to avoid any stimulus for regrowth, there is a high rate of restenosis in both primary and secondary forms of pediatric PVS. Therefore, continued noninvasive imaging follow-up is warranted in this pediatric patient population. In severe cases, lung transplantation or combined heart–lung transplantation may be necessary.[91,101]

Pulmonary Varix

Pulmonary varix is a relatively rare vascular anomaly that manifests as the focal aneurysmal dilatation of a segment of a pulmonary vein. Pulmonary varices should not be confused with the more common pulmonary AVM.[102,103] Unlike pulmonary AVM, pulmonary varices do not result in right-to-left shunting. The condition may be congenital or acquired; the latter is seen in pediatric patients who have underlying cardiac conditions resulting in pulmonary venous hypertension, such as central PVS, mitral valve disease, and aortic coarctation.[103] In most instances, pulmonary varices are incidental findings in otherwise asymptomatic pediatric patients and characteristically regress following correction of the underlying abnormality. Seldom, the varix may serve as a thrombogenic nidus, and affected pediatric patients may become symptomatic as a result of complications such as rupture and thromboembolism.[47,50,58]

On chest radiographs, pulmonary varices may appear as well-defined pulmonary or mediastinal lesions in close proximity to the cardiac silhouette and should be differentiated from other etiologies for space-occupying lesions in the pediatric patient, such as a congenital lung anomaly, round pneumonia, or a neoplasm. CT with 3D reconstruction is particularly useful for characterization of these vascular lesions. The imaging features that support a diagnosis of pulmonary varix include the following: (1) contiguity between the pulmonary vein and varix with concomitant enhancement of both structures, (2) draining of the varix into the left atrium with no evidence of shunting between the systemic and pulmonary circulations, (3) delayed emptying of the varix compared to the remaining normal pulmonary veins, (4) tortuosity involving the central portion of the affected pulmonary varix, and (5) lack of a feeding artery contiguous with the pulmonary artery.[47,58,104] Some authors advocate the use of modalities that demonstrate the flow direction and pattern within the lesion, such as US, MR, or conventional angiography, to differentiate pulmonary varix from pulmonary AVM.[102,103,105]

For managing pulmonary varix, surgical resection is only indicated for symptomatic pediatric patients or in cases of complications such as rupture or thromboembolism.[47,105]

Partial Anomalous Pulmonary Venous Return (Including Scimitar Syndrome)

Partial anomalous pulmonary venous return (PAPVR) results from the failure of one or several, but not all, of the pulmonary veins to be incorporated into the left atrium. The anomalous vein drains into the systemic circulation, ultimately resulting in a left-to-right shunt. PAPVR is usually an isolated finding and is more frequently seen on the right side. The right pulmonary veins are involved twice as often as the left pulmonary veins. Anomalous drainage of the right pulmonary veins occurs most frequently into the SVC (Fig. 10.24), right atrium (Fig. 10.25), and IVC, whereas anomalous drainage of the left pulmonary veins into the left brachiocephalic vein (Fig. 10.26) and coronary sinus is more common.

In pediatric patients with PAPVR, pulmonary to systemic flow is increased proportionally to the anomalous number of connected veins and to the presence of an associated atrial septal defect (ASD), usually a sinus venosus defect, which is seen in ~50% of patients with PAPVR.[106] A sinus venosus defect is the end product of a deficient sinus venosus septum, which ultimately results in contiguity of the anomalous right pulmonary vein with the SVC or the posterior aspect of the right atrium. The right cardiac chambers and pulmonary vasculature are frequently enlarged due to volume overload. However, in the pure forms of PAPVR, pulmonary hypertension and right heart failure rarely develop. Other forms of PAPVR are sometimes associated with a secundum type of ASD or a PFO.

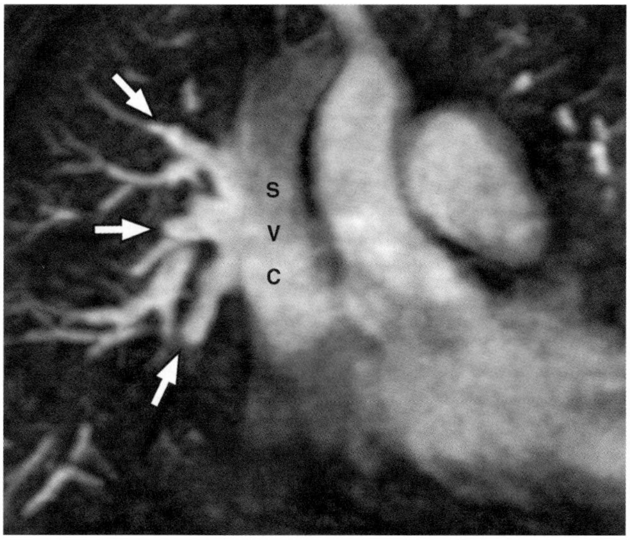

FIGURE 10.24 **Right-sided partial anomalous pulmonary venous return in a 9-year-old boy with a history of abnormal echocardiogram showing poor visualization of the right pulmonary veins, right ventricular dilatation, and a sinus venosus atrial septal defect.** Coronal maximum intensity projection MRA image shows partial anomalous pulmonary venous return of at least three right-sided pulmonary veins (*arrows*) to the right superior vena cava (*SVC*).

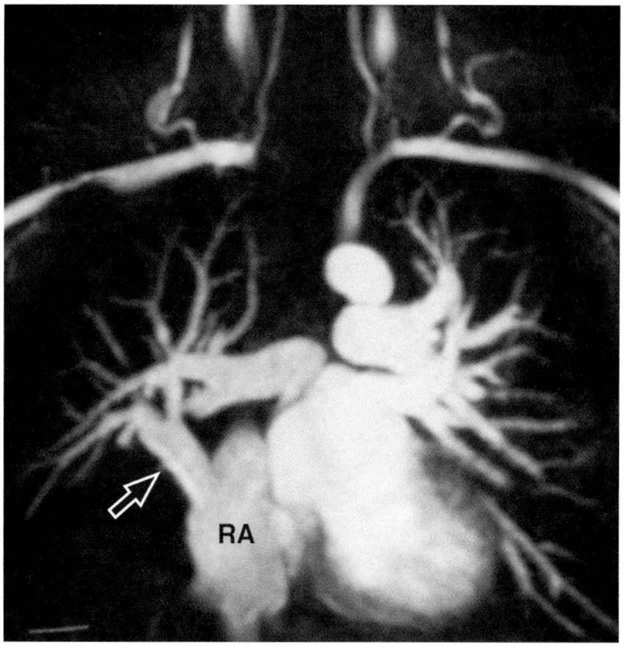

FIGURE 10.25 **Right-sided partial pulmonary venous return in an 8-year-old boy who presented with persistent dyspnea after exercising at school.** Coronal maximum intensity projection MRA image shows the right pulmonary vein (*arrow*) draining into the right atrium (*RA*).

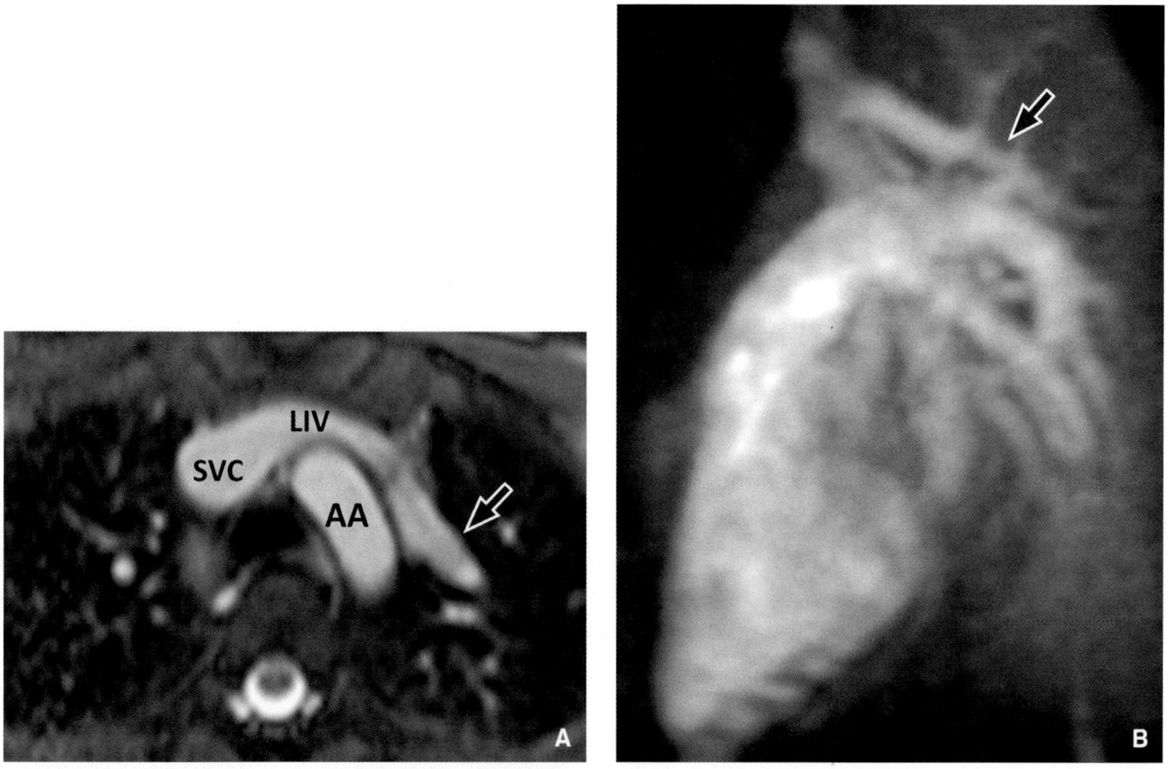

FIGURE 10.26 **Left upper lobe partial anomalous pulmonary venous return in a 14-year-old boy with abnormal chest radiographic findings of widened superior mediastinum obtained for evaluation of pneumonia.** Axial white-blood MR image **(A)** and sagittal maximum intensity projection MR image **(B)** show an anomalous left upper lobe pulmonary vein (*arrow*) draining into the left innominate vein (*LIV*). *AA*, aortic arch; *SVC*, superior vena cava.

The most common type of PAPVR involves a right upper lobe pulmonary vein returning anomalously into the SVC with or without an associated sinus venosus defect, followed by PAPVR of a left upper lobe pulmonary vein into the left innominate vein. Unlike total anomalous pulmonary venous return, obstruction to drainage is rare in PAPVR, and the majority of affected pediatric patients are either mildly symptomatic or asymptomatic.[5,60,107,108]

The scimitar syndrome, hypogenetic lung syndrome, or congenital pulmonary venolobar syndrome is a form of PAPVR in which an anomalous pulmonary vein drains a portion of or the entire right lung, typically into the IVC, and manifests on imaging as a crescent-like shadow in the right lower lung zone (Fig. 10.27). The anomalous vein may drain into the hepatic veins, portal veins, azygos vein, coronary sinus, or right atrium and often resembles a scimitar (a curved Turkish sword), hence the name "scimitar syndrome." Scimitar syndrome nearly always occurs on the right side and is usually associated with a hypoplastic RPA and varying degrees of right lung hypoplasia ensuing from heart dextroposition. Approximately 25% of affected pediatric patients have associated CHD, most often a sinus venosus ASD. Female preponderance is a classic feature of this syndrome, and frequently associated anomalies include bronchogenic cyst, horseshoe lung, pulmonary sequestration, accessory diaphragm, cardiac dextroposition, and aberrant arterial supply to portions of the right lung, characteristically from the descending aorta.[47,50,60,109]

The hemodynamic sequelae of PAPVR are contingent on the number and size of anomalous pulmonary veins and on the duration of shunting. When the shunt is significant, flow across the right heart is increased, and there is increased pulmonary blood flow. Pulmonary hypertension and right heart failure may subsequently develop. Although pediatric patients with PAPVR are most often asymptomatic, because of its common association with other forms of CHD, PAPVR may occasionally be diagnosed during the workup. Similarly, an incidentally found cardiac murmur may trigger imaging studies disclosing the PAPVR.[47,58] For infants with scimitar syndrome, a high prevalence of respiratory complications is often present. Lung function tests may show reduced lung volumes and airflows that are indicative of persistent pulmonary hypoplasia, which is a marker of severity, as are cardiac defects and pulmonary hypertension. On the other end of the spectrum, scimitar syndrome may be seen as an incidental finding in older patients.[109]

Imaging findings of PAPVR vary relative to the site of anomalous connection and the presence or absence of obstruction. On chest radiographs, variable degrees of increased pulmonary blood flow with a pattern of overcirculation may be seen. If shunting is severe enough and sufficient time has elapsed, mild to moderate right-sided cardiomegaly may be observed. Cross-sectional imaging and in particular cardiac MRI are the imaging modalities of choice for accurate depiction of the anomalous venous connections. MRI can also provide further physiologic information with quantification of the pulmonary-to-systemic flow ratio, the Qp/Qs ratio, which is necessary to determine whether surgical repair is warranted.[50,95] CT and MRI can also provide accurate information regarding postoperative pulmonary vein obstruction or narrowing.

In pediatric patients with scimitar syndrome, the typical vertically oriented curvilinear opacity representing the scimitar vein may be seen projecting over the right lower hemithorax in association with a hypoplastic right lung on

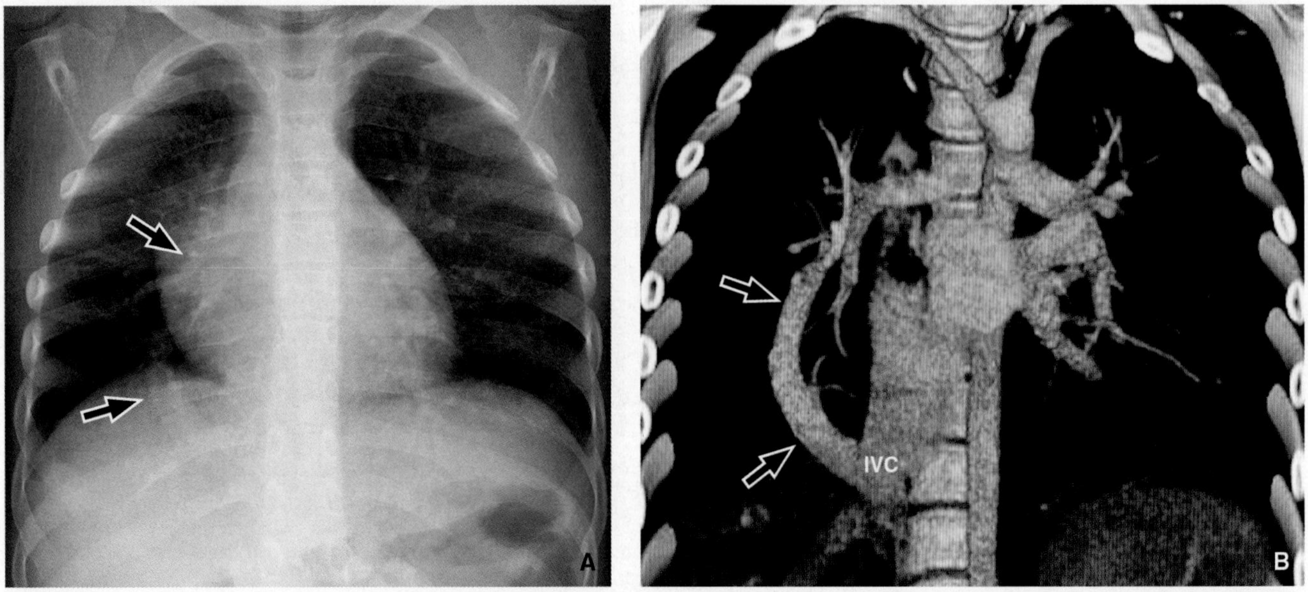

FIGURE 10.27 **Scimitar syndrome in a 6-year-old girl who presented with fever and cough. A:** Frontal chest radiograph shows a scimitar vein (*arrows*) and mild heart dextroposition consistent with hypogenetic lung syndrome. **B:** Coronal 3D volume-rendered CT image demonstrates anomalous pulmonary venous drainage of a vast portion of a hypoplastic right lung via the scimitar vein (*arrows*) into the inferior vena cava (*IVC*).

frontal chest radiographs.[107,110,111] CT and MR are currently the favored imaging modalities for corroborating and illustrating the constellation of findings related to scimitar syndrome in the pediatric patient. Three-dimensional imaging has been reported to be particularly useful for conveying the entire course of the anomalous scimitar vein as a preprocedural or preoperative assessment.[58,60] Given the associated abnormal lung parenchymal changes, abnormal lung lobulation, and anomalous bronchial branching patterns often seen in patients with scimitar syndrome, this syndrome can be particularly well evaluated with CT.[58,60] The absence of an ipsilateral inferior pulmonary vein is a helpful clue that supports the diagnosis of scimitar syndrome on cross-sectional imaging studies.

In the experience of Alsoufi et al.,[112] surgical management of PAPVR is recommended when patients fail to respond to medical treatment or in the presence of a continuous, large left-to-right shunt (Qp/Qs > 2:1). The surgery is associated with excellent outcomes and low time-related morbidity. Conversely, the management of scimitar syndrome is complex, with a high incidence of postoperative pulmonary venous obstruction and abnormally decreased perfusion of the right lung. Indications for surgical repair of scimitar syndrome are controversial, but they are usually recommended in cases of volume-loaded right ventricle and are typically performed within the same time frame as ASD repair. Surgery is not deemed necessary when a single anomalously draining vein has not produced right ventricular volume loading. The type of surgery is determined by the location of the anomalous connection and generally consists of reconnection of the anomalous veins to the left atrium either by direct anastomosis or, in most instances, utilizing a baffle. In cases of scimitar syndrome, occlusion of the collateral arteries may be also necessary.[111,112]

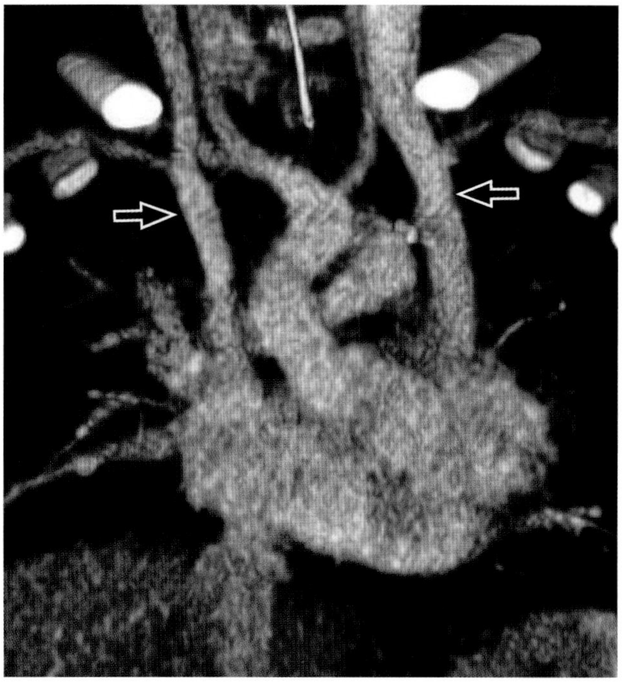

FIGURE 10.28 **Duplicated superior vena cava in a 10-month-old girl with congenital heart disease.** Coronal 3D volume-rendered CT image shows bilateral superior vena cava (*arrows*). Contrast was injected from the left upper extremity and delineates a left-sided superior vena cava draining into a prominent coronary sinus (*not shown*). No bridging vein is seen joining the left and the right superior vena cava.

Superior Vena Cava

Left Superior Vena Cava and Duplicated Superior Vena Cava

Persistent left SVC has a prevalence of 0.3% in the general population; however, the reported prevalence in patients with CHD may be as high as 4.4%.[5,113–116] A higher incidence (13.5%) of these anomalies has been reported in patients of Middle Eastern descent.[113] Embryologically, a persistent left SVC results from failure of the left anterior cardinal vein to involute.[117] Concomitant persistence of the right anterior and common cardinal veins yields bilateral SVCs with or without a bridging, communicating brachiocephalic vein (Fig. 10.28). In most instances, the persistent left SVC drains into the right atrium via a dilated coronary sinus. However, in some instances, it may drain into the left atrium and result in a right-to-left shunt.[115,116]

Anomalies frequently associated with left SVC include septal defects (ventricular and atrioventricular), tetralogy of Fallot, double outlet right ventricle, heterotaxy, and mitral abnormalities.[5,113,116] Commonly associated extracardiac disorders include VACTERL association (vertebral defects, anal atresia, cardiac defects, tracheo-esophageal fistula, renal anomalies, and limb abnormalities), trisomy 21, 22q11 deletion, CHARGE syndrome, and Turner syndrome.[114]

Identification of SVC anomalies is of paramount importance because the technique for the venous cannulation of the cardiopulmonary bypass and other surgical techniques may be radically changed depending on whether an innominate vein that bridges to a right-sided SVC is present.[113,116,118] Therefore, it is of particular importance to actively investigate for these anomalies in cardiac surgery candidates. In addition, when the right atrium is entered through the left SVC and coronary sinus, it is highly unlikely that the catheter will traverse the RV to the PA because the direction of flow is unfavorable. Furthermore, coronary sinus catheterization in patients with left SVC has been reported to be associated with chest pain, collapse, and electrocardiographic changes consistent with myocardial ischemia.[117]

Imaging clues suggesting the presence of a left-sided SVC include the presence of an enlarged coronary sinus and the absence of the left innominate vein.[5,114] If a bridging vein is present, constituting a so-called duplicated SVC, the usual direct cannulation of the SVC and IVC is sufficient to provide suitable venous return. If the bridging vein is absent, other, more complicated tactics are needed to ensure satisfactory venous return.[118] Similarly, if a cavopulmonary anastomosis (bidirectional Glenn) is needed and the bridging vein is not present, bilateral bidirectional Glenn surgeries are needed.[113,116]

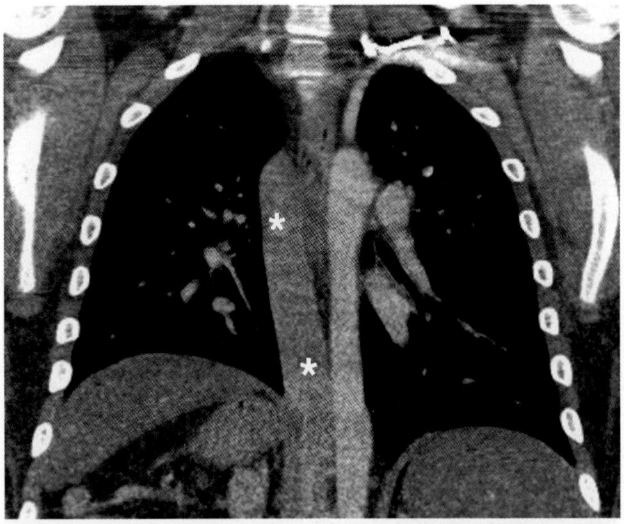

FIGURE 10.29 **Interrupted inferior vena cava with azygos continuation in a 15-year-old girl with a history of heterotaxy.** Coronal reformatted CT image shows a prominent azygos vein (*asterisks*) in this patient with interrupted inferior vena cava and azygos continuation, not an uncommon finding in pediatric patients with heterotaxy.

Inferior Vena Cava

Interrupted Inferior Vena Cava with Azygos Continuation

The reported incidence of IVC interruption with azygos or hemiazygos continuation ranges between 0.15% and 1.3%.[113,119] This vascular anomaly is usually seen in association with complex CHD, right or left isomerism, and anomalous pulmonary venous connections.[113,119] Diagnosis of this venous vascular anomaly is important because it can result in technical difficulties during interventional or surgical procedures. Reported associations include bilateral recurrent lower extremity deep venous thrombosis, sick sinus syndrome, and atrial flutter[119–121] (Fig. 10.29).

Acquired Great Vascular Abnormalities

Infectious Disorders (Including Mycotic Aortic Aneurysm)

Mycotic aortic aneurysm refers to any arterial dilatation of infectious etiology, irrespective of size or etiology. Mycotic aortic aneurysms represent <3% of all aortic aneurysms[122,123] and are uncommon in pediatric patients[124] (Fig. 10.30). Reported etiologies in the pediatric population include umbilical artery catheterization, mediastinitis, tuberculous para-aortic lymphadenitis, previous aortic or mediastinal surgery, bacterial endocarditis, and hematogenous seeding from distant sites of infection. The mechanisms of infection include contiguous spread from neighboring infected structures, such as may occur in cases of mediastinitis, infectious pericarditis, empyema, paravertebral abscess, septic emboli to the aortic vasa vasorum, bacteremic seeding of an intimal injury, and direct bacterial inoculation at the time of trauma.[122,123,125–127] *Staphylococcus aureus*, salmonellae, and enterococci are the three most common causative organisms.[122,123,125]

On imaging studies, most mycotic aortic aneurysms are saccular in shape and show irregular, thickened walls. Periaortic fluid and fat stranding of the surrounding soft tissues may be seen at early stages of infection. Rapid progression or change in shape of a saccular aneurysm is highly suggestive of superimposed infection. At later stages, air may occasionally be seen trapped in the walls of the mycotic aneurysm.[122,123,125] The literature on pediatric mycotic aortic aneurysm repair is scarce, precluding adequate evaluation of outcomes or conclusions concerning recommended management or preferred surgical technique.

Traumatic Disorders

Acute Traumatic Aortic Injury (Including Dissection and Pseudoaneurysm)

Trauma is the primary cause of death in pediatric patients older than 1 year. Although traumatic vascular injury is relatively uncommon in this population, it results in significant morbidity and mortality. The mechanism of injury to the thoracic aorta is violent deceleration, causing movement of the aorta and shearing forces at the sites of relative immobility, typically the ligamentum arteriosum, aortic root, and diaphragmatic hiatus,[128] with the aortic isthmus being the most common site of injury in clinical practice (Fig. 10.31). On autopsy series, injury to the ascending aorta has been reported in 20% to 25% of cases; however, 80% of these injuries are fatal, resulting in hemopericardium with tamponade, aortic valve rupture, or coronary artery dissection.[129]

In an epidemiologic study of pediatric vascular trauma using nationwide data,[130] it was shown that ~40% of pediatric vascular thoracic injuries are penetrating vascular injuries, usually produced by a firearm or stabbing. Nearly 50% of the pediatric patients who sustained an intrathoracic vascular injury owing to a penetrating trauma did not survive.

The most common traumatic aortic injuries are transverse tears; these may range from intimal laceration to complete transection depending on how many layers of the aortic wall are involved. Partial tears result in a contained rupture and usually involve only the inner two layers, whereas complete transections, which are generally fatal because of exsanguination, typically involve all three layers.[128] CT with CTA technique is the most important imaging modality and technique for evaluating traumatic aortic injury; it has a sensitivity and a negative predictive value approaching 100% for the detection of traumatic aortic injury.[128,131]

Periaortic mediastinal hematoma is an indirect sign of aortic trauma, which may result from hemorrhage of the aorta vasa vasorum, hemothorax, and hemopericardium.[132,133]

Direct signs of aortic trauma include pseudoaneurysm formation, intimal flap, irregular contour, mural thrombus, sudden change in aortic caliber, and rarely, direct extravasation of contrast, especially if located in the juxtaductal regions.[128,131–134] Traumatic pseudoaneurysms manifest as rounded bulges with irregular margins projecting anteriorly and originating from the isthmus region. These features indicate a rupture that is contained by the adventitia, resulting

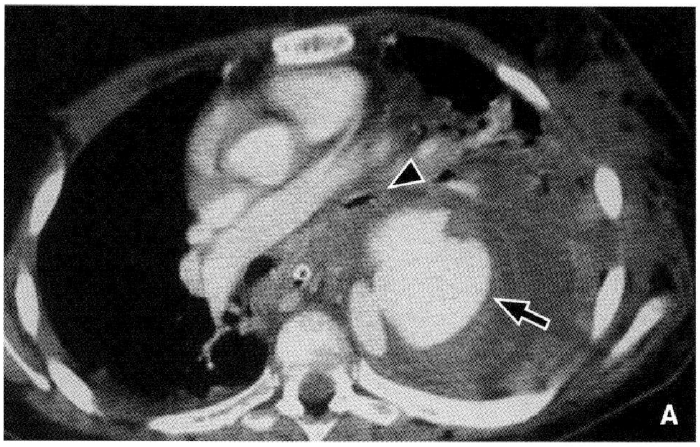

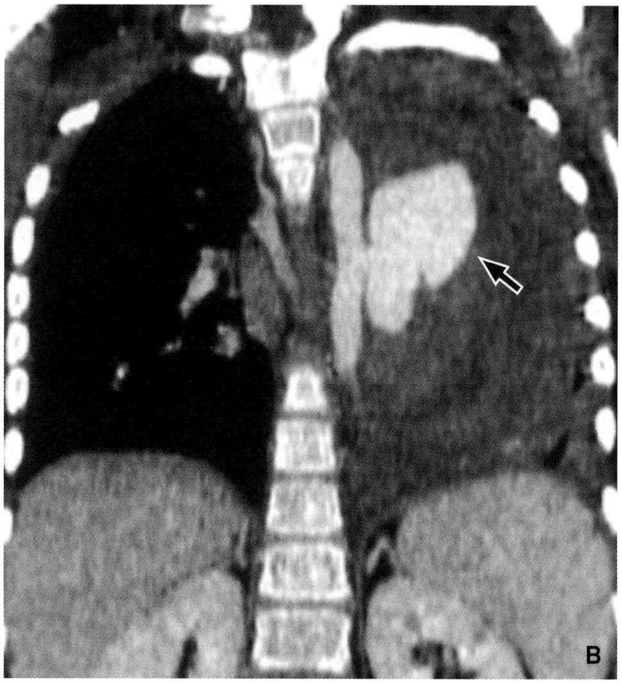

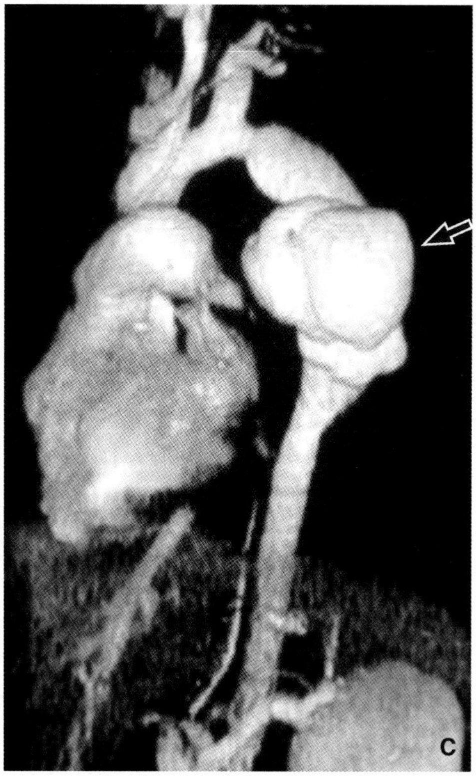

FIGURE 10.30 **Mycotic aortic aneurysm in an 8-year-old boy who presented with fever, pneumonia, and worsening respiratory distress.** Chest radiograph (not shown) demonstrated complete opacification of the left hemithorax and CT was subsequently obtained for further evaluation. Axial **(A)** and coronal reformatted **(B)** CT images show irregular contours to the left mid-thoracic aorta with focal aneurysmatic dilation with irregular contours (*arrow*) exerting compression on the left mainstem bronchus (*arrowhead*). Also seen is the increased heterogeneous density surrounding the aorta and the left lung parenchyma related to pneumonia. **C:** Volume-rendered 3D CT image demonstrates the location, extension, and entire shape of the mycotic aortic aneurysm (*arrow*).

in bulging as a result of the dissection of blood through an intimal and medial tear. The torn intima may present as a flap across the base of the pseudoaneurysm. The finding of a juxtaductal pseudoaneurysm nearly always indicates aortic injury.

An aortic intimal tear must be differentiated from the normal ductus diverticulum or ductus bump, which is an embryologic remnant at the site of the ligamentum arteriosum in the aortic isthmus and manifests as a focal bulge along the anteromedial aspect of the aortic isthmus.[135,136] This is a normal variant that can easily be mistaken for a posttraumatic pseudoaneurysm, which can also occur at the aortic isthmus. The ductus bump has smooth contours and exhibits obtuse angles, whereas a tear usually has irregular contours and more acute angles. Multiplanar, MIP, volume-rendered, and virtual angioscopic 3D images can aid in determining the precise anatomy of such irregularities because of the ability to align the reconstructions with the planes of the vessel.[5,134]

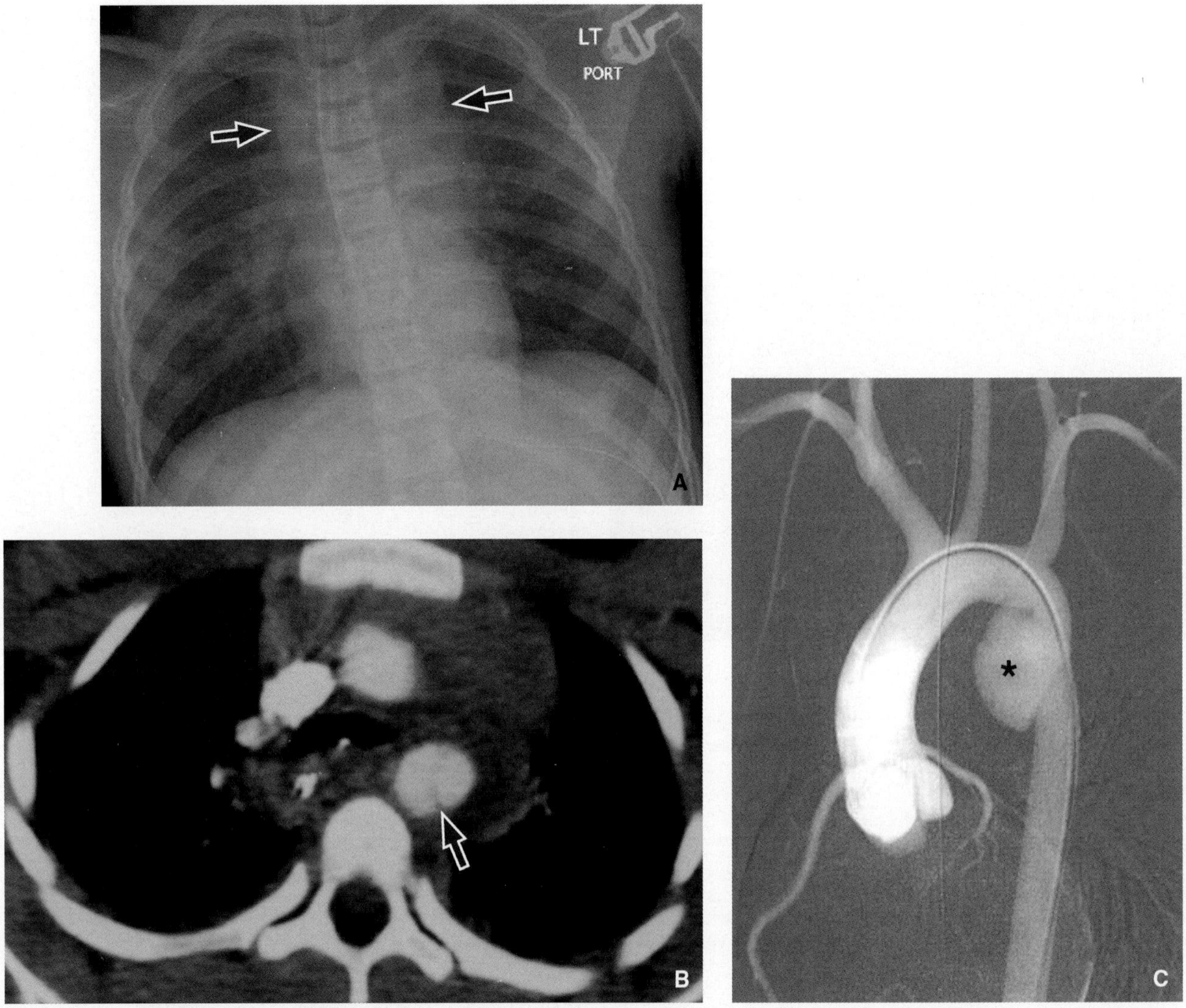

FIGURE 10.31 **Acute traumatic aortic injury in a 15-year-old boy status post motor vehicle accident. A:** Frontal chest radiograph shows a widened mediastinum (*arrows*). The trachea is slightly deviated to the right. **B:** Axial enhanced CT image shows traumatic aortic injury (dissection) at the typical location of the aortic isthmus. Note the intimal flap (*arrow*) and the surrounding mediastinal hematoma. **C:** Angiogram demonstrates the resultant pseudoaneurysm formation (*asterisk*).

One specific type of traumatic aortic injury and complication is an aortoesophageal fistula, which can result in fatal hemorrhage. This condition has been reported in infants following ingestion of button batteries. The aortoesophageal fistula results from a combination of mechanical pressure, corrosive hydroxyl ions produced by electric currents, and leakage of alkaline contents resulting in corrosive damage.[137] If lodging of a battery in the esophagus is suspected, this should be confirmed on chest radiographs; endoscopic removal must be carried out immediately because perforation has been described as soon as 5 hours after ingestion.[137]

Depending on the type of injury, treatment of traumatic aortic injury may include medical, percutaneous, or operative approaches. In general, surgical repair remains the mainstay of therapy, although in recent years, the use of percutaneous endovascular stent grafting as an alternative to surgery has been expanded in many trauma centers. Given the scarcity of long-term follow-up data, however, the latter choice must be tempered.[128,138]

Vascular Disorders

Takayasu Arteritis

Childhood vasculitis encompasses a group of unusual multisystemic disorders that are characterized by the presence of inflammation in the blood vessel walls. If it is left untreated, this condition may potentially result in tissue ischemia from vascular stenosis, occlusion, aneurysm, or rupture.[139,140] Vasculitis in children may occur secondary to infection, malignancy, or drug or radiation exposure or secondary to other rheumatologic disorders such as lupus or juvenile dermatomyositis.[141] The classification of vasculitis in children is primarily based on the size of the affected vessels and the presence or absence of granulomatous changes.[142]

Takayasu arteritis is a large- and medium-sized vessel granulomatous vasculitis that primarily affects the aorta and its major branches, and the pulmonary arteries. There is a strong female predilection for this condition. Its etiology is currently unknown, but it is believed to involve a T-cell–mediated autoimmune process that results in a panarteritis extending from the adventitial vasa vasorum inward. Early diagnosis is challenging because the clinical manifestations are often nonspecific. The most common presentations are hypertension, headaches, dizziness, abdominal pain, lower extremity claudication, fever, and weight loss.[139–141,143]

Clinically, Takayasu arteritis is divided into two phases, an early, systemic, "prepulseless" phase and a late, occlusive, "pulseless" phase. During the early "prepulseless" phase, constitutional systemic symptoms, including malaise, fever, night sweats, and weight loss, are common. On physical examination, hypertension is present in nearly 90% of patients, and bruits or weakened blood pulses may be detected in the involved vessels. The symptoms of Takayasu arteritis during the chronic phase depend on the vessels involved, and symptoms of ischemia are present once vascular occlusions or high-grade stenosis develop. Depending on the vascular territories involved, affected pediatric patients may show hypertension, ischemic heart disease, abdominal pain, hematuria, or proteinuria.[122,123,125,141]

Cross-sectional imaging, preferably MR angiography, is used to evaluate Takayasu arteritis because MRI can show contrast enhancement of the thickened wall, a finding that correlates well with disease activity, which is difficult to adequately evaluate clinically[144] (Figs. 10.32 and 10.33). MIP and volume-rendered 3D reconstructions are particularly helpful in delineating the degree of stenosis or aneurysmatic dilata-

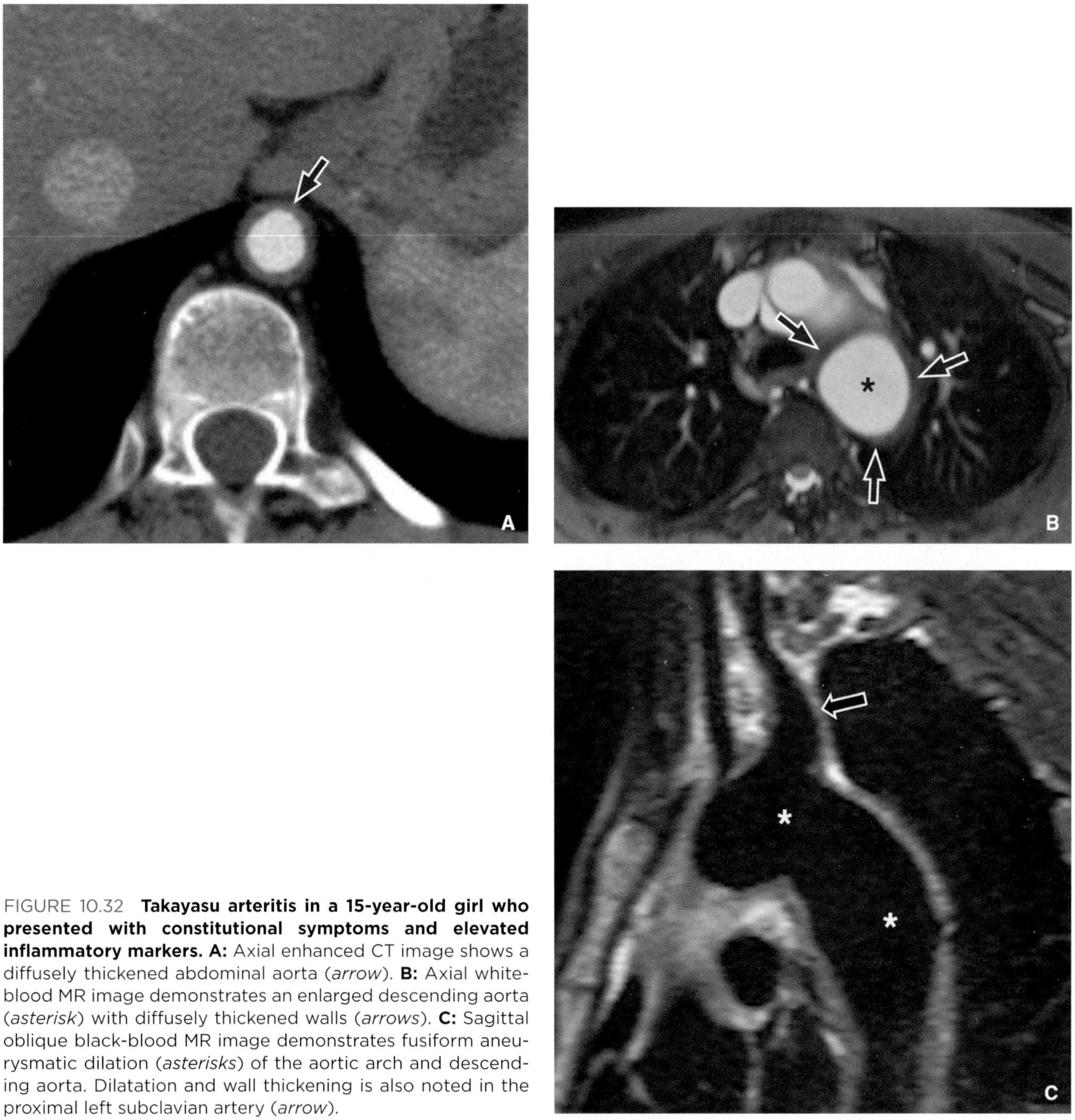

FIGURE 10.32 **Takayasu arteritis in a 15-year-old girl who presented with constitutional symptoms and elevated inflammatory markers. A:** Axial enhanced CT image shows a diffusely thickened abdominal aorta (*arrow*). **B:** Axial white-blood MR image demonstrates an enlarged descending aorta (*asterisk*) with diffusely thickened walls (*arrows*). **C:** Sagittal oblique black-blood MR image demonstrates fusiform aneurysmatic dilation (*asterisks*) of the aortic arch and descending aorta. Dilatation and wall thickening is also noted in the proximal left subclavian artery (*arrow*).

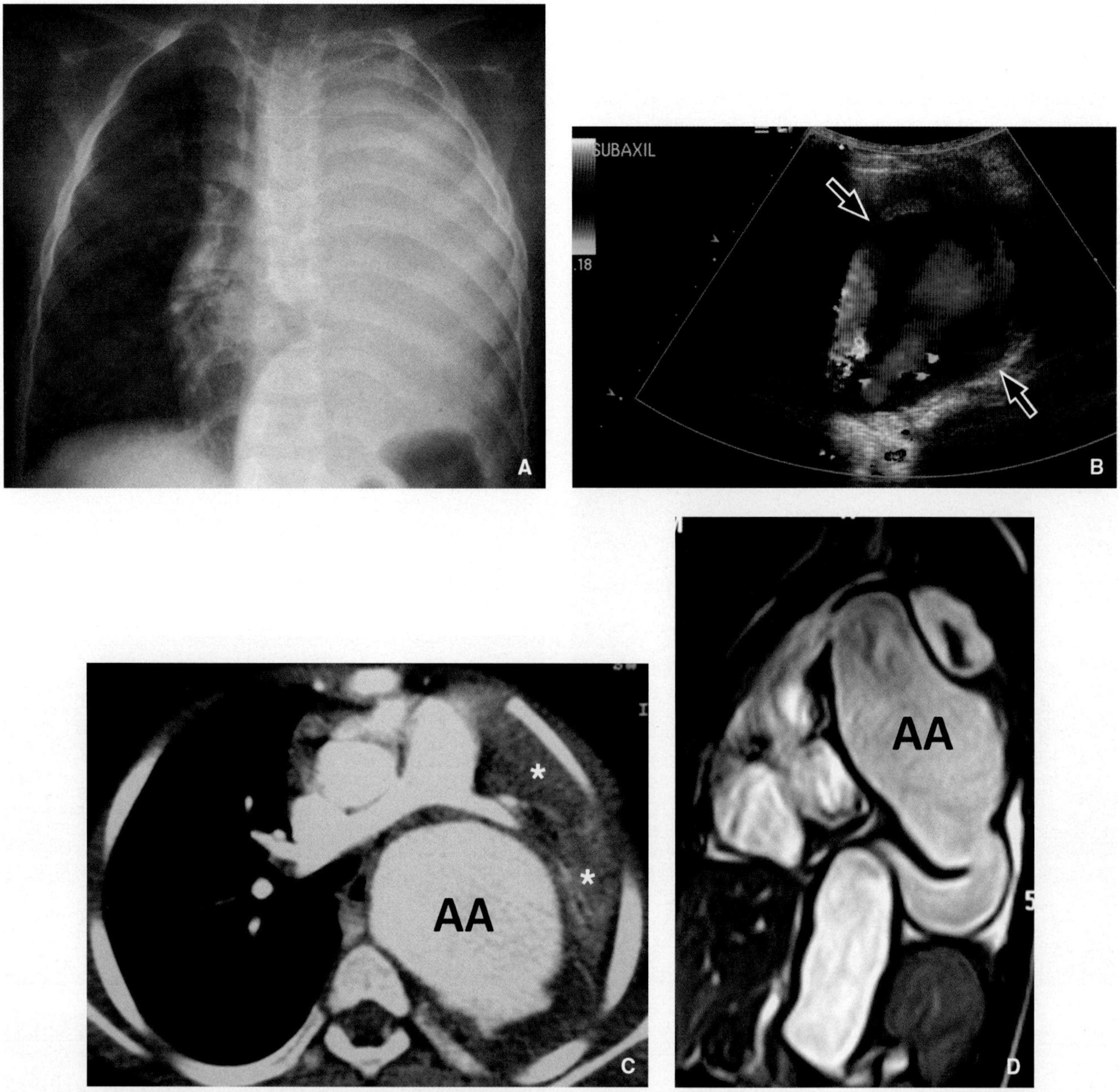

FIGURE 10.33 **Takayasu arteritis in a 5-year-old girl who presented with 6 months of low-grade fevers of unknown origin.** **A:** Frontal chest radiograph shows complete opacification of the left hemithorax with mild deviation of the trachea to the right. **B:** Doppler ultrasound image demonstrates a hypoechoic lesion (*arrows*) with internal blood flow. **C:** Axial enhanced CT image shows an aortic aneurysm (*AA*). Left lung atelectasis (*asterisks*) and a small left pleural effusion are also seen. **D:** Sagittal white blood MR image demonstrates a tortuous, redundant, markedly dilated aorta (*AA*).

tion of the vessels involved. Furthermore, mural edema may occasionally be seen on T2-weighted MR images as a concentric rim of high signal intensity.[123,125] The limitations of MRI include its limited depiction of vascular branch points, which may be misinterpreted as vascular occlusions, poor depiction of calcifications that may occur in late-stage Takayasu arteritis, and relatively low sensitivity for the evaluation of smaller vessels as well as the limited areas that can be scanned in each station as opposed to CTA.[125,145,146]

Steroids are the mainstay of therapy in pediatric patients with Takayasu arteritis. Alternative therapy is used in patients who fail to respond to 3 months' of steroids or show a flare of the disease while on tapering steroid dosage. Alternative agents include methotrexate, cyclophosphamide, and mycophenolate mofetil.[147] Azathioprine and infliximab have also been used in children.[140,141] Revascularization procedures should be considered in pediatric patients with any of the following conditions: (1) hypertension secondary to significant aortic coarctation or renovascular disease, (2) peripheral limb ischemia, (3) cerebral ischemia, and (4) aortic or arterial aneurysms, or aortic insufficiency.[147]

Ehlers-Danlos Syndrome

Ehlers-Danlos syndrome is an inherited connective tissue disorder characterized by joint and skin hyperextensibility, excessive bruising, blood vessel fragility, and poor wound healing. Currently, six types of Ehlers-Danlos syndrome are recognized. The vascular type, formerly known as type IV, is an autosomal dominant disorder of type II collagen resulting from a mutation in the COL3A1 gene on chromosome 2. The clinical diagnosis of vascular Ehlers-Danlos syndrome is made on the basis of at least two of four major diagnostic criteria including arterial, intestinal, or uterine fragility or rupture, thin translucent skin, easy bruising, and characteristic facial appearance.[11,148,149]

The most common sites of vascular disease in Ehlers-Danlos syndrome include the abdominal visceral arteries, iliac arteries, and thoracic and abdominal aorta. In half of the affected patients, more than one site may be seen.[148–150] Aortic aneurysms in these pediatric patients are fusiform, and over time they may progress or new aneurysms may develop. These aortic aneurysms are at risk of spontaneous rupture, and dissection may result in vascular compromise and infarcts. Therefore, these patients should be kept under routine surveillance to assess the expansion rate. CA and endoscopy are usually avoided in these patients due to the high risk of associated complications.[149,150] Vascular disease in Ehlers-Danlos syndrome patients can be evaluated either by CT or MR angiography depending on local expertise and preferences (Fig. 10.34).

A clinical trial is ongoing to determine the utility of β-blockers with vasodilating drugs as a preventive measure in these patients.[150] Traditionally, Ehlers-Danlos syndrome was managed conservatively, with surgery being reserved for life-threatening complications. However, it has recently been suggested that elective surgical management of aneurysms could be associated with favorable outcomes and should not be deferred until complications such as rupture or dissection occur.[149]

Marfan Syndrome

Marfan syndrome is an autosomal dominant connective tissue disorder demonstrating complete penetrance but variable expression. The vast majority of cases result from mutations in the fibrillin 1 (*FBN1*) gene located on chromosome 15.[151] In the absence of fibrillin 1, elastin is more speedily degraded by matrix metalloproteinases, and dissociation of smooth muscle cells from the medial matrix components occurs. The diagnosis of Marfan syndrome is clinical and is based on the revised Ghent nosology.[152,153]

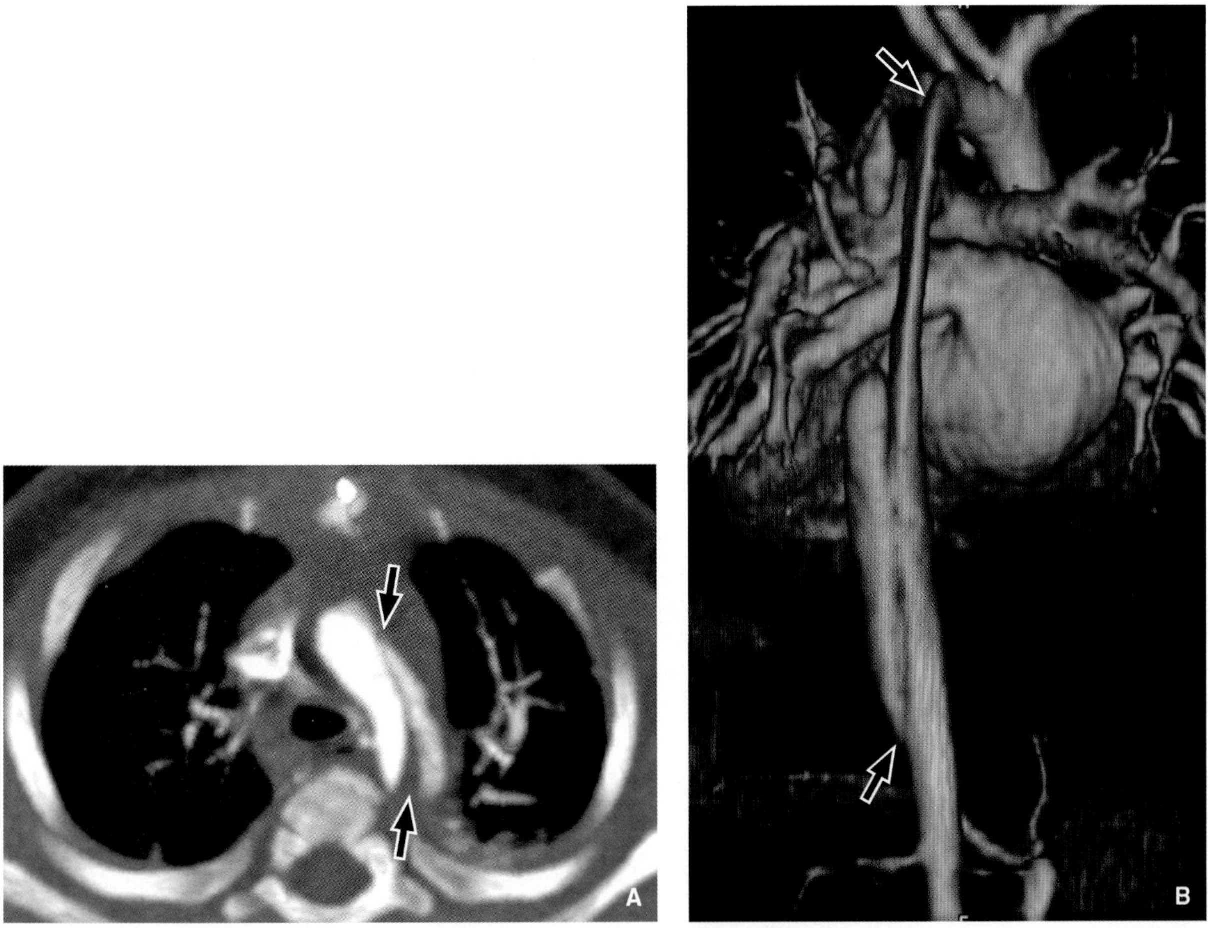

FIGURE 10.34 **Aortic dissection in a 4-month-old boy with Ehlers-Danlos syndrome. A:** Axial enhanced CT image shows an aortic dissection (*arrows*). **B:** Posterior view of 3D volume-rendered CT image better demonstrates the entire length of the aortic dissection (*arrows*).

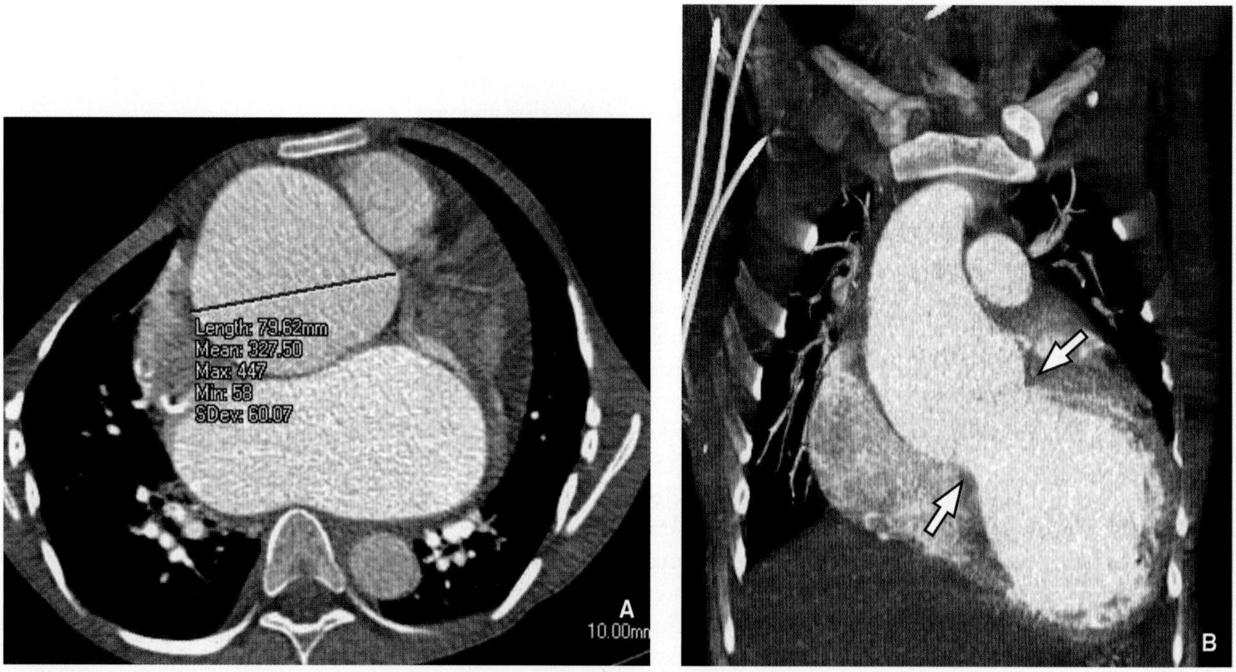

FIGURE 10.35 **Aortic aneurysm in a 16-year-old boy with Marfan syndrome.** Axial enhanced **(A)** and coronal 3D volume-rendered enhanced **(B)** CT images show a pear-shaped aortic root (*arrows*) with aneurysmatic dilatation up to 7.9 cm.

The cardinal clinical features of this entity include ectopia lentis and aortic root aneurysm[153,154] (Fig. 10.35). Cardiovascular complications are the major source of morbidity and early mortality in Marfan syndrome and include aortic, mitral, and tricuspid valve involvement. Marfan syndrome is characterized by progressive aneurysmal dilatation of the aortic root (Fig. 10.36) that is most pronounced at the level of the sinuses of Valsalva and ultimately results in fatal aortic rupture or dissection, usually in early adult life.[153] Myocardial involvement is also well recognized, and affected pediatric patients may present with a combination of systolic and diastolic dysfunctions unrelated to valvular abnormalities.[151,154,155]

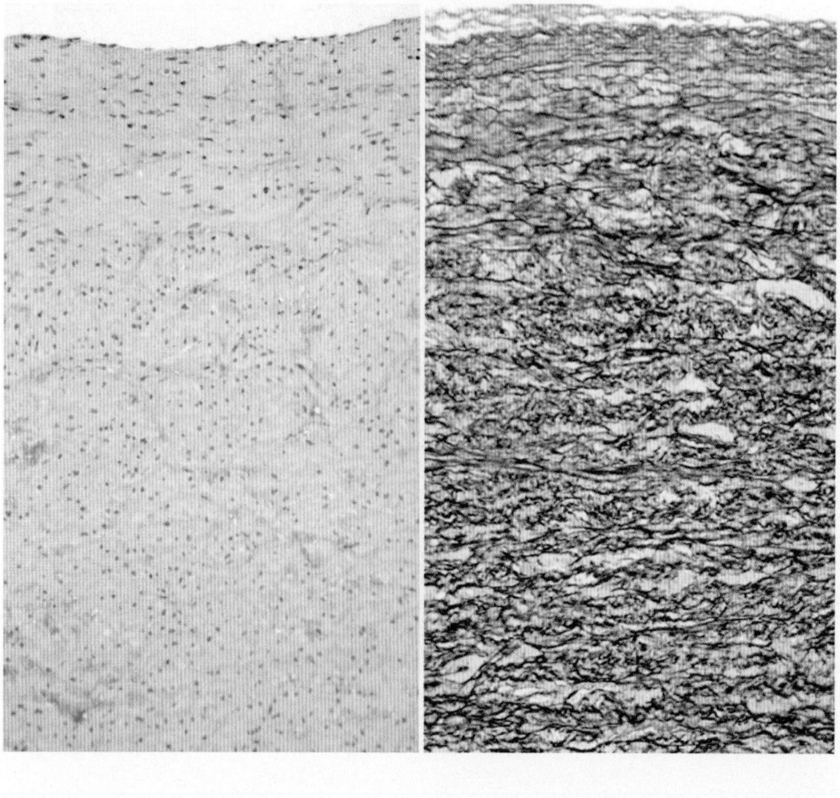

FIGURE 10.36 **Marfan disease causing aortic root aneurysm in a 1-year-old boy.** Microscopic examination showed a segment of aorta (**left**, hematoxylin and eosin) with loss of the typically organized parallel elastic lamellae (**right**, elastic stain; both original magnification, 200x).

Surgical repair is recommended in affected patients when the external diameter of a dilated aortic root/ascending aorta is > 5.0 cm.[15]

Neurofibromatosis Type 1

NF1 is an autosomal dominant neurocutaneous disorder caused by mutations in a tumor suppression gene (NF1) on chromosome 17 encoding the protein neurofibromin.[156,157] NF1 is characterized by the presence of multiple hyperpigmented macules (café au lait spots) and neurofibromas. The diagnosis of NF1 is based on the National Institutes of Health (NIH) diagnostic criteria[158] and is made in individuals with at least 2 of the following features: (1) café au lait spots, (2) intertriginous freckling, (3) Lisch nodules, (4) neurofibromas, (5) optic pathway gliomas, (6) characteristic bony lesions, and (7) a first-degree family relative with NF1.[157]

NF1 is also associated with cardiovascular abnormalities including CHD, vasculopathy (particularly middle aortic syndrome), and hypertension. Pulmonic stenosis is the most common CHD, followed by aortic coarctation.[159] The potential etiologies of hypertension in children with NF1 include renal artery stenosis and pheochromocytoma. The vasculopathy that occurs in NF1 most characteristically affects the abdominal aorta and its branches, especially the renal arteries[160,161] (Fig. 10.37). The histologic features of renal disease in NF1 are those of an arterial dysplasia. Although there is potential for encroachment of neurofibromas on the renal arteries, this is unrelated to the underlying vasculopathy of NF1.[162] Like fibromuscular dysplasia (FMD), the main features of extraparenchymal disease in NF1 include stenosis, beading, and aneurysms; however, ostial renal artery stenosis and midaortic syndrome are more common in NF1 than in FMD.[160] Intraparenchymal renal artery disease is less common in NF1 than in FMD.[163]

At the time of diagnosis, a thorough cardiac examination with blood pressure measurement should be made. If a murmur is detected, the affected pediatric patient should be referred to a cardiologist and imaged with ECHO.[157,164,165] In addition, annual blood pressure monitoring for hypertension is recommended. If abnormal, these pediatric patients should be referred to a nephrologist, and urinary catecholamines and renal Doppler US should be obtained.[165] For more detailed evaluation of the vessels, CTA or MRA can be used.[166]

Treatment of the lesions can be accomplished with medical, endovascular, or surgical interventions, but the feasibility of these interventions depends on the type and anatomical distribution of the lesion.[160]

Thromboembolic Disorders

Pulmonary Thromboembolism

In the past, pulmonary thromboembolism or pulmonary embolism (PE) was considered relatively rare in the pediatric population. However, recent studies show a prevalence of 14% to 15.5% among children with clinically suspected PE who underwent pulmonary CTA studies.[167–171] The most common symptoms of PE are chest pain, dyspnea, and cough. Hemoptysis is rarely seen in pediatric patients. Five independent risk factors, including immobilization, hypercoagulable state, excess estrogen state, indwelling central venous line, and prior PE and/or deep venous thrombosis, are found to be associated with PE in the pediatric population.[167–169]

In most pediatric institutions in the United States, computed tomography pulmonary angiography is the imaging modality of choice for the diagnosis and evaluation of PE. In this setting, radiation-dose reduction strategies,[170] such as lowering the tube voltage and current, should be used in the

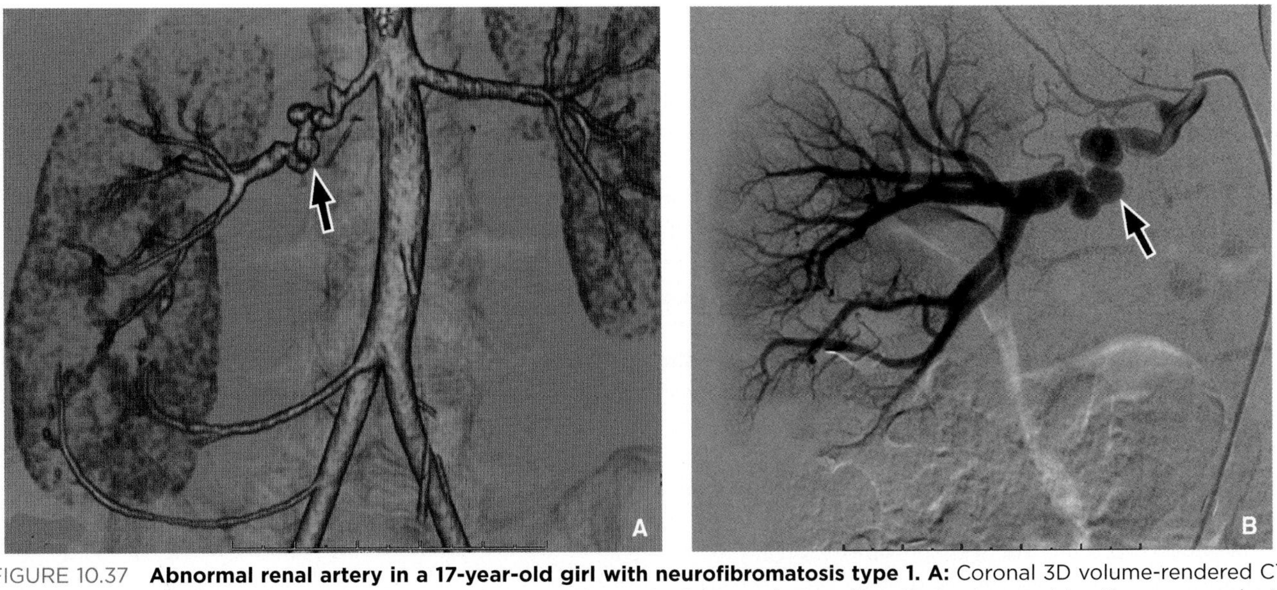

FIGURE 10.37 **Abnormal renal artery in a 17-year-old girl with neurofibromatosis type 1. A:** Coronal 3D volume-rendered CT image shows a duplex configuration to the right kidney with a main right renal artery from the aorta supplying the upper and mid right kidney and two accessory renal arteries originating from the right common iliac artery supplying the lower moiety. The main right renal artery shows multiple grape-like aneurysms and a beaded appearance (*arrow*). **B:** Digital subtraction angiography image confirms the CT findings (*arrow*).

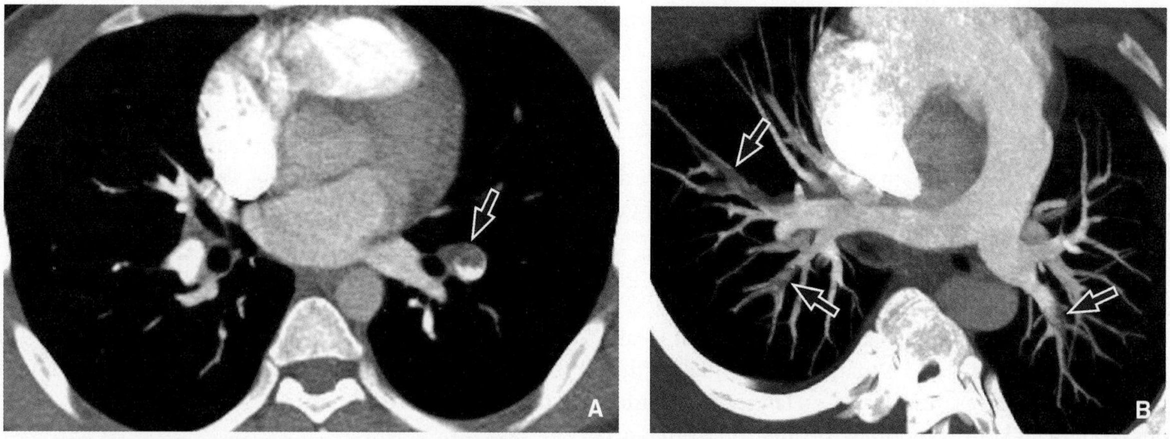

FIGURE 10.38 **Pulmonary embolism in a 17-year-old girl on oral contraceptive use who presented with shortness of breath and leg swelling. A:** Axial enhanced CT image shows an eccentric filling defect (*arrow*) in a left lower lobe pulmonary artery. Note the relative large size of the artery when compared to the adjacent bronchus. **B:** Axial-oblique maximum intensity projection reformatted CT image demonstrates intraluminal filling defects (*arrows*) in right and left lower lobe pulmonary artery branches consistent with pulmonary embolism.

pediatric population. As in adults, PE in children especially affects lobar and segmental arteries. In children, however, the subsegmental branches of these arteries may be not well visualized in up to 80% of cases.[171] PE manifests as complete or partial pulmonary arterial filling defects that are either located centrally in the vessel or are eccentric in location but form acute angles with the vessel wall. If the occlusion is complete, the artery is typically larger in caliber than the accompanying bronchus.[172,173] The use of multiplanar reformatting aids significantly in the diagnosis of PE in children by increasing the confidence level of the radiologists interpreting the study, although at the expense of a longer interpretation time[173] (Fig. 10.38).

Among all lung parenchymal and pleural abnormalities, wedge-shaped peripheral consolidation is highly associated with the presence of PE and is typically present in the same vascular distribution as the PE.[174] Once lodged within a pulmonary artery, the fate of a PE may be to lyse completely or to undergo eventual recanalization. Recanalized thrombi identified histologically in the setting of PAH suggest PE as a cause. When a PE leads to pulmonary infarct, it is seen grossly and microscopically as wedge-shaped, pleural-based areas of hemorrhage (Fig. 10.39). Depending on the age of the infarct, the affected lung tissue may have undergone coagulative necrosis or organization/resorption from the periphery with eventual fibrous scarring.

The mainstay of therapy for PE is anticoagulation, with thrombolytic therapy reserved for hemodynamic unstable pediatric patients. In cases of saddle emboli, surgical pulmonary thrombectomy may be needed.

Paget-Schroetter Disease

Effort-induced thrombosis, also known as Paget-Schroetter syndrome, is characterized by the development of axillary–subclavian vein thrombosis, usually occurring in young, otherwise healthy individuals (Fig. 10.40). It most commonly affects the dominant upper extremity following vigorous sports activities involving sustained upper extremity movements such as wrestling, weight lifting, pitching, rowing, gymnastics, and swimming or after execution of repetitive overhead activities such as painting. The condition is believed to represent the result of microtrauma to the vascular endothelium with activation of the coagulation cascade following retroversion, hyperabduction, and extension of the arm in these activities. Affected pediatric patients are usually quite symptomatic and present with a blue, heavy, painful, swollen upper extremity.[175–178]

For evaluation of Paget-Schroetter syndrome, the presence of a mediastinal mass or any osseous abnormality such as a cervical rib should be excluded on chest radiographs. US with Doppler is the first-line imaging modality for this condition.

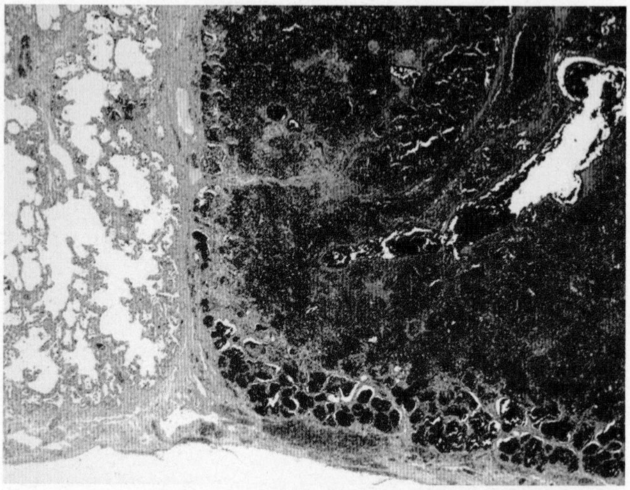

FIGURE 10.39 **Pulmonary infarct, identified in donor lung tissue at the time of transplant into a 13-year-old girl with cystic fibrosis.** The affected tissue extends to the pleura and shows extensive bleeding (attributed to an unobstructed bronchial arterial circulation) into an area showing coagulative necrosis (hematoxylin and eosin, original magnification, 40x).

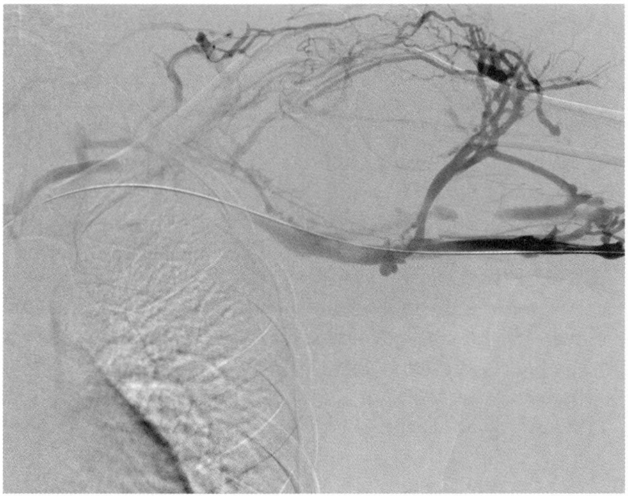

FIGURE 10.40 **Left subclavian vein thrombosis in a 17-year-old boy who is a tennis player with Paget-Schroetter syndrome.** Venography image shows occlusive thrombosis of the left central subclavian vein with multiple collaterals.

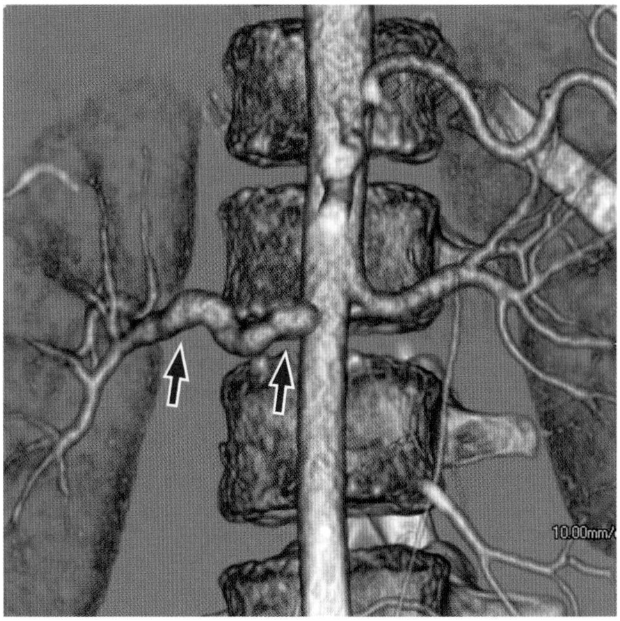

FIGURE 10.41 **Renal artery abnormality in a 15-year-old girl with fibromuscular dysplasia who presented with severe hypertension.** Volume-rendered 3D CT image demonstrates beaded contours (*arrows*) of the extraparenchymal portion of the right main renal artery.

Significant venous compression during hyperabduction may be inferred when there is interruption of flow or flattening of the waveforms with loss of the transmitted cardiac and respiratory dynamics on spectral display.[179] The contralateral extremity should be also evaluated. If significant arterial or venous compression is also noted, an anatomical predisposition may be inferred. CT or MR venography performed during neutral and provocative maneuvers and with the arms at rest and in the "surrender" position are useful because they may reveal the vascular anatomy as well as any other causes of extra-anatomical vascular compression.[180] The drawbacks of using these methods are the need for double doses of contrast material and the need for a second additional scan, which doubles the time required for the study as well as the radiation dose in the case of CT.

Management of Paget-Schroetter syndrome is currently aimed at preventing irreversible fibrotic changes to the vein, which may result in chronic edema and significant disability. Based on current management algorithms, treatment consists of anticoagulation therapy, thrombolysis, and subsequent surgical decompression.[175–178]

Idiopathic Disorders

Fibromuscular Dysplasia

Fibromuscular dysplasia (FMD) is an idiopathic, noninflammatory, nonatheromatous vasculopathy that results in fibrodysplastic narrowing of medium-sized arteries.[181] FMD is the most common cause of renal artery stenosis in pediatric patients. The three major histologic types of FMD are intimal, medial, and perimedial/subadventitial. The intimal type is the most common type in children and is highly associated with stroke.[160,181,182] Medial type is the most common type overall, typically affecting young adult females and manifesting the classical "string of beads" sign on conventional angiography.[183] Extraparenchymal disease in FMD manifests most commonly as focal postostial stenoses involving the main or segmental renal arteries, beading, and aneurysms[160,166] (Fig. 10.41). Intraparenchymal disease results in tiny aneurysms and stenotic and tortuous interlobar, arcuate, or intralobular arteries.[160] Affected patients with FMD should also be evaluated for carotid and intracranial involvement.

The angiographic as well as the histologic features of FMD, neurofibromatosis type 1 (NF1), and middle aortic syndrome (MAS) overlap and may be indistinguishable in some instances. Middle aortic syndrome and mesenteric artery and renal artery stenosis can be seen in all three entities.[160] Additional clinical features, if present, may provide a clue enabling the clinician to differentiate between these entities. In patients without syndromic features, the etiology is usually presumed to be FMD, although some cases could be due to an unknown underlying pathologic process.[160,184]

Renal angioplasty is considered the treatment of choice in FMD. Stenosis recurs in ~10% of cases.[185]

Middle Aortic Syndrome

Middle aortic syndrome (MAS) is a dysplastic process of unknown etiology resulting in narrowing of the midthoracoabdominal aorta (Fig. 10.42). It is characterized by hypertension with weakened or absent femoral pulses. MAS frequently involves visceral arterial branches such as the renal and superior mesenteric arteries. The term "middle aortic syndrome" is also applied to the acquired aortic narrowing seen in other vasculopathies such as NF1 and Takayasu arteritis.[186]

Clinically, MAS is characterized by systemic hypertension, a change in blood pressure proximal and distal to the stenosis, abdominal angina, and lower extremity claudication.

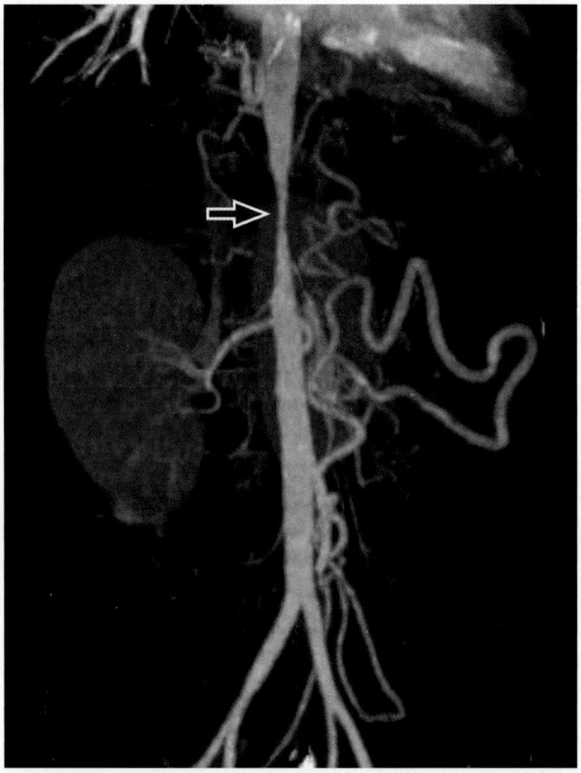

FIGURE 10.42 **Middle aortic syndrome in a 4-year-old boy who presented with hypertension.** Right anterior oblique maximum intensity projection CT image shows high-grade abdominal coarctation (*arrow*) involving the upper abdominal aorta from the supraceliac segment to just above the renal arteries over a 5 cm length with associated celiac artery origin occlusion and high grade superior mesenteric artery ostial stenosis. Mesenteric arterial flow is dependent on collateral vessels.

The aortic stenosis of MAS can be diffuse or segmental and can involve any portion of the distal thoracic aorta and the abdominal aorta; the inter-renal aorta is the most common site of involvement.[186,187] Concurrent renal artery stenosis is seen in ~60% of cases, whereas stenosis of the mesenteric artery is seen in ~30% of instances.[187]

Aortic revascularization by means of prosthetic or autologous venous grafts can provide long-term relief from hypertension and its deleterious effects.[188]

References

1. Kondrachuk O, Yalynska T, Tammo R, et al. Multidetector computed tomography evaluation of congenital mediastinal vascular anomalies in children. *Sem Roentgenol.* 2012;47(2):127–134.
2. Lee EY, Zurakowski D, Waltz DA, et al. MDCT evaluation of the prevalence of tracheomalacia in children with mediastinal aortic vascular anomalies. *J Thorac Imaging.* 2008;23(4):258–265.
3. Epelman M, Kreiger PA, Servaes S, et al. Current imaging of prenatally diagnosed congenital lung lesions. *Semin Ultrasound CT MR.* 2010;31(2):141–157.
4. Hellinger JC, Pena A, Poon M, et al. Pediatric computed tomographic angiography: imaging the cardiovascular system gently. *Radiol Clin North Am.* 2010;48(2):439–467.
5. Hellinger JC, Daubert M, Lee EY, et al. Congenital thoracic vascular anomalies: evaluation with state-of-the-art MR imaging and MDCT. *Radiol Clin North Am.* 2011;49(5):969–996.
6. Hellinger JC, Medina LS, Epelman M. Pediatric advanced imaging and informatics: state of the art. *Semin Ultrasound CT MR.* 2010;31(2):171–193.
7. Kalva SP, Sahani DV, Hahn PF, et al. Using the K-edge to improve contrast conspicuity and to lower radiation dose with a 16-MDCT: a phantom and human study. *J Comput Assist Tomogr.* 2006;30(3):391–397.
8. Weininger M, Barraza JM, Kemper CA, et al. Cardiothoracic CT angiography: current contrast medium delivery strategies. *AJR Am J Roentgenol.* 2011;196(3):W260–W272.
9. Barmeir E, Tann M, Zur S, et al. Improving CT angiography of the carotid artery using the "right" arm. *AJR Am J Roentgenol.* 1998;170(6):1657–1658.
10. Fleischmann D, Kamaya A. Optimal vascular and parenchymal contrast enhancement: the current state of the art. *Radiol Clin North Am.* 2009;47(1):13–26.
11. Epelman M, Johnson C, Hellinger JC, et al. Vascular lesions—congenital, acquired, and iatrogenic: imaging in the neonate. *Semin Ultrasound CT MR.* 2015;36(2):193–215.
12. Krishnamurthy R. Neonatal cardiac imaging. *Pediatr Radiol.* 2010;40(4):518–527.
13. Krishnamurthy R, Lee EY. Congenital cardiovascular malformations: noninvasive imaging by MRI in neonates. *Magn Reson Imaging Clin N Am.* 2011;19(4):813–822; viii.
14. Ginat DT, Fong MW, Tuttle DJ, et al. Cardiac imaging: Part 1, MR pulse sequences, imaging planes, and basic anatomy. *AJR Am J Roentgenol.* 2011;197(4):808–815.
15. Hiratzka LF, Bakris GL, Beckman JA, et al. 2010 ACCF/AHA/AATS/ACR/ASA/SCA/SCAI/SIR/STS/SVM guidelines for the diagnosis and management of patients with thoracic aortic disease: executive summary. A report of the American College of Cardiology Foundation/American Heart Association Task Force on Practice Guidelines, American Association for Thoracic Surgery, American College of Radiology, American Stroke Association, Society of Cardiovascular Anesthesiologists, Society for Cardiovascular Angiography and Interventions, Society of Interventional Radiology, Society of Thoracic Surgeons, and Society for Vascular Medicine. *Catheter Cardiovasc Interv.* 2010;76(2):E43–E86.
16. Kellenberger CJ, Yoo SJ, Buchel ER. Cardiovascular MR imaging in neonates and infants with congenital heart disease. *Radiographics.* 2007;27(1):5–18.
17. Lee EY, Browne LP, Lam W. Noninvasive magnetic resonance imaging of thoracic large vessels in children. *Semin Roentgenol.* 2012;47(1):45–55.
18. Nael K, Krishnam M, Ruehm SG, et al. Time-Resolved MR Angiography in the evaluation of central thoracic venous occlusive disease. *AJR Am J Roentgenol.* 2009;192(6):1731–1738.
19. Goldberg A, Jha S. Phase-contrast MRI and applications in congenital heart disease. *Clin Radiol.* 2012;67(5):399–410.
20. Grant FD, Treves ST. Nuclear medicine and molecular imaging of the pediatric chest: current practical imaging assessment. *Radiol Clin North Am.* 2011;49(5):1025–1051.
21. Braverman AC, Thompson RW, Sanchez LA. Diseases of the aorta. In: Bonow RO, Mann DL, Zipes DP, et al., eds. *Braunwald's Heart Disease—A Textbook of Cardiovascular Medicine.* 9th ed. Philadelphia, PA: Elsevier Saunders; 2011, Chapter 60.
22. Kirby A, Kirsch J, Williamson EE. Arterial anatomy of the thorax. In: Ho VB, Reddy GP, eds. *Cardiovascular Imaging.* St. Louis, MO: Elsevier Saunders; 2011.

23. Murillo H, Lane MJ, Punn R, et al. Imaging of the aorta: embryology and anatomy. *Semin Ultrasound CT MR.* 2012;33(3):169–190.
24. Backer CL, Mavroudis C. Congenital heart surgery nomenclature and database project: patent ductus arteriosus, coarctation of the aorta, interrupted aortic arch. *Ann Thorac Surg.* 2000;69(4):S298–S307.
25. Restrepo CS, Melendez-Ramirez G, Kimura-Hayama E. Multidetector computed tomography of congenital anomalies of the thoracic aorta. *Semin Ultrasound CT MR.* 2012;33(3):191–206.
26. Gray H. VI. The arteries; 2. The aorta. In: Gray H, ed. *Anatomy of the Human Body*, 20th ed., thoroughly rev and re-edited by Warren H. Lewis. Philadelphia, PA: Lea & Febiger 1918; Bartleby.com, 2000.
27. Kaiser T, Kellenberger CJ, Albisetti M, et al. Normal values for aortic diameters in children and adolescents—assessment in vivo by contrast-enhanced CMR-angiography. *J Cardiovasc Magn Reson.* 2008;10:56.
28. Madan N, Yau JL, Srivastava S, et al. Comparison between proximal thoracic vascular measurements obtained by contrast-enhanced magnetic resonance angiography and by transthoracic echocardiography in infants and children with congenital heart disease. *Pediatr Cardiol.* 2013;34(3):492–497.
29. Murillo H, Cutalo MJ, Jones RP, et al. Pulmonary circulation imaging: embryology and normal anatomy. *Semin Ultrasound CT MR.* 2012;33(6):473–484.
30. Frazier AA, Galvin JR, Franks TJ, et al. From the archives of the AFIP. *Radiographics.* 2000;20(2):491–524.
31. Krishnan AS, Babar JL, Gopalan D. Imaging of congenital and acquired disorders of the pulmonary artery. *Curr Probl Diagn Radiol.* 2012;41(5):165–178.
32. Marom EM, Herndon JE, Kim YH, et al. Variations in pulmonary venous drainage to the left atrium: implications for radiofrequency ablation. *Radiology.* 2004;230(3):824–829.
33. Kirsch J, Kirby A, Williamson EE. Venous anatomy of the thorax. In: Ho VB, Reddy GP, eds. *Cardiovascular Imaging.* St. Louis, MO: Elsevier Saunders; 2011, Chapter 75.
34. Lawler LP, Fishman EK. Thoracic venous anatomy multidetector row CT evaluation. *Radiol Clin North Am.* 2003;41(3):545–560.
35. Demos TC, Posniak HV, Pierce KL, et al. Venous anomalies of the thorax. *AJR Am J Roentgenol.* 2004;182(5):1139–1150.
36. Gaynor JW, Weinberg PM, Spray TL. Congenital Heart Surgery Nomenclature and Database Project: systemic venous anomalies. *Ann Thorac Surg.* 2000;69(4 suppl):S70–S76.
37. Weinberg PM, Natarajan S, Rogers L. Aortic arch and vascular anomalies. In: Allen HD, Driscoll DJ, Shaddy RE, et al., eds. *Moss & Adams' Heart Disease in Infants, Children, and Adolescents: Including the Fetus and Young Adult.* Philadelphia, PA: Lippincott Williams & Wilkins; 2012.
38. Weinberg PM. Aortic arch anomalies. *J Cardiovasc Magn Reson.* 2006;8(4):633–643.
39. Weinberg PM, Whitehead KK. Aortic arch anomalies. In: Fogel MA, ed. *Principles and Practice of Cardiac Magnetic Resonance in Congenital Heart Disease: Form, Function and Flow.* 1st ed. Wiley-Blackwell; 2010;183–208.
40. Kellenberger C. Aortic arch malformations. *Pediatr Radiol.* 2010;40(6):876–884.
41. Hernanz-Schulman M. Vascular rings: a practical approach to imaging diagnosis. *Pediatr Radiol.* 2005;35(10):961–979.
42. Weinberg PM, Hubbard AM, Fogel MA. Aortic arch and pulmonary artery anomalies in children. *Semin Roentgenol.* 1998; 33(3):262–280.
43. Dillman JR, Attili AK, Agarwal PP, et al. Common and uncommon vascular rings and slings: a multi-modality review. *Pediatr Radiol.* 2011;41(11):1440–1454; quiz 89–90.
44. McElhinney DB, Clark BJ III, Weinberg PM, et al. Association of chromosome 22q11 deletion with isolated anomalies of aortic arch laterality and branching. *J Am Coll Cardiol.* 2001;37(8):2114–2119.
45. Berdon WE. Rings, slings, and other things: vascular compression of the infant trachea updated from the midcentury to the millennium—the legacy of Robert E. Gross, MD, and Edward B. D. Neuhauser, MD. *Radiology.* 2000;216(3):624–632.
46. Gould SW, Rigsby CK, Donnelly LF, et al. Useful signs for the assessment of vascular rings on cross-sectional imaging. *Pediatr Radiol.* 2015.
47. Lee EY, Dorkin H, Vargas SO. Congenital pulmonary malformations in pediatric patients: review and update on etiology, classification, and imaging findings. *Radiol Clin North Am.* 2011;49(5):921–948.
48. Berrocal T, Madrid C, Novo S, et al. Congenital anomalies of the tracheobronchial tree, lung, and mediastinum: embryology, radiology, and pathology. *Radiographics.* 2004;24(1):e17.
49. Kayemba-Kay's S, Couvrat-Carcauzon V, Goua V, et al. Unilateral pulmonary agenesis: A report of four cases, two diagnosed antenatally and literature review. *Pediatr Pulmonol.* 2014;49(3):E96–102.
50. Epelman M, Daltro P, Soto G, et al. Congenital lung anomalies. In: Coley BD, ed. *Caffey's Pediatric Diagnostic Imaging*, 2-Volume Set, 12th ed. Philadelphia, PA: Saunders, an imprint of Elsevier Inc.; 2013; 550–566, Chapter 53.
51. Knowles S, Thomas RM, Lindenbaum RH, et al. Pulmonary agenesis as part of the VACTERL sequence. *Arch Dis Child.* 1988;63(7 Spec No):723–726.
52. Cunningham ML, Mann N. Pulmonary agenesis: a predictor of ipsilateral malformations. *Am J Med Genet.* 1997;70(4):391–398.
53. Gilbert EF, Opitz JM. The pathology of some malformations and hereditary diseases of the respiratory tract. *Birth Defects Orig Artic Ser.* 1976;12(6):239–270.
54. Eroglu A, Alper F, Turkyilmaz A, et al. Pulmonary agenesis associated with dextrocardia, sternal defects, and ectopic kidney. *Pediatr Pulmonol.* 2005;40(6):547–549.
55. Castañer E, Gallardo X, Rimola J, et al. Congenital and acquired pulmonary artery anomalies in the adult: radiologic overview. *Radiographics.* 2006;26(2):349–371.
56. Newman B, Cho Ya. Left pulmonary artery sling—anatomy and imaging. *Semin Ultrasound CT MR.* 2010;31(2):158–170.
57. Newman B. Congenital bronchopulmonary foregut malformations: concepts and controversies. *Pediatr Radiol.* 2006;36(8): 773–791.
58. Lee EY, Boiselle PM, Cleveland RH. Multidetector CT evaluation of congenital lung anomalies. *Radiology.* 2008;247(3):632–648.
59. Newman B, Cho Y. Left pulmonary artery sling—anatomy and imaging. *Semin Ultrasound CT MR.* 2010;31(2):158–170.
60. Konen E, Raviv-Zilka L, Cohen RA, et al. Congenital pulmonary venolobar syndrome: spectrum of helical CT findings with emphasis on computerized reformatting. *Radiographics.* 2003;23(5):1175–1184.
61. Cox D, Quinn R, Moran A, et al. Ductal origin of the pulmonary artery in isolation: a case series. *Pediatr Cardiol.* 2010;31(7):997–1001.
62. Trivedi KR, Karamlou T, Yoo S-J, et al. Outcomes in 45 children with ductal origin of the distal pulmonary artery. *Ann Thorac Surg.* 2006;81(3):950–957.
63. Butera G, Santoro G, Calabro R, et al. Percutaneous treatment of ductal origin of the distal pulmonary artery in low-weight newborns. *J Invasive Cardiol.* 2008;20(7):354, 356.

64. Dillman JR, Sanchez R, Ladino-Torres MF, et al. Expanding upon the unilateral hyperlucent hemithorax in children. *Radiographics.* 2011;31(3):723–741.
65. Ryu DS, Spirn PW, Trotman-Dickenson B, et al. HRCT findings of proximal interruption of the right pulmonary artery. *J Thorac Imaging.* 2004;19(3):171–175.
66. Apostolopoulou SC, Kelekis NL, Brountzos EN, et al. "Absent" pulmonary artery in one adult and five pediatric patients: imaging, embryology, and therapeutic implications. *AJR Am J Roentgenol.* 2002;179(5):1253–1260.
67. Cartin-Ceba R, Swanson KL, Krowka MJ. Pulmonary arteriovenous malformations. *Chest.* 2013;144(3):1033–1044.
68. Shovlin CL, Guttmacher AE, Buscarini E, et al. Diagnostic criteria for hereditary hemorrhagic telangiectasia (Rendu-Osler-Weber syndrome). *Am J Med Genet.* 2000;91(1):66–67.
69. Guttmacher A, Pyeritz R. Hereditary hemorrhagic telangiectasia. In: Rimoin DL, Pyeritz RE, Korf B, eds. *Principles and Practice of Medical Genetics.* 5th ed. Philadelphia, PA: Churchill Livingstone; 2007:1200–1213.
70. Lacombe P, Lacout A, Marcy PY, et al. Diagnosis and treatment of pulmonary arteriovenous malformations in hereditary hemorrhagic telangiectasia: an overview. *Diagn Interv Imaging.* 2013;94(9):835–848.
71. Osler-Weber-Rendu. HHT Foundation International. 2012; Available from http://hht.org/living-with-hht/screening-and-treatment/
72. Trerotola SO, Pyeritz RE. PAVM embolization: an update. *AJR Am J Roentgenol.* 2010;195(4):837–845.
73. Schneider G, Uder M, Koehler M, et al. MR angiography for detection of pulmonary arteriovenous malformations in patients with hereditary hemorrhagic telangiectasia. *AJR Am J Roentgenol.* 2008;190(4):892–901.
74. Faughnan ME, Thabet A, Mei-Zahav M, et al. Pulmonary arteriovenous malformations in children: outcomes of transcatheter embolotherapy. *J Pediatr.* 2004;145(6):826–831.
75. Pollak JS, Saluja S, Thabet A, et al. Clinical and anatomic outcomes after embolotherapy of pulmonary arteriovenous malformations. *J Vasc Interv Radiol.* 2006;17(1):35–44; quiz 5.
76. Faughnan ME, Palda VA, Garcia-Tsao G, et al. International guidelines for the diagnosis and management of hereditary haemorrhagic telangiectasia. *J Med Genet.* 2011;48(2):73–87.
77. Simonneau G, Gatzoulis MA, Adatia I, et al. Updated clinical classification of pulmonary hypertension. *J Am Coll Cardiol.* 2013;62(25 suppl):D34–D41.
78. Ivy DD, Abman SH, Barst RJ, et al. Pediatric pulmonary hypertension. *J Am Coll Cardiol.* 2013;62(25 suppl):D117–D126.
79. Healy F, Hanna BD, Zinman R. Pulmonary complications of congenital heart disease. *Paediatr Respir Rev.* 2012;13(1):10–15.
80. Cerro MJ, Abman S, Diaz G, et al. A consensus approach to the classification of pediatric pulmonary hypertensive vascular disease: Report from the PVRI Pediatric Taskforce, Panama 2011. *Pulm Circ.* 2011;1(2):286–298.
81. Takatsuki S, Ivy DD. Current challenges in pediatric pulmonary hypertension. *Semin Respir Crit Care Med.* 2013;34(5): 627–644.
82. Frazier AA, Burke AP. The imaging of pulmonary hypertension. *Semin Ultrasound CT MR.* 2012;33(6):535–551.
83. Abman SH, Kinsella JP, Rosenzweig EB, et al. Implications of the U.S. Food and Drug Administration warning against the use of sildenafil for the treatment of pediatric pulmonary hypertension. *Am J Respir Crit Care Med.* 2013;187(6):572–575.
84. Brown K, Gutierrez AJ, Mohammed TL, et al. ACR Appropriateness Criteria(R) pulmonary hypertension. *J Thorac Imaging.* 2013;28(4):W57–W60.
85. Grosse C, Grosse A. CT findings in diseases associated with pulmonary hypertension: a current review. *Radiographics.* 2010;30(7):1753–1777.
86. Bernus A, Wagner BD, Accurso F, et al. Brain natriuretic peptide levels in managing pediatric patients with pulmonary arterial hypertension. *Chest.* 2009;135(3):745–751.
87. Robbins IM, Moore TM, Blaisdell CJ, et al. National Heart, Lung, and Blood Institute Workshop: improving outcomes for pulmonary vascular disease. *Circulation.* 2012;125(17):2165–2170.
88. Friesen RH, Williams GD. Anesthetic management of children with pulmonary arterial hypertension. *Paediatr Anaesth.* 2008;18(3):208–216.
89. Lee EY, Jenkins KJ, Muneeb M, et al. Proximal pulmonary vein stenosis detection in pediatric patients: value of multiplanar and 3-D VR imaging evaluation. *Pediatr Radiol.* 2013;43(8):929–936.
90. Riedlinger WF, Juraszek AL, Jenkins KJ, et al. Pulmonary vein stenosis: expression of receptor tyrosine kinases by lesional cells. *Cardiovasc Pathol.* 2006;15(2):91–99.
91. Latson LA, Prieto LR. Congenital and acquired pulmonary vein stenosis. *Circulation.* 2007;115(1):103–108.
92. Grosse-Wortmann L, Al-Otay A, Goo HW, et al. Anatomical and functional evaluation of pulmonary veins in children by magnetic resonance imaging. *J Am Coll Cardiol.* 2007;49(9): 993–1002.
93. Breinholt JP, Hawkins JA, Minich L, et al. Pulmonary vein stenosis with normal connection: associated cardiac abnormalities and variable outcome. *Ann Thorac Surg.* 1999;68(1):164–168.
94. Drossner DM, Kim DW, Maher KO, et al. Pulmonary vein stenosis: prematurity and associated conditions. *Pediatrics.* 2008;122(3):e656–e661.
95. Vyas HV, Greenberg SB, Krishnamurthy R. MR Imaging and CT evaluation of congenital pulmonary vein abnormalities in neonates and infants. *Radiographics.* 2012;32(1):87–98.
96. Smallhorn JF, Pauperio H, Benson L, et al. Pulsed doppler assessment of pulmonary vein obstruction. *Am Heart J.* 1985;110(2):483–486.
97. Miller C. Pulmonary veno-occlusive disease: a misnomer? *Pediatr Radiol.* 2012;42(6):647–652.
98. Dillman JR, Yarram SG, Hernandez RJ. Imaging of pulmonary venous developmental anomalies. *AJR Am J Roentgenol.* 2009;192(5):1272–1285.
99. Swensen SJ, Tashjian JH, Myers JL, et al. Pulmonary veno-occlusive disease: CT findings in eight patients. *AJR Am J Roentgenol.* 1996;167(4):937–940.
100. Bailey CL, Channick RN, Auger WR, et al. "High probability" perfusion lung scans in pulmonary venoocclusive disease. *Am J Respir Crit Care Med.* 2000;162(5):1974–1978.
101. O'Callaghan DS, Dorfmuller P, Jaïs X, et al. Pulmonary veno-occlusive disease: the bête noire of pulmonary hypertension in connective tissue diseases? *Presse Méd.* 2011;40 (1, pt 2):e87–e100.
102. Maillard JO, Cottin V, Etienne-Mastroïanni B, et al. Pulmonary varix mimicking pulmonary arteriovenous malformation in a patient with turner syndrome. *Respiration.* 2007;74(1): 110–113.
103. Kumazoe H, Komori M, Ochiai R, et al. Pulmonary varix mimicking arteriovenous malformation. *Clin Imaging.* 2008; 32(1):61–64.

104. Berecova Z, Neuschl V, Boruta P, et al. A complex pulmonary vein varix—diagnosis with ECG gated MDCT, MRI and invasive pulmonary angiography. *J Radiol Case Rep.* 2012; 6(12):9–16.
105. Abujudeh H. Pulmonary varix: blood flow is essential in the diagnosis. *Pediatr Radiol.* 2004;34(7):567–569.
106. Kafka H, Mohiaddin RH. Cardiac MRI and pulmonary MR angiography of sinus venosus defect and partial anomalous pulmonary venous connection in cause of right undiagnosed ventricular enlargement. *AJR Am J Roentgenol.* 2009;192(1):259–266.
107. Epelman M. Partial and total anomalous pulmonary venous connections. In: Yoo SJ, McDonald C, et al., eds. *Chest Radiographic Interpretation in Pediatric Cardiac Patients.* New York, NY: Thieme Medical Publishers; 2010:206–214.
108. Keane JF, Fyler DC, Lock JE. *Atrial Septal Defect. Keane: Nadas' Pediatric Cardiology*. 2nd ed. WB Saunders; 2006:603–616.
109. Chemin A, Bonnet D, Le Bourgeois M, et al. Respiratory outcome in children with scimitar syndrome. *J Pediatr.* 2013; 162(2):275–279.e1.
110. Mata JM, Cáceres J, Lucaya J, et al. CT of congenital malformations of the lung. *Radiographics.* 1990;10(4):651–674.
111. Webb GD, Smallhorn JF, Therrien J, et al. Congenital heart disease. In: *Bonow: Braunwald's Heart Disease—A Textbook of Cardiovascular Medicine.* 9th ed. WB Saunders; 2011:1141–1467, Chapter 65.
112. Alsoufi B, Cai S, Van Arsdell GS, et al. Outcomes after surgical treatment of children with partial anomalous pulmonary venous connection. *Ann Thorac Surg.* 2007;84(6):2020–2026.
113. Corno AF, Alahdal SA, Das KM. Systemic venous anomalies in the Middle East. *Front Pediatr.* 2013;1:1.
114. Postema PG, Rammeloo LA, van Litsenburg R, et al. Left superior vena cava in pediatric cardiology associated with extracardiac anomalies. *Int J Cardiol.* 2008;123(3):302–306.
115. Gonzalez-Juanatey C, Testa A, Vidan J, et al. Persistent left superior vena cava draining into the coronary sinus: report of 10 cases and literature review. *Clin Cardiol.* 2004;27(9):515–518.
116. Corno AF, Pierluigi F. Anomalous systemic venous connections. In: Corno AF, Pierluigi F, eds. *Congenital Heart Defects: Decision Making for Surgery.* Wurzburg, Germany: Springer; 2009:18–22.
117. Colman AL. Diagnosis of left superior vena cava by clinical inspection, a new physical sign. *Am Heart J.* 1967;73(1):115–120.
118. Corno AF. Systemic venous drainage: can we help Newton? *Eur J Cardiol Thorac Surg.* 2007;31(6):1044–1051.
119. Mamidipally S, Rashba E, McBrearty T, et al. Azygous continuation of inferior vena cava. *J Am Coll Cardiol.* 2010;56(21):e41.
120. Hamoud S, Nitecky S, Engel A, et al. Hypoplasia of the inferior vena cava with azygous continuation presenting as recurrent leg deep vein thrombosis. *Am J Med Sci.* 2000;319(6):414–416.
121. Tsuji Y, Inoue T, Murakami H, et al. Deep vein thrombosis caused by congenial interruption of the inferior vena cava—a case report. *Angiology.* 2001;52(10):721–725.
122. Restrepo CS, Ocazionez D, Suri R, et al. Aortitis: imaging spectrum of the infectious and inflammatory conditions of the aorta. *Radiographics.* 2011;31(2):435–451.
123. Katabathina VS, Restrepo CS. Infectious and noninfectious aortitis: cross-sectional imaging findings. *Semin Ultrasound CT MR.* 2012;33(3):207–221.
124. Mengozzi E, Sartoni Galloni S, Giovannini G, et al. Mycotic aneurysm of the thoracic aorta presenting as pneumonia. *Pediatr Radiol.* 2001;31(7):488–490.
125. Litmanovich D, Yıldırım A, Bankier A. Insights into imaging of aortitis. *Insights Imaging.* 2012;3(6):545–560.
126. Lopes RJ, Almeida J, Dias PJ, et al. Infectious thoracic aortitis: a literature review. *Clin Cardiol.* 2009;32(9):488–490.
127. Knyshov GV, Sitar LL, Glagola MD, et al. Aortic aneurysms at the site of the repair of coarctation of the aorta: a review of 48 patients. *Ann Thorac Surg.* 1996;61(3):935–939.
128. Steenburg SD, Ravenel JG, Ikonomidis JS, et al. Acute traumatic aortic injury: imaging evaluation and management. *Radiology.* 2008;248(3):748–762.
129. Groskin SA. Selected topics in chest trauma. *Radiology.* 1992; 183(3):605–617.
130. Barmparas G, Inaba K, Talving P, et al. Pediatric vs adult vascular trauma: a National Trauma Databank review. *J Pediatr Surg.* 2010;45(7):1404–1412.
131. Dyer DS, Moore EE, Mestek MF, et al. Can chest CT be used to exclude aortic injury? *Radiology.* 1999;213(1):195–202.
132. Mirka H, Ferda J, Baxa J. Multidetector computed tomography of chest trauma: indications, technique and interpretation. *Insights Imaging.* 2012;3(5):433–449.
133. Mirvis SE, Shanmuganathan K. Diagnosis of blunt traumatic aortic injury 2007: Still a nemesis. *Eur J Radiol.* 2007; 64(1):27–40.
134. Mirvis SE. Imaging of acute thoracic injury: the advent of MDCT screening. *Semin Ultrasound CT MR.* 2005;26(5):305–331.
135. Berko NS, Haramati LB. Simple cardiac shunts in adults. *Semin Roentgenol.* 2012;47(3):277–288.
136. Fisher RG, Sanchez-Torres M, Whigham CJ, et al. "Lumps" and "bumps" that mimic acute aortic and brachiocephalic vessel injury. *Radiographics.* 1997;17(4):825–834.
137. Mortensen A, Hansen NF, Schiodt OM. Fatal aortoesophageal fistula caused by button battery ingestion in a 1-year-old child. *Am J Emerg Med.* 2010;28(8):984.e5–984.e6.
138. Karmy-Jones R, Hoffer E, Meissner M, et al. Management of traumatic rupture of the thoracic aorta in pediatric patients. *Ann Thorac Surg.* 2003;75(5):1513–1517.
139. Eleftheriou D, Brogan PA. Vasculitis in children. *Best Pract Res Clin Rheumatol.* 2009;23(3):309–323.
140. Eleftheriou D, Dillon MJ, Brogan PA. Advances in childhood vasculitis. *Curr Opin Rheumatol.* 2009;21(4):411–418.
141. Weiss PF. Pediatric vasculitis. *Pediatr Clin North Am.* 2012; 59(2):407–423.
142. Ozen S, Ruperto N, Dillon MJ, et al. EULAR/PReS endorsed consensus criteria for the classification of childhood vasculitides. *Ann Rheum Dis.* 2006;65(7):936–941.
143. Cakar N, Yalcinkaya F, Duzova A, et al. Takayasu arteritis in children. *J Rheumatol.* 2008;35(5):913–919.
144. Nastri MV, Baptista LP, Baroni RH, et al. Gadolinium-enhanced three-dimensional MR angiography of Takayasu arteritis. *Radiographics.* 2004;24(3):773–786.
145. Gotway MB, Araoz PA, Macedo TA, et al. Imaging findings in Takayasu's arteritis. *AJR Am J Roentgenol.* 2005;184(6): 1945–1950.
146. Papa M, De Cobelli F, Baldissera E, et al. Takayasu arteritis: intravascular contrast medium for MR angiography in the evaluation of disease activity. *AJR Am J Roentgenol.* 2012; 198(3):W279–W284.
147. Gulati A, Bagga A. Large vessel vasculitis. *Pediatr Nephrol.* 2010;25(6):1037–1048.
148. Cury M, Zeidan F, Lobato AC. Aortic disease in the young: genetic aneurysm syndromes, connective tissue disorders,

and familial aortic aneurysms and dissections. *Int J Vasc Med.* 2013;2013:267215.
149. Chu LC, Johnson PT, Dietz HC, et al. Vascular complications of Ehlers-Danlos syndrome: CT findings. *AJR Am J Roentgenol.* 2012;198(2):482–487.
150. Germain DP. The vascular Ehlers-Danlos syndrome. *Curr Treat Options Cardiovasc Med.* 2006;8(2):121–127.
151. Dormand H, Mohiaddin RH. Cardiovascular magnetic resonance in Marfan syndrome. *J Cardiovasc Magn Reson.* 2013;15:33.
152. De Paepe A, Devereux RB, Dietz HC, et al. Revised diagnostic criteria for the Marfan syndrome. *Am J Med Genet.* 1996;62(4):417–426.
153. Loeys BL, Dietz HC, Braverman AC, et al. The revised Ghent nosology for the Marfan syndrome. *J Med Genet.* 2010;47(7): 476–485.
154. Radonic T, de Witte P, Groenink M, et al. Critical appraisal of the revised Ghent criteria for diagnosis of Marfan syndrome. *Clin Genet.* 2011;80(4):346–353.
155. Dietz HC. Marfan syndrome. In: Pagon RA, Adam MP, Bird TD, et al., eds. *GeneReviews*. Seattle, WA: University of Washington; 1993.
156. Pasmant E, Vidaud M, Vidaud D, et al. Neurofibromatosis type 1: from genotype to phenotype. *J Med Genet.* 2012;49(8): 483–489.
157. Williams VC, Lucas J, Babcock MA, et al. Neurofibromatosis type 1 revisited. *Pediatrics.* 2009;123(1):124–133.
158. National Institutes of Health Consensus Development Conference Statement: neurofibromatosis. Bethesda, MD, USA, July 13–15, 1987. *Neurofibromatosis.* 1988;1(3):172–178.
159. Lin AE, Birch PH, Korf BR, et al. Cardiovascular malformations and other cardiovascular abnormalities in neurofibromatosis. *Am J Med Genet.* 2000;95(2):108–117.
160. Srinivasan A, Krishnamurthy G, Fontalvo-Herazo L, et al. Spectrum of renal findings in pediatric fibromuscular dysplasia and neurofibromatosis type. *Pediatr Radiol.* 2011; 41(3):308–316.
161. Fossali E, Signorini E, Intermite RC, et al. Renovascular disease and hypertension in children with neurofibromatosis. *Pediatr Nephrol (Berlin, Germany).* 2000;14(8–9):806–810.
162. Hamilton SJ, Friedman JM. Insights into the pathogenesis of neurofibromatosis 1 vasculopathy. *Clin Genet.* 2000;58(5):341–344.
163. Srinivasan A, Krishnamurthy G, Fontalvo-Herazo L, et al. Angioplasty for renal artery stenosis in pediatric patients: an 11-year retrospective experience. *J Vasc Interv Radiol.* 2010;21(11):1672–1680.
164. Lama G, Graziano L, Calabrese E, et al. Blood pressure and cardiovascular involvement in children with neurofibromatosis type1. *Pediatr Nephrol (Berlin, Germany).* 2004;19(4):413–418.
165. Ardern-Holmes SL, North KN. Therapeutics for childhood neurofibromatosis type 1 and type 2. *Curr Treat Options Neurol.* 2011;13(6):529–543.
166. Kurian J, Epelman M, Darge K, et al. The role of CT angiography in the evaluation of pediatric renovascular hypertension. *Pediatr Radiol.* 2013;43(4):490–501; quiz 487–489.
167. Lee EY, Tse SK, Zurakowski D, et al. Children suspected of having pulmonary embolism: multidetector CT pulmonary angiography—thromboembolic risk factors and implications for appropriate use. *Radiology.* 2012;262(1):242–251.
168. Agha BS, Sturm JJ, Simon HK, et al. Pulmonary embolism in the pediatric emergency department. *Pediatrics.* 2013; 132(4):663–667.
169. Victoria T, Mong A, Altes T, et al. Evaluation of pulmonary embolism in a pediatric population with high clinical suspicion. *Pediatr Radiol.* 2009;39(1):35–41.
170. Lee EY, Zurakowski D, Boiselle PM. Pulmonary embolism in pediatric patients survey of CT pulmonary angiography practices and policies. *Acad Radiol.* 2010;17(12):1543–1549.
171. Kritsaneepaiboon S, Lee EY, Zurakowski D, et al. MDCT pulmonary angiography evaluation of pulmonary embolism in children. *AJR Am J Roentgenol.* 2009;192(5):1246–1252.
172. Pena E, Dennie C. Acute and chronic pulmonary embolism: an in-depth review for radiologists through the use of frequently asked questions. *Semin Ultrasound CT MR.* 2012; 33(6):500–521.
173. Lee EY, Zucker EJ, Tsai J, et al. Pulmonary MDCT angiography: value of multiplanar reformatted images in detecting pulmonary embolism in children. *AJR Am J Roentgenol.* 2011;197(6):1460–1465.
174. Lee EY, Zurakowski D, Diperna S, et al. Parenchymal and pleural abnormalities in children with and without pulmonary embolism at MDCT pulmonary angiography. *Pediatr Radiol.* 2010;40(2):173–181.
175. Engelberger RP, Kucher N. Management of deep vein thrombosis of the upper extremity. *Circulation.* 2012;126(6):768–773.
176. Alla VM, Natarajan N, Kaushik M, et al. Paget-Schroetter syndrome: review of pathogenesis and treatment of effort thrombosis. *West J Emerg Med.* 2010;11(4):358–362.
177. Thompson JF, Winterborn RJ, Bays S, et al. Venous thoracic outlet compression and the Paget-Schroetter syndrome: a review and recommendations for management. *Cardiovasc Intervent Radiol.* 2011;34(5):903–910.
178. Illig KA, Doyle AJ. A comprehensive review of Paget-Schroetter syndrome. *J Vasc Surg.* 2010;51(6):1538–1547.
179. Longley DG, Yedlicka JW, Molina EJ, et al. Thoracic outlet syndrome: evaluation of the subclavian vessels by color duplex sonography. *AJR Am J Roentgenol.* 1992;158(3):623–630.
180. Ersoy H, Steigner ML, Coyner KB, et al. Vascular thoracic outlet syndrome: protocol design and diagnostic value of contrast-enhanced 3D MR angiography and equilibrium phase imaging on 1.5- and 3-T MRI scanners. *AJR Am J Roentgenol.* 2012;198(5):1180–1187.
181. Slovut DP, Olin JW. Fibromuscular dysplasia. *N Engl J Med.* 2004;350(18):1862–1871.
182. Kirton A, Crone M, Benseler S, et al. Fibromuscular dysplasia and childhood stroke. *Brain.* 2013;136(pt 6):1846–1856.
183. Tullus K. Renovascular hypertension—is it fibromuscular dysplasia or Takayasu arteritis. *Pediatr Nephrol.* 2013;28(2):191–196.
184. Vo NJ, Hammelman BD, Racadio JM, et al. Anatomic distribution of renal artery stenosis in children: implications for imaging. *Pediatr Radiol.* 2006;36(10):1032–1036.
185. Baumgartner I, Lerman LO. Renovascular hypertension: screening and modern management. *Eur Heart J.* 2011;32(13): 1590–1598.
186. Connolly JE, Wilson SE, Lawrence PL, et al. Middle aortic syndrome: distal thoracic and abdominal coarctation, a disorder with multiple etiologies. *J Am Coll Surg.* 2002;194(6):774–781.
187. Delis KT, Gloviczki P. Middle aortic syndrome: from presentation to contemporary open surgical and endovascular treatment. *Perspect Vasc Surg Endovasc Ther.* 2005;17(3):187–203.
188. Sebastia C, Quiroga S, Boye R, et al. Aortic stenosis: spectrum of diseases depicted at multisection CT. *Radiographics.* 2003; 23 (Spec No):S79–S91.

CHAPTER 11

Mediastinum

Paul G. Thacker • Kushaljit S. Sodhi • I. Nimala A. Gooneratne • Claudio Fonda • Pierluigi Ciet • Edward Y. Lee

INTRODUCTION

The mediastinum represents the intrathoracic compartment bounded by the sternum anteriorly, the vertebral column posteriorly, the parietal pleura laterally, the thoracic inlet superiorly, and the diaphragm inferiorly. It is the most common location of chest masses in the pediatric population.[1,2] In addition to various normal variants, a wide spectrum of disorders affects the mediastinum including congenital vascular and nonvascular anomalies, infectious and inflammatory diseases, and benign and malignant neoplastic lesions.[1,2] Furthermore, traumatic injury may also affect mediastinal structures in pediatric patients.

It is, thus, imperative for the radiologist to have an up-to-date knowledge of the various imaging techniques currently available for optimal evaluation of both normal anatomy and pathologic mediastinal processes. In addition, the radiologist should be aware of characteristic imaging appearances of this broad spectrum of normal variants as well as congenital and acquired abnormalities. This chapter presents a comprehensive review of the pediatric mediastinum including currently available imaging techniques, the normal mediastinal anatomy, and the broad spectrum of mediastinal disorders that occur in infants and children.

IMAGING TECHNIQUES

Understanding the various modalities available for imaging the mediastinum, their strengths and weaknesses, as well as the most appropriate modality for assessing various mediastinal entities is of paramount importance for developing an accurate and cost-effective diagnostic imaging plan. In general, there are four primary goals for imaging mediastinal abnormalities: (1) identifying mediastinal pathology, (2) characterizing identified pathology, (3) providing a succinct and accurate differential diagnosis, and (4) generating a cost-effective strategy for additional imaging and patient management. All of the radiology modalities currently available, that is, radiography, ultrasound, computed tomography (CT), magnetic resonance imaging (MRI), and nuclear medicine imaging, have utility for the evaluation of the mediastinum.

Radiography

The first diagnostic modality for the evaluation of the mediastinum in infants and children is generally a frontal and lateral chest radiograph. Relative to other modalities, chest radiography has a widespread availability, low cost, and ease of acquisition. However, one disadvantage that should be considered is the ionizing radiation associated with chest radiographs, particularly in the pediatric population who are vulnerable to potentially harmful ionizing radiation. Exact technique varies depending on the patient age and size, but fields of view of chest radiographs generally extend from the base of the neck to the proximal upper abdomen. In the very young and the very sick, only a supine frontal radiograph may be obtainable and suffice. Occasionally, a cross-table lateral radiograph may be added in these situations if necessary. Nevertheless, if feasible, upright frontal and lateral radiographs should be obtained for optimal assessment and characterization of mediastinum in pediatric patients.

Ultrasound

With respect to the mediastinum, the role of ultrasound is limited in older children who are generally older than 5 years because of a suboptimal acoustic window. Conversely, in the young child and infant, ultrasound can be particularly helpful and may be the next imaging modality of choice after an initial radiograph. Advantages of ultrasound include its widespread availability, portability, capability for real-time evaluation of the mediastinum, and its lack of ionizing radiation.

The optimal transducer used for evaluation of the mediastinum varies with age. In neonates and infants, 5- to 10-MHz linear array transducers are generally used whereas older children and adolescents may require 2- to 4- or 4- to 7-MHz sector or linear array transducers for adequate tissue penetration.[3] Depending on the age of the child and the location of the process, suprasternal, sternal, parasternal, intercostal, or subxiphoid transducer positions may be used.[3] In a young child, the unossified sternal and costal cartilage provides an adequate acoustic window for the evaluation of the mediastinum.[1] Imaging is generally performed in the supine position, but additional prone and decubitus positions may be of value. Doppler interrogation may be helpful for the complete evaluation and characterization of both solid and cystic mediastinal lesion.

Computed Tomography

Because of its high spatial resolution and capacity for multiplanar reformations and three-dimensional reconstruction, CT plays a pivotal role in the evaluation of the pediatric mediastinum, particularly in the setting of mediastinal masses. CT has been shown to have a very high diagnostic accuracy for the characterization of mediastinal masses in terms of size, location, nature, and additional organs of involvement.[1,4] Furthermore, outside of the primary lesion, CT has been shown to provide additional diagnostic information in 82% and affected clinical management in 65%.[1,4,5]

Typical CT parameters for mediastinal evaluation should closely adhere to the ALARA (As Low As Reasonably Achievable) principle by using the lowest possible radiation dose to achieve diagnostic value. Given the variance in patient sizes for different age groups in the pediatric protocol, CT parameters can be either weight based or girth based. Thin collimation (<1 mm) and fast table speeds of <1 second are available for use on most modern multidetector computed tomography (MDCT) scanners. In evaluation of mediastinal masses in the pediatric population, obtaining noncontrast CT images is not necessary because it does not typically provide additional information. Intravenous contrast is useful particularly in pediatric patients given the lack of mediastinal fat and the advantage over noncontrast images for the full assessment of mediastinal masses. If at all possible, power injection technique, which provides more homogeneous contrast enhancement, is preferred. However, this often depends on the type, location and stability of venous access available. Postprocessing techniques such as 2D multiplanar reformations and 3D reconstructions have been shown to be beneficial in the characterization of mediastinal vessels, central airway anomalies, and mediastinal mass associated abnormalities.

Magnetic Resonance Imaging

MRI is uniquely suited for the evaluation of the mediastinum given its high tissue contrast resolution relative to other techniques and its lack of ionizing radiation. However, it has several important disadvantages that deserve consideration including high cost, susceptibility to motion artifact, need for sedation in young children, and limited spatial resolution of the lungs.[1,6–14] MRI is particularly advantageous for the evaluation of thymic neoplasms with adjacent mediastinal structure and chest wall involvement, characterization of thoracic lymphatic malformations (LMs), foregut duplication cysts with high proteinaceous content, and intraspinal extent in neurogenic tumors.[1]

MRI protocols for the evaluation of mediastinal lesions vary somewhat based on the scanner type and institutional preferences. However, some general principles and sequences should be employed. Commonly, an eight-channel cardiac coil is recommended for mediastinal evaluation if available. Sedation is often required in younger patients (<6 to 8 years old) with the exception of neonates who can often be swaddled. Specific MR sequences that are useful include axial fast recovery fast spin-echo (FRFSE) T2-weighted imaging with fat saturation; coronal FRFSE T2-weighted imaging with fat saturation; axial T1 or double inversion recovery sequences; coronal gadolinium-enhanced 3D MR angiography spoiled gradient-recalled echo sequences; and axial and coronal postgadolinium T1-weighted imaging with fat-saturation. For the FRFSE T2-weighted MR sequences, a breath-hold or respiratory triggering is recommended to reduce motion artifact. Likewise, ECG gating and a breath-hold are needed for optimal, diagnostic quality double inversion recovery sequences.

Nuclear Medicine

Nuclear medicine imaging of the pediatric mediastinum is primarily limited to positron emission tomography (PET) often co-registered with CT (PET–CT) and metaiodobenzyguanidine (MIBG) imaging with gallium-67 imaging in lymphoma, primarily of historical interest.

Although not currently a first-line modality for the evaluation of all mediastinal masses, PET–CT has become a near first-line modality for staging, response to treatment, and postcompletion therapy assessment in lymphoma patients in recent years.[1,15–24] Specifically, PET is superior to other imaging techniques for the discrimination of viable tumor from scar and necrotic/nonviable residual tissue, the detection of tumor within normal-sized lymph nodes, and the presence of disease within extranodal sites.[1] Typically, the patient is asked to fast for at least 6 hours prior to the administration of 2-fluoro-2-deoxy (18 fluorine)-D-glucose (18FDG). Depending on the Institution, intravenous and oral contrast may be administered. Additionally, co-registered CT technique may vary from full, diagnostic quality technique to very-low-radiation technique, which simply functions for anatomic localization. Although primarily used in the setting of lymphoma, PET–CT may one day find uses in the mediastinum for diseases other than lymphoma, particularly in malignant or metastatic tumors.

A guanethidine analog similar to norepinephrine, MIBG, when tagged to the radioisotope iodine-123, is taken up by chromaffin cells and helpful in the imaging of abnormal sympathetic adrenergic tissue. For the pediatric population, MIBG is mainly employed for the evaluation of suspected or known

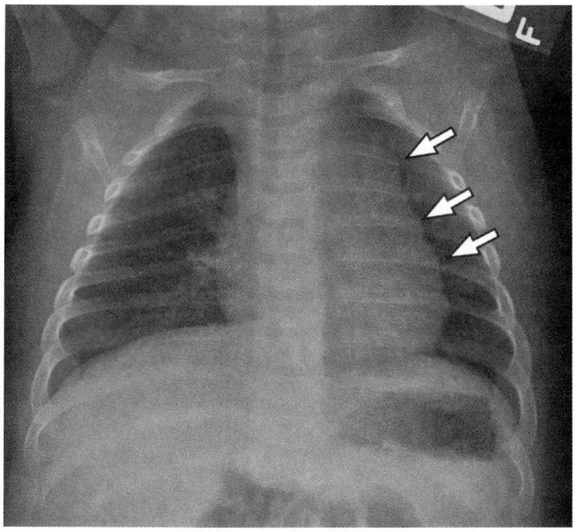

FIGURE 11.1 **A 2-month-old girl with normal thymus on frontal chest radiograph.** Frontal chest radiograph demonstrates an undulating contour of the left lateral thymic border (*arrows*). This represents the normal thymus interleaving into the adjacent rib interspaces giving the so-called "thymic wave" sign and should not be mistaken for a mass.

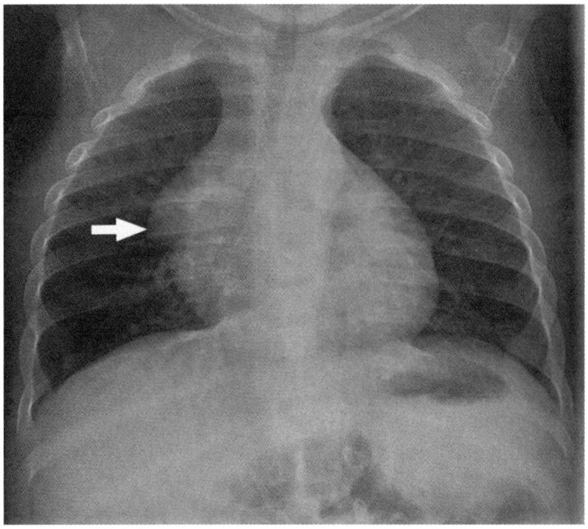

FIGURE 11.2 **A 3-month-old boy with normal thymus on frontal chest radiograph.** Frontal chest radiograph demonstrates the "thymic sail" sign representing the lateral triangular extension (*arrow*) of the normal thymus. This should not be confused for the "spinnaker sail" sign (Fig. 11.50) whereby the thymus is uplifted by pneumomediastinum giving the contour of a spinnaker sail.

sympathetic chain tumors such as neuroblastoma. MIBG imaging has a high detection rate (> 90%) for neuroblastoma. The patient is typically given a dose of 3 to 10 mCi of radioiodinated MIBG radiopharmaceutical. Whole-body planar images are performed 24 to 48 hours after administration.[25]

NORMAL ANATOMY AND VARIATIONS

Thymus

The thymus is a bilobed encapsulated organ located anterior to the pericardium and great vessels. It serves as an important immune system organ with its primary function being the maturation of T lymphocytes. Its appearance varies as the patient ages, which can lead the unwary radiologist to mistake the normal thymus for an abnormal mass. This is particularly troublesome in pediatric patients with lymphoma who are receiving chemotherapy because the thymus often involutes while on therapy with subsequent thymic rebound simulating tumor recurrence at the cessation of therapy. Furthermore, ectopic thymic tissue and thymic variants may also introduce diagnostic dilemma (Figs. 11.1 and 11.2). The two most common thymic variants are superior extension of the thymus to the level of the lower neck (Fig. 11.3) and posterior extension

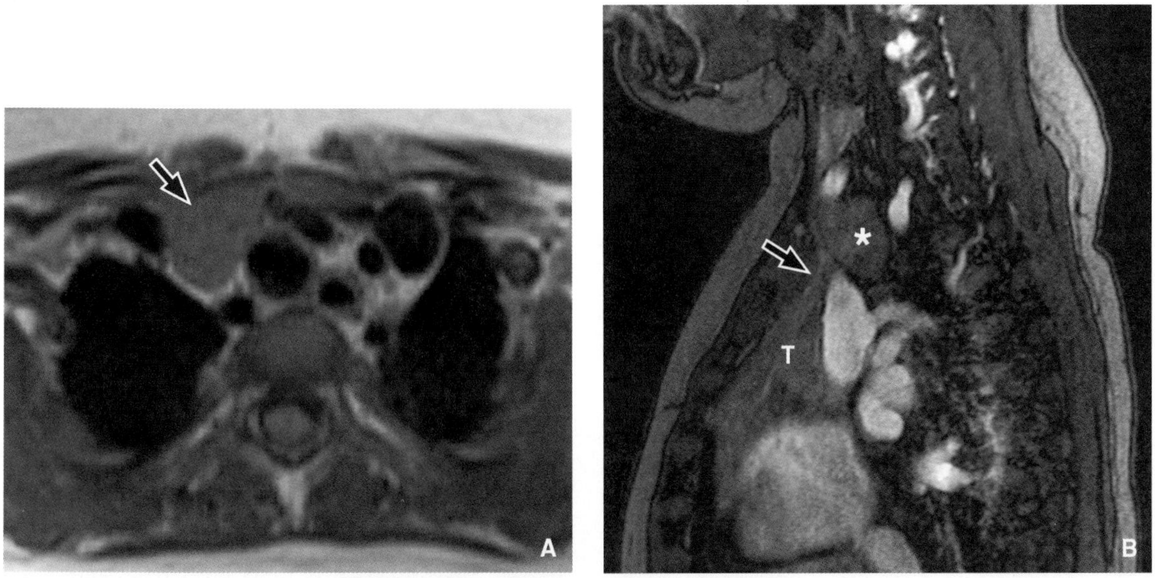

FIGURE 11.3 **A 5-year-old boy who underwent chest MRI for chest wall asymmetry. A:** Axial T1-weighted MR image shows a soft tissue, mass-like structure (*arrow*) located at the level of thoracic inlet. **B:** Sagittal postcontrast T1-weighted MR image demonstrates an ectopically located portion (*asterisk*) of the thymus, which is connected (*arrow*) to the normally positioned thymus (*T*), consistent with superior extension of the thymus.

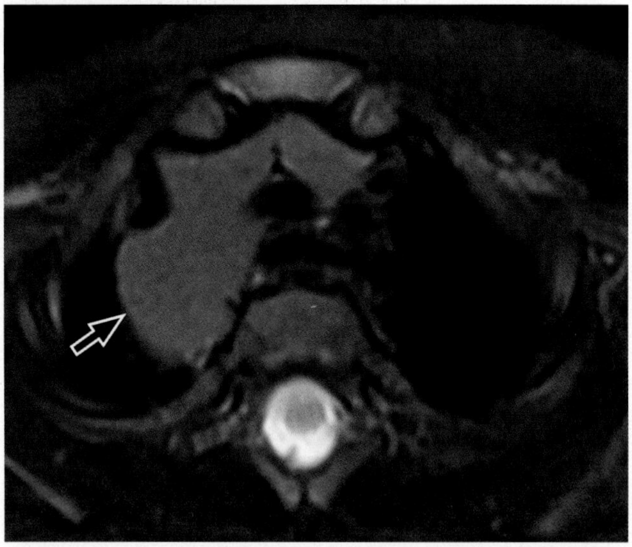

FIGURE 11.4 **A 3-month-old boy who underwent MRI examination for possible mediastinal mass.** Axial T2-weighted MR image shows posterior extension (*arrow*) of the normal thymus.

of the thymus generally posterior to the superior vena cava or posterior to the aortic arch (Fig. 11.4). Recognition of the connection between the ectopically located portion of the thymus and normally positioned portion of the thymus as well as the lack of mass effect upon adjacent mediastinal structures are two helpful clues to confirm the diagnosis of ectopically located but normal thymus.

On chest radiography, the appearance of the thymus varies by patient age (Fig. 11.5). During infancy, the thymus is typically quadrilateral in shape with convex outer margins. After around age 5, the thymus becomes more triangular in shape with straightening of its margins. After approximately age 15, the margins of the triangular-shaped thymus begin to become more convex with the thymus slowly involuting over time into adulthood. Any outward, particularly mass-like, convexity of the margins after approximately age 5 should raise the suspicion for an abnormal thymic mass. However, thymic rebound related to the relief of certain stressors such as the cessation of chemotherapy, recent surgery, or intubation must also be considered (Fig. 11.6).

If question remains after review of the initial chest radiograph, ultrasound may be utilized in children <5 years of age to confirm the presence of a normal thymus. On ultrasound, the normal thymus appears as a smoothly marginated, sharply defined anterior mediastinal organ, which closely molds to the underlying structures (Fig. 11.7). The pliable thymus typically deforms with cardiac and vascular pulsations. There is uniform echogenicity throughout the thymus, which most closely resembles that of the liver with hyperechoic septations interspersed throughout the gland.

Generally, the normal thymus does not require CT or MRI for evaluation. However, the normal thymus is quite frequently demonstrated on these modalities when imaging is performed for alternative indications. Therefore, it is important to understand the CT and MRI appearance of the normal thymus. The macrostructure of the thymus on CT and MRI correlates closely with that on ultrasound, that is, smoothly marginated, homogeneous glandular tissue, which conforms to the adjacent structures. There should be no associated compression or displacement of the surrounding anatomy. On CT, the normal thymus shows a homogeneous attenuation value similar to that of chest wall musculature (Fig. 11.5). On MRI, the signal intensity of the normal thymus is typically slightly higher than that of adjacent thoracic muscle on T1-weighted MR images (Fig. 11.3) and slightly less than or equal to that of fat on T2-weighted and fat-saturated MR images (Fig. 11.4).

Lymph Nodes

Lymph nodes are oval, bean-shaped, or rounded soft tissue structures located along the course of lymphatic chains and consist of a fibrous capsule with multiple internal trabeculae, which help to support and contain lymphatic tissue. They are present throughout the mediastinum. For accurate localization, lymph nodes have been regionally classified by the American Thoracic Society into four nodal regions, that is, superior mediastinal nodes, aortic nodes, inferior mediastinal nodes, and N_1 nodes, with a total of 14 nodal stations.[26]

Unlike in adults, there are currently no established size criteria for normal mediastinal lymph nodes in children.[27] As a general rule, normal mediastinal lymph nodes should not be viewable on imaging, particularly chest radiography, prior to puberty. However, as more and more children are receiving advanced cross-sectional imaging with ever improving spatial resolution, it is conceivable that tiny mediastinal lymph nodes become viewable in the absence of disease. However, at present, any mediastinal lymph nodes seen on imaging should be noted, and any underlying causes of lymphadenopathy should be excluded.[28]

Azygoesophageal Recess

The azygoesophageal recess (AER) is a mediastinal space representing protrusion of the medial border of the right lower lobe into the mediastinum from the level of the azygos arch inferiorly to the level of the aortic hiatus and right hemidiaphragm.[29]

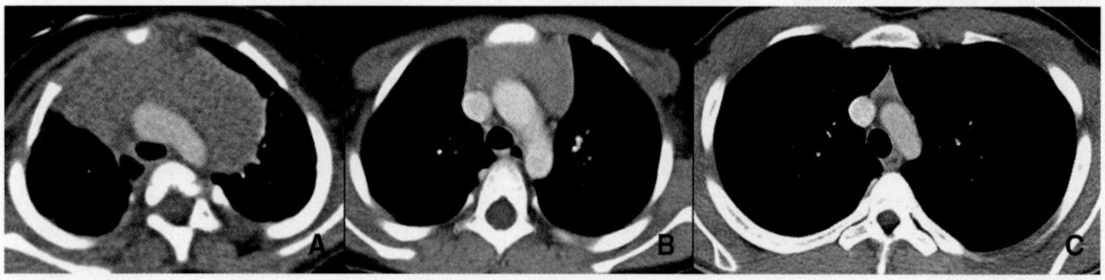

FIGURE 11.5 Three axial CT images of a normal thymus in patients aged 6 months **(A)**, 5 years **(B)**, and 17 years **(C)**.

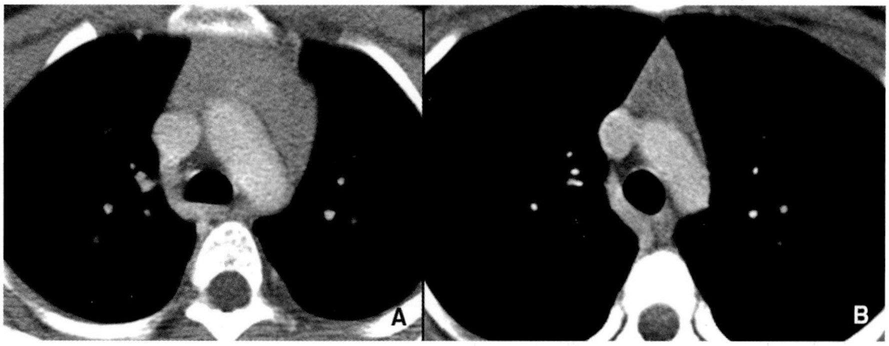

FIGURE 11.6 **Thymic rebound in a 10-year-old girl status post chemotherapy. A:** Axial enhanced CT image through the upper chest demonstrates a quadrilateral-shaped, smooth, and homogeneous thymus consistent with thymic rebound. **B:** Axial enhanced follow-up CT image in the same patient through the thymus demonstrates return of normal triangular thymic shape and size.

On frontal chest radiographs, the AER appears as a vertically oriented interface projected over the thoracic spine. On cross-sectional imaging, the AER appears as a focus of aerated lung protruding and extending across the spine a variable distance and bordered anteriorly and medially by the esophagus, the left atrium, and the azygos vein (Fig. 11.8). In adults, it is most often convex to the left (dextroconcave).[29] However, children demonstrate a more varied appearance ranging from dextroconvex, to straight, to dextroconcave. Multiple abnormalities affect the AER including developmental anomalies such as foregut duplication cysts, esophageal abnormalities particularly inflammation, vascular anomalies, lymphadenopathy, and neurogenic tumors.[29]

Mediastinal Compartments

The mediastinum compartmental division is classically based on the lateral chest radiograph and artificially divided into three compartments, that is, anterior, middle, and posterior (Fig. 11.9). These compartments are important because localizing mediastinal pathology to a particular compartment is often the first step in imaging evaluation. It also substantially helps in limiting the differential diagnosis and aiding in the decision of which additional imaging modality or modalities need(s) to be subsequently obtained in reaching the definitive diagnosis.[1]

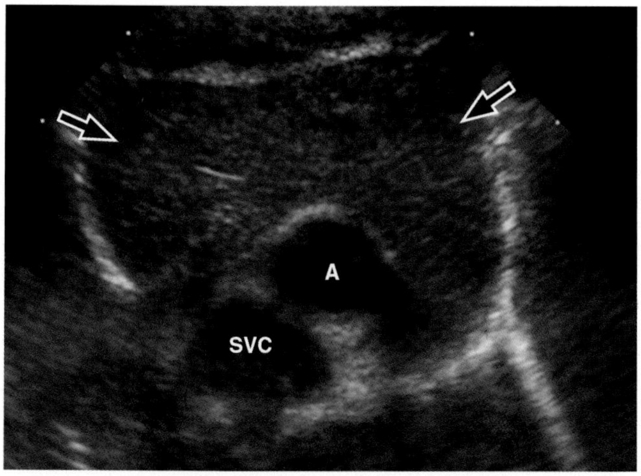

FIGURE 11.7 **Normal thymus in a 6-week-old girl.** The normal thymus (*arrows*) is located anterior to the mediastinal vessels and demonstrates a homogeneous appearance with linear and punctate echogenic foci. No mass effect upon adjacent aorta (*A*) or superior vena cava (*SVC*) is seen.

Recently, the International Thymic Malignancy Interest Group (ITMIG) developed and published a three compartmental mediastinal classification system based on axial CT anatomic divisions.[30] This three compartmental system includes the prevascular compartment, the visceral compartment, and the paravertebral compartment. These three compartments are similar to the radiographically based anterior, middle, and

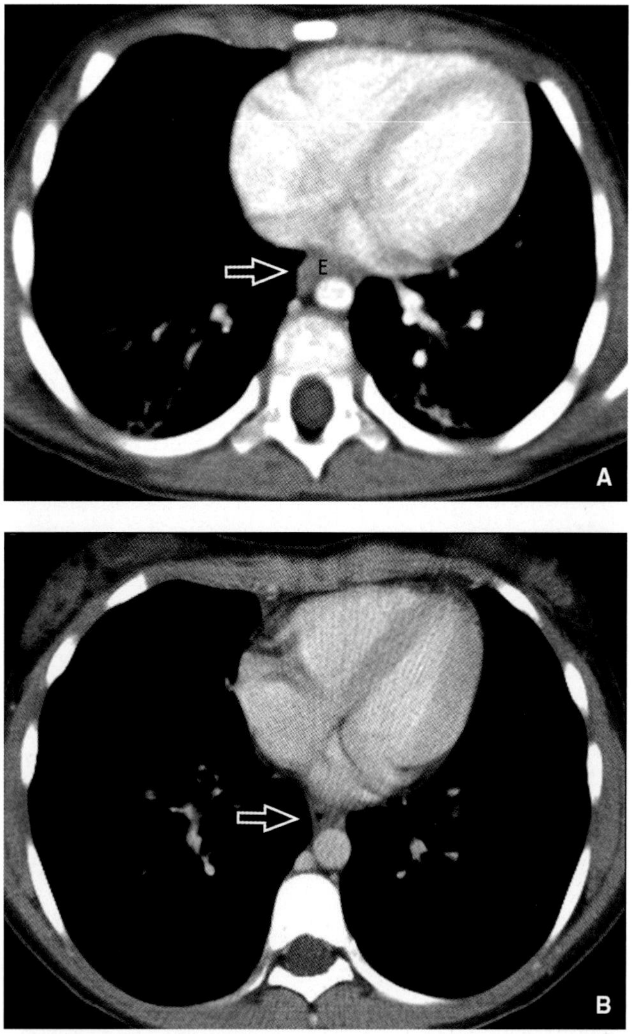

FIGURE 11.8 **Azygoesophageal recess (AER) in two different pediatric patients. A:** Axial enhanced CT image from a 4-year-old girl demonstrates the AER (*arrow*) with a convex lateral shape, resulting from intrusion of the esophagus (*E*) into the AER. **B:** Axial enhanced CT image from a 11-year-old girl shows the AER (*arrow*) with a straight border.

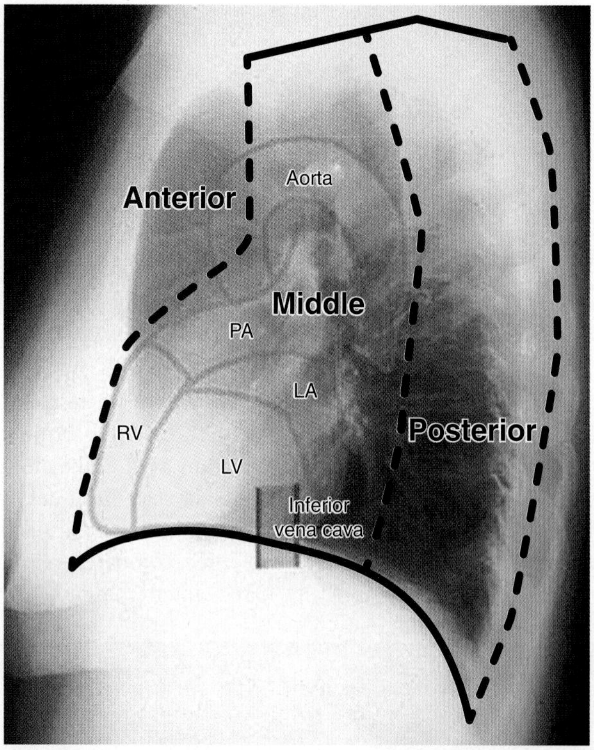

FIGURE 11.9 **Lateral radiograph with three mediastinal compartments.** Anterior, anterior mediastinal compartment; Middle, middle mediastinal compartment; Posterior, posterior mediastinal compartment.

posterior compartment. For the purposes of this chapter, we refer to the classic classification system, as, for our purpose, the compartmental classifications are roughly interchangeable.

The anterior mediastinal compartment is a lenticular space bordered by the sternum anteriorly and the pericardium posteriorly. Often times, it is helpful to consider which normal structures lay within a particular mediastinal compartment because this can aid in formulating the most likely differential diagnosis. Normal structures within the anterior mediastinal compartment include the thymus and lymphatic tissue. The middle mediastinum constitutes the largest mediastinal compartment. It lies between the anterior pericardial border and an imaginary line drawn ~1 cm posterior to the anterior border of the vertebral bodies. The superior border is formed by the thoracic inlet, whereas the diaphragm represents the inferior border. Normal structures within the middle mediastinal compartment include the heart, great vessels, trachea, esophagus, and lymph nodes. The posterior mediastinal compartment is anteriorly bordered by an imaginary line drawn ~1 cm posterior to the anterior border of the vertebral bodies, posteriorly by the posterior paravertebral gutters, superiorly by the thoracic inlet, and inferiorly by the posteromedial slips of the diaphragm. The normal structures of the posterior mediastinal compartment consist predominately of parasympathetic and sympathetic nerve chains and the osseous structures of the vertebral column (Table 11.1).

SPECTRUM OF MEDIASTINAL DISORDERS

Anterior Mediastinal Lesions

Thymic Hyperplasia

Also known as thymic rebound, thymic hyperplasia represents enlargement of the thymus after a period of atrophy induced by medications or severe illness. In the setting of chemotherapy, the thymus atrophies in 90% of patients.[2] After the illness has subsided or the medication administration has ceased, the thymus slowly recovers in volume with the total size possibly exceeding its baseline value. Imaging clearly demonstrates this pattern of involution and subsequent regrowth.

TABLE 11.1 Spectrum of Non-vascular Mediastinal Masses in the Pediatric Population

Anterior Mediastinum	Middle Mediastinum	Posterior Mediastinum
Thymic hyperplasia	Congenital foregut duplication cyst • Bronchogenic cyst • Esophageal duplication cyst • Neurenteric cyst	Neuroblastic tumor • Neuroblastoma • Ganglioneuroblastoma • Ganglioneuroma
Lymphoma • Hodgkin lymphoma • Non-Hodgkin lymphoma	Lymphadenopathy • Infectious lymphadenopathy • Neoplastic lymphadenopathy • Castleman disease	Peripheral nerve sheath tumor • Neurofibroma • Schwannoma
Thymic cyst		
Thymoma • Invasive type • Noninvasive type		
Thymic carcinoma		
Germ cell tumor		
Thymolipoma and lipoma		
Lymphatic malformation		

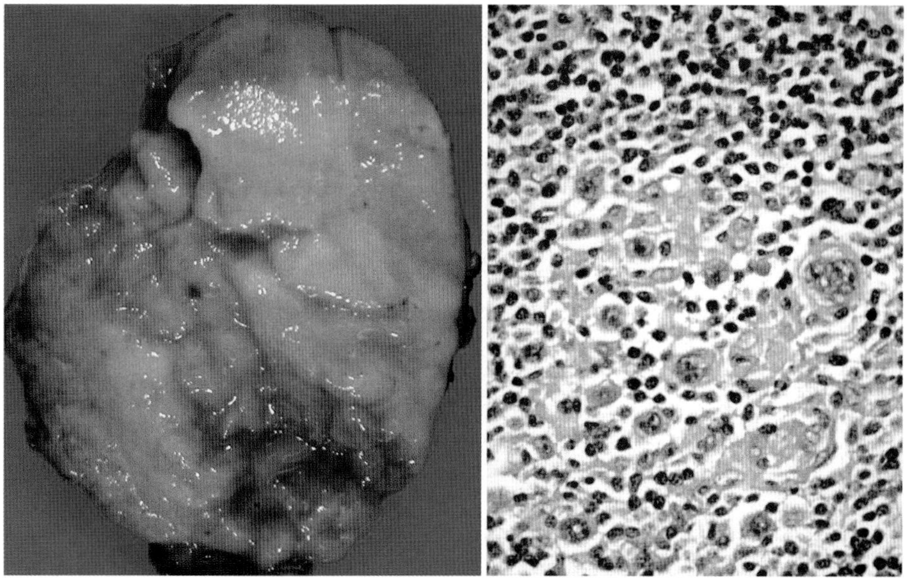

FIGURE 11.10 **Hodgkin lymphoma of the mediastinum in a 13-year-old girl, forming a mass with a fleshy cut surface (left).** Microscopically, large atypical cells ("Reed-Sternberg cells") are present within a background of mixed inflammatory cells (**right**; hematoxylin and eosin; original magnification, 600×).

On chest radiographs, the thymic shadow significantly diminishes in size or completely disappears during the associated stressor. Once the illness or medication stress has subsided, the thymic shadow rebounds and may demonstrate lobulated and convex contours, which can be disconcerting for the imager. Similarly, cross-section imaging demonstrates thymic hyperplasia to best advantage (Fig. 11.6). The hyperplastic thymus typically demonstrates homogeneous soft tissue attenuation and signal on CT and MRI, respectively, helping to differentiate it from more ominous processes. On PET imaging, thymic rebound is quite frequently encountered and should be distinguishable from persistent or recurrent neoplasm. In addition to uniform soft tissue attenuation on co-registered CT, homogeneous rather than masslike focal uptake is a supporting finding for thymic rebound on PET. Additionally, the rebounding thymus typically should not have a standardized uptake value (SUV) of more than 4.[2]

No specific treatment and follow-up is needed for thymic hyperplasia other than distinguishing it from more ominous diseases.

Lymphoma (Hodgkin and Non-Hodgkin Lymphoma)

Lymphoma represents the most common anterior mediastinal mass in childhood, arising from abnormal proliferation of lymphocytes.[1,2] Lymphoma is the third most common malignancy in children with only leukemia and central nervous system tumors being more common. Traditionally, lymphoma is subdivided into Hodgkin, histologically characterized by Reed-Sternberg cells and variants (Fig. 11.10), and non-Hodgkin lymphoma (NHL), resulting from clonal proliferation of lymphocytes (Table 11.2).

TABLE 11.2 Lymphomas Occurring in the Pediatric Mediastinum
T lymphoblastic leukemia/lymphoma
Classical Hodgkin lymphoma
Primary mediastinal large B-cell lymphoma
Anaplastic large cell lymphoma
B-cell lymphoma, unclassifiable, with features intermediate between diffuse large B-cell lymphoma and classical Hodgkin lymphoma
Other mature B-cell lymphoma

Hodgkin lymphoma in children typically occurs after the age of 10 years. It more often affects boys than girls by a ratio of 2:1.[31] It is divided into classical Hodgkin lymphoma and nodular lymphocyte–predominant Hodgkin lymphoma. In classical Hodgkin lymphoma, Reed-Sternberg cells and variants are the characteristic malignant cell (Fig. 11.10); they are present in a background rich in benign lymphocytes and other inflammatory cells with variable amounts of fibrosis. Nodular sclerosis subtype, most often showing prominent interspersed fibrous bands, is the most common subtype in the pediatric mediastinum. Nodular lymphocyte–predominant Hodgkin lymphoma is rare in children.[32] Generally, Hodgkin lymphoma carries a good prognosis with a cure rate of ~90%.[2,31] The majority of affected pediatric patients present with chest pain and discomfort related to enlarged mediastinal lymph nodes with associated compressive effects on the adjacent airway and vascular structures. However, affected children occasionally present with asymptomatic cervical or axillary lymphadenopathy. Additional signs and symptoms include fever, night sweat, and unexplained weight loss. These constitutional symptoms are known as B symptoms, and they affect the disease staging. Based on the Ann Arbor staging classification, both Hodgkin lymphoma and NHL (discussed below) are categorized into four stages (Table 11.3).[33]

NHL, which is more common than Hodgkin lymphoma, typically presents in the first and second decades of life but generally occurs in the pediatric patients younger than 5 years of age.[1,6,31] Similar to Hodgkin lymphoma, boys are affected more commonly, with a male-to-female ratio of 3:1.[31] Four subtypes of NHL are particularly prevalent in children: (1)

TABLE 11.3 Ann Arbor Staging Classification for Hodgkin and Non-Hodgkin Lymphomas

Stage 1	Involvement of a single lymph node region or a single extralymphatic organ
Stage II	Involvement of 2 or more lymph node regions on the same side of the diaphragm or localized involvement of a single extralymphatic organ in association with regional lymph node involvement on the same side of the diaphragm
Stage III	Involvement of lymph node regions on both sides of the diaphragm (III), which may have accompanying extralymphatic extension in association with adjacent lymph node involvement (IIIE) or splenic involvement (IIIS) or both (IIIE, S)
Stage IV	Diffuse involvement affecting one or more tissues or organs outside of the lymphatic system, with or without nearby lymph node involvement A: Without B symptoms B: Fever, night sweats, weight loss of >10% body weight over the last 6 months

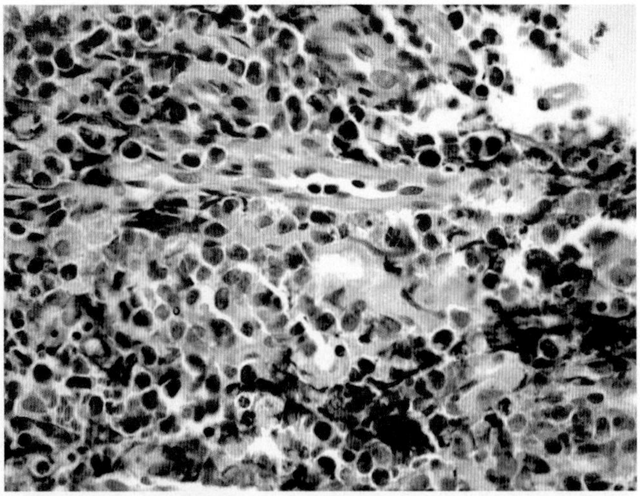

FIGURE 11.11 **Lymphoblastic lymphoma (T-cell phenotype) presenting as a mediastinal mass in a 7-year-old boy.** Cells are small, round, and monotonous (hematoxylin and eosin; original magnification, 600×). Flow cytometry (not shown) confirmed a T-cell phenotype.

lymphoblastic lymphoma (most commonly with a T-cell phenotype) (Fig. 11.11), (2) Burkitt lymphoma, (3) diffuse large B-cell lymphoma (Fig. 11.12), and (4) anaplastic large cell lymphoma. With T-cell lymphoblastic lymphoma, affected pediatric patients commonly present with a mediastinal mass. In contrast, Burkitt lymphoma commonly presents in the abdomen, most frequently around the terminal ileum.

Diffuse large B-cell lymphoma presents variably and may involve the mediastinum, often with fibrosis that imparts nodularity.[31,34] Symptoms of mediastinal NHL are often related to compression or obstruction of adjacent airway and vascular structures.

Imaging features of pediatric lymphoma rely heavily on the underlying histology. For Hodgkin lymphoma, chest radiographic findings are variable, ranging from completely normal with minimal mediastinal lymph node enlargement to a very large anterior mediastinal mass (Fig. 11.13A). Following chest radiography, cross-sectional imaging is typically

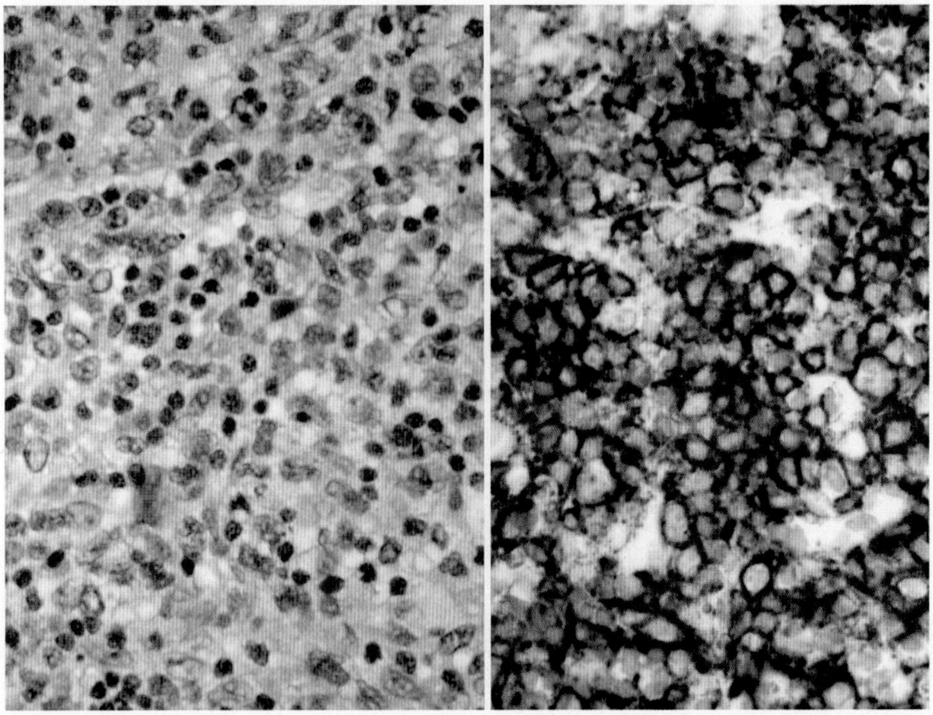

FIGURE 11.12 **Diffuse large B-cell lymphoma, in the mediastinum of a 17-year-old boy.** Cells are large with irregular nuclear contours (**left**; hematoxylin and eosin) and show immunohistochemical expression of the B-cell marker CD20 (**right**; original magnification, 600×).

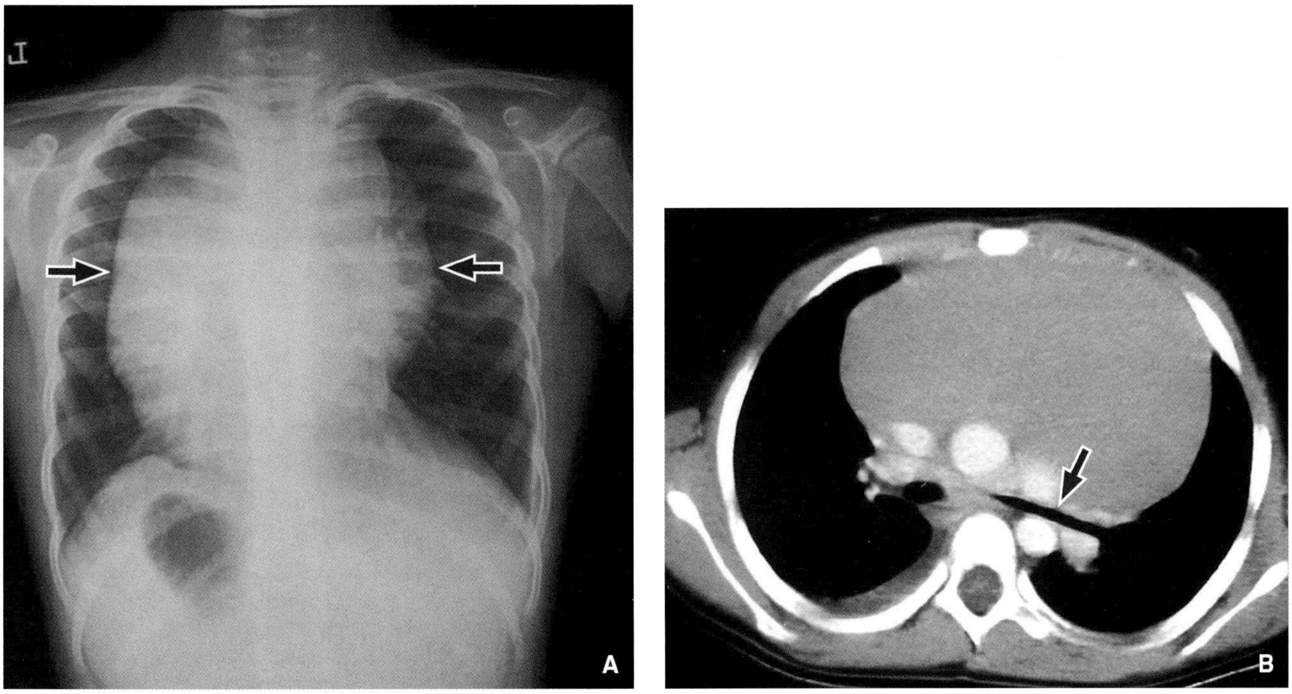

FIGURE 11.13 **Hodgkin lymphoma in a 7-year-old boy who presented with fever, weight loss, and chest pain. A:** Frontal chest radiograph demonstrates a large, smoothly marginated mediastinal mass (*arrows*). The hilum and spine are clearly visible through the mass localizing it to the anterior mediastinum. **B:** Axial enhanced CT image demonstrates a homogeneous, well-defined anterior mediastinal mass. The aorta and pulmonary arteries are displaced posteriorly. The left mainstem bronchus (*arrow*) is elongated, compressed, and narrowed. There is a partially visualized small right pleural effusion.

performed, usually contrast-enhanced chest CT (Fig. 11.13B). Here, the CT serves the purpose of confirming the presence of an anterior mediastinal mass while allowing for the assessment of adjacent nodal involvement, which helps in disease staging (Table 11.3). Imaging appearance of affected nodes ranges from small individually discernible lymph nodes most commonly in the prevascular and pretracheal region to large or conglomerated, lobulated masses that displace adjacent mediastinal structures.[2,31] Hodgkin lymphoma demonstrates variable signal characteristics on MRI, although involved lymph nodes usually have hyperintense signal on T2-weighted and intermediate signal on T1-weighted MR images.

Over the past several years, PET and PET/CT are transitioning into the forefront for lymphoma imaging as they provide useful physiologic data in addition to traditional anatomic evaluation. Active lymphoma demonstrates marked increased FDG activity (Fig. 11.14) relative to the mediastinal blood pool, whereas fibrosis and necrotic tissue in the region of prior disease demonstrates no appreciable FDG activity.

Unlike HL, the site of involvement of NHL is more variable than that of HL; common sites include the abdomen, thorax, and head and neck. Thoracic involvement occurs in ~50% of cases.[2,31] On chest radiograph, thoracic NHL presents as a large anterior mediastinal mass with convex outer margins and often displacement of the mediastinal structures such as mediastinal vessels and trachea (Fig. 11.15A). Discrete or large conglomerated mediastinal lymphadenopathy may be seen on CT and MRI. With contrast administration, NHL may demonstrate heterogeneity (Fig. 11.15B) or central irregular nonenhancing regions representing focal areas of necrosis. Adjacent hilar and subcarinal lymph node chains are frequently involved. Also, pleural-based masses or effusions may be seen, a feature not commonly seen with Hodgkin lymphoma. Like Hodgkin lymphoma, PET is particularly helpful in the assessment of staging, disease activity, and treatment response. Particularly instructive is PET's ability to discriminate viable tumor from scar and its ability to detect disease within otherwise normal-appearing lymph nodes.

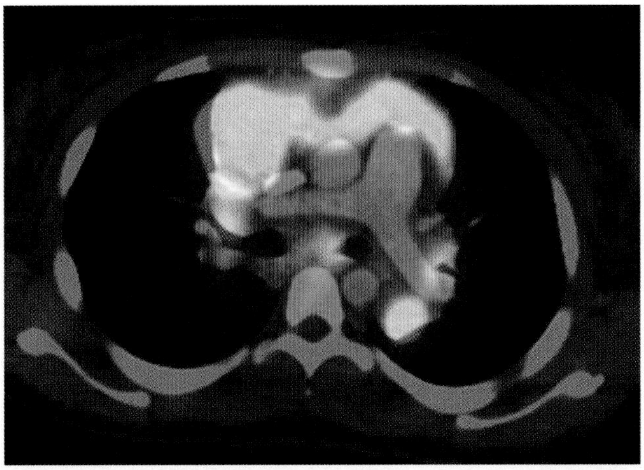

FIGURE 11.14 **Initial PET/CT of a 16-year-old girl with newly diagnosed Hodgkin lymphoma.** Axial fused PET/CT image demonstrates marked FDG avidity seen best within the anterior mediastinal lymphadenopathy with an SUV value of 13.3.

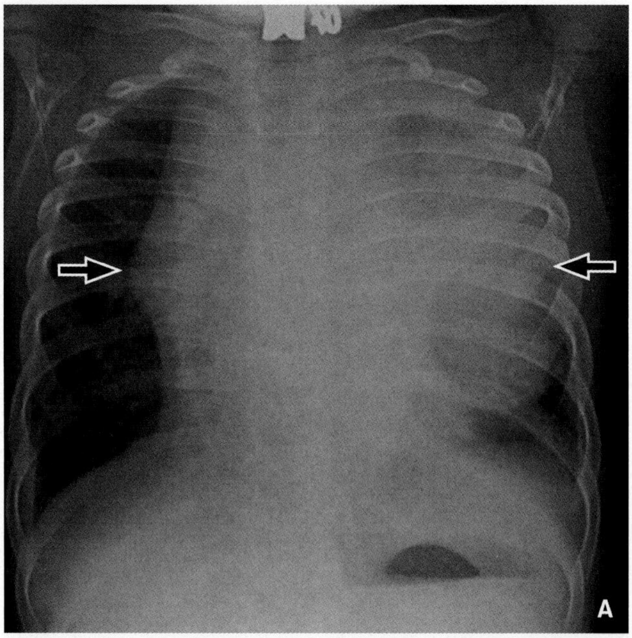

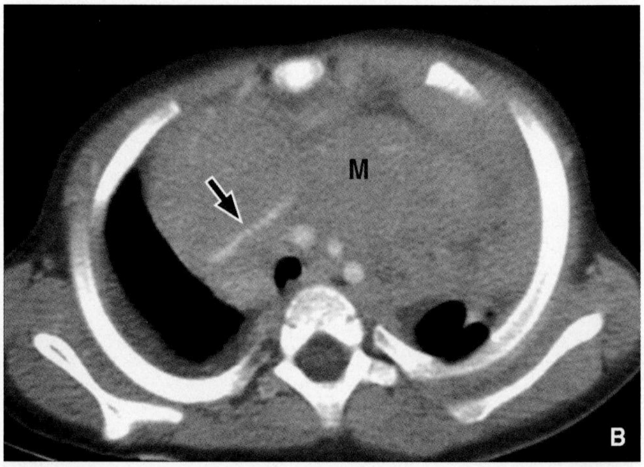

FIGURE 11.15 **Non-Hodgkin lymphoma in a 4-year-old boy who presented with face swelling and respiratory distress. A:** Frontal chest radiograph shows a large anterior mediastinal mass (*arrows*) nearly obscuring the entire left hemithorax. **B:** Corresponding axial enhanced CT image shows a large, heterogeneous soft tissue mass (*M*) nearly occupying the entire chest with an epicenter within the anterior mediastinum. The superior vena cava (*arrow*) is compressed and displaced posteriorly, and the trachea is displaced posteriorly and to the right. There is a partially visualized right pleural effusion.

Treatment for both Hodgkin lymphoma and NHL relies primarily on chemotherapy, sometimes with concurrent radiation therapy. After treatment, coarse calcification at the site of prior disease may develop (Fig. 11.16). Comparatively, the cure rate is higher for Hodgkin lymphoma at 90% with a cure rate among pediatric patients with NHL being 80%.[31,35] For NHL, bone marrow transplantation may also be utilized as a treatment option.

Thymic Cyst

A rare fluid-filled mass within the anterior mediastinum, thymic cysts most commonly represent a remnant of the thymopharyngeal duct. Thymic cysts have been described rarely in patients with human immunodeficiency virus and Langerhans cell histiocytosis.[31,36,37]Generally, thymic cysts are found in the lateral infrahyoid neck intimately associated with the carotid sheath. However, thymic cysts may occur anywhere from the pyriform sinus to the anterior mediastinum. When large, thymic cysts affecting pediatric patients may present with symptoms of respiratory distress or dysphagia in the presence of a slowly enlarging neck mass.

Thymic cysts are generally occult on chest radiograph as they are often obscured by the normal thymus. In infants and very young children, ultrasound may be utilized and yields a fluid-filled, spherical mass with thin or imperceptible walls. Multiple septations and loculations may be seen. On CT,

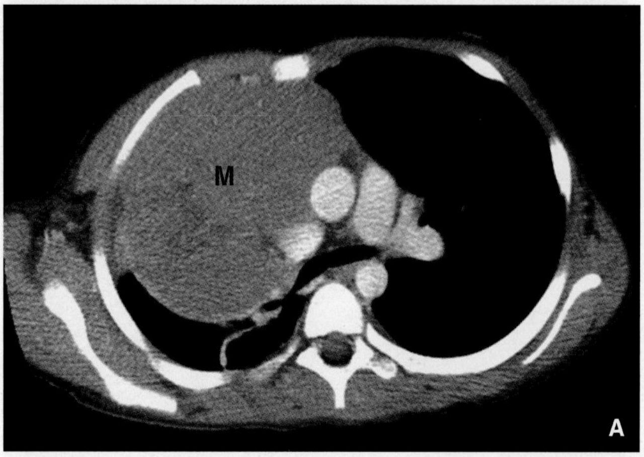

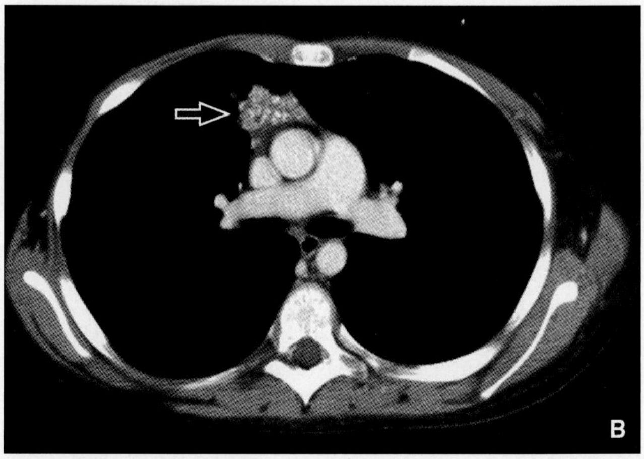

FIGURE 11.16 **A 12-year-old boy with Hodgkin lymphoma with posttreatment calcification. A:** Pretreatment axial enhanced CT image demonstrates a heterogeneous anterior mediastinal mass (*M*). **B:** Posttreatment axial enhanced CT image shows coarse calcifications (*arrow*) at the site of prior disease.

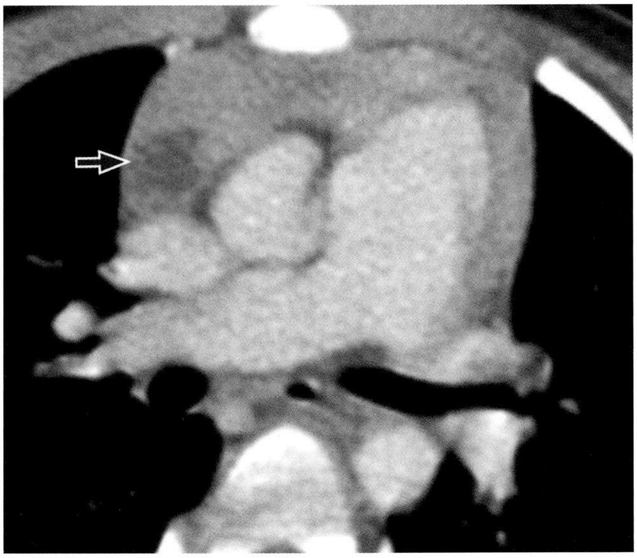

FIGURE 11.17 **A 2-year-old girl with incidentally detected thymic cyst on CT study obtained for evaluation of recurrent pneumonia.** Axial enhanced CT image shows a low-attenuation lesion (*arrow*) located within the thymus.

thymic cysts typically present as a smooth-walled, nonenhancing cystic mass within the anterior mediastinum (Fig. 11.17). MRI signal characteristics are variable depending on the cyst contents, that is, simple fluid versus proteinaceous or hemorrhagic fluid. Given its rather nondescript appearance as a cystic anterior mediastinal mass, a differential must often be entertained, which includes a LM, a branchial cleft cyst, thyroglossal duct cyst, foregut duplication cyst, teratoma, and dermoid cyst in the pediatric population. Cystic change in Hodgkin lymphoma, thymoma, Langerhans cell histiocytosis, or other pediatric neoplasm may also be a consideration.

Surgical resection is the mainstay of treatment for thymic cysts, particularly in the symptomatic pediatric patient. Prognosis is excellent after surgical resection.

Thymoma

Thymomas are rare pediatric anterior mediastinal tumors arising from thymic epithelial cells.[1,31] Representing only 1% to 2% of pediatric anterior mediastinal masses, thymomas are classically categorized into two types, that is, invasive and noninvasive. This division is predicated primarily on gross pathologic analysis with noninvasive thymomas demonstrating well-defined margins without extension through the surrounding fibrous capsule (Fig. 11.18). However, although minimal or local invasion may not be readily ascertained, gross invasion can be readily identified and characterized with presurgical imaging and should be evaluated for in all cases. Affected pediatric patients often present clinically not as a result of the mass itself but as a result of associated autoimmune or paraneoplastic conditions, for example, myasthenia gravis, hypogammaglobulinemia, and pure red cell aplasia. In all, patients with thymoma have concurrent myasthenia gravis in 15% to 30% of cases.[31,36,38,39]

On chest radiography, thymomas appear most often as a smoothly marginated, anterior mediastinal mass occasionally with a thinly calcified peripheral capsule. In cases of invasive thymoma, the borders may become more irregular with loss of the interface between the mass and the adjacent lung or chest wall and associated pleural nodules. On CT, thymomas appear as a soft tissue density, well-defined, lobulated, or rounded lesion with minimal or mild contrast enhancement (Fig. 11.19). Central areas of low attenuation within the lesion suggest cystic necrosis. With invasive thymomas, CT may demonstrate extension outside of the mediastinum

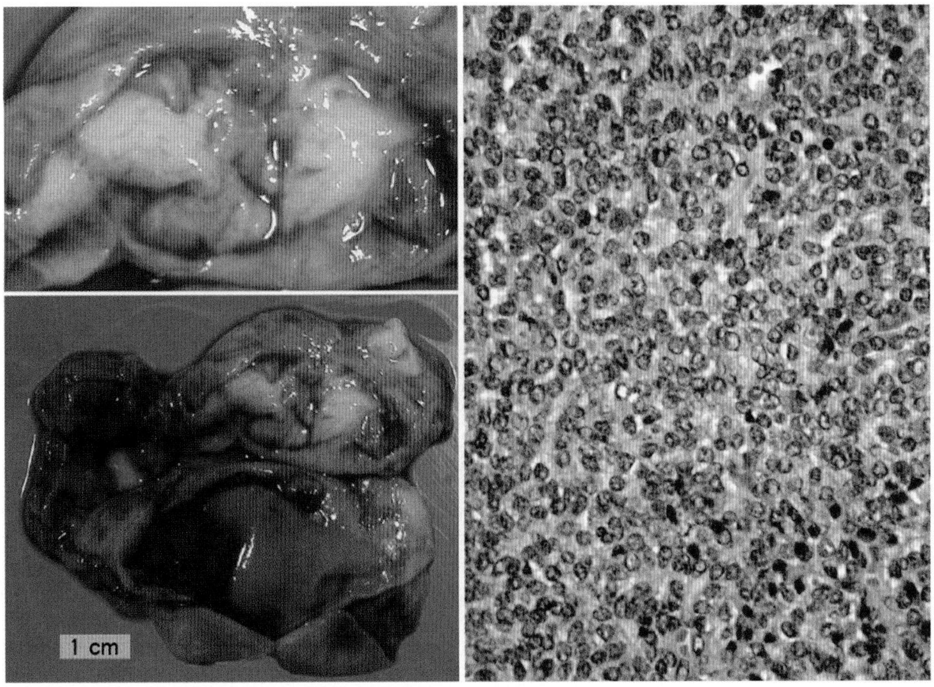

FIGURE 11.18 Thymoma showing a large cystic component **(left upper and lower),** occupying the anterior mediastinum of a 14-year-old girl. Solid areas of densely packed monotonous cells with interspersed lymphocytes are seen microscopically (**right**; hematoxylin and eosin; original magnification, 600x).

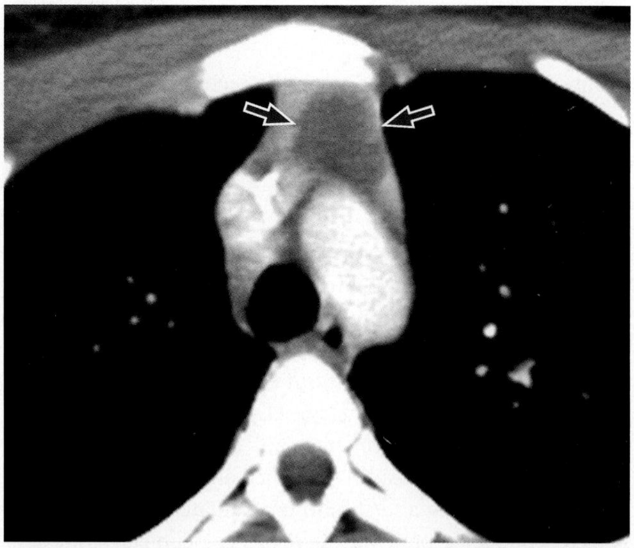

FIGURE 11.19 **A 12-year-old girl who presented with myasthenia gravis.** Axial enhanced CT image demonstrates a relatively nonenhancing and low-attenuation mass (*arrows*) within the thymus. Surgical pathology confirmed the diagnosis of thymoma.

with invasion of the adjacent pleura or chest wall (Fig. 11.20). Again, these lesions may have pleural-based metastatic lesions that are important to note for treatment prognosis and surgical planning. On MRI, thymomas generally demonstrate hyperintense T2 signal with MRI providing little advantage over CT for the evaluation of thymomas.[2]

Most thymomas require radiation and/or chemotherapy. If deemed resectable, all thymomas are ultimately surgically removed.

Thymic Carcinoma

Thymic carcinomas are aggressive epithelial tumors of the thymus characterized by overt histologic malignancy.[31] Normally, these lesions are seen in the fifth to sixth decades of life. However, very rarely, they may occur in the pediatric population. Thus, familiarity with thymic carcinomas and their imaging characteristics is warranted for the pediatric imager. Often affected pediatric patients present with nonspecific constitutional symptoms of night sweats, weight loss, and fatigue in addition to chest pain. Unlike thymomas, thymic carcinomas are rarely associated with myasthenia gravis.[40,41] Metastatic disease or invasion into adjacent structures often exists on presentation leading to an overall poor prognosis for thymic carcinomas.

With chest radiography, thymic carcinomas appear as a large, ill-defined anterior mediastinal mass. CT and MRI demonstrate the extent and characterization of these lesions to best advantage often showing diffuse and heterogeneous contrast enhancement with invasion of the adjacent mediastinal structures and chest wall (Fig. 11.21). Differentiation of these lesions from invasive thymoma may be difficult on imaging alone. However, findings such as distant metastatic lesions and lymphadenopathy favor thymic carcinoma.

Given its poor prognosis with metastatic disease often present on initial evaluation, thymic carcinoma in the pediatric patient is often treated with a combination of neoadjuvant chemotherapy, surgery, and postoperative radiation therapy.[31,42]

Germ Cell Tumor

Anterior mediastinal germ cell tumors are typically located within or near the thymus and represent the third most common pediatric mediastinal mass, accounting for 6% to 18% of all pediatric mediastinal tumors.[1,6,43] These lesions have been attributed to ectopic primitive germ cell rests.[2]

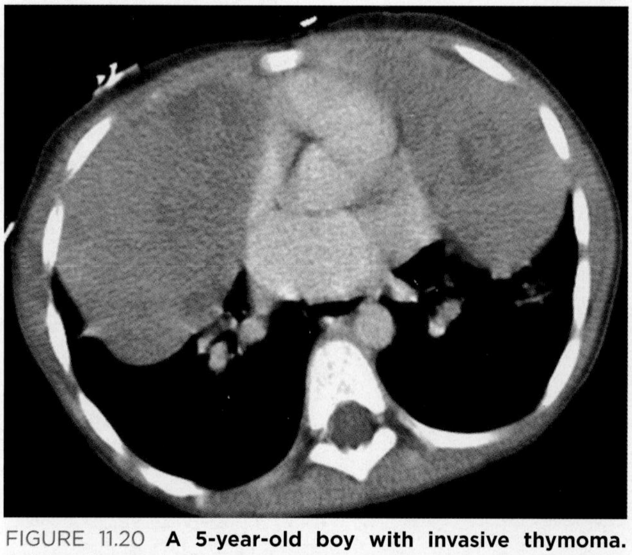

FIGURE 11.20 **A 5-year-old boy with invasive thymoma.** Axial enhanced CT image demonstrates a large, heterogeneous anterior mediastinal mass extending across both hemithoraces and compressing the heart. Surgical resection was consistent with an invasive thymoma.

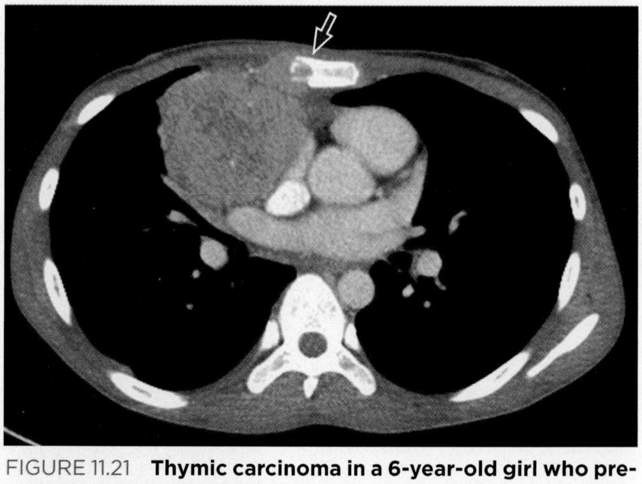

FIGURE 11.21 **Thymic carcinoma in a 6-year-old girl who presented with anterior chest wall pain and shortness of breath.** Axial enhanced CT image demonstrates a heterogeneously enhancing, anterior mediastinal mass with invasion of anterior chest wall and destruction of adjacent sternum (*arrow*).

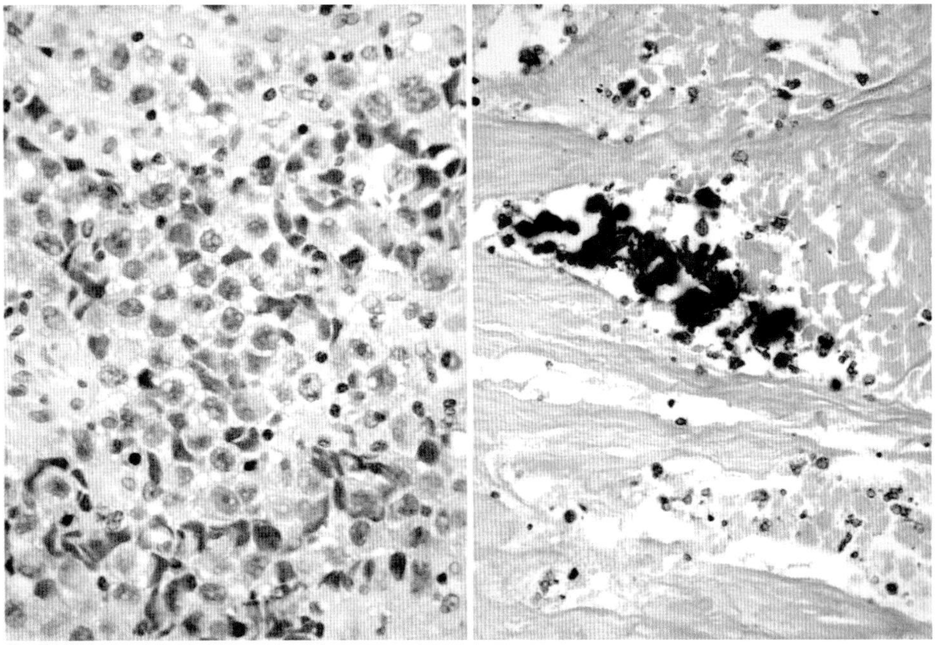

FIGURE 11.22 **Seminoma, diagnosed in needle biopsy material from a primary mediastinal mass in a 19-year-old male; cells are round with prominent nucleoli and frequent interspersed lymphocytes (left).** After therapy, resection showed necrotic cells, basophilic calcifications, and fibrosis (**right**; hematoxylin and eosin; original magnification, 600x).

The epidemiology of mediastinal germ cell tumors in newborns and prepubertal children differs from that in postpubertal children. In infants and young children, teratoma (congenital teratoma) and yolk sac tumor are most common; in congenital teratoma, immature neuroepithelial elements are considered benign, and only the presence of a yolk sac tumor element confers malignant potential. In postpubertal children, mediastinal germ cell tumors are virtually exclusively restricted to males; both seminomatous (Fig. 11.22) and nonseminomatous (embryonal carcinoma, yolk sac tumor, mature/immature teratoma (Fig. 11.23), choriocarcinoma, and occasionally somatic-type malignant components) can be seen. When malignant mediastinal germ cell tumor is suspected, the patient's gonads must be imaged to exclude a primary gonadal tumor.[2] A GCT in a primary mediastinal site is associated with a worse prognosis than one in a primary gonadal or other extragonadal site. Overall, teratomas are the most common pediatric mediastinal germ cell tumor, representing 60% of cases.[2]

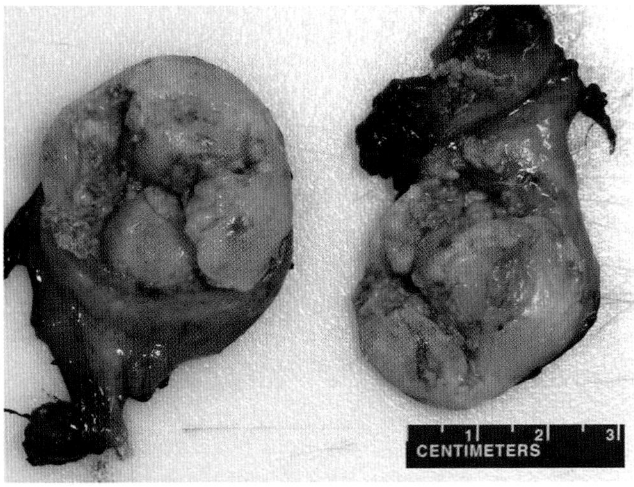

FIGURE 11.23 **Mediastinal mature teratoma in a 5-year-old boy.** Bisected surgical specimen of mediastinal mature teratoma is partially cystic with sebaceous luminal material.

On chest radiographs, germ cell tumors appear as large, well-circumscribed, rounded masses within the anterior mediastinum (Fig. 11.24). Calcifications occur in 25% of teratomas and may occasionally be evident on radiographs as areas of curvilinear density within the mass (Fig. 11.24A).[2] After initial detection on radiographs, CT or MRI generally is utilized for definitive diagnosis. Both imaging modalities demonstrate the lesion well as a complex cystic and solid mass within the anterior mediastinum (Figs. 11.24 to 11.26). Fat, fluid, and calcific components are hallmarks of teratomas at all ages.[1,2,44–47] Another useful feature on cross-sectional imaging is the presence of enhancing solid components, which are seen more often in immature teratomas than in mature teratomas.[2] Malignant germ cell tumors, like other aggressive mediastinal lesions, tend to invade adjacent structures including the lungs, pleura, pericardium, and chest wall, whereas benign teratomas tend to displace adjacent anatomy.[2] Rarely, teratoma may rupture in the mediastinum with involvement of the intrapulmonary bronchus, resulting in obstructive pneumonitis (Fig. 11.26).

Treatment and prognosis is largely dependent on the underlying histology of the mediastinal germ cell tumors. All are generally treated operatively. Mature teratomas tend to have an excellent prognosis with complete surgical excision. Conversely, malignant germ cell tumors tend to require the addition of chemotherapy and radiation with an overall poor prognosis.[2]

Thymolipoma and Lipoma

Thymolipomas represent an uncommon anterior mediastinal mass pathologically composed predominately of fat

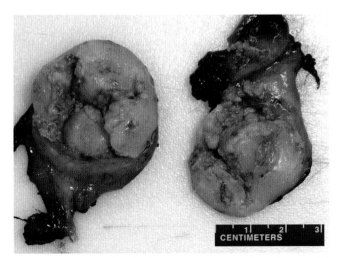

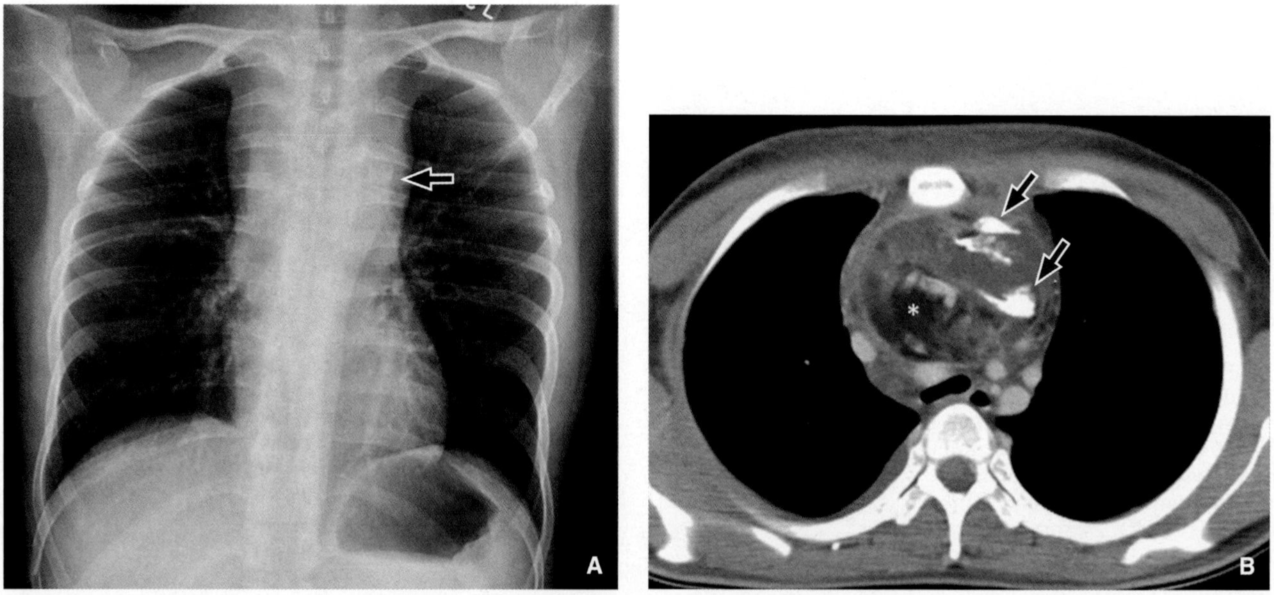

FIGURE 11.24 **Mediastinal mature teratoma in a 9-year-old girl who presented with shortness of breath and chest pain. A:** Frontal chest radiograph demonstrates widening of the superior mediastinum with convex lateral margins consistent with an underlying mass lesion. There are conglomerated areas of calcification (*arrow*) seen best in the interspace between the fourth and fifth left posterior ribs. **B:** Corresponding axial enhanced CT image demonstrates the complex internal constituents of the mediastinal teratoma including focal areas of calcification (*arrows*), fat (*asterisk*), and soft tissue components.

with interspersed thymic tissue. Similarly, lipomas are well-encapsulated fatty masses with a composition identical to subcutaneous fat and can occur in any region of the body including the mediastinum. Pediatric patients with either of these lesions are generally asymptomatic because of the mass's pliability.

On chest radiography, thymolipomas appear as large, sharply marginated, anterior mediastinal masses and are of low density relative to the adjacent soft tissues in one-half of cases.[2] On CT and MRI, thymolipomas are well circumscribed with an internal whorled appearance of nonenhancing soft tissue interwoven between fatty density/fat intensity tissue.

Likewise, depending on their size and location, lipomas may appear as a focus of relative radiolucency compared to adjacent soft tissue. Cross-sectional imaging (CT or MRI) is typically then utilized confirming the fatty character of the mass (Fig. 11.27).

Both lipomas and thymolipomas require no additional treatment or workup once imaging has confirmed the diagnosis. However, if the lesion becomes massive with compression of adjacent structures resulting in respiratory or vascular compromise, surgical resection may be warranted.

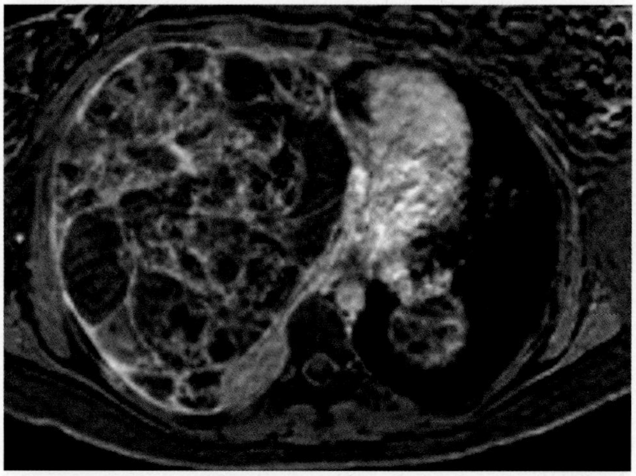

FIGURE 11.25 **A 13-year-old girl with mediastinal malignant teratoma.** Axial enhanced T1-weighted fat-saturated MR image demonstrates a very large and heterogeneous anterior mediastinal mass, filling the entire right hemithorax and displacing the heart to the left.

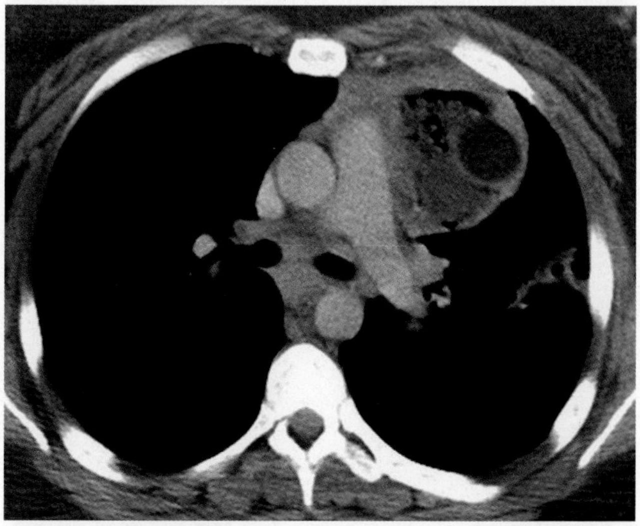

FIGURE 11.26 **A 16-year-old girl with ruptured teratoma.** Axial enhanced CT image demonstrates a heterogeneous lesion within the anterior mediastinum with a focal area of macroscopic fat. There are irregular foci of gas within the lesion in this patient with a ruptured teratoma.

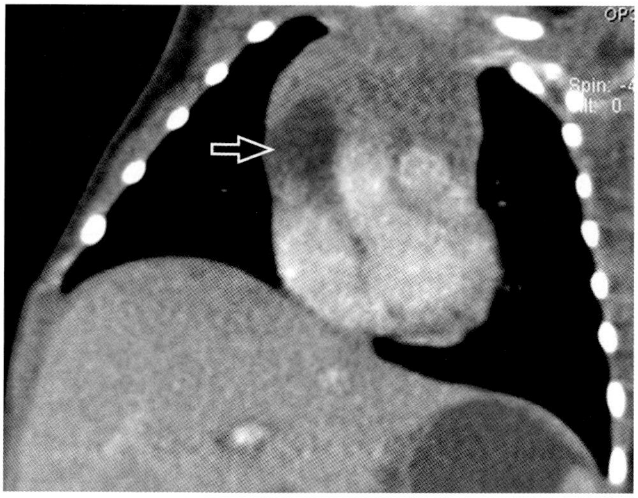

FIGURE 11.27 **A 1-day-old girl with thymic lipoma.** Coronal enhanced CT image demonstrates a well-circumscribed, fatty mass (*arrow*) in the right inferior thymus.

Lymphatic Malformation

Embryologically, LMs result from a congenital malformation of the lymphatic system producing a lymph-containing cystic or multicystic mass. Histologically, the mass is composed of multiple malformed lymphatic channels lined with variably thick smooth muscle coats. LM is often accompanied by excess fibroconnective tissue.[48] LMs may occur anywhere in the body but are most commonly found in the cervicofacial region, axilla, mediastinum, presacral region, and retroperitoneum. Completely intrathoracic LMs, however, are very rare and represent <1% of all LMs.[49]

Most affected pediatric patients present at <2 years of age with the lesion detected on physical examination.[48] The lesion generally enlarges as the patient grows. Often affected children are asymptomatic. However, they may develop dyspnea with infiltration and compression of the airway or mediastinal vascular structures.

When intrathoracic, LMs may be found in any mediastinal compartment but are generally located within the anterior mediastinum. Here, LMs may be demonstrated on chest radiograph as enlargement of the anterior mediastinum with or without a discernible/well-defined mass (Fig. 11.28A). Cross-sectional imaging is imperative for the full evaluation and accurate characterization of these lesions. Regardless of cross-sectional study utilized, for example, US, CT, or MRI, LMs appear as multiloculated cystic, trans-spatial masses with variable thickness of internal septations and the surrounding walls (Fig. 11.28B). However, of the modalities available, MRI is the imaging modality of choice given its superior contrast resolution and soft tissue characterization relative to other modalities.

On MRI, LMs demonstrate hyperintense T2 signal within the cystic portion of the lesion with variable enhancement of its walls and septations (Fig. 11.29). In the setting of intracystic hemorrhage or infection, the fluid within the cysts becomes more complex and may be associated with a variable degree of internal enhancement.[2] LMs often infiltrate through adjacent mediastinal structures and can encase and narrow the trachea or great vessels. Rarely, LMs may also extend into the distal lung interstitium.

Treatment for LMs consists primarily of surgical resection and sclerotherapy, with sclerotherapy commonly used in the

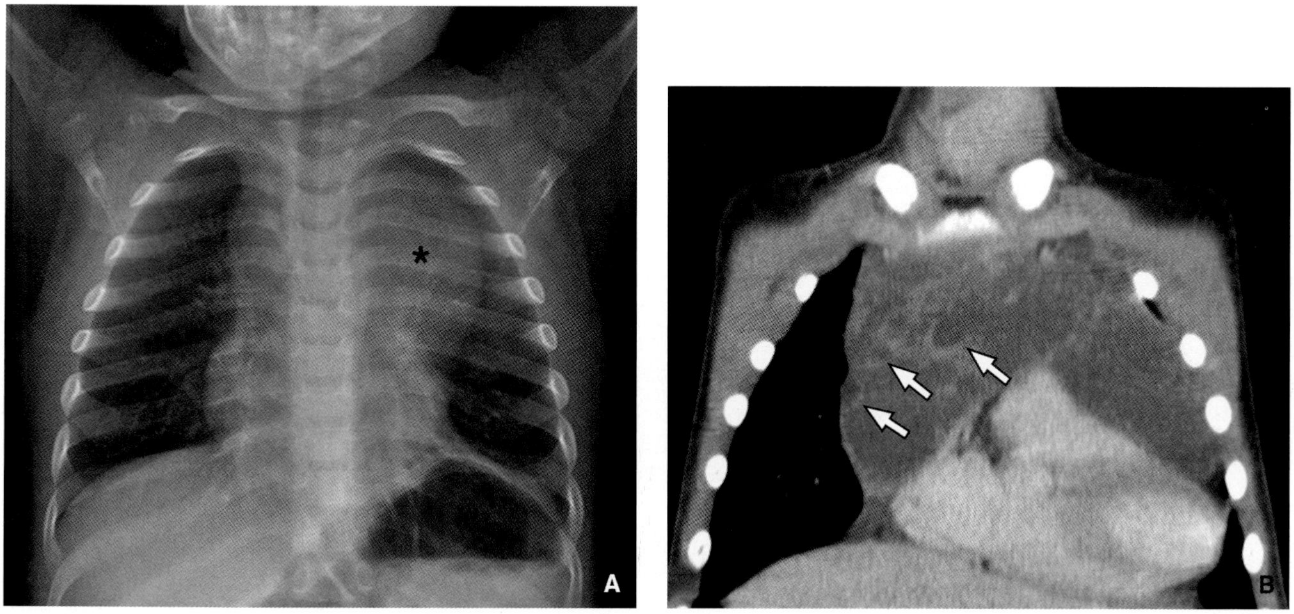

FIGURE 11.28 **A 4-year-old girl with mediastinal lymphatic malformaton (LM) who presented with respiratory distress.** **A:** Frontal chest radiograph demonstrates a smooth mediastinal mass (*asterisk*) with well-defined lateral margins. The margins of the hilum and the spine are both well-defined suggesting that the mass is located in the anterior mediastinum. **B:** Coronal enhanced CT image shows a well-defined anterior mediastinal mass, which is predominately nonenhancing with central water attenuation. There are faint, thin enhancing internal septations (*arrows*) within this macrocystic LM.

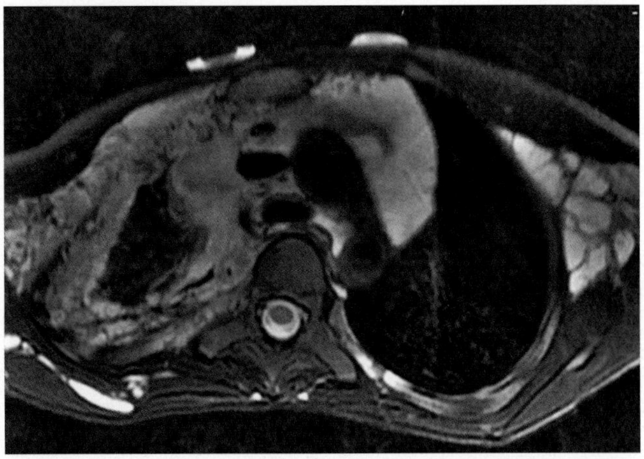

FIGURE 11.29 **A 10-year-old girl with an extensive lymphatic malformation of the chest wall and mediastinum.** Axial T2-weighted fat-saturated MR image demonstrates a multicystic, trans-spatial mass predominately located within the right hemithorax with invasion of the anterior mediastinum. Portions of the mass are seen along the both lateral chest walls and posteriorly on the right.

macrocystic variety of LMs. Given the infiltrative characteristic of LMs, surgical resection may be difficult or in some instances impossible. Thus, it is important for accurate characterization and description of involved or encased normal adjacent structures on preoperative MRI.

Middle Mediastinal Lesions

Congenital Foregut Duplication Cyst

Foregut duplication cysts are congenital anomalies arising from developmental malformations of the embryonic foregut. There are three main types: bronchogenic, esophageal, and neurenteric cysts. Foregut duplication cysts account for 11% of all pediatric mediastinal masses and are the most common primary middle mediastinal mass.[1,6,44,50] Differentiation between the three types of foregut duplication cysts is based on the underlying histology with bronchogenic cysts demonstrating respiratory mucosa and often cartilage, esophageal duplication cysts having squamous mucosa, and neurenteric cysts having a mixture of neural elements and gastrointestinal epithelium. Histologically, many of these lesions demonstrate hybrid features, and the general term foregut duplication cyst may be most apt. For all practical purposes, it is probably prudent for the imager to refer to these entities in the generic term as foregut duplication cysts. There are very few imaging features that can accurately subcategorize these lesions with a few exceptions, such as the presence of a vertebral cleft in neurenteric cysts.

Bronchogenic cysts result from abnormal lung budding during ventral foregut development in the first trimester. They may be located anywhere along the tracheoesophageal tree but are most commonly found in the subcarinal and right paratracheal regions (Fig. 11.30).[2] In 20% of cases, bronchogenic cysts may be intraparenchymal.[2] Most affected pediatric patients are asymptomatic. However, in larger lesions, patients may present with dyspnea related to compression of adjacent airway structures.

Esophageal duplication cysts result from maldevelopment of the posterior division of the embryonic foregut. They are typically located adjacent to the upper third of the esophagus but may be found anywhere along the course of the esophagus and even within the lung parenchyma (Fig. 11.31). Most commonly, affected pediatric patients with esophageal duplication cysts present with dysphagia.[2]

Neurenteric cysts result from failure of complete separation of the gastrointestinal tract from the primitive neural crest, representing one variant of the split notochord syndrome. Most neurenteric cysts are located within the posterior mediastinum and may extend into or communicate

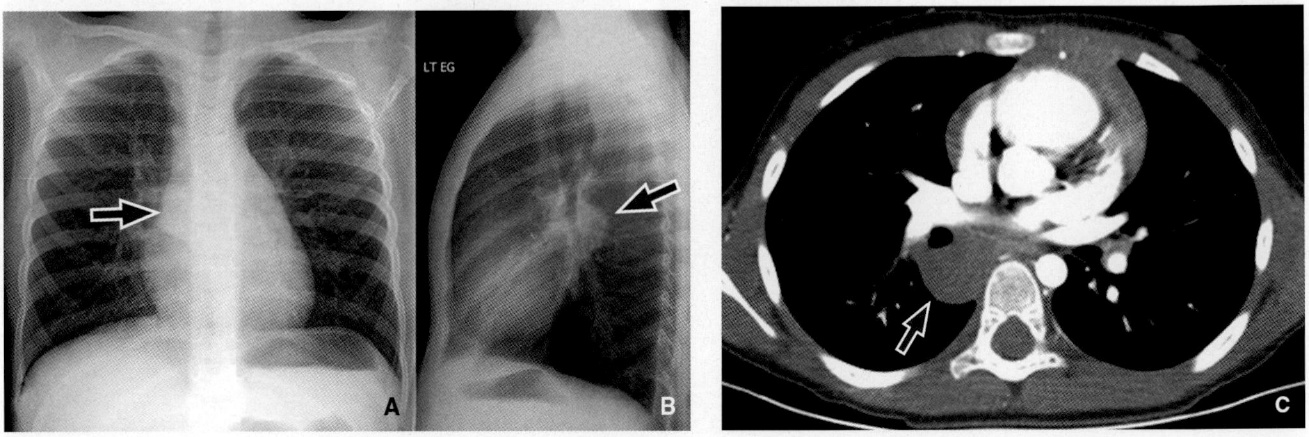

FIGURE 11.30 **A 5-year-old girl with bronchogenic cyst who presented with respiratory distress. A, B:** Frontal chest radiograph **(A)** demonstrates a smoothly marginated mass (*arrow*) visible just to the right of the spine, overlying the right superior aspect of the heart. Lateral chest radiograph **(B)** shows the mass (*arrow*) to be located within the middle mediastinum in a subcarinal location. **C:** Axial enhanced CT image demonstrates the middle mediastinal mass (*arrow*) to be smoothly marginated and of water attenuation consistent with an uncomplicated foregut duplication cyst, pathologically proven to be a bronchogenic cyst.

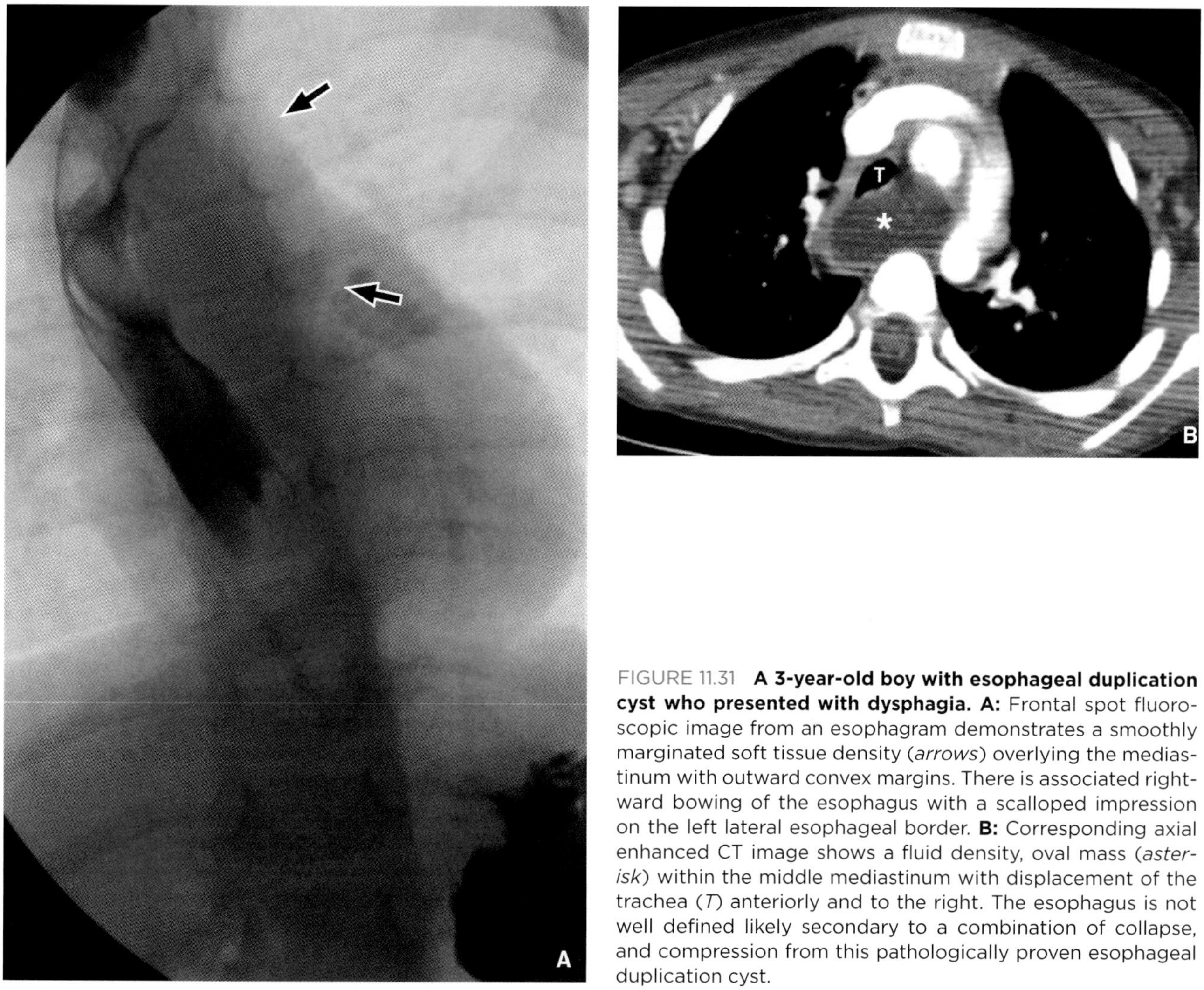

FIGURE 11.31 **A 3-year-old boy with esophageal duplication cyst who presented with dysphagia. A:** Frontal spot fluoroscopic image from an esophagram demonstrates a smoothly marginated soft tissue density (*arrows*) overlying the mediastinum with outward convex margins. There is associated rightward bowing of the esophagus with a scalloped impression on the left lateral esophageal border. **B:** Corresponding axial enhanced CT image shows a fluid density, oval mass (*asterisk*) within the middle mediastinum with displacement of the trachea (*T*) anteriorly and to the right. The esophagus is not well defined likely secondary to a combination of collapse, and compression from this pathologically proven esophageal duplication cyst.

with the adjacent spinal canal (Fig. 11.32). In such cases, neurenteric cysts are often associated with a congenital defect within the adjacent vertebral body through which portions of the cyst pass to communicate with the spinal cord. Affected pediatric patients usually present with pain leading to imaging evaluation.[2]

On chest radiography, all three foregut duplication cyst types present as smoothly marginated, oval or rounded middle mediastinal masses (Fig. 11.30). With neurenteric cysts, an adjacent vertebral anomaly may be demonstrated (Fig. 11.32A). Location may be helpful in suggesting the ultimate histologic diagnosis but is in no way definitive given the substantial overlap in lesion location and intracystic epithelial elements.

On cross-sectional imaging, foregut duplication cysts are nonenhancing, cystic lesions with well-marginated borders (Figs. 11.30 to 11.32). Approximately one-half will have simple fluid attenuation value (~0 HU) at CT (Fig. 11.30B) and uniform T2 hyperintensity on MRI (Fig. 11.32B).[2] However, with increased intracystic proteinaceous contents, superimposed infection or hemorrhage, the intracystic contents may be more complex with higher attenuation value on CT and hyperintense T1 signal on MRI. Such higher attenuation value on CT and hyperintense T1 signal on MRI of these foregut duplication cysts may cause diagnostic dilemma due to similar imaging findings that can be seen in solid mediastinal masses. In this situation, T2-weighted MR imaging is helpful because complex foregut duplication cysts show hyperintense T2 signal on MRI, confirming the cystic nature of the lesion. In addition to increased attenuation value on CT and hyperintense T2 signal on MRI, with superimposed infection, the foregut duplication cysts wall may become more irregular and thickened with associated contrast enhancement.

Surgical resection is currently the management of choice for all three types of foregut duplication cysts, particularly in the symptomatic pediatric patient. Additionally, endoscopic ultrasound-guided aspiration has been utilized in some institutions preoperatively to confirm the diagnosis and is generally considered safe.[51] However, this procedure is not without complications such as infection and is not routinely performed at all institutions.[52]

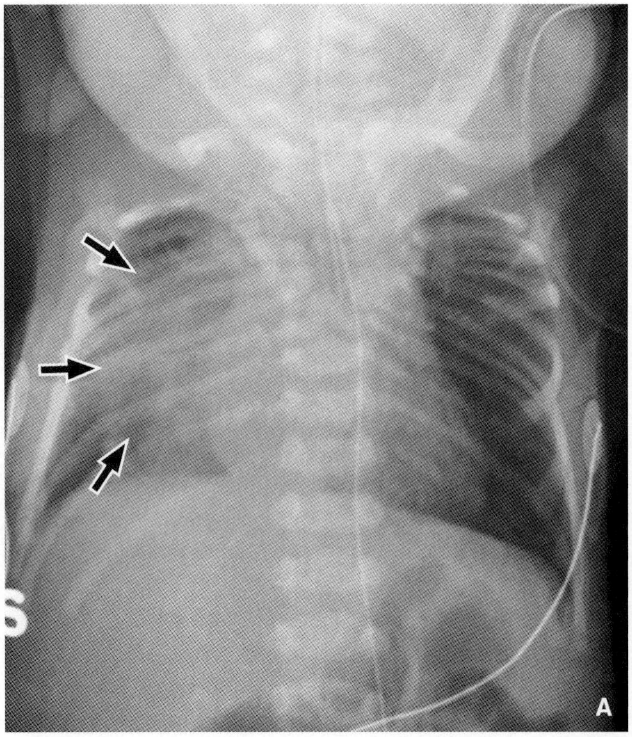

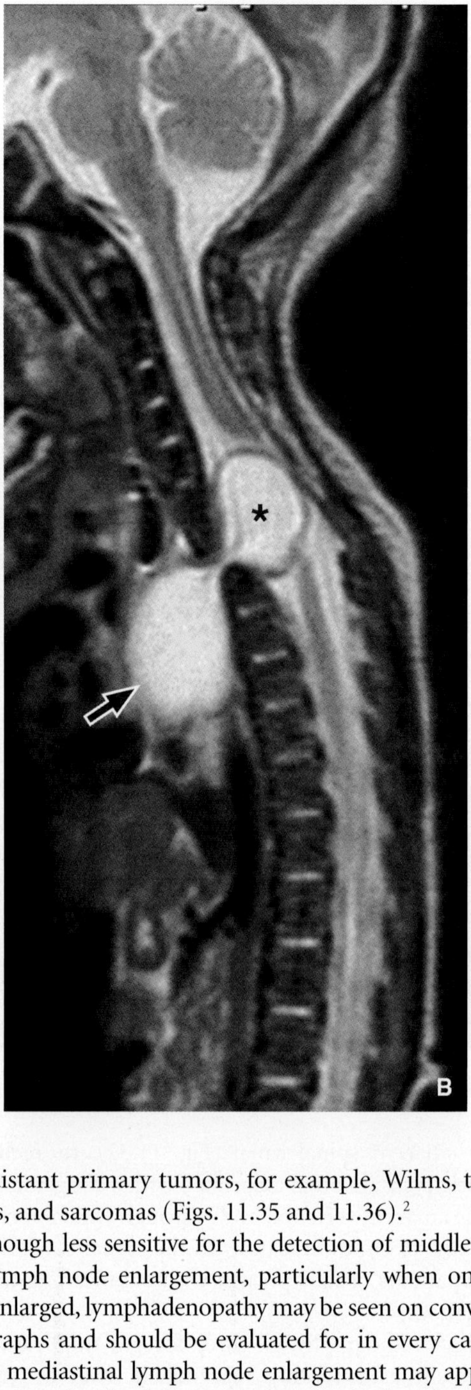

FIGURE 11.32 **A 5-day-old boy with neurenteric cyst. A:** Frontal chest radiograph demonstrates multiple segmentation anomalies of the upper thoracic spine with widely splayed vertebral body analogs and associated crowding of the rib interspaces with deformity of the upper chest wall. Additionally, there is hazy opacity through the right hemithorax (*arrows*). **B:** Sagittal T2-weighted MR image of the thoracic spine demonstrates a well-circumscribed posterior mediastinal cystic mass (*arrow*) extending through a defect in the thoracic spine with a large intracanalicular component (*asterisk*). The spinal canal is widened by the cystic mass, and the spinal cord is significantly compressed.

Lymphadenopathy

Although lymphadenopathy may occur in any of the mediastinal compartments, it is most prevalent in the middle mediastinum in both pediatric and adult populations. Here, the vast majority of pediatric middle mediastinal lymph node enlargement is reactive in nature with the most common infectious causes resulting from granulomatous diseases such as tuberculosis (Fig. 11.33) and histoplasmosis.[1,6,31,44,53] However, neoplastic processes may also afflict the middle mediastinal lymph nodes, with lymphoma being the most common. Because lymphoma has already been discussed earlier in the chapter, it is not further considered in this section.

A recently characterized primary neoplasm, which typically occurs in the midline, commonly in the head, neck, or mediastinum in the pediatric population, is the nuclear protein in testis (NUT) carcinoma. This rare but highly lethal neoplasm is characterized by a chromosomal rearrangement involving the gene NUT. The gene BRD4 is its most common translocation partner, forming a BRAD4-NUT fusion oncogene (Fig. 11.34).[54,55] Secondary neoplastic involvement of the mediastinal lymph nodes often results from metastatic spread from distant primary tumors, for example, Wilms, testicular tumors, and sarcomas (Figs. 11.35 and 11.36).[2]

Although less sensitive for the detection of middle mediastinal lymph node enlargement, particularly when only minimally enlarged, lymphadenopathy may be seen on conventional radiographs and should be evaluated for in every case. Here, middle mediastinal lymph node enlargement may appear as a round or lobulated soft tissue density often in the subcarinal and hilar regions (Fig. 11.33A). Calcification may be seen in cases of granulomatous disease, with ossifying metastatic lesions, such as osteosarcoma metastasis, and with treated lymphoma.

Nevertheless, the majority of middle mediastinal lymphadenopathy is detected and characterized by CT or MRI. With either modality, enlarged lymph nodes appear as a homogeneous soft tissue mass with generally well-defined borders (Fig. 11.33B). Necrotic areas may be demonstrated as areas of low density on CT and heterogeneous signal intensity on MRI (Fig. 11.33B). With both modalities, postcontrast imaging demonstrates no associated enhancement within these necrotic foci. Areas of calcification may be seen on CT as areas of increased density and on MRI as hypointense foci. Both calcification and

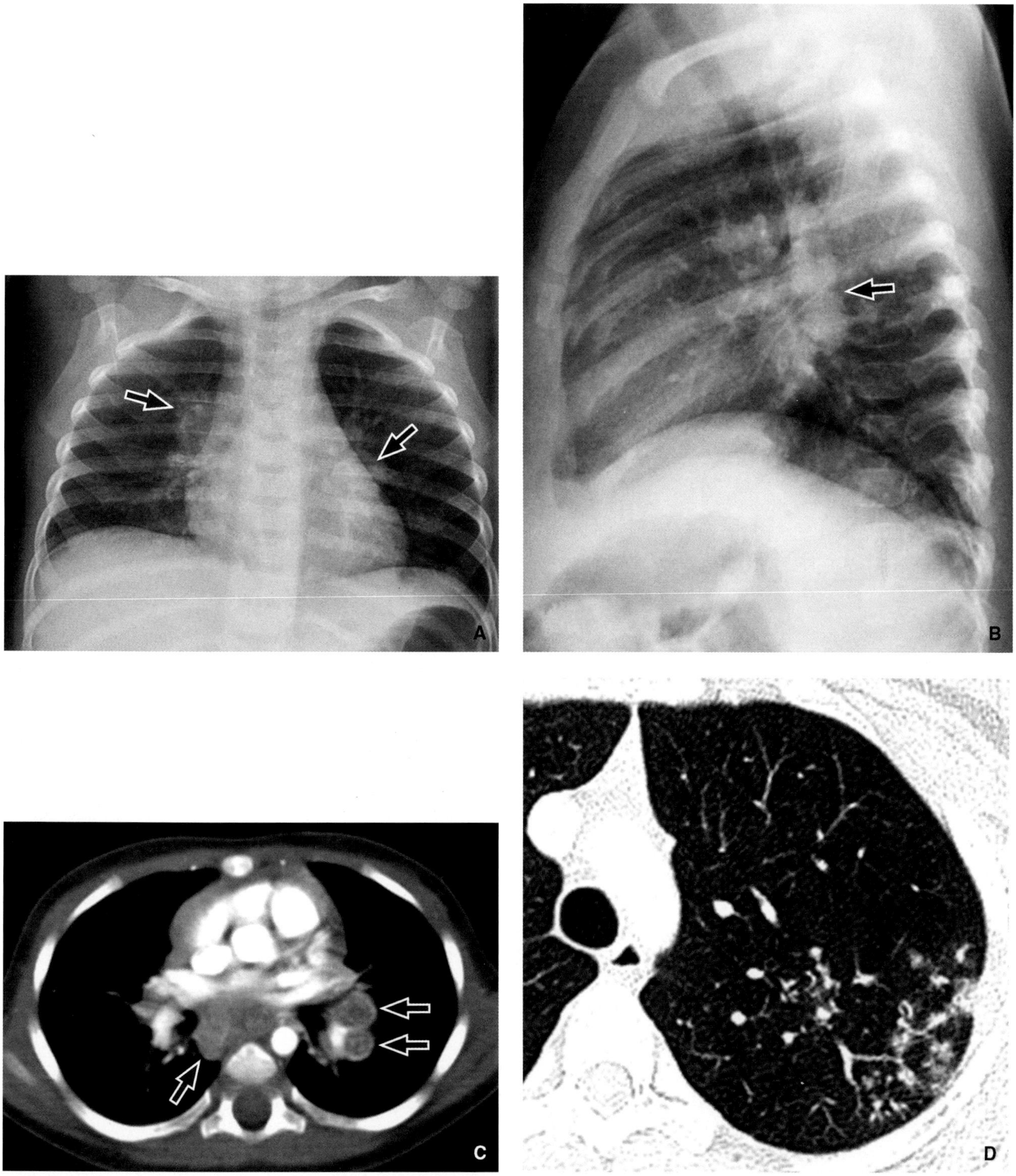

FIGURE 11.33 **A 2-year-old boy with middle mediastinal hypodense lymphadenopathy due to tuberculosis. A, B:** Frontal **(A)** and lateral **(B)** chest radiographs demonstrate multiple, lobulated soft tissue densities (*arrows*) near the bilateral hilar regions and within the middle mediastinum. **C:** Axial enhanced CT image shows multiple, well-defined, round, and oval lymph nodes (*arrows*) within the hilar, right paratracheal, and subcarinal regions. There is minimal associated enhancement, and overall the lymph nodes are hypodense, a finding that is typically associated with tuberculosis as was the final diagnosis in this patient. **D:** Axial lung window CT image demonstrates tree-and-bud opacification of the posterolateral left lung in a different pediatric patient diagnosed with tuberculosis.

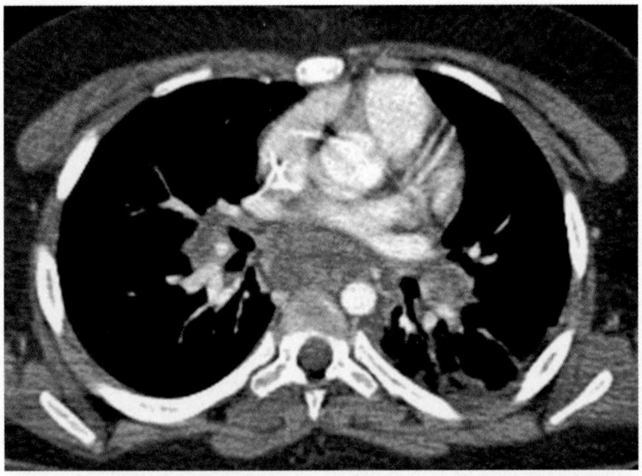

FIGURE 11.34 **An 18-year-old male with NUT midline carcinoma of the mediastinum.** Axial enhanced CT image demonstrates an infiltrative, heterogeneously enhancing soft tissue mass encasing multiple mediastinal structures, compressing the posterior left atrium, and extending laterally and encasing both hila.

necrosis should raise the possibility of prior granulomatous infection in the pediatric population, particularly tuberculosis.

A unique, nonneoplastic cause of middle mediastinal lymphadenopathy, typically along the right paratracheal and hilar regions, is Castleman disease (Fig. 11.37). Castleman disease represents a form of nonclonal lymph node hyperplasia and is associated with concurrent disease processes including human herpesvirus 8, human immunodeficiency virus, lymphoma, paraneoplastic pemphigus, plasma cell dyscrasia, and POEMS (polyneuropathy, organomegaly, endocrinopathy, M protein, and skin changes). Most commonly, Castleman disease manifests in the third and fourth decades of life, but rarely, it manifests in the pediatric population.[56–58] In children, Castleman disease may be mistaken for neoplastic and/or reactive adenopathy. However, unlike the aforementioned entities, Castleman disease classically presents with hyperenhancing, enlarged lymph nodes on CT and MRI, a feature not common for other entities to the extent seen in Castleman disease. The only exception to this classic presentation is in the case of the

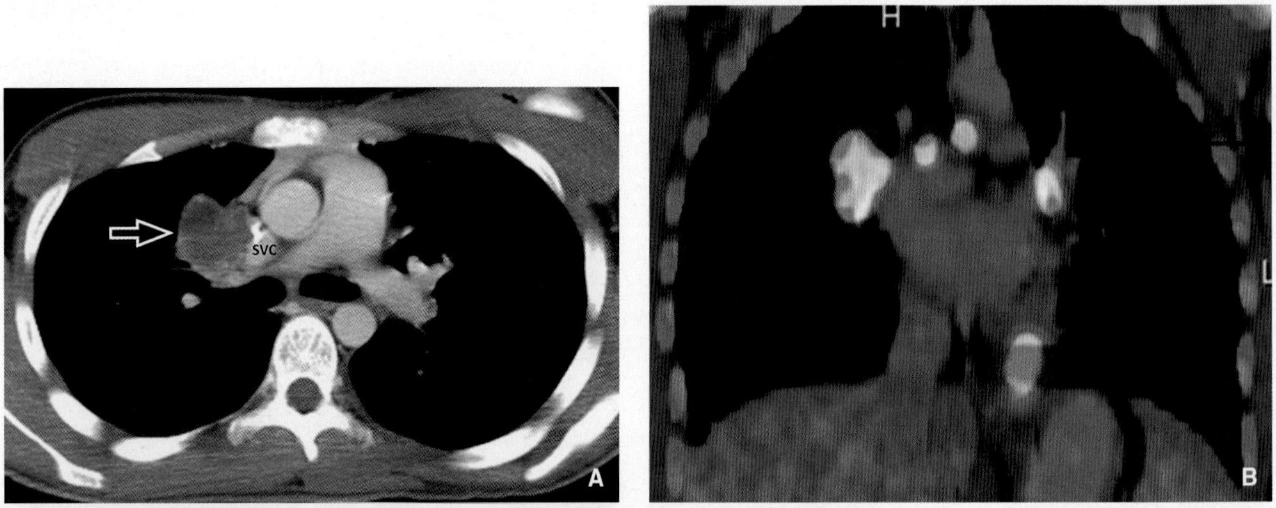

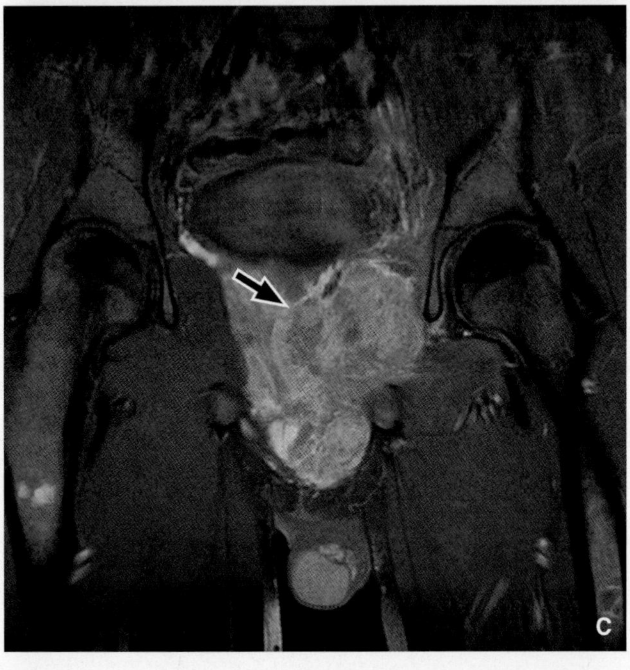

FIGURE 11.35 **A 13-year-old boy with metastatic pelvic rhabdomyosarcoma. A:** Axial enhanced CT image demonstrates a relatively low-density, lobulated mass (*arrow*) in the lateral right anterior mediastinum compressing the superior vena cava (*SVC*). **B:** Corresponding coronal fused PET/CT image demonstrates marked FDG avidity within multiple mediastinal regions in this patient with metastatic lymphadenopathy from his known pelvic rhabdomyosarcoma. **C:** Coronal enhanced T1-weighted fat-saturated MR image of the pelvis shows a large, heterogeneously enhancing low pelvic mass (*arrow*). There are partially visualized small abnormal foci of marrow enhancement in the proximal right femur consistent with osseous metastases.

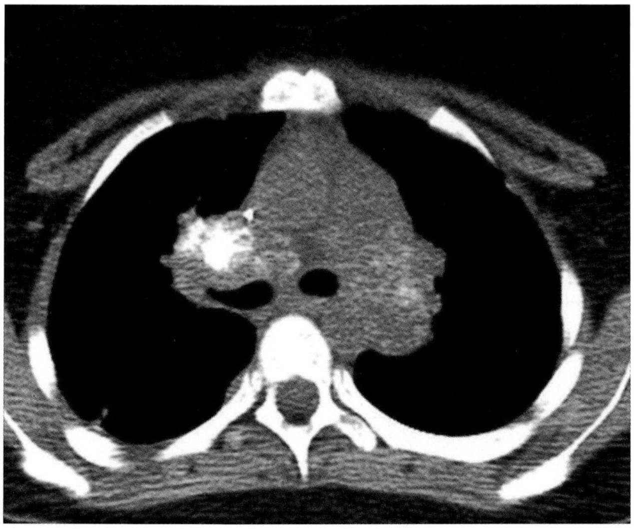

FIGURE 11.36 **A 13-year-old girl with metastatic osteosarcoma from the left femur.** Axial noncontrast chest CT image shows conglomerated, calcified lymph nodes anterior to the right mainstem bronchus. Additionally, there are faint calcifications with an irregular soft tissue conglomerate lateral to the left mainstem bronchus.

plasma cell variant, which demonstrates less avid enhancement compares with the hyaline vascular variant of Castleman disease.[58] Internal calcifications may be seen in up to 10% of cases and is best demonstrated on chest radiography and CT.[58] Central hypoattenuation on CT can be seen rarely.[58]

Treatment for nonlymphomatous middle mediastinal lymphadenopathy is predicated on the underlying etiology. For reactive/infectious disease, microbiologic confirmation and treatment of the underlying organism is often needed except in previously treated tuberculosis with residual calcified lymphadenopathy. For neoplastic lymphadenopathy, surgical resection may be an option. However, often this is in additional to neoadjuvant chemotherapy. Treatment for Castleman disease depends on histopathogenic classification.

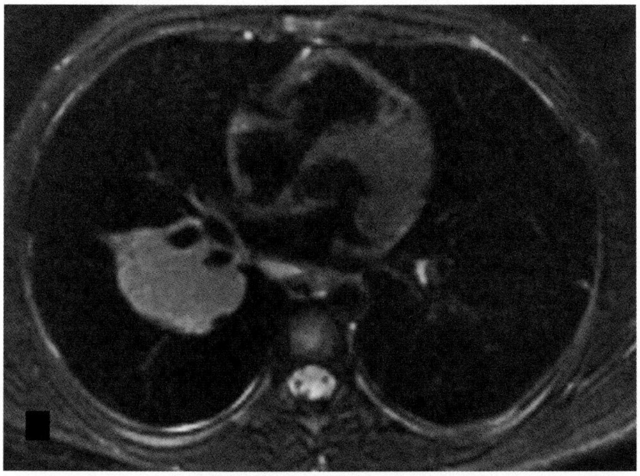

FIGURE 11.37 **A 15-year-old girl with Castleman disease.** Axial T2-weighted fat-saturated MR image demonstrates a mostly well-circumscribed, homogeneously T2 hyperintense mass within the right hila.

Unicentric hyaline vascular Castleman disease may be cured with surgical resection alone. On the contrary, multicentric Castleman disease may require chemotherapy, steroids, antiviral medications, or extensive antiproliferative regimens.[58]

Posterior Mediastinal Lesions

Neuroblastic Tumors

Posterior mediastinal masses compose 34% of pediatric mediastinal tumors with 88% to 90% of neuroblastic origin.[1,2,31] In the pediatric population, the vast majority are neuroblastomas (Fig. 11.38) with the remainder including ganglioneuroblastoma (Fig. 11.39) and ganglioneuroma. These three tumors form a spectrum of neoplastic disease with ganglioneuromas representing the type with the most cellular differentiation and neuroblastomas having the least cellular differentiation and being the most malignant. Imaging alone is incapable of differentiating among these tumors types, with the exception that the detection of a discrete nodule within a neuroblastic tumor can help to suggest the nodular subtype of ganglioneuroblastoma. Nevertheless, imaging plays a important role in identifying and characterizing the mass and its extent.

Neuroblastic tumors typically develop in children <5 years of age, arising in the mediastinum in only 10% to 16% of cases.[31] Mediastinal location is associated with older patient age and mature/benign subtype (Fig. 11.40). Affected pediatric patients often present with constitutional symptoms including irritability, fever, anemia, and weight loss.[2] Other rare but characteristic presentations of neuroblastoma include opsoclonus myoclonus syndrome, Horner syndrome (due to tumor compression of the cervical or thoracic sympathetic chain), transverse myelopathy (due to tumor spinal cord compression), treatment-resistant diarrhea (due to tumor vasoactive intestinal peptide secretion), and hypertension (due to catecholamine secretion). However, some affected pediatric patients are asymptomatic, particularly those with ganglioneuromas, which are typically discovered incidentally on imaging acquired for an alternative purpose. Once discovered, urinary analysis may be undertaken, with urinary catecholamines positive in 76% of neuroblastoma patients.[31,59]

Chest radiographs typically demonstrate a well-defined soft tissue opacity in the paraspinal posterior mediastinum (Fig. 11.38A). Intratumoral calcifications are present in up to 30% of cases.[2] Additionally, erosions of adjacent vertebral bodies and ribs or splaying of the intercostal spaces may be seen and is highly suggestive of an underlying neurogenic tumor.[1,6,44,45,53] Once demonstrated on chest radiographs, CT and MRI are usually indicated for further characterization and evaluation of disease extent.

On CT, neuroblastomas appear as well-circumscribed lenticular paraspinal masses with punctate or curvilinear calcifications (Fig. 11.38B). Encasement of blood vessels and extension into the adjacent neural foramina can be seen on CT but is better characterized by MRI (Fig. 11.38C). Given this fact, MRI is the modality of choice for the evaluation of local tumor spread and the detection of intraspinal canal extension. On MRI, neuroblastomas appear as a well-defined

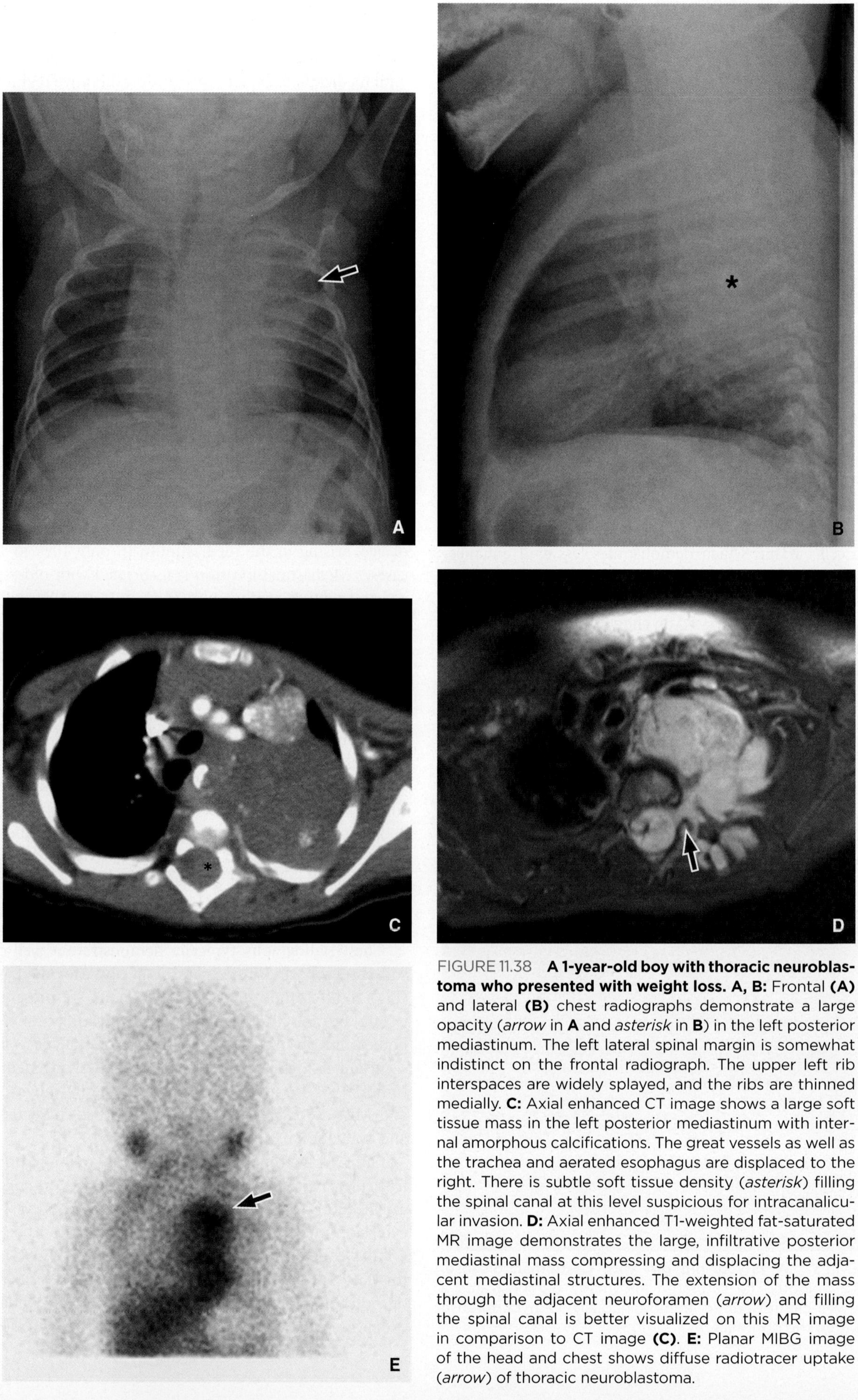

FIGURE 11.38 **A 1-year-old boy with thoracic neuroblastoma who presented with weight loss. A, B:** Frontal **(A)** and lateral **(B)** chest radiographs demonstrate a large opacity (*arrow* in **A** and *asterisk* in **B**) in the left posterior mediastinum. The left lateral spinal margin is somewhat indistinct on the frontal radiograph. The upper left rib interspaces are widely splayed, and the ribs are thinned medially. **C:** Axial enhanced CT image shows a large soft tissue mass in the left posterior mediastinum with internal amorphous calcifications. The great vessels as well as the trachea and aerated esophagus are displaced to the right. There is subtle soft tissue density (*asterisk*) filling the spinal canal at this level suspicious for intracanalicular invasion. **D:** Axial enhanced T1-weighted fat-saturated MR image demonstrates the large, infiltrative posterior mediastinal mass compressing and displacing the adjacent mediastinal structures. The extension of the mass through the adjacent neuroforamen (*arrow*) and filling the spinal canal is better visualized on this MR image in comparison to CT image **(C)**. **E:** Planar MIBG image of the head and chest shows diffuse radiotracer uptake (*arrow*) of thoracic neuroblastoma.

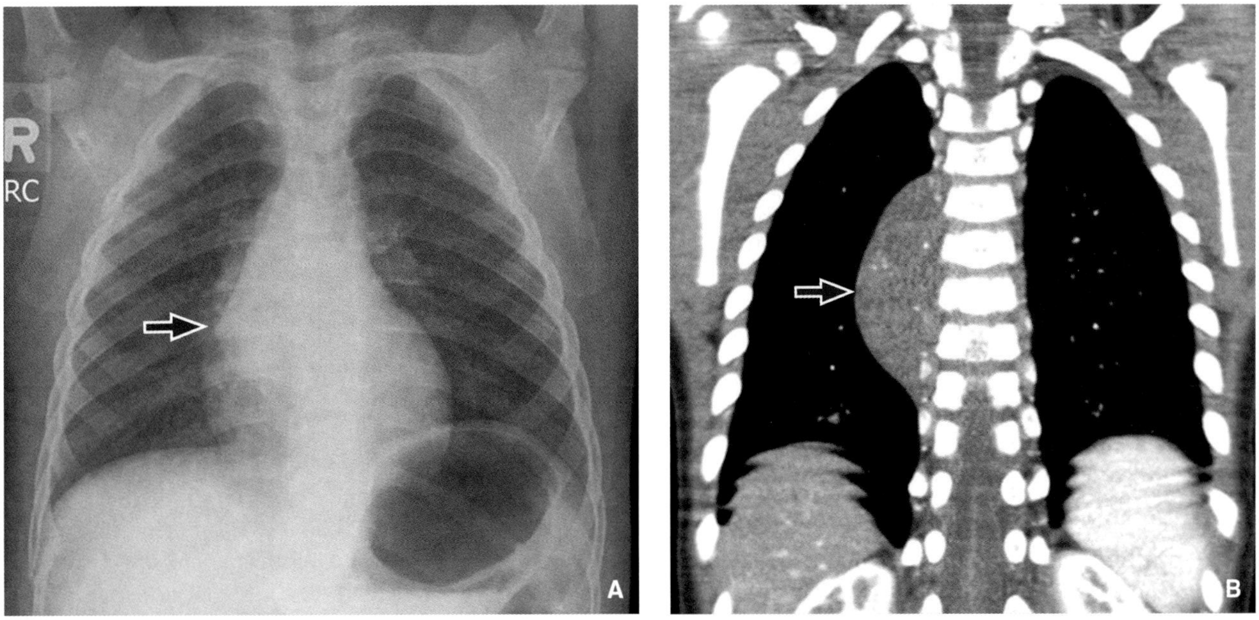

FIGURE 11.39 **A 6-year-old boy with a thoracic ganglioneuroblastoma who presented with chest pain. A:** Frontal chest radiograph demonstrates a well-defined, lenticular-shaped, soft tissue mass (*arrow*) along the right paraspinal region. **B:** Coronal enhanced CT image shows this posterior mediastinal mass (*arrow*) to contain punctate calcification with minimal associated contrast-enhancement.

T2 hyperintense mass with low signal on T1. After the administration of contrast, there is usually rapid and homogeneous enhancement reflecting the highly vascular nature of the mass. Four usual locations of metastatic disease from neuroblastoma include the bone (cortical or marrow), local and distant lymph nodes, liver, and skin. Osseous metastasis to the vertebral bodies and chest wall show a permeative or lytic destructive pattern. Hepatic metastasis presents as either focal or multiple masses or hepatomegaly in the setting of diffuse involvement. Neuroblastoma skin metastasis is usually only seen in infants and has characteristic bluish discoloration.

Neuroblastoma represents an area in which nuclear medicine techniques, particularly MIBG, are very helpful in workup and treatment evaluation. On MIBG, thoracic neuroblastomas demonstrate a focus of abnormal radiotracer uptake within the paravertebral posterior mediastinum (Fig. 11.38D). Metastases are identifiable and should be searched for on MIBG imaging. Generally, MIBG imaging is performed prior to surgical and medical intervention as it is helpful in prognosis and treatment evaluation. It is important to note on pretreatment imaging whether or not neuroblastomas are MIBG positive. If initially positive, neuroblastomas may subsequently become MIBG

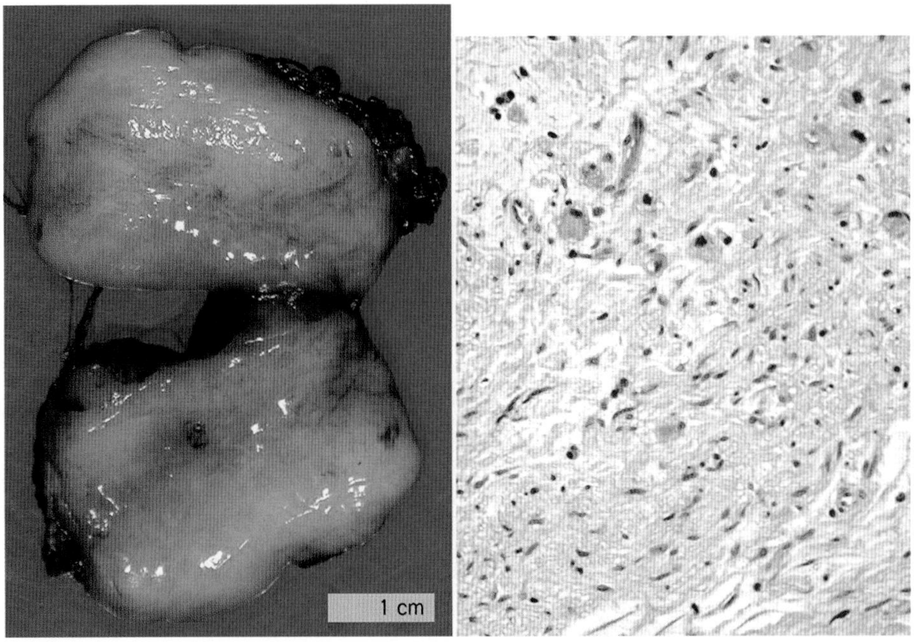

FIGURE 11.40 **Ganglioneuroma from the thoracic paraspinal region of a 5-year-old boy.** The tumor is grossly tan and homogeneous (**left**). Microscopically, abundant schwannian-type stroma contains admixed mature ganglion cells (**right**; hematoxylin and eosin, original magnification, 400×). Nests of primitive neuroblasts characteristic of neuroblastoma and ganglioneuroblastoma are absent.

negative as the mass involutes during chemotherapy. However, in cases of recurrent or unresponsive neuroblastoma, an initially MIBG-positive tumor that is found on follow-up imaging to not have MIBG avidity denotes a poor prognostic sign as it indicates dedifferentiation of the mass, yielding a more primitive and aggressive variant.

For the benign neuroblastic tumors such as ganglioneuromas and most ganglioneuroblastomas, simple excision is curative. Treatment for neuroblastomas relies on a combination of chemotherapy and surgical resection. For the "favorable histology" tumors on this spectrum, prognosis is usually good.[60,61] Conversely, "unfavorable histology" neuroblastomas have the poorest prognosis, particularly if metastatic. One exception to this rule lies in stage 4S neuroblastoma pediatric patients who have isolated metastatic lesions to the skin, liver, and/or bone marrow. Age less than 1 year is one of the conditions for diagnosis of stage 4S, which has an excellent prognosis.

Peripheral Nerve Sheath Tumors

In the pediatric population, peripheral nerve sheath tumors (PNSTs) are much less common than neuroblastic tumors. The two most common PNSTs are neurofibroma and Schwannoma.[2,31,62–64] When intrathoracic, these generally arise from intercostal nerves within the superior and posterior mediastinum and are composed of spindle cells, collagen, and variably myxoid extracellular matrix.[31] Plexiform neurofibromas are virtually pathognomonic for neurofibromatosis type 1. Plexiform neurofibromas, particularly those that are deep-seated, may give rise/degenerate into a malignant peripheral nerve sheath tumor (MPNST), which demonstrates cellular pleomorphism, increased cellular density, and sometimes necrosis and mitotic figures on histologic analysis (Fig. 11.41). Malignant peripheral nerve sheath tumors (MPNSTs) may also arise de novo or rarely from a preexisting schwannoma.[2]

With imaging, benign PNSTs appear as well-marginated, elliptical or rounded lesions within the paravertebral posterior mediastinal compartment.[62] These tumors are often localized to a single or two contiguous vertebral body interspaces, sometimes distinguishing them from sympathetic chain tumors that tend to course over several vertebral body levels (Fig. 11.42). On CT, PNSTs typically present as a soft tissue mass extending along the course of the corresponding intercostal nerve with homogeneous or heterogeneous attenuation (Fig. 11.42B). As with neuroblastic tumors, areas of calcification may be present, and neuroforaminal enlargement and intraspinal extension may be seen. MRI signal characteristics are what would be expected based on the previously described CT pattern with variation from homogeneous increased T2 signal to a heterogeneous appearance (Fig. 11.43). Most commonly, a peripheral pattern of enhancement is seen on CT and MRI after contrast administration. With plexiform neurofibromas, the pattern of peripheral enhancement gives a targetoid pattern of enhancement, which is classically and nearly pathognomonically associated with this lesion.

MPNSTs in contrast to their benign counterparts appear more aggressive on imaging with intraspinal extension and areas of decreased attenuation and variable enhancement related to cystic degeneration or lipid content.[2] However, the predominant imaging findings that help distinguish a malignant PNST from a benign PNST are local invasion, osseous destruction, rapid growth on serial imaging, and an associated pleural effusion (Fig. 11.44).[2] Additionally, FDG–PET imaging has been suggested to help distinguish in type 1 neurofibromatosis MPNST from benign neurofibromas with higher SUV values correlating with MPNST.[65]

Treatment for PNSTs relies generally on surgical resection if symptomatic and if imaging suggests findings concerning for malignant degeneration. However, for small lesions, no direct intervention is necessary other than imaging surveillance.

Infectious Disorders

Acute Mediastinitis

Acute mediastinal infection is a life-threatening and rapidly progressive infection of one or multiple mediastinal compartments often resulting from contiguous spread from adjacent regions, postoperative infection, or from posttraumatic causes.[66] Infection of the superior mediastinum is often from direct spread caudally from a concurrent cervical infection or from direct extension from sternoclavicular osteomyelitis (Fig. 11.45).[31,67–69] Much like infections in the superior mediastinum, infections within the posterior mediastinum

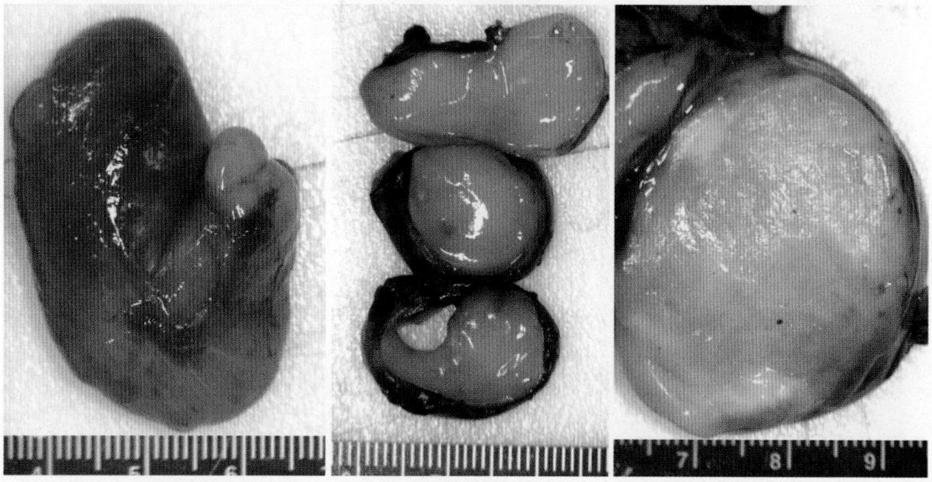

FIGURE 11.41 **Low-grade malignant peripheral nerve sheath tumor, arising in a mediastinal plexiform neurofibroma in a 17-year-old girl with known neurofibromatosis type 1.** The uncut specimen **(left)** resembles the "bag of worms" configuration of plexiform neurofibroma. The cut surfaces were focally soft and gelatinous **(middle)** and focally firm with yellow areas suspicious for necrosis **(right).** Microscopic examination (not shown) showed areas of increased cellularity, nuclear atypia, and occasional mitoses diagnostic of malignant transformation.

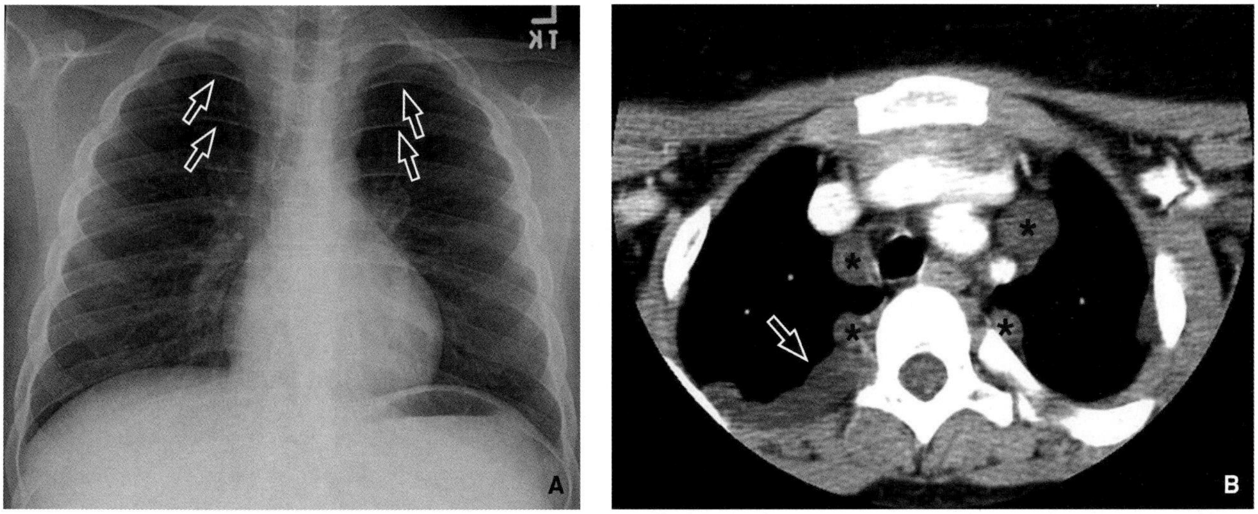

FIGURE 11.42 **Superior mediastinal widening due to multiple neurofibromas in a 15-year-old boy. A:** Frontal chest radiograph demonstrates widening of the superior mediastinum with lobulated lateral margins. There is widening of the upper thoracic rib interspaces bilaterally with subtle undersurface erosions (*arrows*). **B:** Axial enhanced CT image demonstrates multiple well-defined soft tissue masses (*asterisks*) with the larger right posterior mass (*arrow*) tracking along the course of the rib interspace in this patient with multiple mediastinal neurofibromas.

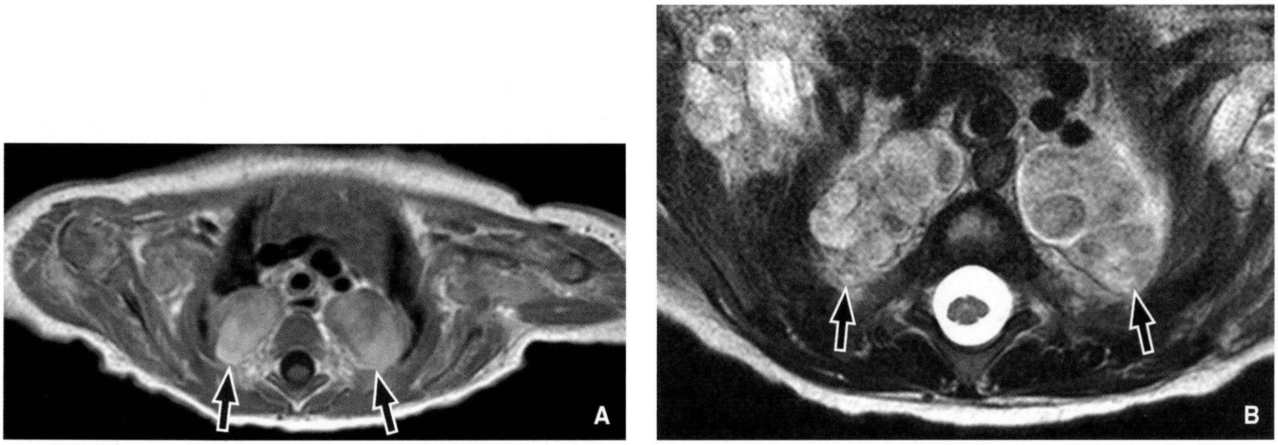

FIGURE 11.43 **A 2-year-old boy with neurofibromatosis. A:** Axial enhanced T1-weighted MR image demonstrates two oval, well-defined posterior mediastinal masses (*arrows*) with patchy internal enhancement. Findings are consistent with neurofibromas in this patient with known neurofibromatosis. Of note, there are partially visualized neurofibromas in both axillas. **B:** Axial T2-weighted MR image shows the bilateral posterior mediastinal/paravertebral masses (*arrows*) with the characteristic targetoid appearance.

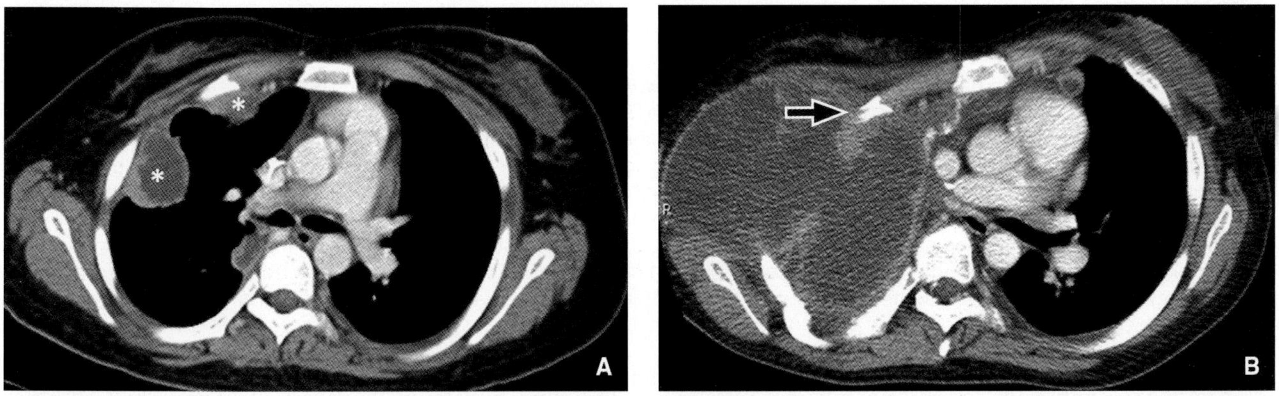

FIGURE 11.44 **A 19-year-old girl with malignant peripheral nerve sheath tumor. A:** Initial axial enhanced CT image demonstrates multiple heterogeneous nodular lesions (*asterisks*) within the anterolateral and posteromedial right chest. **B:** Follow-up axial enhanced CT image demonstrates progressive enlargement of the right chest mass with infiltration of the adjacent chest wall and ribs (*arrow*).

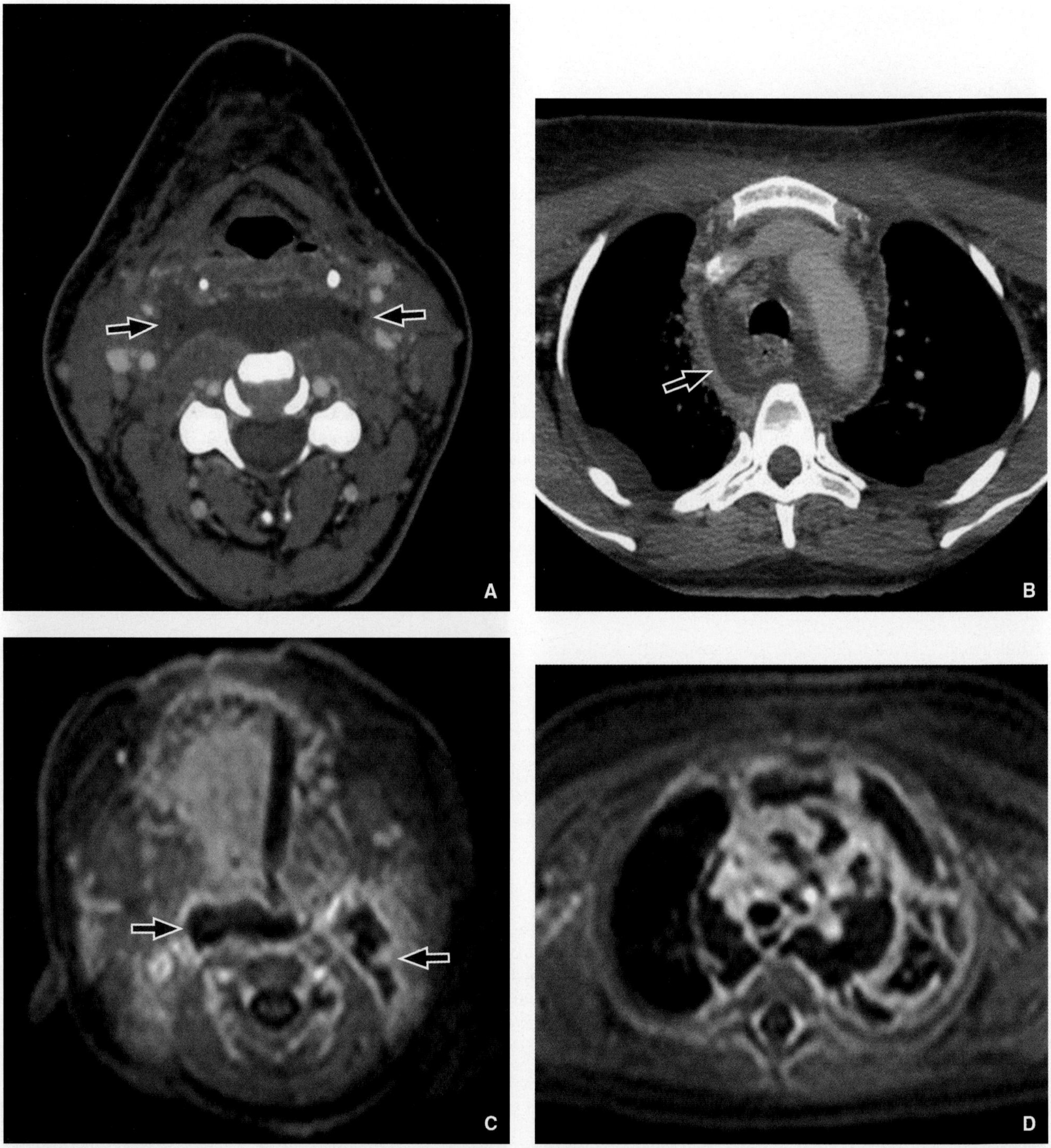

FIGURE 11.45 **Two pediatric patients with acute mediastinitis. A:** Axial enhanced CT image demonstrates an irregular, peripherally enhancing retropharyngeal fluid collecting (*arrows*) in a 13-year-old boy. There are also subtle tiny locules of air within the fluid collection. **B:** Axial enhanced CT image in the same patient as in **(A)** shows fluid (*arrow*) tracking into the mediastinum nearly circumferentially around the esophagus and trachea and adjacent to the medial margin of the aorta. There is an associated thick peripheral rind of enhancement and adjacent inflammatory change. **C:** Axial enhanced T1-weighted fat-saturated MR image in a 2-year-old girl demonstrates an irregular peripherally enhancing retropharyngeal fluid collection (*arrows*). There is extensive irregular enhancement in the adjacent subcutaneous soft tissues consistent with inflammatory edema. **D:** Axial enhanced T1-weighted fat-saturated MR image in the same patient as **(C)** shows a multiloculated fluid collection with thick internal septations. Findings are consistent with acute mediastinitis with multiloculated mediastinal abscess resulting from direct spread from a retropharyngeal abscess.

are often due to contiguous spread from adjacent vertebral osteomyelitis.[31] Anterior and middle mediastinal infections, by contrast, have a greater number of underlying etiologies including postoperative infection, misplaced instrumentation, and posttraumatic causes including child abuse and esophageal rupture from an impacted foreign body. Affected pediatric patients typically present with elevated laboratory infectious/inflammatory markers, fever, and pain.

Although findings on chest radiography are often nonspecific, radiographs are often the first modality utilized and may demonstrate loss of the normal mediastinal contours, mediastinal widening, and narrowing of the trachea in affected pediatric patients. Mediastinal gas may rarely be demonstrated but is highly worrisome for underlying mediastinitis. Nonetheless, contrast-enhanced CT is the current imaging modality of choice for the accurate and complete evaluation of mediastinal infection. Here, primary findings of mediastinitis include focal mediastinal fluid collections and gas. Additional CT findings of mediastinitis include mediastinal widening, lymphadenopathy, pleural and pericardial effusions, and hyperattenuation of the mediastinal fat.[66]

Acute mediastinitis represents a true emergency with aggressive treatment consisting of a combination of intravenous antibiotics and surgical irrigation necessary in order to avoid its substantial impact on patient morbidity and mortality. Continuous mediastinal irrigation and vacuum-assisted closure have also been recently shown to be efficacious.[31,70,71]

Fibrosing Mediastinitis

Fibrosing mediastinitis, which results from proliferation of acellular collagen and fibrous tissue, is rare in the pediatric population.[31,72,73] Underlying etiologies of fibrosing mediastinitis are varied and include sequelae of autoimmune disease, radiotherapy, medications, and sequelae of infection, for example, tuberculosis and histoplasmosis. Affected pediatric patients often present with symptoms related to narrowing of mediastinal structures. Respiratory distress is often resulted from tracheobronchial narrowing whereas dysphagia may present in patients with esophageal narrowing. In addition, facial and neck swelling from obstruction of the superior vena cava may occur.

On chest radiography, fibrosing mediastinitis typically presents as mediastinal widening with an associated paratracheal or subcarinal mass. Associated calcifications may be present within this mass particularly with underlying granulomatous disease. On cross-sectional imaging, specifically CT, fibrosing mediastinitis is categorized as either focal or diffuse (Fig. 11.46).[31,74] Focal fibrosing mediastinitis demonstrates a soft tissue mass within the paratracheal, subcarinal, or hilar regions, which is calcified in 63% of cases.[31,74] In the diffuse type, fibrosing mediastinitis presents on CT as an infiltrative soft tissue lesion, which may spread into multiple mediastinal compartments, surrounding and narrowing multiple mediastinal structures. Calcifications are typically not present in the diffuse type of fibrosing mediastinitis.

Treatment for fibrosing mediastinitis currently remains controversial. Medical therapies include systemic antifungal administration and corticosteroid therapies. Surgical treatment may be utilized in both the localized and diffuse forms. Surgery may be particularly necessary in the diffuse type when associated narrowing of the great vessels and airway is present.

Traumatic Disorders

Pneumomediastinum

Pneumomediastinum is defined as the abnormal presence of air within the mediastinum occurring in the pediatric population most frequently in infants.[75,76] Underlying etiologies may be categorized as those resulting iatrogenically, those that are spontaneous, and those with posttraumatic causes. Iatrogenic causes include changes related to prior surgery, mechanical ventilation with associated barotrauma, and intravascular catheter placement or cardiac catheterization. With forceful inhalation and Valsalva maneuvers, the intra-alveolar pressure may suddenly increase substantially resulting in rupture, air tracking along the bronchovascular tree, and subsequent spontaneous pneumomediastinum.[31] Lastly, pneumomediastinum may result from posttraumatic causes including penetrating trauma, esophageal rupture from an impacted foreign body, and focal tear or rupture of the esophagus related to forceful vomiting such as Boerhaave syndrome.[76]

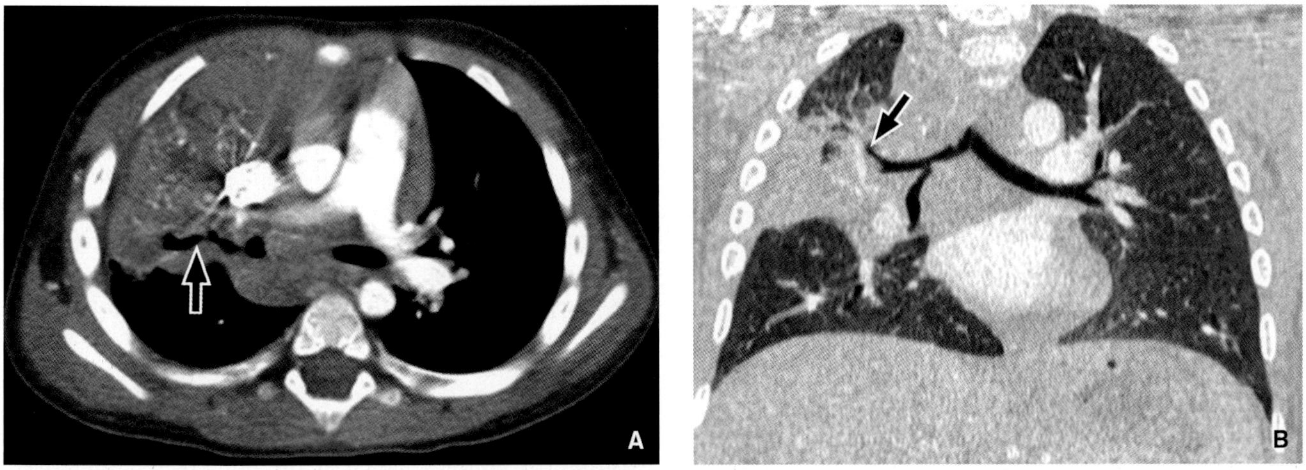

FIGURE 11.46 **A 7-year-old girl with tuberculosis-associated fibrosing mediastinitis. A:** Axial enhanced CT image demonstrates a large infiltrative soft tissue mass with amorphous internal calcifications within the right anterior mediastinum with extension into the subcarinal middle mediastinum. The right middle lobe bronchus (*arrow*) is partially visualized and irregular in contour related to retraction and narrowing in this patient with fibrosing mediastinitis. **B:** Corresponding coronal lung window CT image again demonstrates the infiltrative soft tissue lesion surrounding the carina, both mainstem bronchi, the bronchus intermedius, and the right middle lobe bronchus (*arrow*), which is retracted superiorly with multiple focal areas of narrowing.

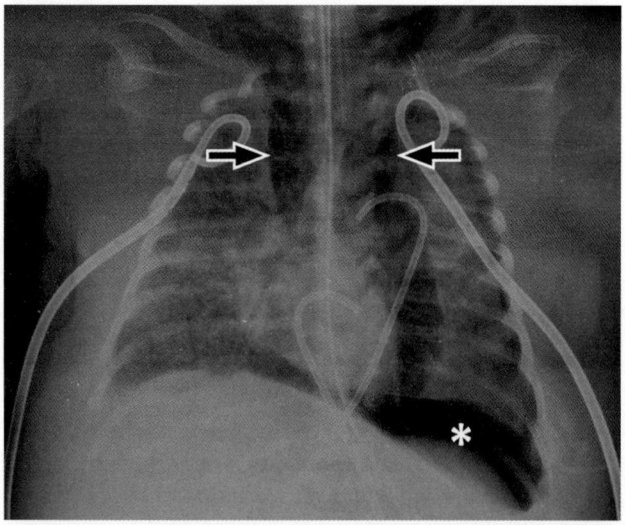

FIGURE 11.47 **A 1-week-old girl with pneumomediastinum.** Frontal chest radiograph demonstrates air filling (*arrows*) the mediastinum and tracking into the neck and along the left heart border. There is also a moderate-sized left pneumothorax (*asterisk*) with diffuse pulmonary opacities throughout the lungs. Also noted are endotracheal tube, nasogastric tube, and bilateral chest tubes.

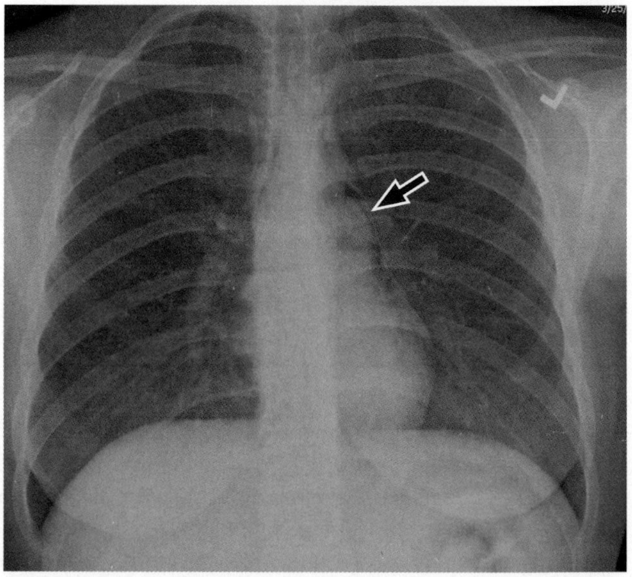

FIGURE 11.49 **A 16-year-old girl with pneumomediastinum who presented with left-sided chest pain.** Frontal chest radiograph shows a small amount of pneumomediastinum extending as a linear lucency (*arrow*) along the lateral margins of the left hilar region.

Patient presentation often is dependent largely on the underlying etiology. However, affected pediatric patients typically present with chest pain, retrosternal pressure, dysphagia, and dyspnea, particularly in the setting of spontaneous pneumomediastinum.

Chest radiography is the initial imaging modality of choice for identifying and evaluating pneumomediastinum (Figs. 11.47 to 11.49). Radiographic findings are largely predicated on the amount of air within the mediastinum.

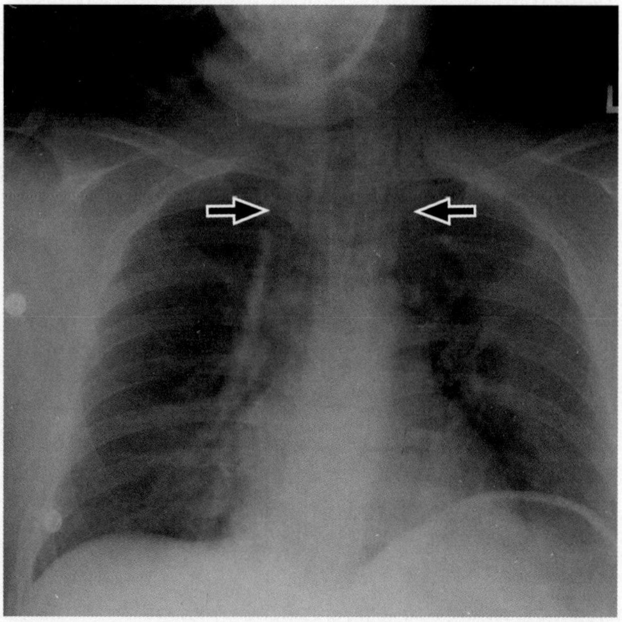

FIGURE 11.48 **A 17-year-old boy with asthma who presented with acute chest pain.** Frontal chest radiograph demonstrates diffuse, spontaneous pneumomediastinum (*arrows*) with air tracking into the base of the neck.

When only a small amount is present, pneumomediastinum appears as a focal curvilinear lucency most often along the left cardiac border. If around only the aorta, a thin lucency may be seen along the lateral margins of the aortic arch or descending aorta sharply outlining these structures. The so-called continuous diaphragm sign is due to air tracking between the pericardium and the diaphragm, resulting in the appearance of the diaphragm as a single continuous structure across the lower chest. With increasing volume of pneumomediastinum, air may be seen outlining the margins of structures on both sides of the mediastinum and may dissect along fascial planes into the neck or inferiorly into the abdomen resulting in pneumoperitoneum. With a moderate amount of pneumomediastinum, the classic "spinnaker sail" sign may be seen with the thymus conforming to the shape of a spinnaker sail as it is uplifted by the pneumomediastinum from more inferior mediastinal structures (Fig. 11.50).

Depending on the suspected underlying etiology, further imaging evaluation in addition to the chest radiograph may be necessary. For instance, with esophageal perforation, fluoroscopic esophagography may be necessary to determine the extent and location of the underlying esophageal defect. With penetrating trauma, in addition to an esophagram, CT may be necessary to demonstrate injury to vital mediastinal structures. Much like chest radiographs, CT demonstrates various amounts of air attenuation with the mediastinum, outlining the margins of mediastinal structures (Fig. 11.51).

Treatment for pediatric patients with pneumomediastinum is typically aimed at the underlying etiology. For esophageal perforation or rupture, treatment can include surgery, endoscopic covered stent placement, or nasogastric tube placement with prohibition of oral intake in the case of small perforations. In spontaneous pneumomediastinum,

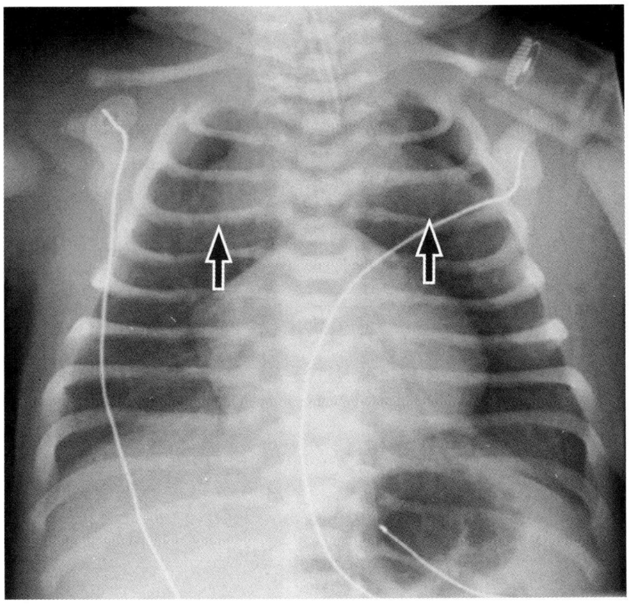

FIGURE 11.50 **A 2-day-old premature boy with acute respiratory distress.** Frontal radiograph shows the "spinnaker sail" sign, which refers to the thymus being outlined by air (i.e., pneumomediastinum) with each lobe (*arrows*) displaced laterally and appearing like spinnaker sails.

supportive therapy may be all that is required. Very rarely, with a large pneumomediastinum, tension pneumomediastinum may result requiring prompt decompression.

Mediastinal Hemorrhage and Hematoma

In the pediatric population, mediastinal hemorrhage often results from blunt force trauma with associated venous rupture.[31] With larger bleeds, the underlying etiology is generally due to rupture of larger caliber venous or arterial vessels from iatrogenic causes related to surgery or catheter placement and

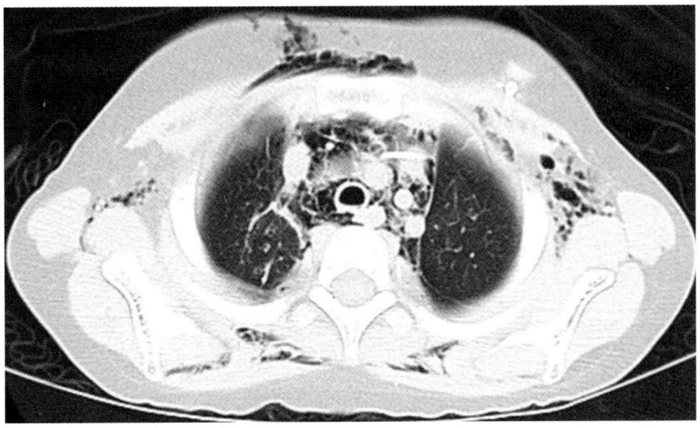

FIGURE 11.51 **An 8-year-old boy with posttraumatic pneumomediastinum.** Axial lung window CT image shows diffuse pneumomediastinum surrounding the trachea, esophagus, and great vessels. There is also extensive subcutaneous emphysema.

from penetrating trauma. Occasionally, underlying medical conditions such as hemophilia may result in spontaneous hemorrhage or rarely in the newborn, thymic hemorrhage thought to result from vitamin K deficiency.[31,77] Pediatric patients with mediastinal hemorrhage generally present with symptoms of dyspnea related to compression of mediastinal airway and vascular structures.

On chest radiography, mediastinal hemorrhage presents as nonspecific mediastinal widening and blurring of the aortic margins with displacement of the trachea or esophagus seen with increasing amounts of hemorrhage (Fig. 11.52). Opacity extending from the mediastinum over the left lung apex referred to as the "apical cap" sign may be a useful finding to suggest mediastinal hemorrhage.

Cross-sectional imaging is very sensitive for the evaluation of mediastinal hemorrhage and is often utilized following the initial chest radiograph. CT is by far the most widely

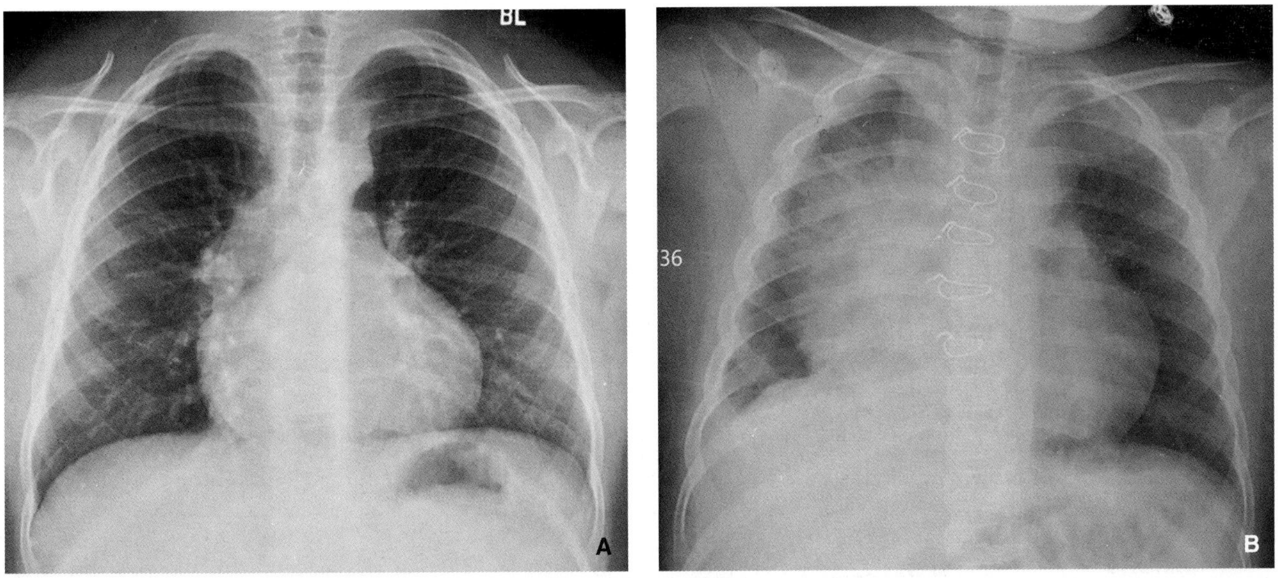

FIGURE 11.52 **A 6-year-old girl with mediastinal hematoma after heart transplant. A, B:** Preoperative **(A)** and postoperative **(B)** frontal chest radiographs demonstrate changes of a sternotomy and heart transplant with diffuse widening and outer convex borders of the superior mediastinum on the postoperative radiograph **(B).**

(*Continued*)

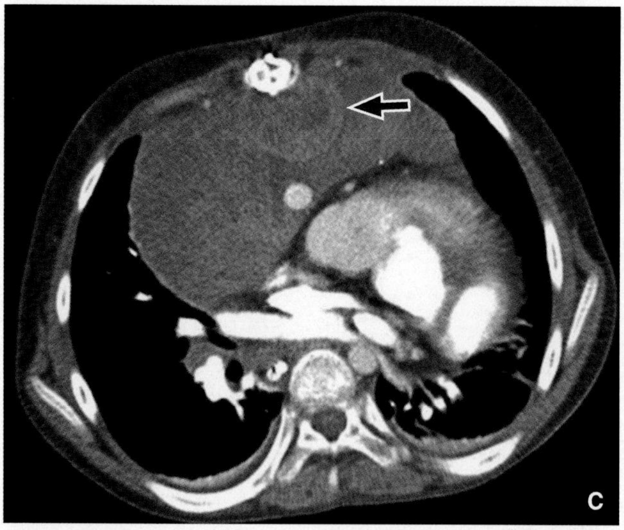

FIGURE 11.52 *(Continued)* **C:** Corresponding axial enhanced CT image shows a very large heterogeneous, mass-like opacity with amorphous areas of increased attenuation (*arrow*) consistent with blood products in this patient who developed a postoperative mediastinal hematoma.

employed of the cross-sectional modalities and superbly demonstrates mediastinal hemorrhage as a well-defined collection of mediastinal fluid with a density >20 Hounsfield units (Fig. 11.52C). Occasionally, active areas of hemorrhage may be seen with angiographic technique. The MRI appearance of mediastinal hemorrhage depends on the age of the hematoma but generally is of increased intensity on T1 in the acute setting. Ultrasound is less often utilized but may be of benefit in the neonate where it may demonstrate focal or diffuse enlargement of the thymus with heterogeneity of thymic echotexture in the region of hemorrhage.[78]

Treatment of mediastinal hemorrhage ranges from supportive care for a small amount of hemorrhage to urgent surgical exploration for large or symptomatic hemorrhages.

References

1. Lee EY. Evaluation of non-vascular mediastinal masses in infants and children: an evidence-based practical approach. *Pediatr Radiol.* 2009;39(suppl 2):S184–S190.
2. Ranganath SH, et al. Mediastinal masses in children. *AJR Am J Roentgenol.* 2012;198(3):W197–W216.
3. Kim OH, et al. US in the diagnosis of pediatric chest diseases. *Radiographics.* 2000;20(3):653–671.
4. Graeber GM, et al. The use of computed tomography in the evaluation of mediastinal masses. *J Thorac Cardiovasc Surg.* 1986;91(5):662–666.
5. Siegel MJ, Sagel SS, Reed K. The value of computed tomography in the diagnosis and management of pediatric mediastinal abnormalities. *Radiology.* 1982;142(1):149–155.
6. Williams HJ, Alton HM. Imaging of paediatric mediastinal abnormalities. *Paediatr Respir Rev.* 2003;4(1):55–66.
7. Gamsu G, et al. Magnetic resonance imaging of benign mediastinal masses. *Radiology.* 1984;151(3):709–713.
8. Webb WR, et al. Evaluation of magnetic resonance sequences in imaging mediastinal tumors. *AJR Am J Roentgenol.* 1984; 143(4):723–727.
9. von Schulthess GK, et al. Mediastinal masses: MR imaging. *Radiology.* 1986;158(2):289–296.
10. Siegel MJ, et al. Mediastinal lesions in children: comparison of CT and MR. *Radiology.* 1986;160(1):241–244.
11. Kornreich L, et al. Cystic mediastinal lesions in children: evaluation by magnetic resonance and conventional imaging. *Eur J Pediatr.* 1992;151(1):38–41.
12. Murayama S, et al. Signal intensity characteristics of mediastinal cystic masses on T1-weighted MRI. *J Comput Assist Tomogr.* 1995;19(2):188–191.
13. Nakata H, et al. MRI of bronchogenic cysts. *J Comput Assist Tomogr.* 1993;17(2):267–270.
14. Jeung MY, et al. Imaging of cystic masses of the mediastinum. *Radiographics.* 2002;22 Spec No:S79–S93.
15. Gawande RS, et al. Differentiation of normal thymus from anterior mediastinal lymphoma and lymphoma recurrence at pediatric PET/CT. *Radiology.* 2012;262(2):613–622.
16. Hudson MM, Krasin MJ, Kaste SC. PET imaging in pediatric Hodgkin's lymphoma. *Pediatr Radiol.* 2004;34(3):190–198.
17. Shankar A, Fiumara F, Pinkerton R. Role of FDG PET in the management of childhood lymphomas—case proven or is the jury still out? *Eur J Cancer.* 2008;44(5):663–673.
18. Montravers F, et al. [(18)F]FDG in childhood lymphoma: clinical utility and impact on management. *Eur J Nucl Med Mol Imaging.* 2002;29(9):1155–1165.
19. Wegner EA, et al. The impact of PET scanning on management of paediatric oncology patients. *Eur J Nucl Med Mol Imaging.* 2005;32(1):23–30.
20. Depas G, et al. 18F-FDG PET in children with lymphomas. *Eur J Nucl Med Mol Imaging.* 2005;32(1):31–38.
21. Hermann S, et al. Staging in childhood lymphoma: differences between FDG-PET and CT. *Nuklearmedizin.* 2005;44(1):1–7.
22. Tatsumi M, et al. Direct comparison of FDG PET and CT findings in patients with lymphoma: initial experience. *Radiology.* 2005;237(3):1038–1045.
23. Kabickova E, et al. Comparison of 18F-FDG-PET and standard procedures for the pretreatment staging of children and adolescents with Hodgkin's disease. *Eur J Nucl Med Mol Imaging.* 2006;33(9):1025–1031.
24. Jerusalem G, et al. Whole-body positron emission tomography using 18F-fluorodeoxyglucose for posttreatment evaluation in Hodgkin's disease and non-Hodgkin's lymphoma has higher diagnostic and prognostic value than classical computed tomography scan imaging. *Blood.* 1999;94(2):429–433.
25. Mettler FA, Guiberteau MJ. *Essentials of Nuclear Medicine Imaging [Electronic Resource].* 6th ed. Philadelphia, PA: Elsevier/Saunders; 2012:607. xii.
26. Mountain CF, Dresler CM. Regional lymph node classification for lung cancer staging. *Chest.* 1997;111(6):1718–1723.
27. Andronikou S. Pathological correlation of CT-detected mediastinal lymphadenopathy in children: the lack of size threshold criteria for abnormality. *Pediatr Radiol.* 2002;32(12): 912.
28. Siegel MJ. *Pediatric Body CT.* 2nd ed. Philadelphia, PA/London: Lippincott Williams & Wilkins; 2008:467. xi.
29. Miller FH, Fitzgerald SW, Donaldson JS. CT of the azygoesophageal recess in infants and children. *Radiographics.* 1993; 13(3):623–634.
30. Carter BW, et al. A modern definition of mediastinal compartments. *J Thorac Oncol.* 2014;9(9 suppl 2):S97–S101.
31. Coley BD. *Caffey's Pediatric Diagnostic Imaging.* 12th ed. Philadelphia, PA: Saunders; 2013. 2 v. (xxix, 1616, 52 p.).

32. Piccaluga PP, et al. Pathobiology of hodgkin lymphoma. *Adv Hematol.* 2011;2011:920898.
33. Zelenetz AD, Jaffe ES, Advani RH, et al. Hodgkin and non-Hodgkin lymphoma. In: Amin MB, Edge S, Greene F, et al., eds., AJCC Cancer Staging Manual, 8th ed. New York: Springer, 2017, p. 937–958.
34. Franco A, Mody NS, Meza MP. Imaging evaluation of pediatric mediastinal masses. *Radiol Clin North Am.* 2005;43(2):325–353.
35. Hamrick-Turner JE, et al. Imaging of childhood non-Hodgkin lymphoma: assessment by histologic subtype. *Radiographics.* 1994;14(1):11–28.
36. Leonidas JC. The thymus: from past misconception to present recognition. *Pediatr Radiol.* 1998;28(5):275–282.
37. Leonidas JC, et al. Human immunodeficiency virus infection and multilocular thymic cysts. *Radiology.* 1996;198(2):377–379.
38. Liang X, et al. Thymoma in children: report of 2 cases and review of the literature. *Pediatr Dev Pathol.* 2010;13(3):202–208.
39. Rocha MM, et al. Invasive thymoma in a child: a rare case report. *J Pediatr Surg.* 2012;47(2):e23–e25.
40. Jung KJ, et al. Malignant thymic epithelial tumors: CT-pathologic correlation. *AJR Am J Roentgenol.* 2001;176(2):433–439.
41. Truong LD, et al. Thymic carcinoma. A clinicopathologic study of 13 cases. *Am J Surg Pathol.* 1990;14(2):151–166.
42. Stachowicz-Stencel T, et al. Thymic carcinoma in children: a report from the Polish Pediatric Rare Tumors Study. *Pediatr Blood Cancer.* 2010;54(7):916–920.
43. Billmire DF. Germ cell, mesenchymal, and thymic tumors of the mediastinum. *Semin Pediatr Surg.* 1999;8(2):85–91.
44. Merten DF. Diagnostic imaging of mediastinal masses in children. *AJR Am J Roentgenol.* 1992;158(4):825–832.
45. Meza MP, Benson M, Slovis TL. Imaging of mediastinal masses in children. *Radiol Clin North Am.* 1993;31(3):583–604.
46. Moeller KH, Rosado-de-Christenson ML, Templeton PA. Mediastinal mature teratoma: imaging features. *AJR Am J Roentgenol.* 1997;169(4):985–990.
47. Rosado-de-Christenson ML, Templeton PA, Moran CA. From the archives of the AFIP. Mediastinal germ cell tumors: radiologic and pathologic correlation. *Radiographics.* 1992;12(5):1013–1030.
48. Mulliken JB, Fishman SJ, Burrows PE. Vascular anomalies. *Curr Probl Surg.* 2000;37(8):517–584.
49. Brown LR, et al. Intrathoracic lymphangioma. *Mayo Clin Proc.* 1986;61(11):882–892.
50. King RM, et al. Primary mediastinal tumors in children. *J Pediatr Surg.* 1982;17(5):512–520.
51. Wildi SM, et al. Diagnosis of benign cysts of the mediastinum: the role and risks of EUS and FNA. *Gastrointest Endosc.* 2003; 58(3):362–368.
52. Diehl DL, et al. Infection after endoscopic ultrasound-guided aspiration of mediastinal cysts. *Interact Cardiovasc Thorac Surg.* 2010;10(2):338–340.
53. Laurent F, et al. Mediastinal masses: diagnostic approach. *Eur Radiol.* 1998;8(7):1148–1159.
54. Nelson BA, et al. BRD4-NUT carcinoma of the mediastinum in a pediatric patient: multidetector computed tomography imaging findings. *J Thorac Imaging.* 2010;25(3):W93–W96.
55. Rosenbaum DG, et al. Radiologic features of NUT midline carcinoma in an adolescent. *Pediatr Radiol.* 2012;42(2):249–252.
56. Moon WK, et al. Mediastinal Castleman disease: CT findings. *J Comput Assist Tomogr.* 1994;18(1):43–46.
57. Moon WK, et al. Castleman disease in the child: CT and ultrasound findings. *Pediatr Radiol.* 1994;24(3):182–184.
58. Bonekamp D, et al. Castleman disease: the great mimic. *Radiographics.* 2011;31(6):1793–1807.
59. Adams GA, et al. Thoracic neuroblastoma: a Pediatric Oncology Group study. *J Pediatr Surg.* 1993;28(3):372–377; discussion 377–378.
60. Shimada H, et al. Terminology and morphologic criteria of neuroblastic tumors: recommendations by the International Neuroblastoma Pathology Committee. *Cancer.* 1999;86(2): 349–363.
61. Shimada H, et al. The international neuroblastoma pathology classification (the Shimada system). *Cancer.* 1999;86(2): 364–372.
62. Strollo DC, Rosado-de-Christenson ML, Jett JR. Primary mediastinal tumors: part II. Tumors of the middle and posterior mediastinum. *Chest.* 1997;112(5):1344–1357.
63. Davis RD Jr, Oldham HN Jr, Sabiston DC Jr. Primary cysts and neoplasms of the mediastinum: recent changes in clinical presentation, methods of diagnosis, management, and results. *Ann Thorac Surg.* 1987;44(3):229–237.
64. Reed JC, Hallet KK, Feigin DS. Neural tumors of the thorax: subject review from the AFIP. *Radiology.* 1978;126(1):9–17.
65. Bredella MA, et al. Value of PET in the assessment of patients with neurofibromatosis type 1. *AJR Am J Roentgenol.* 2007; 189(4):928–935.
66. Exarhos DN, et al. Acute mediastinitis: spectrum of computed tomography findings. *Eur Radiol.* 2005;15(8):1569–1574.
67. Restrepo CS, et al. Imaging appearances of the sternum and sternoclavicular joints. *Radiographics.* 2009;29(3):839–859.
68. Kono T, et al. CT findings of descending necrotising mediastinitis via the carotid space ('Lincoln Highway'). *Pediatr Radiol.* 2001; 31(2):84–86.
69. Santos Gorjon P, et al. Deep neck infection. Review of 286 cases. *Acta Otorrinolaringol Esp.* 2012;63(1):31–41.
70. Argenta LC, et al. Vacuum-assisted closure: state of clinic art. *Plast Reconstr Surg.* 2006;117(7 suppl):127S–142S.
71. Athanassiadi KA. Infections of the mediastinum. *Thorac Surg Clin.* 2009;19(1):37–45, vi.
72. Devaraj A, et al. Computed tomography findings in fibrosing mediastinitis. *Clin Radiol.*2007;62(8):781–786.
73. Rodriguez E, et al. Fibrosing mediastinitis: CT and MR findings. *Clin Radiol.* 1998;53(12):907–910.
74. Sherrick AD, et al. The radiographic findings of fibrosing mediastinitis. *Chest.* 1994;106(2):484–489.
75. Bejvan SM, Godwin JD, Pneumomediastinum: old signs and new signs. *AJR Am J Roentgenol.* 1996;166(5):1041–1048.
76. Johnson NN, Toledo A, Endom EE, Pneumothorax, pneumomediastinum, and pulmonary embolism. *Pediatr Clin North Am.* 2010;57(6):1357–1383.
77. Bees NR, et al. Neonatal thymic haemorrhage. *Br J Radiol.* 1997; 70:210–212.
78. Urvoas E, et al. Ultrasound diagnosis of thymic hemorrhage in an infant with late-onset hemorrhagic disease. *Pediatr Radiol.* 1994;24(2):96–97.

CHAPTER 12

Chest Wall

Dawn R. Engelkemier • Peter G. Kruk • John Naheedy • Yeun-Chung Chang • Pilar Dies-Suarez • Edward Y. Lee

INTRODUCTION

Pediatric chest wall lesions are common. Abnormalities may arise from any component of the chest wall and from a vast array of conditions including congenital and developmental anomalies, infectious disorders, neoplastic disorders, traumatic lesions, and vascular anomalies. Although there is some overlap with adult pathology, many of these entities are unique to the pediatric population. Imaging plays a critical role in detection, characterization, and management of pediatric chest wall lesions (Table 12.1). This chapter reviews imaging techniques for evaluating the pediatric chest wall and briefly discusses normal anatomy and variants. The remainder of the chapter classifies and describes a spectrum of pediatric chest wall lesions with attention to clinical features, imaging characteristics, and treatment options.

IMAGING TECHNIQUES

Various imaging modalities are currently used for evaluation of chest wall lesions in pediatric patients. The imaging techniques as well as unique advantages and disadvantages of these imaging modalities are discussed in this section and summarized in Table 12.2.

Radiography

After clinical evaluation has been performed, chest radiographs are most commonly the first imaging modality employed to evaluate chest wall lesions in pediatric patients. Radiography is a rapid, widely available, low-cost technique that is relatively easy to acquire.[1] Evaluation typically consists of a two-view chest radiograph. In infants, an anterior–posterior (AP) projection is obtained with the patient recumbent, and a cross-table lateral technique is used for the lateral view. Once the child is able to sit with minimal support (around 1 year of age), standard posterior–anterior (PA) and lateral views can be obtained. A grid is used for imaging of adolescent, adult, and large patients.

In addition to standard chest radiographs, dedicated oblique views of the ribs may facilitate characterization of chest wall lesions. Placing a radiopaque marker in the area of concern prior to imaging can help correlate imaging findings with patient symptoms (Fig. 12.1). The patient is positioned erect for imaging of ribs projecting above the diaphragm and recumbent for ribs projecting below the diaphragm. Imaging may include 45-degree right anterior oblique projection for left anterior ribs, 45-degree left anterior oblique projection for right anterior ribs, 30- to 45-degree left posterior oblique for imaging the left axially border, and 30- to 45-degree oblique for imaging the right axillary border.

Some pediatric chest wall lesions have characteristic radiographic findings, and radiographs may be diagnostic. In other cases, radiographs provide valuable information, such as whether a lesion is primarily osseous or soft tissue, and can guide further imaging evaluation.

Ultrasound

Ultrasound (US) may follow radiographs for further evaluation and characterization, or it may be used as a primary modality for superficial lesions, particularly those that are visible or palpable. It has many benefits as an imaging modality, particularly in the pediatric population. US can be performed at the bedside and provides dynamic, real-time information. Sedation and intravenous access are typically unnecessary.

TABLE 12.1 Practical Evaluation of Pediatric Chest Wall Lesions

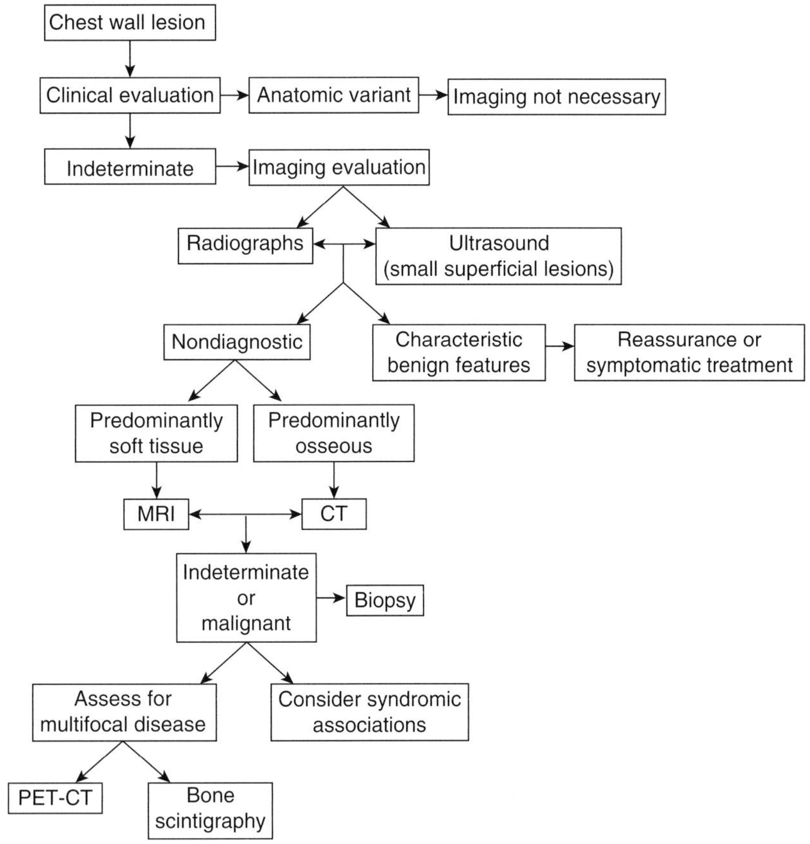

Adapted from Karmazyn B, Davis MM, Davey MS, et al. Imaging evaluation of chest wall tumors in children. Acad Radiol. 1998;5(9):642–654, Ref.[86]

TABLE 12.2 Advantages and Disadvantages of Imaging Modalities for Evaluation of Pediatric Chest Wall Lesions

Modality	Advantages	Disadvantages
Radiography	• Rapid • Accessible • Low cost	• Radiation • Limited evaluation of soft tissues
Ultrasound	• No radiation • Dynamic • Portable	• Limited field of view and depth visibility • Operator dependent
CT	• Fast • Excellent assessment of lung parenchyma and osseous lesions	• Radiation • May require sedation in young children
MRI	• Excellent soft tissue characterization • No radiation	• Relatively long acquisition time • May require sedation • Susceptible to artifacts

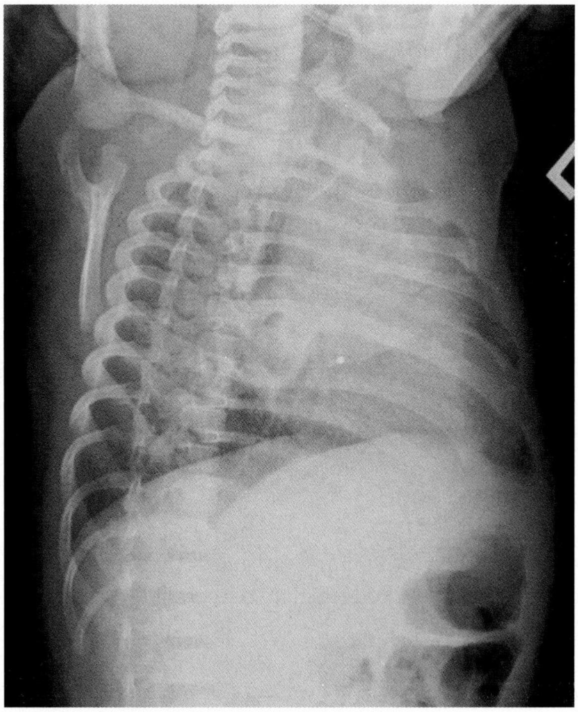

FIGURE 12.1 **Oblique rib radiograph with a radiopaque marker placed in area of palpable mass.**

Additionally, patients are not exposed to the potentially harmful effects of ionizing radiation.

The ultrasound technique should be tailored to the child and to the clinical question. Patient positioning is critical for optimizing the acoustic window and maximizing patient comfort, thereby minimizing motion.[2–5] The anatomic area of interest and patient age and size determine transducer selection. Curved or linear array transducers are commonly utilized. Curved transducer probes provide a wide field of view. Linear probes yield superior resolution at shallow depths. High-frequency (7.5 to 15 MHz) transducers are usually appropriate for evaluation of pediatric chest wall lesions as they provide superior spatial resolution but decreased penetration compared to lower frequency transducers. Tissue equivalent standoff material may improve visualization of superficial lesions.

US may identify the location and extent of a lesion including the chest wall layers involved. The cystic, solid, or vascular nature can be evaluated with gray scale and color Doppler imaging. Some benign lesions have a characteristic US appearance that negates the need for further workup.

Computed Tomography

Computed tomography (CT) is a valuable noninvasive diagnostic tool when radiography and/or US is not sufficient, particularly in evaluation of lesions with an osseous component. CT may be necessary for preoperative planning. A simultaneous assessment of the lung parenchyma can be performed.[1] Modern multidetector CT (MDCT) provides fast acquisition, high spatial resolution, and excellent image quality. Multiplanar and three-dimensional (3D) reformatted images allow evaluation from many perspectives. In recent years, the need for sedation has decreased in light of the fast scanning times of MDCT. Infants and children younger than 5 years or who are unable to lay still or follow breath holding (BH) instructions may still require sedation.[6] Oral chloral hydrate and intravenous pentobarbital are commonly used for moderate (conscious) sedation.[7] Thorough presedation evaluation, monitoring, and cardiorespiratory support by trained providers are critical for performing safe sedated imaging.[8]

In accordance with the "as-low-as-reasonably-achievable" (ALARA) principle, CT in pediatric patients should be performed with the lowest possible radiation dose that maintains diagnostic imaging quality.[1] For some indications, such as pectus excavatum or focal rib lesions, limiting the anatomic coverage to the area of concern can decrease radiation exposure. Specific technical parameters depend on the protocol and type of MDCT scanner used; however, in general, tube current and kilovoltage peak should be adjusted based on patient weight.[6] MDCT should be performed with a fast table speed, thin detector collimation, and a thin reconstruction interval in order to produce high-quality multiplanar and 3D reconstruction images[9] (Table 12.3). Both bone and soft tissue algorithms should be used for reconstruction. Noncontrast examinations are useful to evaluate osseous lesions and identify calcifications. Intravenous contrast is typically used to evaluate soft tissue lesions.[1]

TABLE 12-3 CT Protocol for Chest Wall Lesions

Anatomic coverage (extent)	From sternal notch to below the diaphragm
Scanner settings	See Table 6.1 in this book
Detector collimation	16 row: ~0.75 mm 64 row or higher row: ~0.6 mm
Pitch	1–1.5
Intravenous contrast type	Nonionic: 280–320 mg iodine/mL
Intravenous contrast volume	1–2 mL/kg (up to 100 mL)
Intravenous contrast injection rate	Hand injection: rapid push (~1 mL/s) Mechanical (power) injector: 22 gauge: 1.5–2.5 mL/s 20 gauge: 3–4 mL/s
Scan initiation	~30–40 s after start of contrast injection
Reconstructions (routine viewing)	5 mm x 5 mm
Window width (W) and level (L)	Mediastinum: 400 W and 40 L Lung: 1,250 W and -500 L Bone: 1,500 W and 300 L
Reconstructions (3D imaging)	3 mm x 2 mm or 3 mm x 3 mm
Postprocessing techniques	Multiplanar reconstruction and volume-rendered reformation

Magnetic Resonance Imaging

Magnetic resonance imaging (MRI) is complimentary to radiographs, US, and CT when questions remain unanswered. MRI provides excellent soft tissue characterization without radiation exposure and is particularly useful in evaluating potential spinal involvement. Infants and young children ($\leq$5 years) usually require sedation.

The specific technique should be tailored to the patient and clinical question. A multichannel cardiac coil is typically used for infants and children under the age of 5 years. A phased array torso coil is used in older children and adolescents. Respiratory triggering (RT) and breath holding (BH) techniques can decrease artifact from respiratory motion. Prone positioning may be useful for anterior chest wall lesions to decrease respiratory motion in the area of interest.[10] Flow compensation and flow presaturation techniques can minimize artifact from vascular motion.

The basic protocol for imaging chest wall masses begins with axial and coronal T2-weighted fat saturation (FS) fast relaxation fast spin-echo sequence with BH or RT followed by axial T1-weighted fast spin-echo sequence. Sagittal inversion recovery MR images may be particularly useful for evaluating paraspinal lesions. Diffusion-weighted sequence help characterize soft tissue lesions. Dynamic 3D MR angiogram and postcontrast T1-weighted FS sequence provide information about the vascularity of soft tissue masses and vascular anomalies.

Nuclear Medicine

Nuclear medicine studies may occasionally be used for evaluation of pediatric chest wall lesions and as with other imaging modalities should be appropriately tailored. Radiopharmaceutical doses should be kept as low as possible; a balance must be achieved between minimizing radiation and obtaining a quality diagnostic exam in a reasonable amount of time. Longer acquisition times are more susceptible to patient motion. The length of time the child has to lie still can be decreased by separating long dynamic studies into sequential static images to allow the child to move between acquisitions.[11]

Pediatric administered activity is usually calculated by multiplying the adult reference activity by one of several dose formulas. Body surface area and Webster's formulas have been commonly used; however, these calculations result in significantly larger administered activities per kilogram for infants and small children who are most susceptible to the effects of ionizing radiation. The North American Consensus Guidelines for Administered Radiopharmaceutical Activities in Children and Adolescents recommend weight-based calculations for most common pediatric nuclear medicine studies in children over 1 year of age. In infants, minimum total doses necessary for an adequate study regardless of weight can be used.[12]

Bone scintigraphy and fluorodeoxyglucose (FDG) positron emission tomography (PET) may be of particular use in evaluating a variety of pediatric chest wall disorders including infectious, inflammatory, neoplastic, and traumatic lesions and can aid in diagnosis of multifocal disease. More recently, ^{18}F-NaF PET has been used for detection of new bone formation in a variety of skeletal disorders including identification of skeletal metastasis and skeletal injuries in child abuse.[13,14]

NORMAL ANATOMY AND VARIANTS

The chest wall extends from the skin to the parietal pleural. It provides vital functions including protection of underlying viscera, support for respiratory function, and framework for the shoulders and arms. The normal chest wall is symmetric and broadens cranially to caudally. The skeleton of the chest wall is composed of the sternum anteriorly and the spinal column posteriorly with twelve thoracic vertebrae and paired ribs (Fig. 12.2). The first seven pairs of ribs extend from the costovertebral articulations posteriorly to the sternocostal articulations anteriorly. The eighth through tenth ribs attach to each other anteriorly by costal cartilage; the eleventh and twelve ribs float anteriorly unattached. The internal mammary, posterior intercostal, lateral thoracic, thoracoacromial, and transverse cervical arteries provide the main blood supply to the chest wall.[15]

The configuration of the chest wall changes with age. In infancy, the ribs are oriented horizontally. When an upright position is adopted, the ribs begin to slope downward. The adult rib configuration is reached by ~10 years of age.

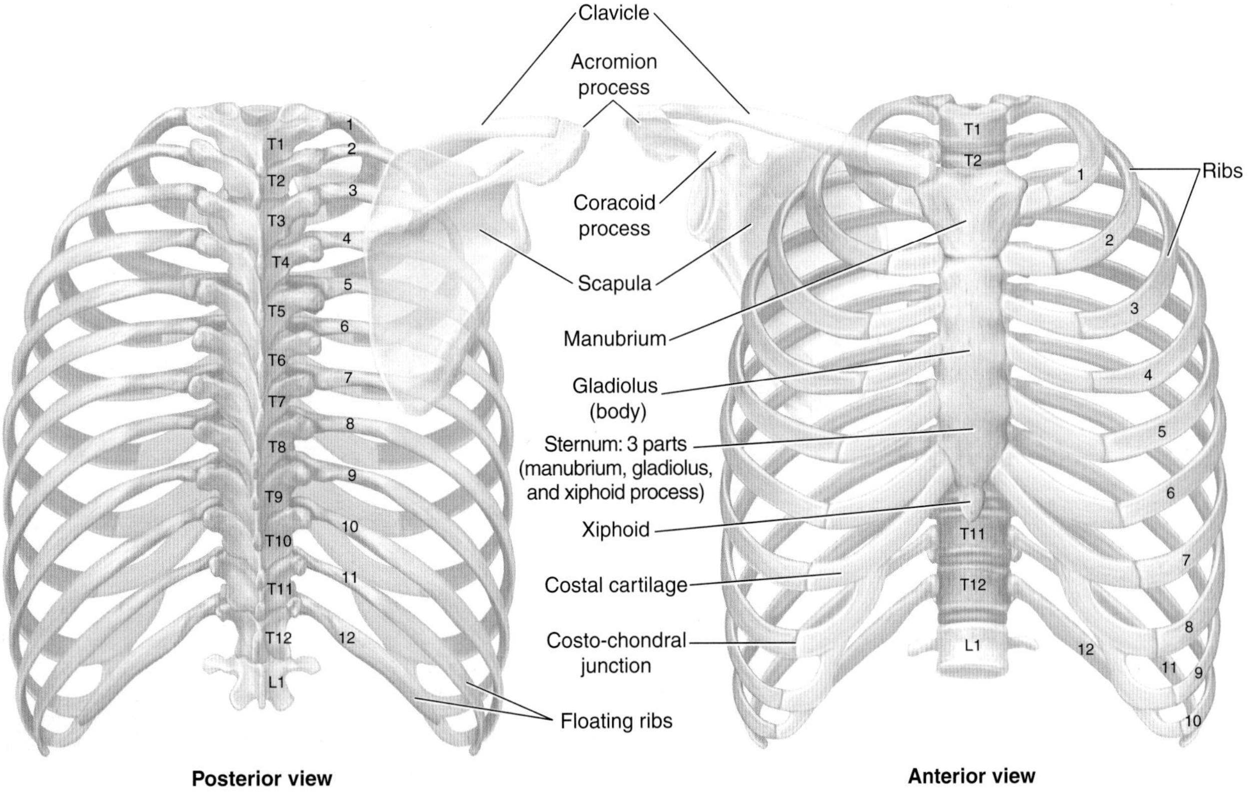

FIGURE 12.2 **Skeletal chest wall anatomy.**

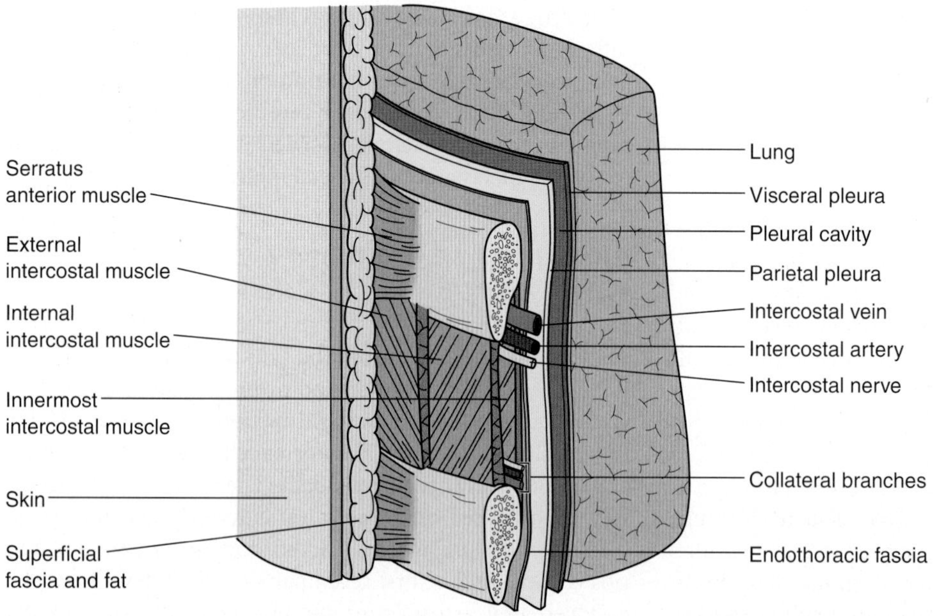

FIGURE 12.3 **Layers of the chest wall.**

Ossification of the skeletal elements begins in utero and continues until the 25th year of life. Due to differences in muscle mass and ossification, the chest wall of infants and children is more elastic and compliant than in adults. This results in lower resting lung volumes and a less efficient respiratory mechanism that predisposes infants and young children to atelectasis. The osseous and soft tissue components gradually become stiffer with age.[16]

The chest wall can be divided into three layers: a superficial layer of skin and subcutaneous fat; an intermediate layer containing the shoulder girdle and pectoralis muscles; and a deep layer including the sternum, ribs, intercostal space, spine, fascia, and parietal pleural[17] (Figs. 12.3 and 12.4). Lesions may arise from any of these layers and their components including the vessels and nerves that course through them.

SPECTRUM OF CHEST WALL DISORDERS

Congenital and Developmental Anomalies

Congenital and developmental anomalies of the pediatric chest wall are common. Mild chest wall asymmetries occur in approximately one third of children.[18] Palpable, but otherwise asymptomatic anterior chest bumps are usually due to anatomic variations; however, they may prompt imaging evaluation for a possible underlying true mass.[19] If the lesion is small, nontender, and stable, radiographs likely provide adequate evaluation. In young children, a predominance of nonossified cartilage in the anterior chest wall may make radiographic evaluation difficult; US can be very useful in these cases.

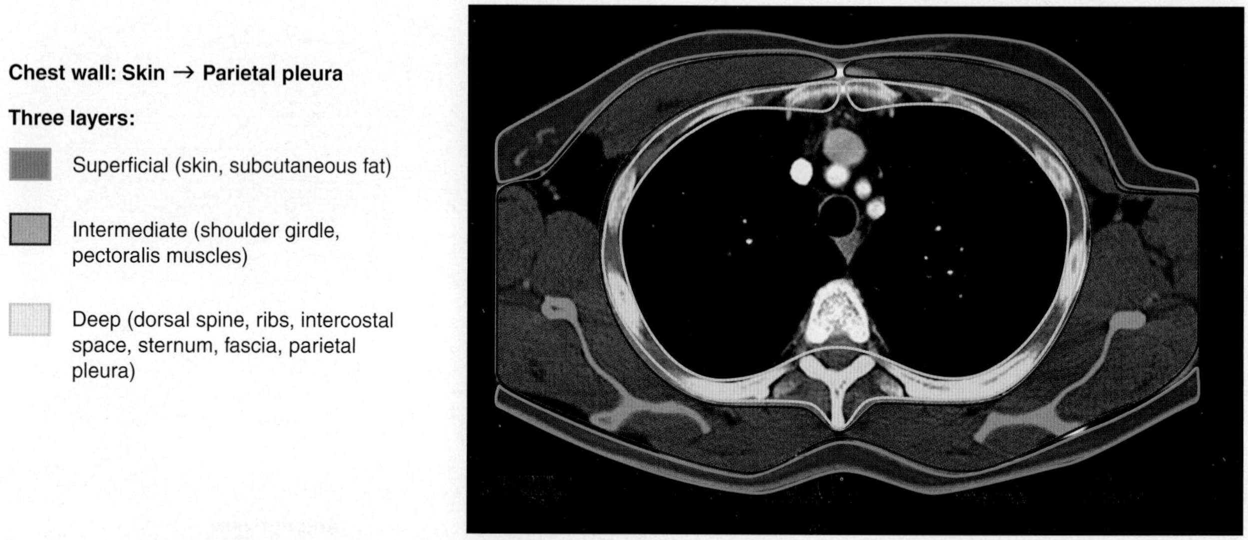

FIGURE 12.4 **Chest wall layers as seen on axial CT image.**

Congenital chest wall anomalies are frequently seen in association with congenital scoliosis. When the scoliosis is due to unilateral vertebral segmentation failure, the chest wall abnormality occurs on the concave side of the scoliosis ipsilateral to the vertebral anomaly.[20]

Chest Wall Asymmetry

Pectus Excavatum

Pectus excavatum is the most common congenital chest wall deformity with a prevalence of 1.3% to 2.6% in school-age children and a male to female ratio of 5:1.[21–23] It is characterized by prominent indentation of the lower sternum, which is usually asymmetric to the right, and resulting decrease in AP diameter of the rib cage[24] (Table 12.4). The etiology has not been clearly elucidated but may be related to abnormal development of costal cartilages.[25] The defect may be noticeable at birth or within the first year, increases in severity during puberty, and stabilizes in adulthood. Associated musculoskeletal abnormalities, particularly scoliosis, are common. Congenital heart disease, osteogenesis imperfecta, muscular dystrophy, and various syndromes including Poland, Pierre Robin, Turner, Ehlers-Danlos, and prune belly syndrome are associated.[26] Two-thirds of patients with Marfan syndrome have pectus excavatum; in these cases the deformity tends to present later and is more progressive.[27]

Although pectus excavatum is usually evident on physical exam, evaluation of the severity of the deformity and associated abnormalities requires imaging. Two-view chest radiographs and chest CT have traditionally been obtained. Frontal radiograph may demonstrate shifting and rotation of the heart to the left. The resulting increased conspicuity of the right-sided hilar vessels and silhouetting of the right heart border by the ventral soft tissue indentation may mimic right middle lobe consolidation.[28] Lateral radiograph demonstrates the sternal depression and narrowed AP thoracic diameter (Fig. 12.5). The pectus or Haller index is calculated by dividing the maximum transverse diameter of the chest by the AP diameter.[29] The pectus index was described using CT; however, significant correlation has been demonstrated with measurements obtained using two-view chest radiograph.[30,31] Due to increasing concern over the use of ionizing radiation, the use of chest radiographs alone, limited CT through the area of interest, or chest MRI has been advocated. Fast chest MRI using balanced gradient-echo

TABLE 12.4 Key Features of Common Primary Pediatric Chest Wall Lesions

Lesion	Classification	Key Features
Pectus excavatum	Congenital/ developmental	• Lower sternal indentation • Decreased anteroposterior diameter rib cage • Syndromic associations
Lipoma	Soft tissue benign neoplasm	• Homogeneous fat density on CT and signal intensity on MRI
Osteochondroma	Osseous benign neoplasm	• Metaphyseal location • Corticomedullary continuity with underlying bone • Cartilaginous cap
Ewing sarcoma	Malignant neoplasm	• Rib location most common • Osseous destruction with periosteal reaction and large soft tissue mass • Heterogeneous enhancement
Rhabdomyosarcoma	Soft tissue malignant neoplasm	• Large painful soft tissue mass • Osseous erosion • Heterogeneous enhancement
Rib fracture	Traumatic	• May appear more aggressive during healing due to periosteal reaction • Suspicious for child abuse without appropriate traumatic history
Venous malformation	Vascular malformation	• Low flow • Soft • Compressible • Phleboliths • Gradual diffuse enhancement
Lymphatic malformation	Vascular malformation	• Low flow • Rubbery • Noncompressible • Septated cysts with fluid–fluid levels • Mild mural enhancement
Hemangioma	Vascular tumor	• High-flow vascular channels • Typical pattern of growth and regression

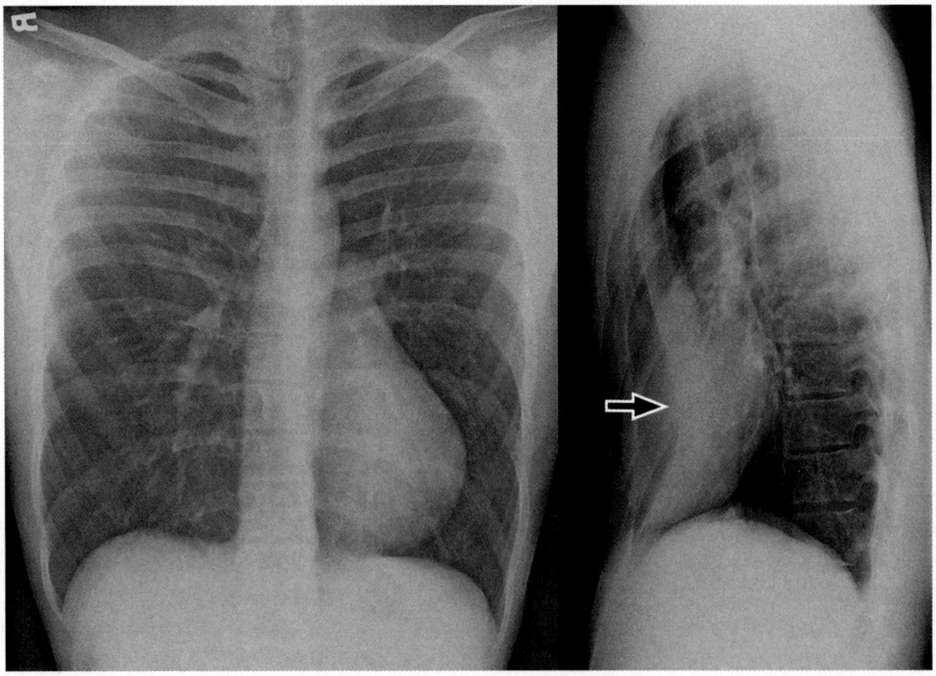

FIGURE 12.5 **Pectus excavatum in a 10-year-old boy.** PA **(left)** and lateral **(right)** radiographs of the chest demonstrate posterior depression (*arrow*) of the sternum with a narrowed anteroposterior diameter of the thorax and leftward shifting of the mediastinal structures.

sequences may negate the need for ionizing radiation in preoperative evaluation[32] (Fig. 12.6).

Structural compression, cardiopulmonary compromise, and significant cosmetic deformity are indications for surgical correction.[33] The mean pectus index in a normal population is around 2.56; surgical correction is usually necessary when the pectus index is >3.24.[29] A steel bar may be placed to brace the sternum and anterior chest wall (Nuss procedure), which may be combined with more invasive resection of costal cartilage and sternal manipulation (modified Ravitch procedure). The later may not be necessary in pediatric patients as recent meta-analysis shows greater improvement in pulmonary function after pectus bar removal from Nuss procedure than from modified Ravitch procedure.[34]

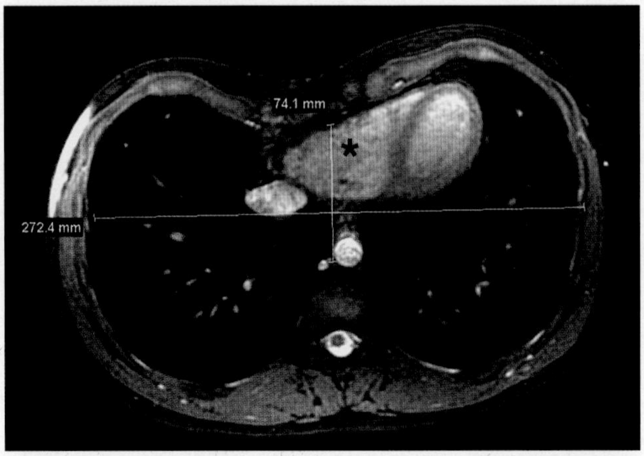

FIGURE 12.6 **Pectus excavatum in a 16-year-old boy with chest asymmetry.** Axial 2D balanced gradient-echo T2-weighted fat-saturated MR image demonstrates rightward tilt and depression of the lower sternum with compression of the right atrium (*asterisk*). The heart is slightly deviated to the left. Haller index is 3.7 (272.4/74.1).

Pectus Carinatum

In contrast to pectus excavatum, pectus carinatum is an outward protrusion of the sternum resulting in increased AP diameter of the thorax. It is the second most common congenital chest wall deformity with a prevalence of ~0.6% in school-age children and a male to female ratio of 4:1.[21–23] The chondrogladiolar variant with protrusion of the body of the sternum is most common. The chondromanubrial variant with protrusion of the manubrium is rare but may be associated with sternal body depression resulting in a "mixed" defect. As with pectus excavatum, the pathogenesis of pectus carinatum remains unclear. Most cases are isolated and asymptomatic other than the cosmetic deformity, which may lead patients to seek treatment.[35,36] Occasionally, the deformity may cause pain, recurrent injury, reduced exercise endurance, and abnormal pulmonary function tests.[37] Scoliosis, congenital heart disease, Marfan syndrome, and Noonan syndrome are associated.[26]

Similar to pectus excavatum, pectus carinatum is often identified on physical exam; however, a prominent anterior bulge may result in workup for an underlying true mass. AP and lateral radiographs are usually sufficient for diagnostic confirmation and pretreatment evaluation. CT or MRI may be useful for surgical planning in patients with mixed defects or a significant rotatory component (Fig. 12.7).

Treatment has historically been operative with resection of abnormal costal cartilage; however, conservative management with bracing has been shown to be successful and is recommended as first-line therapy in most pediatric patients with typical chondrogladiolar pectus carinatum.[38]

Rib Anomalies

Prominent Convexity

Prominent convexity of a rib or costal cartilage is one of the most common anatomic variations resulting in a palpable

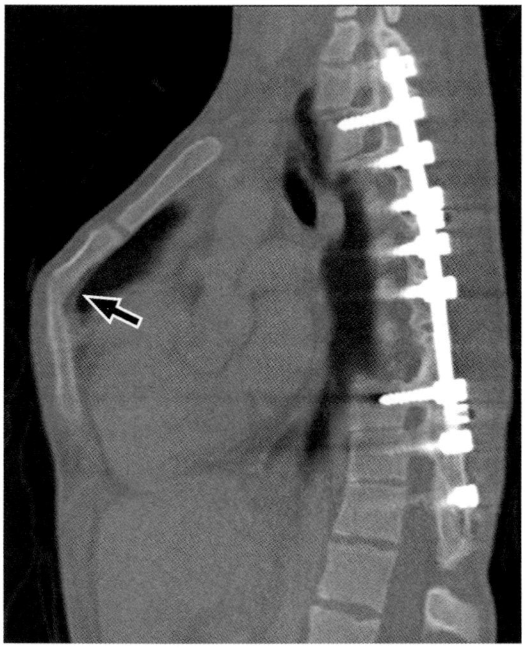

FIGURE 12.7 **Pectus carinatum in a 10-year-old boy with neurofibromatosis type 1 and prior spinal fixation for scoliosis.** Sagittal CT image shows anterior protrusion of the sternum (*arrow*) resulting in increased anteroposterior diameter of the chest.

anterior chest wall "mass"[19] (Fig. 12.8). When the etiology is not evident on physical exam, chest radiographs with a BB marker placed at the area of concern are usually sufficient. US may also provide adequate evaluation, especially for cartilaginous lesions. If CT is performed, 3D reformatted images are useful to clearly depict the prominent contour. Management is reassurance.

Segmentation and Fusion Anomalies

Rib segmentation and fusion anomalies may prompt evaluation due to visible or palpable abnormality, or they may be incidental on imaging (Fig. 12.9).

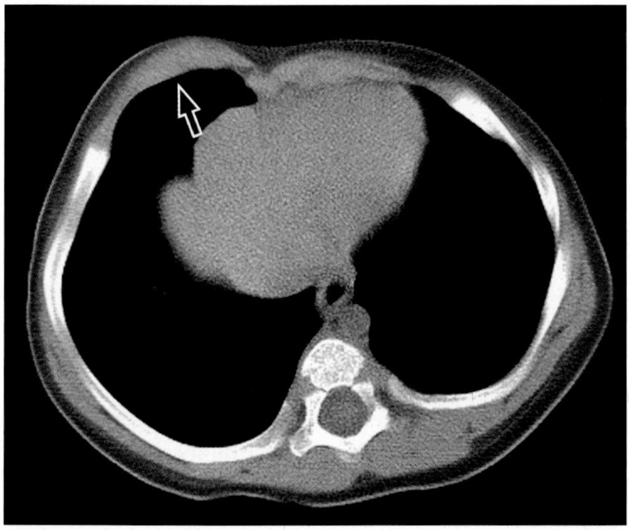

FIGURE 12.8 **Prominent convexity in a 6-month-old boy with a chest wall "mass."** Axial CT image shows asymmetric prominence of the right anterior seventh costal cartilage (*arrow*), which accounted for the palpable abnormality.

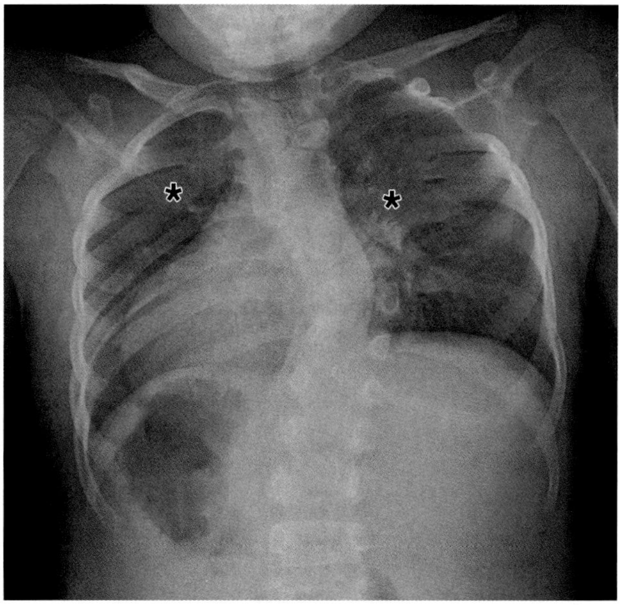

FIGURE 12.9 **Rib fusion in a 4-year-old boy.** Chest radiograph shows complex scoliosis with multiple thoracic vertebral anomalies and bilateral posterior rib fusions (*asterisks*).

Bifid Ribs

Bifid rib describes cleavage of the anterior aspect of the rib or costal cartilage and is most frequently seen in the upper right-sided ribs. It is usually an isolated finding and asymptomatic.[39] Bifid ribs can be syndromic and have been reported in 26% of a series of 82 patients with nevoid basal cell carcinoma syndrome (Gorlin syndrome).[40] If other malformations are present, a thorough clinical assessment should be conducted. If radiographs are not diagnostic, limited CT or MRI can demonstrate the anomaly (Fig. 12.10).

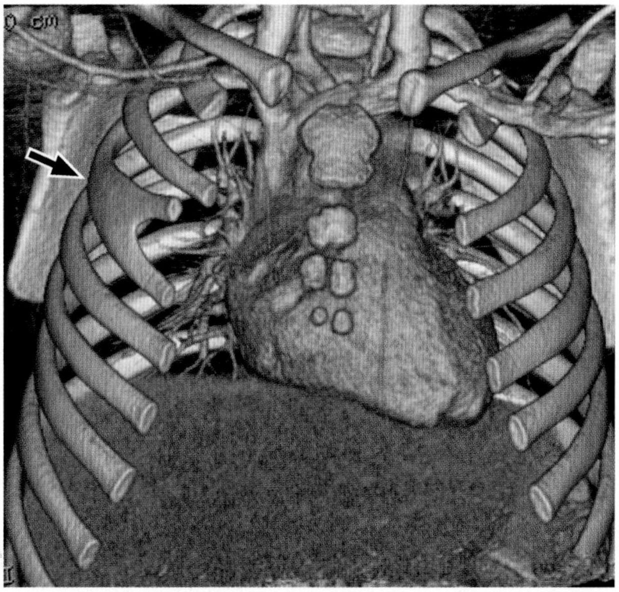

FIGURE 12.10 **Bifid rib in a 2-year-old boy referred for a chest mass.** Three-dimensional reformatted CT image shows the right third bifid rib (*arrow*), which accounted for the palpable mass.

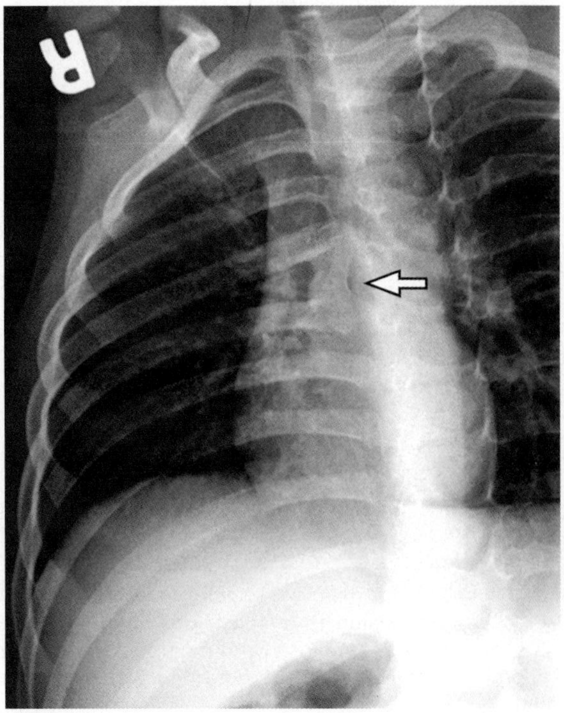

FIGURE 12.11 **Intrathoracic rib in a 3-year-old boy.** Oblique radiograph of the ribs shows a vertically oriented osseous structure (*arrow*) coursing from the right posterior fifth costovertebral junction to the posterior sixth rib.

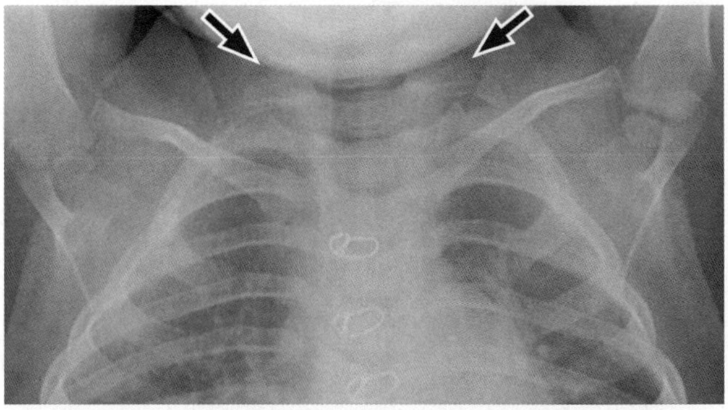

FIGURE 12.12 **Cervical ribs in a 2-year-old girl with prior sternotomy for truncus arteriosus repair.** Coned chest radiograph shows bilateral cervical ribs (*arrows*) articulating with the transverse processes of C7.

Intrathoracic Rib

Intrathoracic rib is a rare anomaly in which a normonumerary or supernumerary rib courses abnormally through the thorax. The rib is usually right sided and originates posteriorly from the third through eighth ribs or vertebral bodies and extends inferior toward the diaphragm in an extrapleural location. The rib may have fibrous attachments to the diaphragmatic pleura and associated intrathoracic fat.[41,42] Most affected pediatric patients are asymptomatic. Radiographs are usually diagnostic; however, the band-like opacity may mimic an anomalous pulmonary vein, pleural calcification, or a foreign body[43] (Fig. 12.11). In these cases, MDCT with 2D or 3D reconstruction can provide the appropriate diagnosis. No treatment is necessary in most asymptomatic pediatric patients.

Cervical Rib

Cervical rib is a supernumerary rib that articulates with an upward sloping cervical-type transverse process from the seventh cervical vertebrae. The reported incidence ranges up to 1.0%, and the vast majority (90%) are asymptomatic.[44,45] Radiographs are diagnostic (Fig. 12.12). Klippel-Feil anomaly may be associated.[46] Large cervical ribs and those fused to the first thoracic rib are more likely to cause neurogenic or vascular thoracic outlet syndrome.[47] In symptomatic patients, cross-sectional imaging and/or angiography can identify complications of vascular thoracic outlet syndrome such as aneurysm or thrombosis of the subclavian vessels. The cervical rib and the first thoracic rib are usually resected for treatment of thoracic outlet syndrome.[47]

Cleidocranial Dysostosis

Cleidocranial dysostosis or dysplasia is a rare autosomal dominant disorder resulting in delayed ossification of midline structures such as the clavicle, calvarium, spine, and pelvis. The *RUNX2* gene on chromosome 6p21, which affects the differentiation of osteoblasts and chondrocytes, is responsible in most cases, but the resulting phenotype is variable.[48]

Diagnosis may be apparent at birth; however, many patients are asymptomatic, and diagnosis may be delayed or incidental. Hypoplasia or absence of the acromial ends of the clavicles is characteristic and results in hypermobility allowing the shoulders to be approximated anteriorly. Cranial manifestations include Wormian bones, delayed or failed suture closure, and delayed or failed eruption of permanent teeth. Skeletal manifestations are manifold including posterior thoracic vertebral body wedging, narrow iliac wings, pubic bone absence or hypoplasia, tapered distal phalanges, and proximal and distal metacarpal and phalangeal epiphyses.[49]

Radiographs of the calvarium, chest, and pelvis are usually diagnostic (Fig. 12.13). Genetic analysis is confirmatory in subtle cases. When necessary, treatment is usually directed toward improving dentition and may require multiple orthodontic procedures.[50]

Poland Syndrome

Poland syndrome is a rare congenital anomaly involving absence of the pectoralis minor muscle and costosternal portion of the pectoralis major muscle, typically on the right side. It is more common in males. Proposed etiologies included disruption of the lateral plate mesoderm and embryonic blood supply resulting in hypoplasia of the ipsilateral subclavian artery or its branches.[51] The phenotype is variable. The ipsilateral breast, areola, ribs, costal cartilages, and sweat glands may be affected. Hypoplasia of the ipsilateral hand with syndactyly and brachydactyly is characteristic.

Chest wall hypoplasia results in relative lucency of the affected hemithorax on radiographs (Fig. 12.14A). CT and MRI are diagnostic, show the extent of the defect, and are useful for surgical planning (Fig. 12.14B).

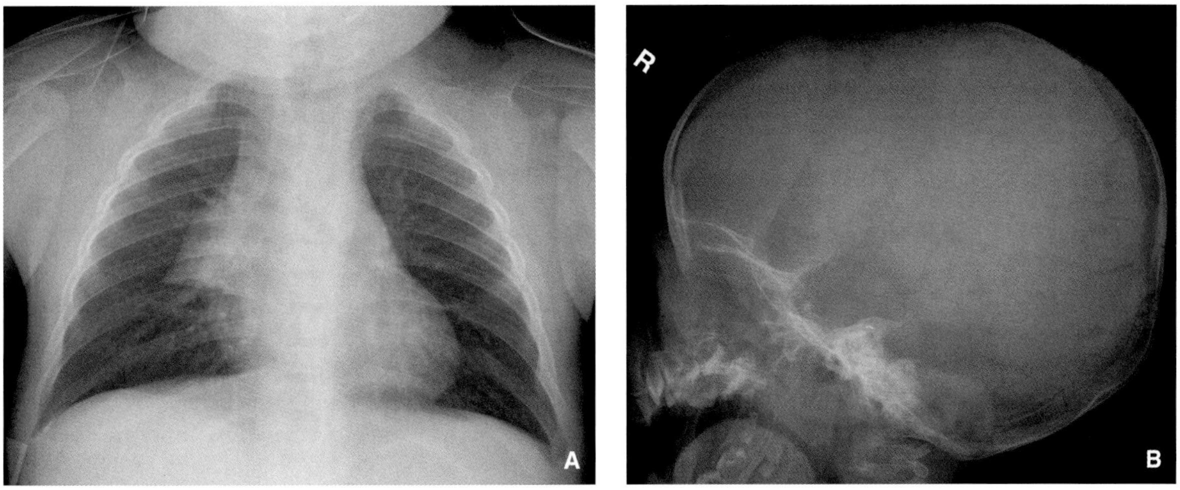

FIGURE 12.13 **Cleidocranial dysostosis in a 3-year-old boy. A:** Chest radiograph shows absent bilateral clavicles. **B:** Lateral skull radiograph shows open skull sutures, large fontanelles, multiple wormian bones, and underdeveloped paranasal sinuses.

Reconstructive surgery may be necessary to provide adequate protection of the underlying visceral organs and/or to improve the cosmetic appearance.[37] A variety of prostheses and surgical flaps have been described; however, more recently less invasive techniques with fat grafting (lipomodeling) have been successfully used for treatment.[52]

Infectious Disorders

Chest wall infections are a relatively uncommon cause of chest wall lesions in children. The ribs and sternum are most affected. Infection in the chest wall may manifest as cellulitis, fasciitis, pyomyositis, osteomyelitis, arthritis, or abscess. Osteomyelitis most commonly presents in infants and young children, usually due to bacterial infection either from hematogenous spread or direct extension. *Staphylococcus, Mycobacterium tuberculosis, Pseudomonas, Actinomyces*, and *Nocardia* have been reported most frequently.[53] Fungal infection with *Aspergillus* and *Candida* may affect immunocompromised pediatric patients. Pain and fever, local edema and erythema, and leukocytosis are typical.

Pyogenic Bacterial Osteomyelitis

The imaging appearance of pyogenic bacterial osteomyelitis is often aggressive and may resemble a wide variety of entities, including neoplasms; however, the clinical findings usually guide appropriate diagnosis (Table 12.5). Classic biopsy findings include necrotic bone serving as a scaffolding for new bone formation ("sequestrum") and variable amounts of marrow fibrosis, plasma cell infiltration, and neutrophils.

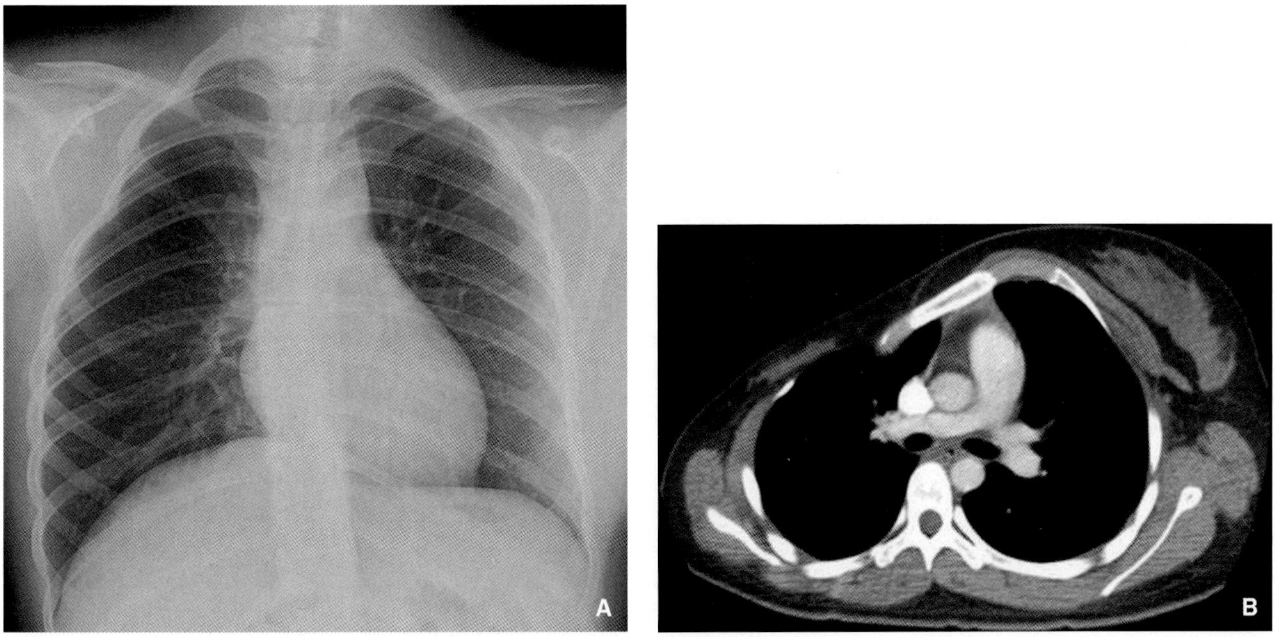

FIGURE 12.14 **Poland syndrome in a 15-year-old girl with chest deformity. A:** Frontal chest radiograph demonstrates diffuse lucency of the right hemithorax. **B:** Axial enhanced CT image shows absent pectoralis muscles and severely diminished breast tissue on the right.

TABLE 12.5 Differential Diagnosis of Aggressive-Appearing Pediatric Chest Wall Lesions

Underlying Etiologies	Disorders
Infection	Bacterial and fungal osteomyelitis
Benign soft tissue neoplasm	Plexiform neurofibroma
Benign osseous neoplasm	Osteoblastoma, fibrous dysplasia, and Langerhans cell histiocytosis
Malignant osseous neoplasm	Ewing sarcoma/primitive neuroectodermal tumor, osteosarcoma, and plasmacytoma
Metastasis	Neuroblastoma, rhabdomyosarcoma, leukemia, and lymphoma
Trauma	Subacute healing pathologic fracture in a benign osseous lesion
Vascular malformation	Kaposiform hemangioendothelioma

Radiographs and CT may show focal osteopenia, cortical irregularity, periosteal reaction, and contiguous soft tissue swelling. Findings are apparent on radiographs only after 7 to 10 days. Cortical irregularity and fluid adjacent to the bone and within the joint can be seen with US. Associated soft tissue changes on US include increased subcutaneous echogenicity, loss of normal soft tissue architecture, and reticular anechoic subcutaneous edema.[54,55] US can be used to identify and guide drainage of superficial abscesses, which appear as hypoechoic or anechoic collections with posterior acoustic enhancement and peripheral hyperemia. Deep infection is better evaluated with CT or MRI. Although CT is superior at demonstrating osseous erosion, MRI best depicts the early changes of osteomyelitis. Abnormal marrow edema is evidenced by high T2-weighted and low T1-weighted signal intensity. Intravenous contrast may clarify regions of abscess formation (Fig. 12.15). Bone scintigraphy is sensitive for early detection but lacks anatomic detail.

Treatment consists of intravenous antibiotics and drainage of focal fluid collections.

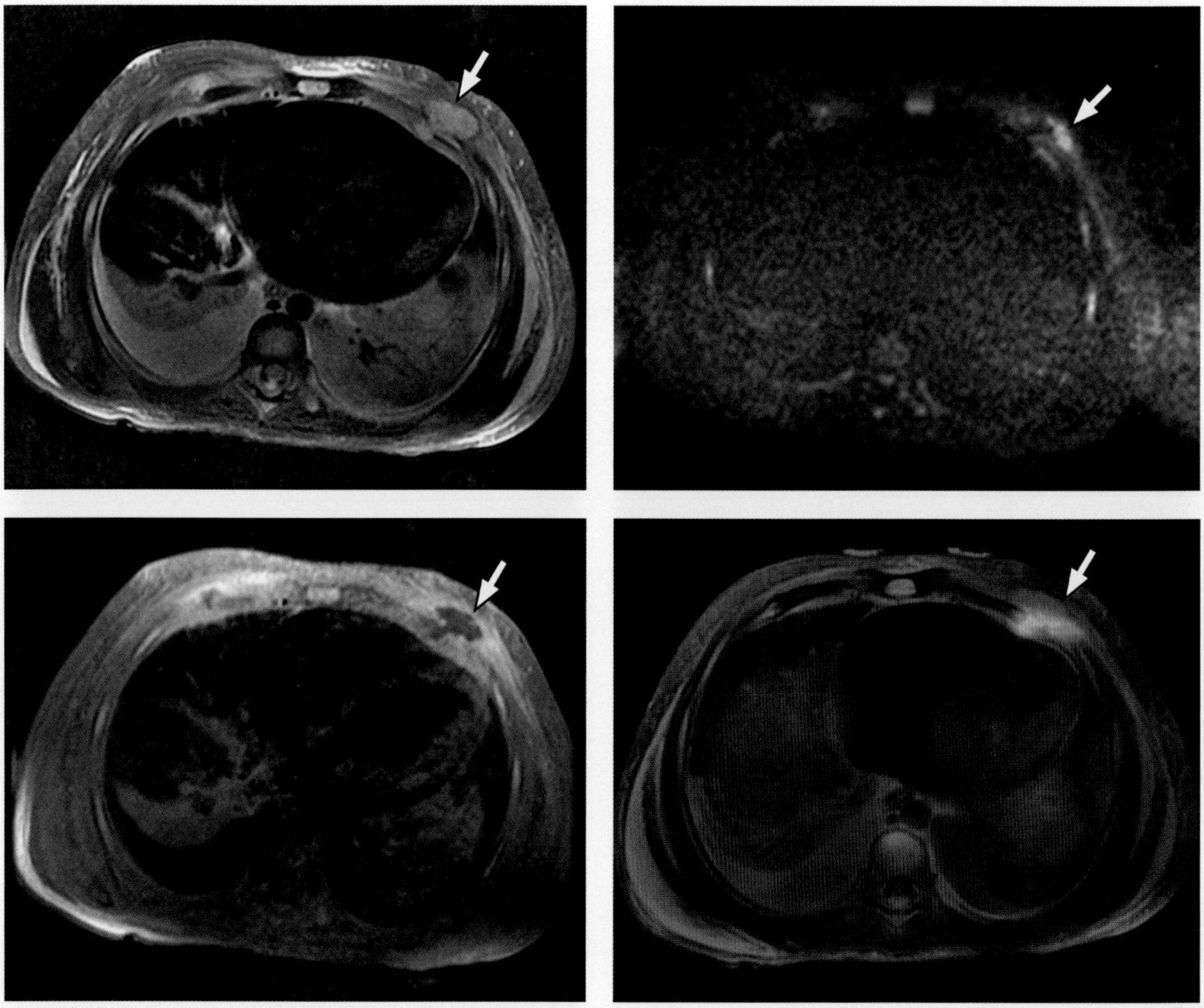

FIGURE 12.15 ***Staphylococcus aureus* abscess and osteomyelitis in a 10-year-old boy with leukemia and disseminated infection.** Axial T2-weighted MR image **(top left)**, T1-weighted postcontrast fat-saturated MR image **(bottom left)**, diffusion-weighted MR image **(top right)**, and fused PET-MR image **(bottom right)** show a focal collection (*arrows*) with high T2 signal, peripheral enhancement, restricted diffusion, and hypermetabolic activity at the left anterior sixth costochondral junction with abnormal signal in the adjacent rib and soft tissues. A smaller collection is present on the right. Abnormal marrow signal in the spine was related to leukemic involvement.

Tuberculosis

Chest wall infection is a relatively rare manifestation of childhood tuberculosis. However, it should be considered in children with undiagnosed chest wall lesions, especially in endemic areas. The potential underlying mechanisms of chest wall tuberculous infection include direct extension from underlying pulmonary or pleural disease, direct extension from lymphadenitis of the chest wall, direct skin inoculation, and hematogenous dissemination. Tuberculous infection is usually more insidious than pyogenic bacterial infection. The presence of soft tissue calcification, abscess, osteolysis, and sequestra is suggestive[56,57] (Fig. 12.16).

Actinomycosis

Actinomycosis results in a chronic granulomatous infection in immunocompromised pediatric patients. The thorax is affected in ~15% of cases.[58] Chest wall infection usually extends from pulmonary disease. Culture is negative in more than 50%; biopsy is frequently necessary for diagnosis.[59]

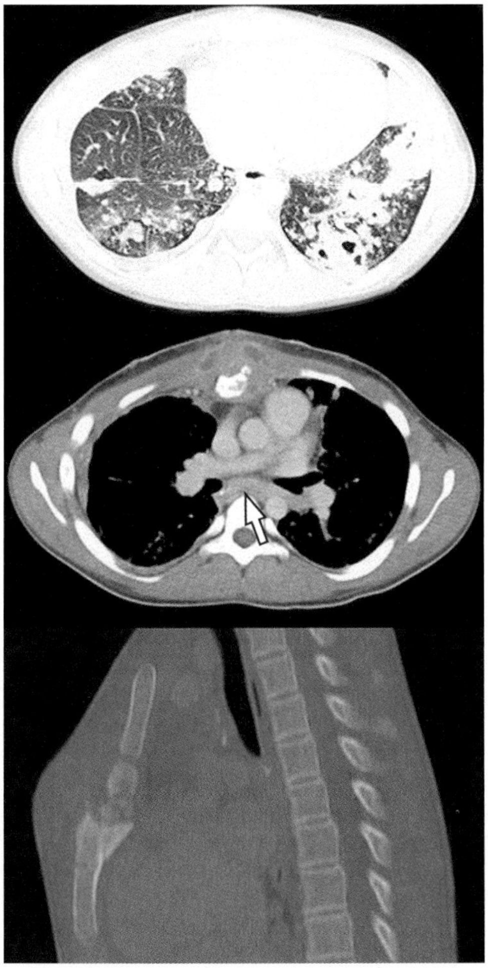

FIGURE 12.16 **Pulmonary tuberculosis with sternal osteomyelitis and abscess in a 15-year-old boy.** Axial enhanced lung window CT image **(top)** shows nodular and tree-in-bud pattern opacities with areas of cavitation. Axial enhanced soft tissue window CT image **(middle)** shows partially calcified subcarinal lymph nodes (*arrow*) and sternal destruction with surrounding soft tissue thickening and fluid collections. Sagittal bone window CT image **(bottom)** more clearly demonstrates the sternal osteolysis with adjacent sclerosis and cortical thickening.

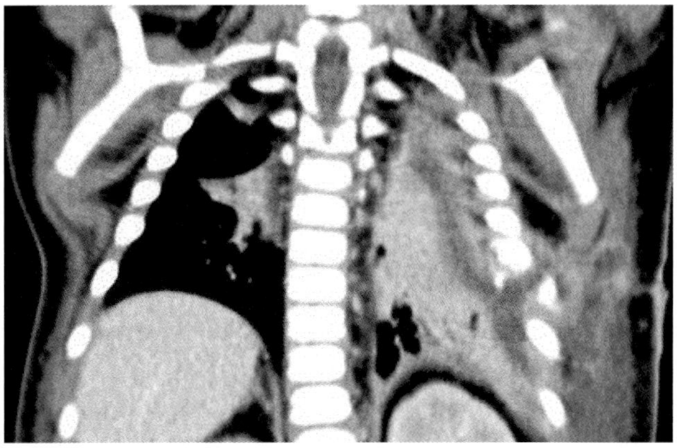

FIGURE 12.17 **Empyema necessitates in a 1-year-old girl with a history of gastropleural fistula and empyema.** Coronal enhanced soft tissue window CT image shows a left pleural collection with surrounding pleural thickening and enhancement. The collection extends laterally through the eighth intercostal space into the subcutaneous tissues of the left lateral chest wall. There is significant atelectasis of the left lung. Pleural fluid culture showed multimicrobial infection.

Empyema Necessitates

Rarely, pleural empyema may directly extend into the soft tissues of the chest wall, usually anteriorly, resulting in empyema necessitates (Fig. 12.17). This is most commonly due to *Mycobacterium tuberculosis* and *Actinomyces* species.[60]

Neoplastic Disorders

Benign Neoplasms

Soft Tissue Tumors

Lipoma

Lipomas are proliferations of mature adipose tissue most commonly found in the upper back, neck, extremities, and abdomen.[61] Other than causing a focal mass, they are usually asymptomatic. Grossly, they are soft, yellow, lobulated, and variably encapsulated. Microscopically, they consist of mature adipose tissue and variably prominent fibrous septa (Fig. 12.18). Genetically, a large proportion are characterized by dysregulation of the *HMGA2* gene on the long arm of chromosome 12.

Radiographs may reveal a fat density mass without osseous erosion (Table 12.4). US shows an echogenic avascular mass with circumscribed or imperceptible borders.[55] Homogenous fat attenuation (−100 Hounsfield units) is characteristic on CT (Fig. 12.19). MRI signal follows that of subcutaneous fat; fat-saturation technique can be applied for confirmation. A thin, fibrous capsule may surround subcutaneous and intermuscular lipomas but is usually absent in intramuscular lipomas, which tend to be infiltrative.[62] Thin septa may be visible. Minimal or no enhancement is present. Fat necrosis can cause heterogeneity, in which case differentiation from liposarcoma cannot be definitively made, and biopsy is necessary.[63]

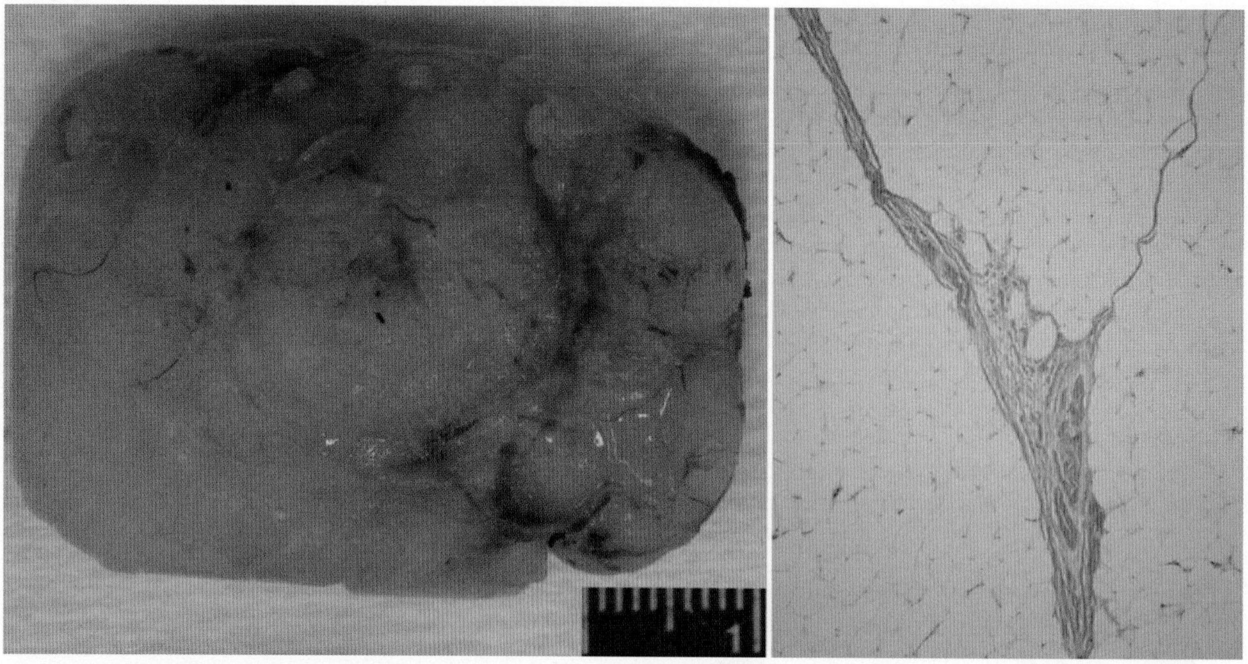

FIGURE 12.18 **Lipoma in a 13-year-old girl.** This 4 cm lesion resected from the chest subcutis consists grossly of pale yellow lobulated adipose tissue **(left)**. Microscopically, the adipose tissue is traversed by thin septa containing mature fibroblasts (**right**, hematoxylin and eosin, original magnification, 100×).

Symptomatic lesions can be excised. Newer surgical techniques such as axillary approach subcutaneous endoscopic excision minimize scarring.[64]

Lipoblastoma/Lipoblastomatosis

In contrast to lipomas, lipoblastomas contain variable numbers of immature fat cells (lipoblasts), often with a myxoid extracellular matrix and highly vascular septa. The myxoid change can impart a shiny gelatinous quality to the gross specimen. However, variability in the maturity of lipoblasts can make lipoblastomas difficult to distinguish from lipoma, both grossly and microscopically (Fig. 12.20). The term "lipoblastomatosis" may be used for a lipoblastoma that exhibits diffuse involvement. Chromosomal rearrangements involving the *PLAG1* gene are characteristic.[65] Lipoblastomas present in infants and young children as painless masses in the extremities or trunk.[62] They may recur after excision.

Imaging features reflect the amount of fat within the lesion. Radiographs may demonstrate a fat and soft tissue

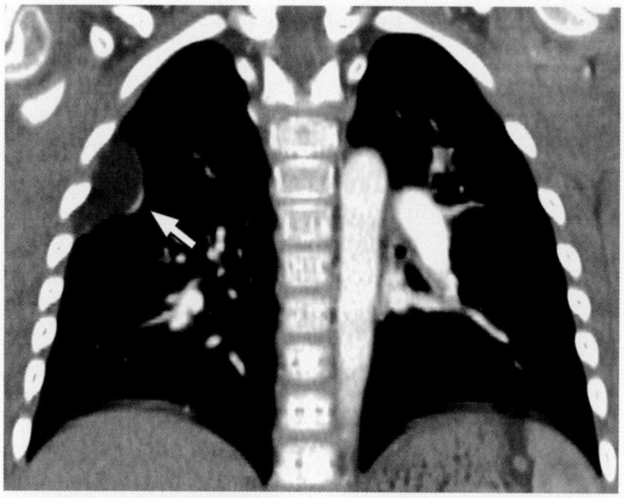

FIGURE 12.19 **Lipoma in a 4-year-old boy who presented with right sided chest discomfort.** Coronal enhanced CT image shows a well-defined, homogeneous fat attenuation mass (*arrow*) along the right lateral chest that extending into the fourth and fifth intercostal space.

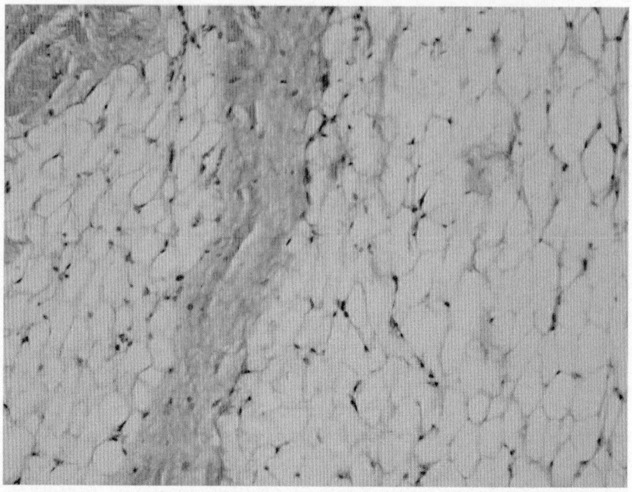

FIGURE 12.20 **Lipoblastoma in a 5-year-old boy.** There was longstanding diffuse involvement (lipoblastomatosis) of the chest wall, axilla, and brachial plexus. Here, the features are of a "mature" lipoblastoma with adipose tissue, prominent fibrous septa, and only rare lipoblasts (hematoxylin and eosin, original magnification, 200×).

density mass. CT and MRI appearance is heterogeneous with fatty and nonfatty elements and occasionally a combination of nonenhancing cystic areas and enhancing soft tissue[66] (Fig. 12.21).

Definitive diagnosis of lipoblastoma requires biopsy and subsequent pathologic evaluation.

Desmoid Fibromatosis

Fibromatosis refers to a proliferation of fibroblasts or myofibroblasts, which tends to invade surrounding tissue and recur after incomplete excision. Desmoid fibromatosis (desmoid tumor) is the most common type of fibromatosis and presents as a painless mass in infants or young children, more commonly in males. It occurs in the deep or superficial soft tissue, most commonly in the trunk or extremities. Thoracic desmoids are usually isolated entities, whereas intra-abdominal desmoids are more frequently associated with Gardner syndrome. Young age and large tumor size are associated with increased risk of recurrence.[67,68] Grossly, desmoid fibromatosis is firm, white gray and fairly well circumscribed, but not encapsulated. Microscopically, it shows plump active-appearing fibroblasts in fascicles or sheets[68] (Fig. 12.22).

A nonspecific soft tissue mass is seen on radiography, often with erosion and deformity of adjacent bone (Fig. 12.23A). The attenuation on contrast-enhanced CT is usually greater than that of skeletal muscle. MRI usually shows homogeneous intermediate or low T1 and variable T2 signal intensity. Collagen-rich regions appear as curvilinear areas of low signal intensity on T2-weighted MR images (Fig. 12.23B). Enhancement after contrast is moderate to marked.[69] Both an infiltrative and well-circumscribed pattern is seen in the pediatric population.[70]

Management is complex. Surgical resection has been a traditional approach. Adjuvant systemic chemotherapy and radiation may be used for rapidly growing symptomatic lesions. Due to treatment-associated morbidity, watchful waiting may be appropriate initial management. Recent study shows event-free survival does not significantly differ in children undergoing a period of observation compared to patients receiving surgical resection or systemic therapy.[71]

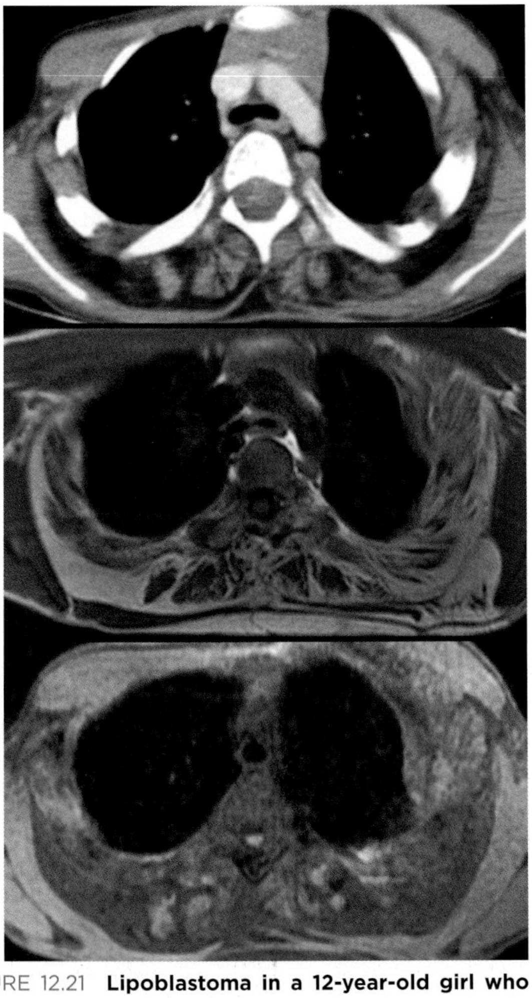

FIGURE 12.21 **Lipoblastoma in a 12-year-old girl who presented with posterior chest wall deformity.** Axial enhanced CT image **(top)**, T1-weighted MR image **(middle)**, and T1-weighted fat-saturated MR image **(bottom)** demonstrate a predominantly fatty lesion insinuating throughout paraspinal musculature, axilla, and intercostal regions bilaterally.

Myofibroma/Myofibromatosis

Myofibroma is a proliferation of fibroblasts and myofibroblasts that usually presents before 2 years of age with firm fleshy nodules. Though rare, it is the most common fibrous tumor of infancy. Three forms are described: solitary myofibroma, multicentric myofibroma in soft tissues, and multicentric myofibroma with visceral involvement. Solitary and multicentric myofibromas (myofibromatosis) typically occur in the head and neck, followed by the trunk and extremities. Lesions may increase in size and number or regress and even resolve. Nonvisceral lesions can be found in skin, subcutaneous tissue, muscle, or bone and have an excellent prognosis; however, reported mortality is up to 70% with visceral

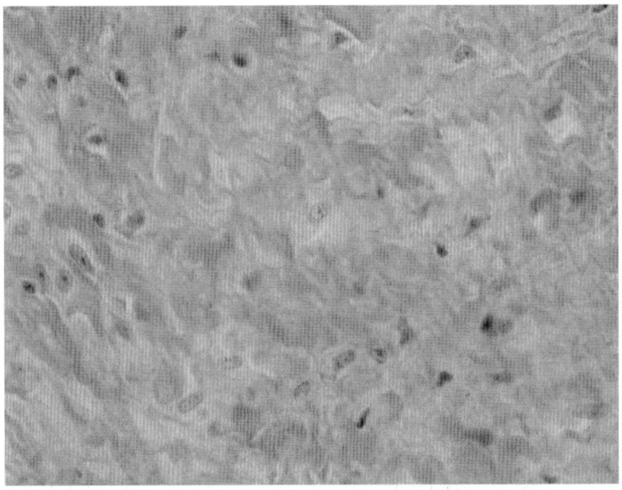

FIGURE 12.22 **Desmoid fibromatosis in a 19-year-old male with a history of chest wall mass and bone marrow transplantation.** Core biopsy shows fibroblastic cells with plump nuclei embedded in a fibrillar collagenous matrix (hematoxylin and eosin, original magnification, 400×). Positive nuclear staining for beta-catenin (not shown) helped to confirm the diagnosis.

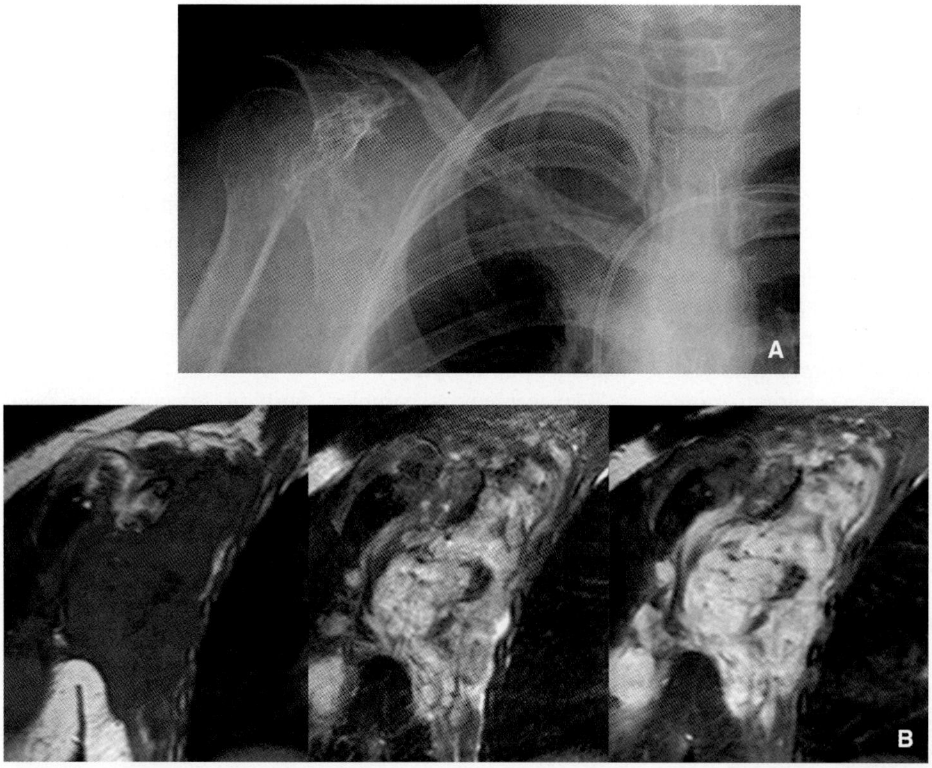

FIGURE 12.23 **Desmoid fibromatosis in a 15-year-old boy with chest mass. A:** Frontal radiograph shows multiple lytic lesions in the right scapula. **B:** Coronal T1-weighted **(left)**, T1-weighted postcontrast fat-saturated **(middle)**, and T2-weighted fat-saturated **(right)** MR images show avidly enhancing right axillary mass with T2 prolongation. Focal areas of low T2 signal and lack of enhancement likely represent collagen-rich areas.

involvement, which is most common in the lungs, gastrointestinal tract, and heart.[68,72,73] Grossly, myofibroma/myofibromatosis is a firm white mass and variably well circumscribed. Microscopically, whorled bundles of fibroblastic cells are seen. A characteristic feature is the involvement of vessel walls (Fig. 12.24).

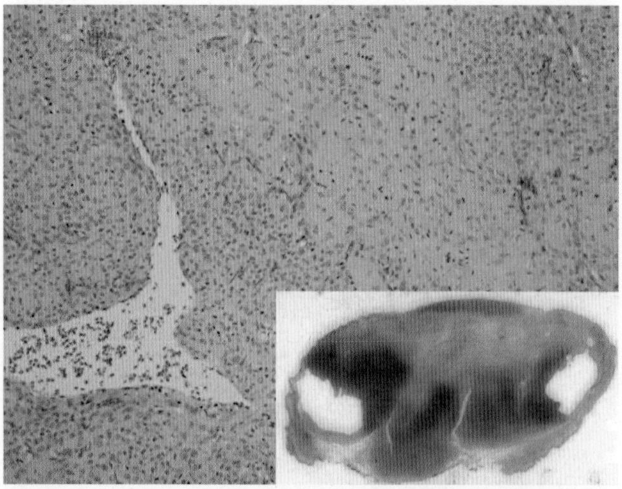

FIGURE 12.24 **Infantile myofibroma/myofibromatosis in a 2-week old boy.** This protuberant 4.5 cm myofibroma with overlying skin ulceration was resected from the left flank with the clinical suspicion of a vascular lesion. Occasional large channels are seen grossly (**inset**, hematoxylin and eosin stain, original magnification, 1×). Microscopically, areas show spindled to round (pericytic or glomoid) cells with smooth muscle differentiation forming solid areas that merge with the walls of variably sized vascular channels (hematoxylin and eosin, original magnification, 200×).

Radiographs may demonstrate multiple soft tissue masses, lytic osseous lesions with a narrow zone of transition, and occasionally vertebra plana. Calcification and ossification may develop. A typical targetoid pattern on US and MRI is due to central hemorrhage, cystic degeneration, and necrosis[70] (Fig. 12.25). MRI best depicts the lesions; however, the appearance is usually nonspecific.

When possible, complete surgical excision provides the best treatment. Watchful waiting is also reasonable in cases of limited involvement. Chemotherapy, typically with vinblastine and methotrexate, is used in multicentric forms and for life-threatening tumors in inoperable sites.[72] Genetic mutations have recently been discovered in platelet-derived growth factor B and one of its regulatory proteins, *NOTCH3*, which could serve as targets for future therapy.[73]

Fibrous Hamartoma of Infancy

Fibrous hamartoma of infancy (subdermal fibromatous tumor of infancy) is a rare tumor of mature fibrous and adipose tissue and immature mesenchymal tissue that presents in infants and young children, more commonly in males (Fig. 12.26). The mass is usually painless and mobile within the subcutaneous tissues of the shoulder girdle; however, local infiltration can occur. Lesions usually remain asymptomatic despite rapid initial growth.[74] No characteristic genetic alterations have been identified, and there are no known syndromic or familial disease associations.[68]

Radiographs show a nonspecific soft tissue mass. Displacement of local structures, osseous erosion, and calcifications are common. US appearance is heterogeneous. CT and MRI more clearly define the extent of the mass. T1- and

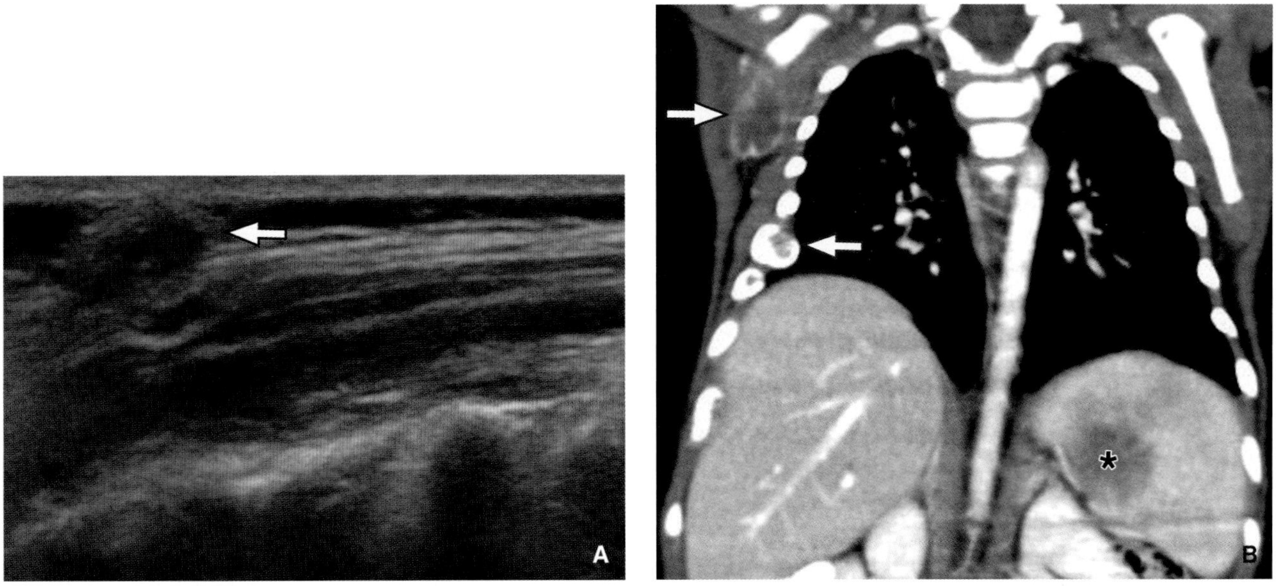

FIGURE 12.25 **Myofibromatosis in the lateral chest wall of a 5-year-old boy. A:** Ultrasound shows a mildly heterogeneous, hypoechoic mass (*arrow*) within and extending deep to the subcutaneous fat and superficial to the ribs. **B:** Coronal enhanced CT image shows multiple lesions (*arrows*) involving the right lateral chest wall and ribs as well as the spleen (*asterisk*).

T2-weighted MR images demonstrate high signal intensity fat intermixed with linear/curvilinear areas of intermediate to low signal intensity fibrous tissue[70] (Fig. 12.27).

Definitive diagnosis requires histologic examination. The treatment of choice is local excision. Approximately 12% to 15% of cases recur.[74]

Neurofibroma

Neurofibroma is the most common peripheral nerve sheath tumor in the pediatric population. Solitary lesions are usually sporadic. The presence of multiple lesions is strongly associated with neurofibromatosis type 1 (NF1). In the chest, intercostal and paraspinal locations are most common. Pain or a palpable mass may develop, and growth can occur, but malignant degeneration in classic neurofibromas is rare.

On radiographs, secondary signs such as thinning, splaying, and undersurface notching of the ribs or neuroforaminal widening may be apparent. Neurofibromas are

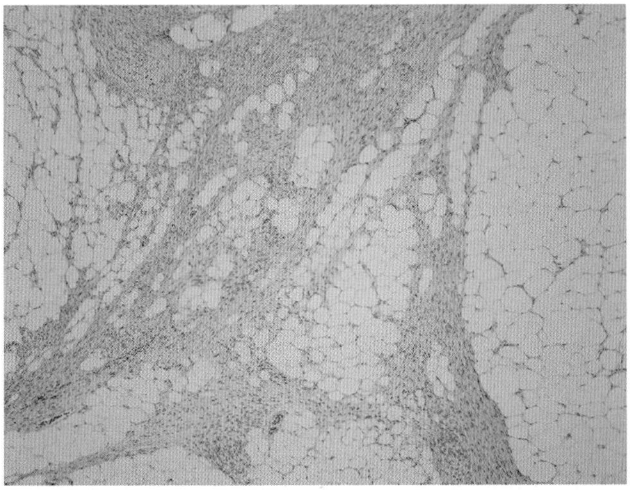

FIGURE 12.26 **Fibrous hamartoma of infancy in an 11-month-old boy.** This 5 cm mass from the shoulder shows the classic triphasic histologic appearance. Mature adipose tissue is coursed by septa of fibrous tissue as well as aggregates of somewhat primitive mesenchymal cells in a myxoid background (hematoxylin and eosin, original magnification, 100×).

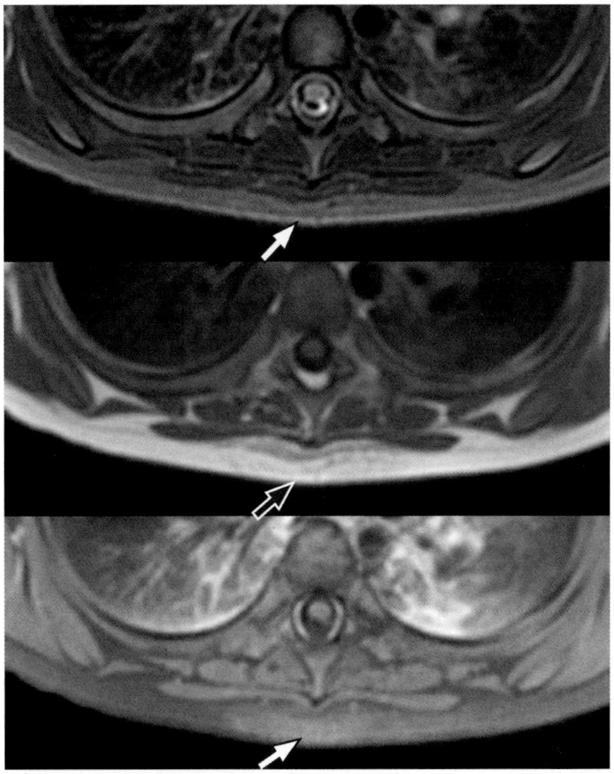

FIGURE 12.27 **Fibrous hamartoma of infancy in a 3-month-old boy with tuberous sclerosis.** Axial T2-weighted fat-saturated **(top)**, T1-weighted **(middle)**, and postcontrast T1-weighted fat-saturated MR images show subtle ill-defined heterogeneous subcutaneous signal abnormality with mild enhancement (*arrows*).

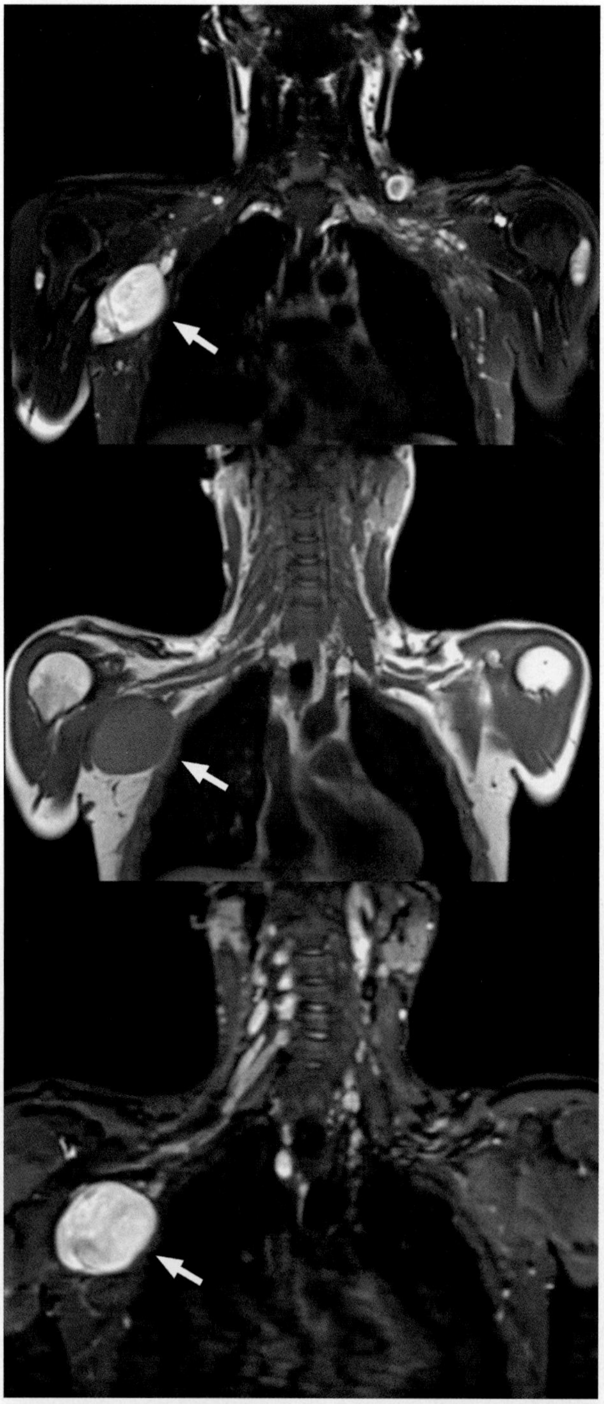

FIGURE 12.28 **Neurofibromas in a 14-year-old boy with neurofibromatosis type 1.** Coronal T2-weighted fat-saturated **(top)**, T1-weighted **(middle)**, and postcontrast T1-weighted fat-saturated **(bottom)** MR images show a dominant neurofibroma (*arrow*) in the right axilla with high T2 and low T1 signal and enhancement. There is suggestion of a "split-fat" sign on precontrast T1-weighted sequence and target appearance on the postcontrast sequence. Multiple smaller cervical neurofibromas are also present.

well demarcated and hypoechoic with or without posterior acoustic enhancement on US and low attenuation soft tissue masses on CT. Signal is isointense to muscle on T1-weighted MR images and hyperintense on T2-weighted MR images with heterogeneous enhancement on postcontrast MR images (Fig. 12.28). A target appearance with central low signal on T2 and postcontrast T1 sequences is characteristic.[75] A rim of fat surrounding the lesion, the "split-fat" sign, indicates a tumor of nerve sheath origin.

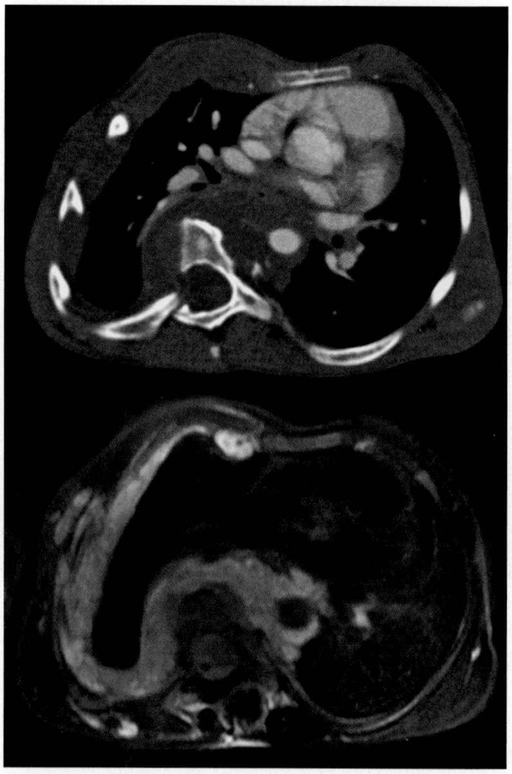

FIGURE 12.29 **Plexiform neurofibroma in a 5-year-old boy with neurofibromatosis type 1.** Axial enhanced CT image **(top)** and STIR MR image **(bottom)** show the mass displacing the aorta and insinuating along the spine and ribs. The lesion is low attenuation on enhanced CT image and demonstrates T2 prolongation on MRI.

Plexiform neurofibromas are less organized and more diffuse than classic neurofibromas and are considered pathognomonic of NF1. They are locally aggressive with increased potential for malignant degeneration, which occurs in ~5% of patients. Imaging characteristics are similar to classic neurofibromas, but with a more disorganized, tortuous appearance along the course of a nerve with ill-defined margins and inhomogeneous signal intensity[75] (Fig. 12.29). This corresponds to the gross pathologic appearance of a dumbbell-shaped lesion or even a "bag of worms" in which preexisting nerves are diffusely expanded by the neurofibromatous growth (Fig. 12.30). Microscopically, neurofibromas consist of cells with oval to spindle-shaped nuclei with indistinct cytoplasm in a background of fine collagen, myxoid material, and scattered mast cells.

Treatment is surgical resection of symptomatic lesions. Plexiform lesions that are increasing in size or becoming symptomatic should be excised; however, complete resection may be challenging.[76]

Osseous Tumors

Osteoblastoma

Osteoblastomas are rare osteoid producing tumors that resemble osteoid osteomas histologically, but are more variable in

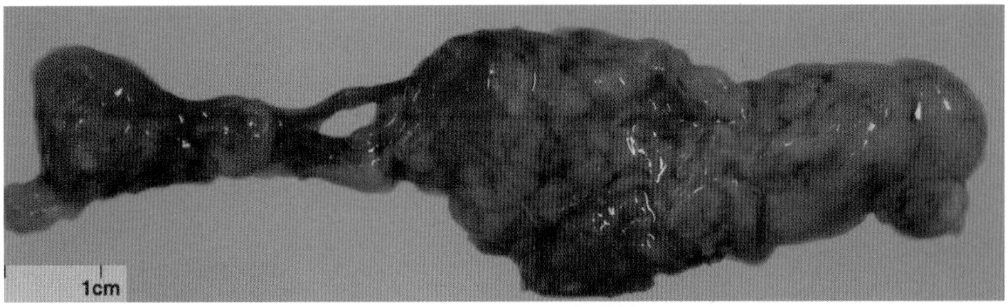

FIGURE 12.30 **Plexiform neurofibroma from a 15-year-old girl with neurofibromatosis type 1.** This superficial chest wall mass has a plexiform appearance accounted for by expansion along the course of preexisting nerves.

appearance and have a larger nidus (>1.5 to 2 cm).[77,78] They have a predilection for the posterior elements of the spine, which may result in scoliosis. Affected pediatric patients may be asymptomatic or complain of dull pain and swelling.

On imaging, osteoblastomas may be centrally lytic with surrounding sclerosis resembling an osteoid osteoma, predominantly lytic with expansion similar to an aneurysmal bone cyst (ABC), or aggressive mimicking a malignant neoplasm. CT is useful to evaluate the extent of the lesion and osteoid matrix (Fig. 12.31). MRI usually reveals low to intermediate T1 and intermediate to high T2 signal with prominent surrounding edema and enhancement.[77,79] Intense focal uptake is present on bone scintigraphy.

Resected osteoblastomas are often red, due to a rich vascular supply, and show a fairly well-circumscribed border. Microscopically, innumerable small foci of mineralizing osteoid matrix are cuffed by plump osteoblasts (Fig. 12.32).

Treatment traditionally involves surgical resection; however, less invasive techniques such as CT-guided radiofrequency ablation have demonstrated success.[80]

Enchondroma

Enchondromas are neoplasms of hyaline cartilage that arise within the medullary cavity. They are the second most common benign bone tumor in children, commonly present in the second decade, and are usually asymptomatic.[81] Within the chest, the costochondral junction is most frequently affected.[82] Multiple enchondromas occur in Ollier syndrome and in association with venous malformations in Maffucci syndrome. Heterozygous somatic mutations in the *IDH1* and *IDH2* genes are present in many enchondromas, particularly those from syndromic patients.[83,84] Malignant transformation in enchondroma is rare.[85]

Radiographs demonstrate lytic lesions with endosteal scalloping, mild expansion, and partially calcified chondroid matrix[86] (Fig. 12.33). On MRI, chondromas are usually low to intermediate signal intensity on T1-weighted MR images with areas of high T2 signal and variable contrast enhancement. Foci of low T2 signal intensity reflect calcification of chondroid matrix. Differentiation from low-grade chondrosarcoma can be difficult on imaging; both may demonstrate increased uptake on bone scintigraphy.[87]

No treatment is necessary in asymptomatic lesions with classic imaging features. Resection may be performed when diagnostic confirmation is needed particularly in

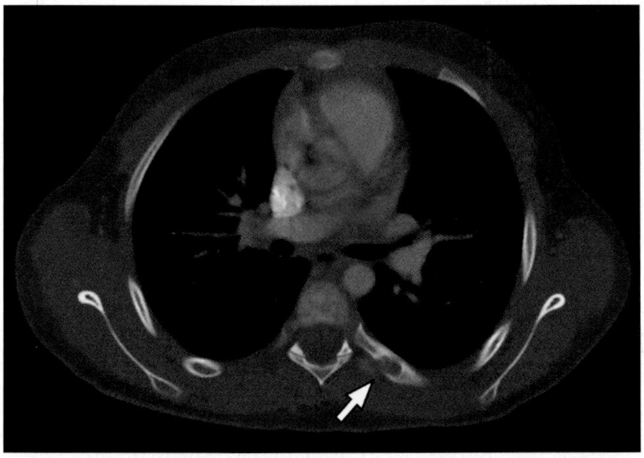

FIGURE 12.31 **Osteoblastoma in an 8-year-old girl with back pain.** Axial enhanced bone window CT image shows a mildly expansile lytic lesion (*arrow*) with surrounding sclerosis in the posterior medial left rib.

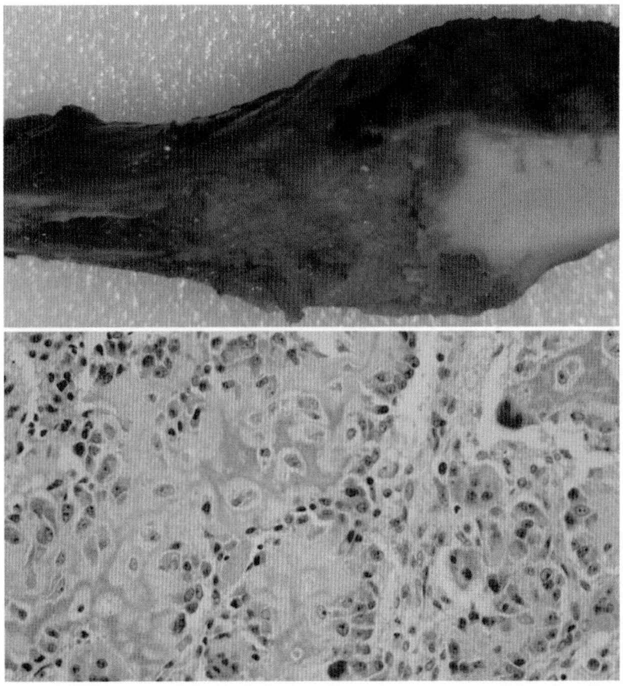

FIGURE 12.32 **Osteoblastoma from a 16-year-old girl with a rib mass.** The en bloc resection specimen shows a 1.5-cm expansile area of soft, gritty homogeneous pale tissue (**upper**). Microscopically, areas of pink woven bone are lined by plump osteoblasts and occasional multinucleate giant cells (**lower**, hematoxylin and eosin, original magnification, 400x).

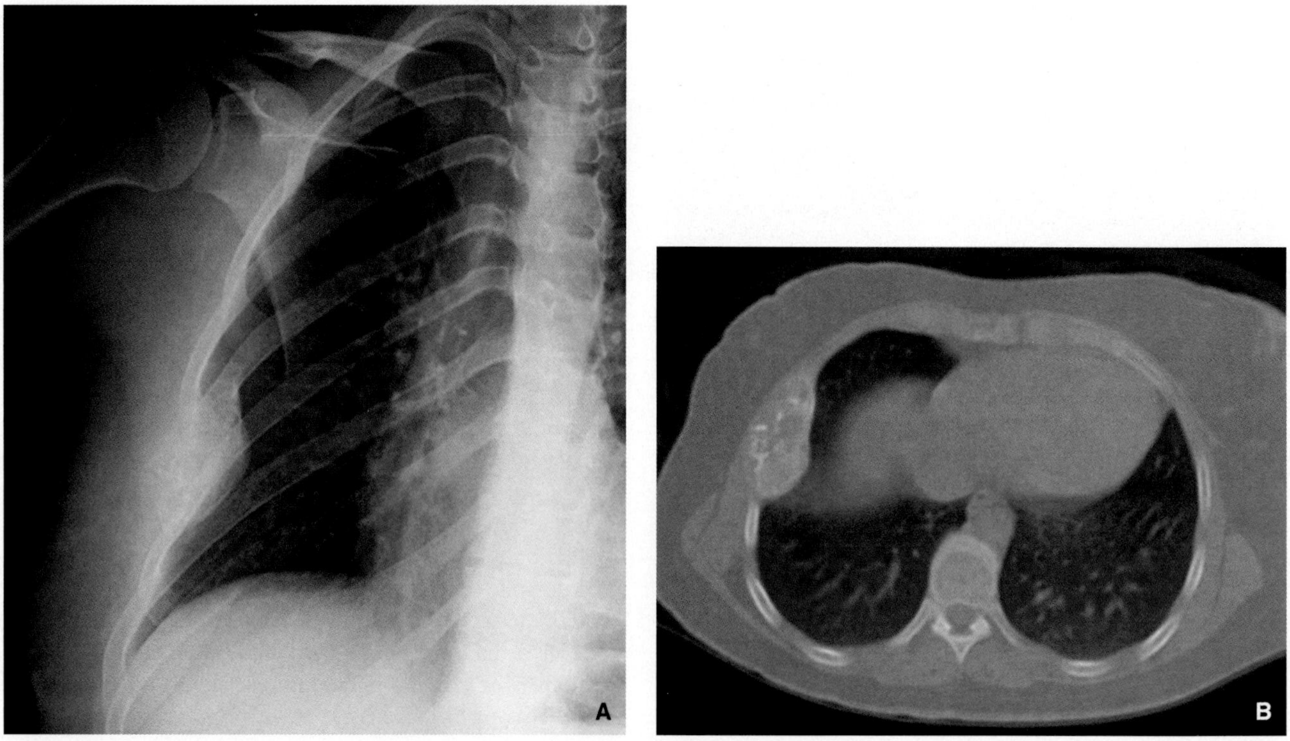

FIGURE 12.33 **Enchondroma in a 17-year-old boy with right sided chest discomfort. A:** Rib radiograph shows an expansile lesion with chondroid matrix in the right anterolateral fifth rib. **B:** Axial bone window CT image more clearly demonstrates the chondroid matrix.

symptomatic pediatric patients. Resection specimens show a well-delineated area of firm, gray-white opalescent tissue with focal gritty calcification (Fig. 12.34). Microscopically, histologically bland chondrocytes are embedded in a variably mineralized hyaline cartilage matrix.[85]

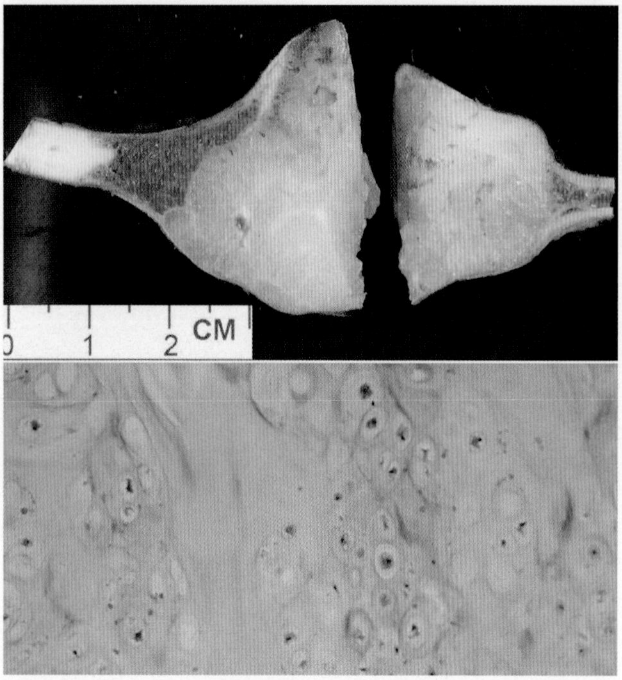

FIGURE 12.34 **Enchondroma in a 15-year old girl.** The anterior fifth rib is expanded circumferentially by a vaguely lobulated, white, well-circumscribed mass **(upper panel)**. Microscopic examination shows histologically bland chondrocytes in a hyaline matrix (**lower panel**, hematoxylin and eosin, original magnification, 200×).

Osteochondroma

Osteochondroma is an outgrowth of histologically normal bone with a cartilaginous cap. It is the most common benign chest wall tumor in the pediatric population, has a male predilection, and usually presents at 2 to 10 years of age as a slowly growing, painless mass.[77] Growth continues until the bone is mature. Metaphyseal location is classic; in the chest wall, lesions occur most frequently at the costochondral junction.[82] Compression of adjacent structures or trauma may cause symptoms. Malignant degeneration, typically to chondrosarcoma, is seen in <1% of solitary lesions overall and is less frequent in skeletally immature patients. Sarcomatous transformation is more common in axial lesions and in the syndrome of multiple hereditary exostosis.[88]

Radiographs are usually diagnostic demonstrating a pedunculated or sessile osseous lesion in continuity with the bone of origin (Table 12.4). CT and MRI may be used for confirmation of the corticomedullary continuity, surgical planning in symptomatic lesions, or evaluation of malignant transformation (Fig. 12.35). MRI most clearly demonstrates the high T2 signal intensity cartilaginous cap. Irregularity and thickening of the cartilaginous cap >3 cm in children, associated soft tissue mass, development of pain, and growth after skeletal maturity are concerning for malignant transformation.[77,81,88]

Microscopically, osteochondromas show fairly organized projections of perichondrium and cartilage with a growth zone and bone. Treatment is surgical resection of

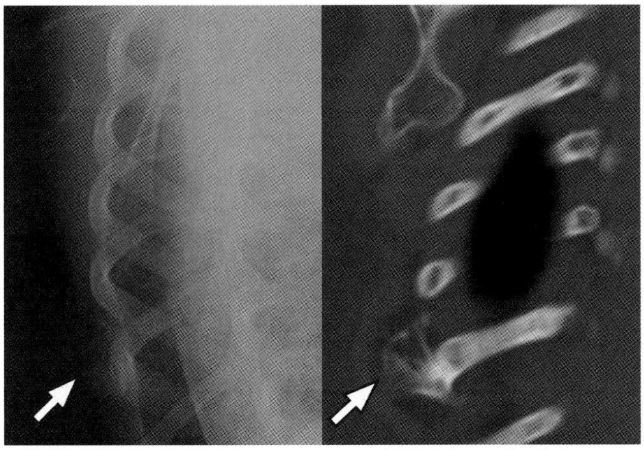

FIGURE 12.35 **Osteochondroma in a 14-year-old girl who presented with a painless and palpable back mass.** Lateral chest radiograph **(left)** and coronal CT image **(right)** demonstrate an exophytic cauliflower-like lesion (*arrows*) arising from the right posterior 8th rib with cortical and marrow continuity with the adjacent bone.

symptomatic lesions or those with concerning imaging features. Close clinical and radiographic follow-up is advised for syndromic lesions.[88]

Aneurysmal Bone Cyst

An ABC is an expansile growth of thin-walled, blood-filled cavities. The discovery of a clonal chromosomal rearrangement involving the *USP6* gene as a consistent abnormality in ABC[89] has ended controversy as to whether primary ABCs represent true neoplasms. "Secondary ABC," occurring in conjunction with a separate type of bone lesion, may also occur, and whether it represents the same biologic phenomenon is unclear. Presentation is typically pain and swelling in patients under 20 years of age.

Radiographs demonstrate an eccentric, lytic, expansile metaphyseal lesion with a narrow zone of transition. On cross-sectional imaging, multiple cysts with thin septations and fluid–fluid levels are characteristic (Fig. 12.36A, B). Surrounding edema and septal enhancement may be evident on MRI. Bone scintigraphy demonstrates increased uptake.[90]

Although imaging features are highly suggestive, histologic examination is required before definitive treatment, mainly to exclude a telangiectatic osteosarcoma. Histologic diagnosis is based on the identification of blood-filled cystic spaces interspersed among mononuclear fibroblast-like cells with scattered giant cells and variable amounts of hemosiderin (Fig. 12.37). Close correlation with the radiologic imaging is required because other benign and malignant tumor types may have overlapping histologic features. When the cystic component is minor or absent, the lesion may be termed "solid-variant ABC."

Treatment may involve curettage with bone grafting or en bloc resection.[91] Local recurrence occurs in up to 20%. Success in treatment has been demonstrated with cryotherapy, sclerotherapy, radionuclide ablation, and embolization.[92]

Fibrous Dysplasia

Fibrous dysplasia is a benign fibro-osseous lesion of bone that can be monostotic or polyostotic. It occurs in children and adults, most commonly in the femur and craniofacial bones.[93] The rib is the most common site of chest wall involvement, particularly the lateral or posterior arc. Occasionally pain, pathologic fracture, and cosmetic deformity result. Polyostotic fibrous dysplasia is associated with several syndromes. McCune-Albright syndrome is characterized by a triad of fibrous dysplasia, café au lait spots, and endocrine dysfunction. Mazabraud syndrome is a rare association of intramuscular myxomas and polyostotic fibrous dysplasia.[82]

Radiographs demonstrate an expansile, intramedullary lesion with a ground-glass appearance and sclerotic rim. More focally lucent or sclerotic areas may intervene. CT may be necessary for lesions that are not well visualized radiographically

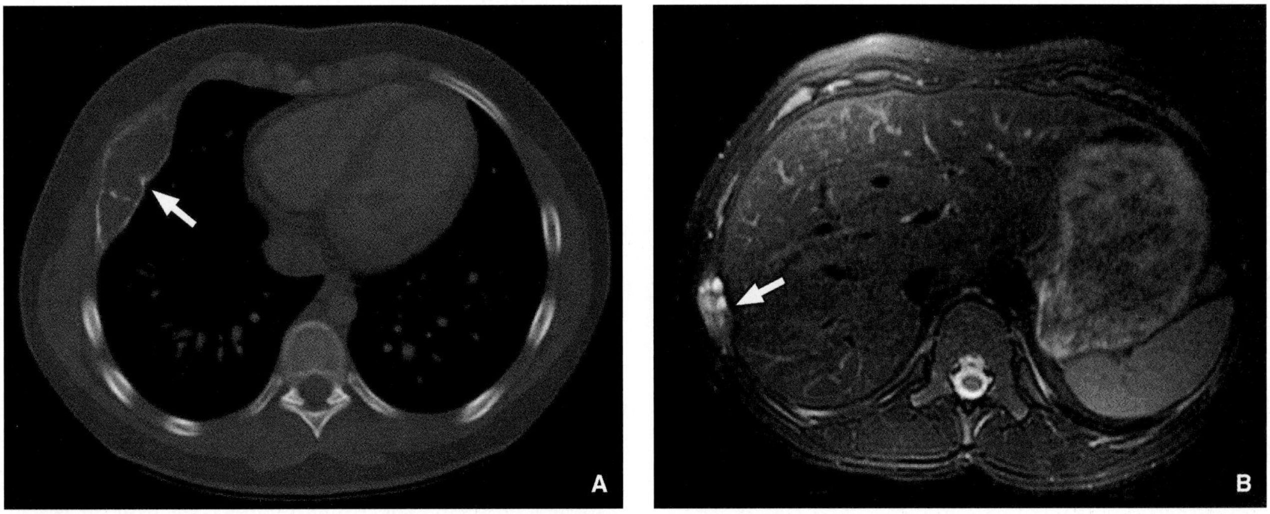

FIGURE 12.36 **Aneurysmal bone cyst in two pediatric patients. A:** Axial bone window CT image from a 3-year-old boy who presented with palpable chest bump shows an expansile, lytic lesion (*arrow*) arising from right anterior 5th rib with thinning of the cortex and thin bony septa, but no appreciable matrix. **B:** Axial T2-weighted fat-saturated MR image from a 12-year-old boy shows a well-defined, expansile lesion (*arrow*) in the lateral right ninth rib with fluid-fluid levels.

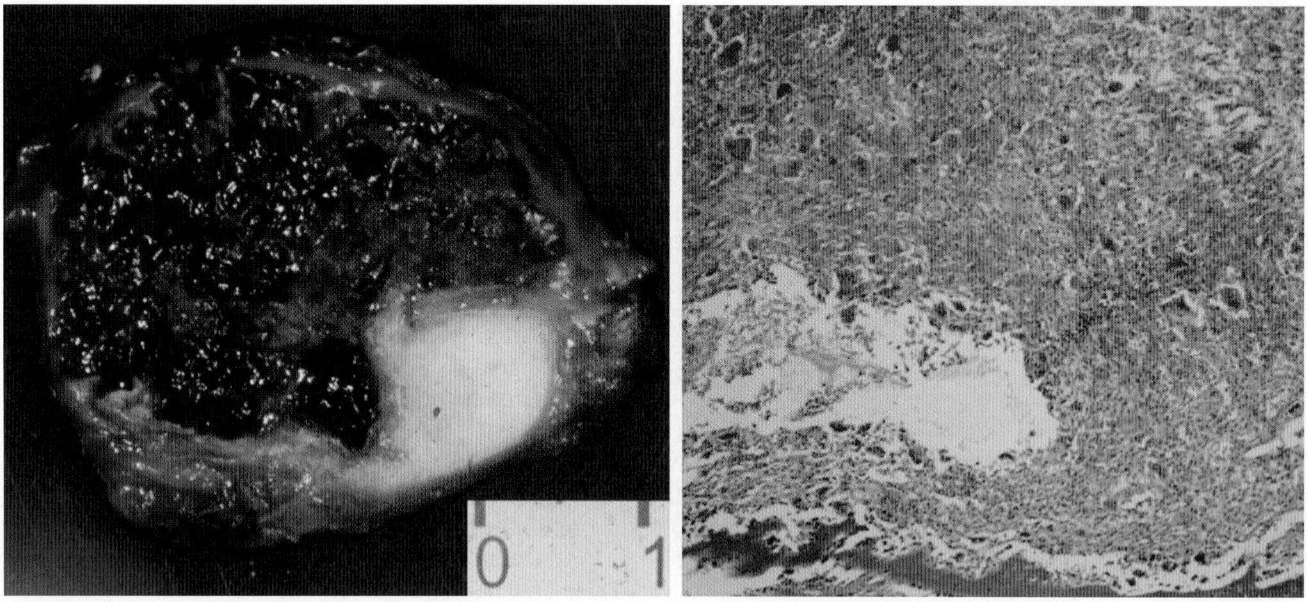

FIGURE 12.37 **Aneurysmal bone cyst from a 12-year-old boy.** A cross-section of affected rib shows expansion of the bone with thinning and destruction of the cortex by a bloody mass containing blood-filled spaces **(left)**. Microscopically, the lesion consists of mononuclear and giant cells with abundant blood and blood-filled spaces (**right**, hematoxylin and eosin, original magnification, 100×).

(Figs. 12.38 and 12.39A, B). MRI demonstrates a sharply defined intramedullary lesion that is isointense to skeletal muscle on T1-weighted MR images and heterogeneously hyperintense on T2-weighted MR images with variable contrast enhancement on postcontrast MR images. A low signal intensity rim corresponds to the sclerotic rim on radiographs.[77]

In most cases, no treatment is indicated. Follow-up imaging confirms stability. Curettage and bone grafting can be used to reinforce the abnormal bone and reduce the risk of fracture. Resection is performed for persistent symptoms or indeterminate features.[94] In resection specimens, an expansile pale tan lesion is seen. Microscopic examination shows bland fibroblastic cells with embedded spicules of bone (Fig. 12.40). Genetically, activating mutations in the *GNAS* gene are characteristic.[93]

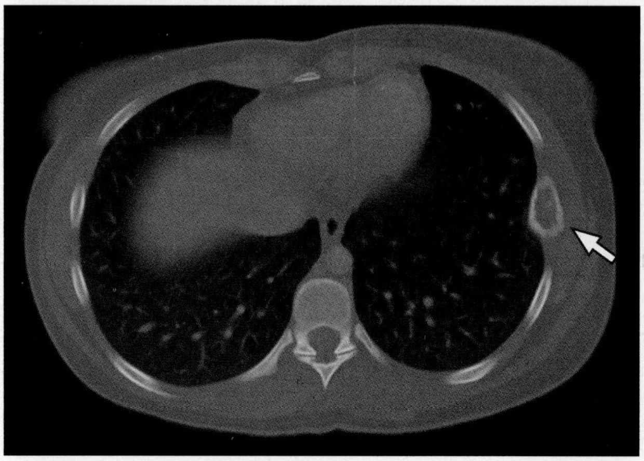

FIGURE 12.38 **Fibrous dysplasia in a 15-year-old girl with left lateral chest pain.** Axial bone window CT image shows a mildly expansile lesion (*arrow*) in the lateral left seventh rib with faint internal mineralization.

Langerhans Cell Histiocytosis

Langerhans cell histiocytosis (LCH) is a proliferation of bone marrow-derived Langerhans cells that usually presents as a painful mass. It can occur at any age, but most commonly presents in the first two decades. Traditionally, LCH has been classified as unifocal (eosinophilic granuloma), multifocal monosystem (Hand-Schüller-Christian syndrome), and multifocal multisystem (Letterer-Siwe disease). The skull, femora, mandible, pelvis, ribs, and spine are often involved. The prognosis is good if the disease is limited to the skeleton; lesions may regress on their own or with mild treatment.[95]

Initial workup for suspected osseous LCH involves radiographs of the area of interest. LCH has a variable appearance ranging from a permeative pattern with associated periostitis early in the disease to well-defined lytic lesions with beveled borders during the healing phase (Fig. 12.41A). Rib lesions are usually lytic and may have a large associated soft tissue mass, which can raise concern for a more aggressive process. Vertebral plana with preservation of the adjacent intervertebral disks is the classic appearance in the spine. CT is useful to assess intrathoracic extension and lung involvement (Fig. 12.41B). MRI demonstrates low T1 and high T2 signal intensity and enhancement when the lesion is in an active phase. Older or treated lesions are dark on T1-weighted and T2-weighted MR images with decreased surrounding marrow and soft tissue edema.[77,96]

Histologic examination confirms the characteristic Langerhans cells (Fig. 12.42). Given the availability and ease of immunohistochemical confirmation of Langerhans cells (using CD1a and Langerin antibodies), electron microscopic examination for Birbeck granules is mainly of historical interest. The identification of clonal mutations in the *BRAF* gene in most LCH has provided insights into the pathobiology of

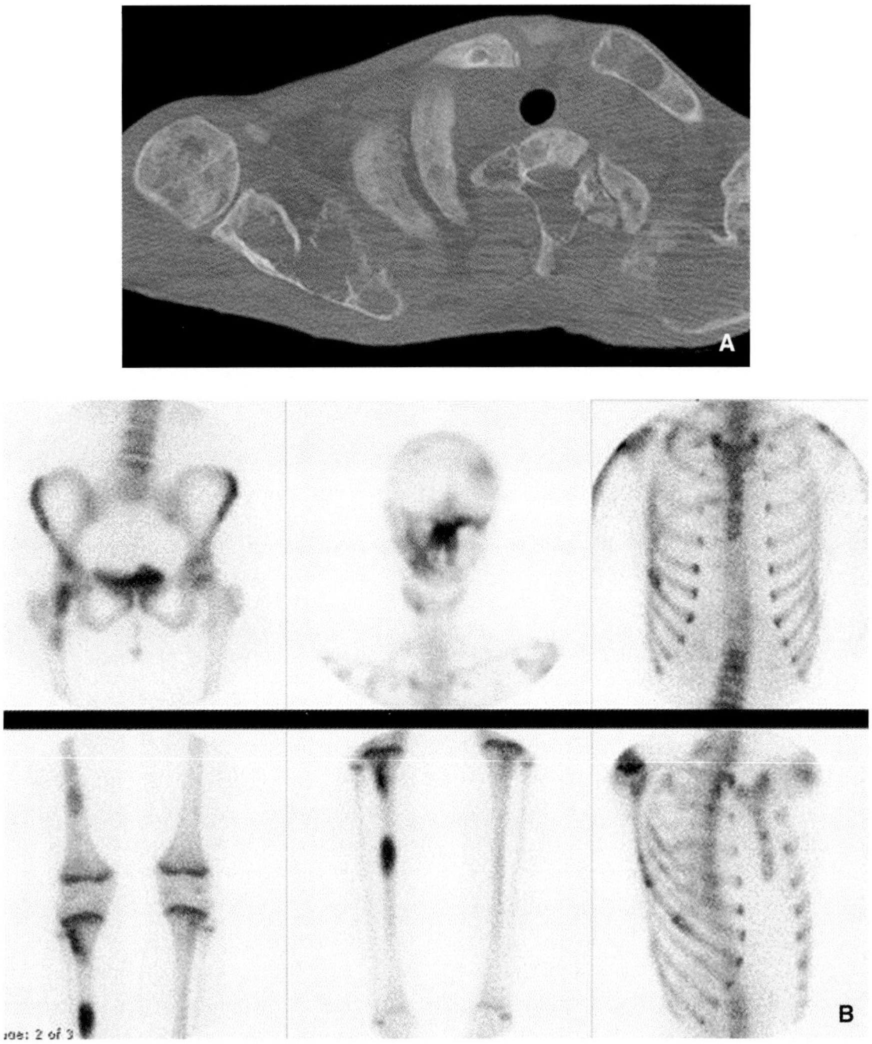

FIGURE 12.39 **Polyostotic fibrous dysplasia in two pediatric patients. A:** Axial CT image from a 17-year-old boy with McCune-Albright syndrome shows the ground-glass matrix as well as more lytic areas of involvement. **B:** MDP bone scan in an 18-year-old female with McCune-Albright syndrome demonstrates multifocal areas of increased bone turnover in the calvarium, facial bones, ribs, lumbar vertebrae, right humerus, right femur, and right tibia corresponding sites of fibrous dysplasia involvement.

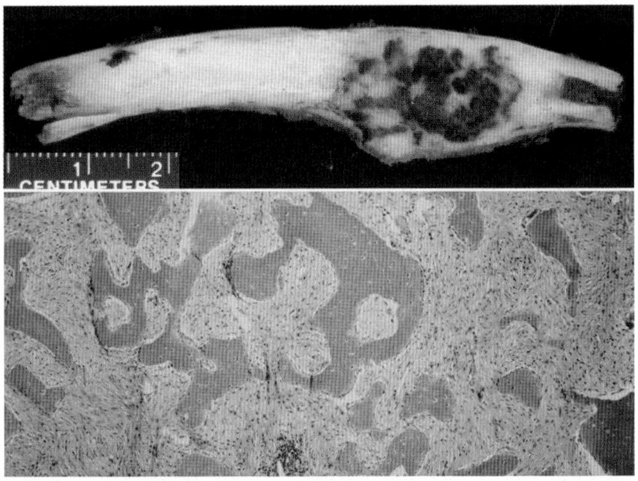

FIGURE 12.40 **Fibrous dysplasia from a 17-year-old boy with polyostotic disease.** Here, a rib shows bony expansion and cortical thinning by a tan and focally hemorrhagic mass **(upper panel)**. Microscopically, small islands of bone are embedded in a background of fibrous tissue (**lower panel**, hematoxylin and eosin, original magnification, 100×).

LCH, suggesting that it is a neoplastic disease, at least in a subset of patients.[97]

Traditionally, skeletal survey and bone scintigraphy have been performed to evaluate the extent of osseous involvement; however, whole-body coronal MR with STIR and T1 sequences has been shown to be more sensitive.[98,99] PET-CT has also emerged as an alternative or complimentary assessment tool; however, the associated radiation remains of concern. Treatment is variable depending on the extent of disease and ranges from conservative management to systemic therapy with chemotherapy, corticosteroids, and stem cell transplantation.[100]

Chondromesenchymal Hamartoma

It is debatable whether chondromesenchymal hamartoma (also known as chest wall hamartoma of infancy or mesenchymal hamartoma of chest wall) is a true neoplasm or an extremely rare overgrowth of normal skeletal components. Visible chest wall deformity usually leads to diagnosis in infancy. Significant mass effect and cardiopulmonary

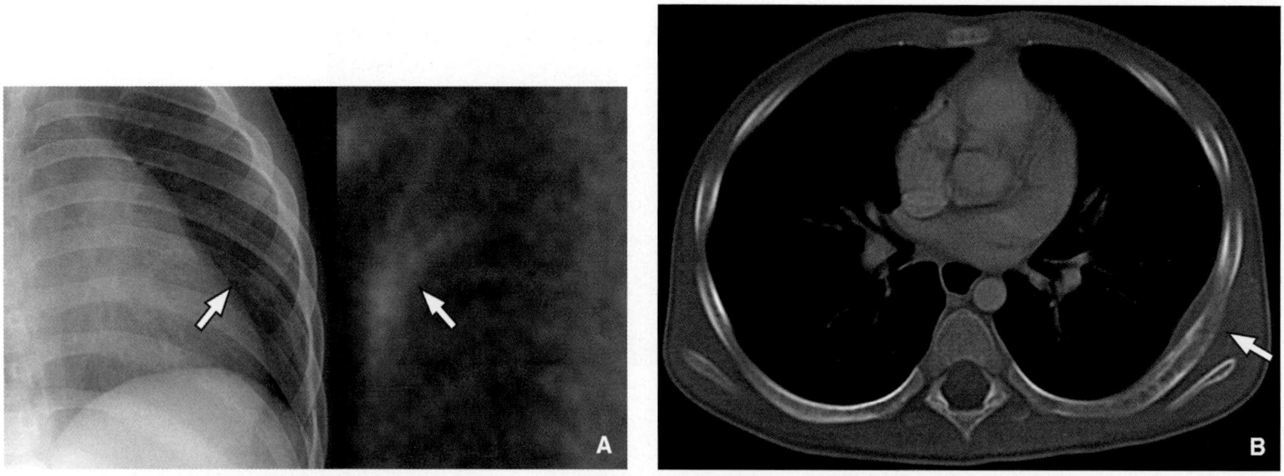

FIGURE 12.41 **Langerhans cell histiocytosis (LCH) in a 3-year-old boy who presented with cough and fever. A:** Coned-down chest radiograph **(left)** shows irregularity and expansion of left posterior 7th rib with multiple lytic areas and mild periosteal reaction (*arrow*). Posterior view bone scintigraphy **(right)** demonstrates increased uptake in the same region (*arrow*). **B:** Axial bone window CT image shows mild pleural thickening adjacent to osseous LCH lesion (*arrow*). No pulmonary parenchymal involvement is present.

compromise can occur. Histologically, the components include lobules of cartilage, immature mesenchymal cells, fibroblast-like areas, and bone, often with enchondral ossification (Fig. 12.43). The fibroblast-like areas can contain giant cells and cysts, bearing a strong resemblance to ABC.

Radiographs demonstrate an extrapleural soft tissue mass with expanded and partially destroyed ribs of origin and deformity of adjacent ribs (Fig. 12.44A). Parenchymal compression and mediastinal shift are common. Calcification is detected in the majority of lesions on radiographs and in nearly all lesions on CT. Both CT and MRI are useful to confirm the rib origin, lesion extent, and mass effect (Fig. 12.44B). Chondromesenchymal hamartomas are heterogeneous on MRI with predominantly intermediate T1 and high T2 signal. Solid components enhance with contrast. Hemorrhagic cavities are common. Calcification may cause areas of low T1 signal, whereas hemorrhage may result in focal high T1 signal.[101]

Imaging features are suggestive, but biopsy is usually required for definitive diagnosis. Growth usually stops in the first year of life and spontaneously regression can occur. Observation is adequate in asymptomatic pediatric patients. Surgical resection with chest wall reconstruction is effective in patients with symptoms or significant cosmetic deformity.[102]

Malignant Neoplasms

Malignant tumors tend to present with painful chest wall enlargement, which may be related to osseous destruction and pleural involvement. Their appearance is usually aggressive, but nonspecific on imaging, and biopsy is required for definitive diagnosis. Workup of concerning tumors

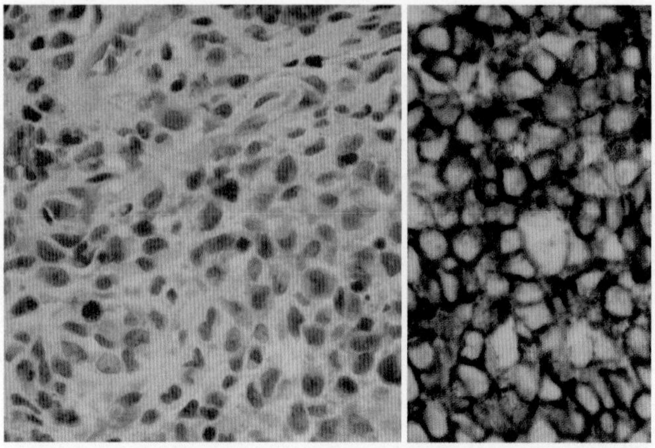

FIGURE 12.42 **Langerhans cell histiocytosis involving the rib in a 5-year-old boy.** Microscopic examination shows the characteristic Langerhans cell features of large nuclei, often with indentations or folds and abundant eosinophilic cytoplasm. An admixed eosinophil is pictured here (**left panel**, hematoxylin and eosin, original magnification, 600×). Immunostaining for CD1a is strongly positive, confirming the diagnosis (**right panel**, original magnification, 600×).

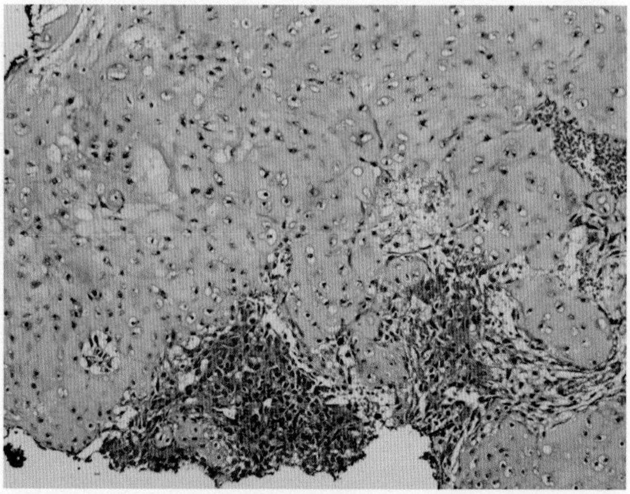

FIGURE 12.43 **Chondromesenchymal hamartoma (also known as chest wall hamartoma of infancy or mesenchymal hamartoma of chest wall) in a 4-month-old boy.** This large congenital mass involving two ribs shows a characteristic area of myxoid cartilage merging with immature mesenchymal cells (hematoxylin and eosin, original magnification, 600×). Elsewhere, aneurysmal bone cyst-like areas were seen.

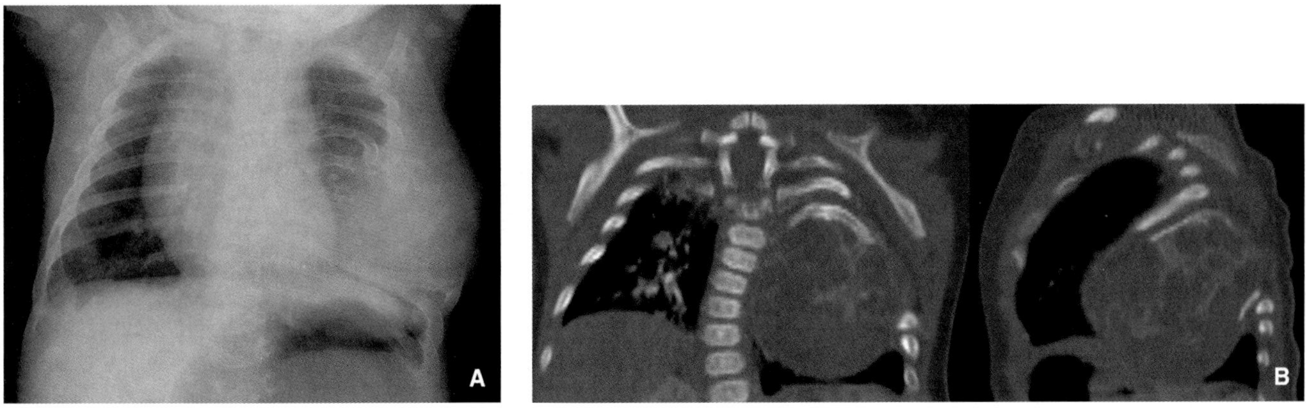

FIGURE 12.44 **Chondromesenchymal hamartoma (also known as chest wall hamartoma of infancy or mesenchymal hamartoma of chest wall) in a 3-year-old boy who presented with palpable chest lump. A:** Frontal radiograph shows a large left chest wall mass deforming, displacing, and eroding left 6th to 8th ribs. **B:** Coronal and sagittal bone window CT images confirm the rib origin and better define the partially calcified soft tissue mass. Associated scoliosis is also present.

traditionally used bone scintigraphy to evaluate for metastatic disease; however, the role of whole-body MRI and PET-CT in initial staging and posttreatment monitoring of pediatric malignancies is expanding.[103]

Soft Tissue Tumors

Rhabdomyosarcoma

Rhabdomyosarcoma is a high-grade tumor of primitive mesenchymal rhabdomyoblasts. It is the most common pediatric soft tissue sarcoma overall, but second to Ewing in the chest wall.[17] Males are affected more often than females. Presentation is usually with a large painful mass.[104] Prognosis is variable based upon histology, tumor site and size, node involvement, and patient age. Of the three types of rhabdomyosarcoma (embryonal, alveolar, and pleomorphic), the alveolar subtype is most commonly seen in the chest wall and typically presents in adolescence.[103]

A nonspecific soft tissue mass with osseous erosion may be seen radiographically (Fig. 12.45A). US shows a heterogeneous soft tissue mass with increased flow. CT is useful to evaluate for pulmonary and osseous metastatic disease. MRI can demonstrate the extent of disease, but is nonspecific with intermediate T1 signal, intermediate to high T2 signal, and avid enhancement[105] (Fig. 12.45B).

Standard of care is surgical resection and chemotherapy. Radiotherapy is frequently used for local control.[103]

Malignant Peripheral Nerve Sheath Tumor

Malignant peripheral nerve sheath tumor (MPNST) can occur sporadically or within plexiform neurofibromas in NF1. Malignant lesions are more commonly symptomatic; rapid growth and development of pain are suspicious.[75] In the thorax, the intercostal nerves are frequently involved.

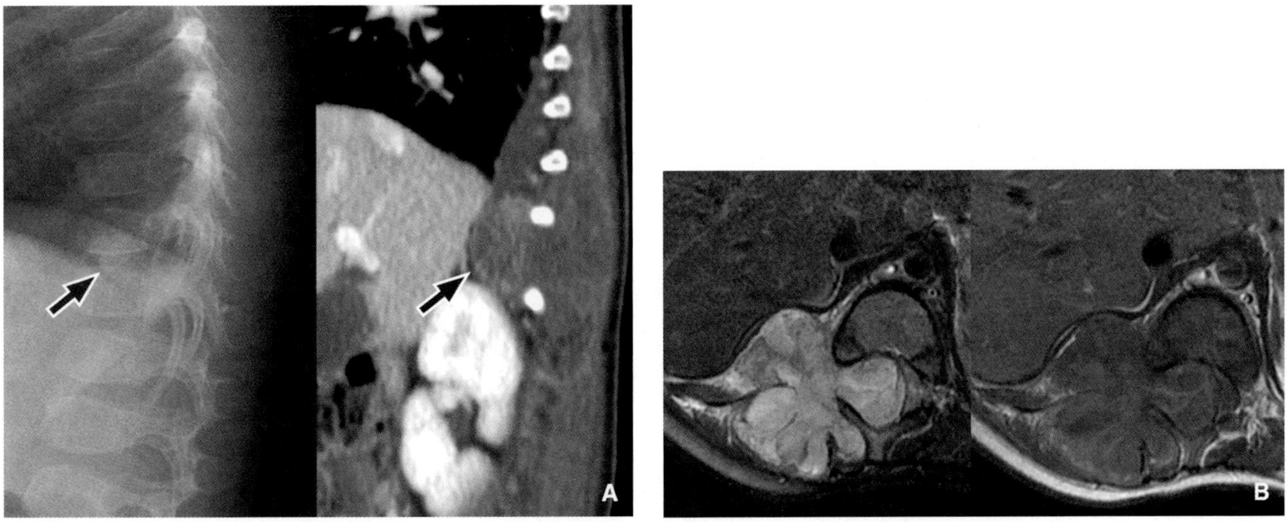

FIGURE 12.45 **Rhabdomyosarcoma in a 2-year-old girl who presented with painful back mass. A:** Lateral chest radiograph **(left)** shows abnormal soft tissue opacity (*arrow*) in the posterior costophrenic sulcus region. Sagittal enhanced CT image (**right**) shows heterogeneously enhancing paraspinal mass (*arrow*) extending through the chest wall and splaying the right posterior 11th and 12th ribs. **B:** Axial postcontrast T2-weighted fat-saturated MR image (**left**) and postcontrast T1-weighted MR image (**right**) show a heterogeneous lesion with T2 prolongation and irregular enhancement extending through right T11-12 neuroforamen into the central spinal canal.

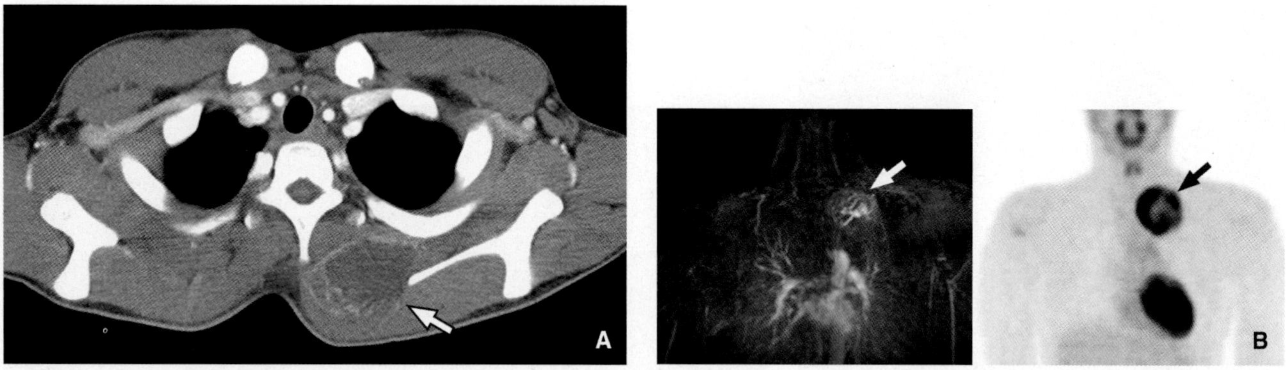

FIGURE 12.46 **Malignant peripheral nerve sheath tumor in a 17-year-old boy who presented with a new shoulder mass. A:** Axial enhanced CT image shows a somewhat ill-defined low attenuation soft tissue mass (*arrow*) with heterogeneous peripheral enhancement in the left paraspinal region. **B:** Coronal time-resolved imaging of contrast kinetic MR image **(left)** and FDG PET image **(right)** demonstrate intense early enhancement and intense uptake (*arrows*), respectively. Central photopenia on FDG PET image corresponds to necrosis.

The imaging appearance of MPNST can be similar to their benign counterparts. Radiographs may show a soft tissue mass with rib space widening and bony erosion. CT shows a heterogeneous soft tissue mass following the course of a peripheral nerve (Fig. 12.46A). The MRI appearance is usually heterogeneous due to necrosis and hemorrhage. Iso- to hyperintensity to muscle on T1-weighted MR imaging and high signal on T2-weighted sequences with heterogeneous enhancement is most common. The target and split fat signs characteristic of benign nerve sheath tumors are less common in MPNST.[106] Size >5 cm, prominent vascularity and enhancement, heterogeneity, necrosis, ill-defined infiltrative margins in nonplexiform lesions, and perilesional edema favor malignancy.[75,107,108] FDG-PET may be used for screening for malignant transformation of peripheral nerve sheath tumors[109] (Fig. 12.46B).

Wide surgical resection in conjunction with adjuvant chemotherapy and radiation is the standard of care.[76]

Synovial Sarcoma

Synovial sarcoma arises from primitive mesenchymal cells and is characterized by a specific chromosomal translocation, t(X;18)(p11;q11) leading to the fusion of the *SS18* gene on chromosome 18 with one of the *SSX* genes on chromosome X. It is the second most common pediatric soft tissue sarcoma[110] and usually does not appear until the second decade of life. Affected pediatric patients tend to present with a painful slowly growing bump. The tumor classically develops near large joints in the extremities but may occur in any soft tissue site and may occasionally arise within viscera such as the lung, heart, and kidney. Large tumor size, especially greater than 10 cm, increased tumor depth, invasion, grade, and truncal location are poor prognostic factors.[111,112] Microscopic examination shows short fascicles of primitive spindle-shaped cells. Variable stromal hyalinization and calcification are seen. Monophasic and biphasic subtypes, based on whether or not epithelial differentiation is present, have no prognostic importance.

Radiographs and CT demonstrate soft tissue mass with or without calcification. On MRI, the tumor usually appears well circumscribed with predominantly fluid signal characteristics on T1-weighted and T2-weighted MR images. Contrast may be required to distinguish the lesion from benign cystic entities, such as ganglions cysts or old hematoma.

Surgical excision is the primary treatment and may be followed by chemotherapy with or without radiation.[111]

Infantile Fibrosarcoma

Fibrosarcoma is a malignant tumor of spindle cells. Infantile fibrosarcoma (congenital fibrosarcoma) is distinct from adult-type fibrosarcoma. It is characterized by a t(12:15) translocation resulting in a fusion of the *ETV6* and *NTRK3* genes.[68,103] Infantile fibrosarcoma usually presents as a large solitary mass in infants and has a male predominance. Metastatic disease is uncommon, and prognosis is good.[103] Adult-type fibrosarcoma presents later, usually during the second decade in the pediatric population. Microscopically, fascicles of closely packed spindle cells are seen (Fig. 12.47). Mitotic figures may be frequent, and necrosis and calcification may occur.

On imaging, the tumor appears aggressive, but nonspecific as a heterogeneous soft tissue mass with osseous destruction

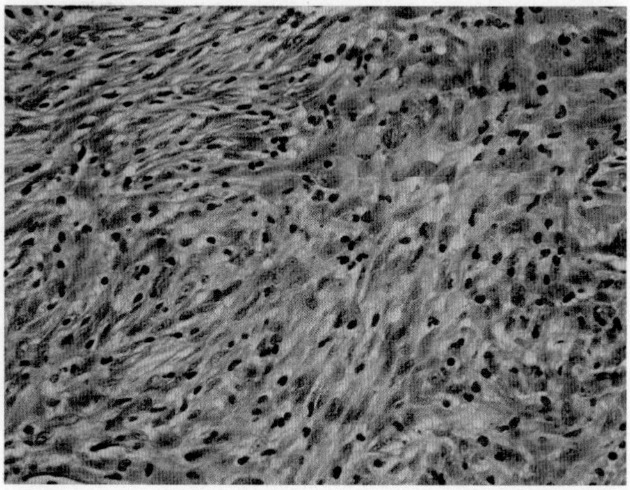

FIGURE 12.47 **Infantile fibrosarcoma in a 6-month-old girl.** Histologically, this 6 cm thigh mass shows a fascicular arrangement of densely spaced spindle cells (hematoxylin and eosin, original magnification, 400x).

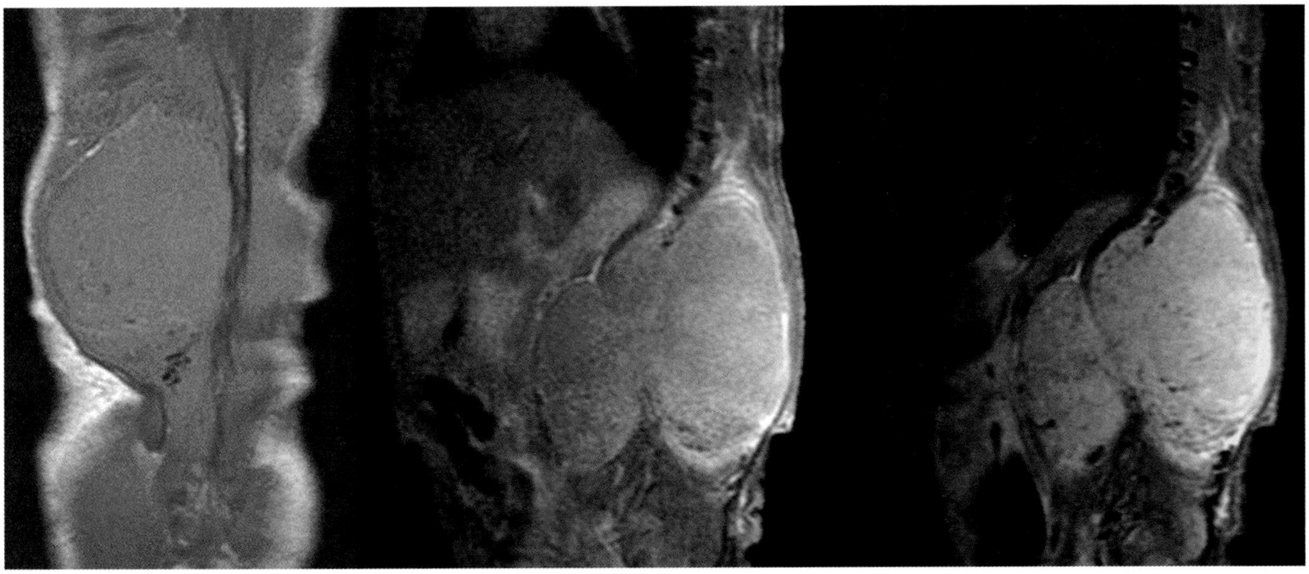

FIGURE 12.48 **Infantile fibrosarcoma in a newborn boy.** Coronal T1-weighted MR image **(left)** shows a large paraspinal mass isointense to muscle extending into the posterior inferior thoracic wall. The mass demonstrates high signal intensity on sagittal STIR MR image **(middle)** and diffuse heterogeneous enhancement on postcontrast T1-weighted fat-saturated MR image **(right)**. Sagittal MR images show extension of the mass into the psoas muscle.

and deformity.[70] Calcification or ossification may be present. Tumors are generally isointense to muscle on T1-weighted MR images and variable signal on T2-weighted MR images with heterogeneous postcontrast enhancement (Fig. 12.48). Rapid growth may result in hemorrhage and necrosis.[108]

Chemotherapy and surgery are the mainstays of treatment.[103] Radiotherapy may be added in older children.[103]

Chondrosarcoma

Chondrosarcoma is the third most common primary malignant tumor of bone, but it is rare in the pediatric population. It is characterized by infiltrating cartilage matrix forming tumor cells.[81] Presentation is usually a palpable painful mass. Within the chest wall, chondrosarcomas most commonly arise from the anterior upper five ribs near the costochondral junction or from the sternum.[108,113] Lesions may arise de novo or from a preexisting enchondroma or osteochondroma.

The radiographic appearance may be difficult to differentiate from a benign cartilage lesion or it may be more aggressive with a poorly defined mass and cortical destruction. CT more clearly demonstrates chondroid matrix calcification and any associated osseous destruction (Fig. 12.49). MRI is useful to evaluate the extent of marrow involvement and extraosseous extension. Signal intensity is similar to muscle on T1-weighted MR images and hyperintense on T2-weighted MR images with dark calcifications. Contrast enhancement is heterogeneous.[108]

Diagnosis requires histologic demonstration of tumor infiltration.[81] Resection is the primary method of treatment.[76]

Osseous Tumors

Ewing Sarcoma/Primitive Neuroectodermal Tumor

The most common malignant tumor of the chest wall in the pediatric population is the Ewing sarcoma/primitive neuroectodermal tumor (EWS/PNET). This tumor type combines entities formerly known as PNET, Askin tumor, classic EWS of bone, and extraosseous EWS,[106,114] tumors that are recognized as genetically and biologically similar. EWS/PNET is composed of small, round, blue-stained cells of neural crest origin (Fig. 12.50). EWS/PNET is one of several different tumor types that is most often characterized by a chromosomal translocation involving the *EWSR1* gene on the long arm of chromosome 22.[115] EWS/PNET is more common in males and frequently presents in the second decade with a rapidly growing mass or pain. Presentation may mimic osteomyelitis with fever and leukocytosis.[116] Within the chest wall, the rib is the most common primary location accounting for ~50% cases.[117] Overall, ~6% to 11% of primary tumors involve the chest wall.[118,119]

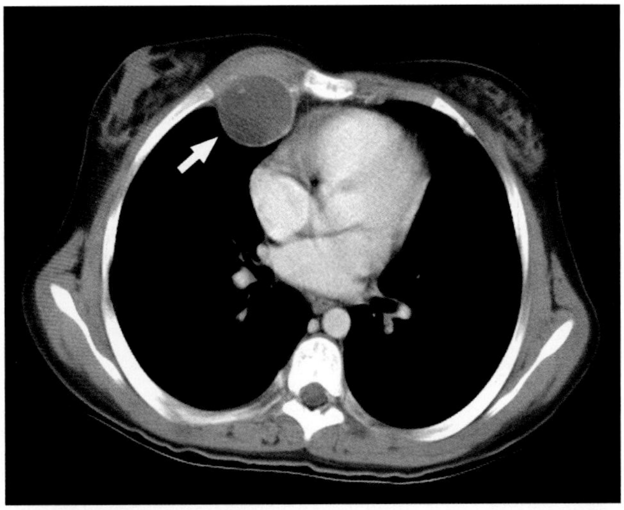

FIGURE 12.49 **Chondrosarcoma in a 11-year-old girl who presented with a painful and palpable right anterior chest wall mass.** Axial enhanced CT image demonstrates a low attenuation mass (*arrow*) with a small focus of mineralization arising from the right anterior costal cartilage.

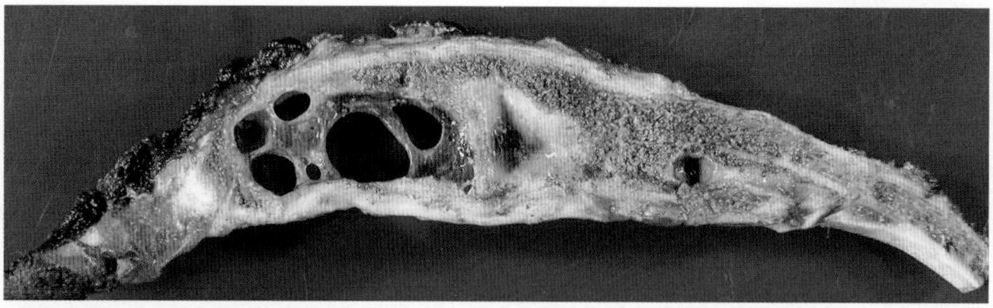

FIGURE 12.50 **Ewing sarcoma/primitive neuroectodermal tumor in an 11-year-old boy.** In the postchemotherapy resection specimen of the 10th rib and surrounding soft tissue (pictured here), the extensive cystic change and fibrosis reflect treatment effect. Only scant residual tumor cells were identified microscopically (not shown).

Lesions may be lytic, sclerotic, or mixed. Radiographs typically demonstrate a permeative pattern of osseous destruction and expansion with aggressive, classically lamellated, periosteal reaction and a large soft tissue mass[120] (Fig. 12.51A) (Table 12.4). US may readily show the soft tissue mass but is not as reliable as CT in demonstrating the extent of cortical bone involvement (Fig. 12.51B). CT is superior for identifying early pulmonary metastases. The soft tissue characteristics, marrow involvement, and spread to adjacent structures are best depicted on MRI. Signal intensity of the mass is usually hyperintense to muscle on T1-weighted MR images and heterogeneously hyperintense on T2-weighted MR images. The soft tissue tumor and involved marrow show heterogeneous enhancement.

Extraskeletal EWS/PNET tends to present in slightly older patients in paravertebral and intercostal locations.[121] Radiographs and CT typically demonstrate a well-circumscribed, noncalcified soft tissue mass with osseous erosion.[122] On MRI, the tumors demonstrate low to intermediate signal on T1-weighted MR images and heterogeneous high signal on T2-weighted MR images with heterogeneous enhancement.[121]

Surgery and neoadjuvant chemotherapy are standard. Radiation may be used for local control in metastatic disease. Overall, prognosis is variable with event-free survival ranging from 33% to 75%.[123]

Osteosarcoma

Osteosarcomas are high-grade tumors of bone. They are the most common primary malignant bone tumor in children and adolescents, but only 1% of osteosarcomas arise in the chest wall and spine.[103] Ribs (especially the costochondral junction), scapulae, and clavicles are the most common chest wall sites of origin.[76] They occur more commonly in males and may arise de novo, in a site of prior radiation, or within a preexisting lesion. There is an increased risk in patients with retinoblastoma and Li-Fraumeni syndrome. Most osteosarcomas in children are conventional high-grade type.[77] Pain is the most common presenting symptom. Chest wall lesions are more likely to result in pulmonary and lymph node metastases compared to extremity lesions.[108] Tumor burden and histologic responses to preoperative chemotherapy (indicated by necrosis) are prognostic.[77]

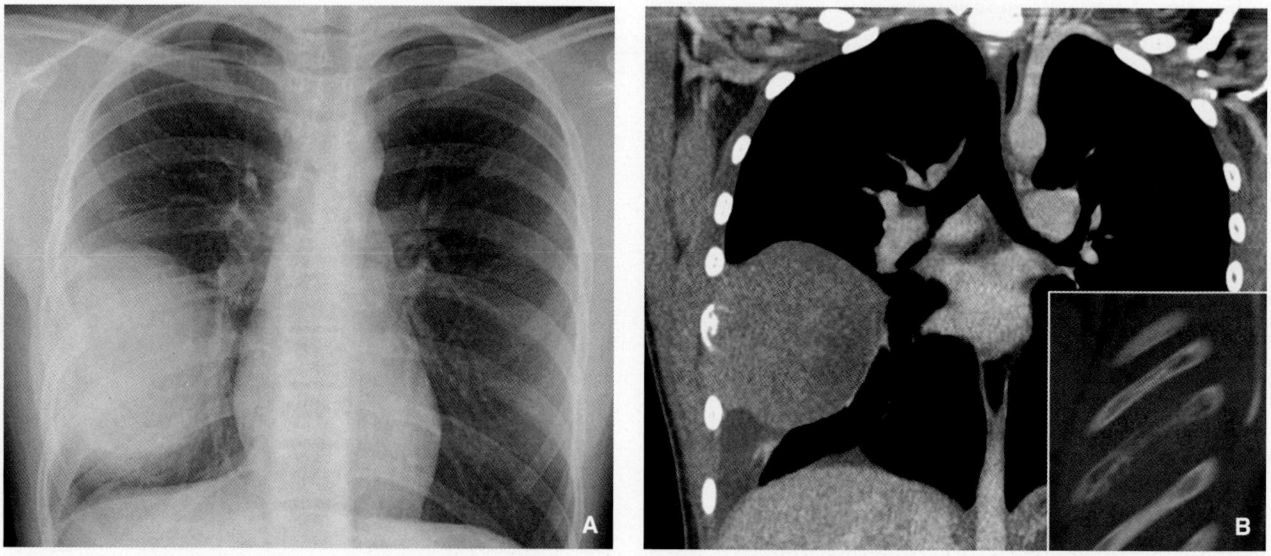

FIGURE 12.51 **Ewing sarcoma in a 15-year-old boy who presented with right axillary pain. A:** Frontal radiograph shows a large mass in the right hemithorax with adjacent pleural thickening and moth-eaten appearance of the lateral right sixth rib. **B:** Coronal enhanced CT image demonstrates heterogeneous enhancement of the mass, which extends into the chest wall between the fifth through seventh ribs. Right sixth rib (**inset**) demonstrates permeative destruction with periosteal reaction.

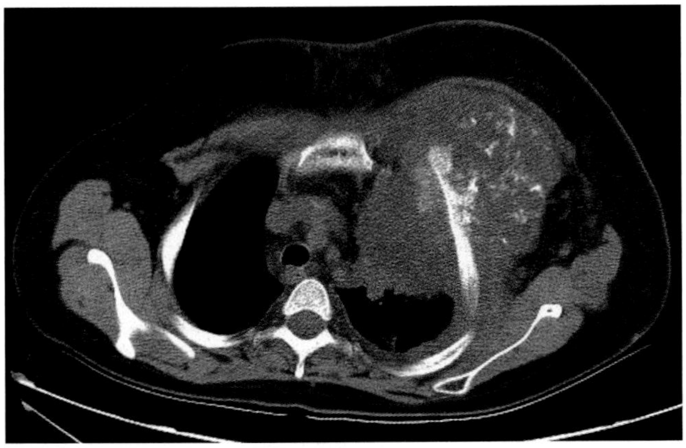

FIGURE 12.52 **Osteosarcoma in a 15-year-old boy who presented with a painful and enlarging left chest wall mass.** Axial nonenhanced CT image shows a large mass arising from a left rib with associated extensive ossification.

Imaging demonstrates a destructive bone lesion with osteoid matrix and associated soft tissue mass.[113] The classic sunburst pattern of periosteal reaction in extremity osteosarcomas is not commonly seen in the chest wall.[108] CT best demonstrates cortical involvement, whereas MRI is superior in demonstrating marrow and soft tissue components (Fig. 12.52). The associated soft tissue mass is hyperintense to muscle on T1- and T2-weighted sequences with heterogeneous enhancement. Low signal intensity foci represent calcification. Intense FDG uptake is demonstrated on PET.[108]

Gross examination of osteosarcoma typically reveals a tan focally hemorrhagic and necrotic mass within the medullary cavity, permeating the cortex, and extending into soft tissue. Microscopically, malignant cells may show osteoblastic, chondroblastic, and fibroblastic differentiation in varying proportions. In the appropriate radiographic context, the histologic identification of "malignant osteoid" is diagnostic of osteosarcoma (Fig. 12.53).

Treatment involves surgical resection and chemotherapy. Osteosarcomas are relatively insensitive to radiotherapy.[103]

Plasmacytoma

Plasmacytomas are a localized proliferation of monoclonal plasma B cells. They are more common in males and may present as a slowly growing, painful mass. The lesions are often recurrent and may precede systemic disease (multiple myeloma) by 10 years. The axial skeleton, especially the vertebrae, is most commonly affected.[124] Neurologic deficit may occur from spinal cord compression.[125] Plasmacytoma-like posttransplant lymphoproliferative disorder has recently been reported in pediatric renal and combined liver and intestinal transplant recipients.[126]

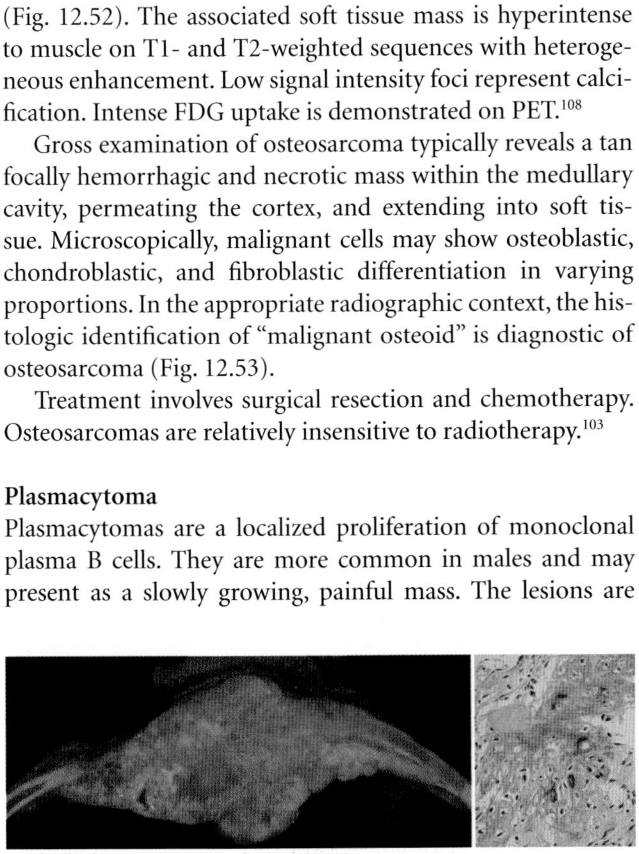

FIGURE 12.53 **Osteosarcoma in a 15-year-old girl.** Tumor expands the fifth rib, destroying cortex, and extending into soft tissue. The cut surface (**left**) is hard and focally white and shiny, reflecting a component of cartilaginous differentiation. Microscopically (**right**), the tumor shows areas with large atypical malignant cells lying in an osteoid extracellular matrix, diagnostic of osteosarcoma (hematoxylin and eosin, original magnification 400×).

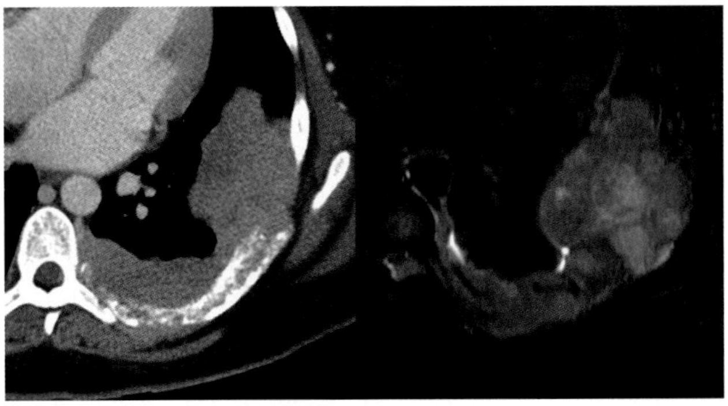

FIGURE 12.54 **Plasmacytoma in a 16-year-old boy who presented with chest pain.** Axial enhanced CT image (**left**) shows a heterogeneously enhancing mass with permeative destruction of adjacent posterior lateral seventh rib. STIR MR image (**right**) shows heterogeneous T2 prolongation.

Radiographs typically show a well-defined lytic lesion with soft tissue mass; marked osseous erosion and expansion are seen in advanced cases. A "soap bubble appearance" may be present. MRI demonstrates low T1 and high T2 signal and homogeneous enhancement[125] (Fig. 12.54).

Treatment is primarily with radiation.[76] Treatment of PTLD-associated lesions may require chemotherapy, steroids, and reduced immunosuppression.[126]

Metastasis

Metastatic involvement of the chest wall from tumors such as neuroblastoma, rhabdomyosarcoma, lymphoma, and leukemia occurs more frequently than primary chest wall malignancy.[127] Although the imaging appearance is often nonspecific, the development of a focal chest wall lesion should raise concern for metastatic disease in any pediatric patient with a known diagnosis of malignancy. Chest wall involvement may result from direct extension or hematogenous spread. Metastatic lesions are typically lytic with cortical destruction and periosteal reaction. Treatment is generally palliative.

Neuroblastoma originates from neural crest cells in the adrenal glands or sympathetic chain (Fig. 12.55). It is one of the most common childhood malignancies and usually presents before age five with mass and pain.[128] Tumor behavior and prognosis are extremely variable depending on patient age, histology, and tumor genetics.[103] Calcifications are commonly seen on radiographs and CT. MR is useful to evaluate extension through the neural foramina and spinal canal. The tumor demonstrates high T2 signal and enhancement. Metaiodobenzylguanidine (MIBG) scans are used for metastatic workup and treatment response evaluation. Therapy ranges from observation to aggressive management with surgery, chemotherapy, radiation, and stem cell transplantation.[103]

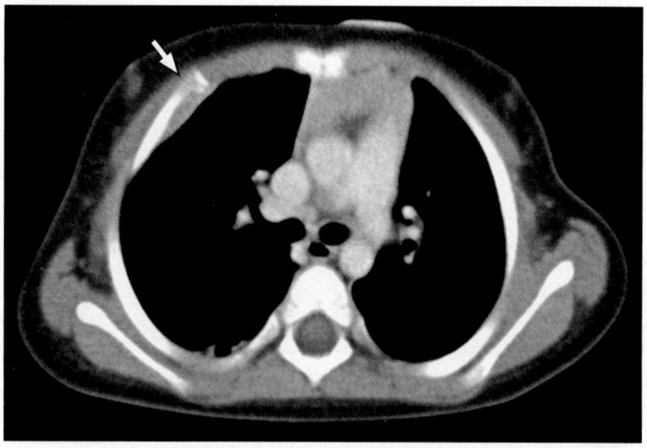

FIGURE 12.55 **Neuroblastoma metastasis in a 4-year-old boy with primary adrenal neuroblastoma.** Axial enhanced CT image shows ill-defined soft tissue surrounding the right anterior third rib with osseous destruction (*arrow*).

Approximately 14% of pediatric patients with rhabdomyosarcoma have metastatic disease at the time of diagnosis. Lung and bone are common locations for rhabdomyosarcoma metastasis (Fig. 12.56). Chest CT, bone scintigraphy, and marrow aspirate and biopsy are usually performed in newly diagnosed cases. MRI is useful to demonstrate marrow metastases not evident on bone scintigraphy.[129]

Bone lesions are most common in the acute lymphoblastic form of leukemia.[128] Chest wall involvement may manifest as bone pain and multiple lytic, destructive lesions with periosteal reaction. MRI is useful to identify more subtle diffuse marrow changes.

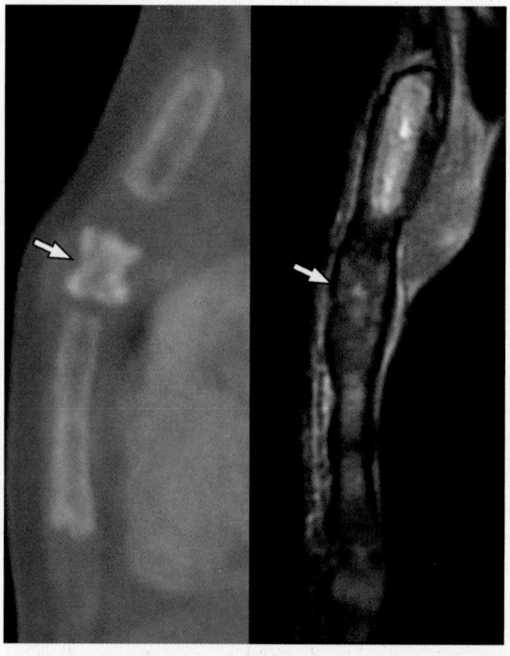

FIGURE 12.56 **Metastatic rhabdomyosarcoma in a 4-year-old boy who presented with fever, anemia, and cough.** Metastasis (*arrow*) to the sternum on sagittal bone window CT image (**left**) as evidenced by sclerosis and irregularity of the midsternal segment. Sagittal T2-weighted fat-saturated MR image (**right**) shows irregular and abnormal heterogeneous low signal (*arrow*) in the corresponding sternal segment.

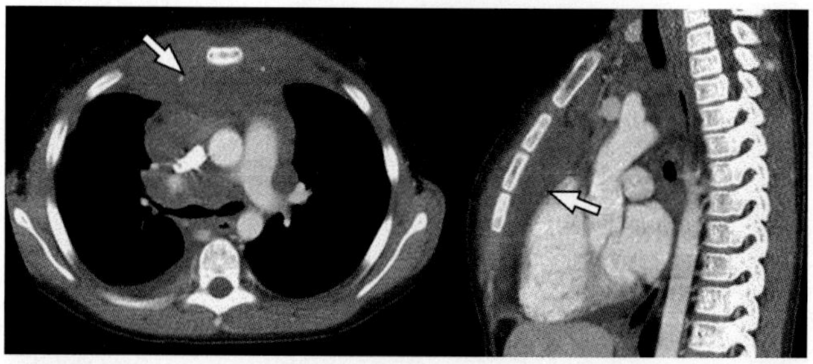

FIGURE 12.57 **Lymphoma in an 11-year-old boy who presented with chest wall swelling.** Axial **(left)** and sagittal **(right)** enhanced CT images show a low attenuation anterior mediastinal mass (*arrows*) directly extending into the anterior chest wall.

Lymphoma occasionally involves the chest wall by direct extension from the mediastinum[28] (Fig. 12.57). Involvement of the chest wall in primary extranodal soft tissue lymphoma and primary lymphoma of bone is uncommon. Soft tissue disease may appear as subtle loss of tissue planes or a focal enhancing soft tissue mass. Affected osseous structures may demonstrate a permeative pattern of destruction. Extent of marrow involvement is more clearly seen on MRI as abnormal low T1 signal intensity.[130]

Traumatic Disorders

Accidental Traumatic Injuries

Posttraumatic abnormalities may cause concern for an aggressive lesion on physical exam or imaging. History usually provides clarity; however, in some cases, no history of trauma can be elicited.

Hematoma may resemble a soft tissue mass on radiographs. On US, acute hematomas are hyperechoic with ill-defined borders, and no internal flow, subacute hematomas are more defined with central hypoechogenicity and echogenic borders, and chronic hematomas are anechoic and well circumscribed[55] (Fig. 12.58A). CT shows a hyperattenuated collection in the acute setting. MRI is not usually indicated unless there is no clear history of trauma. The appearance is variable depending on the acuity, but areas of high T1 and low T2 signal with blooming on gradient-echo sequences are characteristic[62] (Fig. 12.58B).

Fat necrosis may result from mechanical injury; however, a clear history of trauma is often infrequent.[131] In the neonatal period, hypoxia and hypothermia contribute.[132] Resulting hemorrhage and fibrosis may create superficial, palpable masses.[131] CT demonstrates subcutaneous nodular areas of increased attenuation.[132] MR confirms lack of a true mass and demonstrates characteristic linear signal abnormalities (high T2 or low T1 or T2 signal intensity) confined to the subcutaneous fat.[131]

Traumatic rib and sternal fractures occur less frequently in children due to the elasticity of the chest wall. Radiographs demonstrate acute displaced fractures and healing fractures; nondisplaced acute fractures are often occult. Exuberant or unusual callous may cause concern on physical exam or radiographs; correlation with history and evolution over time guides proper diagnosis. CT more clearly shows acute nondisplaced fractures; however, due to the radiation exposure, it is typically reserved for evaluation of parenchymal or cardiovascular injury in patients with severe trauma

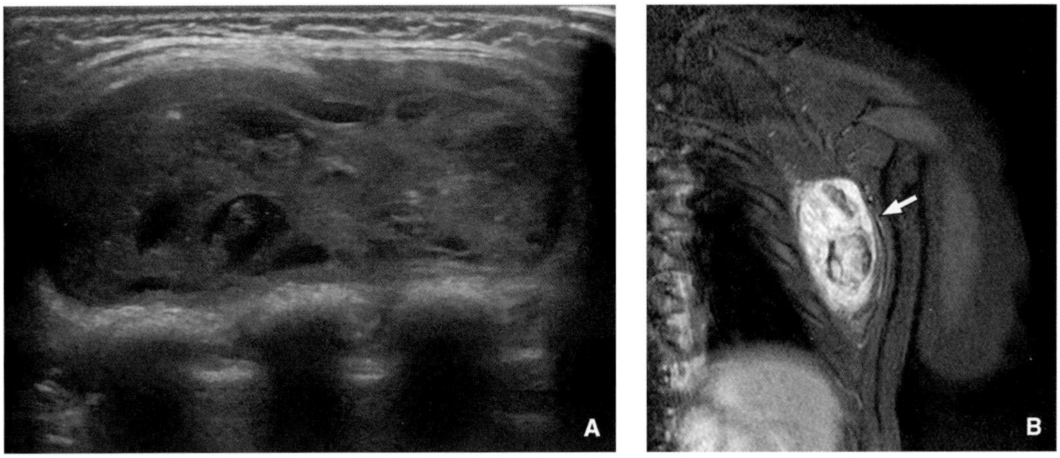

FIGURE 12.58 **Chest wall hematoma in a 4-year-old boy status post motor vehicle accident. A:** Ultrasound shows a slightly echogenic mass with small cystic spaces consistent with an evolving hematoma overlying the ribs after blunt trauma. **B:** Coronal T2-weighted fat-saturated MR image shows a hyperintense round lesion (*arrow*) with hypointense elements likely due to hemosiderin.

(Fig. 12.59). A low signal intensity fracture line with marrow edema can be seen on MRI; however, it is not routinely indicated. Cortical disruption with hematoma can be demonstrated on US. Treatment of rib fractures is supportive. In rare cases, multiple consecutive rib fractures can cause a flail chest necessitating ventilatory support.

Nonaccidental Fracture

The imaging appearance of the fracture itself is the same for accidental and inflicted rib fractures; clinical history and fracture location aid diagnosis. Rib fractures are unusual in pediatrics in the absence of major trauma and should be regarded with a high level of suspicion (Table 12.4). Multiple fractures of various ages are of moderate specificity for inflicted injury. Metaphyseal corner fractures, posteromedial rib fractures, and sternal, scapular, and spinous process fractures are considered highly specific[133,134] (Fig. 12.60A, B).

Radiographic skeletal survey is the initial imaging modality of choice in cases of suspected abuse. A follow-up skeletal survey may be needed for confirmation of findings. Tc-99 MDP bone scan may be performed as a compliment to the skeletal survey. More recently, ^{18}F-NaF PET has been shown to have a higher overall sensitivity for detection of fractures in children younger than 2 years than the initial skeletal survey. However, detection of classic metaphyseal fractures is limited due to physiologic physeal uptake: consequently, initial radiographic survey remains necessary.[14]

Vascular Disorders

Vascular anomalies, including malformations and tumors, are the most common cause of pediatric soft tissue masses.[62] In general, superficial lesions may be well evaluated by US, which can discriminate between high and low flow lesions.

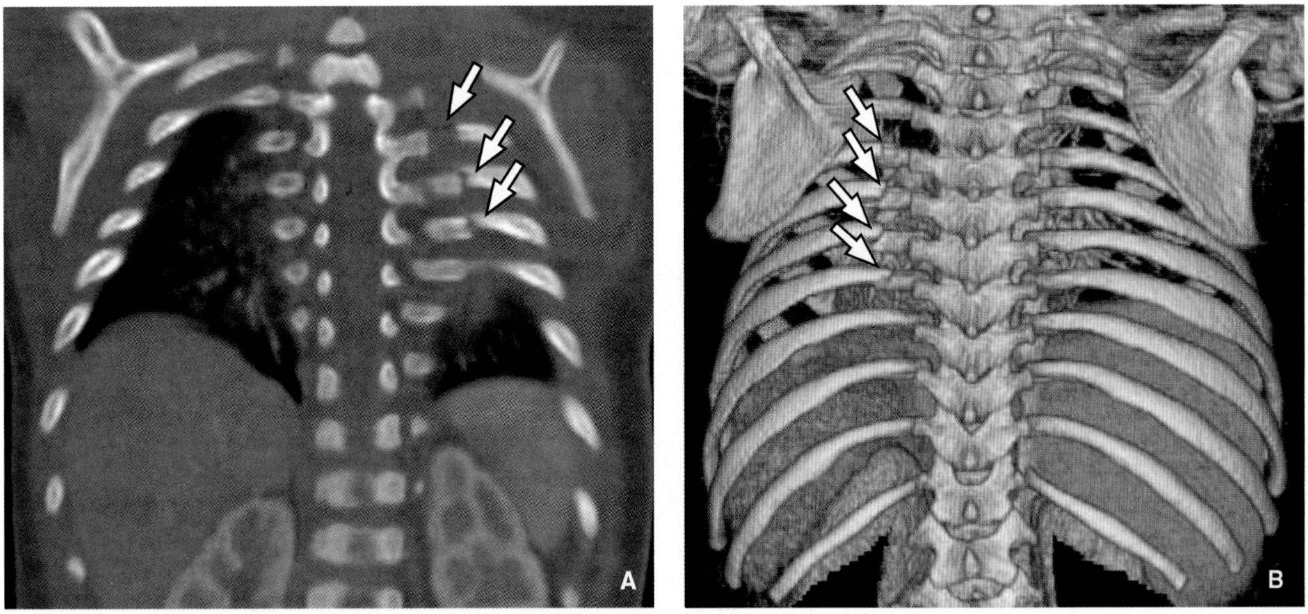

FIGURE 12.59 **Traumatic rib fractures in a 5-year-old boy after a car accident.** Coronal bone window CT image **(A)** and posterior view of 3D volume-rendered CT image **(B)** show four consecutive rib fractures (*arrows*) of the fifth through eighth posterior medial ribs.

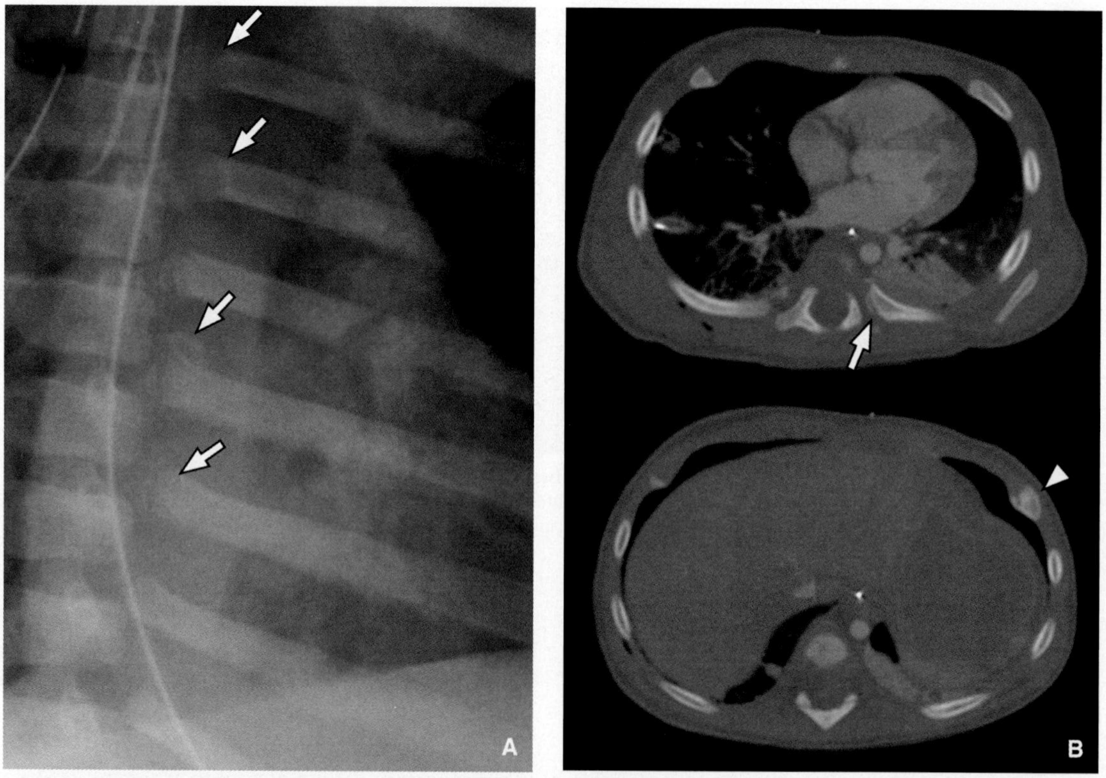

FIGURE 12.60 **Nonaccidental rib fractures in a 9-month-old boy. A:** Coned rib radiograph shows multiple healing left posterior medial rib fractures (*arrows*) with periosteal reaction. **B:** Axial bone window CT images show the left posterior medial rib fracture (*arrow*), more chronic appearing left anterior costochondral junction fracture (*arrowhead*), and pulmonary contusion and atelectasis.

For deeper and more extensive lesions, cross-sectional imaging, particularly, MRI, provides superior evaluation. Heavily T2-weighted MRI sequences are highly accurate in demonstrating the extent of vascular anomalies.[135]

Vascular Malformations

Vascular malformations are developmental anomalies with normal cell turnover. Although not always visible, they are present at birth and typically grow commensurate with the child. Rapid expansion can result from trauma, infection, or hormonal influence.[136] No gender predilection has been identified. Transpatial involvement is typical. Skeletal and soft tissue overgrowth and significant disfigurement may result. Vascular malformations are divided into high-flow malformations (e.g., arteriovenous malformation and arteriovenous fistula) and low-flow malformations (e.g., venous malformation and lymphatic malformation). The distinction is critical to guide appropriate management. Chest wall vascular malformations that occur in pediatric patients are typically low-flow malformations.

Venous Malformation

Venous malformations (VMs) are composed of dysplastic, thin-walled, tortuous postcapillary channels that connect with physiologic veins. They are the most common vascular malformation outside of the central nervous system. A bluish lesion may be visible on the skin (Fig. 12.61A). Lesions are soft and compressible unless complicated by thrombosis.

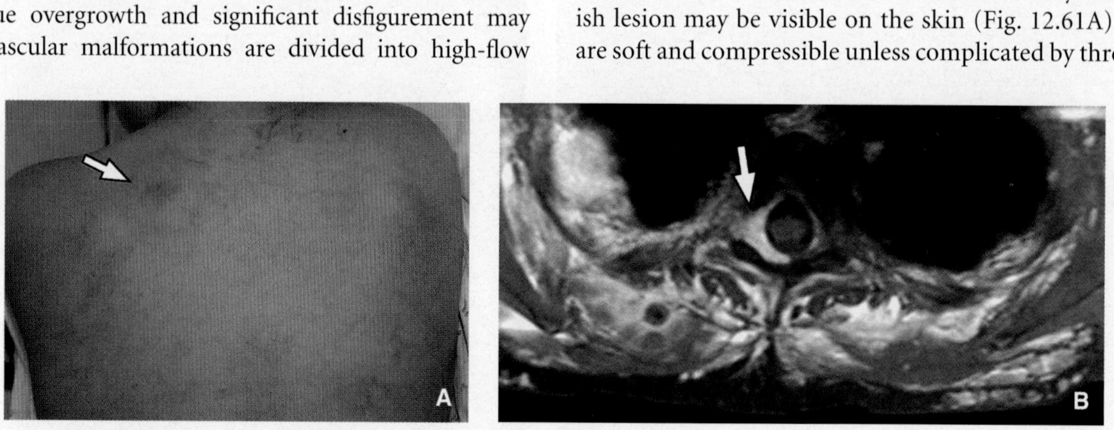

FIGURE 12.61 **Venous malformation (VM) in a 9-year-old boy. A:** Photograph shows blue soft tissue mass (*arrow*) in the upper back. Multiple dilated superficial veins are also visible. **B:** Axial postcontrast T1-weighted fat-saturated MR image in the same patient shows contrast enhancement of the lobulated left posterior chest wall lesion involving the subcutaneous tissues and extending intramuscularly. Additionally, there is more infiltrative VM involving deeper portions of the posterior chest wall bilaterally extending into the right neuroforamen (*arrow*).

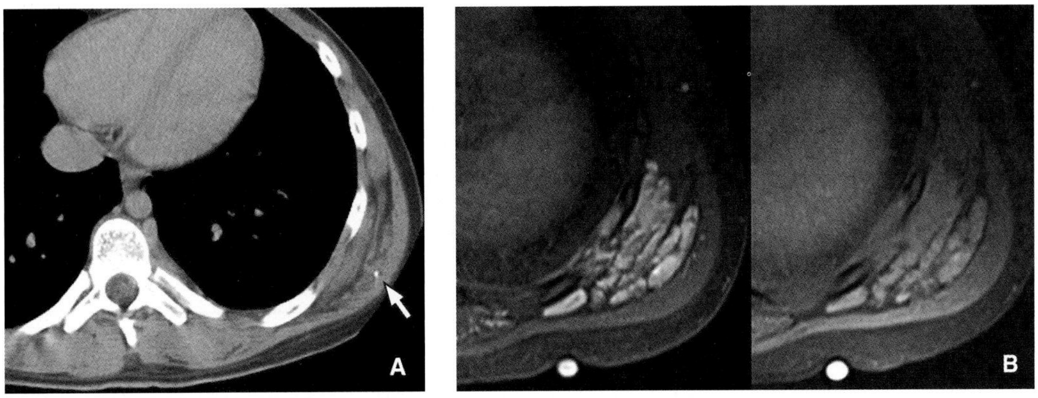

FIGURE 12.62 **Venous malformation in a 17-year-old girl with left back pain and swelling. A:** Axial CT image demonstrates lobulated left posterior-lateral chest wall soft tissue mass isointense to adjacent skeletal muscle with small phlebolith (*arrow*). **B:** Axial T2-weighted fat-saturated MR image **(left)** and axial postcontrast T1-weighted fat-saturated MR image **(right)** show lobulated high T2 signal and enhancement.

Large and/or deep VMs are associated with localized intravascular coagulopathy (LIC), which can lead to pain from thrombosis and hemorrhage.[137] The vast majority of VMs are sporadic and unifocal. Multiple cutaneous VMs may be associated with visceral VMs in blue rubber bleb nevus syndrome.[138]

On radiographs, VMs appear as soft tissue masses sometimes containing phleboliths (Table 12.4). They demonstrate mixed echogenicity on US with sponge-like anechoic vascular spaces, which are usually compressible.[139] Doppler may show slow venous flow or no flow. Echogenic shadowing foci correspond to phleboliths. Phleboliths associated with VMs are better visualized on CT (Fig. 12.62A). MRI demonstrates lobulated, septated high T2 signal with well circumscribed hypointense phleboliths, slow gradual diffuse contrast enhancement, and absence of flow voids[140] (Fig. 12.62B).

Pathologic examination of VM typically shows blood-filled spaces, often with thrombi and phleboliths (Fig. 12.63). Sclerotherapy, typically with ethanol or foamed detergent, has become the treatment of choice for symptomatic lesions.[141]

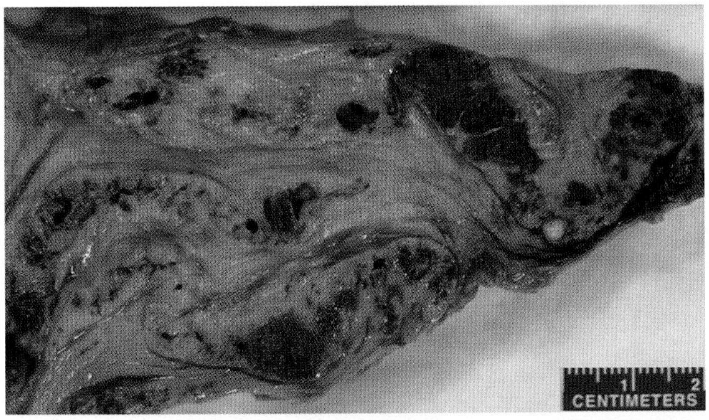

FIGURE 12.63 **Venous malformation.** Long-standing congenital venous malformation of the chest wall resected at age 27, years after sclerotherapy and embolization therapy. Numerous thrombi and phleboliths are seen grossly within the fibroadipose tissue.

Low molecular weight heparin can be used to treat LIC and to prevent severe LIC from progressing to disseminated intravascular coagulopathy.[137]

Lymphatic Malformation

Lymphatic malformations (LMs) are composed of endothelial-lined, chyle-filled sequestered lymphatic sacs. They are the second most common vascular malformation. Axillary, chest, and cervicofacial regions are most commonly affected.[28] LMs lack communication with draining lymphatic channels and thus are typically rubbery and noncompressible. Turner syndrome, Noonan syndrome, and trisomies 13, 18, and 21 are associated with LMs.[142]

The imaging appearance of LMs is variable depending upon the predominance of microcystic or macrocystic components. Microcystic lesions may mimic solid soft tissue masses. Infiltrative foci of high T2 signal may be seen on MRI. Macrocystic lesions demonstrate discrete cysts without internal flow on US. Low-level echoes and fluid–fluid levels may result from blood or proteinaceous material (Table 12.4). MRI shows septated cysts with septal and mural enhancement, but no internal enhancement[28] (Fig. 12.64).

Reaccumulation is typical after drainage unless complete surgical excision or sclerotherapy is performed. Sclerotherapy has become the treatment of choice for symptomatic lesions.

Vascular Tumors

Infantile Hemangioma

Hemangiomas are benign high flow vascular neoplasms resulting from endothelial cell proliferation (Table 12.4). They are the most common soft tissue tumors of childhood, affecting ~10% of Caucasian infants.[143] Lesions are visualized at birth or within the first few months of life (Fig. 12.65A). Diagnosis is often made clinically by the appearance and typical growth pattern characterized by an early proliferative phase in the first few months of life, growth plateau, and spontaneous involution over several years.

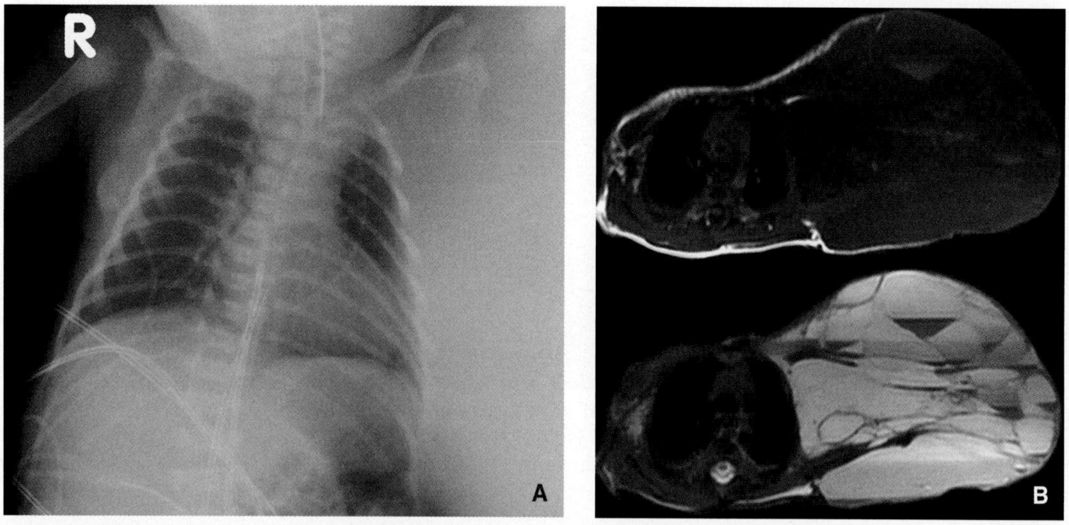

FIGURE 12.64 **Lymphatic malformation in a newborn boy with axillary mass. A:** Chest radiograph demonstrates a massive soft tissue mass extending from the left chest wall. **B:** Axial T1-weighted (**top**) and T2-weighted fat-saturated (**bottom**) MR images demonstrate large left chest wall mass composed of multiple cystic areas with fluid–fluid levels. High T1 and low T2 signal intensity within dependent portions of cystic areas represents blood products and/or proteinaceous material.

Most lesions never present for imaging; however, occasionally, the extent of a lesion or presence of a deep lesion cannot be determined clinically. US should be the first-line imaging and typically reveals a homogeneous soft tissue mass hypoechoic or isoechoic to adjacent muscle with high velocity arterial and venous spectra (Fig. 12.65B). Vessel density >5 vessels/cm^2 and maximum systolic Doppler shift of >2 kHz has a specificity of 98%.[144] Arterial flow may be more difficult to identify in involuting lesions making distinction from low flow lesions difficult. Hemangiomas can be distinguished from arteriovenous malformations by presence of a solid parenchyma component.[139] CT demonstrates a well-defined soft tissue mass with diffuse, intense contrast enhancement. On MRI, hemangioma is a well-defined lobulated mass of intermediate to low signal intensity on T1-weighted MR images and high signal intensity on T2-weighted MR images with diffuse arterial phase enhancement and flow voids. Areas of fibrofatty deposition develop in the involutional phase with corresponding heterogeneously increased T1 signal, decreased T2 signal, and decreased enhancement.[142]

The microscopic appearance of infantile hemangioma depends on the stage at which it is biopsied. In early lesions, the vessels are tightly packed, and the cells are plump and proliferative (Fig. 12.66). In late-stage lesions, the vessels are widely spaced with flat, inactive endothelial lining. Infantile hemangiomas usually spontaneously regress, and no treatment is needed. If lesions are symptomatic due to location, large size, compromise of adjacent structures, or altered vascular dynamics, medical therapy with propranolol is the initial treatment of choice.[145]

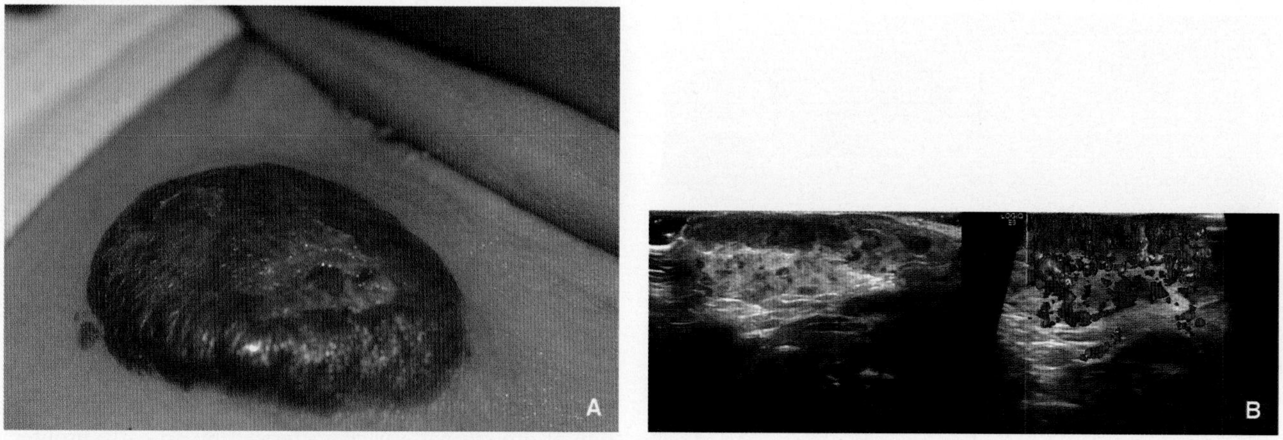

FIGURE 12.65 **Infantile hemangioma in a 2-week-old boy. A:** Photograph of a typical superficial infantile hemangioma shows a raised, red, "strawberry-like" lesion. **B:** Gray scale ultrasound **(left)** demonstrates a heterogeneous superficial soft tissue mass with numerous vascular channels. Color Doppler **(right)** shows the high vessel density of the mass.

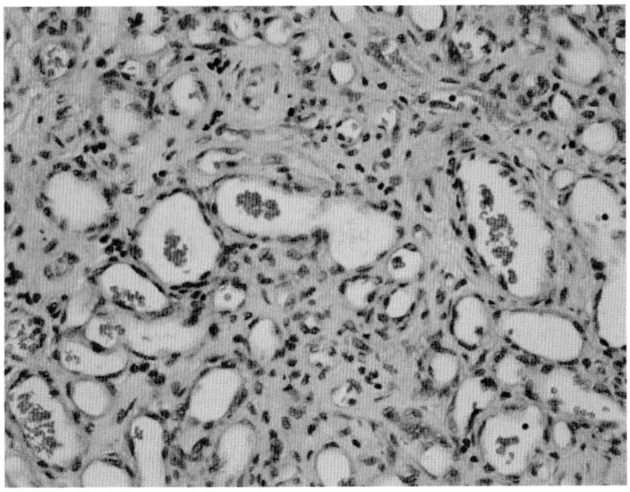

FIGURE 12.66 **Infantile hemangioma in a 4-year-old girl.** Still at a fairly cellular stage, this infantile hemangioma shows plump endothelial cells lining closely spaced blood vessels (hematoxylin and eosin, original magnification, 400×).

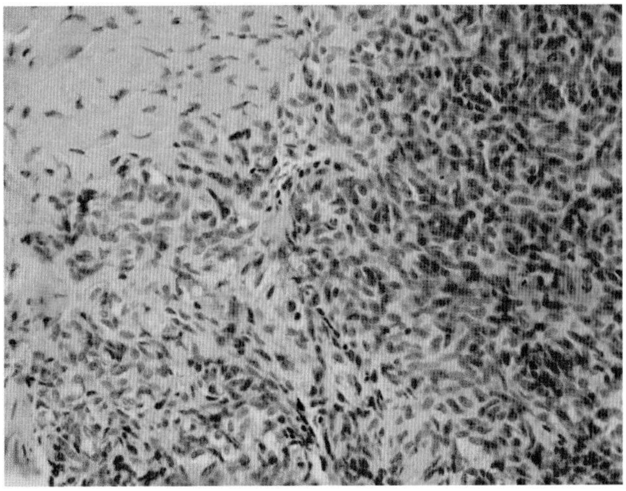

FIGURE 12.67 **Kaposiform hemangioendothelioma in a 6-month-old girl.** Densely packed spindle-shaped cells forming occasional slit-like vascular lumens in a Kaposiform hemangioendothelioma of the shoulder. Occasional brown hemosiderin particles are seen (hematoxylin and eosin, original magnification, 400×).

Kaposiform Hemangioendothelioma

Kaposiform hemangioendothelioma (KHE) is a rare, aggressive neoplasm with borderline malignant potential composed of convoluted vessels. KHE presents in early childhood as a blue-red skin lesion and often has a progressive course. It involves the superficial and deep soft tissue and, rarely, internal organs. Regional lymph node metastases are rare, and no distant metastases have been reported. The Kasabach-Merritt phenomenon (KMP) of profound thrombocytopenia and consumptive coagulopathy occurs in ~50% of cases.[146] Grossly, the lesion shows a poorly circumscribed border and variably bloody cut surface. Microscopic examination shows a densely cellular collection of plump vascular cells with slit-like lumens (Fig. 12.67). Positive D2-40 immunostaining, reflecting a degree of lymphothelial differentiation, is characteristic.[147]

KHE has similarities on imaging to hemangiomas and other high-flow vascular lesions, but is more aggressive with ill-defined margins, perilesional fat stranding, and osseous destruction or remodeling.[142] Radiographs and CT may demonstrate a nonspecific soft tissue mass. US can show a heterogeneous, hyperechoic mass with high resistive arterial waveforms (Fig. 12.68A). MRI is the preferred imaging modality to evaluate the full extent of disease. Infiltrating high T2 and low T1 signal with intense enhancement, ectatic flow voids, and overlying skin thickening is typical[148] (Fig. 12.68B).

KHE may undergo spontaneous partial regression, but complete regression is rare. Surgical resection has historically been the gold standard for cure; however, complete resection is often not possible due to the associated morbidity. A recent consensus-derived treatment plan advocates oral prednisolone as first line therapy for KHE with symptoms or progressive growth but without KMP; the addition of intravenous vincristine is recommended for KHE with KMP.[148]

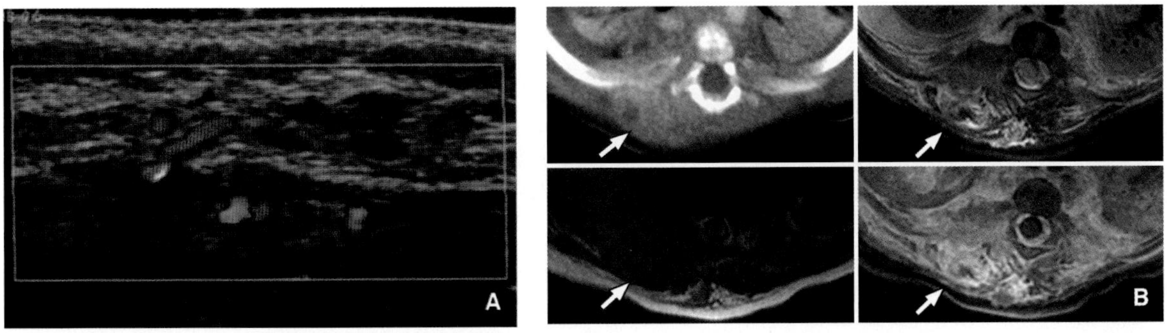

FIGURE 12.68 **Kaposiform hemangioendothelioma in a 2-month-old girl with thrombocytopenia. A:** Color Doppler ultrasound image shows an ill-defined lesion with anechoic vascular spaces and significant flow. **B:** Axial enhanced CT image (**top left**) shows heterogeneous, ill-defined enhancing mass (*arrow*) in the right paraspinal region. Axial T1-weighted (**bottom left**), T2-weighted fat-saturated (**top right**), and postcontrast T1-weighted fat-saturated (**bottom right**) MR images show irregular, ill-defined areas (*arrows*) of T2 prolongation and enhancement within enlarged paraspinal muscles. Low signal intensity flow voids are present.

References

1. Restrepo R, Lee EY. Updates on imaging of chest wall lesions in pediatric patients. *Semin Roentgenol.* 2012;47(1):79–89.
2. Coley BD. Pediatric chest ultrasound. *Radiol Clin North Am.* Mar 2005;43(2):405–418.
3. Ben-Ami TE, O'Donovan JC, Yousefzadeh DK. Sonography of the chest in children. *Radiol Clin North Am.* 1993;31(3):517–531.
4. Koh DM, Burke S, Davies N, et al. Transthoracic US of the chest: clinical uses and applications. *Radiographics.* 2002;22(1):e1.
5. Kim OH, Kim WS, Kim MJ, et al. US in the diagnosis of pediatric chest diseases. *Radiographics.* 2000;20(3):653–671.
6. Lee EY, Boiselle PM, Cleveland RH. Multidetector CT evaluation of congenital lung anomalies. *Radiology.* 2008;247(3):632–648.
7. Cravero JP, Blike GT. Review of pediatric sedation. *Anesth Analg.* 2004;99(5):1355–1364.
8. American Academy of Pediatrics and the American Academy of Pediatric Dentistry. Guideline for monitoring and management of pediatric patients during and after sedation for diagnostic and therapeutic procedures. 2006;118(6):194–210.
9. Lee E, Siegel P. *Pediatric Airways Disorders: Large Airways.* Totowa, NJ: Humana; 2008.
10. Knisely BL, Broderick LS, Kuhlman JE. MR imaging of the pleura and chest wall. *Magn Reson Imaging Clin N Am.* 2000;8(1):125–141.
11. Gilday D. Pediatric nuclear medicine. In: Leslie WD, Greenberg ID, eds. *Nuclear Medicine.* Georgetown, TX: Landes Bioscience; 2003:385–883.
12. Gelfand MJ, Parisi MT, Treves ST. Pediatric radiopharmaceutical administered doses: 2010 North American consensus guidelines. *J Nucl Med.* 2011;52(2):318–322.
13. Segall G, Delbeke D, Stabin MG, et al. SNM practice guideline for sodium 18F-fluoride PET/CT bone scans 1.0. *J Nucl Med.* 2010;51(11):1813–1820.
14. Drubach LA, Johnston PR, Newton AW, et al. Skeletal trauma in child abuse: detection with 18F-NaF PET. *Radiology.* 2010;255(1):173–181.
15. Clemens MW, Evans KK, Mardini S, et al. Introduction to chest wall reconstruction: anatomy and physiology of the chest and indications for chest wall reconstruction. *Semin Plast Surg.* 2011;25(1):5–15.
16. Mortola J. Comparative apects of neonatal respiratory mechanisms. In: Haddad G, Abman S, Chernick V, eds. *Chernick-Mellins Basic Mechanisms of Pediatric Respiratory Disease.* 2nd ed. Hamilton, ON: Decker; 2002:171–178.
17. Eich GF, Kellenberger CJ, Willi UV. Radiology of the chest wall. In: Lucaya J, Strife JL, eds. *Pediatric Chest Imaging: Chest Imaging in Infants and Children.* 2nd ed. New York: Springer; 2008:313–336.
18. Donnelly LF, Frush DP, Foss JN, et al. Anterior chest wall: frequency of anatomic variations in children. *Radiology.* 1999; 212(3):837–840.
19. Donnelly LF, Taylor CN, Emery KH, et al. Asymptomatic, palpable, anterior chest wall lesions in children: is cross-sectional imaging necessary? *Radiology.* 1997;202(3):829–831.
20. Tsirikos AI, McMaster MJ. Congenital anomalies of the ribs and chest wall associated with congenital deformities of the spine. *J Bone Joint Surg Am.* 2005;87(11):2523–2536.
21. Westphal FL, Lima LC, Lima Neto JC, et al. Prevalence of pectus carinatum and pectus excavatum in students in the city of Manaus, Brazil. *J Bras Pneumol.* 2009;35(3):221–226.
22. Coskun ZK, Turgut HB, Demirsoy S, et al. The prevalence and effects of Pectus Excavatum and Pectus Carinatum on the respiratory function in children between 7–14 years old. *Indian J Pediatr.* 2010;77(9):1017–1019.
23. Shamberger RC, Welch KJ. Surgical repair of pectus excavatum. *J Pediatr Surg.* 1988;23(7):615–622.
24. Koumbourlis AC, Stolar CJ. Lung growth and function in children and adolescents with idiopathic pectus excavatum. *Pediatr Pulmonol.* 2004;38(4):339–343.
25. Feng J, Hu T, Liu W, et al. The biomechanical, morphologic, and histochemical properties of the costal cartilages in children with pectus excavatum. *J Pediatr Surg.* 2001;36(12):1770–1776.
26. Shamberger RC, Welch KJ, Castaneda AR, et al. Anterior chest wall deformities and congenital heart disease. *J Thorac Cardiovasc Surg.* 1988;96(3):427–432.
27. Golladay ES, Char F, Mollitt DL. Children with Marfan's syndrome and pectus excavatum. *South Med J.* 1985;78(11):1319–1323.
28. Fefferman NR, Pinkney LP. Imaging evaluation of chest wall disorders in children. *Radiol Clin North Am.* 2005;43(2):355–370.
29. Haller JA, Jr., Kramer SS, Lietman SA. Use of CT scans in selection of patients for pectus excavatum surgery: a preliminary report. *J Pediatr Surg.* 1987;22(10):904–906.
30. Mueller C, Saint-Vil D, Bouchard S. Chest x-ray as a primary modality for preoperative imaging of pectus excavatum. *J Pediatr Surg.* 2008;43(1):71–73.
31. Khanna G, Jaju A, Don S, et al. Comparison of Haller index values calculated with chest radiographs versus CT for pectus excavatum evaluation. *Pediatr Radiol.* 2010;40(11):1763–1767.
32. Marcovici PA, Losasso BE, Kruk P, et al. MRI for the evaluation of pectus excavatum. *Pediatr Radiol.* 2011;41(6):757–758.
33. Haller JA Jr, Scherer LR, Turner CS, et al. Evolving management of pectus excavatum based on a single institutional experience of 664 patients. *Ann Surg.* 1989;209(5):578–582; discussion 582–573.
34. Chen Z, Amos EB, Luo H, et al. Comparative pulmonary functional recovery after Nuss and Ravitch procedures for pectus excavatum repair: a meta-analysis. *J Cardiothorac Surg* 2012;7:101.
35. Steinmann C, Krille S, Mueller A, et al. Pectus excavatum and pectus carinatum patients suffer from lower quality of life and impaired body image: a control group comparison of psychological characteristics prior to surgical correction. *Eur J Cardiothorac Surg.* 2011;40(5):1138–1145.
36. Bostanci K, Ozalper MH, Eldem B, et al. Quality of life of patients who have undergone the minimally invasive repair of pectus carinatum. *Eur J Cardiothorac Surg.* 2013;43(1):122–126.
37. Colombani PM. Preoperative assessment of chest wall deformities. *Semin Thorac Cardiovasc Surg.* 2009;21(1):58–63.
38. Desmarais TJ, Keller MS. Pectus carinatum. *Curr Opin Pediatr.* 2013;25(3):375–381.
39. Kaneko H, Kitoh H, Mabuchi A, et al. Isolated bifid rib: clinical and radiological findings in children. *Pediatr Int.* 2012; 54(6):820–823.
40. Kimonis VE, Mehta SG, Digiovanna JJ, et al. Radiological features in 82 patients with nevoid basal cell carcinoma (NBCC or Gorlin) syndrome. *Genet Med.* 2004;6(6):495–502.
41. Watkins TW, Wilkinson AG, Greer ML. Atypical intrathoracic rib in a pediatric patient requiring helical CT scan with 3-D reconstruction for diagnosis. *Pediatr Radiol.* 2008;38(9):1003–1005.
42. Hawass NE, Bahakim H, al-Boukai AA.Intrathoracic fat. A new CT feature of intrathoracic rib. Case report. *Clin Imaging.* 1991;15(1):31–34.
43. Kamaruddin K, Wright NB, Pilling DW. Intrathoracic rib. *Pediatr Radiol.* 1995;25(1):60–61.

44. Jeung MY, Gangi A, Gasser B, et al. Imaging of chest wall disorders. *Radiographics*. 1999;19(3):617–637.
45. Adson AW, Coffey JR. Cervical rib: a method of anterior approach for relief of symptoms by division of the scalenus anticus. *Ann Surg*. 1927;85(6):839–857.
46. Glass RB, Norton KI, Mitre SA, et al. Pediatric ribs: a spectrum of abnormalities. *Radiographics*. 2002;22(1):87–104.
47. Chang KZ, Likes K, Davis K, et al. The significance of cervical ribs in thoracic outlet syndrome. *J Vasc Surg*. 2013;57(3):771–775.
48. Mundlos S, Mulliken JB, Abramson DL, et al. Genetic mapping of cleidocranial dysplasia and evidence of a microdeletion in one family. *Hum Mol Genet*. 1995;4(1):71–75.
49. Rhinehart B. Cleidocranial dysostosis (mutational dysostosis). *Radiology*. 1936(26):741–748.
50. Roberts T, Stephen L, Beighton P. Cleidocranial dysplasia: a review of the dental, historical, and practical implications with an overview of the South African experience. *Oral Surg Oral Med Oral Pathol Oral Radiol*. 2013;115(1):46–55.
51. Fokin AA, Robicsek F. Poland's syndrome revisited. *Ann Thorac Surg*. 2002;74(6):2218–2225.
52. La Marca S, Delay E, Toussoun G, et al. [Treatment of Poland syndrome thorax deformity with the lipomodeling technique: about ten cases]. *Ann Chir Plast Esthet*. 2013;58(1):60–68.
53. Wong KS, Hung IJ, Wang CR, et al. Thoracic wall lesions in children. *Pediatr Pulmonol*. 2004;37(3):257–263.
54. Riebel TW, Nasir R, Nazarenko O. The value of sonography in the detection of osteomyelitis. *Pediatr Radiol*. 1996;26(4):291–297.
55. Siegel MJ. Chest. In: Siegel MJ, ed. *Pediatric Sonography*. Philadelphia, PA: Lippincott Williams & Wilkins; 2002:167–211.
56. Adler BD, Padley SP, Muller NL. Tuberculosis of the chest wall: CT findings. *J Comput Assist Tomogr*. 1993;17(2):271–273.
57. Khalil A, Le Breton C, Tassart M, et al. Utility of CT scan for the diagnosis of chest wall tuberculosis. *Eur Radiol*. 1999;9(8):1638–1642.
58. Cheon JE, Im JG, Kim MY, et al. Thoracic actinomycosis: CT findings. *Radiology*. 1998;209(1):229–233.
59. Chelli Bouaziz M, Jelassi H, Chaabane S, et al. Imaging of chest wall infections. *Skeletal Radiol*. 2009;38(12):1127–1135.
60. Freeman AF, Ben-Ami T, Shulman ST. Streptococcus pneumoniae empyema necessitatis. *Pediatr Infect Dis J*. 2004;23(2):177–179.
61. Murphey MD, Carroll JF, Flemming DJ, et al. From the archives of the AFIP: benign musculoskeletal lipomatous lesions. *Radiographics*. 2004;24(5):1433–1466.
62. Navarro OM, Laffan EE, Ngan BY. Pediatric soft-tissue tumors and pseudo-tumors: MR imaging features with pathologic correlation: part 1. Imaging approach, pseudotumors, vascular lesions, and adipocytic tumors. *Radiographics*. 2009;29(3):887–906.
63. Toirkens J, De Schepper AM, Vanhoenacker F, et al. A comparison between histopathology and findings on magnetic resonance imaging of subcutaneous lipomatous soft-tissue tumors. *Insights Imaging*. 2011;2(5):599–607.
64. Pricola KL, Dutta S. Stealth surgery: subcutaneous endoscopic excision of benign lesions of the trunk and lower extremity. *J Pediatr Surg*. 2010;45(4):840–844.
65. Hibbard MK, Kozakewich HP, Dal Cin P, et al. PLAG1 fusion oncogenes in lipoblastoma. *Cancer Res*. 2000;60(17):4869–4872.
66. Chen CW, Chang WC, Lee HS, et al. MRI features of lipoblastoma: differentiating from other palpable lipomatous tumor in pediatric patients. *Clin Imaging*. 2010;34(6):453–457.
67. Crago AM, Denton B, Salas S, et al. A prognostic nomogram for prediction of recurrence in desmoid fibromatosis. *Ann Surg*. 2013;258(2):347–353.
68. Coffin CM, Alaggio R. Fibroblastic and myofibroblastic tumors in children and adolescents. *Pediatr Dev Pathol*. 2012;15(1 suppl):127–180.
69. Vandevenne JE, De Schepper AM, De Beuckeleer L, et al. New concepts in understanding evolution of desmoid tumors: MR imaging of 30 lesions. *Eur Radiol*. 1997;7(7):1013–1019.
70. Eich GF, Hoeffel JC, Tschappeler H, et al. Fibrous tumours in children: imaging features of a heterogeneous group of disorders. *Pediatr Radiol*. 1998;28(7):500–509.
71. Honeyman JN, Theilen TM, Knowles MA, et al. Desmoid fibromatosis in children and adolescents: a conservative approach to management. *J Pediatr Surg*. 2013;48(1):62–66.
72. Levine E, Freneaux P, Schleiermacher G, et al. Risk-adapted therapy for infantile myofibromatosis in children. *Pediatr Blood Cancer*. 2012;59(1):115–120.
73. Lee J. Mutations in PDGFRB and NOTCH3 are the first genetic causes identified for autosomal dominant infantile myofibromatosis. *Clin Genet*. 2013;84(4):340–341.
74. Carretto E, Dall'Igna P, Alaggio R, et al. Fibrous hamartoma of infancy: an Italian multi-institutional experience. *J Am Acad Dermatol*. 2006;54(5):800–803.
75. Murphey MD, Smith WS, Smith SE, et al. From the archives of the AFIP. Imaging of musculoskeletal neurogenic tumors: radiologic-pathologic correlation. *Radiographics*. 1999;19(5):1253–1280.
76. David EA, Marshall MB. Review of chest wall tumors: a diagnostic, therapeutic, and reconstructive challenge. *Semin Plast Surg*. 2011;25(1):16–24.
77. Wootton-Gorges SL. MR imaging of primary bone tumors and tumor-like conditions in children. *Magn Reson Imaging Clin N Am*. 2009;17(3):469–487, vi.
78. De Andrea C, Bridge J, Schiller A. Osteoblastoma. In: Fletcher CDM, Bridge JA, Hogendoorn P, et al., eds. *WHO Classification of Tumours of Soft Tissue and Bone*. 4th ed. Lyon, France: IARC; 2013:185, Vol. 5.
79. Kroon HM, Schurmans J. Osteoblastoma: clinical and radiologic findings in 98 new cases. *Radiology*. 1990;175(3):783–790.
80. Rehnitz C, Sprengel SD, Lehner B, et al. CT-guided radiofrequency ablation of osteoid osteoma and osteoblastoma: clinical success and long-term follow up in 77 patients. *Eur J Radiol*. 2012;81(11):3426–3434.
81. Vlychou M, Athanasou NA. Radiological and pathological diagnosis of paediatric bone tumours and tumour-like lesions. *Pathology*. 2008;40(2):196–216.
82. Nam SJ, Kim S, Lim BJ, et al. Imaging of primary chest wall tumors with radiologic-pathologic correlation. *Radiographics*. 2011;31(3):749–770.
83. Amary MF, Bacsi K, Maggiani F, et al. IDH1 and IDH2 mutations are frequent events in central chondrosarcoma and central and periosteal chondromas but not in other mesenchymal tumours. *J Pathol*. 2011;224(3):334–343.
84. Pansuriya TC, van Eijk R, d'Adamo P, et al. Somatic mosaic IDH1 and IDH2 mutations are associated with enchondroma and spindle cell hemangioma in Ollier disease and Maffucci syndrome. *Nat Genet*. 2011;43(12):1256–1261.
85. Lucas D, Bridge J. Chondromas: enchondroma, periosteal chondroma. In: Fletcher C, Bridge J, Hogendoorn P, et al., eds. *WHO Classification of Tumours of Soft Tissue and Bone*. 4th ed. Lyon, France: IARC; 2013:252–254, Vol 5.

86. Karmazyn B, Davis MM, Davey MS, et al. Imaging evaluation of chest wall tumors in children. *Acad Radiol.* 1998;5(9):642–654.
87. Brien EW, Mirra JM, Kerr R. Benign and malignant cartilage tumors of bone and joint: their anatomic and theoretical basis with an emphasis on radiology, pathology and clinical biology. I. The intramedullary cartilage tumors. *Skeletal Radiol.* 1997;26(6):325–353.
88. Lee KC, Davies AM, Cassar-Pullicino VN. Imaging the complications of osteochondromas. *Clin Radiol.* 2002;57(1):18–28.
89. Oliveira AM, Perez-Atayde AR, Inwards CY, et al. USP6 and CDH11 oncogenes identify the neoplastic cell in primary aneurysmal bone cysts and are absent in so-called secondary aneurysmal bone cysts. *Am J Pathol.* 2004;165(5):1773–1780.
90. Kransdorf MJ, Sweet DE. Aneurysmal bone cyst: concept, controversy, clinical presentation, and imaging. *AJR Am J Roentgenol.* 1995;164(3):573–580.
91. Rapp TB, Ward JP, Alaia MJ. Aneurysmal bone cyst. *J Am Acad Orthop Surg.* 2012;20(4):233–241.
92. Shiels WE II, Mayerson JL. Percutaneous doxycycline treatment of aneurysmal bone cysts with low recurrence rate: a preliminary report. *Clin Orthop Relat Res.* 2013;471(8):2675–2683.
93. Siegal GP, Bianco P, Dal CP. Fibrous dysplasia. In: Fletcher C, Bridge J, Hogendoorn P, et al., eds. *WHO Classification of Tumours of Soft Tissue and Bone.* 4th ed. IARC: Lyon, France; 2013:352–353, Vol 5.
94. De Mattos CB, Binitie O, Dormans JP. Pathological fractures in children. *Bone Joint Res.* 2012;1(10):272–280.
95. Howarth DM, Gilchrist GS, Mullan BP, et al. Langerhans cell histiocytosis: diagnosis, natural history, management, and outcome. *Cancer.* 1999;85(10):2278–2290.
96. George JC, Buckwalter KA, Cohen MD, et al. Langerhans cell histiocytosis of bone: MR imaging. *Pediatr Radiol.* 1994;24(1):29–32.
97. Badalian-Very G, Vergilio JA, Fleming M, et al. Pathogenesis of Langerhans cell histiocytosis. *Annu Rev Pathol* 2013;8:1–20.
98. Goo HW, Yang DH, Ra YS, et al. Whole-body MRI of Langerhans cell histiocytosis: comparison with radiography and bone scintigraphy. *Pediatr Radiol.* 2006;36(10):1019–1031.
99. Steinborn M, Wortler K, Nathrath M, et al. [Whole-body MRI in children with langerhans cell histiocytosis for the evaluation of the skeletal system]. *Rofo.* 2008;180(7):646–653.
100. Khung S, Budzik JF, Amzallag-Bellenger E, et al. Skeletal involvement in Langerhans cell histiocytosis. *Insights Imaging.* 2013;4:569.
101. Groom KR, Murphey MD, Howard LM, et al. Mesenchymal hamartoma of the chest wall: radiologic manifestations with emphasis on cross-sectional imaging and histopathologic comparison. *Radiology.* 2002;222(1):205–211.
102. Jozaghi Y, Emil S, Albuquerque P, et al. Prenatal and postnatal features of mesenchymal hamartoma of the chest wall: case report and literature review. *Pediatr Surg Int.* 2013;29(7):735–740.
103. van den Berg H, van Rijn RR, Merks JH. Management of tumors of the chest wall in childhood: a review. *J Pediatr Hematol Oncol.* 2008;30(3):214–221.
104. Saenz NC, Ghavimi F, Gerald W, et al. Chest wall rhabdomyosarcoma. *Cancer.* 1997;80(8):1513–1517.
105. Van Rijn RR, Wilde JC, Bras J, et al. Imaging findings in noncraniofacial childhood rhabdomyosarcoma. *Pediatr Radiol.* 2008;38(6):617–634.
106. Laffan EE, Ngan BY, Navarro OM. Pediatric soft-tissue tumors and pseudotumors: MR imaging features with pathologic correlation: part 2. Tumors of fibroblastic/myofibroblastic, so-called fibrohistiocytic, muscular, lymphomatous, neurogenic, hair matrix, and uncertain origin. *Radiographics.* 2009;29(4):e36.
107. Kransdorf MJ, Murphey MD. Neurogenic tumors. In: Kransdorf MJ, Murphey MD, eds. *Imaging of soft tissue tumors.* 2nd ed. Philadelphia, PA: Lippincott Williams & Wilkins; 2006:328–380.
108. Foran P, Colleran G, Madewell J, et al. Imaging of thoracic sarcomas of the chest wall, pleura, and lung. *Semin Ultrasound CT MR.* 2011;32(5):365–376.
109. Solomon SB, Semih Dogan A, Nicol TL, et al. Positron emission tomography in the detection and management of sarcomatous transformation in neurofibromatosis. *Clin Nucl Med.* 2001;26(6):525–528.
110. McCarville MB, Spunt SL, Skapek SX, et al. Synovial sarcoma in pediatric patients. *AJR Am J Roentgenol.* 2002;179(3):797–801.
111. Speth BM, Krieg AH, Kaelin A, et al. Synovial sarcoma in patients under 20 years of age: a multicenter study with a minimum follow-up of 10 years. *J Child Orthop.* 2011;5(5):335–342.
112. Stanelle EJ, Christison-Lagay ER, Healey JH, et al. Pediatric and adolescent synovial sarcoma: multivariate analysis of prognostic factors and survival outcomes. *Ann Surg Oncol.* 2013;20(1):73–79.
113. Gladish GW, Sabloff BM, Munden RF, et al. Primary thoracic sarcomas. *Radiographics.* 2002;22(3):621–637.
114. Franken EA Jr, Smith JA, Smith WL. Tumors of the chest wall in infants and children. *Pediatr Radiol.* 1977;6(1):13–18.
115. Tsokos M, Alaggio RD, Dehner LP, et al. Ewing sarcoma/peripheral primitive neuroectodermal tumor and related tumors. *Pediatr Dev Pathol.* 2012;15(1 Suppl):108–126.
116. Maygarden SJ, Askin FB, Siegal GP, et al. Ewing sarcoma of bone in infants and toddlers. A clinicopathologic report from the Intergroup Ewing's Study. *Cancer.* 1993;71(6):2109–2118.
117. Schuck A, Hofmann J, Rube C, et al. Radiotherapy in Ewing's sarcoma and PNET of the chest wall: results of the trials CESS 81, CESS 86 and EICESS 92. *Int J Radiat Oncol Biol Phys.* 1998;42(5):1001–1006.
118. Thomas PR, Foulkes MA, Gilula LA, et al. Primary Ewing's sarcoma of the ribs. A report from the intergroup Ewing's sarcoma study. *Cancer.* 1983;51(6):1021–1027.
119. Shamberger RC, LaQuaglia MP, Gebhardt MC, et al. Ewing sarcoma/primitive neuroectodermal tumor of the chest wall: impact of initial versus delayed resection on tumor margins, survival, and use of radiation therapy. *Ann Surg.* 2003;238(4):563–567; discussion 567–568.
120. Levine E, Levine C. Ewing tumor of rib: radiologic findings and computed tomography contribution. *Skeletal Radiol.* 1983;9(4):227–233.
121. Vilanova JC, Woertler K, Narvaez JA, et al. Soft-tissue tumors update: MR imaging features according to the WHO classification. *Eur Radiol.* 2007;17(1):125–138.
122. Sallustio G, Pirronti T, Lasorella A, et al. Diagnostic imaging of primitive neuroectodermal tumour of the chest wall (Askin tumour). *Pediatr Radiol.* 1998;28(9):697–702.
123. Indelicato DJ, Keole SR, Lagmay JP, et al. Chest wall Ewing sarcoma family of tumors: long-term outcomes. *Int J Radiat Oncol Biol Phys.* 2011;81(1):158–166.
124. Dimopoulos MA, Moulopoulos LA, Maniatis A, et al. Solitary plasmacytoma of bone and asymptomatic multiple myeloma. *Blood.* 2000;96(6):2037–2044.

125. Ropper AE, Cahill KS, Hanna JW, et al. Primary vertebral tumors: a review of epidemiologic, histological, and imaging findings, Part I: benign tumors. *Neurosurgery*. 2011;69(6): 1171–1180.
126. Plant AS, Venick RS, Farmer DG, et al. Plasmacytoma-like post-transplant lymphoproliferative disorder seen in pediatric combined liver and intestinal transplant recipients. *Pediatr Blood Cancer*. 2013;60(11):E137–E139.
127. Donnelly LF. *Fundamentals of Pediatric Radiology*. Philadelphia, PA: Saunders Elsevier; 2001.
128. Watt AJ. Chest wall lesions. *Paediatr Respir Rev*. 2002;3(4): 328–338.
129. McCarville MB, Spunt SL, Pappo AS. Rhabdomyosarcoma in pediatric patients: the good, the bad, and the unusual. *AJR Am J Roentgenol*. 2001;176(6):1563–1569.
130. Lee WK, Duddalwar VA, Rouse HC, et al. Extranodal lymphoma in the thorax: cross-sectional imaging findings. *Clin Radiol*. 2009;64(5):542–549.
131. Tsai TS, Evans HA, Donnelly LF, et al. Fat necrosis after trauma: a benign cause of palpable lumps in children. *AJR Am J Roentgenol*. 1997;169(6):1623–1626.
132. Norton KI, Som PM, Shugar JM, et al. Subcutaneous fat necrosis of the newborn: CT findings of head and neck involvement. *AJNR Am J Neuroradiol*. 1997;18(3):547–550.
133. Dwek JR. The radiographic approach to child abuse. *Clin Orthop Relat Res*. 2011;469(3):776–789.
134. Kleinman PK. Skeletal trauma: General considerations. In: Kleinman PK, ed. *Diagnostic Imaging of Child Abuse*. 2nd ed. St. Louis, MO: Mosby Inc.; 1998.
135. Flors L, Leiva-Salinas C, Maged IM, et al. MR imaging of soft-tissue vascular malformations: diagnosis, classification, and therapy follow-up. *Radiographics*. 2011;31(5):1321–1340; discussion 1340–1321.
136. Dubois J, Garel L. Imaging and therapeutic approach of hemangiomas and vascular malformations in the pediatric age group. *Pediatr Radiol*. 1999;29(12):879–893.
137. Dompmartin A, Acher A, Thibon P, et al. Association of localized intravascular coagulopathy with venous malformations. *Arch Dermatol*. 2008;144(7):873–877.
138. Dompmartin A, Vikkula M, Boon LM. Venous malformation: update on aetiopathogenesis, diagnosis and management. *Phlebology*. 2010;25(5):224–235.
139. Paltiel HJ, Burrows PE, Kozakewich HP, et al. Soft-tissue vascular anomalies: utility of US for diagnosis. *Radiology*. 2000;214(3):747–754.
140. Laor T. MR imaging of soft tissue tumors and tumor-like lesions. *Pediatr Radiol*. 2004;34(1):24–37.
141. Burrows PE. Endovascular treatment of slow-flow vascular malformations. *Tech Vasc Interv Radiol*. 2013;16(1):12–21.
142. Mulliken JB, Fishman SJ, Burrows PE. Vascular anomalies. *Curr Probl Surg*. 2000;37(8):517–584.
143. Hochman M, Adams DM, Reeves TD. Current knowledge and management of vascular anomalies: I. Hemangiomas. *Arch Facial Plast Surg*. 2011;13(3):145–151.
144. Dubois J, Patriquin HB, Garel L, et al. Soft-tissue hemangiomas in infants and children: diagnosis using Doppler sonography. *AJR Am J Roentgenol*. 1998;171(1):247–252.
145. Drolet BA, Frommelt PC, Chamlin SL, et al. Initiation and use of propranolol for infantile hemangioma: report of a consensus conference. *Pediatrics*. 2013;131(1):128–140.
146. Lyons LL, North PE, Mac-Moune Lai F, et al. Kaposiform hemangioendothelioma: a study of 33 cases emphasizing its pathologic, immunophenotypic, and biologic uniqueness from juvenile hemangioma. *Am J Surg Pathol*. 2004;28(5): 559–568.
147. Debelenko LV, Perez-Atayde AR, Mulliken JB, et al. D2-40 immunohistochemical analysis of pediatric vascular tumors reveals positivity in kaposiform hemangioendothelioma. *Mod Pathol*. 2005;18(11):1454–1460.
148. Drolet BA, Trenor CC, III, Brandao LR, et al. Consensus-derived practice standards plan for complicated Kaposiform hemangioendothelioma. *J Pediatr*. 2013;163(1):285–291.

CHAPTER 13

Diaphragm

Mark C. Liszewski • Pedro Daltro • Celia Ferrari • Gloria Soto Giordani • Fred E. Avni • Edward Y. Lee

INTRODUCTION

The diaphragm is a musculofibrous structure that separates the thoracic and abdominal cavities and is integral to respiratory function. In the pediatric population, several important pathologic conditions can affect the diaphragm, which include congenital and developmental anomalies, neoplasms, and trauma. In this chapter, imaging techniques to evaluate the diaphragm are discussed, the normal anatomy of the pediatric diaphragm is reviewed, and the spectrum of diaphragmatic disorders is presented.

IMAGING TECHNIQUES

Several currently available imaging modalities, alone or in combination, can be used to effectively evaluate the diaphragm in infants and children. Each modality's utility depends largely on the pathologic condition in question. The current imaging techniques of various imaging modalities used for evaluating the diaphragm are discussed in the following section.

Radiography

Chest radiography often serves as the first-line imaging modality to evaluate the diaphragm. Whenever possible, both frontal and lateral chest radiographs are recommended for a complete assessment of the diaphragm in pediatric patients. Normally, the upper aspect of the diaphragm is seen adjacent to the aerated lung, and the lower aspect is silhouetted by the abdominal viscera on frontal chest radiograph (Fig. 13.1).[1] The position of the diaphragm is determined by the phase of respiration at the time of imaging. When imaging at end inspiration, the superior aspect of the right hemidiaphragm normally projects at approximately the level of the anterior sixth rib,[2] and the dome of the left hemidiaphragm projects approximately one intercostal space lower.[1] However, there is wide variability in the position of the normal diaphragm.[3] On the lateral radiograph, the domed right hemidiaphragm is seen in its entirety, whereas the anterior left hemidiaphragm is silhouetted by the mediastinum superiorly (Fig. 13.2).[1]

Although radiographs do not provide detailed information about the diaphragm, secondary radiographic signs may suggest a pathologic condition of the diaphragm and can guide the appropriate next imaging studies for further evaluation. For example, herniated abdominal viscera may be seen within the thorax in cases of congenital diaphragmatic hernia (CDH), though the actual diaphragmatic defect may be poorly visualized radiographically. Similarly, persistent elevation of the diaphragm may suggest a diagnosis of diaphragmatic paralysis, though other modalities, such as ultrasound (US) and fluoroscopy that can provide real-time assessment, are often needed for definitive diagnosis.

Ultrasound

Because of its ability to visualize structures in real time without the use of ionizing radiation, US is an attractive and useful noninvasive imaging modality in the evaluation of the diaphragm. Curved or linear array US transducers are typically used for evaluation of the diaphragm. Higher-frequency US transducers (7.5 to 15.0 MHz) provide higher-resolution images but have less soft tissue penetration. Therefore, high-frequency transducers are often the best tool for evaluating the diaphragm in infants and young children with small amounts

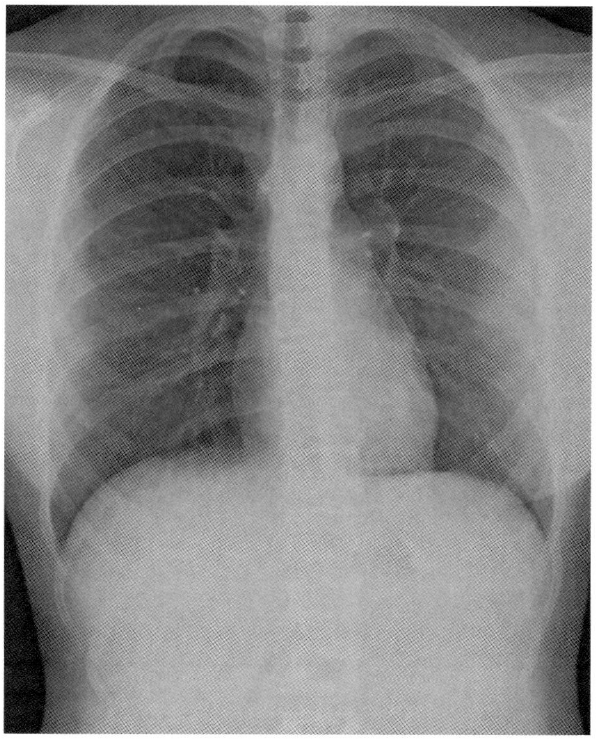

FIGURE 13.1 **Normal posteroanterior chest radiograph in a 13-year-old girl.** Note the upper aspect of the diaphragm is seen adjacent to the aerated lung, and the lower aspect is silhouetted by the abdominal viscera on frontal chest radiograph.

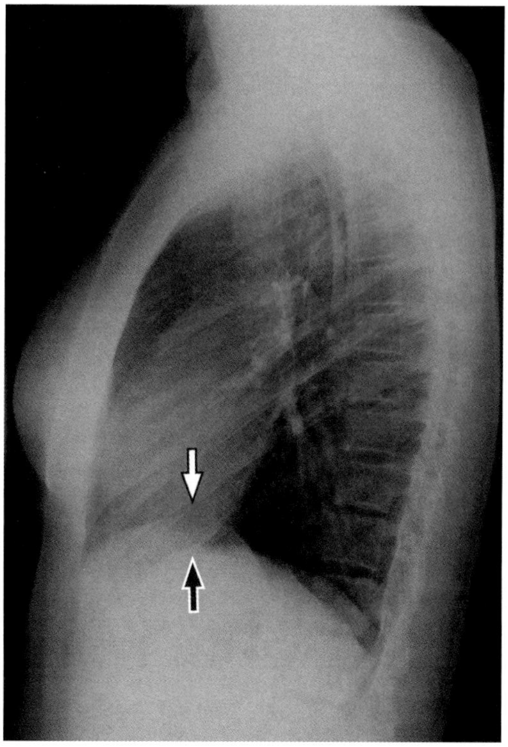

FIGURE 13.2 **Normal lateral chest radiograph in a 13-year-old girl.** The domed right hemidiaphragm (*white arrow*) is seen in its entirety, whereas the anterior left hemidiaphragm (*black arrow*) is silhouetted by the mediastinum superiorly.

of subcutaneous fat but can be less helpful in larger children with less optimal acoustic windows. Lower-frequency US transducers (<5 MHz) produce lower-resolution images but provide better soft tissue penetration and are more suitable for larger children with greater amounts of subcutaneous fat.[4]

The diaphragm is a specular reflector and is seen as an echogenic linear structure on US (Fig. 13.3). Each hemidiaphragm can be imaged individually in axial, sagittal, and/or oblique planes, or both hemidiaphragms may be visualized simultaneously utilizing a transverse subxiphoid view in infants and young children with an available acoustic window.[1] US is particularly useful in the evaluation of diaphragmatic paralysis, as it can visualize movement in real time. The use of M-mode imaging allows for accurate quantification of this movement.[5,6] High spatial resolution and portability make US particularly useful in the evaluation of diaphragmatic hernias[7] and eventration.[5,8] US may also be helpful in selected cases of late-presenting CDH[9] and traumatic diaphragmatic rupture,[10,11] though a multimodality approach is often employed in the diagnosis of these conditions. Additionally, US may be useful in the evaluation of diaphragmatic tumors, though localization of the mass to the diaphragm as opposed to an adjacent abdominal organ is often challenging without additional cross-sectional imaging assessment.[12,13]

Fluoroscopy

Before the increased use of US, fluoroscopy was the primary imaging tool used to evaluate diaphragmatic movement, particularly in the pediatric population. In selected cases, fluoroscopy can be a useful tool to evaluate diaphragmatic motion when US may be unavailable or suboptimal. Imaging can be performed during quiet breathing, deep breathing, coughing, and/or sniffing in infants and children in frontal and lateral projections. As with all studies

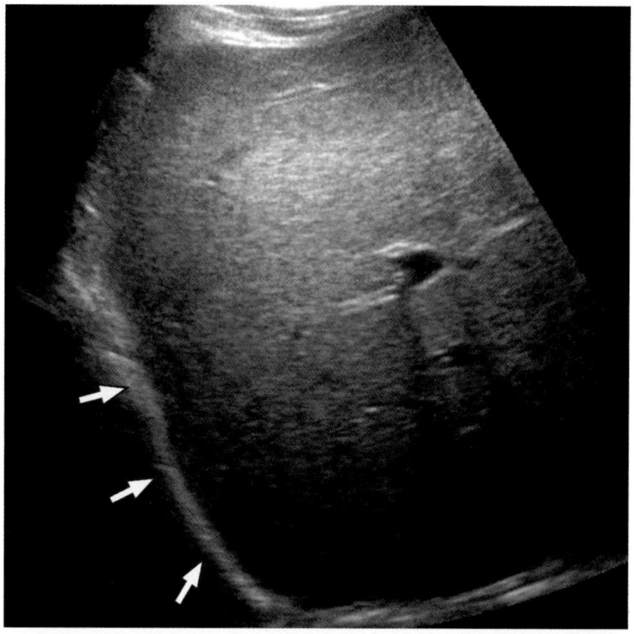

FIGURE 13.3 **A 6-year-old girl with a normal right hemidiaphragm.** Sagittal ultrasound image shows that the normal diaphragm is a specular reflector and appears as a continuous dome-shaped linear echogenic structure (*arrows*).

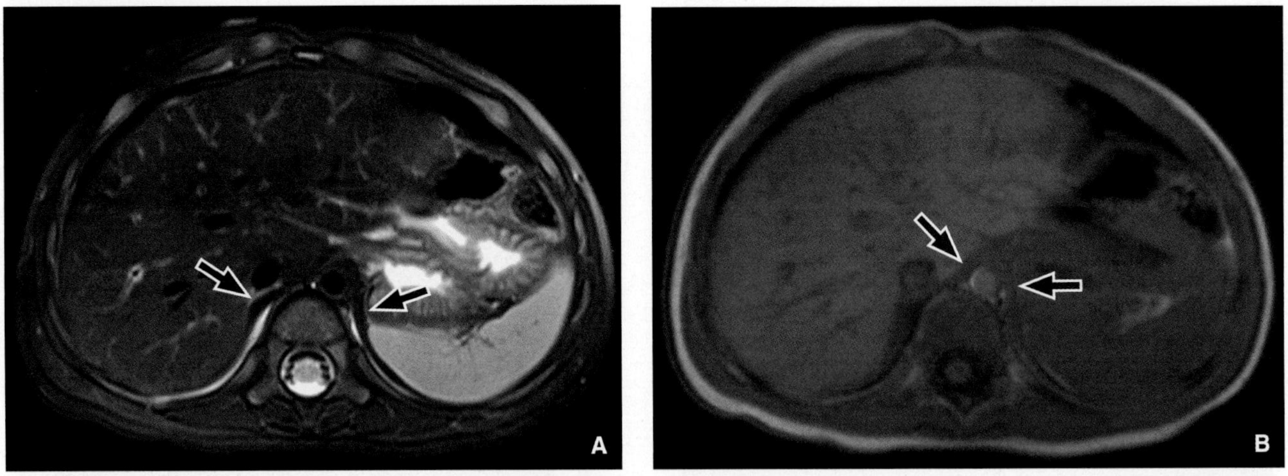

FIGURE 13.4 **A 12-month-old boy with a normal diaphragm on MRI.** The diaphragm is seen as a thin muscular sheet that is lower in signal intensity than other skeletal muscles on T2-weighted MR image with fat saturation (**A**, *arrows*) and T1-weighted MR image (**B**, *arrows*).

that utilize ionizing radiation, the ALARA (As Low As Reasonably Achievable) principle of radiation dose management should be closely followed.[14] Helpful methods that can be employed to reduce overall radiation dose during fluoroscopy include (1) removing the antiscatter grid when imaging small patients (<18 kg and <4 years old), (2) using the largest fields of view (i.e., smallest electronic magnification) possible, and (3) collimating to the area of interest.[14] Diaphragmatic paralysis is suggested when there is absent or paradoxical movement of a hemidiaphragm. Diaphragmatic eventration may be suggested when there is a lag at inspiration, followed by delayed inferior movement, though differentiation from diaphragmatic paralysis is often challenging.

Computed Tomography and Magnetic Resonance Imaging

Because of its excellent contrast resolution and multiplanar imaging capability, computed tomography (CT), particularly multidetector CT (MDCT), and magnetic resonance imaging (MRI) are both excellent tools for evaluating the diaphragm.[1,8,15] Additionally, specialized MR imaging can be performed to evaluate diaphragmatic motion by employing fast gradient-recalled-echo (GRE) pulse sequences[16] or utilizing steady-state acquisition sequences (FIESTA; GE Medical Systems).[17] The excellent soft tissue resolution of MRI allows the diaphragm to be visualized as a thin muscular sheet that is lower in signal intensity than other skeletal muscles on all sequences (Fig. 13.4).[1]

CT and MR can be useful in evaluating pathologic conditions of the diaphragm. For example, CT and MRI are helpful in the diagnosis and management of diaphragmatic tumors, though attributing an origin from the diaphragm as opposed to an adjacent abdominal organ can be challenging.[12,13] CT is useful in the diagnosis of traumatic diaphragmatic injury.[10] The large majority of CDHs are diagnosed and managed based on antenatal US and MRI findings as well as postnatal radiographs, but in selected cases, CT or MRI can provide important information about hernia contents, particularly in cases of late presentation or when findings are unclear.[1,8,9]

NORMAL ANATOMY AND DEVELOPMENT

The diaphragm begins development in the 4th week of gestation.[7] Bilateral pleuroperitoneal membranes fuse with the horizontal septum transversum, the mesentery of the esophagus, and the musculature of the lateral body wall to form the diaphragm.[18] The septum transversum forms the central tendon, which is the central fibrous portion of the diaphragm (Fig. 13.5). The majority of the muscular diaphragm is derived from the pleuroperitoneal membranes, with the peripheral portions derived from the lateral body wall and midline portions, including the crura, formed by the dorsal

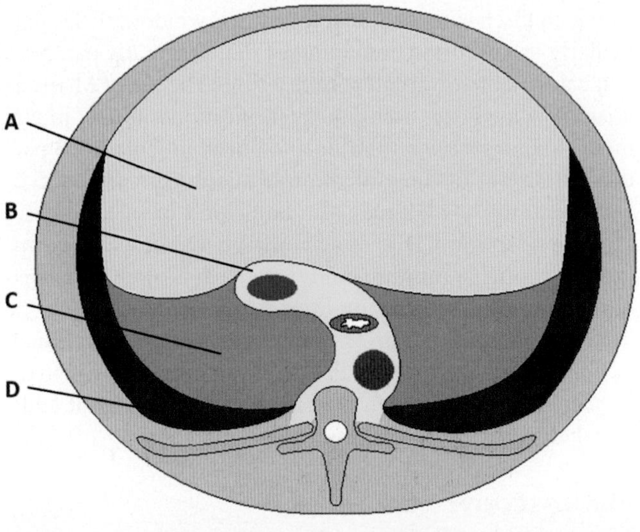

FIGURE 13.5 **Embryology of the diaphragm.** The diaphragm forms from the fusion of the septum transversum (*A*), dorsal mesentery of the esophagus (*B*), pleuroperitoneal membrane (*C*), and the musculature of the lateral body wall (*D*).

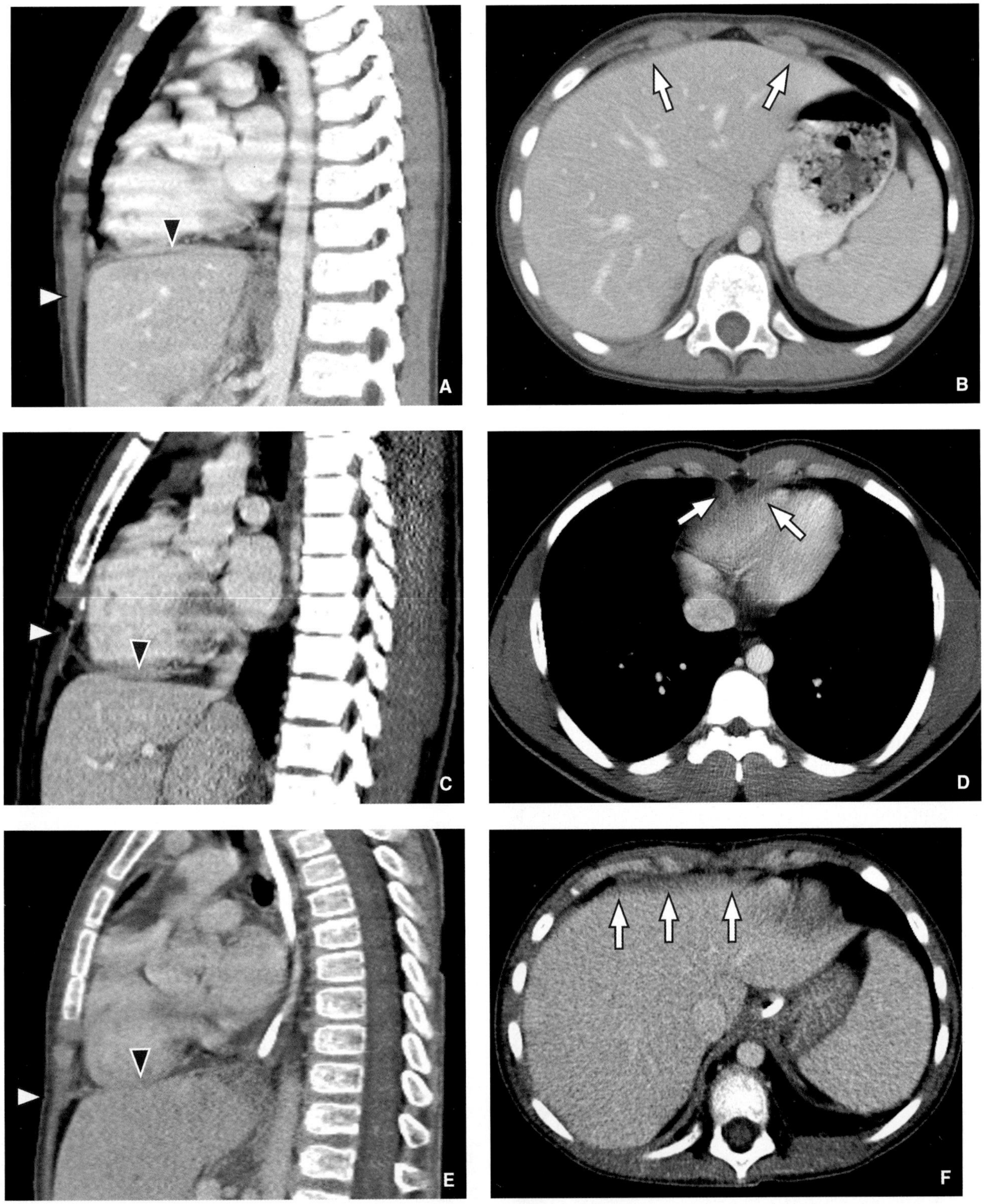

FIGURE 13.6 **Three normal configurations of the anterior diaphragm.** Sagittal **(A)** and axial **(B)** enhanced CT images in a type I configuration demonstrate the central tendon (*black arrowhead*) superior to the xiphoid process (*white arrowhead*) and continuity between the anterior and anterolateral fibers (*arrows*). Sagittal **(C)** and axial **(D)** enhanced CT images in a type II configuration show the central tendon (*black arrowhead*) located inferior to the xiphoid process (*white arrowhead*) and discontinuity of the anterior diaphragm (*arrows*) in the midline. Sagittal **(E)** and axial **(F)** enhanced CT images in a type III configuration demonstrate the central tendon (*black arrowhead*) and the xiphoid process (*white arrowhead*) in the same axial plane, leading the anterior diaphragm to have poorly defined margins (*arrows*) on the axial CT image.

mesentery of the esophagus.[1] A fibrous lumbocostal trigone remains at the posterior lateral junction of each hemidiaphragm, where the pleuroperitoneal membranes fuse with the lateral body wall muscle fibers.[7]

The mature diaphragm is characterized by anterolateral muscle fibers that originate from the sternum and ribs and posteromedial fibers that originate from the right aspect of the upper three lumbar vertebrae and the left aspect of the upper two lumbar vertebrae as the crura.[1,18] The three major openings in the normal diaphragm are the aortic hiatus, esophageal hiatus, and inferior vena caval hiatus. The aortic hiatus is at the level of T12 and contains the aorta, thoracic duct, azygos vein, and hemiazygos vein.[18] The esophageal hiatus is at the level of T10 and contains the esophagus, vagus nerve, sympathetic nerves, and esophageal branches of the left gastric vessels.[18] The inferior vena caval hiatus is located at the level of T8-9 and contains the inferior vena cava and branches of the right phrenic nerve.[18]

The anterior diaphragm can have a variable appearance on cross-sectional imaging depending on the position of the middle leaflet of the central tendon relative to the xiphoid.[19] Familiarity with the normal variations in diaphragmatic morphology is essential, particularly when evaluating for Morgagni hernias.[19] Three normal configurations of the anterior diaphragm have been described (Fig. 13.6).[1,18,19] In type I, the middle leaflet of the central tendon is located superior to the xiphoid process with posterior concavity of the anterior portion and continuity between the anterior and anterolateral fibers (Fig. 13.6A, B). In type II, the middle leaflet of the central tendon is located inferior to the xiphoid process, and the anterior diaphragm is discontinuous in the midline, with the anterior fibers oriented at an angle to the lateral fibers (Fig. 13.6C, D). In type III, the middle leaflet of the central tendon and the xiphoid process are at the same level causing the anterior diaphragm to appear broad and angular on axial images with poorly defined margins because it runs in the plane of the axial image (Fig. 13.6E, F). M. Elon Gale described the incidence of each configuration, finding type I in 48%, type II in 28%, and type III in 11%.[19]

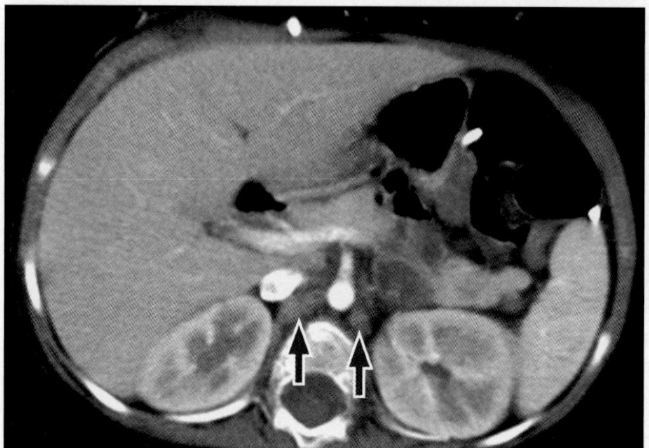

FIGURE 13.7 **A 28-month-old girl with a normal diaphragm.** Axial enhanced CT image shows a normal nodular appearance of bilateral diaphragmatic crura (*arrows*).

Familiarity with the normal appearance of the diaphragmatic crura is also essential to avoid potential delayed diagnosis or misdiagnosis. Because crural width does not change substantially with age, the crura appear relatively larger in children.[20] This may lead the normal crura to have a more nodular appearance in the pediatric patient population, which should not be mistaken for pathology (Fig. 13.7).

SPECTRUM OF DIAPHRAGMATIC DISORDERS

Congenital and Developmental Anomalies

Three main congenital anomalies of the diaphragm include diaphragmatic hernias, diaphragmatic eventration, and duplication of the diaphragm (Table 13.1). These conditions are encountered with varying frequency, and familiarity with these anomalies is essential to avoid confusion and misdiagnosis.

Diaphragmatic Hernia

Diaphragmatic hernias can occur as a result of a defect in the diaphragmatic musculature, as in CDH, or because of protrusion of the stomach through the esophageal hiatus, as in hiatal hernia. CDHs are potentially serious congenital anomalies with a high morbidity and mortality and frequent associations with additional malformations, syndromes, and chromosomal anomalies.[7] CDH occurs in ~1 in 4,000 births[21] and is traditionally classified based on location. Posterolateral hernias that pass through the foramen of Bochdalek (i.e., Bochdalek hernias [BHs]) are the most common type, accounting for ~90% of all CDHs (Fig. 13.8).[22] Parasternal hernias that pass through the foramen of Morgagni (i.e., Morgagni hernias) are the next most common type, accounting for 9% to 12% of CDHs (Figs. 13.9 and 13.10).[7]

TABLE 13.1 Congenital Anomalies of the Diaphragm
Diaphragmatic Hernia
Bochdalek hernia
Morgagni hernia
Hiatal hernia
Diaphragmatic Eventration
Complete eventration
Partial eventration
Duplication of the Diaphragm

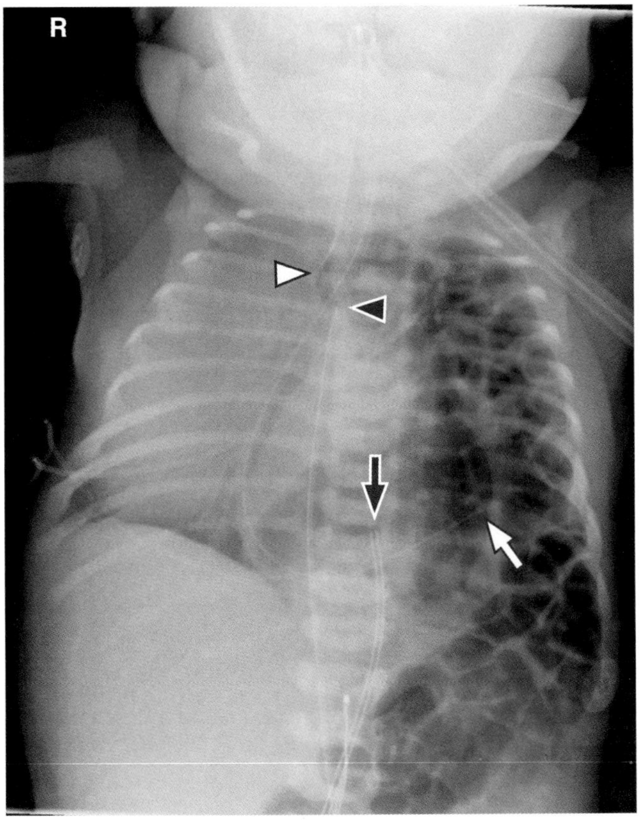

FIGURE 13.8 **Newborn girl with left Bochdalek congenital diaphragmatic hernia.** Frontal chest and upper abdomen radiograph shows bowel loops herniating into the left hemithorax and causing rightward mediastinal shift. Nasogastric tube is deviated to the right as it passes through the esophagus, and the tip (*white arrow*) projects over the left thorax, likely within an intrathoracic stomach. Umbilical venous catheter (*black arrow*) is deviated to the left because of liver herniation. Umbilical artery catheter (*black arrowhead*) and endotracheal tube (*white arrowhead*) are deviated to the right.

A recent classification scheme proposes new categories and definitions for diaphragmatic hernia and eventration and provides opportunities for more detailed subtyping based on such parameters as size, location, presence, or absence of a "sac" or dividing membrane and other anatomic factors.[23] Improving the precision of phenotypic diagnosis may pave the way for better genotype–phenotype correlation as more genetic causes of CDH are understood. However, many of the detailed parameters involved in the new classification scheme are better addressed by the type of gross inspection available at surgery and autopsy than by radiographic study, and this classification scheme has not been widely adopted by the radiology community to date. Nevertheless, the limitations of categorizing the traditional "Bochdalek" and "Morgagni" hernias are recognized, and therefore, the following classifications should be utilized only as a guideline for interpretation.

Bochdalek Hernia

The pathogenesis of Bochdalek hernias (BHs) is poorly understood. It has been suggested that the primary inciting event in this condition is failure of the septum transversum and pleuroperitoneal fold to fuse with the musculature of the lateral body wall at ~8 weeks of gestation, though more recent studies have shown that the defect may occur earlier, during the development of the pleuroperitoneal folds.[24] Because Bochdalek hernia (BH) is associated with additional malformations of the heart, lungs, and other organ systems, it has been postulated that the defect in the development of the pleuroperitoneal fold arises from a disruption of a common signaling pathway that triggers mesenchymal differentiation of several different organ systems, leading to a global embryopathy with CDH being one of several manifestations.[25] This has led to the hypothesis that the diaphragmatic defect and pulmonary hypoplasia seen in patients with CDH arise from a single "mesenchymal hit" rather than purely from a cause–effect relationship.[7] Approximately 80% of BHs are left sided, and bilateral hernias occur rarely.[7] A hernia sac may be present in up to 15% of cases.[7]

CDHs are frequently diagnosed on prenatal imaging. In general, patients with CDH have a survival rate of 70%, but rates are lower among patients with chromosomal and genetic syndromes, organ malformations, and severe isolated CDH.[26] Survival rates are higher among patients diagnosed postnatally as compared with patients diagnosed prenatally, reflecting the fact that prenatally diagnosed patients generally have more severe disease.[27] Fetal US and MRI can evaluate for severity of CDH and provide important prognostic information before birth. Parameters measured on fetal US include lung-to-head ratio and presence/absence of liver herniation. Parameters measured on fetal MRI include total lung volume and percent liver herniation. These parameters help assess the severity of disease and help predict mortality.[26] Because of MRI's superior contrast resolution, MRI parameters have proven more accurate in predicting survival than US parameters, and fetal MRI is therefore being more widely adopted (Fig. 13.11).[28–30]

The first imaging study in a newborn with BH most frequently is a chest radiograph. The initial radiograph may show opacification of a hemithorax with contralateral mediastinal shift. If bowel loops have herniated into the thorax, follow-up radiographs will show gas-filled bowel in the thorax as the infant swallows air (Fig. 13.8). Abdominal radiographs may demonstrate a paucity of intra-abdominal bowel loops if a large amount of bowel has herniated into the thorax.[31] If intra-abdominal organs have herniated into the thorax, opacity will persist on follow-up radiographs. Nasogastric tube (NGT) and umbilical venous catheter (UVC) position can be helpful in determining hernia contents and degree of mass effect (Fig. 13.8). As the NGT passes through the esophagus, it will deviate away from the side of the hernia because of mass effect. If the stomach has herniated into the chest, the tip of the NGT will be located within the thorax. In cases of liver herniation, UVCs will often have an altered position. The position of umbilical artery catheters can also be altered, but they are frequently less affected than UVCs and NGTs because of the aorta's location within the retroperitoneum and posterior mediastinum.[7] Identification of these findings on chest radiographs is essential for

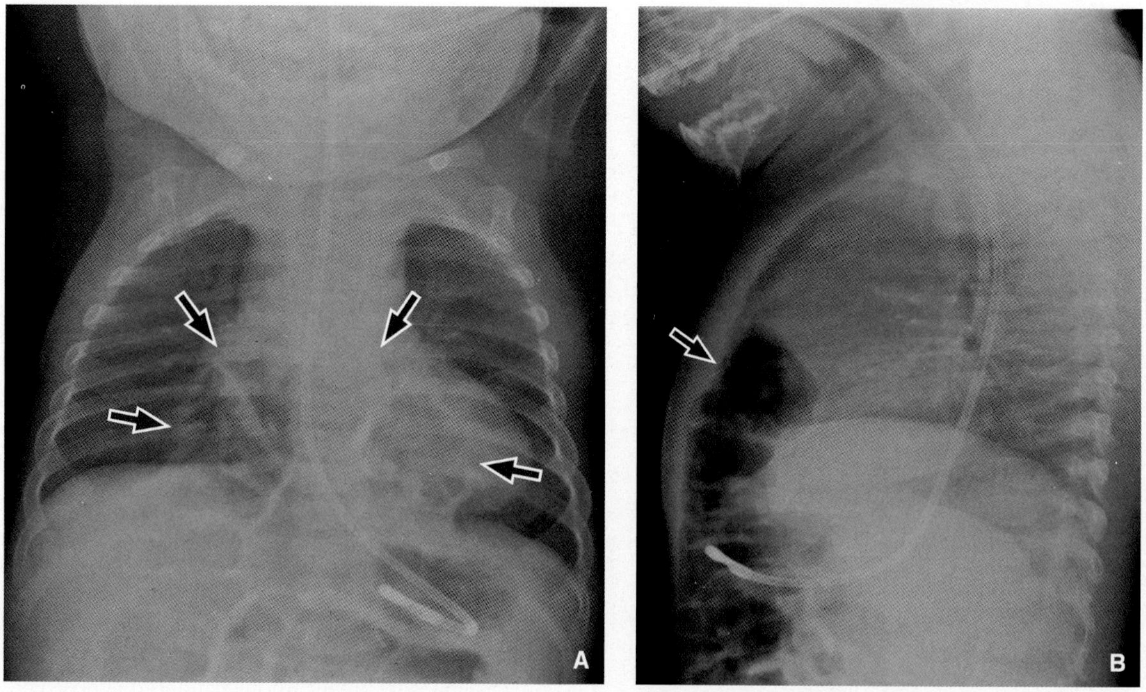

FIGURE 13.9 **A 5-month-old girl with poor weight gain, atrial septal defect, and Morgagni congenital diaphragmatic hernia. A:** Frontal radiograph demonstrates intrathoracic bowel loops (*arrows*). **B:** Lateral radiograph demonstrates that herniated bowel loops (*arrow*) are located within the anterior chest.

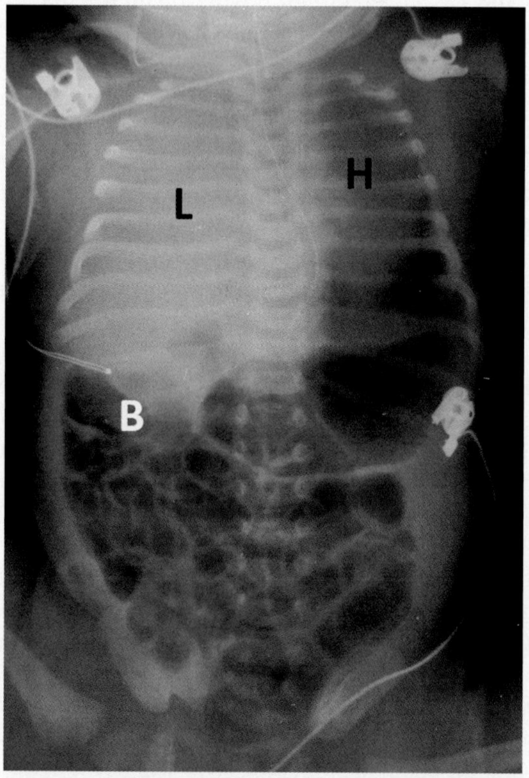

FIGURE 13.10 **Newborn baby girl with a prenatal diagnosis of a right-sided Morgagni congenital diaphragmatic hernia who presented with severe perinatal respiratory distress.** Frontal chest and abdomen radiograph shows complete opacification of the right hemithorax because of a complete liver (*L*) herniation causing shift of the heart (*H*) to the left and displacement of the nasogastric tube. There is bowel (*B*) in the right upper quadrant with a lack of a hepatic shadow.

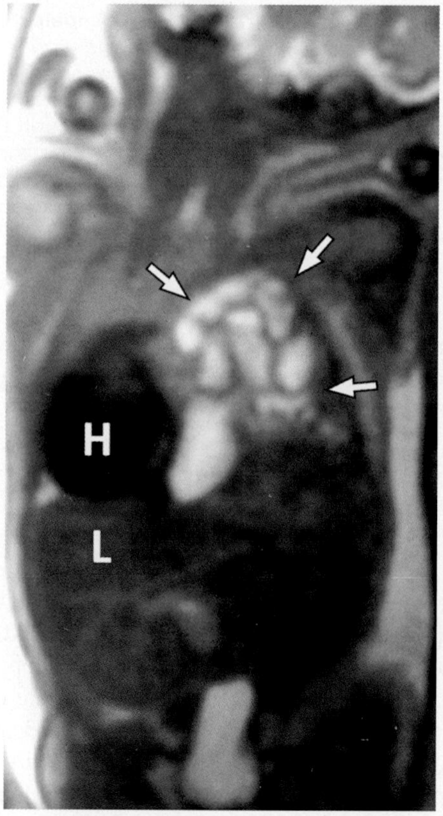

FIGURE 13.11 **Prenatal diagnosis of congenital diaphragmatic hernia.** Coronal T2-weighted MR image shows bowel loops (*arrows*) located in the left hemithorax, consistent with left-sided congenital diaphragmatic hernia. *H*, heart; *L*, liver.

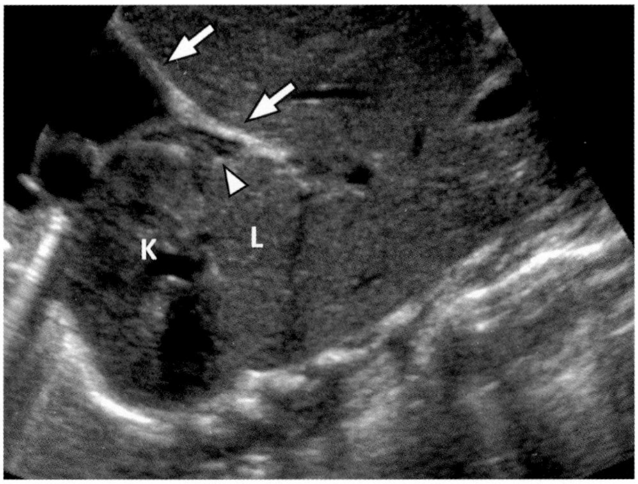

FIGURE 13.12 **Newborn baby girl with a prenatal diagnosis of a right diaphragmatic hernia who presented with perinatal respiratory distress.** Sagittal ultrasound image of the right hemidiaphragm (*arrows*) shows interruption of the posterior diaphragm. The right kidney (*K*), adrenal gland (*arrowhead*), and a segment of the liver (*L*) are herniating through the diaphragmatic defect.

confirmation of CDH, though specific findings on radiographs are not predictive of overall outcome.[32] US may be helpful to confirm or characterize solid organ position prior to surgery (Fig. 13.12).

Though usually not necessary, in rare instances, CT and MRI may be utilized as problem-solving tools in unclear cases and can be useful in diagnosing associated malformations.[1] If CT is considered, oral contrast should be administered very cautiously because it can cause a sudden increase in mass effect within the thorax, leading to increased mediastinal shift and worsening respiratory compromise.[7]

Pathologic features of CDH are appreciated well at autopsy in patients without previous surgical repair (Fig. 13.13). Reflecting the sternum downward permits examination of all diaphragmatic attachments to the chest wall. A membranous covering overlying the superiorly herniated abdominal organs may or may not be identified. Typically, the lungs are small, particularly the ipsilateral lung (Fig. 13.14); the mediastinum is displaced to the contralateral side; and the herniated viscera such as the liver may show a notched contour (Fig. 13.15).

In the past few decades, the philosophy driving treatment strategies in CDH has shifted from emergent surgical repair to initial medical management followed by elective repair. Studies have shown improved outcomes when patients are medically optimized by treating underlying pulmonary hypoplasia and pulmonary hypertension prior to repair.[33–35] This treatment focuses on hemodynamic and ventilatory support and correction of metabolic abnormalities utilizing permissive hypercapnia, extracorporeal membrane oxygenation, high-frequency oscillatory ventilation, and inhaled nitric oxide.[36] Once medically optimized, surgical repair is performed utilizing a transabdominal approach,[37] or in more stable patients, a thoracoscopic approach has been used.[1] The herniated abdominal viscera are repositioned within the abdomen, and the posterolateral diaphragmatic defect is closed (Fig. 13.16).

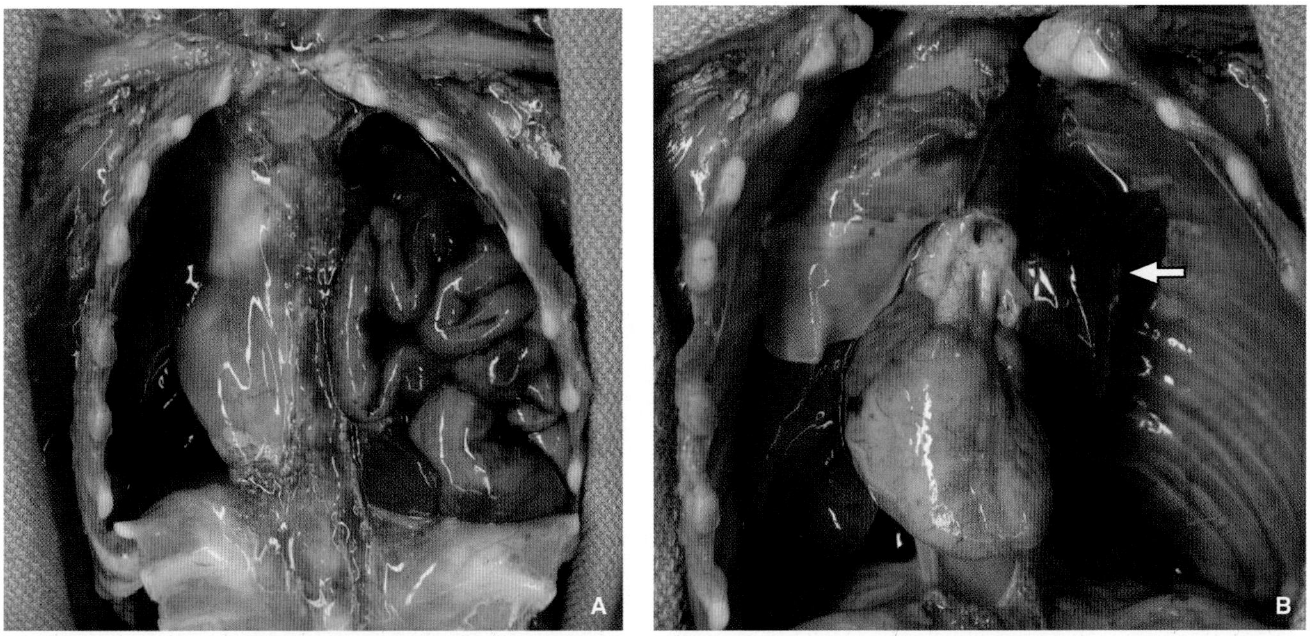

FIGURE 13.13 **Large posterolateral diaphragmatic defect (Bochdalek hernia) in a 2-day-old boy. A:** Downward reflection of the sternum reveals a right-shifted mediastinum and herniated abdominal organs including the intestines, pancreas, and spleen. **B:** After removal of the herniated organs, pulmonary hypoplasia, which is severe on the left (*arrow*), is better visualized.

(*Continued*)

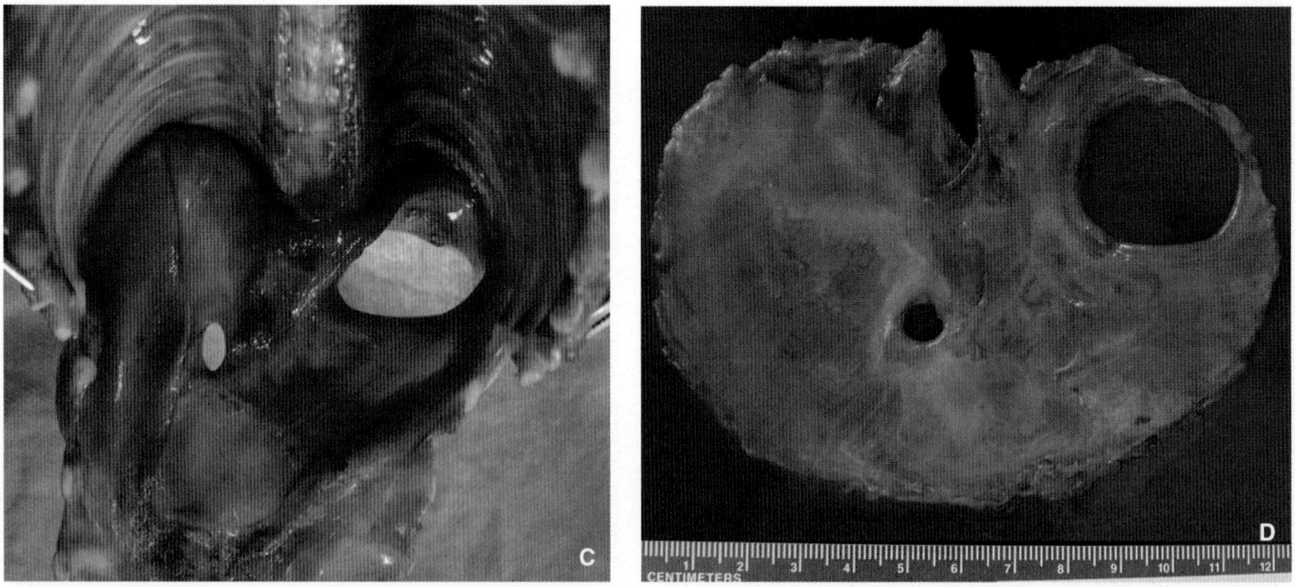

FIGURE 13.13 (*Continued*) The diaphragm as seen from its superior surface before **(C)** and after **(D)** its evisceration shows a large posterolateral defect. (Photographs courtesy of Harry P.W. Kozakewich, MD, Boston Children's Hospital and Harvard Medical School, Boston, MA.)

The defect is closed using nonabsorbable sutures when small, but when larger than ~5 cm, a prosthetic patch may be utilized[38] (Fig. 13.17). Occasionally, a split abdominal wall muscle flap is employed.[39]

Following repair, postoperative pneumothorax is a common finding (Fig. 13.18). Even if the pneumothorax is large, rapid evacuation should be avoided because the neonatal mediastinum is mobile, and rapid evacuation can lead to mediastinal rotation with torsion and obstruction of the inferior vena cava.[7] Therefore, pneumothoraces should be allowed to slowly resorb, and pleural fluid can often be seen replacing the air on serial radiographs. Additional findings on postoperative chest radiographs in pediatric patients with prior repaired CDH include lung hypoplasia, decreased pulmonary vasculature, and persistent mediastinal shift (Fig. 13.19). Recurrent hernia can be seen in 3% to 22% of cases[40] and may be seen on chest radiograph, US, fluoroscopic contrast studies, CT, and/or MRI (Fig. 13.20). Patch repairs are at greatest risk of recurrence and infection (Fig. 13.21).[1] Poor growth and decreased motility of the repaired diaphragm can occur and may be evaluated with M-mode US.[41] Pulmonary scintigraphy may demonstrate decreased perfusion within the ipsilateral lung (Fig. 13.22).[42] Long-term musculoskeletal conditions including pectus excavatum, pectus carinatum, and scoliosis occur in ~46% of pediatric patients with prior CDH.[43]

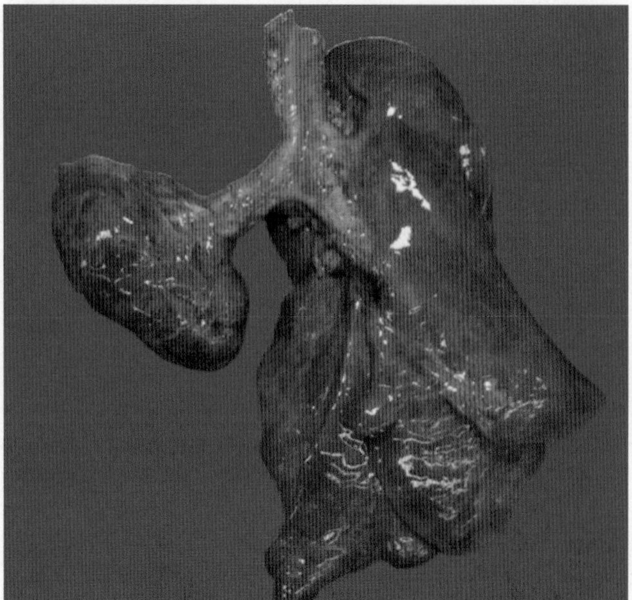

FIGURE 13.14 **Pulmonary hypoplasia in a 7-week-old girl with multiple congenital anomalies.** The left lung (posterior aspect shown) is markedly smaller than the right in the setting of a left-sided congenital diaphragmatic defect.

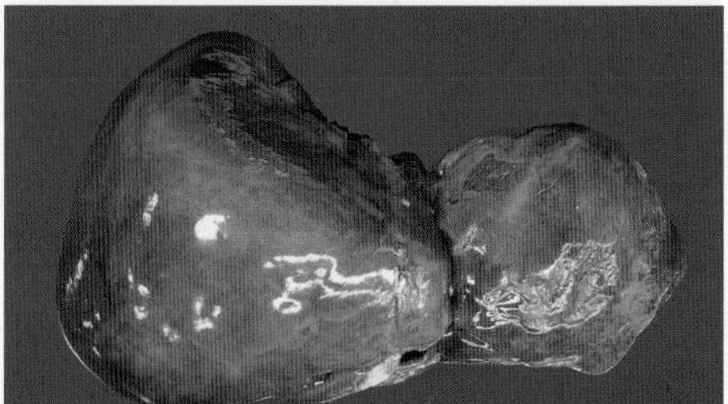

FIGURE 13.15 **Notched liver in a 5-week-old girl with history of surgically repaired congenital diaphragmatic hernia.** The liver has fibrous adhesions as well as an abnormal scalloped external contour.

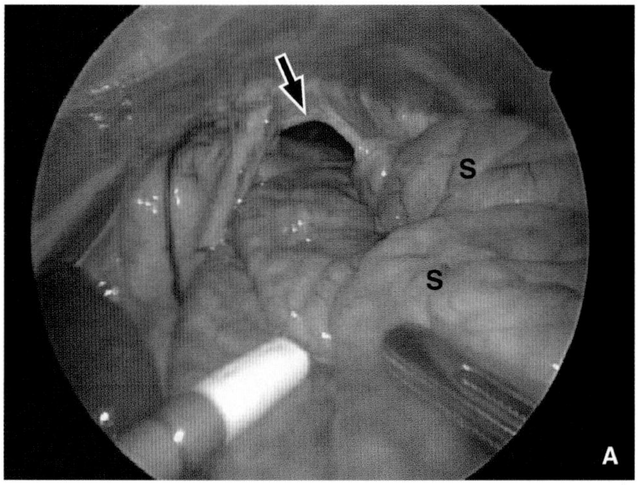

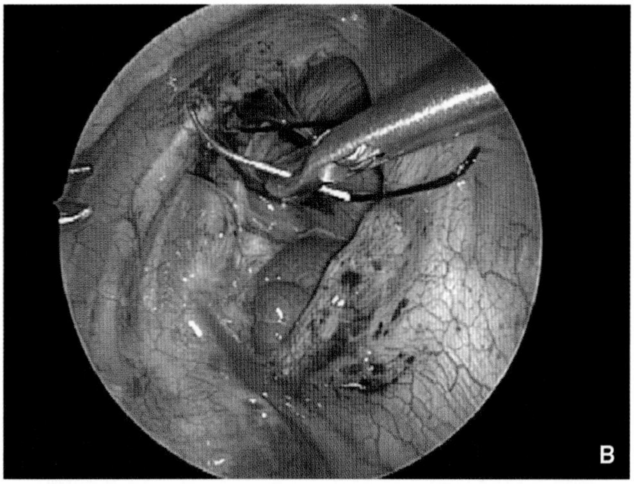

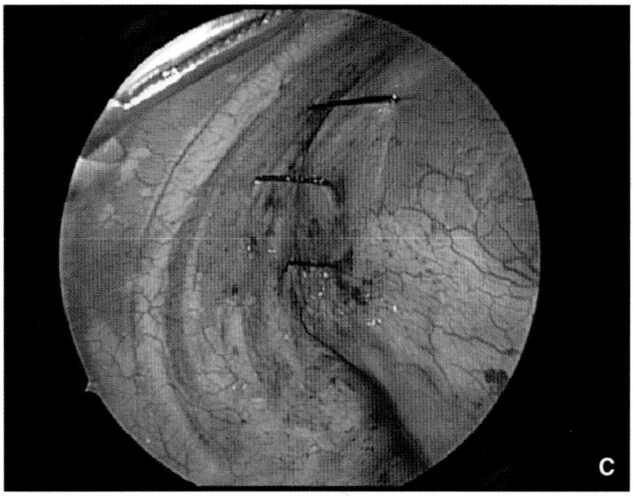

FIGURE 13.16 **Thoracoscopic Bochdalek congenital diaphragmatic hernia (CDH) repair. A:** Thoracoscopic image shows herniated small bowel loops (*S*) through left Bochdalek CDH (*arrow*). **B:** Thoracoscopic repair of the left Bochdalek CDH using nonabsorbable sutures. **C:** Complete closure of the left Bochdalek CDH. (Case courtesy of Craig Lillehei, MD, Boston Children's Hospital and Harvard Medical School, Boston, MA.)

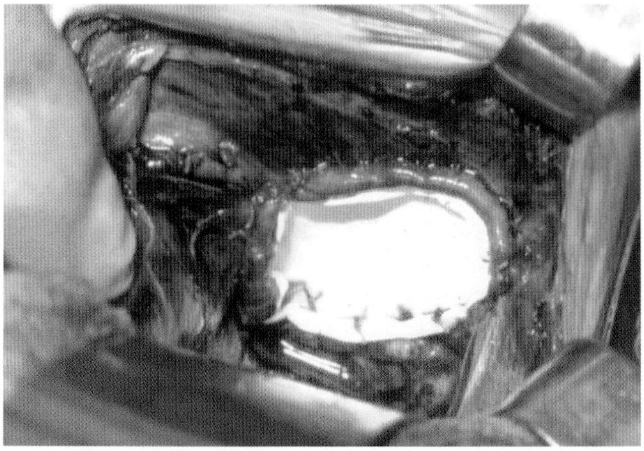

FIGURE 13.17 **Surgical closure of the left Bochdalek congenital diaphragmatic hernia using a prosthetic patch.** (Image courtesy of Craig Lillehei, MD, Boston Children's Hospital and Harvard Medical School, Boston, MA.)

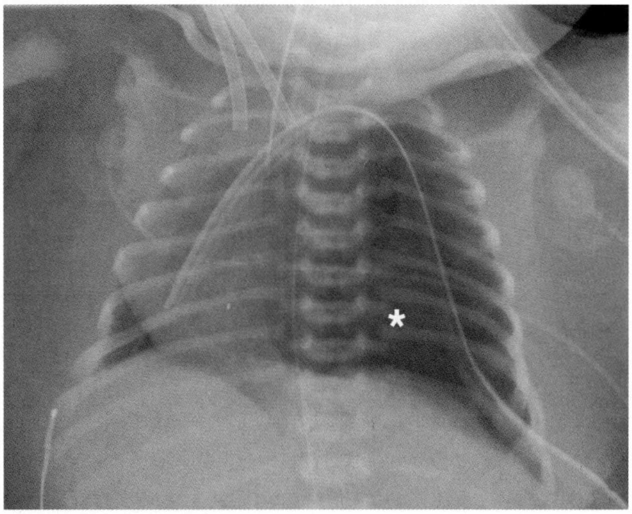

FIGURE 13.18 **A 6-day-old girl status post repair of left-sided congenital diaphragmatic hernia with Gore-Tex patch.** Frontal chest radiograph demonstrates a large left pneumothorax (*asterisk*) with persistent rightward mediastinal shift, which is allowed to slowly resorb in order to limit risk of mediastinal torsion.

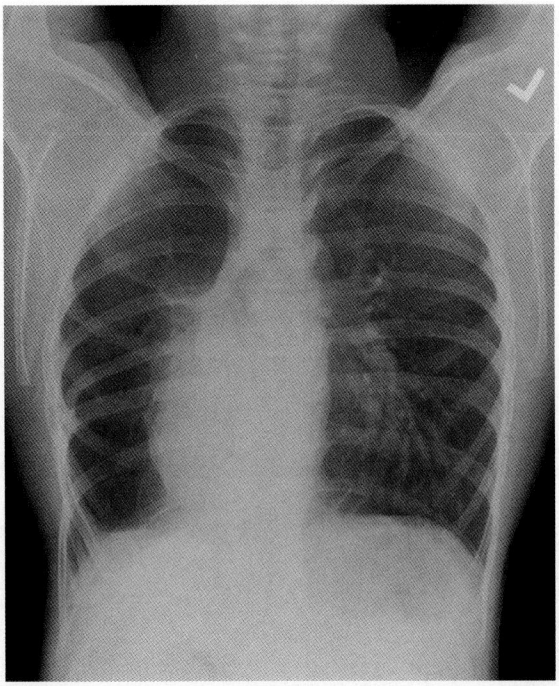

FIGURE 13.19 **A 9-year-old girl with right sided congenital diaphragmatic hernia (CDH) repair as a newborn who presented with chronic changes after CDH repair.** Frontal chest radiograph shows right lung hypoplasia leading to chronic rightward mediastinal shift and decreased right pulmonary vascularity. Chronic right pleural thickening and mild scoliosis are also noted.

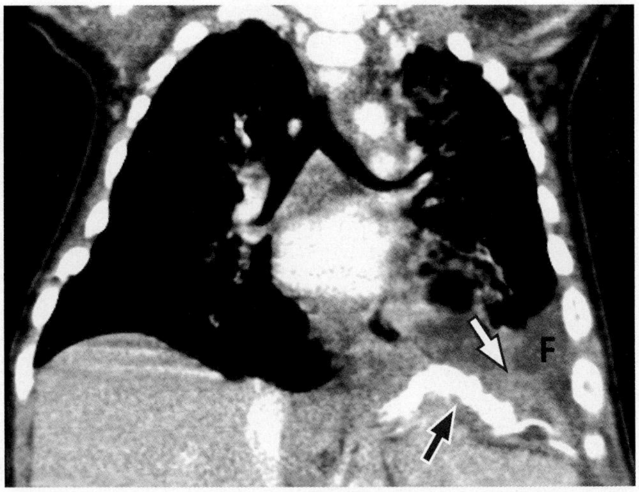

FIGURE 13.21 **A 6-month-old girl with history of left-sided congenital diaphragmatic hernia patch repair as a newborn who presented with new fever and elevated white blood cell count.** Coronal enhanced CT image demonstrates complex fluid (*F*) and soft tissue density (*white arrow*) adjacent to the dense left diaphragmatic patch (*black arrow*). Subsequent drainage demonstrated an infectious fluid collection adjacent to the patch.

Morgagni Hernia

Morgagni hernias (MHs) occur when the transverse septum and the lateral body wall fail to fuse at the level where the internal mammary artery crosses the diaphragm.[7] MHs account for 9% to 12% of all CDHs, occur on the right in 90% of cases, and are most commonly unilateral.[7] MHs typically have a hernia sac.[7] They are associated with trisomy 21 in 14% of cases and congenital heart disease in 58% of cases.[7,44] A similar type of retrosternal hernia can occur as a component of the pentalogy of Cantrell, which also includes omphalocele, inferior sternal cleft, cardiac defects, ectopia cordis, and pericardial defects (Fig. 13.23). Rarely, patients with right-sided CDH can have associated hepatopulmonary

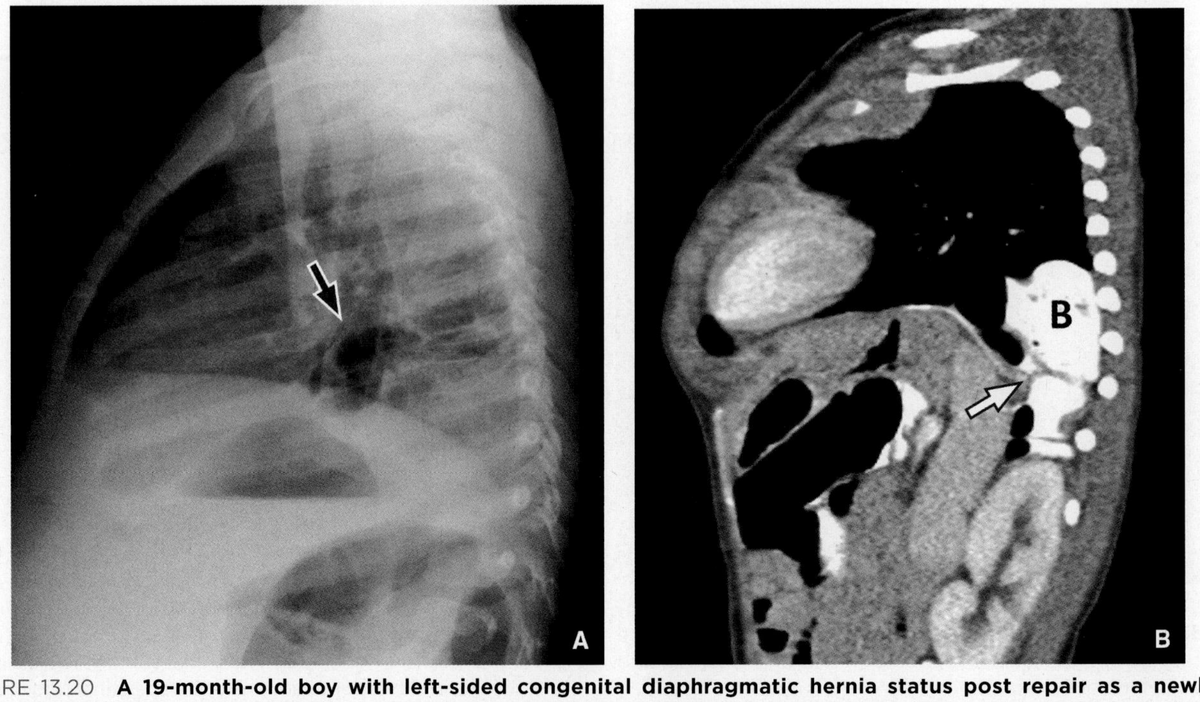

FIGURE 13.20 **A 19-month-old boy with left-sided congenital diaphragmatic hernia status post repair as a newborn who presented with recurrent hernia. A:** Lateral radiograph demonstrates intrathoracic bowel loops (*black arrow*). **B:** Sagittal enhanced CT image obtained with oral contrast demonstrates a diaphragmatic defect (*white arrow*) posterior to the dense diaphragmatic patch, with bowel loops (*B*) herniating into the posterior chest.

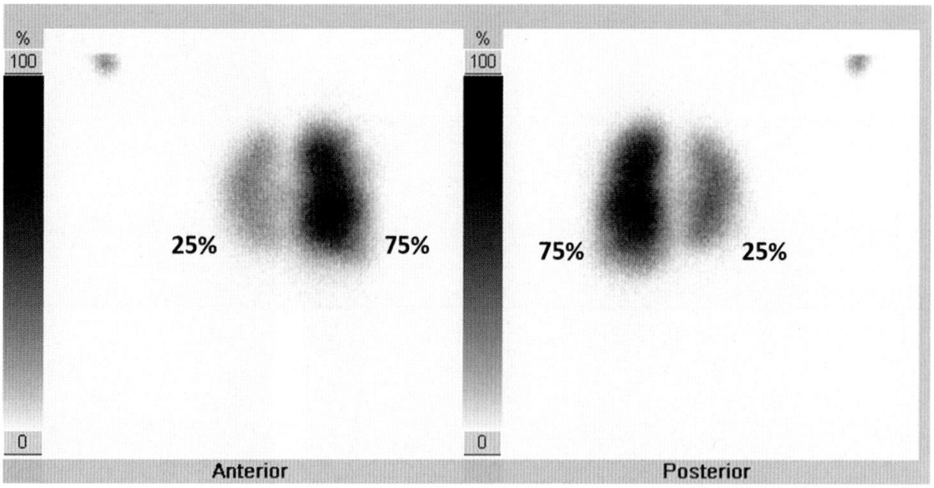

FIGURE 13.22 **A 3-year-old boy with history of right-sided congenital diaphragmatic hernia status post repair as a neonate.** Anterior and posterior projections from a Tc-99m macroaggregated albumin pulmonary perfusion study demonstrate differential pulmonary perfusion of 75% on the *left* and 25% on the *right*.

fusion, a condition in which a dense adhesion forms between the right lung and the herniated hepatic parenchyma.[45–47]

Unlike BHs, most MHs are detected in older children or adults.[1] They are often found incidentally on chest radiograph when herniated bowel loops (most commonly the colon) are seen in the anterior thorax (Fig. 13.9). Alternatively, they may present with bowel obstruction.[1] When solid intra-abdominal organs herniate through the defect, the appearance on chest radiograph may mimic focal eventration, a mass, lymphadenopathy, or foregut duplication cyst (Fig. 13.24), and, US, CT, or MRI is often helpful for better characterization.[1,7] In rare cases of CDH with hepatopulmonary fusion, chest radio-

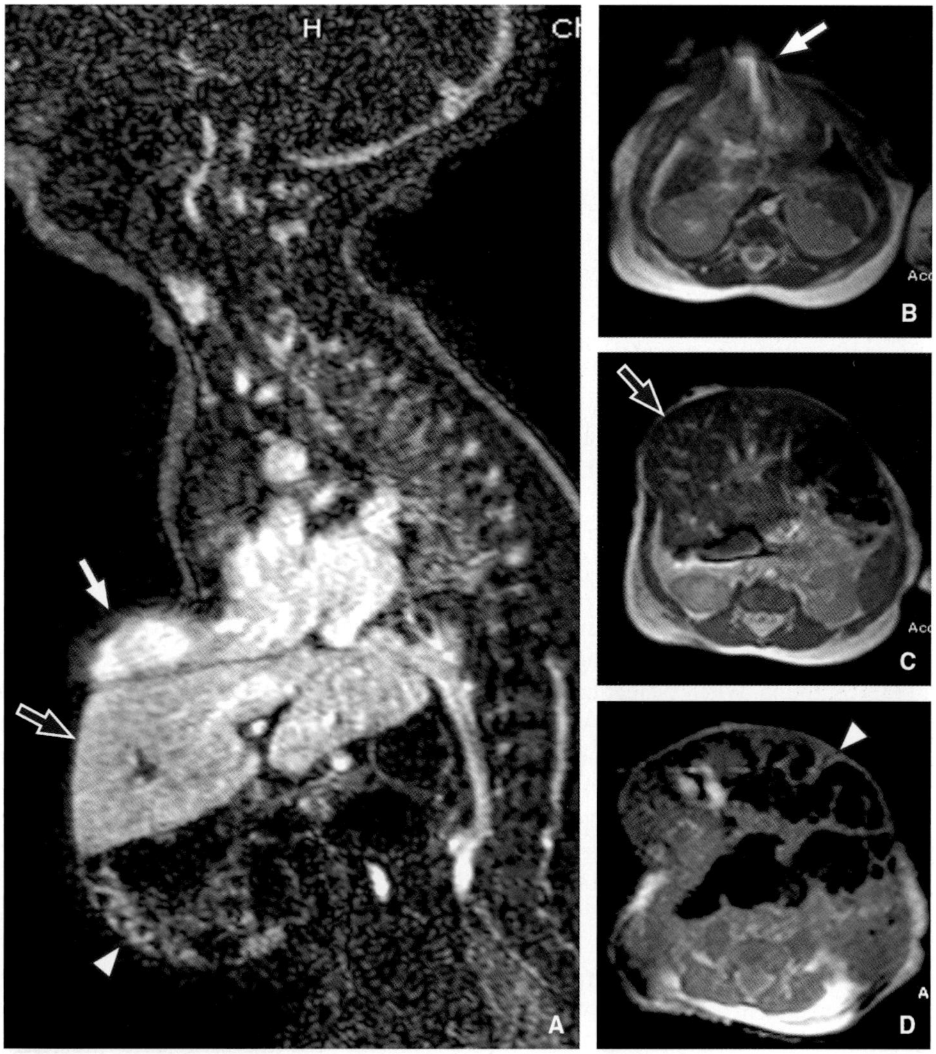

FIGURE 13.23 **A 2-day-old girl with pentalogy of Cantrell.** Sagittal postcontrast T1-weighted **(A)** and serial axial postcontrast T2-weighted **(B–D)** MR images demonstrate ectopia cordis (*white arrows*) and large omphalocele containing the liver (*black arrows*) and bowel (*arrowheads*).

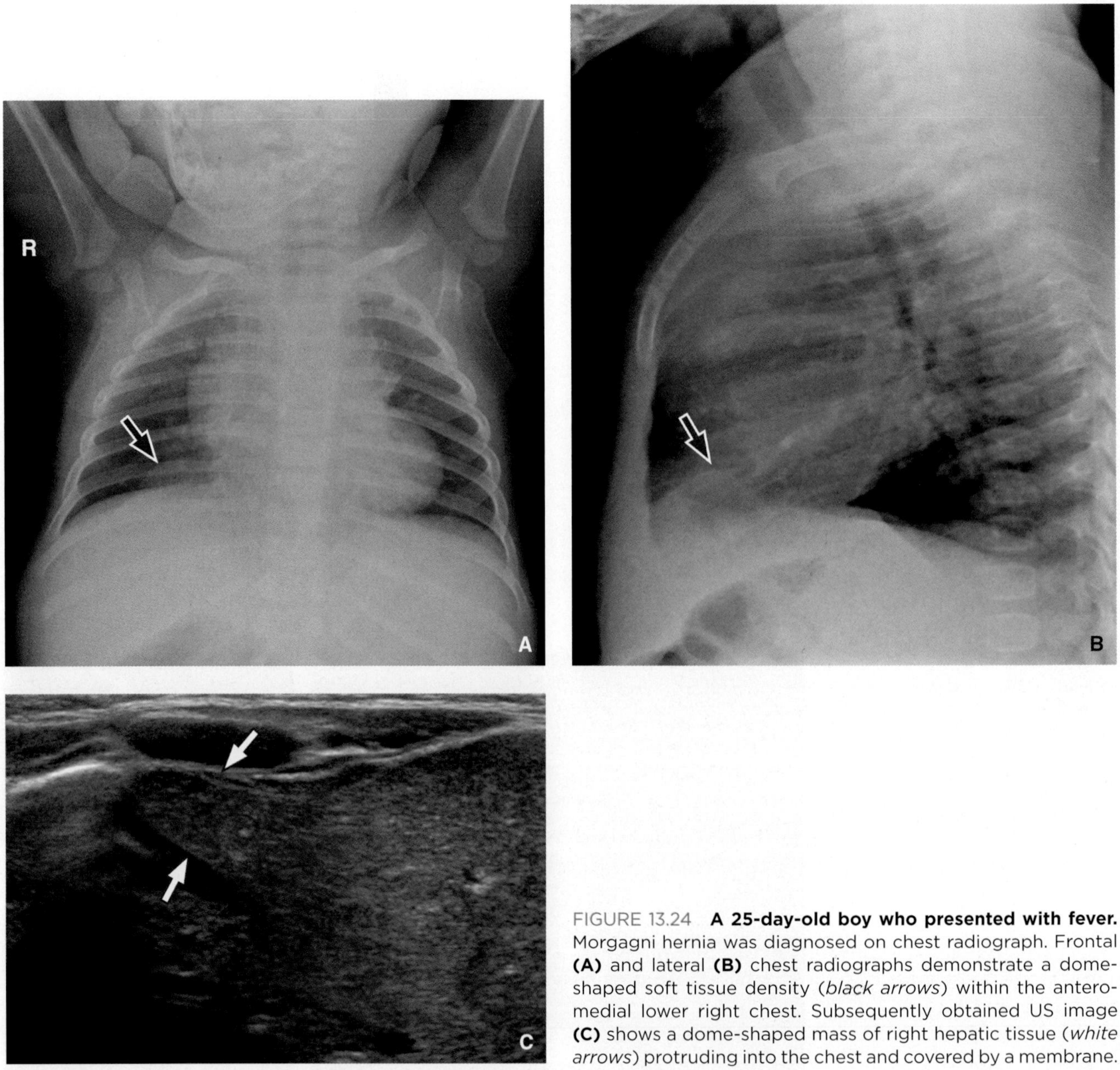

FIGURE 13.24 **A 25-day-old boy who presented with fever.** Morgagni hernia was diagnosed on chest radiograph. Frontal **(A)** and lateral **(B)** chest radiographs demonstrate a dome-shaped soft tissue density (*black arrows*) within the anteromedial lower right chest. Subsequently obtained US image **(C)** shows a dome-shaped mass of right hepatic tissue (*white arrows*) protruding into the chest and covered by a membrane.

graphs may demonstrate right hemithorax opacification without the leftward mediastinal shift that would be expected in a typical CDH. A dense adhesion between the right lung and herniated hepatic parenchyma prevents mediastinal shift in this condition. When evaluating hepatopulmonary fusion, CT or MRI with multiplanar two-dimensional and three-dimensional reconstructions is helpful to delineate the precise anatomy before surgical repair[48,49] (Fig. 13.25). Because of a high risk of strangulation associated with MHs, surgical repair is currently recommended even in asymptomatic pediatric patients. Most MHs can be repaired utilizing a laparoscopic-assisted approach.[50]

Delayed Presentation of Congenital Diaphragmatic Hernia CDHs can present later in life, with estimates of the incidence of delayed diagnosis ranging from 2.6%[51] to 45.5%.[52] It is often unclear whether the diaphragmatic defects in these cases are congenital or acquired. Some have postulated that the defects may be congenital, but were temporarily occluded by a solid organ such as the liver or spleen in the prenatal and neonatal period.[51,52] It has been shown that the patient population with delayed presentation of CDH is demographically similar to the patient population with neonatal CDH,[52] which supports this theory.

Two distinct patient groups are seen with delayed presentation of CDH. The first group consists of older infants who present with respiratory symptoms, and the second group is older children who present with gastrointestinal symptoms.[53,54] When CDH presents in younger children with respiratory symptoms, group B streptococcal (GBS) pneumonia is often associated. The cause and effect relationship between GBS pneumonia and late diagnosis of CDH is not clearly understood,

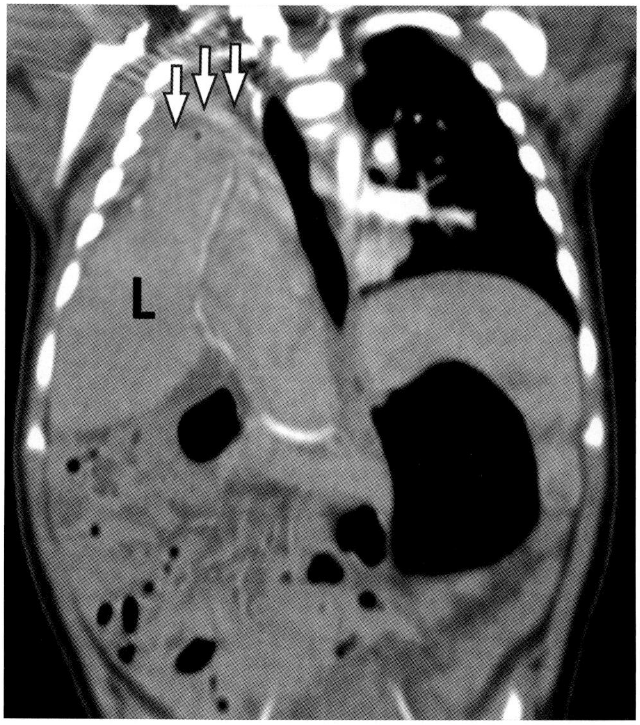

FIGURE 13.25 **Newborn girl with right-sided congenital diaphragmatic hernia and hepatopulmonary fusion.** Coronal enhanced CT image shows a right-sided diaphragmatic hernia containing a large amount of liver (*L*) but without substantial mediastinal shift to the contralateral left hemithorax, due to a dense adhesion (*arrows*) between the right lung and herniated hepatic parenchyma.

but lung consolidation may obscure herniated bowel loops in these cases.[55] When CDH is diagnosed in older children, affected pediatric patients often present with recurrent vomiting and abdominal pain because of bowel obstruction.

Imaging findings in patients with delayed presentation of CDH are variable. Studies have shown that, in patients with delayed presentation of CDH, the diagnosis is often missed or not apparent on initial chest radiographs.[51] If the hernia contains only solid organs, the findings on chest radiographs may mimic pneumonia, pleural effusion, or foregut duplication cyst. If gas-filled bowel loops have herniated into the chest, the findings may mimic pneumothorax or pneumatocele. If misinterpreted as pneumothorax, complications of gastrointestinal perforation because of chest tube placement to evacuate these "pneumothoraces" can occur. Therefore, when the diagnosis of CDH is in doubt, US, upper gastrointestinal imaging study, CT, and/or MRI are often helpful for confirmation and characterization (Fig. 13.26).[9]

Hiatal Hernia

Unlike CDHs, which involve abdominal viscera herniating through an abnormal opening in the diaphragm, hiatal hernias occur when a portion of the stomach protrudes through the esophageal hiatus. There are three types of hiatal hernia: sliding hiatal hernia, paraesophageal hernia, and congenital short esophagus.[7] In sliding hiatal hernia, the esophagus and upper stomach move freely through the hiatus, and as a result, the gastroesophageal junction and a portion of the stomach become intrathoracic in position. In paraesophageal hernia, the gastroesophageal junction remains in a normal position below the hiatus, and a portion of the stomach herniates through the hiatus. In cases of paraesophageal hernia, the gastrosplenic and gastrocolic ligaments are often absent, which increases risk of serious complications including gastric volvulus and colonic herniation.[56] In congenital short esophagus, the stomach is fixed in the thorax.

Hiatal hernias are frequently encountered incidentally as a solid- or gas-filled retrocardiac mass on chest radiograph (Fig. 13.27A). In cases of congenital short esophagus, radiographs may demonstrate a space-occupying lesion in the chest, and visualization of a nasoenteric tube within the lesion may suggest the diagnosis.[7] Upper gastrointestinal series is the definitive imaging modality for evaluation of all three types of hiatal hernia in affected pediatric patients (Fig. 13.27B).[1] Hiatal hernias may lead to altered locations of nasoenteric tubes on radiographs (Fig. 13.28A). Hiatal hernias are easily demonstrated on CT or MRI (Fig. 13.28B), though cross-sectional imaging is rarely needed for the management of hiatal hernia.

Surgical repair of sliding hiatal hernia is often performed laparoscopically, and fundoplication is often performed to control gastroesophageal reflux. Surgical repair is especially important in cases of paraesophageal hernia given the risks of gastric volvulus and colonic herniation. In paraesophageal hernia repair, the herniated viscera are reduced into the abdomen, the hernia sack is excised, and the crura of the esophageal hiatus are tightened.[57]

Diaphragmatic Eventration

Diaphragmatic eventration is a condition in which all or a portion of the diaphragm is abnormally elevated. Eventration can occur because of a paucity of muscle fibers leaving only fibrous tissue, pleura, and peritoneum or because of focal dyskinesia within all or a portion of the diaphragm.[58] Eventration may be congenital or acquired because of muscle infarct or phrenic nerve dysfunction.[58] It has been described in association with poliomyelitis, herpes zoster, diphtheria, lead poisoning, and infantile cortical hyperostosis. In both congenital and acquired causes of diaphragmatic eventration, the weakened or thinned portion of diaphragm bulges superiorly into the chest cavity. Partial diaphragmatic eventration most frequently occurs in the anteromedial right hemidiaphragm and usually contains the liver.[59] Complete eventration occurs more frequently on the left and is more common in males.[1]

Partial diaphragmatic eventration is most commonly encountered as an incidental finding on chest radiograph (Fig. 13.29). The most common appearance of partial diaphragmatic eventration is a focal bulge within the anteromedial right hemidiaphragm. Further imaging with US, CT, or MRI may be sought in symptomatic patients and may visualize a thin sheet overlying an area of scalloping.[1,58] It is often not possible to differentiate

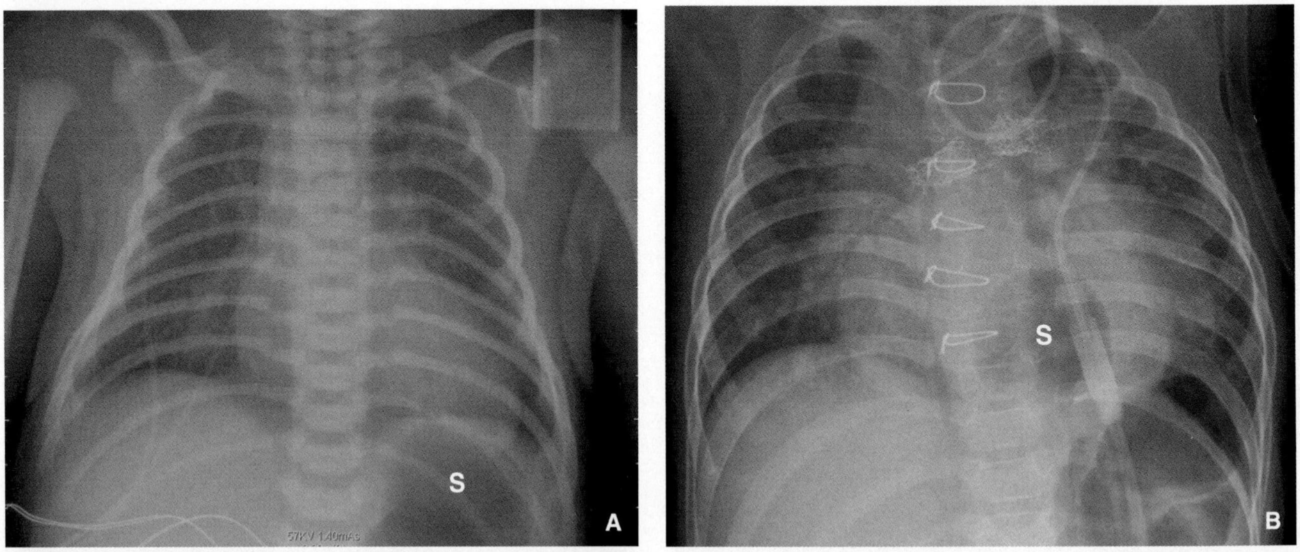

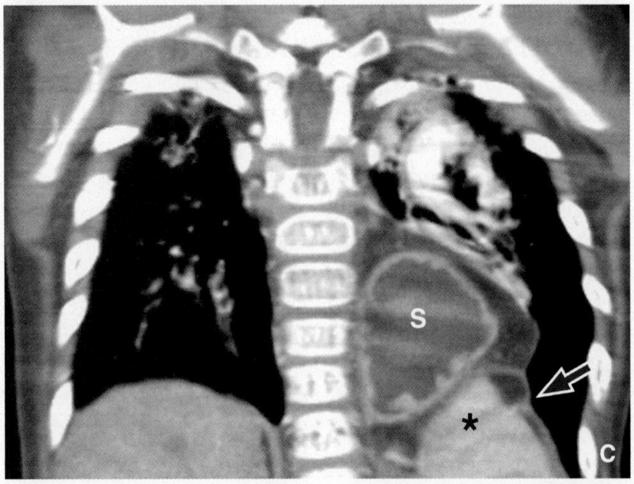

FIGURE 13.26 **A 2-year-old baby boy who underwent a Norwood procedure for a hypoplastic left heart syndrome.** **A:** Initial chest radiograph as a newborn shows intact diaphragm. The gastric bubble (*S*) is clearly visualized in the left upper abdomen. **B:** Chest radiograph obtained at 2 years of age at the time of the Fontan operation shows an interval development of lucency in the left retrocardiac region corresponding to a herniated stomach (*S*). **C:** Coronal enhanced CT image of the posterior chest shows interruption of the left hemidiaphragm (*arrow*) with medial herniation of the stomach (*S*) and spleen (*asterisk*) into the left hemithorax.

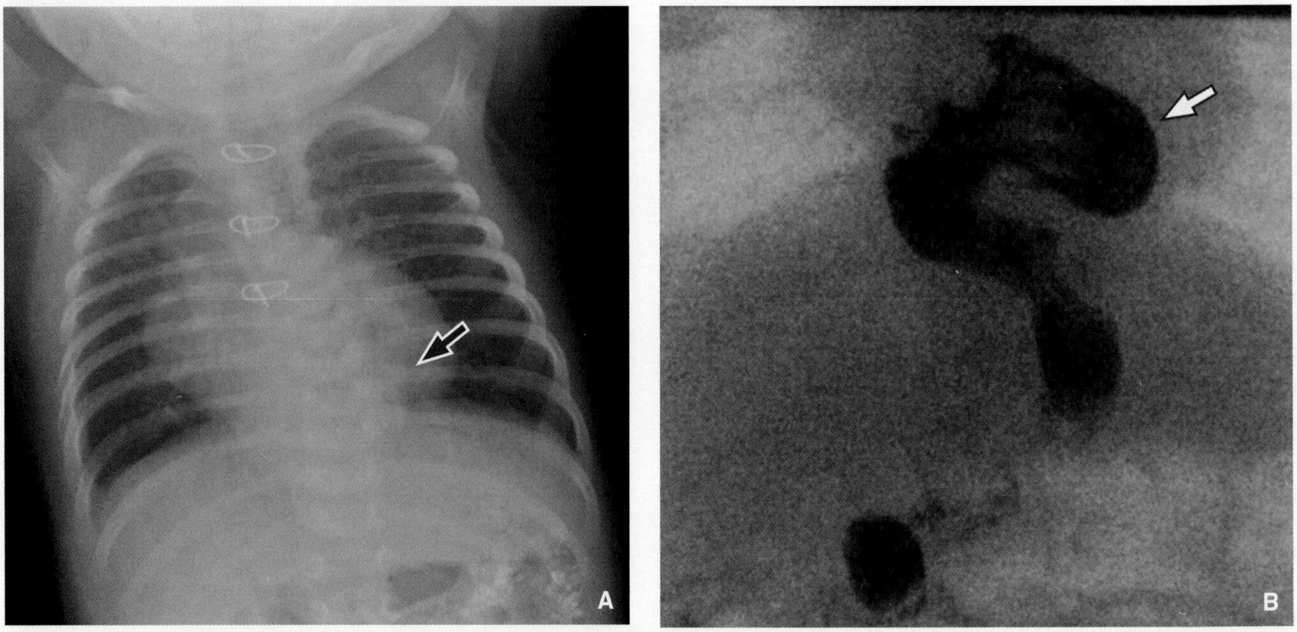

FIGURE 13.27 **A 33-day-old girl with complete atrioventricular canal defect and tetralogy of Fallot with hiatal hernia.** **A:** Frontal chest radiograph demonstrates a paraspinal density (*black arrow*). **B:** Upper gastrointestinal study shows a sliding hiatal hernia (*white arrow*), with the gastroesophageal junction noted to be above the diaphragm.

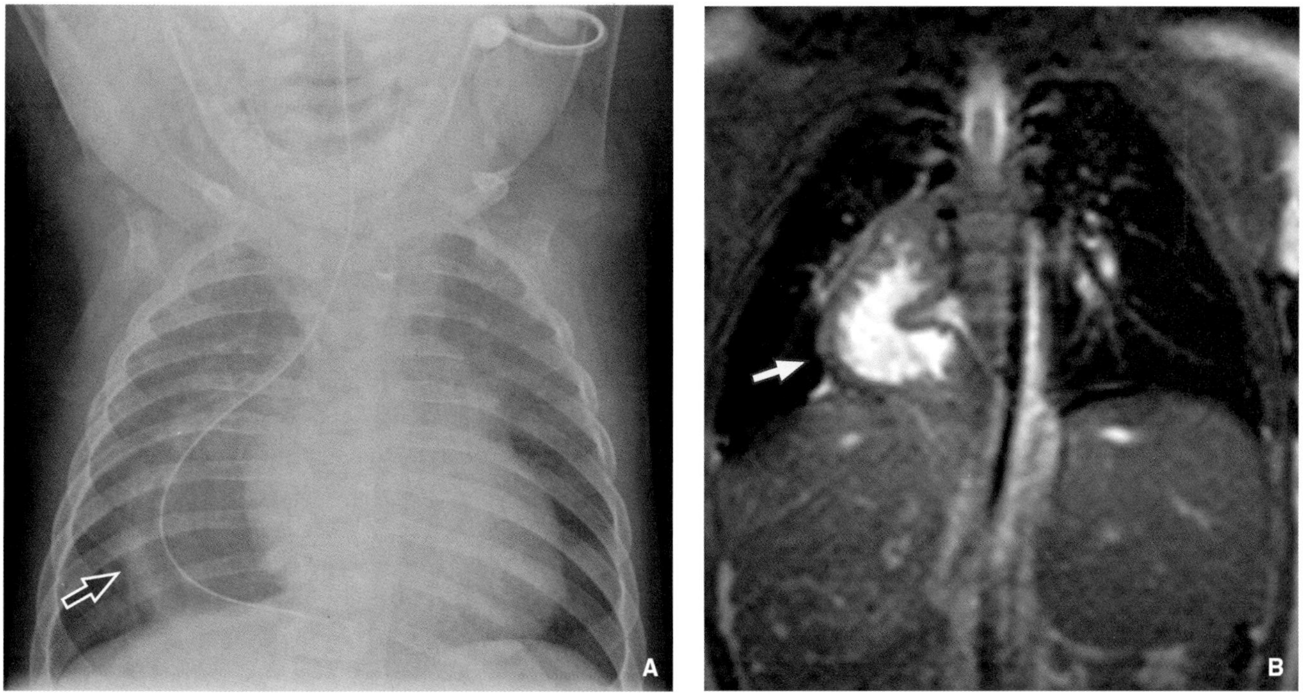

FIGURE 13.28 **An 8-month-old girl with large right-sided hiatal hernia. A:** Frontal chest radiograph demonstrates a large air-filled hiatal hernia (*black arrow*) within the right hemithorax containing a nasogastric tube. **B:** Coronal T2-weighted MR image also demonstrates the large hiatal hernia (*white arrow*) within the right hemithorax.

between partial eventration and CDH with a sac on radiographic studies or on gross pathologic inspection as both are lined with a thin membrane.[1,23] Complete eventration results in an elevated hemidiaphragm on chest radiography. Imaging with US, CT, and/or MRI demonstrate a thinned nonmotile diaphragm. It is often impossible to radiographically differentiate complete eventration from diaphragmatic paralysis, as both conditions have identical imaging findings.[1]

Partial eventration is usually asymptomatic and requires no follow-up or treatment. Symptomatic partial eventration and symptomatic complete eventration can be treated with plication or phrenic nerve stimulation.[8]

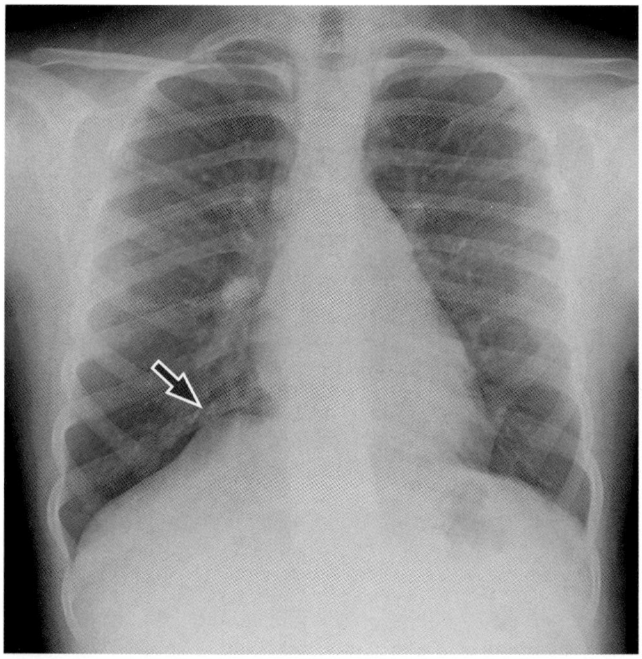

FIGURE 13.29 **An 8-year-old girl with diaphragmatic eventration.** Frontal chest radiograph shows incidentally noted focal eventration (*arrow*) of the right hemidiaphragm.

Duplication of the Diaphragm (Accessory Diaphragm)

Duplication of the diaphragm is a very rare congenital condition in which an accessory fibromuscular membrane parallels the diaphragm. The accessory diaphragm has a serosal lining and is located superior to the diaphragm, fusing with the chest wall posterosuperiorly and the diaphragm anteriorly, leaving an opening (or central hiatus) medially.[1] The duplicated diaphragm is almost exclusively found on the right side and can be associated with lobar agenesis–aplasia complex, extralobar pulmonary sequestration, and unilateral single pulmonary vein.[60,61] This anomaly is theorized to occur as a result of asynchrony between the caudal migration of the septum transversum and the bronchial system.[60,62] Vessels and bronchial structures passing through the central hiatus may become entrapped, leading to respiratory distress in affected patients.

The imaging appearance depends on the degree of air trapping caused at the level of the central hiatus. If the central hiatus is narrow, the lung interposed between the accessory diaphragm and the true diaphragm becomes trapped and nonaerated. This leads to a mass-like appearance on chest radiographs and CT. If the central hiatus

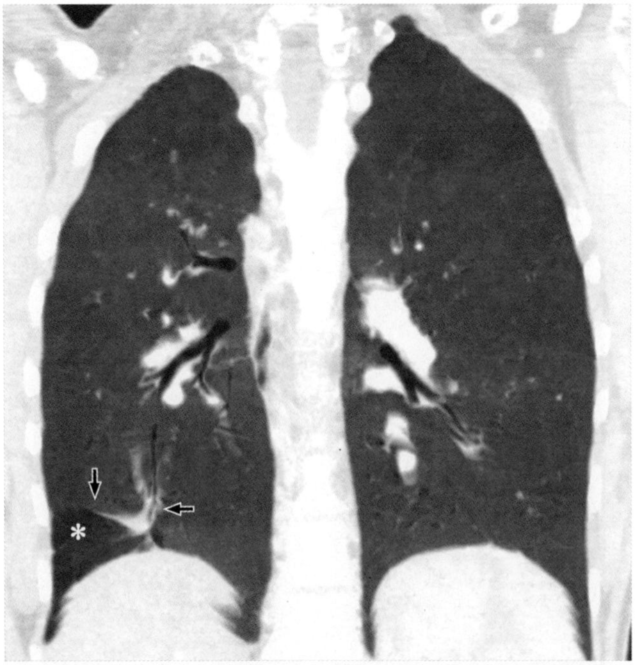

FIGURE 13.30 **A 14-year-old boy with hypogenetic lung syndrome and duplicated diaphragm.** Coronal lung window CT image using minimal intensity projection technique shows an oblique thin linear density in the right pulmonary base touching the right diaphragmatic dome corresponding to a duplicated hemidiaphragm (*vertical arrow*). Lucency in the lung lateral to the duplicated diaphragm indicates air trapping (*asterisk*). There is a bronchus crossing the duplicated diaphragm (*horizontal arrow*).

is large and the lung is not trapped, the accessory diaphragm appears as a crescentic band superior to the diaphragm (Fig. 13.30). CT often demonstrates crowding of the pulmonary vessels and bronchi as they pass medial to the central hiatus, and there may be differential aeration between the lung superior and inferior to the accessory diaphragm.[60,61]

TABLE 13.2 Pediatric Primary Tumors of the Diaphragm

Malignant Diaphragmatic Tumors
Rhabdomyosarcoma
Undifferentiated sarcoma
Extraosseous Ewing sarcoma
Primary germ cell tumor
Benign Diaphragmatic Tumors
Neurofibroma
Lipoma
Myofibroblastic tumor
Hemangioma

Management of the duplicated diaphragm is usually conservative. Surgical resection can be performed in affected patients with substantial dyspnea.[60]

Malignant and Benign Neoplasms of the Diaphragm

Primary malignant tumors of the diaphragm are very rare in children, with only 41 cases reported in the literature between 1968 and 2005[12] (Table 13.2). Seventy-eight percent of primary pediatric diaphragmatic tumors are malignant, most commonly rhabdomyosarcoma.[12,63] Other malignant tumors include undifferentiated sarcoma, extraosseous Ewing sarcoma, and primary germ cell tumor (Fig. 13.31).[13,63] Benign diaphragmatic neoplasms include neurofibromas, lipomas, myofibroblastic tumors, and hemangiomas. Benign cystic lesions of the diaphragm include bronchogenic cysts, hydatid cysts, and mesothelial cysts (Fig. 13.32).[1,64]

Primary tumors of the diaphragm have an equal incidence in males and females and occur with equal frequency on the right and left.[12] Affected patients more frequently complain of "chest-associated symptoms" than "abdomen-associated symptoms."[12] Secondary involvement of the diaphragm from an adjacent tumor or metastasis may also occur (Fig. 13.33).[1]

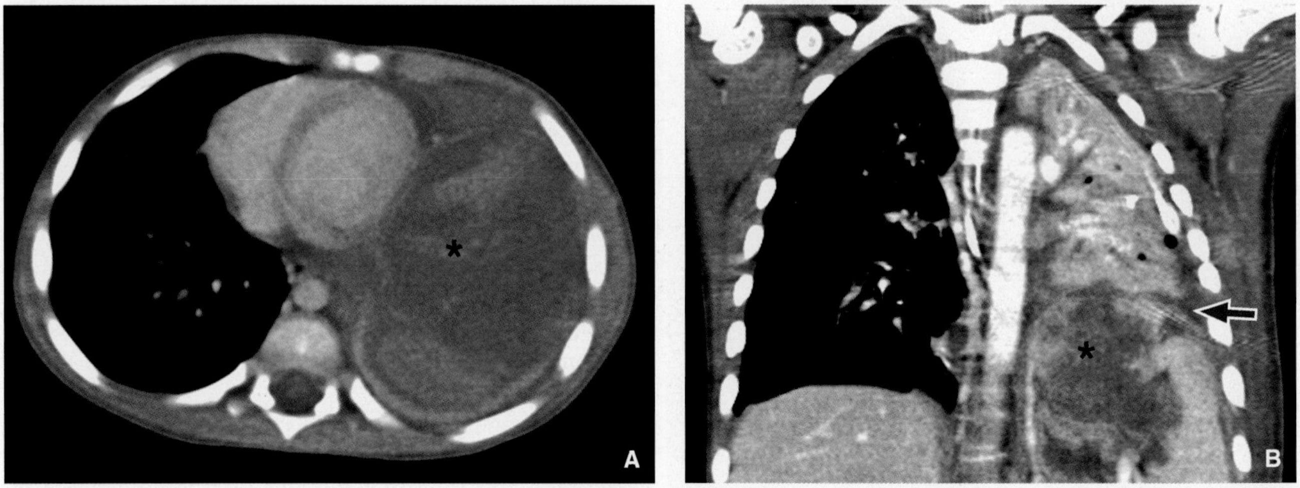

FIGURE 13.31 **A 4-year-old boy with a 2-month history of worsening dyspnea and chest pain. A:** Axial enhanced CT image shows a large solid heterogeneous mass (*asterisk*) occupying most of the left hemithorax. **B:** Coronal enhanced CT image obtained after debulking of tumor demonstrates more clearly the diaphragmatic origin (*arrow*) of the histologically proven residual germ cell tumor (*asterisk*).

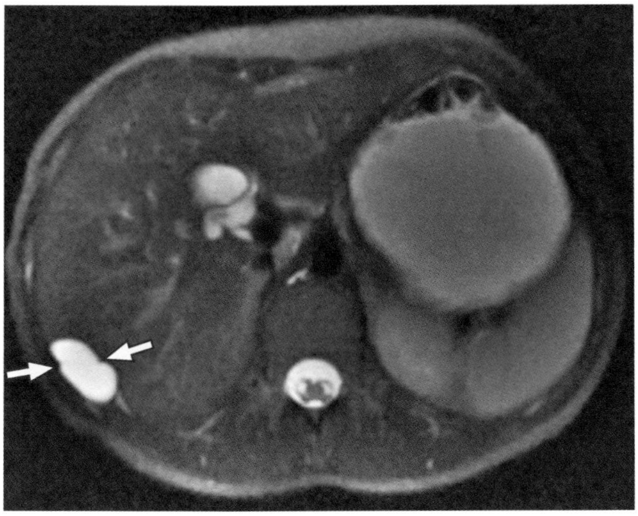

FIGURE 13.32 **A 14-year-old girl with incidentally detected diaphragmatic mesothelial cyst.** Axial T2-weighted MR image shows a bilobed hyperintense lesion (*arrows*) between the diaphragm and right lobe of the liver.

The major challenge when imaging diaphragmatic tumors is identifying that they originate from the diaphragm. Multimodality imaging is often required, including radiography, US, CT, and MRI. Even when utilizing a multimodality approach, mischaracterization is common, with one series reporting that only 33% of pediatric diaphragmatic tumors were correctly identified as originating from the diaphragm.[12] Identification of a claw sign, attention to organ displacement, and recognition of obtuse margins with the body wall are helpful in proper diagnosis and characterization of these lesions.[1,13]

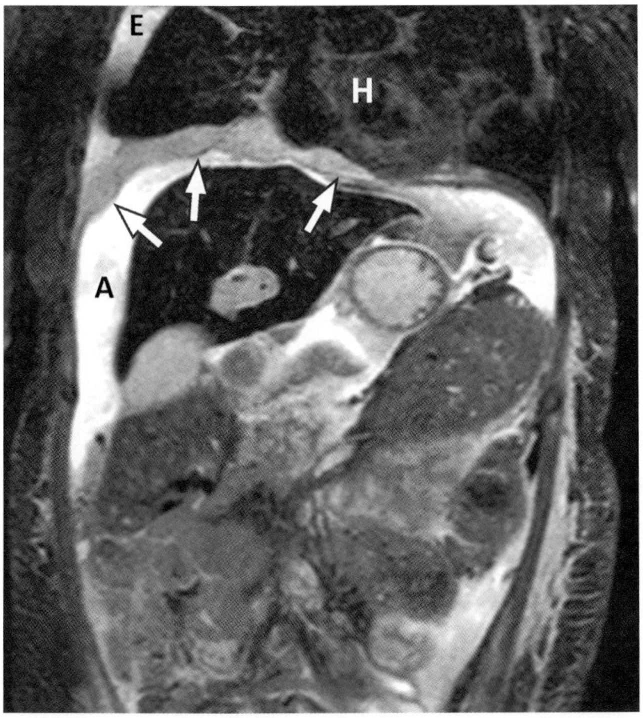

FIGURE 13.33 **A 9-year-old girl with a metastatic retroperitoneal rhabdomyosarcoma involvement of the diaphragm.** Coronal FSE T2-weighted MR image shows thickening and nodularity of the diaphragm (*arrows*) crossing the midline under the heart (*H*). Ascites (*A*) and a right pleural effusion (*E*) are also present.

Management and treatment of malignant diaphragmatic tumors follow the same principles as all malignant tumors. After biopsy and staging, treatment is tailored to the specific histopathology and extent of disease. Treatment usually consists of surgical resection and chemotherapy, often with the addition of radiation therapy.[13] Chemosensitive germ cell tumors may only require chemotherapy.[13]

Traumatic Disorders of the Diaphragm

Traumatic Diaphragmatic Rupture

Traumatic diaphragmatic rupture is very rare in children. In a large retrospective review of 20,500 patients admitted to a large pediatric trauma center, only 0.07% had confirmed traumatic diaphragmatic rupture.[11] Rupture can occur as a result of either blunt or penetrating trauma. Diaphragmatic rupture is most often associated with several other injuries, including liver, spleen, and renal laceration, osseous fracture, major vessel tear, bowel perforation, and/or closed head injury.[11] Isolated diaphragmatic injury can occur and is encountered more frequently in children than in adults.[65] Studies have shown traumatic diaphragmatic rupture to be more common on the left, with the liver thought to shield the right hemidiaphragm from injury,[1,65] though others have found a similar incidence of diaphragmatic rupture on the right and left sides.[11] If the diagnosis is delayed, life-threatening complications from bowel herniation and strangulation can occur.[1]

Chest radiographs have findings suggestive of traumatic diaphragmatic rupture in the majority of cases,[66] though radiographs alone are often not diagnostic.[67] Suggestive findings on chest radiographs include unilateral hemidiaphragm elevation, distortion of the smooth diaphragmatic margin, and contralateral mediastinal shift.[1] Specific findings on chest radiograph include visualization of an intrathoracic bowel loop passing through a diaphragmatic defect (aka "collar sign") or a nasogastric tube passing through the diaphragm.[1,68] CT has a reported sensitivity and specificity of 78% and 100% in the detection of left-sided traumatic diaphragmatic rupture and 50% and 100% in the detection of right-sided traumatic diaphragmatic rupture.[69] Findings on CT may include irregularity and thickening of the diaphragmatic leaflet, herniated abdominal organs, and/or the "CT collar sign" (Figs. 13.34 and 13.35).[68]

Traumatic diaphragmatic rupture is treated surgically. If the defect is small, it is treated with sutures, but, if the defect is larger, mesh may be needed.

Traumatic Diaphragmatic Paralysis

Traumatic diaphragmatic paralysis occurs because of phrenic nerve injury. The most common causes of phrenic nerve injury in the child are birth trauma and

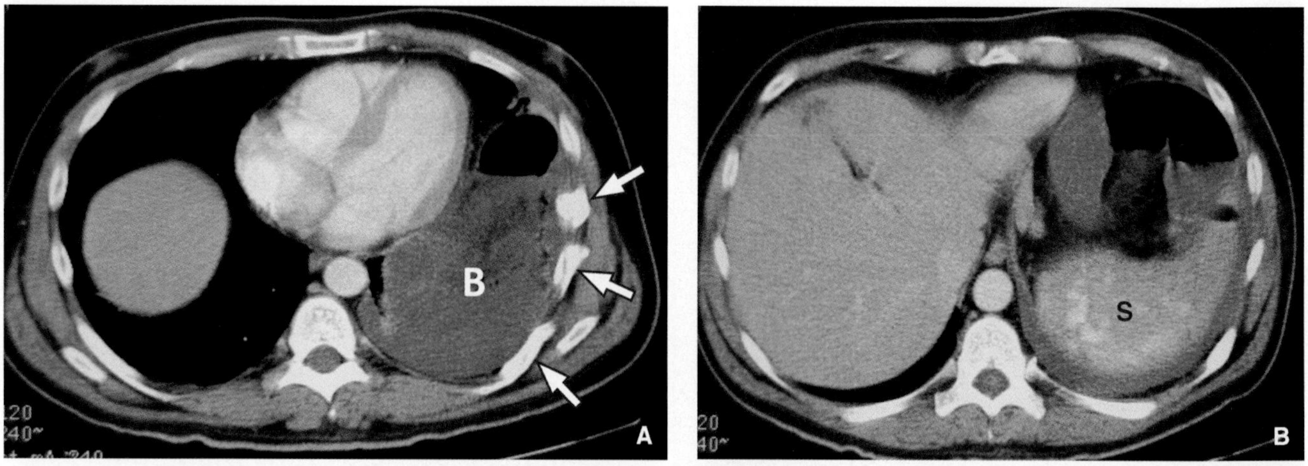

FIGURE 13.34 **Delayed presentation of diaphragmatic rupture in a 17-year-old boy with a history of falling from a ladder several years earlier and who presented with worsening chest pain. A and B:** Axial enhanced CT images show bowel (*B*) and the stomach (*S*) herniated into the left hemithorax through a traumatic defect in the diaphragm. Focal cortical thickening and deformity (*arrows*) of three consecutive ribs on the left are also seen, compatible with healed fractures likely obtained at the time of injury.

thoracotomy,[6] with more rare causes including Lyme disease, West Nile virus, and tumors of the mediastinum or neck.[1,70] The reported prevalence of diaphragmatic paralysis in neonates is 0.03% to 0.5%, and the prevalence following thoracic surgery is between 0.5% and 1.5%.[71] Infants often have more significant respiratory symptoms from diaphragmatic paralysis than adults because their intercostal muscles are weaker, making their ventilation almost entirely dependent on the diaphragm and their mediastinum are more mobile.[72] Differences in anatomy also make the diaphragm function less efficiently in the infant, including the circular shape of the thorax, horizontal orientation of the ribs, and greater compliance of the ribs.[72] Diaphragmatic paralysis should be considered when there is unexplained difficulty weaning from mechanical ventilation, unexplained respiratory distress, asymmetric chest and epigastrium movement with breathing, recurrent pneumonia, recurrent lung collapse, and/or tachypnea.[6,73]

The imaging evaluation of traumatic diaphragmatic paralysis often begins with chest radiographs, which may demonstrate

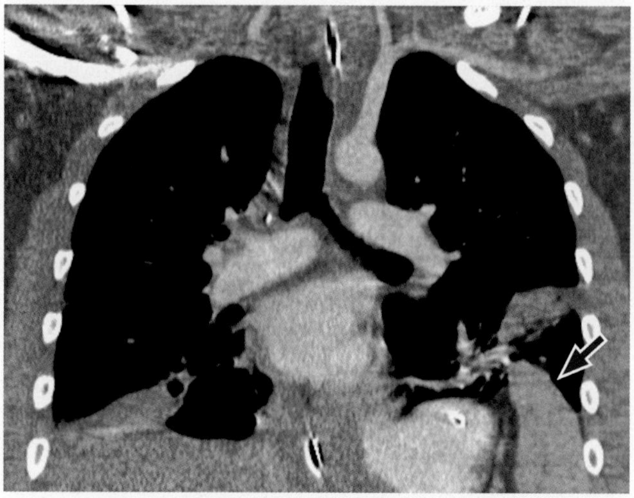

FIGURE 13.35 **A 19-year-old male with left lower chest pain after motor vehicle accident.** Coronal enhanced CT image shows left-sided traumatic diaphragmatic rupture with a herniated spleen (*arrow*) in the left lower hemithorax.

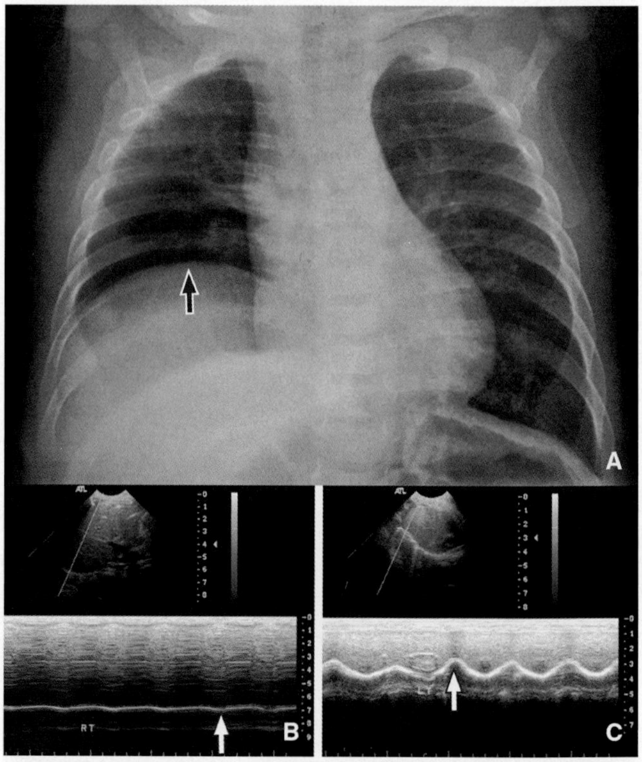

FIGURE 13.36 **A 2-year-old girl with perinatal brachial plexus injury. A:** Frontal chest radiograph shows marked elevation of the right hemidiaphragm (*arrow*). **B:** Ultrasound image of the right hemidiaphragm using M-mode demonstrates a flat diaphragmatic curve (*arrow*) indicating paralysis. **C:** Ultrasound image of the normal left hemidiaphragm of the same patient shows normal excursion (*arrow*) of the hemidiaphragm.

persistent elevation of a hemidiaphragm (Fig. 13.36A). Historically, fluoroscopy was the gold standard for real-time evaluation of diaphragmatic movement, but US has largely supplanted its use because of its portability, lack of ionizing radiation, and ability to visualize the entire diaphragm.[5,6] The use of M-mode US allows for accurate quantification of diaphragmatic movement, with the normal diaphragm moving >4 mm during inspiration and a difference of <50% between each hemidiaphragm (Fig. 13.36B).[5,6] Specialized MR imaging techniques that utilize fast GRE pulse sequences[16] and steady-state acquisition sequences (FIESTA; GE Medical Systems)[17] may also be used to evaluate diaphragmatic motion.

Initial treatment of diaphragmatic paralysis is usually supportive. If function does not return, affected patients often require plication. Plication has been shown to reduce complications from prolonged ventilation because it allows for earlier extubation.[73]

References

1. Chavhan GB, et al. Multimodality imaging of the pediatric diaphragm: anatomy and pathologic. *Radiographics.* 2010; 30(7):1797–1817.
2. Bramson RT, Griscom NT, Cleveland RH. Interpretation of chest radiographs in infants with cough and fever. *Radiology.* 2005;236(1):22–29.
3. Suwatanapongched T, et al. Variation in diaphragm position and shape in adults with normal pulmonary. *Chest.* 2003; 123(6):2019–2027.
4. Lee E, Siegel M. Ultrasound evaluation of pediatric chest. In: Allan P, Baxter G, Weston M, eds. *Clinical Ultrasound.* London, UK: Elsevier; 2011.
5. Urvoas E, et al. Diaphragmatic paralysis in children: diagnosis by TM-mode ultrasound. *Pediatr Radiol.* 1994;24(8): 564–568.
6. Epelman M, et al. M-mode sonography of diaphragmatic motion: description of technique and experience in 278 pediatric patients. *Pediatr Radiol.* 2005;35(7):661–667.
7. Taylor GA, Atalabi OM, Estroff JA. Imaging of congenital diaphragmatic hernias. *Pediatr Radiol.* 2009;39(1):1–16.
8. Nason LK, et al. Imaging of the diaphragm: anatomy and function. *Radiographics.* 2012;32(2):E51–E70.
9. Baglaj M, Dorobisz U. Late-presenting congenital diaphragmatic hernia in children: a literature review. *Pediatr Radiol.* 2005;35(5): 478–488.
10. Shackleton KL, Stewart ET, Taylor AJ. Traumatic diaphragmatic injuries: spectrum of radiographic findings. *Radiographics.* 1998;18(1):49–59.
11. Ramos CT, et al. What have we learned about traumatic diaphragmatic hernias in children *J Pediatr Surg.* 2000;35(4): 601–604.
12. Cada M, et al. Approach to diagnosis and treatment of pediatric primary tumors of the diaphragm. *J Pediatr Surg.* 2006;41(10): 1722–1726.
13. Traubici J, et al. Primary germ cell tumor of the diaphragm. *J Pediatr Surg.* 2004;39(10):1578–1580.
14. Hernanz-Schulman M, et al. Pause and pulse: ten steps that help manage radiation dose during pediatric fluoroscopy. *AJR Am J Roentgenol.* 2011;197(2):475–481.
15. Gierada DS, et al. Fast gradient echo magnetic resonance imaging of the normal diaphragm. *J Thorac Imaging.* 1997;12(1):70–74.
16. Gierada DS, et al. Diaphragmatic motion: fast gradient-recalled-echo MR imaging in healthy subjects. *Radiology.* 1995; 194(3):879–884.
17. Kiryu S, et al. Quantitative analysis of the velocity and synchronicity of diaphragmatic motion. *Magn Reson Imaging.* 2006;24(10):1325–1332.
18. Panicek DM, et al. The diaphragm: anatomic, pathologic, and radiologic considerations. *Radiographics.* 1988;8(3):385–425.
19. Gale ME. Anterior diaphragm: variations in the CT appearance. *Radiology.* 1986;161(3):635–639.
20. Brengle M, Cohen MD, Katz B. Normal appearance and size of the diaphragmatic crura in children: CT evaluation. *Pediatr Radiol.* 1996;26(11):811–814.
21. Keijzer R, Puri P. Congenital diaphragmatic hernia. *Semin Pediatr Surg.* 2010;19(3):180–185.
22. Skari H, et al. Congenital diaphragmatic hernia: a meta-analysis of mortality factors. *J Pediatr Surg.* 2000;35(8):1187–1197.
23. Ackerman KG, et al. Congenital diaphragmatic defects: proposal for a new classification based on observations in 234 patients. *Pediatr Dev Pathol.* 2012;15(4):265–274.
24. Clugston RD, et al. Teratogen-induced, dietary and genetic models of congenital diaphragmatic hernia share a common mechanism of pathogenesis. *Am J Pathol.* 2006;169(5):1541–1549.
25. Bielinska M, et al. Molecular genetics of congenital diaphragmatic defects. *Ann Med.* 2007;39(4):261–274.
26. Coughlin MA, et al. Prenatally diagnosed severe CDH: mortality and morbidity remain high. *J Pediatr Surg.* 2016;51(7): 1091–1095.
27. Mesas Burgos C, et al. Differences in outcomes in prenatally diagnosed congenital diaphragmatic hernia compared to postnatal detection: a single-center experience. *Fetal Diagn Ther.* 2016; 39(4):241–247.
28. Ruano R, et al. Fetal lung volume and quantification of liver herniation by magnetic resonance imaging in isolated congenital diaphragmatic hernia. *Ultrasound Obstet Gynecol.* 2014;43(6): 662–669.
29. Bebbington M, et al. Comparison of ultrasound and magnetic resonance imaging parameters in predicting survival in isolated left-sided congenital diaphragmatic hernia. *Ultrasound Obstet Gynecol.* 2014;43(6):670–674.
30. Benachi A, et al. Advances in prenatal diagnosis of congenital diaphragmatic hernia. *Semin Fetal Neonatal Med.* 2014;19(6): 331–337.
31. Sakurai M, et al. Congenital diaphragmatic hernia in neonates: variations in umbilical catheter and enteric tube position. *Radiology.* 2000;216(1):112–116.
32. Holt PD, et al. Newborns with diaphragmatic hernia: initial chest radiography does not have a role in predicting clinical outcome. *Pediatr Radiol.* 2004;34(6):462–464.
33. Downard CD, et al. Analysis of an improved survival rate for congenital diaphragmatic hernia. *J Pediatr Surg.* 2003;38(5): 729–732.
34. Frenckner B, et al. Improved results in patients who have congenital diaphragmatic hernia using preoperative stabilization, extracorporeal membrane oxygenation, and delayed surgery. *J Pediatr Surg.* 1997;32(8):1185–1189.
35. Boloker J, et al. Congenital diaphragmatic hernia in 120 infants treated consecutively with permissive hypercapnea/spontaneous respiration/elective repair. *J Pediatr Surg.* 2002;37(3):357–366.

36. Brown RA, Bosenberg AT. Evolving management of congenital diaphragmatic hernia. *Paediatr Anaesth.* 2007;17(8):713–719.
37. Chiu PP, Langer JC. Surgical conditions of the diaphragm: posterior diaphragmatic hernias in infants. *Thorac Surg Clin.* 2009;19(4):451–461.
38. Bagolan P, Morini F. Long-term follow up of infants with congenital diaphragmatic hernia. *Semin Pediatr Surg.* 2007;16(2):134–144.
39. Brant-Zawadzki PB, et al. The split abdominal wall muscle flap repair for large congenital diaphragmatic hernias on extracorporeal membrane oxygenation. *J Pediatr Surg.* 2007;42(6):1047–1050; discussion 1051.
40. Rowe DH, Stolar CJ. Recurrent diaphragmatic hernia. *Semin Pediatr Surg.* 2003;12(2):107–109.
41. Arena F, et al. Long-term functional evaluation of diaphragmatic motility after repair of congenital diaphragmatic hernia. *J Pediatr Surg.* 2005;40(7):1078–1081.
42. Kamata S, et al. Radiographic changes in the diaphragm after repair of congenital diaphragmatic hernia. *J Pediatr Surg.* 2008;43(12):2156–2160.
43. Trachsel D, et al. Long-term pulmonary morbidity in survivors of congenital diaphragmatic hernia. *Pediatr Pulmonol.* 2005;39(5):433–439.
44. Pokorny WJ, McGill CW, Harberg FJ. Morgagni hernias during infancy: presentation and associated anomalies. *J Pediatr Surg.* 1984;19(4):394–397.
45. Robertson DJ, Harmon CM, Goldberg S. Right congenital diaphragmatic hernia associated with fusion of the liver and the lung. *J Pediatr Surg.* 2006;41(6):e9–e10.
46. Slovis TL, et al. Hepatic pulmonary fusion in neonates. *AJR Am J Roentgenol.* 2000;174(1):229–233.
47. Katz S, et al. Fibrous fusion between the liver and the lung: an unusual complication of right congenital diaphragmatic hernia. *J Pediatr Surg.* 1998;33(5):766–767.
48. Keller RL, et al. MR imaging of hepatic pulmonary fusion in neonates. *AJR Am J Roentgenol.* 2003;180(2):438–440.
49. Khatwa U, Lee EY. Multidetector computed tomography evaluation of secondary hepatopulmonary fusion in a neonate. *Clin Imaging.* 2010;34(3):234–238.
50. Mallick MS, Alqahtani A. Laparoscopic-assisted repair of Morgagni hernia in children. *J Pediatr Surg.* 2009;44(8):1621–1624.
51. Kitano Y, Lally KP, Lally PA. Late-presenting congenital diaphragmatic hernia. *J Pediatr Surg.* 2005;40(12):1839–1843.
52. Elhalaby EA, Abo Sikeena MH. Delayed presentation of congenital diaphragmatic hernia. *Pediatr Surg Int.* 2002;18(5–6):480–485.
53. Newman BM, et al. Presentation of congenital diaphragmatic hernia past the neonatal period. *Arch Surg.* 1986;121(7):813–816.
54. Numanoglu A, et al. Delayed presentation of congenital diaphragmatic hernia. *S Afr J Surg.* 1997;35(2):74–76.
55. Strunk T, et al. Late-onset right-sided diaphragmatic hernia in neonates—case report and review of the literature. *Eur J Pediatr.* 2007;166(6):521–526.
56. Imamoglu M, et al. Congenital paraesophageal hiatal hernia: pitfalls in the diagnosis and treatment. *J Pediatr Surg.* 2005;40(7):1128–1133.
57. Al-Salem AH. Congenital paraesophageal hernia in infancy and childhood. *Saudi Med J.* 2000;21(2):164–167.
58. Yeh HC, Halton KP, Gray CE. Anatomic variations and abnormalities in the diaphragm seen with US. *Radiographics.* 1990;10(6):1019–1030.
59. Eren S, Ceviz N, Alper F. Congenital diaphragmatic eventration as a cause of anterior mediastinal mass in the children: imaging modalities and literature review. *Eur J Radiol.* 2004;51(1):85–90.
60. Hidalgo A, Franquet T, Gimenez A. 16-MDCT and MR angiography of accessory diaphragm. *AJR Am J Roentgenol.* 2006;187(1):149–152.
61. Mata JM, Caceres J. The dysmorphic lung: imaging findings. *Eur Radiol.* 1996;6(4):403–414.
62. Pober BR. Overview of epidemiology, genetics, birth defects, and chromosome abnormalities associated with CDH. *Am J Med Genet C Semin Med Genet.* 2007;145c(2):158–171.
63. Raney RB, et al. Soft-tissue sarcomas of the diaphragm: a report from the Intergroup Rhabdomyosarcoma Study Group from 1972 to 1997. *J Pediatr Hematol Oncol.* 2000;22(6):510–514.
64. Akinci D, et al. Diaphragmatic mesothelial cysts in children: radiologic findings and percutaneous ethanol sclerotherapy. *AJR Am J Roentgenol.* 2005;185(4):873–877.
65. Shehata SM, Shabaan BS. Diaphragmatic injuries in children after blunt abdominal trauma. *J Pediatr Surg.* 2006;41(10):1727–1731.
66. Koplewitz BZ, et al. Traumatic diaphragmatic injuries in infants and children: imaging findings. *Pediatr Radiol.* 2000;30(7):471–479.
67. Iochum S, et al. Imaging of diaphragmatic injury: a diagnostic challenge *Radiographics.* 2002;22(Spec No):S103–S116; discussion S116–S118.
68. Shanmuganathan K, et al. Imaging of diaphragmatic injuries. *J Thorac Imaging.* 2000;15(2):104–111.
69. Killeen KL, Mirvis SE, Shanmuganathan K. Helical CT of diaphragmatic rupture caused by blunt trauma. *AJR Am J Roentgenol.* 1999;173(6):1611–1616.
70. Betensley AD, et al. Bilateral diaphragmatic paralysis and related respiratory complications in a patient with West Nile virus infection. *Thorax.* 2004;59(3):268–269.
71. Schumpelick V, et al. Surgical embryology and anatomy of the diaphragm with surgical applications. *Surg Clin North Am.* 2000;80(1):213–239, xi.
72. Mok Q, et al. Phrenic nerve injury in infants and children undergoing cardiac surgery. *Br Heart J.* 1991;65(5):287–292.
73. de Leeuw M, et al. Impact of diaphragmatic paralysis after cardiothoracic surgery in children. *J Thorac Cardiovasc Surg.* 1999;118(3):510–517.

PART III

PEDIATRIC ABDOMINOPELVIC RADIOLOGY

Jonathan R. Dillman

CHAPTER 14

Liver, Bile Ducts, and Gallbladder

Andrew T. Trout • Daniel B. Wallihan • Alexander J. Towbin • Daniel J. Podberesky

INTRODUCTION

Imaging plays a crucial role in the assessment of disorders of the pediatric liver and biliary system. Radiologic studies not only can provide anatomic and morphologic information but can characterize tissues and assess hepatobiliary function. In this chapter, the most commonly employed imaging modalities, including state-of-the-art techniques are reviewed. Disorders of the liver are presented first, followed by disorders of the biliary tree and gallbladder. Normal anatomy of each of these systems is discussed because anatomic understanding is critical for accurate interpretation of imaging findings and effective communication with clinicians. Subsequently, the imaging appearances of common as well as unusual but important hepatobiliary abnormalities in the pediatric population are reviewed.

IMAGING TECHNIQUES

Radiography

Radiography is of little value in the primary assessment of the liver and biliary system. Findings that are visible by radiography (such as right upper quadrant calcification or gas) can suggest an underlying hepatic or biliary abnormality and may require further workup.

Ultrasound

The liver and biliary system are ideally suited for evaluation by ultrasound because of their position in the abdomen, the relative homogeneity of the hepatic parenchyma, and the high contrast between the hepatic parenchyma and biliary and vascular structures. As such, ultrasound is the initial modality of choice in the assessment of most hepatic and biliary abnormalities. Ultrasound provides primarily anatomic information but is ideally suited for the real-time assessment of the hepatic vasculature. Ultrasound elastography, including acoustic radiation force imaging (ARFI), is an emerging technique for noninvasive assessment of liver stiffness (Fig. 14.1).

Computed Tomography and Magnetic Resonance Imaging

Computed tomography (CT) and magnetic resonance imaging (MRI) provide high-resolution anatomic images of the liver and biliary tree. They are commonly employed following identification of an abnormality by ultrasound. In general, MRI is favored over CT in the pediatric population because of the lack of ionizing radiation and because it provides high soft tissue contrast. Additionally, advanced MR techniques, including diffusion-weighted imaging, chemical shift imaging, spectroscopy, elastography, and use of hepatobiliary-specific contrast agents, allow assessment of specific tissue characteristics. However, CT remains of particular value in the acute setting.

Nuclear Medicine

Hepatobiliary scintigraphy with iminodiacetic acid (HIDA) derivatives is the dominant nuclear medicine study employed for the assessment of the liver and biliary systems. HIDA allows dynamic assessment of hepatic function and evaluation of biliary system integrity and function. Today, sulfur colloid imaging is only rarely used to assess the liver in the pediatric population. ^{18}F-fluorodeoxyglucose positron emission tomography (^{18}F-FDG-PET) plays a minor but important role in evaluating primary and secondary liver tumors.

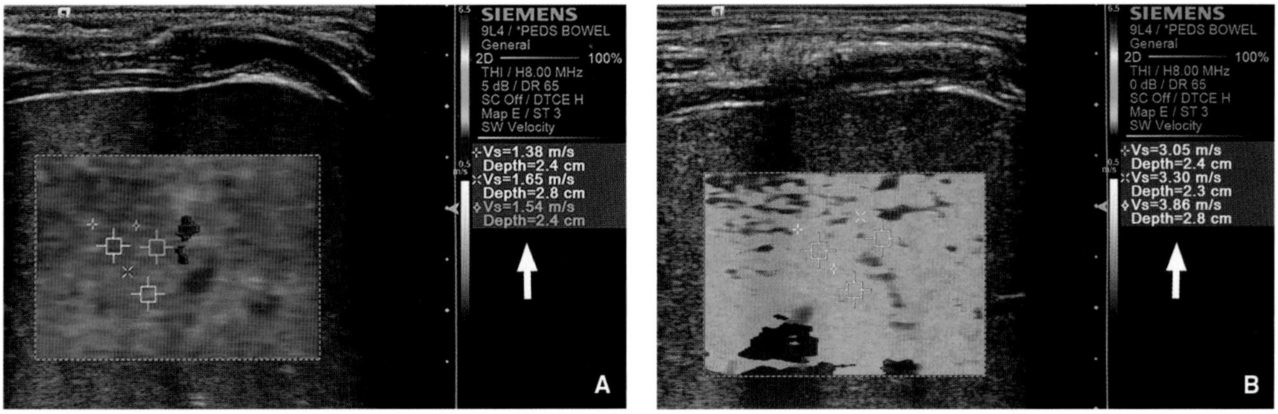

FIGURE 14.1 **Acoustic Radiation Force Imaging (ARFI) of the liver.** ARFI is a noninvasive means of assessing tissue stiffness through measurement of shear wave speed. Color maps (elastograms) show relative differences in tissue stiffness based on shear wave speed. Regions of interest allow quantitation of shear wave speed. **A:** An 8-week-old boy with paucity of intrahepatic bile ducts and Ishak grade 1 hepatic fibrosis. Shear wave speeds (*arrow*) are normal to minimally elevated between 1.38 and 1.65 m/s. **B:** An 8-week-old boy with extrahepatic biliary atresia and Ishak grade 6 hepatic fibrosis. Shear wave speeds (*arrow*) are markedly elevated between 3.05 and 3.86 m/s. (Case courtesy of Jonathan R. Dillman, MD, MSc, Cincinnati Children's Hospital Medical Center, Cincinnati, OH.)

Interventional Diagnostic Imaging

Catheter angiography and percutaneous transhepatic cholangiography are typically employed in children when an abnormality has been identified with noninvasive imaging (e.g., ultrasound or MRI) and additional evaluation is required or intervention is likely to be performed. These techniques are particularly valuable in the management of transplanted livers.

NORMAL ANATOMY

Normal Hepatic Anatomy and Vascular Variants

Knowledge of hepatic segmental anatomy is important to the accurate interpretation of hepatic imaging in the child, as this often guides surgical and therapeutic planning. The liver consists of left and right hepatic lobes, separated by the middle

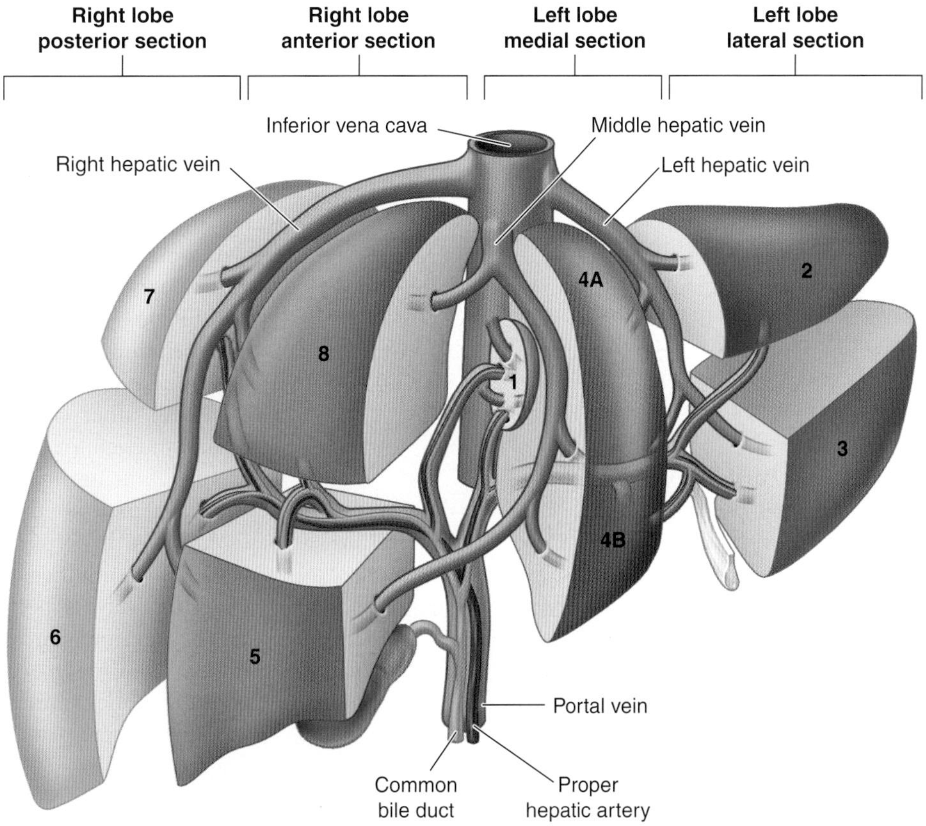

FIGURE 14.2 **Hepatic sectional and segmental anatomy.** Under the Anglo-Saxon system, the liver is divided into four sections by the three hepatic veins (anterior and posterior sections of the right lobe and medial and lateral sections of the left lobe). Under the Couinaud system, the liver is divided into eight segments based on vascular and biliary boundaries. Under this system, the portal vein divides the liver in the horizontal plane and the three hepatic veins divide the liver in the vertical plane.

hepatic vein. The right and left lobes can be divided into a total of four sections or eight segments based on the Anglo-Saxon or Couinaud systems respectively (Fig. 14.2). These divisions are based on typical vascular and biliary boundaries that determine planes of hepatic resection. The most typical and thus the standard pattern of vasculature is as follows:

Portal vein: The main portal vein branches in the porta hepatis into the right and left portal veins, which supply their respective lobes. The right portal vein subsequently branches into anterior and posterior segmental branches.

Hepatic artery: The common hepatic artery arises as a branch of the celiac axis and branches into the gastroduodenal and proper hepatic arteries. In the porta hepatis, the proper hepatic artery branches into the right and left hepatic arteries, which supply their respective lobes.

Hepatic vein: The bulk of the liver is drained to the inferior vena cava (IVC) by the right, middle, and left hepatic veins. Often the middle and left hepatic veins form a common trunk prior to draining into the IVC. The caudate has separate venous drainage via multiple perforating caudate veins to the IVC.

Normal variants are common in all three hepatic vascular systems and are important to recognize and describe in the setting of hepatic disease because of their implications on therapeutic planning. Patterns of variation have been described and classified in detail in the literature.[1–5]

SPECTRUM OF HEPATIC DISORDERS

Congenital and Developmental Anomalies

Preduodenal Portal Vein, Abernethy Malformation, and Other Congenital Portosystemic Shunts

The normal development of the portal vein involves a process of selective involution of a network of interconnections between paired embryonic vitelline veins (Fig. 14.3). This process results in the development of a portal vein that receives splanchnic inflow and courses posterior to the second portion of the duodenum to enter the liver hilum. When this process occurs abnormally, the position and drainage of the portal vein can become abnormal. The most extensively described of these portal venous developmental anomalies are the preduodenal portal vein and Abernethy malformation.

Preduodenal Portal Vein

A preduodenal portal vein receives normal inflow from the splenic vein (SV) and superior mesenteric vein (SMV). Instead of taking its normal course posterior to the second portion of the duodenum, the preduodenal portal vein passes anterior to the second portion of the duodenum. The radiologic and clinical significance of the preduodenal portal vein mostly relates not to the vein itself but to associated developmental anomalies. These include abnormal situs (including heterotaxy syndromes), intestinal malrotation, duodenal webs, biliary atresia, preduodenal common bile duct (CBD), annular pancreas, and congenital heart disease.[6,7] An association has also been described with Down syndrome.[8] Preduodenal portal veins can be diagnosed pre- or postnatally with the majority diagnosed in childhood.[6] Partial duodenal obstruction is a possible clinical presentation. Importantly, the observed obstruction commonly relates to an associated anomaly (e.g., duodenal web) and not to the abnormally positioned portal vein.[7]

The abnormally positioned preduodenal portal vein can be identified by ultrasound, CT, or MRI based on its location relative to the second portion of the duodenum (Fig. 14.4). The aberrant portal vein may cause an impression on the anterior surface of the duodenum that is visible on a fluoroscopic upper GI examination, but sequelae of partial duodenal obstruction related to associated anomalies, such as duodenal webs, are more commonly observed manifesting as dilatation of the first portion of the duodenum (the so-called megacap).[7]

Abernethy Malformation and Other Congenital Portosystemic Shunts

The term "Abernethy malformation" is often used to describe any extrahepatic portosystemic shunt with an associated portal venous anomaly. Congenital extrahepatic portosystemic shunts (CEPS) is a more appropriate term for this broader group, which can be classified as detailed in Table 14.1.[9] True Abernethy malformations relate to shunts between the splanchnic or portal venous system and the systemic venous system that arise during abnormal vitelline venous development. Shunts typically develop to the IVC, azygos vein, or right atrium.[10,11] Although the effect is the same, extrahepatic portosystemic shunts via the renal and iliac veins are likely of a distinct origin.[11]

The effect of CEPS is to allow compounds that would normally be metabolized by the liver to enter the systemic system. Affected pediatric patients are variably symptomatic with clinical presentations ranging from no symptoms to mild hepatic dysfunction, hyperammonemia/hepatic encephalopathy, pulmonary hypertension, and/or hepatopulmonary syndrome.[10] CEPS may be identified prenatally but can also go undiagnosed into adulthood.

CEPS may exist in coincidence with other vascular anomalies, including the spectrum of IVC anomalies. Additionally, the type I Abernethy malformations are known to be associated with other congenital anomalies of the heart, spleen, biliary and genitourinary systems.[10,12] Aberrations in hepatic vascular flow are known to predispose to the development of focal hepatic abnormalities; regenerative nodules, nodular regenerative hyperplasia, focal nodular hyperplasia (FNH), hepatic adenoma, hepatocellular carcinoma (HCC), and hepatoblastoma have all been described in patients with CEPS.[10,12,13]

The key imaging finding in extrahepatic portosystemic shunts is an absent or diminutive portal vein at the level of the hepatic hilum with a venous collateral connecting the splanchnic/portal venous and system venous systems (Fig. 14.5). There is often associated enlargement of the hepatic artery. These findings can be identified by ultrasound,

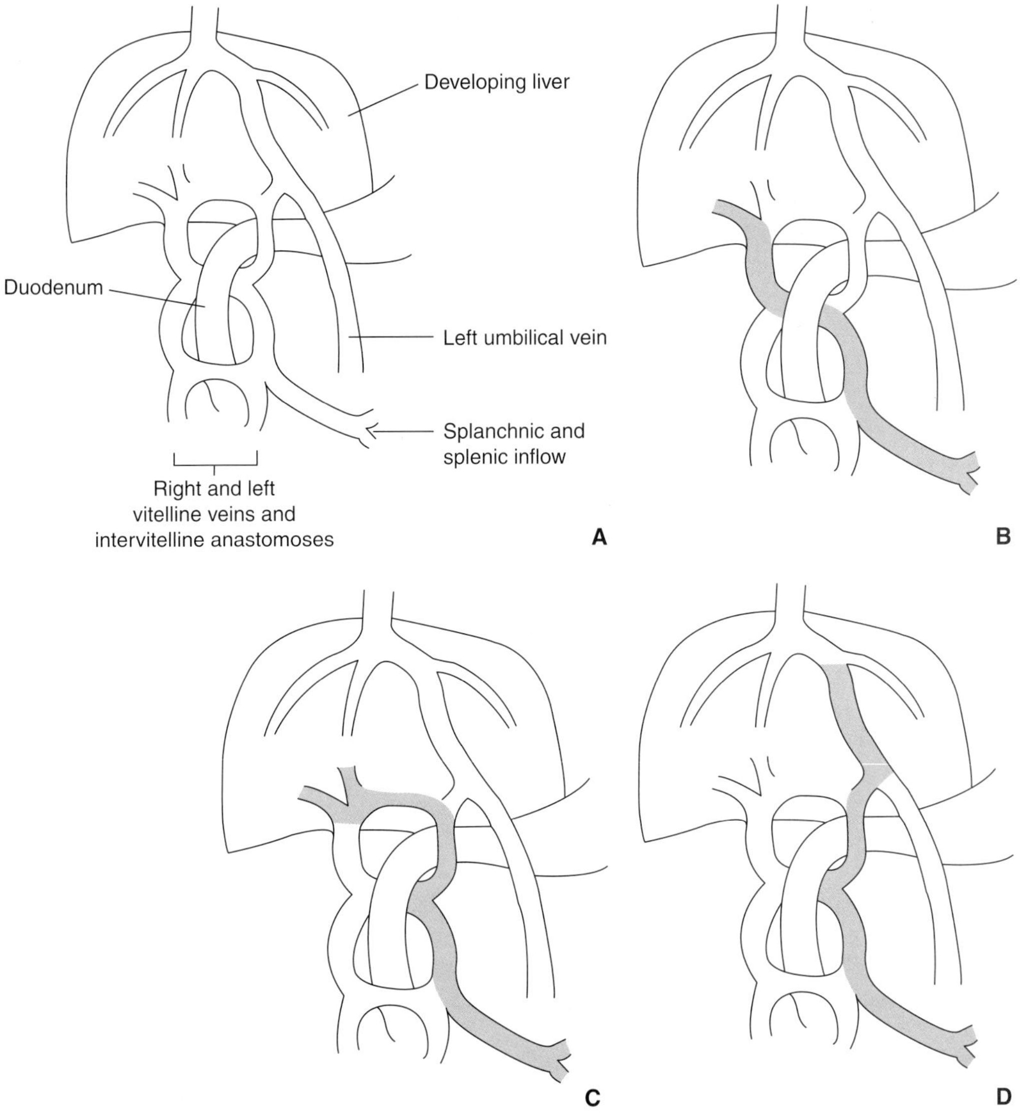

FIGURE 14.3 **Portal vein development. A:** Development of the portal vein is based on selective involution of interconnections of the embryonic vitelline veins. **B:** With normal development, the portal vein receives the bulk of splanchnic inflow and courses posterior to the second portion of the duodenum (gray segment). **C:** A preduodenal portal vein develops based on aberrant involution of the vitelline venous interconnections such that the portal vein courses anterior to the second portion of the duodenum (gray segment). **D:** In the Abernethy malformations, aberrant involution of vitelline venous interconnections result in a diminutive or absent portal vein with portosystemic shunting of splanchnic blood flow (gray segment). Shunts typically drain to the inferior vena cava, azygos venous system, or right atrium based on preexisting embryonic interconnections. (Adapted from Esscher T. Preduodenal portal vein—a cause of intestinal obstruction? *J Pediatr Surg.* 1980;15[5]:609–612; Stringer MD. The clinical anatomy of congenital portosystemic venous shunts. *Clin Anat.* 2008;21[2]:147–157.)

CT, MRI, or catheter angiography. CT and MRI can help map the overall vascular anatomy and provide the broadest field of view for identification of the shunt and associated anomalies. Differentiation of CEPS from acquired portosystemic shunts can be difficult. Imaging findings of portal or splanchnic hypertension, including ascites, splenomegaly, and gastroesophageal varices, are rarely seen in CEPS because of low pressure gradients across the shunt.[12,13] Cavernous transformation of the main portal vein also suggests an acquired portosystemic shunt.

Management of congenital portosystemic shunts depends on the identification of intrahepatic portal venous branches. The presence of any identifiable portal venous blood flow allows staged closure of the portosystemic shunt, thereby rerouting blood flow through the portal venous system.[14,15] Catheter angiography, including direct shunt interrogation, is considered the imaging test of choice in this assessment, although biopsy may ultimately be required.[12,14] Screening, diagnosis, and follow-up of hepatic masses in the setting of CEPS is an important function of imaging. Ultrasound can be used to screen for and follow up known lesions, whereas MRI is ideal for characterization of identified lesions. Of note, caution should be exercised in the diagnosis of specific lesions based on dynamic contrast enhancement characteristics, as

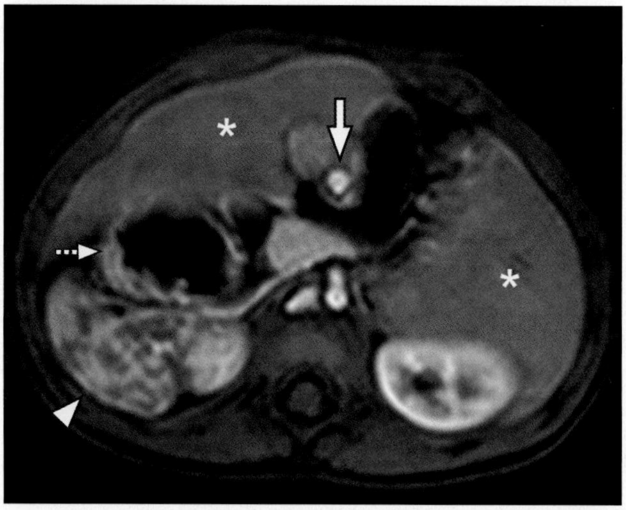

FIGURE 14.4 **A 19-month-old girl with heterotaxy syndrome and preduodenal portal vein.** Axial postcontrast T1-weighted fat-suppressed MR image in the early portal venous phase shows the liver on the left (*asterisk*), stomach on the right (*dashed arrow*), and multiple right upper quadrant spleens (*arrowhead*), compatible with heterotaxy syndrome (polysplenia). The main portal vein (*arrow*) passes anterior to the second portion of the duodenum consistent with preduodenal portal vein. The pancreas is hypoplastic, and there is azygos continuation of the inferior vena cava as well. (Image courtesy of Jonathan R. Dillman, MD, MSc, Cincinnati Children's Hospital Medical Center, Cincinnati, OH.)

the effect of absent portal venous blood flow on enhancement patterns has not been well characterized. Enhancement patterns in the hepatocyte phase with hepatocyte-specific contrast agents are likely unaffected by the altered blood flow.

TABLE 14.1 Classification Scheme for Congenital Extrahepatic Portosystemic Shunts

Congenital Extrahepatic Portosystemic Shunts
• Abernethy malformation, type I: Complete absence of the portal vein and intrahepatic portal vein branches (end-to-side shunt)
Type Ia: SMV and SV do not join prior to draining into the IVC
Type Ib: SMV and SV form a common trunk prior to draining into the IVC
• Abernethy malformation, type II: Hypoplastic extrahepatic portal vein with partial shunting of splanchnic flow (side-to-side shunt)
• Other congenital portosystemic shunts

IVC, inferior vena cava; SMV, superior mesenteric vein; SV, splenic vein. Adapted from Morgan G, Superina R. Congenital absence of the portal vein: two cases and a proposed classification system for portasystemic vascular anomalies. J Pediatr Surg. 1994;29(9):1239–1241, Ref. 9.

Infectious and Inflammatory Disorders

Infectious Disorders

Infectious diseases of the liver in children consist of viral hepatitis, pyogenic (bacterial) and amebic abscesses, parasitic diseases (e.g., hydatid disease and schistosomiasis), as well as fungal and other granulomatous diseases (e.g., tuberculosis, cat-scratch disease).

Viral hepatitis outside of the neonatal period is most commonly caused by hepatitis A, B, and C viruses, but a vast array of other viruses can infect the liver in childhood, including coxsackie, rubella, Epstein-Barr, varicella–zoster, herpes simplex,

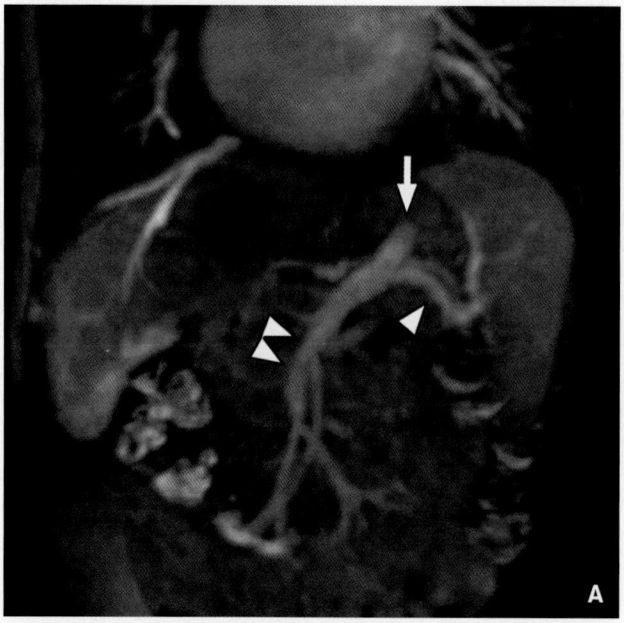

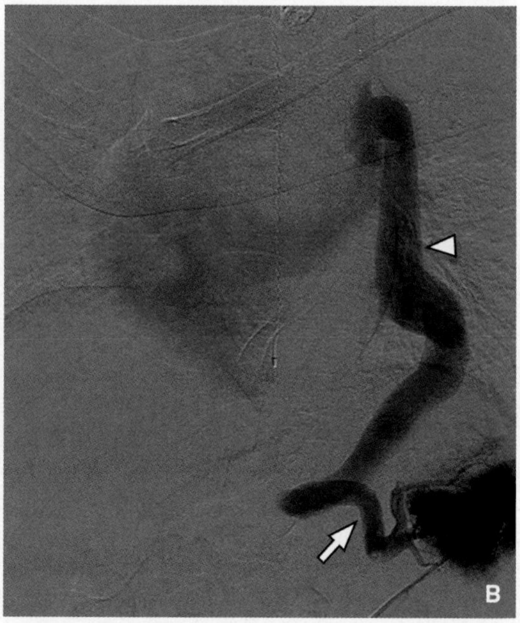

FIGURE 14.5 **A 2-year-old boy with Abernethy malformation. A:** Postcontrast T1-weighted maximum-intensity projection (MIP) MR image shows that the superior mesenteric vein (*double arrowhead*) and the splenic vein (*single arrowhead*) join together and drain via a partially visualized shunt to the right atrium (*arrow*). There is no visible normal main portal vein. **B:** Left anterior oblique digital subtraction image from splenic portography shows a vascular blush in the spleen with contrast filling the splenic vein (*arrow*) and then draining via a large shunt (*arrowhead*) to the right atrium. There is no visible normal main portal vein.

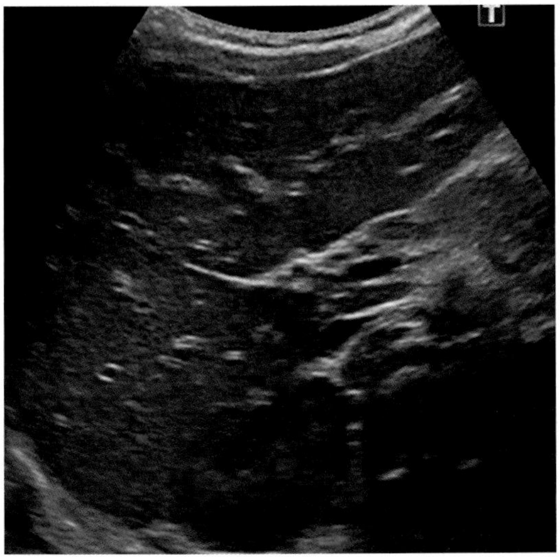

FIGURE 14.6 **A 16-year-old boy status post bone marrow transplant with viral hepatitis.** Transverse gray-scale ultrasound image shows classic "starry sky" appearance of the liver with diffusely decreased parenchymal echogenicity and relatively increased echogenicity of the portal vein walls.

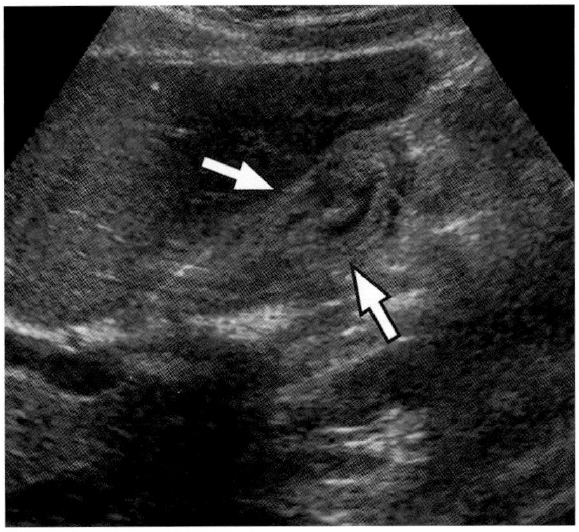

FIGURE 14.7 **A 17-year-old girl with Epstein-Barr viral hepatitis.** Transverse gray-scale ultrasound image shows diffuse and marked gallbladder wall thickening (*arrows*). Although nonspecific, this finding is commonly seen in pediatric patients with viral hepatitis.

adenovirus, and cytomegalovirus. The diagnosis of viral hepatitis is typically clinical. Ultrasound may show hepatomegaly, heterogeneous parenchymal echotexture, "starry sky" appearance (diffuse decrease in hepatic echogenicity with resultant relative increase in echogenicity of the portal vein walls) (Fig. 14.6), gallbladder wall thickening (Fig. 14.7), and periportal lymph node enlargement. Chronic viral hepatitis conveys an increased risk of cirrhosis and resultant complications, such as portal hypertension and malignancy. Ultrasound is frequently used to screen for these complications.

Pyogenic (bacterial) liver abscesses may occur secondary to ascending cholangitis, hematogenous spread, or direct spread from an adjacent organ. Immunocompromised children are at increased risk of pyogenic liver abscess formation. *Escherichia coli* is the most common offending bacterium.[16] Abscesses <5 cm in diameter are generally treated with antibiotic therapy alone, whereas larger abscesses often require a combination of antibiotic therapy and percutaneous drainage.[16] On ultrasound, pyogenic abscesses typically present as focal liver lesions with variable echogenicity, increased posterior acoustic through transmission, and lack of internal Doppler flow; a multiloculated appearance is common (Fig. 14.8). On contrast-enhanced CT and MR, pyogenic liver abscesses are typically well-defined, lobular, often multiseptated hypoattenuating/fluid signal lesions that may demonstrate rim enhancement and perilesional edema (Fig. 14.8).

Amebic liver abscesses are caused by *Entamoeba histolytica*, and are the most common extraintestinal complication of amebiasis, occurring in approximately 8.5% of cases.[16] Infection is typically secondary to ingestion of contaminated food or water. Treatment of amebic abscesses with amebicidal therapy is highly effective, and percutaneous drainage is rarely required.[16] On ultrasound, amebic abscesses are typically peripherally located, hypoechoic

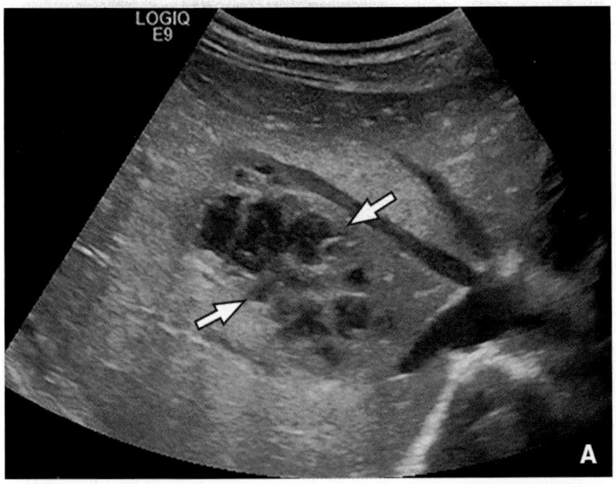

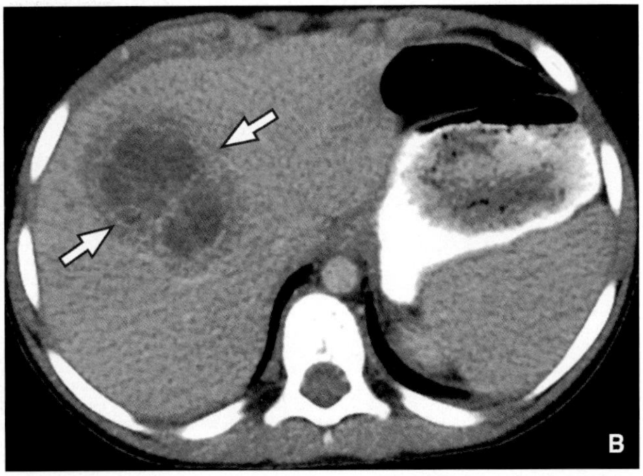

FIGURE 14.8 **A 9-year-old boy with a pyogenic liver abscess who presented with fever and right upper quadrant abdominal pain. A:** Transverse gray-scale ultrasound image demonstrates a complex, mixed-echogenicity lesion (*arrows*) in the right hepatic lobe between the right and middle hepatic veins. **B:** Axial contrast-enhanced CT image in the same patient demonstrates a complex, predominantly hypoattenuating lesion (*arrows*) with surrounding edema, consistent with a liver abscess.

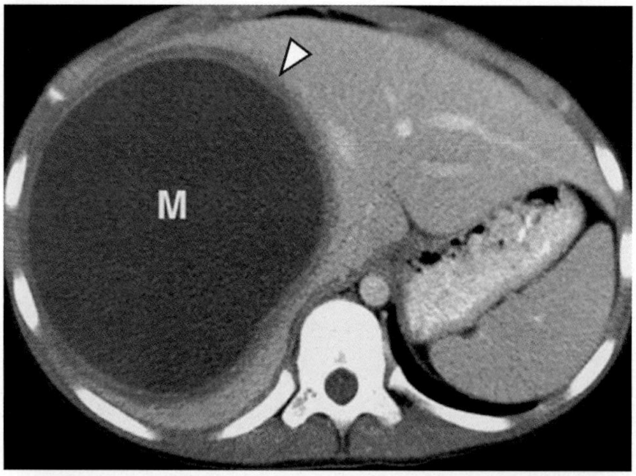

FIGURE 14.9 **Amebic abscess.** Axial contrast-enhanced CT image shows a large, low-attenuation mass (*M*) with a surrounding hypoattenuating rim of edema (*arrowhead*) in the right lobe of the liver. (From Siegel MJ. *Pediatric Body CT*. Philadelphia, PA: Lippincott Williams & Wilkins; 2007, with permission.)

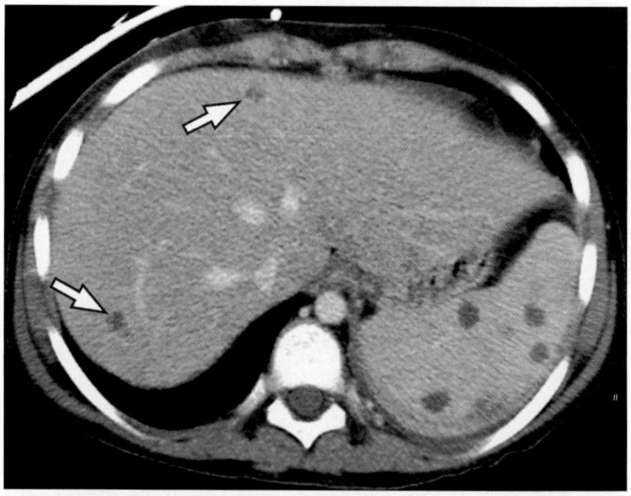

FIGURE 14.11 **An 11-year-old immunocompromised boy with hepatic fungal microabscesses.** Axial contrast-enhanced CT image demonstrates two representative small hypoattenuating foci (*arrows*) within the liver and multiple small hypoattenuating foci in the spleen, consistent with fungal microabscesses.

lesions with increased posterior acoustic through transmission and no internal Doppler flow. On contrast-enhanced CT, amebic abscesses typically appear as unilocular, homogenous fluid attenuation masses with an enhancing rim and a surrounding halo of low-attenuation edema (Fig. 14.9).

Fungal infections of the liver in children most frequently occur in immunocompromised patients, often those with neutropenia, and in patients with lymphoma/leukemia. *Candida*, *Aspergillus*, *Histoplasma*, *Cryptococcus*, *Coccidioides*, *Nocardia*, and *Mucor* are all known causative agents. Several ultrasound patterns of fungal microabscesses have been described: "wheel-within-a-wheel" pattern (central hypoechoic focus surrounded by echogenic rim), target appearance (central echogenic focus surrounded by hypoechoic rim), diffuse uniform hypoechoic foci, and finally, calcified, hyperechoic foci in the healing/healed phase (Fig. 14.10). On CT, both with and without intravenous contrast material, fungal microabscesses present as multiple, small, hypoattenuating lesions scattered throughout the liver (Fig. 14.11). On MRI, fungal microabscesses appear as multiple, small lesions that are hypointense on T1-weighted MR images and hyperintense on T2-weighted MR images with variable enhancement following intravenous contrast material administration.

Hydatid disease, schistosomiasis, tuberculosis, cat-scratch disease, visceral larva migrans, and HIV infections of the liver may also be uncommonly encountered, and the reader is directed to several excellent imaging reviews on the less common etiologies of liver infection in children.[16–18]

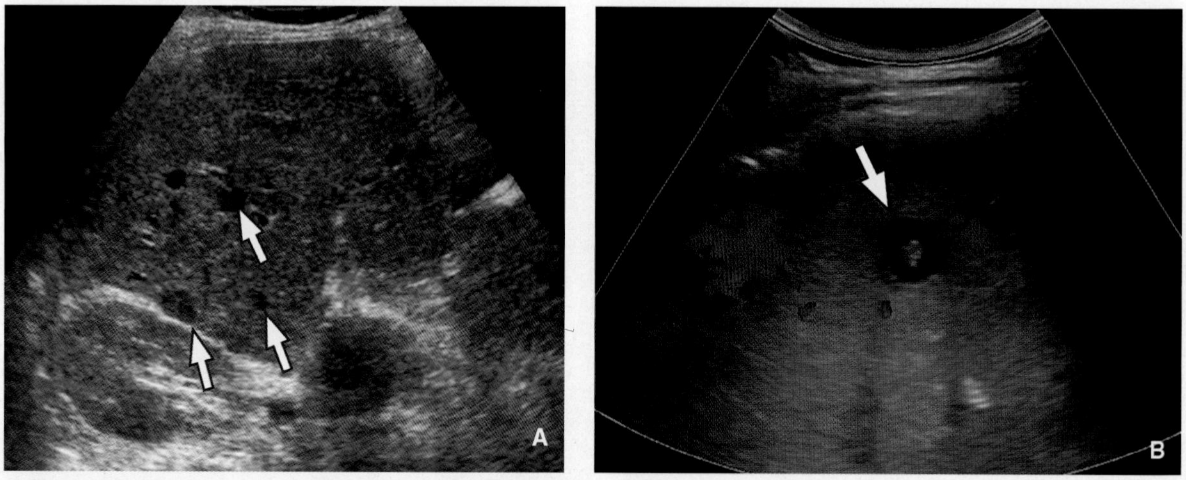

FIGURE 14.10 **Two pediatric patients with hepatic Candida microabscess. A:** A 15-year-old boy post cardiac transplantation on chronic immunosuppression. Transverse gray-scale ultrasound image shows several small, uniformly hypoechoic foci (*arrows*) within the liver determined to be Candida microabscesses. **B:** A 10-year-old boy with acute leukemia and candidemia. Transverse color Doppler ultrasound image shows a target-appearing lesion (*arrow*) in the liver that is centrally hyperechoic and peripherally hypoechoic.

Inflammatory Disorders

Neonatal Hepatitis

Neonatal hepatitis refers to the clinical presentation of a neonate with conjugated hyperbilirubinemia related to underlying liver disease.[19] Hepatic inflammation does not need to be present but frequently is. Causes of the underlying liver disease are numerous, including infection (e.g., toxoplasmosis, rubella, cytomegalovirus, herpes), metabolic (e.g., α-1-antitypsin deficiency), neoplastic, vascular (e.g., Budd-Chiari syndrome), toxic (e.g., total parenteral nutrition (TPN)-associated cholestasis, drug related), immune (i.e., gestational alloimmune liver disease/neonatal hemochromatosis), structural (e.g., choledochal cyst), and idiopathic.

The role of imaging in neonatal hepatitis is not necessarily to identify the exact etiology of the hepatitis but rather to confirm the diagnosis, exclude extrahepatic biliary atresia, and identify structural abnormalities. Ultrasound is typically the initial imaging modality of choice in this scenario. On ultrasound, the liver may be normal in appearance, although hepatomegaly and increased parenchymal echogenicity may be seen. It is important to identify features of biliary atresia, as this condition requires urgent surgical intervention.

Magnetic resonance cholangiopancreatography (MRCP) and hepatobiliary scintigraphy can also be used in the evaluation of a patient with neonatal hepatitis. Visualization of the extrahepatic bile ducts by MRCP has a sensitivity and specificity of 90% and 77%, respectively, for excluding biliary atresia.[20] On hepatobiliary scintigraphy using a ^{99m}Tc-labeled iminodiacetic acid (IDA) analogue, imaging features consistent with neonatal hepatitis include delayed hepatocyte uptake and washout of the radiotracer with identifiable bowel activity. Delayed images at 4 to 6 and 24 hours should be performed to confirm the presence of excreted radiotracer in the bowel (Fig. 14.12). Hepatobiliary scintigraphy with single photon emission computed tomography (SPECT) was recently shown to have an accuracy of 91.3% in this clinical scenario.[21] Ultimately, liver biopsy is often required to add in differentiating neonatal hepatitis from biliary atresia.

Autoimmune Hepatitis

Autoimmune hepatitis is a rare chronic inflammatory disease of the liver that can lead to cirrhosis with a peak incidence in patients 10 to 30 years old.[22] In children, the condition sometimes presents along with autoimmune cholangitis. The etiology is uncertain, but is thought to be a combination of genetic, immunologic, and environmental factors.

Imaging studies in general are not helpful in making the specific diagnosis of autoimmune hepatitis but are often helpful in excluding other underlying liver pathology that can result in similar clinical presentations. On ultrasound, the liver may demonstrate nonspecific heterogeneous increased echogenicity (Fig. 14.13), and on contrast-enhanced CT or MR, the liver may demonstrate heterogeneous enhancement. If the disease progresses to cirrhosis, the typical imaging features of cirrhosis and its complications can be seen on cross-sectional imaging modalities. MR elastography and ultrasound elastography may soon play a role in noninvasively detecting progression of fibrosis, thus limiting serial percutaneous liver biopsies (Fig. 14.14).

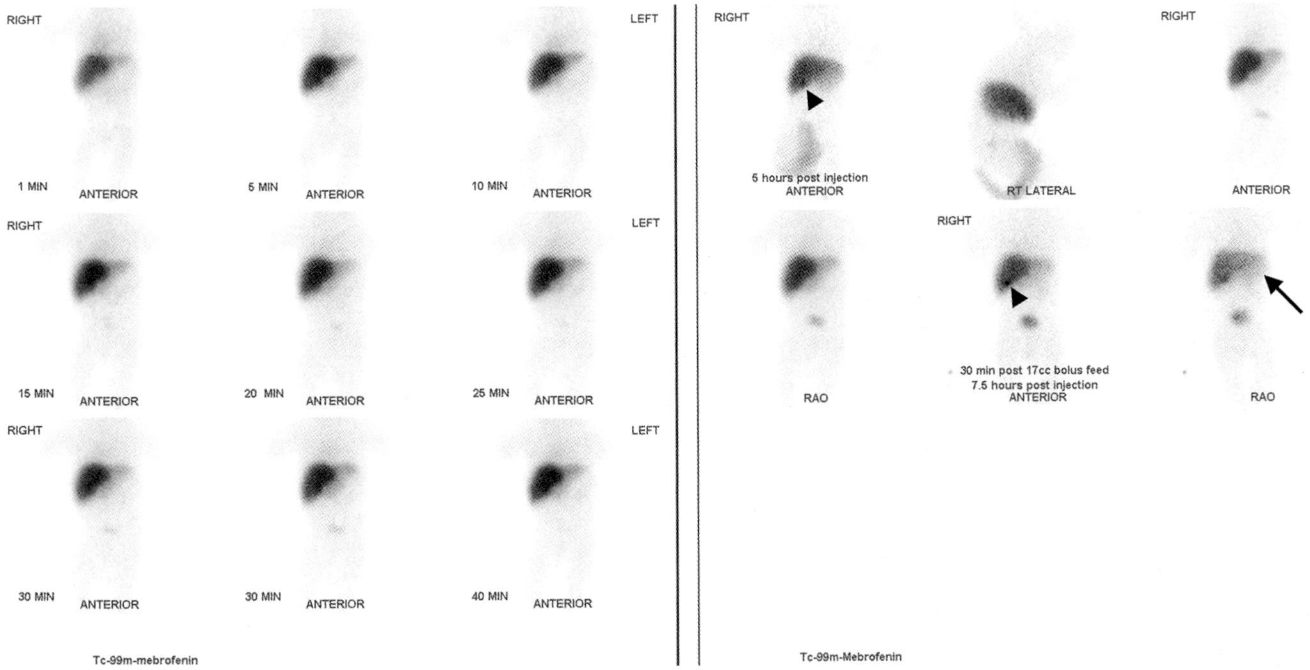

FIGURE 14.12 **A 6-week-old boy with neonatal hepatitis.** Hepatobiliary scan with ^{99m}Tc-mebrofenin demonstrates delayed washout of radiotracer from the liver with some accumulation in the gallbladder (*arrowheads*). There is eventual subtle radiotracer accumulation in bowel (*arrow*) on the 7.5-hour postinjection images that eliminates biliary atresia as a diagnostic possibility. Excreted radiotracer in urine is visible in the patient's diaper on the 5 hour post-injection images.

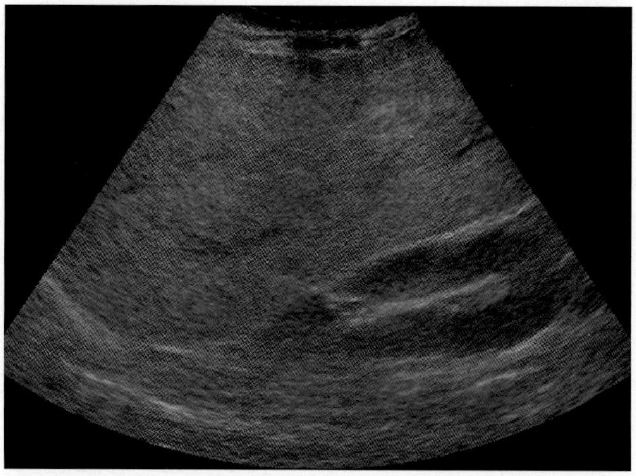

FIGURE 14.13 **An 11-year-old girl with autoimmune hepatitis.** Longitudinal gray-scale ultrasound image of the liver demonstrates nonspecific increased echogenicity. Normal portal venous structures are not visible.

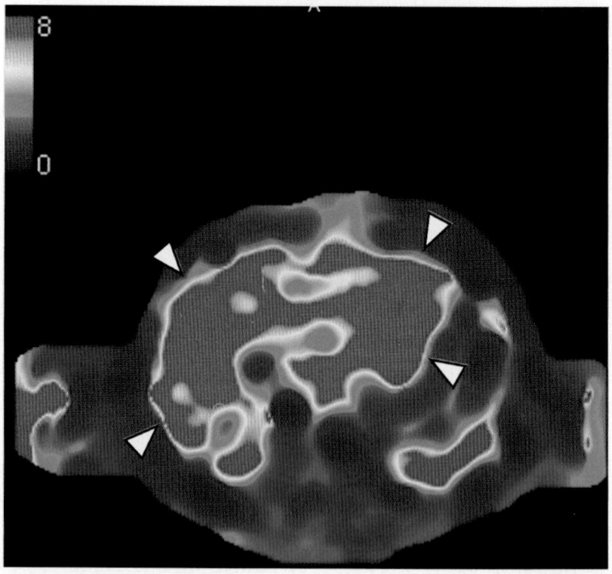

FIGURE 14.14 **A 12-year-old girl with autoimmune hepatitis.** Representative elastogram image from a liver MR elastography exam demonstrates markedly elevated stiffness (*red and orange on the color scale*) throughout the liver (*arrowheads*). Mean liver stiffness was 7.8 kPa.

Neoplastic Disorders

The liver is the third most common site for primary solid abdominal tumors in the pediatric population after the kidneys and adrenal glands.[23] Two-thirds of primary pediatric liver tumors are malignant; hepatoblastoma, HCC, and undifferentiated embryonal sarcoma of the liver are the most common.[24–26] One-third of primary pediatric liver tumors are benign, the most common of which are infantile hepatic hemangioma, FNH, and mesenchymal hamartoma.[23,24,26,27]

Benign Primary Neoplasms

Infantile Hepatic Hemangiomas

Infantile hepatic hemangiomas (IHHs), sometimes inappropriately called hemangioendotheliomas, are the most common liver tumor in infancy and the third most common liver tumor in children.[23,28,29] IHHs are true neoplasms, composed of a network of capillary-sized endothelium-lined vessels, and are distinct from the misnamed adult "hemangiomas," which are venous malformations.[28,29] Most IHHs are asymptomatic.[30] Rare complications include high-output congestive heart failure, consumptive coagulopathy (Kasabach-Merritt syndrome), jaundice, hepatic failure, bleeding, abdominal compartment syndrome, and hypothyroidism.[24,28]

IHHs are classified based on distribution as focal, multifocal, or diffuse (Figs. 14.15 to 14.17). Focal IHHs have many of the same characteristics of cutaneous rapidly involuting congenital hemangiomas (RICH). Unlike multifocal and diffuse IHHs that present in the first weeks of life, focal lesions can present in the prenatal period and are congenital. Focal lesions may regress without therapy within the first 12 to 14 months

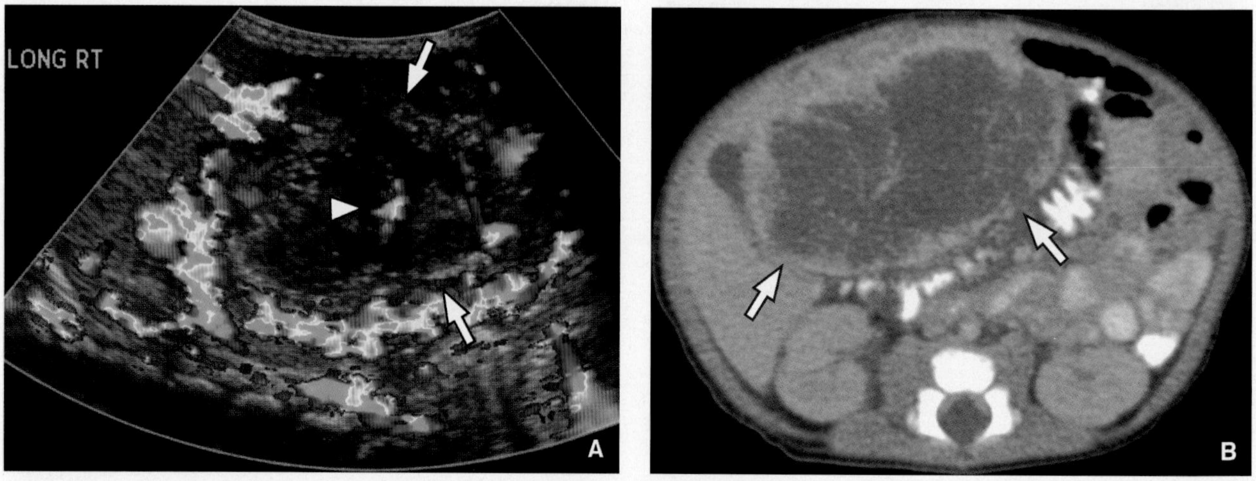

FIGURE 14.15 **A 1-month-old boy with a large focal infantile hepatic hemangioma. A:** Color Doppler ultrasound image of the liver shows a mixed echogenicity mass (*arrows*) with considerably increased vascularity along the periphery of the mass and mildly increased vascularity within the mass (*arrowhead*). **B:** Axial contrast-enhanced CT image of the abdomen shows a large heterogeneous mass (*arrows*) with irregular, peripheral, nodular enhancement.

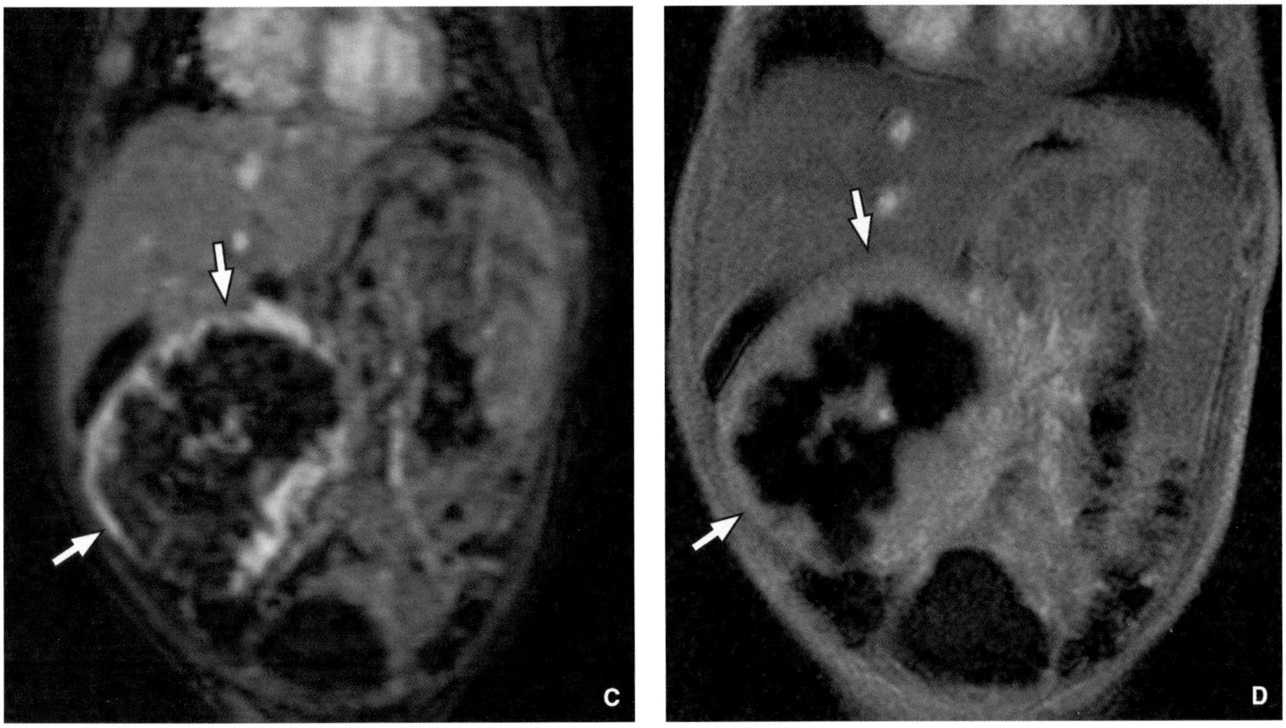

FIGURE 14.15 *(Continued)* **C:** Coronal postcontrast fat-suppressed T1-weighted MR images in the **(C)** hepatic arterial and **(D)** delayed portal venous phases show the mass (*arrows*) with peripheral, nodular enhancement that partially fills in on the more delayed image.

of life.[31] Multifocal and diffuse IHHs are frequently associated with cutaneous infantile hemangiomas.[29] Like cutaneous infantile hemangiomas, multifocal and diffuse IHHs appear in the first weeks of life, grow rapidly over the first year, and then slowly involute.[29]

Imaging can be used to distinguish the subtypes of IHHs and identify sequelae in symptomatic cases. In general, focal and multifocal IHHs appear as well-defined, spherical liver mass(es) (Figs. 14.15 and 14.16). Diffuse IHHs manifest as total or near-total replacement of the liver parenchyma (Fig. 14.17).[31,32] Calcifications may be seen in up to 50% of lesions.[24] Findings of vascular steal and shunting may be visible as enlarged supplying arteries (celiac and hepatic), tapering of the infraceliac abdominal aorta, enlarged portal veins, early draining hepatic veins, and sequelae of congestive heart failure (e.g., cardiomegaly and pulmonary edema).[24,31]

On ultrasound, IHHs appear hypoechoic or of mixed echogenicity reflecting central hemorrhage, necrosis or calcification (Fig. 14.15).[24] Diffuse IHHs may present as an enlarged heterogeneous liver.[24] Doppler interrogation typically demonstrates lesional hypervascularity with variable spectral waveforms.[24] IHHs are typically hypoattenuating on nonenhanced CT. On noncontrast MR images, lesions are typically T1-weighted hypointense and T2-weighted

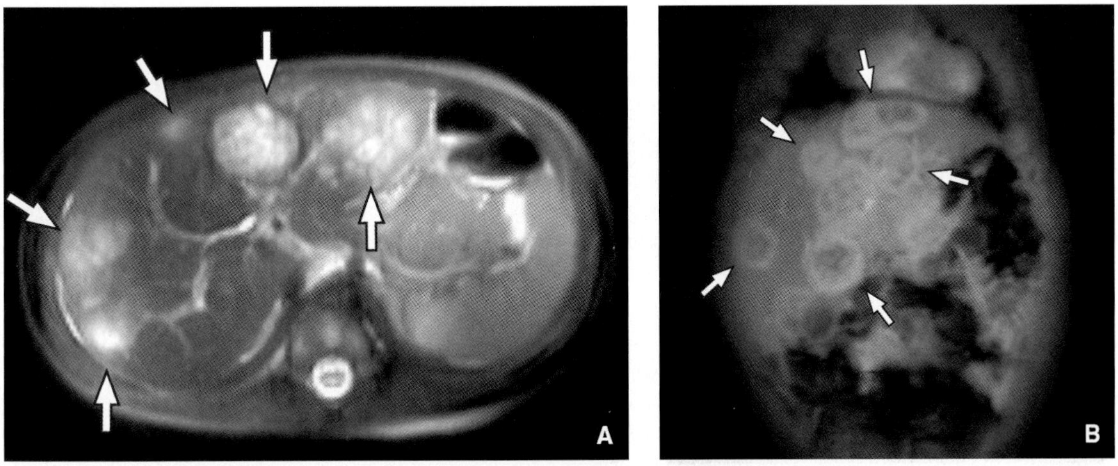

FIGURE 14.16 **An 8-month-old girl with multiple infantile hepatic hemangiomas. A:** Axial T2-weighted fat-suppressed MR image shows multiple lobulated, hyperintense liver masses (*arrows*). **B:** Coronal postcontrast fat-suppressed T2-weighted MR image shows that all of the masses peripherally enhance (*arrows*), and some contain contrast material centrally.

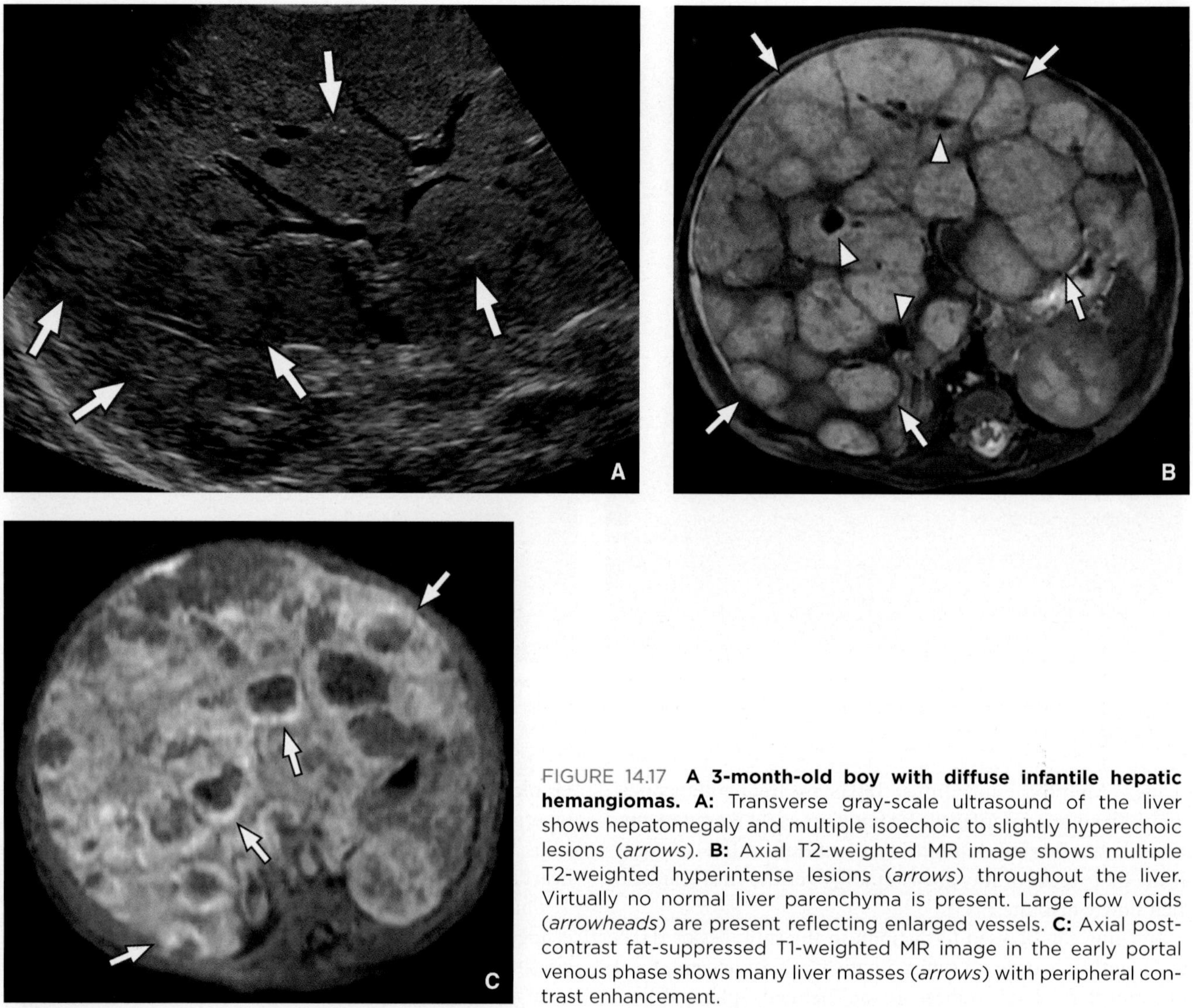

FIGURE 14.17 **A 3-month-old boy with diffuse infantile hepatic hemangiomas. A:** Transverse gray-scale ultrasound of the liver shows hepatomegaly and multiple isoechoic to slightly hyperechoic lesions (*arrows*). **B:** Axial T2-weighted MR image shows multiple T2-weighted hyperintense lesions (*arrows*) throughout the liver. Virtually no normal liver parenchyma is present. Large flow voids (*arrowheads*) are present reflecting enlarged vessels. **C:** Axial post-contrast fat-suppressed T1-weighted MR image in the early portal venous phase shows many liver masses (*arrows*) with peripheral contrast enhancement.

hyperintense (Fig. 14.15).[24,31] Internal heterogeneity, including T1-weighted hyperintensity, may be present reflecting hemorrhage or necrosis. Flow voids in and around the IHH reflect high flow within feeding vessels. Postcontrast imaging with CT or MRI is characteristic with peripheral, continuous, or discontinuous arterial enhancement that centripetally fills the lesion over the portal venous phase and more delayed imaging (Figs. 14.15, 14.16, 14.17). Smaller lesions typically enhance homogenously, whereas larger lesions may never enhance completely because of central hemorrhage or necrosis.[24] Rare reports of IHHs evaluated with hepatocyte-specific contrast agents have described the lesions to be variable in their retention of contrast on the hepatocyte phase of imaging.[33]

IHH is a benign tumor with a good prognosis. Asymptomatic pediatric patients should be followed with ultrasound to document regression.[31] Symptomatic pediatric patients may be treated pharmacologically (e.g., propranolol) to promote lesion regression.[31] Hepatic artery embolization, partial liver resection, or liver transplant may be needed in rare complicated cases.[31]

Focal Nodular Hyperplasia

Focal nodular hyperplasia (FNH) accounts for 2% of pediatric liver tumors.[34] This tumor-like cellular proliferation occurs both sporadically and at an increased rate in long-term survivors of pediatric malignancies (e.g., neuroblastoma, leukemia).[34–40] Sporadic FNH are typically solitary, whereas multiple lesions are common in cancer survivors.[34] FNH is possibly induced by local abnormalities in blood flow. Grossly and microscopically, FNH resembles a localized form of cirrhosis with fibrous bands and nodular collections of hepatocytes accompanied by proliferating bile ductules. Sporadic FNH are generally larger and more likely to have the classic central stellate scar compared with those arising after treatment for a pediatric malignancy (Fig. 14.18).[34]

On ultrasound, FNH typically appears homogeneous with variable echogenicity (Fig. 14.19).[24] The central scar, if present, generally appears hyperechoic compared to the mass. Doppler interrogation may show internal vessels with arterial waveforms, which has been described as a distinguishing feature versus hepatic (hepatocellular) adenoma.[24] On noncontrast CT, FNH is typically iso- or slightly hypoattenuating compared to normal liver with the central scar appearing

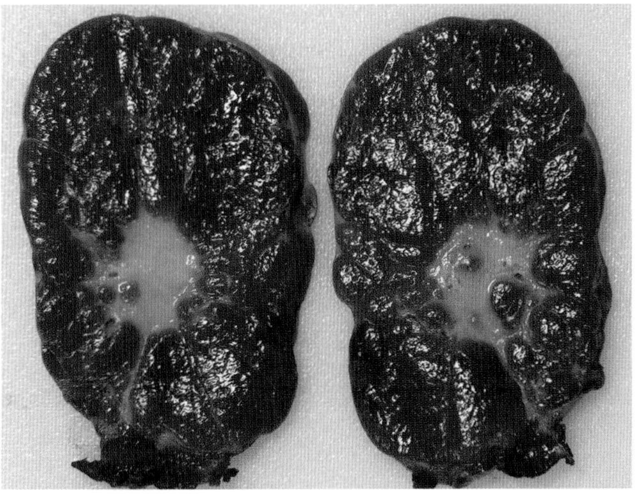

FIGURE 14.18 **Focal nodular hyperplasia, manifesting as a 7 cm mass with a characteristic central white fibrous scar in an otherwise healthy adolescent girl.**

hypoattenuating compared to the mass. On MRI, FNH is typically iso- to slightly hypointense on T1-weighted MR images and iso- to slightly hyperintense on T2-weighted MR images (Fig. 14.19). The central scar is typically hypointense to the mass on T1-weighted MR images and slightly hyperintense on T2-weighted MR images. This differs from the central scar seen in fibrolamellar HCC (FLH), which is commonly hypointense on T2-weighted MR images.

The enhancement pattern of FNH on CT and MRI is characteristic with early, intense arterial enhancement with the lesion becoming isointense to the liver in the portal venous and delayed phases (Fig. 14.19). The central scar typically enhances on the delayed phase of imaging (versus the nonenhancing scar of FLH). Hepatocyte-specific contrast agents provide specificity for the diagnosis of FNH as it is one of the few lesions to retain contrast material on the hepatocyte phase of imaging (Fig. 14.19).[33] The central scar does not retain contrast during the hepatocyte phase, appearing

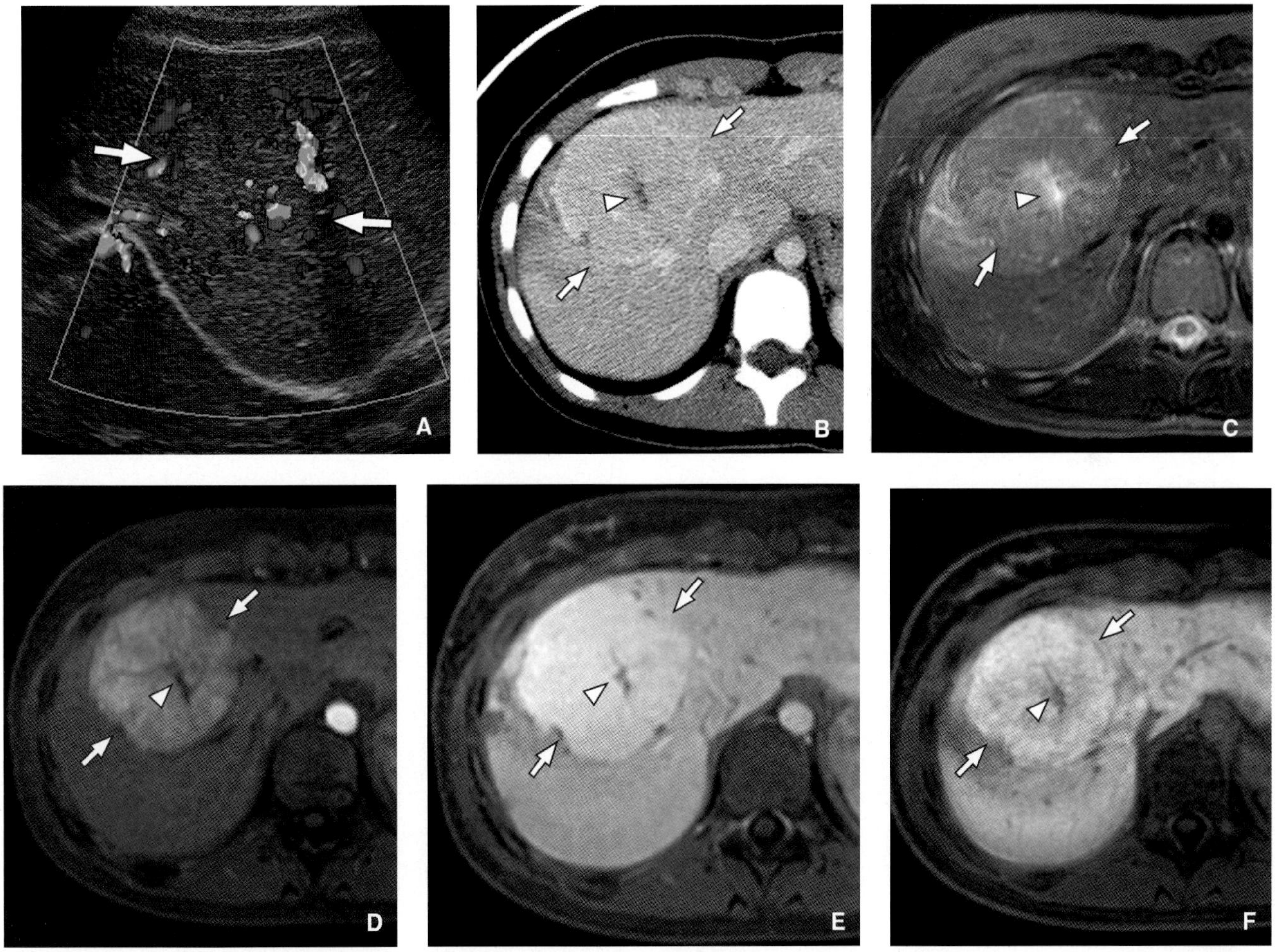

FIGURE 14.19 **A 15-year-old girl with focal nodular hyperplasia (FNH). A:** Longitudinal color Doppler ultrasound image of the liver shows a slightly hyperechoic mass (*arrows*) within the right lobe of the liver. Vascularity is present within the mass with suggestion of a "spoke-wheel" pattern. **B:** Axial contrast-enhanced CT image shows the mass (*arrows*) is mildly hyperenhancing relative to the background liver. There is a central hypoattenuating scar (*arrowhead*) within the mass that does not enhance. **C:** Axial T2-weighted fat-suppressed MR image shows that the mass (*arrows*) is hyperintense in comparison to the liver. The central scar (*arrowhead*) is hyperintense as well. Axial postcontrast fat-suppressed MR images performed with a hepatocyte-specific contrast agent in the **(D)** hepatic arterial, **(E)** portal venous, and **(F)** hepatocyte phases of imaging show that the mass (*arrows*) is hyperenhancing relative to the background liver on the arterial and portal venous phases and retains contrast material on the hepatocyte phase. The central scar (*arrowhead*) does not enhance.

hypointense to the surrounding lesion.[33] Large FNHs may demonstrate evidence of arteriovenous shunting on CT and MRI, including enlarged hepatic artery branches in and surrounding the lesion and early hepatic venous opacification.

Asymptomatic lesions require no follow-up. Surgical resection or hepatic artery embolization of symptomatic lesions can be considered.

Mesenchymal Hamartoma

Mesenchymal hamartoma of the liver is the second most common benign pediatric liver tumor, accounting for 5% to 8% all liver masses.[41] Eighty percent are diagnosed before 2 years of age and ninety-five percent before 5 years of age[24,41]; in utero development has been described. Affected pediatric patients typically present with a rapidly enlarging, painless abdominal mass.[42] Ascites, jaundice, and congestive heart failure can occur if the mass compresses adjacent structures.[41] Mild elevation of alpha fetoprotein (AFP) level has been described, but there is no specific laboratory marker for mesenchymal hamartoma.[24]

Imaging features depend on tumor composition. Lesions can range in appearance from predominantly cystic to predominantly solid with 80% to 85% of tumors having macroscopic cysts.[24,42] These tumors are typically large at presentation, with an average diameter of 16 cm, and they are more likely to arise in the right lobe of the liver than the left.[41,42] If identified on prenatal ultrasound, mesenchymal hamartomas typically appear anechoic to hypoechoic. There may be associated placental thickening, multicystic enlargement, or mesenchymal stem villous hyperplasia.[41] Postnatally, the cystic portions of mesenchymal hamartomas appear anechoic with echogenic septations on ultrasound. Low-level echoes can be seen within the cysts, reflecting the gelatinous content.[24] Solid portions of the mass are generally hyperechoic compared to background liver. Doppler ultrasound typically shows little blood flow.

On CT, mesenchymal hamartoma typically appears as a complex cystic mass with the cystic components similar in attenuation to water (10–20 HU) (Fig. 14.20).[24] On noncontrast CT, the stromal components of the mass are generally hypoattenuating compared to normal liver, but hyperattenuating compared to the cystic portions. Calcifications are rare. Following intravenous contrast material administration, the septations and stromal components enhance (Fig. 14.20). On MRI, the cystic components of the lesion are usually hypointense on T1-weighted MR images and hyperintense on T2-weighted MR images (Fig. 14.20). Cysts may have variable signal intensity, particularly on T1-weighted MR images, depending on the proteinaceous content of the fluid.[24] The solid component of the mass is typically hypointense on T1-weighted and T2-weighted MR images reflecting fibrous tissue[24] and enhances on postcontrast imaging (Fig. 14.20).

Histologically, mesenchymal hamartoma is composed of primitive stellate mesenchymal cells in a myxoid matrix with admixed hepatocytes, ductular structures, and islands of hematopoietic cells; cysts are frequently seen (Fig. 14.21).[41,42] Recurrent clonal cytogenetic abnormalities, in particular a t(11;19) chromosomal translocation, are thought to reflect a neoplastic biology.[43,44] The natural history of mesenchymal hamartoma is to rapidly enlarge in the first several months of life before stabilizing or transitioning to a phase of slow growth.[24] Spontaneous regression has been described, but observation is discouraged because of the small risk of "malignant transformation" to undifferentiated embryonal sarcoma.[24,41] Surgical resection is considered definitive therapy.

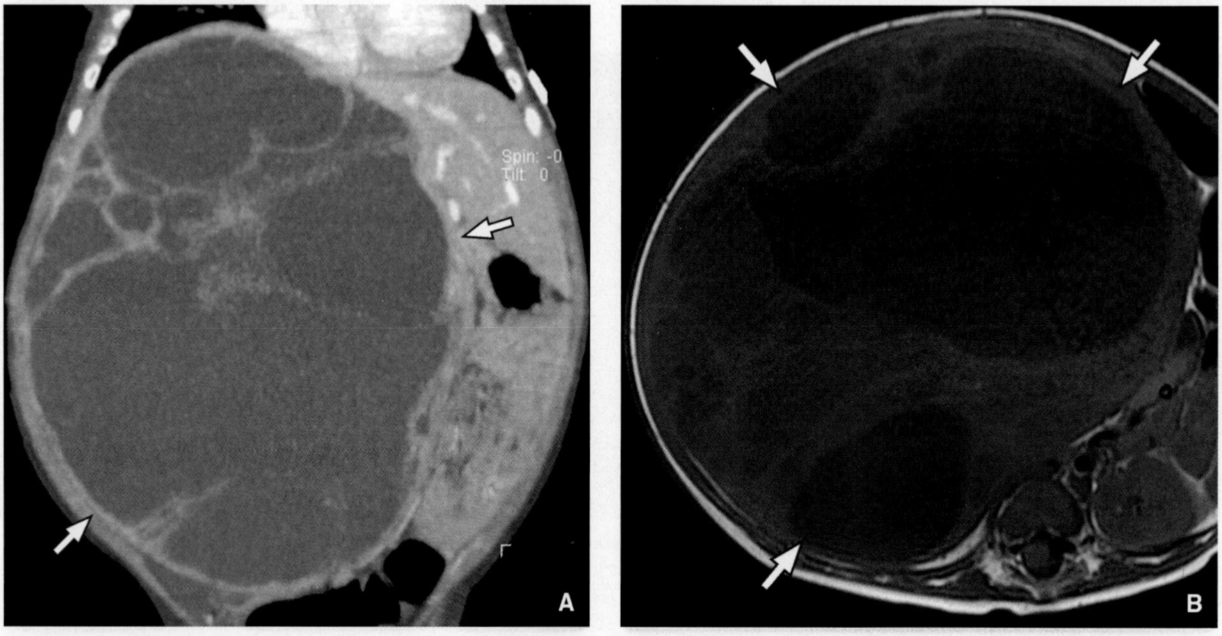

FIGURE 14.20 **An 8-month-old boy with large mesenchymal hamartoma. A:** Coronal contrast-enhanced CT image of the abdomen shows a large, multiseptated cystic mass (*arrows*) arising from the right lobe of the liver. The mass is primarily of fluid attenuation with enhancing septations. **B:** Axial T1-weighted MR image shows a large, multiseptated cystic mass (*arrows*) in the liver. The cystic portions are hypointense relative to the septations and background liver.

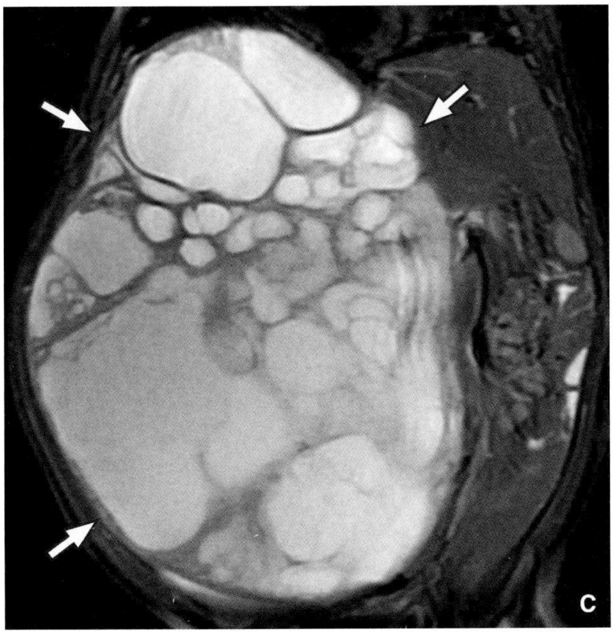

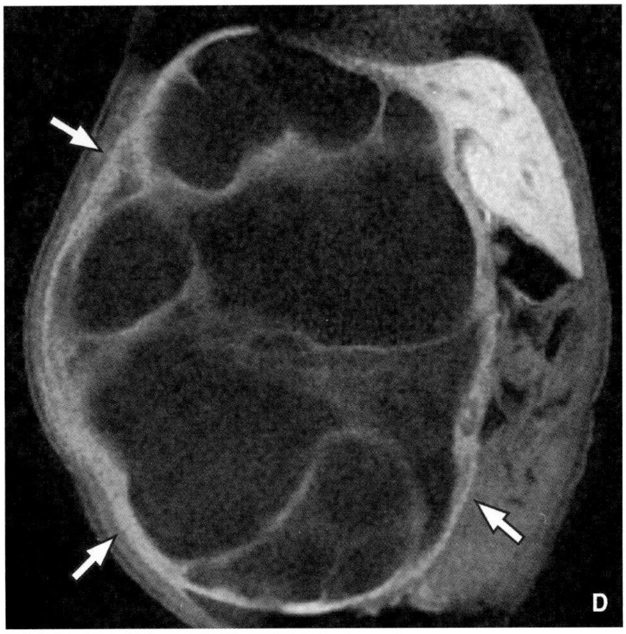

FIGURE 14.20 *(Continued)* **C:** Coronal T2-weighted fat-suppressed MR image shows that the cystic portions of the mass (*arrows*) are hyperintense relative to the liver while septations are iso- to hypointense. **D:** Coronal postcontrast fat-suppressed T1-weighted MR image using a hepatocyte-specific contrast agent obtained in the hepatocyte phase of imaging shows enhancement of the septations and the periphery of the large cystic mass (*arrows*).

Hepatic Adenoma

Hepatic (hepatocellular) adenomas are uncommon in the pediatric population. Lesions can be seen in young women on oral contraceptives and in obese patients. In addition, hepatic adenomas can present in association with altered hepatic blood flow and systemic diseases, such as Fanconi anemia (related to androgen therapy), glycogen storage disease types I and III, galactosemia, familial diabetes mellitus, and familial adenomatous polyposis.[24] Patients with more than nine hepatic adenomas are said to have hepatic adenomatosis, which can be unilobar, massive, or multifocal.[45] Hepatic adenomas are most often asymptomatic. Tumor rupture, however, occurs in 10% to 35% of affected patients manifesting as acute pain, intraperitoneal hemorrhage, or hypovolemic shock.[24,45]

Hepatic adenomas are composed of sheets of hepatocytes without portal tracts or normal bile ducts (Fig. 14.22), and they are supplied by the hepatic artery. Recent studies have subclassified hepatic adenomas based on the presence of genetic mutations (HNF-1α or β-catenin mutation) or histologically based on the presence or absence of inflammation. Inflammatory hepatic adenomas are the most common subtype (40% to 50%) and occur more commonly in association with oral

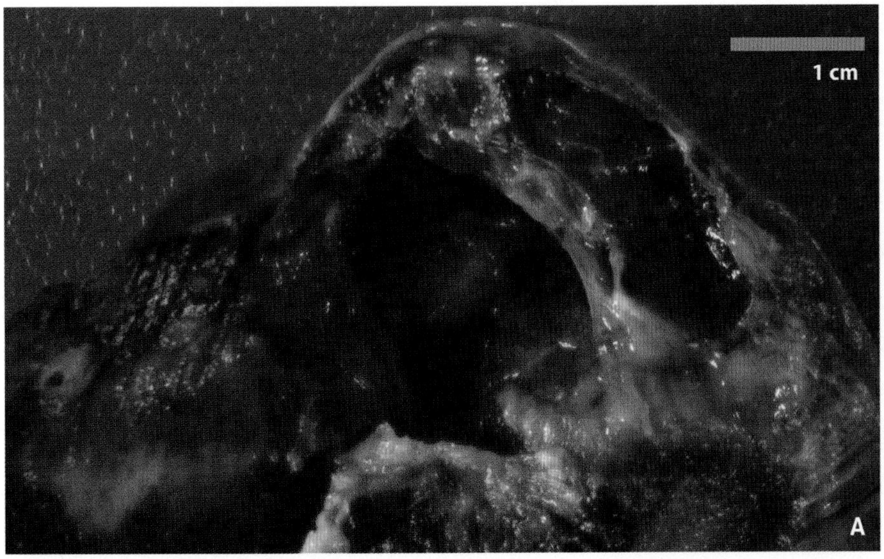

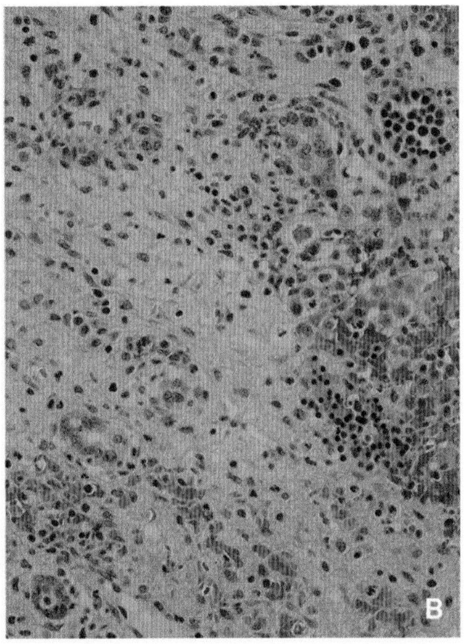

FIGURE 14.21 **Hepatic mesenchymal hamartoma from a 3-month-old boy. A:** The cut surface of a hepatic mesenchymal hamartoma shows heterogeneous cystic and solid tissue. **B:** Microscopically, fibrous stromal tissue containing occasional hepatocytes, cholangiolar epithelium, and areas of extramedullary hematopoiesis is seen (hematoxylin and eosin, original magnification, 400×).

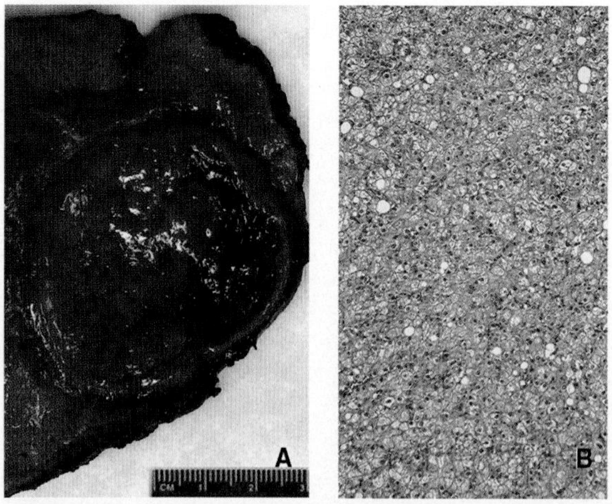

FIGURE 14.22 **Hepatic adenoma from an 18-year-old boy with glycogen storage disease type 1. A:** The cut surface of a hepatic adenoma appears as a well-circumscribed mass with an area of softening corresponding to necrosis. **B:** Microscopically, the mass consists of hepatocytes virtually identical to those in surrounding liver but lacking acinar arrangement around portal triads (hematoxylin and eosin, original magnification, 200x).

contraceptive use and obesity.[46] Systemic symptoms of chronic anemia and a systemic inflammatory syndrome (fever, leukocytosis, and elevated serum levels of C-reactive protein) have been reported.[46] HNF-1α mutated hepatic adenomas (30% to 35%) occur exclusively in girls, with many having a history of oral contraceptive use.[46] A background of steatosis is common, and 50% are multiple.[46] This mutation results in promotion of lipogenesis and accumulation of lesional intracellular lipid, which is apparent by imaging. β-catenin mutated hepatic adenomas (10% to 15%) occur more commonly in boys and are associated with male hormone administration, glycogen storage disease, and familial adenomatous polyposis.[46] Unclassified adenomas have no specific associations.

In general, hepatic adenomas appear well-defined by ultrasound with variable echogenicity depending on the amount of intralesional lipid, hemorrhage, and glycogen as well as the echogenicity of adjacent liver (Fig. 14.23).[24] On noncontrast CT, hepatic adenomas appear as well-defined, homogeneously hypoattenuating lesions (Fig. 14.23). Lesions that have bled may show internal hyperattenuation (Fig. 14.24). Calcifications are uncommon (5% to 15%).[24] On postcontrast imaging, hepatic adenomas show arterial enhancement with a variable appearance on delayed phase imaging. By MRI, the classic appearance of a hepatic adenoma is a lesion that is heterogeneously T1-weighted hyperintense and mildly T2-weighted hyperintense, and that shows loss of signal on T1-weighted gradient-recalled echo out-of-phase (opposed phase) imaging (Fig. 14.23). On postcontrast imaging, hepatic adenomas classically show arterial enhancement reflecting hepatic arterial supply and no uptake of hepatocyte-specific contrast agents during the hepatocyte phase of imaging (Fig. 14.23). Loss of signal on T1-weighted gradient-recalled echo opposed phase imaging can be seen in some subtypes of hepatic adenomas (HNF-1α) (Fig. 14.23)

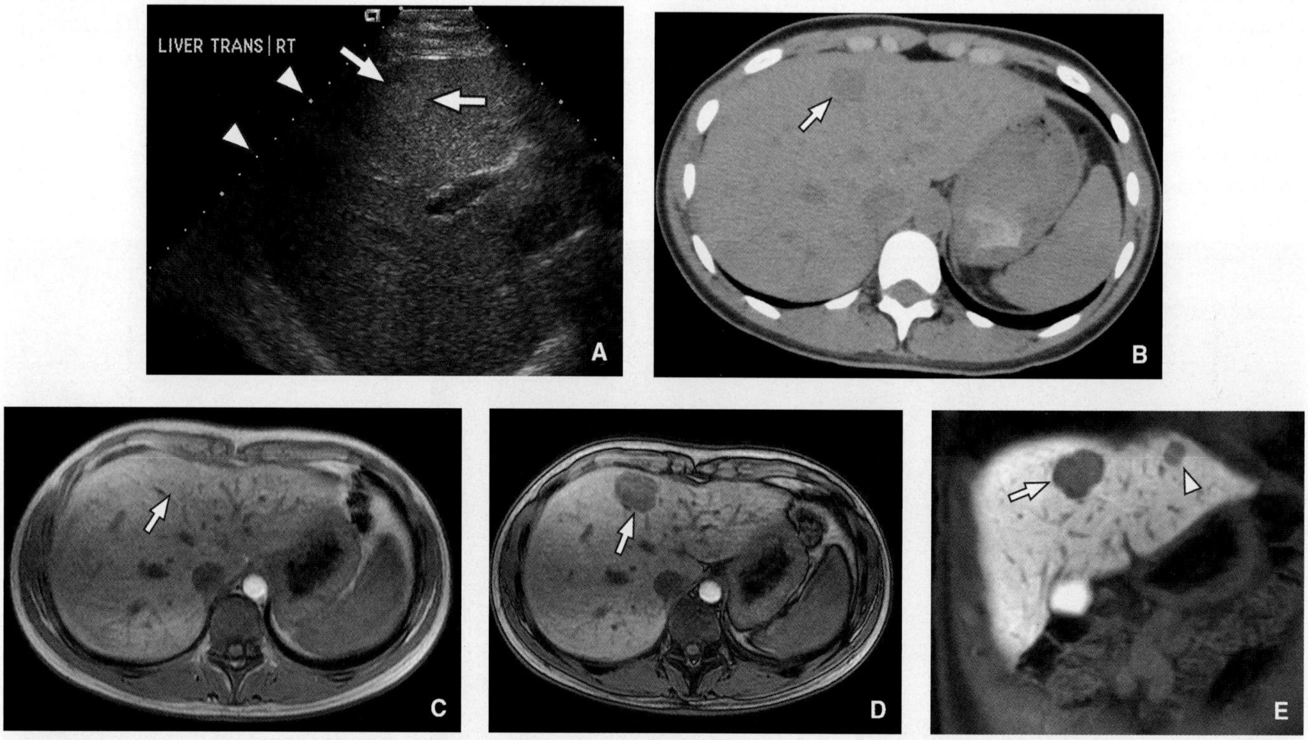

FIGURE 14.23 **A 17-year-old girl with hepatic adenomatosis. A:** Transverse gray-scale ultrasound image of the liver shows a hyperechoic lesion (*arrows*) within the medial section of the left hepatic lobe. **B:** Axial noncontrast CT image shows that the lesion is hypoattenuating (*arrow*). Axial **(C)** in- and **(D)** out-of-phase T1-weighted gradient-recalled echo MR images show signal dropout within the lesion (*arrow*) reflecting intracellular lipid. After the administration of a hepatocyte-specific contrast agent **(E)**, the lesion (*arrow*) appears hypointense compared to normally enhancing background liver in the hepatocyte phase (*arrow*). More than 20 additional lesions (*arrowhead*) were visible throughout the liver on hepatocyte phase images.

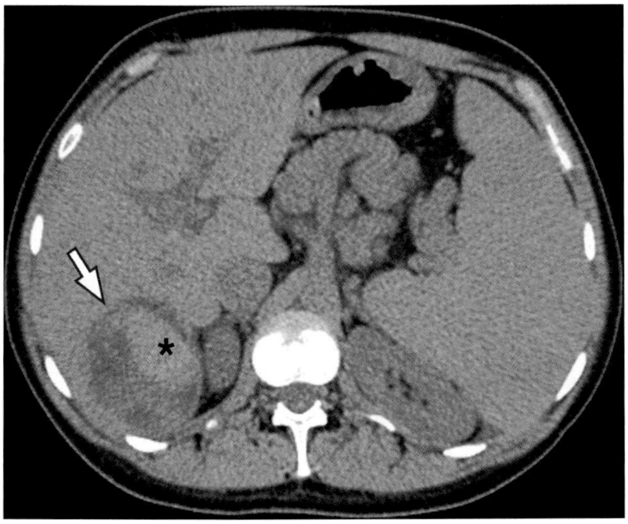

FIGURE 14.24 **A 22-year-old woman with a history of congenital heart disease, portal hypertension, and acute abdominal pain.** The patient was diagnosed with a ruptured hepatic adenoma. Axial noncontrast CT image of the abdomen shows a heterogeneous mass (*arrow*) within the posterior section of the right hepatic lobe. Mixed attenuation within the lesion is due to hemorrhage, with acute hemorrhage (*asterisk*) appearing as focal high attenuation.

and some hepatic adenomas can retain contrast (though generally less than normal background liver) on the hepatocyte phase of imaging (β-catenin mutated). Specific imaging features have not been well-defined for β-catenin mutated and unclassified hepatic adenomas; however, there is some evidence to suggest that MRI can distinguish the inflammatory and HNF-1α mutated hepatic adenoma subtypes.[46]

The two main complications of hepatic adenomas are bleeding and degeneration to HCC (Fig. 14.24). The risk of these complications depends on the subtype. Inflammatory hepatic adenomas are the most likely to bleed, with the risk of hemorrhage increasing with the size of the tumor.[46] HNF-1α mutated hepatic adenomas are the least aggressive and have the smallest risk of hemorrhage or malignant degeneration. β-catenin mutated hepatic adenomas have the highest risk of malignant transformation to HCC. Risk factors that increase the likelihood of malignant transformation include male gender, glycogen storage disease, anabolic steroid use, β-catenin subtype, and size larger than 5 cm.[46]

Hepatic adenomas are first treated with discontinuation of hormonal therapy (e.g., oral contraceptives).[24] Lesions larger than 5 cm and those that enlarge or fail to regress are typically surgically resected. Radiofrequency ablation has been used to treat small hepatic adenomas.[47] Depending on the size, location, and number of hepatic adenomas, orthotopic liver transplant may be performed.[45]

Malignant Neoplasms

Hepatic Metastasis

Metastases are the most common malignant tumor to involve the liver in children and are most commonly seen with neuroblastoma and Wilms tumor. Metastases can be solitary or multifocal, and their appearance on imaging is variable. On MRI, if hepatocyte-specific contrast agents are used, metastases show no uptake of contrast material during the hepatocyte phase because of the absence of functioning hepatocytes in the lesions (Fig. 14.25). Hepatic metastases also commonly restrict diffusion of water on diffusion-weighted imaging (Fig. 14.25). Although uncommon, lymphoma can also involve the pediatric liver (Fig. 14.26).

Hepatoblastoma

Hepatoblastoma is the most common primary hepatic malignancy in childhood, accounting for between 65% and 80% of all pediatric liver tumors.[27,48,49] Median age at diagnosis is 18 months,[48] and 90% to 95% of cases are diagnosed before 4 years of age.[26,48] Risk factors for hepatoblastoma include male gender, genetic syndromes (familial adenomatous polyposis coli, Beckwith-Wiedemann, hemihypertrophy,

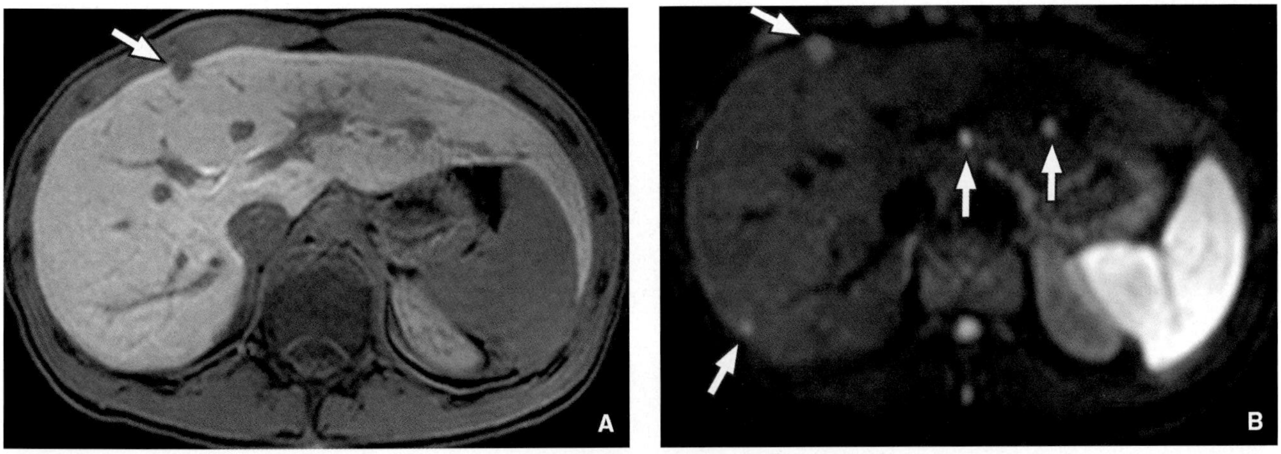

FIGURE 14.25 **A 15-year-old boy with metastatic nasopharyngeal carcinoma. A:** Axial postcontrast T1-weighted fat-suppressed MR image using a hepatocyte-specific contrast agent in the hepatocyte phase shows a peripheral hypointense metastasis (*arrow*) in the anterior section of the right hepatic lobe. **B:** Axial diffusion-weighted MR image shows additional metastatic lesions, which appear hyperintense (*arrows*). Several metastatic lesions in this patient were only seen on postcontrast hepatocyte phase and diffusion-weighted imaging. (Case courtesy of Jonathan R. Dillman, MD, MSc, Cincinnati Children's Hospital Medical Center, Cincinnati, OH.)

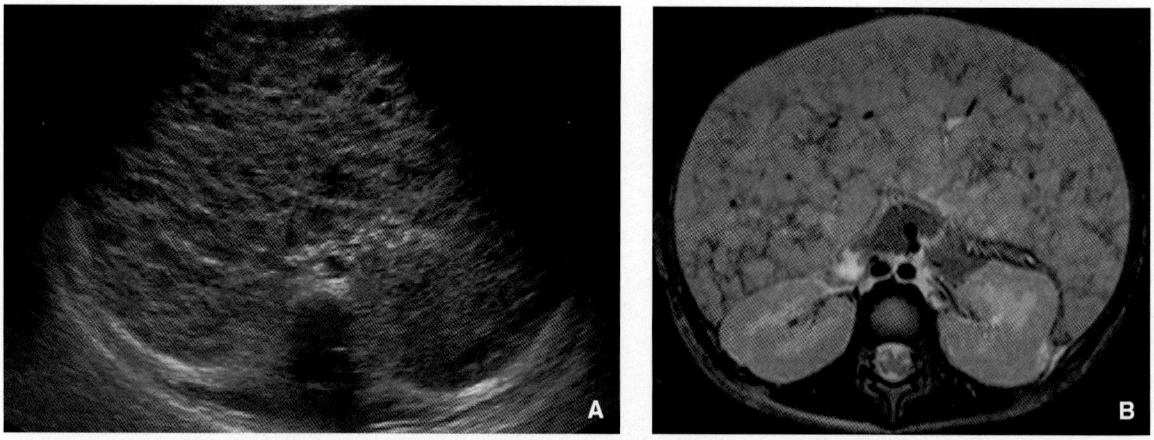

FIGURE 14.26 **A 3-year-old girl with large B-cell lymphoma. A:** Transverse gray-scale ultrasound image shows an enlarged liver containing many hypoechoic lesions. **B:** Axial T2-weighted MR image confirms hepatomegaly due to innumerable small hyperintense masses. Bilateral renal masses were also evident on postcontrast imaging. Liver biopsy confirmed the presence of hepatic lymphoma. (Case courtesy of Jonathan R. Dillman, MD, MSc, Cincinnati Children's Hospital Medical Center, Cincinnati, OH.)

and trisomy 18), low birth weight, and prematurity.[25,50,51] Of pediatric patients with hepatoblastoma, 6.4% have an associated congenital anomaly.[50] Children with hepatoblastoma usually present with a palpable abdominal mass, and sometimes with nonspecific anorexia and weight loss.[25,27] Rarely, affected pediatric patients present with precocious puberty/virilization due to secretion of human chorionic gonadotropin (β-HCG).[27] Serum AFP is elevated in 90% of patients; tumors that do not express AFP have a worse prognosis.[25,26]

Histologically, hepatoblastoma is classified into two types, epithelial and mixed.[25] The epithelial type of hepatoblastoma is the most common and consists of primitive hepatocytes mimicking those seen in embryonal or fetal life (Fig. 14.27). When mesenchymal elements, such as bone, cartilage, or adipose tissue, are admixed, the tumor is termed a mixed type. In general, tumor behavior is linked to the degree of hepatocyte differentiation, with the most "mature" tumors (pure fetal pattern) having a better prognosis and small cell undifferentiated pattern correlating with a worse prognosis.

The role of imaging in hepatoblastoma is to confirm the diagnosis, stage the disease, and assist in surgical planning. Attention should be paid to hepatic sectional and vascular anatomy as these determine disease stage and resectability. CT of the chest should be performed in all cases, as lung is the most common site of metastatic disease.[52]

On ultrasound, the appearance of hepatoblastoma is variable. The tumor is usually heterogeneously hyperechoic compared to background liver (Fig. 14.28).[52] Calcifications and necrosis may be identifiable.[52] Color Doppler can be useful to assess location and involvement of vascular structures. On noncontrast CT, hepatoblastoma typically appears as a well-defined hypoattenuating mass compared to normal background liver.[25] Calcifications are visible in approximately 50% and are usually small and fine in epithelial tumors and

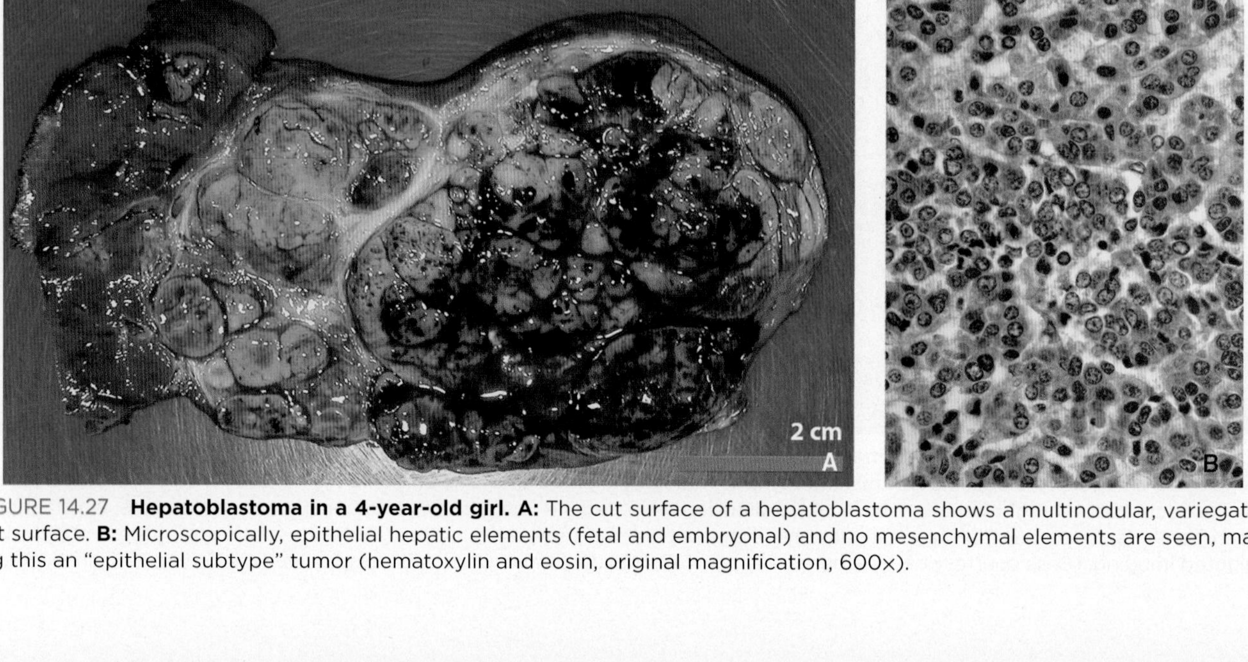

FIGURE 14.27 **Hepatoblastoma in a 4-year-old girl. A:** The cut surface of a hepatoblastoma shows a multinodular, variegated cut surface. **B:** Microscopically, epithelial hepatic elements (fetal and embryonal) and no mesenchymal elements are seen, making this an "epithelial subtype" tumor (hematoxylin and eosin, original magnification, 600×).

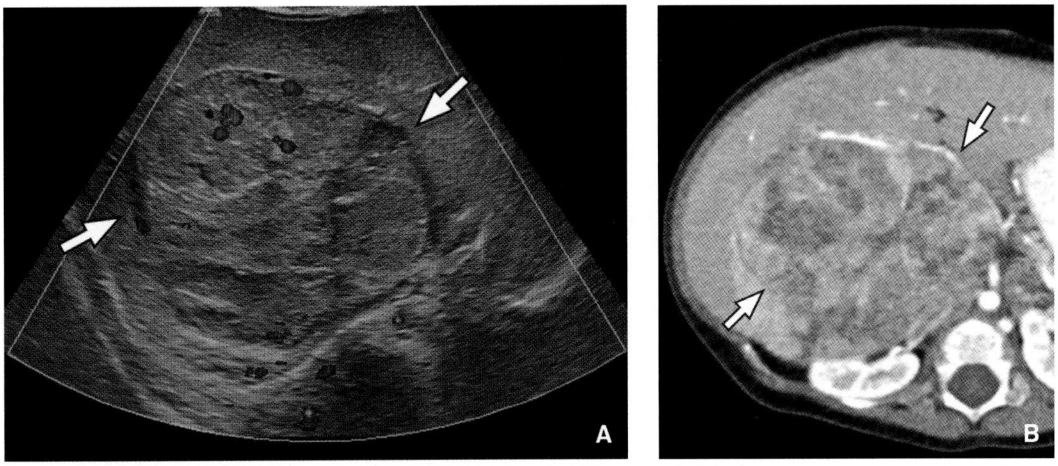

FIGURE 14.28 **A 15-month-old boy with hepatoblastoma. A:** Transverse color Doppler ultrasound image shows a heterogeneous mass (*arrows*) arising from the liver with internal vascularity. **B:** Axial contrast-enhanced CT image in the hepatic arterial phase of imaging shows a heterogeneous mass (*arrows*) with areas of hyperenhancement relative to normal liver arising from the inferior aspect of the right lobe of the liver. There is mass effect on the right kidney.

coarse in mixed mesenchymal–epithelial tumors.[25,52] The MRI appearance of hepatoblastoma depends on the histologic subtype. Epithelial tumors typically appear homogeneously hypointense on T1-weighted MR images and hyperintense on T2-weighted MR images.[52] Mixed epithelial–mesenchymal tumors are more often heterogeneous because of the presence of intralesional calcification, cartilage, and fibrous septa (Fig. 14.29).[52]

Following intravenous contrast material administration, rim and septal enhancement may be seen early on CT and MRI (Fig. 14.28), with the tumor appearing hypoenhancing relative to background liver during the delayed phases (Fig. 14.29).[25,52] Attention should be paid to the hepatic vasculature and IVC to exclude bland or tumor thrombus. Hepatoblastoma can have a variable appearance on the hepatocyte phase of imaging if hepatocyte-specific contrast agents are used.[33] The majority of tumors show decreased uptake with a small number showing variable retention of contrast.[35] Intrahepatic satellite lesions can occur.

The most commonly used staging system is the pretreatment extent of disease (PRETEXT) system. Primary tumor staging under this system reflects the number of liver sections that need to be resected to completely excise the tumor. The PRETEXT number is obtained by subtracting the number of contiguous tumor-free sections of the liver from four.[53,54] In addition to describing the anatomic extent of the tumor, the PRETEXT staging system includes other criteria defining involvement of the IVC or hepatic veins, portal vein, extrahepatic disease, and distant metastases.[53]

Pediatric patients with hepatoblastoma are treated with either up-front surgical resection or neoadjuvant chemotherapy followed by surgery.[55] Patients treated with cisplatin-based chemotherapy and complete surgical resection have a 5-year survival rate of 80% to 90%.[56] Ten to twenty percent of tumors are unresectable and are treated with neoadjuvant chemotherapy followed by liver transplantation.[56] Overall survival in this group ranges from 82% to 100%.[56]

Hepatocellular Carcinoma

HCC is the second most common primary pediatric liver malignancy, accounting for <25% of hepatic malignancies.[25] HCC generally occurs in older children and adolescents (>10 years of age).[48] Known risk factors for developing HCC during childhood include cirrhosis, chronic hepatitis B or C infection, type 1 glycogen storage disease, tyrosinemia, hemochromatosis, alpha-1 antitrypsin deficiency, autoimmune hepatitis, primary sclerosing cholangitis (PSC), biliary atresia, familial cholestatic jaundice, Wilson disease, Alagille syndrome, neurofibromatosis, ataxia–telangiectasia, and Fanconi anemia.[25,26,48] Preexisting liver disease, however, is present in only 30% to 50% of patients.[25,57] Children with HCC usually present with a large abdominal mass and elevated serum AFP levels.[25,58]

Like in hepatoblastoma, the role of imaging in HCC is to confirm the diagnosis, stage the disease, and assist in surgical planning. In general, there are three patterns of primary tumor growth in HCC: a solitary mass, multinodular tumor, and diffuse infiltrative tumor [6]. Metastatic disease is present in 25% to 50% of patients at the time of diagnosis and most commonly occurs in the lungs.[58,59]

Small HCCs are generally hypoechoic by ultrasound, but can be variable in appearance.[25] On noncontrast CT, hypoattenuation is typical. On MRI, lesions are typically predominantly hypo- to isointense on T1-weighted MR images and slightly hyperintense on T2-weighted MR images. However, large lesions can appear homogeneous or heterogeneous by any of these modalities depending on the presence of internal macro- and microscopic fat, hemorrhage, and/or necrosis.[25]

HCCs are supplied by the hepatic artery, and, thus, show arterial phase hyperenhancement.[25,58] On the portal venous phase of imaging, HCC can be variable in appearance.[25,58] With hepatocyte-specific contrast agents, HCC typically shows decreased uptake on the hepatocyte phase, although well-differentiated HCC may appear hyperintense relative

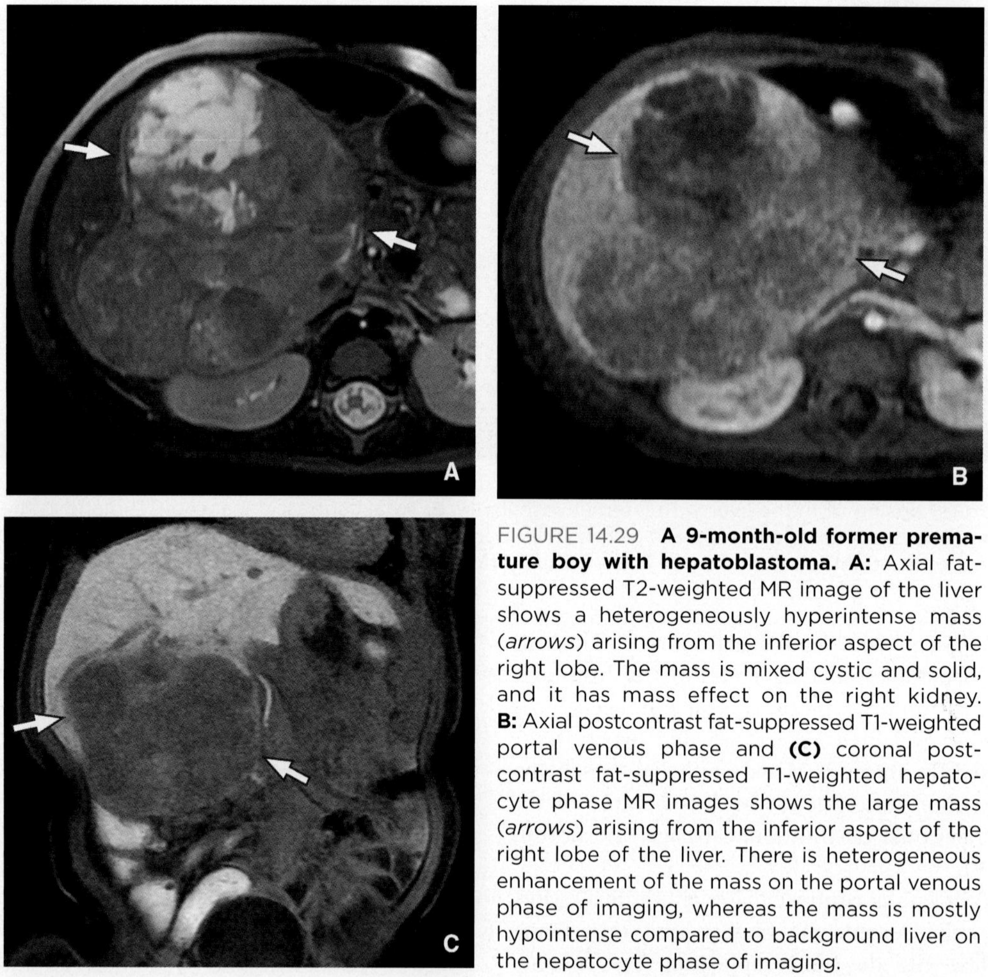

FIGURE 14.29 **A 9-month-old former premature boy with hepatoblastoma. A:** Axial fat-suppressed T2-weighted MR image of the liver shows a heterogeneously hyperintense mass (*arrows*) arising from the inferior aspect of the right lobe. The mass is mixed cystic and solid, and it has mass effect on the right kidney. **B:** Axial postcontrast fat-suppressed T1-weighted portal venous phase and **(C)** coronal postcontrast fat-suppressed T1-weighted hepatocyte phase MR images shows the large mass (*arrows*) arising from the inferior aspect of the right lobe of the liver. There is heterogeneous enhancement of the mass on the portal venous phase of imaging, whereas the mass is mostly hypointense compared to background liver on the hepatocyte phase of imaging.

to background liver.[33] Careful attention must be paid to the hepatic vasculature to exclude tumor invasion (Fig. 14.30).

Children with HCC have a poor prognosis with an overall survival rate of 10% to 30%.[25,59] Survival is largely dependent on tumor resectability, but two-thirds of patients have unresectable disease at diagnosis.[25] HCC is relatively chemotherapy resistant with 30% to 50% of affected pediatric patients showing some response.[57,60] Alternative treatment strategies include radiofrequency ablation, transarterial chemoembolization, 90Y radioembolization, and liver transplantation. The 5-year survival rate of childhood HCC treated with liver transplantation is 63% to 83%.[61,62]

Fibrolamellar Hepatocellular Carcinoma

Fibrolamellar hepatocellular carcinoma (FLH) is a rare (0.85% of all primary liver malignancies) variant of HCC with unique clinical, imaging, and histologic features. The tumor is more common in adolescents and young adults with a peak incidence near 25 years of age.[63] Pediatric patients with FLH typically present with an abdominal mass with occasional gynecomastia or jaundice.[25] Most affected pediatric patients do not have underlying liver disease.[64] Serum AFP is usually not elevated, but serum B12, unsaturated B12-binding capacity, and serum neurotensin are elevated.[64–66] FLH most often occurs as a solitary mass, more commonly in the left lobe of the liver.[64] A central stellate or amorphous scar is present in 33% to 60%[25,63,66] (Fig. 14.31). Lymph node metastases are common.

On ultrasound, FLH usually appears as a solitary, well-circumscribed mass with heterogeneous echotexture (Fig. 14.32).[25,66] If a central scar is present, it appears hyperechoic. On noncontrast CT, FLHs are heterogeneously hypoattenuating with a lobular contour.[63,66] Calcifications are present in 35% to 68% of tumors and tend to be centrally located, small, and fewer than three in number.[63] On MRI, FLHs are usually hypointense on T1-weighted MR images and slightly hyperintense on T2-weighted MR images.[25] The central scar, if present, is hypointense on all sequences, distinguishing this lesion from FNH, which has a T2-weighted hyperintense scar (Fig. 14.32).[63] FLHs show arterial hyperenhancement in 80% of cases.[63] On the portal venous phase, the enhancement pattern of FLH is variable. The central scar does not enhance on delayed postcontrast imaging, further distinguishing this tumor from FNH.[25,63,66] Intrahepatic satellite lesions can occur.

The current concept is that there is no difference in prognosis between FLH and HCC.[63,65] Overall 5-year survival for patients with FLH is 45%.[65] Surgical resection is the mainstay of treatment and the only chance for cure. Unresectable disease has a 5-year survival of 0%.[63] Multifocality, vascular invasion, tumors larger than 5 cm, serum AFP >2,000 μg/mL,

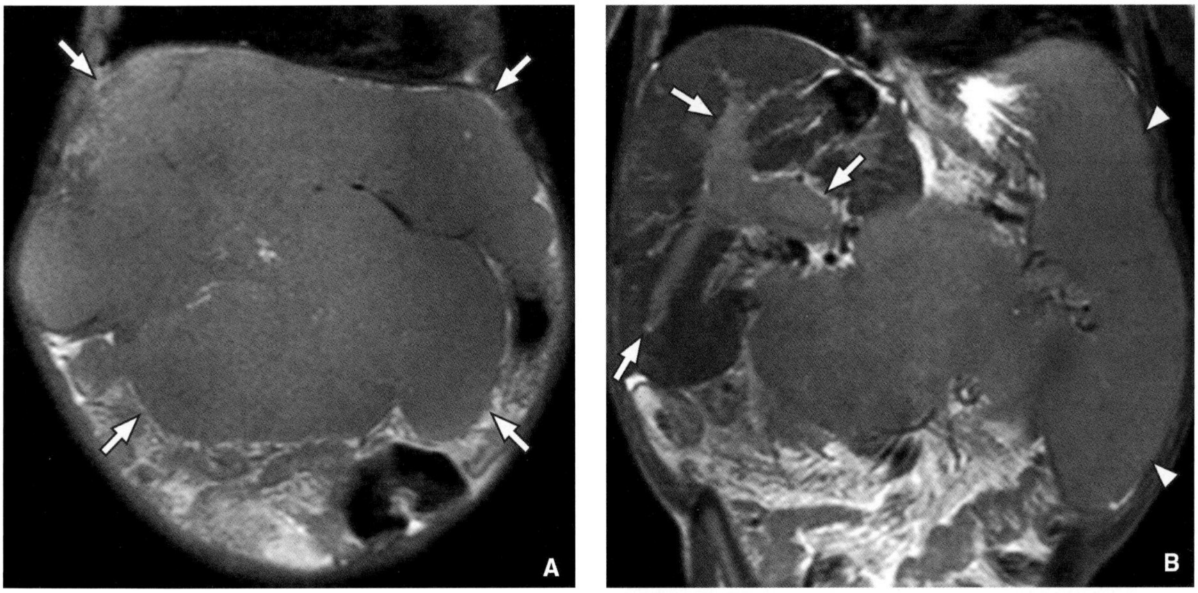

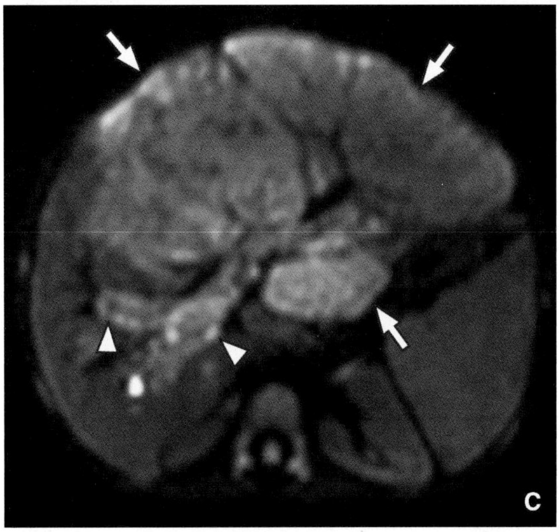

FIGURE 14.30 **A 5-year-old girl with Alagille syndrome, hepatocellular carcinoma, and tumor thrombus in the portal veins. A:** Coronal T2-weighted fat-suppressed MR image shows a large mildly hyperintense mass (*arrows*) occupying the entire left lobe of the liver. **B:** A more posterior image shows tumor thrombus (*arrows*) filling the main portal vein and its branches. Tumor thrombus has identical signal intensity to the primary mass. The spleen (*arrowheads*) is enlarged because of chronic liver disease and portal hypertension. **C:** Axial diffusion-weighted MR image shows that both the primary mass (*arrows*) and tumor thrombus (*arrowheads*) restrict (impede) diffusion of water.

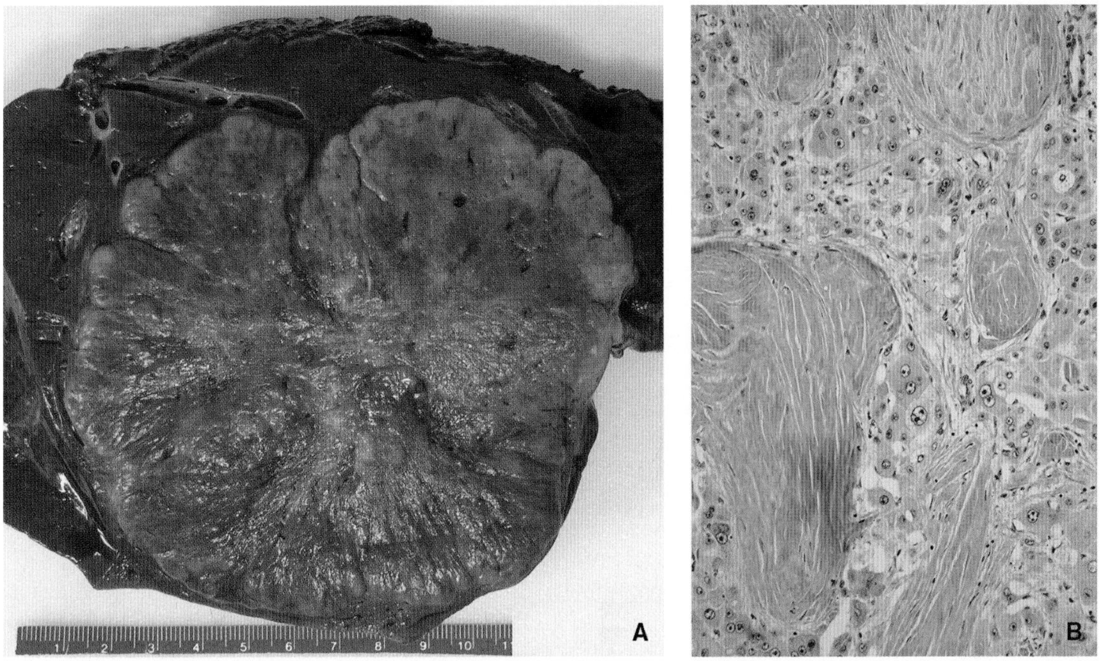

FIGURE 14.31 **Fibrolamellar hepatocelluar carcinoma. A:** The cut surface of a fibrolamellar hepatocellular carcinoma shows a firm and somewhat lobuar mass which stands out from the surrounding liver as more pale and gray. **B:** Microscopically, tumor cells are large with prominent nucleoli and copious pink cytoplasm, and prominent short fibrous bands ("lamellar fibrosis") are interspersed (hematoxylin and eosin, original magnification, 200×).

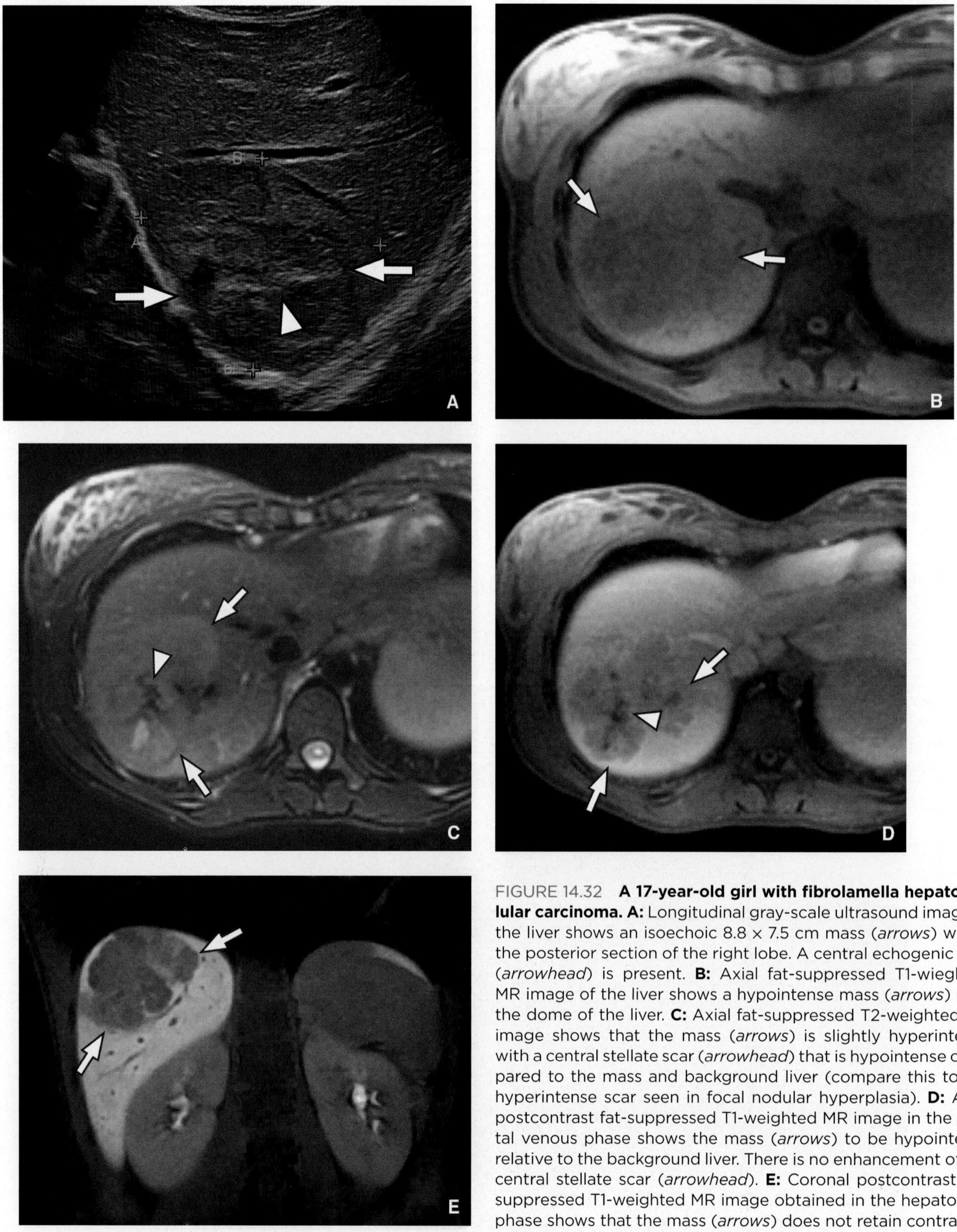

FIGURE 14.32 **A 17-year-old girl with fibrolamella hepatocellular carcinoma. A:** Longitudinal gray-scale ultrasound image of the liver shows an isoechoic 8.8 × 7.5 cm mass (*arrows*) within the posterior section of the right lobe. A central echogenic scar (*arrowhead*) is present. **B:** Axial fat-suppressed T1-wieghted MR image of the liver shows a hypointense mass (*arrows*) near the dome of the liver. **C:** Axial fat-suppressed T2-weighted MR image shows that the mass (*arrows*) is slightly hyperintense with a central stellate scar (*arrowhead*) that is hypointense compared to the mass and background liver (compare this to the hyperintense scar seen in focal nodular hyperplasia). **D:** Axial postcontrast fat-suppressed T1-weighted MR image in the portal venous phase shows the mass (*arrows*) to be hypointense relative to the background liver. There is no enhancement of the central stellate scar (*arrowhead*). **E:** Coronal postcontrast fat-suppressed T1-weighted MR image obtained in the hepatocyte phase shows that the mass (*arrows*) does not retain contrast.

positive resection margins, and positive lymph nodes all portend worse outcomes.[63,67] After surgical resection, relapse rates are high (36% to 100%).[65] Sites of recurrence for FLH include the liver, regional lymph nodes, peritoneum, and lungs.[67] Aggressive surgical and medical treatment for relapsed disease can help to prolong survival.[65]

Undifferentiated Embryonal Sarcoma

Undifferentiated embryonal sarcoma of the liver is a rare malignant hepatic neoplasm composed of malignant mesenchymal cells that are frequently pleomorphic and bizarre.[68,69] Embryonal sarcoma is the third most common primary pediatric hepatic malignancy (9% to 13%), with a peak incidence

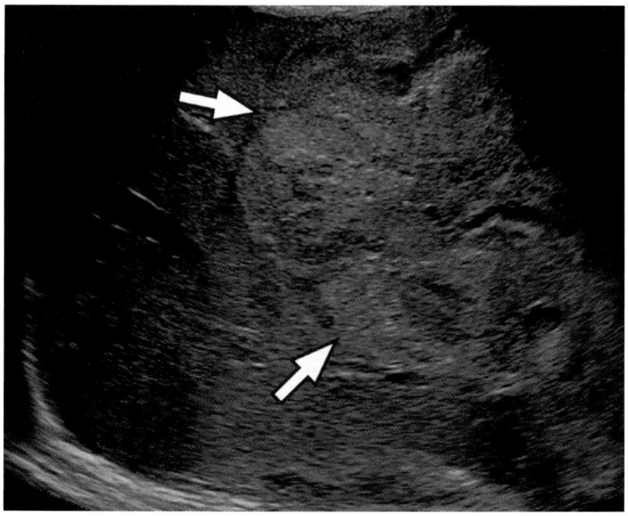

FIGURE 14.33 **A 12-year-old girl with hepatic undifferentiated embryonal sarcoma.** Longitudinal gray-scale ultrasound image of the liver shows a large slightly hyperechoic lobulated predominantly solid mass (*arrows*).

in patients between 5 and 10 years of age.[69,70] Affected pediatric patients typically present with an abdominal mass, abdominal pain, nausea, and/or anorexia.[68,71] There is a predilection for the right lobe of the liver.[68] Metastases, if present, typically involve the lungs, pleura, and peritoneum.[25] Genetically, many embryonal sarcomas harbor the chromosomal translocation t(15;19)(q13;q13.4), which has also been identified in mesenchymal hamartoma of the liver, a neoplasm that may occasionally coexist with embryonal sarcoma.[43,44]

On ultrasound, embryonal sarcoma typically appears solid and iso- to hyperechoic compared to background liver (Fig. 14.33).[25,68,71] Small anechoic or hypoechoic spaces corresponding to foci of necrosis, hemorrhage, and cystic degeneration may be present.[25] On CT and MRI, embryonal sarcoma commonly appears as a mixed solid and cystic mass, often with internal debris and hemorrhage that appear as high attenuation on CT and increased T1-weighted signal on MRI[25,68,71] (Fig. 14.34). Hematocrit levels may be seen on MRI (Fig. 14.34); calcifications are rare.[25] On MRI, a surrounding

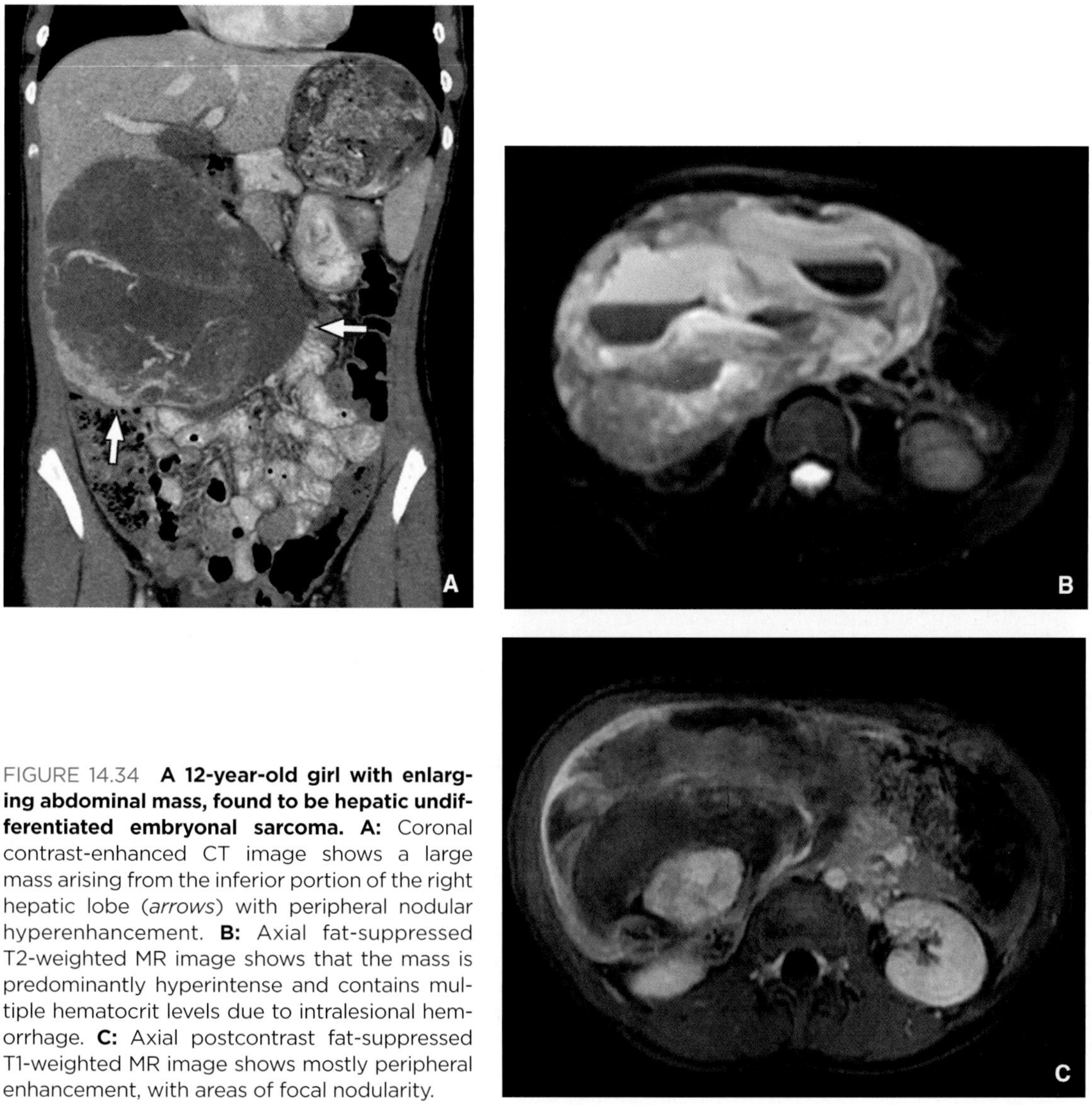

FIGURE 14.34 **A 12-year-old girl with enlarging abdominal mass, found to be hepatic undifferentiated embryonal sarcoma. A:** Coronal contrast-enhanced CT image shows a large mass arising from the inferior portion of the right hepatic lobe (*arrows*) with peripheral nodular hyperenhancement. **B:** Axial fat-suppressed T2-weighted MR image shows that the mass is predominantly hyperintense and contains multiple hematocrit levels due to intralesional hemorrhage. **C:** Axial postcontrast fat-suppressed T1-weighted MR image shows mostly peripheral enhancement, with areas of focal nodularity.

fibrous pseudocapsule can appear hypointense on both T1- and T2-weighted MR images.[25] Following intravenous contrast material administration, embryonal sarcoma does not substantially enhance in the arterial phase. Peripheral and solid nodular components of the lesion generally show heterogeneous enhancement on later postcontrast phases[25,68,71] (Fig. 14.34). If hepatocyte-specific contrast agents are used, embryonal sarcoma appears hypointense compared to background liver on the hepatocyte phase images.[33]

Although prognosis of this neoplasm has been historically dismal, embryonal sarcoma is now considered potentially curable and is typically treated with neoadjuvant chemotherapy followed by surgical resection or transplant.[25,68,72,73]

Traumatic Disorders

Trauma is the number one cause of death in children worldwide, accounting for more than 500,000 hospital admissions and 20,000 deaths per year in the United States.[74,75] The abdomen is the second most common site of injury after the head. Children are at increased risk of traumatic abdominal injuries due to an incompletely ossified rib cage, underdeveloped chest and abdominal wall musculature, proportionally larger visceral organs relative to total body size, and less intra-abdominal fat to cushion blows.[76]

The liver is the most frequently injured organ in children following abdominal trauma.[77] The right hepatic lobe is injured more often than the left, and blunt injuries are more common than penetrating injuries. Iatrogenic liver injury may also occur related to percutaneous biopsy, laparoscopic surgery, or open surgery. Injuries of other visceral organs, as well as fractures, may be seen in association with liver injuries. Indications for imaging after suspected trauma to the liver include physical examination or laboratory findings of injury, including abdominal distention, abdominal wall ecchymosis, absence of bowel sounds, pain, vomiting, decreased hematocrit, and elevated liver enzymes.

Imaging in the pediatric abdominal trauma patient is typically limited to ultrasound and/or CT in the acute setting. Ultrasound can be rapidly performed, including at the bedside. Although a recent meta-analysis of the efficacy of abdominal ultrasound in pediatric trauma patients showed a sensitivity of 80% and specificity of 96%, other studies have shown that up to one-third of solid organ injuries may be missed with ultrasound.[78,79] At pediatric institutions, the "focused abdominal sonography for trauma" (FAST) exam is variably used to evaluate the upper quadrants and pelvis for evidence of hemoperitoneum in trauma patients.

In hemodynamically stable pediatric trauma patients, CT remains the imaging modality of choice. Intravenous iodinated contrast material administration is essential as it allows for visualization of solid organ lacerations, hematomas, and active hemorrhage. Multiphase imaging for the evaluation of liver injury is generally not necessary. The administration of oral contrast material in the setting of an abdominal CT for trauma is controversial, and is not currently performed at multiple large level I pediatric trauma centers mostly because of concern about delay in patient management.[79]

Types of Traumatic Hepatic Injury

Types of liver injuries detected on CT include lacerations, contusions/hematomas, and vascular injuries. Lacerations typically manifest as hypoattenuating linear and branching defects in the liver parenchyma. Hematomas can be intraparenchymal and/or subcapsular in location. Vascular injuries can manifest as pseudoaneurysms, active hemorrhage, or geographic areas of decreased attenuation reflecting devascularization. Pseudoaneurysms and active hemorrhage both appear as focal areas of hyperattenuation (typically similar in attenuation to arterial blood pool). Pseudoaneurysms are generally well-defined and contained, whereas active extravasation appears more irregular, poorly defined, and to be present in association with hematoma. Hemoperitoneum and/or hemoretroperitoneum may or may not be present with liver injuries depending on whether or not there is disruption of the liver capsule, or injury to the bare area of the liver (which communicates with the retroperitoneal space). Periportal low attenuation is frequently encountered on pediatric trauma CT examinations and is thought to reflect distended periportal lymphatics related to fluid resuscitation.[79]

Grading Scale of Traumatic Hepatic Injury

The most widely used injury grading scale for liver trauma is from the American Association for the Surgery of Trauma (AAST).[80] There are six grades of injury that depend on the size of subcapsular collection, the depth of parenchymal injury, the integrity of the liver capsule, and the state of the vascular

TABLE 14.2 American Association for the Surgery of Trauma Liver Injury Scale (1994 Revision)

Grade	Injury Description
I	Subcapsular hematoma <10% surface area OR laceration <1 cm parenchymal depth, capsular tear
II	Subcapsular hematoma 10%–50% surface area OR intraparenchymal hematoma <10 cm diameter OR laceration <10 cm in length, capsular tear 1–3 cm parenchymal depth
III	Subcapsular hematoma >50% surface area OR ruptured subcapsular or parenchymal hematoma OR intraparenchymal hematoma > 10 cm or expanding OR laceration > 3 cm parenchymal depth
IV	Laceration/parenchymal disruption involving 25%–75% of hepatic lobe OR 1–3 Couinaud segments
V	Parenchymal disruption involving >75% of hepatic lobe OR >3 Couinaud segments within a single lobe OR juxtahepatic venous injuries (retrohepatic IVC/central major hepatic veins)
VI	Hepatic avulsion

Adapted from http://www.aast.org/Library/TraumaTools/InjuryScorigScalesaspx#liver. Ref. 80.

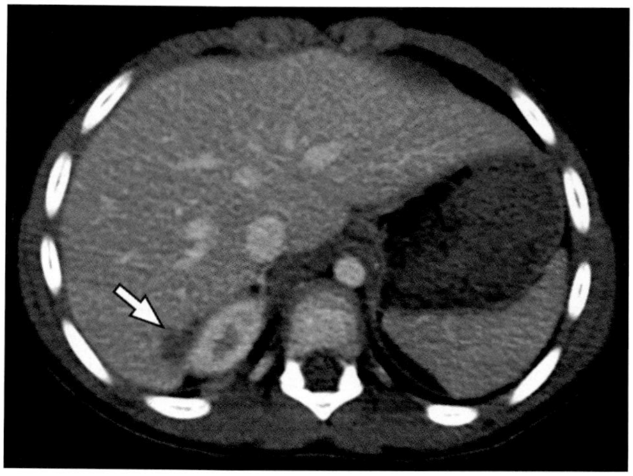

FIGURE 14.35 **A 6-year-old pedestrian girl hit by a motor vehicle.** Axial contrast-enhanced CT image shows focal subcapsular low attenuation consistent with hematoma (*arrow*) involving <10% of the liver surface area, consistent with a grade I injury.

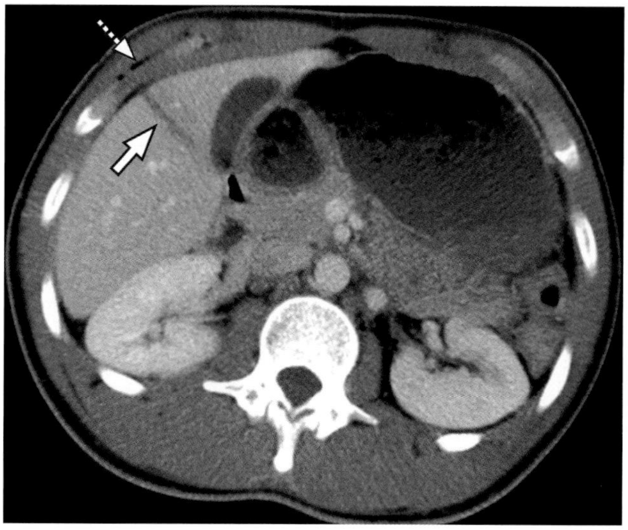

FIGURE 14.37 **A 17-year-old boy with right upper abdominal trauma.** Axial contrast-enhanced CT image shows linear hypoattenuation involving the capsule and extending >3 cm in parenchymal depth (*solid arrow*), consistent with a laceration. Air bubbles in the anterior abdominal wall (*dashed arrow*) are also posttraumatic. This is consistent with a grade III injury.

pedicle and juxtahepatic veins (Table 14.2). Examples of the various grades of traumatic liver injuries seen in children are seen in Figures 14.35 to 14.39. Complications that can arise following hepatic trauma and may be detected on surveillance imaging include bilomas (Fig. 14.40), infarcts, pseudoaneurysms, and arteriovenous fistulas.

Hepatic Injury Related to Non-accidental Trauma (Child Abuse)

Liver injury related to child abuse deserves specific mention. Abdominal injuries are second to only head injuries as the leading cause of death in the setting of child abuse, with mortality rates ranging from 13% to 30%.[81,82] Hepatic injury is the most frequent intra-abdominal injury seen in this population.[81,83] Indications for when to perform abdominal CT imaging in a child suspected of being abused remain controversial. The literature suggests that children suspected of being abused who have liver transaminase levels >80 IU/L should undergo CT imaging.[84] Others have suggested CT imaging for those children suspected of being abused who have absent/hypoactive bowel sounds, liver transaminases greater than twice normal, or multiple physical exam or laboratory abnormalities.[82] CT findings of abusive liver injury are similar to those seen in other forms of blunt trauma,[81] although left hepatic lobe trauma along with other signs of compressive injury against the spine, such as pancreatic and duodenal (hematoma or perforation) injury, should raise suspicion for abuse in the correct clinical setting (Fig. 14.41).

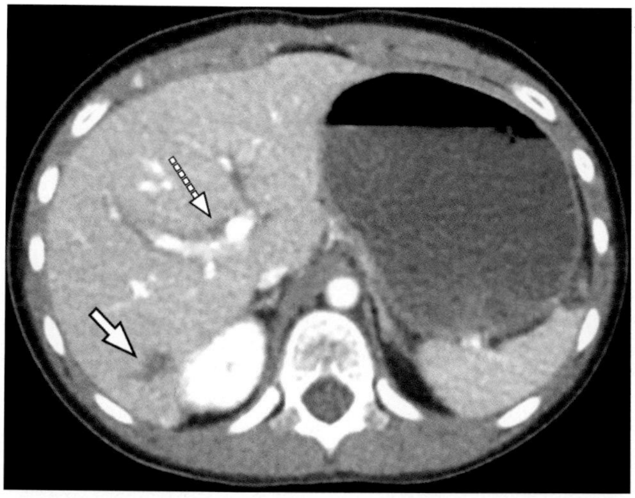

FIGURE 14.36 **A 9-year-old girl involved in a motor vehicle collision.** Axial contrast-enhanced CT image shows a small laceration (*solid arrow*) that is <10 cm in length, and extends 1 to 3 cm in parenchymal depth, consistent with a grade II injury. Note also the periportal edema (*dashed arrow*), a finding commonly seen in trauma patients related to fluid resuscitation.

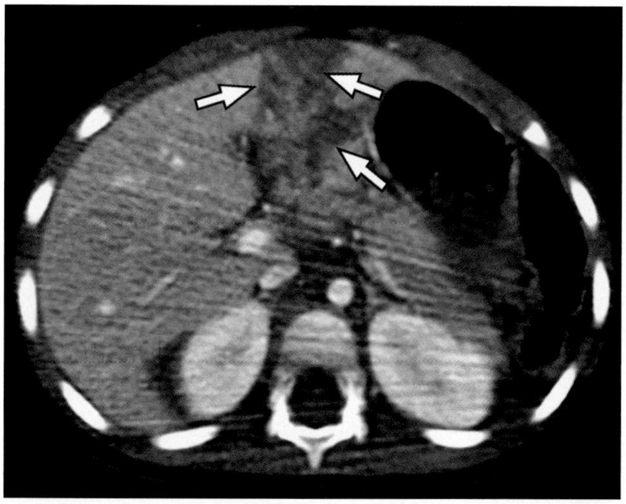

FIGURE 14.38 **A 3-year-old girl ejected from a car because of motor vehicle accident.** Axial contrast-enhanced CT image shows a complex laceration/parenchymal hematoma (*arrows*) involving a large percentage of the left hepatic lobe, consistent with a grade IV injury. Extensive streak artifact is due to the child's left arm which could not be repositioned.

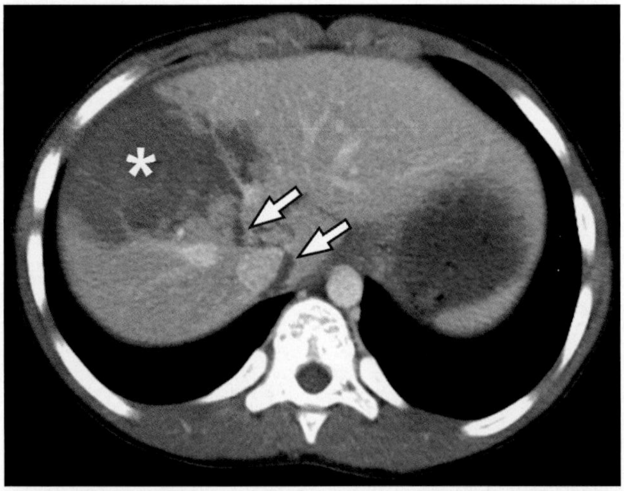

FIGURE 14.39 **A 10-year-old girl who suffered a handlebar injury while bicycle riding.** Axial contrast-enhanced CT image shows a large parenchymal hematoma in the right lobe (*asterisk*), as well a laceration (*arrows*) extending to the IVC and left hepatic vein, consistent with a grade V injury.

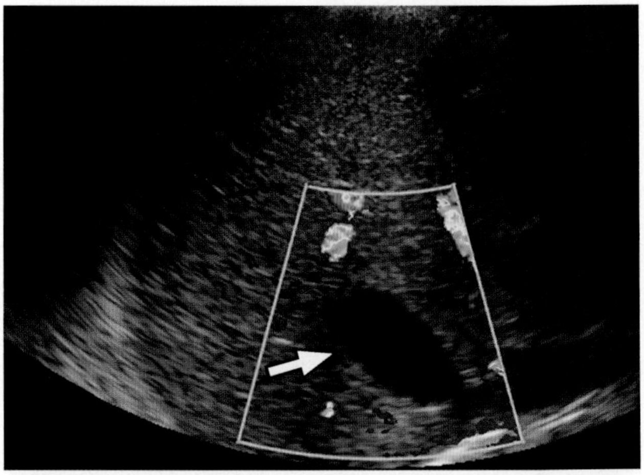

FIGURE 14.40 **A 16-year-old boy who was involved in a motor vehicle accident.** Five weeks after the accident, the patient continued to have right upper quadrant pain. Transverse color Doppler ultrasound image demonstrates a well-circumscribed, anechoic, avascular fluid collection (*arrow*) within the posterior right hepatic lobe, which was subsequently drained and determined to be a biloma.

Hepatic Cirrhosis and Portal Hypertension

Hepatic Cirrhosis

Hepatic Cirrhosis is the result of chronic liver disease and is characterized by progressive fibrosis and nodular regeneration.[85] In children, the most common causes of chronic liver disease are hepatitis, genetic/metabolic disorders, and biliary disorders (Table 14.3).[86,87] Specific diseases that cause cirrhosis in children are detailed in the following sections.

Morphologic findings of cirrhosis that are apparent by imaging include heterogeneously coarsened hepatic echotexture by ultrasound, parenchymal and surface nodularity, small right hepatic lobe with enlargement of the left and caudate lobes, and widening of the hepatic fissure (Figs. 14.42 and 14.43).[85] MRI commonly reveals reticular or band-like areas of T2-weighted signal hyperintensity that show delayed enhancement when using conventional gadolinium contrast agents or hypoenhancement compared to normal liver when using a hepatocyte-specific contrast agent. Complications of cirrhosis, including HCC and sequelae of portal hypertension (see following section), are also apparent by imaging.

Traditionally, liver biopsy has been considered the gold standard for the diagnosis and staging of cirrhosis. Biopsy, however, is an imperfect standard. Percutaneous core needle biopsy is invasive and carries risks of pain, bleeding, pneumothorax, and rarely death. Children also commonly require deep sedation or general anesthesia and an overnight hospital admission when undergoing a liver biopsy, adding both cost and risk.[85,88] Liver biopsy samples only a small portion of the liver and is thus subject to sampling error.[85] Other limitations of biopsy include subjective grading systems for parenchymal fibrosis, high degree of interobserver variability, and poor patient acceptance.[88]

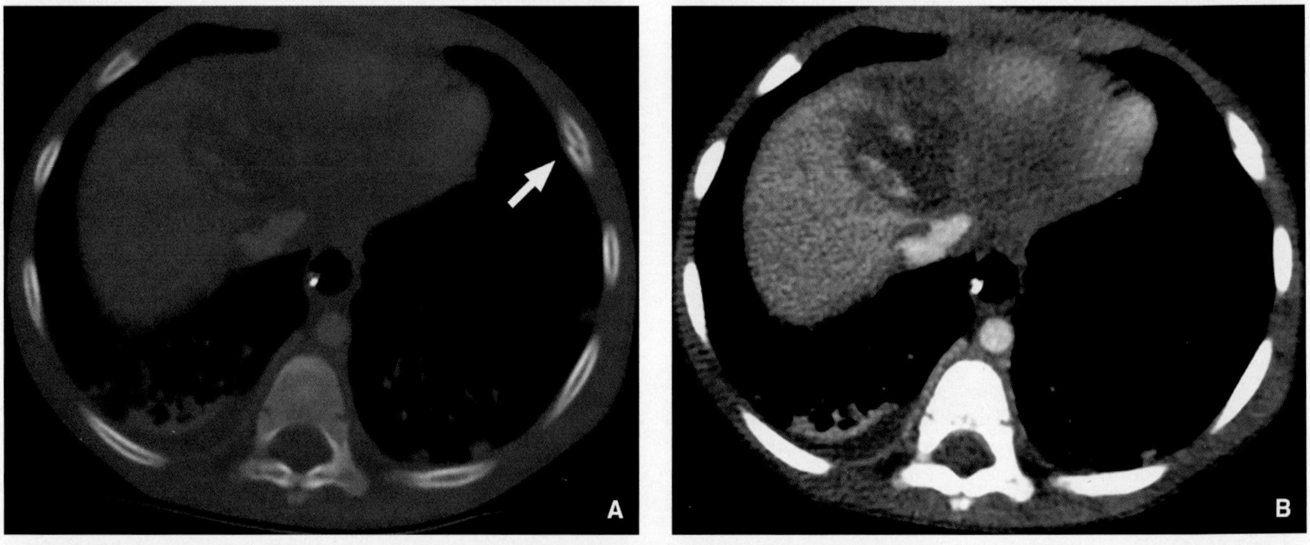

FIGURE 14.41 **A 1-year-old boy who suffered multiple abusive injuries.** Axial contrast-enhanced CT images in bone **(A)** and soft tissue **(B)** windows demonstrate a grade V liver injury (parenchymal hematoma/laceration extending to the inferior vena cava and hepatic veins) as well as a left anterolateral 8th rib fracture (*arrow*).

TABLE 14.3 Causes of Chronic Liver Disease in Children

Hepatitis
Infectious (hepatitis B virus, hepatitis C virus)
Autoimmune
Drug-related
Genetic/Metabolic Disorders
Nonalcoholic fatty liver disease (NAFLD)/nonalcoholic steatohepatitis (NASH)
Cystic fibrosis
Wilson disease
Glycogen storage disorders (see Table 14.5)
α-1-antitrypsin deficiency
Tyrosinemia
Progressive familial intrahepatic cholestasis syndromes
Gestational alloimmune liver disease/neonatal hemochromatosis
Biliary Disorders
Biliary atresia
Alagille syndrome
Primary sclerosing cholangitis

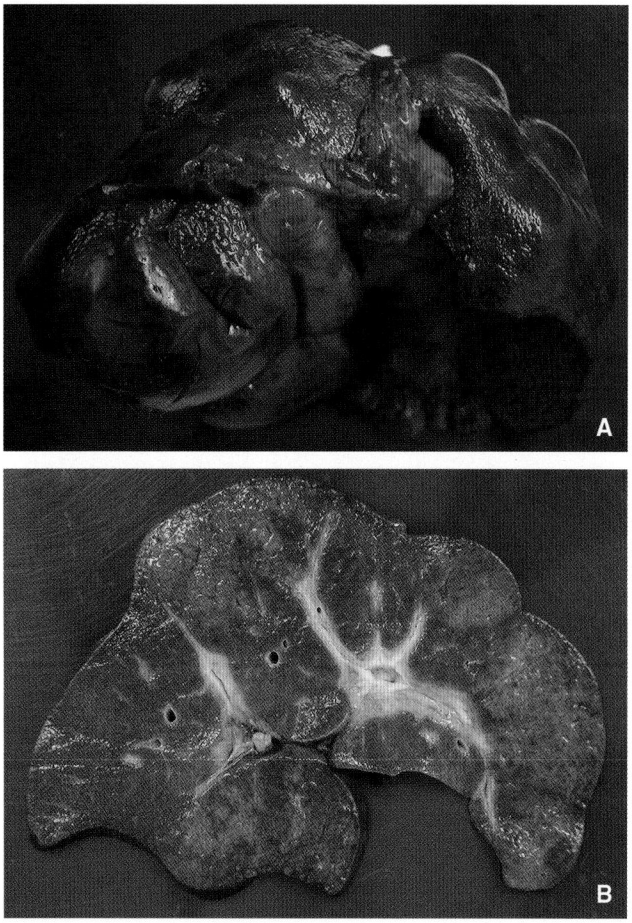

FIGURE 14.42 **Cirrhotic liver from a 10-year-old boy with alpha-1-antitrypsin deficiency. A:** Surgical specimen demonstrates a macronodular external surface. **B:** The cut surface shows both micro- and macronodular changes.

There are a number of noninvasive methods of quantifying liver fibrosis. The most promising techniques are MRI and ultrasound-based shear wave elastography. These techniques measure the speed of propagation of shear waves through the liver to quantify hepatic stiffness (Figs. 14.1, 14.14 and 14.43).[86,88–90] Stiffness measurements obtained by tissue elastography are reproducible and correlate with the degree of liver fibrosis determined histologically.[91–93] Other MRI techniques described for the noninvasive assessment of hepatic fibrosis include diffusion-weighted imaging, magnetization transfer imaging, and spectroscopy, but these have not been extensively studied in pediatric patients.

Portal Hypertension

Portal hypertension is defined as pressure in the portal vein >10 mm Hg.[94] Affected pediatric patients are often diagnosed when splenomegaly and/or portosystemic collateral vessels become apparent based on physical examination or imaging.[95] Complications can be life-threatening and include variceal bleeding, ascites, hepatopulmonary syndrome, portopulmonary hypertension, and hepatic encephalopathy.[95] Portal hypertension can be cirrhotic or noncirrhotic in etiology. The noncirrhotic causes of portal hypertension are typically vascular in nature and are classified based on the site of increased vascular resistance as prehepatic, hepatic, or posthepatic (Table 14.4).[94] The hepatic causes can be further subclassified as presinusoidal, sinusoidal, or postsinusoidal.[94]

Ultrasound is often the preferred imaging modality for assessment of portal hypertension in children as it allows for evaluation of both anatomy and blood flow. On grayscale ultrasound, the liver can have variable echogenicity depending on the underlying cause of disease and the presence of cirrhosis. The spleen is typically enlarged, and ascites may be present. If patent, the portal vein is typically enlarged. Collateral vessels (varices) commonly involve the esophagus and stomach and surrounding tissues, mesentery/omentum, and body wall. The paraumbilical vein may be recanalized, visible in the expected location of the falciform ligament. On Doppler ultrasound, the portal venous waveform varies depending on the severity of portal hypertension. Early in the course of the disorder, portal venous velocities may be normal or slightly decreased. As portal hypertension worsens, velocity continues to decrease until in advanced disease, blood flow reverses (Fig. 14.44). Morphologic imaging findings of portal hypertension, such as splenic enlargement and portosystemic collateral vessels, are similar in appearance by ultrasound, CT, and MRI (Fig. 14.45).

The treatment of portal hypertension depends on its cause and the specific symptoms. Bleeding varices are treated with endoscopic ligation or sclerotherapy.[95] A portosystemic shunt can be created to decrease pressure within the portal venous system and decrease risk of variceal bleeding, although hepatic encephalopathy is a

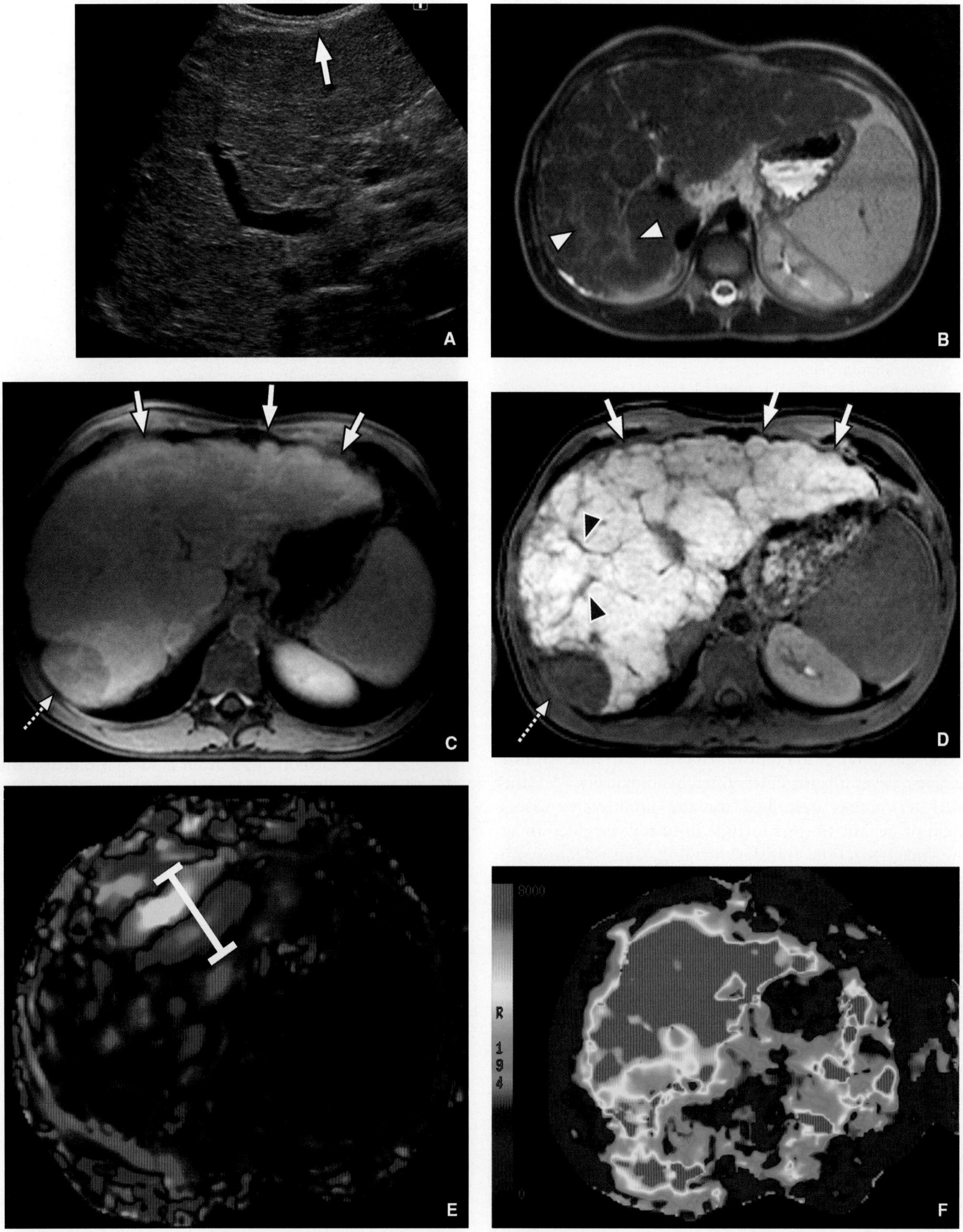

FIGURE 14.43 **An 11-year-old boy with a history of alpha-1 antitrypsin deficiency and cirrhosis. A:** Transverse gray-scale ultrasound of the liver shows a coarsened, heterogenous echotexture. There is mild nodularity (*arrow*) of the liver surface. **B:** Axial T2-weighted MR image of the liver shows nodular liver contour and lace-like areas of increased signal (*arrowheads*) reflecting fibrosis. **C:** Axial postcontrast fat-suppressed T1-weighted MR image obtained in the portal venous phase shows heterogeneous enhancement and nodular liver surface. A lesion in the posterior section of the right hepatic lobe (*dashed arrow*) is hypoenhancing. Based on overall imaging characteristics, this was determined to represent a hepatic adenoma. **D:** Axial postcontrast fat-suppressed T1-weighted MR image obtained in the hepatocyte phase of imaging shows nonenhancement of the lace-like areas of fibrosis (*arrowheads*). The hepatic adenoma (*dashed arrow*) has no retention of contrast material. **E:** Axial color wave image from MR elastogram shows widening of the shear wave (*line*) reflecting increased shear wave speed and increased stiffness. **F:** Axial elastogram based on the shear wave image (scale 0–8 kPa; 0 = purple, 8 = red) shows the liver to be markedly stiffened with an average stiffness of 7.7 kPa.

TABLE 14.4 Causes of Noncirrhotic Portal Hypertension in Children
Prehepatic Causes
Portal vein thrombosis
Splenic causes:
Splenic vein thrombosis
Infiltrative splenic disease (e.g., Gaucher disease, lymphoma)
Hepatic Causes
Presinusoidal:
Idiopathic
Congenital hepatic fibrosis
Inflammatory disorders:
Primary biliary cirrhosis
Primary sclerosing cholangitis
Peliosis hepatis
Early myeloproliferative diseases
Sinusoidal:
Hypervitaminosis A
Nodular regenerative hyperplasia
Postsinusoidal:
Hepatic veno-occlusive disease
Hepatic vein thrombosis/stenosis
Posthepatic Causes
Venous:
Inferior vena cava stenosis/web
Cardiac:
Constrictive pericarditis
Tricuspid regurgitation
Right heart failure

Adapted from Sarin SK, Kumar A. Noncirrhotic portal hypertension. Clin Liver Dis. 2006;10(3):627–651, x. Ref. 94.

possible complication.[96] In patients with end-stage liver disease and portal hypertension, liver transplant may be indicated.

Extrahepatic Portal Venous Obstruction

Extrahepatic portal venous obstruction (commonly due to portal venous thrombosis) represents the second most common cause of portal hypertension in the Western hemisphere. In most pediatric patients, the cause of extrahepatic portal venous obstruction is unknown.[94] When a cause is identified, congenital and infectious etiologies are most common, with umbilical venous catheters increasingly recognized as a contributing etiology.[94] The clinical presentation of extrahepatic portal venous obstruction is variable depending on the acuity with which the obstruction develops. The most common presenting symptoms are those of portal hypertension, including splenomegaly and anemia in the setting of long-standing occlusion.[94] Ascites and hematemesis can occur. Growth retardation is seen in nearly one-third of patients who develop extrahepatic portal venous obstruction before puberty.[94]

Ultrasound is the mainstay of diagnostic imaging modality because of its ability to provide both anatomic and vascular evaluation. In acute obstruction, thrombus occluding the portal vein can be anechoic to hypoechoic compared to the liver. In more chronic obstruction, the main portal vein may not be distinctly visible. Instead, a tangle of collateral vessels representing "cavernous transformation" may be present (Figs 14.45 and 14.46). Sequelae of portal hypertension (described previously) are often apparent (Figs. 14.45 and 14.46). On CT and MRI, the liver may have a characteristic morphologic appearance with a rounded contour reflecting central hypertrophy and peripheral atrophy (Fig. 14.45).[97] Postcontrast images obtained in the portal venous phase can show the thrombosed portal vein and the associated periportal collaterals (so-called cavenoma) (Fig. 14.46). Tumor thrombus, if present, is distinguishable by identification of a liver tumor, expansion of the portal vein, and internal Doppler vascularity/postcontrast enhancement.

In children with obstruction of blood flow through the main portal vein, a surgical shunt is often the treatment of choice, although angioplasty and stenting have been attempted.[98] The most commonly employed surgical shunt is a Rex shunt connecting the SMV to the left portal vein, as this minimizes the risk of portal encephalopathy.[96]

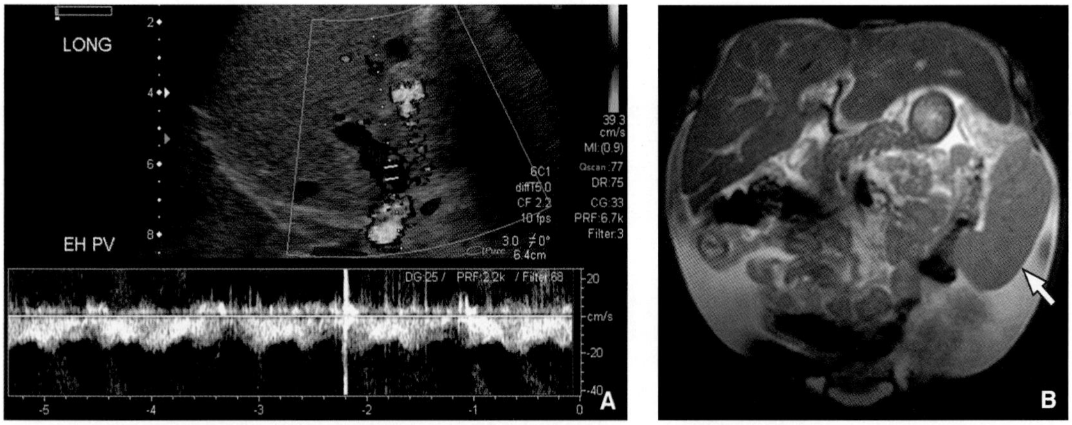

FIGURE 14.44 **An 11-month-old boy with a history of biliary atresia and portal hypertension. A:** Longitudinal ultrasound image of the liver with color and spectral Doppler shows pulsatile and reversed (hepatofugal) portal venous blood flow. **B:** Coronal T2-weighted MR image shows marked ascites and splenomegaly (*arrow*).

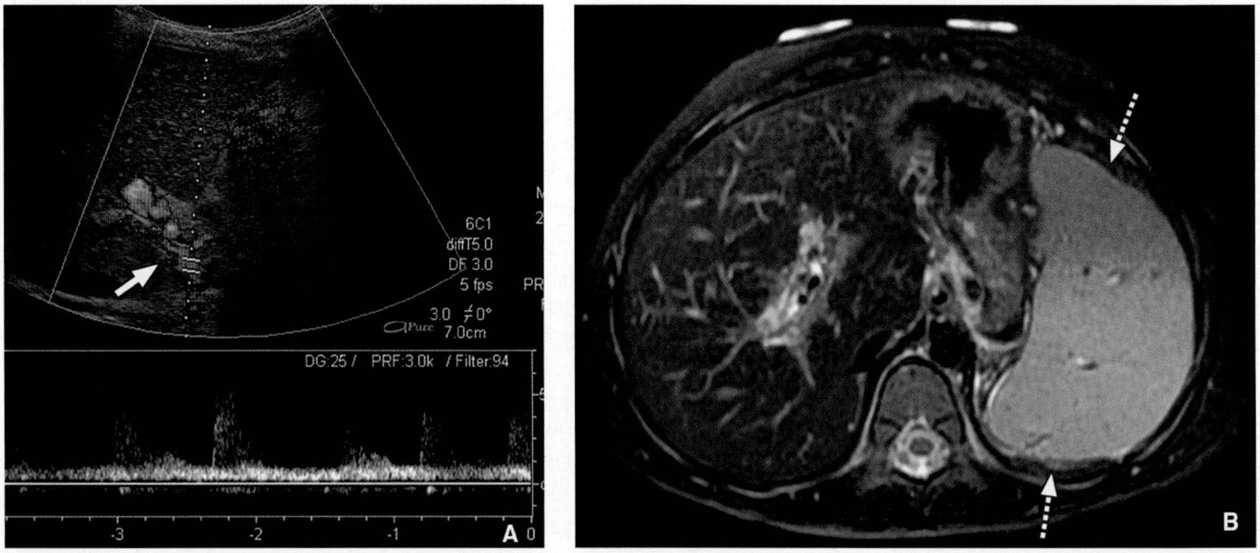

FIGURE 14.45 **A 4-year-old girl with congenital cytomegalovirus infection, chronic portal venous thrombosis, and portal hypertension. A:** Ultrasound image of the liver with color and spectral Doppler shows a tangle of vessels replacing the portal vein in the hepatic hilum (*arrow*) reflecting cavernous transformation. Flow within these vessels is hepatopedal, and velocity is diminished. **B:** Axial fat-suppressed T2-weighted MR image shows absence of normal portal venous structures in the region of the porta hepatis and splenomegaly (*dashed arrows*).

Nonalcoholic Fatty Liver Disease

Nonalcoholic fatty liver disease (NAFLD) is the most common cause of chronic liver disease in children in the United States occurring in up to 9.6%.[88] NAFLD is more common in boys, older children, and obese children.[99] Affected pediatric patients most commonly present with vague abdominal pain, irritability, and fatigue.[99] Pathologically, the liver has a golden yellow gross appearance from the lipid that accumulates intracellularly (Fig. 14.47), and histologic changes range from simple steatosis to steatohepatitis (NASH) to overt cirrhosis.[88]

Findings of steatosis by ultrasound include hyperechogenicity of the liver (compared to the adjacent right kidney) with decreased visibility of the portal triads, poor acoustic penetration, and poor visualization of the hemidiaphragm (Fig. 14.48). By CT, the noncontrast attenuation of the liver is decreased relative to the spleen (normally attenuation of the liver is 8 to 10 Hounsfield units greater than the spleen) (Fig. 14.49). Following

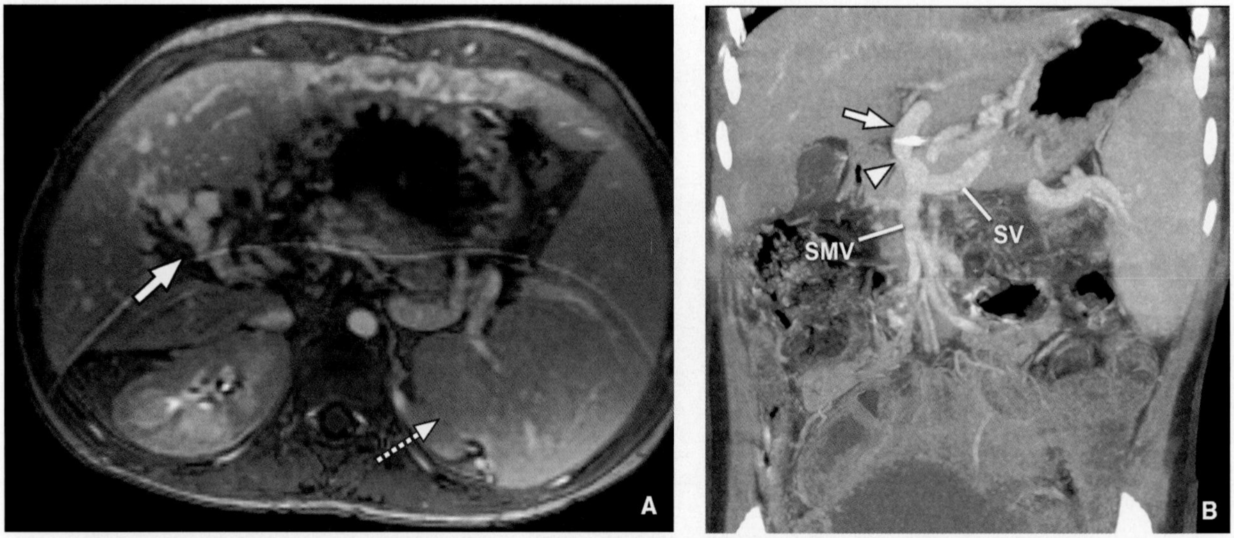

FIGURE 14.46 **An 8-year-old girl with chronic portal vein thrombosis and cavernous transformation of the main portal vein. A:** Axial T1-weighted MR image after the administration of a blood pool contrast agent shows multiple tortuous vessels (*arrow*) in the hepatic hilum. A normal main portal vein is not identified. The spleen is diffusely enlarged (*dashed arrow*). **B:** Coronal contrast-enhanced maximum intensity projection (MIP) CT image shows no normal portal vein. A contrast-filled structure (*arrow*) extending from the confluence of the superior mesenteric vein (*SMV*) and splenic vein (*SV*) toward the left portal vein represents a surgically created Rex shunt. Mild narrowing is present at the shunt origin (*arrowhead*).

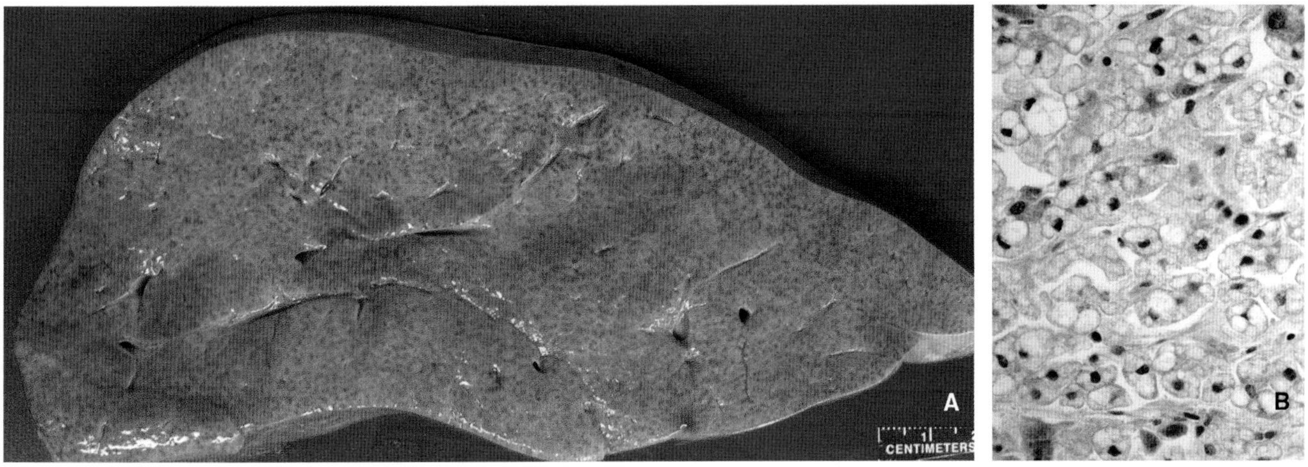

FIGURE 14.47 **Hepatic steatosis in an 18-year-old boy with immune dysregulation, polyendocrinopathy, enteropathy, and X-linked (IPEX) syndrome. A:** Surgical specimen shows hepatic steatosis or intracellular accumulation of fat that lends a diffusely yellow, greasy appearance to the cut surface of the liver. **B:** Microscopically, lipid droplets fill the hepatocyte cytoplasm (hematoxylin and eosin, original magnification, 600×).

intravenous contrast material administration, steatosis is said to be present if the attenuation of the spleen is more than 35 Hounsfield units higher than the liver during the portal venous phase.

Recently, MRI-based methods of hepatic fat quantification, including MR spectroscopy and chemical shift imaging, have been gaining traction.[100] Of the two techniques, MR spectroscopy is considered the gold standard because it is the most direct method of separating the liver parenchyma into its water and fat components.[101,102] MR spectroscopy has several other advantages over chemical shift imaging, including its ability to quantify fat over the entire dynamic range, higher sensitivity and specificity for fat quantitation, and its ability to detect an inflammatory response.[100] Despite these advantages of spectroscopy, chemical shift imaging is preferred at most centers because of its ease of performance, ease of interpretation, and speed of acquisition (Fig. 14.49).[88] While there are multiple methods that can be used to perform chemical shift imaging, each relies on the difference between the procession frequencies of fat and water protons to quantify fat content.[100] Proton-density fat fractionation is favored by some because of its quantitative nature, reproducibility, ease of use and relatively wide availability across MRI scanners.[88]

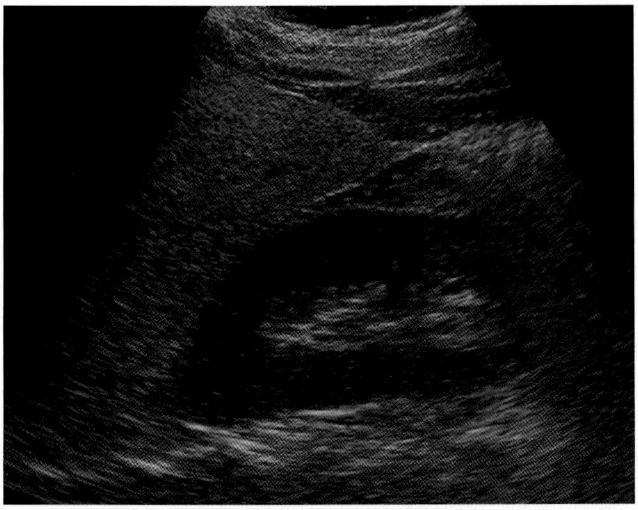

FIGURE 14.48 **A 15-year-old girl with nonalcoholic fatty liver disease.** Longitudinal gray-scale ultrasound image of the liver shows diffusely hyperechoic hepatic parenchyma relative to the right kidney. The portal triads are not visualized.

Hepatic Iron Deposition Disorders

Hepatic iron overload in children can occur through excess absorption or repeated blood transfusions. Excess absorption can occur in utero via gestational alloimmune liver disease (neonatal hemochromatosis, which presents in infancy), or it can accumulate slowly due to inherited dysregulation of intestinal uptake (primary hemochromatosis, which typically presents in adulthood). Although the hepatic imaging findings are similar in patients with either mechanism, secondary findings may differ. In pediatric patients with neonatal hemochromatosis, iron deposition occurs in the liver, heart and pancreas (Fig. 14.50). In pediatric patients with secondary hemochromatosis, iron first accumulates in the reticuloendothelial system including the liver, spleen, bone marrow, and lymph nodes (Fig. 14.51). As the accumulation of iron increases, it can deposit in the pancreas and heart as well.

If CT is performed, the liver can appear hyperattenuating. With progressive disease, the liver can decrease in size and findings of cirrhosis become apparent. On MRI, iron deposition is recognized by decreasing tissue signal intensity with increasing echo time (TE in ms) values (Figs. 14.50 and 14.51).[88] This is typically most apparent in the liver. On standard T1-weighted gradient recalled echo in- and opposed-phase imaging (with the opposed-phase image acquired first), iron deposition appears as signal loss on in-phase imaging as compared to the opposed-phase image.

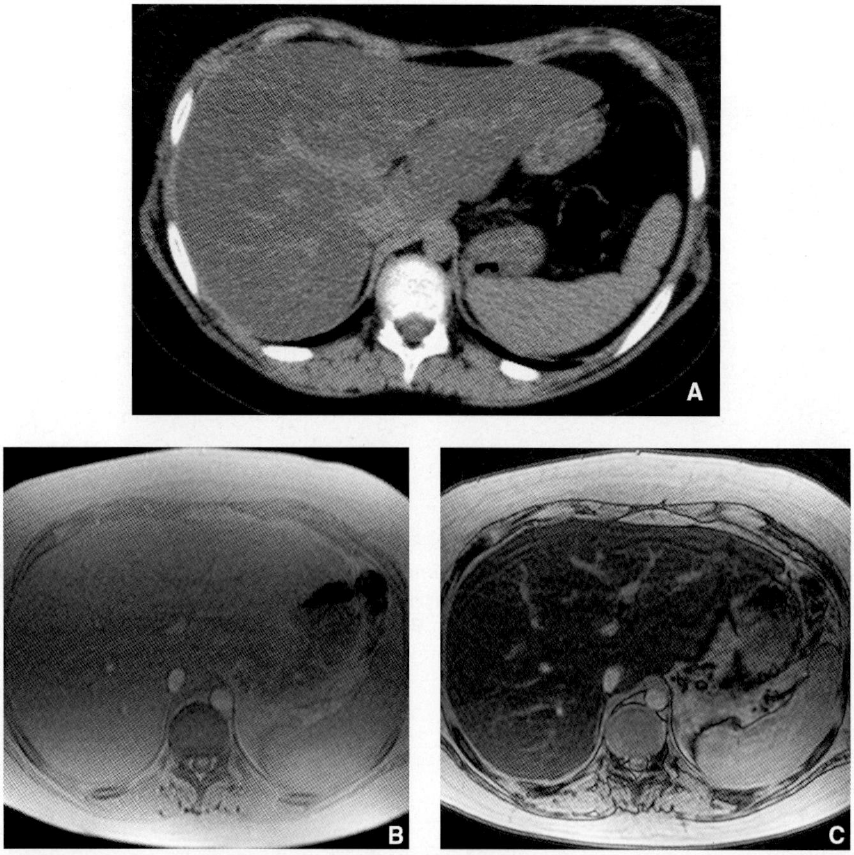

FIGURE 14.49 **A 12-year-old boy with nonalcoholic fatty liver disease. A:** Axial noncontrast CT image shows diffuse low attenuation of the liver parenchyma as compared to the spleen. Because there is diffuse hepatic fatty infiltration, the hepatic vessels appear hyperdense relative to the liver parenchyma. When regions of interest were placed on the liver and spleen, the attenuation values measured 20 Hounsfield units for the liver and 44 Hounsfield units for the spleen. Axial **(B)** in-phase and **(C)** opposed-phase T1-weighted gradient-recalled echo MR images of the abdomen show diffuse hepatic parenchymal signal dropout on the opposed-phase image. Calculated fat fraction is 27.6%.

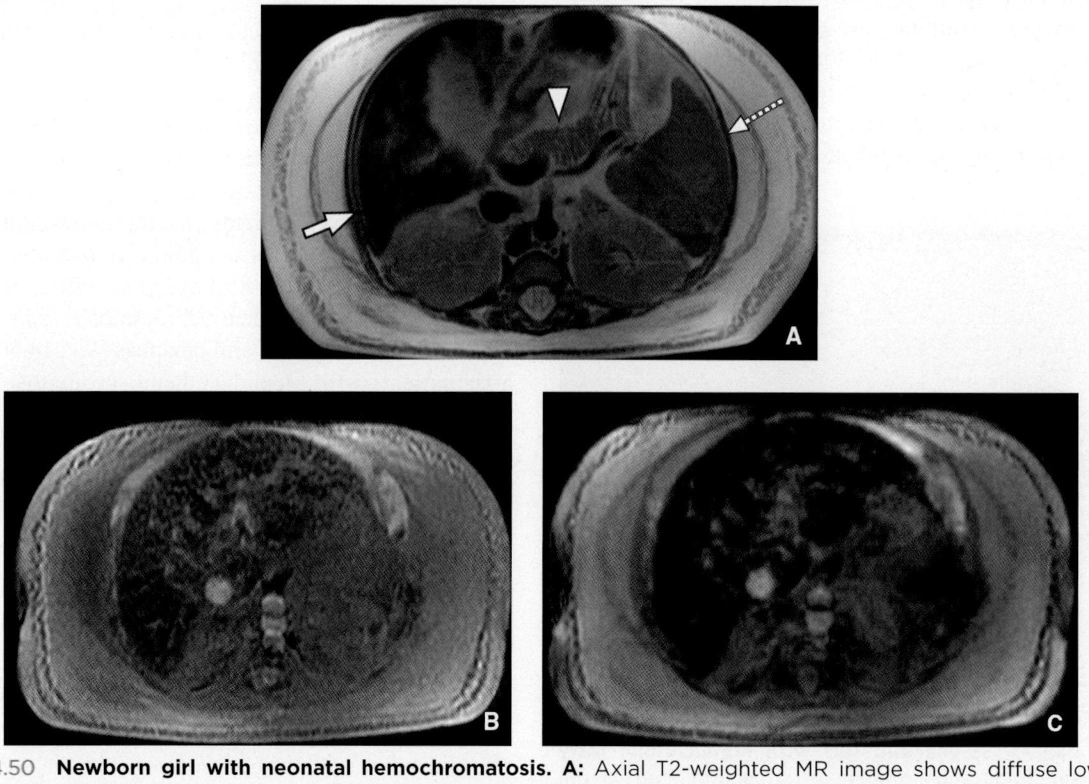

FIGURE 14.50 **Newborn girl with neonatal hemochromatosis. A:** Axial T2-weighted MR image shows diffuse low hepatic (*arrow*), splenic (*dashed arrow*), and pancreatic (*arrowhead*) signal intensity. Lower than expected signal is also present within the renal parenchyma. There is marked body wall edema. **B:** Axial T1-weighted gradient recalled echo MR image with an echo time of 4.5 ms shows low signal intensity throughout the liver. As the echo time increases to 14 ms **(C)**, there is progressive hepatic parenchyma signal loss.

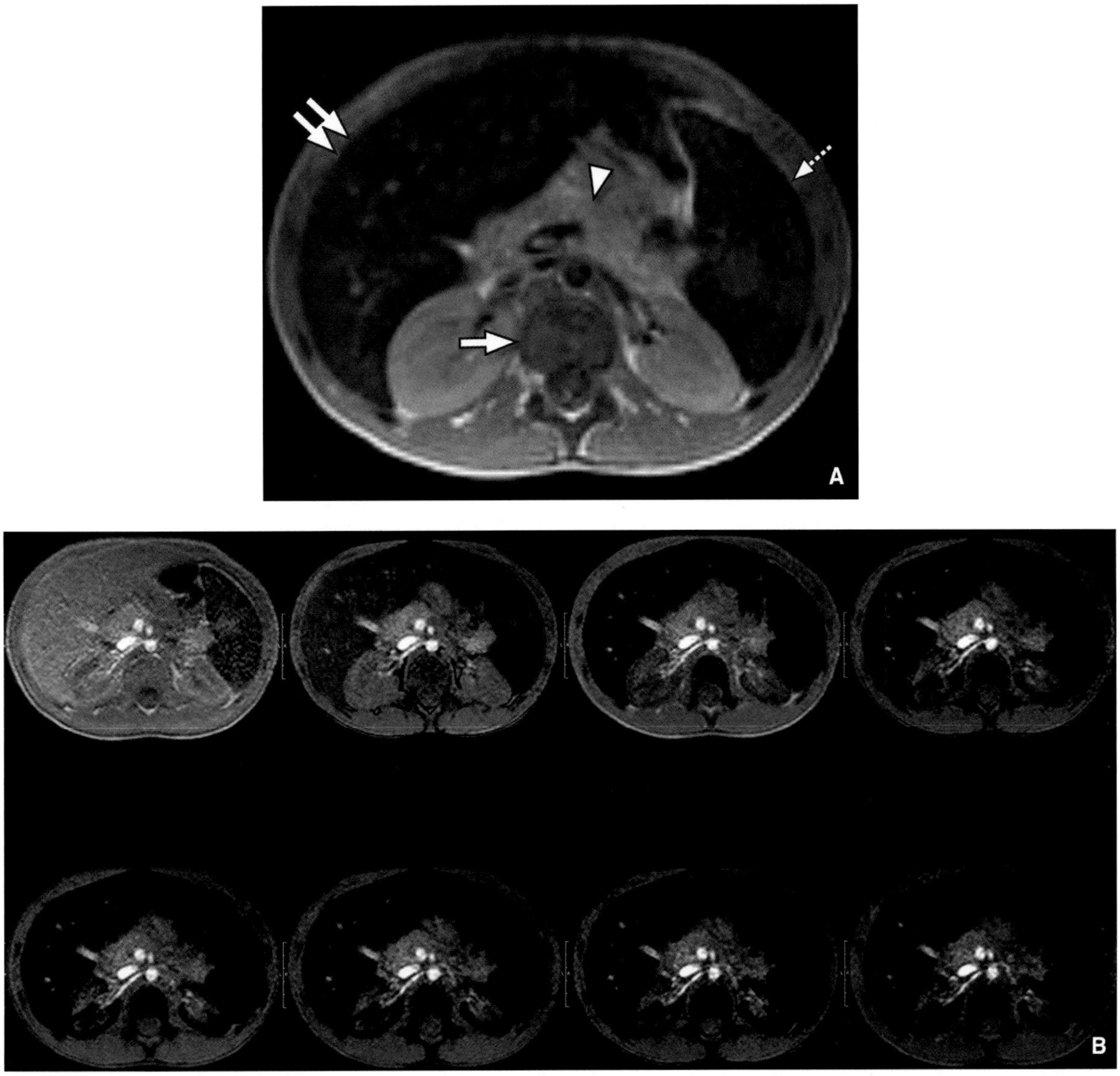

FIGURE 14.51 **A 7-year-old boy with sickle cell anemia and history of multiple blood transfusions leading to secondary hemochromatosis. A:** Axial T1-weighted fast spin-echo MR image of the abdomen shows diffuse signal hypointensity in the liver (*double arrow*), spleen (*dashed arrow*), and bone marrow (*arrow*). Note that the pancreas (*arrowhead*) has normal signal intensity. **B:** Axial gradient-recalled echo MR images with progressively longer echo times show progressive loss of signal in the liver, spleen, bone marrow, and renal cortices (left to right and top to bottom). The liver iron concentration was calculated to be 11,661 μg/g dry weight of the liver.

There are two main MRI methods for determining liver iron content: signal intensity ratio and relaxometry.[103,104] An online calculator has been developed to help radiologists estimate liver iron content using the signal intensity ratio [http://radio.univ-rennes1.fr/Sources/EN/HemoCalc15.html]. Although this method is widely used, the technique saturates with very high iron content (>350 μmol/g), and multiple breath holds are required.[103,104] Relaxometry methods are more complex and require a higher degree of sophistication to perform, but have fewer limitations. With these methods, T2* (ms) and R2* (1/ms) or T2 (ms) and R2 (1/ms) values are calculated that decrease and increase, respectively, with increasing liver iron content. Commercial options are increasingly available providing this technique.[88]

Glycogen Storage Diseases

The glycogen storage diseases are genetic enzyme deficiencies that lead to impaired glycogen synthesis, storage, or degradation.[105,106] The variable phenotypes of the glycogen storage diseases (Table 14.5) depend on the enzyme affected and the specific mutation.[107] Although these disorders primarily affect the liver and skeletal muscle, variants can also affect the heart, central nervous system, and/or kidneys.[107]

TABLE 14.5 Subtypes of Glycogen Storage Diseases

Glycogen Storage Disease Type (Eponym)	Enzyme Deficiency	Liver Effects[107]
O (Aglycogenesis)	Glycogen synthetase	• Normal-sized liver • Small amounts of glycogen and moderate steatosis
I (von Gierke disease)	Glucose-6-phosphatase	• Hepatomegaly • Glycogenated nuclei and steatosis • Hepatic fibrosis • Hepatic adenoma • Hepatocellular carcinoma
II (Pompe disease)	Acid alpha-glucosidase	• Presence of hepatomegaly depends on clinical onset of disease • Distention of liver cells with microvacuolization
III (Cori disease or Forbes disease)	Glycogen debranching enzyme	• Hepatomegaly • Liver symptoms improve with age • Hepatic adenoma in ~25% • Distended hepatocytes, glycogenated nuclei, hepatocytes in mosaic pattern, periportal fibrosis, and micronodular cirrhosis
IV (Anderson disease)	Glycogen branching enzyme	• Hepatosplenomegaly • Portal hypertension • Cirrhosis
V (McArdle disease)	Muscle glycogen phosphorylase	None
VI (Hers disease)	Liver glycogen phosphorylase	• Hepatomegaly • Tends to affect periportal hepatocytes
VII (Tarui disease)	Muscle phosphofructokinase	Unknown
IX	Phosphorylase kinase	• Hepatomegaly • Elevated liver enzymes • Cirrhosis
XI (Fanconi-Bickel syndrome)	Glucose transporter	• Hepatomegaly • Steatosis
XII (aldolase A deficiency)	Aldolase A	None

At cross-sectional imaging, hepatic findings are variable, including hyperechogenicity on ultrasound, hepatomegaly, steatosis, hepatic fibrosis, cirrhosis, portal hypertension, and development of hepatic adenomas or HCC (Fig. 14.52).

With the advent of dietary therapies, including continuous feeds and total parenteral nutrition, pediatric patients with glycogen storage diseases can survive into adulthood.[105] Ultrasound is often used in these pediatric patients for surveillance purposes. If a discrete lesion is identified by ultrasound, it can be further characterized with MRI using a hepatocyte-specific contrast agent.

Hepatic Tyrosinemia

Hereditary tyrosinemia is a group of inherited disorders related to abnormalities in the degradation pathway for tyrosine. Three subtypes have been described based on different enzyme deficiencies. Although still rare (about 1:100,000), type 1 hereditary tyrosinemia is the most common form.[108] Type 1 tyrosinemia is inherited in an autosomal recessive pattern and relates to a deficiency of the enzyme fumarylacetoacetate hydrolase. The clinical presentation of type 1 tyrosinemia is biphasic.[108] In the acute phase, affected pediatric patients present with hepatic failure and neurologic crisis.[108] If the patient survives the acute phase, chronic sequelae include hepatic dysfunction, including cirrhosis, and renal dysfunction.[108] Pediatric patients with hereditary tyrosinemia are at increased risk of developing hepatocellular neoplasms (adenomas and carcinomas) and are more likely to develop a tumor at a young age.[108] Ultrasound, serum AFP, and sometimes MRI are used to screen for malignancy (Fig. 14.53).

Nitisinone is used to treat patients with hereditary tyrosinemia, moderating many of the symptoms in the acute phase as well as decreasing the short and

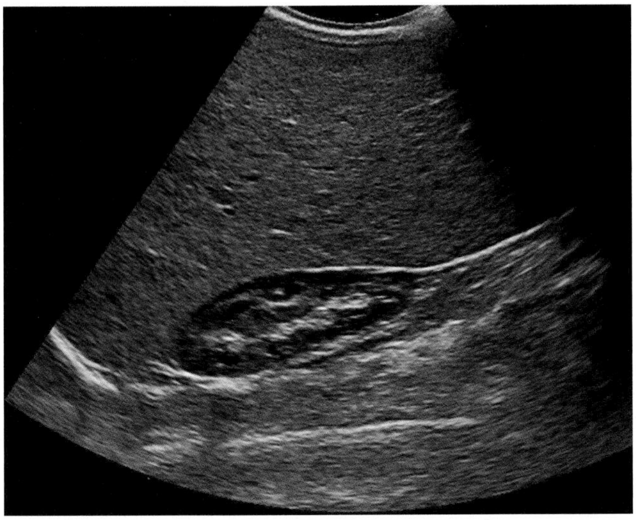

FIGURE 14.52 **A 7-year-old girl with glycogen storage disease type III.** Longitudinal right upper quadrant ultrasound image shows marked hepatomegaly and diffusely increased hepatic echogenicity. The liver extends well below the inferior pole of the right kidney.

medium-term risk of developing HCC.[108] Affected pediatric patients are placed on a low-tyrosine, low-phenylalanine diet.[109]

Hepatic Venoocclusive Disease

Hepatic venoocclusive disease (VOD), also called hepatic sinusoidal obstruction syndrome, is the most common cause of liver disease in the first 3 weeks after hematopoietic stem cell transplantation (HSCT) or bone marrow transplant (BMT).[110] VOD occurs in 10% to 60% of patients and is thought to result from destruction of the hepatic microvasculature (sinusoids and venules) during cytoreductive conditioning.[110,111] Patients with VOD present with ascites, jaundice, and painful hepatomegaly. In severe cases, symptoms can include panvasculitis and multiorgan failure.[110] VOD can be due to other causes as well, including certain medications and radiation therapy.

There are few studies evaluating the ability of modern imaging modalities to diagnose VOD. With previous generations of CT and ultrasound equipment, results were mixed regarding whether VOD could reliably be diagnosed with imaging.[111–113] One of the more recent studies, published in 2001, found that clinical criteria were superior to ultrasound for diagnosing VOD.[113]

Ultrasound is the mainstay of imaging in these patients because of its ability to evaluate the hepatic vasculature. Findings that have been described in the setting of VOD include splenomegaly, gallbladder wall thickening, narrowed hepatic veins, ascites, recanalized paraumbilical vein, increased hepatic echogenicity, and increased periportal echogenicity (Fig. 14.54).[110,111] Findings on Doppler ultrasound interrogation include decreased or reversed blood flow in the portal vein, increased resistive index in the hepatic artery, or monophasic flow in the hepatic veins (Fig. 14.54).[110] Findings by CT and MRI include hepatosplenomegaly, periportal edema, ascites, increased diameter of the portal vein, and narrowed/effaced hepatic veins (Fig. 14.55).[110]

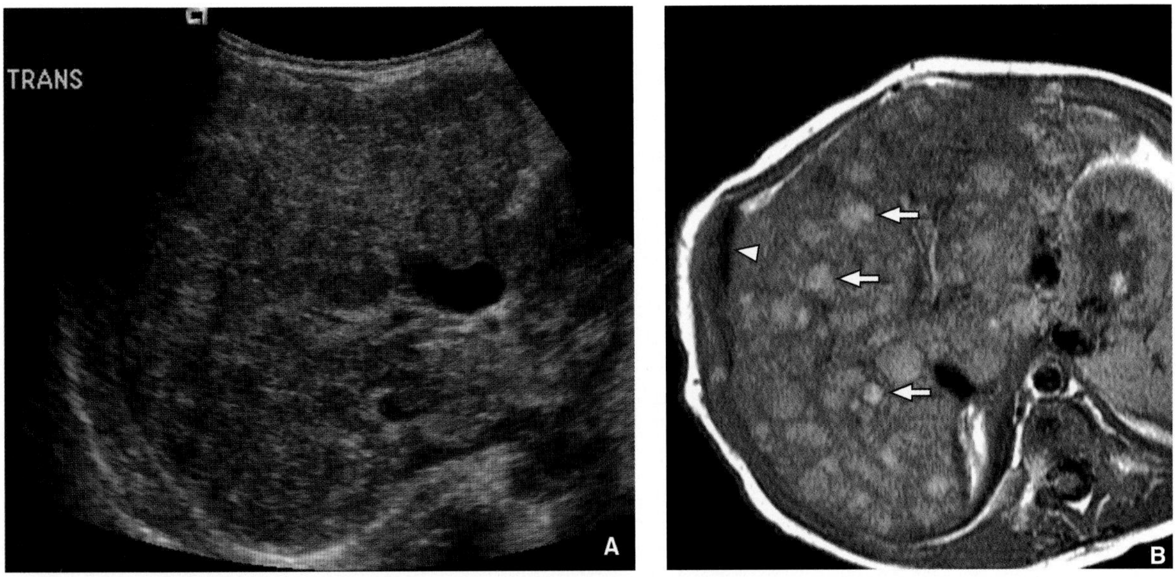

FIGURE 14.53 **A 12-month-old boy with cirrhosis due to tyrosinemia. A:** Transverse gray-scale ultrasound image of the liver shows a coarsened, heterogeneous hepatic echotexture, in part due to many regenerative nodules. The liver has a nodular contour. **B:** Axial T1-weighted MR image of the liver shows innumerable nodules throughout the liver, many of which are hyperintense (*arrows*). Small amount of ascites (*arrowhead*) is present along the hepatic margin.

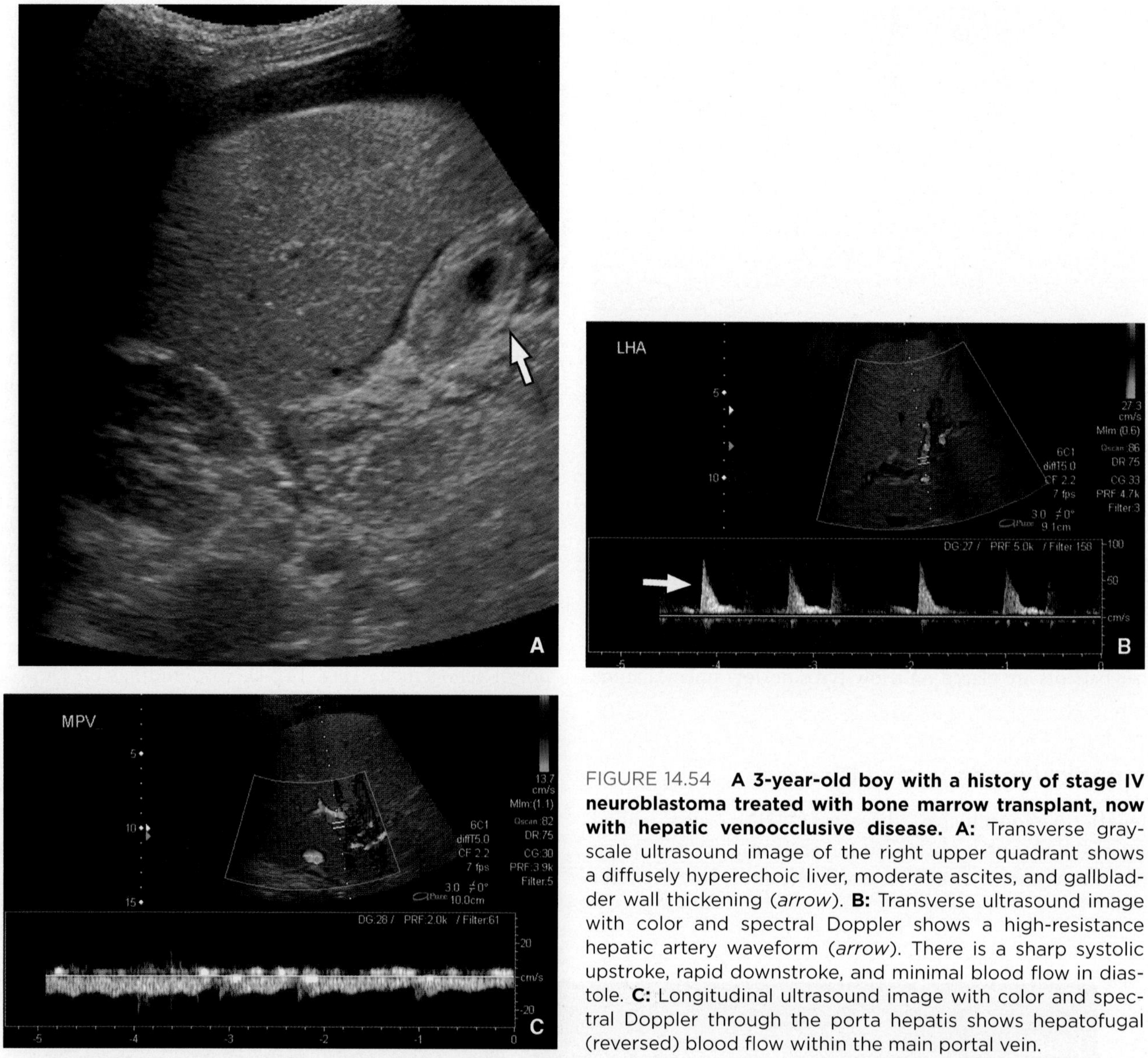

FIGURE 14.54 **A 3-year-old boy with a history of stage IV neuroblastoma treated with bone marrow transplant, now with hepatic venoocclusive disease. A:** Transverse grayscale ultrasound image of the right upper quadrant shows a diffusely hyperechoic liver, moderate ascites, and gallbladder wall thickening (*arrow*). **B:** Transverse ultrasound image with color and spectral Doppler shows a high-resistance hepatic artery waveform (*arrow*). There is a sharp systolic upstroke, rapid downstroke, and minimal blood flow in diastole. **C:** Longitudinal ultrasound image with color and spectral Doppler through the porta hepatis shows hepatofugal (reversed) blood flow within the main portal vein.

If the diagnosis of VOD is in question, it can be confirmed with liver biopsy. The overall prognosis of patients with VOD depends on the severity of disease with mortality ranging from 9% in mild cases to nearly 100% in severe cases.[110]

Hepatic Peliosis

Peliosis hepatis is a rare, benign entity characterized by variably sized, cystic, blood-filled cavities in the liver.[114,115] The pathogenesis of peliosis is unknown.[114] In adults, it has been associated with chronic wasting diseases (e.g., tuberculosis, malignancy, AIDS), medications (e.g., steroids, oral contraceptives), transplantation (e.g., renal, cardiac), and toxin exposure.[114] In children, peliosis has been described in pediatric patients with chronic conditions such as cystic fibrosis, malnutrition, Fanconi anemia, adrenal tumors, Marfan syndrome, and myotubular myopathy.[116] In 20% to 50% of affected patients, no associated process is identified.[114]

On ultrasound, peliosis hepatis appears as multiple well-defined, hypoechoic liver lesions.[117] Larger lesions can display posterior acoustic enhancement. On Doppler ultrasound, there may be peri- and intralesional vascularity.[117] On noncontrast CT, peliosis appears hypoattenuating compared to background liver. On MRI, the signal characteristics of peliosis vary depending on the chronicity of the blood content of the lesion.[118] Most commonly, lesions appear cystic with T1-weighted signal hypointensity and T2-weighted signal hyperintensity (Fig. 14.56).[115] On postcontrast imaging, peliosis lesions show arterial hypoenhancement with progressive enhancement during the portal venous phase of imaging (Fig. 14.56).[114] If the peliosis cavities are thrombosed, enhancement may not be observed.[114]

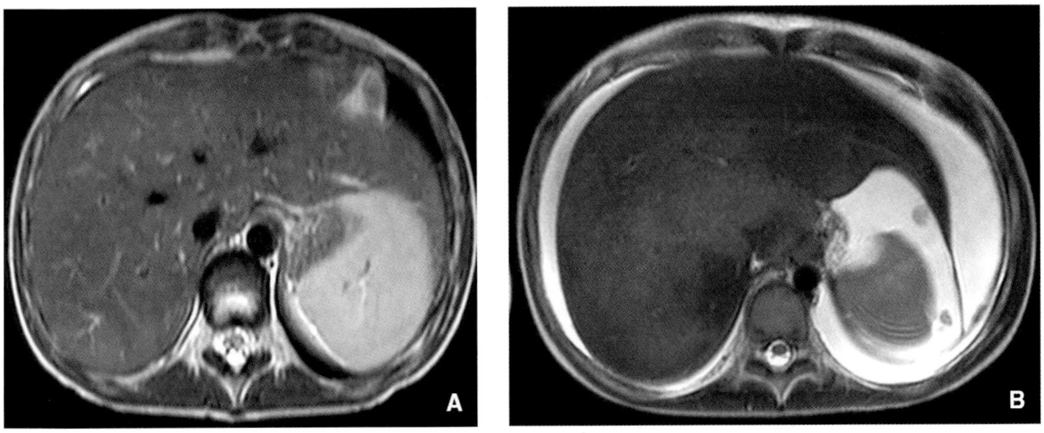

FIGURE 14.55 **A 13-year-old girl with Crohn disease and medication-induced hepatic venoocclusive disease proven by biopsy.** **A:** Axial T2-weighted single-shot fast spin-echo MR image acquired at the time of Crohn disease diagnosis shows that the liver is normal. **B:** Six months later, the liver appears diffusely enlarged and heterogeneous; the hepatic veins are effaced. There is a large amount of ascites.

There is no specific treatment for peliosis. If possible, offending agents are withdrawn. Complications, such as hepatic failure, cholestasis, portal hypertension, or hepatic rupture with intraperitoneal hemorrhage, are managed as they arise.

Orthotopic Liver Transplantation and Complications

An adequate discussion of pediatric liver transplantation, its complications, and the imaging of the transplant liver is beyond the scope of this chapter. The reader is referred to dedicated reviews on the clinical and imaging aspects of pediatric liver transplantation.[119,120]

Briefly, common indications for pediatric liver transplant include diffuse parenchymal liver disease, fulminant liver failure, and unresectable liver tumors. Many of the specific indications are described in other sections of this chapter. Types of liver allografts transplanted in children include whole organ, reduced-size, split-liver, and living-donor. In all but the whole organ transplant, typical hepatic anatomy is altered.

In the pretransplant period, imaging can be used to assess donor and recipient anatomy and vasculature. Following transplant, ultrasound is the dominant modality employed, allowing serial assessment of the transplanted organ, its vasculature (including anastomoses), and potential complications.[120,121] Abnormalities identified by ultrasound can be further evaluated with CT, MRI, scintigraphy, or catheter angiography as indicated.[120,122,123]

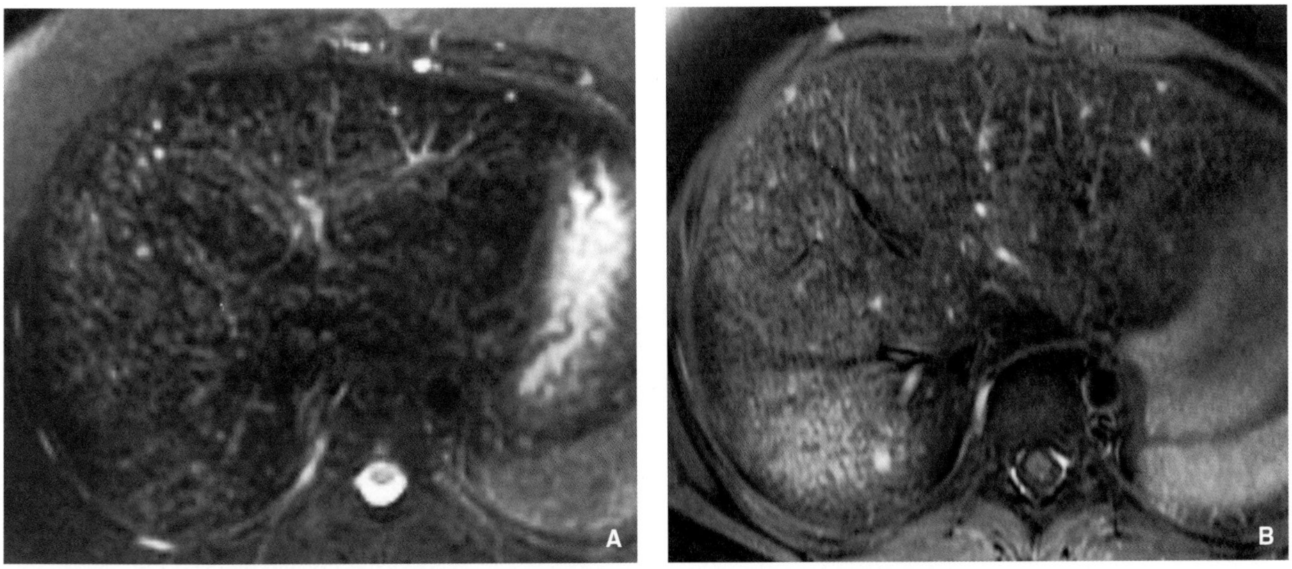

FIGURE 14.56 **A 13-year-old girl with history of Fanconi anemia and peliosis hepatitis.** **A:** Axial fat-suppressed T2-weighted MR image shows many small T2-weighted hyperintense lesions throughout the liver. **B:** Axial postcontrast fat-suppressed T1-weighted MR image shows enhancement of these lesions. The liver is diffusely low in signal on both sequences due to iron deposition.

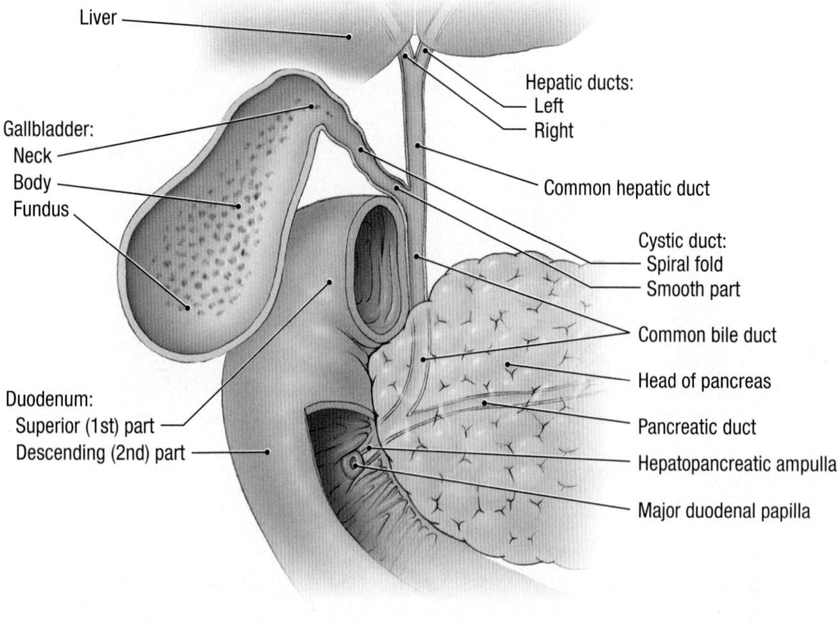

FIGURE 14.57 **Standard biliary anatomy.** Union of the right and left hepatic ducts forms the common hepatic duct. The cystic duct then joins with the common hepatic duct, forming the common bile duct. The caudal aspect of the common bile duct usually joins with the main pancreatic duct (duct of Wirsung) and drains into the duodeunum at the major duodenal papilla.

SPECTRUM OF BILIARY DISORDERS

Normal Anatomy and Common Variants

Major intrahepatic bile ducts parallel the portal veins and conform to the segmental hepatic anatomy previously described. In standard anatomy, the right anterior duct and right posterior duct (RPD) join to form the right hepatic duct, which drains segments 5, 6, 7, and 8. The left hepatic duct (LHD) is formed from smaller branches draining segments 2, 3, and 4. In most cases, the caudate lobe (segment 1) has bile duct branches draining into both the right and LHDs.[124] Union of the right and left hepatic ducts forms the common hepatic duct (CHD) at the liver hilum. The cystic duct then joins with the CHD, forming the common bile duct (CBD) (Fig. 14.57). The caudal aspect of the CBD usually joins with the main pancreatic duct, creating the ampulla of Vater within the duodenal wall, which then drains into the duodenum through the major papilla (Fig. 14.58).

The chief importance of recognizing anatomic variants of the biliary system relates to surgical planning. Biliary ductal variants have been described in detail in prior reviews.[125] Of those described, the most common variant (19%) is when the RPD drains into the LHD (Fig. 14.59).[124] Of the noninvasive imaging modalities, MRCP has the highest sensitivity and specificity for detecting aberrant drainage patterns.[126]

Congenital and Developmental Anomalies

The process of hepatic development is complex and described in detail in prior reviews.[127,128] Important for the radiologist to understand are the distinct origins of the intra- and extrahepatic biliary tree and the concept of the ductal plate.

The liver develops from a diverticulum of the foregut. The cranial component of the diverticulum (pars hepatica) gives rise to the liver parenchyma and intrahepatic bile ducts, and the caudal component (pars cystica) gives rise to the extrahepatic bile ducts, gallbladder, and ventral pancreas. The process of intrahepatic bile duct development relates to progressive development of sheathes of hepatocyte precursor cells (hepatoblasts) surrounding portal vein branches—the so-called ductal plate. Maldevelopment of the ductal plate results in Caroli disease, congenital hepatic fibrosis, biliary

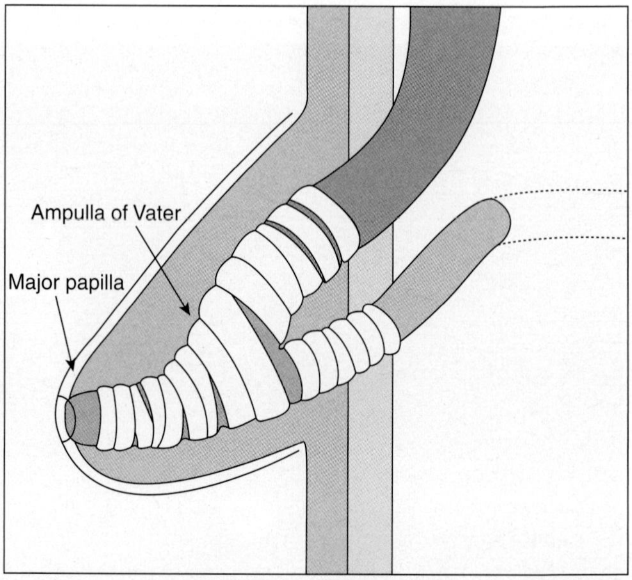

FIGURE 14.58 **Anatomy of the ampulla of Vater.** The ampulla is the junction of the common bile duct and pancreatic duct and is named for a Roman vessel with two handles. Sphincter of Oddi muscle fibers surround the ampulla of Vater and distal segments of the common bile and pancreatic ducts within the duodenal wall.

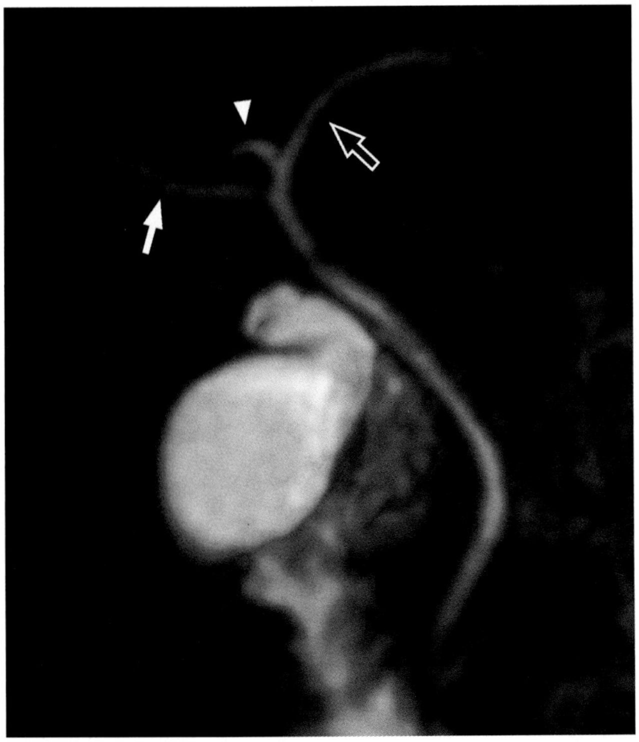

FIGURE 14.59 **A 7-year-old boy with variant biliary anatomy.** Coronal maximum-intensity projection (MIP) image from an MRCP examination shows the right posterior duct (*arrowhead*) joining with the left hepatic duct (*black arrow*), which then joins the right anterior duct (*white arrow*) to form the common hepatic duct.

hamartomas, and polycystic liver disease. Maldevelopment of the pars cystica results in choledochal malformations, anomalous pancreaticobiliary junction, and gallbladder anomalies.

Choledochal Malformations and Anomalous Pancreaticobiliary Junction

Choledochal cysts are rare anomalies characterized by cystic dilation of the intra- and/or extrahepatic bile ducts. Although patients may present at any age, choledochal cysts are usually discovered before 10 years of age. The classic presentation is abdominal pain, jaundice, and palpable abdominal mass, but this triad occurs in <20% of cases.

The most widely accepted classification system for choledochal cysts was developed by Todani et al.[129] (Fig. 14.60). Type I choledochal cysts, representing saccular or fusiform dilation of the CBD, are the most common subtype (Fig. 14.61). One of the most widely held theories for the development of choledochal cysts is that they are associated with pancreaticobiliary maljunction (PBM).[130] PBM is defined as union of the CBD and pancreatic duct outside the duodenal wall, resulting in an abnormally long common channel. The long common channel allows reflux of pancreatic enzymes into the biliary tree that weaken the bile duct wall, resulting in dilation.

Ultrasound may be the initial imaging examination to identify a choledochal abnormality (Fig. 14.61) and can be used to follow known choledochal cysts. MRCP allows visualization of the full extent of the choledochal abnormality and communication of cysts with the biliary tree, especially when multiple cysts are present or when large cysts result in distortion of anatomy (Fig. 14.61). MRCP is also the best noninvasive imaging modality for identifying PBM. PBM should be considered when the CBD and pancreatic duct join outside of the duodenal wall (Fig. 14.62). No normal common channel length has been described for children.

Complications of choledochal abnormalities include stone formation, abscesses, and development of pancreatitis and cholangitis. Large cysts can rupture, potentially resulting in bile peritonitis. Choledochal cysts and PBM are associated with an increased risk of cholangiocarcinoma. Treatment of choledochal abnormalities varies with the type of abnormality and includes cyst excision and liver transplantation.[131,132]

Gallbladder Anomalies

Anomalous Gallbladder Location

The gallbladder is most commonly located along the undersurface of the liver, paralleling the interlobar fissure. Described anomalous positions include intrahepatic (Fig. 14.63), left-sided, transverse, anterior, posterior and suprahepatic.[133] An anomalous location of the gallbladder may be an incidental finding or may result in poor emptying and bile stasis, which predispose to cholelithiasis and cholecystitis. Anomalous location can have surgical implications.

Ultrasound is the first-line modality for imaging the gallbladder and determining its location. MRI or CT may be helpful in select cases, particularly when the gallbladder is far removed from its normal location.

Gallbladder Dysgenesis

Gallbladder dysgenesis results from complete or partial failure of development of the gallbladder and cystic duct resulting in a hypoplastic, atretic, or absent gallbladder. Gallbladder agenesis is rare (0.02%) and most commonly sporadic, but can also be seen in conjunction with other gastrointestinal, cardiovascular and genitourinary disorders, suggesting a genetic predisposition.[134,135] Pediatric patients with isolated gallbladder dysgenesis may be asymptomatic or present with nonspecific biliary symptoms, including right upper quadrant pain, jaundice, nausea and fatty food intolerance. Diagnosis is made by nonvisualization of the gallbladder that is best confirmed by MRCP. Treatment for symptomatic gallbladder dysgenesis may involve smooth muscle relaxants or sphincterotomy of the major papilla rather than surgery, highlighting the importance of an accurate preoperative diagnosis.[136]

Gallbladder Duplication and Septation

Gallbladder duplication (Fig. 14.64) is a rare disorder thought to result from abnormal separation or persistence of outpouchings of the pars cystica.[137] This anomaly has an estimated incidence of 1/4,000.[138] Each gallbladder has its own cystic duct that may drain separately or join forming a Y-shaped duct draining into the CBD. Septate gallbladders are thought to be within the same spectrum as duplicated gallbladders, occurring when there is abnormal vacuolization

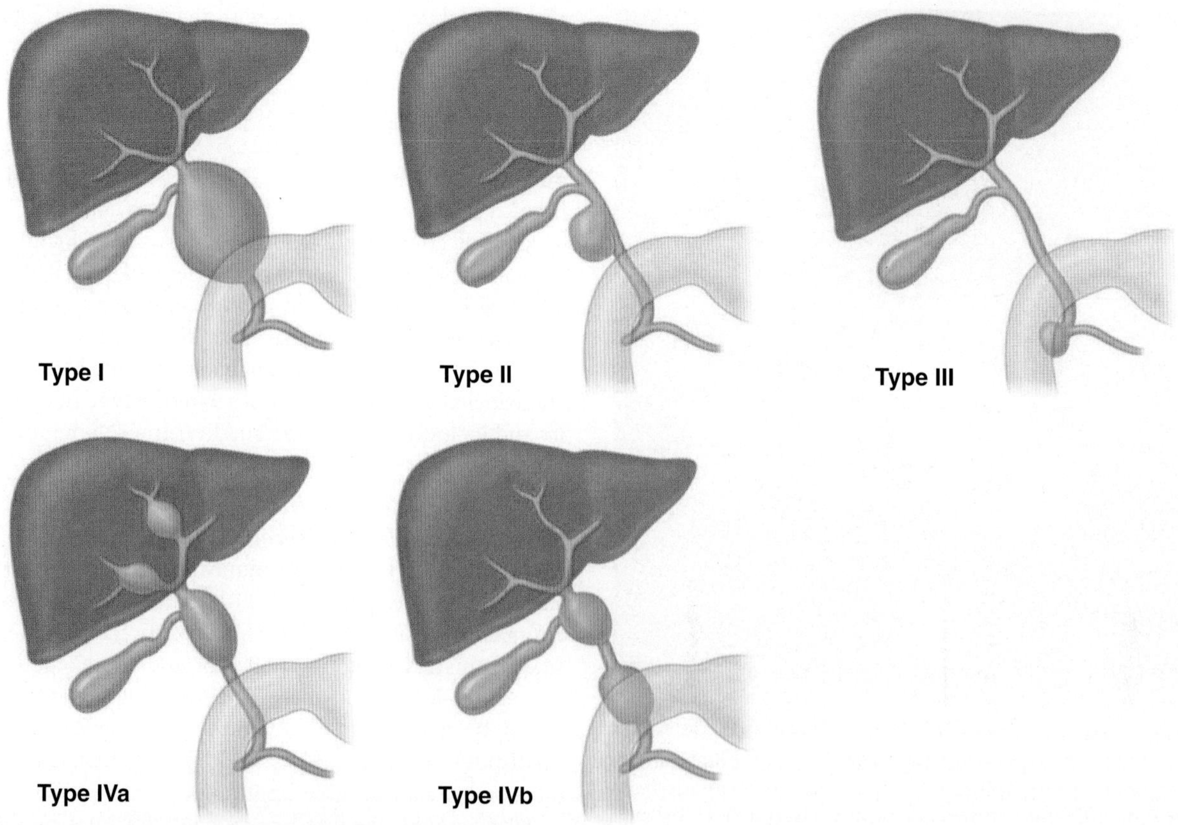

FIGURE 14.60 **Choledochal cyst classification per Todani et al.**[129] A type I cyst is dilation of the extrahepatic bile duct that has three subtypes: Type Ia cysts are diffuse dilation of the entire extrahepatic bile duct, without intrahepatic involvement. Type Ib cysts are focal dilations of the extrahepatic duct, and Type Ic cysts are longer segment fusiform dilations. Type II cysts are eccentric diverticula having a narrow communication with the common bile duct (CBD). Type III cysts, also known as choledochoceles, are focal dilations of the terminal intramural portion of the CBD, often bulging into the duodenal lumen. Type IV cysts are multiple separate dilations of the biliary tree, with type IVA cysts IVa cysts involving both the intrahepatic and extrahepatic ducts and type IVb cysts involving only the extrahepatic duct. Todani et al. previously defined a type V choledochal cyst (Caroli disease), which has since been recognized as a ductal plate malformation rather than a choledochal abnormality.

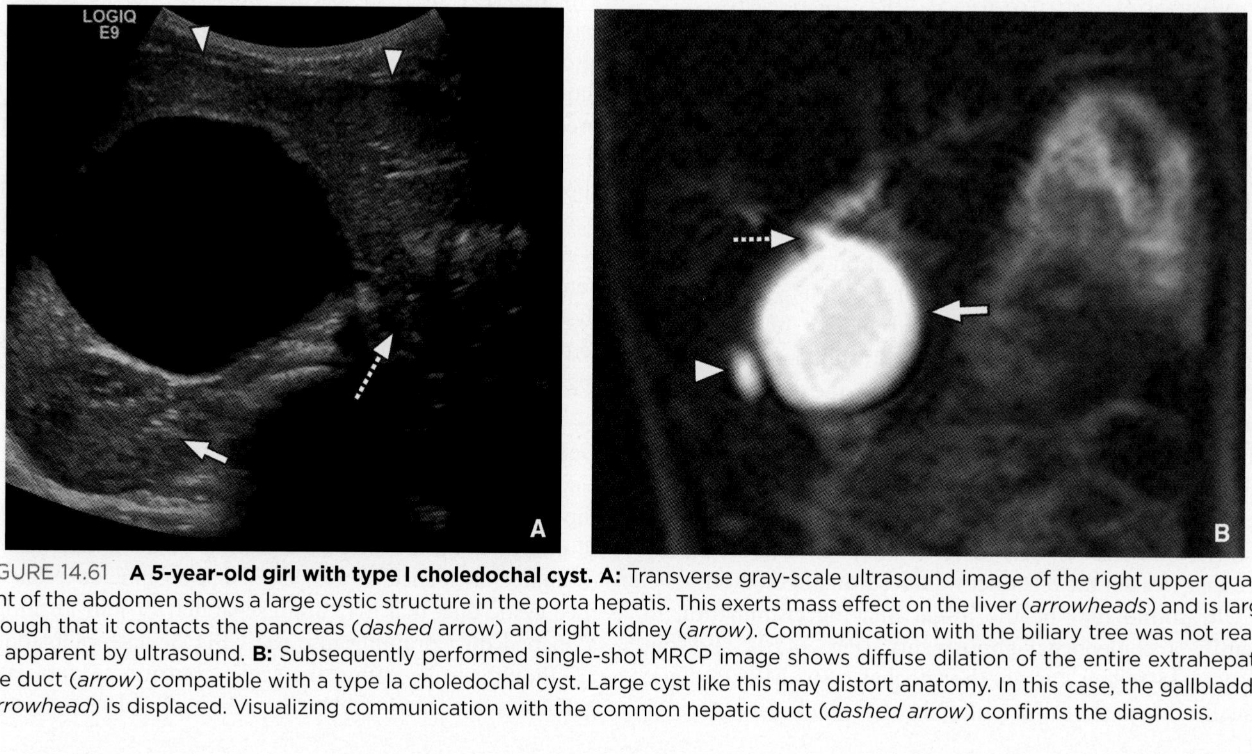

FIGURE 14.61 **A 5-year-old girl with type I choledochal cyst. A:** Transverse gray-scale ultrasound image of the right upper quadrant of the abdomen shows a large cystic structure in the porta hepatis. This exerts mass effect on the liver (*arrowheads*) and is large enough that it contacts the pancreas (*dashed* arrow) and right kidney (*arrow*). Communication with the biliary tree was not readily apparent by ultrasound. **B:** Subsequently performed single-shot MRCP image shows diffuse dilation of the entire extrahepatic bile duct (*arrow*) compatible with a type Ia choledochal cyst. Large cyst like this may distort anatomy. In this case, the gallbladder (*arrowhead*) is displaced. Visualizing communication with the common hepatic duct (*dashed arrow*) confirms the diagnosis.

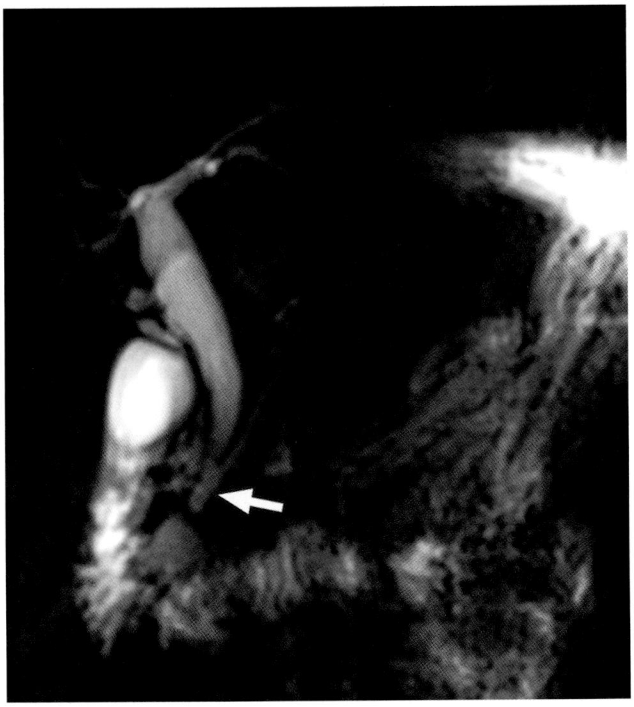

FIGURE 14.62 **A 17-year-old girl with type I choledochal cyst.** Coronal heavily T2-weighted MR image shows diffuse dilatation of the extrahepatic biliary tree. There is pancreaticobiliary maljunction with an abnormally long common channel. (Image courtesy of Jonathan R. Dillman, MD, MSc, Cincinnati Children's Hospital Medical Center, Cincinnati, OH.)

of the primitive gallbladder. In this entity, the gallbladder is drained by a single cystic duct and contains one or more septa dividing the lumen (Fig. 14.65).[139]

Children with duplicated or septate gallbladders may be asymptomatic or present with signs of cholelithiasis or cholecystitis. Ultrasound can identify the duplicated or septate gallbladder and the presence of calculi. MRCP better demonstrates the anatomy of the gallbladder(s), can help identify cystic duct(s) to distinguish duplicated and septate gallbladders, and can exclude mimicking conditions, including choledochal cyst, gallbladder diverticulum, Phrygian cap (a gallbladder with folded fundus), and enteric duplication

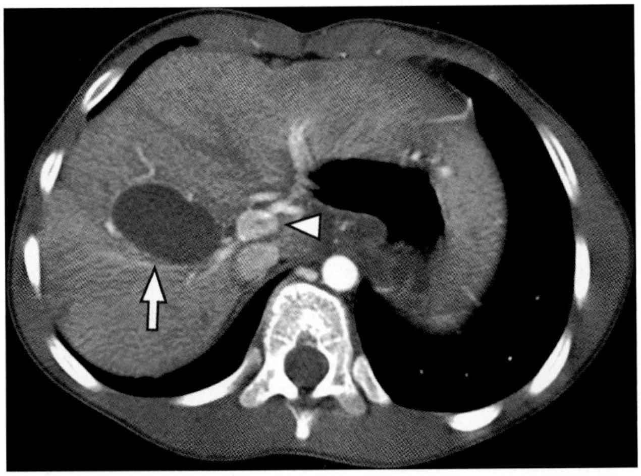

FIGURE 14.63 **An 8-year-old girl with type 1 Abernethy malformation and intrahepatic gallbladder.** Axial contrast-enhanced CT images show the gallbladder (*arrow*) to be completely surrounded by hepatic parenchyma instead of being located along the undersurface of the liver. The patient's large portosystemic shunt is partially visualized immediately anterior to the inferior vena cava (*arrowhead*). (Image courtesy of Jonathan R. Dillman, MD, MSc, Cincinnati Children's Hospital Medical Center, Cincinnati, OH.)

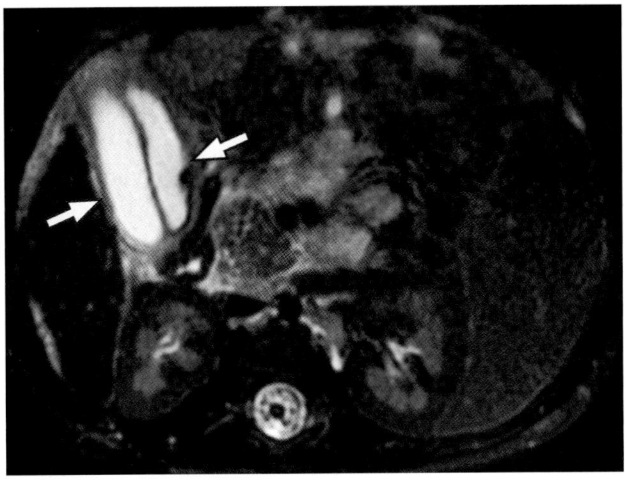

FIGURE 14.64 **A 4-year-old boy with duplicated gallbladder.** Axial T2-weighted fat-suppressed MR image shows two elongated cystic structures in the gallbladder fossa (*arrows*). These did not communicate with each other, and each drained to the common bile duct via separate cystic ducts (not shown).

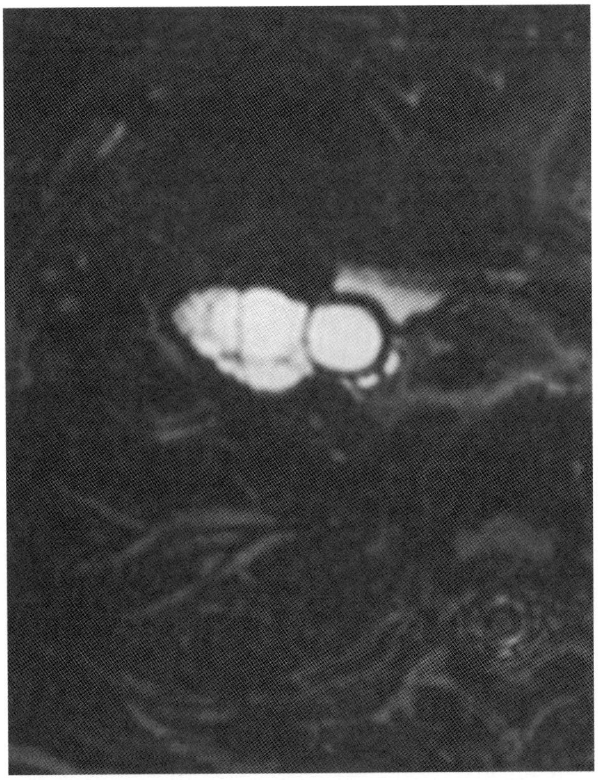

FIGURE 14.65 **A 9-year-old boy with multiseptate gallbladder.** Axial MRCP image shows a multilocular cystic structure in the gallbladder fossa. This was found to represent a gallbladder containing multiple thin septations, creating internal chambers of various sizes.

cyst. Treatment for symptomatic patients usually involves cholecystectomy, including removal of both gallbladders in the case of duplication.[140]

Ductal Plate Malformations

Ductal plate malformations, including Caroli disease, congenital hepatic fibrosis, and biliary hamartomas, are a spectrum of disorders that involve maldevelopment of the ductal plate, a structure present in embryonal and fetal life from which both hepatocytes and bile ducts derive. Many types of ductal plate malformation are the result of gene mutations related to the primary cilium and are thus considered ciliopathies.[141] Because similar processes govern development in the kidney, ductal plate malformations are often accompanied by polycystic disease in the kidney. The common pathogenesis of this broad group of ciliopathies explains the frequent phenotypic overlap between liver and kidney disease and between subtypes of ductal plate malformations. Most of the ductal plate malformations, with the exception of biliary hamartomas, predispose to cholangitis and cholangiocarcinoma.[142,143]

Caroli Disease

Previously classified as a subtype of choledochal cyst (Type V), Caroli disease is the result of a ductal plate malformation involving the large intrahepatic bile ducts.[144] In Caroli disease, there is dilation of the intrahepatic bile ducts that can be segmental, lobar, or diffuse. The extrahepatic ducts, because of their discrete embryologic origin, typically are not involved by the abnormality.

The classic imaging feature of Caroli disease that can be seen on ultrasound, contrast-enhanced CT, and MRI is the "central dot sign," which represents a portal vein branch completely surrounded by the focally dilated bile duct (Fig. 14.66). When Caroli disease occurs in conjunction with congenital hepatic fibrosis, it is termed Caroli syndrome (Fig. 14.67).[145]

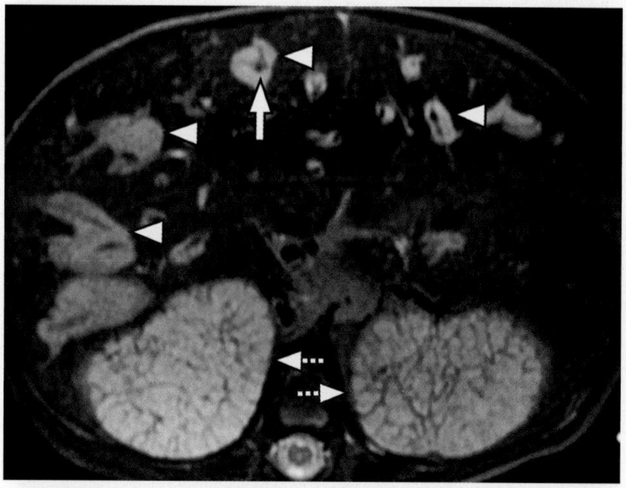

FIGURE 14.66 **A 3-year-old girl with Caroli disease.** Axial T2-weighted fat-suppressed MR image at the level of the liver and kidneys shows dilated bile ducts (*arrowheads*) that surround portal vein branches, giving the "central dot" sign (*arrow*). Enlarged kidneys that are replaced by innumerable small cysts (*dashed arrows*) is consistent with autosomal recessive polycystic kidney disease.

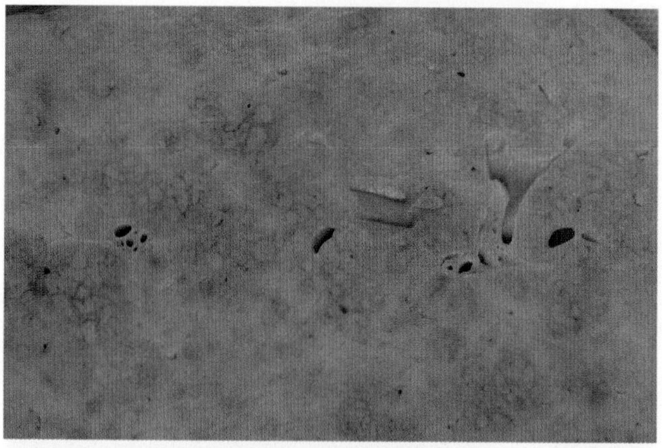

FIGURE 14.67 **A 22-year-old young woman with Caroli syndrome.** Explanted liver shows fibrous bands and green cholestatic discoloration (congenital hepatic fibrosis) as well as diated biliary structures (Caroli disease), the combination of which is known as Caroli syndrome.

Congenital Hepatic Fibrosis

Congenital hepatic fibrosis is a ductal plate malformation involving the intralobular bile ducts that results in dysplastic bile ducts and fibrous enlargement of the periportal tracts.[144] The surrounding hepatic parenchyma is normal, distinguishing this disease from secondary cirrhosis.[146] Congenital hepatic fibrosis is most commonly described in association with autosomal recessive polycystic kidney disease (ARPKD) but can be seen with other ciliopathies. The classic description is of an inverse severity of the renal and hepatic components of the disease, with children having more severe renal disease (and less severe liver disease) presenting in the perinatal/neonatal/infantile periods.[143] Children with more predominant hepatic involvement have a variable onset of symptoms, sometimes presenting in adolescence.[144]

There are four clinically recognized forms of congenital hepatic fibrosis defined by patient symptoms: portal hypertensive (most common), cholangitic, mixed hypertensive/cholangitic, and latent forms.[142] Hepatic synthetic function is typically preserved, and there is generally little deterioration over time.[142,143]

Classic imaging findings of cirrhosis are not present in children with congenital hepatic fibrosis. Periportal thickening may be apparent by ultrasound as increased periportal echogenicity or by MRI as periportal tissue with low T1-weighted and high T2-weighted signal intensity (Fig. 14.68).[144] Sequelae of portal hypertension and irregular intrahepatic bile duct dilatation, including findings of Caroli disease, can be seen.[142,144]

Biliary Hamartoma

Biliary hamartomas, also known as von Meyenburg complexes, are ductal plate malformations of the small interlobular bile ducts. Despite this being a developmental abnormality, the diagnosis is rarely made in the pediatric population.

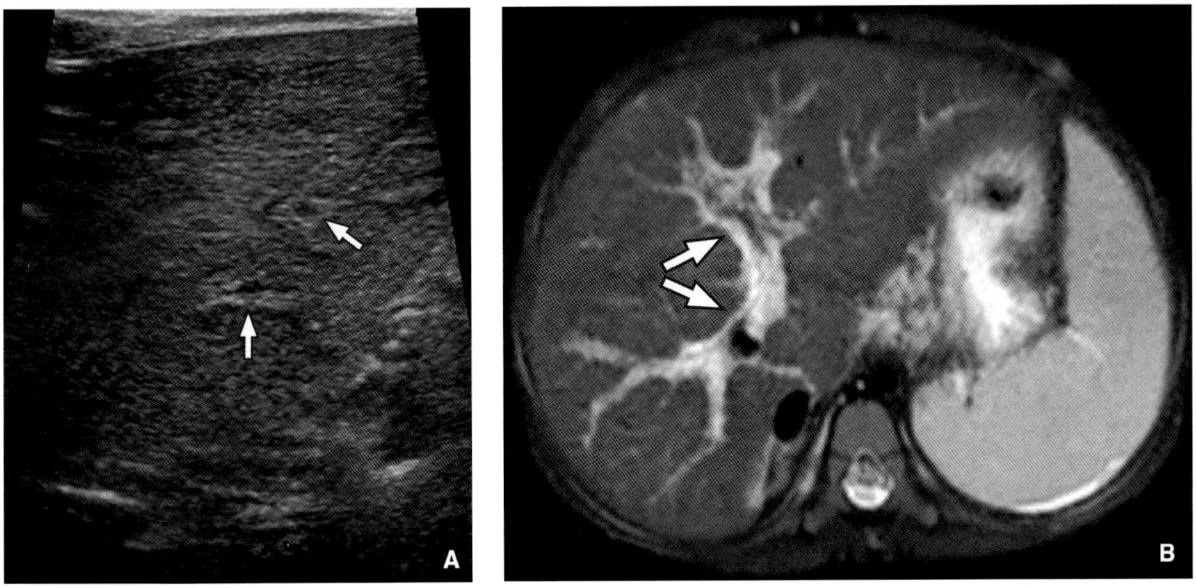

FIGURE 14.68 **A 1-year-old boy with congenital hepatic fibrosis. A:** Longitudinal ultrasound image of the liver shows diffuse coarsening of the hepatic echotexture with increased periportal echoes (*arrows*). **B:** Axial fat-suppressed T2-weighted MR image obtained 4 months later shows periportal increased T2-weighted signal (*arrows*) reflecting fibrosis. Splenomegaly and perisplenic fluid are due to portal hypertension.

Biliary hamartomas are nearly always asymptomatic and usually found incidentally.

On ultrasound, biliary hamartomas appear as numerous, usually cystic foci measuring <1 cm, sometimes having a comet tail artifact. Contrast-enhanced CT typically shows multiple round hypoattenuating structures scattered throughout the liver. At MRI, the lesions appear hypointense on T1-weighted MR images and hyperintense on T2-weighted MR images with no enhancement after intravenous contrast material administration (Fig. 14.69).[147,148] Less commonly, these lesions appear as solid enhancing nodules.

Neonatal Cholestasis

Imaging is often utilized in conjunction with liver biopsy in patients with neonatal cholestasis. In these patients, biliary atresia, which requires surgical intervention, must be distinguished from other causes of neonatal cholestasis, such as neonatal hepatitis (discussed previously) and Alagille syndrome (Table 14.6).

Hepatobiliary scintigraphy utilizing ^{99m}Tc-labeled IDA derivatives may be used to evaluate patients with neonatal cholestasis. Normally, the radiotracer rapidly disappears from the blood pool with uniform hepatic uptake reaching maximum activity by 5 minutes after injection. Subsequently,

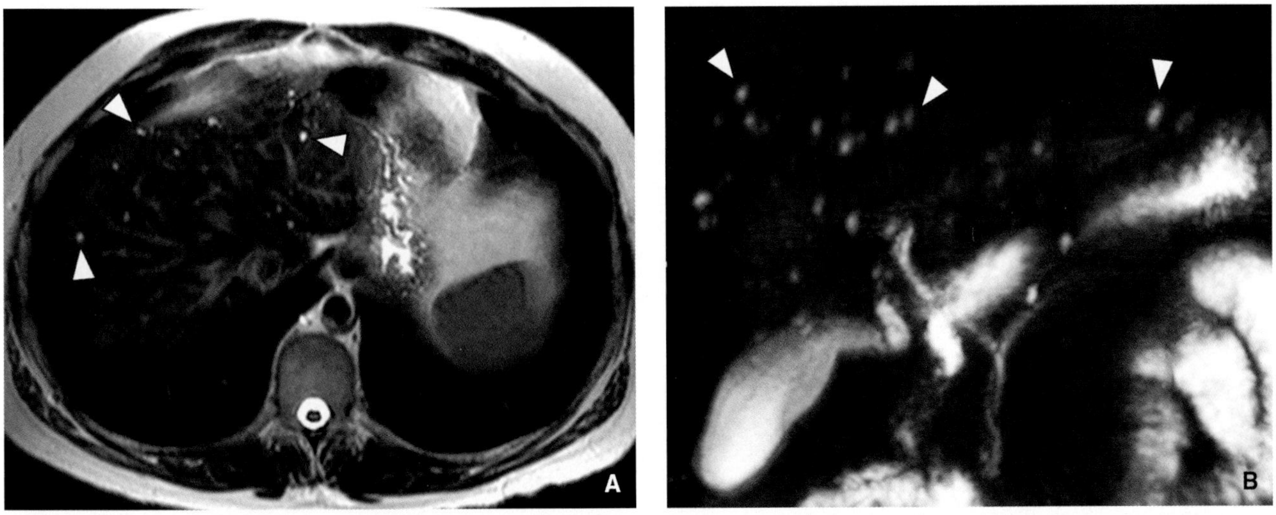

FIGURE 14.69 **A 25-year-old man with biliary hamartomas.** Axial T2-weighted **(A)** and coronal **(B)** MRCP maximum intensity projection MR images show many tiny hyperintense foci scattered throughout the liver (*arrowheads*). (Case courtesy of Jonathan R. Dillman, MD, MSc, Cincinnati Children's Hospital Medical Center, Cincinnati, OH.)

TABLE 14.6 Causes of Neonatal Cholestasis

Obstructive/Biliary Disorders
Biliary atresia
Choledochal malformation
Cystic fibrosis
Choledocholithiasis
Alagille syndrome
Neonatal sclerosing cholangitis
Tumor
Spontaneous common bile duct perforation
Hepatocellular Disorders
Neonatal hepatitis
Infection (e.g., TORCH infections, sepsis)
Metabolic (e.g.,α-1-antitrypsin deficiency)
Chromosomal disorders
Toxic (e.g., total parenteral nutrition, medications)
Endocrinopathy
Vascular (e.g., congestive heart failure)

tracer is excreted into the biliary tree with activity visible within the gallbladder and duodenum within 60 minutes. Proper protocol is important for the differentiation of causes of neonatal cholestasis. Patients should be premedicated with phenobarbital for 5 days prior to the exam to stimulate hepatocyte activity, and delayed images must be obtained through 24 hours to separate absent (biliary atresia) and delayed radiotracer excretion into bowel (e.g., neonatal hepatitis, Alagille syndrome).[149]

Biliary Atresia

Biliary atresia is the most common cause of neonatal cholestasis and the most common reason for pediatric liver transplantation.[150] This obliterative cholangiopathy is caused by an as-yet-unidentified prenatal and perinatal inflammatory process that results in chronic cholestasis and biliary cirrhosis.[151] In most infants, the obliterative process involves both the central intrahepatic ducts and the extrahepatic ducts at the level of the porta hepatis. The majority of cases are isolated (90%) with the remainder occurring in association with syndromes, including heterotaxy.[152]

Classic clinical features are jaundice, pale- or clay-colored stools, and dark urine presenting at birth, or soon thereafter. Kasai portoenterostomy is usually the initial surgical intervention in biliary atresia. The Kasai procedure involves excision of the central fibrotic bile ducts with anastomosis of a Roux-en-Y jejunal limb to the porta hepatis, restoring bile flow in 60% to 70% of patients[153] (Fig. 14.70). Ultimately many patients need liver transplantation.

In the initial assessment of suspected biliary atresia, ultrasound and hepatobiliary scintigraphy are commonly performed. The classic ultrasound finding is the triangular cord sign in which fibrotic remnants of the bile ducts appear as a hyperechoic thickening (≥3 mm) contiguous with the anterior wall of the right portal vein, at or just

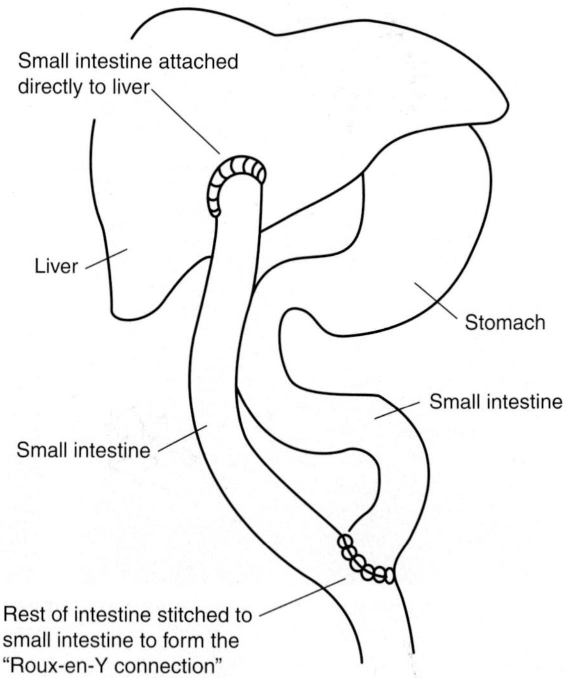

FIGURE 14.70 **Diagram of the Kasai portoenterostomy procedure.** In this operation designed to restore biliary outflow from the liver, the proximal jejunum is divided creating a Roux-en-Y limb that is brought up and anastomosed to the porta hepatis. Enteric continuity is then restored by anastomosing the proximal jejunum to more distal jejunum downstream from the Roux limb.

beyond the bifurcation (Fig. 14.71). This finding is reported to be highly specific for biliary atresia, but sensitivity varies from 60% to 85%.[154–156] Other findings of biliary atresia include nonvisualization of the CBD, an enlarged hepatic artery, and an absent or small gallbladder with abnormal morphology and wall thickness. Importantly, the presence of a relatively normal-appearing gallbladder does not exclude biliary atresia, however, and can be seen in up to 25% of patients.[155,157]

Hepatobiliary scintigraphy is highly (nearly 100%) sensitive for biliary atresia[149] (Fig. 14.72). Hepatocyte uptake of the tracer can be normal or delayed with the diagnosis hinging on absent excretion of radiotracer into the bowel at 24 hours. MRCP is being increasingly described for the diagnosis of biliary atresia, though it has not been shown to have higher diagnostic accuracy than other modalities.[21,158]

Ultrasound and MRI currently are the imaging tests of choice in the longitudinal follow-up of patients after Kasai portoenterostomy. Important findings potentially heralding Kasai failure include recurrent biliary obstruction, ascending cholangitis, and progressive liver disease resulting in cirrhosis. Bile duct dilation also suggests a complication and may be segmental or diffuse, often having a beaded appearance (Fig. 14.73).[159] Superimposed cholangiohepatitis can be suggested when an abscess, other focal parenchymal abnormality, or hyperenhancement is present along the course of the dilated ducts (Fig. 14.74).[160,161] Bile lakes are frequently

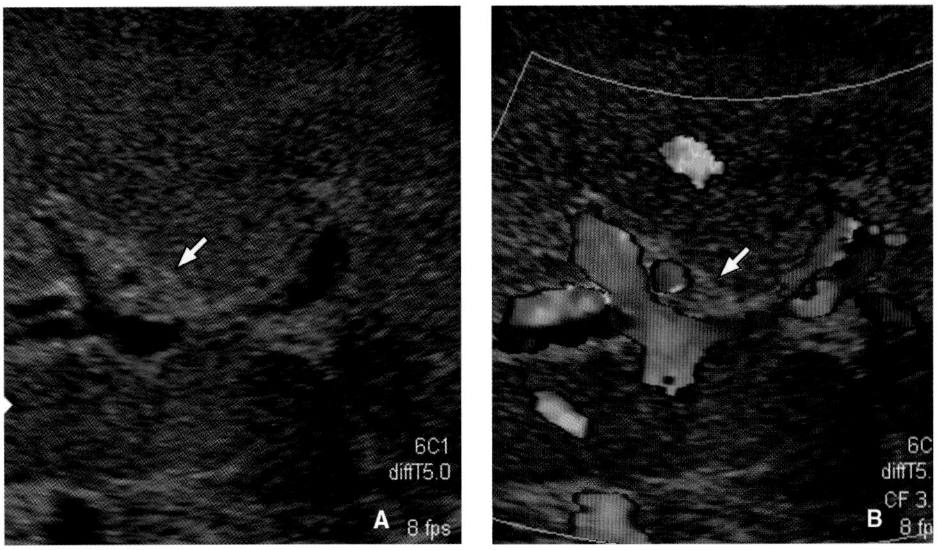

FIGURE 14.71 **A 6-month-old girl with biliary atresia.** Transverse gray-scale **(A)** and color Doppler **(B)** ultrasound images at the level of the liver hilum show echogenic thickening anterior to the portal vein bifurcation (*arrow*) with nonvisualization of the common hepatic duct, consistent with the "triangular cord" sign.

present, representing bile pseudocysts caused by damaged bile ducts.[162] As cirrhosis progresses, regenerative nodules may be identified and must be differentiated from hepatocellular neoplasm (adenoma and carcinoma), for which late-stage Kasai patients are at risk.[163,164]

Alagille Syndrome

Alagille syndrome, also known as arteriohepatic dysplasia, is an autosomal dominant inherited disorder in which a paucity of intrahepatic bile ducts results in chronic cholestasis and potentially progressive biliary cirrhosis. The genetic basis of the disease accounts for its association with other multisystemic developmental anomalies, the most clinically significant of which affect the cardiovascular system (e.g., tetralogy of Fallot).

The primary reason for imaging the liver in suspected Alagille syndrome is to exclude a surgically correctable cause for cholestasis, such as biliary atresia. In the early phase of

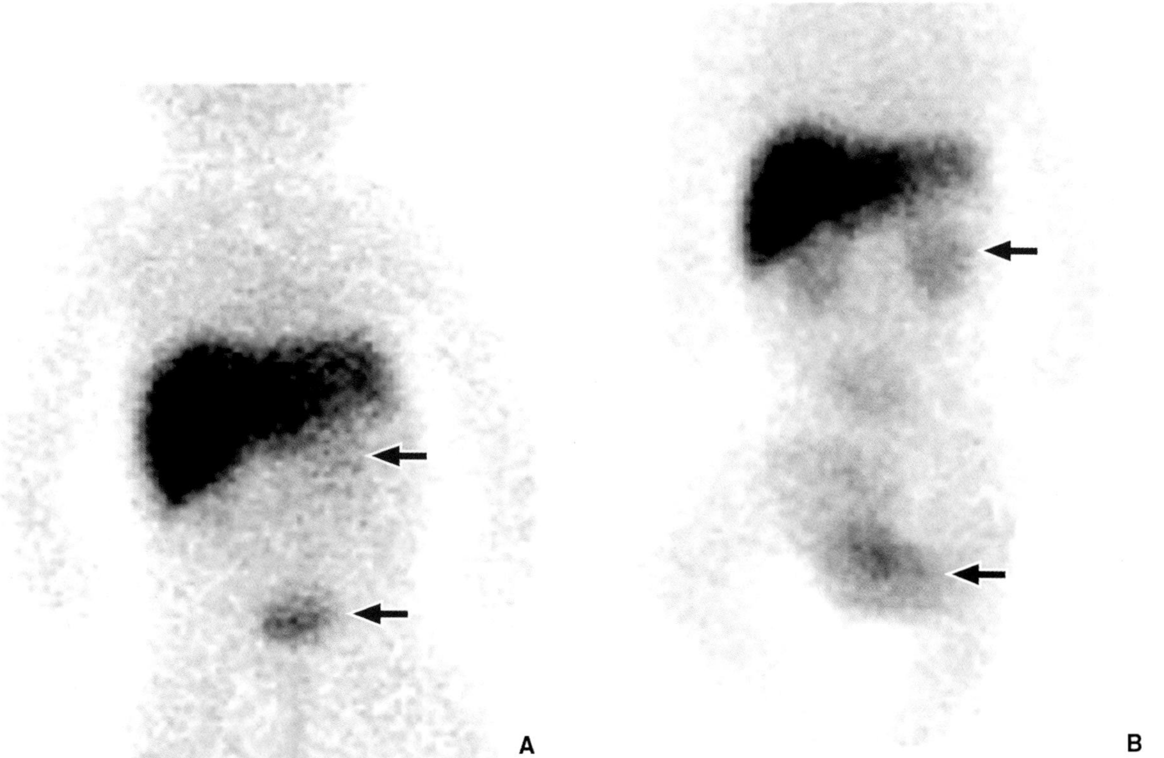

FIGURE 14.72 **A 2-week-old boy with biliary atresia. A:** A 4-hour delayed anterior projection image (**left**) from a HIDA scan with ^{99m}Tc-mebrofenin shows intense radiotracer activity within the liver (delayed clearance) and faint activity in the genitourinary system (*arrows*). No activity is seen in the intestinal tract. **B:** A 24-hour delayed image shows persistent intense radiotracer activity in the liver with continued lack of intestinal activity. Again, activity is seen in the genitourinary system and in the child's diaper (*arrows*).

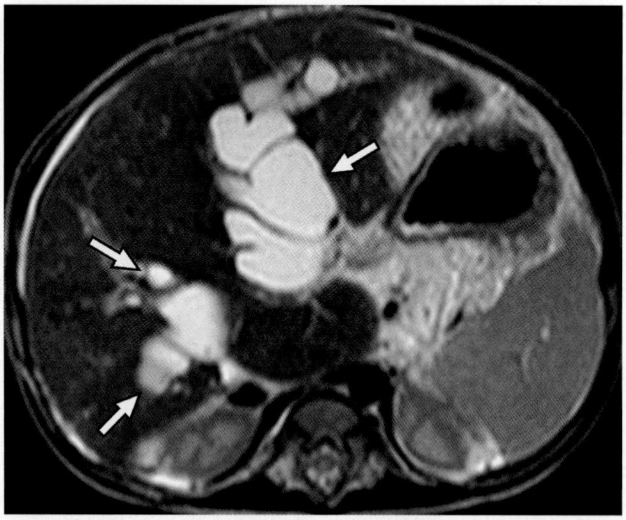

FIGURE 14.73 **An 11-month-old girl with biliary atresia status post Kasai operation.** Axial T2-weighted MR image shows marked cystic enlargement of multiple bile ducts (*arrows*). Associated bile stasis is a risk factor for ascending cholangitis. (Image courtesy of Jonathan R. Dillman, MD, MSc, Cincinnati Children's Hospital Medical Center, Cincinnati, OH.)

disease, ultrasound findings are nonspecific and often normal. As the disease progresses, hepatomegaly and findings of cirrhosis may become apparent; affected children are at some increased risk for hepatocellular neoplasms. On hepatobiliary scintigraphy, bowel excretion may be delayed but should be present, thereby excluding biliary atresia.[165,166] Intraoperative cholangiography and liver biopsy can also be used to confirm

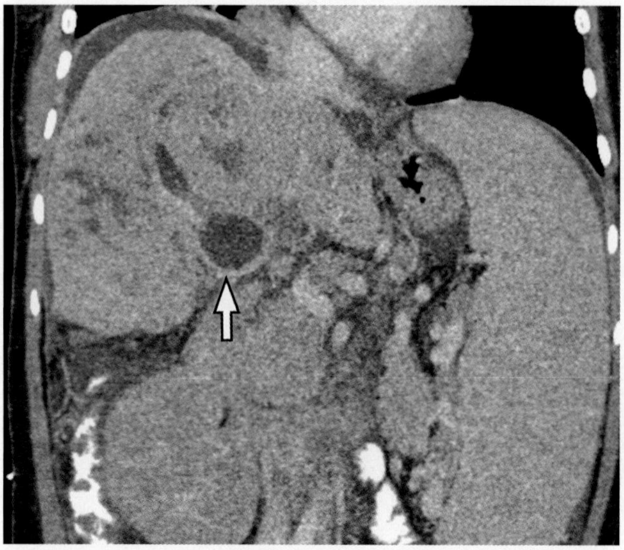

FIGURE 14.74 **An 11-year-old girl with biliary atresia with failing liver after Kasai procedure.** Coronal reformatted CT image 11 years after initial Kasai procedure shows a shrunken cirrhotic liver with findings of portal hypertension, including splenomegaly and ascites. Central bile duct dilation is present at the portoenterosomy anastomosis (*arrow*) with irregular areas of low attenuation throughout the liver. In the setting of fever and leukocytosis, ascending cholangitis is likely due to bile stasis.

this diagnosis. Over time, patients with Alagille syndrome may develop characteristic central macroregenerative tissue/nodules. These pseudolesions should be distinguishable from hepatocellular neoplasms.

Treatment includes medical therapy to improve bile flow and decrease pruritus as well as surgical correction of cardiovascular anomalies.

Acquired Biliary and Gallbladder Disorders

Cholelithiasis and Choledocholithiasis

The two most common types of biliary tract calculi in children are pigmented and cholesterol stones. Pigmented stones containing calcium bilirubinate are typically seen in neonates and children with an underlying abnormality resulting in elevated bilirubin, such as hemolytic anemia (e.g., hereditary spherocytosis) or chronic parenteral nutrition.[167] Cholesterol stones (Fig. 14.75) are caused by oversaturation of bile with cholesterol and are more common in adolescent patients, especially in the setting of obesity.[168]

Cholelithiasis is more common than choledocholithiasis (stones within the bile ducts) in children. Most cases of choledocholithiasis are a complication of cholelithiasis. Less commonly, stones may form primarily within the intra- or extrahepatic bile ducts related to a congenital or acquired disorder resulting in bile stasis. Uncomplicated cholelithiasis presents with biliary colic (pain caused by transient cystic duct obstruction by a stone), nausea, vomiting, and fatty meal intolerance. Choledocholithiasis presents with similar features, although obstructive jaundice is a more frequent occurrence.[169] Choledocholithiasis can be complicated by cholangitis or pancreatitis if the stone obstructs the duct at the ampulla of Vater or major papilla.

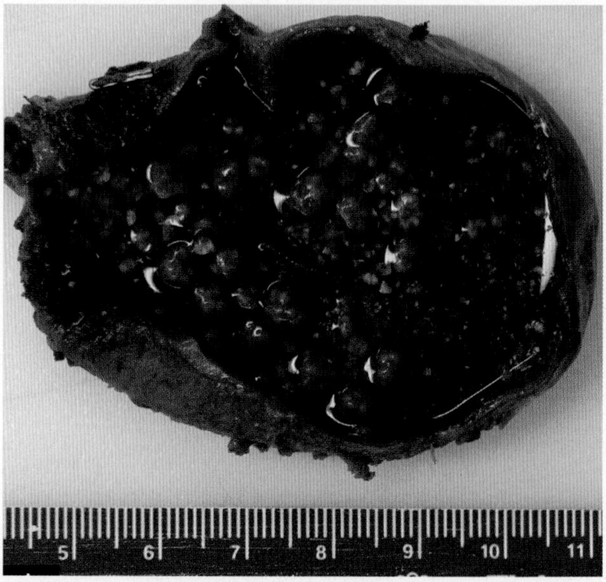

FIGURE 14.75 **Cholelithiasis in a child.** The lumen of this gallbladder is opened to show multiple yellow bosselated stones, characteristic of cholesterol gallstones.

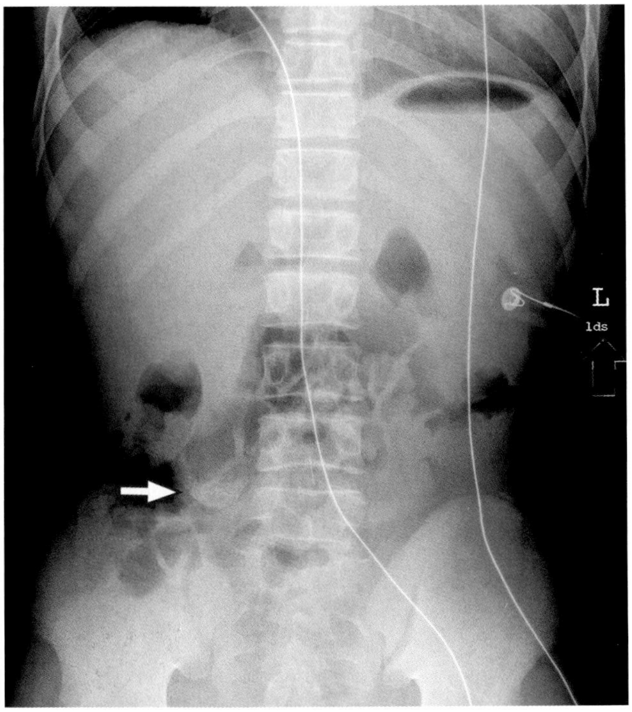

FIGURE 14.76 **A 16-year-old boy with cholelithiasis.** Upright abdominal radiograph shows numerous calcifications (*arrow*) layering dependently in the gallbladder fundus.

Pigmented stones may be heavily calcified and visible on radiographs (Fig. 14.76). Other types of stones are more commonly radiolucent. Ultrasound is the most appropriate initial imaging modality to evaluate for cholelithiasis, having a sensitivity of 98%.[170] Stones are seen as mobile, echogenic foci. Larger calculi typically have posterior acoustic shadowing and may show twinkling artifact on Doppler interrogation (Fig. 14.77). The stones may completely fill the lumen, giving the classic wall-echo-shadow appearance (Fig. 14.78). Sonography

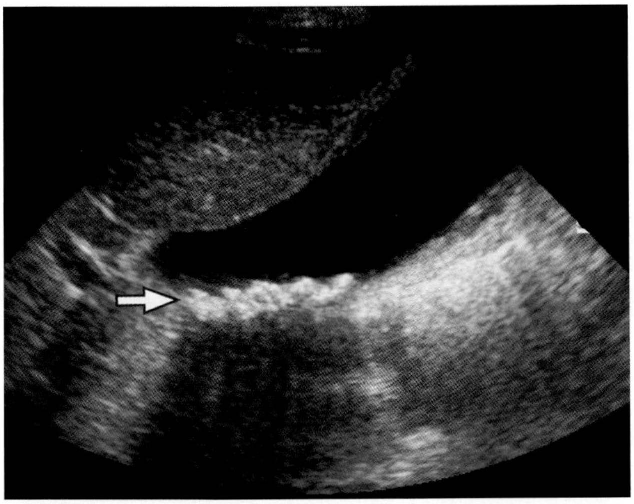

FIGURE 14.77 **A 16-year-old boy with cholelithiasis.** Gray-scale ultrasound image through the gallbladder confirms the presence of multiple dependent, echogenic, shadowing gallstones (*arrow*). There is no gallbladder wall thickening or pericholecystic fluid to suggest acute cholecystitis.

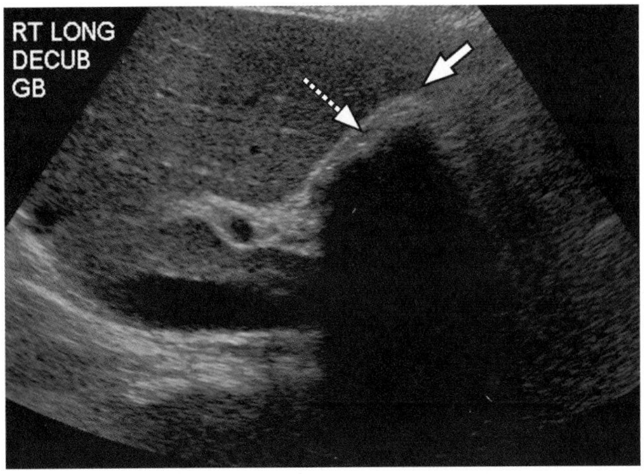

FIGURE 14.78 **A 13-year-old girl with cholelithiasis.** Longitudinal gray-scale ultrasound image shows a gallbladder nearly completely filled with gallstones, giving the characteristic wall-echo-shadow appearance. Other than the anterior wall (*arrow*), the gallbladder is entirely obscured by the shadowing gallstones (*dashed arrow*).

is less reliable in detecting CBD stones, particularly stones lodged in the ampulla of Vater, because of overlying bowel gas. Secondary findings, however, of a dilated CBD (>2.5 mm in infant and >4 mm in older children) in the setting of gallstones should raise suspicion for choledocholithiasis (Fig. 14.79).[171] CT and MRI generally do not add value in uncomplicated cholelithiasis. These modalities may be useful, however, when choledocholithiasis or cholecystitis is suspected. MRCP has been shown to be moderately effective at visualizing stones in the extrahepatic bile duct, which appear as hypointense intraluminal foci on heavily T2-weighted sequences[172] (Fig. 14.80).

Symptomatic cholelithiasis in children is usually an indication for cholecystectomy. Concurrent choledocholithiasis may require endoscopic retrograde cholangiopancreatography (ERCP) with balloon sweep and sphincterotomy.

Acute Cholecystitis

Acute cholecystitis can be calculous or acalculous in origin. In acute calculous cholecystitis, the gallbladder becomes inflamed following obstruction of the cystic duct by a stone or stones. Distinct episodes of acute calculous cholecystitis requiring urgent surgical intervention occur in only a small proportion of patients with cholelithiasis.[173] Instead, studies suggest that children with cholelithiasis may suffer repeated bouts of low-grade or subclinical acute cholecystitis.[174] This is supported by the common pathologic finding of chronic cholecystitis in pediatric patients who undergo cholecystectomy for symptomatic cholelithiasis.

Acalculous cholecystitis is more common in children than adults, accounting for 30% to 50% of all cases.[175] In acute acalculous cholecystitis, gallbladder inflammation occurs in the absence of cholelithiasis. The inciting factor is thought to be at least partially related to bile stasis with bacterial overgrowth, often in patients with a systemic illness, such as septicemia, pneumonia, burn wounds, and viral infections. Clinical signs of acute cholecystitis may include right upper quadrant abdominal

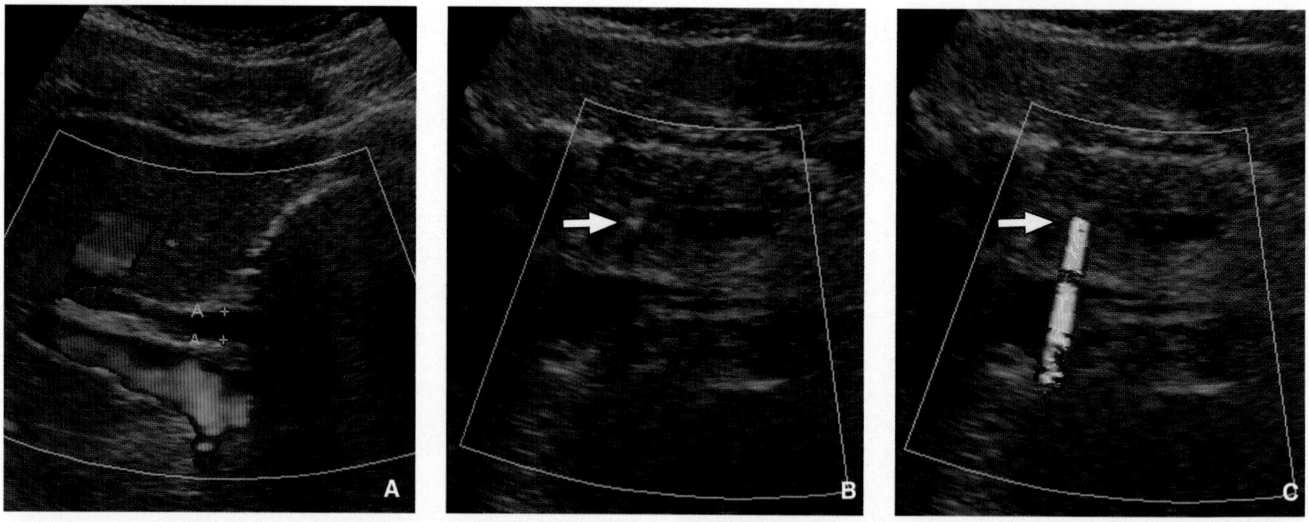

FIGURE 14.79 **A 16-year-old boy with choledocholithiasis. A:** Longitudinal ultrasound image shows a dilated common bile duct (CBD) (*cursors*) measuring 7 mm in diameter. A 4 mm echogenic, shadowing focus [*arrow* in **(B)**] is seen at the level of the pancreatic head, demonstrating twinkling artifact with the application of color Doppler [*arrow* in **(C)**], compatible with a stone in the distal CBD.

pain, nausea, vomiting, fever, and jaundice. The clinical presentation may be unclear in patients with a systemic illness, leading to delayed recognition and increased morbidity and mortality[176]; imaging adds particular value in this subgroup of patients.

Ultrasound and scintigraphy are the primary modalities employed in the assessment of acute cholecystitis. Ultrasound findings include cholelithiasis, gallbladder wall thickening (>3 mm), hyperemia, pericholecystic fluid, gallbladder distention, and sonographic Murphy sign (Fig. 14.81). Wall thickening in the absence of other findings is nonspecific and can be seen in conditions such as hypoalbuminemia, ascites, hepatitis, and diseases resulting in systemic venous hypertension.[177] Hepatobiliary scintigraphy is reported to be the most accurate imaging modality for acute cholecystitis, having a sensitivity and specificity of 96% and 90%, respectively.[178] Dynamic imaging is typically performed for 60 minutes with either delayed imaging at 2 to 4 hours or supplemental imaging over 30 minutes following morphine augmentation. Nonvisualization of the gallbladder during initial imaging and on delayed or morphine augmented images is suggestive of acute cystic duct obstruction and acute cholecystitis (Fig. 14.82). CT and MRI are not first-line modalities for imaging acute cholecystitis, although they may be performed in the workup of abdominal pain, with findings similar to what is seen by ultrasound. These modalities can detect delayed complications, such as abscess formation or gallbladder rupture.

Initial nonoperative treatment (e.g., antibiotic therapy, percutaneous cholecystotomy) is preferred at some institutions with surgery performed after a "cooling down" period. Gallbladder perforation is rare but requires emergent surgery as this complication is potentially fatal.

Functional Biliary Disease

Functional biliary disease is a general term for biliary symptoms (pain, nausea, vomiting) in the absence of biliary calculi. Functional biliary disease encompasses biliary dyskinesia,

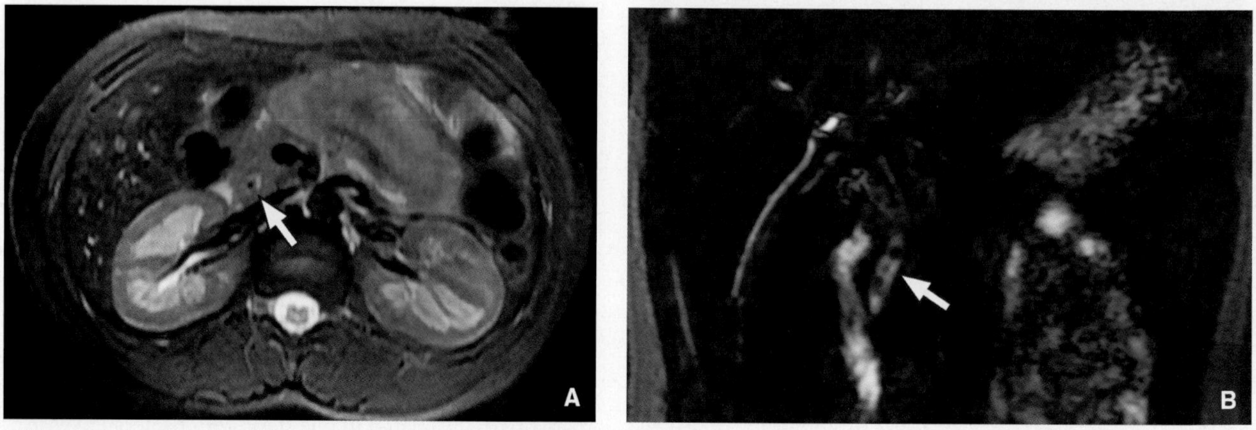

FIGURE 14.80 **A 17-year-old girl with choledocholithiasis. A:** Axial fat-suppressed T2-weighted MR image shows a low signal filling defect in the distal common bile duct (CBD) in the head of the pancreas (*arrow*). Diffuse low signal in the renal cortex reflects iron deposition related to this patient's sickle cell disease. **B:** Coronal MRCP image shows multiple hypointense stones within a mildly dilated distal CBD (*arrow*).

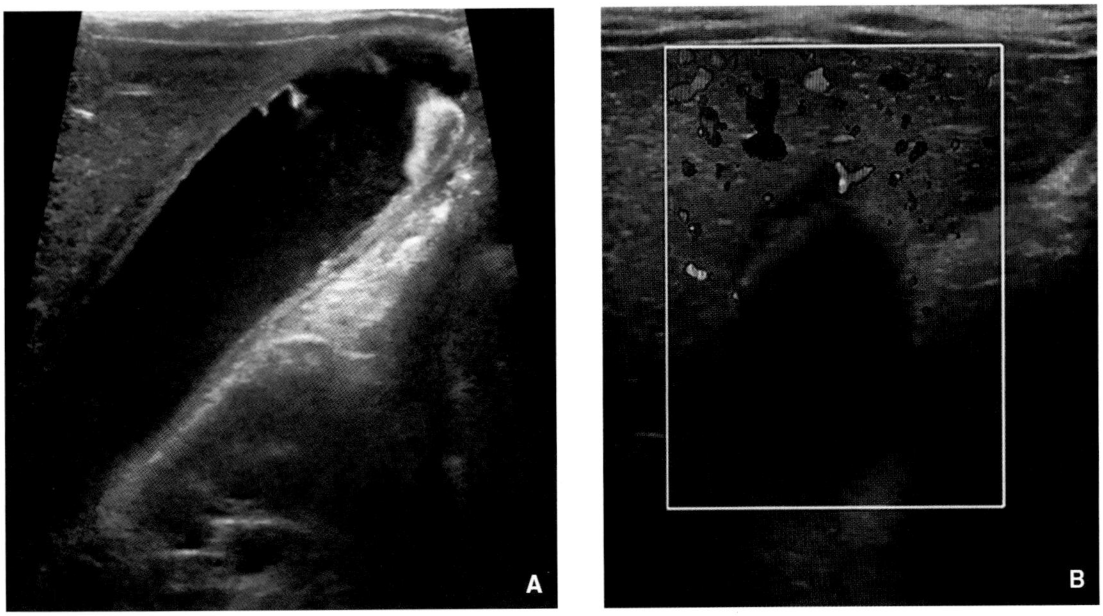

FIGURE 14.81 **A 6-year-old girl with pathology-proven acute acalculous cholecystitis. A:** Longitudinal gray-scale ultrasound image shows gallbladder wall thickening, pericholecystic fluid/edema, and intraluminal debris. No shadowing gallstones were identified. **B:** Transverse color Doppler ultrasound image shows adjacent liver parenchymal hyperemia.

cystic duct syndrome, and gallbladder and cystic duct spasm. This group of disorders has recently become a leading cause of cholecystectomy in children but remains a diagnosis of exclusion.[179] Cholecystokinin (CCK)-stimulated hepatobiliary scintigraphy is well established as a diagnostic method in adults. A gallbladder ejection fraction <39% during a 60 minute continuous infusion of CCK is considered abnormal and suggestive of functional biliary disease.[180] The use of CCK-stimulated hepatobiliary scintigraphy has been extrapolated to children, but normative values for pediatric gallbladder ejection fraction have not been established (Fig. 14.83).

Infectious Cholangitis

Infection of the biliary tree may occur from bacterial, viral, or parasitic sources. Bacteria are the most common cause of infectious cholangitis in Western countries. Bacterial cholangitis typically occurs in the setting of bile stasis or obstruction that diminishes the normal antibacterial properties of bile. Causes of bile stasis/obstruction in children that can predispose to cholangitis include choledocholithiasis, congenital biliary anomalies, inflammatory disorders (e.g., primary sclerosing cholangitis) and postsurgical stenoses. The Charcot triad is the classic symptom complex associated

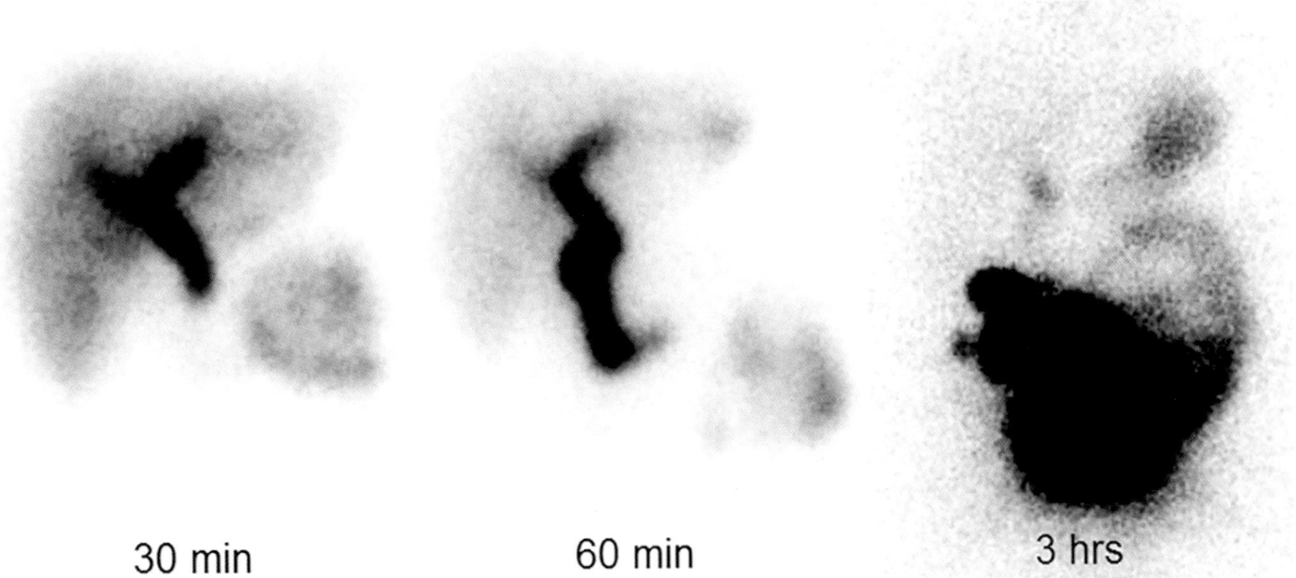

FIGURE 14.82 **A 13-year-old girl with right upper quadrant abdominal pain due to acute calculous cholecystitis.** Selected images from a HIDA scan with ^{99m}Tc-mebrofenin show radiotracer activity in the biliary tree and increasing bowel activity as time progresses. Lack of gallbladder visualization at 60 minutes with persistent absence of gallbladder activity at 3 hours is suggestive of acute cholecystitis.

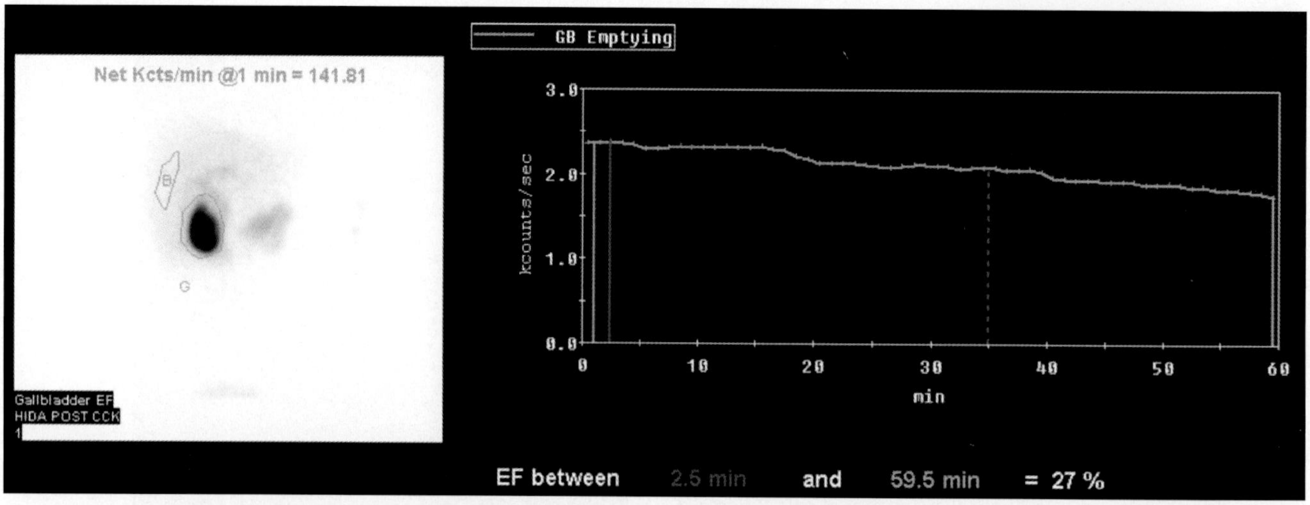

FIGURE 14.83 **A 15-year-old girl with chronic abdominal pain.** Dynamic post-CCK image sequence from a HIDA scan with ^{99m}Tc-mebrofenin to assess gallbladder ejection fraction shows 27% ejection fraction with a 60 minute CCK infusion. This is below the 39% cutoff and is compatible with biliary dyskinesia.

with bacterial cholangitis, composed of fever, right upper quadrant abdominal pain, and jaundice and is present in approximately 70% of patients.[181]

Imaging findings of bacterial cholangitis include diffuse, central, or regional intrahepatic ductal dilation. Debris, purulent material, and calculi within the bile ducts are best demonstrated with ultrasound or MRI. Ductal inflammation can be seen as wall thickening with either increased or decreased periductal echogenicity on ultrasound or as abnormal mural enhancement on MRI with periductal T2-weighted signal hyperintensity. Parenchymal abscesses along a biliary distribution are well seen on US, CT, and MRI. MRI may also show abnormal parenchymal increased T2-weighted signal or heterogeneous enhancement in the absence of a discrete abscess. Pneumobilia can be seen in severe cases.

Early recognition and treatment of cholangitis is necessary as life-threatening sepsis can develop. Treatment includes antibiotic therapy and relieving biliary obstruction, by surgical, percutaneous transhepatic, or endoscopic (e.g., ERCP) methods.

Primary Sclerosing Cholangitis

Primary sclerosing cholangitis (PSC) is a chronic cholestatic disorder characterized by progressive inflammation and fibrosis of the intra- and extrahepatic bile ducts leading to obliteration of the lumen. The etiology of PSC is unknown but is thought to be autoimmune.[182] PSC and autoimmune hepatitis coexist in up to 25% of patients.[183] The most common risk factor (60% to 80%) for developing PSC is inflammatory bowel disease, primarily ulcerative colitis but also Crohn disease.[182] The clinical presentation of PSC is variable, and children are frequently asymptomatic or present with vague symptoms such as fatigue, pruritus, right upper quadrant abdominal pain, direct hyperbilirubinemia, or fever. A frequent complication of PSC is recurrent infectious cholangitis caused by biliary obstruction. Although it is extremely rare in the pediatric population, cholangiocarcinoma may develop.

PSC affects the bile ducts in a heterogeneous pattern, leading to a wide range of appearances at imaging. Involvement of both the intrahepatic and extrahepatic ducts is the most common pattern (40%). Isolated intrahepatic disease is seen in 15%, and isolated extrahepatic involvement in 10%. Up to 35% of patients will have what is termed small-duct PSC.[184] This form is characterized by isolated involvement of the peripheral intrahepatic bile ducts, which are not well seen on imaging.

Dilated and irregular intrahepatic bile ducts can be seen with US and CT. However, MRCP is the mainstay for noninvasive imaging of PSC, allowing high-resolution imaging of both the intra- and extrahepatic biliary tree with the advantage over ERCP of being able to visualize obstructed intrahepatic ducts without risk of pancreatitis. The classic finding is a "beaded" appearance of the intrahepatic ducts in a diffuse or segmental distribution (Fig. 14.84). Isolated or "floating" peripheral ducts may also be seen. Bile duct wall thickening and hyperenhancement are common findings on postcontrast imaging. Diverticular outpouchings resulting from more severe damage to the duct wall are sometimes seen. In long-standing disease, liver parenchyma may show changes of biliary cirrhosis (Fig. 14.84).

Treatment is aimed at palliating the clinical symptoms and slowing progression of the disease. Medical management may include antibiotic therapy and immunosuppression, which is commonly ineffectual. Balloon dilation and stenting of dominant strictures and percutaneous drainage can improve symptoms and delay liver transplantation. Liver transplantation remains the definitive treatment for advanced PSC, although the disease may recur in up to 37% of cases.[185]

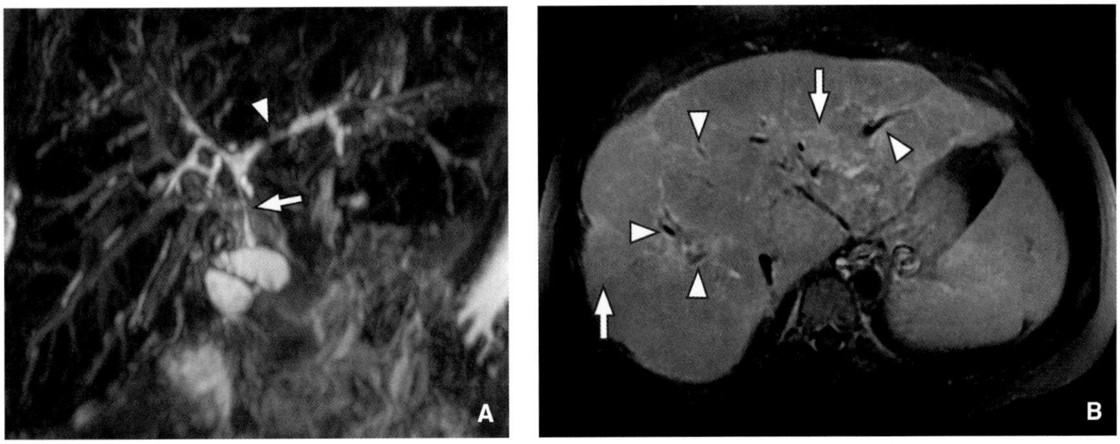

FIGURE 14.84 **A 15-year-old girl with primary sclerosing cholangitis. A:** Coronal maximum intensity projection (MIP) MRCP image shows multifocal areas of bile duct stricturing and luminal irregularity, best seen in the common bile duct (CBD) (*arrow*) and central left intrahepatic duct (*arrowhead*). **B:** Axial postcontrast fat-suppressed T1-weighted MR image shows abnormal enhancement of the thickened bile duct walls (*arrowheads*). Also present are changes of parenchymal fibrosis with capsular retraction and patchy areas of parenchymal delayed hyperenhancement (*arrows*).

Gallbladder Hydrops

Gallbladder hydrops, or gallbladder mucocele, is characterized by marked overdistention of the gallbladder in the absence of gallstones and is a rare cause of abdominal pain in children. Several mechanisms have been suggested, most involving some form of intermittent cystic duct obstruction by bile salts/solids, anatomical narrowing, or extrinsic compression. This entity may present at any age but has been most commonly reported in infants and young children. Gallbladder hydrops has a well-known association with Kawasaki disease, although it can also be seen with other disorders such as infectious hepatitis, polyarteritis nodosa, and systemic streptococcal and staphylococcal infections.

Imaging of this entity is best performed with ultrasound, which typically shows a markedly distended fluid-filled gallbladder without gallstones, wall thickening, or pericholecystic inflammation (Fig. 14.85). Normal maximal gallbladder length is <3.6 cm in infants and ranges up to 7 cm in older children. Similarly, normal maximum gallbladder width can range from 1.3 cm in infants to 2.5 cm in older children.[186]

Management usually includes treating any underlying systemic illness, intravenous fluids, and supportive care as the overdistention is usually transient.

Gallbladder Polyps and Hyperplastic Cholecystoses

Polypoid lesions of the gallbladder are uncommon in children. Histologically, most lesions are cholesterol polyps, but polyps may also be adenomatous, hyperplastic, or inflammatory.[187] Of the different histologic types, only adenomatous polyps are true neoplasms. Gallbladder polyps are usually clinically silent and found incidentally during abdominal ultrasound. On ultrasound, polyps appear as echogenic pedunculated or sessile lesions attached to the gallbladder wall (nonmobile) without a posterior acoustic shadow (Fig. 14.86). As these lesions are generally considered to be benign, no specific treatment is indicated for small polyps. Larger polyps (≥10 mm) are usually treated with cholecystectomy because of the risk of malignancy associated with adenomatous polyps.[188]

Cholesterolosis and adenomyomatosis are considered hyperplastic cholecystoses, both of which are mucosal abnormalities with features of hyperplasia. Cholesterolosis is the abnormal accumulation of cholesterol in macrophages present

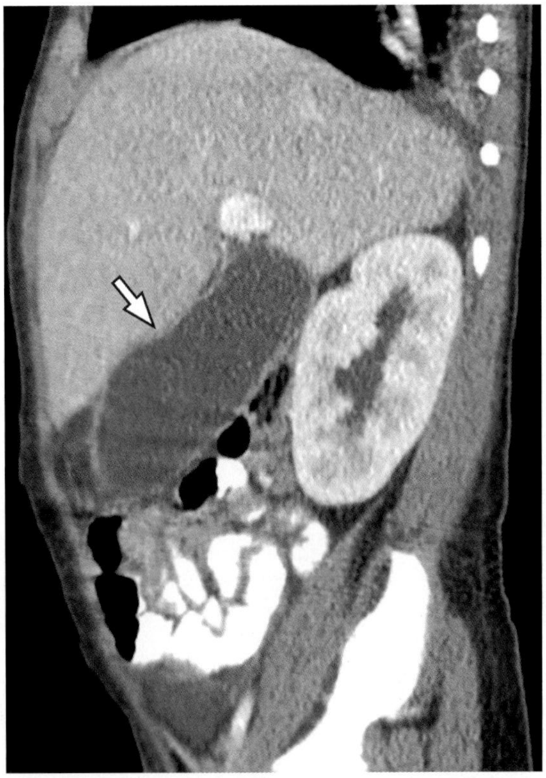

FIGURE 14.85 **A 5-year-old boy with Kawasaki disease and gallbladder hydrops.** Sagittal contrast-enhanced CT image shows a markedly enlarged gallbladder (*arrow*) that is nearly equal in size to the adjacent kidney. There is no gallbladder wall thickening or pericholecystic fluid.

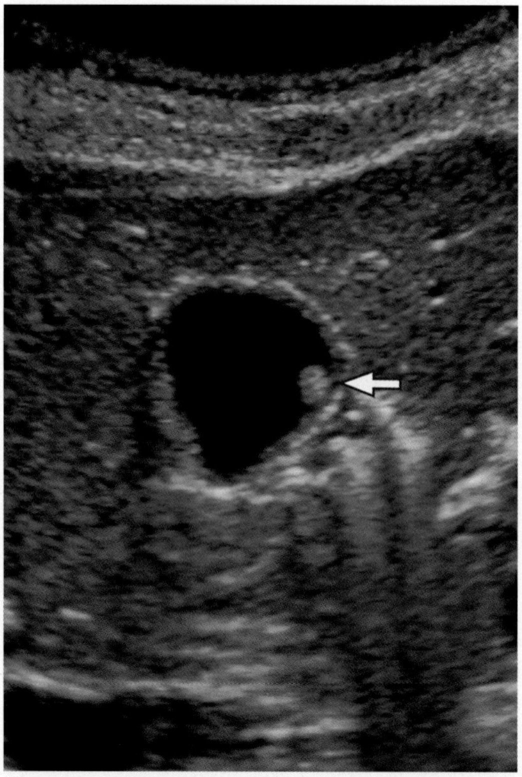

FIGURE 14.86 **An 18-year-old man with a gallbladder polyp.** Transverse gray-scale ultrasound image obtained in right lateral decubitus position shows a nondependent mucosal-based echogenic structure (*arrow*) within the gallbladder with no posterior acoustic shadowing.

in the mucosa. Adenomyomatosis results from mucosal hyperplasia creating intramural invaginations (Rokitansky-Aschoff sinuses) that trap bile salts.[189] Both of these entities are most commonly identified by ultrasound. Cholesterolosis can appear as echogenic gallbladder polyps with no posterior acoustic shadowing. Comet tail (ring down) reverberation and twinkling artifacts may be seen (Fig. 14.87). The polyps usually range in size from 1 to 10 mm with the small polyps sometimes difficult to distinguish.[188] Adenomyomatosis appears as focal or diffuse gallbladder wall thickening, sometimes with small intramural diverticula appearing as cystic spaces within the affected portion (Fig. 14.88). Similar to cholesterolosis, the trapped intramural bile salts may demonstrate reverberation artifact.[190] When it is symptomatic (e.g., right upper quadrant abdominal pain), cholecystectomy may be performed.

Neoplastic Disorders

Biliary Rhabdomyosarcoma

Rhabdomyosarcoma (RMS) is the most common malignancy of the biliary tract in the pediatric population, but this tumor is extremely rare, constituting <1% of all pediatric RMS.[191,192] Most patients present between 1 and 4 years of age with jaundice, abdominal distention, and fever being the most common symptoms.[193] The site of origin is the CBD in most cases, but the tumor can arise from any biliary structure, including the gallbladder. Embryonal histologic subtype is typical. Metastases are present at diagnosis in 30% involving lymph nodes, liver, lung, or bone.[25,194,195]

The primary tumor is usually seen on ultrasound as a heterogeneous mass centered in the porta hepatis with secondary intrahepatic bile duct dilation. Cystic or necrotic areas within the mass are frequently present. On CT, the mass is usually hypoattenuating with variable enhancement. On MRI, RMS usually demonstrates T1-weighted signal hypointensity and heterogeneously hyperintense T2-weighted signal with heterogeneous postcontrast enhancement (Fig. 14.89). MRCP may better depict the intraductal location of the mass.[196] Imaging helps define local tumor extension and identify distant metastatic disease.

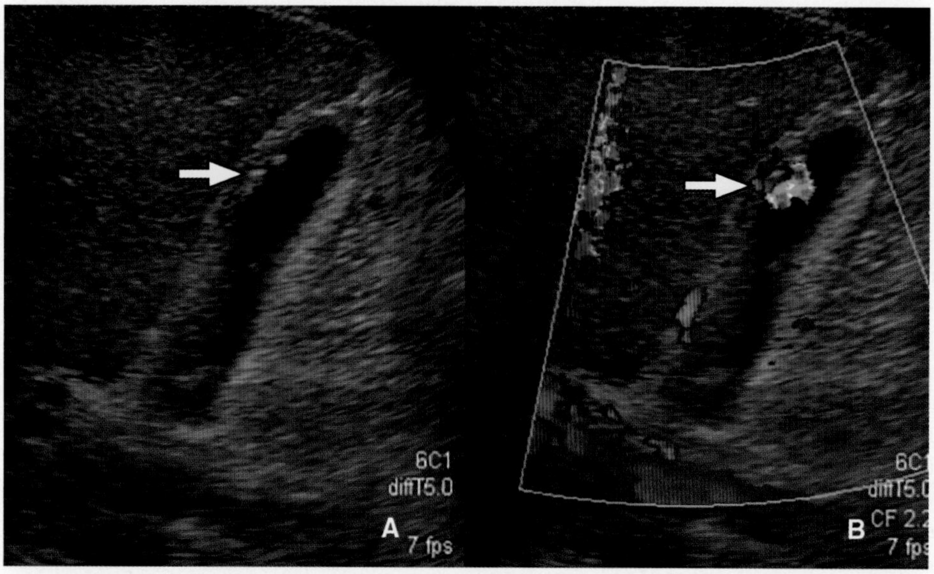

FIGURE 14.87 **A 19-year-old man with gallbladder cholesterolosis. A:** Longitudinal gray-scale ultrasound image shows small echogenic foci along the mucosa of the nondependent gallbladder fundus (*arrow*). There are associated "comet tail" (or "ring down") reverberation artifacts. **B:** With color Doppler ultrasound interrogation, there is twinkling artifact (*arrow*) associated with these foci.

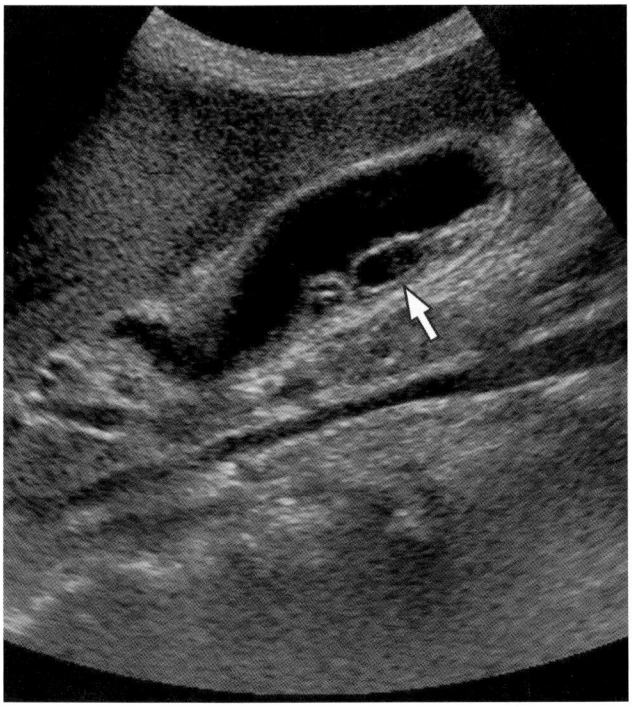

FIGURE 14.88 **A 15-year-old boy with gallbladder adenomyomatosis.** Longitudinal gray-scale ultrasound image demonstrates regional thickening of the gallbladder wall with intramural cystic spaces (*arrow*).

Management typically includes surgical resection of the mass and chemotherapy.

Cholangiocarcinoma and Gallbladder Adenocarcinoma

Cholangiocarcinoma (Fig. 14.90) is exceedingly rare in patients <25 years of age. This neoplasm can be seen in the later stages of many biliary tract disorders, most commonly PSC and choledochal cysts. Associations with PBM, choledocholithiasis, recurrent infectious cholangitis, and biliary atresia following Kasai operation have also been reported.[197] Imaging features in children have not been specifically described but should be similar to those in adults with either an obstructing hilar or a peripheral parenchymal mass with delayed enhancement. Gallbladder adenocarcinoma is even rarer in children but has been associated with several benign gallbladder disorders in adults, primarily cholelithiasis.[198]

Traumatic Disorders

Blunt and Iatrogenic Trauma

Injury to the biliary tract is an infrequent occurrence in blunt abdominal trauma. The most common site of injury is the gallbladder, followed by the extrahepatic and intrahepatic ducts.[199] Injury to these structures may occur because of stretching,

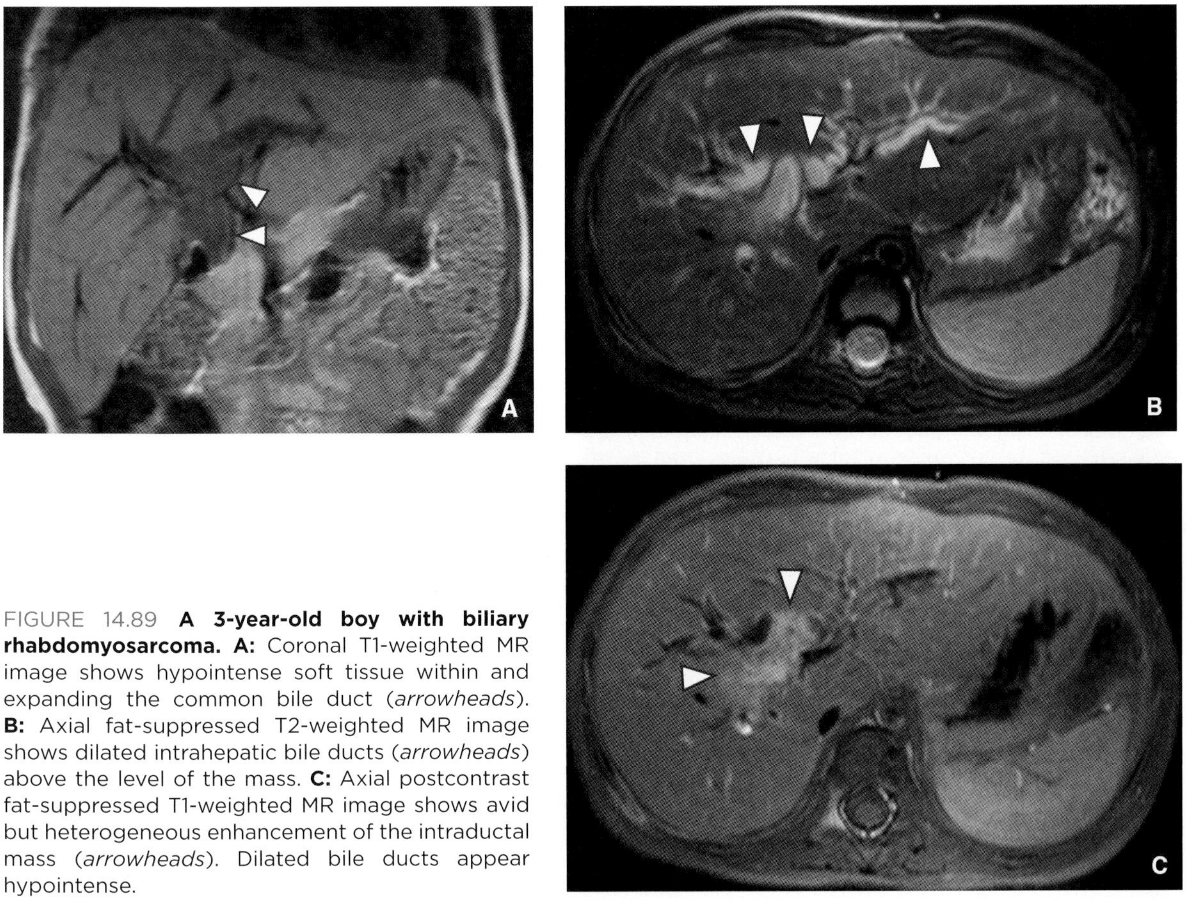

FIGURE 14.89 **A 3-year-old boy with biliary rhabdomyosarcoma. A:** Coronal T1-weighted MR image shows hypointense soft tissue within and expanding the common bile duct (*arrowheads*). **B:** Axial fat-suppressed T2-weighted MR image shows dilated intrahepatic bile ducts (*arrowheads*) above the level of the mass. **C:** Axial postcontrast fat-suppressed T1-weighted MR image shows avid but heterogeneous enhancement of the intraductal mass (*arrowheads*). Dilated bile ducts appear hypointense.

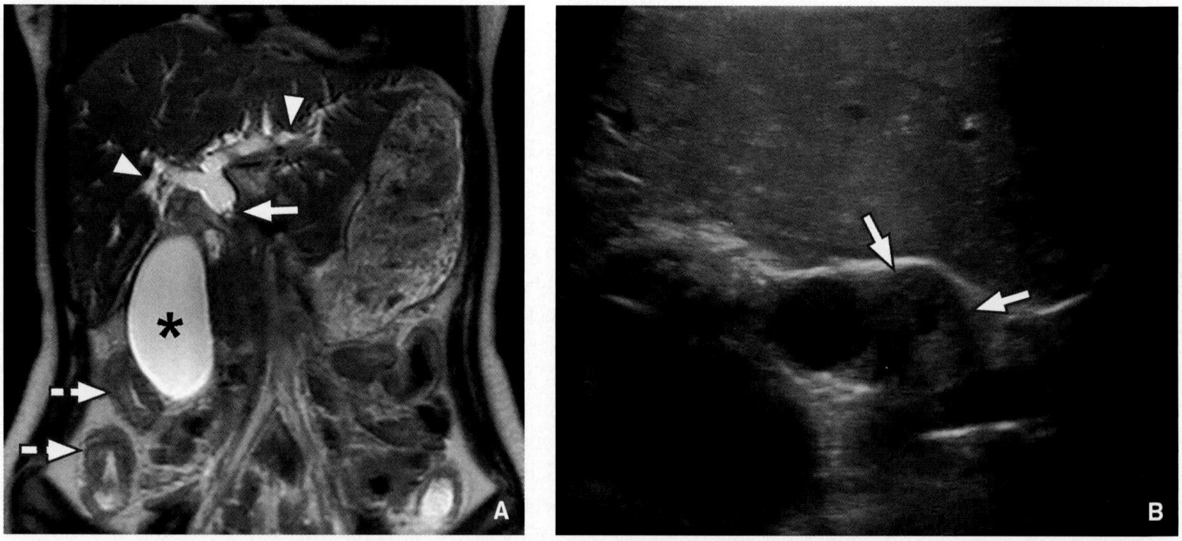

FIGURE 14.90 **A 17-year-old girl with ulcerative colitis and cholangiocarcinoma involving the common bile duct. A:** Coronal T2-weighted MR image of the abdomen shows intrahepatic bile duct and common hepatic duct dilation (*arrowheads*) with an abrupt cutoff at the level of the common bile duct (CBD) (*arrow*) reflecting the obstructing tumor. The gallbladder (*asterisk*) is distended because of obstruction. Colonic wall thickening is due to ulcerative colitis (*dashed arrows*). **B:** Transverse gray-scale ultrasound image shows marked wall thickening of the CBD (*arrows*) due to tumor. (Case courtesy of Jonathan R. Dillman, MD, MSc, Cincinnati Children's Hospital Medical Center, Cincinnati, OH.)

shearing, or compressive forces particularly at sites of anatomic fixation, such as the hepatic duct confluence and intrapancreatic segment of the CBD. Potential biliary injuries include contusion, perforation/ laceration, and complete avulsion.[200]

CT is the imaging modality of choice for evaluating trauma patients in the acute setting, but is of limited utility for assessment of all but the most severe biliary injuries. Gallbladder contusion may appear as a thickened, ill-defined gallbladder wall. Although nonspecific, gallbladder collapse with pericholecystic fluid should raise the suspicion for gallbladder perforation. Complete avulsion is extremely rare appearing as a free-floating or displaced gallbladder. Intra- and extrahepatic bile duct injuries may be seen as focal subhepatic fluid or intrahepatic fluid associated with a liver laceration.

Biliary injury can also be iatrogenic in origin, most commonly occurring in the setting of cholecystectomy (e.g., inadvertent clipping of an anomalous bile duct or thermal injury). Other potential iatrogenic causes of bile duct injury/biliary leak include partial hepatectomy, liver transplantation (living donors and recipients), percutaneous biliary interventions, and ERCP.

Biliary leaks can manifest as contained intra- or extrahepatic leaks (biloma) or as free intraperitoneal leaks. On anatomic imaging, bilomas appear as focal intrahepatic or extrahepatic fluid collections. Free intraperitoneal leaks appear as nonspecific free fluid within the peritoneal cavity. Hepatobiliary scintigraphy and MRI performed with a hepatocyte-specific contrast agent can confirm the biliary origin of loculated or free fluid through the identification of abnormal accumulation of the biliary excreted radiotracer or contrast agent (Fig. 14.91). MRI has the potential advantage of being able to directly localize the source of bile leakage[201–203] (Fig. 14.92). Chronic sequelae of biliary injury include superinfection of bile collections and development of bile duct strictures. MRCP is ideally suited for the assessment of resultant bile duct strictures.[204]

Treatment of biliary trauma depends on the location and severity of the injury. Signs of peritonitis are an indication for immediate laparotomy. Gallbladder perforation and avulsion are treated with cholecystectomy. Extrahepatic duct injuries may be treated surgically, by percutaneous biliary drainage catheters, or with stent placement during ERCP.

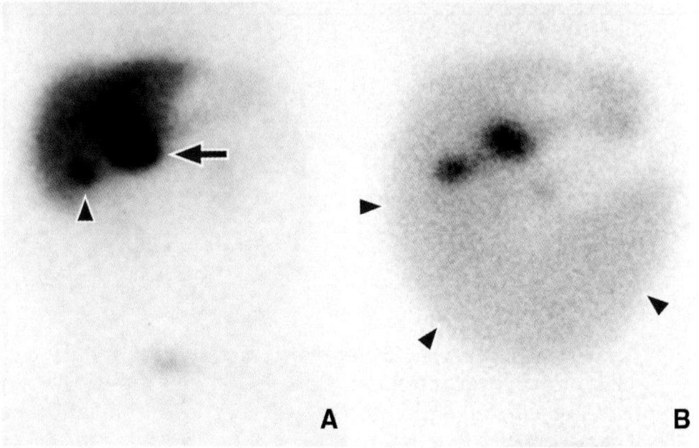

FIGURE 14.91 **A 10-week-old boy with bile leak.** Anterior image from ^{99m}Tc-mebrofenin HIDA scan obtained **(A)** 20 minutes after injection shows normal liver and gallbladder activity (*arrowhead*) and intense activity in the region of the porta hepatis (*arrow*). **B:** At 75 minutes after injection, there is now diffuse activity throughout the peritoneal cavity (*arrowheads*), compatible with a bile leak in this patient who had spontaneous perforation of the common bile duct.

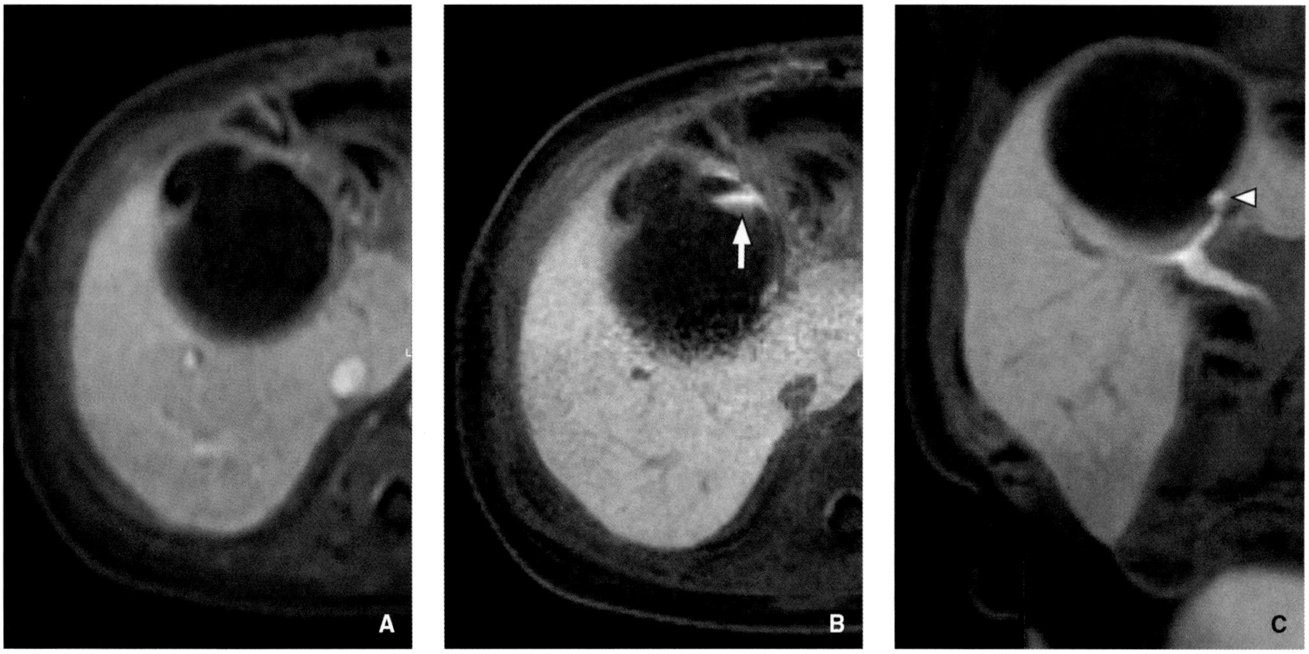

FIGURE 14.92 **A 14-month-old boy with biloma.** Postcontrast fat-suppressed T1-weighted MR images [**(A)** axial portal venous phase, **(B)** axial hepatocyte phase, and **(C)** coronal hepatocyte phase] using a hepatocyte-specific contrast agent obtained after left hepatic lobectomy show a low-signal fluid collection at the cut margin, demonstrating leakage of contrast material (*arrow*) from the biliary system into the collection. The proximal left hepatic duct (*arrowhead*) is shown to be the source of the leak.

References

1. Barbaro B, Soglia G, Alvaro G, et al. Hepatic veins in presurgical planning of hepatic resection: what a radiologist should know. *Abdom Imaging.* 2013;38(3):442–460.
2. Schmidt S, Demartines N, Soler L, et al. Portal vein normal anatomy and variants: implication for liver surgery and portal vein embolization. *Sem Intervent Radiol.* 2008;25(2):86–91.
3. Sahani D, Mehta A, Blake M, et al. Preoperative hepatic vascular evaluation with CT and MR angiography: implications for surgery. *Radiographics.* 2004;24(5):1367–1380.
4. Hiatt JR, Gabbay J, Busuttil RW. Surgical anatomy of the hepatic arteries in 1000 cases. *Ann Surg.* 1994;220(1):50–52.
5. Michels NA. Newer anatomy of the liver and its variant blood supply and collateral circulation. *Am J Surg.* 1966;112(3): 337–347.
6. Esscher T. Preduodenal portal vein—a cause of intestinal obstruction? *J Pediatr Surg.* 1980;15(5):609–612.
7. Johnson GF. Congenital preduodenal portal vein. *Am J Roentgenol Radium Ther Nucl Med.* 1971;112(1):93–99.
8. Fernandes ET, Burton EM, Hixson SD, et al. Preduodenal portal vein: surgery and radiographic appearance. *J Pediatr Surg.* 1990; 25(12):1270–1272.
9. Morgan G, Superina R. Congenital absence of the portal vein: two cases and a proposed classification system for portasystemic vascular anomalies. *J Pediatr Surg.* 1994;29(9):1239–1241.
10. Lisovsky M, Konstas AA, Misdraji J. Congenital extrahepatic portosystemic shunts (Abernethy malformation): a histopathologic evaluation. *Am J Surg Pathol.* 2011;35(9):1381–1390.
11. Stringer MD. The clinical anatomy of congenital portosystemic venous shunts. *Clin Anat.* 2008;21(2):147–157.
12. Alonso-Gamarra E, Parron M, Perez A, et al. Clinical and radiologic manifestations of congenital extrahepatic portosystemic shunts: a comprehensive review. *Radiographics.* 2011;31(3):707–722.
13. Banz V, Olliff S, Taniere P, et al. Liver tumours in patients with Abernethy malformation. *ANZ J Surg.* 2011;81(9):640–641.
14. Lautz TB, Tantemsapya N, Rowell E, et al. Management and classification of type II congenital portosystemic shunts. *J Pediatr Surg.* 2011;46(2):308–314.
15. Murray CP, Yoo SJ, Babyn PS. Congenital extrahepatic portosystemic shunts. *Pediatr Radiol.* 2003;33(9):614–620.
16. Mortele KJ, Segatto E, Ros PR. The infected liver: radiologic-pathologic correlation. *Radiographics.* 2004;24(4):937–955.
17. Benedetti NJ, Desser TS, Jeffrey RB. Imaging of hepatic infections. *Ultrasound Q.* 2008;24(4):267–278.
18. Doyle DJ, Hanbidge AE, O'Malley ME. Imaging of hepatic infections. *Clin Radiol.* 2006;61(9):737–748.
19. Roberts EA. Neonatal hepatitis syndrome. *Sem Neonatol.* 2003; 8(5):357–374.
20. Norton KI, Glass RB, Kogan D, et al. MR cholangiography in the evaluation of neonatal cholestasis: initial results. *Radiology.* 2002;222(3):687–691.
21. Yang JG, Ma DQ, Peng Y, et al. Comparison of different diagnostic methods for differentiating biliary atresia from idiopathic neonatal hepatitis. *Clin Imaging.* 2009;33(6):439–446.
22. Ferri Liu PM, de Miranda DM, Fagundes ED, et al. Autoimmune hepatitis in childhood: the role of genetic and immune factors. *World J Gastroenterol.* 2013;19(28):4455–4463.
23. Kochin IN, Miloh TA, Arnon R, et al. Benign liver masses and lesions in children: 53 cases over 12 years. *Isr Med Assoc J.* 2011; 13(9):542–547.
24. Chung EM, Cube R, Lewis RB, et al. From the archives of the AFIP: Pediatric liver masses: radiologic-pathologic correlation part 1. Benign tumors. *Radiographics.* 2010;30(3):801–826.
25. Chung EM, Lattin GE, Jr, Cube R, et al. From the archives of the AFIP: Pediatric liver masses: radiologic-pathologic correlation. Part 2. Malignant tumors. *Radiographics.* 2011;31(2):483–507.
26. Meyers RL. Tumors of the liver in children. *Surg Oncol.* 2007; 16(3):195–203.
27. Hadzic N, Finegold MJ. Liver neoplasia in children. *Clin Liver Dis.* 2011;15(2):443–462, vii–x.

28. Feng ST, Chan T, Ching AS, et al. CT and MR imaging characteristics of infantile hepatic hemangioendothelioma. *Eur J Radiol.* 2010;76(2):e24–e29.
29. Kulungowski AM, Alomari AI, Chawla A, et al. Lessons from a liver hemangioma registry: subtype classification. *J Pediatr Surg.* 2012;47(1):165–170.
30. Moon SB, Kwon HJ, Park KW, et al. Clinical experience with infantile hepatic hemangioendothelioma. *World J Surg.* 2009; 33(3):597–602.
31. Christison-Lagay ER, Burrows PE, Alomari A, et al. Hepatic hemangiomas: subtype classification and development of a clinical practice algorithm and registry. *J Pediatr Surg.* 2007; 42(1):62–67; discussion 67–68.
32. Yeh I, Bruckner AL, Sanchez R, et al. Diffuse infantile hepatic hemangiomas: a report of four cases successfully managed with medical therapy. *Pediatr Dermatol.* 2011;28(3):267–275.
33. Meyers AB, Towbin AJ, Serai S, et al. Characterization of pediatric liver lesions with gadoxetate disodium. *Pediatr Radiol.* 2011;41(9):1183–1197.
34. Towbin AJ, Luo GG, Yin H, et al. Focal nodular hyperplasia in children, adolescents, and young adults. *Pediatr Radiol.* 2011; 41(3):341–349.
35. Meyers AB, Towbin AJ, Geller JI, et al. Hepatoblastoma imaging with gadoxetate disodium-enhanced MRI—typical, atypical, pre- and post-treatment evaluation. *Pediatr Radiol.* 2012; 42(7):859–866.
36. Smith EA, Salisbury S, Martin R, et al. Incidence and etiology of new liver lesions in pediatric patients previously treated for malignancy. *AJR Am J Roentgenol.* 2012;199(1):186–191.
37. Bouyn CI, Leclere J, Raimondo G, et al. Hepatic focal nodular hyperplasia in children previously treated for a solid tumor. Incidence, risk factors, and outcome. *Cancer.* 2003;97(12): 3107–3113.
38. Do RK, Shaylor SD, Shia J, et al. Variable MR imaging appearances of focal nodular hyperplasia in pediatric cancer patients. *Pediatr Radiol.* 2011;41(3):335–340.
39. Gobbi D, Dall'Igna P, Messina C, et al. Focal nodular hyperplasia in pediatric patients with and without oncologic history. *Pediatr Blood Cancer.* 2010;55(7):1420–1422.
40. Masetti R, Biagi C, Kleinschmidt K, et al. Focal nodular hyperplasia of the liver after intensive treatment for pediatric cancer: is hematopoietic stem cell transplantation a risk factor? *Eur J Pediatr.* 2011;170(6):807–812.
41. Orlowski A, Breborowicz D. Mesenchymal hamartoma of the liver—case report and short literature overview. *Pol J Pathol.* 2011;62(2):108–112.
42. Anil G, Fortier M, Low Y. Cystic hepatic mesenchymal hamartoma: the role of radiology in diagnosis and perioperative management. *Br J Radiol.* 2011;84(1001):e91–e94.
43. Bove KE, Blough RI, Soukup S. Third report of t(19q)(13.4) in mesenchymal hamartoma of liver with comments on link to embryonal sarcoma. *Pediatr Dev Pathol.* 1998;1(5):438–442.
44. Mathews J, Duncavage EJ, Pfeifer JD. Characterization of translocations in mesenchymal hamartoma and undifferentiated embryonal sarcoma of the liver. *Exp Mol Pathol.* 2013;95(3): 319–324.
45. Wellen JR, Anderson CD, Doyle M, et al. The role of liver transplantation for hepatic adenomatosis in the pediatric population: case report and review of the literature. *Pediatr Transplant.* 2010;14(3):E16–E19.
46. Katabathina VS, Menias CO, Shanbhogue AK, et al. Genetics and imaging of hepatocellular adenomas: 2011 update. *Radiographics.* 2011;31(6):1529–1543.
47. Rocourt DV, Shiels WE, Hammond S, et al. Contemporary management of benign hepatic adenoma using percutaneous radiofrequency ablation. *J Pediatr Surg.* 2006;41(6):1149–1152.
48. Litten JB, Tomlinson GE. Liver tumors in children. *Oncologist.* 2008;13(7):812–820.
49. Venkatramani R, Furman WL, Fuchs J, et al. Current and future management strategies for relapsed or progressive hepatoblastoma. *Paediatr Drugs.* 2012;14(4):221–232.
50. Spector LG, Birch J. The epidemiology of hepatoblastoma. *Pediatr Blood Cancer.* 2012;59(5):776–779.
51. Tomlinson GE, Kappler R. Genetics and epigenetics of hepatoblastoma. *Pediatr Blood Cancer.* 2012;59(5):785–792.
52. McCarville MB, Roebuck DJ. Diagnosis and staging of hepatoblastoma: imaging aspects. *Pediatr Blood Cancer.* 2012;59(5):793–799.
53. Roebuck DJ, Aronson D, Clapuyt P, et al. 2005 PRETEXT: a revised staging system for primary malignant liver tumours of childhood developed by the SIOPEL group. *Pediatr Radiol.* 2007;37(2):123–132; quiz 249–150.
54. von Schweinitz D. Hepatoblastoma: recent developments in research and treatment. *Sem Pediatr Surg.* 2012;21(1):21–30.
55. Malogolowkin MH, Katzenstein HM, Krailo M, et al. Treatment of hepatoblastoma: the North American cooperative group experience. *Front Biosci.* 2012;4:1717–1723.
56. Meyers RL, Tiao GM, Dunn SP, et al. Liver transplantation in the management of unresectable hepatoblastoma in children. *Front Biosci.* 2012;4:1293–1302.
57. Ismail H, Broniszczak D, Kalicinski P, et al. Liver transplantation in children with hepatocellular carcinoma. Do Milan criteria apply to pediatric patients? *Pediatr Transplant.* 2009;13(6):682–692.
58. Das CJ, Dhingra S, Gupta AK, et al. Imaging of paediatric liver tumours with pathological correlation. *Clin Radiol.* 2009; 64(10):1015–1025.
59. Agarwala S. Primary malignant liver tumors in children. *Indian J Pediatr.* 2012;79(6):793–800.
60. Schmid I, Haberle B, Albert MH, et al. Sorafenib and cisplatin/doxorubicin (PLADO) in pediatric hepatocellular carcinoma. *Pediatric Blood Cancer.* 2012;58(4):539–544.
61. Beaunoyer M, Vanatta JM, Ogihara M, et al. Outcomes of transplantation in children with primary hepatic malignancy. *Pediatr Transplant.* 2007;11(6):655–660.
62. Kosola S, Lauronen J, Sairanen H, et al. High survival rates after liver transplantation for hepatoblastoma and hepatocellular carcinoma. *Pediatr Transplant.* 2010;14(5):646–650.
63. Smith MT, Blatt ER, Jedlicka P, et al. Best cases from the AFIP: fibrolamellar hepatocellular carcinoma. *Radiographics.* 2008; 28(2):609–613.
64. Ward SC, Waxman S. Fibrolamellar carcinoma: a review with focus on genetics and comparison to other malignant primary liver tumors. *Sem Liver Dis.* 2011;31(1):61–70.
65. Maniaci V, Davidson BR, Rolles K, et al. Fibrolamellar hepatocellular carcinoma: prolonged survival with multimodality therapy. *Eur J Surg Oncol.* 2009;35(6):617–621.
66. Yen JB, Chang KW. Fibrolamellar hepatocellular carcinoma—report of a case. *Chang Gung Med J.* 2009;32(3):336–339.
67. Stipa F, Yoon SS, Liau KH, et al. Outcome of patients with fibrolamellar hepatocellular carcinoma. *Cancer.* 2006;106(6): 1331–1338.
68. Boybeyi O, Karnak I, Orhan D, et al. Undifferentiated (embryonal) sarcoma of the liver: an intriguing diagnosis in a child. *Eur J Pediatr Surg.* 2009;19(5):328–330.
69. Shehata BM, Gupta NA, Katzenstein HM, et al. Undifferentiated embryonal sarcoma of the liver is associated with mesenchymal

hamartoma and multiple chromosomal abnormalities: a review of eleven cases. *Pediatr Dev Pathol.* 2011;14(2):111–116.
70. Ida S, Okajima H, Hayashida S, et al. Undifferentiated sarcoma of the liver. *Am J Surg.* 2009;198(1):e7–e9.
71. Crider MH, Hoggard E, Manivel JC. Undifferentiated (embryonal) sarcoma of the liver. *Radiographics.* 2009;29(6):1665–1668.
72. May LT, Wang M, Albano E, et al. Undifferentiated sarcoma of the liver: a single institution experience using a uniform treatment approach. *J Pediatr Hematol Oncol.* 2012;34(3):e114–e116.
73. Walther A, Geller J, Coots A, et al. Multimodal therapy including liver transplantation for hepatic undifferentiated embryonal sarcoma. *Liver Transplant.* 2014;20(2):191–199.
74. Nellensteijn D, Porte RJ, van Zuuren W, et al. Paediatric blunt liver trauma in a Dutch level 1 trauma center. *Eur J Pediatr Surg.* 2009;19(6):358–361.
75. Wegner S, Colletti JE, Van Wie D. Pediatric blunt abdominal trauma. *Pediatr Clin North Am.* 2006;53(2):243–256.
76. Podberesky DJ, Unsell BJ, Anton CG. Imaging of American football injuries in children. *Pediatr Radiol.* 2009;39(12):1264–1274; quiz 1385–1266.
77. *Caffey's Pediatric Diagnostic Imaging.* 12 ed. Philadelphia, PA: Saunders; 2013.
78. Holmes JF, Gladman A, Chang CH. Performance of abdominal ultrasonography in pediatric blunt trauma patients: a meta-analysis. *J Pediatr Surg.* 2007;42(9):1588–1594.
79. Sivit CJ. Imaging children with abdominal trauma. *AJR Am J Roentgenol.* 2009;192(5):1179–1189.
80. The American Association for the Surgery of Trauma. *Liver Injury Scoring Scale (1994 Revision).* 1994. http://www.aast.org/Library/TraumaTools/InjuryScoringScales.aspx#liver Accessed October 17, 2013.
81. Hilmes MA, Hernanz-Schulman M, Greeley CS, et al. CT identification of abdominal injuries in abused pre-school-age children. *Pediatr Radiol.* 2011;41(5):643–651.
82. Trout AT, Strouse PJ, Mohr BA, et al. Abdominal and pelvic CT in cases of suspected abuse: can clinical and laboratory findings guide its use? *Pediatr Radiol.* 2011;41(1):92–98.
83. Trokel M, Discala C, Terrin NC, et al. Patient and injury characteristics in abusive abdominal injuries. *Pediatr Emerg Care.* 2006;22(10):700–704.
84. Lindberg DM, Shapiro RA, Blood EA, et al. Utility of hepatic transaminases in children with concern for abuse. *Pediatrics.* 2013;131(2):268–275.
85. Rustogi R, Horowitz J, Harmath C, et al. Accuracy of MR elastography and anatomic MR imaging features in the diagnosis of severe hepatic fibrosis and cirrhosis. *J Magn Reson Imaging.* 2012;35(6):1356–1364.
86. Serai SD, Towbin AJ, Podberesky DJ. Pediatric liver MR elastography. *Dig Dis Sci.* 2012;57(10):2713–2719.
87. Pariente D, Franchi-Abella S. Paediatric chronic liver diseases: how to investigate and follow up? Role of imaging in the diagnosis of fibrosis. *Pediatr Radiol.* 2010;40(6):906–919.
88. Towbin AJ, Serai SD, Podberesky DJ. Magnetic resonance imaging of the pediatric liver: imaging of steatosis, iron deposition, and fibrosis. *Magn Reson Imaging Clin N Am.* 2013;21(4):669–680.
89. Binkovitz LA, El-Youssef M, Glaser KJ, et al. Pediatric MR elastography of hepatic fibrosis: principles, technique and early clinical experience. *Pediatr Radiol.* 2012;42(4):402–409.
90. Nobili V, Monti L, Alisi A, et al. Transient elastography for assessment of fibrosis in paediatric liver disease. *Pediatr Radiol.* 2011;41(10):1232–1238.
91. Serai SD, Wallihan DB, Venkatesh SK, et al. Magnetic resonance elastography of the liver in patients status-post fontan procedure: feasibility and preliminary results. *Congenit Heart Dis.* 2014;9(1):7–14.
92. Xanthakos SA, Podberesky DJ, Serai SD, et al. Use of magnetic resonance elastography to assess hepatic fibrosis in children with chronic liver disease. *J Pediatr.* 2014;164(1):186–188.
93. Yin M, Talwalkar JA, Glaser KJ, et al. Assessment of hepatic fibrosis with magnetic resonance elastography. *Clin Gastroenterol Hepatol.* 2007;5(10):1207–1213 e1202.
94. Sarin SK, Kumar A. Noncirrhotic portal hypertension. *Clin Liver Dis.* 2006;10(3):627–651, x.
95. Ling SC. Advances in the evaluation and management of children with portal hypertension. *Sem Liver Dis.* 2012;32(4):288–297.
96. Cardenas AM, Epelman M, Darge K, et al. Pre- and postoperative imaging of the Rex shunt in children: what radiologists should know. *AJR Am J Roentgenol.* 2012;198(5):1032–1037.
97. Tublin ME, Towbin AJ, Federle MP, et al. Altered liver morphology after portal vein thrombosis: not always cirrhosis. *Dig Dis Sci.* 2008;53(10):2784–2788.
98. Cwikiel W, Keussen I, Larsson L, et al. Interventional treatment of children with portal hypertension secondary to portal vein occlusion. *Eur J Pediatr Surg.* 2003;13(5):312–318.
99. Lindback SM, Gabbert C, Johnson BL, et al. Pediatric nonalcoholic fatty liver disease: a comprehensive review. *Adv Pediatr.* 2010;57(1):85–140.
100. Ma X, Holalkere NS, Kambadakone RA, et al. Imaging-based quantification of hepatic fat: methods and clinical applications. *Radiographics.* 2009;29(5):1253–1277.
101. Hu HH, Kim HW, Nayak KS, et al. Comparison of fat-water MRI and single-voxel MRS in the assessment of hepatic and pancreatic fat fractions in humans. *Obesity.* 2010;18(4):841–847.
102. Reeder SB, Cruite I, Hamilton G, et al. Quantitative assessment of liver fat with magnetic resonance imaging and spectroscopy. *J Magn Reson Imaging.* 2011;34(4):spcone.
103. Alustiza Echeverria JM, Castiella A, Emparanza JI. Quantification of iron concentration in the liver by MRI. *Insights imaging.* 2012;3(2):173–180.
104. Sirlin CB, Reeder SB. Magnetic resonance imaging quantification of liver iron. *Magn Reson Imaging Clin N Am.* 2010;18(3):359–381, ix.
105. Maheshwari A, Rankin R, Segev DL, et al. Outcomes of liver transplantation for glycogen storage disease: a matched-control study and a review of literature. *Clin Transplant.* 2012;26(3):432–436.
106. Wang S, Raju BI, Leyvi E, et al. Acoustic accessibility investigation for ultrasound mediated treatment of glycogen storage disease type Ia patients. *Ultrasound Med Biol.* 2011;37(9):1469–1477.
107. Hicks J, Wartchow E, Mierau G. Glycogen storage diseases: a brief review and update on clinical features, genetic abnormalities, pathologic features, and treatment. *Ultrastruct Pathol.* 2011;35(5):183–196.
108. Roy A, Finegold MJ. Hepatic neoplasia and metabolic diseases in children. *Clin Liver Dis.* 2010;14(4):731–746.
109. de Laet C, Dionisi-Vici C, Leonard JV, et al. Recommendations for the management of tyrosinaemia type 1. *Orphanet J Rare Dis.* 2013;8:8.
110. Mahgerefteh SY, Sosna J, Bogot N, et al. Radiologic imaging and intervention for gastrointestinal and hepatic complications of hematopoietic stem cell transplantation. *Radiology.* 2011;258(3):660–671.

111. Teefey SA, Brink JA, Borson RA, et al. Diagnosis of venoocclusive disease of the liver after bone marrow transplantation: value of duplex sonography. *AJR Am J Roentgenol.* 1995;164(6):1397–1401.
112. Herbetko J, Grigg AP, Buckley AR, et al. Venoocclusive liver disease after bone marrow transplantation: findings at duplex sonography. *AJR Am J Roentgenol.* 1992;158(5):1001–1005.
113. McCarville MB, Hoffer FA, Howard SC, et al. Hepatic venoocclusive disease in children undergoing bone-marrow transplantation: usefulness of sonographic findings. *Pediatr Radiol.* 2001;31(2):102–105.
114. Torabi M, Hosseinzadeh K, Federle MP. CT of nonneoplastic hepatic vascular and perfusion disorders. *Radiographics.* 2008;28(7):1967–1982.
115. Kim SH, Lee JM, Kim WH, et al. Focal peliosis hepatis as a mimicker of hepatic tumors: radiological-pathological correlation. *J Comput Assist Tomogr.* 2007;31(1):79–85.
116. Samyn M, Hadzic N, Davenport M, et al. Peliosis hepatis in childhood: case report and review of the literature. *J Pediatr Gastroenterol Nutr.* 2004;39(4):431–434.
117. Xu HX, Xie XY, Lu MD, et al. Unusual benign focal liver lesions: findings on real-time contrast-enhanced sonography. *J Ultrasound Med.* 2008;27(2):243–254.
118. Battal B, Kocaoglu M, Atay AA, et al. Multifocal peliosis hepatis: MR and diffusion-weighted MR-imaging findings of an atypical case. *Upsala J Med Sci.* 2010;115(2):153–156.
119. Tiao GM, Alonso MH, Ryckman FC. Pediatric liver transplantation. *Sem Pediatr Surg.* 2006;15(3):218–227.
120. Babyn PS. Imaging of the transplant liver. *Pediatr Radiol.* 2010;40(4):442–446.
121. Crossin JD, Muradali D, Wilson SR. US of liver transplants: normal and abnormal. *Radiographics.* 2003;23(5):1093–1114.
122. Towbin AJ, Towbin RB. Interventional radiology in the treatment of the complications of organ transplant in the pediatric population-part 2: the liver. *Sem Intervent Radiol.* 2004;21(4):321–333.
123. Singh AK, Nachiappan AC, Verma HA, et al. Postoperative imaging in liver transplantation: what radiologists should know. *Radiographics.* 2010;30(2):339–351.
124. Vakili K, Pomfret EA. Biliary anatomy and embryology. *Surg Clin N Am.* 2008;88(6):1159–1174, vii.
125. Catalano OA, Singh AH, Uppot RN, et al. Vascular and biliary variants in the liver: implications for liver surgery. *Radiographics.* 2008;28(2):359–378.
126. Basaran C, Agildere AM, Donmez FY, et al. MR cholangiopancreatography with T2-weighted prospective acquisition correction turbo spin-echo sequence of the biliary anatomy of potential living liver transplant donors. *AJR Am J Roentgenol.* 2008;190(6):1527–1533.
127. Roskams T, Desmet V. Embryology of extra- and intrahepatic bile ducts, the ductal plate. *Anat Rec.* 2008;291(6):628–635.
128. Strazzabosco M, Fabris L. Development of the bile ducts: essentials for the clinical hepatologist. *J Hepatol.* 2012;56(5):1159–1170.
129. Todani T, Watanabe Y, Narusue M, et al. Congenital bile duct cysts: classification, operative procedures, and review of thirty-seven cases including cancer arising from choledochal cyst. *Am J Surg.* 1977;134(2):263–269.
130. Babbitt DP. [Congenital choledochal cysts: new etiological concept based on anomalous relationships of the common bile duct and pancreatic bulb]. *Ann Radiol (Paris).* 1969;12(3):231–240.
131. Liu YB, Wang JW, Devkota KR, et al. Congenital choledochal cysts in adults: twenty-five-year experience. *Chin Med J.* 2007;120(16):1404–1407.
132. Jordan PH Jr, Goss JA Jr, Rosenberg WR, et al. Some considerations for management of choledochal cysts. *Am J Surg.* 2004;187(6):790–795.
133. Schneider EA, Eisner M, Fridrich R. Scintigraphic demonstration of an intrahepatic gall-bladder presenting as a focal liver lesion. *Br J Radiol.* 1979;52(621):754–755.
134. Hershman MJ, Southern SJ, Rosin RD. Gallbladder agenesis diagnosed at laparoscopy. *J R Soc Med.* 1992;85(11):702–703.
135. Bedi N, Bond-Smith G, Kumar S, et al. Gallbladder agenesis with choledochal cyst—a rare association: a case report and review of possible genetic or embryological links. *BMJ Case Rep.* 2013;2013.
136. Malde S. Gallbladder agenesis diagnosed intra-operatively: a case report. *J Med Case Rep.* 2010;4:285.
137. Causey MW, Miller S, Fernelius CA, et al. Gallbladder duplication: evaluation, treatment, and classification. *J Pediatr Surg.* 2010;45(2):443–446.
138. Roldan-Valadez E, Osorio-Peralta S, Vivas-Bonilla I, et al. Asymptomatic true gallbladder duplication: a case report and review of the literature. *Acta Radiol.* 2004;45(8):810–814.
139. Karaca T, Yoldas O, Bilgin BC, et al. Diagnosis and treatment of multiseptate gallbladder with recurrent abdominal pain. *Case Rep Med.* 2011;2011:162853.
140. Gigot J, Van Beers B, Goncette L, et al. Laparoscopic treatment of gallbladder duplication. A plea for removal of both gallbladders. *Surg Endosc.* 1997;11(5):479–482.
141. Gunay-Aygun M, Font-Montgomery E, Lukose L, et al. Characteristics of congenital hepatic fibrosis in a large cohort of patients with autosomal recessive polycystic kidney disease. *Gastroenterology.* 2013;144(1):112–121 e112.
142. Ernst O, Gottrand F, Calvo M, et al. Congenital hepatic fibrosis: findings at MR cholangiopancreatography. *AJR Am J Roentgenol.* 1998;170(2):409–412.
143. Srinath A, Shneider BL. Congenital hepatic fibrosis and autosomal recessive polycystic kidney disease. *J Pediatr Gastroenterol Nutr.* 2012;54(5):580–587.
144. Akhan O, Karaosmanoglu AD, Ergen B. Imaging findings in congenital hepatic fibrosis. *Eur J Radiol.* 2007;61(1):18–24.
145. Singham J, Yoshida EM, Scudamore CH. Choledochal cysts: part 1 of 3: classification and pathogenesis. *Can J Surg.* 2009;52(5):434–440.
146. Desmet VJ. What is congenital hepatic fibrosis? *Histopathology.* 1992;20(6):465–477.
147. Markhardt BK, Rubens DJ, Huang J, et al. Sonographic features of biliary hamartomas with histopathologic correlation. *J Ultrasound Med.* 2006;25(12):1631–1633.
148. Zheng RQ, Zhang B, Kudo M, Onda H, Inoue T. Imaging findings of biliary hamartomas. *World J Gastroenterol.* 2005;11(40):6354–6359.
149. Kianifar HR, Tehranian S, Shojaei P, et al. Accuracy of hepatobiliary scintigraphy for differentiation of neonatal hepatitis from biliary atresia: systematic review and meta-analysis of the literature. *Pediatr Radiol.* 2013;43(8):905–919.
150. Benchimol EI, Walsh CM, Ling SC. Early diagnosis of neonatal cholestatic jaundice Test at 2 weeks. *Can Fam Physician.* 2009;55(12):1184–1192.
151. Mieli-Vergani G, Vergani D. Biliary atresia. *Semin Immunopathol.* 2009;31(3):371–381.
152. Rozel C, Garel L, Rypens F, et al. Imaging of biliary disorders in children. *Pediatric Radiol.* 2011;41(2):208–220.

153. Davenport M, De Ville de Goyet J, Stringer MD, et al. Seamless management of biliary atresia in England and Wales (1999–2002). *Lancet.* 2004;363(9418):1354–1357.
154. Lee HJ, Lee SM, Park WH, et al. Objective criteria of triangular cord sign in biliary atresia on US scans. *Radiology.* 2003;229(2):395–400.
155. Humphrey TM, Stringer MD. Biliary atresia: US diagnosis. *Radiology.* 2007;244(3):845–851.
156. Kim MJ, Park YN, Han SJ, et al. Biliary atresia in neonates and infants: triangular area of high signal intensity in the porta hepatis at T2-weighted MR cholangiography with US and histopathologic correlation. *Radiology.* 2000;215(2):395–401.
157. Kanegawa K, Akasaka Y, Kitamura E, et al. Sonographic diagnosis of biliary atresia in pediatric patients using the "triangular cord" sign versus gallbladder length and contraction. *AJR Am J Roentgenol.* 2003;181(5):1387–1390.
158. Han SJ, Kim MJ, Han A, et al. Magnetic resonance cholangiography for the diagnosis of biliary atresia. *J Pediatr Surg.* 2002;37(4):599–604.
159. Matsui A. Immune pathogenesis of sclerosing cholangitis in biliary atresia. *Hepatol Res.* 2007;37(suppl 3):S501.
160. Bader TR, Braga L, Beavers KL, et al. MR imaging findings of infectious cholangitis. *Magn Reson Imaging.* 2001;19(6):781–788.
161. de Bie HM, Kneepkens CM, Vos A, et al. Late cholangitis after kasai procedure detected with magnetic resonance cholangiopancreaticography: a case report. *J Pediatr Gastroenterol Nutr.* 2002;35(3):363–365.
162. Tainaka T, Kaneko K, Seo T, et al. Intrahepatic cystic lesions after hepatic portoenterostomy for biliary atresia with bile lake and dilated bile ducts. *J Pediatr Gastroenterol Nutr.* 2007; 44(1):104–107.
163. Hussein A, Wyatt J, Guthrie A, et al. Kasai portoenterostomy—new insights from hepatic morphology. *J Pediatr Surg.* 2005; 40(2):322–326.
164. Hol L, van den Bos IC, Hussain SM, et al. Hepatocellular carcinoma complicating biliary atresia after Kasai portoenterostomy. *Eur J Gastroenterol Hepatol.* 2008;20(3):227–231.
165. Turnpenny PD, Ellard S. Alagille syndrome: pathogenesis, diagnosis and management. *Eur J Hum Genet.* 2012;20(3):251–257.
166. Hartley JL, Gissen P, Kelly DA. Alagille syndrome and other hereditary causes of cholestasis. *Clin Liver Dis.* 2013; 17(2):279–300.
167. Stringer MD, Soloway RD, Taylor DR, et al. Calcium carbonate gallstones in children. *J Pediatr Surg.* 2007;42(10):1677–1682.
168. Walker SK, Maki AC, Cannon RM, et al. Etiology and incidence of pediatric gallbladder disease. *Surgery.* 2013;154(4):927–933.
169. Kumar R, Nguyen K, Shun A. Gallstones and common bile duct calculi in infancy and childhood. *Aust N Z J Surg.* 2000; 70(3):188–191.
170. Cooperberg PL, Burhenne HJ. Real-time ultrasonography. Diagnostic technique of choice in calculous gallbladder disease. *N Engl J Med.* 1980;302(23):1277–1279.
171. Zhang Y, Wang XL, Li SX, et al. Ultrasonographic dimensions of the common bile duct in Chinese children: results of 343 cases. *J Pediatr Surg.* 2013;48(9):1892–1896.
172. Richard F, Boustany M, Britt LD. Accuracy of magnetic resonance cholangiopancreatography for diagnosing stones in the common bile duct in patients with abnormal intraoperative cholangiograms. *Am J Surg.* 2013;205(4):371–373.
173. Tannuri AC, Leal AJ, Velhote MC, et al. Management of gallstone disease in children: a new protocol based on the experience of a single center. *J Pediatr Surg.* 2012;47(11):2033–2038.
174. Tsai J, Sulkowski JP, Cooper JN, et al. Sensitivity and predictive value of ultrasound in pediatric cholecystitis. *J Surg Res.* 2013;184(1):378–382.
175. Batra V, Ang JY, Asmar BI. *Staphylococcal acalculous* cholecystitis in a child. *South Med J.* 2003;96(2):206–208.
176. Saha A, Batra P, Vilhekar KY, et al. Acute acalculous cholecystitis in a child with Plasmodium falciparum malaria. *Ann Trop Paediatr.* 2005;25(2):141–142.
177. Patriquin HB, DiPietro M, Barber FE, et al. Sonography of thickened gallbladder wall: causes in children. *AJR Am J Roentgenol.* 1983;141(1):57–60.
178. Kiewiet JJ, Leeuwenburgh MM, Bipat S, et al. A systematic review and meta-analysis of diagnostic performance of imaging in acute cholecystitis. *Radiology.* 2012;264(3):708–720.
179. Vegunta RK, Raso M, Pollock J, et al. Biliary dyskinesia: the most common indication for cholecystectomy in children. *Surgery.* 2005;138(4):726–731; discussion 731–723.
180. Ziessman HA, Tulchinsky M, Lavely WC, et al. Sincalide-stimulated cholescintigraphy: a multicenter investigation to determine optimal infusion methodology and gallbladder ejection fraction normal values. *J Nucl Med.* 2010;51(2):277–281.
181. Boey JH, Way LW. Acute cholangitis. *Ann Surg.* 1980;191(3): 264–270.
182. Eaton JE, Talwalkar JA, Lazaridis KN, et al. Pathogenesis of primary sclerosing cholangitis and advances in diagnosis and management. *Gastroenterology.* 2013;145(3):521–536.
183. Mieli-Vergani G, Vergani D. Unique features of primary sclerosing cholangitis in children. *Curr Opin Gastroenterol.* 2010;26(3):265–268.
184. Miloh T, Arnon R, Shneider B, et al. A retrospective single-center review of primary sclerosing cholangitis in children. *Clin Gastroenterol Hepatol.* 2009;7(2):239–245.
185. Ibrahim SH, Lindor KD. Current management of primary sclerosing cholangitis in pediatric patients. *Paediatr Drugs.* 2011;13(2):87–95.
186. Yoo JH, Kwak HJ, Lee MJ, et al. Sonographic measurements of normal gallbladder sizes in children. *J Clin Ultrasound.* 2003;31(2):80–84.
187. Stringer MD, Ceylan H, Ward K, et al. Gallbladder polyps in children—classification and management. *J Pediatr Surg.* 2003; 38(11):1680–1684.
188. Sandri L, Colecchia A, Larocca A, et al. Gallbladder cholesterol polyps and cholesterolosis. *Minerva Gastroenterol Dietol.* 2003; 49(3):217–224.
189. Zani A, Pacilli M, Conforti A, et al. Adenomyomatosis of the gallbladder in childhood: report of a case and review of the literature. *Pediatr Dev Pathol.* 2005;8(5):577–580.
190. Yoon JH, Cha SS, Han SS, et al. Gallbladder adenomyomatosis: imaging findings. *Abdom Imaging.* 2006;31(5):555–563.
191. Ali S, Russo MA, Margraf L. Biliary rhabdomyoscarcoma mimicking choledochal cyst. *J Gastrointest Liver Dis.* 2009;18(1): 95–97.
192. Kitagawa N, Aida N. Biliary rhabdomyosarcoma. *Pediatr Radiol.* 2007;37(10):1059.
193. Ruymann FB, Raney RB Jr, Crist WM, et al. Rhabdomyosarcoma of the biliary tree in childhood. A report from the Intergroup Rhabdomyosarcoma Study. *Cancer.* 1985;56(3): 575–581.
194. Himes RW, Raijman I, Finegold MJ, et al. Diagnostic and therapeutic role of endoscopic retrograde cholangiopancreatography in biliary rhabdomyosarcoma. *World J Gastroenterol.* 2008;14(30):4823–4825.

195. Nemade B, Talapatra K, Shet T, et al. Embryonal rhabdomyosarcoma of the biliary tree mimicking a choledochal cyst. *J Cancer Res Ther.* 2007;3(1):40–42.
196. Roebuck DJ, Yang WT, Lam WW, et al. Hepatobiliary rhabdomyosarcoma in children: diagnostic radiology. *Pediatr Radiol.* 1998;28(2):101–108.
197. Bjornsson E, Angulo P. Cholangiocarcinoma in young individuals with and without primary sclerosing cholangitis. *Am J Gastroenterol.* 2007;102(8):1677–1682.
198. Kiran RP, Pokala N, Dudrick SJ. Incidence pattern and survival for gallbladder cancer over three decades—an analysis of 10301 patients. *Ann Surg Oncol.* 2007;14(2):827–832.
199. Sharif K, Pimpalwar AP, John P, et al. Benefits of early diagnosis and preemptive treatment of biliary tract complications after major blunt liver trauma in children. *J Pediatr Surg.* 2002;37(9): 1287–1292.
200. Gupta A, Stuhlfaut JW, Fleming KW, et al. Blunt trauma of the pancreas and biliary tract: a multimodality imaging approach to diagnosis. *Radiographics.* 2004;24(5):1381–1395.
201. Cieszanowski A, Stadnik A, Lezak A, et al. Detection of active bile leak with Gd-EOB-DTPA enhanced MR cholangiography: comparison of 20-25 min delayed and 60-180 min delayed images. *Eur J Radiol.* 2013;82(12):2176–2182.
202. Tana C, D'Alessandro P, Tartaro A, et al. Sonographic assessment of a suspected biloma: a case report and review of the literature. *World J Radiol.* 2013;5(5):220–225.
203. Mungai F, Berti V, Colagrande S. Bile leak after elective laparoscopic cholecystectomy: role of MR imaging. *J Radiol Case Rep.* 2013;7(1):25–32.
204. Kelly MD, Armstrong CP, Longstaff A. Characterization of biliary injury from blunt liver trauma by MRCP: case report. *J Trauma.* 2008;64(5):1363–1365.

CHAPTER 15

Spleen, Pancreas, and Adrenal Glands

Ethan A. Smith • Jonathan R. Dillman • Sara O. Vargas • Peter J. Strouse

INTRODUCTION

Disorders of the spleen, pancreas, and adrenal glands are less common in children than are gastrointestinal, hepatobiliary, and genitourinary abnormalities, but nonetheless make up an important group of pediatric diagnoses. Radiologic imaging plays a critical role in evaluating a wide variety of splenic, pancreatic, and adrenal pathologies, including developmental, infectious, inflammatory, and neoplastic entities. In this chapter, the normal anatomy of the spleen, pancreas, and adrenal glands are discussed, followed by a description of common and selected rare pathologic processes that affect each of these organs.

SPLEEN

Imaging Techniques

Radiography

Radiography of the spleen is of limited value. Radiographs can be used to evaluate splenic size in the setting of suspected or known splenomegaly. The absence of a normal splenic shadow can be seen in children with sickle cell disease who have suffered autosplenectomy due to splenic infarction. Radiographs may detect splenic calcifications in sickle cell disease and granulomatous diseases, such as histoplasmosis and tuberculosis.

Ultrasound

Ultrasound is an excellent noninvasive, nonionizing modality for evaluation of the spleen. The spleen is usually readily imaged given its superficial position in the left upper quadrant of the abdomen. Sonography provides detailed information regarding splenic size, position, and vascularity, including assessment of the splenic artery and vein using Doppler sonography. The normal spleen is crescent shaped, demonstrates homogenous echotexture, and is usually slightly hyperechoic relative to the normal liver[1] (Fig. 15.1). With higher frequency transducers, the spleen may have a somewhat granular or reticular appearance related to areas of red and white pulp that should not be confused with pathology.[2]

Both solid and cystic focal splenic lesions and their associated vascularity are also readily evaluated using ultrasound. Calcifications may be seen as hyperechoic foci with associated artifacts (twinkling artifact and/or posterior acoustic shadowing). Structures adjacent to the spleen also may be seen, for example, abnormal perisplenic portosystemic collateral vessels in the setting of portal hypertension.

Computed Tomography

Computed tomography (CT) is the most widely used imaging modality in the evaluation of pediatric splenic trauma. CT is also useful in assessment of the spleen in children with oncologic diseases and in suspected infectious splenic conditions. On noncontrast CT, the normal spleen demonstrates homogenous soft tissue attenuation. After intravenous administration of iodinated contrast material, the spleen typically demonstrates inhomogeneous enhancement on early (arterial) phase postcontrast images, with arc-like, striated, or focal areas of enhancement.[3] This pattern of inhomogeneous enhancement is of unclear etiology, although some have attributed this appearance to differential rates of blood flow through the architecture of the spleen with alternating cords of red pulp and white pulp.[3] On later postcontrast imaging phases, the normal spleen demonstrates homogeneous parenchymal enhancement.[4]

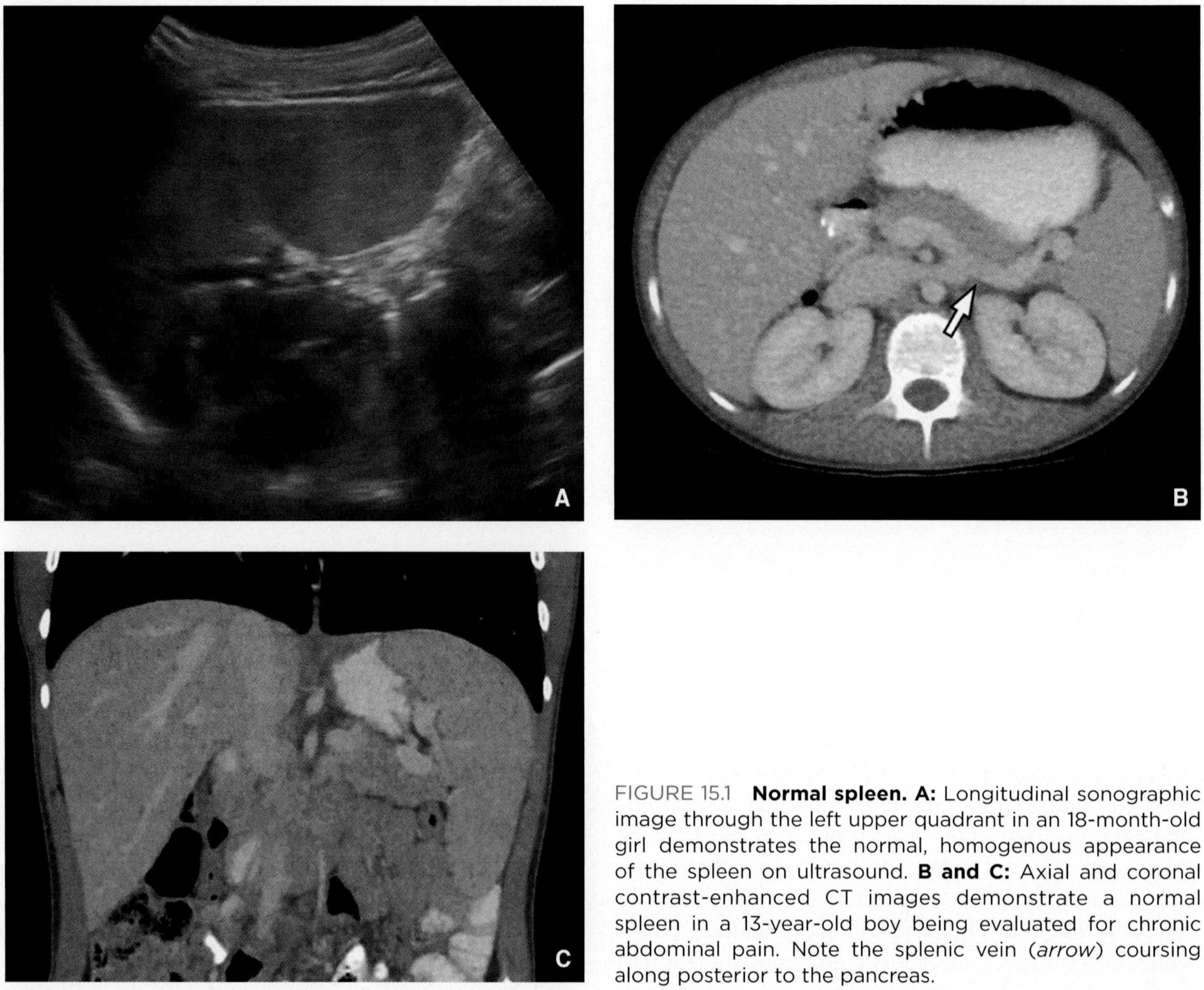

FIGURE 15.1 **Normal spleen. A:** Longitudinal sonographic image through the left upper quadrant in an 18-month-old girl demonstrates the normal, homogenous appearance of the spleen on ultrasound. **B and C:** Axial and coronal contrast-enhanced CT images demonstrate a normal spleen in a 13-year-old boy being evaluated for chronic abdominal pain. Note the splenic vein (*arrow*) coursing along posterior to the pancreas.

Magnetic Resonance Imaging

Similar to CT, MRI provides detailed evaluation of the spleen and splenic pathology. The normal spleen is homogeneously hyperintense on T2-weighted images and also demonstrates hyperintense signal on diffusion-weighted imaging. As with CT, on dynamic postcontrast images, the normal spleen demonstrates inhomogeneous enhancement on early phases and becomes more homogeneous on later phases[3,4] (Fig. 15.2).

The superior tissue contrast of MRI related to the availability of various pulse sequences allows for detailed evaluation of focal splenic lesions, including solid masses, cystic lesions, and vascular abnormalities. Pulse sequences obtained both before and after the intravenous administration of gadolinium-containing contrast material generally are useful. In addition, MRI allows for characterization of diffuse splenic processes, such as splenic iron deposition in secondary hemochromatosis. Finally, dynamic contrast-enhanced MRI (DCE-MRI) excellently depicts the splenic arterial and venous vasculature, including aneurysms, thromboses, and perisplenic portosystemic collateral vessels in the setting of portal hypertension.

Nuclear Medicine

Several nuclear medicine techniques are available for imaging the spleen. Normal, functional splenic tissue can be identified using radiolabeled damaged red blood cells that are filtered and stored in the spleen. Radiolabeled sulfur colloid also localizes to the normal liver and spleen. In pediatric oncology patients, ^{18}F-fluorodeoxyglucose positron emission tomography (^{18}F-FDG-PET) imaging, often performed in conjunction with CT, has proven to be useful in evaluating the spleen for focal metastases as well as for diffuse involvement in lymphoma and other hematologic malignancies.[5]

Normal Anatomy

The spleen is the largest lymphatic organ in the human body and also functions as the primary hematopoietic organ during fetal development.[6] The spleen contains two primary histologic elements: red pulp and white pulp. The red pulp of the spleen acts as a filter for damaged hematopoietic elements (mainly red blood cells) and also plays an important role in immunologic response.[7] The white pulp serves as an important component of the lymphatic system.[7] The spleen is derived from mesenchymal cells arising from the left side of the dorsal mesogastrum.[6] The mesenchymal cells enlarge, develop vascularity, and subsequently fuse to become the trabeculae and capsule of the spleen, after which they are covered by a peritoneal lining derived from the coelomic epithelium.

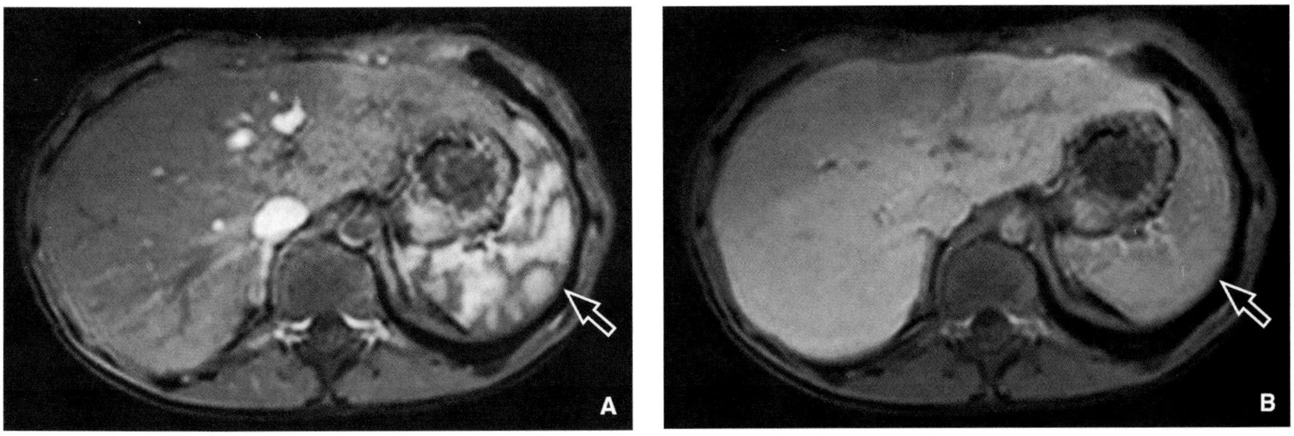

FIGURE 15.2 **Normal splenic enhancement pattern in a 12-year-old girl undergoing evaluation for a liver mass. A:** Arterial phase axial postcontrast T1-weighted 3D spoiled gradient-recalled echo (SPGR) image demonstrates the striated appearance of the spleen (*arrow*) commonly seen on early postcontrast images. **B:** Delayed phase axial postcontrast 3D SPGR image demonstrates normal homogeneous enhancement of the spleen (*arrow*).

Fusion of the individual mesenchymal elements is what gives rise to splenic clefts and the sometimes lobulated appearance of the spleen.[6] The final position of the spleen in the left upper quadrant is determined by rotation of the stomach, with the spleen being posterior to the stomach and anterior to the tail of the pancreas.[6] The spleen is attached to adjacent structures by the gastrosplenic ligament anteriorly, and the splenorenal and splenopancreatic ligaments medially.[6]

The blood flow to the spleen is provided by the splenic artery, which is a branch of the celiac artery. The splenic artery bifurcates into segmental branches near the splenic hilum. The venous outflow from the spleen is provided by the splenic vein, which courses along the inferior and posterior aspect of the pancreas and then joins the superior mesenteric vein to form the main portal vein.

The spleen increases in size with age until puberty. Graphs and tables describing normal spleen sizes for both male and female pediatric patients as a function of age are available.[8]

Congenital Anomalies

Heterotaxy Syndromes (Asplenia and Polysplenia)

Asplenia and polysplenia are part of a complex association with visceral heterotaxy syndromes (i.e., situs ambiguous) and are associated with variable cardiac and other visceral congenital anomalies resulting from discordance of the normal left–right asymmetry of various organ systems, vascular structures, and cardiac chambers.[7,9] The spleen is nearly universally involved in heterotaxy syndromes.

Imaging findings vary depending on the type of abnormality present. The spleen may be absent (asplenia), multiple (polysplenia), or unusually lobulated, or there may be single spleen located in the right upper quadrant.[10] In polysplenia, the multiple spleens are often located in the right upper quadrant[10] (Fig 15.3). Congenital heart disease is common in patients with heterotaxy syndromes. Importantly, in pediatric patients with heterotaxy with polysplenia, the incidence of congenital heart disease is ~50% to 90%, whereas in patients with asplenia, the incidence

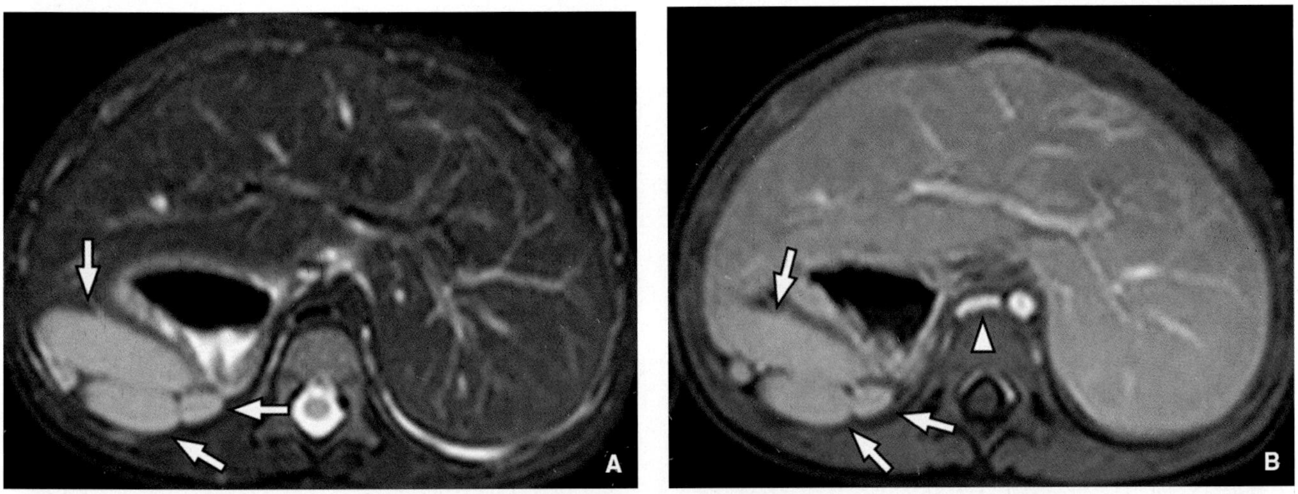

FIGURE 15.3 **Polysplenia in a 6-month-old boy with heterotaxy syndrome and complex congenital heart disease. A:** Axial T2-weighted fat-saturated fast spin-echo MR image shows multiple spleens in the right upper quadrant (*arrows*). Note the midline position of the liver. **B:** Axial postcontrast T1-weighted fat-saturated MR image again shows multiple right upper quadrant spleens (*arrows*). The large vascular structure behind the crus of the diaphragm represents an enlarged azygos vein (*arrowhead*) because of the absence (interruption) of the hepatic portion of the inferior vena cava. Note the gas-filled stomach on the right side of the abdomen.

of congenital heart disease is 99% to 100%.[11] Congenital heart disease in asplenia is often more complex and is commonly associated with anomalous pulmonary venous return. Additional congenital anomalies associated with heterotaxy with polysplenia include interruption of the inferior vena cava, a truncated pancreas, and a preduodenal location of the portal vein.[10,12]

Accessory Spleen

Accessory or supernumerary spleens, sometimes called splenules, are a common normal variant, occurring in between 10% and 30% of the population.[6,9,13,14] Accessory spleens are usually located near the splenic hilum, but can also be found along the supporting splenic ligaments, along the splenic vessels, or even within the pancreas (most often the tail) or in the wall of the stomach.[9] .

On imaging, accessory spleens are often solitary, but can be multiple. Accessory spleens vary in size, but are usually around 1 cm in diameter.[9] They are usually smooth and rounded or oval in shape and have identical echogenicity, CT attenuation, and MR signal characteristics to the spleen itself.[13] Accessory spleens are typically of no clinical significance, except in certain uncommon instances. For example, in hereditary spherocytosis, splenectomy may be ineffective if an accessory spleen is left behind at surgery.[14] Intrapancreatic accessory spleens can cause diagnostic confusion as the intrapancreatic splenic tissue can be confused with a pancreatic neoplasm

Wandering Spleen

Failure of development of the normal gastrosplenic and splenorenal ligaments, which fix the spleen in its normal anatomic position in the left upper quadrant, can result in an abnormally elongated splenic attachment.[9,13,14] The end result is a hypermobile spleen that can change position within the abdomen and may be confused with a mass. Wandering spleen is most common in children and young women.[9] Clinically, wandering spleen may be an incidental finding, although in some cases this entity can be symptomatic because of chronic or intermittent torsion of the spleen resulting in ischemia and occasionally infarction. Gastric outlet obstruction due to gastric volvulus or mass effect on the stomach has also been described.[15]

Plain radiography may demonstrate the absence of a normal splenic opacity in the left upper quadrant. Ultrasound, CT, and MRI can demonstrate otherwise normal spleen in an ectopic location, with a lack of spleen in the normal anatomic position (Fig 15.4).

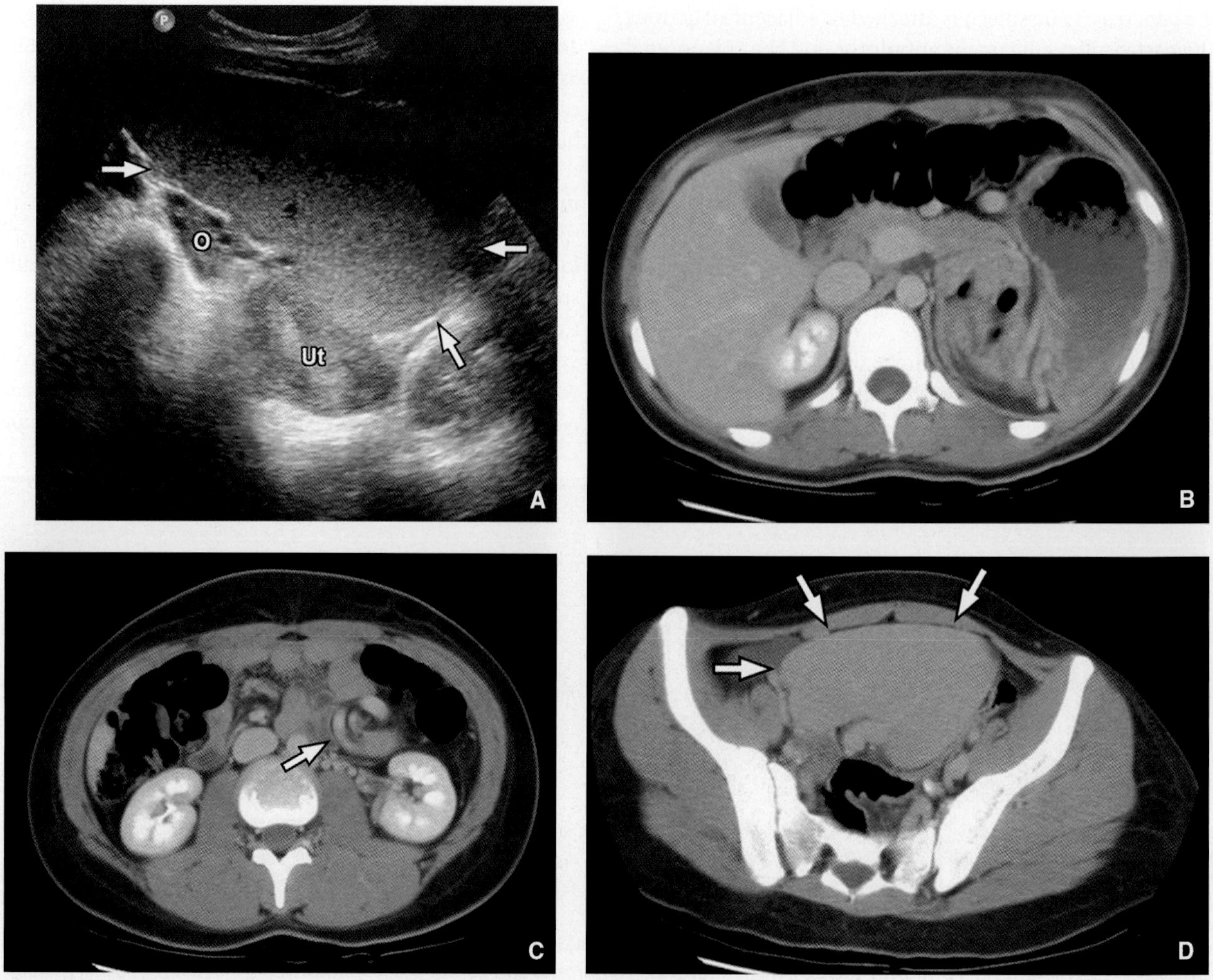

FIGURE 15.4 **Wandering spleen in a 15-year-old girl with sudden onset of abdominal pain. A:** Longitudinal ultrasound image shows a homogenous soft tissue structure (*arrows*) within the pelvis adjacent to the normal-appearing uterus (*Ut*) and ovary (*O*). Axial contrast-enhanced CT images show absence of the normal spleen in the left upper quadrant **(B)**, swirling of the splenic artery and vein (*arrow*) in the left mid-abdomen **(C)**, and the spleen (*arrows*) located in the mid-pelvis **(D)**.

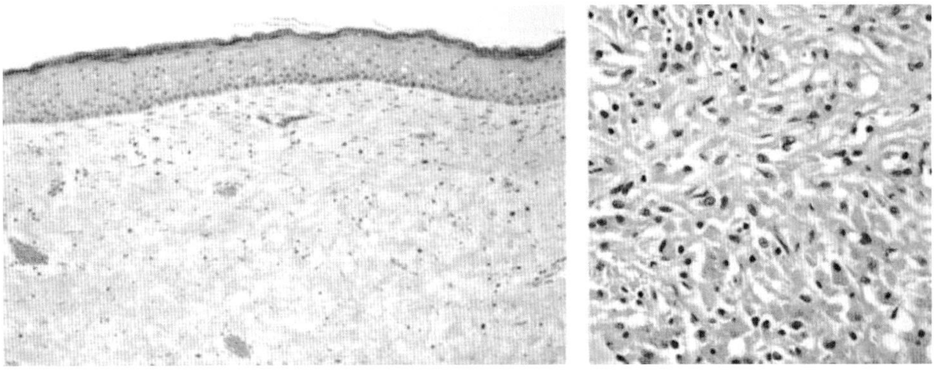

FIGURE 15.5 **Two different resected specimens of splenic cysts.** The wall of a congenital splenic cyst is typically lined by epithelium (**left**, hematoxylin and eosin, original magnification, 200x). The wall of a posttraumatic splenic cyst is fibrous, often with prominent hemosiderosis (**right**, hematoxylin and eosin, original magnification, 600x).

In cases of wandering spleen with torsion, patients present clinically with either acute or chronic abdominal pain.[16] Imaging findings suggestive of torsion include twisting or swirling of the splenic vessels, lack of enhancement or Doppler flow in the spleen in cases of infarction, and adjacent reactive inflammatory changes.[9] Treatment consists of either surgical fixation of the spleen (splenopexy) or splenectomy.[16]

Congenital Splenic Cyst

Also known as epithelial cysts, congenital splenic cysts are relatively uncommon. Differentiation of congenital splenic cysts from the more common splenic pseudocysts is not possible on imaging. Only upon histologic examination can the distinction be made by demonstrating an epithelial lining in the congenital splenic or epithelial cyst (Fig. 15.5).

Congenital splenic cysts demonstrate typical imaging features of simple cysts. On ultrasound, they are well-defined and homogeneously anechoic, whereas, at CT, they measure fluid attenuation. On MRI, congenital splenic cysts are homogeneously low in signal on T1-weighted sequences and high in signal on T2-weighted sequences (Fig. 15.6). Occasionally, these lesions may contain thin septations or debris.[1] Cysts should not enhance after the administration of intravenous contrast material. Clinically, congenital splenic cysts are most often of no clinical significance and generally do not require treatment or resection. The differential diagnosis for a cystic lesion within the spleen includes splenic pseudocysts (most often posttraumatic), infectious cystic lesions, and lymphatic malformations.[4]

Infectious and Inflammatory Disorders

Fungal Infection

Fungal infections in the spleen are encountered almost exclusively in immunocompromised children.[17] *Candida* are the most common species, followed by *Aspergillus* and *Cryptococcus*.[18,19] Clinical presentation is usually nonspecific, with variable signs and symptoms of infection depending on the patient's immune status. As opposed to bacterial abscesses, which are often larger and solitary, fungal infection commonly demonstrates multiple small (1 cm or less) splenic lesions, often termed *microabscesses*.[18,20]

On ultrasound, fungal microabscesses are typically hypoechoic and may have a target or "bull's-eye" appearance[17]

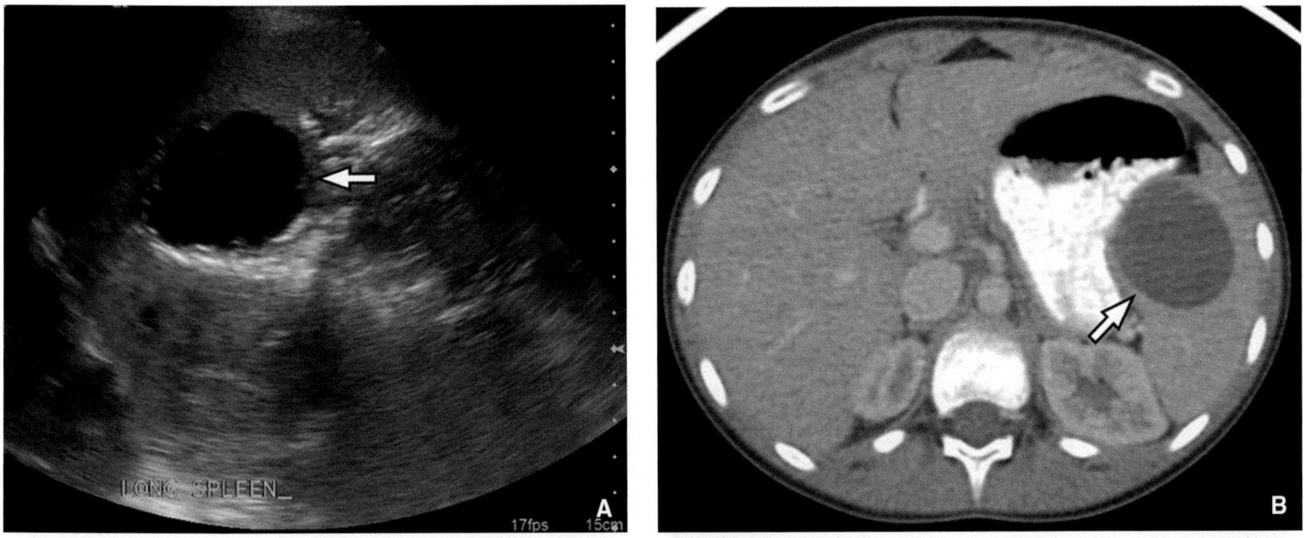

FIGURE 15.6 **Congenital splenic cyst in an 11-year-old girl with abdominal pain. A:** Longitudinal ultrasound image of the spleen shows an anechoic rounded lesion (*arrow*) in the mid spleen. The wall of the cyst appears slightly irregular. **B:** Axial contrast-enhanced CT image demonstrates a fluid-attenuation, circumscribed lesion (*arrow*) in the spleen, consistent with a cyst.

(Fig. 15.7). They may be difficult to visualize on noncontrast CT, but after intravenous contrast material administration, the lesions are typically multiple and low in attenuation relative to the spleen.[19] MRI may be the most sensitive method for detecting small microabscesses.[20] The lesions may be inconspicuous on precontrast T1-weighted sequences, but are typically hyperintense on T2-weighted sequences and enhance less than the adjacent spleen after intravenous gadolinium-based contrast material administration.[20] Affected pediatric patients commonly have hepatic lesions as well.

Splenic calcifications may be a manifestation of subacute or remote infection, including prior infection with the endemic fungal pathogen *Histoplasma capsulatum*. Histoplasmosis is the most common systemic fungal infection in the United States.[21] *Blastomyces dermatitidis* and *Coccidioides sp.* are the other common endemic fungal pathogens found in the United States.[22] Acute splenic involvement is rare in the immunocompetent child but can present as splenic enlargement and multiple hypoechoic or low-attenuation splenic lesions, accompanied by systemic symptoms (Fig 15.8). Calcifications are the most common manifestation of remote infection and are usually punctate and multiple (Fig. 15.9). Occasionally, calcifications can be identified on abdominal radiography, but they are best demonstrated as hyperechoic foci on ultrasound, or round, punctate high-attenuation foci on CT.

Bacterial Infection

The most frequent manifestation of bacterial infection in the spleen is a pyogenic abscess. The majority of splenic abscesses are due to hematogenous spread of infection. Other, less common etiologies include penetrating trauma, direct extension from adjacent organs, or superinfection after splenic infarction.[18,19] Clinically, affected pediatric patient with signs of infection, including fevers and abdominal pain, usually localized to the left upper quadrant.

Plain radiographs are not useful in evaluation of a suspected splenic abscess. Sonography is the diagnostic test of choice in children, given the lack of ionizing radiation and noninvasive nature. Ultrasound typically shows a hypoechoic or anechoic focal lesion, depending on the complexity of internal contents. The lesion may have mural irregularity or septations. Doppler evaluation often shows adjacent hyperemia due to an

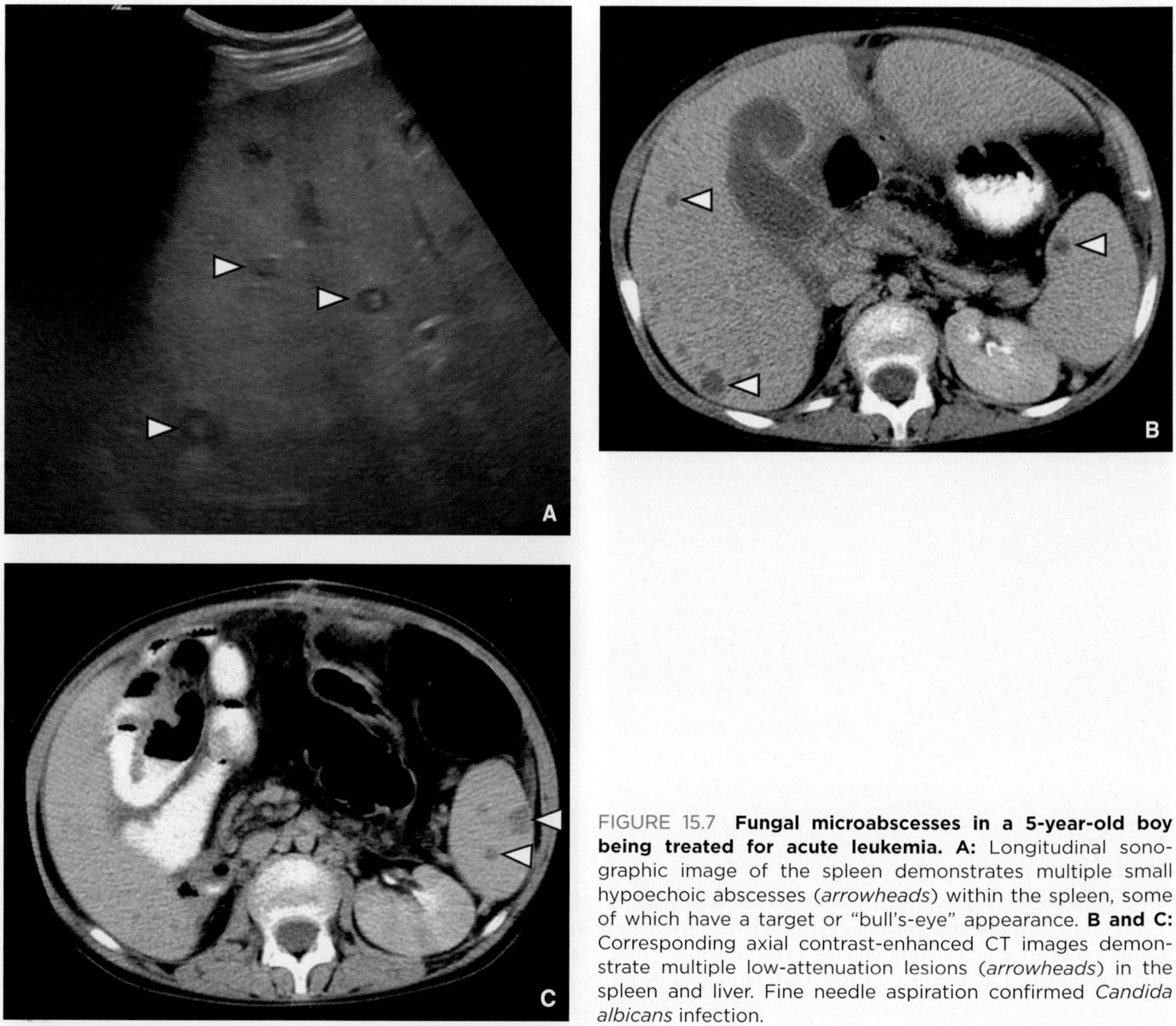

FIGURE 15.7 **Fungal microabscesses in a 5-year-old boy being treated for acute leukemia. A:** Longitudinal sonographic image of the spleen demonstrates multiple small hypoechoic abscesses (*arrowheads*) within the spleen, some of which have a target or "bull's-eye" appearance. **B and C:** Corresponding axial contrast-enhanced CT images demonstrate multiple low-attenuation lesions (*arrowheads*) in the spleen and liver. Fine needle aspiration confirmed *Candida albicans* infection.

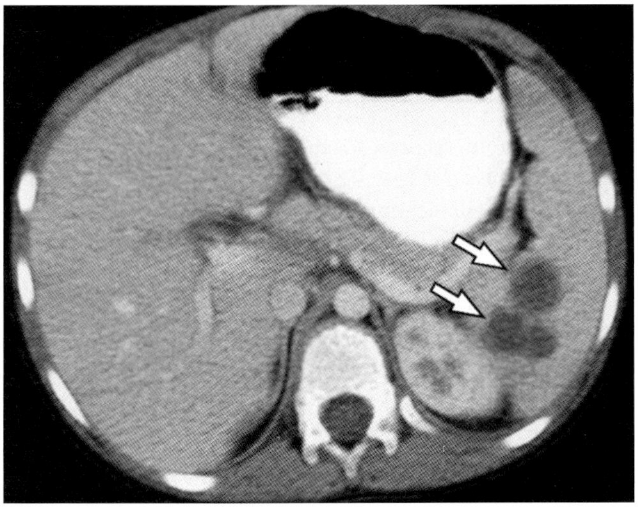

FIGURE 15.8 **Blastomycosis infection in a 16-year-old boy.** Axial contrast-enhanced CT image shows multiple low-attenuation lesions (*arrows*) in the spleen. The patient was later proven to have acute blastomycosis based on biopsy and culture of an osseous lesion.

inflammatory response. If needed, CT or MRI can be performed and demonstrate a complex cystic lesion, appearing relatively low in attenuation on CT and hyperintense in T2-weighted signal on MRI. After intravenous contrast material administration, there is usually a thick or irregular enhancing rim, but no central enhancement.[19] Foci of gas may be evident, most readily demonstrated on CT.[18] On MRI, diffusion-weighted imaging may be helpful by demonstrating restricted diffusion on high b-value images, indicating an abscess.

Treatment is with antibiotic therapy, with or without percutaneous image-guided drainage. Rarely, surgical splenectomy may be required.[18]

Another relatively common bacterial infection that can rarely affect the spleen is *Bartonella sp.*, which is the pathogen responsible for "cat-scratch disease." Patients present clinically with fever and lymph node enlargement, and occasionally the spleen may become enlarged or may demonstrate multiple small *microabscesses*, which appear hypoechoic on ultrasound, low attenuation on CT, and hyperintense on T2-weighted MRI sequences.[18]

Mycobacterium

Mycobacterium species, most commonly *M. avium-intracellulare* and *M. tuberculosis*, can also affect the spleen. Similar to fungal infections, acute involvement of the spleen is rare in the immunocompetent host, but can be seen in immunocompromised children with disseminated disease, manifesting on imaging as either nonspecific splenic enlargement or multiple small splenic lesions. Adjacent lymph nodes may also be enlarged, and they may appear relatively low in attenuation on CT.[18]

Echinococcal Infection

Infection with *Echinococcus sp.* is rare in the developed world but continues to be a common source of disease worldwide.[23] Dogs and similar carnivorous species are the definitive hosts. Humans are secondarily infected by ingesting water that is contaminated by feces containing the parasite. Once ingested, the parasite is absorbed through the duodenal mucosa and passes into the portal vein. Most echinococcal infections involve the liver, but spread to other organ systems also occurs, often secondary to rupture of hepatic lesion with secondary dissemination.[18] Splenic involvement is relatively rare, with a reported prevalence of between 0.9% and 8% of cases.[23]

The most common appearance on imaging is that of a solitary cystic lesion which may or may not demonstrate mural calcification. Occasionally separation of the cyst layers may result in a visible floating membrane within the cyst. Smaller "daughter cysts" may also be present adjacent to the primary lesion.[18,23]

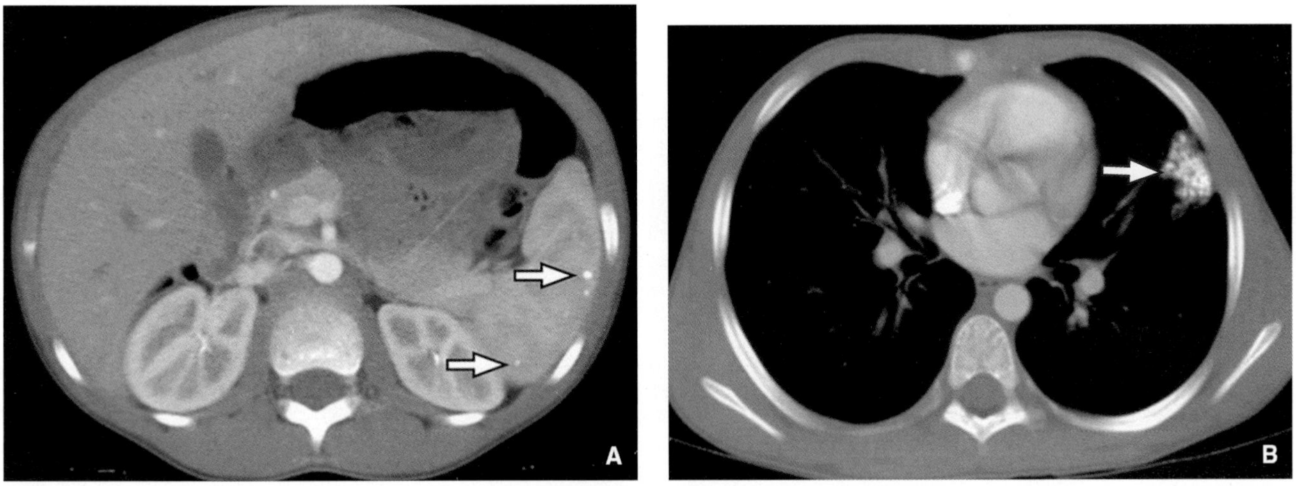

FIGURE 15.9 **A 14-year-old boy with splenic calcifications secondary to prior *Histoplasma sp.* exposure. A:** Axial contrast-enhanced CT image demonstrates multiple punctate calcifications (*arrows*) in the spleen. **B:** Axial contrast-enhanced CT image demonstrates a large, heavily calcified, lobulated nodule (*arrow*) in the lingula.

TABLE 15.1 Splenic Neoplasms in Children

Benign	
	Hamartoma
Malignant	
	Angiosarcoma
	Lymphoma
	Leukemia
	Metastases

Neoplastic Disorders

Splenic neoplasms, both benign and malignant, are rare in children, and they can be categorized by their site of origin into hematolymphoid tumors, nonhematolymphoid tumors, and tumor-like lesions.[24] Lymphoid tumors arise from the white pulp and are the most common type of splenic neoplasm. Vascular neoplasms, such as angiosarcoma, arise from the red pulp and are less common[24] (Table 15.1).

Benign Neoplasms

Hamartoma

Splenic hamartomas are rare, benign lesions consisting of a proliferation of elements resembling red pulp. Hamartomas occur at all ages and do not demonstrate a gender predilection.[24] There is an association between splenic hamartomas and genetic conditions that predispose to other hamartomatous lesions, most commonly tuberous sclerosis.[24] Most splenic hamartomas are asymptomatic and discovered incidentally. Occasionally, large hamartomas may be palpable on physical examination and cause mass effect. Pathologically, splenic hamartomas are well-circumscribed nodules characterized histologically by disorganized red pulp, often in a fibrotic background, without intervening malpighian corpuscles (Fig. 15.10).

Ultrasound is usually the primary imaging modality for assessing suspected or known splenic hamartomas. These lesions typically appear as circumscribed, usually round masses, which are typically with homogeneously isoechoic or hyperechoic relative to the adjacent normal spleen.[24] Occasionally lesions may be heterogenous, have cystic areas, or even have calcifications.[24] On Doppler ultrasound, hamartomas often demonstrate increased blood flow relative to adjacent spleen.[25] Splenic hamartomas may be difficult to identify on CT, as the lesions are generally isoattenuating or slightly hypoattenuating to adjacent normal spleen on both noncontrast and postcontrast images. The only clue to the presence of a splenic hamartoma may be focal distortion of the contour of the spleen. At MRI, these lesions may be similar in signal intensity to normal spleen on T1-weighted images, but can be heterogeneously isotense or slightly hyperintense on T2-weighted images[4,24] (Fig. 15.11).

Malignant Neoplasms

Angiosarcoma

Angiosarcoma is a rare, aggressive malignant neoplasm that can arise within the spleen. This tumor is most common in adults, with most cases presenting in the sixth and seventh decades of life; however, cases have been reported in pediatric patients, including young children.[26,27] Affected pediatric patients typically present with nonspecific left upper quadrant pain and splenomegaly. Metastases are often present at the time of diagnosis.[28] Treatment is focused on splenectomy to remove the tumor and postoperative chemotherapy. The prognosis is generally poor, with only 20% of patients surviving >6 months after diagnosis.[26]

Ultrasound, CT, and MRI all demonstrate an aggressive splenic mass, usually with marked enlargement of the spleen.[28] On ultrasound, the mass is usually heterogeneous, with areas of cystic change reflecting necrosis and

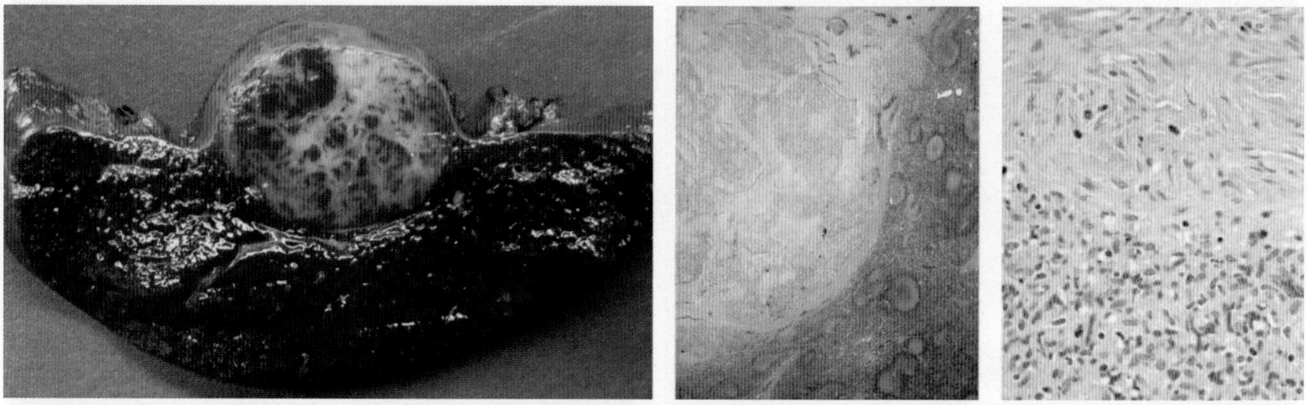

FIGURE 15.10 **This 3.5 cm splenic hamartoma presented as a subcapsular mass in a 9-year-old boy.** It is well circumscribed with a bulging cut surface that was red with intersecting white slightly gelatinous fibrous bands **(left)**. Microscopically, the tumor is paler than the adjacent spleen (**middle**, hematoxylin and eosin, original magnification, 20×). It is composed of closely packed vascular channels resembling sinusoids in collections traversed by pale blue fibromyxoid tissue (**right**, hematoxylin and eosin, original magnification, 400×).

internal hemorrhage.[24] CT may demonstrate multiple heterogeneous and hypervascular masses replacing the spleen. Areas of hemorrhage and calcification may also be present.[24,28] At MRI, these lesions are often heterogeneous on both T1-weighted and T2-weighted sequences with heterogeneous enhancement after intravenous contrast material administration.[28]

Lymphoma

The spleen is the largest lymphatic organ in the body, and, as such, it is commonly involved in both Hodgkin and non-Hodgkin lymphoma. Splenic involvement is present in up to 35% of children with Hodgkin lymphoma at the time of diagnosis.[29] Accordingly, surgical splenectomy with pathologic evaluation of the spleen used to be a standard part of the initial diagnostic staging.[30] The spleen is less commonly involved in non-Hodgkin lymphoma, but certain subtypes frequently involve the spleen.[29] Current imaging techniques have obviated the need for surgical staging of the abdomen, but defining the extent of disease within the abdomen remains a critical part of radiologic disease evaluation at diagnosis and follow-up.

Radiologically, four different patterns of splenic involvement by lymphoma have been described, including diffuse infiltration, tiny nodules (miliary pattern), multiple larger nodules, and solid bulky masses[28] (Fig. 15.12). Diffuse infiltration may only be apparent as splenomegaly at imaging. Discrete lymphomatous masses are generally hypoechoic on ultrasound and low attenuation relative to the normal spleen on contrast-enhanced CT,[28] but both ultrasound and CT have been shown to have suboptimal sensitivity. As such, both ^{18}F-FDG-PET/CT and MRI have emerged as important imaging tools to evaluate for splenic lymphoma. The sensitivity and specificity of ^{18}F-FDG-PET/CT are excellent, with lymphomatous involvement appearing as foci of increased metabolic activity, although the ionizing radiation used for imaging is a drawback, especially in pediatric patients. At MRI, T2-weighted sequences alone have been shown to have high specificity, but relatively low sensitivity. Diffusion-weighted imaging can be helpful but also can be

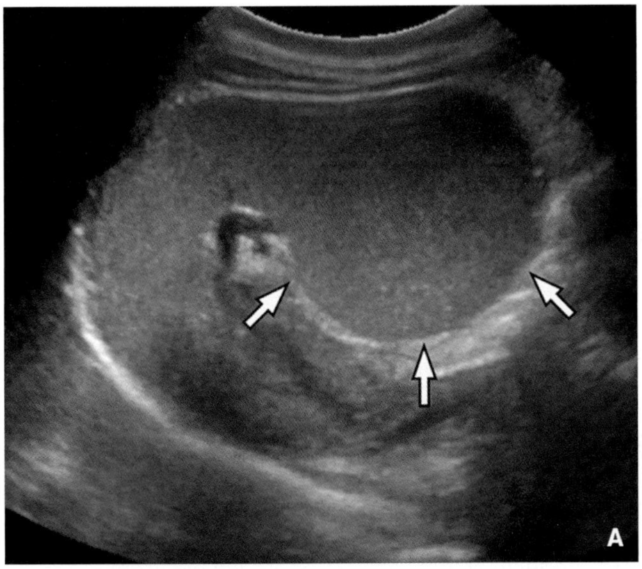

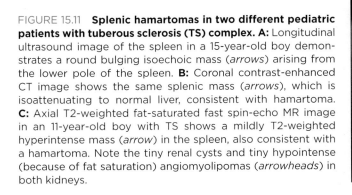

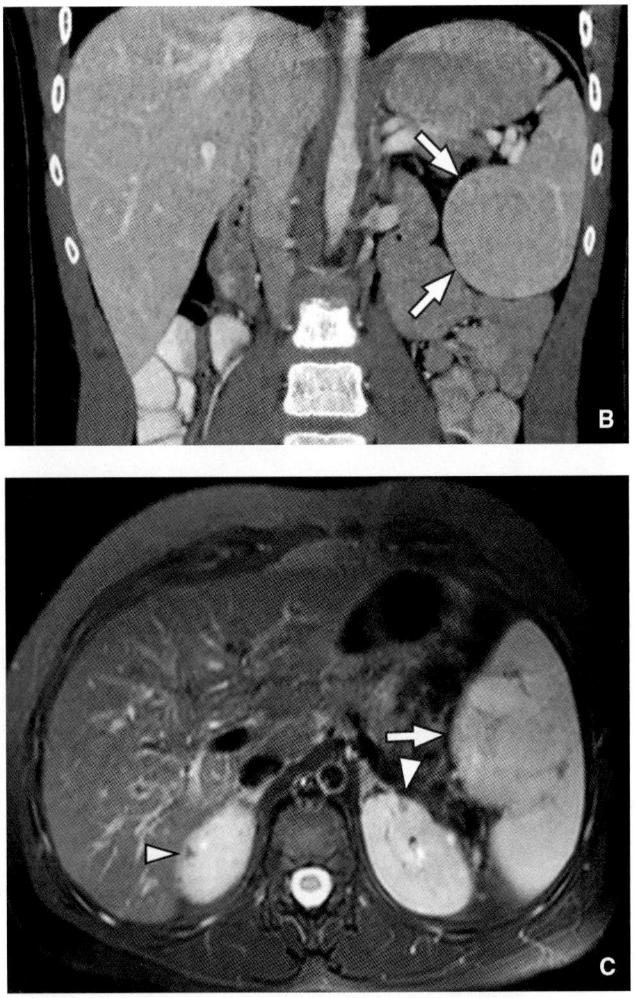

FIGURE 15.11 **Splenic hamartomas in two different pediatric patients with tuberous sclerosis (TS) complex. A:** Longitudinal ultrasound image of the spleen in a 15-year-old boy demonstrates a round bulging isoechoic mass (*arrows*) arising from the lower pole of the spleen. **B:** Coronal contrast-enhanced CT image shows the same splenic mass (*arrows*), which is isoattenuating to normal liver, consistent with hamartoma. **C:** Axial T2-weighted fat-saturated fast spin-echo MR image in an 11-year-old boy with TS shows a mildly T2-weighted hyperintense mass (*arrow*) in the spleen, also consistent with a hamartoma. Note the tiny renal cysts and tiny hypointense (because of fat saturation) angiomyolipomas (*arrowheads*) in both kidneys.

limited because the normal spleen is relatively high in signal intensity making hyperintense lymphomatous deposits less conspicuous.[31] However, the addition of DCE-MRI has shown promise in delineating splenic involvement.[31] During DCE-MRI, lymphomatous deposits are seen as areas of focal signal hypointensity on the earlier phases of contrast enhancement.[31]

Leukemia

The most common splenic manifestation of pediatric leukemia is diffuse enlargement of the spleen. Other relatively common splenic manifestations in leukemia are that of infection due to immunocompromise, as described previously. There are reports of pathologic splenic rupture as a presenting manifestation of leukemia or as a complication in patients with known leukemia.[32]

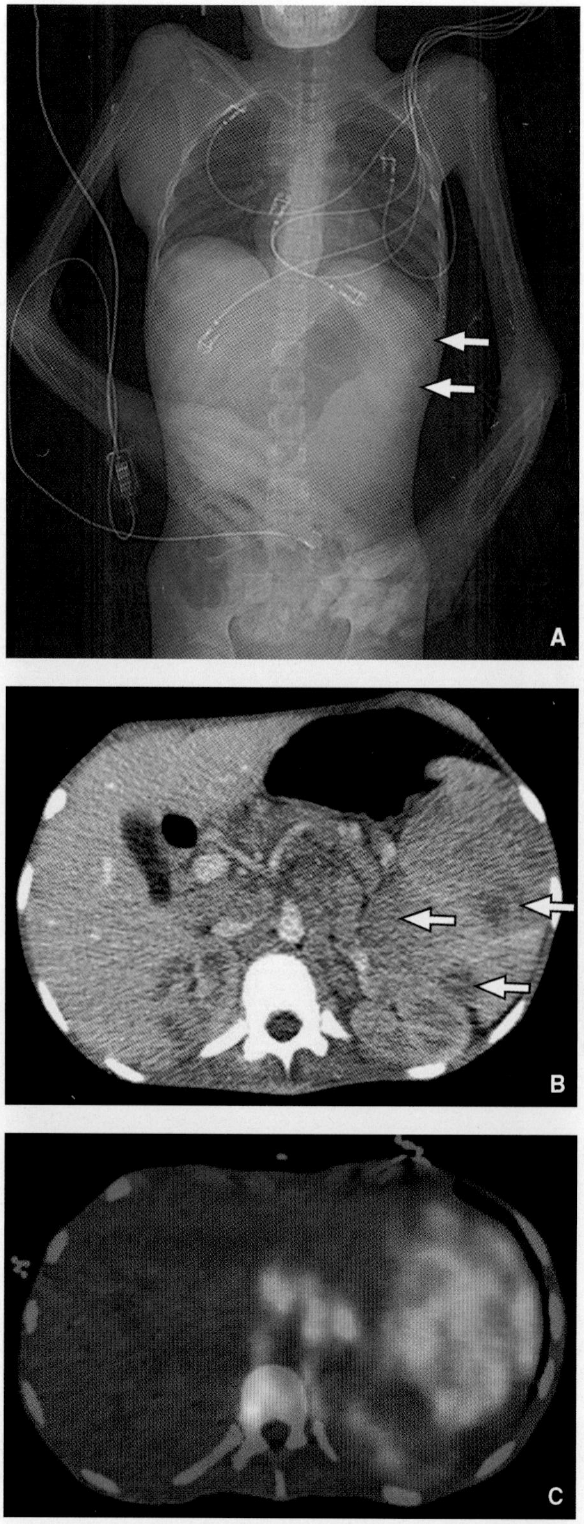

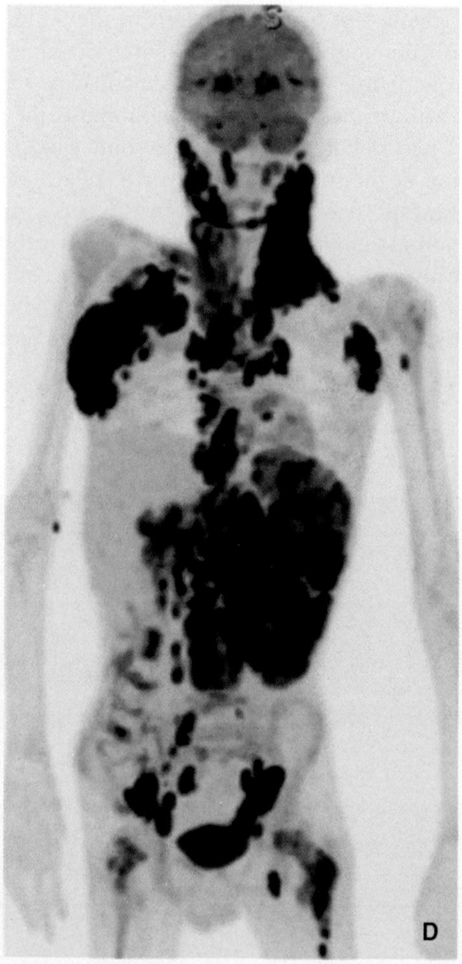

FIGURE 15.12 **Lymphoma involving the spleen in a 13-year-old boy with relapsed Hodgkin lymphoma. A:** Scout image from a CT shows soft tissue density (*arrows*) in the left upper quadrant consistent with an enlarged spleen. The stomach is displaced medially. Because of the patient's medical condition, he was unable to raise his arms for imaging. **B:** Axial contrast-enhanced CT image demonstrates splenic enlargement and multiple low-attenuation masses (*arrows*). There are also multiple enlarged upper abdominal and retroperitoneal lymph nodes. **C:** Fused ^{18}F-FDG-PET/CT image shows marked uptake of radiotracer within the spleen and multiple lymph nodes. **D:** Maximum intensity projection image from an ^{18}F-FDG-PET scan shows extensive FDG uptake in many abnormal cervical, thoracic, and abdominopelvic lymph nodes, in bone, and throughout the spleen.

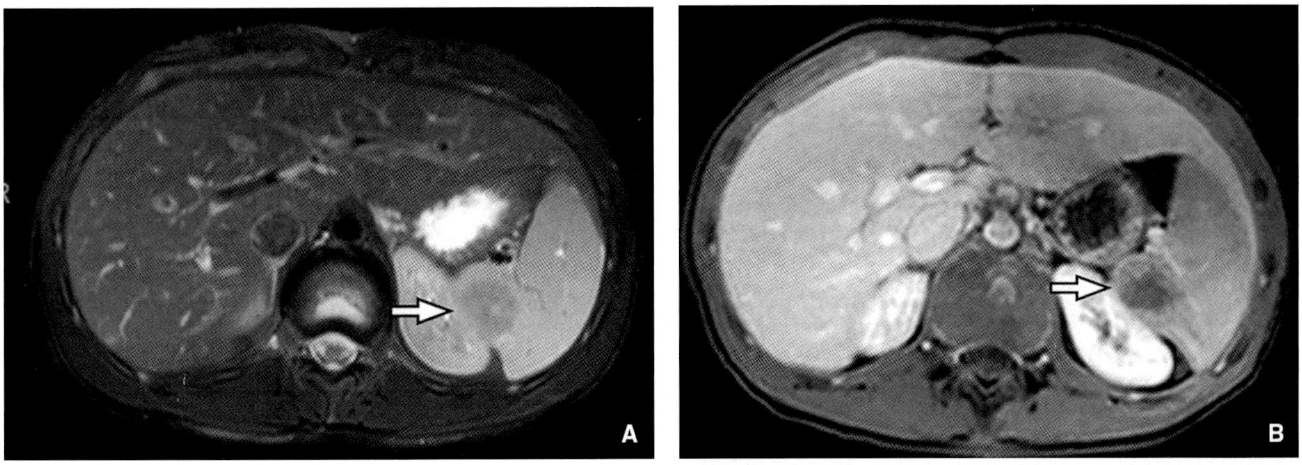

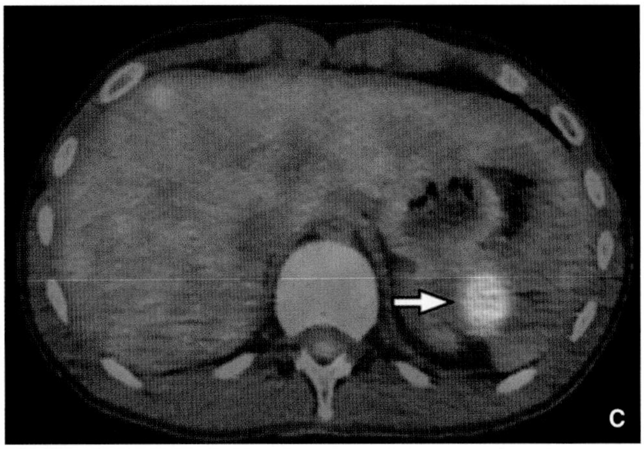

FIGURE 15.13 **Splenic metastasis in a 15-year-old boy with nasopharyngeal carcinoma.** Axial T2-weighted fat-saturated fast spin-echo **(A)** and axial postcontrast 3D T1-weighted SPGR MR **(B)** images demonstrate a focal lesion (*arrow*) in the spleen posteriorly, biopsy proven to be a metastasis. **C:** Fused ^{18}F-FDG-PET/CT image demonstrates that the same lesion (*arrow*) in the spleen is hypermetabolic.

Metastases

Splenic metastases are relatively rare, occurring in 2% to 9% of all cancer patients, and are much less common in children than adults.[28,33] Tumors that metastasize to the spleen tend to be the more aggressive malignancies, such as sarcomas or advanced neoplasms with widespread metastatic disease. In general, splenic metastases present as focal splenic lesions, generally hypoechoic on ultrasound and low attenuation on contrast-enhanced CT. At MRI, lesions are usually iso- to hypointense on T1-weighted images and variable signal intensity on T2-weighted images and demonstrate relative hypoenhancement after intravenous gadolinium-based contrast material administration[28] (Fig. 15.13). Additional sites of metastatic disease within the abdomen are often present as well.

Traumatic Disorders

In blunt trauma, the spleen is the most commonly injured abdominal solid organ in both children and adults.[34,35] The location of the spleen in the left upper quadrant as well as its highly vascular nature predispose the organ to injury during blunt thoracoabdominal trauma. Contrast-enhanced CT is the primary imaging modality used in suspected splenic trauma.[34,36] Occasionally ultrasound may be considered, but has been shown to have relatively low sensitivity in children.[36,37] The use of contrast-enhanced ultrasound for evaluation of pediatric splenic trauma has been reported, but this technique is not yet widely available for use in the United States.[38] Nuclear medicine studies and MRI do not generally play a role in the workup of suspected pediatric splenic trauma. Angiography may be utilized for treatment but is generally no longer used for diagnostic purposes.

Types of Splenic Injuries

Specific types of splenic injuries in blunt trauma include subcapsular and perisplenic hematomas, lacerations, contusions, infarctions, and vascular injuries. Although most splenic injuries have accompanying free intra-abdominal fluid (often blood) or hematoma, up to 25% of pediatric splenic trauma patients do not have fluid or blood elsewhere in their abdomen.[39]

A subcapsular hematoma implies extraparenchymal hemorrhage that is confined within the capsule of the spleen. At CT, a subcapsular hematoma appears as a lenticular or crescentic collection of blood along the periphery of the spleen with mass effect upon the adjacent parenchyma.[34] The blood products can be variable in attenuation, depending on the timing of imaging relative to the trauma, but are usually higher in attenuation than simple fluid (35 to 80 HU) in the setting of acute trauma. Extracapsular, perisplenic hematoma

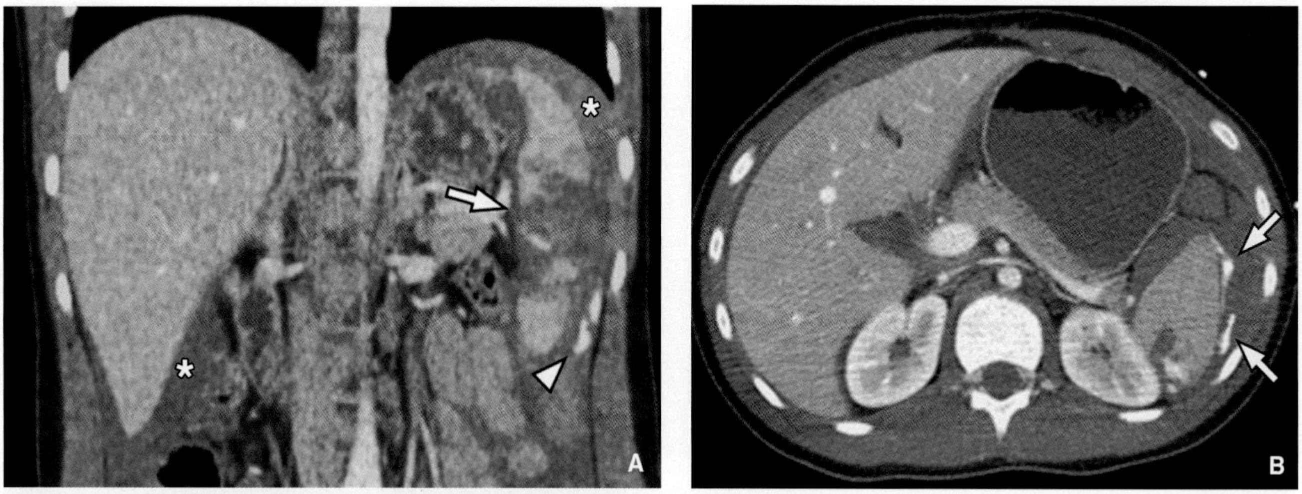

FIGURE 15.14 **Splenic trauma in two different pediatric patients. A:** Coronal contrast-enhanced CT image in a 9-year-old girl after blunt abdominal trauma demonstrates low-attenuation clefts through the spleen, consistent with an extensive splenic laceration (*arrow*). Note the high-attenuation free fluid consistent with hemoperitoneum (*asterisk*) and a small amount of extravasated contrast material (*arrowhead*). **B:** Axial contrast-enhanced CT image in a 13-year-old boy after a motor vehicle collision demonstrates a splenic laceration with perisplenic hematoma and active extravasation of contrast material (*arrows*).

implies blood products adjacent to the spleen and indicates that the splenic capsule has been disrupted.

A splenic laceration appears as discrete linear, branching, or stellate low-attenuation area extending through the splenic parenchyma[34] (Fig. 15.14). If there is active bleeding, there may be high-attenuation iodinated contrast material pooling in or near the laceration, implying active extravasation of blood and contrast material. Lacerations can disrupt the vascular supply to the spleen resulting in splenic infarction (devascularization). Infarcted areas of spleen typically appear as geographic areas of low attenuation on contrast-enhanced CT (Fig. 15.15).

It is important to look for other associated injuries as well. In adults, up to 35% of patients with splenic injuries have other intra-abdominal injuries apparent on CT, and up to 80% have extra-abdominal injuries, including rib fractures and body wall injuries.[34]

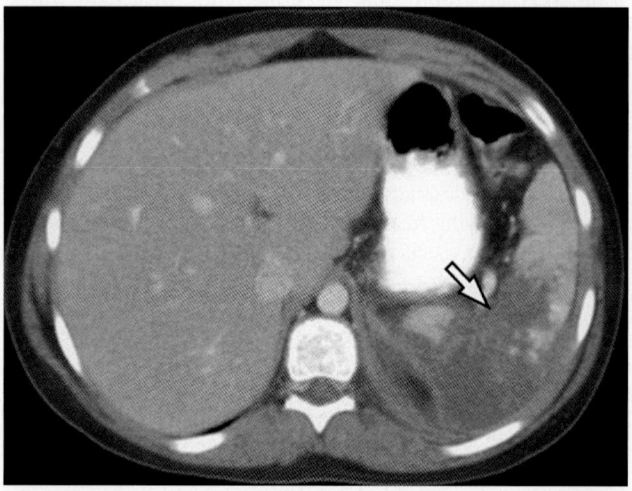

FIGURE 15.15 **Splenic trauma in a 12-year-old girl after a snowboarding accident.** Axial contrast-enhanced CT image shows a large splenic laceration (*arrow*) with devascularization of a portion of the splenic parenchyma.

Grading Splenic Injuries

Grading splenic injuries allows clinicians caring for pediatric trauma patients to have a standardized reference for injury severity and is increasingly being used to guide nonoperative management in pediatric splenic blunt trauma.[34] A commonly used grading system for the severity of splenic trauma was created by the American Association for the Surgery of Trauma (AAST), which takes into account the types of injuries, number of injuries, depth of specific injuries, and any associated infarction, and results in a severity grade of 1–5 (1 = least severe; 5 = most severe).[40]

Complications from Splenic Injuries

Nonoperative management is now the standard of care for pediatric patients with blunt splenic trauma who are hemodynamically stable.[41] Although rare, a few patients may develop delayed complications, including vascular injury with pseudoaneurysm formation, infection of posttraumatic fluid collections, and pseudocyst formation.

Pseudoaneurysms, or contained vascular rupture, occur as the result of arterial wall injury. Splenic artery pseudoaneurysms have been reported to occur in up to 5% of pediatric splenic injuries.[42] Although rare, these lesions are clinically significant as there is a small risk of rupture with resultant life-threatening hemorrhage. On ultrasound, a splenic artery pseudoaneursym typically appears as a rounded hypo- or anechoic cystic structure, often located near the splenic hilum. With color Doppler ultrasound, there can be variable amounts of internal blood flow depending on any associated thrombus. Doppler ultrasound sometimes may reveal an alternating pattern of color signal, sometimes referred to as a "yin-yang" sign. Spectral Doppler ultrasound sampling of the neck of the pseudoaneurysm can confirm the diagnosis

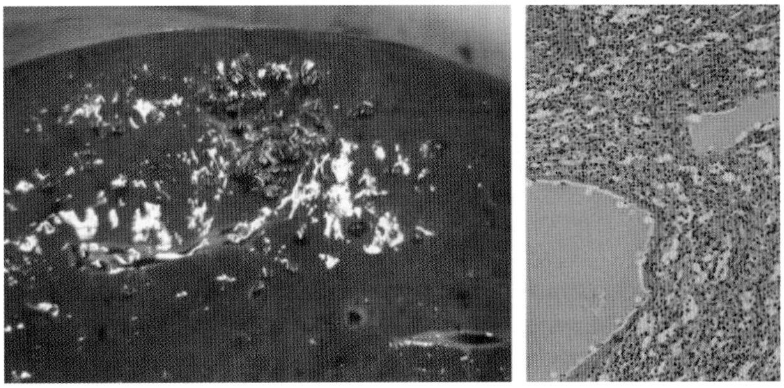

FIGURE. 15.16 **A 10-year-old girl with Klippel-Trenaunay syndrome and portal hypertension.** Resected spleen shows numerous small cyst-like spaces (**left**) that microscopically proved to represent lymphatic channels (**right**, hematoxylin and eosin, original magnification, 200x).

by demonstrating to-and-fro blood flow going into and coming out of the pseudoaneurysm. On CT and MRI, the lesion appears as an avidly enhancing structure that should be similar in attenuation or signal intensity to adjacent enhanced vascular structures.

Perisplenic and intrasplenic fluid collections are relatively common after blunt splenic trauma due to liquefaction and degradation of blood products. Occasionally, these collections can become infected and form abscesses with similar imaging features to abscesses elsewhere in the body, including an irregular enhancing wall, internal locules of gas, and adjacent inflammatory changes. As mentioned previously, splenic pseudocysts can be the result of trauma. These lesions lack an epithelial lining, differentiating them from epithelial or congenital splenic cysts. Imaging features are indistinguishable from other benign cystic lesions at ultrasound, CT, and MRI. Occasionally, large pseudocysts may require percutaneous drainage.[4]

Vascular Malformations

Vascular malformations can occur within the spleen and may be either isolated or associated with an underlying syndrome, such as Klippel-Trenaunay syndrome[43] (Fig. 15.16). Imaging features of splenic vascular malformations are similar to those elsewhere in the body. On ultrasound, slow-flow vascular malformations are usually well-defined, anechoic, or hypoechoic lesions that may have lobulations or septations. Internal Doppler blood flow is variable depending on whether the lesion is predominantly venous or lymphatic. On CT, postcontrast enhancement of the lesion depends on the exact histologic nature of the lesions (venous versus lymphatic) as well as the phase of contrast enhancement.

MRI is the imaging modality of choice for characterizing splenic vascular malformations. The lesions are usually predominantly hyperintense on T2-weighted images with variable signal intensity on T1-weighted images (Fig. 15.17). In venous malformations, phleboliths may be identified as rounded T2-weighted hypointense filling defects, or rounded hypointense structures on gradient-recalled echo sequences. Predominantly venous malformations show enhancement, especially on more delayed postcontrast images. Predominantly lymphatic malformations generally only show thin, uniform enhancement of the walls and any internal septations. If there has been prior hemorrhage or infection, thin mural calcifications may be present, most easily seen on CT but also potentially visible on plain radiographs, ultrasound, and MRI.[24]

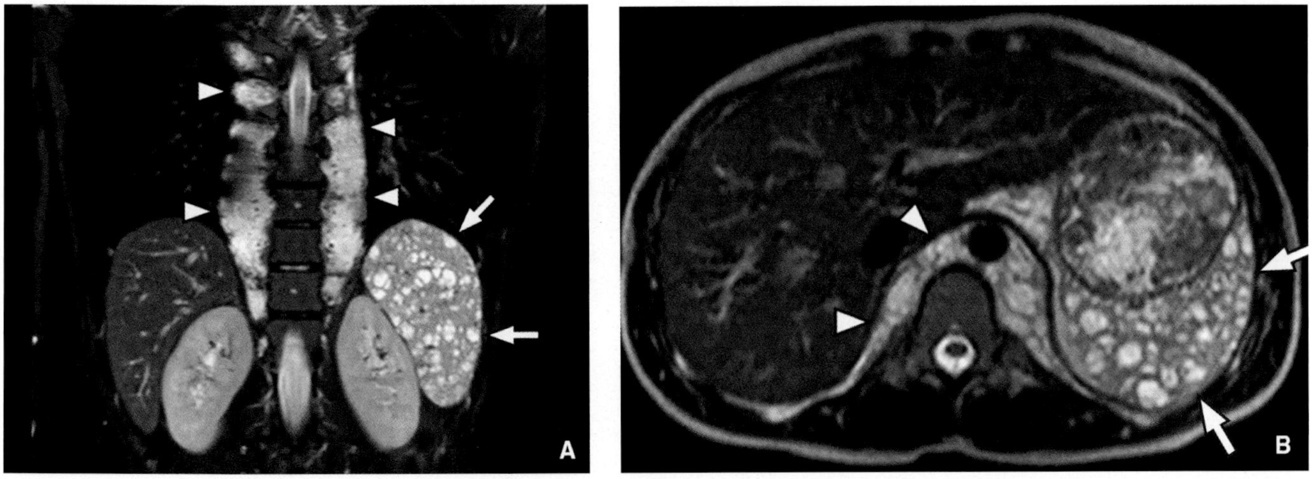

FIGURE 15.17 **Extensive splenic venolymphatic malformation in a 17-year-old girl.** Coronal fat-saturated **(A)** and axial T2-weighted fast spin-echo MR **(B)** images show multiple hyperintense lesions (*arrows*) within the spleen. On delayed contrast-enhanced images (not shown), many of the lesions demonstrate enhancement suggesting venous elements. Note the accompanying extensive venolymphatic malformations (*arrowheads*) in the bilateral paraspinal and retrocrural regions.

Splenomegaly

The spleen normally increases in size throughout childhood, becoming larger as the child grows. There are published normal values for pediatric splenic length based on age and gender.[8] Splenomegaly is often defined as enlargement of the spleen >2 standard deviations above the mean expected length for patient age and gender (Fig. 15.18). The causes of splenomegaly are multiple, including portal hypertension (e.g., due to cirrhosis or chronic portal vein occlusion), infiltrative splenic disorders, neoplastic conditions, hyperfunction of the spleen (i.e., hypersplenism), infections (e.g., mononucleosis), and congenital disorders.[4]

Hemoglobinopathies

The red pulp of the spleen acts as a filter for damaged or abnormal red blood cells, to remove them from circulation and begin to recycle their components into new red blood cells. As such, several congenital conditions that affect red blood cells can affect the spleen. Examples of these conditions include congenital hemoglobinopathies, such as sickle cell disease and hereditary spherocytosis.

Sickle Cell Disease

Sickle cell disease is an autosomal recessive condition that results in abnormal hemoglobin molecules (HbS) that are prone to polymerize when in their deoxygenated state. This polymerization results in morphologically abnormal red blood cells, limiting the erythrocytes' ability to deform and resulting in vascular occlusions.[44] Sickle cell disease affects the spleen in two discrete ways. First, the spleen has to function to remove the abnormal red blood cells, which accumulate and fill the red pulp. In younger patients, this relative hyperfunction of the spleen can result in anemia and thrombocytopenia, a syndrome termed "splenic sequestration."[44] Second, the spleen, as an end-organ, has little or no collateral blood flow, making it vulnerable to vascular occlusions and infarction.

Imaging manifestations of splenic involvement with sickle cell disease are variable. In acute splenic sequestration, the spleen is diffusely enlarged. Variable findings of splenic infarction can occur over time. Infarcted areas generally appear as wedge-shaped or geographic areas of capsular-based hypoenhancement on CT or MRI.[4] Occasionally, preserved islands of normal spleen can simulate splenic masses[45] (Figs. 15.19 and 15.20). The end result of splenic infarction is a small calcified spleen, or in cases of complete infarction, the spleen may be nonvisualized.

Patients with hemoglobinopathies often undergo multiple blood transfusions. The iron associated with multiple blood transfusions can be deposited in the reticuloendothelial system and results in secondary hemochromatosis. Imaging manifestations of iron deposition are best evaluated using MRI, based on the principle that sequences with longer echo times (TE) result in susceptibility artifact and greater loss of signal than is normal. The amount of parenchymal iron can be quantified in the form of a T2* (or R2*) value. The most

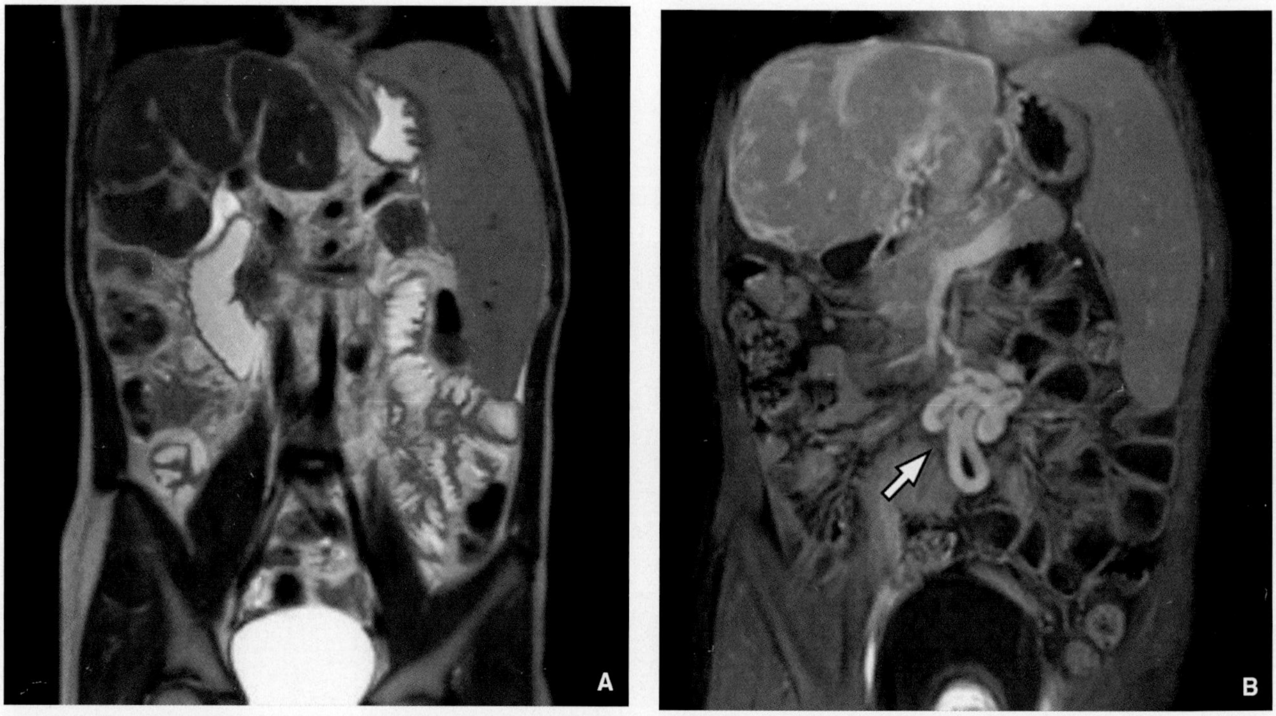

FIGURE 15.18 **Splenomegaly due to portal hypertension in a 6-year-old boy with a history of biliary atresia, status post Kasai portoenterostomy. A:** Coronal T2-weighted image shows an enlarged spleen and a shrunken, nodular liver contour consistent with cirrhosis. **B:** Coronal T1-weighted 3D SPGR postcontrast image shows an enlarged spleen and multiple collateral venous structures (*arrow*) in the mid-abdomen secondary to portal hypertension.

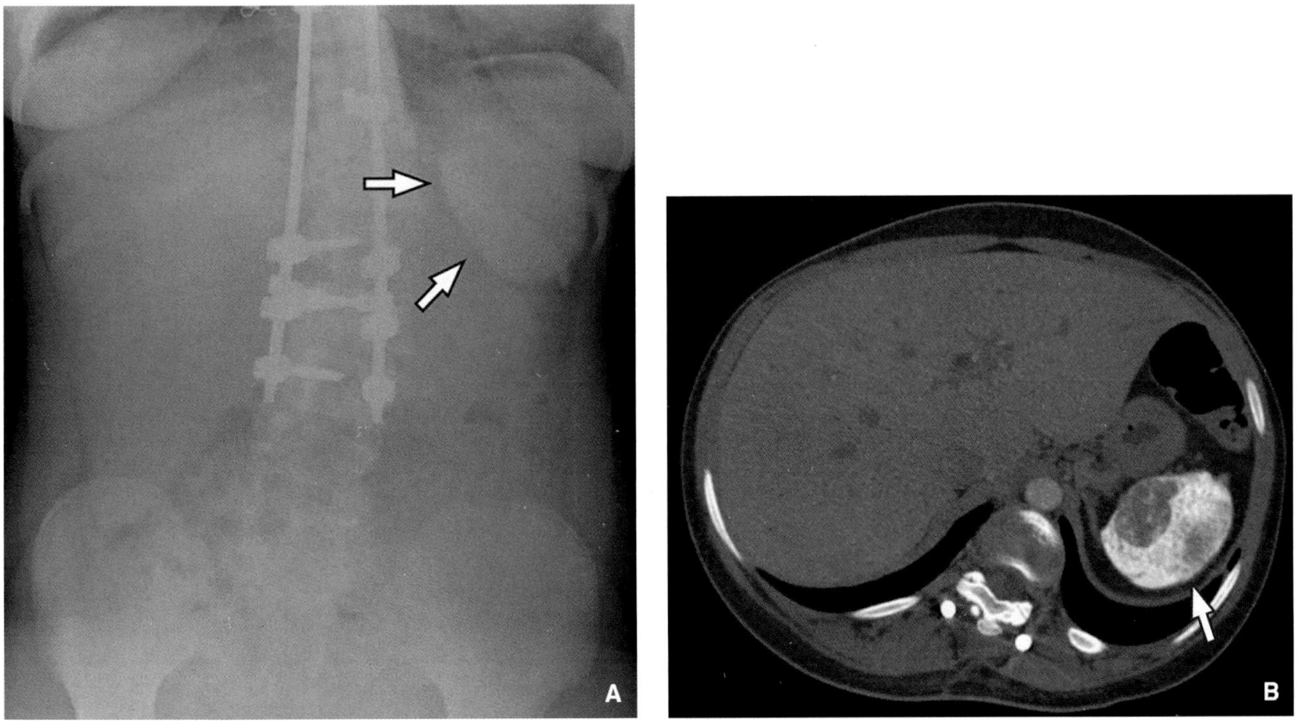

FIGURE 15.19 **Splenic manifestations of sickle cell disease in an 18-year-old girl. A:** Abdominal radiograph demonstrates an opacity (*arrows*) in the left upper quadrant representing the heavily calcified spleen. **B:** Axial noncontrast CT image in the same patient shows a small spleen with extensive calcification (*arrow*) and a few relatively preserved islands of noncalcified splenic tissue.

commonly affected organs in secondary hemochromatosis include the liver, spleen, pancreas and bone marrow.

Hereditary Spherocytosis

Hereditary spherocytosis is a common heritable disorder of red blood cells in which the erythrocytes have an abnormal spherical shape with resultant decreased surface area and lack of the ability of the cell to deform, all due to abnormal surface protein expression and disruption of normal phospholipid chains in the cell membrane.[46] Affected pediatric patients present clinically with variable degrees of anemia and splenomegaly as a result of sequestration of the abnormal erythrocytes within the spleen with subsequent phagocytosis of abnormal erythrocyte membranes by splenic macrophages.

The most common imaging finding in hereditary spherocytosis is splenomegaly, which can range from mild to severe.

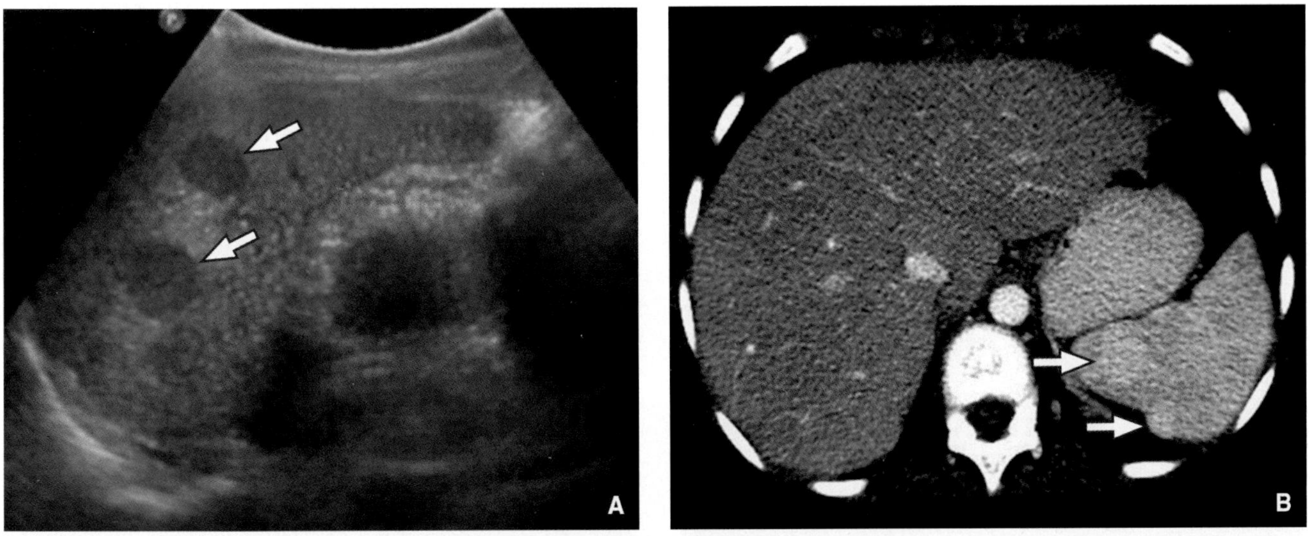

FIGURE 15.20 **Sickle cell disease with preserved islands of tissue in a 14-year-old girl. A:** Longitudinal ultrasound image shows rounded, hypoechoic lesions (*arrows*) within the spleen. **B:** Axial contrast-enhanced CT image demonstrates rounded areas of higher attenuation (*arrows*) simulating focal masses within the spleen. The findings on both ultrasound and CT are likely due to areas of relatively preserved splenic parenchyma in the setting of sickle cell disease.

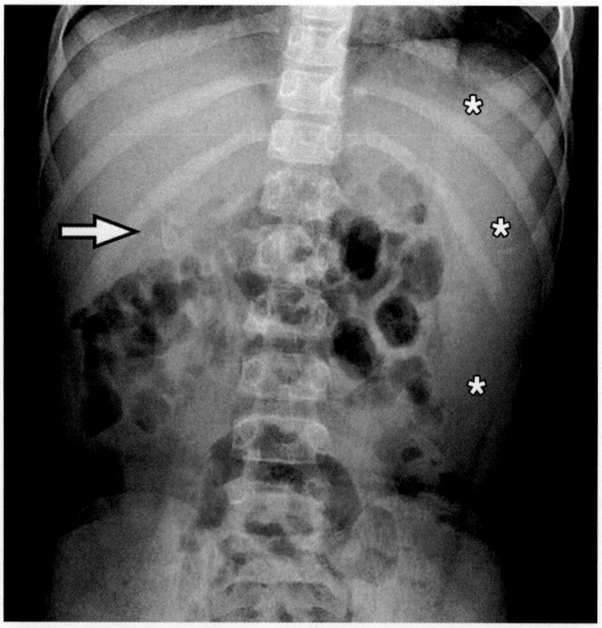

FIGURE 15.21 **Hereditary spherocytosis.** Supine abdominal radiograph is a 16-year-old boy with hereditary spherocytosis shows splenomegaly (*asterisk*) and calcified gallstones (*arrow*).

Children may also have gallstones as a result of increased red blood cell turnover[47] (Fig. 15.21).

Treatment is usually supportive, with close monitoring of anemia and transfusions when necessary, although, in some cases, splenectomy may be performed to prevent red blood cell sequestration.[46] Occasionally, partial splenectomy or partial splenic embolization may be performed to reduce the future risk of infectious complications related to asplenia. Splenectomy specimens are usually large and show an expanded red pulp (Fig. 15.22).

PANCREAS

Imaging Techniques

Radiography

The normal pancreas is not visible on plain radiographs. Occasionally, radiography may demonstrate pancreatic calcifications in chronic pancreatitis, or mass effect in the setting of a large pancreatic mass or pseudocyst.

Ultrasound

Portions of the pancreas may be difficult to visualize with sonography because of its retroperitoneal location and artifacts from overlying gas-filled stomach and loops of bowel. However, the pancreatic head and uncinate process are usually readily visualized adjacent to the duodenum. With appropriate graded compression, the entire pancreas often can be visualized, especially in younger children. Pancreatic parenchymal echogenicity, focal lesions, and ductal dilation can all be assessed by ultrasound.

Computed Tomography

Contrast-enhanced CT is the primary imaging modality in the setting of suspected pancreatic trauma and in acute conditions of the pancreas, such as acute necrotizing pancreatitis. CT can also readily demonstrate pancreatic atrophy, parenchymal calcifications, and ductal dilation in the setting of chronic pancreatitis or ductal obstruction. In the setting of suspected pancreatic masses, CT allows assessment of the size of the mass, its relationship to adjacent structures, and any evidence of local or distant abdominal metastatic spread. Detailed anatomic assessment of the pancreatic duct can be difficult given the limited contrast resolution of CT compared to MRI.

Magnetic Resonance Imaging

MRI, with its excellent contrast resolution, provides a detailed assessment of both the pancreatic parenchyma and the pancreatic ductal system. T2-weighted sequences, especially when fat saturation is applied, readily depict pancreatic inflammation, peripancreatic edema/fluid, and a variety of cystic lesions. Multiphase postcontrast imaging after intravenous administration of gadolinium-based contrast material can evaluate enhancement of the pancreatic parenchyma as well as characterize focal pancreatic lesions.

Magnetic resonance cholangiopancreatography (MRCP) can be used to evaluate the anatomy of the pancreatic ductal system. MRCP utilizes heavily T2-weighted pulse sequences in order to take advantage of the intrinsically long T2 relaxation times of fluid-containing structures, including bile ducts and pancreatic ducts.[48] A variety of 2D and 3D MRCP techniques exist; however, 3D techniques are most commonly employed in modern MRCP protocols. When specifically

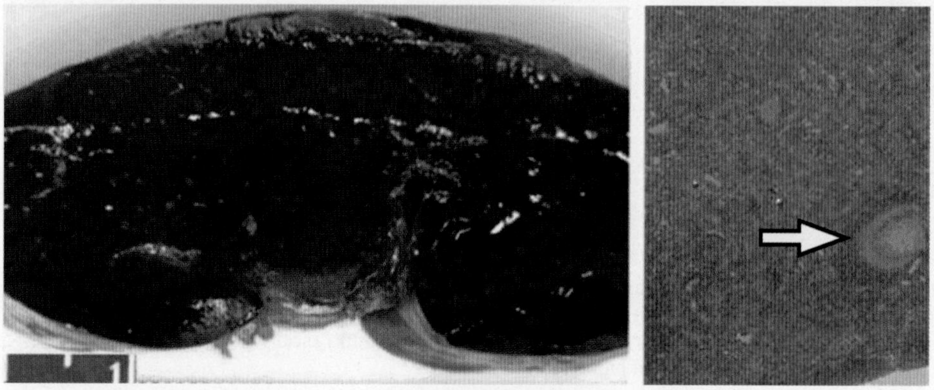

FIGURE 15.22 **Spleen from a 9-year-old boy with hereditary spherocytosis and splenic sequestration syndrome.** The spleen is large (235 g, versus the expected 70 g) with an expanded red pulp **(left)**. Microscopically, red blood cells fill the red pulp and the malpighian corpuscles of the white pulp (*arrow*) are sparse (**right**, hematoxylin and eosin, original magnification, 100×).

imaging the pancreatic duct, some have advocated the use of secretin, a hormone that causes increased production and secretion of pancreatic fluid, in order to dilate the duct and make the anatomy more evident; however, recently the utility of this technique has been called into question.[49]

Nuclear Medicine

Nuclear medicine imaging plays a limited role in evaluation of pediatric pancreatic abnormalities. In patients with suspected neuroendocrine tumors, somatostatin receptor (octreotide) scintigraphy may play a role in characterizing the tumor and in the evaluation for metastatic disease. In malignant tumors of the pancreas, ^{18}F-FDG-PET/CT may play a role in disease staging and surveillance.

Normal Anatomy

The pancreas has both endocrine and exocrine functions, with its primary endocrine role in control of glucose homeostasis and its primary exocrine function being to assist in the digestion of food.[50] Pancreatic endocrine function is carried out by five distinct cell types organized into functional units termed "islet of Langerhans."[50] These five cell types include β-cells, which produce insulin; α-cells, which produce glucagon; δ-cells, which produce somatostatin; pancreatic polypeptide–producing PP cells; and ghrelin-producing ε-cells.[51] These endocrine hormones are secreted into the body via the bloodstream. Pancreatic exocrine function is carried out in acinar cells, which produce amylase and lipase that is secreted into the small bowel via the pancreatic duct.[52]

Developmentally, the pancreas arises from two separate structures located on either side of the duodenum called the dorsal and ventral buds, both of which arise from the endodermal lining of the duodenum.[52] Around the 6th week of fetal development, the ventral bud rotates counterclockwise posterior to the duodenum and fuses with the dorsal bud, with the ducts of the both the dorsal bud and the ventral bud also fusing.[51,52] The fused duct now extends the entire length of the pancreas and becomes the main pancreatic duct of Wirsung.[51] A smaller remnant of a portion of the prior dorsal bud duct persists as the accessory duct of Santorini.[51] In its final configuration, the pancreas retains these two ducts, the main duct (of Wirsung) and the smaller accessory duct (of Santorini) (Fig. 15.23). The main pancreatic duct drains into the duodenum via the major papilla, or ampulla of Vater, whereas the smaller duct drains into the duodenum via the minor papilla.

Anatomically, the pancreas is an elongated, lobular organ located in the retroperitoneum. Growth of the pancreas is accelerated during the first year of life and slows thereafter; thus, the pancreas in a young child is larger relative to body size than in an older child or adult.[52] The head of the pancreas and the triangle-shaped uncinate process,

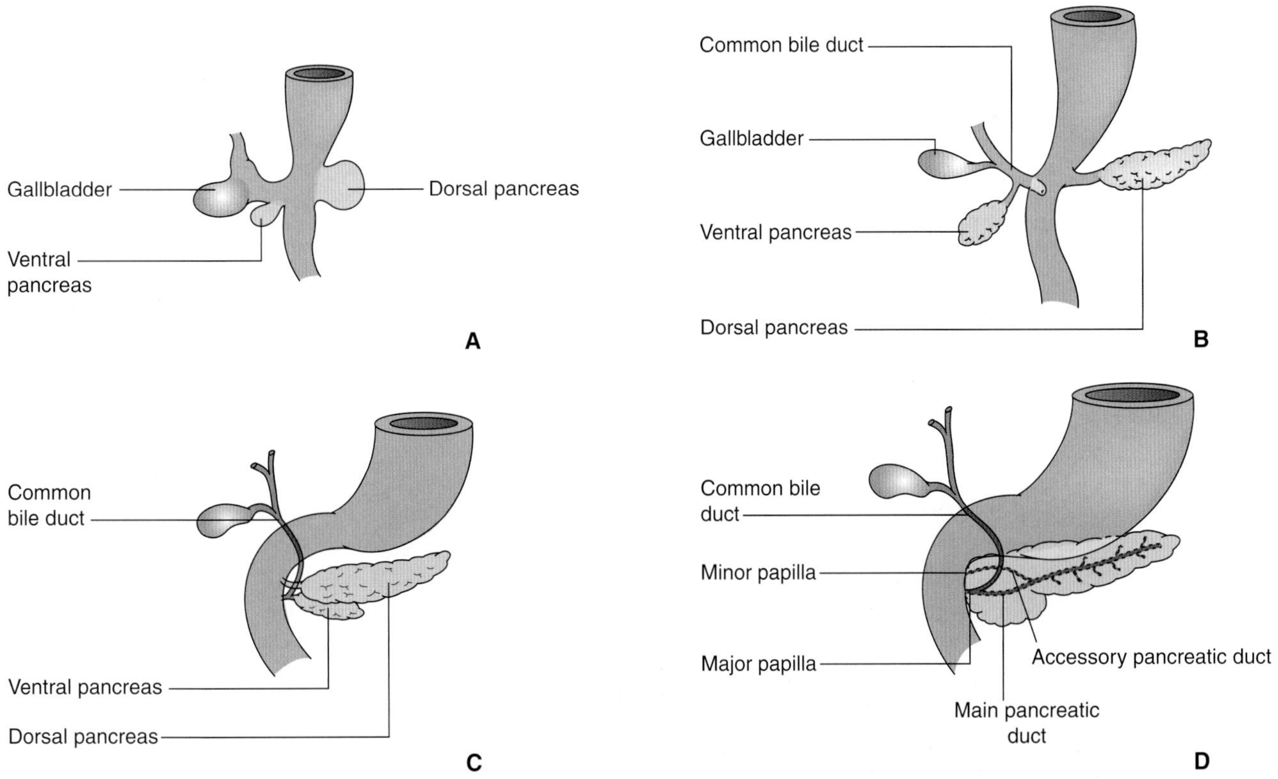

FIGURE 15.23 **Normal development of the pancreas.** The pancreas develops as separate ventral and dorsal pancreatic buds, located on either side of the duodenum **(A and B)**. During the 6th week of fetal development, the ventral bud rotates counterclockwise around the duodenum and fuses with the dorsal bud **(C)**. Subsequently, the ventral and dorsal ducts fuse, giving rise to the normal configuration with a main pancreatic duct (of Wirsung) derived from components of the both the embryologic ventral and dorsal ducts and the medial portion of the embryologic dorsal duct persisting as the accessory pancreatic duct (of Santorini) **(D)**.

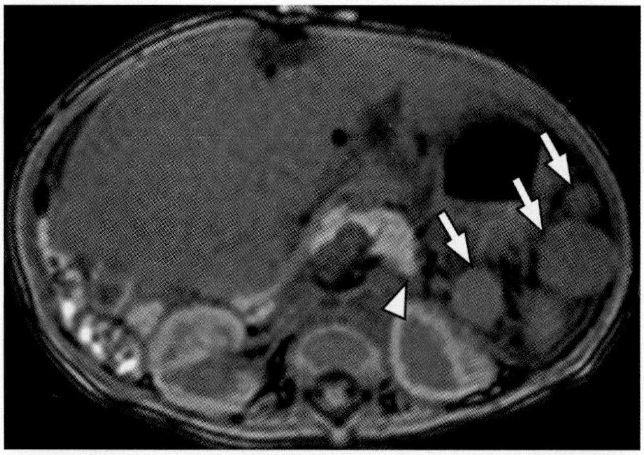

FIGURE 15.24 **Partial pancreatic agenesis in a 6-month-old boy with heterotaxy syndrome and polysplenia.** Precontrast axial T1-weighted fat saturated MR image shows truncation of the normally hyperintense pancreas with absence of the distal body and tail of the pancreas (*arrowhead*). Note the multiple left upper quadrant spleens (*arrows*).

which protrudes posteriorly, are located to the right of midline and are closely associated with the C loop of the duodenum.[53] The tail of the pancreas lies to the left and is located near the hilum of the spleen, within the layers of peritoneum that form the splenorenal ligament.[53] The pancreas is invested in connective tissue but does not have a true capsule. Arterial supply to the pancreas arises from both the celiac axis and the superior mesenteric artery via the pancreaticoduodenal arteries and branches of the splenic artery.[53] Venous drainage from the pancreas is via the splenic vein and other smaller branches that ultimately empty into the portal vein.[53]

At ultrasound, the normal pancreas appears as a homogeneous structure of slightly increased echogenicity relative to the liver.[52] At CT, the gland appears homogenous and similar in attenuation to the liver, with homogeneous enhancement after the administration of intravenous iodinated contrast material. Peak parenchymal enhancement is often in the late arterial phase. At MRI, the pancreas is usually hyperintense compared to liver on T1-weighted pulse sequences.[52] The gland is homogeneously isointense to liver on T2-weighted sequences and enhances after intravenous gadolinium-based contrast material administration. The normal main pancreatic duct may or may not be visible at routine imaging. If visible, the main pancreatic duct should measure between 1 and 2 mm and should not be greater than 2.5 to 3 mm in diameter.[52]

Congenital Abnormalities

Pancreatic Agenesis

Complete pancreatic agenesis occurs when there is complete failure of pancreatic development, resulting in absence of the pancreas. This is a very rare congenital anomaly and is often incompatible with life.[54] More frequently, partial pancreatic agenesis occurs, also referred to as pancreatic hypoplasia. In this entity, either the dorsal or ventral pancreatic bud fails to develop; failure of the dorsal bud is more common.[54] At imaging, the most common appearance is a prominent, rounded pancreatic head near the duodenum with absence of the pancreatic body and tail.[54] There is an association between partial pancreatic agenesis and heterotaxy syndromes with polysplenia[54] (Fig 15.24).

Ectopic Pancreas

Ectopic pancreatic tissue is defined as normal pancreatic tissue that is located in an abnormal location and anatomically separate from the normal pancreas. The most common location is the stomach, followed by the duodenum and jejunum[55] (Fig 15.25). The reported incidence in autopsy series ranges from 2% to 14%.[55,56] Ectopic pancreas is more commonly diagnosed in adults, but has been reported in all ages. The lesions are often small and asymptomatic but can rarely cause complications, such as gastric outlet or bowel obstruction, pancreatitis, or pseudocysts.[57]

Ectopic pancreatic tissue is often difficult to visualize in younger children. In older children and young adults, the lesions are usually small, often measuring <1 cm.[55] Occasionally, ectopic pancreas may be visualized on an upper GI series as a small mucosal-based filling defect, usually in

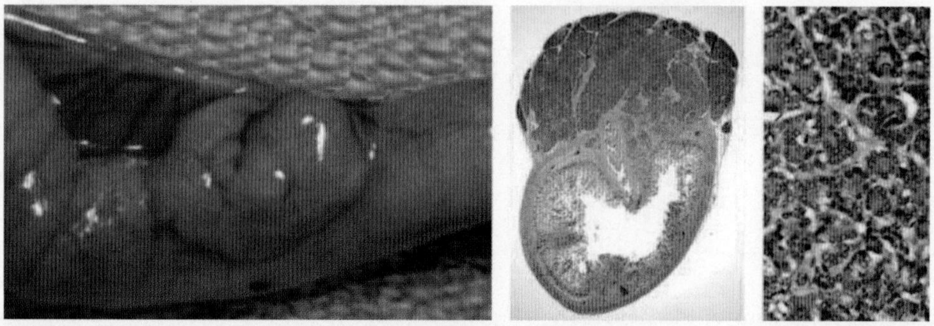

FIGURE 15.25 **Nodule of ectopic pancreas on the serosal surface of the jejunum (left)**, observed during autopsy of a 2-week-old girl who died of complex congenital heart disease. Microscopically, the mass extended into the bowel wall, connected by a duct-like structure (**middle**, hematoxylin and eosin, original magnification, 20×) and was composed of well-developed pancreatic acinar and endocrine tissue (**right**, hematoxylin and eosin, original magnification, 600×).

the antropyloric region of the stomach.[55] These lesions may be very difficult to visualize with cross-sectional imaging, including ultrasound, CT, and MRI. CT findings that have been described include a rounded or oval-shaped well-defined mass with serrated margins and similar CT attenuation and postcontrast enhancement to that of the normal pancreas.[56,57]

Annular Pancreas

Annular pancreas occurs when the ventral pancreatic bud fails to rotate in the normal fashion, leaving a segment of the pancreas that encircles the second portion of the duodenum and causes varying degrees of duodenal obstruction[54,58] (Fig 15.26). There is often some degree of intrinsic duodenal stenosis as well.[59] The incidence of annular pancreas is ~1 in 1,000.[58,59] Affected patients present clinically at all ages, with varying presentations depending on the age of the patient and the degree of duodenal obstruction. Neonates and infants typically present with vomiting, which is usually nonbilious, and feeding intolerance.[58,60] These patients may also have associated congenital anomalies. In contrast, older children and adults typically present with abdominal pain and are unlikely to have associated congenital anomalies.[58] The treatment of patients with annular pancreas is typically surgical bypass of the narrowed portion of the duodenum.[58]

The imaging evaluation of affected pediatric patients often begins with plain radiographs, which may be normal or may demonstrate varying degrees of proximal obstruction, including dilation of the stomach and duodenal bulb (so-called double bubble sign) that can mimic duodenal atresia.[54] In infants and young children, a fluoroscopic upper gastrointestinal series may be performed and will demonstrate focal narrowing at the second portion of the duodenum (Fig. 15.27). The duodenum may or may not be completely obstructed. Ultrasound, CT, and MRI can all demonstrate similar findings with varying degrees of duodenal obstruction and enlargement of the pancreatic head with soft tissue that is identical in appearance to the pancreas surrounding the second portion of the duodenum.[54]

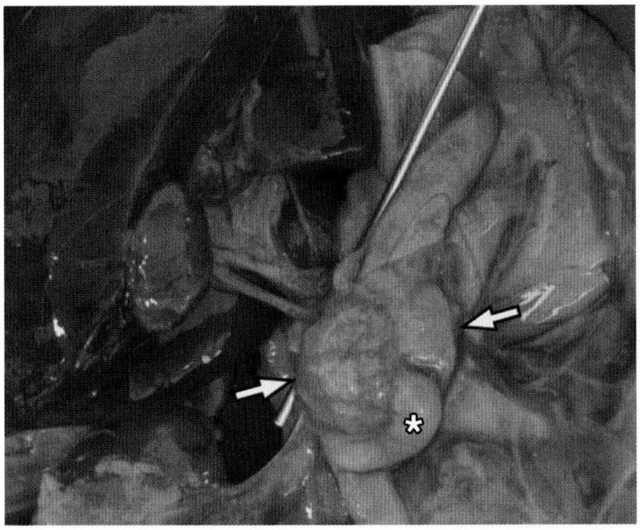

FIGURE 15.26 **Annular pancreas in a 9-month-old boy who died because of congenital heart disease.** Photographic image from the autopsy shows that pink-tan lobulated tissue of the pancreas (*arrows*) completely surrounds the duodenum (*asterisk*).

Pancreas Divisum

Pancreas divisum is a relatively common congenital anomaly of the pancreatic ductal system, occurring in 4% to 14% of the population.[54] Pancreas divisum results from abnormal fusion of the dorsal and ventral pancreatic buds such that the embryologic dorsal duct persists and does not fuse with the embryologic ventral duct to form a normal main pancreatic duct (Wirsung) that drains through the major papilla (ampulla of Vater). Instead, the dorsal and ventral ducts remain separate, and the result is that the majority of the pancreatic exocrine drainage is through the dorsal duct (Santorini) that drains through the minor papilla, proximal to the ampulla of Vater.[54] Pancreas divisum can be complete, where the ducts remain completely separate, or incomplete in which there is partial fusion of the ducts.[61] The clinical importance of this abnormality is an associated increased incidence of pancreatitis, which sometimes occurs during childhood, especially in children with complete divisum.[61]

Pancreas divisum is usually not detectable by ultrasound. Contrast-enhanced CT on occasion may allow visualization of the main pancreatic duct and delineation of the anomalous ductal drainage. MRI, and specifically high-resolution 3D MRCP, generally allows optimal visualization of pancreatic ductal anatomy[52] (Fig. 15.28). Cross-sectional imaging may also demonstrate associated acute or chronic pancreatitis. Endoscopic retrograde cholangiopancreatography (ERCP) also readily depicts pancreatic ductal anatomy, although this imaging technique is much more invasive and can cause procedure-related acute pancreatitis.

Infectious and Inflammatory Disorders

Acute Pancreatitis

Acute pancreatitis is defined as acute, reversible inflammation involving the pancreas.[62] Clinically, patients with acute pancreatitis present with acute onset of abdominal or back pain, and elevated pancreatic enzymes.[63] Although acute pancreatitis is less common in pediatric patients than in adults, its incidence in children has increased considerably over the past few decades.[62,64] The reported incidence of acute pancreatitis in children ranges from 2 to 13 cases per 100,000 children, with a mortality rate of as high as 4%.[64]

The etiology of acute pancreatitis in children is often different than in adults. Whereas, in adults, most cases of pancreatitis are related to either cholelithiasis or alcohol abuse, acute trauma, congenital anomalies, and genetic factors are much more important in children. Hereditary pancreatitis has been linked to defects in the genes encoding for the pancreatic enzyme trypsin.[62] Other etiologies include medications, endocrine abnormalities, and autoimmune pancreatitis.[64]

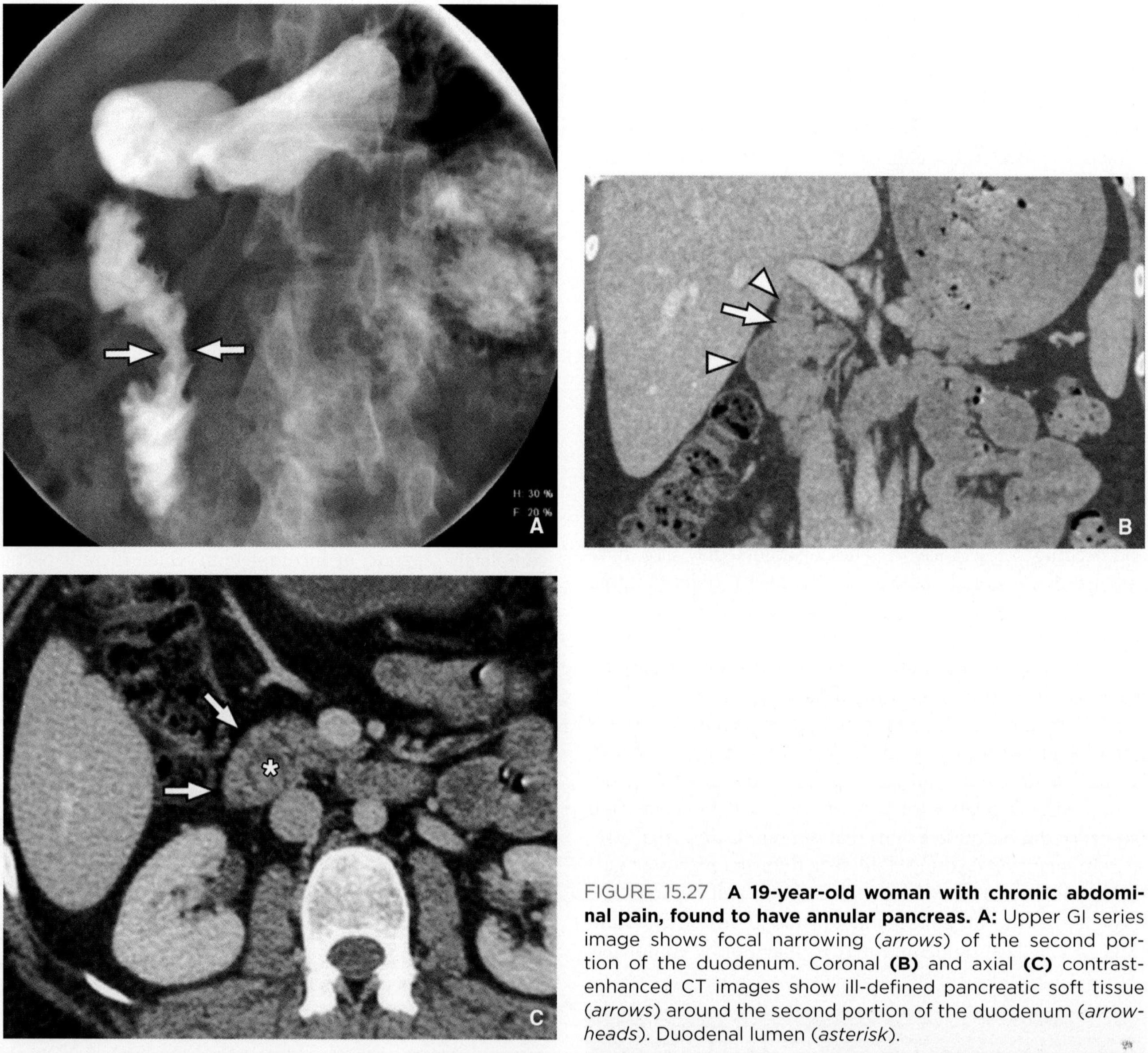

FIGURE 15.27 **A 19-year-old woman with chronic abdominal pain, found to have annular pancreas. A:** Upper GI series image shows focal narrowing (*arrows*) of the second portion of the duodenum. Coronal **(B)** and axial **(C)** contrast-enhanced CT images show ill-defined pancreatic soft tissue (*arrows*) around the second portion of the duodenum (*arrowheads*). Duodenal lumen (*asterisk*).

An important cause of acute pancreatitis in younger children that should not be overlooked is nonaccidental trauma, in which inflicted abdominal injuries lead to pancreatic duct damage and pancreatitis.[65]

Imaging generally is not required for the diagnosis of acute pancreatitis, as the clinical and laboratory findings are usually conclusive. Instead, imaging is usually reserved for evaluation of suspected associated complications or to investigate for an underlying anatomic cause for recurrent pancreatitis. In the setting of acute pancreatitis, ultrasound may demonstrate diffuse or focal pancreatic enlargement with variable echogenicity of the gland, ranging from hyperechoic to hypoechoic relative to the liver.[63] The main pancreatic duct may be dilated, measuring over 2.5 to 3 mm in diameter.[63] CT findings of acute pancreatitis in children are similar to those seen in adults, including diffuse or focal pancreatic enlargement and adjacent inflammatory stranding, edema, or fluid (Fig. 15.29). The pancreas may appear abnormally heterogeneous on postcontrast imaging, and absent parenchymal enhancement indicates pancreatic necrosis. MRI and MRCP are not usually performed in the acute setting. If MR is performed, the pancreas generally appears enlarged, hyperintense on T2-weighted sequences because of parenchymal edema, and demonstrates variable postcontrast enhancement depending on the presence of necrosis[63] (Fig. 15.30). Peripancreatic inflammatory stranding, edema, and fluid are also commonly present on T2-weighted images (Fig. 15.31). MRCP can be used to define pancreatic ductal anatomy and to exclude choledocholithiasis (and pancreatic ductal stones), ductal disruption, or pancreas divisum, all of which may be the inciting etiology.[63]

Chronic Pancreatitis

Chronic pancreatitis usually occurs in the setting of recurrent episodes of acute pancreatitis and results in irreversible damage to the pancreas with variable loss of both exocrine and endocrine function.[66] In children, the most common causes

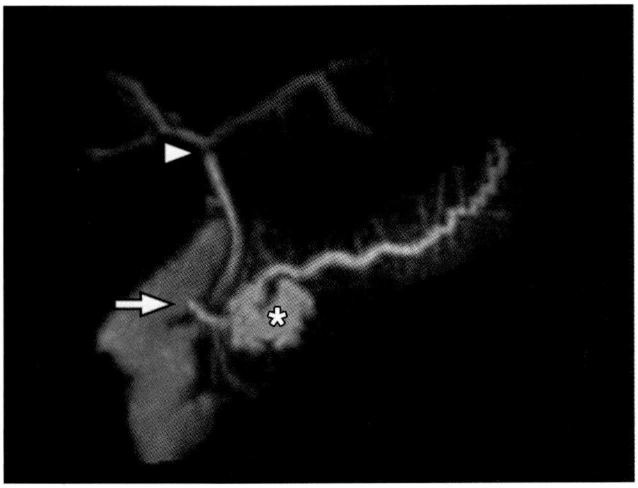

FIGURE 15.28 **Pancreas divisum in a 17-year-old girl with recurrent pancreatitis.** Coronal maximum intensity projection image from MRCP exam demonstrates the main pancreatic duct draining to the minor papilla (*arrow*), separate from the common bile duct. A small pseudocyst (*asterisk*) from prior pancreatitis is present. There is artifact (*arrowhead*) obscuring the proximal common hepatic duct due to an overlying vessel.

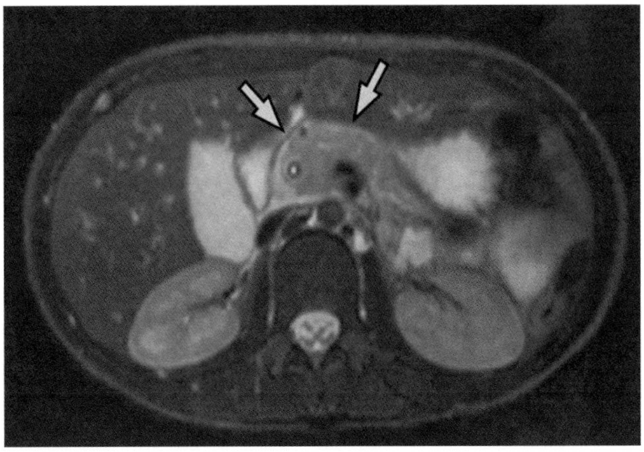

FIGURE 15.30 **Acute pancreatitis in a 15-year-old girl.** Axial T2W-weighted fat-saturated fast spin-echo MR image shows diffuse enlargement of the pancreas with parenchymal T2-weighted signal hyperintensity indicating parenchymal edema (*arrows*). Normally, the pancreas should be similar signal intensity as the liver on T2-weighted imaging.

of chronic pancreatitis are genetic, including hereditary pancreatitis and cystic fibrosis (CF), although many cases remain idiopathic.[66,67] Chronic pancreatitis in children is associated with significant morbidity, with many patients developing diabetes and other endocrine abnormalities, as well as needing digestive enzyme supplementation. Recurring abdominal pain is also a cause of significant morbidity. In severe cases, some patients require complete or subtotal pancreatectomy,

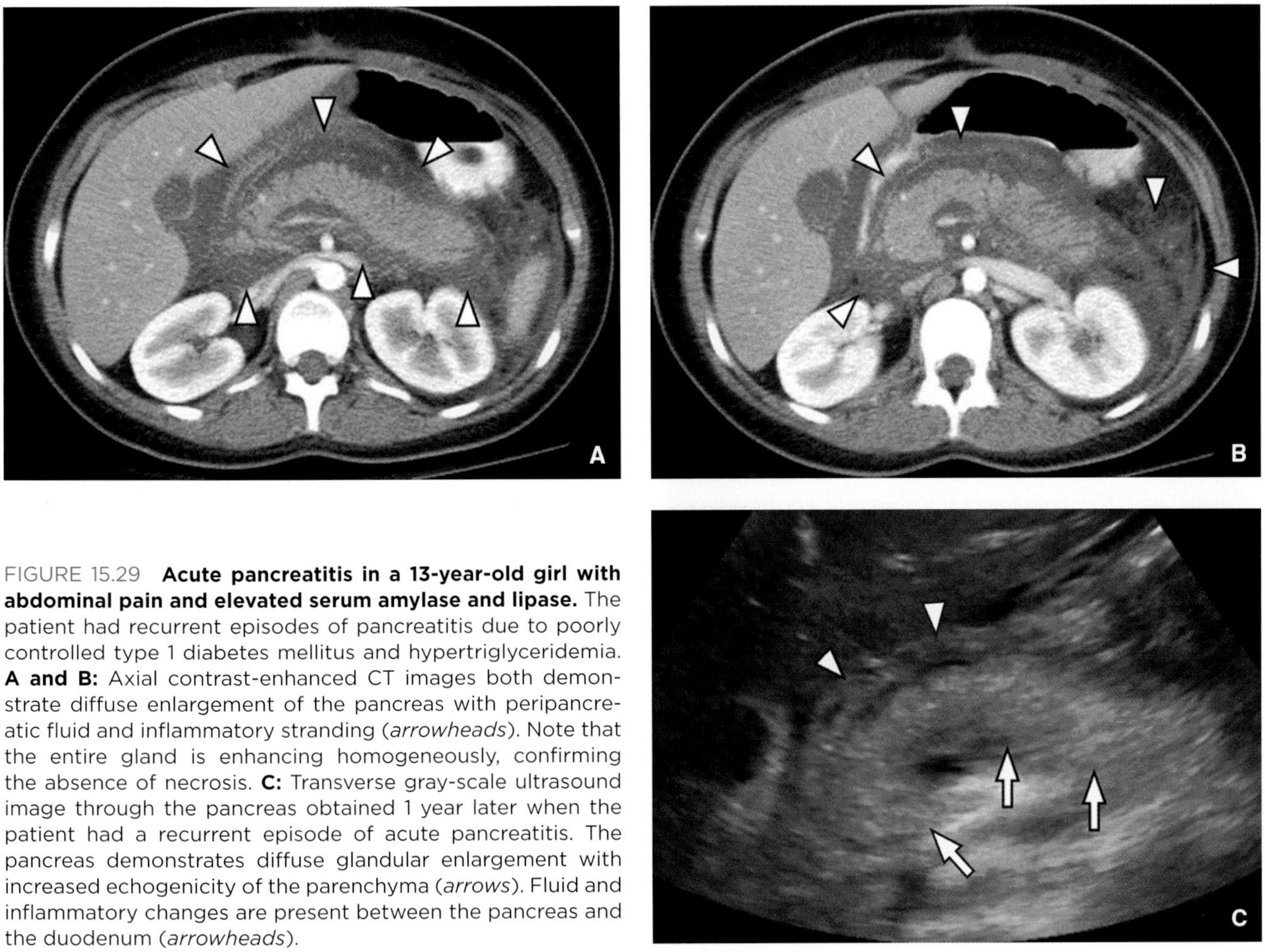

FIGURE 15.29 **Acute pancreatitis in a 13-year-old girl with abdominal pain and elevated serum amylase and lipase.** The patient had recurrent episodes of pancreatitis due to poorly controlled type 1 diabetes mellitus and hypertriglyceridemia. **A and B:** Axial contrast-enhanced CT images both demonstrate diffuse enlargement of the pancreas with peripancreatic fluid and inflammatory stranding (*arrowheads*). Note that the entire gland is enhancing homogeneously, confirming the absence of necrosis. **C:** Transverse gray-scale ultrasound image through the pancreas obtained 1 year later when the patient had a recurrent episode of acute pancreatitis. The pancreas demonstrates diffuse glandular enlargement with increased echogenicity of the parenchyma (*arrows*). Fluid and inflammatory changes are present between the pancreas and the duodenum (*arrowheads*).

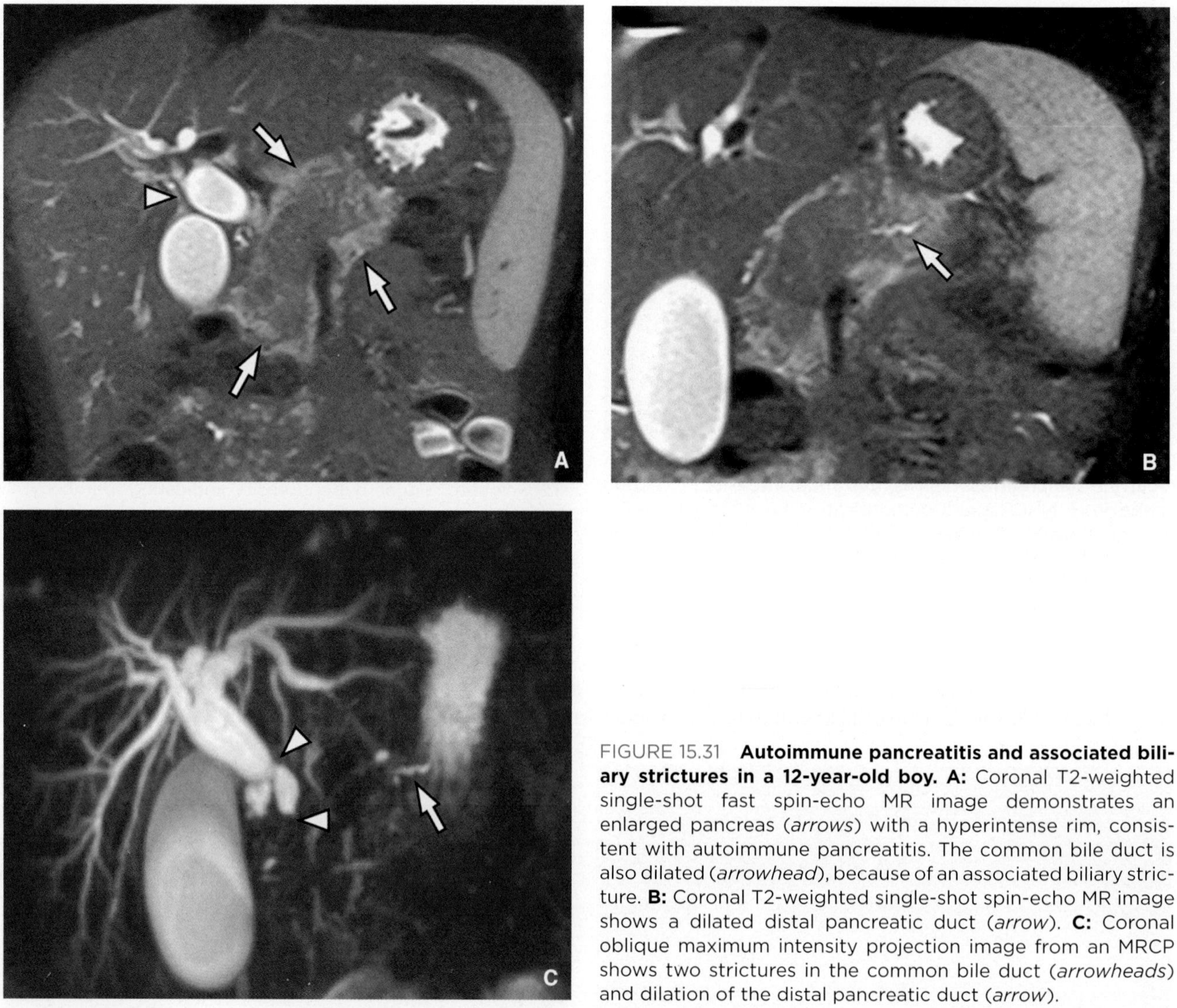

FIGURE 15.31 **Autoimmune pancreatitis and associated biliary strictures in a 12-year-old boy. A:** Coronal T2-weighted single-shot fast spin-echo MR image demonstrates an enlarged pancreas (*arrows*) with a hyperintense rim, consistent with autoimmune pancreatitis. The common bile duct is also dilated (*arrowhead*), because of an associated biliary stricture. **B:** Coronal T2-weighted single-shot spin-echo MR image shows a dilated distal pancreatic duct (*arrow*). **C:** Coronal oblique maximum intensity projection image from an MRCP shows two strictures in the common bile duct (*arrowheads*) and dilation of the distal pancreatic duct (*arrow*).

with or without allogenic pancreatic transplantation, for control of symptoms.[68]

Imaging features of chronic pancreatitis include atrophy of the pancreas, calcifications either within the gland or within the pancreatic duct, and pancreatic ductal dilation involving both the main pancreatic duct and side branches[63,67] (Fig. 15.32). Occasionally, calcifications may be visible on plain radiographs. Ultrasound, CT, and MRI all excellently depict the imaging findings of chronic pancreatitis, although visualization of calcifications may be limited on MRI.[63] MRCP allows noninvasive evaluation of the pancreatic ductal system and is of value in idiopathic chronic pancreatitis, permitting evaluation for filling defects (e.g., pancreatic duct stones), strictures, and ductal anatomic variants[67] (Fig. 15.33).

Complications of Pancreatitis

Complications of pancreatitis are relatively rare in children, occurring in about 5% of pediatric patients with pancreatitis.[69] Both acute and delayed complications have been described. Common complications include pseudocyst formation, pancreatic necrosis, hemorrhage, vascular abnormalities, and pancreatic endocrine and exocrine dysfunction (Figs. 15.34 and 15.35).

Pancreatic pseudocysts are relatively uncommon in children, but do occur in the setting of severe acute pancreatitis or pancreatic trauma. A pseudocyst is defined as a fluid collection without a true epithelial lining. Pseudocysts occur in the setting of acute pancreatitis as a result of injury to the pancreatic parenchyma or to the pancreatic duct itself.[69] At ultrasound, pseudocysts appear as well-defined hypoechoic or anechoic cystic lesions of varying size. Pseudocysts may be unilocular, or they may contain multiple septations.[52] On CT, pseudocysts appear as well-defined low attenuation structures; septations may be difficult to visualize on CT. At MRI, pseudocysts are usually hypointense on T1-weighted images and hyperintense on T2-weighted images, although the signal characteristics may vary depending on the complexity of the fluid. Septations are readily seen with MRI.

The treatment of pseudocysts varies with their size and location. In general, treatment consists of drainage, either

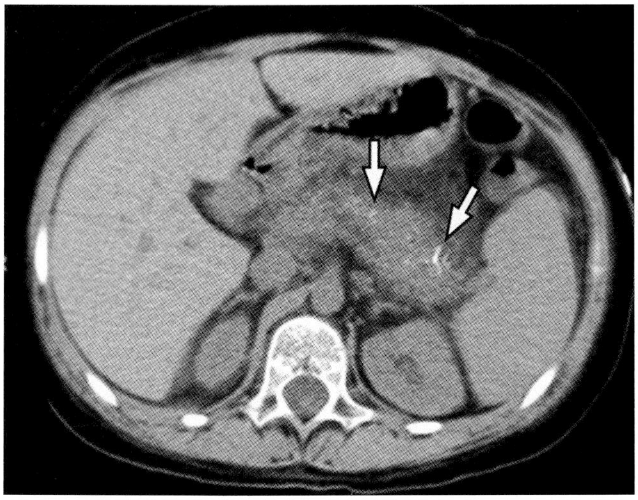

FIGURE 15.32 **Chronic pancreatitis in an 8-year-old girl with mitochondrial disorder and severe developmental delay.** Axial noncontrast CT image demonstrates scattered pancreatic parenchymal calcifications (*arrows*) due to chronic pancreatitis. The pancreatic body and tail are also enlarged with adjacent fat stranding due to superimposed acute pancreatitis.

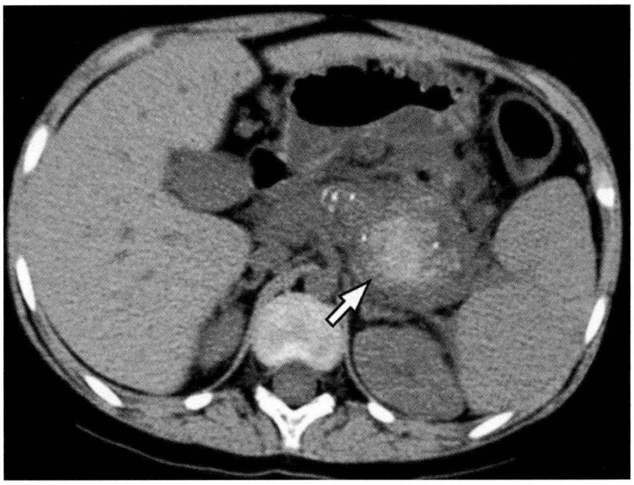

FIGURE 15.34 **A 10-year-old boy with acute hemorrhagic pancreatitis in the setting of chronic pancreatitis related to cytochrome c oxidase deficiency.** Axial noncontrast CT image demonstrates enlargement of the pancreatic body and tail with scattered parenchymal calcifications. Focal high attenuation (*arrow*) in the pancreatic body and tail is due to hemorrhage.

surgical, endoscopic, or percutaneous. Some lesions may be amenable to a cystogastrostomy, in which the pseudocyst is connected to the stomach in order to allow drainage and prevent reaccumulation.

Pancreatic necrosis can occur in patients with severe acute pancreatitis, and can be focal or diffuse. Pancreatic necrosis is rare in children, occurring in an estimated 1% of cases of acute pancreatitis.[70] At imaging, pancreatic necrosis manifests as areas of nonenhancement of the gland on postcontrast CT or MRI. Pancreatic necrosis is associated with a worse prognosis and higher rate of major complications, such as pseudocyst formation and pancreatic dysfunction.[70,71]

Vascular complications also can occur in the setting of acute pancreatitis and include vascular thrombosis, pseudoaneurysm formation, and hemorrhage.[72] The most commonly affected vascular structures include the splenic artery and vein, given their close proximity to the pancreas.[72] The pancreaticoduodenal artery and its pancreatic branches are also susceptible to injury from contact with pancreatic exocrine enzymes. At imaging, vascular thrombosis manifests as lack of blood flow on Doppler ultrasound, as well as lack of enhancement on postcontrast CT and MRI. Hemorrhage and pseudoaneurysm formation occur as the result of injury to the vessel wall by pancreatic enzymes. Pancreatitis-related pseuodaneurysms appear as anechoic or hypoechoic cystic structures adjacent to the

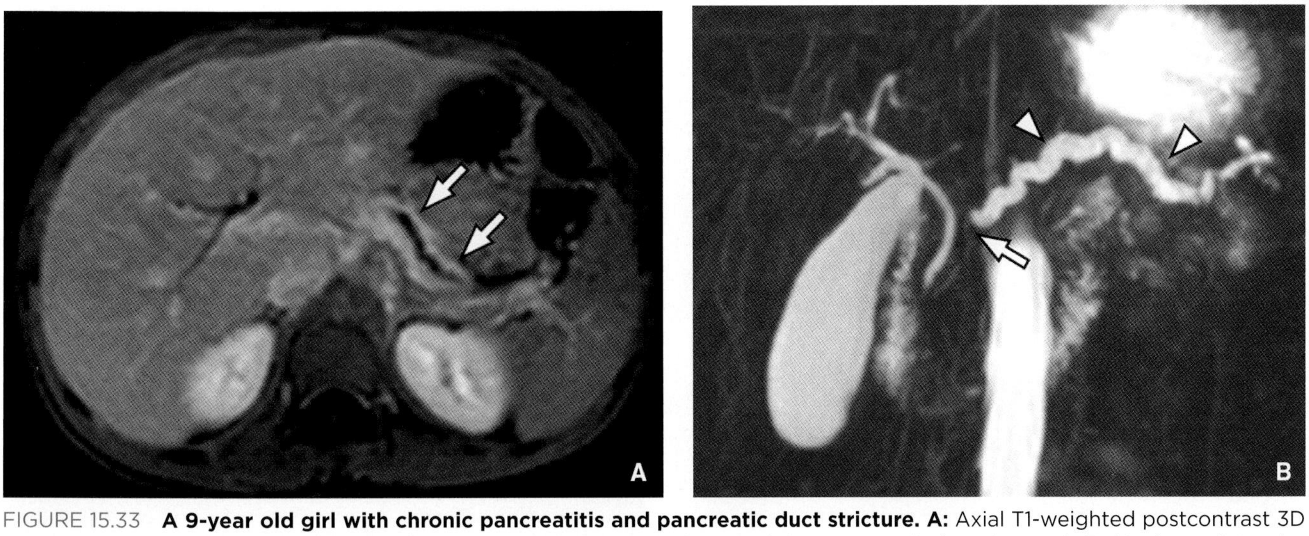

FIGURE 15.33 **A 9-year old girl with chronic pancreatitis and pancreatic duct stricture. A:** Axial T1-weighted postcontrast 3D SPGR image shows atrophy of the pancreatic parenchyma and dilation of the pancreatic duct (*arrows*). **B:** Maximum intensity projection image from and MRCP shows a dilated pancreatic duct (*arrowheads*) with abrupt change in caliber at the level of a pancreatic duct stricture (*arrow*).

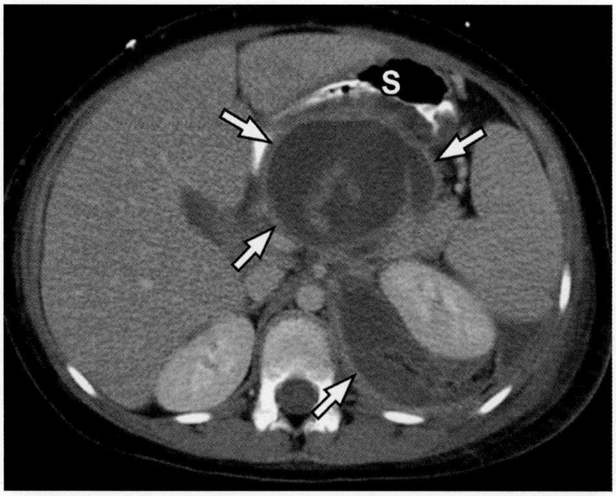

FIGURE 15.35 **A 12-year-old girl with prolonged acute pancreatitis and pseudocyst formation.** Axial contrast-enhanced CT image shows multiple peripancreatic fluid collections (*arrows*). A fluid collection in the lesser sac displaces the stomach (*S*) anteriorly, while a left perirenal collection displaces the left kidney anteriorly.

pancreas with internal blood flow on color Doppler ultrasound. Postcontrast CT and MR imaging should demonstrate focal aneurysmal dilatation of the affected vessel or a contrast-filled outpouching arising from the affected vessel wall.

Neoplastic Disorders (Table 15.2)

Benign Neoplasms

Solid Pseudopapillary Neoplasm

Solid pseudopapillary neoplasm (SPN), also called solid and papillary epithelial neoplasm (SPEN), is a primary pancreatic tumor of low malignant potential.[73] Although uncommon, recent studies have shown that SPN may be the most common primary pancreatic tumor in children.[74,75] This tumor is most frequently encountered in adolescent and young adult females.[52]

TABLE 15.2 Pancreatic Neoplasms in Children

Benign
Solid pseudopapillary neoplasm (SPN)
Pancreatic cystic neoplasms
Malignant
Pancreatoblastoma
Adenocarcinoma
Neuroendocrine tumors
Lymphoma
Leukemia
Metastases

Affected pediatric patients often present with nonspecific abdominal complaints and normal laboratory findings.[76] Although classically described in pancreatic head, SPN can be located anywhere within the pancreas.[77] Metastatic disease to the liver has been reported but is rare.[77] Surgical resection is the treatment of choice, when anatomically feasible.

Certain imaging features are highly suggestive of SPN. First, the finding of a solitary solid pancreatic mass in a young female patient makes SPN the most likely diagnosis, no matter what the imaging appearance. The most common imaging appearance of this tumor is that of a relatively large, well-circumscribed pancreatic mass. At ultrasound, the tumor is typically solid but may have both solid and cystic components.[74] The mass is usually surrounded by a pseudocapsule, which may be visible with ultrasound, CT, or MRI.[76,77] At CT, the lesion is typically low in attenuation, although internal heterogeneity often occurs secondary to internal hemorrhage (Fig. 15.36). Calcifications may be present in up to 30% of these tumors.[76] At MRI, the mass is typically heterogeneously hypo- to isointense on T1-weighted images and hyperintense on T2-weighted images.[77] The pseudocapsule may show early and more intense enhancement than the rest of the tumor after intravenous gadolinium-based contrast material administration.[77] Pathologic examination shows solid and pseudopapillary

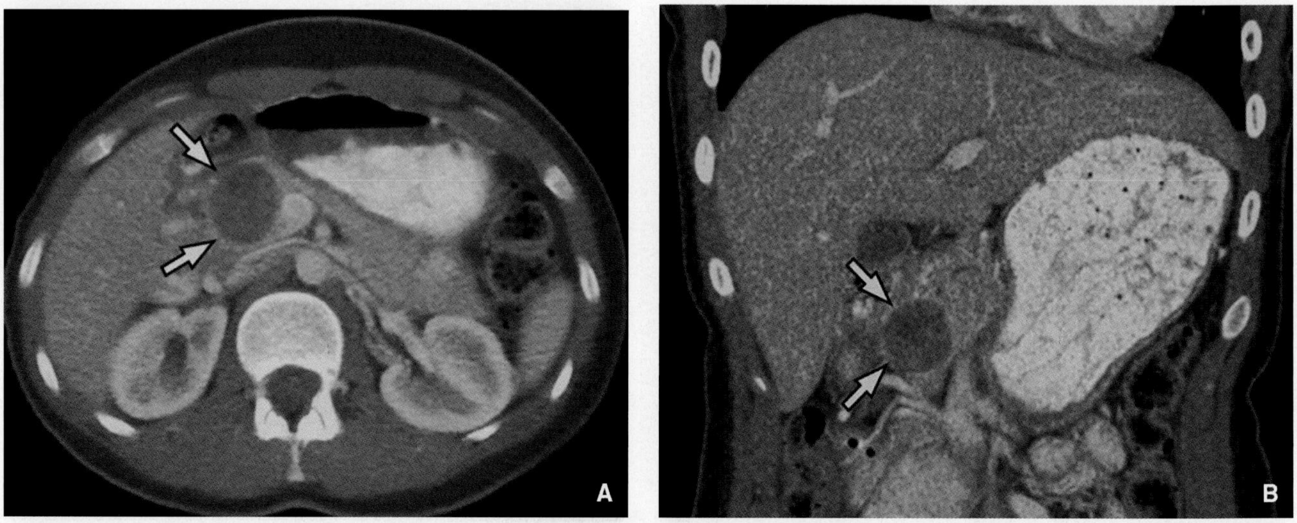

FIGURE 15.36 **Solid pseudopapillary neoplasm of the pancreas in a 16-year-old girl who presented with abdominal pain.** Axial **(A)** and coronal contrast-enhanced CT **(B)** images show a well-defined, slightly heterogeneous, predominantly low-attenuation mass (*arrows*) in the head of the pancreas. Note the absence of intrahepatic biliary dilation.

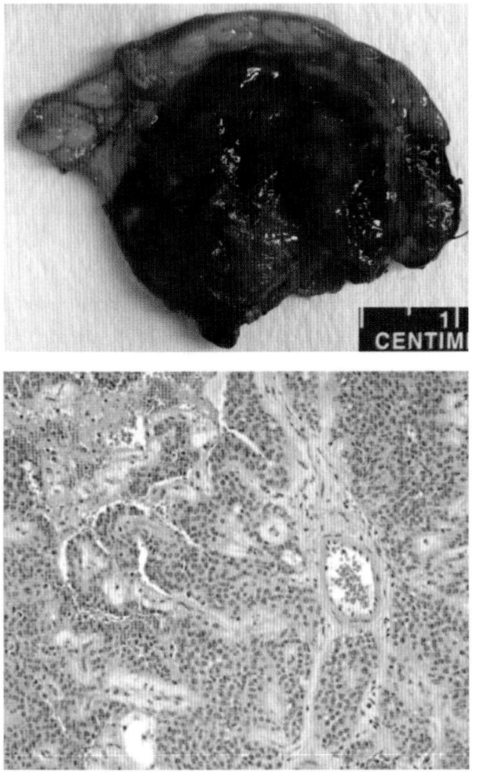

FIGURE 15.37 **A 4 cm solid pseudopapillary neoplasm from the body of the pancreas in a 10-year-old girl shows a rim of yellow lobulated pancreatic tissue partially surrounding the reddish predominantly solid tumor (top).** Microscopically, monotonous round cells line pseudopapillary structures. Here, the structures radiate around a central fibrovascular core in a rosette-like pattern (**bottom**, hematoxylin and eosin, original magnification, 200x).

structures lined by monomorphic round to ovoid cells with pink cytoplasm (Fig. 15.37). Immunohistochemical staining usually reveals expression of alpha-1-antitrypsin, and there is variable expression of epithelial and/or neuroendocrine markers. Mutations in the gene for beta-catenin (exon 3) are seen in the large majority of SPN.[73]

Serous and Mucinous Cystic Pancreatic Neoplasms

Cystic tumors of the pancreas are exceedingly rare in children and include serous cystadenoma and mucinous cystic neoplasm.[78] Serous cystadenoma is benign and appears at imaging as a small lesion, usually <2 cm in size, with multiple tiny cystic spaces.[78] Mucinous cystic neoplasm, on the other hand, represents a spectrum from benign to malignant. These tumors usually present on imaging as larger tumors containing multilocular or unilocular fluid attenuation cystic spaces.[78]

Malignant Neoplasms

Pancreatoblastoma

Pancreatoblastoma is a rare neoplasm in children, but is the most common primary pancreatic malignant tumor in children during the first decade of life, with a mean age at presentation of about 4.5 years.[79,80] There is a slight male predominance, as well as an association with Beckwith-Wiedemann syndrome.[52,79,80] The most common clinical presentation is a palpable abdominal mass, although some patients present with vague abdominal complaints.[80] Serum alpha-fetoprotein (AFP) level may be elevated.[79] Pancreatoblastomas tend to be large and advanced in stage at diagnosis.[79] The head and the tail of the pancreas are affected in equal proportion. Histologically, pancreatoblastoma has primitive cells with a variably organoid appearance, as they may show areas of differentiation toward primitive acinar cells, squamous nests, endocrine cells, ductal structures, and cellular stroma, somewhat resembling the pancreas of a developing embryo (Fig. 15.38). The treatment of pancreatoblastoma commonly involves both surgical resection and chemotherapy. Prognosis is dependent on the stage of disease at presentation and resectability. In a large European series, 5-year event-free survival for stage 1 disease was 75%, whereas, for stage 3 and 4 disease, 5-year event-free survival dropped to about 53%.[79]

The typical imaging appearance of pancreatoblastoma is that of a large, lobulated mass usually replacing either all or a portion of the pancreas, although the tumor can also grow exophytically from the pancreas[52] (Fig. 15.39). The tumor may cause dilation of the main pancreatic duct.[52] Calcifications are frequently present. The typical ultrasound appearance is that of a heterogenous mass with areas of hypoechogenicity

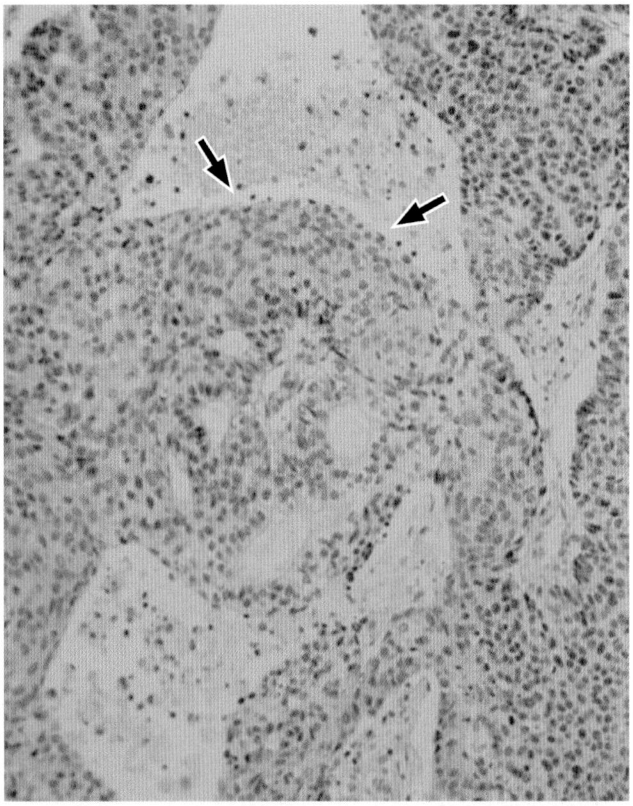

FIGURE 15.38 **Pancreatoblastoma from a 6-month-old girl.** Primitive tumor cells show solid and acinar growth patterns, frequently accompanied by squamous metaplasia (*arrows*) (hematoxylin and eosin, original magnification, 200x).

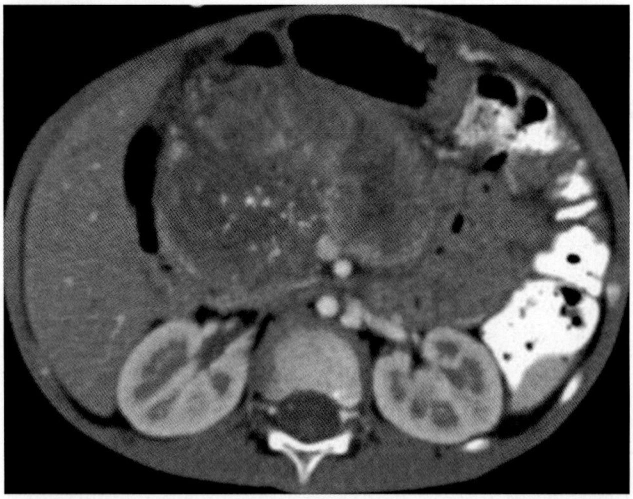

FIGURE 15.39 **Pancreatoblastoma in a 2-year-old boy.** Axial contrast-enhanced CT image demonstrates a large, heterogeneous mass with scattered calcifications replacing the pancreas. (Courtesy of Sudha Anupindi, MD, Children's Hospital of Philadelphia, Philadelphia, PA.)

centrally.[52,80] At CT and MRI, the mass typically enhances mildly and has a lobulated appearance with central areas of decreased enhancement corresponding to necrosis.[80] The mass is typically predominantly high in signal on T2-weighted images and low to intermediate in signal on T1-weighted images.[52,80] There usually is mass effect on adjacent structures due to the size of the tumor. Adjacent lymph nodes may be enlarged, reflecting spread of the tumor.[52] The most common sites of distant metastatic disease include the liver and lungs.[79]

Adenocarcinoma

Pancreatic adenocarcinoma arises from the pancreatic ducts or acini and is very rare in children.[52] When these tumors do occur in children, the most commonly affected age groups are adolescents and young adults.[81] Patients typically present with abdominal pain and anorexia and may have obstructive jaundice. The tumor is most commonly located in the pancreatic head and typically appears as a small hypoenhancing mass on CT and MRI.[52] Ultrasound may show a focal hypoechoic mass with associated dilated biliary and pancreatic ductal dilation.[52] Treatment is generally with surgical resection, if feasible. The prognosis is very poor, with 5-year survival rates under 5%.[80]

Neuroendocrine Tumors

Islet cell tumors, or neuroendocrine tumors, arise from the endocrine cells of the pancreas.[80] These tumors are rare in children but account for about 20% of malignant pancreatic tumors in pediatric patients.[52] There is an association between these tumors and von Hippel–Lindau disease, tuberous sclerosis, and multiple endocrine neoplasia type 1 (MEN-1).[80] Neuroendocrine tumors can be classified as functional or nonfunctional, depending on their ability to secrete hormones.[52,78] Functional tumors often present with clinical symptoms related to hormone overproduction. The two most common types of functional neuroendocrine tumors in children are the insulinoma and gastrinoma.[80]

Functional neuroendocrine tumors tend to present at an earlier stage because of clinical symptoms related to hormonal activity, and therefore the tumors are usually smaller at presentation. Histologically, tumor cells are generally round and uniform; their arrangement may take on a variety of architectural patterns (Fig. 15.40). The tumors are considered malignant only if they show invasion of adjacent organs or metastasis to regional lymph nodes or other sites.

The typical imaging appearance is that of a small (<3 cm) well-circumscribed pancreatic mass.[78] Nonfunctional tumors tend to have delayed presentation due to the lack of hormonal symptoms and may be larger at presentation.[80] Most insulinomas are located in the body or tail of the pancreas, whereas gastrinomas and nonfunctional tumors tend to be located in the pancreatic head.[80] With ultrasound, the tumors are typically hypoechoic.[52] CT or MRI are frequently performed and commonly demonstrate a small hyperenhancing mass (Fig. 15.41). With MRI, the tumor is usually low in signal on T1-weighted images and homogenously high in signal on T2-weighted images.[52] Hyperenhancement on arterial phase images may aid in the detection of these tumors, and therefore MRI is preferable to CT because of the capability of performing multi-phase dynamic postcontrast imaging. Metastatic disease may be identified in the liver and adjacent peripancreatic lymph nodes. Nuclear medicine also may play a role in diagnosis, with hormonally active tumors demonstrating increased uptake of the somatostatin receptor scintigraphy using radio-labeled octreotide[82] (Fig. 15.42).

Lymphoma and Leukemia

Most commonly, lymphoma involves the peripancreatic lymph nodes with direct extension into the pancreas or

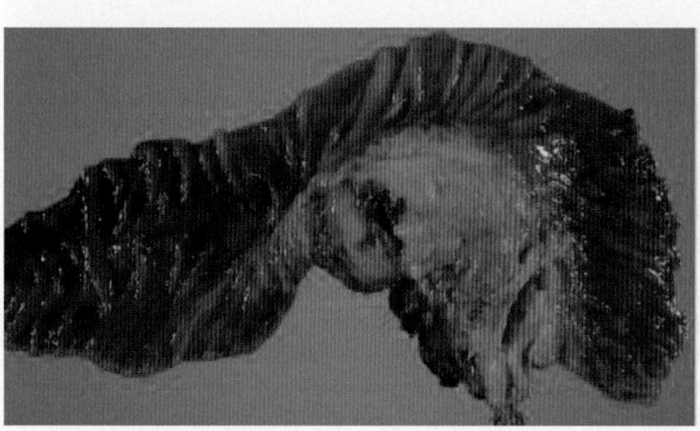

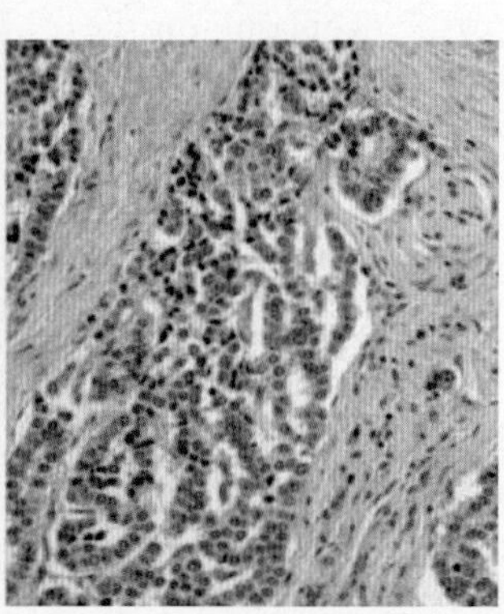

FIGURE 15.40 Pancreatic neuroendocrine neoplasm, infiltrating the wall of the duodenum **(left)**, in a 17-year-old girl who presented with pancreatitis. Microscopically, nests of round regular cells resembling islet cells here show a tubuloacinar architecture (**right**, hematoxylin and eosin, original magnification, 400x). In this patient, metastasis to a lymph node (not shown) confirmed malignancy.

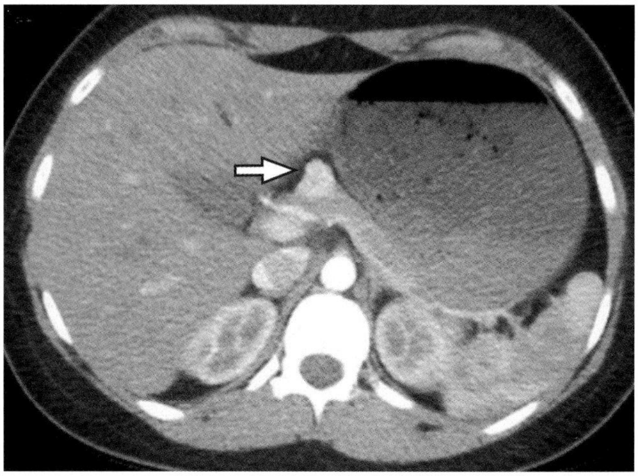

FIGURE 15.41 **Insulinoma in a 16-year-old girl with hypoglycemia.** Axial contrast-enhanced CT image shows a round, hyperenhancing pancreatic mass (*arrow*).

distortion of the pancreatic parenchyma, all in the setting of widespread abdominal disease.[80] Rarely non-Hodgkin lymphoma may arise primarily within the pancreas. Large cell lymphoma and sporadic Burkitt lymphoma are the two most common subtypes to involve the pancreas.[80] Typical imaging features include multiple homogeneous pancreatic masses that are usually hypoechoic on ultrasound and demonstrate hypoenhancement relative to the pancreatic parenchyma with contrast-enhanced CT and MRI.[83] Adjacent peripancreatic lymph nodes are often enlarged. Rarely, leukemia may present with similar findings of multiple pancreatic masses or diffuse infiltration of the pancreatic parenchyma (Fig. 15.43).

Metastases

Metastatic disease to the pancreas occurs in the setting of aggressive neoplasms, such as rhabdomyosarcoma, or in the setting of advanced disease with widespread metastatic disease elsewhere in the abdomen. Pancreatic involvement can occur because of direct extension of a large intra-abdominal tumor, such as neuroblastoma, or by hematogenous metastatic spread.[84] In general, metastatic disease manifests at imaging as multiple hypoechoic masses on ultrasound, or as multiple hypoenhancing masses on postcontrast CT or MRI (Fig. 15.44).

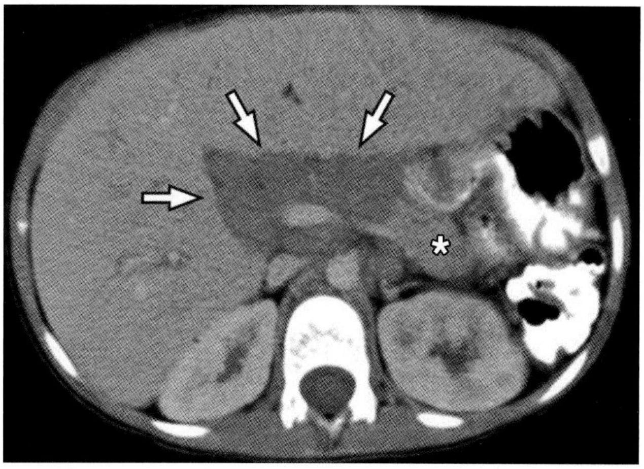

FIGURE 15.43 **Leukemia involving the pancreas in a 6-year-old boy with juvenile myelomonocytic leukemia.** Axial contrast-enhanced CT image shows lobulated, low-attenuation masses (*arrows*) replacing the head and neck of the pancreas. Portions of the pancreatic body and tail (*asterisk*) were normal.

Syndromes Affecting the Pancreas

Cystic Fibrosis

Pancreatic insufficiency is extremely common in CF, occurring in 85% to 90% of patients by 1 year of age.[85] Abnormal pancreatic function is a significant cause of morbidity in these patients, resulting in malabsorbtion, nutritional deficiencies,

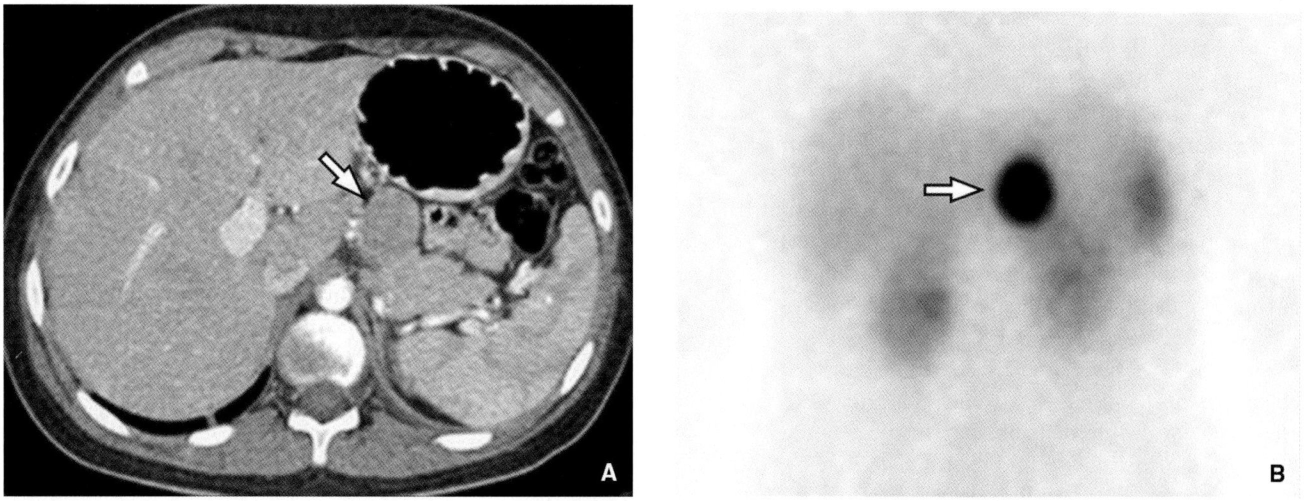

FIGURE 15.42 **Pancreatic neuroendocrine tumor in a 14-year-old boy with recurrent, severe gastritis and a markedly elevated serum gastrin level. A:** Axial contrast-enhanced CT image demonstrates a round, heterogeneously enhancing mass (*arrow*) in the pancreatic body. **B:** Planar image from an ^{111}In-octreotide scan shows focal uptake within the mass (*arrow*). The mass was histologically proven to be a gastrinoma at surgical resection. (Courtesy of William H. McAlister, MD, St. Louis Children's Hospital, St. Louis, MO.)

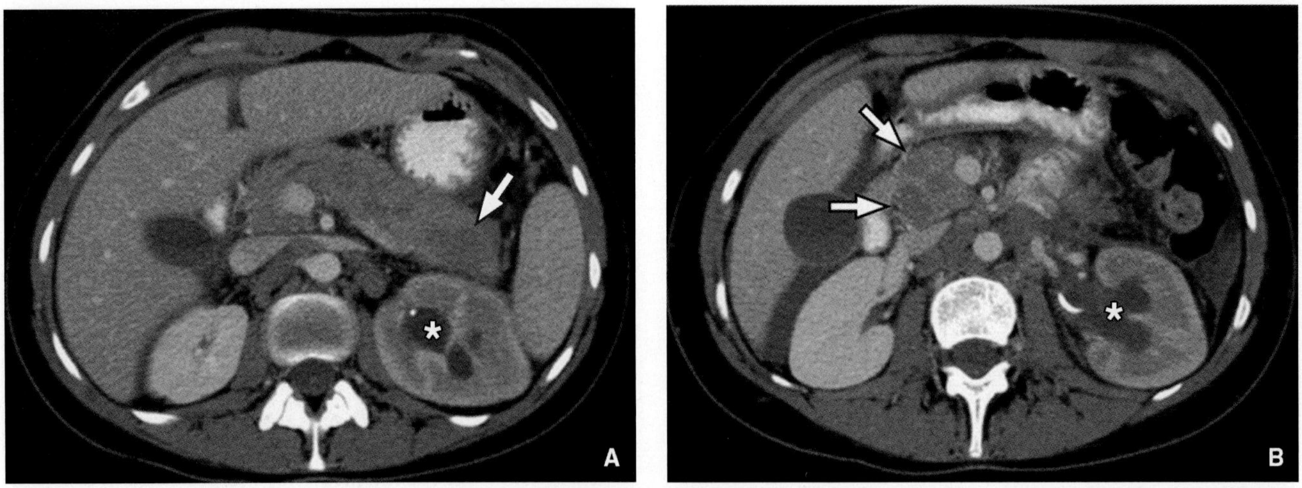

FIGURE 15.44 **Pancreatic metastasis in a 17-year-old girl with advanced metastatic alveolar rhabdomyosarcoma. A and B:** Axial contrast-enhanced CT images demonstrate diffuse enlargement of the pancreas with multiple low-attenuation masses (*arrows*) within the pancreas consistent with metastases. The left kidney is obstructed (*asterisk*) and required a ureteral stent because of a large retroperitoneal metastatic deposit (not shown).

and poor growth.[86] In these patients, pancreatic exocrine dysfunction is the result of abnormal epithelial chloride ion transporters, which in turn result in thickened, inspissated pancreatic secretions that ultimately lead to pancreatic ductal obstruction and subsequent irreversible pancreatic parenchymal damage.[87] A significant minority of affected patients eventually develop endocrine dysfunction as well because of progressive pancreatic fibrosis, atrophy, and replacement by adipose tissue.[87]

Plain radiographs in patients with CF-related pancreatic dysfunction are usually unrevealing, other than showing other manifestations of CF, such as lung and bowel-related abnormalities. Occasionally, patients may have pancreatic parenchymal calcifications visible on radiographs.[87] Findings on cross-sectional imaging, including ultrasound, CT, and MRI, are generally secondary to fatty replacement and fibrosis of the pancreatic parenchyma.[86] On ultrasound, the pancreas may be small and diffusely echogenic, appearing similar in echogenicity to the adjacent retroperitoneal fat.[87] Similarly, CT and MRI may demonstrate diffuse fatty replacement and atrophy of the pancreas, which occasionally may be indistinguishable from the adjacent retroperitoneal fat. Pancreatic cysts may also be seen, thought to be secondary to dilation of the smaller duct branches secondary to obstruction.[86] Pancreatic cystosis is a rare manifestation that occurs when the pancreatic parenchyma is replaced by innumerable 1- to 3-mm cysts.[86]

Shwachman-Diamond Syndrome

Shwachman-Diamond syndrome was first described in 1964 as a syndrome of pancreatic insufficiency and hematologic abnormalities secondary to bone marrow dysfunction.[88] Patients present clinically with pancreatic exocrine dysfunction, anemia, thrombocytopenia, and a variety of skeletal, cardiac, hepatic, and immunologic manifestations. The condition is inherited in an autosomal recessive pattern. Pancreatic exocrine dysfunction occurs as a result of absent acinar cells.[89] On imaging, the pancreas will demonstrate varying degrees of fatty replacement[90] (Fig. 15.45). In the most severely affected individuals, the pancreas is completely replaced with fat and indistinguishable from adjacent retroperitoneal fat.

von Hippel–Lindau Disease

von Hippel–Lindau (VHL) disease is a genetic multisystem cancer syndrome that occurs secondary to abnormalities of the VHL tumor suppressor gene.[91] Affected patients present

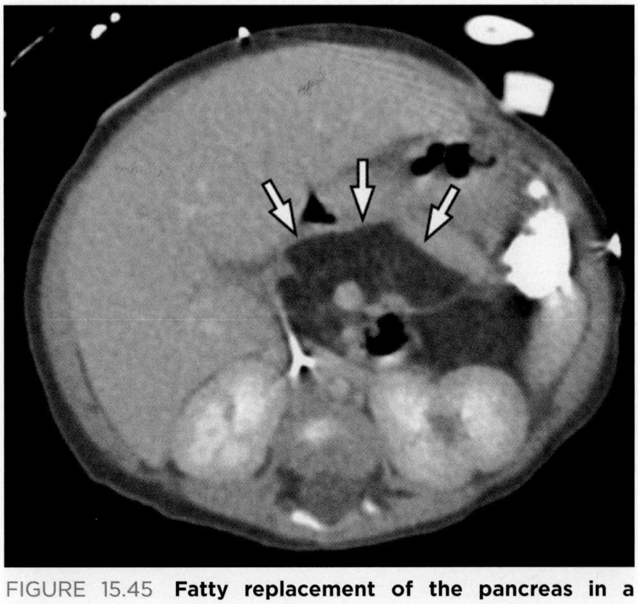

FIGURE 15.45 **Fatty replacement of the pancreas in a 1-year-old boy with Shwachman-Diamond syndrome.** Axial contrast-enhanced CT image reveals only minimal soft tissue remaining in the pancreatic bed, with the majority of the gland being completely replaced by fat (*arrows*).

with multiple cysts, benign tumors, and malignant neoplasms involving the central nervous system and abdominal viscera.[91] Patients with VHL disease manifest a variety of pancreatic abnormalities, the most common being benign pancreatic cysts and serous cystadenomas[92,93] (Fig. 15.46). Malignant lesions also can occur, including neuroendocrine tumors and adenocarcinoma.[92]

Hemochromatosis

In patients with iron overload due to primary hemochromatosis, excess iron can manifest as pancreatic signal abnormality on MRI, especially on gradient-recalled echo sequences with increasing echo times, due to susceptibility artifact. Neonatal hemochromatosis, which presents in the perinatal period with severe liver disease and secondary iron deposition, is thought to be a result of gestational alloimmune liver disease, a cause of in utero hepatic failure.[94] In these patients, MRI reveals iron deposition in pattern similar to primary hemochromatosis, including the liver and pancreas. The pancreas is diffusely low in signal on gradient-recalled echo and T2-weighted sequences. Pancreas also demonstrates progressive greater than expected signal loss with increasing echo time.[95] Neonatal hemochromatosis is usually fatal unless there is prompt treatment with chelation therapy, high-dose intravenous immunoglobulin therapy, and, in some cases, liver transplantation.[94]

Traumatic Disorders

Although injury to the pancreas in blunt abdominal trauma is relatively rare, the pancreas is still the 4th most commonly injured abdominal solid organ behind the spleen, liver and kidneys.[96] In one large series, pancreatic injury was present in 2% of patients treated for acute traumatic injury.[96] Others have reported the incidence to be between 0.3% and 0.7% of all pediatric trauma admissions.[97] Typical mechanisms of injury include focal blunt force trauma to the epigastrium that compresses the pancreas between the abdominal wall and the lumbar vertebra.[97] An example of this type of injury is a so-called handlebar injury when a child falls forward with the mid-to-upper abdomen striking the handlebars of a bicycle. Another important mechanism of pancreatic injury is blunt force trauma to the abdomen in the setting of nonaccidental trauma (child abuse). It is estimated that a substantial percentage of all posttraumatic pancreatitis cases in young children are secondary to child abuse.[65]

Imaging of abdominal trauma in the acute setting is most commonly performed with contrast-enhanced CT. Ultrasound may also be performed in selected settings. MRI, and specifically MRCP, is commonly performed to evaluate for complications of pancreatic injury, such as ductal disruption. Traumatic pancreatic injuries range from contusions to lacerations to complete pancreatic transection. A grading system has been developed by the AAST, which is based on the size of any pancreatic contusion or laceration, as well as involvement of the pancreatic duct and the ampulla.[98] At CT, posttraumatic pancreatic contusion usually presents as focal or diffuse glandular enlargement, parenchymal edema, and peripancreatic edema/fluid, whereas pancreatic lacerations manifest as low-attenuation, linear clefts within the enhancing pancreatic parenchyma. Transection occurs when there is complete disruption of the pancreatic parenchyma with associated disruption of the main pancreatic duct (Fig. 15.47). Peripancreatic fluid collections are common in the setting of acute trauma.[99] Pancreatic trauma is also associated with injuries to other abdominal viscera[99] (Fig. 15.48).

Assessment of the integrity of the main pancreatic duct is important for management and prognosis in patients with pancreatic trauma. Disruption of the duct can lead to a variety of complications, including acute and chronic pancreatitis, pseudocyst formation, and pancreatic dysfunction. The pancreatic duct can be evaluated noninvasively using MRCP.

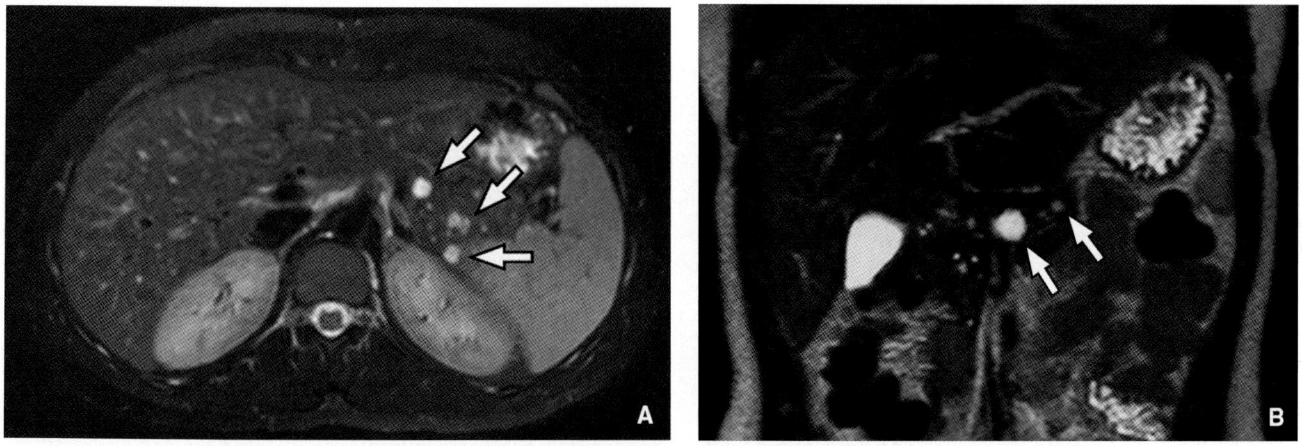

FIGURE 15.46 **Pancreatic cysts in a 12-year-old girl with von Hippel-Lindau disease.** Axial T2-weighted fat-saturated **(A)** and coronal T2-weighted fast spin-echo **(B)** MR images demonstrate multiple small hyperintense cystic lesions (*arrows*) throughout the pancreas.

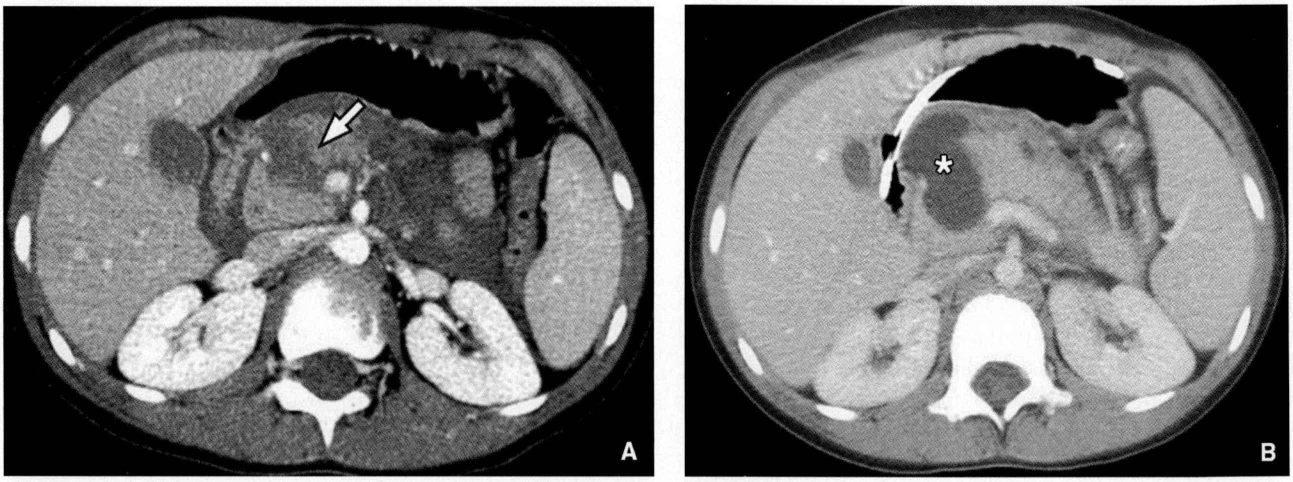

FIGURE 15.47 **Pancreatic trauma in an 8-year-old boy after a bicycle accident. A:** Axial contrast-enhanced CT image demonstrates a low-attenuation cleft (*arrow*) in the pancreatic neck consistent with a pancreatic transection. Adjacent free fluid and inflammatory stranding are also present. **B:** Axial contrast-enhanced CT obtained 1 week after the injury demonstrates a pancreatic fluid collection (*asterisk*) at the site of the prior pancreatic injury due to main pancreatic duct disruption.

Disruption of the duct can be visualized at MRCP as discontinuity of the duct at the site of the pancreatic injury. In more chronic cases, pancreatic parenchyma distal to the injury may appear atrophied. Increasingly, suspected pancreatic duct injury is being evaluated using ERCP, which allows direct assessment of the integrity of the duct as well as the potential for intervention, such as pancreatic duct stent placement.[96,97]

Management of pancreatic trauma is usually conservative, with interventions reserved for treatment of complications related to trauma. Emergent surgery may be indicated in the setting of shock or in the treatment of known pancreatic duct injury or other intra-abdominal injuries.[100] Percutaneous or surgical drainage of fluid collections may be required in the setting of posttraumatic pseudocyst formation.

ADRENAL GLANDS

Imaging Techniques

Radiography

As with the spleen and pancreas, radiography is generally not performed in the evaluation of the adrenal glands. Adrenal calcifications may be detected in patients with prior adrenal hemorrhage or infection, in certain adrenal tumors, and in rare systemic processes, such as Wolman disease.

Ultrasound

In the neonate, ultrasound is useful for evaluating the adrenal glands because of their relatively large size, and the excellent spatial resolution of ultrasound when using a linear,

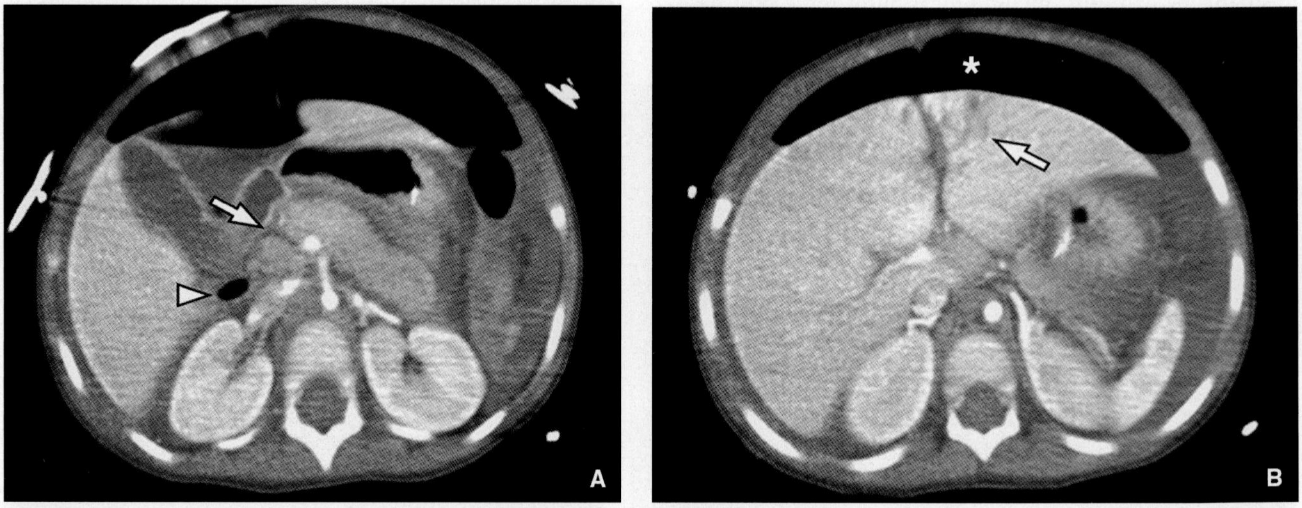

FIGURE 15.48 **Pancreatic, duodenal, and liver injuries due to nonaccidental trauma in an 18-month-old boy. A:** Axial contrast-enhanced CT image demonstrates a low-attenuation cleft (*arrow*) through the pancreas consistent with pancreatic transection. A small amount of extraluminal retroperitoneal gas (*arrowhead*) is present because of a focal traumatic duodenal perforation. **B:** Axial contrast-enhanced CT image demonstrates a laceration (*arrow*) in the left lobe of the liver. Free intraperitoneal air (*asterisk*) is present from an associated bowel injury.

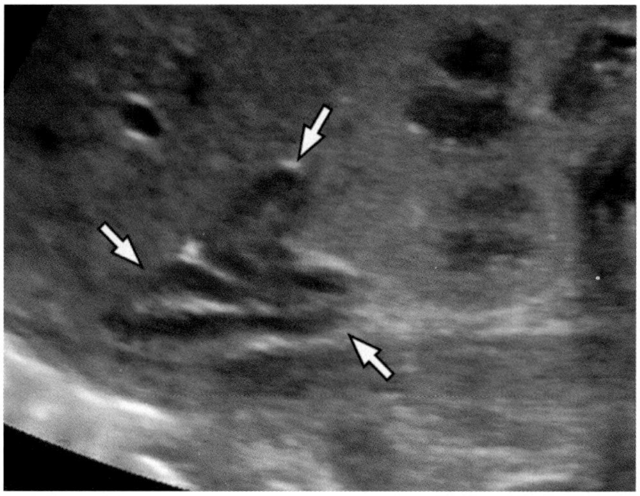

FIGURE 15.49 **Normal neonatal adrenal gland on ultrasound.** Longitudinal gray-scale ultrasound image shows a normal adrenal gland (*arrows*) in the located above the kidney with an inverted Y-configuration. The cortex is hypoechoic, whereas the medulla is echogenic.

high-frequency transducer (Fig. 15.49). Congenital adrenal abnormalities, adrenal hemorrhage, and adrenal masses can all be excellently visualized by ultrasound. In older children and adolescents, the normal adrenal glands are more difficult to visualize; however, adrenal masses and other lesions in the suprarenal fossa can still be assessed by ultrasound.

Computed Tomography

CT excellently depicts the adrenal glands in children of all ages. The lack of significant abdominal fat in children occasionally limits the discrete visualization of the adrenal glands, but, in general, both adrenal glands can be visualized and masses in the adrenal fossa can be excluded. CT also readily depicts adrenal calcifications and fat/lipid, which may be important in the setting of some adrenal tumors.

Magnetic Resonance Imaging

MRI is an excellent modality for evaluating the adrenal glands in pediatric patients of all ages. Although the spatial resolution of MRI is generally less than that of CT, improved contrast resolution and the ability to use a variety of pulse sequences to characterize specific tissues make MRI ideal for evaluating adrenal masses, the most common indication for adrenal imaging in children.

Nuclear Medicine

Nuclear medicine plays an important role in adrenal imaging, especially in the workup and staging of certain adrenal tumors. ^{131}Iodine-metaiodobenzylguanidine (MIBG) is taken up by both normal adrenal tissue and by tumors with adrenergic activity, such as pheochromocytoma and neuroblastoma. MIBG scanning is used extensively in the initial diagnosis, staging, and follow-up of adrenal tumors of sympathetic origin, as these neoplasms generally demonstrate substantial ^{131}I-MIBG uptake.

Normal Anatomy and Development

The adrenal glands are paired retroperitoneal structures located superior to each kidney. The right adrenal gland is located between the liver, inferior vena cava, and the right crus of the diaphragm.[101] The left adrenal gland is located lateral to the left crus of the diaphragm and superomedial to the tail of the pancreas.[101] The adrenal glands usually have an inverted "Y" or "V" shape on imaging, with a linear body superiorly and medial and lateral limbs located anterior and inferior. Arterial blood supply to the adrenal glands is from the inferior adrenal artery (a branch of the renal artery), the middle adrenal artery (a branch directly off the aorta), and the superior adrenal artery (a branch of the inferior phrenic artery).[102] Venous drainage is via the adrenal veins; the right adrenal vein drains directly into the inferior vena cava, whereas the left adrenal vein drains into the left renal vein.[102]

Each adrenal gland has two distinct functional units, an outer cortex and an inner medulla,[102] which arise from separate embryologic structures. The adrenal cortex develops from the coelomic mesoderm of the urogenital ridge during the 5th week of development, when mesothelial cells from the posterior abdominal wall proliferate to form the primitive adrenal cortex.[101] The medulla, on the other hand, develops when neural crest cells from the adjacent sympathetic ganglion (called chromaffin cells because of their distinct staining pattern) migrate towards the adrenal cortex in the 7th week of gestation.[101] These cells gradually invade the adrenal cortex and migrate along the central vein, orienting them in a central position within the gland, a process that continues until approximately the 18th week of gestation.[101,102] At birth, the adrenal glands are between 10 and 20 times larger relative to body size than in the adult.[101]

Congenital Abnormalities

Absent or Ectopic Adrenal Gland

Adrenal agenesis is extremely rare. Affected pediatric patients usually present at birth with clinical evidence of severe adrenal insufficiency. Ectopic or accessory adrenal tissue, on the other hand, is relatively common and is likely the result of fragments of adrenal tissue that break off during development.[101] These so-called adrenal rests are commonly located near the celiac axis but can also be found within intra-abdominal solid organs, the retroperitoneum, the broad ligament, and even the testes.[101] Depending on the developmental stage, adrenal rests may contain cortical tissue only or may contain both cortical and medullary tissue.[101,102] Ectopic adrenal tissue is found in up to 50% of neonates but is only rarely found in adults, suggesting most ectopic adrenal rests undergo atrophy.[101]

On imaging, the rests are usually small soft tissue nodules, measuring 3 to 5 mm. Rests are usually hypoechoic on ultrasound and soft tissue attenuation on CT. Adrenal rests can have a variable appearance on MRI, but are usually isointense to other solid organs on T1-weighted images and intermediate to mildly hyperintense on T2-weighted images and demonstrate diffuse, homogeneous enhancement.[103] Although of little clinical

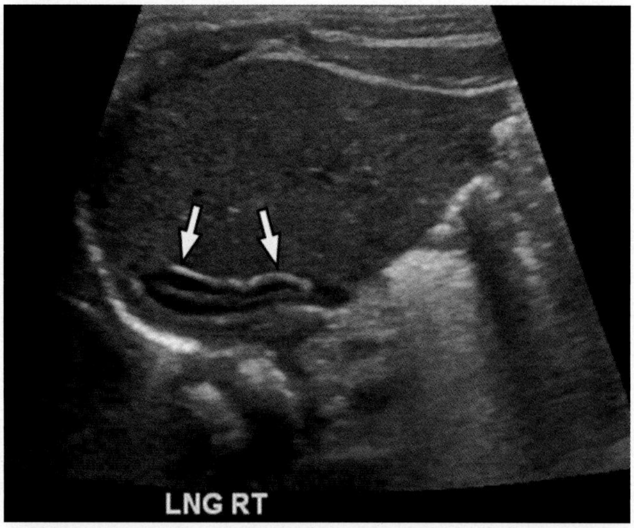

FIGURE 15.50 **Elongated adrenal gland in a newborn girl with absent right kidney.** Longitudinal gray-scale ultrasound image of the right suprarenal fossa demonstrates a linear, elongated configuration of the otherwise normal-appearing right adrenal gland (*arrows*). No right kidney is seen.

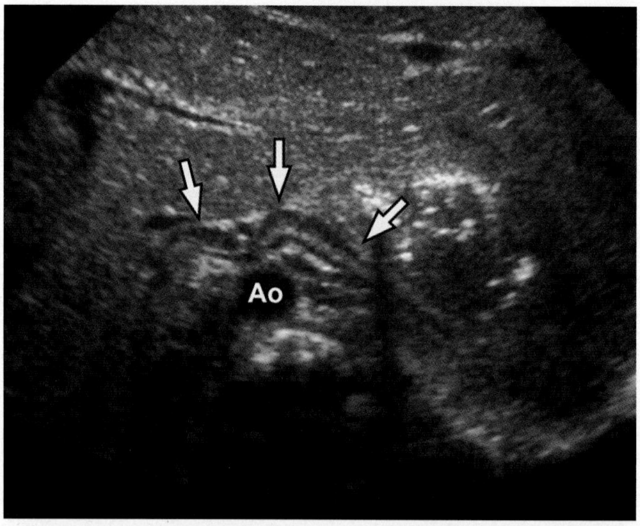

FIGURE 15.51 **Newborn boy with a horseshoe adrenal gland.** Midline transverse ultrasound image demonstrates adrenal tissue (*arrows*) extending across the midline anterior to the spine. (*Ao*, aorta.)

significance, adrenal rests can occasionally be mistaken for solid malignancy (e.g., in the testes), and can also undergo hypertrophy if stimulated by ACTH or other hormonal factors.[101,102]

Linear Adrenal Gland

The kidneys and adrenal glands, although closely anatomically associated, have different embryologic and developmental pathways. However, if a kidney does not develop or develops in an ectopic location, the ipsilateral adrenal gland usually has a linear or "discoid" morphology[101] (Fig. 15.50). This is thought to be secondary to the lack of extrinsic pressure on the adrenal gland by the normal kidney, allowing the adrenal gland to form an elongated linear shape as opposed to the more compact normal "Y" or "V" shape.[101,102] On imaging, the adrenal gland may be longer than usual, and appears as a single linear structure or may even have a slightly ovoid shape. The elongated linear adrenal gland should not be mistaken for a kidney during sonography in neonates with renal agenesis.[104]

Horseshoe Adrenal Gland

A horseshoe adrenal gland is a rare congenital anomaly in which there is midline fusion of the adrenal glands. The etiology is unclear, but proposed mechanisms include disruption of an intervening layer of coelomic epithelium that normally separates the glands, a single anomalous midline primordial gland associated with other midline defects, and a defect of laterality, such as in heterotaxy syndromes.[105,106] Imaging demonstrates fusion of the left and right adrenal glands in the midline in a preaortic location[105,106] (Figs. 15.51 and 15.52). Horseshoe adrenal has been associated with multiple other congenital anomalies, from central nervous system defects to heterotaxy syndromes.[105]

Wolman Disease

Wolman disease is a rare autosomal recessive condition in which a deficiency in a lysosomal enzyme lipase results in excessive deposition of cholesterol esters and triglycerides[107,108] (Fig. 15.53). Clinically, affected pediatric patients present with hepatomegaly, failure to thrive, and gastrointestinal symptoms.[107] The disease is fatal, usually within the first few months of life. Imaging findings include diffuse calcification of the adrenal glands, although rare cases without adrenal calcifications have been reported. The adrenal glands are usually enlarged. Hepatomegaly may also be apparent. The differential diagnosis for adrenal gland calcifications includes prior adrenal hemorrhage, granulomatous disease, Addison disease, or calcifications related to a tumor[108] (Fig. 15.54).

Infectious Disorders

Granulomatous Infection

Tuberculosis, although rare, is the most common infectious cause of adrenal insufficiency worldwide.[109] Imaging findings depend on the chronicity of the infection. In the early phases,

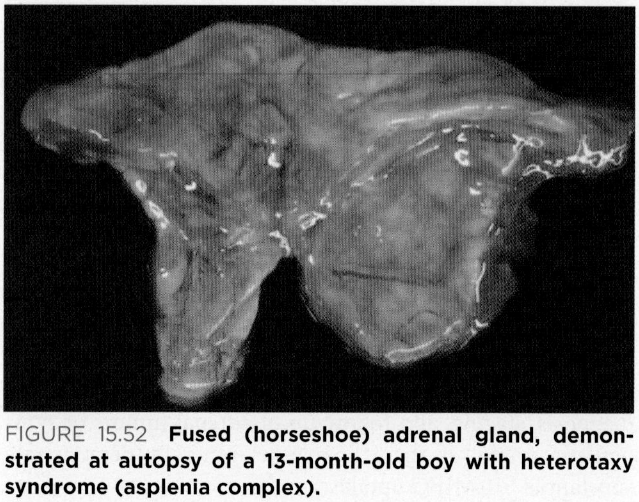

FIGURE 15.52 **Fused (horseshoe) adrenal gland, demonstrated at autopsy of a 13-month-old boy with heterotaxy syndrome (asplenia complex).**

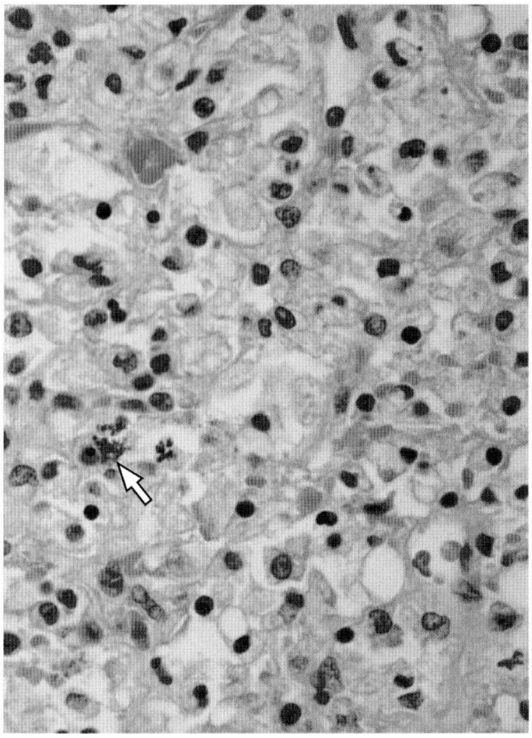

FIGURE 15.53 **Specimen from a 9-day-old boy who died in the setting of suspected Wolman disease.** The fetal cortex of the adrenal gland shows intracellular accumulation of lipid and focal calcification (*arrow*) (hematoxylin and eosin, original magnification, 600×).

ultrasound, CT, and MRI may show diffuse adrenal gland enlargement, sometimes with central areas of necrosis visible on CT and MRI as areas of fluid attenuation or T1-weighted hypointense, T2-weighted hyperintense signal with a peripheral rim of enhancement. Later in the course of infection, the adrenal glands may become atrophic, commonly with associated calcification.[109]

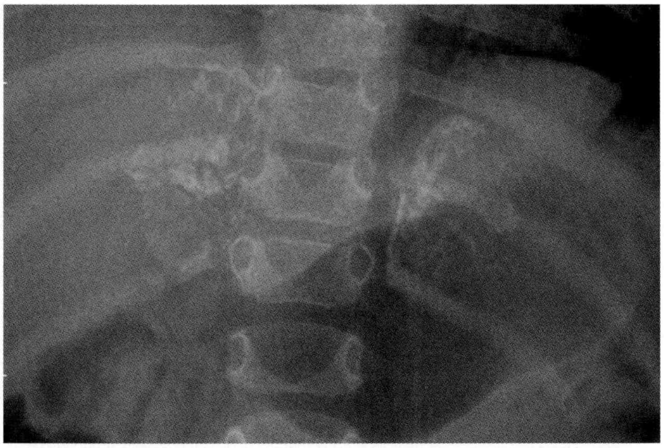

FIGURE 15.54 **Bilateral adrenal calcifications in a 6-month-old boy.** Abdominal radiograph demonstrates bilateral symmetric adrenal calcifications. Adrenal calcifications were thought to be due to prior adrenal hemorrhages. Other etiologies for adrenal calcifications, including Wolman disease, could appear similar. (Courtesy of Christopher Anton, MD, Cincinnati Children's Hospital Medical Center, Cincinnati, OH.)

Disseminated histoplasmosis infection, usually seen in immunocompromised patients, can also affect the adrenal glands and may result in adrenal insufficiency. In the acute setting, the adrenal glands may be enlarged with peripheral enhancement on CT and MRI. Variable amounts of calcifications and adrenal gland atrophy may be present depending on the chronicity of the disease.[109]

Abscess

Adrenal gland abscesses are rare and are most frequently encountered in neonates with a history of a prior adrenal hemorrhage.[109] If a neonatal adrenal hemorrhage fails to resolve, and if the patient exhibits clinical signs of infection, an abscess can be suspected. Imaging findings are similar to abscesses elsewhere in the body. Ultrasound can demonstrate a focal fluid collection, often with a thick and irregular wall. CT and MRI show peripheral enhancement of the fluid collection after intravenous contrast material administration. On MRI, an abscess generally demonstrates hyperintense signal on diffusion-weighted imaging because of impeded diffusion of water.

Other Infection

Rarely, congenital and neonatal herpes simplex virus infection can affect the adrenal glands. The imaging manifestations occasionally include nonspecific adrenal calcifications. Calcifications are usually also found within the liver. In general, affected patients have evidence of infection involving other organ systems allowing for the diagnosis.[110]

In immunocompromised patients, *Pneumocystis jirovecii* (formerly known as *Pneumocystis carinii*) infection affecting the adrenal glands has been reported. The most frequent imaging finding is nonspecific adrenal calcifications. There are usually calcifications elsewhere in the abdomen as well, including the liver, spleen, kidneys, and lymph nodes.[109]

Neoplastic Disorders (Table 15.3)

Primary Neoplasms

Adrenocortical Neoplasms

Adrenocortical neoplasms are primary adrenal tumors that, as their name implies, arise from the adrenal cortex. The lesions can be divided based on malignant potential into

TABLE 15.3 Adrenal Neoplasms in Children
Adrenocortical neoplasms Benign adenoma Adrenocortical carcinoma Adrenocortical neoplasm of uncertain malignant potential
Neurogenic tumors Neuroblastoma Ganglioneuroblastoma Ganglioneuroma
Pheochromocytoma
Teratoma
Metastases

benign adenoma, malignant adrenocortical carcinoma, and adrenocortical neoplasm of uncertain malignant potential. Adrenocortical tumors are rare in children, with a worldwide incidence of between 0.3 and 3 per million, and are most common in young girls under the age of 5 years.[111–113] These tumors are also found with increased frequency in association with certain syndromes, including Beckwith-Wiedemann and Li-Fraumeni.[111] Both benign and malignant adrenocortical tumors are commonly hormonally active, and the majority of patients present with clinical evidence of excess adrenal hormone production, such as Cushing syndrome, virilization in girls, or precocious puberty in boys.[111,113] Aside from frank lymphovascular invasion or metastasis, there is no single pathologic criterion that can reliably distinguish benign (adrenocortical adenoma) from malignant (adrenocortical carcinoma) tumors. Pathologic features that may help predict benign versus malignant behavior in children include tumor size, mitotic activity, and the presence or absence of necrosis.[114]

Radiographs are of little utility in evaluation of patients with suspected adrenocortical neoplasms. Rarely, adrenal calcifications or mass effect from a large adrenal soft tissue mass can be identified. Ultrasound shows a round or oval-shaped solid mass of varying size and echogenicity. Both benign and malignant adrenal masses may be homogeneous or heterogeneous, depending on the amount of internal hemorrhage and necrosis (although malignant lesions are more often heterogenous than adenomas). The size of the mass can vary from small to very large.[111] Malignant adrenocortical tumors frequently invade adjacent structures, such as the liver and inferior vena cava. MRI is the most useful imaging test to further define the mass and its relationship with adjacent structures, as well as to characterize the mass itself (Fig. 15.55). There is significant overlap between the features of benign and malignant adrenocortical neoplasms. MRI can show a suprarenal soft tissue mass that is usually intermediate signal on T1-weighted images and relatively hyperintense on T2-weighted images.[111] Enhancement of at least portions of the mass is usually present after intravenous contrast material administration. CT can also be used to evaluate pediatric adrenal masses, their relationships to adjacent structures, and any vascular invasions or occlusions (Fig. 15.56). CT may demonstrate calcifications better than MRI. Methods for determining lipid content and assessment of contrast material "wash-out" to differentiate benign from malignant tumors that have been described in adult adrenal masses have not been validated in children.[111]

In the end, differentiation of benign and malignant but nonmetastatic adrenocortical neoplasms with imaging may not be possible, although smaller lesions are more likely to be benign (Fig. 15.57). However, because of the hormonally active nature of these tumors, they are almost universally surgically resected. Complete surgical resection is the treatment of choice. Chest CT should be performed in malignant adrenocortical tumors to evaluate for pulmonary metastases. Children with very large tumors, residual disease after surgical resection, and metastatic malignant tumors have a poor prognosis.[113]

Neurogenic Tumors

Neuroblastic tumors (neuroblastoma, ganglioneuroblastoma, and ganglioneuroma) are the most common type of neurogenic tumors to involve the pediatric adrenal gland. They consist of variably differentiated neuroepithelial cells admixed with variable proportions of mature Schwannian stroma. These tumors are the most common extracranial solid tumors of childhood.[115] The malignant potential of these tumors is defined by the degree of cellular differentiation.[112] The least differentiated, and therefore most malignant, tumor in this group is neuroblastoma. In contrast, ganglioneuroblastoma demonstrates intermediate malignant potential, whereas ganglioneuroma is the most mature and demonstrates generally benign behavior and imaging features.

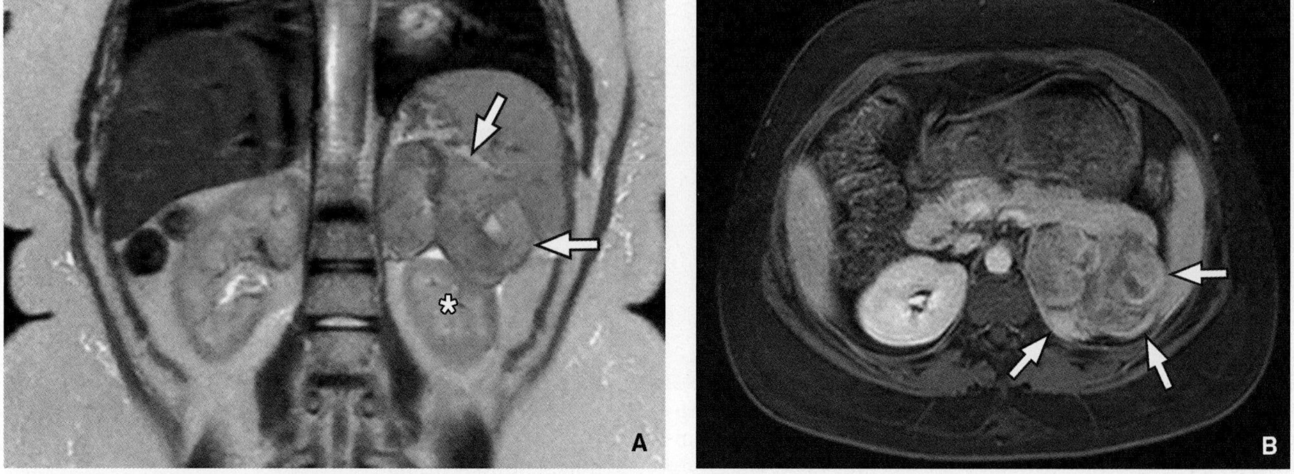

FIGURE 15.55 **Adrenocortical carcinoma in a 13-year-old girl with rapid-onset weight gain and Cushing syndrome. A:** Coronal T2-weighted single-shot fast spin-echo MR image demonstrates a heterogeneous left suprarenal mass (*arrows*) with mass effect on the left kidney (*asterisk*). There is a small amount of adjacent fluid. **B:** Axial T1-weighted postcontrast 3D SPGR fat-saturated MR image shows heterogeneous enhancement of the left adrenal mass (*arrows*).

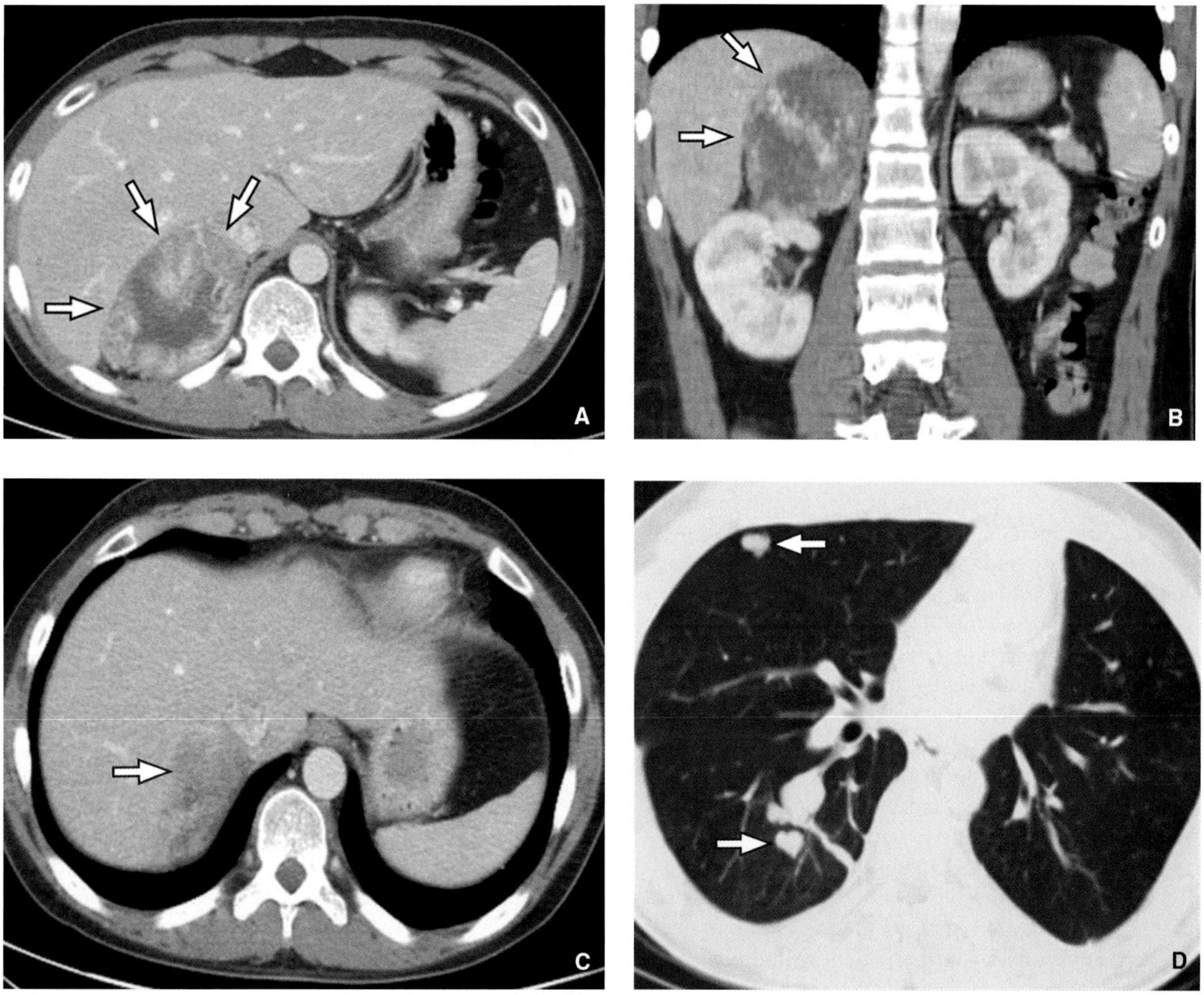

FIGURE 15.56 **Adrenocortical carcinoma in an 18-year-old boy with Cushing syndrome.** Axial **(A)** and coronal **(B)** contrast-enhanced CT images demonstrate a heterogeneous right suprarenal mass (*arrows*) with central areas of nonenhancement suggesting necrosis. **C:** A slightly higher CT image shows direct invasion of the liver by the mass (*arrow*). **D:** Axial lung window CT image demonstrates pulmonary metastatic disease (*arrows*).

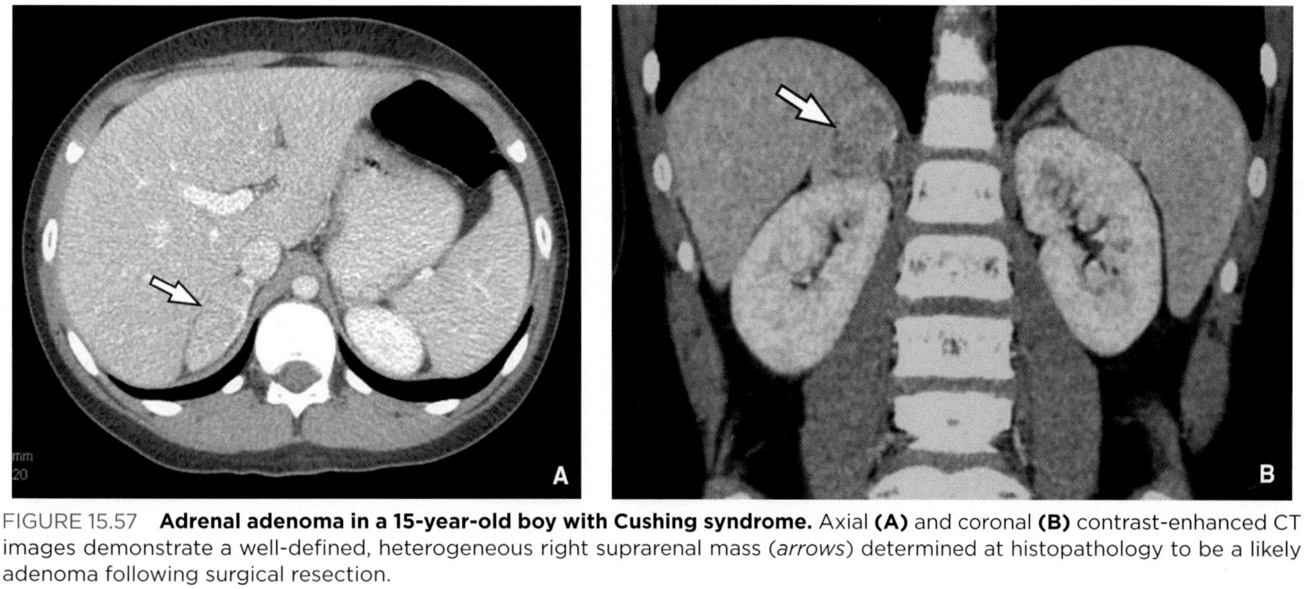

FIGURE 15.57 **Adrenal adenoma in a 15-year-old boy with Cushing syndrome.** Axial **(A)** and coronal **(B)** contrast-enhanced CT images demonstrate a well-defined, heterogeneous right suprarenal mass (*arrows*) determined at histopathology to be a likely adenoma following surgical resection.

Neuroblastoma

Neuroblastoma represents the most undifferentiated and aggressive malignant tumor of neural crest cells, and is the most common pediatric extracranial solid malignancy, accounting for about 8% of childhood malignancies.[112,116,117] Neuroblastoma is also the most common malignancy encountered in infancy.[112,118] The tumor most commonly arises from the medulla of the adrenal glands (30% to 40% of cases) but can arise anywhere along the sympathetic chain, including in the thorax.[115,117] Important prognostic factors include the histologic grade (which incorporates the age at diagnosis) and the initial stage; younger patients with "favorable histology" and lower stage disease tend to have the best prognosis.[112] Increasingly, genetic testing of the tumor for amplification of the oncogene N-MYC, DNA ploidy, and abnormalities of chromosomes 1p and 11q is used to determine therapy and predict prognosis.[115] Approximately 50% of affected pediatric patients have metastatic disease at the time of diagnosis.[108] The most common sites of metastases include local lymph nodes, liver, and bone.

Different staging systems for neuroblastoma exist, including the original International Neuroblastoma Staging System (INSS) and the more recent International Neuroblastoma Risk Group (INRG) staging system.[113] The INSS staging system ranges from 1 to 4, based on the resectability of the primary tumor, whether the tumor crosses midline, the status of local lymph nodes, and the presence of metastatic disease.[119] The INRG staging system is based on localization of the primary tumor, resectability based on proximity to vital structures, and the presence of metastatic disease.[120] Both staging systems account for a unique variant of neuroblastoma that occurs in younger patient with limited metastatic disease, termed stage 4S (INSS) or stage MS (INRG) disease.[119,120]

The clinical presentation of neuroblastoma is variable, ranging from an asymptomatic abdominal mass or nonspecific abdominal pain to various neurologic findings related to intraspinal extension of the tumor. Opsoclonus–myoclonus syndrome is a paraneoplastic phenomenon that occasionally occurs with neuroblastic tumors and involves involuntary ocular movements and ataxia.[121] The presence of opsoclonus–myoclonus in a child should prompt imaging to investigate for occult neuroblastoma.[121] Laboratory findings in patients with neuroblastoma usually include elevation of urine catecholamines.[117] Histologically, neuroblastoma shows nests of primitive neuroblastic cells with varying amounts of neuropil. Schwannian stroma represents a minority of the tumor (Fig. 15.58). Grading involves factoring the patient age with the degree of neuroblast differentiation (undifferentiated, poorly differentiated, or differentiating) and the "mitosis–karyorrhexis index."[122]

Imaging features of neuroblastoma vary, depending on tumor size and location. The most common presentation is a solid retroperitoneal mass (Fig. 15.59). Neuroblastoma tends to surround vascular structures without invading or occluding them. A classic imaging finding described in retroperitoneal neuroblastoma is a tumor that surrounds the abdominal aorta and lifts the aorta away from the spine (Fig. 15.60). Up to 50% of these tumors have visible calcifications, which can help differentiate neuroblastoma from lymphoma at imaging. Ultrasound is often the first imaging test obtained in the setting of a pediatric abdominal mass, and can demonstrate a heterogeneous solid mass with mass effect on adjacent structures, often the ipsilateral kidney.[112,115] Calcifications may be visible as punctate or coarse echogenic foci with or without posterior acoustic shadowing.

Comprehensive evaluation of suspected neuroblastoma requires additional imaging with either CT or MRI. CT excellently depicts the primary tumor and its relationship to adjacent structures, including encasement of adjacent vessels such as the abdominal aorta. CT also readily shows calcifications within the tumor. MRI also plays an important role in both the initial staging and follow-up of neuroblastoma. At presentation, neuroblastoma appears as a solid mass that is usually iso- to hypointense on T1-weighted images, heterogeneously hyperintense on T2-weighted images, and shows variable enhancement after intravenous gadolinium-based contrast material.[123] Calcifications are more difficult to identify on MRI than on CT, but may appear as foci of hypointense signal on T2-weighted and gradient-recalled echo sequences.[123] On diffusion-weighted imaging, the mass is usually hyperintense showing impeded diffusion due to its cellularity.[124] MRI is better than

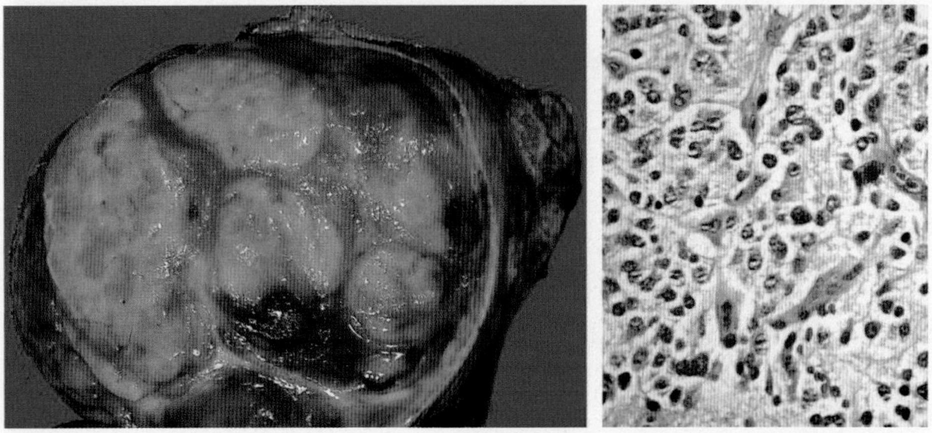

FIGURE 15.58 **Neuroblastoma of the adrenal gland of a 12-year-old boy.** The cut surface is variegated with areas of hard calcification **(left)**. Microscopically, nests of primitive neuroblastic cells lie in a pink fibrillar material ("neuropil") composed of the neoplastic cells' neuritic processes (**right**, hematoxylin and eosin, original magnification, 600×).

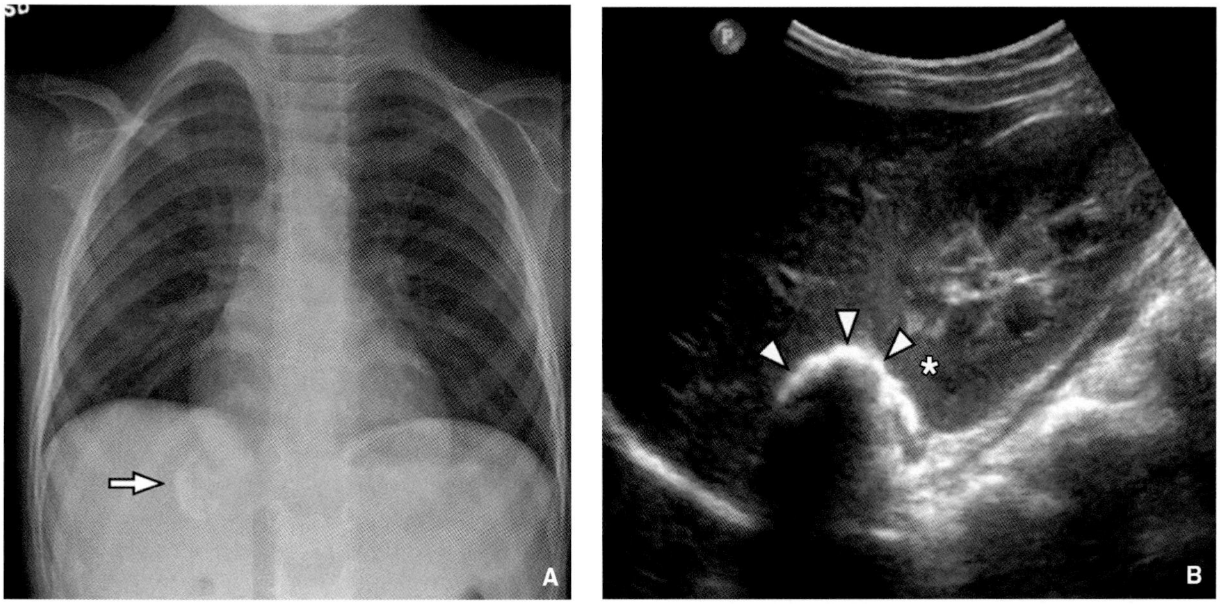

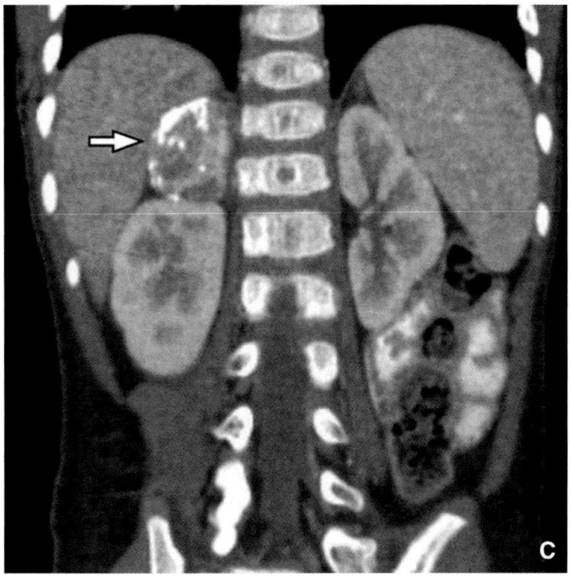

FIGURE 15.59 **Neuroblastoma discovered incidentally in a 3-year-old girl. A:** Chest radiograph performed to evaluate for suspected pneumonia demonstrates a calcified mass (*arrow*) in the right suprarenal fossa. **B:** Subsequent longitudinal gray-scale ultrasound image demonstrates posterior acoustic shadowing from the calcified mass (*arrowheads*). Note the mass effect on upper pole of the right kidney (*asterisk*). **C:** Coronal contrast-enhanced CT image shows similar findings to the ultrasound, with a heterogeneous, partially calcified mass (*arrow*) superior to the right kidney. A normal right adrenal gland was not visualized. The mass was surgically resected and was proven by histopathology to be neuroblastoma.

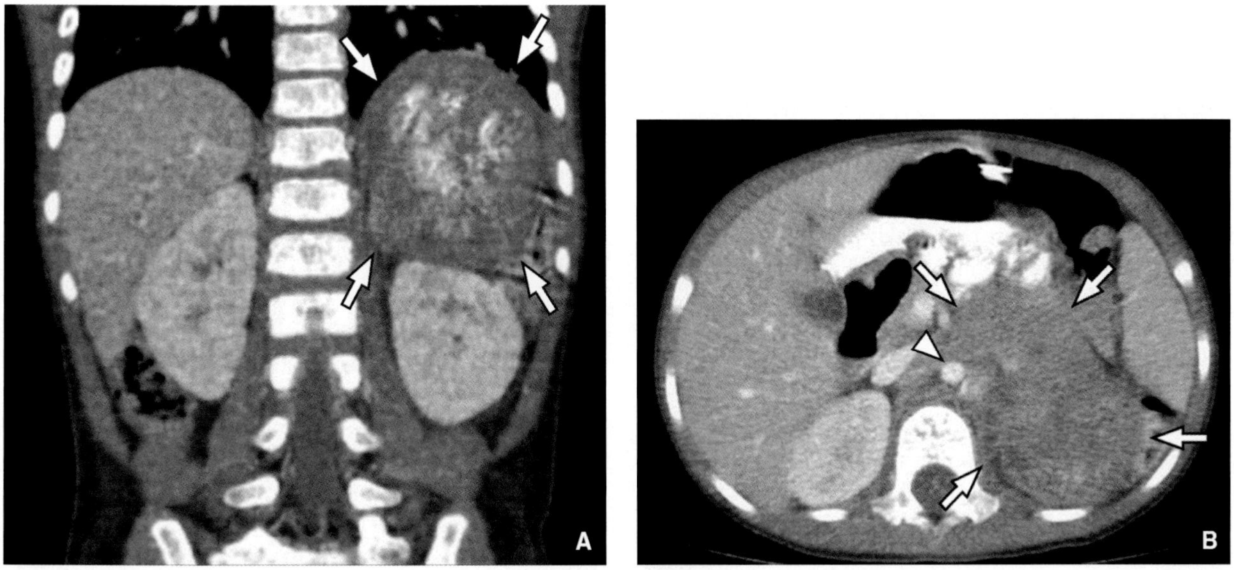

FIGURE 15.60 **Neuroblastoma in a 5-year-old girl.** Coronal **(A)** and axial **(B)** contrast-enhanced CT images demonstrate left suprarenal and retroperitoneal mass (*arrows*) that encase and displace vascular structures and "lift" the aorta off the spine (*arrowhead*), a classic finding in retroperitoneal neuroblastoma. Speckled calcifications are present within the mass, which also has mass effect on the left kidney.

(*Continued*)

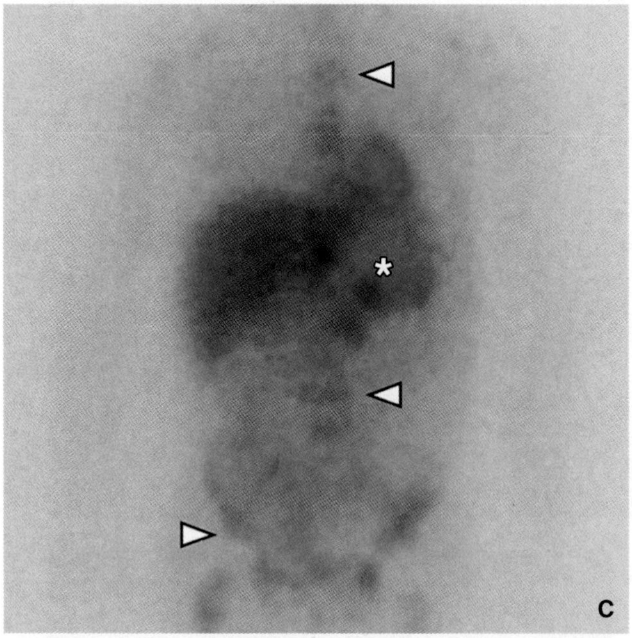

FIGURE 15.60 (*Continued*) **C:** ^{131}I-meta-iodobenzylguanidine (MIBG) scan shows increased radiotracer uptake within the primary mass (*asterisk*). Uptake (*arrowheads*) in the spine and other osseous structures, including the pelvis and proximal femora, is consistent with metastatic disease.

CT at depicting intraspinal extension of the tumor.[123] Another advantage of MRI is the excellent depiction of the bone marrow, which may aid in detection of osseous metastatic disease. As such, whole body MRI is playing an increasing role in detection of skeletal metastases in neuroblastoma.[125,126]

Nuclear medicine also plays an important role in the imaging of neuroblastoma, both at initial staging and at follow-up. MIBG scintigraphy is used to characterize the primary tumor and to perform whole body evaluation for metastasis. Normal distribution of MIBG includes the nasal mucosa, salivary glands, myocardium, liver, bowel, and urinary tract.[118] Any additional uptake of MIBG, including any uptake within the osseous structures, is consistent with either primary tumor or metastatic disease[115,118] (Fig. 15.60). ^{18}F-FDG-PET/CT has also been shown to be useful in imaging of neuroblastoma, although MIBG has been shown to be more sensitive and specific, especially in the evaluation of osseous metastatic disease.[118] ^{18}F-FDG-PET/CT may have role in tumors that are MIBG negative or are only weakly positive on MIBG.[117]

Two important neuroblastoma variants are congenital neuroblastoma and stage 4S disease. Congenital or neonatal neuroblastoma is detected early in infancy and may even be present prenatally (Fig. 15.61). These tumors tend to be less aggressive and may even spontaneously regress.[127] Rarely, affected pediatric patients present with massive hepatic metastatic disease that may lead to respiratory compromise.[128] Stage 4S disease refers to patients <1 year of age with a localized primary tumor and other sites of disease limited to the liver, skin, or bone marrow, but without distant osseous metastatic disease.[112] Both congenital neuroblastoma and stage 4S patients have an excellent prognosis.

Treatment of neuroblastoma generally consists of chemotherapy followed by removal of any surgically resectable disease. Some patients require bone marrow transplantation in the setting of diffuse bone marrow involvement. Targeted therapies, such as I-131 MIBG therapy, are also employed.[129] Prognosis and survival depends on the stage of disease and genetic features of the tumor, ranging from an excellent prognosis in congenital and stage 1 disease to long-term survival rates of 30% to 40% in high-risk disease.[118]

Ganglioneuroblastoma and Ganglioneuroma

Ganglioneuroblastoma and ganglioneuroma represent "favorable histology" type tumors with the exception of the nodular subtype of ganglioneuroma, which may be unfavorable. Similar to neuroblastoma, these tumors are derived from the primordial neural crest cells; however, in distinction from neuroblastoma, which contains primarily primitive neuroblasts with only a minor component of schwannian stroma, ganglioneuroblastoma and ganglioneuroma are stroma-rich neoplasms that contain a preponderance (>50%) of schwannian stroma; neuroblasts and/or gangliocytes are admixed in varying patterns[122]

The intermixed type of ganglioneuroblastoma is less differentiated than ganglioneuroma, and it contains nests of neuroblasts. Clinical presentation, workup, and staging of these tumors are similar to that of neuroblastoma.[128] Imaging features of ganglioneuroblastoma can be similar to those of neuroblastoma, and these tumors often cannot be reliably differentiated by standard imaging techniques (Fig. 15.62). Special note should be made of the nodular type of ganglioneuroblastoma, which is distinguished by the presence of a localized nodule of stroma-poor neuroblastoma within an otherwise stroma-rich tumor. In this subtype, which is viewed conceptually as a composite tumor, the prognosis and therapy are based on the histologic and genetic features of the neuroblastic "clone," and thus the prognosis may be worse than in the more common intermixed type of ganglioneuroblastoma.[122]

Ganglioneuroma represents the benign end of the spectrum, composed of mature or "maturing" neuroblasts (ganglion cells) occurring singly or in clusters within abundant schwannian stroma (Fig. 15.63). Either with therapy, or spontaneously, some neuroblastomas and ganglioneuroblastomas may mature into ganglioneuroma.[124,128] Ganglioneuroma typically occurs in older patients, with a mean age of ~7 years.[128] In distinction from neuroblastoma and ganglioneuroblastoma, ganglioneuroma is more likely to be located in the posterior mediastinum; only about 20% of tumors are located in the adrenal glands[128] (Fig. 15.64). Commonly, ganglioneuroma and ganglioneuroblastoma are asymptomatic and incidentally detected on imaging performed for other reasons. CT imaging typically demonstrates a well-defined, homogeneous soft tissue mass, with fine or speckled calcifications in 40% to 60% of tumors.[128] On MRI, these lesions are often low signal on T1-weighted images and heterogeneous signal on T2-weighted images, thought to reflect mature stromal elements.[128] Variable enhancement is seen after intravenous administration of gadolinium-containing contrast material. Ganglioneuromas can accumulate MIBG, with activity seen in almost 60% of tumors.[128] Management of these tumors includes either surgical resection or observation.

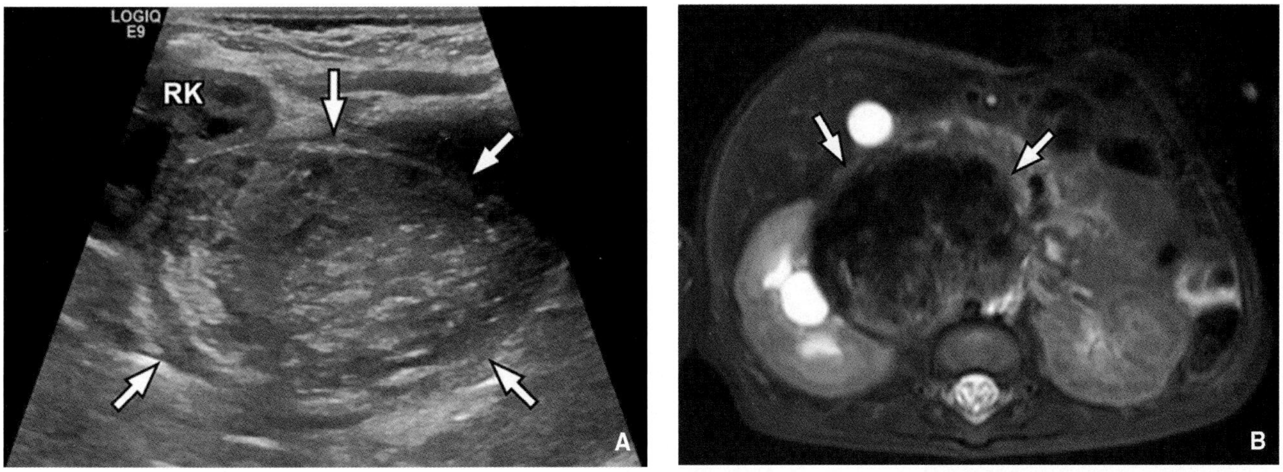

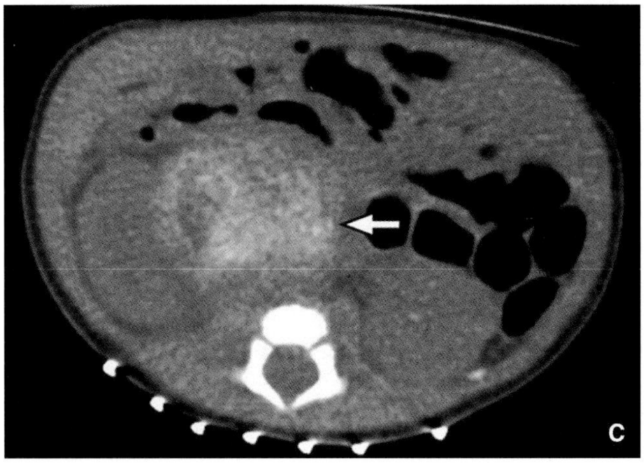

FIGURE 15.61 **Congenital neuroblastoma in a 1-day-old boy. A:** Transverse gray-scale ultrasound image obtained from a posterior approach demonstrates a mass (*arrows*) adjacent to the right kidney (*RK*) with obstructive dilation of the right renal collecting system. The mass contains multiple echogenic foci representing calcifications. **B:** Axial T2-weighted fat-saturated MR image also shows the large retroperitoneal mass (*arrows*) adjacent to the right kidney with associated obstructive renal collecting system dilation. Low signal intensity within the mass is due to the extensive calcifications. **C:** Axial noncontrast CT image performed as part of a percutaneous biopsy shows extensive high attenuation (*arrow*) within the mass due to calcifications.

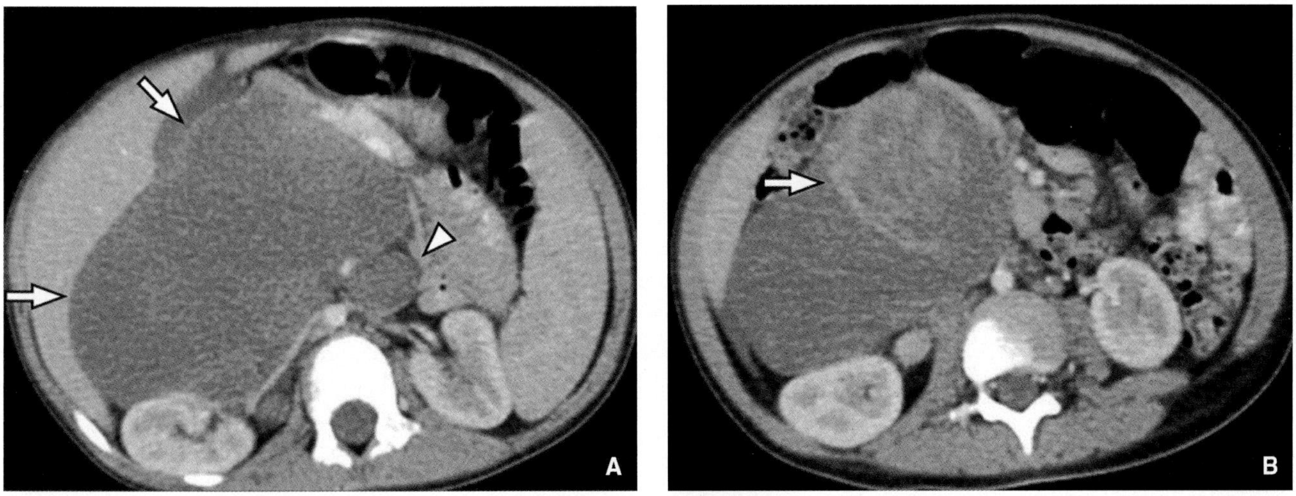

FIGURE 15.62 **Ganglioneuroblastoma in a 4-year-old boy. A and B:** Axial contrast-enhanced CT images demonstrate a large right suprarenal mass (*arrows*). The mass is predominantly homogeneous and low in attenuation, although some areas demonstrate heterogeneous enhancement (*arrow* in **B**). An enlarged retroperitoneal lymph node was confirmed to contain tumor at histopathology (*arrowhead*). The mass exerts substantial mass effect upon the liver, right kidney, right renal artery, bowel, and mesentery.

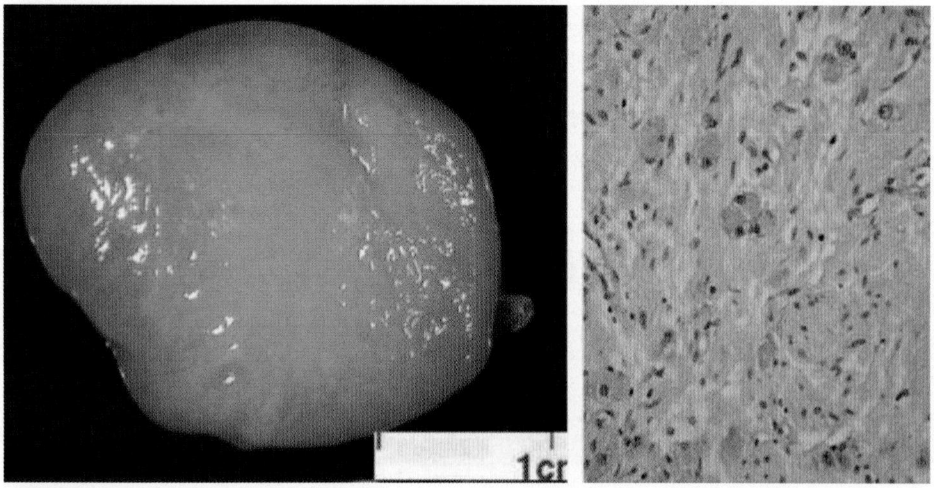

FIGURE 15.63 **Incidentally discovered ganglioneuroma from near the adrenal gland of an 11-year-old girl.** Grossly, the tumor was pale tan, firm, and homogeneous **(left)**. Microscopically, ganglion cells appear singly and in clusters within an abundant stroma composed of spindle-shaped Schwannian cells (**right**, hematoxylin and eosin, original magnification, 400×).

Pheochromocytoma

Pheochromocytoma is an uncommon tumor that originates from neural crest cells, most commonly in the adrenal medulla.[112] When these tumors are extra-adrenal, they are called paragangliomas. Up to 20% of pheochromocytomas occur in children, with an increased incidence in children with certain cancer predisposition syndromes, including multiple endocrine neoplasia type 2 (MEN-2), von Hippel–Lindau disease, Carney-Stratakis syndrome, Carney triad, and other familial paraganglioma-pheochromocytoma syndromes.[130] The average age at diagnosis in pediatric patients is 11 years.[130] The majority of these tumors synthesize and secrete catecholamines, which can result in hypertension, although some tumors are metabolically inactive.[130] Patients with hormonally active tumors have elevated plasma or urine metanephrines.[130] Treatment is generally with surgical resection.

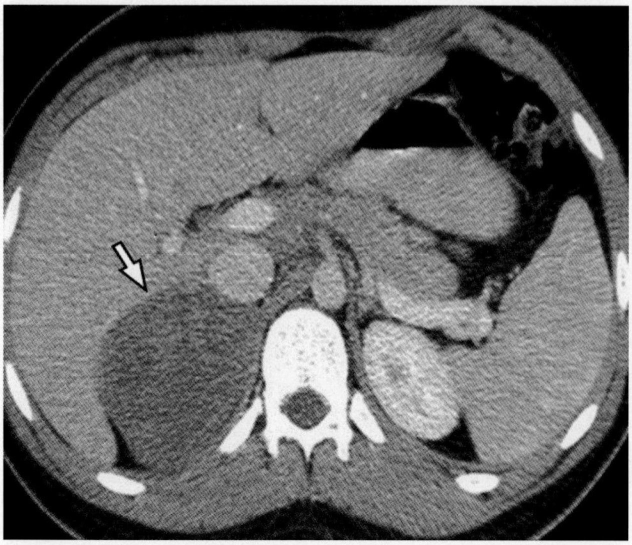

FIGURE 15.64 **Ganglioneuroma discovered incidentally in a 15-year-old boy who underwent CT to investigate abdominal pain.** Axial contrast-enhanced CT image demonstrates a mostly homogeneous right suprarenal mass (*arrow*) histologically confirmed to be a ganglioneuroma after surgical resection.

The most common imaging finding in pheochromocytoma is that of an adrenal mass. The mass may replace all or part of the adrenal gland and, depending on the size of the mass, may cause displacement of the ipsilateral kidney. Ultrasound typically demonstrates a nonspecific solid adrenal mass. Contrast-enhanced CT or MRI often demonstrates avid enhancement of the mass[131] (Fig. 15.65). On MRI, pheochromocytoma may be strikingly hyperintense on T2-weighted sequences, although this appearance is not consistently present.[112,130] MIBG scintigraphy can confirm the diagnosis of a tumor of neural crest origin but is not specific, as other paragangliomas as well as neuroblastic tumors can also take up MIBG (Fig. 15.66). Scintigraphy using somatostatin receptor analogs (e.g., ^{111}In-octreotide) is less sensitive than MIBG, but may be more specific.[132]

Teratoma

Teratomas are the third most common retroperitoneal neoplasm in children and have a bimodal age distribution, with peaks occurring at 6 months and late adolescence.[133] These lesions can be encountered in the suprarenal fossa and may be located adjacent to, or rarely within, the adrenal gland.[133] Histologically, these tumors are composed of elements derived from all three germ cell layers. Congenital/infantile teratomas, even those that contain immature neuroepithelial tissue, are regarded as benign unless they contain frankly malignant elements, such as yolk sac tumor. Teratomas are usually asymptomatic and are discovered incidentally on imaging. These tumors may have a nonspecific, heterogeneous appearance on ultrasound, with mixed cystic and solid components.[133] CT and MRI can readily demonstrate macroscopic fat and calcium within the adrenal mass, which is highly suggestive of a mature teratoma[134] (Fig. 15.67). The differential diagnosis for macroscopic fat in an adrenal lesion includes adrenal myelolipoma, which is extremely rare in children. Angiomyolipoma can also arise in the adrenal gland. In patients with mature teratomas arising from the adrenal gland, surgical resection is curative.

Metastases

Metastatic spread to the adrenal glands is uncommon in pediatric patients, but can occur in aggressive malignancies,

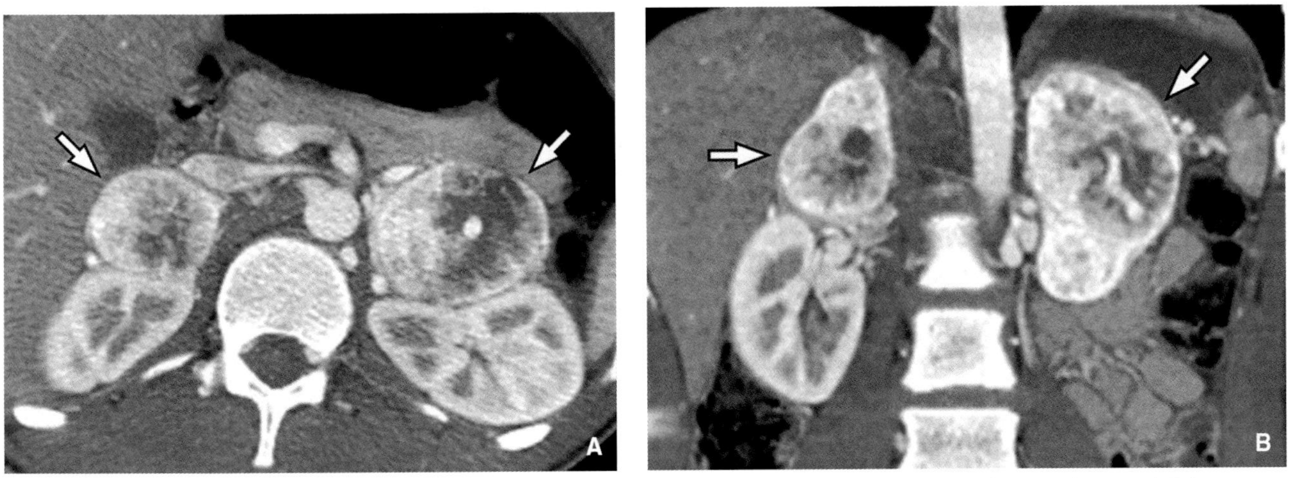

FIGURE 15.65 **Bilateral pheochromocytomas in a 15-year-old boy with hypertensive crisis.** Axial **(A)** and coronal **(B)** contrast-enhanced CT images demonstrate bilateral avidly enhancing adrenal masses (*arrows*) with areas of central nonenhancement, possibly necrosis. At surgical resection, both masses were consistent with pheochromocytomas, and the patient was subsequently diagnosed with von Hippel–Lindau disease.

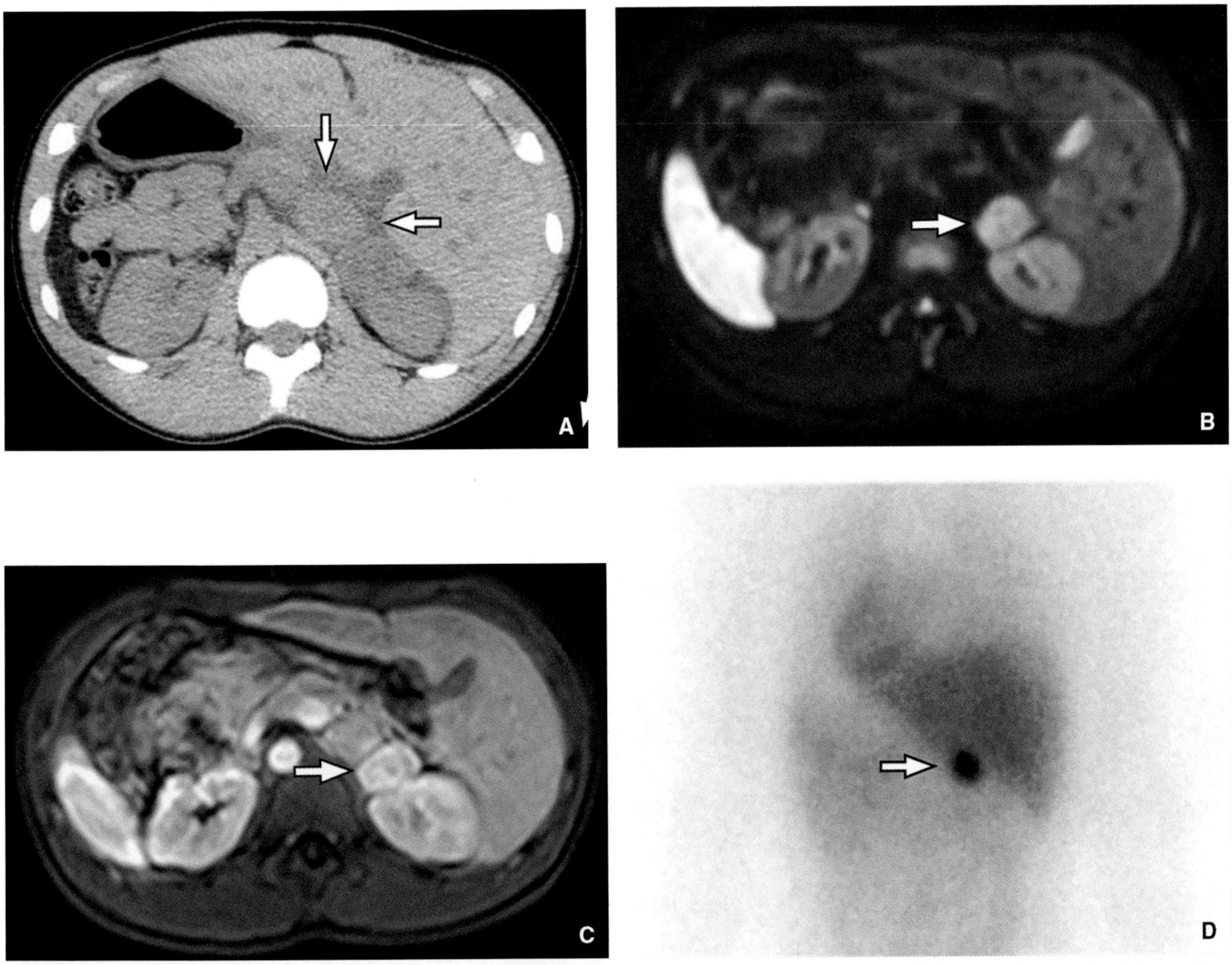

FIGURE 15.66 **Unilateral pheochromocytoma in a 17-year-old boy with abdominal pain after riding a roller coaster. The patient was also found to have situs inversus totalis. A:** Axial noncontrast CT image obtained on the day of presentation demonstrates high attenuation fluid (*arrows*) in the left suprarenal fossa consistent with hemorrhage/hematoma. Axial diffusion-weighted **(B)** and axial T1-weighted postcontrast fat-saturated **(C)** MR images obtained 2 weeks later demonstrate a left adrenal mass (*arrow*) that impedes diffusion and avidly enhances. **D:** Planar scintigraphic image after injection of I-123 MIBG demonstrates avid uptake within the mass (*arrow*). At surgical resection, the mass was confirmed to be a pheochromocytoma.

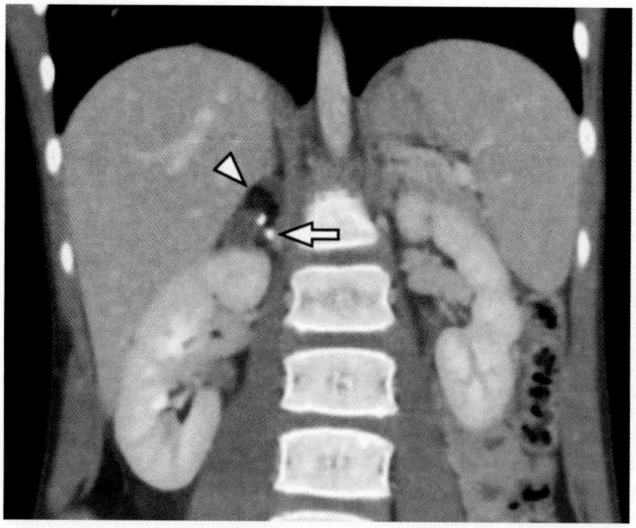

FIGURE 15.67 **Adrenal teratoma, incidentally discovered in a 12-year-old boy.** Coronal contrast-enhanced CT image demonstrates a right suprarenal mass (*arrow*) with areas of calcification and a central area of very low attenuation, consistent with fat (*arrowhead*).

TABLE 15.4 Causes of Adrenal Hemorrhage in Children
Neonatal stress
Difficult or prolonged delivery
Sepsis
Hypoxia
Extracorporeal membrane oxygenation (ECMO)
Physiologic stress
Sepsis
Burns
Hypotension
Surgery
Coagulopathy
Medications (Anticoagulants)
Tumors
Benign tumors
Malignant tumors
Metastasis
Trauma
Idiopathic

such as rhabdomyosarcoma. Imaging typically demonstrates a heterogeneous adrenal mass, and there is often evidence of widespread metastatic disease elsewhere.

Adrenal Hemorrhage

Adrenal hemorrhage refers to hemorrhage originating in the adrenal gland itself, and can be either traumatic or nontraumatic. A variety of causes of adrenal hemorrhage are listed in Table 15.4.

In the setting of blunt abdominal trauma, adrenal gland injury is rare, accounting for about 1% of injuries in children, and is almost always associated with other intra-abdominal solid organ injuries.[135] Traumatic adrenal hemorrhage is usually unilateral and most commonly affects the right adrenal gland[136] (Fig. 15.68). On ultrasound, traumatic adrenal hemorrhage appears as nonspecific fluid in the suprarenal fossa, often obscuring the normal adrenal gland. CT is the imaging modality of choice in blunt abdominal trauma. The injured adrenal gland can have a variable appearance at contrast-enhanced CT. The adrenal gland may be relatively low in attenuation (compared to enhancing liver and spleen), although the hemorrhage itself is usually high attenuation in the acute setting.[137] Hemorrhage within the gland may be focal or diffuse and may alter the normal shape of the gland, causing the affected adrenal to be oval or rounded in shape, or may obscure visualization of one or more of the limbs of the adrenal gland.[136] MRI is infrequently used to evaluate acute trauma but may demonstrate abnormal morphology of the gland and increased T1-weighted signal due to hemorrhage.

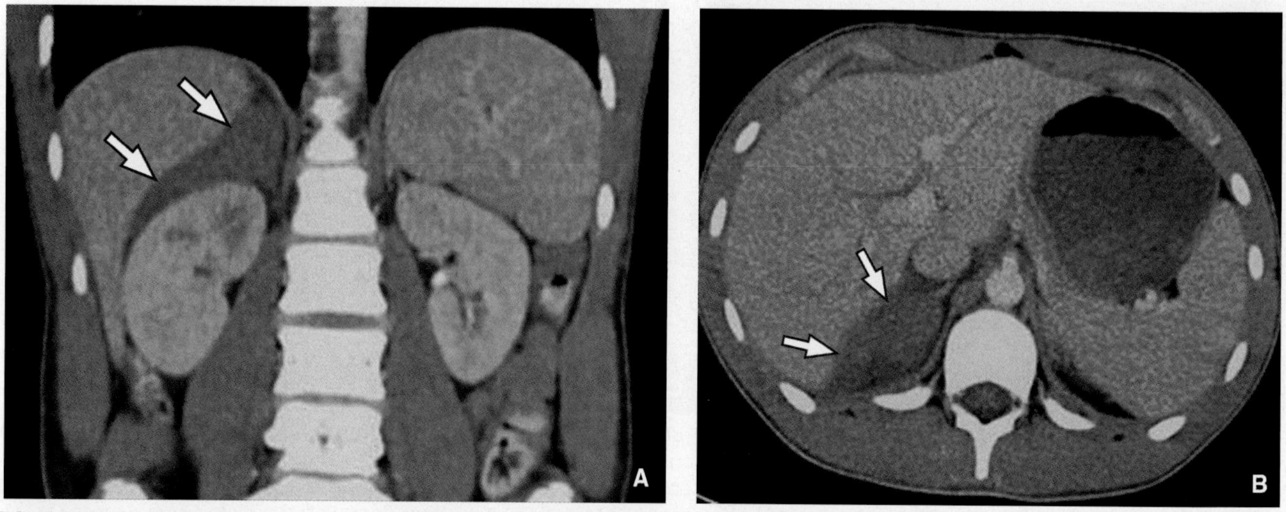

FIGURE 15.68 **Traumatic adrenal hemorrhage in a 14-year-old boy.** Coronal **(A)** and axial **(B)** contrast-enhanced CT images demonstrate triangular hyperdense fluid (*arrows*) in the right suprarenal fossa with adjacent fat stranding, consistent with acute adrenal hemorrhage.

More commonly, adrenal hemorrhage occurs in the nontraumatic setting. The adrenal gland is susceptible to hemorrhage because of a unique blood supply, consisting of three main adrenal arteries that branch into dozens of tiny perforating branches. The gland is drained by relatively few venous structures, creating a relative holdup of blood within the gland. Physiologic stress stimulates increased blood flow to the adrenal glands, exacerbating the relative backup of blood within the glands and predisposing to vascular damage and hemorrhage.[137]

One of the most commonly encountered clinical scenarios involving adrenal hemorrhage in pediatric radiology practices is the incidental discovery of a suspected adrenal hemorrhage in a newborn, often during abdominal sonography performed for unrelated indications. Hemorrhage is the most common adrenal mass-like abnormality in the neonate and is more common in the right adrenal gland.[137] The relatively large size of the neonatal adrenal gland, coupled with the physiologic stress of birth, predisposes to adrenal hemorrhage. Hemorrhage is more common in neonates with underlying conditions, such as those requiring respiratory support. The hemorrhage itself is usually of little or no clinical significance, although in rare instances the hemorrhage can manifest clinically with a palpable mass, jaundice, anemia, and even hypovolemic shock.[137] More commonly, the task of the radiologist is to differentiate hemorrhage from less common adrenal masses, such as congenital neuroblastoma. Initial ultrasound imaging usually demonstrates a hypoechoic, heterogenous mass that may be large enough to displace the kidney.[137] CT and MRI are rarely performed, but may show a mass or fluid collection with characteristics typical of hemorrhage. If needed, serial follow-up ultrasounds can be performed to assess for degradation of blood products and hematoma regression over the course of a period of weeks.[137] Urine catecholamines are also negative in the setting of hemorrhage.

Cystic Adrenal Gland Lesions

Benign cystic lesions of the adrenal gland are very rare in children. Pseudocysts may be encountered in the setting of prior adrenal hemorrhage.[138] Imaging features are typical of cysts elsewhere in the body. Ultrasound typically demonstrates an anechoic structure with a thin, uniform wall if not previously complicated by hemorrhage or infection. Contrast-enhanced CT shows a low-attenuation lesion within the adrenal gland, often with a thin uniform enhancing wall. MRI can characterize internal contents of the cyst and allows for multiphase postcontrast imaging with subtraction images to confirm the lack of central enhancement within the cyst (Fig. 15.69). Calcifications, irregularity of the cyst wall, septations, and enhancement should prompt

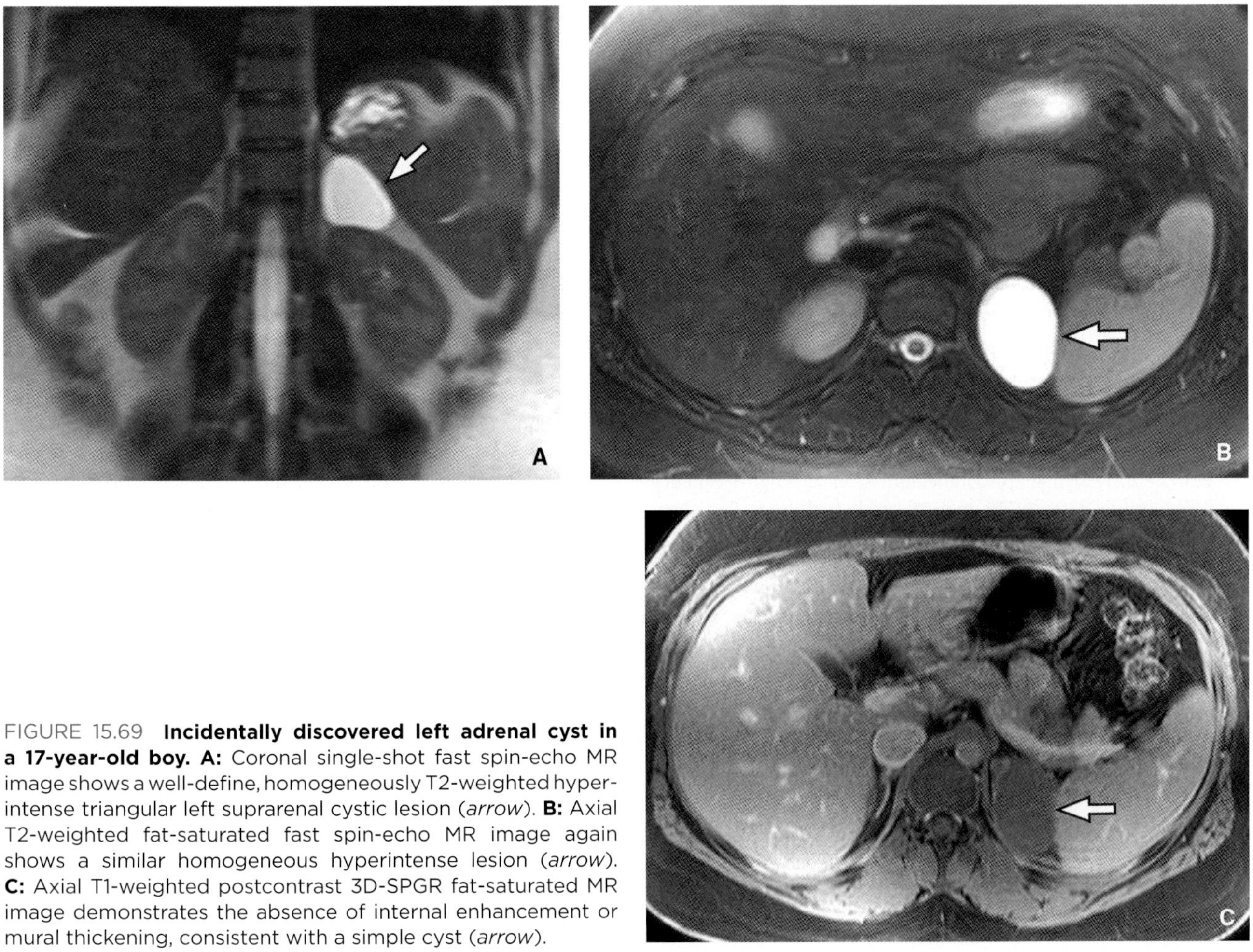

FIGURE 15.69 **Incidentally discovered left adrenal cyst in a 17-year-old boy. A:** Coronal single-shot fast spin-echo MR image shows a well-define, homogeneously T2-weighted hyperintense triangular left suprarenal cystic lesion (*arrow*). **B:** Axial T2-weighted fat-saturated fast spin-echo MR image again shows a similar homogeneous hyperintense lesion (*arrow*). **C:** Axial T1-weighted postcontrast 3D-SPGR fat-saturated MR image demonstrates the absence of internal enhancement or mural thickening, consistent with a simple cyst (*arrow*).

the consideration of an alternative diagnosis, including a complicated pseudocyst or even adrenal neoplasm.[131] The importance of imaging is to differentiate nonneoplastic cysts from cystic neoplasms, such as cystic neuroblastoma.

Congenital Adrenal Hyperplasia

Congenital adrenal hyperplasia (CAH) is inherited as an autosomal recessive condition caused by a deficiency in at least one of the five enzymes needed to synthesize cortisol in the adrenal cortex.[139] The most frequent abnormality is a deficiency in the enzyme 21-hydroxylase.[140] Abnormal enzyme function leads to deficiency of some adrenal hormones and overproduction of others, usually androgens. In milder forms, affected pediatric patients are still able to make cortisol. However, the hyperstimulation of the adrenal glands needed for adequate cortisol production results in androgen excess so that female infant presents with ambiguous genitalia.[140] In more severe forms, cortisol levels are low and other adrenal hormones such as aldosterone are also deficient, leading to salt wasting.[140] The incidence of the most classic form is between 1 in 15,000–16,000 live births,[139,140] with an increased incidence in certain ethnic groups.[139]

The diagnosis of CAH is based on clinical and laboratory findings, although one study demonstrated that a majority of patients have an identifiable abnormality related to CAH on imaging.[141] Ultrasound, CT, and MRI may show diffuse enlargement of the adrenal glands. In male patients, there is an increased incidence of intratesticular adrenal rests, which may be visible on ultrasound as hypoechoic foci within the testicles.[141] Interestingly, there is an increased incidence of benign adrenal tumors in adult patients with CAH, especially myelolipoma.[141,142]

Treatment of CAH is usually medical, with appropriate hormone replacement therapy. In rare patients, bilateral adrenalectomy is performed to aid in stabilizing hormone levels during exogenous hormonal therapy.[139]

References

1. Benter T, Kluhs L, Teichgraber U. Sonography of the spleen. *J Ultrasound Med.* 2011;30:1281–1293.
2. Doria AS, Daneman A, Moineddin R, et al. High-frequency sonographic patterns of the spleen in children. *Radiology.* 2006;240:821–827.
3. Paterson A, Frush DP, Donnelly LF, et al. A pattern-oriented approach to splenic imaging in infants and children. *Radiographics.* 1999;19:1465–1485.
4. Robertson F, Leander P, Ekberg O. Radiology of the spleen. *Eur Radiol.* 2001;11:80–95.
5. Paes FM, Kalkanis DG, Sideras PA, et al. FDG PET/CT of extranodal involvement in non-Hodgkin lymphoma and Hodgkin disease. *Radiographics.* 2010;30:269–291.
6. Catalano Q. Spleen anatomy, function and development. In: Hamm B, Ros PR, eds. *Abdominal Imaging Volume III.* Heidelberg, New York, Dordrecht, London: Springer; 2013.
7. Mebius RE, Kraal G. Structure and function of the spleen. *Nat Rev Immunol.* 2005;5:606–616.
8. Megremis SD, Vlachonikolis IG, Tsilimigaki AM. Spleen length in childhood with US: normal values based on age, sex, and somatometric parameters. *Radiology.* 2004;231:129–134.
9. Gayer G, Zissin R, Apter S, et al. CT findings in congenital anomalies of the spleen. *Br J Radiol.* 2001;74:767–772.
10. Bartram U, Wirbelauer J, Speer CP. Heterotaxy syndrome—asplenia and polysplenia as indicators of visceral malposition and complex congenital heart disease. *Biol Neonate.* 2005;88:278–290.
11. Fulcher AS, Turner MA. Abdominal manifestations of situs anomalies in adults. *Radiographics.* 2002;22:1439–1456.
12. Applegate KE, Goske MJ, Pierce G, et al. Situs revisited: imaging of the heterotaxy syndrome. *Radiographics.* 1999;19:837–852; discussion 853–834.
13. Dodds WJ, Taylor AJ, Erickson SJ, et al. Radiologic imaging of splenic anomalies. *AJR Am J Roentgenol.* 1990;155:805–810.
14. Freeman JL, Jafri SZ, Roberts JL, et al. CT of congenital and acquired abnormalities of the spleen. *Radiographics.* 1993;13:597–610.
15. Sanchez R, Lobert P, Herman R, et al. Wandering spleen causing gastric outlet obstruction and pancreatitis. *Pediatr Radiol.* 2010;40(suppl 1):S89–S91.
16. Allen KB, Andrews G. Pediatric wandering spleen—the case for splenopexy: review of 35 reported cases in the literature. *J Pediatr Surg.* 1989;24:432–435.
17. Miller JH, Greenfield LD, Wald BR. Candidiasis of the liver and spleen in childhood. *Radiology.* 1982;142:375–380.
18. Chun J, Kim Y. Spleen infectious and inflammatory disorders. In: Hamm B, Ros PR, eds. *Abdominal Imaging Volume III.* Heidelberg, New York, Dordrecht, London: Springer; 2013.
19. Urrutia M, Mergo PJ, Ros LH, et al. Cystic masses of the spleen: radiologic-pathologic correlation. *Radiographics.* 1996;16:107–129.
20. Semelka RC, Kelekis NL, Sallah S, et al. Hepatosplenic fungal disease: diagnostic accuracy and spectrum of appearances on MR imaging. *AJR Am J Roentgenol.* 1997;169:1311–1316.
21. Radin DR. Disseminated histoplasmosis: abdominal CT findings in 16 patients. *AJR Am J Roentgenol.* 1991;157:955–958.
22. Hage CA, Knox KS, Wheat LJ. Endemic mycoses: overlooked causes of community acquired pneumonia. *Respir Med.* 2012;106:769–776.
23. Polat P, Kantarci M, Alper F, et al. Hydatid disease from head to toe. *Radiographics.* 2003;23:475–494; quiz 536–477.
24. Abbott RM, Levy AD, Aguilera NS, et al. From the archives of the AFIP: primary vascular neoplasms of the spleen: radiologic-pathologic correlation. *Radiographics.* 2004;24:1137–1163.
25. Lee H, Maeda K. Hamartoma of the spleen. *Arch Pathol Lab Med.* 2009;133:147–151.
26. Chen G, Li M, Wu D, et al. Primary splenic angiosarcoma in a 2.5-year-old boy with hepatic metastasis. *Pediatr Surg Int.* 2012;28:1147–1150.
27. Hsu JT, Ueng SH, Hwang TL, et al. Primary angiosarcoma of the spleen in a child with long-term survival. *Pediatr Surg Int.* 2007;23:807–810.
28. Kaza RK, Azar S, Al-Hawary MM, et al. Primary and secondary neoplasms of the spleen. *Cancer Imaging.* 2010;10:173–182.
29. Abramson SJ, Price AP. Imaging of pediatric lymphomas. *Radiol Clin North Am.* 2008;46:313–338, ix.
30. Rueffer U, Sieber M, Stemberg M, et al. Spleen involvement in Hodgkin's lymphoma: assessment and risk profile. *Ann Hematol.* 2003;82:390–396.

31. Punwani S, Cheung KK, Skipper N, et al. Dynamic contrast-enhanced MRI improves accuracy for detecting focal splenic involvement in children and adolescents with Hodgkin disease. *Pediatr Radiol.* 2013;43:941–949.
32. Athale UH, Kaste SC, Bodner SM, et al. Splenic rupture in children with hematologic malignancies. *Cancer.* 2000;88:480–490.
33. Lam KY, Tang V. Metastatic tumors to the spleen: a 25-year clinicopathologic study. *Arch Pathol Lab Med.* 2000;124:526–530.
34. Boscak A, Shanmuganathan K. Splenic trauma: what is new? *Radiol Clin North Am.* 2012;50:105–122.
35. Cirocchi R, Boselli C, Corsi A, et al. Is non-operative management safe and effective for all splenic blunt trauma? A systematic review. *Crit Care.* 2013;17:R185.
36. Benya EC, Lim-Dunham JE, Landrum O, et al. Abdominal sonography in examination of children with blunt abdominal trauma. *AJR Am J Roentgenol.* 2000;174:1613–1616.
37. Sivit CJ. Pediatric abdominal trauma imaging; Imaging choices and appropriateness. *Appl Radiol.* 2013:8–13.
38. Valentino M, Serra C, Pavlica P, et al. Blunt abdominal trauma: diagnostic performance of contrast-enhanced US in children—initial experience. *Radiology.* 2008;246:903–909.
39. Taylor GA, Sivit CJ. Posttraumatic peritoneal fluid: is it a reliable indicator of intraabdominal injury in children? *J Pediatr Surg.* 1995;30:1644–1648.
40. http://www.aast.org/library/traumatools/injuryscoringscales.aspx#spleen. Injury Scoring Scale. *Trauma Source*: The American Association for the Surgery of Trauma; 2013.
41. Ein S. Evidence based guidelines for children with isolated spleen or liver injury. *J Pediatr Surg.* 2005;40:1217–1218.
42. Safavi A, Beaudry P, Jamieson D, et al. Traumatic pseudoaneurysms of the liver and spleen in children: is routine screening warranted? *J Pediatr Surg.* 2011;46:938–941.
43. Jindal R, Sullivan R, Rodda B, et al. Splenic malformation in a patient with Klippel-Trenaunay syndrome: a case report. *J Vasc Surg.* 2006;43:848–850.
44. Stuart MJ, Nagel RL. Sickle-cell disease. *Lancet.* 2004;364:1343–1360.
45. Levin TL, Berdon WE, Haller JO, et al. Intrasplenic masses of "preserved" functioning splenic tissue in sickle cell disease: correlation of imaging findings (CT, ultrasound, MRI, and nuclear scintigraphy). *Pediatr Radiol.* 1996;26:646–649.
46. Da Costa L, Galimand J, Fenneteau O, et al. Hereditary spherocytosis, elliptocytosis, and other red cell membrane disorders. *Blood Rev.* 2013;27:167–178.
47. Perrotta S, Gallagher PG, Mohandas N. Hereditary spherocytosis. *Lancet.* 2008;372:1411–1426.
48. Egbert ND, Bloom DA, Dillman JR. Magnetic resonance imaging of the pediatric pancreaticobiliary system. *Magn Reson Imaging Clin N Am.* 2013;21:681–696.
49. Trout AT, Podberesky DJ, Serai SD, et al. Does secretin add value in pediatric magnetic resonance cholangiopancreatography? *Pediatr Radiol.* 2013;43:479–486.
50. Cano DA, Hebrok M, Zenker M. Pancreatic development and disease. *Gastroenterology.* 2007;132:745–762.
51. Gittes GK. Developmental biology of the pancreas: a comprehensive review. *Dev Biol.* 2009;326:4–35.
52. Nijs E, Callahan MJ, Taylor GA. Disorders of the pediatric pancreas: imaging features. *Pediatr Radiol.* 2005;35:358–373; quiz 457.
53. Heidt D, Mulholland M, Simeone D. Pancreas: anatomy and structural anomalies. In: Yamada T, ed. *Yamada's Textbook of Gastroenterology*. Hoboken: Wiley; 2009:1745–1760.
54. Borghei P, Sokhandon F, Shirkhoda A, et al. Anomalies, anatomic variants, and sources of diagnostic pitfalls in pancreatic imaging. *Radiology.* 2013;266:28–36.
55. Thoeni RF, Gedgaudas RK. Ectopic pancreas: usual and unusual features. *Gastrointest Radiol.* 1980;5:37–42.
56. Cho JS, Shin KS, Kwon ST, et al. Heterotopic pancreas in the stomach: CT findings. *Radiology.* 2000;217:139–144.
57. Kim JY, Lee JM, Kim KW, et al. Ectopic pancreas: CT findings with emphasis on differentiation from small gastrointestinal stromal tumor and leiomyoma. *Radiology.* 2009;252:92–100.
58. Zyromski NJ, Sandoval JA, Pitt HA, et al. Annular pancreas: dramatic differences between children and adults. *J Am Coll Surg.* 2008;206:1019–1025; discussion 1025–1017.
59. Etienne D, John A, Menias CO, et al. Annular pancreas: a review of its molecular embryology, genetic basis and clinical considerations. *Ann Anat.* 2012;194:422–428.
60. Jimenez JC, Emil S, Podnos Y, et al. Annular pancreas in children: a recent decade's experience. *J Pediatr Surg.* 2004;39:1654–1657.
61. Takuma K, Kamisawa T, Tabata T, et al. Pancreatic diseases associated with pancreas divisum. *Dig Surg.* 2010;27:144–148.
62. Kandula L, Whitcomb DC, Lowe ME. Genetic issues in pediatric pancreatitis. *Curr Gastroenterol Rep.* 2006;8:248–253.
63. Darge K, Anupindi S. Pancreatitis and the role of US, MRCP and ERCP. *Pediatr Radiol.* 2009;39(suppl 2):S153–S157.
64. Lautz TB, Chin AC, Radhakrishnan J. Acute pancreatitis in children: spectrum of disease and predictors of severity. *J Pediatr Surg.* 2011;46:1144–1149.
65. Lonergan GJ, Baker AM, Morey MK, et al. From the archives of the AFIP. Child abuse: radiologic-pathologic correlation. *Radiographics.* 2003;23:811–845.
66. Uc A. Chronic pancreatitits in children: Current knowledge in diagnosis and treatment. *J Pediatr Sci.* 2011;3:e98.
67. Manfredi R, Lucidi V, Gui B, et al. Idiopathic chronic pancreatitis in children: MR cholangiopancreatography after secretin administration. *Radiology.* 2002;224:675–682.
68. Bellin MD, Blondet JJ, Beilman GJ, et al. Predicting islet yield in pediatric patients undergoing pancreatectomy and autoislet transplantation for chronic pancreatitis. *Pediatr Diab.* 2010;11:227–234.
69. Teh SH, Pham TH, Lee A, et al. Pancreatic pseudocyst in children: the impact of management strategies on outcome. *J Pediatr Surg.* 2006;41:1889–1893.
70. Raizner A, Phatak UP, Baker K, et al. Acute necrotizing pancreatitis in children. *J Pediatr.* 2013;162:788–792.
71. Lautz TB, Turkel G, Radhakrishnan J, et al. Utility of the computed tomography severity index (Balthazar score) in children with acute pancreatitis. *J Pediatr Surg.* 2012;47:1185–1191.
72. Vujic I. Vascular complications of pancreatitis. *Radiol Clin North Am.* 1989;27:81–91.
73. Hruban RH, Pitman MB, Klimstra DS. *Tumors of the Pancreas (AFIP Atlas of Tumor Pathology; 4th Series Fascicle 6)*. Washington, DC: American Registry of Pathology; 2007.
74. Ahmed TS, Chavhan GB, Navarro OM, et al. Imaging features of pancreatic tumors in children: 13-year experience at a pediatric tertiary hospital. *Pediatr Radiol.* 2013;43:1435–1443.
75. Park M, Koh KN, Kim BE, et al. Pancreatic neoplasms in childhood and adolescence. *J Pediatr Hematol Oncol.* 2011;33:295–300.
76. Al-Qahtani S, Gudinchet F, Laswed T, et al. Solid pseudopapillary tumor of the pancreas in children: typical radiological findings and pathological correlation. *Clin Imaging.* 2010;34:152–156.

77. Cantisani V, Mortele KJ, Levy A, et al. MR imaging features of solid pseudopapillary tumor of the pancreas in adult and pediatric patients. *AJR Am J Roentgenol.* 2003;181:395–401.
78. Arellano CM, Kritsaneepaiboon S, Lee EY. CT Imaging findings of malignant neoplasms arising in the epigastric region in children. *Clin Imaging.* 2011;35:10–20.
79. Bien E, Godzinski J, Dall'igna P, et al. Pancreatoblastoma: a report from the European cooperative study group for paediatric rare tumours (EXPeRT). *Eur J Cancer.* 2011;47:2347–2352.
80. Chung EM, Travis MD, Conran RM. Pancreatic tumors in children: radiologic-pathologic correlation. *Radiographics.* 2006;26:1211–1238.
81. Chung EM, Travis MD, Conran RM. From the archives of the AFIP—pancreatic tumors in children: Radiologic-Pathologic correlation. *Radiographics.* 2006;26:1211–1238.
82. Rufini V, Calcagni ML, Baum RP. Imaging of neuroendocrine tumors. *Semin Nucl Med.* 2006;36:228–247.
83. Merkle EM, Bender GN, Brambs HJ. Imaging findings in pancreatic lymphoma: differential aspects. *AJR Am J Roentgenol.* 2000;174:671–675.
84. Vaughn DD, Jabra AA, Fishman EK. Pancreatic disease in children and young adults: evaluation with CT. *Radiographics.* 1998;18:1171–1187.
85. Bronstein MN, Sokol RJ, Abman SH, et al. Pancreatic insufficiency, growth, and nutrition in infants identified by newborn screening as having cystic fibrosis. *J Pediatr.* 1992;120:533–540.
86. Chaudry G, Navarro OM, Levine DS, et al. Abdominal manifestations of cystic fibrosis in children. *Pediatr Radiol.* 2006;36:233–240.
87. Agrons GA, Corse WR, Markowitz RI, et al. Gastrointestinal manifestations of cystic fibrosis: radiologic-pathologic correlation. *Radiographics.* 1996;16:871–893.
88. Shwachman H, Diamond LK, Oski FA, et al. The syndrome of pancreatic insufficiency and bone marrow dysfunction. *J Pediatr.* 1964;65:645–663.
89. Burroughs L, Woolfrey A, Shimamura A. Shwachman-Diamond syndrome: a review of the clinical presentation, molecular pathogenesis, diagnosis, and treatment. *Hematol Oncol Clin North Am.* 2009;23:233–248.
90. Berrocal T, Simon MJ, al-Assir I, et al. Shwachman-Diamond syndrome: clinical, radiological and sonographic findings. *Pediatr Radiol.* 1995;25:356–359.
91. Lonser RR, Glenn GM, Walther M, et al. von Hippel-Lindau disease. *Lancet.* 2003;361:2059–2067.
92. Choyke PL, Glenn GM, Walther MM, et al. von Hippel-Lindau disease: genetic, clinical, and imaging features. *Radiology.* 1995;194:629–642.
93. Hough DM, Stephens DH, Johnson CD, et al. Pancreatic lesions in von Hippel-Lindau disease: prevalence, clinical significance, and CT findings. *AJR Am J Roentgenol.* 1994;162:1091–1094.
94. Whitington PF. Gestational alloimmune liver disease and neonatal hemochromatosis. *Semin Liver Dis.* 2012;32:325–332.
95. Hayes AM, Jaramillo D, Levy HL, et al. Neonatal hemochromatosis: diagnosis with MR imaging. *AJR Am J Roentgenol.* 1992;159:623–625.
96. Jacombs AS, Wines M, Holland A, et al. Pancreatic trauma in children. *J Pediatr Surg.* 2004;39:96–99.
97. Houben CH, Ade-Ajayi N, Patel S, et al. Traumatic pancreatic duct injury in children: minimally invasive approach to management. *J Pediatr Surg.* 2007;42:629–635.
98. http://www.aast.org/library/traumatools/injuryscoringscales.aspx#pancreas. Injury Scoring Scale. *Trauma Source*: The American Association for the Surgery of Trauma; 2013.
99. Sivit CJ, Eichelberger MR, Taylor GA, et al. Blunt pancreatic trauma in children: CT diagnosis. *AJR Am J Roentgenol.* 1992;158:1097–1100.
100. Paul MD, Mooney DP. The management of pancreatic injuries in children: operate or observe. *J Pediatr Surg.* 2011;46:1140–1143.
101. Barwick TD, Malhotra A, Webb JA, et al. Embryology of the adrenal glands and its relevance to diagnostic imaging. *Clin Radiol.* 2005;60:953–959.
102. Mitty HA. Embryology, anatomy, and anomalies of the adrenal gland. *Semin Roentgenol.* 1988;23:271–279.
103. Avila NA, Premkumar A, Merke DP. Testicular adrenal rest tissue in congenital adrenal hyperplasia: comparison of MR imaging and sonographic findings. *AJR Am J Roentgenol.* 1999;172:1003–1006.
104. Silverman PM, Carroll BA, Moskowitz PS. Adrenal sonography in renal agenesis and dysplasia. *AJR Am J Roentgenol.* 1980;134:600–602.
105. Shafaie FF, Katz ME, Hannaway CD. A horseshoe adrenal gland in an infant with asplenia. *Pediatr Radiol.* 1997;27:591–593.
106. Strouse PJ, Haller JO, Berdon WE, et al. Horseshoe adrenal gland in association with asplenia: presentation of six new cases and review of the literature. *Pediatr Radiol.* 2002;32:778–782.
107. Dutton RV. Wolman's disease. Ultrasound and CT diagnosis. *Pediatr Radiol.* 1985;15:144–146.
108. Ozmen MN, Aygun N, Kilic I, et al. Wolman's disease: ultrasonographic and computed tomographic findings. *Pediatr Radiol.* 1992;22:541–542.
109. Kawashima A, Sandler CM, Fishman EK, et al. Spectrum of CT findings in nonmalignant disease of the adrenal gland. *Radiographics.* 1998;18:393–412.
110. Morrison SC, Comisky E, Fletcher BD. Calcification in the adrenal glands associated with disseminated herpes simplex infection. *Pediatr Radiol.* 1988;18:240–241.
111. Agrons GA, Lonergan GJ, Dickey GE, et al. Adrenocortical neoplasms in children: radiologic-pathologic correlation. *Radiographics.* 1999;19:989–1008.
112. McHugh K. Renal and adrenal tumours in children. *Cancer Imaging.* 2007;7:41–51.
113. Michalkiewicz E, Sandrini R, Figueiredo B, et al. Clinical and outcome characteristics of children with adrenocortical tumors: a report from the International Pediatric Adrenocortical Tumor Registry. *J Clin Oncol.* 2004;22:838–845.
114. Klein JD, Turner CG, Gray FL, et al. Adrenal cortical tumors in children: factors associated with poor outcome. *J Pediatr Surg.* 2011;46:1201–1207.
115. Brisse HJ, McCarville MB, Granata C, et al. Guidelines for imaging and staging of neuroblastic tumors: consensus report from the International Neuroblastoma Risk Group Project. *Radiology.* 2011;261:243–257.
116. McCarville MB. Imaging neuroblastoma: what the radiologist needs to know. *Cancer Imaging.* 2011;11(Spec No A):S44–S47.
117. Mueller WP, Coppenrath E, Pfluger T. Nuclear medicine and multimodality imaging of pediatric neuroblastoma. *Pediatr Radiol.* 2013;43:418–427.
118. Sharp SE, Gelfand MJ, Shulkin BL. Pediatrics: diagnosis of neuroblastoma. *Semin Nucl Med.* 2011;41:345–353.

119. Brodeur GM, Pritchard J, Berthold F, et al. Revisions of the international criteria for neuroblastoma diagnosis, staging, and response to treatment. *J Clin Oncol.* 1993;11:1466–1477
120. Monclair T, Brodeur GM, Ambros PF, et al. The International Neuroblastoma Risk Group (INRG) staging system: an INRG Task Force report. *J Clin Oncol.* 2009;27:298–303.
121. Brunklaus A, Pohl K, Zuberi SM, et al. Investigating neuroblastoma in childhood opsoclonus-myoclonus syndrome. *Arch Dis Child.* 2012;97:461–463.
122. Shimada H, Ambros IM, Dehner LP, et al. Terminology and morphologic criteria of neuroblastic tumors: recommendations by the International Neuroblastoma Pathology Committee. *Cancer.* 1999;86:349–363.
123. Nour-Eldin NE, Abdelmonem O, Tawfik AM, et al. Pediatric primary and metastatic neuroblastoma: MRI findings: pictorial review. *Magn Reson Imaging.* 2012;30:893–906.
124. Gahr N, Darge K, Hahn G, et al. Diffusion-weighted MRI for differentiation of neuroblastoma and ganglioneuroblastoma/ganglioneuroma. *Eur J Radiol.* 2011;79:443–446.
125. Goo HW. Whole-body MRI of neuroblastoma. *Eur J Radiol.* 2010;75:306–314.
126. Siegel MJ, Acharyya S, Hoffer FA, et al. Whole-body MR imaging for staging of malignant tumors in pediatric patients: results of the American College of Radiology Imaging Network 6660 Trial. *Radiology.* 2013;266:599–609.
127. Forman HP, Leonidas JC, Berdon WE, et al. Congenital neuroblastoma: evaluation with multimodality imaging. *Radiology.* 1990;175:365–368.
128. Lonergan GJ, Schwab CM, Suarez ES, et al. Neuroblastoma, ganglioneuroblastoma, and ganglioneuroma: radiologic-pathologic correlation. *Radiographics.* 2002;22:911–934.
129. DuBois SG, Matthay KK. 131I-Metaiodobenzylguanidine therapy in children with advanced neuroblastoma. *Q J Nucl Med Mol Imaging.* 2013;57:53–65.
130. Waguespack SG, Rich T, Grubbs E, et al. A current review of the etiology, diagnosis, and treatment of pediatric pheochromocytoma and paraganglioma. *J Clin Endocrinol Metab.* 2010;95:2023–2037.
131. Bittman ME, Lee EY, Restrepo R, et al. Focal adrenal lesions in pediatric patients. *AJR Am J Roentgenol.* 2013;200: W542–W556.
132. van der Harst E, de Herder WW, Bruining HA, et al. [(123)I] metaiodobenzylguanidine and [(111)In]octreotide uptake in benign and malignant pheochromocytomas. *J Clin Endocrinol Metab.* 2001;86:685–693.
133. Gatcombe HG, Assikis V, Kooby D, et al. Primary retroperitoneal teratomas: a review of the literature. *J Surg Oncol.* 2004;86:107–113.
134. Davidson AJ, Hartman DS, Goldman SM. Mature teratoma of the retroperitoneum: radiologic, pathologic, and clinical correlation. *Radiology.* 1989;172:421–425.
135. Gabal-Shehab L, Alagiri M. Traumatic adrenal injuries. *J Urol.* 2005;173:1330–1331.
136. Sivit CJ, Ingram JD, Taylor GA, et al. Posttraumatic adrenal hemorrhage in children: CT findings in 34 patients. *AJR Am J Roentgenol.* 1992;158:1299–1302.
137. Kawashima A, Sandler CM, Ernst RD, et al. Imaging of nontraumatic hemorrhage of the adrenal gland. *Radiographics.* 1999;19:949–963.
138. Elsayes KM, Mukundan G, Narra VR, et al. Adrenal masses: MR imaging features with pathologic correlation. *Radiographics.* 2004;24(suppl 1):S73–S86.
139. Speiser PW, White PC. Congenital adrenal hyperplasia. *N Engl J Med.* 2003;349:776–788.
140. Merke DP, Bornstein SR. Congenital adrenal hyperplasia. *Lancet.* 2005;365:2125–2136.
141. Nermoen I, Rorvik J, Holmedal SH, et al. High frequency of adrenal myelolipomas and testicular adrenal rest tumours in adult Norwegian patients with classical congenital adrenal hyperplasia because of 21-hydroxylase deficiency. *Clin Endocrinol (Oxf).* 2011;75:753–759.
142. German-Mena E, Zibari GB, Levine SN. Adrenal myelolipomas in patients with congenital adrenal hyperplasia: review of the literature and a case report. *Endocr Pract.* 2011; 17:441–447.

CHAPTER 16

Gastrointestinal Tract

Sudha A. Anupindi • Andria M. Powers • Suma Kannabiran • Jonathan R. Dillman • Michael S. Gee • Asef Khwaja

INTRODUCTION

Pediatric gastrointestinal (GI) disorders include a wide spectrum of entities involving structures from the level of the esophagus to the rectum. Imaging of these structures can provide both anatomic and functional information, which can help managing pediatric patients with congenital and acquired GI disorders. In this chapter, the currently available imaging modalities used to evaluate the pediatric GI tract are reviewed. In addition, various abnormalities of the pediatric GI tract that can be encountered in clinical practice are discussed, including congenital, infectious, inflammatory, and neoplastic processes, focusing on key clinical and imaging features as well as treatment for each entity and providing a differential diagnosis where appropriate.

IMAGING TECHNIQUES

Radiography

Radiography of the chest and/or abdomen (including the pelvis) is the most simple, least expensive, and most widely available imaging examination performed in children presenting with signs and symptoms related to the GI tract, such as dysphagia, chest pain, abdominal pain, or constipation. Although often insensitive, radiographs in some settings can be very specific.

Abdominal radiographs should be appropriately collimated and have a technique (e.g., tube current, tube potential, exposure time) that enables one to clearly visualize the bowel gas pattern, intraperitoneal free air (when present), and viscera. When performing abdominal radiography, two views (commonly supine frontal and cross-table lateral radiographs in young children) are often acquired. Cross-table lateral, decubitus, and upright radiographs of the abdomen help assess for air–fluid levels within the bowel as well as intraperitoneal free air, which can be easily overlooked on supine frontal views. Cross-table lateral radiography is particularly useful in very ill children who cannot tolerate decubitus or upright imaging, with intraperitoneal free air, when present, accumulating anteriorly within the abdomen, often anterior to the liver.

Abdominal radiography is especially helpful when assessing for bowel obstruction, thereby helping localize the obstructing process to the upper or lower GI tract. In the postoperative setting, radiographs can evaluate for a variety of complications as well as provide clues to what surgery has been performed (in the absence of such knowledge). In the setting of suspected or known ingested foreign body, radiographs of the chest and/or abdomen can be obtained to further characterize the ingested object (if radiopaque), establish its location in the GI tract and potential complications, and guide management.

Fluoroscopy

Fluoroscopy is still widely used to assess the pediatric GI tract because of its diagnostic capabilities, availability, and relative low cost compared to computed tomography (CT) and magnetic resonance imaging (MRI). Fluoroscopic studies of the GI tract require administration of an enteric contrast material; common contrast agents used in children include barium, water-soluble iodinated contrast material, and air. Barium can be used to assess most conditions, whereas water-soluble iodinated contrast materials (such as iohexol, a low-osmolality iodinated contrast material that is commonly administered intravenously for CT, or iothalamate meglumine) are usually employed in cases where bowel perforation is of concern, such as in the setting of acute trauma or the recent postoperative child. Dilute hyperosmolar iodinated contrast materials, such as diatrizoate meglumine and diatrizoate sodium, are less often used in current practice and are reserved for cases where therapeutic cleanout is desired (e.g., in adolescents with cystic fibrosis and distal intestinal obstruction). Hyperosmolar contrast agents have the potential to cause fluid shifts and electrolyte imbalances, and thus should be used with caution. Oral administration of hyperosmolar contrast agents can also cause severe pulmonary complications (e.g., chemical pneumonitis or pulmonary edema) in children if aspirated and should probably be avoided. Instead, a low-osmolality iodinated contrast material should be considered.

In general, low-dose fluoroscopic techniques in accordance with the As Low As Reasonably Achievable (ALARA) principle should always be utilized. This includes (1) using pulse fluoroscopy; (2) maximizing collimation; (3) minimizing magnification; (4) keeping the image intensifier close to the patient; (5) using as little fluoroscopy time as possible to answer the specific clinical question at hand; and (6) minimizing the number of true radiographic exposures and instead using last image capture technique that sufficiently evaluates many conditions.[1] With current generation fluoroscopy systems, last image capture technique can also be used to grab multiple images and document dynamic processes, such as GI tract motility.

Esophagography

The esophagram is a focused examination evaluating the anatomy and motility of the esophagus from the level of the hypopharynx through the proximal stomach, including the gastroesophageal (GE) junction. Typical clinical indications for performing esophagography in the pediatric population include evaluation of suspected or known vascular rings and sling, tracheoesophageal fistula (TEF), dysphagia, and foreign body. This study is also frequently used to evaluate the postoperative appearance of the esophagus, most often following TEF (esophageal atresia) repair.

Esophagography is performed by having the patient drink oral contrast material by cup, syringe, or bottle and acquiring fluoroscopic images in the lateral, oblique, and supine positions. When there is high suspicion for N (also known as H)-type TEF, a pull-back esophagram can be performed by placing a feeding tube into the stomach and gradually pulling back the tube and simultaneously injecting contrast material under direct visualization.[2] However, care should be taken to not inject contrast material too high within the esophagus or too vigorously, as tracheal aspiration can occur. This can be sometimes mistaken for an N-type TEF. It is important to provide measurements of areas of narrowing, including stricture length and minimum luminal diameter. Occasionally, in older children, swallowed barium tablets may be used to estimate of the size of the esophageal lumen.

Upper Gastrointestinal Series and Small Bowel Follow-Through

Esophagography is often followed by assessment of the stomach and duodenum as part of the same examination; this can be referred to as an upper gastrointestinal (UGI) series. UGI series may also refer to evaluation of the stomach and duodenum when contrast material is delivered directly into the stomach through a gastrostomy tube or nasogastric tube. Typical clinical indications for the UGI series in the pediatric population include the following: (1) vomiting including suspected malrotation with volvulus, gastric outlet obstruction, and duodenal/proximal jejunal obstruction; (2) assessment of upper GI tract anatomy prior to gastrostomy tube placement; and (3) evaluation of gastric emptying and suspected gastroesophageal reflux although other diagnostic tests may be more sensitive for these conditions.

Common UGI series images include the following: (1) supine frontal and left lateral decubitus views of the esophagus; (2) supine and oblique views of the stomach; and (3) right lateral decubitus imaging of the distal stomach and duodenum. Lateral imaging is used to confirm a normal retroperitoneal course of the second through fourth portions of the duodenum, just anterior to the spine. Finally, the child is placed supine to capture the location of the duodenojejunal junction (DJJ), which is normally positioned just to the left of the spine and at the level of the duodenum bulb.

In recent years, although the small bowel follow-through (SBFT) examination largely has been replaced by CT and MRI (cross-sectional enterography), particularly in the evaluation of known or suspected inflammatory bowel disease (IBD), it is still a useful study in the pediatric population. Typical clinical indications for SBFT in children include evaluation of obstruction, feeding intolerance, dysmotility/small bowel transit time, polyposis syndrome, and suspected malabsorption syndrome. This study requires enteric contrast material to be orally ingested by the child or administered through a gastrostomy tube or nasogastric tube. Multiple radiographic images are then acquired (typically at 30- to 60-minute intervals) as contrast material passes through the small bowel until it reaches the proximal colon. Compressive fluoroscopic spot images may also beneficial in some children, especially when there is concern for small bowel polyps or Crohn disease. Occasionally, in the inpatient setting, markedly delayed portable radiographs may provide additional value when assessing dysmotility/small bowel transit time and obstruction.

Contrast Enema

Typical clinical indications for performing a contrast enema in the pediatric population include the following: (1) evaluation of obstruction including distal GI tract obstruction in neonates and post–necrotizing enterocolitis strictures; (2) therapeutic clean-out of colonic fecal material, and (3) ileocolic intussusception reduction. Single-contrast technique is generally sufficient in the large majority of children, with double-contrast technique only very rarely performed. When a colonic polyp (e.g., symptomatic juvenile polyp) is suspected, assessment may include contrast enema, CT, and/or colonoscopy.[3] In the setting of neonatal distal GI tract obstruction, water-soluble iodinated contrast material (such as iothalamate meglumine) is preferred because there is slightly increased risk of bowel perforation. Air is preferred by many institutions for identifying and reducing ileocolic intussusceptions.[4]

The contrast enema should be started with the child in the left lateral decubitus position with the tip of the catheter in the lower rectum. Contrast material is delivered into the colon via gravity drip. After fluoroscopic imaging the rectum in the lateral position, supine frontal and oblique images are generally acquired along the course of the colon to the level of the cecum and appendix. Reflux of contrast material into the terminal ileum occurs in some children and can help evaluate the distal small bowel. Imaging with compression can sometimes help further characterize focal abnormalities.

Other Special Fluoroscopy Examinations

Fistulography and ostomy studies performed to assess complex GI anatomy (e.g., in the setting of cloacal and anorectal malformations) require careful review of the child's medical and surgical history to determine the exact imaging procedure to be performed. These studies often serve as a road map for the surgeon prior to definitive surgical treatment. Therefore, it is generally helpful for the radiologist and surgeon to directly communicate prior to the study. These studies are performed using water-soluble iodinated contrast materials such as iothalamate meglumine. When there is concern for a fistula (e.g., between the rectum and genitourinary tract), actual radiographic exposures (in addition to captured images) may provide added value because of increased image detail.

Ultrasound

Ultrasound is a well-established first-line imaging study for evaluation of hypertrophic pyloric stenosis (HPS), appendicitis, and ileocolic intussusception. There is also increasing literature supporting the use of this imaging modality for assessment of children with known or suspected IBD, because it has numerous advantages compared to CT and MRI, including lower cost, no need for sedation/general anesthesia, and no ionizing radiation (when compared specifically to CT).[5,6]

Linear high-frequency (9 to 18 MHz) transducers provide high-resolution gray-scale images of the pediatric GI tract. Cine, panoramic, and color and power Doppler techniques are also important for assessing the pediatric GI tract. When imaging larger children or when bowel loops are located well posterior to the anterior abdominal wall, lower-frequency curved transducers can be used to improve visualization. Graded compression technique allows improved visualization of both the small and large bowel as well as the appendix by displacing/effacing overlying bowel loops and bringing abnormal bowel closer to the transducer[7]; abnormal bowel segments (e.g., the appendix when inflamed, terminal ileitis in Crohn disease) are often noncompressible and become readily apparent.

A systematic approach to scanning is helpful when evaluating the bowel (e.g., for intussusception or IBD). When a gastroduodenal abnormality is suspected, the patient can drink water to distend and improve visualization of the stomach and duodenum.[5,8] Intravenous ultrasound microbubble contrast agents have been shown to be safe when used in children; however, the availability of contrast-enhanced ultrasound is currently limited in the United States.[9]

Computed Tomography

Typical clinical reasons for CT imaging of the abdominopelvic GI tract in the pediatric population include the following: bowel and mesenteric injury in the setting of acute trauma, bowel obstruction, tumor involving the bowel, concern for postoperative complication following intestinal surgery, and suspected or known intestinal infection/inflammation. Intravenous and oral contrast materials are often valuable and are typically used by most institutions unless specifically contraindicated. Positive (high attenuation) oral contrast material is appropriate for most indications, with one notable exception being acute trauma where time is critical. In the setting of acute bowel obstruction, children may not tolerate oral contrast material, and this is generally not a major issue as obstructed bowel is frequently already distended with fluid. CT enterography (CTE) requires a neutral (attenuation near water) oral contrast material that allows improved visualization of bowel wall/mucosal postcontrast hyperenhancment. CTE technique in children has been described in multiple publications[10,11]

Pediatric CT scans of the abdomen and pelvis are typically performed using helical technique in order to acquire an isotropic data set that enables a variety of 2D multiplanar reformations (and 3D reconstructions, if indicated). Similar to fluoroscopy, the ALARA principle should be closely followed when performing pediatric CT. This includes using the lowest tube current (mA) and tube potential (kVp) possible. Recent advances in CT technology, including tube current modulation and iterative image reconstruction techniques, have substantially lowered CT doses while maintaining image quality.[12] In special select cases, CT colonography (which includes colonic air insufflation and intravenous contrast material) can be performed safely in children to assess for colonic polyps and masses.[3]

Magnetic Resonance Imaging

MRI of the GI tract, or MR enterography (MRE), has become a primary imaging modality for evaluating children with known or suspected IBD. MRE can also be used for other indications, such as polyp detection, tumor evaluation, and assessment of non-IBD inflammatory processes.[13] Similar to CTE, MRE requires that children drink a substantial volume of biphasic (T1-weighted hypointense/T2-weighted hyperintense) oral contrast material as well as receive intravenous contrast material (gadolinium chelate). Typical MRI pulse sequences used to image the bowel include single-shot fast spin-echo, balanced steady-state free precession, and postcontrast T1-weighted 3D gradient-recalled echo.[13]

Advantages of MRE versus CTE include lack of ionizing radiation and superior soft tissue contrast resolution. Disadvantages of MRE versus CTE and ultrasound include longer scan times, artifacts due to patient motion/breathing and bowel peristalsis, and the regular need for sedation/general anesthesia. A variety of techniques are available that decrease artifacts related to breathing and motion, including respiratory triggering (or navigator gating) and radial filling of k-space.[14] Antispasmolytic medications (e.g., glucagon) can reduce bowel peristalsis.[15] Recently, MRI also has been used to image suspected appendicitis as an alternative to CT, especially when ultrasound is nondiagnostic or equivocal. MRI for appendicitis can be performed with or without intravenous contrast material, and it has high sensitivity and specificity.[16]

Nuclear Medicine

A variety of nuclear medicine studies are currently available and can be used to assess the pediatric GI tract. Radiopharmaceutical doses should be adjusted for patient size (e.g., weight), in accordance with published guidelines. Similar to fluoroscopy and CT, the ALARA principle should be closely followed with patient exposure to radiation kept to a minimum while maintaining diagnostic quality.

Radionuclide Salivagram

The radionuclide salivagram shows the flow of saliva from the mouth to the stomach and can be used to identify tracheal (pulmonary) aspiration. This imaging test is a particularly effective tool for identifying aspiration of oral contents and can provide complementary information to the more frequently performed videofluoroscopic swallowing study.[17] During this study, the child is positioned supine and a tiny amount of water (or saline) mixed ^{99m}Tc-labeled sulfur colloid is placed in the mouth. Imaging of the neck, chest, and upper abdomen is performed for ~1 hour. Any radioactivity seen in the lungs, bronchi, or trachea is abnormal and considered evidence of aspiration.

Gastroesophageal Reflux Scintigraphy

Gastroesophageal reflux can be detected with higher sensitivity than UGI series using scintigraphy. During this study, ^{99m}Tc-labeled sulfur colloid is delivered into the stomach after the radionuclide is mixed with breast milk, formula, or other meal and ingested. Then, supine imaging of the chest and upper abdomen is performed for ~30 minutes. Any radioactivity seen in the expected location of the esophagus is considered evidence of gastroesophageal reflux, and the number of episodes can be counted.[18,19]

Gastric Emptying Scintigraphy

Scintigraphy is considered the gold standard for the assessment of gastric emptying.[20] Gastric emptying scintigraphy technique varies across institutions. After an NPO period of several hours, patients are asked to ingest a liquid or solid meal mixed with ^{99m}Tc-labeled sulfur colloid. Imaging of the upper abdomen in the left anterior oblique position is performed for ~90 to 120 minutes. A computer program is used to quantify gastric emptying, including generation of time–radioactivity curves from the region of the stomach and calculation of gastric emptying half-time (time required for 50% of radioactivity to leave the stomach).[20]

Meckel Scan

Pertechnetate scintigraphy (Meckel scan) is generally considered the test of choice for evaluating the child with unexplained GI tract bleeding due to a suspected Meckel diverticulum. Meckel diverticula are remnants of the omphalomesenteric duct that commonly accumulate ^{99m}Tc-pertechnetate because of the presence of gastric mucosa. These structures characteristically appear at the same time gastric mucosa is visualized, and are seen as a focally increased area of radioactivity in the lower abdomen usually in the right lower quadrant. Following the intravenous injection of radionuclide, supine imaging is performed for 30 to 60 minutes. Dynamic and static (including lateral imaging) images are usually acquired. With the advent of single photon emission computed tomography differentiating a true Meckel diverticulum from artifact is possible. The sensitivity of pertechnetate scintigraphy for Meckel diverticulum detection is ~85%.[21]

Gastrointestinal Bleeding Scan

GI bleeding scan can be used to evaluate active bleeding from the lower pediatric GI tract. A small aliquot of the child's own blood is labeled with Tc-99m and reinjected into the patient. A dynamic perfusion study can be performed during the first 1 minute after reinjection of labeled red blood cells, followed by static images every few minutes for 30 to 60 minutes. A positive scan shows abnormal radioactivity emanating from the area of active bleeding conforming to a bowel segment. Delayed imaging also can be performed up to 24 hours after reinjection if initial images are unrevealing and GI tract bleeding continues.[19] This test helps by quickly localizing the area of bleeding, which can guide the endoscopist or angiographer to target diagnosis and treatment.

NORMAL ANATOMY

Esophagus

The esophagus is a muscular tube arising from the foregut that extends from the C7 to T10–T11 vertebral levels. The upper one-third contains striated muscle and is innervated by the vagus nerve, and the lower two-thirds contains smooth muscle and is innervated by the splanchnic plexus. The esophagus normally has smooth mucosa and lacks an outer serosa. There are two esophageal sphincters (upper and lower, respectively); the lower sphincter tends to be immature in infants and contributes to gastroesophageal reflux. The descending thoracic aorta and left mainstem bronchus normally have mild mass effect upon the esophagus that can be appreciated at esophagography. Blood supply to the esophagus is provided by branches of the inferior thyroid, bronchial, left gastric, and left phrenic arteries as well as esophageal branches of the thoracic aorta. Periesophageal and submucosal venous plexi provide venous drainage.

Stomach

The stomach also arises from the foregut and is made up of five major parts: cardia, fundus, body, antrum, and pylorus. The cardia is a small portion of the stomach located near the gastroesophageal junction. The fundus is the rounded proximal portion of the stomach located below the left hemidiaphragm that also borders the spleen. The body represents the majority of the stomach and is bordered by the lesser (superiorly) and greater (inferiorly) curvatures. The distal portions of the stomach include the antrum and pylorus; the pylorus acting as a sphincter that opens allowing the stomach to empty and closes preventing small bowel contents from reentering the stomach. The stomach is held in place by four major ligaments: gastrophrenic, gastrohepatic, gastrosplenic, and gastrocolic ligaments. Primary blood supply to the stomach is via the left gastric, right gastric, gastroduodenal, and splenic arteries. Primary gastric venous drainage is via the left gastric (coronary), right gastric, and gastroepiploic veins, which all drain to the portal vein. In infants, the stomach can be horizontal, whereas in older children it can assume a J-shape. Prominent folds (rugae) make the stomach easily recognizable on UGI series, CT, and MRI.

Small Intestine

The small intestine is made up of the duodenum, jejunum and ileum. It grows from about 200 cm at birth to a total of about 600 cm (19.8 feet) into adulthood.[19] The duodenum is very short in length and is derived from both the foregut and midgut. It has a characteristic c-shape and is composed of four portions. The first portion of the duodenum includes the duodenal bulb and extends from the pylorus to the level of the gallbladder. The second or descending portion of the duodenum is located just lateral to the pancreatic head and includes the major ampulla that drains pancreaticobiliary ducts. The third or horizontal portion of the duodenum normally crosses from right to left just anterior to the spine, whereas the fourth or ascending portion extends to the DJJ, where the small bowel should be fixed by the ligament of Treitz. The second through fourth portions of the duodenum should be retroperitoneal in location. Primary blood supply to the duodenum is via the gastroduodenal and pancreaticoduodenal arteries.

The jejunum makes up about 40% of the small bowel, whereas the more distal ileum composes the remainder. The jejunum is most often located in the left upper quadrant of the abdomen, although in some children it may reside in the right upper quadrant (this is normal as long as the ligament of Treitz is appropriately located). The jejunum has visible circular folds, so-called valvulae conniventes, which often have a feathery appearance at ultrasound, SBFT, CT, and MRI. At CT and MRI, it is common for the jejunum to enhance more than ileum. The ileum is primarily located in the lower abdomen and pelvis before ending in the right lower quadrant as the terminal ileum. Normal ileum appears relatively featureless. The primary blood supply to the small bowel is via the superior mesenteric artery (SMA). Mesenteric arterial branches anastomose to form a complex vascular arcade that eventually terminates as the vasa recta. Small bowel venous drainage is via portal venous system (superior mesenteric vein).

Colon

The colon arises from both the midgut and hindgut, and it has multiple segments, including cecum, ascending colon, transverse, descending colon, and sigmoid colon. It grows from about 30 to 40 cm at birth to about 150 cm by adulthood.[19] The most proximal portion of the colon, the cecum, is normally located in the right lower quadrant and may be mobile in infants. The appendix arises from the cecum, varies in length, and blind ends. Three longitudinal bands of smooth muscle (taeniae coli) extend from the cecum to the sigmoid colon and are responsible for colonic sacculations called haustra. Numerous peritoneum-lined fat and blood vessel–containing pouches called epiploic appendages line much of the colon. The colon takes two 90 degree bends called flexures, the hepatic flexure in the right upper quadrant and the splenic flexure in the left upper quadrant. The ascending and descending portions of the colon are retroperitoneal in location, whereas the appendix, cecum, transverse, and sigmoid colon are intraperitoneal and have mesenteries. Blood supply to the colon is provided by the right and middle colic branches of the SMA as well as by the left colic artery, which arises from the inferior mesenteric artery (IMA). Venous drainage is via the portal venous system (superior and inferior mesenteric veins).

Rectum

The rectum is vertically oriented with the rectosigmoid junction located at approximately the level of the sacral promontory. The rectum subsequently gives rise to the anal canal about 4 cm from the anal verge.[22] Importantly, the dentate line is located within the anal canal and this undulating demarcation marks the transition from columnar to squamous epithelium.[23] The distal rectum and anal canal are extraperitoneal in location and bordered laterally by the ischiorectal fossae.[22] Rectal blood supply is via the superior rectal artery arising from the IMA and middle rectal artery arising from the internal iliac artery. Venous drainage above the dentate line is via the portal system, whereas venous drainage below the dentate line is via systemic veins.[22]

SPECTRUM OF GASTROINTESTINAL TRACT DISORDERS

Congenital and Developmental Anomalies

Esophagus

Esophageal Atresia and Tracheoesophageal Fistula

Esophageal atresia is part of a spectrum of anomalies involving the foregut that can occur either in isolation or in association with TEF. The reported incidence of esophageal atresia is about 1:3,500 births, with a slight male predominance.[24] The exact underlying cause is currently unclear, although it is thought to be due to abnormal formation and separation of primitive foregut into the esophagus and trachea,[19] perhaps because of a vascular insult. There are four types of TEF, the most common being proximal esophageal atresia with an associated fistula between the trachea and distal esophagus, occurring in nearly 85% of cases (Table 16.1). Esophageal atresia/TEF sometimes occurs in conjunction with other anomalies, such as DiGeorge syndrome or as a part of the VACTERL association (vertebral, anorectal, cardiac, tracheoesophageal, renal, and limb anomalies).

Prenatal imaging may suggest esophageal atresia based on polyhydramnios and nonvisualization of the stomach, although some affected pediatric patients present initially in the neonatal period. Presenting symptoms after birth include difficulty handling secretions, regurgitation, choking, respiratory distress, and recurrent pneumonia especially in the setting of H or N-type TEF. Radiography often reveals a distended air-filled blind-ending proximal esophagus. In addition, a nasogastric tube may be seen coiled in the proximal esophageal pouch. The presence of bowel gas confirms the presence of a TEF (Fig. 16.1). Fluoroscopic pouchogram performed by instilling a very small volume of contrast material into the proximal esophagus through an end-hole catheter can confirm esophageal atresia. It may also help to identify the presence of a proximal TEF. In addition, esophagram can be performed to identify a suspected H or N-type TEF (Fig. 16.2).

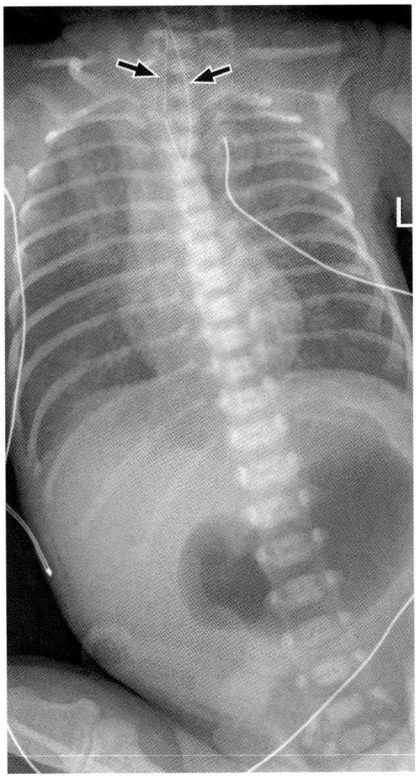

FIGURE 16.1 **Chest and abdominal radiograph in a neonate boy.** Nasogastric tube (*arrows*) is coiled in esophageal pouch, reflecting esophageal atresia. Bowel gas in the stomach indicates presence of tracheoesophageal fistula (TEF).

The current treatment is surgical, with most affected pediatric patients undergoing primary esophageal repair and TEF takedown. Gastric pull-through may be required in children

TABLE 16.1 Classification of Tracheoesophageal Fistulas

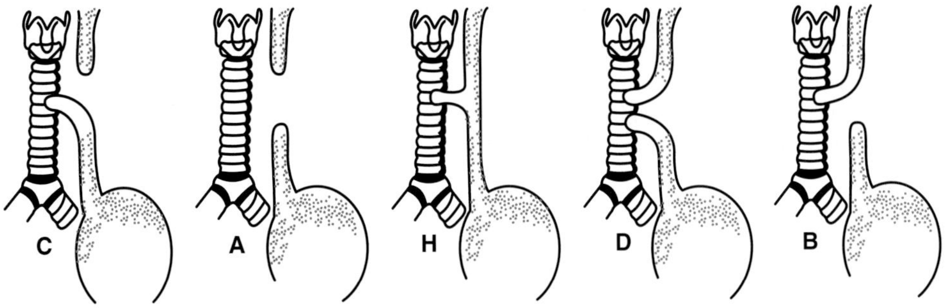

Five types of tracheoesophageal fistula (TEF). Type C, esophageal atresia with distal TEF, is the most common form of TEF, representing more than ~80% of cases. Type A refers to esophageal atresia with no TEF fistula, occurring ~6% of the time. Type H (or N) represents isolated TEF without esophageal atresia (~4%). Type D refers to esophageal atresia with both proximal and distal TEFs (~1%), and Type B represents esophageal atresia with a single proximal fistula (~1%–5%).

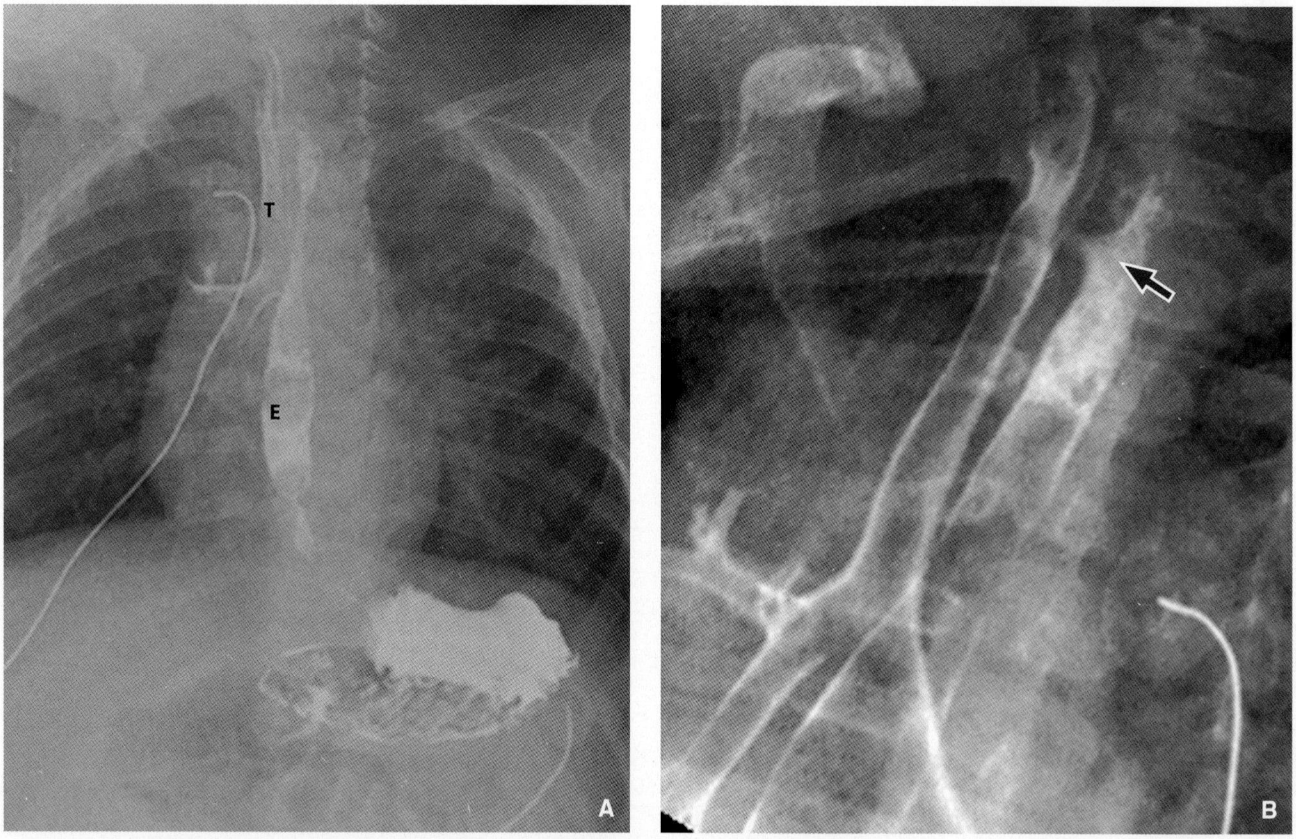

FIGURE 16.2 **Esophagram showing a tracheoesophageal fistula in a newborn girl. A:** Frontal esophagram view shows barium contrast material filling esophagus (*E*), distal trachea (*T*), and right bronchi. **B:** Magnified image better depicts the linear H (or N) type communication (*arrow*) between esophagus and trachea, which fills with contrast material.

with long-gap esophageal atresia. Prognosis depends on the length of the atretic esophageal segment and presence of other congenital abnormalities.[25] Anastomotic esophageal strictures are common and can be readily identified by esophagography.

Esophageal Duplication Cyst

Esophageal duplication cysts are the second most common GI tract duplication anomaly, after ileal duplication cysts.[26] These cysts most often arise from the mid- to lower portion of the esophagus[26] and contain foregut-derived tissues. Esophageal duplication anomalies are most often cystic, presenting as eccentric round or spherical (and less often tubular) lesions in or adjacent to the esophageal wall.[27] Histologically, these lesions typically have a muscular wall and can be lined by a variety of types of epithelium.[28] Although commonly asymptomatic and incidentally detected, some affected children may report dysphagia or other symptoms including chest pain and respiratory distress.

At radiography, esophageal duplication cysts either are imperceptible or appear as middle or posterior mediastinal masses. Esophagography may reveal an intramural mass or extrinsic mass effect upon the esophagus; these anomalies rarely communicate with the esophageal lumen. If visible at ultrasound, esophageal duplication cysts appear as discrete cystic masses with a layered wall.[19] At CT, they are circumscribed, homogeneous, near-water attenuation lesions lacking postcontrast enhancement associated with the esophageal wall[27] (Fig. 16.3). At MRI, they are usually thin-walled, hypointense on T1-weighted sequences and hyperintense on T2-weighted sequences, unless complicated.

Treatment, especially if symptomatic, is surgical resection.

Stomach

Agastria/Microgastria

Complete absence of the stomach, known as agastria, is extremely rare.[27] Such anomalies are frequently associated with other anomalies, including heterotaxy syndromes. Radiography can demonstrate a dilated air-filled esophagus, and the stomach bubble may or may not be seen. Microgastria is a rare developmental anomaly in which the stomach is diminutive, often having a dysmorphic tubular shape (Fig. 16.4). In the setting of microgastria, upper GI series shows a small, sometimes midline stomach with associated esophageal dilatation secondary to poor stomach capacity (Fig. 16.5). Gastroesophageal reflux is common and severe in affected pediatric patients.

Gastric Duplication Cyst

Gastric duplication cysts are rare, accounting for <10% of GI tract duplications.[19] These cysts are more common in girls, and most are located along the greater curvature.[27] Gastric

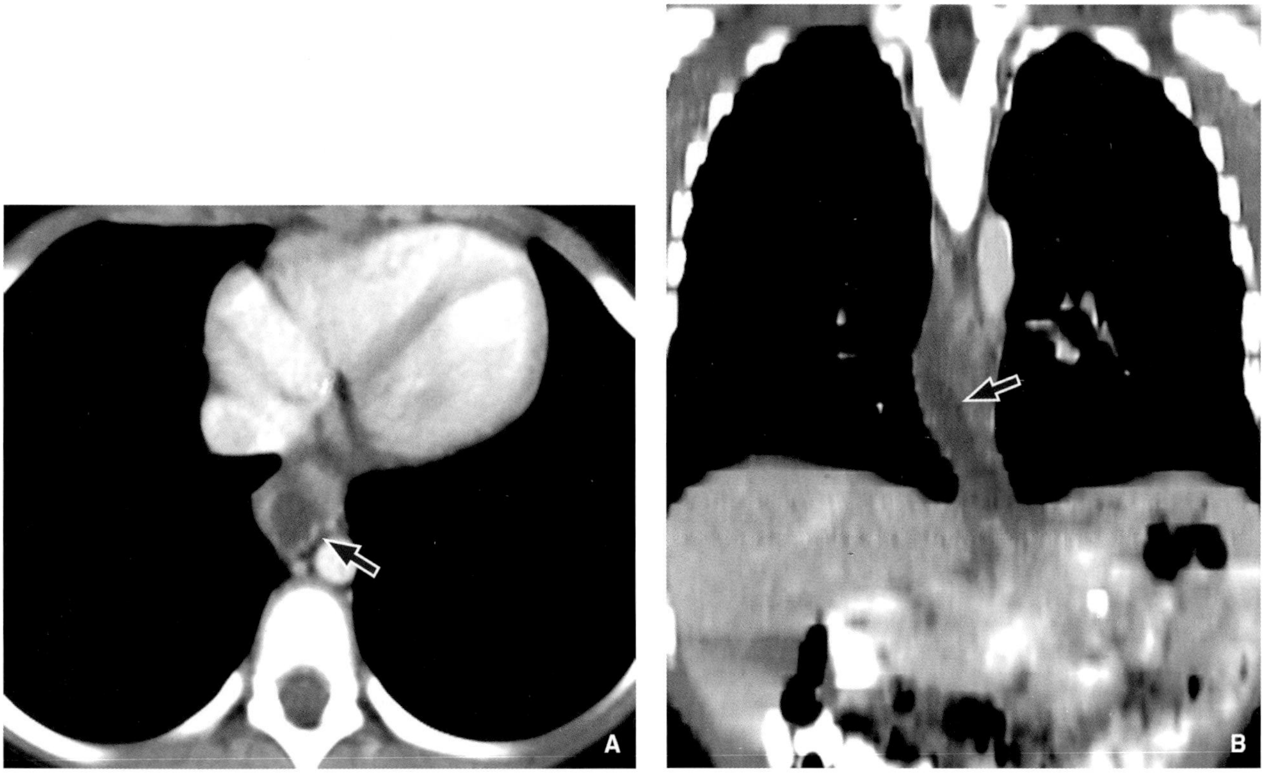

FIGURE 16.3 **Esophageal duplication cyst in an 4-month-old infant girl. A:** Axial contrast-enhanced CT image shows a well-circumscribed, fluid attenuation tubular lesion (*arrow*) adjacent to wall of the esophagus. **B:** Coronal reformatted CT image shows an elongated low-attenuation structure (*arrow*) that was surgically proven as an esophageal duplication cyst.

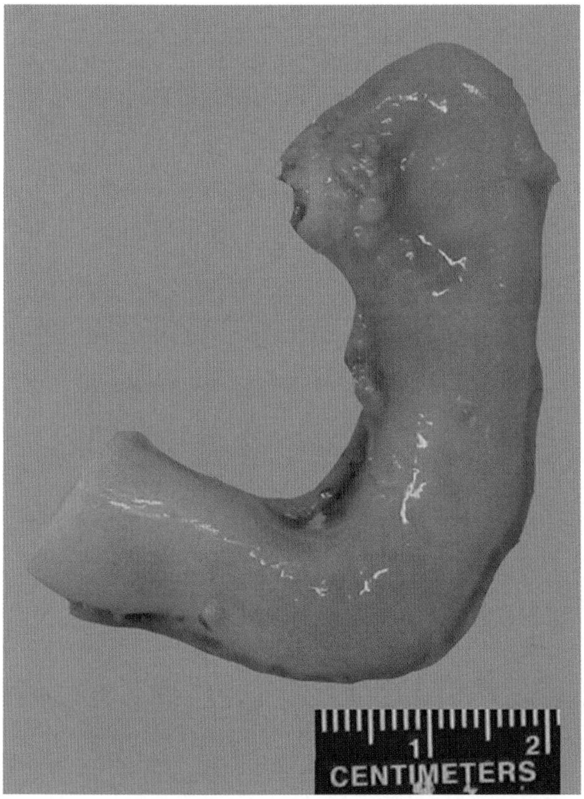

FIGURE 16.4 **Microgastria.** This severely small stomach from a 5-week-old neonate girl who presented with multiple congenital anomalies shows a markedly narrowed antrum, characteristic of a "tubular stomach.")

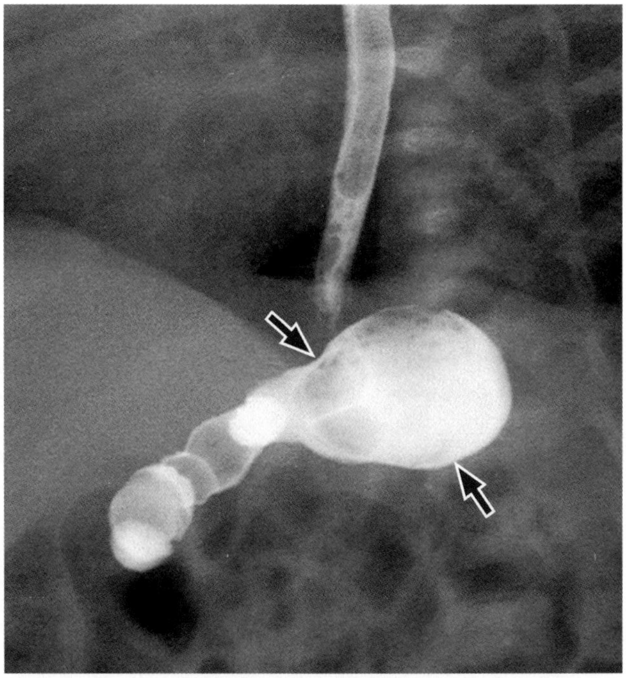

FIGURE 16.5 **Microgastria in a neonatal boy.** Upper GI series image shows an abnormally small stomach with tubular morphology (*arrows*).

duplications are most often asymptomatic, although some affected children may present with obstructive symptoms if large or located near the gastric outlet. Uncommonly, gastric duplications can be associated with ectopic pancreatic tissue leading to pancreatitis, and they can mimic other fluid collections, such as pancreatic pseudocysts.[29]

Radiography may demonstrate mass-like soft tissue opacity in the gastric or perigastric region. These lesions are more likely to be seen by ultrasound, appearing as circumscribed anechoic or complicated cystic mass with a layered wall because of underlying echogenic mucosa and hypoechoic muscularis.[19,27] At CT, gastric duplication cysts appear as well-circumscribed, homogeneous, low-attenuation masses associated with the stomach wall that lack postcontrast enhancement. At MRI, they are usually thin-walled, T1-weighted hypointense, and T2-weighted hyperintense, unless complicated (Fig. 16.6).[19]

The current treatment is surgical resection, especially if symptomatic.

Gastric Volvulus

Gastric volvulus refers to abnormal twisting of the stomach that can be either organoaxial (along its long axis) or mesenteroaxial (along its short axis). Gastric volvulus may be idiopathic (related to incomplete fixation of the stomach due to absent or lax ligaments) or it can occur secondary to paraesophageal hiatal hernia, congenital diaphragmatic hernia/eventration of the diaphragm, or wandering spleen.[30] In organoaxial volvulus, the greater curvature is located above the lesser curvature[19] (Fig. 16.7). In mesenteroaxial volvulus, the pylorus and antrum can be located superior to the proximal stomach. Presentation of gastric volvulus can be acute or chronic.[19] Acutely, affected children present with abdominal pain and gastric outlet obstruction, including persistent vomiting. Chronic gastric volvulus may manifest as intermittent abdominal pain or vomiting. Ischemia can develop if volvulus persists. Radiography can suggest this diagnosis, showing severe gastric distension with little to no distal bowel gas.[19] Other features include abnormal gastric morphology, two air–fluid gastric levels (mesenteroaxial), convex superior contour of the gastric body (organoaxial), or visualization of the pylorus at or above the level of the gastric fundus (mesenteroaxial). Upper GI series can confirm the diagnosis, including the exact type of volvulus.[30]

The current treatment of gastric volvulus is surgical gastropexy.

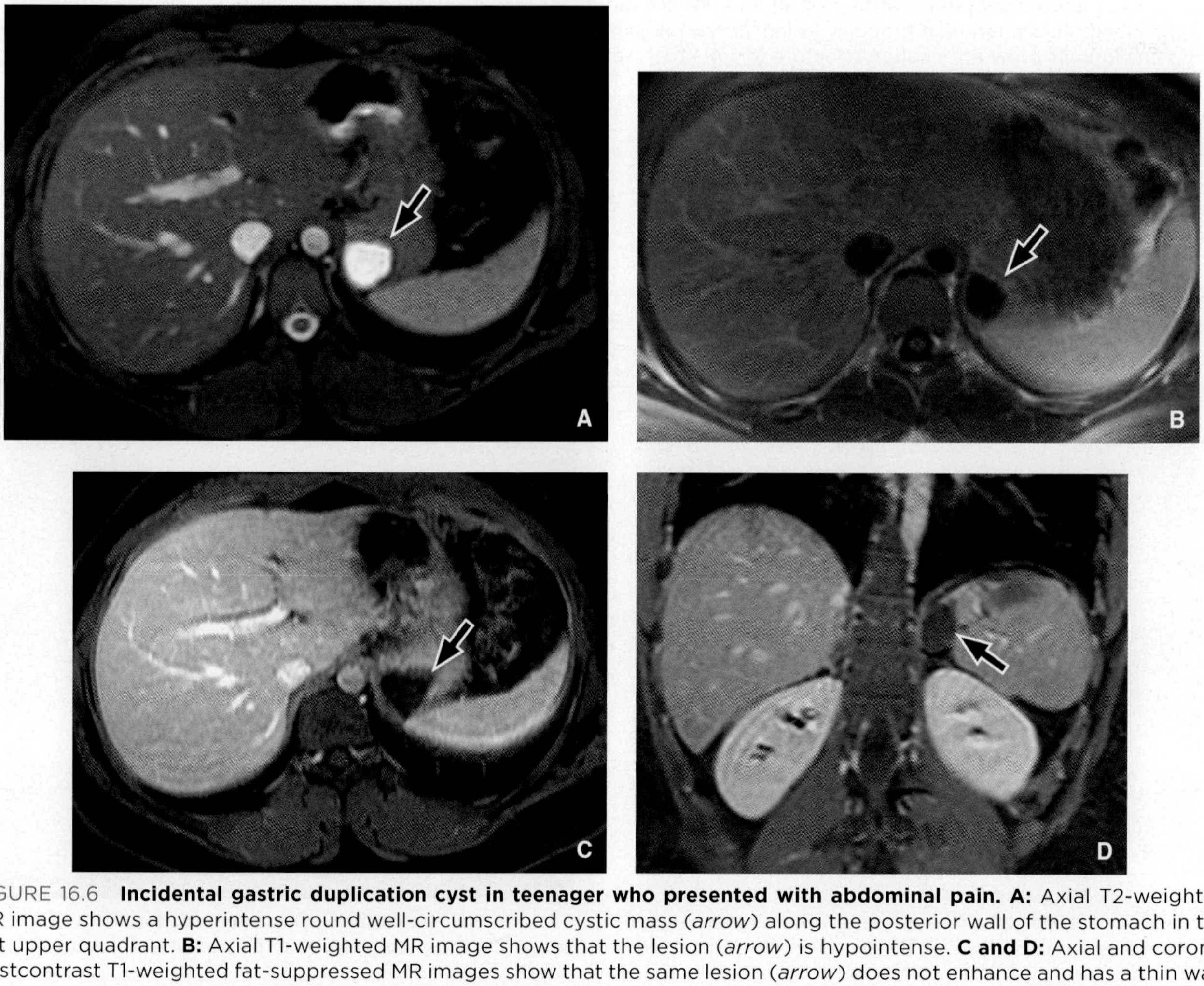

FIGURE 16.6 **Incidental gastric duplication cyst in teenager who presented with abdominal pain. A:** Axial T2-weighted MR image shows a hyperintense round well-circumscribed cystic mass (*arrow*) along the posterior wall of the stomach in the left upper quadrant. **B:** Axial T1-weighted MR image shows that the lesion (*arrow*) is hypointense. **C and D:** Axial and coronal postcontrast T1-weighted fat-suppressed MR images show that the same lesion (*arrow*) does not enhance and has a thin wall.

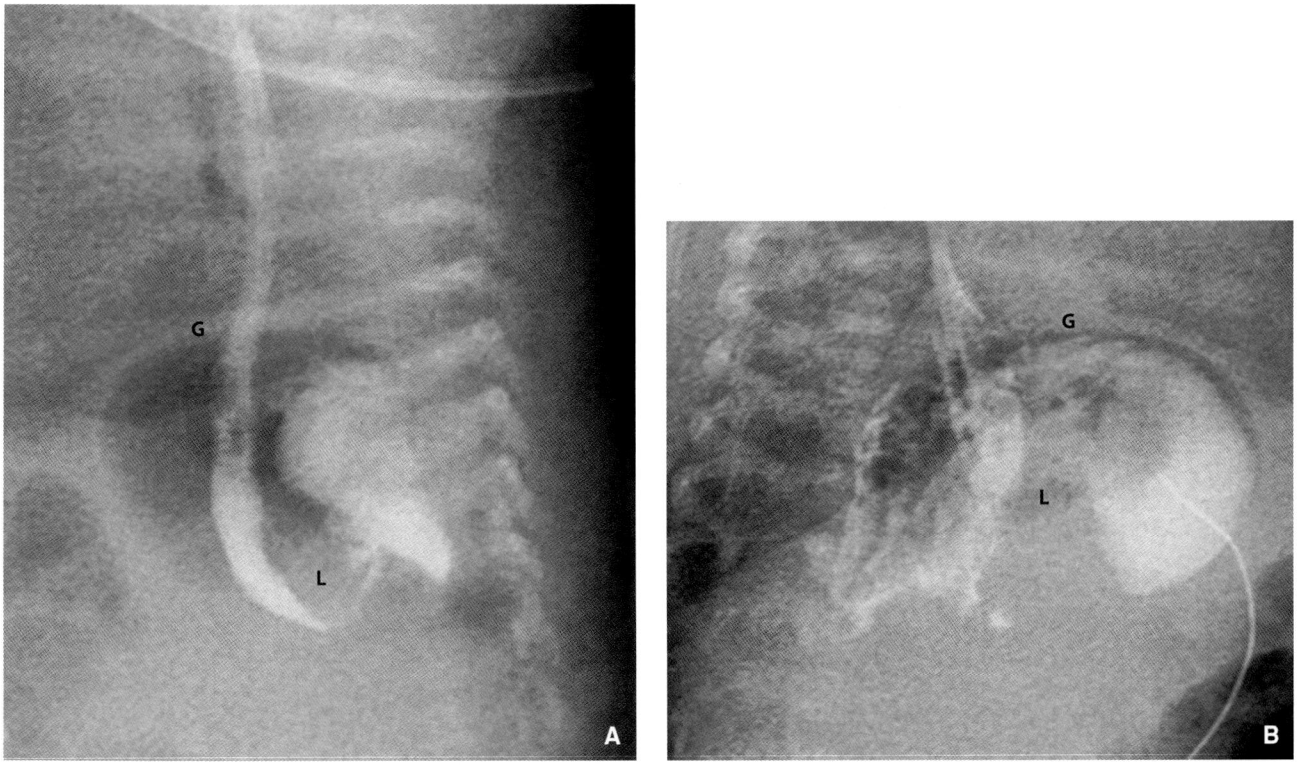

FIGURE 16.7 **Organoaxial gastric volvulus in two different neonates—7-day-old boy (A) and 17-day-old girl (B), respectively. A:** Right lateral image from an upper GI series shows barium in the esophagus and distended stomach, with the greater curve (*G*) located above the lesser curve (*L*). **B:** Left lateral view from an upper GI series show barium in the esophagus and distended stomach, with the greater curve (*G*) superior to the lesser (*L*) curve.

Antral Web

Antral webs are a cause of partial gastric outlet obstruction and gastroesophageal reflux.[27] In this entity, a thin diaphragm or membrane circumferentially lines the gastric antrum, usually within 2 cm of the pylorus. The web is composed of mucosa and submucosa.[19] Radiography may reveal proximal gastric distention. Upper GI series shows a thin linear circumferential filling defect involving the distal stomach (Fig. 16.8). It is important to understand that early and careful gastric imaging is a key because the web can be obscured by contrast material.

The symptomatic antral web requires surgical antroplasty or web excision with or without pyloroplasty.

Hiatal Hernia

Hiatal hernia is diagnosed when a portion of the stomach extends through the diaphragmatic hiatus into the thorax. The hernia can be sliding (Type I), in which the gastroesophageal junction is located above the diaphragm, or paraesophageal (Type II), in which the gastroesophageal junction remains below the diaphragm but a portion of the stomach herniates into the thorax. Type III hiatal hernia has both sliding and paraesophageal components, whereas Type IV is diagnosed when other abdominal contents herniate into the chest. Sliding hiatal hernias are most common and make up over 95%.[31] This condition is due to widening of the diaphragmatic hiatus and weakening of the phrenicoesophageal membrane.[31] When symptomatic, sliding hiatal hernias tend to present with gastroesophageal reflux. Paraesophageal hernias can present with vomiting, dysphagia, and more serious complications, such as gastric obstruction or volvulus.[32]

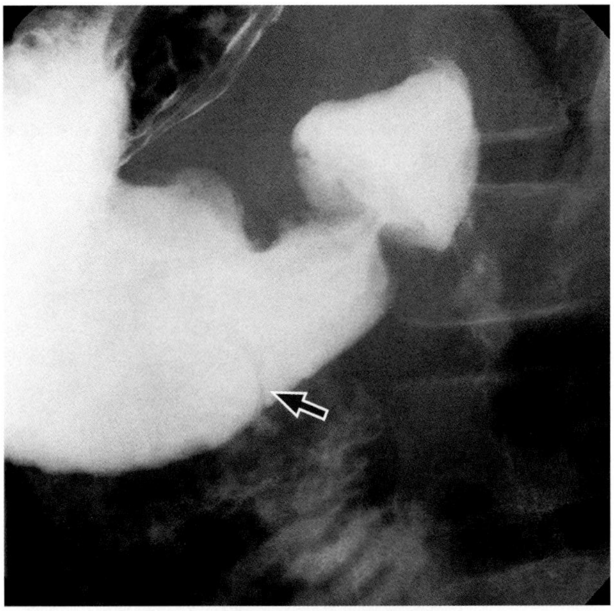

FIGURE 16.8 **Antral web in a 4-year-old boy.** Spot film from an upper GI series outlines a linear filling defect (*arrow*) in gastric antrum representing the web.

Radiographs are commonly normal, although the gastric air bubble or an air–fluid level may be observed in the lower posterior mediastinum.[31] Fluoroscopic imaging (upper GI series or esophagography) can confirm the locations of the gastroesophageal junction and stomach as well as characterize the type of hiatal hernia (Fig. 16.9).[31]

Treatment of sliding and paraesophageal hiatal hernias is surgical, and can include Nissen fundoplication

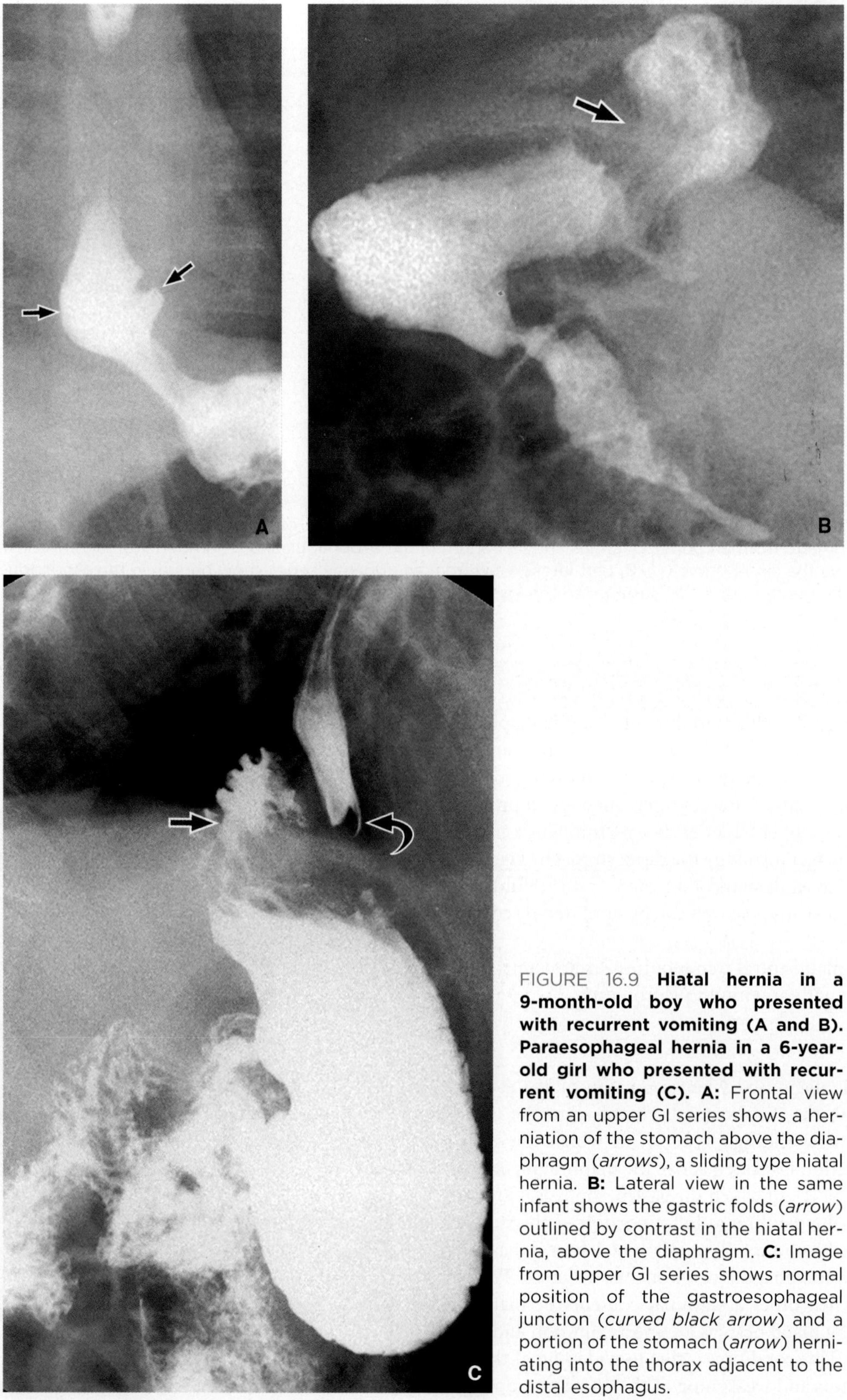

FIGURE 16.9 **Hiatal hernia in a 9-month-old boy who presented with recurrent vomiting (A and B). Paraesophageal hernia in a 6-year-old girl who presented with recurrent vomiting (C). A:** Frontal view from an upper GI series shows a herniation of the stomach above the diaphragm (*arrows*), a sliding type hiatal hernia. **B:** Lateral view in the same infant shows the gastric folds (*arrow*) outlined by contrast in the hiatal hernia, above the diaphragm. **C:** Image from upper GI series shows normal position of the gastroesophageal junction (*curved black arrow*) and a portion of the stomach (*arrow*) herniating into the thorax adjacent to the distal esophagus.

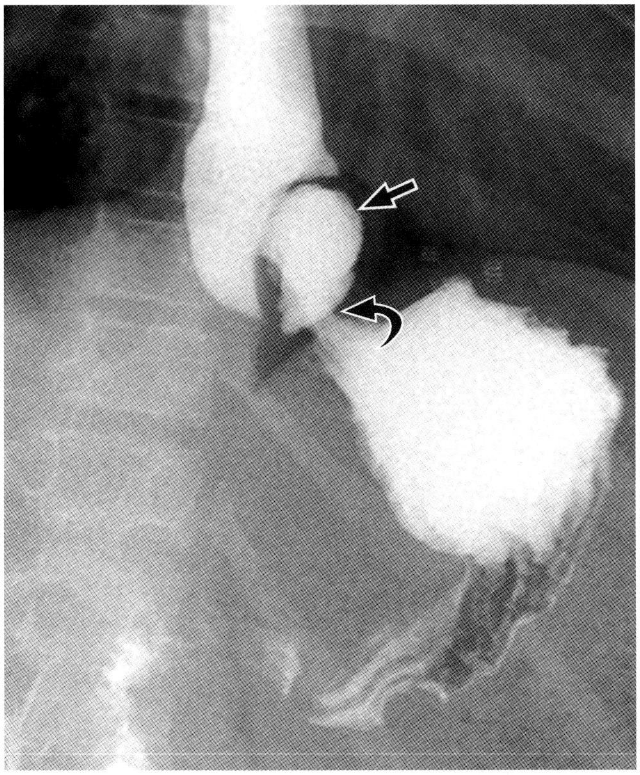

FIGURE 16.10 **Herniation of the Nissen fundoplication in a 7-year-old boy.** Anterior image from upper GI series shows Nissen fundoplication with a portion of the wrap filled with contrast material (*straight arrow*). The proximal stomach (*curved arrow*) and wrap are located above the diaphragm.

(a procedure in which the gastric fundus is partially or completely wrapped around the distal esophagus to reestablish competency at the gastroesophageal sphincter[33]). Post–Nissen fundoplication imaging should show smooth narrowing (about 2 to 3 cm) of the distal esophagus (at the location of the wrap), and the gastric fundus should be located below the diaphragm.[33] The complications of Nissen fundoplication are important to recognize which include esophageal obstruction from an overly tight wrap, wrap migration above the diaphragm, and wrap loosening[33] (Fig. 16.10).

Small Intestine

Duodenal and Other Small Bowel Atresias

Small bowel atresias are a common source of neonatal intestinal obstruction, with their clinical and radiologic presentations varying depending on location. Duodenal atresia is due to failed intestinal recanalization in utero, is most often preampullary, and often occurs in association with other anomalies,[34] including trisomy 21 and VACTERL association (including esophageal atresia). Concurrent malrotation and annular pancreas also have been described. Fetal imaging (ultrasound and MRI) may suggest duodenal atresia based on polyhydramnios and the presence of dilated fluid-filled stomach and duodenum ("double bubble" sign) (Fig. 16.11). Affected neonates present very early in life with vomiting and marked gastric distention. Radiography shows proximal GI tract obstruction, often having the characteristic "double bubble" appearance due to gaseous distention of the stomach and duodenum[34]; no distal bowel gas should be present except in very rare cases where gas may be seen distally because of passage through pancreatic ducts. Upper GI series can be used to confirm the diagnosis, if necessary. Treatment is surgical, most often duodenoduodenostomy.

Jejunal and ileal atresias are other causes of neonatal intestinal obstruction that are more common than duodenal atresia.[19] Such intestinal atresias may be due to intrauterine disruption of blood flow, and there is an association with cystic fibrosis. Uncommonly, intestinal atresias may be both multiple and hereditary.[35] Jejunal atresias are most often proximal, whereas ileal atresias are most often distal in location. Jejunal and ileal atresias can be associated with other congenital anomalies, but are not associated with trisomy 21. Affected pediatric patients typically present with vomiting (possibly bilious) and abdominal distention. Pathologic examination shows one or more areas of absent small bowel lumen (Fig. 16.12).

Radiography reveals evidence of proximal GI tract obstruction in the setting of jejunal atresia (few dilated bowel loops) (Fig. 16.13), whereas ileal atresia appears as a distal GI tract obstruction (numerous dilated bowel loops) (Fig. 16.14).[34] Gaseous distention of the stomach, duodenum, and proximal jejunum, the "triple bubble" sign, is characteristic of proximal jejunal atresia[34] (Fig. 16.13). Upper GI series can be used to confirm suspected jejunal atresia (Fig. 16.13). When ileal atresia is suspected, contrast enema is usually performed. Imaging findings consistent with ileal atresia include an unused microcolon and nondilated small bowel loops distal to the site of atresia[34] (Fig. 16.14).

All intestinal atresias are treated surgically, with the exact surgical approach depending on the location of the involved bowel segment, number of intestinal atresias, and association with other abnormalities, such as malrotation.

Duodenal Stenosis and Web

Congenital duodenal stenosis is a cause of partial proximal small bowel obstruction and is thought to be due to abnormal intestinal recanalization in utero. Similar to duodenal atresia, there is an association with other congenital anomalies, including trisomy 21. Duodenal stenosis is associated with annular pancreas or malrotation in up to one-third of affected children.[19] Clinical presentation can be because of signs and symptoms of partial small bowel obstruction or related to associated anomalies if the stenosis is mild.

Radiography can show findings similar to duodenal atresia, although bowel gas is generally seen distal to the duodenum (Fig. 16.15). Upper GI series reveals contrast in dilated stomach and proximal duodenum, with eventual passage of contrast material through the area of narrowed duodenum into more distal small bowel.[27] A duodenal web is a thin

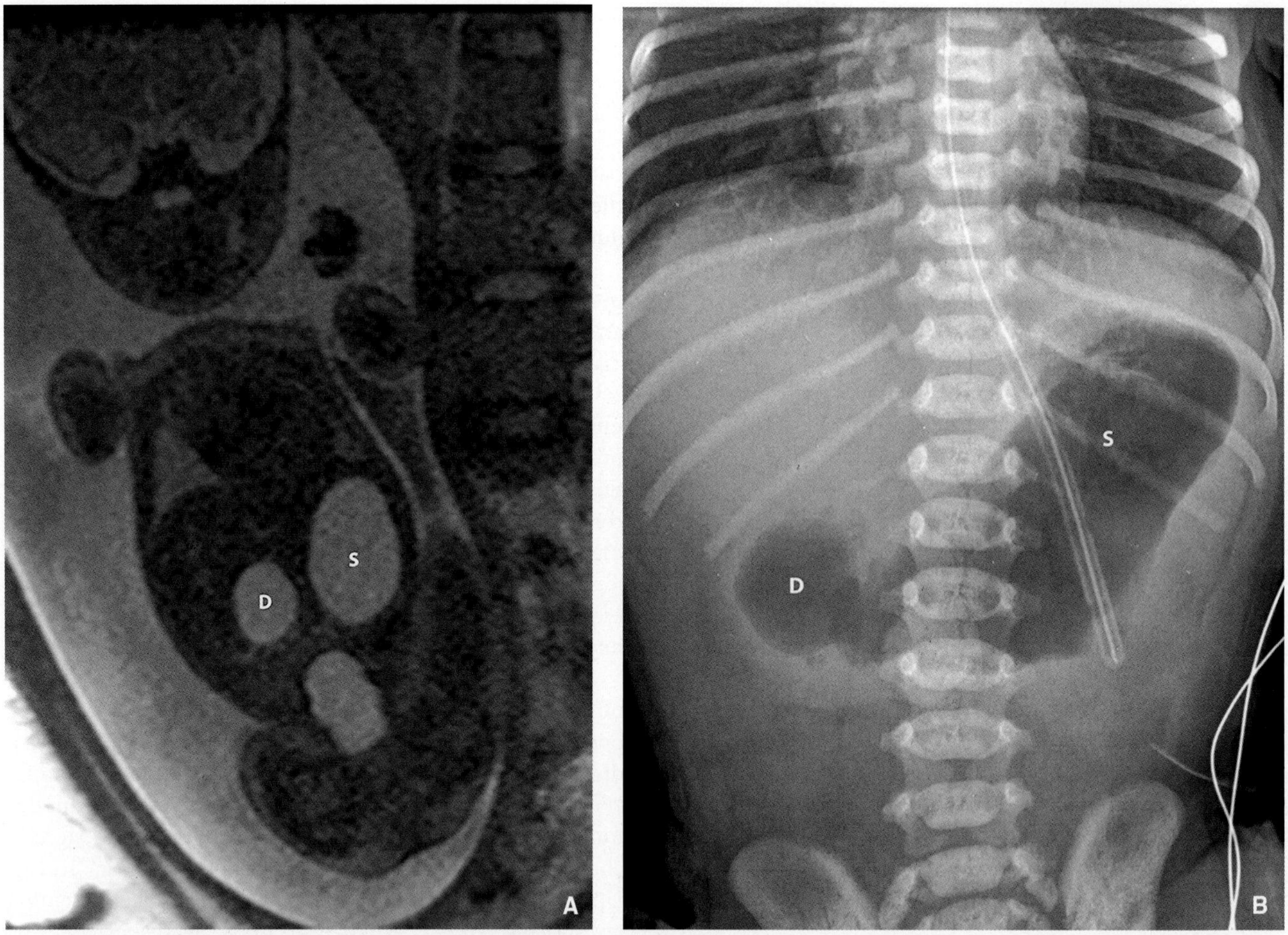

FIGURE 16.11 **Neonate girl with duodenal atresia. A:** Fluid sensitive image from a fetal MRI shows two fluid-filled structures in the upper abdomen of the fetus representing dilated stomach (*S*) and duodenal bulb (*D*). **B:** Postnatal abdominal radiograph shows gaseous distension of stomach (*S*) and duodenal bulb (*D*), the classic radiographic double bubble sign, without any distal bowel gas.

obstructing membrane with a central aperture within the duodenum that can appear as a filling defect or "windsock" when surrounded by contrast material (Fig. 16.16).

Symptomatic duodenal stenoses and webs are most often treated surgically.

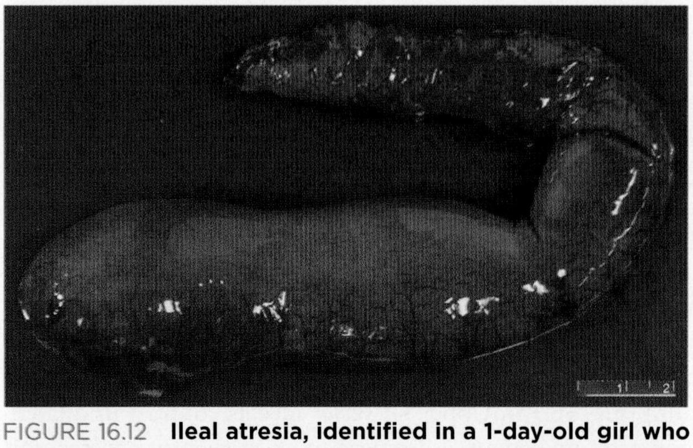

FIGURE 16.12 **Ileal atresia, identified in a 1-day-old girl who presented with abdominal distension and bilious vomiting upon birth.** The resected segment is most dilated near its blind end (lower left).

Malrotation and Midgut Volvulus

Malrotation refers to abnormal in utero rotation of the bowel with associated mesenteric bands and abnormal mesenteric fixation that can lead to volvulus and subsequent intestinal ischemia and infarction. Numerous anomalies are associated with malrotation, including chromosomal abnormalities. Malrotation in the absence of volvulus is commonly asymptomatic, whereas neonates with volvulus generally present with bilious emesis due to proximal small bowel obstruction.[19,36] Older children with malrotation can present with sudden abdominal pain and vomiting due to acute obstruction[19] or have milder intermittent symptoms if the bowel is only intermittently twisting and untwisting.

Radiography can be normal, and on occasion may show evidence of proximal small bowel obstruction. Careful evaluation of the bowel gas pattern may reveal abnormal location of the jejunum and proximal colon. The upper GI series is the diagnostic test of choice to evaluate for malrotation. Frontal imaging should show abnormal location of the DJJ (ligament of Treitz), which is normally located at the level of the duodenal bulb and lateral to the left vertebral pedicle

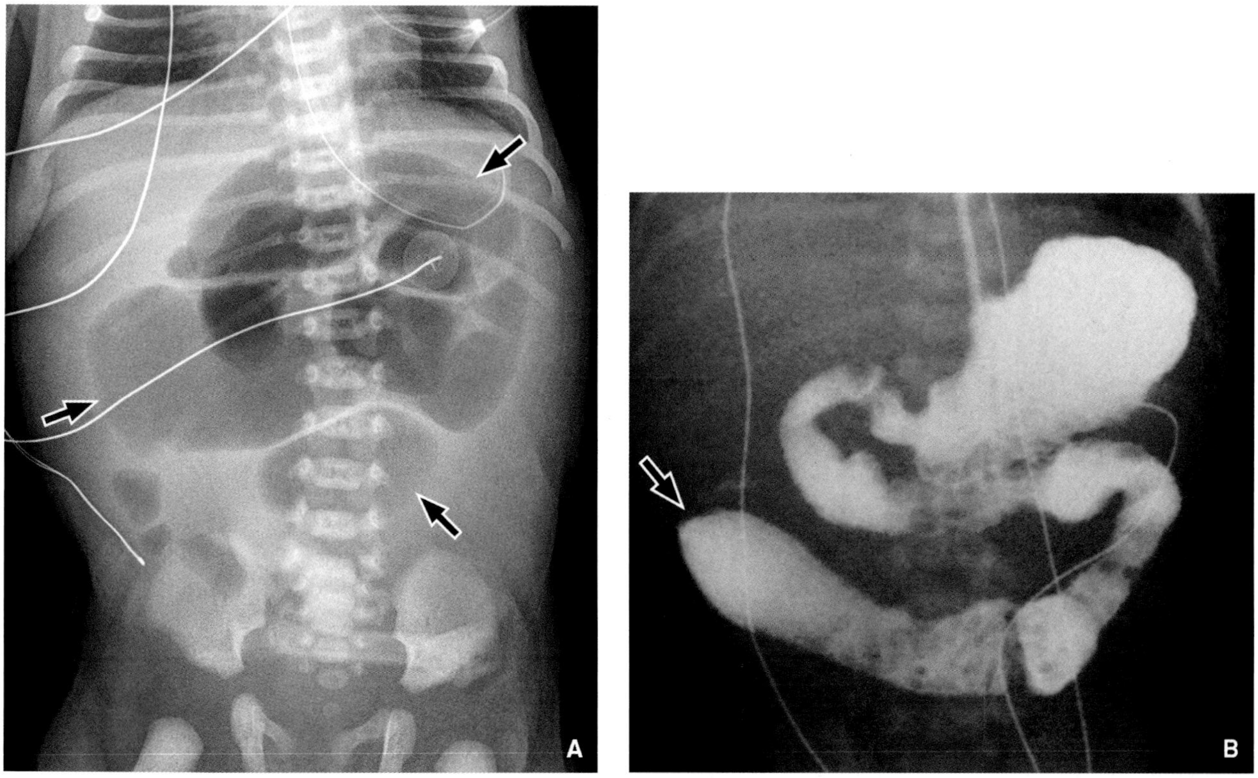

FIGURE 16.13 **Neonate girl who presented with bilious emesis and jejunal atresia. A:** Abdominal radiograph shows multiple upper abdominal dilated, air-filled bowel loops (*arrows*), suggesting proximal GI tract obstruction. **B:** Upper GI series image from the same neonate shows an abrupt cut off of contrast material at the site of atresia (*arrow*).

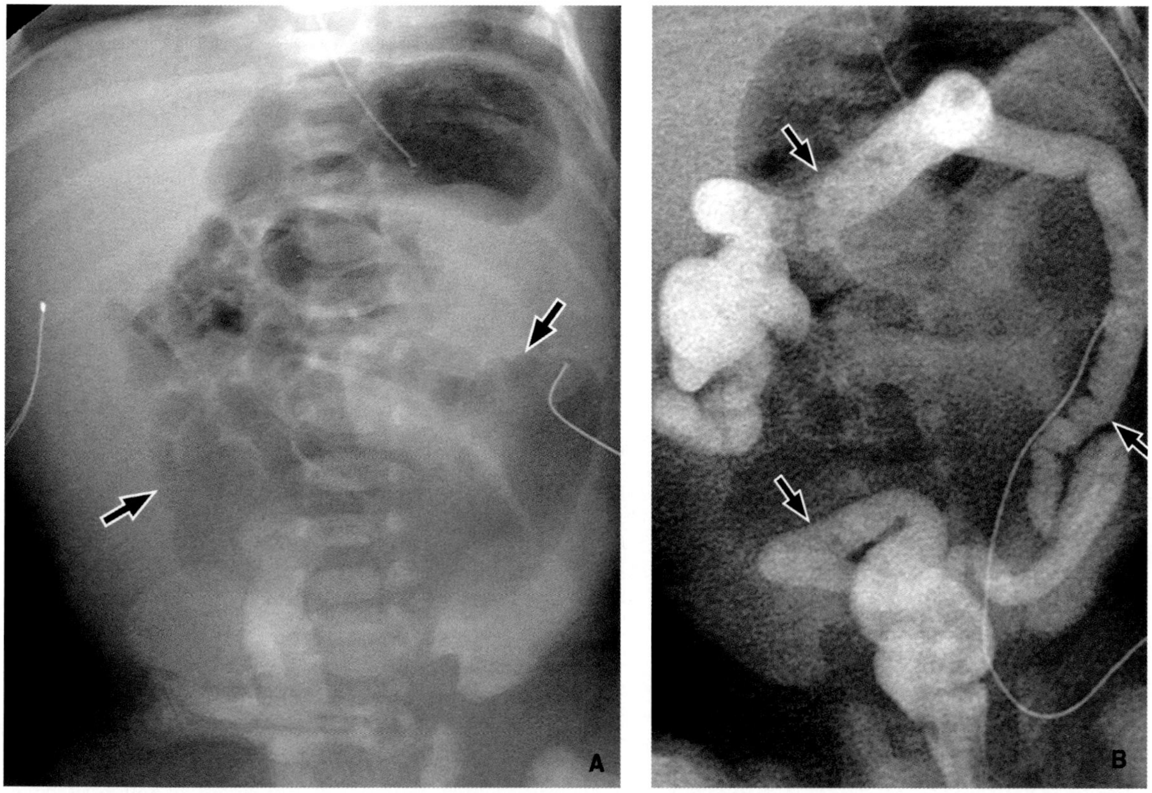

FIGURE 16.14 **Neonate girl who presented with bilious emesis and ileal atresia. A:** Abdominal radiograph shows numerous dilated, air-filled bowel loops (*arrows*), suggesting distal GI tract obstruction. **B:** Contrast enema image shows opacification of a diffusely small caliber microcolon (*arrows*). Contrast could not be refluxed into dilated bowel loops, and atresia of the distal ileum was found at surgery.

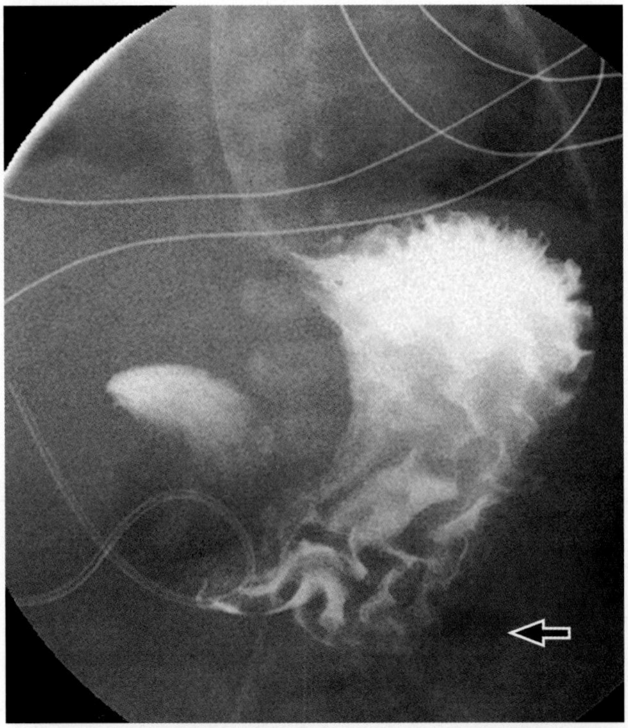

FIGURE 16.15 **Duodenal stenosis in a 10-day-old infant boy who presented with vomiting.** Upper GI series shows opacification of stomach and proximal duodenum, which becomes narrowed and impairs passage of contrast material into more distal intestine. There is bowel gas distally (*arrow*), excluding duodenal atresia.

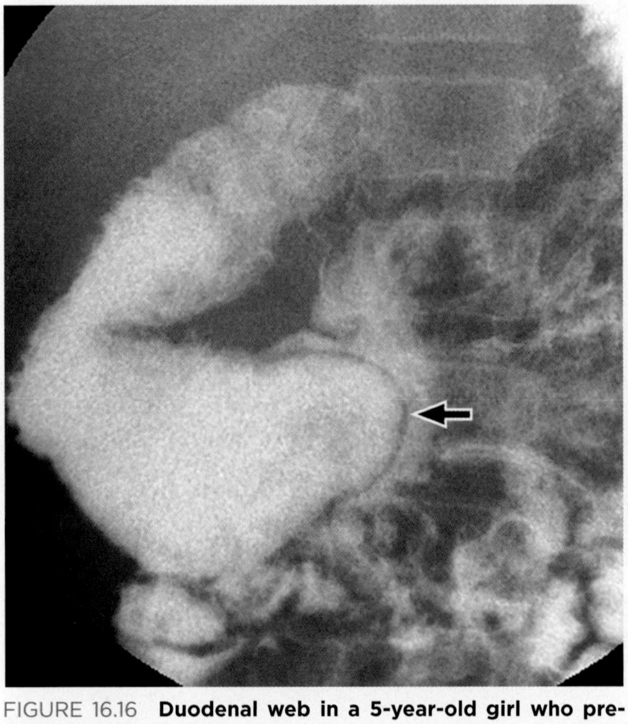

FIGURE 16.16 **Duodenal web in a 5-year-old girl who presented with vomiting.** Upper GI series image shows barium filling the dilated proximal and mid-duodenum. A thin curvilinear filling defect, or web (*arrow*), is present in the third portion of the duodenum.

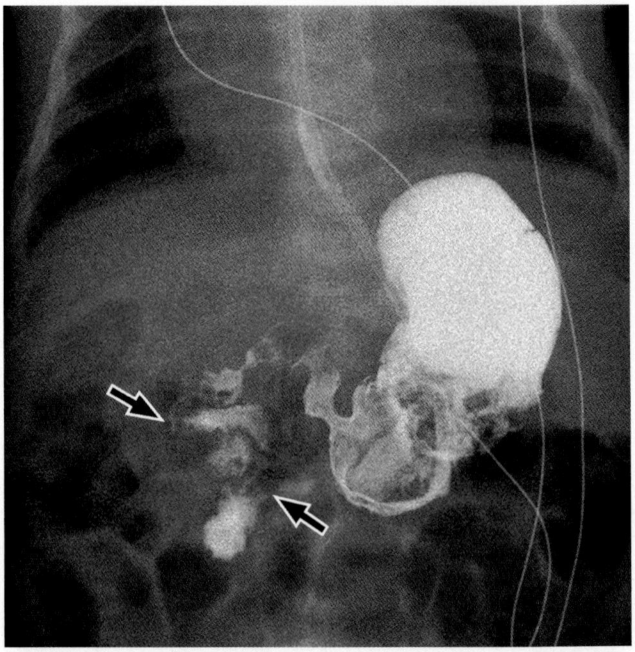

FIGURE 16.17 **Malrotation in a newborn infant girl who presented with intermittent vomiting.** Frontal image from upper GI series shows malposition of duodenal-jejunal junction, which is located to the right of the spine. The proximal small bowel (*arrows*) remains on the right side of the spine in the right upper quadrant.

(Fig. 16.17). When midgut volvulus is concomitantly present, the proximal duodenum may be dilated and abruptly cut-off, similar to duodenal atresia. The duodenum can also have a "corkscrew" appearance in affected children (Fig. 16.18). Lateral imaging should be performed in order to confirm that the duodenal course is abnormal and that there is lack of appropriate duodenal retroperitoneal fixation. When upper GI series findings are equivocal, documentation of position of the cecum can be useful for estimating the length of the small bowel mesentery.

Ultrasound also may be used to diagnose malrotation in children. The normal duodenum should be seen taking a retroperitoneal course, passing between the abdominal aorta and proximal SMA.[37] Ultrasound also can evaluate the relationship of the SMA to the superior mesenteric vein; abnormal swirling ("whirlpool" sign) of these vessels can be seen in the setting of malrotation with volvulus (Fig. 16.18). CT typically is not used to evaluate suspected malrotation or midgut volvulus, although on occasion it can show this diagnosis in children presenting with abdominal pain. Also, CT performed for nonemergent indications may occasionally and incidentally reveal malrotation.

Malrotation is treated surgically with the Ladd's procedure, which consists of untwisting of volvulus (if present), placing the bowel in a nonrotated state to widen the small bowel mesentery, division of any congenital (Ladd's) bands, and appendectomy.

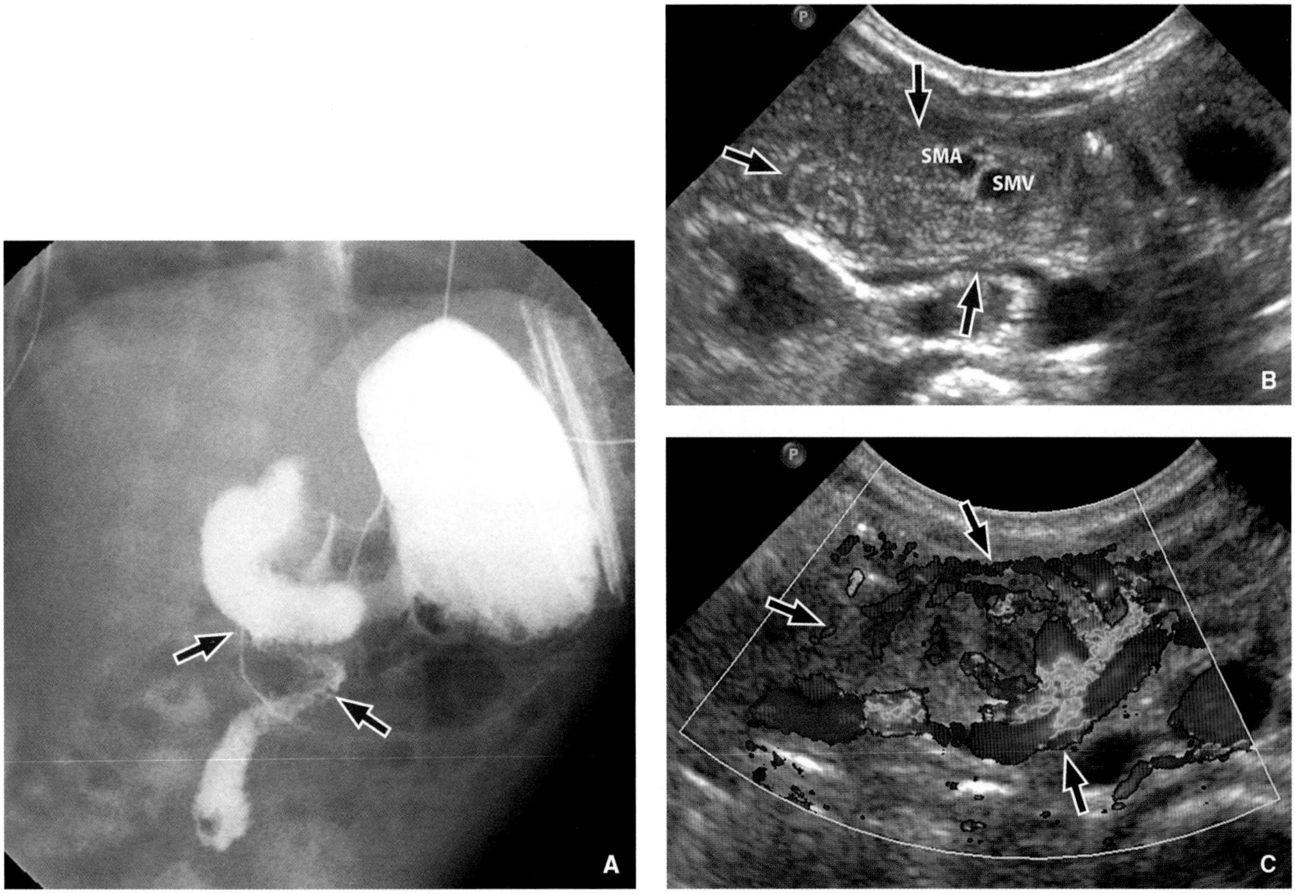

FIGURE 16.18 **Infant girl with malrotation with midgut volvulus who presented with bilious emesis. A:** Upper GI series image shows abnormal position of duodenal-jejunal junction with corkscrew appearance of the contrast material-filled duodenum and proximal jejunum (*arrows*) around the SMA axis. The obstructed duodenum is mildly dilated proximal to the twisted bowel. **B:** Transverse gray-scale ultrasound image shows the classic soft tissue mass (*arrows*) of the bowel around the mesenteric root. The SMA and SMV relationship is abnormal, with the SMA located to the right of the SMV. **C:** Transverse Color Doppler ultrasound image shows the whirlpool sign, or swirling of bowel and vessels (*arrows*) around the SMA axis.

Meconium Ileus

Meconium ileus is a form of neonatal distal small bowel obstruction due to abnormal obstructing viscous, tenacious meconium. This condition is responsible for ~20% of neonatal bowel obstructions and is almost always due to underlying cystic fibrosis.[34] Approximately 15% to 20% of children with cystic fibrosis present with meconium ileus. In utero, meconium ileus can cause bowel perforation with meconium peritonitis, resulting in peritoneal calcifications and meconium pseudocyst formation.[19] Affected infants usually present with failure to pass meconium and symptoms of bowel obstruction, including vomiting and abdominal distension.

Radiography usually shows multiple dilated loops of bowel, consistent with distal GI tract obstruction.[38] Retained meconium in right lower quadrant distal small bowel loops may have a "soap bubble" appearance. If prenatal perforation occurred, peritoneal calcifications can be identified and mass effect can be seen on occasion because of large pseudocysts. Contrast enema findings of meconium ileus include abnormally small caliber of the colon (microcolon) as well as the presence of numerous filling defects in the distal small bowel due to meconium[19] (Fig. 16.19). In some affected children, it is possible to reflux contrast material into dilated small bowel loops located proximal to the site of obstruction. Contrast enema should not be performed on neonates with evidence of complicated meconium ileus (e.g., acute perforation), because this requires urgent surgery.[19] Ultrasound, in addition to radiography, can be used to detect meconium pseudocysts, which often appear as circumscribed round or ovoid cystic lesions with an echogenic rim due to calcification.[19] These collections can be located throughout the peritoneal cavity as well as in the inguinal canal and scrotum of boys (Fig. 16.20).

Simple and uncomplicated meconium ileus often can be successfully treated conservatively with water-soluble contrast enemas as well as fluid and electrolyte monitoring and replacement.[39] Operative treatments, such as enterostomy and decompression, resection and stoma formation, or resection and anastomosis, may be needed when the nonoperative treatment fails.

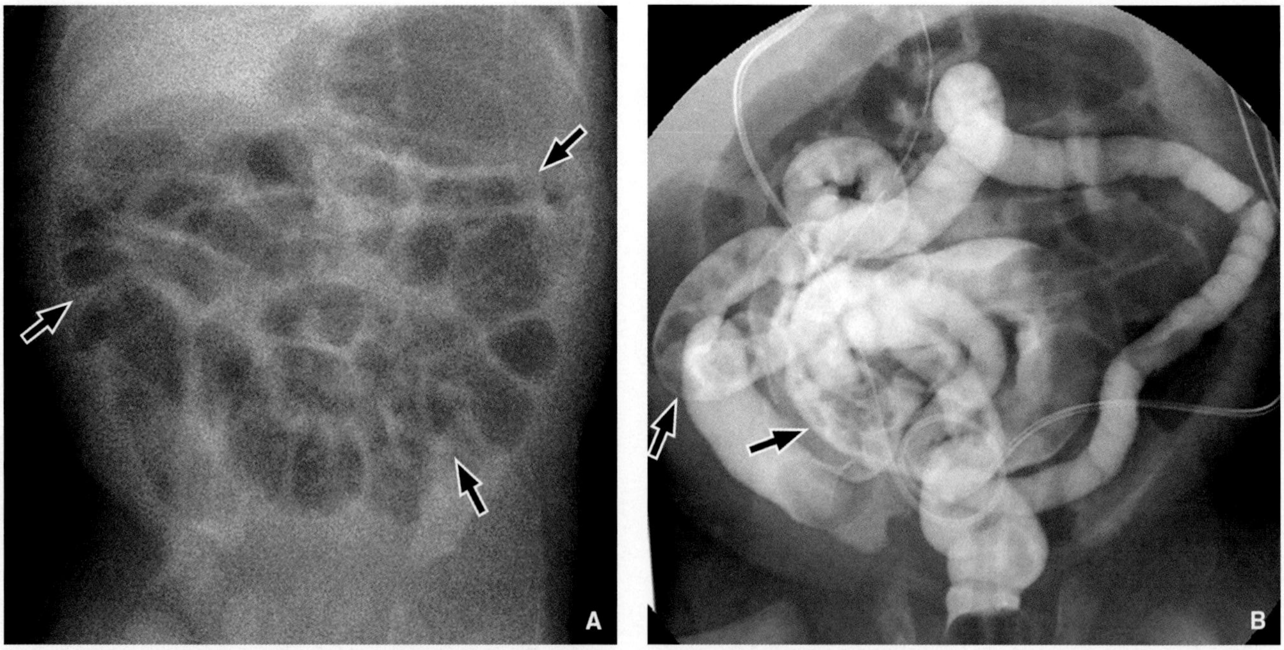

FIGURE 16.19 **Neonate boy who presented with abdominal distention due to meconium ileus. A:** Abdominal radiograph shows multiple dilated, gas-filled loops of bowel (*arrows*) in a distal obstruction pattern. Differential diagnosis includes ileal atresia, meconium ileus, functional immaturity of the left colon (meconium plug syndrome), and Hirschsprung disease. **B:** Water-soluble contrast enema reveals opacification of diffusely small caliber colon with reflux of contrast into the distal ileum. Multiple filling defects (*arrows*) are noted in the proximal colon and distal ileum, reflecting meconium pellets.

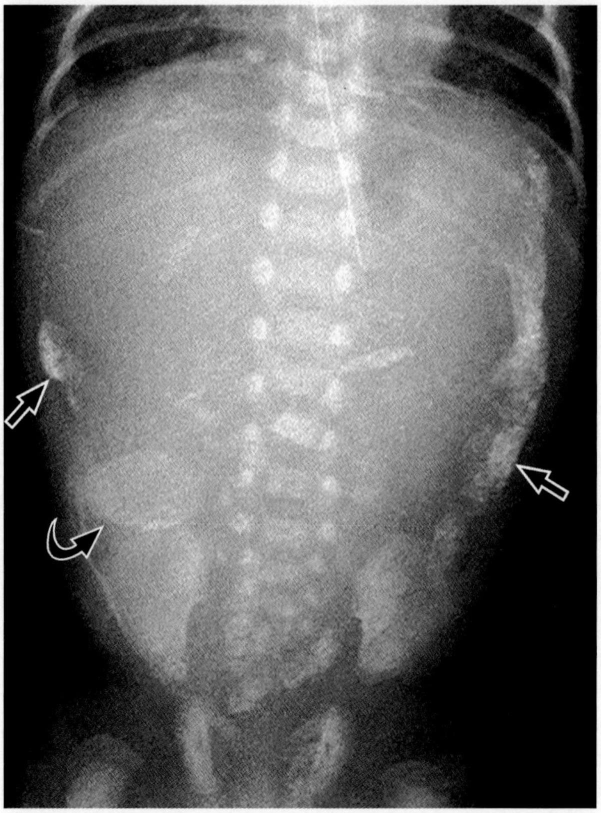

FIGURE 16.20 **Meconium peritonitis in a newborn girl.** Abdominal radiograph shows multiple calcifications (*straight arrows*) in the abdomen and pelvis, outlining peritoneal and mesenteric surfaces. An ovoid hyperdense mass (*curved arrow*) in the right lower quadrant represents meconium pseudocyst.

Small Bowel Duplication Cysts

Most small bowel duplications cysts involve the terminal ileum and fail to communicate with the bowel lumen. Like GI tract duplication cysts located elsewhere, these small bowel duplication cysts have a muscular wall and can be lined by a variety of types of epithelium. They are typically located along the antimesenteric border of the affected small bowel segment.[28] Small bowel duplications are most often asymptomatic, although affected patients can present with abdominal pain or obstructive symptoms because of mass effect or intussusception with the cyst serving as a lead point. Symptoms can also be due to heterotopic mucosa (e.g., gastric mucosa), which may cause GI bleeding.

Most small bowel duplication cysts cannot be seen by radiography, although large cysts may show mass effect appearing as a soft tissue mass (Fig. 16.21). Fluoroscopic studies may show a luminal contour abnormality compatible with an extrinsic mass or less likely obstruction because of mass effect or intussusception. Enteric duplication cysts are most often seen by cross-sectional imaging, appearing as round/ovoid cystic masses associated with bowel wall/mesentery at ultrasound. The wall of these lesions typically has a layered appearance at ultrasound due to hypoechoic muscle and hyperechoic mucosa. At CT and MRI, enteric duplication cysts appear as well-circumscribed, nonenhancing cysts associated with the bowel wall/mesentery (Fig. 16.21). These lesions may appear complicated (thick-walled, attenuation greater than water at CT, increased T1-weighted and decreased T2-wegihted signal at MRI) if they are associated with hemorrhage or infection.

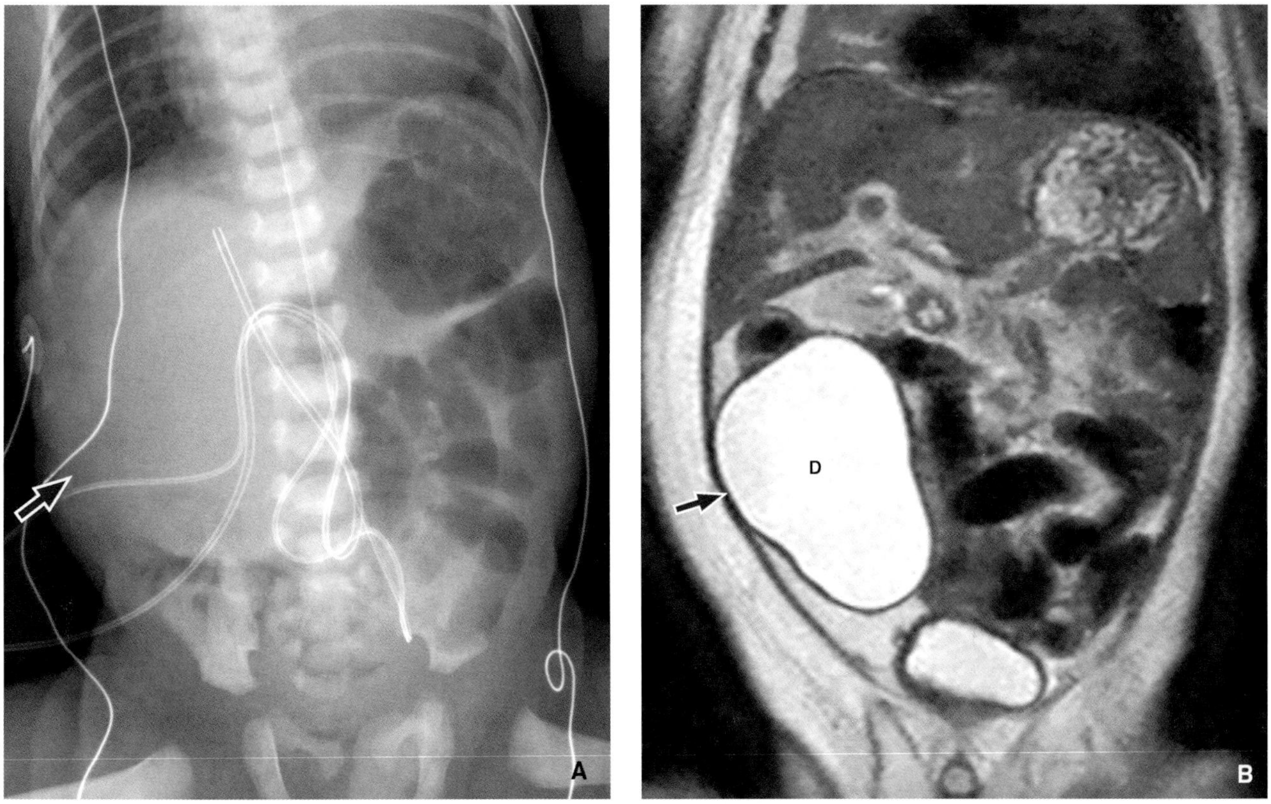

FIGURE 16.21 **Enteric duplication cyst in a neonate boy who presented with bilious emesis. A:** Abdominal radiograph shows a paucity of bowel gas on the right (*arrows*) and mass effect on gas-filled bowel loops. **B:** Coronal T2-weighted MR image shows a large, hyperintense, thin-walled cyst (*D*) associated with a loop of bowel, proven to be a small bowel duplication cyst.

The current treatment is surgically resection, especially if symptomatic.

Meckel Diverticulum

Meckel diverticula are remnants of the omphalomesenteric duct, arising from the antimesenteric border of the distal ileum (Fig. 16.22).[19] The remnant can have a persistent patent or fibrous connection to the umbilicus. Most Meckel diverticula are asymptomatic; however, when symptomatic, most affected children present with painless GI tract bleeding due to heterotopic gastric or pancreatic mucosa within the diverticulum. Inflammation of the diverticulum due to luminal obstruction can clinically and radiologically mimic appendicitis. Small bowel obstruction can occur because of inversion of the diverticulum into the ileal lumen with resultant intussusception or small bowel volvulus around the umbilical connection.

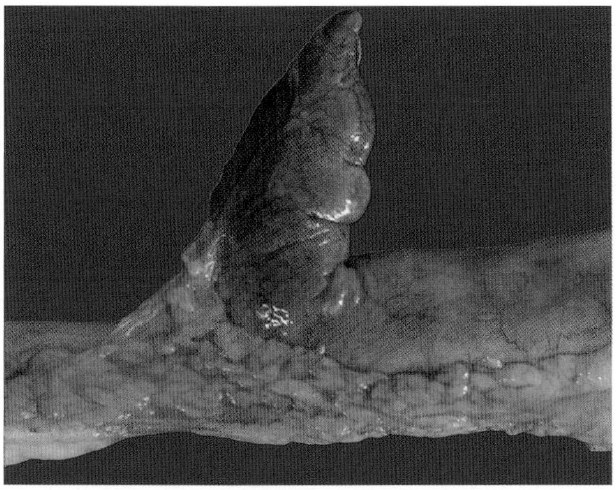

FIGURE 16.22 **Meckel diverticulum.** Meckel diverticulum, projecting from the antimesenteric aspect of the ileum in a 16-year-old boy whose history included abdominal pain.

Meckel diverticula are not usually seen at radiography, although related complications, such as bowel obstruction, may be visualized. Associated enteroliths may also be seen. At fluoroscopic imaging, Meckel diverticula appear as saccular outpouchings from the antimesenteric border of the distal ileum.[21] At ultrasound, CT, and MRI, Meckel diverticula may have an appearance similar to the appendix. These modalities can also identify diverticulum-related inflammation (diverticulitis) and bowel obstruction. The customary imaging examination used to identify Meckel diverticula is the Meckel's scan (^{99m}Tc-pertechnetate scintigraphy). When a Meckel diverticulum that contains gastric mucosa is present, the diverticulum is typically seen as focally increased radiotracer activity in the right mid- to lower abdomen that appears at the same time as the stomach (Fig. 16.23). Meckel's scan is ~90% sensitive and 95% specific for accurately detecting Meckel diverticula that contain gastric mucosa.[21]

Treatment is surgical resection of the Meckel diverticulum.

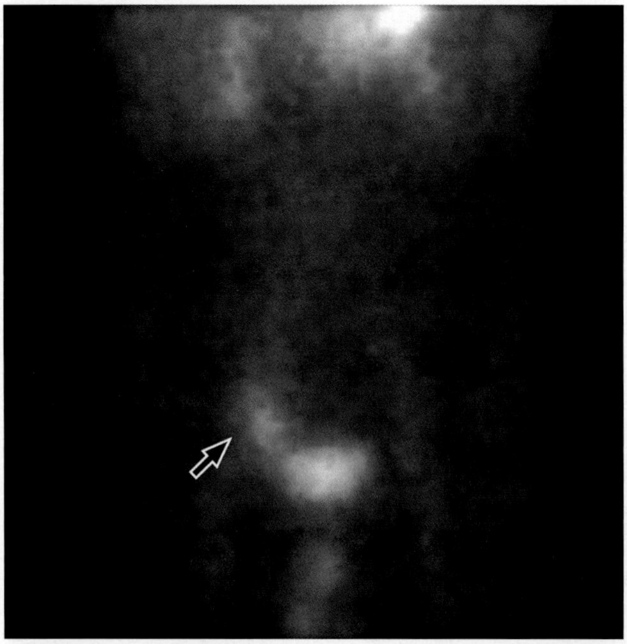

FIGURE 16.23 **Meckel diverticulum in a 5-year-old boy who presented with GI tract bleeding.** Tc-99m pertechnetate scan (Meckel scan) shows abnormal radiotracer uptake (*arrow*) in the right lower quadrant, representing ectopic gastric mucosa in a Meckel diverticulum.

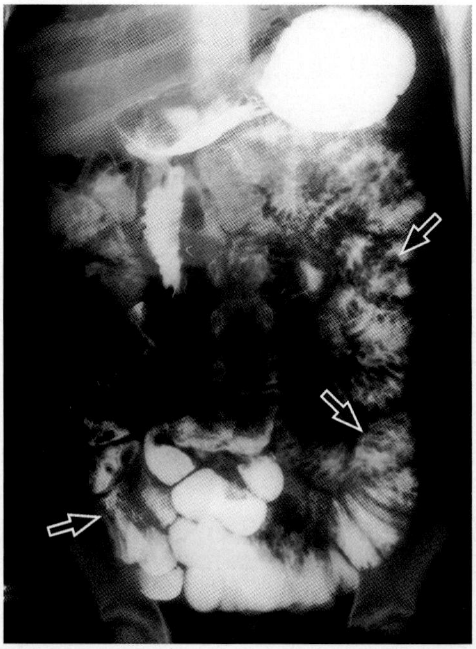

FIGURE 16.24 **Intestinal lymphangiectasia in a 10-year-old girl who presented with failure to thrive and protein losing enteropathy.** SBFT image shows diffuse nodular fold thickening (*arrows*) of the duodenum and small bowel.

Intestinal Lymphangiectasia

Congenital intestinal lymphangiectasia is a primary lymphangiectasia, referring to congenital obstruction and dilatation of the lymphatic drainage of the bowel. Affected pediatric patients may present with soft tissue edema, protein-losing enteropathy, ascites, pleural effusion, and poor weight gain.[40] Imaging features reflect lymphatic congestion and leakage, with SBFT, CT, and MRI demonstrating nodular wall/fold thickening of the jejunum and ileum[41] (Fig. 16.24). Treatment is primarily a low-fat diet with medium-chain triglyceride supplementation.[40]

Colon

Colonic Atresia

Colonic atresia is the least common intestinal atresia, and it can be associated with other congenital anomalies, including Hirschsprung disease. In 15% to 20% of cases, there are other areas of intestinal atresia.[19] Colonic atresia, like jejunal and ileal atresia, is thought to be the result of intrauterine disruption of blood supply. Affected pediatric patients typically present during the neonatal period with lower GI tract obstruction symptoms, including vomiting, abdominal distension, and failure to pass meconium.

Radiography typically shows distal GI tract obstruction, with numerous dilated loops of bowel.[42] Contrast enema reveals a small caliber colon to the point of atresia, which can be located anywhere along the length of the colon, where the contrast column abruptly terminates, without intraluminal filling defects (Fig. 16.25).

Colonic atresia requires surgical management, commonly including an initial diversion operation.

Colonic Duplication Cysts

Large bowel duplication cysts are less common than small bowel duplication cysts and can be classified as appendiceal, colonic, or colorectal tubular duplications.[28] The proximal colon (cecum) is a common location. Although often asymptomatic, colonic duplications can present with bowel obstruction due to the cyst serving as a lead point for intussusception, bowel obstruction from mass effect, or GI tract bleeding due to ectopic gastric mucosa. Colorectal tubular duplications are tubular structures neighboring the involved colon that may or may not communicate with the true colonic lumen (Fig. 16.26). Colorectal tubular duplications can terminate blindly, terminate at a separate perineal anal orifice, or terminate via a fistula to the genitourinary tract.[43]

At ultrasound, colonic duplication cysts are associated with the wall of the colon and appear similar to GI tract duplication cysts located elsewhere, having a layered appearance (Fig. 16.27). CT and MRI demonstrate a well-defined, nonenhancing cystic mass abutting the colon; a communication between the duplication cyst and true colonic lumen may or may not be seen (Fig. 16.27). Also, like duplication cysts elsewhere, colonic duplication cysts on occasion may appear complicated because of internal bleeding or infection. Contrast enemas may reveal extrinsic mass effect on the colon or opacification of the lesion if it communicates with the true lumen of the colon.

Treatment of symptomatic pediatric patients with colonic duplication cysts is surgical resection.

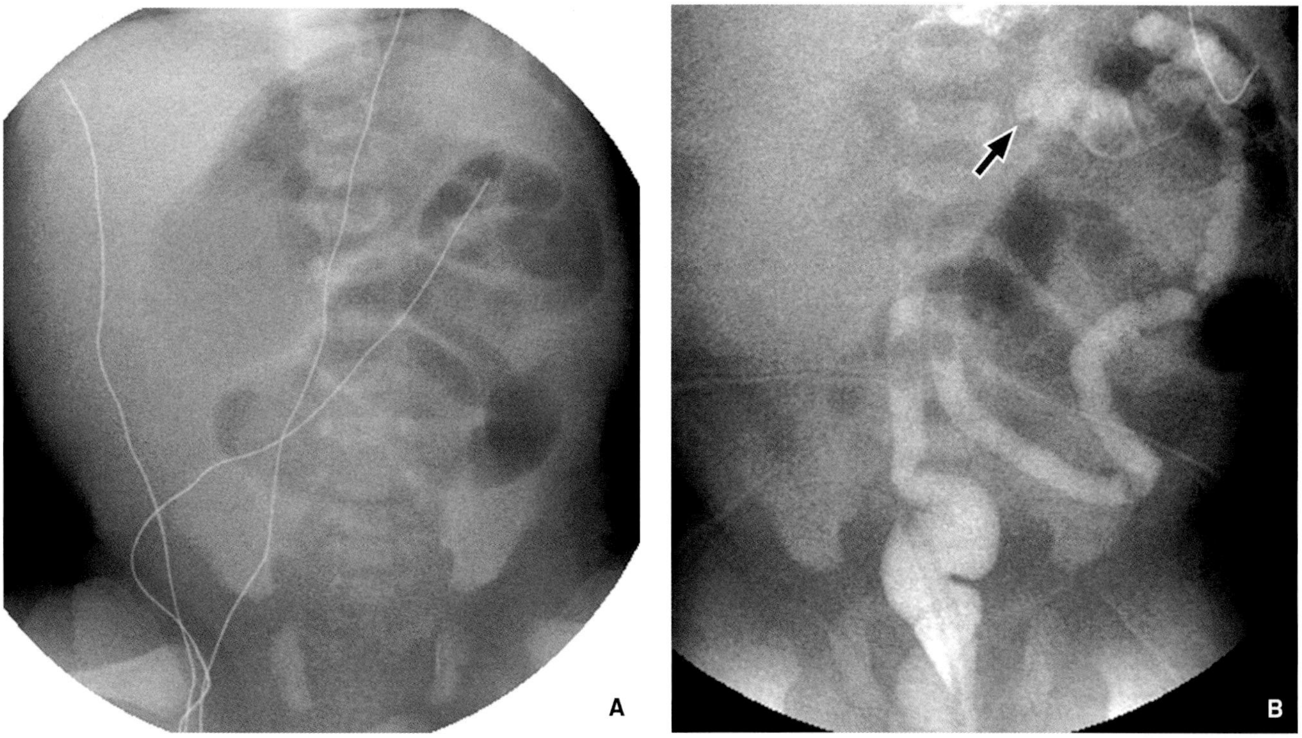

FIGURE 16.25 **Neonate boy who presented with abdominal distention due to colonic atresia. A:** Abdominal radiograph shows a distal obstruction pattern with multiple dilated, gas-filled bowel loops. **B:** Contrast enema reveals opacification of the rectum and a portion of the colon, which is small in caliber. Contrast could not be refluxed beyond the distal transverse colon (*arrow*), which was the site of colonic atresia.

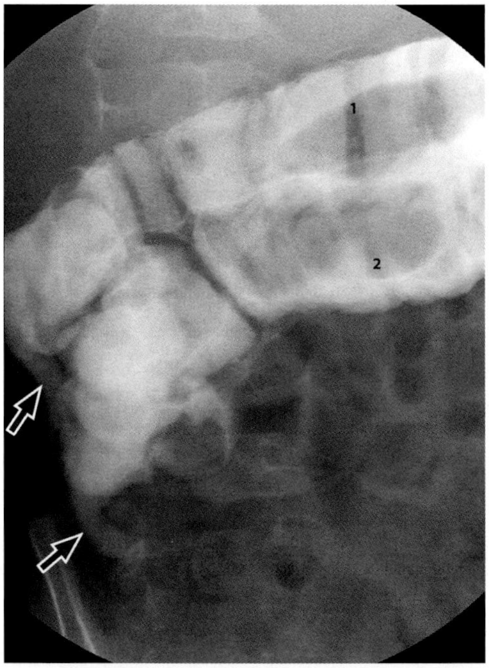

FIGURE 16.26 **A 10-month-old girl with intussusception due to partial colonic duplication serving as lead point.** Contrast enema shows partial colonic duplication with contrast material outlining two separate transverse colons (labeled *1* and *2*) and two separate appendices (*arrows*). The same child also had a duplicated urinary bladder (not shown).

Meconium Plug Syndrome (also known as Small Left Colon Syndrome or Functional Immaturity of the Colon)

Functional obstruction of the distal colon in neonates is called by a variety of names, including meconium plug syndrome, and is likely due to colonic dysmotility.[38] This condition is thought to be due to immature bowel peristalsis and abnormal water reabsorption from the colon.[19] Meconium plug syndrome, in particular, is used to describe a small caliber descending colon in association with retained colonic meconium. Infants of diabetic mothers and very-low-birth-weight infants are at increased risk. Affected infants typically present with evidence of distal bowel obstruction, including vomiting and abdominal distension.[38]

Radiography shows a distal GI tract obstruction with multiple dilated loops of bowel. At contrast enema, the distal colon (descending and sigmoid portions) appear smaller in caliber than expected, and a long luminal filling defect consistent with a meconium plug may be seen (Fig. 16.28). Water-soluble contrast enemas can be both diagnostic and therapeutic.

Rectal biopsy is commonly performed after relief of obstruction to exclude Hirschsprung disease.[44]

Hirschsprung Disease

Hirschsprung disease refers to aganglionosis of the colon, which is more often partial than complete. In this condition, abnormal migration of vagal neural crest cells results in

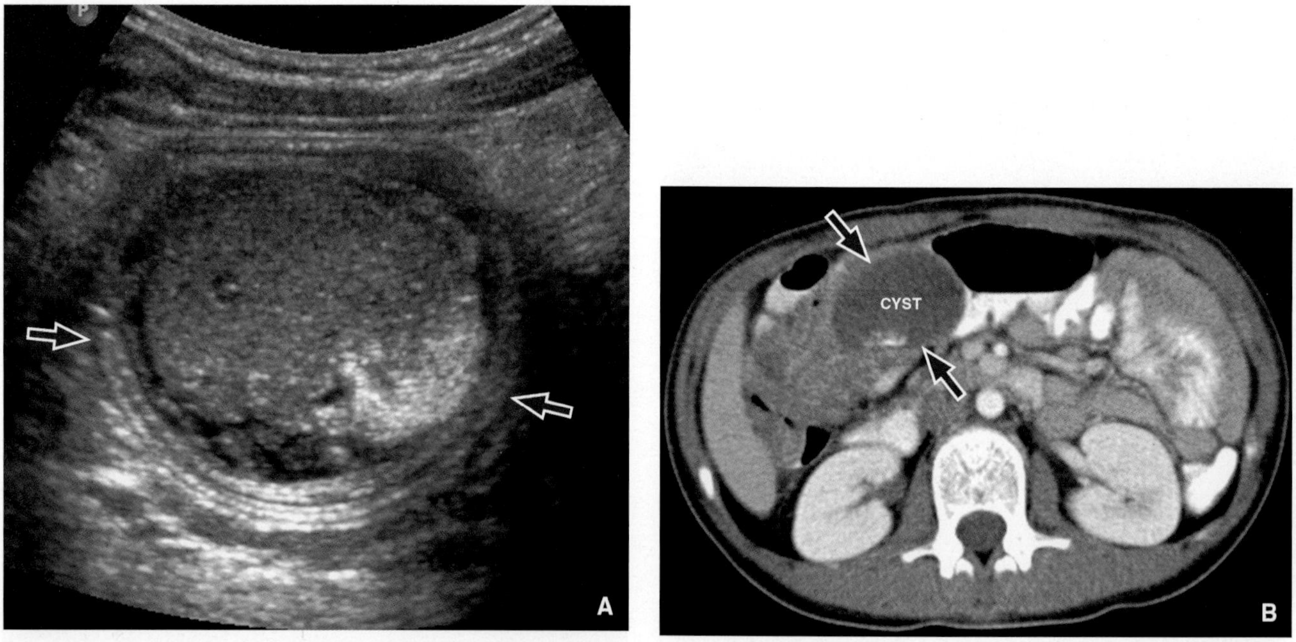

FIGURE 16.27 **A 9-year-old girl with intussusception due to a colonic duplication cyst. A:** Transverse ultrasound image shows a complex, hypoechoic "mass" (*arrows*) associated with the colon in the right upper quadrant; note the layered " gut signature" in the wall, similar to bowel wall. **B:** Axial contrast-enhanced CT image shows a round low-attenuation mass (cyst) associated with the wall of the transverse colon (*arrows*) acting as lead point for an immediately proximal intussusception.

lack of intramural ganglion cells (extending from the pectinate line a variable length proximally) and functional bowel obstruction (Fig. 16.29).[19] Hirschsprung disease is associated with multiple congenital anomalies and syndromes, including trisomy 21. Affected neonates typically present with evidence of distal bowel obstruction, including vomiting and abdominal distension. Hirschsprung disease can also present in older children with severe chronic constipation.

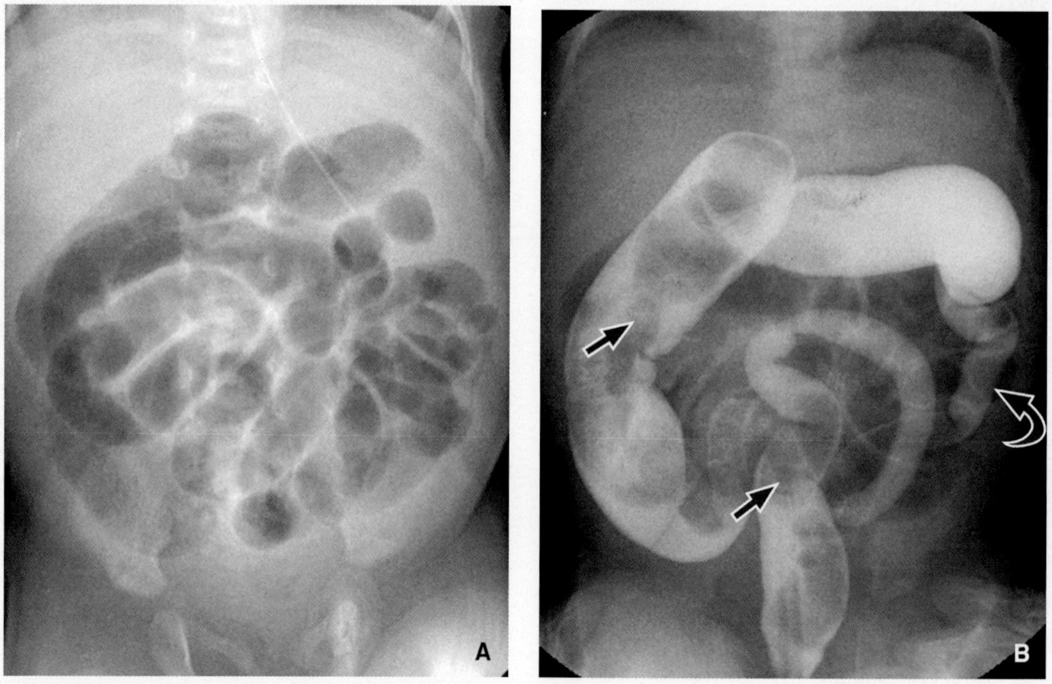

FIGURE 16.28 **A 2-year-old neonate girl who presented with delayed passage of meconium due to meconium plug syndrome (functional immaturity of the colon). A:** Abdominal radiograph shows multiple dilated, gas-filled bowel loops, in a distal obstruction pattern. **B:** Contrast enema shows opacification of the colon, with reflux of contrast material into distal small bowel loops. The descending and sigmoid colon are small in caliber (*curved arrow*), and intraluminal filling defects reflecting meconium plugs (*straight arrows*) are present in rectum as well as portions of the colon.

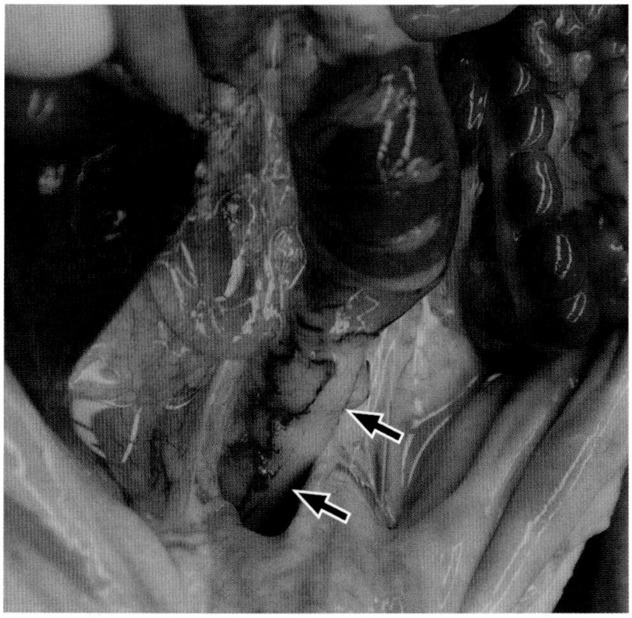

FIGURE 16.29 **Hirschsprung disease, diagnosed at autopsy in a 5-month old girl with trisomy 21 and congenital heart disease.** The rectum (*arrows*) is narrow and pale; proximally, the sigmoid colon is dilated. Microscopically, the distal 6 cm of rectum lacked ganglion cells (not shown).

In neonates, radiography shows evidence of distal GI tract obstruction with multiple dilated bowel loops and air–fluid levels.[38] When Hirschsprung disease is suspected, contrast enema is usually the initial imaging test of choice. Care should be taken to place the enema catheter in the very distal rectum so that the entire rectum can be evaluated. Fluoroscopic imaging is initially performed in the lateral position in order to assess the caliber of the rectum compared to the sigmoid colon. In Hirschsprung disease, the distal aganglionic colonic segment is usually narrowed, and there is dilatation of proximal normal bowel (the rectosigmoid ratio is <1); a distinct "transition zone" strongly supports a diagnosis of Hirschsprung disease (Fig. 16.30). The wall of the abnormal colonic segment may appear irregular having a "saw tooth" appearance. In the setting of total colonic aganglionosis, which can extend to involve the small intestine, the colon can appear normal or may be diffusely small in caliber (i.e., diffuse microcolon). In affected older children who present with chronic constipation, radiography typically shows very large amounts of colonic fecal material with or without colonic dilatation.

Rectal biopsy is performed to confirm the diagnosis of Hirschsprung disease, and treatment is surgical resection of the aganglionic colon.

Megacystis-Microcolon-Intestinal Hypoperistalsis Syndrome

Megacystis-microcolon-intestinal hypoperistalsis (MMIH) syndrome, or Berdon syndrome, is a rare constellation of features, including functional bowel obstruction, marked enlargement of the urinary bladder, microcolon, and malrotation.[45,46] This condition is mostly affects girls, and it shares some radiologic features with prune-belly syndrome.[47] Clinically, affected children present with functional bowel obstruction, decreased bowel sounds, and abdominal distention.[45]

Radiography in the neonate commonly reveals dilated small bowel loops, whereas upper GI series shows malrotation. SBFT examination typically shows diffusely dilated, markedly hypoperistaltic small bowel loops and delayed transit of contrast material to the colon. Contrast enema demonstrates

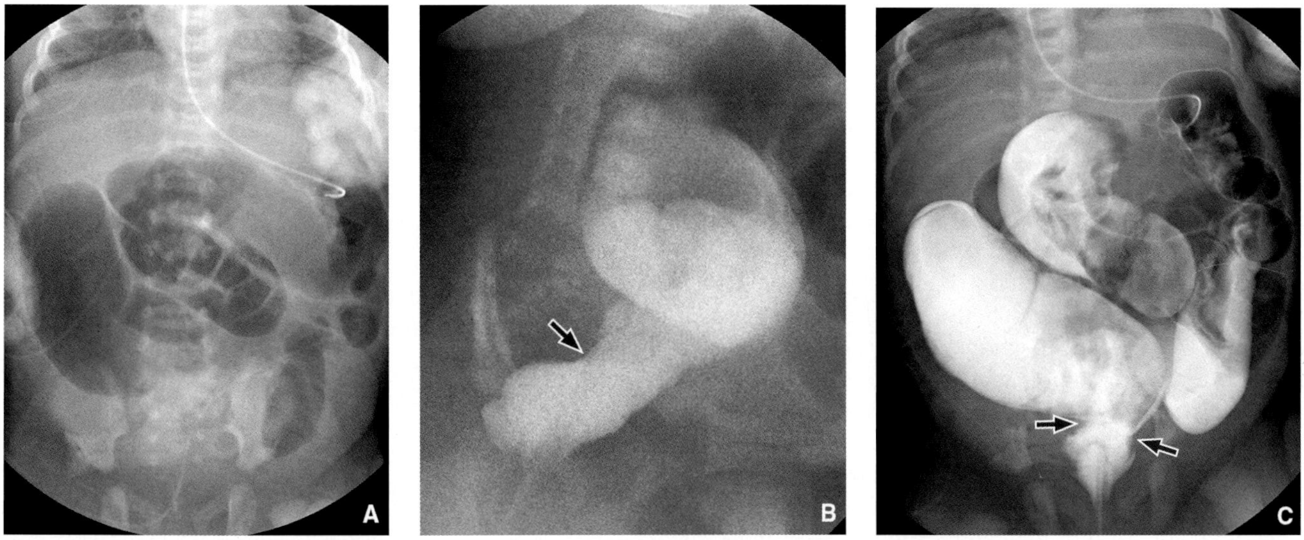

FIGURE 16.30 **Neonate girl who presented with abdominal distension due to Hirschsprung disease. A:** Abdominal radiograph shows multiple dilated, gas-filled bowel loops, in a distal obstruction pattern. **B:** Contrast enema image in the lateral projection shows abnormal rectosigmoid index (<0.9), with the sigmoid colon larger in caliber than the rectum. There is a "transition zone" (*arrow*) near the rectosigmoid junction. **C:** Frontal image confirms the location of the transition zone (*arrows*).

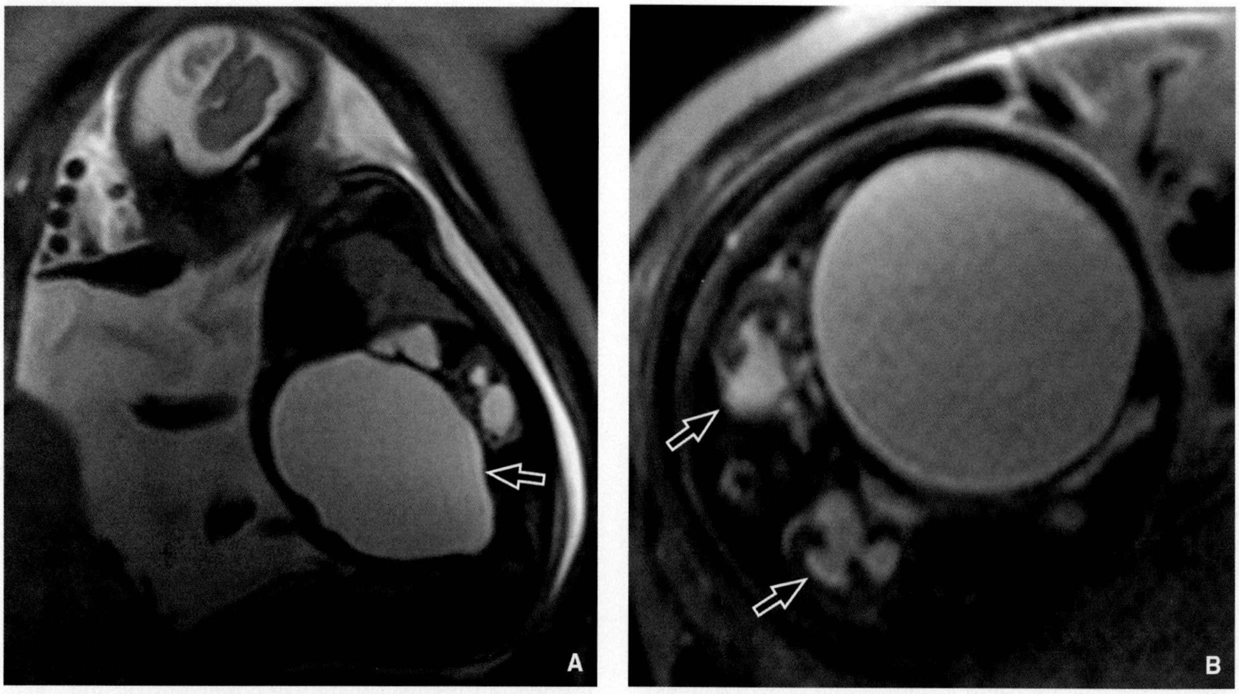

FIGURE 16.31 **Megacystis microcolon–intestinal hypoperistalsis syndrome in a female fetus. A:** Second-trimester prenatal sagittal T2-weighted MR image shows marked distension of the urinary bladder, or megacystis (*arrow*). **B:** Axial T2-weighted MR image shows megacystis as well as bilateral renal pelvicaliectasis (*arrows*).

diffuse microcolon with abnormal location of the cecum. Ultrasound in the neonate reveals marked distention of the urinary bladder and possible hydroureteronephrosis.[45] MMIH syndrome can be suspected based on prenatal imaging because of the presence of megacystis and dilated small bowel loops (Fig. 16.31).

This condition has typically had a dismal prognosis, with described management including total parenteral nutrition and bowel transplantation.[47]

Rectum

Anorectal Malformations

Anorectal malformations represent a spectrum of anomalies involving the rectum and anus, including imperforate anus, anal atresia and stenosis, and rectal atresia. Anorectal malformations frequently coexist with rectourethral fistulas in boys or rectovaginal fistulas in girls. These malformations can be associated with other anomalies, most notably the VACTERL association. Both sporadic and inherited cases occur.[48] Currarino syndrome, which includes anorectal malformation, presacral mass (teratoma or anterior meningocele), and malformed sacrum, is autosomal dominantly inherited.[49] Most anorectal malformations are apparent at birth, except for rectal atresia, which can manifest as distal bowel obstruction. Fistulas may be clinically apparent because of identification of fecal material in the urethra or vagina. Anorectal malformations have been described as high, intermediate, or low in relation to the levator ani muscles.[19] A separate system described by Levitt and Pena classifies these malformations based on the gender of the child and the particular components of the abnormality to provide better prognostic and treatment information.[50]

The role of imaging in anorectal anomalies is to depict relevant anatomy, detect fistula tracts, and identify associated congenital anomalies. Imaging also helps with surgical planning and helps predict prognosis. The imaging appearances of anorectal malformations vary depending on the exact anomaly.[48] Abdominal radiography may show evidence of distal bowel obstruction as well as commonly an anomalous sacrum (Fig. 16.32). Cross-table lateral imaging with the patient prone can be performed to estimate the distance between the lower rectum and skin surface in the setting of imperforate anus. Voiding cystourethrography and augmented-pressure colostogram can be performed to detect and characterize fistulas (Fig. 16.33).[51] Ultrasound also can be performed to evaluate the distal rectum using a transanal approach, especially in the setting of imperforate anus. Currently, MRI is being increasing used in both the preoperative and postoperative settings to characterize pelvic floor musculature, search for fistulas, and identify associated anomalies[48] (Fig. 16.33).

Treatment of anorectal malformations is surgical, most often with a posterior sagittal anorectoplasty (PSARP operation) and can vary based on patient-specific factors, although MRI-assisted rectal pull-through has been described.

Cloacal Exstrophy

Cloacal exstrophy, the most severe anomaly in the bladder exstrophy–epispadias spectrum, is a rare congenital malformation. It is caused by a failure of fusion of the

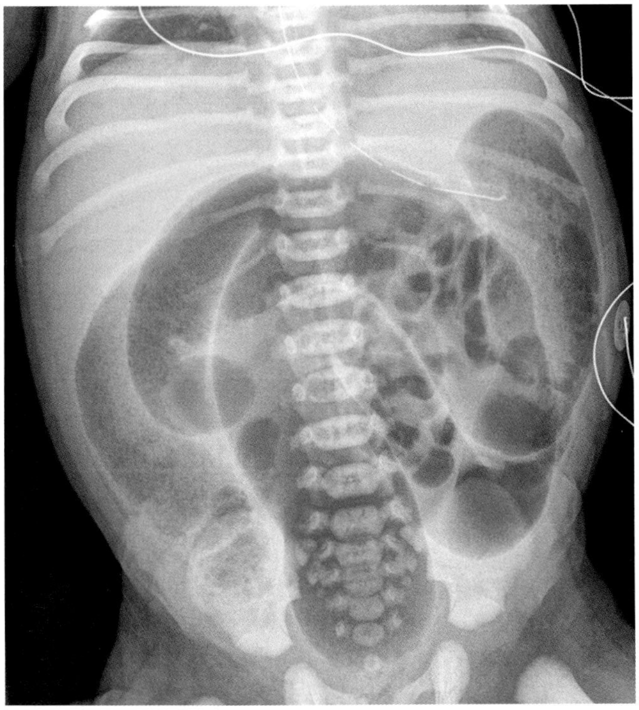

FIGURE 16.32 **Neonate girl with an imperforate anus.** Abdominal radiograph shows multiple dilated and gas-filled loops bowel to the level of rectum. The sacrum is normal.

infraumbilical midline structures at the cloacal stage of embryonic development. Cloacal exstropy is also known as OEIS syndrome (omphalocele-exstrophy-imperforate anus-spinal defects syndrome) because the four features are typically found together, which include **o**mphalocele, **e**xstrophy of the bladder and rectum, **i**mperforate anus, and **s**pinal defects. In affected children, many inner abdominal structures are exposed. In addition, diastatic symphysis pubis, spinal dysraphism, scoliosis, kyphosis, club feet and renal ectopia are also frequently present.

Currently, the diagnosis of cloacal exstrophy can be made by prenatal ultrasound or MRI, which can show the anterior opening of both the bladder and intestine and sometimes posterior opening of the spine. The diagnosis can be later confirmed on physical examination upon birth.

The current management choice of cloacal exstrophy is surgical repair that focuses on separation of the urinary and intestinal tracts, joining of the two hemibladders, colonic pull-through or colostomy, orchiectomy in genetic males, and closure of the abdominal wall defect.

Infectious Disorders

Esophagus

Infection of the esophagus, or esophagitis, occurs most often in immunocompromised children who have either congenital or acquired immunodeficiency. Currently, endoscopy (esophagogastroduodenoscopy [EGD], often with biopsy, has largely replaced esophagography as the preferred method for diagnosing infectious esophagitis. If possible, double-contrast technique should be performed to improve mucosal detail.

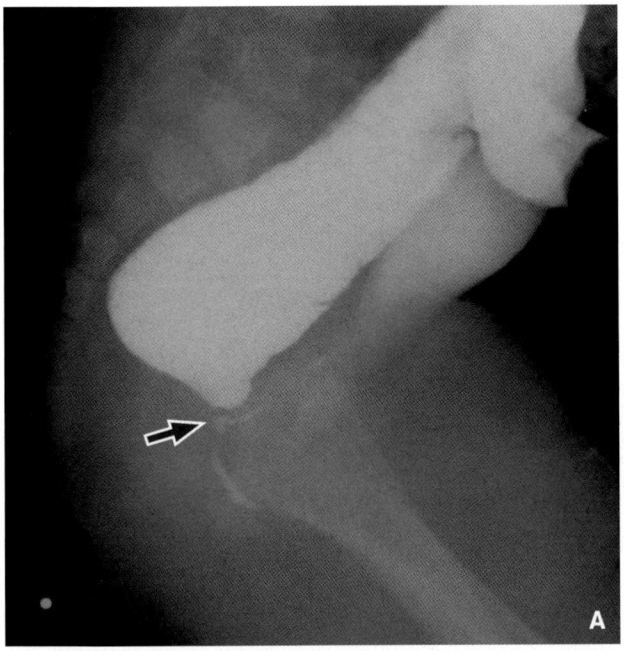

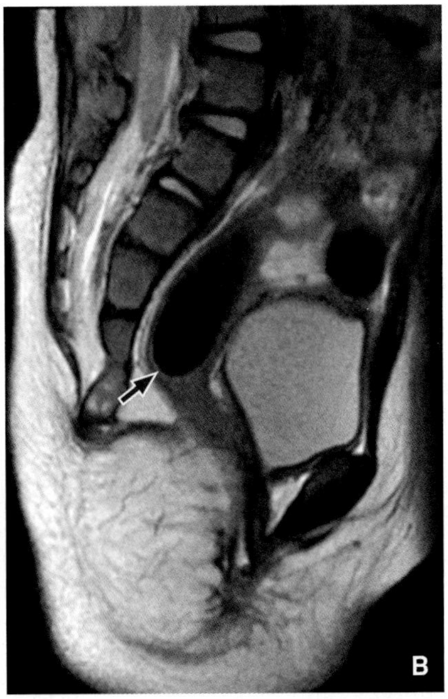

FIGURE 16.33 **Infant girl with an anorectal malformation. A:** Lateral projection from a colostogram study shows opacification of distal colon and proximal rectum with abrupt termination of the contrast column. A BB marks the expected location of the anus. There is a fistula (*arrow*) between the rectum and posterior urethra, with contrast material opacifying the posterior urethra and streaming into the urinary bladder. **B:** Correlative sagittal T2-weighted MR image shows abrupt termination of hypointense, air-filled rectum (*arrow*) with isointense soft tissue distally.

Viral Esophagitis

Cytomegalovirus

Cytomegalovirus (CMV) is a very common opportunistic pathogen in immunocompromised children that affects the esophagus and colon when there is GI tract involvement. Children with CMV esophagitis may present with odynophagia.[52] Although EGD is the preferred diagnostic modality, esophagography can demonstrate large (sometimes >1 cm), shallow mid- or distal esophageal ulcers that are characteristic of CMV infection. Treatment is directed towards restoring immune competence and administering antiviral medications.[52]

Human Immunodeficiency Virus

Human immunodeficiency virus (HIV)-related esophageal ulcers are common and can often be attributed to CMV, herpes simplex virus (HSV), *Candida albicans*, and mycobacteria infections.[53] Esophageal ulcers are termed HIV-related or idiopathic giant ulcers when the ulcer cannot be attributed to another cause. Affected patients usually present with odynophagia, dysphagia, and retrosternal chest pain, occasionally accompanied by hematemesis. Although HIV-related ulcers are difficult to differentiate from CMV-related ulcers by imaging, idiopathic lesions are typically larger and have overhanging edges in comparison to "punched-out" ulcers caused by CMV. These lesions usually occur in the mid- and distal esophagus. Medical management of HIV-related ulcers can include corticosteroids along with thalidomide in certain cases.[54]

Herpes Simplex Virus

HSV esophagitis also mostly occurs in immunocompromised children.[55] Clinical symptoms include odynophagia and retrosternal pain. Esophagography usually reveals numerous tiny superficial ulcers, although ulcers can also appear punctate or linear. Severe HSV esophagitis can mimic Candida esophagitis. Treatment includes antiviral medication, such as acyclovir.[56]

Fungal Esophagitis

Candida albicans is the most common cause of infectious esophagitis. Oropharyngeal candidiasis and immunosuppression are common risk factors. Affected children usually present with odynophagia and dysphagia, and EGD often reveals raised white plaques with hyperemia and ulcerations in some cases. At esophagography, severe infection is characterized by a "shaggy" appearance of the esophagus, resulting from confluent longitudinally oriented plaques, pseudomembranes, and ulcers (Fig. 16.34). Treatment includes antifungal medications, such as nystatin and fluconazole. Other medications, such as amphotericin, are reserved for resistant cases in immunocompromised patients with fungemia.[57]

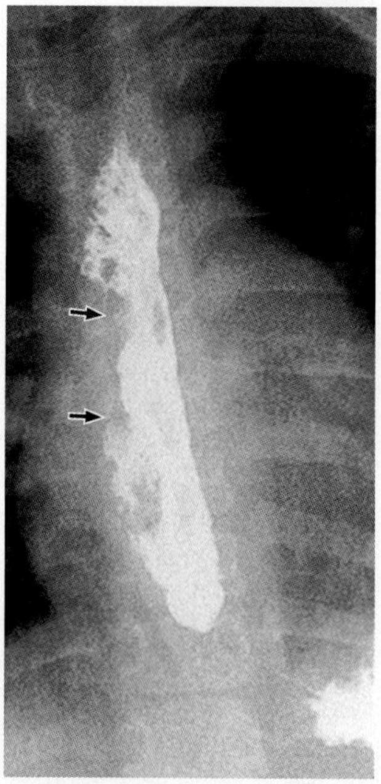

FIGURE 16.34 **A 9-year-old boy with HIV infection and dysphagia due to candida esophagitis.** Frontal esophagram image shows numerous large, irregular persistent filling defects (*arrows*), consistent with plaque-like lesions and ulcerations.

Stomach

Gastritis

Gastritis is a nonspecific term that referring to inflammation of the stomach wall (Fig. 16.35). In children, such changes can result from infection (e.g., *Helicobacter pylori*), chemical ingestion, eosinophilic disease, hypertrophic gastropathy, severe stress, or as the result of chronic conditions, such as Crohn disease and chronic granulomatous disease.

Peptic Ulcer Disease

Peptic ulcers are the result of a breach in the mucosal protective mechanisms of the stomach or duodenum that leads to ulceration. These ulcers may be a primary (secondary to *H. pylori* infection) or secondary (e.g., the result of stress, chemical ingestion, or gastrin-secreting tumor) in children.[58] Peptic ulcers can affect the stomach or duodenum. Typical symptoms of peptic ulcers in young children include difficulty feeding and vomiting, whereas older children may present with GI tract bleeding or peritonitis due to viscus perforation.[58] EGD is currently used to diagnose peptic ulcer disease.

Upper GI series can show large gastric and duodenal ulcers, although this examination lacks sensitivity for small ulcers especially if using single-contrast technique. Large ulcers may sometimes be apparent on CT, appearing as ulceration of the gastric or duodenal wall, adjacent viscus wall thickening, and perigastric or periduodenal inflammation (Figs. 16.36 and 16.37). Perforated ulcers may present with evidence of peritonitis on physical examination as well as pneumoperitoneum on CT (Fig. 16.37).[59,60]

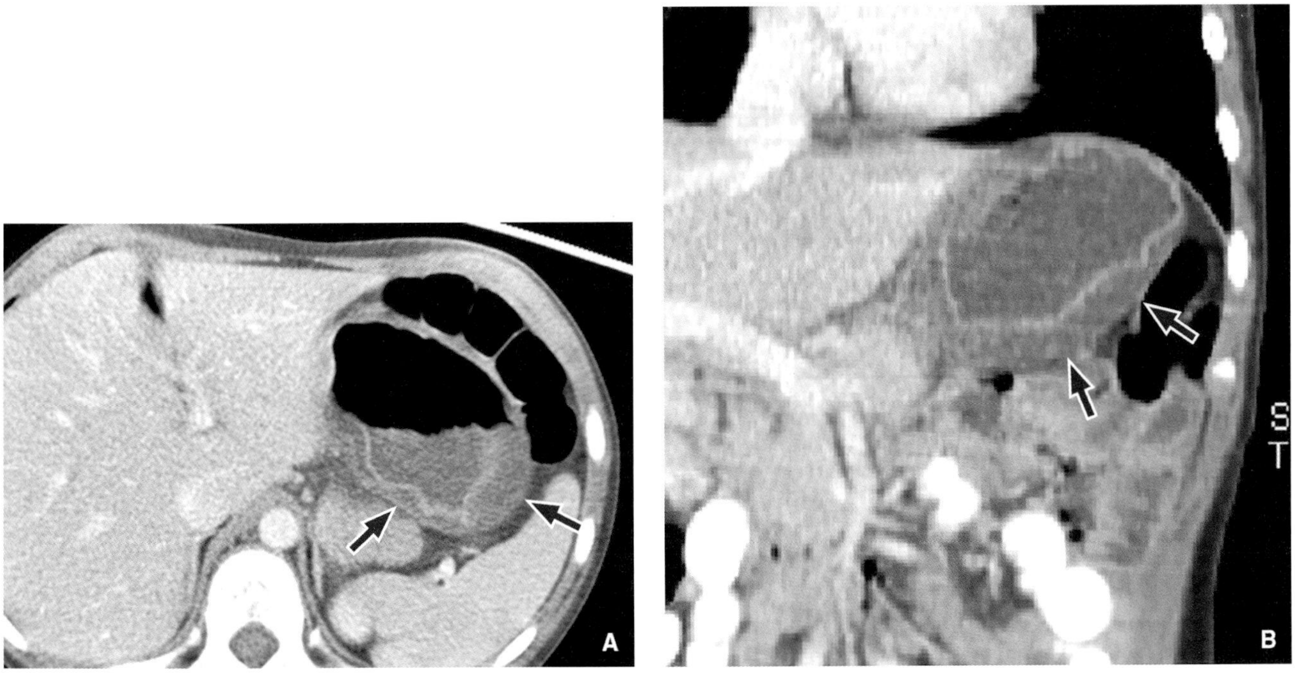

FIGURE 16.35 **A 6-year-old boy with abdominal pain and vomiting. Endoscopy showed severe gastritis. A:** Axial contrast-enhanced CT image shows marked thickening and submucosal edema of the wall of the proximal stomach (*arrows*). **B:** Coronal reformatted contrast-enhanced CT image shows similar findings (*arrows*).

Treatment of infectious peptic ulcer disease involves the eradication of *H. pylori* with antimicrobial agents and decreasing gastric acid production with proton pump inhibitors or histamine blockers.[58]

Small Intestine

Viral Infection

Infectious gastroenteritis due to viral pathogens is common. In the United States, viruses that cause gastroenteritis in the pediatric population are typically rotavirus, norovirus, and adenovirus.[61,62] Viral gastroenteritis typically presents with vomiting followed by watery diarrhea, and in otherwise healthy children is self-limited and managed conservatively.[63] Imaging studies generally are not necessary, because infectious diarrhea in children is usually a clinical diagnosis. However, in certain children where

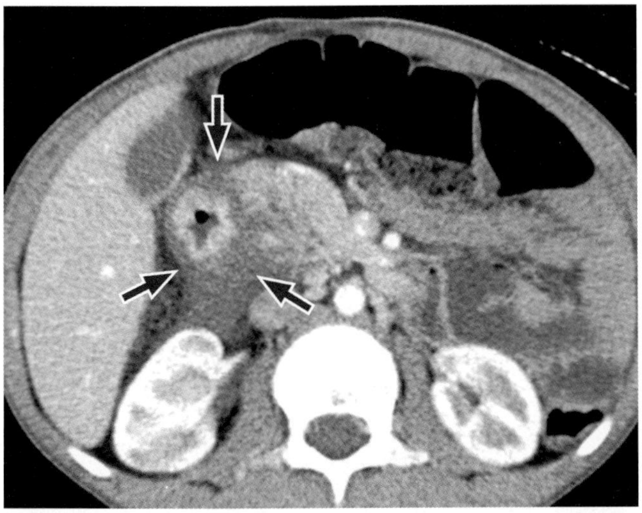

FIGURE 16.36 **A 17-year-old boy with abdominal pain due to endoscopy-confirmed peptic ulcer disease of the duodenum.** Axial contrast-enhanced CT image shows duodenal wall thickening, hyperenhancement, and marked surrounding inflammation (*arrows*).

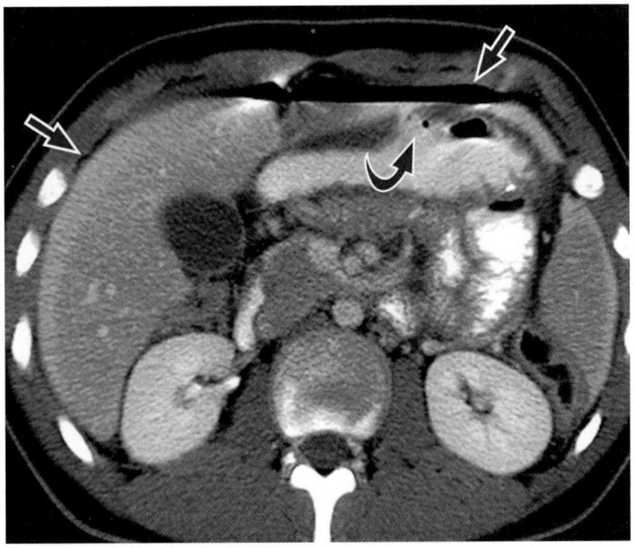

FIGURE 16.37 **A 14-year-old boy with acute abdominal pain and guarding.** Axial contrast-enhanced CT image shows pneumoperitoneum (*straight arrows*) and extraluminal oral contrast material. There is an outpouching arising from the anterior stomach representing a large ulcer (*curved arrow*), which was confirmed at surgery.

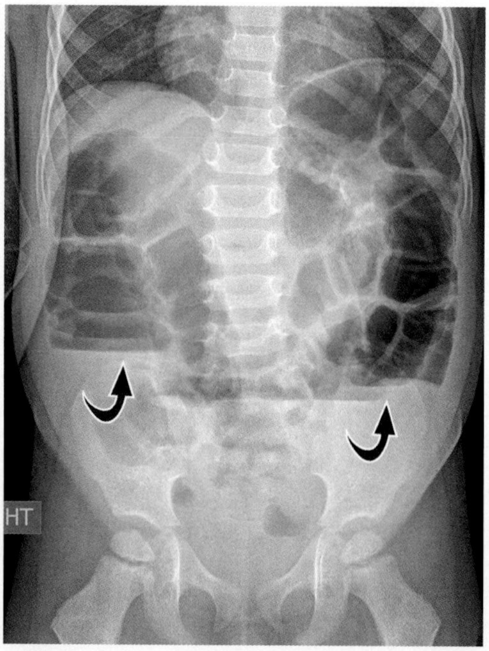

FIGURE 16.38 **A 4-year-old boy with viral gastroenteritis who presented with vomiting and diarrhea.** Upright radiograph of the abdomen shows multiple mildly dilated gas-filled bowel loops and air–fluid levels (*curved arrows*).

symptoms are ambiguous and mimic other medical conditions, imaging may be performed to exclude other diagnoses, such as appendicitis.

Radiographic findings that may be indicative of viral gastroenteritis include nonobstructive bowel loop dilatation, absence of fecal material in the colon, multiple air–fluid levels, and, rarely, pneumatosis intestinalis[64] (Fig. 16.38). Ultrasound and CT may show nonspecific small bowel wall thickening, distended fluid-filled bowel loops,[65,66] and intra-abdominal lymphadenopathy.[62]

Supportive care including oral rehydration is current management choice in children with viral gastroenteritis.

Bacterial Infection

Enteritis due to bacterial pathogens accounts for ~2% to 10% of cases of infectious diarrhea in developed countries. The most common pathogens in the United States responsible for bacterial enteritis include *Shigella, Salmonella, Escherichia coli,* and *Campylobacter.*[66] Common bacterial diarrhea–causing organisms in the developing world include *Yersinia enterocolitica and Vibrio* species. Symptoms of bacterial enteritis are similar to those of viral gastroenteritis, although bloody diarrhea, high fever, and chills are more commonly associated with bacterial pathogens like *E. coli.*[66]

Radiographic findings of bacterial enteritis most often involve the distal small bowel.[65,67] Ultrasound may reveal nonspecific bowel wall thickening, hyperemia, and reactive free fluid. At CT, the small bowel typically shows bowel wall thickening, luminal narrowing, and perienteric inflammatory fat stranding (Fig. 16.39).

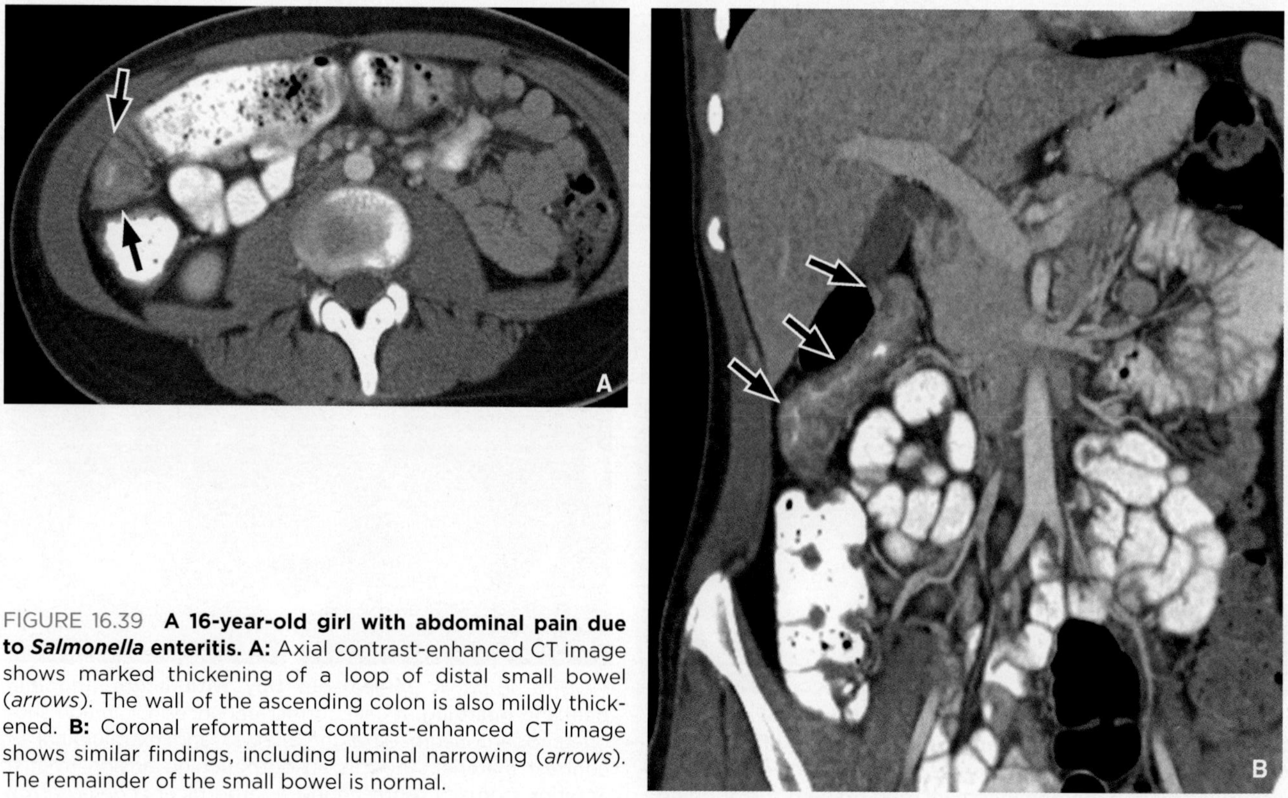

FIGURE 16.39 **A 16-year-old girl with abdominal pain due to *Salmonella* enteritis. A:** Axial contrast-enhanced CT image shows marked thickening of a loop of distal small bowel (*arrows*). The wall of the ascending colon is also mildly thickened. **B:** Coronal reformatted contrast-enhanced CT image shows similar findings, including luminal narrowing (*arrows*). The remainder of the small bowel is normal.

Treatment includes antibiotic therapy as well as fluid and electrolyte management.

Mycobacterial Infection

Abdominal mycobacterial infection is uncommon in the pediatric population, especially in otherwise healthy children. It can be caused by the *Mycobacterium bovis* (because of ingestion of unpasteurized infected milk products) or *Mycobacterium tuberculosis* (because of ingestion of infected sputum) organisms. Peritoneal tuberculosis (TB) is an uncommon extrapulmonary manifestation of *M. tuberculosis* infection that results from lymphohematogenous dissemination from a primary, usually pulmonary lesion. Abdominal TB involvement may present with abdominal distention secondary to ascites, pain, fever, and weight loss.[68]

Intestinal involvement by TB can have different imaging appearances, including ulcerative, hypertrophic, and mixed phenotypes. Among them, the ulcerative form is most common and is characterized by superficial ulcers. The hypertrophic form is characterized by bowel wall thickening and mural fibrosis. Ultrasound can reveal bowel wall thickening, mesenteric thickening, and lymphadenopathy. Affected lymph nodes may have hypoechoic central areas indicative of caseating necrosis.[69] SBFT can be used to demonstrate small bowel and proximal colonic involvement, including associated strictures (Fig. 16.40). SBFT findings of intestinal TB infection include shortening of the ascending colon,

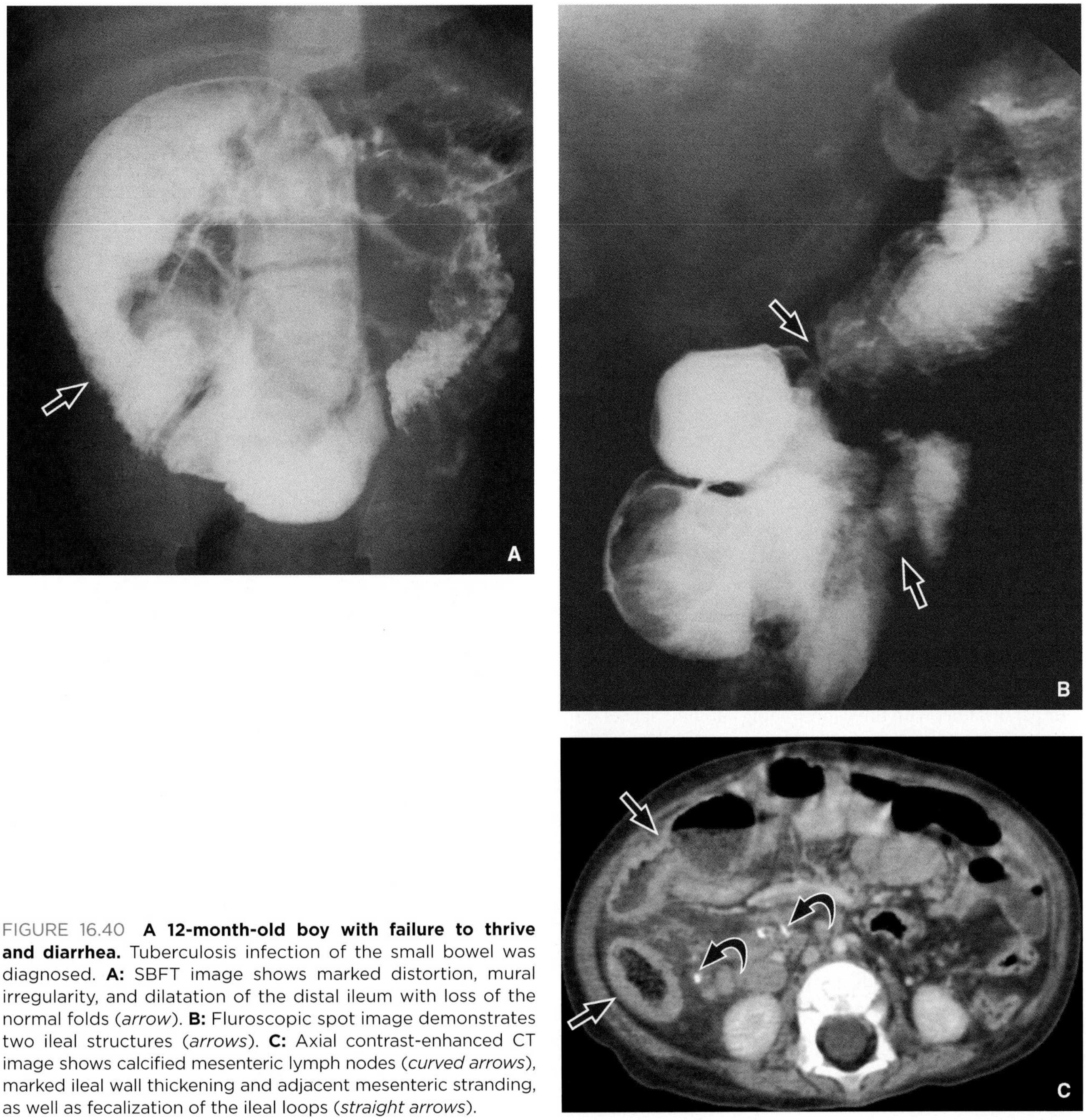

FIGURE 16.40 **A 12-month-old boy with failure to thrive and diarrhea.** Tuberculosis infection of the small bowel was diagnosed. **A:** SBFT image shows marked distortion, mural irregularity, and dilatation of the distal ileum with loss of the normal folds (*arrow*). **B:** Fluroscopic spot image demonstrates two ileal structures (*arrows*). **C:** Axial contrast-enhanced CT image shows calcified mesenteric lymph nodes (*curved arrows*), marked ileal wall thickening and adjacent mesenteric stranding, as well as fecalization of the ileal loops (*straight arrows*).

deformation of the cecum, and ileal thickening with a distorted ileocecal junction.[70,71] Areas of intestinal narrowing and dilatation may also be observed.[70,71] At CT, common findings of intestinal TB infection include distal small bowel wall thickening and right lower quadrant mesenteric lymph node abnormalities, which include enlargement, calcification, or central low attenuation (Fig. 16.40). Overall, imaging features of intestinal TB share substantial overlap with Crohn disease.

Treatment of intestinal TB is directed towards eradication of the infection.

Parasitic Infection

Two most commonly encountered small bowel parasites in the developed world include the protozoa *Giardia lamblia* and *Cryptosporidium*. Transmission generally occurs via the fecal–oral route through contaminated food and water.[64] Parasitic worms, known as helminths, including nematodes (roundworms, such as ascarids, hookworms, and pinworms) and flatworms (such as schistosomes and tapeworms), are common intestinal pathogens in developing countries. These worms are estimated to infect up to one-third of the impoverished world population—most commonly children and adolescents[72].

Small bowel fluoroscopic studies in children with parasitic disease can show dilution of contrast material from fluid retention, mucosal fold thickening, and aberrant transit time, either rapid or delayed, based upon the course of the disease.[73–75] In addition, particular parasites are associated with specific imaging findings. For example, *Giardia* causes thickened duodenal and jejunal mucosal folds, rapid transit time, and dilution of contrast material.[76] In *Ascaris lumbricoides* infection, contrast material may outline the parasitic organisms (Fig. 16.41). Live worms can also ingest contrast material, allowing for visualization of their intestinal tracts as well.[76] *A. lumbricoides* worms also can be seen on ultrasound with the findings dependent on worm orientation, surrounding tissues, part of the worm imaged, and if the worm is alive or dead. Using low frequency transducers, the worm is seen as two parallel echogenic lines separated by anechoic area that represents the fluid-filled alimentary tract of the worm, and when using a high-frequency transducer, worms are seen as four parallel lines with three intervening anechoic spaces.[77] In certain instances, the worms can be seen ingesting fluid during real-time imaging.[77]

Treatment involves antihelmintic medications directed towards eradication of specific parasites.

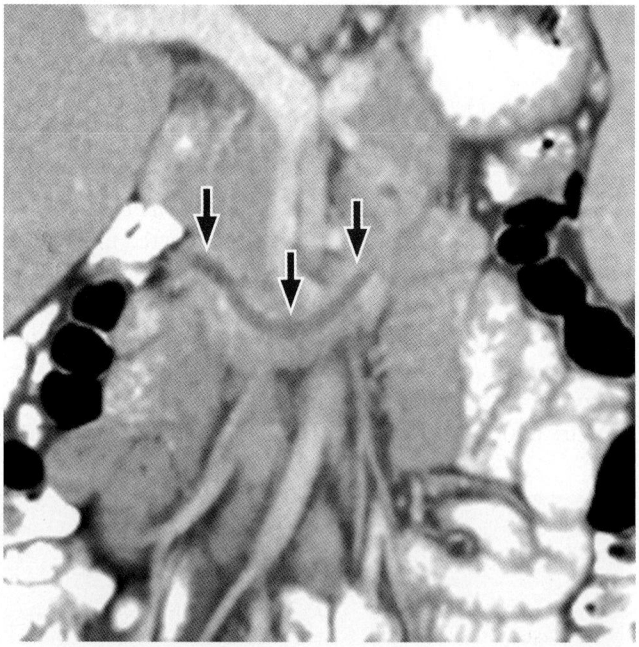

FIGURE 16.41 **A 16-year-old boy with diarrhea due to *Ascaris lumbricoides* infection.** Coronal contrast-enhanced CT image shows a curvilinear low-attenuation filling defect (*arrows*) in the duodenum representing a worm.

Clostridium difficile Infection

Pseudomembranous colitis is most often the result of *Clostridium difficile* infection and toxin production as a result of antibiotic therapy. Other toxin-producing organisms that less commonly cause pseudomembranous colitis include *Clostridium perfringens* and *Staphylococcus aureus*. Affected children typically present with fever, bloody diarrhea, abdominal cramping, and colonic mucositis following antibiotic use. Rarely, pseudomembranous colitis may occur without preceding antibiotic use.[70,71]

Colon

Viral and Bacterial Infections

The organisms that cause infectious colitis are often the same ones that affect the small intestine. Imaging studies are infrequently needed for diagnosis. However, when obtained, they typically show nonspecific colonic inflammation, such as colonic wall thickening, submucosal edema, and prominence of pericolonic blood vessels/pericolonic stranding (Fig. 16.42).

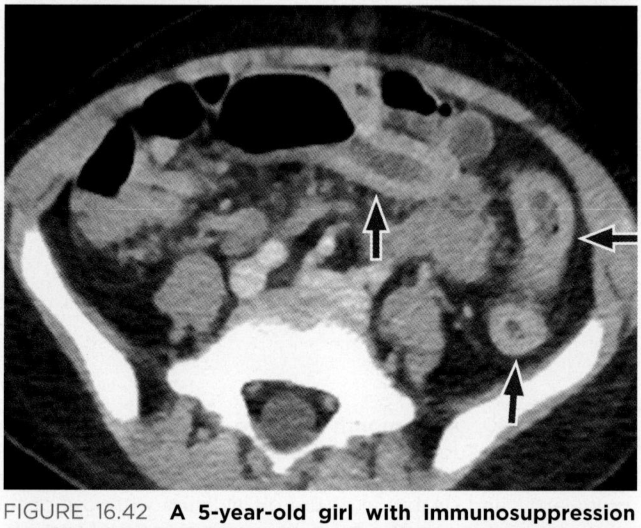

FIGURE 16.42 **A 5-year-old girl with immunosuppression who presented with diarrhea and biopsy-confirmed cytomegalovirus infection.** Axial contrast-enhanced CT image shows wall thickening of the descending and sigmoid colon (*arrows*), with adjacent mild inflammatory changes.

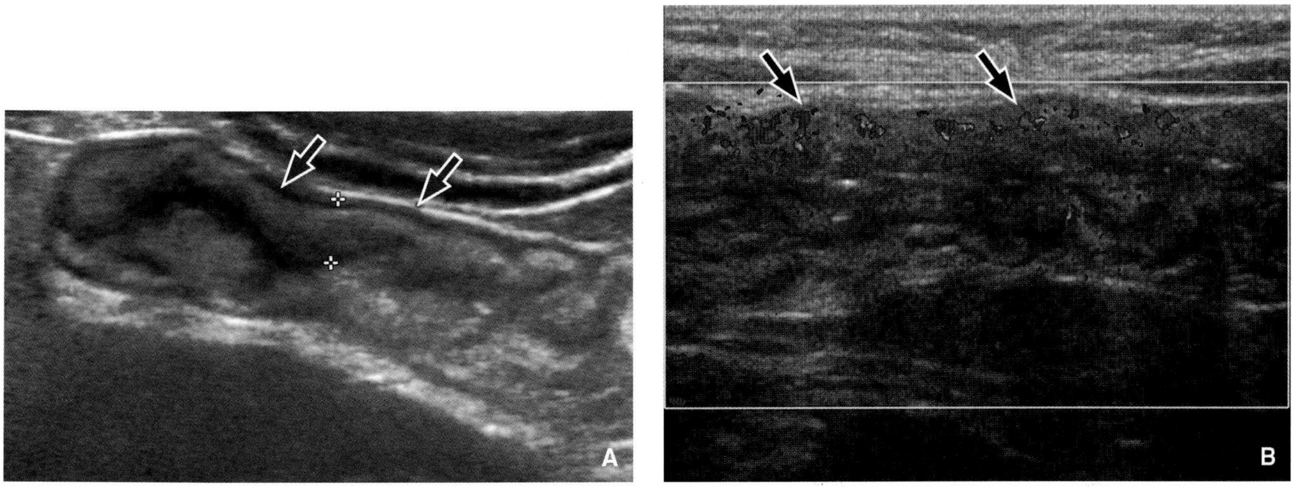

FIGURE 16.43 **A 3-year-old girl with new-onset bloody stools and crampy abdominal pain for 2 days due to *E. coli* infectious colitis. A:** High-resolution gray-scale ultrasound image of the transverse colon shows marked wall thickening (*arrows*), including submucosal edema. **B:** Color Doppler ultrasound image demonstrates bowel wall hyperemia (*arrows*).

Ultrasound (Fig. 16.43) and CT typically show pancolitis, with diffuse colonic wall thickening and submucosal edema (low attenuation at CT). Thickened, edematous haustra may give rise to the "accordion sign" (Figs. 16.44 and 16.45). Post-contrast imaging may reveal mucosal hyperenhancement.

Treatment involves antibiotic therapy directed towards eradication of the *C. difficile* organism, such as oral metronidazole or oral vancomycin.

Neutropenic Colitis (Typhlitis)

Neutropenic colitis, or typhlitis, is a necrotizing colitis seen primarily in children with hematopoietic malignancies, but also in individuals undergoing chemotherapy for other cancers. It is associated with neutropenia and primarily affects the cecum. Clinical presentation can be sometimes mistaken for appendicitis in the pediatric population with symptoms including abdominal pain, fever, nausea, diarrhea, and abdominal distention.[71,78] Peritonitis due intestinal perforation can also occur.[71,78]

Radiography may show a focal ileus or bowel wall thickening in the right lower quadrant.[79] Ultrasound and CT can show cecal and ascending colon (and possibly terminal ileum) wall thickening with adjacent inflammatory changes and free fluid (Fig. 16.46).[79,80] Both pneumatosis and pneumoperitoneum can be also seen.

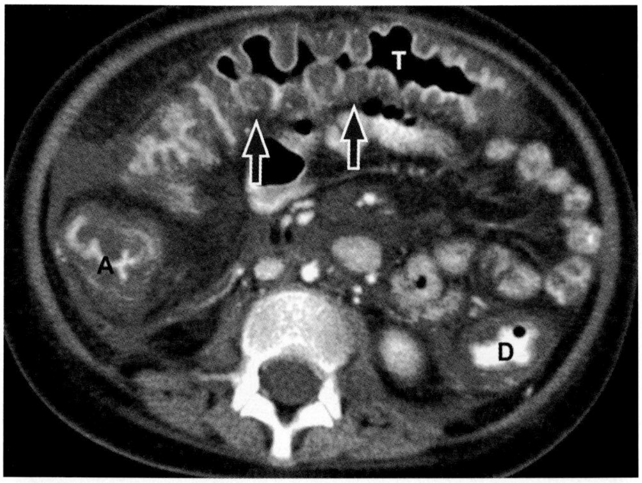

FIGURE 16.44 ***C. difficile* colitis in a 7-year-old girl with abdominal pain and diarrhea.** Axial contrast-enhanced CT image shows marked thickening of the ascending (*A*), transverse (*T*) and descending (*D*) colon with adjacent inflammation and fluid. Note the marked thickening of haustra, including submucosal edema giving the classic "accordion sign" (*arrows*) in the transverse colon; this leads to the "thumb printing" seen on abdominal radiographs.

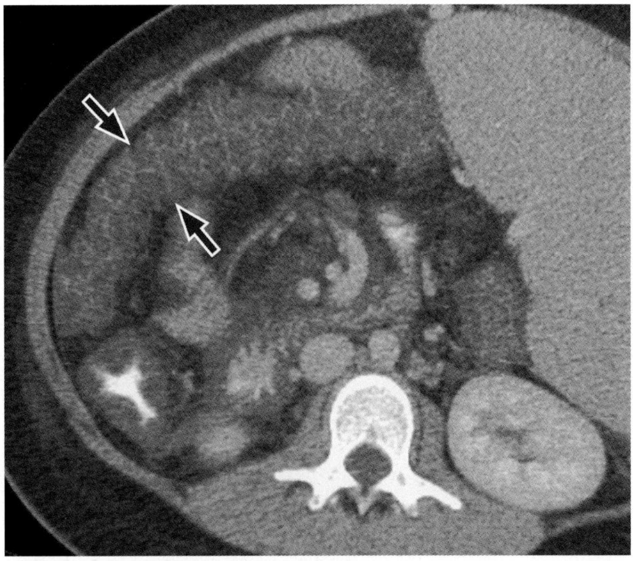

FIGURE 16.45 ***C. difficile* colitis in a 14-year-old girl with acute lymphocytic leukemia.** Axial contrast-enhanced CT image shows colonic wall thickening and mural low attenuation due to submucosal edema; the colonic lumen is narrowed (*arrows*). Splenomegaly is related to the patient's leukemia.

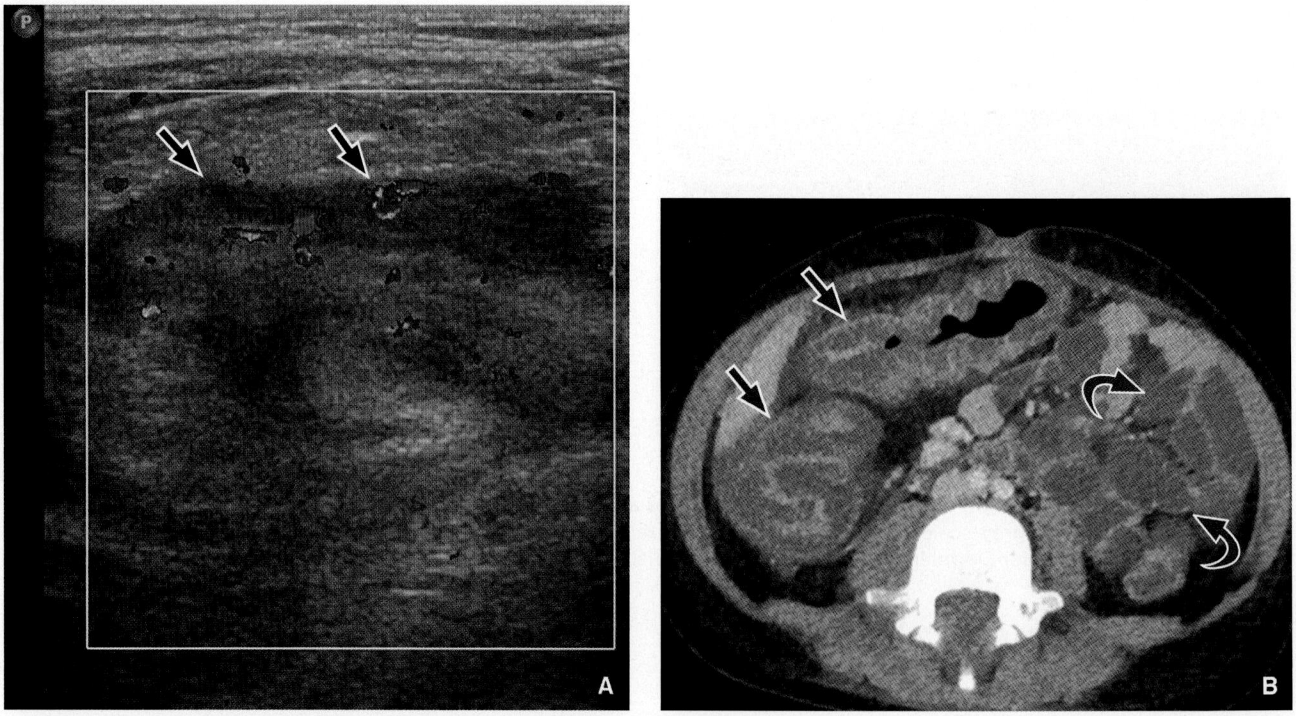

FIGURE 16.46 **Neutropenic colitis (typhlitis) in an 8-year-old boy with acute lymphocytic leukemia status post–stem cell transplant. A:** Color Doppler ultrasound image shows a thick-walled cecum with hyperemia (*arrows*). **B:** Axial contrast-enhanced CT image shows marked wall thickening (including submucosal edema) of the ascending colon and hepatic flexure (*straight arrows*). Normal fluid-filled bowel loops are seen in the left hemiabdomen (*curved arrows*).

Management of uncomplicated neutropenic colitis typically involves antibiotic therapy, whereas complicated cases may require surgery.[80]

Perirectal and Perianal Abscess

Perirectal and perianal abscesses are believed to occur as a result of infection in the crypts of Morgagni (cryptitis) in many instances. In the pediatric population, they are most often a complication of Crohn disease with perianal disease seen in up to 14% of this patient population.[81] In infants and toddlers, skin infections can start as a cellulitis and develop into focal abscess as well (Fig. 16.47). These abscesses may present with perianal/rectal pain or drainage. Physical examination is commonly abnormal, revealing perianal skin inflammation and skin tags in the setting of Crohn disease.

Both ultrasound (conventional and endorectal) and MRI can be used to identify perirectal and perianal abscesses. MRI is particularly useful for determining the exact location and extent of these abscesses including relation to the

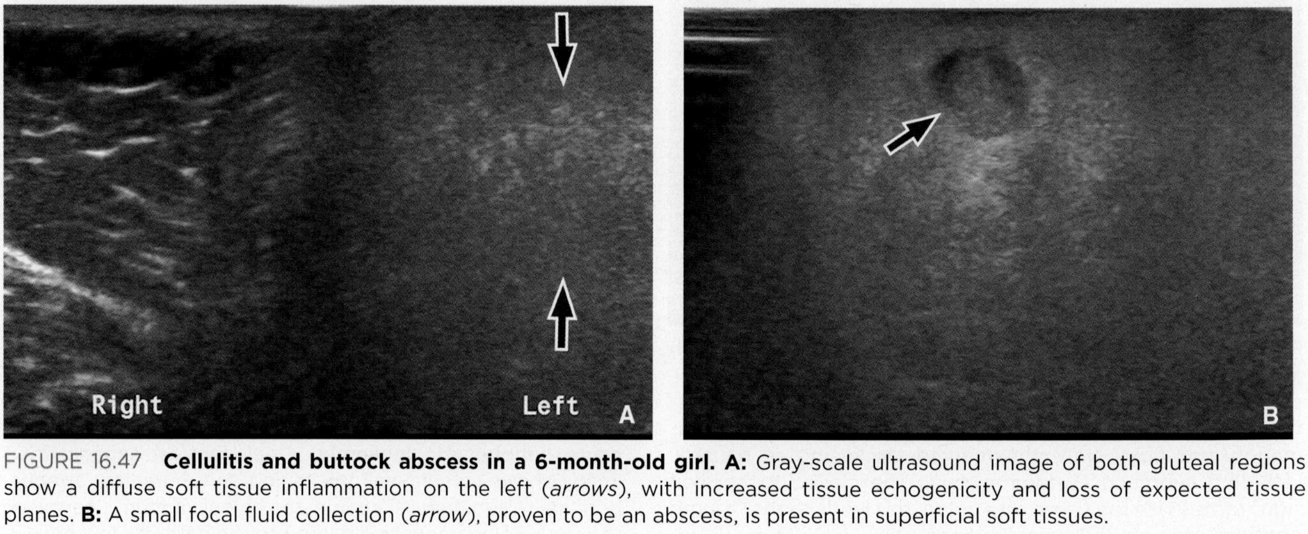

FIGURE 16.47 **Cellulitis and buttock abscess in a 6-month-old girl. A:** Gray-scale ultrasound image of both gluteal regions show a diffuse soft tissue inflammation on the left (*arrows*), with increased tissue echogenicity and loss of expected tissue planes. **B:** A small focal fluid collection (*arrow*), proven to be an abscess, is present in superficial soft tissues.

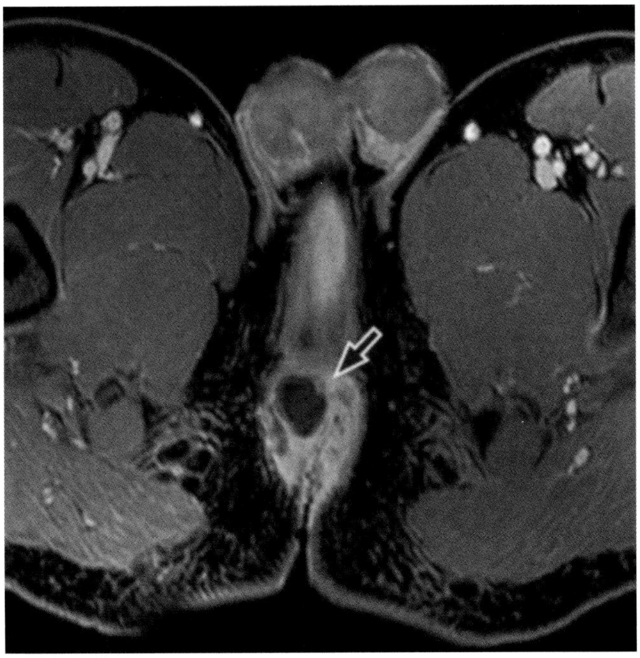

FIGURE 16.48 **A 15-year-old boy with known Crohn disease and perianal involvement.** Axial postcontrast T1-weighted MR image with fat suppression demonstrates a peripherally enhancing perianal abscess (*arrow*). Perianal skin appears hyperenhancing because of inflammation.

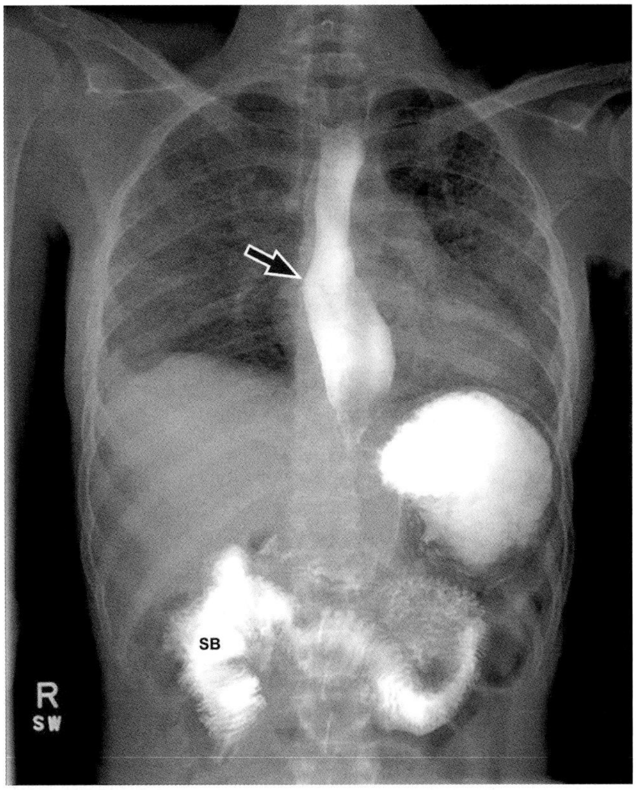

FIGURE 16.49 **A 16-year-old girl with systemic sclerosis (scleroderma).** Radiograph after upper GI series shows a dilated esophagus (megaesophagus) (*straight arrow*); proximal small bowel loops have an increased number of folds (*SB*). The lungs contain widespread opacities due to interstitial lung disease.

internal and external anal sphincters and levator muscles.[82] In addition, MRI is also useful for guiding medical and surgical management[82] (Fig. 16.48). Ultrasound, because of its real-time capability, can provide guidance for drainage procedures.

Perirectal and perianal abscesses may be managed with antibiotic therapy alone when small, although image-guided or surgical intervention may be required for larger fluid collections.[83]

Inflammatory Disorders

Juvenile Systemic Sclerosis

Juvenile systemic sclerosis (JSS), or scleroderma, is a rare connective tissue disorder of unclear etiology that affects the skin, subcutaneous tissues, and internal organs. JSS is one of the most severe rheumatologic conditions affecting children. Esophageal motility is often impaired in pediatric patients with JSS (it affects 75% to 90% of patients). Impaired motility also affects the stomach, small bowel, colon, and anorectal area resulting in substantial morbidity. Esophageal involvement in affected children can be asymptomatic, and other manifestations of rheumatologic disease may be observed.[84] Esophagography may show dilation of the lower esophagus and impaired esophageal motility[85] (Fig. 16.49). SBFT examination may show dilatation of small bowel loops, decreased peristalsis, and "hide bound" because of crowded small bowel folds (Fig. 16.49). Treatment involves immune system suppression and modulation.

Menetrier Disease (Stomach)

Menetrier disease, also known as hypoproteinemic hypertrophic gastropathy, is a rare, acquired condition that is characterized by enlarged gastric folds and associated with protein loss.[86] The childhood form of this disorder often follows a viral infection. Clinical presentation can include soft tissue edema from hypoproteinemia, gastric obstruction, and, in some cases, elevated IgE levels.[87] Endoscopy is the preferred diagnostic modality, showing enlarged, convoluted rugae (Fig. 16.50). These folds are also visible on upper GI series and CT, and may involve the proximal and/or distal portions of the stomach (Fig. 16.50).[88] Histology shows characteristic reduction of chief and parietal cells and cystic areas extending into the muscularis mucosae and submucosal.[87] Unlike in adults, this condition is typically self-limited in children, resolving in weeks or months.

Inflammatory Bowel Disease

Crohn Disease

Crohn disease is a transmural inflammatory condition that can affect the entire GI tract. Onset is commonly insidious. Affected children commonly present with abdominal pain, diarrhea, weight loss, and bloody stools.[89] In addition, they also may present with unexplained anemia, failure to thrive, a variety of skin abnormalities, and perianal pain/drainage

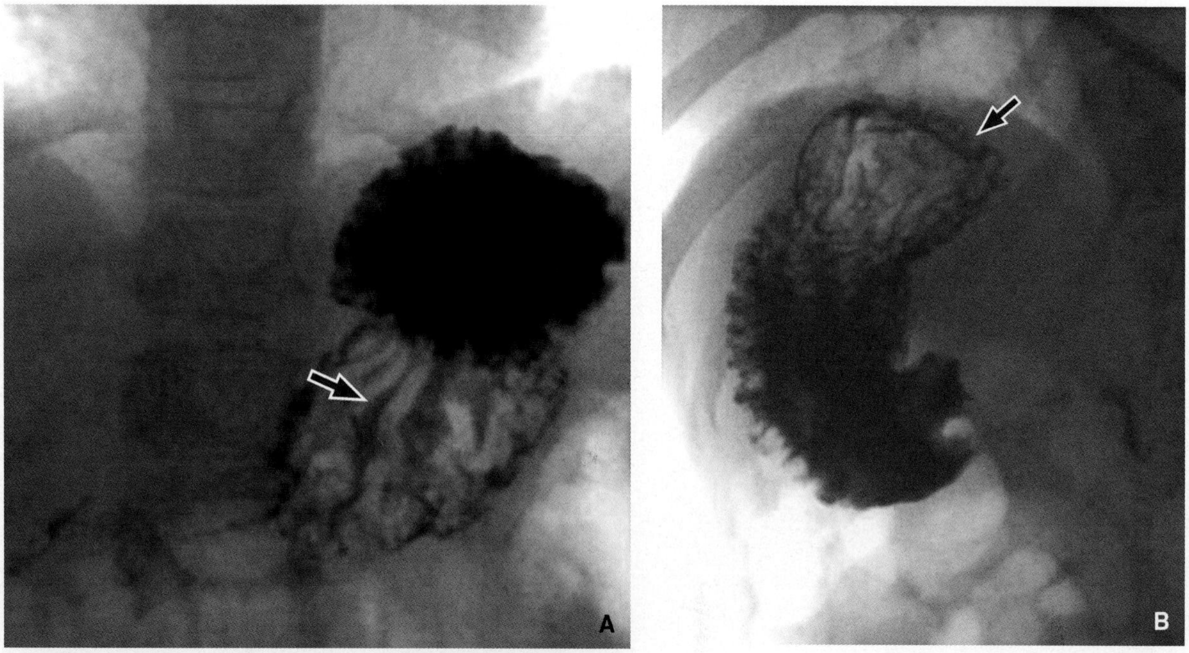

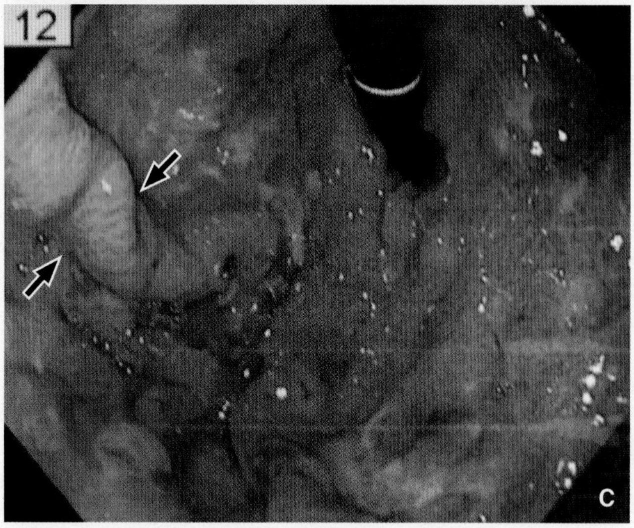

FIGURE 16.50 **Menetrier disease in a 7-year-old boy with aplastic anemia and viral hepatitis who had a CT showing gastric wall thickening. A and B:** Upper GI series images show thickening of gastric folds (*arrows*). **C:** Different child with bilateral lower extremity edema and protein losing enteropathy. Endoscopic photo shows the marked rugal fold thickening (*arrows*), a hallmark of Menetrier disease.

resulting from fistula or abscess formation. Acute presentations can mimic appendicitis. Definitive diagnosis is based on laboratory testing, imaging studies, and endoscopy with biopsy. Distal small bowel and colorectal involvement are most common in the pediatric population.

Imaging is used to identify the presence and extent of Crohn disease as well as complications, such as obstructing strictures and fistulas. Abdominal radiography is generally nonspecific and insensitive. A pathognomonic finding at SBFT is "cobblestone appearance" of the bowel, which corresponds to the presence of numerous linear and transverse ulcers and spared surrounding mucosa (pseudopolyps) (Figs. 16.51 and 16.52). Other findings include bowel wall thickening, luminal narrowing, penetrating disease (fistulas and sinus tracts), "skip lesions," and decreased peristalsis of affected intestine. Compression views of the TI are particularly useful and may show marked luminal narrowing secondary to mural edema and/or fibrosis ("string" sign) (Fig. 16.53). Aphthous ulcers that can be seen at endoscopy are often imaging occult.

Currently, CTE and MRE have largely replaced SBFT and conventional CT examinations for the assessment of suspected or known Crohn disease particularly in the pediatric population. Primary advantages of cross-section enterography are their ability to visualize both the bowel lumen (including abnormal narrowing and dilation) and bowel wall (including thickness and postcontrast enhancement pattern) as well as detect a variety of extraintestinal abnormalities affecting the mesentery, gallbladder, pancreaticobiliary tree, and sacroiliac joints. MRE, like CTE, can be used to diagnose and follow-up pediatric Crohn disease, but has superior contrast resolution, lacks of ionizing radiation, and allows multiphasic postcontrast and cine imaging.[90] Findings suggestive of active inflammation at CTE and MRE

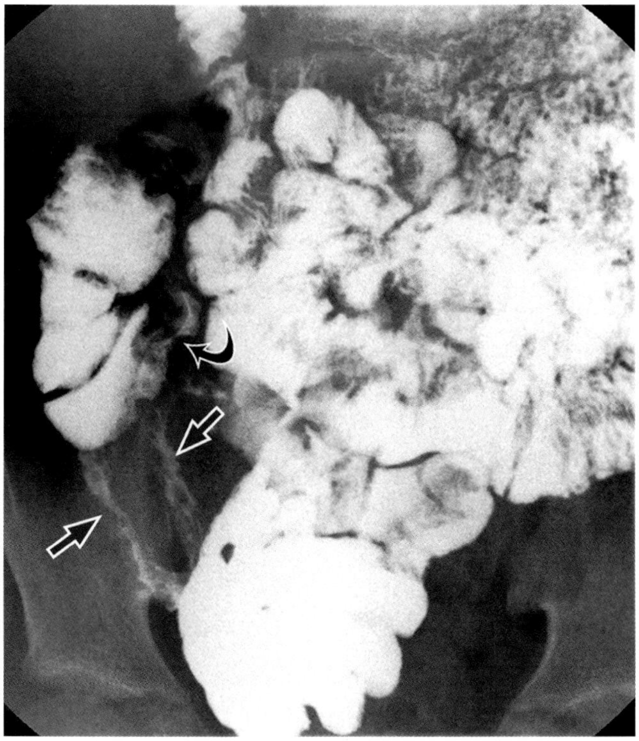

FIGURE 16.51 **A 14-year-old boy with Crohn disease.** SBFT image reveals ulcers, irregular mucosa, and luminal narrowing with separation of bowel loops involving a long segment of ileum (*straight arrows*), including the terminal ileum (*curved arrow*).

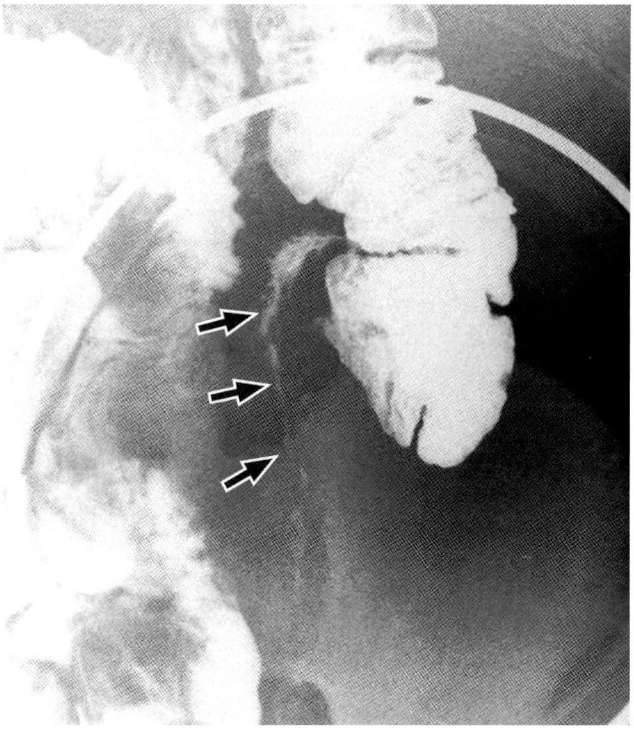

FIGURE 16.53 **A 16-year-old boy with Crohn disease.** SBFT image taken with the patient in a prone position shows severe luminal narrowing (*arrows*) of the terminal ileum, consistent with the classical "string sign."

include bowel wall thickening, avid postcontrast hyperenhancement, and mesenteric stranding and hyperemia (Figs. 16.54 and 16.55). MRE is likely superior to CT for characterizing areas of intestinal narrowing (strictures); hypointense bowel wall signal on T2-weighted MR imaging and increasing enhancement over time can suggest that a stricture is mostly fibrotic.[13] In many instances, however, fibrosis can coexist with inflammation, making it difficult to detect and be fully separated. Intra-abdominal abscesses, areas of phlegmon, and fistulas (types of penetrating complications) can be easily detected by CTE and MRE (Fig. 16.56), whereas MRE is superior for the detection and characterization of perianal involvement (Fig. 16.48).

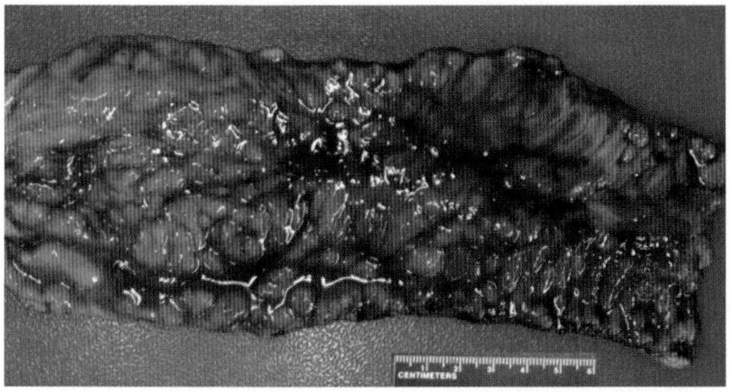

FIGURE 16.52 **Crohn disease in a 16-year-old girl.** The opened colon shows a deep red mucosal surface with pseudopolyps.

Ultrasound of the bowel can also depict the same findings seen on CTE and MRE in many children (Fig. 16.57). Ultrasound provides a low-cost, nonionizing, well-tolerated method to follow-up of pediatric patients with localized TI disease based on assessment of bowel wall thickness and Doppler signal over time.[89,90] Medical management is the preferred first-line therapy and commonly includes immunomodulators and biologic therapies; corticosteroids may also be used, especially in the acute setting. Abscesses may require antibiotic therapy and/or percutaneous drainage depending on size. Persistent, symptomatic strictures and penetrating complications may ultimately require surgical management.

Ulcerative Colitis

Ulcerative colitis (UC) is an inflammatory condition that primarily affects the colon, invariably affects the rectum, and most often in older children and young adults.[91] Affected children typically present with diarrhea and abdominal pain. Ulcerative colitis, like Crohn disease, can be associated with a variety of extraintestinal manifestations, including uveitis, arthritis, sacroileitis, and sclerosing cholangitis.[92] UC also carries a substantial risk of colon cancer, mostly in adulthood[91] .

Abdominal radiography is often normal, although colonic wall thickening or ahaustral appearance may be seen in some children. Contrast enema may show granular ulcerations. With time, the colon can develop a "lead pipe," featureless appearance due to submucosal fibrosis (Fig. 16.58). Although endoscopy and laboratory testing are most often employed to

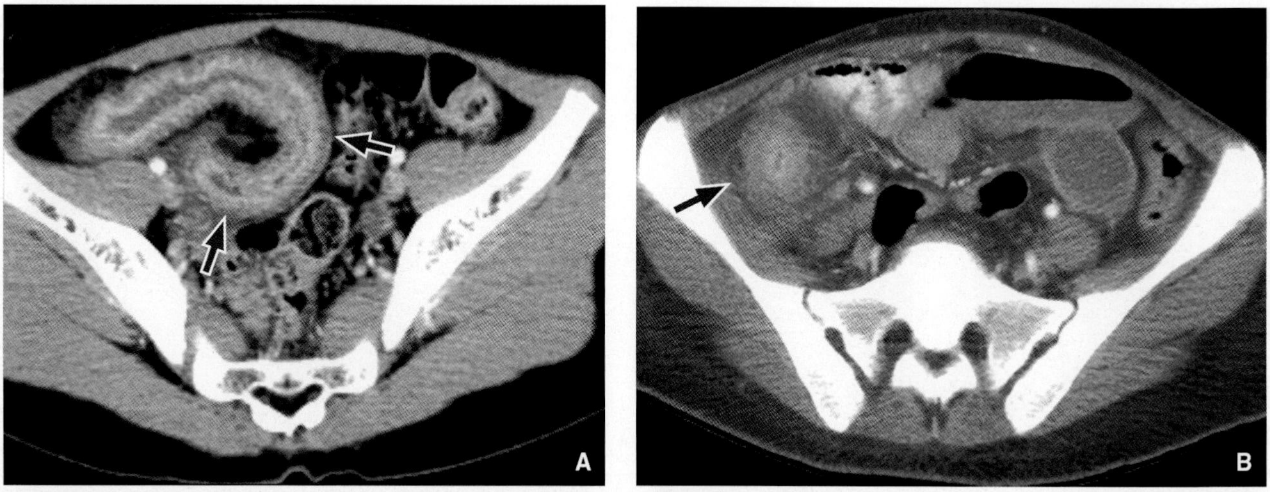

FIGURE 16.54 **CT enterography images from two different adolescents with Crohn disease. A:** Axial contrast-enhanced CT image demonstrates a long segment of ileal wall thickening, stratification, and mucosal contrast hyperenhancement (*arrows*), findings suggestive of active inflammation. **B:** Axial contrast-enhanced CT image demonstrates ileal wall thickening, mucosal contrast enhancement, severe luminal narrowing, and marked perienteric inflammatory changes (*arrow*), findings suggestive of active inflammation. Dilated fluid-filled small bowel loops are due to a partially obstructing stricture.

assess this condition, ultrasound, CTE, and MRE can all be used to evaluate the colon for active inflammation based on wall thickening and contrast hyperenhancement. Pericolonic hypervascularity also can be seen in the setting of active disease (Fig. 16.59). Both ultrasound and MRI can also be used to assess the bile ducts for evidence of sclerosing cholangitis[6,13] (Fig. 16.60).

Affected children are most often initially treated medically with anti-inflammatory or immunosuppressive medications. Pediatric patients with long-standing disease (because of the risk of colon cancer), those refractory to medical management, or who develop complications (such as toxic megacolon or thrombotic storm) require surgery usually employing proctocolectomy (Fig. 16.61).

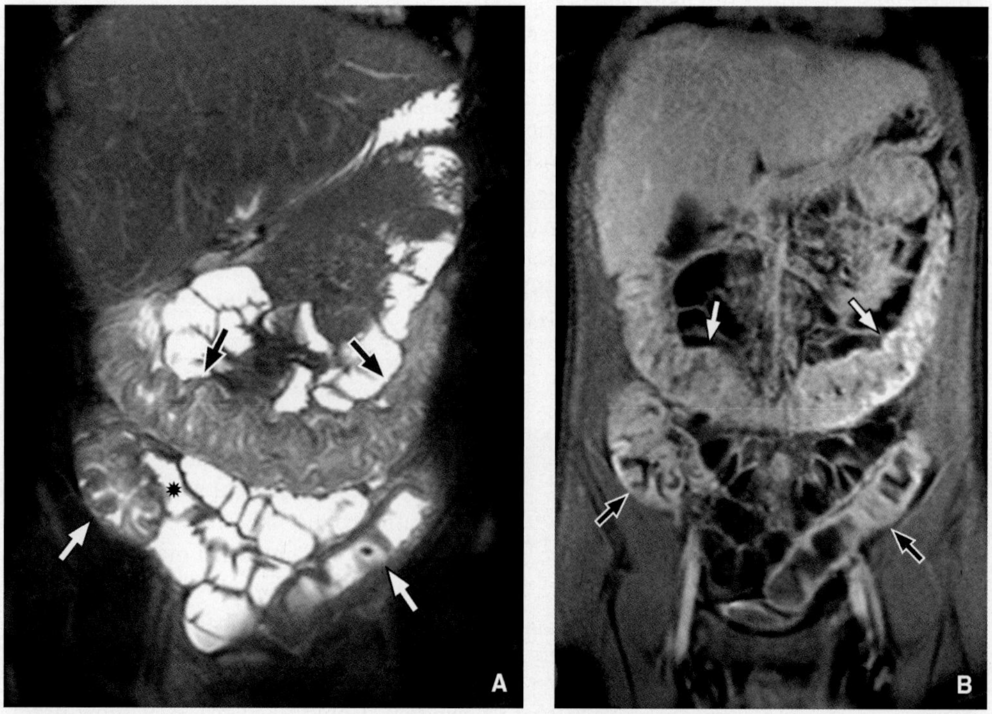

FIGURE 16.55 **A 12-year-old boy with newly diagnosed Crohn colitis. A:** Coronal T2-weighted single-shot fast spin-echo MR image shows diffuse large bowel wall thickening (*arrows*). There is minimal nodularity of the terminal ileum (*asterisk*). **B:** Coronal T1-weighted postcontrast fat suppressed MR image shows intense hyperenhancement of the same segments of bowel (*arrows*), indicative of active inflammation.

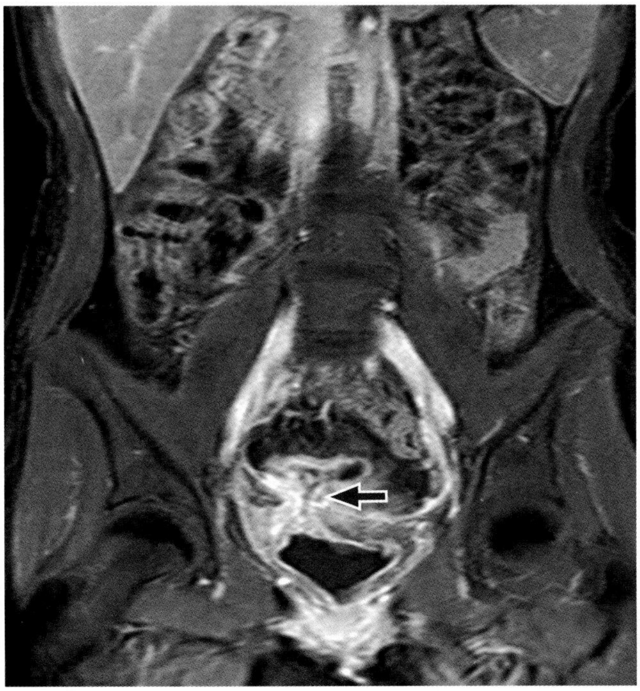

FIGURE 16.56 **A 15-year-old girl with abdominal pain and recurrent urinary tract infections.** Coronal T1-weighted postcontrast fat suppressed MR image shows thick-walled, hyperenhancing distal ileum due to active Crohn disease. There is an enhancing tract between the ileum and urinary bladder dome, due to an ileovesical fistula (*arrow*). The bladder dome is abnormally thickened and hyperenhances.

Henoch-Schonlein Purpura

Henoch-Schonlein purpura (HSP) is a systemic small-vessel vasculitis that most commonly affects children. It may be preceded by an infection or exposure to certain medications, including vancomycin and nonsteroidal anti-inflammatory drugs.[93] HSP commonly presents with purpura rash, arthralgia/arthritis, and abdominal pain due to GI tract involvement. In a majority of cases, GI tract symptoms (abdominal pain and vomiting) come before skin lesions.[93] Hematuria due to glomerulonephritis may also occur.

Ultrasound is the most useful imaging modality for assessing children with HSP. Salient features of HSP include bowel wall thickening (due to inflammation or intramural hemorrhage), hyperemia, decreased peristalsis, multiple enteroenteric intussusceptions (that sometimes persist), and occasional bowel dilatation due to obstruction (Fig. 16.62).[93,94] Rare complications of HSP include severe GI tract bleeding, bowel necrosis, and perforation. Imaging of the kidneys may show renal enlargement, increased echogenicity, and/or altered corticomedullary differentiation.

Treatment is most often conservative and supportive because this condition is generally self-limiting. Corticosteroids and other immunosuppressive agents may be used when there is evidence of more severe disease, such as ongoing kidney injury.[94]

Celiac Disease

Celiac disease (or nontropical sprue) is an immune-mediated condition that is triggered by the gluten in wheat, rye, and barley.[95] Affected children commonly present between the ages of 9 and 24 months when foods containing gluten are initially introduced, causing diarrhea, anorexia, poor weight gain and vomiting.[96] Serologic testing is both sensitive and specific for this condition in children older than 2 years of age.[95] Histology of proximal small bowel biopsy specimens shows effacement of intestinal villi and decreased crypt length.[95] Older children can present with more vague symptoms, including recurrent abdominal pain, nausea, diarrhea and constipation.[95]

SBFT examination may reveal delayed transit of contrast material and dilated small bowel loops containing excess fluid

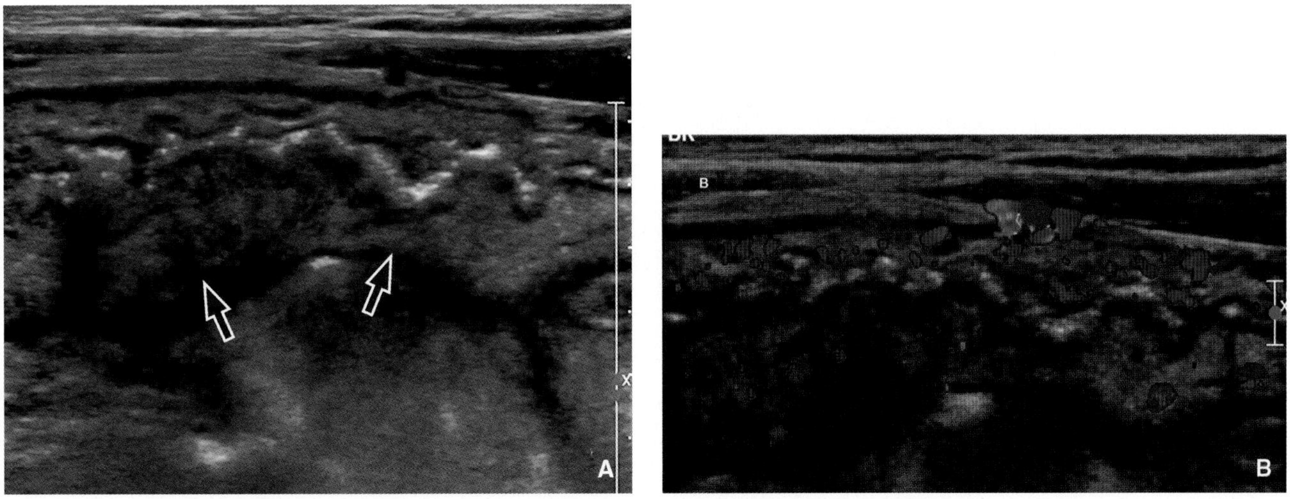

FIGURE 16.57 **Ultrasound images from two different children with Crohn disease. A—C: 14-year old girl:** Gray-scale **(A)** and color Doppler **(B)** ultrasound images show markedly thickened terminal ileum with decreased bowel wall stratification (*arrows*) and hyperemia, indicative of active inflammation.

(*Continued*)

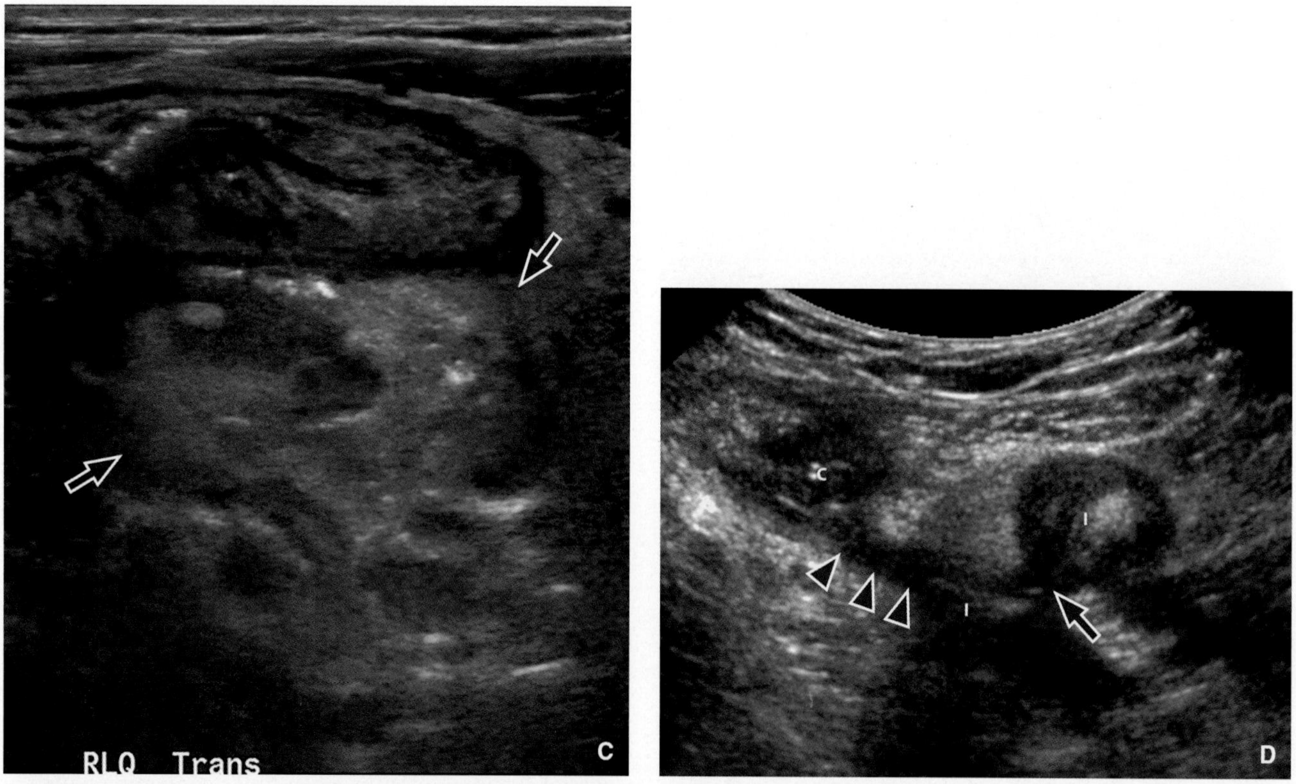

FIGURE 16-57 (*Continued*) Another gray-scale **(C)** ultrasound image shows thickened, echogenic inflamed mesentery (*arrows*). **D:** 15-year old boy: Gray-scale ultrasound image obtained using a sector probe shows a hypoechoic fistula tract (*arrowheads*) between ileum and cecum; cecum (*C*), loop of distal ileum (*I*). Additional fistula tracts arise from the ileum (*arrow*).

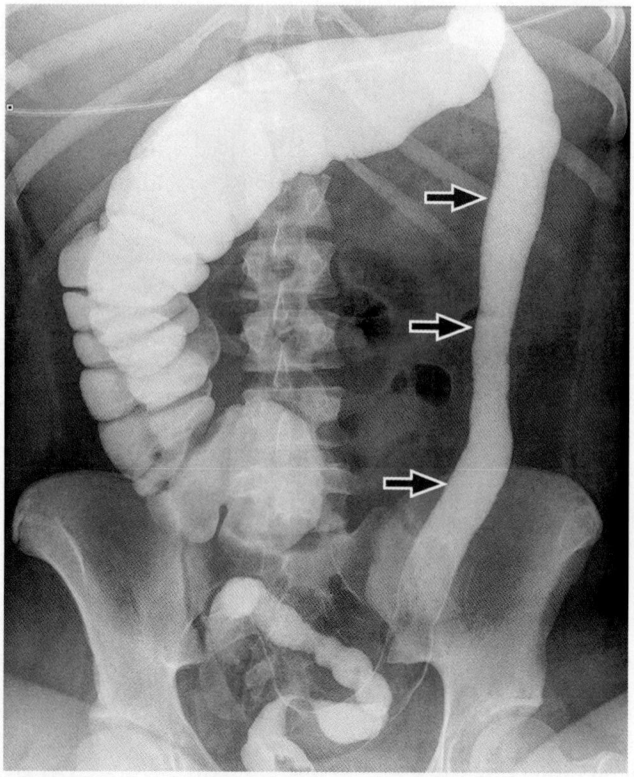

FIGURE 16.58 **Adolescent girl with long-standing ulcerative colitis.** Water soluble contrast enema shows the so-called "lead pipe" appearance of the descending colon with narrowing and loss of haustral markings (*arrows*).

giving barium a "wet" appearance (Fig. 16.63). Additionally, one may see loss of the normal "feathery" folds of the jejunum, whereas the ileum may have more prominent folds (reversal of small bowel fold pattern). Multiple small bowel intussusceptions may be also present.

Initial management of celiac disease is based on diet modification. In some cases, refractory celiac disease can be treated with corticosteroids.[97] In adulthood, there is an increased risk for lymphoma.

Appendicitis

Acute appendicitis is the most common atraumatic surgical disorder in children of 2 years of age and older.[98] It typically occurs in the setting of appendiceal luminal obstruction because of an appendicolith or less commonly carcinoid tumor or foreign body. It is postulated to occur in the setting of appendiceal luminal obstruction; however, it is only a minority of resected appendices that show a fecalith, carcinonoid tumor, or other obstructing body.[99] Children with appendicitis classically present with periumbilical pain that migrates to the right lower quadrant, anorexia, nausea, and fever. However, symptoms can be nonspecific, especially in younger children, making clinical diagnosis challenging and accounting for higher rates of perforation in this population.[98] Granulomatous appendicitis, a rare form of appendicitis, can be due to previous rupture, infection (e.g., *Mycobacterium* species), and Crohn disease.[100,101]

Abdominal radiography can be normal in the setting of uncomplicated acute appendicitis. In some children, a

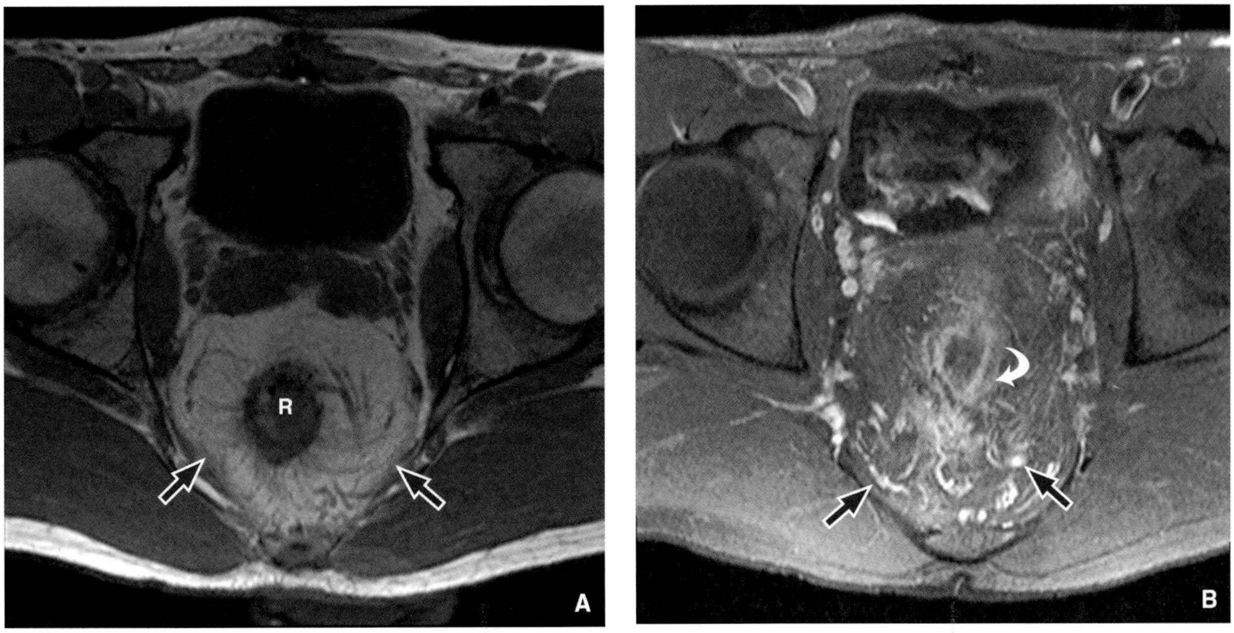

FIGURE 16.59 **A 18-year-old boy with long-standing ulcerative colitis. A:** T1-weighted MR image without fat saturation shows marked perirectal fibrofatty proliferation (*arrows*). The rectal wall thickening has resulted in luminal narrowing of the rectum (*R*). **B:** Axial postcontrast T1-weighted fat-suppressed MR image shows enhancement of the rectal mucosal (*curved arrow*) and engorgement of the perirectal vasculature (*straight arrows*), suggesting active inflammatory disease.

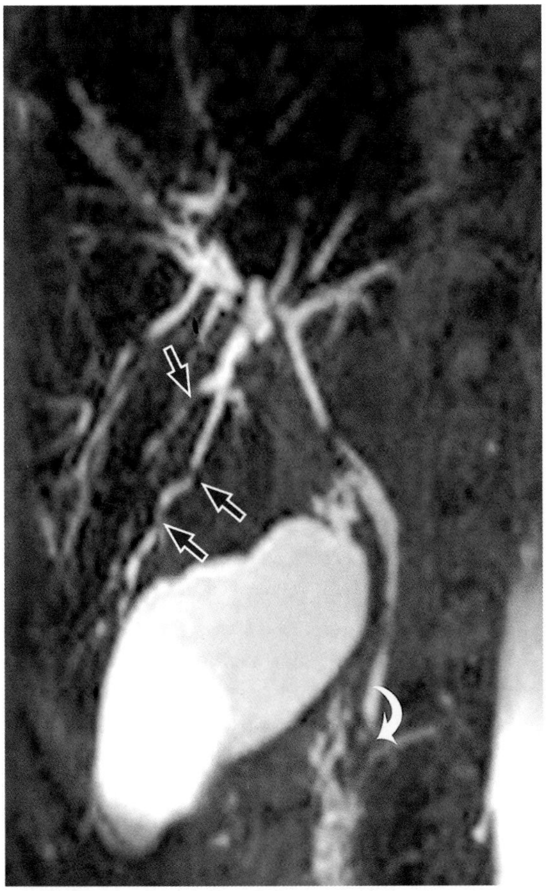

FIGURE 16.60 **Adolescent girl with ulcerative colitis and sclerosing cholangitis.** Maximum intensity projection (MIP) 3D T2-weighted magnetic resonance cholangiopancreatography (MRCP) image shows multiple areas of intra- (*straight arrows*) and extrahepatic (*curved arrow*) bile duct narrowing.

radiopaque appendicolith may be visible in the right lower quadrant.[98,102] In the setting of delayed presentation or appendiceal perforation, small bowel obstruction or ileus may be seen. Ultrasound is a typical first-line imaging test for assessing children with suspected acute appendicitis. Inflamed appendices are characterized by noncompressibility, wall thickening, and a transverse diameter >6 mm. In addition, one or more appendicoliths may be noted (Fig. 16.64).

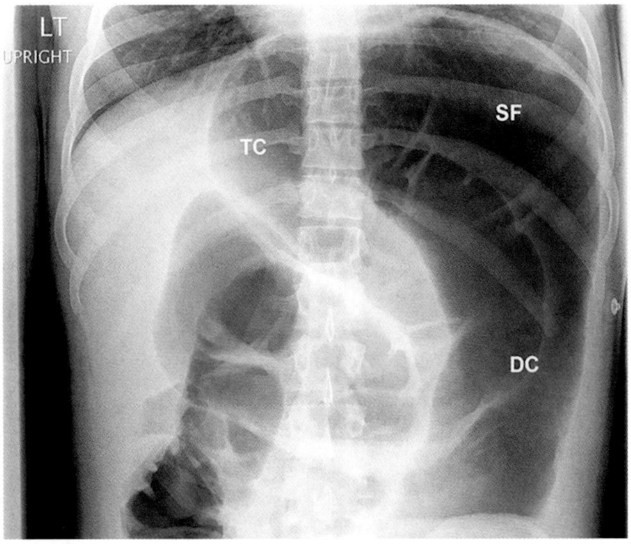

FIGURE 16.61 **Toxic megacolon in a 17-year-old boy with ulcerative colitis.** Abdominal radiograph demonstrates markedly dilated large bowel, with the descending colon (*DC*), splenic flexure (*SF*), and transverse colon (*TC*) most affected. This patient subsequently developed a colonic perforation and required surgical management.

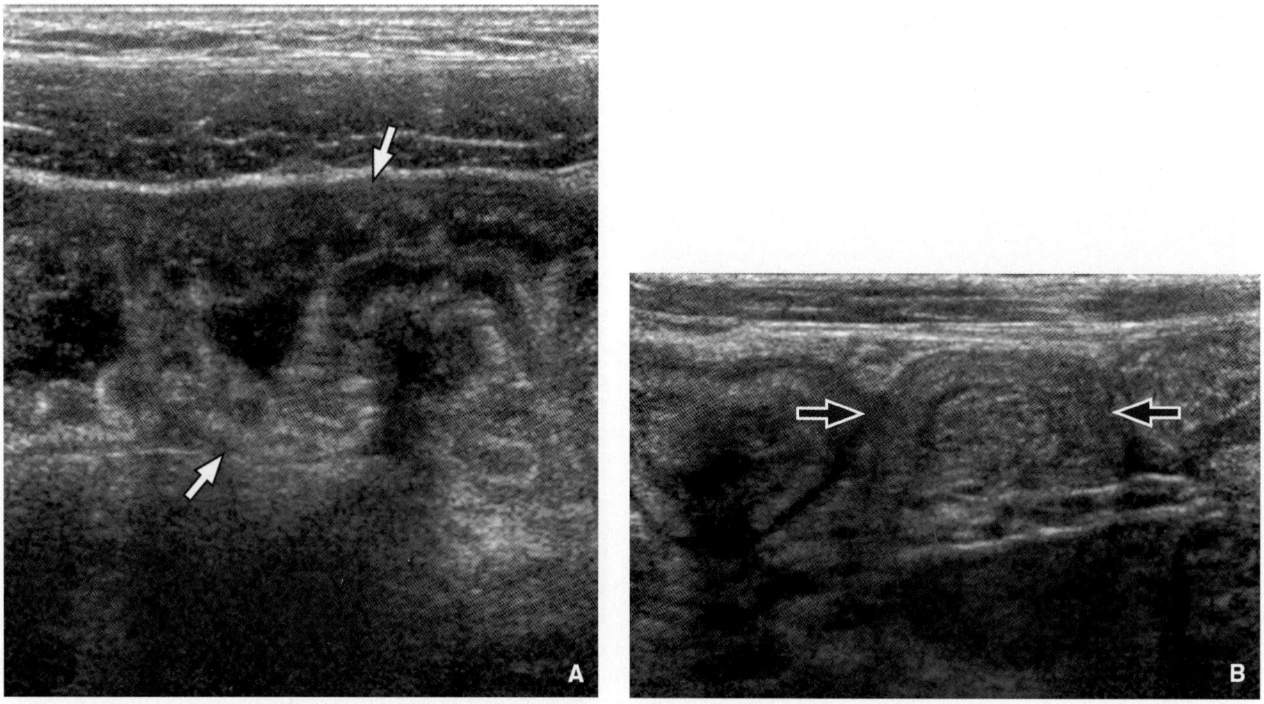

FIGURE 16.62 **A 7-year-old girl with abdominal pain due to Henoch-Schonlein purpura (HSP). A:** Gray-scale ultrasound image shows small bowel wall thickening (*arrows*). **B:** Transverse ultrasound image shows a transient small bowel–small bowel intussusception (*arrows*), which are commonly observed in the setting of HSP.

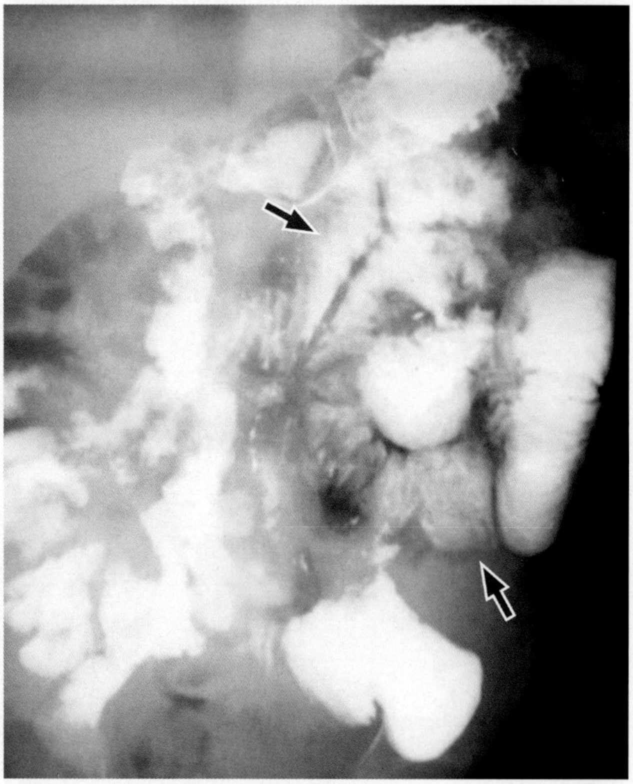

FIGURE 16.63 **A 5-year-old girl with intermittent bloating, abdominal distension, and diarrhea due to celiac disease.** SBFT image reveals dilated loops of jejunum (*arrows*) with a "wet" bowel appearance. There is slight flocculation of the barium, a finding seen in malabsorption conditions because of excess fluid in the bowel lumen.

Doppler evaluation may reveal appendiceal/periappendiceal hyperemia, and periappendiceal fat may appear thickened and echogenic (Fig. 16.64). If the appendix cannot be visualized by ultrasound and clinical suspicion for appendicitis persists, additional imaging such as CT or MRI may be indicated to further assess for appendicitis and other causes of right lower quadrant pain.[103]

CT is both sensitive and specific for the diagnosis of appendicitis. At CT, the inflamed appendix appears as a tubular structure with surrounding inflammatory changes, such as fat stranding, free fluid, and cecal/TI wall thickening (Fig. 16.65).[104–106] Findings suggestive of perforation include observing a focal defect in the wall of the appendix, appendicolith extrusion, abscess formation, and nonvisualization of the appendix with right lower quadrant phlegmon.[106] There is an increasing body of literature in children and adults suggesting that MRI provides comparable sensitivity and specificity to CT for detecting appendicitis and its complications, even when using abbreviated protocols (Fig. 16.66). Disadvantages of MRI include the length of the examination, potential need for sedation to prevent patient motion in very young children, and limited availability.[16]

Children presenting with nonperforated acute appendicitis are typically treated with intravenous antibiotic therapy and urgent appendectomy. In perforated appendicitis, intravenous antibiotic therapy may be followed by delayed appendectomy several weeks to months following presentation. Children who develop an abscess may require image-guided aspiration or percutaneous (or transrectal) drainage catheter placement.[107]

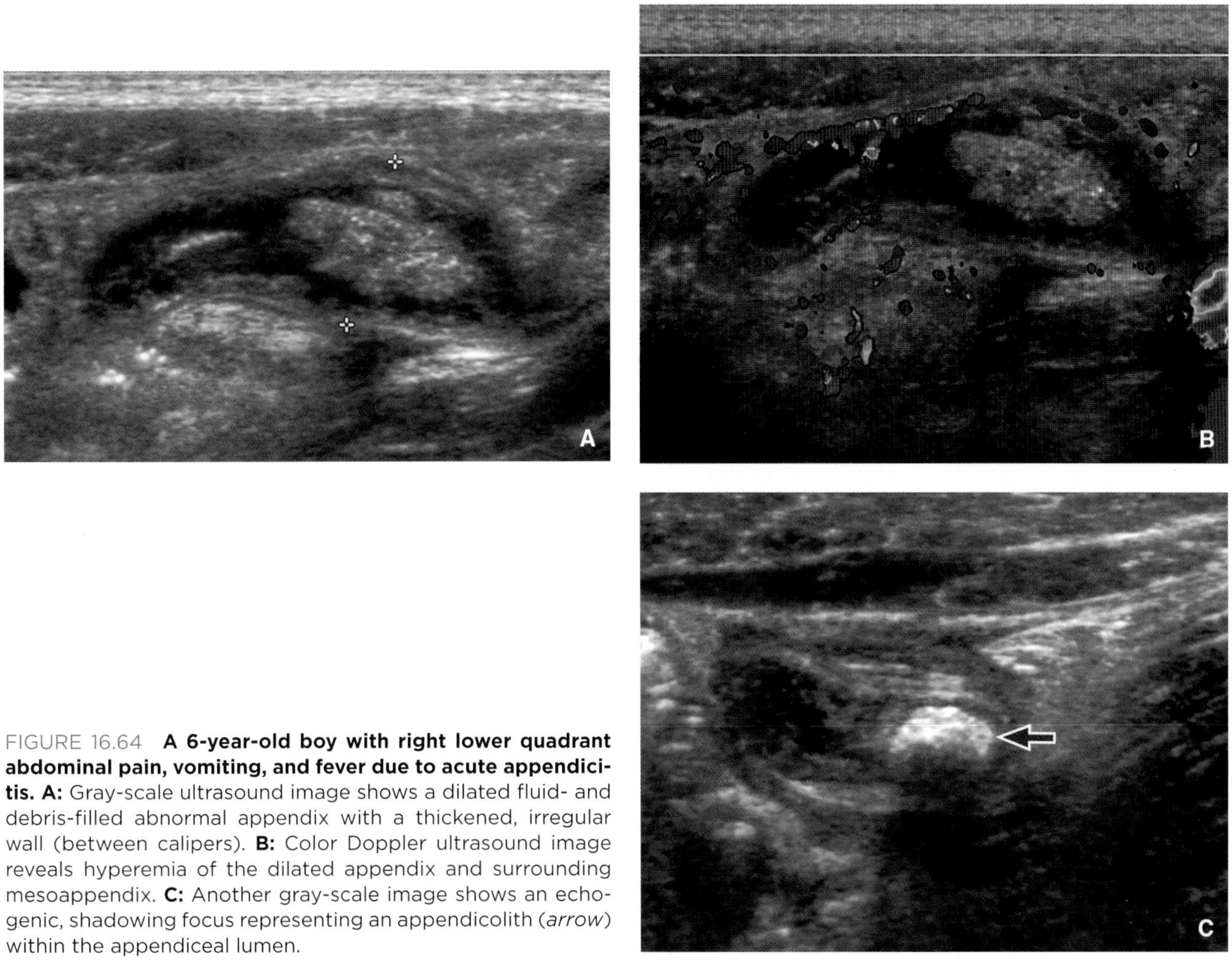

FIGURE 16.64 **A 6-year-old boy with right lower quadrant abdominal pain, vomiting, and fever due to acute appendicitis. A:** Gray-scale ultrasound image shows a dilated fluid- and debris-filled abnormal appendix with a thickened, irregular wall (between calipers). **B:** Color Doppler ultrasound image reveals hyperemia of the dilated appendix and surrounding mesoappendix. **C:** Another gray-scale image shows an echogenic, shadowing focus representing an appendicolith (*arrow*) within the appendiceal lumen.

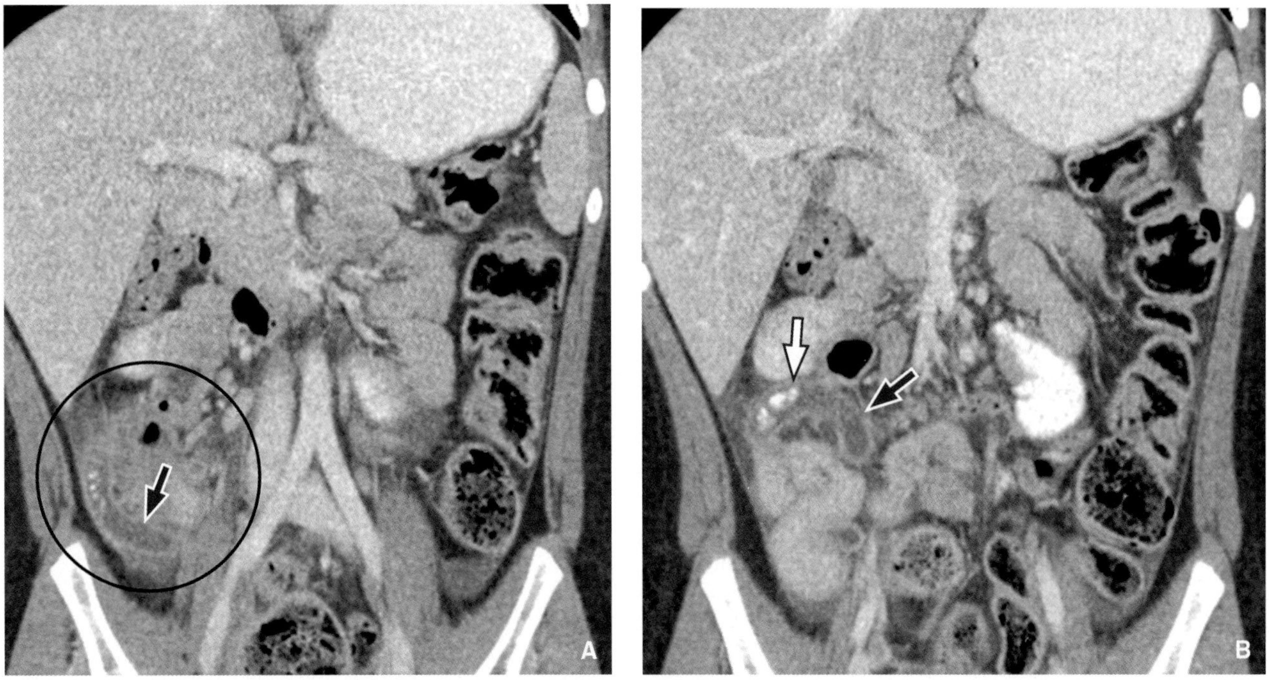

FIGURE 16.65 **A 15-year-old boy with uncomplicated acute appendicitis. A and B** Coronal contrast-enhanced CT images show a dilated, fluid-filled appendix (*black arrows*) with periappendiceal fat stranding (*black circle*) and appendicoliths (*white arrow*). These are classic findings seen acute appendicitis.

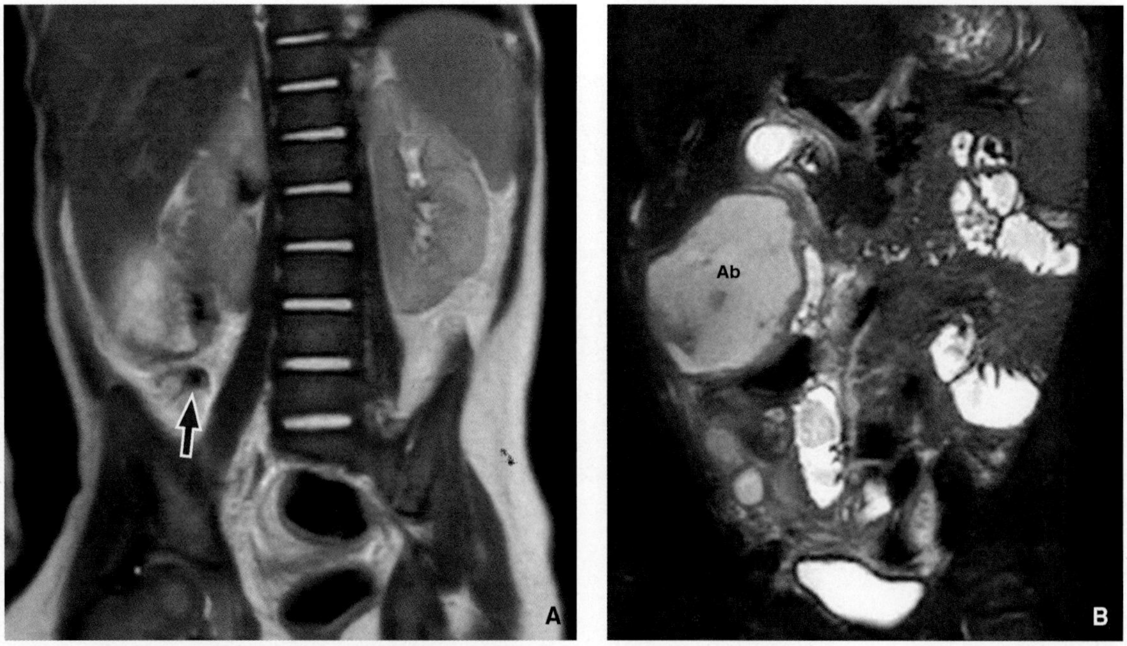

FIGURE 16.66 **A 2-year-old boy with complicated acute appendicitis including abscess formation. A:** Coronal single-shot fast-spin echo MR image acquired without sedation shows a partially seen retrocecal dilated appendix containing a hypointense appendicolith (*arrow*). **B:** Coronal T2-weighted fat suppressed MR image shows a right upper quadrant thick-walled hyperintense fluid collection (*Ab*), consistent with an abscess due to acute appendicitis with perforation.

Eosinophilic Diseases

Eosinophilic gastrointestinal disorders (EGIDs) are uncommon but increasingly recognized chronic inflammatory conditions characterized by dense eosinophilia of the GI tract on histologic examination. These disorders can be subgrouped as eosinophilic esophagitis, eosinophilic gastroenteritis, and eosinophilic colitis.[108] Eosinophilic esophagitis is the most prevalent, and affected children can present with difficulty swallowing, chest pain, vomiting, feeding disturbance, and food impaction. Children with eosinophilic gastroenteritis can present with abdominal pain, diarrhea, bloody stools, and failure to thrive. Eosinophilic colitis is the rarest of the EGIDs and presents similarly to eosinophilic gastroenteritis with diarrhea and weight loss. The diagnosis of eosinophilic esophagitis can be challenging because symptoms are often mistaken for gastroesophageal reflux disease. Of note, gastroesophageal reflux also can cause an increased number of eosinophils in the esophageal wall. Children with EGIDs commonly have other atopic conditions, including asthma, various food allergies, and eczema.[109]

Esophagography is most often normal in children with eosinophilic esophagitis.[110] Findings that can be seen include dysmotility, strictures of variable length (including the small-caliber esophagus), ringed esophagus, and evidence of food bolus impaction (Fig. 16.67).[108,111] At CT, children with eosinophilic gastroenteritis and colitis may show nonspecific intestinal wall thickening (Fig. 16.68).[112] Definitive diagnosis for all of these conditions requires endoscopy with biopsy (Fig. 16.69).[97]

The current treatments in the pediatric population include dietary modifications, corticosteroid therapy, and other anti-inflammatory medications, such as leukotriene modifiers.[97,113]

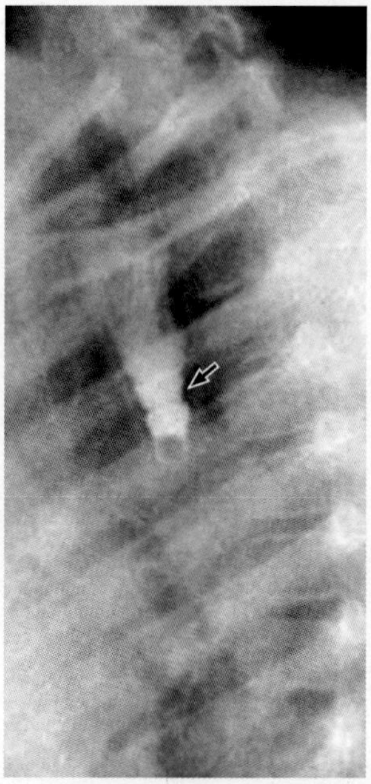

FIGURE 16.67 **A 15-year-old boy with dysphagia due to eosinophilic esophagitis.** Lateral esophagram image shows areas of ring-like narrowing (*arrow*) involving the upper thoracic esophagus, a classic feature seen in eosinophilic esophagitis. A round filling within the esophagus is a stuck pill at a site of severe luminal narrowing.

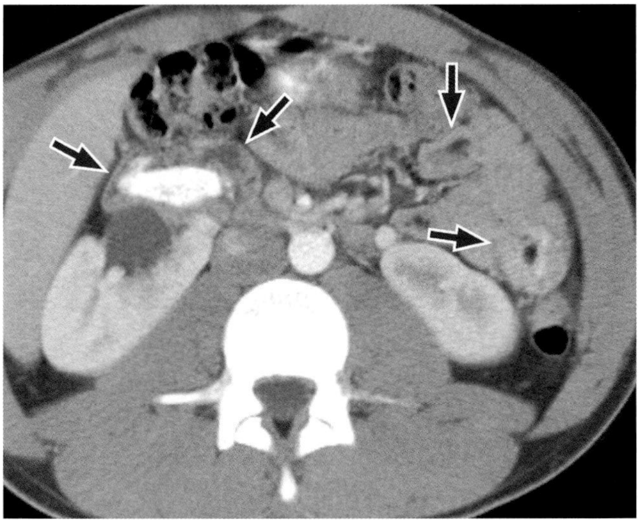

FIGURE 16.68 **A 15-year-old boy with recurrent abdominal pain and biopsy-proven eosinophilic enteritis.** Axial contrast-enhanced CT image shows areas of nonspecific circumferential wall thickening (*arrows*) of the duodenum and jejunum.

Graft versus Host Disease

Graft versus host disease (GVHD) is an immune-mediated complication of allogenic hematopoietic cell transplantation. Acute GVHD describes a unique constellation of signs and symptoms, including skin, hepatobiliary, and intestinal abnormalities that develop within 100 days of transplantation.[79] Affected patients often present with a diarrhea, GI tract bleeding, and abdominal pain.[79] In addition, a pruritic and painful rash that usually results from hepatobiliary involvement of GVHD may also present.[79]

Abdominal radiography may reveal evidence of bowel involvement from GVHD, which includes "ribbon" or "tooth paste" appearance of the small bowel or dilated bowel loops with air–fluid levels. SBFT also may show narrowing of the

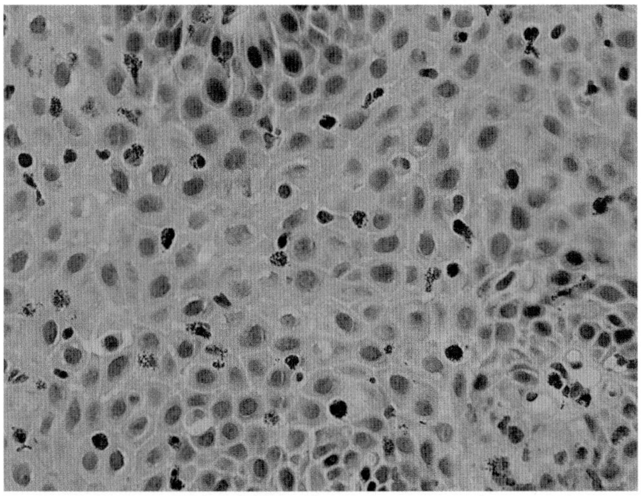

FIGURE 16.69 **Eosinophilic esophagitis a 15-year-old girl with dysphagia and food impaction.** In eosinophilic esophagitis, numerous eosinophils infiltrate the esophageal squamous epithelium (hematoxylin and eosin stain, 600x).

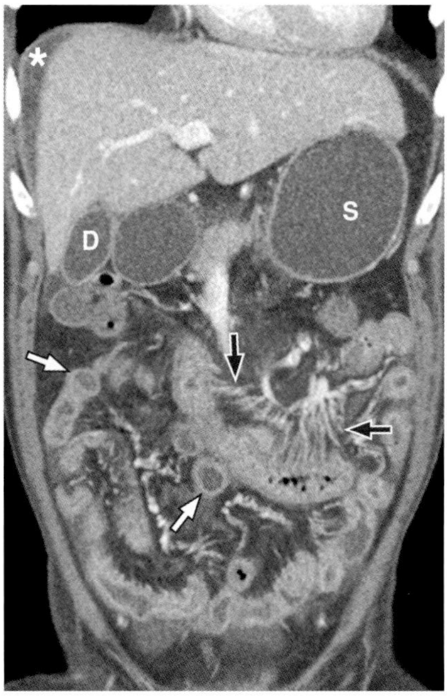

FIGURE 16.70 **A 8-year-old boy status post bone marrow transplant for acute lymphocytic leukemia with GVHD.** Coronal contrast-enhanced CT image shows numerous thick-walled, hyperenhancing small bowel loops (*white arrows*). There are scattered pockets of intraperitoneal free fluid (*asterisk*), mesenteric vascular engorgement (*black arrows*), as well as a dilated fluid-filled stomach (*S*) and duodenum (*D*).

small bowel lumen. On CT, findings of GVHD include dilated fluid-filled small bowel loops with bowel wall thickening and hyperenhancing mucosa. The colon and stomach may also appear abnormal (Fig. 16.70). Intraperitoneal free fluid and mesenteric vascular engorgement are also common findings in children with GVHD (Fig. 16.70).

Management is primarily medical with immunosuppressive GVHD prophylaxis.

Pneumatosis Intestinalis

Pneumatosis intestinalis refers to the radiologic finding of gas in the wall of the small bowel or colon. It can be a benign finding or indicative of a serious underlying process including certain medical and surgical emergencies. Pneumatosis is well known to occur in patients with a variety of "benign" conditions, such as IBD, GVHD, HIV infection, and chronic immunosuppression. In addition, pulmonary diseases such as cystic fibrosis and asthma can also cause pneumatosis in children.[114] However, pneumatosis can also be radiologic evidence of an underlying life-threatening abdominal condition, such as intestinal ischemia/infarction, typhlitis, and necrotizing enterocolitis (NEC).[79]

In the setting of pneumatosis intestinalis, abdominal radiography can show ring-like and small bubbly lucencies in the expected location of the bowel wall of the small or large intestine. In addition, pneumoperitoneum may be also concomitantly present in some children with pneumatosis intestinalis (Fig. 16.71). Pneumatosis intestinalis may be difficult to distinguish from intraluminal bowel contents

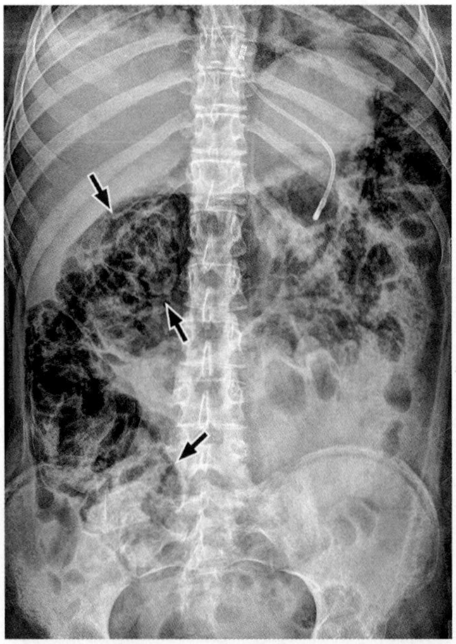

FIGURE 16.71 **Benign, self-limiting pneumatosis in an 16-year-old girl with myelodysplastic syndrome status post stem cell transplant on immunosuppressive medications including corticosteroids.** Abdominal radiograph shows curvilinear lucencies (*arrows*) along the entire colon, most pronounced in the right hemiabdomen.

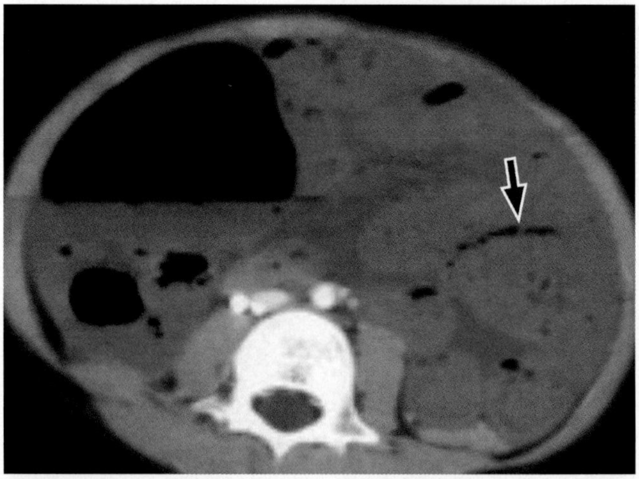

FIGURE 16.73 **A 7-year-old boy with small bowel ischemia due to delayed diagnosis of midgut volvulus.** Axial contrast-enhanced CT image shows decreased perfusion of dilated, fluid-filled small bowel loops secondary to the volvulus. There is pneumatosis (*arrow*) in the wall of one loop of ischemic bowel.

at radiography. CT allows direct visualization of gas foci in the bowel wall and has greater sensitivity than abdominal radiography. Pneumatosis often involves the bowel circumferentially, appearing both dependent and nondependent. CT can also identify causative intra-abdominal processes, including some that may be life threatening[115] (Figs. 16.72 and 16.73).

Benign cases of pneumatosis intestinalis are typically asymptomatic and self-limiting. However, pneumatosis intestinalis due to more serious causes, such as intestinal ischemia/infarctions, may require surgery. Therefore, early detection and accurate diagnosis are essential.

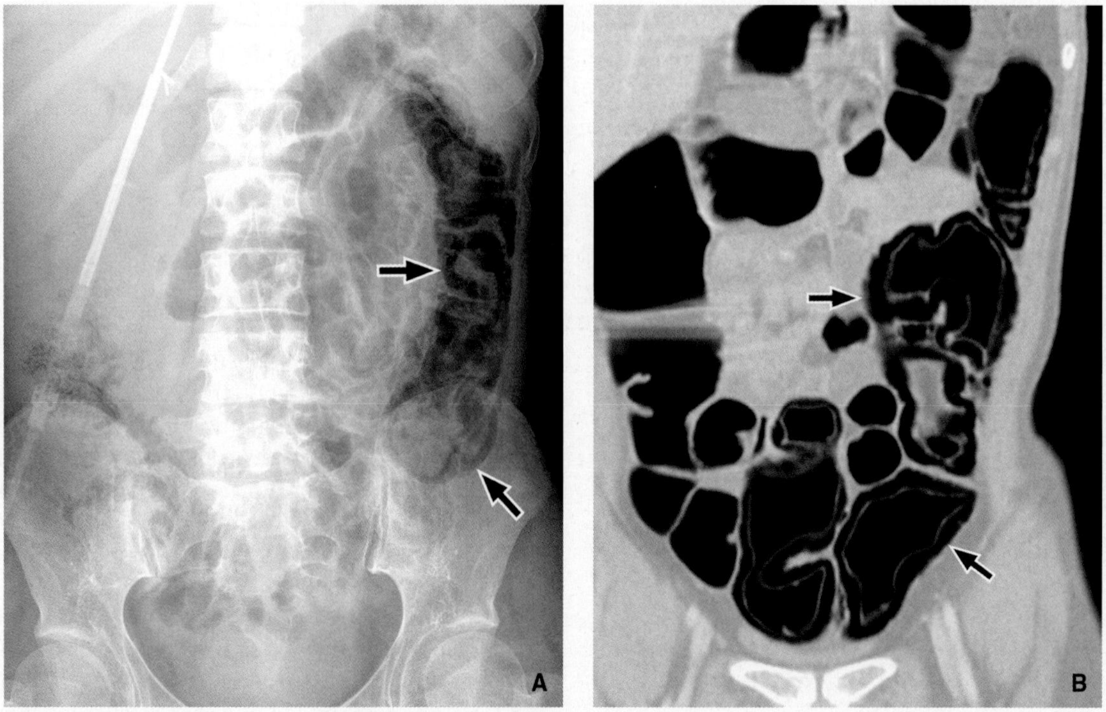

FIGURE 16.72 **A 15-year-old girl with Kabuki syndrome and abdominal pain due to ischemic colitis. A:** Abdominal radiograph shows serpiginous curvilinear collections of air in the wall of the descending colon representing pneumatosis intestinalis (*arrows*). **B:** Coronal lung window CT image confirms the pneumatosis (*arrows*) and shows the extent of involvement to include the sigmoid colon.

Necrotizing Enterocolitis

NEC is a condition that most commonly affects the small bowel and colon of premature neonates but may also affect term infants with congenital heart disease.[116] The exact etiology of NEC remains unclear. Clinical presentations include abdominal distention, bloody bowel movements, and feeding intolerance. Affected bowel initially becomes thick-walled and hyperemic. Then, while over time the bowel wall becomes thin, aperistaltic, hypoperfused, and at risk for perforation. Eventually gas may be seen in the bowel wall and portal venous system. The presence of pneumoperitoneum suggests bowel perforation in patients with NEC.

Serial abdominal radiography and bedside ultrasound are the most useful imaging studies to pediatric patients with suspected NEC.[117] Although abdominal radiographs can be normal, they classically show prominent/mildly dilated featureless bowel loops, most often in the right lower quadrant, with or without pneumatosis and portal venous gas within the liver (Fig. 16.74). Pneumoperitoneum, when present, is best appreciated on erect, lateral decubitus or cross-table lateral imaging. Ultrasound may be sensitive to assess the changes of early NEC, and it can detect pneumatosis and portal venous gas, which may not be see at radiography[117] (Fig. 16.75). In the setting of a gasless abdomen, ultrasound can help assess bowel viability, detect NEC-related complications, and predict outcome.[117]

Management of NEC includes bowel rest, antibiotic therapy, and serial abdominal radiographs to assess for evidence of complications, such as bowel perforation, that may warrant surgical intervention.

Neoplastic Disorders

Benign and malignant tumors of the GI tract in the pediatric population are less common than in adults. When they occur, they can involve all portions of the GI tract.

Esophagus

Benign Tumors

Although rare in children, leiomyomas are the most common benign tumor of the esophagus and are important to recognize because of the obstructive symptoms that can occur, such as dysphagia, vomiting, and odynophagia leading to weight loss.[118] In the pediatric population, leiomyomas are most commonly seen in teenage girls. Most affected children have multiple lesions or diffuse esophageal involvement (i.e., leiomyomatosis).[118–120] Esophageal leiomyomatosis can be associated with Carney triad, Alport syndrome, and multiorgan leiomyomatosis syndromes.[119]

Solitary leiomyomas may present at radiography as a middle mediastinal mass. Leiomyomatosis is more subtle, although deviation of the azygoesophageal stripe has been described.[121] Esophagography can show extrinsic mass effect upon the esophageal lumen because of intramural lesions. More proximal esophagus may be dilated.[90,122] At CT and MRI, leiomyomatosis appears as circumferential wall thickening involving the distal esophagus that can extend into the stomach. More focal masses often appear similar in attenuation and signal intensity to skeletal muscle at CT and MRI, respectively, although avid contrast enhancement may be seen (Fig. 16.76).

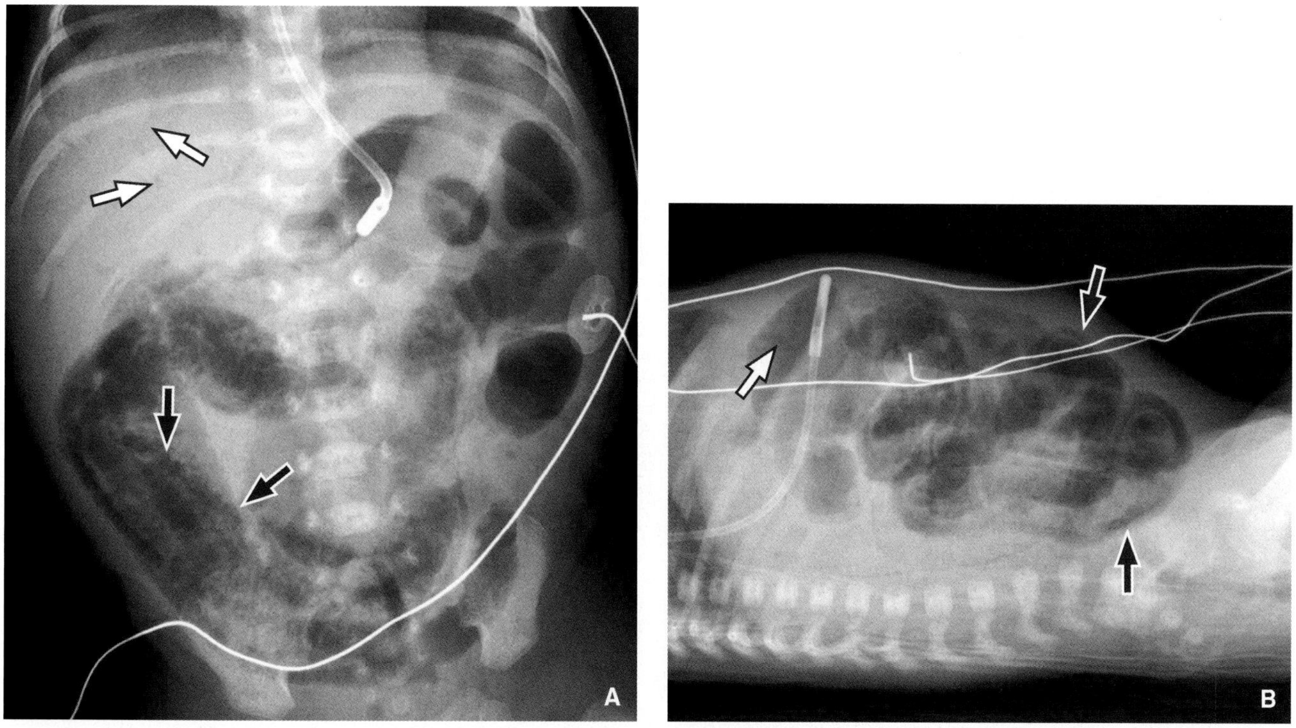

FIGURE 16.74 **Preterm infant boy clinically suspected of necrotizing enterocolitis who presented with bloody stools. A and B:** Supine and cross-table lateral abdominal radiographs show featureless, dilated gas-filled bowel loops with diffuse pneumatosis manifested as curvilinear and round collections of air in the bowel wall (*black arrows*). In the liver, there are branching lucent tracks representing portal venous gas (*white arrows*).

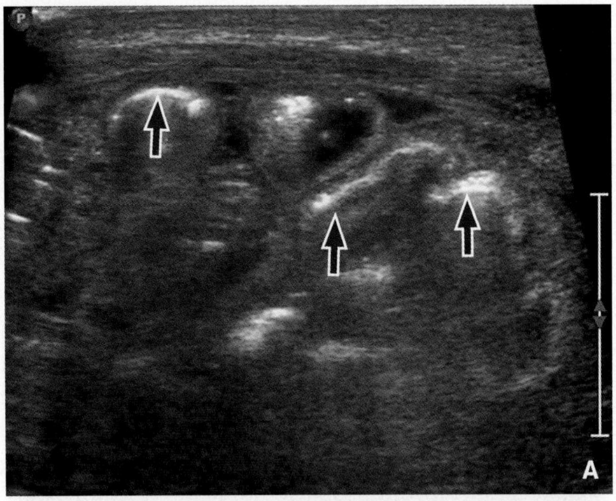

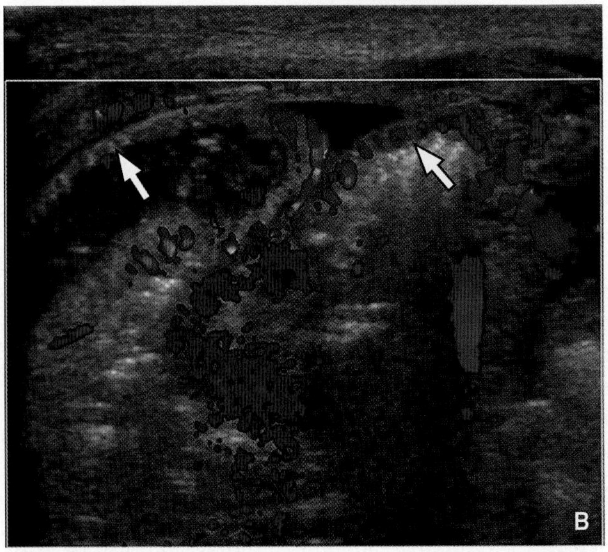

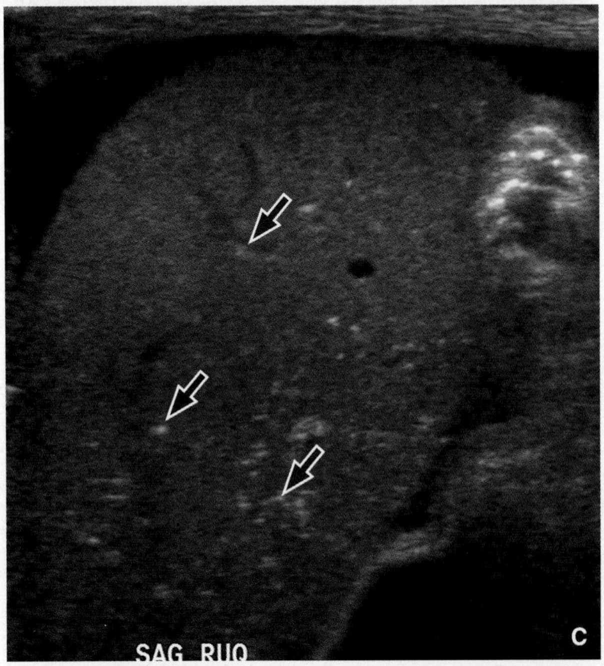

FIGURE 16.75 **Neonate with necrotizing enterocolitis (NEC) on ultrasound. A and B:** Gray-scale and color Doppler ultrasound images show thickened, hyperemic bowel loops (*white arrows*) with echogenic foci with posterior acoustic shadowing in the bowel wall (*black arrows*) that do not change with the position of the infant indicating pneumatosis. **C:** Right upper quadrant ultrasound image shows ascites along the liver surface and tiny echogenic foci moving central to peripheral representing portal venous air (*arrows*).

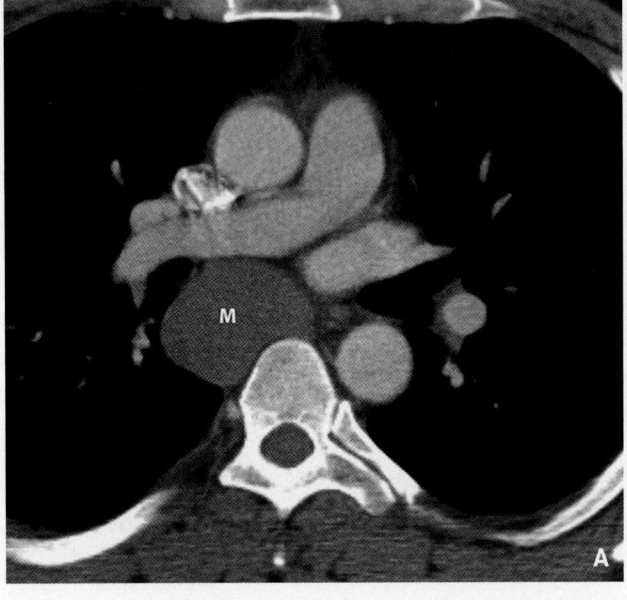

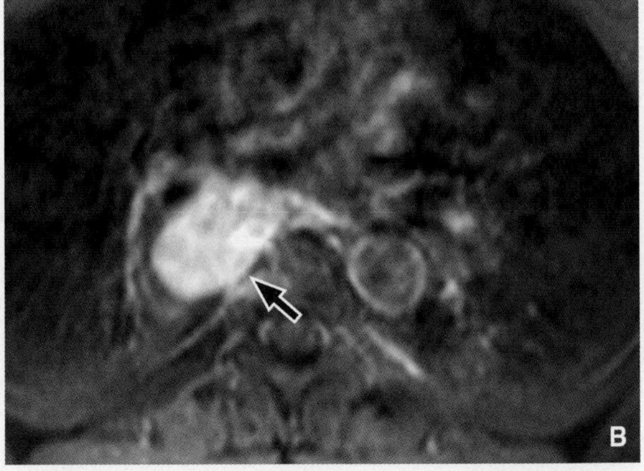

FIGURE 16.76 **A 20-year-old girl with dysphagia due to esophageal leiomyoma. A:** Axial contrast-enhanced CT image shows a middle mediastinal mass (*M*) that is homogeneous in attenuation. The esophagus is not visible as a separate structure. **B:** Axial postcontrast T1-weighted fat-suppressed MR image shows avid enhancement of the mass (*arrow*).

The current treatment is surgical, and some children may require esophagectomy and gastric pull-through.[118,119,121,122]

Malignant Tumors

Adenocarcinoma

Esophageal malignancies are very rare in children and hypothesized to result from chronic irritation after a latent period of carcinogenesis, such as seen with gastroesophageal reflux disease and Barrett esophagitis or in children who have ingested caustic material.[119,123] These tumors are mostly distal in location, presenting with dysphagia and weight loss.[124] Esophagography commonly shows esophageal narrowing with abrupt/irregular margins, nodular and ulcerated mucosal surfaces, or even polypoid masses.[124] At CT, nonspecific focal esophageal wall thickening may be observed with possible soft tissue infiltration of adjacent mediastinal fat (Fig. 16.77). Because this neoplasm is very rare in children, there is no defined management, although treatment is likely to involve surgical resection and chemotherapy.[119,123]

Stomach

Benign Tumors

Gastric Polyps

The detection of gastric polyps in children is increasing because of increased use of endoscopy in recent years.[125,126] These lesions can be hyperplastic, hamartomatous, or adenomatous, with histologic distinction important because of the risk of cancer each subtype carries. Hyperplastic polyps are most common and are considered benign, whereas adenomatous polyps are less common but considered premalignant.[126,127] Polyps can be solitary lesions; however, they are commonly multiple because of polyposis syndromes that affect the GI tract, such as Peutz-Jeghers syndrome (PJS) and familial adenomatous polyposis (FAP).[126,127] Pediatric patients with gastric polyps can present with epigastric pain, vomiting, and GI tract bleeding.[127]

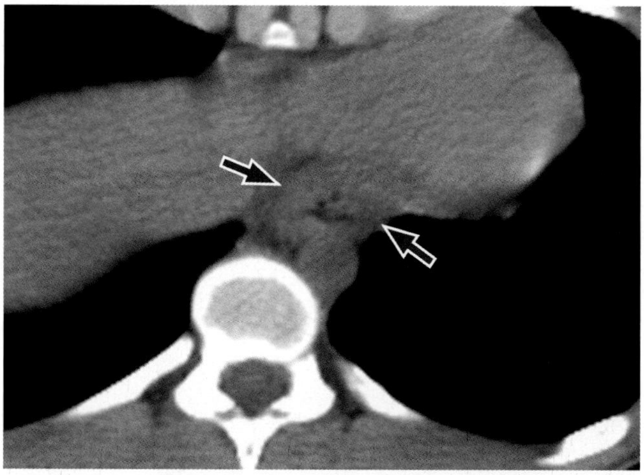

FIGURE 16.77 **Esophageal adenocarcinoma in a 17-year-old boy with progressive dysphagia and 20-pound weight loss.** Axial non-contrast CT image shows marked circumferential thickening (*arrows*) of the lower esophagus with adjacent fat stranding. The mass was markedly hypermetabolic at ^{18}F-FDG-PET imaging.

Gastric polyps typically appear as pedunculated or sessile filling defects arising from the stomach wall at upper GI series, CT, and MRE when surrounded by orally-ingested contrast material. Diagnosis by CT and MRE is much more difficult when the stomach is collapsed. When visualized, however, most hyperplastic polyps are round or oval, commonly sessile, and smooth (Fig. 16.78). Adenomatous polyps tend to be larger, are more commonly pedunculated than hyperplastic polyps, and tend to occur distally within the stomach.[128,129]

Gastric polyps identified by imaging should be evaluated with endoscopy with or without removal.[127]

Gastrointestinal Stromal Tumor

Gastrointestinal stromal tumors (GISTs) are a distinct mesenchymal tumor that was recognized by the World Health Organization in 1990.[130] It comprises tumors formerly diagnosed as smooth muscle tumors (leiomyoma and leiomyosarcoma) and autonomic neural tumors. In adults, GISTs are the most common nonlymphoid, mesenchymal tumors of the GI tract. This tumor is rare in children. However, large pediatric cancer centers typically encounter on average one child with GIST every few years, with the stomach being the most common site.[131,132] Pediatric GISTs are more common in girls than boys, with a mean age of 14 years.[132] Syndromic conditions in which GISTs arise include neurofibromatosis type 1, Carney triad, and Carney-Stratakis syndrome.[130] Clinical presentations of these tumors often relate to nonspecific abdominal symptoms, and lesions may be detected incidentally.[130–132] Histologically, GISTs consist of spindled or epithelioid cells that typically stain with antibodies to CD117, a marker of interstitial cells of Cajal (the pacemaker cells within the GI tract) (Fig. 16.79). Pathologic features used to predict prognosis include tumor size and mitotic rate.

Abdominal radiography of GISTs can show soft tissue opacity indenting or displacing the gas within the stomach when these masses are large. Upper GI series may demonstrate a smoothly circumscribed, intramural mass with obtuse or right angles to the stomach wall. Some GISTs have a focal ulceration, particularly when larger than 2 cm.[130,133] At CT, these lesions appear as a focal enhancing mass arising from the wall of the stomach that may be endophytic or exophytic. The bulk of some tumors can be extragastric (Fig. 16.80).[130] At CT and MRI, GISTs commonly appear heterogeneous because of associated hemorrhage and/or necrosis, and they can show peripheral postcontrast enhancement.[130]

GISTs have variable malignant potential, and a small number of GISTs that are histologically benign recur or have metastatic disease (e.g., to regional lymph nodes or liver). Therefore, surveillance imaging may be indicated.[130] Malignant GISTs tend to recur locally as well as metastasize to liver, lymph nodes, and peritoneal surfaces.[130] Up to one-half of pediatric patients with malignant GISTs have been reported to have metastatic disease at diagnosis.[131] It is important to note that the degree of necrosis, hemorrhage, and postcontrast enhancement do not correlate to malignant potential of GISTs.[130]

Treatment of gastric GISTs is en bloc surgical resection, with adjuvant chemotherapy as needed.[131]

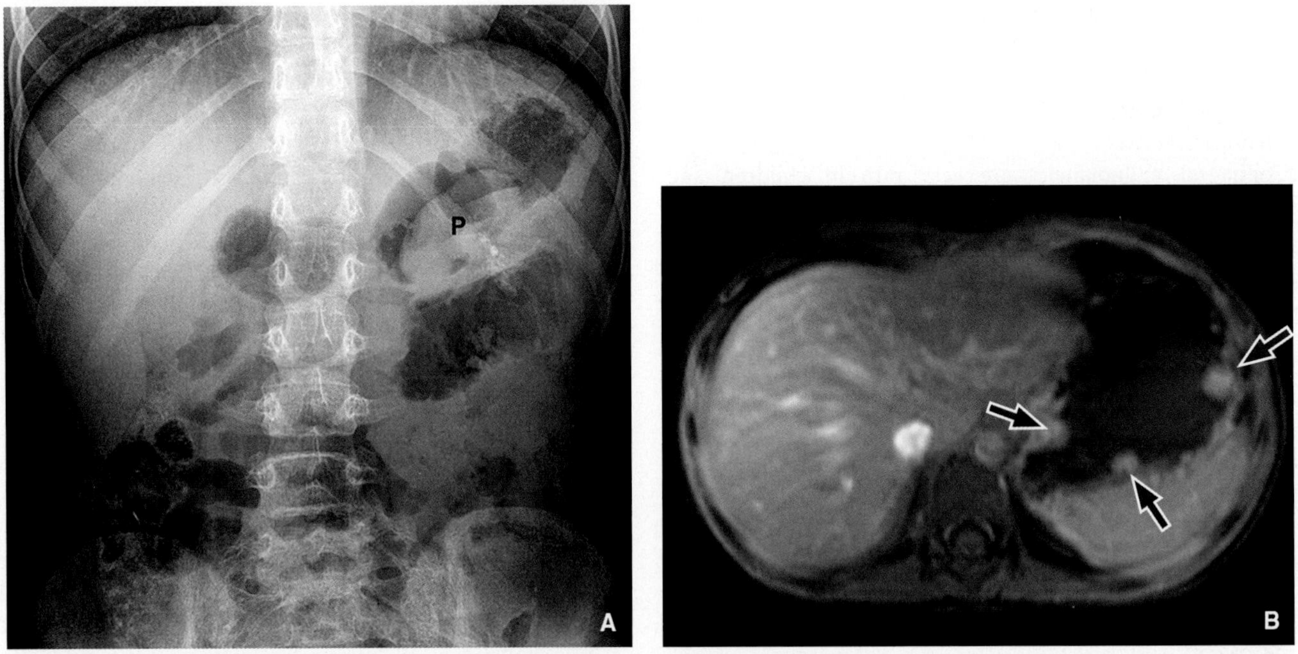

FIGURE 16.78 **A 9-year-old boy with vomiting and gastric polyps due to Peutz-Jeghers syndrome (PJS). A:** Abdominal radiograph shows a large polyp (*P*) in the stomach appearing as a soft tissue mass. **B:** Axial postcontrast T1-weighted fat-suppressed MR image shows additional enhancing round polyps (*arrows*) in the stomach.

Malignant Neoplasm

Lymphoma

Primary lymphomas of the stomach are very rare in children even though non-Hodgkin lymphomas are the most common malignancy of the pediatric GI tract.[131] Gastric lymphoma can be categorized into two forms: mucosa-associated lymphoid tissue (MALT) or non-MALT non-Hodgkin lymphoma. A causal relationship between *H. pylori* and MALT lymphoma is established in adults, but is not definitively proven in children at this time.[131] Posttransplant lymphoproliferative disorder (PTLD) is encountered in children who have received solid organ or stem cell transplants; it is characterized by unregulated expansion of lymphoid cells that is often related to

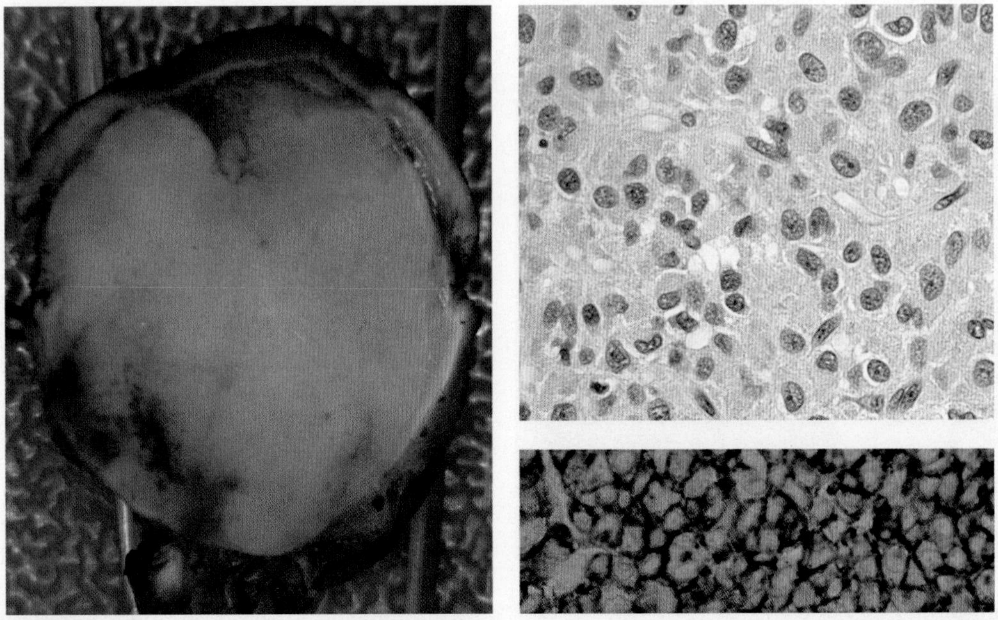

FIGURE 16.79 **Gastrointestinal stromal tumor (GIST).** GIST, from a 12-year-old boy, showing typical nodular growth within the gastric wall (**left panel**), where it arises from the interstitial cells of Cajal of the myenteric plexus. Microscopically, the tumor shows the epithelioid (round-cell) subtype (**right upper**; original magnification, 600×) positive for c-kit (**right lower**, original magnification, 600×).

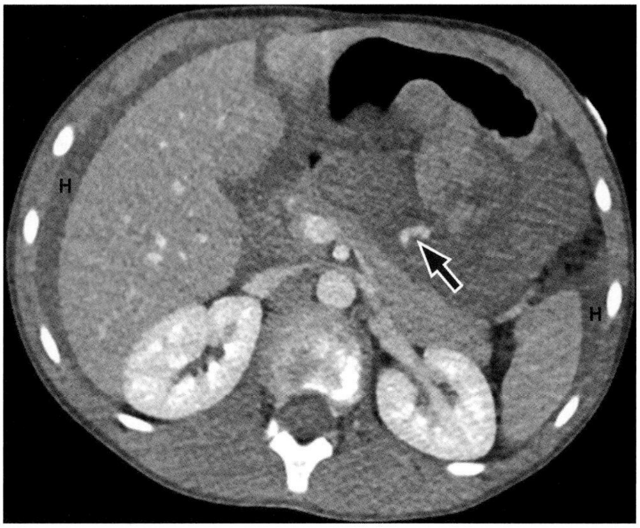

FIGURE 16.80 **A 12-year-old girl with hemoperitoneum due to ruptured gastrointestinal stromal tumor (GIST).** Axial contrast-enhanced CT image shows a large lobulated mass arising from the posterior wall of the stomach. There is active extravasation of contrast material (*arrow*) and related hemoperitoneum (*H*).

Epstein-Barr virus (EBV) infection.[134] PTLD is usually seen within the first 2 years of transplantation, and the abdomen is the most commonly involved site.[134,135] Although GI tract involvement is seen in about one-third of patients, isolated gastric involvement is uncommon.[134] Dyspepsia and epigastric pain are common presenting symptoms for primary gastric lymphoma.[136] PTLD involving the GI tract can present with bleeding, anemia, diarrhea, or weight loss.[134]

UGI series can demonstrate a variety of findings, including gastric nodularity, ulcerations, and focal or diffuse rugal fold enlargement due to infiltrative disease.[135] At CT, gastric lymphomas are usually hypo- or iso-attenuating to muscle with diffuse infiltration of the gastric wall, which is a common findings, particularly with Burkitt lymphoma.[137] Abdominal lymphadenopathy can be also concomitantly seen.[134]

Currently, there is no standard of care for the treatment of these patients with gastric lymphoma.[131] However, the mainstay of treatment for isolated gastric lymphoma lymphoma is complete surgical resection, if possible.[131] Children with more extensive disease typically require combination therapy that includes surgery, chemotherapy, and/or radiation therapy.

Treatment for PTLD relies on four basic principles: reduction of immunosuppression, control of EBV replication, immunotherapy, and chemotherapy.[134]

Metastatic Disease

Neoplasia metastatic to the stomach is very rare in children. In adults, however, primary breast cancer and melanoma can spread to the stomach.[138]

Small Intestine

Benign Tumors

Polyps of the Small Intestine

Small bowel polyps may be solitary or multiple because of a polyposis syndrome. PJS is a cause of multiple hamartomatous polyps of the small bowel and is inherited in an autosomal dominant manner. Affected children can also have mucocutaneous hyperpigmentation affecting the mouth, hands, and feet.[127,139] Although these polyps can be seen from the stomach to the rectum, they are most commonly observed in the small bowel (Fig. 16.81).[139] Individuals with PJS also have an increased lifetime cancer risk when compared to the general population, with the small intestine being the most common site.[139] Abdominal pain due to acute or intermittent small bowel intussusception is a common clinical presentation in children with PJS. Ulceration of the polyps can lead to GI tract bleeding and anemia.[127,139]

Polyps appear as filling defects within the small bowel on SBFT series. The presence of multiple small bowel filling defects should raise suspicion for an underlying polyposis syndrome. Small bowel polyps can also be detected on CT and MRE, especially when oral contrast material surrounds the polyp (Fig. 16.82). A study by Gupta et al. compared MRE to capsule endoscopy for the detection of small bowel polyps in PJS patients and showed that both tests have similar diagnostic performances, although capsule endoscopy missed three polyps larger than 15 mm that were detected by MRE.[140] Ultrasound using graded compression also has been shown to be effective for detecting small bowel hamartomatous polyps, appearing as solid hypoechoic nodules with color Doppler flow and containing small cystic areas, with or without a stalk.[125] Related intussusceptions can be seen by ultrasound, CT, and MRE (Fig. 16.83).[141]

Larger polyps that are at risk for causing intussusception and bowel obstruction require prophylactic polypectomy via endoscopy. Pediatric patients with PJS require monitoring via capsule endoscopy or MRE.[140,141]

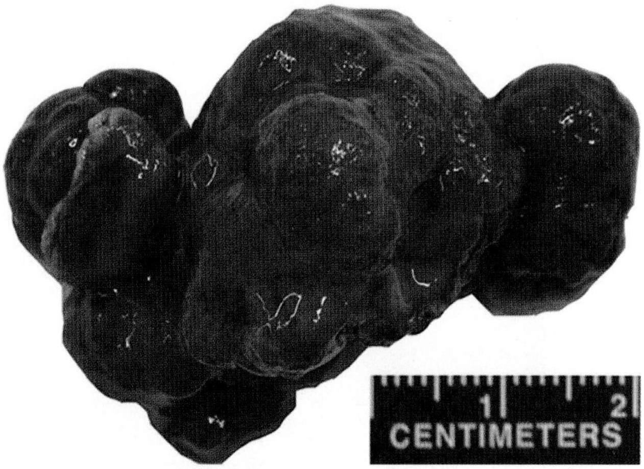

FIGURE 16.81 **Peutz-Jegher-type polyps.** Polyps resected from the jejunum of a 4-year-old girl with Peutz-Jegher syndrome.

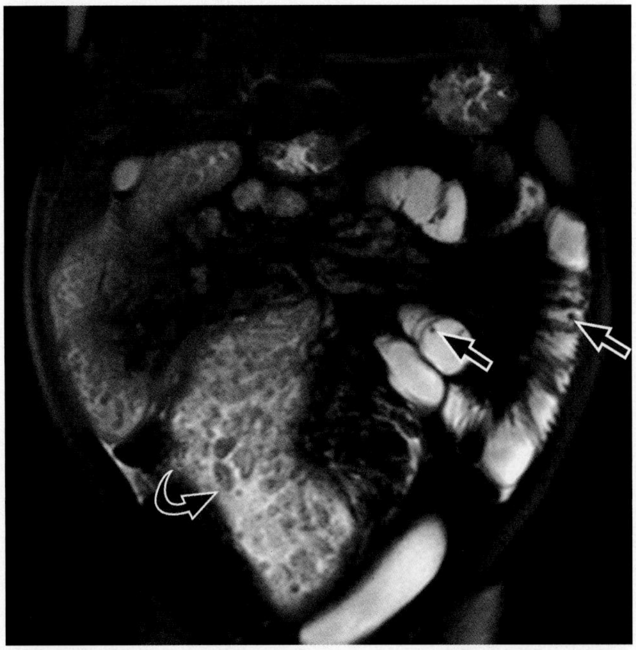

FIGURE 16.82 **A 15-year-old boy with juvenile polyposis syndrome and innumerable colonic polyps.** Coronal T2-weighted fat-suppressed MR image shows many polyps (*curved arrow*) in the colon. A few tiny small bowel polyps (*straight arrows*) are also seen.

Malignant Tumors

Adenoma/Adenocarcinoma

Primary adenomas and adenocarcinomas of the small bowel in children are rare, although predisposing conditions exist, such as Crohn disease-associated and fundic gland polyp-associated dysplasia.[142] These tumors can show intestinal wall thickening that may be eccentric or annular. Bowel obstruction due to luminal narrowing and/or intussusception is possible[142] (Fig. 16.84). Affected children should undergo genetic evaluation to exclude a cancer-predisposing syndrome.

Carcinoid Tumor

Carcinoid tumors arise from the enterochromaffin cells that are widely distributed in the body, including in the small bowel.[143] They are uncommon tumors in children and can be sporadic or due to a syndrome, such as multiple endocrine neoplasia or neurofibromatosis type 1.[143] There is a 3:1 female to male ratio, and they usually occur in older children.[131] GI tract carcinoid tumors can arise from the small bowel (usually ileum) and appendix of children, and rarely from a duplication cyst or Meckel diverticulum.[131] Carcinoid tumors arising from the appendix may present with acute appendicitis due to luminal obstruction (Fig. 16.85). Small bowel lesions may present with hematochezia or anemia due to bleeding, abdominal pain, or vomiting due to obstruction. Carcinoid syndrome, which includes cutaneous flushing, diarrhea, asthma-like respiratory symptoms, and right-sided cardiac failure, is extremely rare in children. Although the large majority pediatric GI tract carcinoid tumors are benign, malignant tumors that can metastasize usually to regional lymph nodes or liver can also occur.[131]

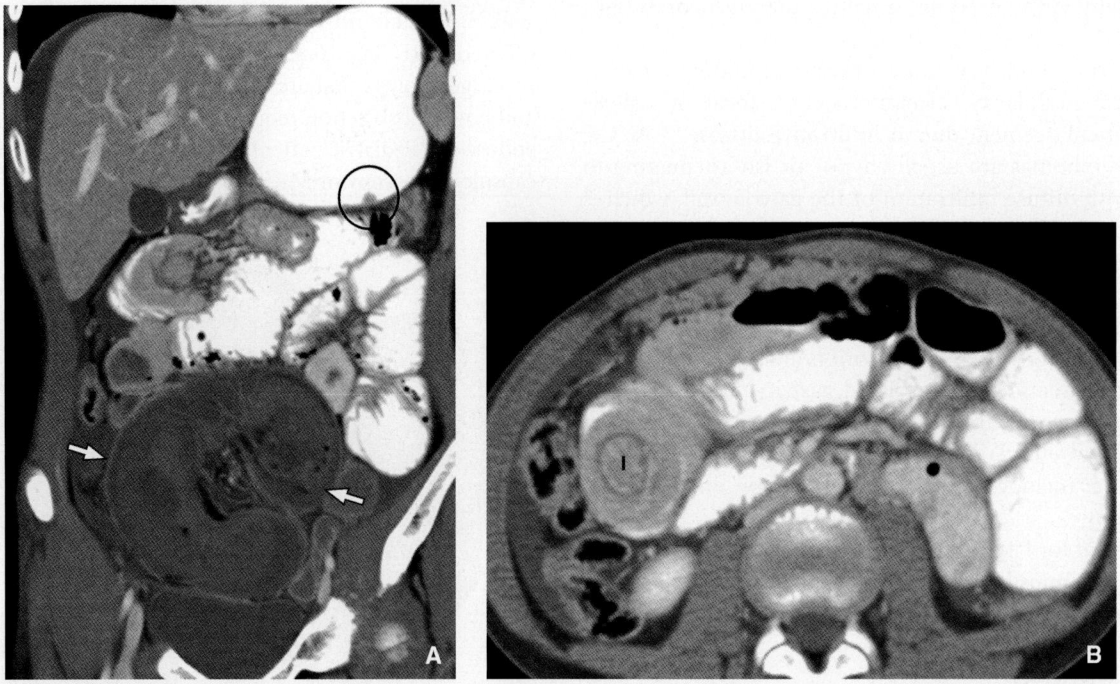

FIGURE 16.83 **A 14-year-old boy with acute abdominal pain and previously unrecognized Peutz-Jegher syndrome. A:** Coronal contrast-enhanced CT image shows a segment of hypoenhancing, infarcted small bowel (*arrows*) in the midabdomen secondary to a large intussusception; a 3.3 cm hamartomatous polyp acted as the lead point. A sessile gastric polyp is also seen (*black circle*). **B:** Axial contrast-enhanced CT image from the same patient shows another small bowel–small bowel intussusception (*I*), with normal bowel wall enhancement.

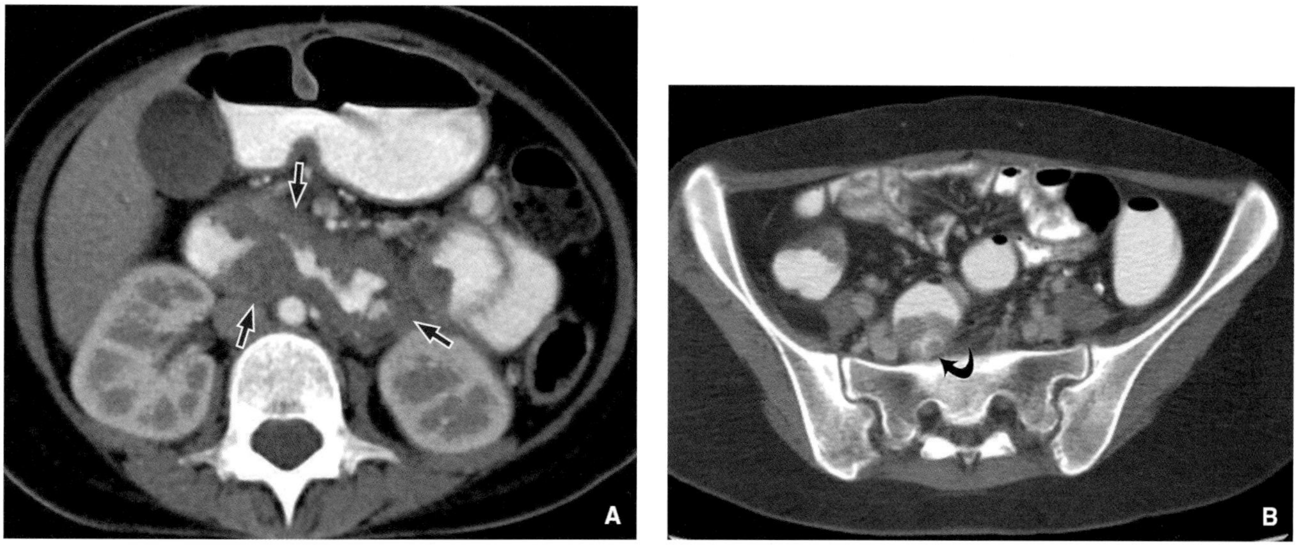

FIGURE 16.84 **A 16-year-old girl with recurrent vomiting and previously unrecognized Lynch syndrome. A:** Axial contrast-enhanced CT image shows a large circumferential mass (*arrows*) resulting in luminal narrowing arising from the second and third portions of the duodenum, proven to be adenocarcinoma of the small bowel. **B:** A more inferior axial CT image shows a soft tissue filling defect in the colon (*arrow*), proven to be an adenoma.

Abdominal radiography may show secondary evidence of carcinoid tumor, such as small bowel obstruction. These small bowel lesions are often small and difficult to appreciate at cross-sectional imaging (Fig. 16.85). When visualized at CT or MRI, the primary tumor may avidly enhance. In some pediatric patients, the only evidence of carcinoid tumor may be subtle focal asymmetric bowel wall thickening or mesenteric desmoplastic reaction and lymphadenopathy.

Incidentally detected histologically benign lesions may be treated with surgery alone, although surveillance imaging may be performed. Malignant carcinoid tumors generally respond poorly to traditional chemotherapies; instead somatostatin analogs and interferon are commonly employed.[143]

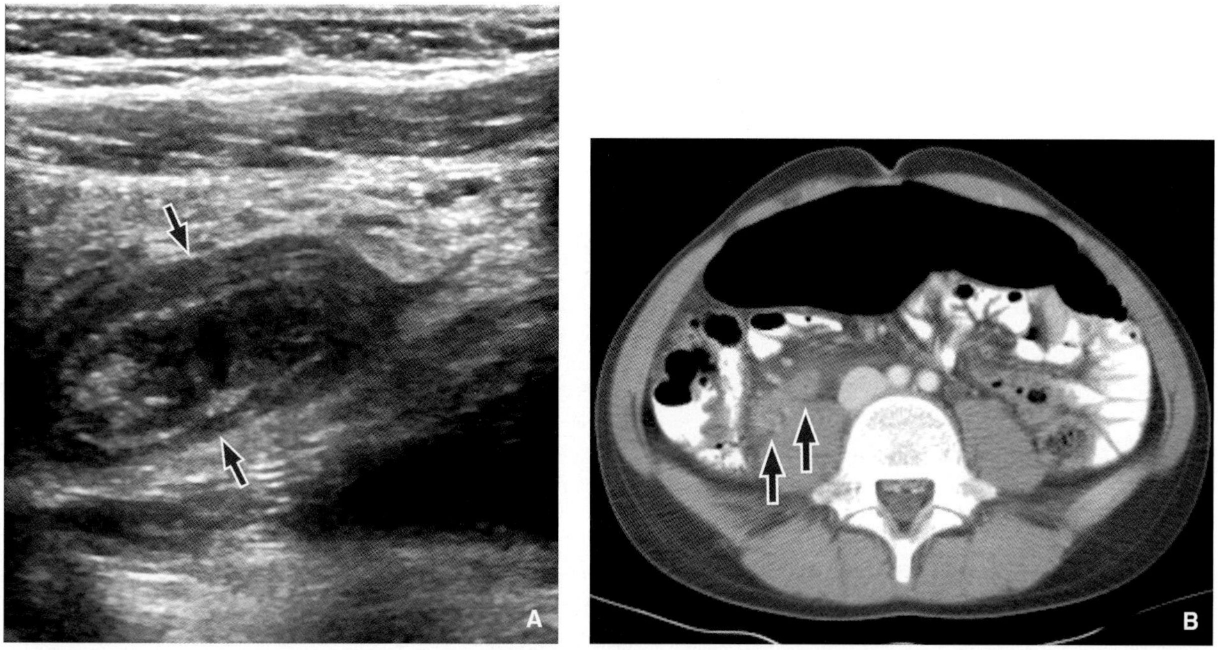

FIGURE 16.85 **A 15-year-old boy with chronic right lower quadrant pain and incidental carcinoid tumor of the appendix. A:** Gray-scale ultrasound image shows a dilated, tubular structure (*arrows*) containing debris thought to represent simple uncomplicated acute appendicitis. On pathology, the appendix was found to be obstructed by a small carcinoid tumor. **B:** Axial contrast-enhanced CT from the same patient shows a dilated, abnormally hyperenhancing appendix (*arrows*) with periappendiceal fat stranding, consistent with acute appendicitis. The known carcinoid tumor cannot be separately identified.

Lymphoma

Burkitt lymphoma, a subtype of non-Hodgkin lymphoma, represents about 50% of GI tract malignancies reported in children, and it is the most common pediatric small bowel tumor.[131] The terminal ileum is most often involved because of its large concentration of intramural lymphoid cells.[137] Intestinal lymphoma can have a variety of presentations, including palpable abdominal mass, obstruction, and perforation. As with other small bowel tumors, lymphoma may act as a lead point for intussusception.[131,137] The small bowel is also the most frequent site of GI tract involvement of PTLD.[134]

Ultrasound typically shows heterogeneous, hypoechoic wall thickening of the small bowel with central hyperechogenicity that represents the apposed mucosal surfaces and intraluminal gas. Small bowel lymphoma can have a "pseudokidney" or target appearance.[137] The bowel should also be assessed for intussusception and proximal dilatation due to obstruction (Fig. 16.86). Mesenteric lymph node enlargement also may be present. CT findings of small bowel lymphoma include mass-like intestinal wall thickening, sometimes with characteristic aneurysmal dilatation of the bowel lumen (Fig. 16.87).[136,137] Intussusception and obstruction may also be seen. Preservation of surrounding fat planes and absence of invasion or obstruction of adjacent structures, despite large tumor size, are important findings to help distinguish lymphoma from other causes of bowel masses.[136] ^{18}F-FDG-PET is helpful for tumor staging and treatment evaluation.[137]

The mainstay of treatment for isolated GI lymphoma is complete surgical resection if possible, whereas those with more extensive disease typically require a combination of therapies, including surgery, radiation therapy, and/or chemotherapy.[131] PTLD is managed using the four basic principles including reduction of immunosuppression, control of EBV replication, immunotherapy, and chemotherapy.[134]

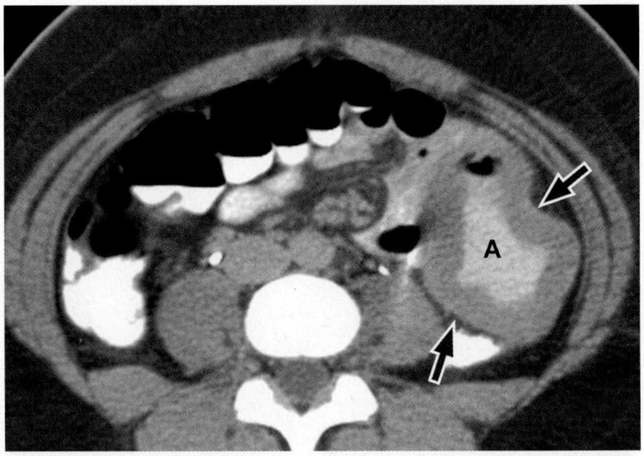

FIGURE 16.87 **A 13-year-old girl with new neck mass confirmed to be Burkitt lymphoma.** Axial contrast-enhanced CT image shows marked wall thickening (*arrows*) of a small bowel loop with aneurysmal (*A*) dilation of the lumen. No adjacent inflammatory changes are seen. Findings are consistent with small bowel lymphomatous involvement.

Colon

Benign Tumors

Juvenile Polyps

Juvenile polyps are hamartomatous lesions that are most often found in the colon and rectum.[125,131] The solitary juvenile polyp is the most common type of polyp encountered in children.[144] Less commonly, juvenile polyps are seen as part of a polyposis syndrome, such as juvenile polyposis syndrome (JPS). JPS is a rare autosomal dominant condition characterized by multiple (>5) juvenile polyps of the GI tract.[139] There is further classification of JPS with the most notable being juvenile polyposis of infancy, which presents with protein losing enteropathy, diarrhea, and hemorrhage with death occurring before 2 years of age.[139]

Colonic juvenile polyps usually appear as filling defects within the bowel lumen on contrast enema, CT, and MRE.

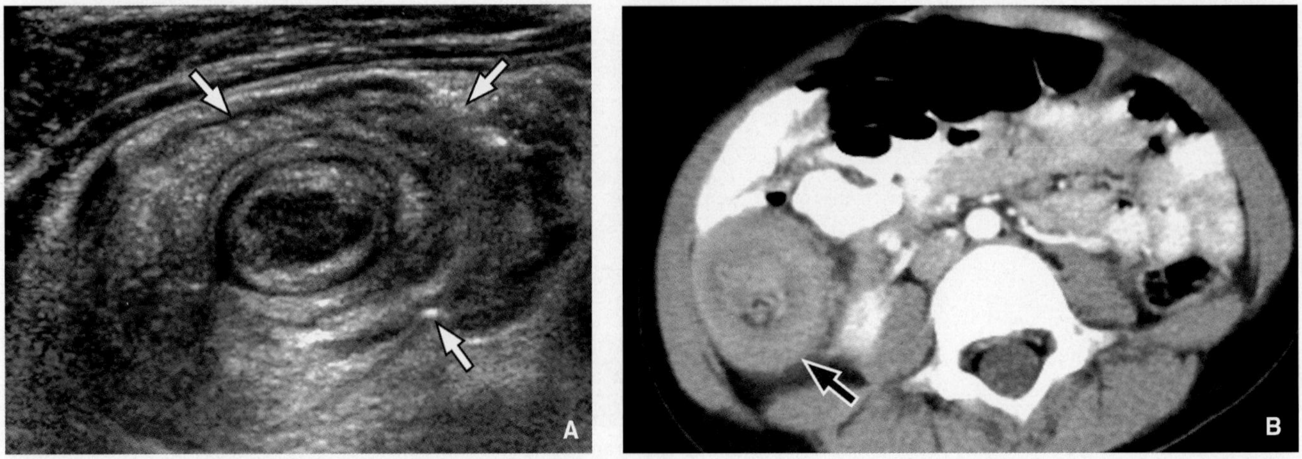

FIGURE 16.86 **A 7-year-old boy with B-cell lymphoma and crampy abdominal pain and vomiting. A:** Gray-scale ultrasound image shows a mass-like structure (*arrows*) in the right hemiabdomen, consistent with an intussusception. **B:** Axial contrast-enhanced CT image shows a persistent intussusception (*arrow*). At surgery, a small bowel lymphomatous mass was confirmed to act as the lead point.

At CT and MRE, they may present as a nonspecific intraluminal mass. Multiple small tiny cystic areas within the lesion are typical at T2-weighted MRI. At ultrasound, juvenile polyps appear as small oval or round solid hypoechoic masses with internal blood flow that can be detected within the colon lumen. They may contain numerous tiny cystic areas and a stalk may be also appreciated (Fig. 16.88).[125] Determining the mass is located in the colon can sometimes be difficult using conventional ultrasound.

The diagnosis of colonic juvenile polyps can be confirmed by endoscopy, with individual polyps treated with polypectomy.[144] Malignancy can be detected in some polyps in older children, with the risk magnified in polyposis syndromes.[131] When polyps are multiple, evaluation for an inherited disorder should be undertaken and routine surveillance performed.[139]

Malignant Neoplasm

Adenoma/Adenocarcinoma

Adenomas and dysplasia of colonic epithelium can be precursor lesions of invasive neoplasms. Although uncommon in children, colorectal adenocarcinoma may be observed in the pediatric population.[131] While a majority of cases are sporadic, some cases are related to an underlying predisposing condition, such as a polyposis syndrome or IBD.[131] FAP syndrome (including Gardner syndrome) is the most common inherited polyposis syndrome, characterized by the development of hundreds of colorectal adenomatous polyps.[145] This disease is inherited in autosomal dominant manner, and polyps tend to develop in the late first or second decade of life.[145] Hereditary nonpolyposis colorectal cancer, or Lynch syndrome, is another autosomal dominant condition that predisposes children to colorectal adenomas and adenocarcinomas.[146] Nonspecific presenting symptoms, such as GI tract bleeding, abdominal pain and vomiting, are common in affected children.[131] Pediatric colorectal adenocarcinomas tend to have a more aggressive histologic appearance when compared to adults and are often more advanced at the time of diagnosis.[146]

Some colorectal cancers in children may be initially detected by CT or MRE in children presenting with bowel

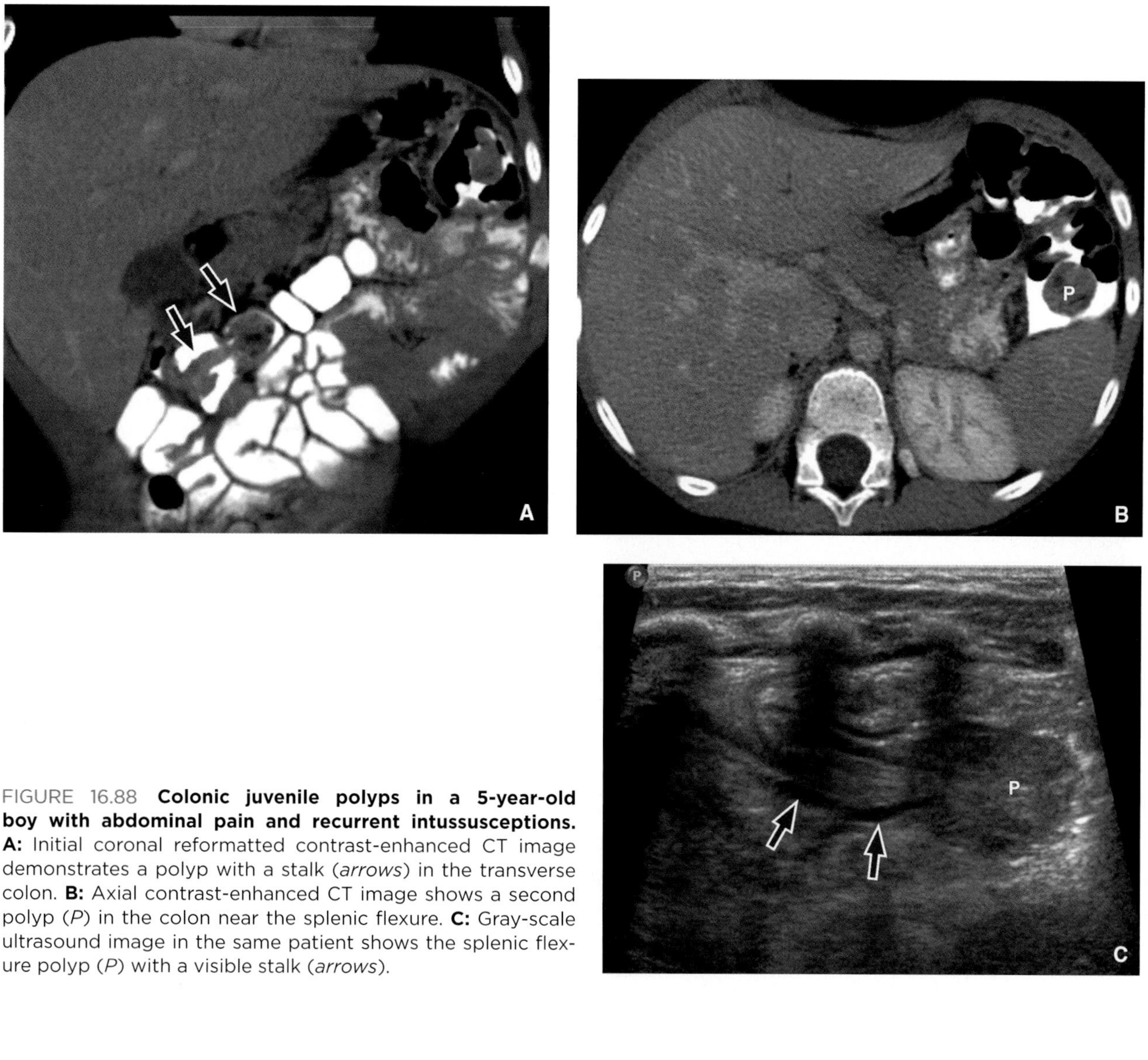

FIGURE 16.88 **Colonic juvenile polyps in a 5-year-old boy with abdominal pain and recurrent intussusceptions. A:** Initial coronal reformatted contrast-enhanced CT image demonstrates a polyp with a stalk (*arrows*) in the transverse colon. **B:** Axial contrast-enhanced CT image shows a second polyp (*P*) in the colon near the splenic flexure. **C:** Gray-scale ultrasound image in the same patient shows the splenic flexure polyp (*P*) with a visible stalk (*arrows*).

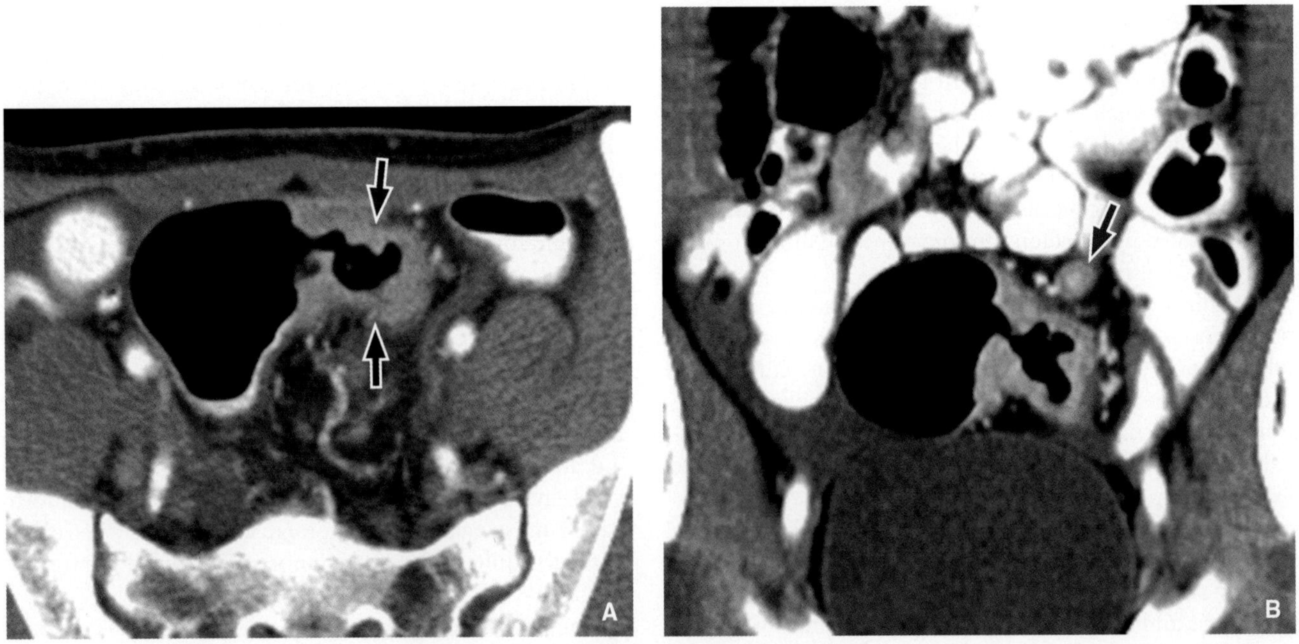

FIGURE 16.89 **A 16-year-old girl with colonic adenocarcinoma. A:** Axial contrast-enhanced CT image through the pelvis shows circumferential wall thickening of the sigmoid colon (*arrows*). **B:** Coronal reformatted contrast-enhanced CT image shows similar findings as well as an enlarged lymph node (*arrow*) in the adjacent sigmoid mesentery.

obstruction or GI tract bleeding. Typical findings include polypoid or mass-like colonic wall thickening and annular, concentric luminal narrowing causing an "apple core" appearance (Fig. 16.89).[146] Images should be also carefully assessed for evidence of metastatic disease. Lymph node, peritoneal, liver, and pulmonary metastases are typical locations (Fig. 16.89). ^{18}F-FDG-PET may be used to detect distant metastatic disease and for staging purposes. Small colorectal adenocarcinomas may be indistinguishable from adenomas by imaging. Therefore, colonoscopy with biopsy is required to confirm the diagnosis. In children with FAP, the colon can be carpeted with many polyps of varying morphologies and sizes.

Treatment of pediatric colorectal adenocarcinoma typically includes surgical resection of the mass and chemotherapy.[146] Prophylactic colectomy is currently performed in many pediatric patients with FAP.

Lymphoma

Primary colonic lymphoma is less common than small bowel lymphoma. When it occurs, the cecum is the most commonly involved site.[137,147] In addition, PTLD can involve the colon in pediatric transplant recipients.[134] Imaging and treatment of colonic lymphoma is similar to that of small bowel lymphoma. Imaging findings may mimic those of colonic adenocarcinoma. The mainstay of treatment for isolated colonic lymphoma is complete surgical resection if possible, whereas those with more extensive disease typically require a combination of therapies, including surgery, radiation therapy, and/or chemotherapy.

Traumatic Disorders

Esophagus

Boerhaave Syndrome

Boerhaave syndrome, or esophageal rupture secondary to severe vomiting, is rare in children. About 50% of pediatric cases occur in neonates.[148] The distal portion of the thoracic esophagus is most susceptible to rupture. Esophageal rupture tends to occur on the right side in children unlike in adults where the left side is more common. Affected children can present with vomiting, thoracic back pain, pneumomediastinum, and subcutaneous emphysema.[148] At imaging, chest radiography may reveal pneumomediastinum, pneumothorax, or pleural effusion. CT may show similar findings and/or focal esophageal abnormality above the gastroesophageal junction. Esophagography can be used to confirm the diagnosis. Treatment is surgical repair.

Iatrogenic Injury

Published literature indicates that 71% to 84% of pediatric esophageal perforations are iatrogenic, and they most commonly result from malpositioned tubes, endoscopy, or dilatation procedures.[149] Common causes of perforation in neonates include nasogastric tube and endotracheal tube insertion as well as pharyngeal suctioning.[149,150] Location of perforation depends on the age of the child. In neonates, perforations tend to occur in the cervical esophagus near the cricopharyngeal muscle, whereas in older children, they commonly occur in the thoracic esophagus. Proximal esophageal perforations tend to result in left-sided pneumothorax and pleural effusion, whereas distal perforations show similar findings on the right.[151] Clinical presentations may include dysphagia, chest or back pain, subcutaneous emphysema, and respiratory distress. If the injury is near the gastroesophageal junction, the affected child may present with abdominal pain or peritonitis.[152]

Chest radiography is typically initially performed and may show pneumothorax, pneumomediastinum, subcutaneous emphysema, pleural effusion, and/or a malpositioned tube. Esophagography using water-soluble iodinated contrast material can be used to confirm esophageal perforation; extraluminal contrast material may be seen in the mediastinum or pleural space. Other findings of esophageal injury include pooling of contrast material posterior to the cervical esophagus and tracking of contrast material in the esophageal wall due to traumatic dissection.[152] On occasion, esophagography may be falsely negative. CT findings suggestive of esophageal injury include pneumomediastinum, focal esophageal wall thickening or mural defect, mediastinal inflammation (mediastinitis), and pleural effusion (Fig. 16.90).

Treatment is generally conservative with esophageal rest, antibiotic therapy, chest tube placement, and gastrostomy or other feeding tube placement. Surgery is reserved for children who fail conservative therapy.

Caustic Ingestion

Accidental caustic ingestion usually occurs in young children, about 3 years of age, with most reported cases due to ingested household cleaners.[153,154] Caustic agents mostly fall into two groups: alkaline and acidic.[154] Alkaline agents are most harmful because they cause greater necrosis and more rapid mural penetration. A child who has consumed a caustic agent may present with chest or back pain, drooling, and respiratory distress with evidence of airway obstruction.[155] There may be skin (including perioral) damage. Esophageal stricture is a delayed complication that can occur as early as 3 weeks after ingestion.

Radiography of the chest can be normal or show evidence of esophageal perforation in affected children. Water-soluble esophagography generally is not useful in the acute phase.[155] Delayed esophagography is useful for detecting ingestion-related complications. Short strictures are the hallmark of ingestion of acidic agents, whereas ingestion of alkaline agents reveals relatively long strictures (Fig. 16.91).[156] Most strictures are located in the upper to midesophagus.

Treatment is generally conservative, including antibiotic therapy and proton pump inhibitors. Endoscopic dilatation eventually may be required to treat symptomatic strictures. In children with severe stricturing, esophagectomy with gastric pull-through or colonic interposition may be required.

Foreign Body Ingestion

Coins

Coins are the most common foreign body ingested by children. There are three locations in the esophagus where coins typically become stuck, which include the thoracic inlet, at the level of the aortic arch, and at the lower esophageal sphincter.[157] The majority of ingested coins become lodged at the thoracic inlet.[157] Children who swallow coins can present variably with dysphagia, cough, gagging, and vomiting. When the coin has been lodged in the esophagus for days to weeks, a child can present with respiratory distress due to the chronic inflammatory changes having mass effect upon adjacent trachea.

Standard assessment for ingested foreign body includes radiography of the neck, chest, abdomen, and pelvis. Only

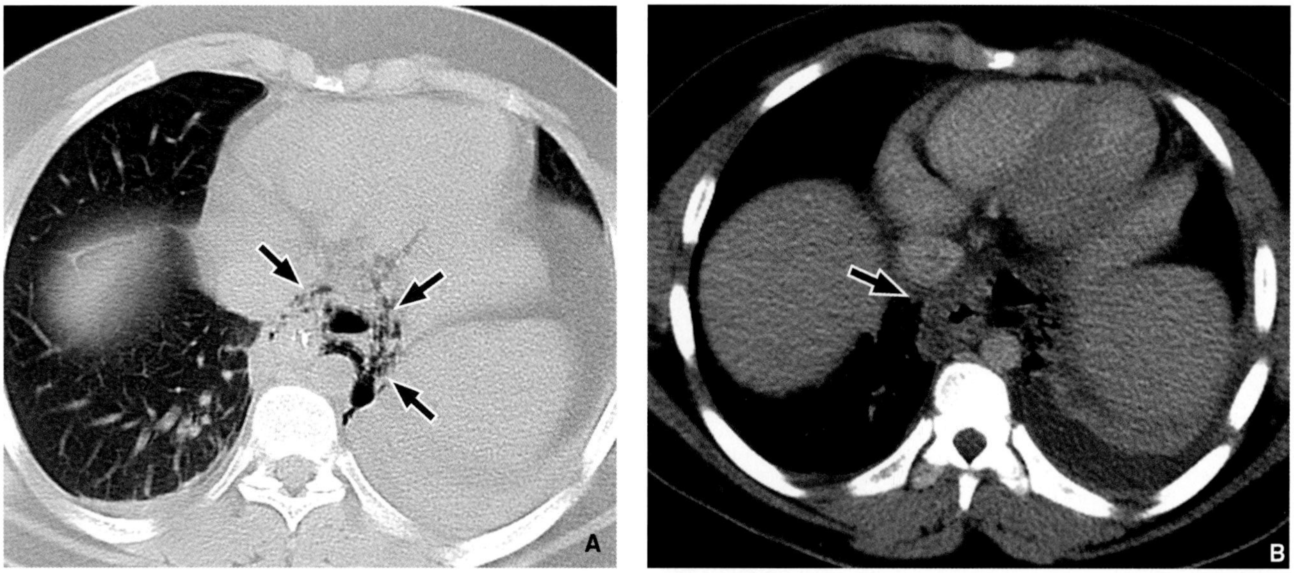

FIGURE 16.90 **A 10-year-old boy with acute chest pain due to esophageal perforation after endoscopic esophageal dilatation. A:** Axial lung window CT image shows air (*arrows*) in the mediastinum surrounding the esophagus and thoracic aorta, consistent with pneumomediastinum. **B:** Axial contrast-enhanced CT image shows circumferential esophageal wall thickening (*arrow*) and adjacent inflammatory stranding. There is also a left pleural effusion.

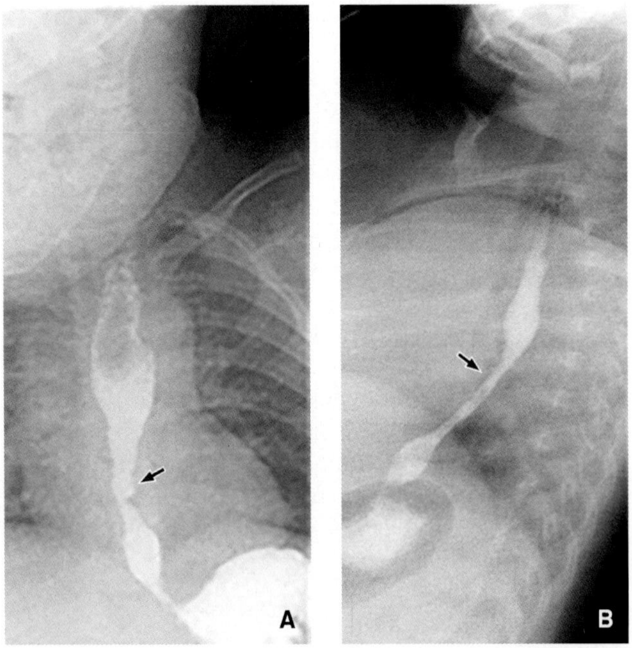

FIGURE 16.91 **A 2-year-old boy with lye-induced stricture 3 weeks after the initial ingestion. A:** Frontal esophagram image shows long segment narrowing (*arrow*) of the distal esophagus. **B:** Lateral view is confirmatory, with the stricture persisting (*arrow*).

radiopaque ingested foreign bodies can be directly seen. On occasion, frontal and lateral images of the chest may be needed to determine if the object is located in the esophagus or airway. A coin seen en face on the frontal and projecting behind the airway on the lateral image is typically esophageal in location (Fig. 16.92). Chronically lodged coins can cause an inflammatory reaction that presents as increased soft tissue opacity between the airway and esophagus, sometimes with mass effect on the airway.[158] Esophagography is only required when there is concern for stricture or perforation (Fig. 16.92).

Ingested coins are generally removed via endoscopy if lodged in the esophagus. Coins in the stomach commonly eventually pass from the GI tract, although on occasion they may become stuck at the pylorus or ileocecal valve.

Button Battery Ingestion

The incidence of button battery ingestion in young children is increasing.[159] More than 3,000 button battery–related emergency room visits occur annually in the United States.[159] Unlike coins, ingestion of a battery can have devastating consequences, especially if presentation is delayed. Early recognition and swift removal is crucial to reduce morbidity and mortality. Esophageal injury may be due to pressure necrosis, electrical current, and/or leakage of battery contents. Injury induced by button batteries can extend beyond the esophagus to involve the adjacent airway or the aorta causing respiratory failure, shock, and even internal hemorrhage.[160]

At radiography, it is imperative that a button battery be distinguished from a coin. The hallmarks of a button battery include seeing a beveled edge on the lateral image and lucent halo or circle near the surface of the battery surface on the frontal image (Fig. 16.93). Radiographs may also show

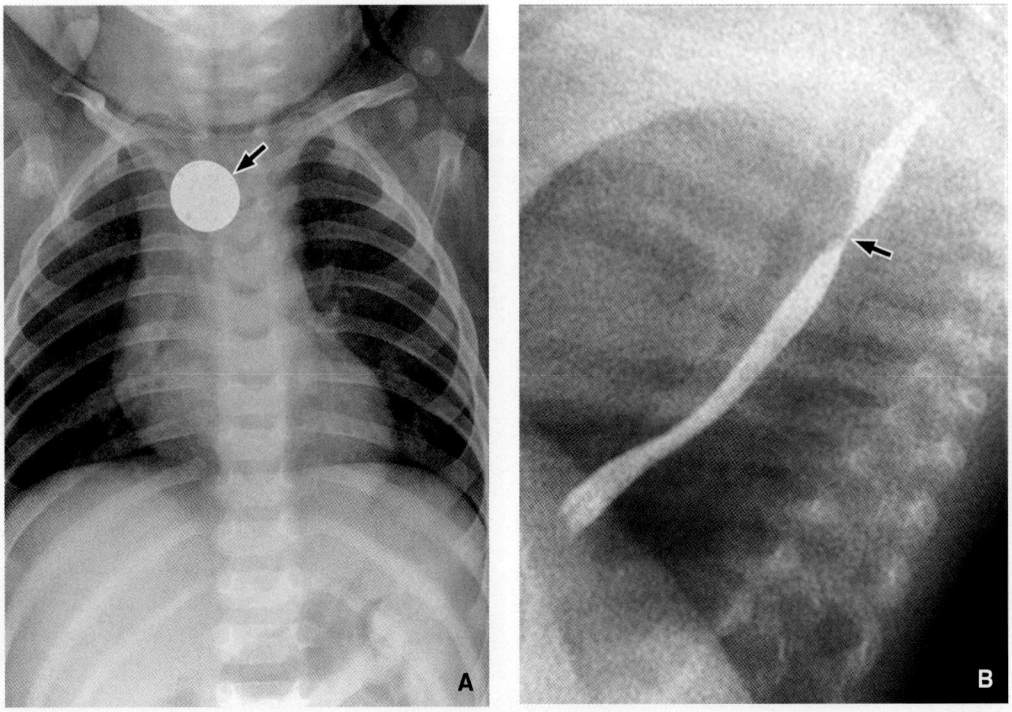

FIGURE 16.92 **A 2-year-old boy with ingested coin lodged in the esophagus. A:** Frontal radiograph shows a coin (*arrow*) in the upper thoracic esophagus. **B:** Lateral esophagram image obtained 3 weeks later because of dysphagia shows a focal esophageal stricture (*arrow*) at the site where coin was lodged.

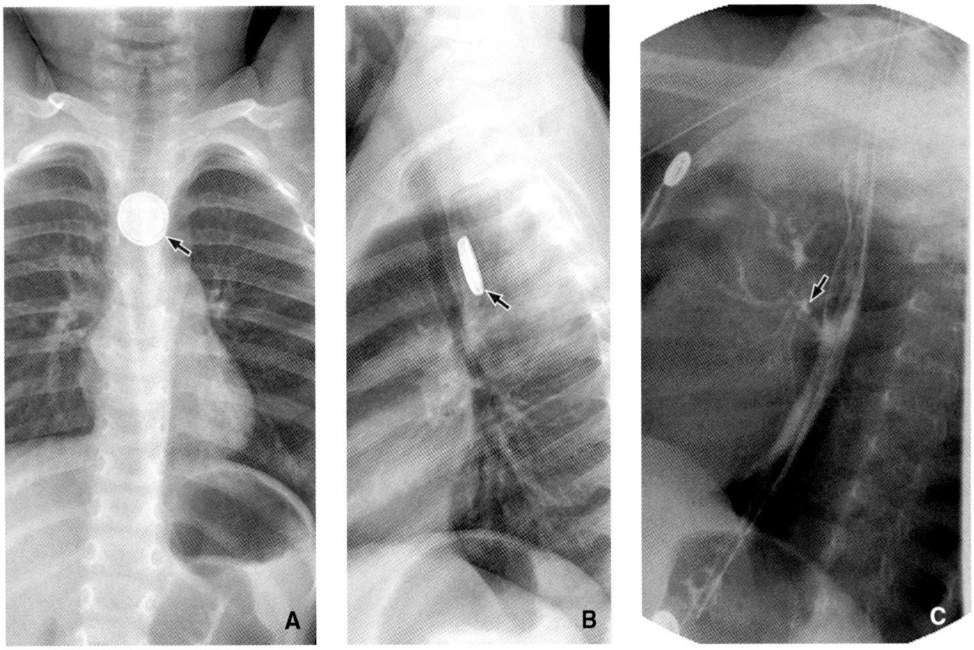

FIGURE 16.93 **A 3-year-old boy with ingested button battery complicated by tracheoesophageal fistula (TEF). A:** Frontal radiograph shows a foreign body projecting over the upper chest with a circle within a *circle* appearance (*arrow*), consistent with an ingested button battery. **B:** Lateral radiograph shows that the ingested foreign body (*arrow*) has a beveled edge and is located posterior to the trachea. **C:** The child developed a chronic cough a few weeks later. Lateral esophagram image shows an abnormal contrast-filled communication between the esophagus and trachea, consistent with an acquired tracheoesophageal fistula (*arrow*).

evidence of esophageal wall thickening and mass effect upon the adjacent airway. Esophagram can be used to assess for esophageal injury, including TEF (Fig. 16.93). MRI and CT angiography can be used to evaluate for related mediastinitis and possible aortic injury.

Treatment is emergent removal of the battery. If it cannot be removed, the battery can be pushed into the stomach. Once the battery reaches the duodenum, about 85% of them pass from the GI tract within 72 hours.[160] Button batteries vary in size, with smaller batteries more likely to pass.

Blunt Trauma

Blunt trauma to the chest rarely results in esophageal injury. However, when it does, esophageal injury can occur in conjunction with tracheal or airway injury.[161] In the setting of blunt chest trauma, the esophagus usually decompresses via the mouth and stomach, thus avoiding significant injury.[161] Pediatric esophageal injuries most frequently present with chest pain, fever, and subcutaneous emphysema, which are nonspecific and often produced by more prevalent injuries of the lung. Consequently, these factors lead to a delay in diagnosis of esophageal injury in the pediatric population.[162]

Chest radiography and CT may demonstrate show pneumomediastinum, subcutaneous emphysema, pneumothorax, and/or pleural effusion.[161] The esophageal wall may appear thickened at CT. Esophagram also can sometimes confirm the diagnosis of perforation, demonstrating contrast material extending beyond the lumen into the esophageal wall or mediastinum. TEF is a rare complication from blunt trauma.

Depending on the exact injury, management may be conservative or surgical.[162]

Small Intestine

Magnet Ingestion

The advent of toy magnets has resulted in an increasing number of magnet ingestions in the pediatric population.[163,164] Like button batteries, ingested magnets can cause substantial morbidity and mortality in children. Swallowing a single small magnet is not usually dangerous because most eventually pass from the GI tract. However, when multiple magnets are swallowed, they can be located in different portions of the bowel and become attracted to one another with ensuing pressure necrosis that can lead to perforation, obstruction, or fistula formation.[163] Small magnets generally are easy to swallow and do not cause esophageal obstructive symptoms. Affected children can present with abdominal pain or signs and symptoms of peritonitis in the event of bowel perforation.

Abdominal radiography typically demonstrates round or oval-shaped metallic foreign bodies within the GI tract (Fig. 16.94). It may be difficult to determine if abutting magnets are in the same bowel loop or adjacent bowel loops, although a thin gap between magnets suggests that they are in adjacent bowel loops.[165] A stack of magnets can also appear to be a single magnet. Upper GI series can be used to show that the magnets are intraluminal and have not eroded through the bowel wall (Fig. 16.94).

Retained magnets in the GI tract typically require endoscopic or surgical removal.[163]

Accidental Trauma

Pediatric abdominal trauma can be due to either blunt or penetrating injury. Penetrating trauma, such as knife or gunshot wounds, accounts for 20% of traumatic injuries to the

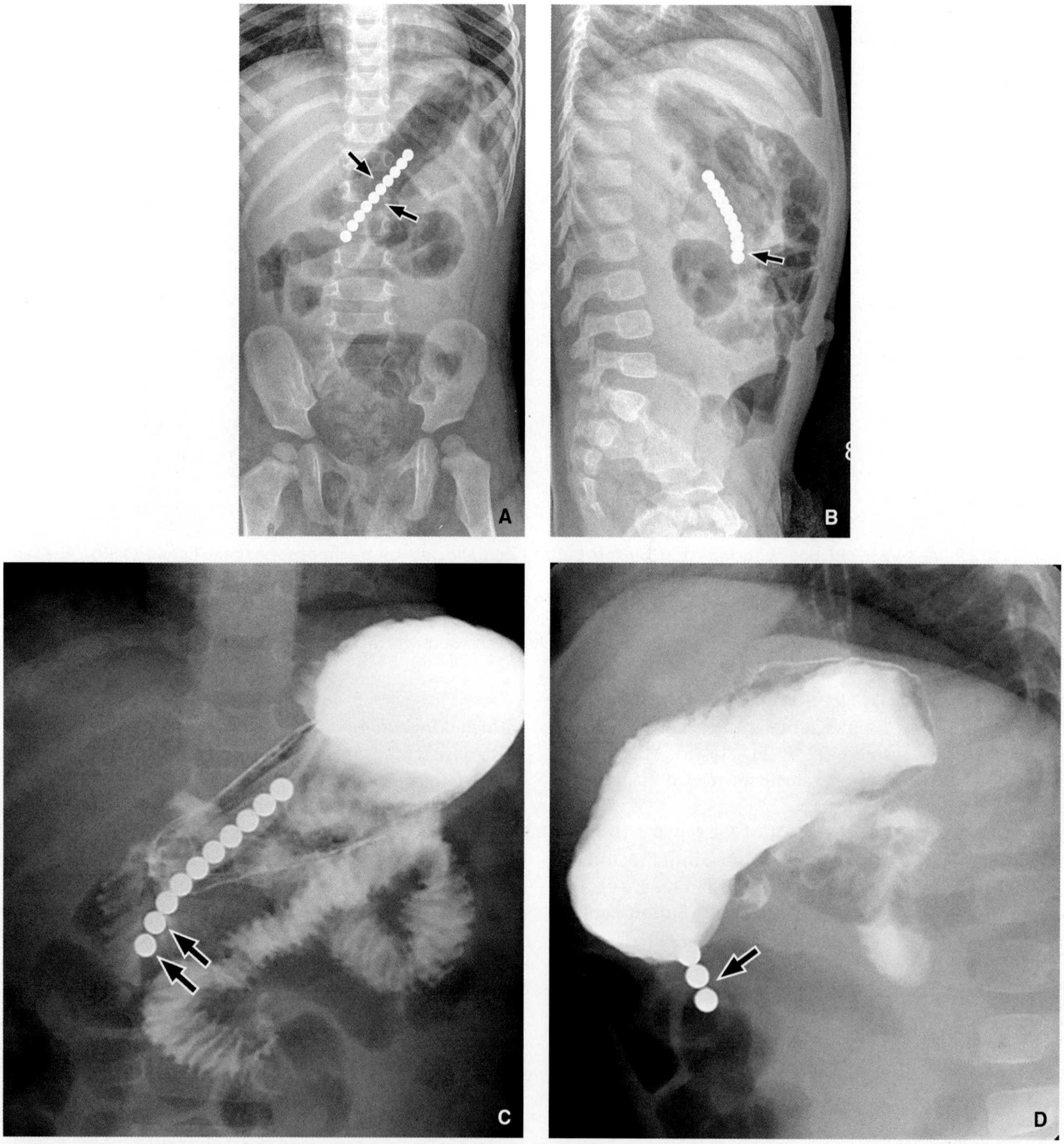

FIGURE 16.94 **A 3-year-old boy who swallowed toy magnets. A:** Abdominal radiograph shows multiple round metallic magnets (*arrows*) adhering to each other in a row within the upper GI tract, thought to be in the stomach. **B:** Cross-table lateral radiograph also confirms the absence of pneumoperitoneum. The magnets (*arrow*) may project beyond the confines of the stomach. **C:** Frontal upper GI series image shows contrast material opacifying the stomach and duodenum. Several magnets are extraluminal (*arrows*), exiting the stomach through the distal antral wall. **D:** Lateral upper GI series image confirms gastric perforation, with at least three magnets (*arrow*) located outside of the stomach. At surgery, there was a gastric perforation, and the magnets were plugging the perforation preventing free spillage of air and contrast into the peritoneal cavity.

abdomen in children.[166] In these cases, children are commonly taken to surgery immediately to control bleeding and assess internal injuries. Blunt trauma, such as occurs with motor vehicle collisions (MVCs), pedestrian versus car accidents, and falls, is much more commonly encountered in clinical practice, accounting for 80% of pediatric abdominal trauma cases. The incidence of intestinal injury in the pediatric population in the trauma setting has been reported to be between 5% and 10%, and most are due to inappropriately restrained children in MVCs.[167]

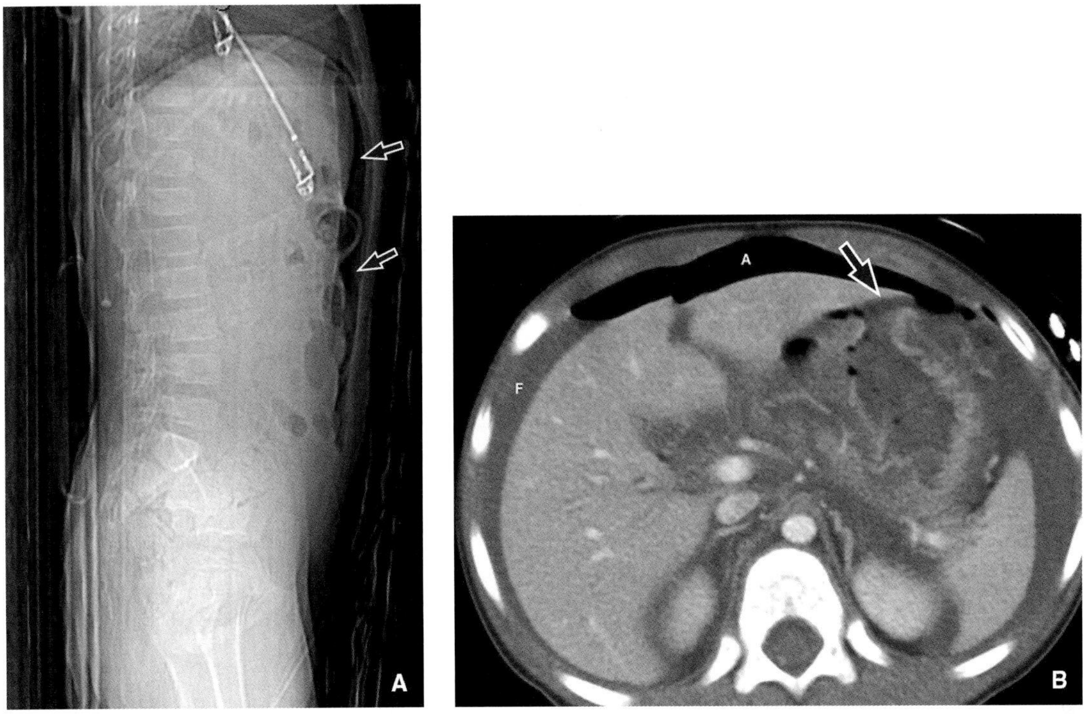

FIGURE 16.95 **A 6-year-old girl with blunt abdominal trauma from a motor vehicle accident with seatbelt-related bruising on the anterior abdominal wall. A:** Lateral CT scout image shows extensive anterior abdominal lucency due to pneumoperitoneum (*arrows*). **B:** Axial contrast-enhanced CT image shows intraperitoneal free fluid (*F*) and air (*A*). There is a disruption of the anterior wall of the stomach, consistent with gastric perforation (*arrow*).

CT with intravenous contrast material is the imaging test of choice for evaluating blunt trauma to the pediatric abdomen, with an overall sensitivity 87% to 95% and a specificity 48% to 84% in the detection bowel injuries.[167] Oral contrast material usually does not provide additional clinical benefit and may delay diagnosis; therefore, it is not typically used in the trauma setting. CT findings suggestive of intestinal (and gastric) trauma include more than physiologic amount of intraperitoneal fluid, focal bowel wall thickening, focally altered bowel wall enhancement, pneumoperitoneum, and focal bowel wall discontinuity with adjacent mesenteric fat stranding (Fig. 16.95). The first three CT findings mentioned are the most common findings seen in a larger pediatric series (Fig. 16.96).[167] Up to one-third of significant bowel injuries are not obvious by CT.[168]

When CT findings are suspicious for bowel perforation, the child is typically surgically explored[167] (Figs. 16.96 and 16.97).

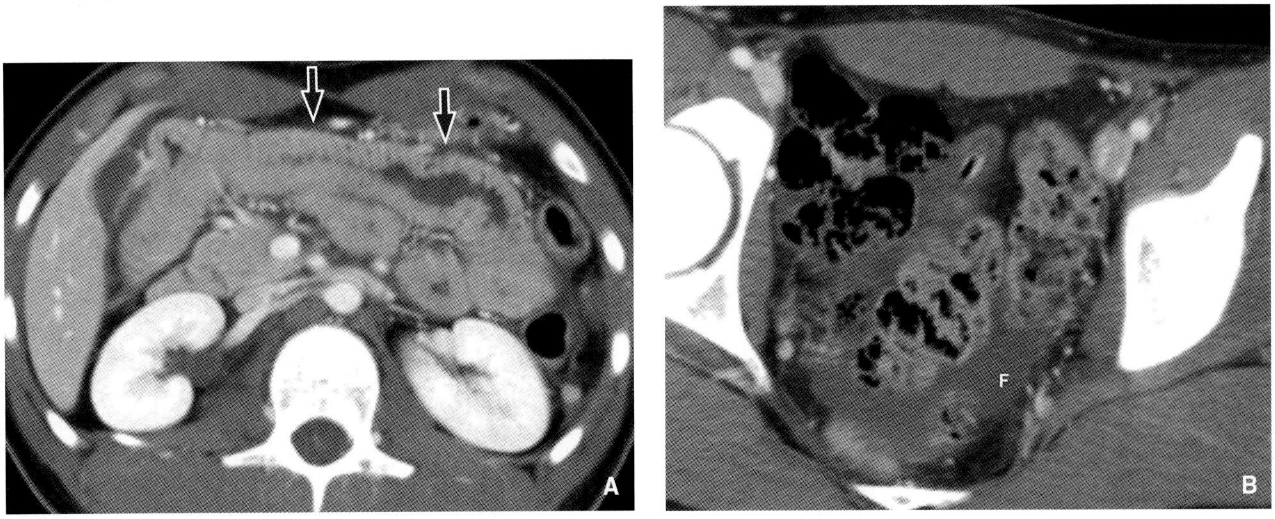

FIGURE 16.96 **A 13-year-old boy with blunt abdominal trauma from a motor vehicle accident. A:** Axial contrast-enhanced CT image shows thick-walled small bowel loops (*arrows*) in the midabdomen, thought to represent contusion. Small bowel loops located elsewhere in the abdomen were normal in thickness. **B:** Axial contrast-enhanced CT image through the pelvis shows free fluid (*F*). At surgical exploration, two areas of small bowel perforation were identified.

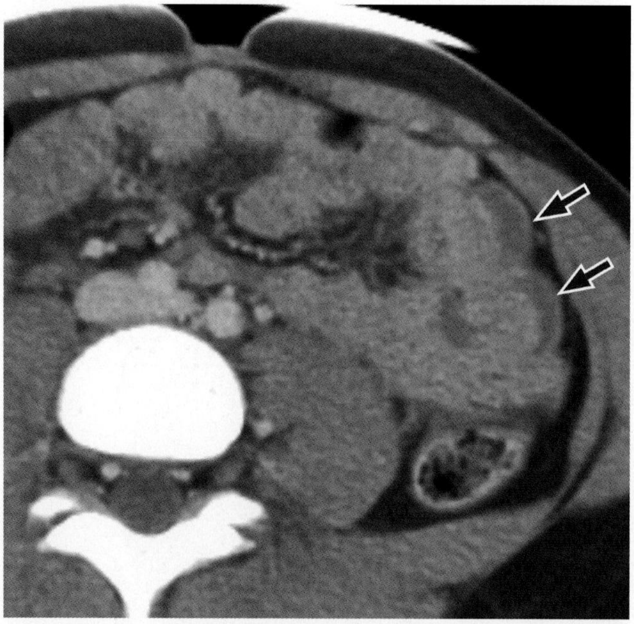

FIGURE 16.97 **A 17-year-old boy with blunt abdominal trauma from a motor vehicle accident.** Axial contrast-enhanced CT image shows jejunal wall thickening with intramural low attenuation (*arrows*). Patient was surgically explored and found to have small bowel contusion without perforation.

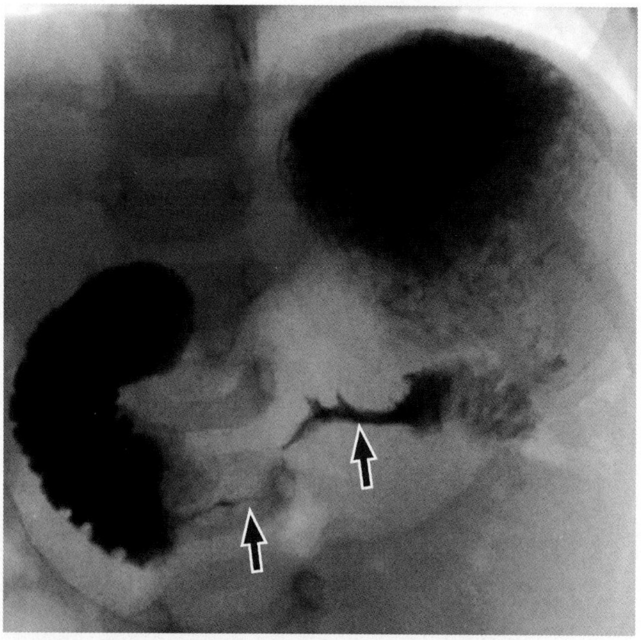

FIGURE 16.98 **A 3-year-old boy with abdominal pain due to nonaccidental (blunt) trauma.** Upper GI series image demonstrates duodenal wall thickening and luminal narrowing (*arrows*) due to intramural hematoma.

Conservative management is generally relied upon if CT imaging is normal or equivocal and the patient is stable. Serial abdominal examinations may be useful if increased suspicion for bowel injury persists and imaging is unremarkable.

Nonaccidental Trauma

In young children (ages 0 to 4 years), nonaccidental trauma (NAT) accounts for about 15% of blunt abdominal trauma cases.[169] Many of these injuries are severe, associated with multiorgan trauma, and have a higher morbidity and mortality when compared to blunt trauma from other causes. The mechanism of NAT injures of the abdomen usually involves punches and kicks to the epigastric and midabdomen regions that result in the intestinal injuries as well as injuries to the liver and pancreas. Affected children may present with abdominal wall bruising or vomiting due to bowel obstruction.

CT is the imaging modality of choice when there is high suspicion for abdominal trauma in the setting of NAT. Findings suggestive of duodenal or other small bowel injury include focal wall thickening, high-attenuation intramural fluid due to hematoma, peribowel fluid/hemorrhage, and peribowel extraluminal gas. In some children, bowel injury, such as duodenal hematoma, may be the first sign of NAT[169] (Fig. 16.98). Duodenal hematomas also can be identified using ultrasound and upper GI series, both showing focal wall thickening and luminal narrowing (Fig. 16.98). No blood flow is seen within the hematoma on Doppler ultrasound. Upper GI series can also be used to assess for associated obstruction based on delayed passage of contrast material and upstream dilatation. It may sometimes be difficult to distinguish intestinal intramural hematoma from perforation by imaging, although findings that confirm perforation include intra- or retroperitoneal air or extraluminal contrast material.[169] This differentiation is important because bowel wall rupture requires surgery, whereas intramural hematomas are managed conservatively.

Shock Bowel/Hypoperfusion Complex

Shock bowel, or hypoperfusion complex, occurs in the setting of hypotension and severe trauma that requires substantial resuscitation efforts. This condition, which occurs in both children and adults, is an indicator of trauma severity, is associated with a high mortality rate, and has distinct CT features. Shock bowel can be seen in a variety of traumatic settings, including intracranial injury.[169] CT findings of shock bowel include diffusely dilated fluid-filled bowel loops that demonstrate intense postcontrast enhancement, diminished caliber of the inferior vena cava (IVC) and abdominal aorta, as well as solid organ altered enhancement (Fig. 16.99).[167] There is no specific treatment for shock bowel other than continued patient resuscitation and standard management of associated traumatic injuries.

Gastrointestinal Tract Obstructive Disorders

Achalasia

Achalasia is due to failure of the lower esophageal sphincter to relax, with resultant esophageal dilatation and hypoperistalsis.[119] Affected children commonly present with dysphagia, chest pain, vomiting, regurgitation, or symptoms of gastroesophageal reflux.[170] The gold standard for diagnosis is esophageal manometry, which can show incomplete relaxation

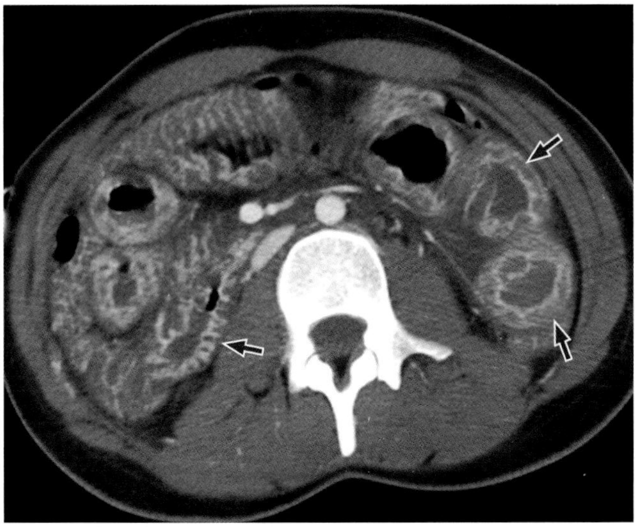

FIGURE 16.99 **A 14-year-old boy with hypotension and shock bowel/hypoperfusion after motor vehicle accident.** Axial contrast-enhanced CT image shows diffuse bowel wall thickening and mucosal hyperenhancement (*arrows*). The inferior vena cava is abnormally flattened, and there is mesenteric low attenuation due to fluid/edema.

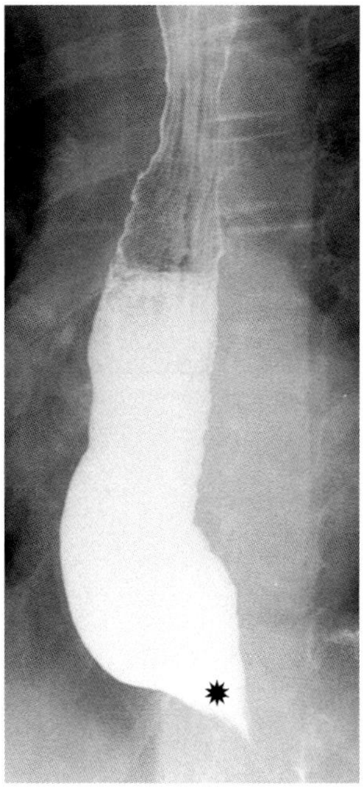

FIGURE 16.100 **A 13-year-old girl with dysphagia due to achalasia.** Esophagram image shows esophageal dilatation (megaesophagus) with "bird's beak" appearance (*asterisk*) of the gastroesophageal junction.

of the lower esophageal sphincter.[170] Chest radiography can show a dilated esophagus containing an air–fluid/debris level. Upper GI series can be performed to confirm the diagnosis, showing a dilated proximal esophagus, decreased peristalsis, and smooth tapering of the distal esophagus to the level of the gastroesophageal junction having the appearance of a "bird's beak" (Fig. 16.100).[119] Occasionally this disorder may be detected by CT in older children presenting with chest pain. Achalasia can be treated with balloon dilation of the narrowed esophagus, botulinum toxin injection, or Heller myotomy.[170]

Abdominal Adhesions

Adhesions are a predictable component of the healing process after abdominal surgery with the adult literature reporting adhesion formation in up to 95% of patients after laparotomy.[171] Clinically, adhesions most often come to attention secondary to small bowel obstruction. Rates of adhesion formation are possibly lower with laparoscopic versus open surgical technique and are increased in children with perforated appendicitis and those undergoing multiple operations.[172,173] There are also two types of adhesions, adhesive bands and matted adhesions, with the former resulting in an increased risk of closed loop obstruction.[173] Affected children typically present with abdominal pain, abdominal distention, and emesis.

In symptomatic children, radiography may demonstrate an obstructive bowel gas pattern, including dilated loops of bowel with differential air–fluid levels and absent or decreased distal bowel gas (Fig. 16.101). As many bowel obstructions are partial, some distal bowel gas may be seen. CT is helpful for determining the exact level of intestinal obstruction because the transition point where the bowel changes caliber can be directly visualized. The offending adhesion is generally unable to be seen.[173]

Small bowel obstructions due to abdominal adhesions can be managed with both conservative and operative approaches. In one study, fever and leukocytosis were clinical findings that predicted the need for operative intervention in this pediatric patient population.[171]

Hypertrophic Pyloric Stenosis

HPS is the most common surgical entity affecting infants in the first 6 months of life.[174] This condition in most common in white populations, is four to five times more common in boys, and has its highest incidence in first-born children.[174] A familial predisposition is also seen with a fivefold increase in risk in first-degree relatives.[175] The cause of HPS remains unknown. However, the common final pathway is that of abnormal hypertrophy of the circular muscle of the pylorus that is unable to relax. As a result, the pyloric lumen becomes obstructed by redundant, thickened mucosa.[174,176] Greater than 95% of affected children present in the 3rd to 12th week of life with projectile, nonbilious vomiting.[175]

Historically, the diagnosis of HPS relied on physical examination with palpation of the hypertrophied pylorus as an "olive"-like mass. However, given a sensitivity and specificity nearing 100%, ultrasound is now widely accepted as the first-line diagnostic test for HPS.[174,175] Ultrasound shows abnormal persistent thickening of the hypoechoic pyloric muscle; a single wall thickness >3 to 4 mm is

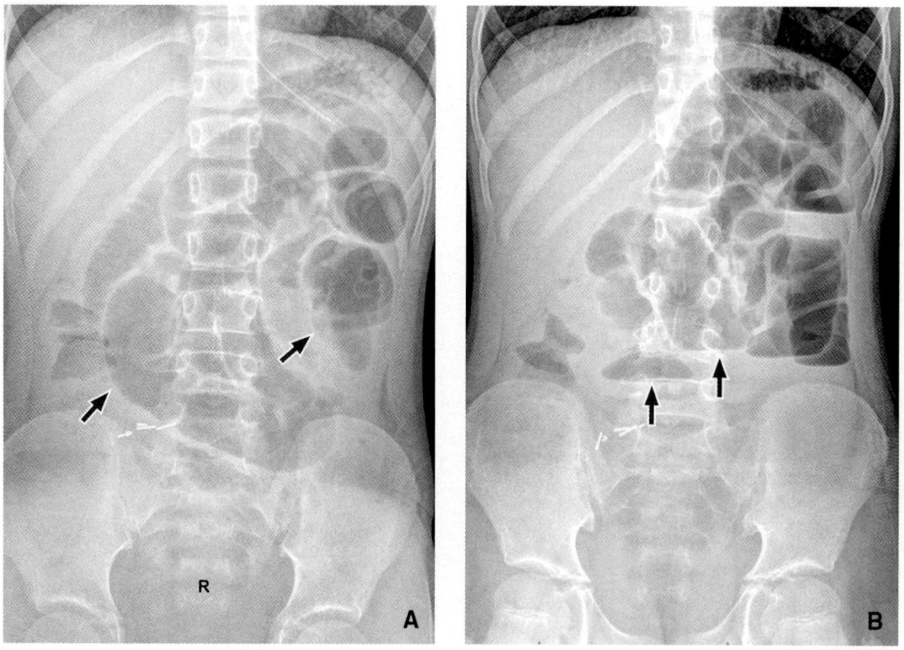

FIGURE 16.101 **A 10-year-old girl with small bowel obstruction 3 months after appendectomy.** Surgical exploration confirmed an obstructing adhesion. **A:** Supine abdominal radiograph shows multiple dilated loops of small bowel (*arrows*) and a paucity of gas within the colon and rectum (*R*). **B:** Upright abdominal radiograph shows numerous small bowel air-fluid levels (*arrows*).

abnormal. The pyloric channel is also abnormally elongated in HPS; a pyloric channel length >14 to 16 mm is abnormal (Fig. 16.102).[175] Other ultrasound findings seen in HPS include distended stomach containing fluid and debris, pyloric muscle and mucosa increased vascularity, hyperperistalsis of the stomach, and thickened mucosa that prolapses into the gastric lumen.[175]

Radiography typically shows gaseous distention of the stomach with prominent peristaltic waves ("caterpillar" sign). Upper GI series, once the mainstay for confirming this diagnosis, can show the "string" sign and "double-track" sign, which relate to one or more thin strings of contrast material coursing through the mucosal interstices of the pyloric channel. Another radiologic sign that can be seen on upper GI series is the "shoulder sign," which is due to hypertrophied pyloric muscle mass protruding into the lumen of the gastric antrum (Fig. 16.103).[174] Gastric obstruction is typically incomplete in patients with HPS as evidenced by small amounts of contrast material passing through the pyloric channel into the duodenum over time. Treatment for HPS consists of surgical pyloromyotomy, which can be performed using laparoscopic technique, and fluid and electrolyte management.[174]

Pylorospasm is an important differential consideration in infants presenting with vomiting. Although pyloric muscle appears persistently thickened and pyloric channel appears persistently elongated in HPS, pylorospasm is intermittent with a more normal appearing pylorus being seen on occasion. A few infants with pylorospasm may go on to develop HPS.[177]

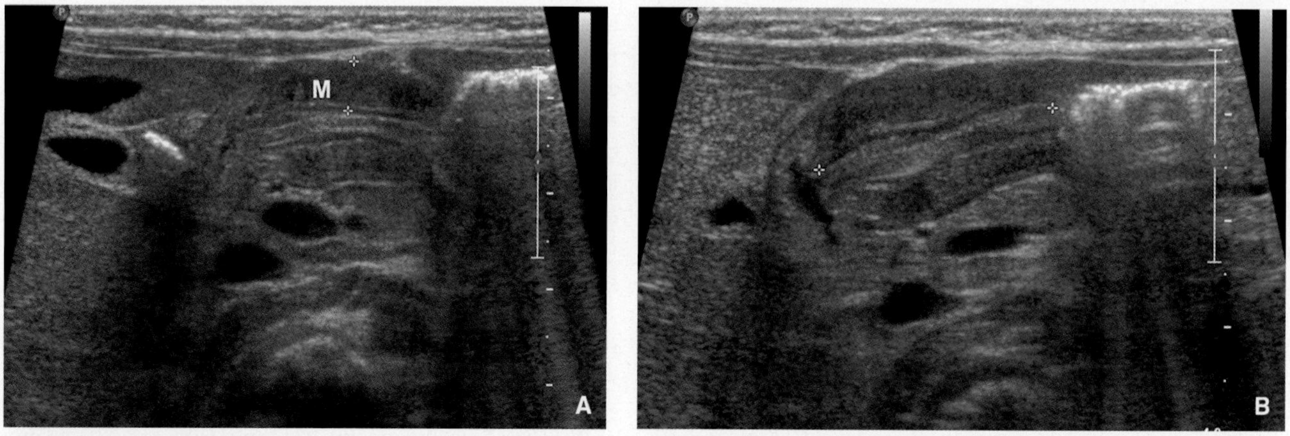

FIGURE 16.102 **A 8-week-old infant boy with vomiting due to hypertrophic pyloric stenosis (HPS). A:** Gray-scale ultrasound image of the pylorus shows abnormally thickened muscularis propria (*M*), measuring 5 mm between the calipers. **B:** Another gray-scale ultrasound image shows abnormal pyloric channel elongation (depicted between the calipers), measuring 23 mm in length.

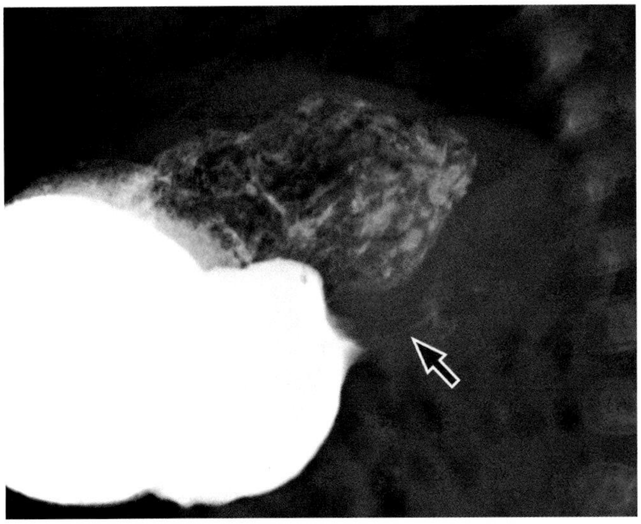

FIGURE 16.103 **A 4-week-old infant boy with vomiting due to hypertrophic pyloric stenosis (HPS).** Upper GI series oblique image shows thin linear tracks (*arrow*) of barium in the pyloric channel, compatible with double-track sign because of redundant mucosa. The pyloric channel never opened during the entire examination.

Bezoars

Bezoars are mass-like foreign bodies in the stomach or other portions of the GI tract that are made of indigestible material and that can increase in size over time.[178] There are many types of bezoar, with the four most common being phytobezoar (the most commonly encountered, and composed of indigestible portions of fruits and vegetables), trichobezoar (composed of hair) (Fig. 16.104), lactobezoar (composed of undigested milk, typically in preterm neonates), and pharmacobezoar (conglomeration of medications or medication vehicles).[178] Predisposing factors for bezoar formation include prior GI tract surgery, poor bowel motility/gastric emptying, cystic fibrosis, intrahepatic cholestasis, and renal failure.[178] Trichobezoar is associated with psychiatric disorders, such as trichotillomania.[179] In this condition, ingested hairs become trapped in gastric folds, resist peristalsis, and then food particles can get stuck within these fibers. "Rapunzel syndrome" is diagnosed when a trichobezoar in the stomach extends into the small bowel; there are case reports of colon extension (Fig. 16.105).[179]

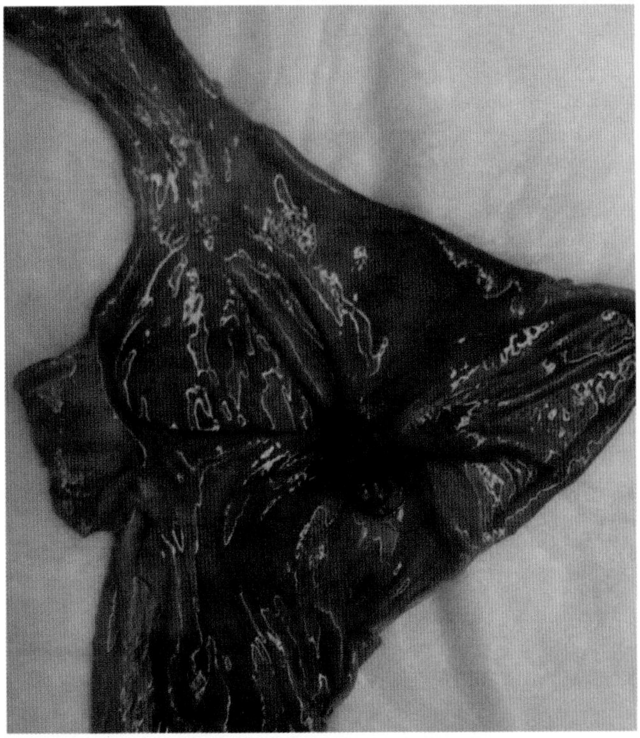

FIGURE 16.104 **Bezoar.** Trichobezoar, entangled within duodenal synechiae in a 6-year-old girl with trisomy 21 and a history of duodenal atresia repaired at birth.

Bezoars can be diagnosed using a variety of imaging modalities. Fluoroscopic studies show bezoars as apparent masses, or filling defects, within the GI tract. CT allows direct visualization of the bezoar that is often surrounded by oral contrast material and can assess for complications, such as bowel or common bile duct obstruction. Trichobezoars commonly demonstrate mixed attenuation with a layered (concentric ring) appearance and may contain gas (Fig. 16.105).

Bezoars typically require endoscopic or surgical removal. Dietary modification, enzymatic therapy, and gastric lavage are other treatment options.[178,179] Any underlying psychiatric issue also should be addressed in order to prevent future recurrent event.

Intussusception

Intussusception refers to one portion of bowel invaginating or "telescoping" into an adjacent portion. The proximal bowel that invaginates into the distal bowel is called the intussusceptum, whereas the distal bowel that receives the more proximal bowel is called the intussuscipiens. Intussusception is the most common cause of small bowel obstruction in children.[180] The classic pediatric intussusception is that of invagination of the terminal ileum into the colon (ileocolic intussusception), although intussusceptions can occur from the duodenum through the colon. The majority of ileocolic intussusceptions are idiopathic, probably related to hypertrophied lymphoid tissue in the wall of the terminal ileum (Peyer patches) or mesenteric lymphadenopathy and recent viral infection.[180,181] Ileocolic intussusception most commonly occurs in infants and toddlers, with an age range of 2 months to 3 years and a peak incidence between 5 and 9 months of age.[181] Intussusceptions can also be caused by a pathologic lead point, such as Meckel diverticulum, intestinal polyp, duplication cyst, and lymphoma.[181] The likelihood of a pathologic lead point increases with age, especially over the age of 5 years.[181]

Children with symptomatic ileocolic intussusceptions may present with the triad of abdominal pain, red currant jelly stool, and palpable abdominal mass. However, this triad is present in <50% of children, with most presenting with nonspecific abdominal signs and symptoms.[182] Intussusception also can present with bowel obstruction or less often peritonitis due to intestinal ischemia/necrosis and perforation.

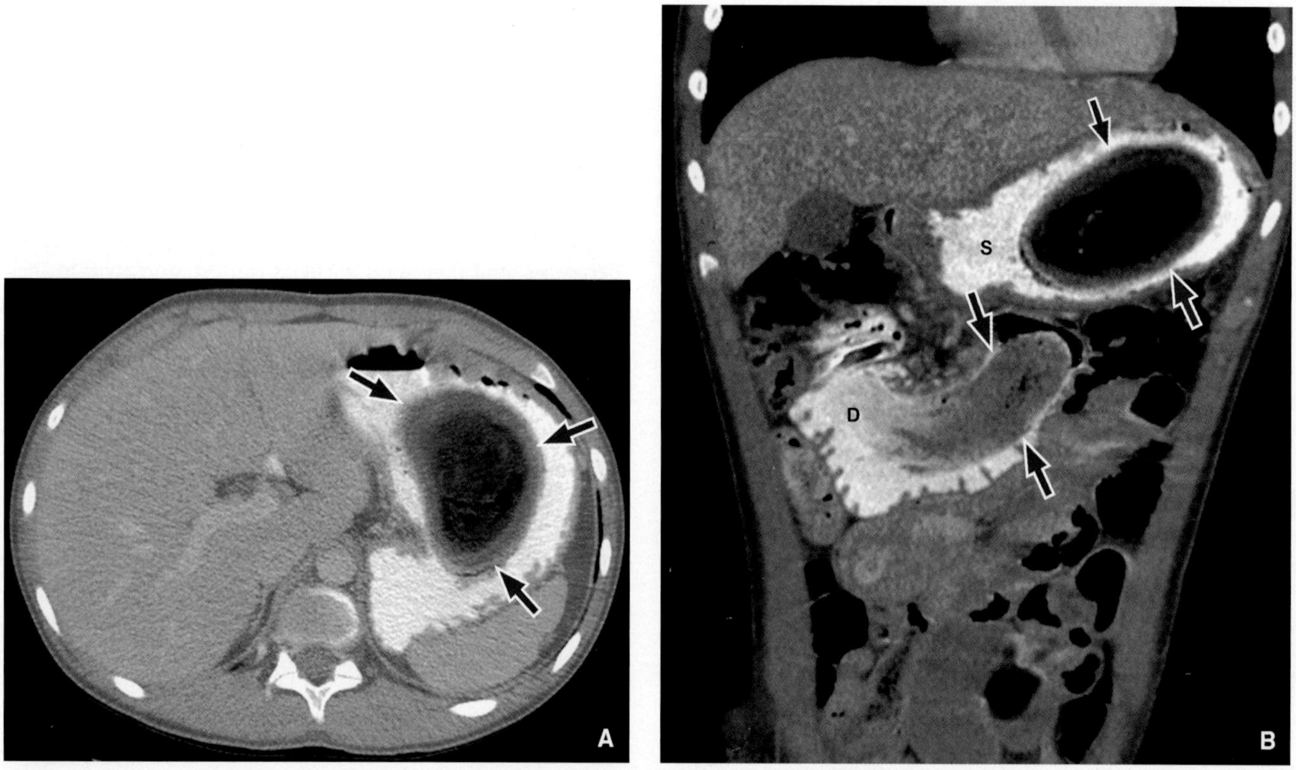

FIGURE 16.105 **A 15-year-old girl with trichobezoar. A:** Axial contrast-enhanced CT image demonstrates a large mass-like structure (*arrows*) in the stomach with a layered appearance, consistent with a trichobezoar. **B:** Coronal reformatted contrast-enhanced CT image confirms that the trichobezoar (*arrows*) in the stomach (*S*) extends into the duodenum (*D*).

Small bowel–small bowel intussusceptions represent 17% of pediatric intussusceptions,[183] and they tend to be transient (spontaneously resolving) and of no clinical significance. This type of intussusception is commonly incidentally noted on cross-sectional imaging,[183,184] appearing round and small (diameter <2 cm) (Fig. 16.106).[184] Multiple small bowel–small bowel intussusceptions can suggest an underlying predisposing condition, such as HSP or celiac disease, which should be further investigated. Persistent, long small bowel–small bowel intussusceptions are more likely to be associated with a lead point, such as a polyp, Meckel diverticulum, or indwelling tube.[184] Small bowel–small bowel intussusception length >3.5 cm is a predictor of need for surgery.[183]

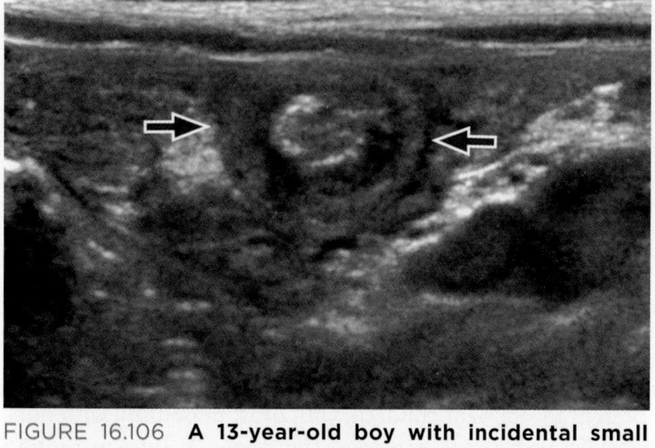

FIGURE 16.106 **A 13-year-old boy with incidental small bowel-small bowel intussusception.** Gray-scale ultrasound image shows a small, round intussusception (*arrows*) in the left upper quadrant that resolved during the imaging examination.

Abdominal radiography generally has a low sensitivity for detecting ileocolic intussusceptions. The presence of a curvilinear soft tissue mass that is partly surrounded by bowel gas along the expected course of the colon ("crescent" sign) is highly specific for ileocolic intussusception (Fig. 16.107).[180] Radiography can also reveal intussusception-related complications, such as small bowel obstruction and perforation. The accuracy of ultrasound for detecting clinically relevant intussusceptions approaches 100% based on the literature.[180,182,185] Ileocolic intussusceptions typically appear as a 3- to 5-cm mass-like abnormality along the expected course of the colon that has a characteristic doughnut, target-like, or "pseudokidney" appearance; these appearances being due to two concentric layers of bowel and intervening mesentery (Fig. 16.107).[182] Ultrasound also plays a role in assessing the potential reducibility of ileocolic intussusceptions by enema and detecting the presence of a pathologic lead point. Findings that suggest decreased likelihood of successful enema reduction include substantial amount of fluid trapped between the intussusception layers and lack of color Doppler blood flow in involved bowel wall.[180] CT is generally not used to diagnose ileocolic intussusception, although this modality commonly detects transient enteroenteric intussusceptions as well as other small bowel intussusceptions that are due to a lead point (e.g., a polyp).

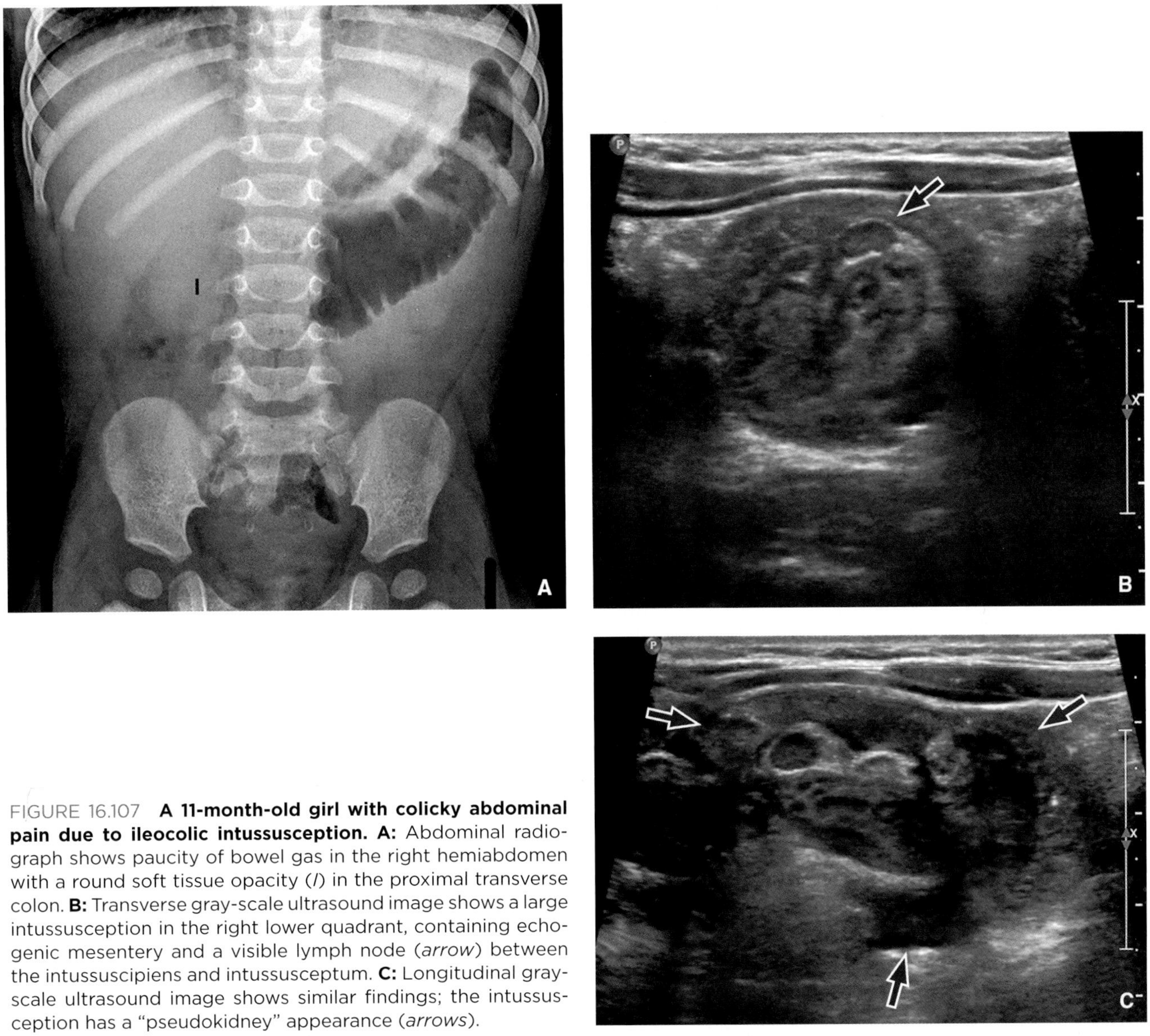

FIGURE 16.107 **A 11-month-old girl with colicky abdominal pain due to ileocolic intussusception. A:** Abdominal radiograph shows paucity of bowel gas in the right hemiabdomen with a round soft tissue opacity (*I*) in the proximal transverse colon. **B:** Transverse gray-scale ultrasound image shows a large intussusception in the right lower quadrant, containing echogenic mesentery and a visible lymph node (*arrow*) between the intussuscipiens and intussusceptum. **C:** Longitudinal gray-scale ultrasound image shows similar findings; the intussusception has a "pseudokidney" appearance (*arrows*).

Fluoroscopically guided enema is the preferred initial treatment for ileocolic intussusceptions. Children with evidence of peritonitis, shock, sepsis, or intraperitoneal free air are not candidates for enema reduction.[180,186] Surgical consultation should occur prior to attempted enema reduction to assess for peritoneal signs on physical examination, and it is preferable to have a surgeon present during the reduction attempt, if possible. A peripheral IV catheter is also a common requirement prior to reduction.[180,186] Both water-soluble iodinated contrast material (hydrostatic) and air (pneumatic) can be used to perform the reduction enema. Advantages of the air enema include a cleaner procedure, potentially faster procedure, potentially higher rate of reduction, and less peritoneal contamination with fecal debris in the case of perforation during the reduction (Fig. 16.108).[180] A primary advantage of the contrast enema is improved visualization of the intussusception when there is a large amount of overlying bowel gas (Fig. 16.109). Perforation rates and rates of intussusception recurrence do not differ substantially between the two techniques, with a mean reported perforation rate of 0.8%.[180,186] Tension pneumoperitoneum is one complication uniquely related to perforation during air reduction[187,188] Air enema intussusception reduction technique is outlined in Table 16.2. Contrast enema technique uses gravity to apply hydrostatic pressure on the intussusception. The "rules of 3" for this technique include three attempts of 3 minutes each and placing the enema bag 3 feet above the table (even though there is no substantial evidence to support these "rules").[180,186] Delayed, repeated enema may be considered if the patient meets specific clinical criteria, and there has been partial reduction of the intussusception on the prior attempt.[180] Ultrasound-guided hydrostatic or pneumatic reduction also has been described in the literature with the clear advantage of this procedure being the lack of ionizing radiation. Reported ileocolic intussusception reduction rates using this technique are similar to fluoroscopic techniques.[186]

Recurrence of ileocolic intussusception following enema reduction occurs in about 10% of successfully reduced

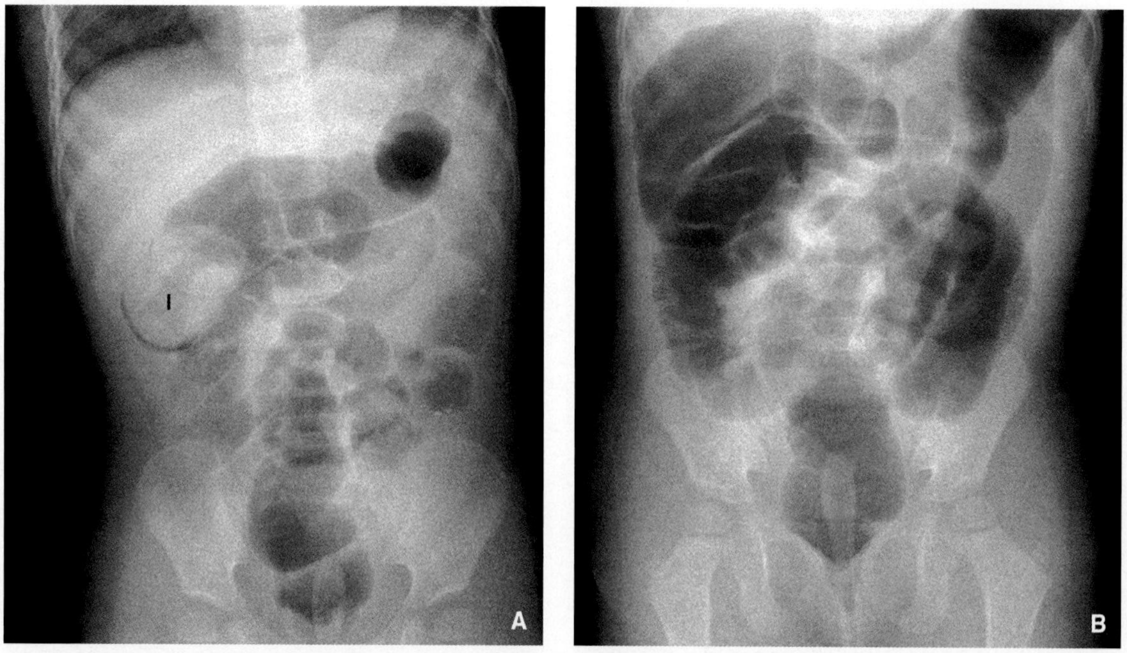

FIGURE 16.108 **An 1-year-old girl with ileocolic intussusception undergoing air (pneumatic) enema reduction. A:** Scout fluoroscopic image shows a right upper quadrant soft tissue mass–like opacity representing an intussusception (*I*) in the transverse colon. **B:** Post-reduction radiographic image shows that the intussusception is no longer visible, and air has been refluxed into distal small bowel loops.

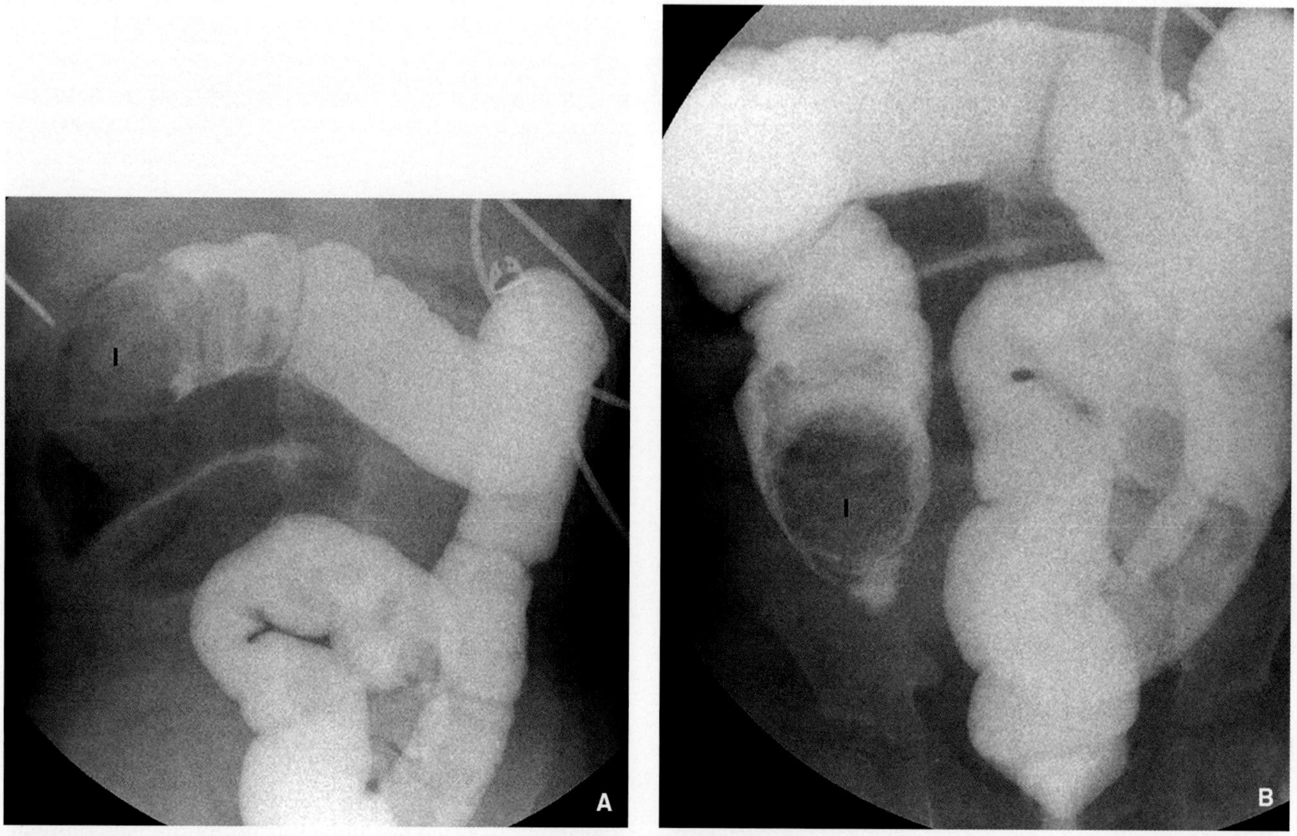

FIGURE 16.109 **A 5-year-old girl with ileocolic intussusception undergoing water-soluble contrast (hydrostatic) enema. A:** Early fluoroscopic image shows the intussusception (*I*) as a filling defect in the proximal transverse colon. **B:** Later fluoroscopic image shows partial reduction of the intussusception (*I*), which is now located in the ascending colon.

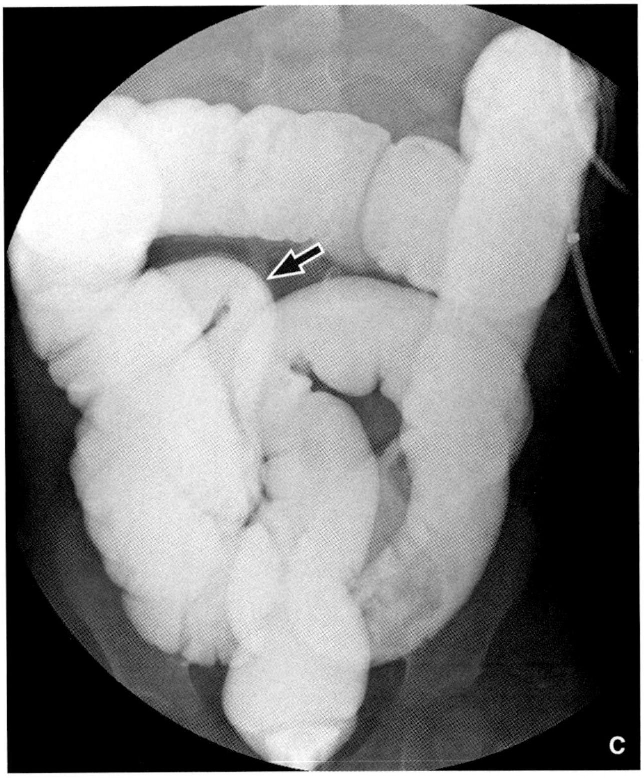

FIGURE 16.109 *(Continued)* **C:** Final fluoroscopic image shows that the filling defect is no longer evident because of complete reduction; contrast material refluxed freely into the distal small bowel (*arrow*).

cases. In these cases, repeated enema reduction is safe and effective as long as the patient remains clinically stable.[186] If the intussusception recurs multiple times, some thought should be given to the possibility of a pathologic lead point. Surgery is reserved for those cases that cannot be reduced by fluoroscopic enema, clinically unstable patients, and when a lead point is identified by imaging.

TABLE 16.2 Step-by-Step Air Enema Procedure for Reduction of Ileocolic Intussusception

1. Insert enema tip (or large Foley catheter [e.g., 22–24 French]) into the child's rectum. Abundant perianal/gluteal tape (or purpose-built device) should be used to ensure air lock/tight seal. Placing the child prone allows one to manually squeeze the buttocks and improve seal.
2. Insufflate air under fluoroscopic observation until intussusception is encountered. Continue air insufflation in order to achieve intussusception reduction. Do not exceed 120 mm Hg mean pressure to minimize risk of bowel perforation.
3. Disappearance of filling defect within the colon caused by intussusceptum and retrograde filling of small bowel with air indicate successful reduction.

Note: An 18-gauge angiocatheter should be present in the procedure room in order to treat tension pneumoperitoneum should bowel perforation occur.

Volvulus

Colonic volvulus, unlike midgut volvulus, is less common in children than adults, and the most common sites are the sigmoid colon and cecum. Etiologies for colonic volvulus include redundancy of the colon, chronic constipation, absent ligamentous attachments, malfixated mesentery, and prior abdominal surgery.[189] Practically speaking, colonic volvulus is commonly seen in severely chronically constipated children with neurologic impairment.[190] Affected children present with signs and symptoms of a bowel obstruction.

Abdominal radiography typically shows marked dilatation of the affected colonic segment, possibly with air–fluid levels (Fig. 16.110). Contrast enema classically demonstrates the "bird's beak" sign where the two loops of bowel meet at the point of torsion[190] (Fig. 16.110). CT generally is not required to make the diagnosis, but when performed can accurately confirm the level of bowel obstruction as well as identify intraperitoneal free air and evidence if ischemia, such as bowel wall thickening.

Treatment options include colonoscopic reduction or surgical reduction with resection of ischemic or redundant bowel.

Hernias

Hernias occur when there is protrusion of abdominal contents through sites of congenital or acquired defects/weakness in the abdominal wall (external) or within the peritoneal cavity (internal).[191,192] There are numerous types of hernias that occur in children. Although many hernias are asymptomatic, others may present with intestinal obstruction or ischemia/infarction. Incarcerated hernias are those that cannot be reduced.[191,193] Strangulation refers to ischemia secondary to impaired blood supply.[193] This section focuses on two common types of hernias that occur in children: indirect inguinal hernias and umbilical hernias (Table 16.3).

Indirect inguinal hernias occur in 4% of infants, and incarcerated inguinal hernia is a common cause of bowel obstruction in children.[191,193] Indirect inguinal hernias develops when the processus vaginalis fails to undergo normal closure, allowing abdominal contents to enter the inguinal canal.[193] The processus vaginalis is often at least partly open in newborns and continues to close postnatally, which explains the increased incidence in premature infants.[194] This type of hernia is much more common in boys and right-sided hernias predominate. Infants weighing <1,000 g also have a particularly increased incidence of inguinal hernias, and there is an increased rate of incarceration in premature infants.[191,194]

Technically, all newborns have a defect in the umbilicus at birth through which the umbilical vessels pass and this defect usually closes spontaneously.[191,194] Umbilical hernias are four times more likely in infants weighing <1,200 g and 6 to 10 times more likely in African American infants.[191] Incarceration and strangulation are infrequent complications of umbilical hernias, because most remain asymptomatic.

At radiography, obstructed hernias may demonstrate proximally dilated bowel loops and with air–fluid levels. Soft

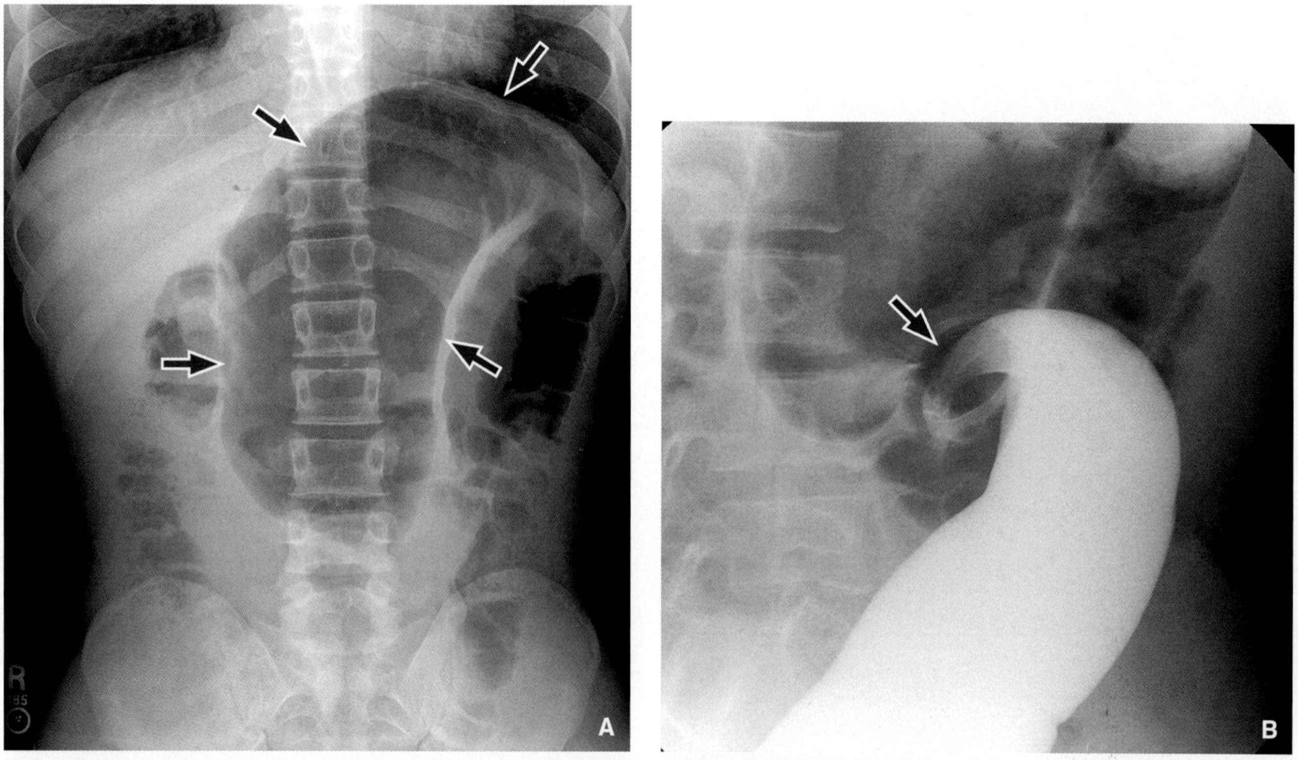

FIGURE 16.110 **A 17-year-old girl with abdominal pain due to sigmoid volvulus. A:** Abdominal radiograph shows a markedly distended sigmoid colon (*arrows*), which extends well above the transverse colon. **B:** Water soluble contrast enema shows obstructed, "beaked" appearance of the sigmoid colon (*arrow*), compatible with sigmoid volvulus.

tissue opacity or gas-filled bowel may be seen in the area of the hernia (Fig. 16.111). Cross-table lateral imaging is helpful for evaluating umbilical hernias. Ultrasound excellently depicts both inguinal and umbilical hernias (Figs. 16.111 and 16.112). CT and MRI also can show these hernias, but are not usually indicated. Incarceration is usually a clinical diagnosis, although imaging can suggest this possibility when the hernia has a very narrow neck.[193] Incarceration also should be suspected when there is free fluid in the hernia sac, fluid in the herniated bowel, and evidence of obstruction.[195] Signs of strangulation include bowel wall thickening, abnormal bowel wall hypo- or hyperenhancement, engorgement of the vasa recta, ascites, and mesenteric fat stranding.[193] Testicular assessment is important for male patients with inguinal hernia

TABLE 16.3 Types of Abdominal Hernias Seen in Children

Hernia Type	Contents
Indirect	Hernia into open deep inguinal ring, through patent processus vaginalis, and exiting superficial inguinal ring
Direct	Hernia through wall of inguinal canal, secondary to weak musculature, and exiting superficial inguinal ring
Umbilical	Hernia through open umbilical ring
Femoral	Hernia through femoral ring
Spigelian	Hernia defect lateral to rectus muscle and medial to semilunar line
Incisional/ventral	Hernia through an abdominal wall defect caused by a surgical incision
Parastomal	Subtype of incisional hernia that occurs adjacent to a stoma
Littre	Hernia containing a Meckel diverticulum
Amyand	Inguinal hernia containing appendix
Richter	Hernia containing only one wall of involved bowel loop
Internal	Protrusion of viscera through a normal or an abnormal aperture within the peritoneal cavity

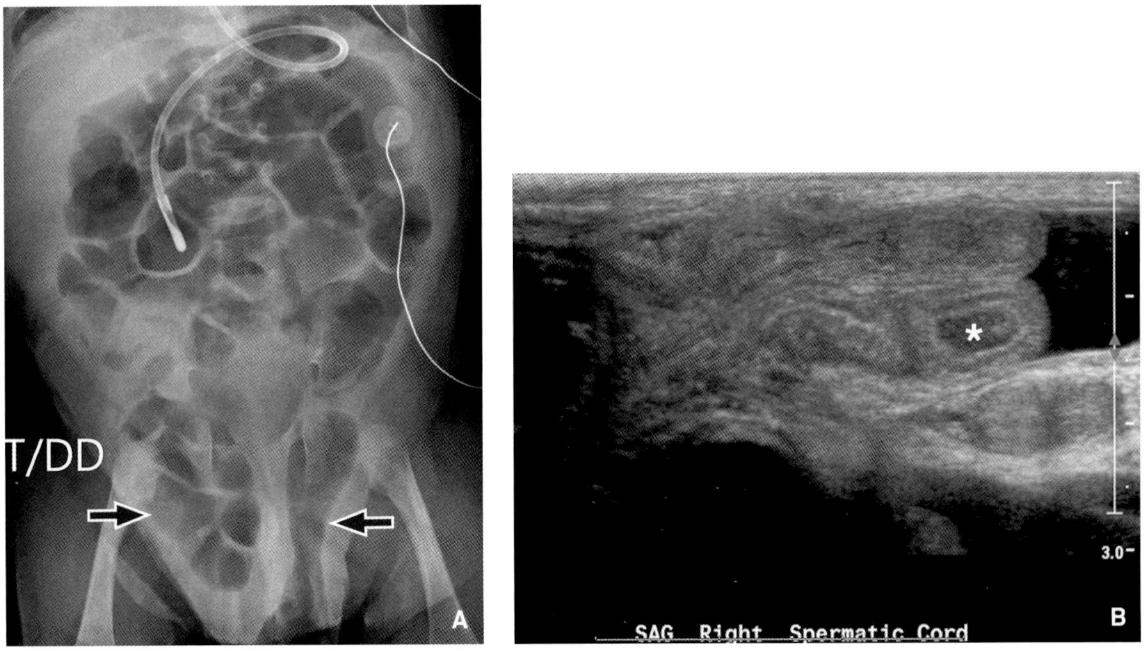

FIGURE 16.111 **A 1-month-old infant boy with bilateral inguinal hernias. A:** Abdominal radiograph shows gas-filled bowel loops (*arrows*) projecting over the bilateral inguinal canals and scrotum. **B:** Longitudinal gray-scale ultrasound image of the right groin shows multiple small bowel loops (*asterisk*) and fluid in the right inguinal canal.

because of the risk of ischemia in the setting of incarcerated hernia. Ultrasound may show asymmetrically decreased flow to the testicle on the side of hernia with or without changes in echogenicity and echotexture.[196]

Treatment of incarcerated or strangulated hernias is surgical resection and/or repair.

Superior Mesenteric Artery Syndrome

SMA syndrome is diagnosed when there is obstruction of the third portion of the duodenum as it crosses midline between the abdominal aorta and SMA secondary to abnormally decreased aortomesenteric angle (angle between the abdominal aorta and SMA).[197] This uncommon disorder is most often seen in females between the ages of 10 and 39 years.[197] SMA syndrome can be associated with severe weight loss, depletion of retroperitoneal fat, anatomic abnormalities (high insertion of the ligament of Treitz or low origin of the SMA), and neurologic conditions, such as cerebral palsy.[197–199] SMA syndrome can also be associated with corrective spinal surgery in the setting of scoliosis; it is thought that the relative lengthening of the spine places traction on the SMA.[199] Children with this condition often have delays in diagnosis, and may present with nonspecific abdominal symptoms, such as postprandial abdominal pain, vomiting, nausea, and anorexia. As the obstruction is generally partial, it can sometimes be relieved by lying prone or in the left lateral decubitus position.[197]

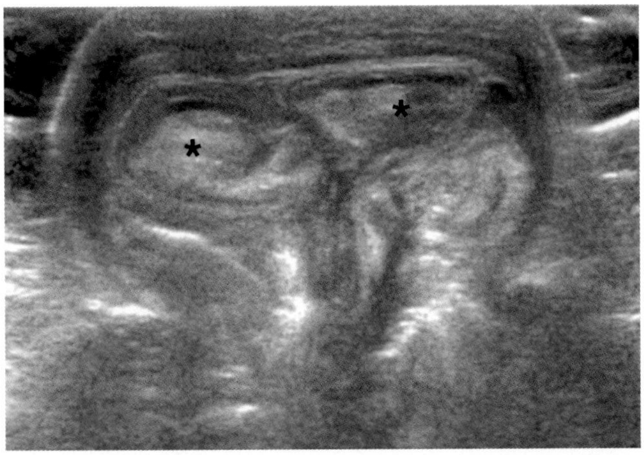

FIGURE 16.112 **A 1-month-old boy with umbilical hernia.** Gray-scale ultrasound image scanning over the umbilicus shows small bowel loops (*asterisks*) protruding through an anterior abdominal wall defect at the level of the umbilicus.

Upper GI series is most often performed when SMA syndrome is suspected. Suspicious findings include delayed passage of contrast material through the third portion of the duodenum, more proximal duodenal dilatation, and normal caliber proximal jejunum. A discrete linear cut-off of the contrast column in the duodenum is often seen at the expected level of the SMA (Fig. 16.113). Imaging in the left lateral decubitus may aid passage of contrast material through the third portion of the duodenum.[198] Ultrasound and CT can aid in diagnosis by allowing measurement of the aortomesenteric angle as well as the distance between the abdominal aorta and SMA (Fig. 16.113). The normal aortomesenteric angle is 25 to 60 degrees, and the mean distance between the SMA and abdominal aorta is 10 to 28 mm. Children with SMA syndrome have abnormally decreased aortomesenteric angles and SMA–abdominal aorta distances.[198,200] One study has shown 100% specificity and sensitivity for the diagnosis of SMA syndrome if a cut-off value of 8 mm is used for the SMA–abdominal aorta distance.[198] Marked dilatation of the proximal duodenum and stomach may also be seen by ultrasound and CT.

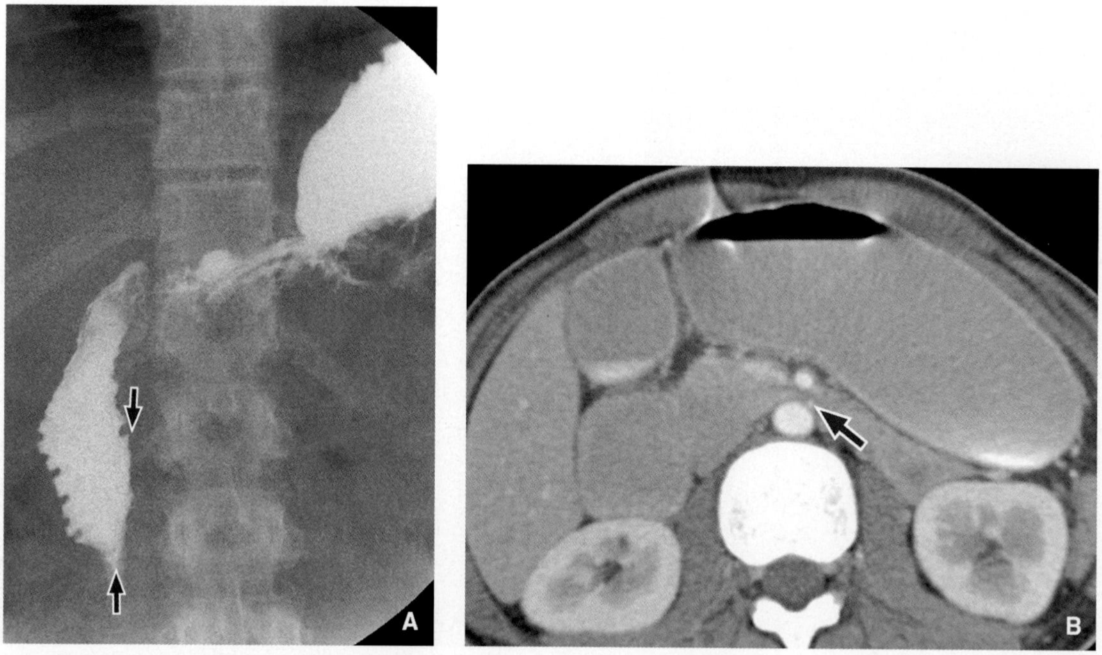

FIGURE 16.113 **Superior mesenteric artery syndrome in two different adolescent girls presenting with vomiting and weight loss. A:** Upper GI series image shows a contrast-opacified proximal duodenum with abrupt linear cutoff/obstruction (*arrows*) at the expected level of the superior mesenteric artery syndrome. There was markedly delayed passage of contrast material into more distal small bowel. **B:** Axial contrast-enhanced CT image shows marked distention of the stomach and duodenum up to the third segment, as the duodenum crosses midline. The superior mesenteric artery–aorta interval (*arrow*) measures 4 mm (anteroposterior dimension).

Initial treatment of SMA syndrome is conservative treatment with the goals of correcting electrolyte and fluid imbalances and providing nutritional support in order to promote weight gain. Nutritional support can be provided by administering tube feeds through a nasojejunal enteric tube or intravenous parenteral feeding.[197,198] Surgical treatment is reserved for refractory cases and may include mobilization of the duodenum after division of the ligament of Treitz (Strong's procedure), duodenojejunostomy, or gastrojejunostomy.[197]

Swallowing Disorders

Normal Swallowing Mechanism

Swallowing is a complex process that requires intact neuromuscular function. The swallowing process is broken down into four phases: *oral preparatory phase, oral phase, pharyngeal phase,* and *esophageal phase.*

Oral Preparatory Phase

During the oral preparatory phase, the food is tasted, chewed, and mixed with saliva to become a bolus that is to be propelled into the pharynx.[201] The tongue spreads food out to expose it to the action of grinding by the teeth. Then, the tongue elevates by the actions of the genioglossus, genohyoid, and mylohyoid muscles[201] to hold the bolus between the hard palate and tongue. This phase is most apparent after 6 to 9 months of age when solid foods are introduced to infants.[202] Prior to this age, the preparatory phase is comprised of sucking from a nipple.

Oral Phase

The oral phase involves transport of the food bolus to the oropharynx that triggers the swallow. The soft palate elevates to protect the food from entering the nasopharynx.[202]

Pharyngeal Phase

The hallmark of the pharyngeal phase is the extensive muscle action and coordination of the swallow reflex stimulated and initiated by the cranial nerves IX and X.[201] Once the swallow starts, the food bolus rapidly passes from the oropharynx, into the hypopharynx, and eventually the esophagus.[202] During this phase, the airway is protected as the palate rises, breathing is ceased, the larynx elevates, the vocal cords adduct, and the epiglottis is pushed posteriorly into a horizontal position to cover the laryngeal passage.[202] To enter the esophagus, the bolus has to pass through the relaxed cricopharyngeal muscle.[201] Newborns are unique in that their suck reflex is maintained without any interruption in breathing during this phase; sucking occurs rapidly and rhythmically as the airway is protected.

Esophageal Phase

This final swallowing phase is under the control of the autonomic nervous system. The cervical esophagus is comprised of skeletal muscle, and food passes through rapidly. The thoracic esophagus is comprised of smooth muscle, and food passes through more slowly.[201] The lower esophageal sphincter must relax to allow food to enter the stomach.

Imaging Assessment of Swallowing

The videofluoroscopic swallow study (VFSS), also known as the modified barium swallow study (MBSS), is the most common test used to assess swallowing. This imaging test is most often performed in radiology department in conjunction with a speech/swallowing therapist using different consistencies of liquid and solid food impregnated with barium. The study is customized to the age of the patient and does not assess the majority of the esophagus.

The examination, which is video recorded (on video tape or digitally), is performed under fluoroscopy with the patient usually upright in a chair. Swallowing is most often examined in the lateral projection, but also can be evaluated in the frontal projection. This examination allows evaluation of swallowing physiology and detection of abnormalities, such as laryngeal penetration or aspiration. Compensatory mechanisms used to improve swallowing can also be evaluated. Disadvantages of VFSS include its use of ionizing radiation (low-dose techniques should be used, including pulse fluoroscopy) and the fact that the test is difficult to perform unless the child is cooperative.

Swallowing Abnormalities

A problem at any of the phases of swallowing can cause dysphagia or other feeding problems in children. Overall, the incidence of feeding issues is on the rise primarily because of an increasing number of premature births and the improved care and life expectancy in these children with comorbidities, such as chronic lung disease, congenital craniofacial anomalies, and neurologic impairment. Assessment of potentially impaired swallowing includes a clinic or bedside feeding evaluation with food and a formal radiologic VFSS using different consistencies of barium. In some cases, additional evaluation with an upper GI series may be indicated, particularly if planning to place percutaneous gastrostomy or gastrojejunostomy.

Nasopharyngeal Reflux

Normally during early swallowing, the soft palate elevates to prevent food from entering the nasopharynx; failure of this mechanism results in nasopharyngeal reflux. This finding can be seen normally in premature and even in some full-term infants because of lack of neuromuscular coordination and is usually of no clinical significance. However, this condition can be symptomatic in children who have cleft palate, soft palate palsy or paralysis, undergone adenoidectomy, or a history of surgery for nasopharyngeal mass.

Penetration/Aspiration

Laryngeal penetration is defined as liquid or solid food entering the upper the larynx without extension below the level of the true vocal cords[203] (Fig. 16.114). This occurs when there is inadequate laryngeal elevation and failure of the epiglottis to tilt posteriorly during the pharyngeal phase of swallowing.[203] Penetration can occur transiently and can be easily missed. VFSS examinations allow radiologists and therapists to review the study in a frame-by-frame manner in order to capture this finding. Laryngeal penetration can be self-limiting; however, it is probable that some children with this finding actually experience aspiration.

Aspiration is defined as liquid or solid food below the level of the true vocal cords[203] (Fig. 16.114). On occasion, it is due to esophageal disorders, such as gastroesophageal reflux, achalasia, H or N-type TEF, esophageal stricture, and other causes of dysmotility. When aspiration occurs, it is important to document the phase of swallowing during which it was observed, the exact liquid or solid, and if a cough reflex is elicited by the patient.[203] Aspiration that elicits a cough means that the body is attempting to clear the material from the airway. Aspiration that does not elicit a cough ("silent aspiration") is worrisome because it can go unnoticed and cause substantial morbidity, such as repeated pneumonia and pulmonary complications such as bronchiectasis.

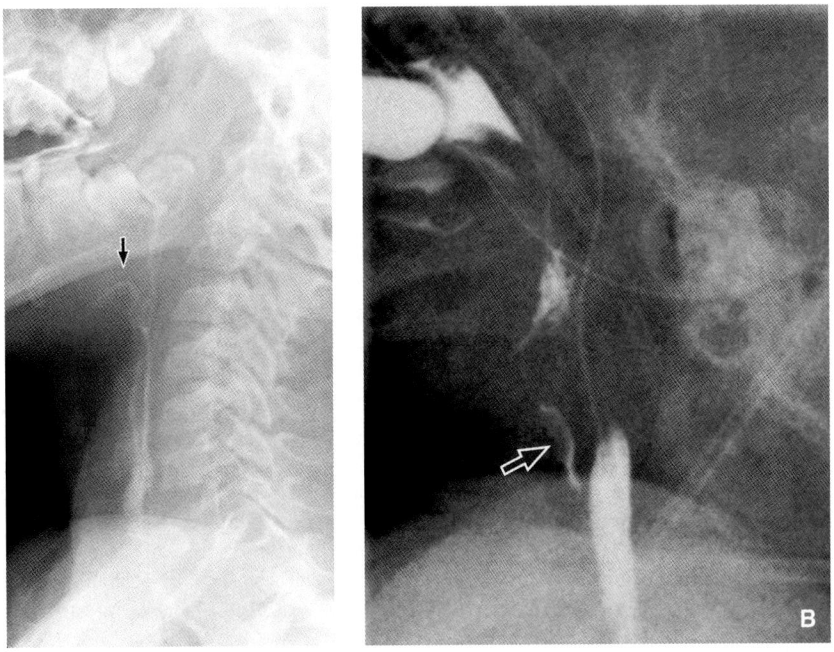

FIGURE 16.114 **Two different pediatric patients with abnormal swallowing studies. A:** An 11-year old boy shows deep penetration (*arrow*) during swallowing as the contrast material extends to the supraglottic larynx. **B:** A 2-month-old boy with left vocal cord paralysis shows contrast material (*arrow*) in the trachea below the level of the vocal cords.

Both penetration and aspiration can be treated by changing the patient's position during swallowing, changing the viscosity or texture of feeds, changing nipple flow rate, and altering the duration/quantity of feeds.[202] These therapies improve the safety of feeding by lowering the risk of aspiration and related pulmonary complications.

References

1. Fefferman NR, et al. The efficacy of digital fluoroscopic image capture in the evaluation of vesicoureteral reflux in children. *Pediatr Radiol.* 2009;39(11):1179–1187.
2. Butterworth SA, Webber EM, Jamieson DH. H-type tracheoesophageal fistula. *J Pediatr Surg.* 2001;36(6):958–959.
3. Anupindi S, et al. Low-dose CT colonography in children: initial experience, technical feasibility, and utility. *Pediatr Radiol.* 2005;35(5):518–524.
4. Schmit P, Rohrschneider WK, Christmann D. Intestinal intussusception survey about diagnostic and nonsurgical therapeutic procedures. *Pediatr Radiol.* 1999;29(10):752–761.
5. Anupindi SA, et al. Common and uncommon applications of bowel ultrasound with pathologic correlation in children. *AJR Am J Roentgenol.* 2014;202(5):946–959.
6. Alison M, et al. Ultrasonography of Crohn disease in children. *Pediatr Radiol.* 2007;37(11):1071–1082.
7. Darge K, et al. Ultrasound of the bowel in children: how we do it. *Pediatr Radiol.* 2010;40(4):528–536.
8. Jeckovic M, et al. Is ultrasound useful in detection and follow-up of gastric foreign bodies in children? *Clin Imaging.* 2013;37(6):1043–1047.
9. Darge K, et al. Safety of contrast-enhanced ultrasound in children for non-cardiac applications: a review by the Society for Pediatric Radiology (SPR) and the International Contrast Ultrasound Society (ICUS). *Pediatr Radiol.* 2013;43(9):1063–1073.
10. Towbin AJ, et al. CT and MR enterography in children and adolescents with inflammatory bowel disease. *Radiographics.* 2013;33(7):1843–1860.
11. Dillman JR, et al. CT enterography of pediatric Crohn disease. *Pediatr Radiol.* 2010;40(1):97–105.
12. Smith EA, et al. Model-based iterative reconstruction: effect on patient radiation dose and image quality in pediatric body CT. *Radiology.* 2014;270(2):526–534.
13. Anupindi SA, Terreblanche O, Courtier J. Magnetic resonance enterography: inflammatory bowel disease and beyond. *Magn Reson Imaging Clin N Am.* 2013;21(4):731–750.
14. Chavhan GB, Babyn PS, Vasanawala SS. Abdominal MR imaging in children: motion compensation, sequence optimization, and protocol organization. *Radiographics.* 2013;33(3): 703–719.
15. Dillman JR, et al. IV glucagon use in pediatric MR enterography: effect on image quality, length of examination, and patient tolerance. *AJR Am J Roentgenol.* 2013;201(1):185–189.
16. Moore M, et al. MRI for clinically suspected pediatric appendicitis: an implemented program. *Pediatr Radiol.* 2012;42(9):1056–1063.
17. Drubach LA, et al. Utility of salivagram in pulmonary aspiration in pediatric patients: comparison of salivagram and chest radiography. *AJR Am J Roentgenol.* 2013;200(2):437–441.
18. Blumhagen JD, Rudd TG, Christie DL. Gastroesophageal reflux in children: radionuclide gastroesophagography. *AJR Am J Roentgenol.* 1980;135(5):1001–1004.
19. Coley BD. Congenital and neonatal disorders. In: Seekins JM, et al., eds. *Caffey's Pediatric Diagnostic Imaging.* Philadelphia, PA: Elsevier; 2013:1004–1013, 1032–1038, 1057–1080, 1107–1121.
20. Heyman S. Gastric emptying in children. *J Nucl Med.* 1998;39(5):865–869.
21. Kotecha M, et al. Multimodality imaging manifestations of the Meckel diverticulum in children. *Pediatr Radiol.* 2012; 42(1):95–103.
22. Kaiser AM, Ortega AE. Anorectal anatomy. *Surg Clin North Am.* 2002;82(6):1125–1138, v.
23. Gordon PH. Anorectal anatomy and physiology. *Gastroenterol Clin North Am.* 2001;30(1):1–13.
24. Coran A, Adzick NEA. *Pediatric Surgery.* 7th ed. Philadelphia, PA: Elsevier; 2012.
25. Konkin DE, et al. Outcomes in esophageal atresia and tracheoesophageal fistula. *J Pediatr Surg.* 2003;38(12):1726–1729.
26. Patterson A. *Pearson's Thoracic and Esophageal Surgery.* 3rd ed. London, England: Churchill Livinigstone; 2008.
27. Berrocal T, et al. Congenital anomalies of the upper gastrointestinal tract. *Radiographics.* 1999;19(4):855–872.
28. Macpherson RI. Gastrointestinal tract duplications: clinical, pathologic, etiologic, and radiologic considerations. *Radiographics.* 1993;13(5):1063–1080.
29. Singh JP, et al. Gastric duplication cyst: two case reports and review of the literature. *Case Rep Surgery.* 2013;2013:605059.
30. Park WH, Choi SO, Suh SJ. Pediatric gastric volvulus: experience with 7 cases. *J Korean Med Sci.* 1992;7(3):258–263.
31. Abbara S, Kalan MM, Lewicki AM. Intrathoracic stomach revisited. *AJR Am J Roentgenol.* 2003;181(2):403–414.
32. Karpelowsky JS, Wieselthaler N, Rode H. Primary paraesophageal hernia in children. *J Pediatr Surg.* 2006;41(9):1588–1593.
33. Raeside MC, et al. Post-fundoplication contrast studies: is there room for improvement? *Br J Radiol.* 2012;85(1014):792–799.
34. Vinocur DN, Lee EY, Eisenberg RL. Neonatal intestinal obstruction. *AJR Am J Roentgenol.* 2012;198(1):W1–W10.
35. Cole C, et al. Hereditary multiple intestinal atresias: 2 new cases and review of the literature. *J Pediatr Surg.* 2010. 45(4): E21–E24.
36. Applegate K. Evidence-based diagnosis of malrotation and volvulus. *Pediatr Radiol.* 2009;39(2):161–163.
37. Yousefzadeh D. The position of the duodenojejunal junction: the wrong horse to bet on in diagnosing or excluding malrotation. *Pediatr Radiol.* 2009;39(2):172–177.
38. Hussain SM, et al. Plain film diagnosis in meconium plug syndrome, meconium ileus and neonatal Hirschsprung's disease. A scoring system. *Pediatr Radiol.* 1991;21(8):556–559.
39. Kao SC, Franken EA Jr. Nonoperative treatment of simple meconium ileus: a survey of the Society for Pediatric Radiology. *Pediatr Radiol.* 1995;25(2):97–100.
40. Vignes S, Bellanger J. Primary intestinal lymphangiectasia (Waldmann's disease). *Orphanet J Rare Dis.* 2008;3:5.
41. Yang DM, Jung DH. Localized intestinal lymphangiectasia: CT findings. *AJR Am J Roentgenol.* 2003;180(1):213–214.
42. Pasto ME, et al. Neonatal colonic atresia: ultrasound findings. *Pediatr Radiol.* 1984;14(5):346–348.
43. Domajnko B, Salloum RM. Duplication cyst of the sigmoid colon. *Gastroenterol Res Pract.* 2009;2009:918401.
44. Keckler SJ, et al. Current significance of meconium plug syndrome. *J Pediatr Surg.* 2008;43(5):896–898.
45. Ballisty M, et al. Imaging findings in megacystis-microcolon-intestinal hypoperistalsis syndrome. *Pediatr Radiol.* 2013; 43(4):454–459.

46. Berdon WE, et al. Megacystis-microcolon-intestinal hypoperistalsis syndrome: a new cause of intestinal obstruction in the newborn. Report of radiologic findings in five newborn girls. *AJR Am J Roentgenol.* 1976;126(5):957–964.
47. Levin T, et al. Megacystis–microcolon–intestinal hypoperistalsis and prune belly: overlapping syndromes. *Pediatr Radiol.* 2004;34(12):995–998.
48. Taccone A, et al. New concepts in preoperative imaging of anorectal malformation. New concepts in imaging of ARM. *Pediatr Radiol.* 1992;22(3):196–199.
49. Belloni E, et al. Involvement of the HLXB9 homeobox gene in Currarino syndrome. *Am J Hum Genet.* 2000;66(1):312–319.
50. Pena A, Hong A. Advances in the management of anorectal malformations. *Am J Surg.* 2000;180(5):370–376.
51. Gross GW, Wolfson PJ, Pena A. Augmented-pressure colostogram in imperforate anus with fistula. *Pediatr Radiol.* 1991;21(8):560–562.
52. Ukarapol N, et al. Cytomegalovirus-associated manifestations involving the digestive tract in children with human immunodeficiency virus infection. *J Pediatr Gastroenterol Nutr.* 2002;35(5):669–673.
53. Blitman NM, Ali M. Idiopathic giant esophageal ulcer in an HIV-positive child. *Pediatr Radiol.* 2002. 32(12):907–909.
54. Epstein DP, Locketz M. Oesophageal ulceration in HIV-infected patients. *S Afr Med J.* 2009;99(2):107–109.
55. Ramanathan J, et al. Herpes simplex virus esophagitis in the immunocompetent host: an overview. *Am J Gastroenterol.* 2000;95(9):2171–2176.
56. Kurahara K, et al. Treatment of herpes simplex esophagitis in an immunocompetent patient with intravenous acyclovir: a case report and review of the literature. *Am J Gastroenterol.* 1998;93(11):2239–2240.
57. Chiou CC, et al. Esophageal candidiasis in pediatric acquired immunodeficiency syndrome: clinical manifestations and risk factors. *Pediatr Infect Dis J.* 2000;19(8):729–734.
58. Gryboski JD. Peptic ulcer disease in children. *Pediatr Rev.* 1990;12(1):15–21.
59. Wallis-Crespo MC, Crespo A. Helicobacter pylori infection in pediatric population: epidemiology, pathophysiology, and therapy. *Fetal Pediatr Pathol.* 2004;23(1):11–28.
60. Wolfe MM, Soll AH. The physiology of gastric acid secretion. *N Engl J Med.* 1988;319(26):1707–1715.
61. Goodgame R. Norovirus gastroenteritis. *Curr Gastroenterol Rep.* 2006;8(5):401–408.
62. Dennehy PH. Acute diarrheal disease in children: epidemiology, prevention, and treatment. *Infect Dis Clin North Am.* 2005;19(3): 585–602.
63. Miller TL, et al. Gastrointestinal and nutritional complications of human immunodeficiency virus infection. *J Pediatr Gastroenterol Nutr.* 2008;47(2):247–253.
64. Ebama N, Wehbeh W, Rubin D. HIV Enteropathy: case report and review of advances in pathogenesis, diagnosis, and treatments. *Infect Dis Clin Pract.* 2010;18(5):293–295.
65. Bollinger RR, et al. Biofilms in the normal human large bowel: fact rather than fiction. *Gut.* 2007;56(10):1481–1482.
66. Loughran CF, Tappin JA, Whitehouse GH. The plain abdominal radiograph in pseudomembranous colitis due to Clostridium difficile. *Clin Radiol.* 1982;33(3):277–281.
67. Tajiri H, et al. Abnormal computed tomography findings among children with viral gastroenteritis and symptoms mimicking acute appendicitis. *Pediatr Emerg Care.* 2008;24(9):601–604.
68. Sanai FM, Bzeizi KI. Systematic review: tuberculous peritonitis—presenting features, diagnostic strategies and treatment. *Aliment Pharmacol Ther.* 2005;22(8):685–700.
69. Pereira JM, et al. Abdominal tuberculosis: imaging features. *Eur J Radiol.* 2005;55(2):173–180.
70. Cruz AT, Starke JR. Clinical manifestations of tuberculosis in children. *Paediatr Respir Rev.* 2007;8(2):107–117.
71. Abramson SJ, Berdon WE, Baker DH. Childhood typhlitis: its increasing association with acute myelogenous leukemia. Report of five cases. *Radiology.* 1983;146(1):61–64.
72. Chan MS. The global burden of intestinal nematode infections—fifty years on. *Parasitol Today.* 1997;13(11):438–443.
73. Levine MS, Rubesin SE, Laufer I. Pattern approach for diseases of mesenteric small bowel on barium studies. *Radiology.* 2008;249(2):445–460.
74. Louis CL, Barton CJ. The radiological diagnosis of Strongyloides stercoralis enteritis. *Radiology.* 1971;98(3):535–541.
75. Reeder MM. Radiological diagnosis of giardiasis. *Semin Roentgenol.* 1997;32(4):291–300.
76. Huang DB, Chappell C, Okhuysen PC. Cryptosporidiosis in children. *Semin Pediatr Infect Dis.* 2004;15(4):253–259.
77. Mahmood T, et al. Ultrasonographic appearance of Ascaris lumbricoides in the small bowel. *J Ultrasound Med.* 2001;20(3): 269–274.
78. Hobson MJ, et al. Appendicitis in childhood hematologic malignancies: analysis and comparison with typhilitis. *J Pediatr Surg.* 2005;40(1):214–220.
79. Lee J-H, et al. Gastrointestinal complications following hematopoietic stem cell transplantation in children. *Korean J Radiol.* 2008;9(5):449–457.
80. Kirkpatrick IDC, Greenberg HM. Gastrointestinal complications in the neutropenic patient: characterization and differentiation with abdominal CT. *Radiology.* 2003;226(3):668–674.
81. Tolia V. Perianal Crohn's disease in children and adolescents. *Am J Gastroenterol.* 1996;91(5):922–926.
82. Essary B, et al. Pelvic MRI in children with Crohn disease and suspected perianal involvement. *Pediatr Radiol.* 2007;37(2): 201–208.
83. Chang HK, Ryu JG, Oh JT. Clinical characteristics and treatment of perianal abscess and fistula-in-ano in infants. *J Pediatr Surg.* 2010;45(9):1832–1836.
84. Guariso G, et al. Esophageal involvement in juvenile localized scleroderma: a pilot study. *Clin Exp Rheumatol.* 2007;25(5):786–789.
85. Ortiz-Alvarez O, et al. Intestinal pseudo-obstruction as an initial presentation of systemic sclerosis in two children. *Rheumatology.* 1997;36(2):280–284.
86. Canan O, Ozcay F, Bilezikci B. Menetrier's disease and severe gastric ulcers associated with cytomegalovirus infection in an immunocompetent child: a case report. *Turk J Pediatr.* 2008;50(3): 291–295.
87. Faure C, et al. Chronic hypertrophic gastropathy in a child resembling adult Menetrier's disease. *J Pediatr Gastroenterol Nutr.* 1996;23(4):419–421.
88. Trout AT, et al. Case 189: pediatric Menetrier disease. *Radiology.* 2013;266(1):357–361.
89. Jacobstein D, Baldassano R. Inflammatory bowel disease. 1st ed. In: Piccoli L, ed. *Pediatric Gastroenterology: Requisites.* Philadelphia, PA: Elsevier; 2007.
90. Carucci LR, Levine MS. Radiographic imaging of inflammatory bowel disease. *Gastroenterol Clin North Am.* 2002;31(1): 93–117, ix.

91. Danese S, Fiocchi C. Ulcerative colitis. *N Engl J Med.* 2011;365(18):1713–1725.
92. Dahnert W. *Radiology Review Manual.* 5th ed. Philadelphia, PA: Lippincott Williams & Wilkins; 2003.
93. Gedalia A. Henoch-Schönlein purpura. *Curr Rheumatol Rep.* 2004;6(3):195–202.
94. Weiss PF, et al. Effects of corticosteroid on Henoch-Schönlein purpura: a systematic review. *Pediatrics.* 2007;120(5):1079–1087.
95. Catassi C, et al. Natural history of celiac disease autoimmunity in a USA cohort followed since 1974. *Ann Med.* 2010;42(7):530–538.
96. Guandalini S, Setty M. Celiac disease. *Curr Opin Gastroenterol.* 2008;24(6):707–712.
97. Guandalini S. *Celiac Disease. Textbook of Pediatric Gastroenterology and Nutrition.* London, UK: Taylor & Francis; 2004:15.
98. Rothrock SG, Pagane J. Acute appendicitis in children: emergency department diagnosis and management. *Ann Emerg Med.* 2000;36(1):39–51.
99. Lamps LW. Appendicitis and infections of the appendix. *Semin Diagn Pathol.* 2004;21(2):86–97.
100. Higgins MJ, et al. Granulomatous appendicitis revisited: report of a case. *Dig Surg.* 2001;18(3):245–248.
101. Bronner MP. Granulomatous appendicitis and the appendix in idiopathic inflammatory bowel disease. *Semin Diagn Pathol.* 2004;21(2):98–107.
102. Larson DB, et al. National trends in CT use in the emergency department: 1995–2007. *Radiology.* 2011;258(1):164–173.
103. Chan L, et al. Pathologic continuum of acute appendicitis: sonographic findings and clinical management implications. *Ultrasound Q.* 2011;27(2):71–79.
104. Sivit CJ, et al. Evaluation of suspected appendicitis in children and young adults: helical CT. *Radiology.* 2000;216(2):430–433.
105. Brennan G. Pediatric appendicitis: pathophysiology and appropriate use of diagnostic imaging. *CJEM.* 2006;8(6):425–432.
106. Lowe LH, et al. Appendicolith revealed on CT in children with suspected appendicitis. *AJR Am J Roentgenol.* 2000;175(4):981–984.
107. Morrow SE, Newman KD. Current management of appendicitis. *Semin Pediatr Surg.* 2007;16(1):34–40.
108. Tien F-M, et al. Clinical features and treatment responses of children with eosinophilic gastroenteritis. *Pediatr Neonatol.* 2011;52(5):272–278.
109. Alfadda AA, Storr MA, Shaffer EA. Eosinophilic colitis: epidemiology, clinical features, and current management. *Therap Adv Gastroenterol.* 2011;4(5):301–309.
110. Diniz LO, Putnum PE, Towbin AJ. Fluoroscopic findings in pediatric eosinophilic esophagitis. *Pediatr Radiol.* 2012;42(6):721–727.
111. White SB, et al. The small-caliber esophagus: radiographic sign of idiopathic eosinophilic esophagitis. *Radiology.* 2010;256(1):127–134.
112. Savino A, et al. Role of ultrasonography in the diagnosis and follow-up of pediatric eosinophilic gastroenteritis: a case report and review of the literature. *Ultraschall Med.* 2011;32(suppl 2):E5–E62.
113. Neustrom MR, Friesen C. Treatment of eosinophilic gastroenteritis with montelukast. *J Allergy Clin Immunol.* 1999;104(2):506.
114. McCarville MB, et al. Clinical and CT features of benign pneumatosis intestinalis in pediatric hematopoietic stem cell transplant and oncology patients. *Pediatr Radiol.* 2008;38(10):1074–1083.
115. Olson DE, et al. CT Predictors for differentiating benign and clinically worrisome pneumatosis intestinalis in children beyond the neonatal period. *Radiology.* 2009;253(2):513–519.
116. McElhinney DB, et al. Necrotizing enterocolitis in neonates with congenital heart disease: risk factors and outcomes. *Pediatrics.* 2000;106(5):1080–1087.
117. Muchantef K, et al. Sonographic and radiographic imaging features of the neonate with necrotizing enterocolitis: correlating findings with outcomes. *Pediatr Radiol.* 2013;43(11):1444–1452.
118. Guest AR, et al. Progressive esophageal leiomyomatosis with respiratory compromise. *Pediatr Radiol.* 2000;30(4):247–250.
119. Hryhorczuk AL, Lee EY, Eisenberg RL. Esophageal abnormalities in pediatric patients. *AJR Am J Roentgenol.* 2013;201(4):W519–W532.
120. Bourque MD, et al. Esophageal leiomyoma in children: two case reports and review of the literature. *J Pediatr Surg.* 1989;24(10):1103–1107.
121. Levine MS, et al. Esophageal leiomyomatosis. *Radiology.* 1996;199(2):533–536.
122. Gupta V, et al. Leiomyomatosis of the esophagus: experience over a decade. *J Gastrointest Surg.* 2009;13(2):206–211.
123. Issaivanan M. et al. Esophageal carcinoma in children and adolescents. *J Pediatr Hematol Oncol.* 2012;34(1):63–67.
124. Iyer R, Dubrow R. Imaging of esophageal cancer. *Cancer Imaging.* 2004;4(2):125–132.
125. Parra DA, Navarro OM. Sonographic diagnosis of intestinal polyps in children. *Pediatr Radiol.* 2008;38(6):680–684.
126. Goedde TA, et al. Gastroduodenal polyps in familial adenomatous polyposis. *Surg Oncol.* 1992;1(5):357–361.
127. Wang LC, et al. Gastrointestinal polyps in children. *Pediatr Neonatol.* 2009;50(5):196–201.
128. Feczko PJ, Halpert RD, Ackerman LV. Gastric polyps: radiological evaluation and clinical significance. *Radiology.* 1985;155(3):581–584.
129. Ba-Ssalamah A, et al. Dedicated multidetector CT of the stomach: spectrum of diseases. *Radiographics.* 2003;23(3):625–644.
130. Levy AD, et al. Gastrointestinal stromal tumors: radiologic features with pathologic correlation. *Radiographics.* 2003;23(2):283–304, 456; quiz 532.
131. Ladd AP, Grosfeld JL. Gastrointestinal tumors in children and adolescents. *Semin Pediatr Surg.* 2006;15(1):37–47.
132. Janeway KA, Weldon CB. Pediatric gastrointestinal stromal tumor. *Semin Pediatr Surg.* 2012;21(1):31–43.
133. Kang HC, et al. Beyond the GIST: mesenchymal tumors of the stomach. *Radiographics.* 2013;33(6):1673–1690.
134. Pickhardt PJ, et al. Posttransplantation lymphoproliferative disorder in children: clinical, histopathologic, and imaging features. *Radiology.* 2000;217(1):16–25.
135. Gross TG, Savoldo B, Punnett A. Posttransplant lymphoproliferative diseases. *Pediatr Clin North Am.* 2010;57(2):481–503.
136. Chang ST, Menias CO. Imaging of primary gastrointestinal lymphoma. *Semin Ultrasound CT MR.* 2013;34(6):558–565.
137. Biko DM, et al. Childhood Burkitt lymphoma: abdominal and pelvic imaging findings. *AJR Am J Roentgenol.* 2009;192(5):1304–1315.
138. Critchley AC, et al. Synchronous gastric and colonic metastases of invasive lobular breast carcinoma: case report and review of the literature. *Ann R Coll Surg Engl.* 2011;93(5):e49–e50.
139. Huang SC, Erdman SH. Pediatric juvenile polyposis syndromes: an update. *Curr Gastroenterol Rep.* 2009;11(3):211–219.

140. Gupta A, et al. A prospective study of MR enterography versus capsule endoscopy for the surveillance of adult patients with Peutz-Jeghers syndrome. *AJR Am J Roentgenol.* 2010;195(1):108–116.
141. Kopacova M, et al. Peutz-Jeghers syndrome: diagnostic and therapeutic approach. *World J Gastroenterol.* 2009;15(43): 5397–5408.
142. Buckley JA, Fishman EK. CT evaluation of small bowel neoplasms: spectrum of disease. *Radiographics.* 1998;18(2): 379–392.
143. Scarsbrook AF, et al. Anatomic and functional imaging of metastatic carcinoid tumors. *Radiographics.* 2007;27(2):455–477.
144. Durno CA. Colonic polyps in children and adolescents. *Can J Gastroenterol.* 2007;21(4):233–239.
145. Alkhouri N, Franciosi JP, Mamula P. Familial adenomatous polyposis in children and adolescents. *J Pediatr Gastroenterol Nutr.* 2010;51(6):727–732.
146. Blumer SL, et al. Sporadic adenocarcinoma of the colon in children: case series and review of the literature. *J Pediatr Hematol Oncol.* 2012;34(4):e137–e141.
147. Wong MT, Eu KW. Primary colorectal lymphomas. *Colorectal Dis.* 2006;8(7):586–591.
148. Antonis JH, Poeze M, Van Heurn LW. Boerhaave's syndrome in children: a case report and review of the literature. *J Pediatr Surg.* 2006;41(9):1620–1623.
149. Garey CL, et al. Esophageal perforation in children: a review of one institution's experience. *J Surg Res.* 2010;164(1): 13–17.
150. Emil SG. Neonatal esophageal perforation. *J Pediatr Surg.* 2004;39(8):1296–1298.
151. Panieri E, et al. Iatrogenic esophageal perforation in children: patterns of injury, presentation, management, and outcome. *J Pediatr Surg.* 1996;31(7):890–895.
152. Gander JW, Berdon WE, and Cowles RA. Iatrogenic esophageal perforation in children. *Pediatr Surg Int.* 2009;25(5): 395–401.
153. Saliakellis E, Borrelli O, Thapar N. Paediatric GI emergencies. *Best Pract Res Clin Gastroenterol.* 2013;27(5):799–817.
154. Dinis-Ribeiro M, Amaro P. Management of gastrointestinal emergencies. *Best Pract Res Clin Gastroenterol.* 2013;27(5): 631–632.
155. Riffat F, Cheng A. Pediatric caustic ingestion: 50 consecutive cases and a review of the literature. *Dis Esophagus.* 2009;22(1): 89–94.
156. Youn BJ, et al. Balloon dilatation for corrosive esophageal strictures in children: radiologic and clinical outcomes. *Korean J Radiol.* 2010;11(2):203–210.
157. Kay M, Wyllie R. Pediatric foreign bodies and their management. *Curr Gastroenterol Rep.* 2005;7(3):212–218.
158. Towbin R, et al. Esophageal edema as a predictor of unsuccessful balloon extraction of esophageal foreign body. *Pediatr Radiol.* 1989;19(6–7):359–360.
159. Sharpe SJ, Rochette LM, Smith GA. Pediatric battery-related emergency department visits in the United States, 1990–2009. *Pediatrics.* 2012;129(6):1111–1117.
160. Brumbaugh D, Kramer RE, Litovitz T. Hemorrhagic complications following esophageal button battery ingestion. *Arch Otolaryngol Head Neck Surg.* 2011;137(4):416; author reply 416–417.
161. Moore M, Wallace EC, Westra S. The imaging of paediatric thoracic trauma. *Pediatr Radiol.* 2009;39(5):485–496.
162. Sartorelli KH, McBride WJ, Vane DW. Perforation of the intrathoracic esophagus from blunt trauma in a child: case report and review of the literature. *J Pediatr Surg.* 1999;34(3):495–497.
163. Uchida K, et al. Ingestion of multiple magnets: hazardous foreign bodies for children. *Pediatr Radiol.* 2006;36(3): 263–264.
164. Oestreich AE. Worldwide survey of damage from swallowing multiple magnets. *Pediatr Radiol.* 2009;39(2):142–147.
165. Otjen JP, Rohrmann CA Jr, Iyer RS. Imaging pediatric magnet ingestion with surgical-pathological correlation. *Pediatr Radiol.* 2013;43(7):851–859.
166. Cotton BA, Nance ML. Penetrating trauma in children. *Semin Pediatr Surg.* 2004;13(2):87–97.
167. Chatoorgoon K, et al. Role of computed tomography and clinical findings in pediatric blunt intestinal injury: a multicenter study. *Pediatr Emerg Care.* 2012;28(12):1338–1342.
168. Schonfeld D, Lee LK. Blunt abdominal trauma in children. *Curr Opin Pediatr.* 2012;24(3):314–318.
169. Sheybani EF, et al. Pediatric nonaccidental abdominal trauma: what the radiologist should know. *Radiographics.* 2014; 34(1):139–153.
170. Hussain SZ, Thomas R, Tolia V. A review of achalasia in 33 children. *Dig Dis Sci.* 2002;47(11):2538–2543.
171. Eeson GA, Wales P, Murphy JJ. Adhesive small bowel obstruction in children: should we still operate? *J Pediatr Surg.* 2010;45(5):969–974.
172. Tsao KJ, et al. Adhesive small bowel obstruction after appendectomy in children: comparison between the laparoscopic and open approach. *J Pediatr Surg.* 2007;42(6):939–942.
173. Delabrousse E, et al. Small-bowel obstruction from adhesive bands and matted adhesions: CT differentiation. *AJR Am J Roentgenol.* 2009;192(3):693–697.
174. Hernanz-Schulman M. Infantile hypertrophic pyloric stenosis. *Radiology.* 2003;227(2):319–331.
175. Cogley JR, et al. Emergent pediatric US: what every radiologist should know. *Radiographics.* 2012;32(3):651–665.
176. Hernanz-Schulman M, et al. Hypertrophic pyloric stenosis in infants: US evaluation of vascularity of the pyloric canal. *Radiology.* 2003;229(2):389–393.
177. Cohen HL, et al. Ultrasonography of pylorospasm: findings may simulate hypertrophic pyloric stenosis. *J Ultrasound Med.* 1998;17(11):705–711.
178. Sanders MK. Bezoars: from mystical charms to medical and nutritional management. *Pract Gastroenterol.* 2004;13:37–50.
179. Western C, Bokhari S, Gould S. Rapunzel syndrome: a case report and review. *J Gastrointest Surg.* 2008;12(9):1612–1614.
180. Applegate K. Intussusception in children: evidence-based diagnosis and treatment. *Pediatr Radiol.* 2009;39(2):140–143.
181. Navarro O, Daneman A. Intussusception. Part 3: diagnosis and management of those with an identifiable or predisposing cause and those that reduce spontaneously. *Pediatr Radiol.* 2004;34(4):305–312.
182. Daneman A, Navarro O. Intussusception. Part 1: a review of diagnostic approaches. *Pediatr Radiol.* 2003;33(2):79–85.
183. Munden MM, et al. Sonography of pediatric small-bowel intussusception: differentiating surgical from nonsurgical cases. *AJR Am J Roentgenol.* 2007;188(1):275–279.
184. Strouse PJ, DiPietro MA, Saez F. Transient small-bowel intussusception in children on CT. *Pediatr Radiol.* 2003;33(5): 316–320.

185. Hryhorczuk AL, Strouse PJ. Validation of US as a first-line diagnostic test for assessment of pediatric ileocolic intussusception. *Pediatr Radiol.* 2009;39(10):1075–1079.
186. Daneman A, Navarro O. Intussusception. Part 2: an update on the evolution of management. *Pediatr Radiol.* 2004;34(2):97–108.
187. Fallon S, et al. Needle decompression to avoid tension pneumoperitoneum and hemodynamic compromise after pneumatic reduction of pediatric intussusception. *Pediatr Radiol.* 2013;43(6):662–667.
188. Shiels WE II. Childhood intussusception: the safety case. *Pediatr Radiol.* 2013;43(6):659–661.
189. Altaf MA, et al. Colonic volvulus in children with intestinal motility disorders. *J Pediatr Gastroenterol Nutr.* 2009;49(1):59–62.
190. Folaranmi SE, et al. Proximal large bowel volvulus in children: 6 new cases and review of the literature. *J Pediatr Surg.* 2012;47(8):1572–1575.
191. Kelly KB, Ponsky TA. Pediatric abdominal wall defects. *Surg Clin North Am.* 2013;93(5):1255–1267.
192. Tang V, et al. Internal hernias in children: spectrum of clinical and imaging findings. *Pediatr Radiol.* 2011;41(12):1559–1568.
193. Aguirre DA, et al. Abdominal wall hernias: imaging features, complications, and diagnostic pitfalls at multi-detector row CT. *Radiographics.* 2005;25(6):1501–1520.
194. Brandt ML. Pediatric hernias. *Surg Clin North Am.* 2008;88(1):27–43.
195. Rettenbacher T, et al. Abdominal wall hernias. *AJR Am J Roentgenol.* 2001;177(5):1061–1066.
196. Orth R, Towbin A. Acute testicular ischemia caused by incarcerated inguinal hernia. *Pediatr Radiol.* 2012;42(2):196–200.
197. Merrett ND, et al. Superior mesenteric artery syndrome: diagnosis and treatment strategies. *J Gastrointest Surg.* 2009;13(2):287–292.
198. Agrawal GA, Johnson PT, Fishman EK. Multidetector row CT of superior mesenteric artery syndrome. *J Clin Gastroenterol.* 2007;41(1):62–65.
199. Zhu ZZ, Qiu Y. Superior mesenteric artery syndrome following scoliosis surgery: its risk indicators and treatment strategy. *World J Gastroenterol.* 2005;11(21):3307–3310.
200. Neri S, et al. Ultrasound imaging in diagnosis of superior mesenteric artery syndrome. *J Intern Med.* 2005;257(4):346–351.
201. Derkay CS, and Schechter GL. Anatomy and physiology of pediatric swallowing disorders. *Otolaryngol Clin North Am.* 1998;31(3):397–404.
202. Kakodkar K, Schroeder JW Jr. Pediatric dysphagia. *Pediatr Clin North Am.* 2013;60(4):969–977.
203. Kramer, SS. Radiologic examination of the swallowing impaired child. *Dysphagia.* 1989;3(3):117–125.

CHAPTER 17

Kidneys and Urinary Tract

Jonathan R. Dillman • Kassa Darge

INTRODUCTION

Congenital and acquired abnormalities of the kidneys and urinary tract are common in the pediatric population. Accurate detection and characterization of such abnormalities are important, as many may be associated with substantial morbidity, such as infection and progressive kidney injury. In this chapter, imaging techniques for evaluating the kidneys and urinary tract are discussed, and normal anatomy is reviewed. In addition, selected disorders affecting the pediatric kidneys and urinary tract are presented, including clinical features, characteristic imaging findings, and treatment approaches.

IMAGING TECHNIQUES

Radiography

Radiography has a limited role in assessment of the kidneys and urinary tract. On occasion, renal enlargement (e.g., due to a mass or severe hydronephrosis) may be first detected by radiography-based mass effect with the epicenter in one of the renal fossae. Urinary tract calculi may be evident on radiographs, though sensitivity may be decreased for small or radiolucent stones. In addition, bowel contents may obscure or simulate stones. Radiography may also depict urinary tract anatomy when obtained after IV contrast administration for preceding computed tomography (CT).

Ultrasound

Ultrasound is generally the first-line imaging modality for assessing the kidneys and urinary tract in the pediatric population. Gray-scale imaging can be used to thoroughly assess the renal parenchyma, renal collecting system, and bladder. The ureters may also be evaluated when dilated. Images through the kidneys and bladder are typically acquired in the longitudinal and transverse planes. Color and power Doppler imaging are useful for detecting blood flow within the kidneys and mass-like abnormalities affecting the kidneys and urinary tract. Color Doppler imaging can also be used to detect urolithiasis based on the presence of "twinkling" artifact.[1,2] Spectral Doppler imaging can be used to assess the renal arteries and veins and to detect conditions such as renovascular hypertension and renal vein thrombosis. Advantages of ultrasound include its widespread availability, low cost, portability, and lack of ionizing radiation.

The intravesical use of ultrasound microbubble contrast agents enables the performance of contrast-enhanced voiding urosonography (ceVUS) for detecting vesicoureteral reflux (VUR). This technique has been shown to be more sensitive for detecting VUR than fluoroscopic voiding cystourethrography (VCUG),[3] and it can be combined with transperineal ultrasound of the urethra.

Computed Tomography

CT may be used to evaluate the kidneys and urinary tract in select situations in the pediatric population. Noncontrast CT is most often used to identify symptomatic urinary tract calculi that cannot be detected by ultrasound.[4] CT imaging with intravenous (IV) contrast material is commonly used to assess renal trauma and masses as well as to evaluate for complications of infection, such as perinephric abscess. When excretory-phase imaging (CT urography) is desired, the IV contrast material bolus can be split into two injections (separated by about 10 minutes).[5] This split-bolus technique provides images with optimal renal parenchymal enhancement as well as excreted contrast material in the urinary tract. The recent development of iterative reconstruction techniques has the potential to allow for reduced dose CT imaging of the kidneys and urinary tracts with preserved image quality.[6]

CT imaging is generally performed using helical technique. The acquisition of an isotropic data set allows for the reconstruction of axial CT images at a variety of section widths and the creation of two-dimensional (2D) multiplanar reformations and three-dimensional (3D) reconstructions. These 2D multiplanar and 3D reconstruction CT images are helpful for evaluation of complex renal and urinary tract anatomic structures and enhance diagnostic accuracy.

Magnetic Resonance Imaging

Magnetic resonance imaging (MRI) is an increasingly utilized imaging modality for evaluating the kidneys and urinary tract, particularly in children. MRI can be used to assess a wide variety of renal parenchymal abnormalities identified but incompletely characterized by ultrasound or CT, such as certain renal masses.

MR urography (MRU) examinations are tailored to assess the kidneys and urinary tract, and this technique can be used to decipher complex urinary tract anatomy, evaluate suspected urinary tract obstruction, and estimate differential renal function. Most MRU examinations utilize multiple T2-weighted pulse sequences to image fluid (urine) in the urinary tract (MR hydrography) as well as postcontrast T1-weighted pulse sequences. Dynamic postcontrast T1-weighted MR imaging (e.g., up to 50 or more 3D image volumes over 8 to 15 minutes) can be used to evaluate for urinary tract obstruction and estimate differential renal function. IV hydration and furosemide injection assist with the acquisition of high-quality MRU images, as these adjunct maneuvers improve urinary tract visualization by increasing distention, allow evaluation of the urinary tract under diuretic "stress," and help minimize T2*-related signal loss of postcontrast images.[7] Volumetric 3D T2-weighted and postcontrast T1-weighted MR image acquisitions allow for 2D multiplanar reformations of the kidneys and urinary tracts as well as 3D reconstructions.

Drawbacks to MRI in children include the need for sedation (or general anesthesia) in some children and long examination times. Also, gadolinium chelate contrast materials should not be administered to pediatric patients with suspected or known acute kidney injury or chronic kidney disease with an estimated glomerular filtration rate <30 mL/min because of risk of nephrogenic systemic fibrosis.[8]

Nuclear Medicine

Several nuclear medicine studies can be used to evaluate the kidneys and urinary tract. Tc-99m dimercaptosuccinic acid (DMSA) is a radiotracer that selectively binds renal cortex and allows detection of pyelonephritis and parenchymal scarring, as well as calculation of differential renal function based on parenchymal mass. Imaging is generally performed 2 to 3 hours after radiotracer injection, and both pinhole collimation and single-photon emission computed tomography technique can be used to acquire higher-quality images.

Dynamic renal scintigraphy is most often performed using Tc-99m mercaptoacetyltriglycine (MAG3) and can be used to estimate differential renal function (based on effective renal plasma flow to the kidneys) and evaluate suspected urinary tract obstruction (based on renal diuretic response following IV furosemide injection). Tc-99m pertechnetate nuclear cystography is highly sensitive for the detection of VUR and can be used to as a first-line imaging test for evaluating suspected VUR in girls or to follow-up known VUR in children of either gender.

The major drawback of nuclear cystography is its inability to clearly depict urinary tract anatomy. This is a particular disadvantage in boys with possible posterior urethral valves where assessment of the urethra is critical. All of these nuclear medicine studies require ionizing radiation for image creation, with DMSA renal scintigraphy imparting the greatest radiation dose.

Fluoroscopy

VCUG is frequently the first-line imaging modality used to evaluate suspected VUR. Water-soluble iodinated contrast material is instilled into the bladder by gravity drip, and fluoroscopic images of the urinary tract are obtained before, during, and after voiding. Routinely acquired VCUG images are presented in Table 17.1. VUR, when present, is graded based on whether refluxed contrast material reaches the renal collecting system, as well as the degree of upper urinary tract dilatation and tortuosity. VCUG can also be used to further assess bladder, urethra, and upper tract anatomy when VUR is present. The radiation dose of VCUG examinations can be substantially reduced by using state-of-the-art fluoroscopy equipment and radiation dose reduction techniques, such as pulsed fluoroscopy and last image hold (grab or capture).[9]

Although the pediatric urethra is usually evaluated using VCUG, retrograde urethrography (RUG) may be necessary when the clinical question pertains specifically to the urethra, particularly in older boys. RUG is most commonly used to

TABLE 17.1 Routine Pediatric Voiding Cystourethrogram Images Acquired in Children with Typical Renal and Urinary Tract Anatomy[a]

1. Scout image (frontal abdominopelvic radiograph or fluoroscopic last image capture)—OPTIONAL
2. Frontal image during early bladder filling
3. Bilateral oblique images during mid–late bladder filling
4. Frontal image with bladder fully distended
5. Image (or cine imaging using last image capture technique) of urethra during voiding (frontal projection in girls; right posterior oblique projection in boys)
6. Frontal images of the renal fossae during peak of voiding and following void

[a]*Imaging should be tailored to the individual child and known/suspected renal and/or urinary tract abnormalities.*

assess the male urethra in the setting of trauma (e.g., pelvic or perineal injury with hematuria) or suspected stricture.

NORMAL ANATOMY AND VARIANTS

Kidneys

The kidneys typically reside in the retroperitoneum just below the liver and spleen (one on each side of the spine) and are surrounded by perinephric fat and Gerota fascia. The renal hila are normally oriented anteromedially, and the long axis of the kidney is typically parallel to the long axis of the ipsilateral psoas muscle. The kidneys should increase in length over time during childhood.[10]

Renal parenchyma is composed of peripheral cortex and deeper medulla. The renal cortex contains glomeruli and tubules, whereas the medulla (medullary pyramids) contains tubules and collecting ducts. Normal kidneys typically demonstrate corticomedullary differentiation at imaging (e.g., ultrasound and MRI), and loss of corticomedullary differentiation may be a sign of parenchymal abnormality (e.g., renal dysplasia or autosomal recessive polycystic kidney disease [ARPKD]). The tips of the renal medullary pyramids, or papillae, empty into the renal collecting system and may be susceptible to certain pathologic processes, such as papillary necrosis because of renal ischemia. Embryologically, the kidney develops from two structures: (1) the metanephric blastema, which gives rise to renal glomeruli and tubules of the nephron and (2) the mesonephric (wolffian) duct (ureteric bud), which gives rise to the renal collecting system and collecting ducts.

Upper Urinary Tract

The renal collecting system and ureter comprise the upper urinary tract. The renal collecting system is made up of numerous calyces, with well-defined papillary impressions and sharp fornices, which empty into a renal pelvis. On occasion, the renal pelvis may extend beyond the contour of the kidney giving rise to an extrarenal pelvis, commonly considered a normal variant. The ureter is muscular-walled tubular structure connecting the renal pelvis to the bladder, normally inserting into the ipsilateral bladder trigone region. The mucosa of the renal collecting system and ureter is difficult to appreciate by imaging unless thickened because of infection, inflammation, or obstruction. Like the renal collecting system, the ureter also arises from the ureteral bud of the mesonephric duct.

Urinary Bladder

The bladder serves as a reservoir for urine produced by the kidneys. Normal bladder volume increases with age during childhood. The Koff formula[11] is commonly employed for estimating bladder capacity and is based on patient age (in years), stating:

$$\text{Capacity in mL} = (\text{Age} + 2) \times 30$$

Appearance and thickness of the bladder wall depend in part on the degree of distention with urine. In utero, the bladder dome communicates with the allantois membrane via a tubular channel coursing through the space of Retzius (the urachus). Much of the bladder develops from the urogenital sinus, whereas the trigone arises from the caudal portions of the mesonephric ducts.

Urethra

The urethra is a tubular channel that transports urine from the bladder to outside the body. Micturition normally occurs after relaxation of the internal (involuntary) and external (voluntary) sphincter mechanisms. The female urethra is short, typically opens just above the vaginal orifice, and is rarely abnormal (other than in developmental abnormalities of the urogenital sinus, such as bladder exstrophy or cloacal malformation). The male urethra is substantially longer and has four parts (Fig. 17.1). The pelvic portion of the urogenital sinus gives rise to the entire female urethra as well as the prostatic and membranous portions of the male urethra. The anterior male urethra arises from the phallic portion of the urogenital sinus.

SPECTRUM OF RENAL DISORDERS

Congenital and Developmental Anomalies

Congenital and developmental anomalies of the kidneys are common. While often isolated, they also regularly occur in the presence of other congenital anomalies. For example, renal anomalies can be associated with congenital heart disease, mullerian anomalies, anorectal malformations, abnormalities of the urogenital sinus, and a variety of chromosomal anomalies (e.g., Turner syndrome [45,X]). In such conditions, detection may occur during the antenatal period, and renal sonography is typically performed early in life. Renal anomalies are also part of the nonrandom VACTERL association of congenital anomalies (Vertebral, Anorectal, Cardiovascular, TracheoEsophageal, Renal, Limb anomalies).[12]

Agenesis

Renal agenesis, or congenital absence of the kidney, is due to in utero failure of development, and it can be either unilateral or bilateral. Bilateral renal agenesis is incompatible with life, a cause of Potter sequence, and results in fetal demise or death very soon after birth, in part due to pulmonary insufficiency. Unilateral renal agenesis can be detected by antenatal ultrasound, and it is commonly associated with other congenital anomalies, including VACTERL association, mullerian anomalies in girls, and seminal vesicle cysts in boys.[13] Renal agenesis is a part of the MURCS association (Mullerian anomaly, Renal agenesis, Cervicothoracic Somite dysplasia).[14] No identifiable renal tissue is found in the ipsilateral renal fossa at ultrasound imaging. Careful imaging assessment of the retroperitoneum and pelvis must be undertaken to exclude the possibility of an ectopic, sometimes dysplastic kidney. The ipsilateral adrenal gland usually appears abnormally elongated ("lying down" appearance)

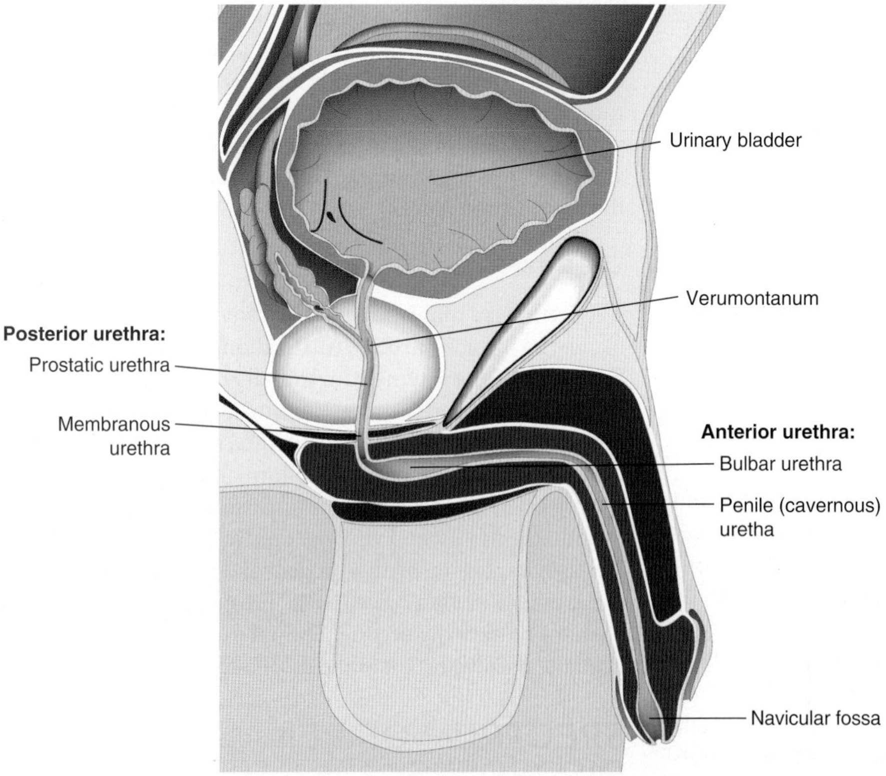

FIGURE 17.1 **Anatomy of the male urethra.**

on longitudinal ultrasound images early in life (Fig. 17.2).[15] Contralateral renal parenchymal hypertrophy is often present, even early in life. CT and MRI demonstrate similar findings and can be used to search for residual renal tissue, if clinically necessary. There is no specific medical or surgical therapy for renal agenesis, and prognosis is generally good assuming the contralateral kidney is normal. Care should be taken to preserve contralateral kidney function.

Hypoplasia and Dysplasia

Abnormal development of the kidney in utero can cause a variety of parenchymal abnormalities. Renal hypoplasia refers to an abnormally small kidney that contains fewer nephrons than expected. This condition is uncommon and in some cases may be the result of decreased blood flow or congenital VUR. At imaging, hypoplastic kidneys appear smaller than expected for patient age but are otherwise morphologically normal without overt evidence of dysplasia (Fig. 17.3).[16]

Renal dysplasia commonly occurs in the setting of in utero urinary tract obstruction (e.g., due to ectopic

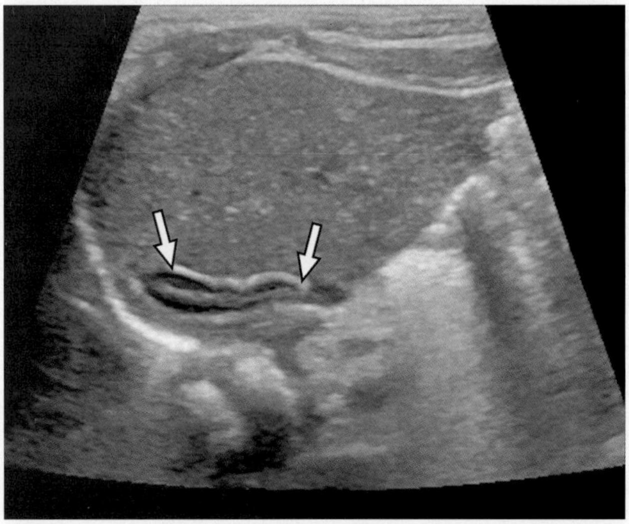

FIGURE 17.2 **1-day-old girl with right renal agenesis.** No kidney is identified in the right renal fossa, and the right adrenal gland (*arrows*) appears abnormally elongated.

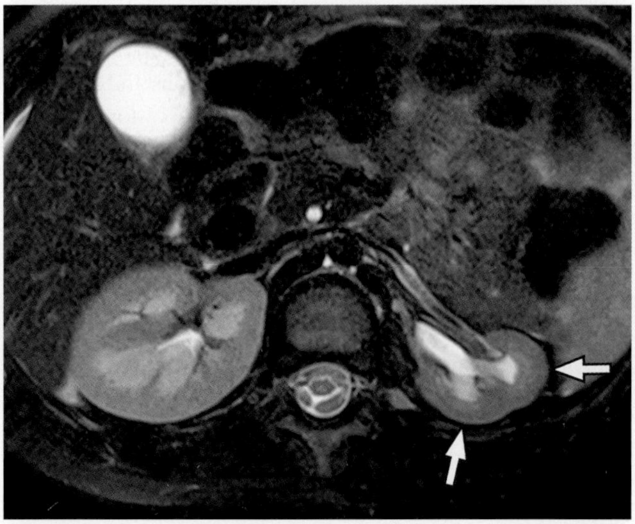

FIGURE 17.3 **7-year-old boy with hypoplastic (vs. mildly dysplastic) left kidney due to congenital vesicoureteral reflux.** Axial T2-weighted fat-saturated MR image shows a small but otherwise morphologically normal left kidney (*arrows*). There is slightly diminished left kidney corticomedullary differentiation and mild pelvicaliectasis. Right kidney is enlarged due to compensatory hypertrophy.

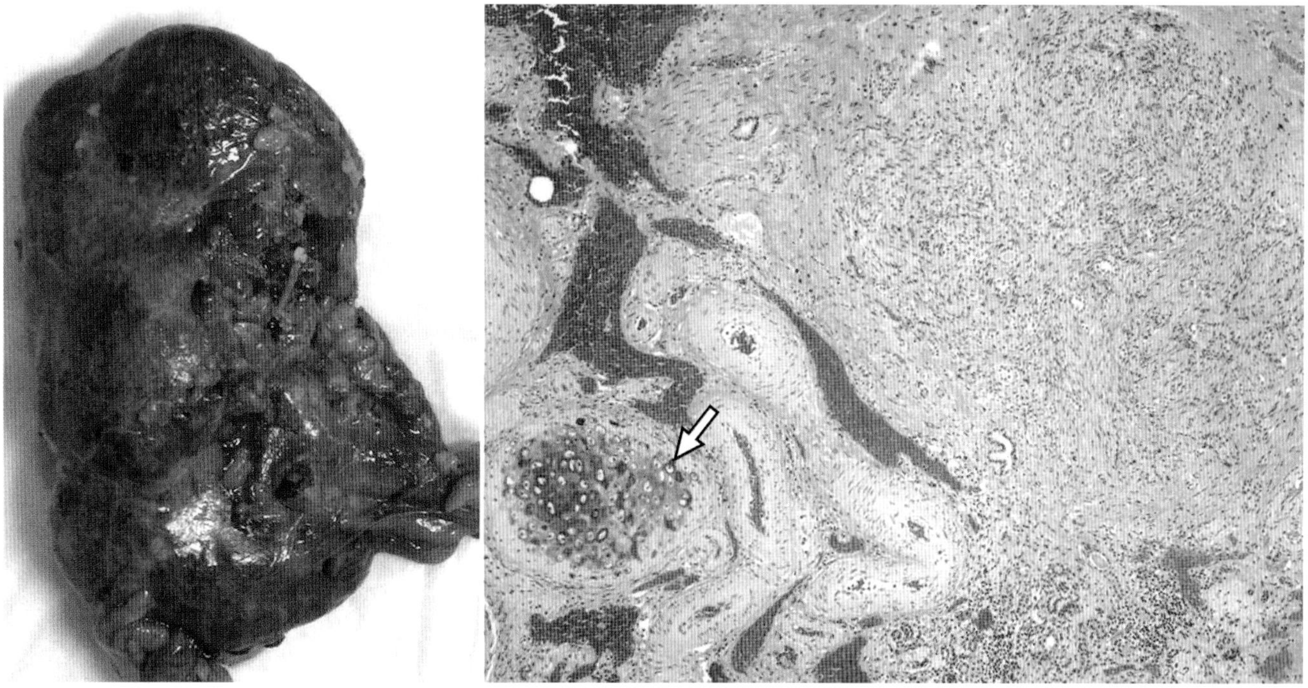

FIGURE 17.4 **Hypoplastic/dysplastic kidney resected from a 9-year-old boy with a history of prune-belly syndrome (left).** Microscopically (**right**), it showed disorganized renal elements characteristic of renal dysplasia, including nodules of abortive tubular structures surrounded by collarettes of stroma, large aberrant blood vessels, and islands of cartilage (*arrow*) (hematoxylin and eosin, original magnification, 200×).

ureteric insertion, ureterocele, or severe upper urinary tract narrowing) with resultant disordered assembly of renal tissue elements. While sometimes isolated, renal dysplasia can be associated with a variety of predisposing conditions, including upper urinary tract duplication (upper moiety parenchyma is most often dysplastic), posterior urethral valves, prune-belly syndrome, and mullerian anomalies.[16,17] Microscopically, immature renal tubules embedded in primitive stroma, islands of cartilage, epithelium-lined cysts, and large aberrant blood vessels may be seen (Fig. 17.4).

At imaging, renal dysplasia can have a spectrum of appearances. Milder forms of dysplasia are associated with abnormal morphologic appearance of renal parenchyma and collecting system, small parenchymal cysts, and loss of corticomedullary differentiation (Fig. 17.5).[18] The most severe form of renal dysplasia, multicystic dysplastic kidney (MCDK), presents as numerous variably sized noncommunicating cysts with no normal intervening renal parenchyma (Fig. 17.6). This entity may be associated with contralateral ureteropelvic junction (UPJ) obstruction and VUR, and it rarely can occur in the setting of pelvic kidney, horseshoe kidney, or crossed renal ectopia. MCDKs commonly decrease in size over time and may involute (based on ultrasound evaluation); rarely, MCDKs may enlarge.[19,20] Asymptomatic dysplastic kidneys are often managed conservatively, whereas symptomatic dysplastic kidneys (e.g., those causing recurrent infections or hypertension) are often surgically removed.[21] Based on recent studies, MCDKs are likely at no significantly increased risk

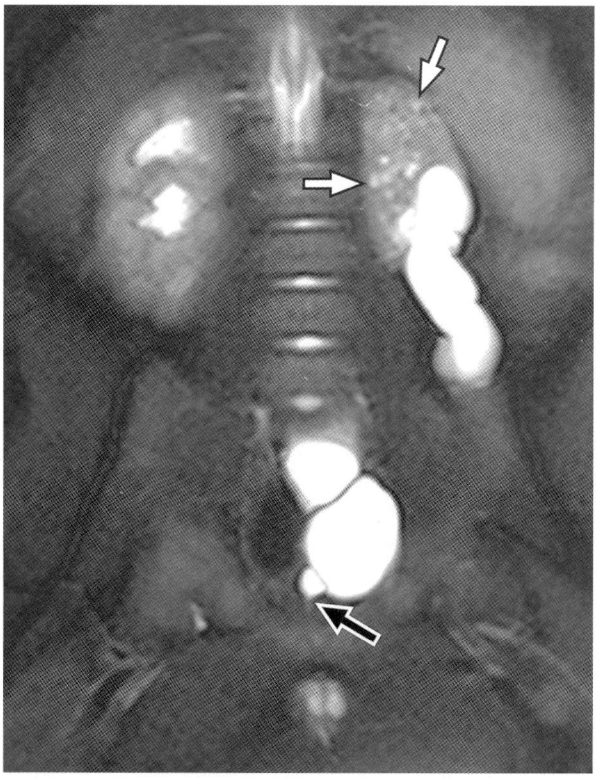

FIGURE 17.5 **6-month-old girl with left kidney dysplasia.** Coronal T2-weighted fat-saturated MR image shows a poorly formed left kidney with absent corticomedullary differentiation and scattered tiny parenchymal cysts (*white arrows*). The left ureter is obstructed due to an ectopic insertion (*black arrow*) and is markedly dilated.

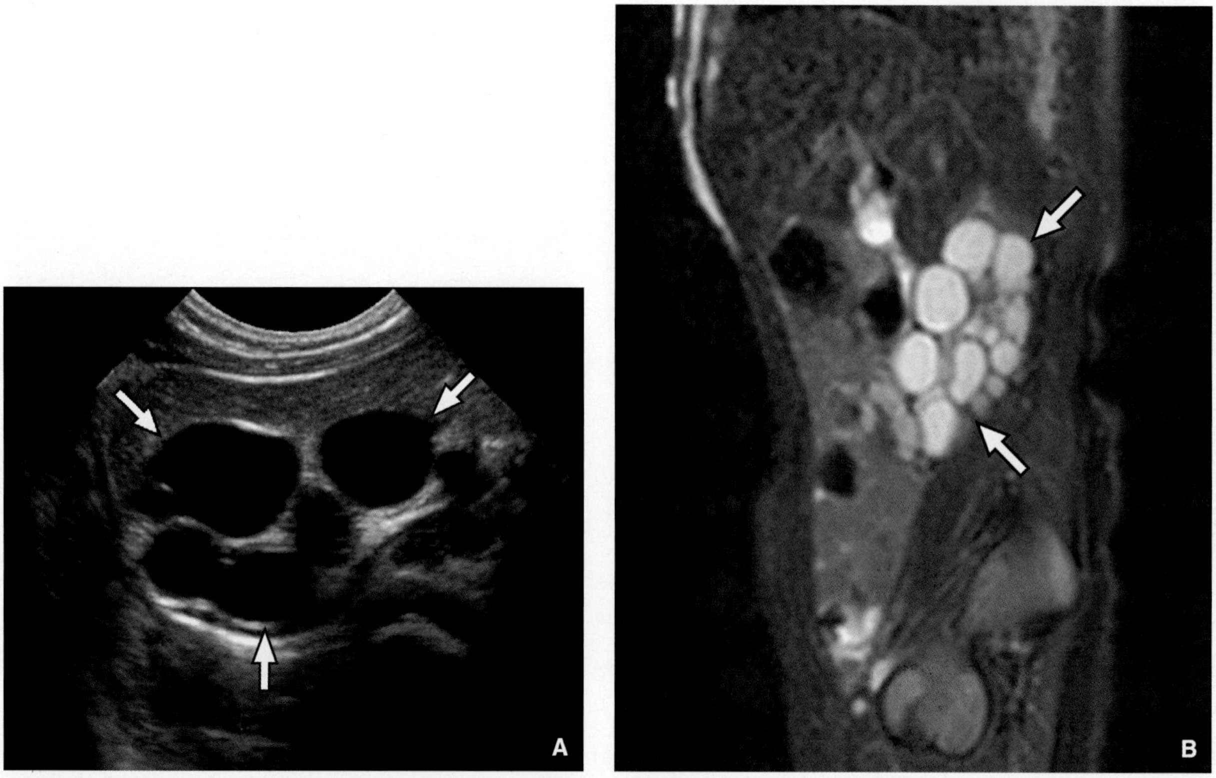

FIGURE 17.6 **2-month-old girl with right multicystic dysplastic kidney. A:** Transverse gray-scale ultrasound image shows multiple variably sized, noncommunicating cysts (*arrows*) in the right renal fossa. Residual right kidney parenchyma is abnormally echogenic. **B:** Sagittal T2-weighted fat-saturated MR image shows similar findings (*arrows*).

of malignancy.[20,21] In the setting of unilateral renal dysplasia, care should be taken to preserve contralateral kidney function.

Abnormal Rotation, Ectopia, and Fusion

Abnormal Rotation

As the fetal kidneys ascend from the pelvis in utero, they normally undergo medial rotation in the transverse plane. As a result, the renal hila and pelves are normally oriented anteromedially. When a kidney fails to completely rotate, it is said to be either nonrotated or malrotated (Fig. 17.7). Much less commonly, the renal hilum and pelvis may be oriented posteriorly or laterally due to either hyperrotation or reverse rotation. Although kidneys that appropriately ascend can be abnormally rotated, this phenomenon is more commonly associated with ectopic or fused kidneys.[22] Abnormal renal rotation can be detected by a variety of imaging modalities (e.g., ultrasound, CT, MRI, and VCUG) and is most often by itself of no clinical significance.

Ectopia

As previously mentioned, the kidneys normally ascend in utero from the pelvis to their expected locations in the retroperitoneum. Consequently, an ectopic kidney can be identified anywhere along its expected course of ascent. Less commonly, an ectopic kidney may cross the midline (crossed ectopia) or may be located superior to the expected location of the renal fossa (e.g., in the setting of a Bochdalek-type congenital diaphragmatic hernia). The majority of ectopic kidneys are located in the pelvis, whereas thoracic kidneys are very rare and most often left sided.[23] Ectopic kidneys in children are usually identifiable using ultrasound and may show absence of the renal sinus echo complex.[24] They can be easily

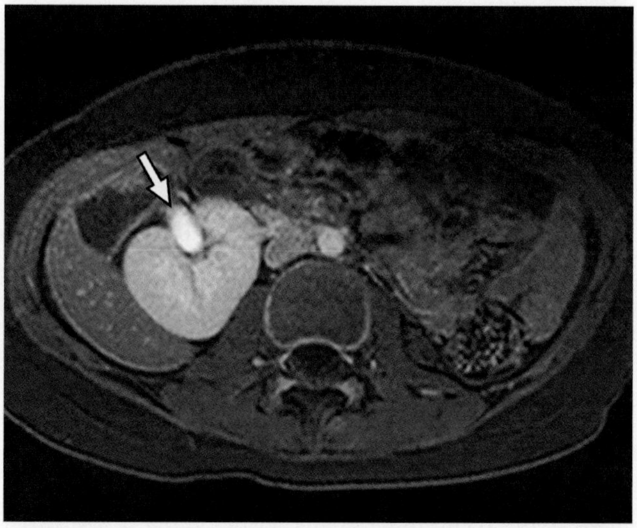

FIGURE 17.7 **3-year-old girl with nonrotated right kidney.** Axial postcontrast T1-weighted fat-saturated MR image shows nonrotation of the right kidney, with an anteriorly oriented renal pelvis (*arrow*). The left renal fossa is empty.

identified by CT and MRI. Suspicion should be high when imaging reveals an empty renal fossa. Ectopic kidneys are commonly nonrotated or malrotated, and they may have mild pelvicaliectasis, even in the absence of urinary tract obstruction or VUR (Fig. 17.8). The arterial supply and venous drainage of ectopic kidneys are usually anomalous, with renal arteries arising from nearby major arterial structures and renal veins draining to nearby major systemic venous structures. Ectopic kidneys are often asymptomatic but may be complicated by ipsilateral VUR, UPJ obstruction, and urolithiasis.[25] Small, poorly functioning malpositioned kidneys rarely can present with urinary dribbling and/or incontinence due to an associated ectopic ureter.[26]

Abnormal Fusion

Anomalies of renal fusion can take on several configurations. The horseshoe kidney is fused in the midline, most often at the lower poles. Both renal moieties are lower in position than expected (as ascent is hindered by the inferior mesenteric artery), and they are abnormally oriented with their lower poles directed medially. Horseshoe kidneys occur with increased frequency in Turner syndrome (45,X).[27] Cross-fused renal ectopia is diagnosed when both kidneys are located on the same side of the midline and fused, whereas pancake kidney refers to bilateral pelvic kidneys that are fused at both the upper and lower poles.

At ultrasound, abnormal long-axis orientation of the kidneys with poor visualization of the lower poles may be the first clue to the presence of a horseshoe kidney.[22] Ultrasound imaging in the transverse and coronal planes can be used to identify either a parenchymal or fibrous isthmus located anterior to the lumbar spine between the abdominal aorta and inferior mesenteric artery (Fig. 17.9). The kidneys are frequently abnormally rotated, nonobstructed pelvicaliectasis may be present, and multiple bilateral renal arteries are typical (arising from the abdominal aorta, iliac arteries, and sometimes the inferior mesenteric artery).[22] CT or MRI can be used to confirm the diagnosis of horseshoe kidney if ultrasound is inconclusive (Fig. 17.10). Horseshoe kidneys may be associated with VUR, UPJ obstruction, and urolithiasis, and they are at increased risk of traumatic injury due to their location adjacent to the spine (Fig. 17.11).[28] Horseshoe kidneys have been reported to be associated with an increased incidence of Wilms tumor; a large study by the National Wilms Tumor Study Group demonstrated 41 of 8,617 (0.48%) Wilms tumors arose in a horseshoe kidney.[29] Horseshoe kidneys require no specific treatment.

Crossed fused renal ectopia can also be readily identified by ultrasound. Both kidneys are located on the same side of the midline (with the ectopic kidney usually inferior). The ectopic kidney's ureterovesical junction is usually orthotopic, on the contralateral side. A notch or indentation is frequently seen at the site of parenchymal fusion (Fig. 17.12).[30] Cross-fused renal moieties are frequently abnormally rotated (e.g., anteriorly or laterally oriented), and they may take on a variety of configurations (e.g., S-shape or L-shape). Similar to horseshoe kidneys, renal arterial supply is typically anomalous, and these

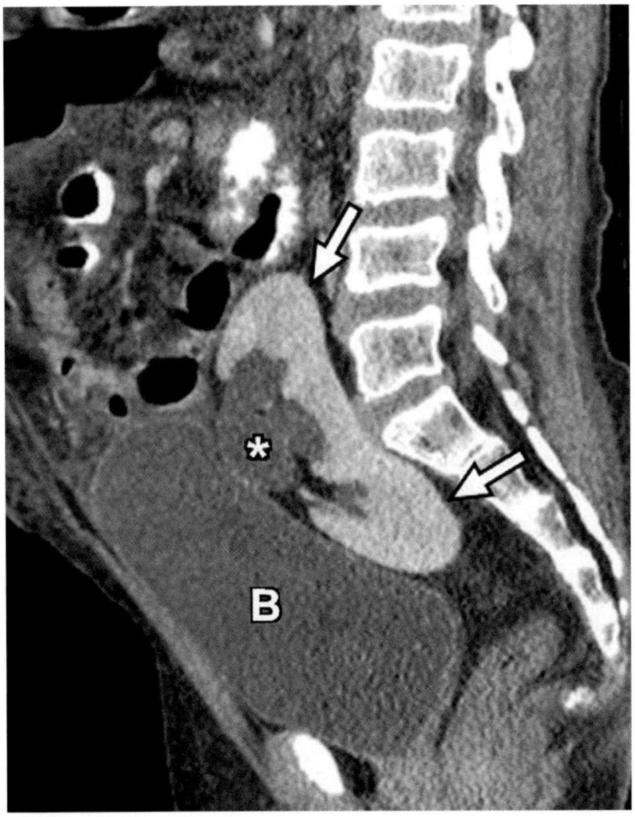

FIGURE 17.8 **11-year-old boy with pelvic kidney.** Sagittal contrast-enhanced CT image shows that the left kidney (*arrows*) is located in the pelvis, posterior to the bladder (*B*). The kidney is nonrotated with its mildly dilated renal collecting system (*asterisk*) facing anteriorly.

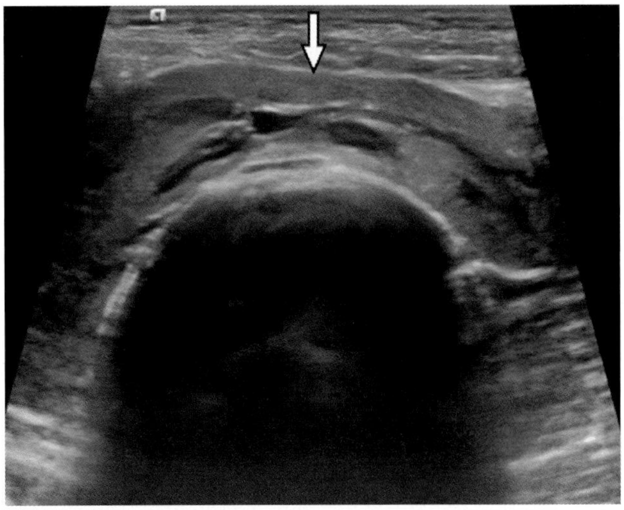

FIGURE 17.9 **3-month-old boy with horseshoe kidney.** Transverse gray-scale ultrasound image through the midabdomen shows fusion of the bilateral lower renal poles in the midline (*arrow*), anterior to the lumbar spine.

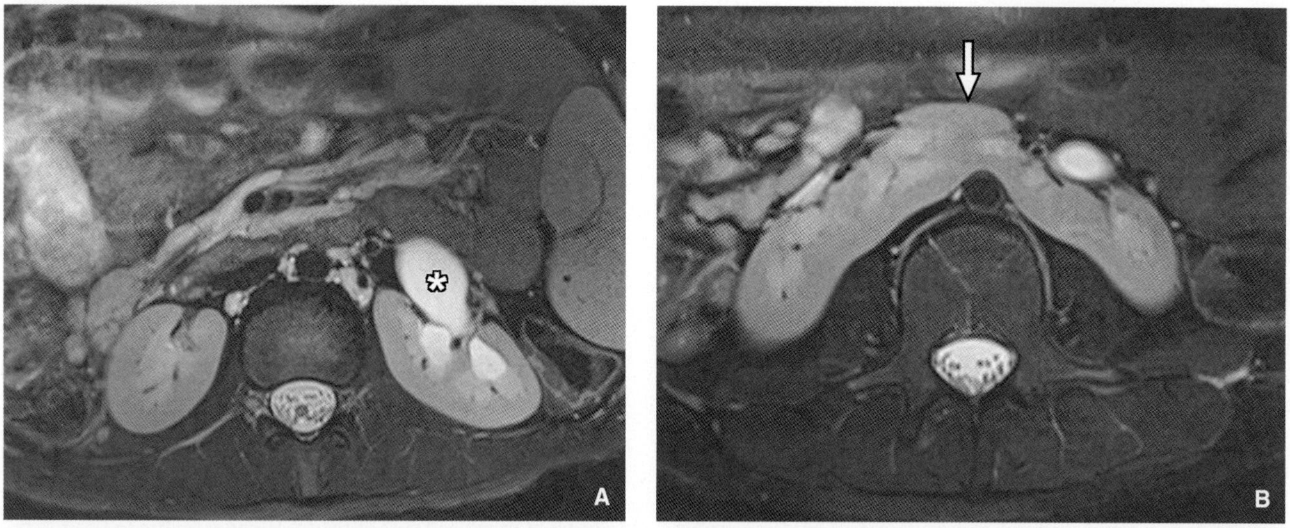

FIGURE 17.10 **7-year-old boy with horseshoe kidney. A:** Axial T2-weighted fat-saturated MR image shows abnormal rotation of the kidneys and mild left pelvicaliectasis (*asterisk*). **B:** More inferior MR image shows that the kidneys are fused in the midline with a thick parenchymal isthmus (*arrow*). (Case courtesy of J. Damien Grattan-Smith, MD, Children's Healthcare of Atlanta, Atlanta, GA.)

kidneys may be associated with VUR, UPJ obstruction, and urolithiasis. Cross-fused renal ectopia also generally requires no specific treatment.

Infectious Disorders

Bacterial Pyelonephritis

Bacterial infection of the kidney, or pyelonephritis, characteristically presents with clinical findings of urinary tract infection. Fever and flank pain are common, but may not be present, particularly in very young children. The source of infection may be either ascending (due to cystitis related to perineal bacterial flora) or hematogenous. *Escherichia coli* is the most frequent causative organism. Urinary tract obstruction, high-grade VUR, and dysfunctional voiding are risk factors.

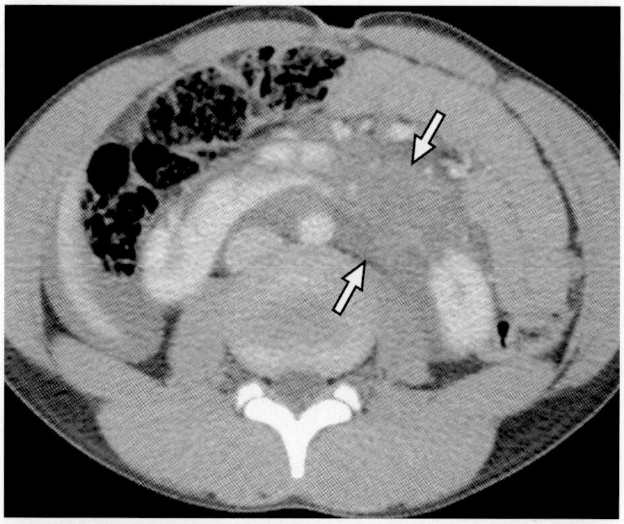

FIGURE 17.11 **13-year-old boy with injured horseshoe kidney due to motor vehicle accident.** Axial contrast-enhanced CT image shows a lacerated horseshoe kidney with adjacent retroperitoneal hematoma (*between arrows*). Renal collecting system disruption was identified on delayed excretory-phase imaging.

At imaging, pyelonephritis may be either focal or widespread and either unilateral or bilateral. Renal infection at ultrasound commonly appears as areas of increased parenchymal echogenicity and decreased corticomedullary differentiation with relatively decreased or absent color or power Doppler signal compared to adjacent normal kidney (Fig. 17.13).[31] At contrast-enhanced CT, pyelonephritis can present as linear, geographic, or mass-like areas of decreased parenchymal attenuation (Fig. 17.13).[32] The involved kidney is frequently enlarged, and perinephric fat stranding due to inflammation may be present.[32] Acute pyelonephritis is usually less conspicuous on unenhanced CT images and may go undetected. Similar findings may be observed at MRI, including linear, geographic, or mass-like areas of signal intensity alteration and hypoenhancement. Interestingly, affected areas can hyperenhance on delayed postcontrast CT or MR imaging due to parenchymal edema and tubular obstruction.[33] Tc-99m DMSA renal scintigraphy can also be used to detect pyelonephritis, appearing as areas of focal photopenia. Unlike MRI, DMSA imaging cannot differentiate acute pyelonephritis from scarring.[34]

Prompt recognition and treatment of children with pyelonephritis can prevent potential complications, such as renal scarring, loss of kidney function, and hypertension. Acute pyelonephritis may also be complicated by abscess formation within the kidney or adjacent perinephric space. Such abscesses appear as peripherally enhancing fluid collections on contrast-enhanced imaging and may be multiloculated, septated, or debris laden at ultrasound (Fig. 17.14).

Xanthogranulomatous pyelonephritis (XGP) is a form of chronic renal parenchymal infection that only rarely occurs in the pediatric population.[35] Clinical presentation may be nonspecific, leading to delayed diagnosis. XGP is

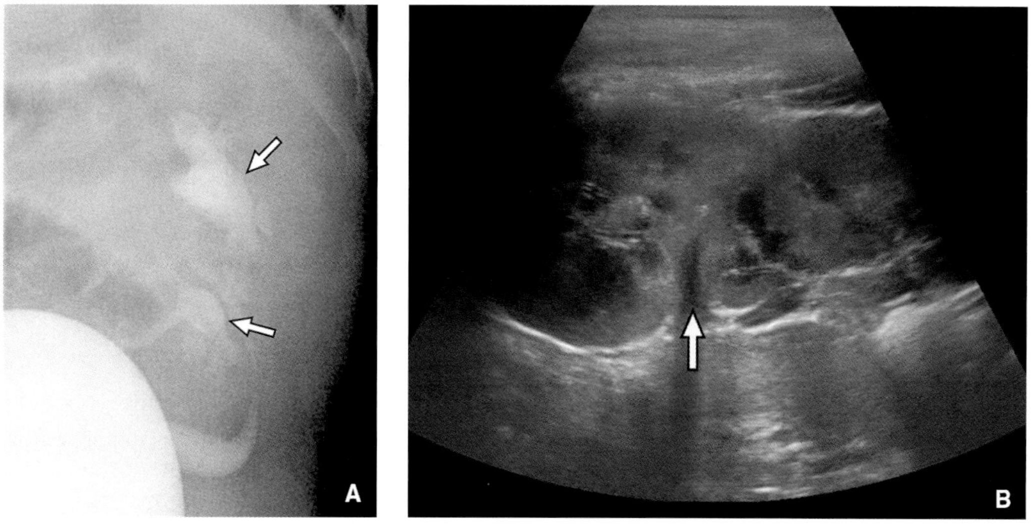

FIGURE 17.12 **3-month-old boy with crossed fused renal ectopia. A:** Voiding cystourethrogram image shows vesicoureteral reflux into two separate renal collecting systems (*arrows*), both located to the left of midline. **B:** Gray-scale ultrasound image confirms that the right kidney is ectopic and fused to the left kidney. A parenchymal notch (*arrow*) can be seen at the site of parenchymal fusion.

often associated with infection by *Proteus mirabilis*, a urea-splitting bacterium that forms struvite calculi. At histology, XGP is characterized by the presence of chronic inflammation, including lipid-laden macrophages. At imaging, a large obstructing calculus, sometimes staghorn in appearance, classically is present in the renal pelvis. The affected kidney usually appears diffusely enlarged and contains numerous round areas of decreased echogenicity at ultrasound or decreased attenuation at CT that are due to severe hydronephrosis ("bear paw" sign) and parenchymal necrosis (Fig. 17.15). Extensive perinephric inflammatory changes are typically present, and abscess formation may occur in the perinephric space, adjacent psoas muscle, and even body wall. Delayed contrast-enhanced CT and renal scintigraphy reveal minimal or no renal function, and radical nephrectomy is generally indicated for definitive treatment. A minority of XGP cases are focal, involving only a portion of the kidney, sometimes appearing mass-like.[36]

Fungal Infection

Fungal infections of the kidneys and urinary tract are most often due to *Candida* species and commonly present with funguria. Involvement of the kidneys and collecting systems can be the result of hematogenous dissemination (often bilateral) or ascending spread from the bladder (often unilateral). Infection in very young children, including premature neonates, has the potential to be serious due to immature neutrophil function.[37] Hematogenous spread of infection (candidemia) to the kidney may present as focal areas of parenchymal low attenuation on contrast-enhanced CT.

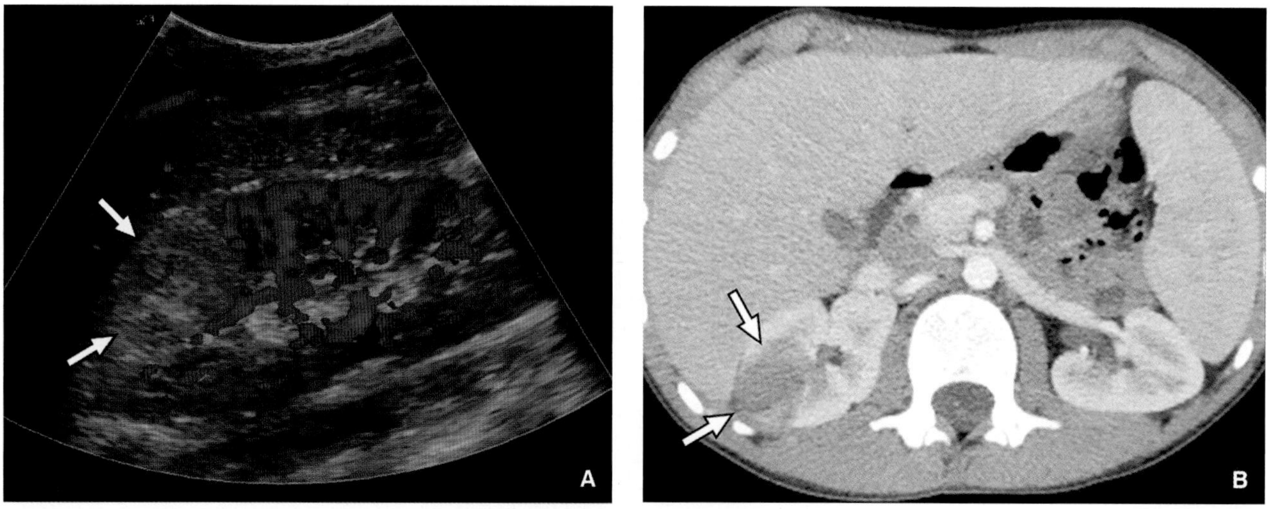

FIGURE 17.13 **13-year-old boy with fever, right flank pain, and hematuria due to pyelonephritis. A:** Longitudinal color Doppler ultrasound image of the right kidney shows a mass-like area of increased echogenicity (*arrows*) in the upper pole that has decreased blood flow compared to adjacent parenchyma. **B:** Axial contrast-enhanced CT image shows an ill-defined low attenuation area (*arrows*) in the right kidney upper pole due to parenchymal infection. This area of acute focal bacterial pyelonephritis resolved on follow-up ultrasound imaging after antibiotic therapy.

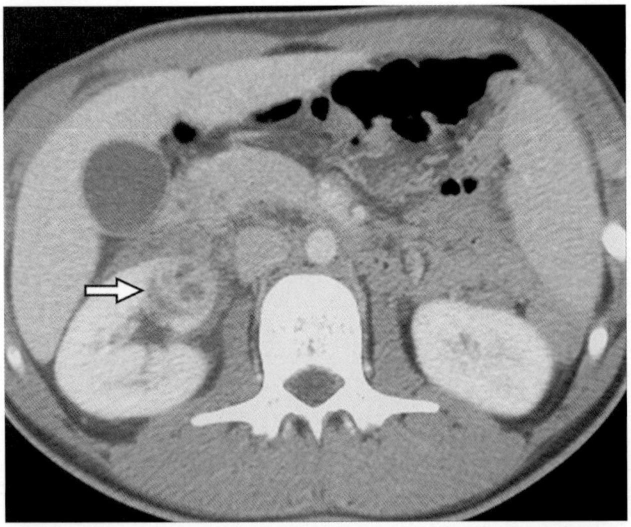

FIGURE 17.14 **13-year-old girl with fever and right flank pain.** Axial contrast-enhanced CT image shows a heterogeneous abscess (*arrow*) in the anterior aspect of the mid right kidney. Perinephric fluid surrounds much of the right kidney.

Ascending fungal infection within the renal collecting system is best appreciated by ultrasound, sometimes presenting as nonspecific echogenic debris in the urine or as an echogenic, circumscribed, sometimes mobile fungus ball (mycetoma) (Fig. 17.16).[38] On occasion, ascending infection can infiltrate the renal medulla. Renal or perinephric abscesses due to fungal infection can rarely occur. Treatment is typically antifungal medical therapy, although, in certain children, asymptomatic funguria is due to colonization and does not require medical therapy. Rarely, such fungal infections can result in urinary tract obstruction or nonresolving abscesses that require percutaneous drainage or surgical management.[39]

Neoplastic Disorders

Benign and Low-Malignant Potential Neoplasms

Congenital Mesoblastic Nephroma

Congenital mesoblastic nephroma is the most common neonatal renal neoplasm and may be present at birth. These tumors may be detected antenatally, and affected children sometimes have a history of maternal polyhydramnios.[40] Ninety-percent of these lesions are diagnosed in children <1 year of age. Affected children can present with a palpable abdominal mass or less commonly hypertension and hematuria. This mesenchymal spindle cell tumor is divided into two histologic variants: (1) classic and (2) cellular.[41] Both consist histologically of fibroblastic cells arranged in fascicles (Fig. 17.17). The cellular variant harbors the same t(12;15) chromosomal translocation as infantile fibrosarcoma and is currently viewed as infantile fibrosarcoma arising within the kidney.

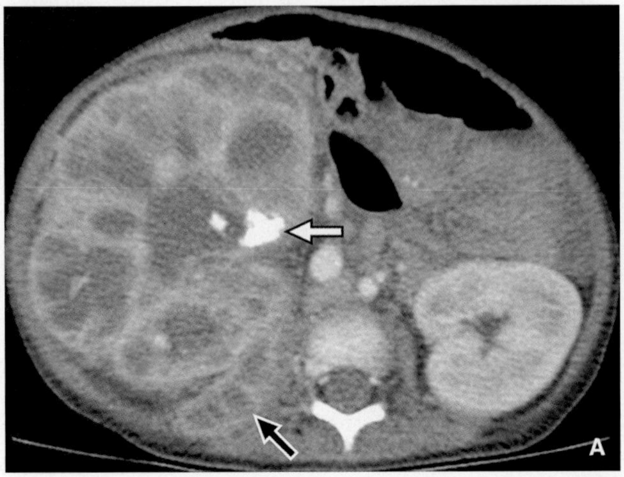

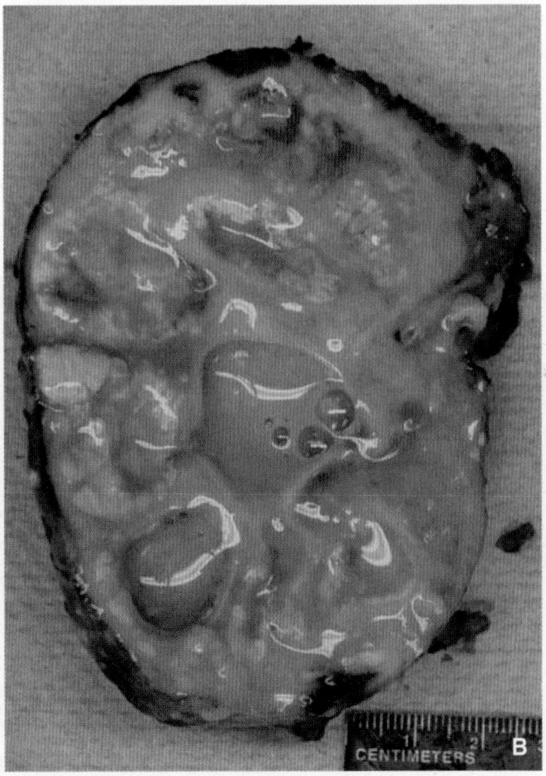

FIGURE 17.15 **1-year-old girl with recurrent fevers due to xanthogranulomatous pyelonephritis. A:** Axial contrast-enhanced CT image shows marked enlargement of the right kidney. Multiple calculi (*white arrow*) are present in the right renal collecting system. Numerous areas of focal low attenuation in the right kidney are due to pelvicaliectasis and parenchymal necrosis. A right retroperitoneal abscess (*black arrow*) is present adjacent to the right psoas muscle. Enlarged retroperitoneal lymph nodes are reactive in etiology. **B:** Bivalved gross pathologic specimen shows extensive renal parenchymal necrosis.

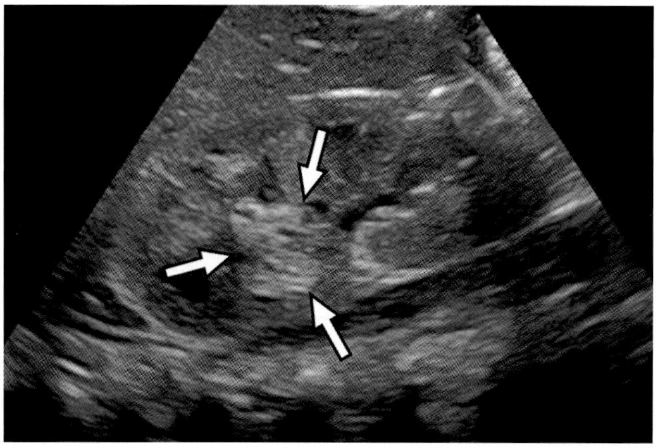

FIGURE 17.16 **4-month-old girl with fungemia and funguria.** Longitudinal gray-scale ultrasound image of the right kidney shows an echogenic, lobulated fungus ball (*arrows*) in upper pole collecting system.

At imaging (ultrasound, CT, and MRI), these lesions commonly present as large, infiltrating masses replacing much of the affected kidney (Fig. 17.18). The classic variant usually appears solid, and it may have a peripheral hypoechoic ring at ultrasound.[41] The cellular variant, which tends to present later in infancy, is often larger and more heterogeneous at imaging due to necrosis, hemorrhage, and/or cyst formation.[42] This form can behave more aggressively with encasement of major vascular structures, recurrence in the setting of positive margins, or distant metastatic disease.[42,43] Prognosis is generally excellent in the setting of nephrectomy with complete surgical resection of the lesion.

Ossifying Renal Tumor of Infancy

Ossifying renal tumor of infancy is a rare, benign pediatric renal neoplasm. This tumor presents with hematuria or, less often, as a palpable abdominal mass, and it occurs in young children under 3 years of age.[44] Histopathologic examination reveals a mass composed of spindle cells and bone (including osteoid and osteoblasts) typically attached to a renal papilla; some have suggested a urothelial origin.[45] At ultrasound, these lesions are typically echogenic with posterior acoustic shadowing, mimicking a large renal calculus. Renal collecting system dilatation can be present due to obstruction.[46] CT typically reveals an ossified renal mass in the central kidney that may be associated with a hypoenhancing soft tissue mass (Fig. 17.19).[47,48] Surgical resection is curative.

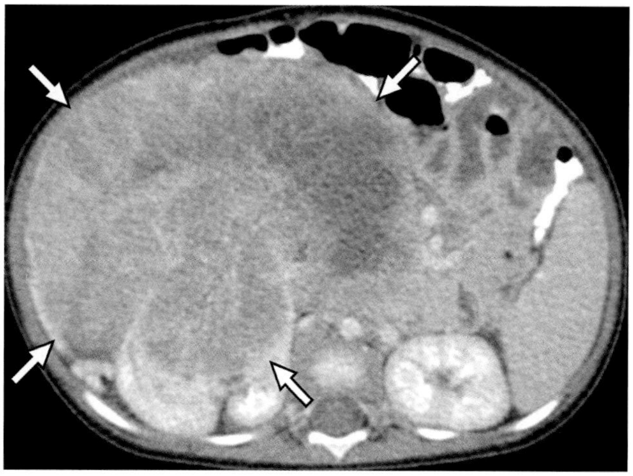

FIGURE 17.18 **7-month-old girl with right congenital mesoblastic nephroma (cellular variant).** Axial contrast-enhanced CT image demonstrates a very large, heterogeneous mass (*arrows*) arising from the right kidney with substantial mass effect upon adjacent structures.

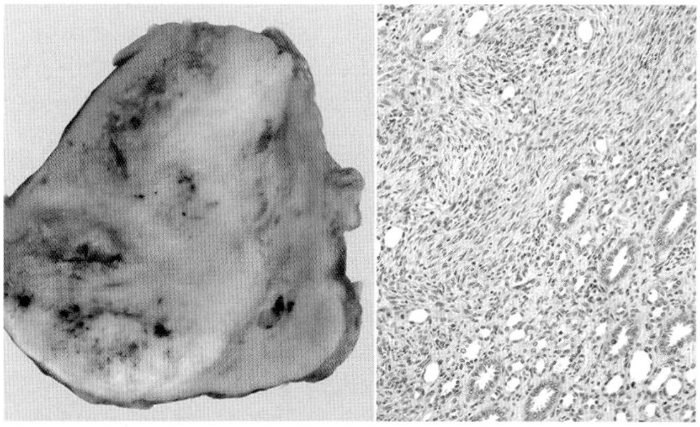

FIGURE 17.17 **Congenital mesoblastic nephroma, resected from a 2-month-old girl.** The 9 cm mass expanded and occupied the majority of the kidney tissue, showing a poorly demarcated border with normal kidney (**left**). Microscopically, the tumor consisted of a cellular fibroblastic proliferation, showing intermixed residual nonneoplastic kidney including the benign medullary tubules depicted here (**right**, hematoxylin and eosin, original magnification, 200×). This tumor harbored an *ETV6* gene rearrangement typical of cellular congenital mesoblastic nephroma, and the patient had a high serum calcium level attributed to paraneoplastic disease.

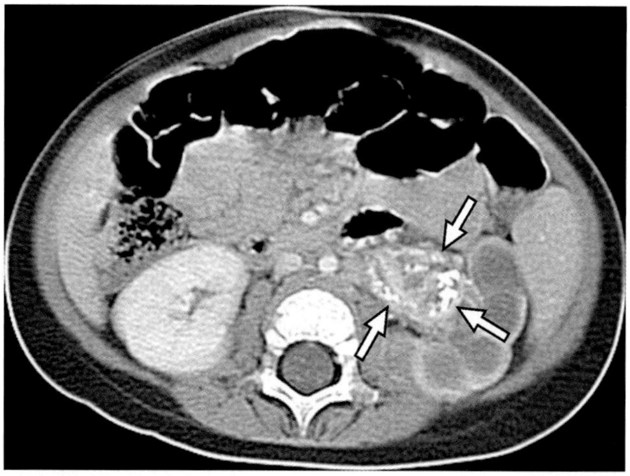

FIGURE 17.19 **10-month-old girl with ossifying renal tumor of infancy.** Axial contrast-enhanced CT image shows a partially calcified mass (*arrows*) centered in the left renal collecting system. Left caliectasis and renal parenchymal thinning are due to chronic obstruction. (Image courtesy of Edward Y. Lee, MD, MPH, Boston Children's Hospital and Harvard Medical School, Boston, MA.)

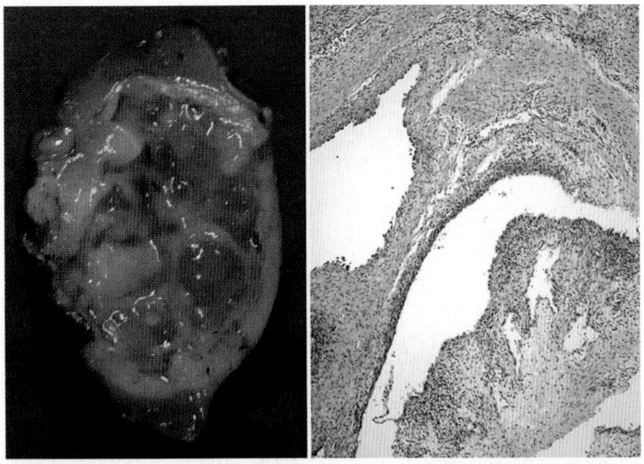

FIGURE 17.20 **Cystic nephroma in a 13-year-old girl with a known *DICER1* gene mutation and previous cervicovaginal rhabdomyosarcoma.** The cut surface (**left**) shows a well-delineated 4.5 cm mass containing multiple cysts filled with clear fluid. Microscopically, the lesion shows epithelium-lined cysts with condensation of stromal cells immediately underlying the epithelium (**right**, hematoxylin and eosin, original magnification, 100x).

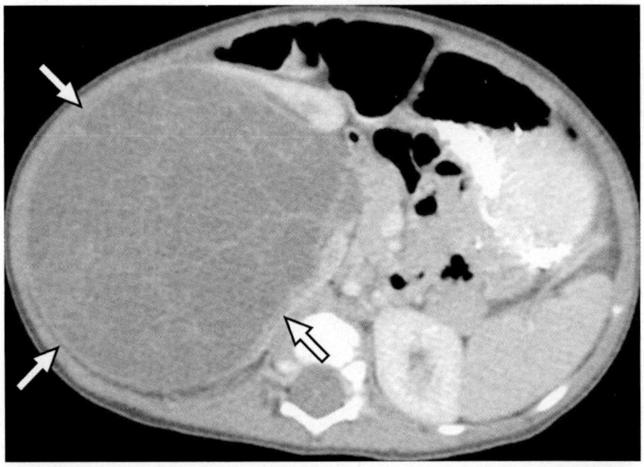

FIGURE 17.21 **Cystic partially-differentiated nephroblastoma in an 11-month-old girl with a palpable abdominal mass.** Axial contrast-enhanced CT image shows a large, cystic, heavily septated, centrally located mass (*arrows*) within the right kidney.

Cystic Nephroma and Cystic Partially Differentiated Nephroblastoma

There are generally two forms of multilocular cystic neoplasm in children: (1) multilocular cystic nephroma (MLCN) and (2) cystic partially differentiated nephroblastoma (CPDN).[49] Clinical presentations in affected children include palpable abdominal mass and hematuria. MLCN, or simply cystic nephroma, is a benign cystic lesion composed of epithelium-lined septated cysts; the childhood form is thought to be distinct from the type that occurs predominantly in adult women and commonly abuts pelvicalyceal structures (Fig. 17.20). CPDN is an intermediate lesion that is distinguished microscopically from MLCN by the presence of very primitive cells called blastema within the septa.[49] Childhood CN is associated with the familial cancer syndrome caused by *DICER1* gene mutations (a syndrome that includes pleuropulmonary blastoma, embryonal rhabdomyosarcoma, and Sertoli-Leydig cell tumor, among other tumors).

At ultrasound, both MLCN and CPDN appear similar, presenting as variably sized cystic renal masses containing numerous thin septations. On contrast-enhanced CT and MRI, mural and septal enhancement are generally present, and the lesion may bulge into the renal hilar region causing mass effect upon the collecting system (Fig. 17.21). These lesions normally have no associated solid elements. The radiologic differential diagnosis in the pediatric population includes the cystic forms of Wilms tumor and renal cell carcinoma.[49] Surgical resection, either radical or partial nephrectomy based on size and location, is generally curative.

Angiomyolipoma

Angiomyolipomas (AMLs) are benign hamartoma-like renal masses that are classified as perivascular epithelioid cell tumors (PEComas) and contain variable amounts of smooth muscle, fat, and abnormal blood vessels.[50] While sporadic lesions occur, many pediatric AMLs arise in the setting of tuberous sclerosis and may be bilateral and numerous.

At ultrasound, AMLs are variably sized and typically echogenic due to the presence of fat (Fig. 17.22). At CT, these lesions may heterogeneously enhance when large, and the presence of macroscopic fat is considered diagnostic (Hounsfield unit measurement less than −20). MRI can also be used to confirm the presence of an AML. Specific findings include loss of signal within the lesion when applying fat saturation and "India ink" artifact (black boundary artifact) on out-of-phase T1-weighted gradient-recalled echo imaging at fat–water interfaces within the mass or at its interface with the kidney (due to signal loss in voxels containing both lipid and water) (Fig. 17.23).[51] However, up to about one-third of AMLs do not contain evidence of fat by imaging, making the diagnosis challenging.[52] As AML may be complicated by life-threatening retroperitoneal hemorrhage (Wunderlich syndrome) (Fig. 17.24), serial ultrasound imaging is commonly performed to evaluate for enlarging lesions. Some recommend prophylactic embolization of large lesions (usually >4 cm) to minimize the risk of life-threatening hemorrhage.[53]

Malignant Neoplasms

Wilms Tumor and Nephroblastomatosis

Wilms tumor, or nephroblastoma, is the most common pediatric abdominal solid neoplasm, representing about 90% of pediatric renal malignancies. These tumors may clinically present with a palpable abdominal mass, abdominal pain, nausea and vomiting, hematuria, and/or hypertension. Histologically, they are triphasic, containing blastema, abortive epithelial tubular elements, and stroma (Fig. 17.25). It is common to see heterologous elements such as rhabdomyoblastic, cartilaginous, osseous, and, less often, adipocytic and neuroglial differentiation. While most Wilms tumors are sporadic (about 75%), there are several predisposing conditions, including Beckwith-Wiedemann syndrome (macroglossia,

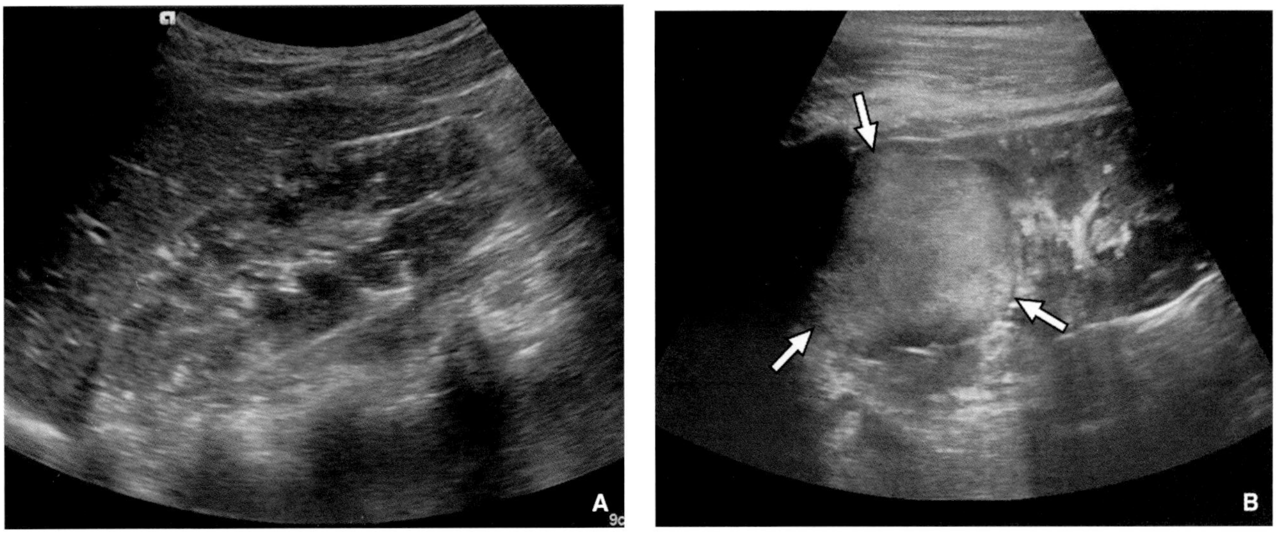

FIGURE 17.22 **7-year-old girl with tuberous sclerosis, numerous bilateral renal angiomyolipomas (AMLs), and left renal cell carcinoma. A:** Longitudinal gray-scale ultrasound image of the right kidney shows many small echogenic parenchymal lesions, consistent with AMLs. **B:** Longitudinal gray-scale ultrasound image through the left kidney shows multiple punctate echogenic AMLs as well as a 3.5 cm dominant echogenic mass (*arrows*) in the upper pole. Image-guided core needle biopsy of the large upper pole lesion revealed renal cell carcinoma, which was confirmed at surgical pathology.

hemihypertrophy, macrosomia, midline abdominal wall defects, ear anomalies, and/or neonatal hypoglycemia), sporadic aniridia, WAGR syndrome (Wilms tumor, Aniridia, Genitourinary anomalies, and mental Retardation), and Denys-Drash syndrome (gonadal dysgenesis, mesangial renal sclerosis leading to nephrotic syndrome and chronic kidney disease). All of these predisposing conditions relate to abnormalities of chromosome 11 and the *WT1* and *WT2* genes.[54,55]

Ultrasound typically reveals a large, heterogeneous mass arising from the kidney. Doppler ultrasound can be used to confirm the presence of blood flow within the mass as well as assess for extension of tumor into the renal vein and inferior vena cava. Contrast-enhanced CT and MRI typically demonstrate a large, heterogeneously enhancing renal mass that may rarely contain fat or calcification (reflecting heterologous adipose or osseous tumor components).[56] Both of these imaging modalities can also be used to assess for tumor thrombus in the renal vein and inferior vena cava (Fig. 17.26).[57] The presence of renal parenchyma wrapping around a portion of the mass ("claw sign") indicates that the lesion is likely originating from the kidney. Tumor may spread to retroperitoneal lymph nodes, lung, and, less commonly, liver. The preoperative detection of Wilms tumor rupture by imaging is challenging. A recent report from the Children's Oncology Group showed that CT has low sensitivity (54% to 70%)

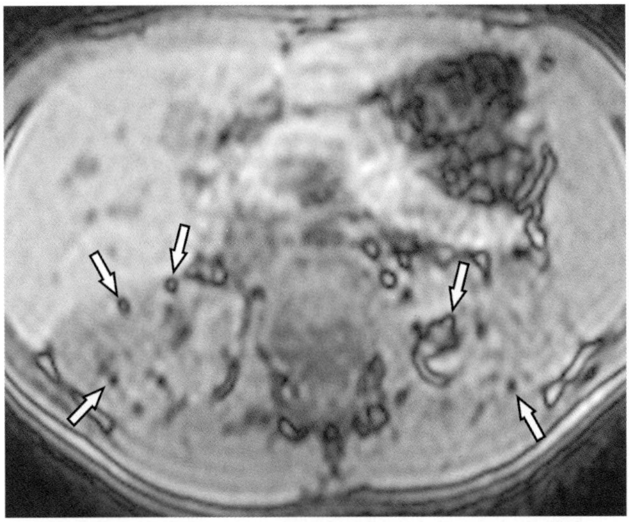

FIGURE 17.23 **13-year-old girl with tuberous sclerosis and numerous bilateral renal angiomyolipomas.** Axial out-of-phase T1-weighted gradient-recalled echo MR image demonstrates numerous areas of signal loss (*arrows*) in the kidneys ("India ink" artifact) due to the presence of lipid and water in the same voxel.

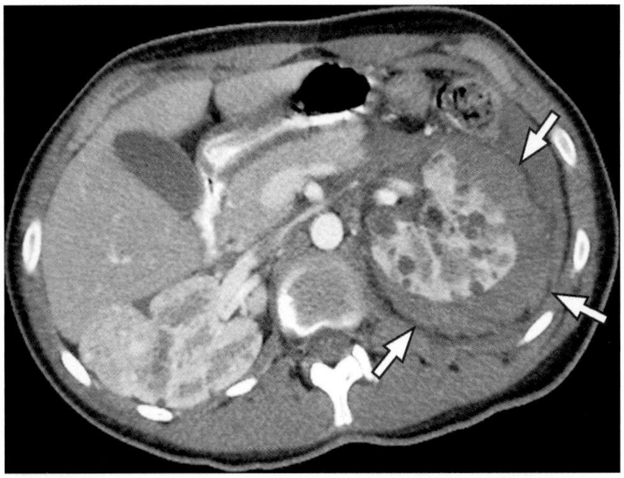

FIGURE 17.24 **17-year-old girl with life-threatening left retroperitoneal hemorrhage.** Multiple bilateral low-attenuation and enhancing renal lesions representing a combination of cysts and angiomyolipomas. High-attenuation perinephric hematoma (*arrows*) is due to a bleeding angiomyolipoma.

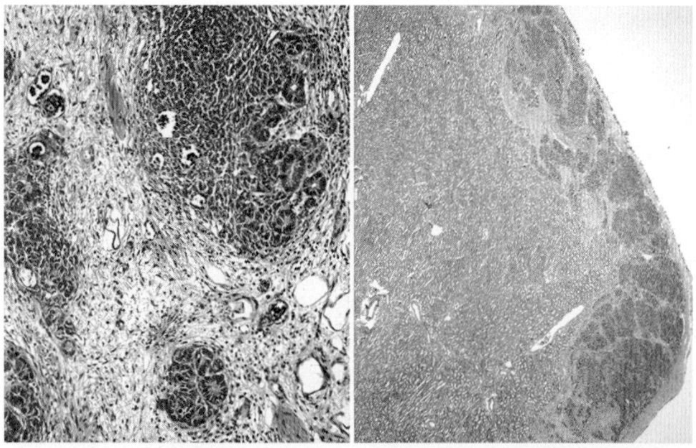

FIGURE 17.25 **3-year-old boy with bilateral Wilms tumors.** The **left image** shows triphasic differentiation, including blastemal, stromal, and epithelial elements, which here are forming abortive tubules and glomeruli (hematoxylin and eosin, original magnification, 200×). These tumors arose in a background of nephroblastomatosis (**right**), illustrated here by a perilobar nephrogenic rest (hematoxylin and eosin, original magnification, 20×).

and moderate specificity for identifying preoperative Wilms tumor rupture, with extension of ascites beyond the pelvic cul-de-sac being the best indicator.[58]

Treatment for unilateral Wilms tumor is generally radical nephrectomy with or without chemotherapy and radiation therapy.[59] Preoperative chemotherapy is generally indicated in the following settings: bilateral Wilms tumor, unilateral Wilms tumor with two or more clearly separated masses, Wilms tumor in a solitary kidney, extension of tumor thrombus above the level of the hepatic veins, tumor involving contiguous vital structures, respiratory failure due to extensive pulmonary metastases, and tumor rupture.[60] Partial nephrectomies or wedge resections may be performed in children with bilateral Wilms tumors or a solitary kidney. With appropriate therapy, 5-year survival is around 90%. Children with the predisposing conditions mentioned above typically undergo ultrasound screening for Wilms tumor every 3 months until ~8 years of age.[55]

Nephrogenic rests have been defined as foci of persistent benign embryonal cells that have the potential to develop into Wilms tumor, and they are found in nearly all bilateral Wilms tumors.[61] Nephroblastomatosis refers to multiple, sometimes diffuse, nephrogenic rests in one or both kidneys. There are two types of nephrogenic rests: (1) intralobar and (2) perilobar. While the intralobar form is at highest risk for giving rise to Wilms tumor due to its association with *WT1* and *WTX* gene mutations, it is much less common than the perilobar form.

At ultrasound, nephroblastomatosis commonly presents as multiple hypoechoic nodules within the kidneys. However, CT or MRI evaluation is preferred, as ultrasound has limited sensitivity for detecting nephrogenic rests under about 1 cm in size. Nephrogenic rests are typically hypoenhancing on contrast-enhanced CT and MR images (Fig. 17.27). Diffuse nephroblastomatosis may present with nephromegaly and a

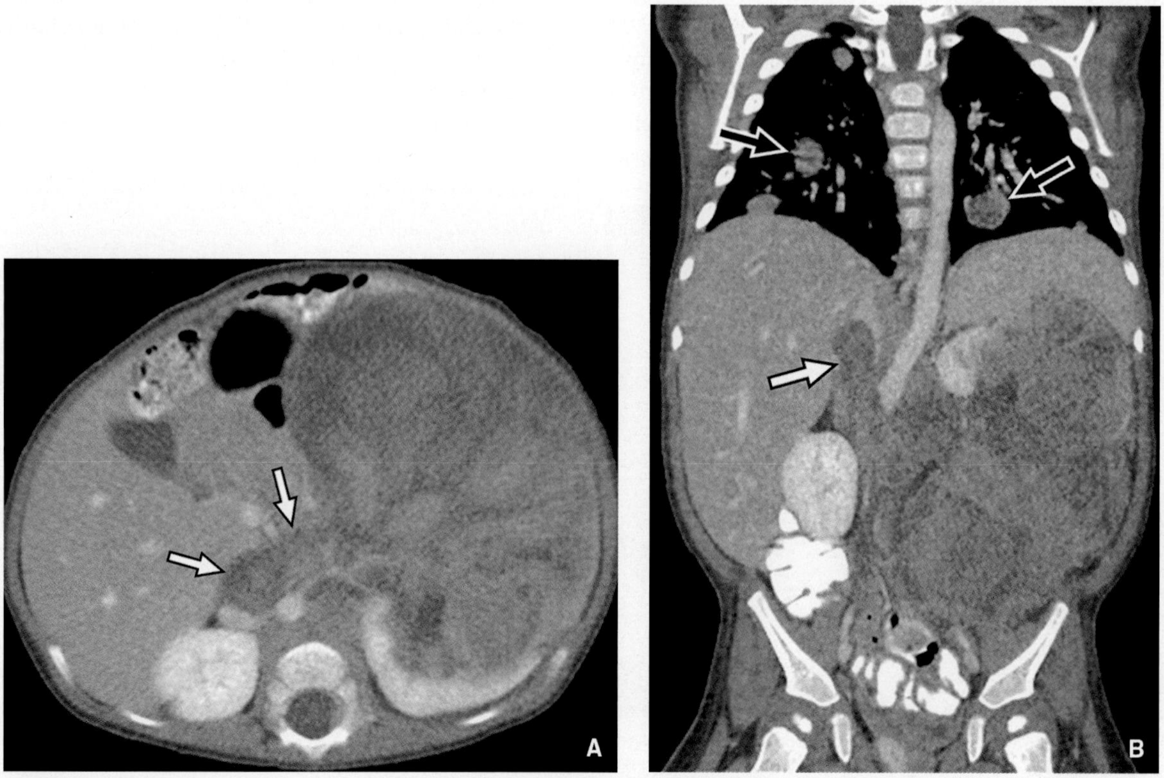

FIGURE 17.26 **14-month-old boy with a palpable abdominal mass due to left Wilms tumor. A:** Axial contrast-enhanced CT image shows a large, heterogeneously enhancing mass arising from the left kidney extending into the left renal vein (*arrows*). The "claw sign" is present. **B:** Coronal contrast-enhanced CT image shows that the mass extends into the inferior vena cava (*white arrow*). There are multiple pulmonary metastases (*black arrows*).

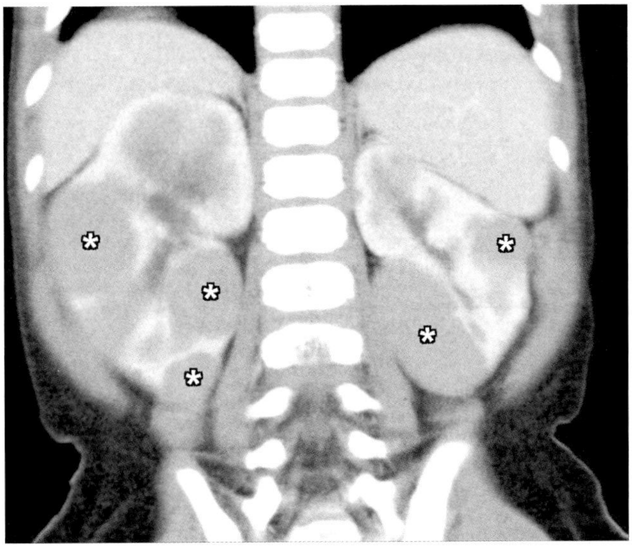

FIGURE 17.27 **11-month-old girl with Beckwith-Wiedemann syndrome, bilateral nephroblastomatosis, and presumed bilateral Wilms tumor.** Coronal contrast-enhanced CT image shows multiple bilateral low-attenuation renal masses (*asterisks*) due to nephrogenic rests and multifocal Wilms tumor.

rind-like soft tissue abnormality replacing the renal cortex (Fig. 17.28).[61,62]

Management is typically conservative with close radiologic observation, as most children with nephroblastomatosis do not develop Wilms tumor. Chemotherapy may be administered in the setting of new, enlarging, or increasingly heterogeneous nephrogenic rests, as such lesions are suspicious for Wilms tumor.[61]

Renal Cell Carcinoma

Renal cell carcinoma is the most common renal malignancy in children over the age of 10 years.[63,64] Common clinical presentations include palpable abdominal mass, flank pain, retroperitoneal hemorrhage, hypertension, and hematuria. The nomenclature of epithelial tumors in the kidney has transformed as increasing knowledge of tumor genetics has been integrated into classification schemes. Renal cell carcinomas have been increasingly subdivided based on their genetic aberrations or their genetic syndromic associations. Some of these "new" tumors occurring in childhood include MiT family translocation renal cell carcinoma (including t(6;11) renal cell carcinoma), succinic dehydrogenase B deficiency–associated renal cell carcinoma, ALK translocation renal cell carcinoma, and hereditary leiomyomatosis renal cell carcinoma syndrome–associated renal cell carcinoma. Von Hippel-Lindau disease and tuberous sclerosis are other syndromes known for conferring a predisposition to renal cell carcinoma.[65,66]

Although pediatric renal cell carcinomas average about 6 cm in size, they can be smaller or larger.[63] Ultrasound may demonstrate a solid or complex cystic renal mass containing internal blood flow upon Doppler evaluation. At CT and MRI, most renal cell carcinomas appear heterogeneous and show the "claw sign." These lesions may contain calcification (about 40%) and show evidence of intralesional or perinephric hemorrhage (about 50%) (Fig. 17.29).[63] Areas of hemorrhage are usually hyperintense on T1-weighted MR images. Renal cell carcinomas and associated metastases frequently avidly enhance on arterial-phase postcontrast CT and MR imaging. Metastatic disease most often involves regional lymph nodes, liver, lung, brain, and bone.

Treatment is typically radical nephrectomy, although partial nephrectomy may be performed in children with solitary kidney, very small lesions, or a predisposing syndrome. Unfortunately, these tumors are generally chemotherapy resistant, resulting in poor outcomes in children with metastatic disease.[67]

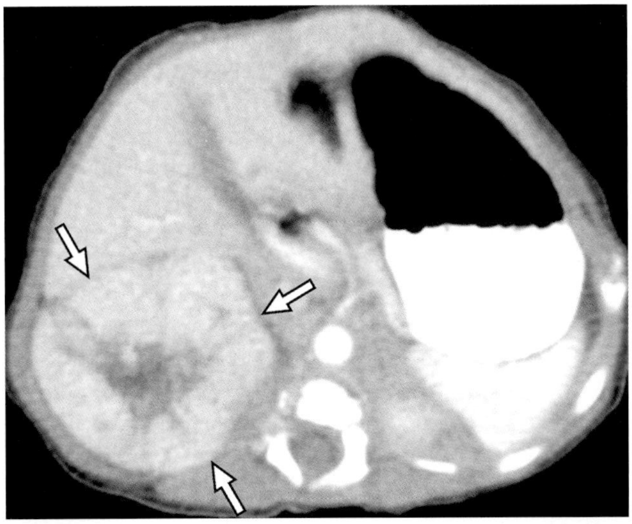

FIGURE 17.28 **2-week-old boy with multiple congenital anomalies.** Axial contrast-enhanced CT image shows right nephromegaly and rind-like parenchymal thickening (*arrows*) due to diffuse nephroblastomatosis. The patient was later treated with chemotherapy for presumed Wilms tumor as this abnormality enlarged during infancy.

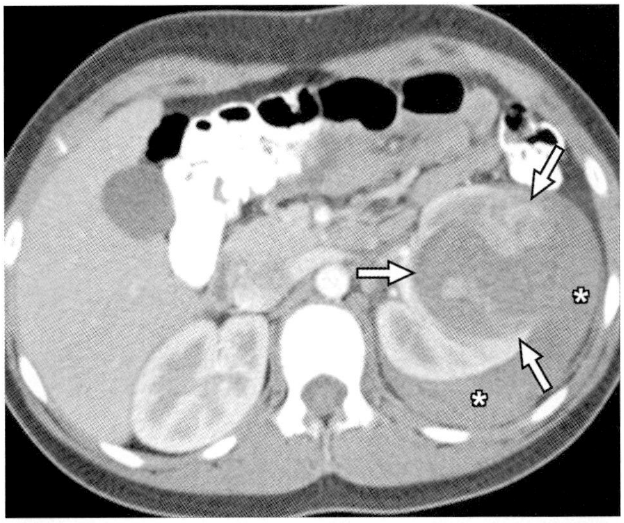

FIGURE 17.29 **11-year-old girl with left flank pain due to renal cell carcinoma.** Axial contrast-enhanced CT image shows a heterogeneously enhancing mass (*arrows*) arising from the left kidney. A large amount of high attenuation fluid (*asterisks*) in the left perinephric space is due to hemorrhage. Mildly enlarged retroperitoneal lymph nodes were proven to contain metastatic neoplasm.

Clear Cell Sarcoma of the Kidney

Clear cell sarcoma of the kidney (CCSK), formerly known as bone metastasizing renal tumor of childhood, is a rare pediatric primary renal malignancy. This tumor affects young children, on average 36 months of age.[68] Clinical presentation may be similar to Wilms tumor, including palpable abdominal mass, hematuria, and hypertension. Microscopically, undifferentiated cells arranged in cords and nests are divided by numerous small blood vessels. A subset of these tumors have been characterized by a t(10;17) translocation resulting in a *YWHAE-FAM22* gene fusion.

This renal tumor is usually very large at presentation (11 cm mean diameter) and indistinguishable from Wilms tumor at ultrasound, CT, and MRI, appearing as a heterogeneous renal mass (Fig. 17.30).[69] The "claw sign" is typically present, and both the renal vein and inferior vena cava should be assessed for tumor thrombus. CCSK has a propensity to metastasize to regional lymph nodes, bone, brain, and lung.[54] Bone scintigraphy and contrast-enhanced CT and MRI of the brain are performed at the time of initial diagnosis. Staging is similar to Wilms tumor. Treatment may include radical nephrectomy, chemotherapy, and radiation therapy and can differ from Wilms tumor, as CCSK has a poorer prognosis with higher recurrence and mortality rates.[69]

Rhabdoid Tumor of the Kidney

Rhabdoid tumor of the kidney (RTK) is a rare, highly malignant primary renal neoplasm that is usually diagnosed under the age of 2 years (11 months mean age).[70] This neoplasm is the most aggressive renal mass of childhood and portends the worst prognosis. Affected children may present with a palpable abdominal mass, hematuria, fever, and hypercalcemia.[70] RTK is associated with the development of synchronous or metachronous posterior fossa brain tumors, ususally atypical teratoid/rhabdoid tumors, in 10% to 15% of children (rhabdoid tumor predisposition syndrome, due to germline SMARC gene alterations).

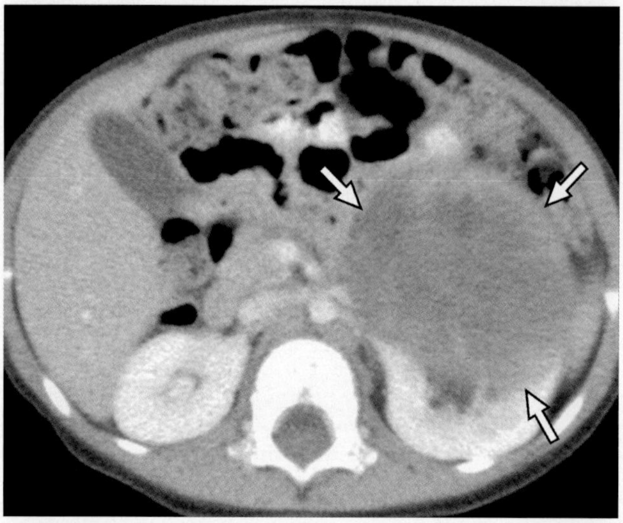

FIGURE 17.30 **1-year-old boy with palpable abdominal mass due to clear cell sarcoma of the kidney.** Axial contrast-enhanced CT image shows a large, heterogeneous mass (*arrows*) arising from the left kidney. The "claw sign" is present.

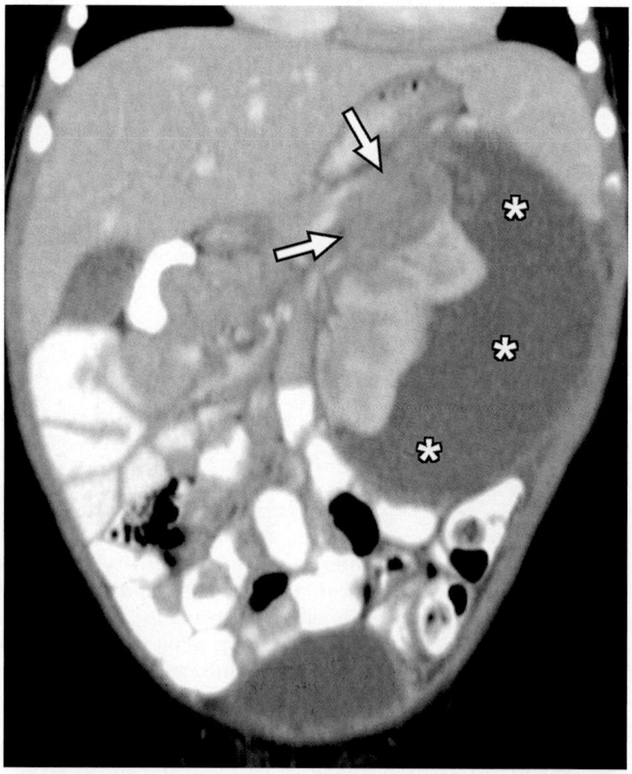

FIGURE 17.31 **1-year-old girl with rhabdoid tumor of the kidney.** Coronal contrast-enhanced CT image shows a heterogeneously enhancing mass (*arrows*) in the upper pole of the left kidney. There is a large subcapsular fluid collection (*asterisks*) that is causing mass effect on normal left kidney parenchyma. (Image courtesy of Edward Y. Lee, MD, MPH, Boston Children's Hospital and Harvard Medical School, Boston, MA.)

At imaging, these lesions are typically large, heterogeneous, and infiltrative. They can be centrally located in the kidney. Calcification, subcapsular fluid collections due to hemorrhage, and vascular invasion can be present in RTK (Fig. 17.31).[71] Metastatic disease is frequently present at the time of diagnosis or soon thereafter, is commonly multicentric, and often involves regional lymph nodes, lung, brain, and bone. Staging is similar to Wilms tumor. Treatment may include radical nephrectomy, chemotherapy, and radiation. Age at diagnosis has prognostic implications, with children <6 months old having only an 8.8% 4-year overall survival.[72]

Medullary Carcinoma of the Kidney

Renal medullary carcinoma is a rare primary renal malignancy that occurs in adolescent and young adult black individuals with sickle cell trait (or less often hemoglobin SC disease). Common clinical presentations include palpable abdominal mass, flank pain, and hematuria. Individuals affected are typically between the age of 10 and 40 years, and, interestingly, only a small percentage of these tumors are left-sided.[73,74]

At imaging, renal medullary carcinomas are generally large (7 cm mean size), heterogeneous, and centrally located within the kidney, arising from the medullary papilla (possibly the collecting duct) (Fig. 17.32). They commonly infiltrate the renal medulla and fill the renal collecting system, may cause calyceal obstruction, and often demonstrate venous and

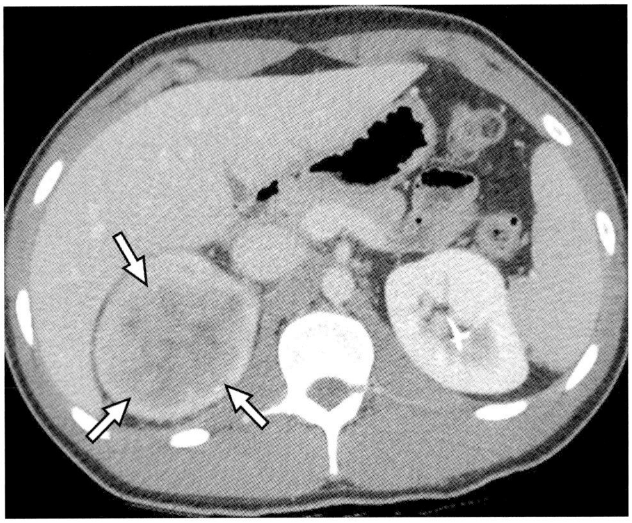

FIGURE 17.32 **21-year-old young man with sickle cell trait and right kidney medullary carcinoma.** Axial contrast-enhanced CT image shows a large, heterogeneous, infiltrative mass (*arrows*) located centrally in the right kidney. Coronal CT images (not shown) revealed extension of tumor into the proximal right ureter.

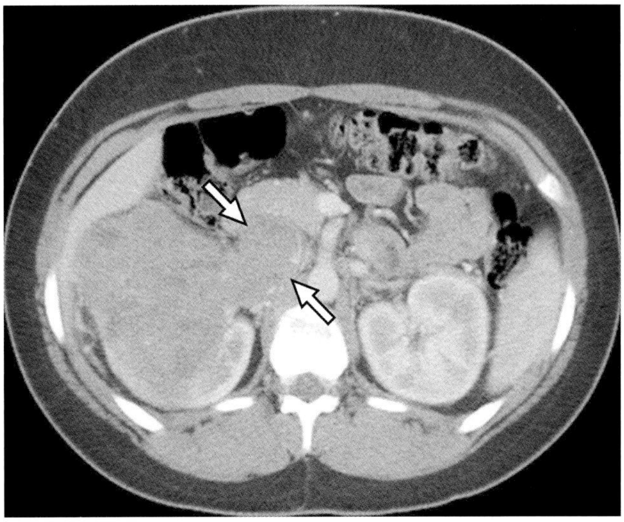

FIGURE 17.33 **14-year-old girl with flank pain and hematuria due to right kidney Ewing sarcoma/primitive neuroectodermal tumor (PNET).** Axial contrast-enhanced CT image shows a large, enhancing mass arising from the right kidney. The mass extends into the right renal vein and inferior vena cava (*arrows*).

lymphatic invasion. Renal parenchymal satellite lesions are also common.[73] This neoplasm has an extremely poor prognosis with survival typically <6 months, and it is frequently metastatic at the time of diagnosis.[74]

Ewing Sarcoma/Primitive Neuroectodermal Tumor

Ewing sarcoma (or primitive neuroectodermal tumor [PNET]) of the kidney is another extremely rare, very aggressive pediatric malignancy. It is a fairly common childhood tumor of bone and soft tissue, and the advent of molecular tissue diagnostics has aided its recognition in visceral organs, such as the kidney. These tumors most commonly arise in adolescents and young adults, although cases have been described in very young children and the elderly. With primary kidney involvement, reported clinical presentations include flank pain and hematuria.[75] This small round blue cell neoplasm classically shows CD99 (MIC2) antigen positivity along tumor cell membranes, and it characteristically contains chromosomal rearrangements in which the *EWSR1* gene is fused to a member of the ETS family of transcription factor genes.[76]

Imaging generally reveals a large, heterogeneous, infiltrative mass arising from the kidney.[77] Tumor may extend to involve the renal vein and inferior vena cava (Fig. 17.33).[78,79] Up to two-thirds of affected individuals have metastatic disease at diagnosis, often involving the lungs and bone marrow.[75] These tumors may mimic other primary renal malignancies of childhood, including Wilms tumor. Preoperative neoadjuvant chemotherapy is commonly administered if Ewing sarcoma of the kidney is diagnosed prior to radical nephrectomy. Median overall survival is about 24 months in patients with metastatic disease.[75]

Renal Lymphoma and Leukemia

Lymphoma

Involvement of the kidneys by lymphoma is relatively common and typically secondary to hematogenous dissemination, or less often, contiguous extension of retroperitoneal disease. Renal involvement in children is most often seen in the Burkitt subtype of non-Hodgkin lymphoma.

At ultrasound and CT, bilateral hypoechoic or low-attenuation renal masses, respectively, are the most common imaging appearance (Fig. 17.34). Less common presentations

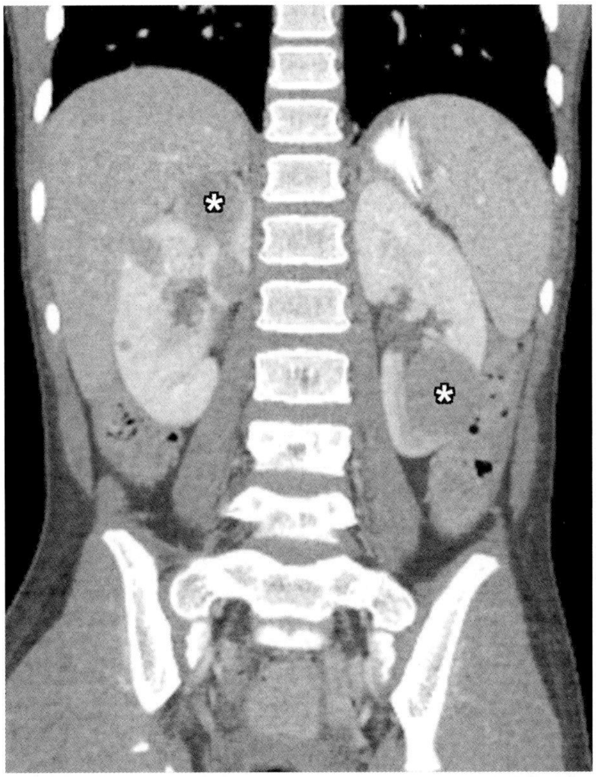

FIGURE 17.34 **5-year-old boy with renal involvement by Burkitt lymphoma, identified after presentation with a palatine tonsillar mass.** Coronal contrast-enhanced CT image shows bilateral hypoenhancing solid renal masses (*asterisks*) due to lymphomatous deposits.

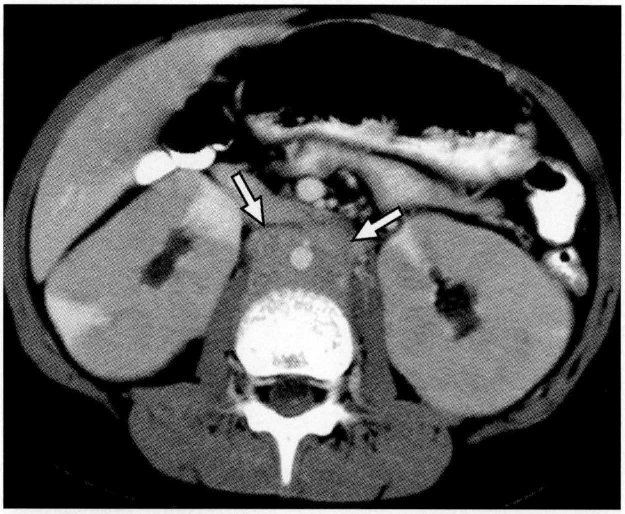

FIGURE 17.35 **12-year-old boy with acute leukemia.** Axial contrast-enhanced CT image shows very large areas of geographic low attenuation in both kidneys due to leukemia. The kidneys are enlarged, and abnormal soft tissue (*arrows*) encases the abdominal aorta.

include a solitary renal mass or large retroperitoneal mass engulfing the kidney.[80] Nearby retroperitoneal lymph node enlargement is common. Renal lymphomatous deposits typically regress with chemotherapy.

Leukemia

The kidneys may also be a site of infiltration by leukemic disease, most often in the setting of acute lymphoblastic leukemia in children. Renal leukemic involvement is relatively infrequently observed by imaging, as most pediatric patients with acute leukemia do not undergo routine CT staging or surveillance (unlike lymphoma).

Multiple bilateral hypoechoic (at ultrasound) or low-attenuation (at CT) masses are the most common imaging appearance of renal leukemia. Other presentations include a solitary renal mass and geographic (or wedge-shaped) renal parenchymal low attenuation at contrast-enhanced CT (Fig. 17.35).[81] Bilateral renal enlargement is also common, even when focal renal parenchymal lesions are not apparent. Similar to lymphoma, renal leukemic deposits usually regress with chemotherapy.

Traumatic Disorders

Renal trauma in the pediatric population most often occurs in the setting of blunt abdominal trauma (e.g., motor vehicle accident or fall from a height); penetrating renal trauma is less common. Grading of renal trauma is commonly performed using the American Association for the Surgery of Trauma classification system based upon extent of parenchymal injury as well as involvement of the collecting system and renal hilum (Table 17.2).[82]

A variety of findings may be seen at ultrasound and contrast-enhanced CT, including focal parenchymal contusion, subcapsular hematoma, and laceration. Renal contusion may appear as focally altered renal parenchymal echogenicity or attenuation at ultrasound and CT, respectively. Lacerations are usually linear parenchymal defects that may contain fluid (urine and/or blood). When lacerations extend into the central kidney, delayed postcontrast CT imaging should be performed to assess for extravasation of contrast material from the renal collecting system into the perinephric space (urinoma) and to determine if the UPJ is intact (Fig. 17.36). "Shattered" kidney and complete devascularization of the kidney due to hilar injury are the most severe forms of renal injury (Fig. 17.37).

TABLE 17.2 American Association for the Surgery of Trauma Kidney Injury Grading Scale

Grade	Injury Pattern
1	Contusion or nonexpanding subcapsular hematoma without parenchymal laceration
2	Nonexpanding perinephric hematoma or parenchymal laceration <1 cm in depth without urinary extravasation
3	Parenchymal laceration >1 cm without urinary extravasation
4	Parenchymal laceration extending through cortex, medulla, and collecting system with urinary extravasation or vascular injury involving the main renal artery (or vein) with contained hematoma or segmental infarctions without associated lacerations
5	Completely shattered kidney or devascularized kidney due to renal hilar avulsion

From http://www.aast.org/Library/TraumaTools/InjuryScoringScales.aspx

In hemodynamically stable children, management is most often conservative.[83] Recent studies in children have shown that nonoperative management is highly successful,[84] with at least partial renal preservation in most patients. Radical nephrectomy is rarely indicated in pediatric renal trauma (e.g., in the setting of irreparable vascular injury and severe hemodynamic instability).

Postprocedure Complications

A variety of complications may be diagnosed following renal percutaneous interventional procedures (e.g., percutaneous needle biopsy, percutaneous nephrostomy) in children. Bleeding along the surface of the kidney into the perinephric space can be easily detected by ultrasound, appearing as a focal fluid collection. Echogenicity of the fluid collection depends on the age of the hematoma. Perinephric hematomas are very common, most often clinically insignificant, and

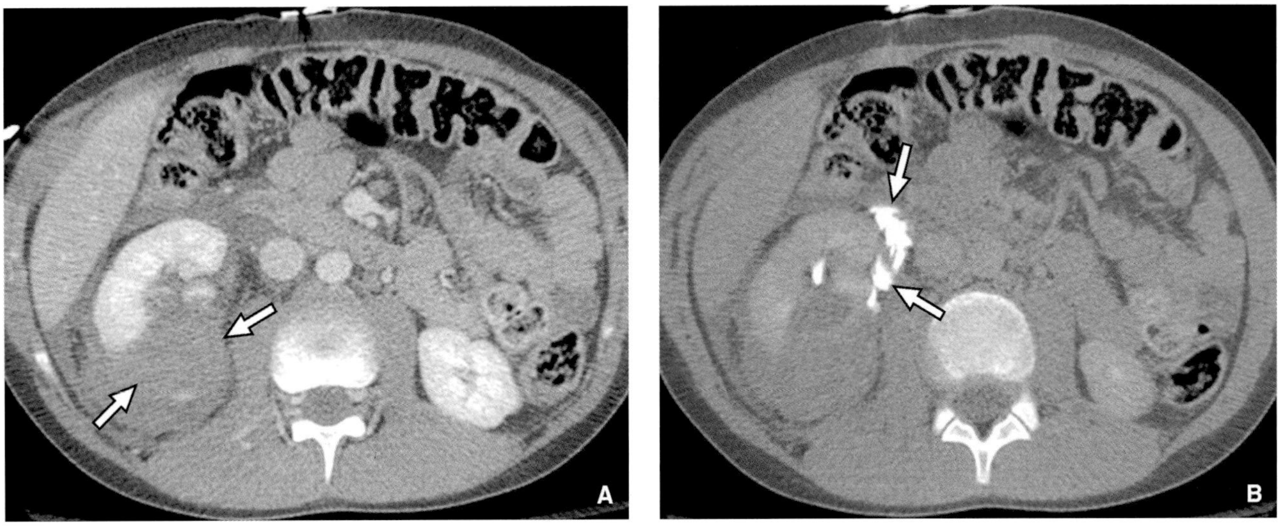

FIGURE 17.36 **12-year-old boy in bicycle accident with right kidney laceration. A:** Axial contrast-enhanced nephrographic phase CT image shows a large area of posterior right kidney hypoenhancement (*between arrows*). A large amount of fluid (blood and/or urine) is present in the right retroperitoneum. **B:** Axial contrast-enhanced excretory-phase CT image shows extravasation of excreted contrast material (*arrows*) into the right perinephric space due to collecting system injury.

vary in size from very small to quite large.[85,86] Extravasation of intravascular contrast material on contrast-enhanced CT suggests active bleeding that may require treatment (e.g., arterial embolization). On occasion, hemorrhage may be confined between the renal capsule and underlying parenchyma. Subcapsular hematomas are generally crescentic or elliptical in shape and exert mass effect upon underlying renal parenchyma (Fig. 17.38). Acute and subacute subcapsular hematomas demonstrate higher attenuation than water at CT. On occasion, subcapsular hematomas and associated renal compression may cause renal failure and renin-mediated hypertension (so-called Page kidney).[87]

Arteriovenous fistulas occur when there is injury to an adjacent artery and vein within the kidney with resultant abnormal communication. These lesions are usually diagnosed by ultrasound and best appreciated on color and spectral Doppler evaluation. Color Doppler imaging reveals focally increased renal vascularity with aliasing. Spectral Doppler typically shows increased arterial systolic velocity and dia-

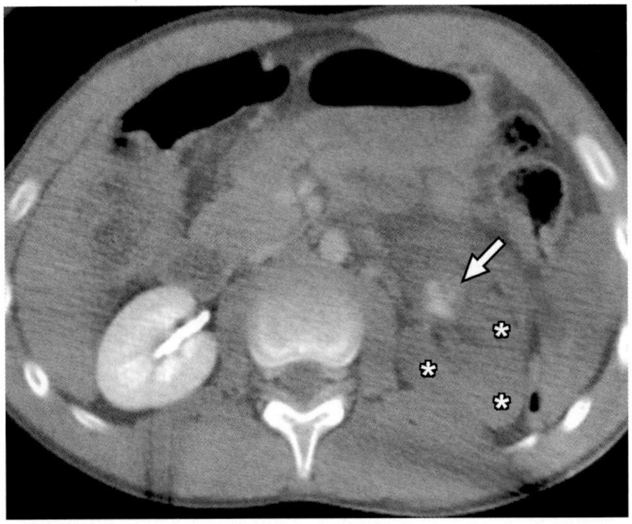

FIGURE 17.37 **13-year-old boy with blunt abdominal trauma and left renal artery injury.** Axial contrast-enhanced excretory-phase CT image shows complete absence of left kidney parenchymal enhancement (*asterisks*). A contrast-filled pseudoaneurysm (*arrow*) is present in the left renal hilar region.

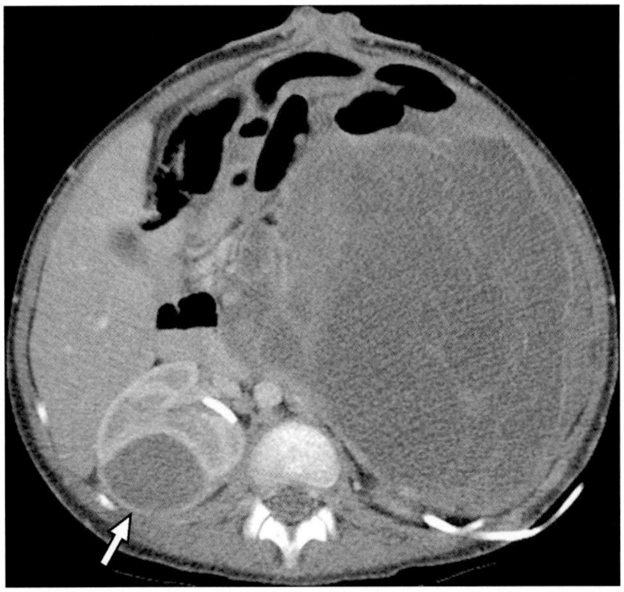

FIGURE 17.38 **8-year-old boy with obstructed right kidney due to large intra-abdominal rhabdomyosarcoma.** Axial contrast-enhanced CT image shows a traumatic right kidney subcapsular hematoma (*arrow*) related to percutaneous nephrostomy tube placement. The hematoma has mass effect upon adjacent renal parenchyma.

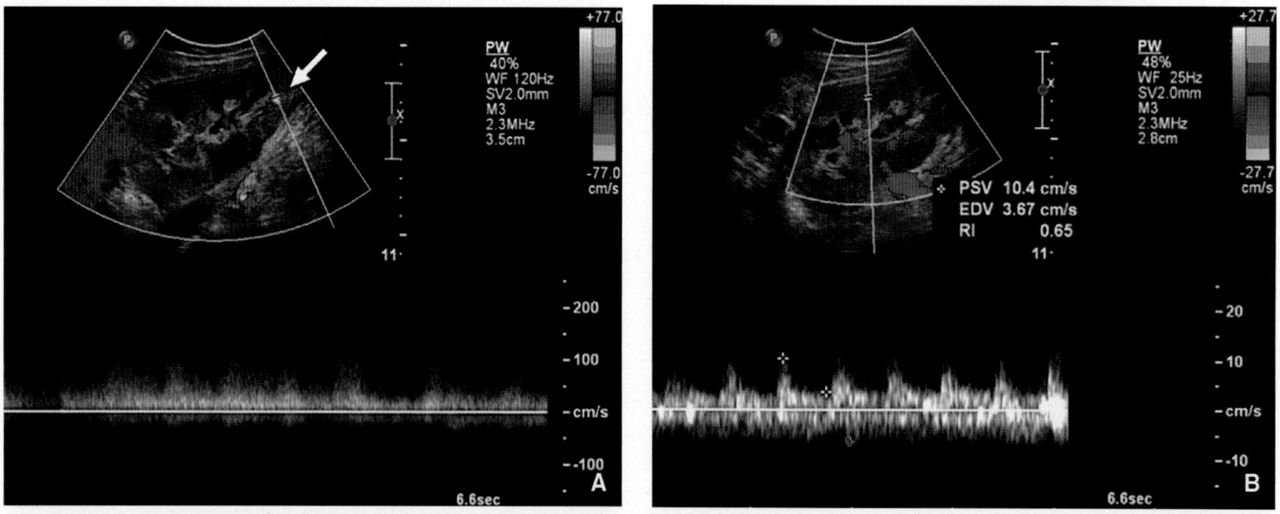

FIGURE 17.39 **11-year-old boy with left lower quadrant renal allograft status post percutaneous biopsy. A:** Longitudinal spectral Doppler ultrasound image shows a focus of very high arterial peak systolic velocity with increased diastolic blood flow in the lower pole of the transplant kidney (*arrow*), consistent with arteriovenous fistula from recent biopsy. **B:** Interrogation of an interpolar arcuate artery shows a normal spectral Doppler waveform.

stolic blood flow as well as "arterialization" of venous blood flow with increased turbulence (Fig. 17.39).[85] Many of these lesions are small and involute without intervention, although large lesions may persist and require arterial embolization.[86]

Pseudoaneurysm is a rare (incidence <1%) complication of percutaneous interventional procedures that is due to focal arterial wall disruption.[88] These lesions most often appear as intrarenal cyst-like structures on gray-scale ultrasound evaluation.[88] However, color Doppler imaging shows swirling blood flow within the lesion, sometimes with a "yin–yang" appearance. Renal pseudoaneurysms can be treated with selective arterial embolization.

Nonneoplastic Cystic Disorders

Benign Epithelial Cysts

While prevalence increases with age, benign epithelial renal cysts are increasingly common in the pediatric population. This likely relates, at least in part, to the rising use of medical imaging in children as well as improvements in ultrasound image quality. At ultrasound, many of these cysts are solitary, simple, and anechoic with thin, imperceptible walls, demonstrating posterior acoustic through-transmission.

Simple renal cysts show no internal complexity or enhancement at CT or MRI (Figs. 17.40 and 17.41). Benign epithelial cysts can sometimes appear complicated, containing thin septations, mural calcification, and/or internal debris (Fig. 17.42). When renal cystic lesions have mural nodularity or solid elements, a diagnosis other than benign epithelial cyst should be considered. Although most benign renal cysts in children are asymptomatic, occasional lesions may be symptomatic due to hemorrhage or very large size. Image-guided percutaneous aspiration or sclerotherapy in children has been described.[89]

The Bosniak classification system for risk assessment, while not validated in the pediatric population, has been shown useful for directing the management of pediatric renal cysts.[90]

Autosomal Dominant Polycystic Kidney Disease

Autosomal dominant polycystic kidney disease (ADPKD) is an inherited disorder that affects the kidneys as well as other organs. In some instances, this condition is noninherited due to a spontaneous genetic mutation. While ADPKD is most

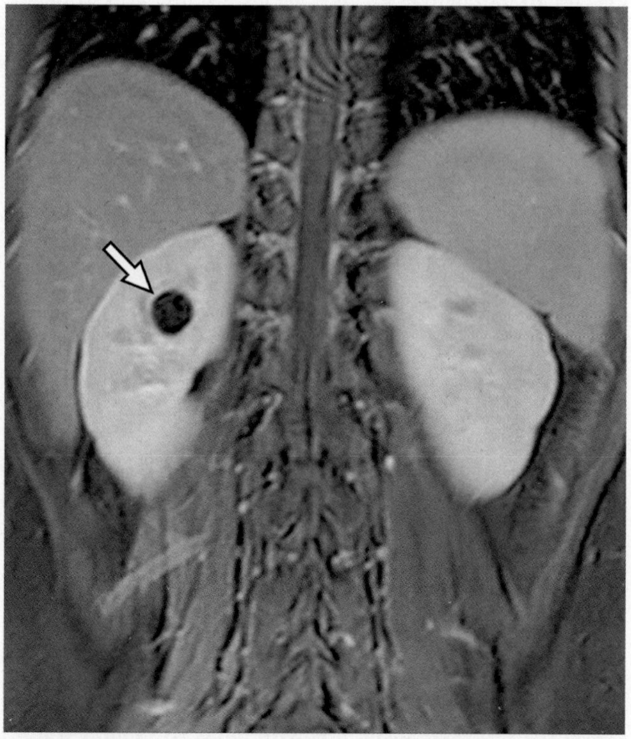

FIGURE 17.40 **16-year-old girl with incidentally detected simple renal cyst.** Coronal postcontrast T1-weighted fat-saturated MR image shows a 1.5-cm circumscribed, nonenhancing lesion (*arrow*) in the right kidney upper pole. There is no internal complexity.

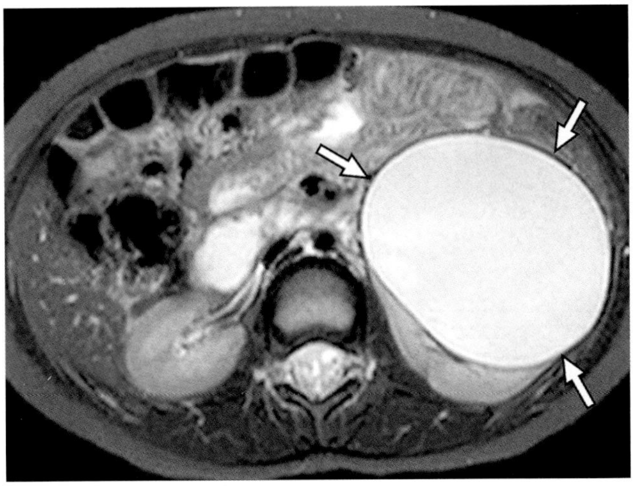

FIGURE 17.41 **3-year-old girl with palpable abdominal mass due to a large left renal simple cyst.** Axial T2-weighted fat-saturated MR image demonstrates a large left kidney cyst (*arrows*) without mural thickening or internal complexity.

often diagnosed during adulthood, it can present during childhood. ADPKD is classified as a "ciliopathy" and can be due to a mutation in either the *PKD1* (85%) or *PKD2* (15%) gene.[91]

Imaging of the kidneys is often normal early in life. Characteristically, over time, the kidneys become enlarged and develop an increasing number of variably sized renal cysts (Fig. 17.43). Although most cysts are simple, they can be complicated, containing debris, septations, and calcifications. Hemorrhagic or infected cysts often appear hyperdense at CT. Ultrasound can demonstrate abnormally echogenic renal parenchyma with loss of corticomedullary differentiation in some children.[92] Cysts may also be detected in numerous other organs, such as the liver, spleen, pancreas, testis, seminal vesicles, and prostate gland. Ultimately, most affected individuals eventually require dialysis or renal transplantation due to end-stage chronic kidney disease. Affected children should be screened for hypertension and early renal dysfunction.[93] While there is an increased frequency of intracranial aneurysms in ADPKD patients, such aneurysms are only rarely symptomatic during childhood.[94]

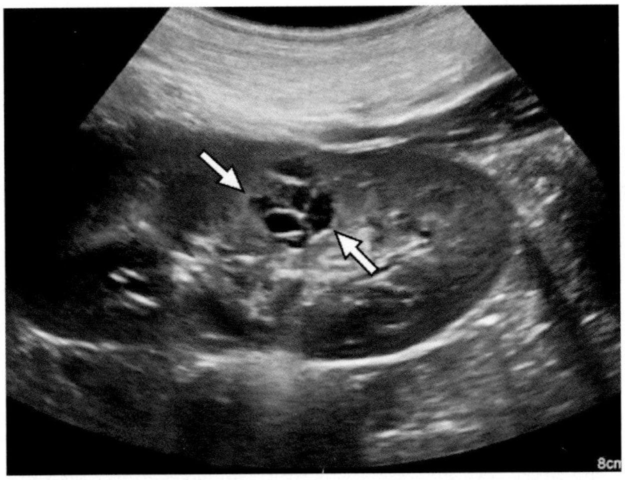

FIGURE 17.42 **9-year-old girl with enuresis.** Longitudinal gray-scale ultrasound image through the left kidney lower pole shows a complicated cyst (*arrows*) containing multiple septations.

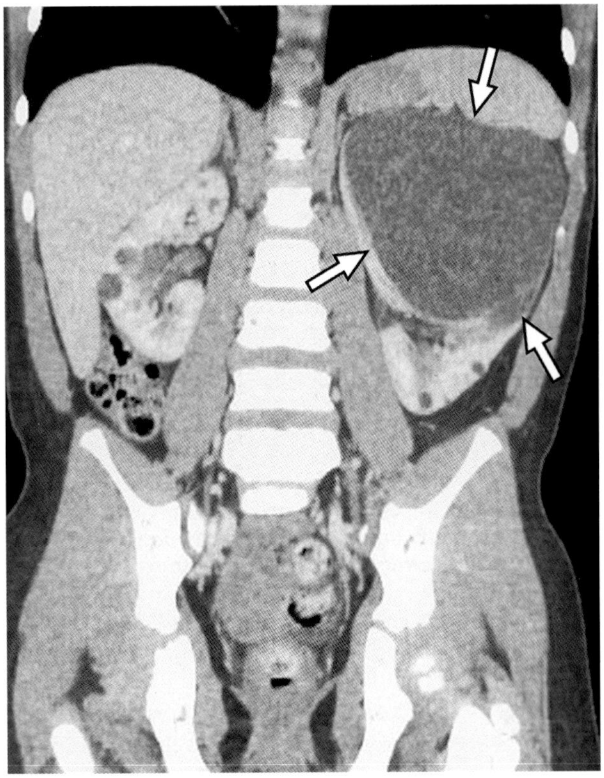

FIGURE 17.43 **7-year-old boy with autosomal dominant polycystic kidney disease.** Coronal contrast-enhanced CT image shows multiple bilateral simple renal cysts. The left kidney is enlarged, and a very large cyst (*arrows*) arises from its upper pole.

Autosomal Recessive Polycystic Kidney Disease

ARPKD is another inheritable ciliopathy that affects the kidneys as well as other organs.[91] As this condition is autosomal recessive, it is much less common than ADPKD. ARPKD most often presents during the neonatal period or infancy and, less often, later in childhood. Antenatal detection has also been described. Common clinical presentations early in life include Potter sequence due to oligohydramnios (including pulmonary hypoplasia) and bilateral palpable abdominal masses.

At ultrasound, the kidneys appear enlarged and echogenic with loss of corticomedullary differentiation.[95] The kidneys contain many tiny cystic structures (ectatic, nonobstructed tubules and ducts) that are best seen using a high-frequency linear transducer, although macrocysts may be observed in some children (Figs. 17.44 and 17.45). Renal cortical sparing has been described in some children, and scattered hyperechoic nonshadowing foci in the kidneys have been associated with the onset of renal failure.[92,95]

A variety of hepatic ductal plate abnormalities are observed in ARPKD. These liver abnormalities may be most severe in children that present with ARPKD later in childhood and that

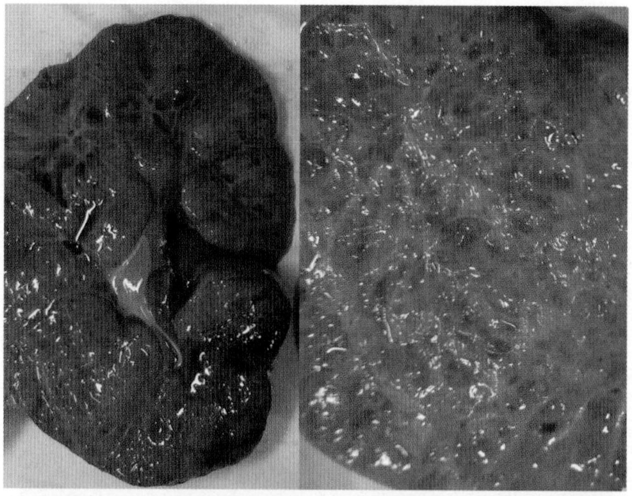

FIGURE 17.44 **Diffusely enlarged (14.5 cm) kidney from a 6-day-old girl with autosomal recessive polycystic kidney disease who underwent bilateral nephrectomy to ameliorate respiratory distress.** Close gross inspection (**right**) shows innumerable small cysts, some oriented with their long axis perpendicular to the kidney capsule.

have less severe renal involvement. Such abnormalities include congenital hepatic fibrosis and bile duct ectasia (Caroli syndrome), with associated splenomegaly, portosystemic varices, and ascites due to portal hypertension.[96] Almost all individuals affected by ARPKD require dialysis or renal transplantation by adulthood, sometimes very early in life.

Renal Cysts Associated with Syndromes

Several other syndromes are associated with renal cysts. Children with von Hippel-Lindau disease and tuberous sclerosis, both autosomal dominant phakomatoses, often

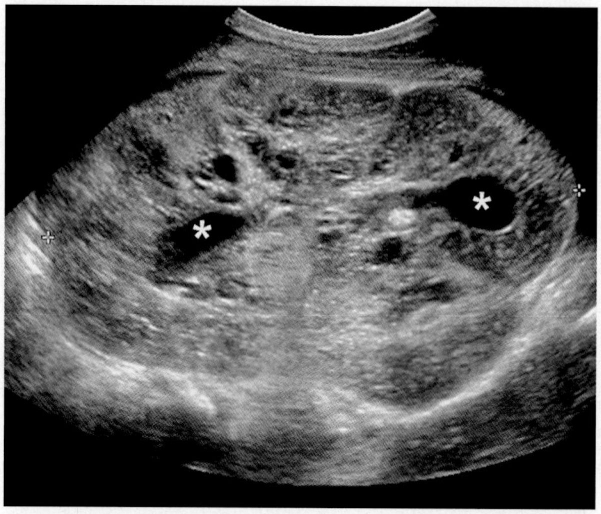

FIGURE 17.45 **6-month-old boy who presented with cardiac arrest, respiratory failure, and marked abdominal distention.** Longitudinal gray-scale ultrasound image through the left kidney reveals nephromegaly and loss of parenchymal corticomedullary differentiation. Numerous tiny cystic structures are present throughout the kidney. Findings are consistent with autosomal recessive polycystic kidney disease. The left renal collecting system is mildly dilated (*asterisks*).

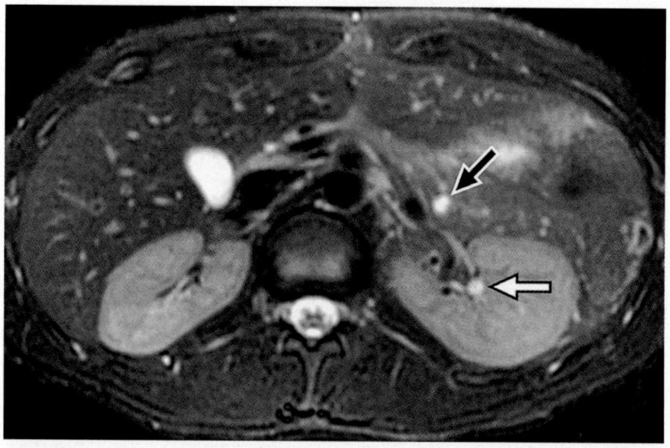

FIGURE 17.46 **19-year-old man with von Hippel-Lindau disease.** Axial T2-weighted fat-saturated MR image shows a centrally located simple cyst in the left kidney (*white arrow*; two other small cysts were also present in the left kidney, not shown). Multiple small cystic lesions (*black arrow*) are also present in the pancreas.

develop renal cysts, commonly bilateral and multiple (Figs. 17.46 and 17.47).[97,98] Some renal cysts in von Hippel-Lindau patients are likely premalignant.[99] Both von Hippel-Lindau disease and tuberous sclerosis are also associated with the development of renal cell carcinoma during childhood (Figs. 17.22 and 17.47), while tuberous sclerosis is also associated with renal AMLs. Renal cysts also arise in children with other syndromes, including Joubert syndrome, Meckel-Gruber syndrome, and asphyxiating thoracic dysplasia (Jeune syndrome), all of which are ciliopathies.[100]

Vascular Disorders

Renal Artery Stenosis

Hypertension is uncommon in the pediatric population, with many cases having an identifiable secondary cause. Renin-mediated hypertension is responsible for 2% to 10% of cases, due to either aortic and/or renal artery narrowing.[101] Clinically, renovascular hypertension is often severe and refractory to medical therapy, and it may be associated with the development of numerous complications, such as hypertensive encephalopathy, stroke, cardiac dysfunction, kidney injury, and retinopathy. There are numerous causes of renal artery narrowing in children, including developmental arteriopathy (sometimes referred to as fibromuscular dysplasia), vasculitis (e.g., Takayasu arteritis), thromboembolic complication of umbilical artery catheterization, and a variety of syndromes (e.g., neurofibromatosis, type 1, and Williams syndrome). Early detection of renovascular hypertension allows for potential endovascular or surgical cure, fewer hypertension-related complications, and decreased need for antihypertensive medications.

Catheter-based digitally subtracted angiography (CBDSA) is the gold standard for detecting and characterizing renal artery narrowings and allows therapeutic intervention in some children. This imaging modality can thoroughly assess extra- and intrarenal (including high-order branch) steno-

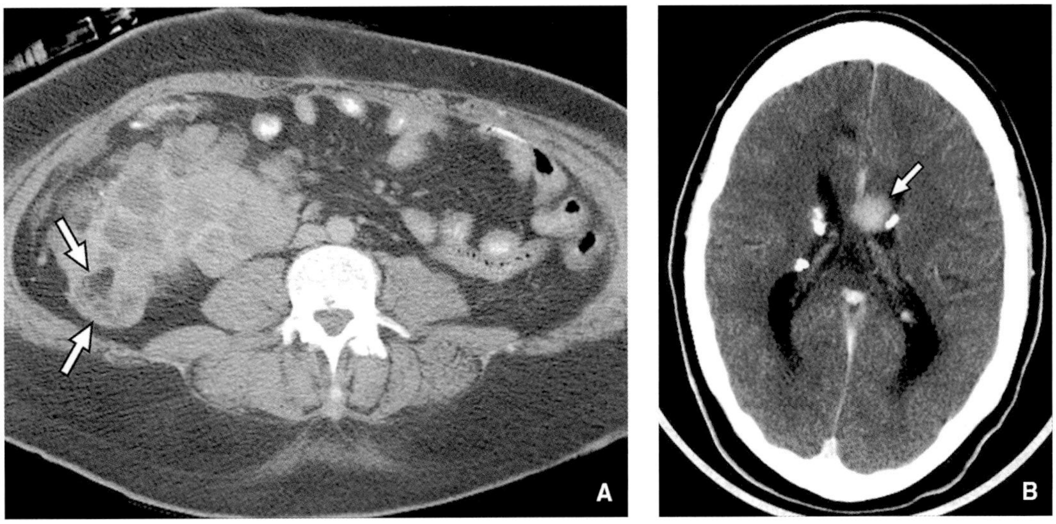

FIGURE 17.47 **16-year-old girl with tuberous sclerosis. A:** Axial contrast-enhanced CT image of the inferior right kidney confirms the presence of numerous renal cysts, several of which are complicated by hemorrhage (high attenuation). A fat-containing angiomyolipoma (*arrows*) is also present. Upon right nephrectomy, multifocal renal cell carcinoma was also discovered. **B:** Axial noncontrast CT image confirms the diagnosis of tuberous sclerosis, demonstrating calcified subependymal nodules and a hyperattenuating subependymal giant cell astrocytoma (*arrow*) arising from the left foramen of Monro.

ses, measure pressure gradients, as well as evaluate the aorta (Figs. 17.48 and 17.49). CBDSA has superior spatial resolution compared to other imaging modalities, detects accessory renal artery stenoses, and allows for simultaneous endovascular therapy of certain lesions.[102] Renal artery stenoses are frequently intrarenal in children,[102] and bilateral lesions occur in about 40%.[103] Aneurysm formation is also common, often poststenotic in location (Fig. 17.49).

While renal Doppler sonography is nonionizing, low cost, and widely available, it is operator dependent and may be limited for the detection of intrarenal and accessory renal artery stenoses. A recent study by Castelli et al., has shown that renal Doppler sonography is sensitive for detecting suprarenal aortic and main renal artery narrowings based on intrarenal spectral Doppler tardus parvus waveforms and/or abnormally low resistive index measurements (<0.5) (Fig. 17.48).[104] CT and MR angiography are also sometimes used to evaluate suspected renovascular hypertension in children, although there are scant data showing the accuracy of these imaging modalities in this age group, particularly for evaluating intrarenal and accessory renal artery stenoses. When renal artery stenosis is identified in a child, other abdominopelvic major arterial structures (including the aorta and splanchnic circulation) also should be carefully evaluated.

Definitive surgical correction may require renal artery reimplantation, bypass of the stenosis (aortorenal or iliorenal), focal renal arterioplasty, or stenosis resection with primary reanastomosis.[103] In a study evaluating renal artery angioplasty in children, clinical benefit was demonstrated in 10 of 18 patients.[105] Radical nephrectomy may be necessary to

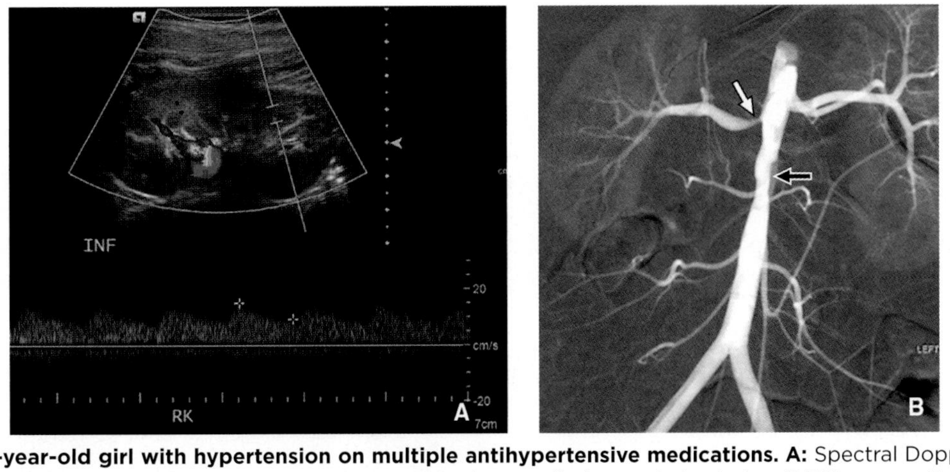

FIGURE 17.48 **8-year-old girl with hypertension on multiple antihypertensive medications. A:** Spectral Doppler image of the right kidney shows intrarenal tardus parvus waveforms with abnormally low resistive index (0.38), suggesting more proximal renal artery or aortic narrowing. **B:** Digitally subtracted conventional angiogram image shows moderate to severe narrowing of the proximal right renal artery (*white arrow*). The infrarenal abdominal aorta is mildly narrowed (*black arrow*), with an irregular contour.

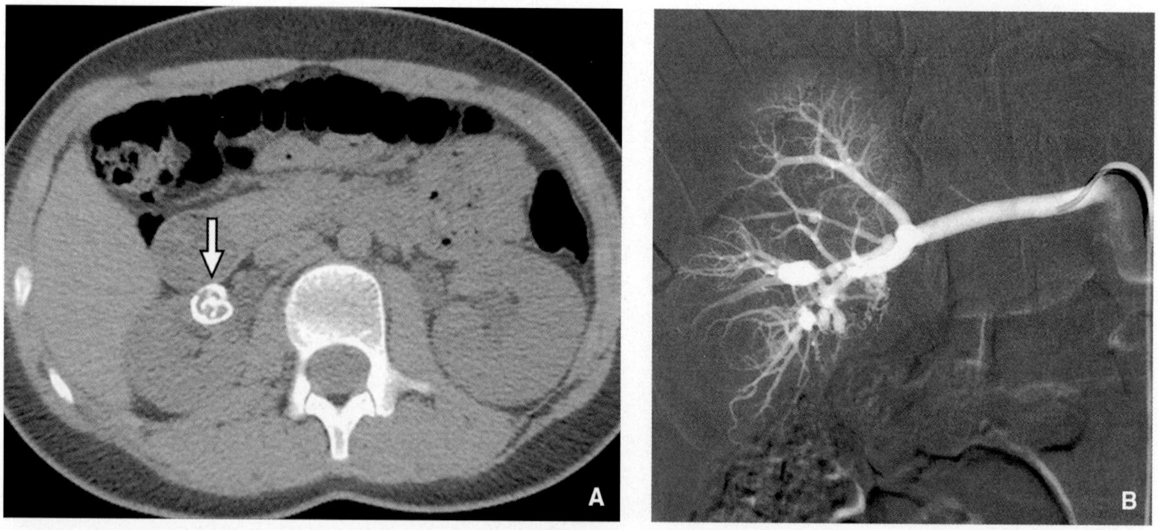

FIGURE 17.49 **12-year-old boy with medical refractory hypertension. A:** Axial noncontrast CT image shows a peripherally calcified, thrombosed aneurysm (*arrow*) in the right renal hilum. **B:** Digitally subtracted conventional angiogram image shows multiple right intrarenal arterial aneurysms, arterial occlusions, and collateral vessels.

control hypertension when vascular lesions are not amenable to surgical repair or endovascular therapy.

Renal Vein Thrombosis

Renal vein thrombosis during childhood most often occurs during the neonatal period. Predisposing factors include dehydration, sepsis, maternal diabetes mellitus, and catheterization of the inferior vena cava.[106] Causes of renal vein thrombosis in older children include renal malignancy and nephrotic syndrome.[107] The ipsilateral kidney is commonly enlarged and heterogeneous at ultrasound, CT, and MRI with loss of corticomedullary differentiation (Fig. 17.50).[108] Renal Doppler ultrasound may reveal absent blood flow in the main renal vein, while intrarenal spectral Doppler evaluation classically shows pandiastolic reversal of arterial blood flow (resistive index >1) in the acute setting. Postcontrast CT and MRI may reveal a filling defect in the renal vein. Bilateral renal vein thrombosis is common.[109] Management typically includes treatment of any underlying condition and anticoagulation. Infarction with subsequent renal atrophy is a potential complication of renal vein thrombosis.[106] Imaging findings that may predict renal atrophy include markedly reduced perfusion at diagnosis, subcapsular collections, patchy cortical echotexture, and profoundly hypoechoic and irregular renal pyramids.[109]

Nutcracker Syndrome

Nutcracker syndrome refers to symptomatic compression of the left renal vein as it passes between the abdominal aorta and superior mesenteric artery. This condition is uncommon in children and may present with abdominal or flank pain, hematuria, and, less often, varicocele in boys and pelvic varices in girls.[110] Spectral Doppler evaluation may reveal left renal vein peak velocity at the aortomesenteric portion,

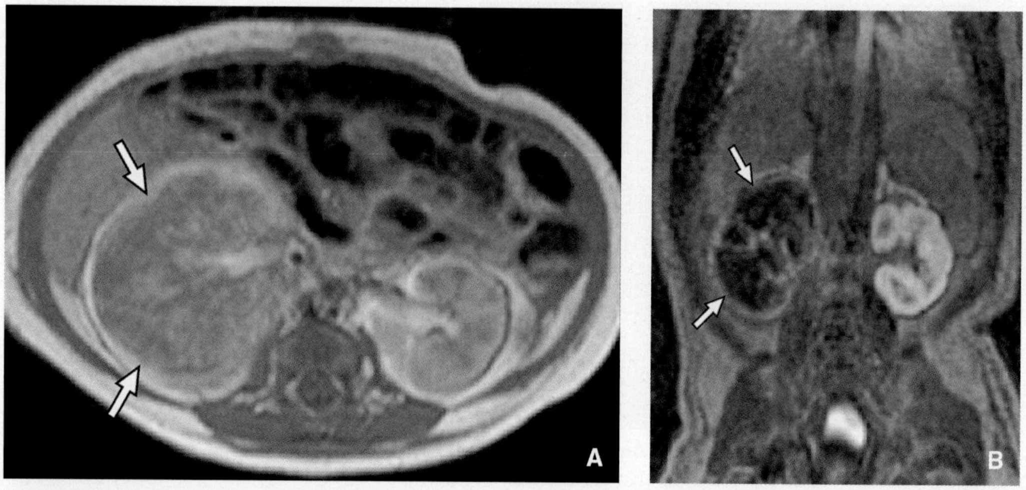

FIGURE 17.50 **3-day-old girl with right renal vein thrombosis. A:** Axial T1-weighted MR image shows a markedly enlarged, heterogeneous right kidney (*arrows*). **B:** Coronal postcontrast T1-weighted MR image shows global hypoenhancement of the right kidney (*arrows*) due to infarction.

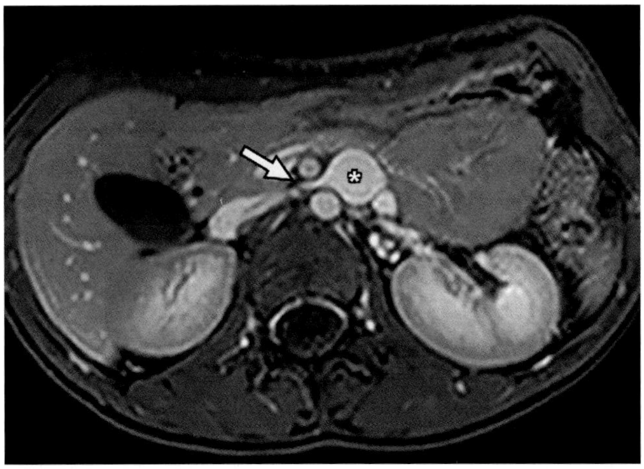

FIGURE 17.51 **16-year-old girl with hematuria and "nutcracker syndrome" anatomy.** Axial postcontrast T1-weighted MR image shows narrowing of the left renal vein (*arrow*) between the abdominal aorta and superior mesenteric artery. The left renal vein (*asterisk*) is dilated peripheral to the level of narrowing.

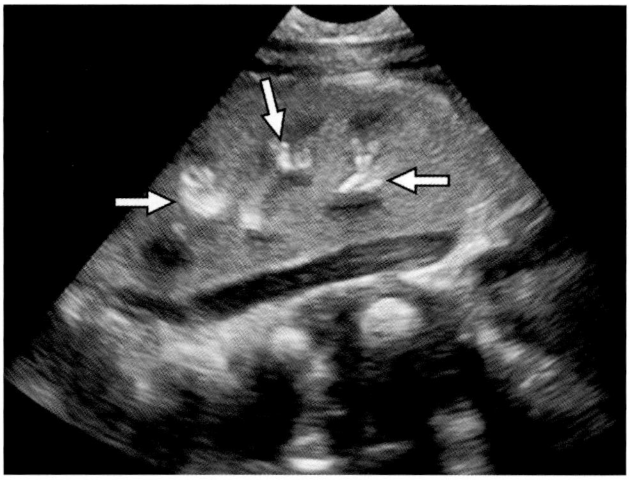

FIGURE 17.52 **2-month-old premature boy on furosemide therapy with medullary nephrocalcinosis.** Longitudinal ultrasound image of the right kidney shows multiple echogenic medullary pyramids (*arrows*).

while CT and MRI demonstrate left renal vein narrowing in the aortomesenteric space (Fig. 17.51).[111] More proximal left renal vein and left gonadal vein are commonly engorged due to venous hypertension (Fig. 17.51). Possible treatment options are reimplantation of the left renal vein and endovascular stenting.[112] These imaging findings can be identified in asymptomatic patients, however, making the diagnosis of true nutcracker syndrome sometimes difficult.[113]

Nephrocalcinosis

Abnormal renal parenchymal calcification, or nephrocalcinosis, more often involves the medulla than the cortex. Common causes of medullary nephrocalcinosis during childhood include prematurity, furosemide therapy, distal renal tubular acidosis, and numerous causes of hypercalcemia and hypercalciuria.[114,115] Nephrocalcinosis is usually asymptomatic, although symptomatic nephrolithiasis may occur in some children.

At ultrasound, nephrocalcinosis classically presents as abnormally echogenic medullary pyramids (Figs. 17.52 and 17.53). Multiple patterns of medullary pyramid calcification have been described when using a linear high-frequency transducer.[116] When involvement is severe, posterior acoustic shadowing and color Doppler "twinkling" artifact can be present (Fig. 17.53). While renal involvement is most often bilateral and symmetric, asymmetry may exist.[117] Severe nephrocalcinosis can present as areas of renal parenchymal hyperattenuation at CT and signal hypointensity at MRI (Fig. 17.53).

Management mainly involves treating any underlying predisposing medical condition or metabolic abnormality. Medullary nephrocalcinosis should not be confused with transient increased echogenicity of the renal medulla that is commonly observed in the neonate during the first week of life and that has been attributed to stasis nephropathy (Tamm-Horsfall protein deposition) by some authors.[118,119]

Renal Transplantation

Renal transplantation is increasingly common in the pediatric population. Postoperative complications similar to those observed in adults occur in children and may be detected by imaging. Peritransplant fluid collections are common in the acute setting and may be due to hematoma, seroma, urinoma, lymphocele, or abscess.[120] These fluid collections can be easily detected and followed using ultrasound. The exact cause of a fluid collection can often be elucidated based on ultrasound appearance and clinical data. If the cause of a fluid collection is uncertain, image-guided aspiration or renal scintigraphy can be performed. In the setting of urinoma, renal scintigraphy reveals extravasation of radiotracer into the fluid collection.

Vascular complications most often occur in the early postoperative period and are a major cause of allograft dysfunction and eventual loss. Common vascular complications include arterial and venous thrombosis and renal artery narrowing due to intrinsic anastomotic stenosis, kinking, extrinsic compression, or twisting of the allograft.[120,121] Rarely, a pseudoaneurysm may be identified at the renal artery anastomosis or within the renal allograft following percutaneous biopsy.

No renal Doppler signal is present in the kidney or renal artery in the setting of transplant artery thrombosis. Renal vein thrombosis commonly presents with absent Doppler signal in the main renal vein and diastolic reversal of arterial blood flow. Spectral Doppler evaluation demonstrates intrarenal tardus parvus waveforms and/or abnormally low resistive index measurements in the setting of renal artery narrowing. Evaluation of the renal artery at the site of narrowing commonly reveals focal disturbance of blood flow, with aliasing and poststenotic increased peak systolic velocity.[120] There is no highly sensitive and highly specific ultrasound appearance of the kidney in the setting of acute rejection, although common

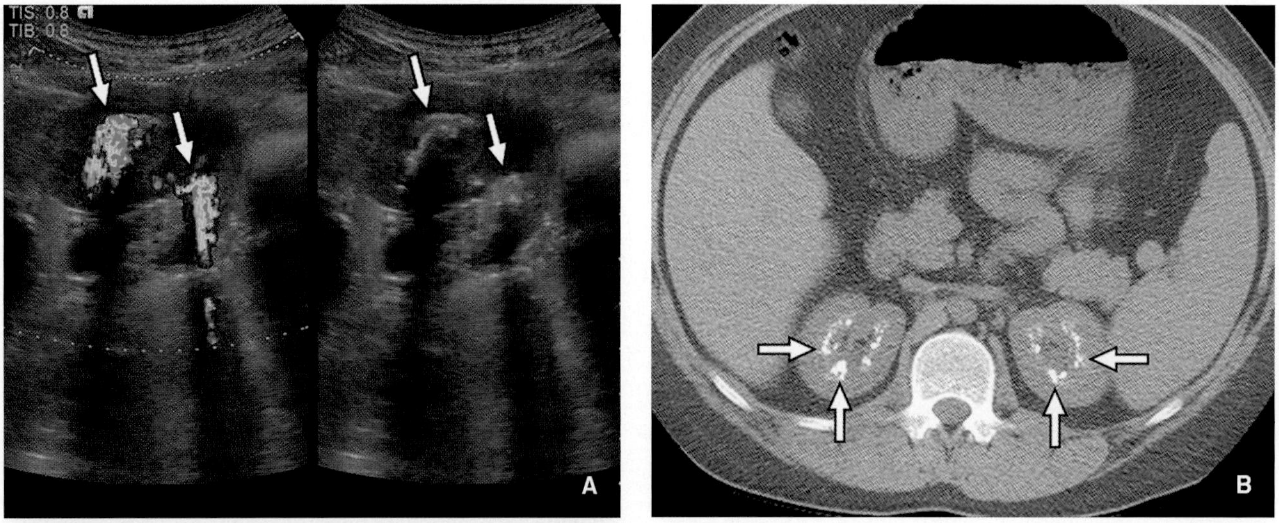

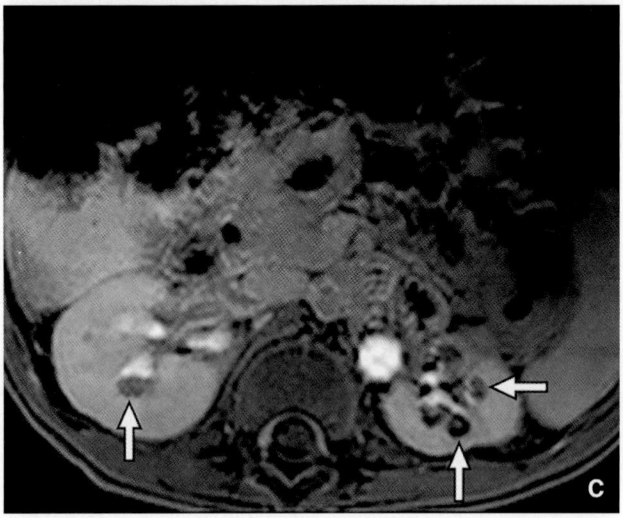

FIGURE 17.53 **14-year-old boy with distal renal tubular acidosis. A:** Transverse side-by-side color Doppler and gray-scale ultrasound images show areas of renal medullary increased echogenicity that demonstrate both posterior acoustic shadowing and "twinkling" artifact (*arrows*). **B:** Axial noncontrast CT image shows extensive bilateral renal medullary calcifications (*arrows*). **C:** Axial postcontrast T1-weighted fat-saturated MR image shows decreased signal intensity involving multiple bilateral renal medullary pyramids (*arrows*).

findings include allograft enlargement, altered parenchymal echogenicity, loss of corticomedullary differentiation, urothelial thickening, and increased resistive index measurements. It may be difficult to distinguish acute rejection from acute tubular necrosis in the immediate postoperative setting.

SPECTRUM OF UPPER URINARY TRACT DISORDERS

Congenital and Developmental Anomalies

Upper Urinary Tract Duplication

Duplication, or duplex kidney, is the most common developmental anomaly of the upper urinary tract. This condition is due to abnormalities of the ureteric buds, which arise from the wolffian duct, and it can be either incomplete (bifid renal collecting system or Y-type duplication; single ureteric orifice) or complete (two or more completely separate upper urinary tracts with separate ureteric orifices). The Weigert-Meyer rule states that lower-moiety ureters have an orthotopic insertion into the bladder, while upper moiety ureters insert ectopically (most often abnormally inferior and medial).

While the majority of children with upper urinary tract duplication are asymptomatic, this anomaly can have a variety of clinical presentations, including urinary tract obstruction and infection. When symptomatic, upper moieties tend to present with obstruction due to either a ureterocele or stenotic ectopic ureteric insertion. Ureteroceles are saccular dilatations of the distal ureter that may be confined to bladder or that may prolapse into the bladder neck or urethra causing bladder outlet obstruction. Ectopic ureteral insertions in boys can involve the bladder base, posterior urethra, or genital tract (e.g., seminal vesicles, vas deferens, or epididymis). Ectopic ureteral insertions in girls can involve the bladder base, bladder neck, urethra (either above or below the external sphincter), uterus, cervix, vagina, or Gartner duct cyst. A unique presentation in girls (when the ureteral orifice involves the infrasphincteric urethra, uterus, cervix, vagina, or Gartner duct cyst) is incontinence with both daytime and nighttime dribbling of urine.[122]

Cross-sectional imaging (ultrasound, CT, and MRI) commonly allows direct visualization of two separate renal

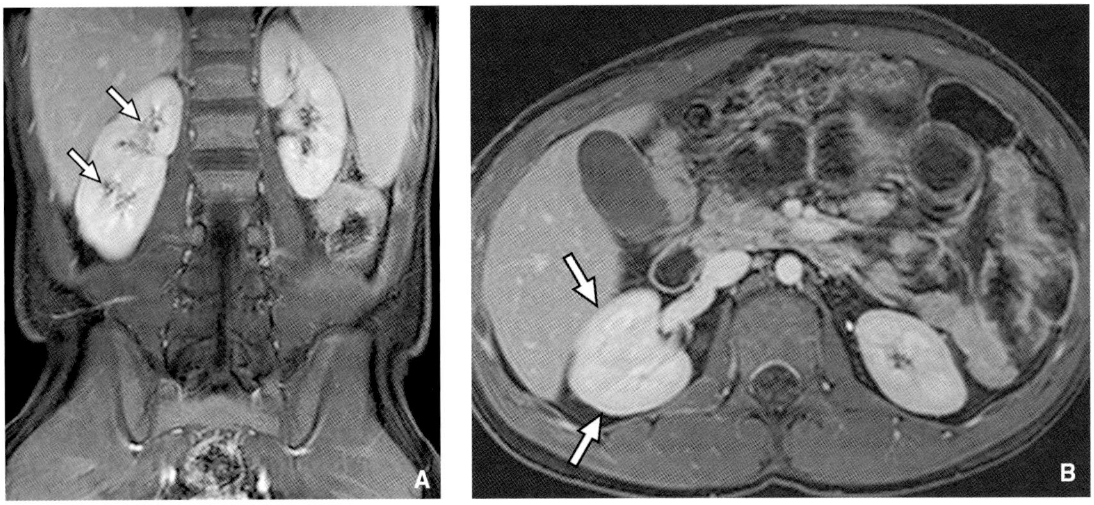

FIGURE 17.54 **13-year-old boy with incidentally detected, uncomplicated right upper urinary tract duplication. A:** Coronal postcontrast T1-weighted fat-saturated MR image shows separate right upper and lower-moiety renal sinuses and collecting systems (*arrows*) with intervening renal parenchyma. **B:** Axial postcontrast T1-weighted fat-saturated MR image through the mid right kidney reveals a "faceless" appearance (*arrows*).

collecting systems or ureters (Fig. 17.54). Other findings suggestive of upper urinary tract duplication include elongation of the affected kidney, focal upper pole caliectasis (sometimes mimicking a renal cyst), prominent parenchymal column dividing the kidney into upper and lower moieties, and so-called faceless kidney (transverse image through the midkidney that fails to demonstrate expected renal sinus fat and collecting system) (Figs. 17.54 and 17.55). Upper moiety parenchymal thickness varies depending on the degree of obstruction, and renal dysplasia (including MCDK) can occur when in utero obstruction is severe (Fig. 17.56).[123] Recognition of a ureterocele, usually appearing as variably sized thin-walled cystic structure in the bladder, is highly suggestive of upper urinary tract duplication (Fig. 17.57), although single-system (orthotopic) ureteroceles occasionally occur. On occasion, a large ureterocele may be associated with a nondilated or small dysplastic upper moiety collecting system, so-called ureterocele disproportion.[124]

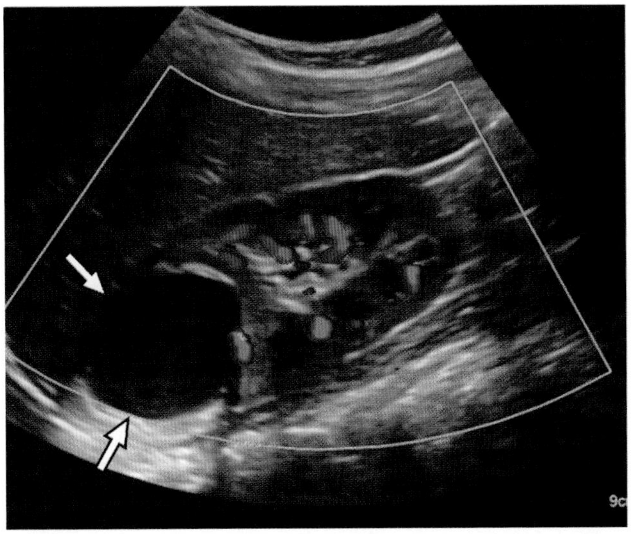

FIGURE 17.55 **2-year-old girl with right duplex kidney.** Longitudinal right kidney color Doppler image shows an apparent cyst (*arrows*) in the upper pole. In reality, this is a dilated right upper moiety pelvicalyceal system with overlying severe parenchymal thinning.

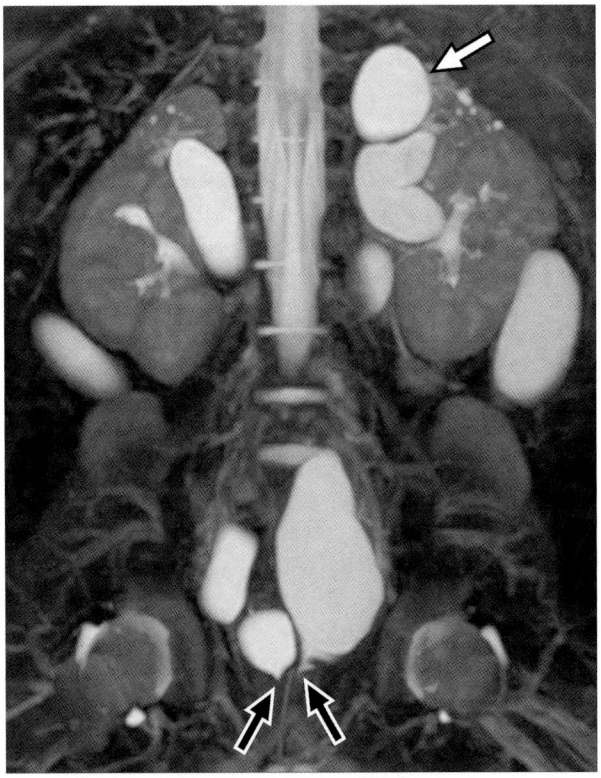

FIGURE 17.56 **3-month-old girl with bilateral duplex kidneys.** Coronal 3D T2-weighted fat-saturated maximum-intensity projection MR image shows bilateral upper moiety hydroureteronephrosis. Bilateral upper moiety renal parenchyma is dysplastic, containing numerous variably sized cysts (*white arrow*). Both upper moiety ureters (*black arrows*) are ectopic, inserting into the urethra.

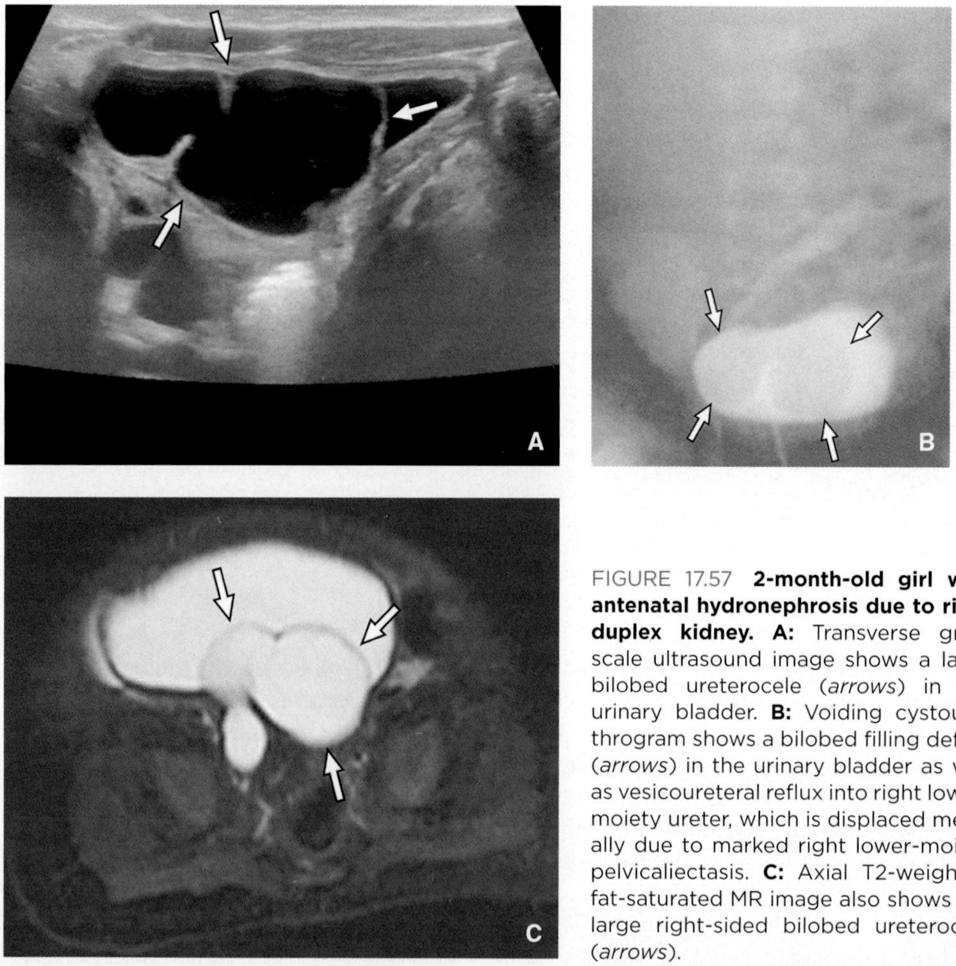

FIGURE 17.57 **2-month-old girl with antenatal hydronephrosis due to right duplex kidney. A:** Transverse gray-scale ultrasound image shows a large bilobed ureterocele (*arrows*) in the urinary bladder. **B:** Voiding cystourethrogram shows a bilobed filling defect (*arrows*) in the urinary bladder as well as vesicoureteral reflux into right lower-moiety ureter, which is displaced medially due to marked right lower-moiety pelvicaliectasis. **C:** Axial T2-weighted fat-saturated MR image also shows the large right-sided bilobed ureterocele (*arrows*).

Lower-moiety pelvicaliectasis may be due to VUR or UPJ obstruction and may require further evaluation with VCUG or a functional imaging study (renal scintigraphy or MRU) (Figs. 17.58 and 17.59).[125] Common VCUG findings include a round or oval filling defect in the bladder due to ureterocele (best seen on early filling-phase imaging) and lower-moiety VUR. The lower-moiety collecting system commonly has too few calyces and an abnormal long axis with inferior calyces deviated inferomedially (so-called "drooping lily" appearance, which can occur both in the presence and absence of upper moiety pelvicaliectasis).[126] MRU can be used to evaluate children with complex duplications when anatomic questions remain after standard evaluation or when an ectopic ureter is suspected (Fig. 17.60).[127] MRU can also be performed to establish upper- and lower-moiety differential function and comprehensively assess the renal parenchyma.

Children with incomplete and asymptomatic complete upper urinary tract duplications commonly require no intervention (Fig. 17.61). Symptomatic upper moieties may require endoscopic ureterocele incision, urinary diversion (cutaneous pyelostomy or ureterostomy), ureteral reimplantation, or heminephrectomy when there is minimal associated functional renal parenchyma. Symptomatic lower moieties may require ureteral reimplantation to treat VUR, pyeloplasty to relieve UPJ obstruction, or heminephrectomy when there is minimal associated functional renal parenchyma.

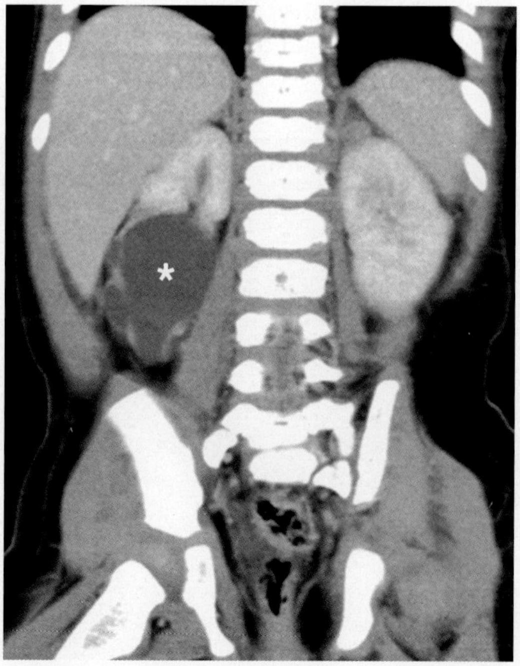

FIGURE 17.58 **11-month-old boy with congenital neuroblastoma and incidentally detected right duplex kidney.** Coronal enhanced CT image shows a right duplex kidney with marked lower moiety pelvicaliectasis (*asterisk*) due to scintigraphy confirmed ureteropelvic junction obstruction. There is severe parenchymal thinning due to long-standing obstruction.

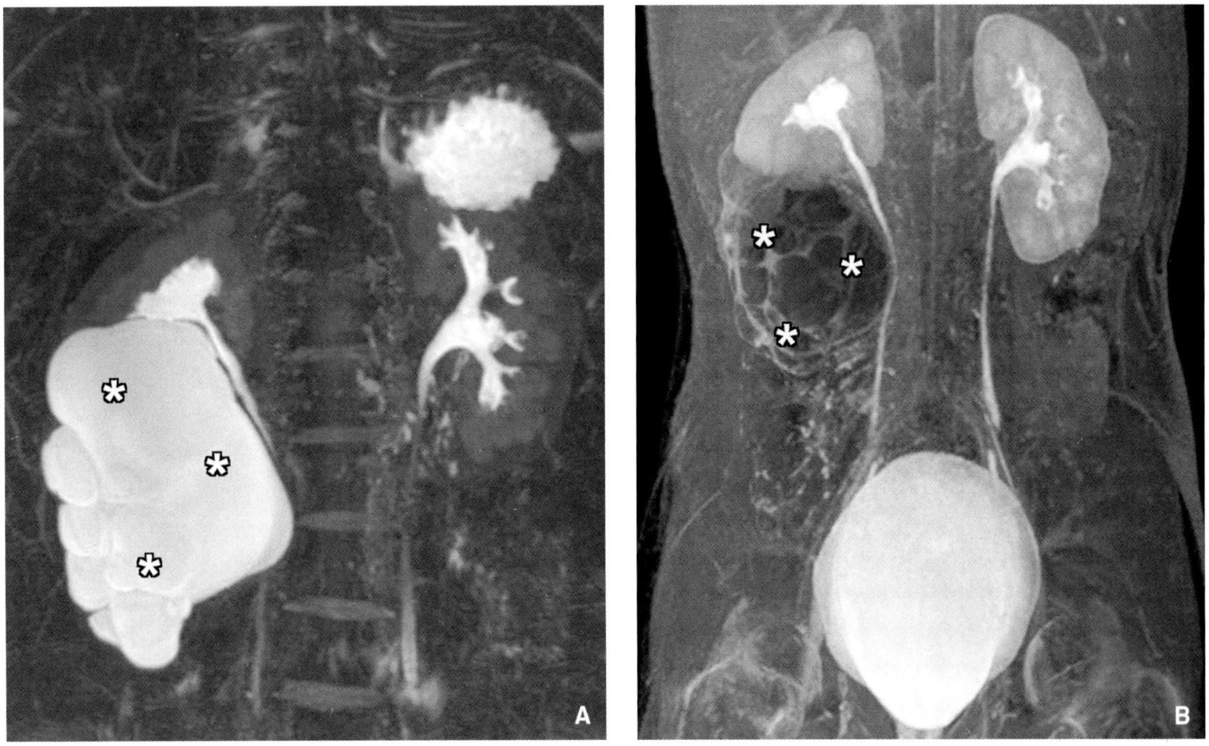

FIGURE 17.59 **8-year-old boy with right flank pain and hydronephrosis on ultrasound. A:** 3D T2-weighted maximum-intensity projection MR image reveals that the right kidney is duplex, with the lower moiety demonstrating marked pelvicaliectasis (*asterisks*). **B:** Delayed-phase postcontrast T1-weighted maximum-intensity projection MR image shows no excretion of contrast material into right lower-moiety collecting system (*asterisks*). Findings are consistent with right lower-moiety ureteropelvic junction obstruction.

Ureteropelvic Junction Obstruction

Abnormal narrowing of the UPJ is the most common congenital cause of urinary tract obstruction. When detected antenatally or presenting very early in life, this condition is most often due to an intrinsic developmental abnormality of the UPJ wall with histopathology usually revealing

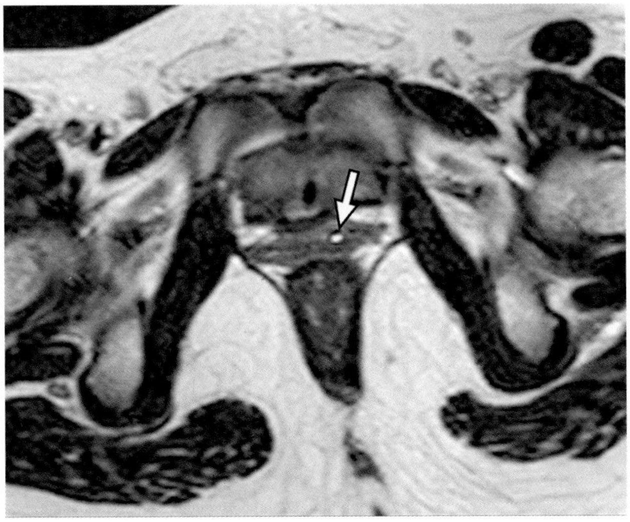

FIGURE 17.60 **10-year-old girl with daytime and nighttime incontinence and normal renal ultrasound examination.** Axial T2-weighted MR image shows a small, round fluid-structure (*arrow*) in the anterior wall of the vagina, consistent with an ectopic ureter.

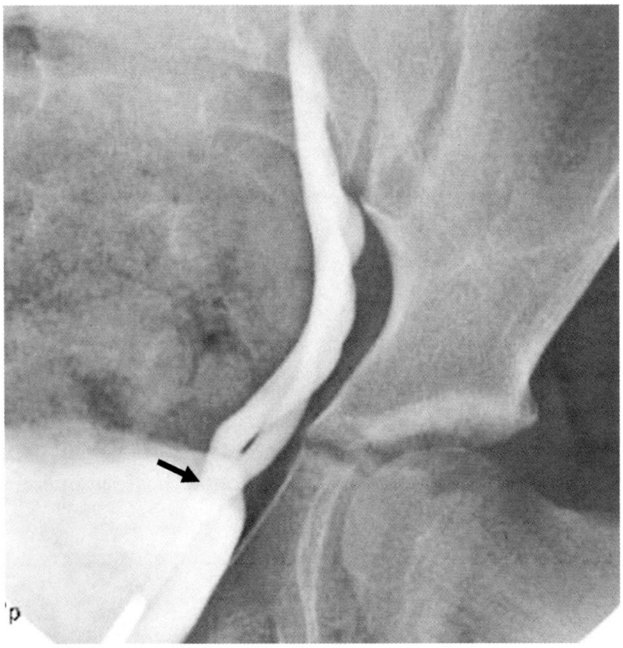

FIGURE 17.61 **9-year-old girl with incomplete y-type duplication of the left upper urinary tract who underwent retrograde pyelography.** Fluoroscopic image shows incomplete y-type duplication of the left upper urinary tract. A single ureter is seen distally (*arrow*).

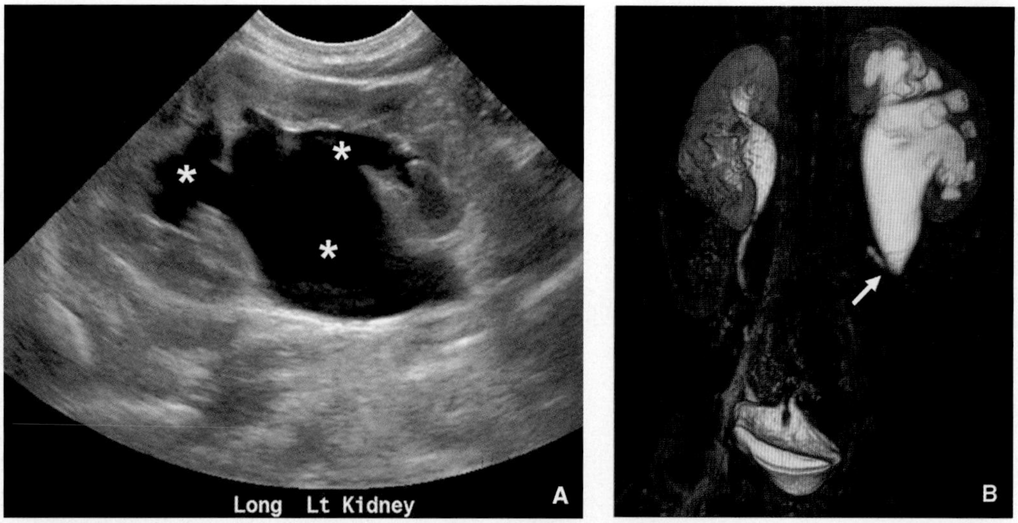

FIGURE 17.62 **1-year-old boy with left ureteropelvic junction (UPJ) obstruction. A:** Longitudinal gray-scale image of the left kidney shows pelvicaliectasis (*asterisks*), with the renal pelvis appearing more dilated than the calyces. **B:** Postcontrast T1-weighted volume-rendered MR image shows excreted contrast material filling the dilated left renal collecting system. There is a severe left UPJ kink (*arrow*), with contrast material seen only in the very proximal left ureter. Left kidney parenchyma is diffusely mildly thinned, while the right kidney and upper urinary tract are normal.

abnormal smooth muscle arrangement or fibrosis and luminal narrowing. UPJ obstruction can also occur in the setting of high-grade VUR (so-called secondary UPJ obstruction) or may be intermittent due to a crossing vessel causing extrinsic compression in older children and adults.[128] Rarely, fibroepithelial polyps can cause UPJ obstruction in children.[129] Clinical presentations of UPJ obstruction include palpable abdominal mass, hematuria, infection, urolithiasis, and abdominal/flank pain. Intermittent abdominal/flank pain may be associated with drinking large volumes of fluid, so-called Dietl crisis.[130] UPJ obstructions are more often left sided, can be bilateral, and may be associated with contralateral MCDK. UPJ obstruction also occurs with increased frequency in horseshoe kidneys and duplex kidney lower moieties.[125]

Ultrasound is most often performed to evaluate suspected UPJ obstruction. Findings suggestive of UPJ obstruction include pelvicaliectasis (with the pelvis appearing more dilated than calyces) and demonstration of a normal caliber ureter (Fig. 17.62). Over time, obstruction may lead to kidney injury with areas of focal scarring or diffuse parenchymal thinning, and corticomedullary differentiation may be lost.[131] Renal scintigraphy (e.g., Tc-99m MAG3) with adjuvant IV hydration and furosemide administration is most often used to confirm the presence of obstruction and assess differential renal function. More recently, MRU has been described for UPJ obstruction evaluation (Figs. 17.62 and 17.63). This imaging technique allows assessment of the upper urinary tract before and after furosemide administration, detailed evaluation of renal parenchyma, and determination of renal function (including transit times, differential function, and time vs. enhancement curves),[132] all without ionizing radiation. MRU also excellently depicts renal parenchymal edema in acute obstruction and causative crossing vessels in older children with intermittent obstruction (Fig. 17.63).[133] VCUG may reveal UPJ obstructions that are associated with VUR. Delayed postvoid imaging is helpful for assessing drainage of the pelvicalyceal system when UPJ obstruction is suspected (Fig. 17.64).[134]

Pediatric UPJ obstructions that are symptomatic or associated with kidney injury are treated surgically with dismembered pyeloplasty (open, laparoscopic, or robot assisted).[135] The UPJ must be transposed anterior to any causative crossing vessel. In the setting of UPJ obstruction and VUR, pyeloplasty is commonly performed prior to ureteral reimplantation.[134]

Congenital Primary Megaureter

Congenital primary megaureter is a form of distal ureter/ureterovesical junction obstruction that is due to a usually short aperistaltic juxtavesical segment of distal ureter that causes variable degrees of urinary tract obstruction, including intermittent obstruction in some children.[136] There is some evidence that this condition may be in part due to a decreased number of interstitial cells of Cajal in the ureter wall.[137] Common clinical presentations include antenatal hydronephrosis and infection.[138,139] Two-thirds of affected children are boys, and two-thirds of those affected have involvement of the left ureter only.[140] The degree and length of ureteral dilatation is variable based on the severity of obstruction, with some patients also having substantial pelvicaliectasis (Fig. 17.65).[139]

Ultrasound classically reveals ureteral dilatation with a sometimes recognizable short segment of very distal ureteral narrowing (Fig. 17.66). Real-time ultrasound imaging of the very distal ureter shows hypo- or aperistalsis, while the more proximal dilated ureter often demonstrates increased but ineffectual peristalsis.[139] Debris may be seen in dilated ureter

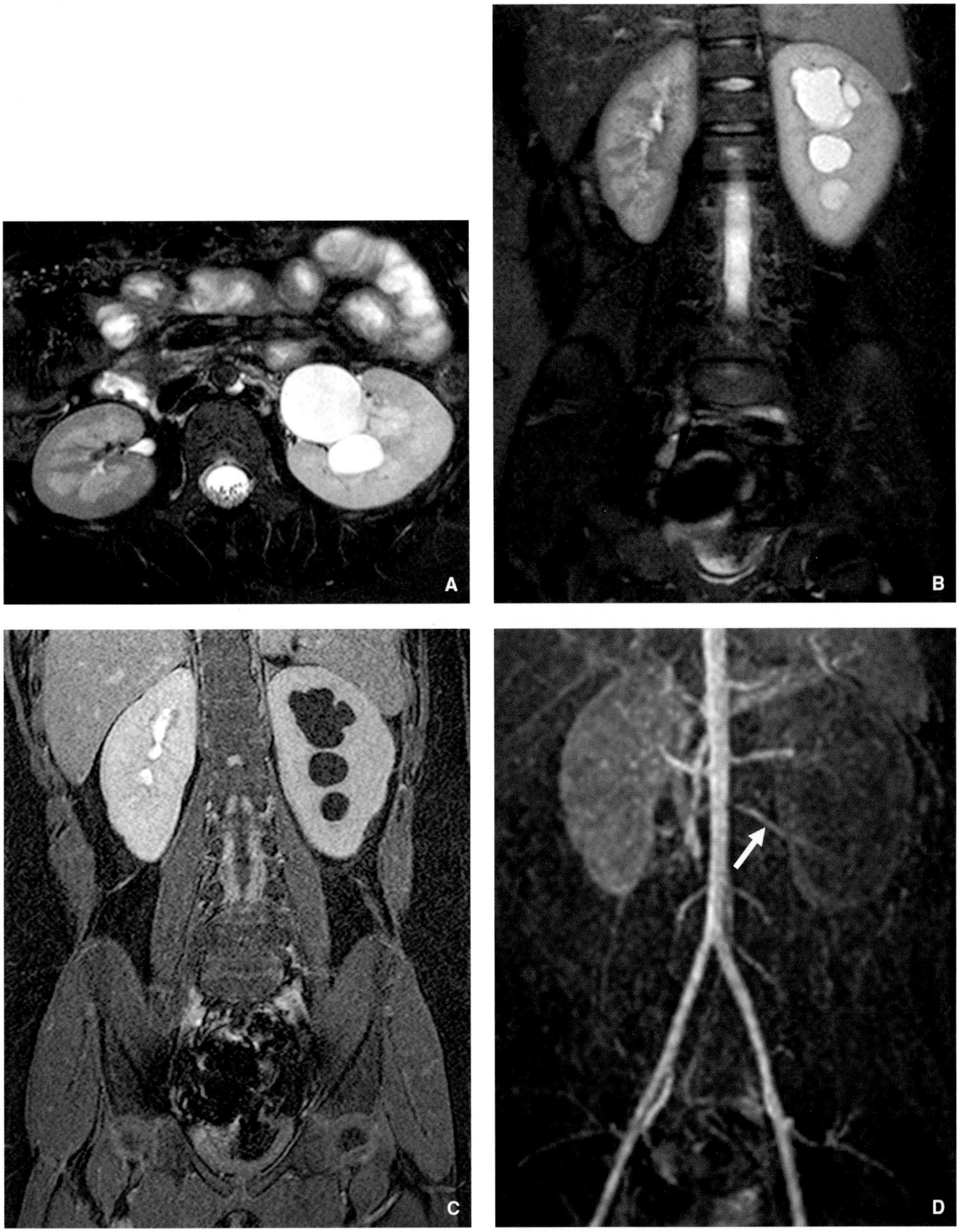

FIGURE 17.63 **8-year-old girl with left flank pain due to intermittent ureteropelvic junction (UPJ) obstruction and normal renal ultrasound. A and B:** Axial and coronal T2-weighted fat-saturated MR images after IV hydration show marked left hydronephrosis and renal parenchymal edema. **C:** Coronal delayed postcontrast T1-weighted MR image shows contrast material filling right renal collecting system. No contrast is present in the left renal collecting system due to decompensated UPJ obstruction. **D:** Coronal postcontrast arterial-phase T1-weighted maximum-intensity projection MR image shows hypoperfusion of the left kidney and an accessory left renal artery (*arrow*) to the lower pole, proven at surgery to be the cause of obstruction. The left UPJ was otherwise normal upon intraoperative inspection, without intrinsic narrowing.

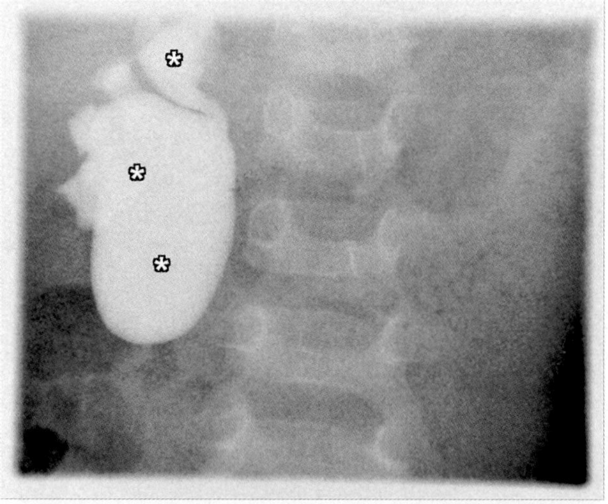

FIGURE 17.64 **5-year-old boy with intermittent right ureteropelvic junction obstruction and vesicoureteral reflux (VUR).** Delayed postvoid voiding cystourethrogram image shows high-grade VUR (*asterisks*) on the right with impaired pelvicalyceal drainage. No contrast material is present in the right ureter, as it is unobstructed and drains freely.

due to stasis or infection. The typical workup of congenital primary megaureter also includes VCUG to exclude VUR as the primary cause of ureterectasis and a functional imaging study to assess the degree of obstruction, such as MRU or renal scintigraphy (Fig. 17.67). In some cases, ipsilateral renal collecting system dilatation may be due to coexistent UPJ obstruction or congenital megacalyces.[141,142] When ureteral dilatation is slight and obstruction is absent or mild, conservative management may be indicated as spontaneous resolution frequently occurs. When symptomatic or associated with deterioration in renal function, surgical repair may be indicated.[143,144]

Congenital Megacalyces

Also known as megacalycosis, congenital megacalyces refers to nonobstructive caliectasis due to developmental medullary hypoplasia.[145] Histopathologic evaluation typically demonstrates

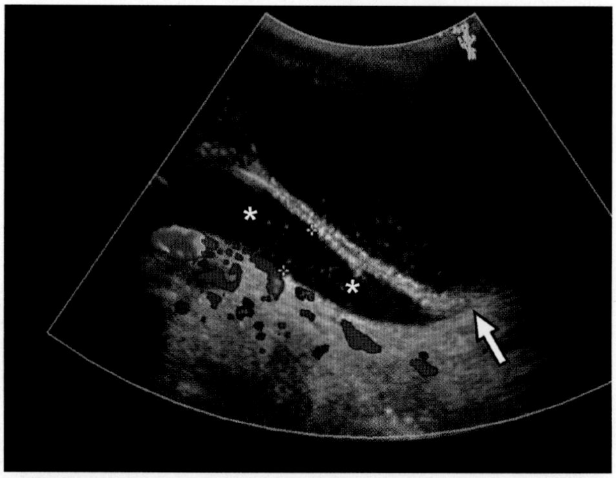

FIGURE 17.66 **6-year-old boy with febrile urinary tract infection and obstructing left congenital primary megaureter.** Longitudinal color Doppler ultrasound image shows a dilated, debris-filled distal left ureter (*asterisks*). The very distal portion of the left ureter is decompressed (*arrow*). Debris is present in the urinary bladder as well.

normal cortical thickness, loss of medullary height, and papillary flattening.[145] While rare, it is important to recognize this condition as being different from other causes of caliectasis that may cause deterioration in renal function and require surgical management, such as that seen with UPJ obstruction or VUR.

This condition is best recognized at MRU (or excretory urography, if MRU is not available), with images showing unilateral or bilateral calyceal dilatation in the absence of pelviectasis (Fig. 17.68). Classically, there appears to be an increased number of polygonal or facet-shape calyces.[145] The ipsilateral renal pelvis and ureter are typically normal in caliber, although this condition can be associated with congenital primary megaureter (Fig. 17.68).[142] Morphologically, affected kidneys are larger than expected for age, and postcontrast imaging typically shows no evidence of urinary tract obstruction. This condition can be difficult to distinguish from other causes of caliectasis at ultrasound.[146] Associated urinary stasis can lead to infection and calculus formation.

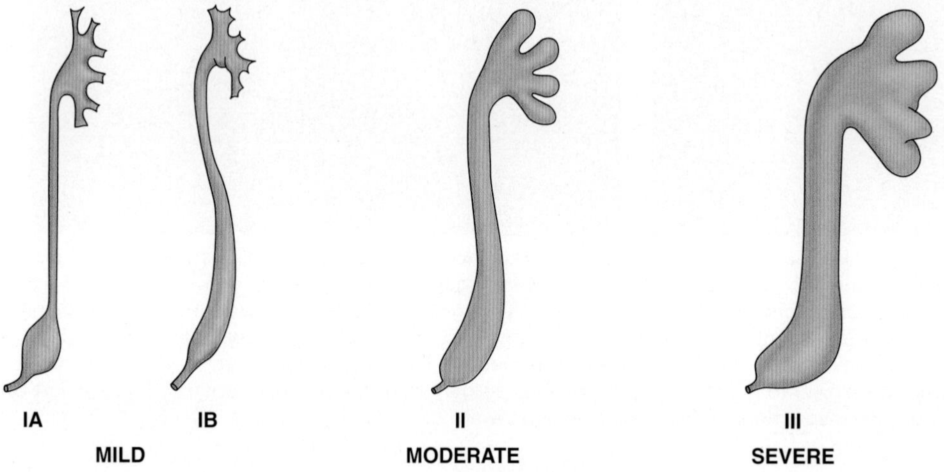

FIGURE 17.65 **Grading of congenital primary megaureter.**

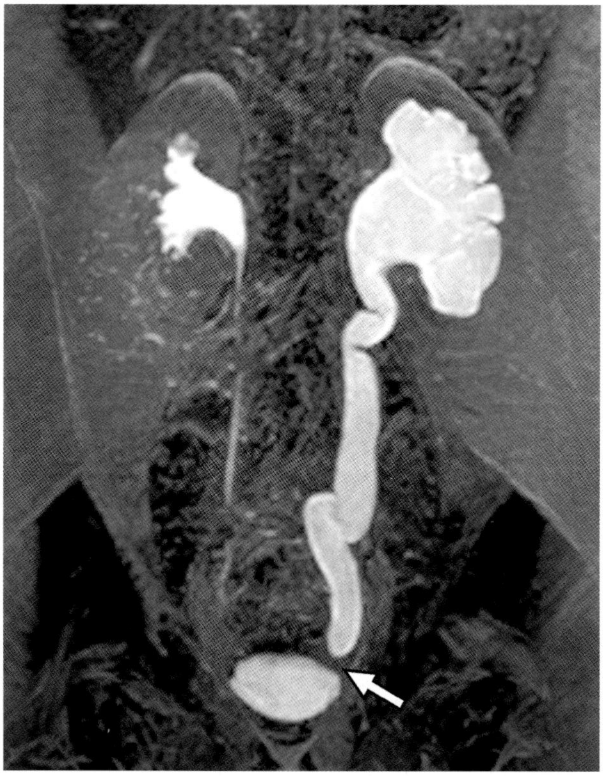

FIGURE 17.67 **11-year-old boy with partially obstructing left congenital primary megaureter.** Postcontrast 3D T1-weighted maximum intensity projection MR image shows left hydroureteronephrosis. The very distal portion of the left ureter (*arrow*) is narrowed and was abnormally fibrotic upon histologic examination.

Calyceal Diverticulum

Calyceal diverticula are outpouchings of the renal collecting system that often mimic simple cysts at ultrasound, CT, and MRI. Both congenital and acquired etiologies have been proposed. However, delayed postcontrast excretory-phase imaging (e.g., CT or MRU) classically shows that these apparent cysts fill with contrast material, thus confirming their communication with the pelvicalyceal system (Fig. 17.69).[147] On occasion, these diverticula contain mobile calculi or dependent milk of calcium, and they may be complicated by infection or rupture.[148] Symptomatic calyceal diverticula may require percutaneous ablation or surgical treatment (diverticulectomy or infundibulotomy).

Midureteric Stricture

Congenital midureteric obstructions, sometimes referred to as strictures or valves, are a rare cause of pediatric upper urinary tract obstruction that has been theorized to be due to failure of ureter recanalization, prenatal vascular insult to the ureter, or persistent ureteral fold.[149] Localizing the site of urinary tract obstruction to the midureter is important as surgical treatment (often ureteroureterostomy) is different from that for UPJ and distal ureter obstructions.[150] Antenatal detection has been described.[150]

Midureteric obstructions may be diagnosed using a variety of imaging modalities, including MRU and antegrade or retrograde pyelography (Fig. 17.70).[149,151] Typical findings include pelvicaliectasis and proximal ureterectasis. The distal ureter is normal in caliber. A transverse filling defect (valve) or abrupt "beak-like" ureteric narrowing is observed. MRU and renal scintigraphy demonstrate variable degrees

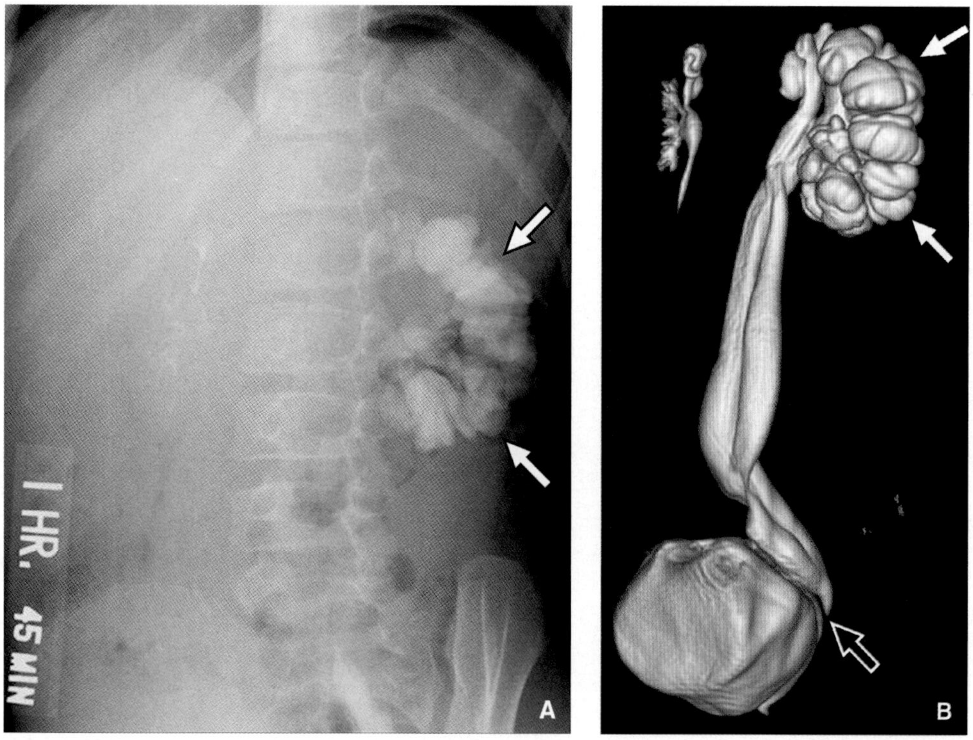

FIGURE 17.68 **6-year-old boy with recurrent urinary tract infections. A:** Excretory urogram image shows an increased number of left-sided dilated, polygonal calyces (*white arrows*), consistent with primary megacalyces. The right renal collecting system appears normal. **B:** 3D T2-weighted volume-rendered MR image shows similar findings (*white arrows*). MRI also reveals previously unknown incomplete duplication of the left upper urinary tract as well as coexisting left primary megaureter. The left distal ureter (*black arrow*) is decompressed.

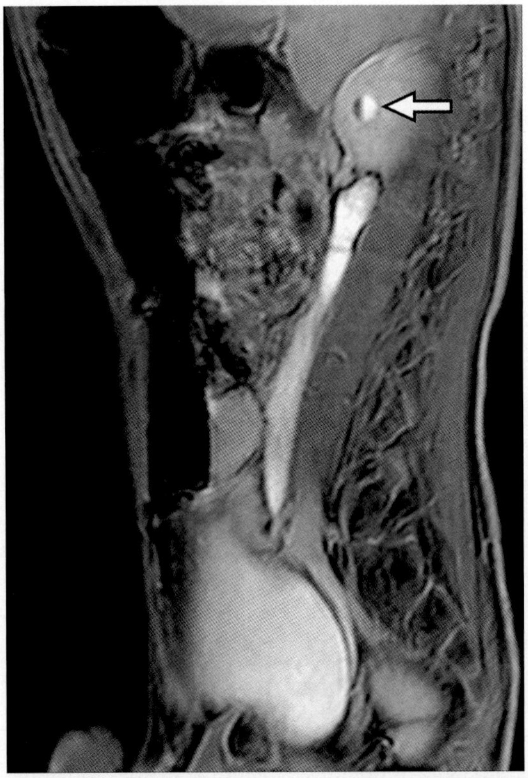

FIGURE 17.69 **14-year-old boy with incidentally detected right kidney calyceal diverticulum.** Sagittal postcontrast T1-weighted fat-saturated excretory-phase MR image shows a cystic structure (*arrow*) that fills with contrast material and that is separate from the renal collecting system.

of obstruction. Unfortunately, ultrasound commonly fails to make this diagnosis, as the midureter is often poorly seen.[150] Contralateral MCDK is common (Fig. 17.70).[149–151]

Retrocaval Ureter

Also known as circumcaval ureter, this uncommon developmental anomaly is the result of abnormal embryogenesis of the inferior vena cava. Consequently, a portion of the right ureter courses posterior and medial to the inferior vena cava, passes anteriorly between the inferior vena cava and abdominal aorta, and then returns to its normal location. This anomaly is most often incidental and asymptomatic, although associated proximal upper urinary tract obstruction or symptoms related to urinary stasis have been described.[152]

This aberrant ureteric course can be directly visualized on excretory-phase postcontrast imaging and may be detected by MR or CT urography.[153,154] Ultrasound may reveal ipsilateral pelvicaliectasis and proximal ureterectasis, although the retrocaval portion of the ureter is unlikely to be appreciated. The presence of a retrocaval ureter may also be inferred at VCUG when there is an abnormally medial course of the right ureter (Fig. 17.71).

When symptomatic, the ureter may be surgically repositioned anterior to the inferior vena cava.[155]

Infectious Disorders

Pyonephrosis refers to purulent infection of the renal collecting system and ureter. This condition is frequently observed in the setting of urinary tract obstruction, is most often unilateral,

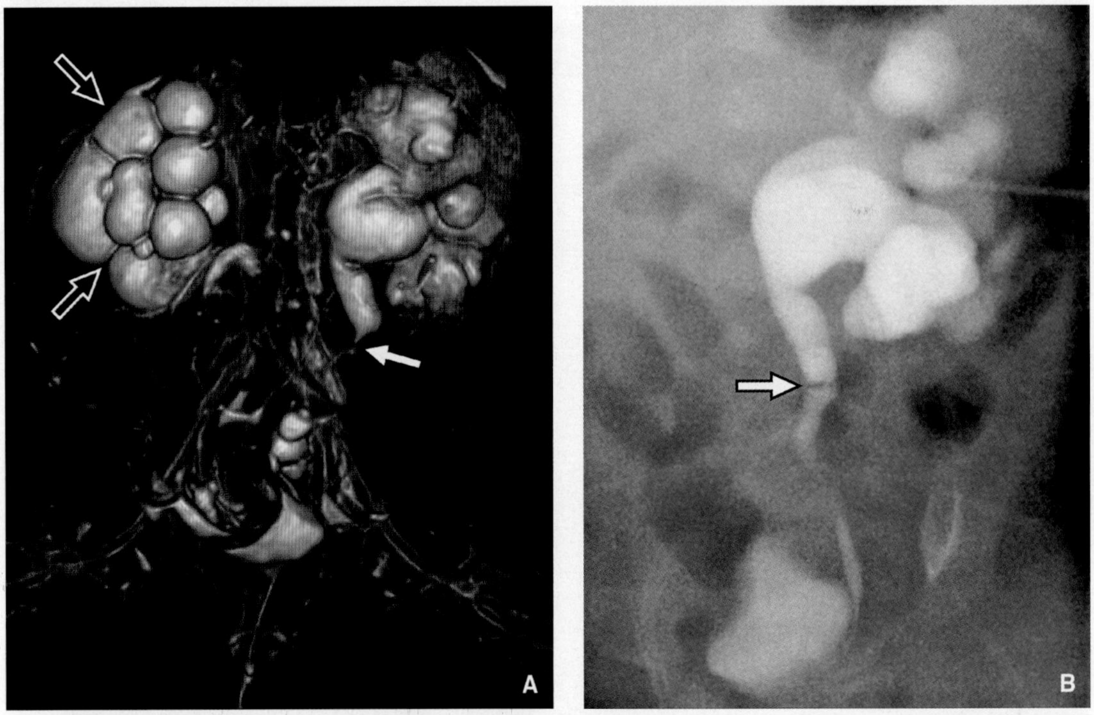

FIGURE 17.70 **2-month-old girl with congenital left midureteric stricture. A:** 3D volume-rendered T2-weighted fast spin-echo MR image shows left pelvicaliectasis and proximal ureterectasis. There is abrupt narrowing of the left midureter due to the presence of a congenital narrowing (*white arrow*). The right kidney contains numerous noncommunicating cysts and no normal renal parenchyma, consistent with multicystic dysplastic kidney (*black arrows*). **B:** Percutaneous antegrade pyelogram confirms abnormal narrowing of the mid left ureter with more proximal hydroureteronephrosis. A transverse filling defect (*arrow*) is consistent with a ureteral valve.

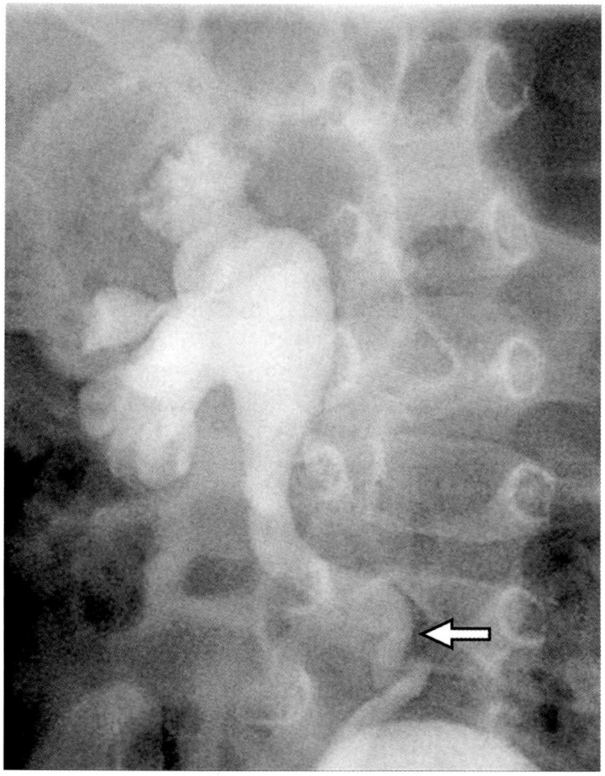

FIGURE 17.71 **4-year-old boy with febrile urinary tract infection.** Voiding cystourethrogram image demonstrates high-grade vesicoureteral reflux. Medial deviation of the right midureter (*arrow*) is consistent with retrocaval course.

and may be complicated by sepsis or kidney injury.[156] Clinical presentations include flank pain, fever, and pyuria, although some affected pediatric patients may be asymptomatic.[157] There are a variety of predisposing conditions in children, such as bladder outlet obstruction (e.g., due to posterior urethral valves in boys), UPJ obstruction, obstructing congenital primary megaureter, and obstructing ureterocele.

Ultrasound often shows renal collecting system dilatation. The ipsilateral ureter may also be dilated if obstruction is present distal to the UPJ. Echogenic urinary tract debris and urothelial thickening are also common (Fig. 17.72).[158] A few studies have suggested that the diagnostic accuracy of ultrasound for this diagnosis is limited.[156]

Treatment includes antibiotic medical therapy and prompt drainage of the infected upper urinary tract (e.g., percutaneous nephrostomy, ureterocele incision).[157]

Neoplastic Disorders

Outside of the kidney, tumors of the upper urinary tract are uncommon in children, with the majority being benign. Fibroepithelial polyps are benign masses composed of a fibrovascular core and urothelial lining. These lesions occur substantially more frequently in boys, and common presentations include flank pain due to UPJ or ureteric obstruction and hematuria.[129] At ultrasound, these polyps appear as echogenic filling defects in the upper urinary tract. When present, hydronephrosis (or hydroureteronephrosis) suggests associated urinary tract obstruction. A recent study has recommended that children drink large amounts of water just prior to ultrasound imaging to aid in the detection of these lesions.[129] Fibroepithelial polyps present as variably sized (<1 cm to >5 cm), mobile filling defects in the upper urinary tract at excretory urography and retrograde pyelography.[159] MRU and CT urography reveal similar upper urinary tract filling defects. Ureteroscopic resection is curative.[160]

Urothelial neoplasms of the upper urinary tract are even less common than fibroepithelial polyps. Such lesions include benign papillomas and carcinomas.[161,162] Clinical presentations include pain due to urinary tract obstruction

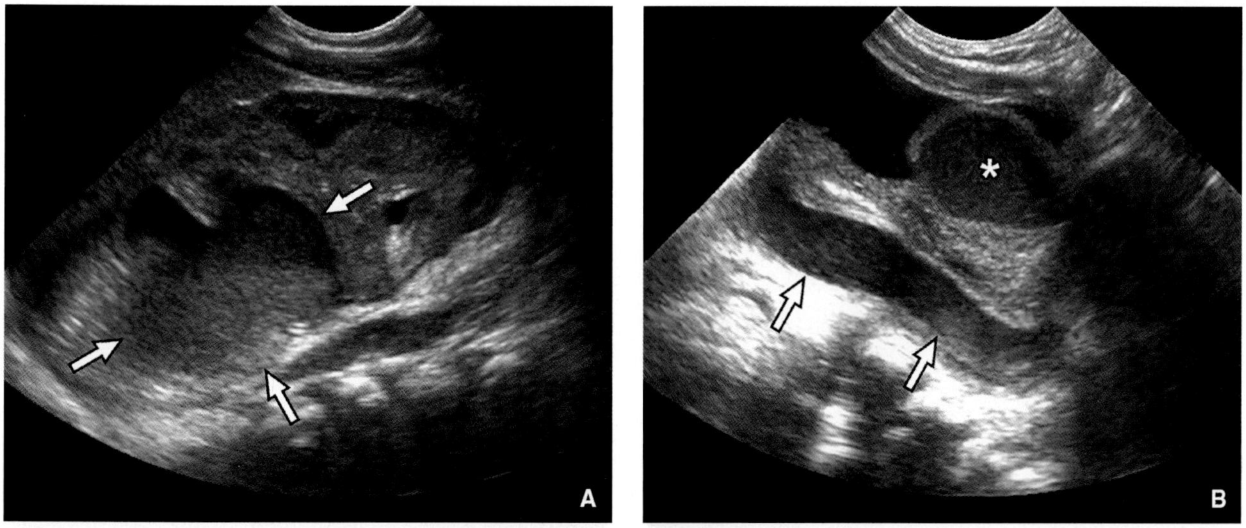

FIGURE 17.72 **3-month-old girl with fever and pyuria due to pyonephrosis. A:** Longitudinal gray-scale ultrasound image demonstrates echogenic fluid (*arrows*) filling the upper moiety collecting system of a duplex right kidney. **B:** Longitudinal gray-scale ultrasound image through the urinary bladder shows similar-appearing complicated fluid within a ureterocele (*asterisk*) and dilated, obstructed right distal ureter (*arrows*).

and hematuria. Ultrasound may reveal hydronephrosis in the setting of urinary tract obstruction. Imaging (including ultrasound, MRU, CT urography, and retrograde pyelography) typically reveals an upper urinary tract filling defect. Benign urothelial lesions may require only ureteroscopic resection, whereas urothelial malignancies may require more aggressive surgical management and/or chemotherapy.

Vesicoureteral Reflux (Including Reflux Nephropathy)

VUR refers to retrograde passage of urine from the bladder into the upper urinary tract. This condition, which is more common in girls, is thought to be due to insufficient length of the very distal ureter's submucosal portion as it passes through the bladder wall. However, VUR is also commonly seen in children with certain predisposing congenital disorders, such as posterior urethral valves, prune-belly syndrome, and upper urinary tract duplication. While many children are asymptomatic (particularly those with low-grade VUR) and have no associated complications, a subset of children (particularly those with high-grade VUR of infected urine) are likely to have symptomatic reflux, which can be complicated by pyelonephritis (febrile urinary tract infection) and so-called acquired reflux nephropathy (severe chronic kidney injury due to parenchymal scarring). Congenital reflux nephropathy commonly presents as antenatal hydronephrosis due to in utero VUR and is more common in boys. This condition is associated with renal hypoplasia/dysplasia and substantially diminished renal function (Fig. 17.73). It is unknown to what degree postnatal VUR and infection (if any) cause additional renal injury in these children, and this population has a propensity to go on to end-stage renal disease.[18,163]

Many children with VUR have normal-appearing kidneys and ureters at ultrasound. Persistent or intermittent ureterectasis (± pelvicaliectasis) may be observed.[164] Ultrasound imaging of the renal parenchyma may uncommonly show evidence of pyelonephritis, or more often, areas of parenchymal scarring (commonly in the polar regions due to compound calyces), and urothelial thickening may be observed.[165] However, ultrasound has been shown to have poor sensitivity

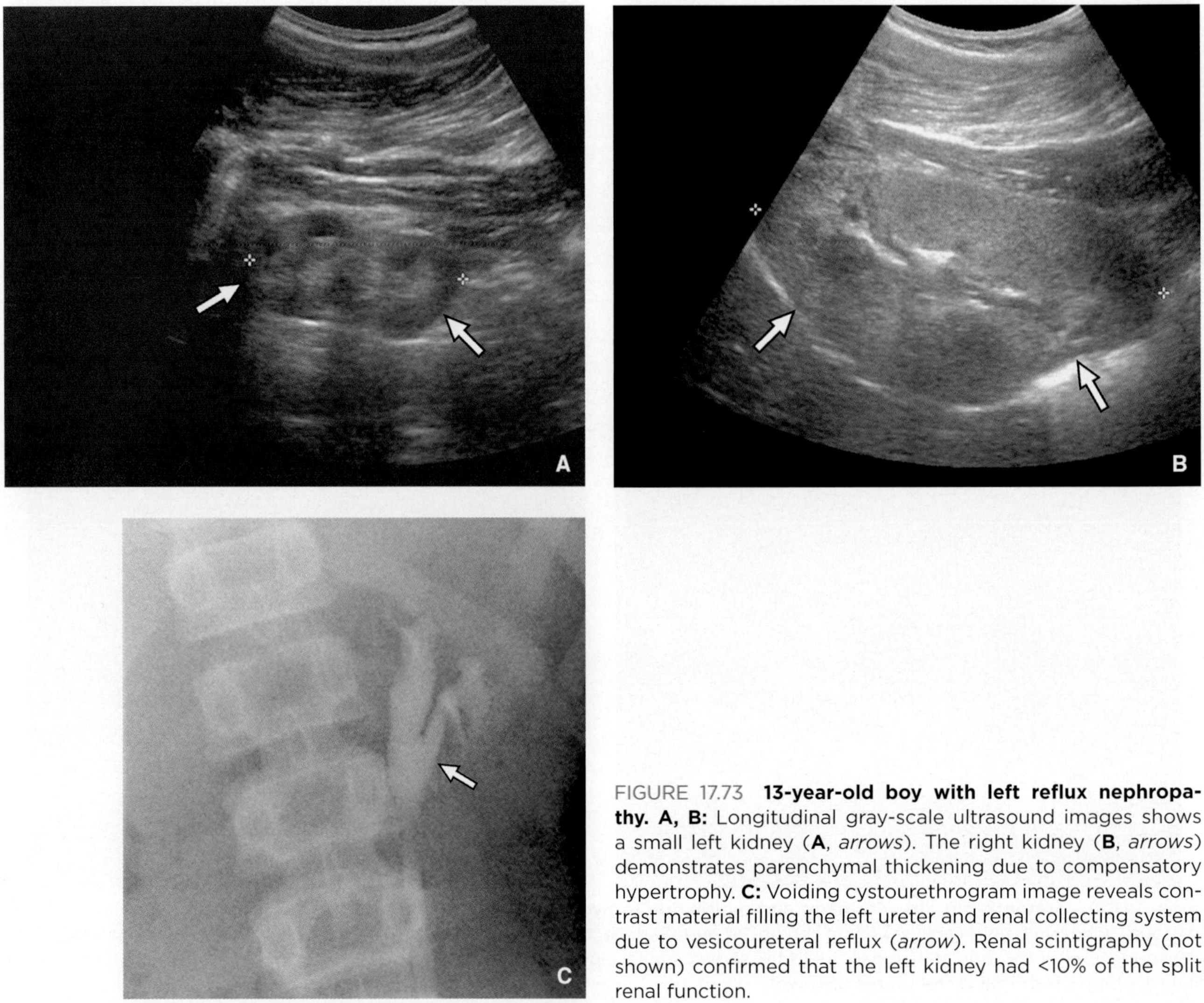

FIGURE 17.73 **13-year-old boy with left reflux nephropathy. A, B:** Longitudinal gray-scale ultrasound images shows a small left kidney (**A**, *arrows*). The right kidney (**B**, *arrows*) demonstrates parenchymal thickening due to compensatory hypertrophy. **C:** Voiding cystourethrogram image reveals contrast material filling the left ureter and renal collecting system due to vesicoureteral reflux (*arrow*). Renal scintigraphy (not shown) confirmed that the left kidney had <10% of the split renal function.

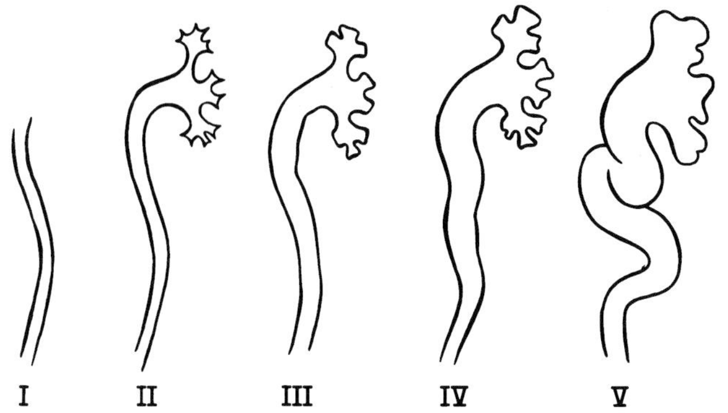

FIGURE 17.74 **Grading of vesicoureteral reflux.**

and negative predictive value for detecting VUR in children under the age of 2 years.[166] VCUG and nuclear cystography are commonly performed to detect VUR, and the use of ceVUS is increasing as an alternative radiation-free modality.[3]

Grading of VUR (1 through 5) by VCUG has prognostic implications and is based on the appearance of refluxed contrast material in the upper urinary tract (Figs. 17.74 to 17.78).[167] This imaging technique also allows anatomic assessment of the urethra and bladder and evaluation for parenchymal opacification due to intrarenal reflux. Nuclear cystography generally correlates with VCUG findings and exposes children to minimal ionizing radiation, although it lacks anatomic detail and allows slightly less precise grading.[168,169] Some recommend using nuclear cystography to

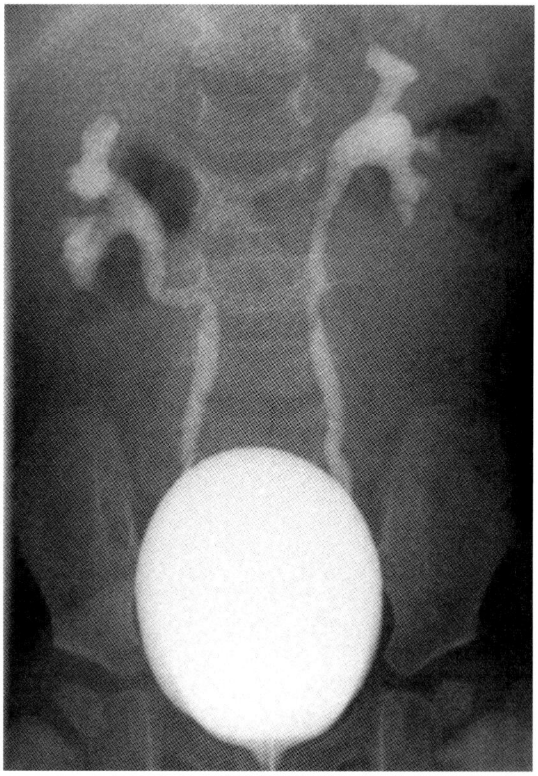
FIGURE 17.76 **11-month-old girl with febrile urinary tract infection and bilateral grade 3 vesicoureteral reflux.** Voiding cystourethrogram image shows bilateral grade 3 vesicoureteral reflux. The ureters are mildly dilated and tortuous while the renal collecting systems are prominent and mildly dilated as well.

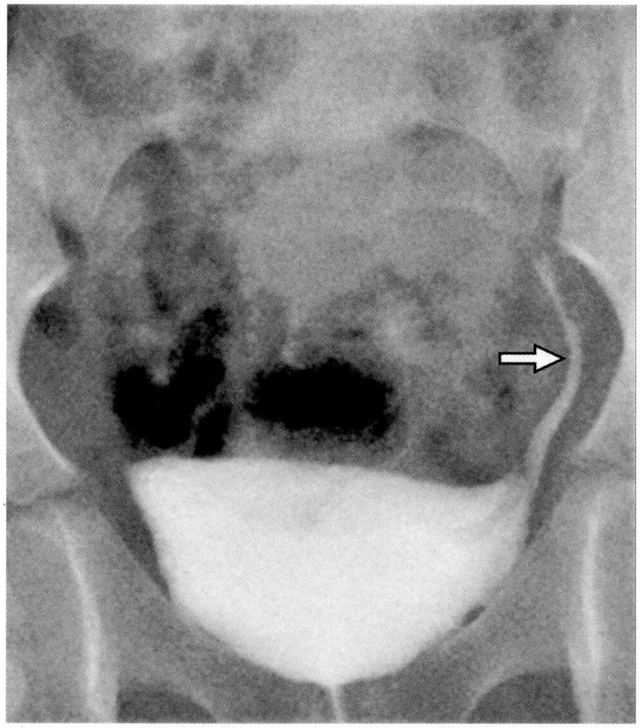
FIGURE 17.75 **6-year-old boy with left grade 1 vesicoureteral reflux.** Voiding cystourethrogram image during filling phase shows refluxed contrast material (*arrow*) in the left distal ureter.

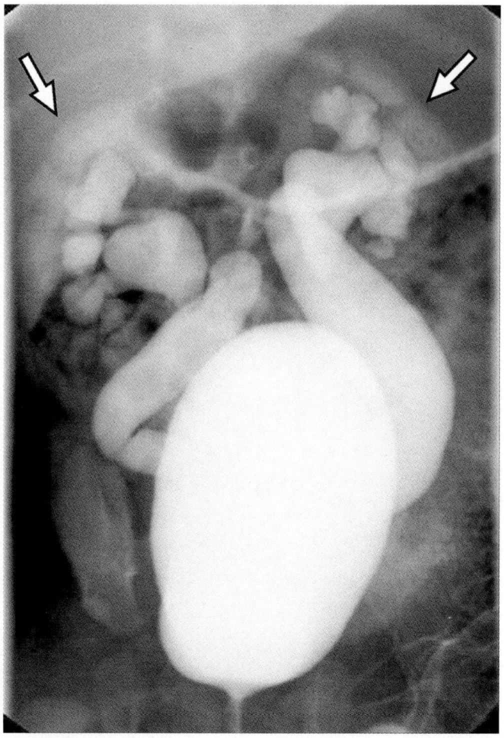
FIGURE 17.77 **4-year-old boy with febrile urinary tract infection and bilateral grade 5 vesicoureteral reflux.** Voiding cystourethrogram image demonstrates high-grade reflux of contrast material into dilated upper urinary tracts. Visualization of renal parenchyma (*arrows*) is due to intrarenal reflux of contrast material.

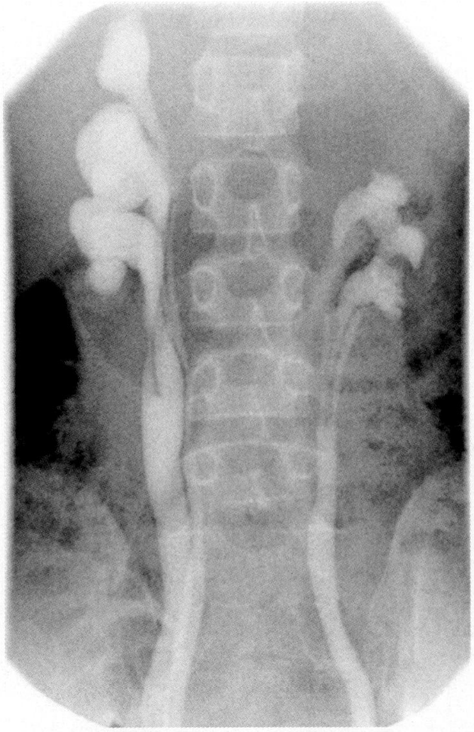

FIGURE 17.78 **9-year-old boy with multiple urinary tract infections and bilateral vesicoureteral reflux.** Voiding cystourethrogram image shows reflux of contrast material into four right and three left proximal ureters and renal collecting systems. Two distal ureters are seen distally on the right, while a single ureter is seen distally on the left. An additional ureter to the left kidney upper pole did not demonstrate reflux but was visualized by MRI (not shown).

follow-up known VUR or when imaging of the urethra is not necessary. More recently, some authors and working groups have recommended initially evaluating febrile urinary tract infections and suspected VUR with DMSA renal scintigraphy in order to show areas of pyelonephritis and/or parenchymal scarring (so-called top-down approach to VUR).[170] If no such areas are identified, then VCUG or nuclear cystography does not need to be performed, although some have cautioned that the sensitivity of this approach for identifying children with high-grade VUR may be limited.[171] Also, unlike at MRI, renal parenchymal acute infection and scarring are difficult to distinguish at DMSA imaging (Fig. 17.79).

Low-grade VUR spontaneously resolves in many children (particularly low-grade VUR). Prophylactic antibiotics may be used in certain children in order to minimize urinary tract infections and possibly prevent renal scarring. If conservative management fails, then surgical reimplantation of the ureter or endoscopic injection of dextranomer/hyaluronic acid copolymer around the ureteral orifice may be performed.

Urolithiasis

Urinary tract calculi are solid, proteinaceous and/or crystalline concretions that form in the renal collecting system and less often elsewhere in the urinary tract or kidney. Calculi can have a variety of chemical compositions and may be calcium, uric acid, cysteine, or struvite based. While many urinary tract calculi are asymptomatic, others may present with hematuria or obstructive symptoms.[4] The incidence of

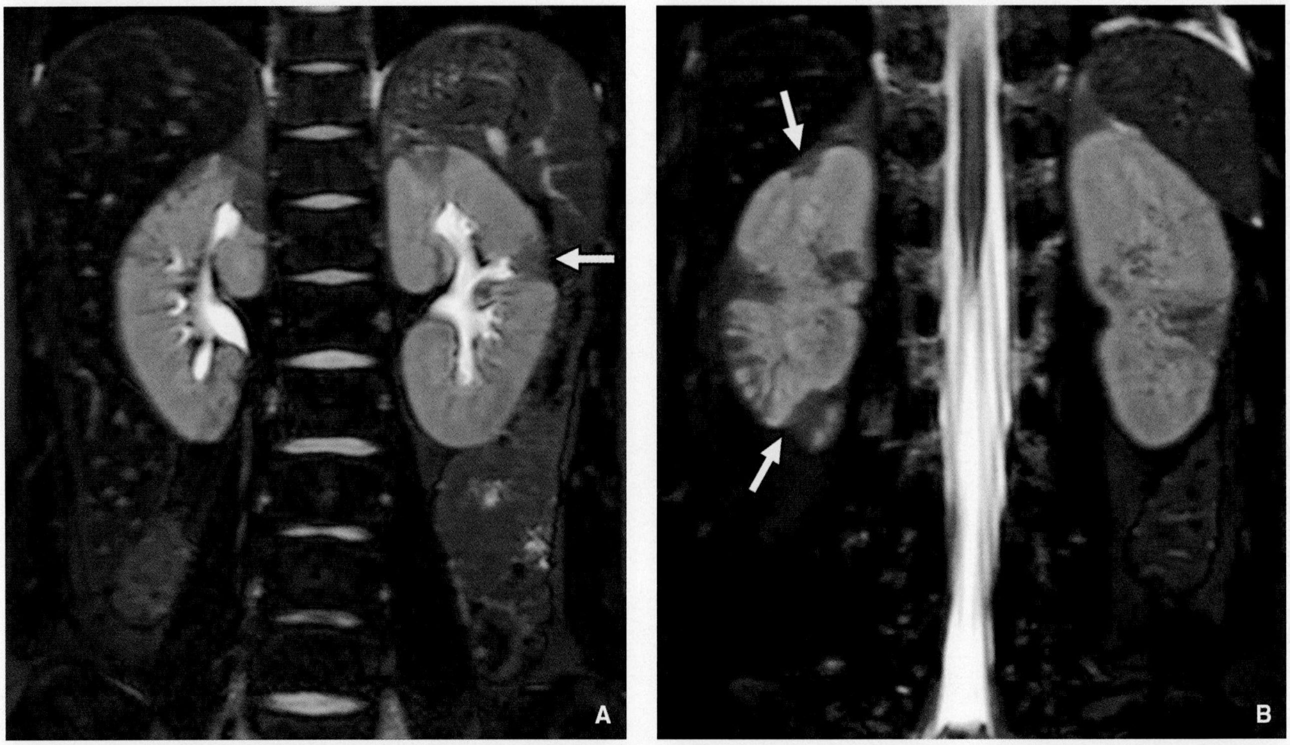

FIGURE 17.79 **8-year-old girl with recurrent pyelonephritis. A, B:** Coronal T2-weighted fat-saturated MR images show multiple bilateral wedge-shaped areas of signal abnormality. Areas of signal abnormality with associated parenchymal volume loss are compatible with developing scars (*arrows*).

pediatric urolithiasis is increasing, and numerous medical conditions predispose children to urolithiasis, such as a variety of metabolic abnormalities (e.g., cystinuria), urinary tract infection, certain urinary tract anomalies that cause urinary stasis (e.g., renal tubular ectasia, UPJ obstruction, congenital megacalyces, congenital primary megaureter), and prematurity.[172–174]

Radiography can reveal large, dense calculi, while smaller and/or less dense calculi (e.g., uric acid calculi) may go undetected (Fig. 17.80).[174] One large study showed that radiography has a sensitivity of only 45% to 59%.[175] Ultrasound has better sensitivity and specificity than radiography in the pediatric population, avoids ionizing radiation, and commonly detects calculi not appreciated at radiography. Gray-scale ultrasound classically shows an abnormal echogenic focus in the urinary tract with associated posterior acoustic shadowing. Pelvicaliectasis and/or ureterectasis may be present in the setting of urinary tract obstruction. Color Doppler imaging can also demonstrate "twinkling" artifact (rapidly alternating color pixels located just deep to the strong reflecting surface of a calculus when adjusting the pulse repetition frequency to its highest setting) (Fig. 17.81).[1] Low-dose noncontrast CT is generally considered to have the highest diagnostic accuracy for the detection of urinary tract calculi,[4] particularly when using thin (<5 mm) reconstructions and multiplanar reformations. CT is particularly adept at identifying symptomatic ureteral calculi that are not detected by radiography or ultrasound. MRI is capable of demonstrating large

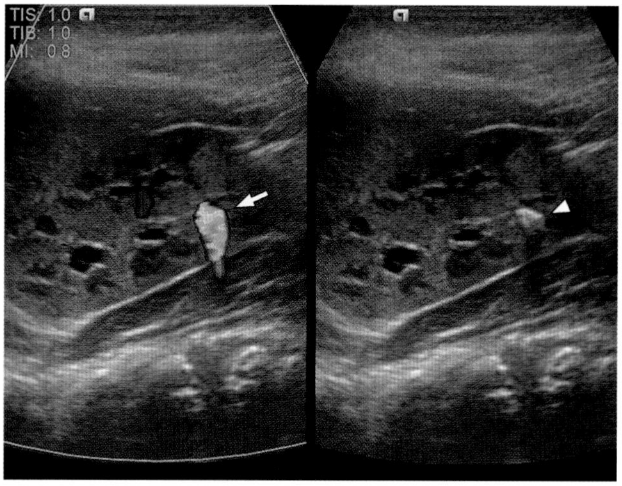

FIGURE 17.81 **2-month-old girl with antenatal hydronephrosis and incidentally detected calculus in the right renal collecting system.** Longitudinal color Doppler and gray-scale ultrasound images demonstrate an echogenic, shadowing calculus (*arrowhead*) in a lower pole calyx with associated "twinkling" artifact (*arrow*).

urinary tract calculi, particularly in the setting of obstruction (Fig. 17.82).

A variety of treatments may be employed, including conservative watchful waiting with pain management, endoscopic intervention, extracorporeal shock wave lithotripsy, or percutaneous lithotomy.[176]

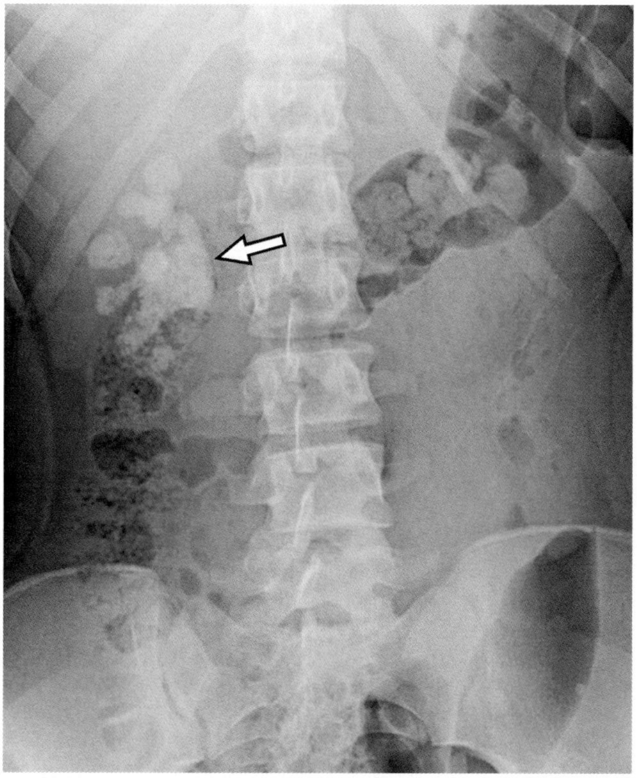

FIGURE 17.80 **15-year-old girl with cystinuria.** Frontal abdominal radiograph shows a large, branching staghorn calculus (*arrow*) filling the right renal collecting system.

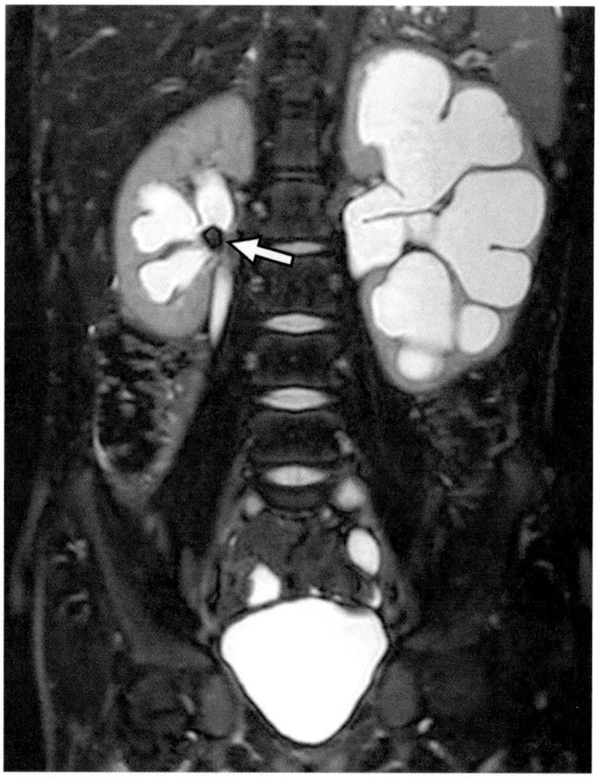

FIGURE 17.82 **7-year-old with gross hematuria and bilateral hydronephrosis.** Coronal 3D T2-weighted fat-saturated MR image shows a 1-cm hypointense structure in the right renal pelvis, consistent with a calculus (*arrow*). There is bilateral renal collecting system dilatation, left greater than right.

SPECTRUM OF URINARY BLADDER DISORDERS

Congenital and Developmental Anomalies

Megacystis–Microcolon–Intestinal Hypoperistalsis Syndrome

Also known as Berdon syndrome, megacystis–microcolon–intestinal hypoperistalsis (MMIH) is a very rare, likely autosomal recessive congenital disorder that usually occurs in girls.[177–179] Historically, this condition, which is associated with gastrointestinal and genitourinary tract muscular deficiencies, has had a very poor prognosis and typically been lethal early in life.[180]

Antenatal imaging may suggest this diagnosis, in part based on bladder enlargement (megacystis).[181] Postnatal ultrasound and VCUG also reveal megacystis; hydroureteronephrosis and VUR are common (Fig. 17.83).[180] Contrast enema confirms the presence of a microcolon (Fig. 17.83). As these children are commonly malrotated, the cecum may be malpositioned. Abdominal radiography generally demonstrates dilated small bowel loops due to hypoperistalsis and functional bowel obstruction. Upper GI series with small bowel follow-through imaging can be used to confirm the presence of malrotation, as well as document abnormally prolonged small bowel transit time.

Treatment is generally supportive, including supplemental enteral or parenteral nutrition. The use of intestinal or multivisceral transplantation has been described.[180]

Prune-Belly Syndrome

Prune-belly syndrome (also known as Eagle-Barrett or triad syndrome) is an uncommon congenital disorder that consists of bilateral cryptorchidism, abdominal wall muscular deficiency, and a variety of urinary tract abnormalities. This condition, which occurs almost exclusively in boys, varies in severity, can be associated with other anomalies (e.g., cardiovascular, gastrointestinal, or musculoskeletal), and has been hypothesized by some to be related to MMIH syndrome.[182,183] The exact cause is unknown.

Radiography demonstrates a protuberant abdomen with redundancy of the abdominal wall due to muscular deficiency (complete or partial absence) (Fig. 17.84). Ultrasound and VCUG are performed to evaluate the kidneys and urinary tract. Common ultrasound findings include hydroureteronephrosis and megacystis; the kidneys may appear dysplastic in some children, a finding that affects overall prognosis. A variety of abnormalities may be noted at VCUG, including bilateral high-grade VUR, megacystis, bladder diverticula (including urachal diverticula), enlarged prostatic utricle, megalourethra, and nonobstructive dilatation of the posterior urethra (Fig. 17.84). Rarely, posterior urethral valves can either be associated with or mimic prune-belly syndrome.[182,184]

Management is surgical and individualized to the particular child, commonly including some combination of abdominal wall reconstruction (abdominoplasty), orchiopexy, urinary tract surgery (e.g., vesicostomy, ureterostomy, ureteral reimplantation), and renal transplantation.[185]

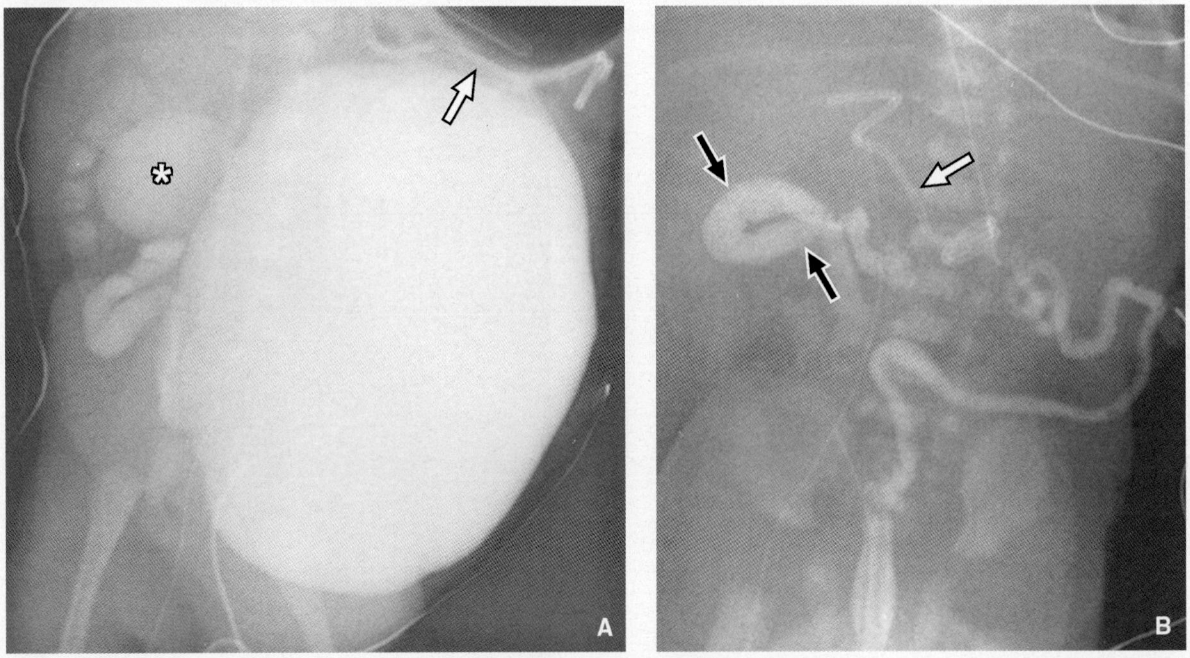

FIGURE 17.83 **Newborn with megacystis-microcolon-intestinal hypoperistalsis syndrome. A:** Voiding cystogram image shows marked enlargement of the urinary bladder. There is high-grade reflux of contrast material into the right upper urinary tract (*asterisk*). A retained peritoneoamniotic shunt (*arrow*) is present. **B:** Contrast enema reveals a microcolon with the cecum likely near the midline due to abnormal bowel rotation. A retained peritoneoamniotic shunt (*white arrow*) is again seen. Contrast material in the right hemiabdomen was retained from a prior upper gastrointestinal tract series (*black arrows*).

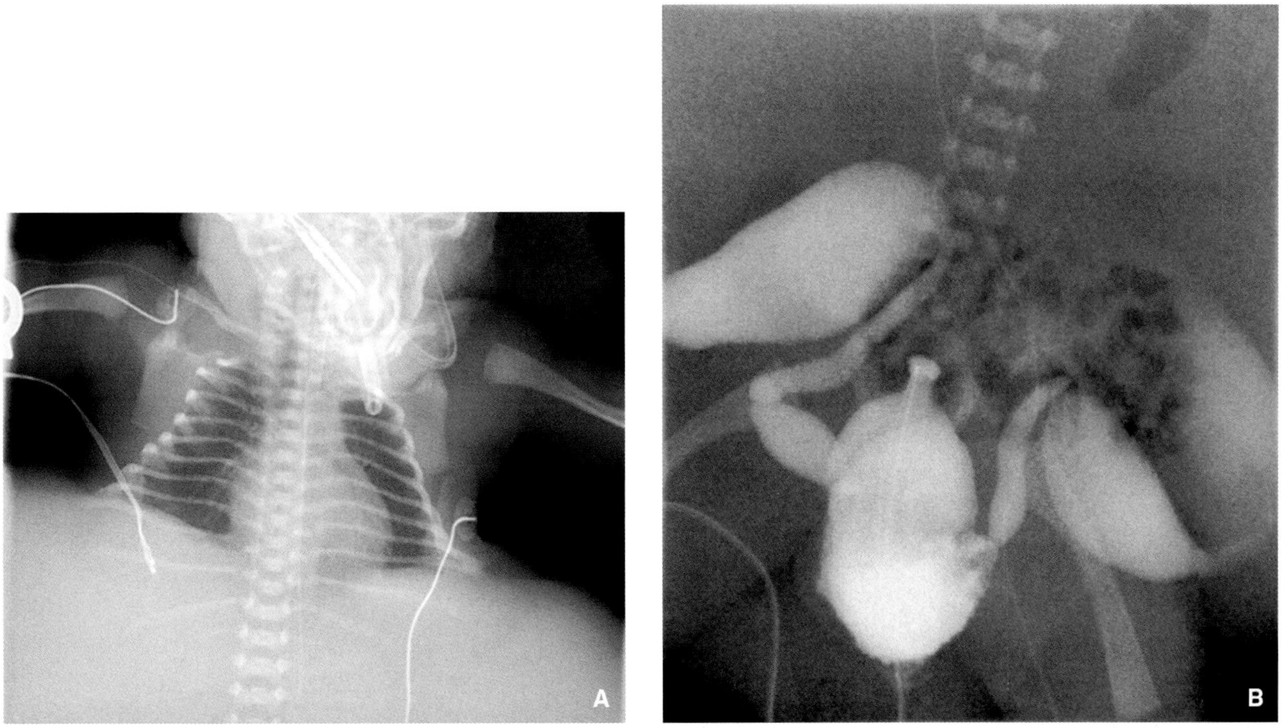

FIGURE 17.84 **Newborn boy with bilateral cryptorchidism and prune-belly syndrome. A:** Frontal abdominal radiograph shows marked laxity of the visualized anterior abdominal wall. **B:** Voiding cystourethrogram image shows high-grade vesicoureteral reflux into markedly dilated and tortuous ureters.

Bladder Exstrophy

Bladder exstrophy is a rare congenital anomaly that more commonly affects boys and that occurs when the lower abdominal wall fails to appropriately close in utero. As a result, bladder mucosa is visible herniating through the anterior abdominal wall in the midline. Epispadias in boys and a bifid clitoris in girls are common associations. Prenatal detection has been described.[186]

Radiography of the pelvis may demonstrate a variety of osseous abnormalities, including widening of the pubic symphysis (Fig. 17.85).[187] An infraumbilical mass-like opacity can also be seen. Ultrasound is commonly used to assess the kidneys in bladder exstrophy. Although a recent study revealed that renal anomalies occur in only 2.8% of affected children, postrepair hydronephrosis and renal parenchymal scarring can occur.[188,189] VUR occurs with increased frequency in children with bladder exstrophy due to altered ureterovesical junction anatomy and increased pressure within the bladder, and it can be assessed using VCUG.[190]

Treatment involves surgical reconstruction of the bladder, bladder neck, anterior abdominal wall, genitalia, and osseous pelvis, often requiring multiple surgeries.[191] Augmentation cystoplasty may be required in some cases when the reconstructed bladder is small and noncompliant.

Cloacal Anomalies

Cloacal Malformation

Cloacal malformation is a very rare congenital anomaly that occurs in girls, where the gastrointestinal, genital, and urinary tracts converge to form a single common channel that opens onto the perineum.[192] Coexisting anomalies may involve the uterus and vagina (e.g., mullerian anomalies), kidneys (e.g., agenesis or MCDK), ureters (e.g., ectopia), spinal cord (e.g., tethering, truncation), and bones (e.g., pubic symphysis diastasis, partial sacral agenesis, spinal dysraphism).[192] Preoperative imaging plays very important roles in delineating the length of the common channel, identifying the exact site of insertion

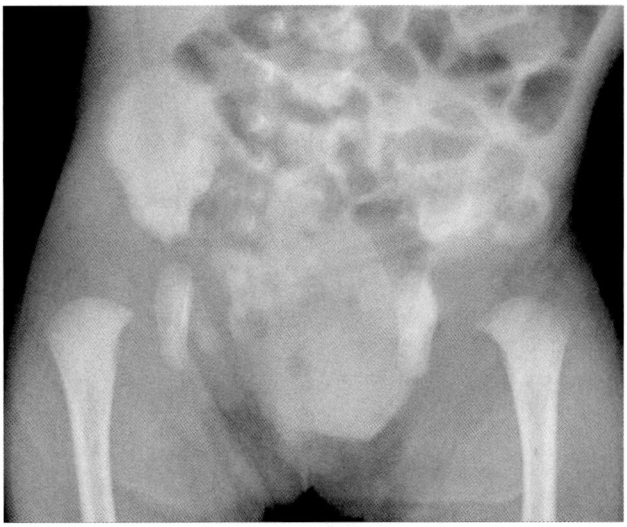

FIGURE 17.85 **3-day-old girl with bladder exstrophy.** Frontal pelvic radiograph shows marked widening of the pubic symphysis. Oval-shaped opacity projecting over the pelvis relates to anterior abdominal wall defect and herniation of the urinary bladder.

and length of the rectal fistula, defining other associated anomalies, and establishing postrepair prognosis.[193] Prenatal MRI may suggest this diagnosis in some instances, based on fluid signal in the bowel and meconium in the bladder.[194]

Ultrasound is commonly performed soon after birth to assess the kidneys and spinal cord. In some instances, pelvic and/or transperineal ultrasound may assist in establishing pelvic anatomy. Traditionally, physical examination, endoscopy, and instillation of iodinated contrast material into the common channel under fluoroscopic observation (genitogram or cloacagram) have been used to further characterize this anomaly. More recently, 3D fluoroscopic and MRI techniques have been described that may involve the use of augmented pressure injections as well as instillation of contrast material into the mucous fistula (many cloacal malformation patients undergo total diverting colostomy soon after birth (Fig. 17.86).[193,195] High-resolution MR imaging, preferably at 3-Tesla, has the potential to allow assessment of the cloacal malformation as well as the kidneys, ureters, uterus and vagina, lumbosacral spine, and spinal cord during

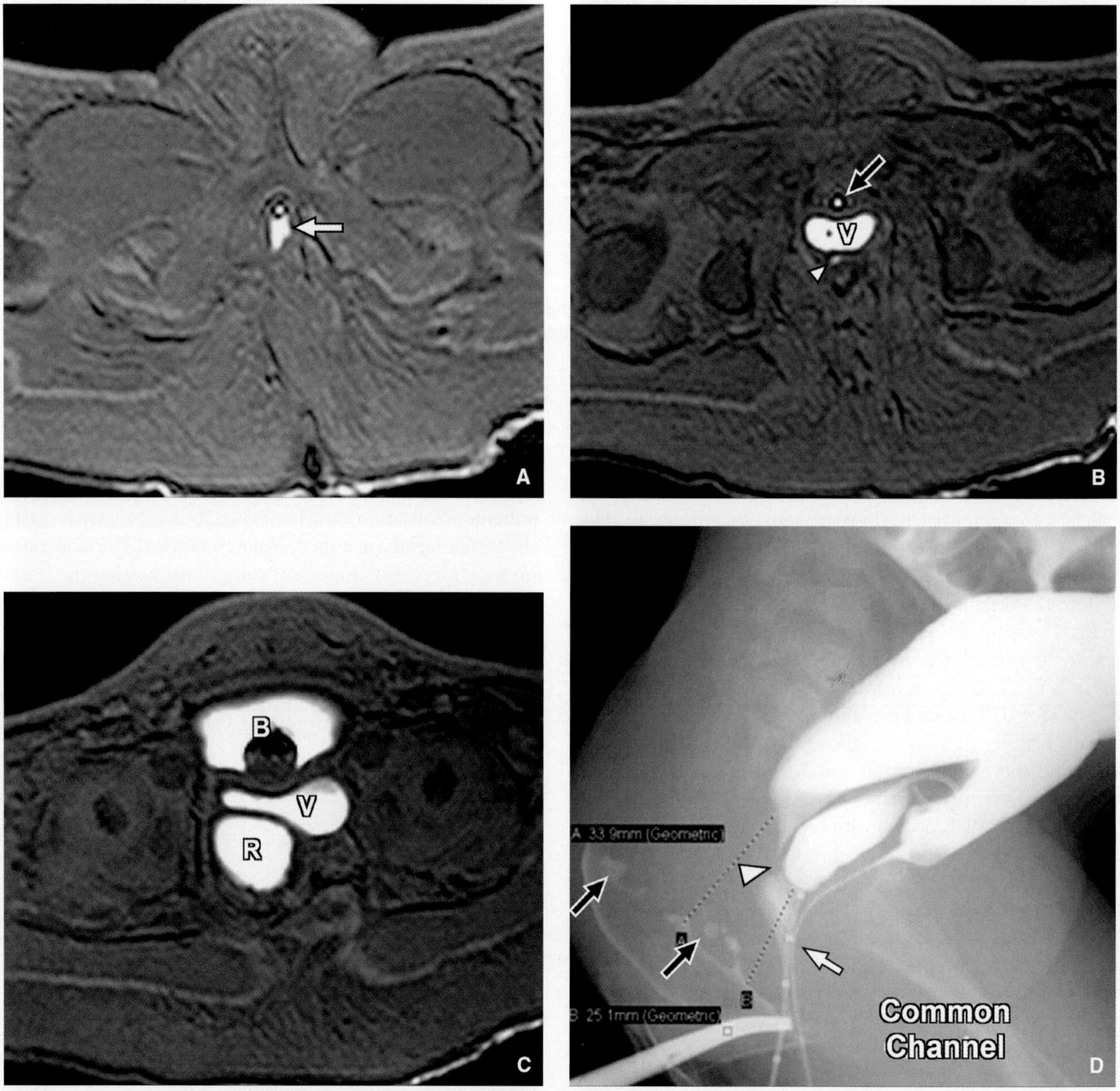

FIGURE 17.86 **7-month-old girl with single perineal opening draining both urine and fecal material.** Diverting colostomy was performed on the 3rd day of life. **A–C:** Axial T1-weighted MR images following intracavitary instillation of dilute gadolinium-based contrast material shows findings consistent with cloacal malformation. Contrast material fills the common channel (*white arrow*), urethra (containing a catheter) (*black arrow*), rectal fistula (*white arrowhead*), urinary bladder (*B*), vagina (*V*), and rectum (*R*). **D:** Fluoroscopic image clearly demonstrates the rectal fistula (*arrowhead*). The common channel (*white arrow*) measures ≈25 mm in length. BB markers are taped to the perineal skin and opening of a dermal sinus (*black arrows*). Hemostat marks the cloacal orifice.

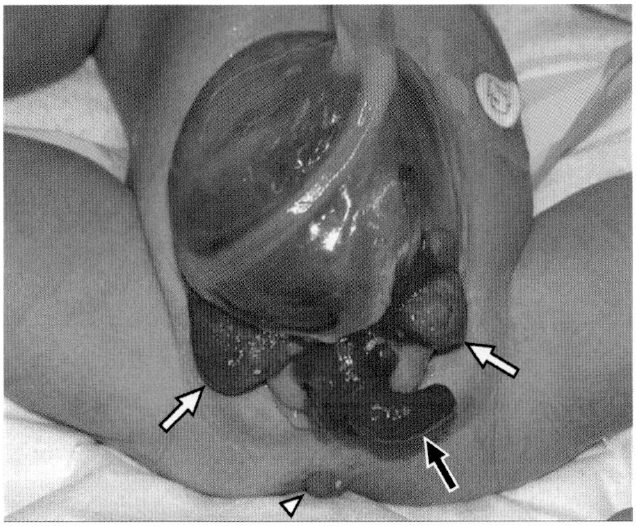

FIGURE 17.87 **Newborn girl with cloacal exstrophy.** Photograph demonstrates a large omphalocele. There are separate hemibladders (*white arrows*) with intervening prolapsed ileum (*black arrow*). The anus is imperforate (*arrowhead*). (Image courtesy of Peter Ehrlich, MD, Section of Pediatric Surgery, C.S. Mott Children's Hospital, University of Michigan Health System, Ann Arbor, MI.)

a single examination. Following diverting colostomy, definitive surgical repair is deferred until later in infancy, using a posterior sagittal approach.[196]

Cloacal Exstrophy

Cloacal exstrophy is a very rare congenital anomaly that affects both boys and girls and that is due to abnormal ventral abdominal wall fusion with resultant omphalocele and bladder exstrophy.[197] Some believe this anomaly is due to failure of migration of the lateral mesodermal folds of the lower abdominal wall and associated rupture of the cloacal membrane prior to the 8th week of gestation.[197,198] Classically, the bladder is divided into two halves with intervening cecal tissue and prolapsed ileum (so-called "elephant trunk" deformity) (Fig. 17.87).[197] Cloacal exstrophy is part of the OEIS complex (omphalocele, bladder exstrophy, imperforate anus, and spinal defect [e.g., dysraphism, vertebral segmentation anomalies]) and is also associated with cryptorchidism, malrotation, renal anomalies, mullerian anomalies, bifid penis in boys and bifid clitoris in girls, developmental hip dysplasia, and clubfoot.[199]

Prenatal diagnosis is possible at MRI based on nonvisualization of the bladder, protuberant abdominopelvic contour, and absence of meconium-filled rectum and colon.[200] Postnatal abdominopelvic radiography may reveal widening of the pubic symphysis, spinal dysraphism, and/or vertebral segmentation anomalies (Fig. 17.88). The omphalocele is often appreciable as an apparent soft tissue mass protruding from the abdomen. Ultrasound is commonly performed soon after birth to assess the kidneys and spinal cord. Associated mullerian anomalies may be detected by ultrasound or MRI early in life when the effects of maternal hormones are still present or postmenarche (Fig. 17.88).

Treatment is surgical and involves abdominal wall closure, bladder reconstruction, as well as individualized management of associated anomalies.

Urachal Anomalies

In utero, the urachus connects the bladder and allantois membrane. This structure, which extends from the bladder dome to the umbilicus in the space of Retzius, typically obliterates very early in life, becoming a thin fibrous cord (median umbilical ligament), and it can sometimes be appreciated on axial CT images along the posterior surface of the anterior abdominal wall, just superficial to the peritoneum.[182] Persistent urachal tissue can give rise to a variety of urachal anomalies that are lined by transitional or metaplastic squamous epithelium. While many urachal anomalies are incidentally detected, others may be symptomatic, presenting with evidence of infection or drainage (urine or purulent material) from the umbilicus.

By imaging, five major forms of urachal anomalies have been described (Fig. 17.89). The most common presentation is an area of focal oval-shaped, hypoechoic bladder

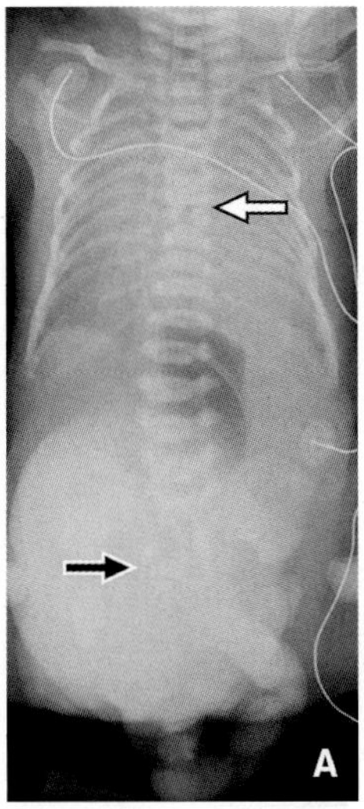

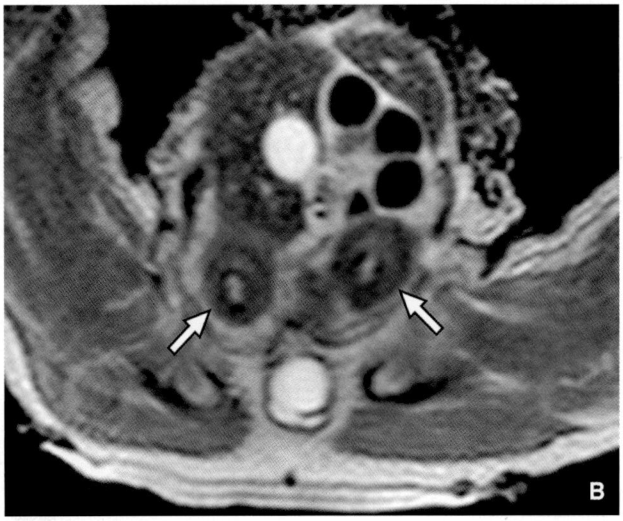

FIGURE 17.88 **1-day-old girl with cloacal exstrophy. A:** Frontal radiograph of the chest, abdomen, and pelvis shows marked widening of the pubic symphysis. A large mass-like opacity projecting over the pelvis represents a large omphalocele and urinary bladder exstrophy. Midthoracic (*white arrow*) and sacral (*black arrow*) spine segmentation anomalies are present. **B:** Axial T2-weighted MR image shows a large omphalocele containing liver and bowel. There are two entirely separate uterine horns (*arrows*), consistent with uterus didelphys.

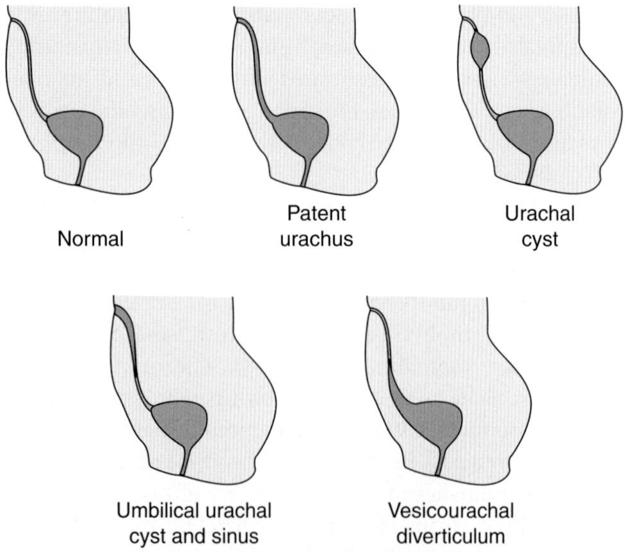

FIGURE 17.89 **Types of urachal anomalies.**

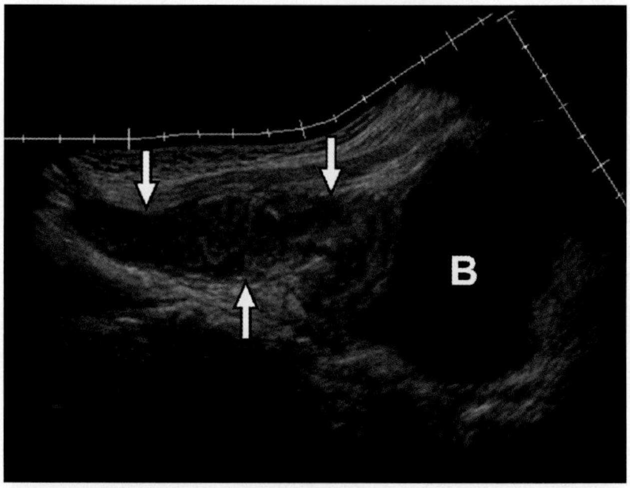

FIGURE 17.91 **8-year-old boy with infected patent urachus.** Longitudinal gray-scale ultrasound image shows a dilated, debris-filled tubular structure (*arrows*) extending from the dome of the urinary bladder (*B*) to the umbilicus in the space of Retzius.

wall thickening detected at ultrasound and located near the dome (Fig. 17.90).[201] This form of urachal remnant is generally asymptomatic and is considered by many to be a normal variant. A patent urachus is often evident during the neonatal period, presenting as urine draining from the umbilicus.[202] VCUG in the lateral projection reveals a contrast material–filled tract extending from the bladder dome to the umbilicus, often with spillage onto anterior abdominal wall skin.[202] Ultrasound may demonstrate a fluid-filled channel between the bladder dome and umbilicus (Fig. 17.91). Urachal diverticula are variably sized bladder outpouchings in the region of the dome that also fill with contrast material at VCUG (Fig. 17.92). This form of urachal anomaly is best seen on lateral or oblique images and is associated with posterior urethral valves and prune-belly syndrome.[202] Urachal sinus is a blind-ending tract with an opening at the umbilicus.[182] These structures should not fill with contrast material at VCUG and can be further evaluated by injection of iodinated contrast material into the umbilical opening. Urachal cysts occur anywhere between the bladder dome and umbilicus along the posterior aspect of the anterior abdominal wall. These cysts do not communicate with either the umbilicus or the bladder, and they can be identified at ultrasound, CT, or MRI (Fig. 17.93). While often simple, urachal cysts can appear complicated containing debris or having a thickened wall due to infection or hemorrhage.[202]

Symptomatic urachal anomalies are typically surgically resected, whereas the management of asymptomatic urachal anomalies in children is somewhat controversial, with some authors recommending excision to prevent problems in adulthood.[203] Adenocarcinoma can arise from persistent urachal tissue but is extremely rare in the pediatric age group.[203]

Infectious and Inflammatory Disorders

The diagnosis of uncomplicated infectious cystitis in children generally does not require imaging but instead relies upon a combination of clinical signs and symptoms as well as urine laboratory analysis. Clinical presentations can include nonspecific pelvic pain, dysuria, urgency, frequency, and hematuria. On occasion, cystitis may be unexpectedly detected when imaging is being performed for another indication.

Ultrasound commonly reveals bladder wall thickening (often circumferential, although sometimes eccentric or lobular) as well as internal debris (dependent or floating) (Fig. 17.94). Color Doppler evaluation may show bladder wall hyperemia. Hemorrhagic cystitis is an uncommon condition

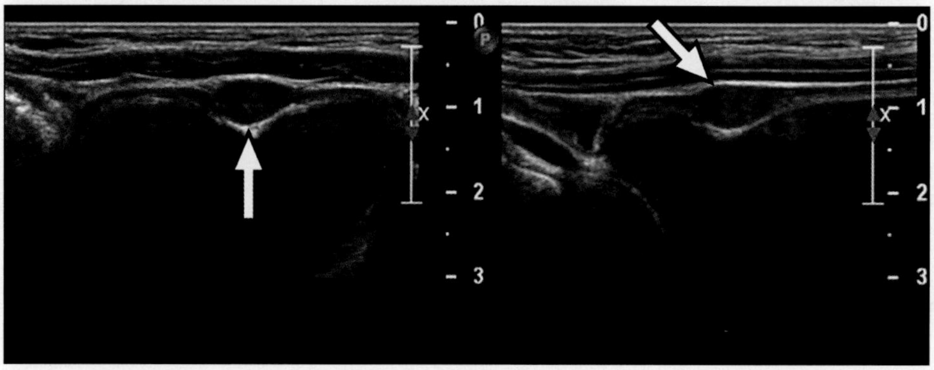

FIGURE 17.90 **3-year-old boy with incidentally detected urachal remnant.** Side-by-side transverse and longitudinal gray-scale ultrasound images using a linear, high-frequency transducer show an oval-shaped, hypoechoic solid-appearing structure (*arrows*) in the urinary bladder wall near the dome.

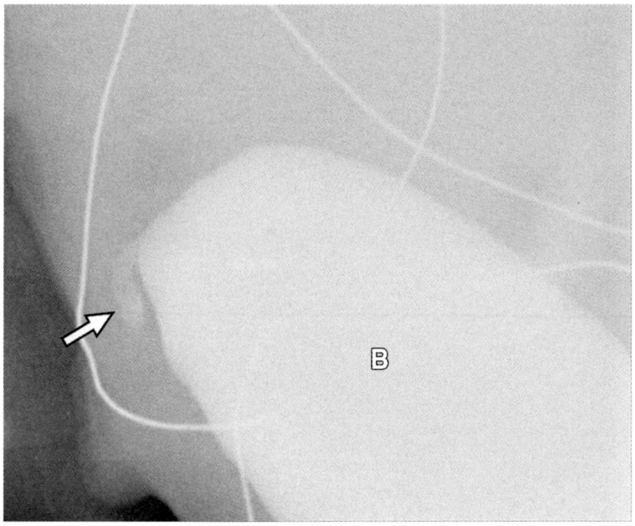

FIGURE 17.92 **7-day-old boy with urachal diverticulum.** Voiding cystourethrogram image in a lateral projection shows a contrast material–filled outpouching (*arrow*) arising from the urinary bladder (*B*) dome.

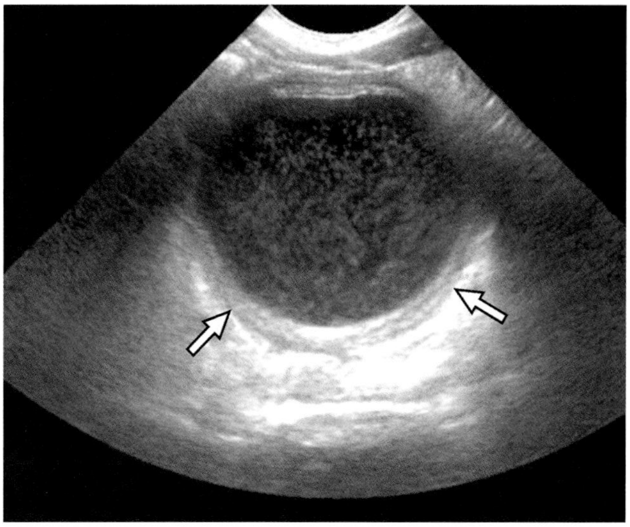

FIGURE 17.94 **19-month-old boy with urinary tract infection.** Transverse gray-scale ultrasound image shows a large amount of debris within the urinary bladder. The urinary bladder also has a thickened wall (*arrows*). Findings are consistent with the clinical diagnosis of infectious cystitis.

that is associated with certain medications, including cyclophosphamide.[204] Associated blood clots in the bladder cavity commonly appear mass-like but lack internal vascularity upon Doppler evaluation (Fig. 17.95). BK virus–associated hemorrhagic cystitis can also occur in pediatric bone marrow transplantation recipients, with the bladder sometimes demonstrating nodular mural thickening.[205]

Neoplastic Disorders

Bladder neoplasms are uncommon in the pediatric population. Pelvic rhabdomyosarcoma commonly arises from or extends into the bladder, is most often of the embryonal subtype, and has a better prognosis than rhabdomyosarcomas found elsewhere in the body.[206,207] Common clinical presentations include hematuria, urinary tract infection, and bladder outlet obstruction. Rhabdomyosarcoma may present as an irregular or lobulated filling defect within the bladder at VCUG.[208]

At ultrasound, these lesions can appear solid or primarily cystic and contain internal blood flow on color Doppler imaging (which excludes hematoma as a cause). CT and MRI can show a solid, enhancing mass arising from the bladder wall or numerous peripherally enhancing mass-like structures occupying the bladder cavity (Fig. 17.96). In some instances, multiple polypoid intraluminal masses may be observed resembling a cluster of grapes.[208]

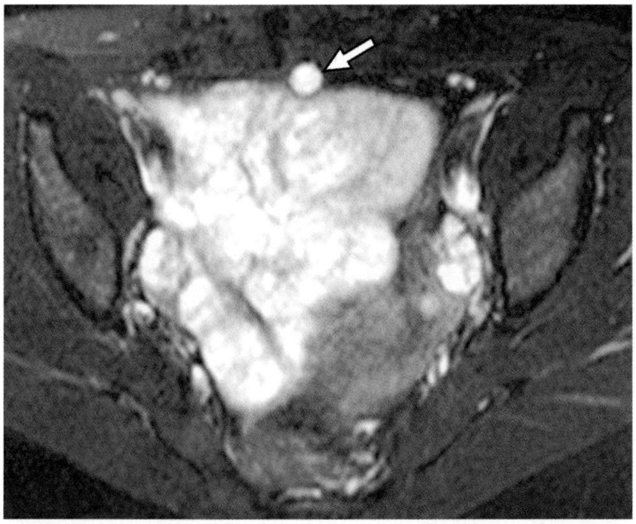

FIGURE 17.93 **13-year-old girl with an asymptomatic incidentally detected urachal cyst.** Axial T2-weighted fat-saturated MR image demonstrates a hyperintense simple cyst (*arrow*) within the prevesical space (space of Retzius), just above the urinary bladder dome.

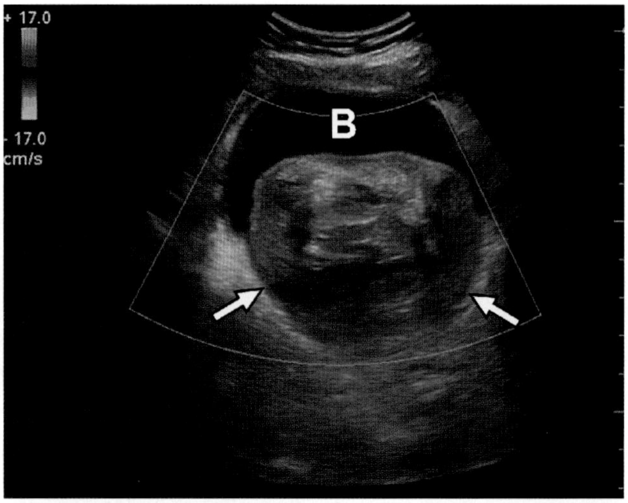

FIGURE 17.95 **10-year-old boy with lymphoma treated with cyclophosphamide.** Transverse color Doppler ultrasound image shows a large mass-like, avascular structure (*arrows*) filling the urinary bladder cavity (*B*). Cystoscopy revealed areas of mucosal bleeding and a large intravesical hematoma due to hemorrhagic cystitis.

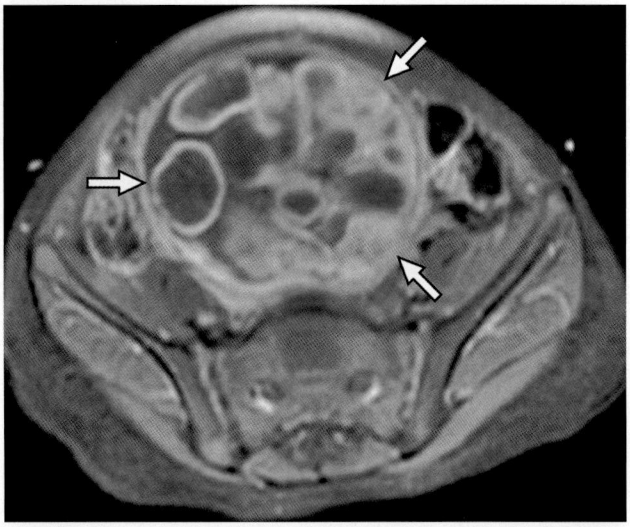

FIGURE 17.96 **2-year-old boy with hematuria and embryonal rhabdomyosarcoma arising from the urinary bladder.** Axial postcontrast T1-weighted fat-saturated MR image shows numerous intravesical cystic masses (*arrows*) that peripherally hyperenhance.

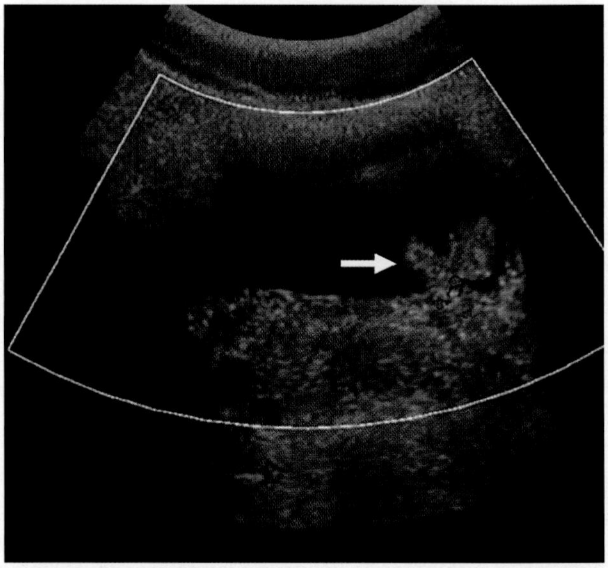

FIGURE 17.97 **15-year-old boy with a urothelial papilloma who presented with hematuria.** Transverse color Doppler ultrasound image shows a papillary lesion (*arrow*) with a vascular stalk arising from the left posterolateral urinary bladder wall. Histologic analysis showed an urothelial papilloma with both inverted and exophytic components.

Urothelial neoplasms also rarely arise from the bladder in children. These lesions are almost always solitary, occur most often in boys, and typically present with gross hematuria. Pediatric urothelial neoplasms of the bladder histologically range from benign papillomas to urothelial neoplasms of low malignant potential (the most common pediatric urothelial lesion) to urothelial carcinomas. Mean age at presentation is about 13 years. These lesions are usually adequately evaluated using ultrasound, appearing as broad-based or pedunculated papillary lesions arising from the bladder mucosa (Fig. 17.97). Color Doppler evaluation may reveal a vascular stalk.[209] In general, pediatric urothelial neoplasms are low grade and have favorable outcomes.[207,210]

Other tumors may very rarely arise from the pediatric bladder. Nephrogenic adenomas are benign masses that occur in the setting of chronic irritation or prior surgery. They are thought to be due to either implanted ectopic renal tubular cells or metaplasia.[206,211] Involvement of the bladder by neurofibromas has been described in the setting of neurofibromatosis, type 1 (Fig 17.98).[212] Inflammatory myofibroblastic tumor (inflammatory pseudotumor) of the bladder also has been described.[213]

Traumatic Disorders

Bladder injury is most often due to blunt trauma, although penetrating injuries can occur. Causes of bladder injury in children include motor vehicle accidents, falls, and occasionally, child abuse.[214] Clinically, affected children may present with hematuria.

Standard CT may reveal pelvic fractures, extraperitoneal fluid, or ascites.[215] Conventional cystography, CT cystography, and delayed CT imaging following Foley catheter occlusion have been used to successfully evaluate suspected pediatric traumatic bladder injuries.[216] Intraperitoneal rupture typically occurs when the bladder is distended at the time of trauma

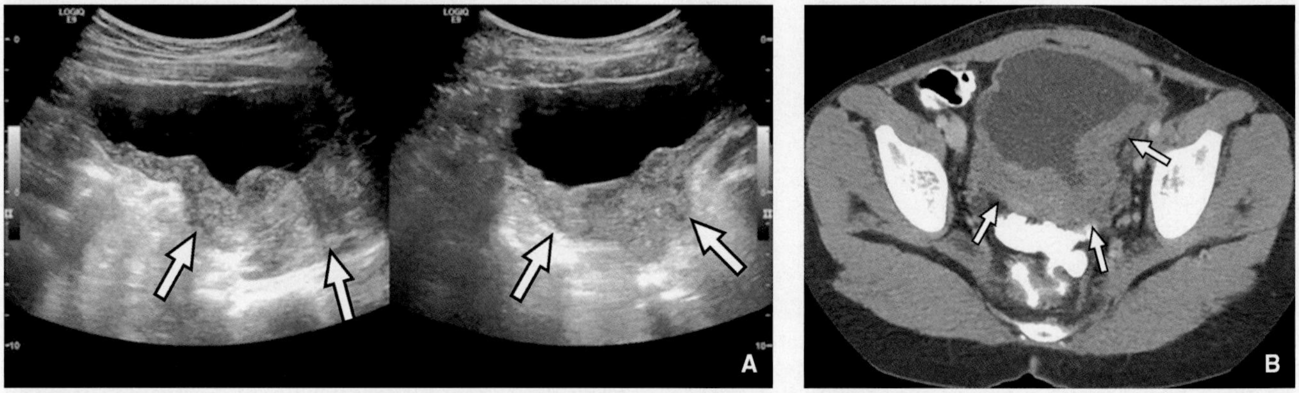

FIGURE 17.98 **8-year-old male with known neurofibromatosis type 1. A:** Longitudinal and transverse gray-scale ultrasound images show lobulated areas of marked bladder wall thickening (*arrows*) due to presumed neurofibromas. **B:** Similar findings are seen at CT (*arrows*). These areas of bladder wall thickening did not significantly change over a 3-year period.

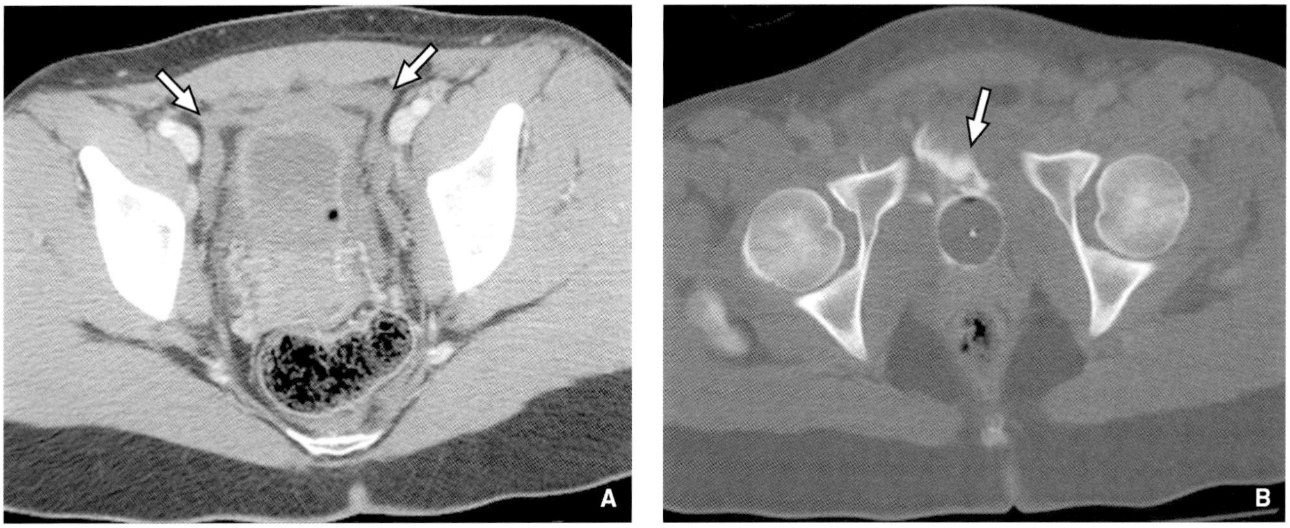

FIGURE 17.99 **17-year-old girl injured in a motor vehicle accident with multiple pelvic fractures. A:** Axial enhanced CT image shows extraperitoneal fluid (either blood and/or urine) anterior and lateral to the urinary bladder (*arrows*). **B:** Axial CT cystogram image confirms extraperitoneal urinary bladder rupture, with extravasation of contrast material (*arrow*) from the anterior urinary bladder base.

and is diagnosed when extravasated contrast material is present in the peritoneal cavity at cystography or CT cystography. Contrast material may be seen surrounding bowel loops, in the paracolic gutters, or in the pelvic cul-de-sac. Extraperitoneal rupture is more common and usually associated with adjacent pelvic fractures. This type of injury is diagnosed at cystography or CT cystography when extraperitoneal contrast material is noted in the perivesical space (Fig. 17.99), sometimes having a "molar tooth" configuration.[217] Extravasated contrast material in extraperitoneal rupture can also cross fascial planes, extending into the body wall, upper thighs, perineum, and scrotum.[217] Combined intra- and extraperitoneal injuries also occur.[218]

Intraperitoneal ruptures commonly require surgical repair, whereas extraperitoneal ruptures can often be managed with catheter drainage alone.[219]

Neurogenic Bladder

Bladder dysfunction due to a central or peripheral nervous system abnormality is referred to as neurogenic bladder. Causes of neurogenic bladder in children include a variety of brain and spinal cord (e.g., spinal dysraphism) disorders. Depending on the location of the nervous system lesion, the bladder may be hyper- or hyporeflexic.

In the setting of lower motor neuron injury, ultrasound and VCUG commonly demonstrate a smooth flaccid bladder with increased capacity. Upper motor neuron injuries more often show a smaller capacity, contracted bladder with wall thickening, and pronounced trabeculations. Bladder diverticula and VUR may also be noted (Fig. 17.100).[220,221] Children with neurogenic bladders have variable difficulty voiding; in some patients, the bladder neck may be abnormally open and there may be intermittent leakage of small amounts of contrast material at VCUG. Resultant bladder dysfunction can cause chronic kidney injury and complications related to urinary stasis, such as infection (including epididymitis) and calculus formation.[222]

Management may include intermittent self-catheterization, medications (e.g., anticholinergic therapy or botulinum toxin injection), and augmentation cystoplasty.[223,224] Augmentation cystoplasty can be performed to increase compliance and capacity of the bladder in the setting of neurogenic bladder in an attempt to preserve renal function (Fig. 17.101).[224] While bladder augmentation using large

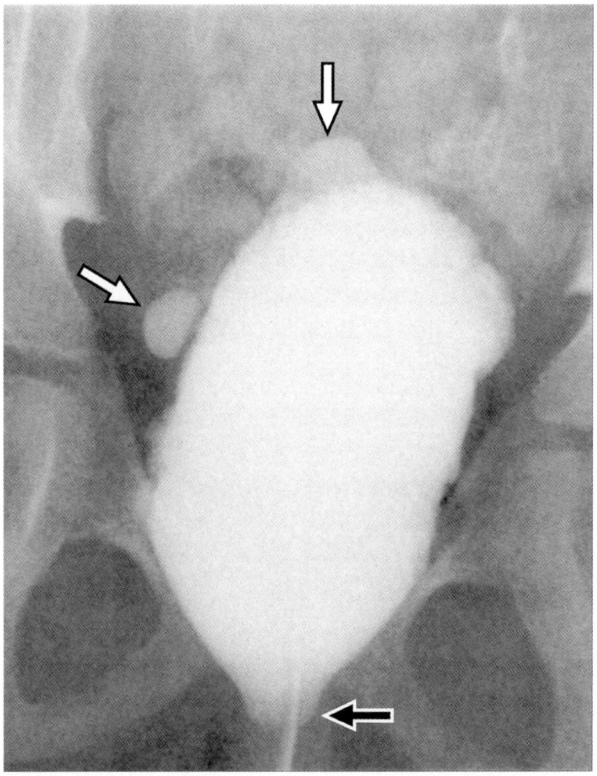

FIGURE 17.100 **5-year-old girl with repaired myelomeningocele and neurogenic bladder.** Voiding cystourethrogram frontal image shows a small capacity urinary bladder with multiple diverticula (*white arrows*). The bladder neck is open (*black arrow*).

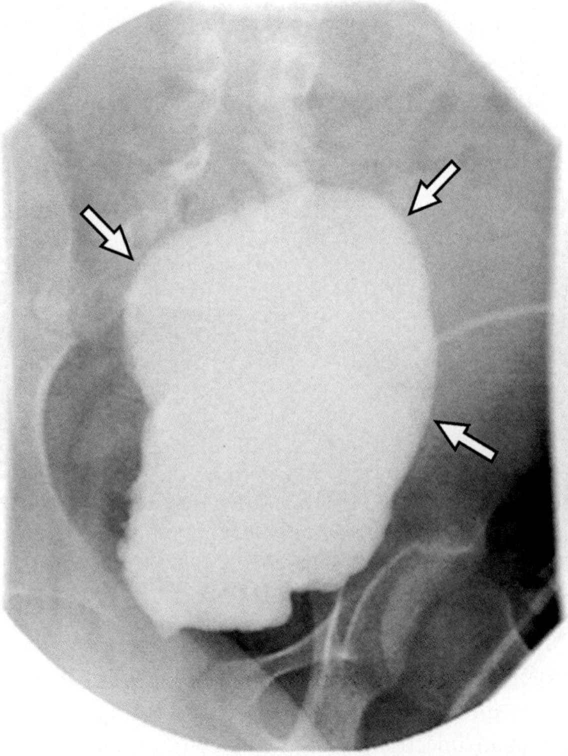

FIGURE 17.101 **16-year-old girl with myelomeningocele status post ileal cystoplasty.** Frontal image following instillation of contrast material into the bladder through a suprapubic catheter shows no leak. The augmented portion of the bladder appears smooth (*arrows*) and demonstrated peristalsis under real-time fluoroscopic observation.

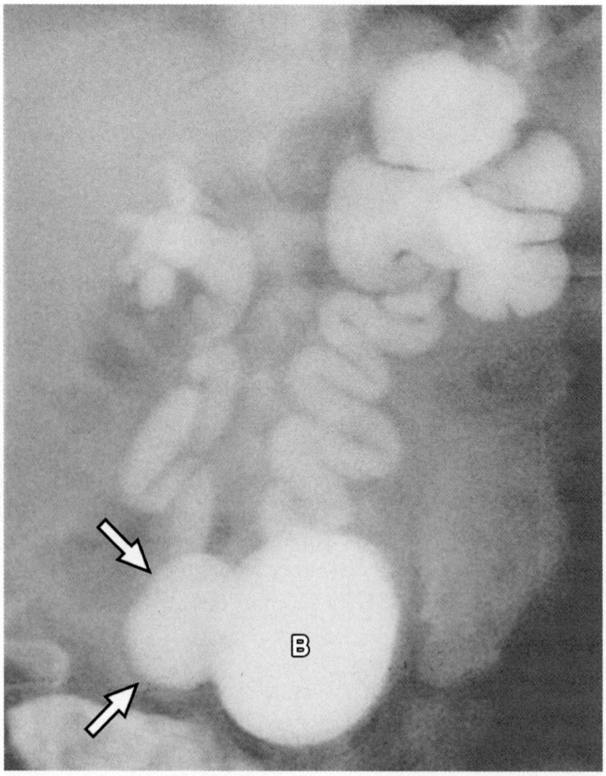

FIGURE 17.102 **9-month-old boy with treated posterior urethral valves.** Voiding cystourethrogram image shows bilateral high-grade vesicoureteral reflux. A large diverticulum (*arrows*) arises from the right posterolateral aspect of the urinary bladder (*B*).

bowel has been preferred in the past, small bowel is now most commonly used. A recent study showed that both ileal and colonic bladder augmentations have similar rates of malignancy (about 5%).[225] A subsequent study from the same institution concluded that in patients with congenital bladder dysfunction, neither ileal nor colonic bladder augmentation increases the risk of bladder malignancy over inherent cancer risk.[226] Intraperitoneal rupture of augmented bladders is an additional uncommon, but recognized complication.[221] Mitrofanoff appendicovesicostomy may also be performed in the setting of bladder augmentation to provide a conduit between the skin and bladder to facilitate self-catheterization.

Bladder Diverticulum

Outpouchings of the bladder, or diverticula, can be congenital or acquired (e.g., due to bladder outlet obstruction, such as posterior urethral valves, or neurogenic bladder) in children.[227] Certain syndromes, such as Williams, Ehlers-Danlos, Menkes kinky-hair, and prune-belly syndromes, are associated with these structures. [220,227] "Hutch" (paraureteral) diverticula occur at or near the ureterovesical junction and are commonly associated with VUR if the diverticulum and ureteral orifice are related.[220]

Large bladder diverticula may be noted at ultrasound, appearing as fluid-filled cystic structures adjacent to the bladder. A discernable neck can be seen in some cases. Bladder diverticula appear as contrast material–filled outpouchings arising from the bladder at VCUG (Fig. 17.102). Diverticula can be solitary or multiple, and they can widely vary in size.[227] Related complications include urinary tract obstruction, retention of urine with resultant calculus formation or infection, and malignancy during adulthood.[228]

When large and symptomatic, surgical diverticulectomy may be performed during childhood.

Calculi and Foreign Bodies

Bladder calculi are uncommon in the pediatric population. Urinary stasis (e.g., due to neurogenic bladder or following augmentation cystoplasty) and chronic urinary tract infection are predisposing factors for many primary calculi (those that form in the bladder).[229,230] Calculi may also enter the bladder from the upper urinary tract. Clinically, bladder calculi occur in children of all ages, and they may be asymptomatic or present with hematuria or pain due to bladder outlet obstruction.[229] Bladder calculi may appear as round- or oval-shaped opacities projecting over the midpelvis at radiography. Larger calculi may appear lamellated (Fig. 17.103). Ultrasound reveals dependent, mobile echogenic foci in the bladder that can show posterior acoustic shadowing or color Doppler twinkling artifact (Fig. 17.104). Calculi can vary in both size and number. Treatment options include surgery and endourologic techniques, such as endoscopic laser lithotripsy.[231]

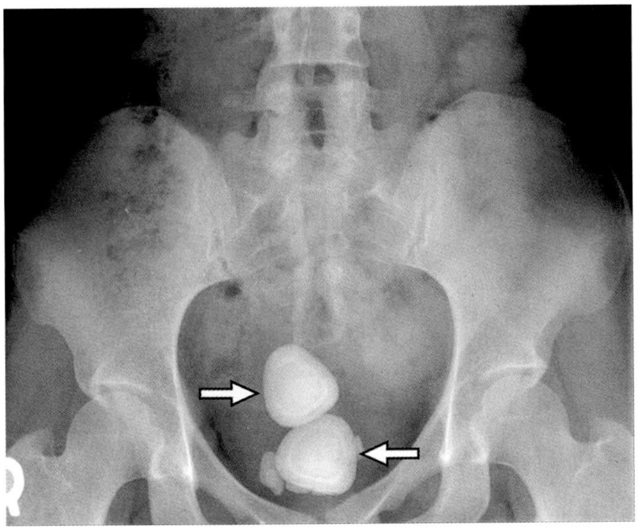

FIGURE 17.103 **18-year-old girl with neurogenic bladder due to spinal dysraphism.** Frontal pelvic radiograph shows multiple opaque calculi projecting over the midpelvis. The larger calculi appear lamellated (*arrows*).

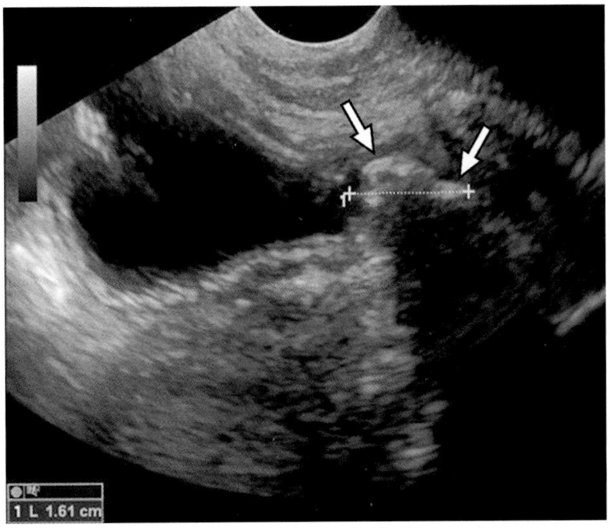

FIGURE 17.104 **12-year-old boy with neurogenic urinary bladder.** Longitudinal gray-scale ultrasound image shows multiple echogenic, shadowing calculi (*arrows*) located near the urinary bladder base.

Bladder calculi may also be the result of encrustation of an intravesical foreign body.[229] While indwelling catheters or stents are common foreign bodies, unsuspected foreign bodies very rarely can gain access to the bladder by transurethral self-insertion.[232] At ultrasound, encrusted foreign bodies in the bladder are typically echogenic and can demonstrate posterior acoustic shadowing or color Doppler twinkling artifact (Fig. 17.105). Certain intravesical foreign bodies may be radiopaque (e.g., those that are metallic or heavily encrusted). Large intravesical foreign bodies may require surgical removal, while others can be removed using transurethral endoscopic techniques.[233] Self-insertion of foreign bodies into the bladder has been attributed to both normal childhood curiosity and psychiatric disturbance.[234]

SPECTRUM OF URETHRAL DISORDERS

Congenital and Developmental Anomalies

Posterior and Anterior Urethral Valves

Posterior urethral valves are the most common form of congenital urethral obstruction. This condition, which is due to a valve-like membrane in the posterior urethra associated with the bottom of the verumontanum, is frequently detected in utero based on the presence of bladder outlet obstruction (oligohydramnios and bilateral hydronephrosis) in a male fetus.[235,236] If not prenatally detected, this condition may present early in life with pulmonary hypoplasia (Potter sequence), decreased urine output, urinary tract infection, or

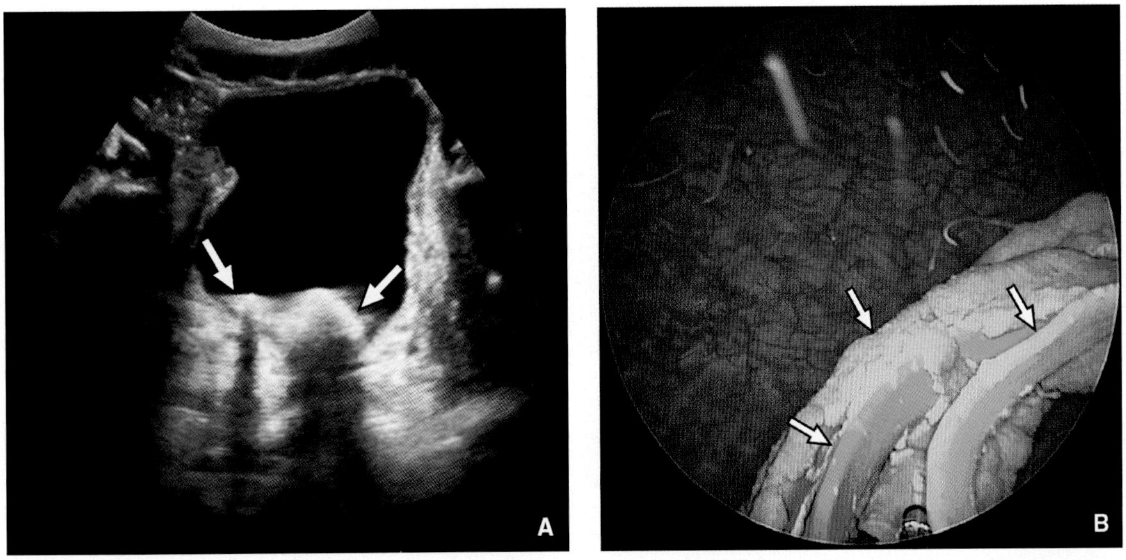

FIGURE 17.105 **14-year-old boy with an intravesical foreign body who presented with hematuria. A:** Transverse gray-scale ultrasound image shows large, echogenic shadowing structures (*arrows*) located posteriorly in the urinary bladder, thought to be calculi. **B:** Cystoscopy revealed that the abnormality was actually a mineralized foreign body (*arrows*; necklace).

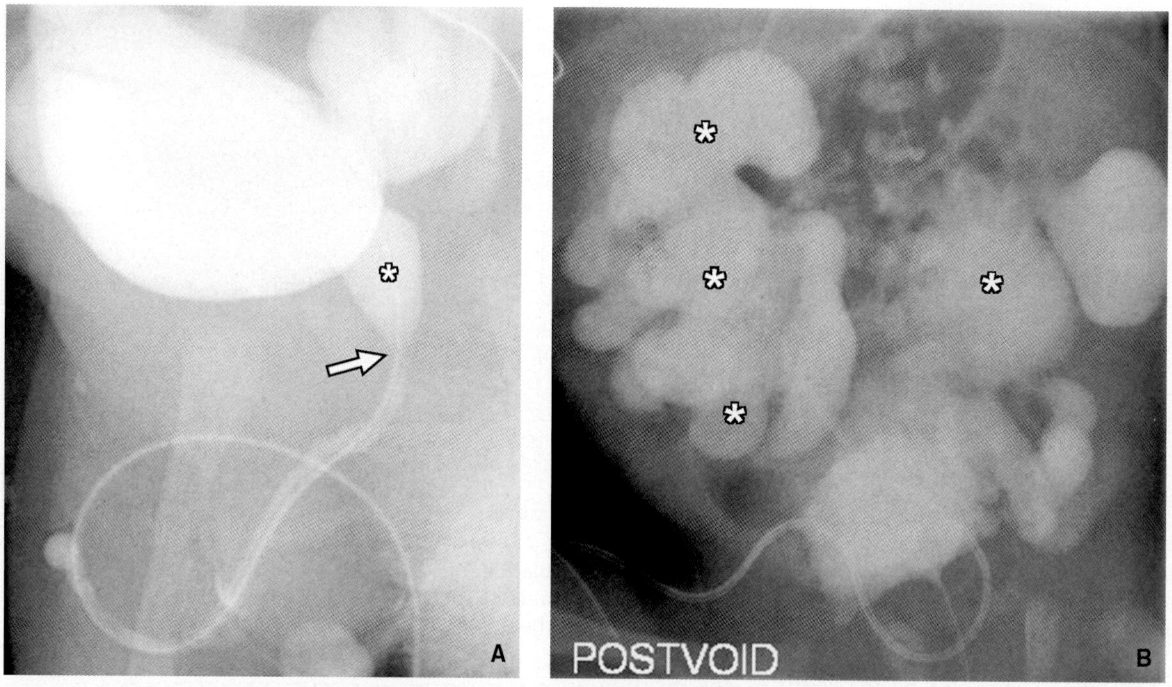

FIGURE 17.106 **1-day-old boy with bladder outlet obstruction due to posterior urethral valves. A:** Voiding cystourethrogram oblique image during micturition shows dilatation of the posterior urethra (*asterisk*), while the anterior urethra is normal in caliber. An abrupt change in urethral caliber is noted (*arrow*). **B:** Postvoid image shows bilateral high-grade vesicoureteral reflux (*asterisks*).

signs and symptoms of renal insufficiency (e.g., electrolyte imbalance).[237]

VCUG is the postnatal imaging study of choice when posterior urethral valves are suspected. Imaging during micturition reveals dilatation of the posterior urethra and normal caliber of the anterior urethra (Fig. 17.106). A thin transverse filling defect in the posterior urethra representing the obstructing membrane may be seen in some children. Bladder wall thickening and diverticula as well as high-grade VUR are common (Figs. 17.106 and 17.107). Multiple studies have demonstrated that urethral catheters do not obscure posterior urethral valves in boys and do need not to be removed routinely during voiding.[238,239] Sonography often shows indirect evidence of posterior urethral valves, including bladder wall thickening, bilateral hydroureteronephrosis, and renal dysplasia (Fig. 17.107). Perinephric fluid collections (urinomas) and urinary ascites suggest urinary tract rupture and in the past have been thought to be renal

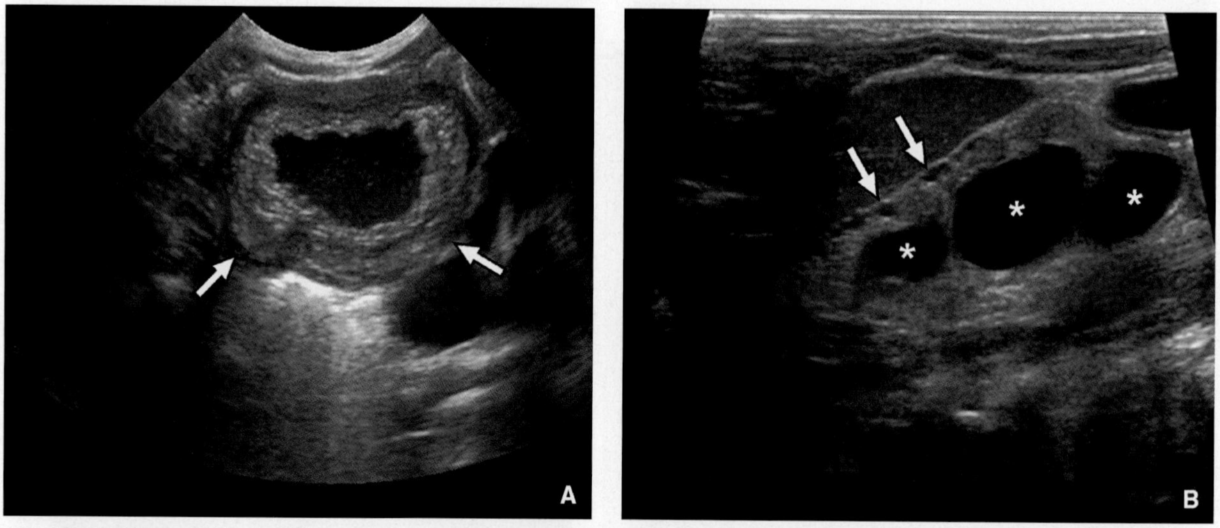

FIGURE 17.107 **Neonatal boy with posterior urethral valves and bilateral renal dysplasia. A:** Transverse gray-scale ultrasound image through the urinary bladder shows marked wall thickening (*arrows*) due to outlet obstruction. Debris is present in the urinary bladder, proven to be pyuria. The left distal ureter is dilated. **B:** Follow-up longitudinal ultrasound image shows findings consistent with renal dysplasia, including echogenic parenchyma, loss of corticomedullary differentiation, and numerous tiny subcapsular cysts (*arrows*). There is moderate hydronephrosis (*asterisks*).

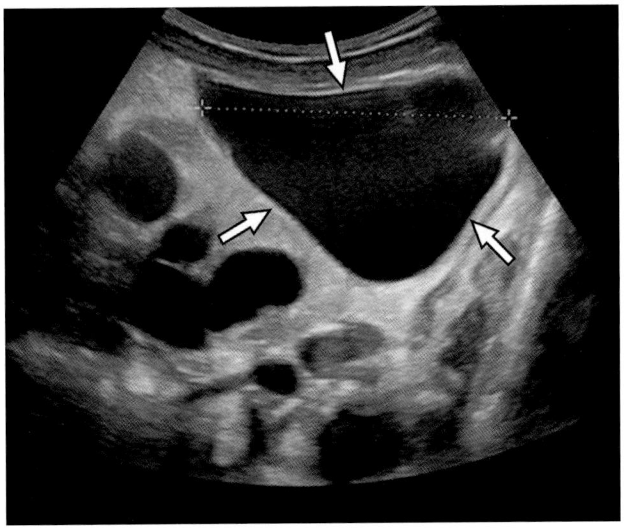

FIGURE 17.108 **Neonatal boy with posterior urethral valves and large left perinephric urinoma.** Transverse ultrasound image shows a large perinephric fluid collection (*arrows*) adjacent to the left kidney. The left kidney is hydronephrotic, and its parenchyma is abnormally echogenic.

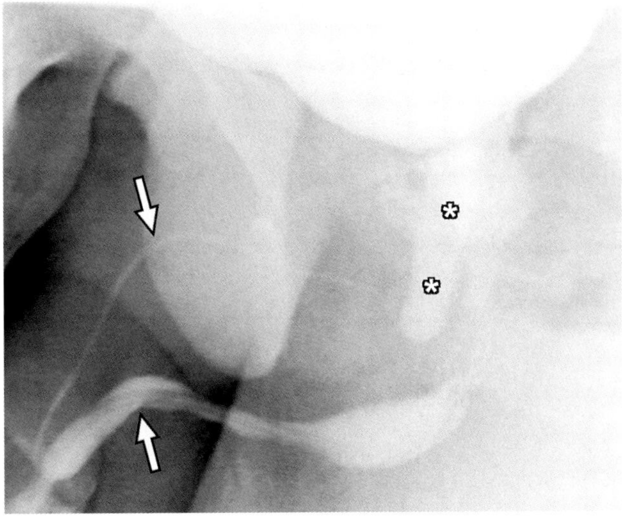

FIGURE 17.109 **18-year-old young man with two urinary streams.** Voiding cystourethrogram oblique image shows two urethras (*arrows*), with the ventral urethra appearing larger in caliber and serving as the functional urethra. The posterior portion of the accessory urethra is dilated (*asterisk*) due to posterior urethral valves.

protective measures, although recent studies have questioned this beneficial effect (Fig. 17.108).[240] Transperineal ultrasound before and during micturition can also be used to show the abnormally dilated posterior urethra.[241,242] Transurethral ablation of the valve is curative. Although prognosis is improving, long-term complications of this condition persist, including bladder dysfunction ("valve bladder" syndrome) and end-stage kidney disease requiring dialysis or renal transplantation.[243,244]

Anterior urethral valves are another cause of congenital urethral obstruction. Anterior urethral valves occur in boys and are much less common than posterior urethral valves. This form of obstruction can involve either the bulbar or penile urethra, and the degree of obstruction is variable. This condition can clinically mimic posterior urethral valves, causing bladder wall thickening and hydroureteronephrosis. Hematuria, infection, and weak urinary stream are other presentations.[245] VCUG shows anterior urethral obstruction to urine flow with dilatation of the more proximal urethra. An associated anterior urethral diverticulum may be present.[246] Transpenile ultrasound has also been shown to detect this condition.[247] Transurethral ablative techniques can be used to alleviate the urethral obstruction.[246]

Urethral Duplication

Duplication (and less often triplication) of the urethra is a rare congenital anomaly typically occurring in boys. This anomaly has also been described in girls in the setting of bladder duplication (typically in the coronal plane).[248]

Clinically, affected children may present with two urinary streams, although some individuals can be asymptomatic. VCUG reveals two separate urethras (either complete or incomplete), usually in the sagittal plane (Fig. 17.109).[249,250] The more ventral urethra is the functional urethra, while the accessory urethra is dorsal in location and smaller in caliber. There may be one or more meatal openings. Urethral duplications can be described using the Effman classification system (Fig. 17.110).[251] Unlike in congenital urethroperineal fistulas, the functional urethra opens onto the perineum in Y-type urethral duplications. There are multiple reports of posterior urethral valves affecting one or both urethras in the setting of urethral duplication (Fig. 17.109).[252]

When symptomatic, current treatment is surgical with resection of the accessory urethra.

Urethral Fistulas

Urethral fistulas in children are most often congenital, almost always occurring in boys. Acquired urethral fistulas are much less common and can be due to infection, other inflammatory process, trauma, iatrogenic injury, or neoplasm.[253] In the setting of imperforate anus in boys, associated fistulas most commonly involve the urethra or, less often, the bladder or perineum. Preoperative detection and characterization of these fistulas are important for optimal surgical outcomes.

VCUG may reveal rectourethral fistulas in some children, either demonstrating the fistula tract itself or showing contrast material within the colon following micturition. When a suspected rectourethral fistula cannot be demonstrated by VCUG, augmented (high-pressure) distal colostogram (typically following diverting colostomy performed in the early neonatal period) can be performed (Fig. 17.111).[254] MRI with intraluminal contrast material (dilute gadolinium-based contrast material) can also be used to detect such fistulas.[255] Incomplete surgical resection of rectourethral fistulas can give rise to posterior urethral diverticula, which can also be detected by MRI,[256] appearing as cystic structures located posterior to the posterior urethra or bladder.

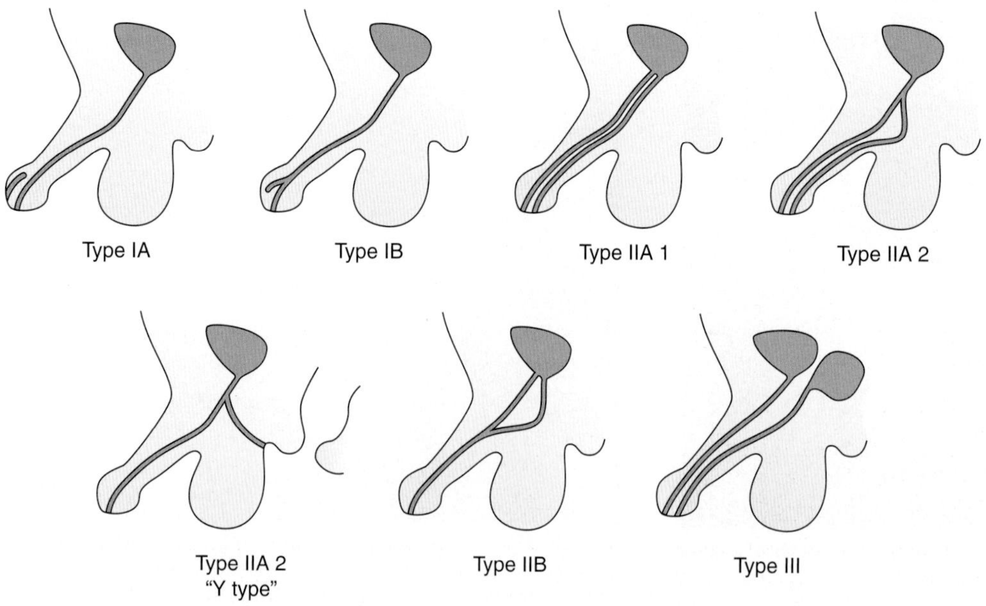

FIGURE 17.110 **Effman's classification system of urethral duplication.**

Congenital urethroperineal fistula is a rare, often isolated anomaly, appearing similar to the Effman IIA 2 "Y type" form of urethral duplication.[257,258] In this condition, there is an epithelium-lined fistula between the posterior urethra and perineum (Fig. 17.112). Only tiny amounts of urine dribble from the fistula opening onto the perineal surface, unlike urethral duplication where the ventral structure serves as the functional urethra. Congenital urethroperineal fistulas are most commonly detected by VCUG, although MRI detection and characterization have been described.[257,258]

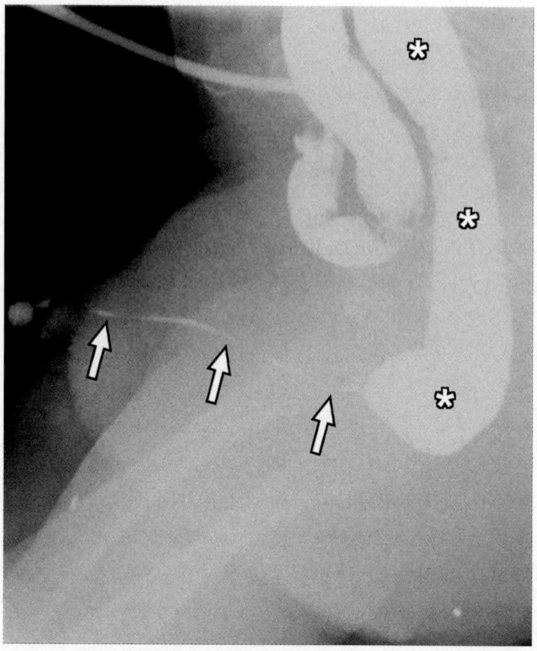

FIGURE 17.111 **3-month-old boy with imperforate anus.** Colostogram image shows contrast material filling the distal colon (*asterisks*) and anterior urethra (*arrows*). There is abnormal communication between the colon and urethra, consistent with rectourethral fistula.

Surgical resection of the fistula tract, often via a perineal approach, is usually performed to eliminate perineal urine leakage and minimize risk of infection and future malignancy.

Hypospadias and Epispadias

Hypospadias refers to abnormal positioning of the urethral meatus along the underside (ventral surface) of the penis, scrotum, or perineum. This condition is most often mild,

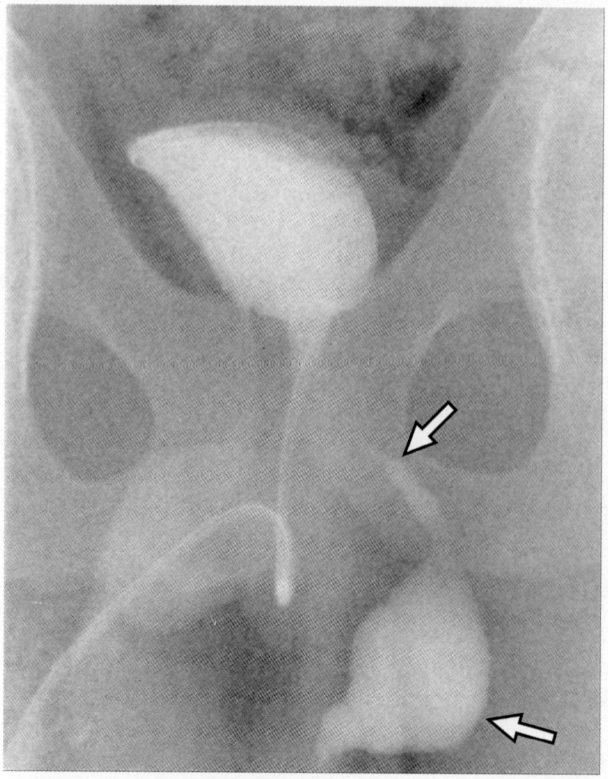

FIGURE 17.112 **12-year-old boy with urinary tract infection and congenital urethroperineal fistula.** Frontal postvoid cystourethrogram image shows a contrast material–filled fistulous tract (*arrows*) extending from the posterior urethra to the perineum.

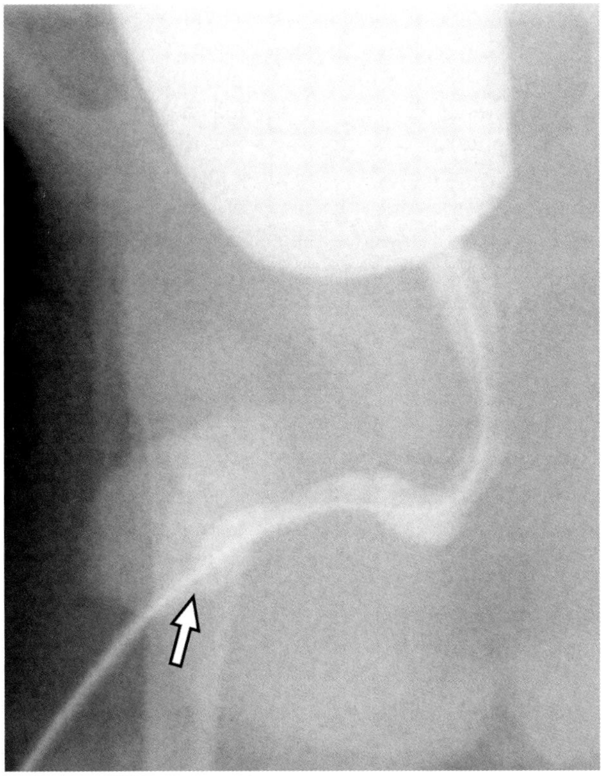

FIGURE 17.113 **Newborn boy with hypospadias.** Voiding cystourethrogram oblique image shows that the urethral meatus (*arrow*) is located more proximally than expected along the ventral surface of the penis.

with the meatus located on the underside of the glans penis (Fig. 17.113). Some authors have suggested that this anomaly is due to in utero testosterone deficiency or end-organ resistance to testosterone, with resultant incomplete fusion of the urogenital folds.[259] This condition is sometimes associated with chordee (downward curvature of the penis), cryptorchidism, enlarged prostatic utricle (size increases with increasing severity of the hypospadias), and inguinal hernia. Imaging is generally not required to diagnose hypospadias. VCUG or RUG can be used to evaluate more severe cases of hypospadias, or in the postoperative setting when complications, such as urethral stricture or aneurysmal dilatation of the neourethra, are suspected.[259] Surgical correction is commonly performed to assure normal urination and sexual function. Chromosomal analysis should be performed when hypospadias is severe to exclude an underlying disorder of sexual differentiation.

Epispadias refers to abnormal positioning of the urethral meatus along the dorsal surface of the penis and is much less common than hypospadias. Female epispadias also occurs (the urethra is short and opens in the region of the clitoris or just above) but is extremely rare. Epispadias may be isolated or part of the exstrophy–epispadias complex (i.e., associated with bladder or cloacal exstrophy). The penis can demonstrate dorsal curvature or have a bifid appearance, while the clitoris in girls is frequently bifid.[260] In severe cases, the bladder sphincter mechanism is deficient, and the bladder neck is abnormally open with resultant incontinence. Pelvic radiography commonly reveals widening of the pubic symphysis. VCUG may be performed to assess the bladder neck and bladder capacity. Treatment is typically surgical with urethral and penile reconstruction in boys.[260] Surgical repair in girls usually entails bladder neck reconstruction and genitoplasty.[261]

Megalourethra

Congenital megalourethra refers to nonobstructive dilatation of the penile urethra due to abnormal development (hypoplasia or absence) of the corpora cavernosa and spongiosum.[262] This condition is seen with increased frequency in prune-belly syndrome and VATER/VACTERL association.[263] Antenatal imaging can reveal this anomaly in some instances.[264] Two forms of congenital megalourethra have been described: (1) scaphoid (milder type in which the corpus spongiosum is abnormal) and (2) fusiform (more severe type in which both the corpus spongiosum and corpora cavernosa are abnormal).[265] VCUG or RUG can be used to confirm the presence of anterior urethral dilatation and exclude an obstructing lesion (Fig. 17.114), although some have described sepsis following instrumentation due to bacterial colonization.[265] Surgical treatment is both functional and cosmetic, and sexual dysfunction is a potential long-term complication.[262,265]

Prostatic Utricle

The prostatic utricle is a typically small structure associated with the posterior urethra in boys. Some authors have suggested that this structure is mullerian in origin and

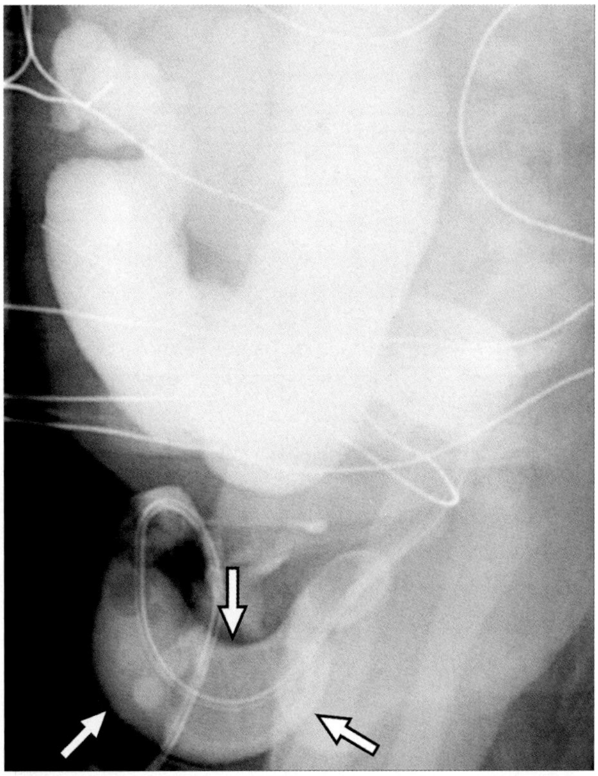

FIGURE 17.114 **3-day-old boy with prune-belly syndrome.** Voiding cystourethrogram image shows fusiform dilatation of the anterior urethra (*arrows*), consistent with megalourethra. Air bubbles are present in the urethra. There is a high-grade vesicoureteral reflux of contrast material as well.

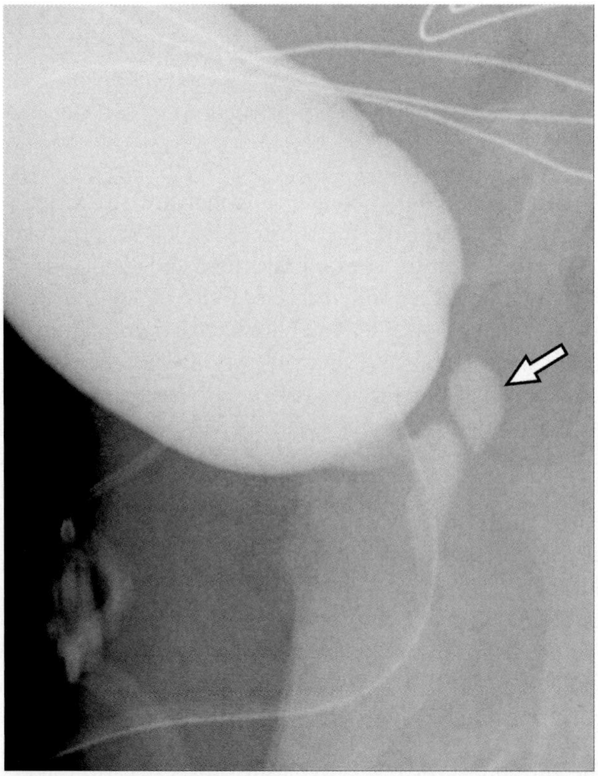

FIGURE 17.115 **2-month-old boy with enlarged prostatic utricle on voiding cystourethrogram.** Oblique image reveals a contrast material–filled outpouching (*arrow*) arising from the posterior urethra in the midline, in the expected location of the prostate gland.

homologous to the female uterus and vagina, although others suggest a urogenital sinus origin.[266] Microscopically, it consists of a hollow mass of smooth muscle with a cavity lined by epithelium. This structure may be enlarged in some children, appearing as a midline cystic diverticulum arising from the prostatic urethra extending into the prostate gland. Symptomatic prostatic utricles may present with urinary dribbling, infection, pelvic pain, and/or hematuria; malignancy can rarely arise from these structures in adults.[267,268]

In the oblique projection, VCUG shows a contrast-filled outpouching arising from the posterior aspect of the verumontanum of the prostatic urethra (Fig. 17.115). These structures vary in size, rarely extend above the prostate gland, and are sometimes visible with transabdominal ultrasound (Fig. 7.116A). MRI can show the precise location and size of the prostate utricle for preoperative assessment (Fig. 7.116B). Enlarged prostatic utricles can sometimes occur in association with other anomalies, including hypospadias, cryptorchidism, prune-belly syndrome, and disorders of sexual differentiation.[268,269] Symptomatic utricles may require surgical resection.

Infectious Disorders

Infection of the urethra during childhood is rare. Sexually transmitted infections, such as chlamydia and gonorrhea, can occur in sexually active adolescents and present with symptomatic urethritis.[270] Imaging is typically not indicated, unless postinfectious urethral stricture is suspected.

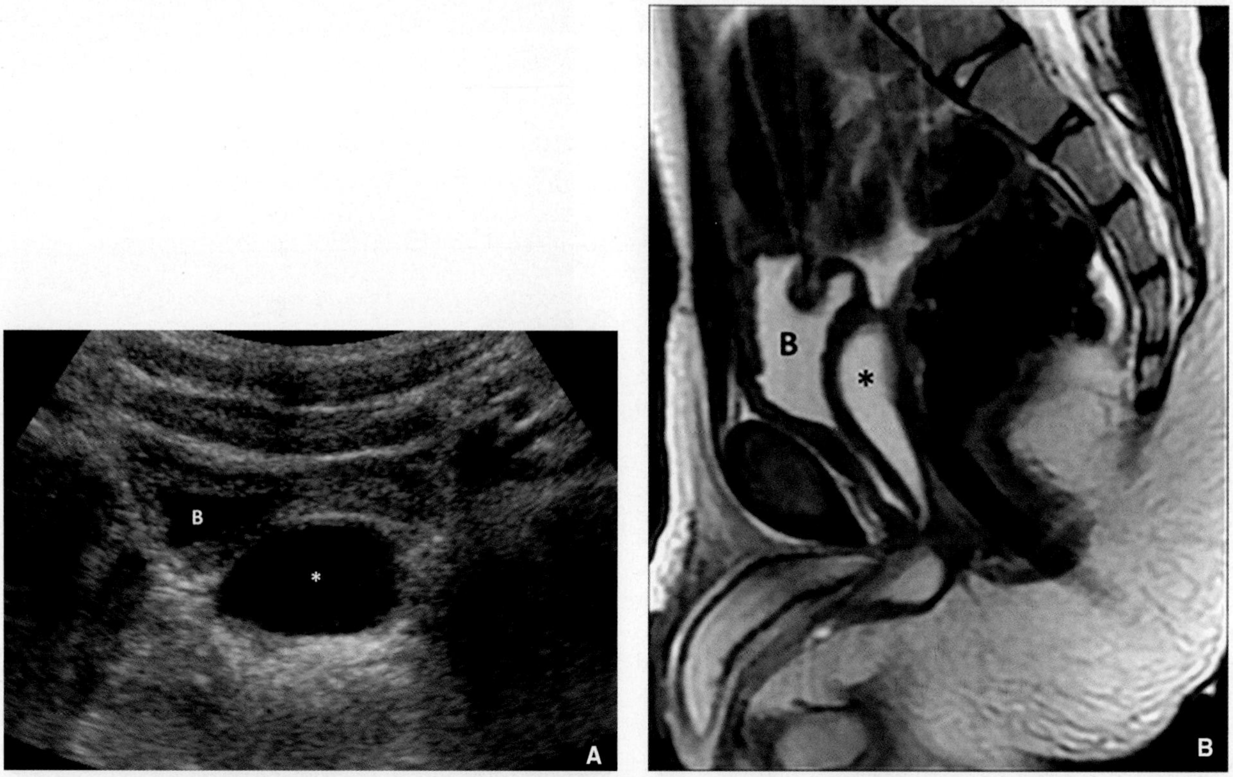

FIGURE 17.116 **8-year-old boy with prostate utricle who presented with multiple urinary tract infections. A:** Transverse abdominal ultrasound shows an anechoic cystic stricture (asterisk) located posterior to the decompressed bladder **(B)**. **B:** Sagittal T2-weighted MR image demonstrates the precise location and size of the prostate utricle (*asterisk*).

Tuberculosis can rarely affect the urethra (sometimes causing urethroperineal fistulas), although involvement of the upper urinary tract is most common in the pediatric population.

Neoplastic Disorders

Urethral neoplasms are very rare in children. Benign urothelial polyps are the most common pediatric urethral mass, affecting children during the first decade of life and presenting with hematuria, dysuria, or obstructive urinary complaints.[271,272] These fibroepithelial lesions usually affect the posterior urethra of boys, and they are best appreciated at RUG or VCUG as a mobile filling defect in the urethral lumen (Fig. 17.117). Imaging findings of bladder outlet obstruction, including hydronephrosis and bladder wall thickening, may be present.[271] The use of ultrasound to evaluate urethral polyps has also been described.[273] Transurethral resection is typically curative.[272] Other benign neoplasms very rarely can affect the urethra. Pediatric urethral malignancy is exceptionally unusual.

Traumatic Disorders

Urethral trauma is less frequently observed in children than in adults, and it is more common in boys.[274] Injury to the female urethra is infrequent because of its short length, internal location, and lack of rigid attachment to the osseous pelvis. Urethral injuries are commonly the result of "straddle injury" or blunt pelvic trauma with pelvic bone fracture(s) (or pelvic diastasis), although injuries due to penetrating trauma occur.[274] Urethral trauma is also frequently iatrogenic, related to catheterization or cystoscopy. Clinical signs of urethral injury include gross hematuria, blood at the urethral meatus in boys and vaginal introitus in girls, and posttraumatic swelling (including hematoma) of the penis or scrotum.

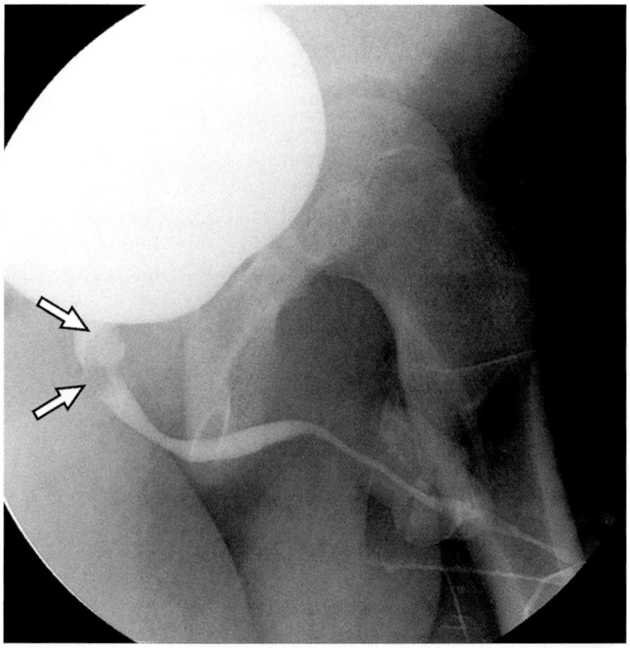

FIGURE 17.117 **15-year-old boy with bladder outlet obstruction due to urethral fibroepithelial polyp.** Voiding cystourethrogram oblique image shows an oval-shaped, circumscribed filling defect (*arrows*) in the posterior urethra.

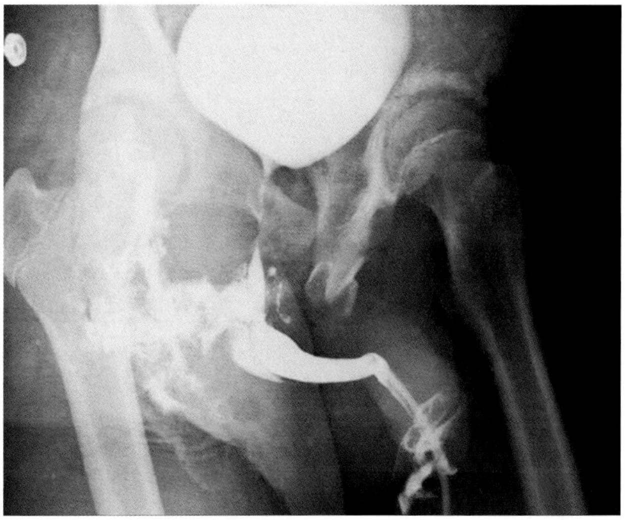

FIGURE 17.118 **13-year-old boy hit by a motor vehicle while riding a bicycle.** Retrograde urethrogram image shows partial urethral disruption with extravasation of contrast material into the perineum and right thigh below the urogenital diaphragm.

Urethral trauma is most commonly evaluated using RUG.[275] Findings suggestive of urethral injury include intraluminal filling defects due to blood clots, abnormal elongation of the urethra, and extraurethral extravasation of contrast material (Fig. 17.118). A urethral injury classification system that is based on injury severity and management is presented in Table 17.3.[82] Injury types 1 to 3 are often managed conservatively, with suprapubic or urethral catheterization, while types 4 and 5 often require endoscopic realignment or delayed graft urethroplasty. Urethral strictures can develop as a result of urethral trauma (most often iatrogenic), including as a complication of previous urethral catheter placement or surgery.[276] Suspected urethral strictures can be evaluated with RUG or VCUG (if a small catheter can be atraumatically advanced into the bladder) (Fig. 17.119).

TABLE 17.3 American Association for the Surgery of Trauma Classification System of Urethral Injuries

Injury Type	Injury Description
1	Contusion
2	Stretch injury—elongation of the urethra without extravasation
3	Partial disruption—contrast still opacifies bladder
4	Complete disruption <2 cm—contrast material fails to opacify bladder
5	Complete disruption >2 cm or extension into prostate/vagina—contrast material fails to opacify bladder

From http://www.aast.org/Library/TraumaTools/InjuryScoringScales.aspx

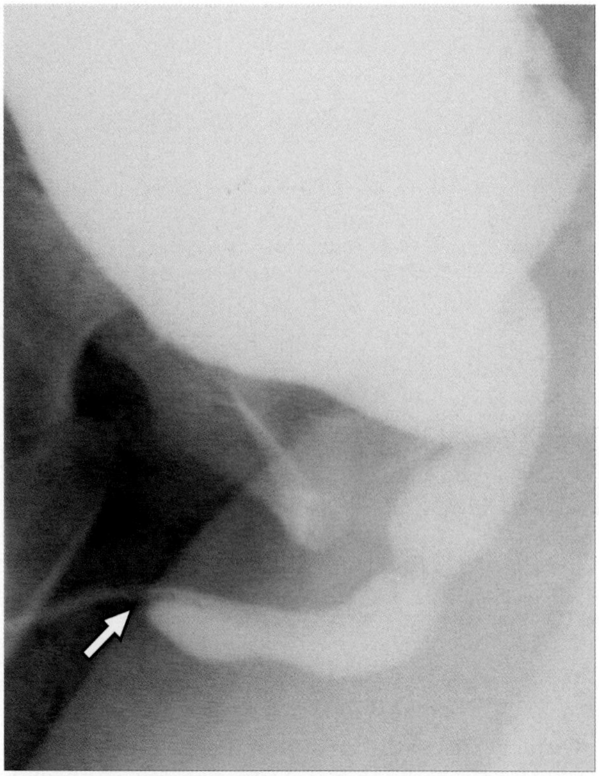

FIGURE 17.119 **6-year-old boy with history of treated posterior urethral valves and poor urinary stream.** Voiding cystourethrogram image confirms a likely acquired urethral stricture (*arrow*) at the penoscrotal junction (junction of the penile and bulbar portions of the urethra). The more proximal urethra is dilated to the site of urethral narrowing.

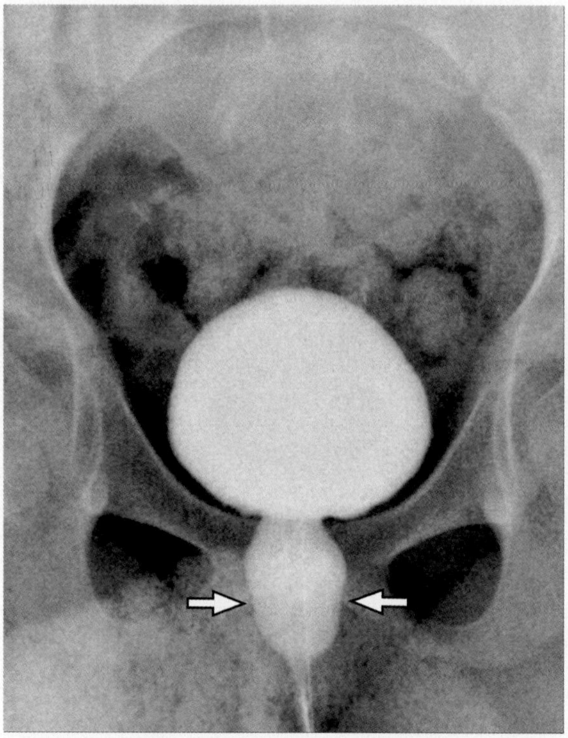

FIGURE 17.120 **7-year-old girl with enuresis and an abnormal urodynamic study.** Voiding cystourethrogram image shows dilatation of the urethra with a "spinning top" configuration (*arrows*).

"Spinning Top" Urethra

"Spinning top" appearance of the female urethra is thought to relate to dysfunctional voiding (e.g., detrusor muscle–external sphincter dyssynergia), although some have suggested that this urethral configuration can be a normal variant in certain children.[277] "Spinning top" urethra is typically observed at VCUG during micturition. Imaging findings include abnormal widening of the bladder neck and dilatation of the urethra (Fig. 17.120). Bladder abnormalities may also be present due to voiding dysfunction, including wall thickening and diverticula.

References

1. Dillman JR, Kappil M, Weadock WJ, et al. Sonographic twinkling artifact for renal calculus detection: correlation with CT. *Radiology.* 2011;259(3):911–916.
2. Darge K, Heidemeier A. Modern ultrasound technologies and their application in pediatric urinary tract imaging. *Radiologe.* 2005;45(12):1101–1111.
3. Darge K. Voiding urosonography with US contrast agent for the diagnosis of vesicoureteric reflux in children: an update. *Pediatr Radiol.* 2010;40(6):956–962.
4. Strouse PJ, Bates DG, Bloom DA, et al. Non-contrast thin-section helical CT of urinary tract calculi in children. *Pediatr Radiol.* 2002;32(5):326–332.
5. Chow LC, Kwan SW, Olcott EW, et al. Split-bolus MDCT urography with synchronous nephrographic and excretory phase enhancement. *AJR Am J Roentgenol.* 2007;189(2):314–322.
6. Smith EA, Dillman JR, Goodsitt MM, et al. Model-based iterative reconstruction: effect on patient radiation dose and image quality in pediatric body CT. *Radiology.* 2014;270(2):526–534.
7. Grattan-Smith JD, Little SB, Jones RA. MR urography in children: how we do it. *Pediatr Radiol.* 2008;38(suppl 1):S3–S17.
8. American College of Radiology. *ACR Manual on Contrast Media.* 2013; Version 9:[ACR Committee on Drugs and Contrast Media]. Available from: http://www.acr.org/~/media/ACR/Documents/PDF/QualitySafety/Resources/Contrast%20Manual/2013_Contrast_Media.pdf
9. Ward VL, Strauss KJ, Barnewolt CE, et al. Pediatric radiation exposure and effective dose reduction during voiding cystourethrography. *Radiology.* 2008;249(3):1002–1009.
10. Han BK, Babcock DS. Sonographic measurements and appearance of normal kidneys in children. *AJR Am J Roentgenol.* 1985;145(3):611–616.
11. Koff SA. Estimating bladder capacity in children. *Urology.* 1983;21(3):248.
12. Khoury MJ, Cordero JF, Greenberg F, et al. A population study of the VACTERL association: evidence for its etiologic heterogeneity. *Pediatrics.* 1983;71(5):815–820.
13. van den Ouden D, Blom JH, Bangma C, et al. Diagnosis and management of seminal vesicle cysts associated with ipsilateral renal agenesis: a pooled analysis of 52 cases. *Eur Urol.* 1998;33(5):433–440.
14. Duncan PA, Shapiro LR, Stangel JJ, et al. The MURCS association: Mullerian duct aplasia, renal aplasia, and cervicothoracic somite dysplasia. *J Pediatr.* 1979;95(3):399–402.
15. Hoffman CK, Filly RA, Callen PW. The "lying down" adrenal sign: a sonographic indicator of renal agenesis or ectopia in fetuses and neonates. *J Ultrasound Med.* 1992;11(10):533–536.

16. Risdon RA, Young LW, Chrispin AR. Renal hypoplasia and dysplasia: a radiological and pathological correlation. *Pediatr Radiol.* 1975;3(4):213–225.
17. Kiechl-Kohlendorfer U, Geley T, Maurer K, et al. Uterus didelphys with unilateral vaginal atresia: multicystic dysplastic kidney is the precursor of "renal agenesis" and the key to early diagnosis of this genital anomaly. *Pediatr Radiol.* 2011;41(9):1112–1116.
18. Grattan-Smith JD, Little SB, Jones RA. Evaluation of reflux nephropathy, pyelonephritis and renal dysplasia. *Pediatr Radiol.* 2008;38(suppl 1):S83–S105.
19. Strife JL, Souza AS, Kirks DR, et al. Multicystic dysplastic kidney in children: US follow-up. *Radiology.* 1993;186(3):785–788.
20. Tiryaki S, Alkac AY, Serdaroglu E, et al. Involution of multicystic dysplastic kidney: is it predictable? *J Pediatr Urol.* 2013;9(3):344–347.
21. Ylinen E, Ahonen S, Ala-Houhala M, et al. Nephrectomy for multicystic dysplastic kidney: if and when? *Urology.* 2004;63(4):768–771; discussion 71–72.
22. Strauss S, Dushnitsky T, Peer A, et al. Sonographic features of horseshoe kidney: review of 34 patients. *J Ultrasound Med.* 2000;19(1):27–31.
23. Liddell RM, Rosenbaum DM, Blumhagen JD. Delayed radiologic appearance of bilateral thoracic ectopic kidneys. *AJR Am J Roentgenol.* 1989;152(1):120–122.
24. Barnewolt CE, Lebowitz RL. Absence of a renal sinus echo complex in the ectopic kidney of a child: a normal finding. *Pediatr Radiol.* 1996;26(5):318–323.
25. Donahoe PK, Hendren WH. Pelvic kidney in infants and children: experience with 16 cases. *J Pediatr Surg.* 1980;15(4):486–495.
26. Gharagozloo AM, Lebowitz RL. Detection of a poorly functioning malpositioned kidney with single ectopic ureter in girls with urinary dribbling: imaging evaluation in five patients. *AJR Am J Roentgenol.* 1995;164(4):957–961.
27. Lippe B, Geffner ME, Dietrich RB, et al. Renal malformations in patients with Turner syndrome: imaging in 141 patients. *Pediatrics.* 1988;82(6):852–856.
28. Gaffney CM. Rupture of horseshoe kidney in a child. Secondary to blunt abdominal trauma. *Urology.* 1974;4(4):446–447.
29. Neville H, Ritchey ML, Shamberger RC, et al. The occurrence of Wilms tumor in horseshoe kidneys: a report from the National Wilms Tumor Study Group (NWTSG). *J Pediatr Surg.* 2002;37(8):1134–1137.
30. McCarthy S, Rosenfield AT. Ultrasonography in crossed renal ectopia. *J Ultrasound Med.* 1984;3(3):107–112.
31. Dacher JN, Pfister C, Monroc M, et al. Power Doppler sonographic pattern of acute pyelonephritis in children: comparison with CT. *AJR Am J Roentgenol.* 1996;166(6):1451–1455.
32. Maturen KE, Blane CE, Strouse PJ. Computed tomographic diagnosis of unsuspected pyelonephritis in children. *Can Assoc Radiol J.* 2002;53(5):279–283.
33. Ishikawa I, Saito Y, Onouchi Z, et al. Delayed contrast enhancement in acute focal bacterial nephritis: CT features. *J Comput Assist Tomogr.* 1985;9(5):894–897.
34. Lavocat MP, Granjon D, Allard D, et al. Imaging of pyelonephritis. *Pediatr Radiol.* 1997;27(2):159–165.
35. Smith EA, Styn N, Wan J, et al. Xanthogranulomatous pyelonephritis: an uncommon pediatric renal mass. *Pediatr Radiol.* 2010;40(8):1421–1425.
36. Rao AG, Eberts PT. Xanthogranulomatous pyelonephritis: an uncommon pediatric renal mass. *Pediatr Radiol.* 2011;41(5):671–672; author reply 3–4.
37. Hitchcock RJ, Pallett A, Hall MA, et al. Urinary tract candidiasis in neonates and infants. *Br J Urol.* 1995;76(2):252–256.
38. Kale H, Narlawar RS, Rathod K. Renal fungal ball: an unusual sonographic finding. *J Clin Ultrasound.* 2002;30(3):178–180.
39. Karlowicz MG. Candidal renal and urinary tract infection in neonates. *Semin Perinatol.* 2003;27(5):393–400.
40. Irsutti M, Puget C, Baunin C, et al. Mesoblastic nephroma: prenatal ultrasonographic and MRI features. *Pediatr Radiol.* 2000;30(3):147–150.
41. Chaudry G, Perez-Atayde AR, Ngan BY, et al. Imaging of congenital mesoblastic nephroma with pathological correlation. *Pediatr Radiol.* 2009;39(10):1080–1086.
42. Bayindir P, Guillerman RP, Hicks MJ, et al. Cellular mesoblastic nephroma (infantile renal fibrosarcoma): institutional review of the clinical, diagnostic imaging, and pathologic features of a distinctive neoplasm of infancy. *Pediatr Radiol.* 2009;39(10):1066–1074.
43. Schlesinger AE, Rosenfield NS, Castle VP, et al. Congenital mesoblastic nephroma metastatic to the brain: a report of two cases. *Pediatr Radiol.* 1995;25(suppl 1):S73–S75.
44. Schelling J, Schroder A, Stein R, et al. Ossifying renal tumor of infancy. *J Pediatr Urol.* 2007;3(3):258–261.
45. Chatten J, Cromie WJ, Duckett JW. Ossifying tumor of infantile kidney: report of two cases. *Cancer.* 1980;45(3):609–612.
46. Vazquez JL, Barnewolt CE, Shamberger RC, et al. Ossifying renal tumor of infancy presenting as a palpable abdominal mass. *Pediatr Radiol.* 1998;28(6):454–457.
47. Lee EY. CT imaging of mass-like renal lesions in children. *Pediatr Radiol.* 2007;37(9):896–907.
48. Son J, Lee EY, Restrepo R, et al. Focal renal lesions in pediatric patients. *AJR Am J Roentgenol.* 2012;199(6):W668–W682.
49. Agrons GA, Wagner BJ, Davidson AJ, et al. Multilocular cystic renal tumor in children: radiologic-pathologic correlation. *Radiographics.* 1995;15(3):653–669.
50. Martignoni G, Pea M, Reghellin D, et al. PEComas: the past, the present and the future. *Virchows Arch.* 2008;452(2):119–132.
51. Israel GM, Hindman N, Hecht E, et al. The use of opposed-phase chemical shift MRI in the diagnosis of renal angiomyolipomas. *AJR Am J Roentgenol.* 2005;184(6):1868–1872.
52. Choyke PL. Imaging of hereditary renal cancer. *Radiol Clin North Am.* 2003;41(5):1037–1051.
53. Kothary N, Soulen MC, Clark TW, et al. Renal angiomyolipoma: long-term results after arterial embolization. *J Vasc Interv Radiol.* 2005;16(1):45–50.
54. Lowe LH, Isuani BH, Heller RM, et al. Pediatric renal masses: Wilms tumor and beyond. *Radiographics.* 2000;20(6):1585–1603.
55. National Cancer Institute. *Wilms Tumor and Other Childhood Kidney Tumors Treatment (PDQ®) General Information* ; 2012. Available from: http://www.cancer.gov/cancertopics/pdq/treatment/wilms/HealthProfessional/page1#Section_558, updated November 27, 2012.
56. Inoue M, Uchida K, Kohei O, et al. Teratoid Wilms' tumor: a case report with literature review. *J Pediatr Surg.* 2006;41(10):1759–1763.
57. Khanna G, Rosen N, Anderson JR, et al. Evaluation of diagnostic performance of CT for detection of tumor thrombus in children with Wilms tumor: a report from the Children's Oncology Group. *Pediatr Blood Cancer.* 2012;58(4):551–555.
58. Khanna G, Naranjo A, Hoffer F, et al. Detection of preoperative wilms tumor rupture with CT: a report from the Children's Oncology Group. *Radiology.* 2013;266(2):610–617.

59. Kaste SC, Dome JS, Babyn PS, et al. Wilms tumour: prognostic factors, staging, therapy and late effects. *Pediatr Radiol.* 2008;38(1):2–17.
60. National Cancer Institute. *Treatment Option Overview Wilms Tumor*; 2012. Available from http://www.cancer.gov/cancertopics/pdq/treatment/wilms/HealthProfessional/page4, updated November 27, 2012.
61. Sethi AT, Narla LD, Fitch SJ, et al. Best cases from the AFIP: Wilms tumor in the setting of bilateral nephroblastomatosis. *Radiographics.* 2010;30(5):1421–1425.
62. Rohrschneider WK, Weirich A, Rieden K, et al. US, CT and MR imaging characteristics of nephroblastomatosis. *Pediatr Radiol.* 1998;28(6):435–443.
63. Downey RT, Dillman JR, Ladino-Torres MF, et al. CT and MRI appearances and radiologic staging of pediatric renal cell carcinoma. *Pediatr Radiol.* 2012;42(4):410–417; quiz 513–514.
64. Spreafico F, Collini P, Terenziani M, et al. Renal cell carcinoma in children and adolescents. *Expert Rev Anticancer Ther.* 2010;10(12):1967–1978.
65. Alrashdi I, Levine S, Paterson J, et al. Hereditary leiomyomatosis and renal cell carcinoma: very early diagnosis of renal cancer in a paediatric patient. *Fam Cancer.* 2010;9(2):239–243.
66. Choyke PL, Glenn GM, Walther MM, et al. Hereditary renal cancers. *Radiology.* 2003;226(1):33–46.
67. Indolfi P, Spreafico F, Collini P, et al. Metastatic renal cell carcinoma in children and adolescents: a 30-year unsuccessful story. *J Pediatr Hematol Oncol.* 2012;34(7):e277–e281.
68. Glass RB, Davidson AJ, Fernbach SK. Clear cell sarcoma of the kidney: CT, sonographic, and pathologic correlation. *Radiology.* 1991;180(3):715–717.
69. Argani P, Perlman EJ, Breslow NE, et al. Clear cell sarcoma of the kidney: a review of 351 cases from the National Wilms Tumor Study Group Pathology Center. *Am J Surg Pathol.* 2000;24(1):4–18.
70. Amar AM, Tomlinson G, Green DM, et al. Clinical presentation of rhabdoid tumors of the kidney. *J Pediatr Hematol Oncol.* 2001;23(2):105–108.
71. Agrons GA, Kingsman KD, Wagner BJ, et al. Rhabdoid tumor of the kidney in children: a comparative study of 21 cases. *AJR Am J Roentgenol.* 1997;168(2):447–451.
72. Tomlinson GE, Breslow NE, Dome J, et al. Rhabdoid tumor of the kidney in the National Wilms' Tumor Study: age at diagnosis as a prognostic factor. *J Clin Oncol.* 2005;23(30):7641–7645.
73. Blitman NM, Berkenblit RG, Rozenblit AM, et al. Renal medullary carcinoma: CT and MRI features. *AJR Am J Roentgenol.* 2005;185(1):268–272.
74. Davis CJ Jr, Mostofi FK, Sesterhenn IA. Renal medullary carcinoma. The seventh sickle cell nephropathy. *Am J Surg Pathol.* 1995;19(1):1–11.
75. Risi E, Iacovelli R, Altavilla A, et al. Clinical and pathological features of primary neuroectodermal tumor/ewing sarcoma of the kidney. *Urology.* 2013;82(2):382–386.
76. Parham DM, Roloson GJ, Feely M, et al. Primary malignant neuroepithelial tumors of the kidney: a clinicopathologic analysis of 146 adult and pediatric cases from the National Wilms' Tumor Study Group Pathology Center. *Am J Surg Pathol.* 2001;25(2):133–146.
77. Ekram T, Elsayes KM, Cohan RH, et al. Computed tomography and magnetic resonance features of renal Ewing sarcoma. *Acta Radiol.* 2008;49(9):1085–1090.
78. Rizzo D, Barone G, Ruggiero A, et al. Massive venous thrombosis of inferior vena cava as primary manifestation of renal Ewing's sarcoma. *Clin Nephrol.* 2011;75(6):560–564.
79. Chu WC, Reznikov B, Lee EY, et al. Primitive neuroectodermal tumour (PNET) of the kidney: a rare renal tumour in adolescents with seemingly characteristic radiological features. *Pediatr Radiol.* 2008;38(10):1089–1094.
80. Chepuri NB, Strouse PJ, Yanik GA. CT of renal lymphoma in children. *AJR Am J Roentgenol.* 2003;180(2):429–431.
81. Hilmes MA, Dillman JR, Mody RJ, et al. Pediatric renal leukemia: spectrum of CT imaging findings. *Pediatr Radiol.* 2008; 38(4):424–430.
82. The American Association for the Surgery of Trauma. *Injury Scoring Scale—A Resource for Trauma Care Professionals. Trauma Source.* Available from http://www.aast.org/library/traumatools/injuryscoringscales.aspx.
83. Bartley JM, Santucci RA. Computed tomography findings in patients with pediatric blunt renal trauma in whom expectant (nonoperative) management failed. *Urology.* 2012;80(6): 1338–1343.
84. Henderson CG, Sedberry-Ross S, Pickard R, et al. Management of high grade renal trauma: 20-year experience at a pediatric level I trauma center. *J Urol.* 2007;178(1):246–250; discussion 50.
85. Gulcu A, Goktay Y, Soylu A, et al. Doppler US evaluation of renal biopsy complications in children. *Diagn Interv Radiol.* 2013;19(1):15–19.
86. Riccabona M, Schwinger W, Ring E. Arteriovenous fistula after renal biopsy in children. *J Ultrasound Med.* 1998;17(8):505–508.
87. Heffernan E, Zwirewich C, Harris A, et al. Page kidney after renal allograft biopsy: sonographic findings. *J Clin Ultrasound.* 2009;37(4):226–229.
88. Xue R, Wang M, Li Q, et al. Successful interventional treatment of post-biopsy renal artery pseudoaneurysm in pediatric patients. *Clin Nephrol.* 2013;79(5):407–413.
89. Akinci D, Gumus B, Ozkan OS, et al. Single-session percutaneous ethanol sclerotherapy in simple renal cysts in children: long-term follow-up. *Pediatr Radiol.* 2005;35(2):155–158.
90. Wallis MC, Lorenzo AJ, Farhat WA, et al. Risk assessment of incidentally detected complex renal cysts in children: potential role for a modification of the Bosniak classification. *J Urol.* 2008;180(1):317–321.
91. Gunay-Aygun M. Liver and kidney disease in ciliopathies. *Am J Med Genet C Semin Med Genet.* 2009;151C(4):296–306.
92. Avni FE, Guissard G, Hall M, et al. Hereditary polycystic kidney diseases in children: changing sonographic patterns through childhood. *Pediatr Radiol.* 2002;32(3):169–174.
93. Selistre L, de Souza V, Ranchin B, et al. Early renal abnormalities in children with postnatally diagnosed autosomal dominant polycystic kidney disease. *Pediatr Nephrol.* 2012;27(9):1589–1593.
94. Kubo S, Nakajima M, Fukuda K, et al. A 4-year-old girl with autosomal dominant polycystic kidney disease complicated by a ruptured intracranial aneurysm. *Eur J Pediatr.* 2004;163(11):675–677.
95. Turkbey B, Ocak I, Daryanani K, et al. Autosomal recessive polycystic kidney disease and congenital hepatic fibrosis (ARPKD/CHF). *Pediatr Radiol.* 2009;39(2):100–111.
96. Gunay-Aygun M, Font-Montgomery E, Lukose L, et al. Characteristics of congenital hepatic fibrosis in a large cohort of patients with autosomal recessive polycystic kidney disease. *Gastroenterology.* 2013;144(1):112–121 e2.
97. Cook JA, Oliver K, Mueller RF, et al. A cross sectional study of renal involvement in tuberous sclerosis. *J Med Genet.* 1996;33(6):480–484.

98. Leung RS, Biswas SV, Duncan M, et al. Imaging features of von Hippel-Lindau disease. *Radiographics.* 2008;28(1):65–79; quiz 323.
99. Choyke PL, Glenn GM, Walther MM, et al. von Hippel-Lindau disease: genetic, clinical, and imaging features. *Radiology.* 1995;194(3):629–642.
100. Hildebrandt F, Benzing T, Katsanis N. Ciliopathies. *N Engl J Med.* 2011;364(16):1533–1543.
101. Tullus K, Brennan E, Hamilton G, et al. Renovascular hypertension in children. *Lancet.* 2008;371(9622):1453–1463.
102. Vo NJ, Hammelman BD, Racadio JM, et al. Anatomic distribution of renal artery stenosis in children: implications for imaging. *Pediatr Radiol.* 2006;36(10):1032–1036.
103. Stanley JC, Criado E, Upchurch GR Jr, et al. Pediatric renovascular hypertension: 132 primary and 30 secondary operations in 97 children. *J Vasc Surg.* 2006;44(6):1219–1228; discussion 28–29.
104. Castelli PK, Dillman JR, Kershaw DB, et al. Renal sonography with Doppler for detecting suspected pediatric renin-mediated hypertension—is it adequate? *Pediatr Radiol.* 2014; 44(1)42–49.
105. Srinivasan A, Krishnamurthy G, Fontalvo-Herazo L, et al. Angioplasty for renal artery stenosis in pediatric patients: an 11-year retrospective experience. *J Vasc Interv Radiol.* 2010;21(11):1672–1680.
106. Messinger Y, Sheaffer JW, Mrozek J, et al. Renal outcome of neonatal renal venous thrombosis: review of 28 patients and effectiveness of fibrinolytics and heparin in 10 patients. *Pediatrics.* 2006;118(5):e1478–e1484.
107. Tinaztepe K, Buyan N, Tinaztepe B, et al. The association of nephrotic syndrome and renal vein thrombosis: a clinicopathological analysis of eight pediatric patients. *Turk J Pediatr.* 1989;31(1):1–18.
108. Elsaify WM. Neonatal renal vein thrombosis: gray-scale and Doppler ultrasonic features. *Abdom Imaging.* 2009; 34(3):413–418.
109. Kraft JK, Brandao LR, Navarro OM. Sonography of renal venous thrombosis in neonates and infants: can we predict outcome? *Pediatr Radiol.* 2011;41(3):299–307.
110. Alaygut D, Bayram M, Soylu A, et al. Clinical course of children with nutcracker syndrome. *Urology.* 2013;82(3):686–690.
111. Cheon JE, Kim WS, Kim IO, et al. Nutcracker syndrome in children with gross haematuria: Doppler sonographic evaluation of the left renal vein. *Pediatr Radiol.* 2006;36(7):682–686.
112. Chen W, Chu J, Yang JY, et al. Endovascular stent placement for the treatment of nutcracker phenomenon in three pediatric patients. *J Vasc Interv Radiol.* 2005;16(11):1529–1533.
113. Zerin JM, Hernandez RJ, Sedman AB, et al. "Dilatation" of the left renal vein on computed tomography in children: a normal variant. *Pediatr Radiol.* 1991;21(4):267–269.
114. Kenney IJ, Aiken CG, Lenney W. Furosemide-induced nephrocalcinosis in very low birth weight infants. *Pediatr Radiol.* 1988;18(4):323–325.
115. Schell-Feith EA, Kist-van Holthe JE, van der Heijden AJ. Nephrocalcinosis in preterm neonates. *Pediatr Nephrol.* 2010;25(2):221–230.
116. Daneman A, Navarro OM, Somers GR, et al. Renal pyramids: focused sonography of normal and pathologic processes. *Radiographics.* 2010;30(5):1287–1307.
117. Navarro O, Daneman A, Kooh SW. Asymmetric medullary nephrocalcinosis in two children. *Pediatr Radiol.* 1998;28(9): 687–690.
118. Riebel TW, Abraham K, Wartner R, et al. Transient renal medullary hyperechogenicity in ultrasound studies of neonates: is it a normal phenomenon and what are the causes? *J Clin Ultrasound.* 1993;21(1):25–31.
119. Starinsky R, Vardi O, Batasch D, et al. Increased renal medullary echogenicity in neonates. *Pediatr Radiol.* 1995;25(suppl 1):S43–S45.
120. Akbar SA, Jafri SZ, Amendola MA, et al. Complications of renal transplantation. *Radiographics.* 2005;25(5):1335–1356.
121. Mutze S, Turk I, Schonberger B, et al. Colour-coded duplex sonography in the diagnostic assessment of vascular complications after kidney transplantation in children. *Pediatr Radiol.* 1997;27(12):898–902.
122. Carrico C, Lebowitz RL. Incontinence due to an infrasphincteric ectopic ureter: why the delay in diagnosis and what the radiologist can do about it. *Pediatr Radiol.* 1998;28(12):942–949.
123. Diard F, Le Dosseur P, Cadier L, et al. Multicystic dysplasia in the upper component of the complete duplex kidney. *Pediatr Radiol.* 1984;14(5):310–313.
124. Share JC, Lebowitz RL. Ectopic ureterocele without ureteral and calyceal dilatation (ureterocele disproportion): findings on urography and sonography. *AJR Am J Roentgenol.* 1989;152(3):567–571.
125. Fernbach SK, Zawin JK, Lebowitz RL. Complete duplication of the ureter with ureteropelvic junction obstruction of the lower pole of the kidney: imaging findings. *AJR Am J Roentgenol.* 1995;164(3):701–704.
126. Callahan MJ. The drooping lily sign. *Radiology.* 2001; 219(1):226–228.
127. Avni FE, Nicaise N, Hall M, et al. The role of MR imaging for the assessment of complicated duplex kidneys in children: preliminary report. *Pediatr Radiol.* 2001;31(4):215–223.
128. Rooks VJ, Lebowitz RL. Extrinsic ureteropelvic junction obstruction from a crossing renal vessel: demography and imaging. *Pediatr Radiol.* 2001;31(2):120–124.
129. Wang XM, Jia LQ, Wang Y, et al. Utilizing ultrasonography in the diagnosis of pediatric fibroepithelial polyps causing ureteropelvic junction obstruction. *Pediatr Radiol.* 2012;42(9):1107–1111.
130. Alagiri M, Polepalle SK. Dietl's crisis: an under-recognized clinical entity in the pediatric population. *Int Braz J Urol.* 2006;32(4):451–453.
131. Chavhan G, Daneman A, Moineddin R, et al. Renal pyramid echogenicity in ureteropelvic junction obstruction: correlation between altered echogenicity and differential renal function. *Pediatr Radiol.* 2008;38(10):1068–1073.
132. McDaniel BB, Jones RA, Scherz H, et al. Dynamic contrast-enhanced MR urography in the evaluation of pediatric hydronephrosis: part 2, anatomic and functional assessment of uteropelvic junction obstruction. *AJR Am J Roentgenol.* 2005;185(6):1608–1614.
133. Calder AD, Hiorns MP, Abhyankar A, et al. Contrast-enhanced magnetic resonance angiography for the detection of crossing renal vessels in children with symptomatic ureteropelvic junction obstruction: comparison with operative findings. *Pediatr Radiol.* 2007;37(4):356–361.
134. Lebowitz RL, Blickman JG. The coexistence of ureteropelvic junction obstruction and reflux. *AJR Am J Roentgenol.* 1983;140(2):231–238.
135. Barbosa JA, Kowal A, Onal B, et al. Comparative evaluation of the resolution of hydronephrosis in children who underwent open and robotic-assisted laparoscopic pyeloplasty. *J Pediatr Urol.* 2013;9(2):199–205.

136. Botelho L, Rincon JA, Nguyen HT, et al. Intermittent ureterovesical junction obstruction in children. *J Pediatr Urol.* 2011;7(5):579–581.
137. Kart Y, Karakus OZ, Ates O, et al. Altered expression of interstitial cells of Cajal in primary obstructive megaureter. *J Pediatr Urol.* 2013;9:1028–1031.
138. Gimpel C, Masioniene L, Djakovic N, et al. Complications and long-term outcome of primary obstructive megaureter in childhood. *Pediatr Nephrol.* 2010;25(9):1679–1686.
139. Pfister RC, Hendren WH. Primary megaureter in children and adults. Clinical and pathophysiologic features of 150 ureters. *Urology.* 1978;12(2):160–176.
140. Meyer JS, Lebowitz RL. Primary megaureter in infants and children: a review. *Urol Radiol.* 1992;14(4):296–305.
141. McGrath MA, Estroff J, Lebowitz RL. The coexistence of obstruction at the ureteropelvic and ureterovesical junctions. *AJR Am J Roentgenol.* 1987;149(2):403–406.
142. Vargas B, Lebowitz RL. The coexistence of congenital megacalyces and primary megaureter. *AJR Am J Roentgenol.* 1986; 147(2):313–316.
143. Liu HY, Dhillon HK, Yeung CK, et al. Clinical outcome and management of prenatally diagnosed primary megaureters. *J Urol.* 1994;152(2 pt 2):614–617.
144. Ranawaka R, Hennayake S. Resolution of primary nonrefluxing megaureter: an observational study. *J Pediatr Surg.* 2013;48(2):380–383.
145. Kozakewich HP, Lebowitz RL. Congenital megacalyces. *Pediatr Radiol.* 1974;2(4):251–257.
146. Zerin JM. Congenital megacalyces. *Pediatr Radiol.* 2010; 40(9):1470.
147. Lin N, Xie L, Zhang P, et al. Computed tomography urography for diagnosis of calyceal diverticulum complicated by urolithiasis: the accuracy and the effect of abdominal compression and prolongation of acquisition delay. *Urology.* 2013;82(4):786–790.
148. Siegel MJ, McAlister WH. Calyceal diverticula in children: unusual features and complications. *Radiology.* 1979; 131(1):79–82.
149. Docimo SG, Lebowitz RL, Retik AB, et al. Congenital midureteral obstruction. *Urol Radiol.* 1989;11(3):156–160.
150. Hwang AH, McAleer IM, Shapiro E, et al. Congenital mid ureteral strictures. *J Urol.* 2005;174(5):1999–2002.
151. Grattan-Smith JD, Jones RA, Little S, et al. Bilateral congenital midureteric strictures associated with multicystic dysplastic kidney and hydronephrosis: evaluation with MR urography. *Pediatr Radiol.* 2011;41(1):117–120.
152. Acharya SK, Jindal B, Yadav DK, et al. Retrocaval ureter: a rare cause of hydronephrosis in children. *J Pediatr Surg.* 2009; 44(4):846–848.
153. Pienkny AJ, Herts B, Streem SB. Contemporary diagnosis of retrocaval ureter. *J Endourol.* 1999;13(10):721–722.
154. Uthappa MC, Anthony D, Allen C. Case report: retrocaval ureter: MR appearances. *Br J Radiol.* 2002;75(890):177–179.
155. Smith KM, Shrivastava D, Ravish IR, et al. Robot-assisted laparoscopic ureteroureterostomy for proximal ureteral obstructions in children. *J Pediatr Urol.* 2009;5(6):475–479.
156. Schneider K, Helmig FJ, Eife R, et al. Pyonephrosis in childhood—is ultrasound sufficient for diagnosis? *Pediatr Radiol.* 1989;19(5):302–307.
157. St Lezin M, Hofmann R, Stoller ML. Pyonephrosis: diagnosis and treatment. *Br J Urol.* 1992;70(4):360–363.
158. Colemen BG, Arger PH, Mulhern CB Jr, et al. Pyonephrosis: sonography in the diagnosis and management. *AJR Am J Roentgenol.* 1981;137(5):939–943.
159. Niu ZB, Yang Y, Hou Y, et al. Ureteral polyps: an etiological factor of hydronephrosis in children that should not be ignored. *Pediatr Surg Int.* 2007;23(4):323–326.
160. Childs MA, Umbreit EC, Krambeck AE, et al. Fibroepithelial polyps of the ureter: a single-institutional experience. *J Endourol.* 2009;23(9):1415–1419.
161. Miranda D, DeAssis AS. Transitional cell papilloma of ureter in young boy. *Urology.* 1975;5(4):559–561.
162. Yanase M, Tsukamoto T, Kumamoto Y, et al. Transitional cell carcinoma of the bladder or renal pelvis in children. *Eur Urol.* 1991;19(4):312–314.
163. Smith EA. Pyelonephritis, renal scarring, and reflux nephropathy: a pediatric urologist's perspective. *Pediatr Radiol.* 2008;38(suppl 1):S76–S82.
164. Schneider K, Jablonski C, Wiessner M, et al. Screening for vesicoureteral reflux in children using real-time sonography. *Pediatr Radiol.* 1984;14(6):400–403.
165. Alton DJ, LeQuesne GW, Gent R, et al. Sonographically demonstrated thickening of the renal pelvis in children. *Pediatr Radiol.* 1992;22(6):426–429.
166. Massanyi EZ, Preece J, Gupta A, et al. Utility of screening ultrasound after first febrile UTI among patients with clinically significant vesicoureteral reflux. *Urology.* 2013;82:905–909.
167. Lebowitz RL, Olbing H, Parkkulainen KV, et al. International system of radiographic grading of vesicoureteric reflux. International Reflux Study in Children. *Pediatr Radiol.* 1985;15(2):105–109.
168. Conway JJ, Belman AB, King LR, et al. Direct and indirect radionuclide cystography. *J Urol.* 1975;113(5):689–693.
169. Fretzayas A, Karpathios T, Dimitriou P, et al. Grading of vesicoureteral reflux by radionuclide cystography. *Pediatr Radiol.* 1984;14(3):148–150.
170. Herz D, Merguerian P, McQuiston L, et al. 5-year prospective results of dimercapto-succinic acid imaging in children with febrile urinary tract infection: proof that the top-down approach works. *J Urol.* 2010;184(4 suppl):1703–1709.
171. Shaikh N, Hoberman A, Rockette HE, et al. Identifying children with vesicoureteral reflux: a comparison of 2 approaches. *J Urol.* 2012;188(5):1895–1899.
172. Cochat P, Pichault V, Bacchetta J, et al. Nephrolithiasis related to inborn metabolic diseases. *Pediatr Nephrol.* 2010;25(3): 415–424.
173. Dwyer ME, Krambeck AE, Bergstralh EJ, et al. Temporal trends in incidence of kidney stones among children: a 25-year population based study. *J Urol.* 2012;188(1):247–252.
174. Kraus SJ, Lebowitz RL, Royal SA. Renal calculi in children: imaging features that lead to diagnoses: a pictorial essay. *Pediatr Radiol.* 1999;29(8):624–630.
175. Levine JA, Neitlich J, Verga M, et al. Ureteral calculi in patients with flank pain: correlation of plain radiography with unenhanced helical CT. *Radiology.* 1997;204(1):27–31.
176. Gnessin E, Chertin L, Chertin B. Current management of paediatric urolithiasis. *Pediatr Surg Int.* 2012;28(7):659–665.
177. Anneren G, Meurling S, Olsen L. Megacystis-microcolon-intestinal hypoperistalsis syndrome (MMIHS), an autosomal recessive disorder: clinical reports and review of the literature. *Am J Med Genet.* 1991;41(2):251–254.

178. Berdon WE, Baker DH, Blanc WA, et al. Megacystis-microcolon-intestinal hypoperistalsis syndrome: a new cause of intestinal obstruction in the newborn. Report of radiologic findings in five newborn girls. *AJR Am J Roentgenol.* 1976;126(5):957–964.
179. Mc Laughlin D, Puri P. Familial megacystis microcolon intestinal hypoperistalsis syndrome: a systematic review. *Pediatr Surg Int.* 2013;29(9):947–951.
180. Ballisty MM, Braithwaite KA, Shehata BM, et al. Imaging findings in megacystis-microcolon-intestinal hypoperistalsis syndrome. *Pediatr Radiol.* 2013;43(4):454–459.
181. Munch EM, Cisek LJ Jr, Roth DR. Magnetic resonance imaging for prenatal diagnosis of multisystem disease: megacystis microcolon intestinal hypoperistalsis syndrome. *Urology.* 2009;74(3):592–594.
182. Berrocal T, Lopez-Pereira P, Arjonilla A, et al. Anomalies of the distal ureter, bladder, and urethra in children: embryologic, radiologic, and pathologic features. *Radiographics.* 2002;22(5):1139–1164.
183. Levin TL, Soghier L, Blitman NM, et al. Megacystis-microcolon-intestinal hypoperistalsis and prune belly: overlapping syndromes. *Pediatr Radiol.* 2004;34(12):995–998.
184. Krueger RP. Posterior urethral valves masquerading as prune belly syndrome. *Urology.* 1981;18(2):182–184.
185. Denes FT, Arap MA, Giron AM, et al. Comprehensive surgical treatment of prune belly syndrome: 17 years' experience with 32 patients. *Urology.* 2004;64(4):789–793; discussion 93–94.
186. Goldman S, Szejnfeld PO, Rondon A, et al. Prenatal diagnosis of bladder exstrophy by fetal MRI. *J Pediatr Urol.* 2013;9(1):3–6.
187. Suson KD, Sponseller PD, Gearhart JP. Bony abnormalities in classic bladder exstrophy: the urologist's perspective. *J Pediatr Urol.* 2013;9(2):112–122.
188. Bolduc S, Capolicchio G, Upadhyay J, et al. The fate of the upper urinary tract in exstrophy. *J Urol.* 2002;168(6):2579–2582; discussion 82.
189. Stec AA, Baradaran N, Gearhart JP. Congenital renal anomalies in patients with classic bladder exstrophy. *Urology.* 2012;79(1):207–209.
190. Garat JM, de la Pena E, Caffaratti J, et al. Prevention of vesicoureteral reflux at the time of complete primary repair of the exstrophy-epispadias complex. *Int Urol Nephrol.* 2004;36(2):211–212.
191. Baird AD, Nelson CP, Gearhart JP. Modern staged repair of bladder exstrophy: a contemporary series. *J Pediatr Urol.* 2007;3(4):311–315.
192. Jaramillo D, Lebowitz RL, Hendren WH. The cloacal malformation: radiologic findings and imaging recommendations. *Radiology.* 1990;177(2):441–448.
193. Patel MN, Racadio JM, Levitt MA, et al. Complex cloacal malformations: use of rotational fluoroscopy and 3-D reconstruction in diagnosis and surgical planning. *Pediatr Radiol.* 2012;42(3):355–363.
194. Calvo-Garcia MA, Kline-Fath BM, Levitt MA, et al. Fetal MRI clues to diagnose cloacal malformations. *Pediatr Radiol.* 2011;41(9):1117–1128.
195. Jarboe MD, Teitelbaum DH, Dillman JR. Combined 3D rotational fluoroscopic-MRI cloacagram procedure defines luminal and extraluminal pelvic anatomy prior to surgical reconstruction of cloacal and other complex pelvic malformations. *Pediatr Surg Int.* 2012;28(8):757–763.
196. Pena A, Levitt MA, Hong A, et al. Surgical management of cloacal malformations: a review of 339 patients. *J Pediatr Surg.* 2004;39(3):470–479; discussion 470–479.
197. Woo LL, Thomas JC, Brock JW. Cloacal exstrophy: a comprehensive review of an uncommon problem. *J Pediatr Urol.* 2010;6(2):102–111.
198. Bruch SW, Adzick NS, Goldstein RB, et al. Challenging the embryogenesis of cloacal exstrophy. *J Pediatr Surg.* 1996;31(6):768–770.
199. Meglin AJ, Balotin RJ, Jelinek JS, et al. Cloacal exstrophy: radiologic findings in 13 patients. *AJR Am J Roentgenol.* 1990;155(6):1267–1272.
200. Calvo-Garcia MA, Kline-Fath BM, Rubio EI, et al. Fetal MRI of cloacal exstrophy. *Pediatr Radiol.* 2013;43(5):593–604.
201. Cacciarelli AA, Kass EJ, Yang SS. Urachal remnants: sonographic demonstration in children. *Radiology.* 1990;174(2):473–475.
202. Fernbach SK, Feinstein KA. Abnormalities of the bladder in children: imaging findings. *AJR Am J Roentgenol.* 1994;162(5):1143–1150.
203. Ashley RA, Inman BA, Routh JC, et al. Urachal anomalies: a longitudinal study of urachal remnants in children and adults. *J Urol.* 2007;178(4 Pt 2):1615–1618.
204. Kumar A, Aggarwal S. The sonographic appearance of cyclophosphamide-induced acute haemorrhagic cystitis. *Clin Radiol.* 1990;41(4):289–290.
205. Schechter T, Liebman M, Gassas A, et al. BK virus-associated hemorrhagic cystitis presenting as mural nodules in the urinary bladder after hematopoietic stem cell transplantation. *Pediatr Radiol.* 2010;40(8):1430–1433.
206. Huppmann AR, Pawel BR. Polyps and masses of the pediatric urinary bladder: a 21-year pathology review. *Pediatr Dev Pathol.* 2011;14(6):438–444.
207. Alanee S, Shukla AR. Bladder malignancies in children aged <18 years: results from the Surveillance, Epidemiology and End Results database. *BJU Int.* 2010;106(4):557–560.
208. Agrons GA, Wagner BJ, Lonergan GJ, et al. From the archives of the AFIP. Genitourinary rhabdomyosarcoma in children: radiologic-pathologic correlation. *Radiographics.* 1997;17(4):919–937.
209. Fine SW, Humphrey PA, Dehner LP, et al. Urothelial neoplasms in patients 20 years or younger: a clinicopathological analysis using the world health organization 2004 bladder consensus classification. *J Urol.* 2005;174(5):1976–1980.
210. Giedl J, Wild PJ, Stoehr R, et al. Urothelial neoplasms in individuals younger than 20 years show very few genetic alterations and have a favourable clinical outcome. *Verh Dtsch Ges Pathol.* 2006;90:253–263.
211. Kao CS, Kum JB, Fan R, et al. Nephrogenic adenomas in pediatric patients: a morphologic and immunohistochemical study of 21 cases. *Pediatr Dev Pathol.* 2013;16(2):80–85.
212. Wilkinson LM, Manson D, Smith CR. Best cases from the AFIP: plexiform neurofibroma of the bladder. *Radiographics.* 2004;24(suppl 1):S237–S242.
213. Netto JM, Perez LM, Kelly DR, et al. Pediatric inflammatory bladder tumors: myofibroblastic and eosinophilic subtypes. *J Urol.* 1999;162(4):1424–1429.
214. Sawyer RW, Hartenberg MA, Benator RM. Intraperitoneal bladder rupture in a battered child. *Int J Pediatr Nephrol.* 1987;8(4):227–230.

215. Morgan DE, Nallamala LK, Kenney PJ, et al, CT cystography: radiographic and clinical predictors of bladder rupture. *AJR Am J Roentgenol.* 2000;174(1):89–95.
216. Sivit CJ, Cutting JP, Eichelberger MR. CT diagnosis and localization of rupture of the bladder in children with blunt abdominal trauma: significance of contrast material extravasation in the pelvis. *AJR Am J Roentgenol.* 1995;164(5):1243–1246.
217. Vaccaro JP, Brody JM. CT cystography in the evaluation of major bladder trauma. *Radiographics.* 2000;20(5):1373–1381.
218. Chan DP, Abujudeh HH, Cushing GL Jr, et al. CT cystography with multiplanar reformation for suspected bladder rupture: experience in 234 cases. *AJR Am J Roentgenol.* 2006;187(5):1296–1302.
219. Hayes EE, Sandler CM, Corriere JN Jr. Management of the ruptured bladder secondary to blunt abdominal trauma. *J Urol.* 1983;129(5):946–948.
220. Boechat MI, Lebowitz RL. Diverticula of the bladder in children. *Pediatr Radiol.* 1978;7(1):22–28.
221. Zawin JK, Lebowitz RL. Neurogenic dysfunction of the bladder in infants and children: recent advances and the role of radiology. *Radiology.* 1992;182(2):297–304.
222. Karmazyn B, Kaefer M, Kauffman S, et al. Ultrasonography and clinical findings in children with epididymitis, with and without associated lower urinary tract abnormalities. *Pediatr Radiol.* 2009;39(10):1054–1058.
223. Game X, Mouracade P, Chartier-Kastler E, et al. Botulinum toxin-A (Botox) intradetrusor injections in children with neurogenic detrusor overactivity/neurogenic overactive bladder: a systematic literature review. *J Pediatr Urol.* 2009;5(3): 156–164.
224. Lopez Pereira P, Moreno Valle JA, Espinosa L, et al. Enterocystoplasty in children with neuropathic bladders: long-term follow-up. *J Pediatr Urol.* 2008;4(1):27–31.
225. Husmann DA, Rathbun SR. Long-term follow up of enteric bladder augmentations: the risk for malignancy. *J Pediatr Urol.* 2008;4(5):381–385; discussion 6.
226. Higuchi TT, Granberg CF, Fox JA, et al. Augmentation cystoplasty and risk of neoplasia: fact, fiction and controversy. *J Urol.* 2010;184(6):2492–2496.
227. Blane CE, Zerin JM, Bloom DA. Bladder diverticula in children. *Radiology.* 1994;190(3):695–697.
228. Bhat A, Bothra R, Bhat MP, et al. Congenital bladder diverticulum presenting as bladder outlet obstruction in infants and children. *J Pediatr Urol.* 2012;8(4):348–353.
229. Lebowitz RL, Vargas B. Stones in the urinary bladder in children and young adults. *AJR Am J Roentgenol.* 1987;148(3): 491–495.
230. Mathoera RB, Kok DJ, Nijman RJ. Bladder calculi in augmentation cystoplasty in children. *Urology.* 2000;56(3):482–487.
231. Uygun I, Okur MH, Aydogdu B, et al. Efficacy and safety of endoscopic laser lithotripsy for urinary stone treatment in children. *Urol Res.* 2012;40(6):751–755.
232. Ceran C, Uguralp S. Self-inflicted urethrovesical foreign bodies in children. *Case Rep Urol.* 2012;2012:134358.
233. Ellimoottil C, Faasse MA, Lindgren BW. Endoscopic management of transurethrally inserted magnetic beads. *Urology.* 2013;81(2):e13–e14.
234. Mukerji G, Rao AR, Hussein A, et al. Self-introduction of foreign body into urinary bladder. *J Endourol.* 2004;18(1):123–125.
235. Chauvin NA, Epelman M, Victoria T, et al. Complex genitourinary abnormalities on fetal MRI: imaging findings and approach to diagnosis. *AJR Am J Roentgenol.* 2012;199(2):W22 2–W231.
236. Chen C, Shih SL, Liu FF, et al. In utero urinary bladder perforation, urinary ascites, and bilateral contained urinomas secondary to posterior urethral valves: clinical and imaging findings. *Pediatr Radiol.* 1997;27(1):3–5.
237. Wolf EL, Berdon WE, Baker DH, et al. Diagnosis oligohydramnios-related pulmonary hypoplasia (Potter syndrome): value of portable voiding cystourethrography in newborns with respiratory distress. *Radiology.* 1977;125(3):769–773.
238. Chaumoitre K, Merrot T, Petit P, et al. Voiding cystourethrography in boys. Does the presence of the catheter during voiding alter the evaluation of the urethra? *J Urol.* 2004;171(3):1280–1281.
239. Ditchfield MR, Grattan-Smith JD, de Campo JF, et al. Voiding cystourethrography in boys: does the presence of the catheter obscure the diagnosis of posterior urethral valves? *AJR Am J Roentgenol.* 1995;164(5):1233–1235.
240. Sarhan OM, El-Ghoneimi AA, Helmy TE, et al. Posterior urethral valves: multivariate analysis of factors affecting the final renal outcome. *J Urol.* 2011;185(6 suppl):2491–2495.
241. Cremin BJ. A review of the ultrasonic appearances of posterior urethral valve and ureteroceles. *Pediatr Radiol.* 1986;16(5):357–364.
242. Good CD, Vinnicombe SJ, Minty IL, et al. Posterior urethral valves in male infants and newborns: detection with US of the urethra before and during voiding. *Radiology.* 1996;198(2):387–391.
243. Ansari MS, Gulia A, Srivastava A, et al. Risk factors for progression to end-stage renal disease in children with posterior urethral valves. *J Pediatr Urol.* 2010;6(3):261–264.
244. Lopez Pereira P, Martinez Urrutia MJ, Espinosa L, et al. Long-term consequences of posterior urethral valves. *J Pediatr Urol.* 2013;9(5):590–596.
245. Kibar Y, Coban H, Irkilata HC, et al. Anterior urethral valves: an uncommon cause of obstructive uropathy in children. *J Pediatr Urol.* 2007;3(5):350–353.
246. Prakash J, Dalela D, Goel A, et al. Congenital anterior urethral valve with or without diverticulum: A single-centre experience. *J Pediatr Urol.* 2013;9(6 Pt B):1183–1187.
247. Bates DG, Coley BD. Ultrasound diagnosis of the anterior urethral valve. *Pediatr Radiol.* 2001;31(9):634–636.
248. Berrocal T, Novak S, Arjonilla A, et al. Complete duplication of bladder and urethra in the coronal plane in a girl: case report and review of the literature. *Pediatr Radiol.* 1999;29(3):171–173.
249. Onofre LS, Gomes AL, Leao JQ, et al. Urethral duplication: a wide spectrum of anomalies. *J Pediatr Urol.* 2013;9(6 Pt B): 1064–1071.
250. Vollman DP, Watts FB Jr. Partial duplication of the posterior urethra. An unusual form of urethral duplication. *Pediatr Radiol.* 1984;14(5):353–355.
251. Effmann EL, Lebowitz RL, Colodny AH. Duplication of the urethra. *Radiology.* 1976;119(1):179–185.
252. Lorenzo RL, Turner WR, Bradford BF, et al. Duplication of the male urethra with posterior urethral valves. *Pediatr Radiol.* 1981;11(1):39–41.

253. Nerli RB, Koura A, Prabha V, et al. Acquired recto-urethral fistula in children: long-term follow-up. *J Pediatr Urol.* 2009; 5(6):485–489.
254. Gross GW, Wolfson PJ, Pena A. Augmented-pressure colostogram in imperforate anus with fistula. *Pediatr Radiol.* 1991; 21(8):560–562.
255. Kavalcova L, Skaba R, Kyncl M, et al. The diagnostic value of MRI fistulogram and MRI distal colostogram in patients with anorectal malformations. *J Pediatr Surg.* 2013;48(8): 1806–1809.
256. Podberesky DJ, Weaver NC, Anton CG, et al. MRI of acquired posterior urethral diverticulum following surgery for anorectal malformations. *Pediatr Radiol.* 2011;41(9):1139–1145.
257. Ghadimi-Mahani M, Dillman JR, Pai D, et al. MRI of congenital urethroperineal fistula. *Pediatr Radiol.* 2010;40(suppl 1): S1–S5.
258. Bates DG, Lebowitz RL. Congenital urethroperineal fistula. *Radiology.* 1995;194(2):501–504.
259. Milla SS, Chow JS, Lebowitz RL. Imaging of hypospadias: pre- and postoperative appearances. *Pediatr Radiol.* 2008;38(2):202–208.
260. Frimberger D. Diagnosis and management of epispadias. *Semin Pediatr Surg.* 2011;20(2):85–90.
261. Lazarus J, van den Heever A, Kortekaas B, et al. Female epispadias managed by bladder neck plication via a perineal approach. *J Pediatr Urol.* 2012;8(3):244–248.
262. Bar-Moshe O, Oboy G, Timmermans C, et al. Megalourethra and abnormalities of the cavernous bodies: cause of erectile dysfunction. *Eur Urol.* 1995;27(3):249–251.
263. Fernbach SK. Urethral abnormalities in male neonates with VATER association. *AJR Am J Roentgenol.* 1991;156(1):137–140.
264. Amsalem H, Fitzgerald B, Keating S, et al. Congenital megalourethra: prenatal diagnosis and postnatal/autopsy findings in 10 cases. *Ultrasound Obstet Gynecol.* 2011;37(6): 678–683.
265. Shrom SH, Cromie WJ, Duckett JW Jr. Megalourethra. *Urology.* 1981;17(2):152–156.
266. Shapiro E, Huang H, McFadden DE, et al. The prostatic utricle is not a Mullerian duct remnant: immunohistochemical evidence for a distinct urogenital sinus origin. *J Urol.* 2004;172(4 Pt 2):1753–1756; discussion 6.
267. Lopatina OA, Berry TT, Spottswood SE. Giant prostatic utricle (utriculus masculinis): diagnostic imaging and surgical implications. *Pediatr Radiol.* 2004;34(2):156–159.
268. Nghiem HT, Kellman GM, Sandberg SA, et al. Cystic lesions of the prostate. *Radiographics.* 1990;10(4):635–650.
269. Devine CJ Jr, Gonzalez-Serva L, Stecker JF Jr, et al. Utricular configuration in hypospadias and intersex. *J Urol.* 1980;123(3):407–411.
270. Beharry MS, Shafii T, Burstein GR. Diagnosis and treatment of chlamydia, gonorrhea, and trichomonas in adolescents. *Pediatr Ann.* 2013;42(2):26–33.
271. Beluffi G, Berton F, Gola G, et al. Urethral polyp in a 1-month-old child. *Pediatr Radiol.* 2005;35(7):691–693.
272. Gleason PE, Kramer SA. Genitourinary polyps in children. *Urology.* 1994;44(1):106–109.
273. de Filippi G, Derchi LE, Coppi M, et al. Sonographic diagnosis of urethral polyp in a child. *Pediatr Radiol.* 1983;13(6): 351–352.
274. Silber JS, Flynn JM, Koffler KM, et al. Analysis of the cause, classification, and associated injuries of 166 consecutive pediatric pelvic fractures. *J Pediatr Orthop.* 2001;21(4):446–450.
275. Pichler R, Fritsch H, Skradski V, et al. Diagnosis and management of pediatric urethral injuries. *Urol Int.* 2012;89(2):136–142.
276. Kaplan GW, Brock WA. Urethral strictures in children. *J Urol.* 1983;129(6):1200–1203.
277. Saxton HM, Borzyskowski M, Mundy AR, et al. Spinning top urethra: not a normal variant. *Radiology.* 1988;168(1): 147–150.

CHAPTER 18

Male Genital Tract

Andrew Phelps • Jesse Courtier • Peter "Buzz" Marcovici • Sara O. Vargas • John D. MacKenzie

INTRODUCTION

Abnormalities of the genital tract in infants and children can be either congenital or acquired and commonly require imaging assessment. In particular, scrotal pain and intrascrotal palpable abnormalities are common indications for imaging in both the emergency department and outpatient settings. This chapter reviews imaging techniques used to evaluate the male genital tract as well as discusses the clinical and radiologic features of various conditions affecting the pediatric scrotum, testicles, epididymides, seminal vesicles, and prostate gland.

IMAGING TECHNIQUES

Radiography

Radiography of the male genital tract is of limited value in the pediatric population. However, in addition to an inguinal hernia containing the intestine, a pediatric genital tract mass such as testicular and paratesticular neoplasm presenting as an enlarged soft tissue mass or other lesions associated with calcification may be incidentally detected on radiographs. Such radiographic information can guide decision making for subsequent imaging study for further evaluation.

Ultrasound

Imaging of the scrotum, like genitourinary imaging in general, relies principally upon ultrasound, with other imaging modalities playing secondary roles. A high-frequency (9 to 18 MHz) linear transducer is ideal for obtaining high-resolution gray-scale images of the testicles, epididymides, and inguinal canals. Testicular volume can be estimated by ultrasound by measuring the longitudinal, transverse, and anteroposterior diameters of the testicle and multiplying by a constant (either 0.52 or 0.71).[1] Testicular volume measurements are useful for identifying subtle size asymmetry and comparing with standardized growth charts.[2,3] Cine sweeps through the testicles help exclude the presence of small testicular lesions that may be missed by representative still ultrasound images.

It is also important to demonstrate symmetric and uniform blood flow in the testicles and surrounding soft tissues (including epididymides) with Doppler ultrasound (color, power, and spectral Doppler); a side-by-side color or power Doppler image of both testicles in the transverse plane is helpful for detailing symmetric blood flow and is preferred by some as the first image obtained in the workup of acute scrotal pain. Dedicated gray-scale and Doppler ultrasound images also should be obtained of the epididymides and inguinal canals. At some institutions, ultrasound images of the urinary bladder and kidneys are also obtained as part of a routine scrotal ultrasound, with the thought that acute renal abnormalities can mimic acute scrotal pathology (e.g., pain from obstructing urolithiasis can cause inguinal or scrotal pain).

A transabdominal approach with ultrasound, when the bladder is adequately distended with urine, is most often used to image the seminal vesicles and prostate gland in children. These structures can also be further evaluated with computed tomography (CT) or magnetic resonance imaging (MRI) when ultrasound is inadequate. In older children, transrectal ultrasound imaging of the prostate gland and seminal vesicles can also be performed.

Computed Tomography

If a testicular mass is identified, cross-sectional imaging of the abdomen and pelvis with contrast-enhanced CT may be employed to facilitate tumor staging, with particular attention paid to retroperitoneal lymph nodes. In general, CT does not aid in the evaluation of the testicular mass itself, except in situations where the mass is larger than the footprint of an ultrasound transducer and local extension may be better defined with the larger field of view afforded by CT. Infrequently, CT may be used to evaluate the prostate gland or seminal vesicles (e.g., in the setting of a known or suspected mass).

Magnetic Resonance Imaging

To eliminate ionizing radiation exposure associated with CT, MRI can also be employed for testicular tumor staging or definition of locoregional tumor extension. In addition, MRI is helpful for characterizing disorders of sex development (DSD) when ultrasound fails to adequately depict or characterize the gonads or uterus. Diffusion-weighted MR imaging, in particular, provides a sensitive means of detecting gonads, which can be otherwise difficult to detect by ultrasound or even CT when they are intra-abdominal in location. MRI also may be used to evaluate the prostate gland or seminal vesicles (e.g., in the setting of a known or suspected mass or cystic abnormality).

Nuclear Medicine

Historically, nuclear medicine evaluation of the scrotum using ^{99m}Tc-pertechnetate scintigraphy was performed to assess for altered testicular perfusion in the setting of suspected torsion; currently, ultrasound has replaced this technique. ^{18}F-fluorodeoxyglucose (FDG)–positron emission tomography (PET) imaging may be used in the initial staging and follow-up of certain male genital tract malignancies.

NORMAL ANATOMY

Embryology

The male genital tract is composed of the scrotum, testicles, epididymides, vas deferentia, seminal vesicles, prostate gland, and penis. In the sexually undifferentiated embryo, the paired gonads are located high in the retroperitoneum. The sex-determining region on the short arm of the Y chromosome (SRY gene) causes germ cells to differentiate into Sertoli cells (which produce Mullerian-inhibiting factor) and Leydig cells (which produce testosterone); together this leads to gonadal transformation into testicles, descent into the scrotal swellings, and near-complete regression of the paramesonephric ducts (discussed more below).[4] Testicular descent is guided by the gubernaculum (also called the caudal genital ligament) in conjunction with an inguinal outpouching of the peritoneal cavity, the processus vaginalis, which ultimately mostly obliterates and no longer communicates with the peritoneal cavity.

Once the testicle has descended into the scrotum, the scrotal portion of the processus vaginalis (also known as the tunica vaginalis) should cover the majority of the testicle, though leaving a broad "uncovered" portion of the testicle which is in direct contact with the internal spermatic fascia (the fascia is an evagination of the transverse abdominal wall fascia).[4] The layer of the tunica vaginalis that contacts the testicle is called the lamina visceralis and the remainder is called the lamina parietalis. All but the caudal most portion of the gubernaculum involutes in males, leaving what is called the gubernaculum testis (also called the scrotal ligament), which serves to anchor the caudal aspect of the testicle to the scrotum.

The epididymides, ejaculatory ducts, and seminal vesicles arise from the paired mesonephric ducts (also known as Wolffian ducts). This is covered in more detail in the kidney chapter (Chapter 17) in this book. The prostate gland arises from a combination of the mesonephric ducts and urogenital sinus. The paramesonephric ducts (also known as Mullerian ducts) give rise to the upper portion of the vagina, uterus, and fallopian tubes in females, but nearly completely regress in males; the only remnant is a tiny midline posterior outpouching of the prostatic urethra (prostatic utricle) located at the verumontanum.[5] In females, the mesonephric ducts nearly completely regress; the paravaginal Gartner ducts (and sometimes seen Gartner duct cysts) are persistent remnants. These gender-specific changes are illustrated in Figure 18.1.

The penis develops from several tissues surrounding the opening of the urogenital sinus.[6] The genital tubercle arises dorsal (superior) to the urogenital sinus opening and becomes the erectile tissue: corpora cavernosa and glans penis (versus clitoris in female). The mesenchyme surrounding the penile urethra gives rise to the corpus spongiosum. The urogenital folds are located to the sides of the urogenital sinus opening and become the foreskin (versus labia minora in females). The labioscrotal folds lie on either side of the urogenital folds and form the external scrotal layer (versus labia majora in females).

Normal Anatomy

The scrotal sac (lined by tunica vaginalis) may contain trace simple fluid in normal children. When the scrotal sac is pathologically fluid filled (e.g., hydrocele), the fluid surrounds the covered portion of the testicle. There should normally be no communication between the scrotal sac and the peritoneal cavity, as the inguinal portion of the processus vaginalis closes. Also, a midline septum divides the scrotum into two portions, further limiting movement of intrascrotal structures and fluid.

The testicles normally have a characteristic ovoid shape and homogeneous echotexture on gray-scale ultrasound (Fig. 18.2). The testicular surface is normally smooth, correlating with the tunica albuginea (a connective tissue layer covering testicular parenchyma and that itself is covered by the tunica vaginalis). Arterial and venous spectral Doppler waveforms should be readily detectable in most children (Fig. 18.3), although Doppler signal can be challenging to detect in the normal testicles of very young boys. Normal testicular volume in the newborn male averages 0.3 mL and increases to 0.5 mL in the first year of life, after which the

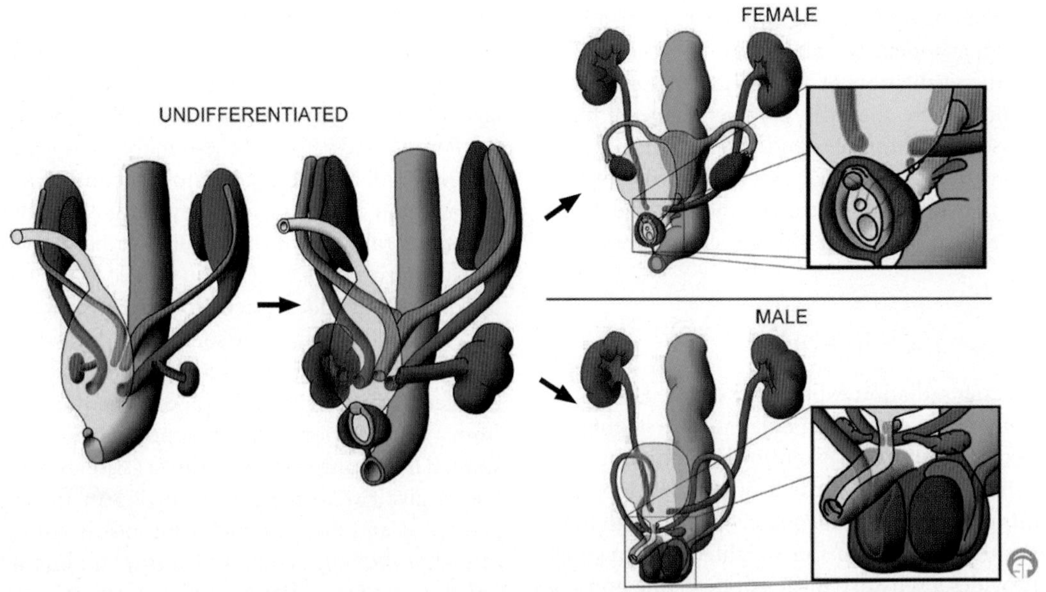

FIGURE 18.1 **Embryology and sexual differentiation of the genitourinary system is schematized.** Color-coded components include urogenital sinus (*yellow*), gastrointestinal tract (*green*), mesonephros/Wolffian ducts (*blue*), metanephros (*red*), paramesonephros/Mullerian ducts (*pink*), gonads (*brown*), genital tubercle (*orange*), and labioscrotal folds (*purple*). (Reproduced with permission from RSNA and the copyright owner.[120])

volume increases minimally until puberty, when the volumes rapidly increase to the adult volume of 13 to 17 mL.[2,3] As the testicle enlarges with puberty, the more hyperechoic testicular mediastinum (a connective tissue structure that contains the rete testis and is the interface between epididymis and testicle) becomes more apparent extending from the superior to inferior portion of the testicle posteriorly. The mediastinum testis gives off fibrous trabeculae that course toward the tunica albuginea dividing the testicle into lobules.

The head of the epididymis is located adjacent to the superior pole of the testicle and is normally smaller than the testicle. The epididymal head is approximately semiovoid, often with a visible small cleft separating it from the testicle (Fig. 18.2). The body and tail of the epididymis are small tubular structures hugging the long axis of the testicle and contiguous with the epididymal head distally and vas deferens proximally. The vas deferens is generally indistinguishable from other spermatic cord contents. The spermatic cord has the ultrasound appearance of a nonperistalsing tight bundle of tubular elements coursing from the scrotum to the internal inguinal ring, with some tubular elements having demonstrable Doppler blood flow.

As mentioned above, a transabdominal approach with ultrasound when the bladder is adequately distended with urine best shows the seminal vesicles and prostate gland in children. Like the testicles, their sizes increase during puberty. The normal prostate gland and seminal vesicles are often difficult to visualize in prepubertal children unless pathologically enlarged.

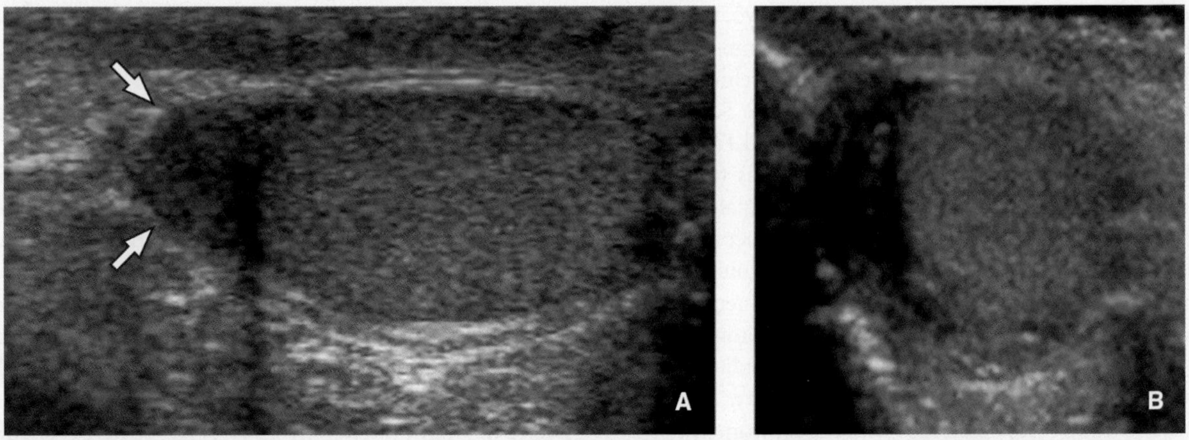

FIGURE 18.2 **Normal gray-scale ultrasound appearance of the neonatal testicle shown in (A) longitudinal and (B) transverse planes.** Testicular echotexture is homogenous and contour is smooth. Longitudinal ultrasound image demonstrates oval-shaped hypoechoic epididymal head (*arrows*).

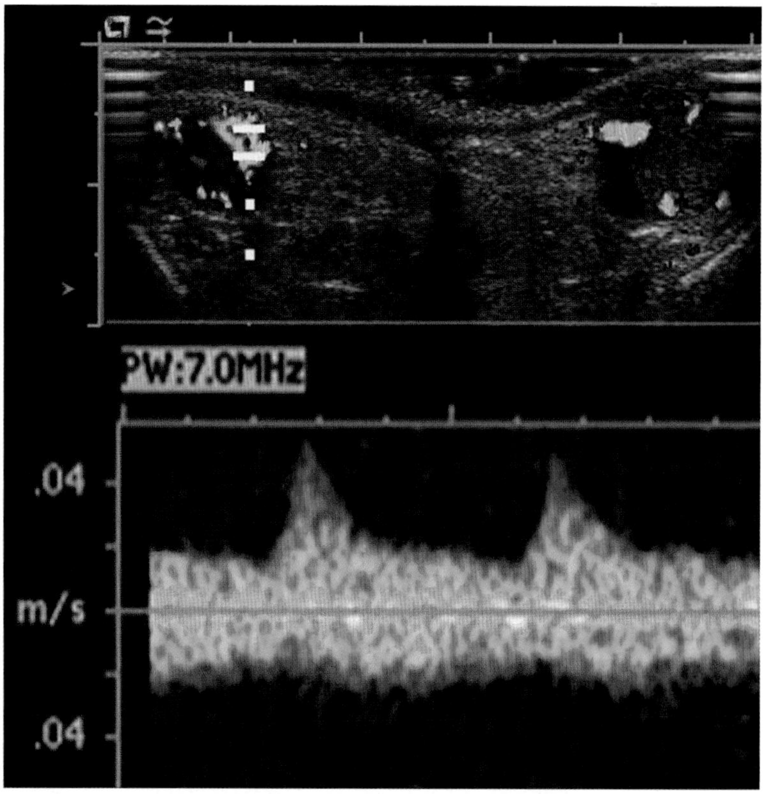

FIGURE 18.3 **Transverse ultrasound image of scrotum.** Pulse wave gate is placed over right testicular parenchyma where Doppler flow is seen. Normal testicular arterial and venous waveforms are demonstrated above and below baseline, respectively.

SPECTRUM OF TESTICULAR AND SCROTAL DISORDERS

Congenital and Developmental Anomalies

Cryptorchidism

Cryptorchidism is defined as the absence of one or both testicles from the scrotum, and the incidence of congenital cryptorchidism in full-term males is estimated at 2% to 4%.[7] Testicles originate in the high retroperitoneum; therefore, ultrasound evaluation for undescended testicles must extend from below the liver and spleen, inferiorly through retroperitoneum and inguinal canals, to the scrotum (Fig. 18.4). Multiple risk factors have been implicated for causing undescended testicles, including prematurity and multiple maternal factors/exposures; however, no single etiology stands out.[8–10]

If undescended testicles are occult to ultrasound, MRI may be helpful, particularly using T2-weighted and diffusion-weighted sequences where they appear hyperintense (Fig. 18.4). The undescended testicle has a higher risk of malignancy (especially seminoma), and it is unclear whether this risk is decreased with surgical repair.[11]

Ambiguous External Genitalia

Ambiguous external genitalia can be a source of great concern and require a multidisciplinary approach to determine the correct diagnosis. The currently accepted term for the spectrum of etiologies is "disorders of sex development" (DSD). It should be noted that not all DSD manifests as ambiguous external genitalia. In the absence of the Y chromosome, the internal and external genitalia develop the "default" female phenotype.

Ultrasound workup of ambiguous genitalia must include evaluation of scrotum/labia, inguinal canals, pelvis, kidneys, and adrenal glands. As shown in Table 18.1, identification of the uterus and characterization of both gonads are critical to classifying the DSD. The most common cause of ambiguous genitalia is congenital adrenal hyperplasia, which is one of the several causes of female pseudohermaphroditism (46,XX).[12] In congenital adrenal hyperplasia, the adrenal glands are often enlarged with a "cerebriform" appearance. The most common cause of ambiguous genitalia with a 46,XX genotype is androgen insensitivity syndrome, which is one of the several causes of male pseudohermaphroditism.[12] In complete androgen insensitivity (Fig. 18.4), the external genitalia are female, whereas in partial androgen insensitivity, the external genitalia are ambiguous. In some children, DSD may be very complex, requiring MRI evaluation and a systematic interdisciplinary approach to fully classify and characterize the disorder (Fig. 18.5).

Adrenal Cortical Rests/Testicular Adrenal Rest Tumors (TARTs)

Heterotopic adrenal cortical tissue can be found in the paratesticular region and sometimes within the testicle. Intratesticular adrenocortical tissue can proliferate into tumor-like masses in patients with congenital adrenal hyperplasia, and Nelson syndrome can sometimes present with detectable intratesticular masses at ultrasound both during childhood and adulthood.[13–15] The adrenal tissue becomes trapped in the testicles in utero prior to migration from the high retroperitoneum and subsequently enlarges in response to elevated adrenocorticotropic hormone.

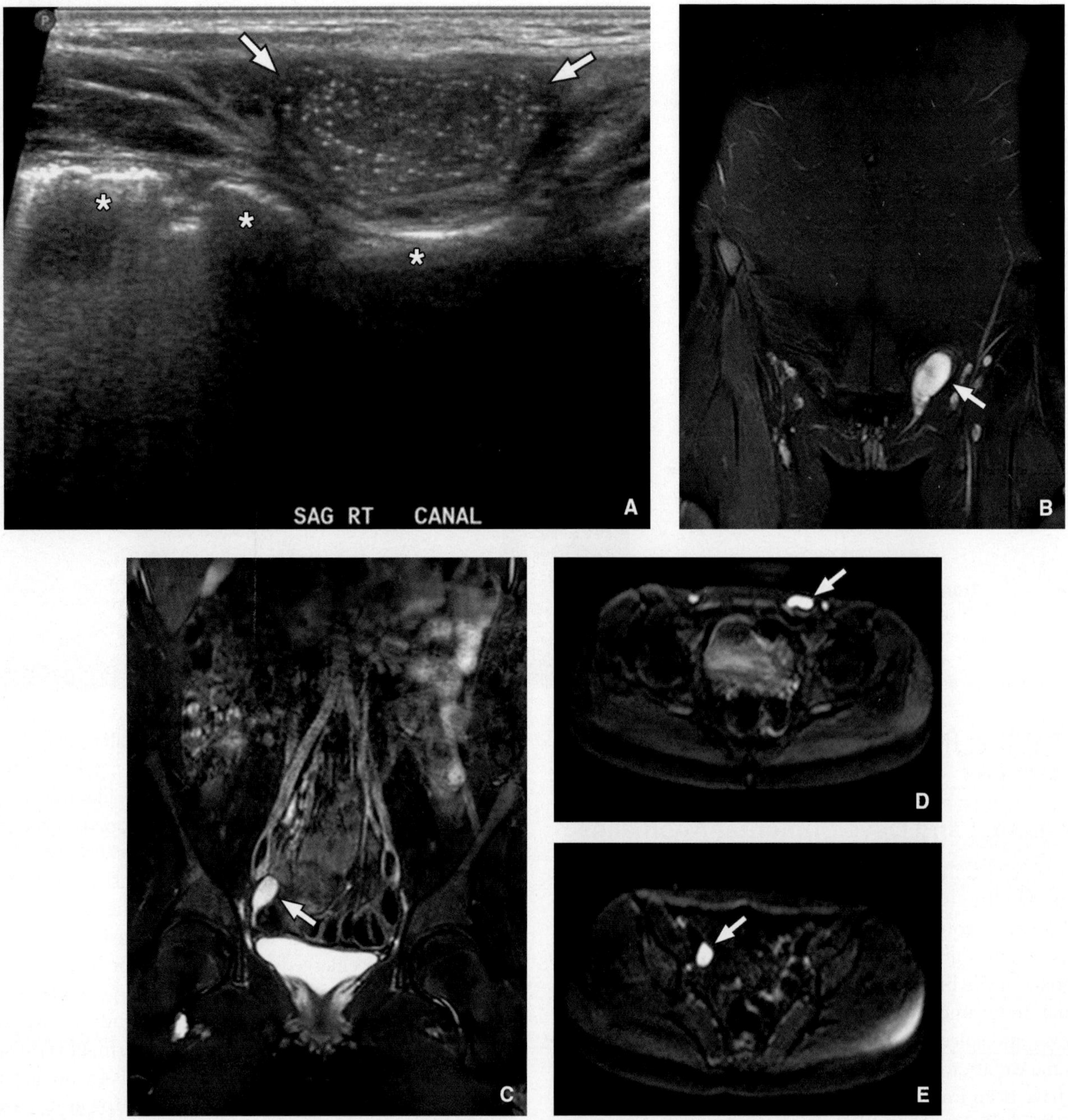

FIGURE 18.4 **A: A 9-year-old boy with undescended testicle.** Longitudinal gray-scale ultrasound image shows that the right testicle (*arrows*) is located in the upper portion of the right inguinal canal and contains diffuse microlithiasis. The testicle is located superficial to gas-containing bowel loops (*asterisks*). **B—E: A 15-year-old phenotypic girl presents with amenorrhea.** Coronal T2-weighted fat-saturated MR images show hyperintense undescended testicles (*arrows*) along the right pelvic sidewall and in the left inguinal region, respectively. The gonads are markedly hyperintense on diffusion-weighted MR imaging. Genetic workup revealed XY sex chromosomes and 17-beta hydroxylase deficiency. (Images B—E courtesy of Jonathan R. Dillman, MD, MSc, Cincinnati Children's Hospital Medical Center, Cincinnati, OH. Reprint with permission from *J Pediatr Adolesc Gynecol.* 2016 Dec;29(6):577—581.)

Although their ultrasound appearance can be variable, these rests most often present as one or more bilateral intratesticular hypoechoic masses (Fig. 18.6).[13] Testicular venous sampling for elevated cortisol levels may confirm the diagnosis.[16]

Splenogonadal Fusion

Splenogonadal fusion is a rare cause of an extratesticular mass that results from the migration of splenic tissue with the testicle.[17] The connection may be *direct* (continuous) with the principle spleen fused to the intrascrotal testicle or *indirect* (discontinuous) with independent (ectopic) splenic tissue traveling into the scrotum with the testicle. Although the involved splenic tissue should have similar imaging features of native spleen at ultrasound, CT, and MRI (Fig. 18.7), there may be overlap in appearance with the testicle. Although scintigraphy (^{99m}Tc-labeled sulfur colloid or damaged red blood cells) could potentially help in the diagnosis,[18] splenogonadal fusion is rare; therefore, most patients go on to surgery for removal of a scrotal mass and the diagnosis is confirmed by histopathology.

TABLE 18.1 Disorders of Sex Development

Diagnosis	Chromosomes	External Genitalia	Gonads	Uterus
Persistent Mullerian duct syndrome	46,XY	Male	Testes	Present
Male pseudohermaphrodite	46,XY	Female or ambiguous	Testes	Absent
Female pseudohermaphrodite	46,XX	Female or ambiguous	Ovaries	Present
Mixed gonadal dysgenesis	46,XY or 45,XO	Ambiguous	Testis and streak	Present
Pure gonadal dysgenesis	Variable	Female	Streak	Present
True hermaphrodite	Variable	Variable	Testis and ovary, or ovotestis	Present

Disorders of Sex Development can be classified using imaging based on presence/appearance of the gonads and uterus.
Adapted from Chavhan G, Parra D, Oudjhane K, et al. Imaging of ambiguous genitalia: classification and diagnostic approach. Radiographics. 2008;28(7):1891–1904.

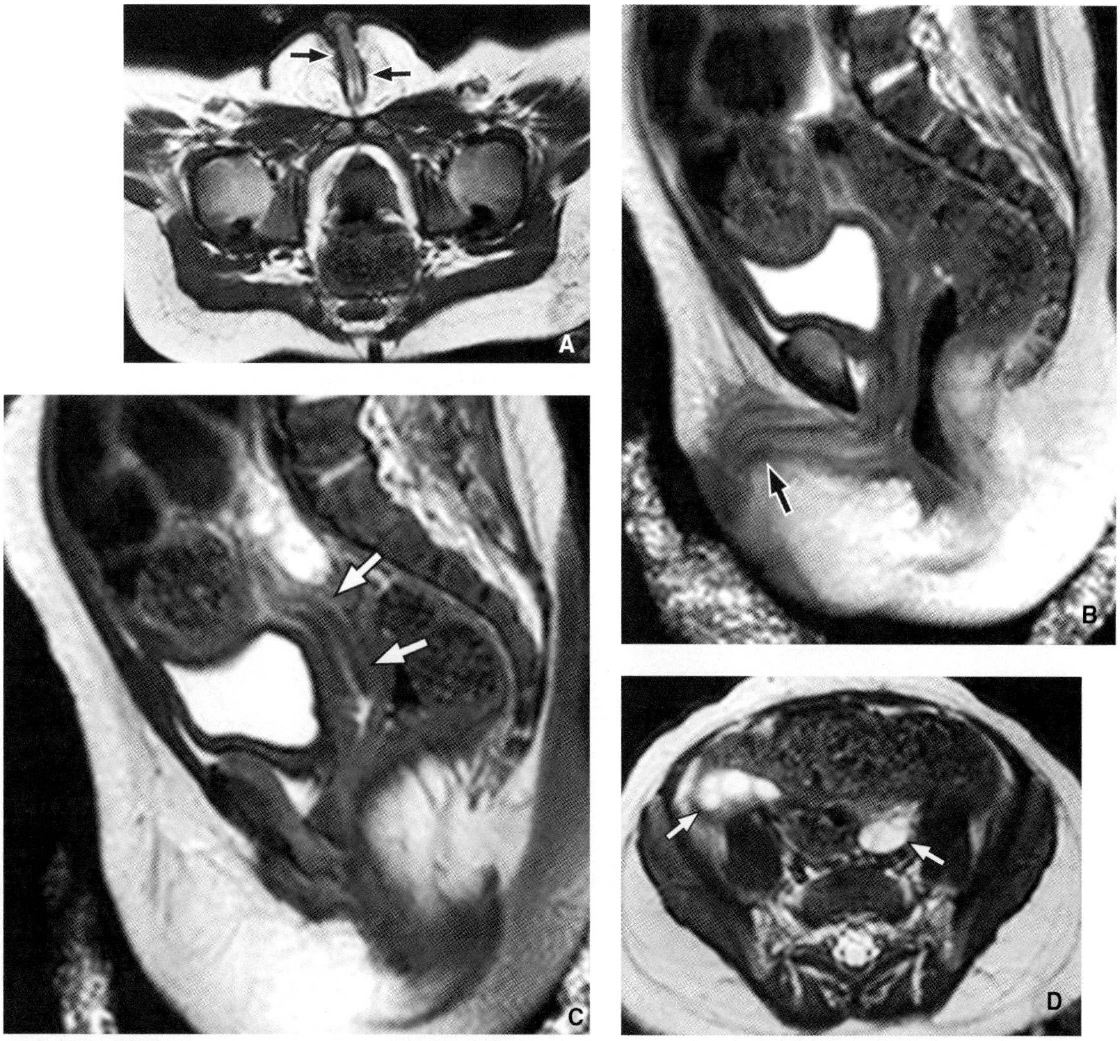

FIGURE 18.5 **A 3-month-old 46XX infant with disorder of sexual differentiation. A and B:** Axial and sagittal T2-weighted MR images show a penis-like structure (*arrows*) with recognizable corpora. A scrotum was present at physical examination, and no perineal orifice was appreciated. **C:** Sagittal T2-weighted MR image shows a uterus (*arrows*) posterior to the bladder. **D:** Higher axial T2-weighted MR image shows normal-appearing ovaries (*arrows*) containing numerous small cysts (follicles). (Case courtesy of Jonathan R. Dillman, MD, MSc, Cincinnati Children's Hospital Medical Center, Cincinnati, OH.)

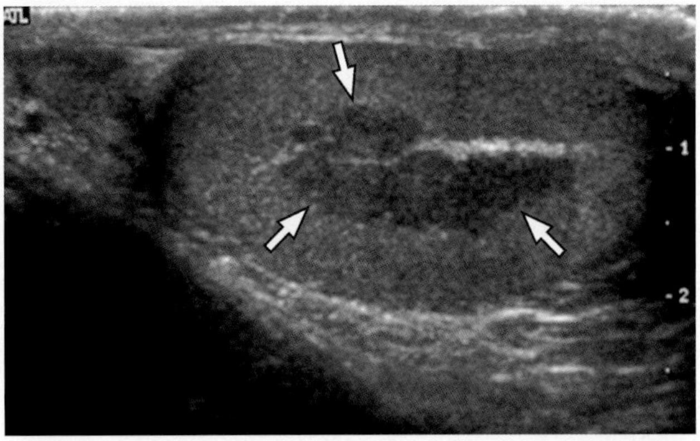

FIGURE 18.6 **A 9-year-old boy with poorly controlled congenital adrenal hyperplasia.** Longitudinal gray-scale ultrasound image shows a geographic area of decreased echogenicity (*arrows*) in the central left testis, consistent with an adrenal rest.

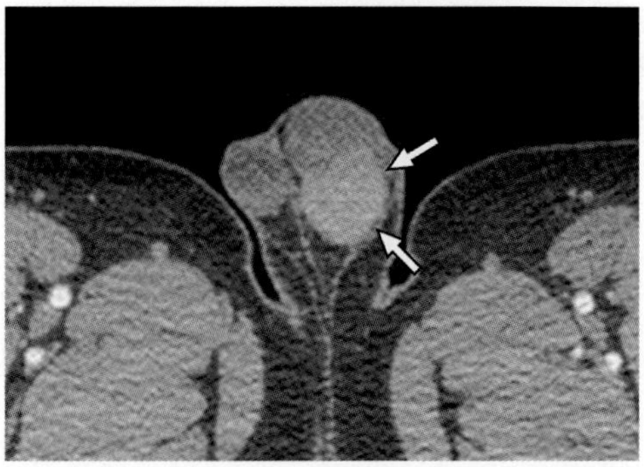

FIGURE 18.7 **A 20-year-old young man with palpable scrotal mass.** Axial contrast-enhanced CT image demonstrates an enhancing left extra-testicular scrotal mass (*arrows*) which was surgically removed and confirmed to be splenic tissue at histopathology.

Tunica Albuginea Cyst

Tunica albuginea cysts are common benign palpable avascular cysts that arise from the tunica albuginea, the fibrous capsule surrounding the testicle. Uncomplicated cysts are anechoic at ultrasound and may exert mass effect on the underlying testicular parenchyma (Fig. 18.8). Complicated cysts may contain debris or calcification. The location of this type of cyst is key to distinguishing it from other cystic abnormalities arising from either the testicle or epididymis.[19]

Bell Clapper Anomaly and Testicular Torsion

If the processus (tunica) vaginalis completely envelopes the testicle and there is failure of normal posterior anchoring of the testicle to the scrotum, the resulting configuration is called a "bell clapper" anomaly. This is because the testicle can freely swing and rotate within the processus vaginalis like a bell clapper in a bell (Fig. 18.9). Normally, a broad base of direct testicular contact with the internal spermatic fascia prevents free mobility. Therefore, children with a bell clapper anomaly are at increased risk of intravaginal testicular torsion.[20] The incidence of bell clapper anomaly has been reported to be 12% in autopsy series,[21] although the frequency of torsion is far less than this[22]; therefore; other factors are likely involved.

Testicular torsion is the twisting of the testicle about the spermatic cord and causes obstructed venous outflow, lack of arterial inflow, and eventual infarction of the testicle (Fig. 18.10). The clinical presentation is most often severe acute unilateral scrotal pain, nausea, and vomiting; physical exam may reveal a high-riding horizontal testicle with an absent cremasteric reflex.[23] The acute presentation should help distinguish torsion from the gradual symptom onset of epididymitis or orchitis; however, intermittent torsion may present more subacutely.[24] The lack of venous outflow leads to testicular congestion (edema), and this presents at ultrasound as an enlarged testicle with decreased echogenicity and heterogeneous echotexture as well as decreased Doppler

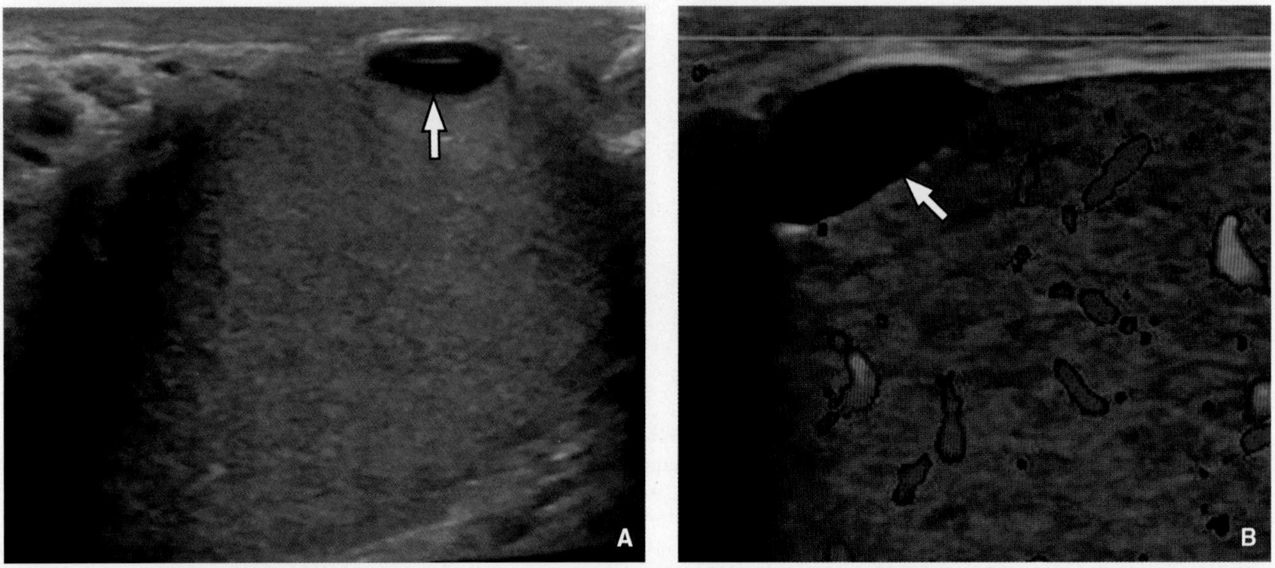

FIGURE 18.8 **A 13-year-old boy with palpable mass in the scrotum due to tunica albuginea cyst.** Transverse gray-scale **(A)** and color Doppler **(B)** ultrasound images demonstrate a well-circumscribed, avascular, anechoic cyst (*arrows*) located along the surface of the testicle.

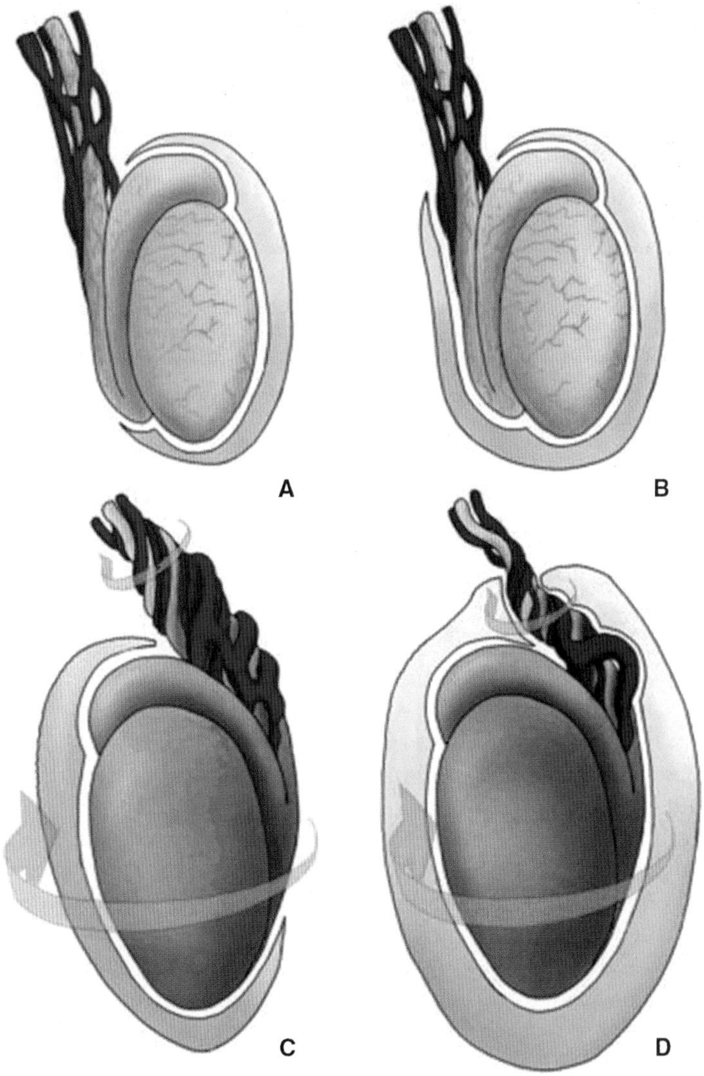

FIGURE 18.9 **A:** Normal posterior fixation of the testicle in the scrotum. **B:** Bell clapper anomaly without torsion. Note the lack of normal posterior fixation. **C:** Extravaginal testicular torsion without bell clapper anomaly. **D:** Intravaginal testicular torsion with bell clapper deformity. Note that fluid is present posterior to the testicle. (Reproduced with permission from RSNA and the copyright owner.[121])

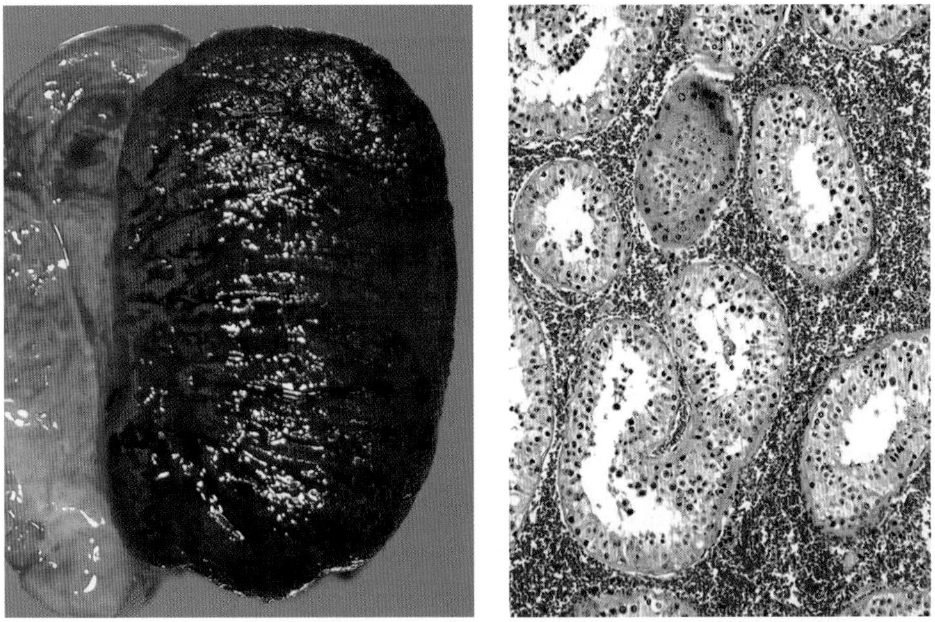

FIGURE 18.10 **A 12-year-old boy with acute scrotal pain due to intravaginal torsion and testicular infarction.** Grossly, the cut surface of the testis is red-maroon and bulging **(left)**. Microscopically, there is hemorrhagic infarction, with extensive interstitial blood; tubular cells show cytoplasmic hypereosinophilia and nuclear pyknosis, characteristic of an evolving infarct (**right**, hematoxylin and eosin, original magnification, 200×).

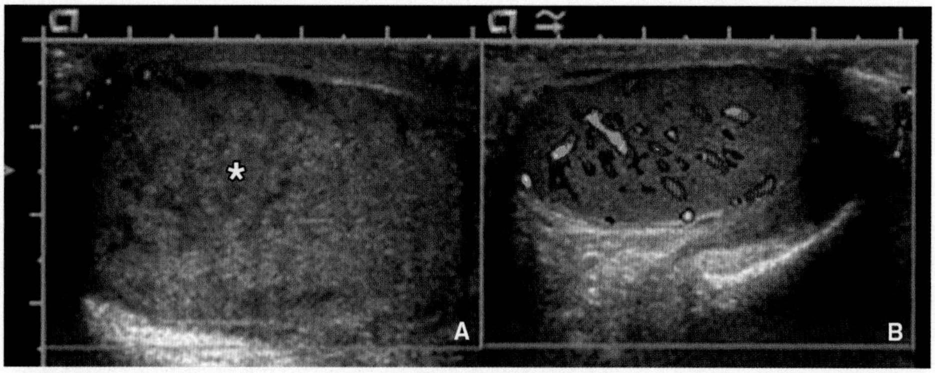

FIGURE 18.11 **An 8-year-old boy with acute testicular pain awaking him from sleep.** Longitudinal color Doppler ultrasound images of the **(A)** right and **(B)** left testicles demonstrate right testicular enlargement and heterogeneity (*asterisk*) as well as absent blood flow, consistent with testicular torsion. The left testicle is normal.

blood flow (Fig. 18.11). Prolonged torsion may result in a markedly enlarged, heterogeneous testicle with areas of geographic increased and decreased echogenicity. However, as abnormally decreased Doppler blood flow is only 84% sensitive for detecting torsion, normal or increased intratesticular Doppler signal should not exclude the diagnosis when clinical suspicion is high.[25] Presumably, a false-negative Doppler ultrasound examination is commonly due to intermittent torsion.

There are two unique types of testicular torsion that occur in children. As discussed above, the bell clapper anomaly is a developmental abnormality where the testicle is inadequately affixed to the posterior scrotum, thus allowing the spermatic cord and testicle to twist within the confines of the processus (tunica) vaginalis. This type of torsion is therefore defined as intravaginal. The diagnosis of a bell clapper anomaly can be confidently made when fluid completely surrounds the testicle without the usual posterior anchoring of the gubernaculum, epididymis, and testis to the scrotum. The "torsion knot" sign may also be observed, appearing as a supratesticular mass–like abnormality, which is due to twisted, edematous spermatic cord.[26] Intravaginal torsion is much more common in adolescents, whereas extravaginal torsion (described below) is more common in neonates.

Very young children (including fetuses and neonates) are susceptible to testicular torsion due to a deficient gubernaculum, which allows the testicle and processus vaginalis to twist together. This type of torsion is referred to as extravaginal, and it most often occurs in utero or soon after birth. At ultrasound, findings suggestive of extravaginal testicular infarction include a small hypoechoic testicle (frequently inguinal in location) with a calcific rim (the rim is echogenic and may show posterior acoustic shadowing) and decreased Doppler blood flow[27] (Fig. 18.12).

Treatment of testicular torsion generally requires surgery; however, there is only about a 4- to 8-hour window after onset before permanent ischemic damage occurs. Delay in treatment may result in infertility or require orchiectomy.[23] In cases where a bell clapper anomaly is present, bilateral orchiopexy is performed. Based on a recent survey of practicing urologists, management of neonatal (including prenatal/perinatal) torsion is inconsistent with children undergoing surgical exploration on emergent, urgent, and elective bases.[28] In the setting of neonatal torsion (when bell clapper anomaly is not the primary mechanism of torsion), many surgeons also still perform bilateral orchiopexy.[28,29]

Infectious and Inflammatory Disorders

Orchitis

Pediatric patients with infectious or inflammation of the testicle and epididymis may present with severe pain, swelling, and hematuria and/or ejaculation of blood, and presenting signs and symptoms overlap considerably with testicular torsion.[25,30–34] The primary cause of orchitis and epididymitis in young children is an underlying genitourinary tract abnormality (e.g., neurogenic bladder or ectopic ureter), whereas a descending or sexually transmitted urinary tract infection from *E. coli*, *N. gonorrhea*, or *Chlamydia* is more common in adolescents. Viruses, including mumps, are another potential infectious cause.[35]

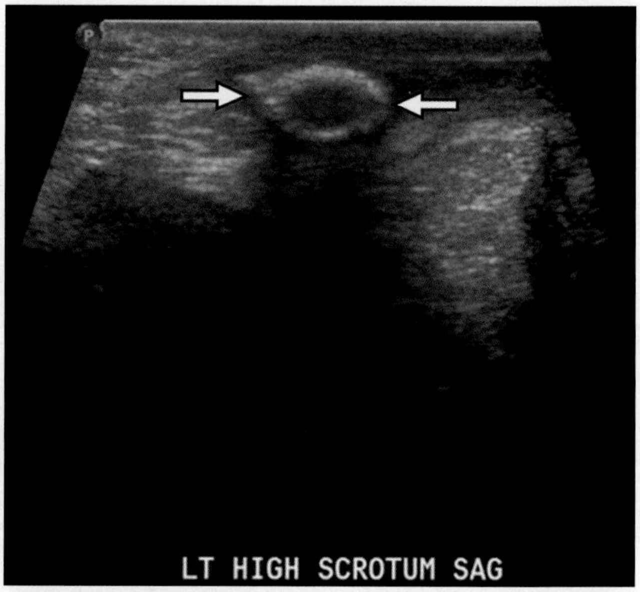

FIGURE 18.12 **A 3-month-old boy with nonpalpable left testicle.** Gray-scale longitudinal ultrasound image through the left inguinal canal demonstrates an oval-shaped structure with an echogenic, shadowing rim (*arrows*). Ultrasound findings are consistent with an infarcted, peripherally calcified testicle due to extravaginal torsion occurring either in utero or during the neonatal period. (Case courtesy of Jonathan R. Dillman, MD, MSc, Cincinnati Children's Hospital Medical Center, Cincinnati, OH.)

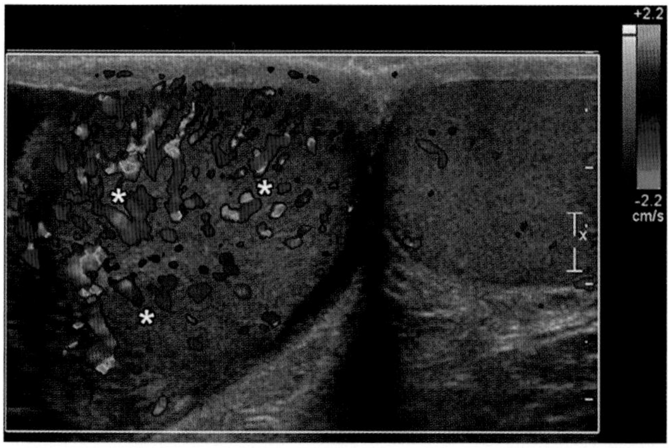

FIGURE 18.13 **A 16-year-old boy with 3 days of acute scrotal pain and swelling due to orchitis.** Transverse color Doppler ultrasound image of the scrotum shows both testicles, with increased blood flow on the right (*asterisks*). The right testicle is also enlarged, and there is a reactive right hydrocele.

Ultrasound can help differentiate between orchitis and testicular torsion. Orchitis frequently shows an enlarged, heterogeneous, hypoechoic testicle with increased color Doppler blood flow[30] (Fig. 18.13), whereas torsion most often has absent or decreased Doppler blood flow. Both echotexture and Doppler blood flow can be variable in appearance with epididymo-orchtis, however: the testes and epididymides have normal echotexture and show only hyperemia in 20% of patients with epididymitis and 40% of patients with orchitis.[36] An enlarged epididymis in children with testicular torsion may lead to a misdiagnosis of epididymitis in cases of partial or intermittent torsion and normal or increased testicular blood flow.[37,38] The sonographic findings of leukemia or lymphoma involving the testicle show considerable overlap with and may be challenging to distinguish from epididymo-orchitis.[39] Once other etiologies are excluded, the management of epididymo-orchitis is directed at the suspected organism with antibiotic therapy, hot or cold packs for analgesia, and scrotal elevation.[40]

Hydrocele, Pyocele, and Hematocele

Increased fluid in the scrotal sac is a common finding on ultrasound and is most often due to a simple hydrocele.[30,41,42] Hydroceles are collections of fluid that develop between the visceral and parietal layers of the tunica vaginalis and/or along the spermatic cord, and at ultrasound they typically appear as thin-walled anechoic fluid collections (Fig. 18.14) or fluid collections with low-level swirling echoes[43]. Children with hydroceles most commonly present with painless scrotal swelling. The etiology is congenital in most neonates and infants as well as some older children, because of a patent processus vaginalis (Fig. 18.15). Hydroceles in older children and adolescents are more likely to be acquired from inflammation/infection, testicular torsion, trauma, or a tumor.[30] In rare cases, very large hydroceles may communicate with the abdominal cavity, having an "hour-glass" configuration, and are called abdominoscrotal hydroceles[44–46] (Fig. 18.16). Spermatic cord hydroceles may be classified into two types: the fluid of an *encysted hydrocele* does not communicate with the peritoneal cavity above or the scrotal sac below, whereas the fluid of a *funicular hydrocele* communicates with the peritoneal cavity at the internal ring but not the scrotum.[47,48]

Other cystic/fluid-filled abnormalities that may occupy the scrotal sac and inguinal canal include infection (pyocele and scrotal abscess), hematocele (usually due to recent trauma), and bowel from an inguinal hernia (Fig. 18.17). Pyoceles and hematoceles are commonly complex in appearance, containing debris, septations, and fluid-fluid levels at ultrasound.

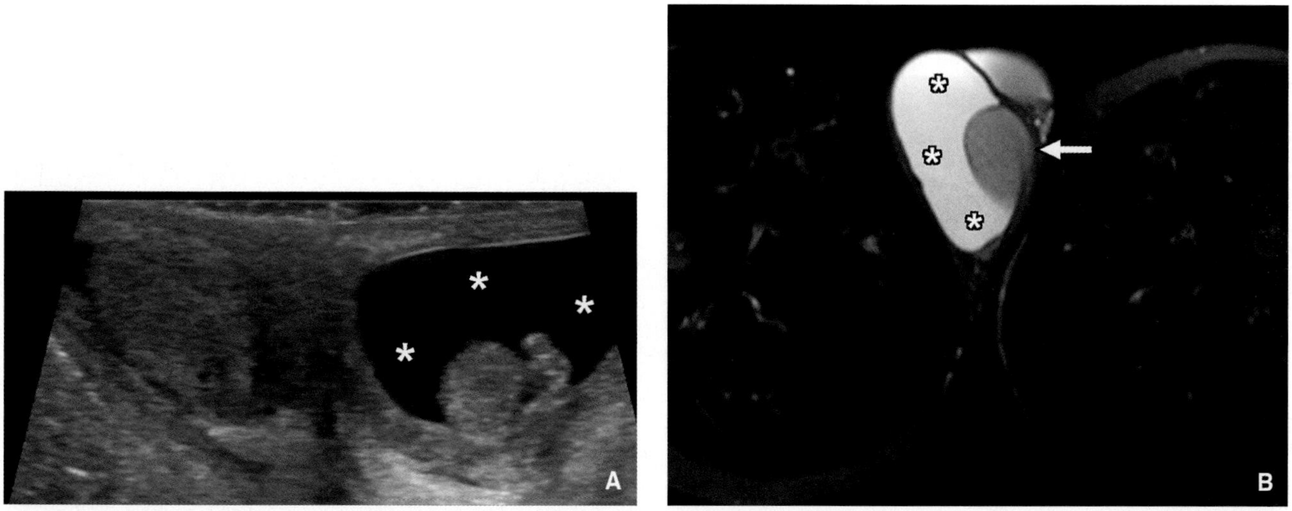

FIGURE 18.14 **A: An 8-day-old boy with scrotal swelling.** Transverse gray-scale ultrasound image of the scrotum shows both testicles. There is increased fluid (*asterisks*) in the left scrotal sac surrounding the left testicle, consistent with a left hydrocele most likely due to a patent processus vaginalis. **B: A 16-year-old boy with right scrotal swelling.** Axial T2-weighted MR image with fat-saturation demonstrates a large right hydrocele (*asterisks*). Note that a portion of the right testicle is fixed to the scrotal wall (*arrow*).

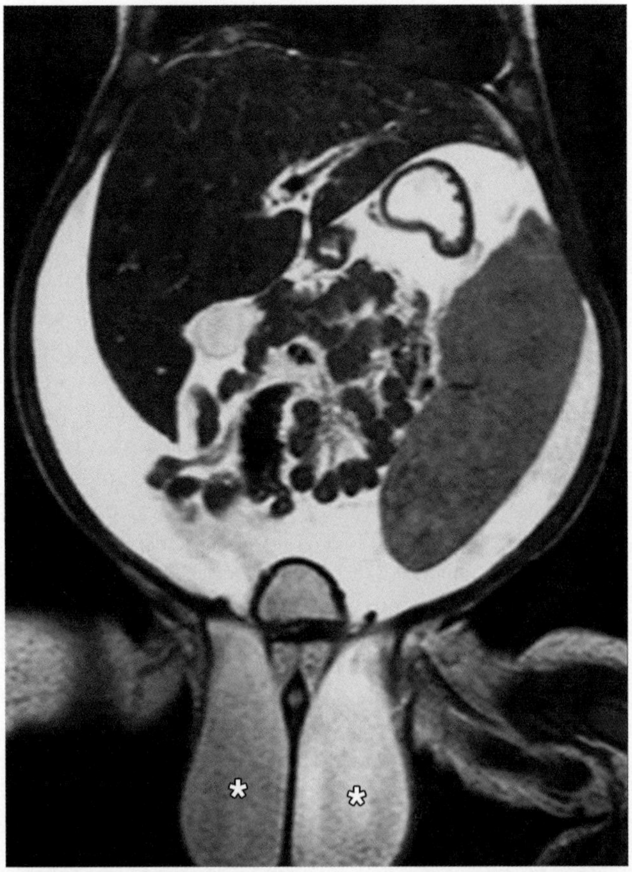

FIGURE 18.15 **A 6-month-old boy with scrotal swelling due to large bilateral communicating hydroceles.** Coronal T2-weighted MR image demonstrates a large amount of ascites extending into the scrotum (*asterisks*) through bilateral patent processus vaginalis.

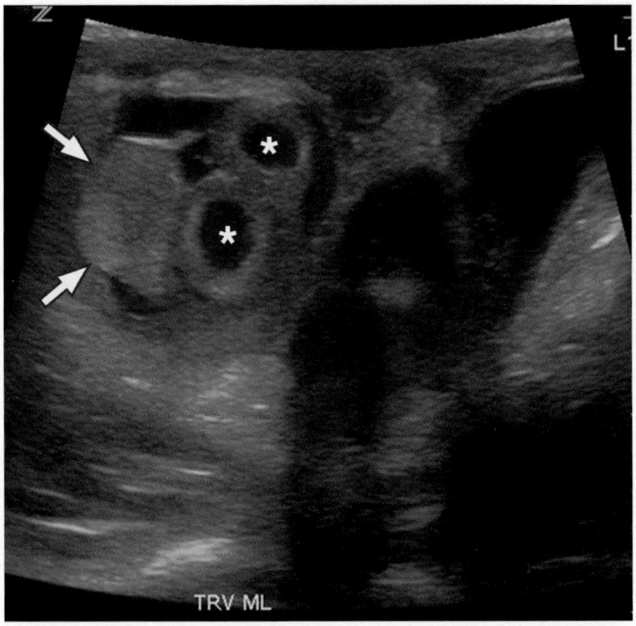

FIGURE 18.17 **A 1-month-old boy with swollen scrotum due to a right inguinal hernia.** Transverse gray-scale ultrasound image of the scrotum shows two bowel loops (*asterisks*) adjacent to the right testicle (*arrows*). Bilateral hydroceles are present, suggesting bilateral patent processus vaginalis. The left testicle is not seen on this image.

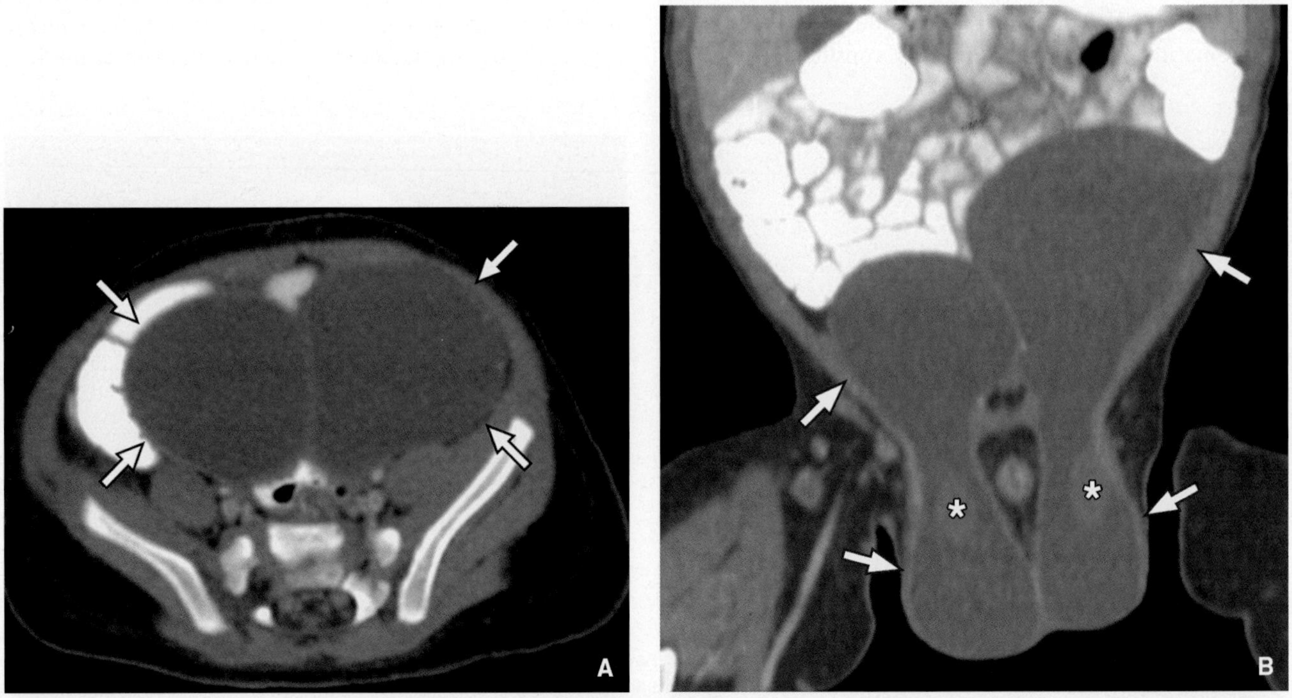

FIGURE 18.16 **A 4-month-old boy with distended abdomen and scrotum on physical examination due to giant abdominoscrotal hydroceles. A:** Axial contrast-enhanced CT image shows large thin-walled fluid collections (*arrows*) in the lower abdomen. **B:** Coronal reformatted CT image demonstrates bilateral fluid-filled structures (*arrows*) extending from the scrotum into the abdominal cavity. Testicles (*asterisks*) can be seen.

Torsion of Intrascrotal Appendages (Appendix Testis and Appendix Epididymis)

Torsion of an intrascrotal appendage is a common cause of acute scrotal pain during the pediatric period.[49] These appendages are embryonic remnants of the paramesonephric (testicular) and mesonephric (epididymis) ducts and are named based on their location.[36,50] Three of five types can be identified on ultrasound and are more readily apparent in the presence of a hydrocele—the appendix testis, appendix epididymis, and appendix of the epididymal tail.[30]

Upon torsion, these appendages become enlarged and devascularized, causing pain, ischemia, and even infarction. Ultrasound demonstrates a round or ovoid mass of variable echogenicity (that can be hypoechoic, echogenic, or even cystic) adjacent to the superior pole of the testicle or epididymal head with no internal vascularity (Fig. 18.18). If the testicular appendage measures larger than 5 to 6 mm in the correct clinical scenario, this carries a very high degree of specificity for torsion.[51] The associated reactive inflammation and hyperemia affecting the surrounding tissues is often robust, and a reactive hydrocele is very common. With time, torsed appendages may calcify, decrease in size, and may be an etiology for small extratesticular mobile calcifications in the scrotum (so-called scrotal pearls or scrotoliths). This diagnosis is managed conservatively once testicular torsion and epididymo-orchitis are excluded.

Vasculitis

Children with small vessel vasculitides from systemic immune-mediated conditions may present with an acutely painful, swollen scrotum. Henoch-Schönlein purpura normally affects the skin, kidneys, joints, and gastrointestinal tract, but has scrotal involvement in 15% to 38% of cases.[52,53] Although the sonographic findings can be indistinguishable from epididymo-orchitis, the testicles most often remain normal on gray-scale and color Doppler ultrasound. In some children, the epididymis may become enlarged, heterogeneously echogenic, and hyperemic secondary to hemorrhage and inflammation. Scrotal skin thickening and a reactive hydrocele also can occur.[54] Behçet disease is another rare immune-mediated small-vessel systemic vasculitis that can involve the testes and produce sonographic findings of orchitis.[55]

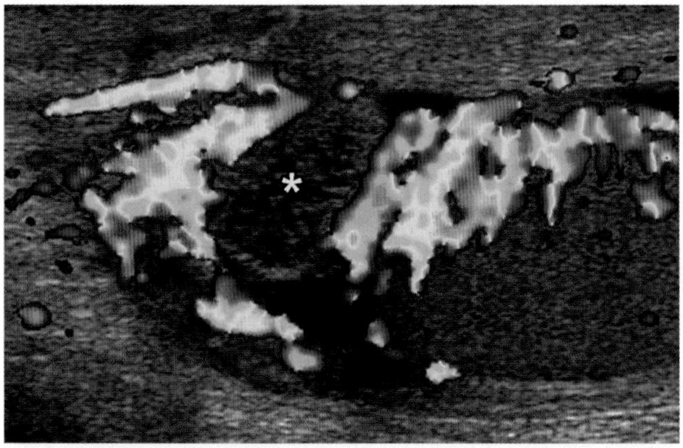

FIGURE 18.18 **An 11-year-old boy with acute testicular pain due to torsed appendage.** Longitudinal color Doppler ultrasound image shows hypoechoic, heterogeneous, avascular ovoid structure (*asterisk*) adjacent to the superior pole of the testicle and separate from epididymis. There is exuberant adjacent reactive hyperemia.

Neoplastic Disorders

Neoplastic disorders of the scrotum primarily arise from the testicular tissues and are categorized as benign or malignant. Prepubertal testicular and paratesticular tumors are a rare and distinct group compared with adult or postpubertal populations with regard to epidemiology, natural history, histologic types, and management[56] (Table 18.2). Prepubertal primary testicular neoplasms are uncommon,[57,58] have a greater chance of being benign, and have better outcomes than postpubertal tumors. Treatment, described in more detail below, depends on the type of tumor and usually involves either orchiectomy or enucleation.[57]

Benign Neoplasms

The two most common benign tumors of the pediatric testicle are epidermoid cyst and mature teratoma.[56,59] Testicular teratomas classically present early in life between birth and 18 months of age.[56] Epidermoid cysts are found in both children and adults. Teratomas have a variable appearance, as would be expected of a tumor containing three germ layers, and they may show a mixture of solid, cystic, and calcified elements (Fig. 18.19). Epidermoid cysts typically have the most specific imaging features of any scrotal or testicular

TABLE 18.2 Prepubescent Testicular and Paratesticular Masses

Tumor Type	Benign	Malignant
Germ cell	Mature teratoma	Yolk sac
	Epidermoid cyst	Embryonal
Sex cord/ stromal[a]	Juvenile granulosa cell	
	Leydig cell	
	Sertoli cell	
Paratesticular	Lipoma	Rhabdomyosarcoma
	Leiomyoma	
	Calcifying fibrous pseudotumor	
	Adenomatoid	
	Vascular malformation	
Other	Gonadoblastoma[a]	

[a]*Rarely can demonstrate malignant behavior.*

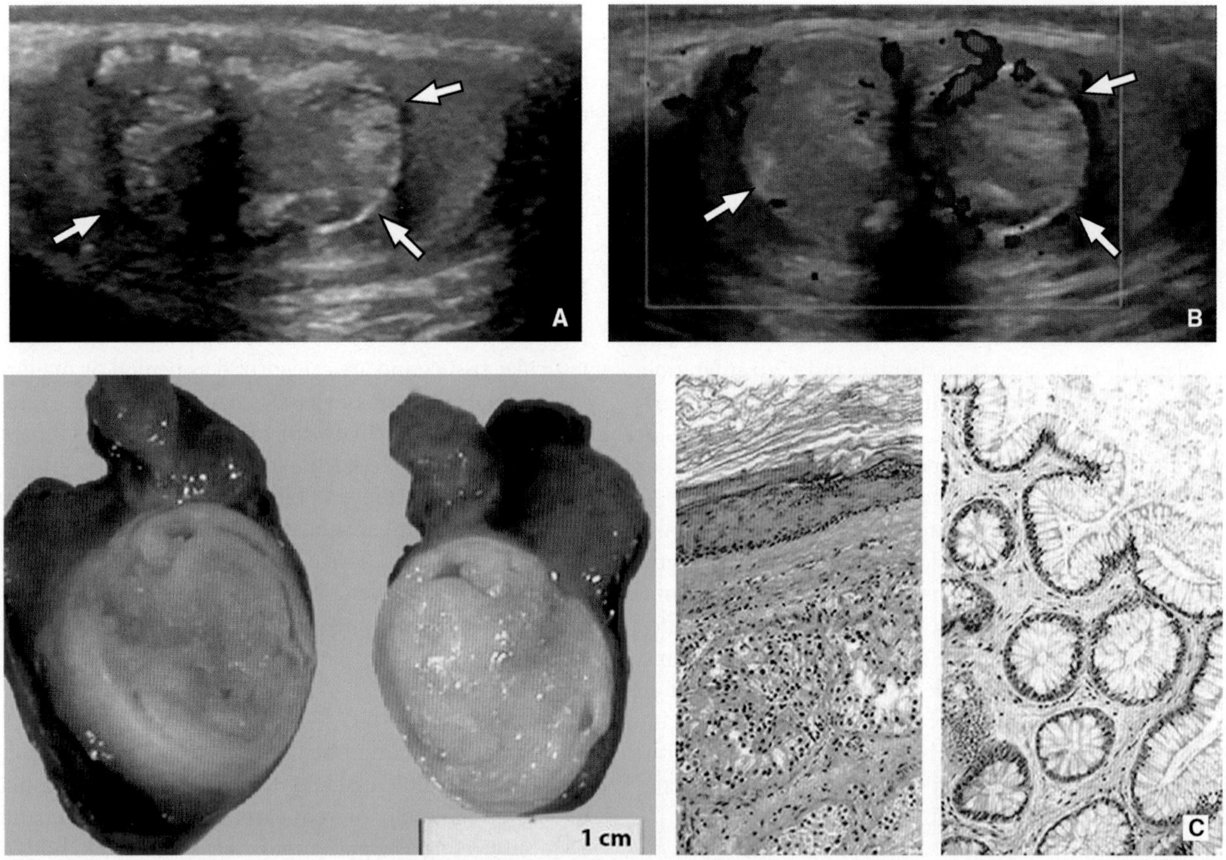

FIGURE 18.19 **A and B: A 10-year-old boy with palpable testicular mass.** Longitudinal gray-scale **(A)** and power Doppler **(B)** ultrasound images show a large, solid, heterogeneous, partly calcified testicular mass (*arrows*), surgically proven to be mature teratoma at histopathology. **C: A 16-year-old boy with palpable testicular mass.** Surgical specimen shows a well-circumscribed, 1 cm mass (*left*) lined by skin (*middle*; hematoxylin and eosin, original magnification, 400×) as well as mucus-secreting cells (*right*; hematoxylin and eosin, original magnification, 400×).

mass, which is a characteristic lamellated or onion-skin appearance at ultrasound[42,60,61] due to the intraluminal accumulation of shed keratin (Fig. 18.20). Testicular epidermoid cysts can have other appearances, however, including that of a solid echogenic mass or large simple cyst (Fig. 18.21). Sex cord–stromal tumors (e.g., juvenile granulosa cell tumor, Leydig cell tumor, Sertoli cell tumor) are rarely malignant, and their imaging appearances are nonspecific (Fig. 18.22).

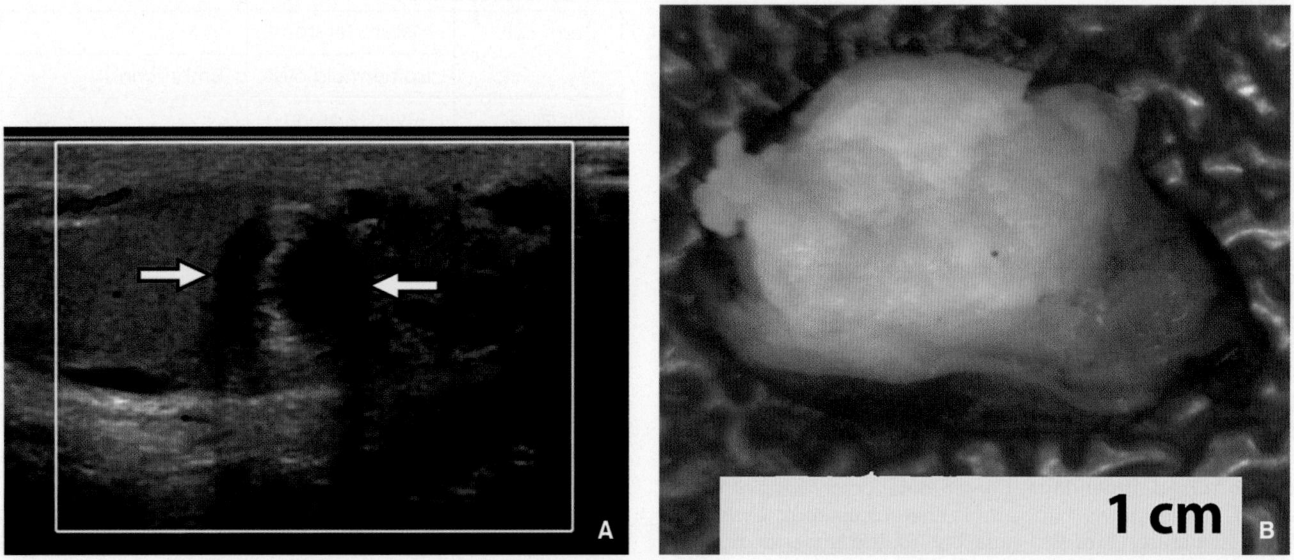

FIGURE 18.20 **A: A 12-year-old boy with palpable left testicular mass.** Longitudinal color Doppler ultrasound image demonstrates an avascular mass with "onion-skin" appearance (*arrows*), consistent with an epidermoid cyst. **B: A 5-year-old boy with testicular epidermoid cyst.** Grossly, the small mass is wholly cystic, filled with friable pale tan keratinous debris.

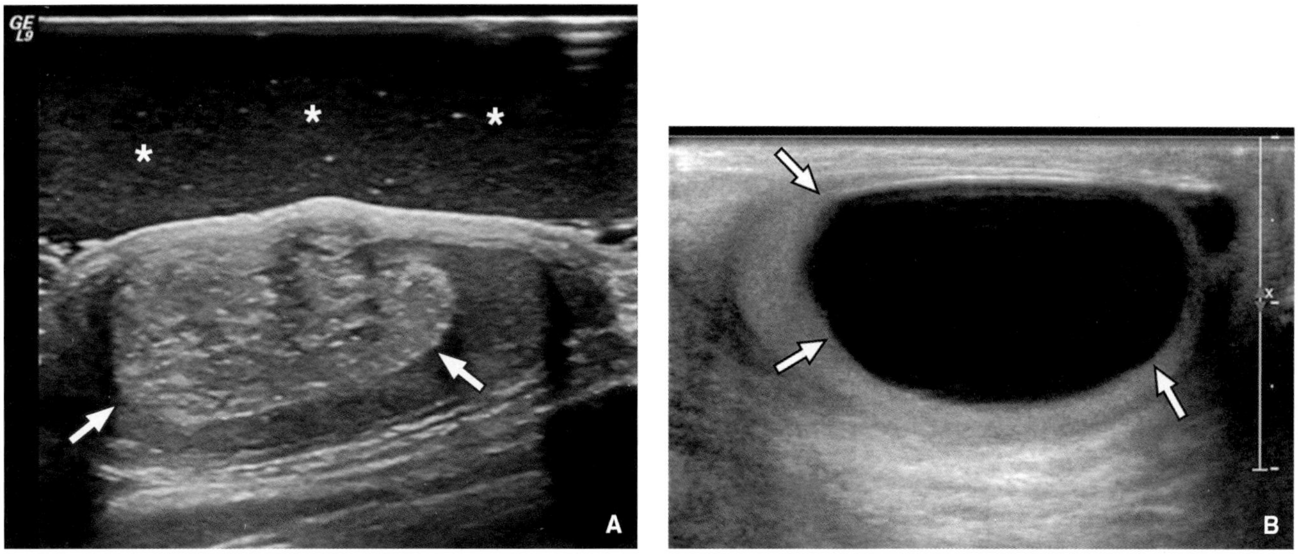

FIGURE 18.21 **A: A 7-year-old boy with palpable testicular mass.** Longitudinal gray-scale ultrasound image demonstrates a large, echogenic mass (*arrows*) occupying most of the testicle, proven to be an epidermoid cyst at histopathology. A large amount of ultrasound gel (*asterisks*) was placed between the transducer and scrotum to act as a stand-off pad. **B: A 6-month-old boy with palpable testicular mass.** Longitudinal gray-scale ultrasound image of the scrotum shows a large cyst (*arrows*) occupying much of the right testicle. Surgical enucleation was performed, and histopathology confirmed epidermoid cyst as well. (Case courtesy of Jonathan R. Dillman, MD, MSc, Cincinnati Children's Hospital Medical Center, Cincinnati, OH.)

No large series are available to guide their management in children; only anecdotal reports and limited published series provide limited experience help guide therapy.[62] These tumors may come to light because of excess hormone secretion.

Testicular-sparing surgery may be considered for suspected benign tumors when the adjacent testicular tissue appears otherwise normal at ultrasound, and the patient has normal alpha-fetoprotein concentration.[56] Suspected epidermoid cysts are commonly enucleated from the surrounding testicle, whereas a testicular mass with imaging features of a teratoma may still require complete orchiectomy.

Malignant Neoplasms

Primary Testicular Neoplasms

A variety of primary testicular neoplasms occur in the pediatric population. Neoplasms affecting prepubescent boys are presented in Table 18.2, and their management may be different from those tumors occurring in adolescents and adults.[63] In prepubertal boys, the most common tumor is pure yolk sac tumor.[56,57,64–66] Testicular malignancies in prepubescent boys

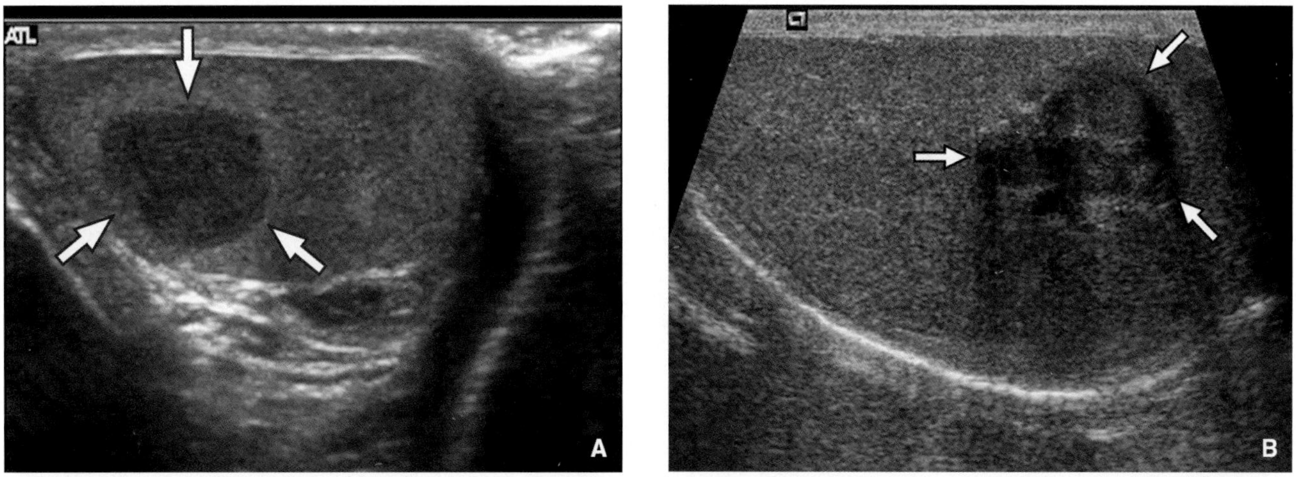

FIGURE 18.22 **A: An 8-year-old boy with precocious puberty due to Leydig cell tumor.** Longitudinal gray-scale ultrasound image shows a nonspecific solid hypoechoic mass (*arrows*) within the right testicle. **B: A 17-year-old boy with palpable testicular mass due to Sertoli cell tumor.** Longitudinal gray-scale ultrasound image shows a nonspecific solid hypoechoic mass (*arrows*) within the left testicle with irregular margins and posterior acoustic shadowing. (Case courtesy of Jonathan R. Dillman, MD, MSc, Cincinnati Children's Hospital Medical Center, Cincinnati, OH.)

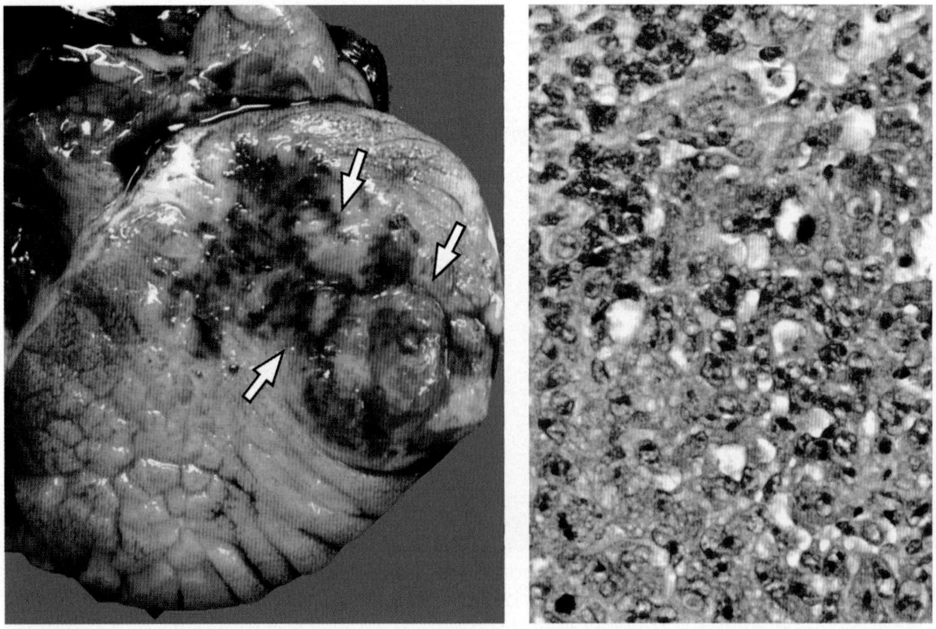

FIGURE 18.23 **An 18-year-old boy with malignant mixed germ cell tumor of the testicle.** A 3.5 cm ill-defined, variegated testicular mass is seen **(left)**. Microscopically, this tumor consisted largely of an embryonal carcinoma component (**right**, hematoxylin and eosin, original magnification, 600×).

most often present with a painless scrotal mass, except when complicated by torsion or hemorrhage. Pure yolk sac tumors are most commonly confined to the testis (stage I) and seen virtually exclusively in prepubertal boys; alpha-fetoprotein levels are usually elevated.[64] Survival for this "malignancy" is nearly 100%, even in the event of recurrence.[67] The overwhelming majority of postpubertal testicular tumors are malignant with histologic features of either seminoma or mixed germ cell tumor (Fig. 18.23).[13] These tumors are uncommon prior to puberty.

The initial imaging evaluation of boys with a known or suspected scrotal mass starts with ultrasound. Primary neoplastic tumors of the testicle have a variable appearance on ultrasound and range from a well-defined mass to diffuse infiltrative enlargement of the entire testis[13,68] (Fig. 18.24). Echogenicity is also variable because of the presence/absence of hemorrhage, necrosis/cystic degeneration, and calcification. Ultrasound provides valuable information regarding the size and location of the mass and usually can distinguish primary testicular tumors from extratesticular lesions.[13] Ultrasound can also be used to identify extension of the tumor beyond the tunica albuginea. After diagnosis of a primary testicular malignancy, CT (or MRI) of the abdomen and pelvis is typically performed to identify any sites of metastatic disease (including retroperitoneal lymph node involvement) (Fig. 18.25), and chest radiography or CT may be obtained to evaluate for pulmonary metastasis and involvement in the mediastinum.[13,63]

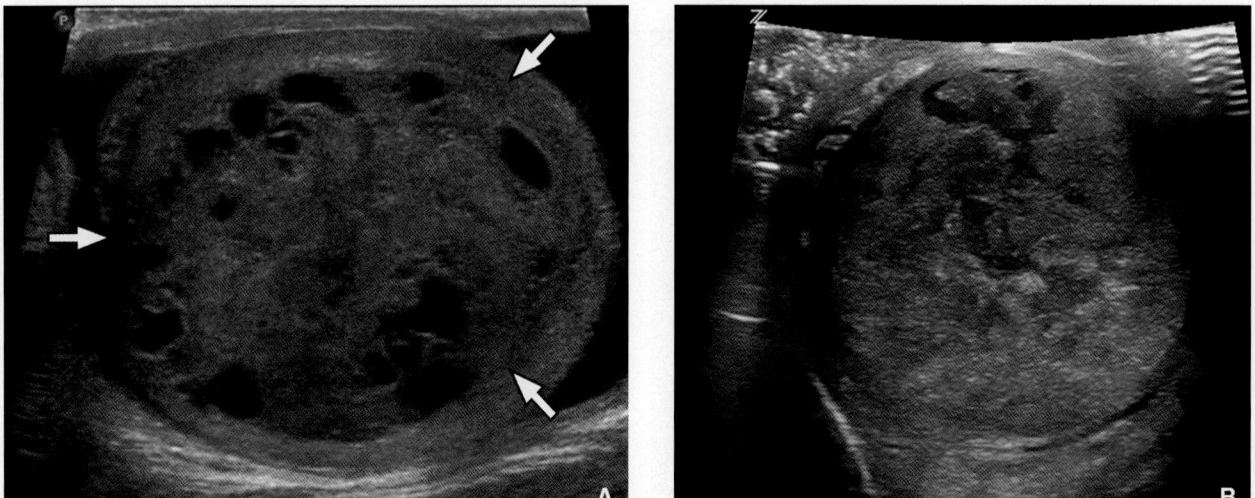

FIGURE 18.24 **A: A 15-year-old boy with palpable scrotal mass due to malignant mixed germ cell tumor.** Longitudinal gray-scale ultrasound image shows an enlarged right testicle containing a mixed solid and cystic mass (*arrows*) that is surrounded by normal parenchyma. **B: A different 15-year-old boy with palpable scrotal mass due to malignant mixed germ cell tumor.** Transverse gray-scale ultrasound image shows that the right testicle is diffusely enlarged and heterogeneous.

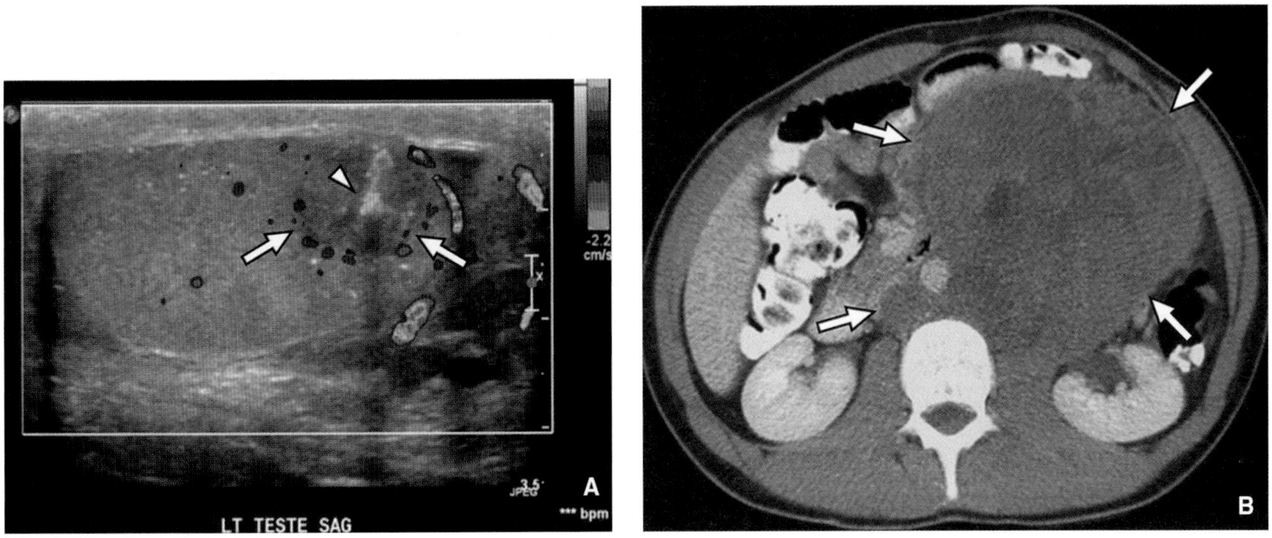

FIGURE 18.25 **A 14-year-old boy with palpable abdominal mass. A:** Longitudinal color Doppler ultrasound image demonstrates a round, heterogeneous, solid intratesticular mass (*arrows*). The mass contains echogenic, shadowing calcification (*arrowhead*), and there is also diffuse microlithiasis. **B:** Axial contrast-enhanced CT image reveals a very large retroperitoneal mass (*arrows*), proven to be metastatic germ cell tumor (embryonal carcinoma). (Case courtesy of Jonathan R. Dillman, MD, MSc, Cincinnati Children's Hospital Medical Center, Cincinnati, OH.)

Gonadoblastomas contain a mixture of gonadal elements (germ cells and sex cord–stromal cells) and are commonly diagnosed in the setting of DSD. The majority of cases occur in children with a Y chromosome, including mosaic Turner syndrome (45,X0/46,XY).[69] Streak gonads in the setting of mixed gonadal dysgenesis are at particular increased risk for developing this neoplasm. As gonadoblastomas can demonstrate malignant transformation, gonadectomy is frequently performed in at-risk children.[69]

Secondary Testicular Neoplasms

Secondary testicular neoplasms are most commonly due to leukemia and lymphoma.[70,71] A common sonographic presentation (other than a normal testicle with involvement that cannot be detected by imaging) is that of an enlarged, hypoechoic testicle because of diffuse infiltration by the tumor, although focal masses also can be seen (Fig. 18.26). Hypervascularity and concomitant enlargement of the epididymis can also be signs for these tumors.[72] Because the

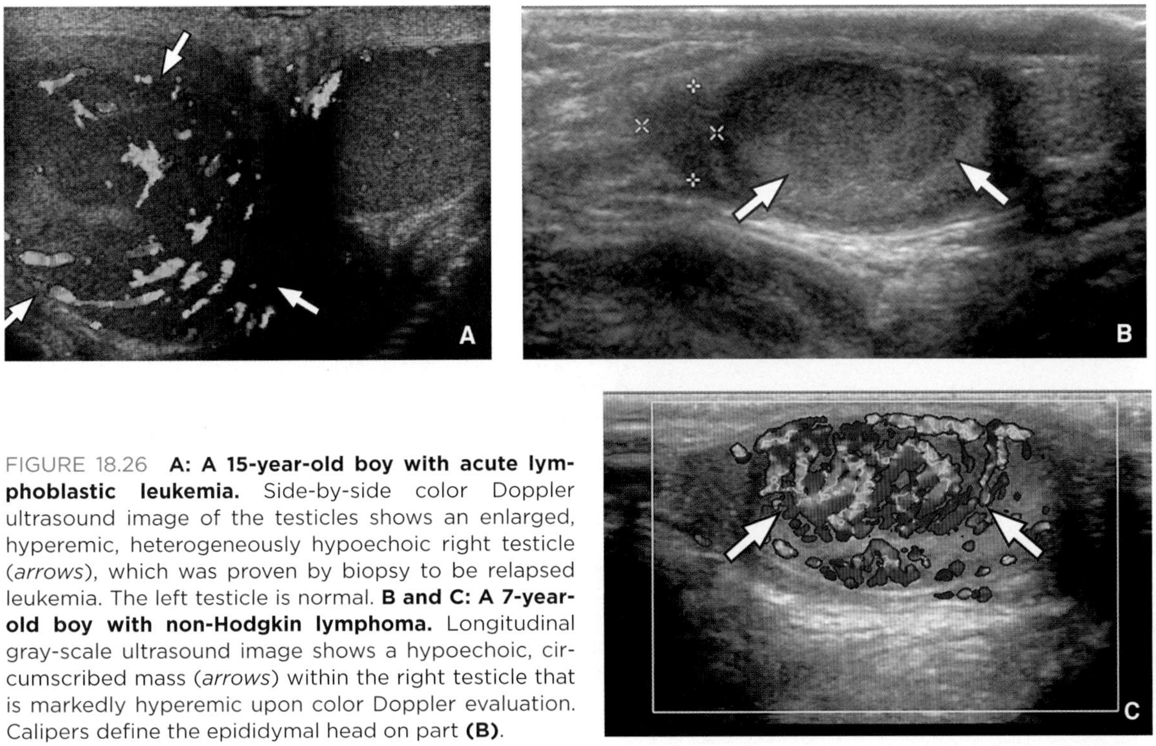

FIGURE 18.26 **A: A 15-year-old boy with acute lymphoblastic leukemia.** Side-by-side color Doppler ultrasound image of the testicles shows an enlarged, hyperemic, heterogeneously hypoechoic right testicle (*arrows*), which was proven by biopsy to be relapsed leukemia. The left testicle is normal. **B and C: A 7-year-old boy with non-Hodgkin lymphoma.** Longitudinal gray-scale ultrasound image shows a hypoechoic, circumscribed mass (*arrows*) within the right testicle that is markedly hyperemic upon color Doppler evaluation. Calipers define the epididymal head on part **(B)**.

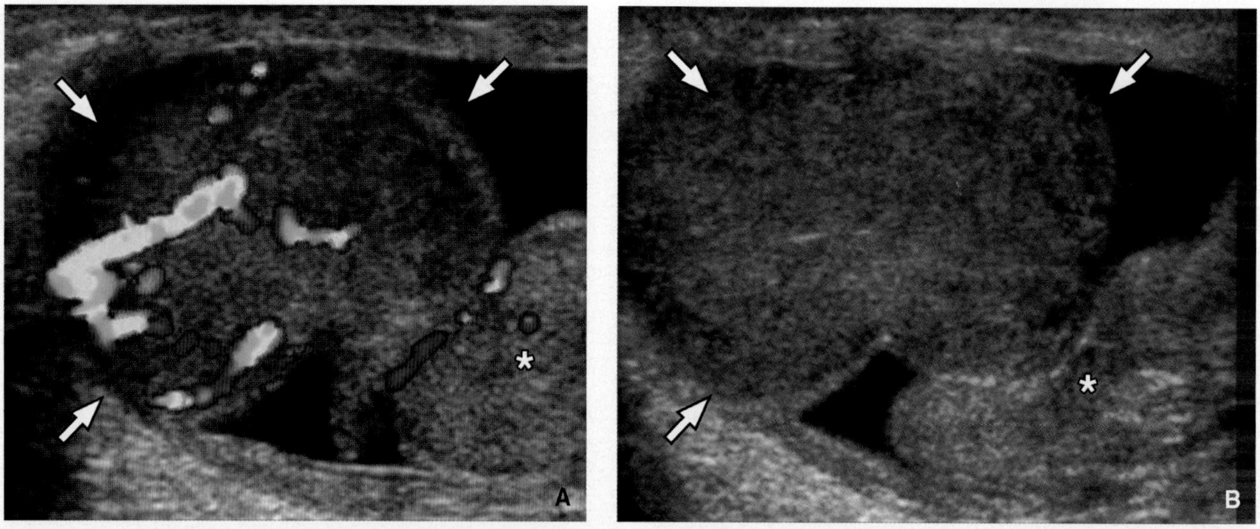

FIGURE 18.27 **A 5-year-old boy with palpable scrotal mass.** Longitudinal color Doppler **(A)** and gray-scale **(B)** ultrasound images show a lobulated, hyperemic extratesticular solid mass (*arrows*) with mass effect on adjacent testicle (*asterisk*), surgically proven to be paratesticular embryonal rhabdomyosarcoma.

blood-testicle barrier limits entry of chemotherapeutic agents into the testicle, the testicle is predisposed to residual disease and relapse. Testicular lymphoma is usually due to secondary involvement from non-Hodgkin lymphoma, especially Burkitt lymphoma.[73] Treatment strategies for testicular lymphoma include systemic chemotherapy, orchiectomy, and radiotherapy directed at the involved testis.[74,75]

Extratesticular Neoplasms

Rhabdomyosarcoma is the most common soft tissue sarcoma in prepubertal children, and 7% to 10% of them arise from the distal spermatic cord[76] (Fig. 18.27). Paratesticular rhabdomyosarcomas range widely in size (up to 20 cm), can invade the testicle, and show a high rate of metastases to the retroperitoneal lymph nodes, lungs, cortical bone, and bone marrow.[56,77,78]

Ultrasound typically shows a heterogeneous scrotal mass arising outside of the testicle; often, no definable features separate rhabdomyosarcoma from other paratesticular tumors (Table 18.2). Radiologic staging includes CT imaging of the chest, CT (or MRI) imaging of abdomen and pelvis, and PET/CT; imaging surveillance during and after therapy is generally standard.[56,79] Pathologically, these tumors are composed of malignant cells with immunohistochemistry evidence of skeletal muscle differentiation (Fig. 18.28).

Combined treatment strategies now confer a relatively good prognosis for this neoplasm, with up to 90% to 95% 3-year survival.[80–82] The dictum that extratesticular scrotal masses are almost always benign is substantially less reliable in children than in adults, on account of paratesticular rhabdomyosarcoma. Other paratesticular neoplasms can occur in children, but are very rare.

Testicular Microlithiasis

Diffuse testicular microlithiasis is defined as the presence of five or more tiny, punctate 1- to 3-mm nonshadowing, echogenic foci on a single ultrasound image of testicle (Fig. 18.29). Microliths are located in seminiferous tubules and may be present very early in testicular development.[83,84] Microlithiasis is encountered in 1% to 2% of men,[85] up to 9% of boys,[86] and around 20% in patients with subfertility.[87]

The clinical significance of this finding depends on the clinical scenario. A large meta-analysis showed an association

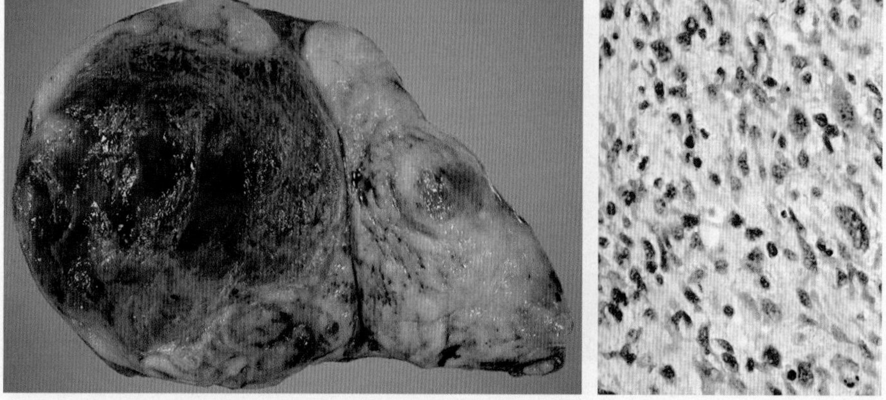

FIGURE 18.28 **A 16-year-old boy with a scrotal mass, found to have a 20 cm embryonal paratesticular rhabdomyosarcoma (left).** Microscopically, the tumor showed pleomorphic mesenchymal cells with frequent eosinophilic cytoplasmic tails indicating rhabdomyoblastic differentiation. Tumor cells were positive for immunohistochemical markers of skeletal muscle differentiation, including desmin and myogenin (not shown).

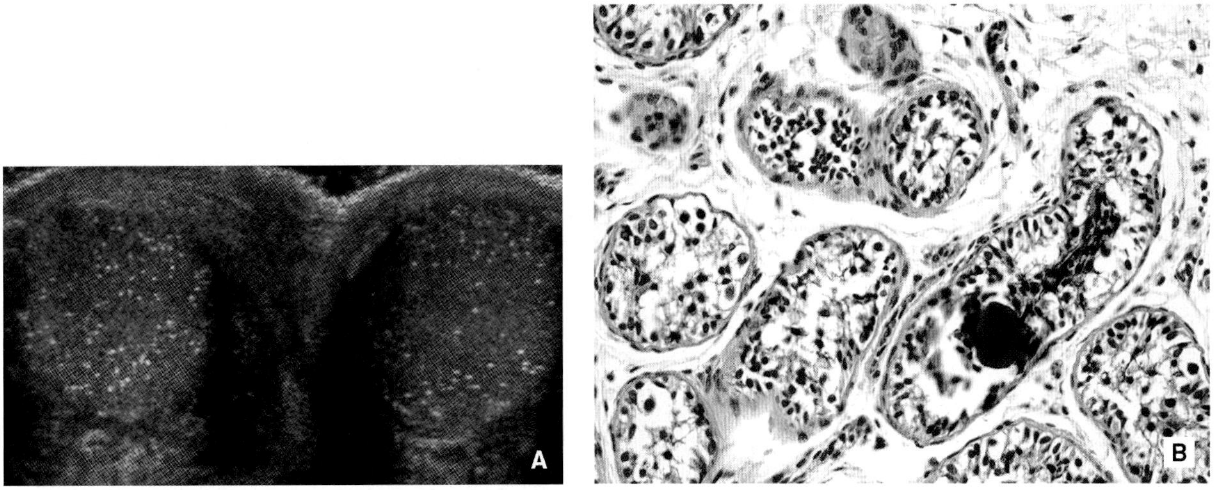

FIGURE 18.29 **A: A 16-year-old boy with acute scrotal pain found to have incidental testicular diffuse microlithiasis.** Transverse gray-scale ultrasound image of the testicles shows many bilateral punctate, echogenic, nonshadowing calcifications. No testicular mass is identified. **B: Microlithiasis from an assigned female with 46, XO/46, XY mosaicism.** This dysplastic testis shows microlithiasis, characterized by spherical dark purple (basophilic) intratubular microcalcifications (hematoxylin and eosin, original magnification, 40×).

between diffuse testicular microlithiasis and risk of testicular cancer in individuals who have other risk factors for testicular germ cell tumors in adults[88]; however, the significance of this finding in individuals without other risk factors remains controversial,[89] and in children the association needs further investigation. Some have suggested that microlithiasis without other risk factors (e.g., previous testicular cancer, history of cryptorchidism) for testicular cancer is unlikely to warrant screening.[85] However, others advocate screening for testicular neoplasm in the setting of diffuse microlithiasis, including physical examination and scrotal ultrasound every 6 to 12 months.[90] Limited testicular microlithiasis (fewer than five microliths on a single ultrasound image) is of doubtful clinical significance.

Traumatic Disorders

Scrotal Trauma Overview and Imaging Approach

Traumatic injuries to the scrotum and its contents are common and can be devastating. Depending on the type of mechanism and the forces applied, the resulting injury can vary from minor superficial contusions to severe testicular rupture. Sports-related blunt injuries account for more than half of testicular trauma in children, whereas motor vehicle accidents cause another 9% to 17%.[91] Ultrasound imaging is the preferred method of interrogation.[92] A stable pediatric patient may be positioned supine, and it is important to provide stabilization and support for the scrotum.

The highest frequency linear-array transducer available that provides adequate tissue penetration is important for depiction of testicular anatomy. Both gray-scale and Doppler ultrasound are critical to evaluating suspected testicular injury. In order to characterize the presence or absence of blood flow within the testicle, Doppler ultrasound settings should be set in order to be sensitive to low-velocity flow (e.g., minimize the pulse repetition frequency). In cases of penetrating injuries (e.g., due to gunshot wounds), ultrasound evaluation has the same diagnostic goals; however, evaluation can be limited by artifacts from air. Ultrasound in the setting of penetrating trauma is also useful for identifying foreign bodies.

Types of Scrotal Injuries

A variety of trauma patterns occur in the scrotum, and the terminology used to describe the type of scrotal injury is important to understand. A hematocele is an intrascrotal collection of blood products located between the visceral and parietal layers of the tunica vaginalis[92] (Fig. 18.30). This may appear as complex fluid collection on ultrasound, possibly with septations. It is important to screen for abdominal trauma because a hematocele can potentially arise from hemoperitoneum entering the scrotum through a patent processus vaginalis.[93]

A hematoma is a nonvascular mass–like collection of blood products localized in the soft tissues of the scrotal wall, epididymis, or testis. A testicular fracture involves disruption of testicular parenchyma with resultant loss of normal architecture, but preservation of the echogenic tunica albuginea (Fig. 18.31). At ultrasound, a linear or stellate cleft may be recognized within the testicle, with disruption of the normal background homogeneous parenchymal appearance.

The most severe form of testicular trauma is a testicular rupture, involving disruption of the tough fibrous echogenic tunica albuginea and loss of testicular parenchymal organization (Fig. 18.32). In cases of rupture, ultrasound may show extrusion of testicular contents through defects of the tunica albuginea with resultant focal contour abnormalities of the testicle. Traumatic dislocation of the testis into the inguinal canal, abdominal cavity, or perineum has also been reported.

Traumatic epididymitis, with inflammation occurring secondary to trauma, results in an enlarged, heterogeneous, and

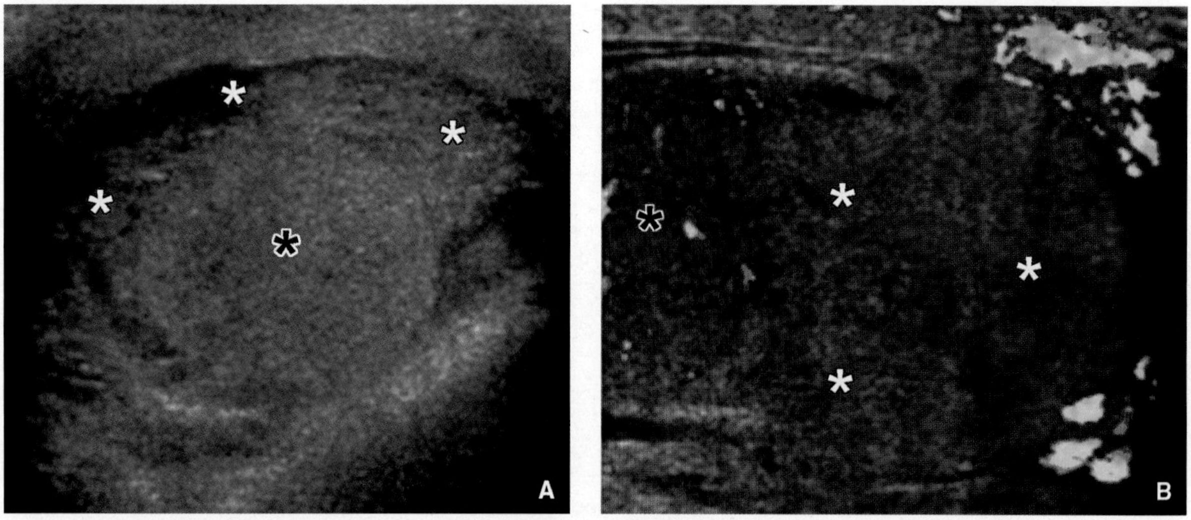

FIGURE 18.30 **A 15-year-old boy with blunt scrotal trauma.** Gray-scale **(A)** and color Doppler **(B)** ultrasound images show echogenic, complex fluid between the layers of the tunica vaginalis, consistent with a hematocele (*white asterisks*). Doppler signal is present in the testicle (*black asterisk*; **B**).

hyperemic epididymis. In addition to blunt traumatic injuries, injuries to the supplying blood vessels can cause a nontwisting "torsion," with resultant ischemia or even infarction of the testicle. Penetrating scrotal injuries are rare and the majority are caused by gunshot wounds (Fig. 18.33).

Varicocele

Varicocele is an abnormal enlargement of the pampiniform plexus of veins that drain the testicles. This condition is typically diagnosed in older children and young men, aged 15 to 30, and may present with scrotal fullness, pain, infertility, or eventually ipsilateral testicular atrophy.[94,95] Primary, or idiopathic, varicocele is caused by failure of the venous valves of the gonadal veins, resulting in backflow of blood into the pampiniform plexus. The vast majority of primary varicoceles (90%) occurs on the left side,[96] thought to be secondary to the left testicular vein draining into the left renal vein at approximately a 90-degree angle. The right testicular vein drains instead directly into the IVC at a more gradual angle. Right-sided varicoceles should prompt a search for causes of venous obstruction, which may be either benign or malignant. Secondary varicoceles develop as a result of obstruction to drainage of the testicular veins and can be secondary to masses (e.g., renal cell carcinoma or lymphoma) or compression by other structures (e.g., nutcracker phenomenon due to compression of the left renal vein between the superior mesenteric artery and the aorta).

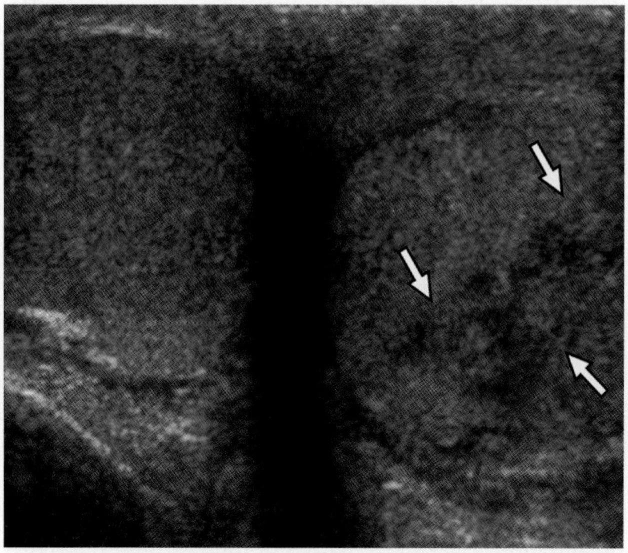

FIGURE 18.31 **A 17-year-old boy with blunt scrotal trauma.** Side-by-side gray-scale ultrasound image of the testicles shows irregular linear areas of decreased echogenicity in the left testicle due to disruption of testicular parenchyma, consistent with fractures (between *arrows*). There was no disruption of the surrounding tunica albuginea to suggest testicular rupture.

At gray-scale ultrasound, varicoceles present as dilatation of the veins of the pampiniform plexus to >2 mm in diameter (Fig. 18.34). These vessels may enlarge with Valsalva maneuver. At Doppler ultrasound, these veins show a venous monophasic waveform and demonstrate increased color Doppler signal with Valsalva maneuver. A rare form of varicocele, intratesticular varicocele, as the name implies, involves enlargement of the intratesticular veins around the mediastinum testis, or along the periphery of the testicle (Fig. 18.34). Generally, this uncommon form of varicocele is observed with an associated extratesticular varicocele.

Treatment of pediatric and adolescent varicocele is somewhat controversial, given that the majority of adult males with the condition do not manifest infertility, which remains the primary concerning clinical outcome.[97] Relative testicular volume loss of 20% or more compared to the nonaffected contralateral testicle, as well as semen analysis, help guide the urologist and patient in determining when intervention is indicated.[97] Currently, there are well-tolerated, effective,

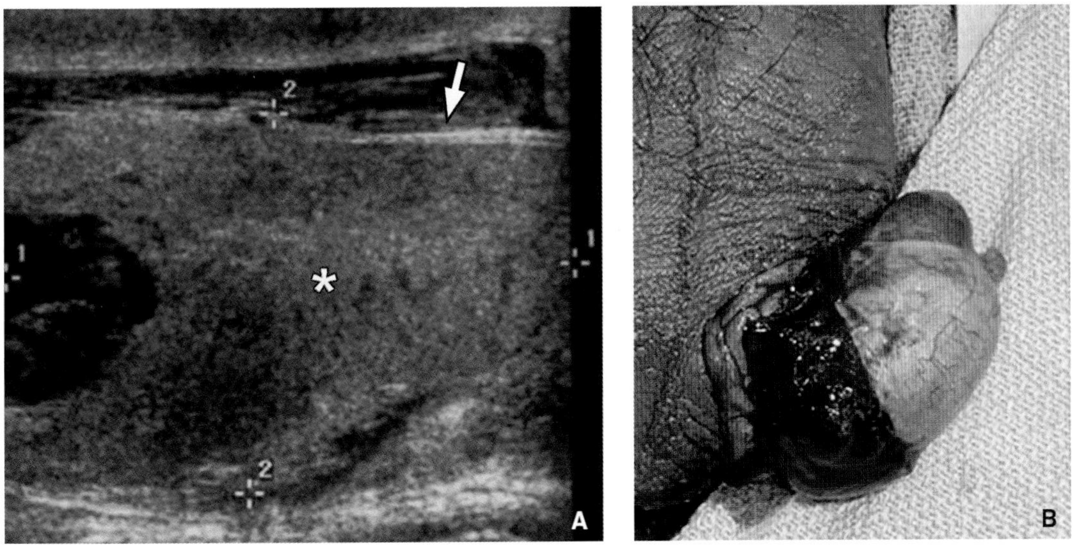

FIGURE 18.32 **A 16-year-old boy with straddle injury on bicycle. A:** Longitudinal gray-scale ultrasound image shows a heterogeneous testicle (*asterisk*) with irregular contours and areas of disruption of testicular capsule/tunica albuginea (*arrow* shows intact tunica albuginea) consistent with testicular rupture. **A 12-year-old boy with skateboard trauma. B:** Intraoperative image shows testicular parenchyma extruding through the capsule. (Image courtesy of Laurence Baskin, MD, UCSF Benioff Children's Hospital, San Francisco, CA.)

and safe surgical and minimally invasive interventional techniques for the treatment of varicocele; the overall best method remains controversial, as large prospective studies comparing these methods are still needed.[97]

SPECTRUM OF EPIDIDYMAL DISORDERS

Congenital and Developmental Anomalies

Epididymal Cyst and Spermatocele

The most common epididymal mass–like abnormality is a cyst, present in 20% to 40% of asymptomatic individuals.[98] Epididymal cysts occur with increased frequency in pediatric patients with von Hippel-Lindau disease and cystic fibrosis. Both epididymal cysts and spermatoceles appear as well-defined cystic epididymal masses, most often in the head. Epididymal cysts may be lymphatic or epithelial, whereas spermatoceles represent dilated efferent ductules and contain sperm (Fig. 18.35).

At ultrasound, both commonly appear as anechoic cysts in the epididymis (Fig. 18.36). Spermatoceles may contain debris (low-level echoes) due to sperm; septations may also be seen. When very large, these cysts can be confused with hydroceles, although hydroceles tend to envelop the testis and cysts arising from the epididymis tend to displace the testis.

Conservative management of these lesions is considered standard; however, surgical excision is performed in large symptomatic cases.[99]

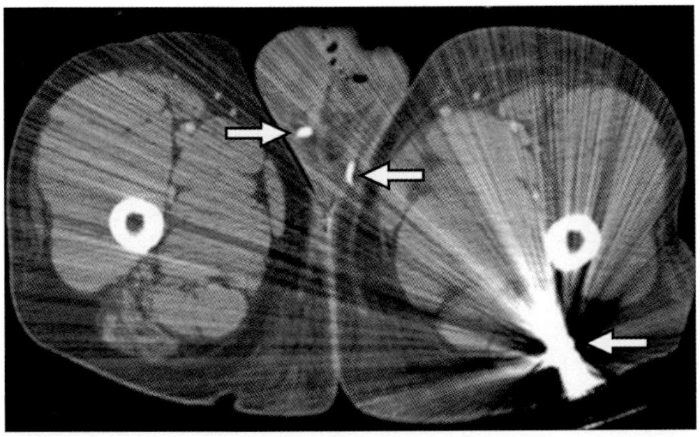

FIGURE 18.33 **A 19-year-old man status post gunshot to the perineum.** Axial contrast-enhanced CT image shows irregularity of the scrotum and intrascrotal gas. Metallic shrapnel (*arrows*) is present in the scrotal wall and left buttock.

Infectious and Inflammatory Disorders

Epididymitis and Epididymo-orchitis

Both epididymitis and epididymo-orchitis are common causes of acute scrotal pain in childhood. Together, these infectious and inflammatory conditions represent the most common cause of acute scrotal pain in older boys and adult men.[100,101]

Bacterial seeding is presumed to occur either via direct extension of pathogens retrograde via the vas deferens or possibly hematogenously in the absence of a demonstrable anatomic predisposition. Several urinary tract abnormalities predispose to retrograde bacterial seeding, including bladder and urethral obstructive anomalies (e.g., hypospadias, neurogenic bladder, functional bladder abnormality, posterior urethral valves) or other anatomic variants (ectopic ureter or vas deferens, fistula, or ureteral duplication).[102] *Neisseria gonorrhoeae* and *Chlamydia trachomatis* are common sexually transmitted disease pathogens that cause both epididymitis and epididymo-orchitis in adolescent boys and younger

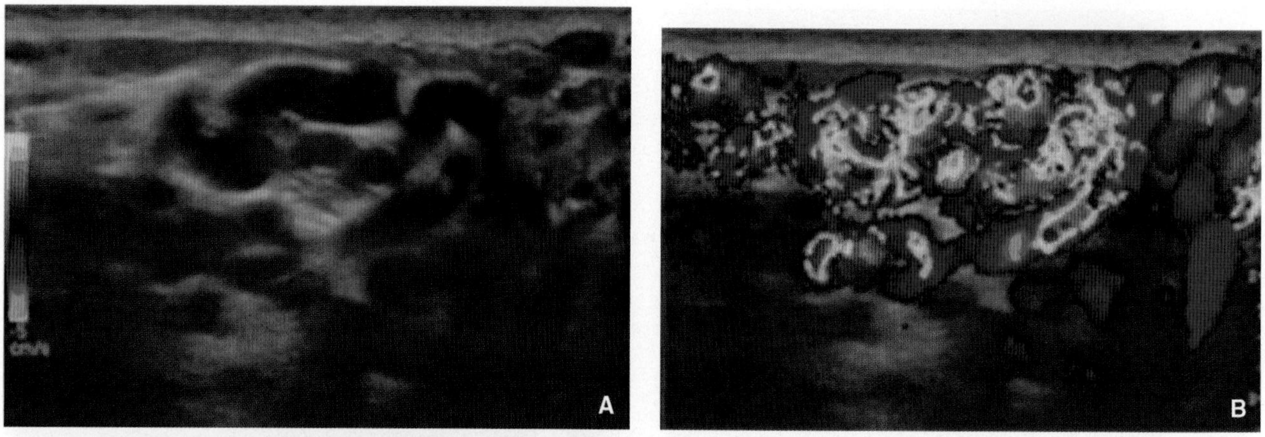

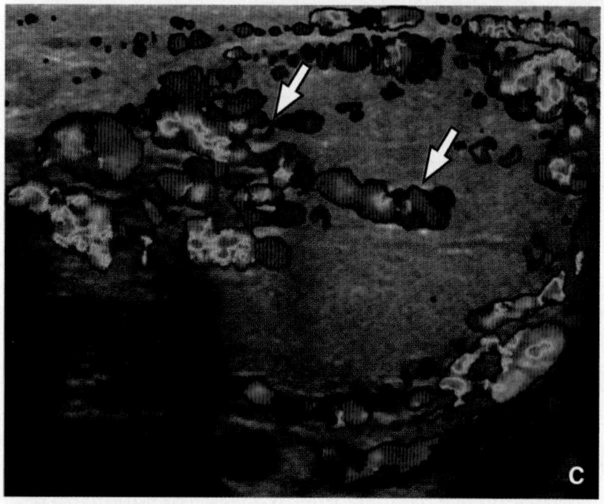

FIGURE 18.34 **A 16-year-old boy with left scrotal fullness. A–B:** Gray-scale and color Doppler ultrasound images of the left inguinal canal show dilatation and tortuosity of the pampiniform plexus that increased in prominence with Valsalva maneuver, consistent with a varicocele. **C:** Doppler ultrasound image demonstrates a large varicocele surrounding the left testicle as well as intratesticular extension (*arrows*).

adult men; older adult men are more frequently affected by *E. coli*. Chemical epididymitis is an acute inflammatory process caused by reflux of sterile urine. Because of the direct exposure, this tends to only affect the vas deferens and epididymal tail, and does not typically reach the more remote epididymal head. Chronic, atypical, and granulomatous forms of epididymitis can occur, but tend to affect older adult men.

The imaging evaluation of epididymitis and epididymo-orchitis involves primarily ultrasound performed with a linear high-frequency transducer.[30] The inflamed epididymis typically shows increased size and hyperemia upon gray-scale and Doppler ultrasound evaluation; orchitis may also be present in some children (Fig. 18.37). Echogenicity of the inflamed

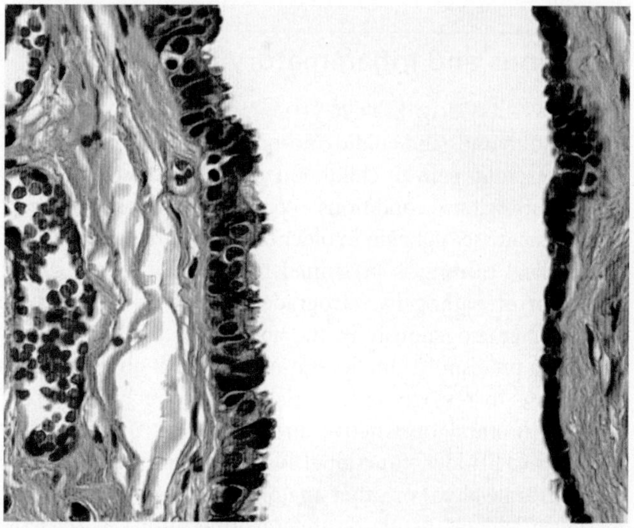

FIGURE 18.35 **A 12-year-old boy with an extratesticular mass found to be an epididymal cyst.** Microscopy shows characteristic cuboidal to columnar epithelial lining with occasional ciliated cells (hematoxylin and eosin, original magnification, 600×).

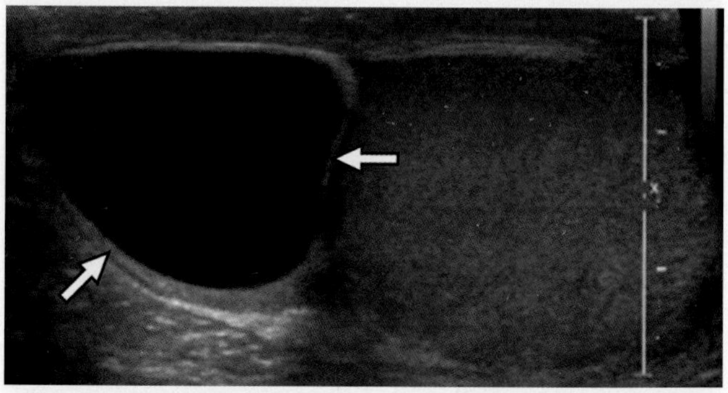

FIGURE 18.36 **A 12-year-old boy with scrotal mass palpated at sports physical exam.** Longitudinal gray-scale ultrasound image demonstrates a large anechoic cyst (*arrows*) centered in the epididymal head with mass effect exerted on the adjacent testicle, consistent with a large spermatocele (vs. epididymal cyst).

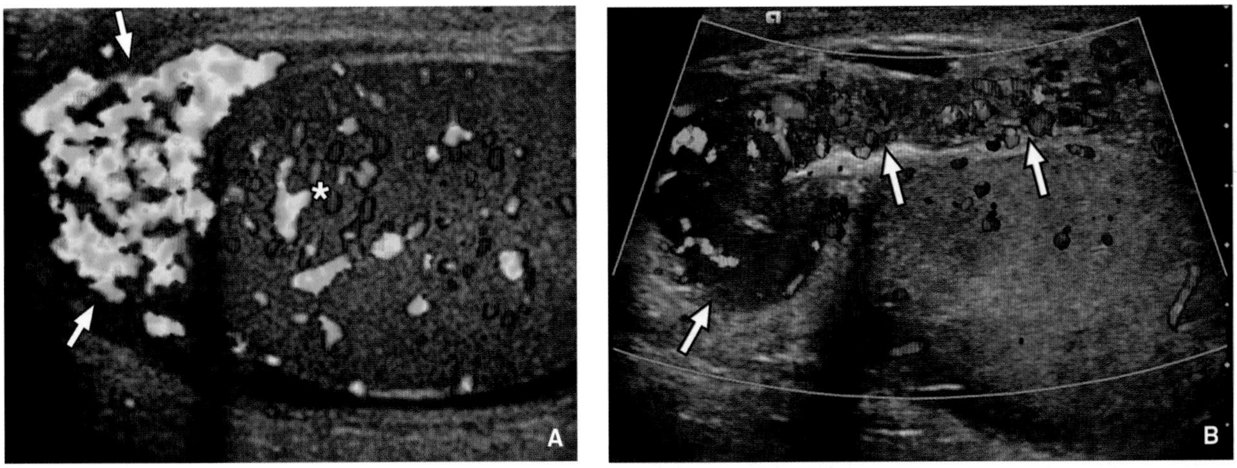

FIGURE 18.37 **A: An 8-year-old boy with acute testicular pain due to epididymo-orchitis.** Longitudinal color Doppler ultrasound image shows an enlarged, hypervascular epididymis (*arrows*) in association with testicular hyperemia (*asterisk*). **B: A 13-year-old boy with acute testicular pain due to epididymitis.** Longitudinal color Doppler ultrasound image shows an enlarged, hypoechoic, hypervascular epididymis (*arrows*).

epididymis is variable. Reactive hydrocele is common, and there may be overlying scrotal wall edema (skin thickening). It is important to exclude rare complications, such as ischemia, infarction, and abscess formation.[101]

The mainstay of therapy is antibiotic therapy. In boys who present with repeated episodes, dedicated search for genitourinary anomalies is indicated.

Neoplastic Disorder

Adenomatoid Tumor

Adenomatoid tumor is the most common epididymal solid mass, generally occurring in adult men.[103] This benign proliferation of mesothelial cells accounts for ~30% of all paratesticular neoplasms, second only to "lipoma" (which in this anatomic site typically represents displaced preperitoneal adipose tissue rather than a true neoplasm).[103] It tends to arise from the lower tail more than upper head of the epididymis, though it can also occur in the testis, testicular tunica (vaginalis or albuginea), and rarely the spermatic cord.[103,104] It classically manifests as a painless, round, well-circumscribed echogenic mass,[103] although the ultrasound appearance is variable.[104] At color Doppler ultrasound, internal vascularity is usually demonstrated.[103] Surgical resection is the current standard of care.[104]

SPECTRUM OF PROSTATE GLAND AND SEMINAL VESICLE DISORDERS

Congenital and Developmental Anomalies

Congenital anomalies of the seminal vesicles range from agenesis (Fig. 18.38) to hypoplasia to duplication.[105] Structural developmental anomalies, such as ectopia, cyst formation, ureteral communication, or urethral communication, may also occur. Overall, the most commonly encountered congenital/developmental anomalies of the seminal vesicles are agenesis and cystic anomalies.[106] Because of their close embryologic relationship, anomalies of the male urinary and genital tracts often coexist.

Seminal Vesicle Cyst

Seminal vesicle cysts are well-defined fluid-filled structures located posterior to the urinary bladder (Fig. 18.39). These cysts are most often identified in patients between 10 and 40 years of age.[5] They can be congenital or acquired (e.g., due to seminal vesicle obstruction) and may be isolated or associated with upper urinary tract anomalies, including ureteral ectopia, ipsilateral renal agenesis, multicystic dysplastic kidney, and autosomal dominant polycystic kidney disease (Figs. 18.39 and 18.40).[5,106] Although cysts are typically small (<5 cm) and asymptomatic, infectious genitourinary-related symptoms, including recurrent prostatitis and epididymitis, can occur.

On MRI, these cysts appear hyperintense on T2-weighted MR images and are of variable signal intensity on T1-weighted MR images. An ectopic ureter inserting into the seminal vesicles

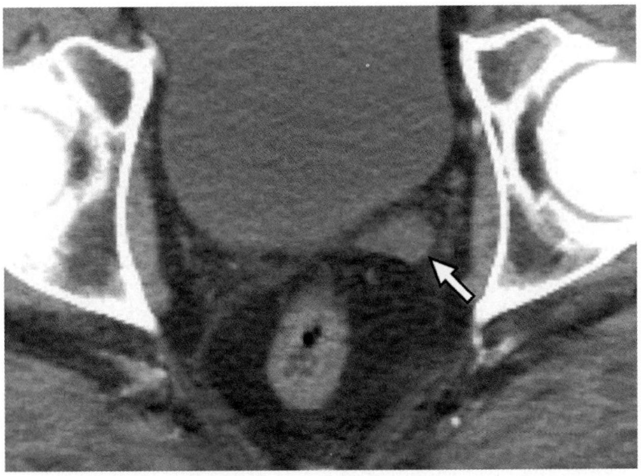

FIGURE 18.38 **A 10-year-old boy with right pelvic kidney being evaluated for renal colic.** Axial noncontrast CT image shows congenital absence of the right seminal vesicle. The left seminal vesicle (*arrow*) appears normal.

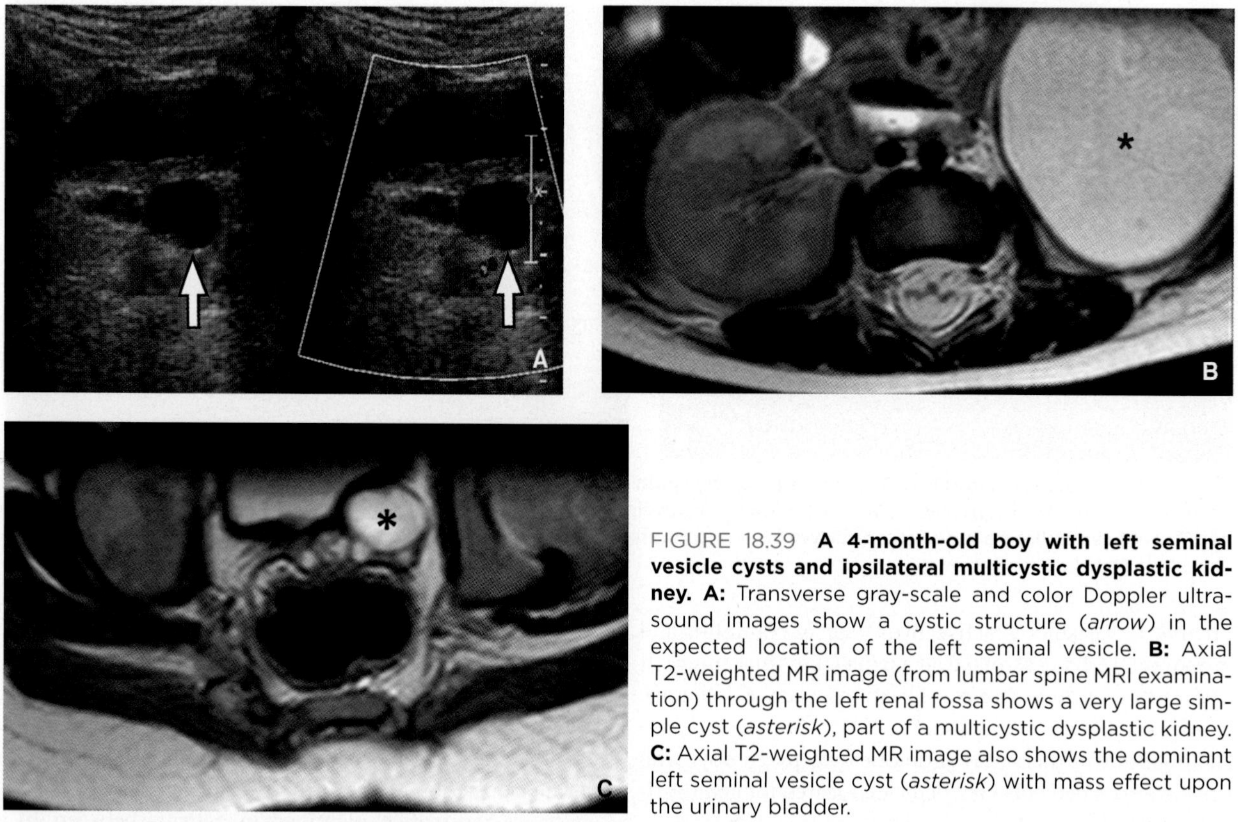

FIGURE 18.39 **A 4-month-old boy with left seminal vesicle cysts and ipsilateral multicystic dysplastic kidney. A:** Transverse gray-scale and color Doppler ultrasound images show a cystic structure (*arrow*) in the expected location of the left seminal vesicle. **B:** Axial T2-weighted MR image (from lumbar spine MRI examination) through the left renal fossa shows a very large simple cyst (*asterisk*), part of a multicystic dysplastic kidney. **C:** Axial T2-weighted MR image also shows the dominant left seminal vesicle cyst (*asterisk*) with mass effect upon the urinary bladder.

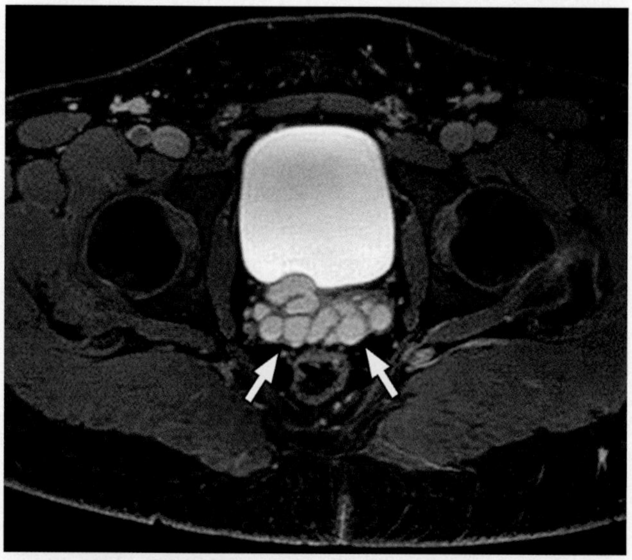

FIGURE 18.40 **A 16-year-old boy with chronic pelvic pain.** Axial postcontrast T1-weighted fat-saturated excretory phase MR image shows cystic dilatation of the seminal vesicles (*arrows*). Excreted contrast material is present in the bladder, whereas hyperintense material in the seminal vesicles is due to blood or proteinaceous material. The patient was found to have a right multicystic dysplastic kidney with some preserved function and an associated ectopic ureter draining into the right seminal vesicle. (Case courtesy of Jonathan R. Dillman, MD, MSc, Cincinnati Children's Hospital Medical Center, Cincinnati, OH.)

is another rare cause of seminal vesicle cyst–like enlargement that can be definitively diagnosed by MRI (Fig. 18.40).

Seminal Vesicle and Prostate Gland Agenesis and Hypoplasia

The seminal vesicles are paired structures that form during the 12th week of gestation from the distal mesonephric duct. Seminal vesicle hypoplasia is described as congenitally small seminal vesicles, although no described diagnostic criteria have been established. Associations with other congenital genitourinary anomalies, including hypogonadism and cryptorchidism, have been described; however, this can also be an isolated finding.[107]

Agenesis of the seminal vesicles can occur from one of the two scenarios: primary insult to the mesonephric duct during embryogenesis or secondary to an underlying cystic fibrosis transmembrane conductance regulator (CFTR) gene.[106] The primary form may be associated with anomalies of the vas deferens (including agenesis or ectopia). When the primary insult occurs before ureteral budding (prior to 7 weeks of gestational age), ipsilateral renal agenesis also occurs. In pediatric patients with underlying CFTR mutations, the seminal vesicle agenesis is thought to be related to blockage of the lumen of the seminal vesicle (and vas deferens) by thick secretions. As the kidneys are often normal in these cases, this process is thought to likely occur after the 7th week of gestation.[106] Complications include infertility and, in cases of ectopic insertion of the vas deferens, hematospermia, epididymitis, and urinary tract infection.[107]

The prostate gland develops separately from the seminal vesicles and is formed from the urogenital sinus.[107] Although complete agenesis of the prostate has not been reported in the literature, hypoplasia of the prostate gland can occur and is one of two proposed mechanisms for the development of prune belly syndrome (PBS). In PBS, affected pediatric patients have abnormally thinned, poorly developed abdominal wall musculature, enlarged floppy urinary bladder, dilated ureters, and bilateral cryptorchidism. It is theorized that the hypoplastic prostate leads to a temporary kinking of the urethra and subsequently causes bladder outlet obstruction.[108] This leads to massive distention of the urinary bladder and upper urinary tracts, and it is this distention that interferes with the development of the abdominal wall musculature. An underlying insult during mesodermal development is the other leading theory for the development of PBS, given that the affected tissues in PBS are of mesodermal origin.[109] The lack of involvement of other organ systems of mesodermal origin is an unresolved question for this theory. Prostate hypoplasia manifests at ultrasound and voiding cystourethrography (VCUG) as an enlarged posterior urethra.

Prostatic Utricle Cyst

Prostatic utricle cysts (enlargement of the prostatic utricle) are thought to be remnants of the Mullerian duct system, occurring in 1% to 5% of the population.[5] They are midline in location and do not extend above the prostate gland. These structures are on average 8 to 10 mm in size (although they can be considerably larger)[5] and are located behind the upper portion of the prostatic urethra. Although sometimes isolated, they can be associated with hypospadias, DSD, PBS, cryptorchidism, and ipsilateral renal agenesis.[110,111] Clinical manifestations include postvoid dribbling (as these cysts communicate with the urethra), recurrent epididymitis, and hematospermia[5]; they can also be complicated by calculus formation.[112]

Prostatic utricle cysts appear as a focal collection of contrast material (diverticulum) arising posterior to the prostatic urethra at the level of the verumontanum on VCUG and as a midline hypoechoic or anechoic structure located posterior to the prostatic urethra at ultrasound (Fig. 18.41). At MRI, utricle cysts are generally hypointense on T1-weighted MR images and hyperintense on T2-weighted MR images unless secondarily infected.

Infectious and Inflammatory Disorder

Prostatitis

Prostatitis is uncommonly reported in the pediatric population, although some studies suggest this condition may be underreported in adolescent males.[113] When prostatitis occurs in younger children, it is typically in association with an underlying congenital anomaly, such as an enlarged prostatic utricle or seminal vesicle cyst.[5]

At ultrasound, findings of acute bacterial prostatitis can include glandular enlargement, a hypoechoic rim surrounding the prostate gland, and increased prostatic blood flow on Doppler imaging.[114] At MRI, the prostate may appear enlarged and heterogeneous; focal T2-weighted signal hyperintensity can be observed (Fig. 18.42).

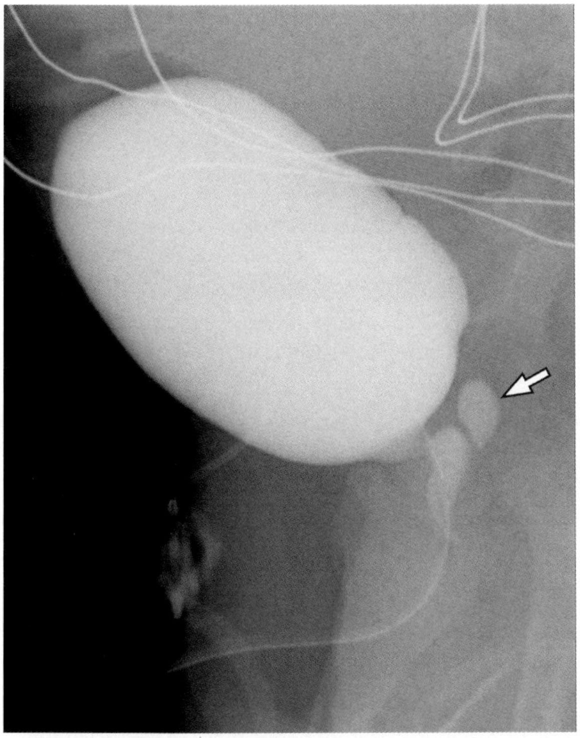

FIGURE 18.41 **A 2-month-old boy with prostatic utricle cyst.** Lateral voiding cystourethrogram image shows a contrast material–filled outpouching (diverticulum; *arrow*) arising from the posterior aspect of the prostatic urethra in the midline.

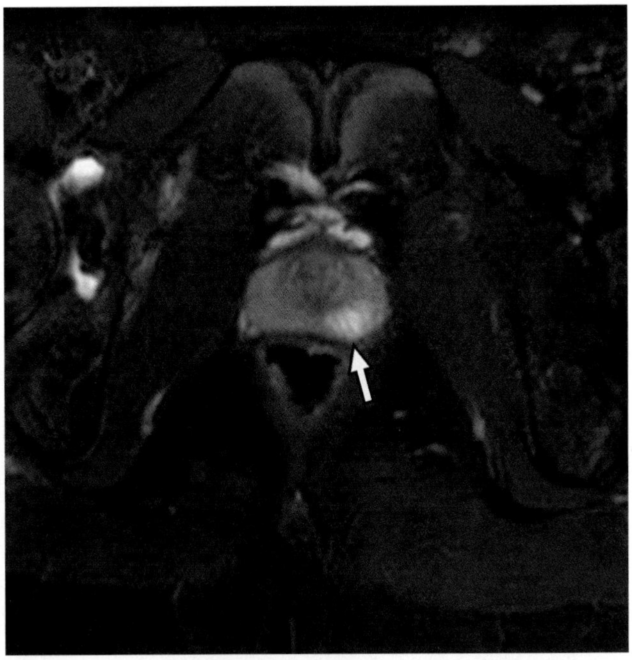

FIGURE 18.42 **A 17-year-old sexually active adolescent boy with pelvic pain and tender prostate gland on rectal examination.** Axial T2-weighted fat-saturated MR image through the prostate gland shows focal signal hyperintensity (*arrow*) in peripheral zone to the left of the midline, consistent with focal prostatitis. (Case courtesy of Jonathan R. Dillman, MD, MSc, Cincinnati Children's Hospital Medical Center, Cincinnati, OH.)

Neoplastic Disorders

Adenocarcinoma

Adenocarcinoma of the prostate gland, although common in older adults, is very rare in childhood with only a small number of pediatric cases reported in the literature.[115,116] Metastatic disease (e.g., to the skeleton and lymph nodes) can occur. There is overall limited data on prognosis of affected pediatric patients, although a single case report followed one patient to 4 years beyond initial resection.[116]

Rhabdomyosarcoma

The most common prostate gland neoplasm in children is rhabdomyosarcoma, usually the embryonal subtype.[117] Most children presenting with prostate gland rhabdomyosarcoma present with symptoms of bladder outlet obstruction; tumors commonly infiltrates the urinary bladder base.[118] Dysuria, urinary tract infection, and hematuria may also be presenting symptoms.[118]

At ultrasound, CT, and MRI, rhabdomyosarcoma of the prostate gland usually appears as a large, heterogeneous, bulky mass with internal vascularity and postcontrast enhancement (Fig. 18.43). Calcifications are uncommon.[118] The urinary bladder may be displaced superiorly and invaded by the tumor. Local recurrence is not uncommon, and MRI provides a useful means of surveillance. Particular care must be paid when imaging after radiation therapy to avoid mistaking posttreatment changes for local recurrence. Local radiologic staging evaluation is typically performed using MRI because of superior contrast resolution and soft tissue assessment.[117] CT imaging of the chest is typically performed to assess for lung metastases and bone scan may be used to search for additional distant metastases. ^{18}F-FDG PET/CT also can be used to perform whole body staging and follow-up.[117]

Numerous factors determine overall prognosis including age, clinical group, and stage.[117] Patients with metastatic disease at presentation have 5-year event-free survival rates of ~20%, whereas patients with nonmetastatic disease at presentation have an overall survival rate of 71%.[117] Surgical excision may be performed if resectability is determined by imaging. In nonresectable cases, chemotherapy and radiation therapy may be first performed in attempt to downstage the tumor to a resectable size.

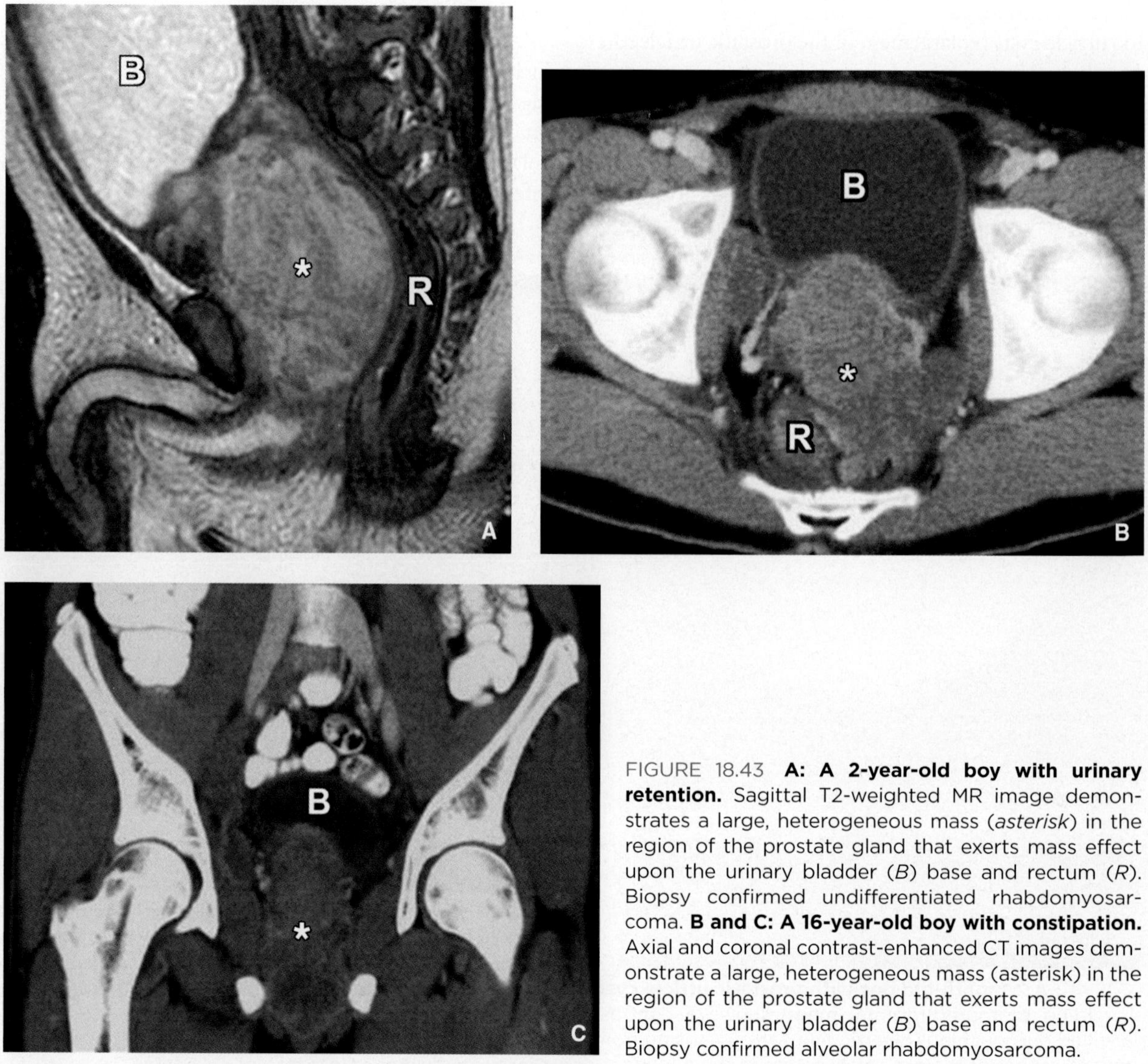

FIGURE 18.43 **A: A 2-year-old boy with urinary retention.** Sagittal T2-weighted MR image demonstrates a large, heterogeneous mass (*asterisk*) in the region of the prostate gland that exerts mass effect upon the urinary bladder (*B*) base and rectum (*R*). Biopsy confirmed undifferentiated rhabdomyosarcoma. **B and C: A 16-year-old boy with constipation.** Axial and coronal contrast-enhanced CT images demonstrate a large, heterogeneous mass (asterisk) in the region of the prostate gland that exerts mass effect upon the urinary bladder (*B*) base and rectum (*R*). Biopsy confirmed alveolar rhabdomyosarcoma.

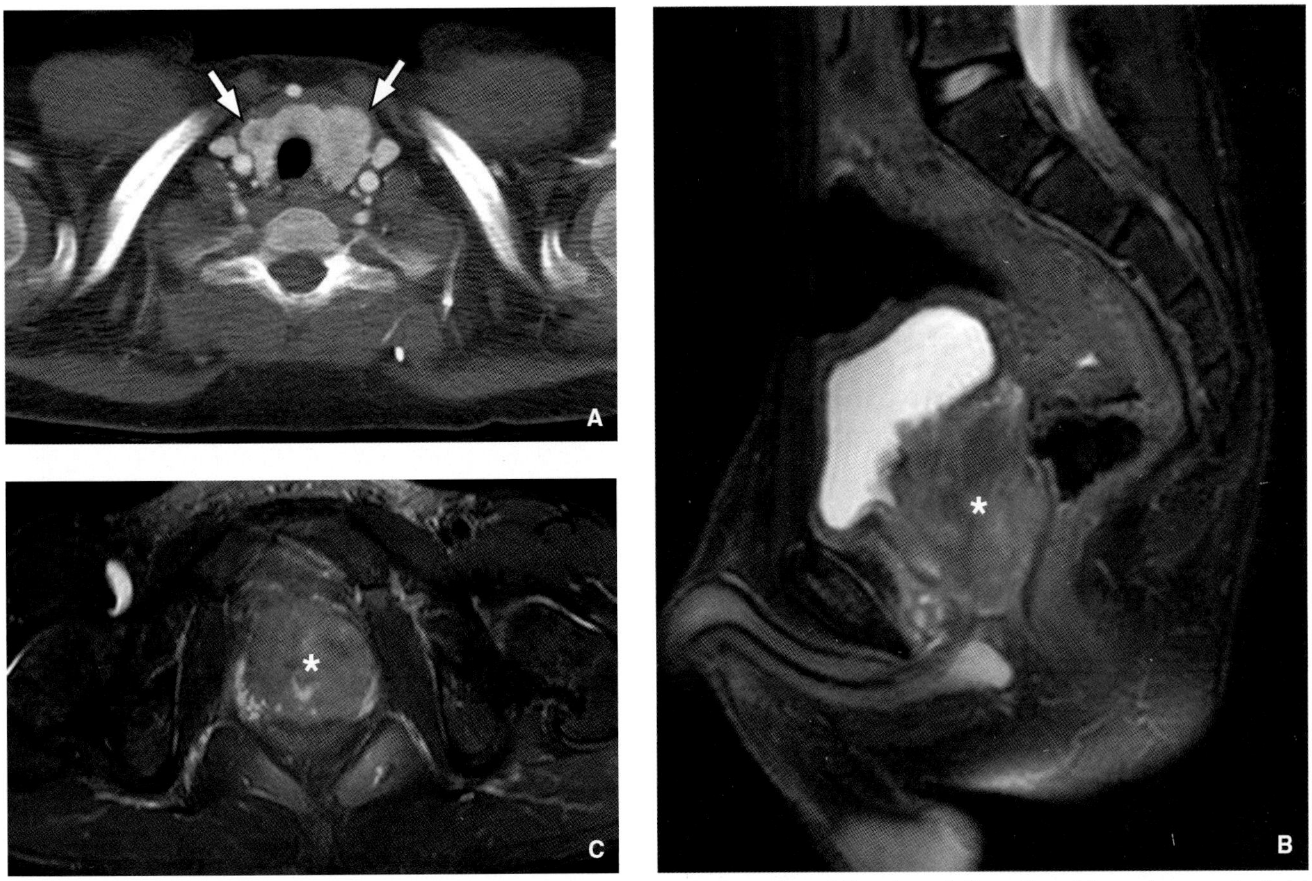

FIGURE 18.44 **A 14-year-old boy with multiple endocrine neoplasia and multifocal medullary thyroid carcinoma. A:** Axial contrast-enhanced CT image shows an enlarged, heterogeneous thyroid gland (*arrows*). **(B)** Sagittal and **(C)** axial T2-weighted fat-saturated MR images obtained 4 years later show marked enlargement of the prostate gland (*asterisk*) with mass effect upon the urinary bladder. Biopsy of the prostate gland confirmed metastatic medullary thyroid carcinoma. (Case courtesy of Jonathan R. Dillman, MD, MSc, Cincinnati Children's Hospital Medical Center, Cincinnati, OH.)

Metastasis

Metastasis to the pediatric prostate gland is very rare (Fig. 18.44). No pediatric tumor has a propensity to metastasize to the prostate gland. Typically, pediatric patients with prostatic metastases have widely disseminated disease and are symptomatic because of pain (from bladder outlet obstruction) or hematuria.[119]

References

1. Sakamoto H, Saito K, Oghta M, et al. Testicular volume measurement: comparison of ultrasonography, orchidometry, and water displacement. *Urology.* 2007;69(1):152–157.
2. Goede J, Hack W, Sijstermans K, et al. Normative values for testicular volume measured by ultrasonography in a normal population from infancy to adolescence. *Horm Res Paediatr.* 2011;76(1):56–64.
3. Kuijper E, VanKooten J, Verbeke J, et al. Ultrasonographically measured testicular volumes in 0- to 6-year-old boys. *Hum Reprod.* 2008;23(4):792–796.
4. Sadler T. *Langman's Medical Embryology*. 8th ed. Philadelphia, PA: Lippincott Williams & Wilkins; 2000:304–344.
5. Shebel H, Farg H, Kolokythas O, et al. Cysts of the lower male genitourinary tract: embryologic and anatomic considerations and differential diagnosis. *Radiographics.* 2013;33(4):1125–1143.
6. Yiee J, Baskin L. Penile embryology and anatomy. *Scientific World Journal.* 2010;10:1174–1179.
7. Barthold J, Gonzalez R. The epidemiology of congenital cryptorchidism, testicular ascent and orchiopexy. *J Urol.* 2003;170: 2396–2401.
8. Ritzen E, Bergh A, Bjerknes R, et al. Nordic consensus on treatment of undescended testes. *Acta Paediatr.* 2007;96:638–643.
9. Virtanen H, Bjerknes R, Cortes D, et al. Cryptorchidism: classification, prevalence and long-term consequences. *Acta Paediatr.* 2007;96:611–616.
10. Mathers M, Sperling H, Rubben H, et al. The undescended testis: diagnosis, treatment and long-term consequences. *Dtsch Arztebl Int.* 2009;106:527–532.
11. Lip S, Murchison L, Cullis P, et al. A meta-analysis of the risk of boys with isolated cryptorchidism developing testicular cancer in later life. *Arch Dis Child.* 2013;98(1):20–26.
12. Chavhan G, Parra D, Oudjhane K, et al. Imaging of ambiguous genitalia: classification and diagnostic approach. *Radiographics.* 2008;28(7):1891–1904.
13. Woodward P, Sohaey R, O'Donoghue M, et al. From the archives of the AFIP: tumors and tumorlike lesions of the testis: radiologic-pathologic correlation. *Radiographics.* 2002;22(1):189–216.
14. Stikkelbroeck N, Otten B, Pasic A, et al. High prevalence of testicular adrenal rest tumours, impaired spermatogenesis, and Leydig cell failure in adolescent and adult males with congenital adrenal hyperplasia. *J Clin Endocrinol Metabol.* 2001;86(12):5721–5728.

15. Nistal M, Paniagua R, Gonzalez-Peramato P, et al. Ectopic and heterotopic tissues in the testis. *Pediatr Dev Pathol.* 2015; 18(6):446–457.
16. Shawker T, Doppman J, Choyke P, et al. Intratesticular masses associated with abnormally functioning adrenal glands. *J Clin Ultrasound.* 1992;20:51–58.
17. Pomara G. Splenogonadal fusion: a rare extratesticular scrotal mass. *Radiographics.* 2004;24(2):417.
18. Guarin U, Dimitrieva Z, Ashley S. Splenogonadal fusion—a rare congenital anomaly demonstrated by 99Tc-sulfur colloid imaging: case report. *J Nucl Med.* 1975;16(10):922–924.
19. Alvarez D, Bhatt S, Dogra V. Sonographic spectrum of tunica albuginea cyst. *J Clin Imaging Sci.* 2011;1:5.
20. Favorito L, Cavalcante A, Costa W. Anatomic aspects of epididymis and tunica vaginalis in patients with testicular torsion. *Int Braz J Urol.* 2004;30(5):420–424.
21. Caesar R, Kaplan G. Incidence of the bell-clapper deformity in an autopsy series. *Urology.* 1994;44(1):114–116.
22. Huang W, Chen Y, Chang H, et al. The incidence rate and characteristics in patients with testicular torsion: a nationwide, population-based study. *Acta Paediatr.* 2013;102(8):363–367.
23. Sharp V, Kieran K, Arlen A. Testicular torsion: diagnosis, evaluation, and management. *Am Fam Physician.* 2013;88(12): 835–840.
24. Trojian T, Lishnak T, Heiman D. Epididymitis and orchitis: an overview. *Am Fam Physician.* 2009;79(7):583–587.
25. Yu K, Wang T, Chen H, et al. The dilemma in the diagnosis of acute scrotum: clinical clues for differentiating between testicular torsion and epididymo-orchitis. *Chang Gung Med J.* 2012;35(1):38–45.
26. Maroto A, Serres X, Torrent N, et al. Sonographic appearance of the torsion knot in spermatic cord torsion. *AJR Am J Roentgenol.* 1992;159(5):1029–1030.
27. Zerin J, DiPietro M, Grignon A, et al. Testicular infarction in the newborn: ultrasound findings. *Pediatr Radiol.* 1990;20(5):329–330.
28. Broderick K, Martin B, Herndon C, et al. The current state of surgical practice for neonatal torsion: a survey of pediatric urologists. *Pediatr Urol.* 2013;9(5):542–545.
29. Nandi B, Murphy F. Neonatal testicular torsion: a systematic literature review. *Pediatr Surg Int.* 2011;27(10):1037–1040.
30. Aso C, Enriquez G, Fite M, et al. Gray-scale and color Doppler sonography of scrotal disorders in children: an update. *Radiographics.* 2005;25(5):1197–1214.
31. Atkinson GJ, Patrick L, Ball TJ, et al. The normal and abnormal scrotum in children: evaluation with color Doppler sonography. *AJR Am J Roentgenol.* 1992;158(3):613–617.
32. Schalamon J, Ainoedhofer H, Schleef J, et al. Management of acute scrotum in children—the impact of Doppler ultrasound. *J Pediatr Surg.* 2006;41(8):1377–1380.
33. Stehr M, Boehm R. Critical validation of colour Doppler ultrasound in diagnostics of acute scrotum in children. *Eur J Pediatr Surg.* 2003;13(6):386–392.
34. Yagil Y, Naroditsky I, Milhem J, et al. Role of Doppler ultrasonography in the triage of acute scrotum in the emergency department. *J Ultrasound Med.* 2010;29(1):11–21.
35. Ternavasio-de la Vega H, Boronat M, Ojeda A, et al. Mumps orchitis in the post-vaccine era (1967–2009): a single-center series of 67 patients and review of clinical outcome and trends. *Medicine (Baltimore).* 2010;89(2):96–116.
36. Dogra V, Gottlieb R, Oka M, et al. Sonography of the scrotum. *Radiology.* 2003;227(1):18–36.
37. Albrecht T, Lotzof K, Hussain H, et al. Power Doppler US of the normal prepubertal testis: does it live up to its promises? *Radiology.* 1997;203(1):227–231.
38. Allen T, Elder J. Shortcomings of color Doppler sonography in the diagnosis of testicular torsion. *J Urol.* 1995;154(4): 1508–1510.
39. Stengel J, Remer E. Sonography of the scrotum: case-based review. *AJR Am J Roentgenol.* 2008;190(6 suppl):S35–S41.
40. Schul M, Keating M. The acute pediatric scrotum. *J Emerg Med.* 1994;12(4):591.
41. Barth R, Teele R, Colodny A, et al. Asymptomatic scrotal masses in children. *Radiology.* 1984;152(1):65–68.
42. Dogra V, Gottlieb R, Rubens D, et al. Benign intratesticular cystic lesions: US features. *Radiographics.* 2001;21(Spec No):S273–S281.
43. Gooding G, Leonhardt W, Marshall G, et al. Cholesterol crystals in hydroceles: sonographic detection and possible significance. *AJR Am J Roentgenol.* 1997;169(2):527–529.
44. Avolio L, Chiari G, Caputo M, et al. Abdominoscrotal hydrocele in childhood: is it really a rare entity? *Urology.* 2000;56(6):1047–1049.
45. Yarram S, Dipietro M, Graziano K, et al. Bilateral giant abdominoscrotal hydroceles complicated by appendicitis. *Pediatr Radiol.* 2005;35(12):1267–1270.
46. Cuervo J, Ibarra H, Molina M. Abdominoscrotal hydrocele: its particular characteristics. *J Pediatr Surg.* 2009;44(9): 1766–1770.
47. Rathaus V, Konen O, Shapiro M, et al. Ultrasound features of spermatic cord hydrocele in children. *Br J Radiol.* 2001; 74(885):818–820.
48. Martin L, Share J, Peters C, et al. Hydrocele of the spermatic cord: embryology and ultrasonographic appearance. *Pediatr Radiol.* 1996;26(8):528–530.
49. Kadish H, Bolte R. A retrospective review of pediatric patients with epididymitis, testicular torsion, and torsion of testicular appendages. *Pediatrics.* 1998;102(1):73–76.
50. Sellars M, Sidhu P. Ultrasound appearances of the testicular appendages: pictorial review. *Eur Radiol.* 2003;13(1):127–135.
51. Singh A, Kao S. Torsion of testicular appendage. *Pediatr Radiol.* 2010;40(3):373.
52. Laor T, Atala A, Teele R. Scrotal ultrasonography in Henoch-Schonlein purpura. *Pediatr Radiol.* 1992;22(7):505–506.
53. Sudakoff GS, Burke M, Rifkin MD. Ultrasonographic and color Doppler imaging of hemorrhagic epididymitis in Henoch-Schonlein purpura. *J Ultrasound Med.* 1992;11(11):619–621.
54. Ben-Sira L, Laor T. Severe scrotal pain in boys with Henoch-Schönlein purpura: incidence and sonography. *Pediatr Radiol.* 2000;30(2):125–128.
55. Pektas A, Devrim I, Besbas N, et al. A child with Behcet's disease presenting with a spectrum of inflammatory manifestations including epididymoorchitis. *Turk J Pediatr.* 2008;50(1):78–80.
56. Ahmed H, Arya M, Muneer A, et al. Testicular and paratesticular tumours in the prepubertal population. *Lancet Oncol.* 2010;11(5):476–483.
57. Agarwal P, Palmer J. Testicular and paratesticular neoplasms in prepubertal males. *J Urol.* 2006;176(3):875–881.
58. Brosman S. Testicular tumors in prepubertal children. *Urology.* 1979;13(6):581–588.
59. Baik K, Kang M, Park K, et al. Prepubertal testicular tumors in Korea: a single surgeon's experience of more than 20 years. *Korean J Urol.* 2013;54(6):399–403.

60. Dogra V, Gottlieb R, Oka M, et al. Testicular epidermoid cysts: sonographic features with histopathologic correlation. *J Clin Ultrasound.* 2001;29(3):192–196.
61. Smith E, Dillman J. Epidermoid cyst: a rare intratesticular tumor in children. *Pediatr Radiol.* 2010;40(8):1450.
62. Thomas JC, Ross JH, Kay R. Stromal testis tumors in children: a report from the prepubertal testis tumor registry. *J Urol.* 2001;166(6):2338–2340.
63. Ross J. Prepubertal testicular tumors. *Urology.* 2009;74:94–99.
64. Ross J, Rybicki L, Kay R. Clinical behavior and a contemporary management algorithm for prepubertal testis tumors: a summary of the Prepubertal Testis Tumor Registry. *J Urol.* 2002;168(4 pt 2):1675–1678; discussion 1678–1679.
65. Schneider D, Calaminus G, Koch S, et al. Epidemiologic analysis of 1,442 children and adolescents registered in the German germ cell tumor protocols. *Pediatr Blood Cancer.* 2004;42(2):169–175.
66. Pohl H, Shukla A, Metcalf P, et al. Prepubertal testis tumors: actual prevalence rate of histological types. *J Urol.* 2004;172(6 pt 1):2370–2372.
67. Wu H, Snyder HR. Pediatric urologic oncology: bladder, prostate, testis. *Urol Clin North Am.* 2004;31(3):619–627, xi.
68. Coley B. Sonography of pediatric scrotal swelling. *Semin Ultrasound CT MR.* 2007;28(4):297–306.
69. Brant WO, Rajimwale A, Lovell MA, et al. Gonadoblastoma and Turner syndrome. *J Urol.* 2006;175(5):1858–1860.
70. Phillips G, Kumari-Subaiya S, Sawitsky A. Ultrasonic evaluation of the scrotum in lymphoproliferative disease. *J Ultrasound Med.* 1987;6(4):169–175.
71. Mazzu D, Jeffrey RJ, Ralls P. Lymphoma and leukemia involving the testicles: findings on gray-scale and color Doppler sonography. *AJR Am J Roentgenol.* 1995;164(3):645–647.
72. Ishigami K, Yousef-Zahra D, Abu-Yousef M. Enlargement and hypervascularity of both the epididymis and testis do not exclude involvement with lymphoma or leukemia. *J Clin Ultrasound.* 2004;32(7):365–369.
73. Zwanger-Mendelsohn S, Shreck E, Doshi V. Burkitt lymphoma involving the epididymis and spermatic cord: sonographic and CT findings. *AJR Am J Roentgenol.* 1989;153(1):85–86.
74. Vitolo U, Chiappella A, Ferreri A, et al. First-line treatment for primary testicular diffuse large B-cell lymphoma with rituximab-CHOP, CNS prophylaxis, and contralateral testis irradiation: final results of an international phase II trial. *J Clin Oncol.* 2011;29(20):2766–2772.
75. Locatelli F, Schrappe M, Bernardo M, et al. How I treat relapsed childhood acute lymphoblastic leukemia. *Blood.* 2012;120(14):2807–2816.
76. Rodary C, Rey A, Olive D, et al. Prognostic factors in 281 children with nonmetastatic rhabdomyosarcoma (RMS) at diagnosis. *Med Pediatr Oncol.* 1988;16(2):71–77.
77. Dang N, Dang P, Samuelian J, et al. Lymph node management in patients with paratesticular rhabdomyosarcoma: a population-based analysis. *Cancer.* 2013;119(17):3228–3233.
78. Shimada H, Newton WAJ, Soule E, et al. Pathology of fatal rhabdomyosarcoma. Report from Intergroup Rhabdomyosarcoma Study (IRS-I and IRS-II). *Cancer.* 1987;59(3):459–465.
79. Federico SM, Spunt SL, Krasin MJ, et al. Comparison of PET-CT and conventional imaging in staging pediatric rhabdomyosarcoma. *Pediatr Blood Cancer.* 2013;60(7):1128–1134.
80. Fan R, Zhang J, Cheng L, et al. Testicular and paratesticular pathology in the pediatric population: a 20 year experience at Riley hospital for children. *Pathol Res Pract.* 2013;209(7):404–408.
81. LaQuaglia M, Ghavimi F, Heller G, et al. Mortality in pediatric paratesticular rhabdomyosarcoma: a multivariate analysis. *J Urol.* 1989;142(2 pt 2):473–478; discussion 489.
82. Raney RJ, Tefft M, Lawrence WJ, et al. Paratesticular sarcoma in childhood and adolescence. A report from the Intergroup Rhabdomyosarcoma Studies I and II, 1973–1983. *Cancer.* 1987;60(9):2337–2343.
83. Nistal M, Paniagua R, González-Peramato P, et al. Perspectives in Pediatric Pathology, Chapter 13. Calcifications in the testis and paratesticular structures. *Pediatr Dev Pathol.* 2016;19(3):173–182.
84. Drut R, Drut R. Testicular microlithiasis: histologic and immunohistochemical findings in 11 pediatric cases. *Pediatr Dev Pathol.* 2002;5(6):544–550.
85. Richenberg J, Brejt N. Testicular microlithiasis: is there a need for surveillance in the absence of other risk factors? *Eur Radiol.* 2012;22(11):2540–2546.
86. Deganello A, Svasti-Salee D, Allen PC, et al. Scrotal calcification in a symptomatic paediatric population: prevalence, location, and appearance in a cohort of 516 patients. *Clin Radiol.* 2012;67(9):862–867.
87. Meissner A, Mamoulakis C, de la Rosette J, et al. Clinical update on testicular microlithiasis. *Curr Opin Urol.* 2009;19(6):615–618.
88. Tan I, Ang K, Ching B, et al. Testicular microlithiasis predicts concurrent testicular germ cell tumors and intratubular germ cell neoplasia of unclassified type in adults: a meta-analysis and systematic review. *Cancer.* 2010;116(19):4520–4532.
89. Volokhina Y, Oyoyo U, Miller J. Ultrasound demonstration of testicular microlithiasis in pediatric patients: is there an association with testicular germ cell tumors? *Pediatr Radiol.* 2014;44(1):50–55.
90. Silveri M, Bassani F, Colajacomo M, et al. Management and follow-up of pediatric asymptomatic testicular microlithiasis: are we doing it well? *Urol J.* 2011;8(4):287–290.
91. Deurdulian C, Mittelstaedt C, Chong W, et al. US of acute scrotal trauma: optimal technique, imaging findings, and management. *Radiographics.* 2007;27(2):357–369.
92. Bhatt S, Dogra V. Role of US in testicular and scrotal trauma. *Radiographics.* 2008;28(6):1617–1629.
93. Bhosale P, Patnana M, Viswanathan C, et al. The inguinal canal: anatomy and imaging features of common and uncommon masses. *Radiographics.* 2008;28(3):819–835; quiz 913.
94. Nistal M, Paniagua R, González-Peramato P, et al. Adolescent varicocele. *Pediatr Dev Pathol.* 2014 Aug 8. [Epub ahead of print] PubMed PMID:25105427.
95. Kessler A, Meirsdorf S, Graif M, et al. Intratesticular varicocele: gray scale and color Doppler sonographic appearance. *J Ultrasound.* 2005;24(12):1711–1716.
96. Wampler S, Llanes M. Common scrotal and testicular problems. *Prim Care.* 2010;37(3):613–626.
97. Diamond D, Gargollo P, Caldamone A. Current management principles for adolescent varicocele. *Fertil Steril.* 2011;96(6):1294–1298.
98. Woodward P, Schwab C, Sesterhenn I. From the archives of the AFIP: extratesticular scrotal masses: radiologic-pathologic correlation. *Radiographics.* 2003;23(1):215–240.
99. Erikci V, Hoşgör M, Aksoy N, et al. Management of epididymal cysts in childhood. *J Pediatr Surg.* 2013;48(10):2153–2156.
100. Luzzi G, O'Brien T. Acute epididymitis. *BJU Int.* 2001;87(8):747–755.

101. Muttarak M, Na Chiangmai W, Kitirattrakarn P. Necrotising epididymo-orchitis with scrotal abscess. *Biomed Imaging Interv J.* 2005;1(2):11.
102. Karmazyn B, Kaefer M, Kauffman S, et al. Ultrasonography and clinical findings in children with epididymitis, with and without associated lower urinary tract abnormalities. *Pediatr Radiol.* 2009;39(10):1054–1058.
103. Akbar S, Sayyed T, Jafri S, et al. Multimodality imaging of paratesticular neoplasms and their rare mimics. *Radiographics.* 2003;23(6):1461–1476.
104. Liu W, Wu R, Yu Q. Adenomatoid tumor of the testis in a child. *J Pediatr Surg.* 2011;46(10):15.
105. Nino-Murcia M, Freidland G, deVries P. *Clinical Urology.* Vol. 1. 2nd ed. Philadelphia, PA: Saunders; 2002.
106. Arora S, Breiman R, Webb E, et al. CT and MRI of congenital anomalies of the seminal vesicles. *AJR Am J Roentgenol.* 2007;189(1):130–135.
107. Kim B, Kawashima A, Ryu J, et al. Imaging of the seminal vesicle and vas deferens. *Radiographics.* 2009;29(4):1105–1121.
108. Moerman P, Fryns J, Goddeeris P, et al. Pathogenesis of the prune-belly syndrome: a functional urethral obstruction caused by prostatic hypoplasia. *Pediatrics.* 1984;74(4):470–475.
109. Ives E. The abdominal muscle deficiency triad syndrome—experience with ten cases. *Birth Defects Orig Artic Ser.* 1974; 10(4):127–135.
110. Parsons R, Fisher A, Bar-Chama N, et al. MR imaging in male infertility. *Radiographics.* 1997;1759:627–637.
111. Trigaux J, Van Beers B, Delchambre F. Male genital tract malformations associated with ipsilateral renal agenesis: sonographic findings. *J Clin Ultrasound.* 1991;19(1):3–10.
112. Song N, Wu H, Xu N, et al. The composition and structure of stones in enlarged prostatic utricles (EPU). *J Androl.* 2012;33(1):45–49.
113. Tripp D, Nickel J, Ross S, et al. Prevalence, symptom impact and predictors of chronic prostatitis-like symptoms in Canadian males aged 16–19 years. *BJU Int.* 2009;103(8):1080–1084.
114. Futterer J, Heijmink S, Spermon J. Imaging the male reproductive tract: current trends and future directions. *Radiol Clin North Am.* 2008;46:133–147.
115. Shimada H, Misugi K, Sasaki Y, et al. Carcinoma of the prostate in childhood and adolescence: report of a case and review of the literature. *Cancer.* 1980;46(11):2534–2542.
116. Chow C, Liu H, Lee K, et al. Carcinoma of the prostate in an 11-year-old child with long survival. *Br J Urol.* 1986; 58(1):100–101.
117. McCarville M, Spunt S, Pappo A. Rhabdomyosarcoma in pediatric patients: the good, the bad, and the unusual. *AJR Am J Roentgenol.* 2001;176(6):1563–1569.
118. Agrons G, Wagner B, Lonergan G, et al. From the archives of the AFIP. Genitourinary rhabdomyosarcoma in children: radiologic-pathologic correlation. *Radiographics.* 1997;17(4): 919–937.
119. Bates A, Baithun S. Secondary solid neoplasms of the prostate: a clinico-pathological series of 51 cases. *Virchows Arch.* 2002; 440(4):392–396.
120. Paltiel HJ, Phelps A. US of the pediatric female pelvis. *Radiology.* 2014;270(3):644–657.
121. Basta AM, Courtier J, Phelps A, et al. Is it a tumor? Scrotal swelling in the neonate. *RSNA/Radiology.* 2015;34(3): 495–505.

CHAPTER 19

Female Genital Tract

Sharon W. Gould • Sabah Servaes • Edward Y. Lee • José Ernesto Lipsich • Mohamed Issa Tawil • Sara O. Vargas • Monica Epelman

INTRODUCTION

Evaluation of the female genital tract in the pediatric population presents a unique set of diagnostic challenges due to the developmental changes that occur during childhood and adolescence as well as to the cyclic changes that occur with the onset of menses. This chapter reviews up-to-date imaging techniques for evaluating the female genital tract in the pediatric population. In addition, the normal appearance of the pediatric female reproductive organs as well as the imaging findings of important congenital and acquired pediatric female genital tract disorders are discussed.

IMAGING TECHNIQUES

Radiography

Although ultrasound is usually the initial imaging modality of choice for evaluating the pediatric female genital tract, radiography may be performed first in the setting of acute pelvic or right lower quadrant abdominal pain.[1] A supine anteroposterior (AP) radiograph from the diaphragm to the upper femurs is most often acquired for evaluating abdominopelvic pain, and it may be complemented with an upright or decubitus view. Radiography may show mass effect on gas-filled bowel loops from pelvic masses and mass-like abnormalities, calcification, or even a tooth in the setting of an ovarian teratoma. Such findings can help generate a differential diagnosis and guide subsequent imaging studies for further evaluation.

Ultrasound

The primary imaging modality for assessment of the pediatric female genital tract is ultrasound due to its multiplanar imaging capability, high soft tissue contrast resolution, and lack of ionizing radiation.[1,2] In addition, sedation is typically not required for ultrasound imaging, even in very young children. The ultrasound examination of the female genital tract is usually performed through a fluid-filled bladder using transabdominal technique.[1,3,4] To achieve optimal bladder filling, cooperative children can be asked to drink water prior to imaging while refraining from voiding. If the child is uncooperative or the need for evaluation is urgent, the bladder can be catheterized and filled retrograde with sterile saline. Although transvaginal ultrasound technique excellently depicts the female genital tract, it is generally not appropriate in younger children or adolescents who are not yet sexually active.[1] Transperineal scanning can assess disorders of the vagina, urethra, and vulva.

A complete ultrasound examination of the pediatric female genital tract includes assessment of the upper portion of the vagina and uterus (including cervix). The width of the endometrial stripe, including both layers, should be recorded; a slightly deeper hypoechoic myometrial layer, rarely seen in pediatric patients, should not be included in the measurement[1,3] (Fig. 19.1). Assessment of the adnexae includes measurements of the ovaries in three planes. Ovarian volumes can be calculated and compared to normative values. Note should be made of the presence, appearance, and amount of fluid in the cul-de-sac (between the uterus and rectum), as well as within each lower quadrant of the abdomen. In the setting of acute pelvic pain and possible ovarian torsion, color and spectral Doppler evaluation of the ovaries should be performed with documentation of arterial and venous spectral waveforms.

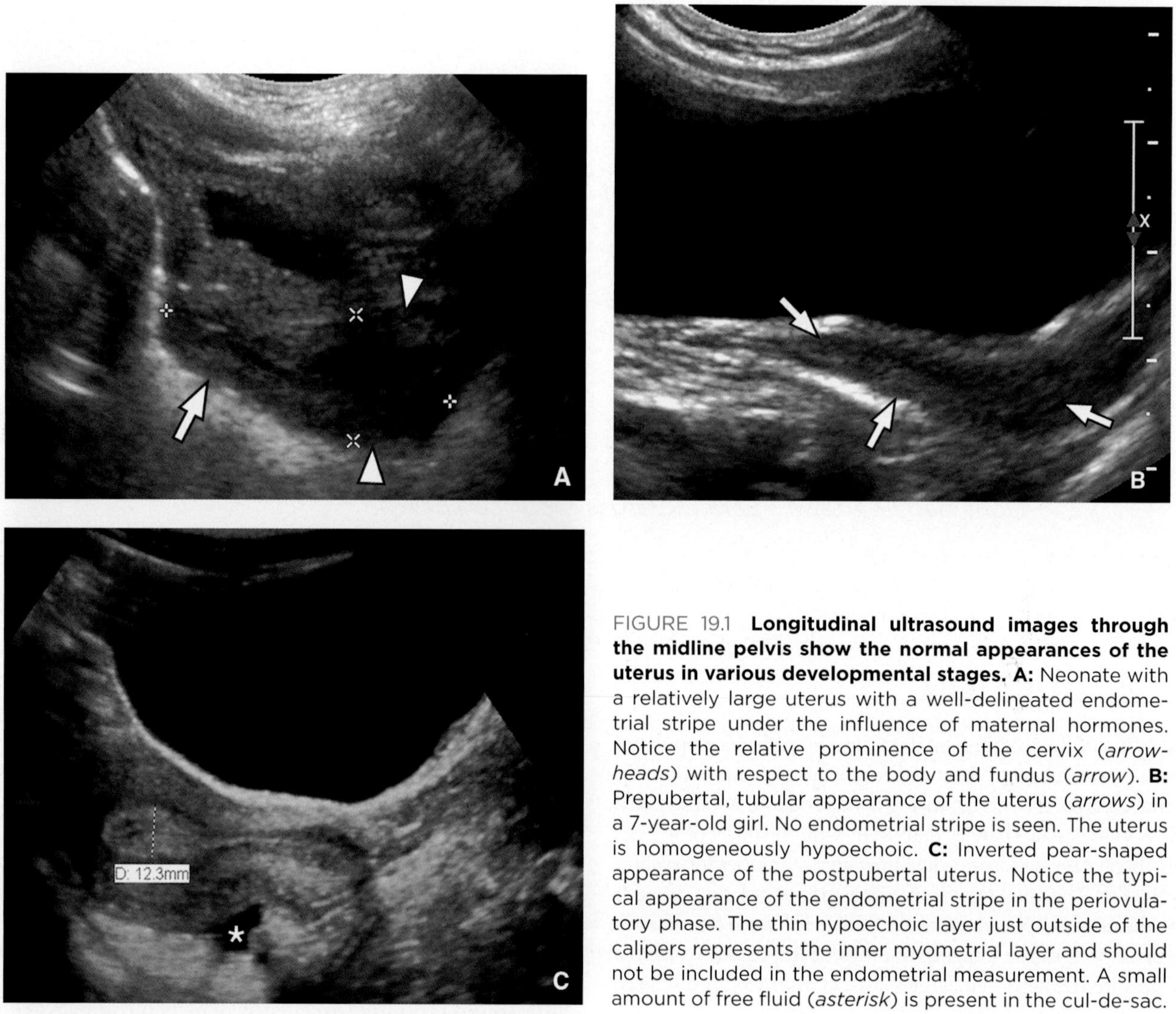

FIGURE 19.1 **Longitudinal ultrasound images through the midline pelvis show the normal appearances of the uterus in various developmental stages. A:** Neonate with a relatively large uterus with a well-delineated endometrial stripe under the influence of maternal hormones. Notice the relative prominence of the cervix (*arrowheads*) with respect to the body and fundus (*arrow*). **B:** Prepubertal, tubular appearance of the uterus (*arrows*) in a 7-year-old girl. No endometrial stripe is seen. The uterus is homogeneously hypoechoic. **C:** Inverted pear-shaped appearance of the postpubertal uterus. Notice the typical appearance of the endometrial stripe in the periovulatory phase. The thin hypoechoic layer just outside of the calipers represents the inner myometrial layer and should not be included in the endometrial measurement. A small amount of free fluid (*asterisk*) is present in the cul-de-sac.

Computed Tomography

Computed tomography (CT) generally provides less soft tissue differentiation than ultrasound or magnetic resonance imaging (MRI) and, therefore, is generally less helpful for evaluating the pediatric female genital tract. Radiation exposure associated with CT is also a limitation in children. In addition, CT lacks the "real-time" capability of ultrasound. However, depending on a child's clinical presentation and institutional protocol, CT may be the first imaging study acquired, especially in the setting of acute right lower quadrant abdominal pain. CT is also used to further characterize and stage masses arising from the pelvis, particularly when malignancy is suspected. In the CT evaluation of pelvic structures, intravenous and oral contrast materials help with lesion characterization as well as distinguishing true pelvic abnormalities from adjacent bowel loops. Single-phase CT imaging is usually sufficient for evaluation of female genital tract anomalies and abnormalities.

Magnetic Resonance Imaging

MRI is an excellent imaging modality for assessing the pediatric female genitourinary tract, particularly for delineation of congenital anomalies[5] and characterization of pelvic masses.[6,7] MRI's inherent multiplanar imaging capability and high soft tissue contrast resolution are especially helpful for evaluating the pelvic organs; however, the need for sedation or general anesthesia in younger pediatric patients because of long imaging times limits MRI to a secondary role after pelvic ultrasound.[1] Imaging of the pediatric female pelvis should be performed in three planes or with an isotropic 3D imaging protocol that allows diagnostic multiplanar reformatted images. An advantage of 3D imaging is that reformatted images can be created in any oblique plane based on the patient's anatomy without additional imaging time.

MRI is the modality of choice for detailed assessment of uterine anatomy because images can be acquired in both the uterine long- and shortaxes.[5] Hence, MRI is ideal for characterizing suspected Mullerian anomalies, although it may need to be performed in the postpubertal period for optimal diagnosis when the uterus is more developed. T2-weighted pulse sequences are most helpful for evaluating uterine zonal anatomy. In the evaluation of adnexal lesions, fat-saturated MR imaging is critical for differentiating fat from hemorrhage/proteinaceous fluid. Postcontrast and diffusion-weighted MR imaging help characterize pelvic masses and inflammatory conditions. When a Mullerian anomaly is known or suspected, limited imaging should be performed through the renal fossae to evaluate for renal agenesis and other anomalies. MR is also an excellent modality for evaluation of vulvar lesions when assessment of deeper structures is required.

Genitography

Genitography (genitogram or cloacagram) is a useful technique for the evaluation of suspected cloacal or urogenital sinus malformations as well as ambiguous genitalia.[8,9] Review of prenatal ultrasound and MRI examinations can help direct the radiologist and limit fluoroscopic exposure.[5] Imaging is initially performed in the lateral projection with the hips flexed. Each perineal opening should be evaluated with water-soluble contrast material and/or air instillation under fluoroscopic observation. It is important to prevent distortion of the relationships of the cavities and their communications; therefore, insertion of a small catheter just inside the orifice of the cavity being examined is suggested.[9] The vagina should be assessed for length and the presence of a cervical impression. Any abnormal communications between pelvic viscera should be documented, and the lengths of associated fistulas should be measured. In cases of ambiguous genitalia, the anatomy of the urethra should be also carefully assessed. CT and MRI genitography techniques have been described and may play increasing roles in the future.[10,11]

NORMAL ANATOMY

Ovary

The ovaries are ellipsoid organs that lie in the ovarian fossae in most children, situated medial and inferior to the external iliac vessels, just caudad to the bifurcation of the common iliac vessels. Located posterior and lateral to the uterine fundus, the ovaries are covered by an epithelial layer under which lies the tunica albuginea, a layer of compressed stroma.[12] The remainder of the ovary consists of follicles with intervening spindle-shaped stromal cells and an abundant vascular supply. In prepubertal girls, the peripheral cortical layer consists of numerous immature follicles measuring ~0.25 mm. In postpubertal girls and adults, the peripheral ovarian cortex contains larger, more mature follicles, corpora lutea, and corpora albicans. In the corpus luteum, the granulosa and theca cells that line the follicle enlarge during the maturational stage and shrink during the regressive stage. The next stage, the corpus albicans, is the replacement of the corpus luteum by fibrous scar tissue, which eventually involutes. The central ovarian medulla contains no follicles in the mature ovary.

Mean ovarian volume is roughly 1 mL at birth[2,13] with an upper limit of 3.6 mL that decreases to 1.7 mL between the first and second years.[1,14] The mean ovarian volume is generally <1 mL until 7 years of age, at which point the ovaries at least double in size by the age of 12 years.[1,2] An ovarian growth spurt may be noted after ~8 years of age related to the onset of puberty.[1]

At ultrasound, ovaries in young girls are mostly homogeneous in echotexture with small subcentimeter cysts sometimes observed, particularly when examined with high-frequency linear ultrasound transducers. These may not necessarily represent true follicles as many times no associated ova are found.[1] In neonates, the size and number of visible follicles is variable and related to maternal hormonal effects; follicles decrease in size as this stimulation subsides. A mature ovarian appearance may be seen after ~7 years of age. As there is considerable overlap in the appearance of the ovaries in normal girls and those with precocious puberty, ovarian appearance is an unreliable indicator of hormonal activity.[13,14] Ovarian development is described in Table 19.1.

Mullerian Derivatives

The Mullerian (or paramesonephric) ducts are the precursors of the female genital tract from which the fallopian tubes,

TABLE 19.1 Normal Uterine and Ovarian Appearances During Childhood

	Neonate	Prepubertal Child	Adolescent
Uterus	Fundus is elongated (longer than cervix) due to maternal hormones. Endometrial stripe may be visible.	Fundus is shorter than cervix. Endometrial stripe measures a few mm and is often not visible. Fundus is no thicker than the cervix.	Fundus and body measure about twice the length of the cervix, and the uterus develops an inverted pear shape. The endometrial stripe can measure from a few mm to 1.6 cm, and zonal anatomy becomes visible.
Ovary	Approximately 1 mL volume average (maximum 3.6 mL) with multiple anechoic follicles. Ovaries decrease in size as maternal hormonal effects subside.	Average volume 1.7 mL between 1 and 2 years of age decreasing to <1 mL up to age 7 years. May enlarge around 8 years due to onset of puberty. Homogeneous appearance. May have subcentimeter cysts. Number and size of ovarian cysts do not correlate well with hormonal activity.	Normal volume 2–10 mL during and after puberty. Multiple follicles of varying size that can measure up to 2.5 cm.

uterus, cervix, and the upper two-thirds of the vagina develop. The lower one-third of the vagina develops from the urogenital sinus, and, therefore, vaginal anomalies and anomalies of the external genitalia are not always associated with Mullerian duct anomalies.[5] Uterine development can be broken down into three stages. The first is organogenesis at 5 to 6 weeks,[15] failure of which results in aplasia/hypoplasia, or if unilateral, a unicornuate uterus. Fusion of the two Mullerian ducts is the second stage occurring at 7 to 9 weeks and when incomplete results in a uterus didelphys or bicornuate uterus. The third stage is septal resorption, and septate and arcuate uteri are the result of at least partial septal persistence.

The lower one-third of the vagina forms from paired outpouchings of the urogenital sinus, the sinovaginal bulbs, after the urorectal septum has grown down to meet the cloacal membrane separating the rectum from the urogenital sinus.[16] The sinovaginal bulbs fuse to form a solid mass that later recanalizes to form the lower vagina. Failure of recanalization results in a transverse septum. The hymen is a vestigial remnant from vaginal canalization forming a distinct membrane in the lower vagina just inside the vestibule.

Fallopian Tube

The fallopian tubes (or oviducts) extend from the lateral margins of the uterine fundus toward the pelvic sidewalls along the superior margins of the broad ligaments. The interstitial portion of the fallopian tube (most medial or distal portion) is encased within the myometrium at the corner of the uterus. The isthmus is the long, narrow portion of the fallopian tube that courses through the broad ligament superior to the mesovarium. The funnel-shaped lateral segment of the tube is the ampulla that curves around the lateral aspect of the ovary and then turns medially. The infundibulum (most proximal portion) with its ostium and fimbriae extends around the posteromedial aspect of the ovary (Fig. 19.2).

Uterus

The uterus is situated in the central pelvis between the rectum and bladder (Fig. 19.2). Although the fundus forms the convex superior portion into which the isthmic portions of the fallopian tubes enter, the body forms the narrower portion between the fundus and cervix. The cervix is the conical, compact lower section of the uterus, the lower 1/3 of which projects into the upper vagina. When the bladder is relatively empty, the uterus is often flexed forward and lies superior to the bladder dome. When the bladder is full, the uterus is displaced into a more coronal plane. Displacement of the uterus slightly to one side of midline is common. Normal variations include anterior and posterior flexion between the uterine cervix and body.

The uterus changes substantially during childhood (Table 19.1; Fig. 19.1). During the neonatal period, the uterine fundus may be elongated because of maternal hormonal influence,[13] although by a few months of age the upper uterus shrinks to about half the length of the cervix.[8] Before puberty, the uterine body and fundus together remain no longer than the cervix,[1] and the endometrium is thin, measuring only a few millimeters. As puberty approaches, the uterus enlarges in size, particularly the body and fundus, and ultimately attains the expected adult configuration.[1,17] In postpubertal girls, the uterus has an inverted pear shape and is densely muscular with a slit-like cavity.[13]

After menarche, there are three phases of the menstrual cycle: the menstrual, proliferative, and luteal (secretory) phases. Ovulation occurs between the proliferative and luteal phases. At the end of the menstrual phase, the endometrium is thin due to recent sloughing.[17] Mediated by estrogen, the endometrium progressively thickens during the proliferative phase to nearly 1 cm in bilayer thickness (uterine midsagittal plane) and appears relatively hypoechoic.[1,17] Under the influence of progesterone during the luteal phase, the endometrium further thickens up to about 1.6 cm and becomes more echogenic.[1,17] As mentioned before, the inner hypoechoic myometrial layer sometimes seen surrounding the endometrium should not be included in the measurement.[1]

Vagina

The vagina extends posterosuperiorly from the vulvar vestibule to the uterus. Situated between the base of the bladder and urethra anteriorly and the rectum posteriorly, the vagina is bounded on either side by the levator ani muscles. Normally, the walls of the vagina are apposed unless fluid is present. Bartholin glands are situated in the lower vagina along either side posteriorly. The vaginal fornices encircle the vaginal portion of the cervix. The hymen is not usually visible radiologically.

Vulva

The vulva extends from the symphysis pubis to the perineum just anterior to the anus. The mons pubis is comprised of fatty tissue overlying the pubic symphysis. The mons extends posteriorly into the labia majora, which are the thicker pads of tissue extending from the mons to the perineum covering the vulvar opening when apposed. The labia minora are the thinner rims of tissue along either side of the vaginal introitus that meet anteriorly at the clitoris.

SPECTRUM OF OVARIAN DISORDERS

Disorders of Sexual Development

The overall incidence of disorders of sexual development (DSDs) is ~1% to 2%.[8] This group of diseases encompasses numerous chromosomal, gonadal, and anatomical abnormalities. DSD can be classified into three groups based on genotype: 46XX, 46XY, and abnormal sex chromosomes, such as 45XO, 47XYY, and mosaic/chimeric genomes.[18,19]

The diagnosis of a DSD may be made prenatally, at birth, or later in childhood. If abnormal external genitalia are suspected on prenatal ultrasound, fetal karyotyping can be performed. Fetal MRI can be a useful adjunct for assessment of the external genitalia and anus as well as additional

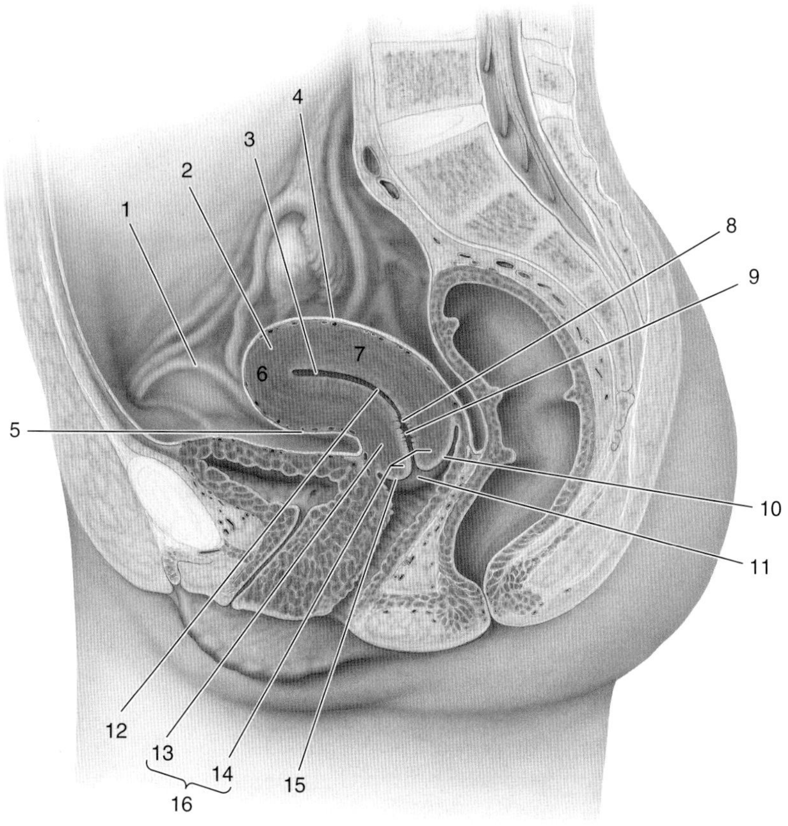

A

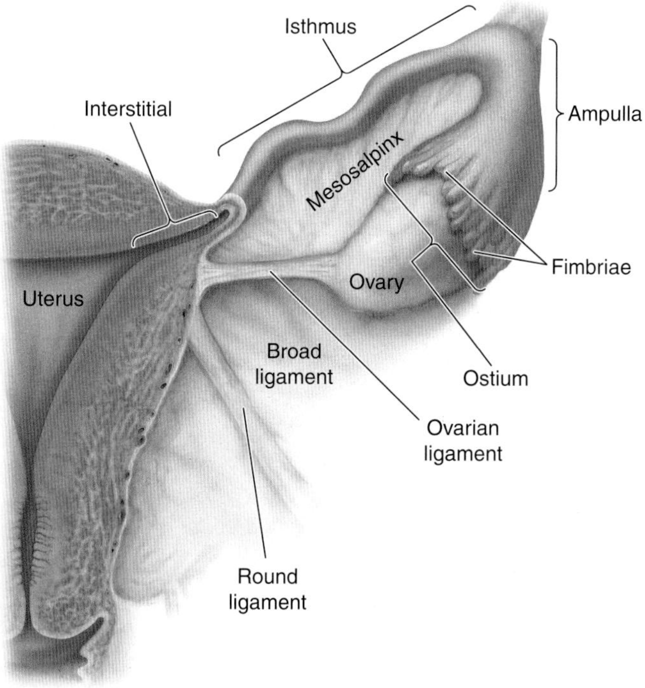

B

FIGURE 19.2 **A:** Schematic drawing of female genital tract anatomy. *1.* Round ligament. *2.* Uterus. *3.* Uterine cavity. *4.* Peritoneal surface of uterus. *5.* Vesical surface of uterus (toward bladder). *6.* Fundus of uterus. *7.* Body of uterus. *8.* Palmate folds of cervical canal. *9.* Cervical canal. *10.* Posterior lip of cervix. *11.* Cervical os (external). *12.* Isthmus of uterus. *13.* Supravaginal portion of cervix. *14.* Vaginal portion of cervix. *15.* Anterior lip of cervix. *16.* Cervix. **B:** Schematic representation of fallopian tube anatomy. The interstitial, isthmic, ampullary, and ostial portions are shown.

anomalies, particularly in the setting of oligohydramnios. At birth, abnormalities of the perineal orifices, urethra, clitoris/penis, scrotum/labia, and palpable gonads at physical examination are indications for imaging investigation of the genitourinary tract.[9] Ambiguous genitalia are found in 4% to 7% of DSD patients in infancy.[8] Congenital adrenal hyperplasia is the most common DSD in 46XX girls and usually presents with ambiguous genitalia and internal female reproductive organs.[8,9,14] The most common defect in congenital adrenal hyperplasia is 21-α-hydroxylase deficiency, and many of these patients have a salt-wasting disorder that may present emergently with an adrenal crisis in the first 2 weeks of life.[20] Older patients with DSD may present with delayed puberty, pelvic pain, inguinal hernia, previously unrecognized genital ambiguity, primary amenorrhea, contrasexual secondary sex characteristics, or menstruation in phenotypic males presenting as recurrent hematuria.[21]

At all ages, imaging evaluation of DSD should be tailored to the abnormalities suspected. Ultrasound is commonly the first-line examination and should assess the kidneys, adrenal glands in the neonate, pelvic organs (is there a uterus?), bladder, and perineum, making note of the location, size, number, and appearance of gonads.[8,9] Genitography can be performed to assess abnormal perineal orifices as well as measure the length of the urethra to determine extent of virilization. MRI is useful for assessment of intra-abdominal gonads and characterization of Mullerian anomalies. In cases of malignancy arising from abnormal gonads (e.g., streak gonads or ovotestes), CT and MRI are useful for staging and surveillance.

The approach to the diagnosis and treatment of DSD is multidisciplinary. Management of these cases includes assigning a sex of rearing as well as surgery to improve genitourinary function, reproductive and sexual health, and cosmesis.[22] One goal in treating children with DSD is to minimize gender dysphoria (the feeling of wanting to live as the opposite sex to one's rearing), and management decisions should take into consideration parental input and cultural background.[8,22]

Congenital and Developmental Anomalies

The undifferentiated gonads arise in utero prior to 7 weeks' gestation from the interaction of primordial germ cells, sex cords (formed from mesenchymal tissue), and epithelium.[9] The Wolffian (mesonephric) structures and Mullerian structures are located lateral to the developing gonads. In girls, the gonads differentiate into ovaries between 7 and 8 weeks' gestation by the complex interaction of several genes, including Wnt4,[23,24] Foxl2,[23] CYP19,[24] RSPO1,[24] Pod1,[23] Dax1,[23,25] and Fst,[23] and under the influence of multiple hormones, including B-catenin[24] and cytochrome P-450 aromatase.[25] Once ovarian differentiation begins, the primordial germ cells develop to form ~2 million primordial follicles by the time of birth, eventually decreasing to around 400,000 by menarche. The sex cord cells become granulosa cells that surround the follicles in the outer, cortical portion of the ovary, whereas the central or medullary portion of the ovary is primarily connective and vascular tissues.

Upon differentiation, the ovary is vertically oriented in the retroperitoneum near the level of the developing kidney. Ovarian descent is partially due to displacement by developing abdominal organs, but is also partly due to fusion of the Mullerian ducts, altering the orientation of the fallopian tubes, broad ligament, and mesovaria. The ovary ultimately attains a horizontal position in the lateral pelvis below the common iliac vessel bifurcation anterior to the ureter.[26]

Ectopic, Supernumerary, and Accessory Ovary

The ovaries have been shown to have a higher incidence of maldescent in association with several Mullerian duct anomalies, specifically didelphys, unicornuate, and bicornuate uteri.[27] Maldescent is defined as the ovarian upper pole at or above the iliac vessel bifurcation (Figs. 19.3 and 19.4). Ectopia of the ovary within the inguinal canal has been reported in a case of Mayer-Rokitansky-Kuster-Hauser syndrome.[28] Supernumerary ovaries are additional loci of ovarian tissue located above the pelvis, distinct from and unconnected to the orthotopic ovaries,[29] and they may be found in the omentum, retroperitoneum, or kidney. Supernumerary ovaries may be the result of disruption of the gonadal ridge tissue or abnormal gonadocyte migration prior to gonadal differentiation. Accessory ovaries are found within adnexal structures connected to the orthotopic ovary by shared blood supply and may be the result of splitting of the developing ovarian primordium.[29] Although rare, ectopic, supernumerary, and accessory ovaries are as equally prone to ovarian pathology as orthotopic ovaries.[29,30] Supernumerary and accessory ovaries can be associated with other genitourinary tract anomalies.

Ovarian Dysgenesis

Ovarian dysgenesis encompasses disorders that result in an abnormal ovarian morphology and function, typically in the setting of DSD. 46XX testicular and ovotesticular dysgenesis are related to genetic mutations that alter gonadal cord development to include purely testicular or mixed ovarian and

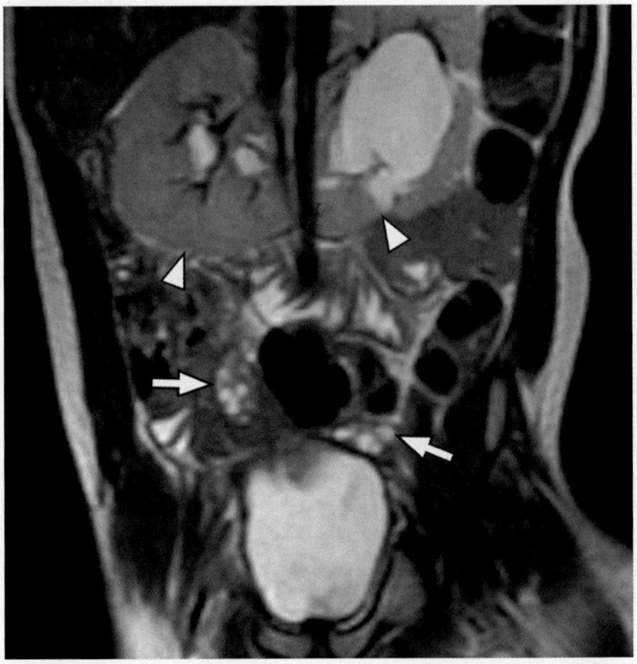

FIGURE 19.3 **A 5-year-old girl with horseshoe kidney (*arrowheads*).** Coronal T2-weighted MR image shows that the ovaries (*arrows*) are abnormally high in position and located close to the midline. Left-sided pelvicaliectasis is due to ureteropelvic junction obstruction. This patient is at increased risk for a Mullerian duct anomaly given the presence of renal and urinary tract anomalies as well as maldescended ovaries.

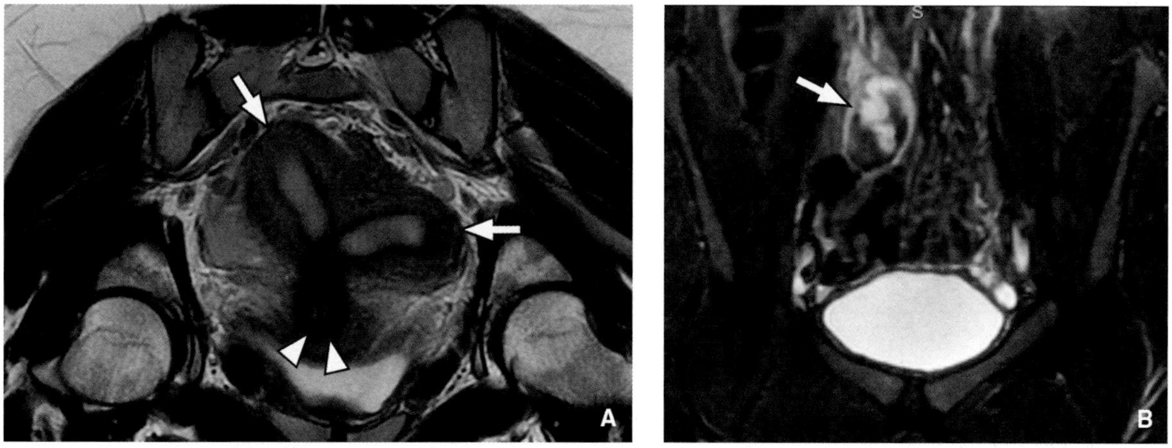

FIGURE 19.4 **Bicornuate bicollis uterus in a 13-year-old girl with a previously repaired cloaca malformation. A:** Coronal-oblique T2-weighted MR image shows two distinct, divergent uterine horns (*arrows*) and two distinct cervices (*arrowheads*). **B:** Coronal T2-weighted fat-saturated MR image demonstrates a malpositioned ovary with a complicated, likely hemorrhagic cyst (*arrow*) located well above the right iliac bifurcation.

testicular tissue in genotypic females.[19] 46XY gonadal dysgenesis may also result in different degrees of ovotesticular dysgenesis with ambiguous internal and external organs. Turner syndrome (45XO) is characterized by streak ovaries due to loss of germ cells after 22 weeks' gestation, despite initially normal ovarian development. Streak ovaries containing no germ cell components can also be found in 46XX ovarian dysgenesis.[31] 45X/46XY mosaicism and 46XX/46XY chimerism result in ovotesticular dysgenesis because of mixed genetic signals during gonadal development.[19]

Dysgenetic and streak gonads (Fig. 19.5) are often not seen at imaging because of their small size and uncharacteristic appearance, having ill-defined margins and lacking the characteristic ellipsoid shape. Ovotesticular or testicular dysgenesis can have normally sized gonads that may be normal or ectopic in position and may be associated with abnormal Mullerian duct development and ambiguous genitalia.[9,19] It is important to note that gonads appearing as morphologically ovarian or testicular tissue may be dysgenetic or can even represent abnormal fallopian tube or epididymis. Surgical biopsy with histologic evaluation is required for definitive gonad characterization.[9,32]

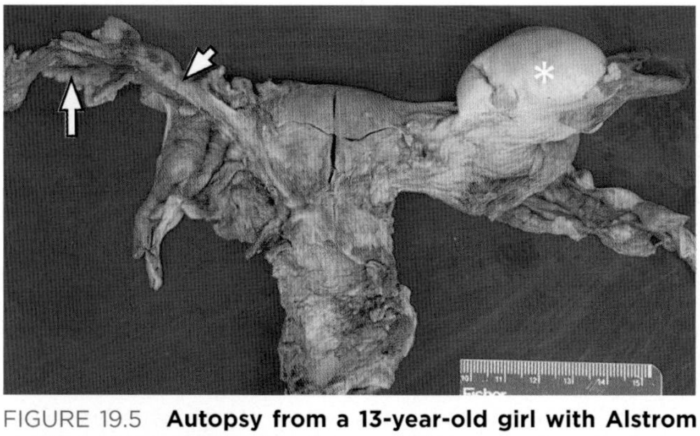

FIGURE 19.5 **Autopsy from a 13-year-old girl with Alstrom syndrome revealed a streak gonad (*long arrow*) and a hypoplastic fallopian tube (*short arrow*) on the left (posterior view).** The right ovary (*asterisk*) is the expected size.

Complications of dysgenetic and streak gonads include premature ovarian failure and primary amenorrhea; patients with a normal physical exam at birth may later present with delayed puberty because of hypoestrogenism.[31] In some cases, the abnormal germ cell derivatives may lack the genetic influence to mature completely, placing the patient at increased risk for malignancy.[8,9,19] Prophylactic removal of dysgenetic gonads is usually recommended in patients raised as girls because of the increased risk of neoplasia, including gonadoblastoma.[32]

Ovarian Cyst and Follicle

A graafian or primordial follicle is tiny, measuring about 0.25 mm; this is the only type of follicle present in prepubertal children. In the neonatal ovary, subcentimeter follicles may be visible, but involute as the effects of maternal hormones subside.[1,33,34] Management of larger neonatal ovarian cysts is somewhat controversial. Lesions larger than 4 cm are prone to torsion[33,34]; however, some authors believe that many of these lesions arise in ovaries that have already infarcted from torsion in utero.[35] The differential diagnosis of these lesions includes mesenteric/omental cyst (lymphatic malformation) and enteric duplication cyst.[33] Ovarian neoplasms, including teratomas, are rare in neonates.

Torsed, infarcted ovaries may appear as abdominal or pelvic cysts or small calcified masses at birth.[2] Imaging evaluation of neonatal ovarian cysts is usually carried out using ultrasound (Fig. 19.6). Some authors advocate intervention to prevent the complications of torsion, hemorrhage, or bowel obstruction with either ultrasound-guided aspiration for optimal ovarian salvage[34] or cystectomy, particularly in cases of suspected acute torsion. Follow-up ultrasound to document cyst involution is an alternative approach for smaller lesions.[35]

In the older child, as follicles mature, their walls thicken and their centers fill with fluid. The mature or dominant follicle can reach a size of up to 3 cm before rupturing and discharging the ovum.[36] After ovum release, follicular lining cells

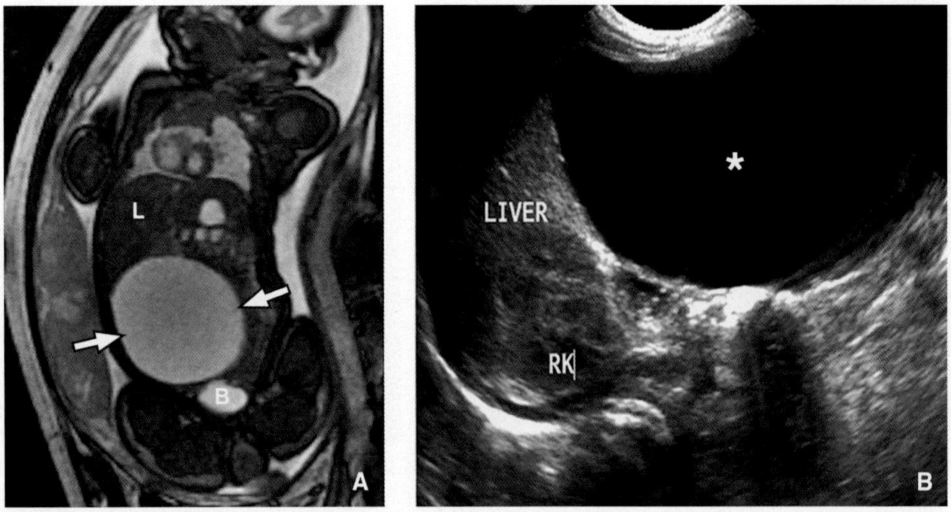

FIGURE 19.6 **Neonatal ovarian cyst. A:** Coronal T2-weighted fetal MR image performed at 34 weeks' gestation shows a round, circumscribed, homogeneously hyperintense cyst (*arrows*) in the right abdomen. The lesion extends from the dome of the bladder (*B*) to the liver (*L*). **B:** Postnatal transverse gray-scale ultrasound image also shows a large simple-appearing cyst (*asterisk*) extending into the right upper quadrant of the abdomen. A 7 cm simple ovarian cyst was found at surgical exploration, and cystectomy was performed. The right ovary was preserved and demonstrated no evidence of torsion. *RK*, right kidney.

luteinize, then regress as vascular tissue grows into the folds of the collapsed follicular walls, eventually involuting to form the corpus albicans.

At ultrasound, a corpus luteum can vary in appearance from an irregular, thick-walled cyst to a more solid appearing, collapsed lesion with low-resistance spectral Doppler waveforms in their wall.[36] At contrast-enhanced CT and MRI, the walls of these cysts usually appear thickened and hyperenhancing with crenated margins. The ovulating ovary and corpora lutea also show increased uptake on ^{18}F-FDG-PET (^{18}F-fluorodeoxyglucose positron emission tomography), simulating pelvic lymphadenopathy or ovarian neoplasm.[37]

Failed ovulation can result in a functional cyst that usually remains simple, but may grow causing pain.[36] In postpubertal girls, simple ovarian cysts up to 3 cm most likely represent a dominant follicle (with rupture either impending or failing to occur) or persistence of the corpus luteum as a cyst after ovulation.[1,36] Although uncommon, autonomously functioning follicular cysts (Fig. 19.7) are a common cause of peripheral precocious puberty.[14] A cyst larger than 9 mm in a girl with precocious puberty should raise a question of an autonomously functioning follicular cyst or hormone-producing tumor[14] requiring resection. Observation is generally sufficient for nonfunctioning cysts; however, aspiration may be needed for large ovarian cysts to minimize the risk of future ovarian torsion.[14]

Hemorrhagic ovarian cysts are generally from corpora lutea, which typically have bloody contents (Fig. 19.8); they vary in appearance depending upon the age of the hemorrhage.[1,36,38] At ultrasound, they may appear echogenic without posterior acoustic shadowing; may contain dependent debris, fluid–debris levels, or retracted, avascular, lobulated blood clot (Figs. 19.9 and 19.10); or may contain lacy or cobweb-appearing fibrinous strands. Retracted blood clot within a cyst does not have blood flow on color Doppler ultrasound and may move with ballottement with the transducer (this is evaluated by applying gentle pressure with the transducer followed by release to assess movement within the fluid), whereas a solid tumor nodule does not. The cyst contents should not have

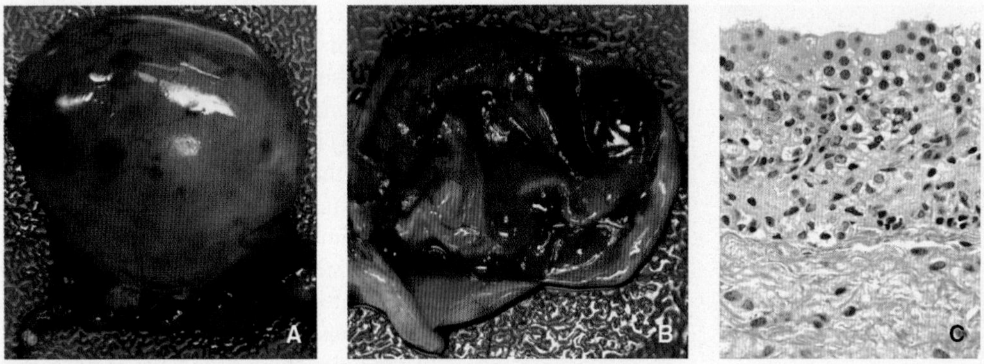

FIGURE 19.7 **This 4.3 cm follicular cyst with luteinization (A) was excised from the ovary of a 6-year-old girl with isosexual precocity.** The luteinized cells impart a yellow color to the cyst lining **(B)**. Microscopically, the cyst lining contains follicular cells with the abundant pink and sometimes vacuolated cytoplasm that typifies "luteinized" cells **(C)** (hematoxylin and eosin, original magnification, 600×).

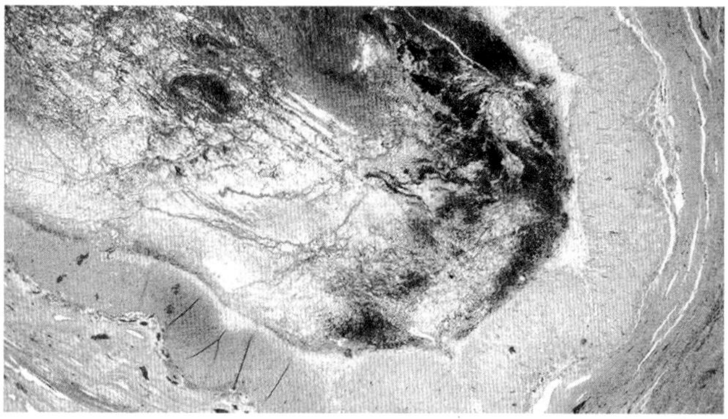

FIGURE 19.8 **Corpus luteum cyst, with a lumen containing a coagulum of blood (hematoxylin and eosin, original magnification, 20×).**

blood flow on Doppler ultrasound evaluation and should not enhance on CT or MRI. At contrast-enhanced CT, a hemorrhagic cyst may appear hyperdense compared to other follicles, but is still less attenuating than surrounding enhanced ovarian stroma. A hematocrit effect may be observed. The MRI appearance depends upon the age of the hemorrhage. Signal hyperintensity on both non–fat-saturated and fat-saturated T1-weighted MR images is a reliable indicator of the presence of hemorrhage. These lesions may show lower than expected signal intensity on T2-weighted MR images, often referred to as "T2 shading," which is the result of evolving blood products (Fig. 19.10). Other causes of blood-filled ovarian cysts besides corpora lutea include posttorsion/infarct and endometriotic cyst, both rare in childhood.

Functional hemorrhagic cysts typically resolve or at least decrease in size over 1 to 2 menstrual cycles.[1] If there is acute and sometimes painful cyst rupture, the cyst may appear collapsed or may be no longer visible with a variable amount of free pelvic fluid that may contain low-level echoes due to hemorrhage. Management is usually conservative. For simple cysts in postmenarchal girls measuring 3 to 5 cm, follow-up is commonly not required.[36] Follow-up ultrasound is recommended for simple cysts measuring >5 cm and less than or

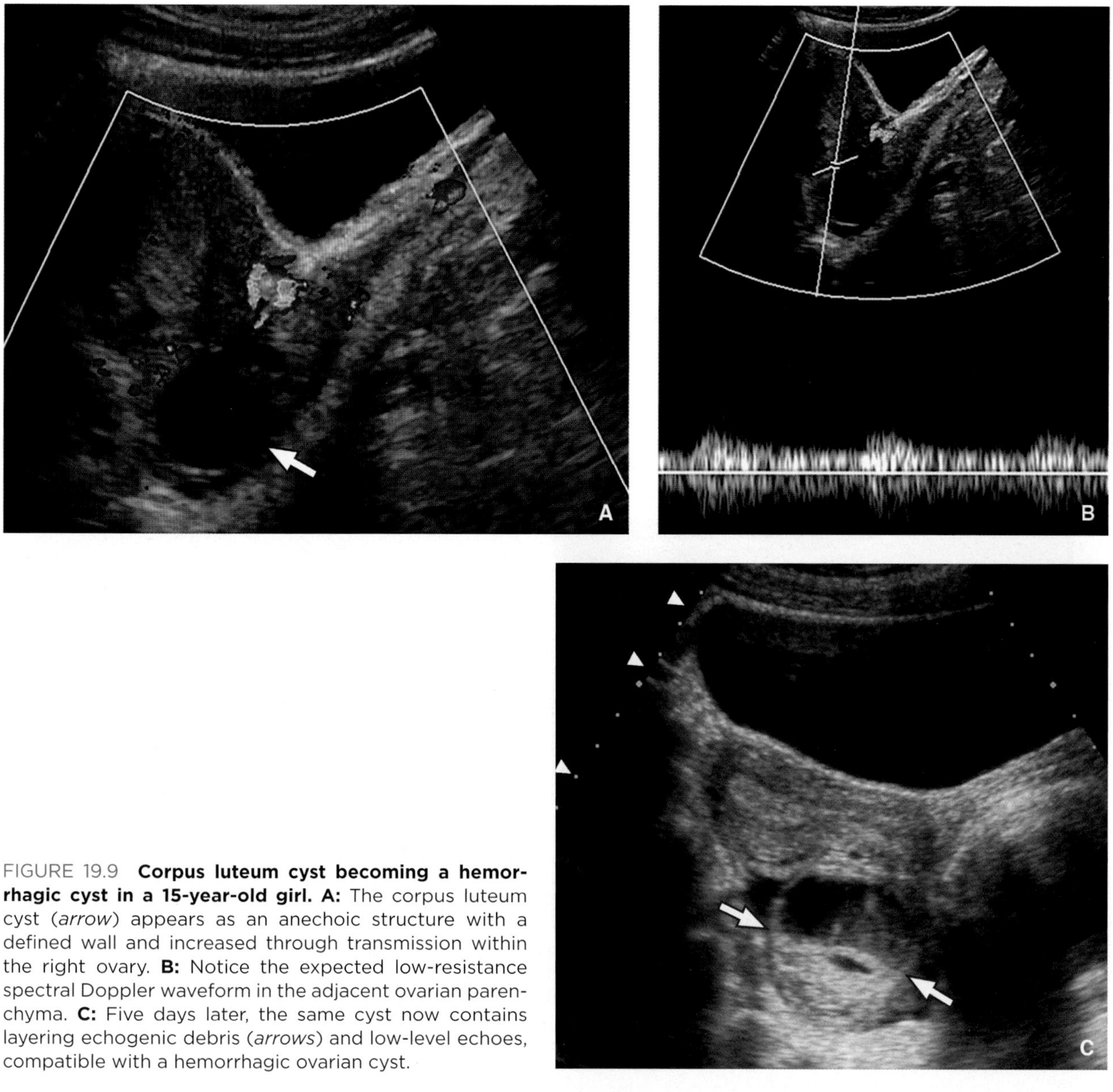

FIGURE 19.9 **Corpus luteum cyst becoming a hemorrhagic cyst in a 15-year-old girl. A:** The corpus luteum cyst (*arrow*) appears as an anechoic structure with a defined wall and increased through transmission within the right ovary. **B:** Notice the expected low-resistance spectral Doppler waveform in the adjacent ovarian parenchyma. **C:** Five days later, the same cyst now contains layering echogenic debris (*arrows*) and low-level echoes, compatible with a hemorrhagic ovarian cyst.

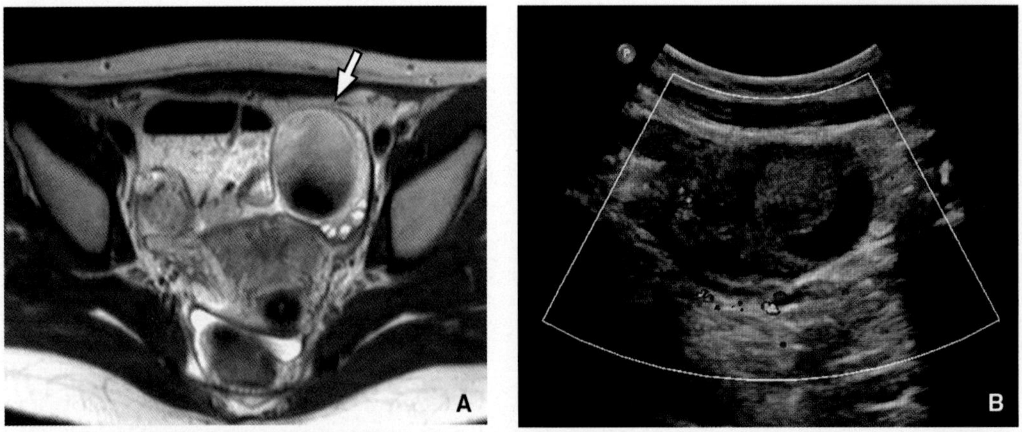

FIGURE 19.10 **A 16-year-old girl with a hemorrhagic left ovarian cyst. A:** Axial T2-weighted MR image shows a hemorrhagic cyst (*arrow*) in the left ovary that demonstrates "T2 shading" phenomenon due to layering blood products within the cyst. This appearance is classically associated with endometriomas, which are typically extraovarian, but can be seen in ovarian hemorrhagic cysts as well. **B:** Longitudinal color Doppler ultrasound image of the left ovary shows internal avascular retractile blood products within the cyst. The cyst resolved on subsequent follow-up ultrasound evaluation. (Case courtesy of Jonathan R. Dillman, MD, MSc, Cincinnati Children's Hospital Medical Center, Cincinnati, OH.)

equal to 7 cm,[36] although aspiration may be warranted to prevent potential torsion. Intervention may also be required for larger cysts for pain control or in case of suspected ovarian torsion, with laparoscopic cyst aspiration or cystectomy most often performed. Simple cysts larger than 7 cm require further evaluation with MR imaging or laparoscopy.[36]

Polycystic Ovarian Syndrome

Polycystic ovarian syndrome (PCOS) consists of hyperandrogenism, enlarged polycystic ovaries, and obesity. Affected patients often present with menstrual cycle irregularity and may have insulin resistance.[39] The incidence of PCOS in adolescents is about 3%,[40] although 16% of girls presenting with menstrual irregularity were diagnosed with PCOS in one study.[41] There is likely a genetic basis for the disease, which has been proposed to represent a form of arrested adrenarche.[40] Given the association of this syndrome with insulin resistance and hypertension, implications for long-term cardiovascular health make PCOS important to detect.

Diagnostic criteria include physical examination evidence of hyperandrogenism; hormonal imbalances, including testosterone elevation and an elevated LH/FSH ratio; oligo- or amenorrhea; insulin resistance or hyperinsulinemia; and polycystic ovarian morphology (PCOM).[40] Accelerated bone maturation may also be present.[42] Because ovaries containing multiple follicles of up to 1 cm can be normal during adolescence,[43] a diagnosis of PCOS should be only be considered if the abnormal ovarian morphology is accompanied by other clinical or laboratory evidence of PCOS.[20,39,40] Normal ovarian morphology does not exclude the diagnosis of PCOS.

The criteria for PCOM include an ovarian volume of more than 10 mL with or without 12 or more follicles in each ovary measuring 2 to 9 mm in diameter[44] (Fig. 19.11). Follicular distribution and stromal hyperechogenicity are not included

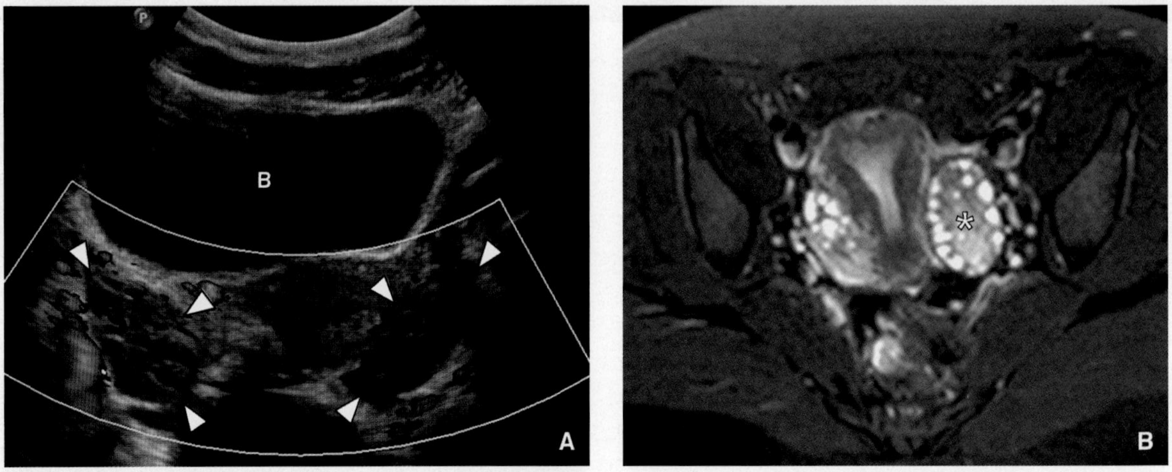

FIGURE 19.11 **A 16-year-old girl with irregular menstrual cycles, severe acne, and hyperandrogenism. A:** Transverse power Doppler ultrasound image of the pelvis shows bilaterally enlarged ovaries (*arrowheads*) containing multiple subcentimeter cysts. Ovarian volumes measure >15 mL. **B:** Axial T2-weighted fat-saturated MR image shows an enlarged left ovary with prominent hypointense central stroma (*asterisk*) and numerous peripherally arranged follicles. These findings can be seen with polycystic ovarian syndrome. Findings are more conspicuous in the left ovary due to the plane of the image.

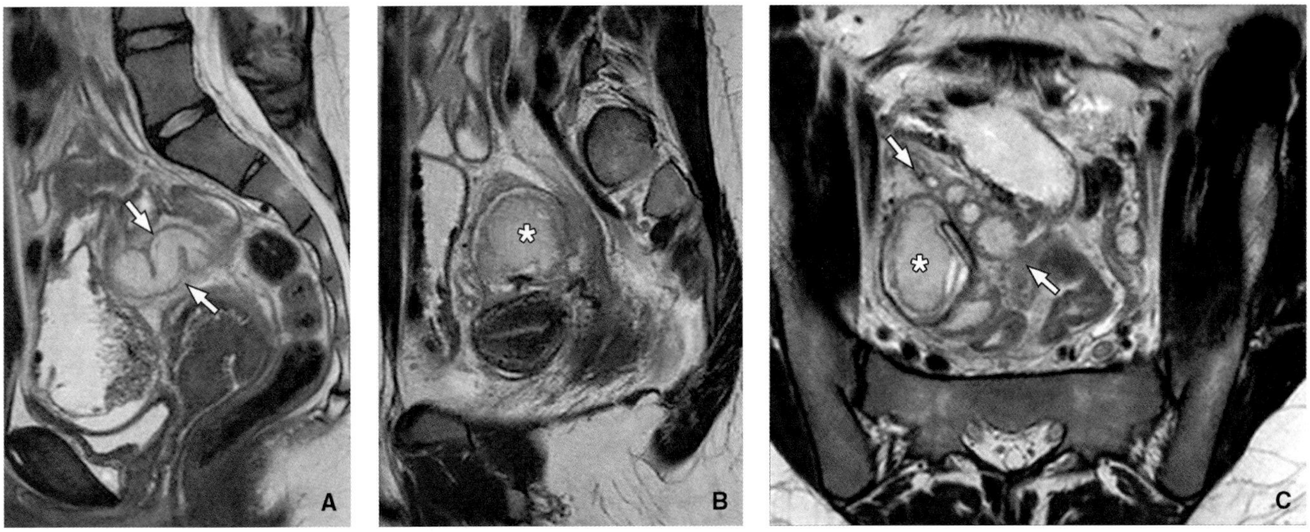

FIGURE 19.12 **A 12-year-old girl with acute pelvic pain. A:** Sagittal T2-weighted MR image shows a dilated, fluid-containing right fallopian tube (*arrows*) with adjacent fluid. **B:** More lateral MR image shows an adjacent focal fluid collection associated with the right ovary (*asterisk*). This collection represents a tubo-ovarian abscess. **C:** Axial-oblique T2-weighted MR image shows the dilated fallopian tube in cross-section appearing as multiple round structures (*arrows*) as well as the adjacent abscess (*asterisk*). (Case courtesy of Jonathan R. Dillman, MD, MSc, Cincinnati Children's Hospital Medical Center, Cincinnati, OH.)

in these criteria. Although both ovaries are typically affected, findings may be seen in only one ovary.

Transvaginal ultrasound is the ideal imaging modality for evaluation of ovaries and ovarian follicles in adolescent pediatric patients with clinically suspected PCOS; however, transvaginal ultrasound may not be appropriate in girls who are not sexually active. When evaluating PCOM with ultrasound, ovarian volumes should be calculated utilizing the simplified formula for a prolate ellipsoid (0.52 × length × width × height).[44] If a dominant follicle (>10 mm) or a corpus luteum is encountered, repeat ultrasound is recommended during the next menstrual cycle. Some authors[36,45] have suggested a threshold of at least 19 or more follicles as criteria for diagnosing PCOS; however, these studies were performed using transvaginal probes.

Current treatments for PCOS include weight reduction, hair growth suppression and/or removal, insulin-sensitizing agents (e.g., metformin), and hormonal therapy with oral contraceptives or antiandrogens.[39,40]

Infectious and Inflammatory Disorder

Tubo-Ovarian Abscess

Twenty percent of adolescents with pelvic inflammatory disease (PID) develop a tubo-ovarian abscess (TOA),[1] presenting with acute or chronic pelvic pain, often associated with fever and an elevated white blood count. At ultrasound, TOAs are typically complex adnexal collections with variable internal echoes and septations, no internal Doppler blood flow, and a thick, hyperemic wall on color Doppler evaluation.[1] TOAs are also well demonstrated by CT and MRI as complex fluid collections with peripheral postcontrast enhancement and adjacent inflammatory changes[46] (Fig. 19.12), although ultrasound is diagnostic in many pediatric cases. The ipsilateral ovary may be indistinguishable, and there may be an associated hydro- or pyosalpinx (Fig. 19.13). The differential diagnosis for TOA includes endometrioma, ectopic pregnancy, and malignancy; however, the clinical findings suggesting acute infection are often helpful in arriving at the correct diagnosis. If the patient denies sexual activity, consideration should be given to secondary adnexal involvement due to other disease, such as a ruptured appendix or inflammatory bowel disease.

Management generally requires intravenous antibiotic therapy. For larger, accessible collections, transvaginal or percutaneous image-guided drainage may be an option. Laparoscopic drainage can be performed if needed.

Neoplastic Disorders

The overall incidence of ovarian neoplasms in childhood is low with ovarian malignancies accounting for up to 30% of ovarian masses, comprising 1% of childhood cancers.[1,7,47] Twenty-five percent of girls between 1 and 8 years of age presenting with an ovarian mass or precocious puberty have an ovarian malignancy, whereas only 10% of girls ages 9 to 19 years with an ovarian mass have a malignant lesion due to the increased incidence of cysts and benign neoplasms in the older age group.[7,48] Ovarian malignancy is very rare under 1 year of age.

The classification of neoplastic ovarian masses is by cell type, including surface epithelial, germ cell, sex cord stromal, metastases, and miscellaneous (Table 19.2). Germ cell tumors comprise 80% of ovarian neoplasms in girls <20 years of age, whereas 95% of ovarian lesions are of epithelial origin in older adults.[7,50,51]

Typical clinical presentations of children with ovarian neoplasms include pelvic or abdominal mass or precocious puberty.[2] Pain due to torsion and/or rupture with hemoperitoneum is also a common presentation,[1,52] but less common in children than adults.[47] As in adults, solid or heterogeneous appearance of an ovarian mass is concerning for malignancy,[2]

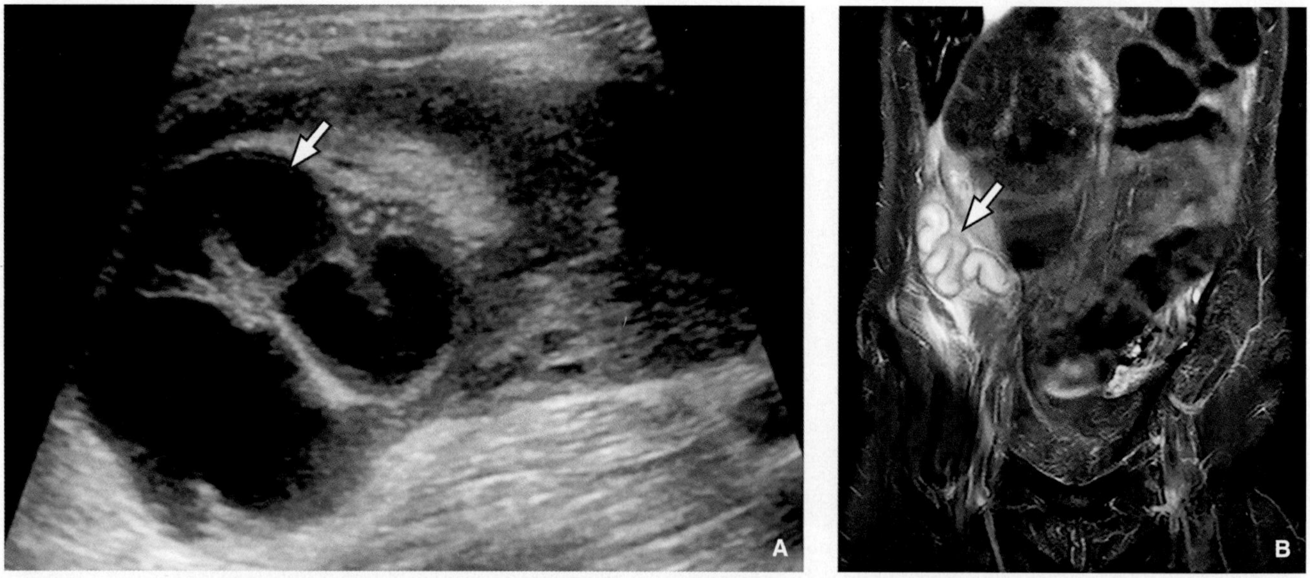

FIGURE 19.13 **A 17-year-old girl presented with a right-sided pyosalpinx.** Transverse ultrasound **(A)** and coronal T2-weighted fat-saturated MR **(B)** images through the right lower quadrant show a dilated fallopian tube (*arrows*) and adjacent inflammation due to pelvic inflammatory disease.

although 5% of simple ovarian cysts over 6 cm in children may contain malignant cells.[7,48] Ovarian lesions over 8 cm are suspicious for malignancy in children.[48]

Ultrasound is considered the first-line imaging modality for assessing pediatric pelvic masses and is typically performed using transabdominal technique. Doppler ultrasound evaluation is a helpful adjunct to gray-scale imaging. MRI often allows for additional tissue characterization and helps confirm the organ of origin for indeterminate pelvic lesions.[6] CT is generally reserved for staging of disease extension in pediatric patients with ovarian neoplasms, although it also depicts intralesional fat and calcification/ossification.

Management of ovarian tumors in children depends upon the likelihood of malignancy with ovarian-sparing procedures commonly attempted for benign lesions.[52,53] A surgical tumor staging workup is performed in cases of suspected malignancy. Additional evaluation includes hormonal assessment in the setting of precocious puberty or virilization. Serum markers, including CA-125, β-hCG (beta-human chorionic gonadotropin), LDH (lactate dehydrogenase), and α-FP (alpha-fetoprotein), are useful at diagnosis as well as at follow-up to monitor response to therapy and relapse.[7,48] Adjuvant chemotherapy and/or radiation therapy may also be indicated for some malignant tumors.[52,54]

Benign Ovarian Neoplasms

Mature teratomas are the only benign germ cell tumor to arise from the ovary,[1] and they are the most common ovarian neoplasm in children, accounting for 67%.[2] By definition, these lesions must contain at least two of the three germ cell layers—endoderm, mesoderm, and ectoderm.[55] These lesions are often called cystic teratomas or dermoid cysts due to their tendency to be mostly cystic and contain dermal elements (Fig. 19.14).[1] About 25% are bilateral.[2,55]

The ultrasound appearance of mature ovarian teratomas is highly variable depending upon the sizes and proportions of cystic, fatty, solid, and calcified components.[1] The classic appearance is a predominantly cystic lesion with a solid echogenic mural nodule representing the Rokitansky nodule (or dermoid plug)[1,55] (Fig. 19.15). This mural nodule may contain fat, skin, hair follicles, teeth, and/or bone. "Dermoid mesh," linear echoes representing hair, may be seen.[7,36] Echogenic nondependent floating sebum, sometimes creating a fat-fluid level, is another distinguishing feature of mature teratomas at ultrasound. An echogenic focus with prominent posterior acoustic shadowing represents the "tip of the iceberg" sign due to absorption/attenuation of sound waves by hair and fat[1,7,36]; however, gas within pelvic bowel loops can also create this appearance and is a pitfall. Ballottement with the transducer is a useful technique to elicit motion as a cohesive mass; bowel loops commonly efface.[36]

At CT, the finding of fat attenuation (<-20 Hounsfield units) in a complex solid or cystic lesion with associated calcification is diagnostic of ovarian teratoma[7] (Fig. 19.15); without pathologic examination, it is difficult to exclude the presence of immature areas. At MRI, fat-containing teratomas can be differentiated from hemorrhagic ovarian cysts by comparison of non–fat-saturated and fat-saturated T1-weighted MR images; the fatty elements of an ovarian teratoma typically show signal loss with fat saturation, whereas hemorrhage remains hyperintense (Fig. 19.16). Complications of mature ovarian teratomas include torsion (Figs. 19.17 and 19.18), seen in 15% of cases,[1] rupture, malignant transformation, and very rarely autoimmune hemolytic anemia[1] and immune-mediated limbic encephalitis.[7,56]

Sex cord-stromal tumors (SCSTs) are reported to account for 5% to 12% of all pediatric ovarian neoplasms.[7,52] Benign

TABLE 19.2 Classification of Ovarian Tumors Found in the Pediatric Age Group (Modified from the WHO Classification of Ovarian Tumors)[49]

Classification	Cell Type	Benign	Borderline	Malignant
Epithelial tumors	Serous	Serous cystadenoma	Serous borderline tumor/atypical proliferative serous tumor Serous borderline tumor—micropapillary variant/noninvasive low-grade serous carcinoma	Low-grade serous carcinoma High-grade serous carcinoma
	Mucinous	Mucinous cystadenoma	Mucinous borderline tumor/atypical proliferative mucinous tumor	Mucinous carcinoma
	Endometrioid	Endometriotic cyst Endometrioid cystadenoma	Endometrioid borderline tumor/atypical proliferative endometrioid tumor	Endometrioid carcinoma
	Seromucinous tumors	Seromucinous cystadenoma Seromucinous adenofibroma	Seromucinous borderline tumor/atypical proliferative seromucinous tumor	Seromucinous carcinoma
	Undifferentiated carcinoma			
Sex cord–stromal tumors	**Cell Type**		**Tumor types**	
	Pure stromal tumors		Fibroma Thecoma Luteinized thecoma associated with sclerosing peritonitis Fibrosarcoma Sclerosing stromal tumor Leydig cell tumor	
	Pure sex cord tumors		Juvenile granulosa cell tumor Sertoli cell tumor Sex cord tumor with annular tubules	
Mixed sex cord-stromal tumors	Sertoli-Leydig cell tumors		Well differentiated Moderately differentiated with heterologous elements Poorly differentiated with heterologous elements Retiform with heterologous elements	
Germ cell tumors	Dysgerminoma Yolk sac tumor Embryonal carcinoma Nongestational choriocarcinoma Mature teratoma Immature teratoma Mixed germ cell tumor			
Monodermal teratoma and somatic-type tumors arising from a dermoid cyst				
Germ cell: sex cord-stromal tumors	Gonadoblastoma including gonadoblastoma with malignant germ cell tumor			
	Mixed germ cell—sex cord-stromal tumor, unclassified			
Miscellaneous	Small cell carcinoma, hypercalcemic type			
	Mesothelioma			
Soft tissue tumors	Rhabdomyosarcoma			
Tumor-like lesions	Follicle cyst Corpus luteum cyst Large solitary luteinized follicle cyst Others			
Lymphoid and myeloid tumors	Burkitt lymphoma			
Secondary tumors				

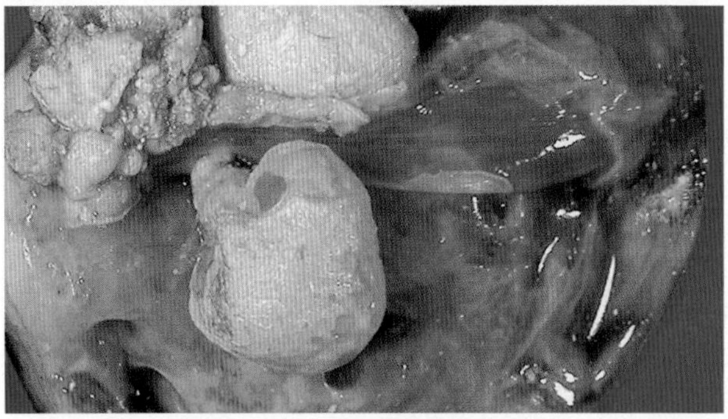

FIGURE 19.14 **This mature ovarian teratoma in a 14-year-old girl is predominantly cystic and shows skin-lined Rokitansky nodules protruding from the cyst wall.**

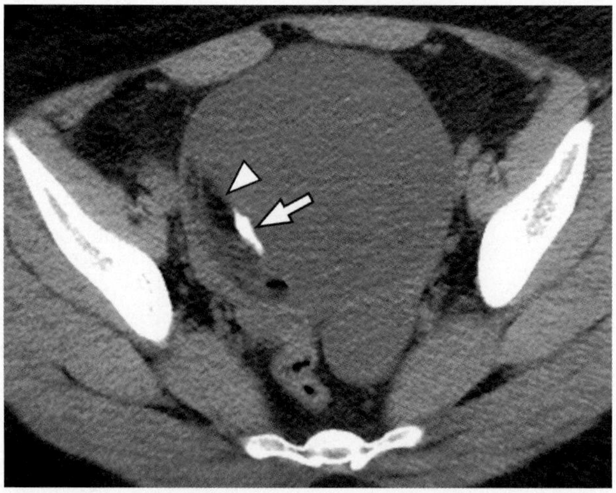

FIGURE 19.15 **Incidentally found large mature ovarian teratoma in a 16-year-old girl being evaluated for nephrolithiasis contains calcification (*arrow*) and fat (*arrowhead*) within the Rokitansky nodule (or dermoid plug) along the wall of the cyst.**

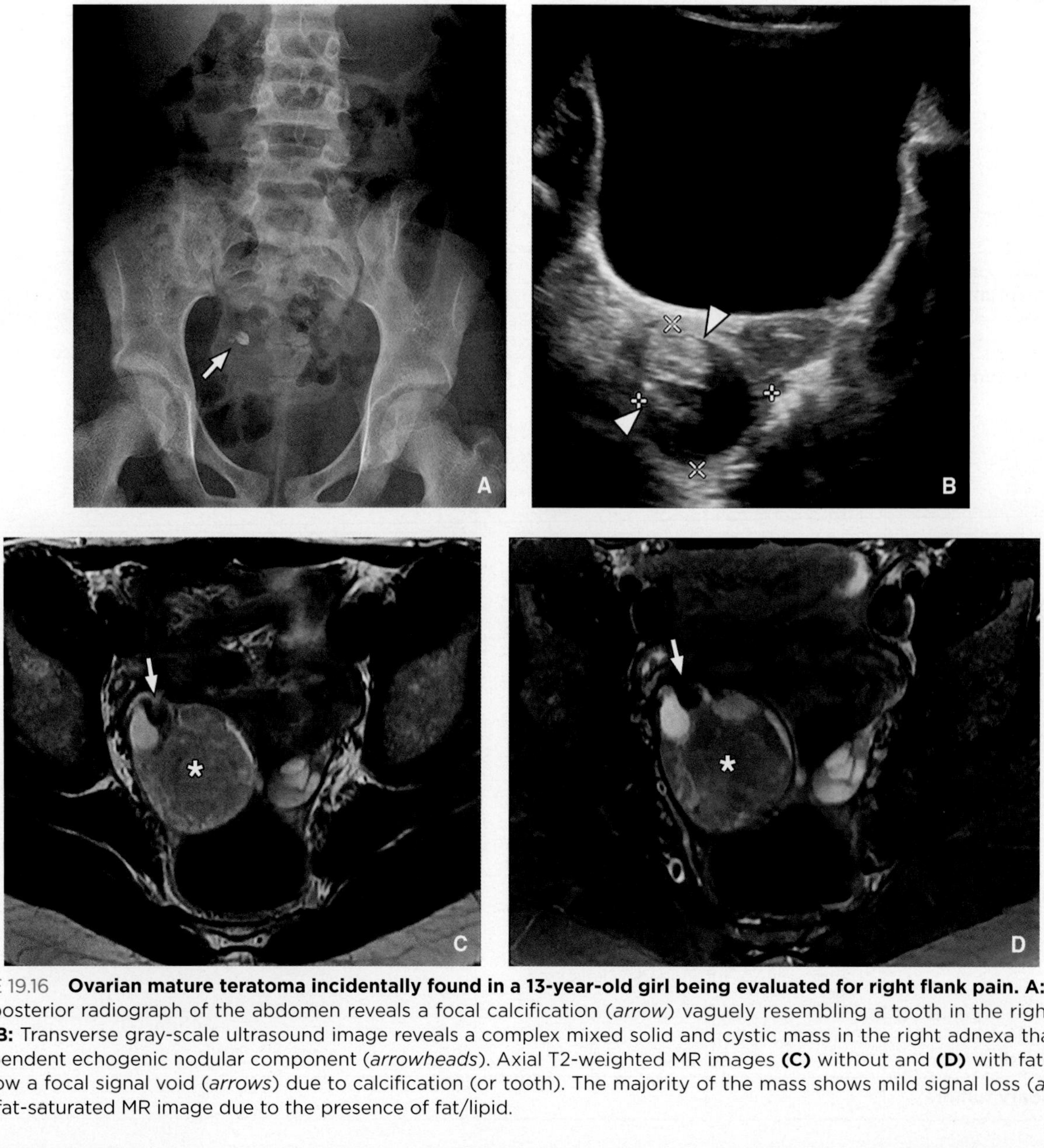

FIGURE 19.16 **Ovarian mature teratoma incidentally found in a 13-year-old girl being evaluated for right flank pain. A:** Supine anteroposterior radiograph of the abdomen reveals a focal calcification (*arrow*) vaguely resembling a tooth in the right hemipelvis. **B:** Transverse gray-scale ultrasound image reveals a complex mixed solid and cystic mass in the right adnexa that has a nondependent echogenic nodular component (*arrowheads*). Axial T2-weighted MR images **(C)** without and **(D)** with fat saturation show a focal signal void (*arrows*) due to calcification (or tooth). The majority of the mass shows mild signal loss (*asterisk*) on the fat-saturated MR image due to the presence of fat/lipid.

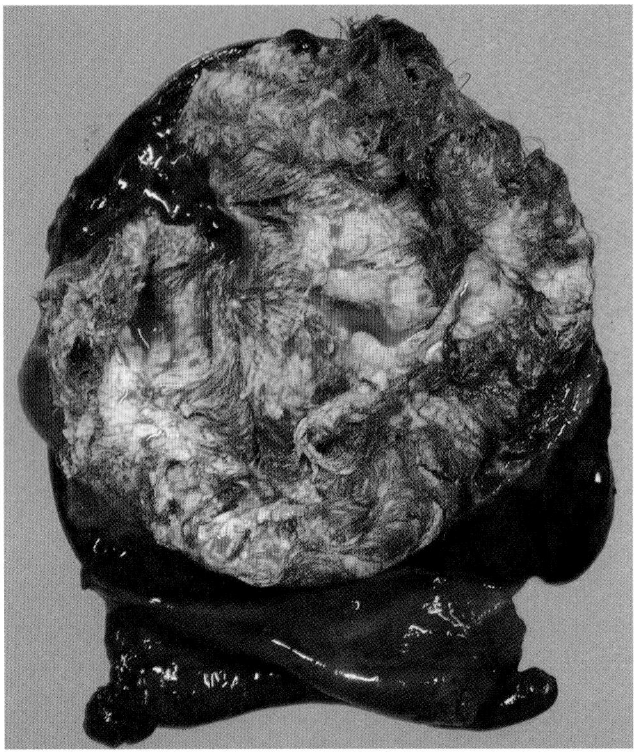

FIGURE 19.17 **This mature cystic teratoma in a 12-year-old girl is lined by hair-bearing skin.** The patient presented with ovarian torsion which is associated with a swollen violaceous necrotic fallopian tube (lower aspect).

types of SCSTs include thecoma, fibroma (Fig. 19.19), fibrothecoma, and sclerosing stromal cell tumors.[2,7] Tumors may be large at presentation,[52] although functioning tumors tend to be smaller.[20] Tumor behavior can be difficult to predict from histology.[57] Thecomas and fibrothecomas are within a spectrum of lesions with varying amounts of fibroblastic and thecal components.[7] These lesions are rare in children and are usually seen in women over 40 years of age. In childhood in particular, fibroma–thecoma group tumors may be associated with basal cell nevus syndrome (Gorlin syndrome).[58] Thecal cells, when present, are associated with increased estrogen production.[7] These tumors are often solid appearing and hypoechoic at ultrasound because of fibrous tissue. Ascites is common. Myxoid degeneration may occur in larger lesions.[7]

Other sometimes benign SCSTs include Sertoli cell tumors, Leydig cell tumors, and stromal luteomas.[20] The latter lesions tend to be smaller and more difficult to detect at imaging.[20] Sclerosing stromal cell tumors are also benign and typically occur in patients <30 years of age.[20] Common presentations for SCSTs include menstrual irregularity and other signs and symptoms related to estrogen and androgen production.

Proliferations of ovarian surface epithelium make up 17% of ovarian neoplasms in children, compared to 95% in adults.[7] Epithelial lesions are classified as benign (cystadenoma), borderline malignant potential, or malignant (carcinoma) based on pathologic features. Serous and mucinous

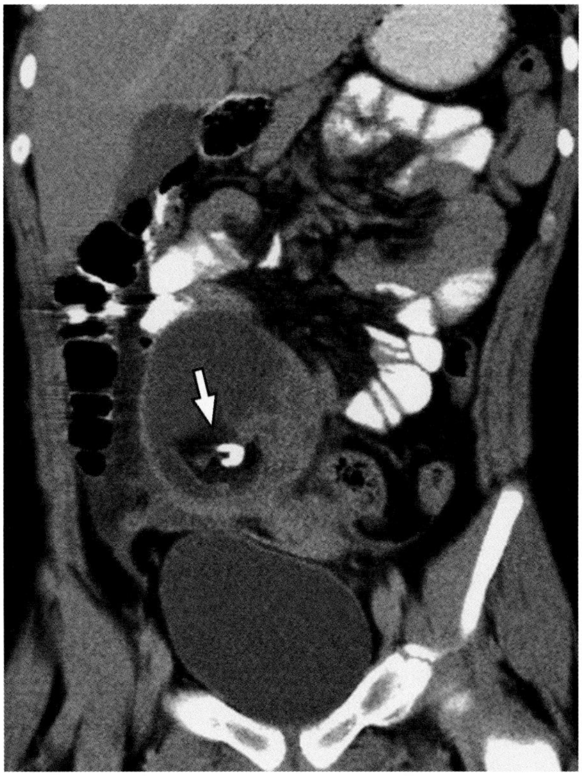

FIGURE 19.18 **A 13-year-old girl with a torsed mature ovarian teratoma.** Contrast-enhanced coronal-reformatted CT image shows a large mature ovarian teratoma arising from the right ovary that contains solid and cystic elements as well as a mural nodule (*arrow*) that contains fat and a probable tooth. Relatively high position of the right ovarian teratoma and adjacent fat stranding raise concern for ovarian torsion. (Image courtesy of Jonathan R. Dillman, MD, MSc, Cincinnati Children's Hospital Medical Center, Cincinnati, OH.)

lesions are the most common epithelial subtypes in children, and they are nearly always benign.[1,7] Lesions between 8 and 10 cm are likely to present with torsion, whereas lesions over 15 cm are unlikely to torse.[7] At ultrasound and MRI, both benign serous and mucinous cysts commonly contain thin

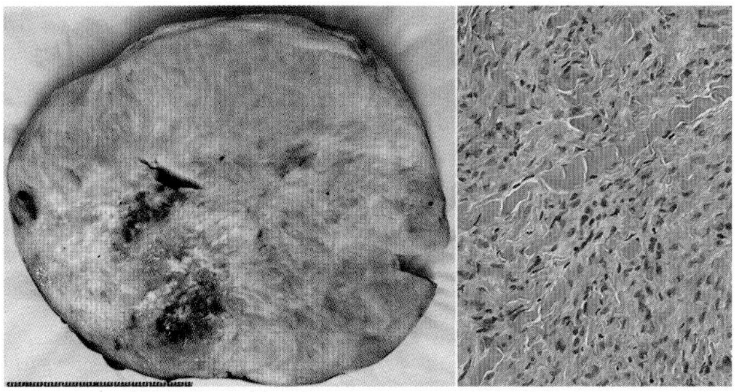

FIGURE 19.19 **This unilateral ovarian fibroma is firm, pale, focally hemorrhagic, and partially calcified (left), triggering a workup for Gorlin syndrome in an otherwise healthy 10-year-old girl.** Microscopic examination shows plump spindle-shaped cells in a background of abundant pink collagen (**right**, hematoxylin and eosin, original magnification, 400×).

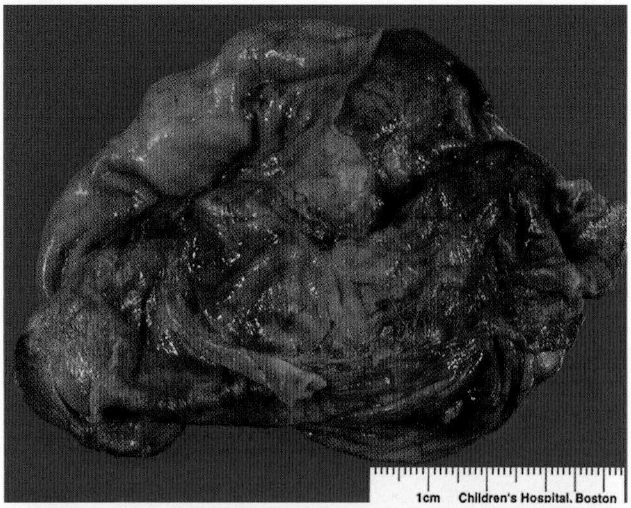

FIGURE 19.20 **This serous cyst from the broad ligament of a 14-year-old girl is thin walled and lined by cells resembling fallopian tube epithelium.**

septations. Serous lesions tend to have fewer cysts and more homogeneous contents, and mucinous lesions tend to have more cysts and more heterogeneous cystic components.[1,7] (Figs. 19.20 to 19.24).

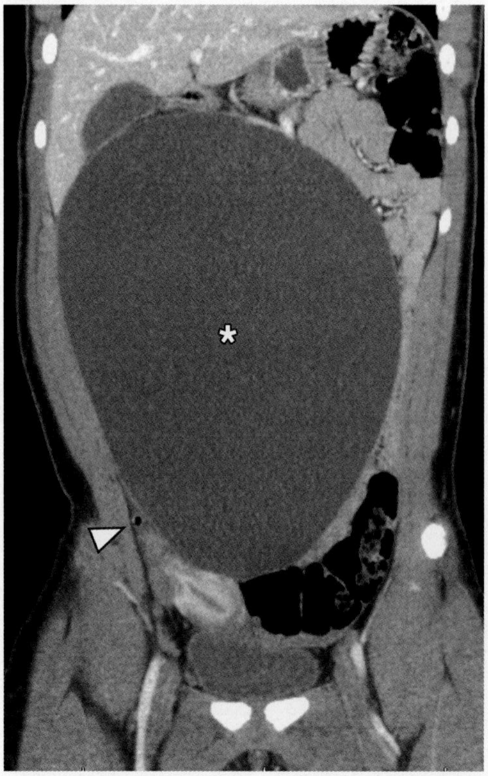

FIGURE 19.21 **Ovarian serous cystadenoma in a 12-year-old girl who presented with a palpable abdominal mass.** Contrast-enhanced coronal-reformatted CT image shows a large simple-appearing cyst (*asterisk*) arising from the right hemipelvis and extending in the upper abdomen. This lesion was determined to be a benign serous cystadenoma by histopathology. Septations are common in these lesions and may be difficult to appreciate by CT; calcifications are unusual. Notice the normal air-filled appendix (*arrowhead*).

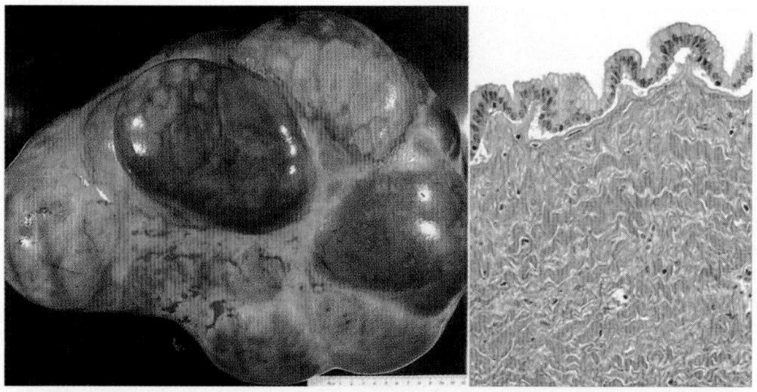

FIGURE 19.22 **Mucinous cystadenoma, typically large, presented as a 40-cm multiloculated mass (left) in this 13-year-old girl.** Microscopically, the cyst is lined by benign mucinous epithelium (**right**, hematoxylin and eosin, original magnification, 400x).

Malignant Ovarian Neoplasms

Dysgerminomas are the most common malignant ovarian neoplasm in children and adolescents.[1,7] Histologically identical to seminomas in boys, they are the least differentiated form of germ cell tumor (Fig. 19.25). At cross-sectional imaging, they are commonly lobulated, solid masses (Fig. 19.26A). On contrast-enhanced CT and MRI, thin, enhancing fibrovascular septa may be seen, and hemorrhage or necrosis may result in small cystic-appearing areas or calcifications. About 10% to 15% are bilateral, and an elevated serum LDH supports the diagnosis.[1] Metastatic disease commonly involves the retroperitoneum (Fig. 19.26B). Similar to seminomas, these tumors are radiosensitive. Dysgerminoma may be seen with other tumor types, particularly in cases of gonadal dysgenesis.

A small subset of ovarian teratomas in childhood may exhibit malignancy, due either to the presence of immature brain components ("immature teratoma") (Fig. 19.27) or to the coexistence of other types of malignancy, for example, rhabdomyosarcoma. Pediatric malignant ovarian teratomas tend to occur in a younger age group than pediatric mature ovarian teratomas. They may be associated with elevated serum β-hCG and α-FP levels. Malignant ovarian teratomas tend to be larger than mature ovarian teratomas, with 7.5 cm considered the threshold of concern.[7] They usually have a larger solid component than mature teratomas (which are often mostly cystic) with less fatty or calcific elements[1] (Fig. 19.28) and are bilateral in 10% of cases.[7] Other types of malignant germ cell tumors include yolk sac tumor (Fig. 19.29) embryonal carcinoma, choriocarcinoma, and mixed patterns.

Granulosa cell tumors (GCTs) are the largest subtype of SCSTs accounting for 7% to 8% of all ovarian neoplasms.[52] Juvenile GCT is the most common subtype of GCT seen in children, accounting for 90% of GCTs in patients <30 years of age.[14] The juvenile variety, which is usually seen in prepubescent girls, is usually less aggressive than the adult form.[52] These lesions can secrete estradiol resulting in precocious puberty or irregular menstruation depending upon patient age.[7,14] Patients with Ollier disease and Maffucci syndrome are at increased risk of developing this type of ovarian tumor.[7]

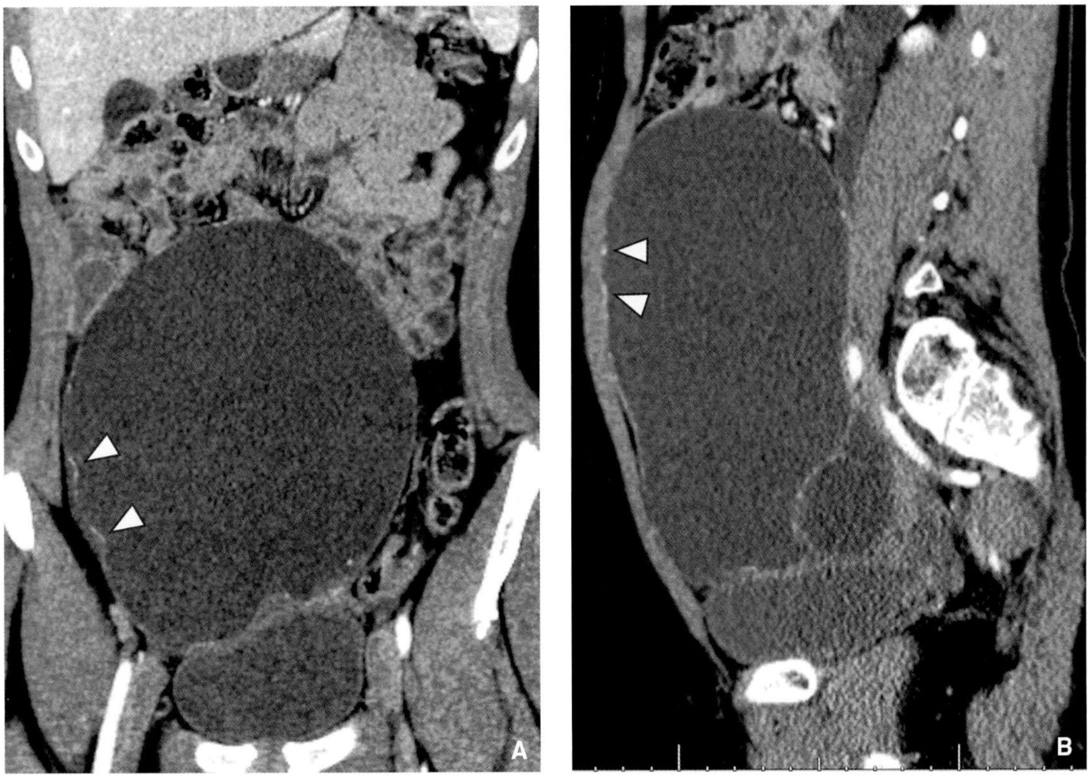

FIGURE 19.23 **Ovarian mucinous cystadenoma in a 11-year-old girl who presented with a palpable abdominal mass.** Contrast-enhanced coronal **(A)** and sagittal **(B)** reformatted CT images show punctate and linear calcifications (*arrowheads*) in the wall of a large cystic lesion arising from the right hemipelvis. At histopathology, this lesion was a benign mucinous cystadenoma containing psammomatous calcifications.

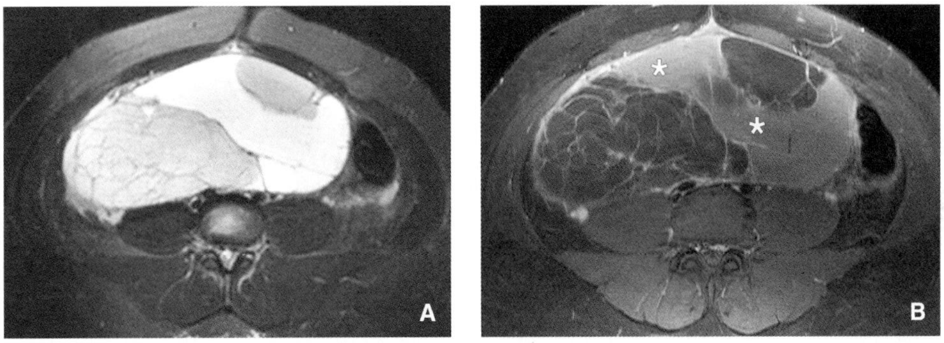

FIGURE 19.24 **A 15-year-old girl with ovarian mucinous cystadenoma.** Axial T2-weighted fat-saturated **(A)** and axial postcontrast T1-weighted fat-saturated **(B)** MR images demonstrate a large multilocular cystic mass in the lower abdomen. The lesion contains numerous small cysts giving rise to a honeycomb-like appearance. The lesion only demonstrates mural and septal postcontrast enhancement; large areas (*asterisks*) of intermediate signal hyperintensity on the postcontrast MR image are due to complicated (proteinaceous or hemorrhagic) fluid.

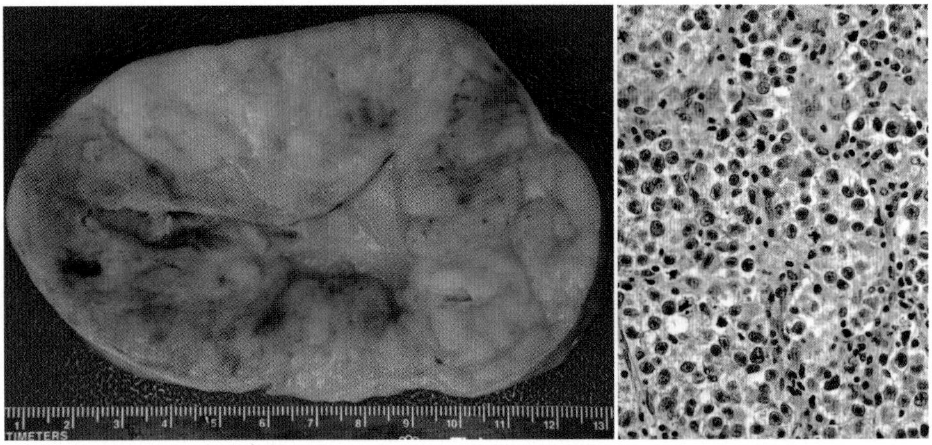

FIGURE 19.25 **This 15-cm ovarian grossly pale and homogeneous (left) germ cell tumor from an 11-year-old girl shows pure dysgerminoma histologically (right, hematoxylin and eosin, original magnification, 600×).**

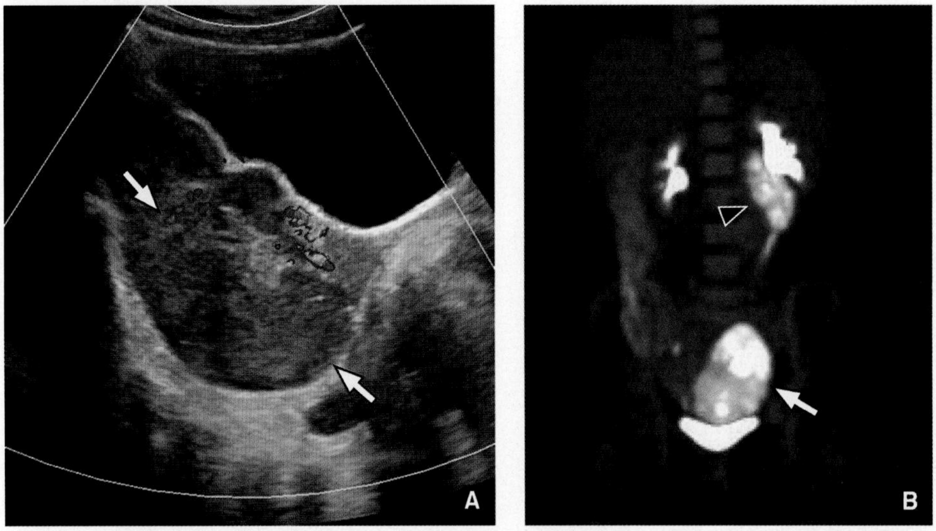

FIGURE 19.26 **Malignant dysgerminoma in a 16-year-old girl who presented with pelvic pain. A:** Longitudinal color Doppler ultrasound image through the pelvis shows a solid, lobular, heterogeneous cul-de-sac mass (*arrows*). **B:** Both the pelvic mass (*arrow*) and left retroperitoneal lymph node metastases (*arrowhead*) are hypermetabolic at ^{18}F-FDG PET imaging. Malignant dysgerminoma was proven at histopathology. (Case courtesy of Jonathan R. Dillman, MD, MSc, Cincinnati Children's Hospital Medical Center, Cincinnati, OH.)

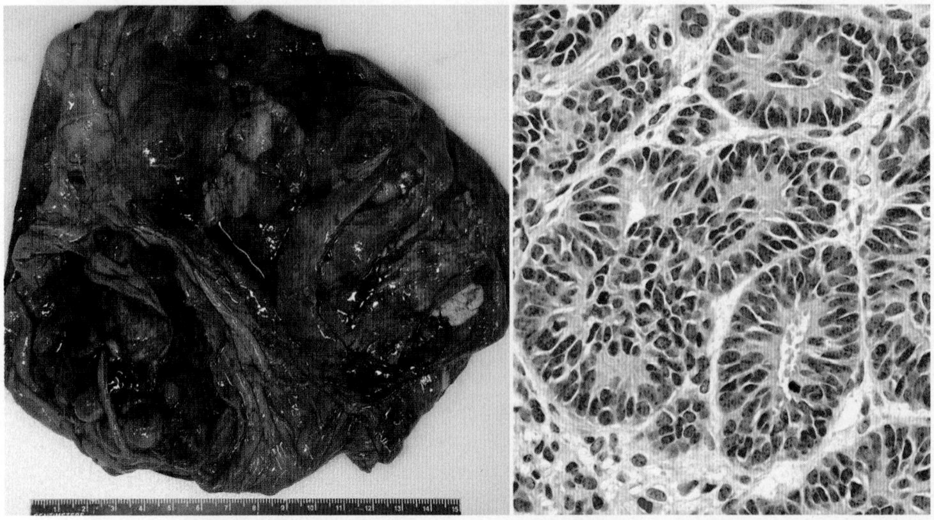

FIGURE 19.27 **This immature teratoma from a 13-year-old's ovary is notable for its large size (left; 22 cm intact).** It was only upon microscopic examination that the presence of small foci of immature brain tissue distinguished it from a mature teratoma (**right**, hematoxylin and eosin, original magnification, 40×).

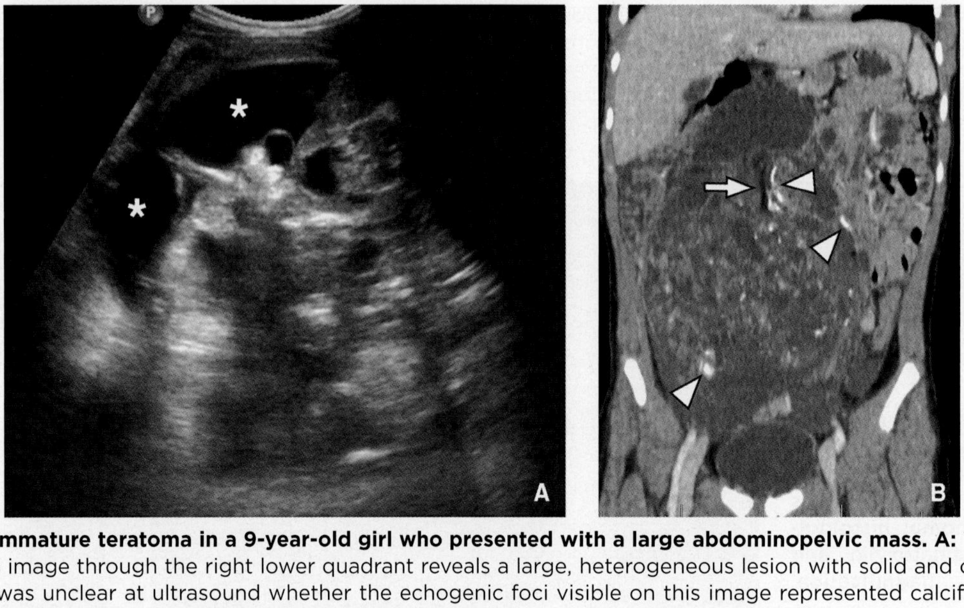

FIGURE 19.28 **Immature teratoma in a 9-year-old girl who presented with a large abdominopelvic mass. A:** Transverse grayscale ultrasound image through the right lower quadrant reveals a large, heterogeneous lesion with solid and cystic (*asterisks*) components. It was unclear at ultrasound whether the echogenic foci visible on this image represented calcification or bowel gas. **B:** Contrast-enhanced coronal-reformatted CT image demonstrates a very large, heterogeneous cystic and solid-appearing mass containing foci of fat (*arrow*) and calcification (*arrowheads*).

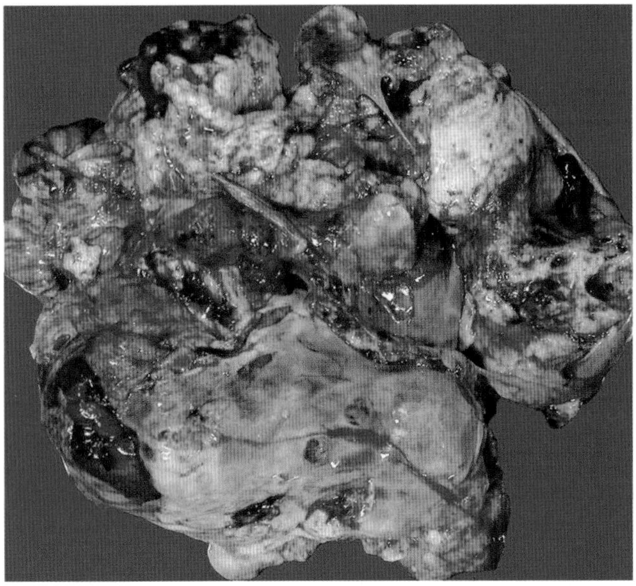

FIGURE 19.29 **This pure yolk sac tumor from a 16-year-old girl's ovary is large (20 cm), multinodular, soft, pale yellow tan, and hemorrhagic.**

Although juvenile GCTs tumors can be large at presentation, averaging 12.5 cm,[14] about 90% carry a good prognosis.[20] They are bilateral in only 2% to 5% of cases.[14] These tumors usually have both solid and cystic components (Figs. 19.30 and 19.31), although completely solid or cystic lesions may occur. At ultrasound, the solid component appears isoechoic to myometrium and contains color Doppler signal.[14] Solid portions enhance at CT and MRI, and they often have a sponge-like appearance on T2-weighted MR imaging with intermediate signal stroma and innumerable internal cysts.[1,14] Hemorrhage is seen in up to 70% of lesions, and calcification is rare. Ascites and peritoneal metastases may be present. Treatment includes salpingo-oophorectomy, which is usually curative. The role of chemotherapy is unclear, but may be warranted as adjuvant therapy for those patients with metastatic disease or residual local disease postoperatively.[52] Follow-up often includes imaging and measurements of serum inhibin, a hormonal marker secreted by granulosa cells.[7]

Sertoli-Leydig cell tumors are rare SCSTs, and though they can be associated with virilization, 60% to 70% are nonfunctional.[7,52] Seventy-five percent of patients with SCST are 30 years of age or younger. These tumors are frequently malignant, and the retiform and heterologous histological types in particular are associated with aggressive behavior.[52] They may be associated with pleuropulmonary blastoma or other tumors associated with DICER1 mutation (Fig. 19.32).[59] Although these tumors are often large,[52] most are stage 1 at diagnosis.[20] They are most commonly solid hypoechoic ovarian masses at ultrasound, have a solid-enhancing appearance at CT, and demonstrate intermediate to low signal intensity on T2-weighted MRI sequences.[60] Cystic components may be present, however, and these lesions may appear indistinguishable from juvenile GCTs[7,60] (Fig. 19.33). Tumors in children with virilization may be too small to identify with imaging.[20] Surgical resection is sufficient for those with stage 1 disease, but adjuvant chemotherapy has been shown to be beneficial for patients with more advanced disease.[61]

Miscellaneous malignant primary pediatric ovarian neoplasms include Burkitt lymphoma and small cell carcinoma of the hypercalcemic type.[7] Burkitt lymphoma is most common in childhood and adolescence. Primary ovarian disease may occur in sporadic, endemic, or immunodeficiency-associated Burkitt lymphoma. Bilateral ovarian disease is more common in Burkitt lymphoma than in other primary ovarian lymphomas.[62] Radiographically, ovarian Burkitt lymphoma appears as enlarged, heterogeneous ovaries with preserved peripheral follicles.[7,63] Small cell carcinoma of the hypercalcemic type is a rare and aggressive malignancy of unclear cell lineage, with intra-abdominal spread often seen. These lesions usually occur in females between the ages of 9 to 43 years and are frequently associated with hypercalcemia.[7,64] Their imaging appearance is nonspecific, most commonly a solid ovarian mass with or without necrosis.[7] Confusion with juvenile GCT may occur.[7]

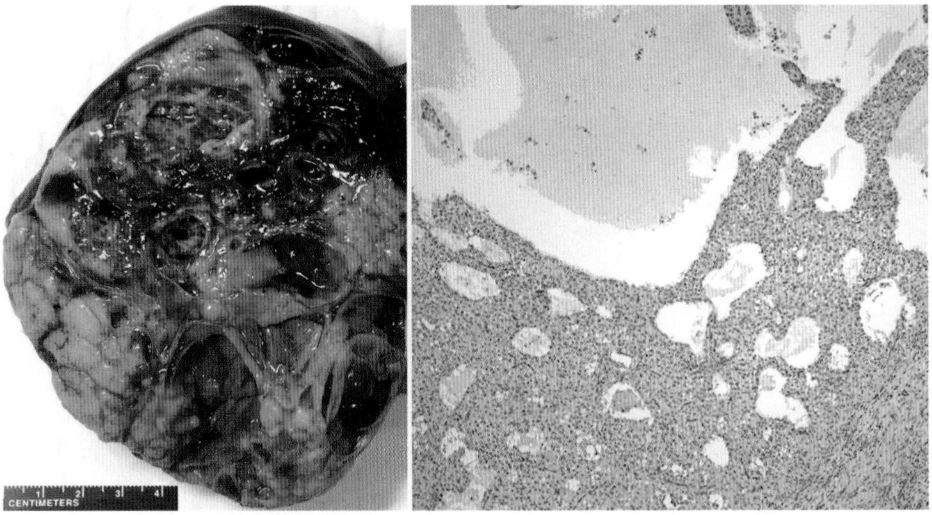

FIGURE 19.30 **This juvenile granulosa cell tumor is a 12.5 cm mass from the ovary of a 2-year-old girl.** Grossly, the mass is soft with cystic and solid components **(left)**. Microscopically, monotonous cells resembling granulosa cells for solid sheets as well as cystic spaces recapitulating follicles are seen (**right**, hematoxylin and eosin, original magnification, 100×).

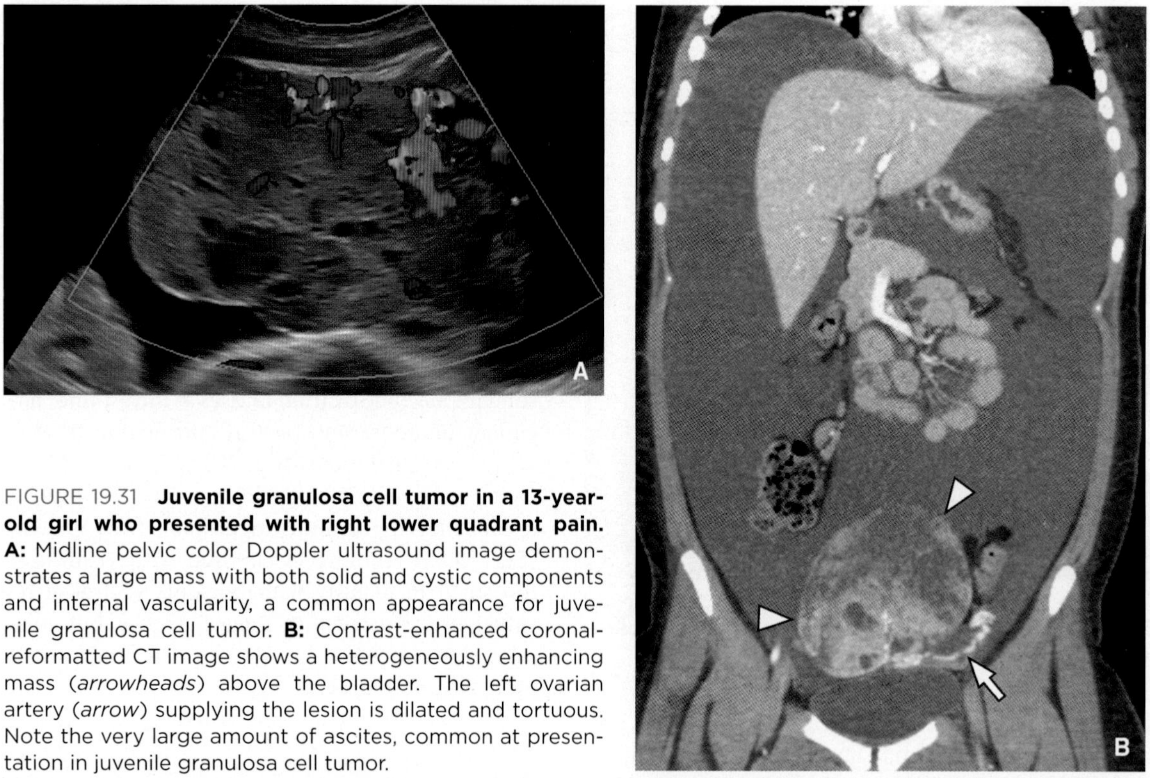

FIGURE 19.31 **Juvenile granulosa cell tumor in a 13-year-old girl who presented with right lower quadrant pain.** **A:** Midline pelvic color Doppler ultrasound image demonstrates a large mass with both solid and cystic components and internal vascularity, a common appearance for juvenile granulosa cell tumor. **B:** Contrast-enhanced coronal-reformatted CT image shows a heterogeneously enhancing mass (*arrowheads*) above the bladder. The left ovarian artery (*arrow*) supplying the lesion is dilated and tortuous. Note the very large amount of ascites, common at presentation in juvenile granulosa cell tumor.

Metastases to the ovary are uncommon in children.[7] Hematogenous spread is the most common mechanism of metastasis to the ovary with intra-abdominal desmoplastic round cell tumor, rhabdomyosarcoma, Wilms tumor, neuroblastoma, and retinoblastoma being among the most common neoplasms.[7] Bilateral lesions are seen in more than half of cases of ovarian metastasis (Fig. 19.34). Evidence of metastases to other abdominal organs helps to confirm the diagnosis.

Ovarian (Adnexal) Torsion

Torsion can involve the ovary, the fallopian tube, or both structures.[1] Ovarian torsion results from twisting of the suspensory ligament of the ovary containing the ovarian artery. An adnexal or ovarian mass commonly serves a lead point in about half of torsion cases. The right ovary is more commonly involved than the left,[1,47] although the reason for the right-sided predilection is unclear. Proposed reasons include that the sigmoid mesentery serves to better anchor the left ovary or that the increased mobility of the cecum and distal ileum allow more adnexal mobility on the right.[1,65] Children are less likely to have an associated mass in the setting of adnexal torsion in comparison to adults because of adnexal hypermobility.[13,38,65] There is a bimodal age distribution for the occurrence of adnexal torsion in children with peaks in the neonatal period and in early adolescence,[1,47,66] presumably related to ovarian hormonal stimulation and associated enlargement/cyst formation. Undetected adnexal torsion in the neonate can lead to autoamputation with involution of the ovary.[1,33,35]

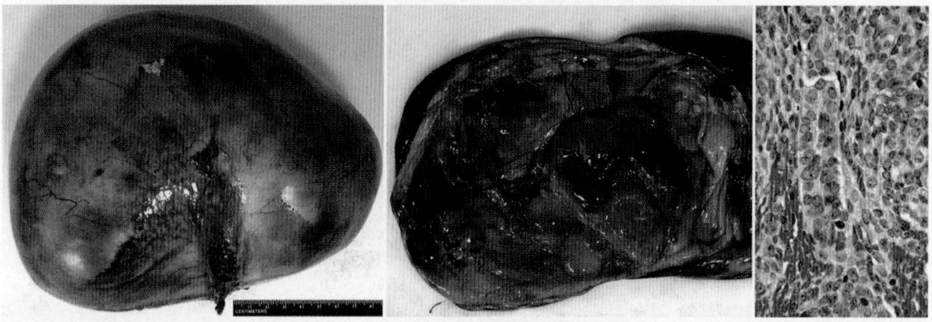

FIGURE 19.32 **This 22 cm Sertoli-Leydig cell tumor from an 18-year-old girl with DICER1 tumor predisposition syndrome is largely cystic (left and middle panels).** Microscopically, tumor cells show areas of tubular architecture (**right** panel, hematoxylin and eosin, original magnification, 600×).

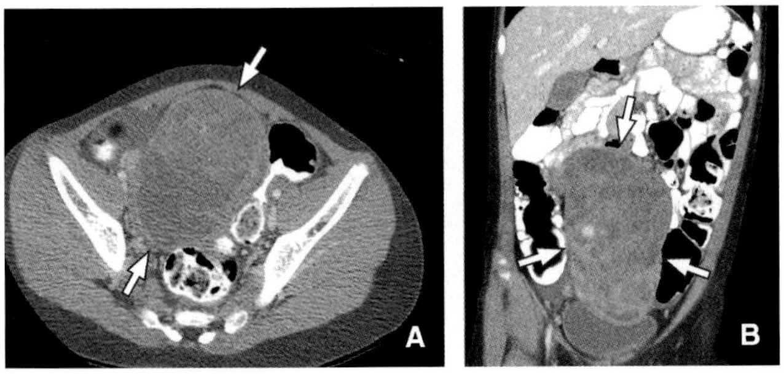

FIGURE 19.33 **An 8-year-old girl with a palpable pelvic mass.** Contrast-enhanced axial **(A)** and coronal **(B)** reformatted CT images show a large, heterogeneously enhancing mostly solid mass (*arrows*) arising from the pelvis that was proven to be a Sertoli-Leydig cell tumor at histopathology. (Case courtesy of Jonathan R. Dillman, MD, MSc, Cincinnati Children's Hospital Medical Center, Cincinnati, OH.)

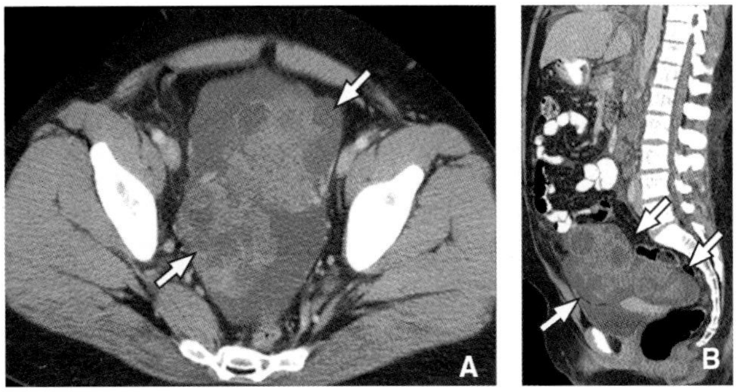

FIGURE 19.34 **A 16-year-old girl with widespread metastatic alveolar rhabdomyosarcoma at initial presentation.** Contrast-enhanced axial **(A)** and coronal **(B)** reformatted CT images reveal bilaterally enlarged, hyperenhancing ovaries (*arrows*) due to biopsy-proven metastatic disease. (Case courtesy of Jonathan R. Dillman, MD, MSc, Cincinnati Children's Hospital Medical Center, Cincinnati, OH.)

In adolescents with adnexal torsion, the clinical presentation is most commonly acute onset of ipsilateral pelvic pain, sometimes accompanied by nausea and vomiting. Pelvic pain can be intermittent because of twisting and untwisting of the involved adnexa with engorgement resulting from obstructed venous outflow.[66] White blood cell count and erythrocyte sedimentation rate may be normal or slightly elevated, and there may be sterile pyuria[66] and low-grade fever.[15,67]

The imaging findings of adnexal torsion are variable. Initially, venous and lymphatic outflow are compromised resulting in ovarian engorgement. With prolonged or progressive torsion, the arterial supply becomes obstructed with vascular thrombosis and eventual ovarian infarction, often with associated hemorrhage.[67] The involved ovary may adopt a midline position because of the twisting of the adnexa.[1] Comparison of ovarian volumes is critical because the affected ovary is usually enlarged, and a difference in size between the ovaries of more than 15-fold is predictive for ovarian torsion[68] (Fig. 19.35). The presence of a pelvic "mass" of 5 cm diameter or more also has a high sensitivity for ovarian torsion.[1,47] Linam et al. found a 100% negative predictive value for ovarian torsion with an adnexal volume of 20 mL or less.[68] A 20-fold difference in the ovarian volumes is predictive an associated ovarian mass.[1]

At ultrasound, a classic finding is that of peripherally arranged small follicles in an enlarged ovary, known as the "string of pearls" sign[67] (Figs. 19.35 and 19.36), while very specific for ovarian torsion, but is seen in <50% of cases.[1] If ovarian arterial and venous blood flow are absent on color and spectral Doppler ultrasound, these findings are also specific for torsion (Fig. 19.35); however, the presence of blood flow within the ovary does not exclude torsion.[1,67] Persistent ovarian blood flow may be seen despite torsion due to the dual blood supply from both the uterine and ovarian circulations or due to partial twisting of the vessels without complete occlusion at the time of imaging.[13] Swirling of the vascular pedicle, the "whirlpool" sign, is a useful finding, and

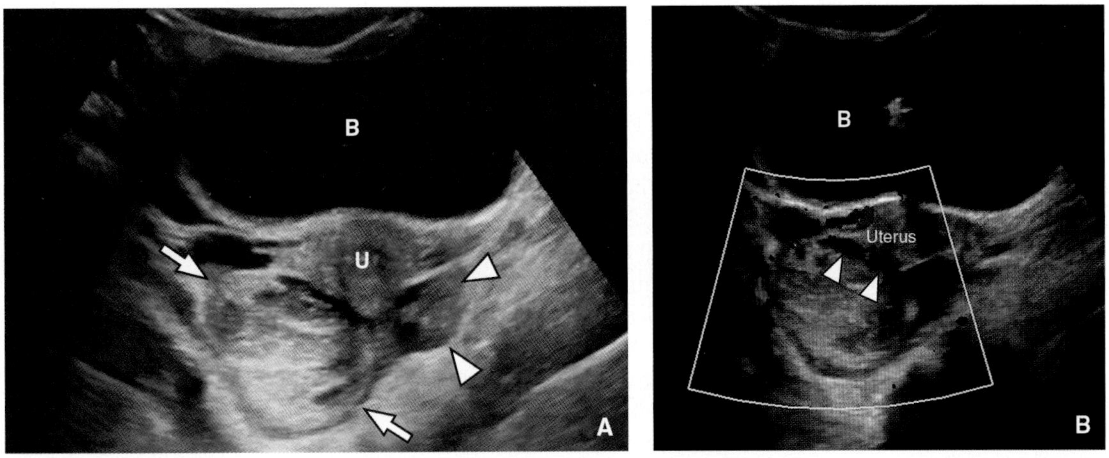

FIGURE 19.35 **Ovarian torsion in a 14-year-old girl with acute pelvic pain. A:** Transverse gray-scale ultrasound image reveals an enlarged, heterogeneous right ovary (*arrows*) that is larger than the left ovary (*arrowheads*) (60 mL vs. 6 mL). **B:** There is a cluster of peripherally arranged follicles (*arrowheads*) in the enlarged, heterogeneous right ovary. There is no color Doppler signal in the right ovary. These findings are specific for ovarian torsion. The right ovary was found to be torsed at surgery, but reperfused upon manual detorsion. *B*, bladder; *U*, uterus.

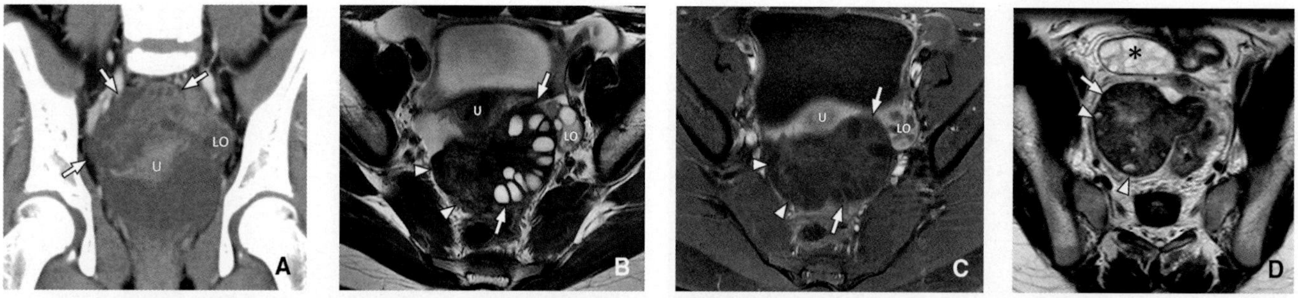

FIGURE 19.36 **Ovarian torsion in a 14-year-old girl with right pelvic pain. A:** Contrast-enhanced coronal-reformatted CT image shows a heterogeneously enhancing pelvic mass with peripheral cysts, consistent with an enlarged, torsed right ovary (*arrows*). **B:** An axial T2-weighted MR image shows the enlarged right ovary (*arrows*) with numerous peripherally arranged follicles—"string of pearls" sign. The thickened fallopian tube (*arrowheads*) is to the right of the torsed ovary. Right ovary parenchyma is abnormally hypointense. **C:** Axial postcontrast T1-weighted fat-saturated MR image shows no enhancement of the torsed right ovary (*arrows*) and fallopian tube (*arrowheads*). Normal enhancement is seen in the left ovary (*LO*) and uterus (*U*). **D:** Axial T2-weighted MR image in a different patient demonstrates heterogeneously low signal in the torsed left ovary (*arrow*) likely due to stromal hemorrhage and edema. Peripheral high T2 signal follicles are visible (*arrowheads*). The right ovary is normal (*asterisk*). This was confirmed to represent a torsed left ovary at laparoscopy, and salpingo-oophorectomy was performed.

when combined with an enlarged ovary is diagnostic of ovarian torsion.[1,67]

CT and MRI findings include ovarian enlargement and decreased or absent postcontrast enhancement from reduced blood flow or infarction.[38,67] Torsed ovaries are also commonly hypointense on T2-weighted MR images. Additional findings include deviation of the uterus to the affected side, ovarian hemorrhage, engorged pelvic blood vessels, twisting of the ovarian vascular pedicle, and fallopian tube wall thickening.[38,65,67] Although CT and MRI are not first-line imaging modalities for evaluating acute pelvic pain in children, the clinical presentation of torsion may mimic acute appendicitis or an obstructing ureteral calculus, and, therefore, CT or MRI may be the initial study performed. Familiarity with the appearance of torsion on these modalities is needed to reach the correct diagnosis in such instances (Fig. 19.36).

Isolated fallopian tube torsion is rare in all age groups. Postulated etiologies of isolated tubal torsion include paraovarian or paratubal masses, infection, adhesions, venous congestion, and trauma.[1,69] Imaging findings include a fusiform, dilated, fluid-filled tubular structure with tapered ends that may have incomplete septa, areas of "beaking," and internal hemorrhage (including fluid–fluid levels)[15] (Fig. 19.37). Adjacent edema and free fluid are also common findings. Identification of a discrete, normal appearing ovary is helpful in confirming the correct diagnosis.

Management of ovarian torsion requires early and accurate diagnosis in order to prevent infarction.[65,66] Although normal ovarian function has been reported up to 72 hours after onset of symptoms, viability decreases after 48 hours of torsion.[70] Because the incidence of underlying malignancy in pediatric ovaries is low, detorsion is generally indicated rather than oophorectomy,[65] with cystectomy if appropriate. Nonviable ovaries are typically resected (Fig. 19.38). Follow-up ultrasound can be used to assess ovarian recovery. The need for oophoropexy of the detorsed ovary is a matter of debate.[66]

SPECTRUM OF FALLOPIAN TUBE, UTERINE, VAGINAL, AND VULVAR DISORDERS

Congenital and Developmental Anomalies

Uterine (Mullerian Duct) Anomalies

The Mullerian (or paramesonephric) ducts are the precursors of the female genital tract from which the fallopian tubes, uterus, cervix, and the upper two-thirds of the vagina develop.[1,5] The lower one-third of the vagina develops from the urogenital sinus,[13] and therefore, vaginal anomalies and anomalies of the external genitalia are not always associated with Mullerian duct anomalies. The incidence of Mullerian duct anomalies (MDAs) as a class of anomalies is reported as 5% to 6% in the general population, but may be as high as 25% in infertility patients.[5] Associated anomalies include renal and urinary tract malformations, anorectal malformations, abnormal ovarian position, and skeletal anomalies. Fetuses with unilateral renal agenesis on prenatal ultrasound should be examined for abnormalities of the reproductive system postnatally[1,71] as the incidence of associated female genital tract anomalies has been reported to be between 37% and 60%.[71]

Ultrasound in the neonatal period sometimes can be helpful for evaluating suspected MDAs due to the uterus' prominent size related to maternal hormonal stimulation.[1] Once the maternal hormonal effects subside, however, the small size of the uterus (and its tubular appearance) limits accurate assessment. Follow-up genital tract evaluation after puberty is often warranted when MDA is suspected.[5] Transabdominal ultrasound may be sufficient for diagnosing MDAs in older children; however, findings may be inconclusive. Transvaginal ultrasound provides more detailed imaging, but is less often employed in the pediatric population. MRI is considered to be the imaging modality of choice for MDA evaluation,[72,73]

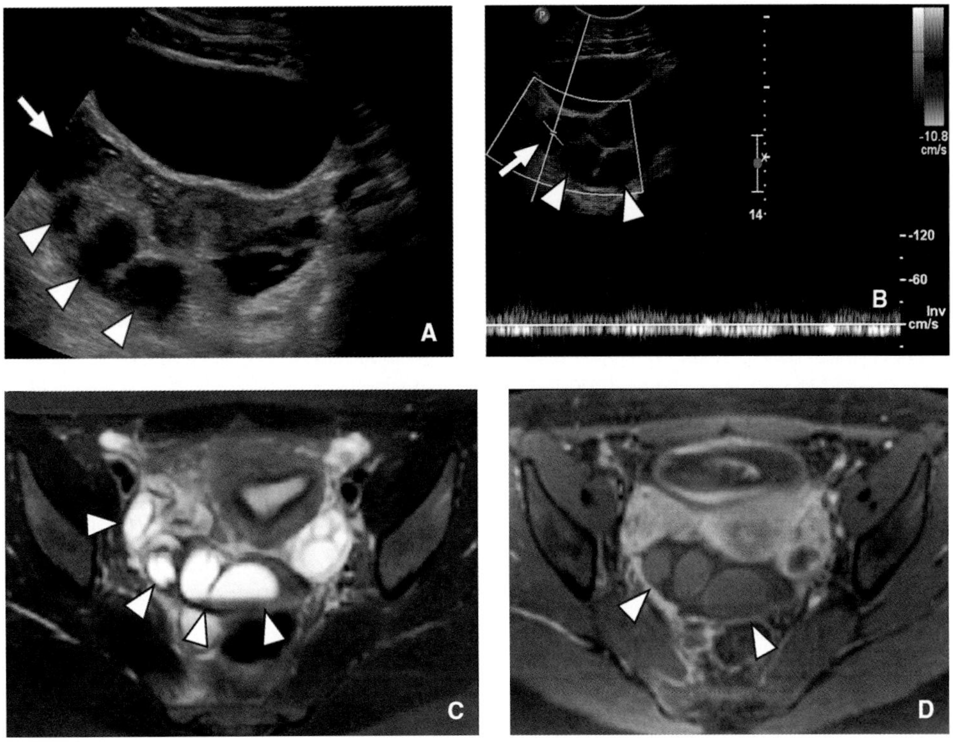

FIGURE 19.37 **Fallopian tube torsion in a 13-year-old girl with acute pelvic pain. A:** Transverse gray-scale ultrasound through the pelvis reveals a serpentine, fluid-filled, thick-walled tubular structure in the right adnexa representing the dilated fallopian tube (*arrowheads*). The right ovary is normal (*arrow*). **B:** Spectral Doppler ultrasound image demonstrates arterial blood flow within the normal right ovary (*arrow*). Again, notice the appearance of the abnormal right fallopian tube (*arrowheads*). **C:** Axial T2-weighted fat-saturated MR image also shows the right fallopian tube to be tortuous and dilated (*arrowheads*), containing a fluid-fluid level. There is ill-defined increased T2-weighted signal in the surrounding adnexal soft tissues due to inflammation. **D:** Axial postcontrast T1-weighted fat-saturated MR image demonstrates absence of mural enhancement in the torsed right fallopian tube (*arrowheads*), whereas the surrounding adnexal soft tissues enhance. At surgery, isolated right fallopian tube torsion was confirmed. The fallopian tube was necrotic, but the right ovary was normal.

with a diagnostic accuracy approaching 100% in adolescents.[5] Advantages of MRI include its multiplanar imaging capability (and its ability to acquire images along the long- and short axes of the uterus) and ability to characterize differing tissues and detect blood products.

Assessment of the kidneys and renal collecting systems is recommended in patients with MDAs because up to 40% of the patients have concomitant renal and urinary tract anomalies, such as unilateral renal agenesis, hypoplasia/dysplasia, ectopia, horseshoe kidney, and hydronephrosis.[1,5,73] Coronal T2-weighted MR imaging of the pelvis and renal fossae is often employed as part of MRI examinations performed to evaluate for MDAs.[5]

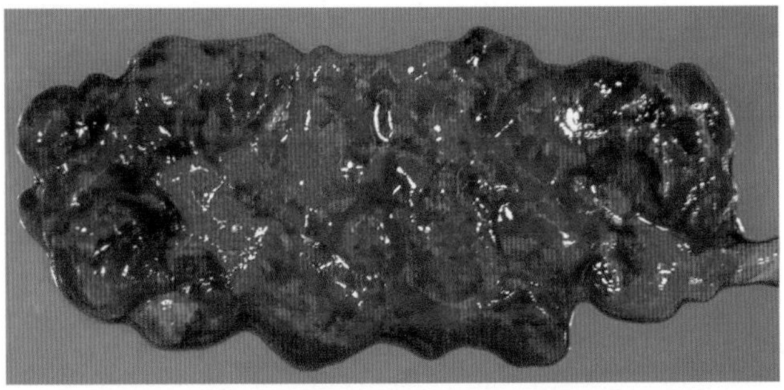

FIGURE 19.38 **Hemorrhagic infarction resulting from ovarian torsion blocking venous outflow in a 7-year-old girl.** The necrotic ovary is enlarged, soft, and maroon.

Uterine congenital anomalies are classified by morphology and prognosis for pregnancy outcome/fetal survival (Table 19.3; Fig. 19.39); however, application of the system proposed by the American Society of Reproductive Medicine (ASRM) may be problematic in children because of organ immaturity. A thorough description of genital tract anatomy and associated anomalies is a recommended approach for radiologists.[5] Discussion with the medical team caring for the child prior to surgical intervention is crucial, as success with the first attempt at genital tract reconstruction and relief of outflow obstruction is associated with best outcomes.[5]

The ASRM classifies congenital uterine anomalies into six categories:

Class I

Failure of development of the Mullerian ducts at 5 weeks' gestation results in aplasia/hypoplasia of the fallopian tubes, uterus, and/or upper vagina, comprising 5% to 10% of MDAs.[1,5] Type I Meyer-Rokitansky-Kuster-Hauser (MRKH) syndrome is complete agenesis of the Mullerian ducts (Fig. 19.40). When there are associated unilateral

TABLE 19.3 American Society of Reproductive Medicine (ASRM) Classification of Mullerian Duct Anomalies[72]

MSRM Classification	Defect/Anomaly	Uterus	Fallopian Tubes	Cervix	Vagina
Class I	1a Vaginal hypoplasia/ agenesis	Present	Present	Present	Hypoplastic or absent upper two-thirds
	1b Cervical hypoplasia/agenesis	Present	Present	Hypoplastic or atretic	Present
	1c Fundal hypoplasia/ agenesis	Hypoplastic or atretic fundus/corpus	Present	Present	Present
	1d Fallopian tube hypoplasia/ agenesis	Present	Hypoplastic or atretic	Present	Present
	1e Combined	Hypoplastic or atretic	Hypoplastic or atretic	Hypoplastic or atretic	Hypoplastic or atretic
Class II	Unicornuate uterus	Type 1: rudimentary horn connects to primary horn	Hypoplastic on the involved side	Single	Normal
		Type 2: rudimentary horn does not communicate			
		Type 3: rudimentary horn has no cavity			
		Type 4: complete absence of one horn			
Class III	Uterus didelphys	2 discrete horns separated by a deep cleft. One side may be obstructed.	One side may be dilated due to obstruction.	2 cervices	Longitudinal septum common. One side may be hypoplastic/ obstructed as in OHVIRA[a]/ Herlyn-Wunder-Werlich syndrome
Class IV	Bicornuate uterus	2 separate horns that fuse at some point in the body above the cervix. Outer contour of the fundus has a cleft of at least 1 cm.	Normal	One (unicollis) or 2 (bicollis)	Normal, usually
Class V	Septate uterus	Persistence of all or part of the septum remaining after Mullerian duct fusion. Uterine fundus has no cleft, but may be subtly concave	Normal	Normal	Normal, usually. Rarely, septum may extend inferiorly into the cervix or vagina
Class VI	Arcuate uterus	Near-complete septal resorption with a residual concavity of the contour of the uterine cavity.	Normal	Normal	Normal

TABLE 19.3 American Society of Reproductive Medicine (ASRM) Classification of Mullerian Duct Anomalies[72] *(Continued)*

MSRM Classification	Defect/Anomaly	Uterus	Fallopian Tubes	Cervix	Vagina
Class VII	T-shaped uterus	Irregular T-shaped endometrial cavity with irregularity and adhesions due to diethylstilbestrol exposure	Normal	Cervical adenosis[74] and increased risk of clear cell carcinoma[75]	Vaginal adenosis[74] and increased risk of clear cell carcinoma[75]

[a]*Obstructed **H**emi-**V**agina, **I**psilateral **R**enal **A**genesis.*

renal agenesis and vertebral anomalies, the term MURCS (**Mu**llerian agenesis, **R**enal agenesis, **C**ervicothoracic **S**omite dysplasia) can be used, also known as MRKH type II.[1,5] These disorders present as primary amenorrhea and are associated with normally developed ovaries, although ovarian position may be abnormal.[28] Although construction of a vagina can be achieved surgically,[72,76] correction of an absent or small uterus (or fallopian tubes) is not performed.[76] Imaging findings include an absent or severely hypoplastic uterus and upper vagina, normal or ectopically located ovaries, and possibly unilateral renal agenesis. Mullerian tissue, if present, appears hypointense on MRI, dysmorphic, and often lacks expected zonal anatomy.[72]

Class II

Failure of one Mullerian duct to normally develop results in a unicornuate uterus, accounting for ~20% of MDAs.[5] There are four subtypes: (1) rudimentary horn communicating with the primary horn, (2) rudimentary horn with a noncommunicating (obstructed) cavity, (3) rudimentary horn with no cavity, and (4) complete absence of one horn. About 40% of patients with unicornuate uteri have anomalies or agenesis of the ipsilateral kidney.[5] These patients may present with a palpable mass due to hematometra and hematosalpinx with dysmenorrhea due to obstruction of the rudimentary horn. Endometriosis is a recognized complication, presumably due to retrograde menstruation. Resection of a rudimentary horn is indicated both to relieve obstruction if noncommunicating and to prevent embryonic implantation in the rudimentary horn if communicating (pregnancies in rudimentary uterine horns are at increased risk of uterine rupture).[76,77]

Imaging findings depend on the subtype of rudimentary horn and include a single tubular off-midline uterine horn with normal zonal anatomy on MRI.[72] Identification of an endometrial canal in the rudimentary horn, if present, is

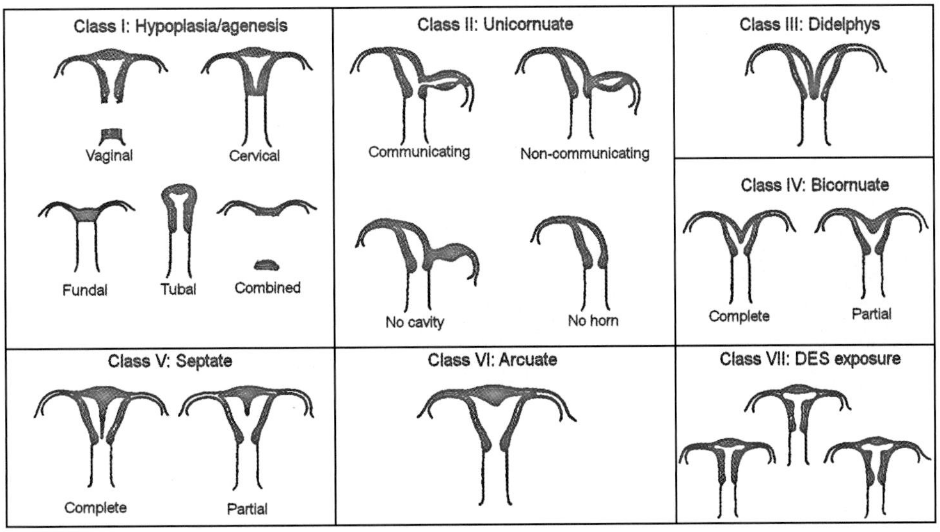

FIGURE 19.39 **Classification system for Mullerian anomalies developed by the American Fertility Society, currently the American Society for Reproductive Medicine.** (Reproduced with permission.

1209 Montgomery Highway, Birmingham, AL 35216.)

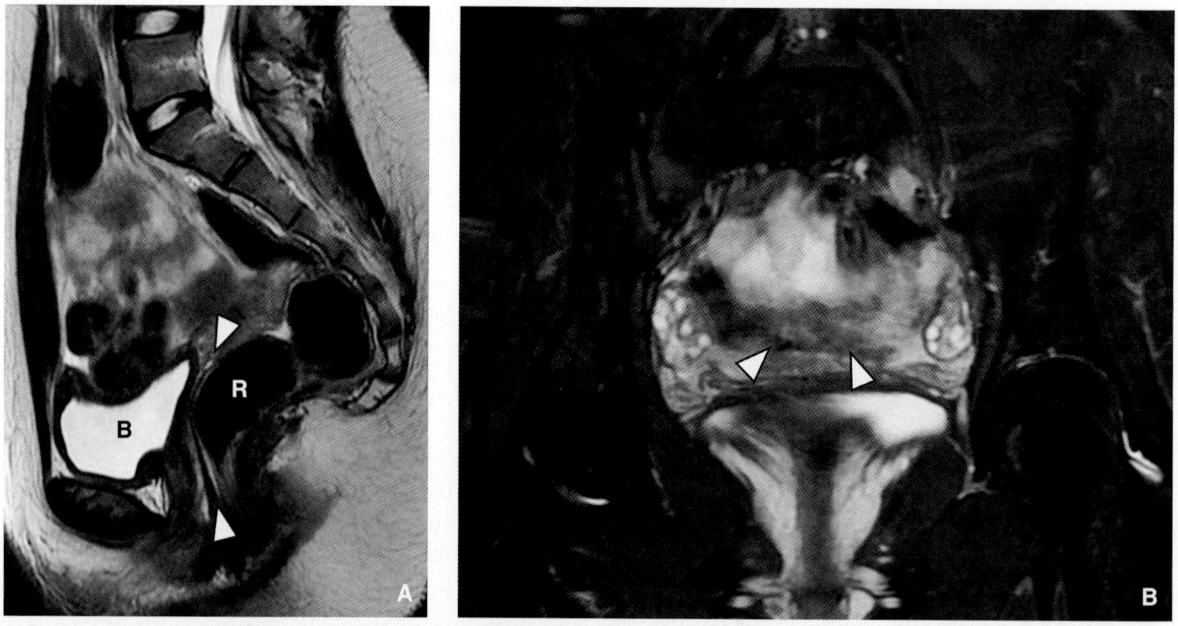

FIGURE 19.40 **A 16-year-old girl with Meyer-Rokitansky-Kuster-Hauser syndrome. A:** Sagittal T2-weighted MR image in the midline demonstrates a hypoplastic, blind-ending vagina (*arrowheads*) between the bladder (*B*) and rectum (*R*). No normal uterine tissue is identified. **B:** Coronal T2-weighted fat-saturated MR image demonstrates absence of expected normal uterine tissue posterior to the bladder; *arrowheads* indicate where the uterus should be located. Normal ovaries are present and are responsible for the normal female phenotype.

critical in correctly identifying the subtype and determines subsequent management. The less well-developed horn may simulate an adnexal mass or appear to be part of the cervix on ultrasound and has low signal intensity on MRI.[72] A more-developed communicating horn has an identifiable endometrium, whereas an obstructed rudimentary horn contains fluid (blood products) on ultrasound and MRI (T1-weighted signal hyperintensity) (Fig. 19.41).[72]

Class III

Failure of fusion of the paired Mullerian ducts results in a uterus didelphys (two separate uterine cavities and

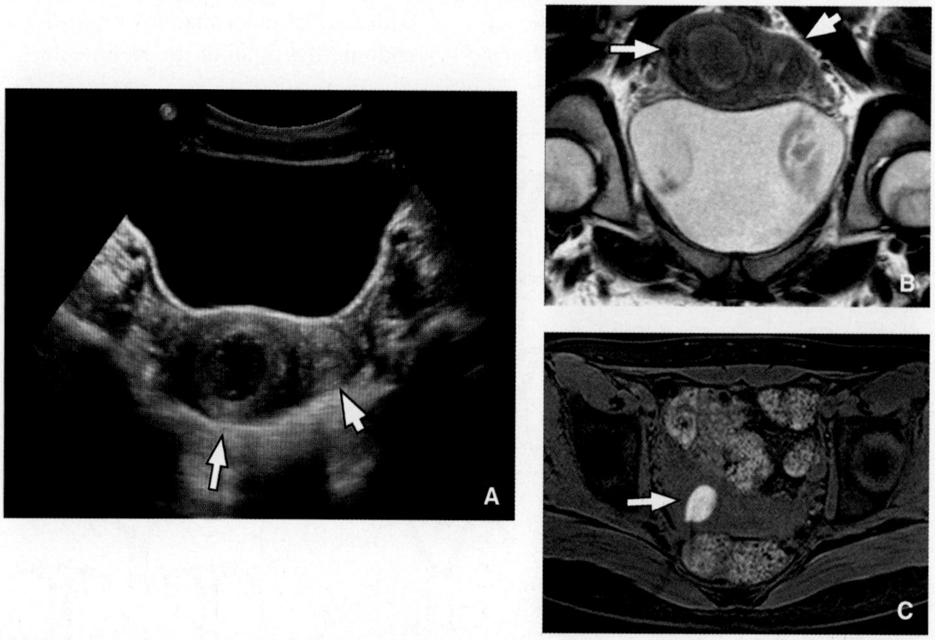

FIGURE 19.41 **An 11-year-old girl with cyclic pelvic pain. A:** Transverse gray-scale ultrasound image shows a left unicornuate uterus (*short arrow*) and an obstructed, noncommunicating right rudimentary uterine horn (*long arrow*) containing complex blood products. **B:** Coronal-oblique T2-weighted MR image shows the unobstructed left uterine horn (*short arrow*). The obstructed right uterine horn (*long arrow*) contains hypointense material, again likely blood products. **C:** Axial T1-weighted fat-saturated MR image reveals hyperintense signal (*arrow*) in the obstructed right uterine cavity confirms the presence of blood products. (Case courtesy of Jonathan R. Dillman, MD, MSc, Cincinnati Children's Hospital Medical Center, Cincinnati, OH.)

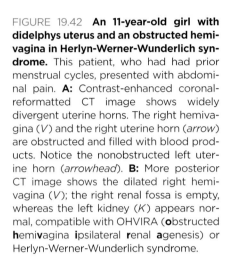

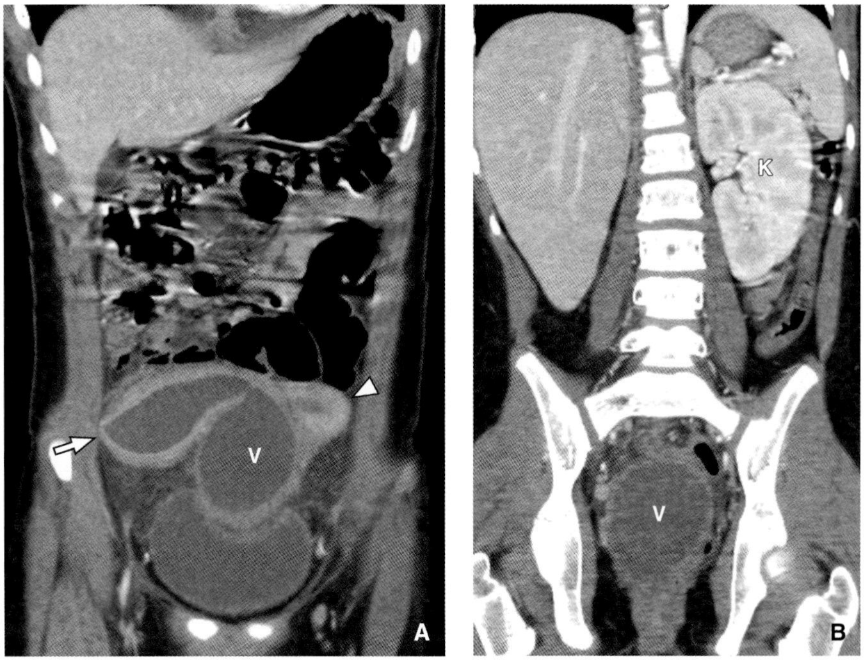

FIGURE 19.42 **An 11-year-old girl with didelphys uterus and an obstructed hemivagina in Herlyn-Werner-Wunderlich syndrome.** This patient, who had had prior menstrual cycles, presented with abdominal pain. **A:** Contrast-enhanced coronal-reformatted CT image shows widely divergent uterine horns. The right hemivagina (*V*) and the right uterine horn (*arrow*) are obstructed and filled with blood products. Notice the nonobstructed left uterine horn (*arrowhead*). **B:** More posterior CT image shows the dilated right hemivagina (*V*); the right renal fossa is empty, whereas the left kidney (*K*) appears normal, compatible with OHVIRA (**o**bstructed **h**emi**v**agina **i**psilateral **r**enal **a**genesis) or Herlyn-Werner-Wunderlich syndrome.

cervices) and often nonfusion of the upper vaginal tracts, commonly with a transverse vaginal septum causing obstruction on one side.[72] A very deep cleft should be present between the uterine horns. This class of anomalies accounts for 5% of uterine anomalies.[5] When associated with obstruction of one hemivagina and ipsilateral renal agenesis, the terms OHVIRA (**o**bstructed **h**emi**v**agina **i**psilateral **r**enal **a**genesis) or Herlyn-Werner-Wunderlich syndrome can be used (Figs. 19.42 and 19.43).[5,72,73] Because of the obstruction at the level of the vagina, hematometrocolpos and hematosalpinx are usually found, and endometriosis is a known complication.[73] Although a patent didelphys may not be detected until later in life, patients with OHVIRA typically present at menarche with nonspecific dysmenorrhea[73] and possibly a palpable mass from the dilated, obstructed vagina, uterus, and fallopian tube.[5] Because menstrual outflow does occur from the nonobstructed side, the diagnosis may not be suspected prior to imaging. Management includes relief of the vaginal obstruction by resection of the obstructing septum[76] as well as surveillance during pregnancy.

At ultrasound, differentiation of a didelphys uterus from bicornuate and septate uteri is based on the appearance of the uterine fundus, which requires a true coronal image.[72] This sometimes can be difficult to achieve with transabdominal imaging; differentiation between a didelphys and bicornuate bicollis uterus may be particularly challenging. MRI allows more detailed inspection of the uterine fundus and any associated cleft and, thus, more accurate assessment of MDAs.[72] Coronal-oblique T2-weighted MR images either acquired or reconstructed through the long axis of the uterine fundus are particularly useful for assessing the external uterine contour.[5] Visualization of the vaginal

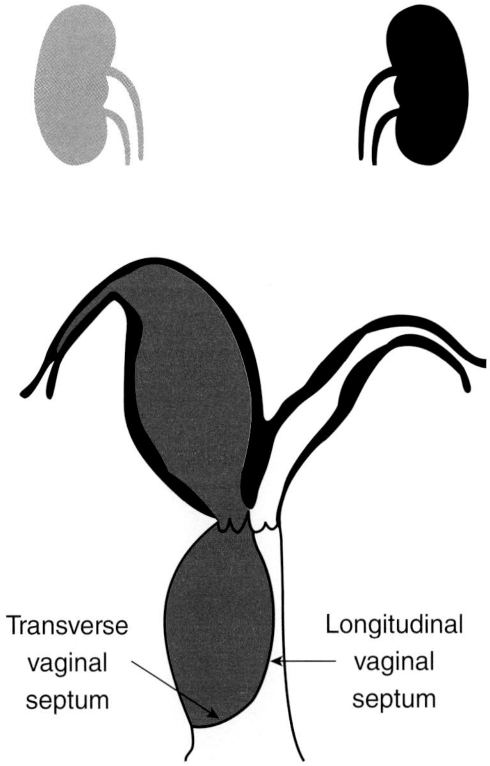

FIGURE 19.43 **Schematic representation of the congenital vaginal septa in OHVIRA (obstructed hemivagina and ipsilateral renal anomaly) or Herlyn-Werner-Wunderlich syndrome.** The longitudinal vaginal septum is the result of failure of lateral fusion of the Mullerian ducts. The transverse vaginal septum results from failure of vertical fusion between the Mullerian duct and the urogenital sinus resulting in vaginal obstruction (*red*), which is typically ipsilateral to the side of renal agenesis. (Reproduced from Epelman M, et al. Mullerian duct and related anomalies in children and adolescents. *Magn Reson Imaging Clin N Am.* 2013;21(4):773–789, with permission.)

septum can be aided by instillation of fluid into the vagina prior to MRI.[72] If there is hemivaginal obstruction, blood products, which are typically T1-weighted hyperintense, may be seen distending the obstructed vagina, ipsilateral uterus, and ipsilateral fallopian tube.

Class IV

Incomplete fusion of the Mullerian ducts results in a bicornuate uterus, accounting for 10% of MDAs.[5] A fundal cleft should be present between uterine horns measuring at least 1cm in depth, and there may be one (unicollis) or two (bicollis) cervices. Longitudinal vaginal septations may also be associated with this anomaly.[72] Surgical intervention is controversial in these cases,[77] although metroplasty may be performed in cases of recurrent miscarriage[76,78] and vaginal septoplasty in cases of outflow obstruction.[72]

At ultrasound and MRI, as with a uterus didelphys, the uterine horns should be widely separated.[72] One or two cervices may be identified. The widely divergent horns have normal MRI zonal anatomy that may fuse at the lower uterine segment[5] (Fig. 19.44) or there may be separate cervices with an "owl eyes" appearance.[72] Bicornuate bicollis uteri can be associated with longitudinal vaginal septations, making differentiation from a didelphys uterus more difficult.[72]

Class V

Failure of resorption of the septum after Mullerian duct fusion resulting in a septate uterus is the most common MDA, comprising 50% to 55% of congenital uterine anomalies.[5,72] This anomaly classically presents in adulthood with recurrent spontaneous pregnancy losses. Management of septate uteri differs greatly from other MDAs, and, therefore, differentiation is essential for proper patient management. While a bicornuate uterus may not require intervention, fibrous septal resection is important in the septate uterus to enhance the likelihood of a successful pregnancy.[76,78] Distinction between a septate uterus and bicornuate uterus is not always possible in younger children, even with MRI.[5] Further imaging may be needed after menarche when the uterus has reached its adult configuration for definitive diagnosis.

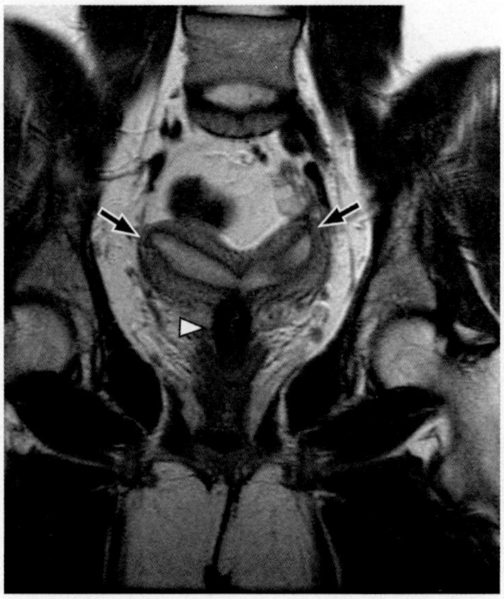

FIGURE 19.44 **A 15-year-old girl with bicornuate uterus.** Coronal T2-weighted MRI image of the pelvis demonstrates widely divergent uterine horns (*arrows*) with a single cervix (*arrowhead*). The depth of the cleft in the external contour of the uterine fundus is diagnostic of a failure of Mullerian duct fusion, either didelphys or bicornuate uterus. The single cervix is compatible with a bicornuate unicollis uterus. (Image courtesy of Jonathan R. Dillman, MD, MSc, Cincinnati Children's Hospital Medical Center, Cincinnati, OH.)

Imaging differentiation between septate and bicornuate uteri requires assessment of the outer uterine fundal contour.[5,72] The fundus may be convex, flat, or subtly concave with a depression of <1 cm in a septate uterus as opposed to the deeper convexity of >1 cm in a bicornuate uterus.[5] Accurate assessment of the external fundal contour requires a true coronal image at ultrasound,[72] which may not be possible without transvaginal ultrasound (again, a technique uncommonly used in pediatric patients[5]). Assessment of the external fundal contour with MRI is reliable in discriminating between septate and bicornuate uteri, as discussed above. At MRI, any muscular component of the septum has a signal intensity on T2-weighted MR images similar to myometrium.[72]The fibrous portion of the septum may be partial or complete and appears hypointense to myometrium.[5,72] Rarely, the septum may extend from the uterine fundus into the vagina and be associated with an obstructing transverse septum or imperforate hymen (Fig. 19.45). Because an abdominal approach is needed for resection of a muscular septum as opposed to a hysteroscopic approach for fibrous septoplasty, identification of a myometrial component of the septum is important.[72]

Class VI

Near-complete septal resorption is the cause of an arcuate uterus, considered by many to be a normal variant requiring no intervention.[5] The uterine cavity has a characteristic saddle-shaped depression at the fundus with no alteration of zonal anatomy and a convex external uterine contour.

Class VII

These anomalies consist of T-shaped uteri related to diethylstilbestrol exposure in utero. This class of abnormality is no longer seen in the pediatric population as maternal exposure to this medication has ceased.

Vaginal Anomalies

Vaginal Agenesis

Vaginal agenesis is an uncommon disorder of the female genital tract affecting ~1 in 5,000 to 10,000 live births.[79] It is characterized by absence or hypoplasia of the vagina, as well as, in most cases, the uterus and fallopian tubes related to Mullerian duct maldevelopment.[5] The vagina may be completely absent; alternatively, a short vaginal pouch or vaginal

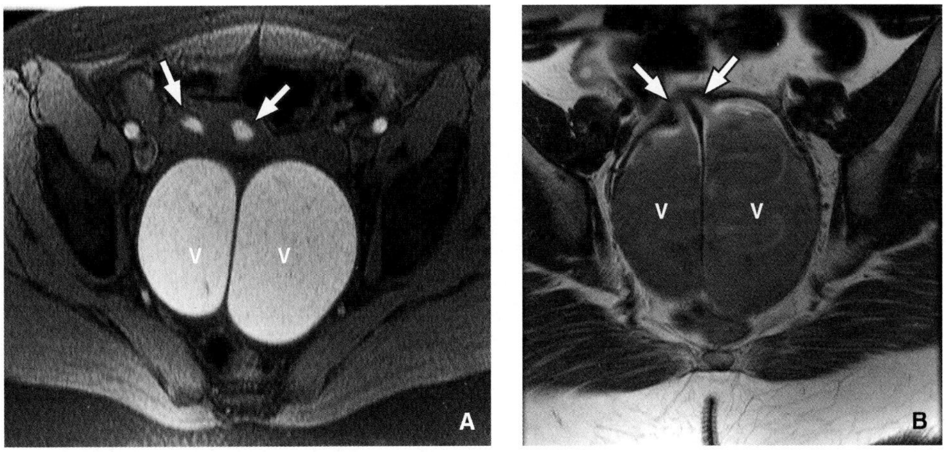

FIGURE 19.45 **An 18-year-old girl with uterocervicovaginal septum.** Axial T1-weighted fat-saturated **(A)** and coronal T2-weighted **(B)** MR images show bilateral obstructed hemivaginas (*V*) and endometrial canals (*arrows*) containing T1-weighted hyperintense and T2-weighted hypointense blood products. A longitudinal septum extends from the uterine fundus into the lower vagina. (Case courtesy of Jonathan R. Dillman, MD, MSc, Cincinnati Children's Hospital Medical Center, Cincinnati, OH.)

dimple 1 to 2 cm superior to the hymenal ring may be noted. In affected patients, the ovaries, and external genitalia are normally developed. Therefore, age-appropriate secondary sexual characteristics are present on physical examination. Complete agenesis of the vagina may be isolated or as part of MRKH syndrome.[5] Other syndromes associated with vaginal (and uterine) agenesis include Turner (45XO), Holt-Oram, Klippel-Feil, and velocardiofacial.

Although vaginal agenesis may be detected at birth, most times it is not diagnosed until puberty when affected patients present with primary amenorrhea. Although imaging evaluation may not be needed, ultrasound findings of an absent uterus and normal ovaries may supplement the clinical diagnosis of vaginal agenesis. At MRI, there is lack of visualization of the vagina and uterus between the bladder base and urethra anteriorly and rectum posteriorly on sagittal and axial images. The current management of vaginal agenesis involves surgical creation of a neovagina, typically during adolescence or adulthood.[8,80]

Vaginal Septa

Septa of the vagina may be transverse or longitudinal. Transverse septa may be due to failure of recanalization of the vaginal plate and are most commonly seen at the junction between the urogenital sinus and Mullerian portion of the vagina.[1,5,81] Transverse septa may uncommonly present in infants or neonates with hydrometrocolpos[17,81] (Fig. 19.46). The vagina, uterus, and fallopian tubes may appear fluid filled at ultrasound and MRI.[5] The more common presentation occurs in older girls at menarche with primary amenorrhea and cyclic pain[81] (Fig. 19.47). In this setting, complex fluid can be seen distending the vagina representing hematocolpos. Hyperintense blood products distend the vagina on T1-weighted MR images. Hematometra and hematosalpinx may be identified as well. Longitudinal septa are related to MDAs and are often clinically silent, but can be associated with symptoms related to menses such as difficulty with tampon insertion or tampon occlusion of only one hemivagina.[1] Obstructive symptoms occur if

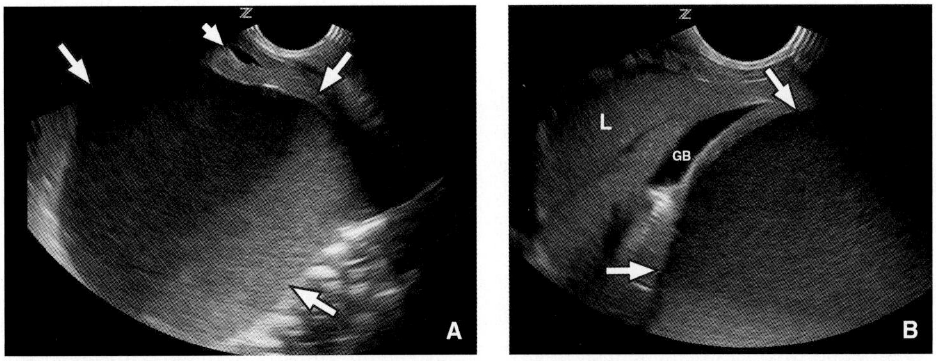

FIGURE 19.46 **A 1-day-old girl with cloaca malformation and vaginal obstruction. A:** Longitudinal gray-scale ultrasound image in the pelvic midline shows a massively dilated vagina (*long arrows*) containing a fluid–debris level posterior to the bladder (*short arrow*). **B:** Longitudinal gray-scale ultrasound image through the right upper quadrant of the abdomen shows that the fluid collection (*arrows*) extends to the inferior margin of the liver (*L*, liver; *GB*, gallbladder). (Case courtesy of Jonathan R. Dillman, MD, MSc, Cincinnati Children's Hospital Medical Center, Cincinnati, OH.)

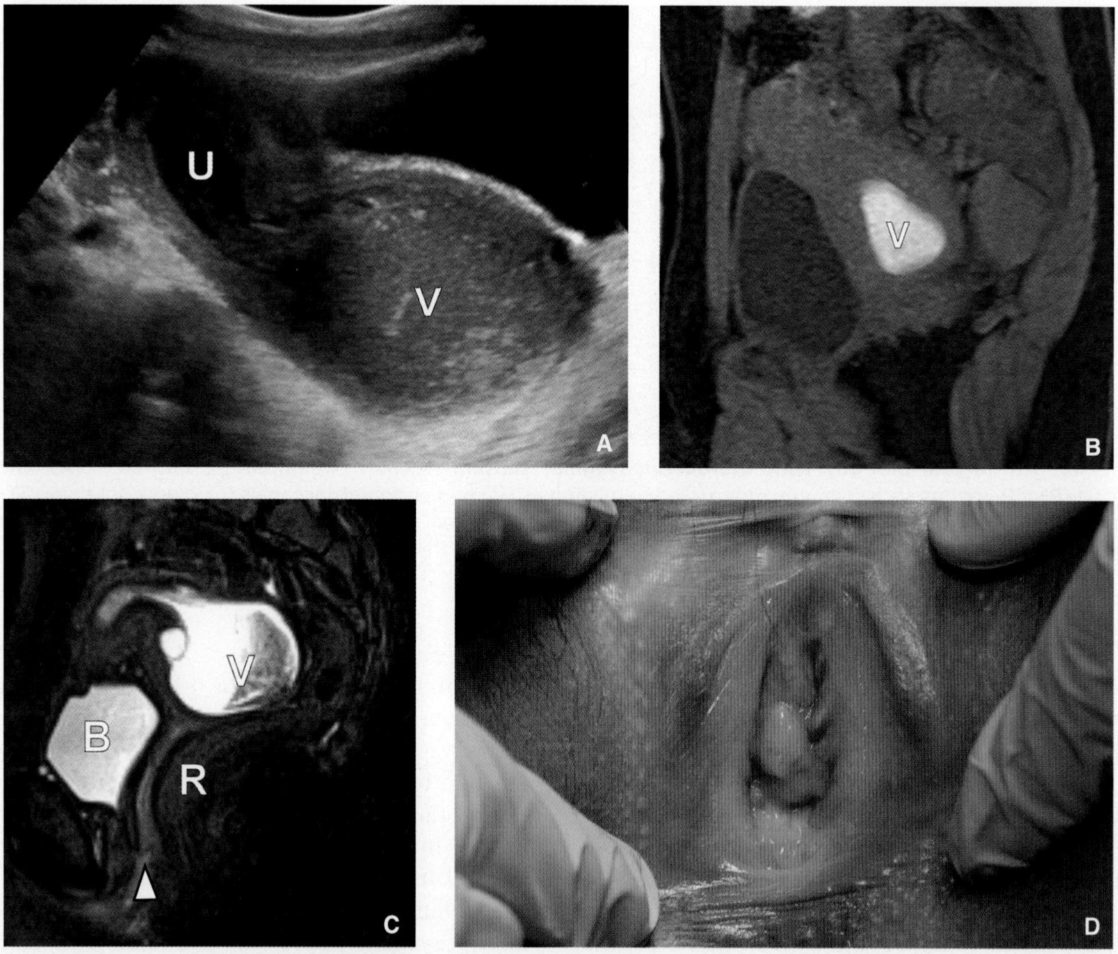

FIGURE 19.47 **A 10-year-old girl with pelvic pain and primary amenorrhea due to a transverse vaginal septum and a severely hypoplastic vagina. A:** Longitudinal ultrasound image shows distention of the vagina (*V*) with complex fluid. There is hypoechoic material in the uterus (*U*) as well. **B:** Sagittal T1-weighted fat-saturated MR image shows hyperintense material filling the upper vagina (*V*), compatible with blood products. **C:** Sagittal T2-weighted fat-saturated MR image shows uncanalized tissue (*arrowhead*) between the bladder (*B*) and rectum (*R*) with a fluid-debris level in the patent upper portion of the vagina (*V*). In this patient, it is the lower portion of the vagina derived from the urogenital sinus that is severely hypoplastic with a transverse septum. **D:** Photograph of the introitus shows no vaginal opening.

there is partial or complete hemivagina obstruction, as in OHVIRA.[5] Resection of vaginal septa is performed to relieve outflow obstruction.

Imperforate Hymen

Imperforate hymen is a common congenital abnormality of the female genital tract with a prevalence of 0.1%.[81] The hymen is a vestigial membrane remaining after recanalization of the vaginal plate. Persistence of an intact membrane generally does not come to attention until menarche when the patient develops cyclic or persistent pelvic pain and primary amenorrhea. As a result, the diagnosis is often delayed until puberty. Imperforate hymen usually occurs in isolation without other associated anomalies.[1,17,81]

Ultrasound classically demonstrates a distended blood-filled vagina (Fig. 19.48), and MRI can be beneficial in cases where the diagnosis is uncertain or the physical examination findings are more consistent with vaginal septum or agenesis.[81] Examination of the external genitalia and vaginal introitus typically reveals a perineal bulge secondary to hematocolpos making imaging often unnecessary.[81] Imperforate hymen is currently managed by partial resection of the hymen (i.e., hymenectomy) to relieve outflow obstruction.

Cloacal and Urogenital Sinus Anomalies

A persistent cloaca results from failure of the urorectal septum to reach the cloacal membrane at 4 to 5 weeks' gestation resulting in communication between the gastrointestinal and genitourinary tracts with a single perineal orifice draining the rectum, vagina, and bladder[1,82,83] (Fig. 19.49). With persistence of the urogenital sinus, there is improper development of the lower one-third of the vagina with persistent communication between the bladder outflow and vagina with one orifice and a normal, separate rectum (Figs. 19.50 and 19.51). Children with these disorders are genotypically female, although ambiguous genitalia may rarely occur.[1,82]

Hydrometrocolpos may occur in these patients, presenting as a central pelvic cystic mass at prenatal ultrasound that may contain fluid–fluid levels from mixed urine and cervical

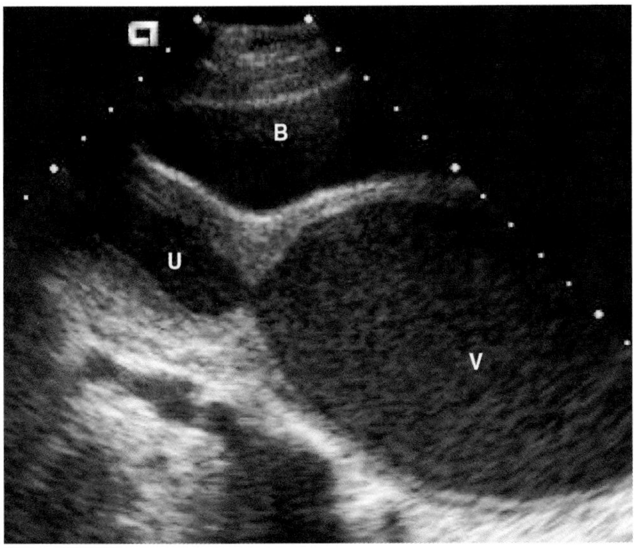

FIGURE 19.48 **A 12-year-old girl with cyclic pelvic pain due to an imperforate hymen.** Longitudinal ultrasound image through the pelvis shows hematometrocolpos. The uterus (*U*) and vagina (*V*) are distended with blood products. *B*, bladder.

secretions[1,82] or even meconium in the setting of a cloacal anomaly.[82] MDAs are common as well. Fetal MRI can be useful in assessing involvement of the rectum due to the high T1-weighted signal of meconium enabling visualization of the rectum as a discrete structure.[1,82,83] It is important to also thoroughly assess kidneys of these patients on prenatal imaging because there is a high association with renal and ureteric anomalies.[82] Postnatal assessment should begin with ultrasound, although MRI and even CT with their multiplanar capabilities may demonstrate the findings and relationships of the pelvic organs better.[82] Genitography helps clarify communications between the bladder, vagina, and rectum[9] (Figs. 19.49C and 19.51).

The goals of management for cloacal and urogenital sinus anomalies are to provide urinary and fecal continence as well as eventual sexual function through division of the urinary, gastrointestinal, and reproductive tracts. The approach to surgical repair depends upon the exact anatomic abnormalities, including the lengths of fistulous connections, as well as the integrity of the pelvic floor musculature and functionality of sacral nerves.

Vaginal Cyst

Congenital vaginal cysts are most commonly derived from Mullerian duct remnants, but can also represent Wolffian duct remnants, so-called Gartner duct cysts.[5,81] Although Mullerian cysts have multiple possible locations, Gartner duct cysts are located anteriorly and laterally in the mid to upper vagina and are above the inferior margin of the symphysis pubis[84] (Fig. 19.52). The differential diagnosis also includes urethral diverticulum (located in the midline between the urethra and vagina) and Bartholin gland cyst (located laterally in the distal vagina or labia majora (Fig. 19.53), which represent inspissated mucous in obstructed glands.[5,81,85]

Congenital vaginal cysts usually have a simple cystic appearance on ultrasound and may be detected with transperineal imaging, although differentiation from urethral diverticula can be problematic with this technique.[84] Vaginal cysts demonstrate low signal intensity on T1-weighted (Fig. 19.52) and high signal intensity on T2-weighted MR pulse sequences when uncomplicated. However, they may appear complex with increased T1-weighted signal intensity if they contain proteinaceous or hemorrhagic contents or become superinfected.[86] When Gartner duct cysts are identified, assessment of the urinary tract should be considered due to an association with renal anomalies and ureteral ectopia.[84]

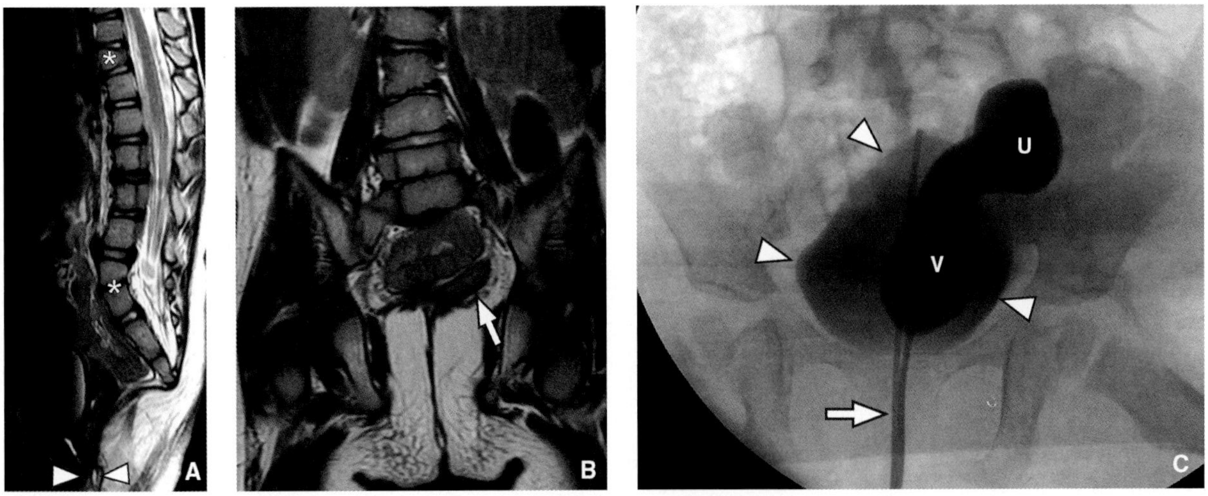

FIGURE 19.49 **Cloacal anomaly in a 2-year-old girl with a single perineal opening. A:** Sagittal T2-weighted MR image shows a single perineal opening (*arrowheads*). There are several vertebral anomalies (*asterisks*), and the sacrum is truncated. **B:** Coronal T2-weighted MR image shows a single horn of a left-sided unicornuate uterus (*arrow*). **C:** Genitogram image shows opacification of the urinary bladder (*arrowheads*) and one hemivagina (*V*) with contrast material. The left-sided unicornuate uterus (*U*) also fills with contrast material. The catheters (*arrow*) were directed anteriorly and posteriorly from the common orifice to achieve opacification of the different cavities.

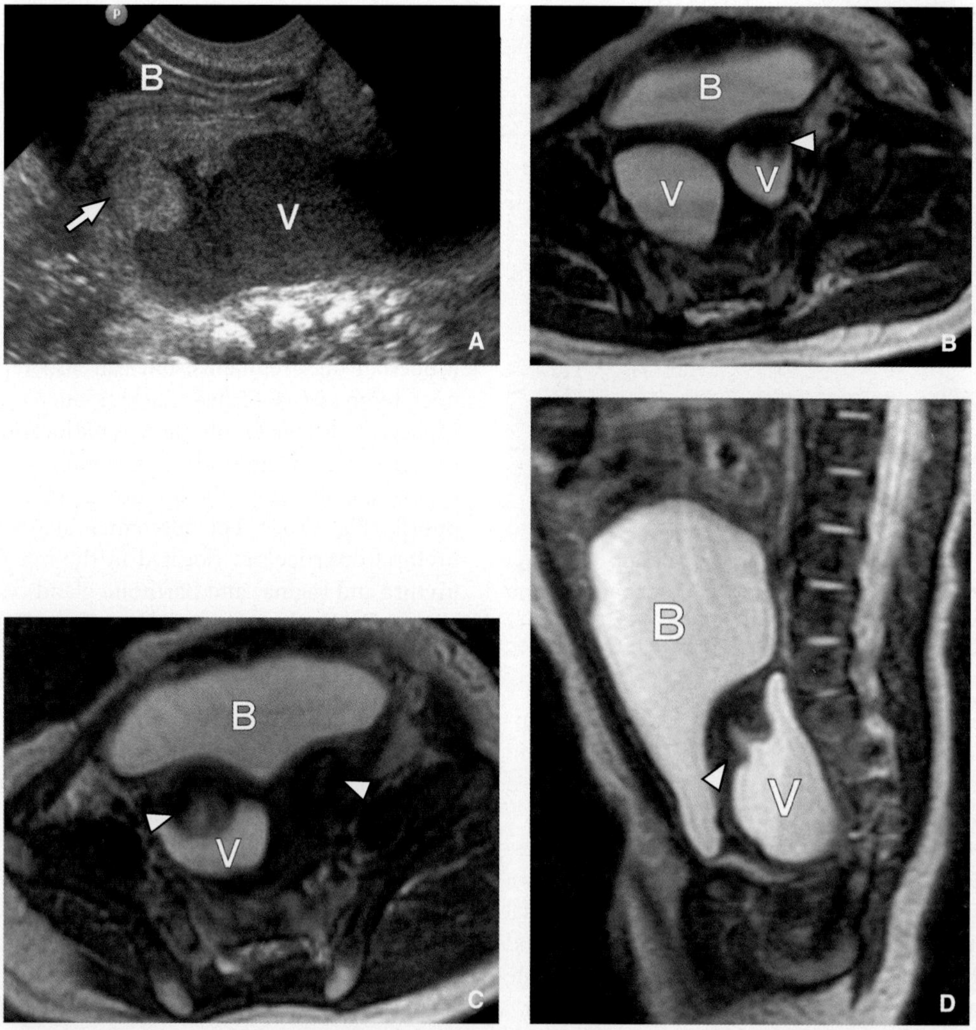

FIGURE 19.50 **Urogenital sinus in a 2-day-old girl. A:** Midline longitudinal gray-scale ultrasound image of the pelvis shows fluid and debris within a distended vagina (*V*), compatible with hydrocolpos. Vaginal obstruction occurs due to stenotic communication with the single perineal opening for the bladder and vagina. Low-level echoes are likely related to urine, cervical secretions, and even meconium in the setting of a cloaca rather than blood products. The uterus (*arrow*) is not dilated, but appears dysmorphic. The bladder (*B*) is anterior to the uterus (*arrow*) and is relatively decompressed. **B** and **C:** Consecutive axial T2-weighted MR images show two hemivaginas (*V*) distended with fluid. Two uterine cervices (*arrowheads*) are also identified in **(C)**. **D:** Sagittal T2-weighted MR image shows anterior superior bladder (*B*) displacement by the hydrocolpos. One of the cervices (*arrowhead*) is visible in the upper, fluid-filled vagina (*V*).

Uncomplicated, asymptomatic vaginal cysts require no intervention. Infected or painful cysts can be excised or marsupialized.[84]

Vulvar Anomalies

The structures of the vulva are derived embryologically from the proliferation of mesoderm and ectoderm around the cloacal membrane.[87] The soft tissue of the vulva shows bilateral swelling at birth attributed to maternal hormones.[88] Canal of Nuck cysts are remnants of the peritoneum that track through the inguinal canal with the round ligament during development similar to the processus vaginalis and gubernaculum in males.[85] After closure of the communication with the peritoneum, retained fluid within the peritoneal remnant creates a canal of Nuck cyst.[5] Lymphatic and vascular malformations can involve the vulva and may also create asymmetry. Congenital cysts of the vagina such as Gartner or Bartholin cysts may deform the labia majora and are discussed in the previous section on the vagina.

Asymmetric swelling of the vulva known as **C**hildhood **A**symmetric **L**abium **M**ajus **E**nlargement (CALME) (Fig. 19.54) is a developmental variant akin to asymmetric budding of the breast.[88,89] Awareness of this benign and usually self-limited entity is important to avoid unnecessary/deforming surgery unless the asymmetry ultimately fails to resolve to cosmetic satisfaction. Imaging findings are variable with increased ill-defined tissue within the involved labium by both US and MRI with slightly increased echogenicity and variable signal intensity.[88] Labium minus hypertrophy is an uncommon entity.[90] The enlargement may be unilateral or bilateral and may not be as relevant for radiologists as no imaging is generally required.

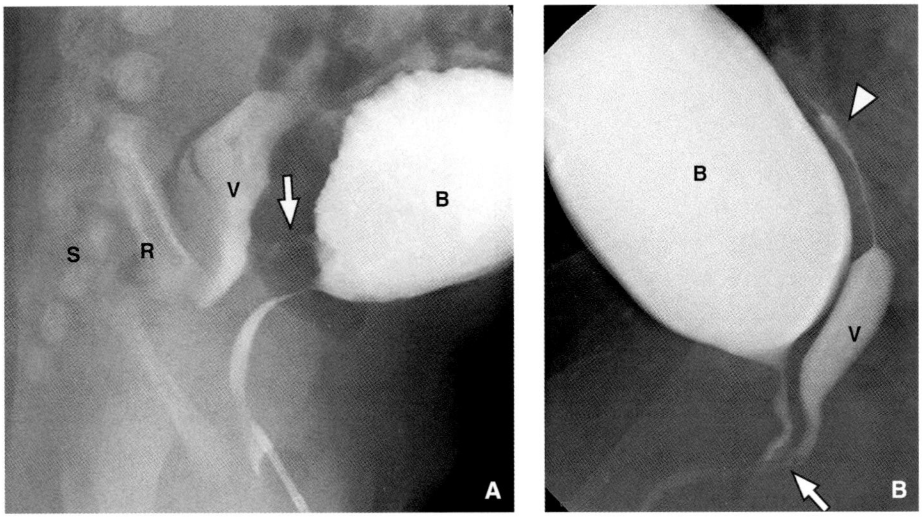

FIGURE 19.51 **Urogenital sinus and ambiguous genitalia in two different infant girls. A:** Retrograde urethrogram in this patient shows a high level of communication (*arrow*) between the bladder (*B*) and vagina (*V*). The rectum (*R*) is air-filled. The sacrum is dysplastic in appearance (*S*). **B:** Voiding cystourethrography image in another patient shows a low level of communication (*arrow*) between the distal urethra and the vagina (*V*). Note contrast opacification of the uterus (*arrowhead*). (Reproduced with permission from Servaes S, et al. Contemporary pediatric gynecologic imaging. *Semin Ultrasound CT MR.* 2010;31[2]:116–140.)

Infectious and Inflammatory Disorders

Pelvic Inflammatory Disease

The etiology of PID is typically ascending infection because of a sexually transmitted organism. The most common pathogens include *Neisseria gonorrhoeae* and *Chlamydia trachomatis*, although a substantial portion of cases are polymicrobial.[15,91] Risk factors include adolescence (opposed to adulthood), high coital frequency, multiple sexual partners, and indwelling uterine or vaginal devices.[15,91] Complications of PID include TOA, hydro- or pyosalpinx, and infertility.

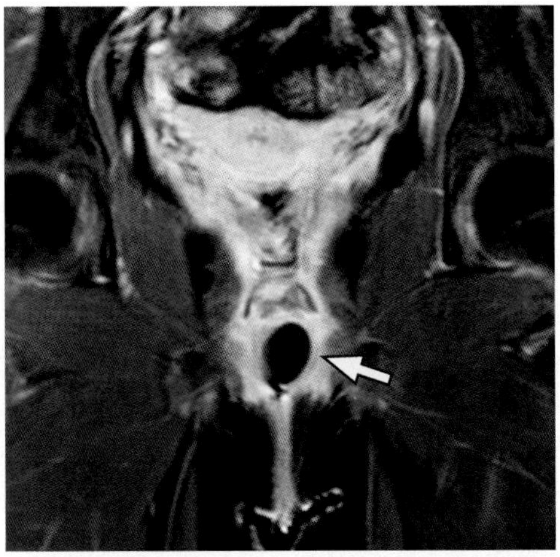

FIGURE 19.52 **A 12-year-old girl with bulging vaginal mass.** Coronal postcontrast T1-weighted fat-saturated MR image of the pelvis shows a presumed Gartner duct cyst (*arrow*) with the anterior wall of the vagina and posterior to the urethra. The lesion demonstrates only thin peripheral enhancement. The differential diagnosis includes urethral diverticulum. (Image courtesy of Jonathan R. Dillman, MD, MSc, Cincinnati Children's Hospital Medical Center, Cincinnati, OH.)

The imaging findings in uncomplicated PID are subtle and may include a loss of tissue planes between the pelvic organs or hyperemia.[91] Adjacent pelvic fat may appear echogenic and thickened at ultrasound because of edema and inflammation.[15] There may be increased endometrial or endocervical fluid as well.[91] The normal fallopian tube is generally not visualized with transabdominal ultrasound and is likely dilated if visible in the absence of ascites.[1] Hydrosalpinx and pyosalpinx are seen as a tortuous fluid-filled structure and apparent incomplete septa because of folding of the tube upon itself[15,36,91] (Figs. 19.13 and 19.55). A "waist" sign can also be seen as diametrically opposed indentations in the tubular walls.[92] The dilated tubular structure also may have a "cog-wheel" appearance due to short nodular intraluminal projections,[15,36,92] and layering debris suggests pyosalpinx in the setting of acute infection. A "bead on a string" appearance of the wall represents chronic inflammation.[36,92] At MRI and CT, pyosalpinx appears as a complex tubular structure with thick, hyperenhancing walls and adjacent inflammatory changes (Fig. 19.13).[15] The signal characteristics of fallopian tube contents at MRI may vary. If the patient denies sexual activity, secondary adnexal involvement from another process, such as ruptured appendicitis or inflammatory bowel disease, should be considered.

Management of PID is generally medical with antibiotic therapy tailored to the organism identified and regional organism sensitivities. As mentioned above, percutaneous or laparoscopic abscess drainage may be necessary in some individuals.

Endometriosis

Endometriosis is defined as the presence of endometrial glandular and stromal tissue outside the uterus, with the ovary and uterosacral ligament, and other pelvic peritoneal sites commonly involved.[38,86] Theories regarding the etiology

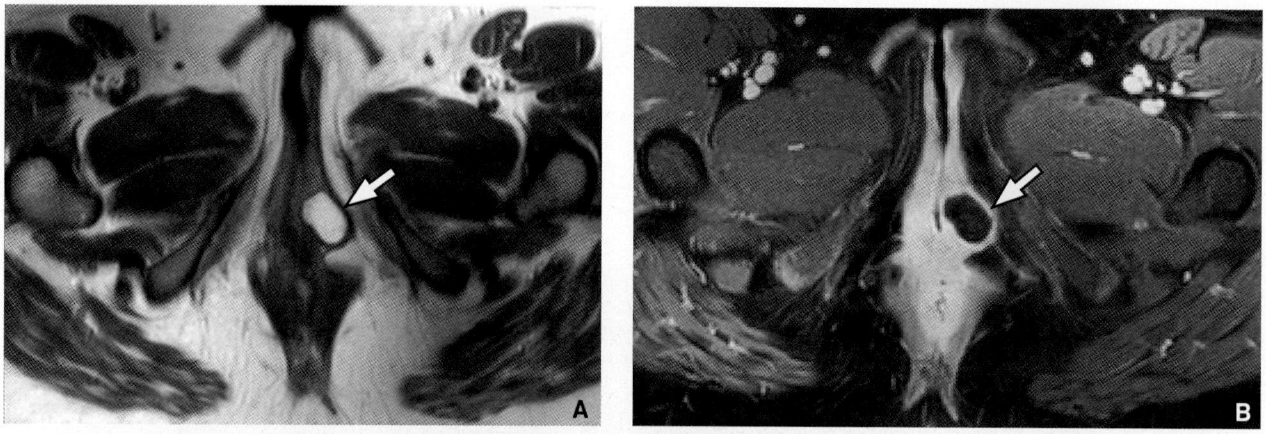

FIGURE 19.53 **A 17-year-old girl with incidental finding of a simple Bartholin gland cyst. A:** Axial single-shot fast spin-echo MR image shows a 2 cm circumscribed, hyperintense lesion (*arrow*) located just to the left of the vaginal introitus. **B:** Axial postcontrast T1-weighted fat-saturated MR image shows that the lesion (*arrow*) peripherally enhances, consistent with a simple Bartholin gland cyst. (Case Image courtesy of Jonathan R. Dillman, MD, MSc, Cincinnati Children's Hospital Medical Center, Cincinnati, OH.)

of endometriosis include retrograde menstruation, coelomic metaplasia, or embryonic rests.[1,86] The presentation of endometriosis is most common in adulthood with chronic pelvic pain or infertility; however, presentation during adolescence is becoming increasingly recognized.[93] If cyclic or acyclic pelvic pain is refractory to nonsteroidal anti-inflammatory agents and oral contraceptives, endometriosis should be considered. The value of imaging is limited unless an endometrioma is suspected.[86]

The appearance of endometriomas is variable depending upon the age of associated hemorrhage. Classic ultrasound appearances include an adnexal lesion with diffuse low-level echoes and ground-glass appearance[1,36] (Fig. 19.56), fluid–fluid levels, and a reticular network of lacy fibrinous strands.[86] Uncommonly, endometriomas may have vascularized, nodular endometrial rests, rendering differentiation from malignancy difficult. Serial ultrasound imaging at 6-week intervals is currently used in adults to assess the changing appearance of the hemorrhage to differentiate from hemorrhagic cyst or endometriomas, although MRI can be used if the US findings of endometrioma remain unclear.[86] Blood products are generally hyperintense on fat-suppressed T1-weighted MR images, and they may lose signal on T2-weighted MR images, so-called "T2 shading," which may be diffuse, dependent/layering, or even focal.[38,86] MRI is 91% to 98% specific for the diagnosis of endometrioma in adults.[86] There is no currently accepted imaging technique for assessment of endometriosis in pediatric patients without endometriomas, however, due to the small size of the lesions and the limits of imaging resolution.[38,86]

Management of endometriosis in adolescents can include laparoscopic ablation or resection by an appropriately trained surgeon and medical management of pain with hormonal therapy.[93]

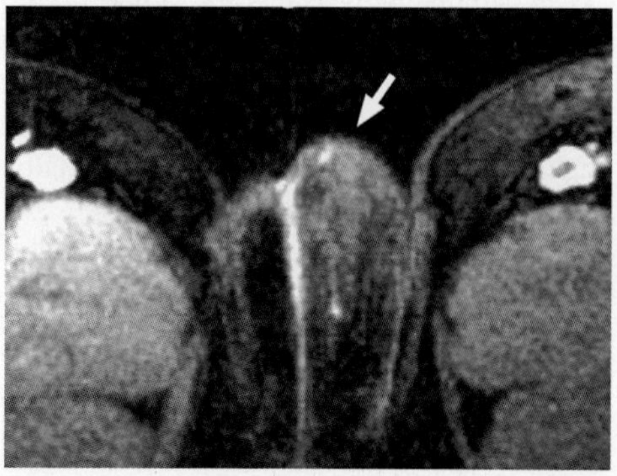

FIGURE 19.54 **An 11-year-old girl who presented with asymmetric enlargement of the left labia majora since the age of 5.** Axial PD MR image shows skin thickening and asymmetrical enlargement of the tissue in the left labia majora (*arrow*) known as CALME (**C**hildhood **A**symmetric **L**abium **M**ajus **E**nlargement).

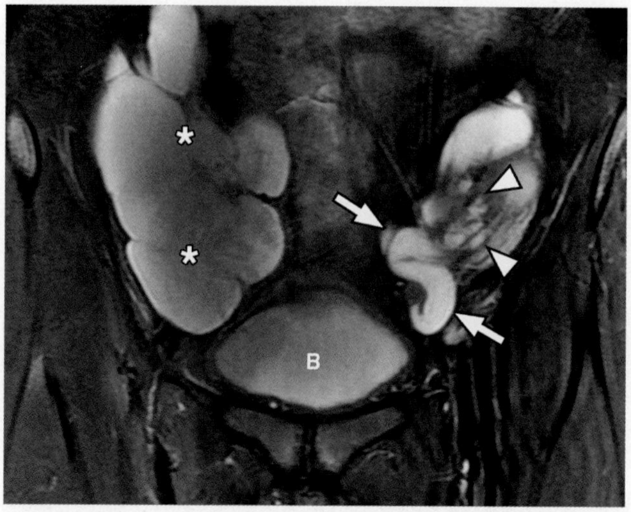

FIGURE 19.55 **A 14-year-old girl with ventriculoperitoneal shunt.** Coronal T2-weighted fat-saturated MR image shows portions of a serpentine fluid-containing tubular structure along the medial aspect of the left ovary (*arrowheads*) representing hydrosalpinx (*arrows*). The fluid collection in the right hemipelvis was a cerebrospinal fluid pseudocyst (CSFoma) (*asterisks*). *B*, bladder.

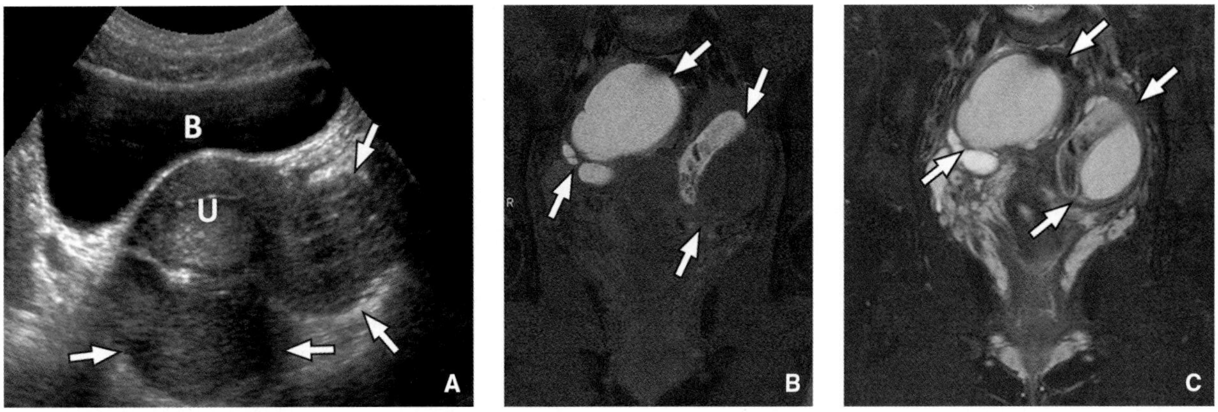

FIGURE 19.56 **Adnexal endometriosis in a 17-year-old girl. A:** Transverse gray-scale ultrasound image shows two hypoechoic pelvic masses (*arrows*) with internal low-level echoes, consistent with endometriomas. Coronal T1-weighted fat-saturated **(B)** and coronal T2-weighted fat-saturated **(C)** MR images show bilateral adnexal lesions (*arrows*) containing T1-weighted hyperintense blood products. The lesion on the left is more heterogeneous and complex in appearance. *B*, bladder; *U*, uterus.

Neoplastic Disorders

Benign Neoplasms

Uterine leiomyomas (also known as fibroids) are the most common gynecologic neoplasm,[92] but they are uncommonly seen in children.[94] Risk factors include being of child-bearing age, having a family history of leiomyomata, and being of African American descent. Histologically, they are composed of benign smooth muscle closely resembling that of the myometrium (Fig. 19.57).

At ultrasound, uterine leiomyomas are usually discrete lesions of variable size containing whorls of smooth muscle cells within a capsule that can appear hypoechoic to normal myometrium, although diffuse leiomyomatosis also has been reported in an adolescent.[94] The tumors can occur anywhere in the myometrium, but it is the submucosal lesions that are the most problematic with the potential to cause dysfunctional uterine bleeding and infertility. Subserosal lesions may be pedunculated and at risk for torsion or can simulate adnexal masses.[92] Ballottement with the transducer during ultrasound imaging may help to demonstrate continuity with the uterus, although MRI may be needed for definitive diagnosis. Leiomyomata are usually isointense on T1-weighted and hypointense to isointense on T2-weighted MR images, unless they are large and/or necrotic (Fig. 19.58). Hormonal medical therapy, such as oral contraceptives, may help reduce abnormal uterine bleeding. Large lesions may require surgical resection.

Benign tumors in the pediatric vulva include tumors of mesenchymal origin such as rhabdomyoma and lipoma or lipoblastoma.[85] Lipomas grow slowly and can be managed conservatively. Vascular malformations as well as hemangiomata, both RICH and NICH, may involve the vulva, as well, and treatment is similar to lesions found elsewhere in the body.[85]

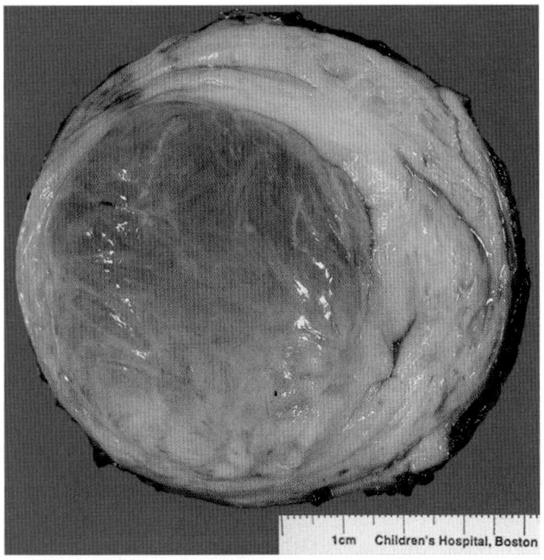

FIGURE 19.57 **Uterine leiomyoma from a 16-year-old girl.** This 10 cm solid tan and vaguely whorled mass excised from the uterus was a leiomyoma, rarely observed in the pediatric age group.

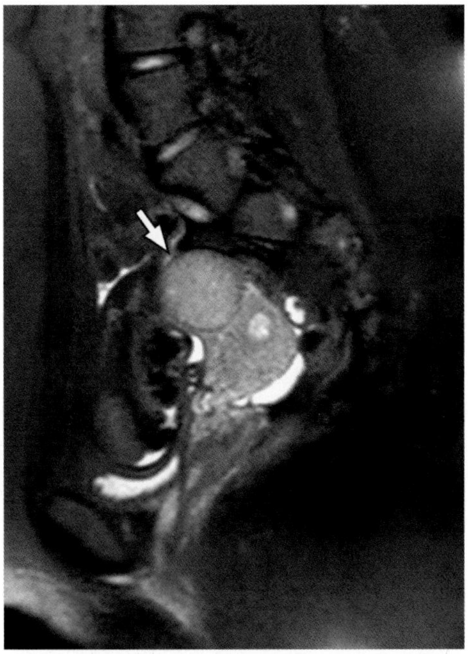

FIGURE 19.58 **Recently postpartum 16-year-old girl with presumed uterine leiomyoma.** Sagittal T2-weighted MR image shows a circumscribed, round, exophytic mass (*arrow*) arising from the uterine fundus serosal surface. (Image courtesy of Jonathan R. Dillman, MD, MSc, Cincinnati Children's Hospital Medical Center, Cincinnati, OH.)

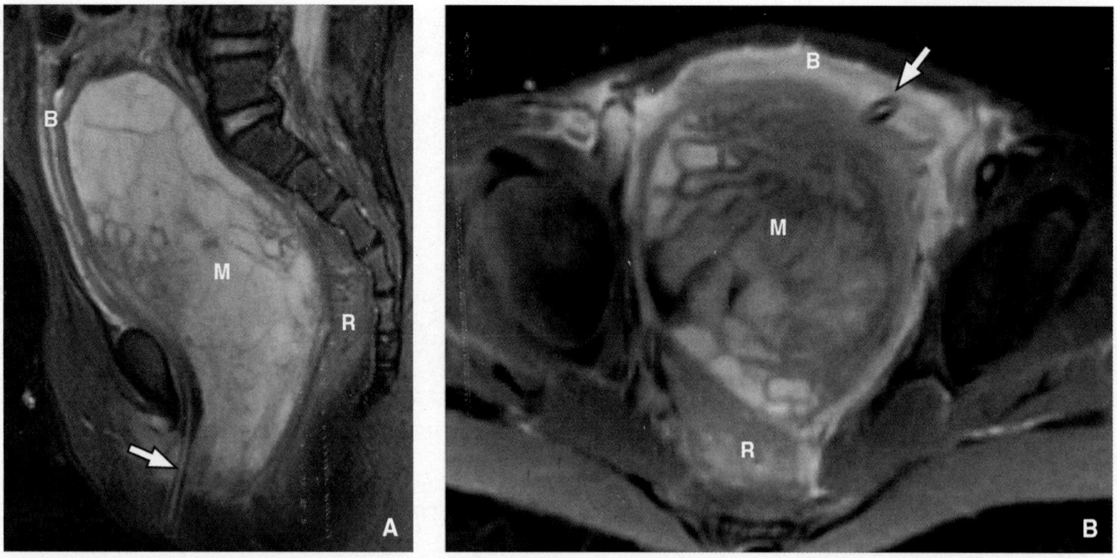

FIGURE 19.59 **A 2-year-old girl with pelvic pain, vaginal bleeding, and a mass extruding from the vaginal introitus. A:** Sagittal T2-weighted fat-saturated MR image shows a markedly dilated vagina secondary to a hyperintense, multiseptated vaginal mass (*M*). The bladder (*B*) is catheterized and markedly displaced anteriorly, whereas the rectum (*R*) is displaced posteriorly. **B:** Axial postcontrast T1-weighted fat-saturated MR image shows that the vaginal mass (*M*) heterogeneously enhances. There is substantial mass effect on the bladder (*B*) and rectum (*R*). Vaginal rhabdomyosarcoma was confirmed microscopically. *Arrow*, bladder catheter.

Malignant Neoplasms

Rhabdomyosarcoma

Rhabdomyosarcoma is the most common soft tissue sarcoma in children and commonly arises from the female pelvis,[64] with the embryonal subtype seen most commonly. It is the most common malignancy of the vagina and uterus in children, with adenocarcinoma and endodermal sinus tumors much less common. This tumor can arise in the vulva, as well. Vaginal rhabdomyosarcoma usually occurs in young children with an age peak at 3 years,[95] and the 5-year survival rate is 91%.[13] Patients with cervicovaginal rhabdomyosarcoma often have a cancer predisposition syndrome related to DICER1 mutation.[96]

Ultrasound is the primary initial imaging modality utilized for visualization of the mass, which can appear as a cystic, solid, or heterogeneous mass (with both solid and cystic elements) located in the expected location of the uterus, cervix, or vagina.[13] The botryoid subtype of embryonal rhabdomyosarcoma classically fills the vagina prolapsing through the introitus,[85] having a characteristic appearance resembling a "bunch of grapes" with high T2-weighted signal intensity and peripheral postcontrast enhancement at MRI (Fig. 19.59).[95] MRI and CT can be utilized to both determine local extent as well as assess for metastatic disease in the abdomen and pelvis. Hydronephrosis is a frequent complication due to spread of tumor into the bladder base and associated obstruction of the distal ureters.

Treatment of rhabdomyosarcoma involves preoperative chemotherapy, wide excision, and adjuvant radiation therapy, which may be employed to prevent local recurrence.[85,97]

Adenocarcinoma

Adenocarcinoma occurs almost exclusively in adult women. Rare pediatric cases have been reported in adolescence, linked to in utero DES exposure.[86] Non-DES exposure cases almost always occur in older women.[95] These tumors can arise from foci of vaginal adenosis, Wolffian rests, endometriosis, and periurethral glands.[95]

Endodermal Sinus Tumor

Endodermal sinus tumor (yolk sac tumor) of the vagina is another rare neoplasm that has a germ cell origin, arising in infants with a peak age of about 10 months.[95] These tumors are heterogeneously hyperintense on T2-weighted MR images, restrict diffusion, and show heterogeneous postcontrast enhancement at CT and MRI.[98,99] The prognosis is worse for vaginal endodermal sinus tumor than for similar neoplasms arising in the gonads due to the more advanced stage at presentation.[99] Endodermal sinus tumor may arise in the vulva and may show lymphatic spread. Treatment involves surgical resection and adjuvant chemotherapy, with a 91% 5-year survival reported.[98]

References

1. Servaes S, et al. Contemporary pediatric gynecologic imaging. *Semin Ultrasound CT MR.* 2010;31(2):116–140.
2. Anthony EY, et al. Adnexal masses in female pediatric patients. *AJR Am J Roentgenol.* 2012;198(5):W426–W431.
3. Lane BF, Wong-You-Cheong JJ. Imaging of endometrial pathology. *Top Magn Reson Imaging.* 2010;21(4):237–245.
4. Lane BF, Wong-You-Cheong JJ. Imaging of endometrial pathology. *Clin Obstet Gynecol.* 2009;52(1):57–72.
5. Epelman M, et al. Mullerian duct and related anomalies in children and adolescents. *Magn Reson Imaging Clin N Am.* 2013; 21(4):773–789.
6. Spencer JA, Ghattanmanani S. MR imaging of the sonographically indetermintae adnexal mass. *Radiology.* 2010;256(3):677–694.
7. Epelman M, et al. Imaging of pediatric ovarian neoplasms. *Pediatr Radiol.* 2011;41(9):1085–1099.
8. Moshiri M, et al. Evaluation and management of disorders of sex development: multidisciplinary approach to a complex diagnosis. *Radiographics.* 2012;32:1599–1618.

9. Chavhan GB, et al. Imaging of ambiguous genitalia: classification and diagnostic approach. *Radiographics.* 2008;28:1891–1904.
10. Jarboe MD, Teitelbaum DH, Dillman JR. Combined 3D rotational fluoroscopic-MRI cloacagram procedure defines luminal and extraluminal pelvic anatomy prior to surgical reconstruction of cloacal and other complex pelvic malformations. *Pediatr Surg Int.* 2012;28(8):757–763.
11. Baughman SM, et al. 3-Dimensional magnetic resonance genitography: a different look at cloacal malformation. *J Urol.* 2007;178(4, pt. 2):1675–1678.
12. Gray H. Anatomy of the human body. Splanchnology: the ovaries [electronic] 1918. *Gray's Anatomy of the Human Body [Online].* 20th ed.; 2002. Available from http://education.yahoo.com/reference/gray/subjects/subject/266 [cited June 20, 2013]
13. Garel L, et al. US of the pediatric female pelvis: a clinical perspective. *Radiographics.* 2001;21:1393–1407.
14. Chung EM, et al. From the radiologic pathology archives: precocious puberty: radiologic-pathologic correltation. *Radiographics.* 2012;32:2071–2099.
15. Rezvani M, Shabaan AM. Fallopian tube disease in the nonpregnant patient. *Radiographics.* 2011;31:527–548.
16. Walker D, et al. Overlooked diseases of the vagina: a directed anatomic-pathologic approach for imaging assessment. *Radiographics.* 2011;31(6):1583–1598.
17. Nalaboff KM, Pellerito JS, Ben-Levi E. Imaging the endometrium: disease and normal variants. *Radiographics.* 2001;21:1409–1424.
18. Hughes IA, et al. Consensus statement on management of intersex disorders. *Arch Dis Child.* 2006;91:554–562.
19. Cools M, et al. Gonadal development and tumor formation at the crossroads of male and female sex determination. *Sex Dev.* 2011;5:167–180.
20. Tanaka YO, et al. Functioning ovarian tumors: direct and indirect findings at MR imaging. *Radiographics.* 2004;24:S147–S166.
21. Houk CP, et al. Summary of consensus statement on intersex disorders and their management. *Pediatrics.* 2006;118(2):753–757.
22. Houk CP, Hughes I, Ahmed SF, et al. Summary of consensus statement on intersex disorders and their management. *Pediatrics.* 2006;118(2):753–757.
23. Barnett KR, et al. Genes controlling ovarian development and follicle growth: studies using transgenic mouse models. Ovarian Kaleidoscope Database [cited November 15, 2013].
24. Chassot AA, et al. Genetics of ovarian differentiation: RSPO1, a major player. *Sex Dev.* 2008;2:219–227.
25. Migeon CJ, Wisniewski AB. Sexual differentiation; from genes to gender. *Horm Res.* 1998;50:245–251.
26. Universities of Friborg, Lausanne and Berne. Human Embryology: Organogenesis. Embryology [Electronic media] 2008 February 20; 2008 [cited May 16, 2013]; Available from: http://www.embryology.ch/anglais/ugenital/diffmorpho01.html
27. Allen JW, et al. Incidence of ovarian maldescent in women with Mullerian duct anomalies: evaluation by MRI. *AJR Am J Roentgenol.* 2012;198(4):W381–W385.
28. Demirel F, Kara O, Esen I. Inguinal ovary as a rare diagnostic sign of Mayer-Rokitansky-Kuster-Hauser syndrome. *J Pediatr Endocrinol Metab.* 2012;25(3–4):383–386.
29. Benbara A, Tigaizin A, Carbillon L. Accessory ovary in the utero-ovarian ligament: an incidental finding. *Arch Gynecol Obstet.* 2011;283(suppl 1):S123–S125.
30. Cheung VYT. Accessory ovary. *J Obstet Gynaecol Can.* 2010; 32(2):107.
31. Meyers CM, et al. Gonadal (ovarian) dysgenesis in 46,XX individuals: frequency of the autosomal recessive form. *Am J Med Genet.* 1996;63:518–524.
32. Griffiths ER, et al. Evaluating failing Fontans for heart transplantation: predictors of death. *Ann Thorac Surg.* 2009;88(2): 558–563; discussion 563–564.
33. Schmahmann S, Haller JO. Neonatal ovarian cysts: pathogenesis, diagnosis and management. *Pediatr Radiol.* 1997;27:101–105.
34. Kessler A, et al. Percutaneous drainage as the treatment of choice for neonatal ovarian cysts. *Pediatr Radiol.* 2006;36(9):954–958.
35. Enriquez G, et al. Conservative versus surgical treatment for complex neonatal ovarian cysts: outcomes study. *AJR Am J Roentgenol.* 2004;185:501–508.
36. Laing FC, Allison SJ. US of the ovary and adnexa: to worry or not to worry? *Radiographics.* 2012;32:1621–1639.
37. Shammas A, Lim R, Charron M. Pediatric FDG PET/CT: physiologic uptake, normal variants, and benign conditions. *Radiographics.* 2009;29(5):1467–1486.
38. Bennett GL, Slywotzky CM, Giovanniello G. Gynecologic causes of acute pelvic pain: spectrum of CT findings. *Radiographics.* 2002;22:785–801.
39. Bremer AA. Polycystic ovary syndrome in the pediatric population. *Metab Syndr Relat Disord.* 2010;8(5):375–394.
40. Pfeifer SM, Kives S. Polycystic ovary syndrome in the adolescent. *Obstet Gynecol Clin North Am.* 2009;36(1):129–152.
41. Chung PW, et al. Menstrual disorders in a paediatric and adolescent gynaecology clinic: patient presentations and longitudinal outcomes. *Hong Kong Med J.* 2011;17:391–397.
42. Choudhary AK, et al. Diseases associated with childhood obesity. *AJR Am J Roentgenol.* 2007;188(4):1118–1130.
43. Lakhani K, et al. Polycystic ovaries. *Br J Radiol.* 2002;75:9–16.
44. The Rotterdam ESHRE/ASRM-sponsored PCOS consensus workshop group. Revised 2003 consensus on diagnostic criteria and long-term health risks related to polycystic ovary syndrome (PCOS). *Hum Reprod.* 2004;19(1):41–47.
45. Dewailly D, et al. Diagnosis of polycystic ovary syndrome (PCOS): revisiting the threshold values of follicle count on ultrasound and of the serum AMH level for the definition of polycystic ovaries. *Hum Reprod.* 2011;26(11):3123–3129.
46. Kim SH, Kim SH, Yang DM, et al. Unusual causes of tubo-ovarian abscess: CT and MR imaging findings. *Radiographics.* 2004;24:1575–1589.
47. Oltmann SC, et al. Cannot exclude torsion—a 15-year review. *J Pediatr Surg.* 2009;44(6):1212–1216; discussion 1217.
48. Oltmann SC, et al. Can we preoperatively risk-stratify ovarian masses for malignancy? *J Pediatr Surg.* 2010;45(1):130–134.
49. Kurman RJ, Carcangiu ML, Herrington CS, Young RH, eds. *WHO Classification of Tumours of Female Reproductive Organs.* Lyon, France: IARC; 2014.
50. Scully R, Young R, Clement P. *Atlas of Tumor Pathology: Tumors of the Ovary, Maldeveloped Gonads, Fallopian Tube, and Broad Ligament, 3rd series, fasc 23.* Washington, DC: Armed Forces Institute of Pathology; 1998.
51. Kaku T, et al. Histological classification of ovarian cancer. *Med Electron Microsc.* 2003;36(1):9–17.
52. Cecchetto G, Ferrari A, Bernini G, et al. Sex cord stromal tumors of the ovary in children: a clinicopathological report from the Italian TREP project. *Pediatr Blood Cancer.* 2011;56:1062–1067.
53. Vaysse C, et al. Ovarian germ cell tumors in children. management, survival, and ovarian prognosis. A report of 75 cases. *J Pediatr Surg.* 2010;45(7):1484–1490.
54. Skinner MA, et al. Ovarian neoplasms in children. *Arch Surg.* 1993;128(8):849–854.
55. Outwater EK, Siegelman E, Hunt JL. Ovarian teratomas: tumor types and imaging characteristics. *Radiographics.* 2001; 21(2):475–490.

56. Shanbhogue AKP, Shanbhogue D, Prasad SR, et al. Clinical syndromes associated with ovarian neoplasms: a comprehensive review. *Radiographics.* 2010;30(3):903–919.
57. Gribbon M, Ein SH, Mancer K. Pediatric malignant ovarian tumors: a 43-year review. *J Pediatr Surg.* 1992;27(3):480–484.
58. Tsuji T, Catasus L, Prat J. Is loss of heterozygosity at 9q22.3 (PTCH gene) and 19p13.3 (STK11 gene) involved in the pathogenesis of ovarian stromal tumors? *Hum Pathol.* 2005;36(7):792–796.
59. Schultz KA, et al. Ovarian sex cord-stromal tumors, pleuropulmonary blastoma and DICER1 mutations: a report from the International Pleuropulmonary Blastoma Registry. *Gynecol Oncol.* 2011;122(2):246–250.
60. Outwater EK, Waqner B, Mannion C, et al. Sex-cord stromal and steroid cell tumors of the ovary. *Radiographics.* 1998; 18(6):1523–1546.
61. Sigismondi C, Gadducci A, Lorusso D, et al. Ovarian sertolileydig cell tumors. a retrospective MITO study. *Gynecol Oncol.* 2012;125(3):673–676.
62. Ferry JA, et al. Lymphoid and myeloid tumours. In: Kurman RJ, et al., eds. *WHO Classification of Tumours of Female Reproductive Organs.* Lyon, France: IARC; 2014.
63. Crawshaw J, Sohaib S, Wotherspoon A, et al. Primary non-Hodgkin's lymphoma of the ovaries: imaging findings. *Br J Radiol.* 2007;80:e155–e158. DOI: 10.1259/bjr/35049074.
64. Agrons GA, Wagner B, Lonergan GJ, et al. Genitourinary rhabdomyosarcoma in children: radiologic-pathologic correlation. *Radiographics.* 1997;17:919-937.
65. Rha SE, Byun J, Jung SE, et al. CT and MR imaging features of adnexal torsion. *Radiographics.* 2002;22:283–294.
66. Poonai N, et al. Pediatric ovarian torsion: case series and review of the literature. *Can J Surg.* 2013;56(2):103–108.
67. Duigenan S, Oliva E, Lee SI. Ovarian torsion: diagnostic features on CT and MRI with pathologic correlation. *AJR Am J Roentgenol.* 2012;198(2):W122–W131.
68. Linam LE, et al. US findings of adnexal torsion in children and adolescents: size really does matter. *Pediatr Radiol.* 2007; 37(10):1013–1019.
69. Orazi C, Inserra A, Lucchetti MC, et al. Isolated tubal torsion: a rare cause of pelvic pain at menarche. Sonographic and MR findings. *Pediatr Radiol.* 2006;36(14):1316–1318.
70. Chen M, Chen M, Yang YS. Torsion of the previously normaluterine adnexa. Evaluation of the correlation between the pathological changes and the clinical characteristics. *Acta Obstet Gynecol Scand.* 2001;80(1):58–61.
71. Barakat AJ. Association of unilateral renal agenesis and genital anomalies. *Case Rep Clin Pract Rev.* 2003;3(2):57–60.
72. Behr SC, Courtier J, Qayyum A. Imaging of müllerian duct anomalies. *Radiographics.* 2012;32:E233–E250. doi: 10.1148/rg.326125515.
73. Del Vescovo R, et al. Herlyn-Werner-Wunderlich syndrome: MRI findings, radiological guide (two cases and literature review), and differential diagnosis. *BMC Med Imaging.* 2012;12:4.
74. Laronda MM, et al. The development of cervical and vaginal adenosis as a result of diethylstilbestrol exposure in utero. *Differentiation.* 2012;84:252.
75. Melnick S, et al. Rates and risks of diethylstilbestrol-related clear-cell adenocarcinoma of the vagina and cervix. An update. *N Engl J Med.* 1987;316:514.
76. Brucker SY, et al. Treatment of congenital malformations. *Semin Reprod Med.* 2011;29(2):101–112.
77. Robbine JE, et al. MRI of pregnancy-related issues: mullarian duct anomalies. *AJR Am J Roentgenol.* 2012;198(2):302–310.
78. Valle RF, Ekpo GE. Hysteroscopic metroplasty for the septate uterus: review and meta-analysis. *J Minim Invasive Gynecol.* 2013;20(1):22–42.
79. Evans TN, Poland ML, Boving RL. Vaginal malformations. *Am J Obstet Gynecol.* 1981;141(8):910–920.
80. Panici PB, Ruscito I, Gasparri ML, et al. Vaginal reconstruction with the Abbè-McIndoe technique: from dermal grafts to autologous in vitro cultured vaginal tissue transplant. *Semin Reprod Med.* 2011;29(1):45–54.
81. Walker DK, et al. Overlooked diseases of the vagina: a directed anatomic-pathologic approach for imaging assessment. *Radiographics.* 2011;31(6):1583–1598.
82. Epelman M, et al. Postnatal imaging of neonates with prenatally diagnosed genitourinary abnormalities: a practical approach. *Pediatr Radiol.* 2012;42(suppl 1):S124–S141.
83. Calvo-Garcia MA, et al. Fetal MRI clues to diagnose cloacal malformations. *Pediatr Radiol.* 2011;41(9):1117–1128.
84. Chaudhari VV, Patel MK, Douek M, et al. MR imaging and US of female urethral and periurethral disease. *Radiographics.* 2010;30:1857–1874.
85. Lowry DLB, Guido RS. The vulvar mass in the prepubertal child. *J Pediatr Adolesc Gynecol.* 2000;13:75–78.
86. Kuligowska E, Deeds L, Lu K. Pelvic pain: overlooked and underdiagnosed gynecologic conditions. *Radiographics.* 2005; 25:3–20.
87. Urogenital Development. Embryology Learning Resources 2013; 2013 [cited December 15, 2014].
88. Vargas SO, et al. Childhood asymmetric labium majus enlargement mimicking a neoplasm. *Am J Surg Pathol.* 2005; 29(8):1007–1016.
89. Quint EH, Smith ER. Vulvar disorders in adolescent patients. *Pediatr Clin North Am.* 1999;46(3):593–608.
90. Schroeder B. Vulvar disorders in adolescents. *Obstet Gynecol Clin North Am.* 2000;27(1):35–48.
91. Sam JW, Jacobs JE, Birnbaum BA. Spectrum of CT findings in acute pyogenic pelvic inflammatory disease. *Radiographics.* 2002;22:1327–1334.
92. Moyle PL, et al. Nonovarian cystic lesions of the pelvis. *Radiographics.* 2010;30:921–938.
93. Batt RE, Mitwally MFM. Endometriosis from thelarche to midteens: pathogenesis and prognosis, prevention and pedagogy. *J Pediatr Adolesc Gynecol.* 2003;16(6):337–347.
94. Pai D, et al. Diffuse uterine leiomyomatosis in a child. *Pediatr Radiol.* 2012;42(1):124–128.
95. Parikh JH, et al. MR imaging features of vaginal malignancies. *Radiographics.* 2008;28:49–63.
96. Dehner LP, Jarzembowski JA, Hill DA. Embryonal rhabdomyosarcoma of the uterine cervix: a report of 14 cases and a discussion of its unusual clinicopathological associations. *Mod Pathol.* 2012;25(4):602–614.
97. Walterhouse DO, et al. Local control and outcome in children with localized vaginal rhabdomyosarcoma: a report from the Soft Tissue Sarcoma committee of the Children's Oncology Group. *Pediatr Blood Cancer.* 2011;57(1):76–83.
98. Liu QY, et al. Clinical manifestations and MRI features of vaginal endodermal sinus tumors in four children. *Pediatr Radiol.* 2013; 43(8):983–990.
99. Chen SJ, Li YW, Tsai WY. Endodermal sinus (yolk sac) tumor of vagina and cervix in an infant. *Pediatr Radiol.* 1993;23:57–58.

CHAPTER 20

Abdominal Wall, Mesentery, Peritoneum, and Vessels

Michael S. Gee • Rahul A. Sheth • Salwa M. Haidar • Dilip Sankhla • Edward Y. Lee

INTRODUCTION

The abdominal wall, mesentery, peritoneum, and blood vessels are often overlooked anatomic regions on imaging studies, particularly in pediatric patients, in whom the focus of imaging studies is frequently the abdominal visceral organs. These regions have their own unique set of disorders with which radiologists should be familiarized. In addition, the spreading pattern of more common abdominal infectious, inflammatory, and neoplastic processes can include these areas, and their involvement may be the only imaging evidence of the underlying disease. This chapter reviews imaging techniques, relevant anatomy, and pathology pertaining to the abdominal wall, mesentery, peritoneum, and vessels in the pediatric population.

IMAGING TECHNIQUES

Radiography

The abdominal radiograph is often the best first-line imaging examination for the evaluation of pediatric abdominal diseases. Air within bowel loops provides intrinsic contrast that can be used to evaluate the caliber and distribution of bowel in diseases that lead to bowel obstruction. In addition, space-occupying lesions in the abdomen can displace bowel and appear on radiographs as regions of absent bowel gas. The radiograph is often an excellent "starting point" to exclude urgent or emergent complications, such as free intraperitoneal air. Although radiographs have poor soft tissue contrast resolution, they have high spatial resolution for detecting the presence of air and calcification within lesions. On a frontal radiograph, free intraperitoneal air is best seen with the patient positioned upright or in a decubitus position. A cross-table lateral radiograph can also be performed in sick infants who need to lie supine. Calcifications of the peritoneum, mesentery, or abdominal wall are also radiographically apparent. Abnormally displaced bowel loops or a localized paucity of bowel gas on an abdominal radiograph can be an indirect sign of ascites or a soft tissue mass in the peritoneum, retroperitoneum, or mesentery. A lateral abdominal radiograph can be helpful for detecting abdominal wall abnormalities, which may manifest as thickening, such as in cellulitis, or calcification. The abdominal vasculature is poorly evaluated on plain radiographs.

Ultrasound

Ultrasound (US) is often an initial imaging modality used in children because it does not require ionizing radiation, sedation, or anesthesia. US is helpful for evaluating children presenting with a palpable abdominal mass to identify the presence, location, and tissue composition of underlying lesions. In children, especially infants, the general lack of internal body fat facilitates imaging of abdominal lesions deep within the peritoneal cavity and retroperitoneum that might not be visible in adults because of acoustic attenuation or shadowing from adjacent bowel gas.

High-frequency (12 to 18 MHz) linear transducers are best for evaluating the subcutaneous tissues and abdominal wall, whereas lower-frequency (4 to 8 MHz) convex transducers are more suitable for evaluating the visceral organs, the peritoneal spaces, and small bowel mesentery.[1] Harmonic imaging and compression technique can also be utilized to facilitate visualization of structures deep in the abdomen. Color and spectral Doppler US detect frequency shifts related to moving blood and are used to evaluate the arteries and veins for anatomic and flow-related abnormalities and to evaluate lesions seen on gray-scale US for internal vascularity to help discriminate complex cysts from solid masses.

Computed Tomography

Computed tomography (CT) is an imaging modality that is ideally suited for evaluating the abdominal wall, peritoneum, and mesentery, because of its high spatial resolution, cross-sectional imaging capability, and ability to provide high-quality images of air-filled or calcified structures. Modern multirow detector CT scanners can image the entire abdomen of a child in ≤1 to 5 seconds and are well suited for imaging awake infants and toddlers who cannot suspend respiration or follow commands. In addition, CT scanners are available in most emergency rooms to evaluate acutely ill children at any time of day. However, an important concern with CT is the use of ionizing radiation, especially in pediatric patients. Prior to CT scanning for each child, an informed analysis that balances the diagnostic benefit of the examination against the potential risk of CT ionizing radiation should be undertaken.

Pediatric CT protocols of the abdomen and pelvis involve modification of a number of scan parameters that reduce radiation dose while still ensuring diagnostic image quality.[2,3] These include setting limits on tube beam current (mA) and potential (kVp) depending on the study indication, increasing scan pitch, and utilizing thick sections (e.g., 2.5 to 5 mm) with retrospective thin collimation for multiplanar reformations. Modern CT scanners utilize adaptive tube current and voltage modulation to decrease radiation dose as a function of patient size. Routine abdominal CT scans are performed with intravenous contrast in the portal venous phase to optimize evaluation of the visceral organs. CT angiography is performed by acquiring images in the arterial phase of enhancement using either contrast bolus tracking or timing. Sagittal reformatted images are especially helpful for evaluating the subcutaneous tissues and abdominal wall as well as the ostia of the abdominal celiac and superior mesenteric arteries.

Magnetic Resonance Imaging

Magnetic resonance imaging (MRI) is being increasingly performed for pediatric abdominal evaluation. Its main advantages include the ability to acquire images in any plane, lack of ionizing radiation, and excellent soft tissue contrast resolution. Because of the lack of ionizing radiation, imaging of the same anatomic region may be performed at multiple time points following intravenous contrast material administration. This is helpful for evaluating blood vessels during combined MR angiography and venography as well as for characterizing the enhancement properties of masses. The superior soft tissue contrast resolution of MRI is ideally suited for tissue characterization of abdominal lesions detected on other imaging modalities, with T1-weighted MR images sensitive for the detection of fatty or hemorrhagic elements and T2-weighted MR images sensitive for cystic or soft tissue components.

Typical pediatric abdominal MRI protocols may include coronal single-shot fast spin-echo and balanced steady-state free precession MR images to provide a motion-free overview of abdominal anatomy as well as axial T1-weighted and fat-suppressed T2-weighted MR images to evaluate for pathology. 3D T1-weighted gradient recalled echo fat-saturated MR images are then acquired before and at multiple time points after intravenous gadolinium chelate administration to evaluate the abdominal vasculature and assess for enhancing lesions. For dedicated evaluation of the abdominal vasculature, time-resolved contrast-enhanced MR angiography/venography can be performed using dynamic acquisition of multiple 3D T1-weighted fast gradient recalled MR images to provide multiphase vascular imaging without the need to suspend respiration.[4] The main disadvantages of MRI are its long scanning time (30 to 60 minutes for a typical examination) and motion-related degradation of image quality, which are both relevant to the pediatric population. Abdominal MRI in young children often requires conscious sedation or general anesthesia for these reasons. Nonetheless, MRI is commonly the study of choice for evaluating most abdominal wall, peritoneal, and vascular lesions prior to biopsy or surgical treatment.

Nuclear Medicine

Nuclear scintigraphy offers the advantage of radiotracer molecule specificity that can be used to characterize lesions based on physiologic properties. For example, ^{18}F-flourodeoxyglucose (FDG) accumulates in cells with increased glucose metabolism and is often used in conjunction with positron emission tomography (PET) to determine malignancy/benignity of soft tissue lesions in the abdominal wall, mesentery, and peritoneum that are detected on other imaging modalities as well as imaging staging of many malignancies. ^{131}I-MIBG is an adrenergic analog that accumulates in neuroblastoma cells and is used for primary neuroblastoma detection and staging. Nuclear scintigraphy using gallium (^{67}Ga)-labeled or ^{111}In-labeled white blood cells can be helpful for abscess detection in pediatric patients with suspected abdominal infection. ^{99m}Tc-labeled red blood cell scanning can help identify a mesenteric arterial bleeding source in pediatric patients with lower gastrointestinal bleeding.

Historically, the major limitations of nuclear scintigraphy have been poor spatial resolution and inability to anatomically localize detected abnormalities. However, the development of tomographic techniques, such as single photon emission computed tomography (SPECT) and PET, has been helpful in this regard, as well as the use of hybrid imaging of SPECT and PET with CT and MRI. Nuclear scintigraphy also involves long scan times similar to MRI and often requires sedation or general anesthesia to be performed in young children.

Conventional Angiography

Although most vascular pathology can be accurately diagnosed with noninvasive vascular imaging, there remains an important role for conventional angiography in the pediatric population. Continuous advancements in interventional techniques have expanded the diagnostic and therapeutic potential for angiography. Increasingly, complex percutaneous arterial interventions can be performed in children for a broad range of conditions including renovascular hypertension, transplant liver hepatic artery stenosis, and abdominal trauma.[5]

Awareness of radiation exposure to the pediatric patient and a commitment to the "ALARA" ("as low as reasonably achievable") principle are vitally important for the pediatric angiographer. Angiography, particularly during lengthy percutaneous interventions, has the potential to deliver the highest radiation dose of any imaging study. Methods to reduce radiation exposure during fluoroscopy include the use of pulse fluoroscopy, last-image hold, copper filtration, optimal collimating, and removal of antiscatter grids while imaging neonates and small infants.

The most commonly accessed vessel in pediatric angiography is the common femoral artery.[6] Arterial access in children can be challenging because of the relatively smaller size of blood vessels in this population; as such, vessel occlusion following catheterization is a more common occurrence in children than in adults. The umbilical artery remains patent for up to 5 days and can serve as suitable arterial access point. Young patients are particularly susceptible to volume overload and nephrotoxicity from iodinated contrast media, and so, the volumes of fluids and contrast media used should be closely monitored.

NORMAL ANATOMY

Abdominal Wall

The anterior abdominal wall extends cranially to the xiphoid process, laterally to the rib cage, and caudally to the iliac and pubic bones. The anterior abdominal wall contributes to respiration as well as urination, defecation, and coughing. The muscles of the anterior abdominal wall also assist with flexion and extension of the body at the hips. These muscles include the rectus abdominis anteriorly and the external oblique, internal oblique, and transversus abdominis laterally/posterolaterally.

Peritoneum, Peritoneal Spaces, and Mesentery

The peritoneum is the largest serous membrane in the body. It is a thin, translucent single sheet of mesothelial tissue. Microscopically, the peritoneum is composed of flat mesothelial cells. The peritoneum that invests abdominal organs is termed the visceral peritoneum, and the peritoneum that lines the abdominal cavity is known as the parietal peritoneum. The potential space between these two layers of the peritoneum is normally filled with a small volume of serous fluid, minimizing friction when the two layers contact. In boys, the peritoneal cavity is a closed space. In girls, however, the peritoneal cavity is pierced laterally by the fallopian tubes.

The peritoneal cavity is segregated into discrete compartments by peritoneal ligaments, structures that represent double layers of the visceral peritoneum and provide suspensory support for abdominal organs (Figs. 20.1 and 20.2). The two major compartments of the peritoneal cavity as defined by

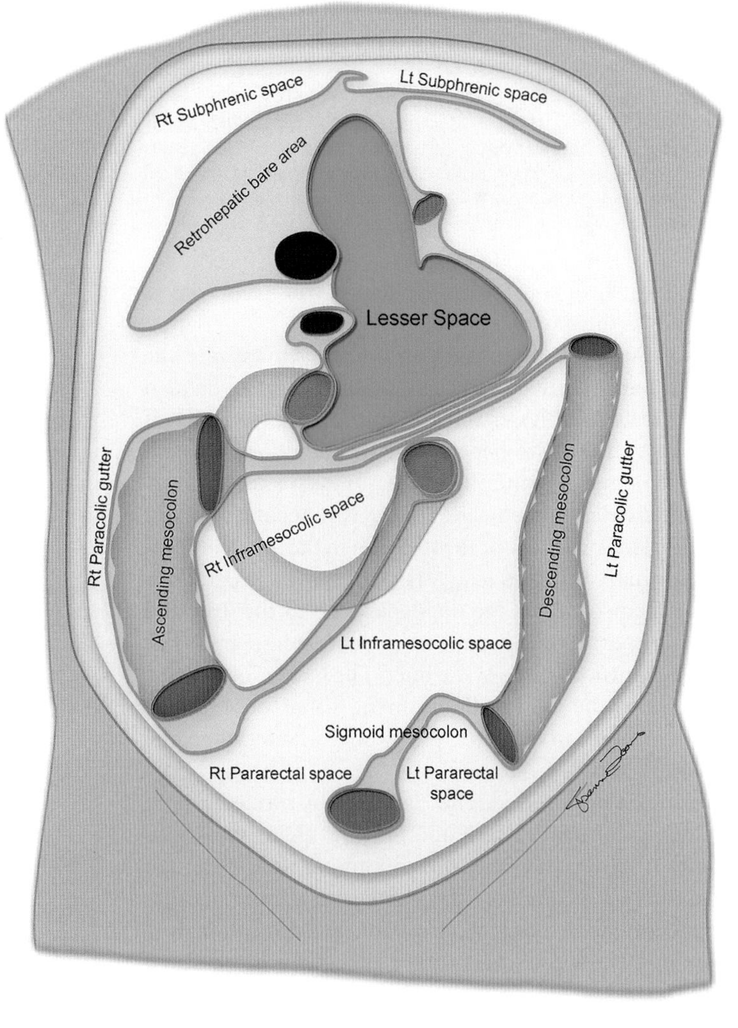

FIGURE 20.1 **Diagram of peritoneal spaces.**

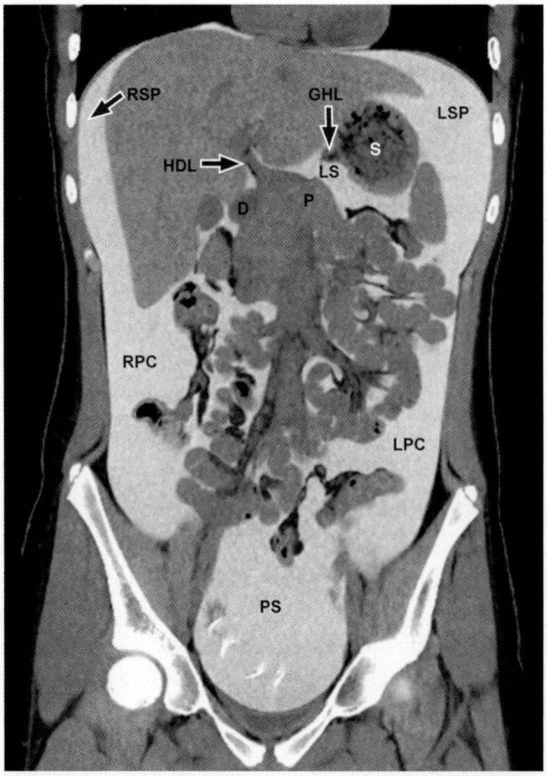

FIGURE 20.2 **A 13-year-old girl on peritoneal dialysis undergoing CT peritoneogram to assess for peritoneal adhesions.** Contrast opacification of the peritoneum identifies the major spaces and ligaments. *RSP*, right subphrenic space; *LSP*, left subphrenic space; *GHL*, gastrohepatic ligament; *HDL*, hepatoduodenal ligament; *LS*, lesser sac; *S*, stomach; *P*, pancreas; *D*, duodenum; *RPC*, right paracolic space; *LPC*, left paracolic space; *PS*, pelvic space. (Image courtesy of Jonathan R. Dillman, MD, MSc, Cincinnati Children's Hospital Medical Center, Cincinnati, OH.)

the peritoneal ligaments are the greater sac and the lesser sac, also known as the omental bursa.

Two of the most important peritoneal ligaments are the omentum and the mesentery. The omentum is subdivided into the greater and lesser omentum, the latter of which is composed of the gastrohepatic and hepatoduodenal ligaments. The lesser omentum fixes the stomach and first portion of the duodenum to the liver. The gastrohepatic ligament binds the lesser curvature of the stomach to the liver, containing the coronary vein and left gastric artery. The hepatoduodenal ligament connects the duodenal bulb to the liver and contains the portal vein, hepatic artery, common hepatic bile duct, and a portion of the cystic duct. The greater omentum, also known as the gastrocolic ligament, hangs dependently from the greater curvature of the stomach, anterior to the small bowel.

The mesentery is a double layer of peritoneum that ensconces abdominal viscera and attaches them to a fixed anatomic structure, typically the abdominal wall. Although the mesentery is a complex three-dimensional structure that undergoes extensive rotation, translation, and resorption during development, it is entirely composed of an uninterrupted sheet of tissue. Nonetheless, by convention, the mesentery is divided into several discrete mesenteries. The small bowel mesentery runs from the ligament of Treitz in the left upper quadrant to the ileocecal valve in the right lower quadrant. It binds the small bowel to the retroperitoneum and contains the superior mesenteric arteries and veins. The transverse mesocolon is a broad fold of peritoneal lining that binds the transverse colon with the posterior abdominal wall. It is continuous with the posterior layers of the greater omentum and contains the middle colic vessels. Similarly, the sigmoid mesocolon binds the sigmoid colon to the posterior pelvic wall, containing the hemorrhoidal and sigmoid arteries and veins.

There are multiple additional peritoneal ligaments. These include the falciform ligament, which represents the vestigial remnant of the embryologic ventral mesentery. It contains the obliterated umbilical vein and separates the subphrenic space into left and right compartments. The gastrosplenic ligament arises from the embryologic dorsal mesentery and connects the greater curvature of the stomach with the spleen. The splenorenal ligament also arises from the embryologic dorsal mesentery and can contain splenorenal shunt vasculature in the setting of portal hypertension.[7]

The omenta, mesenteries, and other ligaments segregate the peritoneal cavity into multiple, somewhat discrete spaces, serving as both barriers and pathways for the spread of disease (Table 20.1). Knowledge of these spaces is indispensable for understanding common patterns of spread of infectious, inflammatory, or neoplastic processes in the abdomen. It should be noted, however, that while the peritoneal ligaments do serve as boundaries for these spaces, the boundaries are not absolute and they can be overcome.

The transverse mesocolon separates the peritoneal cavity into the bilateral supramesocolic and inframesocolic spaces. Laterally, the peritoneal cavity contains the paired paracolic gutters. Inferiorly, the peritoneal cavity is composed of the pelvic space.

TABLE 20.1 Anatomic Spaces of the Peritoneal Cavity

Supramesocolic
Left supramesocolic
Left perihepatic
Left subphrenic
Perisplenic
Right supramesocolic
Right subphrenic
Subhepatic (Morison's pouch)
Lesser sac
Inframesocolic
Left inframesocolic
Right inframesocolic
Paracolic
Left paracolic
Right paracolic
Pelvic

Reference: Tirkes T, Sandrasegaran K, Patel AA, et al. Peritoneal and retroperitoneal anatomy and its relevance for cross-sectional imaging. Radiographics. 2012;32(2):437–451.

The left supramesocolic space is somewhat arbitrarily subdivided into the perihepatic, left subphrenic, and perisplenic spaces. The right supramesocolic space contains the right subphrenic and subhepatic spaces (also known as Morison pouch) and the lesser sac. The bilateral supramesocolic spaces typically communicate freely, with the falciform ligament often representing an incomplete barrier between the left and right subphrenic spaces. The left supramesocolic space also typically communicates with the left paracolic gutter, with the phrenicocolic ligament serving as an incomplete barrier; the right paracolic gutter is a continuation of the right subhepatic space. Both paracolic gutters extend into the pelvic space.

The bilateral inframesocolic spaces, on the other hand, do not communicate with the paracolic gutters because of the right and left colon. The left inframesocolic space is in communication with the pelvic space; the right inframesocolic space, on the other hand, is small and isolated from the pelvis by the small bowel mesentery.

Characterizing lesions as intraperitoneal or extraperitoneal is often highly relevant to the surgeon but can be a challenge for the radiologist. Adding to the challenge is the convention of using "intramesenteric" and "intraperitoneal" interchangeably. Strictly speaking, the intraperitoneal space refers to a thin potential space between the layers of parietal and visceral pleura; the intramesenteric space, on the other hand, describes blood vessels, lymph nodes, and fat that are encased by but not contained within visceral peritoneum. The intramesenteric space is in fact in continuity with the extraperitoneal space including the retroperitoneum. For this reason, the term "subperitoneal space," which includes the intramesenteric space and extraperitoneal space, may be a more helpful term to the surgeon, as accessing lesions in this space does not require violation of the peritoneum.[8]

Abdominal Vessels

Abdominal Aorta

The abdominal aorta extends from the diaphragmatic hiatus at approximately the T12-L1 interspace to the pelvis where it bifurcates into the bilateral common iliac arteries at approximately the L4 level (Fig. 20.3). The diameter of the aorta narrows as it descends in the abdomen and provides mesenteric and visceral branches. The development of the aorta begins in the 3rd week of embryogenesis. Many dorsal and ventral segmental arteries arise from the primitive aorta, some of which regress during development, and others of which persist.[9]

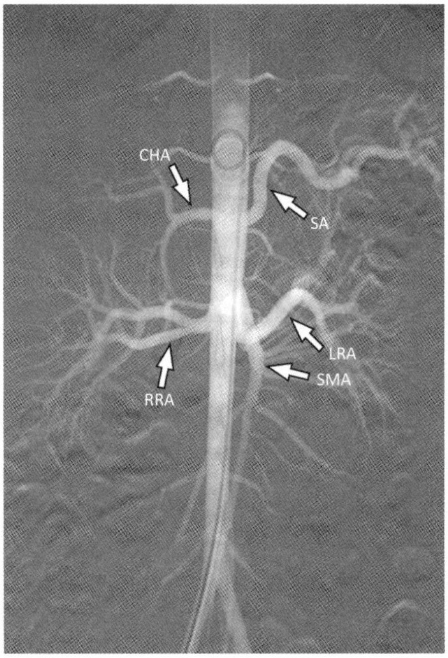

FIGURE 20.3 **Normal angiographic anatomy of the abdominal aorta and its visceral branches.** *Arrows* indicate the major abdominal aortic visceral branches. *CHA*, common hepatic artery; *SA*, splenic artery; *RRA*, right renal artery; *LRA*, left renal artery; *SMA*, superior mesenteric artery.

Inferior Vena Cava

The formation of the inferior vena cava (IVC) (Fig. 20.4) and its major tributaries is a complex process, involving three paired venous systems that selectively regress and fuse. Three retroperitoneal venous systems form chronologically during weeks 6 through 8 of embryogenesis. The posterior cardinal system is the earliest such system, arising in week 6, and does not contribute to the normal IVC. The subcardinal system forms in week 7 and provides the prerenal segment of the IVC. The supracardinal system is the last system to form, arising during week 8, and contributes the postrenal segment of the IVC. Anastomosis between the subcardinal and supracardinal systems form the renal segment of the IVC.[10] An appreciation of this complex embryologic development provides a rational foundation for the array of stereotyped anomalies described subsequently in this chapter.

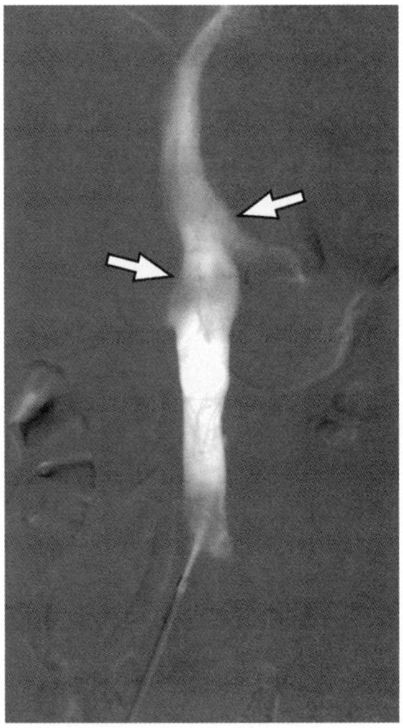

FIGURE 20.4 **Normal inferior vena cavogram.** The ostia of the renal veins are identified as jets of unopacified blood (*arrows*) flowing into the inferior vena cava.

Mesenteric Arteries

The mesenteric arteries develop during embryogenesis from primitive ventral segmental arteries. All but three of these arteries are resorbed and lead to the celiac axis, superior mesenteric artery (SMA), and inferior mesenteric artery (IMA). The celiac axis supplies the foregut and arises from the 10th segmental artery; the SMA supplies the midgut and arises from the 13th segmental artery; the IMA supplies the hindgut and arises from either the 21st or 22nd segmental artery.[9] The majority of vascular anatomic variants involving the mesenteric arteries reflect incomplete resorption of the primitive arteries.

The SMA (Fig. 20.5) arises ~1 cm below the origin of the celiac axis, typically at the level of the L1 vertebral body. It provides blood flow to the duodenum, jejunum, ileum, right colon, and majority of the transverse colon. Several structures normally course between the SMA and the abdominal aorta, including the third portion of the duodenum and the left renal vein. Physical compression of these structures can lead to SMA syndrome and nutcracker syndrome, respectively.

One of the first right-sided branches off the SMA is the inferior pancreaticoduodenal artery, which anastomoses with the superior pancreaticoduodenal artery arising from the gastroduodenal artery, thus providing an important celiac axis–SMA collateral pathway (Table 20.2). This pancreaticoduodenal arcade nourishes the pancreatic head as well as the duodenum. The inferior pancreaticoduodenal artery more commonly arises as two separate branches, namely, the antero- and posteroinferior pancreaticoduodenal arteries, but it can also branch off as a single trunk that subsequently bifurcates.[11]

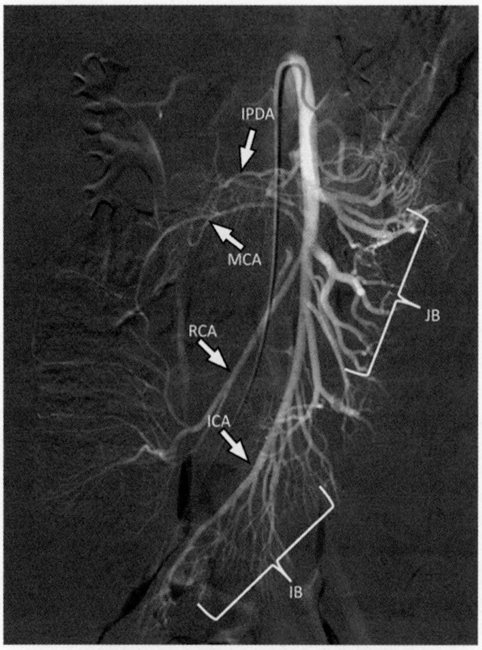

FIGURE 20.5 **Normal angiographic anatomy of the superior mesenteric artery (SMA) and its branches.** On the right, the inferior pancreaticoduodenal artery (*IPDA*) anastomoses with the superior pancreaticoduodenal artery branch of the gastroduodenal artery, forming a collateral pathway between the SMA and celiac axis. There are multiple left-sided jejunal branches (*JB*). On the right are the middle colic (*MCA*), right colic (*RCA*), and ileocolic arteries (*ICA*), and anastomoses among these arteries form a marginal artery (of Drummond) that irrigates the right and transverse colon. Distal to the origin of the ICA, multiple ileal branches (*IB*) supply the ileum.

TABLE 20.2 Collateral Pathways of Mesenteric Arteries

Celiac axis to SMA	1. Arc of Buehler (persistent embryonic communication between celiac axis and SMA) 2. Superior pancreaticoduodenal artery to inferior pancreaticoduodenal artery
SMA to IMA	1. Marginal artery of Drummond (anastomotic connections between middle colic and left colic arteries along the mesenteric margin of the large bowel) 2. Arc of Riolan or meandering mesenteric artery (short direct anastomosis between middle colic and left colic arteries)
IMA to internal iliac artery	1. Superior rectal (hemorrhoidal) to middle and inferior rectal (hemorrhoidal) arteries

SMA, superior mesenteric artery; IMA, inferior mesenteric artery.

Following the inferior pancreaticoduodenal artery, the next right-sided branch is the middle colic artery, followed by the right colic artery and ileocolic artery. The ileocolic artery serves as the landmark beyond which all subsequent small branches off the SMA supply the ileum and no longer the jejunum. The SMA provides ~4 to 6 left-sided jejunal branches and 9 to 13 ileal branches. The middle colic artery nourishes the transverse colon and provides collateral circulation via anastomotic communications with the IMA. It gives rise to a right branch, which anastomoses with the right colic artery, and a left branch, which in some patients anastomoses with the left colic artery (via the arc of Riolan or meandering mesenteric artery) along the root of the small bowel mesentery and as an important SMA-IMA collateral pathway. The middle colic artery typically arises from the SMA before the artery pierces the mesentery. The origin of the middle colic artery, however, can be variable, having been identified as arising from the celiac axis, common hepatic artery, and splenic artery; it may also arise from a replaced right hepatic artery or the gastroduodenal artery. Branches of the middle, right, and ileocolic arteries form a marginal artery (also known as the marginal artery of Drummond) along the inner border of the colon that nourishes the ascending colon and connects with branches of the IMA. Importantly, however, the right colic artery is commonly absent. The middle and right colic artery may share a single trunk off of the SMA.

The IMA (Fig. 20.6) arises from the ventral abdominal aorta below the origin of the SMA at the level of L3.

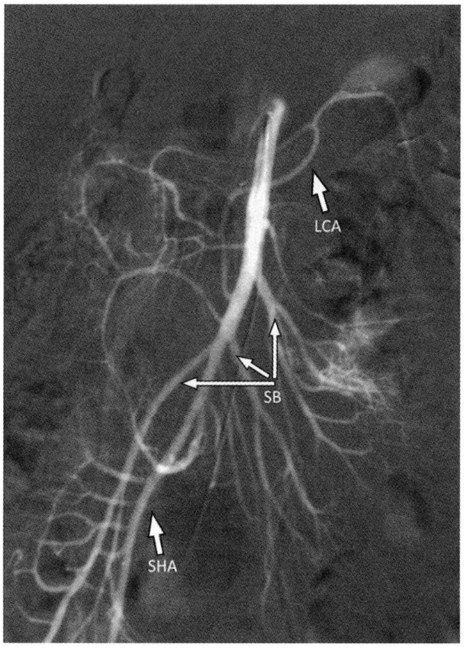

FIGURE 20.6 **Normal angiographic anatomy of the inferior mesenteric artery (IMA).** The left colic artery (*LCA*) anastomoses with the middle colic artery of the superior mesenteric artery (SMA) to provide SMA-IMA collaterals. Multiple sigmoid branches (*SB*) arise from the IMA, and the terminal branch of which is the superior hemorrhoidal artery (*SHA*).

This artery is the smallest of the mesenteric arteries and nourishes the distal transverse colon, descending colon, sigmoid colon, and rectum. The major branches of the IMA are the left colic, sigmoid, and hemorrhoidal arteries, all of which branch off to the left. The left colic ascends from its origin off the IMA to anastomoses with branches from the SMA. In ~12% of individuals, the left colic artery is absent. In this situation, the perfusion of the descending and sigmoid colon is provided by the colosigmoid artery. Occasionally, the left colic artery may arise from the SMA. The left colic artery extends cephalad to the splenic flexure in the majority of patients and reaches the mid-aspect of the transverse colon in ~15% to 20% of patients. However, perfusion of the splenic flexure is highly variable, and in some patients, the middle colic artery may be the only artery irrigating this territory.

Mesenteric Veins

The superior mesenteric vein (SMV) (Fig. 20.7) receives blood from multiple mesenteric veins, including the ileocolic, gastrocolic, right colic, and middle colic veins. These veins typically merge into a single trunk that joins with the splenic vein to form the portal vein. Occasionally, however, the tributaries may not coalesce into a single trunk but rather into right and left mesenteric branches, which then join the splenic vein.[11,12]

The inferior mesenteric vein (IMV) receives blood from the superior hemorrhoidal vein, sigmoid vein, and left colic vein. The IMV may drain into the SMV or continue cephalad to drain into the splenic vein or splenoportal confluence.[11,12]

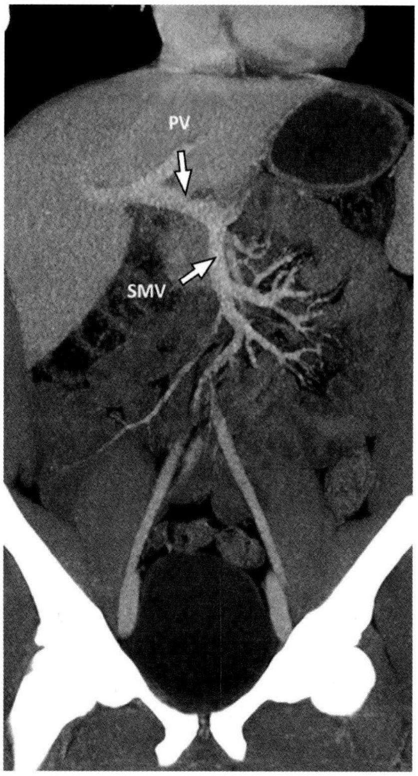

FIGURE 20.7 **Superior mesenteric vein (*SMV*) appearance on CT.** Maximum intensity projection reconstruction CT image demonstrates the normal anatomy of the SMV. This vein receives blood from multiple mesenteric veins, which coalesce most commonly into a single trunk that subsequently joins with the splenic vein to form the portal vein (*PV*).

SPECTRUM OF ABDOMINAL WALL DISORDERS

Congenital and Developmental Anomalies

Omphalocele and Gastroschisis

Omphalocele refers to herniation of the abdominal viscera through the umbilical cord. The most common organs within an omphalocele are the liver and small bowel, with the spleen, stomach, colon, and bladder being less common.[13] It arises from a defect caused by failure of central migration of the lateral mesodermal folds destined to become the anterior abdominal wall. The lining of an omphalocele is composed of peritoneum and amnion with interposed Wharton jelly. Although the majority of omphaloceles are isolated, there is high association with chromosomal abnormalities. Omphaloceles are classified based on size, with size <5 cm associated with higher survival rate (>80%) and having a higher association with chromosomal abnormalities and isolated small bowel herniation, whereas size ≥5 cm is associated with lower survival rate (<50%) and a higher likelihood of having liver herniation and pulmonary hypoplasia.

On physical examination, the umbilical cord is seen at birth to insert into the mass. Plain radiographs show an anterior mass extending from the midline abdominal wall, with herniated bowel loops showing gas within the hernia.

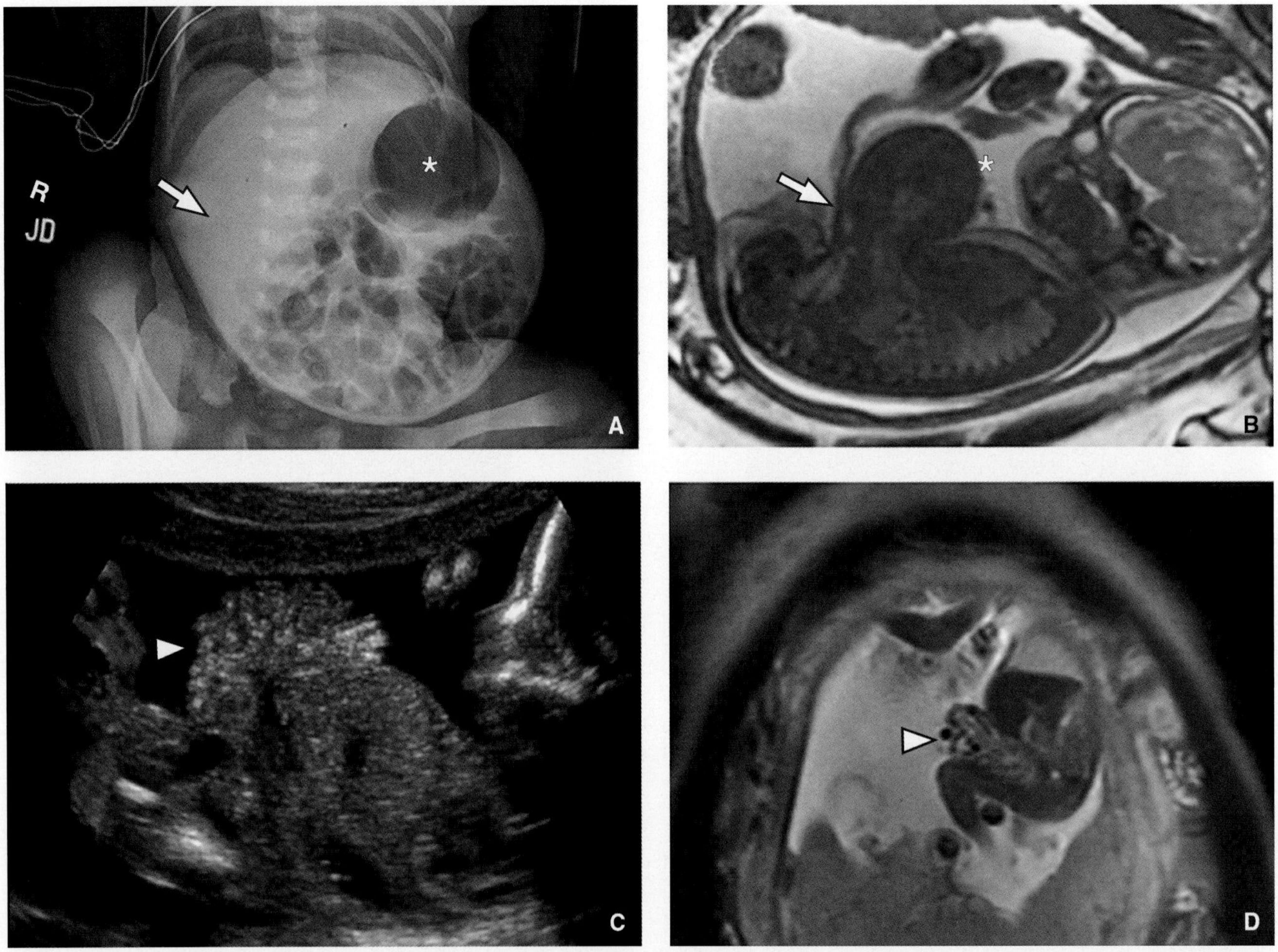

FIGURE 20.8 **Imaging features of omphalocele and gastroschisis. A:** Abdominal radiograph of a neonatal boy with omphalocele demonstrates a large anterior abdominal wall hernia (*arrow*) containing the stomach (*asterisk*) and multiple bowel loops. **B:** Prenatal sagittal T2-weighted MRI of a fetal omphalocele at 32 weeks of gestational age demonstrates an anterior abdominal hernia containing the liver covered by a thin outer membrane (*asterisk*), with the umbilical cord vessels inserting at the hernia base (*arrow*). In contrast, prenatal imaging of a 25-week-gestational-age fetus with gastroschisis on ultrasound **(C)** and sagittal T2-weighted MR image **(D)** demonstrate anterior herniation of small bowel loops (*arrowheads*) with no outer covering membrane. (Radiograph [A] provided by Jonathan R. Dillman, MD, MSc, Cincinnati Children's Hospital Medical Center, Cincinnati, OH. Ultrasound [C] and MRI [B and D] images provided by Sudha Anupindi, MD, and Teresa Victoria, MD, Children's Hospital of Philadelphia, Philadelphia, PA.)

Typically an omphalocele is diagnosed on prenatal US showing an anterior midline herniation with a covering membrane (Fig. 20.8) and the umbilical cord vessels seen inserting at the base of the hernia.

Gastroschisis is a congenital defect in the anterior wall that is off-midline in the paraumbilical location, typically to the right of midline. In contrast to omphalocele, there is a full-thickness defect in the abdominal wall, with herniated abdominal contents contained only in amniotic fluid without a covering membrane. Gastroschisis can produce bowel injury depending on the amount and duration of bowel herniation. Herniated intestine can become edematous and ischemic because of exposure to amniotic fluid, and blood supply can be impaired by the neck of the abdominal wall defect. Gastroschisis is associated with intestinal atresia (usually jejunal or ileal) and gastrointestinal motility disorders. Closed gastroschisis, or "vanishing midgut," refers to midgut infarction resulting from abdominal wall defect closure around herniated bowel.[14]

Prenatal US and MRI show herniated intestine with no covering membrane (Fig. 20.8C, D) and a normal umbilical cord vessel insertion distinct from the site of herniation. Elevated alpha-fetoprotein (AFP) level is present in maternal serum in over 90% of cases.

The current management of omphalocele and gastroschisis is surgical repair, which consists of placing the herniated organs back into the abdomen cavity (often covered by a protective silo) followed by complete closure of the defect via either one operation or gradual staged operations.

Prune Belly Syndrome

Prune belly (Eagle-Barrett) syndrome is characterized by a defect in abdominal wall musculature, urinary system ectasia, and cryptorchidism. It is a rare disorder with a male predominance and estimated incidence of 3 to 4 per 100,000.[15] The etiology is thought to be in utero urethral obstruction due to either a hypoplastic prostate or a failure in

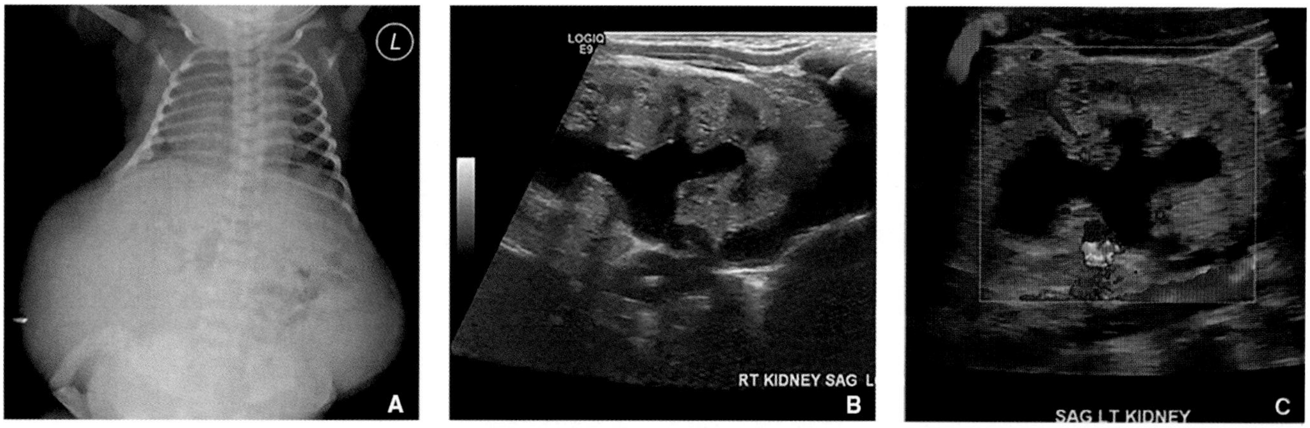

FIGURE 20.9 **Prune belly syndrome in a newborn boy. A:** Radiograph demonstrates marked abdominal wall laxity. **B and C:** Renal ultrasound images show bilateral hydronephrosis. The kidneys are echogenic and contain several small cysts, suggestive of underlying renal dysplasia.

mesodermal development, leading to urinary tract distention, abnormal abdominal wall muscular development, and failure of testicular descent.[16,17] The abdominal wall defect classically consists of disorganized central abdominal wall muscles that are infiltrated with collagen bundles.[18] Cryptorchidism has been attributed to both impeded testicular descent by the distended urinary system as well as atresia of the gubernaculum, which does not pull adequately.[16]

Diagnosis of prune belly syndrome is typically made during the antenatal period, with fetal imaging demonstrating bilateral hydroureteronephrosis, bladder distention, and oligohydramnios. The appearance can be similar to posterior urethral valves, although typically lacking prostatic urethral dilation seen with PUV.[16] Severe renal dysfunction associated with prune belly syndrome is associated with pulmonary hypoplasia and cardiovascular dysfunction, and perinatal mortality rates are in the 10% to 25% range depending on the degree of prematurity and cardiopulmonary compromise.[16] Because of this, antenatal urinary decompression techniques such as vesicoamniotic shunting are considered in some severe cases in an attempt to improve perinatal survival.[19] Postnatal imaging appearance includes severe abdominal distention and wall laxity on radiographs (Fig. 20.9A), as well as hydroureteronephrosis (Fig. 20.9B), renal dysplasia, and cryptorchidism on US.

Treatment of prune belly syndrome includes managing the lower urinary tract, abdominal wall, and cryptorchidism.[16] The goal of urinary management is to preserve renal function and avoid urinary tract infection, via either conservative methods or surgical reconstruction. Premature renal failure is a common long-term complication, with approximately one-third of affected patients requiring renal transplant later in life.[20] Abdominal wall surgical reconstruction aids with abdominal tone and can improve bladder voiding through augmented sensation and contraction.[21] Bilateral orchidopexy is standardly performed as well.

Proteus Syndrome

Proteus syndrome is a tissue overgrowth disorder that is due to a mutation in the AKT1 gene leading to activation of the PI3K-AKT signaling pathway[22] and overgrowth of multiple tissue types. Characteristic lesions include cerebriform connective tissue nevi, vascular malformations, focal gigantism of a digit or limb, facial dysmorphism, dysregulated adipose tissue (lipomas or lipohypoplasia), pulmonary bullae, and deep vein thrombosis.[23] It is a sporadic syndrome that is characterized by mosaic distribution of lesions and progressive disproportionate tissue overgrowth, which in the limbs and digits consists predominantly of bony overgrowth with cortical thinning and relative paucity of overlying soft tissue.[24]

Proteus syndrome is a rare disorder only affecting several hundred patients in the United States and Western Europe, with a male predominance and physical manifestations appearing either at birth or later in childhood.[23,25] Because the mutation is poorly detected in peripheral blood, diagnosis is made predominantly by the presence of multiple disease defining lesions.

Imaging plays an important role in establishing the diagnosis in patients with suspected Proteus syndrome, including a radiographic skeletal survey as well as targeted MRI and/or CT of clinically affected areas or cross-sectional imaging of the chest, abdomen, and pelvis in asymptomatic patients.[23,24] Common abdominal wall abnormalities include vascular malformations and fatty lesions (Fig. 20.10).

Pediatric patients with Proteus syndrome experience numerous disease complications over their lifetime, including large joint arthrosis and scoliosis, visceral organ overgrowth, and development of tumors including ovarian cystadenomas and parotid adenomas.[25] Deep venous thrombosis and pulmonary embolism are other common disease complications.[23] Imaging is helpful for detecting and characterizing these various disease manifestations. The differential diagnosis for Proteus syndrome includes: PTEN hamartoma tumor syndrome, CLOVE syndrome, and Klippel-Trenaunay syndrome.

Infectious and Inflammatory Disorders

Abdominal Wall Cellulitis and Abscess

Cellulitis is acute bacterial infection of the skin and subcutaneous tissues. It is associated with features of acute inflammation including erythema, swelling, warmth, and tenderness to palpation.[26] Often the area of involvement spreads over time and may

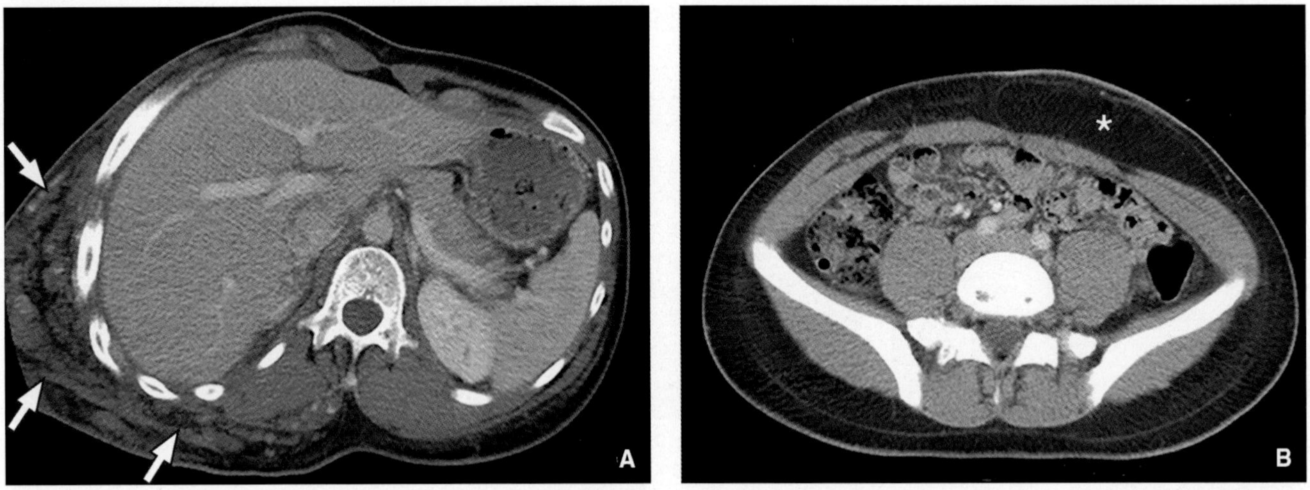

FIGURE 20.10 **Proteus syndrome in an 15-year-old boy.** Axial enhanced CT images demonstrate a vascular malformation (**A**; *arrows*) in the right flank abdominal wall as well as a large abdominal wall lipoma (**B**; *asterisk*).

be accompanied by fever or malaise. Most commonly, cellulitis is a complication of an overlying skin disorder, such as a penetrating wound (including a puncture, abrasion, or bite), ulcer (e.g., varicella lesions or newborn omphalitis), or dermatosis.[27,28] Abdominal wall cellulitis in children may also be a sequela of abdominal surgery, such as appendectomy. Most cases of cellulitis are due to infection by *Streptococcus* and *Staphylococcus* skin flora. Less typical organisms include oral flora in cases of cellulitis secondary to a bite or Gram-negative rods, anaerobic flora, and fungi in immunocompromised patients.[28]

The diagnosis of cellulitis is typically made based on cutaneous examination and clinical history, without the need to perform imaging or obtain a skin culture.[28] Imaging can be performed in two specific clinical scenarios, namely, US to exclude an associated abscess requiring drainage and MRI to exclude necrotizing fasciitis, which would necessitate surgical debridement. CT may also be performed to evaluate for the presence of gas within the soft tissues that can suggest the diagnosis of necrotizing fasciitis. US features of cellulitis include edema and thickening of the skin and subcutaneous tissues, with an associated abscess appearing as a hypoechoic focal fluid collection with posterior acoustic enhancement and often an echogenic rim (Fig. 20.11). The presence of an abscess typically is an indication for surgical or image-guided drainage, as antibiotic therapy is typically inadequate to eradicate the abdominal wall abscess.

MRI is sometimes performed in cases of rapidly progressive skin infection to evaluate for necrotizing fasciitis, which is a surgical emergency. MRI features of necrotizing fasciitis include abnormal thickening, fluid, and enhancement of the deep fasciae.[29] MRI appears to be sensitive but not specific for necrotizing fasciitis, and generally, it is not recommended if there is strong clinical suspicion.[28,29] The typical treatment of uncomplicated abdominal wall cellulitis is antibiotic therapy.

Neoplastic Disorders

Benign Neoplasms

Desmoid Tumor

Desmoid tumors, also known as deep or aggressive fibromatosis, are fibrous mesenchymal neoplasms that are locally aggressive but do not exhibit distant metastasis.[30] These rare tumors

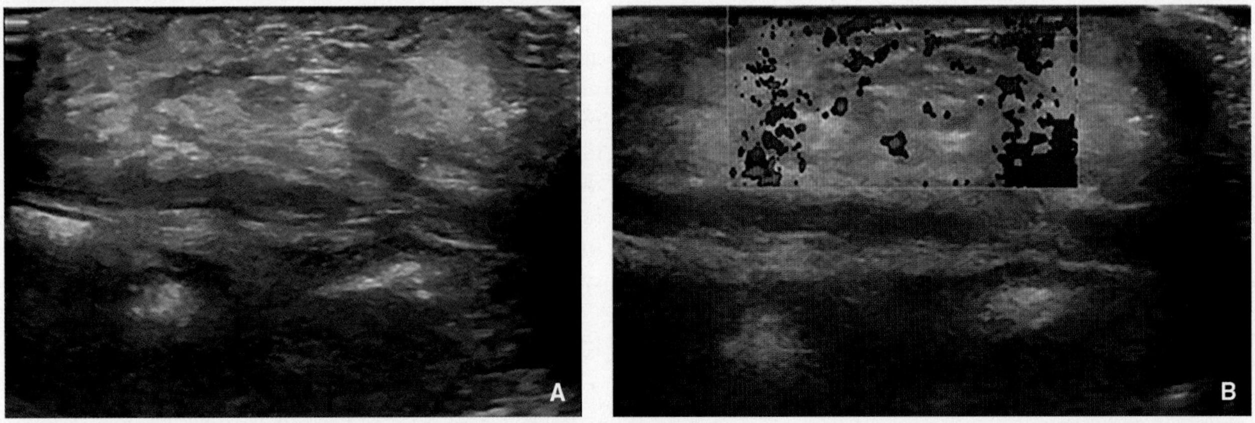

FIGURE 20.11 **Abdominal wall cellulitis in a newborn boy. A:** Gray-scale ultrasound image of the paraumbilical region demonstrates heterogeneous thickening of the paraumbilical abdominal wall soft tissues, consistent with cellulitis. **B:** Color Doppler ultrasound image shows mild hyperemia.

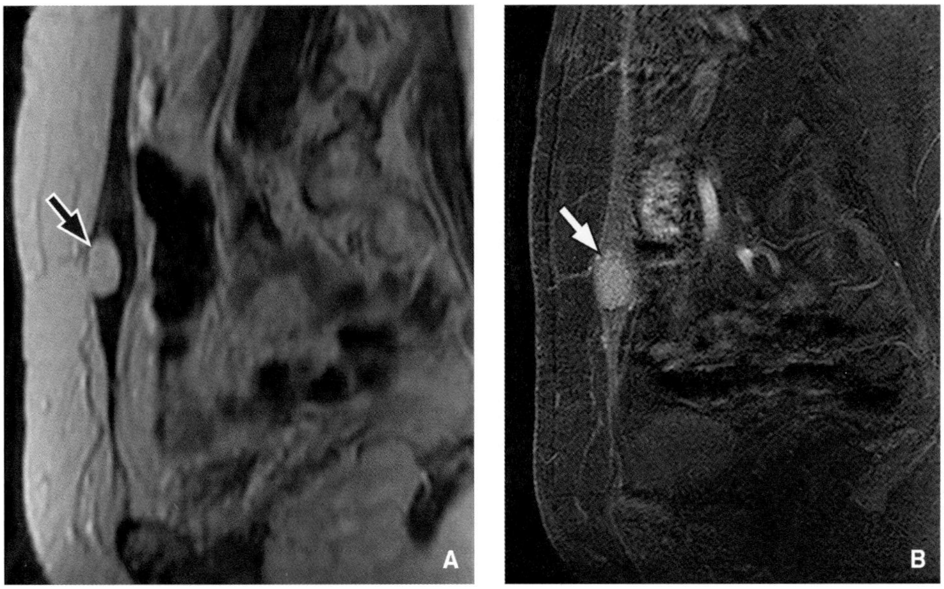

FIGURE 20.12 **Abdominal wall desmoid tumor in a 17-year-old boy with Gardner syndrome.** Sagittal T2-weighted **(A)** and postcontrast T1-weighted fat-saturated **(B)** MR images demonstrate a hyperintense and enhancing mass (*arrows*) centered in the rectus abdominis muscle, consistent with known desmoid tumor.

(<5 per million annual incidence) arise mostly in young adults and less commonly in children, with a slight female predominance and peak incidence in the third and fourth decades.[31] Desmoid tumor locations are traditionally classified as intra-abdominal (mesenteric or pelvic), abdominal wall, or extra-abdominal (most commonly in the proximal extremities, head, and neck). Patients with Gardner-type familial adenomatous polyposis (FAP) have a >800-fold increased incidence of desmoids, which are usually intra-abdominal or mesenteric in location.[32,33] Abdominal wall desmoids occurring in the rectus abdominis or internal oblique muscles have an association with pregnancy.[34] Desmoid tumors usually occur as single tumors, although ~15% are multiple.[34]

Desmoid tumors, especially those in the abdominal wall or extra-abdominal locations in young patients, usually present as a slowly growing palpable mass and often are evaluated initially by US. The sonographic appearance of a desmoid is a well-defined hypoechoic mass with variable internal Doppler vascularity.[35] MRI is frequently performed as the next imaging modality in young patients to define lesion extent and relationship to adjacent structures (Fig. 20.12). Desmoid tumors demonstrate variable T2-weighted signal intensity depending on the degree of collagen and myxoid matrix deposition; collagen-rich tumors are associated with signal hypointensity, and myxoid matrix–rich tumors are associated with signal hyperintensity.[30,36] The lesions demonstrate variable enhancement with intravenous contrast material administration for the same reason.

Grossly, desmoid tumors are firm and usually fairly well circumscribed. They tend to have a white–gray whorled cut surface (Fig. 20.13). Microscopically, fascicles of fibroblasts in a variably collagenized matrix are seen. Genetically, the tumors often show trisomy of chromosome 8; mutations in the beta-catenin or APC gene may also be seen.[37]

Abdominal wall desmoids are often amenable to percutaneous needle biopsy because of their superficial location. Patients diagnosed with desmoid tumor should be screened for FAP, as 2% of all desmoid tumors are FAP associated.[32] Asymptomatic desmoid tumors that are stable over time may be observed, although for abdominal wall desmoids, surgical resection with wide margins with or without abdominal wall reconstruction is the preferred approach and is associated with a very low local recurrence rate.[31,32,38,39] Systemic therapy or radiation can also be considered for cases deemed nonresectable.[31,32]

Malignant Neoplasms

Soft Tissue Sarcoma

Soft tissue sarcomas arising within the abdominal wall are rare and account for only 1% to 5% of total soft tissue sarcomas.[39] Soft tissue sarcomas as a whole are uncommon in the pediatric population, with <1,000 cases in the United States each year.[40] Sarcomas constitute the most common primary abdominal wall malignancy in patients of all ages.[41]

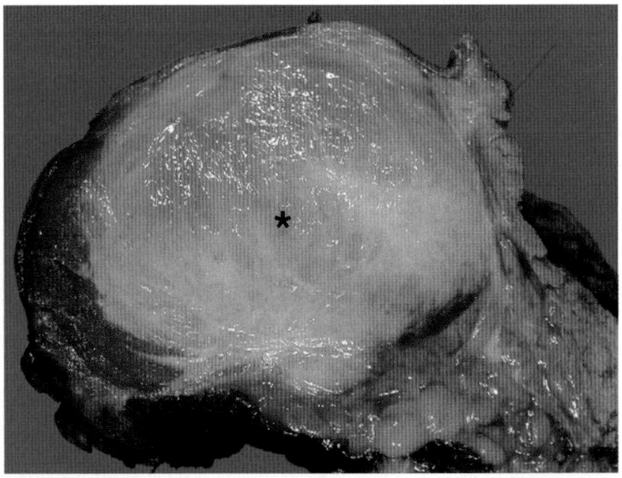

FIGURE 20.13 **Gross appearance of desmoid fibromatosis developing after ileostomy closure in an 18-year-old man with familial adenomatous polyposis.** The 5 cm mass (*asterisk*) is firm and pale tan, distinct from the red-brown abdominal musculature.

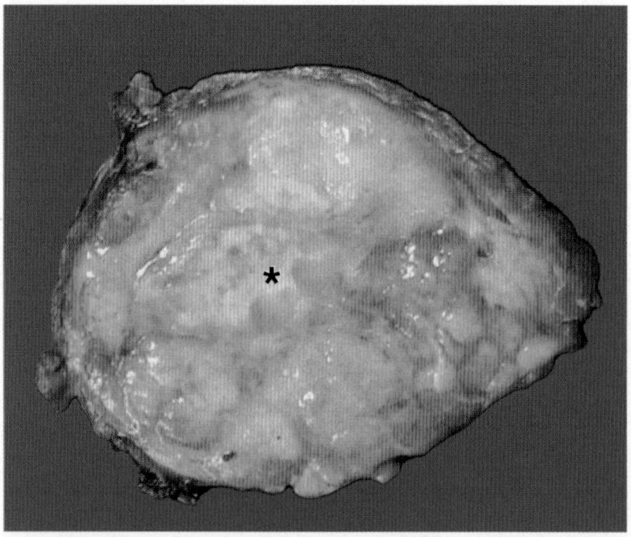

FIGURE 20.14 **Gross appearance of a synovial sarcoma from the abdominal wall of a 13-year-old boy.** This is a 6.5 cm tumor resected after chemotherapy. The tumor (*asterisk*) is multilobular and light tan with soft pale areas of necrosis.

In children, soft tissue sarcomas occurring in the abdominal wall are primarily nonrhabdomyosarcoma soft tissue sarcomas (NRSTS). Such NRSTS are a heterogeneous group of histologic subtypes derived from mesenchymal cells, which often have characteristic genetic translocations that aid in their diagnosis.[40] This includes infantile fibrosarcoma, which is a rare NRSTS that occurs specifically in infants under 2 years of age (median age 3 months) and presents typically as a large infiltrative soft tissue mass with associated skin discoloration that may mimic vascular malformation.[42] Synovial sarcoma (Fig. 20.14) is one of the common sarcomas in older children. All NRSTS typically present as a slowing growing and painless mass.

The initial evaluation of abdominal wall soft tissue sarcoma is similar to the abdominal wall desmoid management, including US[43] to confirm the presence of a solid soft tissue mass and identify its location, followed by CT or MRI to assess extent of invasion and relationship to nearby neurovascular structures, aiding in surgical excision planning (Fig. 20.15).[44] Percutaneous needle or surgical incisional biopsy is the mainstay of histologic diagnosis of soft tissue sarcomas. Once the diagnosis is made, staging CT of the chest, abdomen, and pelvis (with or without ^{18}F-FDG–PET) is routinely performed to assess for metastatic disease.[45] Surgical excision is the mainstay of abdominal wall sarcoma treatment but is often combined with radiation therapy and/or chemotherapy,[44] with potential toxicities to abdominal organs balanced against lower likelihood of local recurrence.[41]

Metastasis

Abdominal wall metastasis in the pediatric population is very rare. Pediatric malignancies that have been shown to metastasize to the skin or subcutaneous soft tissues include neuroblastoma, Wilms tumor, rhabdomyosarcoma, synovial sarcoma, and angiosarcoma[46,47] (Fig. 20.16). Diffuse subcutaneous metastases in neuroblastoma account for the so-called blueberry muffin appearance. Although most cases of abdominal wall metastasis are attributable to hematogenous tumor spread (Figs. 20.16 and 20.17), a few cases of abdominal wall "metastasis" in adults have also been attributable to implantation after surgical resection of an intra-abdominal malignancy.[41] The diagnosis of metastasis should be considered in any pediatric patient with a new abdominal wall mass and a history of prior malignancy.

Traumatic Disorders

Traumatic Abdominal Wall Injuries and Hernias

Traumatic abdominal wall hernia (TAWH) is the disruption of abdominal wall muscle and fascia in the absence of skin penetration, secondary to blunt trauma. This occurs in ~1% of all blunt trauma and up to 9% of blunt trauma patients undergoing abdominal CT.[48] In children, these injuries occur

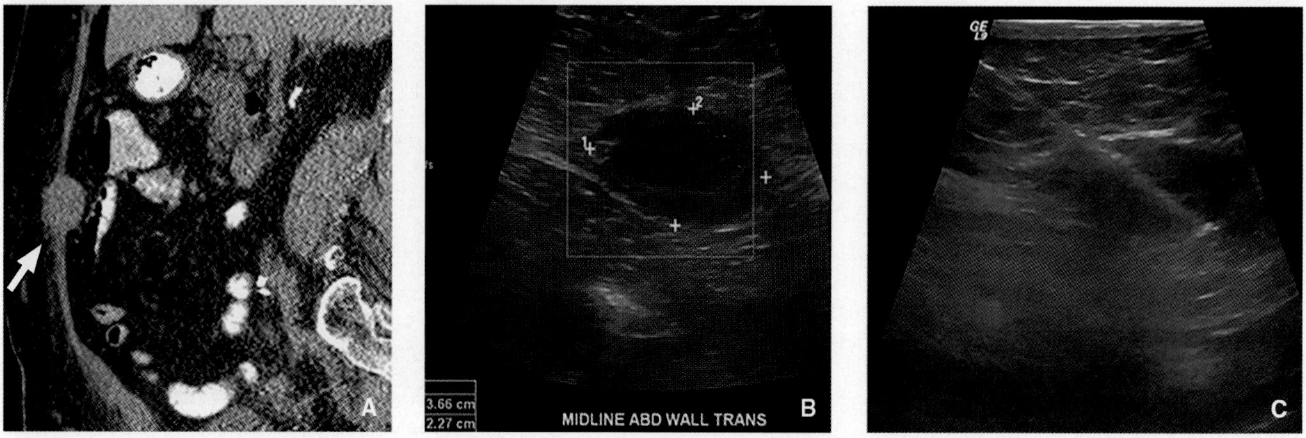

FIGURE 20.15 **Abdominal soft tissue sarcoma in a 17-year-old boy. A:** Sagittal enhanced CT image demonstrates a soft tissue mass (*arrow*) in the abdominal wall. **B:** Ultrasound depicts the lesion as a hypoechoic mass (calipers) with internal Doppler vascularity. **C:** Ultrasound-guided percutaneous core needle biopsy of the lesion established the diagnosis of synovial sarcoma.

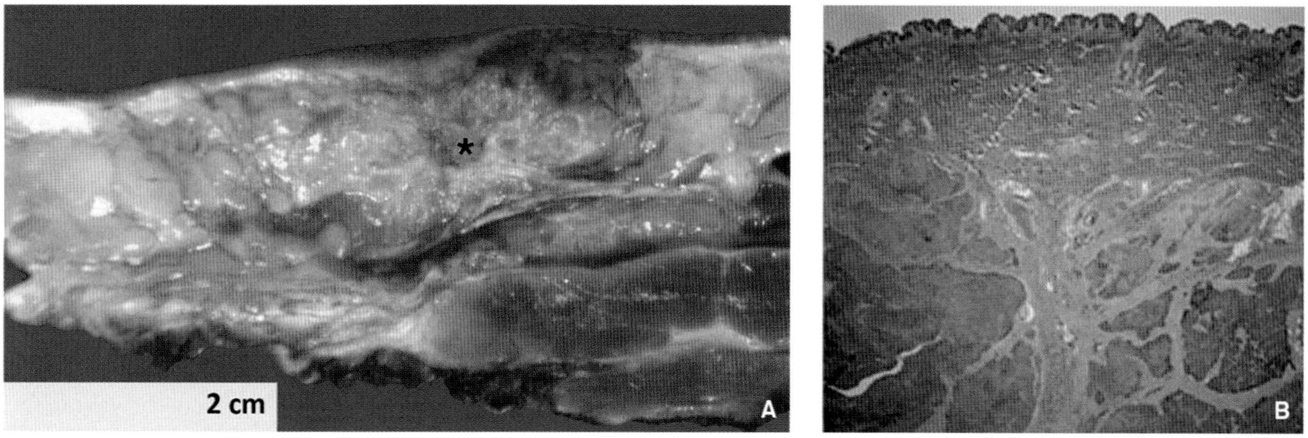

FIGURE 20.16 **Pathologic appearance of a recurrent Wilms tumor metastasis in the abdominal wall of a 14-year-old girl.** Grossly **(A)**, the tumor (*asterisk*) was a gray-tan mass distinct from the surrounding yellow subcutaneous adipose tissue. Microscopically **(B)**, nests of primitive basophilic (*blue*) cells are seen in the subcutis (hematoxylin and eosin; original magnification, 20×).

primarily as a result of high-energy lap-belt trauma during motor vehicle collisions or from low-energy falls onto bicycle handlebars (the so-called handlebar hernia).[49–51] The vast majority of these injuries that are bicycle related are in boys, with a mean age of ~10 years.[51]

The proposed mechanism for low-energy traumatic abdominal wall herniation is a strong force applied to a focal area of the abdominal wall leading to disruption of the underlying muscle and fascia with preservation of the overlying, more elastic skin, which can absorb the force without disruption.[52] The abdominal wall of children is thought to be thinner and less well developed than in adults, which may lead to increased susceptibility to this type of injury.[50] In the case of high-energy abdominal wall herniation, the compressive force of the lap belt can cause either direct or indirect pressure-induced abdominal wall disruption and visceral herniation through the defect.[53] Common sites in these cases include lumbar and anterolateral division hernias.[50,54] The high position of lap belts above the anterior superior iliac spine in children is thought to contribute to this pattern of injury.[50] Associated internal abdominal injuries are commonly present in both high- and low-energy cases of TAWH.[51]

CT is the primary imaging modality to assess for traumatic abdominal wall injuries, as it can evaluate not only for the presence and severity of abdominal wall injury but also for concomitant internal abdominal injuries.[51,55] A grading system has been described for TAWH assessed by CT, which includes depth of involvement, degree of muscular disruption, and presence or absence of abdominal content herniation (Fig. 20.18).[48] Abdominal wall injuries consisting of subcutaneous contusion or intramuscular hematoma, without complete muscle disruption or hernia defect, can typically be managed conservatively. Management of cases with a hernia defect can be either conservative or surgical, with some reports describing spontaneous hernia resolution with no intervention in cases with no evidence of internal injury, and

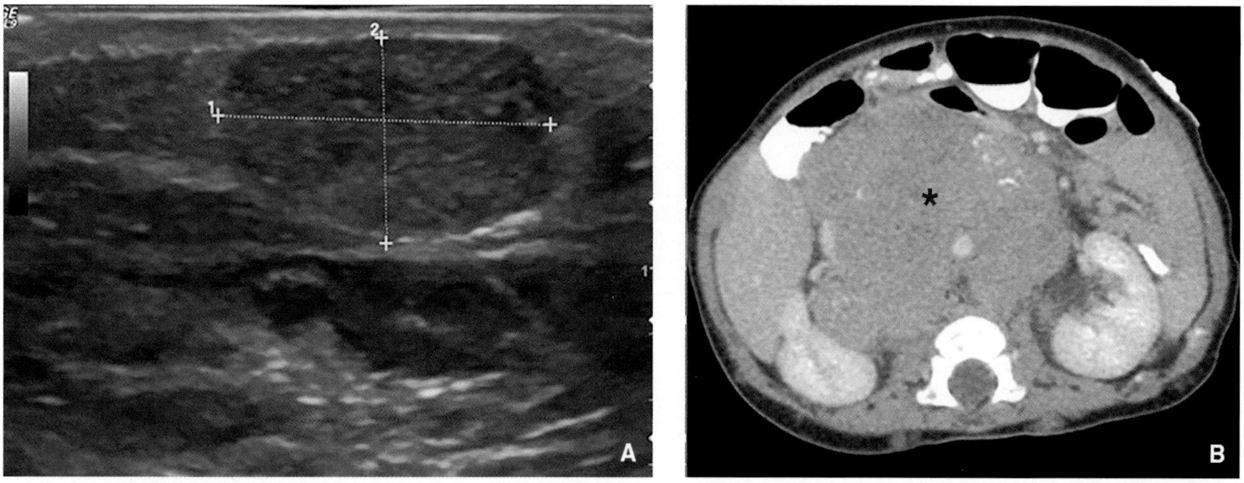

FIGURE 20.17 **Abdominal wall metastasis from neuroblastoma in a 1-year-old boy. A:** Ultrasound image demonstrates a hypoechoic mass (calipers) in the abdominal wall just superficial to musculature. **B:** Axial enhanced CT image from the same patient demonstrates a large confluent retroperitoneal mass (*asterisk*), which was found to be neuroblastoma.

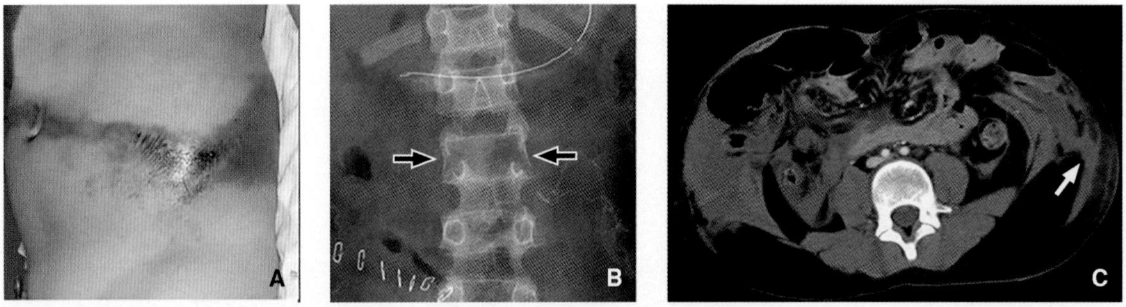

FIGURE 20.18 **Traumatic abdominal wall hernia from lap-belt injury in an 8-year-old boy. A:** Physical exam demonstrates extensive abdominal wall ecchymosis from seat-belt blunt trauma. **B:** Abdominal radiograph shows an L2 lumbar spine Chance fracture (*arrows*) with horizontal fracture lines through both pedicles. **C:** Axial enhanced CT image shows traumatic rupture of the rectus abdominis with bowel and mesenteric herniation. Extensive hemorrhage is also present in the abdominal wall (*arrow*). (Images provided by Jonathan R. Dillman, MD, MSc, Cincinnati Children's Hospital Medical Center, Cincinnati, OH.)

others advocating immediate hernia repair to avoid incarceration, with concomitant exploration for associated internal injuries.[56,57]

SPECTRUM OF MESENTERY AND PERITONEAL DISORDERS

Congenital and Developmental Anomalies

Mesenteric and Omental Cysts and Lymphatic Malformations

Mesenteric and omental cysts are extremely rare in the pediatric population, present in 1 in every 20,000 pediatric hospital admissions.[58] Most commonly, they are located in the small bowel mesentery, although they can also be found along the gastrointestinal tract. These are considered congenital in origin, and the majority of these cysts are diagnosed in children under 5 years of age.[59,60] Historically, the term mesenteric or omental cyst has been a descriptive term for all cystic lesions occurring in these locations; however, there is a histologic distinction between true epithelial enteric cysts (e.g., enteric duplication cysts) lined by cuboidal or columnar epithelium (Fig. 20.19), and cystic lymphatic malformations (Fig. 20.20) containing lymphatic endothelium and smooth muscle that do not communicate with the lymphatic system.[59,61,62] Some studies have categorized mesenteric cysts based on their fluid contents (e.g., chylous vs. serous), which does not appear to correlate with histologic type.[62] The literature overall suggests that, while some mesenteric and omental cysts represent distinct histologic entities from lymphatic malformations (e.g., mesothelial origin), they are not readily distinguishable by imaging.[63]

The most common clinical presentation of mesenteric and omental cysts is abdominal pain, distention, and/or palpable mass.[64] There can also be symptoms related to cyst mass effect such as bowel obstruction and vomiting. Large cysts can be complicated by hemorrhage, rupture, and torsion/volvulus.[64] Some literature suggests that cystic lymphatic malformations are more likely to present earlier in age, have a male predominance, be of larger size, and produce symptoms compared with true mesothelial mesenteric and omental cysts.[59,62]

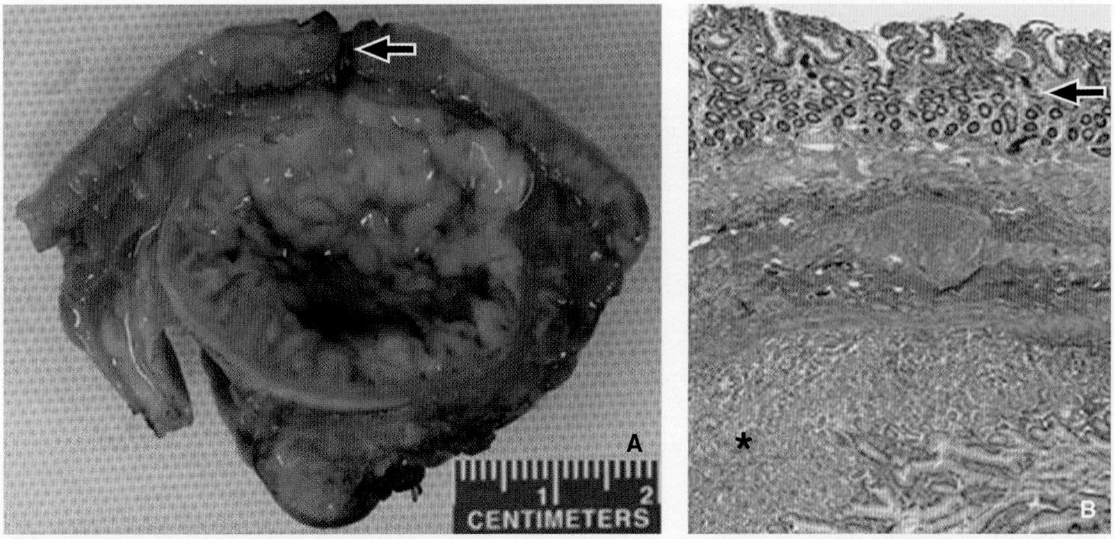

FIGURE 20.19 **Pathologic features of an enteric duplication cyst in a 4-year-old boy with abdominal pain and peritonitis. A:** Gross image demonstrates longitudinally sectioned compressed ileum (*top*) communicating along its mesenteric surface with a spherical structure (*bottom*); the antimesenteric side of the ileum shows a perforation (*arrow*). **B:** Microscopically, a common smooth muscle wall divides the gastric fundic-type mucosa of the duplication cyst (*asterisk*) from the small intestinal–type mucosa (*arrow*) of the bowel (hematoxylin and eosin; original magnification, 400×).

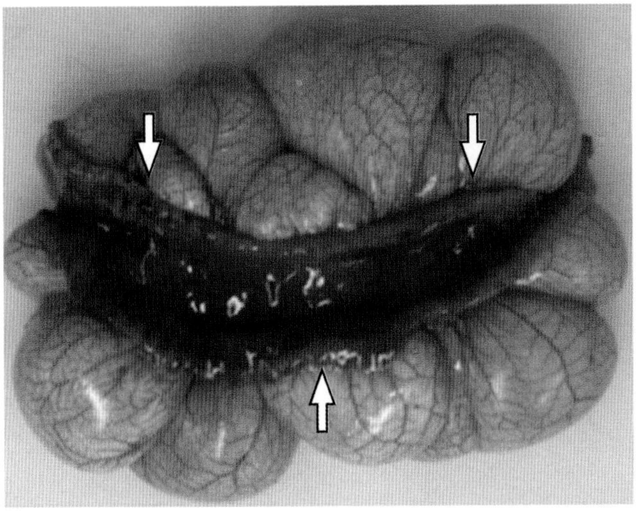

FIGURE 20.20 **Gross appearance of a mesenteric lymphatic malformation in a newborn girl.** The small bowel (*arrows*), opened longitudinally, is encased by a multicystic yellow chyle-filled mass in this newborn with abdominal distention and bloody stools.

On all imaging studies, including US, CT, and MRI, mesenteric and omental cysts appear as well-defined thin-walled cysts with or without thin internal septations in either the small bowel mesentery or the omentum.[65] Imaging provides information regarding cyst location, size, and involvement of abdominal structures as well as its relationship to mesenteric vessels (Fig. 20.21).[60,63] In all cases, surgical resection is standard, typically in a minimally invasive manner, both to alleviate symptoms and prevent rare cases of malignant degeneration.[64]

Mesothelial Cysts and Benign Cystic Mesothelioma

The mesothelium refers to the squamous epithelial lining of the pleura, pericardium, or peritoneum, as well as the serous layer covering the reproductive organs in both males and females.[66] Mesothelial cystic lesions can occur in any of these locations. The most common benign cystic mesothelial-lined lesions are mesothelial cysts and benign multicystic mesothelioma (BCM). A case series has been published describing congenital diaphragmatic mesothelial cysts occurring in children.[67]

Benign cystic mesothelioma most commonly occurs in young adult women with a median age at presentation of 36 years[66,68]; this entity has also been reported to occur within the scrotum of young men.[69] The lack of association with asbestos exposure distinguishes these lesions from malignant mesothelioma.[70] Mesothelial cysts are thought to be congenital, whereas BCM are hypothesized to be inflammatory in nature.[68] It has been suggested that mesothelial cysts and multicystic mesothelioma be classified as a subtype of mesenteric cyst that is distinct from mesenteric cysts and lymphatic malformations.[71]

Most mesothelial cysts and BCM are discovered incidentally, although BCM have been known to produce pain or a palpable mass.[67,68] Mesothelial cysts of the diaphragm appear as thin-walled anechoic cysts in the posterolateral right costophrenic sulcus, interposed between the liver and chest wall,[67] although mesothelial cysts can occur in any mesothelial-lined location (Fig. 20.22). BCM typically appears as a large multiloculated cystic mass that grows along a mesothelial-lined surface, which in the abdomen includes the peritoneum, omentum, and surfaces lining the abdominal viscera.[66]

Asymptomatic mesothelial cysts may be followed by serial imaging to confirm stability or spontaneous resolution.[67] BCM are typically treated by surgical resection and may exhibit local recurrence.[68]

Infectious and Inflammatory Disorders

Peritoneal Inclusion Cyst

Peritoneal inclusion cysts are uncommon pelvic cystic lesions occurring in females of reproductive age and have been described in young female adolescents.[72] The fluid accumulation within the cysts appears related to active ovaries in the presence of peritoneal adhesions.[73,74] Risk factors for development of peritoneal inclusion cysts include prior history of abdominal surgery, pelvic inflammatory disease, inflammatory bowel disease, and endometriosis. Evidence suggests that within the context of inflamed or injured peritoneum, there is diminished clearance of ovarian fluid leading to cyst accumulation.[75] It is unclear whether these cysts form as a reaction to peritoneal injury/inflammation or whether they represent a primary proliferative process.[72] Histologically,

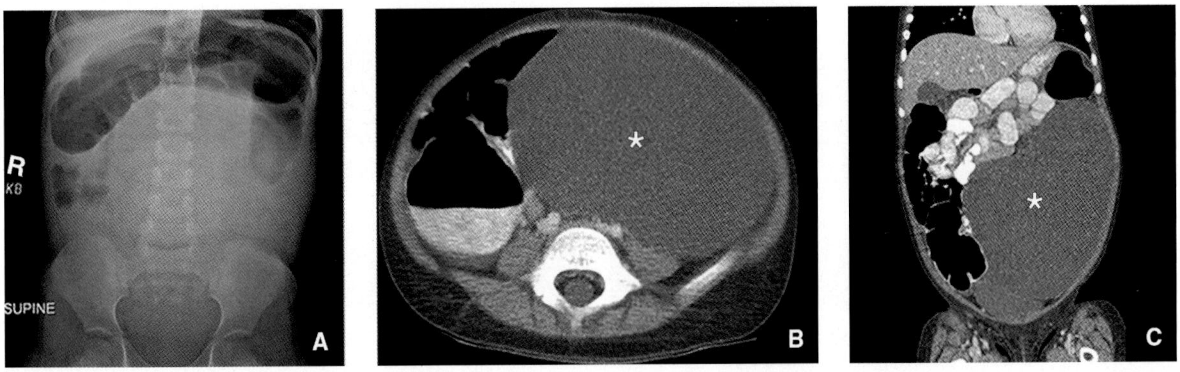

FIGURE 20.21 **Mesenteric cyst in a 4-year-old girl who presented with abdominal pain. A:** Abdominal radiograph demonstrates paucity of bowel gas in the abdomen with displacement of colonic loops. Axial **(B)** and coronal **(C)** images from contrast-enhanced CT demonstrate a large cyst (*asterisk*) filling the abdomen that was shown at surgery to be a mesenteric cyst of lymphatic origin.

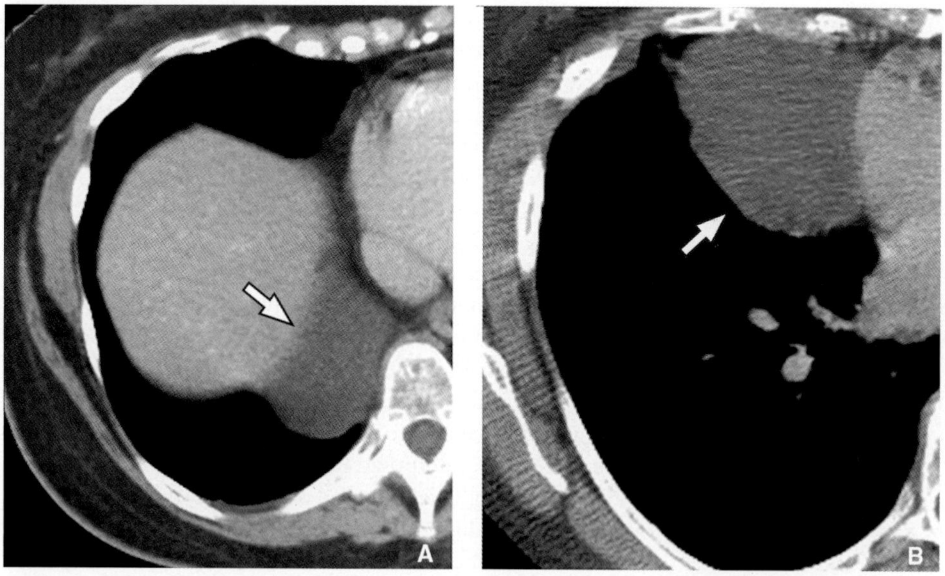

FIGURE 20.22 **Mesothelial cyst in a 17-year-old girl. A and B:** Axial enhanced CT images demonstrate a cyst in the posterolateral right costophrenic sulcus in a typical location of a mesothelial cyst (*arrows*) and which shifts position when the patient is scanned in the prone position **(B)**.

these are lined by mesothelium and can be indistinguishable from benign cystic mesothelioma.[72,76]

Peritoneal inclusion cysts typically present with lower abdominal or pelvic pain or a pelvic mass.[77] Peritoneal inclusion cysts are usually evaluated by US or MRI, where they typically appear as a loculated fluid collection surrounding the ovary, which conforms to the contours of the peritoneum (Fig. 20.23),[78] the so-called spider-in-web appearance.[79] The associated peritoneal adhesions usually appear as thin curvilinear septations associated with the cyst but can coalesce and mimic hydrosalpinx or a solid ovarian mass. Peritoneal inclusion cysts with the classic imaging features can be followed by serial US or MR imaging over 6 to 12 months to confirm stability.[78] Lesions that are symptomatic, enlarging, or demonstrate suspicious imaging features often undergo surgical excision.[72] Recurrence rates following resection are in the 30% to 50% range overall, and there is evidence to suggest that peritoneal inclusion cysts in pediatric patients have a better prognosis and lower recurrence rate compared with those in adults.[72,76] Peritoneal inclusion cysts can undergo metaplasia but do not have malignant potential.[78]

Meconium Peritonitis

Meconium peritonitis is a chemical irritation of the peritoneum secondary to in utero bowel perforation leading to intraperitoneal meconium spillage. The event leading to perforation is believed to occur after 16 weeks of gestation, which is when meconium reaches the ileum. Inciting causes include bowel atresias, meconium ileus, volvulus, peritoneal bands, and internal hernias.[80] Meconium peritonitis is estimated to occur in 1 in every 30,000 live births, with a mortality rate of 10% to 50%. The chemical peritonitis produced by meconium is principally due to a fibroblastic reaction against the digestive enzymes present in meconium.[80]

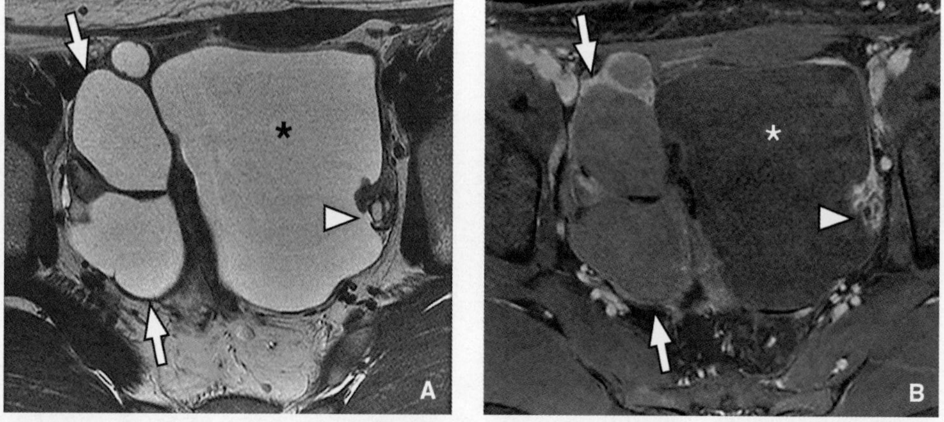

FIGURE 20.23 **Peritoneal inclusion cyst in a 14-year-old girl.** Axial T2-weighted **(A)** and postcontrast T1-weighted fat-saturated **(B)** MR images demonstrate a large cyst (*asterisks*) surrounding the left ovary (*arrowheads*) with boundaries conforming to the peritoneum, which was confirmed at surgery to be a peritoneal inclusion cyst. There is also a tubular structure in the right adnexa (*arrows*) with mildly increased T1-weighted signal intensity that was found to be a hematosalpinx in the same patient.

Three main subtypes of meconium peritonitis have been described: (1) fibroadhesive in which the site of perforation is localized, (2) cystic in which the bowel walls off the spilled meconium within a focal cavity (meconium pseudocyst), and (3) generalized in which meconium is spilled throughout the abdomen because of a late event in the perinatal period.[80,81]

Meconium peritonitis can often be diagnosed on prenatal US as echogenic ascites along with signs of bowel obstruction, including bowel dilation and polyhydramnios.[82] In the postnatal period, affected patients often present with abdominal distention, bilious vomiting, and delayed passage of meconium.[82] Radiographs and US both demonstrate focal calcifications in a peritoneal distribution (Fig. 20.24), including the scrotum in males, and can be associated with either bowel distention or free intraperitoneal air if persistent perforation is present.[83] A meconium pseudocyst typically appears as an abdominal cystic collection with air and fluid along with rim calcification.[80] The majority of patients in whom meconium peritonitis is diagnosed in utero require surgery during the postnatal period.[83]

Mesenteric Adenitis

Mesenteric adenitis is a self-limited benign inflammatory process involving right lower quadrant lymph nodes. It is thought to be a reaction to either a viral or bacterial infectious process involving the terminal ileum and is defined as the presence of at least three lymph nodes ≥5 mm in short-axis diameter, in the absence of an identifiable underlying acute inflammatory process.[84–86]

The clinical presentation of mesenteric adenitis in children is not specific but often consists of fever, right lower quadrant pain, and leukocytosis.[85] Mesenteric adenitis is typically a diagnosis of exclusion in which numerous enlarged right lower quadrant lymph nodes are seen in the absence of appendicitis on US or CT. The enlarged mesenteric lymph nodes are often well depicted by US[86]; however, CT is often the imaging modality of choice (Fig. 20.25) to ensure that the lymphadenopathy is not secondary to another infectious, inflammatory, or malignant process.[85] On CT, mild terminal ileal wall thickening may be present, suggesting an association between mesenteric adenitis and terminal ileitis.[85] Mesenteric adenitis is considered a self-limited process that may be managed either by observation or by antibiotic therapy.

Omental Infarction

Omental infarction is an uncommon cause of acute abdominal pain in children, with the majority of cases occurring in adults.[87] The greater omentum is a four-layered peritoneal reflection that covers the small bowel anteriorly within the peritoneal cavity. Its blood supply is through numerous epiploic (omental) collateral vessels, which makes it relatively resistant to ischemia.[88] There is involvement of the right-sided epiploic vessels supplying the greater omentum in 90%

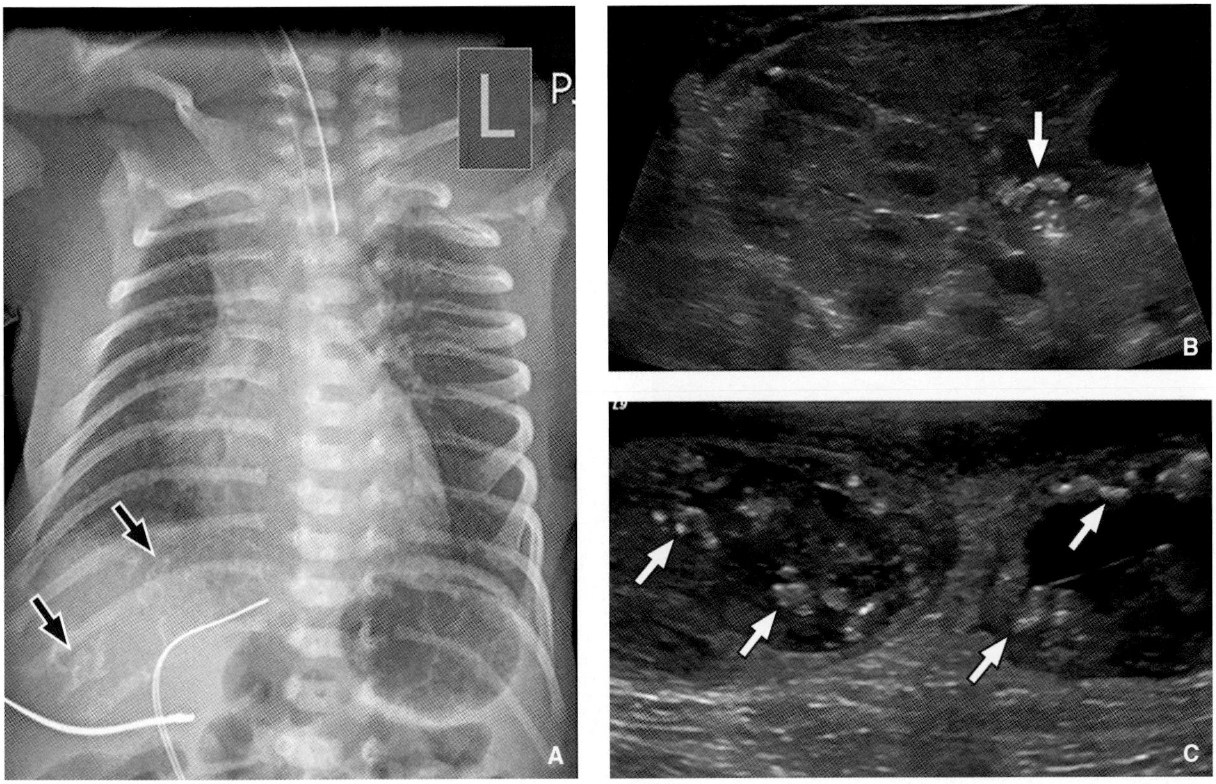

FIGURE 20.24 **Meconium peritonitis in a newborn boy. A:** Frontal radiograph of the chest demonstrates multiple calcifications (*black arrows*) in a peritoneal distribution projecting over the upper abdomen. Gray-scale ultrasound images reveal echogenic calcifications (*arrows*) in the **(B)** subhepatic space and **(C)** scrotum, consistent with meconium peritonitis.

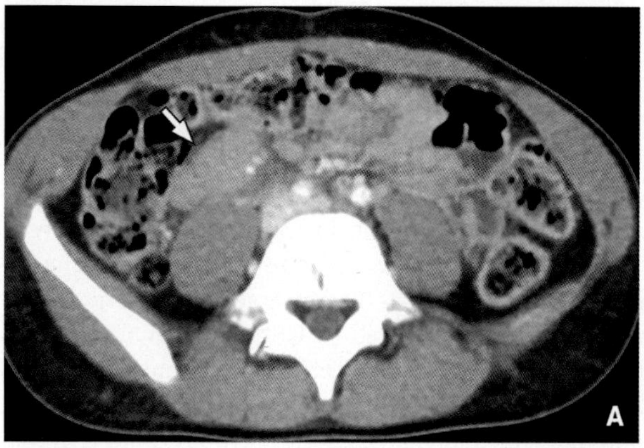
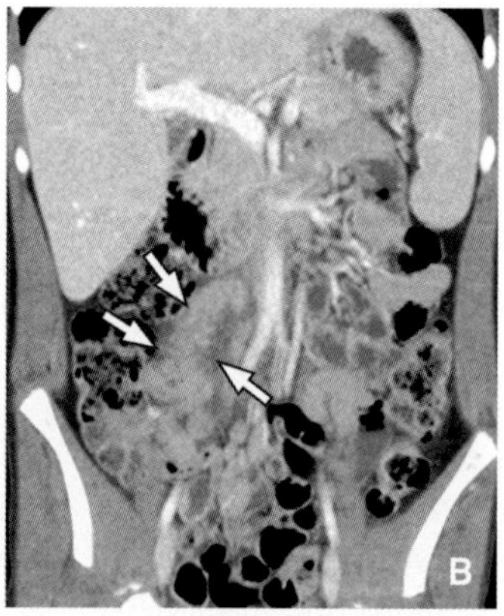

FIGURE 20.25 **Mesenteric adenitis in a 10-year-old girl who presented with right lower quadrant abdominal pain.** Axial **(A)** and coronal **(B)** enhanced CT images show conglomerate nodal enlargement (*arrows*) in the right lower quadrant mesentery with surrounding inflammatory changes most characteristic of mesenteric lymphadenitis. The appendix and adjacent bowel were normal.

of omental infarction cases, which accounts for the typical clinical presentation of right-sided abdominal pain.[87] Current thinking is that mobility along the redundant aspect of the greater omentum may predispose to torsion and ischemia of the small epiploic branch arteries, leading to segmental omental infarction.[89] Risk factors for the development of omental infarction in children include obesity and male gender, with both factors possibly associated with greater omental fat accumulation.[90,91] A separate but similar entity is epiploic appendagitis, which is acute inflammation of the epiploic (omental) appendages of peritoneum that arise from the serosal surface of the colon.[92] Torsion of these appendages causes infarction similar to that of omental infarction; however, this more commonly causes left lower quadrant pain from appendagitis of the sigmoid colon. Omental infarction is much more likely than epiploic appendagitis to be encountered in the pediatric population.[92]

The majority of affected pediatric patients present with acute onset of abdominal pain, especially localized to the right lower quadrant, mimicking acute appendicitis. Of note, omental infarction cases typically do not have preceding periumbilical pain, fever, or gastrointestinal symptoms.[87] US is often the first imaging modality performed. By US, omental infarction classically appears as hypoechoic or hyperechoic mass localized to the omentum that is fixed to the bowel and corresponds to the patient's area of discomfort. US evaluation may miss the area of infarction if it is small or if the adjacent bowel is either collapsed or air filled. CT is currently considered to be the imaging modality of choice for diagnosing omental infarction, as it has been shown to have higher sensitivity than US.[90] On CT, omental infarction classically appears as a focal area of soft tissue inflammation/fat stranding within the omental fat, adjacent to the cecum or ascending colon[90,92] (Fig. 20.26). CT may also be advantageous to exclude acute appendicitis in cases where neither an omental infarction nor appendicitis is seen by US. Omental infarction typically is a benign, self-limiting condition that resolves spontaneously and requires only analgesic medications, usually within 2 weeks.[87,90]

Epiploic appendagitis is also a self-limited process. These finger-like, fat-filled sacs extend from the surface of the colon and rectum and may become inflamed when they torse upon their stalk or when there is thrombosis of the draining vein. Epiploic appendagitis on CT typically appears as a fat

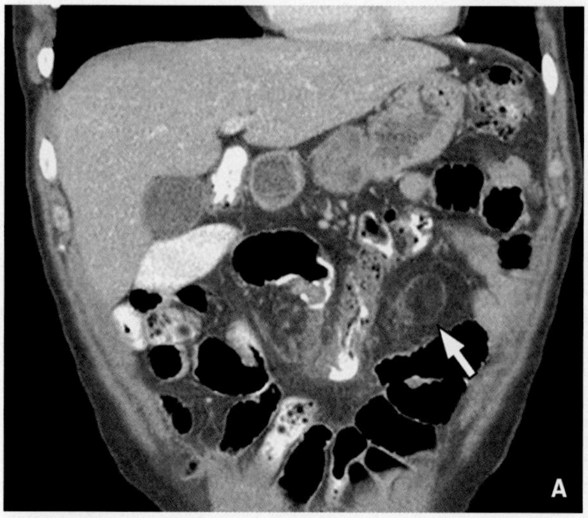
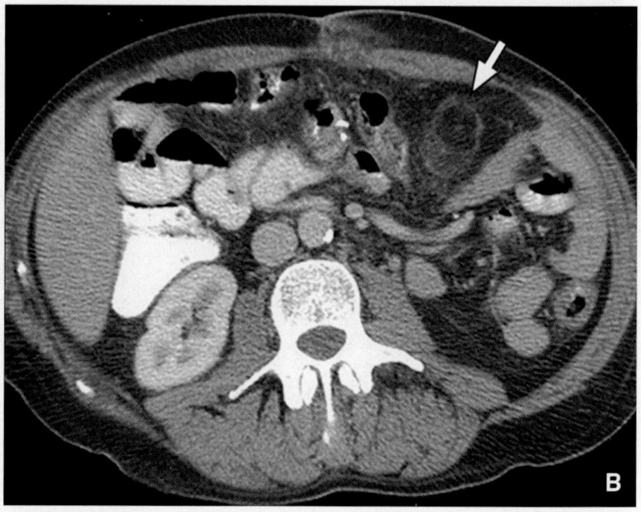

FIGURE 20.26 **Omental infarction in a 17-year-old girl with prior small bowel resection for volvulus.** Coronal **(A)** and axial **(B)** enhanced CT images demonstrate a rounded area of soft tissue inflammation (*arrows*) within the greater omental fat, which spontaneously resolved on subsequent imaging.

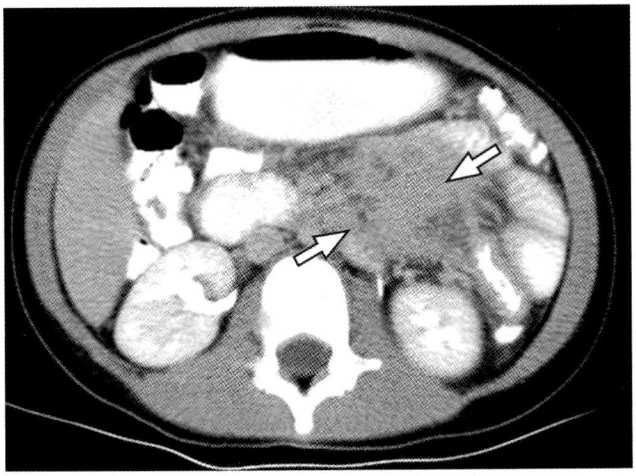

FIGURE 20.27 **Mesenteric desmoid tumor in a 10-year-old boy.** Enhanced axial CT image demonstrates a large spiculated soft tissue mass (*arrows*) in the root of the small bowel mesentery that is characteristic of an intra-abdominal desmoid tumor.

attenuation soft tissue mass abutting the anterior margin of the colon with surrounding inflammatory changes and can be confused for omental infarction. Treatment for this condition is conservative, with pain management and anti-inflammatory medications as first-line therapy. Symptoms typically resolve within 5 to 7 days.[88]

Neoplastic Disorders

Benign Neoplasms

Desmoid-Type Fibromatosis

Desmoid tumors are nonmalignant mesenchymal tumors that often appear locally aggressive on imaging (Fig. 20.27). They typically demonstrate spiculated margins and can invade or surround adjacent structures. Desmoids are commonly mesenteric in location, but they can be found in the abdominal wall, as described above, as well as the extraperitoneal space and nonabdominal locations. Imaging findings for mesenteric desmoids are similar to abdominal wall desmoids described previously within this chapter. Following excision, desmoids tend to locally recur.[30,93] Complete surgical resection, if possible, is the current cornerstone of management of desmoid tumors, whereas unresectable or residual tumors can be treated with chemotherapy or radiotherapy.[94]

Malignant Neoplasms

Rhabdomyosarcoma

Rhabdomyosarcoma represents ~5% of all malignancies in children,[95] the vast majority of whom are <10 years old at diagnosis. It is a malignant soft tissue tumor that arises from primitive mesenchymal cells; given the ubiquity of mesenchymal tissue, primary rhabdomyosarcomas have been found to arise from almost every organ in the body. The most common sites, however, are the head and neck region and the genitourinary tract. Uncommonly, rhabdomyosarcoma can involve the peritoneal cavity (Fig. 20.28), either as a primary malignancy or as a metastatic disease. In a series of 55 pediatric patients with rhabdomyosarcoma by Chung et al.,[96] 11% were found to have intraperitoneal disease during their clinical course.

Imaging findings for intraperitoneal rhabdomyosarcoma are nonspecific, with ascites representing the most common imaging characteristic. Mesenteric nodules and nodules studding the peritoneal lining have also been described; calcification of these nodules has not been reported. Omental nodularity or "caking" is also an imaging feature of intraperitoneal rhabdomyosarcoma. In children, the differential diagnosis of omental modularity includes lymphoma (lymphomatosis), Wilms tumor, and desmoplastic small round cell tumor whereas it is commonly seen in gastrointestinal malignancies in the adult population.

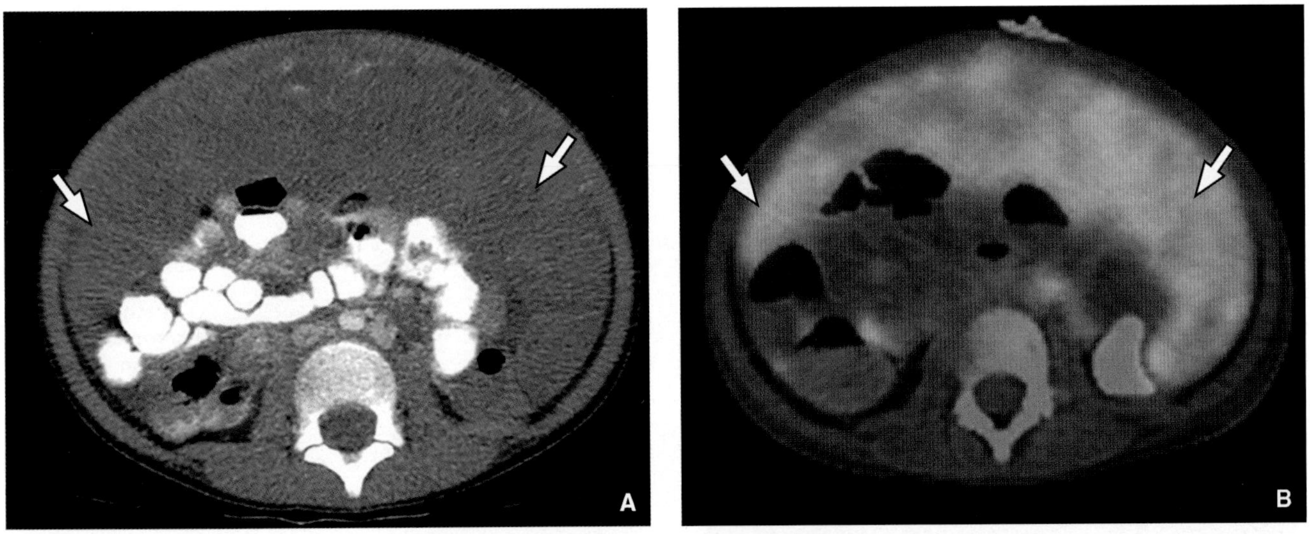

FIGURE 20.28 **Primary peritoneal rhabdomyosarcoma in a 7-year-old girl. A:** Axial enhanced CT image demonstrates extensive soft tissue abnormality (*arrows*) occupying the anterior abdomen with mass effect upon bowel and mesentery. **B:** ^{18}F-FDG–PET/CT shows that the abnormality (*arrows*) is hypermetabolic. Surgery confirmed extensive peritoneal and omental tumor, confirmed by histopathology to be rhabdomyosarcoma.

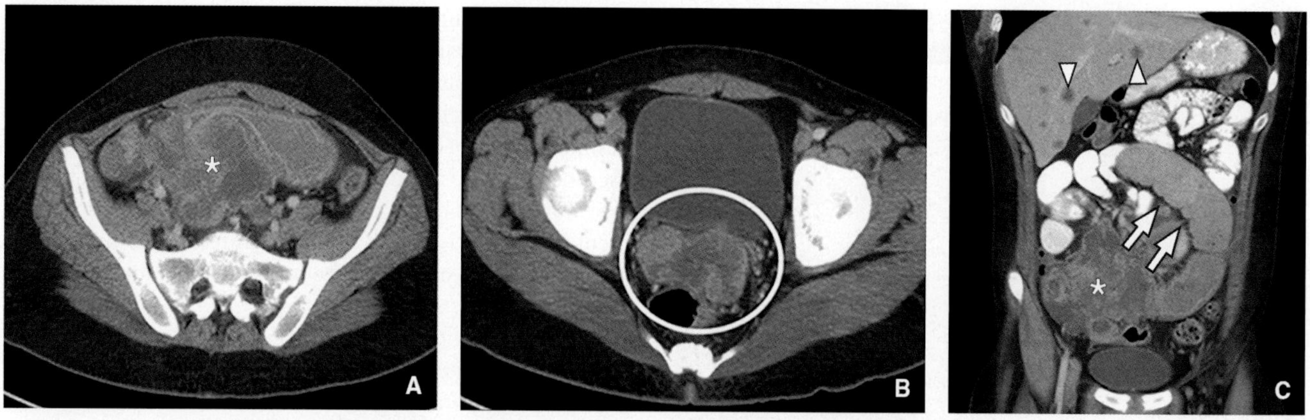

FIGURE 20.29 **Desmoplastic small round cell tumor in a 15-year-old boy.** Axial **(A, B)** and coronal **(C)** enhanced CT images demonstrate a large soft tissue mass (*asterisk*) in the right lower quadrant with central necrosis causing small bowel obstruction (*arrows*). Numerous metastatic lesions (*arrowheads*) in the liver and peritoneal cul-de-sac (*circle*) are also seen.

Desmoplastic Small Round Cell Tumor

Desmoplastic small round cell tumor (Fig. 20.29) is a rare intraperitoneal malignancy that most commonly arises in young males, with a mean age at presentation of 19 years.[97] It is an aggressive malignancy, and the 3-year survival rate is <30%.[98,99] Histologically, the tumor is characterized by nests and cords poorly differentiated round cells embedded in an abundant collagenized ("desmoplastic") stroma (Fig. 20.30). The tumor cells harbor a chromosomal translocation that fuses the *EWSR1* gene on chromosome 22 with the *WT1* gene on chromosome 11.[100]

Desmoplastic small round cell tumors spread throughout the peritoneum and typically present as multiple intraperitoneal nodules and/or bulky masses on imaging. Bellah et al.[101] describe masses >10 cm in the majority of the patients in their 11 patient series. Ascites is commonly present. Punctate or amorphous calcifications within the masses may be seen as well. On CT, large dominant masses demonstrate internal hypoattenuation, reflecting central necrosis; on MR, the masses are typically T1-weighted hypointense and T2-weighted hyperintense, with heterogeneous enhancement following intravenous contrast material administration. Although these imaging features can be shared by other processes, the presence of a single or several large masses in the context of a diffuse intraperitoneal process favors the diagnosis of desmoplastic small round cell tumor.

Desmoplastic small round cell tumors can spread hematogenously or via lymphatic channels, with retroperitoneal lymphadenopathy present in about 50% of cases.[101] Distant metastases at the time of presentation are seen in ~50% of cases.[99] Although there is currently no standardized management, an aggressive approach including surgical resection combined with neoadjuvant chemotherapy and radiotherapy is recommended.[102]

Malignant Mesothelioma

Peritoneal mesothelioma (Fig. 20.31) is the most common primary malignant neoplasm of the peritoneal lining but is extremely rare in the pediatric population. As with pleural mesothelioma, peritoneal mesothelioma is strongly associated with asbestos exposure. Affected patients typically present with nausea, vomiting, abdominal pain, and changes in bowel habits. This malignancy may present as a focal large mass, typically in the upper abdomen. Alternatively, the diffuse form of this disease manifests as multifocal areas of peritoneal thickening, sometimes encasing abdominal organs.

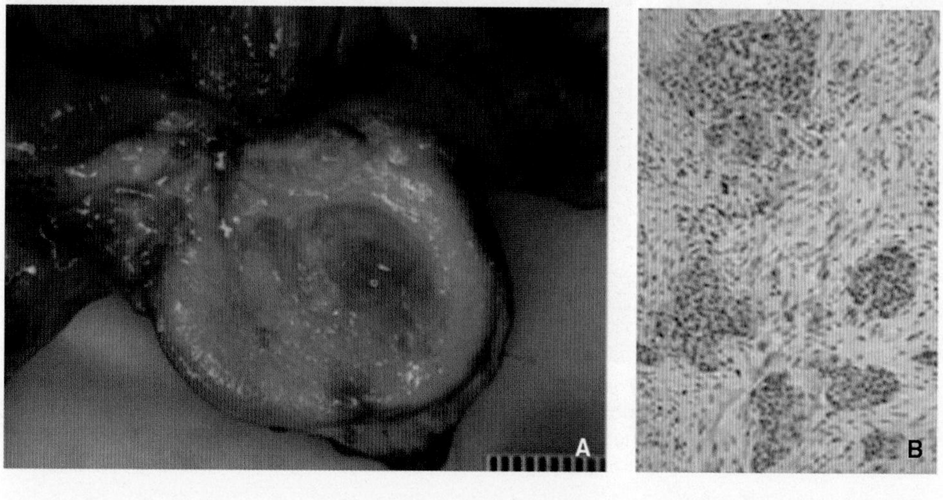

FIGURE 20.30 **Pathologic features of a desmoplastic small round cell tumor in a 3-year-old boy with diffuse peritoneal involvement.** Grossly **(A)**, there is a 4 cm mass adherent to the serosal surface of the jejunum. Microscopically **(B)**, nests of tumor cells are embedded in abundant fibrous tissue ("desmoplasia") (hematoxylin and eosin stain, original magnification, 100×).

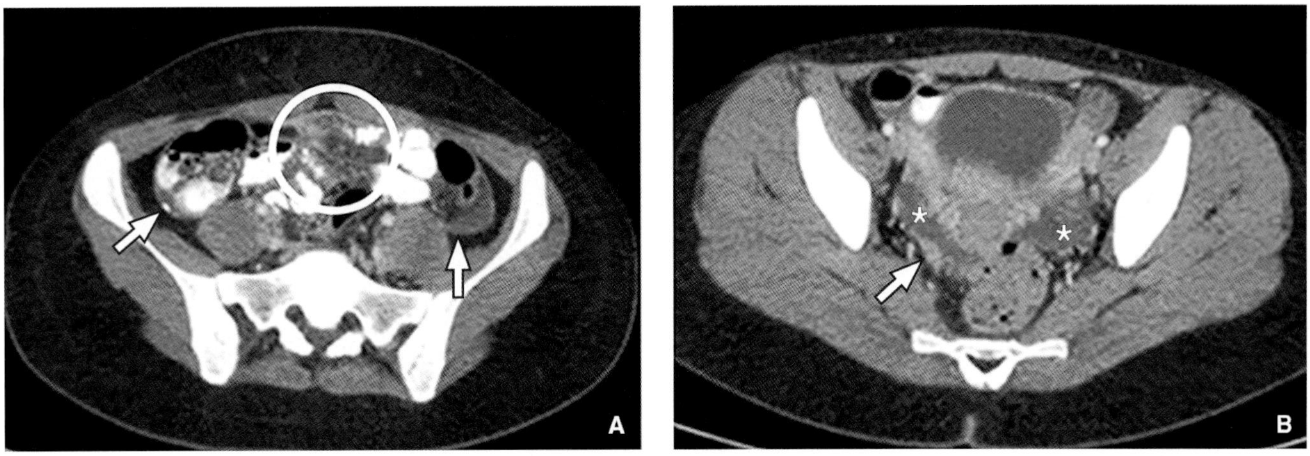

FIGURE 20.31 **Primary peritoneal mesothelioma in a 17-year-old girl who presented with diffuse abdominal pain. A and B:** Axial enhanced CT images demonstrate multiple peritoneal calcified and noncalcified soft tissue plaques (*arrows*), ascites (*asterisks*), as well as mesenteric and omental soft tissue stranding (*circle*). Intraperitoneal fluid is seen separate from the ovaries. (Images provided by Ajaykumar Morani, MD, MD Anderson Cancer Center, Houston, TX.)

Infiltration of the mesenteric fat can result in a stellate-like appearance.[103] If the disease is diagnosed in its early stage, the affected patient may be eligible for surgical resection. However, often palliative methods, such as chemotherapy and radiation therapy, are the only available treatment options for patients with advanced disease.

Peritoneal Dissemination of Malignancy

Diffuse dissemination of malignancy throughout the peritoneal cavity can be seen with metastatic progression. In adults, peritoneal metastasis is most often seen with carcinomatosis from primary epithelial malignancies, such as ovarian, gastrointestinal, pancreas, bladder, and breast cancers. Disseminated peritoneal malignancy in children is not typically related to epithelial malignancies.[104] Wilms tumor (Fig. 20.32) can involve the peritoneum by direct extension through the renal capsule and anterior pararenal space. Intraperitoneal spillage during surgical resection of Wilms tumor is another mechanism of peritoneal involvement. In the latter circumstance, "dropped" metastatic nodules can form in the most dependent portions of the pelvic peritoneal space, which in boys is the rectovesical space and in girls is the rectouterine space (pouch of Douglas).[105] Another source of peritoneal tumoral seeding in children is extracranial extension of brain malignancies through ventriculoperitoneal (VP) shunt catheters. VP shunts can serve as conduits for malignant cells from the cerebrospinal fluid into the peritoneum.[104] Finally, as described above, sarcomas such as rhabdomyosarcomas can diffusely involve the peritoneal space, either as a primary malignancy or as metastatic disease.

On imaging studies, peritoneal tumor dissemination appears as thickening or discrete nodularity of the peritoneal lining. Involvement of the omentum and mesentery is commonly seen. When the omentum is abnormally thickened and diffusely involved by disseminated tumor, the term "omental cake" may be used.

Peritoneal Lymphomatosis

Although mesenteric lymphadenopathy is a common feature of non-Hodgkin lymphoma, the diffuse lymphomatous involvement of the peritoneal cavity, known as peritoneal lymphomatosis, is much less common.[106] Peritoneal lymphomatosis is a radiologic mimic of peritoneal carcinomatosis (Fig. 20.33). Based on imaging alone, differentiating peritoneal lymphomatosis from carcinomatosis can be challenging. This differentiation, however, is clinically important, as the treatment algorithms as well as prognosis are very different.

Common imaging features of peritoneal lymphomatosis include malignant ascites, thickening and enhancement of the various peritoneal surfaces, and "omental caking." Retroperitoneal and mesenteric lymphadenopathy may also be present.[107] These imaging characteristics are shared with

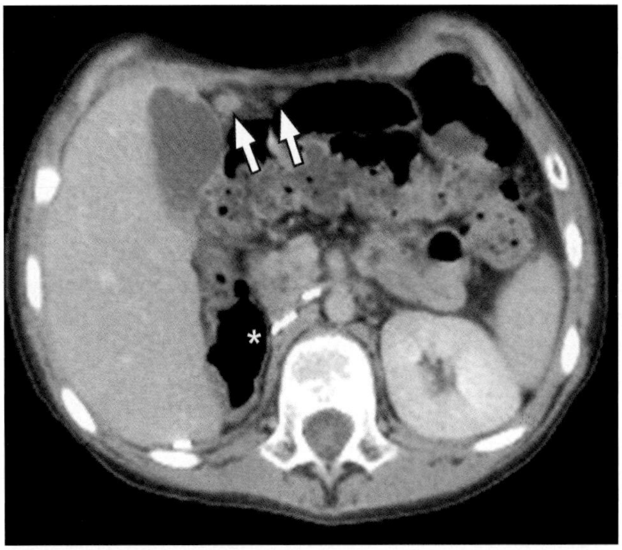

FIGURE 20.32 **Peritoneal dissemination from Wilms tumor in a 4-year-old boy.** Axial enhanced CT image shows two small omental nodules (*arrows*) proven to represent Wilms tumor deposits. The right kidney has been removed (*asterisk*).

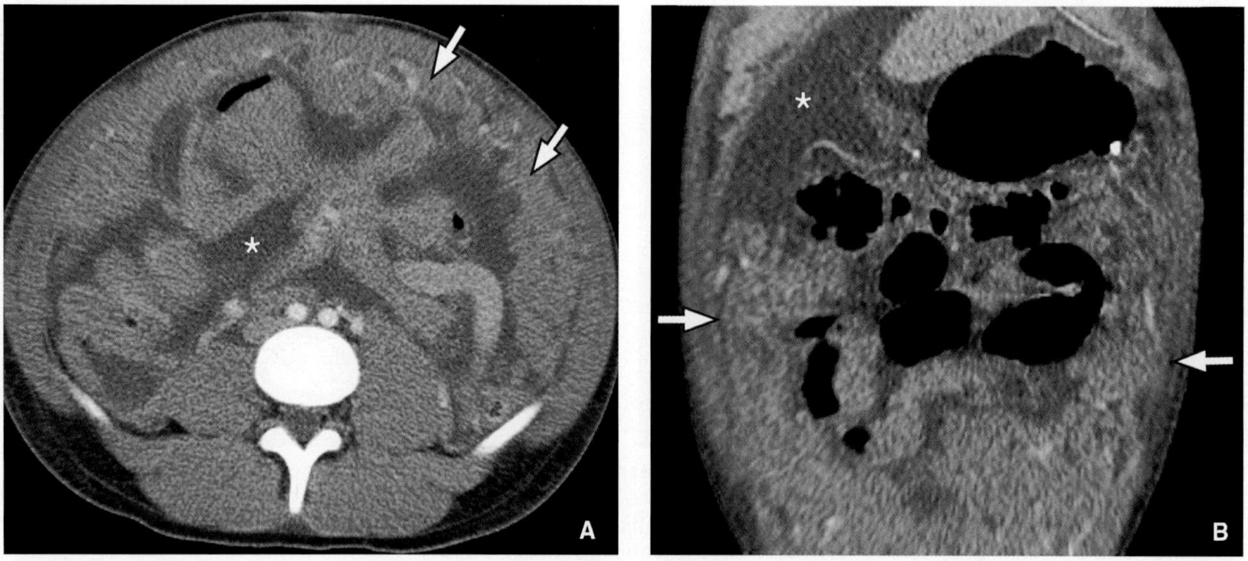

FIGURE 20.33 **Peritoneal lymphomatosis in a 7-year-old girl with Burkitt lymphoma.** Axial **(A)** and coronal **(B)** enhanced CT images demonstrate extensive "omental caking" (*arrows*) and malignant ascites (*asterisks*) due to lymphomatous involvement of the peritoneal cavity.

peritoneal carcinomatosis as well as infectious processes, such as tuberculous peritonitis. However, one distinguishing feature that favors lymphomatosis over infection is the presence of ascites without enhancing septations or loculations.[108]

SPECTRUM OF ABDOMINAL VASCULAR DISORDERS

Congenital and Developmental Anomalies

Abdominal Arterial Anomalies

Abdominal Aortic Coarctation and Hypoplasia (Including Middle Aortic Syndrome)

Developmental anomalies of the abdominal aorta are uncommon but have dramatic clinical ramifications.[109] By convention, narrowing of the abdominal aorta is termed "coarctation" when the narrowing is focal/segmental and is termed "hypoplasia" when the narrowing extends over a long distance (Fig. 20.34). The descriptive diagnosis "middle aortic syndrome" is also applied by some to refer to idiopathic abdominal aortic narrowing, whereas others may use the term when the narrowing is secondary to another disease process (e.g., neurofibromatosis, type 1 [NF1], Takayasu arteritis). In this section, we refer to the congenital and developmental causes of abdominal aortic narrowing as coarctation and hypoplasia; we discuss systemic processes with aortic manifestations individually in subsequent sections.

Abdominal coarctation accounts for fewer than 2% of all cases of aortic coarctation[109] and is believed to occur because of an error in fusion of the primitive aorta during embryogenesis. During the 3rd week of fetal development, two strands of endocardial mesenchyma extend caudally along the neural groove to form two primitive paired dorsal aortas. These exist as discrete vascular channels for ~1 week, after which point they fuse to form a single aorta.[9] Aortic coarctation and hypoplasia are the result of either over fusion or unsuccessful fusion of the primitive dorsal aortas.

There is no specific gender predilection for abdominal aortic coarctation, in distinction to thoracic aortic coarctation, which features a 2:1 male predominance. Congenital narrowing of the aorta is frequently associated with stenoses of the visceral branch arteries, including the renal arteries, and to a lesser degree the celiac axis, SMA, and IMA. These

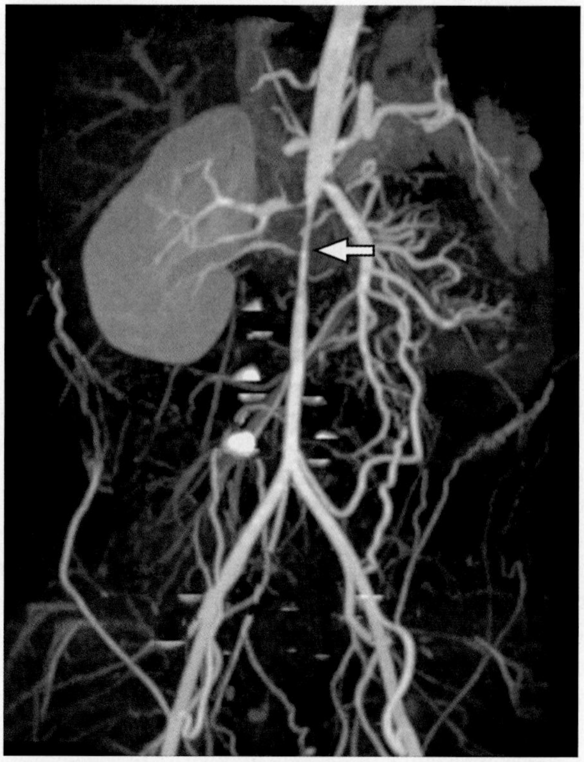

FIGURE 20.34 **Congenital abdominal aortic hypoplasia in a 6-year-old girl.** Coronal enhanced maximum intensity projection CT image demonstrates long segment narrowing (*arrow*) of the abdominal aorta associated with numerous mesenteric and body wall arterial collaterals. There is ostial narrowing of two right renal arteries. Left kidney is absent.

narrowings can result in a prominent arc of Riolan meandering mesenteric artery as a collateral vessel bypassing the areas of stenosis.[110] On imaging, a suprarenal aortic stenosis can manifest as parvus and tardus waveforms in the renal arteries.[111,112] Clinically, affected pediatric patients often present during childhood with severe renovascular hypertension due to stenosis of the suprarenal aorta and renal arteries, as well as diminished perfusion of the lower extremities. Extensive collateral arterial pathways are established over time in order to mitigate lower extremity symptoms, although physical exam is usually notable for diminished or absent pedal pulses and an abdominal bruit from turbulent flow at the site of stenosis. In the setting of abdominal aortic narrowing, CT angiography or MR angiography can be used to assess the entire aorta as well as determine collateral pathways. Conventional angiography is often required to adequately evaluate for narrowings involving the renal and mesenteric arteries.

Life expectancy for congenital narrowing of the aorta is ~30 to 40 years, with the most common cause of death being heart failure or intracranial hemorrhage. Treatment options include aortic reconstruction surgery (aortoplasty), bypass grafting, and angioplasty with or without stent placement. Renal revascularization is an effective intervention for the management of renovascular hypertension when narrowing is extra-renal. Because of the presence of collaterals, lower extremity claudication is a relatively uncommon symptom.

Abdominal Aortic Aneurysm

Although multiple secondary causes of abdominal aortic aneurysms have been identified, including umbilical artery catheterization, connective tissue disorders, and vasculitis, congenital abdominal aortic aneurysms, while extremely uncommon (Fig. 20.35), can occur in the pediatric population.[113–115] Abdominal aortic aneurysms are a rare but well-described manifestation of tuberous sclerosis. These aneurysms range from relatively small to up to 11 cm.[114] Surgical repair has been successful in some cases.

Persistent Sciatic Artery

A persistent sciatic artery (Fig. 20.36) is an anatomic variant that was first described in 1832.[116] During fetal development, the sciatic artery serves as the major artery to the lower limb bud. As the femoral arteries develop, the sciatic artery normally regresses. However, in 0.01% to 0.05% of patients, the sciatic artery persists; when present, ~12% of cases are bilateral.[116] The clinical significance of this anatomic variant is because of its proclivity for early atherosclerosis and aneurysm formation. Affected patients typically present with claudication or other ischemic symptoms due to emboli originating from partially thrombosed sciatic artery aneurysms.

The sciatic artery courses from the internal iliac artery to the popliteal artery, passing through the greater sciatic foramen to enter the thigh. The artery courses along the posterior aspect of the adductor magnus and may lie within or adjacent to the sheath of the sciatic nerve; alternatively, it may run alongside the posterior cutaneous nerve.[117,118]

With a "completely" persistent sciatic artery, which is the most common scenario, the sciatic artery serves as the principal arterial supply to the lower extremity. In this circumstance, the superficial femoral artery is diminutive and terminates in the mid- to lower thigh. Hypoplasia of the superficial femoral artery can be misinterpreted as occlusive disease, for which surgical revascularization may be inappropriately performed. CT angiography, MR angiography, and conventional angiography can all detect this arterial anomaly.

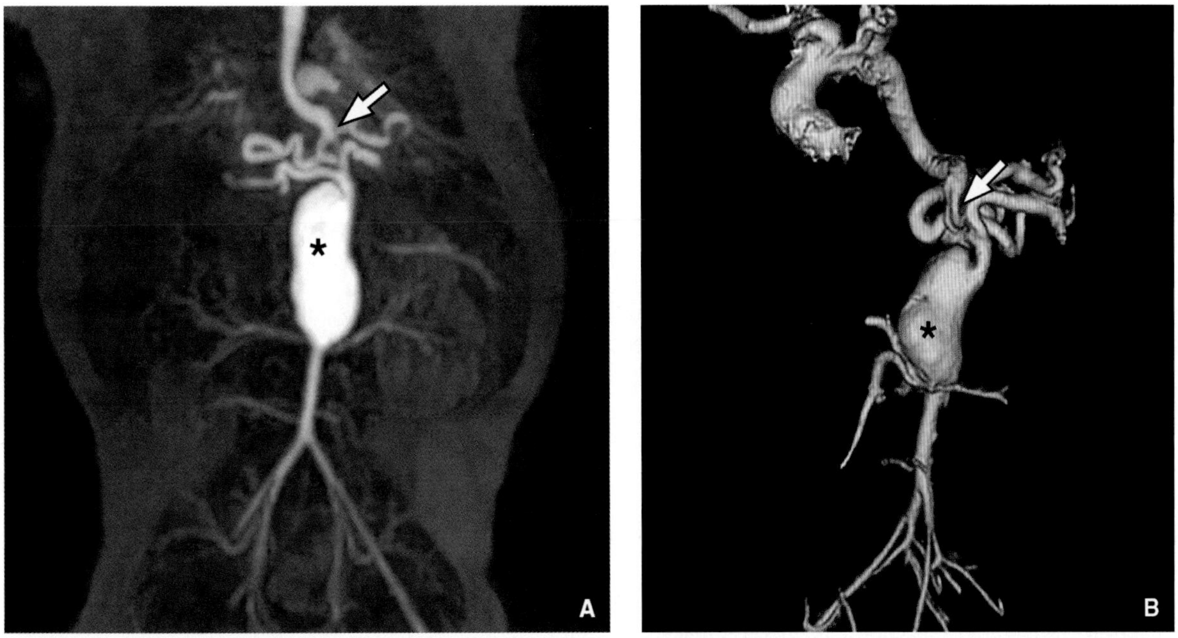

FIGURE 20.35 **Congenital abdominal aortic aneurysm in a 3-month-old boy.** Coronal maximum intensity projection **(A)** and volume rendered **(B)** MR images from postcontrast T1-weighted fat-saturated MR images demonstrate congenital descending thoracic aortic interruption (*arrows*) associated with numerous collateral vessels feeding into an abdominal aortic aneurysm (*asterisks*).

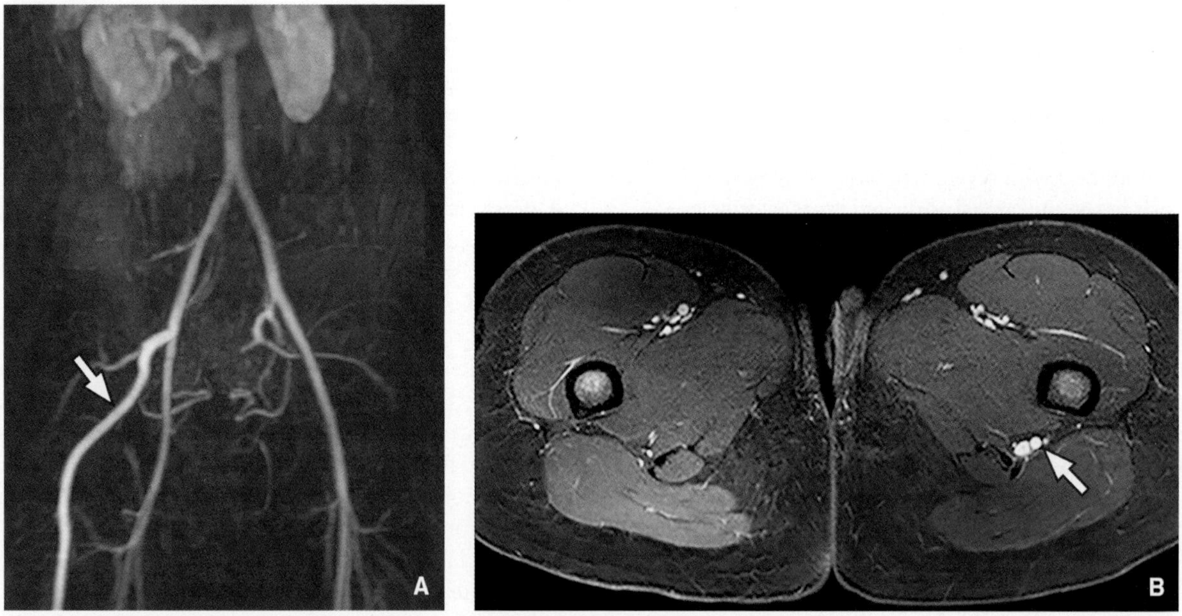

FIGURE 20.36 **Persistent sciatic artery in a 15-year-old girl with claudication.** Posterior maximum intensity projection **(A)** and axial postcontrast T1-weighted fat-saturated **(B)** MR images demonstrate a left-sided persistent sciatic artery (*arrows*) as a dominant branch of the left internal iliac artery feeding the left lower extremity, in its typical location along the posterior aspect of the adductor magnus **(B)**.

Abdominal Venous Anomalies

Many anatomic variants of the IVC and renal veins have been identified. A heuristic appreciation for the development of the IVC provides a useful logical framework and classification system for these anomalies.

Venous drainage in the fetus develops initially as paired anterior and posterior cardinal veins, with the former draining the cranial half of the fetus and the latter draining the caudal half of the fetus. These veins coalesce into the common cardinal veins, which then deliver blood to the sinus venosus. The cardinal veins subsequently involute with the development of the paired subcardinal veins. Notably, however, the caudal ends of the posterior cardinal veins do not involute but rather form the common iliac veins. The cranial aspect of the right subcardinal vein develops communications with coalescent hepatic sinusoids to form the intrahepatic segment of the IVC. The right subcardinal vein also forms the suprarenal segment of the IVC, whereas the cranial aspect of the left subcarinal vein forms the left adrenal gland. The subcardinal veins then begin to involute, with the formation of the supracardinal veins during the 7th week of development. The cranial aspect of the right supracardinal vein forms the azygos vein, and the cranial aspect of the left supracardinal vein forms the hemiazygos vein. The right supracardinal vein forms the infrarenal IVC. Anastomoses between the supracardinal and subcardinal veins form the renal segment of the IVC as well as the renal veins.[119,120]

Double Inferior Vena Cava

Double IVC is the end result of persistence of both supracardinal veins (Fig. 20.37). Typically, the right vena cava is larger than the left, with the latter joining the former at the level of the renal veins or emptying into the left renal vein. It is commonly associated with other congenital anomalies.

Left-Sided Inferior Vena Cava

The right supracardinal vein normally forms the infrarenal IVC, whereas the left supracardinal vein involutes. However, in situations where the opposite occurs, a persistent left

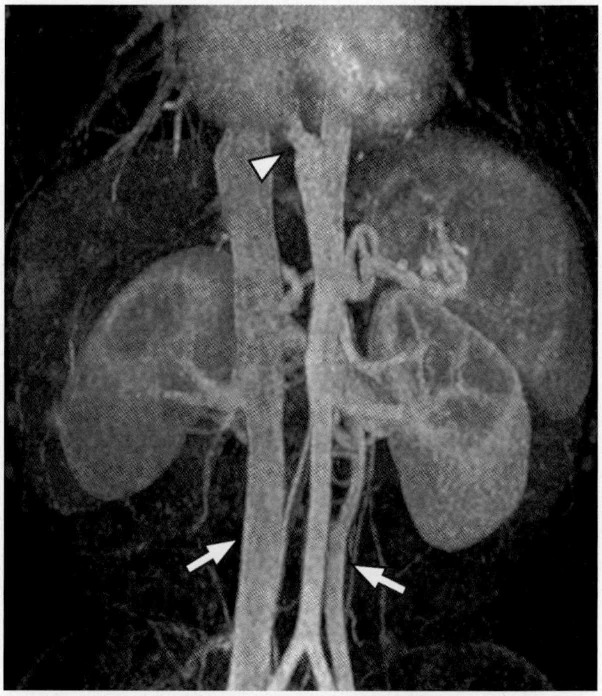

FIGURE 20.37 **Double inferior venae cavae in a 13-year-old boy.** Coronal image from an MR angiogram demonstrates persistence of the left and right supracardinal veins resulting in duplicated inferior venae cavae (*arrows*) on either side of the aorta, as well as associated absence of the portal vein. The portal vein drains directly to the suprahepatic IVC-right atrium junction (*arrowhead*), consistent with Abernethy malformation.

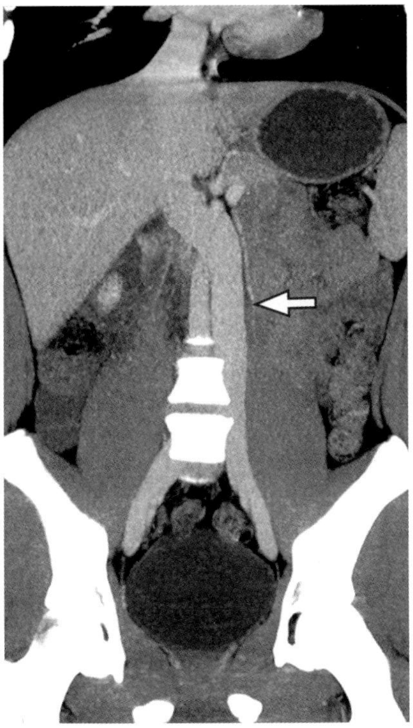

FIGURE 20.38 **Left-sided inferior vena cava in a 7-year-old boy.** Coronal enhanced maximum intensity projection CT image demonstrates persistence of the left supracardinal vein and involution of the right supracardinal vein resulting in a left-sided inferior vena cava (*arrow*) below the level of the renal veins.

supracardinal vein would result in a left-sided IVC below the level of the renal veins (Fig. 20.38). Given that the suprarenal IVC is formed by the subcardinal veins, left-sided IVC joins the left renal vein and crosses anterior to the aorta and assumes a conventional right-sided course above the renal veins. The left gonadal and adrenal veins drain directly into a left-sided IVC, with the right gonadal and adrenal veins draining into the right renal vein.

Interruption of the Inferior Vena Cava with Azygos/Hemiazygos Continuation

If the right subcardinal vein fails to develop communication with hepatic sinusoids, blood return is redirected through the azygos and/or hemiazygos systems, both of which arise from the cranial ends of the supracardinal veins (Fig. 20.39). The hepatic veins drain directly into the right atrium. This anomaly of the IVC is associated with left-sided isomerism (polysplenia).[121]

Retrocaval Ureter

Persistence of the right posterior cardinal vein resulting in an anomalous formation of the IVC impedes the normal ascent of the developing kidneys. The ureter courses in a retrocaval manner and partially encircles the IVC, assuming a dorsolateral position cranially and a ventromedial position caudally. Retrocaval ureter essentially only occurs on the right side. Excretory urography, CT urography, and MR urography reveal a classic hairpin turn or "J-shaped" appearance of the mid right ureter (Fig. 20.40).

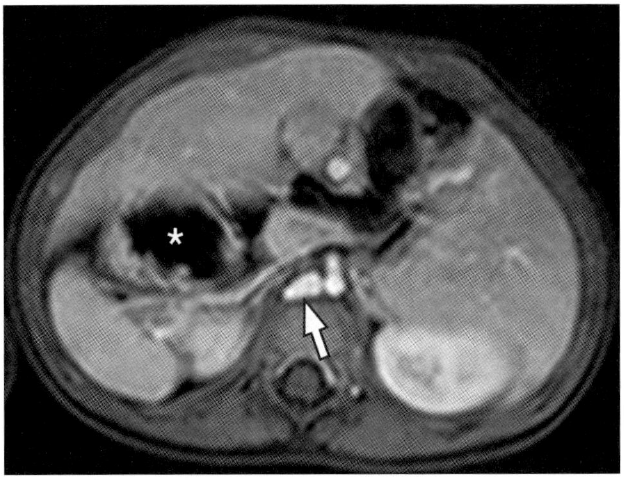

FIGURE 20.39 **Interruption of the inferior vena cava (IVC) with azygous continuation in a 1-year-old girl with polysplenia.** Axial postcontrast T1-weighted fat-suppressed MR image demonstrates an absent intrahepatic IVC with an enlarged azygos vein (*arrow*) anterior to the spine, as well as a stomach (*asterisk*) to the right of midline.

Infectious Disorders

Mycotic Aneurysm

The pathogenesis of mycotic, or infectious, aneurysms is similar in children as it is in adults. Infectious agents, typically bacteria, within the bloodstream cause an endarteritis. This in turn leads to weakening of the arterial wall integrity and can result in either a "true" aneurysm that involves all three mural layers or a "false" or pseudoaneurysm in which an arterial rupture is contained by surrounding adventitia. Mycotic aneurysms are associated with a high mortality rate given the risk of rupture.

One established etiology for mycotic aneurysms in infants is as a delayed complication of umbilical arterial catheter placement. Iatrogenic injury to the aortic wall by the catheter tip coupled with bacteremia can lead to pseudoaneurysm formation.[122–125] Other causes of mycotic aneurysms in the abdomen include direct extension into an artery from a primary focus of infection. Congenital heart disease and immunodeficiencies are risk factors for mycotic aneurysm formation.[126]

Rubella

Rubella infection occurring early in fetal development results in myriad malformations, including congenital heart disease, cataracts, and deafness. In addition, congenital rubella infection is also a recognized infectious cause of abdominal aortic hypoplasia.[127]

Vasculitides

Vasculitis is a nonspecific term describing a spectrum of inflammatory disorders that affect the full gamut of blood vessels in the body. These vasculitides are typically classified by the size of the blood vessel that they most commonly involve. Large-vessel vasculitides such as giant cell arteritis and Takayasu arteritis affect the aorta and its major branches. Medium-vessel vasculitides such as polyarteritis nodosa

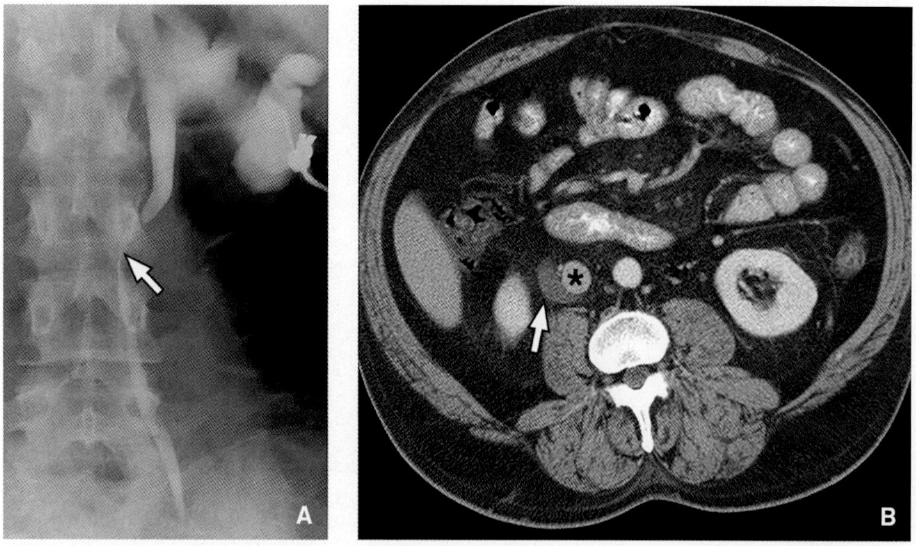

FIGURE 20.40 **Retrocaval ureter in an 18-year-old female. A:** Antegrade pyeloureterogram (posterior view) demonstrates a classic "hairpin" course of the right ureter (*arrow*), diagnostic of retrocaval ureter. **B:** Axial enhanced CT image in a different patient demonstrates a mildly dilated proximal right ureter (*arrow*) coursing posterior to the inferior vena cava (*asterisk*).

and Kawasaki disease affect major visceral arteries and their branches, and small-vessel vasculitides such as microscopic polyangiitis and granulomatosis with polyangiitis (formerly known as Wegener granulomatosis) affect arterioles and capillaries.[128] Manifestations of these disorders can be found in organ systems throughout the body; their involvement of the abdominal vasculature is discussed in this section.

Takayasu Arteritis

Takayasu arteritis is a large-vessel vasculitis that involves the aorta, its branches, and sometimes the pulmonary arteries. Takayasu arteritis demonstrates a female predominance and results in both aneurysm formation as well as arterial narrowings (Figs. 20.41 and 20.42). Histologically, this disorder is a panarteritis, involving all layers of the arterial wall.[129] The clinical presentation of Takayasu arteritis is divided into an early systemic phase, characterized by nonspecific constitutional symptoms such as fever, myalgias and weight loss, and a late occlusive phase, characterized by ischemic symptoms, such as angina and claudication.[130] In the latter phase, vascular imaging typically shows long, smooth, tapered narrowings that may range in severity from mild stenoses to complete occlusions. The stenoses are often multifocal. When stenosis involves the suprarenal abdominal aorta, renovascular hypertension may result; likewise, involvement of the mesenteric arteries can cause mesenteric ischemia. CT and MRI may reveal concentric thickening of the affected arterial wall with associated enhancement on postcontrast imaging.[131] Fusiform aneurysmal dilatation of the large arteries is also a feature of this disease, with mural thrombus often identified within the aneurysms.

Kawasaki Disease

Kawasaki disease is a panarteritis with numerous clinical manifestations, including conjunctival injection, fever, peripheral edema, rash, cervical lymphadenopathy, and gallbladder hydrops.[132] The most common vascular manifestation is aneurysm formation in the coronary arteries, which is discussed in Chapter 9. Aneurysms of the abdominal aorta and iliac arteries can also occur in patients with Kawasaki disease[133] and can be evaluated using CT angiography or MR angiography. Given the risk of delayed aneurysm development after the diagnosis of Kawasaki disease, follow-up imaging for 2 years is currently recommended.[134]

Traumatic Disorders

Vascular trauma in patients younger than 5 years is typically iatrogenic in nature, as may occur during catheter placement. However, for children older than 5 years, traumatic

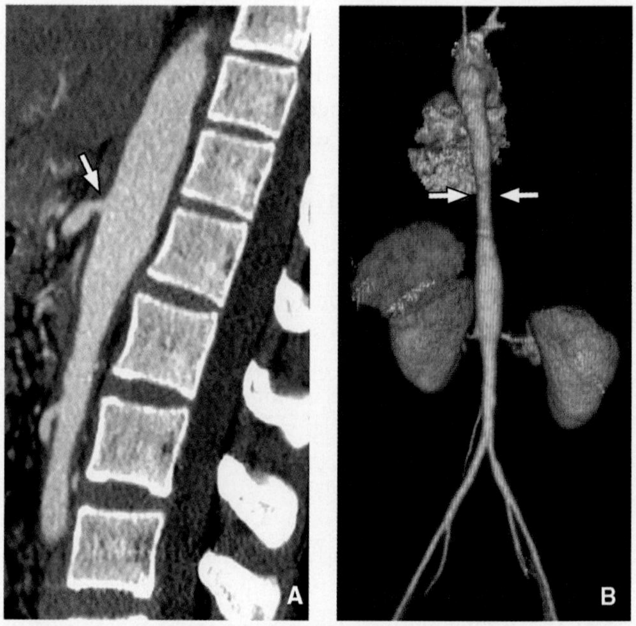

FIGURE 20.41 **Takayasu arteritis in a 16-year-old girl with hypertension. A:** Sagittal enhanced CT image demonstrates abnormal thickening of the abdominal aortic wall associated with narrowing (*arrow*) of the superior mesenteric artery origin. **B:** 3D volume rendered CT image (posterior view) shows long segment narrowing (*arrows*) of the distal thoracic and infrarenal abdominal aorta.

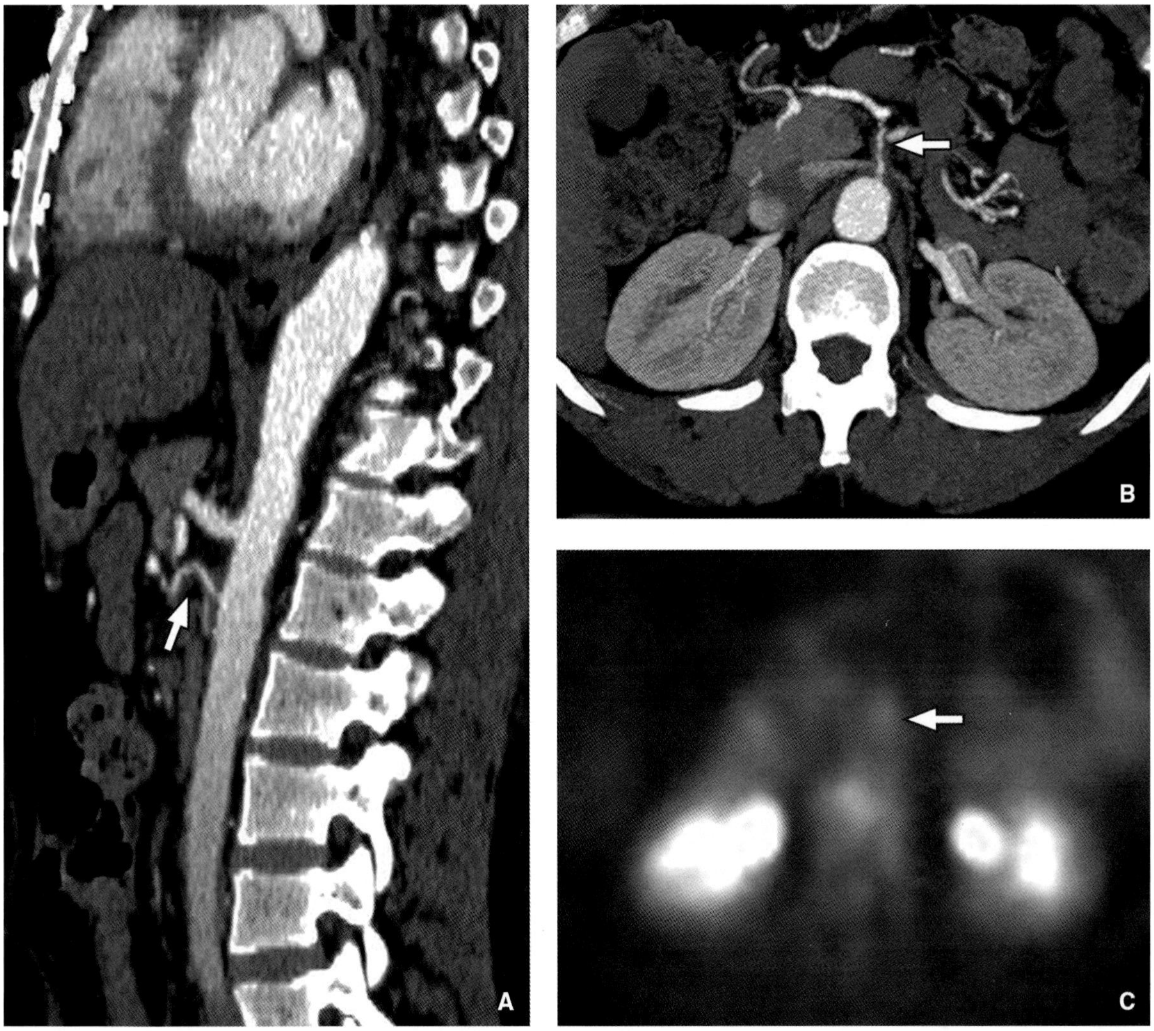

FIGURE 20.42 **Takayasu arteritis in a 17-year-old girl with postprandial pain.** Sagittal enhanced CT image **(A)** and axial enhanced maximum intensity projection CT image **(B)** demonstrate mural thickening and irregular narrowing (*arrows*) of the superior mesenteric artery. Abdominal aortic irregular wall thickening is also present. **C:** Concurrently obtained ^{18}F-FDG–PET image reveals increased metabolism (*arrow*) in the wall of the superior mesenteric artery.

etiologies predominate. Common causes of blunt and penetrating trauma resulting in abdominal vascular injury include motor vehicle accidents, gunshot wounds, and knife wounds. Lap-belt injuries are an important cause of blunt abdominal trauma. The pediatric population is particularly susceptible for lap-belt injuries due to improper positioning of the lap belt over the mid or upper abdomen rather than over the pelvis. Lap-belt injuries often affect the bowel and abdominal wall, but they can also result in major vascular injury.[135]

Mesenteric vascular injuries may manifest in a number of ways at CT and conventional angiography. Traumatic pseudoaneurysms (Fig. 20.43) are most commonly diagnosed more than 48 hours after the traumatic episode.[124] On arterial phase CT imaging, pseudoaneurysms appear as focal areas of abnormal contrast enhancement similar to the attenuation of blood pool, often with surrounding hematoma. Active extravasation of contrast material is less likely to be observed. However, in milder forms of vascular injury, the only apparent finding on CT may be subtle increased attenuation fluid within the leaves of mesentery representing mesenteric hemorrhage. Although this finding does not independently indicate a severe injury requiring surgical exploration, when it is present in the setting of focal bowel thickening, surgical repair is likely necessary.[136]

Finally, in any child with evidence of traumatic injuries without a commensurate clinical history, child abuse must always be considered.

Connective Tissue Disorders Associated with Abdominal Vascular Abnormalities (See Chapter 9 for Additional Discussion)

Ehlers-Danlos Syndrome

Ehlers-Danlos syndrome (EDS) describes a category of inherited disorders that involve impaired synthesis of collagen. Of the different subtypes of EDS, type IV is known as the "vascular" form as it can affect major arteries. In EDS type IV, mutations in the *COL3A1* gene, which encodes type III procollagen,[137] weaken the walls of major arteries, resulting in aneurysmal

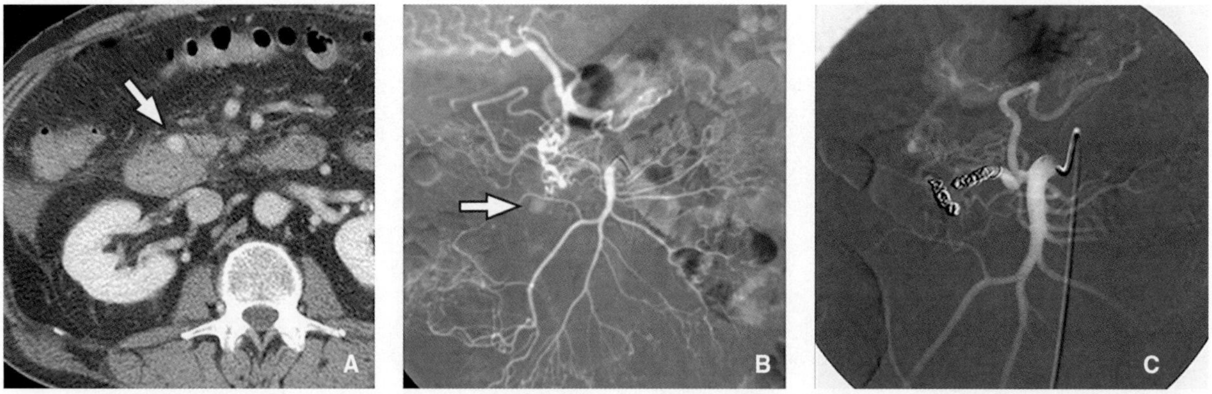

FIGURE 20.43 **Traumatic superior mesenteric artery (SMA) pseudoaneurysm in an 18-year-old male following motor vehicle accident. A:** Axial enhanced CT image demonstrates a rounded area of enhancement (*arrow*) adjacent to the second portion of the duodenum with attenuation similar to blood pool. **B:** Digitally subtracted conventional angiographic image in the frontal projection after SMA injection shows a focal blush (*arrow*) originating from a pancreaticoduodenal branch, consistent with pseudoaneurysm. **C:** Repeat right anterior oblique angiographic image after coil embolization shows that the pseudoaneurysm is no long present.

dilatation of the aortic root as well as aneurysms of the thoracic and abdominal aorta (Fig. 20.44). Arterial rupture, sometimes due to dissection, is the most common cause of death in these patients. Other manifestations typically seen in other types of EDS, such as ligamentous laxity, hypermobile joints, and hyperextensible skin, are not commonly seen in EDS type IV.[137]

Marfan Syndrome

Marfan syndrome is an autosomal dominant connective tissue disorder caused by a mutation in *FBN1*, the gene that encodes for the protein fibrillin-1.[121] Many different mutations affecting *FBN1* have been identified, accounting for the broad spectrum of clinical manifestations of Marfan syndrome. The most common cause of morbidity and mortality in patients with Marfan syndrome is aortic root dilatation,[121] which can result in aortic insufficiency and aortic dissection (Fig. 20.45). Although annual imaging of the aortic root through the aortic arch, typically with US, is recommended for patients with Marfan syndrome, there are no specific guidelines regarding routine screening for abdominal aortic pathology in these patients.[138]

Loeys-Dietz Syndrome

Loeys-Dietz syndrome results from a disruption in connective tissue development arising from loss-of-function mutations in the genes *TGFBR1, TGFBR2, TGFB2, or SMAD3*. Some of the main manifestations include aortic root dilation, craniosynostosis, scoliosis, pectus excavatum or carinatum, clubfoot, pes planus, elongated limbs with joint contractures, intervertebral disc degeneration, osteoarthritis, easy bruising, cutaneous striae, hypertelorism, bifid uvula and cleft palate. Immune problems such as food allergy, asthma, eczema, or inflammatory bowel disease may also result. First identified in 2005, this syndrome is characterized by a pattern of multisystemic abnormalities similar to EDS and Marfan syndrome.[139] For example, both Loeys-Dietz and Marfan syndromes feature aneurysmal dilatation of the aortic root that may lead to aortic dissection. However, the aneurysms of Loeys-Dietz tend to dissect at smaller sizes and

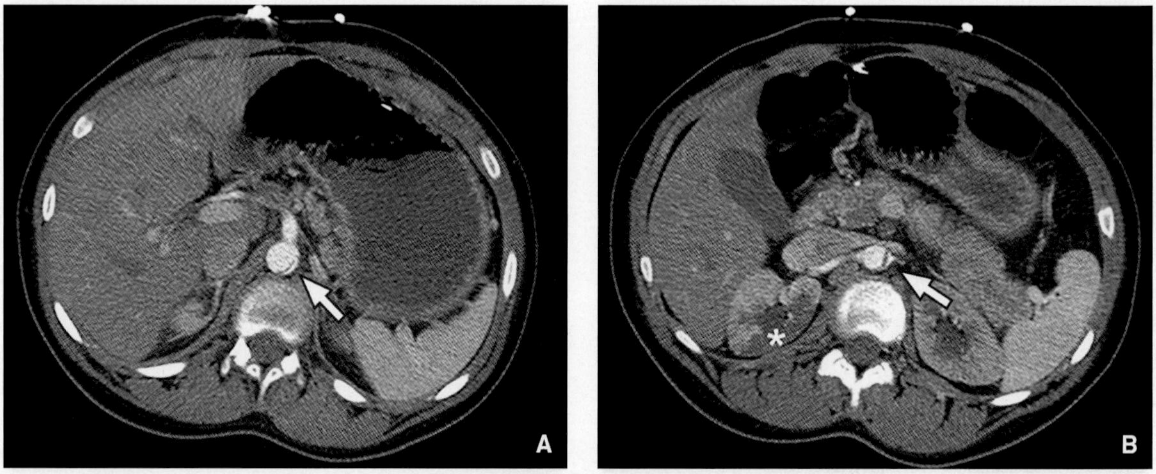

FIGURE 20.44 **Ehlers-Danlos syndrome (type IV) causing aortic dissection in a 15-year-old boy. A and B:** Axial enhanced CT images show a dissection flap in the abdominal aorta as well as right renal infarcts (**B**, *asterisk*).

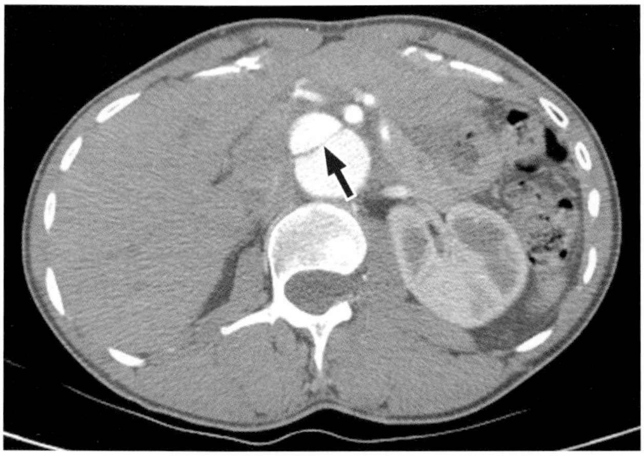

FIGURE 20.45 **Marfan syndrome causing abdominal aortic dissection in a 14-year-old boy.** Axial enhanced CT image demonstrates aneurysmal dilatation of the abdominal aorta and an associated dissection flap (*arrow*).

at an earlier age. Moreover, unlike Marfan syndrome, in which aneurysm formation typically only involves the aortic root, Loeys-Dietz syndrome patients almost always develop multifocal aneurysms (Fig. 20.46). Abdominal aortic aneurysms occur in ~10% of patients.[140] The fragility of these aneurysms, similar to the aneurysms of vascular EDS, renders them very susceptible to rupture. Patients with Loeys-Dietz are recommended to undergo complete aortic imaging at the time of initial diagnosis and at 6 months following the diagnosis, to determine if any aneurysms have increased in size in a short time interval. Subsequently, patients are recommended to undergo yearly MR angiographic imaging from the skull to the pelvis.[141]

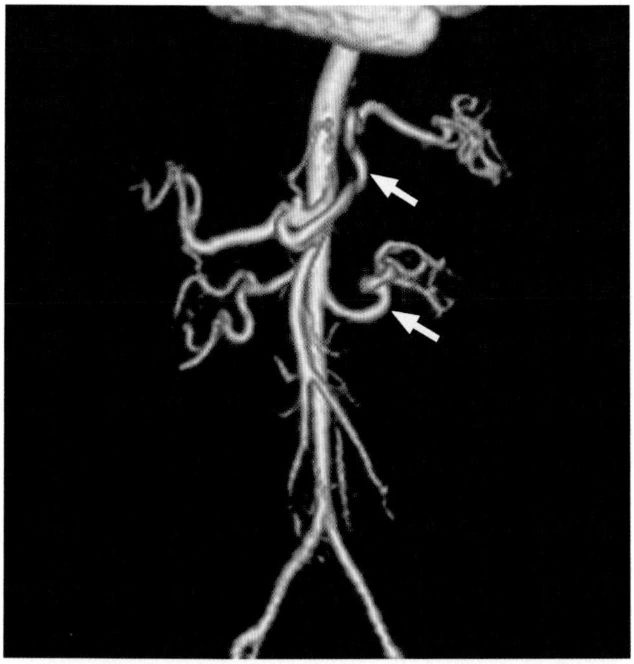

FIGURE 20.46 **Loeys-Dietz syndrome affecting abdominal arteries in an 8-year-old boy.** 3D volume-rendered CT image demonstrates dilation and tortuosity (*arrows*) of the splenic and left renal arteries.

Phakomatoses Associated with Abdominal Vascular Abnormalities

Neurofibromatosis, Type 1

Neurofibromatosis, type 1 (NF1) affects multiple organ systems, including the vascular tree. The renal arteries are the most common abdominal site for NF1 vascular lesions, although vascular narrowings are often multifocal in distribution. These lesions do not represent neurofibromas, but rather an arteriopathy (Fig. 20.47). The disease is characterized predominantly by intimal proliferation, but aneurysm formation may also occur.[142]

The distribution of NF1 vascular lesions is similar to that of abominal atherosclerosis in adults. These lesions are typically found in large- (including the abdominal aorta) and medium-sized vessels (Fig. 20.48) and are one important cause of renovascular hypertension as well as "middle aortic syndrome." CT angiography, MR angiography, and conventional angiography may all prove useful in the evaluation of these children. In some children, many areas of arterial narrowing and associated aneurysm formation may be observed.

Tuberous Sclerosis Complex

As with NF1, tuberous sclerosis complex (TSC) affects a multitude of organ systems, including the vascular tree. Aortic aneurysms have been reported in patients with TSC from infancy onward; the aneurysms can grow to large sizes as well (Fig. 20.49), with the mean size of abdominal aortic aneurysms measuring 5.4 cm.[143] The risk of rupture with these lesions is very high. The pathogenesis of aneurysms in TSC patients is not well understood, but several theories have been proposed, including a collagenopathy or the loss of elastin fibers similar to Marfan syndrome.[143] US, CT angiography, MR angiography, and conventional angiography can all be used to evaluate the aorta for aneurysms and associated branch artery narrowings.

Idiopathic Causes of Abdominal Vascular Abnormalities

Arterial Dysplasia/Fibromuscular Dysplasia

Idiopathic arterial dysplasias, including fibromuscular dysplasia (FMD), represent a heterogeneous group of noninflammatory developmental vascular disorders that typically affect children and young adult women. Following primary renal disease and congenital aortic narrowing, arterial dysplasias (including FMD) are the third most common cause of renovascular hypertension.[144] Commonly involved arteries include the renal arteries followed by the carotid arteries. The mesenteric arteries and iliac arteries are less often affected.

Medial fibroplasia is a common form of arterial dysplasia and on CT angiography, MR angiography, and conventional angiography manifests as a classic "string of beads" appearance, with multifocal areas of stenosis and dilatation (Fig. 20.50). Intimal fibroplasia is a less common form of arterial dysplasia that may present as a focal stenosis or as a long, tapered, smooth narrowing. Patients with arterial dysplasias are at an increased risk for aneurysm formation, arterial dissections, and thromboembolic occlusions.[145]

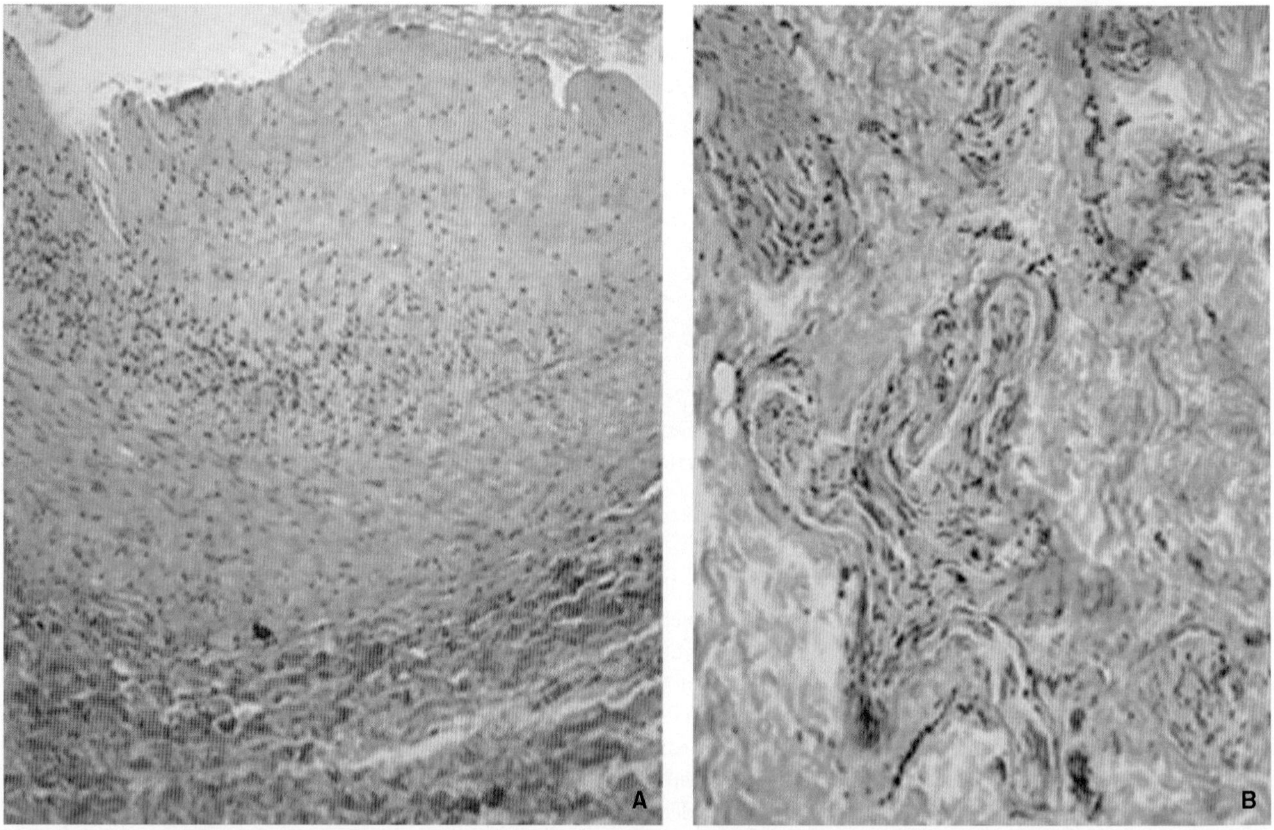

FIGURE 20.47 **Microscopic appearance of middle aortic syndrome involving the celiac artery of an 8-year-old boy with neurofibromatosis, type 1. A:** The artery wall shows fibrous intimal proliferation and degeneration of medial elastic fibers (**left**, hematoxylin and eosin stain, original magnification, 100x). **B:** The adventitial nerves show plexiform changes (**right**, hematoxylin and eosin stain, original magnification, 200x). Whether the adventitial neurofibromatous changes is causative in middle aortic syndrome has not been determined.

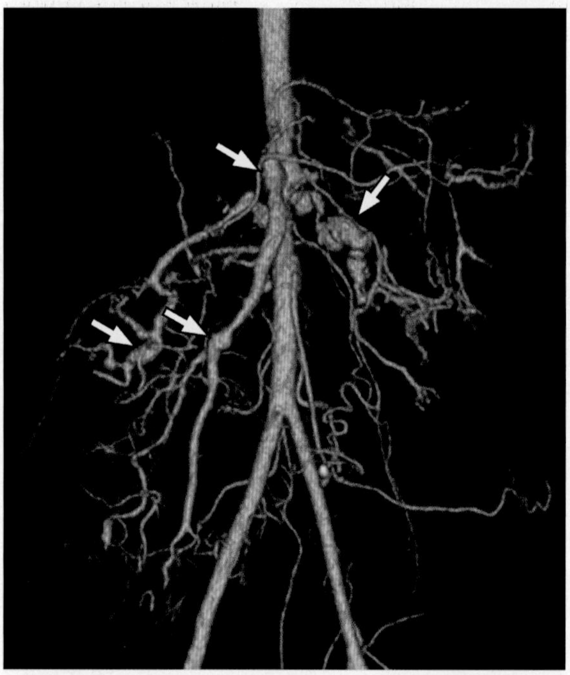

FIGURE 20.48 **Arterial dysplasia in a 9-year-old boy with neurofibromatosis, type 1 (NF1).** 3D volume-rendered CT image demonstrates numerous areas of narrowing and aneurysmal dilation (*arrows*) of the mesenteric and renal arteries consistent with NF1 arterial dysplasia.

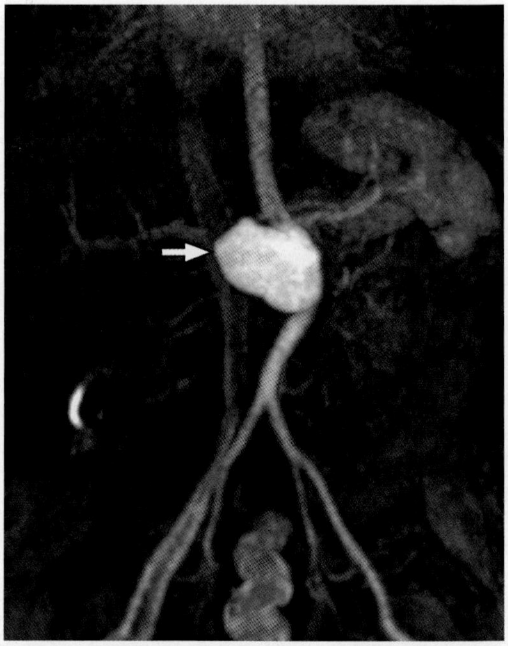

FIGURE 20.49 **Abdominal aortic aneurysm from tuberous sclerosis in a 4-month-old boy with hypertension.** 3D postcontrast maximum intensity projection magnetic resonance image demonstrates a large upper abdominal aortic aneurysm (*arrow*). The thoracic aorta and infrarenal abdominal aorta are normal in caliber.

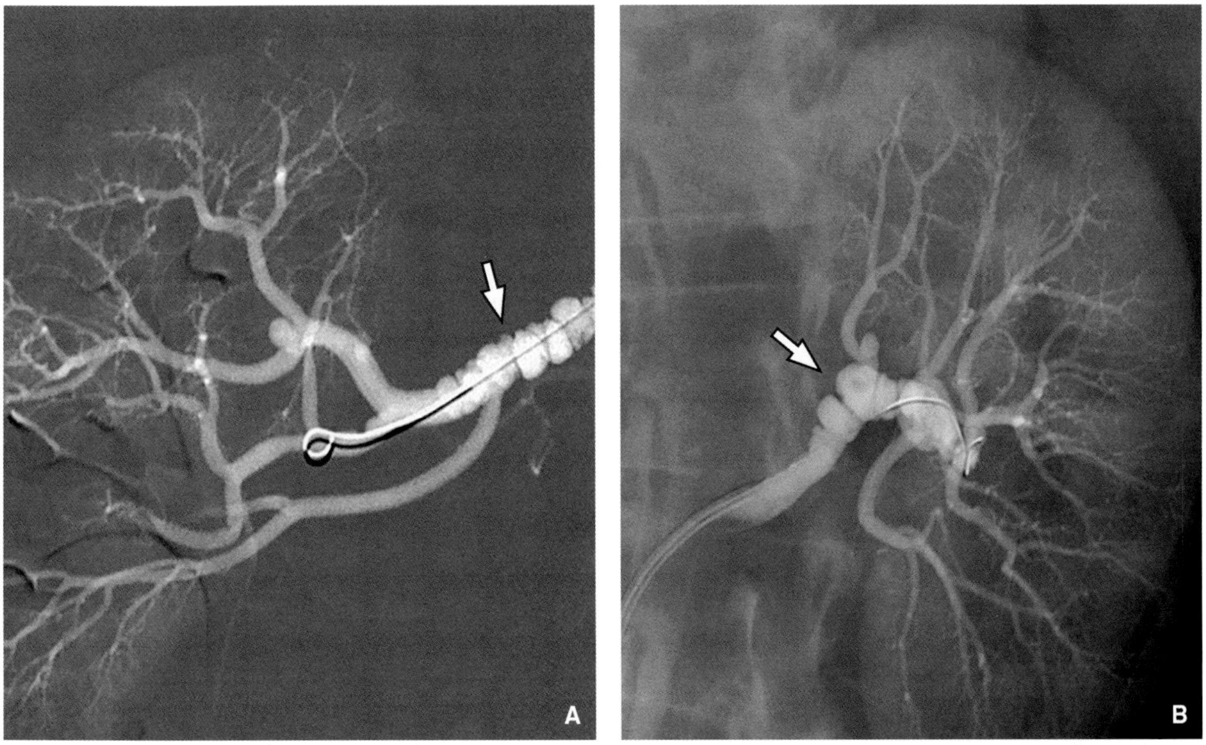

FIGURE 20.50 **Hypertension due to fibromuscular dysplasia in a 20-year-old female.** Right **(A)** and left **(B)** renal artery digitally subtracted conventional angiographic images demonstrate a classic "string of beads" appearance (*arrows*) of both arteries with areas of alternating, narrowing, and aneurysmal dilatation.

In the setting of hypertension and known or suspected pediatric arterial dysplasia affecting the renal arteries, conventional angiography is generally required to determine the true extent of disease, including intrarenal involvement. Depending on the number and location of lesions, management strategies may include transcatheter balloon angioplasty, renal artery reimplantation, arterioplasty, surgical bypass, transcatheter arterial embolization, partial nephrectomy, or radical nephrectomy.

Williams Syndrome

Williams syndrome (also known as Williams-Beuren syndrome) is a genetic disorder discussed in Chapter 9. Its vascular manifestations most commonly involve stenosis of the supravalvular thoracic aorta and pulmonary arteries.[146] These patients may also develop hypoplasia or stenosis of the abdominal aorta (Fig. 20.51), resulting in "middle aortic syndrome." CT angiography and MR angiography

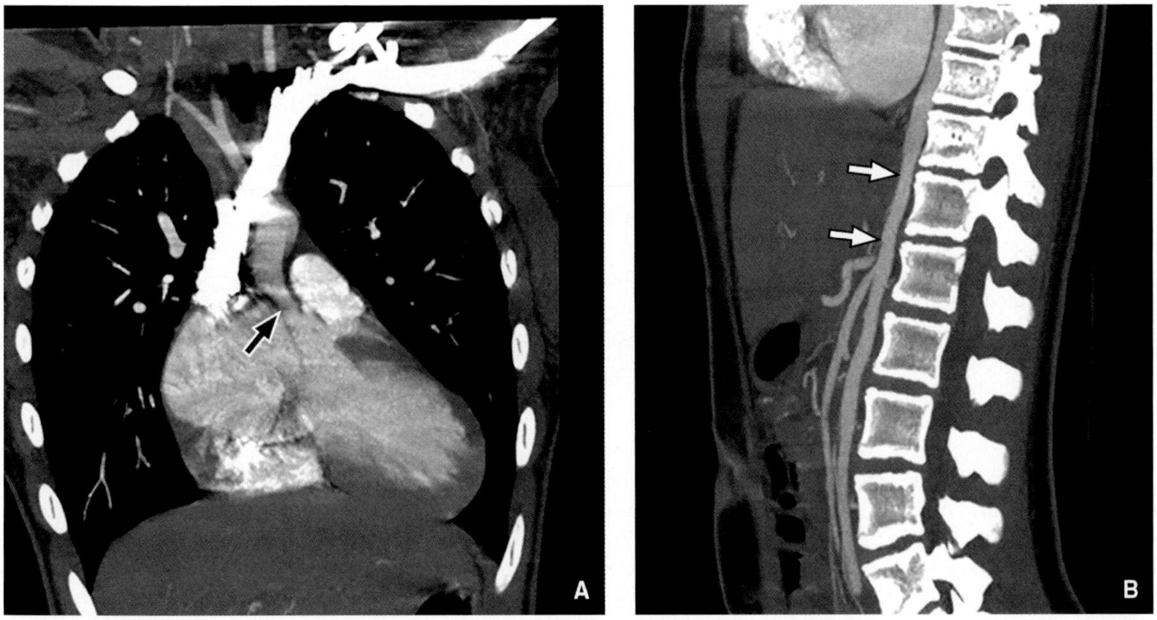

FIGURE 20.51 **Abdominal aortic narrowing in a 13-year-old girl with Williams syndrome. A:** Coronal CT angiography image demonstrates supravalvular aortic narrowing (*black arrow*). **B:** Sagittal maximum intensity projection CT image shows that the abdominal aorta is diffusely narrowed (*white arrows*).

demonstrate narrowed, thick-walled, inelastic vessels.[147] In some children, diffuse aortic hypoplasia may involve the entire thoracoabdominal aorta and may be a relatively subtle finding. The degree of stenosis is believed to progress over time, and renovascular hypertension is a common feature in teenagers.[147]

References

1. Anupindi SA, Janitz E, Darge K. Bowel imaging in children: a comprehensive look using US and MRI. *Semin Roentgenol.* 2012;47(2):118–126.
2. Singh S, Kalra MK, Moore MA, et al. Dose reduction and compliance with pediatric CT protocols adapted to patient size, clinical indication, and number of prior studies. *Radiology.* 2009;252(1):200–208.
3. Zacharias C, Alessio AM, Otto RK, et al. Pediatric CT: strategies to lower radiation dose. *AJR Am J Roentgenol.* 2013;200(5): 950–956.
4. Krishnamurthy R, Guillerman RP. Pediatric abdominal magnetic resonance angiography. *Semin Roentgenol.* 2008;43(1):60–71.
5. Marshalleck F. Pediatric arterial interventions. *Tech Vasc Interv Radiol.* 2010;13(4):238–243.
6. Heran MK, Marshalleck F, Temple M, et al. Joint quality improvement guidelines for pediatric arterial access and arteriography: from the Societies of Interventional Radiology and Pediatric Radiology. *Pediatr Radiol.* 2010;40(2):237–250.
7. Tirkes T, Sandrasegaran K, Patel AA, et al. Peritoneal and retroperitoneal anatomy and its relevance for cross-sectional imaging. *Radiographics.* 2012;32(2):437–451.
8. Coakley FV, Hricak H. Imaging of peritoneal and mesenteric disease: key concepts for the clinical radiologist. *Clin Radiol.* 1999;54(9):563–574.
9. Lin PH, Chaikof EL. Embryology, anatomy, and surgical exposure of the great abdominal vessels. *Surg Clin North Am.* 2000;80(1):417–433, xiv.
10. Mayo J, Gray R, St. Louis E, et al. Anomalies of the inferior vena cava. *AJR Am J Roentgenol.* 1983;140(2):339–345.
11. Horton KM, Fishman EK. Volume-rendered 3D CT of the mesenteric vasculature: normal anatomy, anatomic variants, and pathologic conditions. *Radiographics.* 2002;22(1):161–172.
12. Graf O, Boland GW, Kaufman JA, et al. Anatomic variants of mesenteric veins: depiction with helical CT venography. *AJR Am J Roentgenol.* 1997;168(5):1209–1213.
13. Salihu HM, Boos R, Schmidt W. Omphalocele and gastroschisis. *J Obstet Gynaecol.* 2002;22(5):489–492.
14. Vogler SA, Fenton SJ, Scaife ER, et al. Closed gastroschisis: total parenteral nutrition-free survival with aggressive attempts at bowel preservation and intestinal adaptation. *J Pediatr Surg.* 2008;43(6):1006–1010.
15. Routh JC, Huang L, Retik AB, et al. Contemporary epidemiology and characterization of newborn males with prune belly syndrome. *Urology.* 2010;76(1):44–48.
16. Hassett S, Smith GH, Holland AJ. Prune belly syndrome. *Pediatr Surg Int.* 2012;28(3):219–228.
17. Manivel JC, Pettinato G, Reinberg Y, et al. Prune belly syndrome: clinicopathologic study of 29 cases. *Pediatr Pathol.* 1989; 9(6):691–711.
18. Mininberg DT, Montoya F, Okada K, et al. Subcellular muscle studies in the prune belly syndrome. *J Urol.* 1973;109(3): 524–526.
19. Clark TJ, Martin WL, Divakaran TG, et al. Prenatal bladder drainage in the management of fetal lower urinary tract obstruction: a systematic review and meta-analysis. *Obstet Gynecol.* 2003;102(2):367–382.
20. Fontaine E, Salomon L, Gagnadoux MF, et al. Long-term results of renal transplantation in children with the prune-belly syndrome. *J Urol.* 1997;158(3 Pt 1):892–894.
21. Smith CA, Smith EA, Parrott TS, et al. Voiding function in patients with the prune-belly syndrome after Monfort abdominoplasty. *J Urol.* 1998;159(5):1675–1679.
22. Lindhurst MJ, Sapp JC, Teer JK, et al. A mosaic activating mutation in AKT1 associated with the Proteus syndrome. *N Engl J Med.* 2011;365(7):611–619.
23. Cohen MM Jr. Proteus syndrome review: molecular, clinical, and pathologic features. *Clin Genet.* 2014;85(2):111–119.
24. Biesecker LG, Happle R, Mulliken JB, et al. Proteus syndrome: diagnostic criteria, differential diagnosis, and patient evaluation. *Am J Med Genet.* 1999;84(5):389–395.
25. Biesecker LG. The multifaceted challenges of Proteus syndrome. *JAMA.* 2001;285(17):2240–2243.
26. Lio PA. The many faces of cellulitis. *Arch Dis Child Educ Pract Ed.* 2009;94(2):50–54.
27. Bingol-Kologlu M, Yildiz RV, Alper B, et al. Necrotizing fasciitis in children: diagnostic and therapeutic aspects. *J Pediatr Surg.* 2007;42(11):1892–1897.
28. Swartz MN. Clinical practice. Cellulitis. *N Engl J Med.* 2004; 350(9):904–912.
29. Schmid MR, Kossmann T, Duewell S. Differentiation of necrotizing fasciitis and cellulitis using MR imaging. *AJR Am J Roentgenol.* 1998;170(3):615–620.
30. Shinagare AB, Ramaiya NH, Jagannathan JP, et al. A to Z of desmoid tumors. *Am J Roentgenol.* 2011;197(6):W1008–W1014.
31. Shields CJ, Winter DC, Kirwan WO, et al. Desmoid tumours. *Eur J Surg Oncol.* 2001;27(8):701–706.
32. Berri RN, Baumann DP, Madewell JE, et al. Desmoid tumor: current multidisciplinary approaches. *Ann Plast Surg.* 2011; 67(5):551–564.
33. Lindor NM, Greene MH. The concise handbook of family cancer syndromes. Mayo Familial Cancer Program. *J Natl Cancer Inst.* 1998;90(14):1039–1071.
34. Dinauer PA, Brixey CJ, Moncur JT, et al. Pathologic and MR imaging features of benign fibrous soft-tissue tumors in adults. *Radiographics.* 2007;27(1):173–187.
35. Murphey MD, Ruble CM, Tyszko SM, et al. From the archives of the AFIP: musculoskeletal fibromatoses: radiologic-pathologic correlation. *Radiographics.* 2009;29(7):2143–2173.
36. Kransdorf MJ, Jelinek JS, Moser RP Jr, et al. Magnetic resonance appearance of fibromatosis. A report of 14 cases and review of the literature. *Skeletal Radiol.* 1990;19(7):495–499.
37. Coffin CM, Alaggio R. Fibroblastic and myofibroblastic tumors in children and adolescents. *Pediatr Dev Pathol.* 2012;15(1 Suppl):127–180.
38. Bertani E, Chiappa A, Testori A, et al. Desmoid tumors of the anterior abdominal wall: results from a monocentric surgical experience and review of the literature. *Ann Surg Oncol.* 2009; 16(6):1642–1649.
39. Stojadinovic A, Hoos A, Karpoff HM, et al. Soft tissue tumors of the abdominal wall: analysis of disease patterns and treatment. *Arch Surg.* 2001;136(1):70–79.
40. Loeb DM, Thornton K, Shokek O. Pediatric soft tissue sarcomas. *Surg Clin North Am.* 2008;88(3):615–627, vii.

41. Pencavel T, Strauss DC, Thomas JM, et al. The surgical management of soft tissue tumours arising in the abdominal wall. *Eur J Surg Oncol.* 2010;36(5):489–495.
42. Stein-Wexler R. Pediatric soft tissue sarcomas. *Semin Ultrasound CT MR.* 2011;32(5):470–488.
43. Lakkaraju A, Sinha R, Garikipati R, et al. Ultrasound for initial evaluation and triage of clinically suspicious soft-tissue masses. *Clin Radiol.* 2009;64(6):615–621.
44. Williams KJ, Hayes AJ. A guide to oncological management of soft tissue tumours of the abdominal wall. *Hernia.* 2014;18(1): 91–97.
45. Volker T, Denecke T, Steffen I, et al. Positron emission tomography for staging of pediatric sarcoma patients: results of a prospective multicenter trial. *J Clin Oncol.* 2007;25(34):5435–5441.
46. Fernandez-Pineda I, Bahrami A, Green JF, et al. Isolated subcutaneous metastasis of osteosarcoma 5 years after initial diagnosis. *J Pediatr Surg.* 2011;46(10):2029–2031.
47. Wesche WA, Khare VK, Chesney TM, et al. Non-hematopoietic cutaneous metastases in children and adolescents: thirty years experience at St. Jude Children's Research Hospital. *J Cutan Pathol.* 2000;27(10):485–492.
48. Dennis RW, Marshall A, Deshmukh H, et al. Abdominal wall injuries occurring after blunt trauma: incidence and grading system. *Am J Surg.* 2009;197(3):413–417.
49. Dimyan W, Robb J, MacKay C. Handlebar hernia. *J Trauma.* 1980;20(9):812–813.
50. Moremen JR, Nakayama DK, Ashley DW, et al. Traumatic disruption of the abdominal wall: lap-belt injuries in children. *J Pediatr Surg.* 2013;48(4):e21–e24.
51. Rathore A, Simpson BJ, Diefenbach KA. Traumatic abdominal wall hernias: an emerging trend in handlebar injuries. *J Pediatr Surg.* 2012;47(7):1410–1413.
52. Chen HY, Sheu MH, Tseng LM. Bicycle-handlebar hernia: a rare traumatic abdominal wall hernia. *J Chin Med Assoc.* 2005;68(6):283–285.
53. Ganchi PA, Orgill DP. Autopenetrating hernia: a novel form of traumatic abdominal wall hernia—case report and review of the literature. *J Trauma.* 1996;41(6):1064–1066.
54. Netto FA, Hamilton P, Rizoli SB, et al. Traumatic abdominal wall hernia: epidemiology and clinical implications. *J Trauma.* 2006;61(5):1058–1061.
55. Mitchiner JC. Handlebar hernia: diagnosis by abdominal computed tomography. *Ann Emerg Med.* 1990;19(7):812–813.
56. Litton K, Izzidien AY, Hussien O, et al. Conservative management of a traumatic abdominal wall hernia after a bicycle handlebar injury (case report and literature review). *J Pediatr Surg.* 2008;43(4):e31–e32.
57. van Bemmel AJ, van Marle AG, Schlejen PM, et al. Handlebar hernia: a case report and literature review on traumatic abdominal wall hernia in children. *Hernia.* 2011;15(4): 439–442.
58. Kurtz RJ, Heimann TM, Holt J, et al. Mesenteric and retroperitoneal cysts. *Ann Surg.* 1986;203(1):109–112.
59. Ros PR, Olmsted WW, Moser RP Jr, et al. Mesenteric and omental cysts: histologic classification with imaging correlation. *Radiology.* 1987;164(2):327–332.
60. Weeda VB, Booij KA, Aronson DC. Mesenteric cystic lymphangioma: a congenital and an acquired anomaly? Two cases and a review of the literature. *J Pediatr Surg.* 2008;43(6): 1206–1208.
61. Carpenter HA, Lancaster JR, Lee RA. Multilocular cysts of the peritoneum. *Mayo Clin Proc.* 1982;57(10):634–638.
62. Takiff H, Calabria R, Yin L, et al. Mesenteric cysts and intra-abdominal cystic lymphangiomas. *Arch Surg.* 1985;120(11): 1266–1269.
63. Pampal A, Yagmurlu A. Successful laparoscopic removal of mesenteric and omental cysts in toddlers: 3 cases with a literature review. *J Pediatr Surg.* 2012;47(8):e5–e8.
64. Chang TS, Ricketts R, Abramowsky CR, et al. Mesenteric cystic masses: a series of 21 pediatric cases and review of the literature. *Fetal Pediatr Pathol.* 2011;30(1):40–44.
65. Konen O, Rathaus V, Dlugy E, et al. Childhood abdominal cystic lymphangioma. *Pediatr Radiol.* 2002;32(2):88–94.
66. O'Neil JD, Ros PR, Storm BL, et al. Cystic mesothelioma of the peritoneum. *Radiology.* 1989;170(2):333–337.
67. Esparza Estaun J, Gonzalez Alfageme A, Saenz Banuelos J. Radiological appearance of diaphragmatic mesothelial cysts. *Pediatr Radiol.* 2003;33(12):855–858.
68. Shakya VC, Agrawal CS, Karki S, et al. Benign cystic mesothelioma of the peritoneum in a child-case report and review of the literature. *J Pediatr Surg.* 2011;46(4):e23–e26.
69. Chien AJ, Strouse PJ, Koo HP. Cystic mesothelioma of the testis in an adolescent patient. *J Ultrasound Med.* 2000;19(6):423–425.
70. Niggli FK, Gray TJ, Raafat F, et al. Spectrum of peritoneal mesothelioma in childhood: clinical and histopathologic features, including DNA cytometry. *Pediatr Hematol Oncol.* 1994; 11(4):399–408.
71. de Perrot M, Brundler M, Totsch M, et al. Mesenteric cysts. Toward less confusion? *Dig Surg.* 2000;17(4):323–328.
72. Amesse LS, Gibbs P, Hardy J, et al. Peritoneal inclusion cysts in adolescent females: a clinicopathological characterization of four cases. *J Pediatr Adolesc Gynecol.* 2009;22(1):41–48.
73. Kim JS, Lee HJ, Woo SK, et al. Peritoneal inclusion cysts and their relationship to the ovaries: evaluation with sonography. *Radiology.* 1997;204(2):481–484.
74. Tamai K, Koyama T, Saga T, et al. MR features of physiologic and benign conditions of the ovary. *Eur Radiol.* 2006;16(12): 2700–2711.
75. Hoffer FA, Kozakewich H, Colodny A, et al. Peritoneal inclusion cysts: ovarian fluid in peritoneal adhesions. *Radiology.* 1988; 169(1):189–191.
76. Ross MJ, Welch WR, Scully RE. Multilocular peritoneal inclusion cysts (so-called cystic mesotheliomas). *Cancer.* 1989;64(6): 1336–1346.
77. Sohaey R, Gardner TL, Woodward PJ, et al. Sonographic diagnosis of peritoneal inclusion cysts. *J Ultrasound Med.* 1995; 14(12):913–917.
78. Jain KA. Imaging of peritoneal inclusion cysts. *AJR Am J Roentgenol.* 2000;174(6):1559–1563.
79. Dillman JR, DiPietro MA. Hemorrhagic 'spider-in-web': atypical appearance of a peritoneal inclusion cyst. *Pediatr Radiol.* 2009; 39(11):1252.
80. Minato M, Okada T, Miyagi H, et al. Meconium pseudocyst with particular pathologic findings: a case report and review of the literature. *J Pediatr Surg.* 2012;47(4):e9–e12.
81. Lorimer WS Jr, Ellis DG. Meconium peritonitis. *Surgery.* 1966; 60(2):470–475.
82. Eckoldt F, Heling KS, Woderich R, et al. Meconium peritonitis and pseudo-cyst formation: prenatal diagnosis and post-natal course. *Prenat Diagn.* 2003;23(11):904–908.
83. Estroff JA, Bromley B, Benacerraf BR. Fetal meconium peritonitis without sequelae. *Pediatr Radiol.* 1992;22(4):277–278.
84. Carty HM. Paediatric emergencies: non-traumatic abdominal emergencies. *Eur Radiol.* 2002;12(12):2835–2848.

85. Macari M, Hines J, Balthazar E, et al. Mesenteric adenitis: CT diagnosis of primary versus secondary causes, incidence, and clinical significance in pediatric and adult patients. *AJR Am J Roentgenol.* 2002;178(4):853–858.
86. Simanovsky N, Hiller N. Importance of sonographic detection of enlarged abdominal lymph nodes in children. *J Ultrasound Med.* 2007;26(5):581–584.
87. Helmrath MA, Dorfman SR, Minifee PK, et al. Right lower quadrant pain in children caused by omental infarction. *Am J Surg.* 2001;182(6):729–732.
88. Almeida AT, Melao L, Viamonte B, et al. Epiploic appendagitis: an entity frequently unknown to clinicians—diagnostic imaging, pitfalls, and look-alikes. *AJR Am J Roentgenol.* 2009;193(5): 1243–1251.
89. Schlesinger AE, Dorfman SR, Braverman RM. Sonographic appearance of omental infarction in children. *Pediatr Radiol.* 1999;29(8):598–601.
90. Rimon A, Daneman A, Gerstle JT, et al. Omental infarction in children. *J Pediatr.* 2009;155(3):427–431e1.
91. Theriot JA, Sayat J, Franco S, et al. Childhood obesity: a risk factor for omental torsion. *Pediatrics.* 2003;112(6 Pt 1):e460.
92. Singh AK, Gervais DA, Hahn PF, et al. Acute epiploic appendagitis and its mimics. *Radiographics.* 2005;25(6):1521–1534.
93. Casillas J, Sais GJ, Greve JL, et al. Imaging of intra- and extraabdominal desmoid tumors. *Radiographics.* 1991;11(6):959–968.
94. Ballo MT, Zagars GK, Pollack A, et al. Desmoid tumor: prognostic factors and outcome after surgery, radiation therapy, or combined surgery and radiation therapy. *J Clin Oncol.* 1999; 17(1):158–167.
95. Van Rijn RR, Wilde JCH, Bras J, et al. Imaging findings in noncraniofacial childhood rhabdomyosarcoma. *Pediatr Radiol.* 2008;38(6):617–634.
96. Chung CJ, Fordham L, Little S, et al. Intraperitoneal rhabdomyosarcoma in children: incidence and imaging characteristics on CT. *AJR Am J Roentgenol.* 1998;170(5):1385–1387.
97. Gerald WL, Ladanyi M, de Alava E, et al. Clinical, pathologic, and molecular spectrum of tumors associated with t(11;22) (p13;q12): desmoplastic small round-cell tumor and its variants. *J Clin Oncol.* 1998;16(9):3028–3036.
98. Kushner BH, LaQuaglia MP, Wollner N, et al. Desmoplastic small round-cell tumor: prolonged progression-free survival with aggressive multimodality therapy. *J Clin Oncol.* 1996;14(5): 1526–1531.
99. Quaglia MP, Brennan MF. The clinical approach to desmoplastic small round cell tumor. *Surg Oncol.* 2000;9(2):77–81.
100. Tsokos M, Alaggio RD, Dehner LP, et al. Ewing sarcoma/ peripheral primitive neuroectodermal tumor and related tumors. *Pediatr Dev Pathol.* 2012;15(1 Suppl):108–126.
101. Bellah R, Suzuki-Bordalo L, Brecher E, et al. Desmoplastic small round cell tumor in the abdomen and pelvis: report of CT findings in 11 affected children and young adults. *AJR Am J Roentgenol.* 2005;184(6):1910–1914.
102. Hayes-Jordan A, Anderson PM. The diagnosis and management of desmoplastic small round cell tumor: a review. *Curr Opin Oncol.* 2011;23(4):385–389.
103. Jeong YJ, Kim S, Kwak SW, et al. Neoplastic and nonneoplastic conditions of serosal membrane origin: CT findings. *Radiographics.* 2008;28(3):801–817. discussion 17–18—quiz 912.
104. Dentino CM, Frush DP, Bisset GS. Pediatric radiology case of the day. Peritoneal carcinomatosis. *AJR Am J Roentgenol.* 1995; 165(1):207–208.
105. Slasky BS, Bar-Ziv J, Freeman AI, et al. CT appearances of involvement of the peritoneum, mesentery and omentum in Wilms' tumor. *Pediatr Radiol.* 1997;27(1):14–17.
106. Pickhardt PJ, Bhalla S. Primary neoplasms of peritoneal and sub-peritoneal origin: CT findings. *Radiographics.* 2005;25(4): 983–995.
107. Kim Y, Cho O, Song S, et al. Peritoneal lymphomatosis: CT findings. *Abdom Imaging.* 1998;23(1):87–90.
108. Yoo E, Kim JH, Kim M-J, et al. Greater and lesser omenta: normal anatomy and pathologic processes. *Radiographics.* 2007;27(3):707–720.
109. de Albuquerque FJ, Coutinho AC, Castro Netto EC, et al. Infrarenal abdominal aorta agenesis: a case report with emphasis on MR angiography findings. *Br J Radiol.* 2008;81(967): e179–e183.
110. Bergamini TM, Bernard JD, Mavroudis C, et al. Coarctation of the abdominal aorta. *Ann Vasc Surg.* 1995;9(4):352–356.
111. Castelli PK, Dillman JR, Kershaw DB, et al. Renal sonography with Doppler for detecting suspected pediatric renin-mediated hypertension—is it adequate? *Pediatr Radiol.* 2014; 44(1):42–49.
112. Stein MW, Koenigsberg M, Grigoropoulos J, et al. Aortic coarctation diagnosed in a hypertensive child undergoing Doppler sonography for suspected renal artery stenosis. *Pediatr Radiol.* 2002;32(5):384–386.
113. Howorth MB. Aneurysm of abdominal aorta in the newborn infant. Report of case. *N Engl J Med.* 1967;276(20):1133–1134.
114. Mehall JR, Saltzman DA, Chandler JC, et al. Congenital abdominal aortic aneurysm in the infant: case report and review of the literature. *J Pediatr Surg.* 2001;36(4):657–658.
115. Millar AJ, Gilbert RD, Brown RA, et al. Abdominal aortic aneurysms in children. *J Pediatr Surg.* 1996;31(12):1624–1628.
116. Brantley SK, Rigdon EE, Raju S. Persistent sciatic artery: embryology, pathology, and treatment. *J Vasc Surg.* 1993; 18(2):242–248.
117. Kircher MF, Lee EY, Alomari AI. MRI findings of persistent sciatic artery associated with pelvic infantile hemangioma. *Clin Radiol.* 2010;65(2):172–175.
118. Mandell VS, Jaques PF, Delany DJ, et al. Persistent sciatic artery: clinical, embryologic, and angiographic features. *AJR Am J Roentgenol.* 1985;144(2):245–249.
119. Friedland GW, deVries PA, Nino-Murcia M, et al. Congenital anomalies of the inferior vena cava: embryogenesis and MR features. *Urol Radiol.* 1992;13(4):237–248.
120. Mathews R, Smith PA, Fishman EK, et al. Anomalies of the inferior vena cava and renal veins: embryologic and surgical considerations. *Urology.* 1999;53(5):873–880.
121. Chan FP, Rubin GD. MDCT angiography of pediatric vascular diseases of the abdomen, pelvis, and extremities. *Pediatr Radiol.* 2005;35(1):40–53.
122. Bergsland J, Kawaguchi A, Roland JM, et al. Mycotic aortic aneurysms in children. *Ann Thorac Surg.* 1984;37(4):314–318.
123. Brill PW, Winchester P, Levin AR, et al. Aortic aneurysm secondary to umbilical artery catheterization. *Pediatr Radiol.* 1985;15(3):199–201.
124. Restrepo R, Ranson M, Chait PG, et al. Extracranial aneurysms in children: practical classification and correlative imaging. *AJR Am J Roentgenol.* 2003;181(3):867–878.
125. Wind ES, Wisoff BG, Baron MG, et al. Mycotic aneurysm in infancy: a complication of umbilical artery catheterization. *J Pediatr Surg.* 1982;17(3):324–325.

126. Barth H, Moosdorf R, Bauer J, et al. Mycotic pseudoaneurysm of the aorta in children. *Pediatr Cardiol.* 2000;21(3):263–266.
127. Siassi B, Klyman G, Emmanouilides GC. Hypoplasia of the abdominal aorta associated with the rubella syndrome. *Am J Dis Child.* 1970;120(5):476–479.
128. Ha HK, Lee SH, Rha SE, et al. Radiologic features of vasculitis involving the gastrointestinal tract. *Radiographics.* 2000;20(3):779–794.
129. Yamato M, Lecky JW, Hiramatsu K, et al. Takayasu arteritis: radiographic and angiographic findings in 59 patients. *Radiology.* 1986;161(2):329–334.
130. Gotway MB, Araoz PA, Macedo TA, et al. Imaging findings in Takayasu's arteritis. *AJR Am J Roentgenol.* 2005;184(6):1945–1950.
131. Park JH. Conventional and CT angiographic diagnosis of Takayasu arteritis. *Int J Cardiol.* 1996;54(Suppl):S165–S171.
132. Chung CJ, Stein L. Kawasaki disease: a review. *Radiology.* 1998;208(1):25–33.
133. Canter CE, Bower RJ, Strauss AW. Atypical Kawasaki disease with aortic aneurysm. *Pediatrics.* 1981;68(6):885–888.
134. Sarkar R, Coran AG, Cilley RE, et al. Arterial aneurysms in children: clinicopathologic classification. *J Vasc Surg.* 1991;13(1):47–56, discussion-7.
135. DeCou JM, Abrams RS, Gauderer MW. Seat-belt transection of the pararenal vena cava in a 5-year-old child: survival with caval ligation. *J Pediatr Surg.* 1999;34(7):1074–1076.
136. Strouse PJ, Close BJ, Marshall KW, et al. CT of bowel and mesenteric trauma in children. *Radiographics.* 1999;19(5):1237–1250.
137. Pepin M, Schwarze U, Superti-Furga A, et al. Clinical and genetic features of Ehlers-Danlos syndrome type IV, the vascular type. *New Engl J Med.* 2000;342(10):673–680.
138. Keane MG, Pyeritz RE. Medical management of Marfan syndrome. *Circulation.* 2008;117(21):2802–2813.
139. Johnson PT, Chen JK, Loeys BL, et al. Loeys-Dietz syndrome: MDCT angiography findings. *Am J Roentgenol.* 2007;189(1):W29–W35.
140. Loeys BL, Chen J, Neptune ER, et al. A syndrome of altered cardiovascular, craniofacial, neurocognitive and skeletal development caused by mutations in TGFBR1 or TGFBR2. *Nat Genet.* 2005;37(3):275–281.
141. Hiratzka LF, Bakris GL, Beckman JA, et al. 2010 ACCF/AHA/AATS/ACR/ASA/SCA/SCAI/SIR/STS/SVM Guidelines for the diagnosis and management of patients with thoracic aortic disease. A Report of the American College of Cardiology Foundation/American Heart Association Task Force on Practice Guidelines, American Association for Thoracic Surgery, American College of Radiology, American Stroke Association, Society of Cardiovascular Anesthesiologists, Society for Cardiovascular Angiography and Interventions, Society of Interventional Radiology, Society of Thoracic Surgeons, and Society for Vascular Medicine. *J Am Coll Cardiol.* 2010;55(14):e27–e129.
142. Hamilton SJ, Friedman JM. Insights into the pathogenesis of neurofibromatosis 1 vasculopathy. *Clin Genet.* 2000;58(5):341–344.
143. Jost CJ, Gloviczki P, Edwards WD, et al. Aortic aneurysms in children and young adults with tuberous sclerosis: report of two cases and review of the literature. *J Vasc Surg.* 2001;33(3):639–642.
144. Sandmann W, Schulte KM. Multivisceral fibromuscular dysplasia in childhood: case report and review of the literature. *Ann Vasc Surg.* 2000;14(5):496–502.
145. Slovut DP, Olin JW. Fibromuscular dysplasia. *N Engl J Med.* 2004;350(18):1862–1871.
146. Rose C, Wessel A, Pankau R, et al. Anomalies of the abdominal aorta in Williams-Beuren syndrome—another cause of arterial hypertension. *Eur J Pediatr.* 2001;160(11):655–658.
147. Radford DJ, Pohlner PG. The middle aortic syndrome: an important feature of Williams' syndrome. *Cardiol Young.* 2000;10(6):597–602.

PART IV
PEDIATRIC MUSCULOSKELETAL RADIOLOGY

Andrea S. Doria

CHAPTER 21

Normal Growth, Normal Development, and Congenital Disorders

Victor Ho-Fung • Adji Saptogino • Timothy Cain • Karuna M. Das • Selim Doganay • Diego Jaramillo

INTRODUCTION

The understanding of normal growth and development of the musculoskeletal system is fundamental for the evaluation of the wide spectrum of congenital and developmental abnormalities in children. This knowledge is essential for accurate identification of imaging findings, differential diagnosis, classification, and therapeutic guidance. In this chapter, the currently available various imaging modalities and their main uses in pediatric patients are discussed. The normal anatomy of the developing skeleton is reviewed. An overview of the important imaging characteristics of skeletal abnormalities and syndromes related to skeletal growth and development is provided. In addition, a concise description of the underlying pathophysiology, imaging diagnosis, and therapeutic approaches are also presented.

IMAGING TECHNIQUES

Radiography

Conventional radiographs remain the principal imaging modality for the diagnosis of skeletal abnormalities and skeletal dysplasias. The evaluation of congenital and developmental abnormalities in neonates and infants is based upon the identification of specific morphologic patterns in the different components of the developing skeleton. In the case of skeletal dysplasia, both axial and appendicular skeletal features require a complete assessment using skeletal survey protocols. There are useful comprehensive textbooks dedicated to the evaluation of skeletal dysplasias[1] and anatomic variants.[2]

Ultrasound

The role of ultrasound (US) in musculoskeletal imaging is currently expanding beyond the evaluation of the infant hips. The lack of ionizing radiation exposure or need for sedation, wide availability of US equipment, and the advantage of tailored examinations with both static and dynamic components are all strengths of US, in particular for neonates and young children with abundant hyaline cartilage. Prenatal US is the primary method for evaluation of the fetus and is not unusual to first suspect a potential skeletal dysplasia during routine US examination following identification of shortened long bones or other abnormal skeletal findings.[3,4] However, the accurate prenatal diagnosis of skeletal dysplasias remains challenging because of the heterogeneity of this group of relatively rare disorders, variability in the time of manifestation of clinical findings, and frequent lack of a corroborating genetic and molecular diagnosis.[5–7] A multidisciplinary approach among radiologists, clinicians, pathologists, and geneticists is crucial for the correct diagnosis of skeletal dysplasias and to maximize the usefulness of genetic counseling to the parents.

Computed Tomography

Computer tomography (CT) with multiplanar and three-dimensional (3D) reformation is an ancillary tool to conventional radiography for assessment of skeletal abnormalities, particularly during surgical planning as in the case of tarsal coalitions and transitional fractures.[8,9] The risks of radiation exposure versus the clinical benefits of CT examinations should always be carefully considered in the pediatric population.[10,11] In the case of the long bones in the extremities, potential radiation risks are lower than in the axial skeleton, which is located near more radiosensitive mediastinal, abdominal, and pelvic organs.[12] More recently, selective use of fetal CT with 3D reformations has been described in cases in which US and genetic data are inconclusive to either diagnose or exclude a suspected skeletal dysplasia with impact on accurate counseling of families.[5,12–15]

Magnetic Resonance Imaging

Magnetic resonance imaging (MRI) allows comprehensive evaluation of bone marrow, cartilage, and soft tissues in children with its inherent superior contrast resolution. The capacity to confidently identify different types of hyaline cartilage (physeal, epiphyseal, articular) and their abnormalities in growing children is one of the main advantages of MRI.[16]

The bone marrow is the main site for hematopoiesis. The two normal types of bone marrow consist of red (hematopoietic marrow) and yellow (fatty marrow). The cellular composition of normal marrow changes in an orderly fashion with age (from red to yellow marrow), a process known as marrow conversion (Fig. 21.1).

MRI allows for identification of expected age-related changes through the skeleton. At birth, hematopoietic marrow is present in the entire skeleton. Subsequently, marrow conversion begins in the periphery of the skeleton. This occurs first along distal phalanges (fingers and toes), in a symmetric, centripetal distribution into the axial skeleton. Following the appearance of the secondary center of ossification, both epiphyseal and apophyseal regions are the first to developed fatty marrow within months of ossification (showing signal characteristics of fat tissue on both T1 and fluid-sensitive sequences), an important observation when evaluating marrow signal intensity on infants and young children. In the long bones, marrow conversion occurs during the first decade of life. In these areas, the process begins along the diaphysis and progresses to the distal metaphysis and finally into the proximal metaphysis. Small residual areas of hematopoietic marrow with typical straight margins or feathery-shape appearance can be seen in the metaphyseal regions, particularly in the proximal femur of adolescents. Persistence of large amounts of hematopoietic marrow in the diaphysis after 10 years of age is considered abnormal. The marrow conversion process continues into the mid to late third decade of life, when bone marrow distribution reaches adult state (Fig. 21.1).[17]

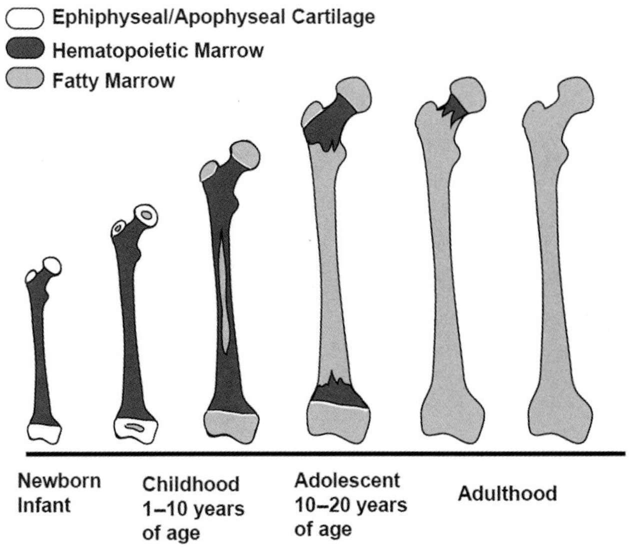

FIGURE 21.1 **Normal bone marrow conversion in long bones.** Sequential age-related changes in hematopoietic marrow to fatty marrow distribution are illustrated in this figure representing a femur.

Multiple factors requiring increased hematopoiesis can cause marrow reconversion (from yellow to red marrow) such as anemias (sickle cell and thalassemia), physiologic stress (high altitude, endurance training, obesity), and chemotherapy with granulocyte colony-stimulating factor therapy. Also, abnormal marrow replacement can be seen with neoplastic disease (leukemia and metastatic disease).

Potential limitations of MRI include cost, availability, and the need for sedation in younger children. However, the role of MRI for prenatal characterization of skeletal dysplasia is limited, primarily because of difficulty in displaying a panoramic image of a fetus and obtaining adequate images for visualization of the main axis of individual bones.[13]

Nuclear Medicine

Nuclear medicine is a useful imaging modality for specific skeletal dysplasias related to metabolically active bone and soft tissue lesions. For example, the use of bone scintigraphy has been described for identification of bone lesions in polyostotic fibrous dysplasia.[18] Also, the role of hybrid imaging combining positron emission tomography (PET) functional imaging with the anatomic detail of CT (PET–CT) in children is expanding, particularly in the characterization and staging of neoplastic disease.[19–21]

NORMAL ANATOMY

The skeletal system develops in utero from a condensation of primitive mesenchymal cells that are precursors of cartilage or membranous bone. Membranous ossification refers to bone formation through mesenchymal differentiation directly into osteoblasts without a cartilaginous precursor. Membranous ossification is responsible for the development of the facial bones and cranium. In the long bones, the periosteal membrane envelopes the outer layer of the bone and is responsible for membranous ossification resulting in axial growth.

The structure of the tubular bones is similar through the body. A synchondrosis refers to a joint in which the connecting medium is hyaline cartilage, such as the epiphysis of long bones and sternocostal joints. The epiphyses are at both ends of most long bones, with each epiphysis located between the joint and the primary physis. The epiphyses are initially completely cartilaginous, followed by the development of a secondary ossification center and progressive conversion into bone.

Endochondral ossification refers to bone formation through a cartilaginous model. It is responsible for the development of the skull base, long bones, clavicles, and vertebral column. In the long bones, endochondral ossification allows longitudinal growth with formation of columns of cartilage in the primary physis with sequential morphologic changes and transformation of the chondrocytes in new bone at the metaphysis.[22]

The apophyses do not contribute to the longitudinal growth of long bones but provide important structural support to the insertion of muscles, tendons, and ligaments. The apophyseal formation is similar to the epiphyses; it is initially entirely cartilaginous with subsequent conversion into bone because of the development of a secondary ossification center and a physeal equivalent.

The epiphyseal cartilage is a vascularized structure supplied by vascular canals. The epiphyseal vascular canals are composed of nonanastomotic arterioles, venules, and sinusoidal capillaries that are radially arranged around the secondary center of ossification.[23] The physeal cartilage is only vascular during the first 18 months of life and then becomes avascular. These changes also determine the pathologic changes seen at different stages of skeletal maturation. For example, vascular canals are prominent in diseases that result in inflamed synovium, such as juvenile idiopathic arthritis, and when infection invades the epiphyseal cartilage. They are attenuated when there is ischemia of the cartilage, such as that resulting from excessive abduction in spica casts for developmental hip dysplasia treatment or that related to large-joint septic arthritis.

The metaphysis is the most vascularized structure of the growing skeleton. Systemic processes are manifested first in these regions along the appendicular skeleton, in particular in rapidly growing bones such as distal femur and proximal tibia. The interaction of the metaphysis on the adjacent physis allows formation of new bone from the cartilaginous template of the physis. Both physiologic and pathologic processes can have similar appearance along the metaphyseal regions, and knowledge of these variants is important for the imaging evaluation in children.

The differential diagnosis for dense metaphyseal transverse bands is extensive, but among the most important considerations are normal dense zones of provisional calcification (most common in neonates), treated leukemia, chronic lead poisoning, hypoparathyroidism, healing rickets, scurvy, and "growth recovery lines" (seen in patients with generalized systemic disease causing periods of chronic illness and recovery).

The differential diagnosis for lucent metaphyseal transverse bands includes normal variation, leukemia and metastatic neuroblastoma, and TORCH (toxoplasmosis, rubella, cytomegalovirus, herpes simplex, and HIV) infection in the neonate. The presence of perpendicular linear bands of metaphyseal lucency and sclerosis (striations) can be seen as a normal variant along the proximal femurs.

DEVELOPMENTAL AND ANATOMIC VARIANTS

Metaphyseal Beaking and Genu Varum

Metaphyseal beaking, particularly in the medial aspect of the proximal tibia, and lower extremity bowing (genu varum) are not uncommon in young children. Genu varum usually is seen in walking children under 2 years of age with physiologic resolution after this age (Fig. 21.2 and **Schematic N**).[24] The differential diagnosis for pathologic genu varum includes trauma, skeletal dysplasia (achondroplasia), rickets, fibrous dysplasia, and Blount disease. Metaphyseal fragmentation with physiologic bowing has also been described in young children and considered physiologic in children after ~18 months of age.[25]

Physiologic Periosteal Reaction

Physiologic periosteal reaction is an important developmental variant in young infants between 1 and 6 months. The typical features of physiologic reaction include smooth, thin (<2 mm), and symmetric distribution along rapidly growing long bones, particularly the humeri, femurs, and tibias (Fig. 21.3). The periosteum, which is responsible for the membranous ossification

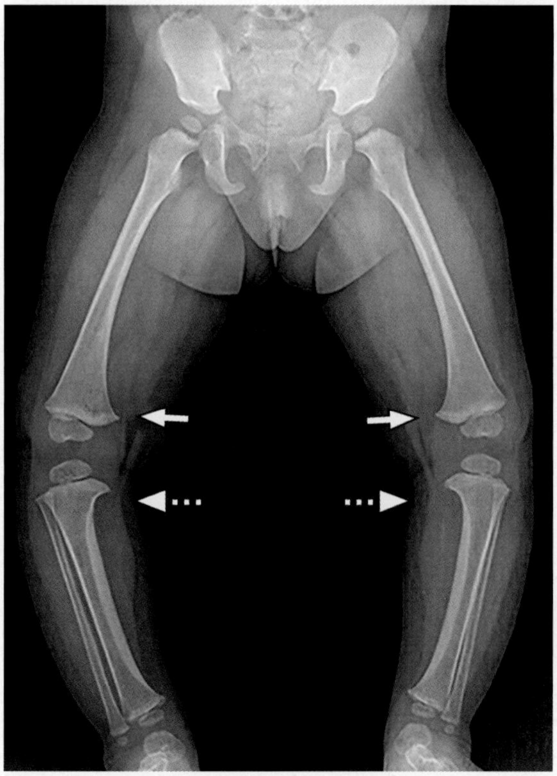

FIGURE 21.2 **Physiologic genu varum and metaphyseal beaking in a 19-month-old girl.** Frontal radiograph of bilateral lower extremities shows symmetric genu varum with medial metaphyseal beaking in both distal femurs (*arrows*) and proximal tibias (*interrupted arrows*). Patient was asymptomatic and genu varum resolved 1 year after radiographic evaluation.

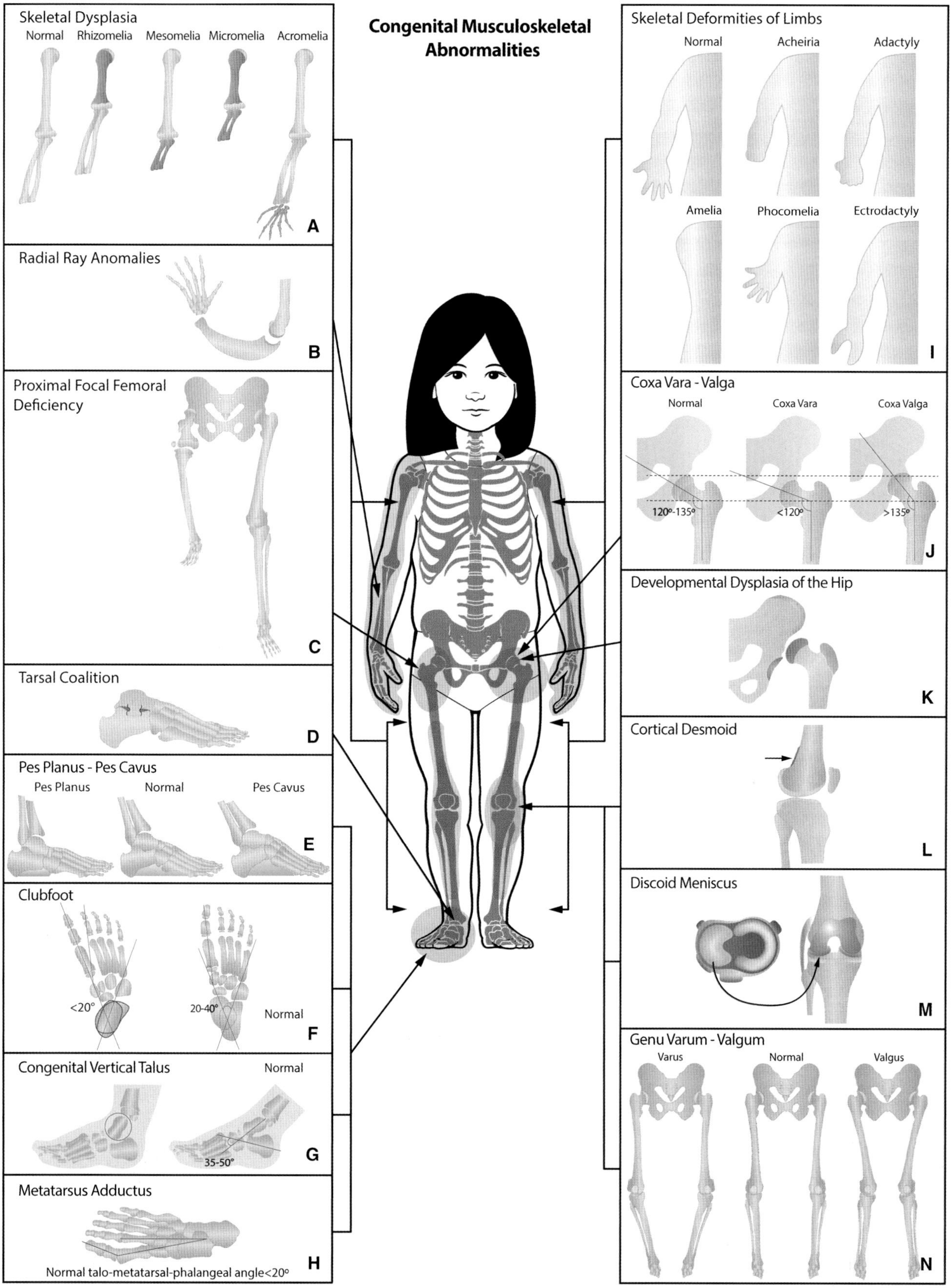
Congenital Musculoskeletal Abnormalities
Skeletal Dysplasia
Normal
Rhizomelia
Mesomelia
Micromelia
Acromelia
A
Radial Ray Anomalies
B
Proximal Focal Femoral Deficiency
C
Tarsal Coalition
D
Pes Planus - Pes Cavus
Pes Planus
Normal
Pes Cavus
E
Clubfoot
<20°
20-40°
Normal
F
Congenital Vertical Talus
Normal
35-50°
G
Metatarsus Adductus
Normal talo-metatarsal-phalangeal angle<20°
H
Skeletal Deformities of Limbs
Normal
Acheiria
Adactyly
Amelia
Phocomelia
Ectrodactyly
I
Coxa Vara - Valga
Normal
Coxa Vara
Coxa Valga
120°-135°
<120°
>135°
J
Developmental Dysplasia of the Hip
K
Cortical Desmoid
L
Discoid Meniscus
M
Genu Varum - Valgum
Varus
Normal
Valgus
N

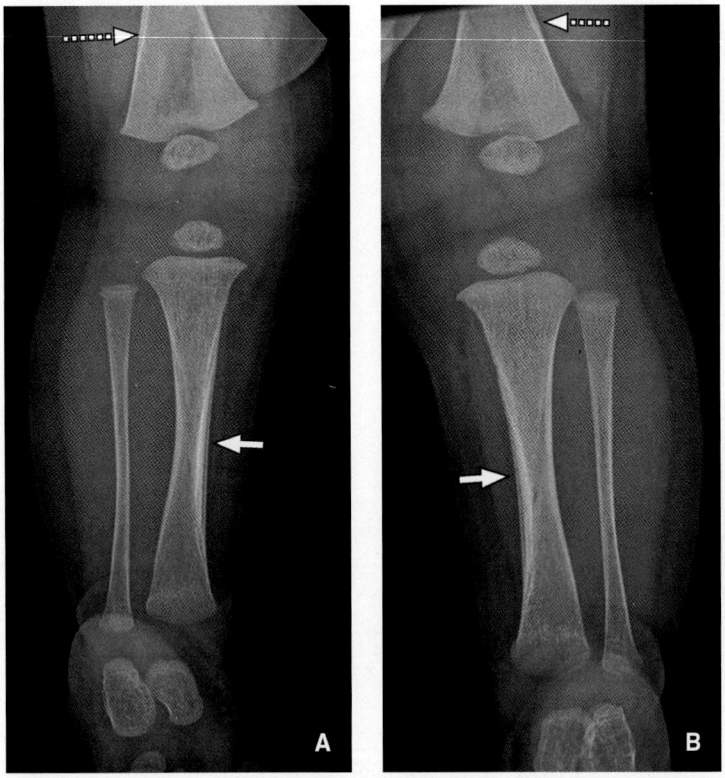

FIGURE 21.3 **Physiologic periosteal reaction in a 2-month-old boy. A:** Frontal radiograph of the right tibia. **B:** Frontal radiograph of the left tibia. Both images show thin, smooth, continuous, symmetric periosteal reaction (*arrows*) along the medial diaphyseal cortex of both tibias. Included portions of the distal femurs also show physiologic periosteal reaction (*interrupted arrows*).

of long bones, also guides the reparative response to stimuli (e.g., trauma, infection, neoplasm, metabolic disorder, and nutritional status). In children, the periosteum is physiologically more active and less adherent to the cortex than in adults, allowing for earlier and more aggressive appearance of the periosteal reaction.[26] The differential diagnosis for benign periosteal reaction in the pediatric population is summarized in Table 21.1.

Cortical Desmoid

A very common developmental variant in older children is a cortical desmoid (also known as distal femoral cortical irregularity) (Fig. 21.4 and **Schematic L**). This lesion is a self-limiting fibrous or fibroosseous lesion most commonly located in the medial supracondylar region, believed to be a tug lesion at the insertion of the adductor magnus aponeurosis or the origin of the medial head of the gastrocnemius.[27,28] Prevalence is highest in boys age 10 to 15 years. The majority of affected pediatric patients are asymptomatic, although some have a history of knee pain secondary to trauma.

Radiographic evaluation typically demonstrates a cortical irregularity or erosion with a sclerotic base at the posteromedial distal femur in the lateral view and occasionally a well-circumscribed lucent region with a sclerotic thin rim in the frontal view. MRI typically demonstrates a cortical irregularity along the posteromedial distal femur with increased T2 signal intensity within the adjacent bone marrow. Occasionally, associated traumatic periostitis and swelling with soft tissue edema at the origin of the medial head of the gastrocnemius can be seen.[27] Typical radiographic features are diagnostic for this entity, and in the presence of a benign clinical course, further workup and biopsy can be avoided.[29]

TABLE 21.1 Differential Diagnosis of Physiologic Periosteal Reaction (1–6 Months of Age)
Healing fracture
Infection
Drugs (prostaglandins, hypervitaminosis A)
Hypertrophic osteoarthropathy (cardiopulmonary diseases, malignancy)
Infantile cortical hyperostosis (Caffey disease)

Discoid Meniscus

Discoid meniscus is a congenital anatomic variant seen more commonly in the lateral meniscus (Fig. 21.5 and **Schematic M**). The incidence varies from 0.4% to 16.6% on arthroscopic studies.[30] A discoid meniscus is more disc shaped than semilunar shaped in configuration with a portion of the meniscus extending to the central portion of the tibial plateau.[31] The majority of affected pediatric patients are asymptomatic; however, the abnormal configuration of the discoid meniscus alters biomechanics and causes a predisposition for increased meniscal tears and intrasubstance degeneration. Symptomatic pediatric patients present with a "snapping knee" and, when torn, can be a cause of locking and knee pain.

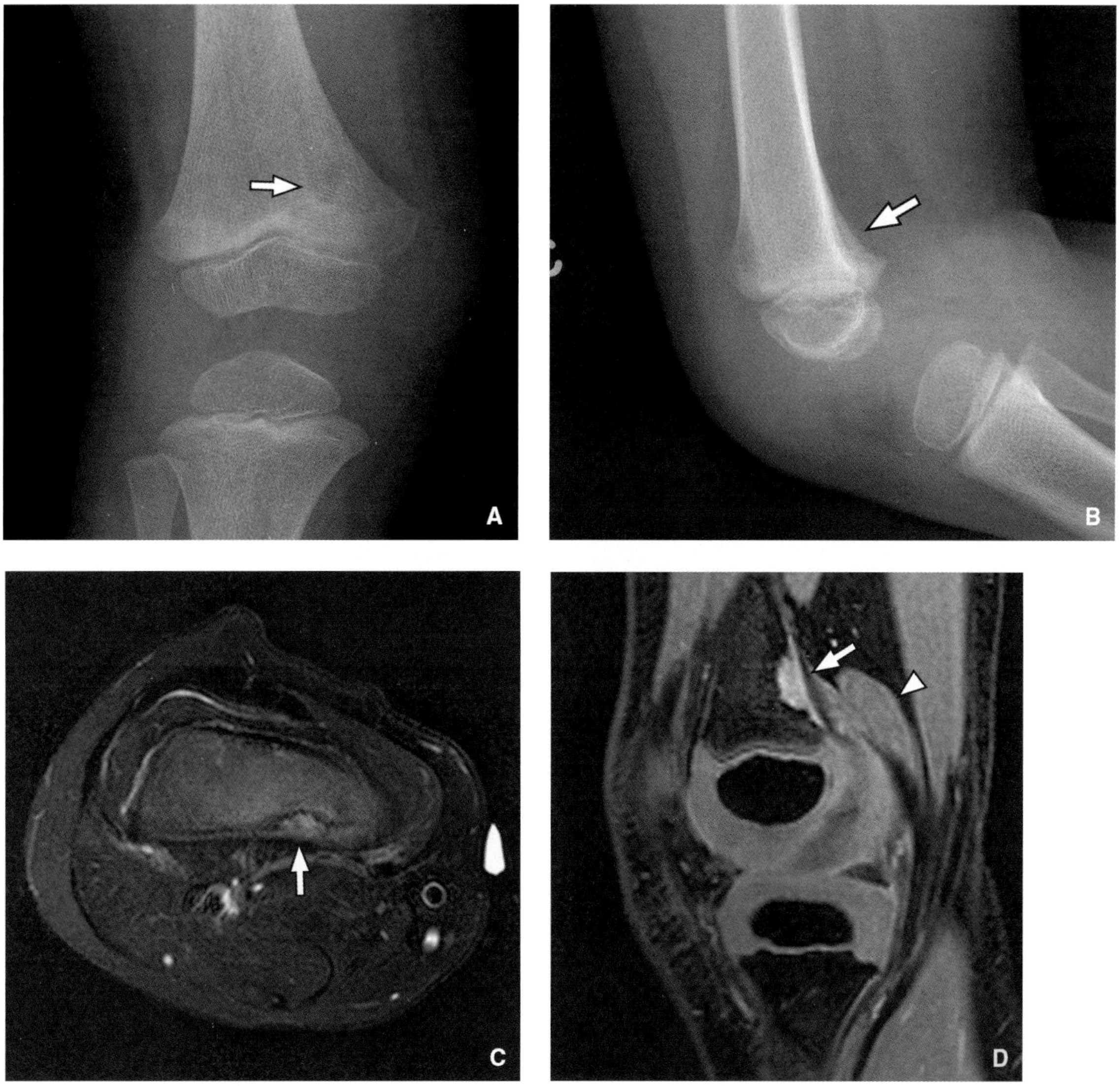

FIGURE 21.4 **Cortical desmoid in a 4-year-old boy. A:** Frontal radiograph of the right knee shows a lucent lesion (*arrow*) with well-marginated sclerotic borders in the medial femoral metadiaphysis. **B:** Lateral radiograph of the right knee shows the typical posterior location with sclerosis and mild irregularity (*arrow*). **C:** Axial fat-saturated T2-weighted MR image shows subperiosteal location of the lesion (*arrow*) with increased signal intensity and sclerotic borders. **D:** Sagittal fat-saturated intermediate gradient-echo sequence MR image shows homogeneous hyperintense signal intensity (*arrow*) consistent with fibrous tissue and anatomic relationship to the insertion of the medial head of the gastrocnemius (*arrowhead*).

Diagnosis of discoid meniscus is performed with MRI, and measurements for diagnosis of discoid meniscus include medial extension of the lateral meniscus into the tibial spines (transverse width >13 mm or height 2 mm greater than the medial meniscus).[32] Incidentally detected discoid meniscus in asymptomatic pediatric patients can be managed with observation alone. However, surgical intervention is often needed to manage intrasubstance tears or instability of the discoid meniscus in symptomatic pediatric patients.

SPECTRUM OF DISORDERS

Congenital Anomalies and Abnormalities

The skeletal dysplasias or osteochondrodysplasias are a heterogeneous group of congenital abnormalities characterized by generalized disorders of bone growth and development. More than 250 dysplasias have been described.[33] Additional dysplasias and specific variants continue to be discovered with new advances in genetic evaluation. Most of the skeletal dysplasias are characterized by disproportionate short stature (micromelia). Useful terms for describing micromelia are summarized in **Schematic A** with the red parts of the figure representing short limb segments.

A helpful catalog for the skeletal dysplasias and most known diseases with a genetic component is the Web site database "Online Mendelian Inheritance in Man" (OMIM).[33,34] OMIM provides a compilation of human genes and genetic disorders. Through this chapter, a six-digit number corresponding to the OMIM disease numbering system is included when appropriate.

The definitive diagnosis of skeletal dysplasias solely based on imaging studies is often challenging. The role of the radiologist is to provide adequate descriptions of the specific

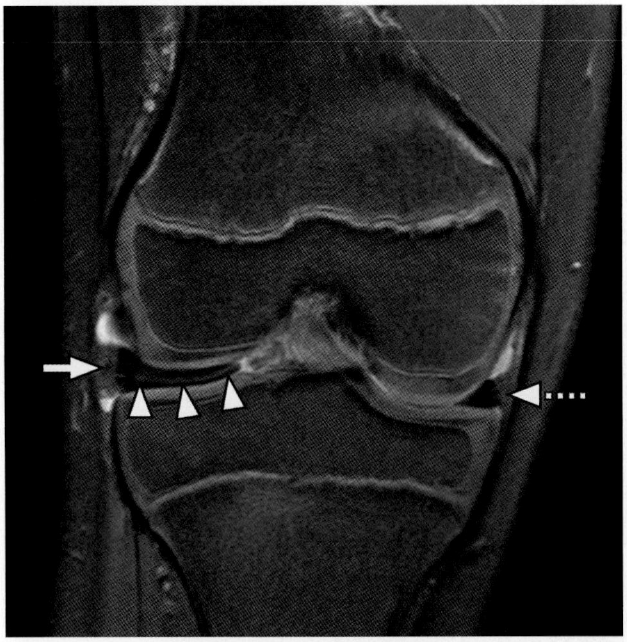

FIGURE 21.5 **Discoid lateral meniscus in a 7-year-old girl with knee pain and locking.** Coronal fat-saturated intermediate sequence MR image demonstrates diffuse enlargement of the lateral meniscus (*arrow*) completely occupying the central portion of the lateral compartment. Linear increased intrasubstance signal intensity is noted along the width of the discoid lateral meniscus (*arrowheads*); however, there is no meniscal tear extending along the articular surface. Normal size medial meniscus is noted (*interrupted arrow*).

bony abnormalities in the axial and appendicular skeleton of affected pediatric patients. This information should be integrated with the rest of the information provided by a multidisciplinary team approach in order to reach a correct diagnosis. A comprehensive analysis of imaging findings in skeletal dysplasias is beyond the scope of this chapter. However, the most common skeletal dysplasias identifiable through imaging at birth or later in life are summarized in this chapter. In addition, the most common disorders of limb reduction, congenital bowing of the legs, and congenital foot deformities are reviewed. Finally, syndromic skeletal abnormalities, developmental hip dysplasia, and skeletal abnormalities associated with neuromuscular disorders are discussed (Table 21.2).

Skeletal Dysplasias Affecting Growth of Tubular Bones and Spine (Identifiable at Birth)

Thanatophoric Dysplasia

Thanatophoric dysplasia (TD) is one of the most common neonatal lethal skeletal dysplasias affecting ~1 of 20,000 live births (Fig. 21.6). It is caused by autosomal dominant mutations in the gene for fibroblast growth factor (FGFR3, at 4p16.3) in one of two sites, corresponding to the two recognized variants, TD type I (OMIM 187600) and TD type II (OMIM 187601).[35,36] TD is characterized clinically by micromelic limbs, marked limb curvature, relative macrocephaly, near-normal trunk length, and small thoracic cage.

Radiographic features include large calvarium (TD type I) and cloverleaf skull (TD type II), long narrow trunk with short ribs, wide-cupped costochondral junctions, small abnormally formed scapula, severe platyspondyly, anterior rounded vertebral bodies, apparent wide disc spaces, diffuse interpedicular narrowing, very characteristic short and small iliac bones, horizontal acetabular roofs with medial and lateral spikes ("trident acetabulum"—however, this can also be seen in other dysplasias), marked shortening, and bowing of the long bones with either a "French telephone receiver femurs" (TD type I) or straight micromelic femurs (TD type II).[37] Prenatal diagnosis with US in the second trimester has been described with demonstration of micromelic features, in particular the short femurs, small narrow thorax, and large or cloverleaf skull. Recent literature describes improved accuracy of antenatal diagnosis of TD using molecular genetic confirmation with cell-free fetal DNA in maternal plasma and the potential role of 3D US.[38,39]

The management of TD is predominantly supportive (e.g., ventilator support, tracheostomy, and ventriculoperitoneal shunt), as most cases are lethal in the perinatal period with occasional reports of longer survival into young childhood.[40,41]

Chondrodysplasia Punctata

Chondrodysplasia punctata (CD) is a rare clinically and genetically diverse group of skeletal dysplasias. There are sporadic, X-linked recessive, X-linked dominant, autosomal recessive, and autosomal dominant forms. The shared feature among the different variants is the presence of stippled epiphyses (Fig. 21.7). One of the most frequent types of CD is the rhizomelic type (OMIM 600121), which is characterized by a symmetric rhizomelic dwarfism, craniofacial dysmorphism (micrognathia, flat face, microcephaly), cataracts, skin lesions, joint contractures, growth failure, and severe psychomotor retardation. The mode of inheritance of CD rhizomelic type is autosomal recessive with metabolic abnormalities related to peroxisomal enzyme deficiencies. The majority of affected patients with CD rhizomelic type do not survive the first few weeks of life, and those who survive beyond this period uniformly present with severe developmental delays, infections, seizures, and growth failure.[42]

Radiographic features include symmetric shortening of proximal and other long bones, punctate calcification in cartilaginous regions of the growing skeleton and periarticular regions with mild or absent stippling of the axial skeleton, and gradual diminution or disappearance of stippling in first year of life and coronal clefts dividing the vertebral bodies.[43] Prenatal diagnosis with US has been described in few case reports, with demonstration of disproportionately short femurs and humeri and possible epiphyseal stippling.[44]

TABLE 21.2 Selected Spectrum of Skeletal Dysplasias with Identifiable Imaging Findings at Birth and Later in Life

Skeletal Dysplasias Identifiable at Birth			
Name	**Pattern of Inheritance**	**Clinical Importance**	**Main Radiographic Findings**
Thanatophoric dysplasia (TD)	AD	Most common lethal skeletal dysplasia	Large calvarium (TD type I) Cloverleaf skull (TD type II) Long narrow trunk with short ribs Severe platyspondyly Diffuse interpedicular narrowing Short small iliac bones Horizontal acetabular roofs with medial and lateral spikes ("trident acetabulum") Bowing of the long bones, particularly the femurs ("French telephone receiver")
Chondrodysplasia punctata	SP X-LR X-LD AR AD	Stippled Epiphysis	Rhizomelia Stippled calcifications on epiphyseal cartilage of long bones (gradual diminution or disappearance) in the 1st year of life Coronal clefts dividing the vertebral bodies
Achondroplasia	SP AD	Most common nonlethal skeletal dysplasia	Rhizomelia with thick tubular bones Progressive craniocaudal interpedicular space narrowing Bullet-shaped vertebra Narrow chest with short ribs V-shaped growth plates Horizontal acetabular roof Squared iliac wings
Asphyxiating thoracic dystrophy	AR	Thoracic insufficiency early in life. If survival, chronic renal failure later in life	Small "bell-shaped" thorax Horizontally oriented ribs "Handlebar clavicles" Small "squared" iliac bones Horizontal acetabular roof with medial and lateral spikes "trident" configuration
Skeletal Dysplasias Identifiable Later in Life			
Name	**Pattern of Inheritance**	**Main Clinical Findings**	**Main Radiographic Findings**
Metaphyseal chondrodysplasia Schmid type	AD	Waddling gait, bowed legs, short stature in the 2nd year of life	Diffuse metaphyseal flaring Physeal widening and irregularity Coxa vara and enlarged capital femoral epiphyses Genu varum Femoral bowing
Multiple epiphyseal dysplasia	AD AR	Present with fatigue and joint pain (mimics rheumatologic disease) Short stature and limb shortening can be very subtle	Delayed appearance of secondary ossification centers of the long bones, hands, and wrists. Abnormal small, irregular, fragmented epiphyses (mainly hips and lower limbs) Can present with avascular necrosis of the femoral heads Mild irregularity of the endplates, anterior wedging, and Schmorl nodes in second decade of life

AD, autosomal dominant; AR, autosomal recessive; SP, sporadic; X-LD; X-linked dominant; X-LR, X-linked recessive.

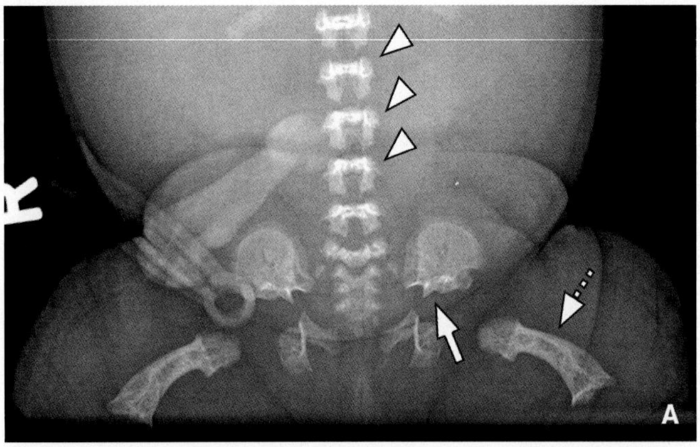

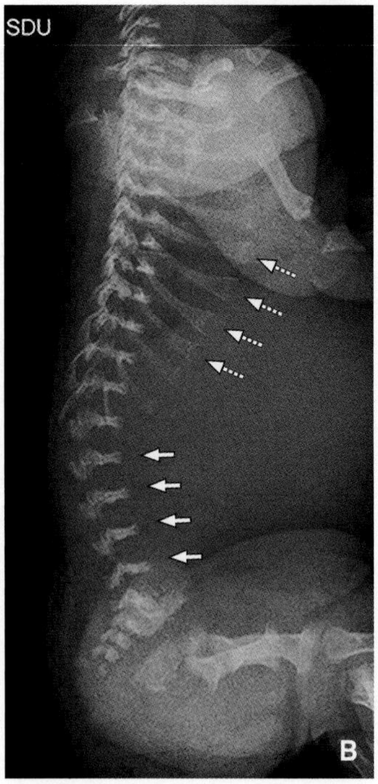

FIGURE 21.6 **Thanatophoric dysplasia in a newborn girl. A:** Frontal radiograph of the pelvis demonstrates bilateral small iliac bones with "trident acetabulum" (*arrow*), shortening and bowing of the femurs "French telephone receiver" (*interrupted arrow*), and diffuse narrowing of the interpedicular spaces (*arrowheads*). **B:** Lateral radiograph of the thoracolumbar spine demonstrates severe platyspondyly (*arrows*) and short ribs with anterior cupping (*interrupted arrows*). Short upper and lower limbs are also noted.

Achondroplasia

Achondroplasia is the most common nonlethal short limb skeletal dysplasia (OMIM 100800) affecting ~1 in 15,000 live births. An autosomal dominant mutation in the FGFR3 gene at locus 4p16.3 causes impaired endochondral bone formation. More than 90% of cases are sporadic.[45] The clinical features of achondroplasia are short stature, rhizomelic shortening of the limbs, characteristics facies with frontal bossing and midface hypoplasia, increased lumbar lordosis, genu varum, elbow contractures, and trident hand. Neurologic complications include hydrocephalus, spinal cord compression, syringomyelia, recurrent ear infections, and dental malocclusion.

Radiographic features include large calvarium with small skull base, narrow foramen magnum, frontal bossing, narrowed lumbar spinal canal, progressive craniocaudal interpedicular space narrowing, bullet-shaped vertebra during infancy and early childhood, short vertebral pedicles,

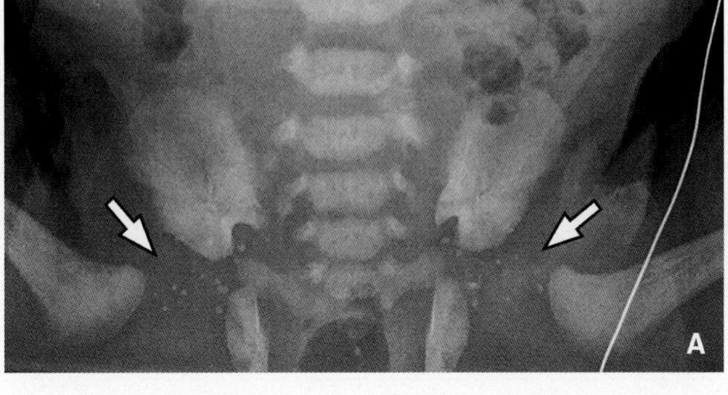

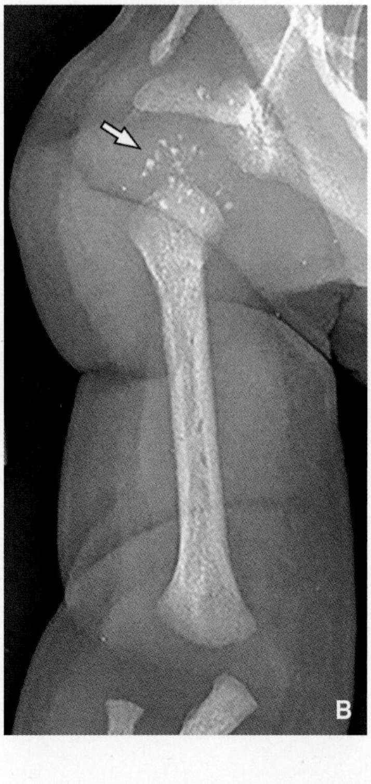

FIGURE 21.7 **Chondrodysplasia punctata in a 5-day-old girl. A:** Frontal radiograph of the abdomen demonstrates stippled calcifications in both proximal femoral epiphyses (*arrows*). **B:** Lateral radiograph of the right humerus demonstrates similar stippled calcifications in the proximal humeral epiphysis (*arrow*).

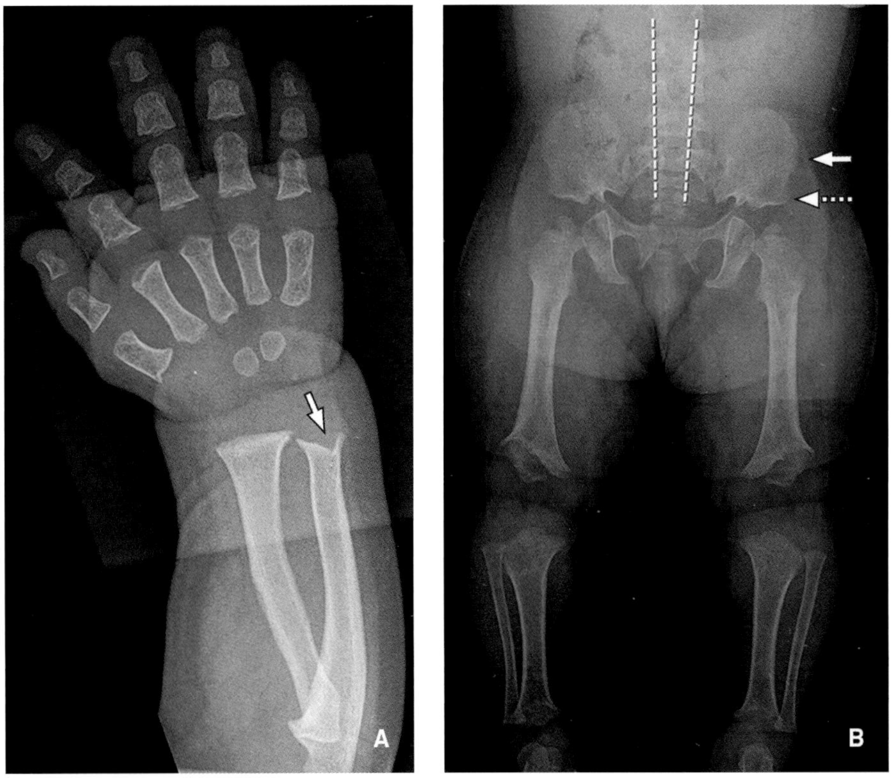

FIGURE 21.8 **Achondroplasia in a 1-year-old girl. A:** Frontal radiograph of the hand demonstrates short, broad, long bones of the forearm and hand. There is V-shape configuration of the distal ulnar physis (*arrow*) and "trident" configuration of the hand. **B:** Frontal radiograph of the pelvis and lower extremities demonstrates squared iliac bones or "tombstone configuration" (*arrow*), horizontal acetabular roofs (*interrupted arrow*), decreased interpedicular space in the lumbar spine (interrupted lines), and short tubular long bones with metaphyseal flaring in bilateral lower extremities.

posterior vertebral scalloping, narrow chest with short ribs, rhizomelia with short thick tubular bones and metaphyseal flaring, notched physis (V shaped), short metacarpals and phalanges in "trident" configuration (separation between third and fourth fingers), horizontal acetabular roof, and squared iliac wings ("tombstone configuration") (Fig. 21.8). Prenatal US demonstrates short long bones, particularly femurs and humeri, flat vertebral bodies, and large skull. In addition, small chest, short fingers, and polyhydramnios have been described.[46]

The management of achondroplasia includes management of spinal cord complications including decompression of lumbar stenosis and craniocervical decompression.[47,48] Upper and lower limb lengthening procedures are well-established techniques for those who elect this treatment.[49,50]

Asphyxiating Thoracic Dystrophy

Asphyxiating thoracic dystrophy (ATD), also known as short rib thoracic dysplasia or Jeune syndrome, is a rare skeletal dysplasia characterized by a narrow and elongated "bell-shaped" thorax causing variable degrees of lung hypoplasia secondary to impaired thoracic expansion.[51] The incidence is ~1 in 100,000 to 130,000 live births. Inheritance is usually autosomal recessive, with the most common disease locus mapped to chromosome 15q13 (OMIM 208500). The clinical features of ATD include short stature, short limbs, and polydactyly. Death in infancy because of respiratory insufficiency is noted in 70% of cases; however, the degree of severity can range from lethal to latent forms.[52] Affected individuals who survive early childhood present with chronic cystic renal disease and hepatic fibrosis.

Radiographic findings of ATD include narrow, small, "bell-shaped thorax" with horizontally oriented ribs, "handlebar" clavicles, hypoplastic "squared" iliac wings, "trident" acetabular roofs, polydactyly, and brachydactyly of long bones. The radiographic findings of ATD can be highly suggestive of the diagnosis. The main differential diagnosis of ATD is chondroectodermal dysplasia (Ellis-van Creveld syndrome) in which polydactyly and nail hypoplasia are seen more frequently and in which ~60% of patients present with congenital heart disease.[53] US, CT, or MRI studies in patients with ATD can demonstrate the following complications: lung hypoplasia, cirrhosis, hepatic portal fibrosis, and microcystic renal disease. Prenatal US diagnosis can be suggested by severely shortened ribs, brachydactyly, small thorax, and renal cystic change.[54]

Therapeutic management focuses on stabilization and support of respiratory function. Vertical expandable prosthetic titanium rib (VEPTR) has been used for treatment of the thoracic insufficiency seen in ATD.[55] In few reported cases of older children with ATD and chronic renal failure, renal transplantation has been used as a therapeutic option.[56]

Skeletal Dysplasias Affecting Growth of Tubular Bones and Spine (Identifiable in Later Life)

Metaphyseal Chondrodysplasia

Metaphyseal chondrodysplasias are a group of rare skeletal dysplasias characterized by metaphyseal deformity and irregularity adjacent to the physes with little or no epiphyseal involvement. Their clinical presentation is variable; however, the onset of symptoms ranges from infancy to early childhood rather than at birth. The most common types of metaphyseal chondrodysplasia are Schmid, McKusick, and Jansen variants.

The Schmid-type metaphyseal chondrodysplasia (OMIM 156500) has been well-delineated clinically. The pattern of inheritance is autosomal dominant with mutations in COL10A1 of type X collagen in locus 6q21-22. This disease is characterized by short limbs, short stature in the second year of life, and bowed legs with waddling gait.[57,58] Radiographic findings of Schmid-type metaphyseal chondrodysplasia are diffuse metaphyseal flaring, growth plate widening particularly at the knees, enlarged capital femoral epiphyses, coxa vara, genu varum, femoral bowing, anterior rib cupping and sclerosis, and less frequently irregular acetabular roofs and mild vertebral body changes (Fig. 21.9).

Therapeutic management of Schmid-type metaphyseal chondrodysplasia is mainly focused on orthopedic management of lower extremity deformities (coxa valga and genu varum realignment).

Multiple Epiphyseal Dysplasia

Multiple epiphyseal dysplasia is one of the most common forms of nonlethal skeletal dysplasia. It can be autosomal dominant or recessive, with at least six different gene mutations described. The diagnosis is usually made in late childhood or adolescence. Clinical manifestations are often related to joint pain and easy fatigue, prompting rheumatologic evaluation. The short stature and limb shortening in affected patients can be very mild.[59]

Radiographic features include delayed appearance of the secondary ossification centers of the long bones of the hands and wrists with abnormal small epiphyses that appear irregular and fragmented, particularly in the hips and lower limbs. During the prepubescent period, affected patients can present with avascular necrosis (AVN) of the femoral heads. Mild irregularity of the endplates, anterior wedging, and Schmorl nodes are seen in the second decade of life.

Therapeutic management of multiple epiphyseal dysplasia is mainly focused on orthopedic management of lower and upper extremity acquired deformities.[59]

Skeletal Dysplasias with Disorganized Development of Cartilage and Fibrous Components of the Skeleton

Multiple Cartilaginous Exostoses

Multiple cartilaginous exostoses or osteochondromatosis is a relatively common skeletal dysplasia. The prevalence is ~1 in 50,000 with a male predilection. The pattern of inheritance is autosomal dominant with multiple mutation loci in the EXT genes (OMIM 133700, 133701).[60,61] The disease is characterized by multiple osteochondromas, the majority located within long bones of the extremities. Clinical manifestations are related to lumps and bumps in early childhood, nerve impingement syndromes, progressive skeletal deformities in the upper and lower extremities related to asymmetrical growth of two bone segments (short ulnas and fibulas), and disproportionate shortening of the limbs. Radiographic evaluation demonstrates typical morphology of the osteochondromas as an exostosis originating from the metadiaphysis

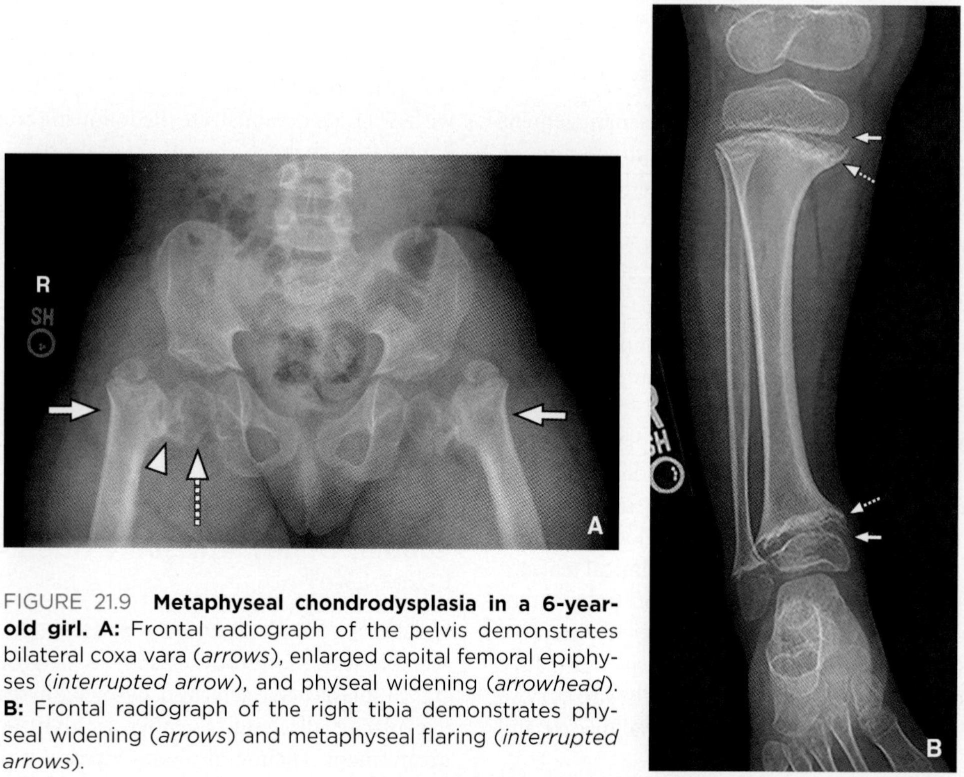

FIGURE 21.9 **Metaphyseal chondrodysplasia in a 6-year-old girl. A:** Frontal radiograph of the pelvis demonstrates bilateral coxa vara (*arrows*), enlarged capital femoral epiphyses (*interrupted arrow*), and physeal widening (*arrowhead*). **B:** Frontal radiograph of the right tibia demonstrates physeal widening (*arrows*) and metaphyseal flaring (*interrupted arrows*).

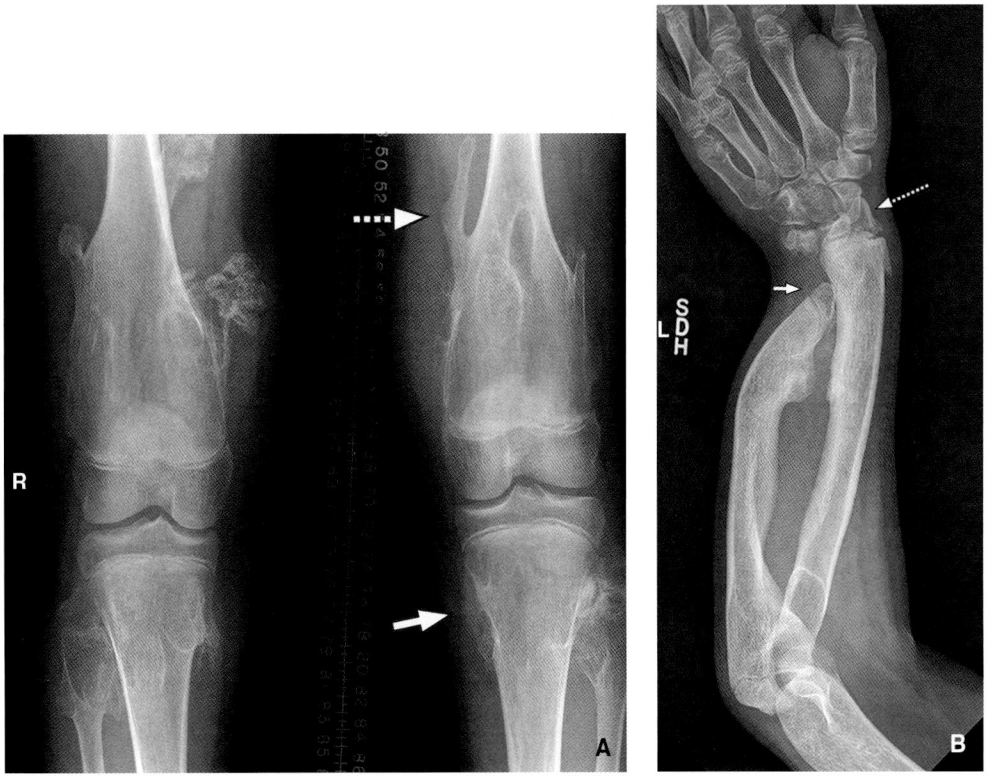

FIGURE 21.10 **Multiple cartilaginous exostoses in a 14-year-old boy. A:** Frontal radiograph of both knees as part of scanogram examination for leg length discrepancy demonstrates numerous bilateral sessile (*arrow*) and exophytic osteochondromas (*interrupted arrow*). Note predominant metadiaphyseal distribution with growth directing away from the joint. **B:** Frontal radiograph of the left forearm with multiple osteochondromas of the proximal and distal radial and ulnar metadiaphysis. There is characteristic shortening and bowing of the distal ulna (*arrow*) with medial angulation of the distal radial epiphysis (*interrupted arrow*).

with apex extending away from the joint (Fig. 21.10). The osteochondromas can also be seen in flat bones, hands, ribs, and spine. There is the potential risk for malignant transformation in ~5% of affected patients with multiple cartilaginous exostoses, most commonly chondrosarcoma.[62]

Therapeutic management of multiple cartilaginous exostoses requires excision of lesions for reasonable indications such as pain, growth disturbance with angular deformity or limb discrepancy, joint motion compromised by juxta-articular lesions, soft tissue impingement, and painful bursa.

Enchondromatosis

Enchondromatosis or Ollier disease is characterized by multiple intraosseous benign cartilaginous tumors (OMIM 166000). The occurrence of multiple enchondromas and hemangiomas is named Maffucci syndrome (Fig. 21.11). Ollier disease and Maffucci syndrome are rare and usually not inherited. In a series of 3,067 primary bone tumors, Ollier disease accounted for 0.90% and Maffucci disease accounted for 0.07%.[63] The clinical manifestations of Ollier disease include palpable masses in fingers and toes, asymmetric shortening

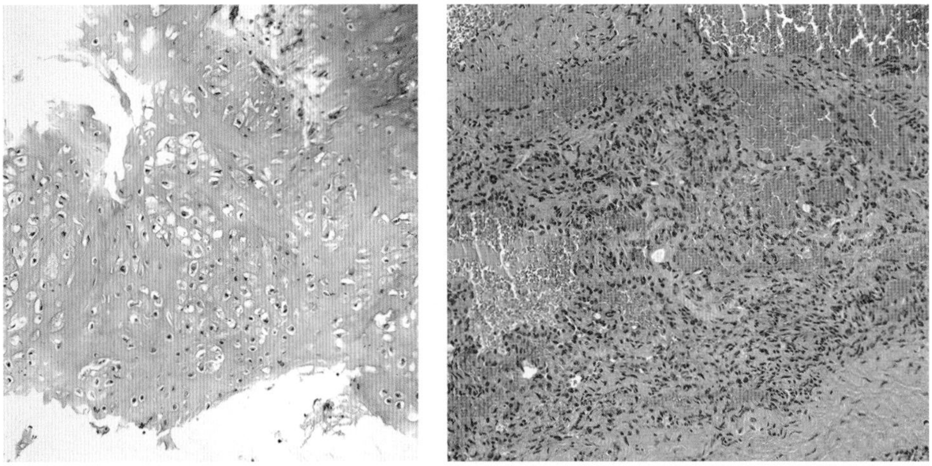

FIGURE 21.11 **Maffucci syndrome.** This 15-year-old boy had a history of multiple enchondromas, all showing benign lobulated cartilage **(left)**. Biopsy of a vascular lesion with cavernous spaces resembling venous malformation as well as solid areas resembling spindle cell hemangioma **(right)** confirmed the diagnosis of Maffucci syndrome. (Both hematoxylin and eosin, original magnification, 200×.)

of an extremity with limping, and osseous deformities with possible pathologic fractures.[64]

Radiographic features of enchondromas in Ollier disease and Maffucci syndrome demonstrate radiolucent expansion and deformity of the long bones (more prominent in tubular bones of hands and feet, ribs, and pelvic bones) secondary to the enchondromas with irregular cartilaginous matrix (ring and arcs pattern) (Fig. 21.12). There is occasional demonstration of phleboliths occurring in the vascular lesions of Maffucci syndrome. The carpal and tarsal bones, vertebral bodies, and base of the skull are seldom involved. Pathologic examination of the cartilaginous lesions shows enchondromas or osteochondromas histologically indistinguishable from nonsyndromic lesions. The vascular lesions are often spindle cell hemangiomas. Both the cartilaginous and vascular tumors are often characterized by mutations in the isocitrate dehydrogenase genes IDH1 and IDH2.[65] Development of chondrosarcoma in Ollier disease is estimated to occur in 25% to 40% of patients.[66,67] The risk for malignant transformation in Maffucci syndrome may be higher.

Therapeutic management of enchondromatosis requires management of limb length discrepancy and joint deformities, particularly of the hands. The risk of malignant transformation in both Ollier and Maffucci syndromes warrants close oncologic surveillance.

Polyostotic Fibrous Dysplasia

Polyostotic fibrous dysplasia refers to the presence of fibrous dysplasia lesions in multiple bones. McCune-Albright syndrome (OMIM 174800) is diagnosed in patients with polyostotic fibrous dysplasia, skin lesions (café au lait spots) and endocrine abnormalities (predominantly precocious puberty).[68,69] Patients have postzygotic activating mutations in the *GNAS1* gene (at 20q13.2) in the affected tissue. The clinical manifestations of the disease include pathologic fractures and limb deformity secondary to the polyostotic fibrous dysplasia as well as endocrinologic abnormalities ranging from precocious puberty to hyperthyroidism, hyperparathyroidism, Cushing syndrome, acromegaly, toxic goiter, hyperprolactinemia, and gynecomastia. The potential for malignant transformation in McCune-Albright syndrome is considered rare, probably occurring in <1% of cases.[68,70] Mazabraud syndrome is a rarer condition characterized by the combination of fibrous dysplasia (usually polyostotic) and soft tissue myxomas. The potential for malignant transformation in Mazabraud syndrome is considered higher than that in McCune-Albright syndrome.

Radiographic manifestations of McCune-Albright syndrome include polyostotic fibrous dysplasia usually in a unilateral distribution and most commonly seen in the pelvis, spine, and femurs. The skull and facial bones can be involved causing cranial nerve impingement and facial deformity. The characteristic "shepherd's crook" deformity refers to the progressive bowing and varus angulation of the proximal femurs (Fig. 21.13). Bone scintigraphy can demonstrate increased radiotracer uptake in axial and appendicular fibrous dysplasia lesions. MRI can be helpful to delineate extent of the lesions and potential fractures in patients with pain.

Therapeutic managements of polyostotic fibrous dysplasia include clinical management of underlying endocrinopathies and management of orthopedic complications related to limb length discrepancy and joint deformities.

Neurofibromatosis

Neurofibromatosis type 1 (NF1) and type 2 (NF2) are distinct genetic disorders characterized by an increased incidence of tumor development.[71] The major tumors arising in NF1 are neurofibromas, malignant peripheral nerve sheath tumors (MPNSTs), and gliomas (Fig. 21.14). The tumors arising in NF2 are schwannomas, meningiomas, and ependymomas.[72] More in-depth discussion of NF2 is provided in the Neuroradiology chapter, as the musculoskeletal manifestations of NF1 are more common in NF1 than in NF2.

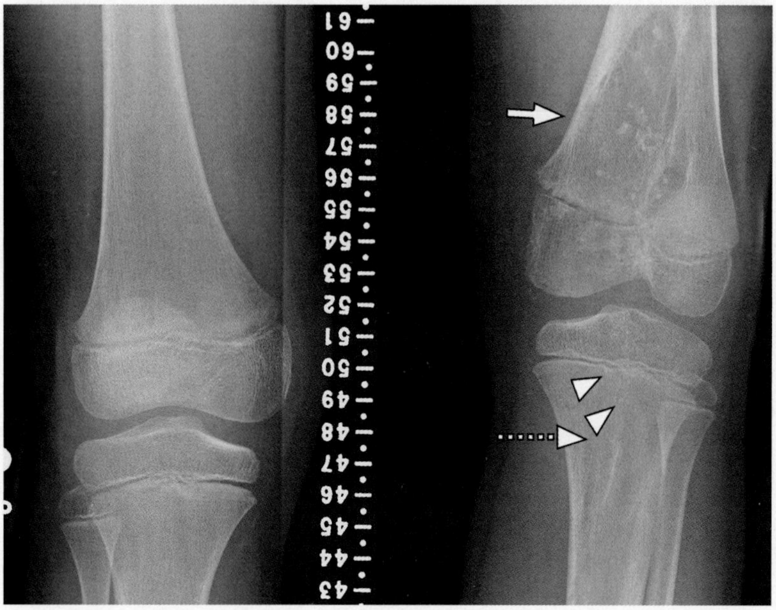

FIGURE 21.12 **Enchondromatosis in an 8-year-old boy with leg length discrepancy.** Frontal view of both knees as part of scanogram examination demonstrates a radiolucent lesion with calcific matrix ("ring-and-arc" pattern) in the left distal femoral metadiaphysis (*arrow*) abutting the physis consistent with a large enchondroma. A subtle linear enchondroma is seen in the left proximal tibial metadiaphysis (*interrupted arrow*) with tiny regions of chondroid matrix (*arrowheads*). Shortening of ~4 cm in the left lower extremity relative to the right secondary to enchondromatosis is also noted (not shown).

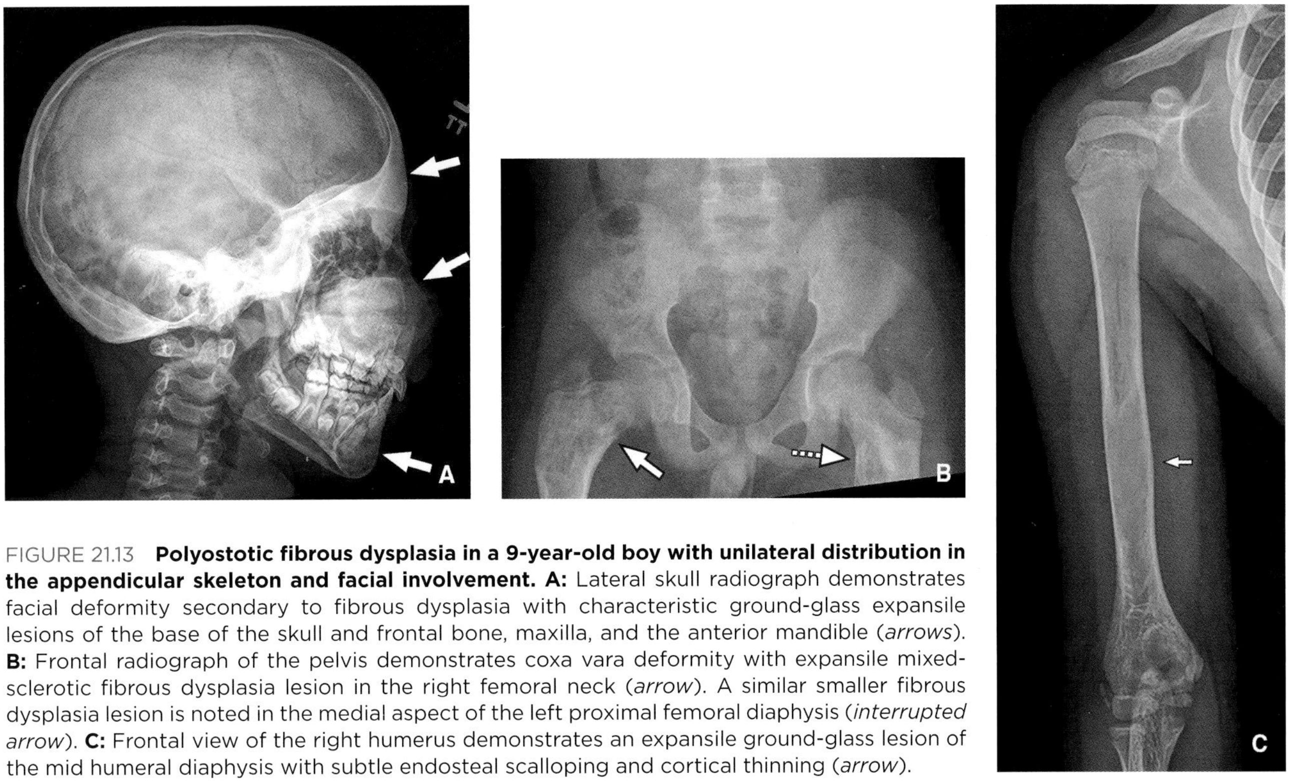

FIGURE 21.13 **Polyostotic fibrous dysplasia in a 9-year-old boy with unilateral distribution in the appendicular skeleton and facial involvement. A:** Lateral skull radiograph demonstrates facial deformity secondary to fibrous dysplasia with characteristic ground-glass expansile lesions of the base of the skull and frontal bone, maxilla, and the anterior mandible (*arrows*). **B:** Frontal radiograph of the pelvis demonstrates coxa vara deformity with expansile mixed-sclerotic fibrous dysplasia lesion in the right femoral neck (*arrow*). A similar smaller fibrous dysplasia lesion is noted in the medial aspect of the left proximal femoral diaphysis (*interrupted arrow*). **C:** Frontal view of the right humerus demonstrates an expansile ground-glass lesion of the mid humeral diaphysis with subtle endosteal scalloping and cortical thinning (*arrow*).

NF1 or von Recklinghausen disease has an incidence of 1 of 2,500 to 3,000 individuals.[73,74] The disease is caused by an autosomal dominant mutation in the neurofibromin gene at 17q11.2 (OMIM 162200). The clinical manifestations of NF1 are extensive and involve multiple organ systems. The most common features include café-au-lait spots, Lisch nodules in the eye, cutaneous and deep plexiform neurofibromas, macrocephaly, optic glioma, and other neoplasms (both benign

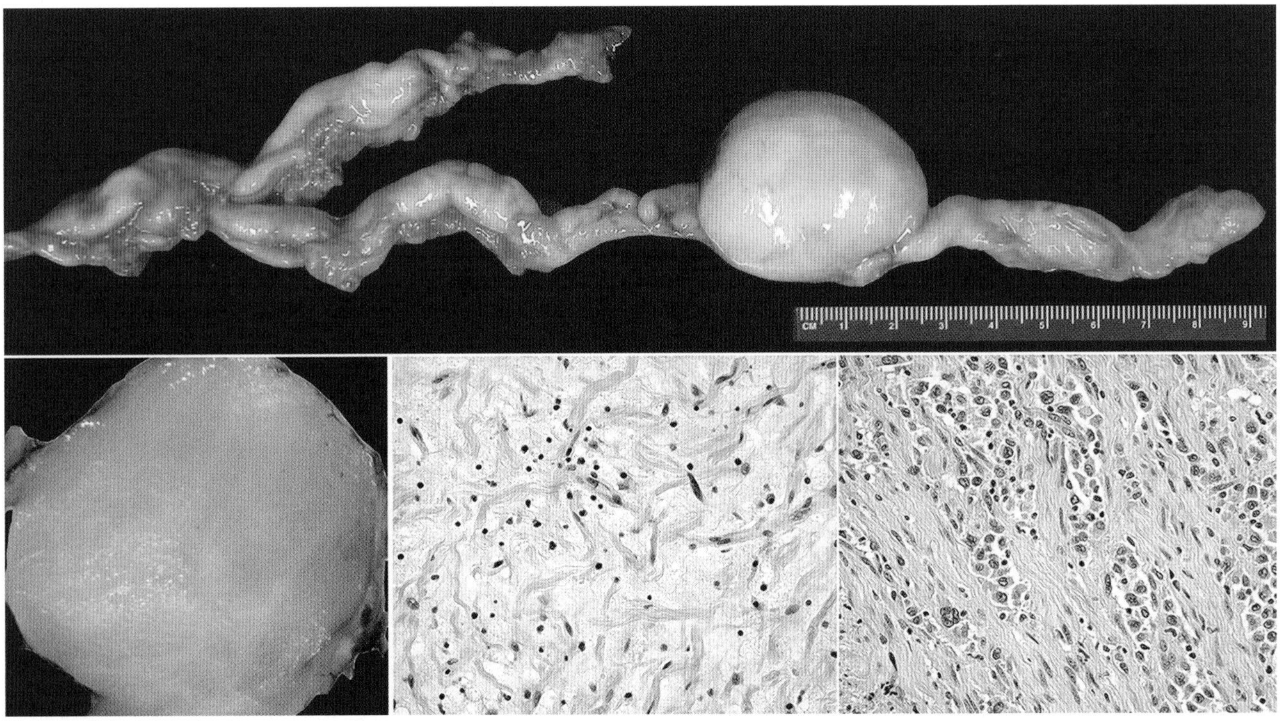

FIGURE 21.14 **Neurofibromatosis type 1.** Plexiform neurofibroma, diffusely expanding a peripheral nerve and its branches **(upper panel),** is seen. The cut surface **(lower left)** is tan white and firm, resembling fibrous tissue. In this example, the majority of the mass has the histologic appearance of neurofibroma **(lower center)**, whereas areas of increased cell density and round "epithelioid" cells characterize a component of malignant peripheral nerve sheath tumor **(lower right)**. (Hematoxylin and eosin, original magnification, 400×.)

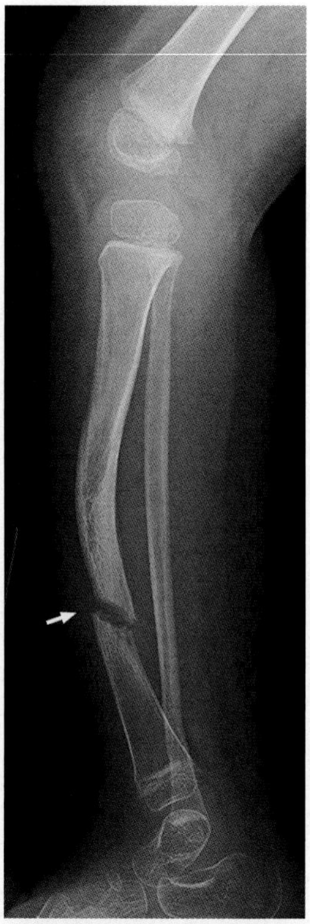

FIGURE 21.15 **Neurofibromatosis type I in a 3-year-old boy with right tibial pseudarthrosis.** Lateral radiograph of the right tibia shows anterior bowing deformity, distal diaphyseal pseudarthrosis with surrounding sclerosis (*arrow*). Normal alignment of the fibula is noted.

and malignant). Musculoskeletal manifestations of NF1 include skull abnormalities (sphenoid wing dysplasia, erosions, and enlargement of foramina), scoliosis and kyphosis, pseudarthrosis of long bones (tibia most common), osteoporosis, and short stature (Fig. 21.15).[72]

Neurofibromas are the most common type of tumor in NF1, and in this disease, they are often "plexiform" (expanding multiple fascicles of a nerve or plexus), a configuration that is pathognomonic for NF1. Radiographic manifestations of plexiform neurofibromas include smooth cortical scalloping and thinning of adjacent bones (particularly ribs) and widening of the intervertebral foramina. MRI of plexiform neurofibromas in NF1 demonstrates tortuous masses of thickened nerve branches extending along the surrounding tissues and described as a "bag of worms." The lesions are usually isointense to muscle on T1-weighted MR images and show heterogeneous high signal intensity on T2-weighted MR images. The presence of a "target sign" (central low to intermediate signal intensity and peripheral high signal intensity on fluid-sensitive sequences) is commonly present in plexiform neurofibromas, but can also be seen with schwannomas.[75] Deep neurofibromas harbor the greatest risk of transformation into MPNSTs.[76] The frequency of MPNSTs in NF1 patients is ~8% to 13%.

MRI diagnosis of patients with NF1 and malignant transformation of plexiform neurofibromas can be challenging and should always be correlated with clinical findings (enlarging mass, persistent pain, new neurologic deficit).[77] The use of [18F]-FDG PET in children with NF1 can be helpful in predicting malignant transformation of plexiform neurofibromas and guide the need for biopsy and surgical resection.[78]

Therapeutic management includes clinical and orthopedic assessment of orthopedic complications related to limb length discrepancy and joint deformities.

Abnormalities of Density of Cortical Diaphyseal Structure and Metaphyseal Modeling

Osteogenesis Imperfecta

Osteogenesis imperfecta (OI) encompasses a group of genetic disorders characterized by skeletal fragility and recurrent fractures caused by low bone density mass. The disease is typically autosomal dominant (95% of cases), but autosomal recessive OI has been described.[79] Most autosomal dominant mutations affect COL1A1 and COL1A2 genes encoding type I collagen, the main component of the bone matrix. The clinical manifestations of OI include fractures, short stature with bone deformity, blue-gray sclera, dentinogenesis imperfecta (weak and discolored teeth), progressive hearing loss, and ligamentous laxity. There is a wide spectrum of clinical severity, ranging from the very mild to lethal forms of the disease.[80]

The Sillence classification was the first systemic classification of OI phenotype: classic nondeforming OI with blue sclera or mild OI (type I), perinatally lethal OI (type II), progressively deforming or severe OI (type III) (Fig. 21.16), and common variable with normal sclera or moderate OI (type IV).[81] Additional types and subtypes of OI have been described based on additional phenotypes and genetic variability.[82,83] Among the different OI types, OI type I (mild) and type IV (moderate) account for more than half of all OI cases.[84]

OI is an important differential diagnosis in the evaluation of young children with fractures and the possibility of nonaccidental trauma (NAI). In particular, the most prevalent forms of OI (types I and IV) can be difficult to diagnose in the absence of few or no obvious extraskeletal manifestations and no family history of bone fragility.[80] Radiologists and clinicians evaluating these patients should look for features of bone demineralization and constitutional bone fragility (cortical bone thinning, trabecular bone rarefaction) and exclude fractures with high specificity for NAI (posteromedial rib fractures, scapular fractures, and metaphyseal fractures in young infants).[85,86]

Radiographic characteristics of OI type I (mild) in the neonatal/infantile period include lack of congenital fractures and normal appearance of the bones at birth with the exception of wormian bones. These intrasutural bones can be seen in normal infants until ~6 months of age. Later in life, patients with OI type IV demonstrates increased fractures with minor deformities and vertebral compression fractures. Radiographic characteristics of OI type II (lethal) in the neonatal/infantile period include wormian bones, severe demineralization, abnormal thin/short ribs with fractures, platyspondyly at birth, and short deformed tubular bones.

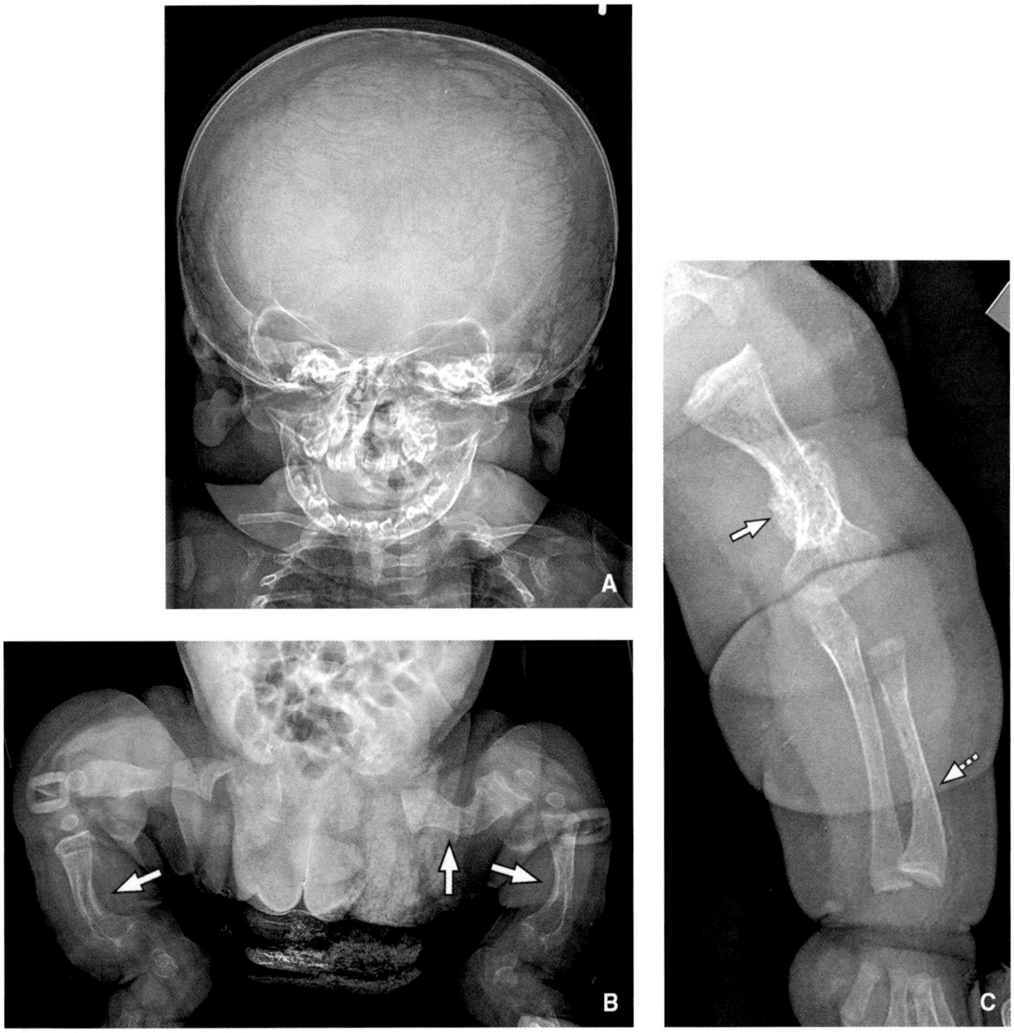

FIGURE 21.16 **Osteogenesis imperfecta type III in a 24-day-old boy with fractures detected in prenatal ultrasound. A:** Frontal radiograph of the skull demonstrates extensive wormian bones in the calvarium. **B:** Frontal view of the lower extremities of this patient in harness demonstrates diffuse and decreased bony mineralization with bowing fracture deformities of multiple long bones (*arrows*). **C:** Frontal view of the left upper extremity demonstrates callus formation across a mid-diaphyseal humeral fracture (*arrow*) and bowing of the distal radius (*interrupted arrow*).

Radiographic characteristics of OI type IV (moderate) in the neonatal period/infantile period include diminished mineralization, occasionally wormian bones, usually lack of congenital fractures, and bowing of long bones. Later in life, patients with OI type IV demonstrate increased fractures with progressive bowing deformities in some patients, vertebral compression fractures, and coxa vara, causing small stature.[80,87] A common radiographic pattern seen in patients treated with bisphosphonates is the presence of dense metaphyseal lines or "zebra lines" paralleling the physis, with each line temporally related to the administration of bisphosphonates and the space between lines to the bone growth between courses of the medication.[80,88] Prenatal US diagnosis of OI can be suspected in cases in which either short femurs with or without bowing and progressive development of fractures are seen (OI type II and III, IV).[89]

Therapeutic management of children with OI includes physiotherapy, rehabilitation, and orthopedic correction of fracture and skeletal deformities. Bisphosphonate therapy augments bone turnover and increase bone density in OI; however, efficacy in preventing fractures, pain reduction, and function improvement remains controversial.[90,91]

Osteopetrosis

Osteopetrosis encompasses a heterogeneous group of genetic disorders characterized by failure of normal endochondral ossification resulting in abnormal accumulation of calcified cartilage matrix within the medullary cavity (Fig. 21.17).[92] Despite the increased bone density, the patients are at higher risk of fractures, potentially because of decreased elasticity and impaired reparative bone capability.[93] Radiographically osteopetrosis is one of the hereditary sclerosing bone dysplasias, which also include pycnodysostosis, osteopoikilosis, osteopathia striata, diaphyseal dysplasia, hereditary multiple diaphyseal sclerosis, and hyperostosis corticalis generalisata.[94]

The clinical course of osteopetrosis can be highly variable; however, high risk of low trauma fractures because of bone fragility is present in almost all cases despite the increased

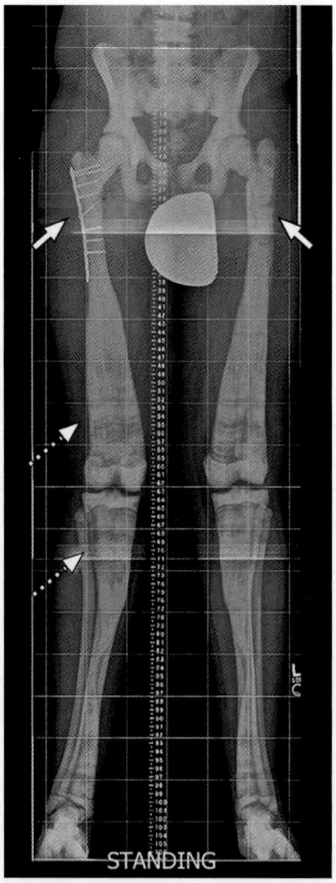

FIGURE 21.17 **Osteopetrosis in a 17-year-old boy.** Frontal view of the lower extremities for assessment of leg length discrepancy demonstrates diffuse increased sclerosis of the bones (particularly within the medullary canals). There is surgical hardware for treatment of a right proximal femoral diaphysis fracture (*arrow*). "Bone-within-bone" appearance was noted after removal of the surgical hardware for an additional fracture in the left proximal femoral diaphysis (*arrow*). Bilateral undertubularization of the distal femurs ("Erlenmeyer flask" deformity) and proximal tibias is noted (*interrupted arrows*).

sclerosis of the bones. Clinical manifestations include life-threatening anemia, pancytopenia, osteomyelitis, and sepsis because of poorly developed bone marrow and impaired medullary hematopoiesis.[95] Different patterns of inheritance have been described in osteopetrosis, including autosomal dominant and recessive and X-linked.

Two of the more distinctive types of osteopetrosis are the precocious type and the delayed type, based in their mode of inheritance, clinical, and radiographic features. The precocious type (also known as congenital, infantile, malignant type) is autosomal recessive and presents at birth or at infancy causing death in early childhood because of severe anemia and infections. The delayed type (also known as benign, adult or Albers-Schönberg type) is autosomal dominant and is a much milder subtype. Most affected patients are asymptomatic and only incidentally discovered by the increased bone density in radiologic examination. Mild anemia has been also described due to decreased size of the medullary canals.[96]

Radiographic evaluation of osteopetrosis is characterized by increased density predominantly within the medullary portions and relative sparing of the cortices. Two phenotypes of delayed type or autosomal dominant osteopetrosis are seen. Type I is characterized by uniform sclerosis of the long bones, skull, and spine. Type II is characterized by the "bone-within-bone" appearance, noted in the pelvis and spine ("sandwich vertebra" or "rugger jersey spine," a pattern of dense endplate sclerosis with sharp margins).[94] An "Erlenmeyer flask" deformity, characterized by metaphyseal widening and blunting of long bones that progressively involves the diaphysis, is also seen in osteopetrosis, particularly in the distal femurs. Of note, an Erlenmeyer flask deformity can be seen in multiple other disorders including other hereditary and metabolic syndromes.[97]

Therapeutic management in osteopetrosis is largely symptomatic, although hematopoietic stem cell transplantation has been used for the most severe forms of osteopetrosis associated with bone marrow failure.[98]

Pycnodysostosis

Pycnodysostosis is a rare sclerosing bone dysplasia characterized by short stature, short limbs, and bone fragility (OMIM 265800). The pattern of inheritance is autosomal recessive with locus in 1q21 causing abnormalities in cathepsin K, a protease expressed by osteoclast and required for degradation of collagen type I.[96] Thus, the bones are brittle and prone to fracture. Typically, generalized osteosclerosis is present, but contrary to osteopetrosis, the medullary canals are usually preserved in the long bones.

Radiographic manifestations of pycnodysostosis are characteristic and include short stature, pectus excavatum, kyphoscoliosis, short fingers and acrosteolysis, dental abnormalities, and dysmorphic facial features (frontal and occipital bossing, wormian bones, delayed closure of fontanelles and sutures, paranasal sinuses underdevelopment, and micrognathia) (Fig. 21.18).

Therapeutic management includes orthopedic treatment of fractures and associated skeletal deformities. Management of mandibular fractures with recurrent osteomyelitis has been described.[99,100] The maxillofacial features of the disease create a dysmorphic facial appearance, and some authors advocate for early-age treatment.[101]

Progressive Diaphyseal Dysplasia

Progressive diaphyseal dysplasia or Camurati-Engelmann disease is rare sclerosing dysplasia that is considered a disorder of intramembranous ossification. Affected patients carry a mutation in the *TGB1* gene at 19q13.1 encoding the transforming growth factor ß1 (TGF-ß1) molecule. TGF-ß1 is responsible for stimulation of bone formation by osteoblasts in the periosteal side and suppression of bone resorption by osteoclasts at the endosteal side and mutations of the molecule causes premature activation and ultimately increase in bone formation.[102] The onset of the disease is usually during early childhood with a highly variable clinical course. The clinical manifestations include muscle weakness, leg pain, and waddling gait, mimicking a muscular dystrophy.[103] Also, exophthalmos, hearing loss, cranial nerve palsies related to foraminal stenosis, and diverse ocular abnormalities have been described.

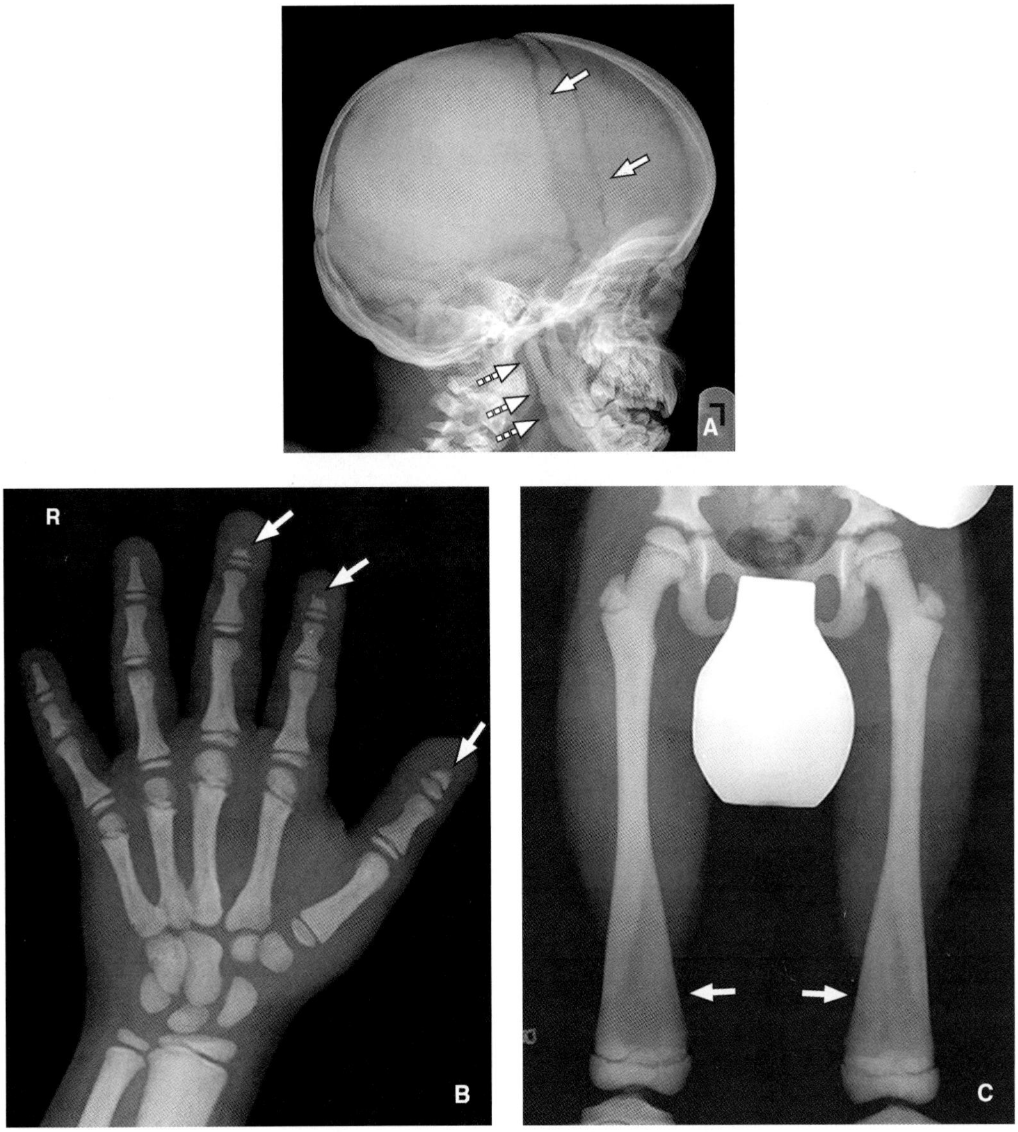

FIGURE 21.18 **Pycnodysostosis in a 9-year-old boy. A:** Lateral skull radiograph demonstrates abnormal patency of the coronal sutures for age (*arrows*), frontal bossing, and abnormally flattened antegonial angle of the mandible (*interrupted arrows*). **B:** Frontal view of the right hand demonstrates acrosteolysis of the distal tufts of the first through third digits (*arrows*). **C:** Frontal view of the pelvis and femurs demonstrates diffuse osteosclerosis and "Erlenmeyer flask" deformity of the distal femurs (*arrows*).

Radiographic manifestations include symmetric, bilateral, fusiform enlargement of the long bones and narrowing of the medullary cavity because of lack of normal endosteal bone resorption. Usually, diaphyseal involvement in long bones is present, but metaphyseal involvement has been described.[92] The base of the skull can be involved with associated nerve palsies.[102] Occasionally, there is sclerosis of the cervical vertebra, scapula, clavicles, and pelvis.

Therapeutic management includes glucocorticoid therapy to reduce bone pain with correction of radiographic abnormalities described in some cases.[103]

Metaphyseal Dysplasia

Metaphyseal dysplasia or Pyle dysplasia is a very rare disease with few reports in the literature (OMIM 265900). The pattern of inheritance is autosomal recessive, and affected pediatric patients are usually asymptomatic. The clinical manifestations of metaphyseal dysplasia when present include genu valgum (most common feature), muscle weakness, joint pain, scoliosis, and decreased range motion in the elbows. In addition, dental caries, mandibular prognathism, and leg length discrepancy are seen occasionally. Fractures are not a common feature of the disease.[104]

The radiographic manifestations of metaphyseal dysplasia are predominantly related to marked undertubulation of the long bones, particularly distal femurs (Erlenmeyer flask deformity) with genu valgum, flaring of the metacarpals distally and phalanges proximally, mild platyspondyly, osteoporosis (codfish vertebral bodies), and infrequently bone fragility (Fig. 21.19). Mild skull sclerosis, thickened clavicles, ribs, and ischiopubic bones have been described.[105]

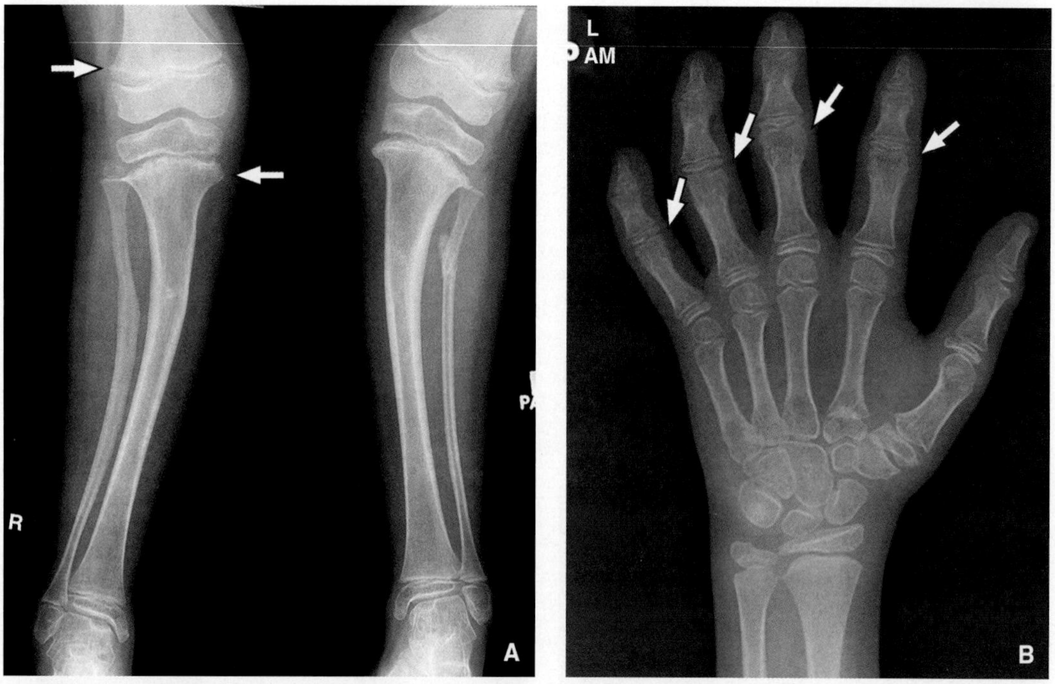

FIGURE 21.19 **Metaphyseal dysplasia in a 10-year-old boy. A:** Frontal radiograph of both knees demonstrates bilateral genu valgum and bowing deformity of both tibias. Metaphyseal flaring (*arrows*) is noted in the distal femoral and proximal tibial regions. **B:** Frontal left hand radiograph demonstrates subtle undertubularization of the distal portions of the second through fifth phalanges and mild flexion contraction of the proximal interphalangeal joints (*arrows*).

Therapeutic management includes epiphysiodesis with or without osteotomies for correction of genu valgum deformity.[106]

Limb Reduction Anomalies

Skeletal deformities of the limbs encompass a heterogeneous group of congenital disorders, which can involve either or both upper and lower extremities. They can be symmetric or asymmetric and unilateral or bilateral. Limb formation occurs during early embryogenesis (4 to 8 weeks of gestation) followed by the formation of primary ossification centers in the long bones (12 weeks of gestation). Molecular regulation of limb formation is a complex process regulated by different gene families: homeobox (HOX) gene regulates position of limbs in the craniocaudal axis, fibroblast growth factor (FGF) genes and bone morphogenetic proteins (BMPs) regulate limb outgrowth, and sonic hedgehog (SHH) genes contribute to the pattern of anteroposterior axis of the limb and correct appearance of the digits.[107] The incidence of limb abnormalities is ~6 in 10,000 live births with a higher incidence in the upper limbs and unilateral presentation. These defects are frequently acquired or multifactorial in etiology but some are occasionally inherited. However, in many cases, the etiology remains unknown.[107]

Prenatal diagnosis of limb abnormalities is possible with fetal US. Subsequent radiographic characterization can be performed in the newborn for assessment of potential associations or syndromes with musculoskeletal involvement. A brief summary of limb reduction anomalies is provided in Table 21.3 and **Schematic I**. Consistent nomenclature describing limb abnormalities is helpful to guide clinical workup. The following terms are useful when defining the type of limb defect:

- **Acheiria**: Absence of hand(s)
- **Adactyly**: Absence of finger(s) or toe(s)
- **Amelia**: Absence of limb(s)
- **Phocomelia**: Hypoplasia and marked shortening of the limb(s) (Fig. 21.20)
- **Ectrodactyly (split hand/foot or "lobster claw")**: Absence of central digits with or without absence of central metacarpal/metatarsal bones; usually associated with syndactyly (webbing) of other digits (Fig. 21.21)

Proximal Focal Femoral Deficiency

Proximal focal femoral deficiency (PFFD) is a rare congenital disorder characterized by variable degrees of proximal femoral hypoplasia (Fig. 21.22 and **Schematic C**). PFFD is predominantly unilateral and can be associated to congenital coxa vara and acetabular abnormalities. Affected pediatric patients with PFFD typically present with an extremely short and bulky thigh, a flexed and abducted hip, and a laterally rotated limb.

The most widely known radiographic classification is the Aitken classification, which divides PFFD into four categories based on the morphology of the femoral head, acetabulum, and femur.[108] However, cartilaginous connections are not well defined radiographically and may underestimate

TABLE 21.3 Summary of Limb Reduction Anomalies

Anomaly	Clinical Manifestations	Imaging Goals
Proximal focal femoral deficiency	Variable degrees of proximal femoral hypoplasia Leg length discrepancy, with affected extremity being short and externally rotated	Aitken classification based on radiographic findings MRI more useful for assessment of cartilage and surgical planning
Radial ray anomalies	Variable degrees of radial hypoplasia to complete absence Important associations to drugs (thalidomide), syndromes (TAR, Holt-Oram, Fanconi anemia), and VACTERL association	Identification of a radial ray anomaly should prompt the radiologist to investigate clinical manifestations and exclude associated abnormalities
Amniotic band syndrome	Nonhereditary skeletal malformation with variable presentation among affected individuals secondary to prenatal injury (entanglement of limbs with amniotic bands)	Accurate description of limb anomalies should be provided for surgical planning

TAR, thrombocytopenia absent radius; VACTERL, vertebral defects, anal atresia, cardiac malformations, tracheoesophageal fistula, esophageal atresia, renal anomalies and limb anomalies.

the extent of cartilage present in PFFD.[108] Hip US can identify morphologic changes of PFFD in the infant; however, detailed anatomic bony characterization can be challenging with this modality. MR imaging of PFFD has been described in preoperative planning and provides more accurate evaluation of cartilaginous and soft tissue abnormalities in PFFD and is most useful in the immature skeleton. Accurate depiction of the hip anatomy can potentially aid surgical planning.

Therapeutic management of PFFD includes amputation with prosthetic replacement or limb lengthening reconstructive surgery.[109]

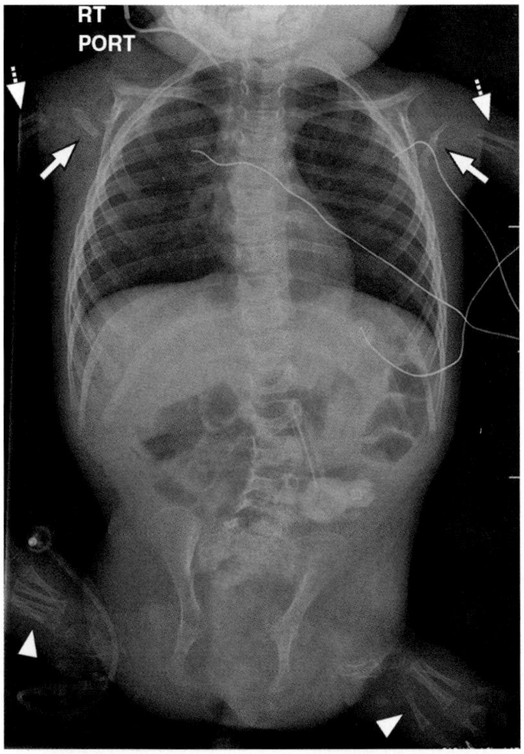

FIGURE 21.20 **Phocomelia in a 3-year-old girl.** Frontal radiograph of the chest and abdomen demonstrates markedly hypoplastic and rudimentary humerus (*arrows*) with shortening of bilateral radius and ulna (*interrupted arrows*). Absent femurs and tibias are seen and rudimentary tarsal bones with only four distal rays are noted (*arrowheads*). Normal thoracic and abdominal body wall proportions with dysplastic appearance of the pelvis and levoconvex thoracolumbar scoliosis are also present.

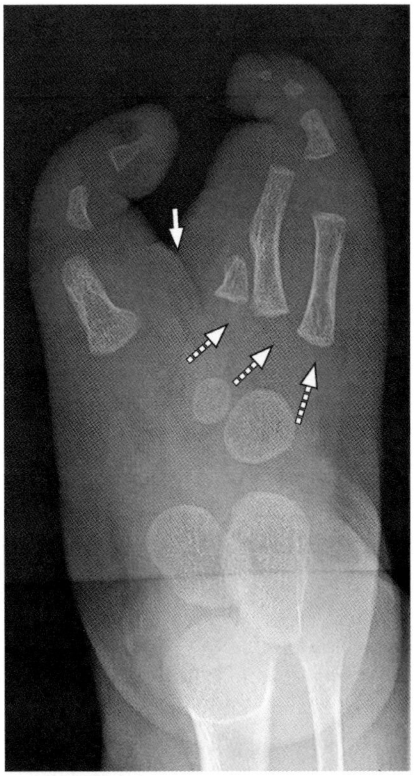

FIGURE 21.21 **Ectrodactyly ("lobster-claw" foot) in an 8-month old boy.** Frontal radiograph of the left foot demonstrates central cleft in the foot (*arrow*) because of the absence of the second ray and rudimentary third and fourth rays with syndactyly of the lateral rays (*interrupted arrows*) giving the foot the appearance of a "lobster claw." Similar deformities were present in the contralateral foot and both hands of the patient (not shown).

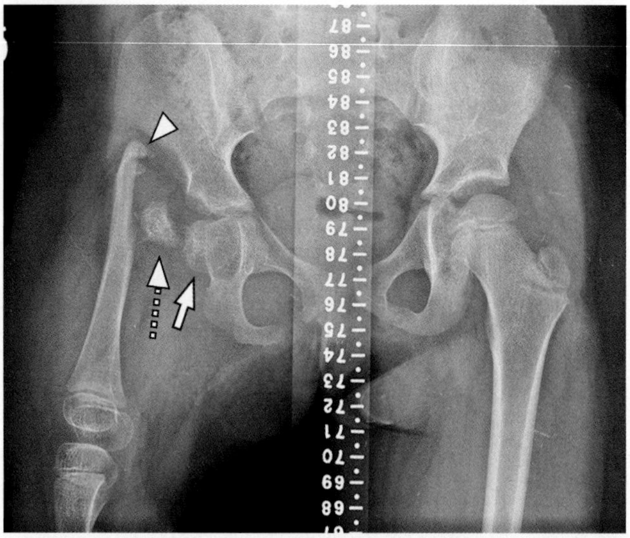

FIGURE 21.22 **Proximal focal femoral deficiency (PFFD) in a 6-year-old girl.** Frontal radiograph of the pelvis as part of leg length discrepancy evaluation demonstrates unilateral shortening of the right lower extremity with right coxa vara and external rotation of the hip secondary to PFFD. The right femoral head (*arrow*) is present and articulates with the acetabulum, the right acetabulum is mildly dysplastic with an increased acetabular index, and the proximal bony tuft (femoral ossicle; *interrupted arrow*) is noted in the region of the proximal femur. Nevertheless, there is lack of ossified bridging between the proximal femoral ossicle and the distal femur (*arrowhead*). A normal left femur is noted.

Radial Ray Anomalies

Radial ray anomalies (RRA) or radial longitudinal deficiency includes a spectrum of osseous, musculotendinous, and neurovascular deficiencies of the radial border of the upper limb (**Schematic B**).[110]

Radiographically, variable degrees of radial hypoplasia or complete absence are present. The thumb is usually involved and approximately half of the patients present with bilateral involvement.[109] The condition is considered sporadic except when associated to well-established systemic and musculoskeletal disorders.[109,111] In addition, RRA and other limb reduction anomalies have been linked to teratogenic effects of thalidomide, used 50 years ago for the treatment of morning sickness in pregnant patients.[112]

The most common associations of RRA are thrombocytopenia absent radius (TAR) syndrome (Fig. 21.23), VACTERL association (vertebral defects, anal atresia, cardiac malformation, tracheoesophageal fistula, esophageal atresia, renal anomalies and limb anomalies), Fanconi anemia (autosomal recessive disease with bone marrow failure with associated limb, heart, and kidney anomalies), and Holt-Oram syndrome (autosomal dominant disease with RRA and heart abnormalities, mainly atrial or ventricular septal defects).[109]

The presence of RRA in a newborn should warrant further investigation of possible additional musculoskeletal or systemic abnormalities. Therapeutic management of RRA is determined by the level of severity of radial and thumb hypoplasia and primarily focuses on the correction of radial angulation and flexed position of the carpus to improve function and appearance of the hand.[110]

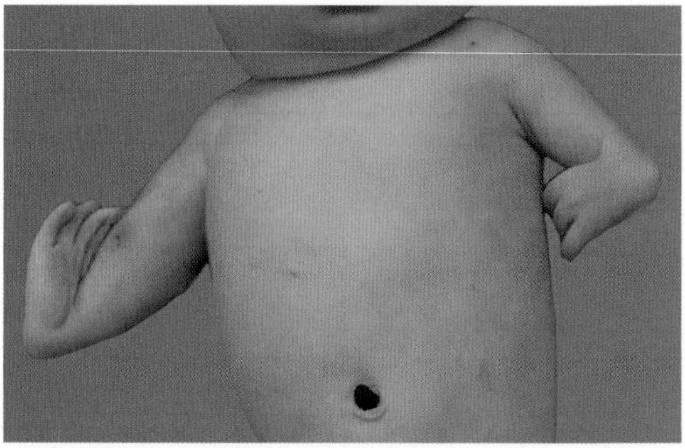

FIGURE 21.23 **Absent radii and thumbs.** Absent radii and thumbs in an infant who had multiple congenital anomalies and negative genetic testing for Fanconi anemia and Holt-Oram syndrome.

Amniotic Band Syndrome

Amniotic band syndrome (ABS) is a rare condition in which fetal parts become entangled in constricting the amniotic membrane, leading to deformation and deletion. ABS is not considered a hereditary syndrome but is rather produced by prenatal environmental factors[113] (Fig. 21.24). "Constriction bands"

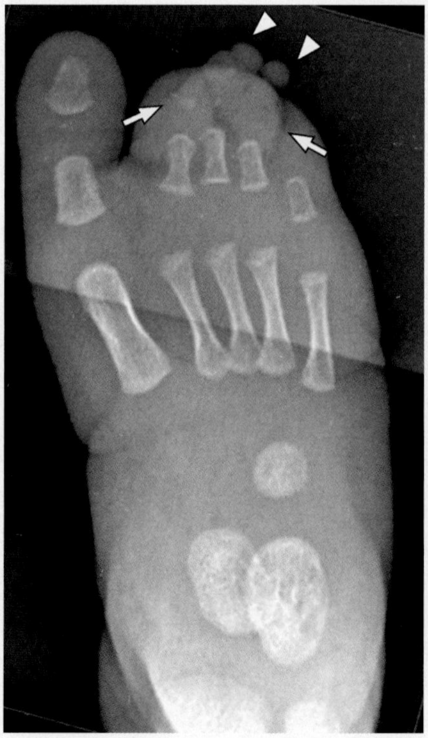

FIGURE 21.24 **Amniotic band syndrome in a 1-month-old baby girl with maternal history of oligohydramnios.** Frontal radiograph of the right foot demonstrates amputation of the second through fifth middle and distal phalanges and syndactyly of these segments (*arrows*). Tiny remnant soft tissue nubbins are noted (*arrowheads*). Normal appearance of the first ray, metatarsal, and proximal phalanges is noted.

consisting of amnionic membrane may produce a spectrum of disease ranging from skin dimpling and soft tissue constriction rings to complete limb or digit deletion. Protruding fetal structures are vulnerable and more likely to be entrapped than other anatomic structures. Upper extremities (distal segment of the hand) are most often affected. Middle digits are more commonly involved with relative sparing of the thumb. This pattern probably relates to fetal positioning, with either outstretched fingers or a clenched thumb in the palm, protected by other digits.[114] The spectrum includes amputation, syndactyly (webbing of fingers and toes), and soft tissue rings around the skin of the arms and legs. Other anomalies stemming from ABS include clubfoot deformity, cleft palate and cleft lip, and occasionally severe craniofacial and visceral deformities.[115]

Therapeutic management requires individualized surgical planning. Multiple procedures including finger and toe transfers, lengthening procedures, composite toe transfer, and bone grafting have been used to restore function in patients with amputation. Patients with acrosyndactyly (fused digits) can be treated with separation of digits and web reconstruction.[114]

Congenital Foot Deformities

Evaluation of congenital foot deformities must include description of the location and plane of abnormal rotation. The foot is divided into the forefoot (metatarsals and phalanges), midfoot (tarsal bones), and hindfoot (talus and calcaneus). Radiographic examinations must be performed using standing weight-bearing techniques for optimal assessment of foot abnormalities.

The following nomenclature, which describes motion of the different components of the foot, is important for the understanding of abnormalities:

- Hindfoot: Coronal plane rotation is described as varus (medial) and valgus (lateral). Sagittal rotation produces equinus (plantar flexion) and calcaneus (dorsiflexion).
- Midfoot and forefoot: Coronal rotation is described as adduction (medial) or abduction (lateral) deviation relative to the foot. Axial rotation is described as pronation (plantar flexion) and supination (dorsiflexion) relative to the midfoot and midfoot–forefoot articulation.

The following angles and lines are important in the assessment of foot deformities (Table 21.4):

Lateral view:

- Lateral talocalcaneal angle (LTCA): A normal LTCA ranges from 30 to 55 degrees in children.[116] The LTCA allows for assessment of hindfoot varus/talipes equinovarus (decreased LTCA) or hindfoot valgus (increased LTCA).
- Long-axis line across talus: The long-axis line of the talus normally transects long axis of the first metatarsal. Pes cavus is suspected when first metatarsal long-axis line is more steep in relationship to the horizontal and relative to the long-axis line of the talus.

Frontal (anteroposterior) view:

- Frontal talocalcaneal angle (FTCA): A normal FTCA ranges from 20 to 40 degrees and is ~35 degrees at 6 years of age; however, infants have a higher normal FTCA angle,

TABLE 21.4 Summary of Normal Radiographic Angles and Lines for Congenital Foot Deformities

Lateral View	Definition	Practical Values to Remember
Lateral talocalcaneal angle (LTCA)	Angle defined by longitudinal lines across the long axis of the midtalus and plantar cortex of the calcaneus Normal LTCA range: 35–50 degrees in children	40 degrees; normal at 6 years of age >50 degrees; consider hindfoot valgus <35 degrees; consider hindfoot varus/equinus deformity (talipes equinovarus)
Long-axis line across talus	Long-axis line of the talus normally transects long axis of the first metatarsal	First metatarsal line more steep (forefoot plantar flexion) and high calcaneal pitch; consider pes cavus
Frontal View	**Definition**	**Practical Values to Remember**
Frontal talocalcaneal angle (FTCA)	Angle defined by longitudinal lines across the lateral margin of the calcaneus and midline long axis of the talus Normal FTCA range: 20–40 degrees in children	~35 degrees; normal at 6 years of age >40 degrees; consider hindfoot valgus <20 degrees; consider hindfoot varus
Talus-first metatarsal angle	Long-axis line across talus extends to the base of the first metatarsal shaft Normal talus-first metatarsal angle: 0–20 degrees in children	Linear extension of this line into the base of the first metatarsal shaft is normal First metatarsal axis medial relative to the talus; consider forefoot varus/metatarsus adductus First metatarsal axis lateral relative to the talus; consider forefoot valgus

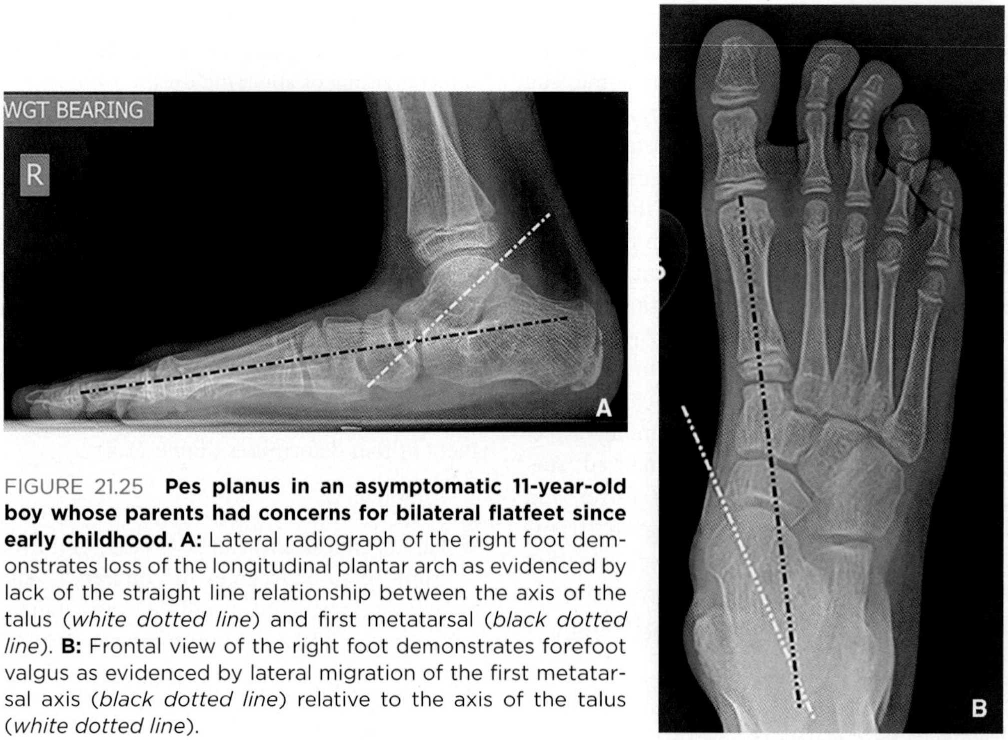

FIGURE 21.25 **Pes planus in an asymptomatic 11-year-old boy whose parents had concerns for bilateral flatfeet since early childhood. A:** Lateral radiograph of the right foot demonstrates loss of the longitudinal plantar arch as evidenced by lack of the straight line relationship between the axis of the talus (*white dotted line*) and first metatarsal (*black dotted line*). **B:** Frontal view of the right foot demonstrates forefoot valgus as evidenced by lateral migration of the first metatarsal axis (*black dotted line*) relative to the axis of the talus (*white dotted line*).

which decreases progressively through the first decade of life.[117] The FTCA allows for assessment of hindfoot varus (calcaneus closer to midline and FTCA <20 degrees) and hindfoot valgus (calcaneus further away from midline and FTCA >40 degrees).

- Talus-first metatarsal angle: The long-axis line across midline talus goes through the base of the first metatarsal base shaft in normal foot. This line allows for evaluation of forefoot varus/metatarsus adductus (axis of first metatarsal directed more medial relative to the talus) and forefoot valgus (axis of the first metatarsal directed more lateral relative to the talus).

Pes Planus

Pes planus or flatfoot is characterized by diminished or absent longitudinal medial arch (Fig. 21.25 and **Schematic E**). Pes planus is a common entity in pediatric patients and encompasses a large spectrum of severity from painless, flexible normal variant of growth to a stiff painful manifestation of tarsal coalition, collagen abnormality, and neurologic disease. Almost all toddlers and children under the age of six have a flexible pes planus and the medial arch typically develops within the first decade of life.[118]

Radiographic evaluation on lateral views demonstrates loss of the normal straight line relationship between talus and first metatarsal. Frontal view allows evaluation of hindfoot valgus (FTCA > 40 degrees), and if present, the combined deformity is called pes planovalgus.

Pes Cavus

Pes cavus is characterized by increased longitudinal medial arch (Fig. 21.26 and **Schematic E**). The biomechanical components of a pes cavus include varus hindfoot, high calcaneal pitch, high-pitched midfoot (increased navicular height), plantar flexion, and adduction of the forefoot. Pes cavus rarely presents in children younger than 3 years of age. It can be secondary to brain, spinal cord, peripheral nerves, or structural problems of the foot. The majority of adults with pes cavus usually have an underlying neurologic condition, most commonly Charcot-Marie-Tooth disease.[116]

Radiographic evaluation in the lateral view demonstrates obvious increased in the plantar arch, manifested as exaggerated plantar flexion of the forefoot and calcaneus position of the calcaneus (high calcaneal pitch) (Fig. 21.26).

Therapeutic management of pes cavus can be complex as the disease progresses from flexible to a fixed bony deformity with arthrosis. Surgical goals are to create a plantigrade, mobile, pain-free, and more stable foot through osteotomies, muscle transfers, and fusions.[116]

Talipes Equinovarus

Talipes equinovarus or congenital clubfoot is one of the most common abnormalities involving the foot (Fig. 21.27). There is a male predominance and ~50% of cases have bilateral involvement.[119] Clubfoot can be classified as congenital versus acquired (usually secondary to neuromuscular disorders). The components of the deformity include hindfoot varus, talipes equinus, and metatarsus adductus (Fig. 21.28 and **Schematic F**).

Radiographic evaluation in the lateral view demonstrates decreased talocalcaneal angle with almost parallel orientation of talus and calcaneus (hindfoot varus) and calcaneus in equinus position (Fig. 21.28A). In the frontal view, decreased talocalcaneal angle with overlapping of the talus and calcaneus again reflects hindfoot varus, and the first metatarsal lies

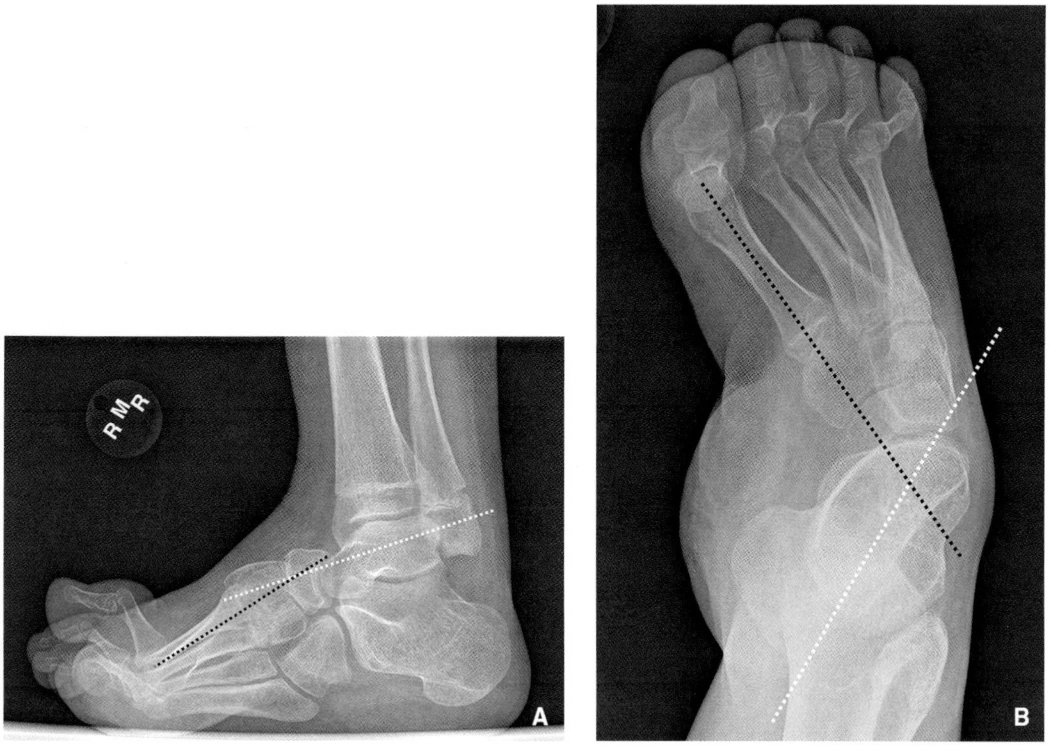

FIGURE 21.26 **Pes cavus in a 14-year-old girl with Charcot-Marie-Tooth disease. A:** Lateral radiograph of the right foot demonstrates increased longitudinal plantar arch as evidenced by a high calcaneal pitch, increased navicular height, and increased plantar flexion of the forefoot. There is loss of the normal straight alignment of the first metatarsal (*black dotted line*) with the talus axis (*white dotted line*). The talar dome appears flattened and the tibiotalar joint is rotated. **B:** Frontal view of the right foot demonstrates forefoot varus as evidenced by medial migration of the first metatarsal axis (*black dotted line*) relative to the axis of the talus (*white dotted line*). Dorsiflexion of all metatarsophalangeal joints and plantar flexion of all proximal and distal interphalangeal joints (claw toe deformity) are noted in both lateral and frontal views, a common finding in a neuropathic foot.

medial relative to the talus (forefoot varus/metatarsus adductus) (Fig. 21.28B).

Therapeutic management of clubfoot includes initial foot manipulation and casting followed by percutaneous tenotomy and continuation of bracing for several months (Ponseti method).[120] A complication of prolonged dorsiflexion without correction of the hindfoot varus and talipes equinus can result in acquired rocker bottom foot deformity.[119]

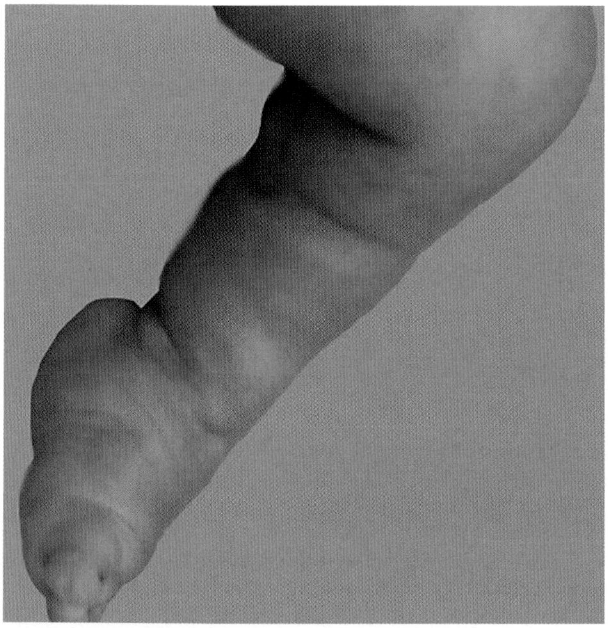

FIGURE 21.27 **Talipes equinovarus.** Congenital talipes equinovarus in a baby girl with Zellweger syndrome.

Congenital Vertical Talus

Congenital vertical talus (CVT) is the most severe form of congenital rigid flatfoot (Fig. 21.29 and **Schematic G**). The characteristic appearance is described as a rocker bottom deformity, which is secondary to a dorsal dislocation of the navicular onto the head of the talus. The talus assumes a vertical position. Both talus and navicular bones have an abnormal contour.[119] Fifty percent of patients demonstrate an isolated CVT disorder, and in the remainder 50%, it occurs in association with neuromuscular disorders or genetic disorders.[121] Some of these conditions include myelomeningocele, arthrogryposis, sacral agenesis, neurofibromatosis, trisomies 13 to 15 and 18, Edwards syndrome, Hurler, and Eagle-Barrett syndrome, among many others.

Radiographic manifestations in the lateral view include steep axis of the talus and convex plantar surface of the foot (rocker bottom foot) (Fig. 21.29).

Therapeutic management is surgical correction of the deformity, as casting is ineffective as a primary method of treatment for the fixed deformity. Preoperative casting is used for stretching and elongation of the talonavicular joint in order to facilitate surgical reduction.

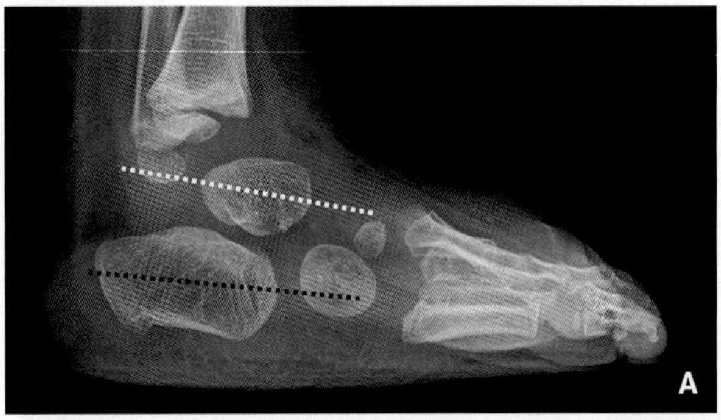

FIGURE 21.28 **Talipes equinovarus in a 3-year-old boy. A:** Lateral radiograph of the right foot demonstrates a parallel relationship between the talus (*white dotted line*) and calcaneus (*black dotted line*) reflecting hindfoot varus. Note increased dorsiflexion of the calcaneus or equinus position and forefoot inversion reflected by the inferior position of the fifth metatarsal relative to the more superior position of the first metatarsal. **B:** Frontal view of the left foot demonstrates increased overlapping of the talus (*white dotted line*) and calcaneus (*black dotted line*) reflecting hindfoot varus. The first metatarsal is medially located relative to the axis of the talus reflecting forefoot varus.

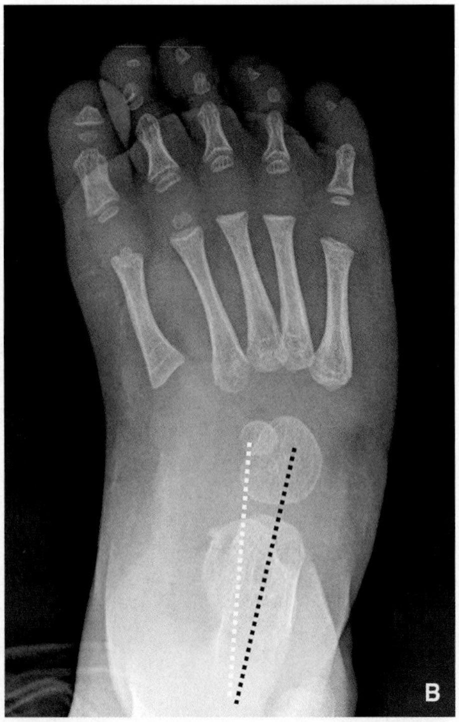

Metatarsus Adductus

Metatarsus adductus is characterized by forefoot adduction and normal alignment of the midfoot and hindfoot (Fig. 21.30 and **Schematic H**).[119] This is one of the most common foot deformities in children. The etiology of metatarsus adductus is unknown and perhaps related to abnormal intrauterine forces applied to the foot (e.g., oligohydramnios). Clinically, the foot has the configuration of a "kidney bean shape" because of the characteristic deep medial crease and convex lateral borders.

The vast majority of patients respond to nonoperative treatment.[122] In severe cases, stretching and sequential casting can be performed. Skewfoot is considered a severe form of metatarsus adductus that requires surgical correction more often than metatarsus adductus. The findings of skewfoot include metatarsus adductus with hindfoot valgus and possible lateral subluxation of the navicular.[119]

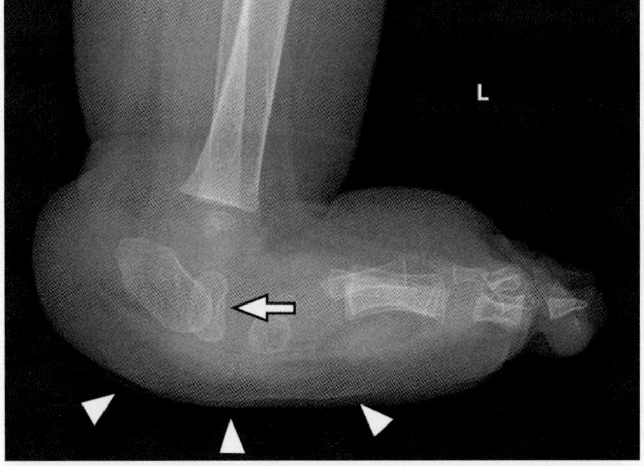

FIGURE 21.29 **Congenital vertical talus in a 5-month-old girl with history of arthrogryposis.** Lateral radiograph of the left foot demonstrates vertical position of the talus (*arrow*) and convex plantar surface or "rocker bottom" deformity (*arrowheads*).

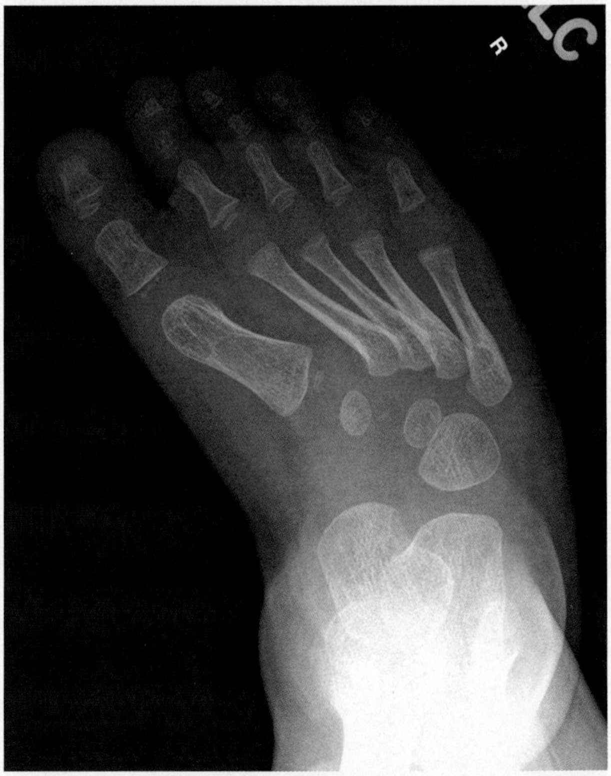

FIGURE 21.30 **Metatarsus adductus in a 2-year-old girl.** Frontal view of the right foot shows forefoot adduction demonstrated by toes "turned in" toward the midline. Normal relationships of the midfoot and hindfoot bones are noted.

Tarsal Coalition

Tarsal coalition is considered a congenital failure of segmentation of the tarsal bones. The aberrant union of two tarsal bones can be classified as osseous, cartilaginous, or fibrous.[123,124] The most common tarsal coalitions are between the talus and calcaneus (talocalcaneal or subtalar coalition) and between the anterior process of the calcaneus and the navicular bone (calcaneonavicular coalition). Other tarsal coalitions can be seen between the bones of the hindfoot and midfoot. The prevalence of tarsal coalition is debated in the literature with most studies reporting a 1% to 3% prevalence in the adult population.[125] Bilateral tarsal coalition is not uncommon.

The presentation of tarsal coalition can be variable. The abnormal joint in the tarsal coalition causes restricted joint motion. Affected pediatric patients are usually asymptomatic in early life; however, pain develops with increased ambulation and physical activity in older children and adolescents. The clinical manifestations of tarsal coalition include medial hindfoot pain by the sustentaculum tali in talocalcaneal coalitions, pain along the sinus tarsi in calcaneonavicular coalitions, lateral heel pain, and restricted subtalar motion in both types of coalitions. Flatfoot deformity (pes planus) secondary to tarsal coalition is common, ranging from flexible to rigid. The progression to rigid flatfoot may correlate with exacerbation of symptoms. Symptomatic tarsal coalitions also present with ankle equinus, posterior tibialis dysfunction, other segmental or pedal misalignment, and potential degenerative arthrosis.[124]

Radiographic findings of talocalcaneal coalition include abnormal overgrowth of the subtalar joint along the sustentaculum tali and adjacent talus (Fig. 21.31 and **Schematic D**). An axial calcaneal weight-bearing image (Harris-Beath view) is used for assessment of the subtalar joint. The C-sign, which can be seen on weighted-bearing lateral view, refers to the radiographic appearance of the continuity of the inferomedial border of the talus with the sustentaculum tali. However, the C-sign is more indicative of a flatfoot deformity than coalition.[126] Occasionally, anterior talar beaking can be seen in lateral radiographs, because of hindfoot motion restriction and increased range of motion at the talonavicular joint in

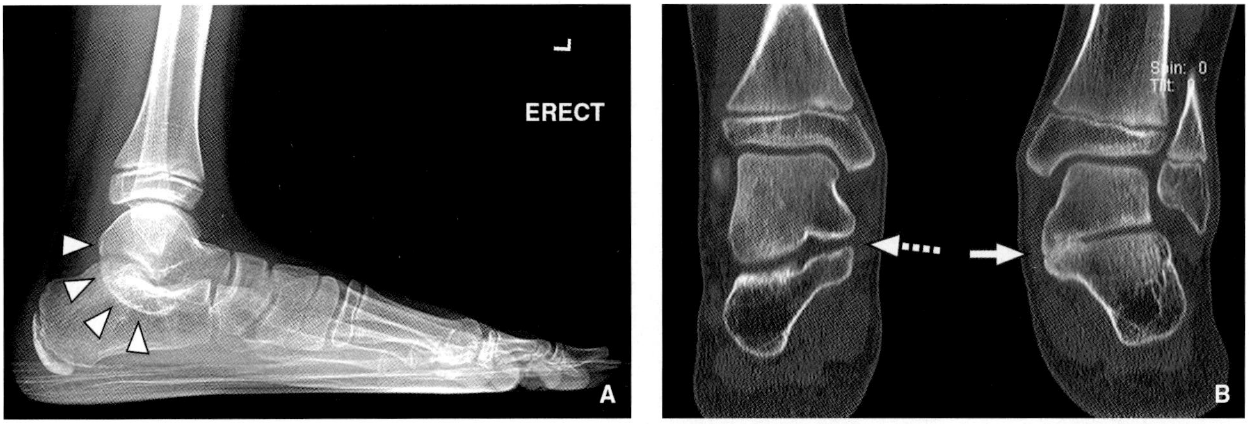

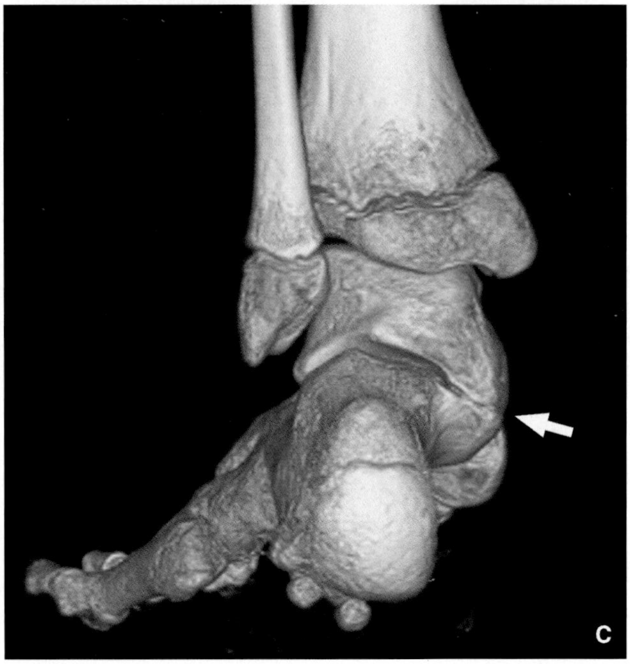

FIGURE 21.31 **Talocalcaneal coalition in an 11-year-old girl with chronic left ankle pain. A:** Lateral view radiograph the left foot demonstrates mild pes planus configuration and continuity of the subtalar joint or "C-sign" (*arrowheads*). **B:** Coronal CT reformat of both subtalar joints demonstrates left bony coalition with sclerosis and irregularity of the subtalar joint (*arrow*). A normal right subtalar joint is shown for comparison (*interrupted arrow*). **C:** Coronal oblique 3D reconstruction CT image demonstrates better visualization of bony coalition and subtalar joint angular deformity (*arrow*).

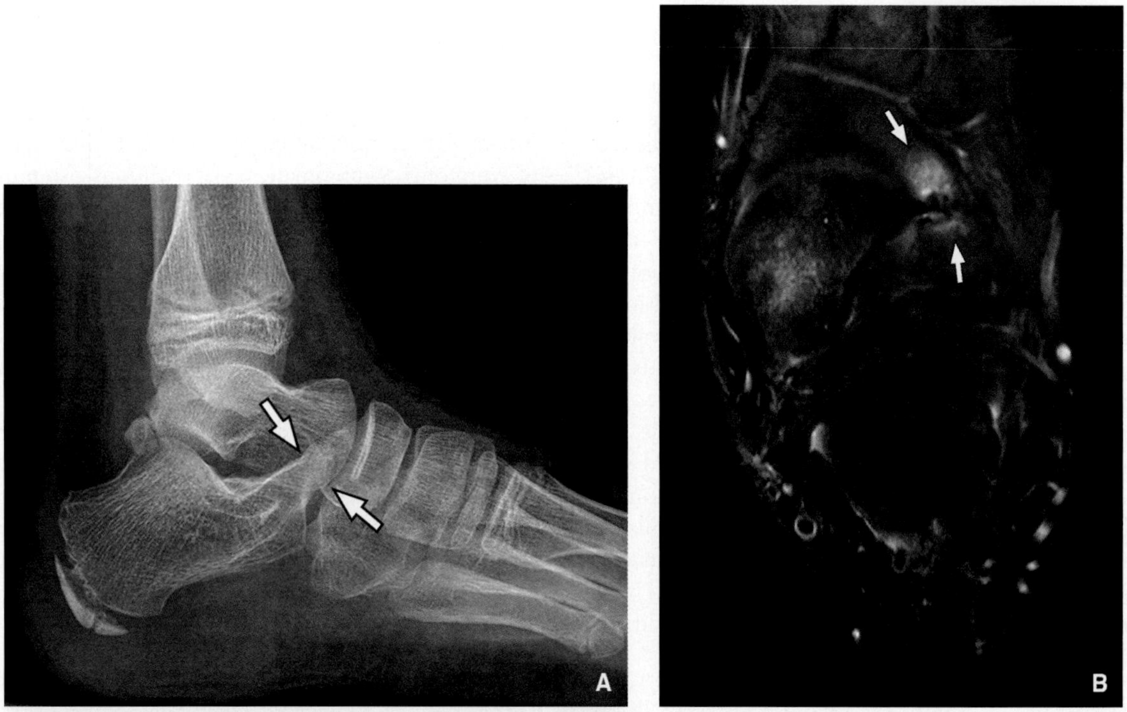

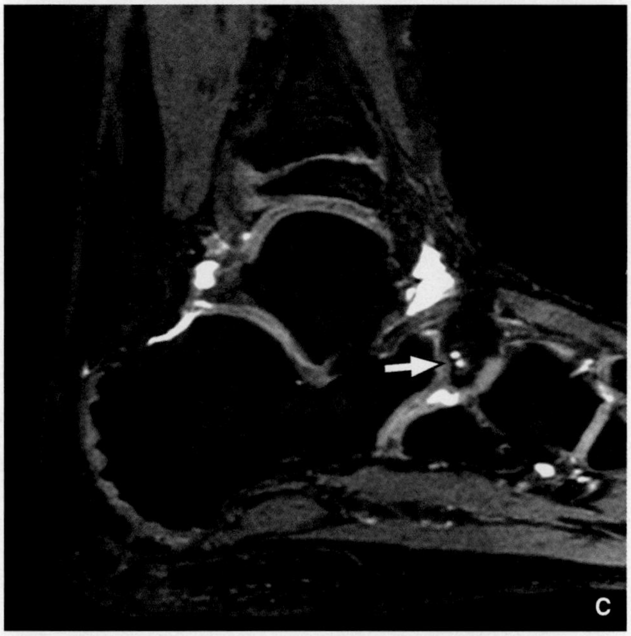

FIGURE 21.32 **Calcaneonavicular coalition in an 11-year-old boy with history of frequently "twisting his ankles." A:** Lateral radiographic view of the ankle demonstrates elongation of the anterior process of the calcaneus, so-called "anteater nose" sign (*arrows*) suggesting calcaneonavicular coalition. **B:** Axial short tau inversion recovery (STIR) MR image demonstrates bony edema and cortical irregularity along both components of the calcaneonavicular coalition (*arrows*). **C:** Coronal gradient-echo (GRE) MR image demonstrates cartilaginous signal intensity bridging the coalition. Small cystic changes (*arrow*) are seen in the navicular bone adjacent to the coalition site.

talocalcaneal coalition; however, this can be seen also in calcaneonavicular coalitions or other degenerative changes not related to tarsal coalition. Radiographic findings of calcaneonavicular coalition include abnormal elongation of the anterior process of the talus ("anteater nose sign") seen on lateral radiographs and abnormal abutment of the lateral margin of the navicular bone, which is better visualized on oblique radiographs of the foot (Fig. 21.32).

CT and MRI are used for confirmation of presence, evaluation of morphology, and preoperative planning of tarsal coalitions. There is currently controversy regarding the superiority of CT versus MR in the evaluation of tarsal coalitions, with CT offering superior depiction of bony and fibrous coalitions and MRI allowing additional assessment of associated tendon pathology and presence of bone marrow edema.[124]

The initial conservative management of tarsal coalitions is aimed at decreasing pain related to subtalar joint motion. Pediatric patients who failed conservative management may require surgical resection (Fig. 21.33) and arthrodesis of the talar coalition.

Skeletal Abnormalities Associated with Syndromes

There is an extensive list of syndromes associated with skeletal abnormalities. A brief discussion of two representative

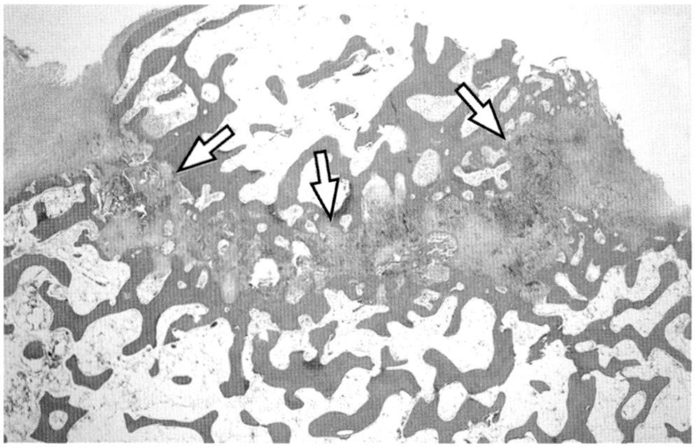

FIGURE 21.33 **Calcaneonavicular coalition.** Calcaneonavicular coalition, excised from a 10-year-old boy, shows the calcaneus and navicular bones connected by a plate of disorganized cartilage (*arrows*) (hematoxylin and eosin, original magnification, 20×).

diseases in this group (trisomy 21 and Marfan disease) is provided.

Trisomy 21

Trisomy 21 or Down syndrome is the most common genetic cause of intellectual disability.[127] Its incidence is ~1 in 650 to 1,000 live births.[128] Associated conditions include hearing loss, otitis media, eye disorders, obstructive sleep apnea, congenital heart defects, gastrointestinal problems, thyroid disease, and hematologic and neurologic disorders.[129]

Musculoskeletal manifestations in Down syndrome are extensive. The presence of 11 pairs of ribs is a common finding. Two manubrial ossification centers can also be seen. There is a characteristic appearance of the pelvis with flared iliac wings and flat acetabular roofs with small acetabular angles. There is increased hypotonia and joint laxity with hip dislocations secondary to developmental dysplasia of the hip (DDH). In the hands, short stubby fingers and clinodactyly with dysplasia of the middle phalanges of the fifth digit can be present (Fig. 21.34). Upper cervical abnormalities include hypoplasia of the odontoid process and hypoplasia of the posterior arch of C1. There is also increased prevalence of atlantoaxial subluxation (>5 mm) and clivus-odontoid misalignment.[130]

Marfan Syndrome

Marfan syndrome is an inherited connective tissue disorder that affects multiple organ systems, most notably the skeletal, cardiovascular, and ocular systems. There is an increased risk of aortic aneurysms and aortic dissections, the primary cause of death in patients with Marfan syndrome. The pattern of inheritance is autosomal dominant.[131]

Affected pediatric patients with Marfan syndrome demonstrate characteristic tall stature (>97th percentile), limb disproportion, classic facial features, high arched palate, and arachnodactyly. The majority of children with Marfan syndrome have an arm span that exceeds their height by 5 cm. Additional skeletal manifestations include pectus carinatum, pectus excavatum (less frequent), scoliosis,

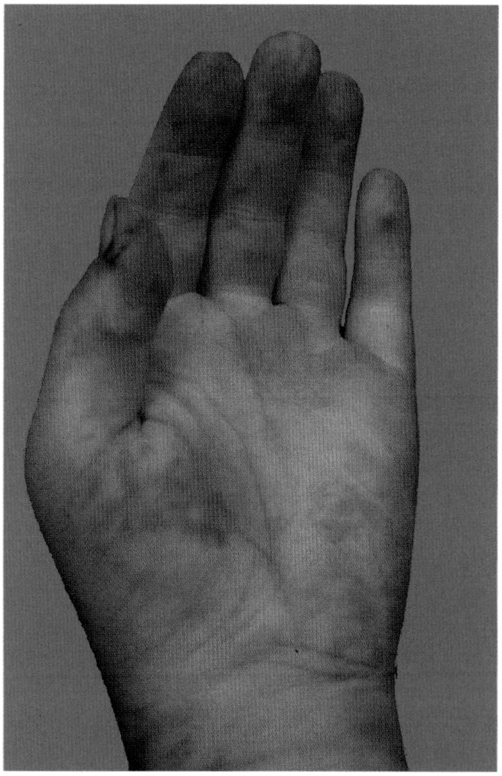

FIGURE 21.34 **Trisomy 21.** Characteristic short stubby fingers, particularly the fifth finger, are present.

spondylolisthesis, pes planus, joint hypermobility, and protrusio acetabuli.[131,132]

Therapeutic management of Marfan syndrome relies in aggressive blood pressure control. This is not curative treatment but delays progressive aortic deterioration.

Developmental Dysplasia of the Hip

Developmental dysplasia of the hip (DDH) includes a spectrum of hip abnormalities describing abnormal relationship between the femoral head and the acetabulum (**Schematic K**). DDH can occur in utero, perinatally, or during infancy and childhood. The affected hip may be dislocated at rest, dislocatable (but normal in position at rest), or subluxable with provocative maneuvers or appear normal on physical examination yet have abnormal configuration by imaging examination (radiographs or US). Normal development of the hip requires a balanced growth of the acetabular and triradiate cartilages as well as a well-located and centered femoral head. In DDH, most abnormalities are in the acetabular side. Secondary femoral head changes related to the anteversion and pressure changes on the femoral head from the acetabulum or ilium (associated to subluxation or dislocation) can be also present.[133,134]

The epidemiology of DDH is variable with known geographic, gender, and ethnic differences with possible environmental and genetic effects. DDH occurs in ~1 in 100 live births and hip dislocation can be present in ~1 to 1.5 in 1,000 live births.[133] Additional risk factors of DDH include female gender, positive family history, and breech presentation.[134]

The presence of torticollis and club foot has been suggested as mechanical changes related to oligohydramnios in prenatal life and potentially associated to DDH.

Physical examination is the primary tool for identification of DDH in the newborn. The examiner looks for asymmetry of thigh creases, leg length discrepancy, range of hip joint motion, and abnormal physical findings on the Barlow and Ortolani maneuvers (up to 8 to 12 weeks of age). The Barlow maneuver is performed with the hip in flexion and adduction applying posterior pressure to the femoral head causing subluxation or dislocation of the unstable femoral head from the acetabulum in DDH. The Ortolani maneuver is the sensation of the dislocated hip reducing, after placing the hip in abduction.

The role of radiologists concerns the early detection and treatment guidance of DDH to avoid morbidity associated to chronic degenerative joint disease and potential early total hip replacement.[135] Hip sonography is an excellent and accurate method for evaluation of the normal hip and abnormalities seen in DDH; however, examinations performed during the first 3 weeks of life are prone to a high number of false-positive examinations secondary to the normal neonatal hip laxity related to maternal hormonal influences. The morphology of the predominantly cartilaginous portions of the acetabular and femoral head epiphyses in young children are well visualized using sonography.

The Graf or static technique is a detailed anatomic classification of the sonographic hip anatomy in normal, immature, and dysplastic hips using alpha and beta angles describing quantitative measures of acetabular bony angle and position of the lateral acetabular labrum in a static hip with standardized coronal views with the patient in the lateral decubitus position (Fig. 21.35).[136]

The alpha angle reflects the depth of the bony acetabular roof and is formed by the intersection of the ilium line (in orange, Fig. 21.35) and acetabular roof line (in blue, Fig. 21.35). In a normal mature hip, the alpha angle is >60 degrees. The beta angle reflects the cartilaginous coverage and is formed by the intersection of the ilium line (in orange, Fig. 21.35) and labrum line (in green, Fig. 21.35). A normal beta angle is <55 degrees.

The Harcke or dynamic technique applies all the morphologic acetabular changes described by Graf using both coronal and transverse planes with the addition of dynamic evaluation during relaxed hip flexion and neutral positions as well as during stress similar to the Barlow maneuver.[137]

In clinical practice, a combination of both static and dynamic hip sonography can be integrated in the evaluation of DDH, which includes qualitative description of the acetabular morphology (normal, immature, dysplastic), coverage of the femoral head in the coronal plane, and dynamic information of the degree of hip instability (normal, laxity, subluxation with stress, frank subluxation, or dislocation at rest). Radiographic evaluation becomes the primary modality for assessment of DDH after 4 to 6 months of age, as the secondary ossification centers of the femoral heads are radiographically evident. An AP view of the hips with the patient in the neutral position is typically performed. Radiographic measurements useful in evaluation of DDH are illustrated in Figure 21.36 and summarized in Table 21.5:

- Hilgenreiner line: Horizontal line drawn between bilateral triradiate cartilages
- Perkin line: Vertical line drawn perpendicular along the Hilgenreiner line at the lateral edge of the acetabulum

The normal location of the secondary ossification center of the femoral heads should be within the medial lower quadrant of the intersection of these two lines.

Other radiographic landmarks include:

- Shenton line: Curved line drawn from the medial aspect of the femoral neck to the lower border of the superior pubic ramus
- Acetabular index: Angle formed between Hilgenreiner line and a line drawn from the depth of the acetabular socket and the most lateral ossified margin of the acetabular roof. This angle is a reflection of the development of the ossified acetabular roof. The values for the acetabular index range from 40 degrees for newborns and no more than 25 degrees after 4 months of age for a normal infant. It should be <25 degrees in patients older than 6 months.

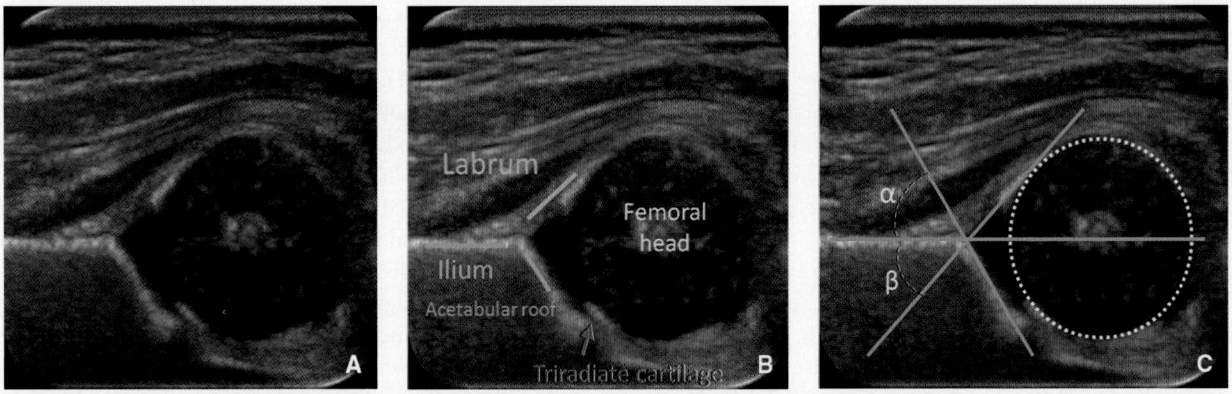

FIGURE 21.35 **Sonographic landmarks in the evaluation of developmental dysplasia of the hip. A:** Normal hip ultrasound image in standard coronal view. **B:** Description of the anatomic structures in **(A)**. **C:** Line drawings used for assessment of acetabular morphology and anatomic relationships as described in the Graf technique.

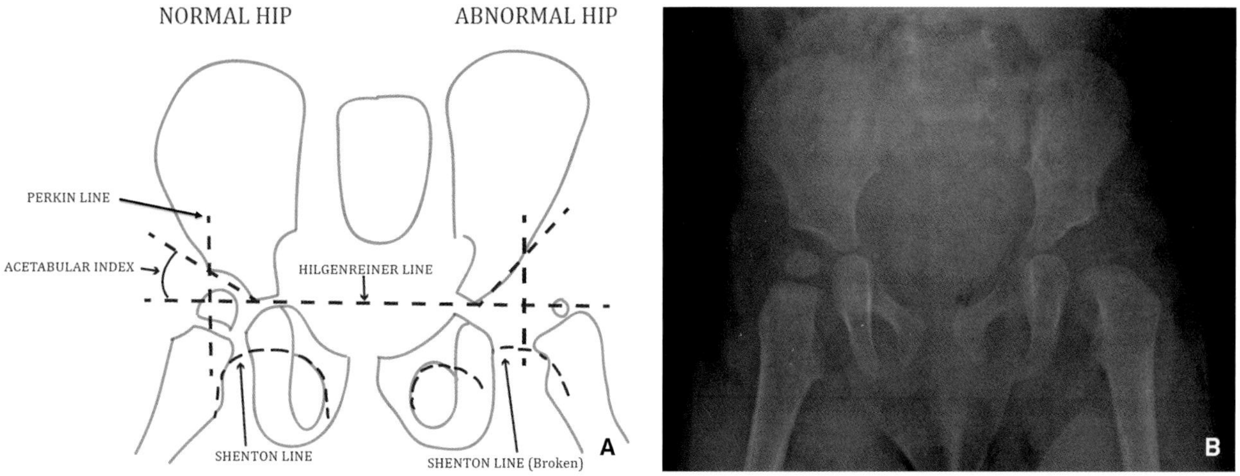

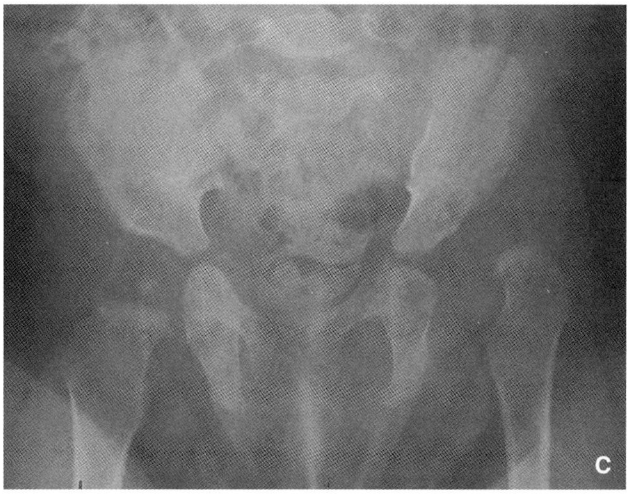

FIGURE 21.36 **Radiographic landmarks in developmental dysplasia of the hip (DDH). A:** Diagram illustrates how to draw hip lines using anatomic landmarks. Right hip depicts normal configuration and left hip demonstrates abnormalities seen in DDH. **B:** Frontal radiograph of the pelvis in a 7-month-old girl with left DDH. Note abnormalities in the left hip including increased acetabular index and small left proximal femoral ossification center localized in the lower outer quadrant (subluxation). **C:** Frontal radiograph of the pelvis in a 5-month-old girl with left DDH. Note more severe abnormalities in the left hip compared to **B**, including increased acetabular index and frank dislocation of the left hip.

TABLE 21.5 Summary of Radiographic Landmarks in the Evaluation of Developmental Dysplasia of the Hip (DDH)

Line/Angle	Definition	Normal	DDH
Hilgenreiner line	Horizontal line drawn between bilateral triradiate cartilages	Normal location of the secondary ossification center of the femoral heads should be along the medial lower quadrant of the intersection of these two lines.	Usually small ossification center displaced superiorly and laterally; degree of displacement dependent on severity of DDH
Perkin line	Vertical line drawn perpendicular along Hilgenreiner line at the lateral edge of the acetabulum		
Shenton line	Curved line drawn from the medial aspect of the femoral neck to the lower border of the superior pubic ramus	Smooth continuous arc	Discontinuous "broken" arc
Acetabular index	Angle formed by the Hilgenreiner line and a line drawn from the depth of the acetabular socket and the most lateral ossified margin of the acetabular roof	This angle is a reflection of the development of the ossified acetabular roof. The values for the acetabular index range from 40 degrees for newborns and no more than 25 degrees after 4 mo of age for a normal infant.	Increased acetabular index in affected hip (shallow hip socket)

Therapeutic management of DDH is guided by the patient's age at the time of diagnosis. Newborn and infants with DDH are usually placed in a hip harness with the hips in flexion and abduction to achieve concentric hip reduction. The harness also allows for stabilization of the hip joints without complete rigidity of the joint allowing for dynamic molding of the acetabulum and femoral head. An observational study noted that patients with DDH in a Pavlik harness for 6 weeks demonstrated resolution of hip instability in 97% of cases.[138] However, it can be argued that the improvement could be influenced by normal maturational improvement rather than the effects of the harness in this observational study, which lacks a control group.[139] The most common complication in the treatment of DDH is AVN of the proximal femoral epiphysis. This is likely related to excessive abduction in a harness or cast causing disruption to the blood supply of the proximal femoral epiphysis and/or physis. The incidence of AVN has been report in ~1% in patients treated with a Pavlik harness.[140]

Patients who failed to improve with a Pavlik harness or older patients (more than 6 months at the time of diagnosis) are candidates for closed reduction under anesthesia in the operating room with placement of a spica cast. During this procedure, the femoral head is manipulated into the acetabulum with flexion, traction, and abduction, usually requiring an arthrogram for confirmation of the reduction and a potential adductor tenotomy to decrease secondary adduction contracture in the hip. Following the performance of a closed reduction, the risk of AVN in the affected hip in patients with DDH can be as high as 47%.[141] For this reason, emphasis in postsurgical imaging has been placed in the perioperative period to confirm the adequacy of the reduction and to identify patients at risk of AVN because of persistent subluxation or dislocation.

Limited CT examinations with appropriate pediatric radiation dose reduction and abbreviated MRI protocols have been used as accurate methods for assessment of anatomic adequacy following close reduction.[142–144] More recently, gadolinium-enhanced (perfusion) MRI protocols in the immediate perioperative following closed reduction in DDH have been described. This technique allows for both accurate anatomical assessment of the closed reduction in addition to provide information about the femoral head perfusion that may be predictive for future AVN.[145] DDH patients with failure to obtain a stable hip with a closed reduction or children older than 2 years of age at the time of diagnosis are usually treated with open reduction and potential pelvic osteotomy.

Femoral Neck Angle Abnormalities (Coxa Vara and Coxa Valga)

The normal configuration of the hip joint is evaluated using the femoral neck–shaft angle, which ranges from 120 to 135 degrees. A coxa vara configuration is defined by a femoral neck–shaft angle of <120 degrees and a coxa valga configuration is defined by a femoral neck–shaft angle of more than 135 degrees in children (**Schematic J**).[146] Changes in the caput–collum–diaphyseal angle are the result of changes in the stress patterns applied to the hip joint, which affects the trabecular patterns inside the bones. Note is made at birth, no difference exists between the hips of children with these disorders and the hips of other children with the deformity manifesting during the development of the child. Coxa vara can be due to congenital disorders such as metaphyseal chondrodysplasia (Fig. 21.9), fibrous dysplasia (Fig. 21.13), PFFD

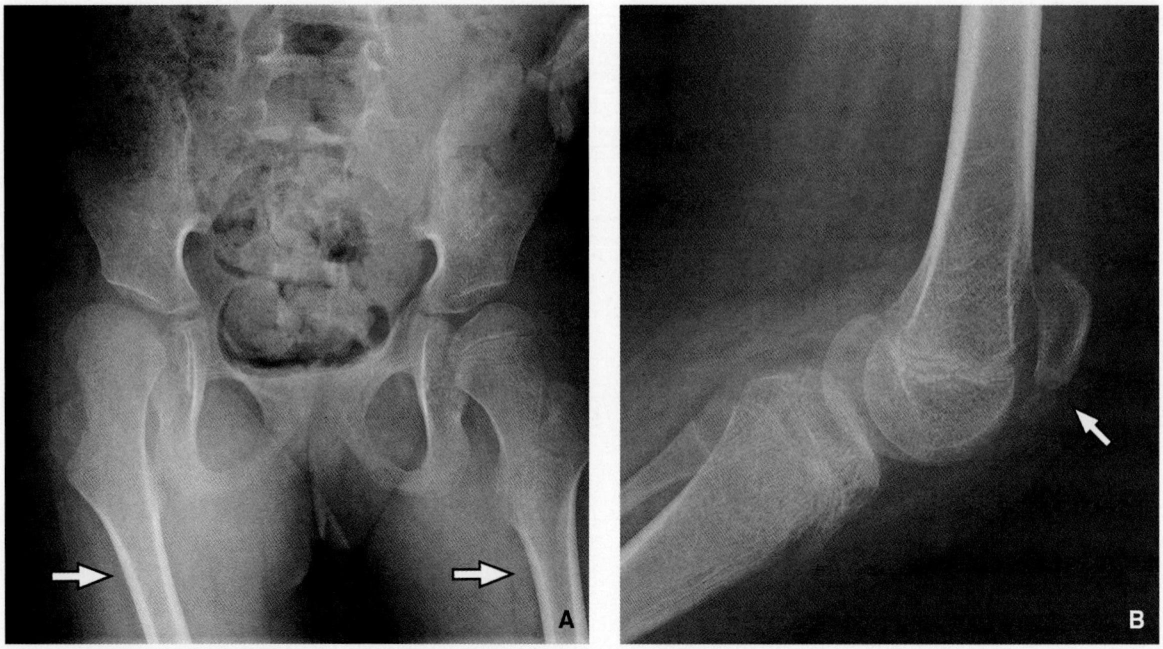

FIGURE 21.37 **Skeletal manifestations of cerebral palsy in an 11-year-old boy. A:** Frontal radiograph of the pelvis demonstrates bilateral coxa valga, partial uncovering of the proximal femoral epiphyses by the acetabula and ipsilateral contracture of the hips or "windswept" deformity (*arrows*). **B:** Lateral view of the knee demonstrates chronic effects of flexion contractures manifested by patella alta and fragmentation (*arrow*) of the lower patellar pole.

(Fig. 21.22), or DDH, and coxa valga can occur due to spastic cerebral palsy (CP) (Fig. 21.37).

Skeletal Abnormalities Associated with Neuromuscular Diseases

The musculoskeletal manifestations of neuromuscular disorders are extensive, and the progressive involvement of multiple joints and muscle groups alter the normal skeletal growth and development of patients. The common denominator among neuromuscular disorders is the loss of central nervous system control over distal motor groups causing progressive skeletal deformity. The most frequently encountered musculoskeletal complications of neuromuscular disorders in children are scoliosis, hip dysplasia, and rotational deformities.[147] The three main neuromuscular conditions causing skeletal abnormalities are meningomyelocele, CP, and muscular dystrophies (Duchenne muscular dystrophy [DMD], Becker muscular dystrophy, and facioscapulohumeral muscular dystrophy).

The care of patients with neuromuscular diseases requires a multidisciplinary approach, and radiologists play a significant role in the recognition of early changes and disease progression for adequate treatment of these complex entities. Therapeutic management for neuromuscular diseases should be individualized to the specific needs of patients; however, conservative and surgical treatments of specific skeletal deformities emphasize preservation of ambulatory status and contracture treatment (orthotics, myotomy, tendon transfer, and osteotomies) and scoliosis treatment (bracing, spinal instrumentation, and arthrodesis).

Meningomyelocele

Meningomyelocele refers to a wide range of neural tube defects affecting the spine and spinal cord. These defects can be classified as either open or closed based on the presence or absence of exposed neural tissue and are described in detail in **Section 1 Pediatric Neuroradiology, Chapter 4**. This chapter focuses on the musculoskeletal sequelae. The distribution and severity of the musculoskeletal sequelae are determined by the level in which the abnormality occurs along the spine, with higher level lesions being more ominous than lower level lesions.

There is a high prevalence of spinal deformities (scoliosis, kyphosis, and lordosis) in patients with myelomeningocele. Scoliosis can be congenital secondary to vertebral anomalies or acquired deformities secondary to asymmetric spinal muscle weakness in meningomyelocele. The term scoliosis is usually reserved for myelomeningocele patients with spinal curves of more than 20 degrees, as spinal curves between 10 and 20 degrees often resolve spontaneously in this population. Scoliosis can develop approximately until 15 years of age in patients with myelomeningocele.[148]

Hip joint contractures, subluxation, and dislocation are very common in patients with myelomeningocele. Presence and severity of hip joint deformity are dependent on the neurologic level of the disorder. For example, patients with a upper thoracic or upper lumbar spinal lesion do not have sensation or muscle control of the lower extremity. Therefore, they can rarely walk independently. Patients with a middle or lower lumbar lesion have sensation distal to the knee and may develop the capacity for independent walking but are at risk of progressive hip dysplasia and dislocation in association to hip flexion contracture. Asymmetric hip contractures can cause compensatory lumbar scoliosis, pelvic obliquity, and abnormal lordosis. Foot deformities are common in patients with myelomeningocele and include calcaneal deformities. Clubfoot is the most common deformity in patients with myelomeningocele and presents in patients with paraplegia at any spinal level. Paralytic pes calcaneus is seen in patients with L4 to L5 nerve root deficit causing weak plantar flexion and stronger dorsiflexion. Affected pediatric patients are prone to developing crouching gait, pressure sores, and osteomyelitis.[146] Myelomeningocele patients are at increased risk of pathologic fractures secondary to diffuse osteopenia and thin bones related to lower extremity paralysis, particularly those with thoracic level paralysis.[149]

Cerebral Palsy

CP is a nonprogressive central nervous system disorder characterized by motion and posture impairment (Fig. 21.37). The incidence is ~1 to 5 per 1,000 live births.[150] No hereditary or specific common disease is related to development of CP. The central motor dysfunction is due to a permanent, nonprogressive insult to the immature brain. The brain injury can occur during the prenatal, perinatal, or postnatal period, but ~70% to 80% of the injuries occur during the prenatal period.[151] Premature delivery and low birth weight are associated to CP. Other risk factors include asphyxia, congenital infection, placental infarction, and occlusion of a cerebral artery or vein.[152]

The most frequent musculoskeletal disorder in patients with CP is joint contracture.[151] Spasticity and muscular imbalance of patients with CP are the primary problem. Progressive musculoskeletal manifestations are secondary. The spine and joints of the lower extremities are most commonly affected. Thoracolumbar scoliosis is seen progressively in patients with CP. Pediatric patients with CP demonstrate increased thoracic kyphosis, lumbar lordosis, spondylolisthesis, and spondylolysis.[153] The hips are commonly involved in patients with CP, and progressive hip dysplasia results from neuromuscular imbalance on the growth and development of the hip. Femoral torsion with or without coxa valga and progressive deformity of the femoral head or acetabulum can be seen. Progressive flexion–adduction contracture shifts the center of rotation of the hip from the femoral head to the lesser trochanter. This results in hip dislocation and femoral head deformity, which radiographically are manifested as the "windswept" deformity of the hips. Around the knee joint, flexion contracture with patella alta and chronic patellar fragmentation have been described. In the ankle and foot, progressive abnormalities are common and include equinovalgus and equinovarus deformities.[154]

Muscular Dystrophy

Muscular dystrophy encompasses a heterogeneous group of primary hereditary myopathies characterized by progressive

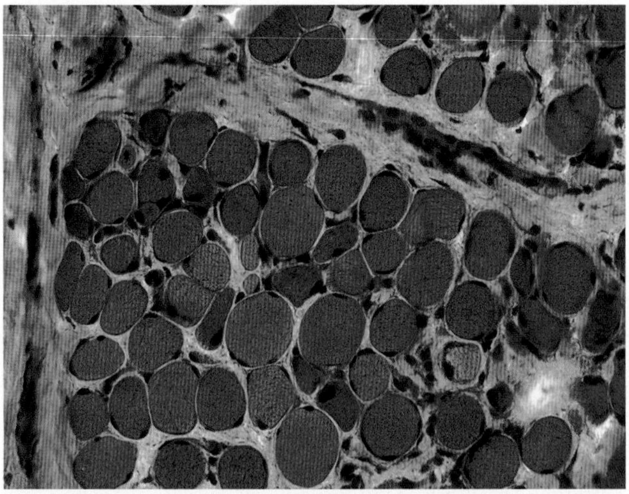

FIGURE 21.38 **Duchenne muscular dystrophy.** Muscle biopsy in Duchenne muscular dystrophy shows variation in myocyte fiber size as well as degenerating/regenerating muscle fibers and increased endomysial connective tissue (hematoxylin and eosin, original magnification, 400×). A negative immunostain for dystrophin (not shown) confirmed the diagnosis.

degeneration of muscle and weakness, occasionally present at birth but evolving over a latent period of apparent normal development and function. Their severity, age of onset, rate of progression, and prognosis vary dramatically among the different types of muscular dystrophy.[155]

DMD is the most common muscular dystrophy. The pattern of inheritance is X-linked recessive and occurs in 1 in 3,600 boys. The disease is characterized by delayed motor milestones, proximal weakness, hypertrophied calves, and elevated creatine kinase.[155] Muscle fibers show dystrophic changes as well as loss of normal dystrophin expression because of a mutation in the corresponding gene (Fig. 21.38).

The skeletal manifestations of DMD are directly related to the proximal muscle weakness such as hips and shoulder girdles with subsequent extension into the more peripheral muscle groups, causing frequent falls and difficulty rising. There is a compensatory hyperlordosis of the spine to compensate for the proximal hip girdle weakness. There is progressive kyphoscoliosis and joint contractures related to the increased muscle weakness and thus more prevalent in nonambulating patients. The typical hip contracture occurs in flexion, abduction, and external rotation. There are also often flexural contractions of the knee and stiff equinovarus of both ankles.

References

1. Lachman RS, Taybi H. *Taybi and Lachman's Radiology of Syndromes, Metabolic Disorders, and Skeletal Dysplasias*. 5th ed. Philadelphia, PA: Mosby Elsevier; 2007.
2. Keats TE, Anderson MW. *Atlas of Normal Roentgen Variants that May Simulate Disease*. 9th ed. Philadelphia, PA: Elsevier/Saunders; 2013.
3. Dighe M, Fligner C, Cheng E, et al. Fetal skeletal dysplasia: an approach to diagnosis with illustrative cases. *Radiographics.* 2008;28(4):1061–1077.
4. Parilla BV, Leeth EA, Kambich MP, et al. Antenatal detection of skeletal dysplasias. *J Ultrasound Med.* 2003;22(3):255–258; quiz 259–261.
5. Cassart M. Suspected fetal skeletal malformations or bone diseases: how to explore. *Pediatr Radiol.* 2010;40(6):1046–1051.
6. Schramm T, Gloning KP, Minderer S, et al. Prenatal sonographic diagnosis of skeletal dysplasias. *Ultrasound Obstet Gynecol.* 2009;34(2):160–170.
7. Krakow D, Lachman RS, Rimoin DL. Guidelines for the prenatal diagnosis of fetal skeletal dysplasias. *Genet Med.* 2009;11(2):127–133.
8. Emery KH, Bisset GS III, Johnson ND, et al. Tarsal coalition: a blinded comparison of MRI and CT. *Pediatr Radiol.* 1998;28(8):612–616.
9. Brown SD, Kasser JR, Zurakowski D, et al. Analysis of 51 tibial triplane fractures using CT with multiplanar reconstruction. *AJR Am J Roentgenol.* 2004;183(5):1489–1495.
10. Miglioretti DL, Johnson E, Williams A, et al. The use of computed tomography in pediatrics and the associated radiation exposure and estimated cancer risk. *JAMA Pediatr.* 2013;167(8):700–707.
11. Goske MJ, Applegate KE, Boylan J, et al. The Image Gently campaign: working together to change practice. *AJR Am J Roentgenol.* 2008;190(2):273–274.
12. Miyazaki O, Nishimura G, Sago H, et al. Prenatal diagnosis of fetal skeletal dysplasia with 3D CT. *Pediatr Radiol.* 2012;42(7):842–852.
13. Victoria T, Epelman M, Coleman BG, et al. Low-dose fetal CT in the prenatal evaluation of skeletal dysplasias and other severe skeletal abnormalities. *AJR Am J Roentgenol.* 2013;200(5):989–1000.
14. Mace G, Sonigo P, Cormier-Daire V, et al. Three-dimensional helical computed tomography in prenatal diagnosis of fetal skeletal dysplasia. *Ultrasound Obstet Gynecol.* 2013;42(2):161–168.
15. Ruano R, Molho M, Roume J, et al. Prenatal diagnosis of fetal skeletal dysplasias by combining two-dimensional and three-dimensional ultrasound and intrauterine three-dimensional helical computer tomography. *Ultrasound Obstet Gynecol.* 2004;24(2):134–140.
16. Ho-Fung VM, Jaramillo D. Cartilage imaging in children: current indications, magnetic resonance imaging techniques, and imaging findings. *Radiol Clin North Am.* 2013;51(4):689–702.
17. Burdiles A, Babyn PS. Pediatric bone marrow MR imaging. *Magn Reson Imaging Clin N Am.* 2009;17(3):391–409.
18. Defilippi C, Chiappetta D, Marzari D, et al. Image diagnosis in McCune-Albright syndrome. *J Pediatr Endocrinol Metab.* 2006;19(Suppl. 2):561–570.
19. Biermann M, Schwarzlmuller T, Fasmer KE, et al. Is there a role for PET-CT and SPECT-CT in pediatric oncology? *Acta Radiol.* 2013;54(9):1037–1045.
20. Eugene T, Corradini N, Carlier T, et al. (1)(8)F-FDG-PET/CT in initial staging and assessment of early response to chemotherapy of pediatric rhabdomyosarcomas. *Nucl Med Commun.* 2012;33(10):1089–1095.
21. Hernandez-Pampaloni M, Takalkar A, Yu JQ, et al. F-18 FDG-PET imaging and correlation with CT in staging and follow-up of pediatric lymphomas. *Pediatr Radiol.* 2006;36(6):524–531.
22. Laor T, Jaramillo D. MR imaging insights into skeletal maturation: what is normal? *Radiology.* 2009;250(1):28–38.
23. Jaramillo D, Villegas-Medina OL, Doty DK, et al. Age-related vascular changes in the epiphysis, physis, and metaphysis: normal findings on gadolinium-enhanced MRI of piglets. *AJR Am J Roentgenol.* 2004;182(2):353–360.
24. Do TT. Clinical and radiographic evaluation of bowlegs. *Curr Opin Pediatr.* 2001;13(1):42–46.

25. Kleinman PK, Sarwar ZU, Newton AW, et al. Metaphyseal fragmentation with physiologic bowing: a finding not to be confused with the classic metaphyseal lesion. *AJR Am J Roentgenol.* 2009;192(5):1266–1268.
26. Rana RS, Wu JS, Eisenberg RL. Periosteal reaction. *AJR Am J Roentgenol.* 2009;193(4):W259–W272.
27. Vieira RL, Bencardino JT, Rosenberg ZS, et al. MRI features of cortical desmoid in acute knee trauma. *AJR Am J Roentgenol.* 2011;196(2):424–428.
28. Gould CF, Ly JQ, Lattin GE Jr, et al. Bone tumor mimics: avoiding misdiagnosis. *Curr Probl Diagn Radiol.* 2007;36(3):124–141.
29. Dunham WK, Marcus NW, Enneking WF, et al. Developmental defects of the distal femoral metaphysis. *J Bone Joint Surg Am.* 1980;62(5):801–806.
30. Kelly BT, Green DW. Discoid lateral meniscus in children. *Curr Opin Pediatr.* 2002;14(1):54–61.
31. Singh K, Helms CA, Jacobs MT, et al. MRI appearance of Wrisberg variant of discoid lateral meniscus. *AJR Am J Roentgenol.* 2006;187(2):384–387.
32. Silverman JM, Mink JH, Deutsch AL. Discoid menisci of the knee: MR imaging appearance. *Radiology.* 1989;173(2):351–354.
33. Hamosh A, Scott AF, Amberger JS, et al. Online Mendelian Inheritance in Man (OMIM), a knowledgebase of human genes and genetic disorders. *Nucleic Acids Res.* 2005;33(Database issue):D514-517.
34. Online Mendelian Inheritance in Man, OMIM®. McKusick-Nathans Institute of Genetic Medicine, Johns Hopkins University (Baltimore, MD). Available from: http://omim.org/. Accessed January 11, 2014.
35. Tavormina PL, Shiang R, Thompson LM, et al. Thanatophoric dysplasia (types I and II) caused by distinct mutations in fibroblast growth factor receptor 3. *Nat Genet.* 1995;9(3):321–328.
36. Kitoh H, Brodie SG, Kupke KG, et al. Lys650Met substitution in the tyrosine kinase domain of the fibroblast growth factor receptor gene causes thanatophoric dysplasia Type I. Mutations in brief no. 199. Online. *Hum Mutat.* 1998;12(5):362–363.
37. Wilcox WR, Tavormina PL, Krakow D, et al. Molecular, radiologic, and histopathologic correlations in thanatophoric dysplasia. *Am J Med Genet.* 1998;78(3):274–281.
38. Chitty LS, Khalil A, Barrett AN, et al. Safe, accurate, prenatal diagnosis of thanatophoric dysplasia using ultrasound and free fetal DNA. *Prenat Diagn.* 2013;33(5):416–423.
39. Machado LE, Bonilla-Musoles F, Raga F, et al. Thanatophoric dysplasia: ultrasound diagnosis. *Ultrasound Q.* 2001;17(4):235–243.
40. Baker KM, Olson DS, Harding CO, et al. Long-term survival in typical thanatophoric dysplasia type 1. *Am J Med Genet.* 1997;70(4):427–436.
41. MacDonald IM, Hunter AG, MacLeod PM, et al. Growth and development in thanatophoric dysplasia. *Am J Med Genet.* 1989;33(4):508–512.
42. Wardinsky TD, Pagon RA, Powell BR, et al. Rhizomelic chondrodysplasia punctata and survival beyond one year: a review of the literature and five case reports. *Clin Genet.* 1990;38(2):84–93.
43. Gilbert EF, Opitz JM, Spranger JW, et al. Chondrodysplasia punctata—rhizomelic form. Pathologic and radiologic studies of three infants. *Eur J Pediatr.* 1976;123(2):89–109.
44. Hertzberg BS, Kliewer MA, Decker M, et al. Antenatal ultrasonographic diagnosis of rhizomelic chondrodysplasia punctata. *J Ultrasound Med.* 1999;18(10):715–718.
45. Rousseau F, Bonaventure J, Legeai-Mallet L, et al. Mutations in the gene encoding fibroblast growth factor receptor-3 in achondroplasia. *Nature.* 1994;371(6494):252–254.
46. Chitty LS, Griffin DR, Meaney C, et al. New aids for the non-invasive prenatal diagnosis of achondroplasia: dysmorphic features, charts of fetal size and molecular confirmation using cell-free fetal DNA in maternal plasma. *Ultrasound Obstet Gynecol.* 2011;37(3):283–289.
47. Baca KE, Abdullah MA, Ting BL, et al. Surgical decompression for lumbar stenosis in pediatric achondroplasia. *J Pediatr Orthop.* 2010;30(5):449–454.
48. Aryanpur J, Hurko O, Francomano C, et al. Craniocervical decompression for cervicomedullary compression in pediatric patients with achondroplasia. *J Neurosurg.* 1990;73(3):375–382.
49. Kim SJ, Agashe MV, Song SH, et al. Comparison between upper and lower limb lengthening in patients with achondroplasia: a retrospective study. *J Bone Joint Surg Br.* 2012;94(1):128–133.
50. Schiedel F, Rodl R. Lower limb lengthening in patients with disproportionate short stature with achondroplasia: a systematic review of the last 20 years. *Disabil Rehabil.* 2012;34(12):982–987.
51. Oberklaid F, Danks DM, Mayne V, et al. Asphyxiating thoracic dysplasia. Clinical, radiological, and pathological information on 10 patients. *Arch Dis Child.* 1977;52(10):758–765.
52. Tuysuz B, Baris S, Aksoy F, et al. Clinical variability of asphyxiating thoracic dystrophy (Jeune) syndrome: Evaluation and classification of 13 patients. *Am J Med Genet A.* 2009;149A(8):1727–1733.
53. Baujat G, Le Merrer M. Ellis-van Creveld syndrome. *Orphanet J Rare Dis.* 2007;2:27.
54. Tongsong T, Chanprapaph P, Thongpadungroj T. Prenatal sonographic findings associated with asphyxiating thoracic dystrophy (Jeune syndrome). *J Ultrasound Med.* 1999;18(8):573–576.
55. Waldhausen JH, Redding GJ, Song KM. Vertical expandable prosthetic titanium rib for thoracic insufficiency syndrome: a new method to treat an old problem. *J Pediatr Surg.* 2007;42(1):76–80.
56. Amirou M, Bourdat-Michel G, Pinel N, et al. Successful renal transplantation in Jeune syndrome type 2. *Pediatr Nephrol.* 1998;12(4):293–294.
57. Savarirayan R, Cormier-Daire V, Lachman RS, et al. Schmid type metaphyseal chondrodysplasia: a spondylometaphyseal dysplasia identical to the "Japanese" type. *Pediatr Radiol.* 2000;30(7):460–463.
58. Lachman RS, Rimoin DL, Spranger J. Metaphyseal chondrodysplasia, Schmid type. Clinical and radiographic delineation with a review of the literature. *Pediatr Radiol.* 1988;18(2):93–102.
59. Unger S, Bonafe L, Superti-Furga A. Multiple epiphyseal dysplasia: clinical and radiographic features, differential diagnosis and molecular basis. *Best Pract Res Clin Rheumatol.* 2008;22(1):19–32.
60. Schmale GA, Conrad EU III, Raskind WH. The natural history of hereditary multiple exostoses. *J Bone Joint Surg Am.* 1994;76(7):986–992.
61. Bovee JV, Sakkers RJ, Geirnaerdt MJ, et al. Intermediate grade osteosarcoma and chondrosarcoma arising in an osteochondroma. A case report of a patient with hereditary multiple exostoses. *J Clin Pathol.* 2002;55(3):226–229.
62. Wicklund CL, Pauli RM, Johnston D, et al. Natural history study of hereditary multiple exostoses. *Am J Med Genet.* 1995;55(1):43–46.

63. Brien EW, Mirra JM, Kerr R. Benign and malignant cartilage tumors of bone and joint: their anatomic and theoretical basis with an emphasis on radiology, pathology and clinical biology. I. The intramedullary cartilage tumors. *Skeletal Radiol.* 1997;26(6):325–353.
64. Silve C, Juppner H. Ollier disease. *Orphanet J Rare Dis* 2006;1:37.
65. Pansuriya TC, van Eijk R, d'Adamo P, et al. Somatic mosaic IDH1 and IDH2 mutations are associated with enchondroma and spindle cell hemangioma in Ollier disease and Maffucci syndrome. *Nat Genet.* 2011;43(12):1256–1261.
66. Schwartz HS, Zimmerman NB, Simon MA, et al. The malignant potential of enchondromatosis. *J Bone Joint Surg Am.* 1987; 69(2):269–274.
67. Verdegaal SH, Bovee JV, Pansuriya TC, et al. Incidence, predictive factors, and prognosis of chondrosarcoma in patients with Ollier disease and Maffucci syndrome: an international multicenter study of 161 patients. *Oncologist.* 2011;16(12):1771–1779.
68. Dumitrescu CE, Collins MT. McCune-Albright syndrome. *Orphanet J Rare Dis.* 2008;3:12.
69. Collins MT, Singer FR, Eugster E. McCune-Albright syndrome and the extraskeletal manifestations of fibrous dysplasia. *Orphanet J Rare Dis.* 2012;7(Suppl. 1):S4.
70. Huvos AG, Higinbotham NL, Miller TR. Bone sarcomas arising in fibrous dysplasia. *J Bone Joint Surg Am.* 1972;54(5): 1047–1056.
71. Lin AL, Gutmann DH. Advances in the treatment of neurofibromatosis-associated tumours. *Nat Rev Clin Oncol.* 2013;10(11):616–624.
72. Ferner RE. The neurofibromatoses. *Pract Neurol.* 2010;10(2): 82–93.
73. Rasmussen SA, Friedman JM. NF1 gene and neurofibromatosis 1. *Am J Epidemiol.* 2000;151(1):33–40.
74. Szudek J, Evans DG, Friedman JM. Patterns of associations of clinical features in neurofibromatosis 1 (NF1). *Hum Genet.* 2003; 112(3):289–297.
75. Ahlawat S, Chhabra A, Blakely J. Magnetic resonance neurography of peripheral nerve tumors and tumorlike conditions. *Neuroimaging Clin N Am.* 2014;24(1):171–192.
76. Jouhilahti EM, Peltonen S, Callens T, et al. The development of cutaneous neurofibromas. *Am J Pathol.* 2011;178(2):500–505.
77. Ducatman BS, Scheithauer BW, Piepgras DG, et al. Malignant peripheral nerve sheath tumors. A clinicopathologic study of 120 cases. *Cancer.* 1986;57(10):2006–2021.
78. Tsai LL, Drubach L, Fahey F, et al. [18F]-Fluorodeoxyglucose positron emission tomography in children with neurofibromatosis type 1 and plexiform neurofibromas: correlation with malignant transformation. *J Neurooncol.* 2012;108(3):469–475.
79. Cundy T. Recent advances in osteogenesis imperfecta. *Calcif Tissue Int.* 2012;90(6):439–449.
80. Renaud A, Aucourt J, Weill J, et al. Radiographic features of osteogenesis imperfecta. *Insights Imaging.* 2013;4(4):417–429.
81. Sillence DO, Senn A, Danks DM. Genetic heterogeneity in osteogenesis imperfecta. *J Med Genet.* 1979;16(2):101–116.
82. Glorieux FH, Moffatt P. Osteogenesis imperfecta, an ever-expanding conundrum. *J Bone Miner Res.* 2013;28(7):1519–1522.
83. Van Dijk FS, Pals G, Van Rijn RR, et al. Classification of Osteogenesis Imperfecta revisited. *Eur J Med Genet.* 2010;53(1): 1–5.
84. Steiner RD, Adsit J, Basel D. COL1A1/2-related osteogenesis imperfecta. In: Pagon RA, Adam MP, Bird TD, et al., eds. *GeneReviews.* Seattle, WA: University of Washington; 1993–2016.
85. Lonergan GJ, Baker AM, Morey MK, et al. From the archives of the AFIP. Child abuse: radiologic-pathologic correlation. *Radiographics.* 2003;23(4):811–845.
86. Offiah A, van Rijn RR, Perez-Rossello JM, et al. Skeletal imaging of child abuse (non-accidental injury). *Pediatr Radiol.* 2009;39(5):461–470.
87. van Dijk FS, Cobben JM, Kariminejad A, et al. Osteogenesis imperfecta: a review with clinical examples. *Mol Syndromol.* 2011;2(1):1–20.
88. Al Muderis M, Azzopardi T, Cundy P. Zebra lines of pamidronate therapy in children. *J Bone Joint Surg Am.* 2007;89(7):1511–1516.
89. Bulas DI, Stern HJ, Rosenbaum KN, et al. Variable prenatal appearance of osteogenesis imperfecta. *J Ultrasound Med.* 1994;13(6):419–427.
90. Phillipi CA, Remmington T, Steiner RD. Bisphosphonate therapy for osteogenesis imperfecta. *Cochrane Database Syst Rev.* 2008(4):CD005088.
91. Laron D, Pandya NK. Advances in the orthopedic management of osteogenesis imperfecta. *Orthop Clin North Am.* 2013; 44(4):565–573.
92. Vanhoenacker FM, De Beuckeleer LH, Van Hul W, et al. Sclerosing bone dysplasias: genetic and radioclinical features. *Eur Radiol.* 2000;10(9):1423–1433.
93. Van Hul W. Lessons from sclerosing bone dysplasias. *Horm Res.* 2007;68(Suppl. 5):37–39.
94. Ihde LL, Forrester DM, Gottsegen CJ, et al. Sclerosing bone dysplasias: review and differentiation from other causes of osteosclerosis. *Radiographics.* 2011;31(7):1865–1882.
95. Del Fattore A, Cappariello A, Teti A. Genetics, pathogenesis and complications of osteopetrosis. *Bone.* 2008;42(1):19–29.
96. Van Hul W, Vanhoenacker F, Balemans W, et al. Molecular and radiological diagnosis of sclerosing bone dysplasias. *Eur J Radiol.* 2001;40(3):198–207.
97. Faden MA, Krakow D, Ezgu F, et al. The Erlenmeyer flask bone deformity in the skeletal dysplasias. *Am J Med Genet A.* 2009;149A(6):1334–1345.
98. Driessen GJ, Gerritsen EJ, Fischer A, et al. Long-term outcome of haematopoietic stem cell transplantation in autosomal recessive osteopetrosis: an EBMT report. *Bone Marrow Transplant.* 2003; 32(7):657–663.
99. Bathi RJ, Masur VN. Pyknodysostosis—a report of two cases with a brief review of the literature. *Int J Oral Maxillofac Surg.* 2000;29(6):439–442.
100. Frota R, Linard RA, de Oliveira e Silva ED, et al. Mandibular osteomyelitis and fracture in a patient with pyknodysostosis. *J Craniofac Surg.* 2010;21(3):787–789.
101. Alves Pereira D, Berini Aytes L, Gay Escoda C. Pycnodysostosis. A report of 3 clinical cases. *Med Oral Patol Oral Cir Bucal.* 2008;13(10):E633–E635.
102. Waterval JJ, Borra VM, Van Hul W, et al. Sclerosing bone dysplasias with involvement of the craniofacial skeleton. *Bone.* 2013;60C:48–67.
103. de Vernejoul MC. Sclerosing bone disorders. *Best Pract Res Clin Rheumatol.* 2008;22(1):71–83.
104. Beighton P. Pyle disease (metaphyseal dysplasia). *J Med Genet.* 1987;24(6):321–324.
105. Heselson NG, Raad MS, Hamersma H, et al. The radiological manifestations of metaphyseal dysplasia (Pyle disease). *Br J Radiol.* 1979;52(618):431–440.
106. Gupta N, Kabra M, Das CJ, et al. Pyle metaphyseal dysplasia. *Indian Pediatr.* 2008;45(4):323–325.

107. Ermito S, Dinatale A, Carrara S, et al. Prenatal diagnosis of limb abnormalities: role of fetal ultrasonography. *J Prenat Med.* 2009;3(2):18–22.
108. Maldjian C, Patel TY, Klein RM, et al. Efficacy of MRI in classifying proximal focal femoral deficiency. *Skeletal Radiol.* 2007;36(3):215–220.
109. Goldfarb CA, Wall L, Manske PR. Radial longitudinal deficiency: the incidence of associated medical and musculoskeletal conditions. *J Hand Surg.* 2006;31(7):1176–1182.
110. Manske PR, Goldfarb CA. Congenital failure of formation of the upper limb. *Hand Clin.* 2009;25(2):157–170.
111. Stoll C, Alembik Y, Dott B, et al. Associated malformations in patients with limb reduction deficiencies. *Eur J Med Genet.* 2010;53(5):286–290.
112. Vargesson N. Thalidomide-induced limb defects: resolving a 50-year-old puzzle. *BioEssays.* 2009;31(12):1327–1336.
113. Kino Y. Clinical and experimental studies of the congenital constriction band syndrome, with an emphasis on its etiology. *J Bone Joint Surg Am.* 1975;57(5):636–643.
114. Moran SL, Jensen M, Bravo C. Amniotic band syndrome of the upper extremity: diagnosis and management. *J Am Acad Orthop Surg.* 2007;15(7):397–407.
115. Walter JH Jr, Goss LR, Lazzara AT. Amniotic band syndrome. *J Foot Ankle Surg.* 1998;37(4):325–333.
116. Vanderwilde R, Staheli LT, Chew DE, et al. Measurements on radiographs of the foot in normal infants and children. *J Bone Joint Surg Am.* 1988;70(3):407–415.
117. Dare DM, Dodwell ER. Pediatric flatfoot: cause, epidemiology, assessment, and treatment. *Curr Opin Pediatr.* 2014;26(1):93–100.
118. Aminian A, Sangeorzan BJ. The anatomy of cavus foot deformity. *Foot Ankle Clin.* 2008;13(2):191–198, v.
119. Harty MP. Imaging of pediatric foot disorders. *Radiol Clin North Am.* 2001;39(4):733–748.
120. Silvani S. The Ponseti technique for treatment of talipes equinovarus. *Clin Podiatr Med Surg.* 2006;23(1):119–135, viii-ix.
121. McKie J, Radomisli T. Congenital vertical talus: a review. *Clin Podiatr Med Surg.* 2010;27(1):145–156.
122. Farsetti P, Weinstein SL, Ponseti IV. The long-term functional and radiographic outcomes of untreated and non-operatively treated metatarsus adductus. *J Bone Joint Surg Am.* 1994;76(2):257–265.
123. Zaw H, Calder JD. Tarsal coalitions. *Foot Ankle Clin.* 2010;15(2):349–364.
124. Kernbach KJ. Tarsal coalitions: etiology, diagnosis, imaging, and stigmata. *Clin Podiatr Med Surg.* 2010;27(1):105–117.
125. Crim J. Imaging of tarsal coalition. *Radiol Clin North Am.* 2008;46(6):1017–1026, vi.
126. Brown RR, Rosenberg ZS, Thornhill BA. The C sign: more specific for flatfoot deformity than subtalar coalition. *Skeletal Radiol.* 2001;30(2):84–87.
127. Bittles AH, Bower C, Hussain R, et al. The four ages of Down syndrome. *Eur J Public Health.* 2007;17(2):221–225.
128. Baird PA, Sadovnick AD. Life expectancy in Down syndrome. *J Pediatr.* 1987;110(6):849–854.
129. Ivan DL, Cromwell P. Clinical practice guidelines for management of children with down syndrome: part I. *J Pediatr Health Care.* 2014;28(1):105–110.
130. Kriss VM. Down syndrome: imaging of multiorgan involvement. *Clin Pediatr.* 1999;38(8):441–449.
131. Iams HD. Diagnosis and management of Marfan syndrome. *Curr Sports Med Rep.* 2010;9(2):93–98.
132. De Paepe A, Devereux RB, Dietz HC, et al. Revised diagnostic criteria for the Marfan syndrome. *Am J Med Genet.* 1996;62(4):417–426.
133. Nemeth BA, Narotam V. Developmental dysplasia of the hip. *Pediatr Rev.* 2012;33(12):553–561.
134. Goldberg MJ. Early detection of developmental hip dysplasia: synopsis of the AAP clinical practice guideline. *Pediatr Rev.* 2001;22(4):131–134.
135. Engesaeter IO, Lie SA, Lehmann TG, et al. Neonatal hip instability and risk of total hip replacement in young adulthood: follow-up of 2,218,596 newborns from the Medical Birth Registry of Norway in the Norwegian Arthroplasty Register. *Acta Orthop.* 2008;79(3):321–326.
136. Graf R. Fundamentals of sonographic diagnosis of infant hip dysplasia. *J Pediatr Orthop.* 1984;4(6):735–740.
137. Clarke NM, Harcke HT, McHugh P, et al. Real-time ultrasound in the diagnosis of congenital dislocation and dysplasia of the hip. *J Bone Joint Surg Br.* 1985;67(3):406–412.
138. Kalamchi A, MacFarlane R 3rd. The Pavlik harness: results in patients over three months of age. *J Pediatr Orthop.* 1982;2(1):3–8.
139. Bracken J, Ditchfield M. Ultrasonography in developmental dysplasia of the hip: what have we learned? *Pediatr Radiol.* 2012;42(12):1418–1431.
140. Cashman JP, Round J, Taylor G, et al. The natural history of developmental dysplasia of the hip after early supervised treatment in the Pavlik harness. A prospective, longitudinal follow-up. *J Bone Joint Surg Br.* 2002;84(3):418–425.
141. Brougham DI, Broughton NS, Cole WG, et al. Avascular necrosis following closed reduction of congenital dislocation of the hip. Review of influencing factors and long-term follow-up. *J Bone Joint Surg Br.* 1990;72(4):557–562.
142. Smith BG, Kasser JR, Hey LA, et al. Postreduction computed tomography in developmental dislocation of the hip: part I: analysis of measurement reliability. *J Pediatr Orthop.* 1997;17(5):626–630.
143. Smith BG, Millis MB, Hey LA, et al. Postreduction computed tomography in developmental dislocation of the hip: part II: predictive value for outcome. *J Pediatr Orthop.* 1997;17(5):631–636.
144. Bachy M, Thevenin-Lemoine C, Rogier A, et al. Utility of magnetic resonance imaging (MRI) after closed reduction of developmental dysplasia of the hip. *J Child Orthop.* 2012;6(1):13–20.
145. Tiderius C, Jaramillo D, Connolly S, et al. Post-closed reduction perfusion magnetic resonance imaging as a predictor of avascular necrosis in developmental hip dysplasia: a preliminary report. *J Pediatr Orthop.* 2009;29(1):14–20.
146. Driscoll SW, Skinner J. Musculoskeletal complications of neuromuscular disease in children. *Phys Med Rehabil Clin N Am.* 2008;19(1):163–194, viii.
147. Trivedi J, Thomson JD, Slakey JB, et al. Clinical and radiographic predictors of scoliosis in patients with myelomeningocele. *J Bone Joint Surg Am.* 2002;84-A(8):1389–1394.
148. Akbar M, Bresch B, Seyler TM, et al. Management of orthopaedic sequelae of congenital spinal disorders. *J Bone Joint Surg Am.* 2009;91(Suppl. 6):87–100.
149. Akbar M, Bresch B, Raiss P, et al. Fractures in myelomeningocele. *J Orthop Traumatol.* 2010;11(3):175–182.

150. DeLuca PA. The musculoskeletal management of children with cerebral palsy. *Pediatr Clin North Am.* 1996;43(5): 1135–1150.
151. Green LB, Hurvitz EA. Cerebral palsy. *Phys Med Rehabil Clin N Am.* 2007;18(4):859–882, vii.
152. Kuban KC, Leviton A. Cerebral palsy. *N Engl J Med.* 1994; 330(3):188–195.
153. Morrell DS, Pearson JM, Sauser DD. Progressive bone and joint abnormalities of the spine and lower extremities in cerebral palsy. *Radiographics.* 2002;22(2):257–268.
154. Spiegel DA, Flynn JM. Evaluation and treatment of hip dysplasia in cerebral palsy. *Orthop Clin North Am.* 2006;37(2):185–196, vi.
155. Shieh PB. Muscular dystrophies and other genetic myopathies. *Neurol Clin.* 2013;31(4):1009–1029.

CHAPTER 22

Musculoskeletal Infectious and Inflammatory Disorders

Clara L. Ortiz-Neira • Jennifer Stimec • Marcia Torre Moreira • Andrea S. Doria

INTRODUCTION

Timely and accurate diagnosis of musculoskeletal infectious and inflammatory disorders remains a challenge in infants and children particularly solely based on clinical grounds. In many cases, mimickers such as malignant tumors or benign but aggressive-appearing bone infarcts may constitute a diagnostic dilemma in the pediatric population. Musculoskeletal infections and inflammatory disorders can affect cartilage, synovium, muscles, bones, and joints.

Imaging evaluation that can visualize abnormalities in all of these anatomic structures is often necessary for reaching a definitive diagnosis in pediatric patients with various underlying congenital and acquired musculoskeletal infectious and inflammatory disorders. In this chapter, currently available imaging modalities and techniques, relevant clinical and laboratory manifestations, characteristic imaging findings, and up-to-date management for pediatric musculoskeletal infectious and inflammatory disorders encountered in clinical practice are discussed.

IMAGING TECHNIQUES

Radiography

Radiography is generally the first imaging modality to be considered when infectious or inflammatory musculoskeletal processes are clinically suspected. It can be often useful for excluding other musculoskeletal causes of patients' symptoms such as fractures and tumors. For evaluation of soft tissue infection, radiography is not necessarily required but may provide valuable information such as demonstrating the presence of soft tissue gas or foreign body. For assessment of bone infection, the sensitivity of radiography ranges from 43% to 75% and its specificity ranges from 75% to 83%.[1] As a result, initial radiographic results are often negative particularly in the early stages of infectious and inflammatory musculoskeletal disorders. For example, radiographic evidence of loss of bone mineralization is not evident on radiographs until the loss reaches 30% to 50%.[2–5] However, radiographs may provide subtle information on early findings of infectious and inflammatory musculoskeletal disorders, which include soft tissue swelling, focal osteopenia, subperiosteal resorption, focal radiolucencies (Fig. 22.1), and periosteal reaction.[2] Therefore, radiographs may provide clues on underlying pathologic conditions and guide subsequent imaging studies for further investigation. In addition, in cases of chronic infectious and inflammatory disorders, radiographs can be helpful in determining the presence, progression, healing, and complications of the process (Figs. 22.2 to 22.4). In more advanced cases, new periosteal bone formation and cortical destruction can also be detected on radiographs.

Ultrasound

Because of its unique ability to clearly visualize soft tissues without potentially harmful radiation, ultrasound (US) is an attractive imaging modality for use in the pediatric population. US examinations are usually easily tolerated even by infants and young children with parents often holding them for maximal comfort. High-resolution musculoskeletal US requires the use of high-frequency linear transducers (10 to 15 MHz), which can provide optimal visualization of superficial and small structures in the pediatric population. If color Doppler is added to the technique, it can help evaluate hyperemia around the periosteum, synovium, and surrounding soft tissue abscesses often associated with infectious and inflammatory disorders.

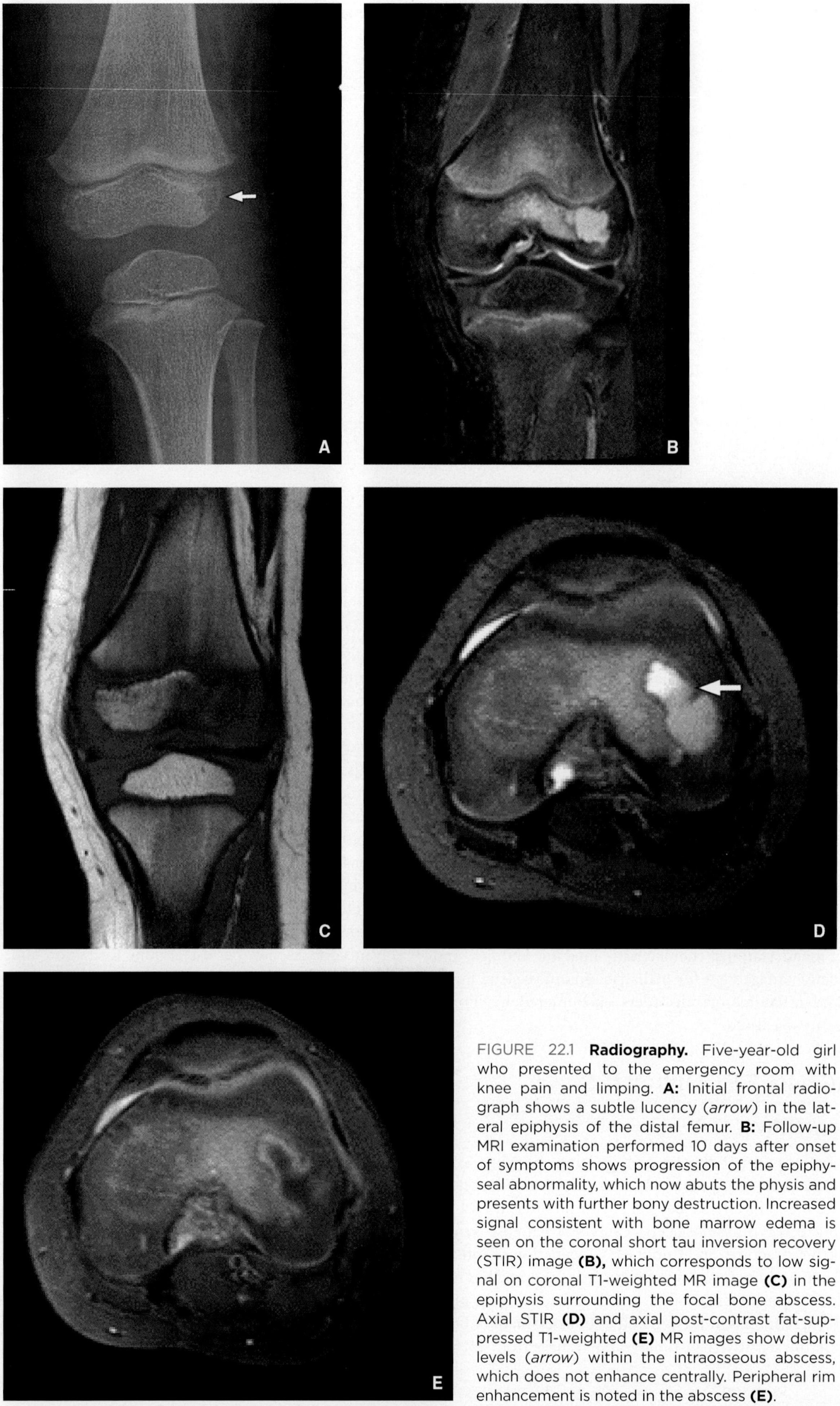

FIGURE 22.1 **Radiography.** Five-year-old girl who presented to the emergency room with knee pain and limping. **A:** Initial frontal radiograph shows a subtle lucency (*arrow*) in the lateral epiphysis of the distal femur. **B:** Follow-up MRI examination performed 10 days after onset of symptoms shows progression of the epiphyseal abnormality, which now abuts the physis and presents with further bony destruction. Increased signal consistent with bone marrow edema is seen on the coronal short tau inversion recovery (STIR) image **(B),** which corresponds to low signal on coronal T1-weighted MR image **(C)** in the epiphysis surrounding the focal bone abscess. Axial STIR **(D)** and axial post-contrast fat-suppressed T1-weighted **(E)** MR images show debris levels (*arrow*) within the intraosseous abscess, which does not enhance centrally. Peripheral rim enhancement is noted in the abscess **(E)**.

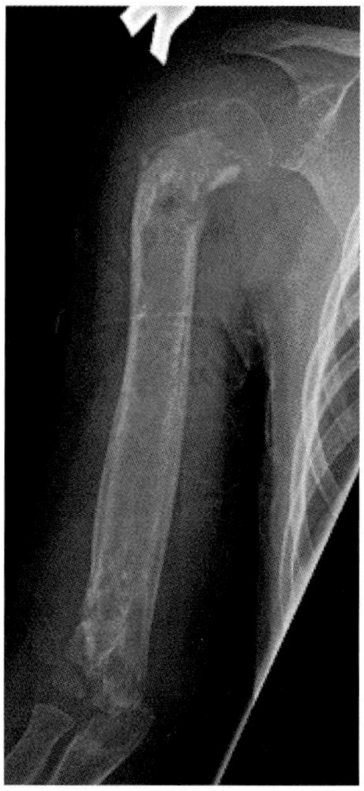

FIGURE 22.2 **Radiographic sequelae of osteomyelitis.** Pathologic fracture through the proximal humerus in a preschool child with sickle cell disease and features of chronic osteomyelitis include diffuse cortical thickening of the diaphysis and bone expansion.

US can show soft tissue abnormalities as early as 2 days after the onset of symptoms.[6] Although US is not typically used for evaluation of cortical bone abnormalities, periosteal elevation or subperiosteal collections presenting as a hypoechoic layer of purulent material can sometimes be evaluated with US (Fig. 22.5). US is useful for diagnosing and following up on soft tissue abscesses, for identifying precipitating factors such as foreign bodies or fistulae, for detecting effusion when transient or septic arthritis is clinically suspected (Fig. 22.6), and for guiding percutaneous drainage of fluid collections associated with infection for therapeutic purposes.[4] In addition, US can be useful for evaluating regions that are complicated by orthopedic instrumentation and therefore might not be well seen with computed tomography (CT) or magnetic resonance imaging (MRI). Furthermore, US can be a valuable imaging modality in pediatric patients for whom MRI is contraindicated.

Computed Tomography

Computed tomography (CT) is an excellent imaging modality for assessing cortical bone and for detecting gas in soft tissues. However, because it is radiation bearing, the use of CT is currently limited in infants and children with underlying musculoskeletal infectious or inflammatory disorders. Overall, MRI is a preferred imaging modality over CT for evaluation of bone or soft tissue infection or inflammation. However, CT may be the only option for infants and young children when sedation is contraindicated and thus, MRI cannot be performed.[4]

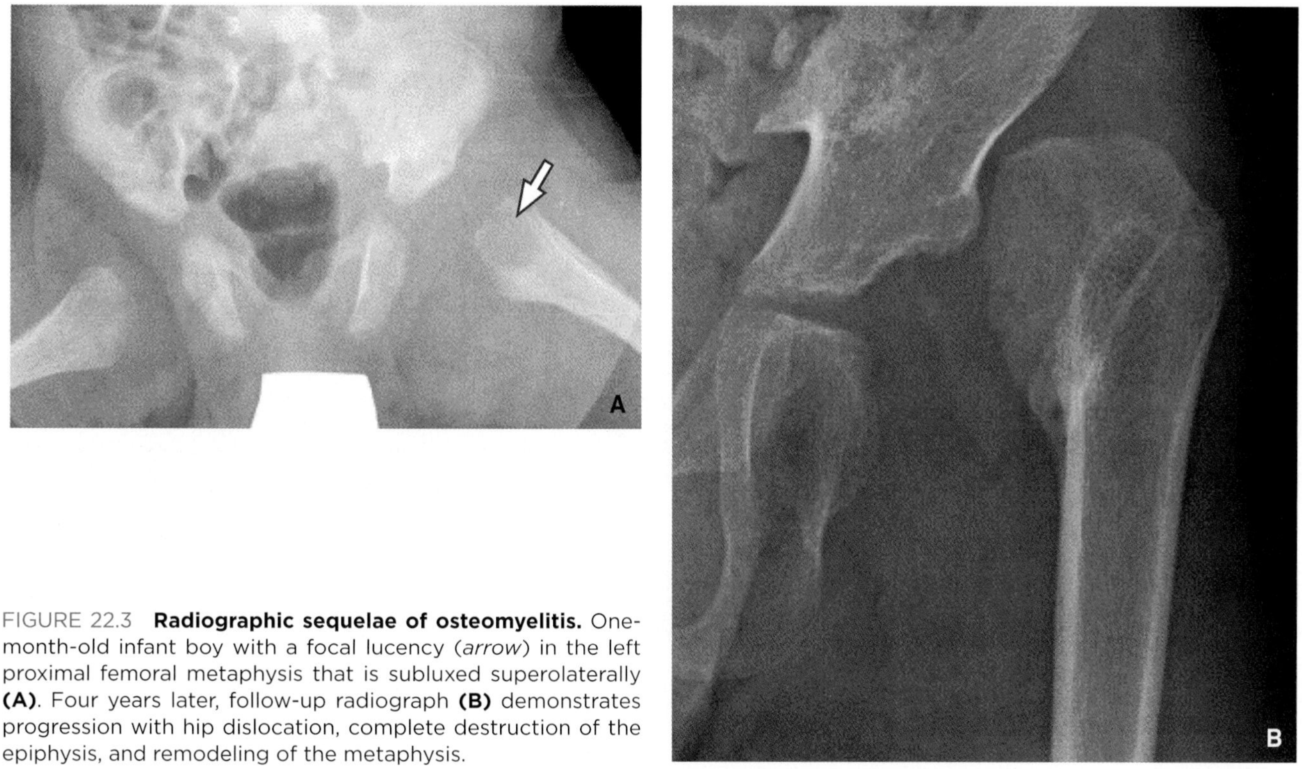

FIGURE 22.3 **Radiographic sequelae of osteomyelitis.** One-month-old infant boy with a focal lucency (*arrow*) in the left proximal femoral metaphysis that is subluxed superolaterally **(A)**. Four years later, follow-up radiograph **(B)** demonstrates progression with hip dislocation, complete destruction of the epiphysis, and remodeling of the metaphysis.

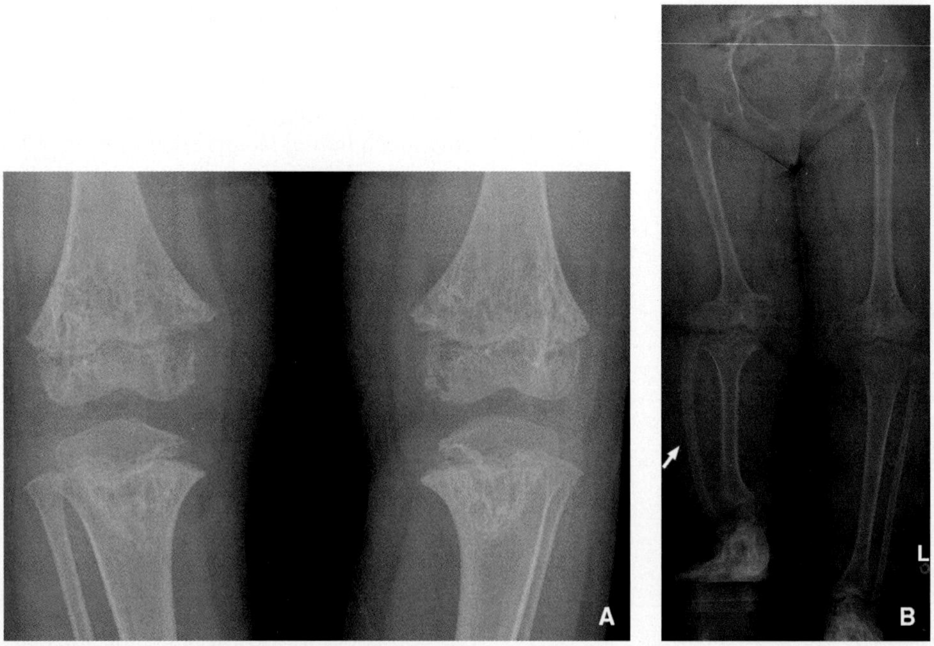

FIGURE 22.4 **Radiographic sequelae of osteomyelitis.** Chronic sequela of meningococcemia in infancy. Frontal radiograph of both knees obtained 3 years after the meningococcemia episode **(A)** shows multiple metaphyseal and epiphyseal lucencies with irregularity of the growth plates. Scanogram of lower extremities obtained a decade later **(B)** shows premature physeal fusion with resultant length discrepancy. Note the fibular bowing (*arrow*) due to tethering from the severely shortened tibia.

The currently available postprocessing techniques including multiplanar and 3D reconstructed CT images allow delineation of even the most subtle osseous changes such as early erosions due to infection or inflammation. CT can also clearly show abnormal thickening of the affected cortical bone, sclerotic changes, encroachment of the medullary cavity, and small draining sinuses in chronic osseous infections. In addition, CT can assist in guiding bone biopsies for diagnosis and draining deep abscesses for treatment. For evaluation of bones alone, intravenous (IV) contrast is not usually needed. However, the use of IV contrast can help better assess the presence and extent of associated soft tissue abnormalities such as abscess formation.

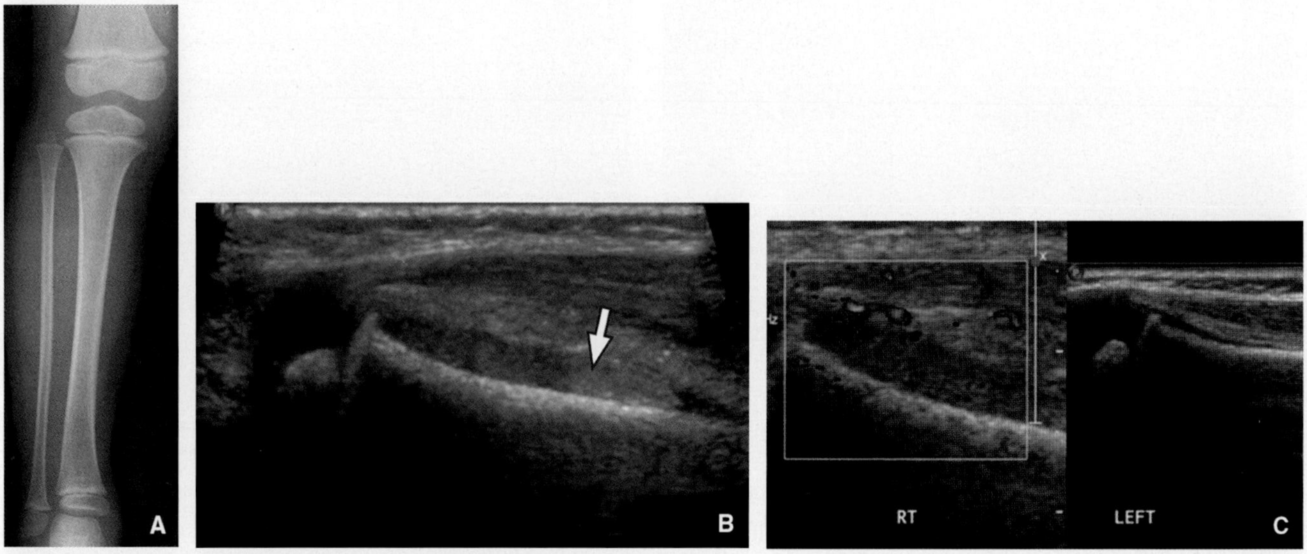

FIGURE 22.5 **Ultrasound.** Normal frontal radiograph of right tibia and fibula in a child with clinical suspicion for osteomyelitis **(A)**. Ultrasound performed on the following day **(B)** shows a large subperiosteal abscess (*arrow*) along the proximal fibular metadiaphysis. Corresponding color Doppler ultrasound imaging **(C)** shows hyperemia in the adjacent soft tissues. The normal contralateral left side is included for comparison.

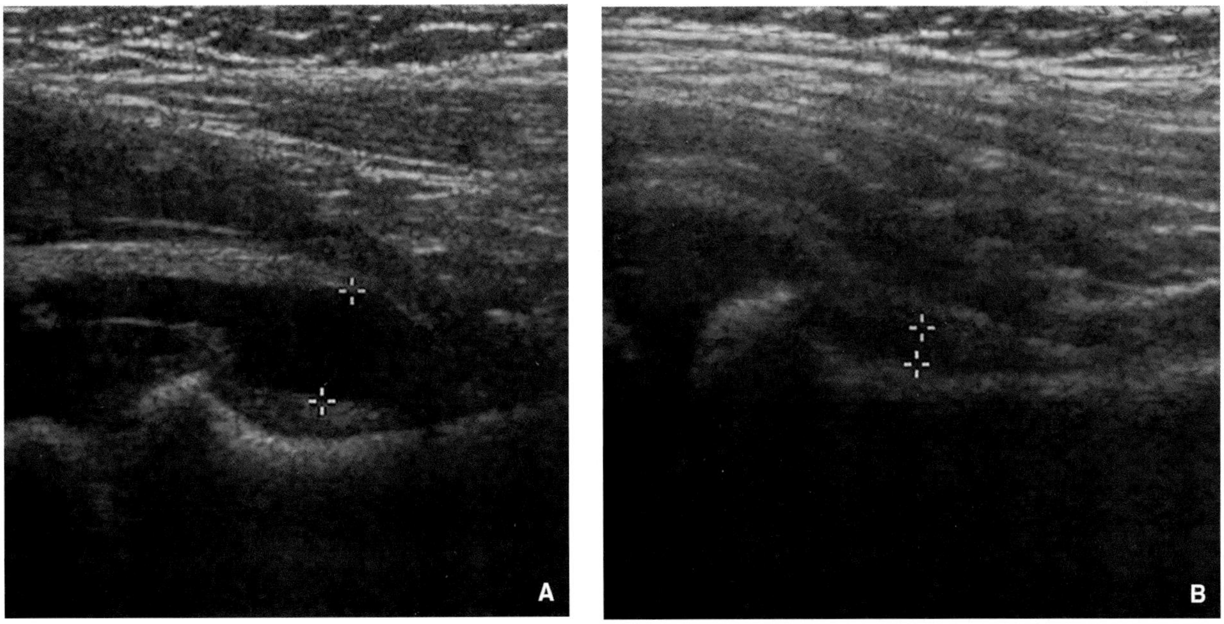

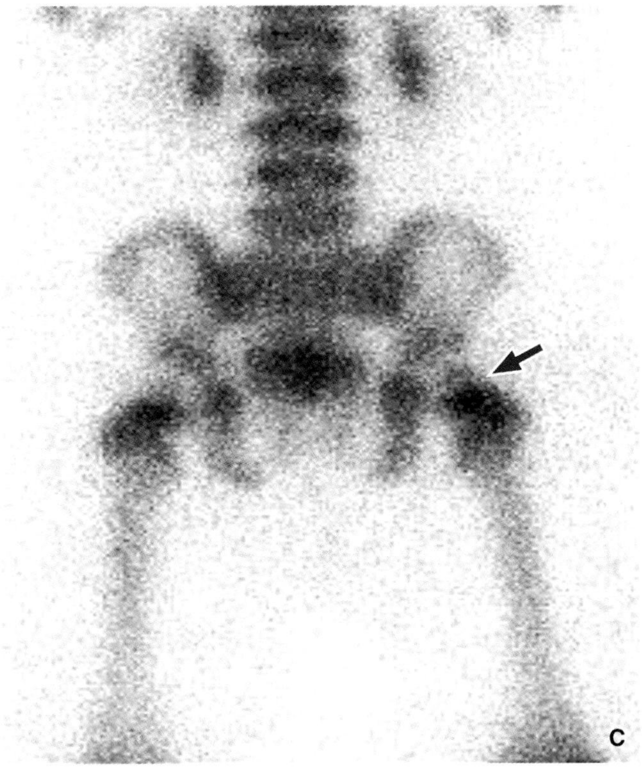

FIGURE 22.6 **Ultrasound and nuclear medicine.** Infant boy who presented with fever, irritability, and lack of mobility of the left lower extremity. Longitudinal gray-scale ultrasound **(A)** shows large effusion (calipers) in the left hip. Ultrasound image of the contralateral asymptomatic hip **(B)** is shown for comparison. Bone scan performed on the same day of the ultrasound scan **(C)** demonstrates increased uptake in the proximal femur and left hip joint (*arrow*) suggesting septic arthritis. Aspiration of pus from the hip joint and culture of the material confirmed the diagnosis.

Magnetic Resonance Imaging

Magnetic resonance imaging (MRI) is currently the only imaging modality with the ability to simultaneously assess all relevant anatomic structures in the setting of musculoskeletal infectious or inflammatory disorders. It is the study of choice when a focal or multifocal area of osteomyelitis is suspected. For detecting soft tissue abnormalities, its specificity is up to 97%[7] and its sensitivity, up to 100%.[8] MRI evaluation can reliably differentiate acute from chronic infection.[9] However, MRI may not be helpful in distinguishing infectious from noninfectious inflammatory processes. Recently, screening for multifocal noninfectious conditions with whole-body MRI has shown promising results.[10] Whole-body MRI has a great potential to become evolved into an established and sensitive imaging modality for the diagnostic workup of pediatric patients with underlying multifocal infectious or inflammatory disorders. With the unique advantage of providing a comprehensive single evaluation of the entire body in a reasonable time without IV contrast or radiation, it is particularly beneficial in the pediatric population. Disadvantages of MRI include its occasional inability to differentiate infectious from reactive inflammation as well as its difficulty with evaluating regions with metallic implants.

The basic MR imaging protocol for investigation of musculoskeletal infectious and inflammatory disorders includes T1 and T2/ short tau inversion recovery (STIR) performed in orthogonal planes. T1-weighted MR imaging is useful for assessment of anatomy and bone marrow. A 3D image acquisition using T1 gradient sequence is useful in the detection of bone erosions, because it allows the generation of multiplanar reconstruction, which adds diagnostic confidence. Fluid-sensitive imaging sequences (T2/STIR) can delineate contrast between normal and abnormal tissue. A gradient echo sequence can be useful to identify hemosiderin, seen as blooming artifacts. The use of gadolinium helps delineate the extent of bone marrow abnormality, differentiate devitalized from vascularized bone, and demonstrate the extent of soft tissue abscesses (Fig. 22.7) and sinus tracts.[11]

Nuclear Medicine

Currently, because of the availability of MRI, nuclear medicine studies are rarely performed for evaluation of infectious or inflammatory disorders particularly in pediatric patients. Nevertheless, they may provide valuable information for children for whom CT or MRI is contraindicated.

Nuclear medicine studies can be of value for evaluating multifocal infections or as a screening imaging modality although they are limited mainly by low spatial resolution. Several nuclear medicine studies are currently available for evaluating pediatric musculoskeletal infectious and inflammatory disorders including technetium-99m methylene diphosphonate (99mTc) bone scan, gallium-67 citrate scan, and indium-111-labeled white blood cell (WBC) scan.

A 99mTc bone scan is usually performed when the area of infection is not well established clinically and the presence of a bone infection is uncertain. It shows elevated blood flow and abnormal increased deposition of tracer at the site of infection (Fig. 22.8). The tracer accumulates in areas of increased vascularity as well as in areas of increased physiologic activity in direct proportion to the destruction of the bone and osteoblastic healing activity. Triple phase (angiographic, blood-pool, delayed-phase) bone scan can be used when the site of acute osteomyelitis is not known or when multifocal points of infection are suspected.[2] A diagnosis of acute osteomyelitis requires tracer activity in all three phases of bone scan.[2] Bone scan is highly sensitive (sensitivity of 85% to 100%) but not particularly specific (specificity of 54% to 96%) for detecting osteomyelitis.[1,12] Both sensitivity and specificity of bone scans can be increased with the use of pinhole collimators and single photon emission computed tomography (SPECT).[13] Because of its variable specificity, bone scan may not be able to distinguish among infection, tumor, and trauma. Furthermore, there can be initial false-negative results secondary to ischemia from vascular compression and thrombosis as well as obscuration of subtle abnormal uptake at the metaphysis by normal high physeal uptake.[11,14]

Indium-111-labeled WBC scan is used in the diagnostic evaluation of occult infections when other imaging modalities are either contraindicated or noninformative. Labeled leukocytes migrate to and accumulate at sites of inflammation, which are then visualized on nuclear medicine imaging.[15] ^{111}In-labeled WBC scans detect localized inflammation but do not clearly distinguish between infectious and noninfectious inflammatory processes.[15] They have been used in the diagnostic evaluation of fever of unknown origin, prosthetic joint infections, and vascular graft infections.

Gallium-67 citrate scan is more specific than 99mTc bone scan for assessment of chronic osteomyelitis, but false positives occur in conditions such as healing fractures, noninfected prosthesis, and tumors.[16] Gallium scan uses radiogallium, which attaches to transferrin and leaks from the bloodstream to the regions of inflammation showing increased isotope uptake in sterile inflammatory conditions, infection, and malignancy.[16] It is often performed in conjunction with bone scan. One limitation of the use of gallium scan is that it does not show bone detail particularly well and may not distinguish well between bone and nearby soft tissue inflammation. In addition, gallium scan involves a higher dose of radiation and requires a longer scanning time than does 99mTc bone scan, making it less appropriate for use in the pediatric population. Gallium scan can take up to 48 hours to be completed, whereas bone scan typically takes up to 3 hours with a delayed view at 24 hours, if necessary.[16]

Fluorodeoxyglucose Positron Emission Tomography

Fluorodeoxyglucose positron emission tomography-CT (FDG PET-CT) is currently widely used for pediatric patients with cancer but is rarely used to diagnose bone infections. However, its use has been demonstrated in evaluating multifocal areas of infection in chronic osteomyelitis.[10]

BONE INFECTIONS

Bacterial Agents

Osteomyelitis

Osteomyelitis is a common pediatric infection that affects cortical bone and bone marrow. It has an incidence of 1 in 5,000 pediatric cases and causes considerable morbidity and sequelae in the pediatric population.[17] Approximately 50% of bone infections occur in patients younger than 5 years.[18–20]

Pathophysiology

The route of infection is usually hematogenous in children, with direct inoculation from trauma or from a surrounding soft tissue infection seen occasionally.[11,20,21] The location

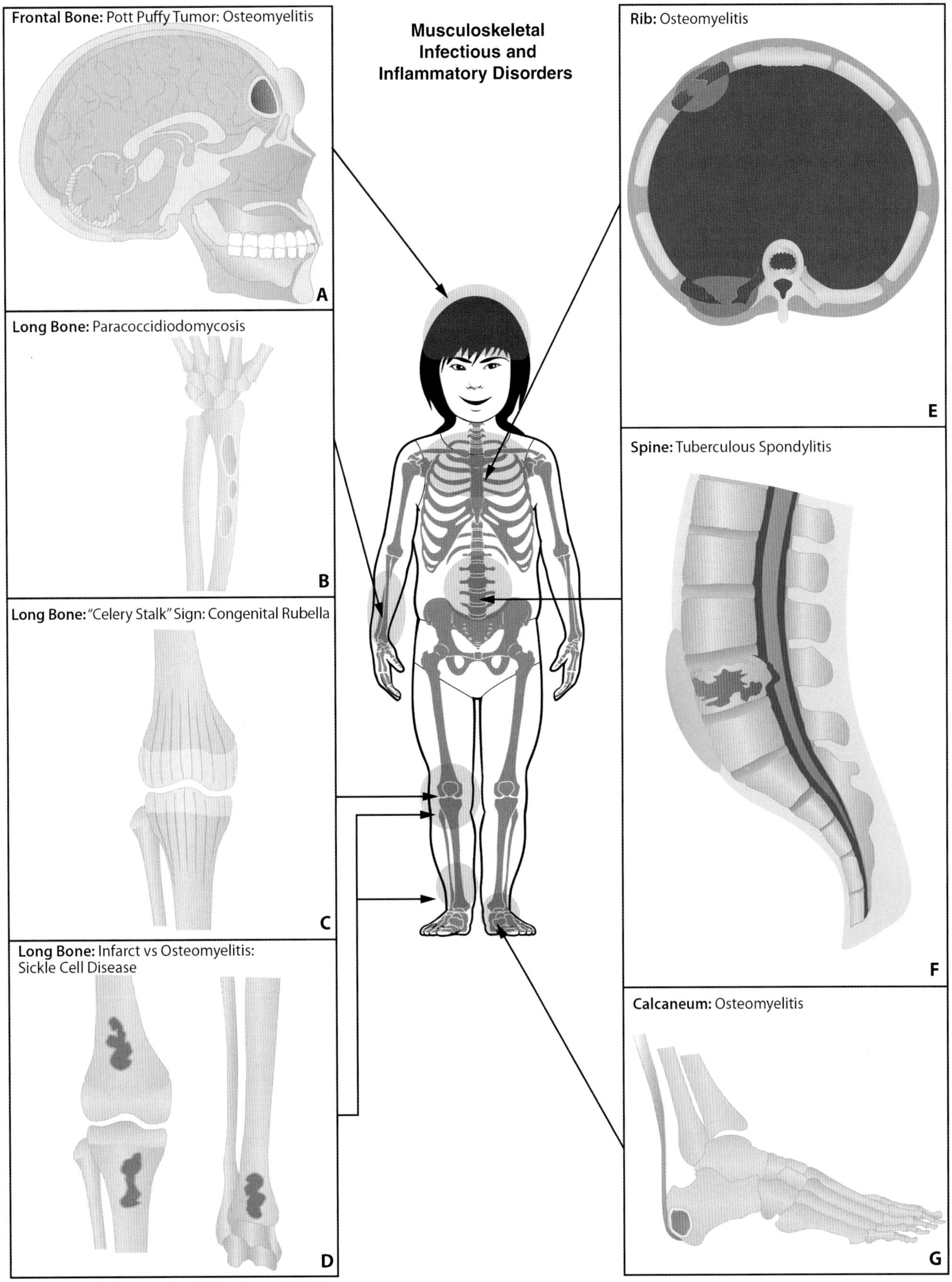
Musculoskeletal Infectious and Inflammatory Disorders
Frontal Bone: Pott Puffy Tumor: Osteomyelitis
A
Long Bone: Paracoccidiodomycosis
B
Long Bone: "Celery Stalk" Sign: Congenital Rubella
C
Long Bone: Infarct vs Osteomyelitis: Sickle Cell Disease
D
Rib: Osteomyelitis
E
Spine: Tuberculous Spondylitis
F
Calcaneum: Osteomyelitis
G

of osteomyelitis depends on the patient's age, affecting most commonly the epiphysis in neonates and infants and the metaphysis in older children. Hematogenous infection typically begins in the metaphysis secondary to its abundant blood supply. Patterns of spread of infection change with varying age groups because of differences in the microanatomy of the vascular supply with growth (Fig. 22.9).[22,23]

Trueta describes three different types of metaphyseal–epiphyseal vascularity according to age groups.[24] In infants younger than 1 year of age (Fig. 22.10), infection can easily spread to the epiphysis (Fig. 22.7) and joint secondary to transphyseal bridging vessels that extend from the metaphysis to the epiphysis. This allows bacteria to spread into the epiphysis and from there into the articular space. Infections in epiphyseal-equivalent regions are also common in this age group for this reason. After 1 year of age, epiphyseal and joint involvement is less commonly seen because the blood supply between the metaphysis and epiphysis is severed. After the transphyseal vessels close (by the time the secondary ossification centers develop), the metaphysis becomes the primary focus of infection, and the infection may then spread into the subperiosteum and adjacent soft tissues. If the infection progresses, it becomes subacute or chronic. After physeal closure occurs in adolescence (Fig. 22.10), the vascular connectivity is restored and the epiphysis and joint become susceptible to infection again.[11,21]

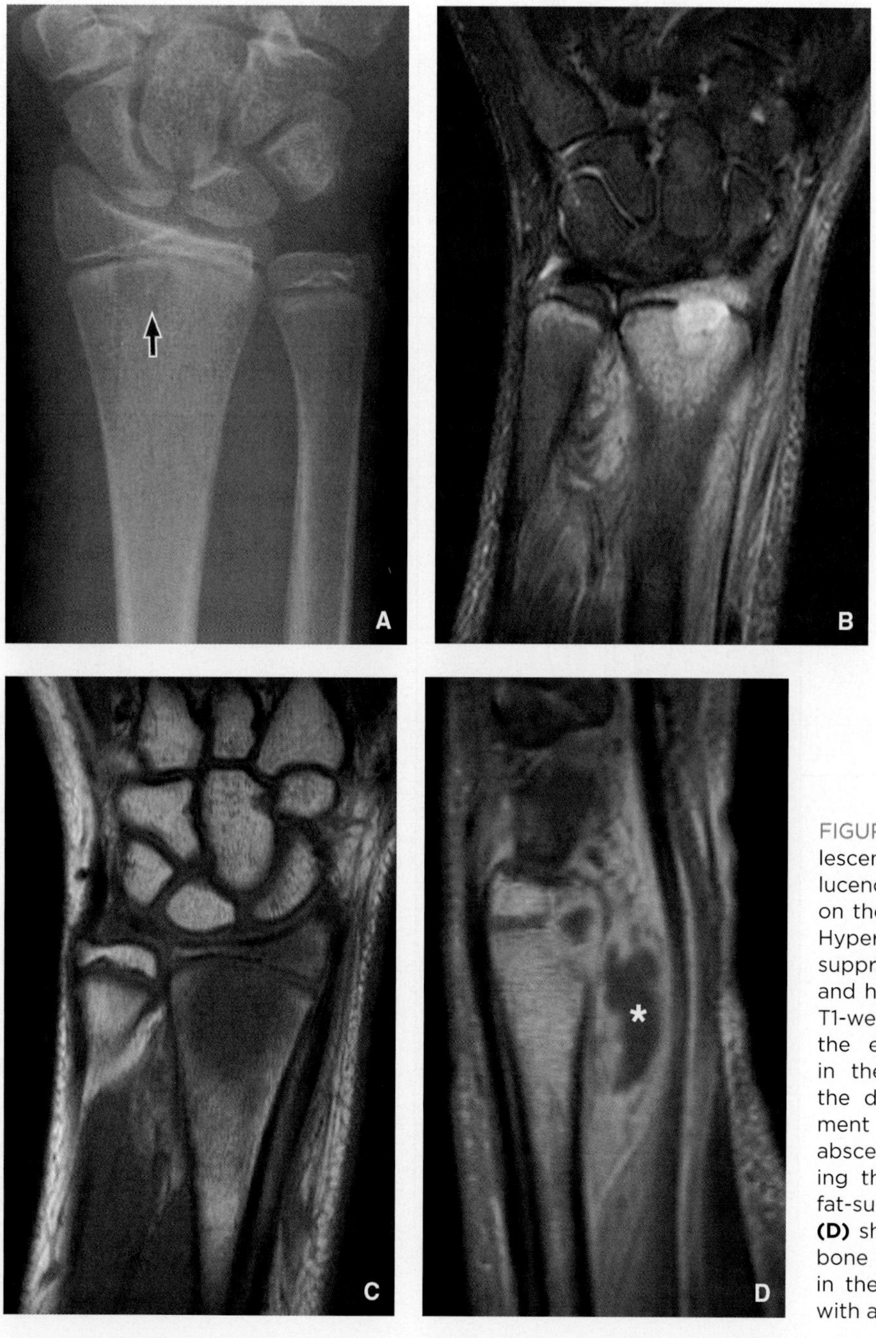

FIGURE 22.7 **MR imaging.** Preadolescent girl with a focal metaphyseal lucency (*arrow*) in the distal radius on the frontal radiograph of wrist **(A)**. Hyperintense signal on the coronal fat-suppressed T2-weighted MR image **(B)** and hypointense signal on the coronal T1-weighted MR image **(C)** highlight the extensive bone marrow edema in the metaphysis and epiphysis of the distal radius. Epiphyseal involvement is related to the metaphyseal abscess, which is also seen penetrating the physis. Sagittal post-contrast fat-suppressed T2-weighted MR image **(D)** shows diffuse enhancement in the bone marrow and rim enhancement in the transphyseal abscess (*asterisk*) with associated pyomyositis.

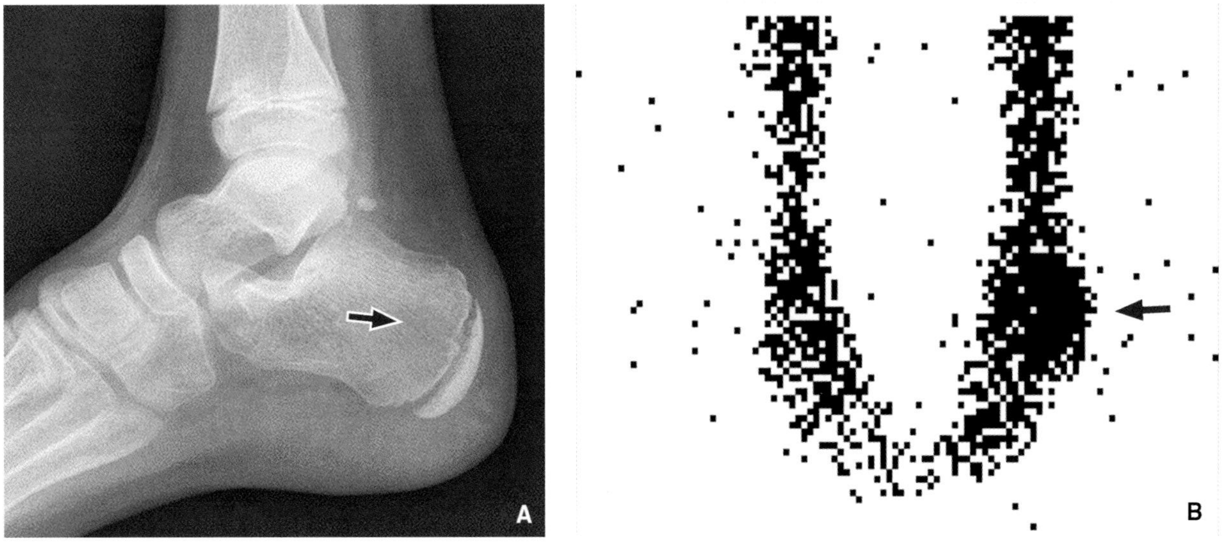

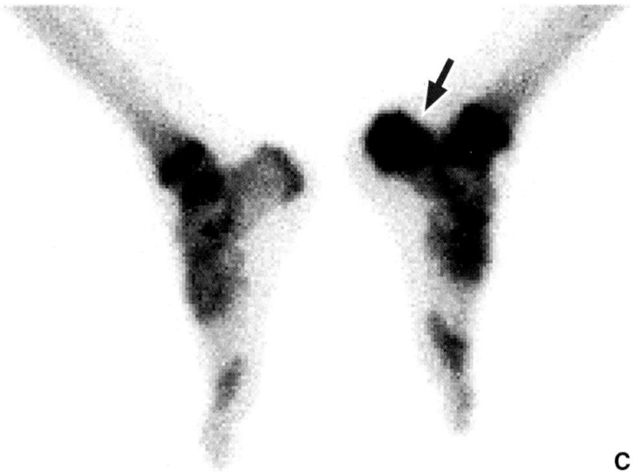

FIGURE 22.8 **Nuclear medicine.** Lateral radiographic view of the foot **(A)** demonstrates a subtle lucency (*arrow*) in the calcaneus in a child who presented with pain and swelling. Flow **(B)** and blood pool **(C)** images from the technetium 99-MDP bone scan confirm increased uptake (*arrow*) in the body of the calcaneus consistent with osteomyelitis.

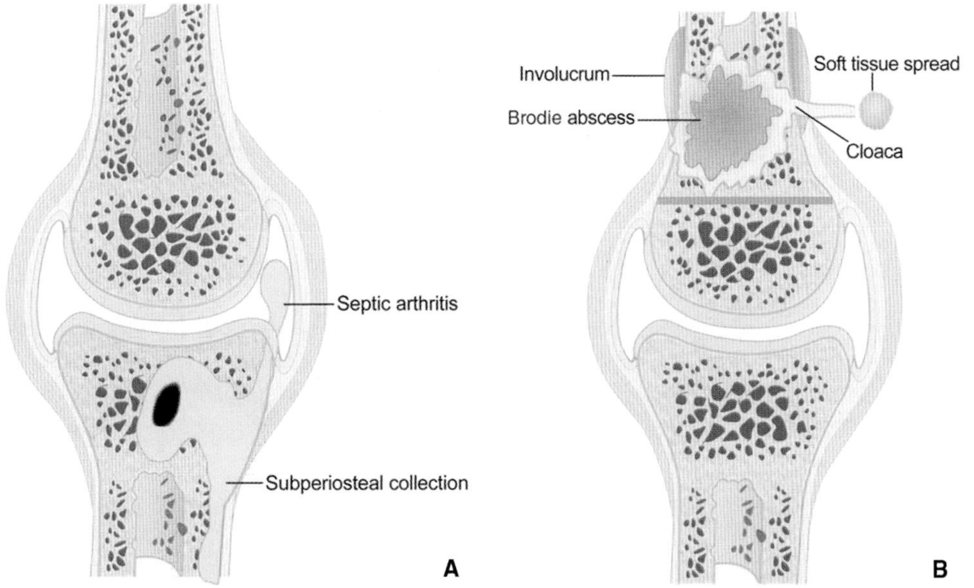

FIGURE 22.9 **Modes of spread of infection. A:** In an infant: Infection originating in the highly vascularized metaphysis can extend into the epiphysis via patent transphyseal vessels. If it spreads into the joint, it results in septic arthritis. If it extends underneath the periosteum, it results in a subperiosteal abscess (collection). **B:** In an older child: Subacute osteomyelitis demonstrates a Brodie abscess surrounded by a local involucrum. In chronic osteomyelitis, spread of infection into the soft tissues following cortical damage can occur through a cloaca.

Clinical and Laboratory Findings

In the pediatric population, the symptoms of acute osteomyelitis generally include fever, local tenderness, and swelling. Symptoms in the neonate may be far more subtle, manifesting only as limited limb motion. Inflammatory markers such as C-reactive protein and erythrocyte sedimentation rate are elevated in 80% to 92% of cases.[19] The WBC count is usually high in musculoskeletal infections but can be normal in 40% of osteomyelitis patients. Biopsy specimens may lack diagnostic findings, and they have variable success in recovering a responsible organism, which occurs in only 48% to 85% of specimens submitted for culture.[19] The low specificity of the clinical and laboratory findings makes imaging a crucial tool in the diagnosis of acute osteomyelitis.

Etiopathogenesis

Hematogenous infections of osteomyelitis are primarily bacterial in origin, with *Staphylococcus aureus (S. aureus)* being the most common organism followed by *Streptococcus* species, pneumococcus species, *Haemophilus influenzae*, and less commonly methicillin-resistant *S. aureus* (MRSA), gram-negative (*Kingella kingae [K. kingae]*) bacteria, mycobacteria (tuberculosis), fungi, parasites, and viruses.[22]

In MRSA infections, affected pediatric patients heal slowly and are more prone to develop sequelae such as limb shortening, coxa plana, and coxa valga.[22] *Pseudomonas* infection is more commonly seen in IV drug users and in patients with diabetes and is usually concurrent with other infections such as those caused by *S. aureus*, *Streptococcus*, *Escherichia coli*, and *Klebsiella*. Other underlying conditions predisposing to bone infections are meningococcemia, sickle cell disease, immunodeficiency, and varicella.[19] In the past, infections by *H. influenzae* were common in children younger than 2 years of age.[23] However, vaccination has significantly decreased the incidence of *H. influenzae*. Emphysematous osteomyelitis has been described in monomicrobial and polymicrobial bone infections and is characterized by the presence of gas in the bone marrow. Monomicrobial infections are usually hematogenous, whereas polymicrobial infections are usually related to the contiguous spread from infected soft tissues.[20]

Acute Osteomyelitis

Acute hematogenous osteomyelitis is the most common form of bone infection in the pediatric population. Acute osseous infection results in extensive inflammatory response and leads to increased intraosseous pressure, blood stasis, thrombosis, and subsequent bone necrosis.[5,21]

In early stages of osteomyelitis, ill-defined bony radiolucencies are often observed on radiographs. Later on, cortical destruction, periosteal elevation, and spread of infection into the adjacent soft tissues are typical. Periosteal elevation accompanying osteomyelitis is more pronounced in children than in adults because of the loose attachment of the periosteum to bone in children.[5]

On MRI, acute osteomyelitis is represented by areas of bone marrow edema, most frequently seen in the metaphysis of the long bones (Table 22.1). Bone marrow edema, which

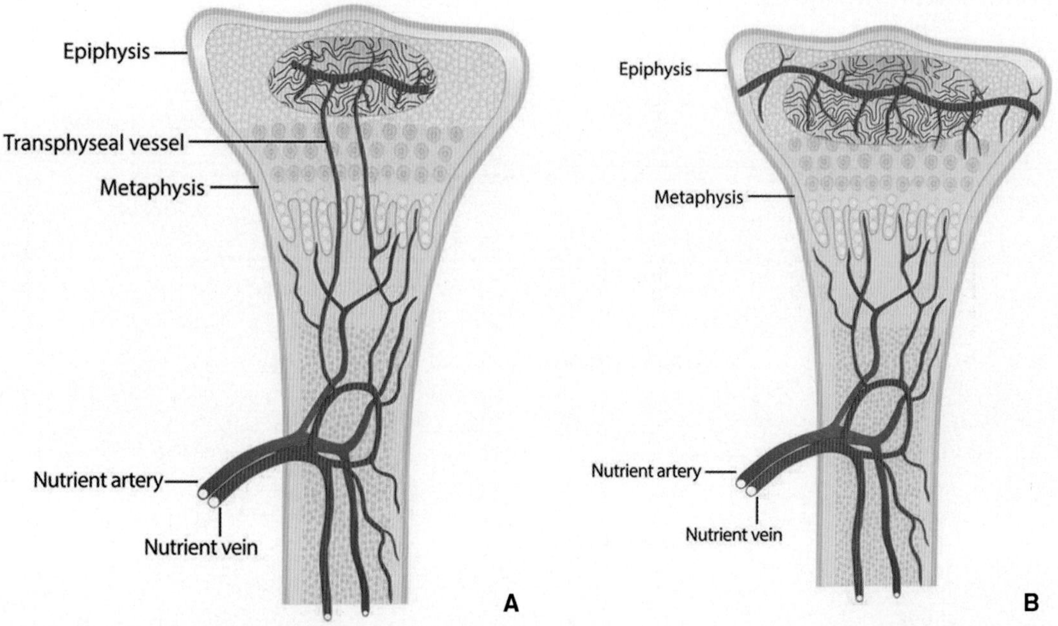

FIGURE 22.10 **Modes of spread of infection. A:** Infant blood supply demonstrates continuity of the metaphyseal and epiphyseal vasculature through the presence of transphyseal vessels, allowing a pathway for spread of infection. **B:** In the preschool child and adolescent, the transphyseal vessels are no longer patent; thus, the physis acts as a barrier to the spread of infection into the epiphysis.

TABLE 22.1 Osteomyelitis: Definitions

Disorder	Definition
Acute osteomyelitis	Acute infection of bone and bone marrow; usually caused by bacteria from hematogenous infection.
Subacute osteomyelitis	Bone infection lasting >4 weeks and <3 months; classic presentation, a Brodie abscess.
Chronic osteomyelitis	Bone infection lasting at least 3 months; sequestrum, involucrum, and cloaca can be present in this phase of the infection.
Brodie abscess	Subacute osteomyelitis; well-defined lytic lesion that corresponds to bone necrosis surrounded by a fibrous granulation tissue.
Sequestrum	A piece of nonresorbed devascularized infarcted bone surrounded by new bone.
Involucrum	Periosteal new bone formation caused by chronic infection or inflammation over necrotic bone.
Cloaca	An opening tract from the cortex of bone.
Chronic recurrent multifocal osteomyelitis (CRMO)	A noninfectious, inflammatory disorder of bone.

can be an initial sign of osteomyelitis, appears hypointense on T1-weighted MR images and hyperintense on T2-weighted MR images. With the administration of contrast, infected bone marrow typically enhances.[16] MRI may also demonstrate regional periosteal reaction, which is caused by disrupted vascular connections that elevate the periosteum and cause new layers of periosteum (involucrum) to form.[24] Spread of infection with involvement of soft tissues is manifested as increased signal intensity on T2-weighted MR images. When an abscess forms within the bone, the marrow signal intensity becomes heterogeneous, and with contrast administration, the rim of the abscess can enhance (Fig. 22.7).

Subacute Osteomyelitis

Subacute osteomyelitis is considered when the diagnosis of infection is made between 1 and 4 weeks from the onset of symptoms.[19] It remains localized either by the low virulence of the organism or increased host resistance.[21] The development of subacute osteomyelitis seems to depend on the interplay between the infecting bacteria and the immune system of the host and represents a favorable host-pathogenic response.[9]

If the infection continuously evolves, it can extend into the bone marrow, generating an intraosseous abscess called Brodie abscess (Table 22.1; Fig. 22.11). Typical radiographic features of Brodie abscess, which is usually located in the metaphysis, consist of a localized destructive lucent bone lesion with a surrounding sclerotic rim with variable thickness. On MRI, Brodie abscess has a characteristic target appearance with four distinct layers. A central abscess cavity appears hypointense on T1-weighted and hyperintense on

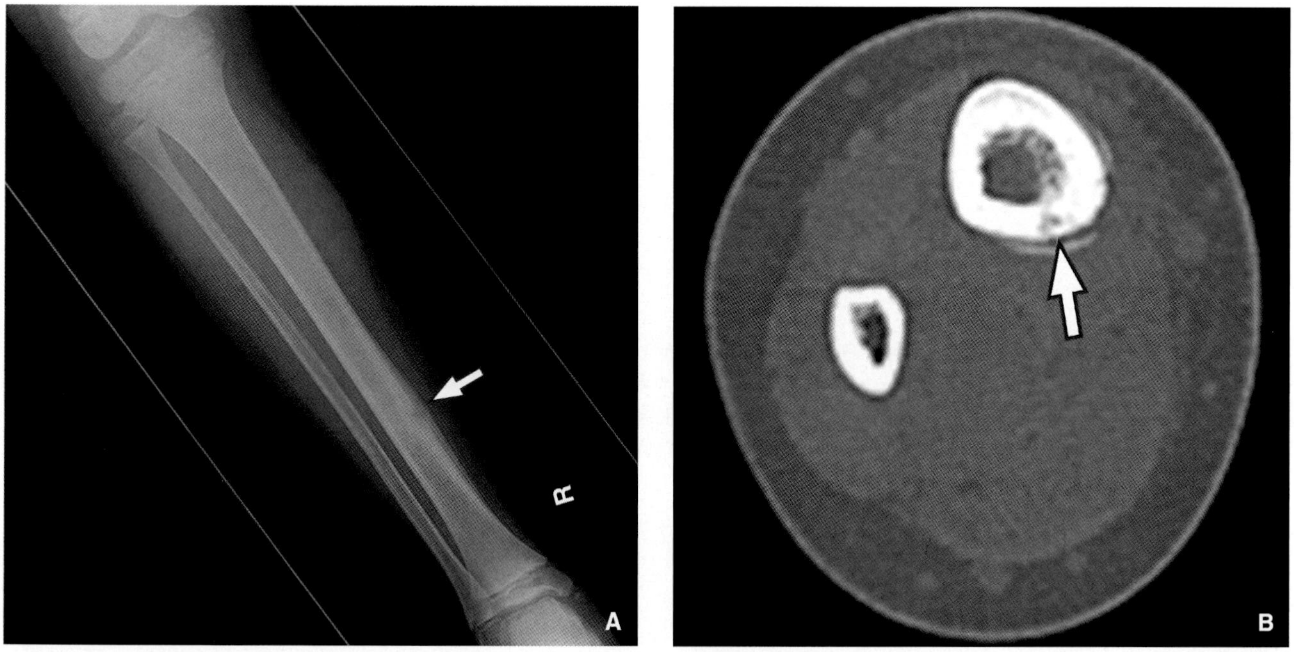

FIGURE 22.11 **Brodie abscess.** Frontal radiograph **(A)** of the tibia and fibula of an 8-year-old boy with a Brodie abscess shows a lytic tibial diaphyseal lesion (*arrow*) with associated periosteal reaction best seen on the axial CT image **(B)**.

(Continued)

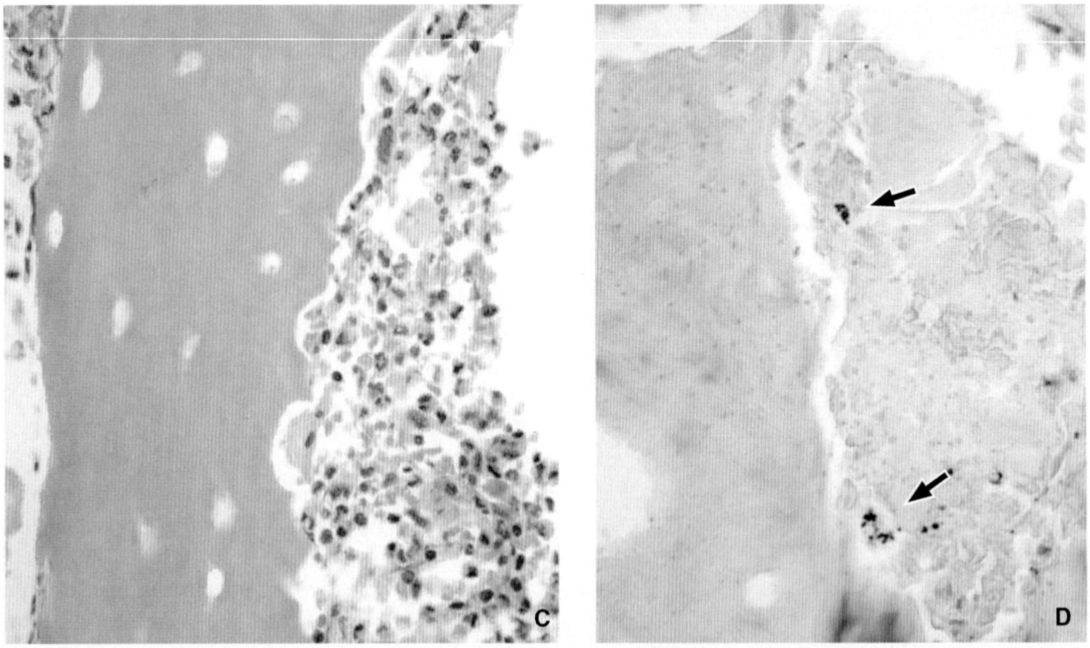

FIGURE 22.11 (*Continued*) Corresponding histologic slides show pus surrounding resorbing scalloped necrotic bone **(C,** hematoxylin and eosin, original magnification, 600×), and clusters of gram-positive cocci (*arrows*) seen within the purulent material **(D,** Brown-Brenn stain, original magnification, 600×). This infection was subacute, having been partially treated by the parents with leftover antibiotics from their medicine cabinet before seeking medical attention.

T2-weighted MR images. Surrounding the cavity is a layer of highly vascularized granulation tissue that appears isointense on T1-weighted and hyperintense on T2-weighted MR images (Fig. 22.12). This layer is best visualized on contrast-enhanced MR images because the halo enhancement corresponds to granulation tissue. Next is a fibrous layer that demonstrates low signal intensity on all MR sequences. The outer halo is composed of a peripheral rim of endosteal reaction and sclerosis that has low signal on T1-weighted and T2-weighted MR images.[25] The halo enhancement on postcontrast MR images corresponds to granulation tissue. The bone marrow edema that usually surrounds the abscess

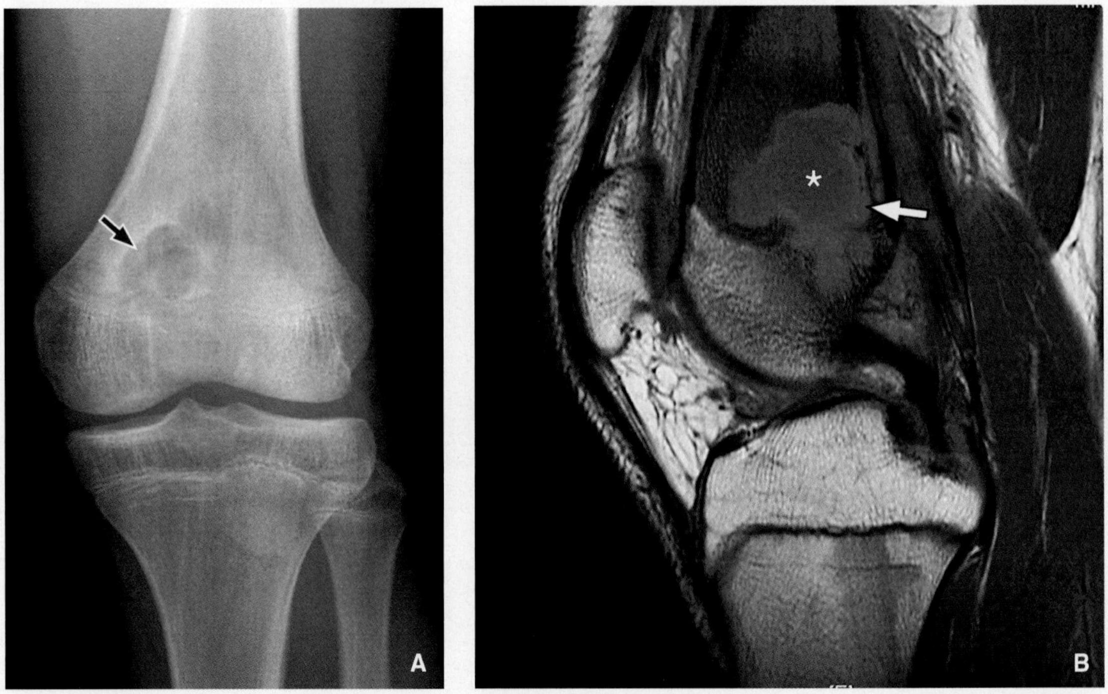

FIGURE 22.12 **Brodie abscess.** Frontal radiograph of the left femur **(A)** shows a geographic lytic lesion (*arrow*) with sclerotic borders in the distal metaphysis. Sagittal proton density-weighted MR image of the corresponding knee **(B)** demonstrates the typical target appearance of a Brodie abscess (*asterisk*) with a hypointnse center (intraosseous abscess), a hyperintense inner ring of vascular granulation tissue (*arrow*) and an outer ring of low signal fibrotic tissue and sclerosis.

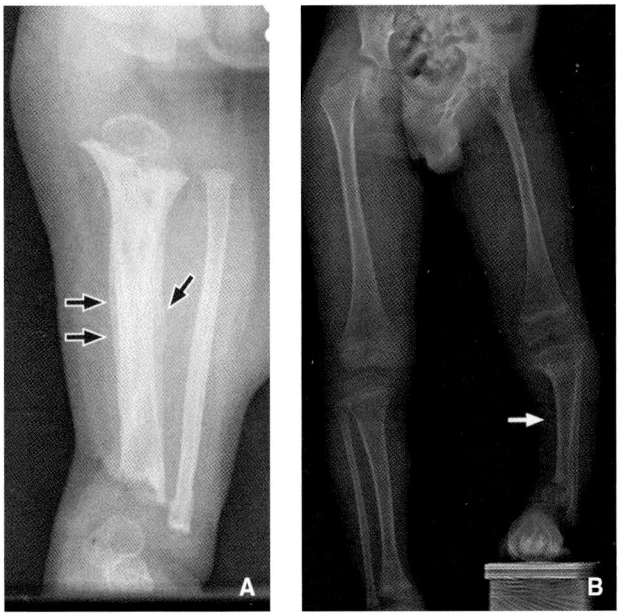

FIGURE 22.13 **Features of chronic osteomyelitis.** Frontal radiograph of the tibia and fibula **(A)** shows diffuse sclerosis, remodeling, and periosteal reaction extensively involving mainly the left tibia (*arrows*) of an 8-month-old infant boy representing chronic osteomyelitis. Frontal radiograph of the region of interest obtained 4 years later **(B)** demonstrates multifocal bone bridging resulting in overall shortening of the left tibia (*arrow*), marked length discrepancy, and varus alignment, as complications.

appears hypointense on T1-weighted and hyperintense on T2-weighted MR images.[10,26] Brodie abscess is managed with curettage and often lengthy antibiotic treatment.[27]

Chronic Osteomyelitis

Chronic osteomyelitis can result from an untreated acute infection or a low-grade continuous infection persistent for at least 3 months, and most frequently, lasting 6 months or longer.[28] It occurs more commonly in developing countries and is associated with significant morbidity and sequelae (Table 22.1).[29] Because of its insidious onset, mild symptoms, lack of systemic reaction, and often inconsistent supportive laboratory data, chronic osteomyelitis may mimic various benign and malignant conditions, resulting in delayed diagnosis and treatment.[30] Sequelae of chronic osteomyelitis include physeal destruction with growth arrest, angular deformities, ankylosis, and leg-length discrepancies (Fig. 22.13).[31]

Imaging features of chronic osteomyelitis include bone sclerosis (Fig. 22.13) with underlying bone resorption and cystic changes.[21] Alternatively, complications such as the formation of a sequestrum (necrotic bone with new bone applied to its surface), involucrum (thick periosteal bone formation surrounding a sequestrum), or cloaca (draining fistula between bone marrow and periosteum) (Fig. 22.14) may occur. At this chronic stage, MRI findings of osteomyelitis include heterogeneity of the bone marrow signal on

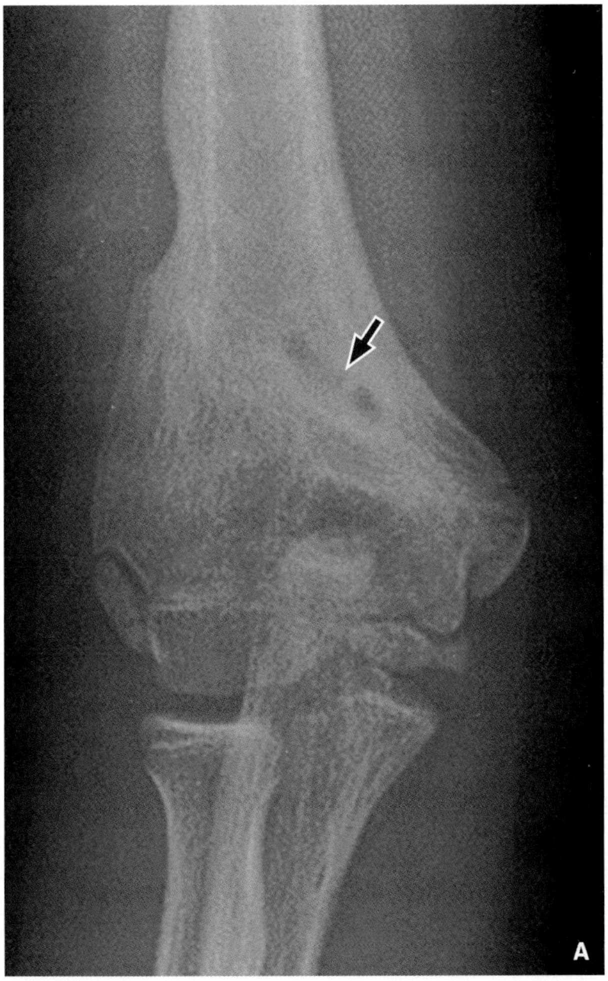

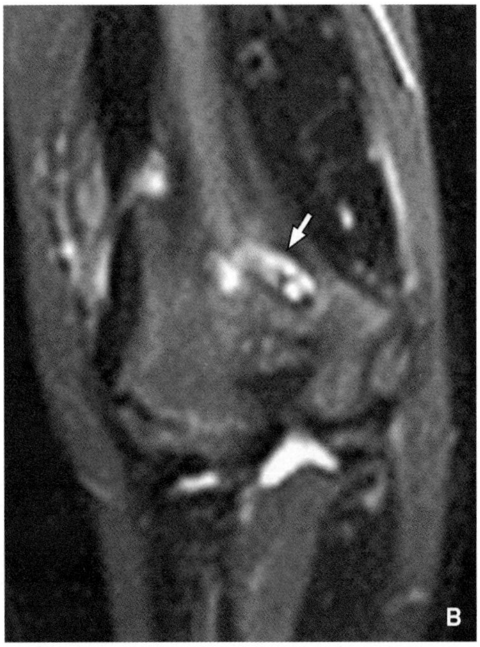

FIGURE 22.14 **Features of chronic osteomyelitis.** Frontal radiograph of the distal humerus of a 12-year-old boy who had undergone pinning of a supracondylar fracture 2 years previously **(A)** shows sclerosis, cortical thickening, and cloaca (*arrow*). Coronal fat-suppressed T2-weighted MR image **(B)** demonstrates an intraosseous abscess with a cloaca (*arrow*) extending superolaterally into a soft tissue abscess.

(Continued)

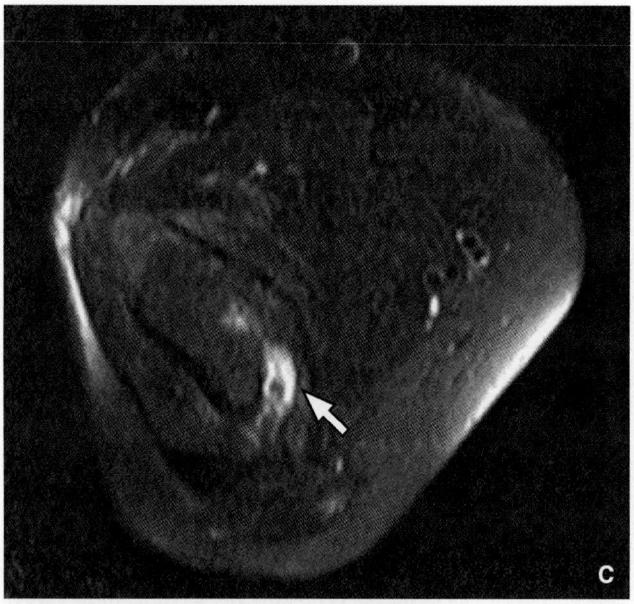

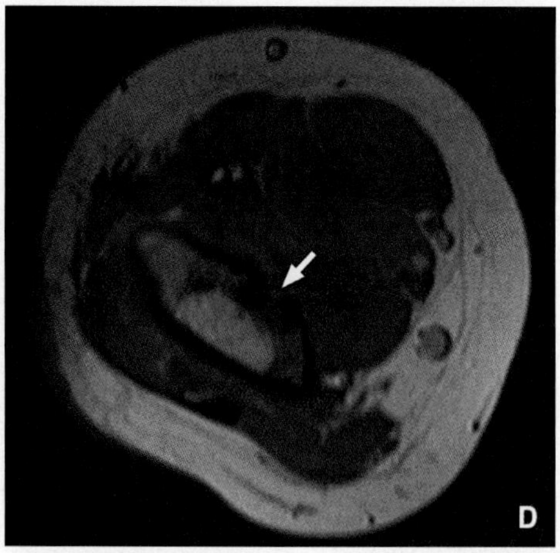

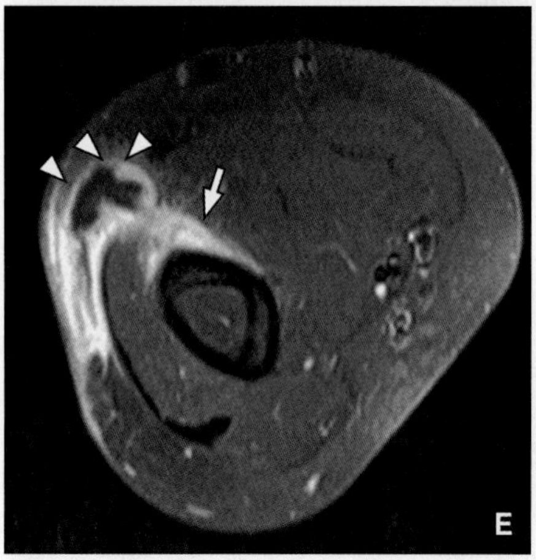

FIGURE 22.14 (*Continued*) A low-signal sequestrum (*arrow*) is seen centrally in the hyperintense osseous abscess on the axial fat-suppressed T2-weighted MR image **(C)**. Axial T1-weighted MR image **(D)** depicts the cloaca (arrow) along the anterior cortex. Axial post-contrast fat-suppressed T1-weighted MR image **(E)** shows the path of the soft tissue component of the abscess (*arrowheads*) tracking through the anterior cortex superficially (*arrow*) dissecting into the subcutaneous soft tissues.

T1- and T2-weighted MR images, with areas of increased and decreased signal intensity. Gradient-echo MR sequences can be helpful for delineation of sequestra, periosteal reaction, and involucrum because susceptibility artifacts from mineralization are exaggerated. Areas of chronic fibrosis or dead bone (including sequestrum) have low signal intensity on both T1- and T2-weighted MR images, which do not enhance with contrast. A sequestrum may be surrounded by tissue that has high-signal intensity on T1- and T2-weighted MR image and enhances with contrast (Fig. 22.14). An involucrum appears as cortical thickening with healing (Table 22.1). If the infection persists, a sinus tract or cloaca can drain pus into the adjacent soft tissues (Fig. 22.15).

Pediatric patients with chronic osteomyelitis usually require further evaluation with bone scan and MRI in order to assess their response to treatment and chronic complications such as soft tissue abscess or fistula formation. In order to detect sequestra or cortical thickening in chronic stages of osteomyelitis for guiding biopsy or debridement, radiologists should consider using CT over MRI.[16]

In summary, MR imaging features of chronic osteomyelitis usually include the following:

1. Bone marrow edema with or without associated enhancement.
2. Focal cortical destruction and associated periosteal elevation.
3. Associated intraosseous or juxtacortical soft tissue abscesses or edema.
4. Cloaca (bone marrow to periosteum) or sinus tract formation.
5. Sequestrum or involucrum formation.

Differential Diagnosis

Clinically acute, subacute, and chronic forms of osteomyelitis may have radiologic features that overlap with each other. The differential diagnosis for all of these forms includes primary bone tumors, particularly Langerhans cell histiocytosis, Ewing sarcoma, and lymphoma.[30] In contrast to osteomyelitis, in the absence of recent pathologic fracture, untreated primary tumors of bone usually do not have loculated fluid collections. Cortical destruction in tumors tends to be diffuse rather than focal. The degree of surrounding edema

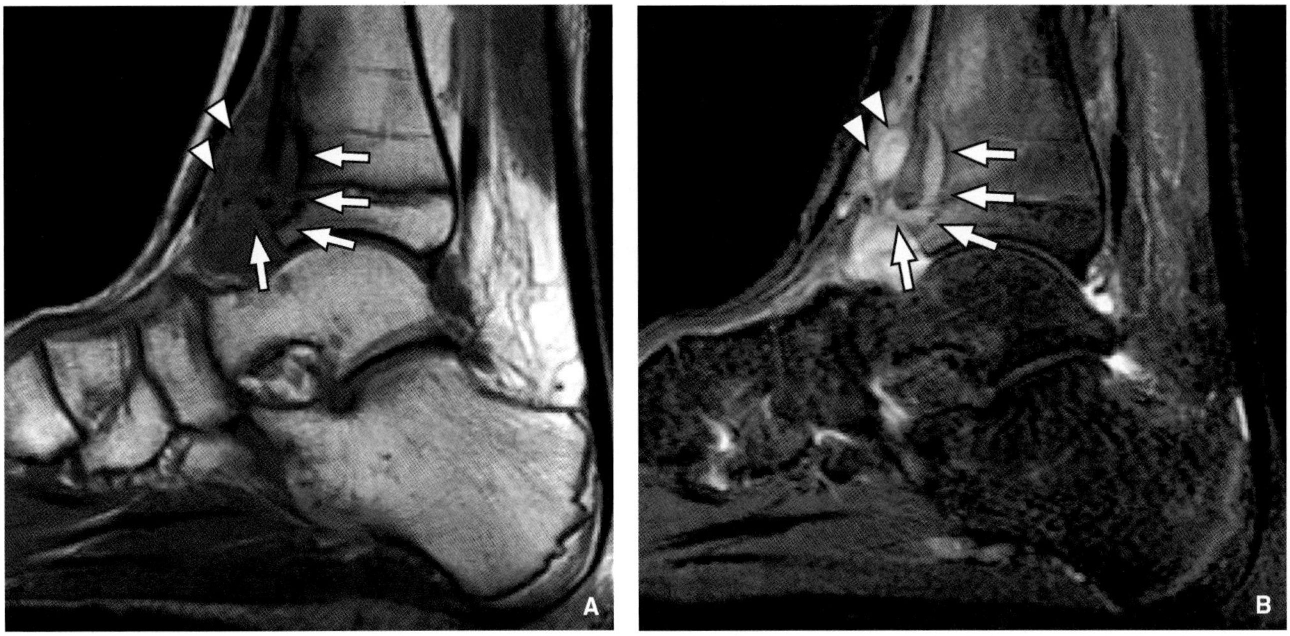

FIGURE 22.15 **Features of chronic osteomyelitis.** Sagittal T1-weighted **(A)** and inversion recovery **(B)** MR images of the ankle of a 10-year-old boy show a sinus tract, which is hypo-/isointense on T1-weighted MR image and hyperintense on T2-weighted MR image with a low signal sclerotic border. It extends from the distal tibial metaphysis into the epiphysis and through the anterior cortex into the soft tissues (*arrows*) with an associated soft tissue collection (*arrowheads*).

related to primary tumors of bone is typically substantially less compared with mass-like edema related to granulation tissue from osteomyelitis.

Treatment

Successful treatment of osteomyelitis is predicated upon timely diagnosis, accurate identification of the offending organism(s), prompt initiation of antibiotic therapy, and surgical debridement if necessary. Although the optimal duration of antibiotic therapy remains undefined, most recommend treatment for ~6 weeks for acute osteomyelitis and for 1 to 2 months, or possibly as long as 2 years, for chronic osteomyelitis.[27,31] In addition to antibiotic treatment, chronic osteomyelitis may require surgery to remove infected tissue and high-dose injectable antibiotic therapy.

Specific Locations of Osteomyelitis

Epiphyseal Osteomyelitis

Epiphyseal osteomyelitis is secondary to transphyseal vascular channels that extend from the metaphysis across the physis into the epiphysis. It is typically seen in patients younger than 18 months of age.[32] Subsequently, the development of the growth plate acts as a barrier to the spread of infection from the metaphysis. Nevertheless, although rare, epiphyseal osteomyelitis can also be seen in older children.[32] In these cases, direct destruction of the growth cartilage can explain contiguous metaphyseal and epiphyseal lesions. The diagnosis of epiphyseal osteomyelitis is often delayed because of slow onset, intermittent pain, and subtle radiologic changes.[33] The most commonly involved site is the epiphysis of the knee; the reasons for this predilection are currently not well established.

MRI can help distinguish classic imaging features of epiphyseal osteomyelitis (Fig. 22.7) from features of other epiphyseal entities such as chondroblastoma, Langerhans cell histiocytosis, osteoid osteoma, and Ewing sarcoma.

Although there is currently no clearly established guideline for managing epiphyseal osteomyelitis in pediatric patients, conservative management with antibiotic therapy is the main option. Surgery should be reserved for persistent infection that does not respond to appropriate antibiotic therapy or when bone lesions cannot be distinguished from bone tumors by use of all available imaging modalities.[34]

Metaphyseal-Equivalent Osteomyelitis

Approximately 30% of cases of hematogenous osteomyelitis in childhood are encountered at sites other than the usual metaphysis.[35] These cases are seen adjacent to cartilage with a vascular arrangement analogous to the metaphysis, known as "metaphyseal-equivalent" sites. "Metaphyseal-equivalent" sites include the acetabulum, sacroiliac joint, ischiopubic synchondrosis, pubic bones, calcaneus, greater trochanter, ischium (Fig. 22.16), vertebrae (Fig. 22.17), tibial tubercle, scapula, and talus.[11] Most of the "metaphyseal-equivalent" sites occur around the pelvis, which are frequently associated with fluid collections and abscesses.[36] Pelvic acute hematogenous osteomyelitis can also be difficult to differentiate clinically from septic arthritis, pyomyositis, and infections of the pelvic organs (e.g., appendicitis and tubo-ovarian abscesses) and may mimic lumbar disc disease.[36] Careful evaluation of osseous structures as well as adjacent soft tissues and pelvic organs with MRI can be helpful for differentiating them and lead to optimal patient care.

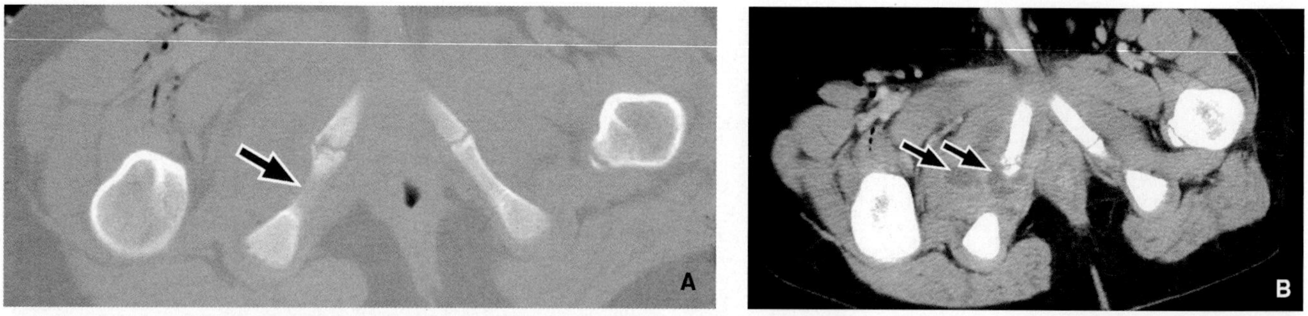

FIGURE 22.16 **Metaphyseal-equivalent osteomyelitis.** Bone **(A)** and soft tissue **(B)** window computed tomography (CT) images of the pelvis of an 11-year-old boy with "metaphyseal-equivalent" osteomyelitis of the right ischium. Bone window CT image **(A)** shows hypodensity (*arrow*) with the ischium. Soft tissue window CT image **(B)** demonstrates fluid collections (*arrows*) within the adjacent musculature suggesting associated pyomyositis.

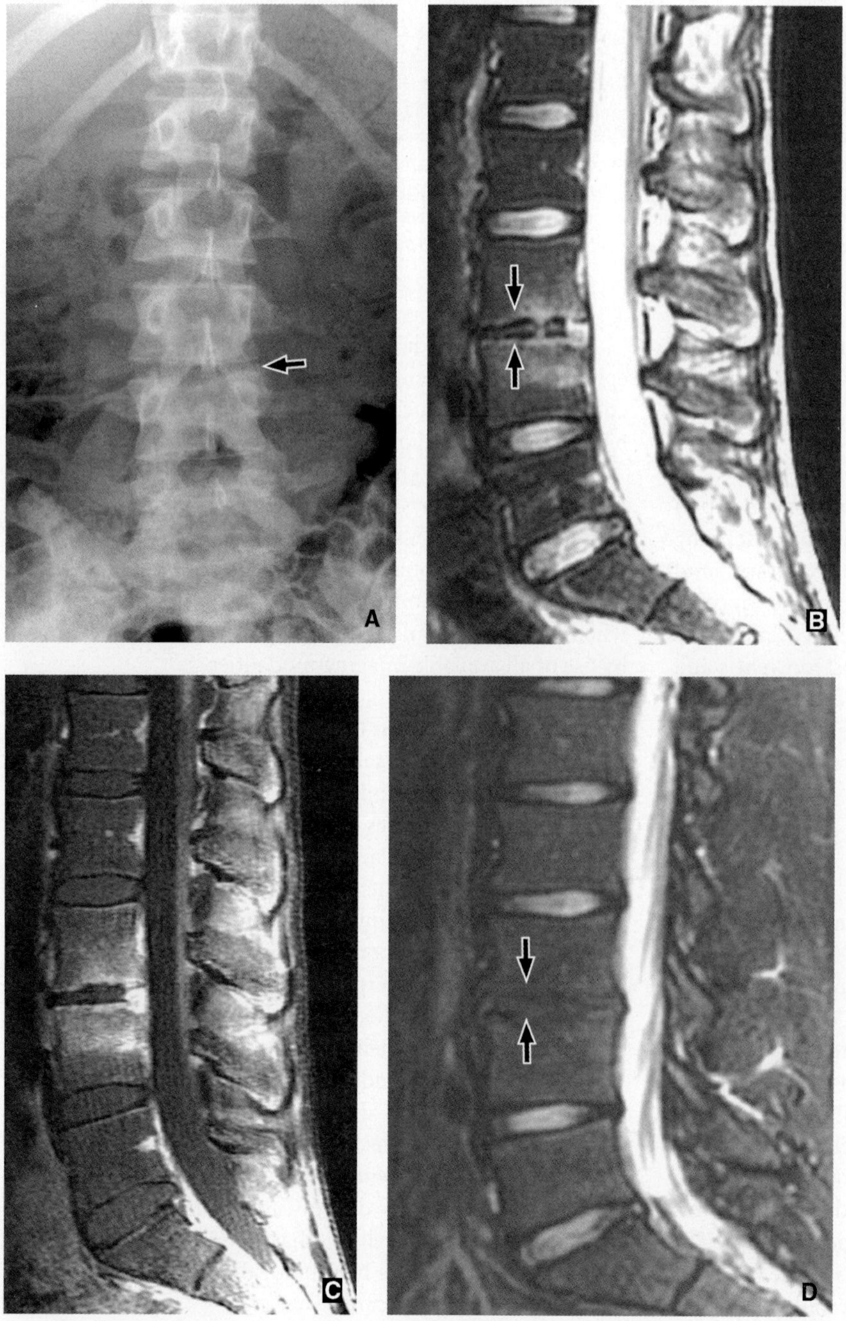

FIGURE 22.17 **Metaphyseal-equivalent osteomyelitis.** Frontal radiograph of the lumbar spine of a 10-year-old girl with vertebral osteomyelitis and diskitis **(A)** shows left-sided intervertebral disk space loss (*arrow*). Sagittal fat-suppressed (FS) T2-weighted MR image **(B)** shows increased signal intensity within the bone marrow of the vertebral bodies of L3 and L4 as well as low signal, irregularity, and compression of the L3–L4 disk space (*arrows*). Sagittal post-contrast FS T1-weighted MR image **(C)** reveals enhancement of the bone marrow of the affected vertebral segments and nonenhancement of the affected disc. Follow-up sagittal FS T2-weighted MR image obtained 6 months after the episode **(D)** shows normalization of the bone marrow signal of L3 and L4 and persistent low signal in the affected disk (*arrows*).

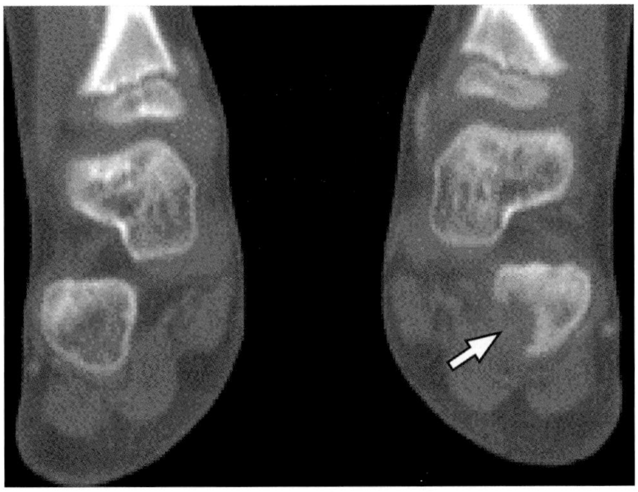

FIGURE 22.18 **Metaphyseal-equivalent osteomyelitis.** Coronal reformatted CT image of the ankles of a 12-year-old girl shows a destructive lesion (*arrow*) in the left calcaneus from blastomycosis osteomyelitis.

Calcaneal Osteomyelitis

Calcaneal osteomyelitis (**Schematic G**) occurs in 3% to 10% of all cases of osteomyelitis.[37] The calcaneus bone is a metaphyseal-equivalent location because it is bordered by the calcaneal apophysis. Typically calcaneal osteomyelitis has an insidious onset with a history of insertion of a foreign body but can also have a hematogenous origin.[38–40] The appearance of calcaneal osteomyelitis on radiographs varies substantially. Radiographs can be normal or present with an area of sclerosis, osteopenia, or osteolysis (Fig. 22.18). It can be associated with effusions. On 99mTc bone scan, high activity can be observed in the entire calcaneus. On MRI, it demonstrates low signal intensity on T1-weighted and high signal intensity on T2-weighted MR images. Bone marrow contrast enhancement is also typically present.[37]

Rib Osteomyelitis

Osteomyelitis of the ribs (**Schematic E**) occurs in areas rich in blood supply, the costochondral junction anteriorly and near the costovertebral angle posteriorly.[41]

Spinal Osteomyelitis

Spinal infections usually involve the disc and endplates of adjacent vertebral bodies (Fig. 22.17). The two most common underlying causative organisms of nontuberculous spondylodiscitis are *S. aureus* and *Streptococcus*. Children with discitis are generally younger and less likely to be ill appearing or febrile, with more frequent involvement of lumbar spine.[42] In contrast, vertebral osteomyelitis is considered a "metaphyseal-equivalent" area of infection. Microorganisms lodge in the low-flow, end-organ vasculature adjacent to the subchondral plate.[42]

The most specific findings of spinal osteomyelitis seen on MRI are bone marrow edema and signal alteration in the disc, as well as epidural or paraspinal abscesses. Although early spinal osteomyelitis can be difficult to be detected on radiographs, radiographic findings become more conspicuous at late stages of spinal osteomyelitis, which include loss of disc height, bone destruction, and focal kyphosis (Fig. 22.17).[43]

Garré Sclerosing Osteomyelitis

Garré sclerosing osteomyelitis, first described by the Swiss surgeon, Carl Garré, in 1893, is a specific type of chronic osteomyelitis that mainly affects children and young adults. It is typically a low-grade infection associated with an odontogenic infection resulting from dental caries. Most cases occur at the lower border of the mandible near the first molar and extend into the mandibular ramus and coronoid process.[44,45] The affected mandible typically shows a thickened bulky cortex caused by the formation of prominent subperiosteal bone (Fig. 22.19).

Pott Puffy Tumor

Pott puffy tumor is characterized by subperiosteal abscess associated with osteomyelitis of the frontal bone (**Schematic A** and Fig. 22.20). It typically results from a complication of frontal sinusitis, either direct or through hematogenous spread. Such complication eventually results in swelling on the forehead, hence the name.[46,47] Pott puffy tumor is more frequently seen in adolescents than in younger children because the former usually have a developed pneumatized frontal sinus.

Pediatric patients with Pott puffy tumor require early evaluation with contrast-enhanced CT or MRI in order to determine the extent of disease and complications, which can include cortical vein thrombosis, epidural abscess, subdural empyema, and brain abscess (Fig. 22.20).[47]

Osteomyelitis-Associated Disorders

Deep Venous Thrombosis

Deep venous thrombosis (DVT), rare in children, is a known complication of acute hematogenous osteomyelitis. It is often reported in pediatric patients affected with MRSA.[48,49] *S. aureus* releases exotoxins that facilitate platelet aggregation and predispose the patient to develop thrombosis. DVT is also associated with the use of central venous lines, surgery, trauma, or infection.[48,49] Radiologists should be aware of pulmonary septic emboli as a potentially life-threatening complication in pediatric patients with acute osteomyelitis.[50,51] Currently, CT pulmonary angiography is the imaging modality of choice for evaluating possible pulmonary septic emboli in pediatric patients with respiratory symptoms in the setting of DVT related to a complication of hematogenous osteomyelitis.

Sickle Cell Disease

Pediatric patients with sickle cell disease are more susceptible to osteomyelitis than the remainder of the population due to multiple factors including splenic hypofunction, opsonophagocytic defects, humoral dysfunction, and an alternate pathway of complement deficiency disorders.[52] Infection by the encapsulated pathogens such as *S. pneumoniae* and

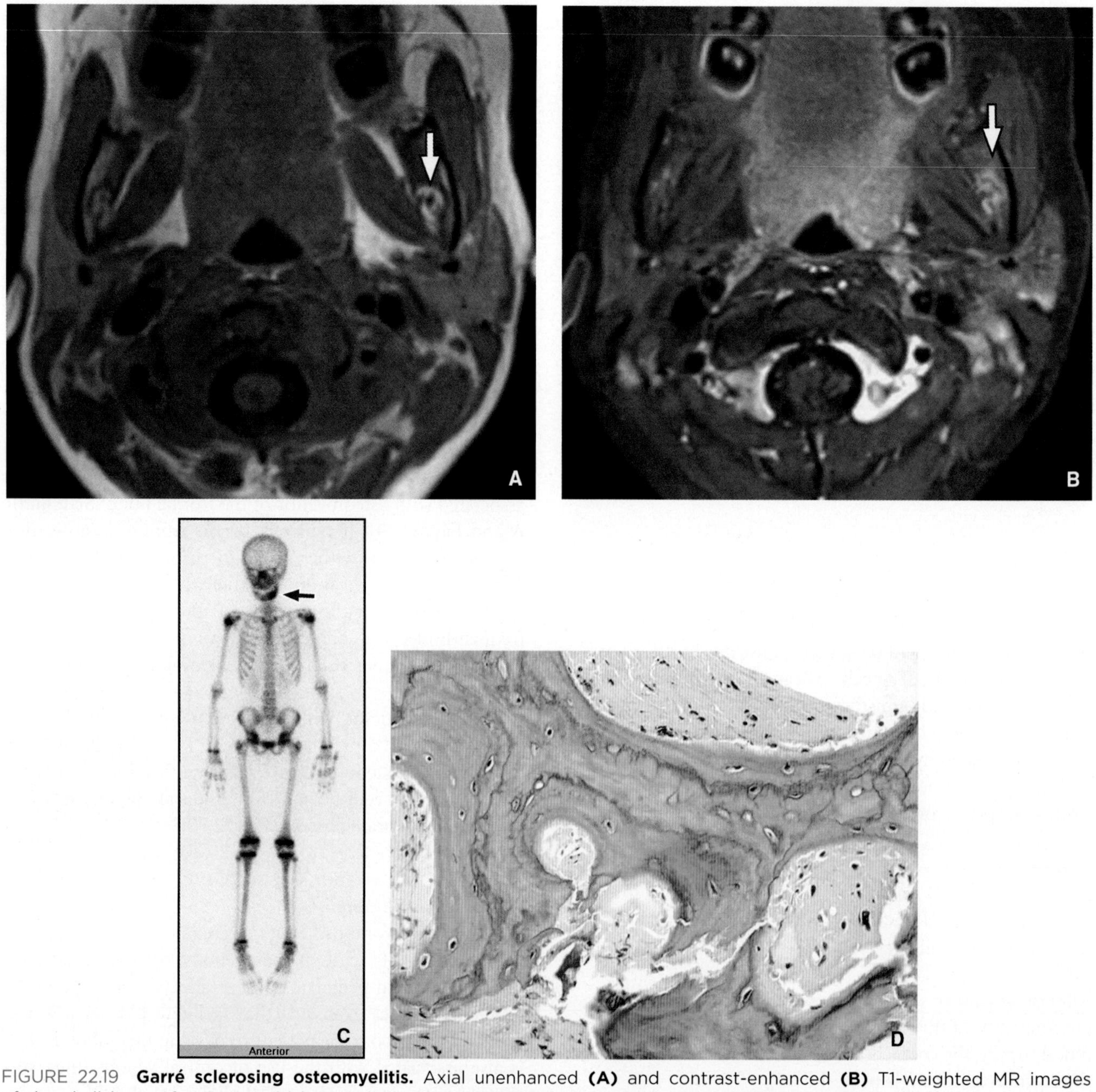

FIGURE 22.19 **Garré sclerosing osteomyelitis.** Axial unenhanced **(A)** and contrast-enhanced **(B)** T1-weighted MR images of the skull base of a 7-year-old boy with Garré sclerosing osteomyelitis of the mandible demonstrate cortical thickening (**A**, *arrow*) and post-gadolinium enhancement (**B**, *arrow*), which present with increased uptake (*arrow*) on ^{99}Tc bone scan **(C)**. Corresponding microscopic examination **(D)** shows exuberant woven bone forming thick trabeculae with scant intervening fibrous tissue (hematoxylin and eosin, original magnification, 400×).

H. influenzae is related to splenic hypofunction. Children with sickle cell anemia can also be infected by *Salmonella* and *S. aureus* and, less frequently, by *E. coli.*[53]

Unique features of osteomyelitis in pediatric patients with sickle cell disease include the involvement of diaphysis of long bones (which are also commonly affected by infarction), multifocal and extensive involvement (Fig. 22.21), and worse prognosis.[54] The high oxygen demand of hyperplastic bone marrow associated with red blood cell sickling predisposes to bone infarction, a contributing factor for osseous infection. The reduced diaphyseal blood supply in comparison with the epiphyseal blood flow also predisposes to infections in the diaphysis of long bones.[55,56]

In pediatric patients with sickle cell disease, differentiating aseptic bone marrow infarcts from infection (**Schematic D**) can be challenging based on clinical grounds alone because pain and fever are common symptoms for both bone infarcts and infections. However, infection is favored if the symptoms persist despite adequate medical management or there is sudden onset of unifocal bone pain.[5] Ischemia may stimulate only osteoblastic activity, which results in increased isotope uptake without a photopenic stage. This feature poses problems in

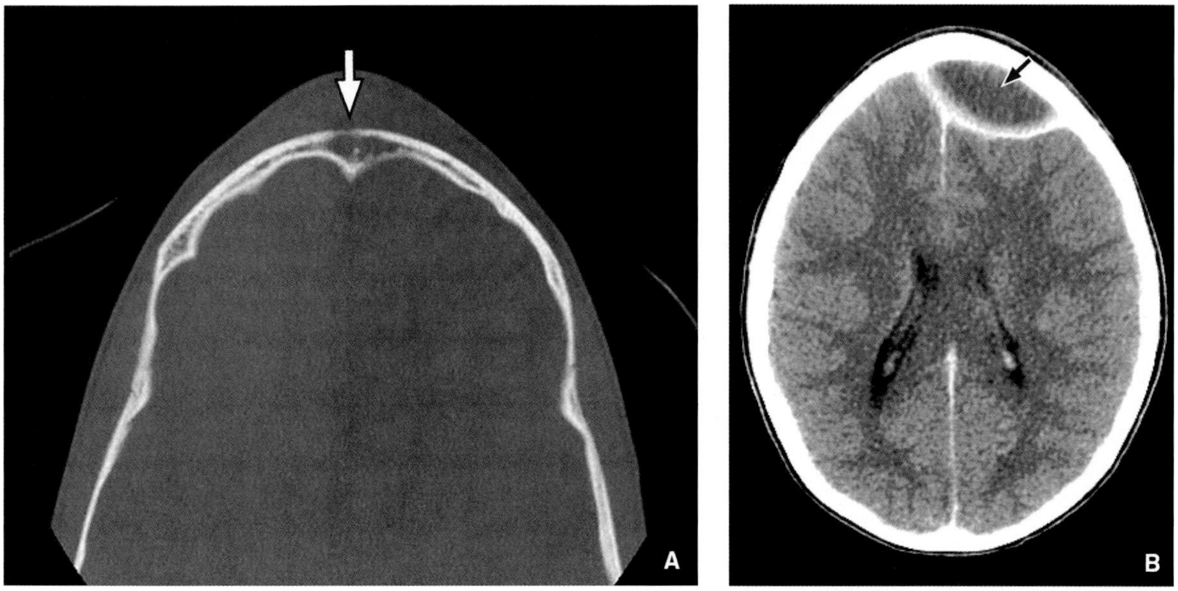

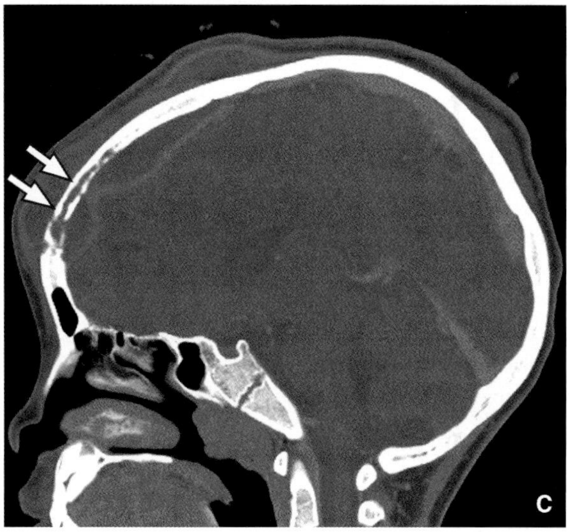

FIGURE 22.20 **Pott puffy tumor.** 5-year-old girl with chronic frontal sinusitis developed further osteomyelitis of the frontal bones with fluctuant swelling over the affected bones, the so-called Pott puffy tumor, accompanied by a subperiosteal pericranial abscess. Bone window computed tomography (CT) image **(A)** shows erosions (*arrow*) and soft tissue swelling in the frontoparietal region centrally. Contrast-enhanced soft tissue window CT image **(B)** reveals an enhancing subperiosteal left frontoparietal collection (*arrow*). Sagittal reformatted contrast-enhanced soft tissue window CT image in a different patient **(C)** shows destructive changes (*arrows*) in the frontal bone with an associated subgaleal abscess and intracranial extension including invasion of the superior sagittal sinus.

differentiating a bone infarct from osteomyelitis in the setting of sickle cell disease. Therefore, discrimination between infarctions and infections based on imaging findings alone can also be challenging, and ^{99m}technetium, ^{67}gallium, and ^{111}indium-labelled leukocyte scans cannot reliably differentiate infections from infarctions in this patient population. Scanning with gallium-67 citrate may be required because its uptake is decreased or absent in acute infarction and is normal or increased in healing infarcts.[55]

For evaluation of osteomyelitis in pediatric patients with sickle cell disease, MRI is currently the imaging modality of choice, which can show classic findings of osteomyelitis, complications such as subperiosteal or soft tissue abscesses, as well as areas of bone infarction (Fig. 22.21).[55,56]

Meningococcal Disease

Meningococcal disease is caused by the bacterium *Neisseria meningitides*, which can result in septicemia and meningitis. Although it is a vaccine-preventable disease, it continues to result in high mortality and morbidity in infants and children in both developed and underdeveloped countries around the world. Pediatric patients with meningococcal infection may end up with bony destruction and subsequent growth disturbances including physeal arrest due to septic arthritis (Fig. 22.22) as well as deep muscle infection, which can be best evaluated with MRI.[57,58]

Bacille Calmette-Guerin Osteomyelitis

Bacille Calmette-Guerin (BCG) is a live mycobacterial vaccine used for preventing tuberculosis and for treating some bladder cancers. Although regional bone infection from BCG, known as BCG osteomyelitis or osteitis, is a rare complication of BCG vaccination, it can be a potentially life-threatening condition in the pediatric population. BCG osteomyelitis usually occurs in the epiphysis and metaphysis and may cross the growth plate. Clinical findings such as a palpable mass, tenderness, limping, and redness usually occur from a few months to 5 years postvaccination in

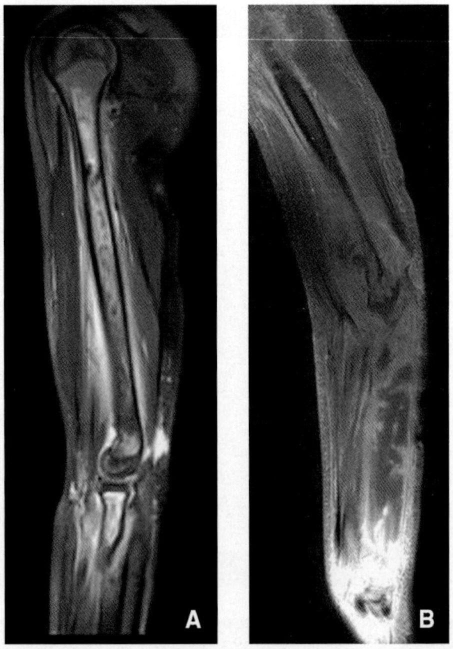

FIGURE 22.21 **Sickle cell disease.** Sagittal fat-suppressed (FS) T2-weighted MR image during a sickle cell crisis in a 15-year-old girl **(A)** shows serpiginous hypointense areas throughout the diaphysis of the humerus corresponding to bone infarcts with diffuse bone marrow and soft tissue edema. A different pediatric patient with sickle cell disease and similar clinical presentation shows septic elbow arthritis and extensive pyomyositis in the forearm on this sagittal post-contrast FS T1-weighted MR image **(B)**.

affected pediatric patients. On imaging studies such as radiography, BCG osteomyelitis has an appearance similar to that of tuberculous (TB) osteomyelitis.[59]

Mycobacterial Agents

Tuberculosis

Despite advances in diagnosis and treatment during the past several decades, TB remains a major global health challenge.

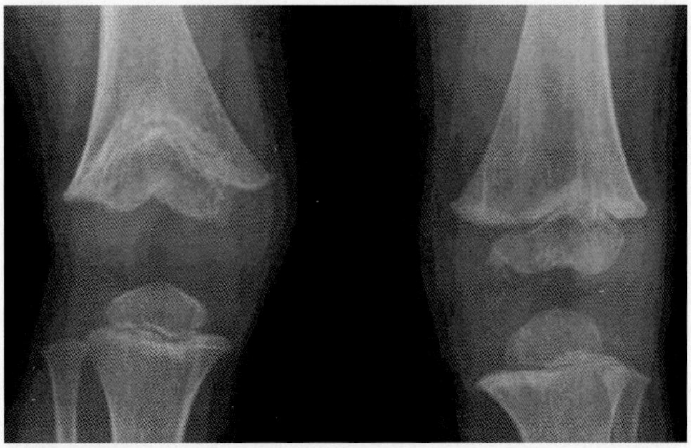

FIGURE 22.22 **Meningococcemia.** Frontal radiograph of the knees of a preschooler with prior diagnosis of meningococcemia shows bilateral metaphyseal cupping deformity and premature physeal fusion of the right distal femur. Milder osteoarticular changes are noted in the left distal femur.

Skeletal TB accounts for one-third of all cases.[60] The main route of infection in skeletal TB is through hematogenous spread from a primary source, which is often unknown in the pediatric population. After initial infection with TB, a granulomatous lesion develops within the bone and this lesion becomes a caseous focus, which causes osseous spread and eventual destruction.

The three most common manifestations of skeletal tuberculosis in children are spondylitis (**Schematic F** and Fig. 22.23), arthritis (Fig. 22.24), and osteomyelitis (Fig. 22.25).[61] Tuberculous spondylitis involves the intervertebral disc only late in the disease progression. Subligamentous spread of the infection may lead to multiple levels of vertebral body involvement that may be either continuous or skipped. Paravertebral

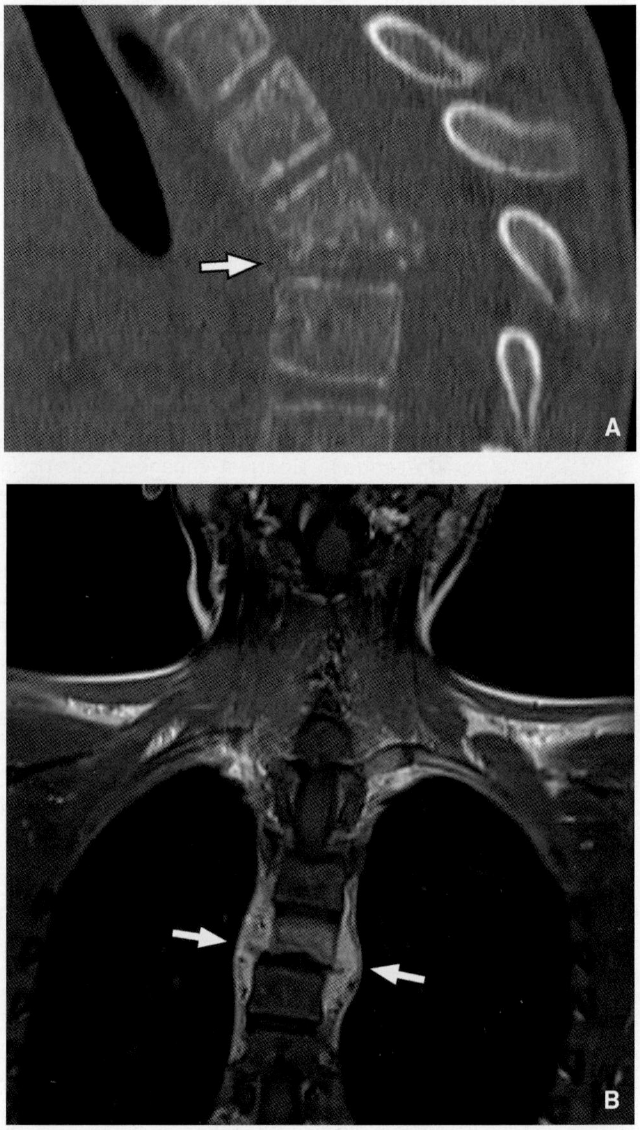

FIGURE 22.23 **Tuberculous spondylitis.** Sagittal bone window (CT) image of the spine **(A)** demonstrates focal kyphosis (*arrow*) in the midthoracic region as a result of tuberculous osteomyelitis and discitis. Coronal post-contrast fat-suppressed T1-weighted MR image **(B)** shows bilateral paraspinal abscesses (*arrows*) at the same level of the diskitis.

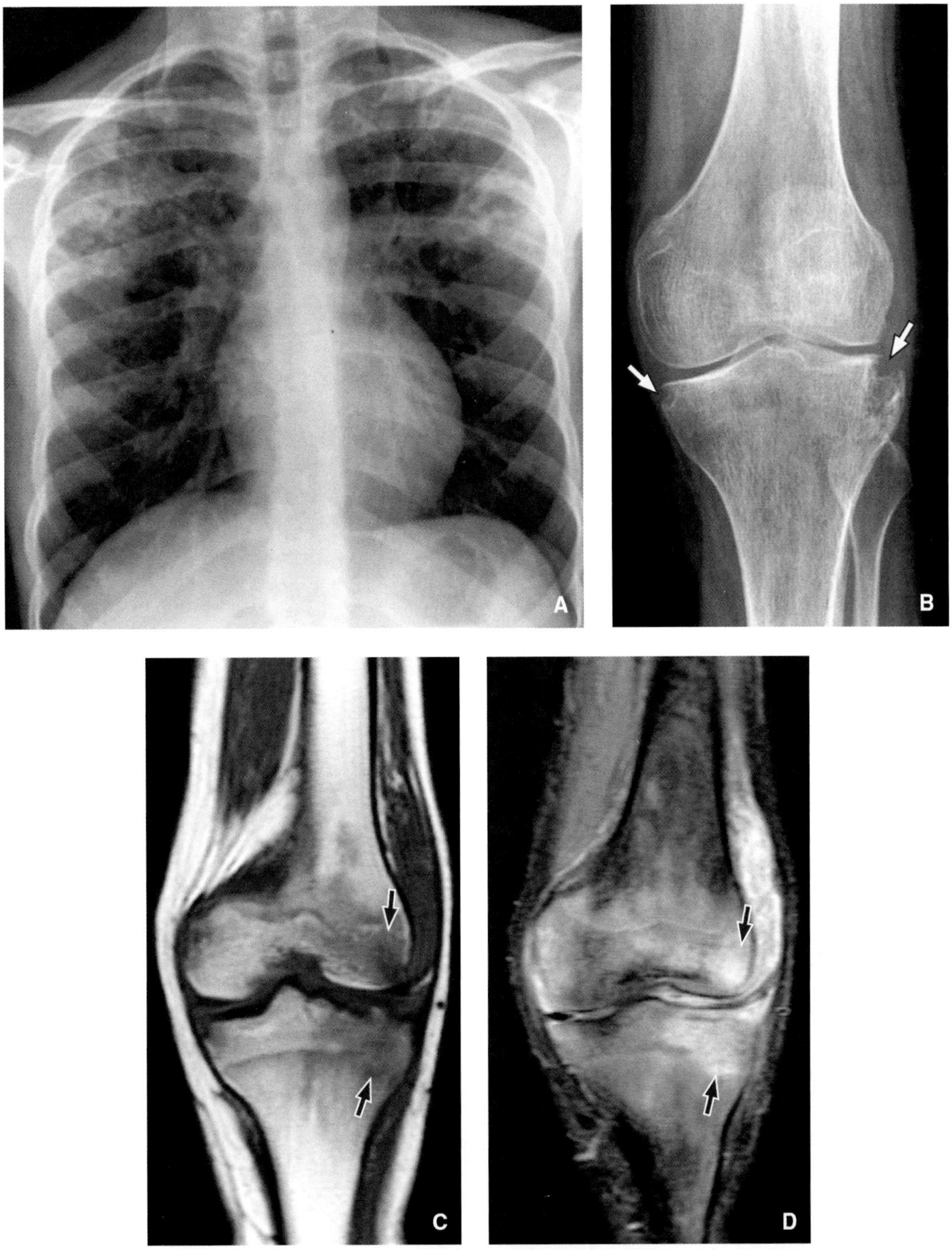

FIGURE 22.24 **Tuberculous arthritis.** Frontal radiograph of the chest **(A)** demonstrates bilateral upper lobe opacities and cavitations. Frontal radiograph of the knee **(B)** shows osteopenia, erosions (*arrows*), and mild joint narrowing. Corresponding coronal T1-weighted **(C)** and inversion recovery **(D)** MR images of the left knee show erosions, joint effusion, and bone marrow edema (*arrows*).

or extradural space extension of the disease may occur.[61] The synovial joint is the second most common site of involvement in skeletal TB. TB arthritis usually occurs as a result of metaphyseal TB osteomyelitis crossing the epiphyseal plate into the joint (Fig. 22.25). Hips and knees are the most common joints affected in TB arthritis.[62] Polyarticular involvement from TB arthritis is rare.[63] Lastly, TB osteomyelitis is less common than TB arthritis. It may appear as well-defined cystic lesions (Fig. 22.25), infiltrative lesions, or spina ventosa, also known as TB dactylitis (a term used to describe a form of tuberculous osteomyelitis characterized by bone destruction, overlying periosteal reaction, and fusiform expansion of the bone resulting in cyst-like cavities with diaphyseal expansion) on MRI.[62]

Viral Agents

Congenital and Acquired Varicella

Congenital varicella infection can result in osseous abnormalities such as limb deformity (Fig. 22.26) and articular effusions in addition to borderline ventriculomegaly,

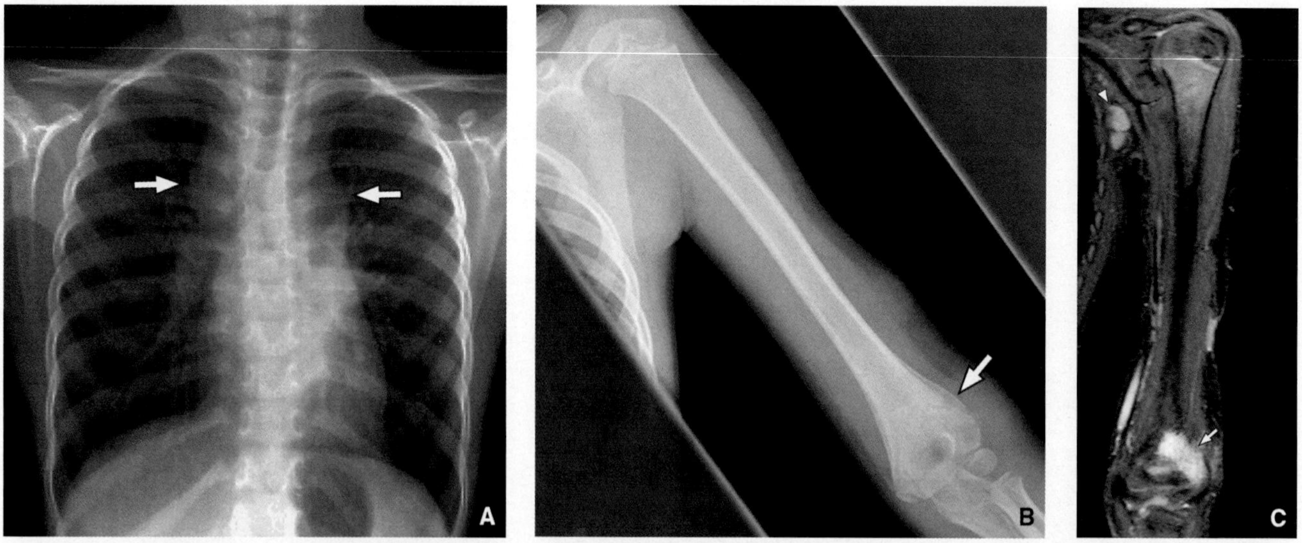

FIGURE 22.25 **Tuberculous osteomyelitis.** Frontal radiograph of the chest **(A)** shows mediastinal adenopathy (*arrows*). Frontal radiograph of the left humerus **(B)** shows a lytic lesion with cortical thickening (*arrow*) in the distal humerus in keeping with osteomyelitis. Soft tissue swelling is noted along the lateral aspect of the mid to distal humerus. Corresponding coronal inversion recovery MR image **(C)** shows increased signal intensity (*arrow*) in the distal humerus, adjacent soft tissue changes, and axillary lymphadenopathy (*arrowhead*). Blood culture confirmed the diagnosis of tuberculosis.

intracerebral, myocardial, and intrahepatic calcifications as well as intrauterine growth retardation, all of which can be detected on prenatal US or MRI.[64]

Acquired varicella infection is a risk factor for osteomyelitis (as well as necrotizing fasciitis/myositis) because the ruptured vesicles can be a point of entry for bacteria, particularly group-A beta-hemolytic *Streptococcus*.[65] Typical sites of osteomyelitis in pediatric patients with varicella include ribs (**Schematic E**), spondylodiscitis, femur (Fig. 22.27), talus, and tibia.[65,66]

Congenital Rubella

Involvement of long bones in congenital rubella has been reported in 25% to 50% of cases.[10] It most commonly affects the distal femur and proximal tibia. A classic finding of congenital rubella is the "celery stalk" sign, which is characterized as longitudinally oriented bands of sclerosis (**Schematic C** and Fig. 22.28).[10] This imaging finding has also been described in syphilis and cytomegalovirus infections.

Congenital Syphilis

Congenital syphilis is caused by transplacental migration of treponemes and subsequent invasion of the perichondrium, periosteum, cartilage, bone marrow, and growth zones.[67] Skeletal involvement is usually multifocal and symmetric. Affected pediatric patients may present with pain in one or more extremities secondary to syphilitic involvement of bone

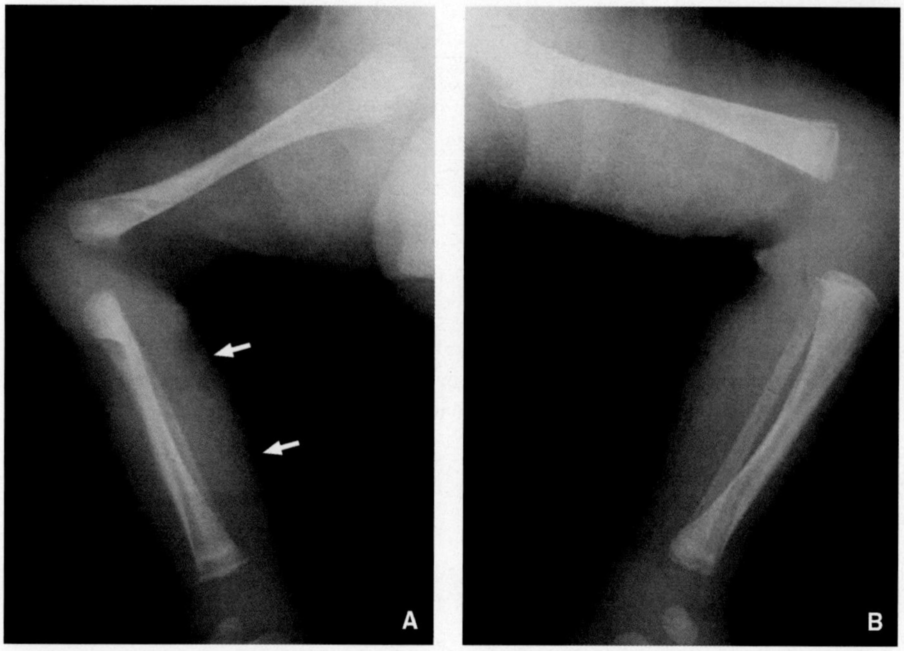

FIGURE 22.26 **Congenital varicella infection.** Lateral radiograph of the right lower limb **(A)** demonstrates hypoplasia and deformity of the right femur and tibia with cutaneous scarring (*arrows*) noted in a dermatome distribution. Lateral radiograph of the unaffected left leg **(B)** for comparison.

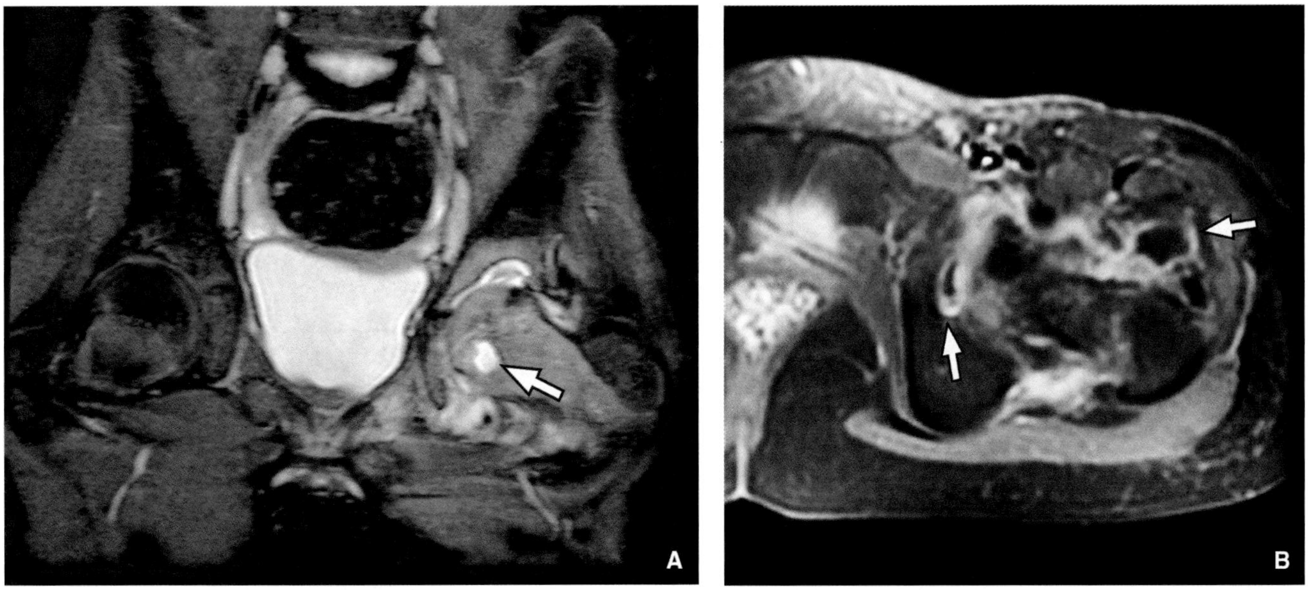

FIGURE 22.27 **Varicella osteomyelitis.** Coronal inversion recovery MR image **(A)** of the pelvis in a child with acquired varicella complicated by streptococcal pneumonia shows left hip effusion and bone marrow edema associated with a focal intraosseous abscess (*arrow*) of the proximal left femur. Axial post-contrast fat-suppressed T2-weighted MR image **(B)** shows low signal effusion with synovial enhancement and soft tissue collections with rim enhancement (*arrows*) consistent with abscess formation adjacent to the intraosseous abscess.

resulting in lack of movement of those extremities. Such physical finding is known as *pseudoparalysis,* first described by Joseph Marie Jules Parrot.[68] Bone abnormalities from congenital syphilis include osteochondritis, diaphyseal osteomyelitis (osteitis), and periostitis[69] (Fig. 22.29). The Wimberger sign refers to localized bilateral metaphyseal destruction of the medial proximal tibias (Fig. 22.29) and is a pathognomonic radiologic sign for congenital syphilis.[68]

Fungal Agents

Cryptococcus neoformans

Immunocompromised patients such as children with human immunodeficiency virus (HIV) and a low CD4 count typically have impaired monocyte and macrophage function. This results in impaired phagocytosis and intracellular killing and predisposition to opportunistic infections such as

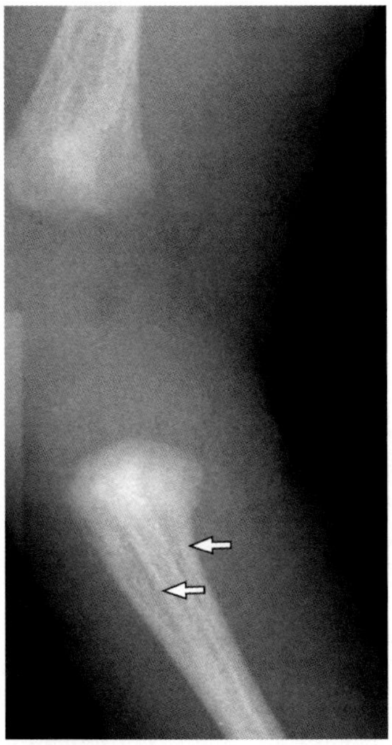

FIGURE 22.28 **Congenital rubella infection.** Lateral radiograph of knee shows "celery stalk" appearance of the metaphyses of the distal femur and tibia with vertical linear areas of lucency and sclerosis (*arrows*).

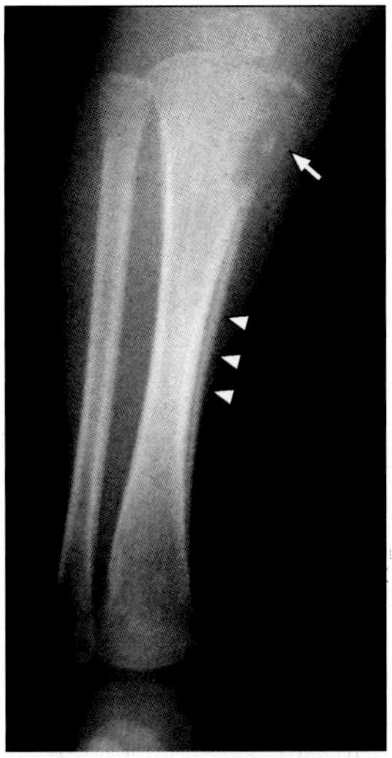

FIGURE 22.29 **Congenital syphilis infection.** Frontal radiograph of tibia and fibula shows metaphyseal changes (*arrow*) and periostitis (*arrowheads*). The focal lytic lesions seen in the proximal medial metaphyses characterize the Wimberger sign (*arrow*).

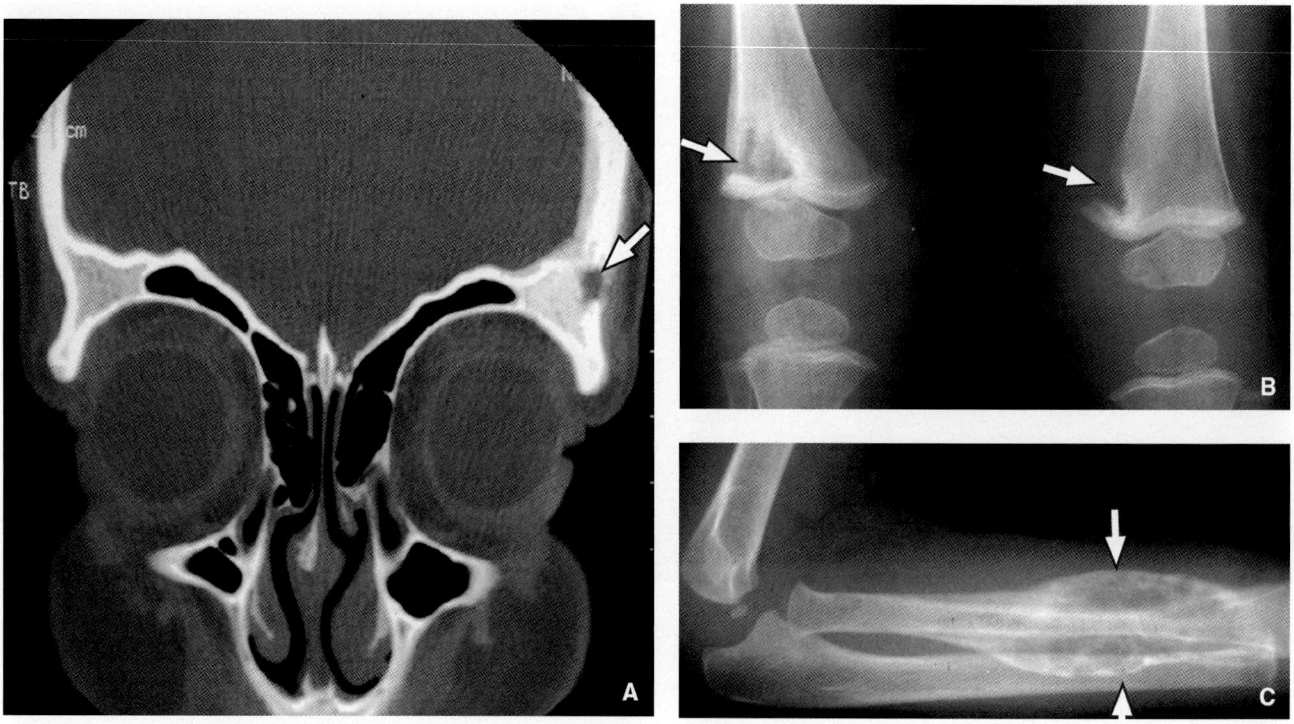

FIGURE 22.30 **Blastomycosis infection.** Coronal CT image of the skull **(A)** demonstrates a lytic lesion (*arrow*) in the left frontal bone. Frontal view of the knees **(B)** shows bilateral lytic lesions (*arrows*) in the distal femoral metaphyses. Lateral view of the elbow **(C)** shows a lytic bubbly lesion (*arrows*) in the radius.

Cryptococcus neoformans that may affect bones. Cryptococcal osteomyelitis is rare, occurring in 5% to 10% of disseminated cryptococcal infections.[70–73] Vertebrae are the most common site of cryptococcal osteomyelitis.[74]

Blastomycosis

Blastomycosis is a rare infection in children, which can result in arthritis and osteomyelitis. It is caused by the fungus named *Blastomyces dermatitidis*, which is endemic around the Great Lakes, and the southeast and south central United States. Bone involvement may occur in vertebrae, skull, ribs, and carpal and tarsal bones[75] (Fig. 22.30). Osseous involvement from blastomycosis is typically asymptomatic and located in the epiphysis or metaphysis. The reported MRI features include (1) eccentrically located lesion in the metaphysis presenting as a slowly growing, geographic, lytic focus[75]; (2) diffuse, rapidly growing lesions that spread into the soft tissue or joints via fistulae; (3) periosteal reaction and sequestra, which are rare; and (4) vertebral lesions, which have an appearance similar to that of tuberculosis.[75]

Paracoccidioidomycosis

Paracoccidioidomycosis (PCM) is a systemic granulomatous disease caused by the dymorphic fungus *Paracoccidioides brasiliensis*, which occurs endemically in Latin American countries.[76,77] PCM can be classified as acute/subacute and chronic forms.[76] Whereas the acute/subacute form of PCM that accounts for 3% to 5% of all cases is frequently seen in children and adolescents, the chronic form is most commonly present in adults.[78] Clinically, it is characterized by fast disease progression associated with cutaneous lesions, lymphadenopathy, gastrointestinal manifestations, hepatosplenomegaly, and osteoarticular involvement (**Schematic B**).

Osteoarticular involvement from PCM occurs by hematogenic dissemination or by direct contiguity. Bone involvement can be solitary or multifocal and is more common in pediatric patients. Metaphyseal or metaepiphyseal location in a long bone is the most common location of osseous PCM infection. Axial skeleton involvement, arthritis, or a disseminated osseous pattern of infection may occasionally occur.[78] On imaging studies, PCM infection typically presents as a well-delineated osteolytic lesion without a surrounding periosteal reaction (Fig. 22.31).[76]

The differential diagnosis for this entity should include bone marrow-infiltrating disorders such as metastases, leukemia, lymphoma, and severe histiocytosis in the pediatric population. Other infectious diseases such as tuberculosis, brucellosis, and coccidioidomycosis should also be considered.[78]

JOINT SPACE INFECTIONS

Transient Synovitis

Transient or toxic synovitis is not an active infection, but it is included here because it can closely mimic one. It is a self-limiting transient inflammation of the synovium that is treated medically with no adverse complications. It is usually seen in pediatric patients between 5 and 10 years of age.[79] It is the most relevant differential diagnosis for septic arthritis in the pediatric population. Diagnosis of transient synovitis is

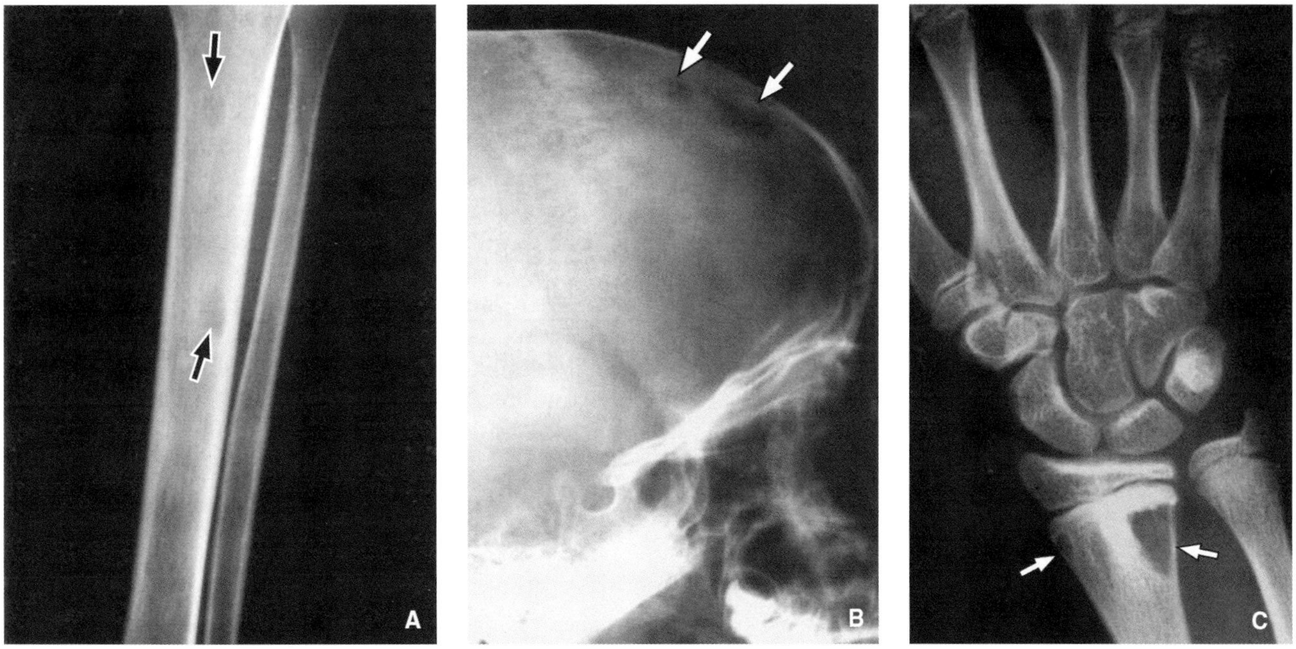

FIGURE 22.31 **Paracoccidioidomycosis infection.** Multifocal infection is demonstrated by multiple geographic lytic foci (*arrows*) seen in radiographs of the tibia **(A)**, skull **(B)**, and radius **(C)** of the same pediatric patient.

suspected clinically when the child is not septic and, usually, has had a preceding viral infection while presenting with hip pain or limping.[79]

In the past, imaging evaluation of transient synovitis used to start with radiographs. However, it has been proposed that radiography should not be used in the primary evaluation of most children with hip pain because the results are generally normal or show only subtle findings of joint effusion. Currently, US is often used as an initial and highly sensitive imaging modality for assessing joint effusion in symptomatic pediatric patients with clinically suspected transient synovitis or septic joint.[80] On US, the presence of simple joint fluid and distension of the joint capsule due to the presence of joint fluid rather than hypertrophy of the synovium are typically present in a child with transient toxic synovitis (Fig. 22.32).[81]

Pediatric patients with transient synovitis can be managed conservatively with rest, non-weight-bearing, and nonsteroidal anti-inflammatory medication, which may shorten the duration of symptoms.[82] Persistent symptoms despite conservative management in conjunction with fever and elevated WBC count should raise other diagnoses including septic arthritis.

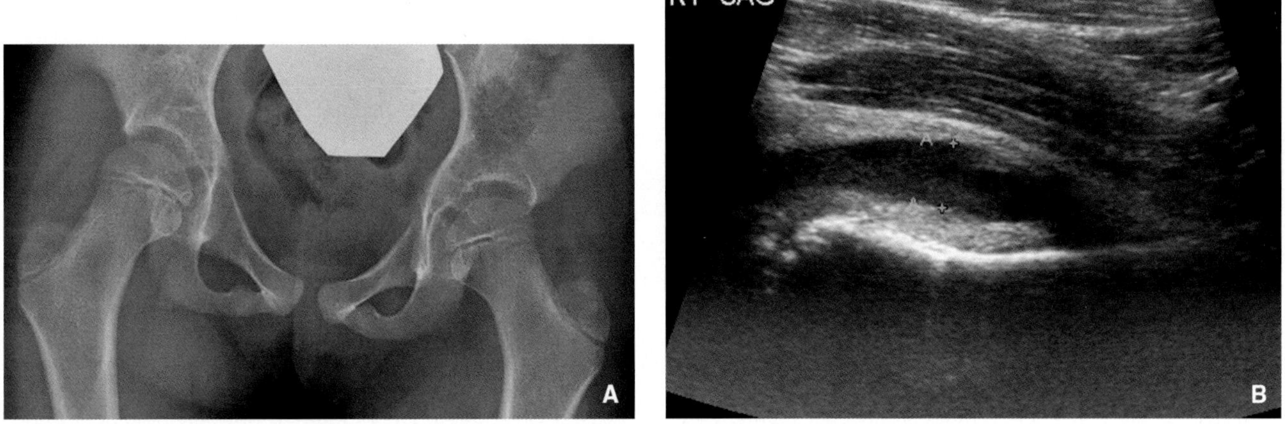

FIGURE 22.32 **Transient synovitis.** Frontal radiograph of hips of a 7-year-old girl with severe right thigh pain and antalgic gait **(A)** shows pelvic tilt but no obvious bone abnormalities. Gray-scale ultrasound obtained on the same day **(B)** shows joint effusion (calipers) in the right hip.

Septic Arthritis

Septic arthritis is a purulent joint infection and is considered a medical emergency because the infection can rapidly destroy the articular cartilage and result in permanent bone deformity (Fig. 22.33). The affected joint needs to be rapidly decompressed and sterilized in order to avoid devastating sequelae.[83] Septic arthritis is frequently encountered in neonates and in children younger than 3 years of age.[5] *S. aureus* is the most common pathogen involved, followed by *S. pyogenes*, *S. pneumoniae,* and *K. kingae.*[26] Other pathogens are *Borrelia burgdorferi* (Lyme disease) and *Neisseria gonorrhoeae* in sexually active adolescents. Acute osteomyelitis is the cause of septic arthritis in 10% to 16% of cases.[19] The most commonly affected joints are the knee (35%) and hip (35%), followed by the shoulder, elbow, and ankle.[9] Routes of spread vary, but in neonates and children younger than 2 years of age, the infection typically spreads from the metaphysis through a patent transphyseal vessel to the epiphysis and joint space (Fig. 22.10).

For evaluation of septic arthritis, radiographic evaluation may be limited during the early phase of the infectious process but can be helpful by showing an indirect sign of joint effusion and excluding other causes of patient's symptoms such as fracture or neoplasm. A later phase of advanced septic arthritis can be assessed with radiographs, which may show joint space widening (due to underlying joint effusion), periarticular osteopenia (due to hyperemia), and sometimes apparent joint dislocation (due to cartilaginous and osseous destruction).[84] For evaluation of underlying joint effusion, US is a sensitive imaging modality (Fig. 22.6); however, it may be insensitive to differentiate infectious joint fluid from noninfectious clear joint effusion.[84] This lack of discriminative capability of US limits its role in the context of septic arthritis in the pediatric population. Nevertheless, US plays an essential role for guiding joint fluid aspiration because surgical drainage and culture of material collected should be immediately conducted for reaching a definitive diagnosis when septic arthritis is clinically suspected. For evaluation of septic arthritis, MRI is indicated when US cannot confirm the presence of joint effusion and clinical concern remains. In addition, MRI may be necessary for completely evaluating the extension of the infection in the joint and adjacent soft tissues.[85] For accurately detecting septic arthritis, the recent study showed that addition of gadolinium-enhanced MR sequences does not seem to significantly change the diagnostic accuracy of MRI for diagnosing septic arthritis in the pediatric population.[86]

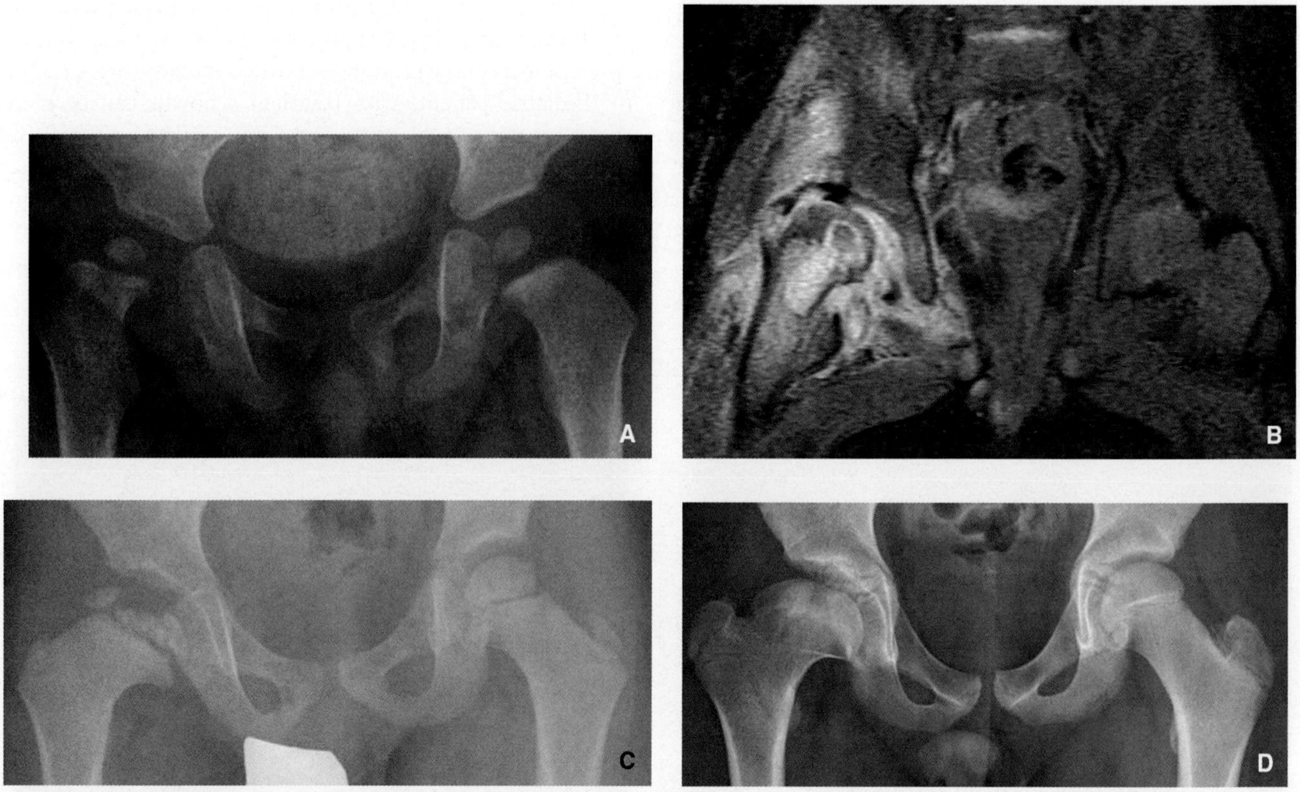

FIGURE 22.33 **Secondary septic arthritis.** Frontal radiograph of hips obtained at the age of 10 months **(A)** fails to show bone abnormalities. However, concurrent coronal post-contrast fat-suppressed T1-weighted MR image **(B)** shows marked abnormality in the signal of the epiphysis and metaphysis of the proximal right femur representing acute osteomyelitis. There is edema in the surrounding muscles and soft tissues, synovial thickening and enhancement, and a fluid collection in the joint space in keeping with secondary septic arthritis. Subsequently obtained frontal radiographs of hips obtained at the age of 5 **(C)** and 13 years **(D)** show sequelae of septic arthritis: fragmentation, irregularity, and remineralization/healing of the right femoral head **(C),** which progressed to "mushroom"-shaped flattening **(D)**, respectively.

SOFT TISSUE INFECTIONS

Cellulitis

Cellulitis is characterized by diffuse inflammation of skin and underlying subcutaneous soft tissues. It is usually caused by gram-positive cocci.[5] Cellulitis is a clinical diagnosis that can be supported by imaging findings.

Radiographs can show soft tissue swelling in children with cellulitis. US can be subsequently obtained for the confirmation of cellulitis and excluding potentially drainable abscess formation. The main US feature of cellulitis includes subcutaneous tissue thickening with increased blood flow.[87] Currently, the main roles of MR imaging in investigating cellulitis are to evaluate cases that do not respond to routine therapy and to assess for associated complications, including soft tissue abscess, pyomyositis, and osteomyelitis. On MRI, cellulitis appears as strands of low signal intensity on T1-weighted MR images and presents with high signal on T2-weighted MR images, extending into muscles or fascial planes with associated mild diffuse enhancement without any associated rim-enhancing fluid collections or underlying bone marrow abnormality.[11] If the cellulitis is extensive, however, bone marrow signal abnormalities are not uncommon. If bone marrow edema and enhancement are seen in the context of deep cellulitis, they may reflect either reactive marrow edema or osteomyelitis.

Abscess

A soft tissue abscess is a walled-off, suppurative fluid collection, which can arise in any of the superficial or deep soft tissues. It can occur via direct inoculation by puncture injury, around a foreign body, in association with an adjacent injection, or via hematogenous dissemination.[88]

It is often challenging to diagnose a soft tissue abscess based on radiographs alone, but the presence of gas within the enlarged soft tissues should suggest the diagnosis in the absence of a prior history of trauma, biopsy, or aspiration. On US, soft tissue abscess typically presents as an anechoic or hypoechoic fluid collection with an increase through transmission and surrounding hyperemic wall. Internal echoes and septations that represent purulent material and debris may present (Fig. 22.34). US can be used for localizing as well as aspirating and draining a soft tissue abscess. On CT, a round- to elliptical-shaped fluid collection with surrounding often irregularly thick and enhancing wall is usually present. The attenuation of abscess is usually low but can be variable depending on the amount of internal cellular debris and proteinaceous material. MRI, which can superbly detect the presence of abscess, delineate the extent of the process, and identify coexisting septic arthritis or osteomyelitis, is a valuable imaging modality. On MRI, soft tissue abscess shows low to intermediate signal intensity on T1-weighted MR images and uniform to slightly heterogeneous high signal intensity on T2-weighted MR images. After contrast administration, peripheral enhancement is usually seen but internal necrotic contents do not enhance (Figs. 22.5 and 22.11). For detecting soft tissue abscess, the sensitivity of MRI is about 89% and its specificity, 80%.[6,89,90]

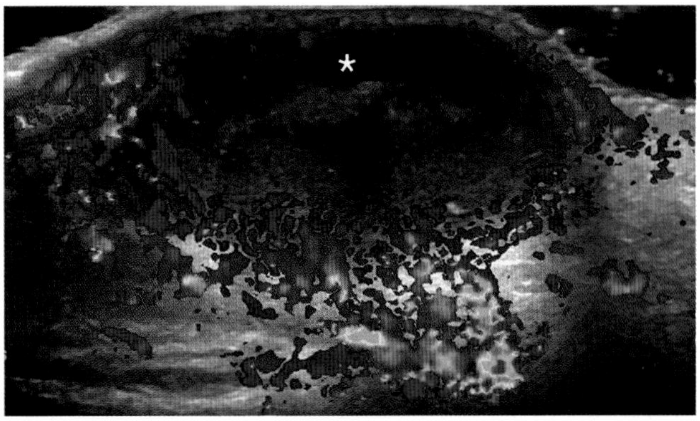

FIGURE 22.34 **Soft tissue abscess.** Transverse color Doppler ultrasound image of a soft tissue abscess in a 3-year-old boy who presented with erythematous and swollen soft tissue of the right distal leg. Ultrasound image shows a hypoechoic fluid collection (*asterisk*) with internal debris and marked peripheral hyperemia.

Necrotizing Fasciitis

Necrotizing fasciitis is a rare but rapidly progressive and potentially life-threatening infection of the subcutaneous tissues and the deeper layers of skin that can spread across the fascial planes. The four most commonly affected sites include the scrotum, perineum, lower extremity, and neck. Diagnosis of necrotizing fasciitis can be challenging solely based on clinical grounds and imaging evaluation can be helpful. Radiographic or CT findings such as soft tissue thickening and the presence of gas are often nonspecific but should raise the possibility of necrotizing fasciitis in the appropriate clinical setting. In advanced disease, adjacent soft tissue including muscles can also be involved. MRI findings of necrotizing fasciitis include involvement of deep fasciae with fluid collections, thickening, and enhancement after contrast administration[6,91] (Fig. 22.35). The current management of necrotizing fasciitis includes emergency surgical debridement, decompression fasciotomy, and IV administration of antibiotics.[92,93]

Pyomyositis

Pyomyositis is a bacterial infection characterized by neutrophilic inflammation of skeletal muscle, often with abscesses. This condition is most commonly seen in tropical climates but can also occur in temperate zones.[94] Pyomyositis is associated with various underlying conditions and disease processes including HIV, intravenous drug abuse, diabetes, leukemia, asplenia, lupus erythematosus, sickle cell anemia, and intramuscular injections.[95] The most typical causative organism is *S. aureus*,[96] and the most common site of involvement is the quadriceps muscle followed by the pelvic musculature. The two most common spreading routes are hematogenous and local from adjacent osteomyelitis or soft tissue infection.[97]

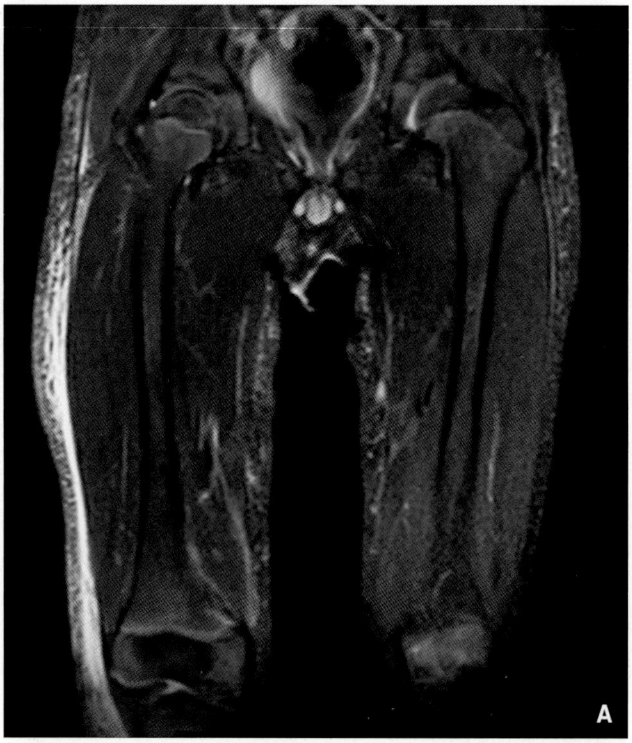

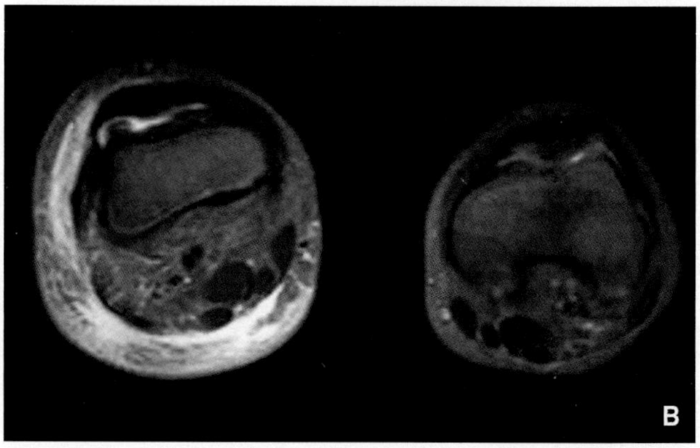

FIGURE 22.35 **Necrotizing fasciitis.** Coronal **(A)** and axial **(B)** inversion-recovery MR images of the lower extremities of a 3-year-old boy with necrotizing fasciitis. MR images show increased reticular signal intensity in the subcutaneous fat and musculature of the popliteal fossa with relative sparing of the medial musculature.

Imaging evaluation of pyomyositis can be performed with US or MRI although MRI is more sensitive than US. For superficially located pyomyositis, US may show enlarged and hyperemic muscles with heterogeneous echotexture as well as abscess formation within the muscles.[98] MRI, with excellent soft tissue characterization capability, is the current imaging modality of choice, which can lead to early diagnosis and detection of complications.[98] MRI findings of pyomyositis include diffuse muscular enlargement with hyperintense signal on STIR/T2-weighted MR images, intermediate signal on T1-weighted MR images, and abscess formation with peripheral rim enhancement around central nonenhancing fluid after gadolinium administration[96,98] (Figs. 22.7 and 22.21).

INFLAMMATORY DISORDERS

Caffey Disease

Caffey disease, also known as infantile cortical hyperostosis, is a genetically inherited autosomal dominant disease with incomplete penetrance. It is due to a mutation in the *COL1A1* gene, which controls type I collagen. The condition can been diagnosed in utero; however, affected neonates can appear well for several weeks after birth before the disease onset.[99,100] Caffey disease is usually self-limiting, begins in the early infancy, and is characterized by unusual irritability, soft tissue swelling, and cortical hyperostosis.[99] There may be involvement of a single or multiple bones. Sequential bone involvement is common, with one area being affected initially followed by other sites. The distribution of lesions is characteristic: mandible (Fig. 22.36), clavicles, and ulnae are the most frequently involved bones, with phalanges, vertebral bodies, and cuboidal bones being rarely affected.[99]

The typical radiologic feature is marked new bone formation (i.e., periostitis and hyperostosis) surrounding the diaphysis of long bones. Although the radiographic abnormalities are virtually diagnostic of Caffey disease, bone scan can be used to further document the extent of skeletal involvement.[101] Occasionally, active disease may persist and recur intermittently for years, resulting in crippling deformities in the extremities and markedly delayed muscular and motor development. Late manifestations of Caffey disease include expansion of the bone marrow cavity and thinning of cortex.

The differential diagnosis of Caffey disease includes nonaccidental trauma, hypervitaminosis A, scurvy, osteomyelitis, syphilis, parotiditis, long-term administration of prostaglandin E, and malignancy in the pediatric population.[99] The majority of these potential alternative diagnoses can be excluded by: (1) age group; (2) absence of mandibular involvement; and (3) triad of irritability, swelling, and osseous lesions, which are characteristic of Caffey disease.

Chronic Recurrent Multifocal Osteomyelitis

Chronic recurrent multifocal osteomyelitis (CRMO) is a well-established skeletal disorder of unknown origin mainly occurring in children and adolescents.[101] It is characterized by multifocal nonpyogenic inflammatory bone lesions, a course of exacerbations and remissions, and an association with other inflammatory disorders.[102] The association of CRMO with dermatologic disorders (such as psoriasis) and inflammatory bowel disease and its response to steroids has led to the suggestion of an autoimmune cause.[103,104]

A typical clinical presentation of children with CRMO includes bone pain, some with concurrent fever and, despite

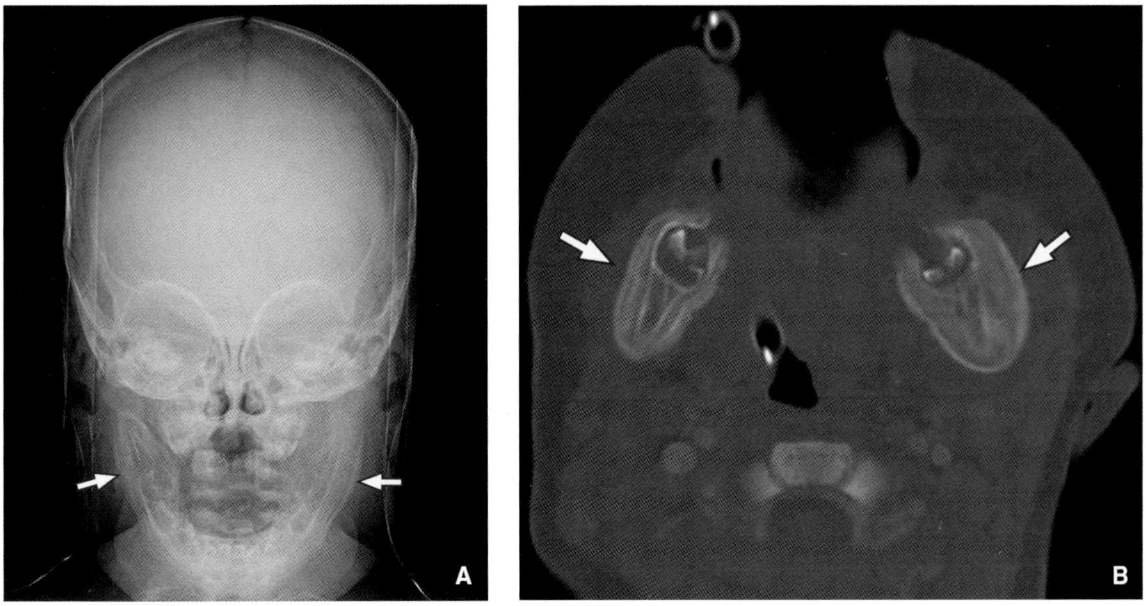

FIGURE 22.36 **Caffey disease.** Frontal radiograph of the skull **(A)** shows extensive sclerosis of the skull bone associated with substantial cortical hyperostosis and enlargement of bilateral mandibles secondary to cortical new bone formation (*arrows*). Axial bone window CT image **(B)** demonstrates cortical hyperostosis and enlargement of bilateral mandibles secondary to cortical new bone formation (*arrows*).

the name, involvement of single or multiple osseous sites.[105] The metaphyseal regions of long bones, particularly the lower extremities are the most commonly involved sites.[106] Vertebral body lesions may resemble spondylodiscitis or lytic lesions leading to collapse. Clavicle and mandibular involvement tends to be more sclerotic or hyperostotic.[106] In addition to these more commonly affected locations, multiple other sites can be involved such as pelvis, mandible, and even small bones of the extremities.[107,108]

SAPHO (synovitis, acne, pustulosis, hyperostosis, osteitis) syndrome may be an adult equivalent of CRMO.[109] Whereas CRMO typically manifests in the first decade of life, the mean age of onset for SAPHO syndrome is 28 years.[110] This clinical entity is a diagnosis of exclusion, distinct from bacterial osteomyelitis, based on the following seven criteria:

1. Bone lesions with a radiographic appearance suggesting subacute or chronic osteomyelitis.
2. An unusual location of lesions when compared with infectious osteomyelitis and frequent multifocality.
3. No abscess formation, fistula, or sequestra.
4. Lack of a causative organism. The diagnosis of CRMO is typically confirmed by bone biopsy.
5. Nonspecific histopathologic and laboratory findings compatible with subacute or chronic osteomyelitis.
6. A characteristic prolonged, fluctuating course with recurrent episodes of pain.
7. Occasional accompanying skin disease.

The imaging evaluation of CRMO should start with focused radiographic evaluation of the symptomatic sites. Radiographic investigation typically shows soft tissue swelling, periosteal reaction, and typical features of a lytic metaphyseal lesion adjacent to the physis in a long bone (Fig. 22.37) as well as progression over time to sclerosis or hyperostosis as the lesion heals.[108] If the radiographs are negative in the presence of substantial clinical symptoms, further evaluation with MRI should be considered to evaluate for abnormality that cannot be evaluated with radiographs such as bone marrow edema (Fig. 22.37). Whole body evaluation for CRMO has traditionally been performed with 99mTc bone scan,[111] although, in recent years, whole-body MRI is being increasingly used for evaluation of multifocal bone lesions in CRMO.[112] It is important to recognize that bone scan may detect focal active lesions but may result in false negatives in cases of bilateral, symmetric lesions, which can be misinterpreted as normal physeal activity.[109,113] On MRI, active lesions usually present as areas of bone marrow edema with high signal intensity on T2-weighted and short tau inversion recovery (STIR) MR images. They are hypointense on T1-weighted MR images and may enhance following gadolinium administration.[107] Because the imaging appearances of CRMO are sometimes highly similar to pyogenic osteomyelitis or malignancy, biopsy may be required for a definitive diagnosis.[107] The differential diagnosis of CRMO includes subacute and chronic infectious osteomyelitis, histiocytosis, hypophosphatasia, and malignancies such as leukemia, lymphoma, and Ewing sarcoma in the pediatric population.[114]

Currently, there are several treatment options for managing CRMO, which include nonsteroidal anti-inflammatory agents (NSAIDs), corticosteroids,[115] azithromycin, tumor necrosis factor-blocker (infliximab),[116] and interferon.[117] In addition, bisphosphonates have been used in CRMO, for pain relief, control of disease progression,[118] and when simple therapies such as anti-inflammatory agents fail to control symptoms or cases in which lesion expansion continues.[118]

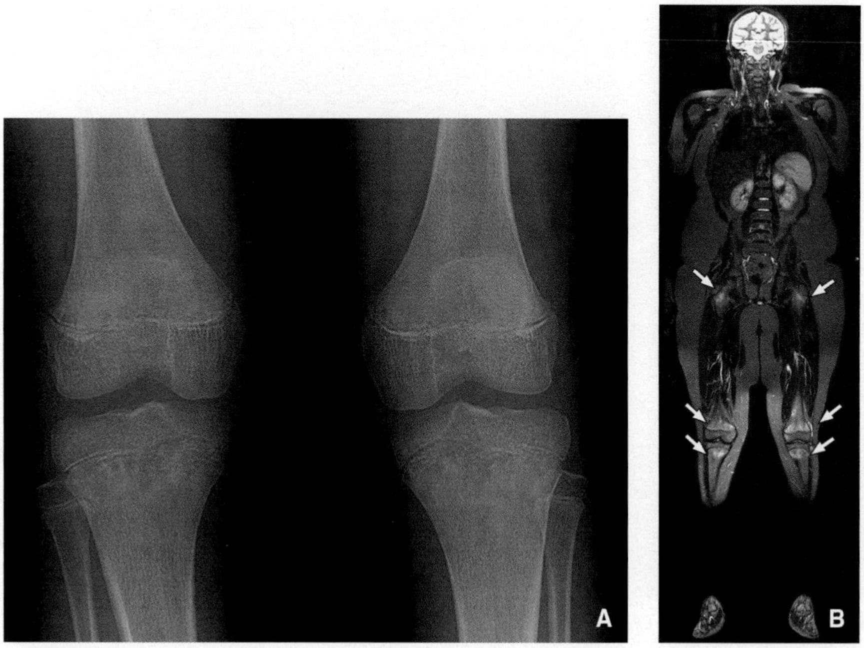

FIGURE 22.37 **Chronic recurrent multifocal osteomyelitis.** Eleven-year-old girl with painful knees. Frontal radiograph of knees **(A)** demonstrates mixed lytic and sclerotic lesions in the metaphyseal regions of bilateral distal femora and tibiae. Whole-body MRI **(B)** shows multifocal sites of bone marrow edema representing multiple lesions, some of them asymptomatic. Note the hyperintense foci (*arrows*) on inversion recovery MR image in a symmetric distribution around the knees but also affecting bilateral proximal femoral metaphyses adjacent to the greater trochanteric apophyses.

References

1. Boutin RD, Brossmann J, Sartoris DJ, et al. Update on imaging of orthopedic infections. *Orthop Clin North Am.* 1998;29(1):41–66.
2. DiPoce J, Jbara ME, Brenner AI. Pediatric osteomyelitis: A scintigraphic case-based review. *Radiographics.* 2012;32(3):865–878.
3. Patel M. Upper extremity radionuclide bone imaging: shoulder, arm, elbow, and forearm. *Semin Nucl Med.* 1998;28(1):3–13.
4. Pineda C, Vargas A, Rodriguez AV. Imaging of osteomyelitis: Current concepts. *Infect Dis Clin North Am.* 2006;20(4):789–825.
5. Kothari NA, Pelchovitz DJ, Meyer JS. Imaging of musculoskeletal infections. *Radiol Clin North Am.* 2001;4:112–117.
6. Guillerman RP. Osteomyelitis and beyond. *Pediatr Radiol.* 2013; 43(suppl 1):S193–S203.
7. Jaramillo D, Treves ST, Kasser JR, et al. Osteomyelitis and septic arthritis in children: appropriate use of imaging to guide treatment. *AJR Am J Roentgenol.* 1995;165(2):399–403.
8. Kaiser S, Jorulf H, Hirsch G. Clinical value of imaging techniques in childhood osteomyelitis. *Acta Radiol.* 1998;39(5):523–531.
9. Pruthi S, Thapa MM. Infectious and inflammatory disorders. *Magn Reson Imaging Clin N Am.* 2009;17(3):423–438.
10. Vial J, Chiavassa-Gandois H. Limb infections in children and adults. *Diagn Interv Imaging.* 2012;93(6):530–546.
11. Gylys-Morin VM. MR imaging of pediatric musculoskeletal inflammatory and infectious disorders. *Magn Reson Imaging Clin N Am.* 1998;6(3):537–559.
12. Gold RH, Tong DJ, Crim JR, et al. Imaging the diabetic foot. *Skeletal Radiol.* 1995;24(8):563–571.
13. Mandell GA. Imaging in the diagnosis of musculoskeletal infections in children. *Curr Probl Pediatr.* 1996;26(7):218–237.
14. Tuscon CE, Hoffman EB, Mann MD. Isotope bone scanning for acute osteomyelitis and septic arthritis in children. *J Bone Joint Surg.* 1994;76:306–310.
15. Lewis SS, Cox GM, Stout JE. Clinical utility of indium 111-labeled white blood cell scintigraphy for evaluation of suspected infection. *Open Forum Infect Dis.* 2014;1(2):ofu089.
16. Saigal G, Azouz EM, Abdenour G. Imaging of osteomyelitis with special reference to children. *Semin Musculoskelet Radiol.* 2004;8(3):255–265.
17. Arnold SR, Elias D, Buckingham SC, et al. Changing patterns of acute hematogenous osteomyelitis and septic arthritis: Emergence of community-associated methicillin-resistant staphylococcus aureus. *J Pediatr Orthop.* 2006;26(6):703–708.
18. Abril Martin JCMD, Rodriguez LAMD, Cilveti JAMD. Flatfoot and calcaneal deformity secondary to osteomyelitis after neonatal heel puncture. *J Pediatr Orthop B.* 1999;8(2):122–124.
19. Song KM, Sloboda JF. Acute hematogenous osteomyelitis in children. *J Am Acad Orthop Surg.* 2001;9(3):166–175.
20. Luey C, Tooley D, Briggs S. Emphysematous osteomyelitis: A case report and review of the literature. *Int J Infect Dis.* 2012;16(3):e216–e220.
21. Schmit P, Glorion C. Osteomyelitis in infant and children. *Eur Radiol.* 2004;14:L44–L54.
22. Martinez-Aguilar G, Avalos-Mishaan A, Hulten K, et al. Community-acquired, methicillin-resistant and methicillin-susceptible staphylococcus aureus musculoskeletal infections in children. *Pediatr Infect Dis J.* 2004;23(8):701–706.
23. Paakkonen M, Kallio PE, Kallio MJ, et al. Management of osteoarticular infections caused by staphylococcus aureus is similar to that of other etiologies: Analysis of 199 staphylococcal bone and joint infections. *Pediatr Infect Dis J.* 2012;31(5):436–438.
24. Trueta J. The three types of acute haematogenous osteomyelitis. *J Bone Joint Surg.* 1959;41B(4):671–680.
25. Martí-Bonmatí L, Aparisi F, Poyatos C, et al. Brodie abscess: MR imaging appearance in 10 patients. *J Magn Reson Imaging.* 1993;3(3):543–546.
26. Ranson M. Imaging of pediatric musculoskeletal infection. *Semin Musculoskelet Radiol.* 2009;13(3):277–299.
27. Lazzarini L, Lipsky BA, Mader JT. Antibiotic treatment of osteomyelitis: what have we learned from 30 years of clinical trials? *Int J Infect Dis.* 2005;9(3):127–138.
28. Termaat MF, Raijmakers PG, Scholten HJ, et al. The accuracy of diagnostic imaging for the assessment of chronic osteomyelitis: a systematic review and meta-analysis. *J Bone Joint Surg Am.* 2005;87(11):2464–2471.
29. Jones HW, Beckles VL, Akinola B, et al. Chronic haematogenous osteomyelitis in children: an unsolved problem. *J Bone Joint Surg Br.* 2011;93(8):1005–1010.

30. Kan JH. Major pitfalls in musculoskeletal imaging-MRI. *Pediatr Radiol.* 2008;38(suppl 2):S251–S255.
31. Armstrong EP, Rush DR. Treatment of osteomyelitis. *Clin Pharm.* 1983;2(3):213–224.
32. Rosenbaum DM, Blumhagen JD. Acute epiphyseal osteomyelitis in children. *Radiology.* 1985;156(1):89–92.
33. Hempfing A, Placzek R, Göttsche T, et al. Primary subacute epiphyseal and metaepiphyseal osteomyelitis in children. Diagnosis and treatment guided by MRI. *J Bone Joint Surg B.* 2003;85(4):559–564.
34. Ezra E, Cohen N, Segev E, et al. Primary subacute epiphyseal osteomyelitis: role of conservative treatment. *J Pediatr Orthop.* 2002;22(3):333–337.
35. Nixon GW. Hematogenous osteomyelitis of metaphyseal-equivalent locations. *AJR Am J Roentgenol.* 1978;130(1):123–129.
36. Connolly SA, Connolly LP, Druback LA, et al. MRI for detection of abscess in acute osteomyelitis of the pelvis in children. *AJR Am J Roentgenol.* 2007 Oct;189(4):867–872.
37. Leigh W, Crawford H, Street M, et al. Pediatric calcaneal osteomyelitis. *J Pediatr Orthop.* 2010;30(8):888–892.
38. Winiker H, Scharli AF. Hematogenous calcaneal osteomyelitis in children. *Eur J Pediatr Surg.* 1991;1(4):216–220.
39. Jaakkola J, Kehl D. Hematogenous calcaneal osteomyelitis in children. *J Pediatr Orthop.* 1999;19(6):699–704.
40. Rasool MN. Hematogenous osteomyelitis of the calcaneus in children. *J Pediatr Orthop.* 2001;21(6):738–743.
41. Nascimento M, Oliveira E, Soares S, et al. Rib osteomyelitis in a pediatric patient case report and literature review. *Pediatr Infect Dis J.* 2012;31(11):1190–1194.
42. Fernandez M, Carrol CL, Baker JC. Discitis and vertebral osteomyelitis in children: an 18-year review. *Pediatrics.* 2000; 105(6):1299–1304.
43. Tsirikos AI, Tome-Bermejo F. Spondylodiscitis in infancy: a potentially fatal condition that can lead to major spinal complications. *J Bone Joint Surg Br.* 2012;94(10):1399–1402.
44. Lincoln TA, Webber SJ. An extremely unusual case of Garre's osteomyelitis of the mandibular condyle after surgical removal of third molars. *J Oral Maxillofac Surg.* 2012;70(12):2748–2751.
45. Belli E, Matteini C, Andreano T. Sclerosing osteomyelitis of Garré periostitis ossificans. *J Craniofac Surg.* 2002;13(6):765–768.
46. Kim HY, Hwang EH, Han YM, et al. Pott's puffy tumor in an adolescent boy. *Pediatr Int.* 2012;54(1):158–160.
47. Vanderveken OM, De Smet K, Dogan-Duyar S, et al. Pott's puffy tumour in a 5-year old boy: the role of ultrasound and contrast-enhanced CT imaging; surgical case report. *B-ENT.* 2012;8(2):127–129.
48. Mantadakis E, Plessa E, Vouloumanou EK, et al. Deep venous thrombosis in children with musculoskeletal infections: the clinical evidence. *Int J Infect Dis.* 2012;16(4):e236–e243.
49. Rodriguez-Fanjul J, Trenchs V, Munoz-Santanach D, et al. Deep vein thrombosis: rare cases of diagnoses in a pediatric emergency department. *Pediatr Emerg Care.* 2011;27(5):417–419.
50. Wright JM, Watts RG. Venous thromboembolism in pediatric patients: Epidemiologic data from a pediatric tertiary care center in alabama. *J Pediatr Hematol Oncol.* 2011;33(4):261–264.
51. Bouchoucha S, Benghachame F, Trifa M, et al. Deep venous thrombosis associated with acute hematogenous osteomyelitis in children. *Orthop Traumatol Surg Res.* 2010;96(8):890–893.
52. Adeyokunnu AA, Hendrickse RG. Salmonella osteomyelitis in childhood. A report of 63 cases seen in nigerian children of whom 57 had sickle cell anaemia. *Arch Dis Child.* 1980;55(3):175–184.
53. Krishnamurthy S, Thimmaiah S, Ramesh A, et al. Osteomyelitis and pyomyositis due to pseudomonas aeruginosa in a child with sickle β^0-thalassemia. *J Pediatr Hematol Oncol.* 2011;33(6):e253–e255.
54. Epps C, Bryant D, Coles M, et al. Osteomyelitis in patients who have sickle cell disease. Diagnosis and management. *J Bone Joint Surg Am.* 1991;73:(9)1281–1294.
55. Wong AL, Sakamoto KM, Johnson EE. Differentiating osteomyelitis from bone infarction in sickle cell disease. *Pediatr Emerg Care.* 2001;17(1):60–63; quiz 64.
56. Ngwube A, Jackson S, Dixon T, et al. Disseminated salmonella osteomyelitis in a 2-year-old with sickle cell disease. *Clin Pediatr (Phila).* 2012;51(6):594–601.
57. Santos E, Boavida JE, Barroso A, et al. Late osteoarticular lesions following meningococcemia with disseminated intravascular coagulation. *Pediatr Radiol.* 1989;19(3):199–202.
58. Buysse CM, Oranje AP, Zuidema E, et al. Long-term skin scarring and orthopaedic sequelae in survivors of meningococcal septic shock. *Arch Dis Child.* 2009;94(5):381–386.
59. Hugosson C, Harfi H. Disseminated BCG-osteomyelitis in congenital immunodeficiency. *Pediatr Radiol.* 1991;21(5):384–385.
60. De Vuyst D, Vanhoenacker F, Gielen J, et al. Imaging features of musculoskeletal tuberculosis. *Eur Radiol.* 2003;13(8):1809–1819.
61. Moore SL, Rafii M. Imaging of musculoskeletal and spinal tuberculosis. *Radiol Clin North Am.* 2001;39(2):329–342.
62. Teo HE, Peh WC. Skeletal tuberculosis in children. *Pediatr Radiol.* 2004;34(11):853–860.
63. Pattamapaspong N, Muttarak M, Sivasomboon C. Tuberculosis arthritis and tenosynovitis. *Semin Musculoskelet Radiol.* 2011; 15(5):459–469.
64. Meyberg-Solomayer GC, Fehm T, Muller-Hansen I, et al. Prenatal ultrasound diagnosis, follow-up, and outcome of congenital varicella syndrome. *Fetal Diagn Ther.* 2006;21(3):296–301.
65. Bozzola E, Krzystofiak A, Lancella L, et al. A severe case of paediatric group A streptococcal osteomyelitis in varicella. *Infection.* 2012;40(3):343–345.
66. Liebergall M, Porat S. Streptococcal osteomyelitis associated with varicella virus infection: a case report and review of the literature. *J Pediatr Orthop.* 1984;4(6):756–758.
67. Resnick D. Osteomyelitis, septic arthritis, and soft tissue infection: organisms. In: Resnick D. *Bone and Joint Imaging.* 2nd ed. Philadelphia, PA: W.B. Saunders Company; 1996:697–699.
68. Woods CR. Congenital syphilis-persisting pestilence. *Pediatr Infect Dis J.* 2009;28(6):536–537.
69. Sharma M, Solanki RN, Gupta A, et al. Different radiological presentations of congenital syphilis: four cases. *Indian J Radiol Imaging.* 2005;15(1):53–57.
70. Winkelstein JA, Marino MC, Johnston RB Jr, et al. Chronic granulomatous disease. Report on a national registry of 368 patients. *Medicine (Baltimore).* 2000;79(3):155–169.
71. Murphy SN, Parnell N. Fluconazole treatment of cryptococcal rib osteomyelitis in an HIV-negative man. A case report and review of the literature. *J Infect.* 2005;51(5):e309–e311.
72. Raftopoulos I, Meller JL, Harris V, et al. Cryptococcal rib osteomyelitis in a pediatric patient. *J Pediatr Surg.* 1998;33(5):771–773.
73. Jirapongsananuruk O, Luangwedchakarn V, Niemela JE, et al. Cryptococcal osteomyelitis in a child with a novel compound mutation of the IL12RB1 gene. *Asian Pac J Allergy Immunol.* 2012;30(1):79–82.
74. Liu PY. Cryptococcal osteomyelitis: case report and review. *Diagn Microbiol Infect Dis.* 1998;30(1):33–35.
75. MacDonald PB, Black GB, MacKenzie R. Orthopaedic manifestations of blastomycosis. *J Bone Joint Surg Am.* 1990; 72(6):860–864.
76. Restrepo A. Paracoccidioidomycosis. In: Feigin RD, Cherry JD, eds. *Textbook of Pediatric Infectious Diseases.* Vol. 2. 3rd ed. Philadelphia, PA: Saunders; 1992:1929–1934.

77. Doria AS, Taylor GA. Bony involvement in paracoccidioidomycosis. *Pediatr Radiol.* 1997;27(1):67–69.
78. Monsignore LM, Martinez R, Simao MN, et al. Radiologic findings of osteoarticular infection in paracoccidioidomycosis. *Skeletal Radiol.* 2012;41(2):203–208.
79. Caird MS, Flynn JM, Leung YL, et al. Factors distinguishing septic arthritis from transient synovitis of the hip in children. A prospective study. *J Bone Joint Surg Am.* 2006;88(6):1251–1257.
80. Merino R, de Inocencio J, Garcia-Consuegra J. [Differentiation between transient synovitis and septic arthritis of the hip with clinical and ultrasound criteria]. *An Pediatr (Barc).* 2010;73(4):189–193.
81. Robben SG, Lequin MH, Diepstraten AF, et al. Anterior joint capsule of the normal hip and in children with transient synovitis: US study with anatomic and histologic correlation. *Radiology.* 1999;210(2):499–507.
82. Kermond S, Fink M, Graham K, et al. A randomized clinical trial: should the child with transient synovitis of the hip be treated with nonsteroidal anti-inflammatory drugs? *Ann Emerg Med.* 2002;40(3):294–299.
83. Shaw BA, Kasser JR. Acute septic arthritis in infancy and childhood. *Clin Orthop Relat Res.* 1990;257:212–225.
84. Blickman JG, van Die CE, de Rooy JWJ. Current imaging concepts in pediatric osteomyelitis. *Eur Radiol.* 2004;14:L55–L64.
85. Browne LP, Guillerman RP, Orth RC, et al. Community-acquired staphylococcal musculoskeletal infection in infants and young children: necessity of contrast-enhanced MRI for the diagnosis of growth cartilage involvement. *AJR Am J Roentgenol.* 2012;198(1):194–199.
86. Kan JH, Young RS, Yu C, et al. Clinical impact of gadolinium in the MRI diagnosis of musculoskeletal infection in children. *Pediatr Radiol.* 2010;40(7):1197–1205.
87. Chao HC, Lin SJ, Huang YC, et al. Sonographic evaluation of cellulitis in children. *J Ultrasound Med.* 2000;19(11):743–749.
88. Turecki MB, Taljanovic MS, Stubbs AY, et al. Imaging of musculoskeletal soft tissue infections. *Skeletal Radiol.* 2010; 39(10):957–971.
89. Hopkins K, Li K, Bergman G. Gadolinium-DTPA-enhanced magnetic resonance imaging of musculoskeletal infectious process. *Skeletal Radiol.* 1995;24(5):325–330.
90. Mazur JM, Ross G, Cummings J, et al. Usefulness of magnetic resonance imaging for the diagnosis of acute musculoskeletal infection in children. *J Ped Orthop.* 1995;15(2):144–147.
91. Schmid MR, Kossmann T, Duewell S. Differentiation of necrotizing fasciitis and cellulitis using MR imaging. *AJR Am J Roentgenol.* 1998;170(3):615–620.
92. Kaiser RE, Cerra FB. Progressive necrotizing surgical infections—a unified approach. *J Trauma.* 1981;21(5):349–355.
93. Majeski JA, Alexander JW. Early diagnosis, nutritional support and immediate extensive debridement improve survival in necrotizing fasciitis. *Am J Surg.* 1983;145(6):784–787.
94. Gubbay AJ, Isaacs D. Pyomyositis in children. *Pediatr Infect Dis J.* 2000;19(10):1009–1012; quiz 1013.
95. Rotman-Pikielny P, Levy Y, Eyal A, et al. Pyomyositis or "injectiositis"—Staphylococcus aureus multiple abscesses following intramuscular injections. *Isr Med Assoc J.* 2003;5(4):295–296.
96. Mitsionis GI, Manoudis GN, Lykissas MG, et al. Pyomyositis in children: early diagnosis and treatment. *J Pediatr Surg.* 2009;44(11):2173–2178.
97. Martínez-Aguilar G, Avalos-Mishaan A, Hulten K, et al. Community-acquired, methicillin-resistant and methicillin-susceptible Staphylococcus aureus musculoskeletal infections in children. *Pediatr Infect Dis J.* 2004;23(8):701–706.
98. Klein-Kremer A, Jassar H, Nachtigal A, et al. Primary pyomyositis in a young boy: clinical and radiologic features. *Isr Med Assoc J.* 2010;12(8):511–513.
99. Phatak S, Kolwadkar P, Phatak M. Pictorial essay: Infantile cortical hyperostosis (caffey's disease). *Indian J Radiol Imaging.* 2004;14(2):185–186.
100. Darmency V, Thauvin-Robinet C, Rousseau T, et al. Contribution of three-dimensional computed tomography in prenatal diagnosis of lethal infantile cortical hyperostosis (caffey disease). *Prenat Diagn.* 2009;29(9):892–894.
101. Jurik AG. Chronic recurrent multifocal osteomyelitis. *Semin Musculoskelet Radiol.* 2004;8(3):243–253.
102. Ferguson PJ, El Shanti HI. Autoinflammatory bone disorders. *Curr Opin Rheumatol.* 2007;19(5):492–498.
103. Laxer RM, Shore AD, Manson D, et al. Chronic recurrent multifocal osteomyelitis and psoriasis—a report of a new association and review of related disorders. *Semin Arthritis Rheum.* 1988;17(4):260–270.
104. Bousvaros A, Marcon M, Treem W, et al. Chronic recurrent multifocal osteomyelitis associated with chronic inflammatory bowel disease in children. *Dig Dis Sci.* 1999;44(12):2500–2507.
105. Jansson A, Renner ED, Ramser J, et al. Classification of non-bacterial osteitis: Retrospective study of clinical, immunological and genetic aspects in 89 patients. *Rheumatology (Oxford).* 2007;46(1):154–160.
106. Ferguson PJ, Sandu M. Current understanding of the pathogenesis and management of chronic recurrent multifocal osteomyelitis. *Curr Rheumatol Rep.* 2012;14(2):130–141.
107. Jurik AG, Egund N. MRI in chronic recurrent multifocal osteomyelitis. *Skeletal Radiol.* 1997;26(4):230–238.
108. Cyrlak D, Pais MJ. Chronic recurrent multifocal osteomyelitis. *Skeletal Radiol.* 1986;15(1):32–39.
109. Khanna G, Sato TS, Ferguson P. Imaging of chronic recurrent multifocal osteomyelitis. *Radiographics.* 2009;29(4): 1159–1177.
110. Hayem G, Bouchaud-Chabot A, Benali K, et al. SAPHO syndrome: a long-term follow-up study of 120 cases. *Semin Arthritis Rheum.* 1999;29(3):159–171.
111. Mandell GA, Contreras SJ, Conard K, et al. Bone scintigraphy in the detection of chronic recurrent multifocal osteomyelitis. *J Nucl Med.* 1998;39(100):1778–1783.
112. Fritz J, Tzaribatchev N, Claussen CD, et al. Chronic recurrent multifocal osteomyelitis: comparison of whole-body MR imaging with radiography and correlation with clinical and laboratory data. *Radiology.* 2009;252(3):842–851.
113. Stern SM, Ferguson PJ. Autoinflammatory bone diseases. *Rheum Dis Clin North Am.* 2013;39(4):735–749.
114. Girschick HJ, Mornet E, Beer M, et al. Chronic multifocal non-bacterial osteomyelitis in hypophosphatasia mimicking malignancy. *BMC Pediatr.* 2007;7:3.
115. Holden W, David J. Chronic recurrent multifocal osteomyelitis: two cases of sacral disease responsive to corticosteroids. *Clin Infect Dis.* 2005;40(4):616–619.
116. Deutschmann A, Mache CJ, Bodo K, et al. Successful treatment of chronic recurrent multifocal osteomyelitis with tumor necrosis factor-alpha blockage. *Pediatrics.* 2005;116(5):1231–1233.
117. Gallagher KT, Roberts RL, MacFarlane JA, et al. Treatment of chronic recurrent multifocal osteomyelitis with interferon gamma. *J Pediatr.* 1997;131(3):470–472.
118. Simm PJ, Allen RC, Zacharin MR. Bisphosphonate treatment in chronic recurrent multifocal osteomyelitis. *J Pediatr.* 2008; 152(4):571–575.

CHAPTER 23

Musculoskeletal Neoplastic Disorders

Hee-Kyung Kim • Jung-Eun Cheon • Sara O. Vargas • Hye-Kyung Yoon

INTRODUCTION

During the past several decades, improved early and accurate diagnosis along with development of new therapeutic regimens for managing childhood musculoskeletal neoplasms have resulted in substantially improved outcomes for pediatric patients with various bone and soft tissue neoplasms. However, musculoskeletal neoplasms continue to cause substantial mortality and morbidity in the pediatric population.[1–3] Imaging evaluation plays an essential role in the initial detection, staging, and follow-up assessment of musculoskeletal neoplasms in infants and children. In this chapter, currently available imaging modalities with up-to-date imaging techniques, clinical presentations, imaging findings, and management of benign and malignant childhood bone and soft tissue neoplasms as classified by the World Health Organization (WHO) are discussed (Table 23.1).[4]

IMAGING TECHNIQUES

Radiography

Radiography is usually the first imaging modality for evaluating bone and soft tissue neoplasms in children. In general, aggressive lesions on radiographs are malignant, and nonaggressive lesions are benign tumors. Osteosarcoma and Ewing sarcoma comprise 90% of malignant bone tumors in children and have an aggressive appearance such as an ill-defined border with a broad zone of transition, periosteal new bone formation, and cortical destruction on radiographs. However, an aggressive radiographic appearance can also be seen with nonmalignant entities such as Langerhans cell histiocytosis (LCH), osteomyelitis, and occasionally with a fracture undergoing the healing process in the pediatric population.[5] Therefore, further evaluation using computed tomography (CT) or magnetic resonance imaging (MRI) may be needed for clarification.

Ultrasound

Ultrasound is often used as the first imaging study in evaluation of palpable mass and useful to differentiate solid from cystic masses. The utilized ultrasound technique usually depends on the depth of the lesions. While superficial masses are often evaluated with high frequency linear transducers (12 to 17 MHz), deep masses are evaluated with lower frequency curved array transducers (5 to 9 MHz) with better soft tissue penetration.[6] Color Doppler imaging is useful for evaluating vascular masses especially vascular malformations and identification of solid masses. However, in most cases, sonographic imaging findings of soft tissue masses are nonspecific and often require further evaluation and characterization with MRI.

Computed Tomography

CT is useful to detect mineralization associated with malignant osseous tumors and nidus in osteoid osteoma. Although CT and MRI have comparable accuracy in local staging of bone and soft tissue tumors, MRI is superior to CT due to its excellent tissue contrast.[7] In addition to evaluation of the primary malignant bone and soft tissue lesions, evaluation of metastases should be also performed. Twenty percent of children with osteosarcoma and 25% of patients with Ewing sarcoma have metastases at presentation.[8] Because the lung is the most common site of metastases, chest CT is currently recommended as a part of initial evaluation and staging.

TABLE 23.1 World Health Organization (WHO) Classification of Bone Tumors

Bone Tumor Origin	Benign	Intermediate	Malignant
Chondrogenic	Osteochondroma Enchondroma Subungual exostosis Synovial chondromatosis	Chondromyxoid fibroma Atypical cartilaginous tumor (chondrosarcoma grade I) Chondroblastoma	Chondrosarcoma (grade II, grade III) Mesenchymal chondrosarcoma
Osteogenic	Osteoma Osteoid osteoma	Osteoblastoma	Osteosarcoma
Fibrogenic	Desmoplastic fibroma of bone		Fibrosarcoma of bone
Fibrohistiocytic	Nonossifying fibroma		
Hematopoietic			Primary lymphoma of bone
Osteoclastic giant cell rich		Giant cell tumor of bone	
Notochordal	Benign notochordal tumor		Chordoma
Vascular	Hemangioma	Epithelioid hemangioma	Epithelioid hemangioendothelioma Angiosarcoma
Miscellaneous			Ewing sarcoma Adamantinoma
Undefined neoplastic nature	Simple bone cyst Fibrous dysplasia Osteofibrous dysplasia	Aneurysmal bone cyst Langerhans cell histiocytosis	

Adapted from: Fletcher CDM, Bridge JA, Hogendoorn PCW, et al., eds. WHO Classification of Tumours of Soft Tissue and Bone. 4th ed. Lyon, France: IARC; 2013.

Magnetic Resonance Imaging

MRI has been used as a standard care imaging modality in evaluation of malignant bone and soft tissue tumors. Staging of malignant bone and soft tissue tumors is summarized in Table 23.2.[9] MRI is an essential step in the preoperative workup because it provides critical information regarding (1) intra- and extraosseous tumor involvement, (2) the extent of bone marrow involvement and skip lesions, (3) invasion of the epiphysis, (4) involvement of the neurovascular or joint structures, and (5) documentation of viable tumor and mineralized matrix to guide biopsy.

Skip metastases are areas of tumor within the bone marrow of the affected bone but separate from the primary lesion. They are associated with an increased incidence of local recurrence and subsequent metastases after ablative surgery. Therefore, MRI with T1-weighted and/or short tau inversion recovery (STIR) sequences should be performed through the entire involved bone to detect skip metastases. In contrast to bone marrow edema from benign entities such as osteomyelitis or trauma, malignant bone tumors typically demonstrate a clear demarcation between normal marrow and tumor involved marrow. The signal intensities of primary bone lesions depend on the tissue components of the tumors. Enhancement after intravenous contrast administration is useful to differentiate peritumoral edema from tumor and to assess tumor necrosis after treatment. At least two planes of postcontrast T1-weighted MR images with fat-suppression are required for a complete assessment.

Nuclear Medicine

Technetium 99m-methylene diphosphonate (MDP) bone scintigraphy can be used to assess the presence of bone metastases and skip lesions, which are represented by increased uptake. Single-photon emission computed tomography (SPECT) can improve sensitivity of the examinations. Whole-body (WB) FDG-PET imaging can be used to detect metastases, assess chemotherapeutic response, and detect tumor recurrence.[10] Whole-body (WB) MRI is currently used in oncology patients. Using a moving tabletop in the scanner and software with automatic direct realignment of the sequential achieved images, imaging the entire body is enabled in a short time. WB MRI is useful to assess tumor extent, follow-up of therapeutic response, as well as detection of complications. Accuracy of WB MRI in detection of skeletal and extraskeletal metastasis is even higher than bone scintigraphy or CT.[11] Integrating WB MRI and PET scan has been recently carried out and enabled metabolic–anatomic combined imaging. This technique might be beneficial to tumor staging with improved accuracy in pediatric oncologic patients.[12]

SPECTRUM OF PEDIATRIC MUSCULOSKELETAL NEOPLASMS

Tumors Arising from Bone

Benign Osseous Tumors

Although the exact incidence is not known, the majority of bone tumors in children are benign.[13] It is common for benign bony lesions to be found incidentally on radiographs obtained for evaluation of traumatic injury or joint pain. For benign bone lesions, such as benign fibrous cortical defects (FCDs), or nonossifying fibromas (NOFs), radiography alone is sufficient for diagnosis, and there is no need for further imaging studies or biopsy.

TABLE 23.2 TNM Classification of Bone and Soft Tissue Tumors

Category Domain	Category Item	TNM Classification of Bone Tumors	TNM Classification of Soft Tissue Tumors
Primary tumor (T)	**TX**	Primary tumor cannot be assessed	Primary tumor cannot be assessed
	T0	No evidence of primary tumor	No evidence of primary tumor
	T1	Tumor ≤8 cm in greatest dimension	Tumor ≤5 cm in greatest dimension[b] T1a: superficial tumor T1b: deep tumor
	T2	Tumor >8 cm in greatest dimension	Tumor >5 cm in greatest dimension[b] T2a: superficial tumor T2b: deep tumor
	T3	Discontinuous tumors in the primary bone site	
Regional lymph nodes (N)	**NX**	Regional lymph nodes cannot be assessed[a]	Regional lymph nodes cannot be assessed[a]
	N0	No regional lymph node metastasis	No regional lymph node metastasis
	N1	Regional lymph node metastasis	Regional lymph node metastasis
Distant metastasis (M)	**MX**	Distant metastasis cannot be assessed	
	M0	No distant metastasis	No distant metastasis
	M1	Distant metastasis M1a: lung M1b: other distant sites	Distant metastasis

[a]Regional node involvement is rare, and cases in which nodal status is not assessed either clinically or pathologically could be considered N0 instead of NX.

[b]Superficial tumor is located exclusively above the superficial fascia without invasion of the fascia; deep tumor is located either exclusively beneath the superficial fascia or superficial to the fascia with invasion of or through the fascia. Retroperitoneal, mediastinal, and pelvic sarcomas are classified as deep tumors.

Edge S, Byrd DR, Compton CC, et al. eds. AJCC Cancer Staging Manual. 7th ed. Chicago, IL: American Joint Commission on Cancer; 2010.

Benign bone lesions are typically well-demarcated, having a narrow transition zone with sclerotic rim and no cortical bone breakdown or soft tissue extension. In some cases, the lesions can have an aggressive radiographic appearance that may mimic malignant bone tumor or osteomyelitis, requiring further evaluation.[14] CT is superior to radiography or MRI in visualizing matrix calcification or ossification and associated fracture. MRI is excellent for showing the cross-sectional intraosseous and extraosseous extent of bone tumors, internal characteristics such as necrosis, hemorrhage, or fluid–fluid levels, adjacent marrow edema, and enhancement pattern.

Benign bone tumors have a tendency to be found in certain bones (**Schematic A**), in specific locations (epiphysis, metaphysis, and diaphysis, **Schematic B**), and in different depths (**Schematic D**) within the bones. Because skeletal growth is ongoing in the pediatric population, benign bone lesions such as bone cysts in the metaphysis may appear to migrate away from the physis. In addition, benign slow-growing tumors can cause substantial deformity of the involved bone or the adjacent joint, for example, Madelung deformity in multiple exostoses and "shepherd crook" deformity in fibrous dysplasia.

Osteochondroma

Osteochondroma, also known as an osteocartilaginous exostosis, is a cartilage-capped bony excrescence that arises from the external surface of the bone and contains a medullary cavity that is continuous with that of the parent bone[15] (Fig. 23.1). It is the most common benign bone tumor, accounting for 20% to 50% of benign bone tumors and affecting 1% of the general population.[1] In most cases, osteochondromas present as a solitary bone lesion (86% of cases) and occur in the first three decades of life with slight male predilection (male: female 1.6 to 3.4:1).[1] They most commonly arise from the metaphyses of the long bones, particularly the distal femur, proximal tibia, and proximal humerus. Less commonly involved locations are the radius, fibula, and flat bones including the ileum, scapula, and ribs. Involvement of small bones of the hand or the foot is seen in 10% of osteochondromas.[16]

Multiple osteochondromas account for 14% of cases and occur in the setting of hereditary multiple exostoses (HME). In ~80% of solitary osteochondromas, homozygous mutations in the *EXT1* gene can be found in the cartilaginous cap. In HME, also known as familial osteochondromatosis or diaphyseal aclasis, germline mutations in the *EXT1* or *EXT2* gene are commonly identified.[17] HME most commonly

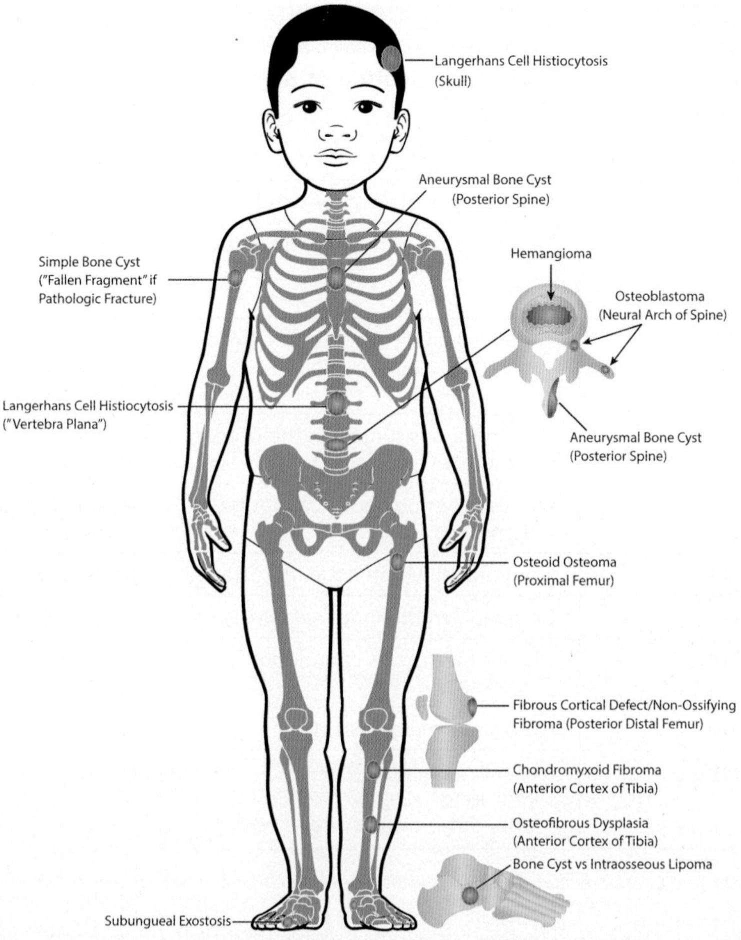

A: Benign Bone Tumors in Characteristic Locations in the Peripheral and Axial Skeletons.

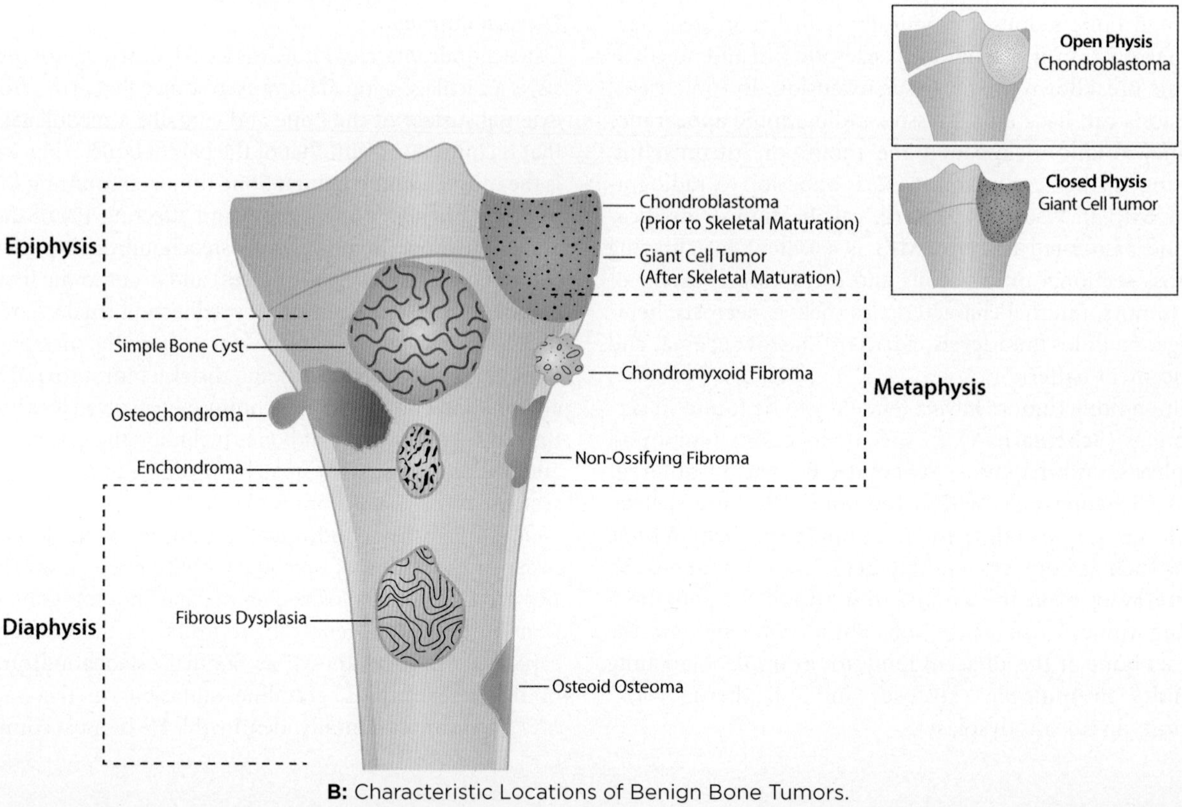

B: Characteristic Locations of Benign Bone Tumors.

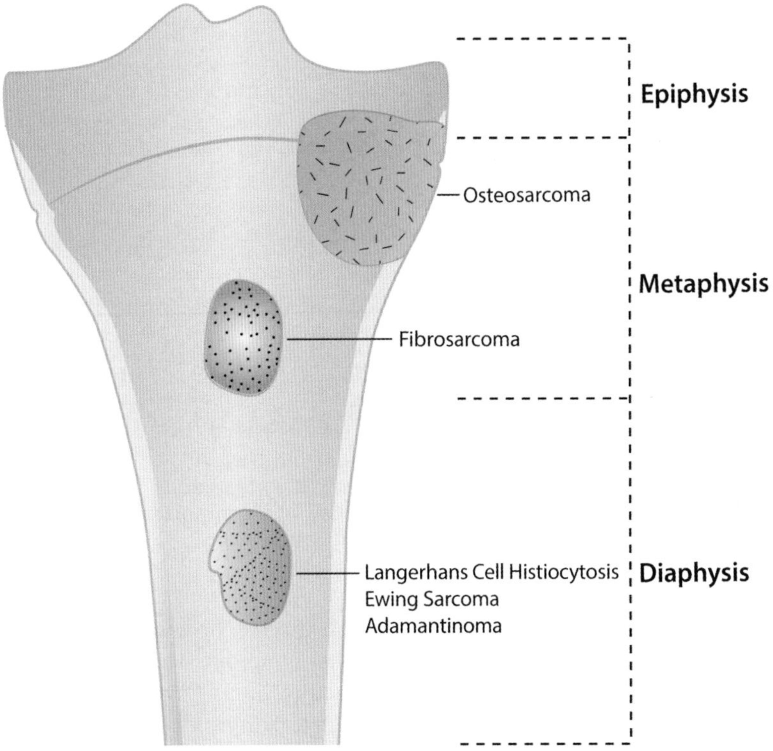

C: Characteristic Locations of Malignant Bone Tumors.

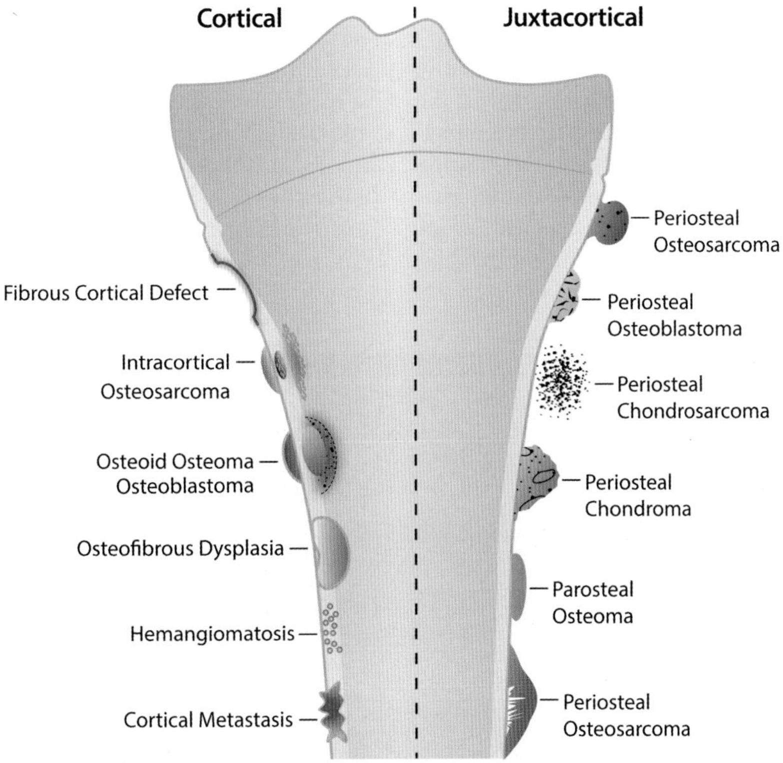

D: Characteristic Locations of Superficial Benign and Malignant Bone Tumors.

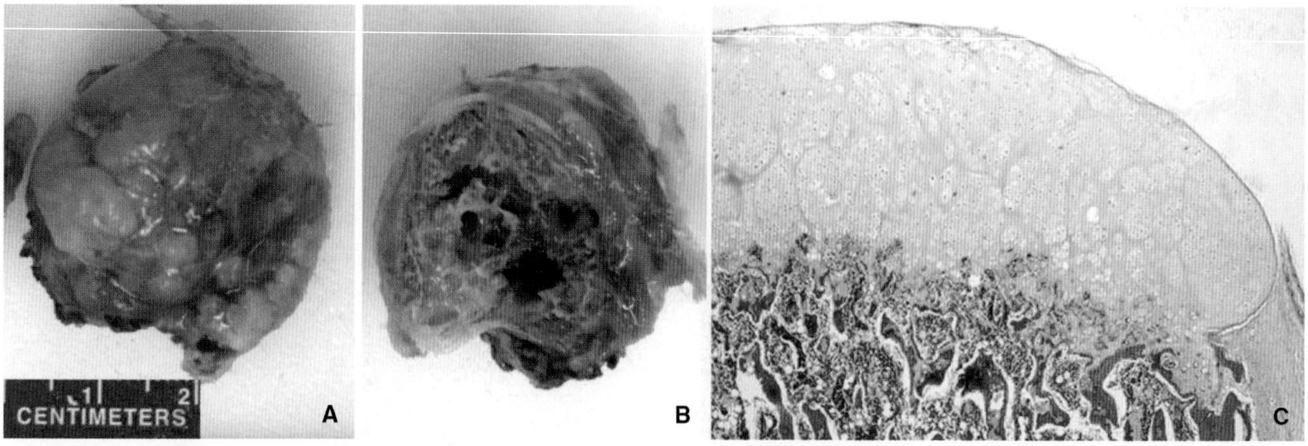

FIGURE 23.1 **Solitary osteochondroma in the humerus of a 13-year-old boy. A:** The outer surface shows knobby cartilaginous protrusions. **B:** The cut surface shows the relationship between the cartilaginous cap and the underlying trabecular bone. **C:** Microscopically, there is a thin fibrous perichondrium overlying a cap of disorganized hyaline cartilage, with enchondral ossification and underlying bone (hematoxylin and eosin, original magnification, 40×).

affects the distal and proximal bones of the lower extremities, and involvement is typically bilateral and symmetrical. Nearly 2% of patients with HME eventually develop a chondrosarcoma.[17]

Osteochondroma is the most common tumor in irradiated skeletons; 6% to 12% of patients who underwent previous radiation at a young age develop osteochondromas, and latent periods are variable with a range of 3 to 16 years.[18,19] Imaging findings and histologic features are the same as those of primary osteochondroma.

In the immature skeleton, osteochondromas continue to increase in size by endochondral ossification occurring at the base of the cartilage cap, which is equivalent to the epiphyseal physis, and growth ceases after skeletal maturation (physeal closure). Spontaneous regression of osteochondromas has been reported after skeletal maturation. In many cases, osteochondromas are asymptomatic and found incidentally, but affected pediatric patients can present with pain and other symptoms. Complications of osteochondromas include fracture, bursa formation, bursitis, vascular injury, and neurologic compromise. Complications and osseous deformities are more common in HME.

The imaging findings of osteochondromas are characteristic and include pedunculated or sessile lesions. Pedunculated osteochondromas have a long and slender appearance with a bony excrescence arising from the surface of the bone (usually long bone metaphyses). Pedunculated osteochondromas grow in the direction of tendon pulling (Fig. 23.2). Sessile osteochondromas have a broad-based and flat appearance. Typically, the medullary portion of the osteochondroma merges into the bone marrow of the parent bone, and the bony cortex and periosteum continuously outline both parent bone and osteochondroma. In contrast to osteochondroma, juxtacortical osteosarcoma

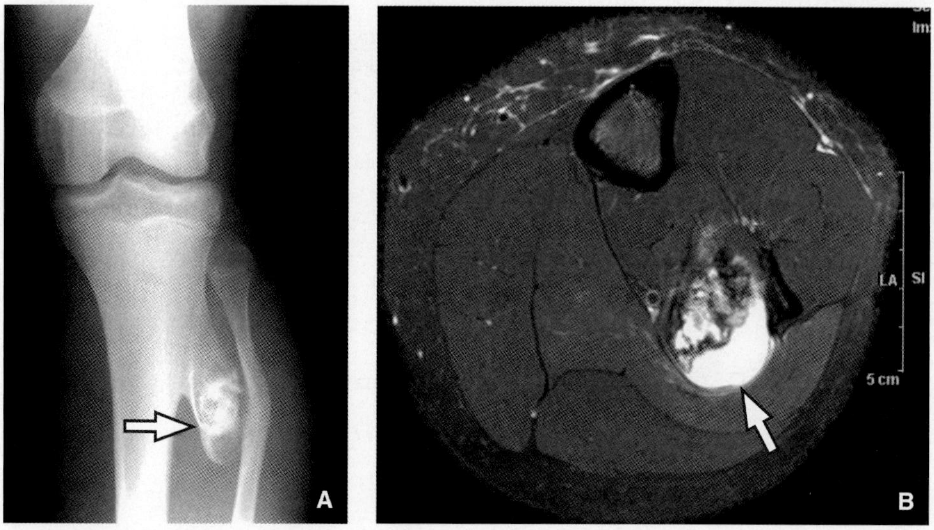

FIGURE 23.2 **Pedunculated osteochondroma in an 11-year-old boy. A:** Frontal radiograph of the left knee shows a solitary osteochondroma (*arrow*) arising from the proximal tibia. The medullary and cortical portions of the lesion are continuous with those of the parent bone. There is bowing of the proximal fibula. **B:** Axial fat-suppressed T2-weighted MR image demonstrates a hyperintensity cartilaginous cap (*arrow*) over the bony mass of the proximal tibia.

has interposed periosteum and cortex between tumor and parent bone.

Imaging findings of individual osteochondromas in HME and solitary osteochondromas are the same. Besides multiple osteochondromas, HME is characterized by abnormal modeling of developing bone, including metaphyseal widening, growth disturbance, and deformities of the joints. Radiographic evaluation is required to delineate the dramatic bone changes.[20] The affected bone is abnormally wide due to failure of normal tubulation. The cartilage cap is not visualized on radiographs except when irregular zones of calcification occur in the cartilage cap. Small stippled calcifications are compatible with a benign growth of the cartilage cap.[21] Osteochondromas arising from the innominate bone tend to be especially large and may exert mass effect, displacing adjacent structures.

Both CT and MRI can show the continuity of the medullary bone between the parent bone and the lesion. MRI is superior to CT in demonstrating the cartilaginous cap, which has a curvilinear area of fluid-like signal intensity (low signal intensity on T1-weighted MR images and high signal intensity on T2-weighted MR images), and can allow accurate measurement of the thickness of the cartilage cap (Fig. 23.2). In children and adolescents, the cartilage cap can be as thick as 3 cm.[22] In adults, the cartilage cap is usually <1 cm in thickness or can be entirely absent. In skeletally mature patients, a cartilage cap presenting with more than 1.5 cm in thickness raises the possibility of underlying malignant change.[23]

Malignant transformation to chondrosarcoma can occur in the cartilage cap and is reported in <1% of solitary osteochondromas and in nearly 2% of HME (Fig. 23.3).[24] Imaging features suggesting malignant transformation include growth of the lesion in a skeletally mature patient or after physeal closure, irregular or indistinct lesion surface, focal areas of radiolucency in the base of the lesion, erosion or destruction of the adjacent bone, and new soft tissue formation with extensive or irregular calcification (Fig. 23.3).[24] Malignant transformation of osteochondroma to chondrosarcoma before the age of 20 years is unusual. Malignant transformation of osteochondroma to osteosarcoma, which usually occurs in the osteochondroma stalk, is even rarer.

Small asymptomatic osteochondromas do not require treatment. Surgical resection is reserved for large solitary lesions or lesions with complications. In pediatric patients with HME, treatment is complex to correct deformities as well as to resect lesions, and often multiple surgical procedures are required.

Osteochondroma Variants

Dysplasia epiphysealis hemimelica (DEH), also known as Trevor disease, is a rare developmental disorder characterized by osteochondromas arising from the epiphysis. DEH is nonhereditary and more commonly seen in boys. The lower extremity is usually affected, and tarsal or carpal bones are also involved in some cases.[25] DEH is caused by asymmetric overgrowth of the medial or lateral aspect of the epiphyseal cartilage or epiphyseal equivalent. Three different types are observed: localized (single epiphyseal involvement), classical (involvement of more than one epiphysis of the same limb), and generalized (involvement of the entire limb).[26]

Radiographs usually demonstrate the characteristic appearance of asymmetric epiphyseal cartilage overgrowth with multiple stippled, irregular, and dense calcifications in the epiphysis.[27] The lesion is more likely to be medial than lateral in a given bone part, and CT can clearly show the continuity of the mass with the mother bone (Fig. 23.4). MRI is helpful for defining epiphyseal overgrowth, which is mainly cartilaginous before ossification. On MRI, the osteochondroma appears incorporated into the epiphysis, and the lesion has the same signal intensity as normal cartilage and may contain internal low signal spots from calcified foci.

Subungual exostosis is a neoplastic overgrowth of cartilage and trabecular bone in the nail bed of the phalanx. Bizarre parosteal osteochondromatous proliferation (BPOP), also known as Nora lesion, is a benign proliferation of bone and cartilage that arises from the bone surface in the hand or foot, or less commonly the long bones. BPOP presents with a nodular mineralized mass arising from the hand and foot bones (Fig. 23.5).[24]

Simple Bone Cyst

A simple bone cyst (SBC), also known as a unicameral cyst, solitary bone cyst, or juvenile bone cyst, is an intramedullary membrane-lined, fluid-filled cavity in the bone. In most cases, SBC remains asymptomatic and is discovered incidentally. However, SBC may present with pain and swelling when there is a pathologic fracture. SBC is most commonly found in the proximal humerus (over two-thirds of cases), followed by the proximal femur. SBC usually involves the metaphysis and is centered in the medullary cavity, in contrast to the eccentric location of a typical aneurysmal bone cyst (ABC). As the child grows, SBC appears to gradually migrate away from the physis into the diaphysis.

On radiograph, SBC appears as a well-demarcated radiolucent lesion with or without septations. There is no or little expansion of the bone. A "fallen-fragment" sign, representing a fractured bone fragment dislodged in the dependent portion of the cyst, is pathognomonic for SBC with pathologic fracture (Fig. 23.6).[28] On MRI, the bone cyst appears as a high signal intensity fluid-filled lesion on T2-weighted MR images and low to iso-signal intensity on T1-weighted MR images. There may be rim or cyst wall enhancement after administration of gadolinium. When complicated by a pathologic fracture, fluid–fluid levels are often demonstrated within a SBC. If the SBC occurs in the calcaneus, mostly in adults, it is typically located near the neck of the calcaneus.[29] Calcaneal pseudocyst and intraosseous lipoma may have a

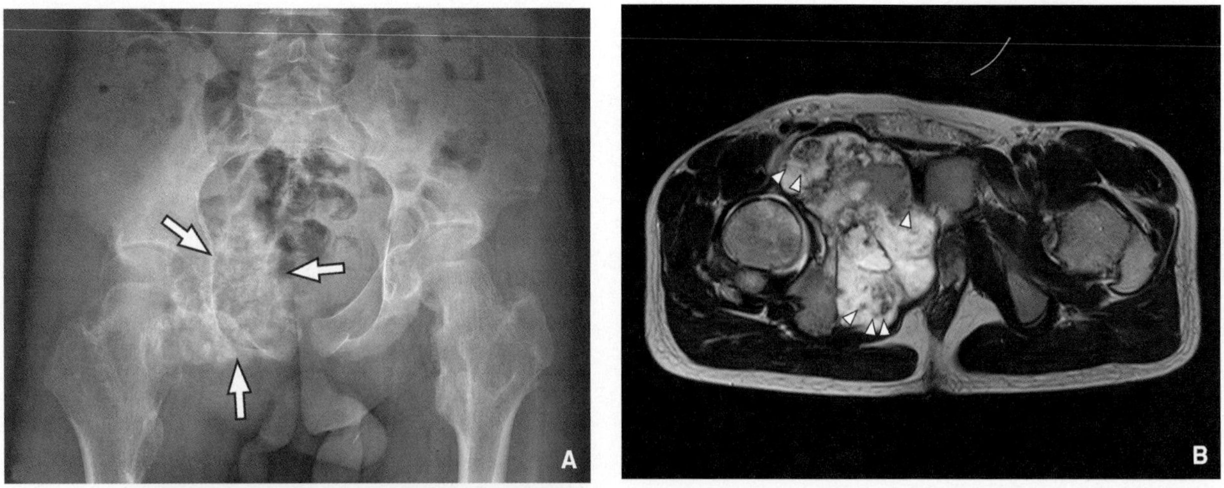

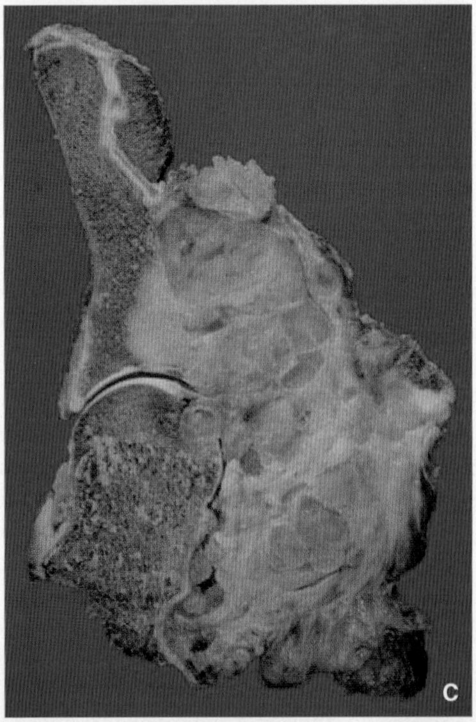

FIGURE 23.3 **Malignant transformation of multiple hereditary exostoses to chondrosarcoma in a 15-year-old boy who presented with a rapidly growing mass. A:** Frontal radiograph of the pelvis shows multiple sessile and bizarre-shaped bony masses and deformities. A calcified mass (*arrows*) is seen arising from the right pelvis. **B:** Axial T2-weighted MR image demonstrates a heterogeneous high-signal mass arising from the right pelvic bones. Multiple areas of dark signal represent calcifications (*arrowheads*). **C:** Gross specimen demonstrates chondrosarcoma arising from the right pelvic bones.

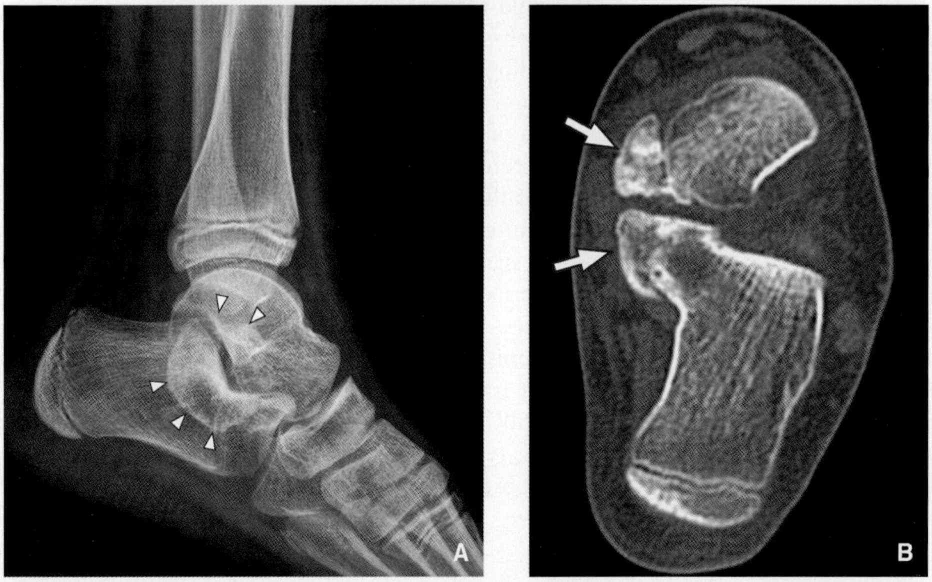

FIGURE 23.4 **Dysplasia epiphysealis hemimelica (Trevor disease) in a 9-year-old girl. A:** Lateral view of the left ankle joint radiograph shows an exuberant bony mass (*arrowheads*) projecting through the calcaneus and talus. **B:** Coronal CT image also demonstrates bony masses (*arrows*) protruding from the medial aspects of the talus and calcaneus around the talocalcaneal joint.

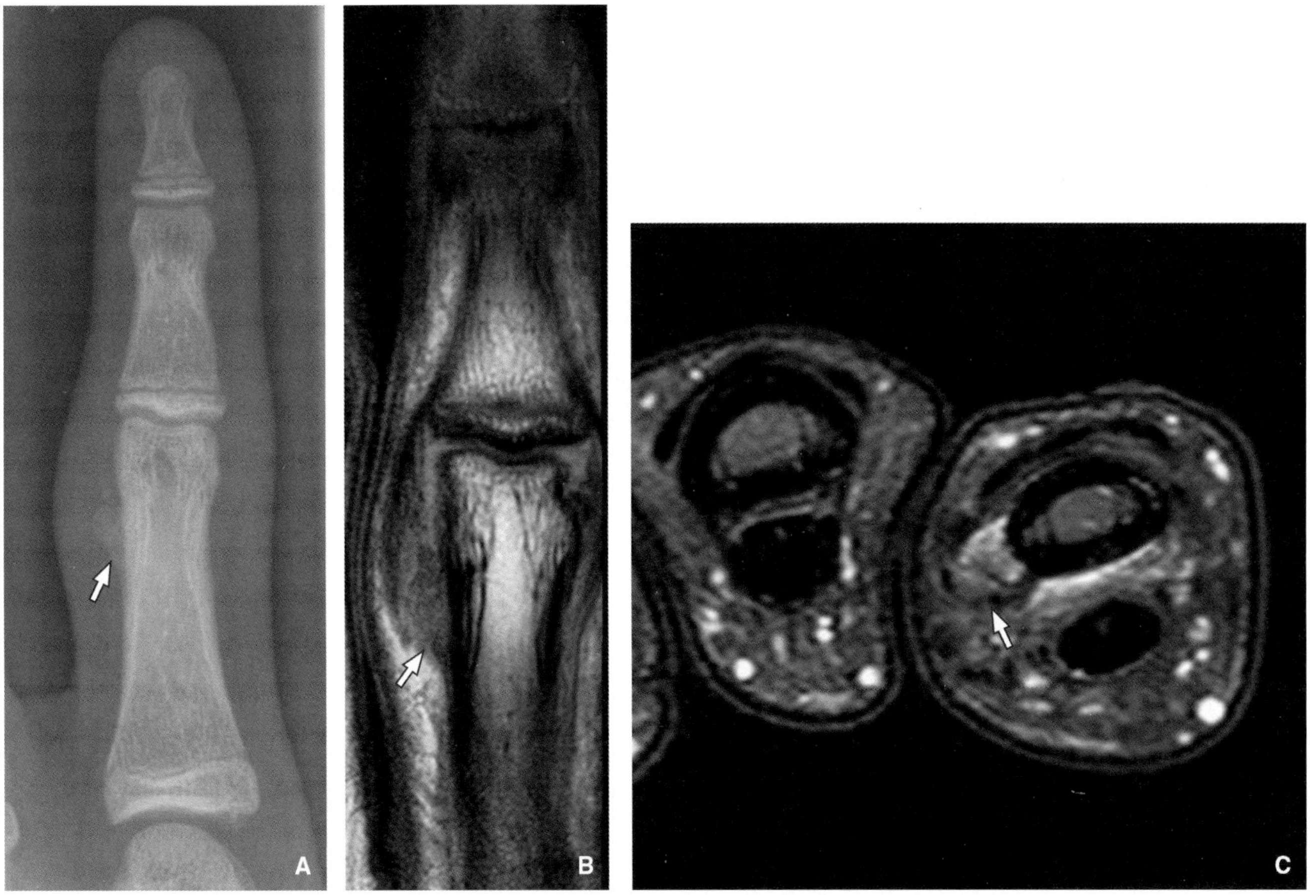

FIGURE 23.5 **Bizarre parosteal osteochondromatous proliferation in a 15-year-old boy. A:** Frontal radiograph of the index finger demonstrates a mineralized mass (*arrow*) arising from the proximal phalanx. **B, C:** Coronal T1-weighted **(B)** and axial fat-suppressed T2-weighted **(C)** MR images demonstrate an intermediate T1, heterogeneous high T2 signal mass (*arrow*) arising from the cortex of the proximal phalanx.

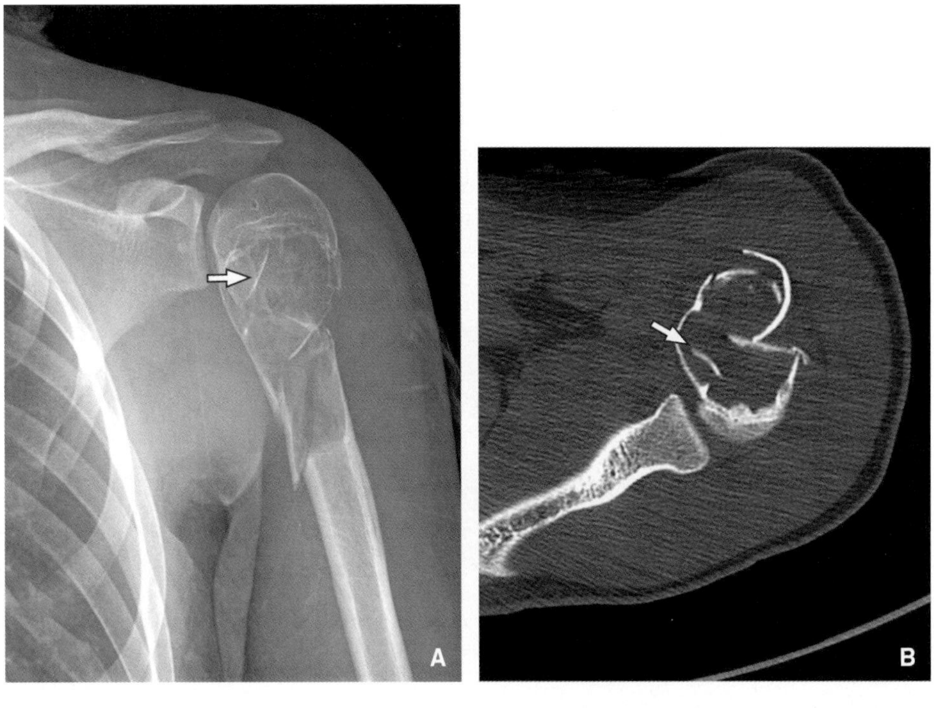

FIGURE 23.6 **Simple bone cyst with a fracture in a 17-year-old boy. A, B:** Frontal radiograph of the proximal left humerus **(A)** and axial CT image **(B)** show an osteolytic bony lesion in the proximal left humerus associated with a pathologic fracture. A detached bone fragment is seen within the bone cyst (*arrows*), which is known as the "fallen fragment" sign.

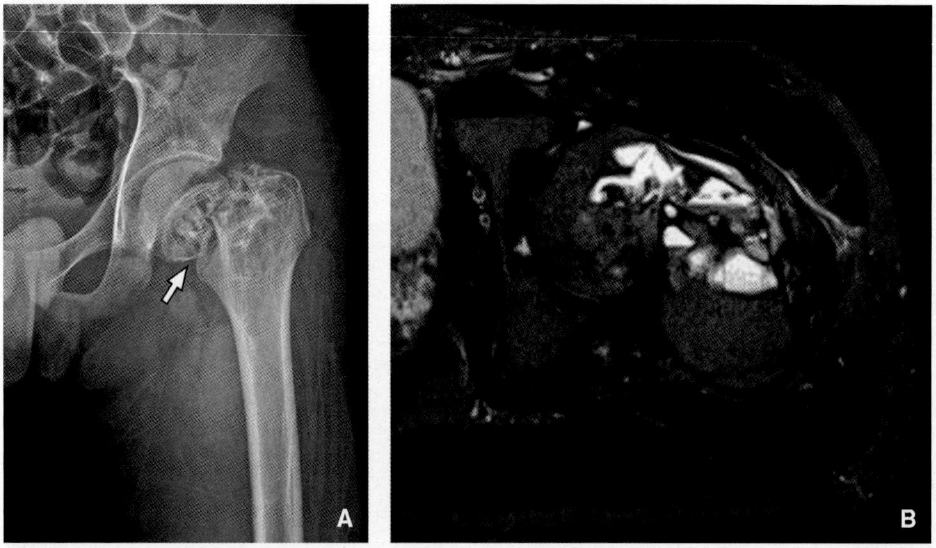

FIGURE 23.7 **Aneurysmal bone cyst (ABC) with an associated fracture in a 16-year-old boy. A:** Frontal radiograph of the left hip shows an expansile bony lesion with a soap-bubble appearance in the left femoral neck. There is a radiolucent line crossing the bony lesion (*arrow*) with angulation representing an associated fracture. **B:** Axial fat-suppressed T2-weighted MR image demonstrates a multilocular cystic mass with fluid–hemorrhage levels, characteristic of an ABC.

similar radiographic appearance with well-demarcated radiolucent lesions.

The current treatment of SBC includes steroid injection after cyst aspiration, sclerotherapy, and curettage with cement engrafting. Posttreatment radiography may show a more complex appearance of the no longer "simple" cyst with sclerosis and deformity.

Aneurysmal Bone Cyst

ABC is a benign bone neoplasm composed of blood-filled spaces separated by multiple thin fibrous septa. Lesions with histologic features of ABC can arise de novo (primary), which accounts for 70% of cases, or they may occur adjacent to other benign or malignant bone tumors (secondary) in the remaining 30%.[4] ABC is most common during the first two decades of life with no gender predilection. The most commonly affected sites are the metaphyses of the long tubular bones, the femur, tibia and humerus, and the posterior aspect of the spine. Typical clinical presentations include pain and swelling and neurologic symptoms in cases of spinal involvement.

Radiographs usually show a well-delineated and expansile osteolytic lesion with thin walls and septa creating a "soap-bubble" appearance. In the long bones, ABC is usually eccentric in location, and the outer cortex is markedly thin (Fig. 23.7). CT and MRI can reveal fluid–fluid levels due to blood products; this finding is nearly diagnostic of ABC (Fig. 23.7). It is important to recognize that secondary ABC components with fluid–fluid levels can be found in various other benign bone lesions such as osteoblastoma, chondroblastoma, giant cell tumor (GCT), NOF, cystic fibrous dysplasia, and SBC. In addition, some of malignant bone lesions such as osteosarcoma, either telangiectatic or even conventional type, can also have an ABC component. Fat-suppressed T2-weighted MR images are best at clearly showing fluid–fluid levels. The bone cortex is preserved in most cases of ABC unless it is associated with a pathologic fracture. The radiologic differential diagnosis of ABC includes GCT, low-grade osteosarcoma, and telangiectatic osteosarcoma in the pediatric population.

Solid-variant ABC, also known as giant cell reparative granuloma when it occurs in the head and neck, is a rare type of ABC that is primarily seen in the craniofacial bones and small tubular bones of the hand and foot. It is uncommonly seen in the long tubular bones.[30] This variant has a wide spectrum of imaging features, from similar to ABC at one end to having aggressive features such as permeative bone destruction and periosteal reaction simulating malignancy at the other end. One-third of the solid-variant ABC lesions are not expansile (nonaneurysmal).[31] MRI shows a persistent solid component with heterogeneous high T1 and T2 signal intensity in an

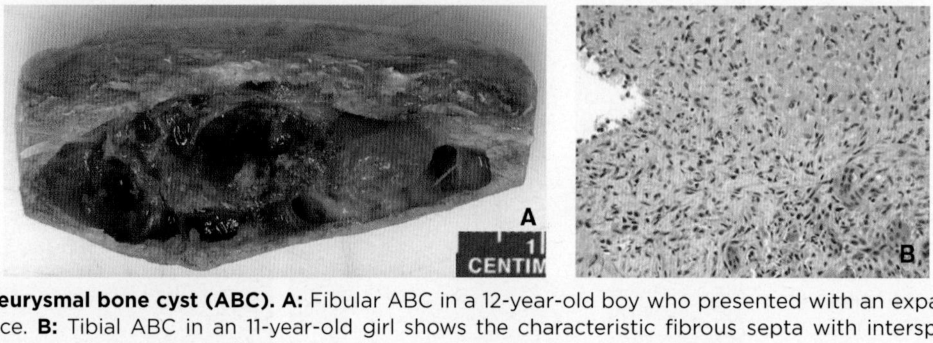

FIGURE 23.8 **Aneurysmal bone cyst (ABC). A:** Fibular ABC in a 12-year-old boy who presented with an expansile mass shows a cystic cut surface. **B:** Tibial ABC in an 11-year-old girl shows the characteristic fibrous septa with interspersed giant cells. Cytogenetic analysis revealed t(1;17), confirming the diagnosis (hematoxylin and eosin, original magnification, 400×).

expansile cystic lesion. Occasional perilesional bone marrow edema can be also observed in the solid-variant ABC.[30]

Grossly and histologically, ABC typically shows blood-filled cysts with intervening septa that contain fibroblasts, multinucleate giant cells, and variable numbers of admixed osteoblasts and inflammatory cells (Fig. 23.8). Chromosomal rearrangement involving the *USP6* gene at chromosome 17p13 is seen in primary ABC, illustrating a relationship between ABC and nodular fasciitis, another fibroblastic proliferation characterized by *USP6* rearrangement.[31] ABC is treated with surgical removal of the entire lesion with bone graft if it is required. Local recurrences after resection are rare.[32]

Osteoid Osteoma

Osteoid osteoma is a benign bone-forming tumor that is characterized by a relatively small-sized lesion with disproportionally severe pain. Osteoid osteomas account for 10% to 12% of all benign bone neoplasms and 2% to 3% of all primary bone tumors.[4] Most cases (over 75%) occur between ages 5 and 24 years with male predilection (3:1).[4] In more than 50% of cases, the femur or tibia is affected, and the proximal femur including the femoral neck is the single most common site.[4] Other locations include the midshaft or metadiaphysis of the long bones and less commonly the tarsal bones, hand phalanges, and the spine. Osteoid osteomas are subclassified into three subtypes based on location: cortical, medullary, or subperiosteal. Of these, cortical osteoid osteomas are the most common, and subperiosteal ones are the least common.[33]

The clinical presentation of an osteoid osteoma is characteristic. Affected pediatric patients experience pain that worsens at night and dramatically improves with salicylates. Unfortunately, the pain is often referred to the adjacent joint and occasionally to a site distant from the lesion, resulting in misdirecting of radiographic studies and incorrect clinical diagnosis.[34]

The characteristic imaging findings of osteoid osteomas include a nidus (core) that is usually located in the cortex and contains a variable degree of mineralization, associated adjacent cortical thickening, and reactive sclerosis in a long bone shaft (Fig. 23.9).[33] The nidus appears as a central radiodense

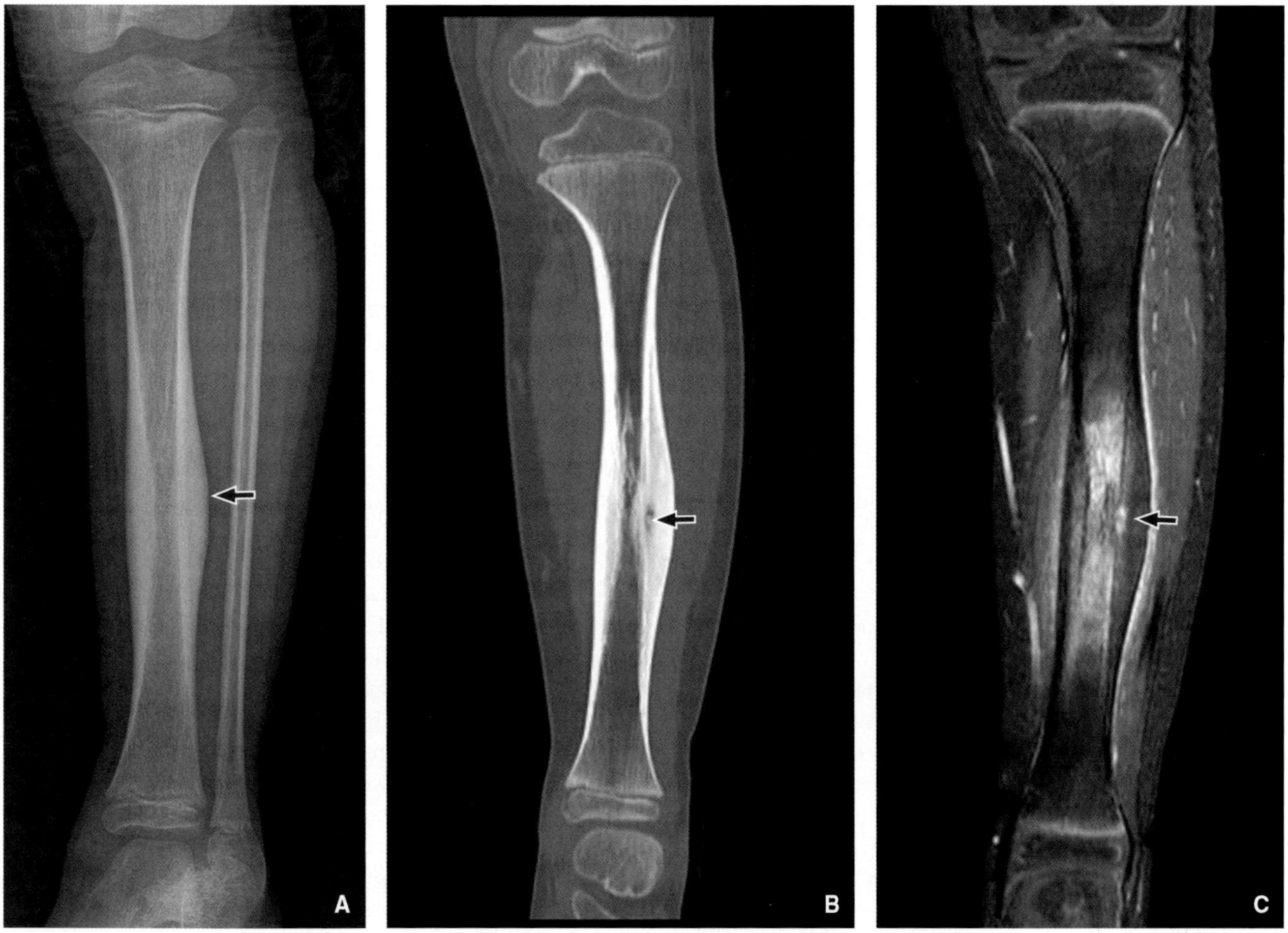

FIGURE 23.9 **Osteoid osteoma in an 8-year-old boy who presented with nocturnal pain. A:** Frontal radiograph shows fusiform cortical thickening and solid periosteal new bone formation (*arrow*) involving the mid- to distal shaft of the left tibia. A radiolucent nidus is not demonstrated on this study. **B:** Coronal reformatted CT image clearly depicts diffuse cortical thickening and a radiolucent nidus (*arrow*). **C:** Coronal postcontrast fat-suppressed T1-weighted MR image shows a central enhancing nidus (*arrow*) with diffuse enhancement of the adjacent bone marrow and soft tissue. The nidus is usually more conspicuous on CT than on MRI, as it is in this case.

area that is surrounded by a lucent rim or a radiolucent focus because it is located in the center of an area of reactive sclerosis. The nidus is round or oval and usually less than 2 cm in size.[33] CT best delineates the nidus; it has a target appearance with a well-defined round or oval area of lucency and a central mineralized area.[35] MRI shows a low to intermediate T1 and variable T2 signal intensity nidus, depending on the mineralization of the central osteoid. The mineralized nidus has a target appearance on T2-weighted MR images; there is a central dark spot (mineralized) surrounded by peripheral high signal (unmineralized area). The nidus may show strong enhancement after administration of gadolinium (Fig. 23.9). With intravenous contrast administration, dynamic CT or MR perfusion imaging technique enables the nidus to be more conspicuously visualized.[36] MRI can also show associated bone marrow edema and surrounding soft tissue changes. With recent advances in MRI techniques, current MRI would be comparable or even better than CT for evaluating osteoid osteoma and has the advantage of showing additional findings such as marrow edema, reactive soft tissue changes, and abnormalities of adjacent joints without associated ionizing radiation exposure.[36]

Intra-articular osteoid osteoma is rare, but somewhat challenging in clinical and imaging diagnosis. An osteoid osteoma near or within the joint typically presents with joint effusion and pain mimicking arthritis. In contrast to osteoid osteoma in usual locations, reactive cortical thickening may be minimal or absent in intra-articular osteoid osteoma. A high level of suspicion is often required, especially when the nidus is small and associated reactive bone changes are minimal.[37,38]

Occurrence in an atypical anatomic location may complicate the diagnosis of osteoid osteomas. Spinal osteoid osteoma, most commonly occurring in the neural arch of the lumbar spine, presents with scoliosis and radicular pain. CT or MRI is required in most cases to detect the nidus in the pedicle and lamina. Imaging and clinical findings of osteoid osteoma in the carpal and tarsal bones may mimic infection or inflammatory arthritis.

The differential diagnosis of an osteoid osteoma includes stress fracture, intracortical abscess, and other tumors such as intracortical hemangioma, osteoblastoma, and compensatory hypertrophy of the pedicle. Osteoid osteoma has a round nidus, as opposed to a stress fracture, which has a linear cortical break in the center of the cortical thickening. On bone scintigraphy, an osteoid osteoma demonstrates the "double density" sign with intense uptake in the nidus and surrounding moderate uptake. In contrast, a stress fracture typically shows linear intense uptake of the tracer.[39] An intracortical osteoid osteoma has a smooth margin with strong enhancement of the nidus; this contrasts with an intracortical abscess or sequestrum, which usually has an irregular shape and margin with peripheral rim enhancement at contrast-enhanced CT.[40] Differentiation between osteoid osteoma and intracortical hemangioma is difficult based on imaging features, although intracortical hemangioma is extremely rare. Compensatory hypertrophy of the vertebral pedicle is seen in unilateral spondylolysis and mimics spinal osteoid osteoma. Lack of a nidus and presence of contralateral spondylolysis in compensatory hypertrophy of the pedicle can differentiate it from spinal osteoid osteoma. The differences between osteoid osteoma and osteoblastoma are discussed in the following section.

Grossly and microscopically, osteoid osteoma shows a nidus rich in osteoblasts and poorly mineralized woven bone (Fig. 23.10). A variably sclerotic bony rim surrounds the nidus. The current treatment of choice for osteoid osteoma is complete excision, which is curative with en bloc resection. Recently, percutaneous radiofrequency ablation of the nidus has become a treatment of choice almost replacing surgical excision. Radiofrequency ablation effectively relieves pain in most cases with few complications and a low recurrence rate.[41]

Osteoblastoma

Osteoblastoma is a rare benign bone-forming neoplasm. It is characterized by loose woven bone bordered by prominent osteoblasts with reactive bone formation. Osteoblastoma is relatively rare, accounting for 3% of all benign bone tumors.[4] It affects patients in the second to fourth decades of life with male predilection (2.5:1).[42]

Histologically, osteoblastomas are identical to osteoid osteomas, but they are quite different regarding imaging findings and clinical manifestations. Compared to osteoid osteoma, osteoblastoma is less painful and less responsive to medication. Osteoblastoma is more expansile, larger (often arbitrarily distinguished from an osteoid osteoma by a measurement of more than 2 cm; mostly in the 3 to 10 cm range), and has less reactive adjacent bone change.[43] Unlike osteoid osteomas that more commonly involve the long tubular bones, osteoblastomas are most frequently found in the spine or flat bones[43]; long tubular bone involvement is seen in 35% of cases, mostly in the diaphysis.

Radiographic features of osteoblastomas are nondiagnostic in most cases; the lesions may appear purely osteolytic or purely osteosclerotic or may demonstrate a combination of the two. In the long tubular bones, osteoblastomas may have an intramedullary or cortical origin. The appearance is usually that of an expansile, predominantly osteolytic lesion with an ossified matrix and reactive sclerosis. While CT is best for showing the calcified matrix and outer bony cortex (Fig. 23.11), MRI is excellent at discriminating the tumor from associated marrow edema and showing soft tissue changes. Osteoblastomas are highly vascularized and demonstrate a dense capillary blush on angiogram. Bone scintigraphy can help pinpoint the tumor site, especially in those occurring in the posterior vertebral column, and shows increased uptake of the radionuclide in the lesion.[44]

Some osteoblastomas, in particular those arising from the posterior elements of the spine, have an ABC-like appearance. In other locations, the appearance of osteoblastoma is variable, and the differential diagnosis includes osteoid osteoma, SBC, ABC, eosinophilic granuloma, enchondroma, chondromyxoid fibroma, and fibrous dysplasia.

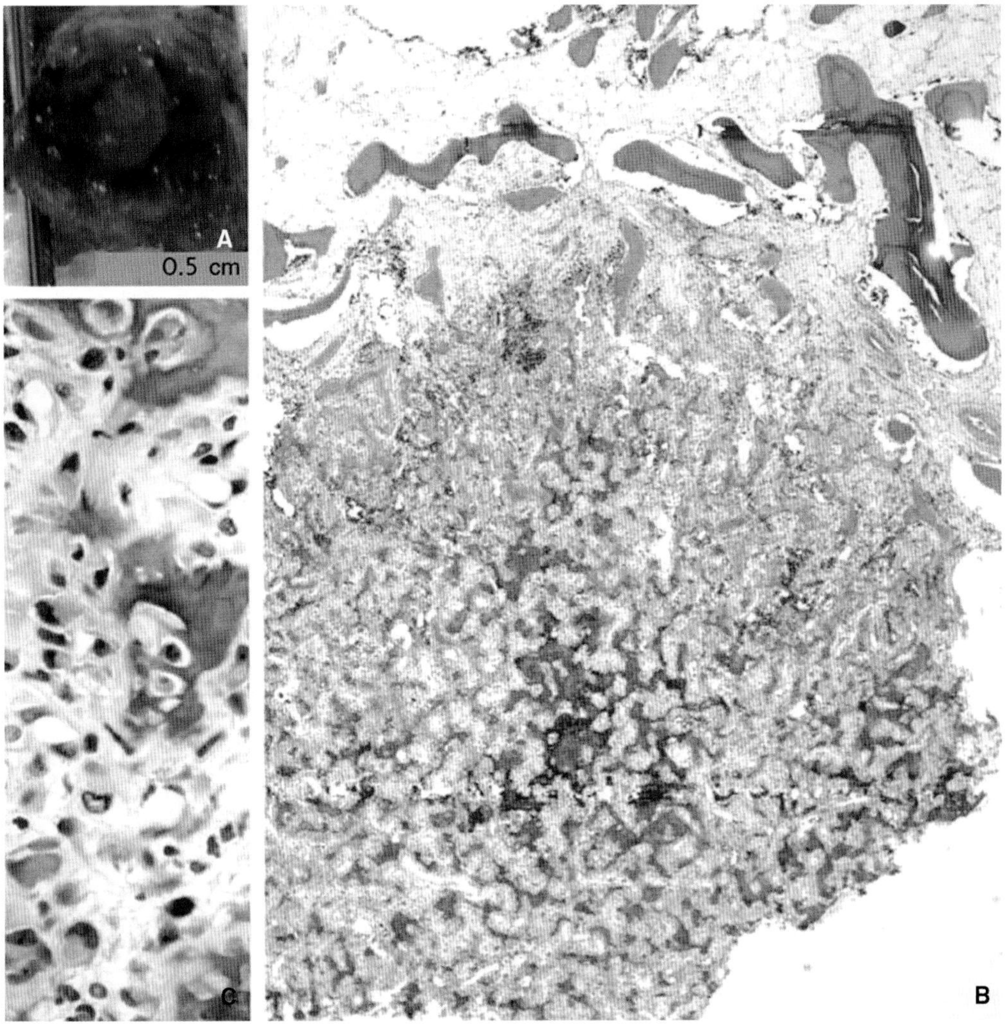

FIGURE 23.10 **Osteoid osteoma of the distal femoral epiphysis in a 9-year-old boy. A:** The en bloc resection specimen shows a nidus surrounded by a bony rim. **B:** The zonal architecture is appreciable microscopically (hematoxylin and eosin, original magnification, 40×). **C:** In the center, the nidus consists of abundant osteoblasts and a poorly mineralized osteoid matrix (hematoxylin and eosin, original magnification, 600×).

Curettage or en bloc surgical resection is the current management of choice for osteoblastomas.

Fibrous Cortical Defect/Nonossifying Fibroma

Fibrous cortical defects (FCDs) and nonossifying fibromas (NOFs) are benign fibrous lesions of bone and are histologically identical to each other. FCD is confined to the cortex of the bone and is smaller than 2 cm in size. NOF, also known as fibroxanthoma, has an eccentric location with medullary extension and is equal or larger than 2 cm in size. FCD is essentially a normal variant and is seen in children during skeletal maturation at age 4 to 8 years. Most (>70%) NOFs occur in teenagers.[4] FCD and NOF are the most common benign bone lesions, seen in up to 40% of children.[4]

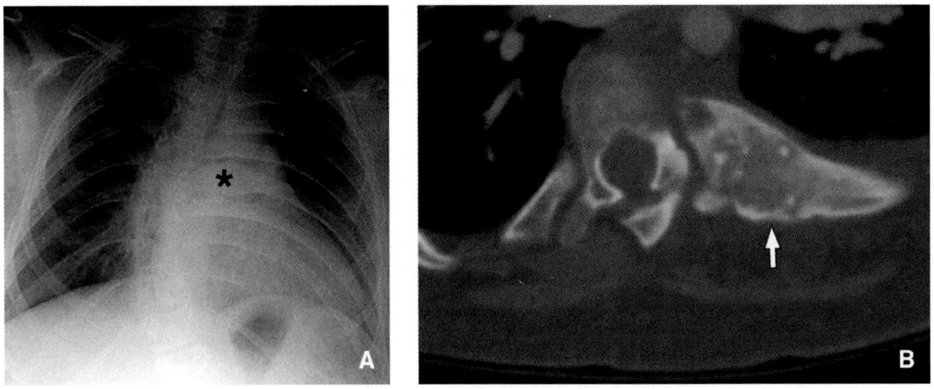

FIGURE 23.11 **Osteoblastoma in an 11-year-old girl. A:** Frontal rib radiograph shows an expansile bony mass (*asterisk*) involving the posterior arc of the left seventh rib near the costovertebral junction. There is right convex thoracic scoliosis, which could be pain related. **B:** Axial CT image demonstrates an ill-defined expansile bony lesion (*arrow*) with mixed lucencies and ossified matrix in the left-sided rib. No cortical breakdown is seen.

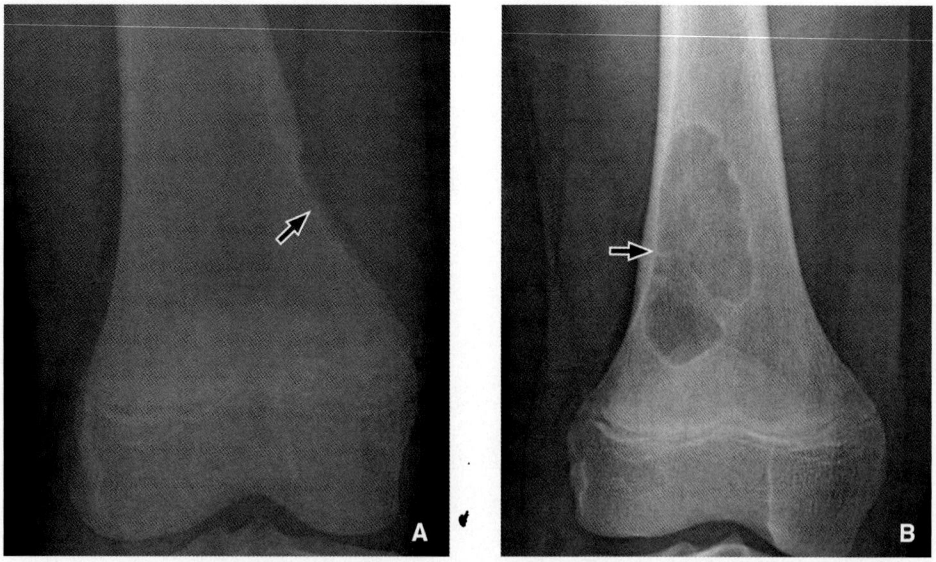

FIGURE 23.12 **Fibrous cortical defect (FCD) versus nonossifying fibroma (NOF). A:** FCD: A small cortical-based elongated radiolucent lesion is noted in the distal femur medially. The lesion is confined to the cortex suggesting a FCD (*arrow*). **B:** NOF: A radiolucent lesion with a well-demarcated thin sclerotic rim is seen in the distal femur. The lesion has an eccentric location with medullary extension suggesting a NOF (*arrow*). There is no periosteal reaction or cortical break.

FCDs are typically asymptomatic and detected incidentally; they spontaneously regress in most cases. NOFs are asymptomatic in most cases, but can present with pain associated with pathologic fractures. Although most NOFs present as a solitary lesion, there have been reported cases of multiple NOFs. Multiple NOFs along with café-au-lait skin lesions and other extraskeletal congenital malformations (mental retardation, ocular anomalies, cardiovascular malformations, hypogonadism) are known as Jaffe-Campanacci syndrome.[45] Some authors have proposed that it could be a different manifestation of neurofibromatosis type 1.[46,47]

Radiography is usually sufficient for the diagnosis of FCDs and NOFs. Both FCDs and NOFs most commonly develop in the metaphyses of the long bones of the lower extremities with a predilection for the posterior cortex. FCD and NOF demonstrate a well-defined and cortex-based (FCD) or eccentrically located (NOF) osteolytic lesion with an adjacent sclerotic rim. In general, the lesions are not accompanied by substantial periosteal reaction. The larger lesions tend to have a more elongated and multiloculated appearance with slight expansion and cortical thinning (Fig. 23.12). Main differential diagnoses include chondromyxoid fibroma, fibrous dysplasia, osteoid osteoma, bone abscess, and periosteal chondroma. FCDs and NOFs located in the metaphyses appear to migrate into the diaphysis with skeletal growth.

CT and MRI are not usually indicated, although CT may be useful in the cases of associated fracture. On MRI, the lesions are well-demarcated, typically in eccentric cortical locations, with low signal intensity on both T1- and T2-weighted MR images with enhancement depending on the evolving stage. As expected, an early active lesion appears hyperintense on T2-weighted MR images and enhances, while a regressing lesion shows a low signal on T2-weighted MR images with a lack of enhancement.[48] Whereas most NOFs can heal spontaneously with reactive sclerosis, some may persist into adulthood with a potential risk of developing a pathologic fracture.

Microscopically, FCD and NOF lesions are characterized by fibroblasts that are arranged in a storiform pattern, along with interspersed multinucleate giant cells and histiocytes (Fig. 23.13). Hemosiderin and lipid may accumulate within the histiocytes. No treatment is required for noncomplicated NOF or FCD.

Fibrous Dysplasia

Fibrous dysplasia is a benign fibroosseous lesion involving the medullary cavity of the bone. It affects children and young adults with an equal gender distribution. Fibrous dysplasia has monostotic and polyostotic forms; the monostotic type accounts for 70% to 80% of cases.[49] The facial bones, in particular the jaw bone, are most commonly affected; other affected sites include the skull, ribs, and long bones including the femur and tibia. The polyostotic form, also known as fibrocartilaginous dysplasia or generalized fibrocystic disease of bone, can be associated with syndromes, such as McCune-Albright syndrome (precocious puberty, cutaneous café-au-lait lesions, unilateral polyostotic fibrous dysplasia) (Fig. 23.14)[50,51] and Mazabraud syndrome (intramuscular myxomas, fibrous dysplasia).[52]

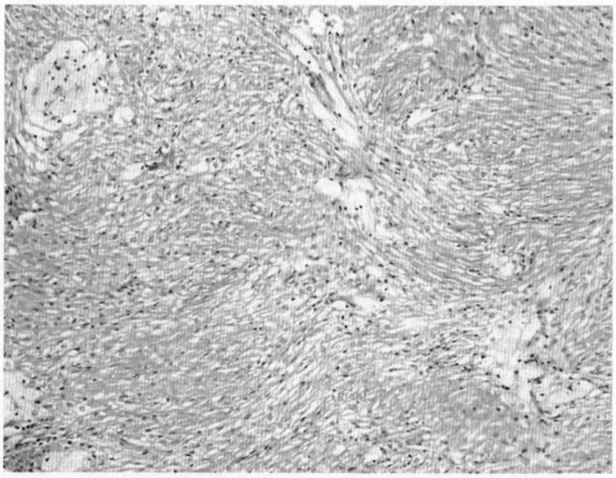

FIGURE 23.13 **Multiple nonossifying fibromas (NOFs) in the femur of an 11-year-old girl with neurofibromatosis type 1.** Histologically, the NOFs show spindle-shaped fibroblasts in a storiform growth pattern; collections of macrophages with pale vacuolated cytoplasm represent lipidization (hematoxylin and eosin, original magnification, 200×).

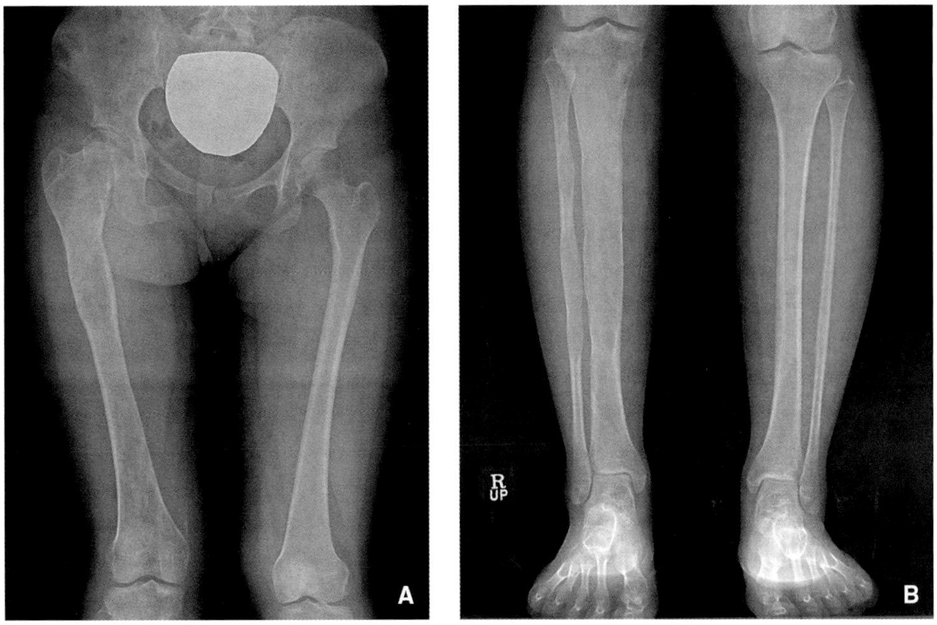

FIGURE 23.14 **Fibrous dysplasia in a 17-year-old girl with McCune-Albright syndrome. A, B:** Frontal radiographs of the lower extremities show multiple bony lesions with a ground-glass matrix in the right femur, tibia, fibula, and talus. There are associated bony expansions, endosteal scalloping, and mild deformity, especially in the right proximal femur. This girl had a past history of precocious puberty and café-au-lait skin lesions.

On radiographs and CT, fibrous dysplasia demonstrates characteristic findings of a well-demarcated intramedullary lesion in a long bone with a ground-glass or hazy matrix. There is also endosteal scalloping with or without bone expansion (Fig. 23.14). "Shepherd crook deformity" is a result of repeated fractures and varus deformity of the proximal femur. There is no periosteal reaction unless it is fractured. Bone scintigraphy may help identify multiple lesions. On MRI, fibrous dysplasia has similar signal intensity to that of muscle on T1-weighted MR images and variable signal on T2-weighted MR images depending on the component (although showing T2 hyperintensity in most cases). After administration of gadolinium-based contrast material, the lesions usually enhance heterogeneously (Fig. 23.15).[53]

Microscopically, fibrous dysplasia shows delicate spindled to stellate fibroblasts with variable amounts of admixed thin bony trabeculae without substantial osteoblastic rimming (Fig. 23.16). The prognosis for this benign disease is excellent.

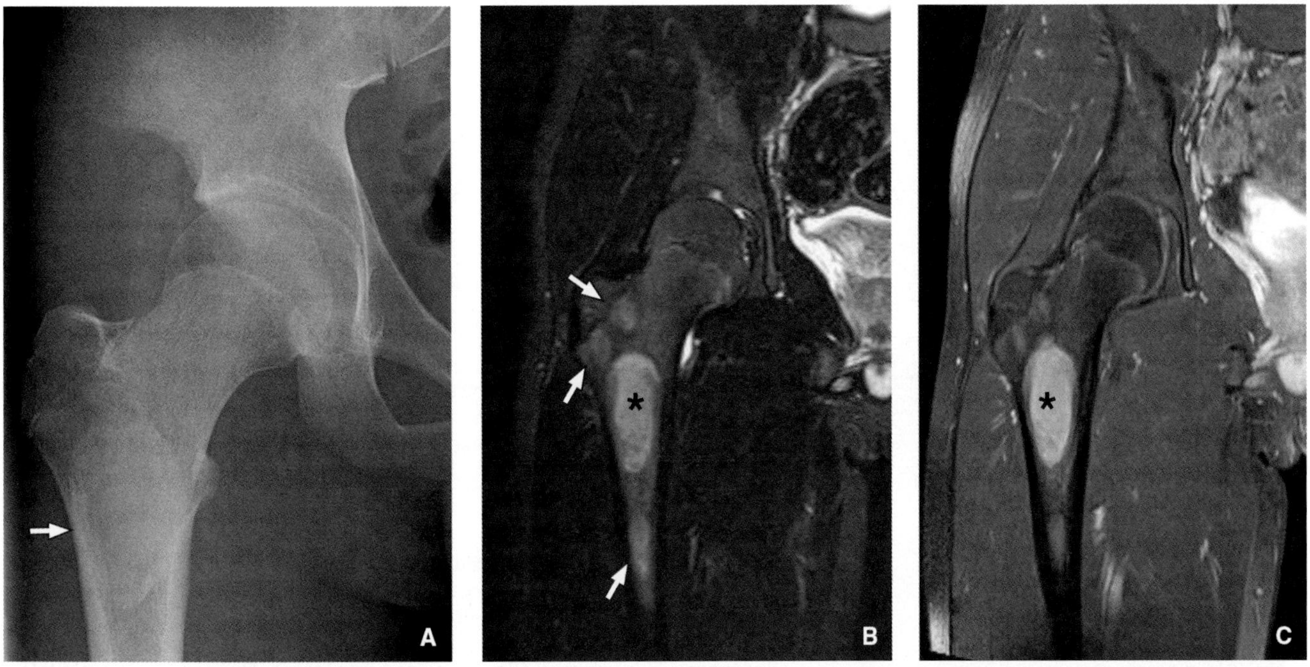

FIGURE 23.15 **Fibrous dysplasia in a 13-year-old boy. A:** Frontal radiograph of right femur shows a well-demarcated ovoid radiopaque lesion (*arrow*) in the right proximal femur with a ground-glass matrix and a thin sclerotic rim. **B, C:** Coronal T2-weighted **(B)** and postcontrast fat-suppressed T1-weighted **(C)** MR images demonstrate an intramedullary hyperintense lesion with homogeneous enhancement (*asterisk*). Several smaller hyperintense T2 lesions are also noted surrounding the larger lesion representing foci of fibrous dysplasia (*arrows*).

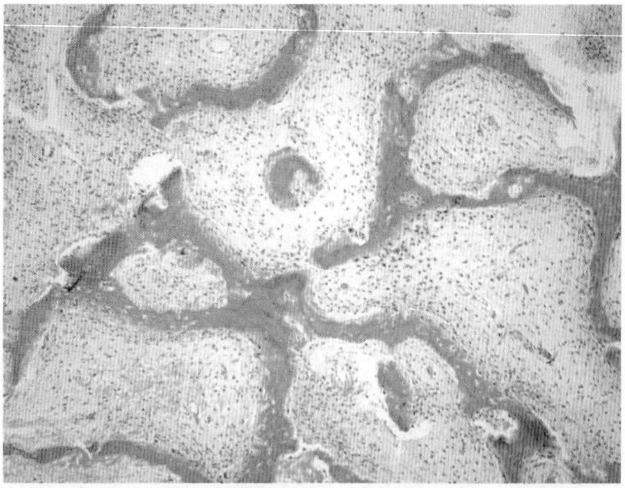

FIGURE 23.16 **Fibrous dysplasia involving the femur of a 10-year-old girl who presented with a pathologic fracture.** Microscopically, elongate and curvilinear bone spicules lie within a background of spindle to stellate fibroblasts (hematoxylin and eosin, original magnification, 100×).

However, affected pediatric patients can occasionally be left with deformities such as leg length discrepancy or bowing. Malignant transformation is exceptionally rare.

Osteofibrous Dysplasia

Osteofibrous dysplasia is a benign fibroosseous lesion of bone. It is confined almost exclusively to the tibia. It occurs mostly during infancy and childhood and is rare after the age of 15 years. Osteofibrous dysplasia shares imaging features with adamantinoma, which has a progressive and malignant nature.[54,55] It has been suggested that osteofibrous dysplasia may represent a precursor to, an incomplete sampling of, or a regression of adamantinoma.[56]

On radiographs, osteofibrous dysplasia is typically seen as a relatively well-circumscribed complex radiolucent lesion with marginal sclerosis involving the anterior cortex of the tibia. There is typically associated cortical thickening and anterior bowing (Fig. 23.17). The eccentric cortical location differentiates it from fibrous dysplasia, which has a medullary location.

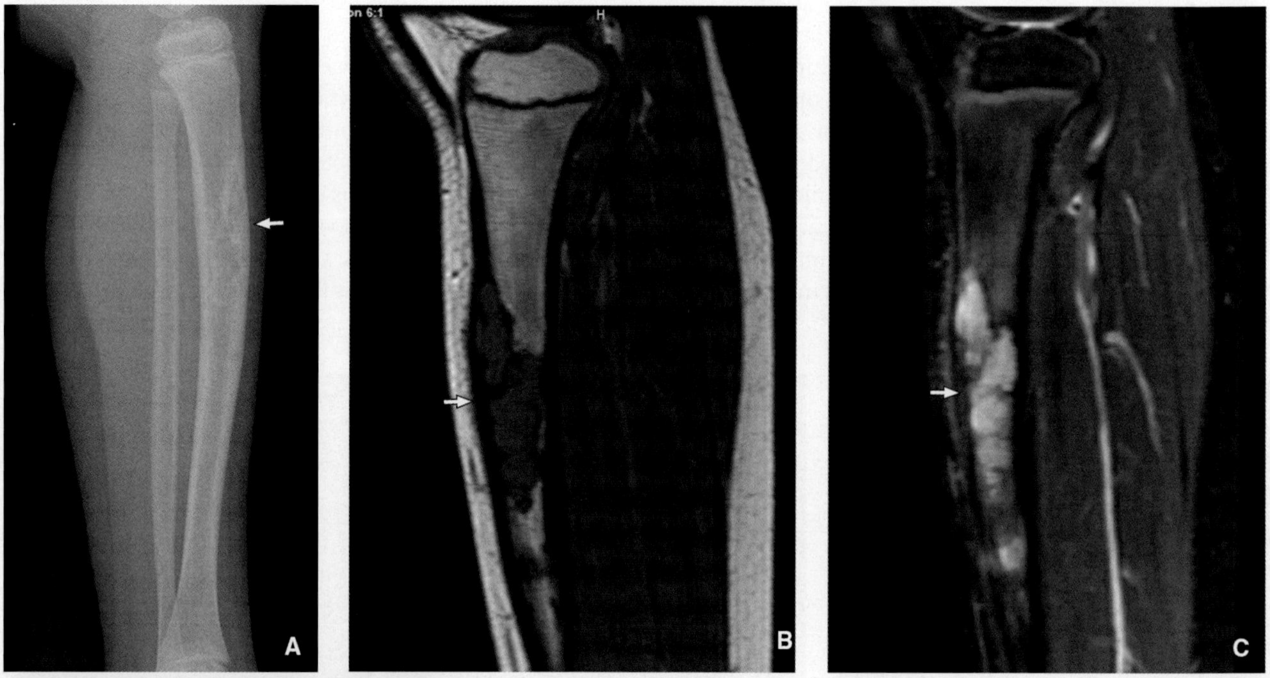

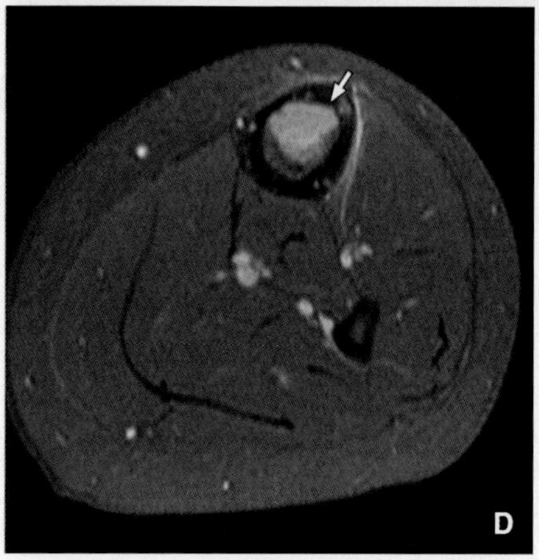

FIGURE 23.17 **Osteofibrous dysplasia in a 10-year-old girl. A:** Lateral radiograph of tibia shows a mixed radiolucent and radiodense lesion (*arrow*) in the anterior aspect of the left proximal tibia, which presents with a sclerotic rim and bone expansion. Anterior bowing of the tibia is seen. **B–D:** Sagittal T1 **(B)**, fat-suppressed T2-weighted **(C)** and axial postcontrast fat-suppressed **(D)** MR images demonstrate an expansile bony lesion (*arrows*) confined to the anterior aspect of the cortex of the tibia. The cortex is thinned out anteriorly, but no definite extraosseous soft tissue mass is formed. Diffuse enhancement of the tumor is seen.

In contrast to adamantinoma, which often has a soft tissue component, osteofibrous dysplasia typically is not accompanied by a soft tissue mass. Pathologic fractures and congenital pseudoarthrosis can be associated with osteofibrous dysplasia. CT and MRI show the extent of the lesions and the degree of narrowing of the medullary cavity as well as the thinned outer cortex. MRI signal intensity of osteofibrous dysplasia is not specific; it is of low to intermediate signal on T1-weighted MR images and high signal on T2-weighted MR images with a varying degree of sclerosis seen as a low signal rim. There is usually strong intralesional enhancement after contrast administration (Fig. 23.17).

Microscopically, osteofibrous dysplasia contains delicate fibroblasts that produce wispy collagen (Fig. 23.18). Bony trabeculae are embedded within the fibrous proliferation. Occasional keratin-positive cells, occurring singly and not well visualized on routine stains, may be highlighted by immunohistochemical stains. Most osteofibrous dysplasias undergo spontaneous healing or regression. In rare cases, they may progress to adamantinoma.

Langerhans Cell Histiocytosis

Langerhans cell histiocytosis (LCH), previously known as eosinophilic granuloma or histiocytosis X, is a neoplastic proliferation of Langerhans cells. LCH is a spectrum of histiocytic disorders in which immature Langerhans cells proliferate in certain parts of the body. The skeletal system is affected in up to 80% of cases.[4] LCH may occur at any age but is mostly seen under the age of 5 years.[57] Systemic involvement is seen in infants and younger pediatric patients. The prognosis is poor in children younger than 2 years.

Traditionally, LCH was divided into three categories according to clinical manifestations: eosinophilic granuloma (skeleton solely involved), Hand-Schuller-Christian disease (cranial lesions, diabetes insipidus, and exophthalmos), and Letterer-Siwe disease (disseminated form that occurs in infants and very young children). More practically, it can be categorized into a restricted (monostotic or polyostotic) or an extensive (visceral organ involvement) form. Clinical symptoms vary with involved organs, and affected pediatric patients often present with low-grade fever and raised inflammatory markers such as erythrocyte sedimentation rate and C-reactive protein.

The skull is most frequently involved, although any of the axial or appendicular bones can be affected by LCH. A punched-out lytic lesion with a beveled edge is characteristic of the skull lesions. Beveled edges are explained by differential destruction of the inner and outer table of the skull (Fig. 23.19). When LCH involves the maxilla or mandible, it can result in "floating teeth." This is the description given to the appearance on imaging of teeth "hanging in the wind" as a result of underlying alveolar bone destruction around the root of the teeth in patients with

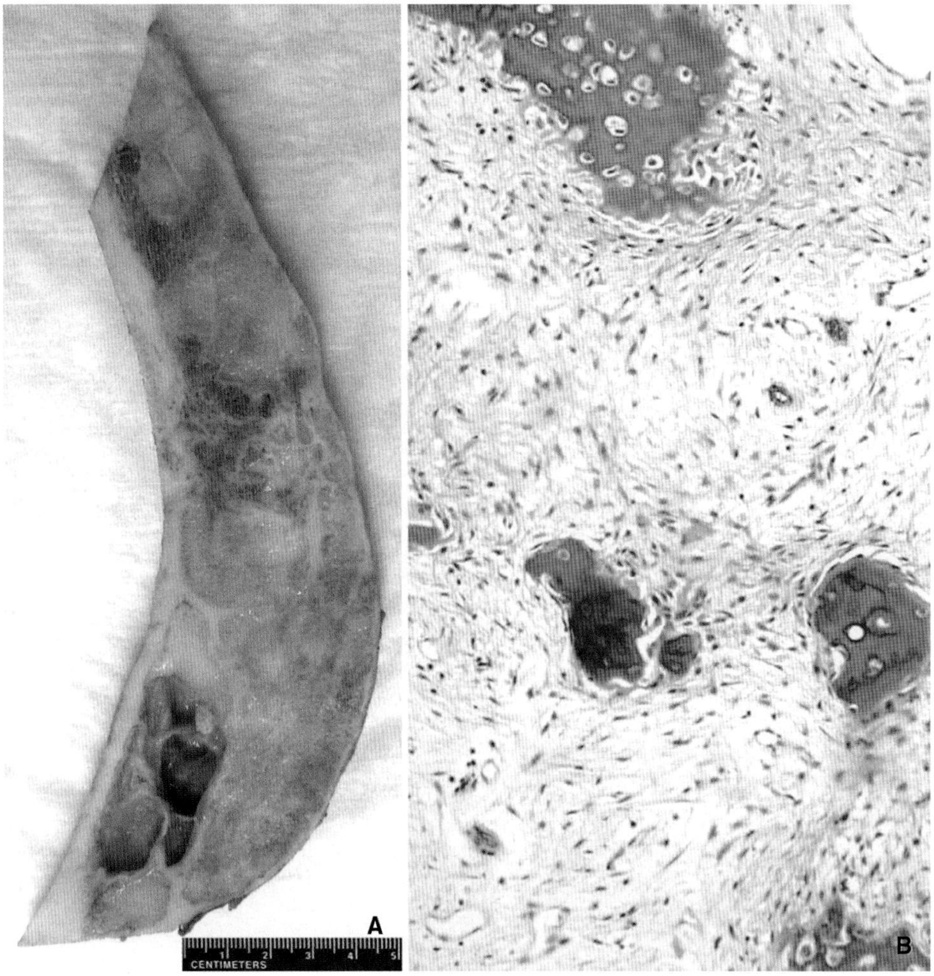

FIGURE 23.18 **Osteofibrous dysplasia in a 14-year-old boy with long-standing tibial bowing. A:** The tibia is bowed, with a cut surface showing pale soft tissue with areas of cystification. **B:** Microscopically, bony spicules with variably prominent osteoblastic rimming lie within a background of fibroblasts and delicate wispy collagen (hematoxylin and eosin, original magnification, 400×).

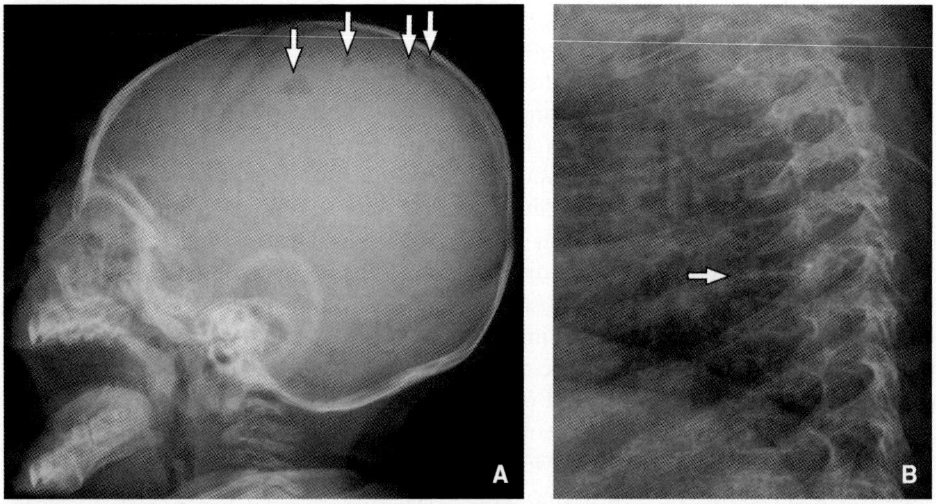

FIGURE 23.19 **Multifocal Langerhans cell histiocytosis in a 6-month-old infant boy. A:** Lateral skull radiograph shows multiple small punched-out bony lesions (*arrows*). **B:** Lateral thoracic spine radiograph shows a midthoracic vertebra plana (*arrow*).

LCH. LCH lesions of the mastoid bone cause ear symptoms. Therefore, the affected children are prone to treatment for otomastoiditis before being diagnosed with LCH. LCH is the most common cause of "vertebra plana" in children (Fig. 23.19). For spinal LCH lesions, MRI is needed to assess the presence of an epidural mass and cord compression. In long tubular bones, the lesions typically develop in the metaphysis or diaphysis. LCH involving uncommon locations such as the clavicle and small tubular bones has also been reported.[58]

A skeletal survey is the first step to be used to investigate bone involvement of LCH despite some controversy regarding its sensitivity in comparison with bone scintigraphy, which is a radiation bearing.[59,60] In children with multiple bone lesions, LCH should be included in the diagnostic considerations. Although radiological findings vary with the stage and disease activity, most LCH bone lesions are well-defined ("punched out") and purely osteolytic with endosteal scalloping (Fig. 23.19). Sometimes, a permeative and aggressive pattern of bone destruction is present in association with either a single or multilayered periosteal reaction (Fig. 23.20), which may mimic findings of malignant bone tumors or osteomyelitis. Spontaneous regression is not

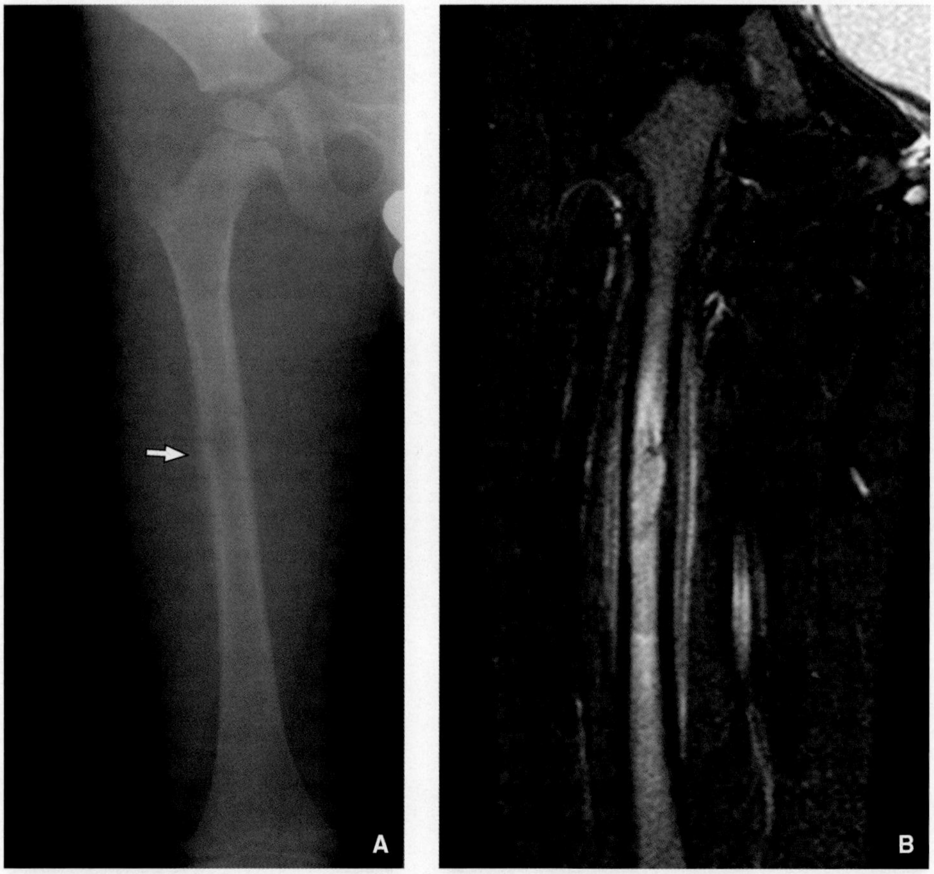

FIGURE 23.20 **Langerhans cell histiocytosis (LCH) in a 3-year-old boy. A:** Frontal right femur radiograph shows a small ill-defined round to ovoid osteolytic lesion (*arrow*) with a relatively wide transition zone. The lesion is intramedullary and diaphyseal in location with multilayered periosteal reaction mimicking a malignant bone tumor such as Ewing sarcoma. **B:** Coronal fat-suppressed T2-weighted MR image demonstrates extensive marrow edema surrounding the femoral lesion. Hyperintense T2 soft tissue edema is noted circumferentially. These findings mimic osteomyelitis.

unusual in LCH, and involuting lesions appear more sclerotic and remodeled.

Cortical breakdown and soft tissue extension of LCH can be well demonstrated on CT; the margins are irregular and tend to be more sharply delineated as compared to those in Ewing sarcoma. On MRI, the bone lesions and soft tissue masses of LCH appear with low signal intensity on T1-weighted MR images, high signal intensity on T2-weighted MR images, and enhance with gadolinium. A soft tissue mass is present in about one-third of lesions. The associated inflammatory reaction causes bone and soft tissue edema, which enhance and may mimic osteomyelitis (Fig. 23.20). Involuting lesions can show low signal intensity on both T1- and T2-weighted MR images. WB MRI using the STIR sequence can provide valuable information in the initial workup as well as for patient monitoring and has many advantages over radiography and bone scintigraphy.[61]

Pathological evaluation of LCH shows sheets of Langerhans-type "histiocytes" as well as variable numbers of admixed eosinophils. LCH localized to the skeletal system carries a favorable prognosis. "Vertebra plana" tends to restore its height, and the involved bones remodel themselves after treatment. Reactivations are relatively common, occurring in about a quarter of the patients with systemic disease. LCH is treated by low-dose chemotherapy in extensive cases.

Chondroblastoma

Chondroblastoma is a benign cartilaginous neoplasm that affects exclusively the epiphyses or apophysis of long bones. It is most common in the second and third decades of life, and almost half of the lesions occur prior to physeal closure.[62] Chondroblasts, chondroid matrix, giant cells, and foci of calcifications are seen on microscopic examination. Chondroblastomas can have a component of ABC. There are two main benign bone lesions that affect the epiphyses: chondroblastoma prior to skeletal maturation and GCT after physeal closure (**Schematic B**). The differential diagnosis for an epiphyseal lesion in a child can also include infectious osteomyelitis (Brodie abscess), which was discussed in Chapter 22.

Chondroblastoma typically presents as an eccentric well-defined osteolytic lesion with a sclerotic rim in the epiphysis or apophysis (epiphysis equivalent) on radiographs (Fig. 23.21). Approximately one-third of cases show calcified chondroid matrix, which is best shown by CT[63,64]. Surrounding inflammatory changes are usually pronounced, resulting in adjacent bone marrow and soft tissue edema. Periosteal reaction is common due to an associated inflammatory response.[63] In contrast to most cartilaginous tumors, which are usually hyperintense on T2-weighted MR imaging, chondroblastoma can present with low- to intermediate-signal intensity on T2-weighted MR images. An ABC component can show cystic areas with or without fluid–fluid levels (Fig. 23.21). Chondroblastoma shows a low signal intensity rim on MRI. The bone marrow edema, soft tissue changes, and/or joint effusions can be pronounced. These findings can be important for differentiating chondroblastoma from other benign tumors. Chondroblastomas variably enhance, while Brodie abscesses typically show enhancement of the granulation tissue around the nonenhancing central abscess. The various signal intensities on T2-weighted MR imaging and enhancement patterns of chondroblastomas correlate well with their underlying histopathologic features, depending on the various amounts of chondroid matrix, calcifications, ABC components, and others.[64]

Microscopically, chondroblastomas show sheets variably mature chondrocytes, often individually outlined by a rim of calcium (so-called "chicken-wire calcification"). Admixed osteoclast-like giant cells are frequently seen. Simple curettage

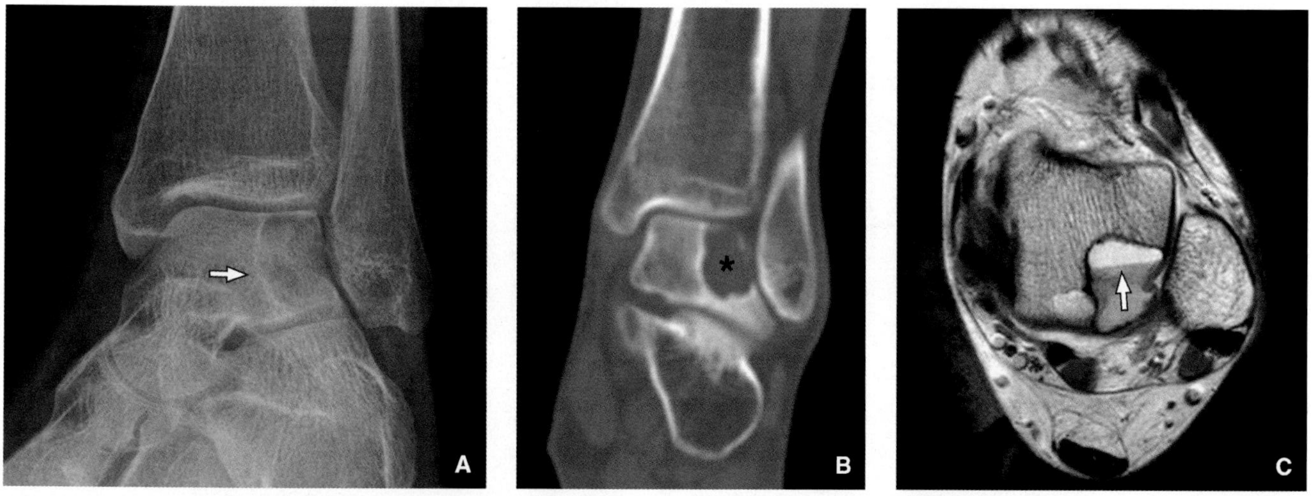

FIGURE 23.21 **Chondroblastoma in a 17-year-old girl. A:** Frontal left ankle mortise view radiograph shows a well-demarcated osteolytic lesion (*arrow*) with a thin sclerotic rim in the lateral aspect of the left talus. **B:** A lytic bony lesion is more clearly seen on the coronal CT image (*asterisk*), which presents with surrounding reactive sclerosis. **C:** Axial T2-weighted MR image demonstrates a talar lesion with a fluid–fluid level (*arrow*) representing secondary aneurysmal bone cyst changes.

is curative in the majority of patients, although recurrence may be observed in 14% to 18%.[65]

Chondromyxoid Fibroma

Chondromyxoid fibroma is a relatively rare benign cartilaginous tumor that usually involves the metaphyses of the extremity bones.[66] The proximal tibia is the most common location, followed by the fibula and the calcaneus.[67] Lesions involving the upper extremity bones, pelvis, and spine have also been described. It is more common in males in the second or third decades of life.[68]

On radiographs, chondromyxoid fibroma shows an eccentric osteolytic lesion with a sclerotic margin in the metaphysis; its elongated shape parallels the axis of the long tubular bone. In small tubular bones, it can occupy the entire width of the medullary cavity with bony expansion and cortical thinning (Fig. 23.22). Calcifications are not usually present. MR signal characteristics are nonspecific and vary depending on the internal composition, but usually show low signal on T1- and high signal on T2-weighted MR images (Fig. 23.22).

The current management of choice for chondromyxoid fibroma is surgical resection. Chondromyxoid fibromas can recur after surgical excision, but there is no known risk of malignant transformation.

Enchondroma

Enchondroma is a type of chondroma that involves the medullary cavity. It is composed of benign hyaline cartilage.

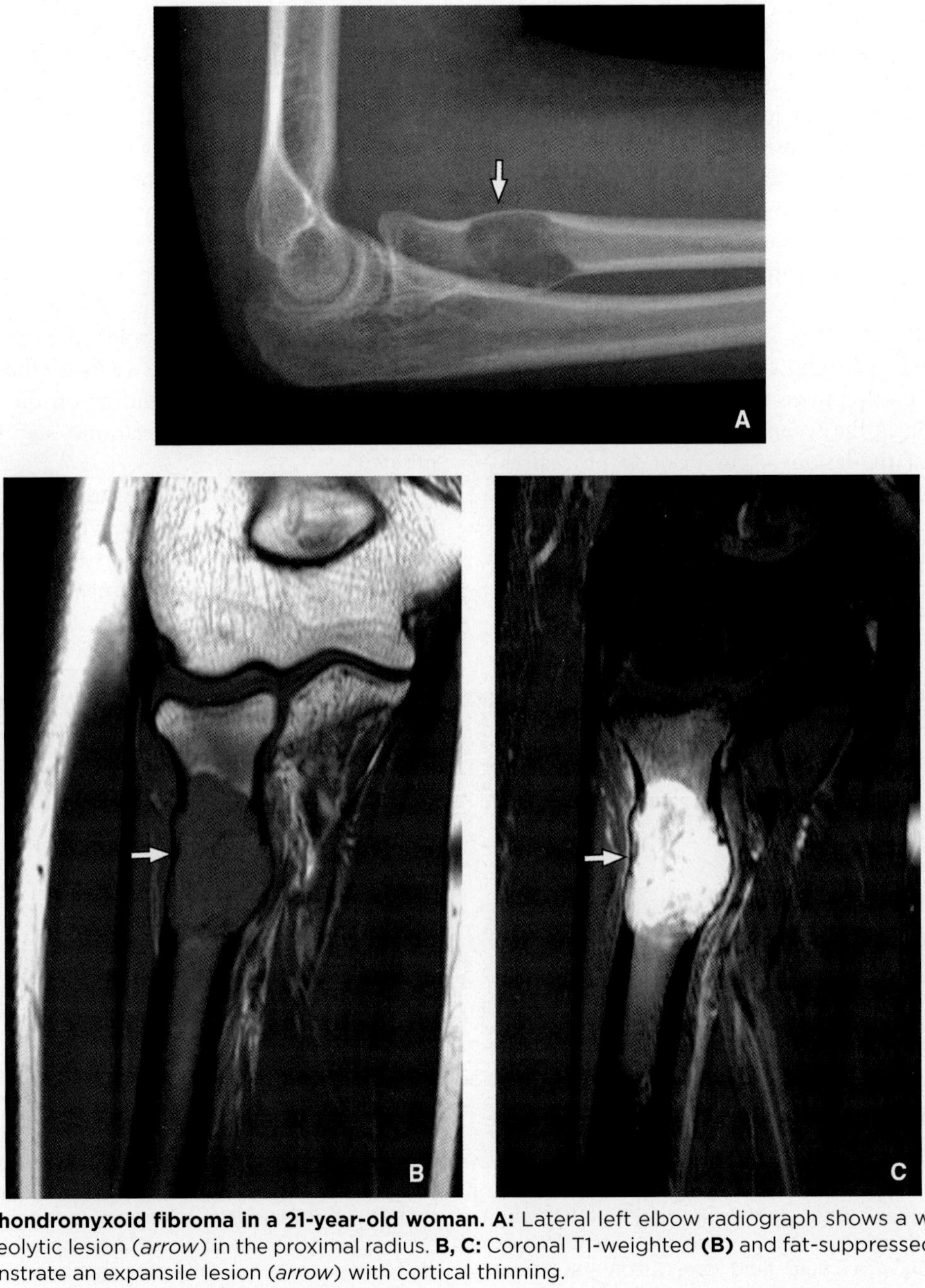

FIGURE 23.22 **Chondromyxoid fibroma in a 21-year-old woman. A:** Lateral left elbow radiograph shows a well-circumscribed and expansile osteolytic lesion (*arrow*) in the proximal radius. **B, C:** Coronal T1-weighted **(B)** and fat-suppressed T2-weighted **(C)** MR images demonstrate an expansile lesion (*arrow*) with cortical thinning.

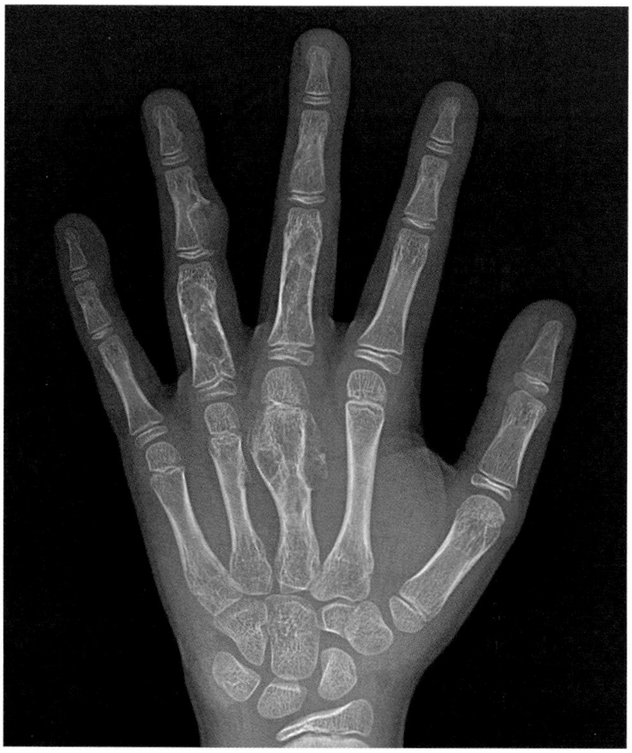

FIGURE 23.23 **Multiple enchondromatosis (Ollier disease) in an 11-year-old boy.** Frontal hand radiograph shows multiple central and eccentric lytic lesions involving the metacarpal and phalangeal bones of the right third and fourth fingers.

Chondromas may also occur in a juxtacortical or periosteal location. The peak age of juxtacortical chondromas is slightly younger than that of enchondromas.[69] Enchondromas commonly occur in the metaphyses or metadiaphyses of the small tubular bones of the hands and feet of children and adults. Enchondroma protuberans has been described as a variant of enchondroma that protrudes outward from one side of the affected bone mimicking an osteochondroma or juxtacortical chondroma.[64]

Ollier disease and Maffucci syndrome are the most common subtypes of endochondromatosis, in which enchondromas can affect both sides of the body, but are random and asymmetric; generally, one side of the body is almost exclusively or more predominantly affected.[70] Enchondromas that arise in the metaphysis near the growth plates may impair physeal bone growth resulting in deformity and limb shortening. The risk of malignant transformation to chondrosarcoma is also a potential complication. Maffucci syndrome refers to multiple enchondromas in association with spindle cell hemangioma (Fig. 23.24). Both Ollier disease and Maffucci syndrome are known to be nonhereditary, usually sporadic disorders. The enchondromas and spindle cell hemangiomas usually harbor somatic mutations in the IDH1 or IDH2 gene.[71]

Radiographic evaluation is often sufficient to make a diagnosis of enchondroma. Typical radiographic findings include multiple expansile, radiolucent lesions with well-defined bony margins in the metaphyses of long bones and small tubular bones. Enchondromas develop in close proximity to the growth plate and then migrate toward the diaphysis (Figs. 23.23 and 23.24). In the long bones, they commonly show longitudinal streaks in the metaphysis that parallel the long bone axis. Metaphyseal widening by clustered enchondromas and variable shortening of metacarpal or phalangeal bones are seen in the hands (Figs. 23.23 and 23.24). On both radiography and CT, punctuate or chondroid calcifications can be seen. On MRI, signal intensity follows that of the cartilage at all sequences, revealing predominantly high signal intensity on T2-weighted MR images. Enhancement after gadolinium administration varies, and some lesions show enhancement in a peripheral, ring-and-arc pattern.

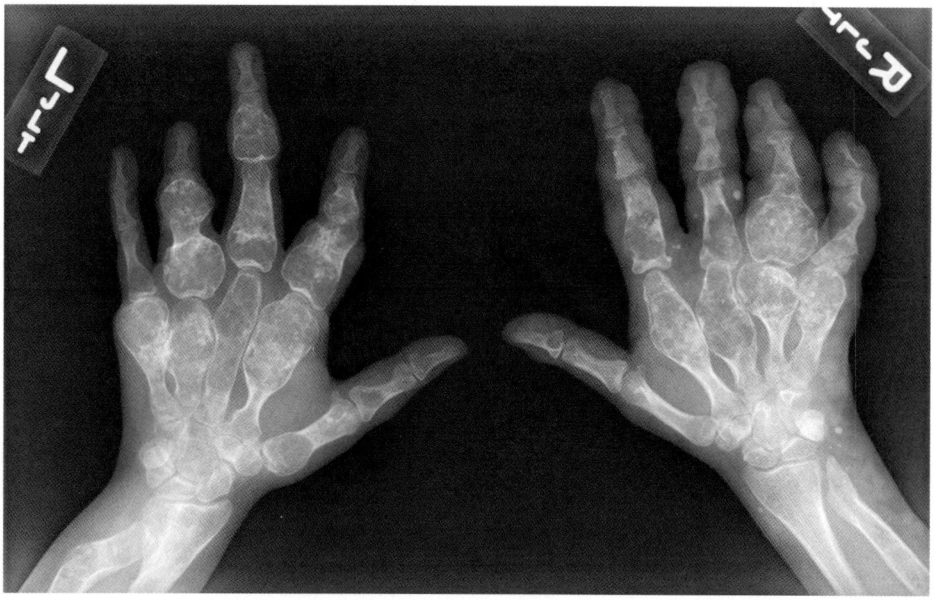

FIGURE 23.24 **Maffucci syndrome in a 21-year-old woman.** Multiple bizarre, expansile lesions are noted involving the bones of both hands, which present with associated soft tissue calcifications (phleboliths) in the right wrist and right second and third fingers representing vascular lesions. Both ulnae are short and deformed, which is a common finding in multiple enchondromatosis.

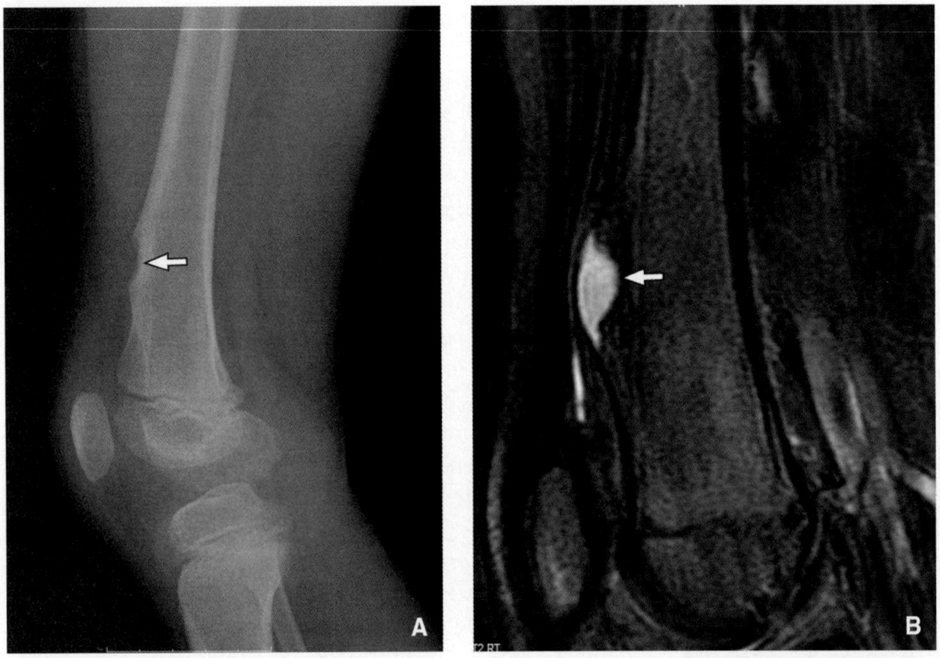

FIGURE 23.25 **Periosteal chondroma in a 9-year-old boy. A:** Lateral radiograph of the femur shows a saucerized cortical defect (*arrow*) with buttresses of solid periosteal new bone and reactive sclerosis. **B:** Sagittal fat-suppressed T2-weighted MR image demonstrates marked hyperintensity of the cortical/periosteal lesion (*arrow*) in keeping with hyaline cartilage in this case of juxta-cortical (periosteal) chondroma.

Periosteal Chondroma

Periosteal or juxtacortical chondroma is a distinctive benign cartilaginous tumor that affects the metaphyseal surface of tubular bones beneath the periosteum. The tumor occurs in children as well as adults younger than 30 years of age.[72] It is a slow-growing tumor that causes erosion and sclerosis at the underlying bony cortex. Because it develops outward from the cortical surface of tubular bones, it can sometimes mimic osteochondroma or other benign or even malignant surface tumor.

The radiographic appearance of periosteal chondroma is often characteristic. A protruding bony mass with or without chondroid matrix is seen causing pressure erosion and remodeling at the cortex (saucerization) (Fig. 23.25). CT shows mineralization of the matrix. The interface between the tumor and the underlying bony cortex helps differentiate periosteal chondroma from sessile osteochondroma. The MRI appearance is similar to that of other cartilaginous tumors with low to iso-signal on T1-weighted MR images and foci of bright high signal on T2-weighted MR images (Fig. 23.25). Peripheral enhancement is typically noted after gadolinium administration (50).

Giant Cell Tumor of Bone

GCT is a benign but locally aggressive bone tumor. It accounts for 4% to 5% of all primary bone tumors and usually affects patients from 20 to 45 years of age with a female predilection.[73,74] Uncommonly, younger pediatric patients are affected. The tumor typically involves the long tubular bones, specifically the distal femur and proximal tibia. Spinal involvement is described in a mainly adult population.[75] Although GCT is rare in skeletally immature patients, GCT can develop in the distal metaphysis and involve the epiphysis before the physis is closed. The tumor is located at the epimetaphysis in most cases, and tumor extension through growth plates may reflect its aggressiveness. Purely metaphyseal GCT has been observed only in the distal radius.[76] Pulmonary "metastasis" occurs rarely; it is indolent, thought to represent tumor emboli rather than true metastasis.

Radiographically, GCT is typically a geographic, expansile, osteolytic lesion with ill-defined or sclerotic margins seen in the epimetaphysis of the tubular bones (Fig. 23.26). Matrix calcification is not a finding in GCT. In cases of expansile bone lesions, there can be cortical breakdown with soft tissue extension. No periosteal reaction is identified unless complicated by a pathologic fracture. MRI shows diverse findings depending on whether the tumor is mainly solid or cystic. A solid tumor shows intermediate signal intensity on both T1- and T2-weighted MR images with diffuse enhancement. There can be associated intratumoral hemorrhage and intratumoral ABC components. Fluid–fluid levels can be demonstrated on both CT and MRI.

Microscopically, GCT of bone shows numerous large multinucleate giant cells embedded in a background of mononuclear fibrohistiocytic cells (Fig. 23.27). En bloc resection is preferred over curettage due to the high recurrence rate of the latter procedure. Local recurrent is not common.

Malignant Osseous Tumors

Malignant bone tumors have a tendency to be found in the specific locations within the bones: the epiphysis, metaphysis, and diaphysis (**Schematic C**).

Osteosarcoma

Osteosarcoma is the most common primary malignant bone tumor in the pediatric population with an overall incidence of 5 per million patients under age 20 years.[77,78] Osteosarcoma is slightly more common in males, and the peak incidence occurs in the 10 to 14 year age range, at the age of the growth

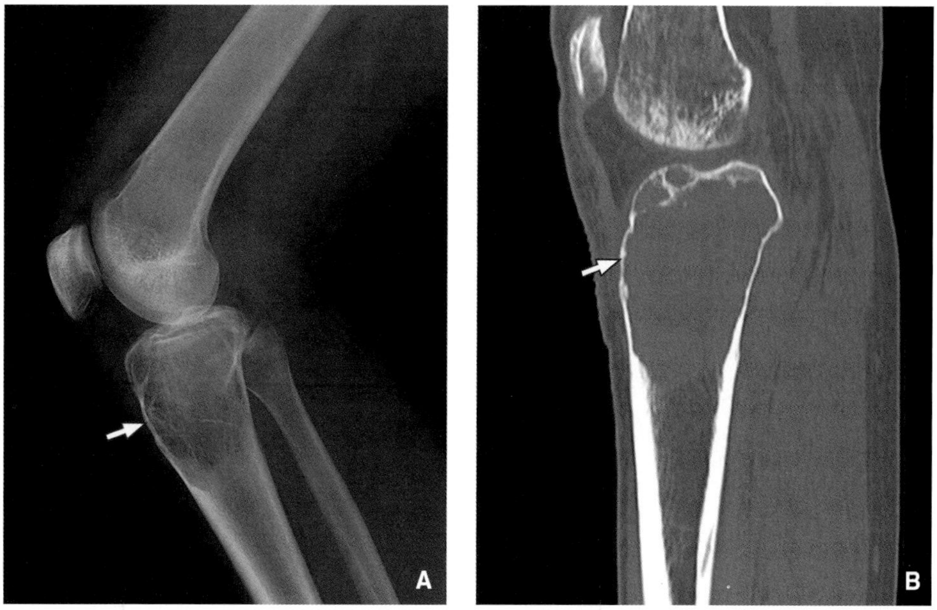

FIGURE 23.26 **Giant cell tumor in a 25-year-old man. A, B:** Lateral knee radiograph **(A)** and sagittal CT image **(B)** show an expansile osteolytic lesion (*arrow*) in the proximal tibia involving the epimetaphysis. The outer cortex is thinned out with endosteal scalloping. Septa-like trabecular structures are noted on radiograph.

spurt.[77,78] The most commonly affected sites are the metaphyses of the long bones, particularly about the knee (42% in femur, 19% in tibia) and the humerus (10%).[77,78] Less commonly affected locations include the skull or jaw (8%) and pelvis (8%).[77,78] Diaphyseal origin is less common, and epiphyseal origin is extremely rare.

The current WHO classification categorizes osteosarcoma into eight subtypes: (1) conventional (chondroblastic, fibroblastic, or osteoblastic), (2) telangiectatic, (3) small cell, (4) low-grade central, (5) parosteal, (6) periosteal, (7) high-grade surface, and (8) secondary osteosarcomas.[4] Conventional osteosarcoma is the most common high-grade type of osteosarcomas. Other high-grade variants include telangiectatic osteosarcoma, small cell osteosarcoma, high-grade surface osteosarcoma, and secondary osteosarcoma. Periosteal osteosarcoma is an intermediate-grade variant. Low-grade variants include low-grade central osteosarcoma and parosteal osteosarcoma.[78,79] Among these eight subtypes of osteosarcoma, parosteal, periosteal, and high-grade surface osteosarcomas are juxtacortical osteosarcomas, which originate from the bone surface.

A few inherited risk factors for osteosarcoma account for a small minority of cases. These include retinoblastoma, Li-Fraumeni, Baller-Gerold, Bloom, McCune-Albright, OSLAM, Rothmund-Thomson, and Werner syndromes.[80,81] Rarely, multicentric osteosarcomas can occur at multiple skeletal sites spontaneously (synchronous) or subsequently that develop at multiple locations after a solitary lesion (metachronous).[82] Extraskeletal osteosarcoma is extremely rare in children.[83] Localized pain and swelling are the most common presentations of osteosarcoma, and pathologic fracture can be the first presenting sign.

Curative treatment for high-grade osteosarcomas consists of surgery and chemotherapy. Most recent protocols for high-grade osteosarcomas include preoperative chemotherapy. The degree of histologic tumor response to preoperative chemotherapy offers the most important prognostic

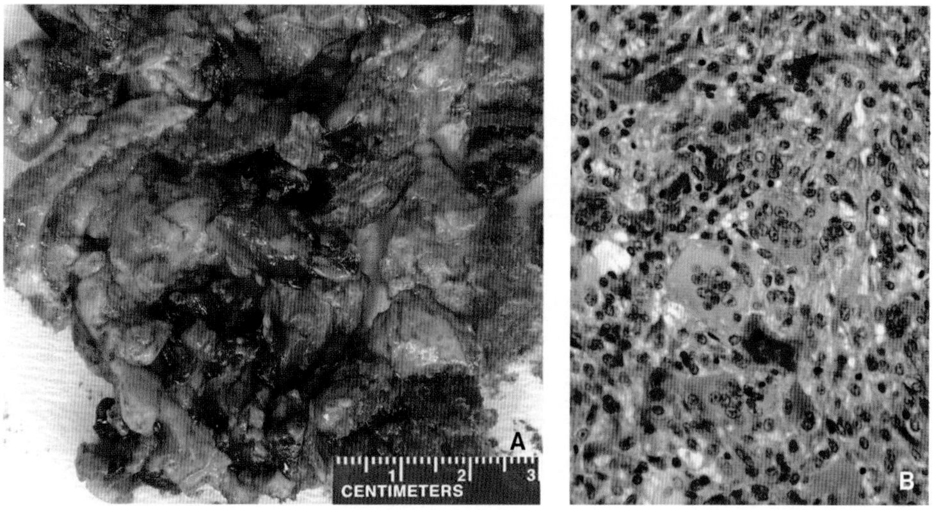

FIGURE 23.27 **Giant cell tumor of bone involving the distal femoral epiphysis in a 17-year-old boy. A:** Grossly, the curetted sample shows soft yellow-tan tissue admixed with blood. **B:** Microscopically, mononuclear cells are admixed with numerous multinucleate giant cells (hematoxylin and eosin, original magnification, 600x).

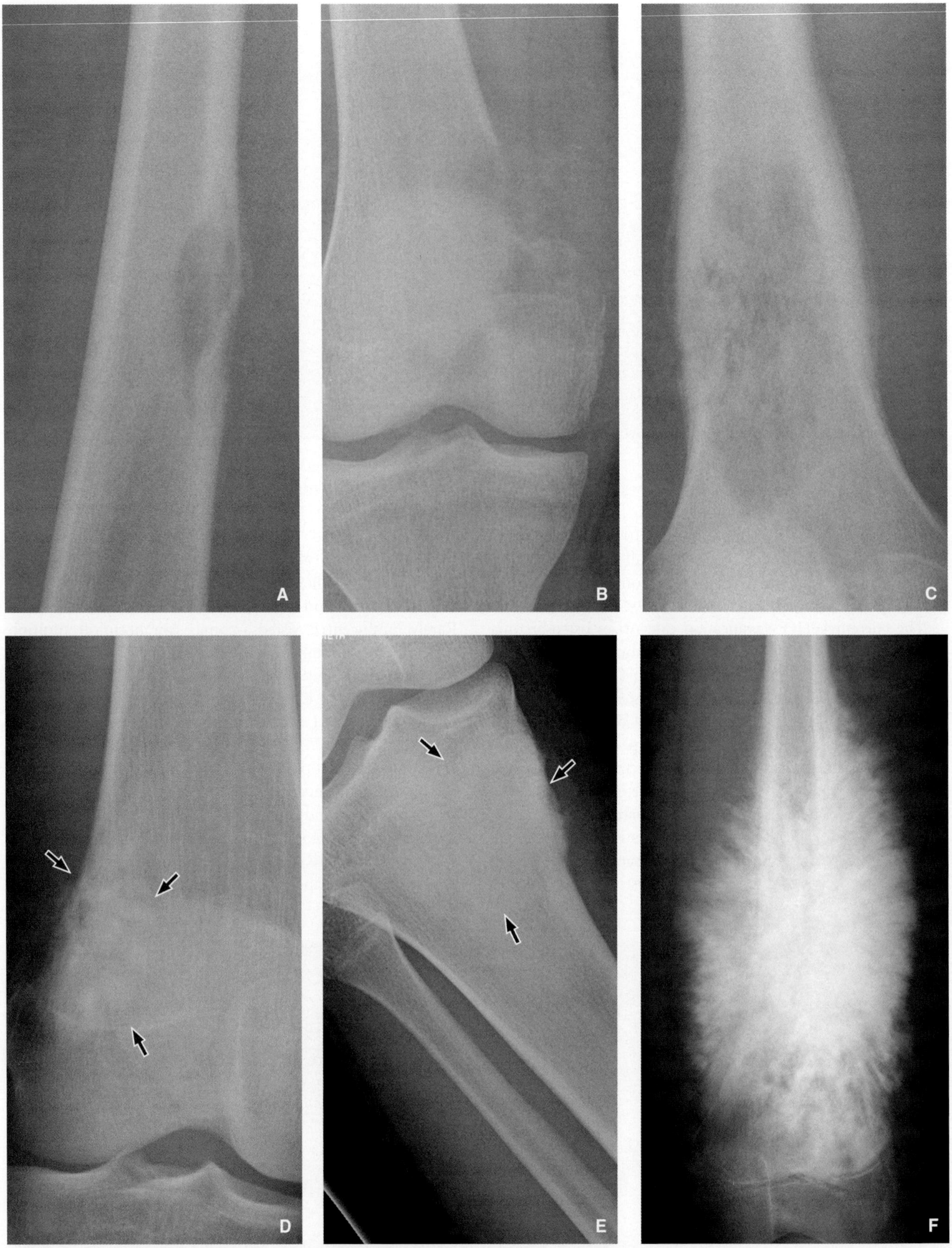

FIGURE 23.28 **Variable radiographic findings of osteosarcoma. A, B:** Pure osteolytic appearance. **C, D:** Mixed osteolytic and sclerotic appearances (*arrows*). **E, F:** Pure sclerotic pattern (*arrows*).

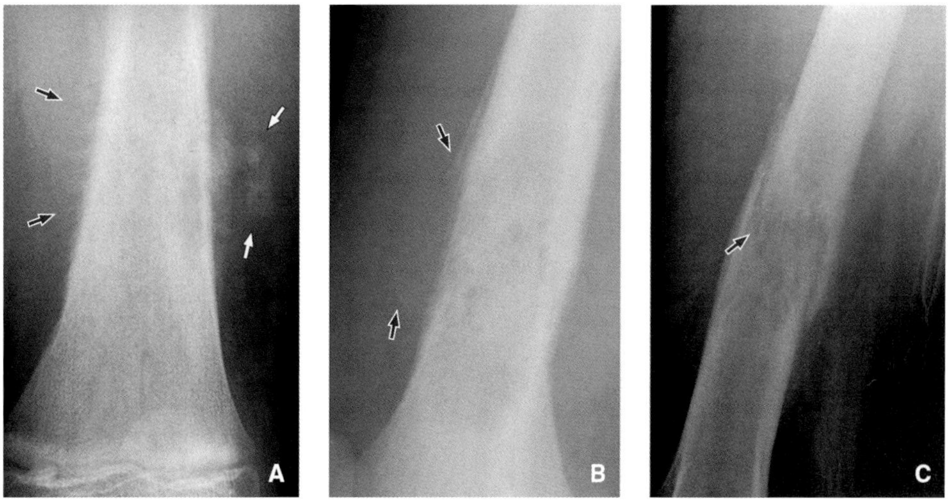

FIGURE 23.29 **Classic radiographic appearances of osteosarcoma (A, B) and associated pathologic fracture. A:** Osteosarcoma with "sunburst" appearance (*black arrows*) and osteoid matrix formation (*white arrows*). **B:** Codman triangle (*arrows*). **C:** Pathologic fracture (*arrow*).

information. Research protocols using diffusion-weighted MR images and dynamic contrast-enhanced MRI allow quantification of tumor necrosis and viable residual tumor.[84] Increased numeric values in apparent diffusion coefficient maps reflect tumor necrosis.[85] Low-grade variants, such as low-grade central or parosteal osteosarcomas, are treated by surgery only. Surgical removal is the primary treatment for metastatic and recurrent osteosarcomas as well. Pulmonary metastases occur most commonly and are seen in 10% to 20% of patients.[77]

Among eight subtypes of osteosarcoma, seven subtypes including conventional, telangiectatic, secondary, small cell, low-grade central, parosteal, periosteal, and high-grade surface osteosarcomas are further discussed in the following section; small cell type, which is exceedingly rare, is omitted in this chapter.

Conventional Osteosarcoma

Conventional osteosarcoma, also known as central high-grade intramedullary osteosarcoma, is the most common subtype and accounts for 80% to 90% of all osteosarcomas. Based on the predominant cell type, conventional osteosarcoma is divided into three subtypes: osteoblastic, chondroblastic, and fibroblastic osteosarcoma.

The radiographic appearance of conventional osteosarcoma varies from purely osteolytic to mixed osteolytic and sclerotic to purely sclerotic (Fig. 23.28). Osteoblastic osteosarcoma is the predominant type seen in 50% to 80% of all cases of osteosarcomas.[86] It demonstrates characteristic osteoid matrix with fluffy or cloud-like calcification in 90% of cases.[86] The chondroblastic type shows predominantly osteolytic lesions. The typical appearance of conventional osteosarcoma is a poorly defined intramedullary mass with metaphyseal origin and mixed osteolysis and sclerosis (Fig. 23.28). Additional radiographic features include cortical destruction, aggressive periosteal reaction such as onion skin, a Codman triangle, and sunburst appearance (Fig. 23.29), features that can also be appreciated upon gross examination of resected tumors (Fig. 23.30). Pathologic fractures are present in 15% to 20% of cases[86] (Fig. 23.29). The radiologic appearance of osteosarcomas in other rare locations is similar to that of long bone osteosarcomas.

MRI of conventional osteosarcoma primarily shows intermediate signal on T1-weighted MR images and areas of high signal intensity on water-sensitive sequences (Fig. 23.31). Epiphyseal extension through an open physis is often seen in metaphyseal osteosarcomas in children (Fig. 23.31).[87] Skip metastases have been reported in 6.5% of osteosarcomas and are associated with a poor prognosis.

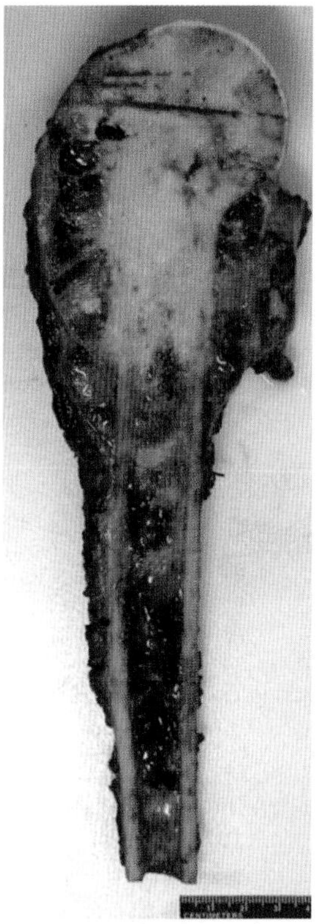

FIGURE 23.30 **Conventional osteosarcoma, involving the proximal humerus in a 16-year-old boy.** Tumor occupies the medullary space, lifts the periosteum (Codman triangle), destroys the cortex, and extends into the soft tissues.

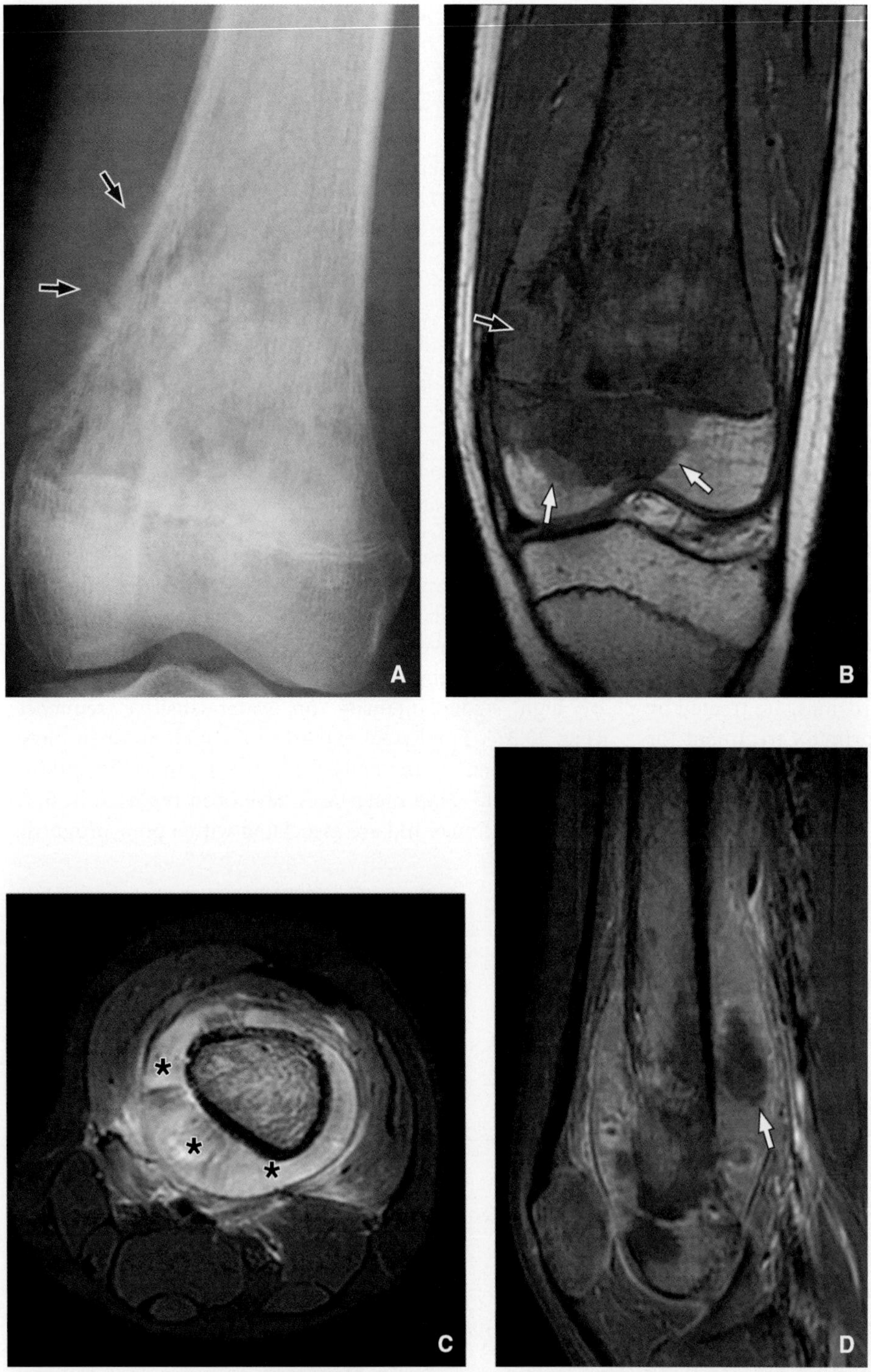

FIGURE 23.31 **Conventional osteosarcoma in a 13-year-old girl. A:** Radiograph demonstrates mixed osteolytic and sclerotic lesions in the distal femur associated with "sunburst" appearance representing periosteal reaction (*arrows*). **B:** Coronal T1-weighted MR image demonstrates cortical disruption (*black arrow*). Epiphyseal extension of tumor (*white arrows*) is seen. **C:** Axial fat-suppressed T2-weighted MR image shows heterogeneous high T2 signal mass replacing bone marrow and an associated extraosseous mass formation (*). **D:** Sagittal postcontrast fat-suppressed T1-weighted MR image shows tumor necrosis (*arrow*).

Areas of necrosis with low T1- and high T2-weighted signal and hemorrhage with high signal on both T1- and T2-weighted MR images are common. Intravenous contrast administration typically shows heterogeneous enhancement of tumor. Mineralized matrix is represented by low-signal intensity on both T1- and T2-weighted MR images. In some cases, differentiation of intra- and extraosseous tumor extension from peritumoral edema is difficult, and tumor enhancement with intravenous contrast can be helpful for differentiation.[86]

Telangiectatic Osteosarcoma

Telangiectatic osteosarcoma is a rare subtype accounting for 2.5% to 12% of all osteosarcomas.[88] The lesion most commonly occurs in the metaphyses of the femur and tibia. Grossly, telangiectatic osteosarcoma is composed predominantly of large blood-filled cavities separated by septations as in an ABC[88] (Fig. 23.32). Therefore, the imaging appearance of a telangiectatic osteosarcoma often simulates an ABC. However, in telangiectatic osteosarcoma, high-grade sarcomatous cells line the septa.

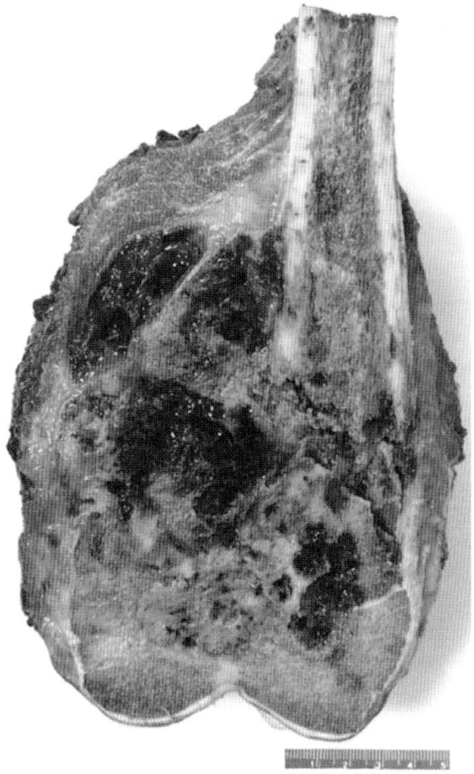

FIGURE 23.32 **Telangiectatic osteosarcoma involving the distal femur in a 15-year-old boy.** This expansile tumor with large blood-filled cysts mimics aneurysmal bone cyst grossly.

On radiographs, geographic bone destruction without appreciable sclerosis and a wide zone of transition are the most common findings (Fig. 23.33). Expansile bone remodeling is observed, and this osseous expansion is often associated with pathologic fractures at initial presentation. Other common findings are aggressive periosteal reaction, cortical destruction, and soft tissue mass formation. Bone scintigraphy and FDG-PET CT demonstrate marked heterogeneous uptake with central photopenia called "donut sign," which is seen in up to 65% of cases (Fig. 23.33).

In all cases, MR imaging evidence of hemorrhage, either as fluid levels or as areas of high signal intensity on both T1- and T2-weighted MR images, is observed. In fact, areas of hemorrhage reflected by high-signal intensity on T1-weighted MR images are seen in 52% of cases of telangiectatic osteosarcoma[88] (Fig. 23.33), but are highly unusual in other types of primary osseous neoplasm in the pediatric population. There are imaging features that favor telangiectatic osteosarcoma as opposed to benign ABCs. The first of these is thick, solid nodular tissue in the septa, which can be best depicted with postcontrast T1-weighted MR images. The second is matrix mineralization in the lesion, recognized in 58% of radiographs, and the third imaging feature is soft tissue formation and cortical destruction reflecting more aggressive growth (Fig. 23.33).[88] Despite these often helpful imaging features, biopsy is required to definitively differentiate telangiectatic osteosarcoma from ABC.

Low-Grade Central Osteosarcoma

Low-grade central osteosarcoma is a rare subtype accounting for 1.9% of all osteosarcomas. Imaging findings are variable; small lesions mimic benign fibrous lesions, and larger lesions display an aggressive nature on radiographs. Low-grade central osteosarcoma can be purely osteolytic or have a mixed appearance with osteolytic and sclerotic portions.[89] MRI typically shows cortical disruption and extraosseous mass formation, but imaging diagnosis is still challenging and requires confirmation with bone biopsy.[90,91]

Parosteal Osteosarcoma

Parosteal osteosarcoma is the most common type of juxtacortical osteosarcoma and accounts for 4% of all

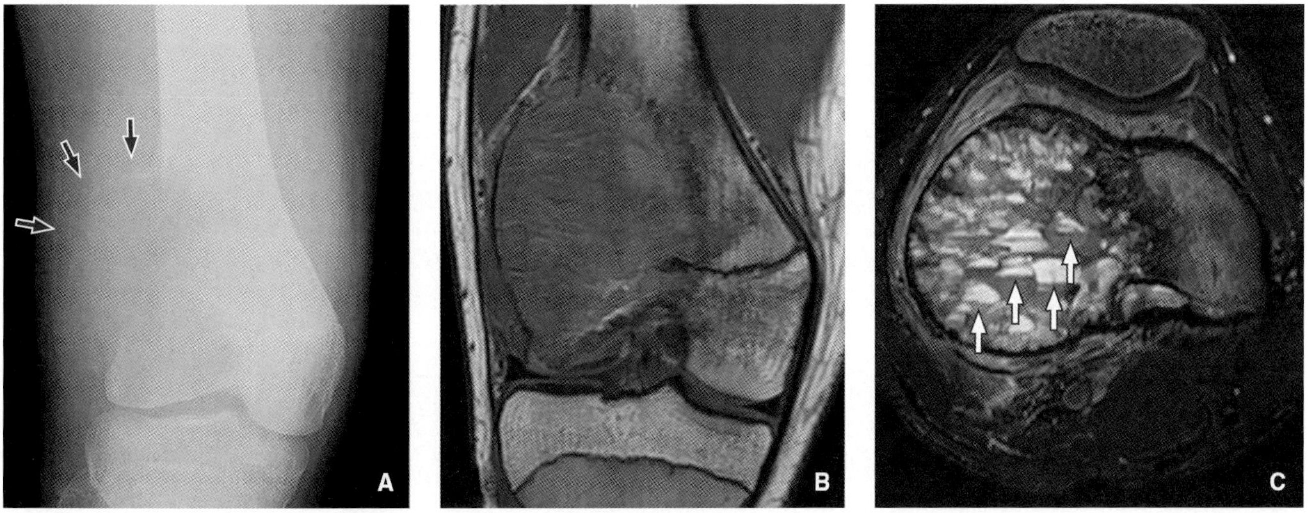

FIGURE 23.33 **Telangiectatic osteosarcoma in a 15-year-old boy. A:** Frontal radiograph demonstrates an osteolytic lesion (*arrows*) with cortical disruption in the distal femur. **B, C:** Coronal T1- **(B)** and axial fat-suppressed T2-weighted **(C)** MR images demonstrate multicystic lesions with fluid–fluid levels (*arrows*, **C**).

(Continued)

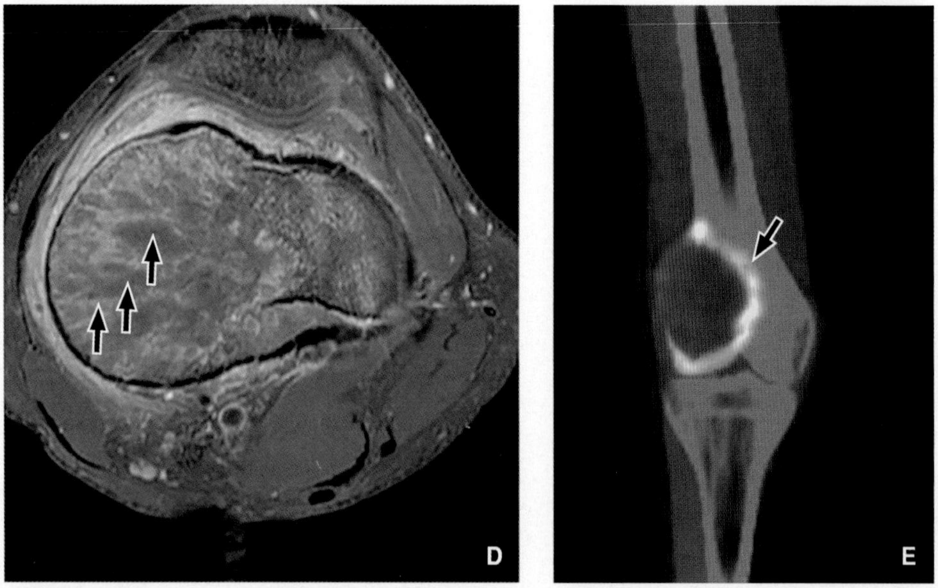

FIGURE 23.33 (*Continued*) **D:** Axial postcontrast fat-suppressed T1-weighted MR image demonstrates thick septal enhancement (*arrows*). **E:** FDG-PET image demonstrates peripheral increased tracer uptake, called "donut" sign (*arrow*).

osteosarcomas.[92] The long bone metaphysis is the primary site with the posterior aspect of the distal femur being most commonly involved. Histologically, parosteal osteosarcoma is usually low grade, but dedifferentiation mixed with high-grade disease is reported in 16% to 43% of cases.[93] Parosteal osteosarcoma originates from the outer layer of the periosteum.

On radiographs, an exophytic lobulated mass with central dense ossification is the classic appearance (Fig. 23.34). A lucent cleavage plane, called the "string sign," is seen in 30% of cases and reflects periosteum interposed between the cortex and the tumor mass (Fig. 23.34).[93–95] Other findings seen in parosteal osteosarcoma include cortical thickening and a relative lack of aggressive periosteal reaction (Fig. 23.34). The MRI appearance depends on cellular contents; low T1 and low T2 signal intensities reflect mineralization, while high T2 signal intensity suggests unmineralized soft tissue (Fig. 23.34). Intramedullary invasion is observed in 22% of cases, and its effect on the prognosis is controversial.[93–95]

Differential diagnostic considerations of parosteal osteosarcoma include myositis ossificans, osteochondroma, and periosteal chondroma. Unlike myositis ossificans, which has dense ossification peripherally, parosteal osteosarcoma

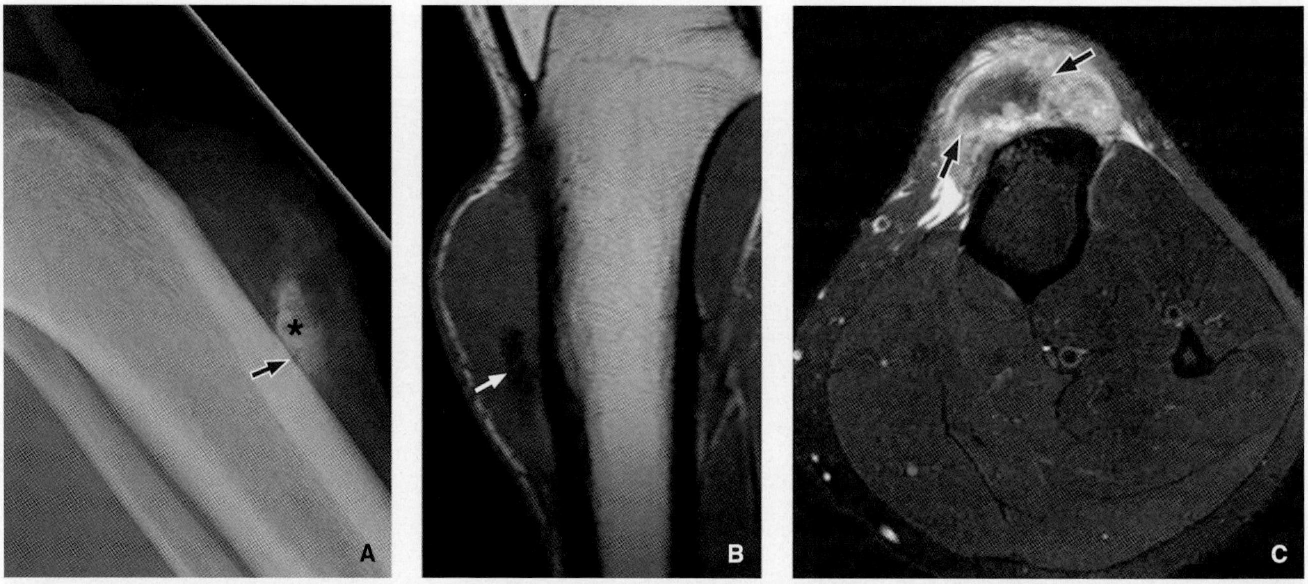

FIGURE 23.34 **Parosteal osteosarcoma in a 26-year-old man. A:** Lateral radiograph view of the tibia demonstrates a lucent cleavage plane, "string" sign (*arrow*) between the cortex and the tumor mass. Note that dense calcification (*) is at the central portion of the mass. **B, C:** Sagittal T1- **(B)** and axial T2-weighted **(C)** MR images demonstrate a tumoral mass with a focal darker T1/T2 signal area suggesting ossification (*arrows*). No intramedullary invasion is seen in this case.

has dense calcification at the central portion of the mass. A broad-based attachment to the cortex is seen in parosteal osteosarcomas, but not in myositis ossificans. In contrast to osteochondroma, in which there is continuity of the bony cortex as well as continuity of the cancellous bone, parosteal osteosarcoma demonstrates disruption between tumor and medullary bone due to interposed cortex. Cartilage tissue in parosteal osteosarcoma is often irregular and thick on MRI and is differentiated from the well-delineated high T2-weighted signal cartilage cap of osteochondromas.[93–95]

Periosteal Osteosarcoma

Periosteal osteosarcoma is the second most common type of juxtacortical osteosarcoma and accounts for 1.5% of all osteosarcomas.[94,95] The most common site is the diaphysis of long bones. The tumor originates from the inner layer of the periosteum.

On radiographs, periosteal osteosarcoma is usually seen as a broad-based soft tissue mass causing an extrinsic erosion on an underlying thickened cortex. Occasional perpendicular periosteal reaction extending into the soft tissue mass may cause a "hair-on-end" appearance (Fig. 23.35). MRI usually demonstrates a well-defined soft tissue mass with heterogeneous low T1 and high T2 signal with variable degree of enhancement with intravenous contrast administration (Fig. 23.35). Intramedullary invasion by periosteal osteosarcoma rarely occurs. When present, it can be seen as areas of abnormal marrow signal intensity continuous with the soft tissue mass.[94]

High-Grade Surface Osteosarcoma

High-grade surface osteosarcoma is the least common type of juxtacortical osteosarcoma, accounting for 0.4% of all osteosarcomas.[94,95] The diaphyses and metaphyses of long bones are common locations, and the femur is the most commonly involved bone. On radiographs, dense ossification with cortical thickening and erosions are observed. There is overlap in the imaging appearance between parosteal and periosteal osteosarcomas. More extensive circumferential bone involvement and medullary invasion are seen in high-grade surface osteosarcomas compared to other forms of juxtacortical osteosarcomas (Fig. 23.36).[94]

Secondary Osteosarcoma

Secondary osteosarcomas can arise in children at an area previously irradiated for the treatment of tumors. Radiation-induced secondary osteosarcoma is usually diagnosed ~10 years after initial treatment and is usually fatal.[96]

Ewing Sarcoma

Ewing sarcoma of bone, also known as Askin tumor when it arises in the chest wall, is the second most common malignant bone tumor after osteosarcoma in the pediatric population. The overall incidence is 3 per 1 million individuals younger than 16 years old.[97] It most often occurs between the ages of 5 and 30 years with a slight male predilection (male: female, 1.6:1) and a predominance in Caucasian patients (95%).[10,98,99] Histologically, Ewing sarcoma is a small round blue cell tumor derived from primitive neural tissue (Fig. 23.37). Both Ewing

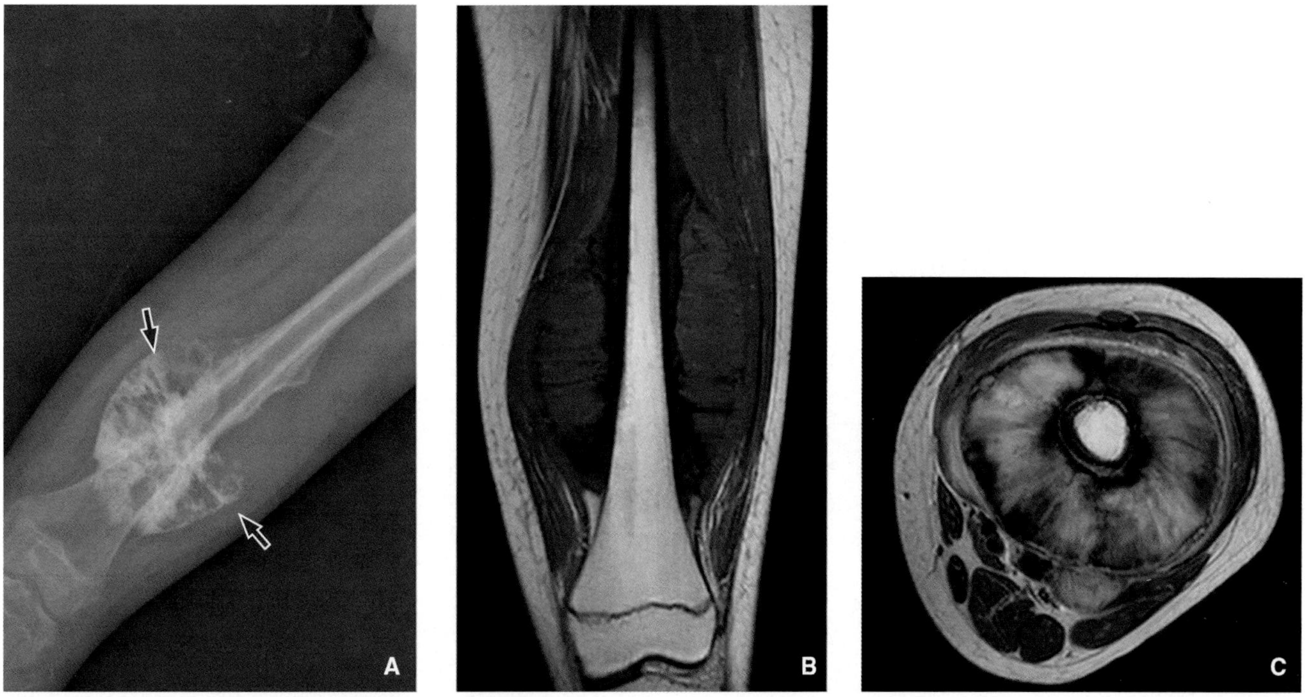

FIGURE 23.35 **Periosteal osteosarcoma in an 11-year-old girl. A:** Frontal radiograph of the femur demonstrates periosteal reaction (*arrows*) perpendicular to the longitudinal bone axis extending into the soft tissue mass, "hair-on-end" appearance (*arrows*). **B, C:** Coronal T1- **(B)** and axial T2-weighted **(C)** MR images demonstrate a circumferential mass in the distal femur. The dark T1/T2 signal foci perpendicular to the longitudinal bone axis correspond to periosteal reaction. No intramedullary invasion is seen.

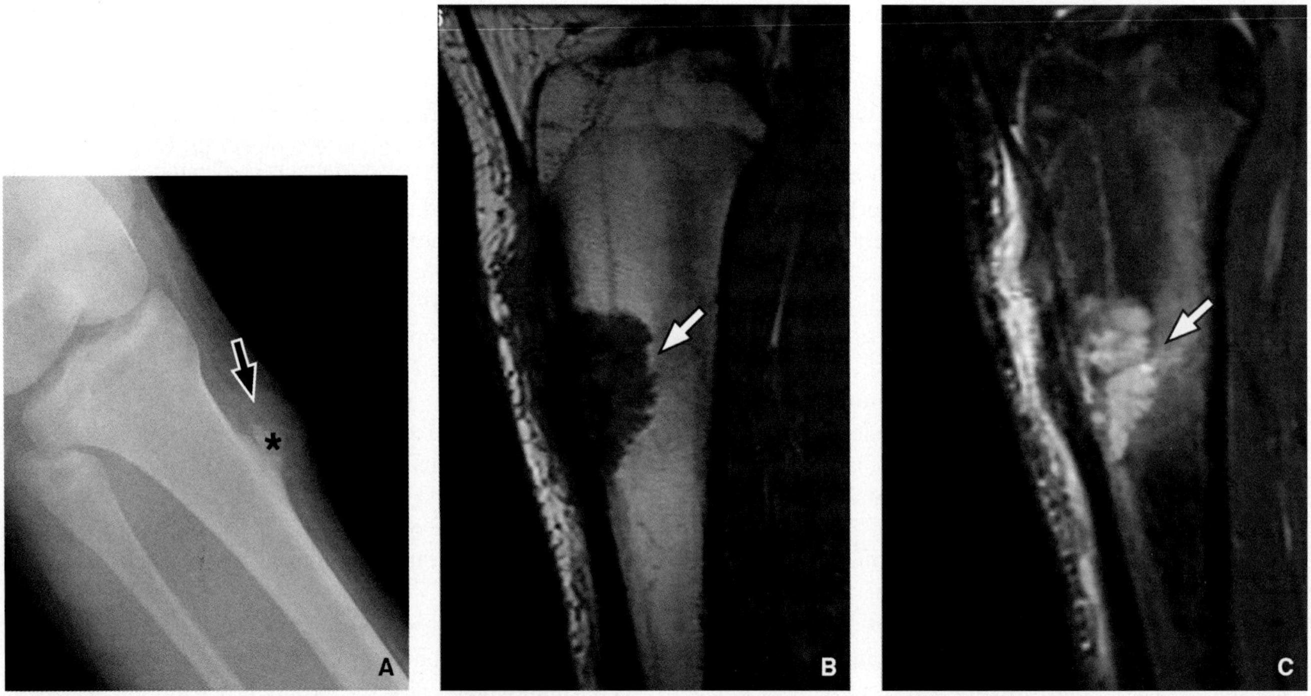

FIGURE 23.36 **High-grade surface osteosarcoma in a 15-year-old boy. A:** Frontal radiograph of the tibia demonstrates dense ossification (*asterisk*) with an associated soft tissue mass formation medially (*arrow*). Note that there is no medullary continuation between the ossification and the parent bone. **B, C:** Sagittal T1- **(B)** and fat-suppressed T2-weighted **(C)** MR images demonstrate intramedullary invasion (*arrow*).

sarcoma and primitive neuroectodermal tumor (PNET) are typically characterized by rearrangements of the EWSR1 gene, most commonly due to a reciprocal translocation of the long arms of chromosomes 11 and 22 (q24; q12), and they are considered to represent the same tumor.[100,101]

Ewing sarcoma of bone affects most commonly the pelvis (21%); femurs; humeri (31%); distal extremity bones including tibia, fibula, radius, and ulna (27%); ribs (7%); and clavicle.[102] The majority of long bone lesions occur in the metadiaphysis (59%).[10,98,99] As opposed to osteosarcoma, Ewing sarcoma commonly occurs in the diaphyses of long tubular bones and in the axial skeleton, as well as in extraosseous sites. The most common presenting symptoms in pediatric patients with Ewing sarcoma are localized pain and swelling, fever, weight loss, anemia, and leukocytosis, which can mislead clinicians toward a diagnosis of osteomyelitis.[103]

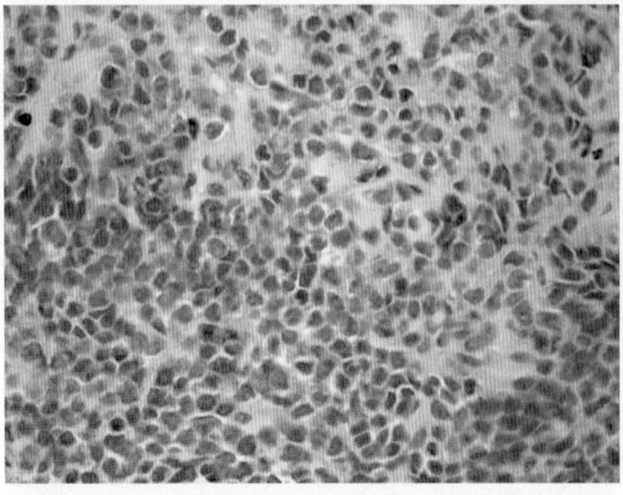

FIGURE 23.37 **Ewing sarcoma of the iliac bone from a 12-year-old girl.** The tumor is composed of small round blue cells with scant cytoplasm (hematoxylin and eosin, original magnification, 600x). In situ hybridization detected an EWSR1 gene rearrangement, confirming the diagnosis.

The radiographic findings of osseous Ewing sarcoma are variable and demonstrate aggressive features. The most common findings are poorly delineated intramedullary bone destruction with soft tissue mass formation in the metadiaphysis or diaphysis of the long bones (>80%).[99] Other common findings include laminated periosteal reaction (onion skin) (57%) and mixed sclerosis (40%)[103] (Fig. 23.38). Less common appearances include spiculated periosteal reaction (sunburst or hair-on-end), cortical thickening and saucerization, pure osteolytic lesions, and rarely soft tissue calcification, honey comb appearance, or vertebra plana.[102] Diffuse sclerosis is the result of reactive bone formation and osteoid deposition on the areas of bone necrosis. In rare cases, Ewing sarcoma arises in the periosteum and is called periosteal Ewing sarcoma. This lesion demonstrates extrinsic erosion of the cortex and a similar radiologic appearance to periosteal osteosarcoma. Periosteal Ewing sarcoma does not involve the medullary cavity and has a better prognosis.[104]

The radiographic appearance of Ewing sarcoma in the innominate bones is similar to that occurring in other skeletal sites. A large soft tissue mass with dysmorphic calcification is usually present in Ewing sarcoma in flat bones, which is better visualized on CT. Ewing sarcoma has homogeneous

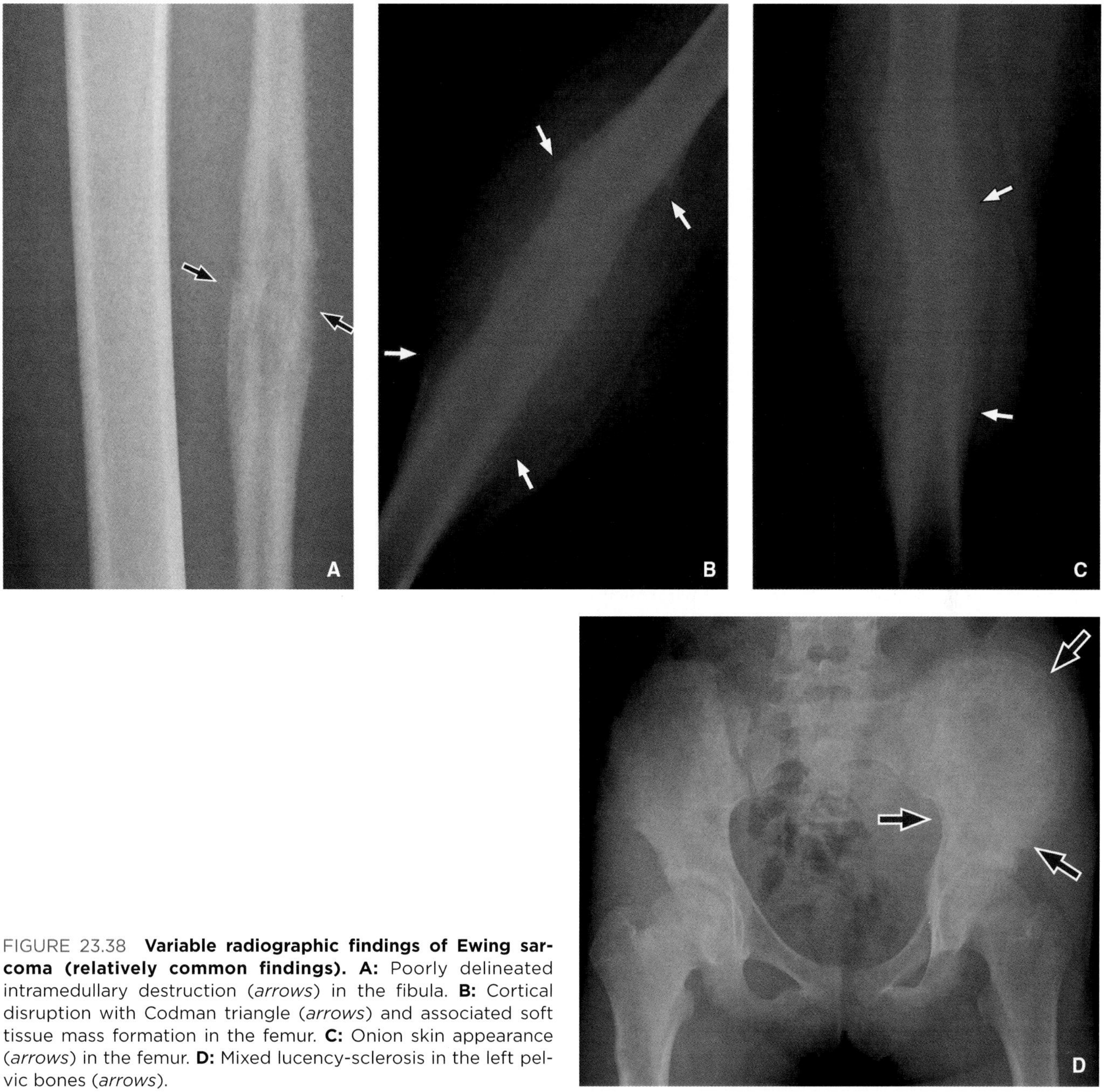

FIGURE 23.38 **Variable radiographic findings of Ewing sarcoma (relatively common findings). A:** Poorly delineated intramedullary destruction (*arrows*) in the fibula. **B:** Cortical disruption with Codman triangle (*arrows*) and associated soft tissue mass formation in the femur. **C:** Onion skin appearance (*arrows*) in the femur. **D:** Mixed lucency-sclerosis in the left pelvic bones (*arrows*).

intermediate T1- (95%) and low to intermediate T2- (68%) or high T2-weighted (32%) signal intensity.[99] Heterogeneous high T2-weighted signal is more common in larger lesions due to hemorrhage or necrosis. Cortical destruction with extraosseous soft tissue continuity is seen in 50% of cases[99] (Fig. 23.39).

Many similar radiologic appearances are observed in both osteosarcoma and Ewing sarcoma. Based on radiologic findings, differentiation of Ewing sarcoma from osteosarcoma is not always possible, and histopathologic examination is required for definitive diagnosis. The differential considerations of long bone lesions that can appear similar to Ewing sarcoma include lymphoma, metastasis, LCH, and osteomyelitis in the pediatric population.

Treatment of Ewing sarcoma is a combination of neoadjuvant chemotherapy followed by surgical resection and supplementary radiation therapy. Factors associated with worse prognosis include older age, tumor size >8 cm, pelvic origin, metastases at presentation or recurrence within 2 years, and most importantly, <90% tumor necrosis after neoadjuvant chemotherapy.[99,100] MRI findings suggesting favorable response to neoadjuvant therapy include extraosseous tumor size reduction and increased tumor necrosis and hemorrhage. To better document a positive response (>90% tumor necrosis after neoadjuvant therapy), dynamic enhanced or diffusion-weighted MRI technique can be used in research protocols.[99]

Extraosseous Ewing Sarcoma

Extraosseous Ewing sarcoma accounts for 15% to 20% of all Ewing sarcomas.[98] Clinically, extraosseous Ewing sarcoma often presents with a rapidly growing large soft

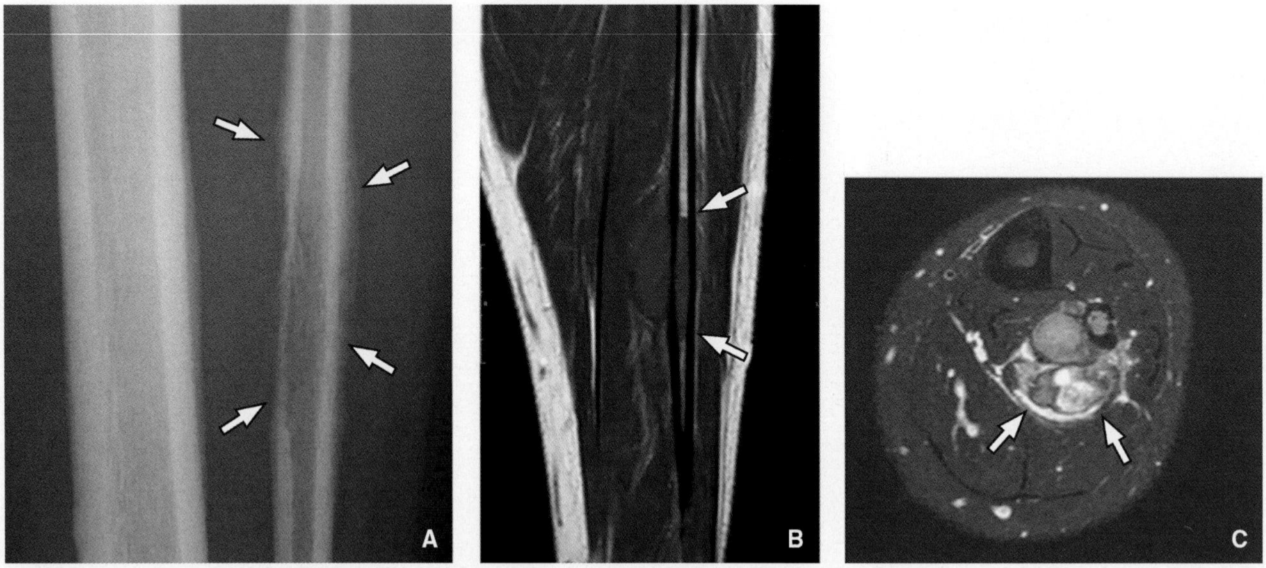

FIGURE 23.39 **Ewing sarcoma in a 14-year-old girl. A:** Frontal radiograph of the fibula demonstrates permeative bone destruction (*arrows*). **B:** Sagittal T1-weighted MR image of the fibula demonstrates a well-demarcated margin of the intramedullary lesion (*arrows*). **C:** Axial fat-suppressed T2-weighted MR image demonstrates an extraosseous soft tissue mass formation (*arrows*).

tissue mass, most commonly involving the paraspinal or lower extremity deep soft tissue. Radiographic findings are nonspecific and may include a normal appearance, a large soft tissue mass, bone scalloping or erosion, cortical thickening, or aggressive periosteal reaction. MRI usually shows an intermediate T1- and intermediate to high T2-weighted signal intensity mass (Fig. 23.40). Signal changes from necrosis or hemorrhage are also frequent. Due to high blood flow in the tumor, serpentine low signal areas can be seen on both T1- and T2-weighted MR images. These MRI findings are not specific for extraosseous Ewing sarcoma and can be seen in other highly vascular tumors such as hemangiopericytoma or hemangioendothelioma, alveolar soft part sarcoma (ASPS), and alveolar rhabdomyosarcoma. Prominent contrast enhancement is also a feature of these lesions. Associated involvement of bone is unusual, and bone scintigraphy is usually normal.[98]

Other Malignant Tumors

Chondrosarcoma

Chondrosarcoma is a malignant cartilaginous matrix-producing neoplasm. It is rare in children, accounting for <2% of pediatric malignant bone tumors.[105] Chondrosarcomas of bone can be classified according to location (central, peripheral, and juxtacortical types), presence of pre-existing lesion (primary vs. secondary), cellular differentiation (low vs. high grade), or cellular variants (clear cell, mesenchymal or dedifferentiated chondrosarcomas). The central type of chondrosarcoma arises in the medullary cavity, whereas the peripheral type arises on the surface of the bone. Primary chondrosarcoma occurs de novo, and secondary chondrosarcoma is superimposed on a pre-existing lesion such as osteochondroma (usually peripheral) or enchondromatosis (usually central type).[88,106] Patients with enchondromatosis, either Ollier disease or Maffucci syndrome, have an increased risk of secondary chondrosarcoma, which is seen in up to 25% and 53% of patients, respectively.[107]

Central primary chondrosarcoma is the most common, accounting for 85% of chondrosarcomas.[88,108] The most common sites are the pelvic bones and proximal femur. Less than 2% of cases involve the epiphysis.[88,108] These lesions can be mimics of chondroblastoma and are usually of the clear cell variant.[109] Chondrosarcoma can occur in previously irradiated skeletons.[108]

On radiographs, a central primary chondrosarcoma is seen as a large, radiolucent lesion with a poorly defined margin. The contour of the bone is enlarged or expanded. Foci of irregular calcifications within the tumor matrix occur in two-third of chondrosarcomas, and characteristic chondroid calcifications, which are ring or popcorn-like calcifications, may be seen in low-grade chondrosarcomas. Distinguishing between a low-grade central chondrosarcoma and an enchondroma can be challenging, although chondrosarcomas are very rare in children (Fig. 23.41). In peripheral chondrosarcomas, cortical destruction and a spiculated periosteal reaction occurs in the soft tissue area adjacent to the peripheral lesions.[110,111] Imaging findings of malignant transformation of osteochondromas to secondary peripheral chondrosarcomas were described in the osteochondroma section of this chapter (Fig. 23.3). Continuing growth of known enchondromatosis in adults, cortical destruction and soft tissue extension are signs of development of secondary central chondrosarcoma (Fig. 23.42). Juxtacortical chondrosarcomas demonstrate an aggressive appearance including Codman triangle and cortical destruction.

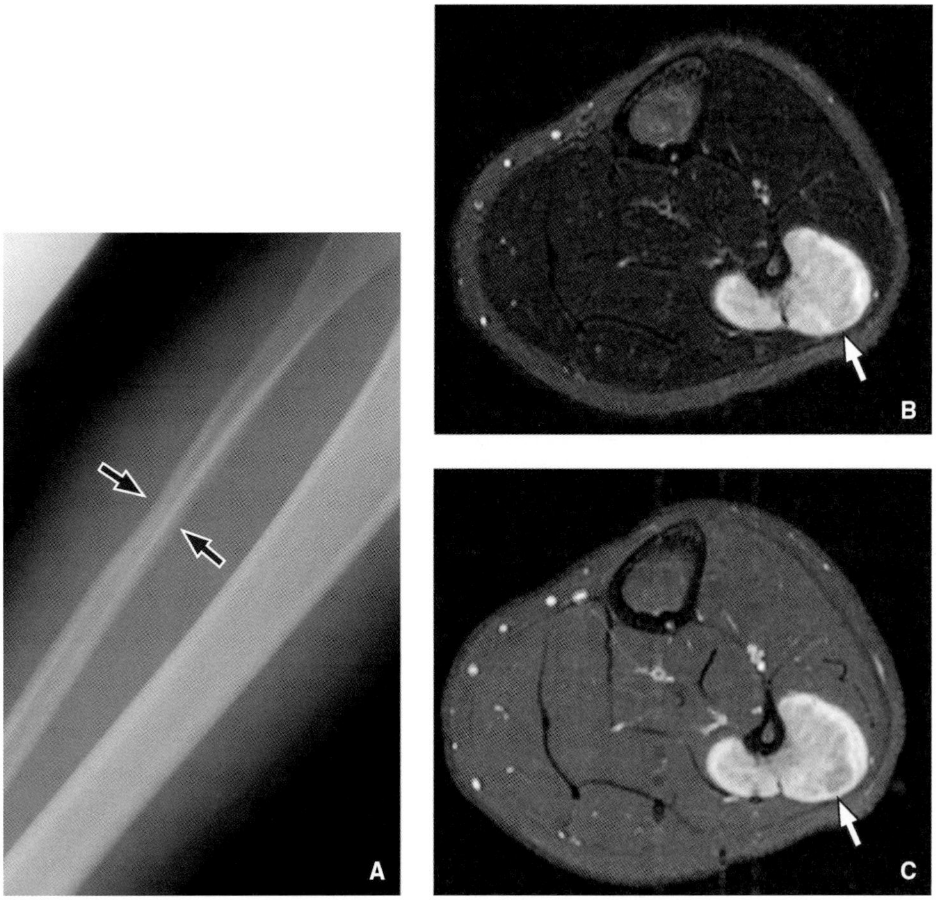

FIGURE 23.40 **Extraosseous Ewing sarcoma in an 8-year-old boy. A:** Frontal radiograph of the fibula demonstrates pressure erosion and saucerization of the bone (*arrows*). **B:** Axial fat-suppressed T2- **(B)** and postcontrast fat-suppressed T1-weighted **(C)** MR images demonstrate a soft tissue mass (*arrow*) formation in keeping with extraosseous Ewing sarcoma.

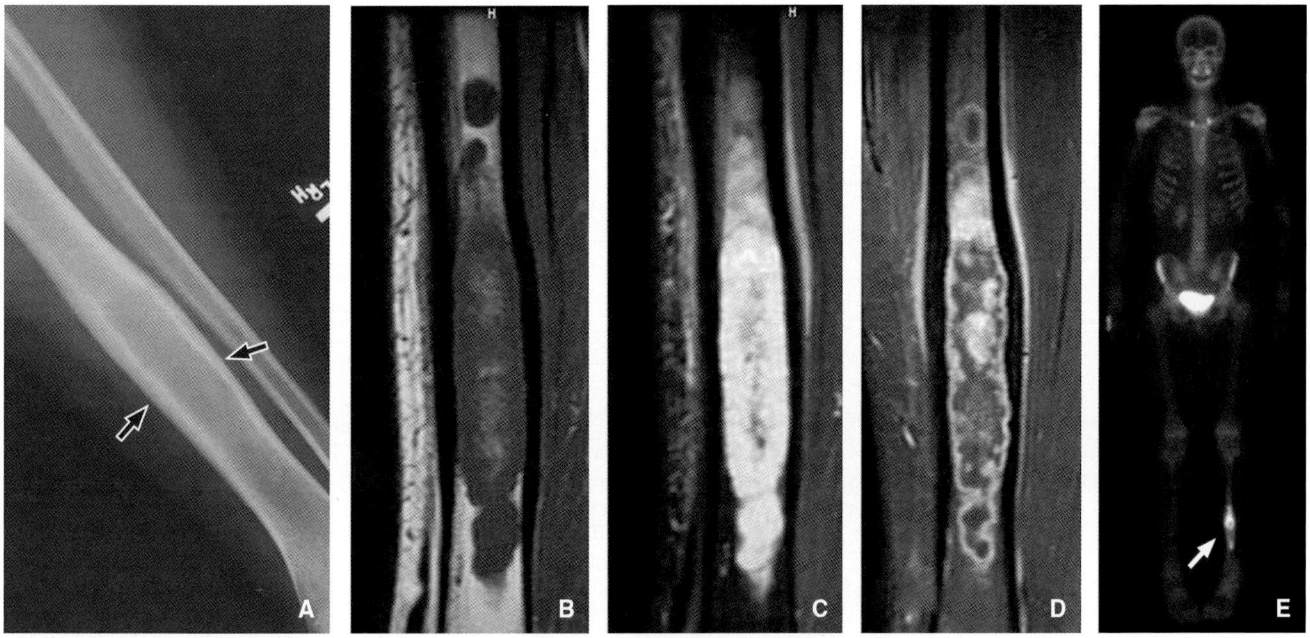

FIGURE 23.41 **Low-grade chondrosarcoma in a 15-year-old girl. A:** Frontal radiograph of the tibia demonstrates an intramedullary lucency with endosteal scalloping (*arrows*). **B–D:** Coronal T1- **(B)**, fat-suppressed T2-weighted **(C)** and postcontrast fat-suppressed T1-weighted **(D)** MR images demonstrate an intramedullary low T1 and high T2 signal mass with peripheral rim enhancement. Findings are similar to those of a benign enchondroma. **E:** 99mTc-MDP bone scan demonstrates increased uptake in the lesion site (*arrow*).

Surgical resection is the primary therapeutic option for chondrosarcomas. Their prognosis for local recurrence and metastases varies with cellular differentiation and variants.

Metastasis

Skeletal metastasis should be also considered in the differential diagnosis of any bone lesion, especially of those that are multifocal or appear aggressive. Skeletal metastases occur from a variety of tumors including lymphoma, leukemia, rhabdomyosarcoma, Wilms tumor, medulloblastoma, neuroblastoma, and multicentered primary bone tumors (Ewing sarcoma and osteosarcoma) in the pediatric population.[105,112,113] Skeletal metastases of neuroblastoma occur in more than 50% of cases.[114] Metastatic neuroblastoma shows permeative involvement of bone and diffuse periosteal reaction. In the skull, metastatic bone lesions have a characteristic appearance with osteolytic lesions and diffuse widening of sutures. A soft tissue mass and a striking sunburst periosteal reaction are also frequently encountered in pediatric patients with metastatic neuroblastoma in the craniofacial bones (Fig. 23.43). Metastatic retinoblastoma often has both osteolytic and osteoblastic lesions.[115,116]

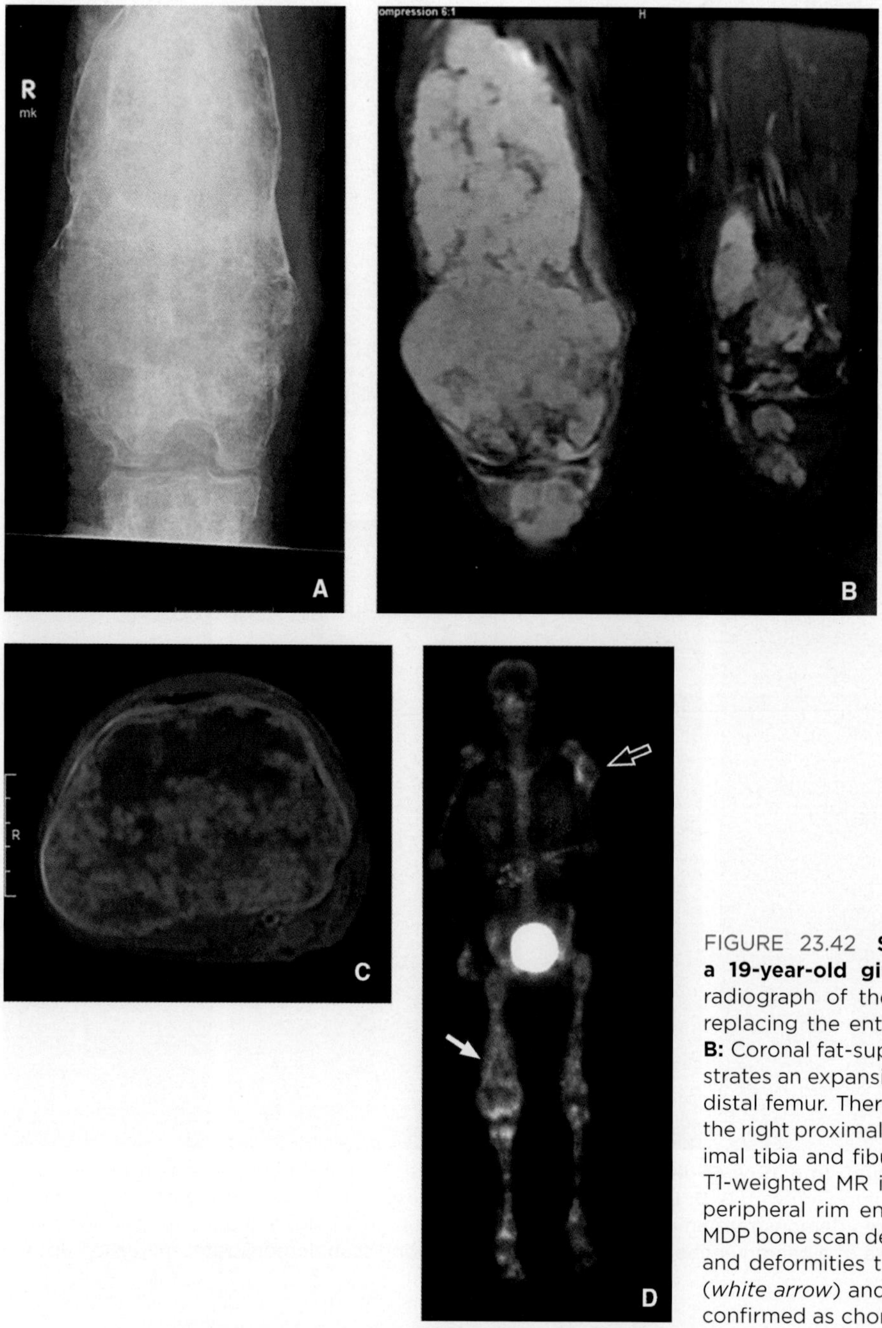

FIGURE 23.42 **Secondary central chondrosarcoma in a 19-year-old girl with Maffucci syndrome. A:** Frontal radiograph of the femur demonstrates extensive lesions replacing the entire right distal femur and proximal tibia. **B:** Coronal fat-suppressed T2-weighted MR image demonstrates an expansile high T2 signal mass replacing the right distal femur. There are multifocal enchondromas involving the right proximal tibia, left distal femur, as well as left proximal tibia and fibula. **C:** Axial postcontrast fat-suppressed T1-weighted MR image demonstrates heterogeneous and peripheral rim enhancement within the mass. **D:** 99mTc-MDP bone scan demonstrates multifocal increased uptakes and deformities throughout the skeleton. The right femur (*white arrow*) and left humerus (*black arrow*) lesions were confirmed as chondrosarcoma.

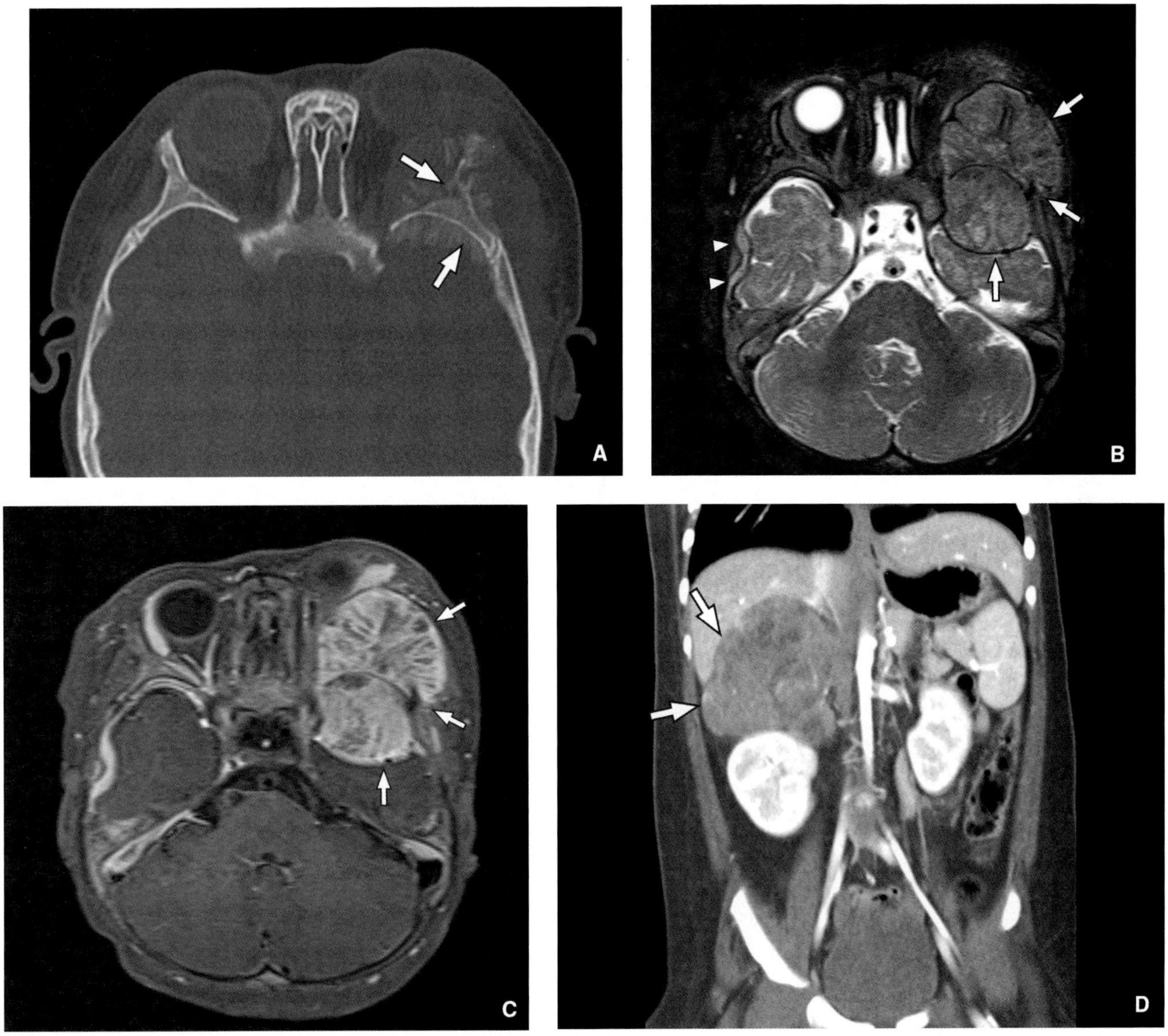

FIGURE 23.43 **Metastatic neuroblastoma in a 12-month-old girl who presented with left exophthalmos and raccoon-eye appearance. A:** Axial CT image shows an irregular osteolytic lesion (*arrows*) with hair-on-end periosteal reaction in the left bony orbit. **B, C:** Corresponding T2-weighted **(B)** and postcontrast T1-weighted **(C)** MR images show a large mass (*arrows*) with a lobulated contour involving the left orbit lateral wall and temporal bone. Note the plaque-like dural mass (*arrowheads*) in the right temporal area. **D:** Coronal post-contrast CT image shows a heterogeneously enhancing right suprarenal mass (*arrows*). Ultrasonography-guided biopsy of the right suprarenal mass confirmed the diagnosis of neuroblastoma.

Leukemia

Leukemia is a common childhood malignancy, and the common sites of bone involvement are the femur, pelvis, spine, humerus, tibia, scapula, and skull. Radiographic features include generalized osteopenia as well as focal osteolytic lesions. Generalized osteopenia may be associated with widespread periosteal reaction. There may be lucent metaphyseal bands, which are often seen around the knee and shoulder.[117,118]

Diffuse and homogeneous decrease in signal intensity of the bone marrow on T1-weighted MR images is commonly seen in pediatric patients with acute leukemia. Abnormal bone marrow shows brighter signal intensities than both red and yellow marrow on T2-weighted MR images and enhances to various degrees depending on the vascularity of the underlying pathologic process (Fig. 23.44).

Lymphoma

Skeletal involvement of lymphomas is usually the result of secondary or metastatic spread of tumors. Primary lymphoma of the bone is an uncommon malignancy that accounts for <5% of primary malignant bone tumors.[119]

Most intraosseous lesions are non-Hodgkin lymphomas, which occur in the medullary cavity as permeative osteolytic lesion(s) (Fig. 23.45). Periosteal reaction is

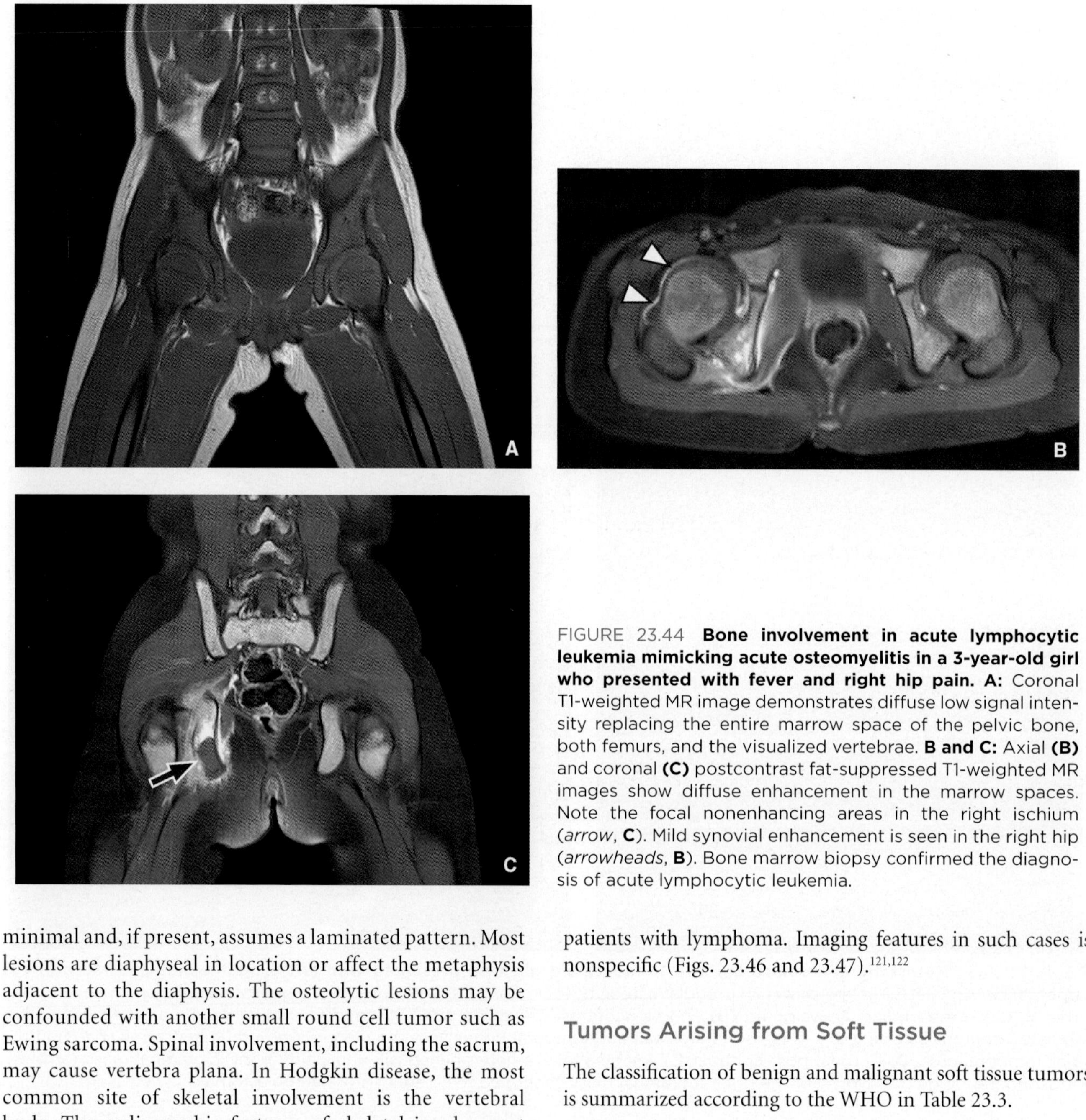

FIGURE 23.44 **Bone involvement in acute lymphocytic leukemia mimicking acute osteomyelitis in a 3-year-old girl who presented with fever and right hip pain. A:** Coronal T1-weighted MR image demonstrates diffuse low signal intensity replacing the entire marrow space of the pelvic bone, both femurs, and the visualized vertebrae. **B and C:** Axial **(B)** and coronal **(C)** postcontrast fat-suppressed T1-weighted MR images show diffuse enhancement in the marrow spaces. Note the focal nonenhancing areas in the right ischium (*arrow*, **C**). Mild synovial enhancement is seen in the right hip (*arrowheads*, **B**). Bone marrow biopsy confirmed the diagnosis of acute lymphocytic leukemia.

minimal and, if present, assumes a laminated pattern. Most lesions are diaphyseal in location or affect the metaphysis adjacent to the diaphysis. The osteolytic lesions may be confounded with another small round cell tumor such as Ewing sarcoma. Spinal involvement, including the sacrum, may cause vertebra plana. In Hodgkin disease, the most common site of skeletal involvement is the vertebral body. The radiographic features of skeletal involvement in Hodgkin disease are similar to those of non-Hodgkin disease, but spinal involvement usually results in ivory vertebrae.[119–121]

Although lymphoma may involve any organ or system, primary lymphoma of soft tissues is extremely rare. Muscle involvement by non-Hodgkin lymphoma usually occurs secondary to metastatic spread via lymphatic and hematogenous routes, although it may be the result of direct extension from primary bone lymphoma (Fig. 23.46). Imaging evaluation usually shows abnormalities in the adjacent osseous structures or lymph nodes, suggesting multifocal involvement (Figs. 23.45 and 23.46). Rarely, an isolated soft tissue or subcutaneous mass may be the presenting symptom in pediatric patients with lymphoma. Imaging features in such cases is nonspecific (Figs. 23.46 and 23.47).[121,122]

Tumors Arising from Soft Tissue

The classification of benign and malignant soft tissue tumors is summarized according to the WHO in Table 23.3.

Benign Soft Tissue Tumors

Benign Soft Tissue Tumors Arising from Synovium

Tenosynovial Giant Cell Tumor

Two main types of tenosynovial giant-cell tumor are giant-cell tumor of tendon sheath (GCTTS) and pigmented villonodular synovitis (PVNS).[123–126]

GCTTS is a type of tenosynovial GCT that typically exhibits localized growth.[123] The hand and wrist are the most commonly involved sites (65% to 89%).[124–126] GCTTS is the second most common soft tissue tumor of the hand and wrist after ganglion cyst.

The radiographic appearance of GCTTS is characterized by either the presence of a soft tissue mass (70%) or the lack of abnormalities (30%).[124–126] Associated calcification

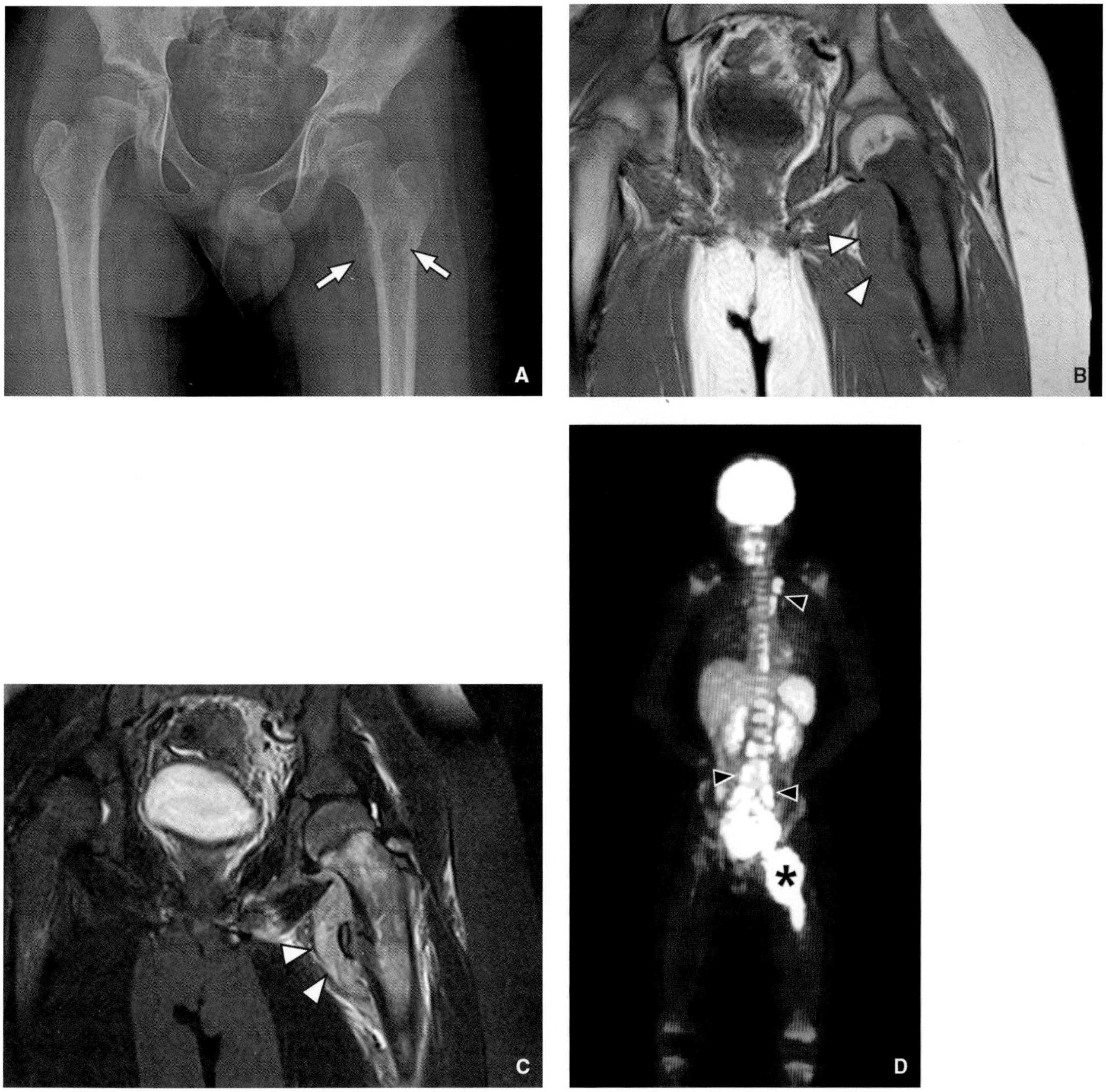

FIGURE 23.45 **Bone involvement of lymphoma in a 12-year-old boy. A:** Frontal radiograph of the hips demonstrates a permeative osteolytic lesion (*arrows*) in the left proximal femur and associated pelvic tilt to the left. **B, C:** Coronal T1-weighted **(B)** and fat-suppressed T2-weighted **(C)** MR images demonstrate localized bone marrow signal abnormalities with soft tissue mass formation (*arrowheads*) in the left proximal femur. **D:** Whole-body PET-CT reveals increased uptake along the lymphatic chains (*arrowheads*) in the mediastinum and abdomen as well as in the left proximal femur (*asterisk*).

is not usually present. MRI typically demonstrates a well-circumscribed soft tissue mass adjacent to or encasing the tendon sheath with low to intermediate signal intensity on both T1- and T2-weighted MR images (Fig. 23.48). The degree of hemosiderin deposition in GCTTS is variable.

PVNS is a type of tenosynovial giant-cell tumor occurring in a large joint and usually exhibiting a diffuse growth pattern. It usually occurs in the third to fifth decades of life, although it can affect the pediatric population.[126] Clinical manifestations can include pain, swelling, and joint dysfunction. The disease course is usually chronic and frequently involves a single joint, most often the knee.

On radiographs, PVNS typically demonstrates joint effusions and soft tissue swelling. The presence of calcification favors synovial osteochondromatosis over PVNS. Extrinsic bone erosions and subchondral lucencies can be seen in the hip, shoulder, elbow, and ankle, but not usually in the knee joint. The joint space is preserved until late disease stage and

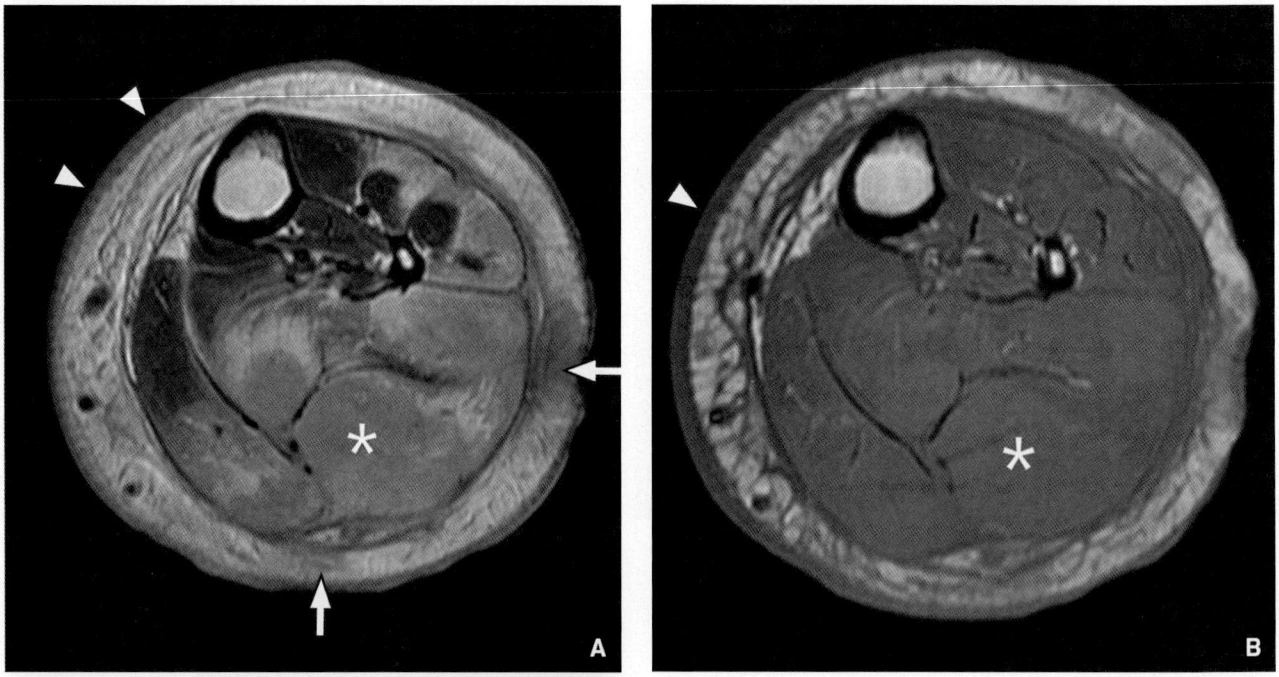

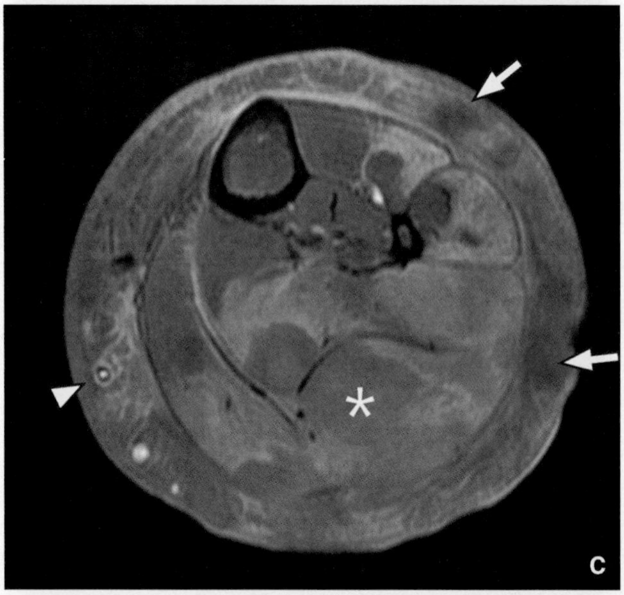

FIGURE 23.46 **T-cell lymphoma in a 9-year-old girl. A:** Axial T2-weighted MR image of the left calf shows multifocal intramuscular hyperintensity lesions (*asterisk*) and diffuse subcutaneous fat infiltration (*arrows*) and skin thickening (*arrowheads*). **B:** Axial T1-weighted MR image shows isointense or slightly hyperintense intramuscular lesions (*asterisk*) in the left calf and skin thickening (*arrowhead*). **C:** Axial post-contrast T1-weighted MR image **(C)** demonstrates heterogeneous signal intensity in the intramuscular lesions (*asterisk*) and heterogeneous enhancement in the subcutaneous lesions (*arrows*). There is also perivascular enhancement in the subcutaneous fat layer (*arrowhead*). Ultrasonography-guided biopsy of the intramuscular lesion confirmed the diagnosis of natural killer T-cell lymphoma.

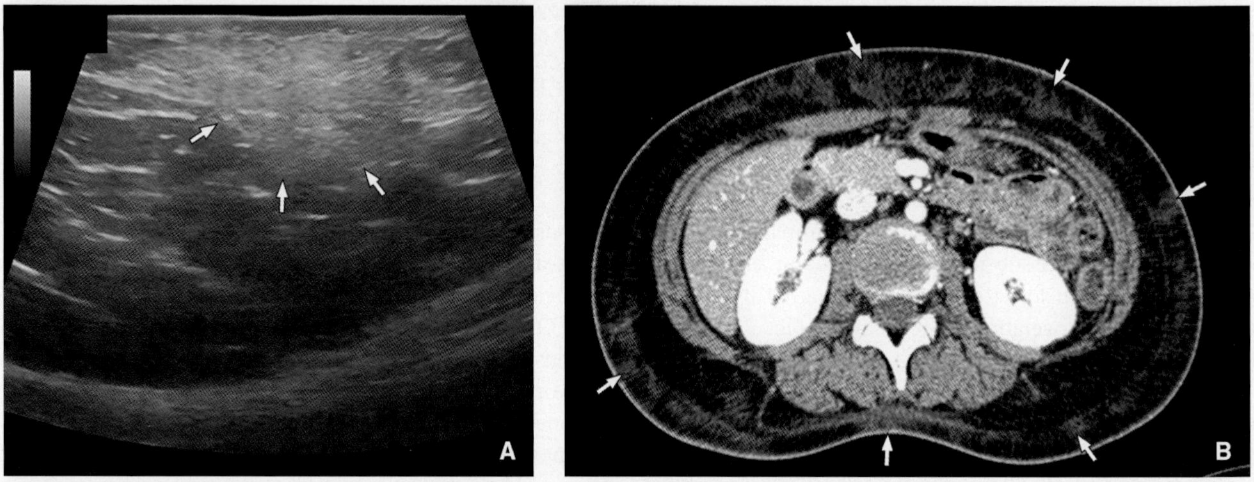

FIGURE 23.47 **Lymphoma presenting as multiple subcutaneous nodules in a 14-year-old girl. A:** Transverse ultrasound image demonstrates an ill-defined hyperechoic nodule (*arrows*) in the subcutaneous layer of the anterior abdominal wall. **B:** Axial post-contrast CT image at the level of the renal hilum demonstrates multifocal, irregularly shaped, enhancing subcutaneous lesions (*arrows*) in the abdomen. Ultrasonography-guided biopsy confirmed lymphoma involving the subcutaneous fat layer.

TABLE 23.3 World Health Organization (WHO) Classification of Soft Tissue Tumors

Soft Tissue Tumor Origin	Benign	Intermediate (Locally Aggressive or Rarely Metastasizing)	Malignant
Adipocytic	Lipoma Lipoblastoma Angiolipoma	Atypical lipomatous tumor	Liposarcoma Myxoid liposarcoma
Fibroblastic	Nodular fasciitis Myositis ossificans Fibrous hamartoma of infancy Fibromatosis colli Juvenile hyaline fibromatosis Inclusion body fibromatosis (infantile digital fibroma) Fibroma of tendon sheath Calcifying aponeurotic fibroma Cellular angiofibroma Nuchal fibroma Gardner fibroma	Palmar/plantar fibromatosis Desmoid-type fibromatosis Lipofibromatosis Giant cell fibroblastoma Dermatofibrosarcoma protuberans Solitary fibrous tumor Inflammatory myofibroblastic tumor Infantile fibrosarcoma	Myxofibrosarcoma Low-grade fibromyxoid sarcoma Sclerosing epithelioid fibrosarcoma
Fibrohistiocytic	Tenosynovial giant cell tumor (pigmented villonodular synovitis, giant cell tumor of tendon sheath) Deep benign fibrous histiocytoma	Plexiform fibrohistiocytic tumor	
Smooth muscle	Deep leiomyoma		Leiomyosarcoma
Pericytic (perivascular)	Glomus tumor Myopericytoma (including myofibroma/myofibromatosis)		
Skeletal muscle	Rhabdomyoma		Rhabdomyosarcoma
Vascular	Hemangioma Epithelioid hemangioma	Kaposiform hemangioendothelioma	Epithelioid hemangioendothelioma
Gastrointestinal stromal (GIST)	Benign GIST	GIST of uncertain malignant potential	Malignant GIST
Nerve sheath	Schwannoma Neurofibroma Perineurioma Ectopic meningioma		Malignant peripheral nerve sheath tumor
Uncertain differentiation	Intramuscular and juxta-articular myxoma Pleomorphic hyalinizing angiectatic tumor Ectopic hamartomatous thymoma	Angiomatoid fibrous histiocytoma Ossifying fibromyxoid tumor Phosphaturic mesenchymal tumor	Synovial sarcoma Epithelioid sarcoma Alveolar soft-part sarcoma Clear cell sarcoma of soft tissue Extraskeletal myxoid chondrosarcoma Extraskeletal Ewing sarcoma Desmoplastic small round cell tumor Rhabdoid tumor Neoplasms with perivascular epithelioid cell differentiation (PEComas)
Undifferentiated/ unclassified			Undifferentiated sarcoma (spindle cell, pleomorphic, round cell, epithelioid, and not otherwise specified)

Adapted from: Fletcher CDM, Bridge JA, Hogendoorn PCW, et al., eds. WHO Classification of Tumours of Soft Tissue and Bone. 4th ed. Lyon, France: IARC; 2013.

the bone mineralization is normal. Hemosiderin deposition in intra-articular PVNS results in a characteristic MR appearance. It can appear as diffuse villonodular synovial thickening (diffuse form) (Fig. 23.49) or a localized mass (localized form) with low signal intensity on both T1- and T2-weighted MR images. Hemosiderin deposition appears more pronounced on gradient-echo sequences due to an enlargement of the area of low signal intensity (blooming) caused by magnetic susceptibility artifact, also seen in any repetitive intra-articular hemorrhage resulting from hemophilic arthropathy or synovial

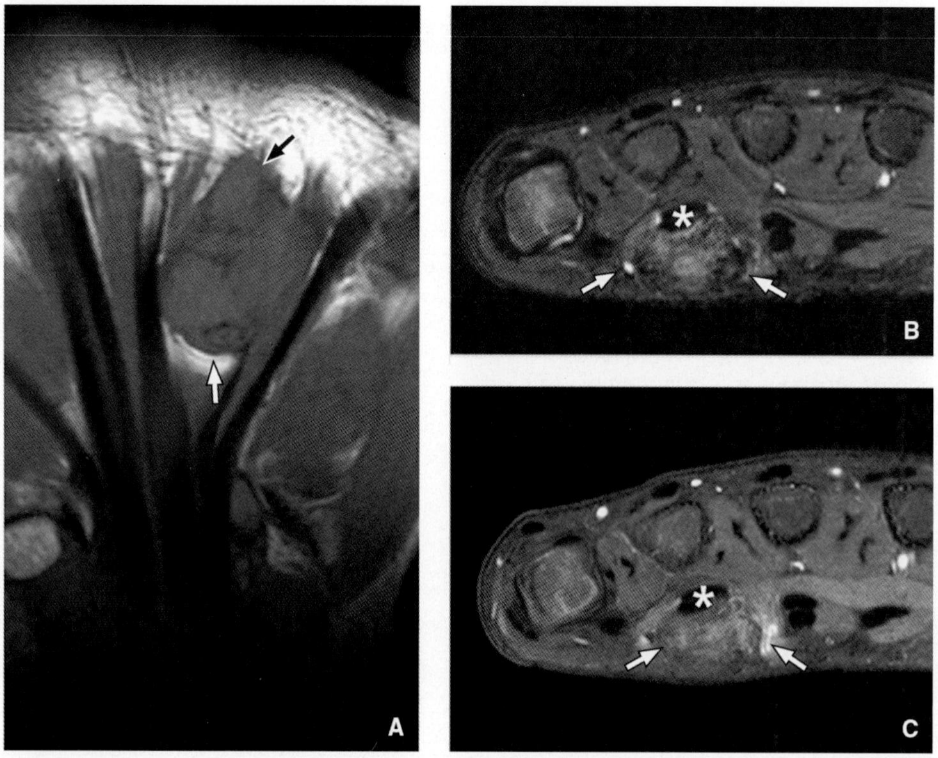

FIGURE 23.48 **Giant cell tumor of tendon sheath in a 9-year-old girl. A, B:** Coronal T1-weighted (A) and axial fat-suppressed T2-weighted (B) MR images demonstrate intermediate- to low signal mass (*arrows*) encasing a hand flexor tendon (*asterisk*). **C.** Postcontrast axial fat-suppressed T1-weighted MR image demonstrates mild enhancement of the lesion (*arrows*) around the flexor tendon (*asterisk*).

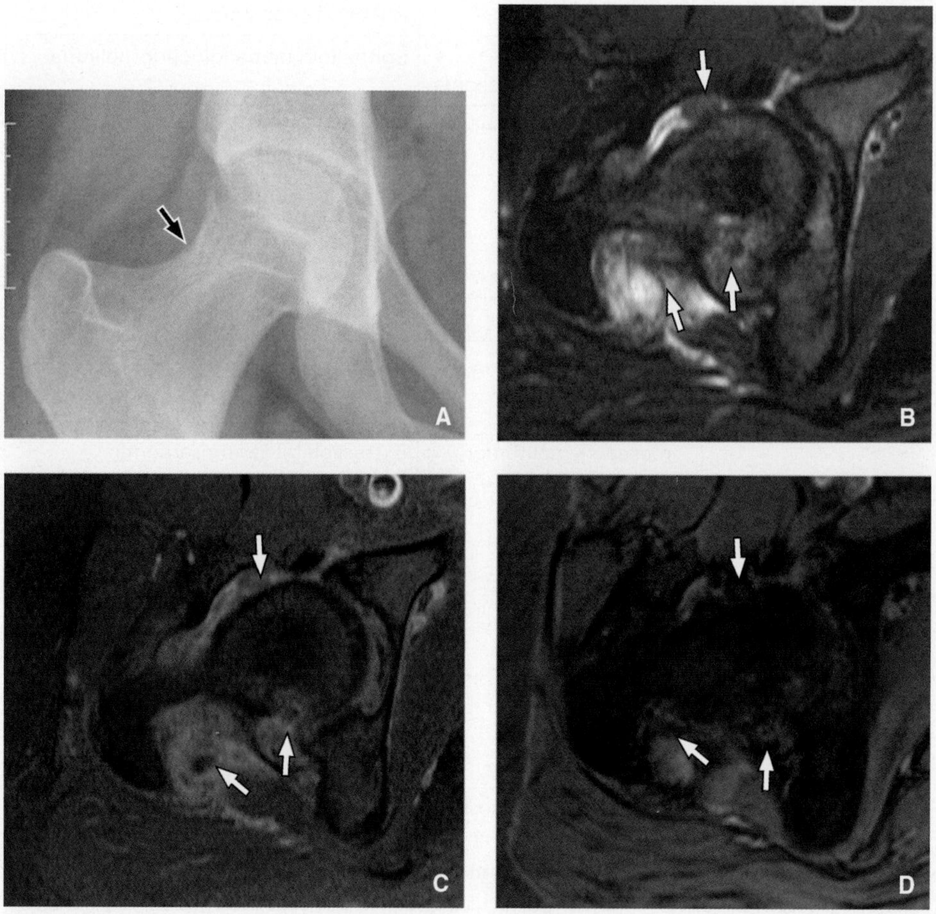

FIGURE 23.49 **Pigmented villonodular synovitis in a 15-year-old girl. A:** Frontal radiograph of the hip demonstrates a subtle erosion along the lateral margin of the femoral neck (*arrow*). **B, C:** Axial fat-suppressed T2-weighted **(B)** and axial postcontrast fat-suppressed T1-weighted **(C)** MR images demonstrate multiple dark signal foci (*arrows*) within the synovial thickening. **D:** Axial gradient-echo MR image demonstrates "blooming artifact" (*arrows*) within synovial areas containing hemosiderin.

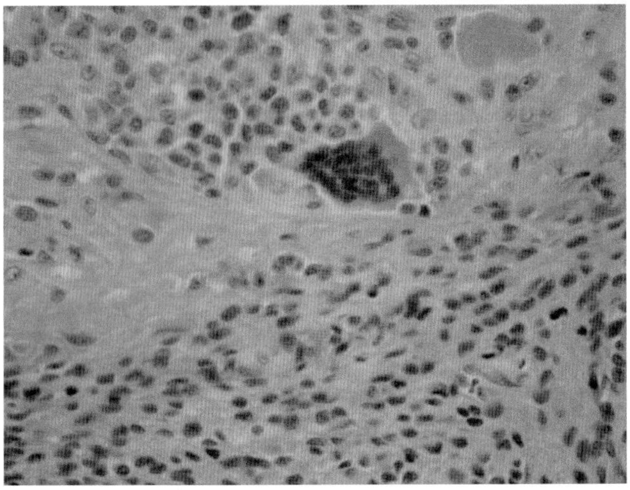

FIGURE 23.50 **Giant cell tumor (GCT) of tendon sheath (localized tenosynovial GCT) involving the ankle of an 11-year-old girl.** Mononuclear histiocyte-like cells are the predominant cell type. Here, there are admixed giant cells and areas of prominent collagen deposition (hematoxylin and eosin, original magnification, 600×).

hemangioma. A variable degree of heterogeneous enhancement is observed after intravenous contrast injection.[125]

Histologically, both localized and diffuse tenosynovial GCTs consist of a proliferation of mononuclear histiocyte-like cells admixed with giant cells and variable numbers of chronic inflammatory cells (Fig. 23.50). Frond-like growth and hemosiderosis are common in PVNS (Fig. 23.51). Both tumors are characterized by a subpopulation of cells with a translocation involving the *CSF1* gene, thought to play a role in the recruitment of an additional population of "reactive" cells.[127]

Surgical resection is the current treatment for tenosynovial GCT in symptomatic pediatric patients. The recurrence rate following resection is extremely low in localized tenosynovial GCT, but relatively high in diffuse intra-articular PVNS, ranging from 8% to 56%.[124–126]

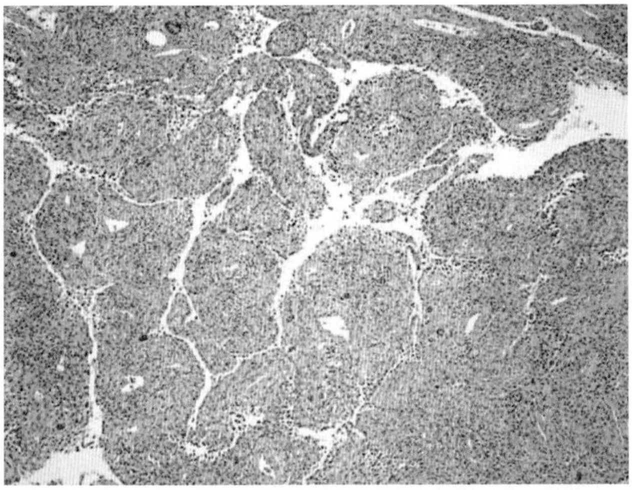

FIGURE 23.51 **Pigmented villonodular synovitis, diffuse-type tenosynovial giant cell tumor, recurring in the knee of a 19-year-old boy.** Histologically, a villiform architecture is observed (hematoxylin and eosin, original magnification, 100×). Cytogenetic analysis showed an abnormal karyotype, with a rearrangement involving 1p13, the site of the *CSF1* gene.

Synovial Chondromatosis

Synovial chondromatosis, also known as synovial osteochondromatosis or osteochondrosis, is a rare benign neoplastic process that produces cartilage nodules in the synovium of a joint or tendon sheath. Patients of all ages can be affected, but most cases occur during the third to fifth decades of life with male predilection (male: female, 2–4:1).[128] The knee is the most commonly affected joint (50% to 65%), followed by the hip.[128] Clinical presentations include pain, swelling, and limited range of motion with insidious onset and slow progression. Synovial chondromatosis usually involves a single joint. However, multiple joint or bilateral involvements are reported in 10% of cases.[128] Extra-articular synovial chondromatosis is rare and can occur in the bursa.[129]

The disease progresses through three different stages. The first phase is characterized by active synovial proliferation with cartilage nodule formation in the synovium without fragmentation. The second phase is characterized by synovial proliferation with cartilage nodules and cartilage bodies that break off into the joint space. The third phase is characterized by intra-articular cartilage bodies without active synovial proliferation. Intra-articular cartilage bodies (known as synovial chondromatosis) undergo calcification and ossification, which may be called synovial osteochondromatosis. The chondrocytes in synovial chondromatosis are typically histologically bland (Fig. 23.52); however, atypical features such as hypercellularity and multinucleation can occur, which can raise suspicion for a malignant cartilage neoplasm if the clinical context is not fully understood.[130] Osteochondral loose bodies (joint mice) may also enter the differential diagnosis.

Radiographs show intra-articular ossifications in 70% to 95% of patients affected with synovial chondromatosis.[128] The calcifications are evenly distributed in the joint space, multiple (more than five in half of cases), and very similar in

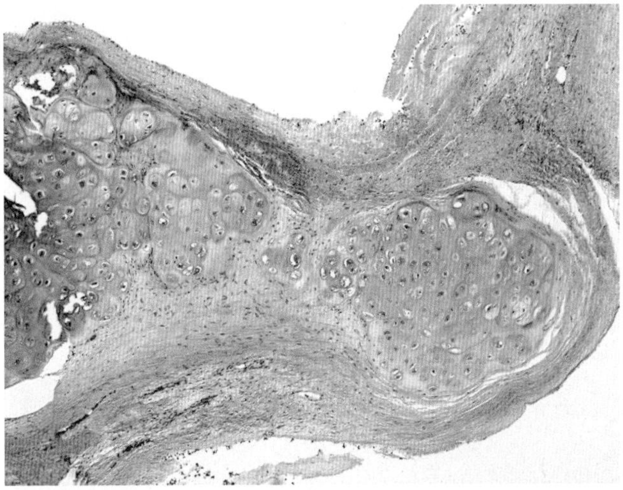

FIGURE 23.52 **Synovial chondromatosis, resected from the hip of a 7-year-old girl.** There is a proliferation of small seed-like nodules of hyaline cartilage (hematoxylin and eosin, original magnification, 100×).

appearance.[128] Characteristic calcification patterns include chondroid mineralization with a *ring-and-arc* appearance, further maturation with endochondral ossification (peripheral rim of cortex and inner trabecular bone), or target appearance (Fig. 23.53). Joint effusion may be seen, and joint space is maintained unless there have been multiple recurrences. Extrinsic erosions on both sides of the joint are seen in 30% of cases, particularly in less capacious joints such as the shoulder and hip. The pattern of mineralization is variable and depends on the stage of disease process, and radiographs can be normal in 5% to 30% of cases.[128] CT is helpful to detect characteristic mineralization.

MRI shows three distinct patterns depending on the presence of ossification of the cartilage bodies. The most common pattern seen in 77% of cases is intra-articular low T1- and high T2-weighted signal bodies with dark signal areas in all pulse sequences (Fig. 23.53). These dark signal areas correspond to ossification and are better visualized on MR gradient echo sequence or on CT. A less common pattern seen in 14% of cases is low T1- and high T2-weighted signal intra-articular bodies without dark signal areas, corresponding to cartilaginous bodies without ossification.[128] The least common pattern, seen in 9% of cases, is represented by intra-articular bodies with internal fatty signal (high T1 and high T2 signal) and sclerotic rim (a dark T1 and T2 peripheral rim). The internal fatty signal corresponds to endochondral ossification with mature fatty marrow.[131] After intravenous contrast administration, synovial enhancement is typically seen.[128]

Surgical resection is the current treatment of choice for synovial osteochondromatosis. Local recurrence in cases of incomplete resection is reported in 3% to 23% cases.[128]

Ganglion Cyst

A ganglion cyst is not a tumor; it is a cystic lesion containing thick gelatinous fluid arising from the juxta-articular soft tissues, intra-articular space, or periosteum.[132] The etiology of ganglion cysts is currently uncertain and may be related to myxoid degeneration of the adjacent soft tissue or synovial herniation. A juxta-articular ganglion is the most common form, seen in 70% of cases.[133] Ganglion cyst is the most common soft tissue mass of the wrist (50% to 70%).[133] Clinically, a ganglion cyst presents with a palpable superficial mass, tenderness, pain, and functional impairment or nerve palsy from compression. Most ganglion cysts are small measuring between 1.5 and 2.5 cm.[133]

Ultrasound is currently the most cost-effective modality to evaluate a ganglion cyst, which can show a well-defined homogeneous anechoic mass.[134] Long-standing ganglion cysts can have a more complex appearance from hemorrhage or infection. The occasional appearance of "pseudopodia," elongated extension into the joint space with communication, has been reported. MRI shows a round or lobulated shaped unilocular or multilocular low T1- and high T2-weighted signal cystic lesion with a fibrous capsule (Fig. 23.54).[133] Rarely, iso- to increased T1 signal is seen due to underlying high-protein content. MRI is also useful to identify the relationship between the ganglion cyst and the adjacent joint, capsule, tendons, nerve, and vessels. Furthermore, MR can show muscle group changes related to compressive neuropathy from nerve compression due to ganglion cyst. Intra-articular ganglion cysts are less common than juxta-articular ganglion cysts. The majority of intra-articular ganglion cysts occur near the anterior or posterior

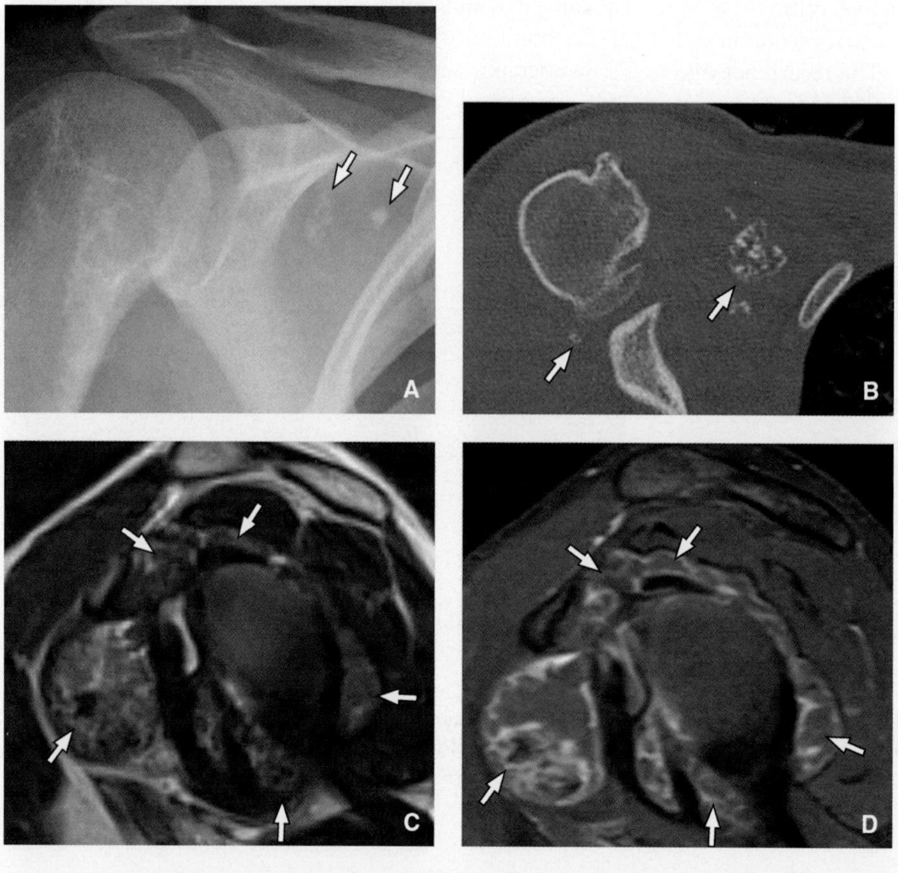

FIGURE 23.53 **Synovial osteochondromatosis in a 15-year-old girl. A:** Frontal radiograph shows multiple ossific foci (*arrows*) in the shoulder. **B:** Axial CT image demonstrates multiple ossific foci (*arrows*) in areas of the shoulder that correspond to the findings seen on radiograph **(A)**. **C, D:** Sagittal T2-weighted **(C)** and sagittal postcontrast fat-suppressed T1-weighted **(D)** MR images demonstrate multiple dark signal foci (*arrows*). Postcontrast MR image also demonstrates synovial thickening.

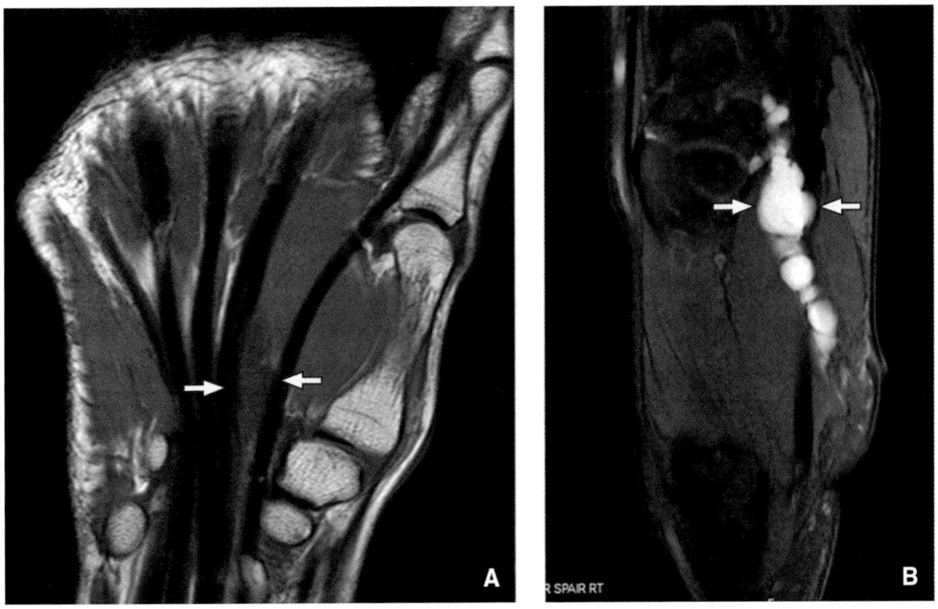

FIGURE 23.54 **Ganglion cyst in a 15-year-old girl who presented with wrist pain. A, B:** Coronal T1- **(A)** and sagittal fat-suppressed T2-weighted **(B)** MR images demonstrate a multiseptated cystic lesion (*arrows*) in the flexor tendon of the wrist.

cruciate ligaments of the knee. Periosteal ganglion cysts have a characteristic radiographic appearance of cortical thickening and bony scalloping from extrinsic compression.

Initially, ganglion cysts are treated nonsurgically including immobilization and aspiration. Surgical removal is performed for symptomatic cases, which are not relieved by nonsurgical treatments.

Soft Tissue Tumors and Tumor-Like Lesions Arising from Fatty Tissue

Fat Necrosis

Fat necrosis is not a neoplasm, but it may present with a palpable superficial mass in the pediatric population. Fat necrosis can occur with minor trauma, and a traumatic event is recalled in only half of cases. Most commonly, fat necrosis is situated in the subcutaneous tissue over the osseous protuberances, which is an area vulnerable to trauma.[135] In addition to preceding trauma, other underlying causes for fat necrosis include collagen vascular disease, myeloproliferative disorders, and complications of pancreatic disorders.

MRI is the best imaging modality for accurately detecting fat necrosis. MRI typically demonstrates a small (usually <3 cm) spiculated linear area of variable signal intensity on T1- and T2-weighted MR images or a fat-containing spiculated lesion surrounded by low T1- and low T2-weighted MR images representing fibrous tissue. An irregular rim enhancement is typically observed after intravenous contrast administration (Fig. 23.55).[136] The characteristic MRI appearance of fat necrosis can be helpful for differentiating it from other

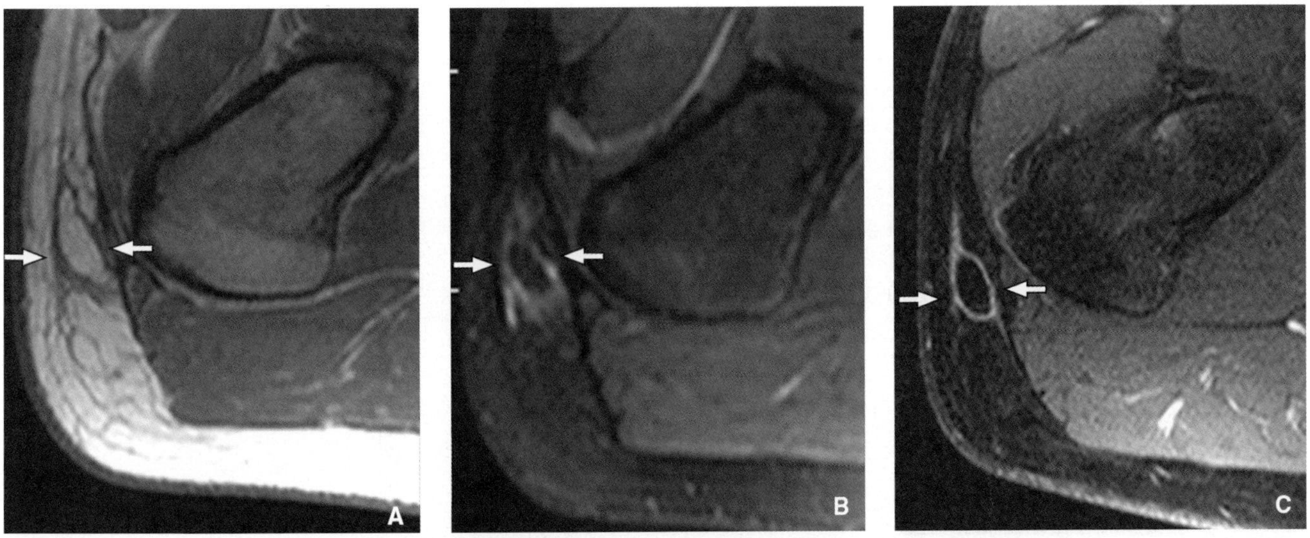

FIGURE 23.55 **15-year-old boy with fat necrosis. A, B:** Axial T1- **(A)** and inversion recovery **(B)** MR images demonstrate a fat-containing lesion (*arrows*) in the subcutaneous tissue. **C:** Axial postcontrast fat-suppressed T1-weighted MR image demonstrates peripheral rim enhancement in the lesion (*arrows*).

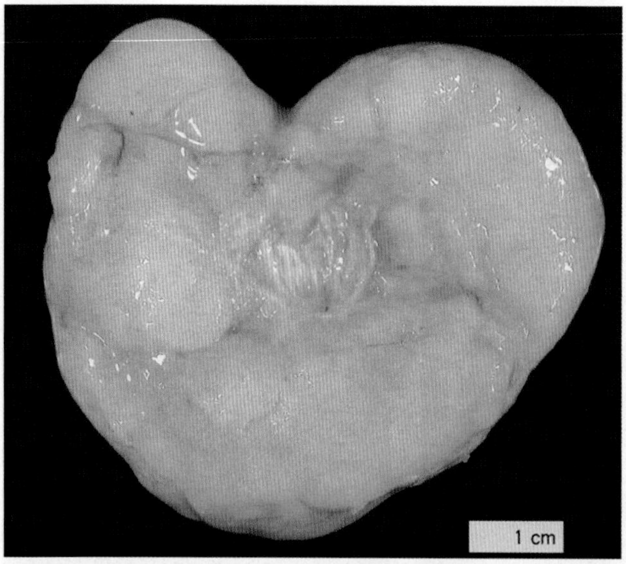

FIGURE 23.56 **Lipoma measuring 6.5 cm, resected from the subcutaneous leg tissue in a 9-year-old girl.** Grossly, a lobulated soft yellow finely encapsulated mass is observed.

aggressive soft tissue masses in order to avoid unnecessary tissue biopsy or surgical resection. Imaging follow-up is not always necessary and may show disappearance of the lesion, decrease in size, or no change.[137]

Benign Adipocytic Tumors

Benign lipomatous lesions are common tumors occurring in both soft tissue and bone. Grossly (Fig. 23.56) and histologically, a lipoma resembles normal fat. Soft tissue lipomas are among the most common soft tissue lesions in children, along with popliteal cysts and vascular malformations. The WHO categorized benign soft tissue adipocytic tumors into: (1) lipoma, (2) lipomatosis, (3) lipomatosis of nerve, (4) lipoblastoma/lipoblastomatosis, (5) angiolipoma, (6) myolipoma, (7) chondroid lipoma, (8) extrarenal angomyolipoma, (9) extra-adrenal myelolipoma, (10) spindle cell/pleomorphic lipoma, and (11) hibernoma.[4] In children, other entities rich in benign adipose tissue include fibroadipose vascular anomaly, phosphatase and tensin homolog (PTEN)-associated soft tissue hamartoma, and "lipofibromatosis".[138–140]

The most common presentation of soft tissue lipomas is a slow-growing mass in the subcutaneous tissue (i.e., superficial lipomas). Superficial lipomas most commonly affect the back, neck, proximal extremities, and abdominal wall. Deep lipomas present as well-delineated or infiltrating masses of the muscle and are less common than superficial lipomas. Deep lipomas most commonly affect the large muscles of the lower extremity (45%).[141,142] Lipomas are usually solitary lesions, but multiple lipomas are reported in 5% to 15%.[141,142] Familial lipomas are reported in 30% of multiple lipomas.[143]

Ultrasound is usually the initial imaging modality for evaluating superficial lipoma in children who present with palpable soft tissue mass, which can be a lipoma. Ultrasound typically shows a hyperechoic mass with similar echogenicity to adjacent subcutaneous fat. CT demonstrates a homogeneous fat-containing mass with Hounsfield units ranging between −65 and −120. MRI shows a mass with signal isointense to subcutaneous fat at all pulse sequences[141,142] (Fig. 23.57). A fibrous capsule can be seen in well-delineated lipomas. A homogeneous fat signal mass or thin fine septations without enhancement can allow confident diagnosis of a lipoma as opposed to a well-differentiated liposarcoma.[141,142] It is important to recognize that lipomas may have an atypical appearance when they contain nonadipose elements; atypical lipomas have a more complex imaging appearance that includes thick septa and nodular soft tissue. An atypical appearance has been reported in 28% to 31% of lipomas and cannot be differentiated from well-differentiated liposarcoma or lipoblastoma based on imaging.[141,142] These lesions therefore require tissue biopsy for differentiation and definitive diagnosis.[142]

Lipoblastoma

Lipoblastoma is a rare benign soft tissue tumor composed of immature adipose tissue. Lipoblastomas occur exclusively in

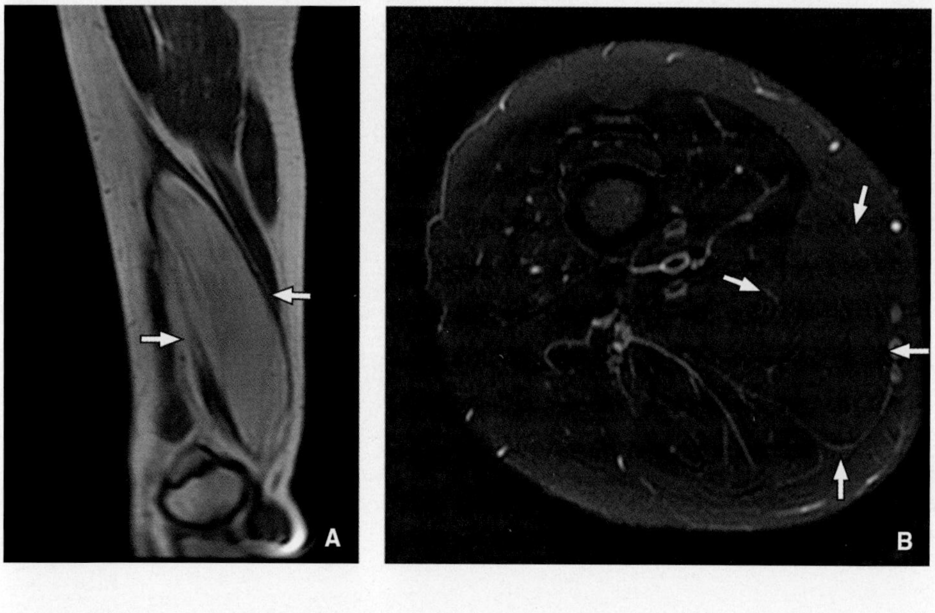

FIGURE 23.57 **Intramuscular lipoma in a 13-year-old boy. A, B:** Sagittal T1- **(A)** and axial fat-suppressed T2-weighted **(B)** MR images demonstrate an intramuscular fat-containing mass (*arrows*).

infants and children younger than 3 years of age.[144] Males are affected two to three times more often than females.[145] Two-thirds to three-quarters of lipoblastomas are solitary well-encapsulated masses referred lipoblastoma. The remaining cases demonstrate diffuse infiltration into the muscle and subcutaneous tissue and are referred to as lipoblastomatosis.[146] Clinically, lipoblastomas present as progressive and painless soft tissue masses. Clinical symptoms depend on the size and anatomic location of the mass.

Imaging findings of lipoblastoma are often characteristic. A well-defined (lipoblastoma) or infiltrative (lipoblastomatosis) mass is seen, which is predominantly fatty due to the presence of mature adipocytes.[147] Within the mass, primitive lipomatous components (myxoid stroma, primitive mesenchymal cells) as well as immature adipocytes coexist. These lipoblastomatous components produce nonspecific soft tissue signal on MR or multiple septations with contrast enhancement. A strong solid component or septal enhancement in the nonlipomatous lesion is seen after intravenous contrast administration due to the rich capillary network (Fig. 23.58).[148] Most lesions become "mature" and fat predominant over time. However, young infants can have predominantly nonlipomatous lesions with a very small amount of fat, which facilitates distinction from lipoma. Liposarcoma, another diagnostic consideration,[149] is extremely rare in children of the young age at which lipoblastoma typically presents.

Complete local excision is the current treatment of choice. The tumors typically do not metastasize, but recurrence is seen in 14% to 25% of cases.[147,148]

Lipoma Arborescens

Lipoma arborescens (tree-like) is a benign intra-articular lesion characterized by frond-like proliferation of the mature fat cells within the subsynovial tissue. Lipoma arborescens is rare in adults and extremely rare in children.[150] The etiology is uncertain and thought to be a nonspecific synovial reaction to trauma or inflammation associated with underlying joint pathology.[151] Lipoma arborescens usually involves a single joint, particularly the knee where the suprapatellar pouch is most commonly affected.[152] Clinically, affected pediatric patients usually present with long-standing progressive joint swelling and effusion. Radiographs show joint effusion. Because of the fatty nature of the lesion, MRI shows a characteristic appearance of villous proliferation of the synovium containing persistent fat signal on all MR pulse sequences (Fig. 23.59).[153] Synovectomy is generally a curative treatment because local recurrence is rare.

Benign Soft Tissue Tumor-Like Mass Arising from Muscle

Myositis Ossificans

Myositis ossificans, also known as myositis ossificans circumscripta, is a benign ossifying soft tissue mass occurring within the skeletal muscle.[154] Although the majority of cases are due to either single or minor repetitive traumas (Fig. 23.60), no prior history of trauma is documented in 25% to 40% of cases.[155,156] Myositis ossificans mostly occurs in the third decade of life and is rare in the first decade.[155–157] The large muscles of the extremities, in particular the thigh muscles, are most commonly affected. Clinically, affected pediatric patients present with pain, tenderness, and palpable soft tissue mass.

Myositis ossificans has an age-related evolution with formation and maturation of a distinct peripheral rim of bone. Due to this progression, imaging findings differ at each stage of development. In the acute phase, immediately or within 2 weeks after onset, no calcification is visualized on radiograph or CT. In this stage, the zonal pattern is not apparent. Ultrasound shows an ill-defined hypoechoic mass. MR demonstrates an ill-defined area of abnormal signal within the muscle with heterogeneous high T2- and low T1-weighted signal intensity with significant or extensive soft tissue edema. Margins are indistinct and can be indirectly appreciated by mass effect and displacement of fascial planes. Curvilinear areas of dark T1- and T2-weighted signal intensity, which

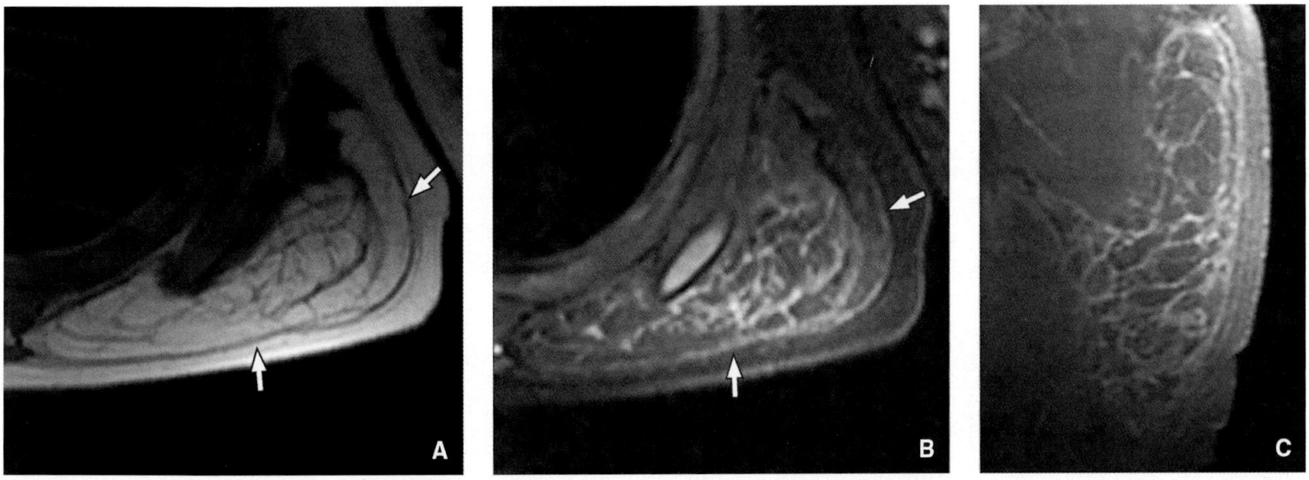

FIGURE 23.58 **Lipoblastoma in a 9-month-old boy. A, B:** Axial T1- **(A)** and fat-suppressed T2-weighted **(B)** MR images demonstrate a well-capsulated fat-containing mass (*arrows*) in the left posterior chest wall. **C:** Postcontrast sagittal fat-suppressed T1-weighted MR image demonstrates multiseptal enhancement.

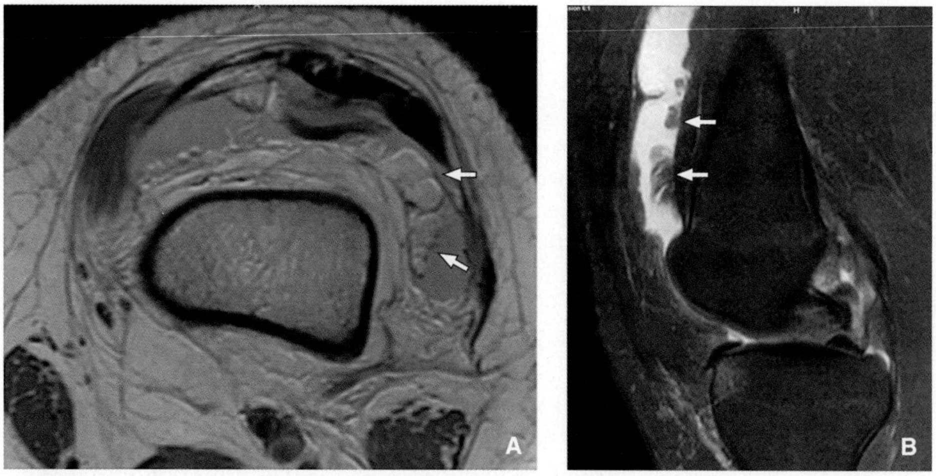

FIGURE 23.59 **Lipoma arborescens in a 16-year-old girl. A, B:** Axial proton-density **(A)** and sagittal fat-suppressed T2-weighted **(B)** MR images demonstrate villous proliferation in the synovium with fat signal intensity (*arrows*).

represent mineralization, can be observed in the periphery of the lesion (Fig. 23.61A, B). In the intermediate phase, 2 weeks to 2 months after a trauma, faint calcification is visualized on radiograph or CT. The lesion at this age demonstrates a zonal pattern with nonossified cells centrally and lamellar bone peripherally. MR demonstrates a well-delineated low T1- and high T2-weighted signal intensity mass with a peripheral dark signal rim suggesting mineralization and diminished soft tissue edema (Fig. 23.61C, D). Fluid–fluid levels from hemorrhage and adjacent bone marrow edema (ill-defined areas of low T1- and high T2-weighted signal) can be detected infrequently. In the late phase, 5 to 6 months after a trauma, the mature lesion is seen as a well-delineated mass with internal mature fat signal (high T1- and high T2-weighted signal intensity) within the trabeculae (Fig. 23.61E, F). The mature lesion has diminished calcifications and is smaller in size. Characteristic radiographic features of myositis ossificans can differentiate it from juxtacortical osteosarcoma that include a lucent zone between the lesion and the adjacent bone, peripheral dense calcification, intact underlying bony cortex, and decrease in volume on serial imaging evaluation.[158]

Histologically, the acute phase of myositis ossificans resembles nodular fasciitis and to an extent, ABC. All of these lesions are characterized by the same genetic aberration, a rearrangement of the USP6 gene. Clinically, myositis ossificans has a benign course with spontaneous regression and eventual resolution.

Benign Vascular Soft Tissue Tumors

Both hemangiomas and vascular malformations are vascular lesions that result from endothelial malformations and are separated based on their biologic natures.[159,160]

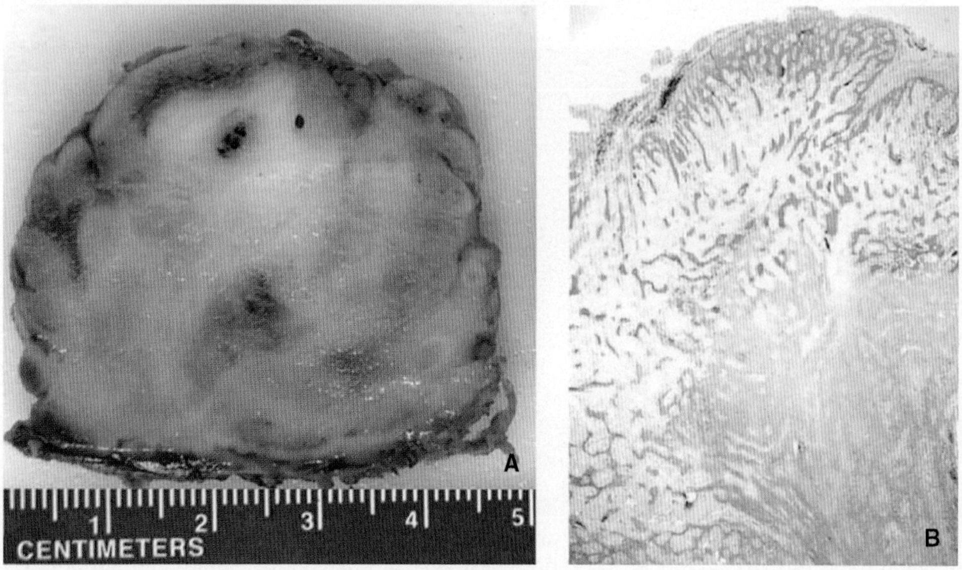

FIGURE 23.60 **Myositis ossificans arising as a rapidly growing painful mass within the vastus medialis muscle in an 13-year-old boy. A:** Grossly, the lesion is rimmed by a pale eggshell-like rim of variably thick bone. **B:** Microscopically, mononuclear cells are admixed with numerous multinucleate giant cells (hematoxylin and eosin, original magnification, 600×).

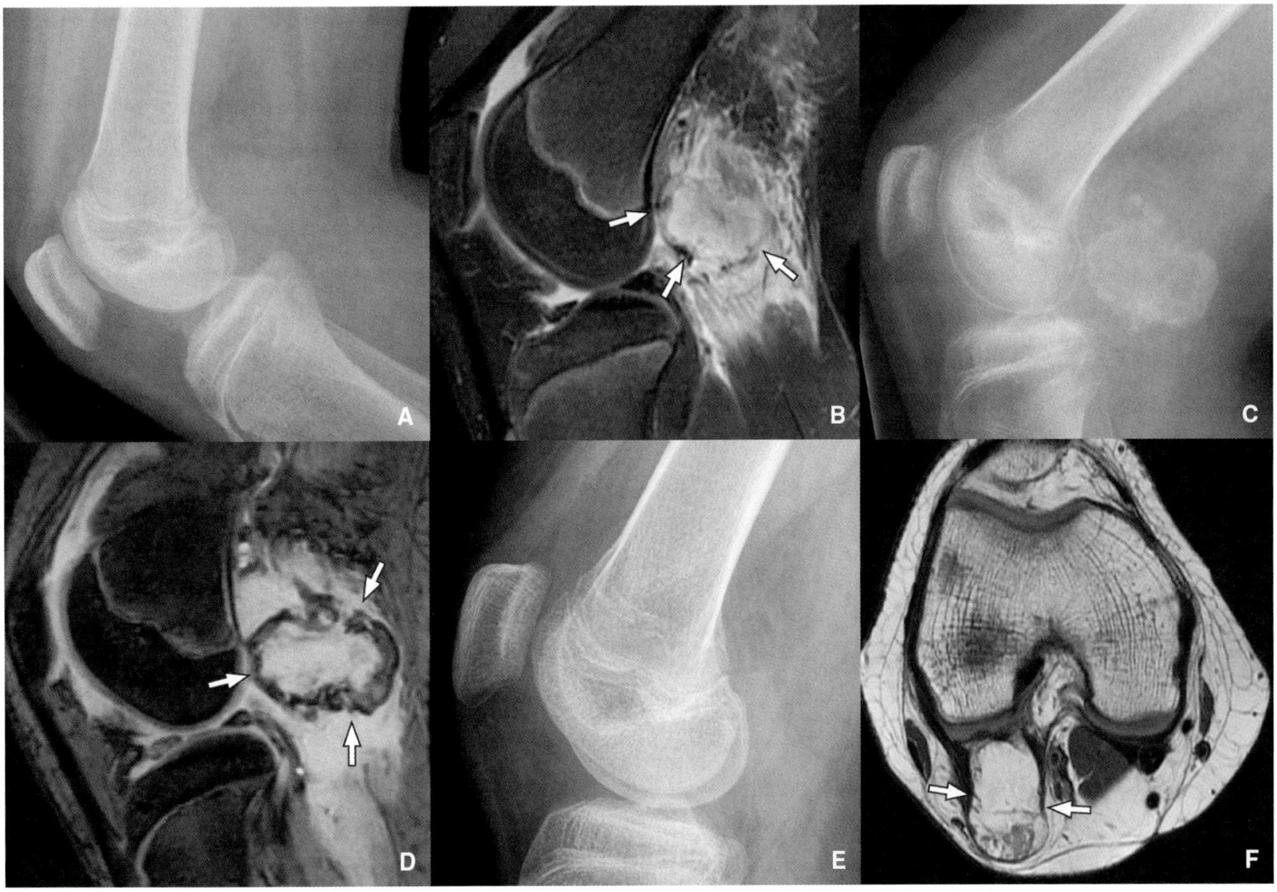

FIGURE 23.61 **Myositis ossificans in different phases in a 14-year-old girl.** ***Acute phase:*** Immediately after trauma. **A, B:** Lateral radiograph **(A)** demonstrates a normal-appearing popliteal fossa without any evidence of calcification. Sagittal fat-suppressed T2-weighted MR image **(B)** demonstrates a faint dark signal rim around an irregular mass in the popliteal fossa suggesting early mineralization (*arrows*) and perilesional edema. ***Intermediate phase:*** 1 month after trauma. **C, D:** Lateral radiograph **(C)** and sagittal gradient-echo MR image **(D)** demonstrate obvious calcification (*arrows*) within and surrounding the popliteal fossa mass. ***Late phase:*** 1 year after trauma. **E:** Lateral radiograph demonstrates disappearance of the calcific mass. **F:** Axial proton-density MR image demonstrates the mass with mature fatty marrow (*arrows*).

Hemangioma

Hemangiomas are benign endothelial neoplasms and are subdivided into congenital, infantile, and other forms. Congenital hemangiomas are less common than infantile hemangiomas and are fully formed at birth. Based on clinical and histologic features, congenital hemangiomas can be divided into rapidly involuting congenital hemangioma and noninvoluting congenital hemangioma. Infantile hemangiomas are the most common soft tissue tumors of infancy and childhood, occurring in about 4% to 10% of infants.[161] They are slightly more frequent in girls, Caucasians, premature infants, and twins.

Hemangiomas present with single or multiple lesions between 2 weeks and 2 months of age. The skin is the most common site, particularly the head and neck (60%), followed by the trunk and extremities.[162–164] Clinical manifestations vary with the degree of skin involvement and depth of the lesion; hemangiomas with skin involvement have a strawberry appearance, and deep hemangiomas below the subcutaneous tissues have a blue appearance. One-third of pediatric patients with multiple cutaneous hemangiomas have other associated anomalies, such as liver hemangiomas; they therefore require abdominal ultrasound at initial workup.[165]

Hemangiomas have three distinct phases: proliferative, plateau, and involution. The proliferative phase is characterized by rapid growth of endothelial cells and high flow. Imaging is performed to characterize the lesions and to evaluate the anatomic extent. Ultrasound is often used as a first imaging modality of choice for evaluating superficial soft tissue lesions. Gray-scale images of hemangiomas are nonspecific and may include a hypo- or mixed echoic mass. Doppler findings of multiple vessels (more than 5 per cm^2) within the lesion and high Doppler shift of more than 2 kHz are useful for diagnosis of hemangiomas. MRI of hemangiomas in the proliferative phase demonstrates a discrete lobulated mass with high T2- and iso- T1-weighted signal intensity. High-flow vessels (dark T1- and T2-weighted signal intensities due to signal void) are seen in the central and peripheral portion of the lesions. Intravenous contrast administration demonstrates diffuse avid enhancement of the mass (Fig. 23.62). However, the MRI appearance of hemangiomas in the proliferative

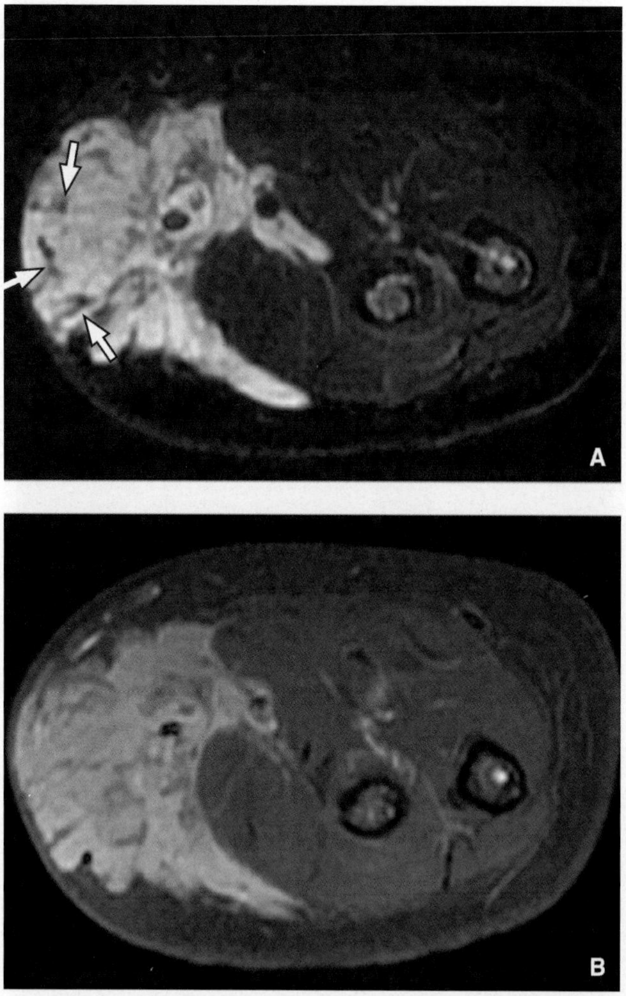

FIGURE 23.62 **Infantile hemangioma in a 4-month-old girl. A:** Axial fat-suppressed T2-weighted MR image demonstrates a lobulated mass in the forearm. Multiple flow voids are seen within the mass (*arrows*). **B:** Axial postcontrast fat-suppressed T1-weighted MR image demonstrates diffuse homogeneous enhancement.

phase is nonspecific. Any high-flow soft tissue mass or malignant soft tissue tumor of infancy including fibrosarcoma and rhabdomyosarcoma can have a similar appearance.[162,164–166] Hemangiomas in the involution phase contain fibrofatty tissue with a characteristic fat signal (high T1- and -T2-weighted signal) on MRI and have less contrast enhancement than in the proliferative phase.

Infantile hemangiomas proliferate rapidly during the first year of life and subsequently involute in early childhood. Thus, in the majority of cases of infantile hemangiomas, treatment is not required.[163] Therapy for complicated cases may include laser therapy, antiangiogenic drugs, embolization, and surgery.

Vascular Malformation

Vascular malformations are not neoplasms per se. They are vessel abnormalities resulting from errors in vascular morphogenesis.[162] Based on the presence of arterial components, vascular malformations are divided into two subtypes: low-flow and high-flow lesions. Vascular malformations grow proportionally to the growth of the child and do not involute. Therefore, they require treatment, which varies according to the subtype of the vascular malformation. Recognition of the imaging characteristics and understanding of the available imaging-guided therapeutic approaches are important topics for radiologists.[164]

Slow-Flow Vascular Malformations. Slow-flow vascular malformations contain venous, lymphatic, or a mixture of venolymphatic vascular channels. Venolymphatic malformations are the most common type with an overall prevalence of 1% in the general population.[162–164] The venous portions have dilated veins with thin walls and the lymphatic portions have collections of lymph vessels filled with serous fluid. The lesions may be present at birth but may also appear later (by 2 years of age) and steadily enlarge with growth. Clinically, venolymphatic malformations present with blue-colored, soft, and easily compressible masses that increase with crying or Valsalva maneuver. The lesions can be small and localized or extensive with infiltration and can affect the face, limbs, trunk, visceral organs, bones, and skeletal muscles.

On ultrasound, the venous components appear as a solid lesion and the lymphatic component as a cystic lesion. MRI is useful to determine the extent of disease and to develop a treatment plan. MRI demonstrates partially solid (venous component) and partially multicystic (lymphatic component) lesions with occasional fluid–fluid levels from hemorrhage. Phleboliths can be observed on radiographs or MR with dark T1- and T2-weighted signal intensity (Fig. 23.63). Klippel-Trenaunay-Weber syndrome is a rare syndrome characterized by port-wine stains of the skin, venolymphatic malformations, and soft tissue hypertrophy of affected limb(s).[159,162–164,167]

Therapeutic options include observation, compression garments, sclerotherapy, and surgical excision and are determined by the extent and location of the lesion.[164]

High-Flow Vascular Malformations. High-flow vascular malformations contain arterial components and include arteriovenous malformations (AVMs) and arteriovenous fistulas (AVF). AVMs are congenital, and AVFs are acquired lesions. Histologically, AVMs are composed of dysplastic arteries, which bypass capillary beds and drain to arterialized veins forming a vascular nidus. On physical examination, AVMs present with warm patches of pink skin with a thrill or murmur. AVMs can be single or multiple or associated with a genetic disorder such as hereditary hemorrhagic telangiectasia syndrome (Osler-Weber-Rendu).[159,162–164,167]

On ultrasound, an AVM is seen as a mutispacial and hypervascular mass on color Doppler study. Due to the high-flow nature, MRI demonstrates a soft tissue mass with numerous flow voids (dark T1- and -T2-weighted signal) (Fig. 23.64).[159,162–164,167]

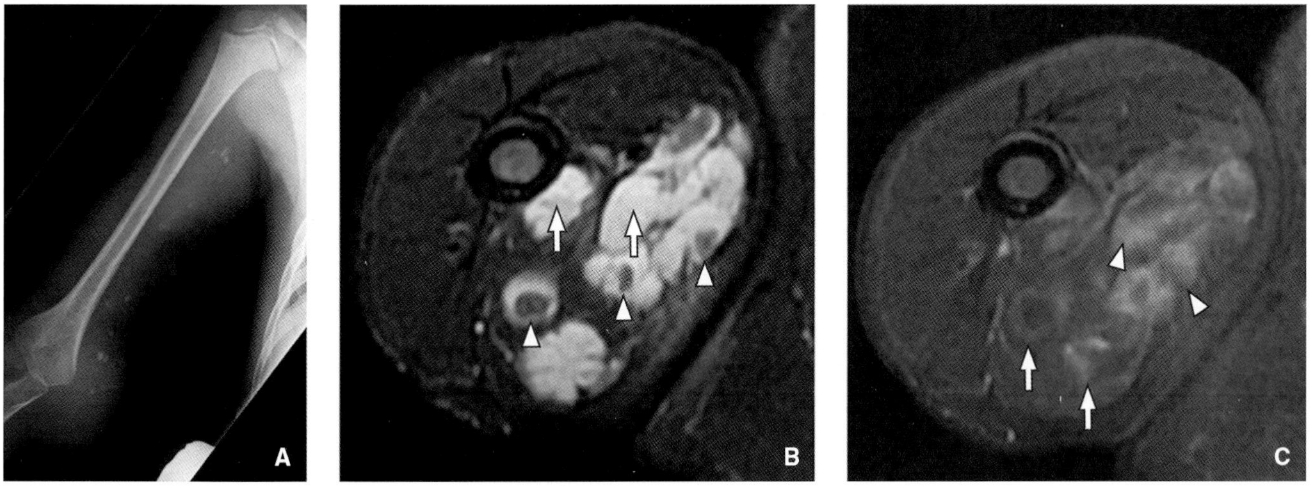

FIGURE 23.63 **Venolymphatic malformation in a 7-year-old boy. A:** Radiograph shows multiple phleboliths within a soft tissue mass in the arm. **B:** Axial fat-suppressed T2-weighted MR image demonstrates fluid–fluid levels (*arrows*) and dark signal from phleboliths (*arrowheads*) within the mass. **C:** Axial postcontrast fat-suppressed T1-weighted MR image demonstrates a mixture of heterogeneous patchy (venous: *arrowheads*) and peripheral (lymphatic: *arrows*) enhancement.

The current treatment for high-flow vascular malformations includes embolization or surgery. Angiography for complete mapping of vessels is typically required before treatment.[164]

Benign Soft Tissue Tumors Arising From Neural Tissue

Neurofibromas and Schwannomas (neurilemomas) are the two most common types of benign nerve sheath tumors in children. Others include perineurioma, granular cell tumor,

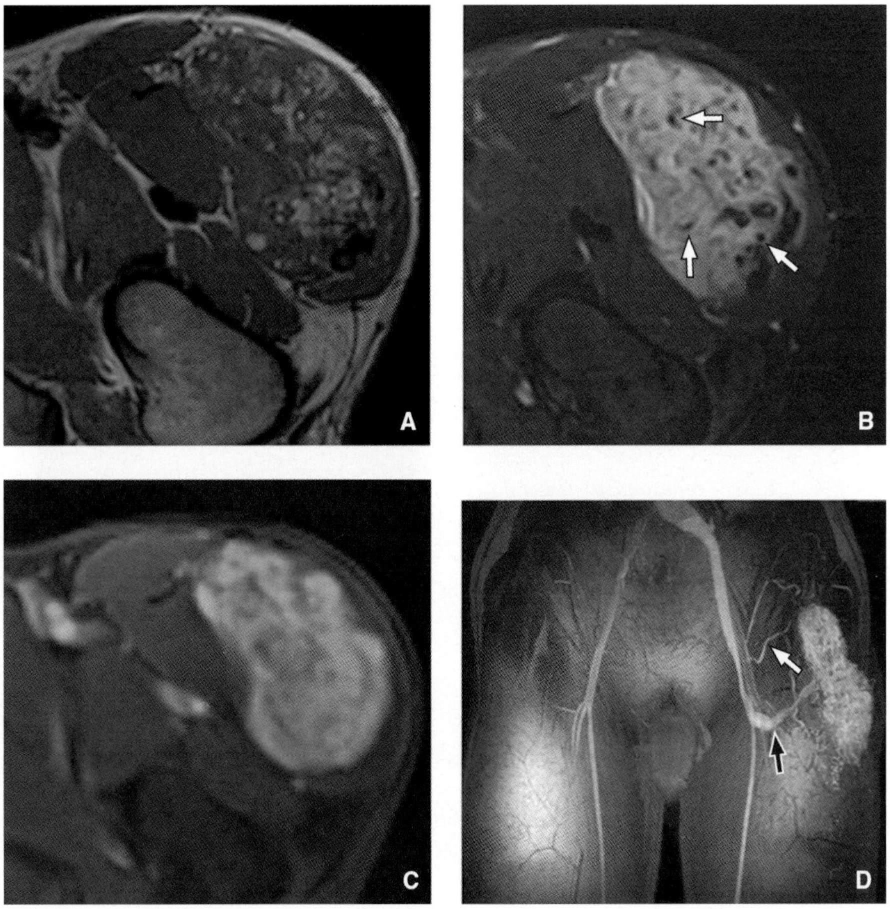

FIGURE 23.64 **Arteriovenous malformation in a 17-year-old boy. A–C:** Axial T1- **(A)**, fat-suppressed T2- **(B)**, and postcontrast fat-suppressed T1-weighted **(C)** MR images demonstrate a soft tissue mass with internal flow voids (*arrows*). **D:** MR angiogram demonstrates a feeding artery (*white arrow*) and draining vein (*black arrow*).

dermal nerve sheath myxoma, solitary circumscribed neuroma, ectopic meningioma, benign Triton tumor, and hybrid nerve sheath tumors.[4]

Localized and Diffuse Neurofibroma

Localized neurofibromas are the most common type comprising 90% of neurofibromas affecting patients 20 to 30 years of age.[46,168] They typically present as a single mass involving a subcutaneous or deep-seated nerve. Diffuse neurofibromas primarily affect children and young adults and present with a plaque-like elevation of the subcutaneous tissue with intense contrast enhancement. The majority (90%) of both localized and diffuse neurofibromas are isolated lesions without association with the genetic syndrome of neurofibromatosis.[169]

Plexiform Neurofibroma Type 1

Neurofibromatosis type 1 (NF1) has a variety of musculoskeletal manifestations. NF1 can present with all three types of neurofibromas (localized, diffuse, and plexiform), but plexiform neurofibroma is the pathognomonic manifestation of NF1. Plexiform neurofibromas develop in early childhood. They present with tortuous expansion of multiple nerve fascicles and network-like tumor growth with a "bag of worms" appearance. Plexiform neurofibromas can have either superficial or deep locations. Superficial plexiform neurofibromas involve cutaneous or subcutaneous nerves and tend to have unilateral and asymmetric involvement.

Superficial plexiform neurofibromas have diffused infiltrative areas of high signal on water-sensitive MR sequences (inversion recovery or fat-suppressed T2-weighted image) (Fig. 23.65). This appearance of infiltrative high T2-weighted signal in the subcutaneous tissue can be similar to vascular malformations (venous, lymphatic, or venolymphatic malformations), hemangiomas, or traumatic or inflammatory lesions of the subcutaneous tissue. This infiltrative signal in the subcutaneous tissue corresponds to a spindle cell infiltration around the normal structures of the subcutaneous tissue.

Deep plexiform neurofibromas involve deep-seated nerves such as nerve plexus, dorsal nerve roots, or major nerves. They have a typical target appearance, which results from the central nerve fiber seen as central dark T2-weighted signal and surrounding myxoid material seen as bright T2-weighted signal on MR images (Fig. 23.65).[168] Malignant transformation to malignant peripheral nerve sheath tumor (MPNST) has been reported in 5% of plexiform neurofibromas, particularly those that are deep-seated.[170]

The therapeutic options for plexiform neurofibromas are limited. Surgical management is still challenging due to the ill-defined and infiltrative nature of the lesions.

Benign Soft Tissue Tumors Arising from Fibrous Tissue

Nodular Fasciitis

Nodular fasciitis is a benign soft tissue lesion composed of fibroblasts. A preceding traumatic event is sometimes documented. Head and neck and extremities, in particular the volar aspect of the forearm, are most commonly affected. Three different forms of nodular fasciitis occur: subcutaneous, fascial, and intramuscular (proliferative myositis), of which subcutaneous nodular fasciitis is the most common.[128]

Clinically, nodular fasciitis presents as a rapidly growing superficial mass with mild pain or tenderness. Most lesions measure 3 to 4 cm although the muscular subtype tends to be larger.[128] Histologically, nodular fasciitis is composed of fibroblasts with a characteristic haphazard loose "tissue culture-like appearance," often accompanied by extravasated red blood cells and cystification (Fig. 23.66). Occasionally, metaplastic ossification can occur within the lesion and is referred as ossifying fasciitis or fasciitis/myositis/periostitis ossificans. Due to rapid growth and high mitotic activity of nodular fasciitis, this benign lesion was historically referred to as a pseudosarcoma.

Radiographs are mostly normal, and visible calcification is rarely observed. The MRI appearance of a "fascial tail sign," linear extension along the fascia extending from each side of the mass, is helpful for diagnosis of nodular fasciitis

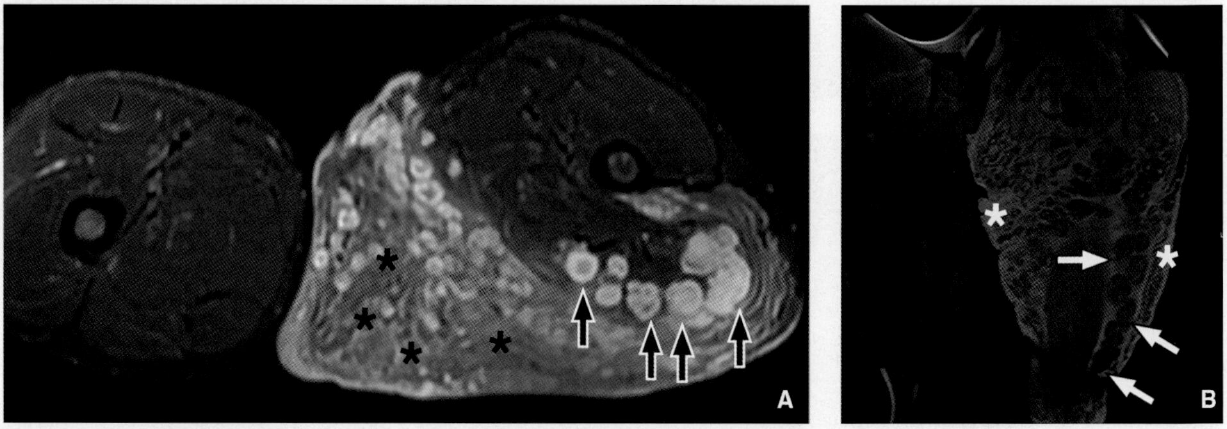

FIGURE 23.65 **Neurofibromatosis type 1 with a plexiform neurofibroma in a 16-year old boy. A:** Axial fat-suppressed T2-weighted MR image demonstrates a target-like appearance (deep plexiform neurofibroma: *arrows*) and diffuse infiltrative high T2 signal in the skin and subcutaneous tissue (superficial plexiform neurofibroma: *asterisks*). **B:** Coronal postcontrast fat-suppressed T1-weighted MR image demonstrates diffuse enhancement within the superficial plexiform neurofibroma (*asterisks*) and lack of enhancement within the deep plexiform neurofibroma (*arrows*).

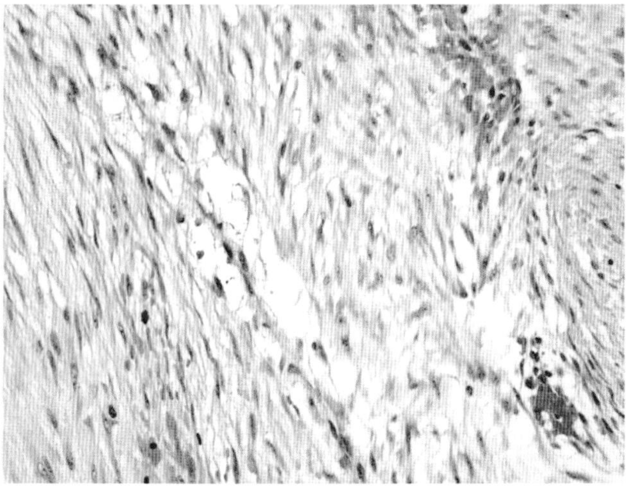

FIGURE 23.66 **Nodular fasciitis involving the neck in an 8-year-old girl.** This 5 cm mass shows a haphazard proliferation of feathery fibroblasts; extravasated red blood cells and microscopic cystification are seen (hematoxylin and eosin, original magnification, 400×).

(Fig. 23.67). MRI signal intensities are variable depending on tissue contents; homogeneous high T2- and low T1-weighted signal are seen in lesions with more myxoid contents, which are more common in the subcutaneous subtype.[171] Lesions containing cellular and fibrotic components, more commonly seen in fascial or muscular subtypes, have heterogeneous and low to intermediate T1- and intermediate T2-weighted signal intensity.[172] Intravenous contrast administration shows diffuse (63%) or peripheral (25%) enhancement.[173]

Nodular fasciitis may be best conceived of as a "transient neoplasia," characterized by clonal rearrangements in the USP6 gene and commonly associated with spontaneous regression. Biopsy or excision can sometimes aggravate the process. Local recurrence is rare.

Fibromatosis

The fibromatoses are a family of soft tissue lesions composed of a proliferation of fibrous tissue with variable degrees of collagen. The fibromatoses range from benign to intermediate in their biologic behavior. Fibromatoses are classified as superficial or deep fibromatosis based on the anatomical location. The superficial group includes plantar (Ledderhose disease) or palmar fibromatosis (Dupuytren contracture), juvenile aponeurotic fibroma, and infantile digital fibroma/fibromatosis.[174] The deep group includes infantile myofibroma/myofibromatosis, infantile fibromatosis, and desmoid-type fibromatosis.[174] Among these, three important types of fibromatosis including infantile myofibroma, myofibromatosis, and desmoid-type fibromatosis are discussed in the following section.

Infantile Myofibroma/Myofibromatosis

Infantile myofibroma/myofibromatosis is the most common fibrous tumor of infancy and is characterized by fibrous tissue proliferation.[175] The WHO designates the lesions as a type of benign perivascular cell tumor (myopericytoma)

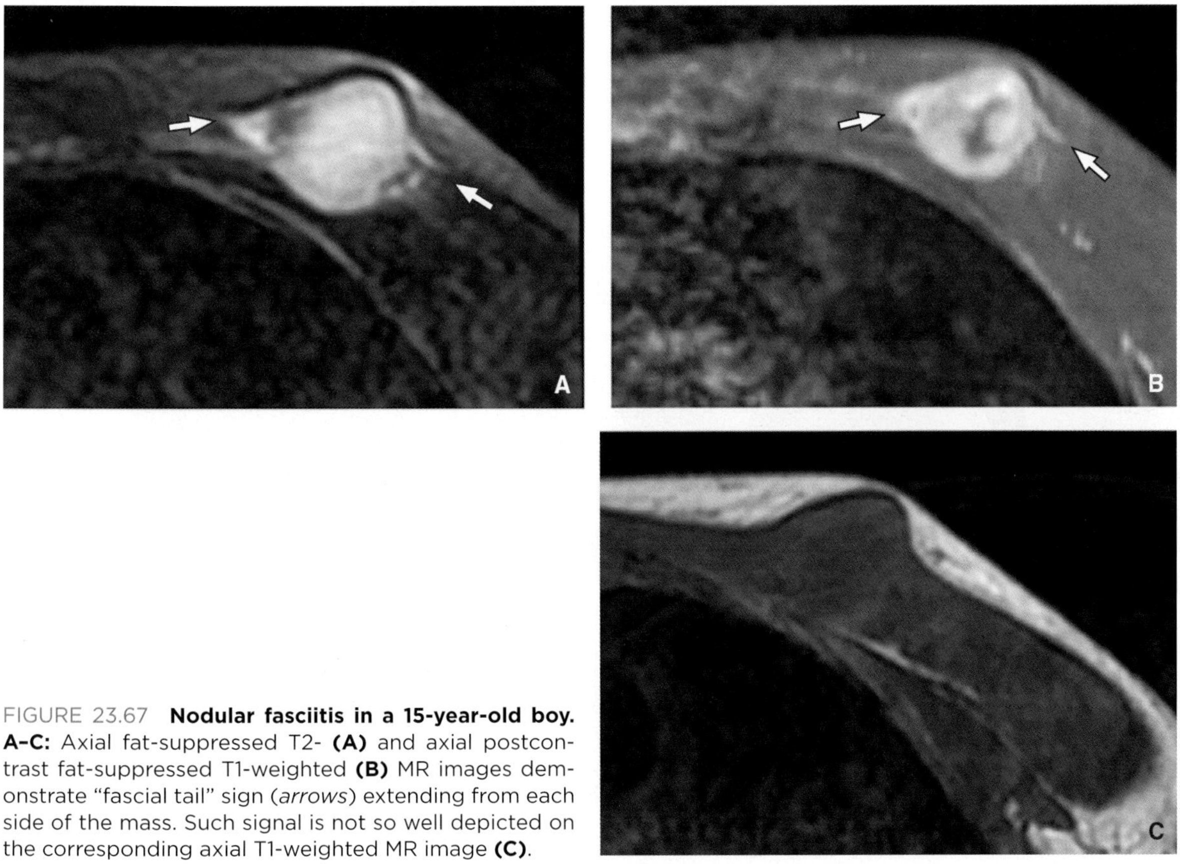

FIGURE 23.67 **Nodular fasciitis in a 15-year-old boy. A–C:** Axial fat-suppressed T2- **(A)** and axial postcontrast fat-suppressed T1-weighted **(B)** MR images demonstrate "fascial tail" sign (*arrows*) extending from each side of the mass. Such signal is not so well depicted on the corresponding axial T1-weighted MR image **(C)**.

rather than as a fibromatosis.[176] They may occur as solitary or multicentric disease. Both forms occur with almost equal frequency and slight male predilection (male: female, 1.6:1). Over 90% of myofibromas/myofibromatosis occur before the age of 2 years. Lesions are present at birth in 70% of cases.[175] The lesions uncommonly occur in children over 10 years and rarely in adults. Infantile hemangiopericytoma is now considered a subtype of infantile myofibroma. The solitary form presents as a subcutaneous mass and has increased vascularity resembling a hemangioma. The multicentric form can involve multiple organs, including skeletal muscle, bone, skin, soft tissue, and visceral organs.

Radiographs in pediatric patients with osseous myofibromatosis have a characteristic appearance that includes multiple eccentric lytic lesions that are relatively well-defined and present with a sclerotic rim. The metaphyses of the long bones (femur and tibia) are commonly affected; other locations of involvement include the ribs, spine, pelvis, and skull, and involvement can be symmetric (Fig. 23.68). Osseous lesions usually heal spontaneously and do not require treatment. The differential diagnosis in young children with multiple osteolytic lesions includes LCH, hematogenous osteomyelitis, metastatic neuroblastoma, lymphangiomatosis, and angiomatosis. Pulmonary involvement can result in interstitial fibrosis, a reticulonodular infiltration, or bronchopneumonia. Gastrointestinal involvement presents with diffuse narrowing and multiple small filling defects on barium studies.

The ultrasound findings of myofibromatosis in soft tissue are nonspecific. They show soft tissue masses that may have partially anechoic centers suggesting necrosis or may have occasional echogenic foci with shadowing from calcification. MRI is the best imaging modality to localize the disease as well as to assess any visceral involvement. MRI typically shows a low T1- and high T2-weighted signal mass. An internal high T2-weighted signal center without contrast enhancement reflecting central necrosis can be observed (Fig. 23.69), but is not specific for myofibromatosis.[177] In young children, multiple soft tissue masses with imaging findings of central necrosis can suggest the diagnosis of multiple myofibromatosis, but tissue sampling is necessary for confirmation of diagnosis.

Histologically, myofibromas are composed of plump to spindled myofibroblastic cells often set in a collagenized matrix with myxohyaline change; the myofibroblastic cells are commonly seen growing within the walls of intralesional blood vessels. The overall prognosis of solitary myofibromas is favorable, and many lesions have spontaneous regression. Approximately one-third of multicentric myofibromatosis lesions undergo

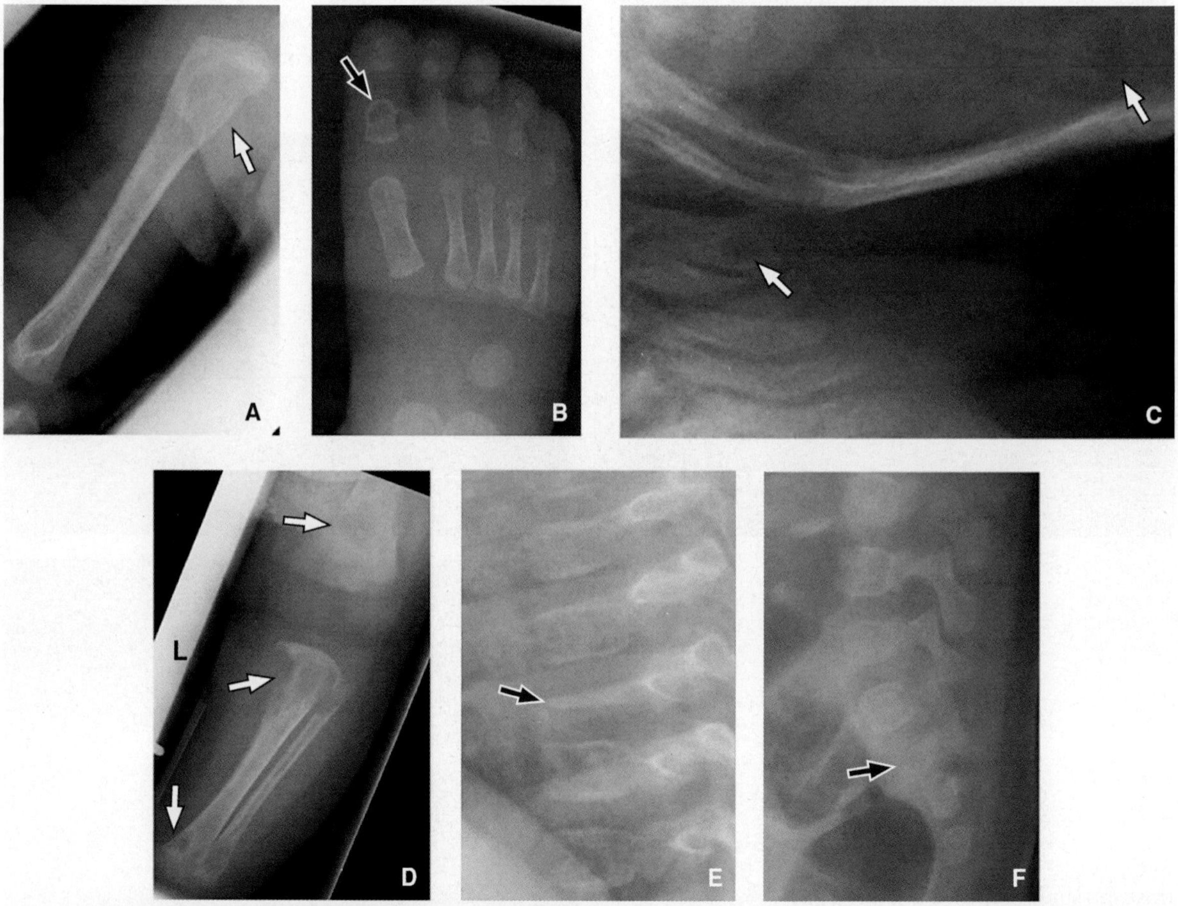

FIGURE 23.68 **Multicentric myofibromatosis in a 3-month-old boy.** Radiographs demonstrate multiple well-defined osteolytic lesions (*arrows*) with sclerotic rim. Bone lesions are symmetric and bilateral. **A:** Right humerus. **B:** Left foot. **C:** Cervical spine. **D:** Left femur, tibia, and fibula. **E:** Vertebra plana of the thoracic spine. **F:** Sacrum.

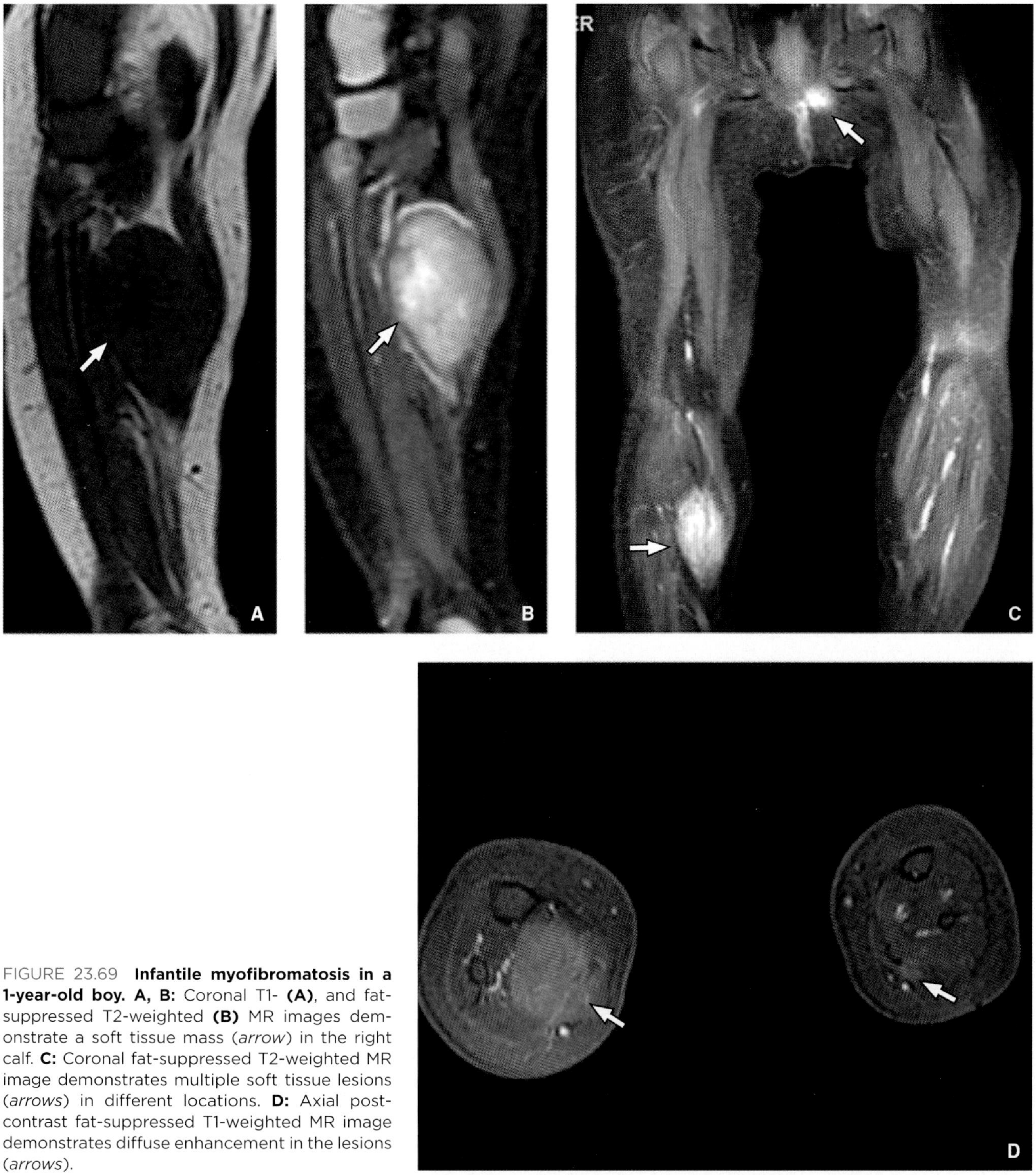

FIGURE 23.69 **Infantile myofibromatosis in a 1-year-old boy. A, B:** Coronal T1- **(A)**, and fat-suppressed T2-weighted **(B)** MR images demonstrate a soft tissue mass (*arrow*) in the right calf. **C:** Coronal fat-suppressed T2-weighted MR image demonstrates multiple soft tissue lesions (*arrows*) in different locations. **D:** Axial post-contrast fat-suppressed T1-weighted MR image demonstrates diffuse enhancement in the lesions (*arrows*).

spontaneous regression. However, when visceral organs are involved, particularly the heart or gastrointestinal system, the mortality from the disease can reach up to 75%.[128,175]

Desmoid-Type Fibromatosis

Desmoid-type fibromatosis is a relatively common soft tissue tumor composed of fibroblasts (Fig. 23.70). Desmoid tumors affect young adults with peak prevalence between 25 and 35 years of age and are less common in children younger than 10 years of age.[174] Extremities are commonly affected (70%); frequently affected sites include the shoulder, chest wall, and back. Clinically, desmoid tumors present with a solitary mass in most cases, but in 10% to 15% of cases, synchronous multicentric lesions in the same extremity can occur.[174] Patients with APC gene mutations (e.g., familial adenomatous polyposis, Gardner syndrome) are prone to develop desmoid-type fibromatosis.

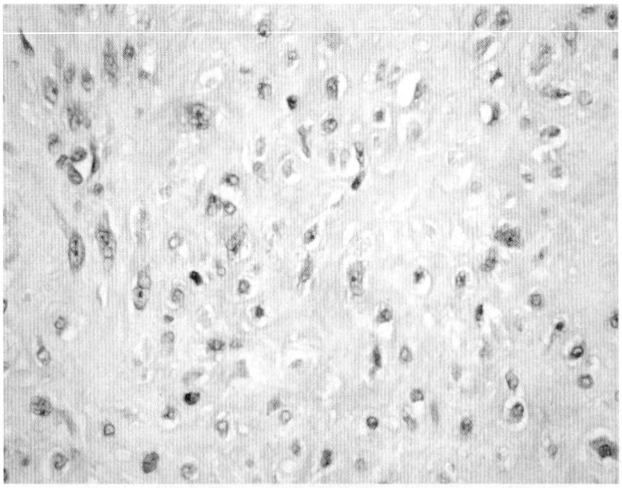

FIGURE 23.70 **Desmoid-type fibromatosis from the gluteal region in a 17-year-old girl.** The fibroblasts show nuclear enlargement and small nucleoli (hematoxylin and eosin, original magnification, 600×).

Infantile fibromatosis is the childhood equivalent of an extra-abdominal desmoid tumor; therefore, the lesions share histologic, biologic, and imaging features. Infantile fibromatosis occurs in the first 2 years of life, is rare after 5 years of age, and has slight male predilection.[174] It presents clinically as a solitary firm mass that occurs in the skeletal muscle and fascia. The head and neck are most commonly affected.

The imaging findings of infantile fibromatosis and desmoid tumor are similar. Radiographs may show a normal appearance or a nonspecific soft tissue mass. Calcifications are uncommon. Osseous changes with pressure erosions and cortical scalloping can be observed. MRI is the best modality for evaluation of deep fibromatosis. Infantile fibromatosis and desmoid tumors are typically intermuscular lesions with occasional muscle invasion. Linear extension along fascial planes is a characteristic manifestation of both lesions (Fig. 23.71) and is not commonly seen in other soft tissue neoplasms. Fibromatosis can be ill-defined or well-demarcated on MRI. MR signal intensities are variable and depend on the components in the lesion; heterogeneous iso- to low T1- and low to high T2-weighted signal intensities are usually present. Lesions with high cellular and myxoid tissue content present with low T1- and high T2-weighted signal due to water content. The dense collagen-containing lesions show low signal intensity bands at all pulse sequences (Fig. 23.71). Low signal intensity bands at all pulse sequences are a characteristic feature for fibromatosis, but are not specific. Moderate to marked contrast enhancement is seen after intravenous contrast administration. Increased contrast enhancement is seen in lesions with increased cellularity.[174]

The current treatment options include wide excision or marginal excision of the lesion followed by postoperative radiation. Although deep fibromatoses are not malignant lesions, they are locally aggressive and can encase neurovascular bundles. The local recurrence rate is high in up to 87% of cases.[174]

Other Benign Soft Tissue Tumors

Subcutaneous Granuloma Annulare

Subcutaneous granuloma annulare (SGA) is an uncommon benign nodule exclusively seen in children.[178] In most cases, SGA presents as a solitary nontender and nonmobile mass in the subcutaneous tissue of children without underlying disease or history of preceding trauma. SGA most commonly occurs in the pretibial region, but can occur in the scalp, upper extremities, foot, or ankle. Atypical manifestations include pain, rapidly growing mass, or mass in an unusual location.

SGA is diagnosed clinically and histologically in most cases and does not require imaging studies. In cases of an atypical clinical manifestation, ultrasound is the first step for assessment of superficial lesions. Ultrasound demonstrates an ill-defined low echoic lesion in the subcutaneous tissue. MRI shows ill-defined areas of iso T1- and heterogeneous high T2-weighted signal in the lesion with the central mass being confined to the subcutaneous tissue without deeper extension to muscle, fascia, or bone (Fig. 23.72).[179] Homogenous or heterogeneous enhancement is observed after intravenous contrast administration.[180] The imaging findings are nonspecific and similar to vascular malformations, fat necrosis, rheumatoid nodules, and foreign body granulomas.[135,181]

Biopsy with pathological evaluation is often needed for a definitive diagnosis of SGA.[179]

Malignant Soft Tissue Tumors

Pediatric soft tissue sarcomas (STSs) are a heterogeneous group of malignant tumors that originate from primitive mesenchymal tissue and account for about 7% of all childhood malignancies.[182–184] These tumors are categorized into two broad groups: rhabdomyosarcomas (RMSs) and nonrhabdomyosarcomatous soft tissue sarcomas (NRSTSs) (Table 23.3).[185] RMS, muscle malignant tumor exhibiting skeletal muscle differentiation, is the most common STS in children, accounting for 50% of soft tissue tumors in children aged 0 to 14 years.[185] Fibrosarcomas are the most common NRSTSs, accounting for 10% to 20% of STS.[182–184] Other pediatric NRSTS include synovial sarcoma, ASPS, liposarcoma, MPNST, and peripheral PNETs. The distribution of STS by histology and age, based on Surveillance Epidemiology and End Results (SEER) information, is summarized in Table 23.4.

The pathologic diagnosis of STS depends on the integration of available clinicoradiographic, histologic, immunohistologic, and genetic studies. Imaging evaluation is essential for staging and surgical management. Staging of malignant soft tissue tumors incorporates the size of the tumor at the primary site, regional lymph node status, and presence of distant metastases. The most common metastatic site from STS is the lung. Certain sarcomas, such as synovial sarcoma, epithelioid sarcoma, and RMS may also spread to the lymph nodes.[184,186,187] MRI is the best imaging modality for assessment of STS because it can define the anatomic location of the tumor, indicate its relationship to important nerves and blood vessels, and demonstrate local involvement of bone or lymph nodes. A chest CT is always necessary to exclude lung metastases.[188–191]

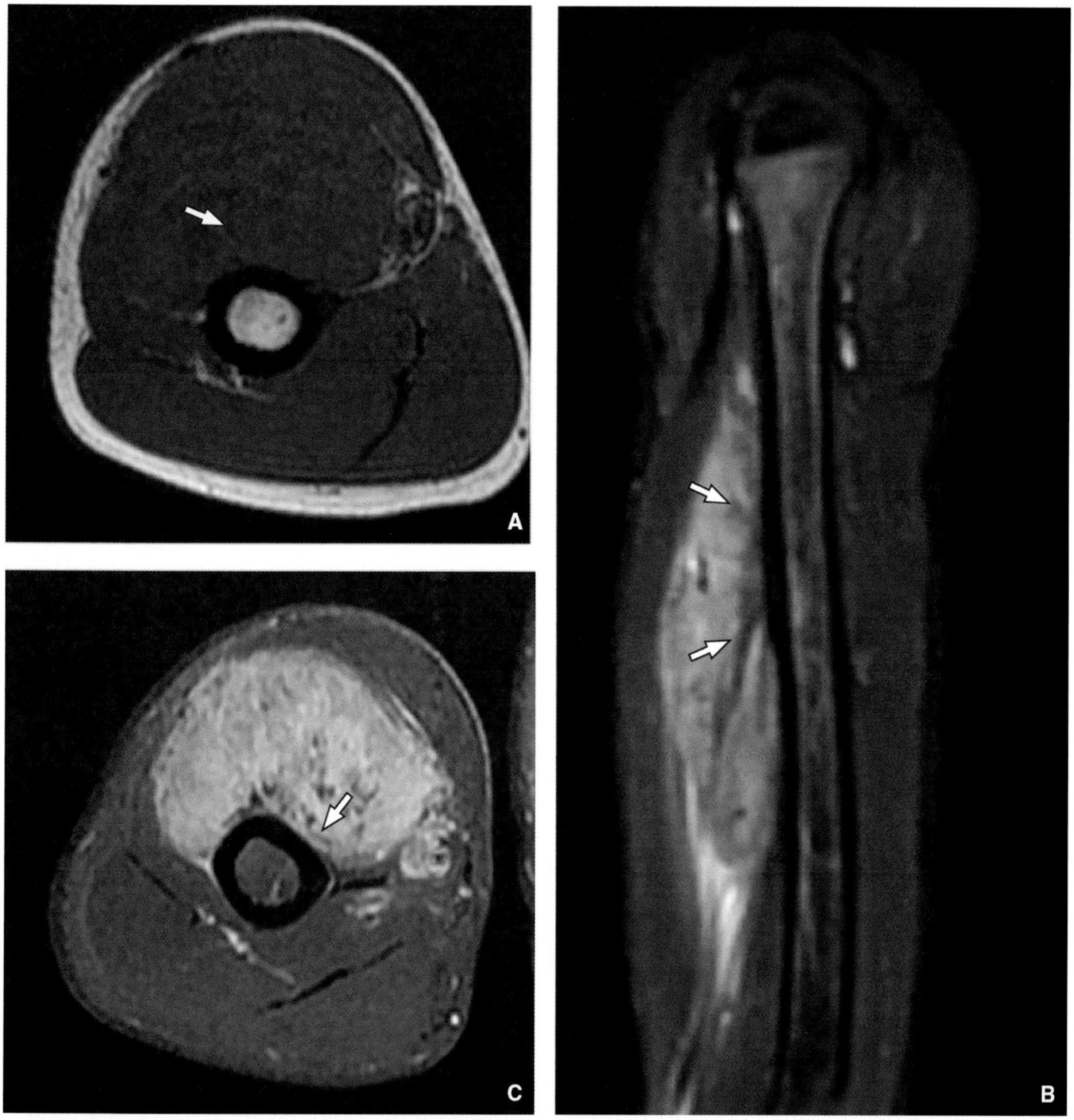

FIGURE 23.71 **Desmoid tumor in the upper arm in a 10-year-old boy. A–C:** Axial T1- **(A)**, coronal fat-suppressed T2- **(B)** and axial postcontrast fat-suppressed T1-weighted **(C)** MR images demonstrate an intramuscular desmoid tumor in the arm. Low-signal intensity bands (*arrows*) are seen on all pulse sequences.

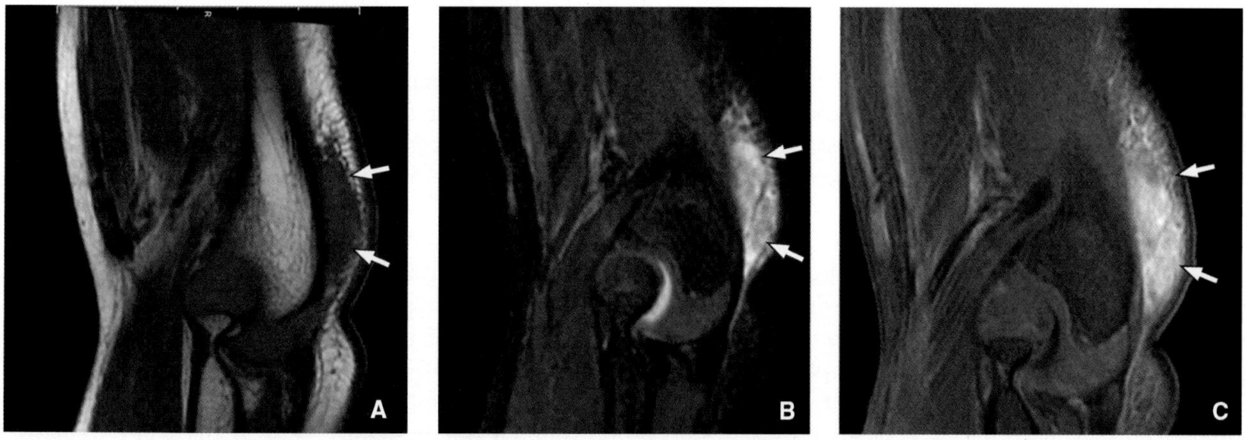

FIGURE 23.72 **Subcutaneous granuloma annulare in a 3-year-old girl. A, B:** Sagittal T1- **(A)**, and fat-suppressed T2-weighted **(B)** MR images demonstrate a soft tissue mass (*arrows*) confined to the subcutaneous tissue in the elbow. **C:** Sagittal postcontrast fat-suppressed T1-weighted MR image demonstrates heterogeneous enhancement within the mass (*arrows*).

TABLE 23.4 Age Distribution of Soft Tissue Sarcomas in Children Aged 0 to 19 Years (SEER 1975–2008)

Types of Tumors	Age <5 y	Age 5–9 y	Age 10–14 y	Age 15–19 y	% of the Total Number of STS Cases <20 y
Soft tissue sarcomas	1,130	810	1,144	1,573	100
Rhabdomyosarcomas	710	466	364	350	41
Fibrosarcomas, peripheral nerve, and other fibrous neoplasms	151	64	132	192	12
Fibroblastic and myofibroblastic tumors	131	31	57	86	6.5
Nerve sheath tumors	19	32	74	104	5
Other fibromatous neoplasms	1	1	1	2	0.1
Kaposi sarcomas	1	2	0	12	0.3
Other specified soft tissue sarcoma subcategories	198	200	512	856	38
Ewing (extraosseous) and Askin tumors of soft tissue	22	28	57	81	4
pPNET of soft tissue	21	19	29	42	2.4
Extrarenal rhabdoid tumors	37	3	8	3	1
Liposarcomas	5	6	22	66	2
Fibrohistiocytic tumors[a]	53	69	171	293	12
Leiomyosarcomas	13	19	22	57	2.4
Synovial sarcomas	12	39	133	204	8.3
Blood vessel tumors	15	7	11	33	1.4
Osseous and chondromatous neoplasms of soft tissue	1	5	9	16	0.6
Alveolar soft part sarcomas	3	7	19	26	1
Miscellaneous soft tissue sarcomas	16	18	31	35	2
Unspecified subcategories	70	58	136	163	9

[a]Dermatofibrosarcoma accounts for 75% of these cases.

pPNET, peripheral primitive neuroectodermal tumors; SEER, Surveillance Epidemiology and End Results; STS, soft tissue sarcoma; y, years.

Intermediate/Malignant Tumor Arising from Fatty Tissue

Liposarcoma

Liposarcoma is a malignant soft tissue tumor composed of primitive mesenchymal cells and malignant lipoblasts. Liposarcoma is rare in children, especially those younger than 5 years of age. It usually occurs in the thigh, gluteal region, retroperitoneum, axilla, neck, back, or behind the knee (popliteal fossa). The tumor tissue has five distinct subtypes: (1) well-differentiated (also known as atypical lipomatous tumor); (2) dedifferentiated; (3) myxoid; (4) pleomorphic, and (5) mixed. Myxoid liposarcomas are the most common type of liposarcoma in the pediatric population.

MRI is currently the best imaging modality to evaluate liposarcoma in the pediatric population. MRI features of liposarcomas are variable with the possible exception of well-differentiated liposarcoma; fat may or may not be present. In the myxoid subtype, the fat component is typically <10% of the overall tumor volume and is often seen as small fatty nodules or septations.[141,192–194] Distinguishing a well-differentiated liposarcoma from a lipoblastoma or a lipoma can be difficult. Although uncommon, multiple thick septations, soft tissue masses, calcification, or ossification may be encountered in well-differentiated liposarcomas.[141,193–195]

The clinical course and prognosis of liposarcomas vary according to subtype. The pleomorphic subtype has the worst prognosis. Large tumors, more than 8 cm in size, usually require preoperative chemotherapy and radiation followed by surgery and postoperative chemotherapy.[193] Local recurrence is common and is seen in ~90% to 100% of retroperitoneal lesions. Metastases most commonly occur in the lung.[193]

Malignant Soft Tissue Tumors Arising from Fibrous Tissue

Infantile Fibrosarcoma

Infantile fibrosarcoma is an intermediate (rarely metastasizing) tumor that nearly always presents in infancy, often at birth or even antenatally.[195] It has a better prognosis than the adolescent and adult forms of fibrosarcoma. Clinically, infantile fibrosarcomas present as enlarging masses, usually in the first year of life. They often occur in the distal extremities and occasionally in the head/neck and trunk. Because of their high degree of vascularization, they may be confused with hemangiomas on imaging and clinical examinations.

Radiographs typically show a nonspecific soft tissue mass. There may be evidence of bone deformity or erosions secondary to the soft tissue mass. Discrete bone destruction is rare.

On MRI, fibrosarcomas are usually isointense to muscle on T1-weighted MR images and hyperintense on T2-weighted MR images. They may contain hypointense foci, which correlate with fibrosis. High-flow, serpentine vascular structures can be found on MR and Doppler sonographic examination (Fig. 23.73).[196,197]

Histologically, fibroblastic cells show a fascicular growth pattern, often with frequent mitoses. A chromosomal translocation resulting in an ETV6-NTRK3 gene

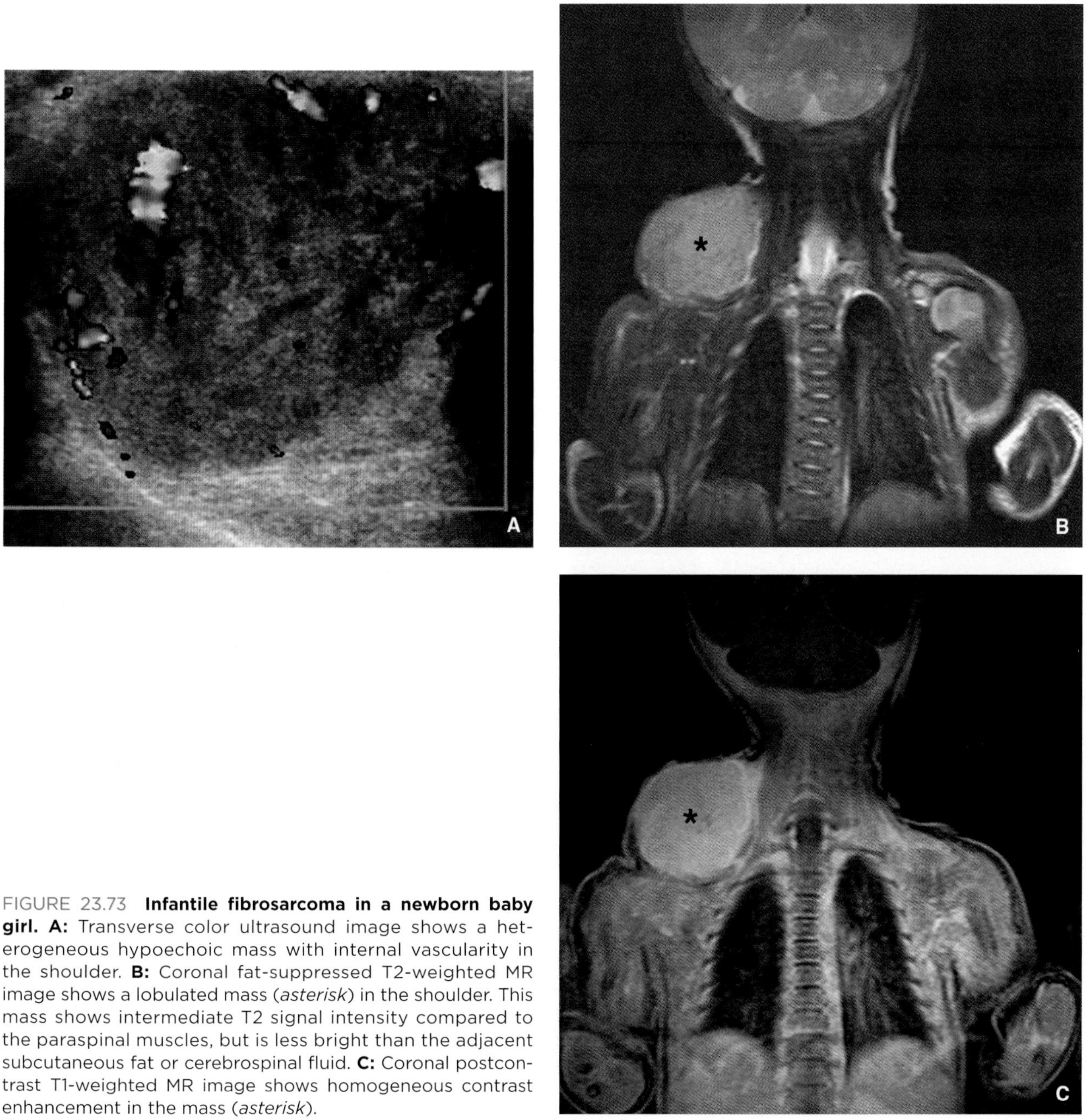

FIGURE 23.73 **Infantile fibrosarcoma in a newborn baby girl. A:** Transverse color ultrasound image shows a heterogeneous hypoechoic mass with internal vascularity in the shoulder. **B:** Coronal fat-suppressed T2-weighted MR image shows a lobulated mass (*asterisk*) in the shoulder. This mass shows intermediate T2 signal intensity compared to the paraspinal muscles, but is less bright than the adjacent subcutaneous fat or cerebrospinal fluid. **C:** Coronal postcontrast T1-weighted MR image shows homogeneous contrast enhancement in the mass (*asterisk*).

fusion is characteristic. The initial treatment of choice is wide local excision. Currently, preoperative chemotherapy has made a more conservative surgical approach possible.

Dermatofibrosarcoma Protuberans

Dermatofibrosarcoma protuberans is a superficial, intermediate grade, locally aggressive fibroblastic neoplasm. It occurs most commonly on the trunk and the proximal extremities. Dermatofibrosarcoma protuberans typically presents as a red-blue or pink plaque that grows slowly and may become nodular. It typically involves skin and subcutaneous adipose tissue, resulting in focal protuberance of the skin. MRI is useful to determine the extent of the disease, but MR signal characteristics are nonspecific (Fig. 23.74).[198,199]

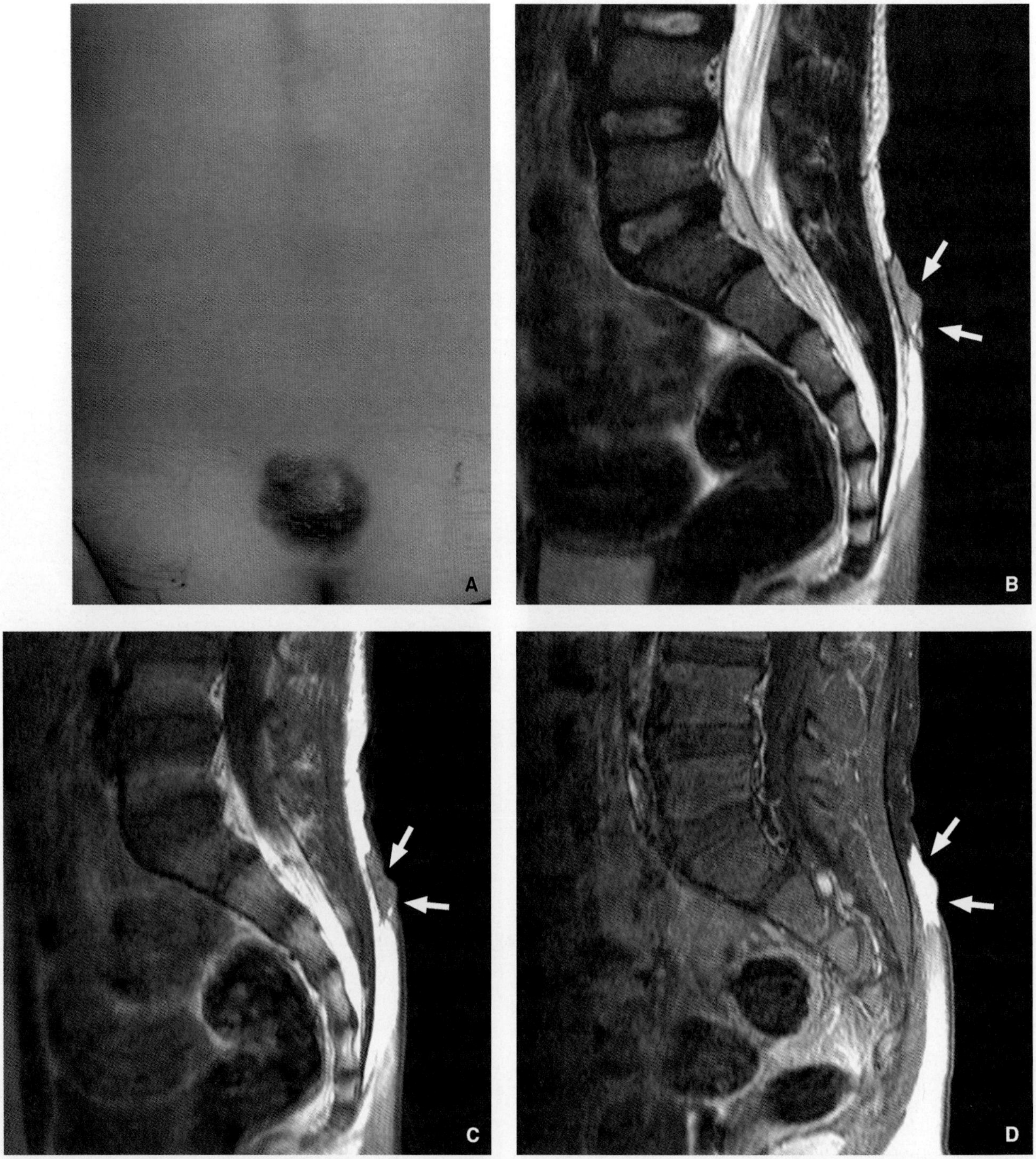

FIGURE 23.74 **Dermatofibrosarcoma protuberans in a 6-year-old boy. A:** Clinical photograph shows a *reddish-brown* nodular lesion in the lower back at midline. **B–D:** Sagittal fat-suppressed T2-weighted **(B)**, T1-weighted **(C)**, and postcontrast fat-suppressed T1-weighted **(D)** MR images show a highly enhancing mass (*arrows*) involving the skin and subcutaneous fat layer that is hypointense compared to the subcutaneous fat layer on T2-weighted **(B)** and T1-weighted **(C)** MR images.

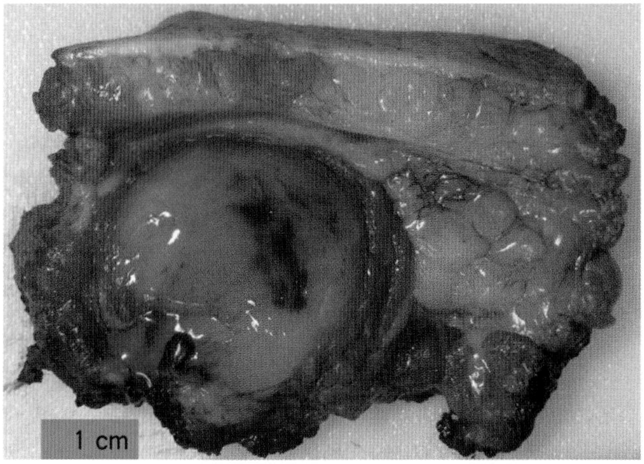

FIGURE 23.75 **Alveolar rhabdomyosarcoma in an 11-month-old girl.** Postchemotherapy resection specimen from a paraspinous muscle mass shows that the tumor is well-circumscribed, pale, and gelatinous.

Most dermatofibrosarcoma protuberans can be treated by complete surgical excision. In retrospective reviews, adjuvant radiation therapy after incomplete excision may have decreased the likelihood of recurrence.[200]

Malignant Soft Tissue Tumors Arising From Skeletal/Smooth Muscle

Rhabdomyosarcoma

Rhabdomyosarcoma (RMS) is a malignant soft tissue tumor with skeletal muscle differentiation. RMS is the most common soft tissue sarcoma in children and adolescents, affecting 4.5 per million persons under age 20 years in the United States of America alone. It has a slight male predilection (males: females, 1.4:1), and 50% of cases are seen in the first decade of life.[201] There are four main histologic types: (1) embryonal (including botryoid and anaplastic subtypes), (2) alveolar (including solid and anaplastic variants) (Fig. 23.75), (3) pleomorphic (virtually never seen in pediatric patients, and (4) spindle cell/sclerosing.[4] Embryonal RMS is the most common type and accounts for ~55% to 70% of all RMS.[201] It most frequently occurs in the first decade of life in the head, neck, and genitourinary regions. The alveolar subtype is the second most common subtype of RMS. Alveolar RMS accounts for ~50% of all extremity lesions and is more common in adolescents and young adults.[201] The pleomorphic subtype is a high-grade sarcoma that occurs almost exclusively in adults. In general, the most favorable histologic type is the botryoid–embryonal type. The alveolar type has a less favorable prognosis than the embryonal type.[182,185]

MR imaging findings of RMS are somewhat nonspecific. However, most tumors are predominantly isointense to skeletal muscle on T1-weighted MR images and hyperintense on T2-weighted MR images. RMS frequently shows prominent vascularity with serpentine signal flow voids and intratumoral hemorrhage. Marked enhancement may be seen following contrast administration[202,203] (Figs. 23.76 and 23.77). Local bone invasion is observed in ~25% of cases.[204–206] Hematogenous metastases are most common in the lung, followed by bone, bone marrow, liver, and lymph nodes. Bone marrow metastases at the time of diagnosis, particularly in alveolar RMS, are not uncommon, occurring in 6% to 16% of affected pediatric patients.[204–206]

The current treatment for extremity RMS includes wide resection and adjuvant chemotherapy and/or radiation.[206]

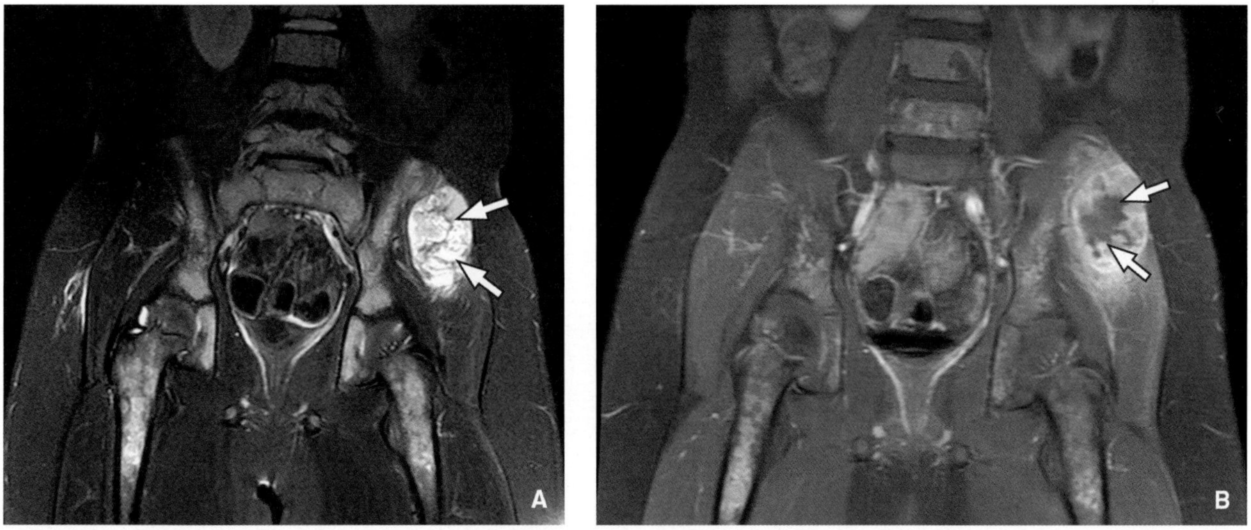

FIGURE 23.76 **Embryonal rhabdomyosarcoma in a 6-year-old boy. A:** Coronal fat-suppressed T2-weighted MR image shows the mass with heterogeneous hyperintensity and multiple internal septa (*arrows*). Note the heterogeneous signal intensity of the bone marrow in both proximal femurs and pelvic bones suggesting tumor infiltration within the bone marrow. **B:** Coronal post-contrast fat-suppressed T1-weighted MR image demonstrates heterogeneous enhancement in the mass, which presents with a central nonenhancing area that suggests central necrosis (*arrows*). Note the heterogeneous enhancement of the bone marrow in the femurs and pelvic bones.

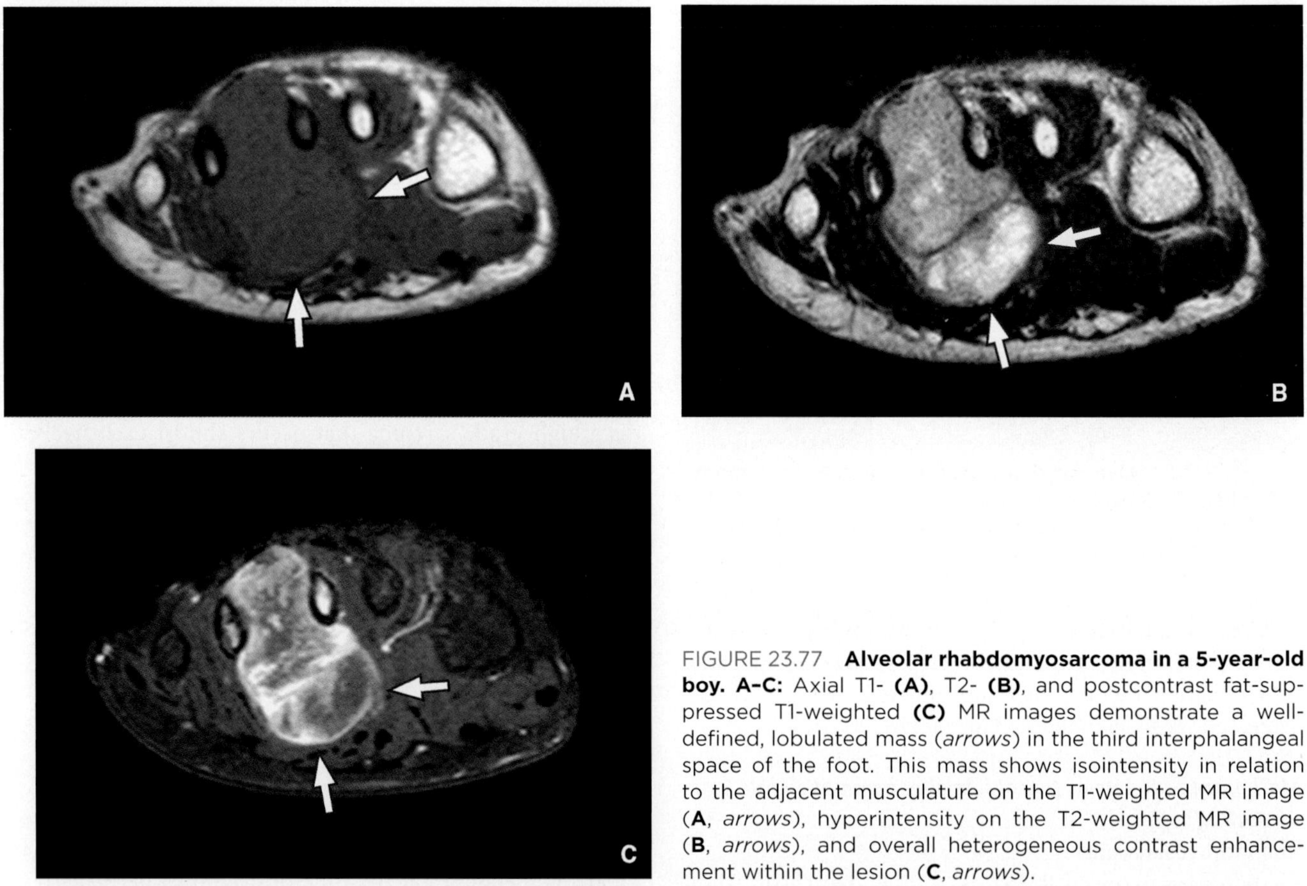

FIGURE 23.77 **Alveolar rhabdomyosarcoma in a 5-year-old boy. A–C:** Axial T1- **(A)**, T2- **(B)**, and postcontrast fat-suppressed T1-weighted **(C)** MR images demonstrate a well-defined, lobulated mass (*arrows*) in the third interphalangeal space of the foot. This mass shows isointensity in relation to the adjacent musculature on the T1-weighted MR image (**A**, *arrows*), hyperintensity on the T2-weighted MR image (**B**, *arrows*), and overall heterogeneous contrast enhancement within the lesion (**C**, *arrows*).

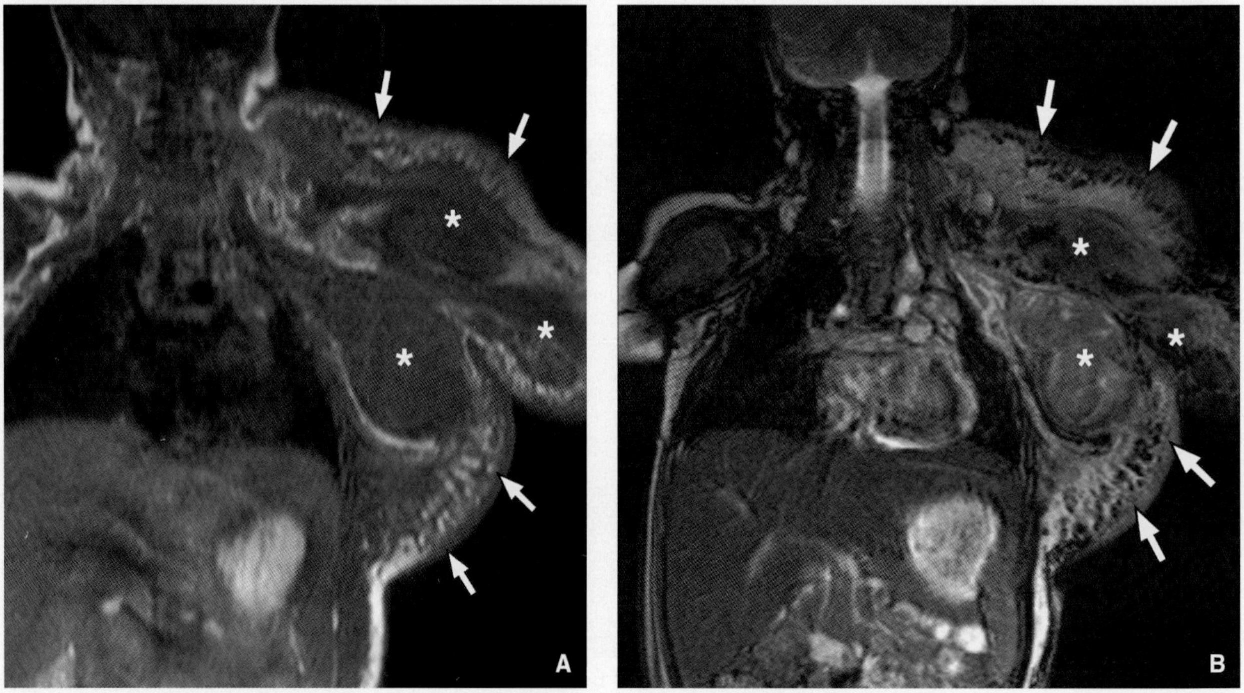

FIGURE 23.78 **Hemangioendothelioma in a 9-month-old-girl with Kasabach-Merritt syndrome. A:** Coronal T1-weighted MR image of the left chest wall and arm shows extensive ill-defined soft tissue lesions (*arrows*) in the subcutaneous fat layer, which present with signal intensity similar to that of adjacent skeletal muscle. Note the mass-like ovoid lesions (*asterisks*) in the left chest wall. **B:** Coronal fat-suppressed T2-weighted MR image shows heterogeneously hyperintense subcutaneous lesions (*arrows*) peripherally and slightly hypointense oval shape lesions (*asterisks*) more centrally in the left chest wall. Poor fat saturation is noted on the right chest wall.

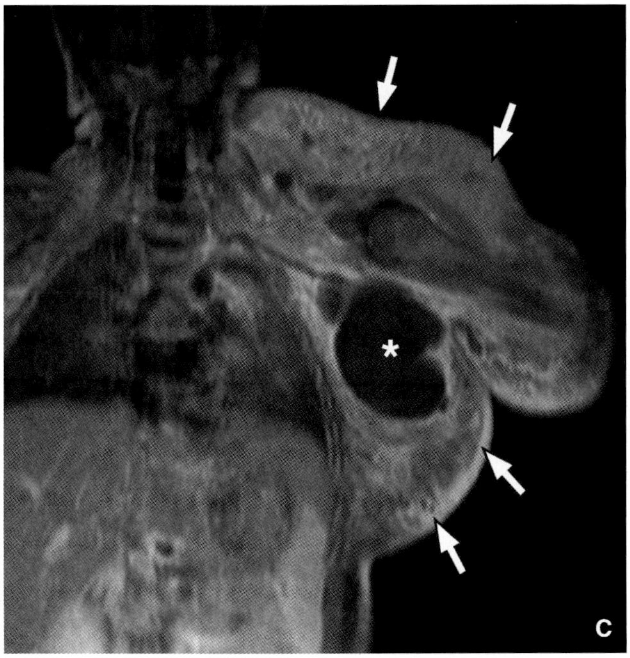

FIGURE 23.78 (*Continued*) **C:** Coronal postcontrast fat-suppressed T1-weighted MR image demonstrates heterogeneously enhancing lesions (*arrows*) in the left chest wall and arm. Note the nonenhancing hypointense lesion (*asterisk*) in the left chest wall suggesting an organizing hematoma. Laboratory studies revealed severe thrombocytopenia (13 × $10^3/\mu L$) and a hemorrhagic diathesis.

Leiomyosarcoma

Leiomyosarcoma is a malignant neoplasm with smooth muscle differentiation. It occurs most often in the middle aged to older adults, and it is extremely rare in children. Pediatric smooth muscle tumors exhibiting histologic features suggestive of malignancy may often represent Epstein-Barr-virus-associated smooth muscle tumors, tumors associated with chronic immunosuppression and uncertain malignant potential.[207]

Malignant Vascular Soft Tissue Tumors

Hemangioendothelioma

Hemangioendotheliomas are vascular neoplasms defined as locally aggressive (Kaposiform hemangioendothelioma, KHE), rarely metastasizing (retiform hemangioendothelioma, papillary intralymphatic angioendothelioma, composite hemangioendothelioma, pseudomyogenic hemangioendothelioma, or malignant (epithelioid hemangioendothelioma).[4] Among these, two most commonly encountered subtypes of hemangioendothelioma in the pediatric population are epithelioid hemangioendothelioma and KHE.

Epithelioid hemangioendothelioma is a rare vascular neoplasm, most frequently involving the deep soft tissues of the extremities (Fig. 23.78). These tumors may also involve bone and viscera (lung and liver). It is considered to be a low- to intermediate-grade angiocentric vascular tumor with metastatic potential. The local recurrence rate is 10% to 15%, and the metastatic rate is 20% to 30%.[208–210]

KHE is a rare locally aggressive vascular neoplasm that may involve the superficial and deep soft tissues and usually affects children and adolescents. The lesion may be associated with Kasabach-Merritt syndrome, which involves a vascular lesion, thrombocytopenia, and purpura. The retroperitoneum, upper and lower extremities, and trunk are the most frequent sites. KHE is usually larger than infantile hemangioma and has a more infiltrative nature (Fig. 23.79).[211–214] KHE may be present at birth and usually becomes apparent before the age of 2 years. It is characterized by a

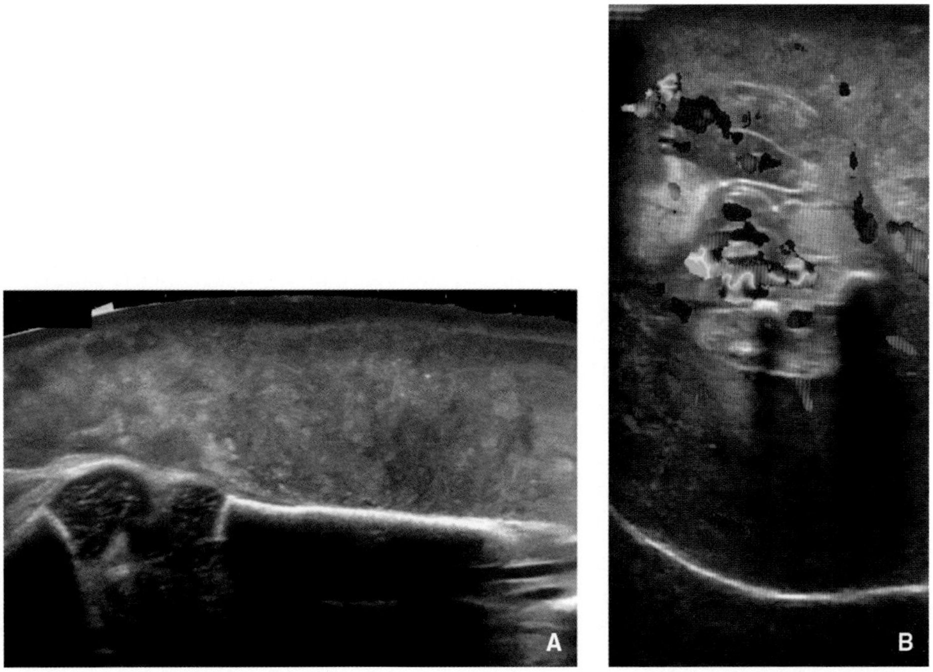

FIGURE 23.79 **Kaposiform hemangioendothelioma in a 2-day-old girl. A:** Longitudinal gray-scale ultrasound image of the leg demonstrates diffuse edema and heterogeneous echogenicity involving the subcutaneous tissue of the upper thigh. **B:** Transverse color Doppler ultrasound image demonstrates increased blood flow within the subcutaneous soft tissue mass.

(*Continued*)

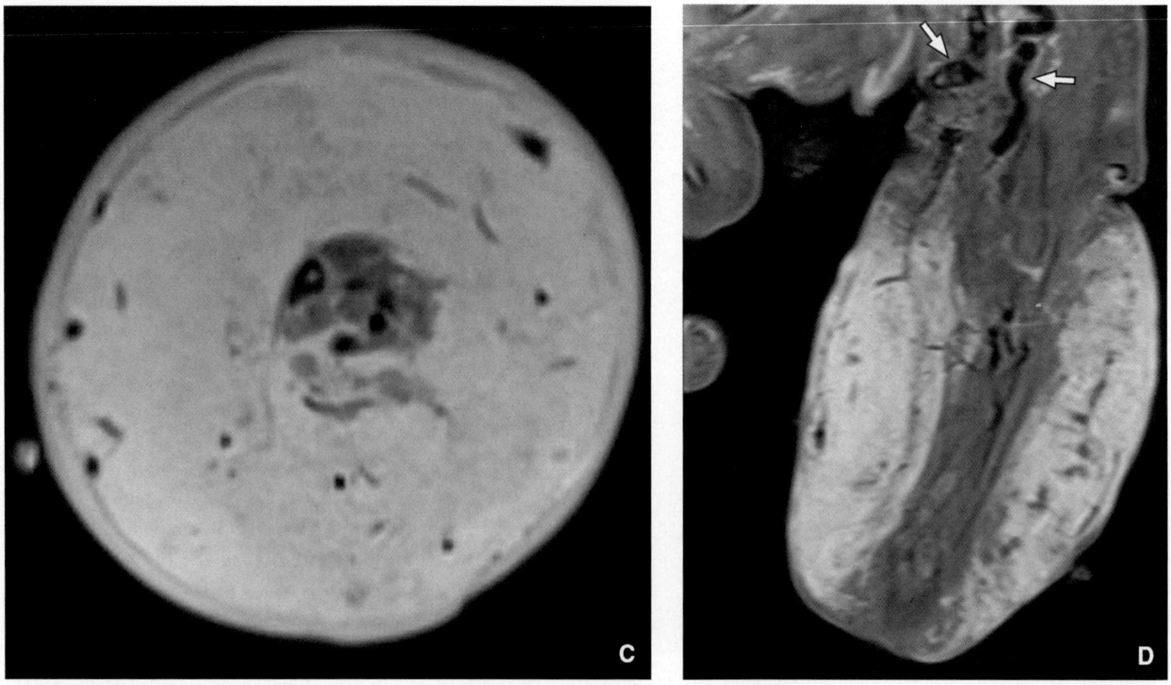

FIGURE 23.79 (*Continued*) **C:** Axial proton density MR image demonstrates a large, infiltrative, poorly defined superficial lesion involving mainly in skin/subcutaneous fat and encasing the entire leg. It relatively spares the underlying muscle and bone. **D:** Coronal fat-suppressed T1-weighted MR image demonstrates diffuse enhancement and large draining and feeding vessels (*arrows*). (Case courtesy of Arnold C. Merrow, MD, Cincinnati, OH.)

disproportionate increase in size, which is different from congenital hemangioma. No complete regression or metastasis is seen in KHE.

Treatment of these lesions has not been satisfactory in the pediatric population. In epithelioid hemangioendothelioma, treatment is complete excision with the goal of negative resection margin.[210] However, in many cases, surgical excision is not feasible because of the local tissue invasion. In KHE, a number of therapeutic options have been published including a multimodality approach with corticosteroids, interferon alpha, or vincristine.[215] Surgical excision is recommended by some for the treatment of KHE with localized cutaneous disease.[210]

Angiosarcoma

Angiosarcoma is a frankly malignant STS composed of cells with endothelial differentiation. It is extremely rare in the pediatric population and most cases occur in adults older than 40 years of age. Angiosarcomas are typically found in the skin, both superficial and deep soft tissue, breast, liver, and bone. The imaging appearance of all aggressive vascular lesions, including hemangioendothelioma, hemangiopericytoma, and angiosarcoma, mainly depends on the lesion location. Superficial lesions involving the cutaneous and subcutaneous layers typically have areas of skin thickening with nodularity and focal soft tissue mass on US, CT, or MR imaging. While prominent vascular channels and spaces are not typically apparent in these superficial lesions, they are frequently seen in deep-seated vascular lesions. The optimal treatment for angiosarcoma in pediatric patients is currently unclear mainly because of the small number of cases reported.

Malignant Soft Tissue Tumor Arising from Nerve Sheath

Malignant Peripheral Nerve Sheath Tumor

Malignant peripheral nerve sheath tumor (MPNST) is a sarcoma that can arise from a peripheral nerve or from a pre-existing benign nerve sheath tumor such as plexiform neurofibroma. Approximately 50% of cases of MPNSTs occur in patients with NF1, particularly in association with plexiform neurofibromas[168,170]; another 10% are related to radiation, and the remaining 40% of cases occur without identifiable predisposing factors.[168,170] MPNSTs are deeply seated STS involving peripheral nerves. They commonly arise in the extremities, followed by the trunk and head/neck region. Examination of the tumor usually shows the nerve entering at the top of the tumor and exiting at the bottom of the tumor. Malignant transformation of benign neurofibroma should be considered when the mass is painful or presents with rapidly growing characteristics and when the typical target appearance of a benign neurofibroma disappears (Fig. 23.80).[216,217]

Wide excision is the mainstay of treatment for MPNST. Adjuvant radiation therapy has yield a significant reduction in the rates of local disease recurrence.

Malignant Soft Tissue Tumors with Uncertain Differentiation

Synovial Sarcoma

Synovial sarcoma is a malignant tumor of uncertain histogenesis. It can arise in the soft tissue and less commonly within viscera. Synovial sarcoma may occur at any age, and

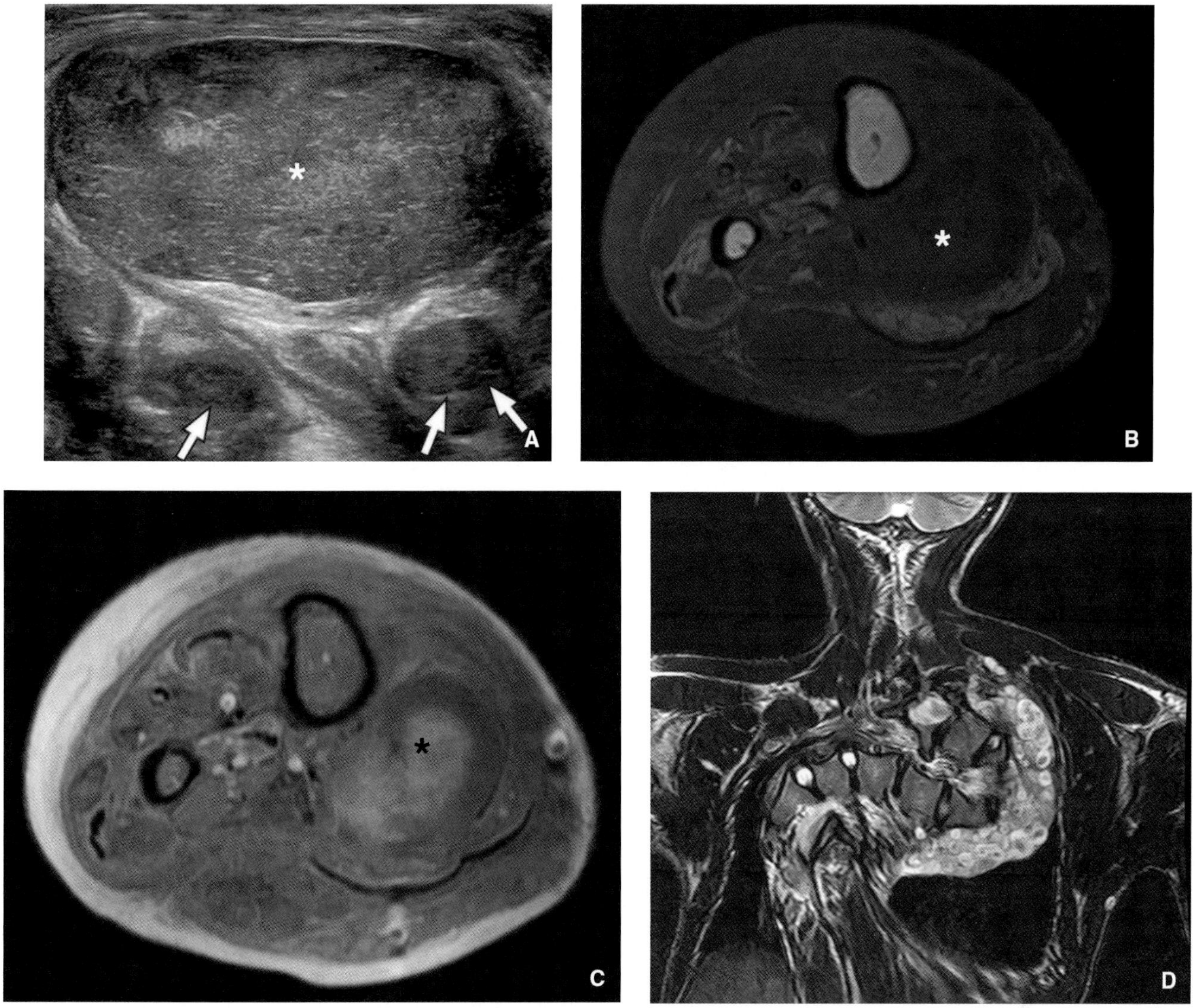

FIGURE 23.80 **Malignant peripheral nerve sheath tumor (MPNST) in a 13-year-old boy. A:** Transverse gray-scale ultrasound image of the right calf shows a heterogeneous hypoechoic mass (*asterisk*) in the proximal intermuscular area. Note other nodules (*arrows*) in the posterior calf. **B:** On the axial fat-suppressed T1-weighted MR image, the largest lesion (*asterisk*) of the right calf shows homogeneous isointensity. **C:** Axial postcontrast T1-weighted MR image demonstrates heterogeneous enhancement in the central portion of the largest lesion (*asterisk*). The other nodular lesions show subtle inhomogeneous enhancement. Fine-needle aspiration biopsy of the mass revealed MPNST arising from a plexiform neurofibroma. **D:** Coronal fat-suppressed T2-weighted MR image of the thoracic spine demonstrates severe scoliosis and numerous paraspinal nodular lesions with target appearance suggesting a plexiform neurofibroma.

more than half of patients are teenagers and young adults. It accounts for about 10% of all pediatric STSs.[218] Synovial sarcoma typically presents as a palpable mass, which is often painful. Initial growth is often slow, and a small circumscribed tumor may clinically simulate a benign process. Most tumors arise in the deep soft tissue of the lower extremities, often in a juxta-articular location. An intra-articular location is very rare. Unusual sites of involvement include kidney, retroperitoneum, lung/mediastinum, various other viscera, central nervous system, and peripheral nerve.

On radiographs, calcifications are present in 30% of synovial sarcomas.[219] On MRI, synovial sarcoma may contain areas of high signal intensity on T1-weighted MR images and fluid–fluid levels that reflect hemorrhage. In a large series of synovial sarcomas reported by Jones et al., 35% of tumors showed a "triple signal pattern": hyperintense, isointense, and hypointense to fat on T2-weighted MR images.[220] These MRI findings are caused by a mixture of cystic (hemorrhage and necrosis) and solid elements resembling that of fibrous tissue (Fig. 23.81). In the appropriate clinical setting, these MR findings may suggest the diagnosis of synovial sarcoma. Some synovial sarcomas may present as a well-circumscribed mass and may mimic a simple cyst or ganglion.[188,221,222] Metastasis or local recurrence is seen in ~80% of affected patients.[190,191,223] The lungs are the most common site of metastasis followed by lymph nodes and bone. Local recurrence may be seen in 20% to 26% of these tumors.[190,191,223]

Microscopically, synovial sarcoma typically shows a cellular proliferation of plump to spindled cells arranged in short

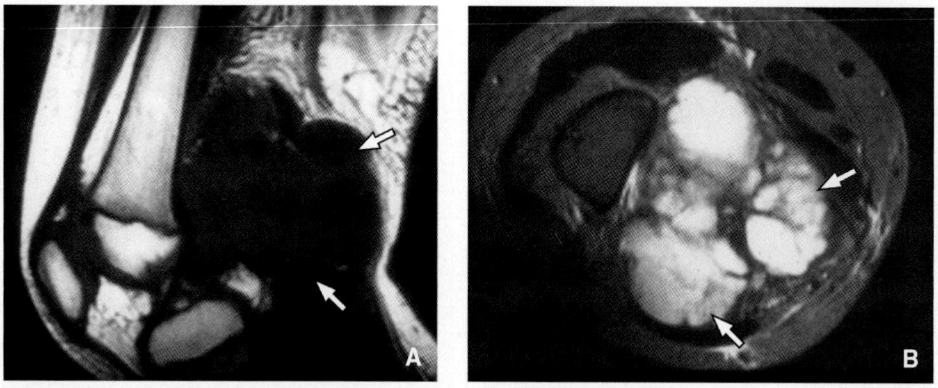

FIGURE 23.81 **Synovial sarcoma in a 10-year-old boy. A:** Sagittal T1-weighted MR image shows a well-defined hypointense intramuscular mass (*arrows*) in the popliteal fossa of the knee. **B:** Axial fat-suppressed T2-weighted MR image shows inhomogeneous signal intensity within the mass (*arrows*).

fascicles (Fig. 23.82). Epithelial differentiation ("biphasic" synovial sarcoma) is common, as are calcifications and cystification. Synovial sarcomas are characterized by a chromosomal rearrangement, t(X;18), involving a fusion between the SS18 gene on chromosome 18 and one of the SSX genes on the X chromosome. The initial treatment for synovial sarcoma is wide local excision with negative resection margin. Chemotherapy might be recommended especially in advanced or metastatic disease.

Alveolar Soft Part Sarcoma

Alveolar soft part sarcoma (ASPS) is a rare tumor in children that may also occur in adolescents and young adults. The tumor consists of a nested ("alveolar") arrangement of large granular cells separated by vascular channels. Because of its high vascularity, ASPS may be erroneously diagnosed as a vascular malformation or hemangioma. ASPS occurs most commonly in the deep soft tissues of the extremities as well as in the head and neck regions. Metastases to the lung or brain are often the first manifestation of the disease.

On MRI, ASPS usually have signal intensity equal to or higher than muscle on T1-weighted MR images and bright signal intensity on T2-weighted MR images. Tubular signal voids at the margin and within the tumors are consistent with enlarged vessels (Fig. 23.83).[224,225]

In addition to distinctive histologic features, ASPS is characterized by an ASPSCR1-TFE3 gene fusion, thought to drive tumor growth via signaling activation of MET and other target genes.[226] Radical resection is the current therapy of choice for localized disease, although molecularly targeted drugs are an emerging modality. Children with ASPS should be followed throughout adolescence and well into adulthood because metastases may occur after several decades have elapsed.

Epithelioid Sarcoma

Epithelioid sarcoma is a malignant mesenchymal neoplasm that is composed of rounded ("epithelioid") cells. Epithelioid sarcoma may involve subcutaneous tissues, as when it presents as an ulcerating nodule, or it may occur in muscles, tendons, tendon sheaths, or fascias. The tumor spreads along neurovascular bundles and may invade vascular structures, but it rarely involves bone. It is one of the few sarcomas that occasionally metastasize to lymph nodes (Fig. 23.84).[227,228]

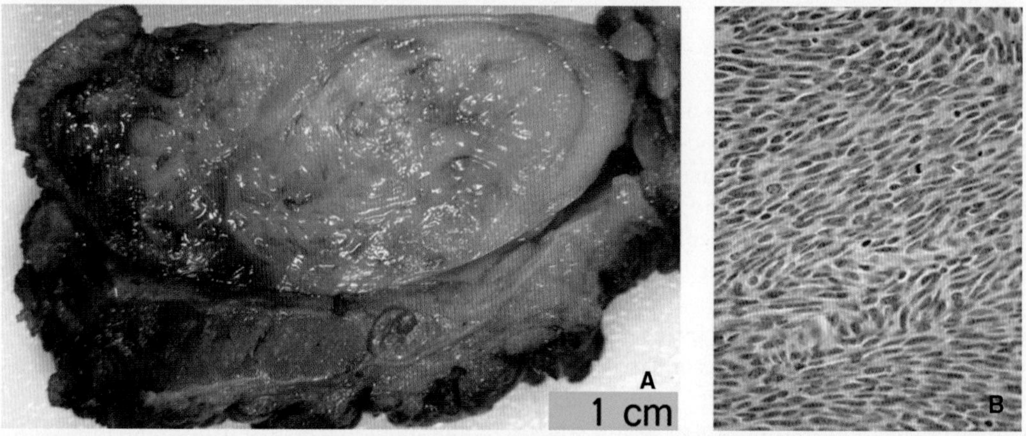

FIGURE 23.82 **Synovial sarcoma, resected from the anterior chest wall in an 18-year-old girl. A:** Grossly, the tumor has a bulging and slightly whorled pale tan cut surface. **B:** Microscopically, there are short fascicles of spindle cells with powdery nuclei (hematoxylin and eosin, original magnification, 600×).

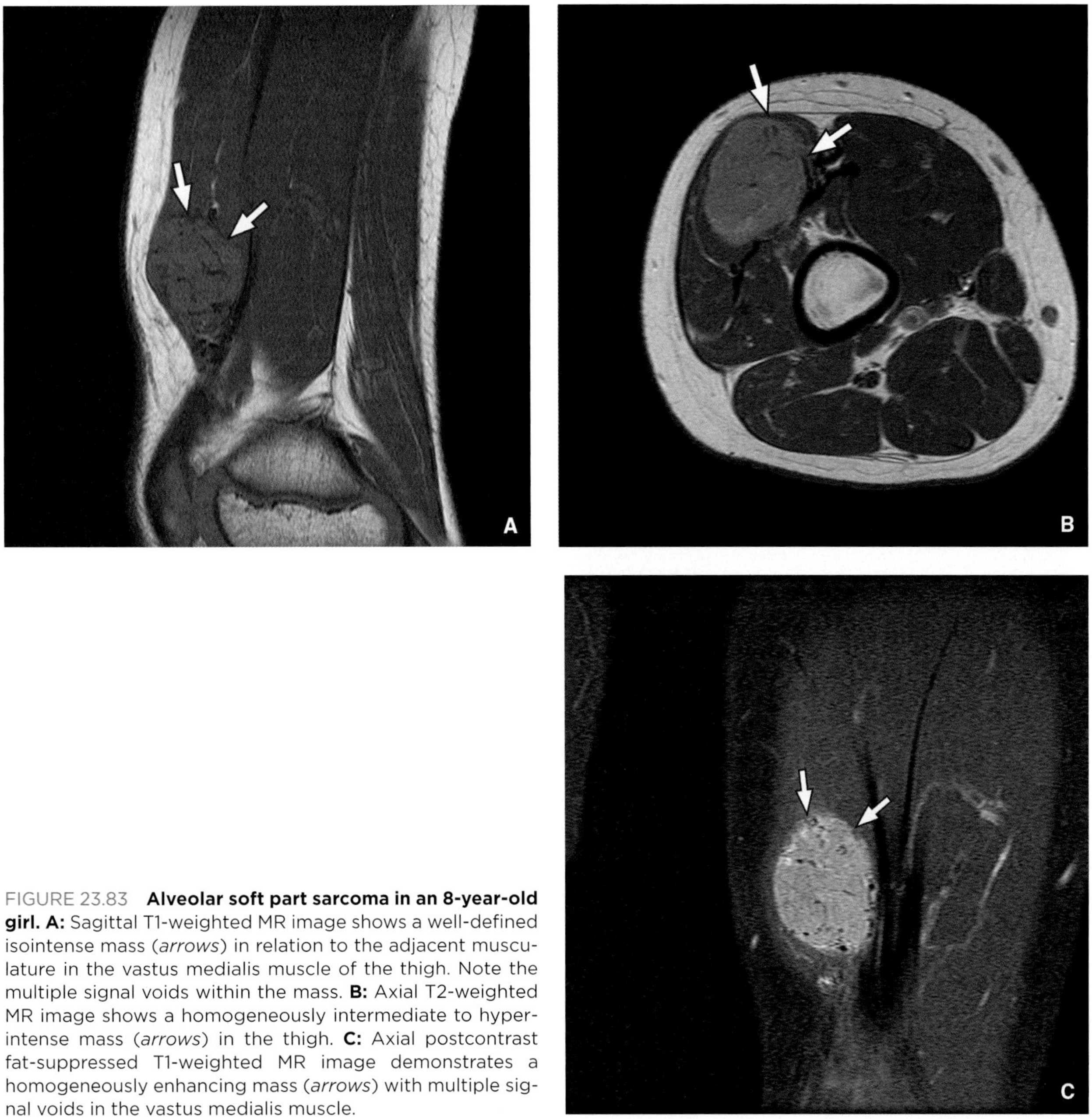

FIGURE 23.83 **Alveolar soft part sarcoma in an 8-year-old girl. A:** Sagittal T1-weighted MR image shows a well-defined isointense mass (*arrows*) in relation to the adjacent musculature in the vastus medialis muscle of the thigh. Note the multiple signal voids within the mass. **B:** Axial T2-weighted MR image shows a homogeneously intermediate to hyperintense mass (*arrows*) in the thigh. **C:** Axial postcontrast fat-suppressed T1-weighted MR image demonstrates a homogeneously enhancing mass (*arrows*) with multiple signal voids in the vastus medialis muscle.

Extrarenal Rhabdoid Tumor

Extrarenal rhabdoid tumor is a highly malignant soft tissue tumor, mainly affecting infants and children. It usually occurs in deep, axial locations such as the neck, paraspinal or perineal regions, abdominal cavity, or retroperitoneum. Lesions in the extremities, especially the thigh, and cutaneous lesions are also well documented. Morphologically and genetically identical tumors also arise in the kidney and brain. Extrarenal rhabdoid tumors frequently demonstrate cytogenetic aberrations involving the SMARCB1 gene at chromosome 22q11 and resulting in the loss of the INI1 protein.[229] Imaging findings of extrarenal rhabdoid tumors have been only rarely reported (Fig. 23.85).[230] The optimal treatment for extrarenal rhabdoid tumor in children is currently unclear because of the small number of cases reported.

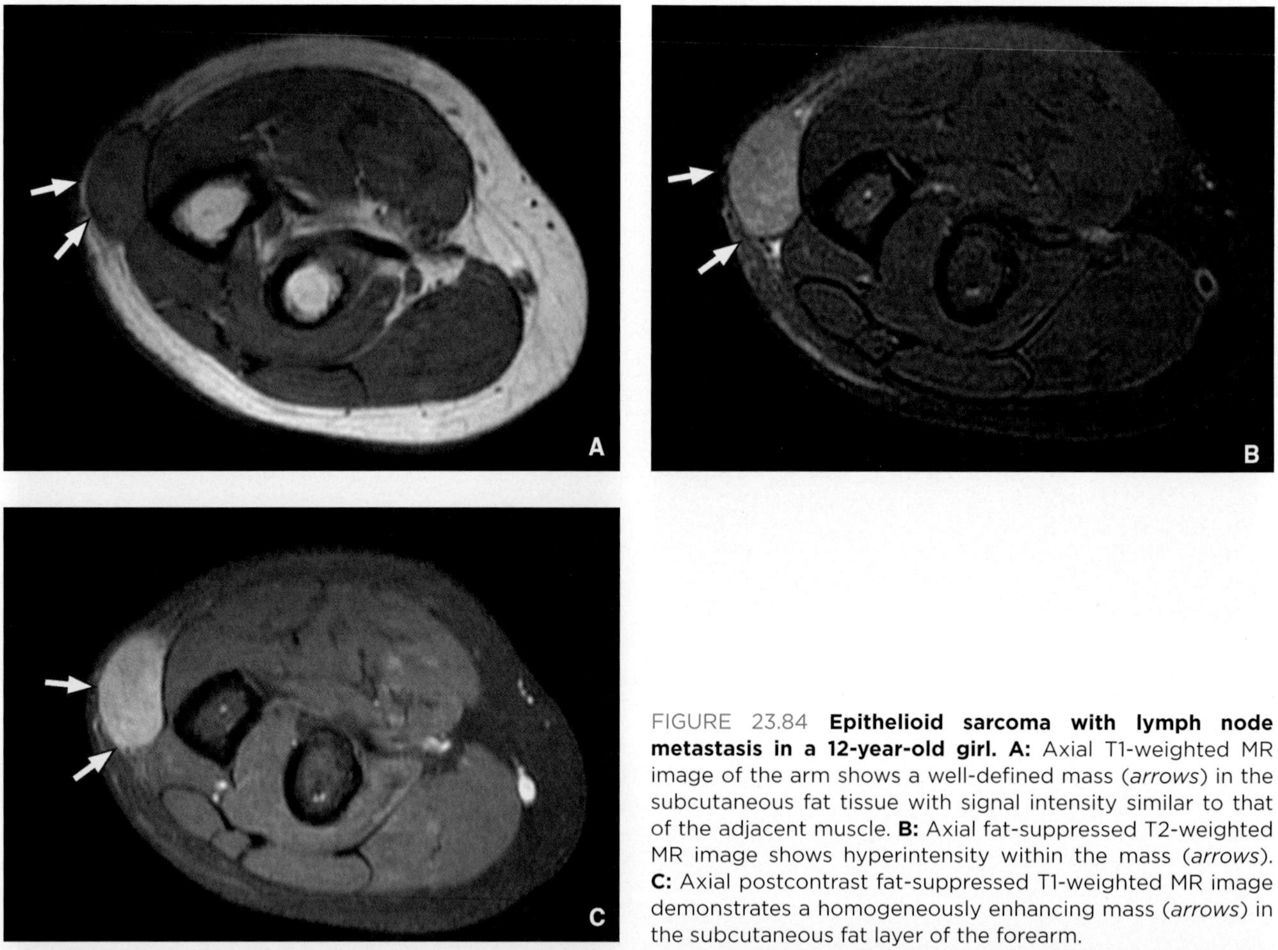

FIGURE 23.84 **Epithelioid sarcoma with lymph node metastasis in a 12-year-old girl. A:** Axial T1-weighted MR image of the arm shows a well-defined mass (*arrows*) in the subcutaneous fat tissue with signal intensity similar to that of the adjacent muscle. **B:** Axial fat-suppressed T2-weighted MR image shows hyperintensity within the mass (*arrows*). **C:** Axial postcontrast fat-suppressed T1-weighted MR image demonstrates a homogeneously enhancing mass (*arrows*) in the subcutaneous fat layer of the forearm.

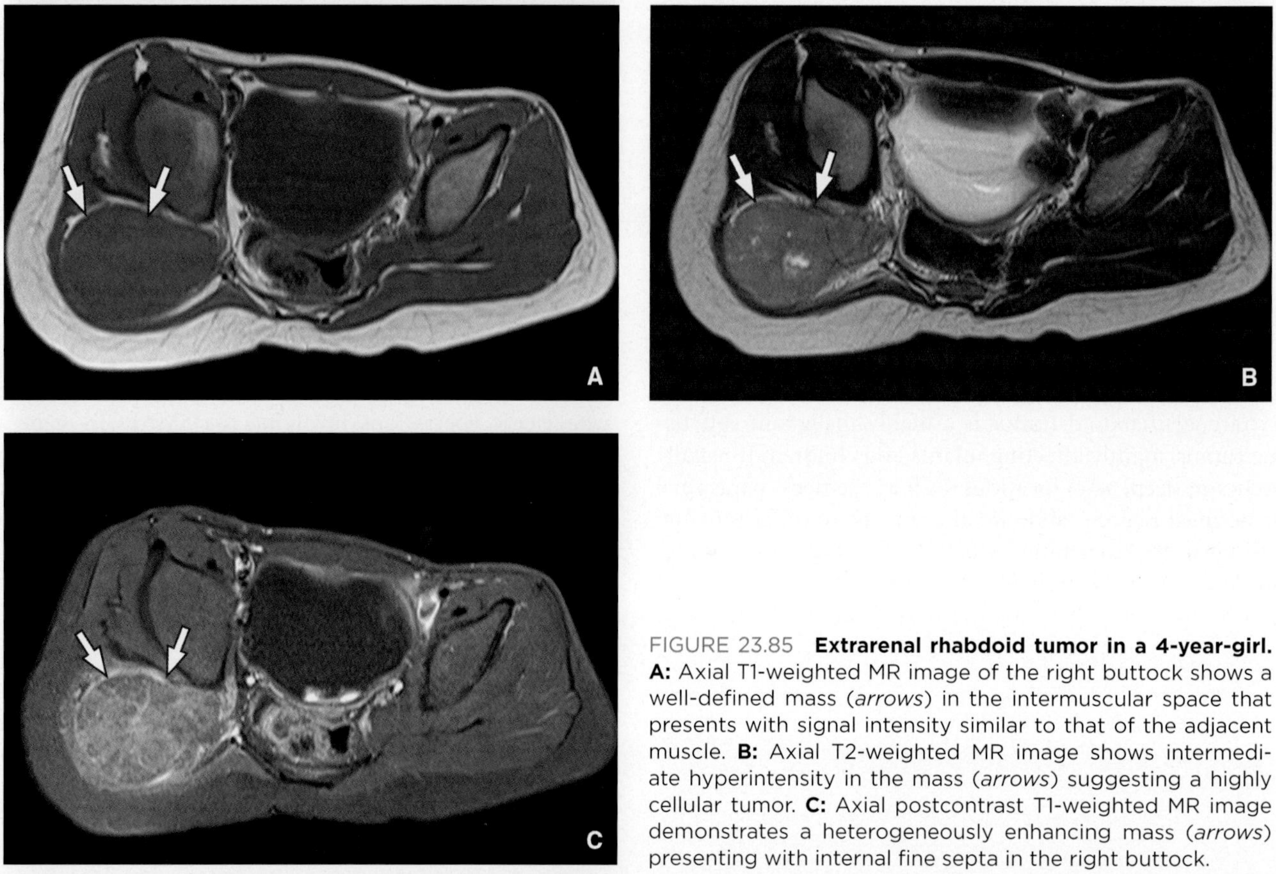

FIGURE 23.85 **Extrarenal rhabdoid tumor in a 4-year-girl. A:** Axial T1-weighted MR image of the right buttock shows a well-defined mass (*arrows*) in the intermuscular space that presents with signal intensity similar to that of the adjacent muscle. **B:** Axial T2-weighted MR image shows intermediate hyperintensity in the mass (*arrows*) suggesting a highly cellular tumor. **C:** Axial postcontrast T1-weighted MR image demonstrates a heterogeneously enhancing mass (*arrows*) presenting with internal fine septa in the right buttock.

References

1. Hayat MJ, Howlader N, Reichman ME, et al. Cancer statistics, trends, and multiple primary cancer analyses from the surveillance, epidemiology, and end results (SEER) program. *Oncologist.* 2007;12:20–37.
2. Murphy SL, Xu J, Kochanek KD. *Deaths: Final Data for 2010. National Vital Statistics Reports.* Vol 61. No. 4. Hyattsville, MD: National Center for Health Statistics; 2013.
3. Howlader N, Noone AM, Krapcho M, et al., eds. *SEER Cancer Statistics Review, 1975–2010.* Bethesda, MD: National Cancer Institute; 2013.
4. Fletcher CDM, Bridge JA, Hogendoorn PCW, et al., eds. *WHO Classification of Tumours of Soft Tissue and Bone.* 4th ed. Lyon, France: IARC; 2013.
5. Rana RS, Wu JS, Eisenberg RL. Periosteal reaction. *AJR Am J Roentgenol.* 2009;193(4):W259–W272.
6. Carra BJ, et al. Sonography of musculoskeletal soft-tissue masses: techniques, pearls, and pitfalls. *AJR Am J Roentgenol.* 2014;202(6):1281–1290.
7. Boyko OB, et al. MR imaging of osteogenic and Ewing's sarcoma. *AJR Am J Roentgenol.* 1987;148(2):317–322.
8. Hogendoorn PC, ESMO/EUROBONET Working Group, Athanasou N, et al. Bone sarcomas: ESMO Clinical Practice Guidelines for diagnosis, treatment and follow-up. *Ann Oncol.* 2014;25(suppl 3):iii113–iii123.
9. Edge S, Byrd DR, Compton CC, et al. eds. *AJCC Cancer Staging Manual.* 7th ed. Chicago, IL: American Joint Commission on Cancer; 2010.
10. Meyer JS, et al. Imaging guidelines for children with Ewing sarcoma and osteosarcoma: a report from the Children's Oncology Group Bone Tumor Committee. *Pediatr Blood Cancer.* 2008;51(2): 163–170.
11. Darge K, Jaramillo D, Siegel KJ. Whole-body MRI in children: current status and future applications. *Eur J Radiol.* 2008;68(2):289–298.
12. Buchbender C, et al. Oncologic PET/MRI, part 2: bone tumors, soft-tissue tumors, melanoma, and lymphoma. *J Nucl Med.* 2012;53(8):1244–1252.
13. Wyers MR. Evaluation of pediatric bone lesions. *Pediatr Radiol.* 2010;40(4):468–473.
14. Hayes CW, Conway WF, Sundaram M. Misleading aggressive MR imaging appearance of some benign musculoskeletal lesions. *Radiographics.* 1992;12(6):1119–1134; discussion 1135–1136.
15. Mirra JM. Benign cartilaginous exostoses: osteochondroma and osteochondromatosis. In: Mirra JM, ed. *Bone Tumors: Clinical, Radiologic, and Pathologic Correlations.* Vol 2. Philadelphia, PA: Lea & Febiger; 1989:1626–1659.
16. Resnick D, Kyriakos M, Greenway GD. Osteochondroma. In: Resnick D, ed. *Diagnosis of Bone and Joint Disorders.* 3rd ed. Vol 5. Philadelphia, PA: Saunders; 1995:3725–3746.
17. Jones KB, Pacifici M, Hilton MJ. Multiple hereditary exostoses (MHE): elucidating the pathogenesis of a rare skeletal disorder through interdisciplinary research. *Connect Tissue Res.* 2014; 55(2):80–88.
18. Bluemke DA, Fishman EK, Scott WW Jr. Skeletal complications of radiation therapy. *Radiographics.* 1994;14(1):111–121.
19. Jaffe N, et al. Radiation induced osteochondroma in long-term survivors of childhood cancer. *Int J Radiat Oncol Biol Phys.* 1983; 9(5):665–670.
20. Solomon L. Hereditary multiple exostosis. *Am J Hum Genet.* 1964;16:351–363.
21. Norman A, Sissons HA. Radiographic hallmarks of peripheral chondrosarcoma. *Radiology.* 1984;151(3):589–596.
22. Woertler K, et al. Osteochondroma: MR imaging of tumor-related complications. *Eur Radiol.* 2000;10(5):832–840.
23. Bernard SA, et al. Improved differentiation of benign osteochondromas from secondary chondrosarcomas with standardized measurement of cartilage cap at CT and MR imaging. *Radiology.* 2010;255(3):857–865.
24. Murphey MD, et al. Imaging of osteochondroma: variants and complications with radiologic-pathologic correlation. *Radiographics.* 2000;20(5):1407–1034.
25. Glick R, et al. Dysplasia epiphysealis hemimelica (Trevor disease): a rare developmental disorder of bone mimicking osteochondroma of long bones. *Hum Pathol.* 2007;38(8):1265–1272.
26. Azouz EM, et al. The variable manifestations of dysplasia epiphysealis hemimelica. *Pediatr Radiol.* 1985;15(1):44–49.
27. Iwasawa T, et al. MRI findings of dysplasia epiphysealis hemimelica. *Pediatr Radiol.* 1996;26(1):65–67.
28. Struhl S, et al. Solitary (unicameral) bone cyst. The fallen fragment sign revisited. *Skeletal Radiol.* 1989;18(4):261–265.
29. Polat O, et al. Our clinical experience on calcaneal bone cysts: 36 cysts in 33 patients. *Arch Orthop Trauma Surg.* 2009;129(11):1489–1494.
30. Ilaslan H, Sundaram M, Unni KK. Solid variant of aneurysmal bone cysts in long tubular bones: giant cell reparative granuloma. *AJR Am J Roentgenol.* 2003;180(6):1681–1687.
31. Oliveira AM, et al. USP6 and CDH11 oncogenes identify the neoplastic cell in primary aneurysmal bone cysts and are absent in so-called secondary aneurysmal bone cysts. *Am J Pathol.* 2004;165(5):1773–1780.
32. Mankin HJ, et al. Aneurysmal bone cyst: a review of 150 patients. *J Clin Oncol.* 2005;23(27):6756–6762.
33. Chai JW, et al. Radiologic diagnosis of osteoid osteoma: from simple to challenging findings. *Radiographics.* 2010;30(3):737–749.
34. Kenzora JE, Abrams RC. Problems encountered in the diagnosis and treatment of osteoid osteoma of the talus. *Foot Ankle.* 1981;2(3):172–178.
35. Assoun J, et al. Osteoid osteoma: MR imaging versus CT. *Radiology.* 1994;191(1):217–223.
36. Liu PT, et al. Imaging of osteoid osteoma with dynamic gadolinium-enhanced MR imaging. *Radiology.* 2003;227(3):691–700.
37. Scalici J, et al. Intra-articular osteoid osteoma of the hip misdiagnosed by MRI: an unusual cause of unexplained hip pain. *Orthop Traumatol Surg Res.* 2011;97(8):881–885.
38. Kattapuram SV, et al. Osteoid osteoma: an unusual cause of articular pain. *Radiology.* 1983;147(2):383–387.
39. Connolly LP, Connolly SA, Treves ST. Differentiation of anterior tibial stress fracture from osteoid osteoma. *Clin Nucl Med.* 2001;26(1):54–56.
40. Mahboubi S. CT appearance of nidus in osteoid osteoma versus sequestration in osteomyelitis. *J Comput Assist Tomogr.* 1986;10(3):457–459.
41. Jankharia B, Burute N. Percutaneous radiofrequency ablation for osteoid osteoma: how we do it. *Indian J Radiol Imaging.* 2009;19(1):36–42.
42. Lucas DR, et al. Osteoblastoma: clinicopathologic study of 306 cases. *Hum Pathol.* 1994;25(2):117–134.
43. Greenspan A. Benign bone-forming lesions: osteoma, osteoid osteoma, and osteoblastoma. Clinical, imaging, pathologic, and differential considerations. *Skeletal Radiol.* 1993;22(7): 485–500.

44. Azouz EM, et al. Osteoid osteoma and osteoblastoma of the spine in children. Report of 22 cases with brief literature review. *Pediatr Radiol.* 1986;16(1):25–31.
45. Campanacci M, Laus M, Boriani S. Multiple non-ossifying fibromata with extraskeletal anomalies: a new syndrome? *J Bone Joint Surg Br.* 1983;65(5):627–632.
46. Colby RS, Saul RA. Is Jaffe-Campanacci syndrome just a manifestation of neurofibromatosis type 1? *Am J Med Genet A.* 2003;123A(1):60–63.
47. Mankin HJ, et al. Non-ossifying fibroma, fibrous cortical defect and Jaffe-Campanacci syndrome: a biologic and clinical review. *Chir Organi Mov.* 2009;93(1):1–7.
48. Jee WH, et al. Nonossifying fibroma: characteristics at MR imaging with pathologic correlation. *Radiology.* 1998;209(1):197–202.
49. Harris WH, Dudley HR Jr, Barry RJ. The natural history of fibrous dysplasia. An orthopaedic, pathological, and roentgenographic study. *J Bone Joint Surg Am.* 1962;44-A:207–233.
50. Lemli L. Fibrous dysplasia of bone. Report of female monozygotic twins with and without the McCune-Albright syndrome. *J Pediatr.* 1977;91(6):947–949.
51. Lightner ES, Penny R, Frasier SD. Growth hormone excess and sexual precocity in polyostotic fibrous dysplasia (McCune-Albright syndrome): evidence for abnormal hypothalamic function. *J Pediatr.* 1975;87(6 Pt 1):922–927.
52. Zoccali C, et al. Mazabraud's syndrome: a new case and review of the literature. *Int Orthop.* 2009;33(3):605–610.
53. Fitzpatrick KA, et al. Imaging findings of fibrous dysplasia with histopathologic and intraoperative correlation. *AJR Am J Roentgenol.* 2004;182(6):1389–1398.
54. Sakamoto A, et al. A comparative study of fibrous dysplasia and osteofibrous dysplasia with regard to expressions of c-fos and c-jun products and bone matrix proteins: a clinicopathologic review and immunohistochemical study of c-fos, c-jun, type I collagen, osteonectin, osteopontin, and osteocalcin. *Hum Pathol.* 1999;30(12):1418–1426.
55. Levine SM, Lambiase RE, Petchprapa CN. Cortical lesions of the tibia: characteristic appearances at conventional radiography. *Radiographics.* 2003;23(1):157–177.
56. Gleason BC, et al. Osteofibrous dysplasia and adamantinoma in children and adolescents: a clinicopathologic reappraisal. *Am J Surg Pathol* 2008;32(3):363–376.
57. Meyer JS, et al. Langerhans cell histiocytosis: presentation and evolution of radiologic findings with clinical correlation. *Radiographics.* 1995;15(5):1135–1146.
58. Mokal NJ, et al. Langerhans cell histiocytosis: orbital involvement as an unusual location. *Plast Reconstr Surg.* 2001;107(3):813–817.
59. Howarth DM, et al. Bone scintigraphy evaluated in diagnosing and staging Langerhans' cell histiocytosis and related disorders. *J Nucl Med.* 1996;37(9):1456–1460.
60. Dogan AS, et al. Detection of bone lesions in Langerhans cell histiocytosis: complementary roles of scintigraphy and conventional radiography. *J Pediatr Hematol Oncol.* 1996;18(1):51–58.
61. Goo HW, et al. Whole-body MRI of Langerhans cell histiocytosis: comparison with radiography and bone scintigraphy. *Pediatr Radiol.* 2006;36(10):1019–1031.
62. Turcotte RE, et al. Chondroblastoma. *Hum Pathol.* 1993;24(9):944–949.
63. Weatherall PT, et al. Chondroblastoma: classic and confusing appearance at MR imaging. *Radiology.* 1994;190(2):467–474.
64. Jee WH, et al. Chondroblastoma: MR characteristics with pathologic correlation. *J Comput Assist Tomogr.* 1999;23(5):721–726.
65. Kilpatrick SE, Romeo S. Chondroblastoma. In: Fletcher CDM, Bridge JA, Hogendoorn PCW, et al., eds. *WHO Classification of Tumours of Soft Tissue and Bone.* 4th ed. Lyon, France: IARC; 2013:262–263.
66. Rouas L, et al. Chondromyxoid fibroma of bone: a rare benign bone tumor in children. *Rev Med Brux.* 2004;25(6):521–524.
67. Schajowicz F, Gallardo H. Chondromyxoid fibroma (fibromyxoid chondroma) of bone. A clinico-pathological study of thirty-two cases. *J Bone Joint Surg Br.* 1971;53(2):198–216.
68. Wu CT, et al. Chondromyxoid fibroma of bone: a clinicopathologic review of 278 cases. *Hum Pathol.* 1998;29(5):438–446.
69. Robinson P, et al. Periosteal chondroid tumors: radiologic evaluation with pathologic correlation. *AJR Am J Roentgenol.* 2001;177(5):1183–1188.
70. Silve C, Juppner H. Ollier disease. *Orphanet J Rare Dis.* 2006;1:37.
71. Pansuriya TC, et al. Somatic mosaic IDH1 and IDH2 mutations are associated with enchondroma and spindle cell hemangioma in Ollier disease and Maffucci syndrome. *Nat Genet.* 2011;43(12):1256–1261.
72. Bauer TW, Dorfman HD, Latham Jr JT. Periosteal chondroma. A clinicopathologic study of 23 cases. *Am J Surg Pathol.* 1982;6(7):631–637.
73. Picci P, et al. Giant-cell tumor of bone in skeletally immature patients. *J Bone Joint Surg Am.* 1983;65(4):486–490.
74. Kransdorf MJ, et al. Giant cell tumor in skeletally immature patients. *Radiology.* 1992;184(1):233–237.
75. Kwon JW, et al. MRI findings of giant cell tumors of the spine. *AJR Am J Roentgenol.* 2007;189(1):246–250.
76. Puri A, et al. Giant cell tumor of bone in children and adolescents. *J Pediatr Orthop.* 2007;27(6):635–639.
77. Bielack S, et al. Osteosarcoma: ESMO clinical recommendations for diagnosis, treatment and follow-up. *Ann Oncol.* 2009; 20(suppl 4):137–139.
78. Mirabello L, Troisi RJ, Savage SA. Osteosarcoma incidence and survival rates from 1973 to 2004: data from the Surveillance, Epidemiology, and End Results Program. *Cancer.* 2009;115(7):1531–1543.
79. Choong PF, et al. Low grade central osteogenic sarcoma. A long-term followup of 20 patients. *Clin Orthop Relat Res.* 1996(322):198–206.
80. Sandberg AA, Bridge JA. Updates on the cytogenetics and molecular genetics of bone and soft tissue tumors: osteosarcoma and related tumors. *Cancer Genet Cytogenet.* 2003;145(1):1–30.
81. Bridge JA, Mertons F. Tumour syndromes: introduction. In: Fletcher CDM, Bridge JA, Hogendoorn PCW, et al., eds. *WHO Classification of Tumours of Soft Tissue and Bone.* 4th ed. Lyon, France: IARC; 2013:368–371.
82. Corradi D, et al. Multicentric osteosarcoma: clinicopathologic and radiographic study of 56 cases. *Am J Clin Pathol.* 2011; 136(5):799–807.
83. Lee JS, et al. A review of 40 patients with extraskeletal osteosarcoma. *Cancer.* 1995;76(11):2253–2259.
84. Uhl M, et al. Osteosarcoma: preliminary results of in vivo assessment of tumor necrosis after chemotherapy with diffusion- and perfusion-weighted magnetic resonance imaging. *Invest Radiol.* 2006;41(8):618–623.
85. Uhl M, et al. Evaluation of tumour necrosis during chemotherapy with diffusion-weighted MR imaging: preliminary results in osteosarcomas. *Pediatr Radiol.* 2006;36(12):1306–1311.
86. Murphey MD, et al. The many faces of osteosarcoma. *Radiographics.* 1997;17(5):1205–1231.

87. Norton KI, et al. Epiphyseal involvement in osteosarcoma. *Radiology.* 1991;180(3):813–816.
88. Murphey MD, et al. From the archives of the AFIP: imaging of primary chondrosarcoma: radiologic-pathologic correlation. *Radiographics.* 2003;23(5):1245–1278.
89. Kurt AM, et al. Low-grade intraosseous osteosarcoma. *Cancer.* 1990;65(6):1418–1428.
90. Bertoni F, et al. Osteosarcoma. Low-grade intraosseous-type osteosarcoma, histologically resembling parosteal osteosarcoma, fibrous dysplasia, and desmoplastic fibroma. *Cancer.* 1993; 71(2):338–345.
91. Malhas AM, et al. Low-grade central osteosarcoma: a difficult condition to diagnose. *Sarcoma.* 2012;2012:764796.
92. Lazar A, Mertens F. Parosteal osteosarcoma. In: Fletcher CDM, Bridge JA, Hogendoorn PCW, et al., eds. *WHO Classification of Tumours of Soft Tissue and Bone.* 4th ed. Lyon, France: IARC; 2013:292–293.
93. Okada K, et al. Parosteal osteosarcoma. A clinicopathological study. *J Bone Joint Surg Am.* 1994;76(3):366–3178.
94. Murphey MD, et al. Imaging of periosteal osteosarcoma: radiologic-pathologic comparison. *Radiology.* 2004;233(1):129–138.
95. Yarmish G, et al. Imaging characteristics of primary osteosarcoma: nonconventional subtypes. *Radiographics.* 2010;30(6):1653–1672.
96. Bechler JR, et al. Osteosarcoma as a second malignant neoplasm in children. *J Bone Joint Surg Am.* 1992;74(7):1079–1083.
97. Young JL Jr, et al. Cancer incidence, survival, and mortality for children younger than age 15 years. *Cancer.* 1986;58(2 suppl):598–602.
98. Javery O, et al. A to Z of extraskeletal Ewing sarcoma family of tumors in adults: imaging features of primary disease, metastatic patterns, and treatment responses. *AJR Am J Roentgenol.* 2011;197(6):W1015–W1022.
99. Murphey MD, et al. From the radiologic pathology archives: ewing sarcoma family of tumors: radiologic-pathologic correlation. *Radiographics.* 2013;33(3):803–831.
100. Qureshi SS, et al. Prognostic factors in primary nonmetastatic Ewing sarcoma of the rib in children and young adults. *J Pediatr Surg.* 2013;48(4):764–770.
101. Granowetter L, West DC. The Ewing's sarcoma family of tumors: Ewing's sarcoma and peripheral primitive neuroectodermal tumor of bone and soft tissue. *Cancer Treat Res.* 1997;92: 253–308.
102. Reinus WR, Gilula LA. Radiology of Ewing's sarcoma; intergroup Ewing's sarcoma study (IESS). *Radiographics.* 1984;4: 929–944.
103. Crist WM, Kun LE. Common solid tumors of childhood. *N Engl J Med.* 1991;324(7):461–471.
104. Shapeero LG, et al. Periosteal Ewing sarcoma. *Radiology.* 1994;191(3):825–831.
105. Stiller CA, et al. Bone tumours in European children and adolescents, 1978–1997;Report from the Automated Childhood Cancer Information System project. *Eur J Cancer.* 2006; 42(13):2124–2135.
106. Kaste SC. Imaging pediatric bone sarcomas. *Radiol Clin North Am.* 2011;49(4):749–765, vi–vii.
107. Schwartz HS, et al. The malignant potential of enchondromatosis. *J Bone Joint Surg Am.* 1987;69(2):269–274.
108. Aprin H, Riseborough EJ, Hall JE. Chondrosarcoma in children and adolescents. *Clin Orthop Relat Res.* 1982(166):226–232.
109. Memis A, et al. Clear cell chondrosarcoma: unusual radiologic appearances with histologic correlation. *Eur Radiol.* 2002;12(2):427–430.
110. Douis H, Saifuddin A. The imaging of cartilaginous bone tumours. II Chondrosarcoma. *Skeletal Radiol.* 2013;42(5): 611–626.
111. Dantonello TM, et al. Mesenchymal chondrosarcoma of soft tissues and bone in children, adolescents, and young adults: experiences of the CWS and COSS study groups. *Cancer.* 2008;112(11):2424–2431.
112. Barai S, et al. Role of skeletal scintigraphy in advanced retinoblastomas. *Acta Radiol.* 2004;45(3):313–316.
113. Lee HJ, et al. Metachronous multifocal osteosarcoma: a case report and literature review. *Clin Imaging.* 2002;26(1):63–68.
114. DuBois SG, et al. Metastatic sites in stage IV and IVS neuroblastoma correlate with age, tumor biology, and survival. *J Pediatr Hematol Oncol.* 1999;21(3):181–189.
115. Meyer JS, et al. Which MRI sequence of the spine best reveals bone-marrow metastases of neuroblastoma? *Pediatr Radiol.* 2005;35(8):778–785.
116. Hahn K, Charron M, Shulkin BL. Role of MR imaging and iodine 123 MIBG scintigraphy in staging of pediatric neuroblastoma. *Radiology.* 2003;227(3):908; author reply 908–909.
117. Merrow AC, Laor T. Leukemia and treatment: imprint on the growing skeleton. *Pediatr Radiol.* 2008;38(5):594.
118. Pui MH, Fletcher BD, Langston JW. Granulocytic sarcoma in childhood leukemia: imaging features. *Radiology.* 1994;190(3):698–702.
119. Krishnan A, et al. Primary bone lymphoma: radiographic-MR imaging correlation. *Radiographics.* 2003;23(6):1371–1383; discussion 1384–1387.
120. Sato TS, Ferguson PJ, Khanna G. Primary multifocal osseous lymphoma in a child. *Pediatr Radiol.* 2008;38(12):1338–1341.
121. Kirsch J, et al. The incidence of imaging findings, and the distribution of skeletal lymphoma in a consecutive patient population seen over 5 years. *Skeletal Radiol.* 2006;35(8):590–594.
122. Chew FS, Schellingerhout D, Keel SB. Primary lymphoma of skeletal muscle. *AJR Am J Roentgenol.* 1999;172(5):1370.
123. Goldblum JR, Folpe AL, Weiss SW. *Enzinger and Weiss's Soft Tissue Tumors*, 6th ed. Philadelphia: Elsevier Saunders, 2014, pp. 766–783.
124. Bravo SM, Winalski CS, Weissman BN. Pigmented villonodular synovitis. *Radiol Clin North Am.* 1996;34(2):311–326, x–xi.
125. Murphey MD, et al. Pigmented villonodular synovitis: radiologic-pathologic correlation. *Radiographics.* 2008;28(5):1493–1518.
126. Myers BW, Masi AT. Pigmented villonodular synovitis and tenosynovitis: a clinical epidemiologic study of 166 cases and literature review. *Medicine (Baltimore).* 1980;59(3):223–238.
127. West RB, Rubin BP, Miller MA, et al. A landscape effect in tenosynovial giant-cell tumor from activation of CSF1 expression by a translocation in a minority of tumor cells. *Proc Natl Acad Sci U S A.* 2006;103(3):690–695.
128. Dinauer PA, et al. Pathologic and MR imaging features of benign fibrous soft-tissue tumors in adults. *Radiographics.* 2007;27(1):173–187.
129. Crotty JM, Monu JU, Pope TL. Synovial osteochondromatosis. *Radiol Clin North Am.* 1996;34:327–342.
130. Resnick D. Tumors and tumor-like lesions of soft tissues. In: Resnick D, ed. *Diagnosis of Bone and Joint Disorders.* 4th ed. Philadelphia, PA: Saunders; 2002:4204–4273.
131. Kramer J, et al. MR appearance of idiopathic synovial osteochondromatosis. *J Comput Assist Tomogr.* 1993;17(5): 772–776.
132. Conrad EU III, Enneking WF. Common soft tissue tumors. *Clin Symp.* 1990;42(1):2–32.

133. Cardinal E, et al. Occult dorsal carpal ganglion: comparison of US and MR imaging. *Radiology.* 1994;193(1):259–262.
134. Fornage BD, Rifkin MD. Ultrasound examination of the hand and foot. *Radiol Clin North Am.* 1988;26(1):109–129.
135. Tsai TS, et al. Fat necrosis after trauma: a benign cause of palpable lumps in children. *AJR Am J Roentgenol.* 1997; 169(6):1623–1626.
136. Chan LP, et al. Imaging features of fat necrosis. *AJR Am J Roentgenol.* 2003;181(4):955–959.
137. Lopez JA, et al. MRI diagnosis and follow-up of subcutaneous fat necrosis. *J Magn Reson Imaging.* 1997;7(5):929–932.
138. Alomari AI, Spencer SA, Arnold RW, et al. Fibro-adipose vascular anomaly: clinical-radiologic-pathologic features of a newly delineated disorder of the extremity. *J Pediatr Ortho.* 2014;34(1):109–117.
139. Fetsch JF, Miettinen M, Laskin WB, et al. A clinicopathologic study of 45 pediatric soft tissue tumors with an admixture of adipose tissue and fibroblastic elements, and a proposal for classification as lipofibromatosis. *Am J Surg Pathol.* 2000; 24(11):1491–1500.
140. Kurek KC, Howard E, Tennant LB, et al. PTEN hamartoma of soft tissue: a distinctive lesion in PTEN syndromes. *Am J Surg Pathol.* 2012;36(5):671–687.
141. Kransdorf MJ, et al. Imaging of fatty tumors: distinction of lipoma and well-differentiated liposarcoma. *Radiology.* 2002;224(1):99–104.
142. Murphey MD, et al. From the archives of the AFIP: benign musculoskeletal lipomatous lesions. *Radiographics.* 2004; 24(5):1433–1466.
143. Leffell DJ, Braverman IM. Familial multiple lipomatosis. Report of a case and a review of the literature. *J Am Acad Dermatol.* 1986;15(2 Pt 1):275–279.
144. Vellios F, Baez J, Shumacker HB. Lipoblastomatosis: a tumor of fetal fat different from hibernoma; report of a case, with observations on the embryogenesis of human adipose tissue. *Am J Pathol.* 1958;34(6):1149–1159.
145. Kransdorf MJ. Benign soft-tissue tumors in a large referral population: distribution of specific diagnoses by age, sex, and location. *AJR Am J Roentgenol.* 1995;164(2):395–402.
146. Chung EB, Enzinger FM. Benign lipoblastomatosis. An analysis of 35 cases. *Cancer.* 1973;32(2):482–492.
147. Kransdorf MJ, et al. Fat-containing soft-tissue masses of the extremities. *Radiographics.* 1991;11(1):81–106.
148. Reiseter T, et al. Lipoblastoma: MRI appearances of a rare paediatric soft tissue tumour. *Pediatr Radiol.* 1999;29(7):542–545.
149. Silverman JS, Hamilton J, Tamsen A. Benign recurring lipoblastoma in an adult versus well differentiated subcutaneous myxoid liposarcoma: clinicopathologic, immunohistochemical and molecular analysis of a unique case. *Pathol Res Pract.* 1999;195(11):787–792; discussion 793.
150. Donnelly LF, Bisset GS III, Passo MH. MRI findings of lipoma arborescens of the knee in a child: case report. *Pediatr Radiol.* 1994;24(4):258–259.
151. Vilanova JC, et al. MR imaging of lipoma arborescens and the associated lesions. *Skeletal Radiol.* 2003;32(9):504–509.
152. Sheldon PJ, Forrester DM, Learch TJ. Imaging of intraarticular masses. *Radiographics.* 2005;25(1):105–119.
153. Martin S, et al. Diagnostic imaging of lipoma arborescens. *Skeletal Radiol.* 1998;27(6):325–329.
154. Kransdorf MJ, Murphey MD. *Imaging of soft tissue tumors.* 2nd ed. Philadelphia, PA: Saunders; 2006:437–477.
155. Beiner JM, Jokl P. Muscle contusion injury and myositis ossificans traumatica. *Clin Orthop Relat Res.* 2002;(403 suppl):S110–S119.
156. Parikh J, Hyare H, Saifuddin A. The imaging features of post-traumatic myositis ossificans, with emphasis on MRI. *Clin Radiol.* 2002;57(12):1058–1066.
157. de Silva MV, Reid R. Myositis ossificans and fibroosseous pseudotumor of digits: a clinicopathological review of 64 cases with emphasis on diagnostic pitfalls. *Int J Surg Pathol.* 2003;11(3):187–195.
158. Goldman AB. Myositis ossificans circumscripta: a benign lesion with a malignant differential diagnosis. *AJR Am J Roentgenol.* 1976;126(1):32–40.
159. Lee BB, et al. Terminology and classification of congenital vascular malformations. *Phlebology.* 2007;22(6):249–252.
160. Mulliken JB, Burrows PE, Fishman SJ, eds. *Mulliken and Young's Vascular Anomalies: Hemangiomas and Malformations.* 2nd ed. New York: Oxford University Press; 2013.
161. Weiss S, Goldblum J. Benign tumors and tumor-like lesions of blood vessels. In: *Enzinger and Weiss's Soft Tissue Tumors.* 4th ed. St Louis: CV Mosby; 2001:837–890.
162. Mulliken JB, Glowacki J. Hemangiomas and vascular malformations in infants and children: a classification based on endothelial characteristics. *Plast Reconstr Surg.* 1982;69(3):412–422.
163. Lowe LH, et al. Vascular malformations: classification and terminology the radiologist needs to know. *Semin Roentgenol.* 2012;47(2):106–117.
164. Donnelly LF, Adams DM, Bisset GS III. Vascular malformations and hemangiomas: a practical approach in a multidisciplinary clinic. *AJR Am J Roentgenol.* 2000;174(3):597–608.
165. Frieden IJ, et al. Infantile hemangiomas: current knowledge, future directions. Proceedings of a research workshop on infantile hemangiomas, April 7–9, 2005, Bethesda, Maryland, USA. *Pediatr Dermatol.* 2005;22(5):383–406.
166. Teo EL, Strouse PJ, Hernandez RJ. MR imaging differentiation of soft-tissue hemangiomas from malignant soft-tissue masses. *AJR Am J Roentgenol.* 2000;174(6):1623–1628.
167. Legiehn GM, Heran MK. Classification, diagnosis, and interventional radiologic management of vascular malformations. *Orthop Clin North Am.* 2006;37(3):435–474; vii–viii.
168. Lim R, et al. Superficial neurofibroma: a lesion with unique MRI characteristics in patients with neurofibromatosis type 1. *AJR Am J Roentgenol.* 2005;184(3):962–968.
169. Kransdorf MJ, Murphey MD. *Imaging of Soft Tissue Tumors.* 2nd ed. Philadelphia, PA: Saunders; 2006:328–374.
170. Ferner RE, Gutmann DH. International consensus statement on malignant peripheral nerve sheath tumors in neurofibromatosis. *Cancer Res.* 2002;62(5):1573–1577.
171. Meyer CA, et al. MR and CT appearance of nodular fasciitis. *J Comput Assist Tomogr.* 1991;15(2):276–279.
172. Wang XL, et al. Nodular fasciitis: correlation of MRI findings and histopathology. *Skeletal Radiol.* 2002;31(3):155–161.
173. Leung LY, et al. Nodular fasciitis: MRI appearance and literature review. *Skeletal Radiol.* 2002;31(1):9–13.
174. Robbin MR, et al. Imaging of musculoskeletal fibromatosis. *Radiographics.* 2001;21(3):585–600.
175. Chung EB, Enzinger FM. Infantile myofibromatosis. *Cancer.* 1981;48(8):1807–1818.
176. Mentzel T. Bridge JA. Myopericytyoma, including myofibroma. In: Fletcher CDM, Bridge JA, Hogendoorn PCW, et al. eds. *WHO Classification of Tumours of Soft Tissue and Bone.* 4th ed. Lyon, France: IARC Press; 2013.

177. Kransdorf MJ, Murphey MD. *Imaging of Soft Tissue Tumors.* 2nd ed. Philadelphia, PA: Saunders; 2006:189–249.
178. Muhlbauer JE. Granuloma annulare. *J Am Acad Dermatol.* 1980;3(3):217–230.
179. Chung S, et al. Subcutaneous granuloma annulare: MR imaging features in six children and literature review. *Radiology.* 1999; 210(3):845–849.
180. Kransdorf MJ, Murphey MD, Temple HT. Subcutaneous granuloma annulare: radiologic appearance. *Skeletal Radiol.* 1998;27(5):266–270.
181. Yu GV, Farrer AK. Benign rheumatoid nodule versus subcutaneous granuloma annulare: a diagnostic dilemma—are they the same entity? *J Foot Ankle Surg.* 1994;33(2):156–166.
182. Pappo AS, Pratt CB. Soft tissue sarcomas in children. *Cancer Treat Res.* 1997;91:205–222.
183. Pastore G, et al. Childhood soft tissue sarcomas incidence and survival in European children (1978–1997): report from the Automated Childhood Cancer Information System project. *Eur J Cancer.* 2006;42(13):2136–2149.
184. Meyer WH, Spunt SL. Soft tissue sarcomas of childhood. *Cancer Treat Rev.* 2004;30(3):269–280.
185. Fletcher CD. The evolving classification of soft tissue tumours—an update based on the new 2013 WHO classification. *Histopathology.* 2014;64(1):2–11.
186. Brisse HJ, Orbach D, Klijanienko J. Soft tissue tumours: imaging strategy. *Pediatr Radiol.* 2010;40(6):1019–1028.
187. Park K, van Rijn R, McHugh K. The role of radiology in paediatric soft tissue sarcomas. *Cancer Imaging.* 2008;8:102–115.
188. Bixby SD, et al. Synovial sarcoma in children: imaging features and common benign mimics. *AJR Am J Roentgenol.* 2010;195(4):1026–1032.
189. Wu JS, Hochman MG. Soft-tissue tumors and tumorlike lesions: a systematic imaging approach. *Radiology.* 2009;253(2):297–316.
190. van Vliet M, et al. Soft tissue sarcomas at a glance: clinical, histological, and MR imaging features of malignant extremity soft tissue tumors. *Eur Radiol.* 2009;19(6):1499–1511.
191. Laor T. MR imaging of soft tissue tumors and tumor-like lesions. *Pediatr Radiol.* 2004;34(1):24–37.
192. Lowenthal D, et al. Differentiation of myxoid liposarcoma by magnetic resonance imaging: a histopathologic correlation. *Acta Radiol.* 2014;55(8):952–960.
193. O'Regan KN, et al. Imaging of liposarcoma: classification, patterns of tumor recurrence, and response to treatment. *AJR Am J Roentgenol.* 2011;197(1):W37–W43.
194. Murphey MD, Arcara LK, Fanburg-Smith J. From the archives of the AFIP: imaging of musculoskeletal liposarcoma with radiologic-pathologic correlation. *Radiographics.* 2005;25(5):1371–1395.
195. Coffin CM, Sorenson PH. Infantile fibrosarcoma. In: Fletcher CDM, Bridge JA, Hogendoorn PCW, et al., eds. *WHO Classification of Tumours of Soft Tissue and Bone.* 4th ed. Lyon, France: IARC Press; 2013:89–90.
196. Canale S, et al. Infantile fibrosarcoma: magnetic resonance imaging findings in six cases. *Eur J Radiol.* 2009;72(1):30–37.
197. Vinnicombe SJ, Hall CM. Infantile fibrosarcoma: radiological and clinical features. *Skeletal Radiol.* 1994;23(5):337–341.
198. Mendenhall WM, Zlotecki RA, Scarborough MT. Dermatofibrosarcoma protuberans. *Cancer.* 2004;101(11):2503–2508.
199. Torreggiani WC, et al. Dermatofibrosarcoma protuberans: MR imaging features. *AJR Am J Roentgenol.* 2002;178(4):989–993.
200. Dagan R, et al. Radiotherapy in the treatment of dermatofibrosarcoma protuberans. *Am J Clin Oncol.* 2005;28(6):537–539.
201. Ognjanovic S, et al. Trends in childhood rhabdomyosarcoma incidence and survival in the United States, 1975–2005. *Cancer.* 2009;115(18):4218–4226.
202. Van Rijn RR, et al. Imaging findings in noncraniofacial childhood rhabdomyosarcoma. *Pediatr Radiol.* 2008;38(6):617–634.
203. McCarville MB, Spunt SL, Pappo AS. Rhabdomyosarcoma in pediatric patients: the good, the bad, and the unusual. *AJR Am J Roentgenol.* 2001;176(6):1563–1569.
204. Simmons M, Tucker AK. The radiology of bone changes in rhabdomyosarcoma. *Clin Radiol.* 1978;29(1):47–52.
205. Shapeero LG, et al. Bone metastases as the presenting manifestation of rhabdomyosarcoma in childhood. *Skeletal Radiol.* 1993;22(6):433–438.
206. Perez EA, et al. Rhabdomyosarcoma in children: a SEER population based study. *J Surg Res.* 2011;170(2):e243–e251.
207. Hryhorczuk AL, et al. Imaging findings in children with proliferative disorders following multivisceral transplantation. *Pediatr Radiol.* 2015;45(8):1138–1145.
208. Deyrup AT, et al. Epithelioid hemangioendothelioma of soft tissue: a proposal for risk stratification based on 49 cases. *Am J Surg Pathol.* 2008;32(6):924–947.
209. Weiss SW, et al. Epithelioid hemangioendothelioma and related lesions. *Semin Diagn Pathol.* 1986;3(4):259–287.
210. Bruder E, et al. Vascular and perivascular lesions of skin and soft tissues in children and adolescents. *Pediatr Dev Pathol.* 2012;15(1 suppl):26–61.
211. Lalaji TA, Haller JO, Burgess RJ. A case of head and neck kaposiform hemangioendothelioma simulating a malignancy on imaging. *Pediatr Radiol.* 2001;31(12):876–878.
212. Botash RJ, Oliphant M, Capaldo G. Imaging of congenital kaposiform retroperitoneal hemangioendothelioma associated with Kasabach-Merritt syndrome. *Clin Imaging.* 1996;20(1):17–20.
213. Chen YJ, et al. MRI of multifocal kaposiform haemangioendothelioma without Kasabach-Merritt phenomenon. *Br J Radiol.* 2009;82(975):e51–e54.
214. Zukerberg LR, Nickoloff BJ, Weiss SW. Kaposiform hemangioendothelioma of infancy and childhood. An aggressive neoplasm associated with Kasabach-Merritt syndrome and lymphangiomatosis. *Am J Surg Pathol.* 1993;17(4):321–328.
215. Fahrtash F, McCahon E, Arbuckle S. Successful treatment of kaposiform hemangioendothelioma and tufted angioma with vincristine. *J Pediatr Hematol Oncol.* 2010;32(6):506–510.
216. Lang N, Liu XG, Yuan HS. Malignant peripheral nerve sheath tumor in spine: imaging manifestations. *Clin Imaging.* 2012; 36(3):209–215.
217. Carli M, et al. Pediatric malignant peripheral nerve sheath tumor: the Italian and German soft tissue sarcoma cooperative group. *J Clin Oncol.* 2005;23(33):8422–8430.
218. Kerouanton A, et al. Synovial sarcoma in children and adolescents. *J Pediatr Hematol Oncol.* 2014;36(4):257–262.
219. Wilkerson BW, et al. Characterization of synovial sarcoma calcification. *AJR Am J Roentgenol.* 2012;199(6):W730–W734.
220. Jones BC, Sundaram M, Kransdorf MJ. Synovial sarcoma: MR imaging findings in 34 patients. *AJR Am J Roentgenol.* 1993;161(4):827–830.
221. Bakri A, et al. Synovial sarcoma: imaging features of common and uncommon primary sites, metastatic patterns, and treatment response. *AJR Am J Roentgenol.* 2012;199(2):W208–W215.
222. McCarville MB, et al. Synovial sarcoma in pediatric patients. *AJR Am J Roentgenol.* 2002;179(3):797–801.

223. Gielen JL, et al. Accuracy of MRI in characterization of soft tissue tumors and tumor-like lesions. A prospective study in 548 patients. *Eur Radiol.* 2004;14(12):2320–2330.
224. Viry F, et al. Alveolar soft part sarcoma-radiologic patterns in children and adolescents. *Pediatr Radiol.* 2013;43(9):1174–1181.
225. Pang LM, et al. Alveolar soft-part sarcoma: a rare soft-tissue malignancy with distinctive clinical and radiological features. *Pediatr Radiol.* 2001;31(3):196–199.
226. Kobos R, et al. Combining integrated genomics and functional genomics to dissect the biology of a cancer-associated, aberrant transcription factor, the ASPSCR1-TFE3 fusion oncoprotein. *J Pathol.* 2013;229(5):743–754.
227. Casanova M, et al. Epithelioid sarcoma in children and adolescents: a report from the Italian Soft Tissue Sarcoma Committee. *Cancer.* 2006;106(3):708–717.
228. Tateishi U, et al. Radiologic manifestations of proximal-type epithelioid sarcoma of the soft tissues. *AJR Am J Roentgenol.* 2002;179(4):973–977.
229. Sredni ST, Tomita T. Rhabdoid tumor predisposition syndrome. *Pediatr Dev Pathol.* 2015;18(1):49–58.
230. Dobbs MD, et al. Extrarenal rhabdoid tumor mimicking a sacral peripheral nerve sheath tumor. *Skeletal Radiol.* 2011;40(10):1363–1368.

CHAPTER 24

Musculoskeletal Traumatic Disorders

Mark E. Bittman • Jeannette M. Peréz-Rosselló • Donald A. Tracy • Abdusamea Shabani • Edward Y. Lee

INTRODUCTION

Trauma to the musculoskeletal system is common, and imaging plays a crucial role in the evaluation of the injured child. Knowledge of the normal appearance of the immature skeleton and familiarity with variants of normal anatomy are essential when evaluating the imaging of a pediatric patient with suspected traumatic injuries. The presence of growth plates in infants and children results in different fracture patterns and healing processes compared with those of adults. The physical properties of the skeletally immature bone are also different from those of adult bones. Skeletally immature bones are more porous and less mineralized than are mature bones, allowing for elasticity and plastic deformation prior to fracturing. Additionally, the periosteum of children's bones is thicker and stronger than the periosteum of adult bones, which limits displacement of fracture fragments.[1–3]

In this chapter, the current imaging techniques and protocol guidelines for assessing the pediatric musculoskeletal trauma are reviewed. This chapter also discusses common injuries of pediatric patients on a bone-by-bone assessment including imaging findings, complications of healing, and treatment of injuries. In addition, an overview of accidental and nonaccidental musculoskeletal trauma is provided, with specific discussions on common mimickers of musculoskeletal injuries related to child abuse. Finally, common sports injuries in children are presented.

IMAGING TECHNIQUES

Radiography

Radiographs are typically the initial examination in the evaluation of a pediatric patient with trauma to the musculoskeletal system. Radiographs are readily available, cost effective, and highly sensitive to the detection of fractures and malalignment. However, one should minimize radiation exposure to children by using radiography judiciously and paying close attention to technical factors including collimation and exposure parameters.

The main utility of radiographs in the setting of trauma is to detect fractures. Radiographs define the anatomic relationship between a fracture line and the joint space or growth plate. This information determines fracture classification and has prognostic and treatment implications. Radiographs readily demonstrate displacement and angulation of fracture fragments. Joint subluxations and dislocations are often easily detected with radiographic evaluation. Follow-up radiographs are used to assess healing, to determine anatomic alignment after open or closed reduction of displaced fractures, and to evaluate for potential complications of orthopedic hardware.

A minimum of two orthogonal views is recommended to fully assess a suspected long bone fracture. The proximal and distal joints on either side of a long bone should be included in the field of view to ensure adequate anatomic coverage. Injuries to joints usually require a minimum of three views, namely, anteroposterior (AP), oblique, and lateral views. When specific types of injuries are clinically suspected, specialized views can be obtained, and it is helpful to tailor the examination based on the clinical query. For example, a 30-degree ulnar deviated view of the wrist is helpful in the detection of an early and subtle nondisplaced scaphoid fracture, which has important clinical implications if not diagnosed and managed in a timely fashion. In select cases where the radiographic diagnosis of a fracture is equivocal, obtaining a comparison view of the contralateral asymptomatic side may be helpful to ascertain whether a finding represents an injury or a normal variation of the anatomy.

Radiographic evaluation of soft tissues is limited and lacks the capability for discrimination of fluid from synovium in joints. However, the presence of soft tissue edema and/or joint effusion may guide additional imaging workup. Radiopaque foreign bodies can be detected on radiographs depending on their composition.

Ultrasound

At present, musculoskeletal ultrasound (US) is not commonly used in the evaluation of musculoskeletal injuries to the pediatric patient. However, in recent years, its use is gaining popularity because it can complement radiography in select cases and may add important information about soft tissue, bony, and cartilaginous injuries in children.[4]

A main advantage of US is the real-time dynamic assessment of the injured area without ionizing radiation. Also, because sedation is not usually required, US may be an alternative to magnetic resonance imaging (MRI) in very young pediatric patients who would otherwise have to undergo an MRI with sedation or anesthesia. Portability and rapid acquisition of images obtained at the bedside are other attractive features of US in the pediatric trauma patient.

High-frequency linear transducers (7.5 to 15 MHz) are typically used to assess superficial musculoskeletal structures. Lower frequency curved or vector transducers can be used to increase tissue penetration and improve visualization of deeper structures, especially in a child with a large body habitus. For demonstrating large continuous areas of anatomy, extended field-of-view software is useful. The split-screen function can provide side-by-side comparisons of the affected and normal contralateral sides. Such comparison is often valuable in situations where a finding is subtle in the symptomatic side. Color, power, and pulsed Doppler techniques are useful for assessing alterations of blood flow to injured tissue such as muscular hematomas and reactive synovitis.

US can be used for evaluation of fractures as well as injuries involving the soft tissues, tendons, and ligaments in the setting of trauma. Evaluation of fractures may be limited with US; however, an unsuspected fracture may be detected incidentally when US is used for assessment of adjacent soft tissue injury. US can detect disruption of ligaments and tendons that are superficially located. In addition, radial head dislocation, posterior shoulder subluxation, and upper extremity birth trauma are other potential clinical scenarios where US may be beneficial.[4–9] Furthermore, when a radiopaque foreign body such as wood is suspected, a targeted US may identify the foreign body or the soft tissue reaction around it.[9]

Computed Tomography

Although a powerful imaging tool, multidetector computed tomography (MDCT) should be used judiciously because of the ionizing effects to the radiosensitive child.[10] MDCT with multiplanar reformation (MPR) and three-dimensional (3D) imaging offers diagnostic advantages over radiographs in areas of complex orthopedic injury.[11] MDCT can define or exclude a fracture that is occult or equivocal on radiographs. The administration of contrast media may be indicated when concomitant vascular injury is suspected.[11,12]

MDCT allows for faster scan speeds and thinner collimation, resulting in submillimeter slice thickness. Thin-slice volume acquisition of data enables isotropic voxels resulting in excellent spatial resolution and multiplanar reformation without degradation in imaging quality. Rapid acquisition decreases the need for sedation and minimizes motion artifact in the pediatric patient who may have difficulties for remaining motionless. Scan parameters depend on whether high detail is necessary for small areas of anatomy or if large areas of anatomy are to be scanned. Specific scan parameters for imaging the musculoskeletal system include 100 kVp, range of 25 to 200 mA, and scan time of 0.5 s/rotation.[13] Radiation dose reduction techniques are rapidly evolving, and frequent revision of scan parameters and imaging protocols is recommended to ensure compliance with the principle of as low as reasonable achievable (ALARA).

The degree of displacement and relationship of fracture fragments influence the decision for surgical management. Multiplanar 2D and 3D CT reformations can define the relationship of fracture planes to the joint space and growth plate. On occasion, pathologic fractures through underlying bony lesions can be better characterized with MDCT. Fracture healing and complications of fractures, such as bony bars, are well depicted on MDCT.[11] However, the evaluation of soft tissue structures, such as ligaments, muscles, and tendons, is limited with MDCT and is best achieved with US or MRI.

Magnetic Resonance Imaging

MRI is a powerful imaging tool for the evaluation of musculoskeletal trauma. It provides excellent contrast resolution, superior depiction of soft tissue structures, and visualization of hyaline cartilage without ionizing radiation. In the acute setting, MRI can identify radiographically occult injuries such as osseous contusions, chondral and osteochondral fractures, and tendon and ligamentous injuries.[14,15] In the subacute and chronic setting, MRI can assess for complications such as growth plate arrest or superimposed infection.

For MRI techniques, the pediatric patient should be placed in a comfortable position with passive restraints applied to the region of interest to minimize motion artifacts. A body coil may be used when a large field of view is needed. However, when possible, a phased array coil or surface coil, which can be optimally fit into the area of interest and provide better quality MR images, should be used. The main MR pulse sequences currently used for evaluating musculoskeletal injuries include T1-weighted, inversion recovery (STIR), fast spin-echo T2–weighted, gradient-echo, and proton density sequences.

Inversion recovery (STIR) sequences are the most sensitive for detecting abnormal bone marrow signal due to trauma. Fast spin-echo T2–weighted sequences are also sensitive to detect abnormal marrow signal, but incomplete fat suppression may occur, potentially mimicking pathology. Gradient-echo sequences can be employed to evaluate cartilage injuries. Proton density sequences are helpful to evaluate ligaments and tendons. Intravenous contrast material is not routinely administered in the setting of acute trauma. However, it is useful for evaluating complications of trauma such as infections.

Nuclear Medicine

Bone scintigraphy, also known as "bone scan," is performed after the injection of bone-seeking radiotracers such as Tc-99m disphosphonates or 18-labeled sodium fluoride (18F-NaF). Planar, pinhole, SPECT, SPECT-CR, or PET-CT images are typically obtained. The role of bone scintigraphy in the setting of musculoskeletal trauma is somewhat limited, particularly in the pediatric population. Typical indications include the detection of occult fractures, stress injury, fracture healing, and bone fragment viability.[16–20] When orthopedic hardware limits fracture assessment on radiographs, bone scintigraphy may be performed as an alternative method of assessing healing. Hardware does not interfere with bone scintigraphy. The two types of nonunion—hypervascular and avascular—can be readily differentiated with a bone scan. Bone scintigraphy has been used in the postoperative setting following bone graft to assess bone graft viability.[21] For the detection of stress reaction, it is important to recognize that bone scintigraphy, once the gold standard, is highly sensitive but lacks specificity.

Correlation with contemporaneous anatomic studies often adds clinically useful diagnostic information. The functional information provided by bone scintigraphy can be complementary to the anatomic information from radiography, CT, or MRI.

Fluoroscopy

Fluoroscopically guided studies, which use real-time moving images of the internal structures, are often provided to orthopedic surgery colleagues during operative reduction of misaligned fractures. Fluoroscopy offers real-time guidance for the surgeon during orthopedic hardware placement.[22] Similarly, fluoroscopy can also help guide closed reduction of fractures prior to cast placement.

SPECTRUM OF PEDIATRIC FRACTURES

Physeal Fractures (Salter-Harris Fractures)

The presence of growth plates in children results in patterns of injuries different from those of adults. Growth plates or physes contribute to the longitudinal growth of long bones. Therefore, physeal injuries can result in growth disturbances. Trauma to the physis has important therapeutic and prognostic implications. Physeal injuries occur in 21% to 30% of pediatric long bone fractures.[23]

Although there are several classification systems to characterize a fracture involving the growth plate,[24] the most widely accepted is the Salter-Harris classification system (**Schematic P**), which enables an effective method of communication among health care professionals.[25] This classification system grades fractures as type I through V according to the risk increase for complications such as growth arrest. A type I fracture is a transverse fracture through the growth plate, with the fracture line traversing the zone of hypertrophic calcification. The epiphysis may separate from the intact metaphysis, or radiographs may be unremarkable (Fig. 24.1). The type II fracture is the most common growth plate injury accounting for ~75% of physeal fractures[26] (Fig. 24.2). The fracture plane involves a

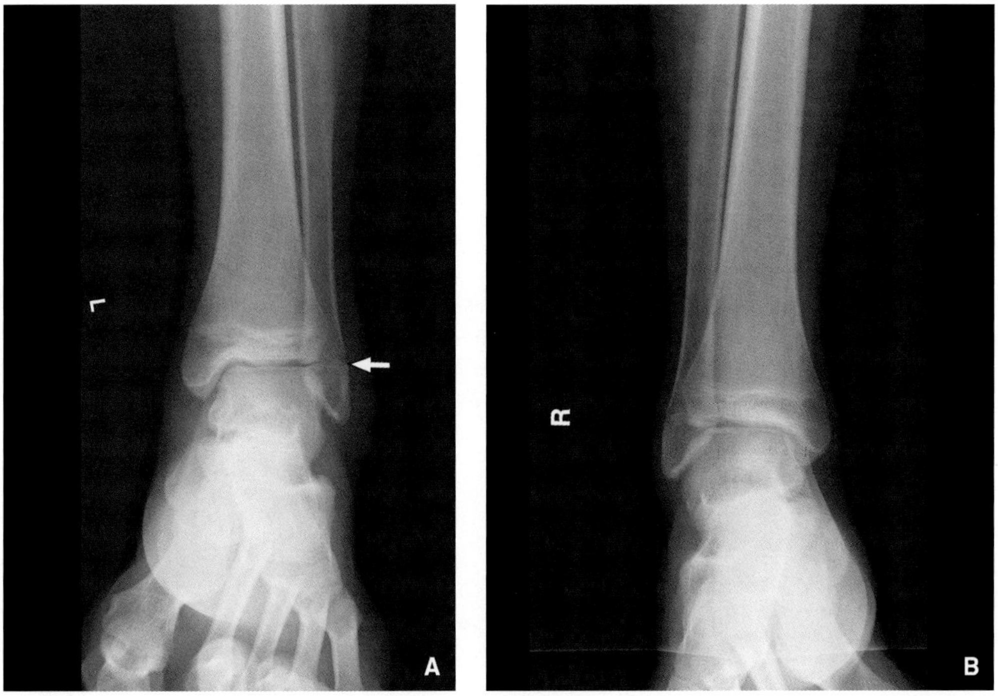

FIGURE 24.1 **Salter-Harris type I fracture of the distal fibula in a 16-year-old boy who presented with left ankle pain and swelling after an inversion injury.** **A:** Frontal radiograph of the left ankle demonstrates subtle widening of the distal fibular physis (*arrow*) with associated lateral soft tissue swelling. **B:** Comparison view of the asymptomatic right side reveals the normal appearance of the fibula increasing the confidence of a Salter-Harris I fracture on the left.

portion of the metaphysis and then propagates though the physis. The type III fracture involves a portion of the physis with the fracture line exiting the epiphysis into the articular surface (Fig. 24.3). A type IV fracture has an intra-articular fracture line through the epiphysis, physis, and metaphysis. The type V fracture is a crush injury to the growth plate and is the least common type. Fractures in the lower extremity usually have a worse prognosis than do those in other locations.[24,27]

Accidental Trauma

Musculoskeletal injuries of the appendicular skeleton by location is presented below (**Schematics I and II**).

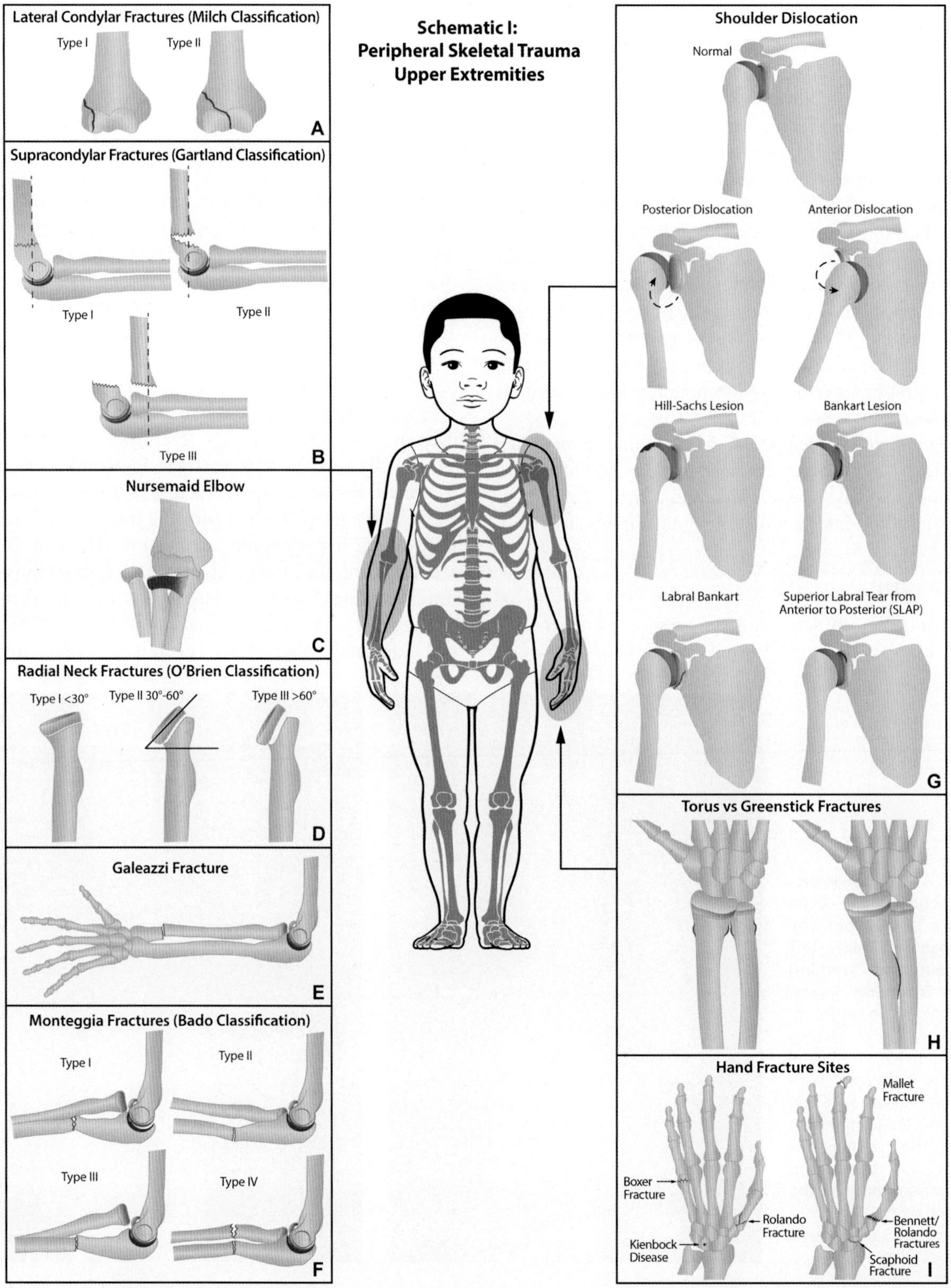

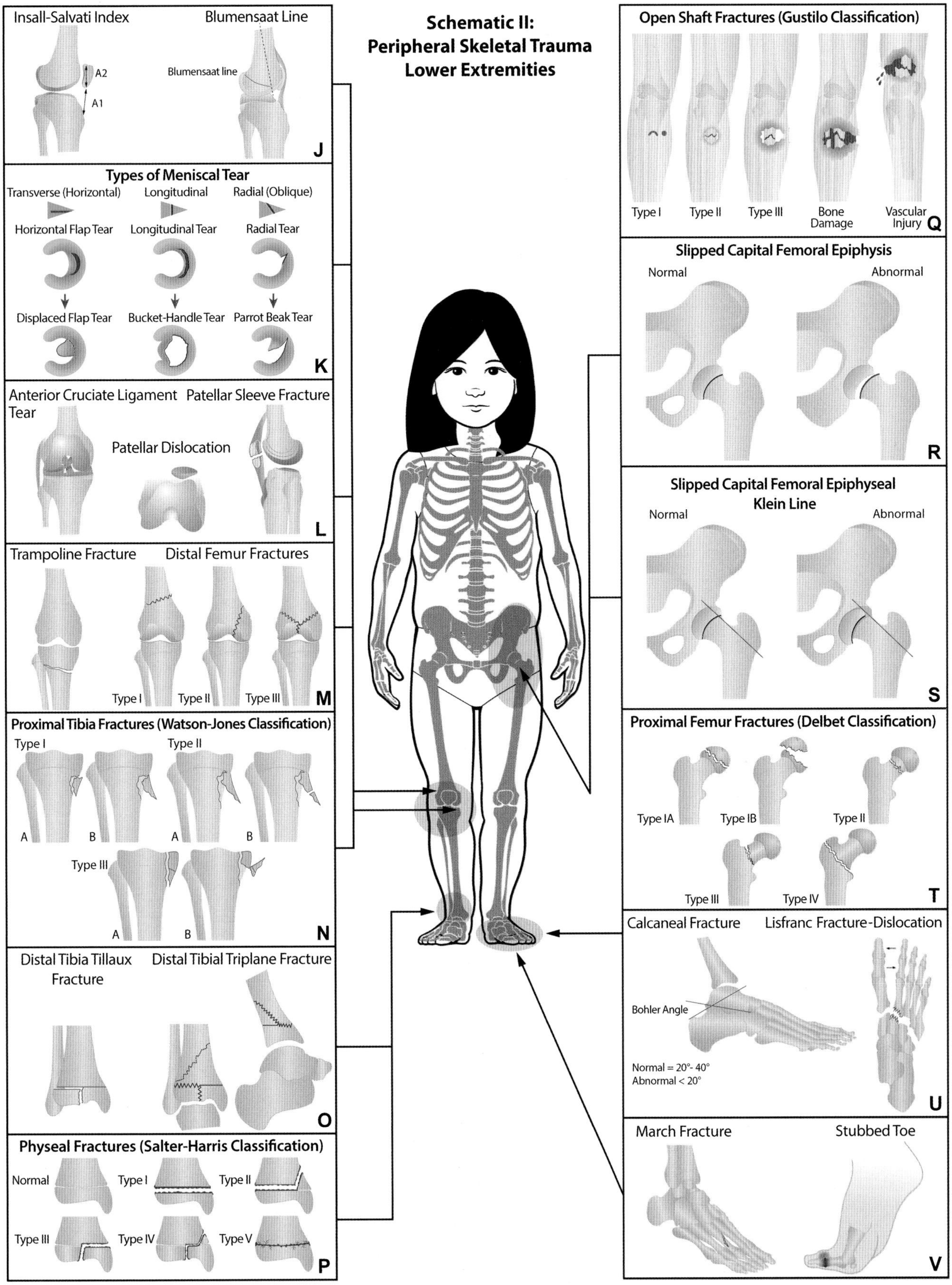
Schematic II: Peripheral Skeletal Trauma Lower Extremities
Insall-Salvati Index
Blumensaat Line
A2
A1
Blumensaat line
J
Types of Meniscal Tear
Transverse (Horizontal)
Longitudinal
Radial (Oblique)
Horizontal Flap Tear
Longitudinal Tear
Radial Tear
Displaced Flap Tear
Bucket-Handle Tear
Parrot Beak Tear
K
Anterior Cruciate Ligament Tear
Patellar Sleeve Fracture
Patellar Dislocation
L
Trampoline Fracture
Distal Femur Fractures
Type I
Type II
Type III
M
Proximal Tibia Fractures (Watson-Jones Classification)
Type I
Type II
A
B
A
B
Type III
A
B
N
Distal Tibia Tillaux Fracture
Distal Tibial Triplane Fracture
O
Physeal Fractures (Salter-Harris Classification)
Normal
Type I
Type II
Type III
Type IV
Type V
P
Open Shaft Fractures (Gustilo Classification)
Type I
Type II
Type III
Bone Damage
Vascular Injury
Q
Slipped Capital Femoral Epiphysis
Normal
Abnormal
R
Slipped Capital Femoral Epiphyseal Klein Line
Normal
Abnormal
S
Proximal Femur Fractures (Delbet Classification)
Type IA
Type IB
Type II
Type III
Type IV
T
Calcaneal Fracture
Lisfranc Fracture-Dislocation
Bohler Angle
Normal = 20°- 40°
Abnormal < 20°
U
March Fracture
Stubbed Toe
V

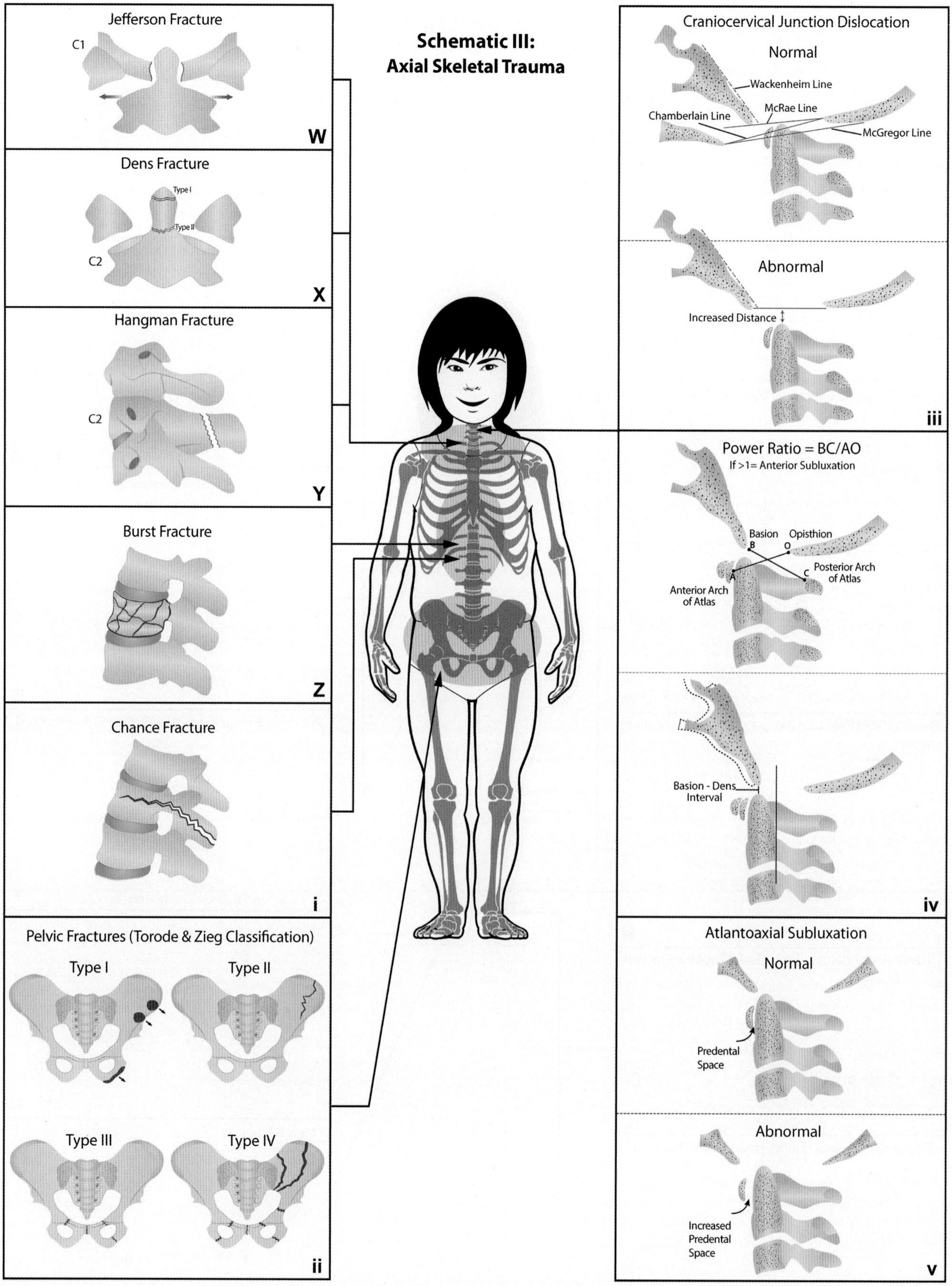
Schematic III:
Axial Skeletal Trauma
Jefferson Fracture
C1
W
Dens Fracture
Type I
Type II
C2
X
Hangman Fracture
C2
Y
Burst Fracture
Z
Chance Fracture
i
Pelvic Fractures (Torode & Zieg Classification)
Type I
Type II
Type III
Type IV
ii
Craniocervical Junction Dislocation
Normal
Wackenheim Line
McRae Line
Chamberlain Line
McGregor Line
Abnormal
Increased Distance
iii
Power Ratio = BC/AO
If >1= Anterior Subluxation
Basion
Opisthion
B
O
A
C
Posterior Arch of Atlas
Anterior Arch of Atlas
Basion - Dens Interval
iv
Atlantoaxial Subluxation
Normal
Predental Space
Abnormal
Increased Predental Space
v

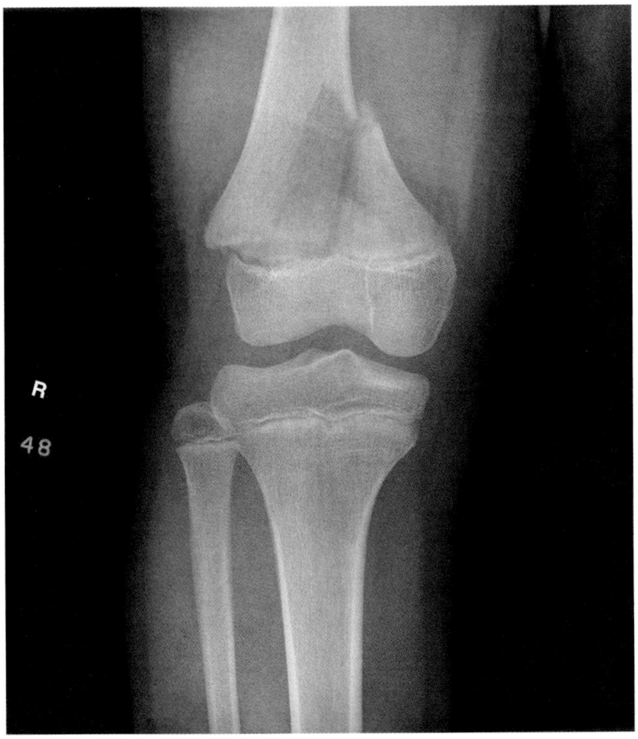

FIGURE 24.2 **Salter-Harris type II fracture of the distal femur in a 15-year-old girl.** Frontal radiograph of the right knee shows a fracture line through the metaphysis of the distal femur that exits the lateral aspect of the physis consistent with a Salter-Harris type II fracture.

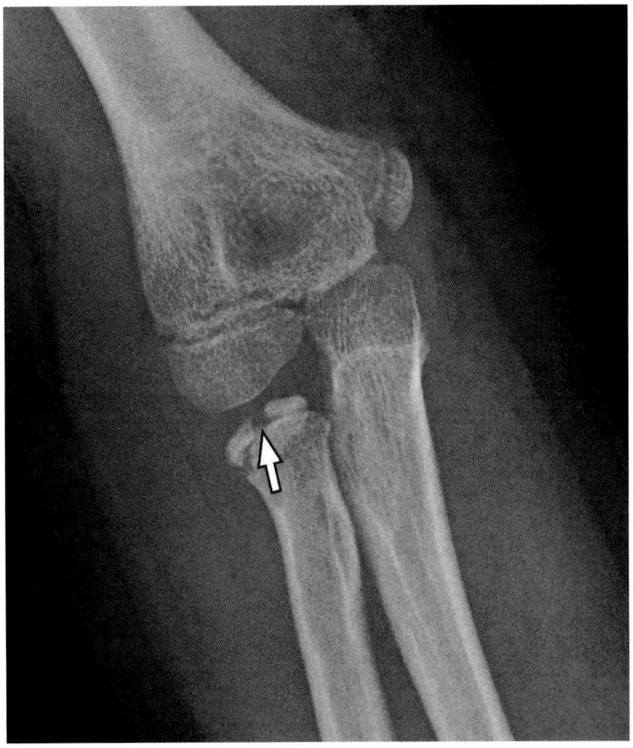

FIGURE 24.3 **Salter-Harris type III fracture of the proximal radius in a 13-year-old boy.** Frontal radiograph of the elbow shows a fracture (*arrow*) through the epiphysis of the proximal radius with extension into the physis.

Appendicular Skeleton

Upper Extremities

Long Bones

Humerus

Proximal Humeral Fracture. Fractures of the proximal humerus are uncommon injuries and may occur at any age.[26,28] In newborns, the proximal humerus is the second most common site of birth trauma following clavicle fractures. The underlying mechanism of injury is rotation and hyperextension of the upper extremity during birth.[29,30] Fractures of the proximal humerus may also occur in both accidental and nonaccidental trauma. In children who ambulate, fractures of the proximal humerus are often sustained because of fall onto an outstretched arm or a direct blow to the lateral aspect of the shoulder girdle. A mechanism not consistent with the injury observed should alert the clinician of possible child abuse. The proximal humeral metaphysis is a common location for underlying bony lesions such as bone cysts, and therefore, pathologic fractures may coexist with minor trauma (Fig. 24.4).

Infants and toddlers more often sustain Salter-Harris type I fracture through the physis. In infants, the proximal humeral epiphysis may not be ossified or may be only partially ossified. As such, radiographic findings may mimic a shoulder dislocation because displacement of the metaphysis may be the only finding. Because the relationship of the humeral epiphysis and glenoid is not visible, one may falsely attribute inferior displacement of the humeral metaphysis to

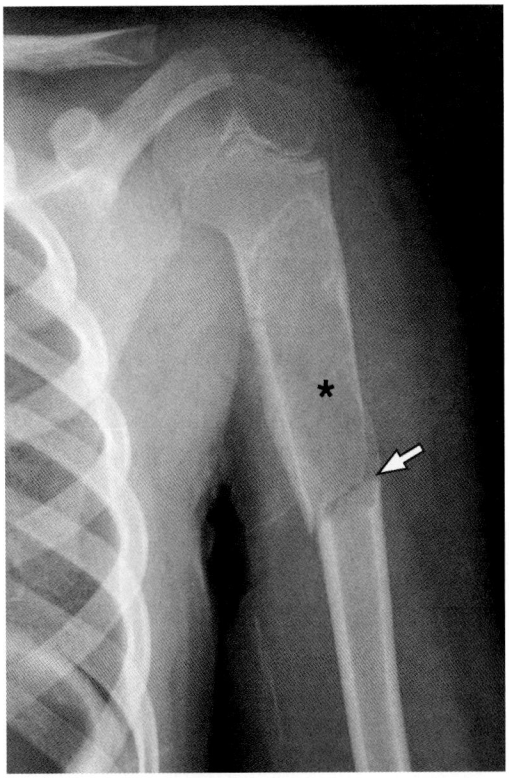

FIGURE 24.4 **Pathologic fracture of the proximal humerus sustained after minor trauma in an 11-year-old boy.** A frontal radiograph of the left shoulder shows a fracture line (*arrow*) traversing the inferior aspect of a unicameral bone cyst (*asterisk*) in the proximal humerus.

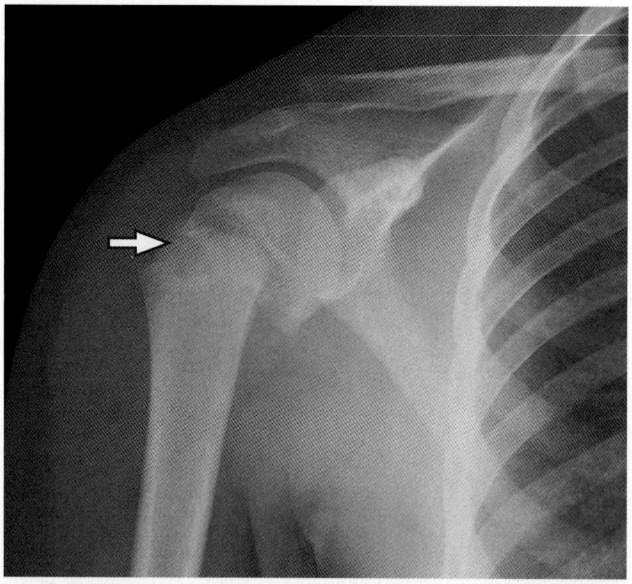

FIGURE 24.5 **Proximal humerus fracture in a 14-year-old boy.** Frontal radiograph of the right shoulder demonstrates an acute fracture (*arrow*) through the physis of the proximal humerus. There is lateral displacement of the humeral shaft with respect to the humeral head.

a dislocation rather than to an epiphyseal separation. US and MRI are particularly useful in this setting in order to directly visualize the nonossified epiphysis and define its relationship with the metaphysis.[4,31] Proximal humeral fractures in older children are more commonly Salter-Harris type II fractures with variable degrees of displacement. Other Salter-Harris fractures occur less frequently (Fig. 24.5). Buckle fractures (discussed in detail below) can also occur in the proximal humeral metaphysis, in a fashion similar to that of the distal radius. Acute avulsion fracture of the lesser tuberosity is rare in adolescents and may cause disability if not recognized in a timely manner.

The majority of the proximal humeral fractures with minimal displacement are treated nonoperatively given their high remodeling potential.[32] However, humeral fractures with substantial displacement often require surgical reduction.

Midshaft Humeral Fracture. Fractures to the midshaft of the humerus are uncommon in the pediatric population. Transverse or oblique fractures typically occur because of direct impact, whereas spiral fractures usually require a torsional force. Comminuted fractures require high-energy forces and are often seen with motor vehicle accidents (MVAs) and are sometimes associated with other injuries. Displacement of fracture fragments depends on the fracture alignment with the adjacent musculotendinous attachment. In fractures located proximal to the attachment of the pectoralis major muscle, the proximal fracture fragment is abducted and rotated by the rotator cuff, and the distal fragment is adducted and pulled proximally by the deltoid and pectoralis major muscles. When the fracture line is located between the insertions of the pectoralis major and the deltoid muscles, the proximal fragment is adducted and the distal fragment is pulled up and outward by the deltoid muscle. Fractures distal to the deltoid muscle result in abduction of the proximal fragment.[33] Because of the high remodeling capability of the humerus, most humeral shaft fractures are managed nonoperatively, and affected pediatric patients typically recuperate without associated complications.

Distal Humeral Fracture. The supracondylar fracture of the distal humerus is the most common pediatric elbow fracture and accounts for ~60% of elbow fractures.[33] The mechanism of injury is usually a fall onto an outstretched hand with the elbow in extension. The axial load of the child is transmitted to the olecranon process of the ulna, which impinges the posterior aspect of the distal humerus leading to a fracture. The olecranon fossa is the thinnest and weakest portion of the distal humerus, likely accounting for the frequency of this injury.[34–36] A minority of distal humeral fractures result from a direct blow to a flexed elbow.[37] There is a wide range of severity of supracondylar fractures ranging from radiographically occult fracture lines to markedly displaced and angulated fractures.

Radiographs are usually sufficient to diagnose a supracondylar fracture. A minimum of two views is obtained, which include an AP projection view and a true lateral view with the elbow in 90 degrees of flexion. The evaluation of the anterior humeral line is a helpful guideline to assess for a supracondylar fracture. On a well-positioned lateral radiograph of the elbow, a line drawn tangential to the anterior cortex of the humerus should bisect the middle third of the capitellum. In the setting of a fracture, there is usually posterior angulation of the distal fracture fragment, and the anterior humeral line course through the anterior aspect of the capitellum or anterior to the capitellum[38] (Fig. 24.6). Lateral radiographs

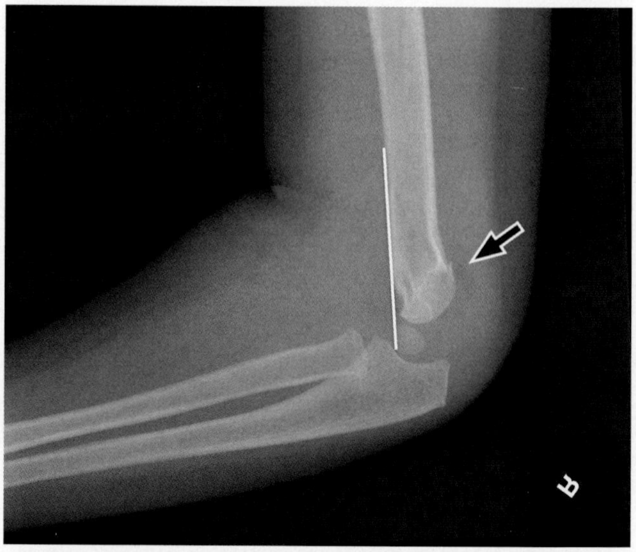

FIGURE 24.6 **Distal humeral supracondylar fracture in a 7-year-old boy.** Lateral radiograph of the right elbow demonstrates a contour abnormality of the posterior cortex of the distal humerus with mild dorsal angulation of the distal fracture fragment. The anterior humeral line (*white line*) courses through the anterior aspect of the capitellum. There is visualization of the posterior fat pad (*arrow*) and bulging of the anterior fat pad, consistent with hemarthrosis.

degraded by suboptimal positioning may falsely reassure, therefore underscoring the importance to critically assess the technical quality of the examination. In some instances, a fracture line is not seen, but there is a joint effusion raising the concern for an underlying occult fracture. Short-interval follow-up radiographs (10 to 14 days) can confirm the presence of a nondisplaced fracture by identifying the fracture line or showing healing in the form of periosteal new bone formation. In these instances, there is usually a joint effusion but no fracture line is identifiable.

The Gartland classification (**Schematic B**) describes supracondylar fractures based on the degree of separation of the fractured fragments.[39] Type I is a nondisplaced or minimally displaced fracture, typically treated with casting. Type II involves the anterior cortex with dorsal angulation, but an intact posterior cortex, resulting in partial displacement. Type III is a fracture involving the anterior and posterior cortex (i.e., no cortical contiguity) resulting in full displacement[40] (Fig. 24.7). The majority of type II and type III fractures are treated with percutaneous pin fixation and casting. Open reduction may be performed if closed reduction does not achieve satisfactory results.[35,37,40] Complications of humeral supracondylar fractures are rare but include neurovascular injuries to the brachial artery or median nerve, compartment syndrome, Volkmann contracture, and cubitus varus.

Medial Epicondylar Fracture. Fractures of the medial epicondyle of the distal humerus represent ~10% of all pediatric elbow fractures. They occur in a slightly older age group, typically 7 to 15 years old, than pediatric patients sustaining supracondylar or lateral condylar fractures.[37,41–43] They are considered Salter-Harris type III or IV fractures and are extra-articular. The mechanism of injury is a valgus stress causing avulsion of the medial epicondyle from the attachment of the forearm flexors and supinators. This injury can occur in isolation or in association with an elbow dislocation.[43,44] Isolated fractures occur in the setting of overuse in overhead-throwing athletes. Throwing athletes can sustain either an acute fracture or a chronic overuse injury from the valgus loading and distraction associated with the throwing motion. In the setting of elbow dislocation, the radius and ulna are usually displaced posteriorly, and there is a high incidence of associated medial epicondyle fractures.

Understanding the orderly progression of the appearance of the elbow ossification centers is important when assessing a pediatric patient with a medial epicondyle fracture. The ossification of the medial epicondyle typically occurs at 6 to 7 years of age and should be accounted for in this age group. Furthermore, when an ossification center is seen in the expected location of the trochlea, but a medial epicondyle ossification center is not present, then a displaced intra-articular avulsion fracture of the medial epicondyle should be suggested[37] (Fig. 24.8).

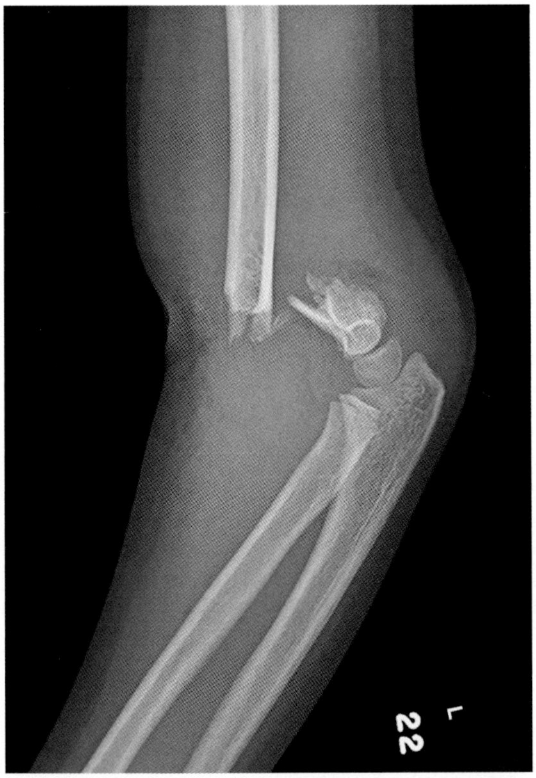

FIGURE 24.7 **Gartland type III distal humeral supracondylar fracture in a 14-year-old boy after fall from a height.** Lateral radiograph of the elbow demonstrates a complete fracture through the supracondylar region of the distal humerus with breach of both the anterior and posterior cortex resulting in full displacement.

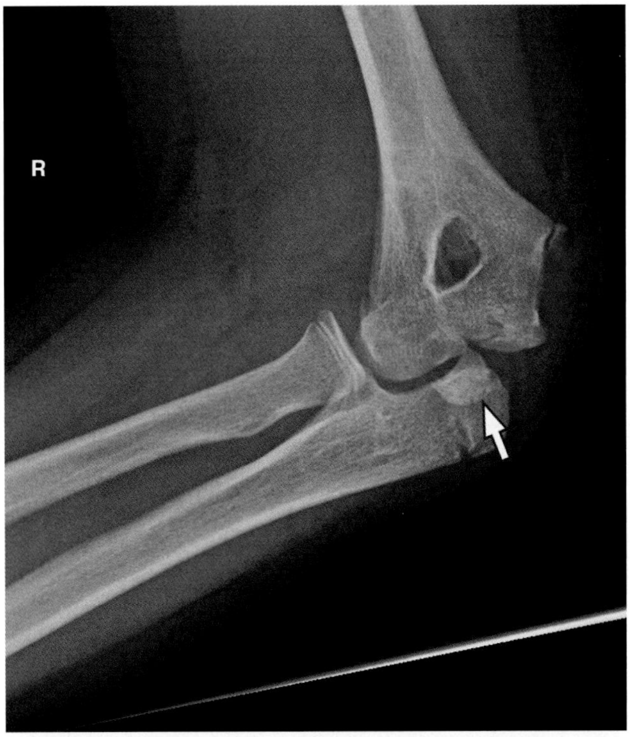

FIGURE 24.8 **Entrapped medial epicondylar fracture of the distal humerus in a 12-year-old girl with associated elbow dislocation.** Frontal radiograph of the elbow shows marked deformity of the elbow characterized by misalignment of the elbow joint and an intra-articular ossific body, which represents the avulsed medial epicondyle (*arrow*).

Entrapped intra-articular fractures require reduction. Open reduction and screw fixation are indicated if closed reduction is unsuccessful.[44] Nonincarcerated fractures that are displaced by >5 mm are usually treated surgically and those that are distracted by ≤5 mm are treated nonoperatively.[45]

Lateral Condylar Fracture. The lateral condylar fracture is the second most common pediatric elbow fracture. This injury accounts for 10% to 15% of the elbow fractures and usually occurs in children 6 to 10 years of age.[42] The mechanism of injury includes varus force applied to a hyperextended elbow.[46] Affected pediatric patients usually present with pain but lack the deformity typically seen with supracondylar fractures. Missed or delayed diagnosis of these fractures can often lead to a high incidence of nonunion or malunion.

Nondisplaced lateral condylar fractures of the distal humerus can be difficult to detect radiographically, with only a subtle fracture line abutting the margin of the metaphysis (Fig. 24.9). An internal oblique view most accurately shows a fracture line and displacement. Typically, there is an associated hemarthrosis with visualization of the posterior fat pad and elevation of the anterior fat pad. US and/or MRI examinations of the elbow can assess for fractures involving the cartilaginous epiphysis.

Lateral condylar fractures are usually Salter-Harris type II fractures involving the metaphysis of the lateral condyle extending to the physis. Less frequently, lateral condylar fractures can be Salter-Harris type IV intra-articular fractures with the fracture line coursing through the capitellum (Fig. 24.10). The Milch classification system (**Schematic A**) is used to characterize the location of the distal fracture line.[47] The Milch type I fractures involve the capitellum, and the fracture line exists lateral to the capitellotrochlear groove. In contrast, the Milch type II fractures exit medial to the capitellotrochlear groove and involve the cartilaginous trochlea.[34,37]

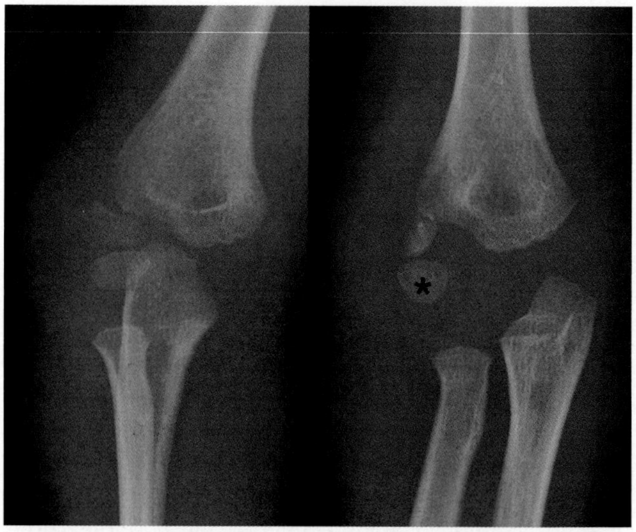

FIGURE 24.10 **Salter-Harris type IV lateral condylar fracture of the distal humerus.** Frontal and oblique radiographs of the elbow demonstrate a Salter-Harris type IV fracture through the lateral condyle with radial displacement of the capitellar ossification center (*asterisk*).

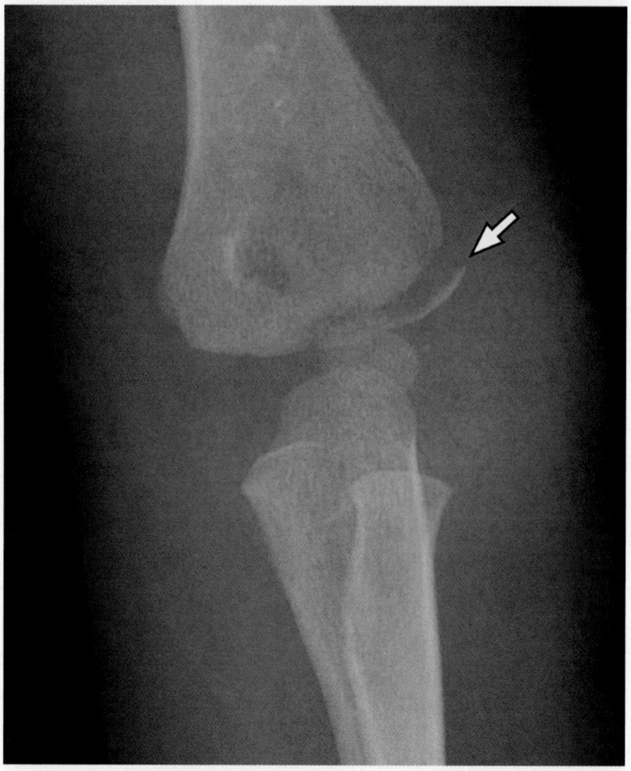

FIGURE 24.9 **Lateral condylar fracture of the distal humerus in an 8-year-old boy after trauma.** Anteroposterior radiograph of the left elbow shows a crescentic fracture fragment (*arrow*) along the lateral aspect of the distal humeral metaphysis.

Nondisplaced fractures are usually treated conservatively with a posterior splint. More than 2 mm displacement of the lateral epicondyle is an indication for operative management.[48,49]

Physeal Fracture. Distal humeral growth plate fractures are uncommon injuries seen in the setting of birth trauma, accidental trauma, and child abuse. A transphyseal fracture of the distal humerus generally occurs in patients 2 to 3 years old before the distal humeral ossification center appears.[50,51] This fracture can be mistaken for an elbow dislocation because the displacement of the ossified distal humerus metaphysis is malaligned in relation to the radius and ulna. In the case of a dislocation, the radiocapitellar congruency is not maintained. US can be useful in evaluating elbow fractures by visualizing the fracture through the nonossified cartilaginous epiphysis.[52] Displaced fractures are treated with closed reduction and pinning.[37]

Radius

Proximal Radial Fracture. Fractures of the radial head and neck account for ~4% to 5% of the pediatric elbow fractures.[34] Affected children usually present with point tenderness over the radial head and lateral elbow pain with pronation and supination. The mechanism is a fall onto an outstretched hand with an extended elbow and associated valgus force.[42] The proximal radius impacts the capitellum and results in a fracture. Proximal radius fractures are usually Salter-Harris type II, with type I fracture being much less common. In contrast to adults, radial neck fractures are more common in pediatric patients than are radial head fractures.[53] Up to half of patients with proximal radial fractures have associated

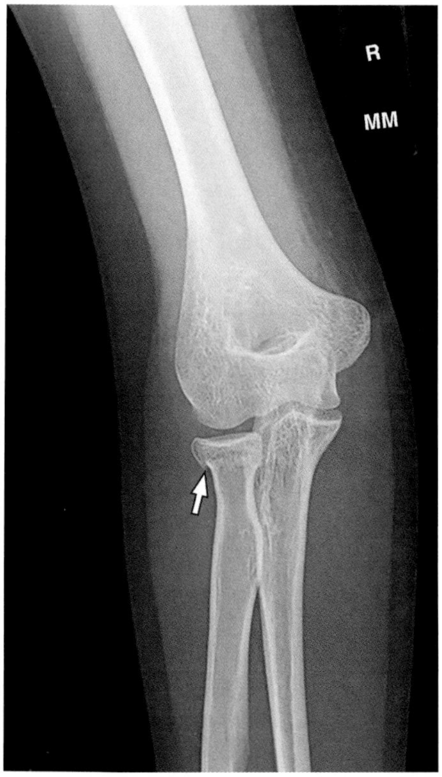

FIGURE 24.11 **Radial neck fracture in a 16-year-old boy.** Frontal radiograph of the right elbow shows subtle contour abnormality of the radial neck (*arrow*), which is diagnostic of a nondisplaced fracture.

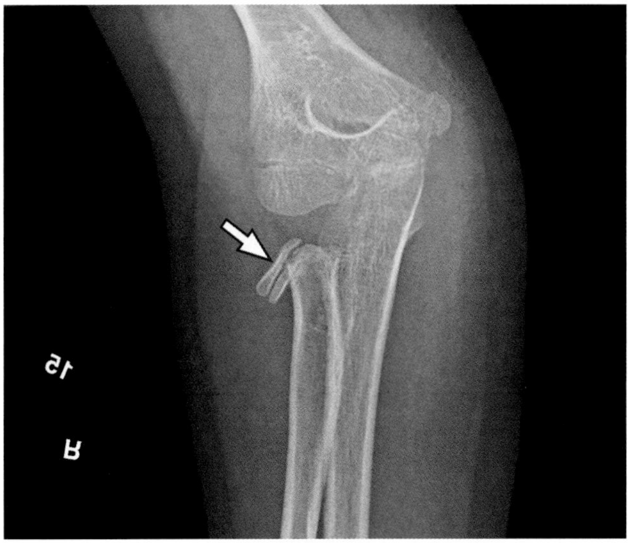

FIGURE 24.12 **O'Brien type III radial neck fracture in an 11-year-old girl after fall onto an outstretched hand.** Frontal radiograph demonstrates a Salter-Harris type II fracture (*arrow*) through the radial neck with >60 degrees of angulation.

ligamentous injury and fractures of the medial epicondyle, olecranon, and proximal ulna.

The findings of a proximal radial fracture on radiographs may be subtle presenting with only mild contour abnormality of the metaphysis (Fig. 24.11). A radiocapitellar view may be helpful to diagnose subtle proximal radial fractures. The O'Brien classification system (**Schematic D**) is used to quantify the degree of angulation.[54] Type I is <30 degrees; type II is between 30 and 60 degrees; and type III is >60 degrees of angulation (Fig. 24.12).

Treatment of radial head or neck osseous injures depends on the degree of angulation. Less than 30 degrees of angulation is acceptable, and these injuries are usually treated conservatively with a cast or a long arm splint. Angulation between 30 and 60 degrees is controversial with regard to open or closed reduction management. With angulation of >60 degrees, operative reduction is required.[55]

Distal Radial Fracture. Fractures of the distal radius are common, accounting for 25% of the pediatric fractures.[56–59] Children are at increased risk because of the rapidly growing skeletal structures and because of their increased level of activity. During rapid longitudinal growth, the mineralization is unable to keep up with the bone growth and makes the skeleton susceptible to fractures.[60] Additionally, some authors suggest that bones prior to the adolescent growth spurt are relatively more porous, which may also contribute to the higher fracture risk.[61] The incidence of distal radial fractures in the United States is increasing, which may be due to increased participation of sports when children fall onto an outstretched hand.[62] Boys more commonly sustain distal radius fractures than do girls.[62–66]

On radiographs, a distal radial fracture with displacement, which is usually dorsal in direction, is relatively easy to diagnose. However, the "torus" fracture of the distal radius, which manifests as a subtle contour abnormality ("buckle") along the compression side of the cortex most often involving the metaphysis, can be often overlooked and missed (Fig. 24.13). The lateral view or additional oblique views of the wrist may be helpful. Such views can distinguish a "torus" fracture from

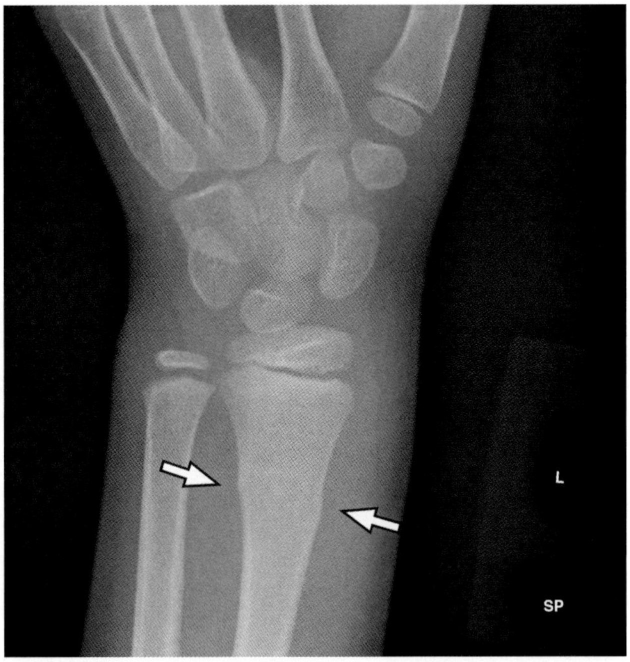

FIGURE 24.13 **Torus fracture in a 2-year-old boy.** Frontal radiograph of the wrist shows contour abnormality (*arrows*) of the distal radius consistent with a torus fracture.

a "greenstick" injury, which comprises a bend in the bone on one side and a visible break in the bone cortex on the other side. Details on these fractures are available at the end of the appendicular skeleton part of this chapter.

Operative treatment for distal radial fractures is rarely indicated because of the ability of the growing skeleton to remodel in the pediatric population. Most distal radial fractures heal with casting and immobilization. Orthopedists advocate closed reduction of distal radial fractures when there is complete displacement, >1 cm of shortening because of bayonet apposition or >15 degrees of angulation.[67]

Galeazzi Fracture. Galeazzi fracture (**Schematic E**) is a fracture of the distal radius, usually involving the diaphysis, with associated subluxation or dislocation of the distal radioulnar joint (DRUJ).[68] The incidence of Galeazzi fractures in children is 0.3% to 2.7% of all forearm fractures.[68,69] The radial fracture typically occurs 4 to 5 cm proximal to the DRUJ. If the radial fracture is <7.5 cm from the articular surface, there is a high incidence of instability of the DRUJ. Galeazzi fractures are seen during a high-energy impact such as MVA or fall from a height onto an outstretched hand with hyperpronation of the forearm.

On frontal radiographs, an angulated radial diaphyseal fracture with shortening of radius and widening of the space between the radius and ulna is seen. On the lateral view, there is dorsal displacement of the ulna with respect to the radius.

In order to restore the alignment and function, open reduction and internal fixation of the radius fracture and reduction and stabilization of the DRUJ is often performed although conservative management with good outcomes has been also reported in pediatric patients.[70] Previous studies have shown that nonoperative management of Galeazzi fracture is associated with increased risk of complications such as malunion of the fracture and residual subluxation of the DRUJ.[71]

Ulna

Olecranon Fracture. Olecranon fractures constitute ~4% to 7% of pediatric elbow fractures. These fractures are uncommon because of the relatively short size and higher strength of the olecranon compared to the distal humerus. The mechanism of injury is a fall onto an outstretched hand or direct impact to the posterior elbow.[72] Stress injury to the olecranon due to overuse has been reported in overhead-throwing adolescent athletes. Avulsion-type fractures occur from strong pull of the triceps. Olecranon fractures are often associated with other elbow injuries such as fractures of the medial or lateral condyle, radial neck, and supracondylar region and may also occur in association with radial head dislocation.[72]

Radiographically, fractures involving the olecranon can be longitudinal, horizontal, or obliquely oriented. These fractures are best evaluated on a true lateral view of the elbow. The fracture may involve the growth plate of the apophysis or the articular surface.[53] It is important to recognize that there is a variable appearance of the olecranon apophysis, which can sometimes simulate a true fracture. Similarly, the growth plate can mimic a nondisplaced fracture. In these situations, obtaining a comparison view of the contralateral asymptomatic side elbow may be beneficial for differentiation (Fig. 24.14).

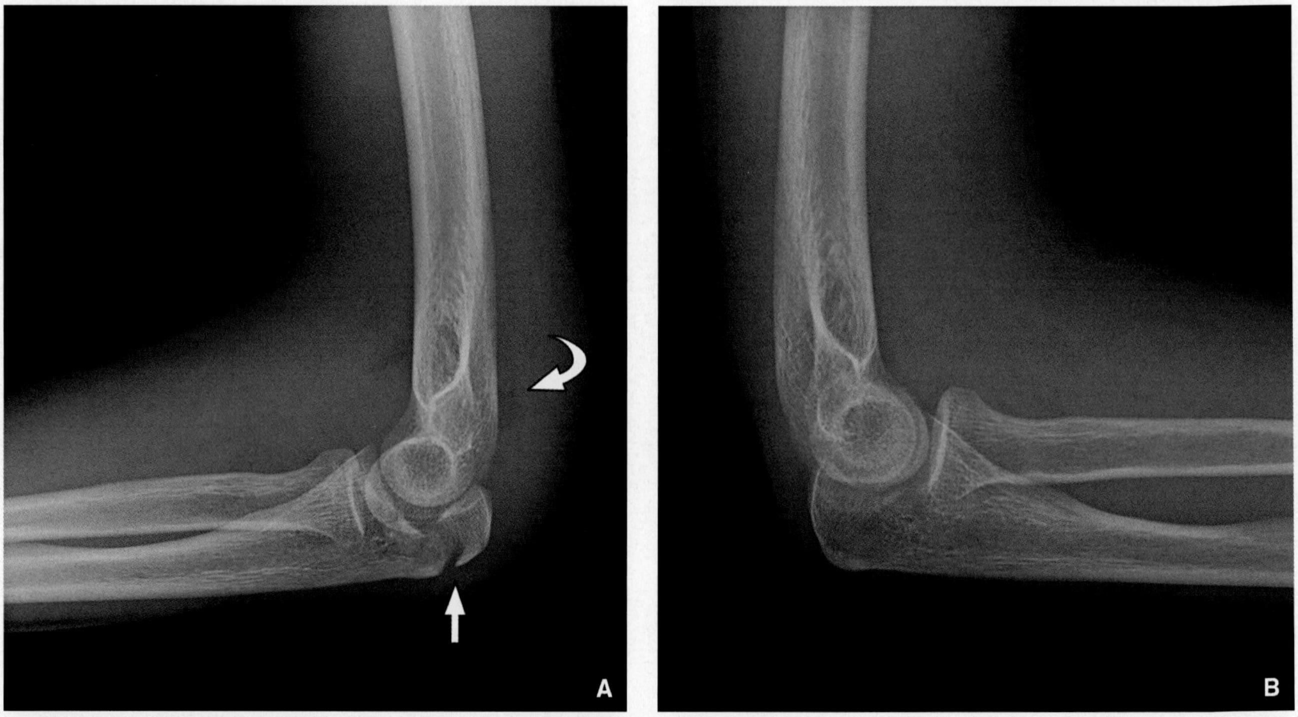

FIGURE 24.14 **Olecranon fracture in a 12-year-old boy who presented with posterior elbow pain after fall. A:** Lateral radiograph of the left elbow demonstrates an intra-articular linear lucency (*straight arrow*) through the olecranon process of the ulna. There is an associated hemarthrosis with visualization of the posterior fat pad (*curved arrow*) and displacement of the anterior fat pad. **B:** Comparison view of the right elbow shows a normal olecranon.

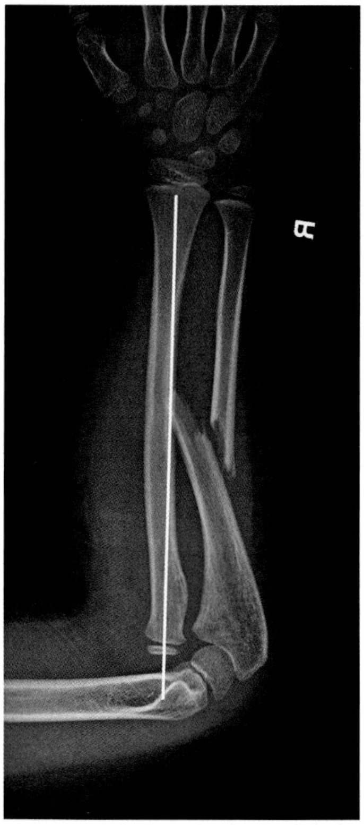

FIGURE 24.15 **Monteggia fracture dislocation in a 5-year-old boy.** Frontal radiograph of the forearm demonstrates an obliquely oriented fracture through the ulna with an associated dislocation of the radiocapitellar joint with misalignment of the radiocapitellar line (*white line*).

Nondisplaced or minimally displaced fractures of the olecranon are treated with immobilization for 4 to 6 weeks, whereas displaced fractures require surgical fixation with pins, wires, screws, or plates.[73]

Monteggia Fracture. The Monteggia fracture represents a dislocation of the radial head with an associated proximal ulna fracture. Typically, the apex of the ulnar fracture and the direction of the radial dislocation are the same. This injury occurs in children who fall on an outstretched hand with the forearm in excessive pronation. The Bado classification (**Schematic F**) categorizes Monteggia fractures based on the displacement of the radial head.[74] Type I (extension type) is the most common, with ulnar fracture and anterior dislocation of the radial head[75,76] (Fig. 24.15). Type II (flexion type) is characterized by the ulnar fracture and posterior or posterolateral dislocation of the radial head. Type III (lateral type) describes the ulnar fracture and posterior or posterolateral dislocation of the radial head. The type IV (combined type) shows ulnar and radius fractures and anterior dislocation of the radius. Pediatric equivalent Monteggia fracture is a proximal ulnar fracture and a radial head or neck fracture without dislocation of the radial head (Fig. 24.16). In children, one can also see a bowing fracture of the ulna with radial head fracture.[77,78]

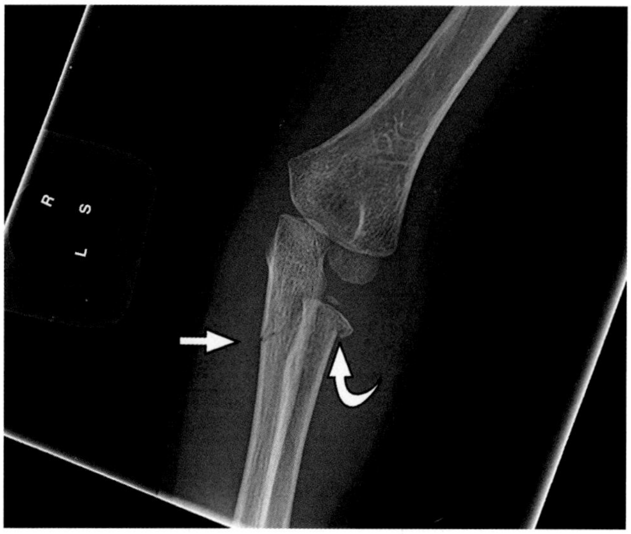

FIGURE 24.16 **Monteggia fracture in a 3-year-old girl.** Frontal radiograph of the left elbow shows a proximal ulnar fracture (*straight arrow*) and an associated radial neck fracture (*curved arrow*).

Closed reduction is the first line of management of Monteggia fractures. A recent study of 40 pediatric patients with Monteggia fracture showed that conservative management of Monteggia fractures, when indicated, may result in excellent outcome.[79] Open reduction with internal fixation is reserved for complicated cases or when closed reduction fails.

Hands

Hand fractures (**Schematic I**) are relatively common in the pediatric population. In comparison to other bone fractures, the incidence of epiphyseal injury is 34% higher than reported elsewhere in the skeletal system in children.[80] Although the majority of hand fractures heal without complication, potentially problematic hand fractures include displaced intra-articular fractures, Salter-Harris type I distal phalangeal fractures due to crushing injuries, and open fractures.

Mallet Finger. The mallet finger, also known as "baseball finger" or "dropped finger," is the most common tendon injury of the hand that typically occurs during sport activities in children. The injury is characterized by avulsion of the bony or ligamentous attachment of the extensor mechanism to the distal phalanx. This injury occurs when the distal finger is "jammed" or struck against an object. Other mechanisms include a direct blow or a hyperextension injury.[81,82] Affected pediatric patients usually present with pain and soft tissue swelling at the dorsum of the finger with inability to extend the distal interphalangeal joint (DIP).[83]

The small triangular avulsed bone fragment at the dorsal aspect of the distal phalanx near the DIP joint is best seen in lateral radiographs of the finger (Fig. 24.17). The distal phalanx may be fixed in flexion because of deficiency of the extensor tendon and unopposed action of the flexor tendon.

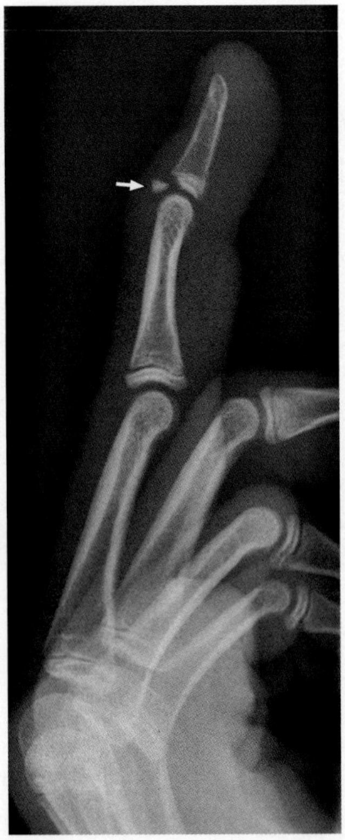

FIGURE 24.17 **Mallet finger in a 13-year-old boy with flexion injury.** Lateral radiograph of the middle finger demonstrates an intra-articular fracture (*arrow*) involving the base of the distal phalanx. There is mild dorsal displacement and rotation of the avulsed fracture fragment. No volar displacement of the distal phalanx is noted.

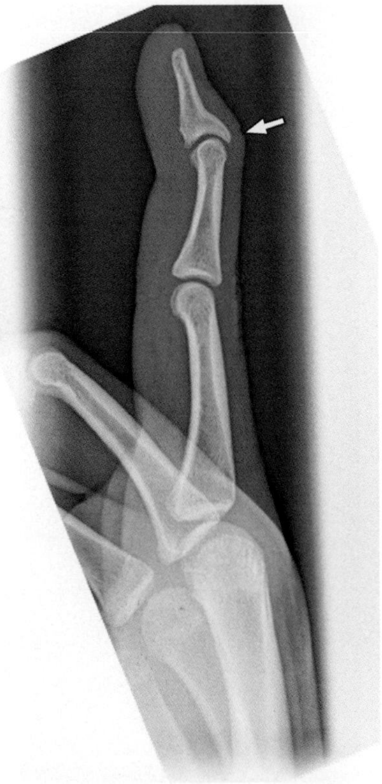

FIGURE 24.18 **Swan-neck deformity of the second distal phalanx in a 17-year-old boy with history of mallet finger.** Lateral radiograph of the finger demonstrates a flexion deformity (*arrow*) of the distal interphalangeal joint with abnormal morphology of the base of the distal phalanx.

Cross-sectional imaging is usually not necessary. However, sagittal MR images can detect injuries to the extensor tendon when no bony injury is present.[83]

Fractures involving less than one-third of the joint surface may be treated nonoperatively with splint immobilization of the finger in extension.[81,84] Greater than 50% of joint surface involvement is often treated surgically.[85,86] Failure to treat a mallet finger in a timely manner may result in a "swan-neck" deformity or early secondary osteoarthritis (Fig. 24.18). A chronic mallet finger with permanent deformity requires surgical management.[87]

Boxer Fracture. The "boxer fracture" is a transverse fracture through the neck of the metacarpal, with apex dorsal angulation and external rotation of the distal fragment. The fifth metacarpal is most often affected. The mechanism of injury is typically a direct blow of the clenched fist against a hard object. Physical examination findings include point tenderness, swelling, and ecchymosis suggesting an underlying fracture. Loss of contour of the knuckle may be seen because of angulation of the fracture fragment.

Radiographs are usually diagnostic for detecting a boxer fracture. The AP radiograph usually shows a fracture line and foreshortening of the affected metacarpal. The lateral view demonstrates the typical volar angulation of the distal fracture fragment[88] (Fig. 24.19).

The management depends on the degree of fracture angulation. The fourth and fifth metacarpals can tolerate a greater degree of angulation compared to the second and third metacarpals. Less than 40 degrees of angulation of the fourth and fifth metacarpal is generally acceptable. Nonoperative management includes splinting with or without closed reduction.[89]

First Metacarpal Fractures. Bennett and Rolando fractures are intra-articular metacarpal fractures/dislocations of the thumb. In the Bennett fracture, there is dorsal and radial dislocation of the distal fragment by the abductor pollicis longus muscle, whereas in the Rolando fracture, bone comminution is noted (Fig. 24.20). Note is made of the fact that both Bennett and Rolando fractures typically require open reduction and internal fixation.

Skier Thumb. The "skier thumb" is a fracture of the base of the proximal phalanx of the thumb with disruption of the ulnar collateral ligament (Fig. 24.21). This type of fracture is commonly seen in children whose thumbs are stressed by entrapment in a ski pole handle during alpine skiing.

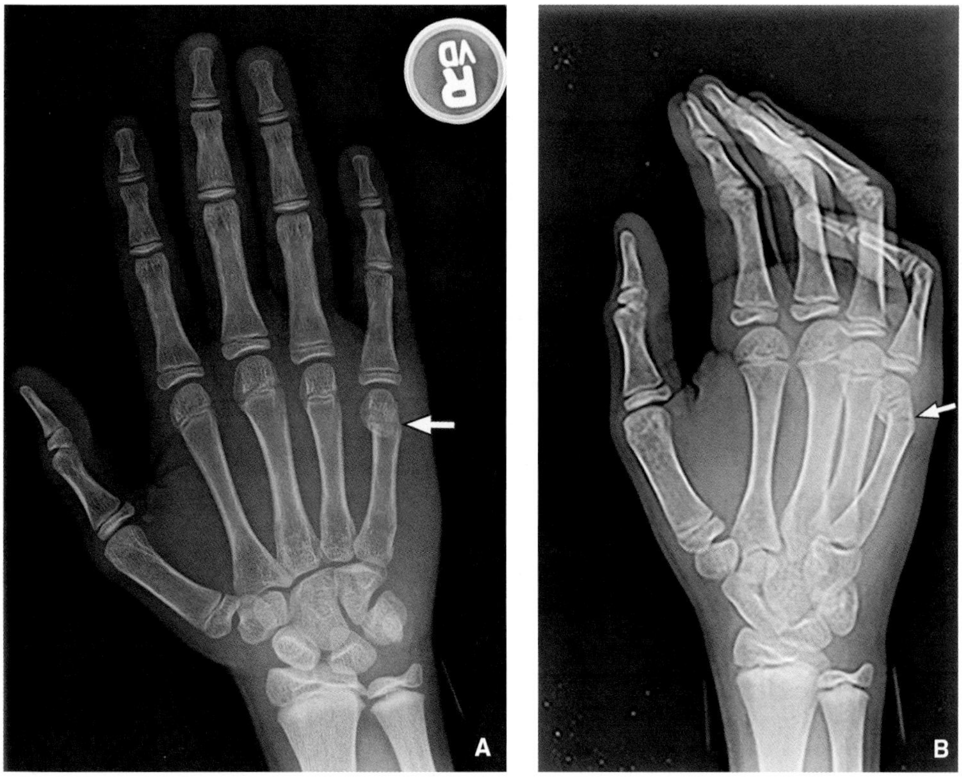

FIGURE 24.19 **Boxer fracture in a 15-year-old boy who presented with pain and swelling after punching a hard object.** Anteroposterior **(A)** and oblique **(B)** radiographs of the hand demonstrate a fracture (*arrow*) though the distal fifth metacarpal with volar angulation of the distal fracture fragment.

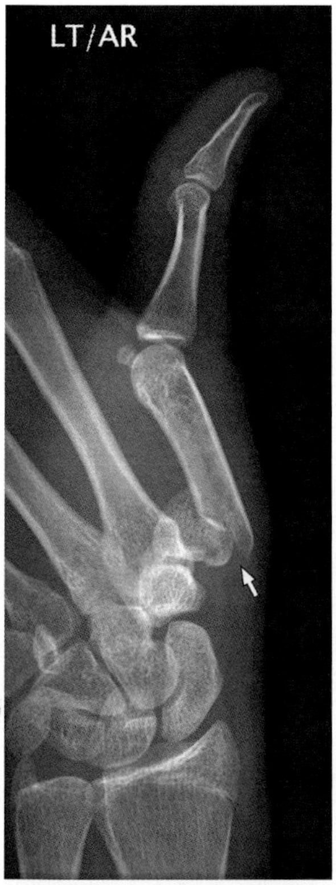

FIGURE 24.20 **Rolando fracture in a 16-year-old boy.** Oblique radiograph of the thumb demonstrates a comminuted intra-articular fracture (*arrow*) involving the base of the thumb.

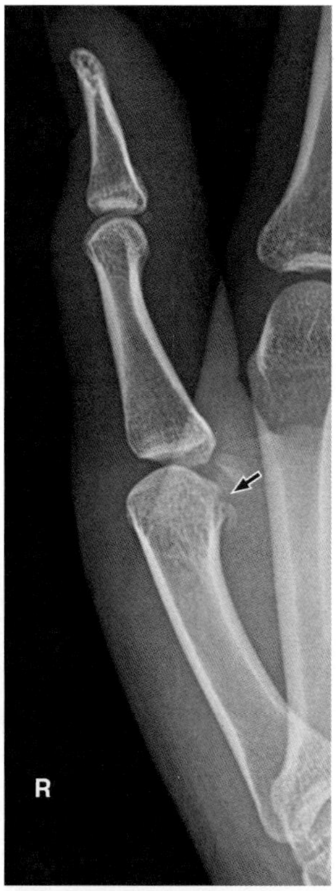

FIGURE 24.21 **Skier thumb fracture in a 15-year-old girl who had an injury to her right thumb while skiing downhill.** Lateral radiograph of the thumb shows a fracture (*arrow*) of the base of the proximal phalanx of the thumb with disruption of the ulnar collateral ligament.

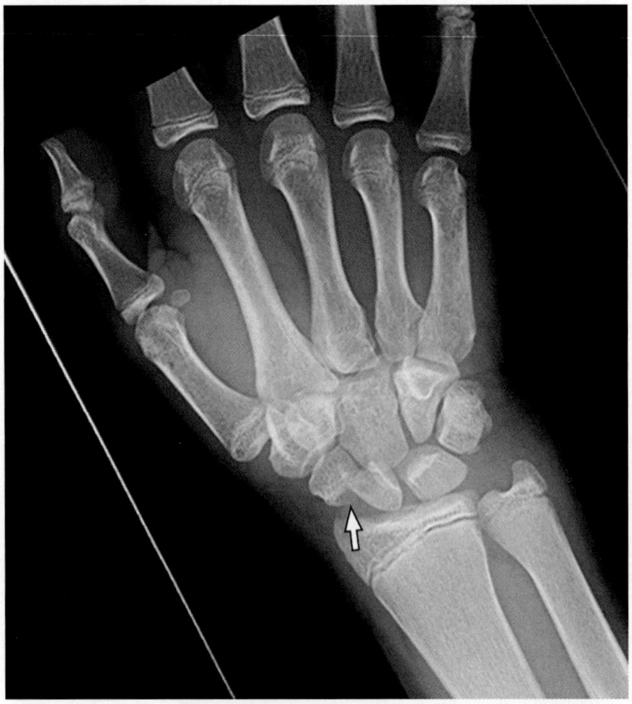

FIGURE 24.22 **Scaphoid waist fracture in a 6-year-old boy with snuffbox tenderness after a fall onto an outstretched hand.** Frontal radiograph of the wrist demonstrates an acute fracture (*arrow*) through the scaphoid waist with radial displacement of the distal pole in relation with the proximal pole.

Scaphoid Fracture. The scaphoid is the most commonly fractured carpal bone, accounting for 3% of hand and carpal bone fractures in pediatric patients.[90,91]

Affected children often complain of radial-sided wrist pain after falling onto an outstretched hand. On physical examination, there is point tenderness elicited in the anatomic snuffbox and diminished range of motion with wrist flexion and extension. Scaphoid fractures can be classified by anatomic location, based on whether they involve the proximal pole, waist (midportion), or distal pole.[91] The scaphoid waist is the most common location (Fig. 24.22).

A complete assessment of scaphoid fracture requires AP, lateral, and scaphoid views. A 30-degree ulnar deviated AP radiograph of the wrist, which is also known as "scaphoid view," is particularly helpful for the detection of subtle and nondisplaced fractures. In addition to fracture line detection, displacement or obliteration of the navicular fat stripe often associated with scaphoid fracture may be seen on radiographs. Although radiographs usually are the initial imaging study for evaluation of clinically suspected scaphoid fractures, radiographs may be unremarkable in the acute setting in 13% to 30% of cases.[90,92] MDCT or MRI can detect scaphoid fractures when clinical suspicion is high and radiographs are normal (Fig. 24.23).

The current management of scaphoid fractures is cast immobilization for a nondisplaced fracture and internal fixation for a displaced fracture with more than 1 mm step-off or angulation.[86] Because of the tenuous blood supply of the proximal pole of the scaphoid, nonunion and avascular necrosis are two common complications in patients with delayed diagnosis.

Kienbock Disease. Although lunate fractures are rare, avascular necrosis of the lunate secondary to trauma can cause lunatomalacia or Kienbock disease.

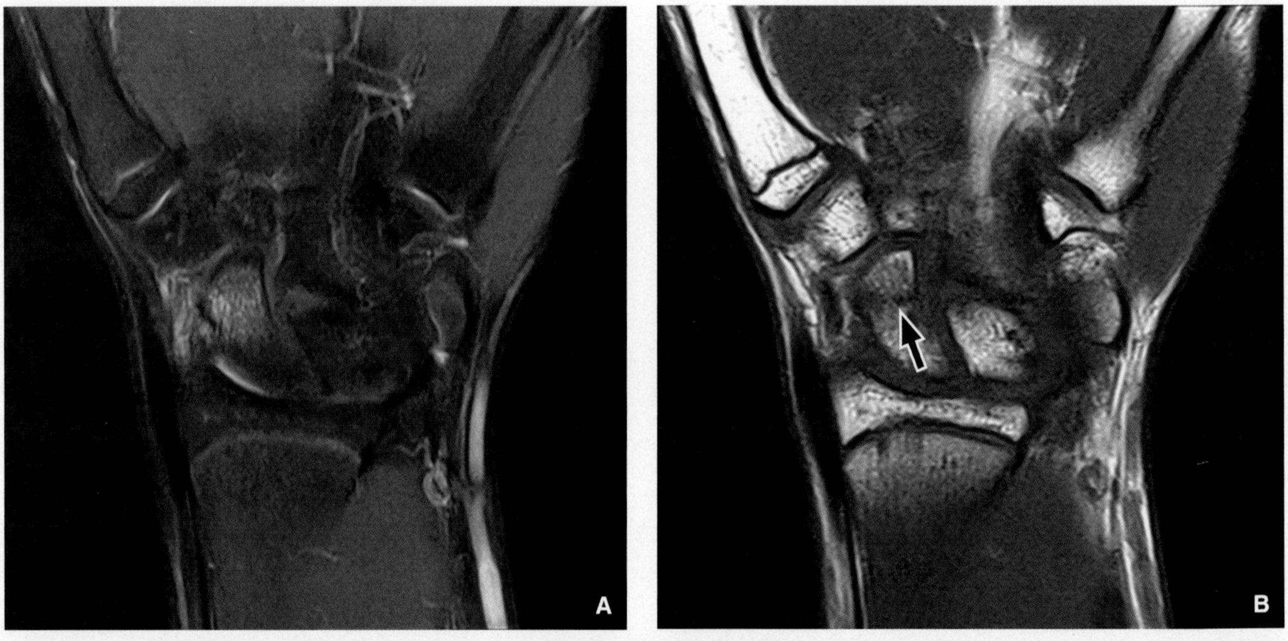

FIGURE 24.23 **Scaphoid waist fracture in a 7-year-old girl with normal radiographs (not shown).** Coronal T2 fat-suppressed **(A)** and coronal T1-weighted MR **(B)** images of the wrist show a fracture line (*arrow*) through the scaphoid waist and marrow edema in the distal scaphoid.

Dislocations

Among various osseous dislocations that occur in the pediatric population, radial head, humeral head, and patella are the three most common bones prone to dislocation.

Nursemaid Elbow. Nursemaid elbow or pulled elbow (**Schematic C**) is anterior subluxation or dislocation of the radial head in relation to the capitellum. The annular ligament, which holds the radial head in place, may be disrupted or displaced in this injury. The mechanism of injury is longitudinal traction of an extended elbow while in supination. This may occur when caretakers are attempting to pull a child away from something or lifting a child by the hands during play.[93] Children aged between 6 months and 3 years are most commonly affected. Affected children present with pain, a telltale history, and the arm is often held in flexion and pronation.

Imaging is not usually necessary because of the classic history but can be useful in excluding possible underling osseous fracture. Often, by the time the requested radiographs are obtained for evaluation, the radial head may be already relocated within the capitellum because the radiographer often reduces the subluxation or dislocation while supinating the patient's elbow for the AP view acquisition.[53] Sonographic findings may show widening of the radiocapitellar joint, increase joint echogenicity, interposition of the displaced annular ligament between the capitellum and the radial head, and the edge of a torn annular ligament.

Shoulder Dislocation. Shoulder dislocation is characterized by dissociation of the humeral head from the glenoid fossa. The shoulder is the most commonly dislocated joint in the body, and the four different types include anterior, posterior, inferior, and superior (**Schematic G**).

Anterior dislocations are the most common, accounting for over 95% of all cases.[94] The mechanism of injury of an anterior dislocation includes a direct blow to the arm that is abducted, externally rotated, and extended at the time of impact. Direct trauma to the posterior humerus and a fall onto an outstretched arm may also result in anterior shoulder dislocation. Posterior dislocations are uncommon, accounting for 2% to 4% of shoulder dislocations.[95] They may be caused by violent muscle contraction during seizure activity, electrocution, or electroconvulsive shock therapy.[96] A direct anterior blow to the anterior aspect of the humerus or axial loading of an adducted and internally rotated arm can result in posterior shoulder dislocation. Inferior dislocation, also known as luxatio erecta, is the least common type and is caused by axial loading of an abducted arm. Conditions that predispose pediatric patients to shoulder dislocation include connective tissue disorders that result in ligamentous laxity, such as Ehlers-Danlos syndrome and Marfan syndrome, and glenoid dysplasia.

When shoulder dislocation is suspected, plain radiographs of the shoulder in the AP, transcapular, and axillary projections should be obtained. In anterior dislocation, the AP view demonstrates loss of congruency of the humeral head with the glenoid fossa, and the humerus lies in a subcoracoid position with the greater tuberosity abutting the anterior glenoid rim (Fig. 24.24). The transcapular view shows the humeral head displaced medial to the scapula. Posterior dislocations can be subtle on radiographs and are underdiagnosed in up to 50% of cases.[97] The AP view shows widening of the glenohumeral distance of >6 mm, humeral head fixed in internal rotation ("lightbulb" sign), and compression fracture of the anteromedial humeral head ("trough line" sign). On the transcapular view, the humeral head can be seen displaced posteriorly with respect to the scapula. With inferior dislocation, the extremity is held over the head in a fixed position and the humeral head is seen beneath the coracoid process.

Postreduction radiographs are typically performed to assess for successful repositioning and to evaluate for concomitant fractures. Associated fractures following an anterior dislocation include Hill-Sachs deformity, bony Bankart lesions, and greater tuberosity fractures (**Schematic G**). A Hill-Sachs deformity is a cortical depression in the superolateral humeral head created by impaction with the inferior glenoid rim. Bony Bankart lesions are avulsions fractures of the anteroinferior glenoid rim. With posterior dislocation, a "reverse Hill-Sachs" deformity can occur in the medial humeral head.

MR imaging in shoulder instability is useful to demonstrate pathology in the osseous, cartilaginous, ligamentous, and labral structures (**Schematic G**). MR criteria for labral

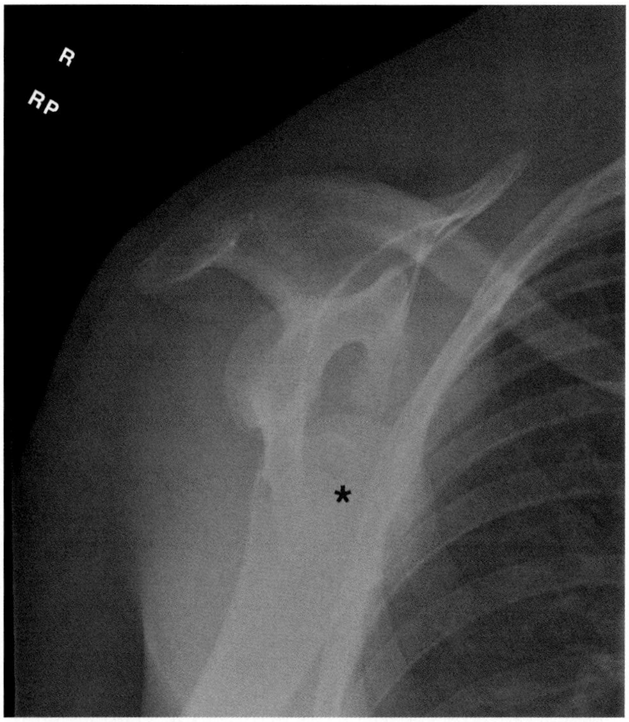

FIGURE 24.24 **Anterior shoulder dislocation in a 16-year-old boy after blunt trauma.** Frontal view of the shoulder demonstrates a subcoracoid position of the humeral head (*asterisk*) in relationship with the glenoid consistent with an anterior dislocation.

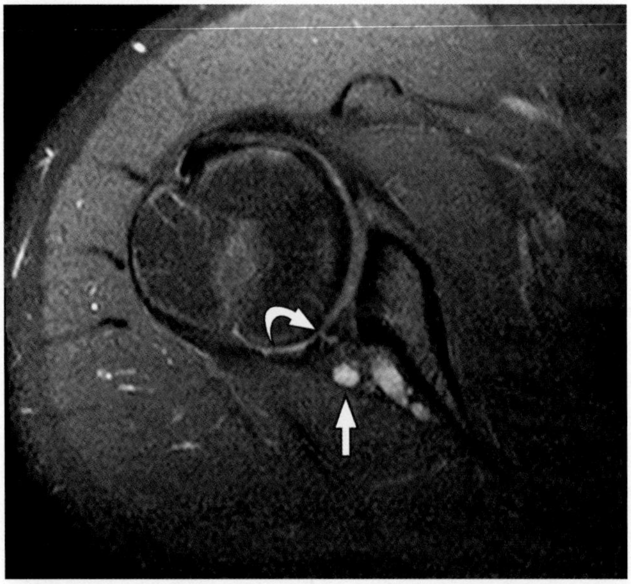

FIGURE 24.25 **Labral tear and glenoid dysplasia in a 15-year-old girl with repeated shoulder dislocations and should pain.** Axial T2 fat-suppressed MR image of the right shoulder demonstrates an abnormal blunted morphology of the glenoid and a fluid signal cleft (*curved arrow*) through the posterior labrum consistent with a tear. A paralabral cyst is also present (*straight arrow*).

tears include increased signal within the substance of the labrum that extends to the surface of the labrum (Fig. 24.25). Secondary findings include paralabral cysts, periosteal stripping, and bony injuries commonly seen with labral tears such as Hill-Sachs and bony Bankart lesions. In Hill-Sachs deformity, there is cortical depression of the superolateral humeral head. Associated bone marrow edema is seen in the acute setting. MRI is also useful to assess the integrity of the hyaline cartilage of the glenohumeral joint. The Bankart lesion describes a tear of the anteroinferior labrum with associated tear of the anterior periosteum. MR arthrogram may be helpful for detection and characterization of labrum and glenohumeral ligaments injuries. CT is useful to detect a shoulder dislocation that is subtle on radiographs and for preoperative planning.

Management includes reduction of the dislocation followed by immobilization and physical therapy. Operative treatment is reserved for irreducible dislocations, displaced fractures, and labral tears.

Lower Extremities

Long Bones

Femur. Pediatric femur fractures can be subdivided into fractures of the proximal femur (hip), femoral shaft, and distal femur. Classification schemes for each location exist and help guide treatment and prognosis. Many important differences exist between pediatric and adult femur fractures. For example, pediatric fractures heal rapidly and remodel quickly because of abundant vascularity and properties of the periosteum. In the pediatric population, high-energy trauma is typically required to cause proximal femur fractures, whereas elderly adults can sustain hip fractures with relatively minor trauma. The presence of growth plates results in injuries unique to the immature skeleton. Additionally, growth plate injuries may predispose children to growth disturbances and angular deformities. In contrast to adult patients with multiple trauma and femur fractures, the risk of pulmonary complications such as fat embolism in children is lower.

Proximal Femur Fracture. Hip or proximal femur fractures are much less common in children than in adults and account for <1% of all pediatric fractures.[98–101] Early detection and treatment of proximal femur fractures are critical because of the risk of femoral head avascular necrosis.

The Delbet classification (**Schematic T**) divides pediatric hip fractures into four types.[102] Type I is a transepiphyseal fracture with a transverse fracture through the proximal physis. Type IA is without dislocation and type IB is with dislocation. These fractures occur most frequently in infants, often resulting from difficult birth delivery. Type I fractures have the worst prognosis and highest association of avascular necrosis. Type II is called the transcervical type and is the most common, accounting for 40% to 50% of hip fractures.[98,100,101,103–107] The fracture line traverses the midfemoral neck. Type III is termed cervicotrochanteric with the fracture line occurring through the base of the femoral neck. Type IV fractures are intertrochanteric and have the best outcome. As the name implies, the fracture line occurs in between the greater and lesser trochanters. If the fracture line involves the greater trochanter, premature closure of the apophysis may occur and subsequent coxa valga deformity.

Treatment of proximal femur fracture is emergent decompression of the intracapsular hematoma and reduction of displaced fracture fragments.

Femoral Shaft Fracture. The femur is the largest bone in the body and one of the most common long bones fractured in children. Femoral fractures are the most common cause for hospitalization in pediatric orthopedic injuries.[108] Epidemiologic studies have shown a bimodal age distribution with regard to peak incidence of femoral shaft fractures. There is an early peak in the toddler age group with falls being the most common underlying mechanism of injury. The second peak occurs in adolescence when motor vehicle trauma is the most common cause. Because of the strength of the femur, usually a high-energy force is required to result in a fracture. Up to 30% of femur shaft fractures in pediatric patients <3 years may be the result of child abuse.[109] Conditions that may predispose a pediatric patient to a femur fracture include osteogenesis imperfecta, as well as additional causes of osteopenia such as cerebral palsy, spina bifida, and other neuromuscular disorders.[41,110–113]

Femoral shaft fractures can be open, with breach of the soft tissues, or closed with intact soft tissues. The Gustilo classification system (**Schematic Q**) is the most commonly accepted classification of open fractures.[114] Type I is an open fracture with a clean wound and a wound size smaller than 1 cm in length. Type II is an open fracture with a wound >1 cm in length but without extensive soft tissue damage, flaps, or avulsions. Type III is a greater degree of soft tissue damage characterized by extensive laceration, damage, or soft tissue loss. Included in type III injuries are fractures requiring vascular repair and fractures that have been open for 8 hours prior to treatment.

Typically, prophylactic antibiotics are administered to all open fractures to prevent osteomyelitis. Gustilo type I and II fractures are treated with immediate intramedullary nail fixation. Grade III fractures with arterial injuries are treated with external fixation. For unstable patients, amputation may be lifesaving.

Distal Femur Fracture. Fractures of the distal end of the femur (**Schematic M**) are less common than are shaft fractures and account for ~12% to 18% of all pediatric femur fractures.[41,108] Boys are more commonly affected than are girls. Common underlying mechanisms of injury include MVAs, pedestrians struck by a vehicle, sports injuries, and sometimes child abuse. Affected pediatric patients typically present with pain, swelling, and inability to bear weight. Concomitant vascular compromise may occur because of injury of the femoral artery. Therefore, a careful neurovascular physical examination is important in the setting of distal femur fractures.

Distal femur fractures are classified as supracondylar or physeal (condylar or intercondylar). Supracondylar fractures are more common in infants and young children, whereas physeal fractures occur more frequently in older children and adolescents. On radiographs, supracondylar fractures are located in the distal femoral metaphysis and do not extend into the growth plate. These fractures are typically transversely oriented and have varying degrees of displacement. Physeal fractures are classified according to the Salter-Harris classification system (previously described) (**Schematic P**).

Growth disturbance and leg length discrepancies are common complications of distal femur fractures in the pediatric population. A large meta-analysis study reported growth arrest in up to 50% of physeal fractures of the distal femur. Of these, 22% had leg length discrepancy of >1.5 cm.[115] In another large series of physeal fractures, the incidence of distal femur fractures was low, accounting for 1.4% of all injuries; however, 25% of these developed physeal bone bridge formation.[116] A large central bone bridge is the most common pattern of growth arrest in the distal femur.[117] Distal femur fractures are typically treated with immobilization and closed reduction of the displaced or angulated fractures.

Patellar Sleeve Fracture. Patellar sleeve avulsion is the most common patellar fracture of the growing skeleton, accounting for 1% of all pediatric fractures.[118] It is caused by cartilage avulsion from the lower pole of the patella from forceful contraction of the quadriceps muscle against a partially flexed knee. A "sleeve" of periosteum is pulled off the patella and continues to form bone if not treated, thus enlarging or even duplicating the patella (Fig. 24.26) (**Schematic L**).

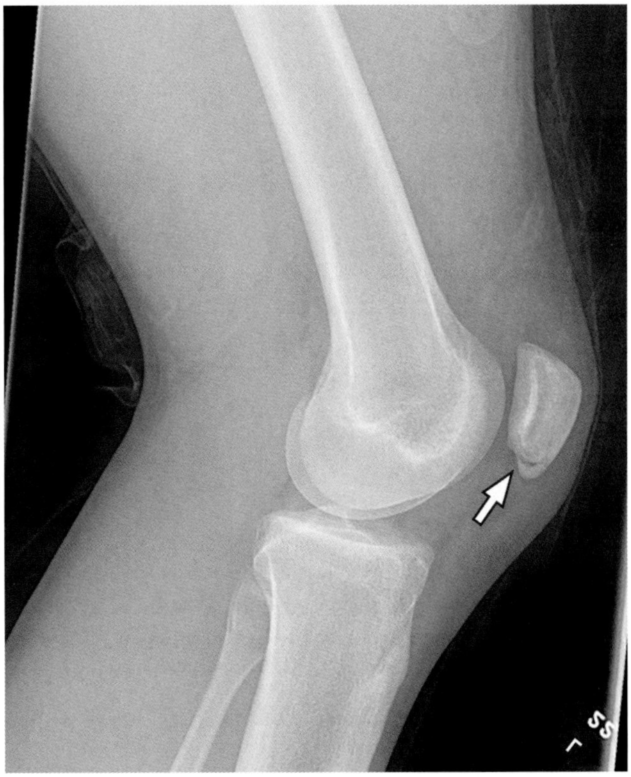

FIGURE 24.26 **Patellar sleeve avulsion fracture in a 16-year-old boy.** Lateral radiograph of the left knee shows a cresentic ossific density (*arrow*) along the inferior margin of the patella at the origin of the patella tendon. Associated soft tissue swelling is also present.

This fracture usually prompts surgical reduction with internal fixation of the patellar tendon.[118]

Patellar Dislocation. Lateral patellar dislocation is a relatively common injury that can occur in the setting of direct trauma. This injury occurs more commonly in active adolescent females.[119] The mechanism of injury in transient lateral patellar dislocation is either a direct medial blow to the knee while the knee is in mild flexion, typically <30 degrees, or, alternatively, a valgus angulation and twisting with the knee in mild flexion, which can also result in lateral dislocation (**Schematic L**).

Lateral patellar dislocation can occur in pediatric patients with variant anatomy that predisposes to maltracking of the patella in the trochlear groove. Risk factors include patella alta, trochlear dysplasia, and excessive lateral position of the tibial tubercle.[120] The Insall-Salvati index (**Schematic J**) is commonly used to assess patella alta, an important predisposing factor that leads to decreased contact of the patella and instability.[121] The length of the patellar tendon divided by the length of the patella should normally be <1.3. If the Insall-Salvati index is >1.3, patella alta is suggested. Morphologic features of trochlear dysplasia that are associated with patellar dislocation include flattening or convexity of the joint surface, shallow femoral sulcus, lateral trochlear inclination,

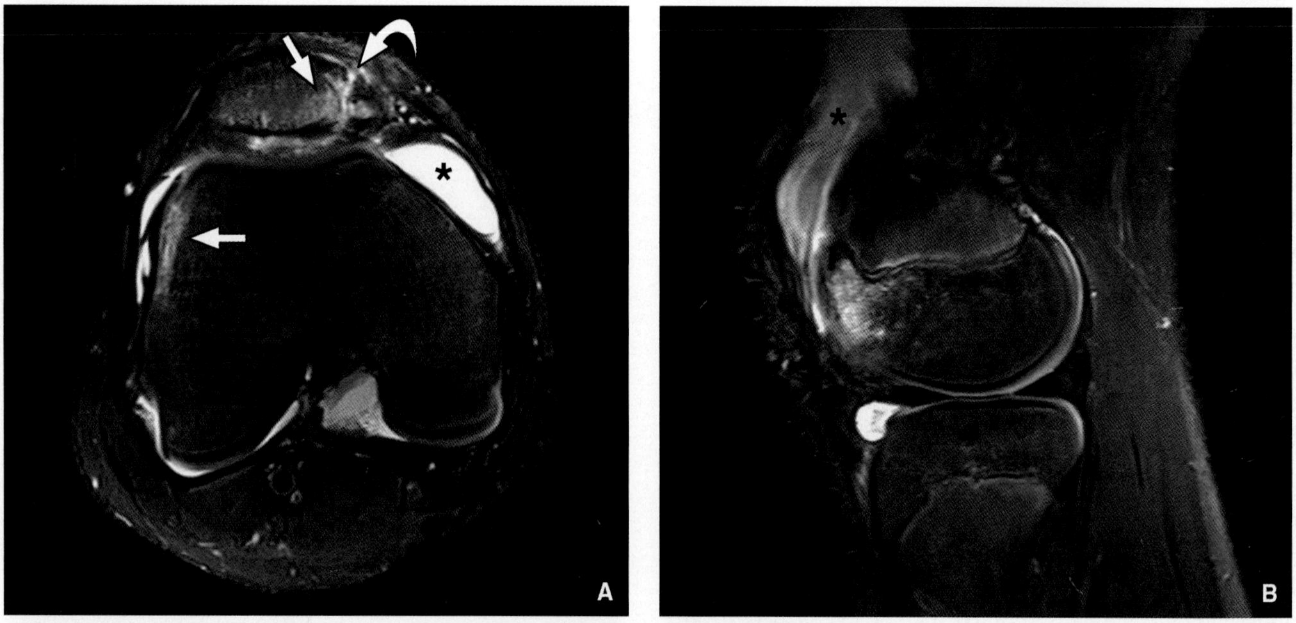

FIGURE 24.27 **Transient patellar dislocation in a 12-year-old girl with knee pain.** Axial **(A)** and sagittal **(B)** T2-weighted fat-suppressed MR images demonstrate characteristic bone contusions (*straight arrows*) in the medial pole of the patella and periphery of the lateral femoral condyle consistent with a recent lateral patellar dislocation. There is a nondisplaced osteochondral fracture (*curved arrow*) involving the medial pole of the patella. A joint effusion is also present (*asterisk*).

and trochlear facet asymmetry.[122] Excessive lateralization of the tibial tubercle in relation to the femoral sulcus can also predispose a patient to lateral dislocation.

In the setting of suspected patellar dislocation, plain radiographs of the knee should be acquired in the AP and lateral planes as well as with sunrise and tunnel views. The position of the patella is assessed in relation to the trochlea on all views and may be laterally positioned.[123] The sunrise view may demonstrate an avulsion fracture fragment adjacent to the medial pole of the patella. On the lateral view, patella alta or superior location of the patella may be seen, a finding that suggests patellar maltracking. Soft tissue swelling and a joint effusion are nonspecific but may be present after patellar dislocation. Note that ~50% to 75% of patellar dislocations are occult and therefore not correctly diagnosed at the time of the initial clinical and radiography evaluation.[124]

MRI is valuable in pediatric patients particularly with recurrent or complicated patellofemoral dislocation. Bone contusions in the medial pole of the patella and anterolateral aspect of the lateral femoral condyle are characteristic of a recent patellar dislocation on MRI (Fig. 24.27). Bone contusion on the lateral femoral condyle is due to the impact of the patella on the femur that occurs during spontaneous relocation. Other frequently encountered findings associated with patellar dislocation include (1) chondral fractures at either the inferomedial patella or the lateral weight-bearing surface of the femur, (2) medial retinaculum and medial patellofemoral ligament injury, and (3) partial- and full-thickness tearing at both the patellar and femoral attachment sites. In addition, in comparison to adults, medial patellar sleeve avulsion fractures are common in children in the setting of patellar dislocation due to the relative weakness of the osteochondral junction.

Conservative management consisting of appropriate rest as well as hip and thigh muscle strengthening exercise may be sufficient for pediatric patients with spontaneously relocated patellar dislocation without fracture or loose fragment. Surgical treatment such as lessening lateral tension and tightening medical restraint after removal of loose fragment may be necessary in recurrent or complicated patellar dislocation.

Tibia

Proximal Tibial Fracture

Trampoline fracture. The trampoline fracture (**Schematic M**) is characterized by a linear transverse fracture through the proximal metaphysis (Fig. 24.28). This injury has been described most often in children ranging between 2 and 5 years of age who engage in the recreational activity of playing on a trampoline.[125] The proposed mechanism is an occurrence when a child is jumping in tandem on a trampoline with a heavier partner. When the heavier partner propels upward, the trampoline mat recoils and the lighter child strikes the mat leading to a compressional force sufficient to cause this characteristic fracture. The outcome of this injury is typically good with immobilization.[125]

Tibial Tuberosity Avulsion Fracture. Acute avulsion fracture of the tibial tuberosity is a rare injury; however, early recognition and treatment is important for optimal outcomes. Athletic adolescent patients between ages 9 years and 17 years, during the transitional phase of physeal closure just prior to completion of growth, are usually affected. The literature reports that many patients who sustain this uncommon

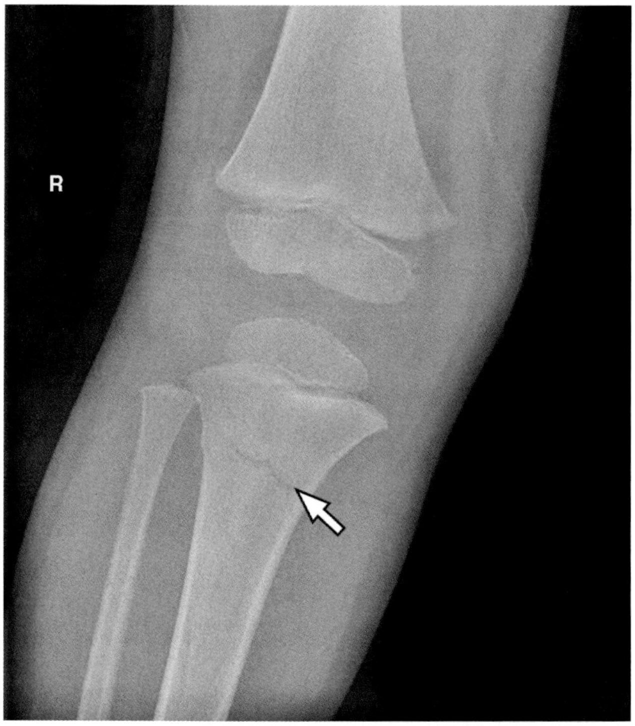

FIGURE 24.28 **Trampoline fracture of the proximal tibia in a 4-year-old boy who injured his leg while playing on a trampoline.** Frontal radiograph of the right knee demonstrates a transverse fracture (*arrow*) through the proximal tibial metaphysis.

injury have a history of Osgood-Schlatter disease, which suggests that chronic avulsive injuries of the tibial tubercles, may also predispose these patients to acute fracture.[126]

There is a strong predominance of male patients. Injuries are typically sustained during sports involving jumping. Two proposed mechanisms of injury include (1) vigorous contraction of the quadriceps during knee extension and (2) rapid passive flexion of the knee against forceful contraction of the quadriceps.[127,128] Pediatric patients sustaining this injury typically present with pain and swelling over the region of the tibial tubercle with difficulty walking and inability to extend the knee on physical examination.

Radiographs are the first-line imaging modality to evaluate fractures of the tibial tubercle. The Watson-Jones classification system (**Schematic N**) modified by Ogden is currently the most accepted classification scheme for tibial tuberosity avulsion fracture with three major subtypes.[129] Type I is a fracture of the secondary ossification center near the attachment of the patellar tendon (Fig. 24.29). Type II is a fracture involving the ossification center with propagation of the fracture into the epiphysis without intra-articular involvement. Type III is further propagation with intra-articular involvement. Subtype A denotes no displacement, and subtype B indicates displacement.[129]

The treatment focuses on restoration of the extensor mechanism and the joint surface. Options for treatment include open reduction and internal fixation or closed reduction and casting depending on the degree of fracture fragment displacement and joint surface involvement.[130]

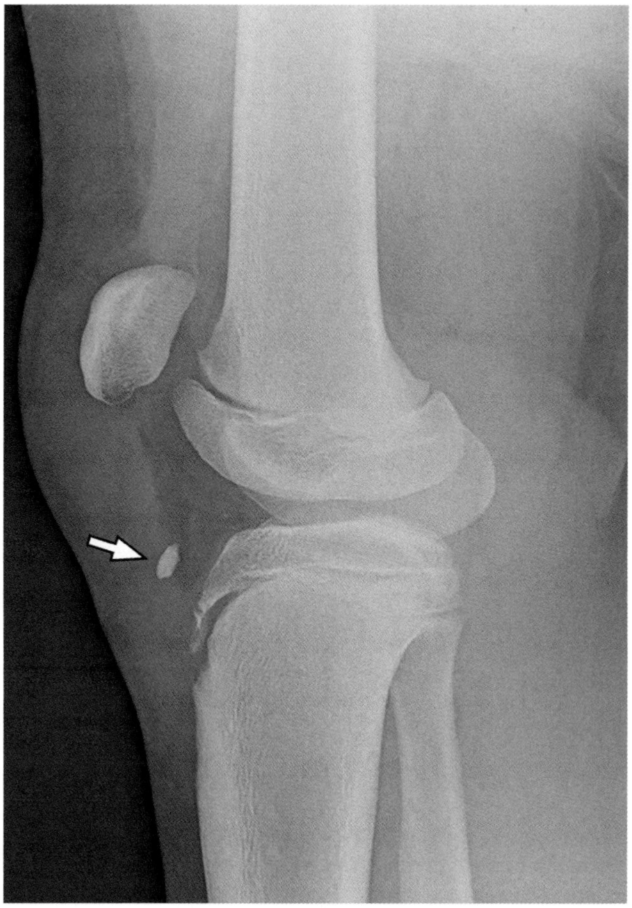

FIGURE 24.29 **Tibial tubercle avulsion fracture in a 13-year-old boy with inability to bear weight after an injury while playing basketball.** Lateral radiograph of the left knee shows an ossific density (*arrow*) adjacent to the tibial tubercle with marked anterior soft tissue swelling and thickening of the patellar tendon shadow.

Tibial spine fracture. This type of fracture occurs more frequently in skeletally immature patients and in boys (in contrast to skeletally mature patients).[131] Because the chondroosseous junction is the weakest component of the anterior cruciate ligament (ACL) complex (**Schematic L**)[132] and given the insertion of the ACL in the medial aspect of the tibial eminence, ACL ligament injuries are commonly associated with tibial spine avulsion fractures (Fig. 24.30).

Anterior cruciate ligament tear. The ACL is the most commonly injured ligament in the knee usually sustained while playing sports in the pediatric population. Mechanisms of injury include a pivot shift injury whereby a valgus load is applied to the knee while in various degrees of flexion. Hyperextension injuries can also result in injuries to the ACL.[133,134]

Plain radiographs are not sensitive in the detection of ACL injuries. However, there are radiographic findings that are suggestive of underlying ACL injury. Avulsion fracture of the lateral capsular ligament (Segond fracture) and "deep lateral femoral condyle sulcus sign" are commonly associated with ACL tears (Fig. 24.31). Joint effusion and soft tissue swelling are also typically present but nonspecific to an ACL injury.

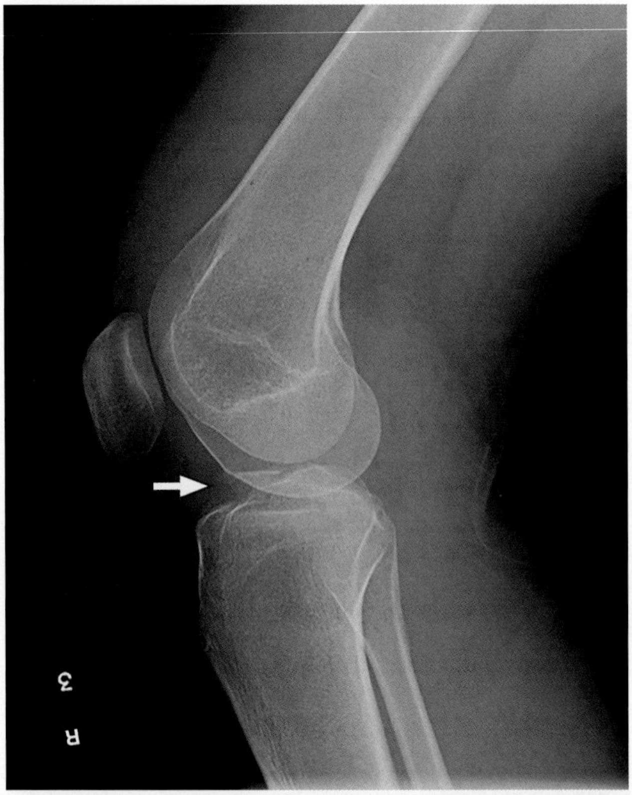

FIGURE 24.30 **Tibial spine fracture in a 17-year-old boy with a twisting injury.** Lateral radiograph of the knee demonstrates a mildly elevated fracture (*arrow*) of the anterior aspect of the intercondylar eminence at the site of ACL attachment.

MRI is the current imaging modality of choice for evaluating ACL tears. Primary MRI findings of ACL injury include focal discontinuity of the ligament, abnormal hyperintense T2 signal within the ligament and an increase in the Blumensaat angle and failure of ACL to parallel Blumensaat line (**Schematic J**). Secondary signs of ACL injuries include posterior cruciate ligament bucking and characteristic bone bruises due to impaction of the tibia against the femur where the tibia is displaced anteriorly and impacts the posterolateral aspect of the lateral femoral condyle resulting in corresponding contusions of the posterolateral tibial plateau and posterolateral femoral condyle, known as "kissing contusions" (Fig. 24.32). Also, there may be uncovering of the posterior horn of the medial meniscus due to anterior tibial translation. MRI readily depicts commonly associated injuries such as meniscal tears and collateral ligament injuries. The medial meniscus and medial collateral ligament are often associated with ACL tears.[135]

Although partial-thickness ACL tears may be managed conservatively, full-thickness ACL tears usually require surgical reconstruction of the ligament with physeal sparing (to avoid future growth disturbance), which should be delayed at least 3 weeks following the injury to prevent the complication of arthrofibrosis. One of the potential sequelae of ACL tears is early osteoarthritis development.

Meniscal injury. Meniscal injury in the pediatric population usually occurs as acute trauma while playing sports. However, chronic overuse can also result in meniscal injuries. Furthermore, a discoid meniscus, which is a normal morphology variant, is also known to be prone to meniscal injury such as tears and degeneration in children. A discoid meniscus is characterized by a thickened and widened appearance (Fig. 24.33). It is seen in ~1% to 3% of the population and is bilateral in up to 79% of cases.[136] The lateral meniscus is most commonly injured if the meniscus is discoid; otherwise, the most common location for a meniscus tear in the knee is the posterior horn of the medial meniscus. Complete and incomplete forms of a discoid meniscus exist and are differentiated by the width of the meniscus. The Wrisberg variant of a discoid meniscus lacks the posterior attachment

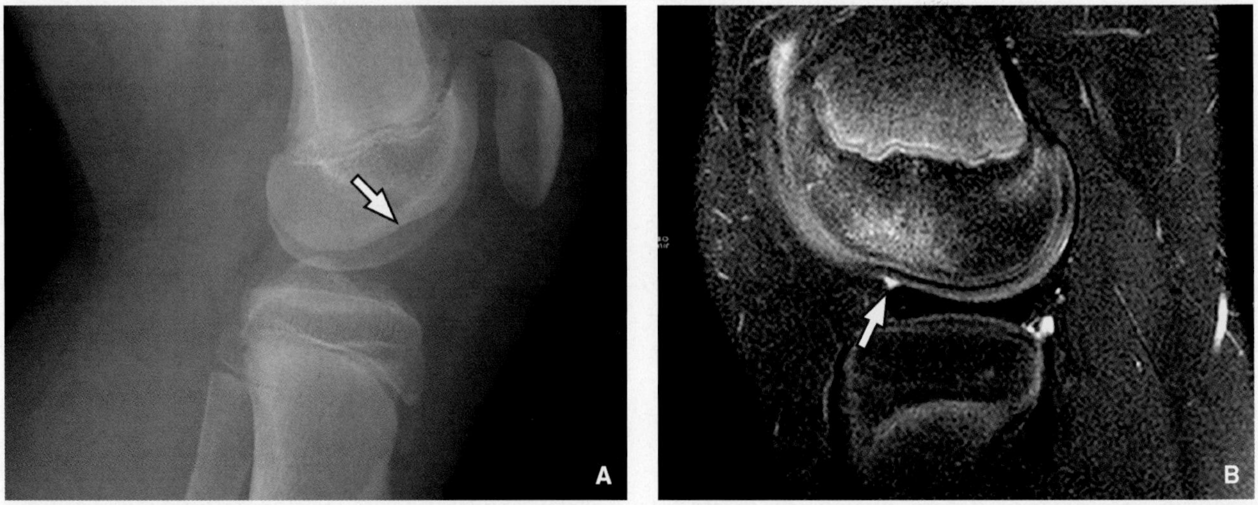

FIGURE 24.31 **Deep lateral femoral condyle sulcus sign in a 14-year-old boy who injured his knee while playing basketball.** **A:** Lateral radiograph of the knee shows a concave contour abnormality (*arrow*) of the lateral femoral condyle. **B:** Sagittal T2-weighted fat-suppressed MR image of the knee demonstrates the same contour abnormality (*arrow*) with associated subchondral bone marrow edema. An ACL tears is highly associated with this type of injury.

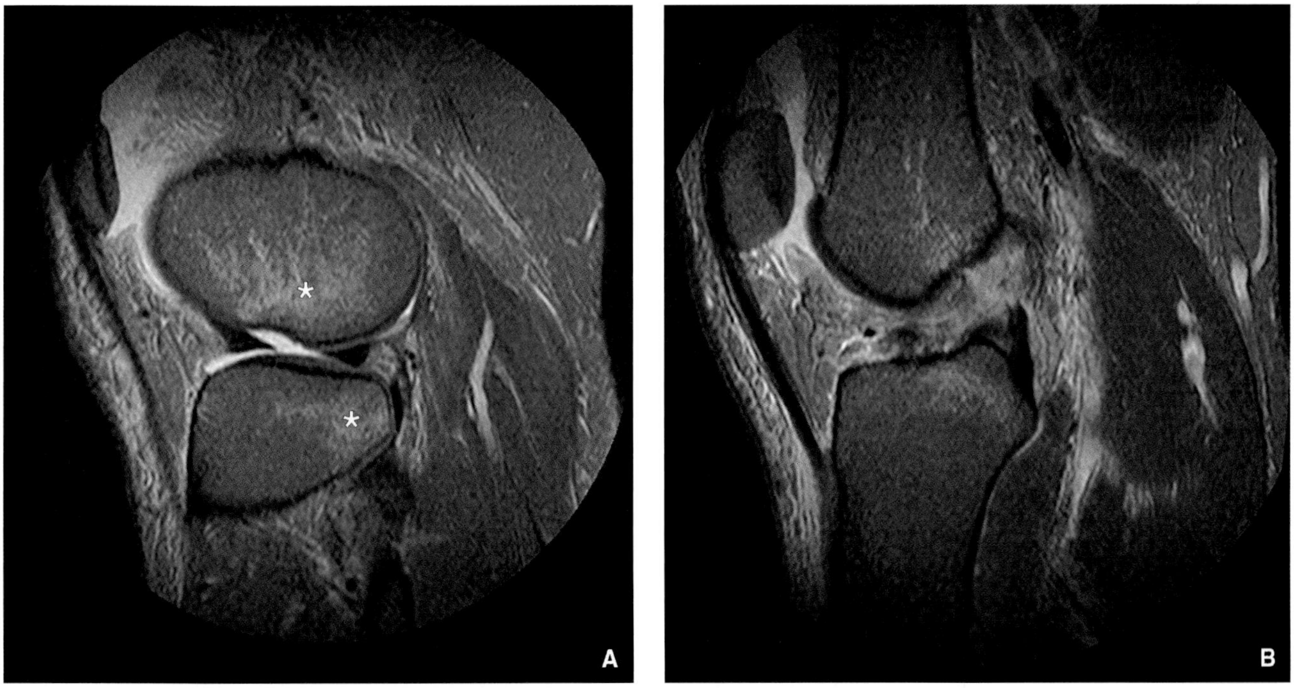

FIGURE 24.32 **Anterior cruciate ligament (ACL) rupture and contusions in a 17-year-old boy with knee pain and instability after soccer injury.** Sagittal T2-weighted fat-suppressed MR images of the knee show **(A)** characteristic bone contusions in the lateral femoral condyle and posterolateral tibial plateau ("kissing contusions," *asterisks*). **(B)** Marked heterogeneity and nonvisualization of the ACL consistent with a full-thickness ACL tear.

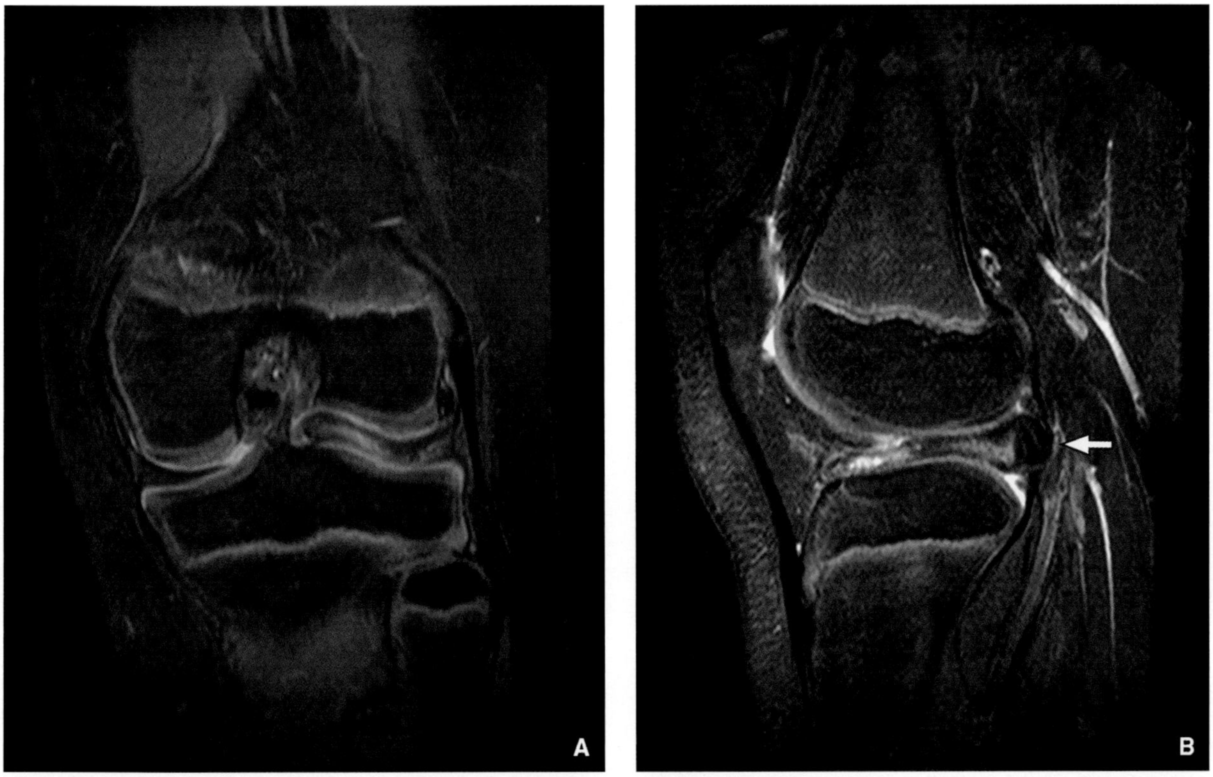

FIGURE 24.33 **Torn discoid meniscus in a 9-year-old girl with knee pain and locking.** Coronal **(A)** and sagittal **(B)** T2-weighted fat-suppressed MR images of the knee demonstrate a thickened discoid lateral meniscus. The anterior horn (*arrow*) of the meniscus is torn and flipped posteriorly.

to the meniscofemoral ligament and is considered unstable. Pediatric patients with meniscal injury can be asymptomatic but typically present with pain (often exacerbated by twisting or rotating the knee), popping sensation, locking stiffness, and difficulty with knee extension.

Radiographs may show widening of the lateral joint space or cupping of the lateral tibial plateau in the setting of discoid menisci. MRI is the imaging modality of choice for evaluating meniscal pathology. Normal menisci are triangular in shape and show low signal on T1-weighted and T2-weighted MR images due to their fibrocartilage composition. Thickening, with or without increase signal intensity, of the body of the meniscus in case of a discoid meniscus is diagnosed by visualizing the body segment on 3 or more contiguous 5 mm cuts on a sagittal MRI sequence. On MRI, tears of the meniscus should meet the following two criteria: (1) contact of intrameniscal signal with the superior or inferior surface and (2) distortion of the normal appearance of the meniscus.[137] Meniscal contusion, in contrast to meniscal tear, demonstrates internal signal equal to fluid on T2-weighted MR imaging in patients with recent trauma,[138] however, without surface contact.

Meniscal tears are often classified into horizontal (transverse), longitudinal, and radial (oblique), which can progress to displaced flap, bucket-handle (Fig. 24.34), and parrot beak types (**Schematic K**). Complex tears combining different types of tears can also occur. Horizontal tears are more common in patients older than 40 and are thought to be degenerative tears. They typically involve the posterior horn and may extend into the body. On MRI, horizontal tears appear as a horizontally oriented line of increased signal through the superior or inferior surface. Longitudinal tears have a vertical orientation on MR and usually involve the posterior horn. Longitudinal tears are often associated with other injuries, most commonly ACL tears.[139] Radial tears are vertically oriented tears from the free edge and extend into the meniscus, perpendicular to the long axis. Radial tears on MRI manifest as a vertical cleft of fluid sign on coronal images and a blunted or absent meniscus on the sagittal MR image. This is known as the "ghost meniscus" sign.[140]

Complex meniscal tears involve more than one plane with multiple separate flaps of meniscus. Displaced flap tears describe meniscal tears resulting in a displaced fragment. Identification of displaced fragments prior to arthroscopy is important. If not removed surgically, fragments can cause persistent knee pain and locking symptoms. In addition to direct meniscal injuries, MRI can also detect indirect signs of meniscal tears, which include subchondral bone marrow edema beneath a meniscus[141] and presence of a parameniscal cyst with a hyperintense fluid collection on T2-weighted MR images directly overlying or adjacent to a meniscus.[142]

Although stable meniscal tears with minimal displacement, degenerative tears, or partial-thickness tears may become asymptomatic with conservative management, surgical management such as partial meniscectomy or meniscus repair is required for patients with persistent symptoms. Pathologic examination typically confirms the traumatic and degenerative changes (Fig. 24.35).

Midtibial Fracture. The tibia is the third most common location for a long bone fracture in the pediatric population, following forearm and femur fractures. There is a high incidence of concomitant fibular fracture, which has been reported in up to 30% of cases.[143] Various mechanisms of injury are implicated such as direct blow to the tibia, high-energy MVAs, sports injuries, and twisting injuries. Affected

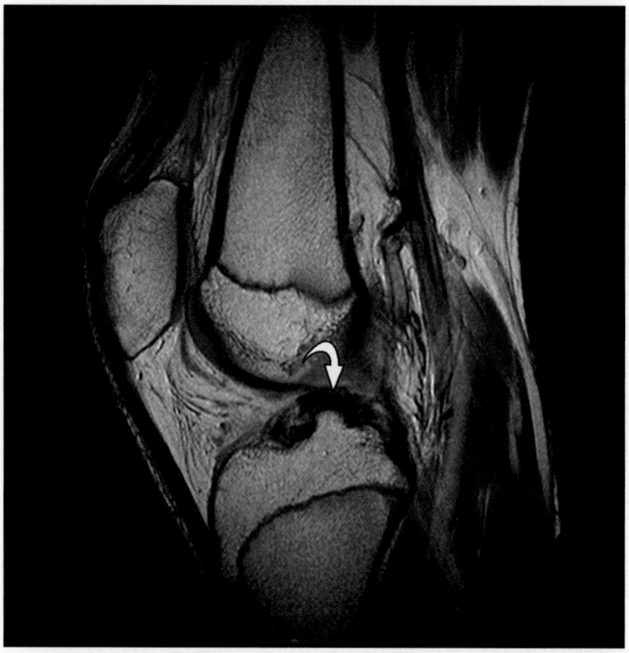

FIGURE 24.34 **Bucket-handle tear of the medial meniscus in a 15-year-old boy with knee pain after twisting injury.** Sagittal proton density MR image of the knee shows a curvilinear hypointense meniscal fragment (*curved arrow*) flipped into the intercondylar notch.

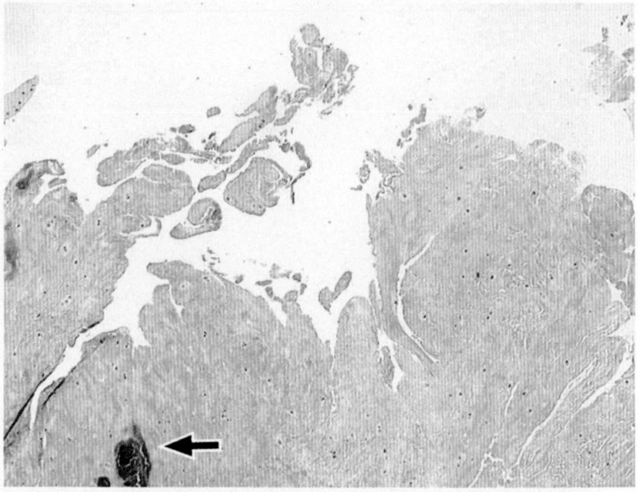

FIGURE 24.35 **Torn meniscus in a 23-year-old female who sustained a knee injury in her teens.** Microscopically, the partial meniscectomy specimen shows fibrillary degeneration and focal calcification (*arrow*) (hematoxylin and eosin, original magnification, 100×).

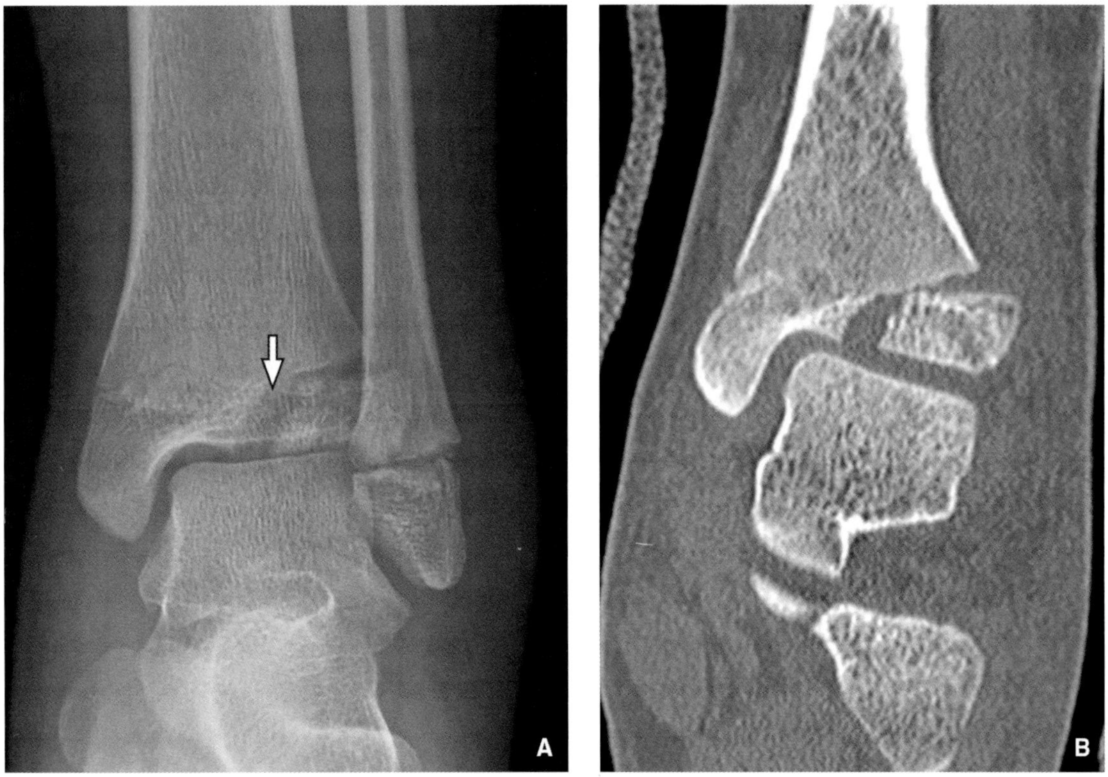

FIGURE 24.36 **Tillaux fracture in a 14-year-old boy with ankle pain after injury. A:** Anteroposterior radiograph of the ankle shows an intra-articular fracture involving the central aspect of the distal tibial epiphysis (*arrow,* Salter-Harris type III fracture) with lateral displacement of the fracture fragment. **B:** Coronal CT reformation image demonstrates the fracture line and accurately delineates the gap between the fracture fragments.

pediatric patients typically present with pain, swelling, inability to walk, and variable degrees of deformity at the fracture site.

Frontal and lateral radiographs of the leg, including the knee and ankle joints, are the initial imaging study of choice for evaluating suspected tibia fracture. Often, the fracture line in the tibial diaphysis is transverse, oblique, or spiral. It is important to assess degree of displacement and/or angulation of the tibial fracture fragment and also to evaluate for associated fibular fractures.[144]

Closed reduction and casting is the mainstay of treatment of tibial fractures with close clinical and radiographic follow-up for confirmation of healing.

Distal Tibial Fracture

Juvenile Tillaux fracture. The juvenile Tillaux fracture is a Salter-Harris type III fracture of the distal tibial physis and a unique pediatric ankle fracture (**Schematic O**). It occurs in children 12 to 15 years of age over a period of 18 months prior to physiologic fusion of the physis.[145] The distal tibial physis usually fuses at about age 15 in girls and age 17 in boys. For this reason, it is called a transitional fracture, because the bone is transitioning to skeletal maturity. The physiologic physeal fusion of the distal tibia occurs in a predictable pattern, starting centrally at "kump's bump," and then progresses medially leaving the lateral aspect of the distal tibial growth plate to be the last to fuse, which makes it vulnerable to injury.

The mechanism of injury includes supination, external rotation, and compression stress. The rotational force causes an avulsion fracture from the attachment of the anterior tibial–fibular ligament. Radiographs typically show a vertical or oblique linear lucency in the sagittal plane through the distal tibia epiphysis (Fig. 24.36A). The oblique or "mortise view" often depicts the fracture line better than do the AP and lateral views. CT with multiplanar reconstruction is often obtained for preoperative planning,[146] demonstrating the degree of fracture fragment displacement and the gap in between the fracture fragments (Fig. 24.36B).

Typically, surgical correction is indicated when the fracture plane results in a 2 mm gap. Although this injury does indeed involve the growth plate, its main complication is posttraumatic ankle arthritis rather than growth arrest given the relatively low remaining growth potential.[147–149]

Triplane fracture. Another transitional fracture of the pediatric ankle is the triplane fracture, so named because the fracture lines occur in all three anatomic planes[150–153] (**Schematic O**). A triplane fracture of the distal tibia typically occurs during adolescence before complete closure of the distal tibial physis. Affected pediatric patients typically present with pain, ankle swelling, and difficulty bearing weight.

This fracture has a multiplanar pattern. There is a sagittally oriented fracture line through the epiphysis, which is best depicted on an AP radiograph and coronal CT reformation. A coronally oriented fracture line through the posterior

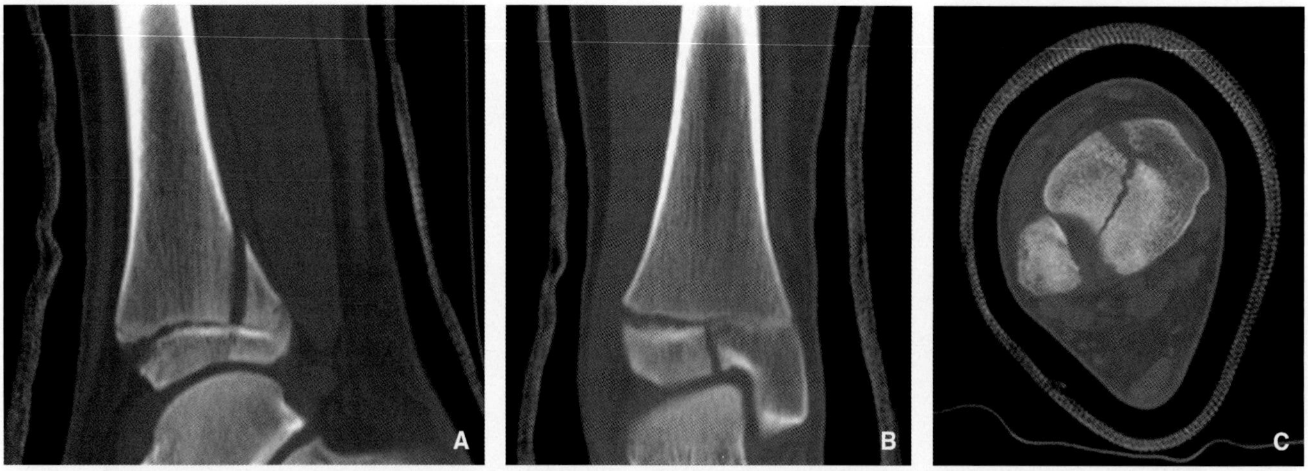

FIGURE 24.37 **Triplane fracture in a 13-year-old girl.** Sagittal **(A)**, coronal **(B)**, and axial **(C)** CT images demonstrate fracture lines in all three planes. **A:** The sagittal CT image shows the posterior malleolar fracture in the coronal plane. **B:** The coronal CT image shows an intra-articular fracture through the epiphysis in the sagittal plane. Both sagittal and coronal CT images depict widening of the physis in the axial plane. **C:** The axial CT image shows the three fragments of this three-part triplane fracture.

aspect of the metaphysis, which is best seen on a lateral radiograph or sagittal reformatted CT, is also present. In addition, there is a transverse fracture through the growth plate (Fig. 24.37). Although these fractures involve the metaphysis, physis, and epiphysis, the fracture lines are not in contiguity with one another; thus, it is generally considered a combination of Salter-Harris types II and III fractures, rather than a true Salter-Harris type IV fracture.[154] A classic configuration of this fracture presents with a posterolateral fragment (consisting of the posterolateral epiphysis and posterior metaphysis) separate from the anteromedial epiphysis (attached to the distal tibia).[154] CT with MPR and surface-rendered 3D imaging is often obtained for preoperative management.[154,155]

Restoration of the articular congruity at the ankle joint is the major concern and the degree of displacement influences the decision between operative and nonoperative management of triplane fractures. Nondisplaced two-part fractures can be treated with closed reduction, whereas three- and four-part fractures and any fracture with >2 mm of displacement are treated with operative reduction and internal fixation.[154–158]

Feet

Foot fractures account for 5% to 8% of the overall pediatric fractures and for 7% of the growth plate fractures.[23,159–161] There is a male predominance on pediatric foot fractures.[162] Although most fractures occur in isolation, with more severe injuries multiple fractures may occur simultaneously.

Talus Fracture. Only 2% of pediatric foot fractures involve the talus.[163] In order of decreasing frequency, talar fractures involve the following sites: talar periphery (avulsion fractures), osteochondral interface, and talar neck and body.[164] Pediatric patients with fractures of the talus usually complain of ankle pain, foot pain, tenderness, and exacerbation of pain with ankle dorsiflexion. Radiographs often make the diagnosis by showing the fracture line, and CT is helpful to assess for the degree of displacement. Whereas nondisplaced fractures are treated conservatively, displaced fractures require close reduction and possibly internal fixation.[165]

Calcaneal Fracture. Calcaneal fractures also account for ~2% of the pediatric fractures. Boys are more commonly affected than are girls.[163] Approximately two-thirds of the pediatric calcaneal fractures are extra-articular in contrast to adult calcaneal fractures, which are usually intra-articular in location. The mechanism of injury includes axial loading, with the talus forcefully driven into the calcaneus. MVAs are the second leading cause of calcaneal fractures.[166,167] There is an increased association of this fracture with lumbar spine injuries given the extra loading mechanism of injury.[168]

Radiographs for evaluation of calcaneal fractures should include a frontal, lateral, and oblique view of the ankle. It is helpful to assess the Bohler angle (**Schematic U**), which is decreased in the setting of a calcaneal fracture (normal values in children range between 14 and 58 degrees; however, in 95% of cases, they are >25 degrees [95% confidence intervals, 25 to 50 degrees])[169] (**Schematic U**). CT is valuable when assessing intra-articular extension of calcaneal fractures. MRI may be used to assess for occult fractures when radiographs are normal.

The management of calcaneal fractures focuses on reestablishment of articular alignment, calcaneal width, and posterior facet. Extra-articular calcaneal fractures are typically treated nonoperatively and long-term sequelae are rare.[162,166] Management of intra-articular fractures is variable; whereas some authors advocate surgical treatment, others favor nonoperative therapy.

Other Tarsal Fracture. Tarsal fractures are rare, accounting for 1% of the pediatric fractures.[23] Most tarsal fractures are avulsion or stress fractures. Displaced fractures of the navicular, cuneiforms, or cuboid bones may result from high-energy trauma and have a high incidence of other associated osseous injuries. Most nondisplaced tarsal fractures are treated conservatively. Displaced and intra-articular fractures often required closed or open reduction and internal fixation.[162]

Metatarsal Fracture. Metatarsal fractures account for ~60% of the pediatric fractures.[163,170] Among pediatric patients <5 years of age, first metatarsal fractures account for 73% of all metatarsal fractures.[170] Approximately 40% of all metatarsal fractures involve the base of the fifth metatarsal.[163] Proximal fifth metatarsal fractures include avulsion fractures of the tuberosity, fractures of the proximal diaphysis (also known as "Jones fracture"), and diaphyseal stress fractures.[171–174]

Fractures of the proximal fifth metatarsal are caused by avulsion by the attachment of the peroneus brevis tendon and lateral band of the plantar fascia. The mechanism of injury is an inversion of the foot and ankle with plantarflexion. Affected pediatric patients typically present with point tenderness and pain while walking. Radiographs of avulsion fractures of the tuberosity show a transverse fracture line perpendicular to the long axis of the metatarsal (Fig. 24.38). Tuberosity avulsion fractures may be intra-articular involving the cuboid–metatarsal joint or extra-articular. In the skeletally immature child, it is important not to confuse the apophysis of the base of the fifth metatarsal for a fracture fragment. The growth plate of the apophysis parallels the long axis of the bone, whereas a true fracture runs perpendicular to the long axis (Fig. 24.38). The apophysis is also prone to avulsion, which is seen as abnormal widening of the apophyseal growth plate and displacement of the apophysis. A comparison contralateral view may be helpful for distinguishing a true avulsion fracture from a normal apophysis of the base of the fifth metatarsal. The treatment of choice is nonoperative with most patients returning to activity after symptomatic therapy.[175–177]

The Jones fracture is a proximal fifth metatarsal fracture that occurs ~1.5 to 2.0 cm distal to tuberosity. The mechanism of injury is due to sudden changes in direction with the heel elevated off the ground. Jones fractures were initially described in dancers but can be seen in pediatric patients involved in other sports such as football, tennis, and basketball. Radiographically, it is important to differentiate the Jones fracture from tuberosity avulsion fracture because the management and prognosis is different. The fracture line of a Jones fracture occurs more proximally, at the junction of the metaphysis and diaphysis at a site of tenuous blood supply.[176] Additionally, the fracture may involve the intermetatarsal joint, a feature not present in avulsion fractures. Jones fractures treated conservatively have a higher incidence of nonunion and refracture. Initial operative management is usually performed and has shown lower incidence of complications compared with conservative management.[177]

Metatarsal stress fractures are caused by increased stress to normal bones. The term "march" fractures (**Schematic V**) has been applied to this injury, because it is common to military recruits involved in increased weight-bearing activities. Young

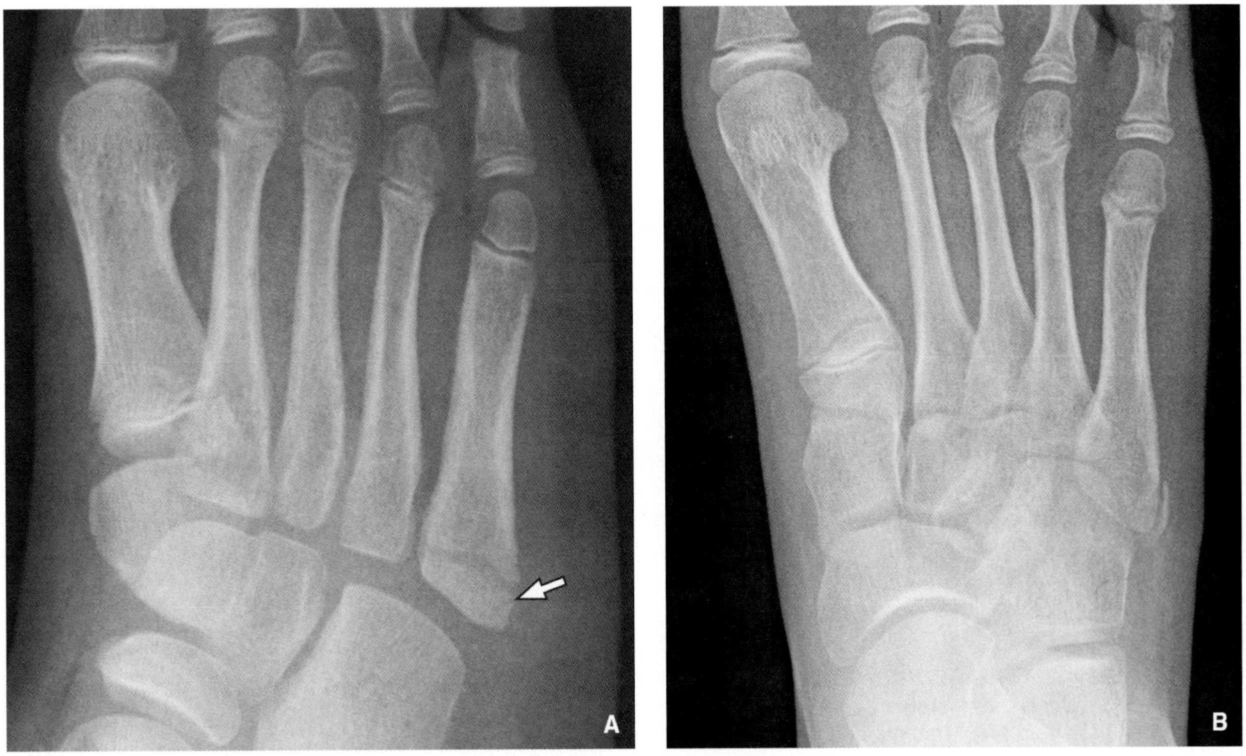

FIGURE 24.38 **Pseudo-Jones fracture and normal fifth metatarsal apophysis. A:** Anteroposterior radiograph shows a transverse fracture (*arrow*) through the base of the fifth metatarsal at the site of the peroneus brevis insertion. **B:** Appearance of the normal apophysis of the base of the fifth metatarsal.

athletes involved in sports such as long-distance running are at increased risk because of the repetitive stress to the forefoot. Poorly fitting shoes, increase in training volume, pes planus (flat foot), and metabolic disorders such as obesity and osteopenia are risk factors for developing a metatarsal stress fracture. The most common location is the second metatarsal. However, they can occur in any of the metatarsals and the diaphysis is most often involved. Stress fractures of the proximal fifth metatarsal are uncommon, but important to recognize because they have a higher incidence of nonunion.

On radiographs, stress fractures in the early stage are often occult. Radiographic findings in later stages include cortical thickening with narrowing of the medullary space, periosteal elevation, and faint fracture lines. MRI is more sensitive than radiography in detecting stress fractures. Findings on MRI include bone marrow edema, cortical thickening, and periosseous soft tissue edema.

Treatment of metatarsal stress fractures typically requires cessation from the causative activity for 4 to 8 weeks. Fifth metatarsal stress fractures are at increased risk for nonunion and may require surgical management in complicated cases.

Phalangeal Fracture. Phalangeal fractures of the foot are common and are likely under reported, accounting for up to 18% of the pediatric foot fractures.[163] Most phalangeal fractures are Salter-Harris type I or II fractures and represent 3% to 7% of all growth plate fractures.[23,159,160] Most phalangeal fractures are treated with buddy taping of the toe. The "stubbed toe" fracture is a Salter-Harris type 1 or 2 injury of the distal phalanx of the great toe (Fig. 24.39) (**Schematic V**). The nail bed is attached to the periosteum, which can predispose the patient to bacterial seeding and subsequent osteomyelitis. Therefore, prophylactic antibiotics are administered for this type of injury.[178]

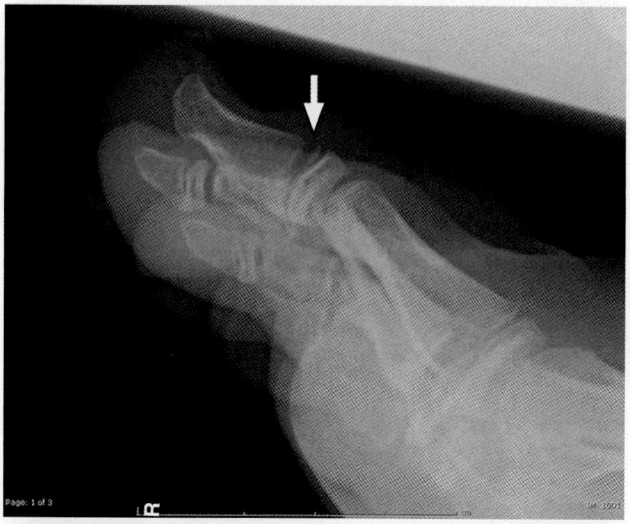

FIGURE 24.39 **Stubbed toe fracture in a 3-year-old boy who complained of foot pain after trauma.** Lateral radiograph of the great toe shows a Salter-Harris type II fracture of the distal phalanx in the subungual region (*arrow*), which predisposes the patient to osteomyelitis.

Lisfranc Fracture. The Lisfranc fracture-dislocation is defined as a midfoot injury whereby one or more of the metatarsal bones are displaced from the tarsus (**Schematic U**). This injury is rare in children and is often misdiagnosed.[179] However, early recognition is essential because of potential severe loss of function and long-term disability from chronic pain and a planovalgus deformity if diagnosis and treatment are delayed. The most common mechanism of this fracture is axial loading with the foot in plantarflexion or a direct crush injury. Associated fractures of the proximal first metatarsal are common. Ligamentous injury of the tarsometatarsal joint complex is also typically associated with Lisfranc fracture-dislocation.

On a frontal radiograph, the medial aspect of the base of the second metatarsal should align with the medial aspect of the middle cuneiform and the medial aspect of the base of the fourth metatarsal should align with the medial aspect of the cuboid. Disruption of these normal relationships suggests underlying ligamentous injury of the tarsometatarsal joint. The most frequent radiographic finding of the Lisfranc fracture-dislocation is diastasis between the first and second metatarsals[180] (Fig. 24.40) (**Schematic U**). Associated fractures of the base of the first metatarsal are also common. MDCT can be used to detect occult Lisfranc fracture-dislocation and additional bony injuries in children with high clinical suspicion but unremarkable radiographs[179,181] (Fig. 24.40).

Lisfranc fracture-dislocation with <2 mm displacement may be treated conservatively,[182] but patients with Lisfranc fracture-dislocation typically need surgical treatment.[183,184]

Specific Types of Appendicular Skeleton Fractures

Toddler Fracture

A classic toddler fracture is a nondisplaced oblique or spiral fracture through the tibial diaphysis.[185] Children 9 months to 3 years of age are usually affected, and the mechanism of injury is often due to a twisting or torsional force applied to the foot or lower leg.[186] Common injuries for this fracture include falls and trapping of the leg between two fixed bars. Affected toddlers typically present with pain, inability to bear weight, and pain localized to the tibia. Clinical signs are often nonspecific and physical exams in patients of this age group can be challenging.[185–187] Therefore, radiographic imaging evaluation is necessary to make an early and accurate diagnosis.

Frontal and lateral radiographs are usually sufficient to detect the hairline oblique or spiral fracture line in the tibial diaphysis (Fig. 24.41). Oblique views may demonstrate a fracture that is occult on the initial radiographs.[186] It is not uncommon for a toddler's fracture to be radiographically occult in the acute setting. In these instances, a short-interval follow-up exam in 10 to 14 days may shows healing in the form of periosteal new bone formation and sclerosis along the fracture line, which confirm the suspected diagnosis.

Toddler fractures and their equivalents are treated conservatively and typically heal without complications.[188]

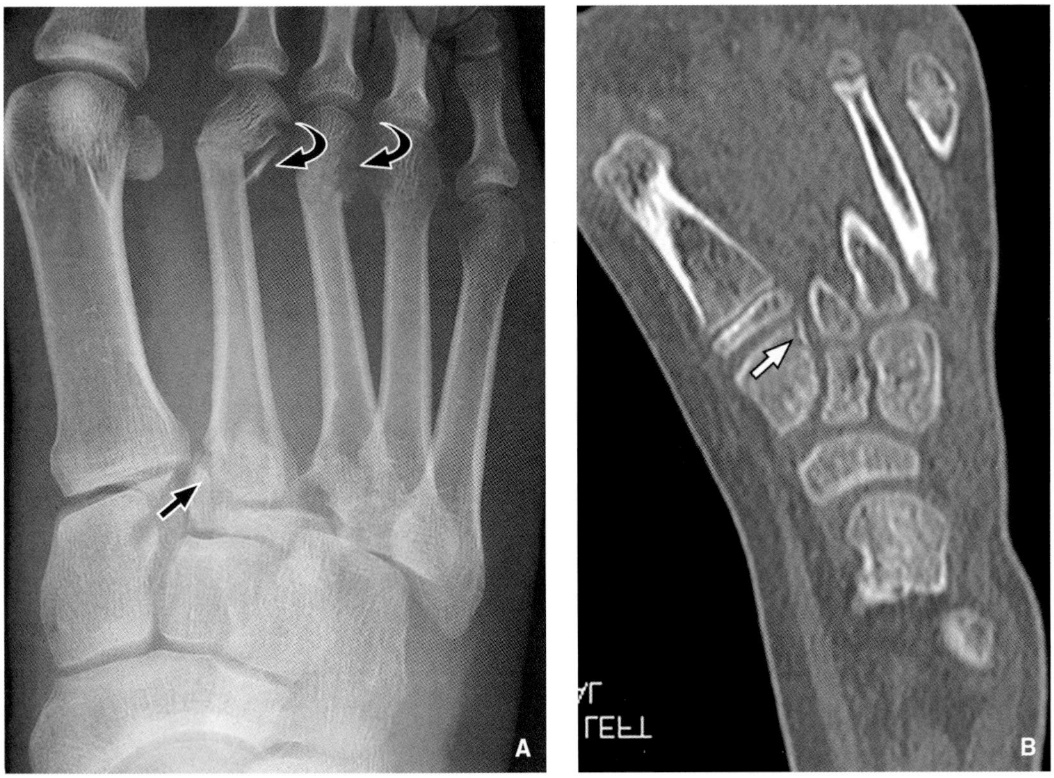

FIGURE 24.40 **Lisfranc fracture-dislocation in a 16-year-old boy. A:** Anteroposterior radiograph of the foot shows an avulsion fracture (*arrow*) of the base of the second metatarsal at the site of attachment of the Lisfranc ligament. There are associated fractures (*curved arrows*) of the distal second and third metatarsals. Lateral displacement of the second through fifth metatarsal bases are present. **B:** Reformatted CT image demonstrates an avulsion fracture (*arrow*) of the lateral aspect of the medial cuneiform at the site of the attachment of the Lisfranc ligament.

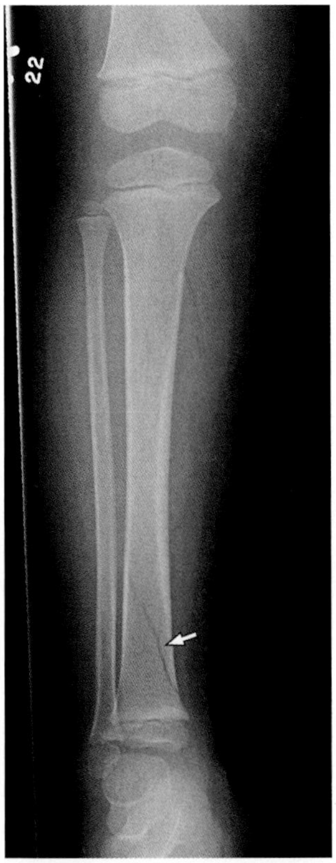

FIGURE 24.41 **Toddler fracture in a 2-year-old boy who presented with pain, limp, and inability to bear weight.** Anteroposterior radiograph of the right leg demonstrates a spiral fracture (*arrow*) through the distal aspect of the tibial diaphysis.

Buckle Fracture

A buckle fracture, also known as a "torus" fracture (**Schematic H**), is an incomplete fracture usually involving the metaphysis or the junction between the metaphysis and diaphysis of a long bone. The wrist, ankle, and elbow are common locations of a buckle fracture, with the distal radius being the most common site. In the upper extremity, the mechanism of injury is axial loading usually due to a fall onto an outstretched hand. Radiographs show the cortical contour abnormality, buckling of the cortex without a visible cortical break (Fig. 24.42). Buckle fractures can be subtle and particular attention to the contour of the metaphysis is required to detect these fractures[189,190] (Fig. 24.42). The lateral views are especially useful in showing this injury. Treatment is immobilization, and complications are uncommon.[191–198]

Greenstick Fracture

A greenstick fracture represents an incomplete fracture of a long bone (Fig. 24.43). This occurs because of underlying soft bone in infants and young children in which the bone bends and partially breaks. The mechanism of injury is typically a force applied perpendicular to the long axis of the bone and commonly involves the diaphysis of the forearm bones.[199,200] A greenstick fracture occurs less frequently than do the torus fractures and is typically located in the middiaphysis of the long bones. In general, greenstick fractures are treated with cast immobilization.[201] On radiographs, there is a cortical

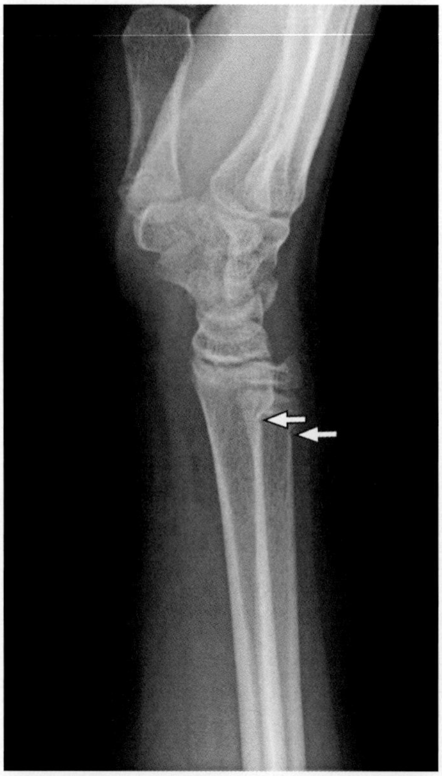

FIGURE 24.42 **Buckle fractures of the distal radius and ulna in a 12-year-old girl after fall onto an outstretched hand.** Lateral radiograph of the wrist shows contour abnormalities (*arrows*) of the dorsal cortex of both the distal radial and ulnar metaphyses.

break involving the tension side of the cortex and plastic deformation of the compression side.

Plastic Fracture

A plastic or bowing fracture is a pediatric fracture that results in bending or bowing of the bone due to a longitudinal force.[202,203] Plastic fractures usually occur in the first decade of life.[204] The physical properties of pediatric bones allow for this unique pattern of injury. Up to a certain point, applied force causes the bone to bend and recoil to its original state. If force continues beyond the elastic limit, the bone deforms resulting in a plastic or bowing fracture with microfractures along the concave surface.[205,206] Increase force beyond the amount causing bowing results in frank fracture. Similar to greenstick fractures, bowing fractures most commonly occur in the radius and ulna although any long bone can be involved.[207,208]

Radiographs show bowing of one or both long bones of the forearm or leg (Fig. 24.44). The degree of bowing is variable, and a comparison view of the contralateral side may be helpful for accurately detecting subtle bowing fractures. Affected pediatric patients with a <20 degrees of fracture angulation are treated with immobilization alone, whereas fractures with greater degrees of angulation are treated with closed reduction or internal fixation.[209,210]

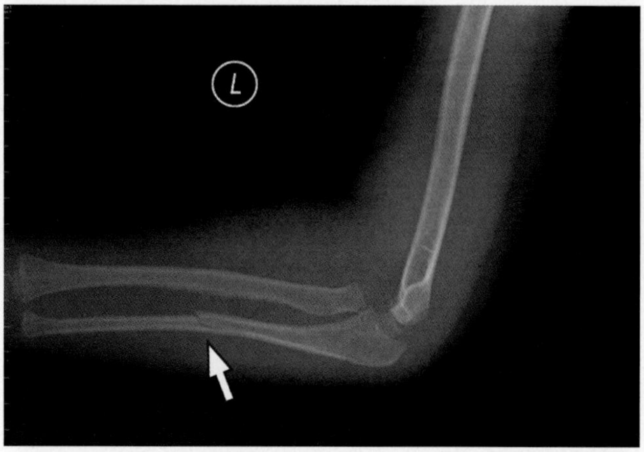

FIGURE 24.43 **Greenstick fracture in a 3-year-old boy.** Lateral radiograph of the left forearm shows an incomplete fracture (*arrow*) through the midshaft of the ulna with breach of the anterior cortex and an intact posterior cortex. There is also radiocapitellar dislocation (Monteggia fracture).

Stress Fracture

A stress fracture is an overuse injury, which results from repetitive stress or muscle tension on normal bone. It typically occurs in highly active children whereby the rate of osteoclastic activity is faster than the body's ability to repair the bone. Bone usually remodels to match increased loading, but without sufficient time to remodel and heal the affected bone subsequently fatigues and fractures. Typical locations and underlying causes of stress fractures in children include (1) tibia, fibula, and tarsals from running; (2) calcaneus from running or jumping; (3) metatarsals from running or ballet; and (4) sesamoids from standing, skiing, or cycling.

Stress changes and fractures typically demonstrate sclerosis and cortical thickening on radiographs. In cases of stress fractures, the stress fracture line is usually transversely oriented but can be longitudinally oriented in the minority of cases[211] (Fig. 24.45). Early or subtle stress injury or fracture may be occult on radiographs but can be detected with bone scintigraphy or MRI. Bone scintigraphy, once considered the gold standard for this diagnosis, is very sensitive in the detection of stress fracture[212] but lacks specificity and exposes the pediatric patient to ionizing radiation. MRI is now the imaging modality of choice in a pediatric patient with suspected stress fracture and can differentiate stress reaction from stress fracture.[213] With stress reaction, there is typically nonspecific bone marrow edema pattern (hyperintense signal on T2-weighted and short tau inversion recovery (STIR) fluid–sensitive sequences and corresponding hypointense signal on T1-weighted MR imaging) without fracture line. Associated periostitis and periosseous soft tissue edema are also commonly encountered findings in case of stress reaction. In contrast, a hypointense band of signal on T1-weighted MR images, representing a fracture line, is seen with stress fractures.

Treatment for stress reaction and stress fractures is usually conservative and affected pediatric patients usually respond well to a period of rest for 4 to 8 weeks. Operative management is currently considered for delayed union of stress fractures.

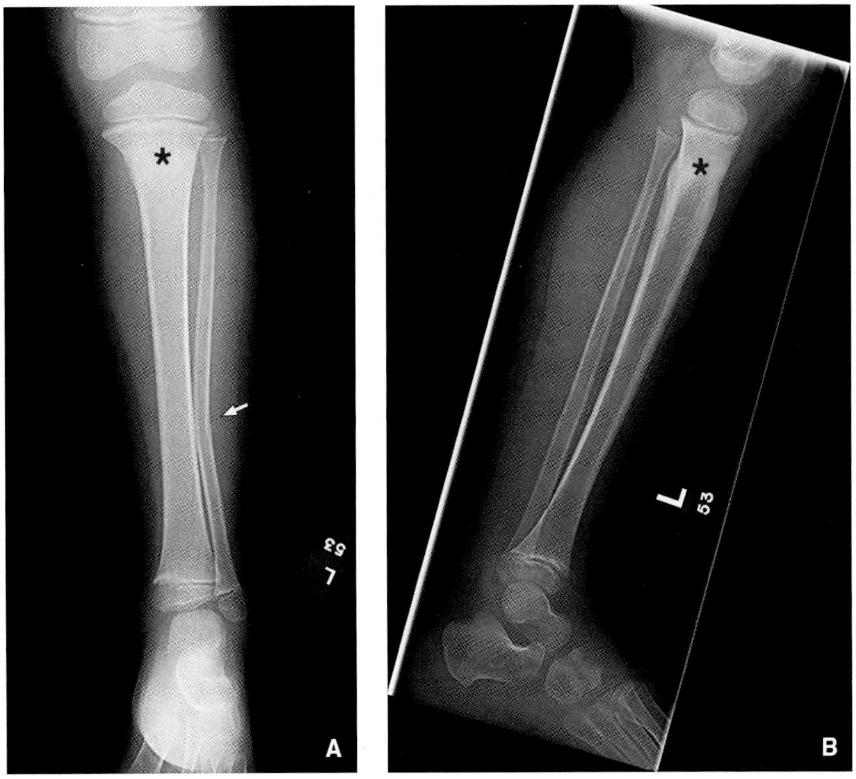

FIGURE 24.44 **Plastic fracture in a 5-year-old boy.** Anteroposterior **(A)** and lateral **(B)** radiographs of the left leg show a medial bowing deformity (*arrow*) of the fibula compatible with a plastic bowing fracture. Note is also made of a healing fracture of the proximal tibia (*asterisk*).

Complications of Fractures

Growth Arrest and Bony Bar Formation

Physeal fractures are relatively common in skeletally immature patients, with an estimated incidence of 3 per 1,000 children.[116] Growth arrest is a common complication of trauma and may result in a growth disturbance due to formation of a bony bridge traversing the physis. However, it may occur from a variety of other insults such as infection, radiation, tumor, thermal injury, and ischemia.[214] Growth arrest occurs more commonly in the injuries involving the lower extremities (distal femur and proximal tibia) than the upper extremities.[215]

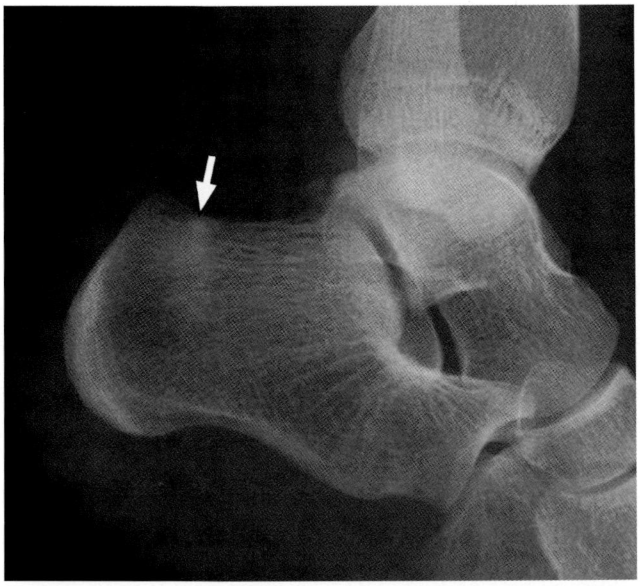

FIGURE 24.45 **Calcaneal stress fracture in a 16-year-old girl who is a runner and presented with heel pain.** Lateral radiograph of the ankle shows a linear band of sclerosis (*arrow*) involving the posterior aspect of the calcaneus consistent with a stress fracture.

In growth arrest, a bridge of bone crosses the physis thereby connecting the metaphysis with the epiphysis. Small, peripheral bone bridges can result in angular deformities. If the bone bridge is large and central, longitudinal growth of the bone is restricted and a limb length discrepancy may ensue. Fractures involving the growth plate should be closely followed clinically and radiographically in order to assess for complications such as growth arrest. Growth arrest usually occurs 3 to 6 months after the initial injury.

Findings on radiographs that raise suspicion for growth arrest include loss of patency of the physis and tethering of a growth recovery line, which usually is parallel to the physis[216] (Fig. 24.46). MRI is the imaging modality of choice to evaluate the growth plate (Fig. 24.46). Gradient-recalled echo sequences can depict the bony bridge in multiple imaging planes. On this sequence, the bony bar is isointense to the bone marrow signal and stands out in contrast to the hyperintense signal of the cartilaginous growth plate.[215] A 3D map can be constructed for preoperative planning. If MRI availability is limited, low-dose MDCT with multiplanar reconstructions and axial maximum-intensity projections of the physis can be used to calculate the area of a physeal bar (Fig. 24.46).

Treatment of growth arrest depends on several factors. The remaining growth potential of the pediatric patient is paramount because children with little remaining growth may tolerate growth arrest relatively well with conservative treatment.

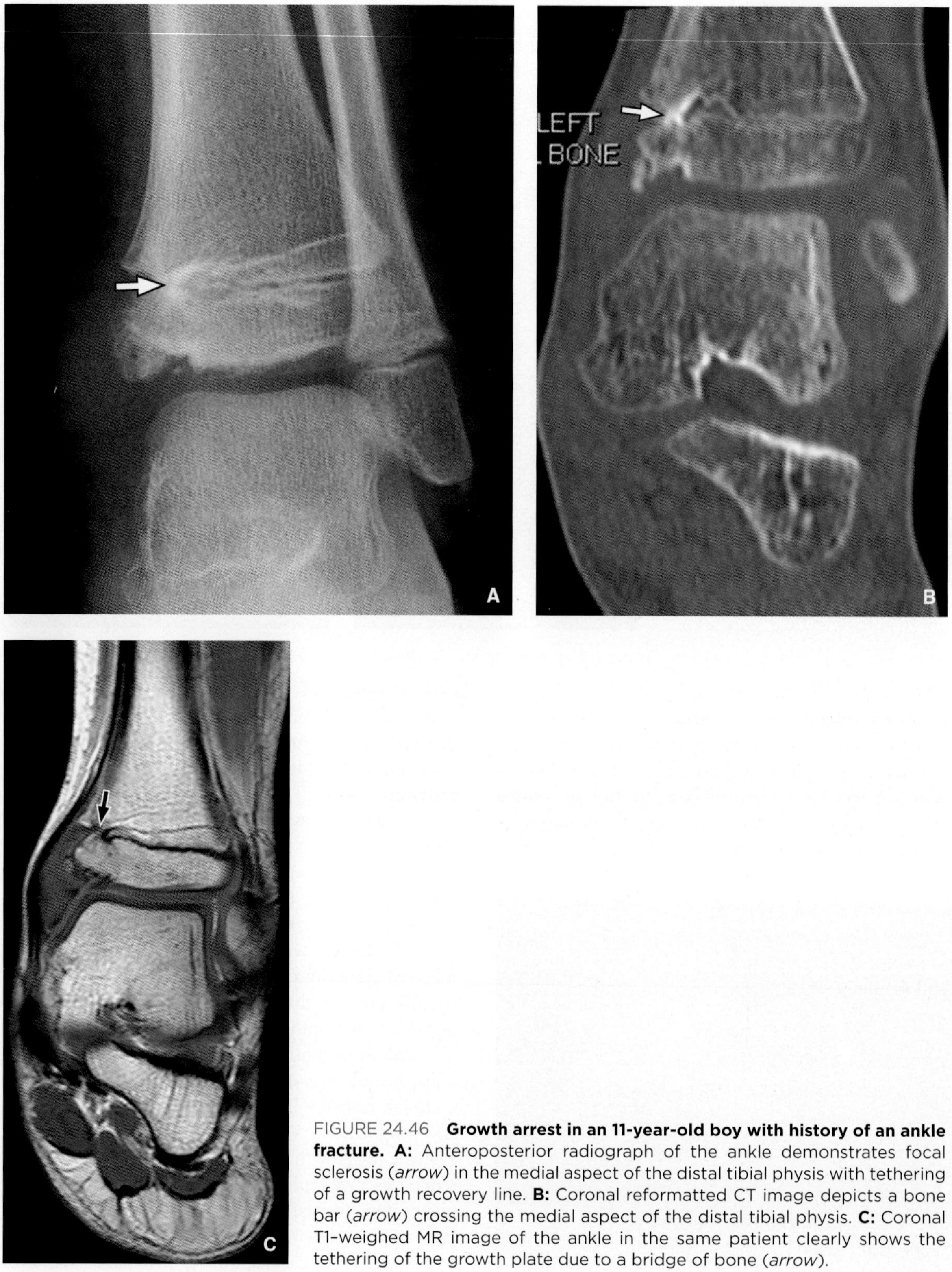

FIGURE 24.46 **Growth arrest in an 11-year-old boy with history of an ankle fracture. A:** Anteroposterior radiograph of the ankle demonstrates focal sclerosis (*arrow*) in the medial aspect of the distal tibial physis with tethering of a growth recovery line. **B:** Coronal reformatted CT image depicts a bone bar (*arrow*) crossing the medial aspect of the distal tibial physis. **C:** Coronal T1-weighed MR image of the ankle in the same patient clearly shows the tethering of the growth plate due to a bridge of bone (*arrow*).

In contrast, younger pediatric patients with substantial growth potential would not tolerate growth arrest because it could result in a disabling limb length discrepancy. The extremity involved, size, and location (central vs. peripheral) of the bar are important considerations when the orthopedic surgeon is planning surgical intervention. Surgical resection of the bone bar with interposition of an inert material such as fat is typically performed when the bone bridge involves <50% of the physis.[217]

Nonunion

Follow-up radiographs are routinely performed in pediatric patients with fractures to assess for appropriate healing.

Subacute or chronic complications of fractures include delayed union, nonunion, and malunion. Delayed union is a term used to describe a fracture that has not healed within the expected time for that particular bone.[218] Nonunion is the endpoint of delayed union when healing fails without bony contiguity of the fracture fragments. Malnutrition, metabolic disorders, medications, and activity level are systemic factors that can impact healing. Local risk factors include comminution, distraction of osseous fragments, open fractures, superimposed infection, insufficient immobilization, and repetitive trauma.[219]

The treatment of nonunion is typically surgical. Fracture malunion is a term applied when a bone heals in an abnormal position. Mild deviations from normal can be functional, whereas greater deformities that are nonfunctional require surgical intervention.

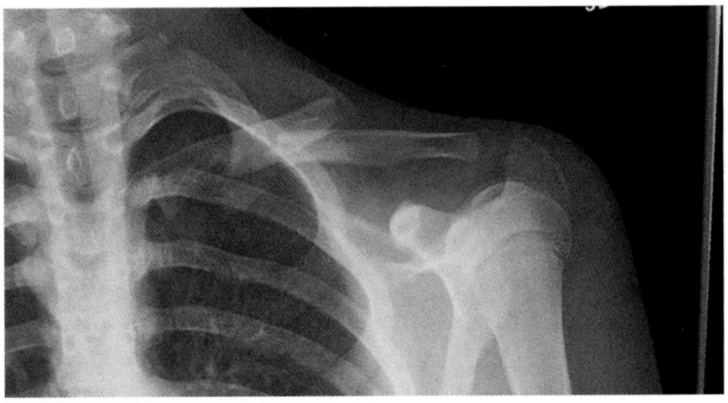

FIGURE 24.47 **Clavicle fracture in a 10-year-old boy after a fall from a height.** Anteroposterior radiograph of the left shoulder shows an acute fracture through the mid left clavicle. There is overlap of the fracture fragments with superior displacement of the proximal fragment from unopposed pull from the sternocleidomastoid muscle.

Axial Skeleton

Clavicle

The clavicle fracture is common in children. The vast majority of clavicle fractures occur in the midshaft (80%), followed by the distal (15%) and medial (5%) aspects of the clavicle. This propensity for the midsegment of the clavicle to fracture is because the middle of the clavicle is the thinnest portion of the bone and is the only part that is not reinforced by muscular and ligamentous attachments.[220] A fall on an outstretched arm, direct impact, and sports injuries are typical mechanisms that can result in a clavicle fracture.[221] The clavicle is also the most commonly fractured bone in newborns during birth and usually heals without sequelae.[222] There is typically pain, deformity, and point tenderness at the site of fracture.

Radiographs are usually sufficient for the diagnosis of a clavicle fracture. It is preferable that two views (AP and cephalad-tilted views) are obtained because the fracture line is usually vertical orientation. With midshaft fractures, the proximal fracture fragment may displace superiorly because of the pull from the attachment of the sternocleidomastoid muscle (Fig. 24.47). The distal fragment may displace inferiorly because of the attachment of the coracoclavicular ligament.

Treatment of clavicle fractures is usually nonoperative consisting of rest and placing the shoulder in a sling. Indications for operative management include open fractures, skin tenting, significant displacement, or >2 cm of overlapping fracture fragments. Distal clavicle fractures involving the acromioclavicular joint and ligaments may require internal fixation. Nonunion is most common with distal clavicle fractures, occurring in up to 30% of cases.[223,224] Degenerative arthritis is a complication when there is joint involvement.

Pelvis

Traumatic Pelvic Fracture

Pelvic fractures are uncommon and often due to high-energy trauma. Fractures of the pelvis account for 1% to 3% of skeletal injuries and for 2.4% to 7.5% of cases of hospitalization for blunt trauma in children.[225,226] Pedestrian struck by a vehicle and a passenger in an MVA are the most common mechanisms of injury.

Pelvic fractures in the skeletally immature child differ from fractures in older children and adults. The elasticity of the sacroiliac joints and symphysis pubis as well as the plasticity of the bones in younger children allow for substantial displacement. Therefore, a higher amount of energy is required to cause a pelvic fracture. Differences in bone composition and joint laxity may result in one fracture of the pelvic ring in the young child, whereas older children and adults typically fracture the pelvic ring in two locations.[227] Because of the high amount of energy required to fracture the pelvis, children with pelvic fractures often have other skeletal and visceral injuries. Long bone fractures are commonly associated with pelvic fractures. Closed head, thoracic, abdominopelvic visceral, and urogenital injuries are common causes of morbidity and mortality in patients with pelvic fractures.[228]

Several classification systems currently exist to categorize pelvic fractures, with the Torode and Zieg (**Schematic ii**) being most widely used. Type 1 pelvic fractures are avulsion fractures (Fig. 24.48). Type II pelvic fractures are iliac wing fractures and are caused by lateral compressive forces. Type III pelvic fractures are the most common and include simple ring fractures such as isolated fractures of the pubic ramus and disruption of the pubic symphysis (with intact sacroiliac joints), and some authors include isolated acetabular fractures in this category. Type IV pelvic fractures are ring disruptions and include fracture or diastasis of both anterior and posterior pelvic structures (Fig. 24.49), such as a pelvic–acetabular fracture and a "straddle fracture," which includes bilateral superior and inferior pubic rami fractures. Both type III and type IV pelvic fractures usually result from anteroposterior compressive forces.[228,229]

Screening AP radiographs of the pelvis are often obtained in patients with blunt abdominal trauma as a part of initial

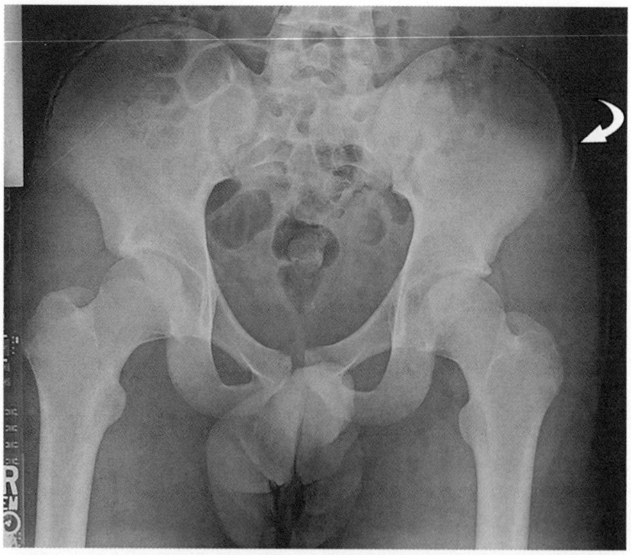

FIGURE 24.48 **Left anterior superior iliac spine avulsion fracture in a 16-year-old boy with left hip pain after sprinting.** Anteroposterior radiograph of the pelvis shows a crescentic ossific density adjacent to the left iliac wing and iliac spine diagnostic of avulsion fractures (*curved arrow*). This is the site of sartorius muscle attachment.

advanced trauma life support evaluation. However, for more accurate assessment of pelvic fractures in the setting of trauma, both inlet and outlet views of the pelvis should be obtained. The inlet view, obtained with x-ray beam angled ~45 degrees caudad, is helpful for evaluation of (1) anterior or posterior translation of the hemipelvis, (2) internal or external rotation of the hemipelvis, (3) widening of the sacroiliac (SI) joint, and (4) sacral ala impaction. The outlet view, obtained with x-ray beam angled ~45-degree cephalad, is useful for evaluation of (1) vertical translation of the hemipelvis, (2) flexion and extension of the hemipelvis, and (3) disruption of sacral foramina and location of sacral fractures. Given the sensitivity of the outlet view for the detection of pelvic fractures, it has become a routine part of pelvic injury evaluation.[230]

CT allows the detection of subtle fractures and displacement of fracture fragments not appreciated on radiographs. CT is particularly helpful for accurately detecting fracture lines relative to sacral foramina, defining comminution and fragment rotation, and characterizing posterior ring injuries. Multiplanar and 3D-reconstructed CT images in bone algorithm can be postprocessed from abdominal and pelvis CT images performed for evaluation of visceral trauma, with special regard to bladder injuries. Up to 57% of children with bladder injury have a pelvic fracture.[231]

The management of pelvic fractures has traditionally been nonoperative.[230,232,233] Operative management is controversial.[234] However, external fixation can be performed in pediatric patients with pelvic ring injuries with an external rotation component or unstable pelvic ring injury with ongoing blood loss. CT angiography may be necessary for evaluation of pelvic vascular injury in the presence of ongoing arterial hemorrhage, which requires embolization.

Pelvic Avulsion Fracture

Pelvic avulsion fractures occur in predictable locations. Adolescent athletes are most commonly affected. In this population, the unfused pelvic apophyses are relatively weak and prone to fracture.[235] If not properly diagnosed and treated, these injuries can be debilitating. Apophyseal avulsion injuries include the ischial tuberosity, anterior superior iliac spine

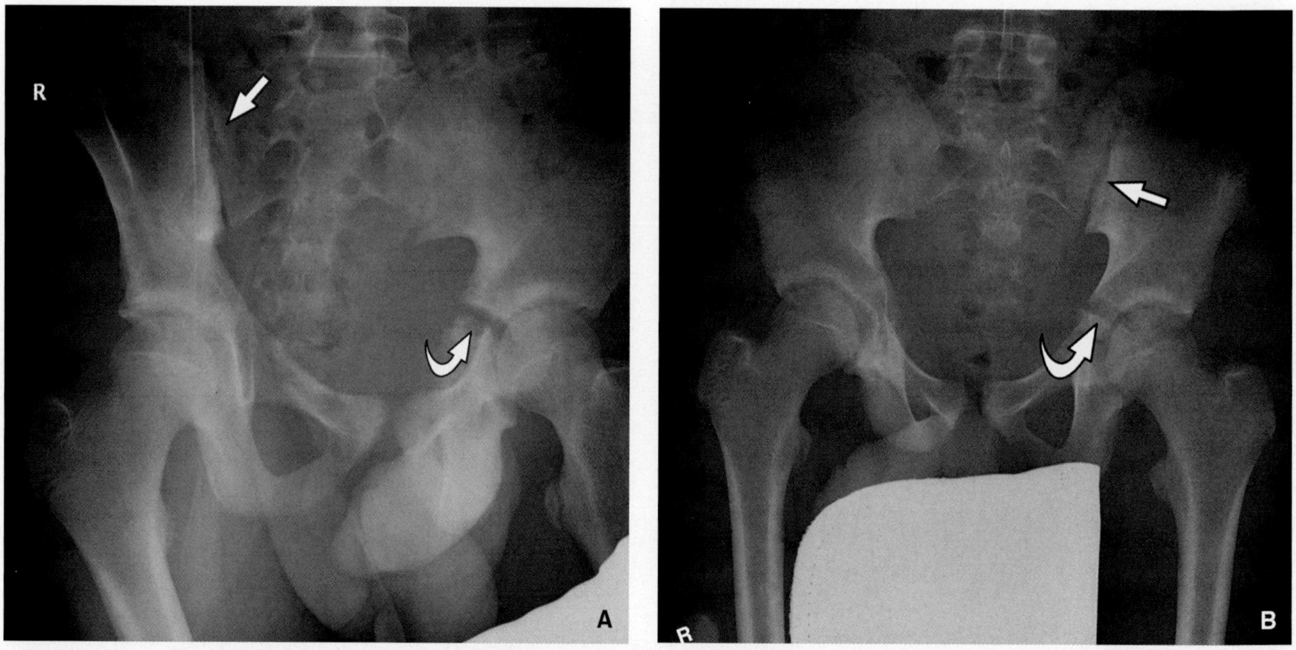

FIGURE 24.49 **Pelvic fractures involving anterior and posterior structures in a 17-year-old boy after car accident.** Oblique **(A)** and frontal **(B)** radiographs of the pelvis demonstrate widening (*curved arrow*) of the left triradiate cartilage and diastasis (*straight arrow*) of the sacroiliac joint.

(ASIS), anterior inferior iliac spine (AIIS), pubis symphysis, and iliac crest. Avulsion of the ischial tuberosity, which is the site of hamstring muscles' attachment, is the most frequent type of pelvic avulsion fracture.[236] This injury usually occurs in forceful contraction of the hamstring muscles during sprinting or passive lengthening of the muscle in activities such as cheerleading or dancing. Avulsion of the ASIS occurs from forceful hip extension at the site of sartorius and tensor fascia lata attachment (Fig. 24.48). Clinically, affected pediatric patients are tender just below the iliac crest and the fracture fragment may be palpable. The straight head of the rectus femoris muscle attaches to the AIIS. Avulsions of the AIIS are less common than are those of the ASIS and are caused by a similar mechanism. Avulsive injuries of the pubic symphysis are uncommon and are usually due to chronic pull of the adductor muscles. Iliac crest avulsions are even less common and are the site of attachment of the abdominal muscles and can occur because of chronic microtrauma or acutely during rapid changes in direction (Fig. 24.48). Avulsions of the greater trochanter, which is the site of attachment of the hip rotators including the gluteal muscles, piriformis muscle, and gemellus muscles, occur with sudden changes in direction of the body.

The diagnosis of pelvic avulsion fractures is usually made with AP pelvic radiograph, sometimes complemented by additional oblique views. When radiographs are unremarkable and clinical suspicion for avulsion fracture persists, CT can be performed. CT is excellent for detecting nondisplaced fractures and fracture fragments. MRI can be also performed to assess for concomitant injury to the muscles, tendons, and ligaments.[237] Findings on MRI include bone marrow edema, injuries to the tendon, and widening of the physis (Fig. 24.50).

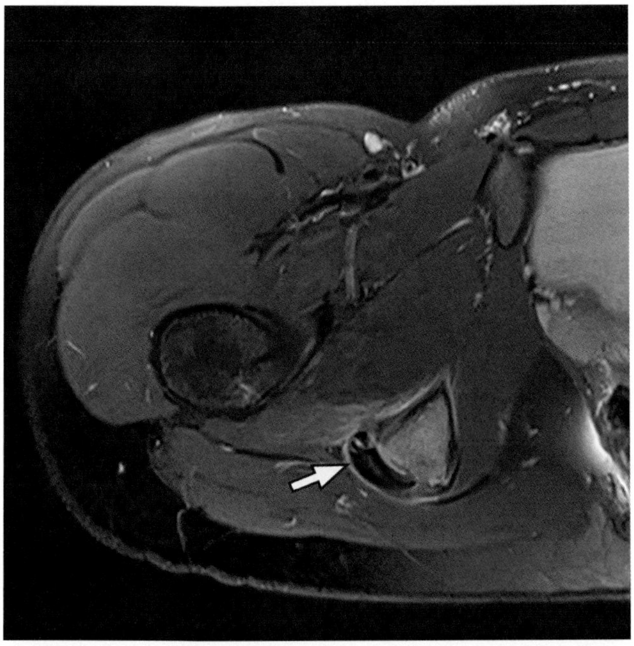

FIGURE 24.50 **Ischial tuberosity avulsion injury in a 15-year-old girl.** Axial T2-weighted fat-suppressed MR image of the right hip demonstrates an avulsion injury (*arrow*) of the ischial tuberosity at the hamstring tendon attachment site. There is marrow edema in the ischium and adjacent soft tissue edema.

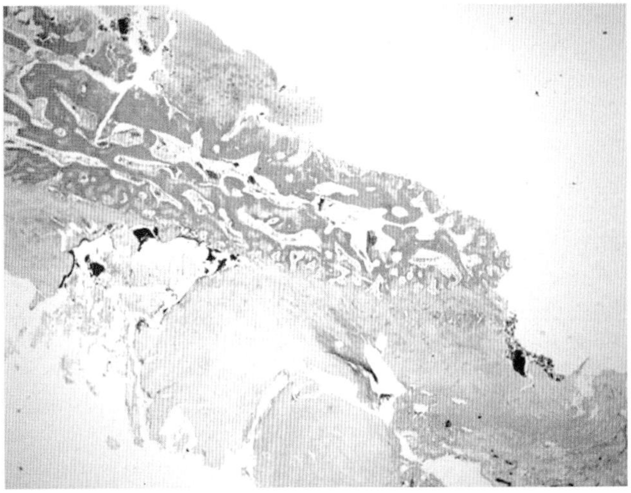

FIGURE 24.51 **Apophyseal avulsion fracture in a 17-year-old boy.** This microscopic image shows an avulsed fragment of ischium, resected because of painful nonunion, with fibrotendinous attachments on one side (lower right) and fracture callus (upper left) on another (hematoxylin and eosin; original magnification, 40×).

In challenging cases, MRI can help differentiate chronic avulsions from neoplasms. It is important not to confuse a healing apophyseal avulsion fracture with a more sinister entity such as infection or sarcoma. Biopsy of a healing avulsion fracture typically shows clear fracture callus and other features of trauma (Fig. 24.51), but it may occasionally be nondiagnostic or misleading and result in additional tests and procedures.

Pelvic apophyseal fractures are treated conservatively with variable amounts of bed rest or restriction of activity in addition to the use of analgesics for pain control. Painful nonunion and exostosis formation may require surgical intervention.

Spine

Cervical Spine

Cervical spinal trauma in pediatric patients is rare but can result in potentially devastating neurologic deficits. Injuries to the cervical spine account for ~1% to 3% of all pediatric trauma patients and represent 37% to 80% of spine injuries occurring after blunt trauma,[238] and ~72% of spine injuries in children <8 years of age occur in the cervical spine.[238–240] In general, pediatric patients <8 years of age sustain injuries to the upper cervical spine, from the occiput to the C2–C3 level, whereas older pediatric patients typically sustain injuries to the lower cervical spine. The propensity of upper cervical spine injuries in the younger age group is thought to result from increased mobility due to incomplete ossification of the spine, increased ligamentous laxity, weaker cervical musculature, and a higher fulcrum of cervical motion at the C2–C3 level, compared to C5–C6 level in older children and adults.[239,241–243]

MVAs are the most common mechanism of injury leading to cervical spinal trauma.[244] Other mechanisms of injury include falls and sports-related injuries. Pediatric patients with Down, Marfan, Morquio, and Grisel syndromes and rheumatoid arthritis are at increased risk for atlantoaxial instability.[245] Cervical spine injuries may be associated with concomitant intracranial injuries.

Determining the imaging modality to be used for assessment of a pediatric patient with known or suspected cervical spine trauma depends on the mechanism of injury and clinical presentation. In general, cervical spine radiographs are performed in children with low-risk injuries and when feasible they should include AP, lateral, and open-mouth views. The use of flexion and extension views is controversial because they can be unsafe to perform and have limitations.[246,247] CT is typically performed in pediatric patients with abnormalities on radiographs and in select patients with high-risk mechanisms of injury.[245,247] In keeping with the principle of ALARA, the radiation dose of the CT examination should be kept as low as possible and collimated to the area of interest. MRI can be performed to assess for spinal cord injury and ligamentous injury.

Pseudosubluxation. One of the challenges in radiographic interpretation of the pediatric spine is due to the range of normal anatomic variants. Pseudosubluxation of the cervical spine can mimic true anterior traumatic subluxation. In children, usually between 1 and 7 years, the C2–C3 or C3–C4 space may have a physiologic displacement mimicking posttraumatic subluxation. On a lateral radiograph of the cervical spine, the spinolaminar line should be contiguous; a >2 mm offset indicates true injury rather than pseudosubluxation[243,248,249] (Fig. 24.52).

Spinal Cord Injury without Radiographic Abnormality (SCIWORA). Spinal cord injury without radiographic abnormality is defined as a spinal cord injury in the setting of normal radiographs and a normal CT.[250] Younger children are at increased risk for this entity, which is thought to be a result of ligamentous laxity and increased mobility of the spine.[239] Another proposed mechanism for this injury is small-vessel damage as a result of hypermobility leading to impaired spinal cord perfusion and subsequent cord ischemia.[251,252] MRI should be performed when clinical symptoms of posttraumatic myelopathy are present despite the absence of radiographic abnormality. MRI may show spinal cord transection or variable degrees of cord edema or hemorrhage (Fig. 24.53). Other MRI findings in SCIWORA include extra-axial hemorrhage and traumatic disc herniation.[253]

Craniocervical Junction Injury. Injuries of the craniocervical junction (**Schematic iii**) are often fatal with pediatric patients suffering from devastating neurologic sequelae. The mechanism of injury is typically a rapid deceleration, which leads to dislocation and reduction of the atlanto-occipital joint. Fortunately, this severe injury is uncommon but more often affects young children because of their relatively small occipital condyles and horizontal orientation of the atlanto-occipital joint.[241,254] Injury to the alar ligaments is common and leads to malalignment.

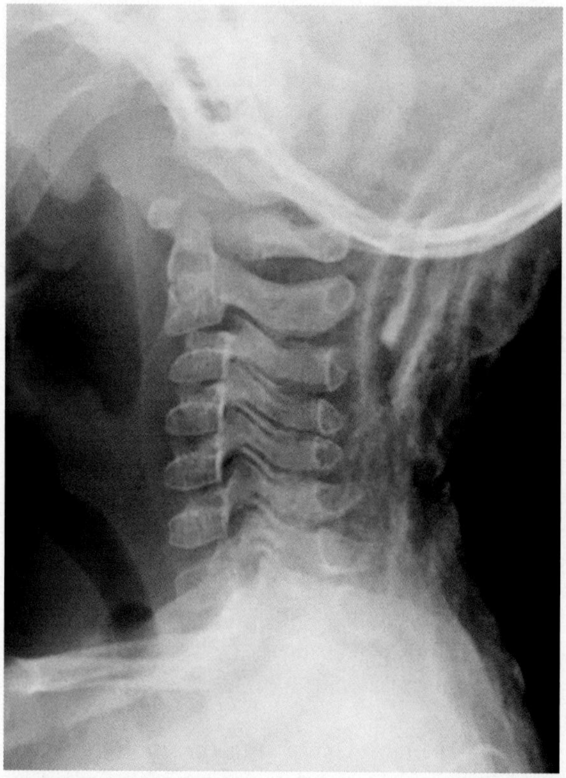

FIGURE 24.52 **Pseudosubluxation in a 3-year-old boy.** There is mild anterolisthesis of C2 on C3 without splaying of the posterior elements.

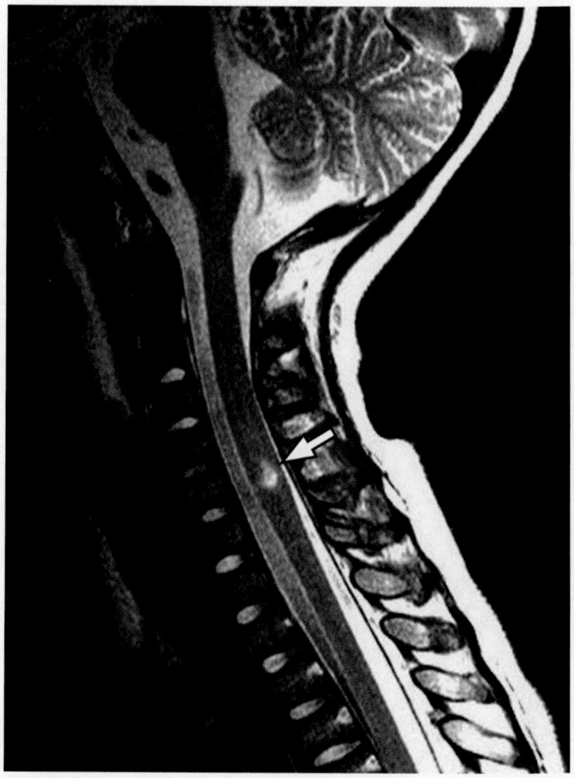

FIGURE 24.53 **Spinal cord injury without radiographic abnormality in a 4-year-old boy with status post motor vehicle accident and normal cervical spine CT (not shown).** Sagittal T2-weighted MR image of the cervical spine shows focal spinal cord contusion (*arrow*).

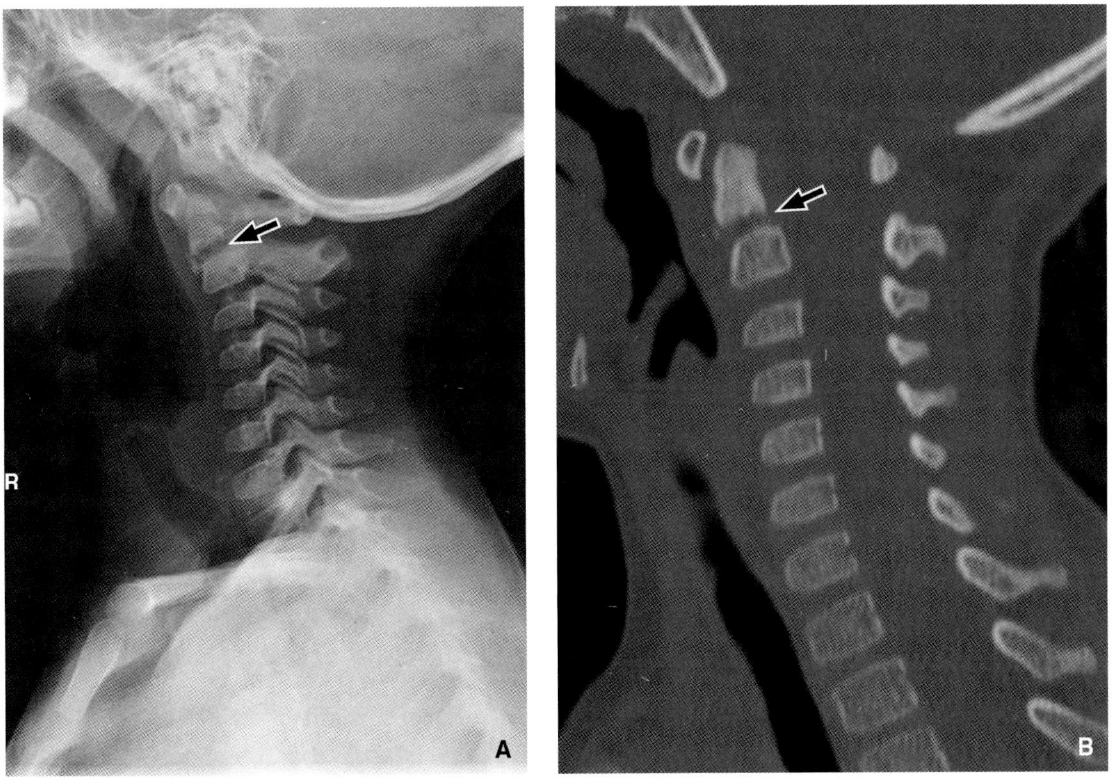

FIGURE 24.54 **Type 2 dens fracture in a 4-year-old boy after a fall.** Lateral radiograph of the cervical spine **(A)** and sagittal reformatted CT image of the cervical spine **(B)** both show a transverse fracture line (*arrow*) through the body of the dens.

On radiographs, retropharyngeal soft tissue swelling is usually present. The Wachenheim clivus line (line drawn along posterior surface of clivus to upper cervical spine), basion-dens interval (distance between the basion and tip of the dens), and power ratio (**Schematic iv**) (described as ratio of BC/OA where BC is the distance from the basion to the midvertical portion of posterior laminar line of the atlas and OA is the distance from opisthion to midvertical portion of posterior surface of anterior ring of atlas; if this ratio is >1, anterior subluxation is strongly suspected) are all helpful measurements that assist in diagnosing distraction injuries. CT should be performed when this injury is suspected.

Craniocervical injuries are often fatal because of brainstem injury.[255] Affected pediatric patients who survive may be treated with fusion of the occiput to C1 or C2.[243]

Atlantoaxial Fracture. A Jefferson fracture (**Schematic W**) is characterized by a fracture of the C1 ring and is caused by axial compression forces in MVAs or diving injuries. Jefferson fractures are almost always associated with fractures in two locations of the C1 ring.[256] Isolated fracture in either the anterior or posterior ring may occur in children, but may be associated with concomitant ligamentous or apophyseal growth plate injuries. On the open-mouth frontal radiograph, there is increased distance between the lateral mass of C1 and the dens. Greater than 8 mm suggests instability.[257,258] Decreased diameter of the spine on a lateral radiograph or sagittal CT suggests spinal cord compression.[259]

The dens fracture (**Schematic X**) is the most common cervical spine fracture in children. There are three types of dens fractures. Type I occurs through the tip of odontoid process. Type II involves the base or the synchondrosis of the odontoid (Fig. 24.54). Type III involves the base with extension into the body. The most common location of dens fractures is through the synchondrosis. On a lateral radiograph of the cervical spine, a fracture line is often demonstrated, and the fragment is usually displaced anteriorly with dorsal tilt of the dens.[249] Accompanying prevertebral soft tissue swelling is commonly present. If the dens is not well visualized on the open-mouth view and clinical suspicion for fracture persists, CT with MPR reformatted images for a complete assessment is necessary.

Hangman fracture is defined as traumatic spondylolisthesis of C2 and is caused by hyperextension of the neck (**Schematic Y**) (Fig. 24.55). This fracture is less common than dens and Jefferson fractures.[243] On the lateral radiograph of the cervical spine, there is anterior displacement of C2 on C3 with associated widening of the spinal canal. Defects through the posterior elements are usually identifiable on radiographs.[241] Further investigation with CT is typically performed for a more detailed assessment of the fractures and degree of displacement.

Atlantoaxial Subluxation. Atlantoaxial subluxation refers to ligamentous instability between the atlas and axis (**Schematic v**). This type of injury occurs more commonly in older children and adolescents. The mechanism of injury is thought to be related to forced rotation of the neck with lateral

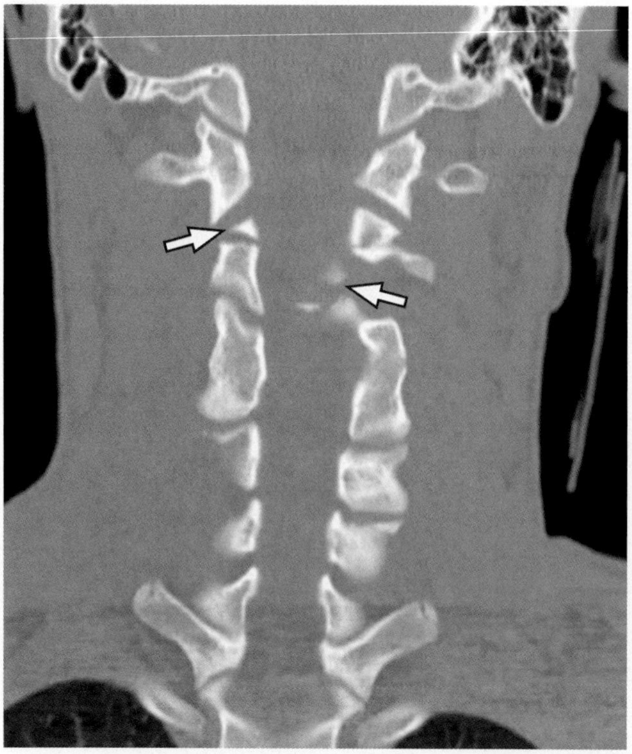

FIGURE 24.55 **Hangman fracture in a 9-year-old girl.** Coronal reformatted CT image through the cervical spine demonstrates a fracture (*arrows*) through lamina and pedicle of C2 on both sides.

tilt. Affected pediatric patients typically present with pain and a neck deformity with the neck tilted toward one side and the head rotated to the opposite side. Associated conditions include trauma, infection, Grisel syndrome, Down syndrome, juvenile idiopathic arthritis, Klippel-Feil syndrome, Morquio syndrome, spondyloepiphyseal dysplasia, achondroplasia, and Larsen syndrome.[260]

Lateral radiographs of the spine usually show loss of the normal superimposition of the posterior arch of C1 and the spinolaminar line of other vertebrae and loss of the atlantodental space. On the AP view, there is typically decreased distance between the dens and lateral mass of C1.[245] Dynamic CT evaluation can be performed with the patient scanned in the neutral position and with the head voluntarily turned in maximal rotation toward each side.[261,262] This examination requires an alert and cooperative child and should never be forced into rotation. Dynamic CT evaluation may help differentiate fixation from rotatory dislocation.[243]

Nonoperative therapy is reserved for pediatric patients in the acute setting without neurologic deficits. Surgical fusion is indicated for affected pediatric patients with neurologic involvement, chronic deformity, or failed conservative management.

Subaxial Fracture. Subaxial fractures (C3–C7) are more commonly seen in older children and adolescents. They range in severity from minor ligamentous strain or spinous process fracture to complete fracture dislocation with bone and ligamentous injury, often resulting in severe spinal cord compromise.[263] Vertebral body compression fractures are caused by axial loading and flexion injuries. On lateral radiograph, there is loss of height of the vertebral body and possible retropulsion of a bony fragment that can cause spinal cord compression. CT for complete assessment of osseous injury and MRI for evaluation of concomitant spinal cord injury may be necessary in affected pediatric patients with neurologic symptoms (Fig. 24.56).

Thoracolumbar Spine

Thoracolumbar spine injuries are less common than cervical spine injuries. Thoracolumbar injuries commonly occur after high-energy MVAs, falls from a height, sports injuries, or penetrating injury such as gunshot wounds. The forces applied to the spine may occur with flexion, extension, rotation, sheering, and distraction each resulting in a different pattern of injury. Most thoracolumbar spinal fractures occur in children 14 to 16 years of age, with boys being more commonly affected.[240,264]

Compression Fracture. Compression fractures result from axial compressive force with associated anterior or lateral flexion.[264] Compression fractures can be caused by accidental or nonaccidental trauma. Predisposing conditions include osteopenia, osteomyelitis, neoplasms (e.g., leukemia, lymphoma, osseous metastasis), and Langerhans cell histiocytosis.

On a lateral radiograph of the thoracolumbar spine, there is loss of height of the vertebral body with variable degrees of anterior wedging (Fig. 24.57). On the AP view of radiograph, vertebral body height loss can be detected and lateral compression may also be seen. A simple compression fracture, which is <50% of height loss or <30 degrees of wedging, is considered a stable fracture and does not usually require surgery. Greater than 50% of vertebral body height loss is considered unstable, and CT is recommended in this setting to completely assess for retropulsed bony fragments into the spinal canal and to evaluate for additional injuries not detected on radiographs. MRI is more useful than radiographs or CT for differentiating thoracolumbar spinal compression fracture caused by trauma from underlying malignancy. Preservation of normal marrow signal and isolated vertebral involvement favor the traumatic cause of compression fracture.

Burst Fracture. Burst fracture represents a more severe injury than vertebral compression fracture (**Schematic Z**). Burst fractures result from hyperflexion and axial loading occurring with falls from a height or high-energy MVAs. Burst fractures usually involve the anterior and middle vertebral columns with retropulsed bony fragments. On radiographs, there is loss of height of the anterior and middle columns of the spine, often with a large fragment involving the posterosuperior spine that is often displaced posteriorly. CT is helpful to assess the bony fragments and their relationship with the spinal canal and also better visualize the posterior elements (Fig. 24.58).

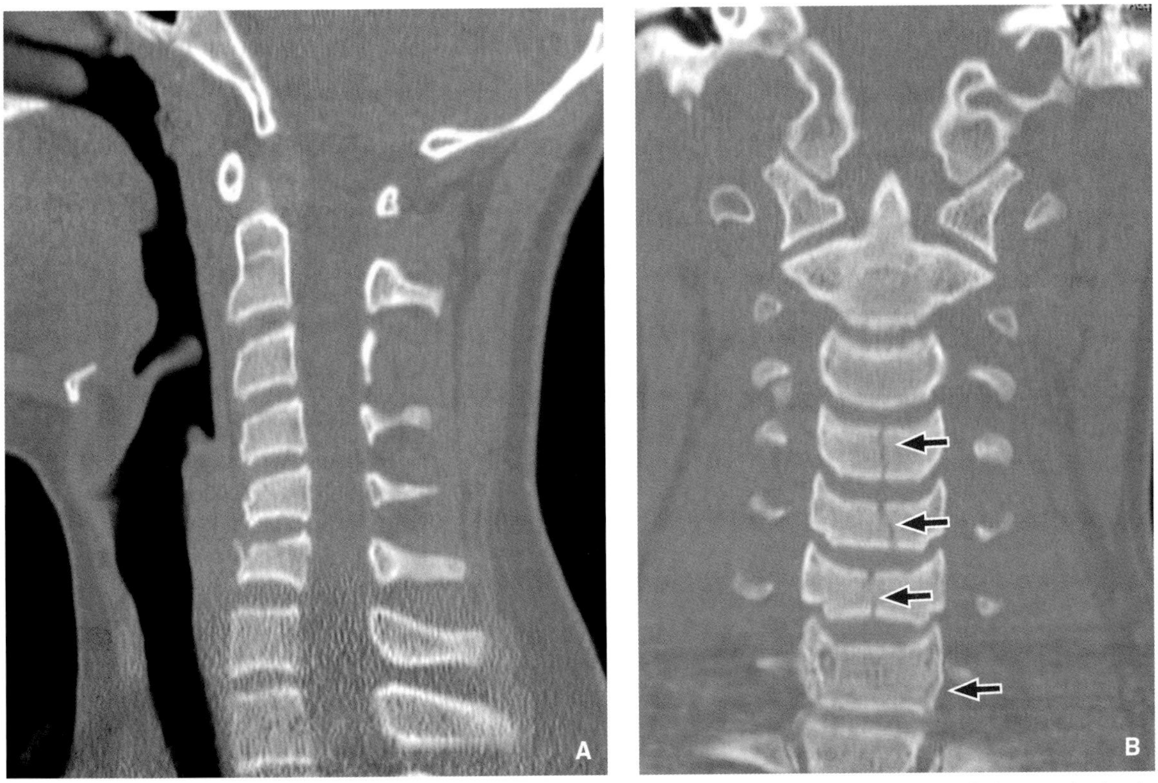

FIGURE 24.56 **Subaxial fractures in an 11-year-old boy.** Sagittal **(A)** and coronal **(B)** CT images of the cervical spine show fractures through the C4 through C7 vertebral bodies (*arrows*). There is straightening (reversal) of the cervical lordosis at these cervical spinal levels.

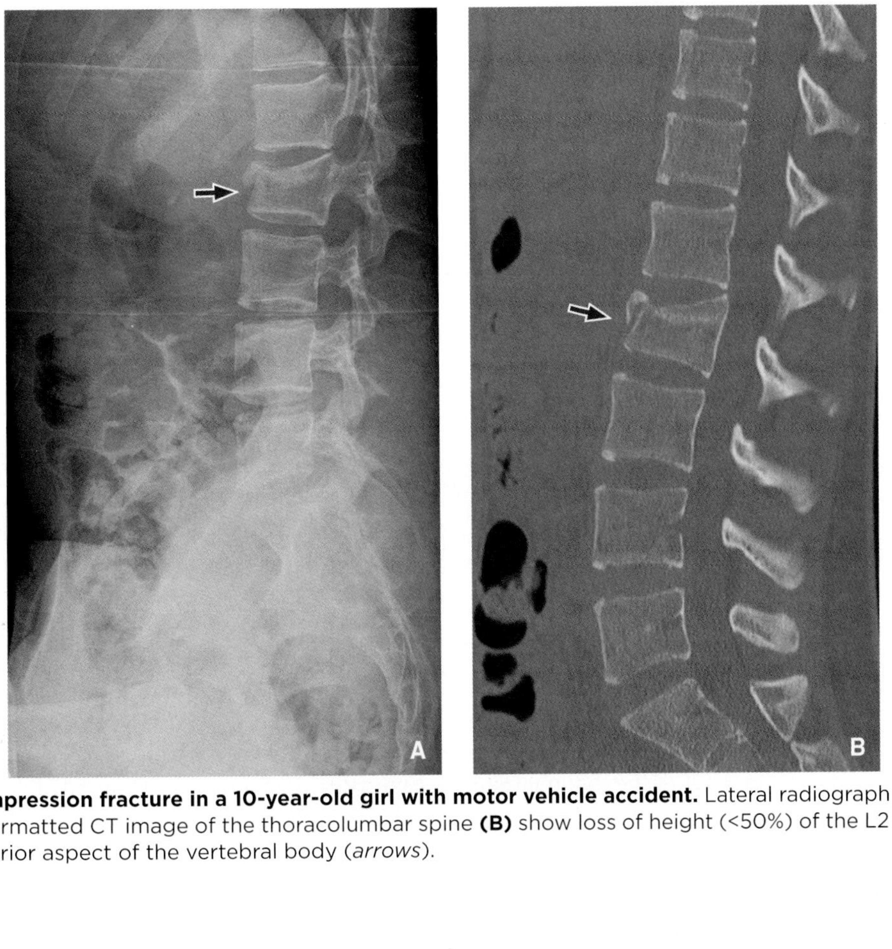

FIGURE 24.57 **Compression fracture in a 10-year-old girl with motor vehicle accident.** Lateral radiograph of the lumbar spine **(A)** and sagittal reformatted CT image of the thoracolumbar spine **(B)** show loss of height (<50%) of the L2 vertebral body with wedging of the anterior aspect of the vertebral body (*arrows*).

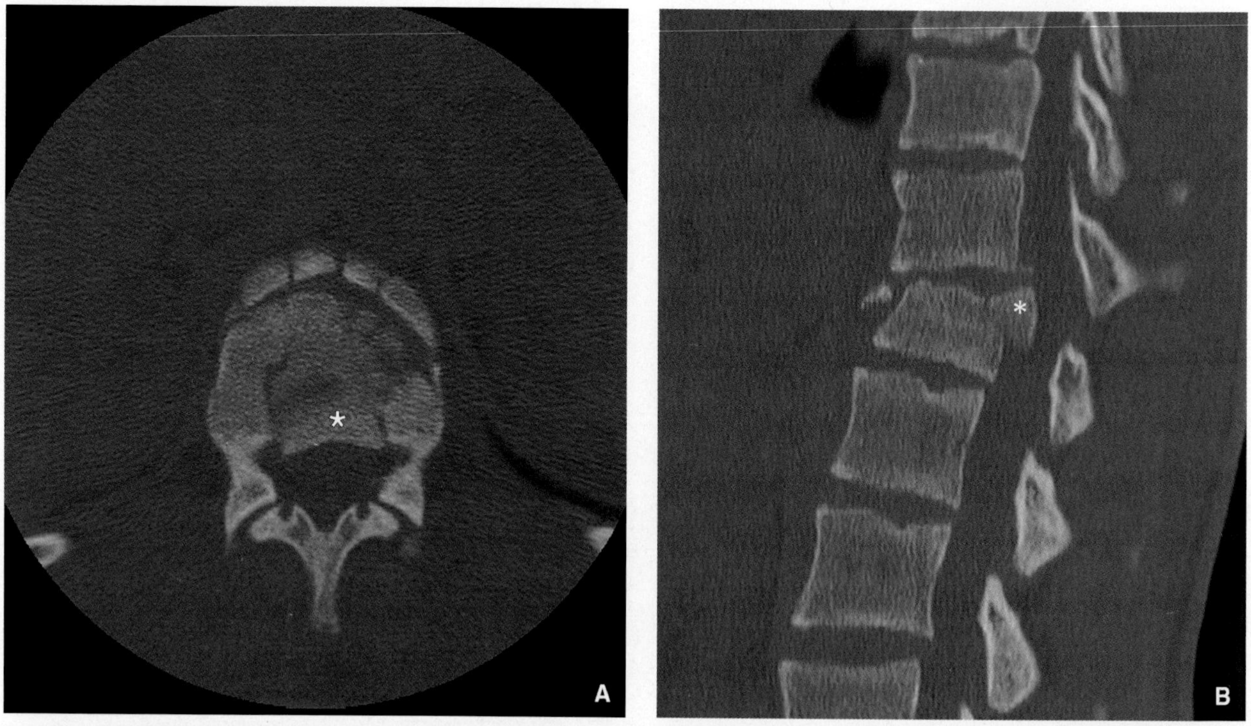

FIGURE 24.58 **Burst fracture in a 15-year-old boy status post fall from a height.** Axial **(A)** and sagittal **(B)** CT images of the thoracic spine show a comminuted vertebral body fracture with loss of height of the anterior and middle columns of the affected vertebral body. There is retropulsion of a fracture fragment (*asterisks*) into the spinal canal.

Management of burst fractures depends on the stability of the fracture and presence or absence of neurologic deficit. Stable fractures without neurologic symptoms may be treated nonoperatively, whereas instability and/or signs or symptoms of neurologic compromise typically require spinal decompression and fusion.[265,266]

Chance Fracture. Also known as "seat-belt" fracture, chance fractures are flexion distraction injuries due to hyperflexion of the back resulting in distraction of the middle and posterior vertebral columns and minor anterior compression (**Schematic i**). Prior to the advent of shoulder straps in seat belts in the 1980s, MVAs were the leading cause of chance fracture. Currently, falls and crush injuries are more frequent causes of this injury. There are two types of chance fracture, those solely involving the bone and those involving the soft tissues and ligaments. Affected pediatric patients typically present with back pain. Ecchymosis of anterior abdominal wall should raise the suspicion for the presence of chance fracture.

Radiographs typically show a horizontal fracture line through the posterior elements of the spine and posterior aspect of the vertebral body (Fig. 24.59). There is usually subtle anterior wedging of the affected vertebral body. The most common locations of chance fractures are the thoracolumbar junction from T12 to L2 and the midlumbar region in pediatric patients. There is an ~50% association with concomitant intra-abdominal injuries.[267] CT of the abdomen and pelvis is indicated to evaluate for potential concomitant solid organ, visceral, and vascular injuries when chance fracture is detected.[268]

Most chance fractures can be managed conservatively with immobilization. However, unstable fractures often associated with a kyphosis of 30 degrees or more usually require internal stabilization with surgical fixation in conjunction with spinal canal decompression.

Nonaccidental Trauma (Child Abuse)

Child abuse, also often referred as nonaccidental trauma, is the second most common cause of brain injury and fractures in infants and young children.[269] In 1946, John Caffey described the association of subdural hematomas and long bone fractures in infants and raised the possibility of maltreatment to explain these injuries.[270] Although optimal evaluation of cases of suspected abuse is accomplished with a multidisciplinary team approach among the radiologist, child abuse pediatrician, orthopedic surgeon, endocrinologists, and pediatric geneticists, the radiologist is usually the first one who is responsible for identifying and documenting the skeletal injures concerning for abuse on imaging studies. In addition, the radiologist has to recognize imaging findings that suggest alternative diagnosis.

Imaging Techniques

For a complete evaluation of nonaccidental trauma, multimodality imaging may be needed to identify and characterize inflicted injuries. Fractures can be missed when

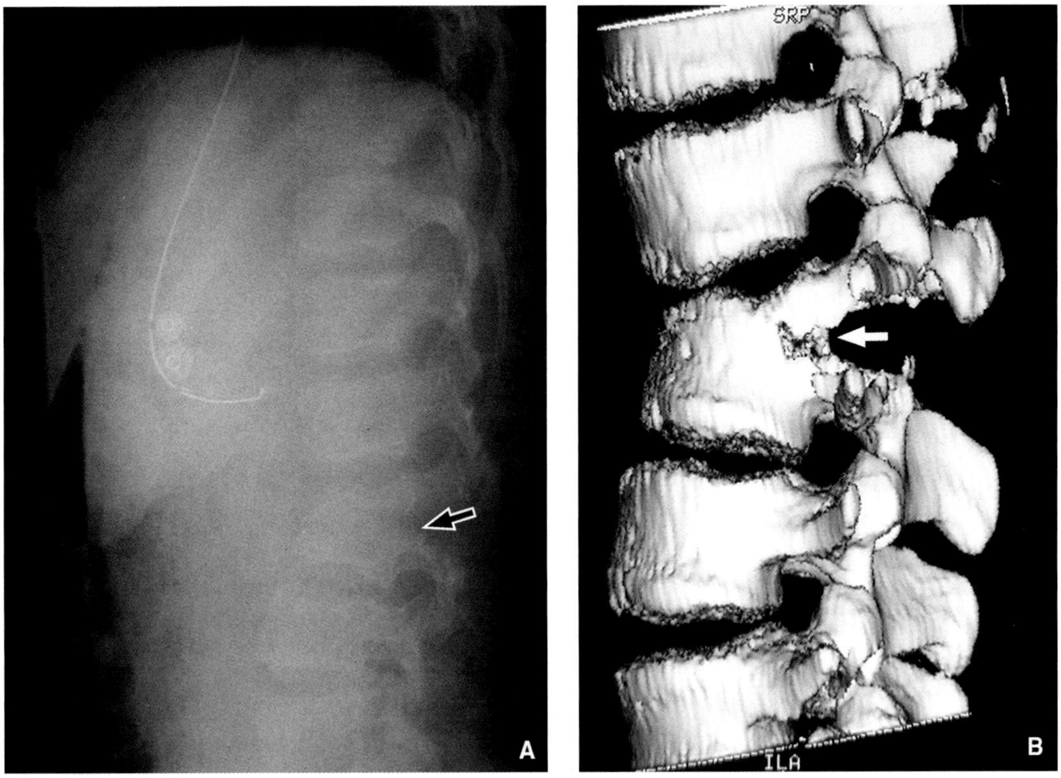

FIGURE 24.59 **Chance fracture in a 5-year-old boy after motor vehicle accident.** Lateral radiograph of the thoracolumbar spine **(A)** and 3D volume-rendered CT image of the spine **(B)** show a transverse fracture (*arrows*) involving the spinous process, laminae, pedicles, and vertebral body of L1 with distraction of the fracture fragments.

proper imaging guidelines and techniques are not followed. Currently, the radiographic skeletal survey is the main imaging modality in cases of suspected abuse. Skeletal surveys are mandatory in all infants and toddlers <2 years of age and recommended in children 2 to 5 years of age when there is suspicion of abuse.[271] In older children, the radiographic evaluation can be limited to the areas of clinical concern. There is little value to global screening for inflicted skeletal injury beyond age 5.

The skeletal survey should be performed following the guidelines of the American College of Radiology (ACR)[272,273] (Table 24.1). The detection of subtle injuries relies on performing digital radiographs with high-detail technique and coned down to the region of interest. Positive or questionable fractures should be imaged in at least two projections. An experienced radiologist should monitor and review all the images prior to completion, and optimally, two experienced radiologists should review the images independently and reach a consensus on equivocal findings. Failure to perform an adequate skeletal survey may result in the return of the child to a dangerous environment. The 2-week follow-up skeletal survey can identify fractures that are subtle initially,

TABLE 24.1 The Skeletal Survey Study Protocol at Boston Children's Hospital

Axial Skeleton	Views Acquired[a]	Appendicular Skeleton	Views Acquired[a]
Skull	AP, lateral (opposite lateral and Towne view if head trauma)	Humerus	AP
Cervical spine	Lateral	Radius, ulna	AP
Chest	AP, lateral, both obliques	Hand	Oblique PA
Pelvis	AP to include lower lumbar spine	Femur	AP
Lumbar spine	Lateral	Tibia, fibula	AP
		Foot	AP

[a]*All views done with high-detail technique.*

AP, anteroposterior; PA, posteroanterior.

but become evident with healing.[274,275] This approach can confirm a suspected fracture, aid in dating the injury, and differentiate fractures from developmental variants that may simulate abuse.

Additional imaging studies may complement the skeletal survey in problematic cases. Skeletal scintigraphy may be performed when a skeletal survey is negative or equivocal in infants and there is high clinical suspicion of abuse. Bone scintigraphy with 18F-NaF PET has better contrast and resolution than does the traditional imaging with Tc-99m–labeled methylene diphosphonate.[276] Bone scintigraphy with 18F-NaF PET has better sensitivity than does a skeletal survey for identification of all fractures and rib fractures, but lower sensitivity for identification of classic metaphyseal lesions (CMLs).[276] MRI and ultrasonography are useful in the evaluation of epiphyseal separations and may have a role in the evaluation of soft tissue injuries such as intramuscular hematomas and joint effusions. Currently, whole-body MRI at 1.5 Tesla is insensitive to the high specificity indicators of abuse, namely, CMLs and rib fractures. Therefore, whole-body MRI cannot replace the skeletal survey.[277] Chest CT can aid in the evaluation of rib fractures in selective cases.[278] CT 3D skull models can complement the four-view skull series and help distinguish skull fractures from normal variants or identifying subtle fractures.[279]

Imaging Findings

After intracranial injury, fractures are the most common injury seen in physical abuse.[280] Skeletal trauma is the strongest indicator that physical abuse has occurred. Skeletal injuries may be minimally symptomatic and rarely life threatening. Bruising is usually not present in infants with fractures.[281] Skeletal injures can be classified according to their relative specificity for abuse based on their imaging pattern and location (Table 24.2).[282,283]

TABLE 24.2 Specificity of Radiologic Findings for Abuse

High specificity[a]
Classic metaphyseal lesions (CMLs)
Posterior rib fractures
Scapular fractures
Spinous process fractures
Sternal fractures
Moderate specificity
Multiple fractures, especially bilateral
Fractures of different ages
Epiphyseal separations
Vertebral body fractures and subluxations
Digital fractures
Complex skull fractures
Pelvic fractures
Common but low specificity
Subperiosteal new bone formation
Clavicular fractures
Long bone shaft fractures
Linear skull fractures

[a]Highest specificity applies in infants.

From Kleinman PK. Diagnostic Imaging of Child Abuse. 2nd ed. St. Louis, MO: Mosby-Year Book Inc.; 1998, with permission.

Rib fractures in infants and young children have the highest association with child abuse and are the most common fracture seen in infant fatalities[284] (Fig. 24.60). In children <3 years of age, the positive predictive value of a rib fracture to indicate abuse is 95%.[285] Rib fractures occur with AP compression of the thorax as can happen during violent shaking.[286] The CML is highly specific and is the most common extremity fracture seen in abuse fatalities.[284,287] The CML is a fracture through the primary spongiosa of the metaphysis and, depending on the projection of the radiographs, may have a corner or bucket-handle appearance (Fig. 24.60C,D). CMLs result from torsional and tractional forces directly applied to the extremities or from acceleration forces during shaking. These fractures are most common in the lower extremity, especially around the knee, including distal femoral and proximal tibial metaphyses. CMLs usually heal without periosteal reaction.

Skull fractures have been reported in 17% of abused infants.[288] Fractures may be simple and linear or multiple and complex. A skull fracture in conjunction with intracranial trauma has a high association with the diagnosis of abuse.[269,289] Simple linear skull fractures can occur with short falls and therefore have a low specificity for abuse.[269,290] Vertebral body fractures are seen in 10% of positive skeletal surveys. Vertebral fractures carry a significantly greater risk of intracranial injury; 71% of children with spinal fractures had evidence of abusive head trauma.[291] Fractures of the hand and feet are present in 11% of positive skeletal surveys, and although usually asymptomatic, their recognition can have an effect on the medical diagnosis of abuse.[292] Long bone diaphyseal fractures have a strong association with abuse in nonambulatory infants. In toddlers and older children, these fractures can occur with household and playground accidents. The patient's age, the mechanism of trauma, and the presence of additional injuries are important factors in raising suspicion of abuse in a child with a long bone diaphyseal fracture.

Patterns of fracture healing vary depending on the patient's age: healing occurs faster in infants than older children. Nonaccidental trauma should be suspected when the pattern of healing of the fracture is not consistent with the mechanism and timing of injury provided by the caretaker. Healing varies depending on the location of the injury, the amount of displacement, and motion of the fracture fragments. Subperiosteal new bone formation usually occurs between 7 and 10 days, soft callus is seen at about 10 to 14 days, and hard callus forms between 14 and 21 days.[293,294] Serial exams are useful in estimating the age of a fracture.

Differential Diagnosis

A number of conditions can be confused with nonaccidental trauma.[282,295] Metaphyseal irregularities mimicking CMLs

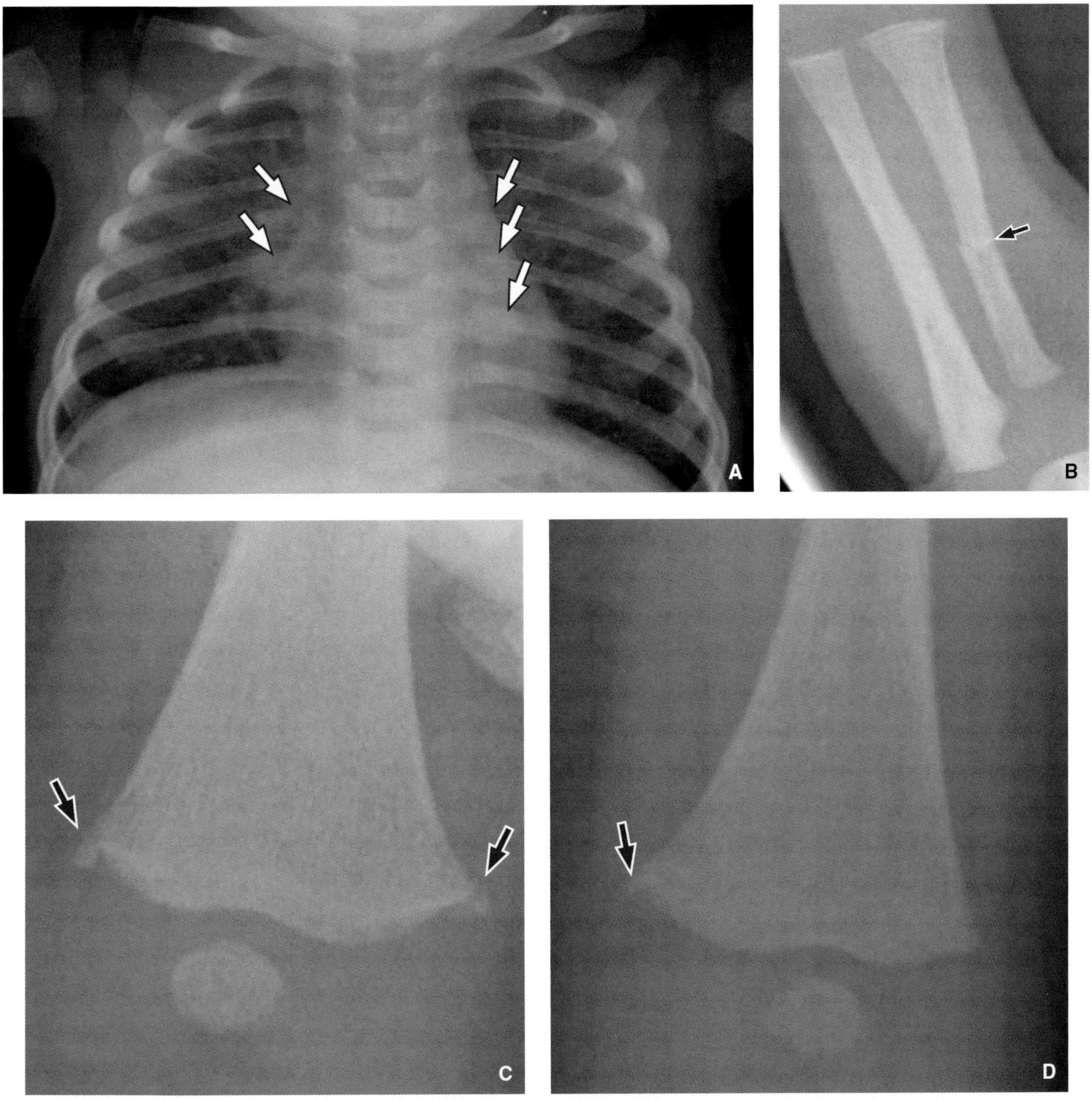

FIGURE 24.60 **Child abuse.** One-month-old girl with a left subdural hematoma and multiple fractures who eventually died. **A:** Frontal chest radiograph demonstrates multiple posterior rib fractures (*arrows*) with advanced healing. **B:** Right forearm radiograph shows an acute transverse fracture (*arrow*) of the right radius diaphysis. **C, D:** Radiographs of the right and left distal femur show classic metaphyseal fractures (*arrows*).

can be seen in osteogenesis imperfecta, rickets, syphilis, and metaphyseal dysplasias. Fractures can also be seen as result of difficult vaginal and caesarian deliveries. Subperiosteal new bone formation can be physiologic or seen in Caffey disease, sickle cell anemia, leukemia, and osteomyelitis. Developmental variants, such as metaphyseal spurs or beaks, can be mistaken for skeletal injury. Careful examination of the imaging findings in conjunction with the clinical history and laboratory data can usually distinguish these entities from child abuse.

Miscellaneous

Slipped Capital Femoral Epiphysis

Slipped capital femoral epiphysis (SCFE) is the most common adolescent hip disorder. SCFE is characterized by displacement of the femoral head epiphysis in relation to the metaphysis (**Schematic R**). It is a Salter-Harris type I fracture. SCFE is common with a male-to-female ratio of ~1.5:1. The average age of presentation is 12 years in girls and 13.5 years

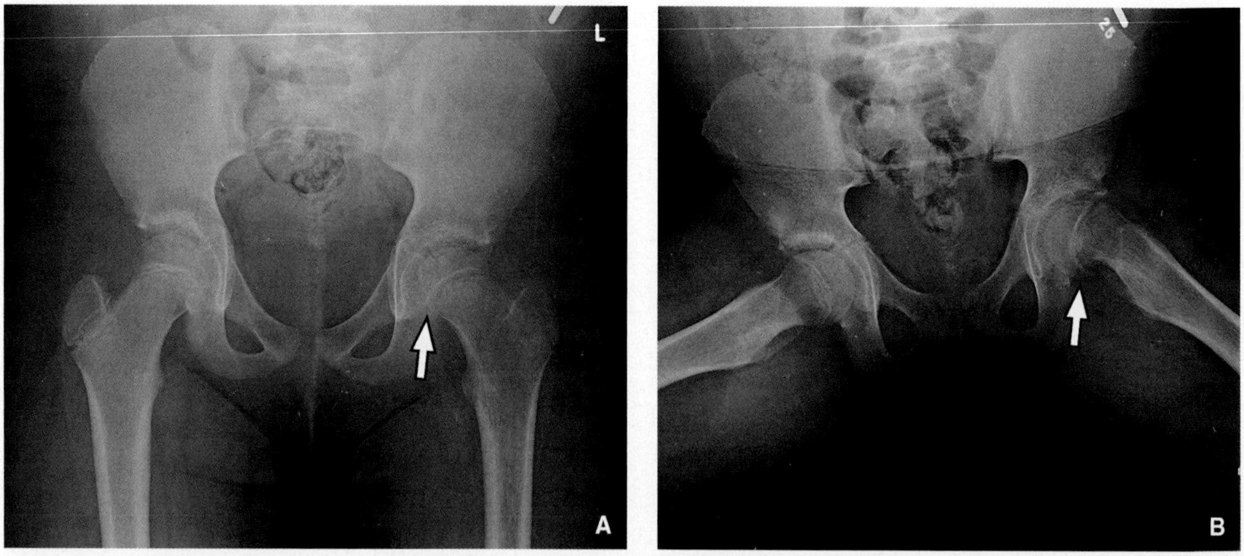

FIGURE 24.61 **Slipped capital femoral epiphysis in an overweight 13-year-old boy who presented with left hip pain.** Anteroposterior **(A)** and frog-leg lateral **(B)** radiographs of the pelvis demonstrate mild medial and inferior displacement (*arrow*) of the capital femoral epiphysis in relationship with the femoral neck. There is mild asymmetric widening of the physis.

in boys.[296] Obesity is the main risk factor for the development of SCFE with 60% of affected patients presenting at the 90th percentile of weight for their age. Other associated underlying risk factors include renal failure, prior history of radiation therapy, and endocrine dysfunction such as hypothyroidism and growth hormone deficiency.[297] Genetic disorders associated with SCFE include trisomy 21 and Rubinstein-Taybi syndrome.[298,299] Affected pediatric patients presenting with SCFE often complain of pain in the hip, groin, thigh, or knee and may have an antalgic gait. A subset of affected patients present with isolated knee or thigh pain. SCFE is bilateral in 20% to 40% of patients.[300]

Radiographs (AP and frog-leg lateral views) are the primary modality used to diagnose SCFE. The frog-leg lateral

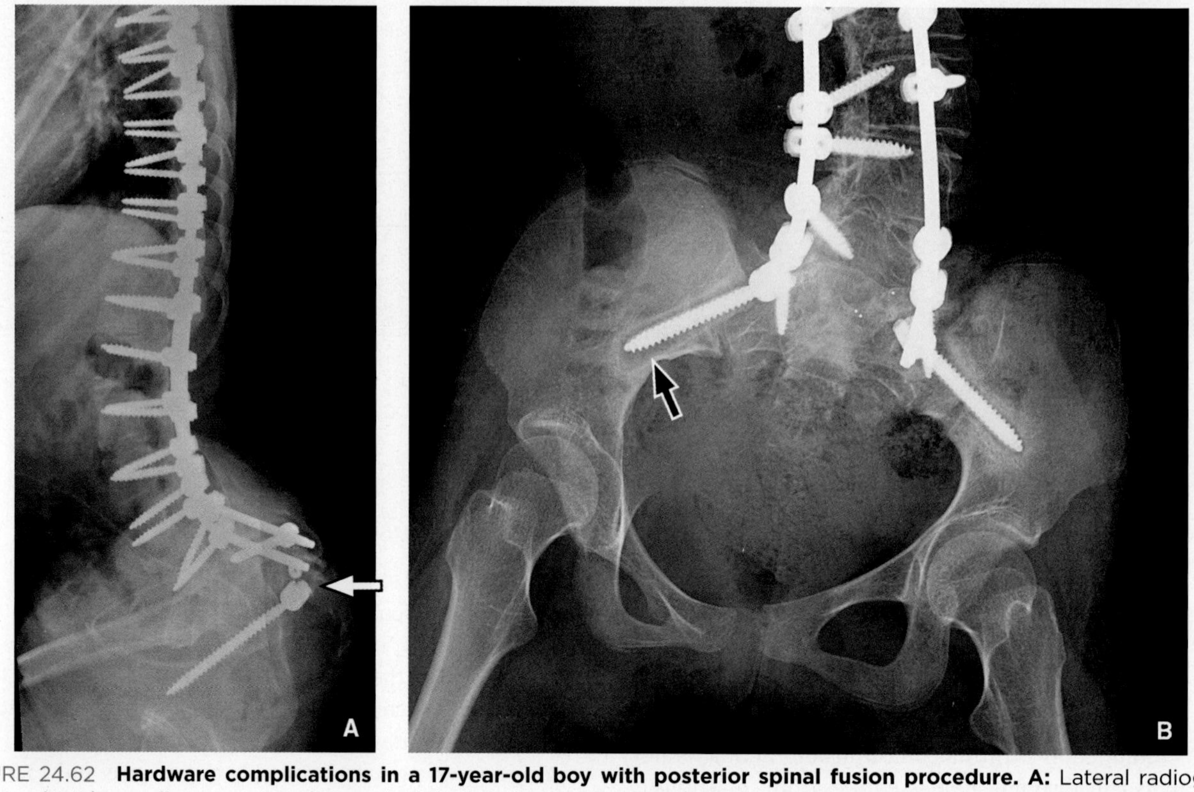

FIGURE 24.62 **Hardware complications in a 17-year-old boy with posterior spinal fusion procedure. A:** Lateral radiograph of the spine shows disengagement (*arrow*) of the left iliac component of the spinal fusion hardware. **B:** Periprosthetic lucency (*arrow*) along the right iliac screw is also seen.

view increases conspicuity of the slippage. The Klein line is a line drawn tangential to the femoral neck on the frontal radiograph. Normally, the Klein line should intersect a portion of the femoral epiphysis (**Schematic S**). With medial slippage, the line does not transect the epiphysis[301] (Fig. 24.61) and suggests SCFE. Posterior displacement of the femoral epiphysis is usually the earliest sign. Other radiographic signs of SCFE include asymmetric physeal widening, diminished craniocaudad height of the epiphysis, and the metaphyseal blanch sign (a double density of the femoral metaphysis due to overlap of the posteriorly displaced epiphysis).[302]

ORTHOPEDIC HARDWARE COMPLICATIONS

Orthopedic hardware is often necessary to properly restore anatomic alignment of displaced, angulated, or rotated fracture fragments. Typically, fractures heal faster and with less deformity when the fragments are in apposition. Intra-articular fractures with >2 mm of displacement are often treated with hardware to prevent posttraumatic osteoarthritis. However, orthopedic hardware is not without risk. Complications may include periprosthetic fracture and hardware loosening from infectious or noninfectious etiology. When pins or screws are used, there is the potential for the screw to penetrate through the cortex and involve the articular surface. In the setting of SCFE, the pin can migrate because of growth of the child and lead to instability of the subcapital epiphysis. Additionally, improper screw placement in SCFE can result in avascular necrosis of the femoral head.[303,304]

Radiography is the initial imaging modality of choice when evaluating orthopedic hardware and potential complications. Typically, a minimum of two orthogonal views is necessary. On radiographs, it is important to evaluate the position of hardware and potential improper positioning (Fig. 24.62). When periprosthetic lucency is seen along the interface between the metal and bone, it is indicative of loosening due to osteolysis. Typically, >2 mm of lucency is considered abnormal (Fig. 24.62). Hardware fractures typically manifest as radiolucencies through the metallic prosthesis.

In cases of overlapping bones, areas of complex anatomy, and complex orientation of the hardware, other imaging modalities such as MDCT, radiolabeled leukocyte scintigraphy, and MRI can be considered. For example, MDCT is superior to radiographs in evaluating hardware complications mainly because of its high spatial and temporal resolution in conjunction with multiplanar and 3D reconstruction capabilities.[305] The advent of MDCT has significantly decreased metallic artifacts that were previously seen with single-detector CT. Radiolabeled leukocyte scintigraphy remains an important imaging examination when an infected prosthesis is suspected, with a reported accuracy of 90%.[306] Because of the metallic artifact, MRI is often limited for direct evaluation of MRI-compatible hardware; however, it has an important role in evaluation of complications such as adjacent soft tissue infection.

References

1. Carson S, Woolridge DP, Colletti J, et al. Pediatric upper extremity injuries. *Pediatr Clin North Am.* 2006;53:41.
2. Specker BL, Brazerol W, Tsang RC, et al. Bone mineral content in children 1 to 6 years of age. Detectable sex differences after 4 years of age. *Am J Dis Child.* 1987;141:343.
3. Frost HM, Schönau E. The "muscle-bone unit" in children and adolescents: a 2000 overview. *J Pediatr Endocrinol Metab.* 2000; 13:571.
4. Pai D, Thapa M. Musculoskeletal ultrasound of the upper extremity in children. *Pediatr Radiol.* 2013;43(suppl 1):S48–S54.
5. Kim MC, Eckhardt B, Craig C, et al. Ultrasonography of the annular ligament and pulled elbow. *Pediatr Radiol.* 2004;24: 999–1004.
6. Konin GP, Nazarian LN, Walz DM. US of the elbow: indications, technique, normal anatomy, and pathologic conditions. *Radiographics.* 2013;33(4):E125–E147.
7. Poyhia TH, Lamminen AE, Peltonen JL, et al. Brachial plexus birth injury: US screening for glenohumeral joint instability. *Radiology.* 2010;254:253–260.
8. Graif M, Stahl-Kent V, Ben-Ami T, et al. Sonographic detection of occult bone fractures. *Pediatr Radiol.* 1998;18:383–385.
9. Peterson JJ, Bancroft LW, Kransdorf MJ. Wooden foreign bodies: imaging appearance. *AJR Am J Roentgenol.* 2002;178(3): 557–562.
10. Brenner DJ. Estimating cancer risks from pediatric CT: going from the qualitative to the quantitative. *Pediatr Radiol.* 2002;32(4):228–231; discussion 242–244. Epub 2002 Mar 7.
11. Salamipour H. Multidetector row CT in pediatric musculoskeletal imaging. *Pediatr Radiol.* 2005;35:555–564.
12. Pretorius ES, Fishman EK. Volume-rendered three-dimensional spiral CT: musculoskeletal application. *Radiographics.* 1999;19: 1143–1160.
13. Society for Pediatric Radiology. *Image Gently.* Retrieved from http://www.imagegently.org/ on March 28, 2105.
14. Jaramillo D, Laor T. Pediatric musculoskeletal MRI: basic principles to optimize success. *Pediatr Radiol.* 2008;38:379–391.
15. Marianne A, et al. Imaging strategies in paediatric musculoskeletal trauma. *Pediatr Radiol.* 2009;39(suppl 3):S414–S421.
16. Tiel-van Buul MM, Roolker W, Verbeeten BW, et al. Magnetic resonance imaging versus bone scintigraphy in suspected scaphoid fracture. *Eur J Nucl Med.* 1996;23(8):971–975.
17. Englaro EE, Gelfand MJ, Paltiel HJ. Bone scintigraphy in preschool children with lower extremity pain of unknown origin. *J Nucl Med.* 1992;33(3):351–354.
18. Park HM, Kernek CB, Robb JA. Early scintigraphic findings of occult femoral and tibial fractures in infants. *Clin Nucl Med.* 1988;13(4):271–275.
19. Monteleone GP Jr. Stress fractures in the athlete. *Orthop Clin North Am.* 1995;26(3):423–432.
20. Campbell RS, Grainger AJ, Hide IG, et al. Juvenile spondylolysis: a comparative analysis of CT, SPECT and MRI. *Skeletal Radiol.* 2005;34(2):63–73.
21. Roca I, Barber I, Fontecha C, et al. Evaluation of bone viability. *Pediatr Radiol.* 2013;43:393–405.

22. Norris BL, Hahn DH, Bosse MJ, et al. Intraoperative fluoroscopy to evaluate fracture reduction and hardware placement during acetabular surgery. *J Orthop Trauma.* 1999;13(6):414–417.
23. Mizuta T, Benson WM, Foster BK, et al. Statistical analysis of the incidence of physeal injuries. *J Pediatr Orthop.* 1987;7:518–523.
24. Chadwick CJ, Bentley G. The classification and prognosis of epiphyseal injuries. *Injury.* 1987;18:157.
25. Salter RB, Harris WR: Injuries involving the epiphyseal plate. *J Bone Joint Surg Am.* 1963;45:587–632.
26. Mizuto T, Benson WM, Foster BK, et al. Statistical analysis of the incidence of physeal injuries. *J Pediatr Orthop.* 1987;7:518–523.
27. Rogers LF, Poznanski AK. Imaging of epiphyseal injuries. *Radiology.* 1994;191(2):297–308.
28. Landin LA. Epidemiology of children's fractures. *J Pediatr Orthop B.* 1997;6:79.
29. Della-Giustina K, Della-Giustina DA. Emergency department evaluation and treatment of pediatric orthopedic injuries. *Emerg Med Clin North Am.* 1999;17:895.
30. Zieger M, Dorr U, Schulz RD. Sonography of the slipped humeral epiphysis due to birth injury. *Pediatr Radiol.* 1987;17:425–426.
31. Broker FH, Burbach T. Ultrasonic diagnosis of separation of the proximal humeral epiphysis in the newborn. *J Bone Joint Surg Am.* 1990;72:187–191.
32. Pandya NK, Behrends D, Hosalkar HS. Open reduction of proximal humerus fractures in the adolescent population. *J Child Orthop.* 2012;6(2):111–118.
33. Alburger PD, Weidner PL, Randal RB. Supracondylar fractures of the humerus in children. *J Pediatr Orthop.* 1992;12:16–19.
34. Jacoby SM, Herman MJ, Morrison WB, et al. Pediatric elbow trauma: an orthopaedic perspective on the importance of radiographic interpretation. *Semin Musculoskelet Radiol.* 2007; 11:48–56.
35. Brubacher JW, Dodds SD. Pediatric supracondylar fractures of the distal humerus. *Curr Rev Musculoskelet Med.* 2008;1:190–196.
36. Skaggs DL. Elbow fractures in children: diagnosis and management. *J Am Acad Orthop Surg.* 1997;5:303–312.
37. Shrader MW. Pediatric supracondylar fractures and pediatric physeal elbow fractures. *Orthop Clin North Am.* 2008;39:163–171.
38. Rogers LF, Malave S, White H, et al. Plastic bowing, torus and greenstick supracondylar fractures of the humerus: radiographic clues to obscure fractures of the elbow in children. *Radiology.* 1978;128:145–150.
39. Gartland JJ. Management of supracondylar fractures of the humerus in children. *Surg Gynecol Obstet.* 1959;109:145–154.
40. Mallo G, Stanat SJ, Ganney J. Use of the Gartland classification system for treatment of pediatric supracondylar humerus fractures. *Orthopedics.* 2010;33:19.
41. Rewers A, Hedegaard H, Lezotte D, et al. Childhood femur fractures, associated injuries, and sociodemographic risk factors: a population-based study. *Pediatrics.* 2005;115(5):e543.
42. Ogden JA. *Skeletal Injury in the Child.* 3rd ed. New York: Springer-Verlag; 2000:456–567.
43. Louahem DM, Bourelle S, Buscayret F, et al. Displaced medial epicondyle fractures on the humerus: surgical treatment and results—a report of 139 cases. *Arch Orthop Trauma Surg.* 2010; 130:649–655.
44. Wilson NI, Ingram R, Rymaszewski L, et al. Treatment of fractures of the medial epicondyle of the humerus. *Injury.* 1988; 19:342–344.
45. Josefsson PO, Danielsson LG. Epicondylar elbow fracture in children: 35-year follow-up of 56 unreduced cases. *Acta Orthop Scand.* 1986;57:313–315.
46. Jakob R, Fowles JV, Rang M, et al. Observations concerning fractures of the lateral humeral condyle in children. *J Bone Joint Surg Br.* 1975;57:430–436.
47. Milch H. Fractures and fracture dislocations of the humeral condyles. *J Trauma.* 1964;4:592–607.
48. Bast SC, Hoffer MM, Aval S. Nonoperative treatment for minimally and nondisplaced lateral condyle fractures in children. *J Pediatr Orthop.* 1998;18:448–450.
49. Mintzer CM, Water PM, Brown DJ, et al. Percutaneous pinning in the treatment of displaced lateral condyle fractures. *J Pediatr Orthop.* 1994;14:462–465.
50. Brown J, Eustace S. Neonatal transphyseal supracondylar fracture detected by ultrasound. *Pediatr Emerg Care.* 1997;13:410–412.
51. Dias JJ, Lamont AC, Jones JM. Ultrasonic diagnosis of neonatal separation of the distal humerus epiphysis. *J Bone Joint Surg Br.* 1988;70:825–828.
52. Ziv N, Litwin A, Katz K, et al. Definitive diagnosis of fracture-separation of the distal humeral epiphysis in neonates by ultrasonography. *Pediatr Radiol.* 1996;26:493–496.
53. Iyer RS, Thapa MM, Khanna PC, et al. Pediatric bone imaging: imaging elbow trauma in children—a review of acute and chronic injuries. *AJR Am J Roentgenol.* 2012;198(5):1053–1068.
54. O'Brien PI. Injuries involving the proximal radial epiphysis. *Clin Orthop Relat Res.* 1965;41:51–58.
55. O'Brien PI. Injuries involving the proximal radial epiphysis. *Clin Orthop Relat Res.* 1965;41:51–58.
56. Landin LA. Fracture patterns in children. Analysis of 8,682 fractures with special reference to incidence, etiology and secular changes in a Swedish urban population 1950–1979. *Acta Orthop Scand Suppl.* 1983;202:1–109.
57. Cooper C, Dennison EM, Leufkens HGM, et al. Epidemiology of childhood fractures in Britain: a study using the general practice research database. *J Bone Miner Res.* 2004;19:1976–1981.
58. Rennie L, Court-Brown CM, Mok JY, et al. The epidemiology of fractures in children. *Injury.* 2007;38:913–922.
59. Ward WT, Rihn JA. The impact of trauma in an urban pediatric orthopaedic practice. *J Bone Joint Surg Am.* 2006;88: 2759–2764.
60. Faulkner RA, Davison KS, Bailey DA, et al. Size-corrected BMD decreases during peak linear growth: implications for fracture incidence during adolescence. *J Bone Miner Res.* 2006;21: 1864–1870.
61. Nishiyama KK, Macdonald HM, Moore SA, et al. Cortical porosity is higher in boys compared with girls at the distal radius and distal tibia during pubertal growth: an HR-pQCT study. *J Bone Miner Res.* 2012;27(2):273–282.
62. Ryan LM, Teach SJ, Searcy K, et al. Epidemiology of pediatric forearm fractures in Washington, DC. *J Trauma.* 2010;69: S200–S205.
63. Nellans KW, Kowalski E, Chung KC. The epidemiology of distal radius fractures. *Hand Clin.* 2012;28(2):113–125.
64. de Putter CE, van Beeck EF, Looman CW, et al. Trends in wrist fractures in children and adolescents, 1997–2009. *J Hand Surg Am.* 2011;36:1810–1815.
65. Khosla S, Melton LJ III, Dekutoski MB, et al. Incidence of childhood distal forearm fractures over 30 years: a population-based study. *JAMA.* 2003;290:1479–1485.
66. Hagino H, Yamamoto K, Ohshiro H, et al. Increasing incidence of distal radius fractures in Japanese children and adolescents. *J Orthop Sci.* 2000;5:356–360.
67. Noonan KJ, Price CT. Forearm and distal radius fractures in children. *J Am Acad Orthop Surg.* 1998;6:146–156.

68. Walsh HP, McLaren CA, Owen R. Galeazzi fractures in children. *J Bone Joint Surg Br.* 1987;69:730–733.
69. Schlickewei W, Oberle M. [Forearm fractures in children][in German]. *Unfallchirurg.* 2005;108:223–232.
70. Rothe M, Rudy T, Stankovic P, et al. [Treatment of Galeazzi's fracture: is the surgical revision of the distal radioulnar joint necessary?] [in German]. *Handchir Mikrochir Plast Chir.* 2001;33:252–257.
71. Mikic ZD. Galeazzi fracture-dislocations. *J Bone Joint Surg Am.* 1975;57:1071–1080.
72. Evans MC, Graham HK. Olecranon fractures in children. Part 1. A clinical review. Part 2. A new classification and management algorithm. *J Pediatr Orthop.* 1999;19:559–569.
73. Gicquel P, Maximin MC, Boutemy P, et al. Biomechanical analysis of olecranon fracture fixation in children. *J Pediatr Orthop.* 2002;22(1):17–21.
74. Bado JL. The Monteggia lesion. *Clin Orthop Relat Res.* 1967;(50):71–86.
75. Reckling FW. Unstable fracture—dislocations of the forearm (Monteggia and Galeazzi lesions). *J Bone Joint Surg Am.* 1982;64:857–863.
76. Olney BW, Menelaus MB. Monteggia and equivalent lesions in childhood. *J Pediatr Orthop.* 1989;9:219–223.
77. Givon U, Pritsch M, Levy O, et al. Monteggia and equivalent lesions. A study of 41 cases. *Clin Orthop Relat Res.* 1997;(337):208–215.
78. Tompkins DG. The anterior Monteggia fracture: observations on etiology and treatment. *J Bone Joint Surg.* 1971;53:1109–1114.
79. Leonidou A, Pagkalos J, Lepetsos P, et al. Pediatric Monteggia fractures: a single-center study of the management of 40 patients. *J Pediatr Orthop.* 2012;32(4):352–356.
80. Hastings H II, Simmons BP. Hand fractures in children. A statistical analysis. *Clin Orthop Relat Res.* 1984;188:120–130.
81. Blair WF, Steyers CM. Extensor tendon injuries. *Orthop Clin North Am.* 1992;23:141–148.
82. Aronowitz ER, Leddy JP. Closed tendon injuries of the hand and wrist in athletes. *Clin Sports Med.* 1998;17:449–467.
83. Clavero JA, Alomar X, Monill JM, et al. MR imaging of ligament and tendon injuries of the fingers. *Radiographics.* 2002;22(2):237–256.
84. Scott SC. Closed injuries to the extension mechanism of the digits. *Hand Clin.* 2000;16:367–373.
85. Pegoli L, Toh S, Arai K, et al. The Ishiguro extension block technique for the treatment of mallet finger fracture: indications and clinical results. *J Hand Surg Br.* 2003;28(1)15–17.
86. Nellans KW, Chung KC. Pediatric hand fracture. *Hand Clin.* 2013;29(4):569–578.
87. Kanaya K, Wada T, Yamashita T. The Thompson procedure for chronic mallet finger deformity. *J Hand Surg Am.* 2013;38(7):1295–1300.
88. Sivit AP, Dupont EP, Sivit CJ. Pediatric hand injuries: essentials you need to know. *Emerg Radiol.* 2014;21(2):197–206.
89. Hofmeister EP, Kim J, Shin AY. Comparison of 2 methods of immobilization of fifth metacarpal neck fractures: a prospective randomized study. *J Hand Surg Am.* 2008;33(8):1362.
90. Christodoulou A, Colton C. Scaphoid fractures in children. *J Pediatr Orthop.* 1986;6(1):37–39.
91. Gholson JJ, Bae DS, Zurakowski D, et al. Scaphoid fractures in children and adolescents: contemporary injury patterns and factors influencing time to union. *J Bone Joint Surg Am.* 2011;93(13):1210–1219.
92. Evenski AJ, Adamczyk MJ, Steiner RP, et al. Clinically suspected scaphoid fractures in children. *J Pediatr Orthop.* 2009;29(4):352–355.
93. Rodts MF. Nursemaid's elbow: a preventable pediatric injury. *Orthop Nurs.* 2009;28:163–166.
94. Westin CD, Gill EA, Noyes ME, et al. Anterior shoulder dislocation. A simple and rapid method for reduction. *Am J Sports Med.* 1995;23(3):369–371.
95. Neviaser JS. Posterior dislocations of the shoulder: diagnosis and treatment. *Surg Clin North Am.* 1963;43:1623–1630.
96. Owens BD, Duffey ML, Nelson BJ, et al. The incidence and characteristics of shoulder instability at the United States Military Academy. *Am J Sports Med.* 2007;35(7):1168–1173.
97. Gor DM. The trough line sign. *Radiology.* 2002;224(2):485–486.
98. Beaty JH. Fractures of the hip in children. *Orthop Clin North Am.* 2006;37(2):223–232.
99. McCarthy J, Noonan K. Fractures and traumatic dislocations of the hip in children. In: Beaty JH, Kasser J, eds. *Rockwood and Wilkins' Fractures in Children.* 7th ed. Philadelphia, PA: Lippincott Williams & Wilkins; 2010:769.
100. Herring JA. Hip fractures. In: *Tachdjian's Pediatric Orthopedics: From the Texas Scottish Rite Hospital for Children.* 4th ed. Philadelphia, PA: Saunders Elsevier; 2008. Vol 3.
101. Mirdad T. Fractures of the neck of femur in children: an experience at the Aseer Central Hospital, Abha, Saudi Arabia. *Injury.* 2002;33(9):823–827.
102. Moon ES, Mehlman CT. Risk factors for avascular necrosis after femoral neck fractures in children: 25 Cincinnati cases and meta-analysis of 360 cases. *J Orthop Trauma.* 2006;20(5):323–329.
103. Davison BL, Weinstein SL. Hip fractures in children: a long-term follow-up study. *J Pediatr Orthop.* 1992;12(3):355–358.
104. Morsy HA. Complications of fracture of the neck of the femur in children. A long-term follow-up study. *Injury.* 2001;32(1):45–51.
105. Pape HC, Krettek C, Friedrich A, et al. Long-term outcome in children with fractures of the proximal femur after high-energy trauma. *J Trauma.* 1999;46(1):58–64.
106. Togrul E, Bayram H, Gulsen M, et al. Fractures of the femoral neck in children: long-term follow-up in 62 hip fractures. *Injury.* 2005;36(1):123–130.
107. Canale ST, Bourland WL. Fracture of the neck and intertrochanteric region of the femur in children. *J Bone Joint Surg Am.* 1977;59(4):431–443.
108. Loder RT, O'Donnell PW, Feinberg JR. Epidemiology and mechanisms of femur fractures in children. *J Pediatr Orthop.* 2006;26(5):561.
109. Thomas SA, Rosenfield NS, Leventhal JM, et al. Long-bone fractures in young children: distinguishing accidental injuries from child abuse. *Pediatrics.* 1991;88(3):471–476.
110. Galano GJ, Vitale MA, Kessler MW, et al. The most frequent traumatic orthopaedic injuries from a national pediatric inpatient population. *J Pediatr Orthop.* 2005;25(1):39.
111. Hinton RY, Lincoln A, Crockett MM, et al. Fractures of the femoral shaft in children. Incidence, mechanisms, and sociodemographic risk factors. *J Bone Joint Surg Am.* 1999;81(4):500.
112. Buess E, Kaelin A. One hundred pediatric femoral fractures: epidemiology, treatment attitudes, and early complications. *J Pediatr Orthop B.* 1998;7(3):186.

113. Schwend RM, Werth C, Johnston A. Femur shaft fractures in toddlers and young children: rarely from child abuse. *J Pediatr Orthop.* 2000;20(4):475.
114. Gustilo RB, Anderson JT. Prevention of infection in the treatment of one thousand and twenty-five open fractures of long bones: retrospective and prospective analyses. *J Bone Joint Surg Am.* 1976;58:453–458.
115. Basener CJ, Mehlman CT, DiPasquale TG. Growth disturbance after distal femoral growth plate fractures in children: a meta-analysis. *J Orthop Trauma.* 2009;23(9):663–667.
116. Peterson HA. Physeal and apophyseal injuries. In: Rockwood J, Wilkins KE, Beaty JH, eds. *Fractures in Children.* 3rd ed. Philadelphia, PA: Lippincott-Raven; 1996:103–165.
117. Ecklund K, Jaramillo D. Patterns of premature physeal arrest: MR imaging of 111 children. *AJR Am J Roentgenol.* 2002;178(4): 967–972.
118. Maripuri SN, Mehta H, Mohanty K. Sleeve fracture of the superior pole of the patella with an intra-articular dislocation. A case report. *J Bone Joint Surg Am.* 2008;90(2):385–389.
119. Fithian DC, Paxton EW, Stone ML, et al. Epidemiology and natural history of acute patellar dislocation. *Am J Sports Med.* 2004;32(5):1114–1121.
120. Hinton RY, Sharma KM. Acute and recurrent patellar instability in the young athlete. *Orthop Clin North Am.* 2003;34:385–396.
121. Insall J, Goldberg V, Salvati E. Recurrent dislocation and the high-ridings patella. *Clin Orthop Relat Res.* 1972;88:67–69.
122. Lippacher S, Dejour S, Elsharkawi M, et al. Observer agreement on the Dejour trochlear dysplasia classification: a comparison of true lateral radiographs and axial magnetic resonance images. *Am J Sports Med.* 2012;40(4):837–844.
123. Dupuis CS, Westra SJ, Makris J, et al. Injuries and conditions of the extensor mechanism of the pediatric knee. *Radiographics.* 2009;29(3):877–886.
124. Zaidi A, Babyn P, Astori I, et al. MRI of traumatic patellar dislocation in children. *Pediatr Radiol.* 2006;36(11):1163–1170.
125. Boyer RS, Jaffe RB, Nixon GW, et al. Trampoline fracture of the proximal tibia in children. *AJR Am J Roentgenol.* 1986;146:83–85.
126. Cohen DA, Hinton RY. Bilateral tibial tubercle avulsion fractures associated with Osgood-Schlatter's disease. *Am J Orthop.* 2008;37(2):92–93.
127. Frankl U, Wasilewski SA, Heary WL. Avulsion fracture of the tibial tubercle with avulsion of the patellar ligament. *J Bone Joint Surg.* 1990;72A:1411–1413.
128. Kaneko K, Miyazaki H, Yamaguchi T. Avulsion fracture of the tibial tubercle with avulsion of the patellar ligament in an adolescent female athlete. *Clin J Sport Med.* 2000;10:144–145.
129. Ogden JA, Tross RB, Murphy MJ. Fractures of the tibial tuberosity in adolescents. *J Bone Joint Surg Am.* 1980;62(2):205–215.
130. Pesl T, Havranek P. Acute tibial tubercle avulsion fractures in children: selective use of the closed reduction and internal fixation method. *J Child Orthop.* 2008;2(5):353–356.
131. Prince JS, Laor T, Bean JA. MRI of anterior cruciate ligament injuries and associated findings in the pediatric knee: changes with skeletal maturation. *AJR Am J Roentgenol.* 2005;185(3): 756–762.
132. Johnston DR, Ganley TJ, Flynn JM, et al. Anterior cruciate ligament injuries in skeletally immature patients. *Orthopedics* 2002;25:864–871; quiz 872–863.
133. Tung GA, Davis LM, Wiggins ME, et al. Tears of the anterior cruciate ligament: primary and secondary signs at MR imaging. *Radiology* 1993;188:661–667.
134. Remer EM, Fitzgerald SW, Friedman H, et al. Anterior cruciate ligament injury: MR imaging diagnosis and patterns of injury. *Radiographics.* 1992;12:901–915.
135. Lee K, Siegel MJ, Lau DM, et al. Anterior cruciate ligament tears: MR imaging-based diagnosis in a pediatric population. *Radiology.* 1999;213(3):697–704.
136. Bae JH, Lim HC, Hwang DH, et al. Incidence of bilateral discoid lateral meniscus in an Asian population: an arthroscopic assessment of contralateral knees. *Arthroscopy.* 2012;28(7): 936–941.
137. De Smet AA. How I diagnose meniscal tears on knee MRI. *AJR Am J Roentgenol.* 2012;199(3):481–499.
138. Cothran RL Jr, Major NM, Helms CA, et al. MR imaging of meniscal contusion in the knee. *AJR Am J Roentgenol.* 2001;177(5):1189–1192.
139. De Smet AA, Graf BK. Meniscal tears missed on MR imaging: relationship to meniscal tear patterns and anterior cruciate ligament tears. *AJR Am J Roentgenol.* 1994;162(4):905–911.
140. Harper KW, Helms CA, Lambert HS III, et al. Radial meniscal tears: significance, incidence, and MR appearance. *AJR Am J Roentgenol.* 2005;185(6):1429–1434.
141. Bergin D, Hochberg H, Zoga AC, et al. Indirect soft-tissue and osseous signs on knee MRI of surgically proven meniscal tears. *AJR Am J Roentgenol.* 2008;191(1):86–92.
142. Janzen DL, Peterfy CG, Forbes JR, et al. Cystic lesions around the knee joint: MR imaging findings. *AJR Am J Roentgenol.* 1994;163(1):155–161.
143. Mashru RP, Herman MJ, Pizzutillo PD. Tibial shaft fractures in children and adolescents. *J Am Acad Orthop Surg.* 2005;13(5):345.
144. Hope PG, Cole WG. Open fractures of the tibia in children. *J Bone Joint Surg Br.* 1992;74(4):546.
145. Koury SI, Stone CK, Harrell G, et al. Recognition and management of Tillaux fractures in adolescents. *Pediatr Emerg Care.* 1999;15(1):37–39.
146. Liporace FA, Yoon RS, Kubiak EN, et al. Does adding computed tomography change the diagnosis and treatment of tillaux and triplane pediatric ankle fractures? *Orthopedics.* 2012;35(2): e208–e212.
147. Kaya A, Altay T, Ozturk H, et al. Open reduction and internal fixation in displaced juvenile Tillaux fractures. *Injury.* 2007; 38(2):201–205.
148. Manderson EL, Ollivierre CO. Closed anatomic reduction of a juvenile Tillaux fracture by dorsiflexion of the ankle. A case report. *Clin Orthop Relat Res.* 1992;276:262–266.
149. Kim JR, Song KH, Song KJ, et al. Treatment outcomes of triplane and tillaux fractures of the ankle in adolescence. *Clin Orthop Surg.* 2010;2(1):34–38.
150. Ogden J. *Distal Epiphyseal and Physeal Injuries.* New York: Springer-Verlag; 2000.
151. Rogers L. *The Ankle.* Philadelphia, PA: Churchill Livingstone; 2002.
152. Spiegel PG, Cooperman DR, Laros GS. Epiphyseal fractures of the distal ends of the tibia and fibula: a retrospective study of two hundred and thirty-seven cases in children. *J Bone Joint Surg Am.* 1978;60:1046–1050.
153. Mac Nealy GA, Rogers LF, Hernandez R, et al. Injuries of the distal tibial epiphysis: systematic radiographic evaluation. *AJR Am J Roentgenol.* 1982;138:683–689.
154. Brown SD, Kasser JR, Zurakowski D, et al. Analysis of 51 tibial triplane fractures using CT with multiplanar reconstruction. *AJR Am J Roentgenol.* 2004;183(5):1489–1495.

155. Jones S, Phillips N, Ali F, et al. Triplane fractures of the distal tibia requiring open reduction and internal fixation: pre-operative planning using computed tomography. *Injury* 2003;34:293–298.
156. Karrholm J. The triplane fracture: four years of follow-up of 21 cases and review of the literature. *J Pediatr Orthop B.* 1997;6:91–102.
157. El-Karef E, Sadek HI, Nairn DS, et al. Triplane fracture of the distal tibia. *Injury.* 2000;31:729–736.
158. Dailiana ZH, Malizos KN, Zacharis K, et al. Distal tibial epiphyseal fractures in adolescents. *Am J Orthop.* 1999;28: 309–312.
159. Peterson CA, Peterson HA. Analysis of the incidence of injuries to the epiphyseal growth plate. *J Trauma.* 1972;12:275–281.
160. Peterson HA, Madhok R, Benson JT, et al. Physeal fractures: Part 1. Epidemiology in Olmsted County, Minnesota, 1979–1988. *J Pediatr Orthop.* 1994;14:423–430.
161. Worlock P, Stower M. Fracture patterns in Nottingham children. *J Pediatr Orthop.* 1986;6:656–660.
162. Kay RM, Tang CW. Pediatric foot fractures: evaluation and treatment. *J Am Acad Orthop Surg.* 2001;9:308–319.
163. Crawford AH. Fractures and dislocations of the foot and ankle. In: Green NE, Swiontkowski MF, eds. *Skeletal Trauma in Children*. Philadelphia, PA: WB Saunders; 1994:449–516.
164. Jensen I, Wester JU, Rasmussen F, et al. Prognosis of fracture of the talus in children: 21 (7–34)-year follow-up of 14 cases. *Acta Orthop Scand.* 1994;65:398–400.
165. Fortin PT, Balazsy JE. Talus fractures: evaluation and treatment. *J Am Acad Orthop Surg.* 2001;9(2):114–127.
166. Schantz K, Rasmussen F. Calcaneus fracture in the child. *Acta Orthop Scand.* 1987;58:507–509.
167. Schmidt TL, Weiner DS. Calcaneal fractures in children: An evaluation of the nature of the injury in 56 children. *Clin Orthop.* 1982;171:150–155.
168. Walters JL, Gangopadhyay P, Malay DS. Association of calcaneal and spinal fractures. *J Foot Ankle Surg.* 2014;53(3):279–281.
169. Boyle MJ, Walker CG, Crawford HA. The paediatric Bohler's angle and crucial angle of Gissane: a case series. *J Orthop Surg Res.* 2011;6:2.
170. Owen RJ, Hickey FG, Finlay DB. A study of metatarsal fractures in children. *Injury.* 1995;26(8):537–538.
171. Polzer H, Polzer S, Mutschler W, et al. Acute fractures to the proximal fifth metatarsal bone: development of classification and treatment recommendations based on the current evidence. *Injury.* 2012;43(10):1626–1632.
172. Lawrence SJ, Botte MJ. Jones' fractures and related fractures of the proximal fifth metatarsal. *Foot Ankle.* 1993;14(6): 358–365.
173. Kavanaugh JH, Brower TD, Mann RV. The Jones fracture revisited. *J Bone Joint Surg Am.* 1978;60:776–782.
174. DeLee JC, Evans JP, Julian J. Stress fracture of the fifth metatarsal. *Am J Sports Med.* 1983;11:349–353.
175. van Aaken J, Berli MC, Noger M, et al. Fritschy Symptomatic treatment of non-displaced avulsion and Jones fractures of the fifth metatarsal: a prospective study. *Rev Med Suisse.* 2007;3:1792–1794.
176. Wiener BD, Linder JF, Giattini JF. Treatment of fractures of the fifth metatarsal: a prospective study. *Foot Ankle Int.* 1997;18:267–269.
177. Herrera-Soto JA, Scherb M, Duffy MF, et al. Fractures of the fifth metatarsal in children and adolescents. *J Pediatr Orthop.* 2007;27(4):427–431.
178. Kensinger DR, Guille JT, Horn BD, et al. The stubbed great toe: importance of early recognition and treatment of open fractures of the distal phalanx. *J Pediatr Orthop.* 2001;21:31–34.
179. Hawkes NC, Flemming DJ, Ho VB. Subtle Lisfranc injury: low energy midfoot sprain. *Mil Med.* 2007;172(9):12–13.
180. Kalia V, Fishman EK, Carrino JA, et al. Epidemiology, imaging, and treatment of Lisfranc fracture-dislocations revisited. *Skeletal Radiol.* 2012;41(2):129–136.
181. Haapamaki V, Kiuru M, Koskinen S. Lisfranc fracture-dislocation in patients with multiple trauma: diagnosis with multidetector computed tomography. *Foot Ankle Int.* 2004;25:614–619.
182. Desmond EA, Chou LB. Current concepts review: Lisfranc injuries. *Foot Ankle Int.* 2006;27:653–660.
183. Sands AK, Grose A. Lisfranc injuries. *Injury.* 2004;35(suppl 2):SB71–SB76.
184. Lattermann C, Goldstein JL, Wukich DK, et al. Practical management of Lisfranc injuries in athletes. *Clin J Sport Med.* 2007;17:311–315.
185. Dunbar JS, Owen HF, Nogrady MB, et al. Obscure tibial fracture of infants—the toddler's fracture. *J Can Assoc Radiol.* 1964;15:136–144.
186. Tenenbein M, Reed MH, Black GB. The toddler's fracture revisited. *Am J Emerg Med.* 1990;8(3):208.
187. Shravat BP, Harrop SN, Kane TP. Toddler's fracture. *J Accid Emerg Med.* 1996;13(1):59.
188. Halsey MF, Finzel KC, Carrion WV, et al. Toddler's fracture: presumptive diagnosis and treatment. *J Pediatr Orthop.* 2001; 21(2):152.
189. Hernandez JA, Swischuk LE, Yngve DA, et al. The angled buckle fracture in pediatrics. A frequently missed fracture. *Emerg Radiol.* 2003;10:71–75.
190. Jadhav SP, Swischuk LE. Commonly missed subtle skeletal injuries in children: a pictorial review. *Emerg Radiol.* 2008;15(6): 391–398.
191. Plint A, Clifford T, Perry J, et al. Wrist buckle fractures: a survey of current practice patterns and attitudes toward immobilization. *CJEM.* 2003;5:95–100.
192. Solan MC, Rees R, Daly K. Current management of torus fractures of the distal radius. *Injury.* 2002;33:503–505.
193. Davidson JS, Brown DJ, Barnes SN, et al. Simple treatment for torus fractures of the distal radius. *J Bone Joint Surg Br.* 2001;83:1173–1175.
194. Symons S, Rowsell M, Bhowal B, et al. Hospital versus home management of children with buckle fractures of the distal radius. A prospective, randomised trial. *J Bone Joint Surg Br.* 2001;83:556–560.
195. Van Bosse HJP, Patel RJ, Thacker M, et al. Minimalistic approach to treating wrist torus fractures. *J Pediatr Orthop.* 2005;25:495–500.
196. West S, Andrews J, Bebbington A, et al. Buckle fractures of the distal radius are safely treated in a soft bandage: a randomized prospective trial of bandage versus plaster cast. *J Pediatr Orthop.* 2005;25:322–325.
197. Plint AC, Perry JJ, Correll R, et al. A randomized, controlled trial of removable splinting versus casting for wrist buckle fractures in children. *Pediatrics.* 2006;117:691–697.
198. Khan KS, Grufferty A, Gallagher O, et al. A randomized trial of 'soft cast' for distal radius buckle fractures in children. *Acta Orthop Belg.* 2007;73:594–597.
199. Lee P, Hunter TB, Taljanovic M. Musculoskeletal colloquialisms: how did we come up with these names? *Radiographics.* 2004;24(4):1009–1027.

200. Mulligan ME. *Classic Radiologic Signs: An Atlas and History.* New York: Parthenon, 1997.
201. Franklin CC, Robinson J, Noonan K, et al. Evidence-based medicine: management of pediatric forearm fractures. *J Pediatr Orthop.* 2012;32(suppl 2):S131–S134.
202. Borden S. Traumatic bowing of the forearm in children. *J Bone Joint Surg Br.* 1974;56:611–616.
203. Borden S. Roentgen recognition of acute plastic bowing of the forearm in children. *AJR Am J Roentgenol.* 1975;125:524–530.
204. Crowe J, Swischuck L. Acute bowing fractures of the forearm in children: a frequently missed injury. *AJR Am J Roentgenol.* 1977;128:9810984.
205. Chamay A. Mechanical and morphological aspects of experimental overload and fatigue in bone. *J Biomech.* 1970;3: 263–270.
206. Chamay A, Tschantz P. Mechanical influences in bone remodeling, experimental research on Wolff's law. *J Biomech.* 1972;5: 173–180.
207. Cail WS, Keats TE, Sussman MD. Plastic bowing fracture of the femur in a child. *AJR Am J Roentgenol.* 1978;130(4): 780–782.
208. Dhillon PS, Currall V, Shannon MN. Traumatic plastic deformation of the tibia: case report and literature review. *Ann R Coll Surg Engl.* 2012;94(1):e30–e32.
209. Mabrey JD, Fitch RD. Plastic deformation in pediatric fractures: mechanism and treatment. *J Pediatr Orthop.* 1989;9(3):310.
210. Price CT, Flynn JM. Management of fractures. In: Morrissy RT, Weinstein SL, eds. *Lovell and Winter's Pediatric Orthopaedics.* 6th ed. Philadelphia, PA: Lippincott Williams & Wilkins; 2006:1463.
211. Jeske JM, Lomasney LM, Demos TC, et al. Longitudinal tibial stress fracture. *Orthopedics.* 1996;19(3):263, 266, 268, 270.
212. Matheson GO, Clement DB, McKenzie DC, et al. Scintigraphic uptake of 99mTc at non-painful sites in athletes with stress fractures: the concept of bone strain. *Sports Med.* 1987;4: 65–75.
213. Fredericson M, Bergman AG, Hoffman KL, et al. Tibial stress reaction in runners: correlation of clinical symptoms and scintigraphy with a new magnetic resonance imaging grading system. *Am J Sports Med.* 1995;23:472–481.
214. Ogden J. Injury to the growth mechanisms. In: Ogden J, ed. *Skeletal Injury in the Child.* Philadelphia, PA: Saunders; 1990: 97–174.
215. Ecklund K, Jaramillo D. Patterns of premature physeal arrest: MR imaging of 111 children. *AJR Am J Roentgenol.* 2002; 178(4):967–972.
216. Hynes D, O'Brien T. Growth disturbance lines after injury of the distal tibial physis: their significance in prognosis. *J Bone Joint Surg Br.* 1988;70:231–233.
217. Williamson RV, Staheli LT. Partial physeal growth arrest: treatment by bridge resection and fat interposition. *J Pediatr Orthop.* 1990;10(6):769–776.
218. Naimark A, Miller K, Segal D, et al. Nonunion. *Skeletal Radiol.* 1981;6:21.
219. Ireland ML, Taleisnik J. Nonunion of metacarpal extra-articular fractures in children: report to two cases and review of the literature. *J Pediatr Orthop.* 1986;6:352.
220. Robinson CM. Fractures of the clavicle in the adult. Epidemiology and classification. *J Bone Joint Surg Br.* 1998;80(3):476.
221. Stanley D, Trowbridge EA, Norris SH. The mechanism of clavicular fracture. A clinical and biomechanical analysis. *J Bone Joint Surg Br.* 1988;70(3):461.
222. Levine MG, Holroyde J, Woods JR Jr, et al. Birth trauma: incidence and predisposing factors. *Obstet Gynecol.* 1984;63(6): 792–795.
223. Kim W, McKee MD. Management of acute clavicle fractures. *Orthop Clin North Am.* 2008;39(4):491–505.
224. Pujalte GG, Housner JA. Management of clavicle fractures. *Curr Sports Med Rep.* 2008;7(5):275–280.
225. Lane-O'Kelly A, Fogarty E, Dowling F. The pelvic fracture in childhood: a report supporting nonoperative management. *Injury* 1995;26:327–329.
226. Quinby WC. Fractures of the pelvis and associated injuries in children. *J Pediatr Surg.* 1966;1:353–364.
227. Silber JS, Flynn JM. Changing patterns of pediatric pelvic fractures with skeletal maturation: implications for classification and management. *J Pediatr Orthop.* 2002;22:22–26.
228. Silber JS, Flynn JM, Koffler KM, et al. Analysis of the cause, classification, and associated injuries of 166 consecutive pediatric pelvic fractures. *J Pediatr Orthop.* 2001;21: 446–450.
229. Torode I, Zeig D. Pelvic fractures in children. *J Pediatr Orthop.* 1985;5:76–84.
230. Silber JS, Flynn JM, Katz MA, et al. Role of computed tomography in the classification and management of pediatric pelvic fractures. *J Pediatr Orthop.* 2001;21(2):148–151.
231. Sivit CJ, Cutting JP, Eichelberger MR. CT diagnosis and localization of rupture of the bladder in children with blunt abdominal trauma: significance of contrast material extravasation in the pelvis. *AJR Am J Roentgenol.* 1995;164(5):1243–1246.
232. Heeg M, Klasen HJ, Visser JD. Acetabular fractures in children and adolescents. *J Bone Joint Surg Br.* 1988;71:34–37.
233. Watts HG. Fractures of the pelvis in children. *Orthop Clin North Am.* 1976;7:615–624.
234. Ziran BH, Towers J. Placement of percutaneous iliosacral screws under computed tomographic guidance. *Oper Tech Orthop.* 2001;11:227–232.
235. Dillon JE, Connolly SA, Connolly LP, et al. MR imaging of congenital/developmental and acquired disorders of the pediatric hip and pelvis. *Magn Reson Imaging Clin N Am.* 2005;13: 783.
236. Rossi F, Dragoni S. Acute avulsion fractures of the pelvis in adolescent competitive athletes: Prevalence, location and sports distribution of 203 cases collected. *Skeletal Radiol.* 2001;30:127–131.
237. Meyers AB, Laor T, Zbojniewicz AM, et al. MRI of radiographically occult ischial apophyseal avulsions. *Pediatr Radiol.* 2012;42:1357.
238. Patel JC, Tepas JJ III, Mollitt DL, et al. Pediatric cervical spine injuries: defining the disease. *J Pediatr Surg.* 2001;36:373–376.
239. Kokoska ER, Keller MS, Rallo MC, et al. Characteristics of pediatric cervical spine injuries. *J Pediatr Surg.* 2001;36: 100–105.
240. Hamilton MG, Myles ST. Pediatric spinal injury: review of 61 deaths. *J Neurosurg.* 1992;77:705–708.
241. Roche C, Carty H. Spinal trauma in children. *Pediatr Radiol.* 2001;31:677–700.
242. Herman MJ, Pizzutillo PD. Cervical spine disorders in children. *Orthop Clin North Am.* 1999;30:457–466.
243. Lustrin ES, Karakas SP, Ortiz AO, et al. Pediatric cervical spine: normal anatomy, variants and trauma. *Radiographics.* 2003;23:539–560.
244. Bilston LE, Brown J. Pediatric spinal injury type and severity are age and mechanism dependent. *Spine.* 2007;32:2339–2347.

245. Egloff AM, Kadom N, Vezina G, et al. Pediatric cervical spine trauma imaging: a practical approach. *Pediatr Radiol.* 2009;39:447–456.
246. Ralston ME, Chung K, Barnes PD, et al. Role of flexion-extension radiographs in blunt pediatric cervical spine injury. *Acad Emerg Med.* 2001;8:237–245.
247. Stiell IG, Clement CM, McKnight RD, et al. The Canadian C-spine rule versus the NEXUS low-risk criteria in patients with trauma. *N Engl J Med.* 2003;349:2510–2518.
248. Cattell HS, Filtzer DL. Pseudosubluxation and other normal variations in the cervical spine in children. *J Bone Joint Surg Am.* 1965;47:1295–1309.
249. Swischuk LE. Emergency imaging of the acutely ill or injured child. In *The Spine and the Spinal Cord.* 4th ed. Philadelphia, PA: Lippincott Williams & Wilkins; 2000;532–587.
250. Pang D, Wilberger JG Jr. Spinal cord injury without radiographic abnormalities in children. *J Neurosurg.* 1982;57:114–129.
251. Akbarnia BA. Pediatric spine fractures. *Orthop Clin North Am.* 1999;30:521–536.
252. Choi J, Hoffman H, Hendrick E, et al. Traumatic infarction of the spinal cord in children. *J Neurosurg.* 1986;65:608–610.
253. Junewick JJ. Cervical spine injuries in pediatrics: are children small adults or not? *Pediatr Radiol.* 2010;40:493–498.
254. Ogden JA. *Skeletal Injury in the Child. Spine.* 2nd ed. Philadelphia, PA: Saunders; 1990;571–562.
255. Pathria MN, Petersilge CA. Spinal trauma. *Radiol Clin North Am.* 1991;29:847–865.
256. Judd DB, Liem LK, Petermann G. Pediatric atlas fracture: a case of fracture through a synchondrosis and review of the literature. *Neurosurgery.* 2000;46:991–994; discussion 994–995.
257. Bonadio WA. Cervical spine trauma in children. II. Mechanisms and manifestations of injury, therapeutic considerations. *Am J Emerg Med.* 1993;11:256–278.
258. Murphey MD, Batnitzky S, Bramble JM. Diagnostic imaging of spinal trauma. *Radiol Clin North Am.* 1989;27:855–872.
259. El-Khoury GY, Kathol MH, Daniel WW. Imaging of acute injuries of the cervical spine: value of plain radiography, CT, and MR imaging. *AJR Am J Roentgenol.* 1995;164:43–50.
260. Kawabe N, Hirotani H, Tanaka O. Pathomechanism of atlantoaxial rotatory fixation in children. *J Pediatr Orthop.* 1989; 9:569–574.
261. Phillips WA, Hensinger RN. The management of rotatory atlanto-axial subluxation in children. *J Bone Joint Surg Am.* 1989; 71:664–668.
262. Roche CJ, O'Malley M, Dorgan JC, et al. A pictorial review of atlanto-axial rotatory fixation: key points for the radiologist. *Clin Radiol.* 2001;56:947–958.
263. Kwon BK, Vaccaro AR, Grauer JN, et al. Subaxial cervical spine trauma. *J Am Acad Orthop Surg.* 2006;14(2):78–89.
264. Clark P, Letts M. Trauma to the thoracic and lumbar spine in the adolescent. *Can J Surg.* 2001;44(5):337–345.
265. Dogan S, et al. Thoracolumbar and sacral spinal injuries in children and adolescents: a review of 89 cases. *J Neurosurg.* 2007;106(suppl 6):426–433.
266. Parisini P, Di Silvestre M, Greggi T. Treatment of spinal fractures in children and adolescents: long-term results in 44 patients. *Spine.* 2002;27(18):1989–1994.
267. Mulpuri K, Reilly CW, Perdios A, et al. The spectrum of abdominal injuries associated with chance fractures in pediatric patients. *Eur J Pediatr Surg.* 2007;17(5):322–327.
268. Reynolds R. Pediatric spinal injury. *Curr Opin Pediatr.* 2000; 12(1):67–71.
269. Leventhal JM, Martin KD, Asnes AG. Fractures and traumatic brain injuries: abuse versus accidents in a US database of hospitalized children. *Pediatrics.* 2010;126:e104–e115.
270. Caffey J. Multiple fractures in the long bones of infants suffering from chronic subdural hematoma. *AJR Am J Roentgenol.* 1946;56:163–173.
271. American Academy of Pediatrics Section on Radiology. Diagnostic imaging of child abuse. *Pediatrics.* 2009;123:1430–1435.
272. American College of Radiology Expert Panel on Pediatric Imaging. ACR appropriateness criteria on suspected physical abuse-child. *J Am Coll Radiol.* 2011;8(2):87–94.
273. American College of Radiology. *ACR–SPR Practice Parameter for Skeletal Surveys in Children Revised 2014 (Resolution 39)*.* Reston, VA: American College of Radiology; 2014:1–8. http://www.acr.org/~/media/ACR/Documents/PGTS/guidelines/Skeletal_Surveys.pdf
274. Kleinman PK, Nimkin K, Spevak MR, et al. Follow-up skeletal surveys in suspected child abuse. *AJR Am J Roentgenol.* 1996;167:893–896.
275. Harlan SR, Nixon GW, Campbell KA, et al. Follow-up skeletal surveys for nonaccidental trauma: can a more limited survey be performed? *Pediatr Radiol.* 2009;39:962–968.
276. Drubach LA, Johnston PR, Newton AW, et al. Skeletal trauma in child abuse: detection with 18F-NaF PET. *Radiology.* 2010;255:173–181.
277. Perez-Rossello JM, Connolly SA, Newton AW, et al. Whole-body MRI in suspected infant abuse. *AJR Am J Roentgenol.* 2010;195:744–750.
278. Wootton-Gorges SL, Stein-Wexler R, Walton JW, et al. Comparison of computed tomography and chest radiography in the detection of rib fractures in abused infants. *Child Abuse Negl.* 2008;32:659–663.
279. Prabhu SP, Newton AW, Perez-Rossello JM, et al. Three-dimensional skull models as a problem-solving tool in suspected child abuse. *Pediatr Radiol.* 2013;43:575–581.
280. Loder RT, Feinberg JR. Orthopaedic injuries in children with nonaccidental trauma: demographics and incidence from the 2000 kids' inpatient database. *J Pediatr Orthop.* 2007;27:421–426.
281. Sugar NF, Taylor JA, Feldman KW. Bruises in infants and toddlers: those who don't cruise rarely bruise. Puget Sound Pediatric Research Network. *Arch Pediatr Adolesc Med.* 1999;153:399–403.
282. Kleinman PK. *Diagnostic Imaging of Child Abuse.* 3rd ed. Cambridge, UK: Cambridge University Press; 2015.
283. Kemp AM, Dunstan F, Harrison S, et al. Patterns of skeletal fractures in child abuse: systematic review. *BMJ.* 2008;337:a1518.
284. Kleinman PK, Marks SC Jr, Richmond JM, et al. Inflicted skeletal injury: A postmortem radiologic-histopathologic study in 31 infants. *AJR Am J Roentgenol.* 1995;165:647–650.
285. Barsness KA, Cha ES, Bensard DD, et al. The positive predictive value of rib fractures as an indicator of nonaccidental trauma in children. *J Trauma.* 2003;54:1107–1110.
286. Tsai A, Coats B, Kleinman PK. Stress profile of infant rib in the setting of child abuse: A finite element parametric study. *J Biomech.* 2012;45:1861–1868.
287. Kleinman PK, Perez-Rossello JM, Newton AW, et al. Prevalence of the classic metaphyseal lesion in infants at low versus high risk for abuse. *AJR Am J Roentgenol.* 2011;197:1005–1008.
288. Leventhal JM, Martin KD, Asnes AG. Incidence of fractures attributable to abuse in young hospitalized children: results from analysis of a United States Database. *Pediatrics.* 2008;122:599–604.

289. Piteau SJ, Ward MG, Barrowman NJ, et al. Clinical and radiographic characteristics associated with abusive and nonabusive head trauma: a systematic review. *Pediatrics.* 2012;130:315–323.
290. Wood JN, Christian CW, Adams CM, et al. Skeletal surveys in infants with isolated skull fractures. *Pediatrics.* 2009;123:e247–e252.
291. Barber I, Perez-Rossello JM, Wilson CR, et al. Prevalence and relevance of pediatric spinal fractures in suspected child abuse. *Pediatr Radiol.* 2013;43:1507–1515.
292. Kleinman PK, Morris NB, Makris J, et al. Yield of radiographic skeletal surveys for detection of hand, foot, and spine fractures in suspected child abuse. *AJR Am J Roentgenol.* 2013;200:641–644.
293. Prosser I, Lawson Z, Evans A, et al. A timetable for the radiologic features of fracture healing in young children. *AJR Am J Roentgenol.* 2012;198:1014–1020.
294. Walters MM, Forbes PW, Buonomo C, et al. Healing patterns of clavicular birth injuries as a guide to fracture dating in cases of possible infant abuse. *Pediatr Radiol.* 2014;44:1224–1229.
295. Flaherty EG, Perez-Rossello JM, Levine MA, et al. Evaluating children with fractures for child physical abuse: clinical report from the American Academy of Pediatrics (AAP) and the Society for Pediatric Radiology (SPR). *Pediatrics.* 2014;133:e477–e489.
296. Loder RT. The demographics of slipped capital femoral epiphysis. An international multicenter study. *Clin Orthop Relat Res.* 1996;322:8–27.
297. Wells D, King JD, Roe TF, et al. Review of slipped capital femoral epiphysis associated with endocrine disease. *J Pediatr Orthop.* 1993;13(5):610–614.
298. Shaw ED, Beals RK. The hip joint in Down's syndrome. A study of its structure and associated disease. *Clin Orthop Relat Res.* 1992;278:101–107.
299. Bonioli E, Bellini C, Sénès FM, et al. Slipped capital femoral epiphysis associated with Rubinstein-Taybi syndrome. *Clin Genet.* 1993;44(2):79–81.
300. Loder RT, Aronson DD, Greenfield ML. The epidemiology of bilateral slipped capital femoral epiphysis. A study of children in Michigan. *J Bone Joint Surg Am.* 1993;75(8):1141–1147.
301. Klein A, Joplin RJ, Reidy JA, et al. Slipped capital femoral epiphysis: early diagnosis and treatment facilitated by normal roentgenograms. *J Bone Joint Surg Am.* 1952;34:233–239.
302. Steel HH. The metaphyseal blanch sign of slipped capital femoral epiphysis. *J Bone Joint Surg Am.* 1986;68:920–922.
303. Lehman WB, Menche D, Grant A, et al. The problem of evaluating in situ pinning of slipped capital femoral epiphysis: an experimental model and a review of 63 consecutive cases. *J Pediatr Orthop.* 1984;4:297–303.
304. Jarrett DY, Matheney T, Kleinman PK. Imaging SCFE: diagnosis, treatment and complications. *Pediatr Radiol.* 2013;43(suppl 1):S71–S82.
305. Ohashi K, El-Khoury GY, Bennett DL, et al. Orthopedic hardware complications diagnosed with multi-detector row CT. *Radiology.* 2005;237(2):570–577.
306. Gemmel F, Van den Wyngaert H, Love C, et al. Prosthetic joint infections: radionuclide state-of-the-art imaging. *Eur J Nucl Med Mol Imaging.* 2012;39(5):892–890.

CHAPTER 25

Musculoskeletal Disorders Due to Endocrinopathy, Metabolic Derangement, and Arthropathy

Ricardo Restrepo • Edward Y. Lee • Paul S. Babyn • Hadeel M. Seif El Dein • Bjorn Lundin • Andrea S. Doria

INTRODUCTION

The pediatric skeleton is an important dynamic system. Bone plays many relevant physiologic roles such as providing hematopoiesis and structural support while helping maintain cellular and chemical blood homeostasis. Endocrine, metabolic, and arthritic diseases often affect the pediatric skeleton as normal bone development in children requires intense anabolic activity. Disorders of hormones, growth and humoral factors, vitamins, and minerals may all lead to changes visible to the radiologist. This chapter reviews the up-to-date imaging techniques and characteristic imaging findings of those bone disorders that occur because of underlying endocrine and metabolic abnormalities as well as arthropathies that can be encountered in the pediatric population.

IMAGING TECHNIQUES

Radiography

Conventional radiography remains the most commonly used initial imaging modality for the evaluation of bone and joint disorders in pediatric patients with clinically suspected endocrine, metabolic, and arthropathic abnormalities. Radiographs are readily available, easy to obtain, and low cost and have minimal radiation exposure.[1] The appearance of the epiphyses, metaphyses, and physes as well as bone density and shape must be carefully assessed.

A typical radiographic series for evaluation of suspected endocrine and metabolic abnormalities includes anterior–posterior views of the wrists/hands and knees, as bone changes are most conspicuous in areas of active growth. Bilateral views are recommended to confirm systemic involvement. Bone age can also be determined on the hand radiograph (or the knee radiograph in children who are younger than 1 year of age) in order to determine delayed maturation.[2] A skeletal survey may be useful in the evaluation of the bones of children with systemic disorders (i.e., metabolic, endocrine) or skeletal dysplasias or when nonaccidental trauma is suspected.

The evaluation of children with suspected osteochondroses also begins with radiographs of the affected area. In children, radiographs of the contralateral side may be helpful to confirm subtle abnormalities and exclude normal developmental variants.[1] There may be the need for two or more views in the imaging assessment of certain osteochondroses such as slipped capital femoral epiphysis or osteochondritis dissecans (OCD) of the knee as described later in this chapter. In children with juvenile idiopathic arthritis (JIA), radiographs are useful at the time of the initial diagnosis to exclude other diagnostic pathologies and in the evaluation of complications occasionally seen late in the disease. In JIA patients, radiographs provide an overall appearance of the disease and information regarding bone mineralization. On the other hand, radiographs have poor sensitivity in detecting early changes of JIA and evaluating JIA activity because of their poor capability of assessment of soft tissues and cartilage.[3]

Ultrasound

Gray-scale as well as color and power Doppler ultrasound (US) may play an important role in evaluating children with underlying endocrine, metabolic, and arthropathic abnormalities. Without requiring sedation or exposing children to ionizing radiation, US can provide information regarding the synovium, marginal articular cartilage, joint effusions, and periarticular soft tissues. In skeletally immature pediatric patients, because of the larger extent of cartilaginous structures, US can be used to evaluate the unossified and superficial portions of bones.

High-frequency (7.5 to 15 MHz) linear array transducers, which can provide excellent spatial resolution of superficial musculoskeletal structures and pathology, are typically used in young children. However, lower-frequency curved or vector US transducers, which can provide increased soft tissue penetration, may be needed in older pediatric patients with larger body habitus. Color and power Doppler US imaging, which can provide information regarding vascularity and blood flow, is useful in the assessment of underlying inflammation. For example, in children with JIA, US is helpful in assessing the extent and severity of joint disease, including early erosions, and in monitoring treatment effectiveness and excluding subclinical disease.[3,4]

Computed Tomography

Computed tomography (CT), which can provide superb visualization of osseous structures, can be a useful imaging modality in children with underlying endocrine and metabolic abnormalities as well as arthropathies. However, as it is associated with ionizing radiation, judicious use is necessary. Multidetector CT (MDCT) with two-dimensional (2D) and three-dimensional (3D) reconstruction capabilities is particularly helpful for assessment of complex anatomic regions such as the face, rib cage, and hip.[1] Such 2D- and 3D-reconstructed CT images can be used as preoperative imaging tool to guide the orthopedic surgeon's interventions in pediatric patients with osseous deformities secondary to Legg-Calve-Perthes (LCP) and Blount disease.[5,6]

Magnetic Resonance Imaging

Magnetic resonance imaging (MRI) provides the most comprehensive evaluation of musculoskeletal structures in pediatric patients clinically suspected of having underlying endocrine, metabolic, and arthropathic abnormalities. Its multiplanar capabilities and the ability to evaluate bone marrow as well as the cortex can be useful in the imaging evaluation of pediatric patients with inflammatory arthropathies and systemic diseases such as sickle cell disease (SCD) and Gaucher disease.[3,7,8] Additionally, MRI is currently the best imaging modality to evaluate cartilage morphology in pediatric patients with inflammatory arthropathies such as JIA or osteochondrosis such as OCD.[4] Disadvantages of MRI include its higher cost and lower availability in comparison to the other imaging modalities, longer duration of the study, and need for intravenous contrast or sedation in young patients. In many cases, because of the long scanning time, MRI only allows the evaluation of a single joint at a time. However, more recent MRI techniques, such as whole-body MRI and parallel imaging, can now allow a relatively fast evaluation of the entire body for systemic diseases such as spondyloarthropathies and childhood inflammatory myopathies.[9,10]

Nuclear Medicine

Bone scintigraphy is a modality that detects the distribution and uptake of a radioactive agent injected into the vascular system throughout the body. The main advantage of bone scintigraphy is its ability to evaluate the entire skeleton at once, which is useful in pediatric patients with underlying systemic and metabolic disorders. It allows the functional evaluation of the soft tissues, cortical bone, and bone marrow. Bone scintigraphy is a sensitive but not specific imaging modality that can help confirm the presence of disease in the early stages. This is critical in pediatric patients with certain osteochondroses, such as early LCP disease and slipped capital femoral epiphysis, that can lead to substantial disability if not accurately diagnosed in a timely fashion. In systemic disorders such as SCD, bone scintigraphy can provide an overall appearance of the entire skeleton. In JIA, bone scintigraphy currently plays no routine role. Disadvantages of bone scintigraphy include its use of radiation, limited spatial resolution which may be improved with SPECT imaging, and the possible need of sedation.[1]

SPECTRUM OF DISORDERS

Musculoskeletal Disorders Due to Endocrinopathy and Metabolic Derangement

Rickets

Rickets results from a disruption of the orderly development and mineralization of the growth plates.[11] Rickets affects the physes by two main mechanisms: (1) deficient mineralization of cartilage and osteoid due to low calcium or phosphate and (2) retarded endochondral ossification, which causes excessive accumulation of cartilage in the physis, growth failure, and skeletal deformities.[12]

The causes of rickets are varied and can be divided into two main groups: calcipenic or phosphopenic, depending on whether the initial problem results in insufficient calcium absorption or excessive phosphate excretion, respectively. Causes of calcipenic rickets include vitamin D abnormalities and calcium deficiency, certain medications such as anticonvulsants (e.g., phenytoin), malabsorption syndromes, and obesity. The latter is due to calcium sequestration in excessive adipose tissue. Dietary calcium deficiency is uncommon in most of the world.[2,12] Rickets can be associated with prematurity and is related to a combination of nutritional, metabolic, and iatrogenic factors, usually manifesting around 12 weeks of age or later in infants who are born younger than 32 weeks of gestational age or weighing <1,500 g (Fig. 25.1).[2,11,13] Phosphopenic rickets is most commonly caused by hereditary or acquired disorders of renal tubular phosphate wasting, the most frequent of which is X-linked hypophosphatemia (familial vitamin D–resistant rickets) (**Schematic D**).[12]

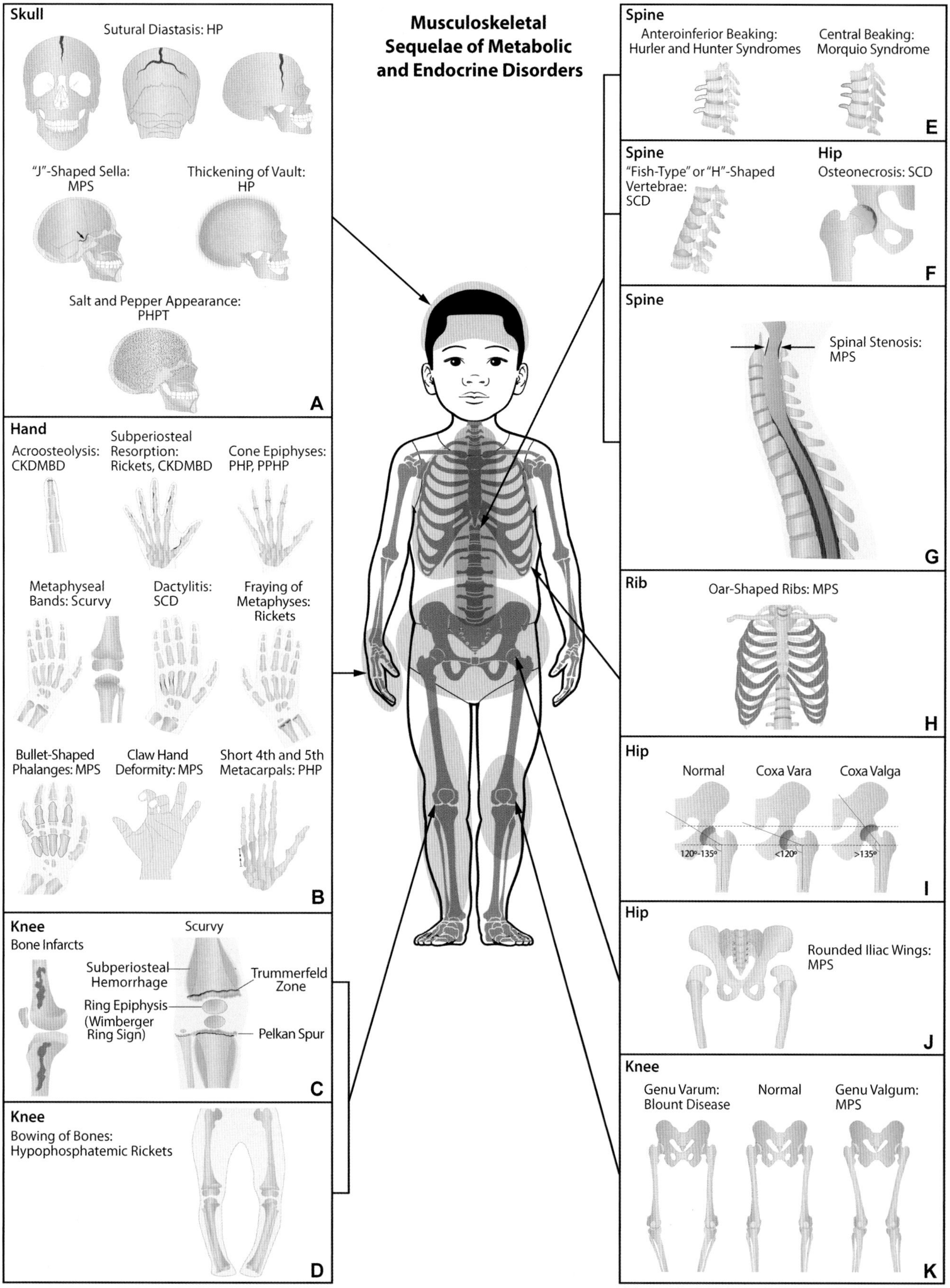

CKDMBD, chronic kidney disease–mineral bone disorder; HP, hypoparathyroidism; MPS, mucopolysaccharidosis; PHP, pseudohypoparathyroidism; PPHP, pseudopseudohypoparathyroidism; PHPT, primary hyperparathyroidism; SCD, sickle cell disease.

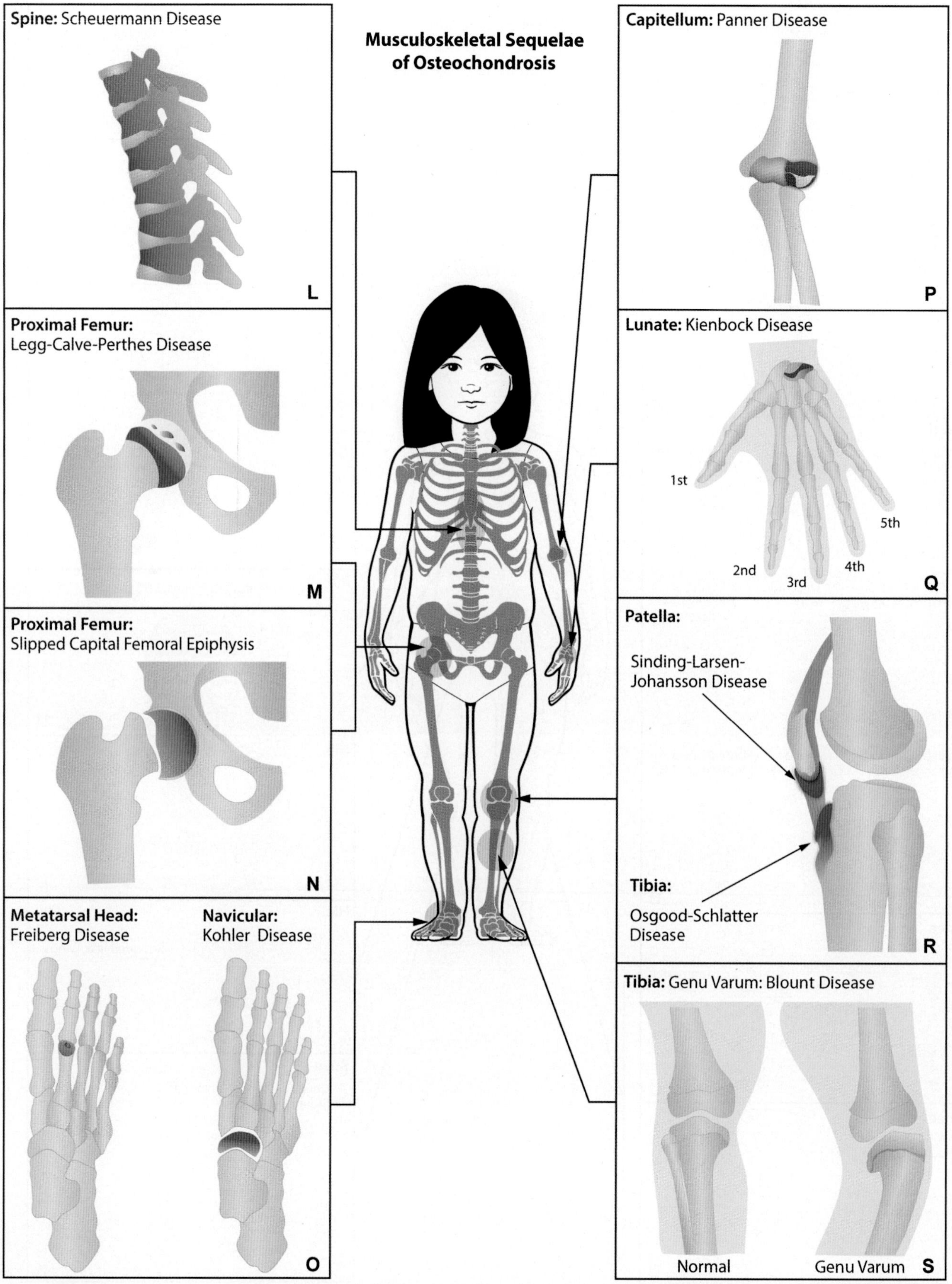
Musculoskeletal Sequelae of Osteochondrosis
Spine: Scheuermann Disease
L
Proximal Femur: Legg-Calve-Perthes Disease
M
Proximal Femur: Slipped Capital Femoral Epiphysis
N
Metatarsal Head: Freiberg Disease
Navicular: Kohler Disease
O
Capitellum: Panner Disease
P
Lunate: Kienbock Disease
1st
2nd
3rd
4th
5th
Q
Patella:
Sinding-Larsen-Johansson Disease
Tibia:
Osgood-Schlatter Disease
R
Tibia: Genu Varum: Blount Disease
Normal
Genu Varum
S

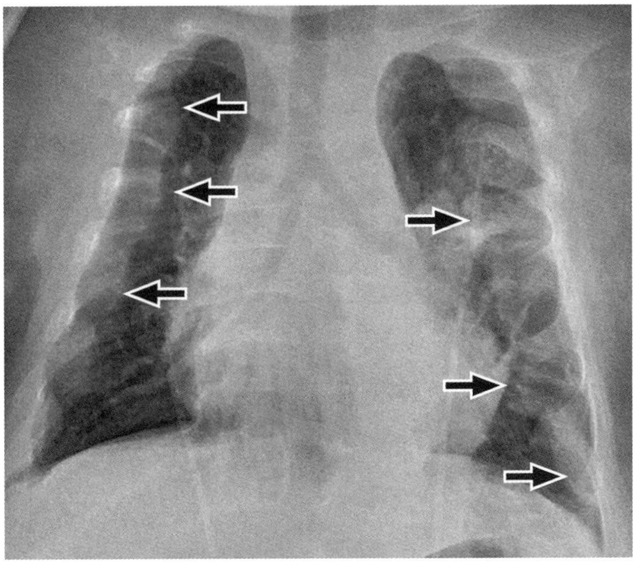

FIGURE 25.1 **A 5-month-old boy with history of severe prematurity and rickets.** Frontal chest radiograph shows severely diffuse osteopenia and a rosary appearance of the costochondral junctions (*arrows*).

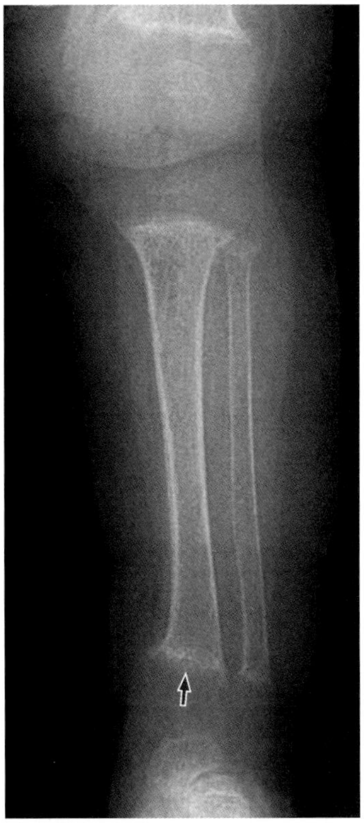

FIGURE 25.2 **A 14-month-old boy with vitamin D deficiency rickets.** Frontal tibia and fibula radiograph shows diffuse osteopenia, metaphyseal splaying, fraying, and cupping of the distal femur, tibia (*arrow*), and fibula.

Radiographs play an important role in the diagnosis of rickets and in the evaluation of treatment response. A typical metabolic radiographic series includes views of the hand and knees, as rachitic changes are more conspicuous in areas of most active growth. Bilateral views are recommended to confirm a systemic involvement. Bone age can also be determined to assess delayed maturation.[2,14] Nonspecific radiographic changes of rickets include diffuse demineralization (osteopenia), coarsening of the trabecular pattern, and the lack of growth that precedes physeal changes. The more typical changes of rickets affect the growth plate, with physeal widening being the first sign to appear. As the disease progresses, the metaphyseal margin, more specifically the zone of provisional calcification, is lost, and the physis widens. Metaphyseal fraying and cupping occur in the affected long bones (Fig. 25.2 and **Schematic B**). Epiphyses progressively become more lucent until their margins are lost. In the shafts, radiographic findings of rickets include subperiosteal resorption, cortical thinning, intracortical tunneling, and endosteal resorption. Additional diaphyseal findings include insufficiency fractures, periosteal reaction, and bowing deformity. Bowing is more pronounced in the lower extremities with weight bearing.[11,14,15]

With healing, radiographic changes are seen by 2 to 3 months, with radiographic changes lagging clinical and laboratory parameters by a few weeks. The earliest radiographic finding of healing rickets is the revisualization of the zone of provisional calcification as an opaque line separated from the rest of the shaft with subsequent mineralization of the underlying physeal cartilage. Periosteal reaction can also be seen in the healing phase. Bowing deformities may persist for a long time.[15]

In hypophosphatemic rickets (Fig. 25.3), bone mineralization is better preserved than it is in vitamin D-deficient rickets. Major clinical differences between these two types of rickets include short stature and bowing, particularly of the lower extremities. Bowing is more frequently present in hypophosphatemic rickets. Insufficiency fractures and looser zones are also more commonly seen in hypophosphatemic rickets than in the vitamin D-deficient type of rickets.[11,15]

The management of rickets aims to treat this disease's underlying cause. Most cases of rickets respond well to vitamin D therapy and, if necessary, calcium supplementation.[15,16]

Hyperparathyroidism

Primary hyperparathyroidism (PHPT) is one of the most common endocrine disorders, with a prevalence of 0.1% to 0.4% and an incidence that increases with age, to peak in the sixth decade.[17] PHPT is uncommon in adolescents and is rare in children, having a prevalence of 3% to 5% in Western countries.[18] PHPT is defined as hypercalcemia secondary to the overproduction of parathormone (PTH) by one or more parathyroid glands in which the negative feedback to regulate calcium is lost, resulting in increased renal absorption of calcium, increased synthesis of vitamin D, phosphaturia, and increased bone resorption.[17] The classic symptoms include bone and abdominal pain, psychiatric symptoms, and fatigue. Affected pediatric patients also often present with renal stones. In comparison to adults with PHPT, affected pediatric patients present with a higher frequency of symptoms and more end organ damage.[17,19,20]

In the pediatric population, PHPT can be divided into two groups by age of onset: neonatal and childhood types.

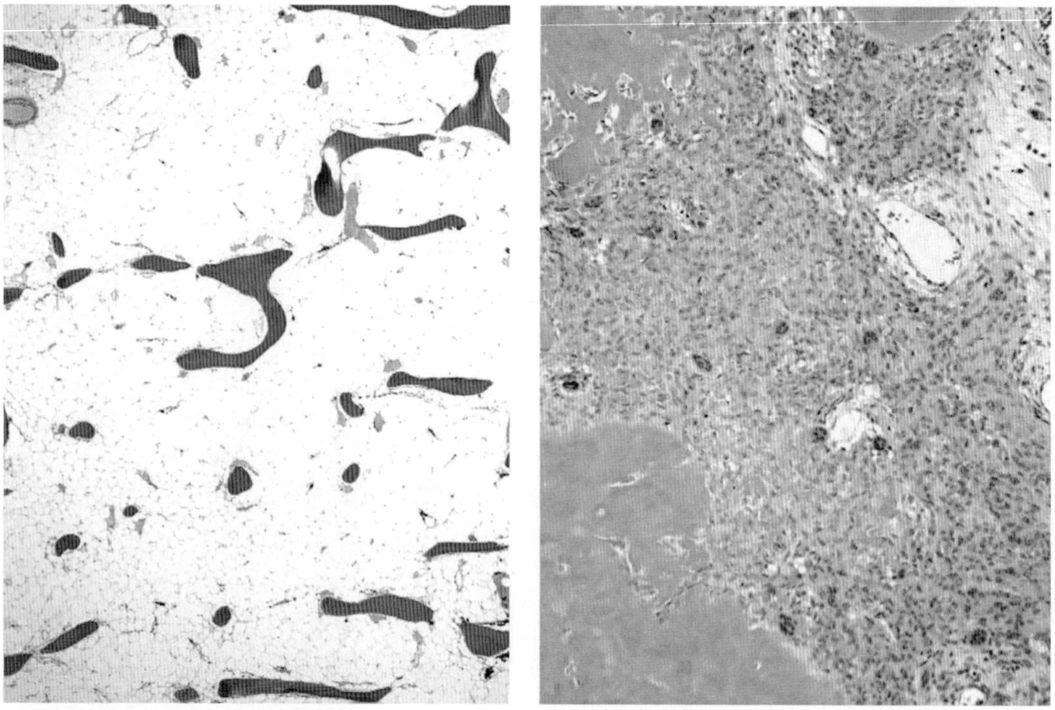

FIGURE 25.3 **Oncogenic hypophosphatemic rickets in an 11-year-old boy.** Bony spicules are markedly diminished in size and number (**left;** hematoxylin and eosin, original magnification, 40×). In this case, the phosphate dysregulation resolved after resection of a phosphaturic mesenchymal tumor occurring in the tibia (**right;** hematoxylin and eosin, original magnification, 200×).

Neonatal HPT has an autosomal recessive inheritance or may be due to maternal hypothyroidism. Neonatal HPT may present in newborns and infants with life-threatening hypercalcemia due to parathyroid hyperplasia.[21,22] In older children and adolescents, most cases of PHPT are sporadic because of a parathyroid adenoma followed by glandular hyperplasia. Some of these pediatric patients have multiple endocrine neoplasia syndrome or familial isolated PHPT.[17,18,20]

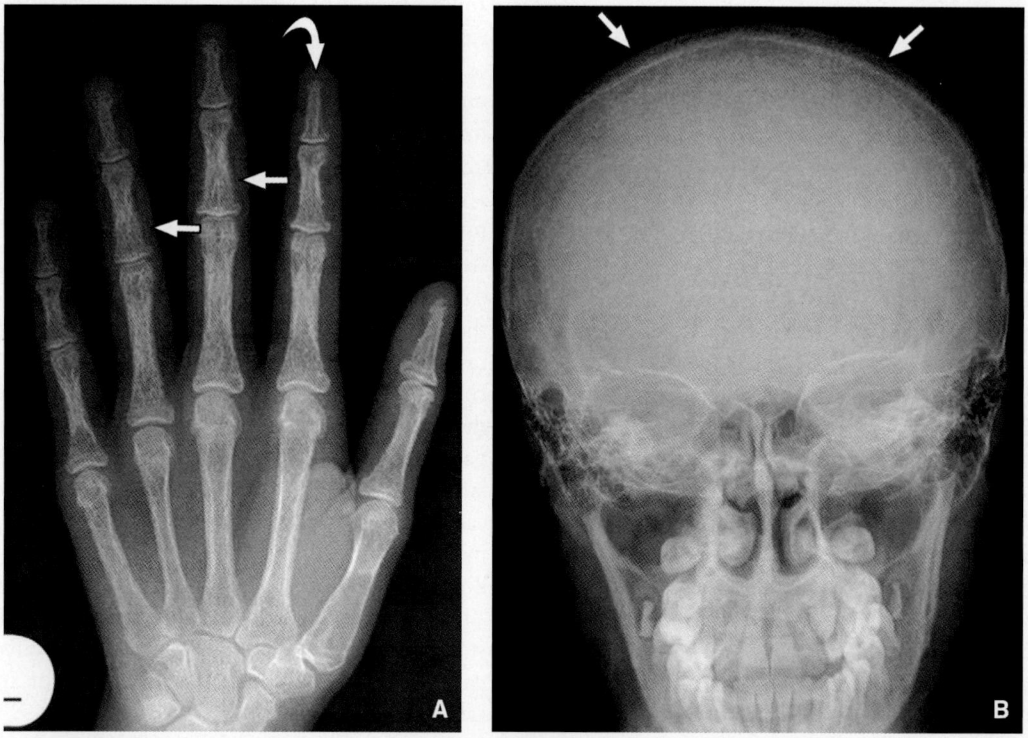

FIGURE 25.4 **Primary hyperparathyroidism in a 15-year-old boy with a parathyroid adenoma. A:** Frontal hand radiograph reveals coarsening of the trabecular pattern and signs of bone resorption such as cortical tunneling (*straight arrows*) and acroosteolysis (*curved arrow*). **B:** Frontal skull radiograph shows the classic "salt and pepper"-appearing skull (*arrows*) indicative of bone resorption.

The imaging modality of choice for evaluating bone involvement in children with PHPT is radiography. Typical radiographic findings include osteopenia, coarsening of the trabeculae, subperiosteal bone resorption, and cortical tunneling (Fig. 25.4A). Subligamentous bone resorption is also common, more typical in the distal femur and proximal tibia. Trabecular bone resorption may occur throughout the skeleton, including the skull, where it produces the "salt and pepper" appearance (Fig. 25.4B and **Schematic A**). Metastatic soft tissue and visceral calcifications, chondrocalcinosis, slipped capital femoral epiphyses, and bone deformities (i.e., genu valgum) may occur as well.[15,21]

Typically, PHPT in the pediatric population has been managed with bilateral neck exploration and biopsy of the parathyroid glands. In cases of confirmed single parathyroid adenoma, exploration and excision of the single affected gland can be performed.[20]

Chronic Kidney Disease–Mineral Bone Disorder

Chronic kidney disease–mineral bone disorder (CKDMBD), formerly known as renal osteodystrophy (ROD), refers to the characteristic musculoskeletal manifestations of hyperparathyroidism secondary to chronic renal failure.[2,15] Both glomerular and tubular dysfunctions contribute to the development of CKDMBD. Tubular dysfunction causes hypocalcemia because of deficient vitamin D synthesis, whereas impaired glomerular function causes phosphorus retention. This results in hypocalcemia that triggers hyperparathyroidism in an effort to restore calcium levels. Secondary hyperparathyroidism is the major metabolic abnormality in ROD. As the disease progresses, rickets and osteomalacia develop.[2,15,23]

Radiographic changes of hyperparathyroidism stem from increased osteoclastic bone resorption. Classic radiographic features include subperiosteal, endosteal, and subligamentous resorption as well as osteopenia with coarsening of the trabecular pattern. Subperiosteal resorption is most frequently seen in the middle phalanges of the hand (Fig. 25.5A and **Schematic B**), distal clavicle (Fig. 25.5B), and distal femur and proximal tibia. Endosteal resorption, also known as cortical tunneling, is seen as a lacy pattern of the inner cortex of the bone. Acroosteolysis, which represents terminal tuft bone resorption, is also a manifestation of CKDMBD (Fig. 25.5A). Subchondral resorption that is adjacent to the physeal cartilage, the so-called osteitis fibrosa, can also be seen causing lucency at the edge of the physis, simulating rickets and predisposing to epiphyseal slippage. Osteosclerosis also is a common manifestation that causes diffuse chalky bone density, which in the spine affects the vertebral end plates, producing the rugger jersey spine.[2,11,15,24] A real measurement of bone mineral density by dual x-ray absorptiometry is currently available to assess bone mass in the pediatric population.[25] Soft tissue and visceral calcification are also a manifestation of CKDMBD because of the deposition of calcium salts.[26]

Histologically, the bone in renal bone disease shows prominent osteoclastic and osteoblastic activity, increased woven bone, and marrow fibrosis that begin as paratrabecular (Fig. 25.5C) and progresses to diffuse (osteitis fibrosa). Control of bone and mineral homeostasis is very challenging in children, with most of the affected patients experiencing signs of hyperparathyroidism to different extents.

The treatment consists of dietary counseling, ergocalciferol and cholecalciferol supplementation, and the use of calcium-free phosphate binders.[23]

Tertiary Hyperparathyroidism

Tertiary hyperparathyroidism (THPT) is rare in children and adolescents, and relatively little is currently known about its radiologic findings. The diagnosis of this entity is mainly based on laboratory findings.[27] The boundary between secondary (nonautonomic function) and tertiary (autonomic function) forms of hyperparathyroidism is sometimes blurry with radiologic findings of THPT representing more advanced stages of ROD (Fig. 25.6). This entity is a manifestation of the uremic state of CKDMBD. Although the characteristic autonomic function of the parathyroid glands in THPT may resemble the metabolic activity of an adenoma, this pathologic entity is in fact rare in THPT. Instead, most cases (94%) of THPT present with marked glandular hyperplasia.[27,28]

^{99m}Tc sestamibi (MIBI) scintigraphy is very sensitive and accurate for preoperative localization of parathyroid lesions in patients with PHPT and has a fair sensitivity and accuracy to detect all abnormal parathyroid glands in multiple hyperplasia.[29] Nevertheless, MIBI is an important diagnostic technique for identifying ectopic parathyroid glands in the mediastinal and thymic regions in patients with THPT.[30]

Hypoparathyroidism, Pseudohypoparathyroidism, and Pseudopseudohypoparathyroidism

Hypoparathyroidism (HP) is an abnormality of the calcium metabolism characterized by low serum levels of PTH in spite of hypocalcemia and secondary hyperphosphatemia.[31] Primary idiopathic HP can be familial or sporadic. It can be associated with several syndromes, including DiGeorge syndrome, which is characterized by congenital absence of the parathyroid glands. Other causes of HP are autoimmune disorders and postsurgical resection. Pseudohypoparathyroidism (PHP) is a hereditary disease characterized by similar findings of HP; however, the parathyroid glands are normal with elevated PTH due to end organ resistance to PTH. Pseudopseudohypoparathyroidism (PPHP) is the normocalcemic form of PHP.[21,31,32]

The musculoskeletal manifestation of HP can be evaluated using radiographs. The most common radiographic feature of HP that occurs in ~20% of affected patients is generalized or focal osteosclerosis, particularly in the calvarium, pelvis, and proximal femora.[21] The face and the skull are areas that are frequently involved in affected pediatric patients. Radiographic findings include thickening of the cranial vault and facial bones, sutural diastasis in cases with associated increased intracranial pressure, and abnormal tooth development with delayed eruption or supernumerary teeth. Other manifestations include premature epiphyseal fusion, dense metaphyseal bands, and calcifications in the soft tissue, tendons, and spinal ligaments.[11,21]

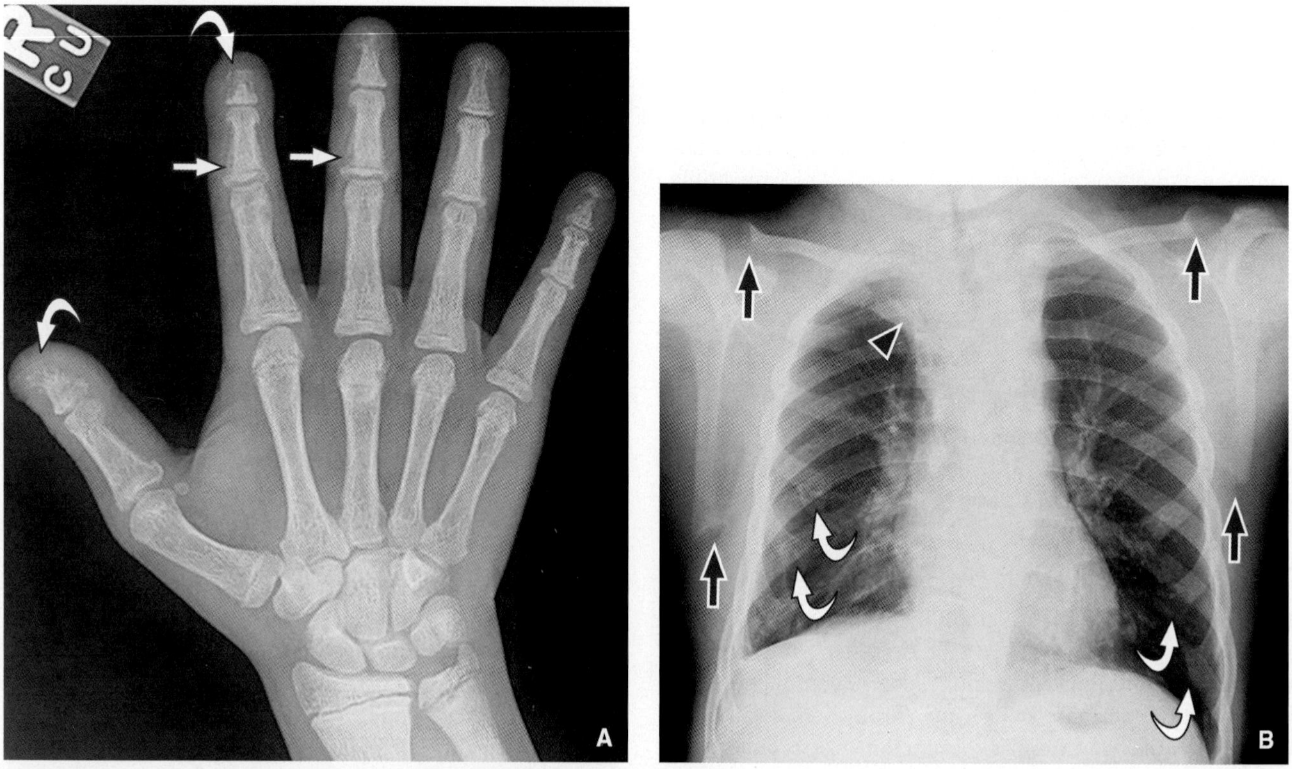

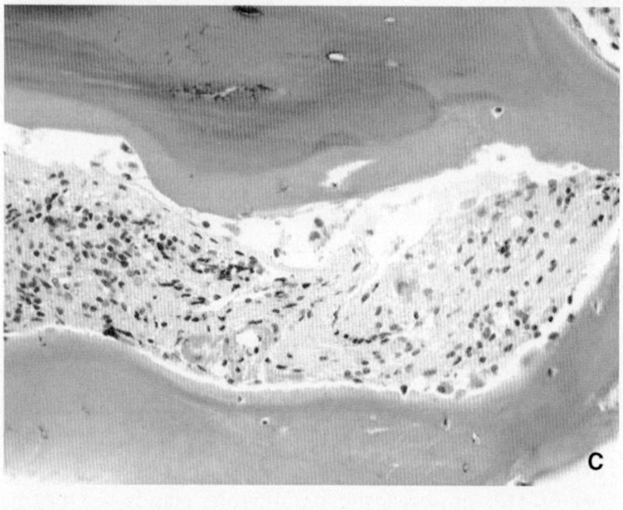

FIGURE 25.5 **A 13-year-old girl with renal osteodystrophy from underlying end-stage renal disease. A:** Frontal hand radiograph shows diffuse osteopenia and signs of bone resorption such as cortical tunneling (*straight arrows*) and acrosteolysis with tuft resorption (*curved arrows*). **B:** Frontal chest radiograph demonstrates resorption of the distal clavicles and scapular tips (*straight arrows*) and widening of the costochondral junctions (*curved arrows*). Note calcified thrombus of the superior vena cava due to previous dialysis catheters (*arrowhead*). **C:** Chronic kidney disease–mineral bone disorder in an 11-year-old girl with renal failure. A posterior iliac crest biopsy shows marrow fibrosis and decreased hematopoiesis (hematoxylin and eosin, original magnification, 400x).

A typical radiographic finding in PHP and PPHP is the shortening of one or more of the metacarpals and metatarsals due to the premature fusion of the physis, most commonly affecting the fourth and fifth rays. This finding occurs more frequently in PPHP and most commonly involves the hands (Fig. 25.7 and **Schematic B**). Other skeletal features of PHP and PPHP include diaphyseal exostoses, coxa valga or vara (**Schematic I**), osseous bowing, cone epiphyses, and accelerated skeletal maturation. Soft tissue calcification similar to HP can also be seen.[21]

The majority of cases of pediatric PHP are well controlled with the administration of calcium and vitamin D analogues. For nonresponding cases, PTH replacement therapy can be used; however, the use of recombinant human PTH is contraindicated in children because of the increased risk of osteosarcoma.[31,32]

Hypophosphatasia

Hypophosphatasia is characterized by a defective bone mineralization caused by insufficient activity of tissue-nonspecific alkaline phosphatase. This eventually leads to the excessive accumulation of inorganic pyrophosphate, resulting in deficient bone mineralization. The four main types of hypophosphatasia are perinatal, infantile, childhood, and adult types.

Similar to rickets, the diagnosis of hypophosphatasia can be made based on radiographs. In hypophosphatasia, there is lack of mineralization of parts of the skeleton which is more severe than the mineralization defect noted in osteogenesis imperfecta. The infantile and childhood forms resemble rickets with less uniform and patchier metaphyseal involvement. The adult form simulates osteomalacia with a coarse trabecular pattern, metatarsal stress fractures, and Looser zones.[33]

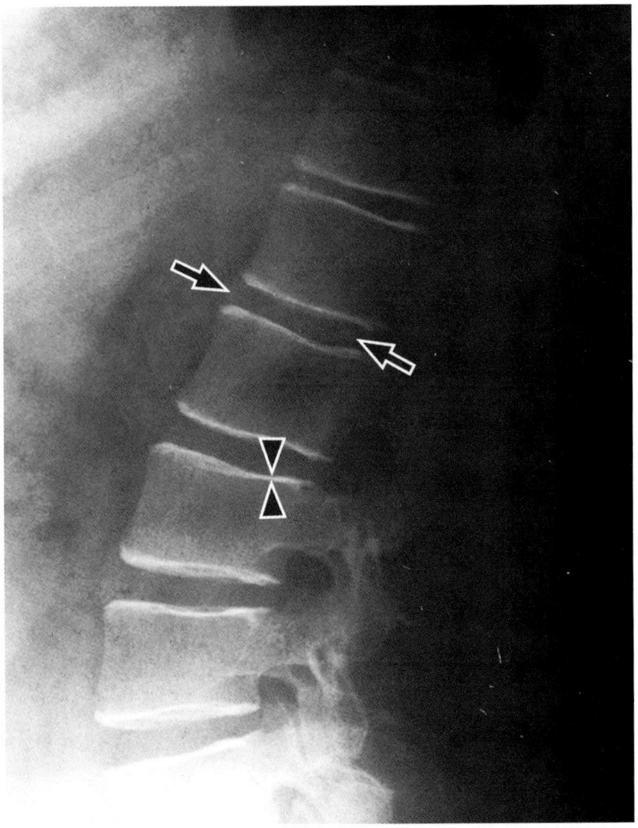

FIGURE 25.6 **A 17-year-old girl with granulomatosis and polyangiitis (previously known as Wegener granulomatosis) and chronic renal failure diagnosed with tertiary hyperparathyroidism on the basis of laboratory findings.** Lateral radiograph of the thoracolumbar spine shows sclerosis of the vertebral endplates (*arrowheads*) with multilevel intervertebral disk calcification foci (*arrows*).

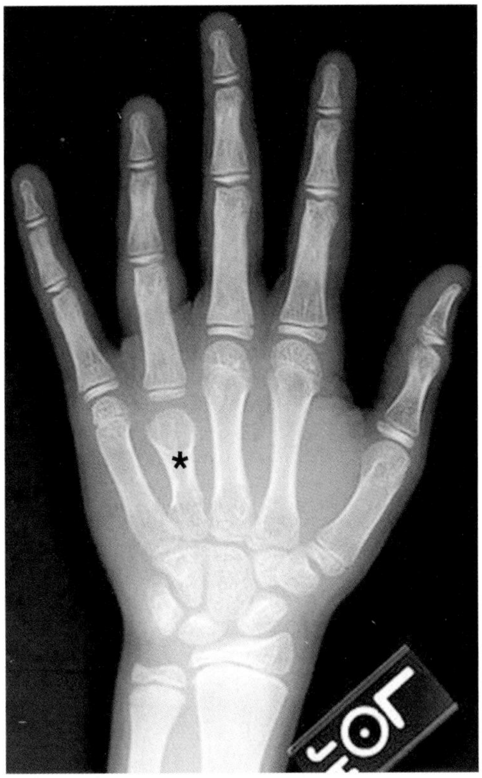

FIGURE 25.7 **A 9-year-old boy with pseudopseudohypoparathyroidsim.** Frontal hand radiograph shows a short fourth metacarpal (*asterisk*).

No effective treatment currently exists for hypophosphatasia. There is only treatment for specific symptoms and supportive measures.[33]

Scurvy

Scurvy is a disease that results from a physiologic deficiency of vitamin C, now rarely seen in the developed world. Humans are dependent on the exogenous intake of vitamin C that is present in vegetables and fruits. Vitamin C is also present in breast milk.[34–36] In children, scurvy is more common in infants who are fed with pasteurized or boiled milk, as heat disrupts the vitamin, and it also is more common in preschool children who have an inadequate intake of vegetables and fruits. Infantile scurvy usually develops after 6 months of age because of the storage of vitamin C built up in utero and during the first few months in life through breast milk.[35] Affected young children present with failure to thrive and gastrointestinal (GI) symptoms. As the disease progresses, affected pediatric patients develop gum bleeding and bone changes. Skin manifestations and bleeding are more common in older children and adults.[35]

The diagnosis of scurvy is made based on serum levels of vitamin C and on the radiographic skeletal manifestations that include osteoporosis and abnormalities in the areas of active endochondral growth, such as at the end of the long bones. Biopsy may occasionally be pursued (Fig. 25.8A). Extensive resorption of cortical and cancellous bone predisposes these areas to fracture (Fig. 25.8A) that often display excessive callus during the healing phase. The Trummerfeld zone is a disrupted metaphyseal zone of osteoporosis that can result in peripheral metaphyseal excrescences if there is associated healing (Fig. 25.8B and **Schematic C**) and osseous malalignment at the metaphyseal–diaphyseal junction due to physeal separation. The Wimberger ring sign is characteristic of the disease and consists of a radiodense line at the edge of an ossification center that corresponds to the normal mineralized cartilaginous zone of provisional calcification, which contrasts more with the demineralized remainder of the center (Fig. 25.8B). Alternating dense and lucent metaphyseal lines can be present along with hemarthrosis and subperiosteal hemorrhage, which is seen as periosteal reaction along the long bones.[11,35,37] More recently, MRI has been used to evaluate scurvy in pediatric patients with autism.[38]

The treatment of scurvy includes vitamin C supplementation, which typically leads to a rapid resolution of the symptoms. For infantile scurvy, avoiding pasteurized or boiled milk and providing vitamin supplementation to the lactating mother is recommended in order to increase the vitamin's level in the breast milk.[36] Radiographically, cortical thickening, dense metaphyseal lines, exaggerated subperiosteal bone formation, and osseous realignment are signs of healing.[11,35]

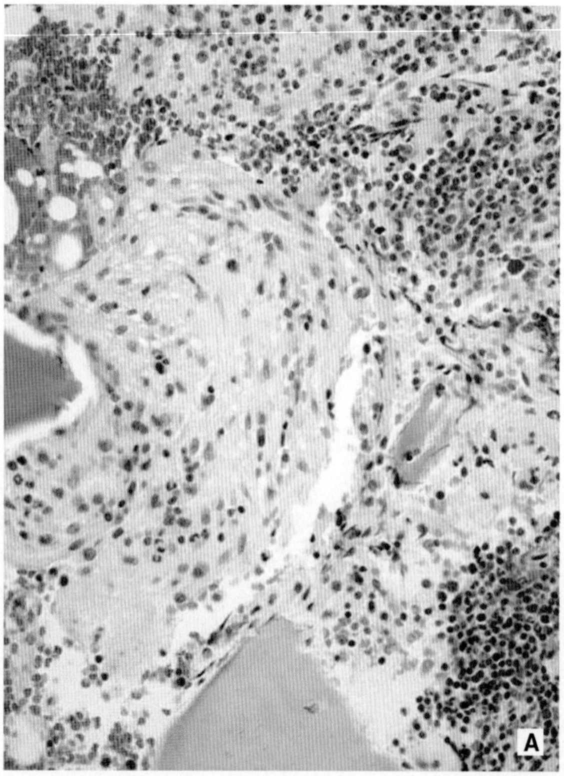

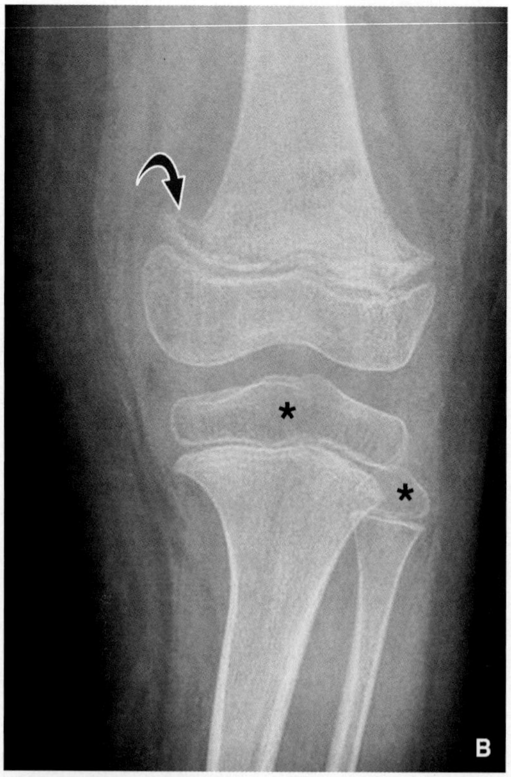

FIGURE 25.8 **A: Scurvy due to vitamin C deficiency in an 11-year-old boy with a history of autism and escalating food aversions.** An iliac crest biopsy shows a paratrabecular spindle cell proliferation (hematoxylin and eosin, original magnification, 400×). **B: Scurvy in a 6-year-old boy.** Frontal knee radiograph shows a linear metaphyseal lucency with an associated fracture and a focal bony excrescence indicating early healing (Trummerfeld zone) (*curved arrow*). Significant osteopenia, more conspicuous in the epiphysis with a peripheral sclerotic line (Wimberger ring sign), is seen (*asterisks*).

Heavy Metal Poisoning

Heavy metals (HM) are defined as those metals that have a specific density of more than 5 g/cm^3, such as lead, mercury, aluminum, arsenic, cadmium, and nickel. They are widely distributed in the earth's crust, and most are normally present at very low concentrations in the body. HM are toxic because of potential cumulative deleterious effects that can cause chronic degenerative changes, especially in the nervous system, liver, kidney, and bones.[39,40]

The mechanisms of toxicity of most of these agents are well known and include enzymatic inhibition, impaired antioxidant metabolism, oxidative stress, and free-radical formation.[39] In modern life, most cases of HM poisoning occur in adults because of occupational hazards; however, lead poisoning still raises serious concern in children.[40–42] Lead has industrial use but no physiologic use; therefore, any evidence of lead in the body should be considered contamination. In children, the mechanism of poisoning is accidental ingestion and most frequently occurs in toddlers. The primary route of lead exposure is through the GI tract, where lead is taken up at calcium absorption sites, which are very active at times of rapid growth. Being an inorganic compound, it is poorly absorbed through the GI tract. Chronic exposure to very small amounts of lead is necessary to cause untoward effects. Lead-based paints in households and toys are common causes of lead intoxication in children.[40,42] The most common childhood presentation of lead poisoning (plumbism) is central neurotoxicity. Other symptoms of lead toxicity include anemia, anorexia, abdominal pain, vomiting, and growth delay.[40–42]

The diagnosis of lead intoxication, as of any other heavy metal toxicity effect, is made by measuring the blood levels of the metal in question. Pediatric patients in high-risk areas should be screened every 1 to 2 years. The skeletal manifestations of lead poisoning can be evaluated using radiographs. Typical features include dense transverse metaphyseal lines due to the increased deposition of calcium along with lead, most prominently around the knee. Dense bands in the femur and tibia can be seen in normal children; thus, the presence of fibular bands supports the diagnosis (Fig. 25.9). Radiodense bands can be seen in other sites of the axial and appendicular skeleton, including the spine. If lead exposure is interrupted, these dense bands slowly migrate to the diaphysis and disappear in a few years. Dense metaphyseal bands are not characteristic of lead poisoning because they can be seen with other types of HM intoxication, scurvy, rickets, and treated leukemia. Abnormal tubular bone remodeling, most pronounced in the distal femur with metaphyseal widening as well as sutural widening in the skull due to increased intracranial pressure, can be seen.[11]

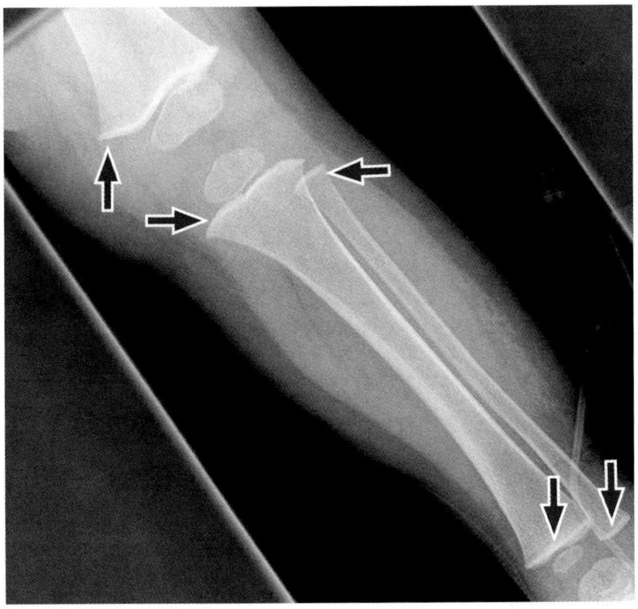

FIGURE 25.9 **Lead poisoning in a toddler boy.** Frontal tibia and fibula radiograph shows a typical dense metaphyseal band (lead band) (*arrows*) around the knee and ankle. The proximal fibular involvement is more supportive of the diagnosis of lead poisoning.

All symptomatic and asymptomatic pediatric patients with markedly elevated blood levels of lead should be handled as emergencies and treated immediately with chelating agents.[42,43]

Sickle Cell Disease

Bone involvement is the most common manifestation of SCD, both acutely and chronically. Acute manifestations of SCD include painful vasoocclusive crisis, osteomyelitis, bone marrow infarcts, stress fractures, and vertebral collapse ("fish-type" or "H-shaped" vertebrae; Fig. 25.10 and **Schematic F**). Chronic manifestations are mainly related to osteonecrosis and secondary bone collapse and deformity.[44] In this chapter, the vasoocclusive crisis and bone infarcts from SCD are discussed.

Vasoocclusive crisis affects virtually all pediatric patients with SCD, often beginning in late infancy and recurring throughout their lives. The pathogenesis of vasoocclusive crisis relates to microvascular occlusion due to the abnormally deformed red cells that may be seen in any organ but occur more frequently in the bone marrow. These microvascular occlusions result in bone marrow infarction, typically in the medullary cavity or epiphyses.[44,45]

Clinically, affected pediatric patients complain of localized or multifocal intense pain, edema and erythema with or without fever and leukocytosis.[44,45] Dactylitis is a fairly classic presentation of vasoocclusive crisis in younger children who are typically between 1 and 2 years; it involves the small bones of the hands and feet, which contain hematopoietic marrow (Fig. 25.11). Affected children present with a swollen and painful digit.[7,44,46] Osteonecrosis occurs when the vasoocclusion results in infarction of the epiphyses and may involve the articular surfaces.[44,45]

The diagnosis of a painful crisis is predominantly clinical. Radiographs are of little value, as the acute changes are usually not seen. Bone scintigraphy or MRI is the imaging modalities of choice during an acute pain crisis. Bone scintigraphy is helpful in assessing multifocal involvement showing increased uptake in areas of acute bone marrow infarction.[44] More recently, whole-body MRI with diffusion-weighted imaging (DWI) sequences has been used successfully not only to evaluate the extent of disease but also to evaluate the acuity of the infarcts.[47,48] In ischemia, DWI shows increased diffusion within the first hours of the insult and remains elevated during the healing process.[47] When the involvement is localized, MRI may be more helpful, as it is very sensitive in detecting bone marrow and soft tissue abnormalities. In the acute setting, bone infarcts are hyperintense on fluid-sensitive sequences and hypointense on T1-weighted MR images. On T1-weighted MR images with fat saturation before contrast, acute lesions tend to be hyperintense and display no enhancement after contrast. When epiphyseal in location, infarcts can be associated with joint effusion. Adjacent soft tissue edema and stranding are findings that support a more acute process.

The more chronic infarcts tend to be predominantly hypointense with a peripheral bright halo on fluid-sensitive sequences and hypointense with fatty elements on T1-weighted MR images (Fig. 25.12A). SCD-related bone marrow infarcts tend to be larger than those from other etiologies, reflecting a more systemic disease. More chronic infarcts can be seen on radiographs as serpiginous lytic lesions with a peripheral sclerotic line (**Schematic C**). On radiographs, diffuse or patchy osteosclerosis is also present (Fig. 25.12B). In the epiphyses, a subchondral crescentic lucency is fairly characteristic on radiographs (**Schematic F**). On MRI, the lucency seen

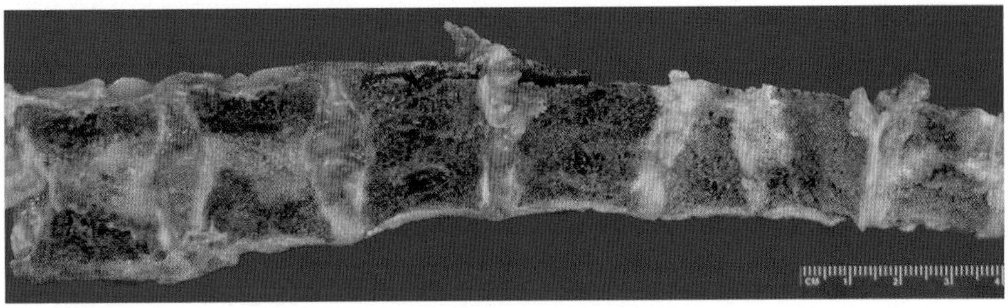

FIGURE 25.10 **Sickle cell disease in a 15-year-old boy.** The vertebral column shows large areas of medullary pallor (infarcts) as well as extensive vertebral body collapse.

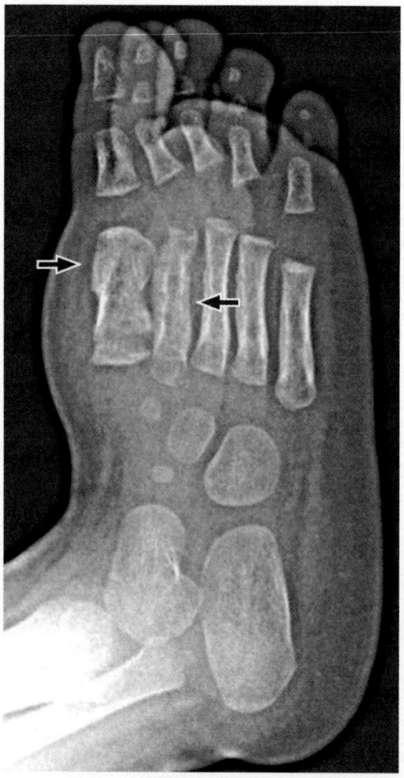

FIGURE 25.11 **An 8-month-old boy with sickle cell disease dactylitis.** The oblique radiograph of foot shows marked periosteal reaction (*arrows*) and adjacent soft tissue swelling involving the first and second metatarsals.

on radiographs has fluid signal on T2-weighted MR images.[7,44–46,49]

The treatment of a vasoocclusive crisis and infarcts from SCD requires the use of analgesics, vasodilators, and aggressive intravenous hydration. If a coexisting infection is suspected, antibiotics are also given.[45,50]

Storage Diseases

Storage diseases are progressive multisystemic metabolic conditions that affect the musculoskeletal system and viscera, such as the lungs, heart, liver, spleen, and in some cases the brain as well. They can be mainly divided into lysosomal and nonlysosomal diseases, with the metabolic substrate determining the involvement of the cell type or organ in the individual storage disease.[51] Individually, lysosomal storage diseases (LSDs) are rare genetic conditions; however, the cumulative incidence of lysosomal diseases is 1:5,000, with more than 50 types described. Most LSDs are inherited as an autosomal recessive pattern.[52] Disorders of the lysosomal type require electron microscopy of the affected tissue for morphologic diagnosis.[51] Lysosomes contain enzymes that degrade cellular macromolecules, and when a specific enzyme is absent, excessive by-products and metabolites accumulate. Typically, LSDs are classified based on the accumulating substrate: mucopolysaccharidoses (MPS), mucolipidoses, sphingolipidoses, glycoprotein storage diseases, and glycogenosis. LSDs are differentiated by clinical features, the age of presentation, and enzyme deficiency. All LSDs affect the skeletal system with overlapping phenotypes; however, some have unique skeletal involvement.[52]

As with any other skeletal dysplasia, a skeletal survey is the first imaging approach, allowing for the evaluation of the entire skeleton. In the MPS, the accumulation of glycosaminoglycans (GAGs) occurs because of a deficiency in different GAG-degrading enzymes, thus causing progressive damage of affected tissues. Seven distinct clinical types of MPS have been identified, caused by 11 different enzymatic deficiencies (Table 25.1).[8,53,54] Mucolipidoses (ML) constitute a more heterogeneous group, with types I and IV being very different from types II and III. Although these conditions are usually grouped together, the enzyme abnormality, stored

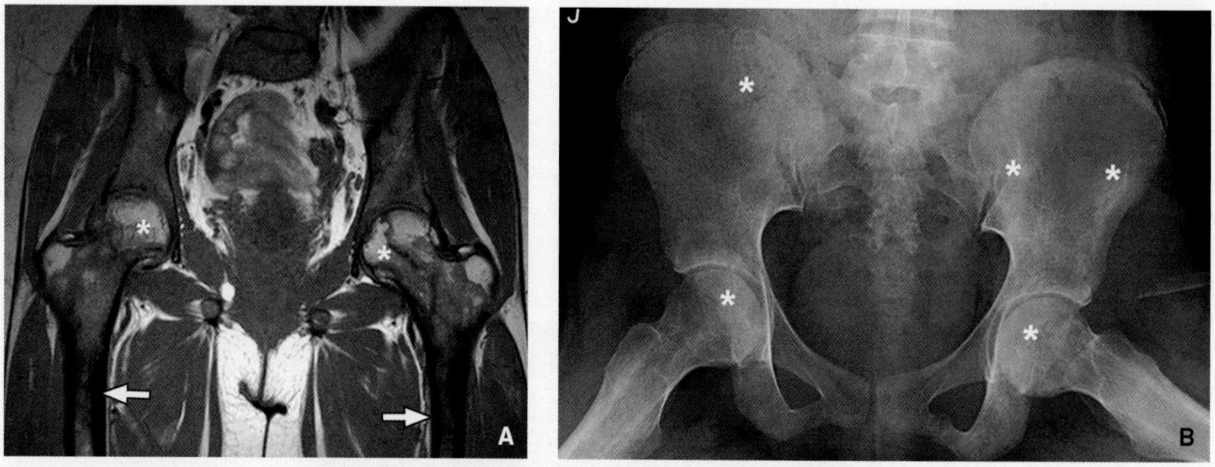

FIGURE 25.12 **A 15-year-old girl with sickle cell disease and multiple painful crisis in the past. A:** Coronal T1-weighted MR image of the pelvis shows bilateral proximal femoral serpiginous lesions with fatty elements and a sclerotic low-signal rim indicative of old bone infarcts (*asterisks*). There is a decreased T1 signal in both proximal femoral diaphyses indicative of bone marrow reconversion (*arrows*). **B:** Frontal radiograph of the pelvis demonstrates patchy increased sclerosis (*asterisks*) in both iliac wings and femoral heads indicating multiple previous bone infarcts. The femoral heads are symmetric in size and shape with preserved sphericity.

TABLE 25.1 Enzyme Deficiency in Mucopolysaccharidoses and Mucolipidoses

Mucopolysaccharidosis (MPS)	Enzyme Deficiency	Mucolipidosis (MLP)	Enzyme Deficiency
MPS I (Hurler/Scheie)	Iduronidase	ML I (sialidosis I)	Alpha-N-acetyl-neuraminidase (sialidase)
MPS II (Hunter)	Iduronate-2-sulfatase	ML II (I-cell)	N-acetylglucosamine-1-phosphate transferase
MPS III (Sanfilippo) IIIA IIIB IIIC IIID	 Heparan-N-sulfatase N-acetyl-glucosaminidase Acetyl-CoA glucosaminidase N-acetyl-glucosamine-6-sulfatase	ML III (pseudo-Hurler)	N-acetylglucosamine-1-phosphate transferase
MPS IV (Morquio) IVA IVB	 Galactose-6-sulfatase Beta-galactosidase	ML IV	Mucolipin/Alpha-N-acetyl-neuraminidase (sialidase)
MPS VI (Maroteaux-Lamy)	Galactosamine-4-sulfatase		
MPS VII (Sly)	Beta-glucuronidase		
MPS IX	Hyaluronidase		

substrate, and clinical features are very different. ML II (I-cell disease) (Fig. 25.13) and ML III (pseudo-Hurler polydystrophy) represent two ends of the same clinical spectrum caused by mutations in the gene encoding for the enzyme UDP-N-acetylglucosamine, the latter being the attenuated form with a late presentation. ML I and ML IV are caused by deficiency of alpha-N-acetyl-neuraminidase (sialidase) and mucolipin/alpha-N-acetyl-neuraminidase (sialidase), respectively.[55]

Dysostosis multiplex is a term used to designate the common radiographic manifestations of MPS and ML.[8,52,53,55] General skeletal manifestations of MPS, including short stature, joint stiffness, and contractures, are seen in all types of MPS except for Morquio syndrome, where hypermobility is common. In the axial skeleton, there is involvement of the skull, thorax, spine, and pelvis. In the skull, thickening of the vault, macrocephaly with dolichocephaly, and a "J"-shape sella are characteristic. In the face, lack of pneumatization of the paranasal sinuses, a short and broad mandible, and unerupted and widely spaced teeth can be found. In the thorax, characteristic findings include oar-shaped ribs because of anterior rib widening (**Schematic H**), small scapulae, a short sternum, and thickened clavicles. Spine involvement is common and includes odontoid hypoplasia, atlantoaxial instability, and spinal stenosis, which are more critical in patients with Morquio syndrome (MPS-type IV), in whom spinal cord compression and cervical myelopathy may exist (Fig. 25.14 and **Schematic G**). The vertebral bodies are oval (bullet shape) and flat (platyspondyly) with anteroinferior beaking in Hurler and Hunter syndromes and central beaking in Morquio syndrome (Fig. 25.14 and **Schematic E**).

The evaluation of the spinal involvement by MPS is best done using CT scan with three-dimensional (3D) reconstructions to assess spinal morphology and craniocervical junction and with MRI to evaluate the spinal cord in cases of suspected cord compression and myelopathy. These spinal cord abnormalities are best seen on sagittal T1- and T2-weighted MR images. In the pelvis rounded iliac wings with an inferior tapering of the ilium and underdevelopment of the acetabula and femoral heads are seen (Fig. 25.15 and **Schematic J**). In the peripheral skeleton, the long bones are

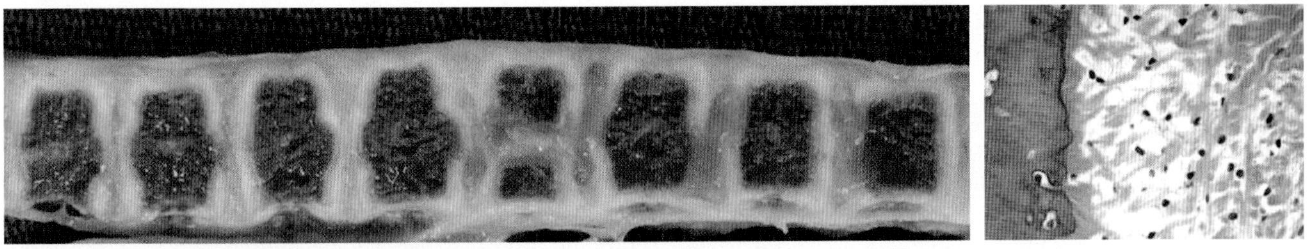

FIGURE 25.13 **Mucolipidosis type II (I-cell disease) in a 3-year-old boy.** The vertebral bodies are misshapen and contain multiple Schmorl nodules **(left)**. Microscopically, the foamy storage cells are particularly prominent lining the periosteum (**right;** hematoxylin and eosin, original magnification, 600×).

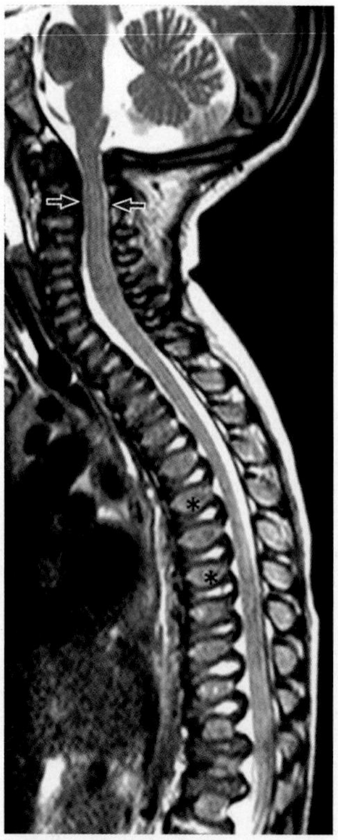

FIGURE 25.14 **An 8-year-old girl with Morquio syndrome and lower extremity weakness.** Sagittal T2-weighted MR image of the spine shows bullet-shaped vertebral bodies with anterior beaking (*asterisks*). There is marked narrowing (*arrows*) of the cervical canal and craniocervical junction with increased T2 signal of the cord at that level indicating mild myelopathy.

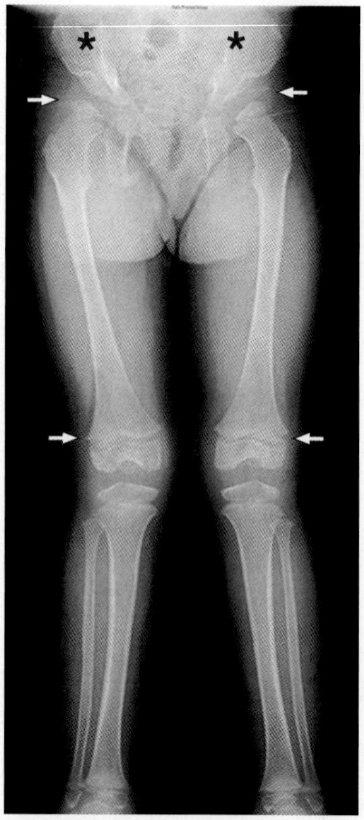

FIGURE 25.15 **Mucolipidosis type II (I-cell disease) in a 3-year-old boy.** Frontal radiograph of the lower extremities shows classic radiographic findings of mucopolysaccharidosis, which include rounded iliac wings (*asterisks*) with inferior iliac tapering, underdeveloped acetabula and femoral heads (*arrows* at the level of hip joint), irregular and widened distal femoral physes (*arrows* at the level of knee joint), and bilateral genu valgum.

notoriously affected with shortening of the diaphysis, hypoplastic epiphyses, irregular and widened physes, proximal humeral notching, and genu valgum due to hypoplasia of the lateral tibial plateaus (Fig. 25.15 and **Schematic K**). All forms of MPS affect the hands and feet. The metacarpal and metatarsal bones are short and squad with a pointy appearance proximally. The distal radius and ulna are underdeveloped and have a "V"-shape appearance, causing wedging of the carpal bones. Thickening of the subcutaneous soft tissues may result in claw hand deformity due to incomplete extension.[8,53,56–58]

Gaucher disease (GD) is an example of glycosphingolipidoses. GD is the most prevalent inherited LSD.[59,60] Even though it is most common in Ashkenazi Jews, it can affect individuals from any racial background. It results from a deficient level of the lysosomal enzyme beta-glucocerebrosidase with accumulation of cerebrosides in monocytes and macrophages, called Gaucher cells.[59–61] Affected pediatric patients frequently complain of bone pain and present with fractures and progressive joint collapse that impair mobility. Osteonecrosis is the most disabling skeletal manifestation of the disease.[52,58,59,61]

Radiographs are readily available and are inexpensive, but they can be insensitive to the marrow changes in GD. Radiographs are helpful in evaluating fractures and osseous deformities, but MRI is the method of choice for evaluating bone marrow involvement and epiphyseal osteonecrosis. The skeletal manifestations of GD are secondary to the infiltration of the bone marrow with Gaucher cells (Fig. 25.16) and include growth retardation; osteopenia that predispose to stress fractures; classic bone deformity called Erlenmeyer flask deformity, which is seen as flaring of the metaphysis of the long bones; osteonecrosis; and bone infarcts. Areas of osteosclerosis can be seen in old healed bone infarcts. Marrow infiltration of Gaucher cells causes a decreased T2 signal in the otherwise normal yellow marrow. Pyogenic osteomyelitis, although it is uncommon in Gaucher disease, can be difficult to differentiate from bone infarcts.[61]

Optimal management of these multisystemic disorders requires the involvement of a multidisciplinary/multispecialty team, including the radiologist. Enzyme replacement therapy is available for MPS I, II, and VI and is in development for types IV and VII. Enzyme therapy is also available for GD. Stem cell transplantation can preserve cognition and prolong survival in very young children with the more severe types, such as MPS I.[54,60]

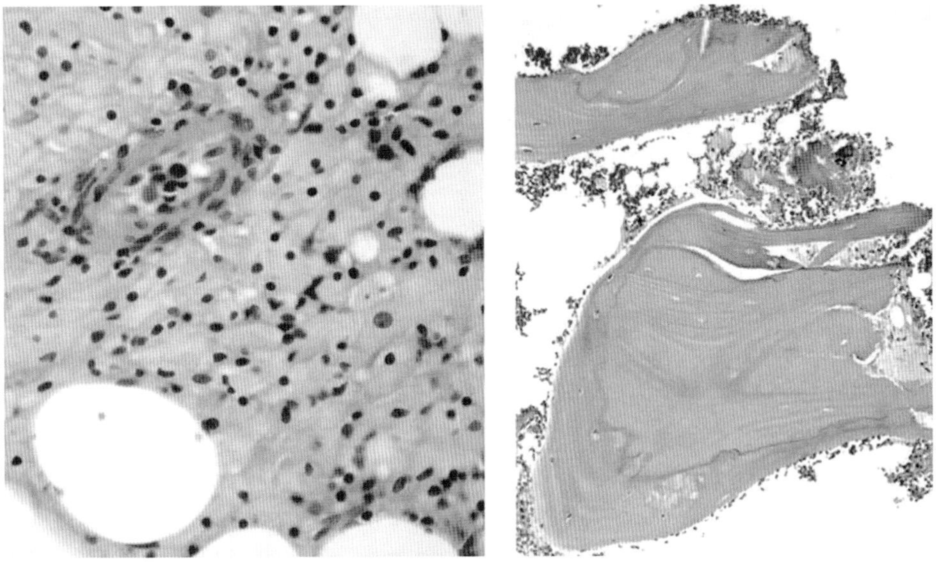

FIGURE 25.16 **Gaucher disease diagnosed via femur and tibia biopsies in an 8-year-old girl who carried a diagnosis of "osteomyelitis" status post multiple debridements.** The storage cells expand the marrow space, compressing blood vessels **(left)** causing osteonecrosis in a manner similar to that seen in osteomyelitis. In this chronic lesion, infarcted bone ("sequestrum") is encased by viable new bone **(right)**. Hematoxylin and eosin, original magnification, 600x **(left)** and 200x **(right)**.

Bone Age Evaluation

Skeletal maturation is marked by an orderly and generally reproducible sequence of recognizable changes in the appearance of the skeleton during childhood. Common indications for evaluating skeletal maturity include suspicion of underlying endocrine disorders, congenital/genetic syndromes, and constitutional short stature and before planning orthopedic procedures, such as scoliosis repair or leg length discrepancy.[62,63]

Radiographic assessment of skeletal maturity is most commonly based on the appearance of the hand and wrist using an anterior–posterior radiograph of the left hand and wrist. In children who are younger than 2 years of age, the use of knee and ankle radiographs are helpful, as the carpal bones are usually not ossified yet, and there is little change in the appearance of the hand and wrist.[62] Skeletal maturity can be estimated by comparing the radiographic appearance of the child's hand and wrist bones with the radiographic appearance of these bones in a healthy group of children of the same age. The most commonly used methods, both based on the recognition of maturity indicators, are the Greulich and Pyle (G&P) atlas and the Tanner-Whitehouse 2 (TW2) methods.[62–64] Maturity indicators are based on the initial onset of ossification of the growth centers, the size and positional relationships of the epiphyses and metaphyses, specific modeling changes that affect the epiphyses and metaphyses, and the closure of the growth plates (Fig. 25.17).[62,63]

The Greulich and Pyle Method

The Greulich and Pyle (G&P) atlas consists of two series of standard plates (i.e., boys and girls) obtained from radiographs of the hands and wrists of upper middle-class Caucasian children from Cleveland, Ohio, obtained between 1931 and 1942.[62,63,65] The standards represent central tendencies, which are modal levels of maturity within chronologic age groups. When using the G&P method, the radiograph in question is compared with the series of standard plates. The chronologic age given to the standard plate that fits most closely is deemed the bone age of the child. The skeletal age is assigned after the normal range is extended to two standard deviations on either side of the fit chronologic age (Fig. 25.17). The standard deviation values are obtained from charts from the Brush Foundation population included in the atlas.[62]

Between the ages of 10 and 14 years, only a relatively slight change occurs in the appearance of the radiographic standards using the G&P atlas, making the assessment sometimes difficult during this period. On occasion, assigning a single standard in the atlas is not possible because of the overlap of two plates. In these cases, the skeletal age can be reported as being between two standards. A disharmonic skeletal maturation can occur because of the considerable variation in the normal sequence in which the secondary ossification centers ossify in healthy children, leading to a discrepant bone age when considering the digits and the carpus. Because the carpal bones are more prone to systemic influences than the tubular bones are, greater weight should be given to the appearance of the more distal bones including metacarpals and phalanges. The presence of disharmony must be also reported.[62]

The Tanner-Whitehouse 2 Method

The Tanner-Whitehouse 2 (TW2) method, based on British children, assesses the maturity of 20 bones: radius, ulna, carpals (with the exception of the pisiform), and metacarpals and phalanges of the first, third, and fifth rays. The individual bones are matched to a series of written criteria that describe eight or nine standard stages through which each bone passes in its progression to maturity. Each stage is defined by several criteria and is assigned a specific point score. The sum of these scores results in a skeletal maturity score (SMS) that can be converted into a skeletal age. The TW2 method differs from the G&P method in two respects: It uses a bone-specific approach, and the results of the assessments are not always expressed as skeletal age "years."[62–64]

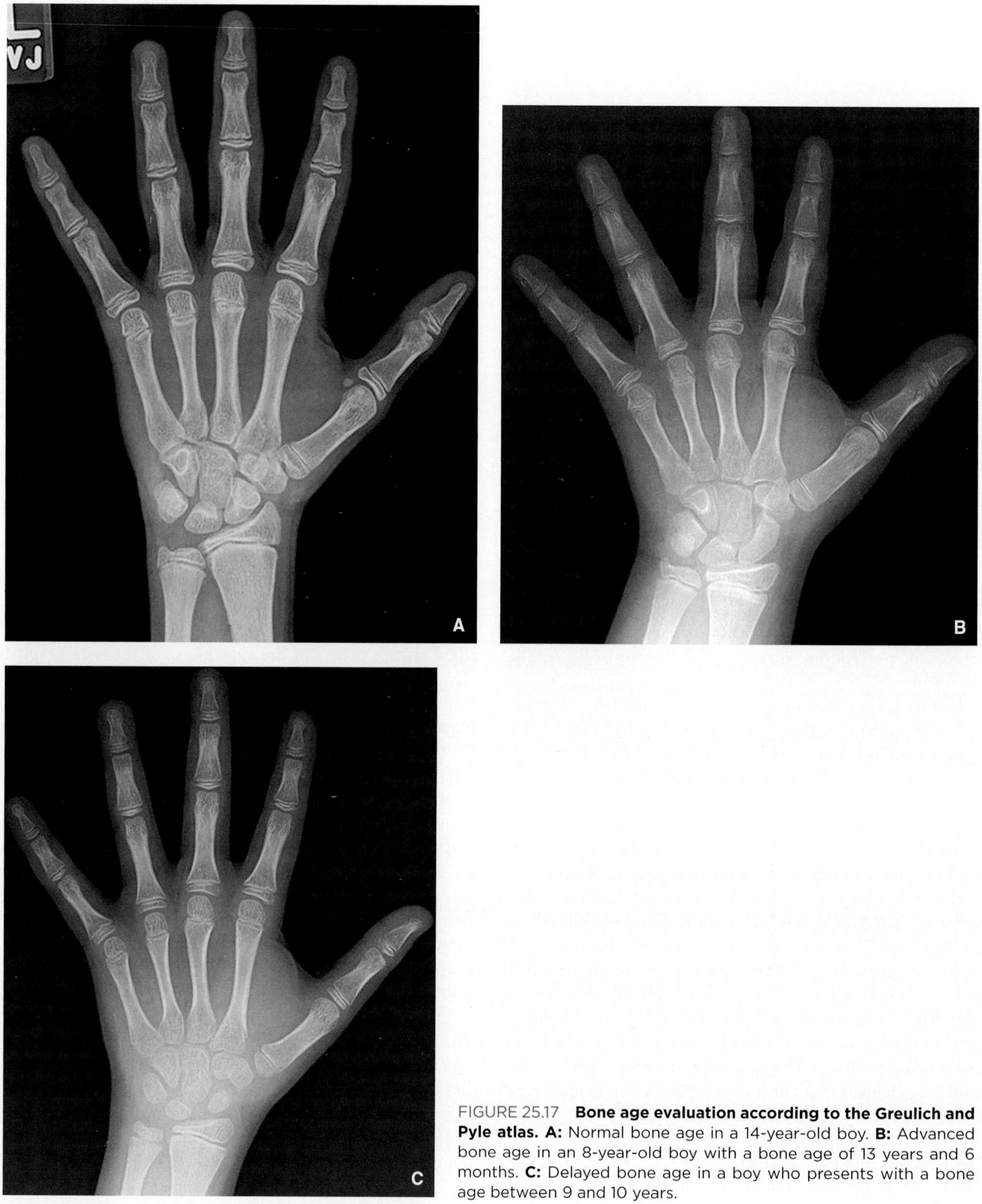

FIGURE 25.17 **Bone age evaluation according to the Greulich and Pyle atlas. A:** Normal bone age in a 14-year-old boy. **B:** Advanced bone age in an 8-year-old boy with a bone age of 13 years and 6 months. **C:** Delayed bone age in a boy who presents with a bone age between 9 and 10 years.

The apparent simplicity and speed with which a bone age can be assigned has made the G&P atlas the most used standard of reference for skeletal maturation worldwide.[63,64] The universal applicability of these methods has been questioned, however, as multiple studies have shown them to be outdated.[65–69] It is well known that children of the 1980s physically matured at younger ages than those of several previous decades.[65] Among the criticisms of the G&P method are that it uses information obtained more than 60 years ago from a pediatric population of upper middle-class children with the inclusion of only Caucasian children causing variability in the assessment of the development of different bones. In addition, there is lack of a specific approach for interpreting the templates.[63–65,69]

When determining bone age, the gender and ethnicity of each child must be considered. The use of standards of G&P to determine bone age must be done with reservations, particularly in adolescent girls of African and Hispanic descent and in adolescent boys of Asian and Hispanic descent.[63,65,69] The two methods used to asses skeletal maturation do not provide equivalent estimates of bone age requiring the selective use of a single method when serial measurements are performed.[64]

Osteochondrosis

The term osteochondrosis is used to designate a heterogeneous group of disorders with common features, which include a predilection for the immature skeleton, involvement of an epiphysis or apophysis with sclerosis, fragmentation, collapse, and, not uncommonly, healing with bone remodeling.[11] The exact underlying etiology of these disorders is currently unknown, but genetic causes, repetitive trauma, vascular abnormalities, mechanical factors, and hormonal imbalance all may play a role.

The osteochondrosis has been classified according to the site of involvement (**Schematics L–S**) or according to their probable pathogenesis. According to their probable pathogenesis, these disorders can be divided into three major groups: (1) conditions characterized by primary or secondary osteonecrosis, (2) conditions related to trauma, and (3) conditions that may represent variations of normal. In general, boys are more affected than girls, possibly because of the greater involvement of boys in sports activity, which results in greater predisposition to trauma.[11,70,71]

Legg-Calve-Perthes Disease

Legg-Calve-Perthes (LCP) disease typically affects children between 2 and 14 years of age, with a peak age of onset of 5 years. LCP disease is more common in boys than in girls, with a ratio of 5:1, and in Caucasians than in Asians or Africans.[70,72] Approximately 15% are bilateral, in which case the involvement is typically metachronous.[11,73,74]

The exact etiology of LCP disease is still unknown; however, there is general consensus that ischemia is the inciting event secondary to disruption of the blood supply to the femoral head, as demonstrated on biopsy results and supported by some imaging studies.[11,71,75] The manifestations vary according to the stage of the disease at which the patient is imaged: ischemic or necrotic, revascularization, and healing or reparative stages.[74,75] Some associations include patients with low birth weight, abnormal birth presentation, family history, higher birth order, and lower socioeconomic status.[71,72] Affected pediatric patients complain of hip pain, referred knee pain, and atraumatic limp. Limited hip abduction and internal rotation are present on a physical exam.[71]

Several imaging modalities are currently available for evaluating LCP disease with their own advantages. Regardless, the first imaging step remains the anterior–posterior and frog leg radiographs of both hips.[5,11] Early radiographic findings include soft tissue swelling of the affected hip due to a hip effusion, decreased size, and lateral displacement of the femoral head ossification center as well as a crescentic subchondral lucency in the femoral head, indicative of a subchondral fracture. As the disease progresses, femoral head fragmentation, sclerosis, and flattening (coxa plana) develop, followed by widening of the femoral metaphysis (coxa magna) (Fig. 25.18 and **Schematic M**).[5,11,76] Subchondral lucencies on the metaphyseal side of the femoral physis are characteristic

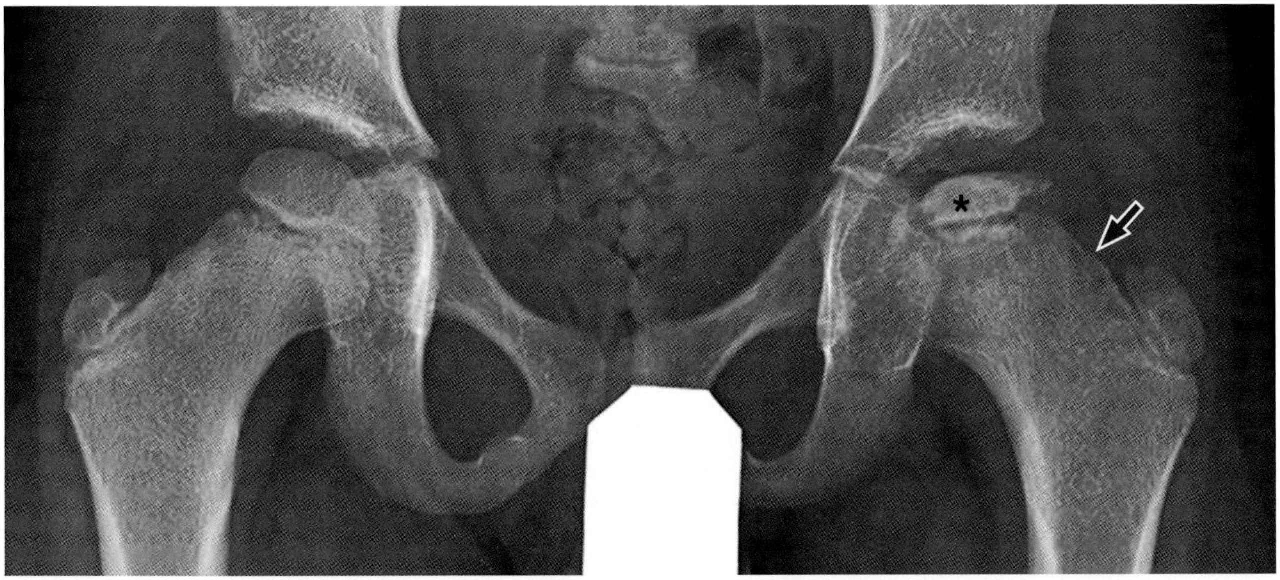

FIGURE 25.18 **A 9-year-old boy with Legg-Calve-Perthes disease who presented with worsening left hip pain.** Frontal pelvic radiograph shows flattening (coxa plana), sclerosis, and fragmentation of the left femoral head (*asterisk*) with secondary widening (*arrow*) of the femoral neck (coxa magna).

and are of an unknown etiology.[76,77] During the healing stage, the femoral head remodels to different degrees. Uncovering of the lateral aspect of the femoral head by the acetabulum, also called extrusion, often starts early in the course of the disease, progressively becoming more apparent. It implies the loss of containment of the femoral head, a very important prognostic factor, as extrusion predisposes to femoral head deformity or loss of sphericity, which, in turn, may lead to secondary degenerative arthritis. Thickening and foreshortening of the femoral neck with secondary hypertrophy of the greater trochanter are manifestations of the disease that can be seen later during adolescence.[5,76]

In addition, bone scintigraphy, CT, and MRI play a role in the evaluation of LCP disease. Early diagnosis of LCP disease is important because it allows prompt initiation of joint-preserving therapies. Triple-phase bone scintigraphy using pinhole collimation can detect ischemic changes to the femoral head at a much earlier phase and more confidently than radiography. Asymmetrically decreased or absent perfusion and uptake of the affected head are diagnostic. A drawback of this modality is the lack of an assessment of the extent of femoral head involvement including fragmentation due to the poor spatial resolution.[5] Likewise, MRI with intravenous contrast, especially with the use of subtraction technique, can accurately diagnose LCP disease early in the course of the disease. MRI has the advantage of evaluating the extent of synovitis, femoral head involvement, complications, and sequelae as well as the differentiation of LCP disease from other pathologies using no ionizing radiation.[5,74] CT, although not routinely used in LCP disease, can provide precise information about the anatomic relationship between the femoral head and acetabulum, allowing for a 3D view of the femoral head.[5] Few studies using contrast-enhanced sonography have shown that the use of contrast agents was effective to demonstrate changes from the revascularization healing process in LCP disease, particularly within the physis, but did not help in differentiating scintigraphic phases of LCP disease.[78,79]

The treatment of LCP disease depends on the patient's age and on the severity of disease as well as the stage of the disease. The goal of all therapeutic alternatives for LCP disease is to prevent femoral head deformity and incongruency that eventually lead to secondary degenerative arthritis.[80] The first line of treatment is usually mechanical stress reduction combined with physical therapy. Very early in the course of the disease, pain management is important until the pain subsides to further stimulate range of motion.[81] A large proportion of children who develop LCP disease heal well with minimal or no sequelae. However, some children eventually develop secondary degenerative arthritis. Poor prognostic factors include an age older than 6 years at the disease's onset; female gender, as there is less time for osseous remodeling because of the faster skeletal maturation in girls; greater epiphyseal collapse, especially that of the lateral pillar; and greater loss of femoral head containment due to the predisposition to sphericity loss.[75,76]

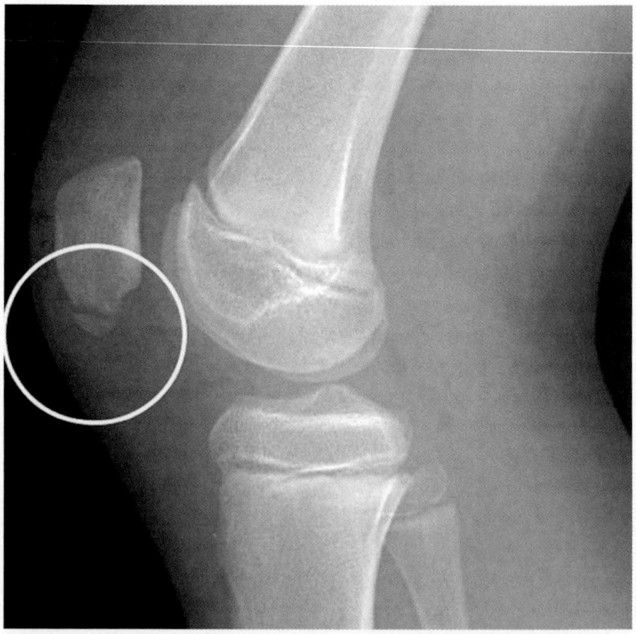

FIGURE 25.19 **Sinding-Larsen-Johansson disease in a 10-year-old boy soccer player with chronic knee pain.** Lateral knee radiograph shows the characteristic fragmentation (*circle*) of the inferior patellar pole with edema of the overlying subcutaneous soft tissues and Hoffa fat pad.

Sinding-Larsen-Johansson Disease

Sinding-Larsen-Johansson (SLJ) disease is a cause of chronic anterior knee pain in children between 10 and 14 years of age, leading to pain and edema around the inferior pole of the immature patella accompanied by fragmentation on radiographs.[11,82–84] A strong association exists with traction activities; thus, affected pediatric patients are usually athletic.[82,84] In the appropriate clinical setting, radiographic findings are confirmatory and fairly characteristic.[84,85] The lateral view is necessary to show the fragmentation of the inferior patellar pole with overlying soft tissue inflammatory changes, such as stranding and thickening (Fig. 25.19 and **Schematic R**).[82,85]

The diagnosis is made clinically and radiographically, but when it is not suspected or is in the very early stages, MRI can be diagnostic, showing edema of the bony fragments at the inferior patellar pole and the adjacent soft tissues (Fig. 25.20), thickening, and increased T2 signal of the proximal patellar tendon and bursitis. MRI can also be helpful in distinguishing SLJ from a patellar avulsion.[86]

The disease is self-limiting, with the majority of cases resolving with rest, anti-inflammatory medications, icing, and activity modification.[82]

Blount Disease

Blount disease is a developmental condition characterized by disordered endochondral ossification of the medial aspect of the proximal tibial physis, which leads to multiplanar deformity; thus, genu varum (**Schematic K**) is an inaccurate term.[87] It has been classified into four types according to the age of onset: (1) infantile, (2) adolescent, (3) late onset, and (4) tibia

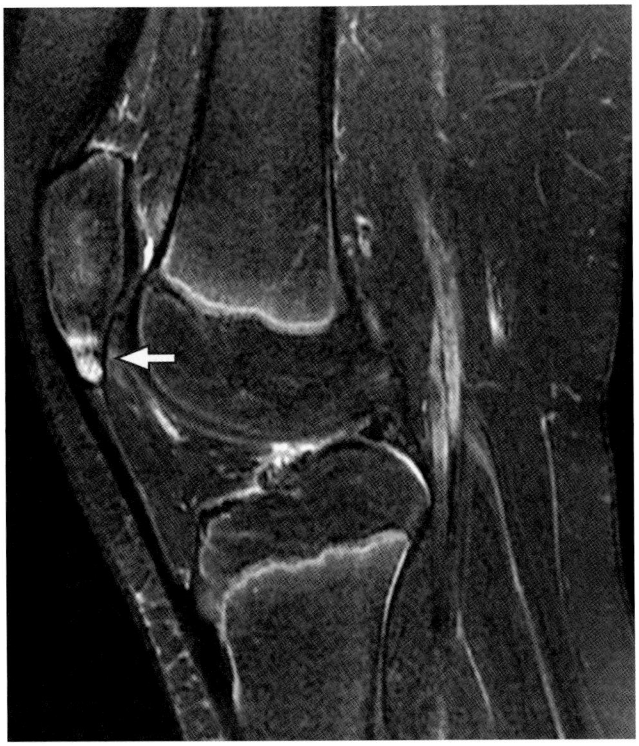

FIGURE 25.20 **A 13-year-old boy with Sinding-Larsen-Johansson disease.** Sagittal shout tau inversion recovery (STIR) MR image shows a fracture line and bone marrow edema at the inferior patellar pole (*arrow*) without significant adjacent soft tissue edema.

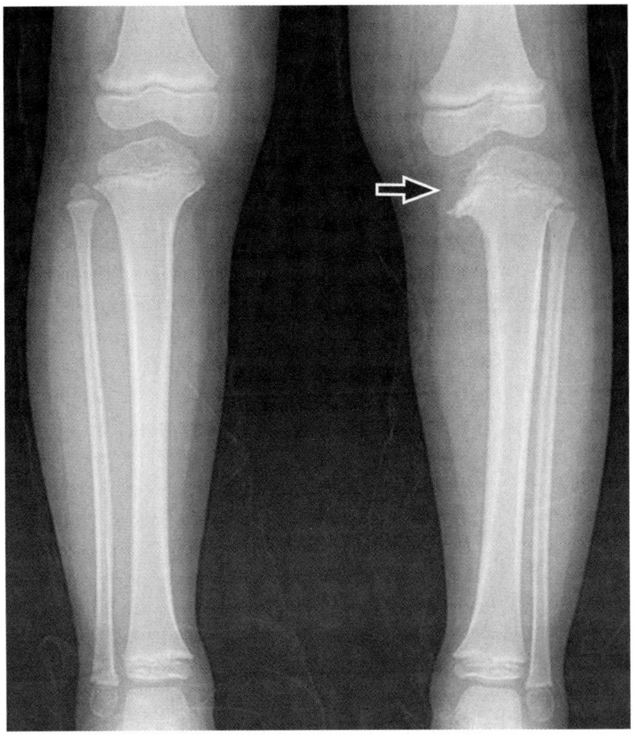

FIGURE 25.21 **A 3-year-old African American boy with Blount disease.** Frontal radiograph of both tibiae and fibulae shows classic findings of Blount disease, which include left genu varum, down-sloping, and mild fragmentation of the medial corner of the proximal tibial metaphysis with underdevelopment of the medial side of the proximal tibia (*arrow*).

vara secondary to focal fibrocartilaginous dysplasia.[11,88] Obese African American children and children of Scandinavian descent are predisposed to all types of Blount disease.[6]

1. Infantile type: It is the most common type of Blount disease, developing between 1 and 3 years of age, most frequently bilateral and symmetric. Affected pediatric patients typically present with pain or knee instability. The etiology is unclear but is probably multifactorial with mechanical and familial etiopathogenic factors including linking to obesity.[6,11,87,88] Radiographs are the main imaging modality for evaluating all types of Blount disease. A standing full-length anterior–posterior radiograph of both lower extremities with the patella forward is crucial for assessing limb alignment. The classic radiographic changes in the proximal tibia include sharp varus angulation and beaking of the proximal metaphysis, widening and irregularity of the medial aspect of the physis, medial down slopping, and irregularity of the epiphysis (Fig. 25.21 and **Schematic S**). Eventually, the bony epiphysis gradually extends and fills in the apparent metaphyseal step and may become fragmented, which are potentially irreversible changes. Additional radiographic parameters, such as the metaphyseal–diaphyseal angle, can help to differentiate physiologic bowing from early-onset Blount disease.[6,11,87,88] MRI is not routinely used; however, it can define intra-articular changes of the knee or detect physeal bars that are not apparent on radiographs.[6,87,89,90] CT is also not routinely required, but it can provide a preoperative 3D image of the existing multiplanar knee deformities in order to avoid incomplete correction and iatrogenic deformities.[6]
2. Adolescent type: The etiology of the less common adolescent tibia vara has been postulated as trauma or infection causing focal premature closure of the proximal tibial physis, thus the typical unilateral occurrence of the disease. Clinically, affected pediatric patients complain of locking, leg length discrepancy, limping, and gait abnormalities. It occurs between the ages of 8 and 15 years. Radiographically, there is narrowing of the proximal tibial physis with only mild epiphyseal wedging and varus angulation of the bone.[6,11,87,88]
3. Late-onset type: Also uncommon, it occurs between the ages of 6 and 14 years with progressing varus deformity. Radiographically, the proximal tibial epiphysis is wedge-shaped owing to medial flattening, and the physis is irregular and widened medially.[11,88,91]
4. Tibia vara secondary to focal fibrocartilaginous dysplasia type: Being the least common, this type presents earlier in life, between 3 and 18 months. Clinically, there is unilateral tibia vara, tibial torsion and limb shortening. On radiographs, a well-defined, oblique radiolucent band is present in the medial cortex of the proximal tibial metadiaphysis with a secondary varus deformity of the tibia. Spontaneous resolution tends to occur between 1 and 4 years of age with this type.[11,88]

Management options include observation with repeat clinical and radiographic examinations, use of orthoses and various surgical procedures that include realignment osteotomies of the tibia and fibula, lateral hemiepiphysiodesis, and proximal tibial distraction and physeal bar resection.[6,88]

Osgood-Schlatter Disease

Osgood-Schlatter (OS) disease is an abnormality of the development of the tibial tuberosity as a consequence of microavulsions caused by repeated traction on the anterior portion of the developing ossification center sparing the growth plate. This is one of the most common forms of the osteochondroses, typically affecting boys, and a history of participation in sports is typical, as physical loading plays a major role in the disease's development.[82,83,92,93] Affected adolescents between the ages of 11 to 15 years present with chronic pain, warmth, edema, and focal deformity in the area of the tibial tuberosity.[67,82]

Radiography is the imaging modality of choice in diagnosing this condition, but signs of inflammation must be present clinically. In order to identify the abnormalities, a true lateral radiograph is necessary. Soft tissue swelling overlying the tibial tuberosity (clinically and radiographically) is the most important diagnostic criterion in addition to irregularity and fragmentation of the tuberosity (Fig. 25.22 and **Schematic R**).[86,92] Stranding and indistinctness of the deep infrapatellar bursa and thickening and indistinctness of the distal patellar tendon are usually present in acute phases.

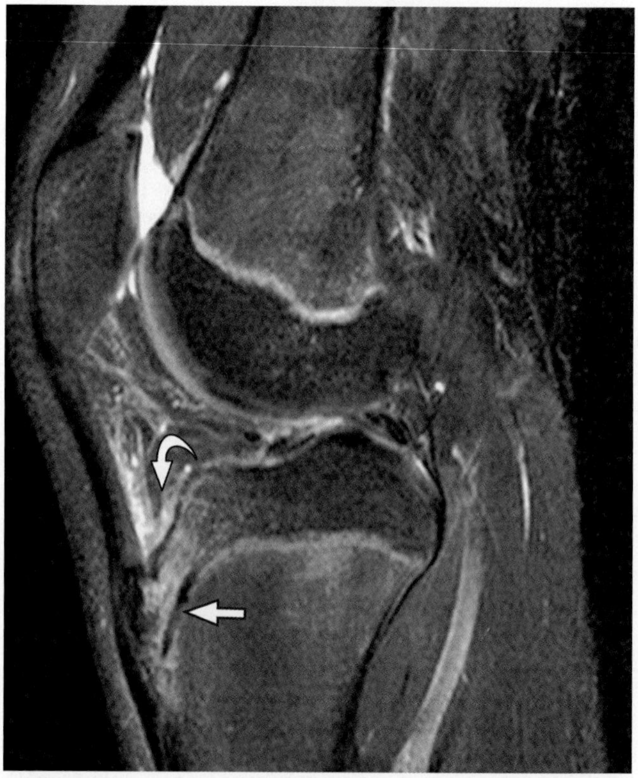

FIGURE 25.23 **A 12-year-old boy with Osgood-Schlatter disease.** Sagittal fat-suppressed T2-weighted MR image shows increased signal intensity within the tibial tuberosity (*straight arrow*), distal aspect of patellar tendon and adjacent soft tissues (*curved arrow*).

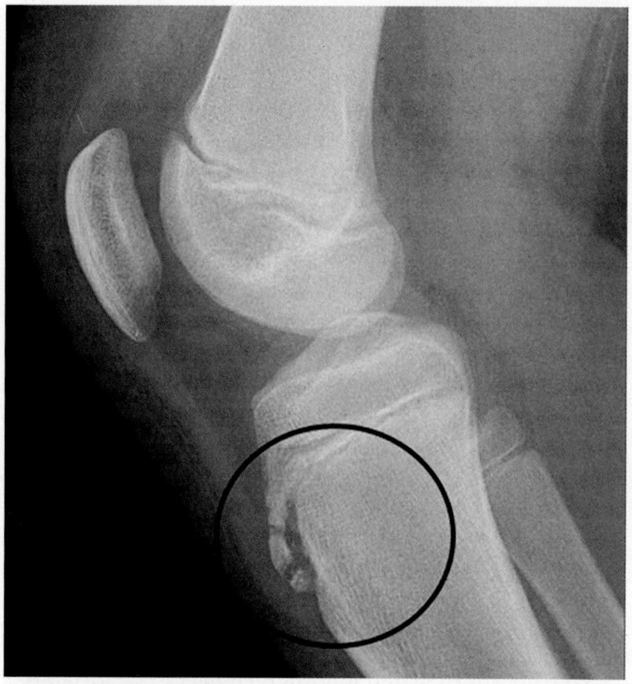

FIGURE 25.22 **A 13-year-old boy with Osgood-Schlatter disease who presented with knee pain.** Lateral knee radiograph shows irregularity and fragmentation (*circle*) of the tibial tuberosity with overlying soft tissue edema.

Several weeks later, several ossification centers may become apparent as they migrate proximally and persist after the inflammatory changes have resolved.[11,86,92] It is most frequently unilateral, but bilateral involvement may occur.[82,92] MRI is not necessary for the diagnosis; however, it can be useful in the very early stages, when the patient's symptoms are vague and when radiographs are negative or in unresolved cases. Features on MRI include multiple ossified centers in the tibial tuberosity with more apparent inflammatory changes of the surrounding soft tissues as well as bone marrow edema that can involve most of the proximal tibial epiphysis and even the metaphysis (Fig. 25.23). Deep infrapatellar bursitis is readily apparent as well. The patellar tendon at its distal attachment is thickened and hyperintense on fluid-sensitive sequences, and occasionally, avulsed ossicles can be seen embedded in the tendon fibers.[94] Almost always, the disease resolves at skeletal maturity, and eventually, the radiographic changes revert, but fragmentation of the tuberosity can remain as an indication of previous involvement.[92,93,95]

The treatment of OSD is usually nonoperative and consists of anti-inflammatory medications, icing, prolonged rest, and activity modification.[82,92,95] In the rare case that requires resection, microscopic examination typically shows avulsion fracture and reactive/reparative bony changes, sometimes with nonunion ("ossicles") (Fig. 25.24).

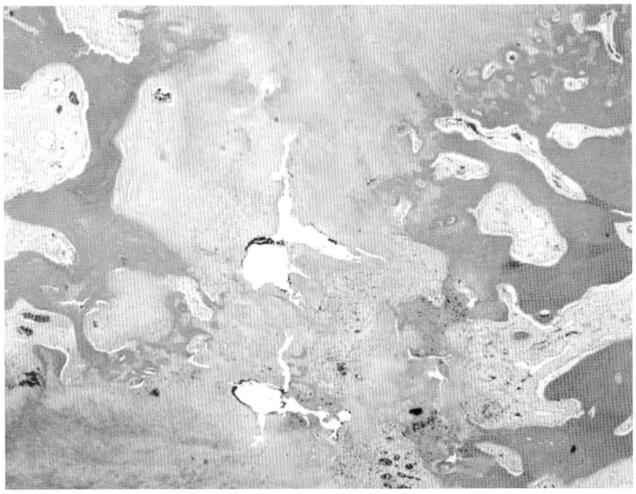

FIGURE 25.24 **Osgood-Schlatter disease in a 13-year-old girl who underwent resection because of persistent pain.** Histologically, the tibial tubercle showed evidence of fracture repair, manifested by a nodular collection of cartilaginous material, woven bone, and granulation tissue separating the residual intact bone (hematoxylin and eosin, original magnification, 20×).

Kohler Disease

Kohler disease is the osteochondrosis that affects the tarsal navicular bone. It occurs in children between 4 and 9 years of age, more frequently in boys. The etiology is unknown, and there is usually no history of previous trauma.[71,96,97] Kohler disease typically presents with limping secondary to midfoot pain that worsens with weight bearing and focal medial tenderness and edema on physical exam.

Radiographs show sclerosis, fragmentation, decreased bone size, and narrowing and flattening of the tarsal navicular bone (Fig. 25.25 and **Schematic O**) with preservation of the adjacent interarticular spaces.[11,96,97] It can be bilateral in approximately one-fourth of patients.[11,96] It is not always symptomatic, as it can be found incidentally on radiographs obtained for other reasons. This overlap with normal variation of the ossification center makes the diagnosis difficult; thus, three criteria must be present in order to establish the diagnosis: (1) changes are detected in a previously normal bone; (2) alterations that are consistent with resorption and reossification must be compatible with osteonecrosis; and (3) clinical manifestation must be present.[11]

Treatment includes rest, icing, and nonsteroidal anti-inflammatories for controlling pain. Immobilization with a short period of casting may be helpful in very symptomatic cases. Most affected pediatric patients heal well without long-term sequelae and good bone remodeling.[96–98]

Freiberg Disease

Freiberg disease is osteonecrosis of the metatarsal heads. The second metatarsal is the most commonly affected; however, it can also be found in other metatarsals. The disorder has been linked to repetitive trauma and stress overloading. It is most frequently seen in athletic adolescent females, being the only

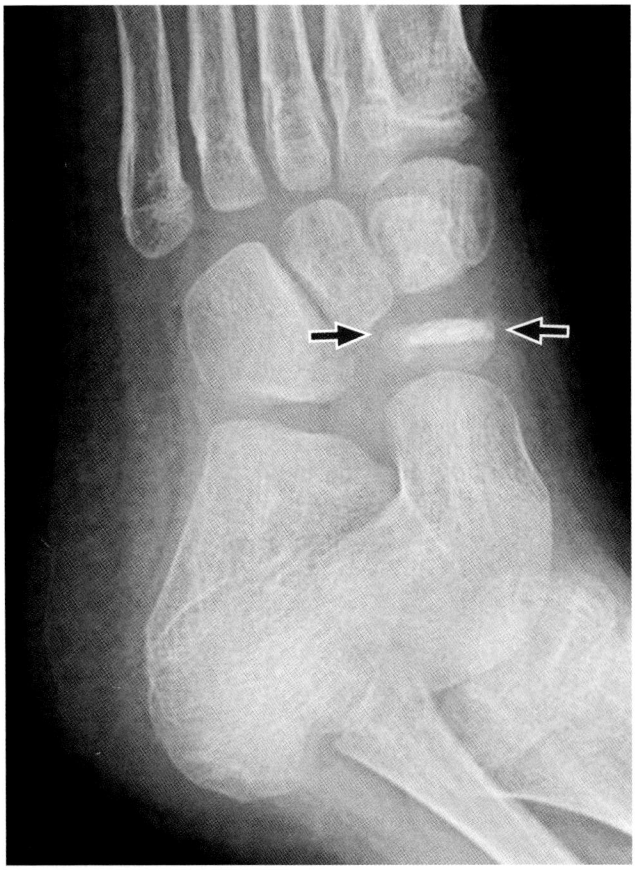

FIGURE 25.25 **A 7-year-old boy with Kohler disease who presented with foot pain.** Oblique radiograph of the foot shows a small, irregular and sclerotic navicular bone (*arrows*) with preservation of the joint spaces.

osteochondrosis that is more prevalent in girls.[1,99–101] On clinical exam, there is localized tenderness of the metatarsophalangeal joint and, occasionally, foreshortening of the involved ray.[96,100,102]

The diagnosis is usually made on radiographs, as the findings are characteristic, showing fissuring, and flattening of the central aspect of the metatarsal head with adjacent soft tissue edema (Fig. 25.26 and **Schematic O**). With progression, the central portion of the metatarsal head collapses, involving the dorsal aspect and exposing the medial and lateral projections of the uninvolved peripheral portions of the metatarsal head. The plantar aspect of the metatarsal head remains intact, better appreciated on the oblique radiographs. Then, joint space widening becomes evident with sclerosis of the femoral head.

The more advanced stage occurs when the peripheral projections of the metatarsal head fracture, separate, and become loose bodies, leaving an incongruent joint. The disease's end-stage corresponds to degenerative arthritis with significant and permanent metatarsal head deformity and hypertrophy as well as secondary thickening of the metatarsal shaft.[11,96,99,100] MRI is not routinely used but could be of value in the early diagnosis of the disease for preventing deformity. MRI findings are those of osteonecrosis in other

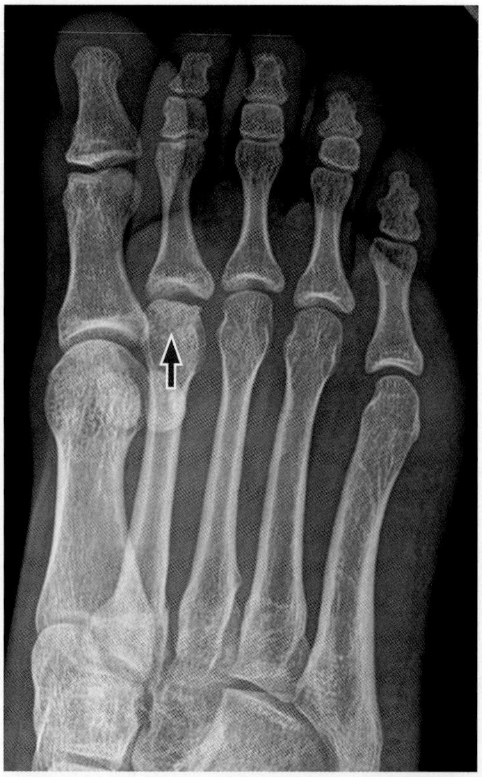

FIGURE 25.26 **A 15-year-old girl with Freiberg disease.** Oblique radiograph of the foot reveals flattening, sclerosis, and mild fragmentation of the head of the second metatarsal (*arrow*).

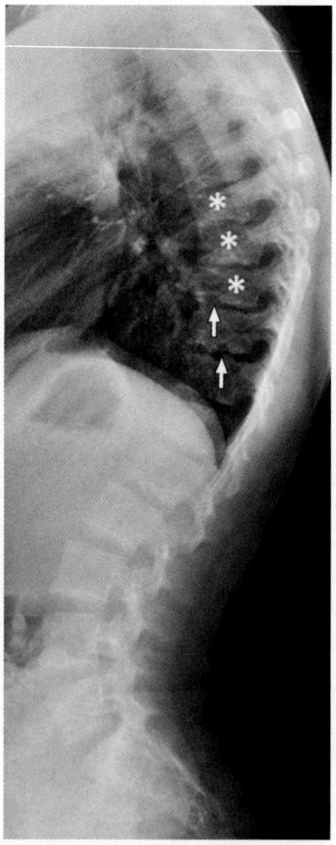

FIGURE 25.27 **Scheuermann disease in a 16-year-old boy with painful kyphosis.** Lateral radiograph of a scoliosis series shows mild anterior wedging of three consecutive thoracic vertebral bodies (*asterisks*), Schmorl nodes (*arrows*), and accentuated thoracic kyphosis.

joints and include joint effusion and synovitis, bone marrow edema of the metatarsal head, and flattening and fragmentation in the disease's later stages. Loose bodies can be readily identified on MRI.[99]

As with other osteochondroses, early management is designed to control symptoms with activity modification, limited weight bearing, and shoe orthotics. Immobilization may be indicated for controlling pain. Most pediatric patients respond to nonsurgical treatment with no sequelae. The surgical treatment of Freiberg infraction is reserved for pediatric patients who do not respond to conservative measures or have disease progression.[96,100]

Scheuermann Disease

Scheuermann disease, also discussed in the spine chapter, is the most common cause of hyperkyphosis in adolescence.[103] It was initially described as rigid kyphosis associated with wedged vertebral bodies occurring during adolescence.[104] The etiology of the disease remains unknown, with ischemic changes affecting the ring apophysis as a possible theory. Repetitive axial loading on the immature spine, osteoporosis, and genetic factors have also been implicated.[103–105] It affects girls and boys equally between the ages of 8 and 12 years.[104] Clinically, affected pediatric patients complain of painful kyphosis secondary to anterior vertebral wedging.

Current diagnostic criteria require the involvement of at least three consecutive thoracic vertebrae with vertebral wedging of at least five degrees in an adolescent with accentuated thoracic or thoracolumbar kyphosis. Other radiographic features include the loss of height of the intervertebral disks as well as irregularity of the end plates and Schmorl nodes of the affected vertebrae (Fig. 25.27 and **Schematic L**).[103–105] Lumbar Scheuermann kyphosis is a subgroup most commonly seen in adolescent males who are involved in activities that require axial loading. Affected pediatric patients present with back pain and similar radiographic vertebral changes at the thoracolumbar junction but do not have clinical kyphosis.[104,106]

The treatment of classic Scheuermann disease is mainly conservative, including activity modification and physical therapy. Bracing can be used primarily in the treatment of deformity. Surgery is reserved for patients with a >75-degree kyphosis or with a >65-degree kyphosis with pain that is not responsive to conservative measurements.[103,104] Lumbar Scheuermann, different from the thoracic type, is nonprogressive, and the symptoms usually resolve with rest and activity modification.[104]

Kienbock Disease

Kienbock disease is osteonecrosis of the carpal lunate which is usually a unilateral disease. It typically occurs between 20 and 40 years of age and rarely seen in children. Clinically, affected pediatric patients present with dorsal wrist pain and decreased grip strength. Kienbock disease often follows a severe or repetitive wrist injury, suggesting trauma as a cause. In addition, many affected pediatric patients have associated negative ulnar variance, possibly rendering the lunate bone more exposed to stress.[107]

The diagnosis is usually made on radiographs with the presence of a fracture line in the lunate initially followed by sclerosis and finally by fragmentation and bone collapse (**Schematic Q**). MRI can detect cases at an earlier stage by identifying bone marrow edema, which should affect the entire bone. Once the diagnosis is made, radiographs are sufficient for follow-up.[107–109]

The initial treatment of Kienbock disease is immobilization and activity modification and anti-inflammatory medications to control pain and inflammation. Although the goals are to relieve pain as well as wrist function specially preserve motion and strength, no single surgical procedure achieves this outcomes. Surgical treatments include first revascularization procedures and procedures to unload the lunate in order to avoid disease progression such radial osteotomy. In cases of lunate collapse, procedures to restore the carpal height may be necessary.[108–110]

Osteochondritis Dissecans

Osteochondritis dissecans (OCD) refers to localized injury to the osteochondral unit that eventually leads to separation of a segment of articular cartilage and subchondral bone. It is most frequently found in the knee, followed by the ankle and elbow in the pediatric population. The exact etiology is unknown, with the most accepted hypothesis as being multifactorial with trauma, genetic predisposition, endocrinopathies, and osteonecrosis as contributing factors. It is more frequently seen in adolescent athlete males, supporting the fact that cumulative stress to the subchondral bone, resulting in stress fracture, is one of the most important etiologic factors.[111–113] The clinical presentation of OCD regardless of the affected joint is similar and depends on the stage of presentation: initially joint pain and swelling that progress to locking and catching.[111–114] Radiographs are the first step in the evaluation of all types of OCD. For further characterization of the lesion and to determine stability or instability, MRI is often necessary.

Osteochondritis Dissecans of the Knee

Osteochondritis dissecans (OCD) of the knee affects two distinct populations differentiated by the status of the physes. The juvenile type occurs in children with open physes, and the adult type occurs in adolescents and young adults with closed physes.[111–113]

On radiographs, lesions are more frequently seen involving the weight-bearing surfaces of the femoral condyles. The posterolateral aspect of the medial femoral condyle is the most common location; thus, tunnel view in addition to frontal, lateral, and sunrise views may improve the detection (Fig. 25.28A). The main roles of radiographs are to confirm and to identify the lesion as well as to evaluate the status of the physis. On radiographs, OCD lesions are seen as elliptical, fairly well-circumscribed, subchondral lucencies (Fig. 25.28A). Sclerotic borders and linear lucencies that

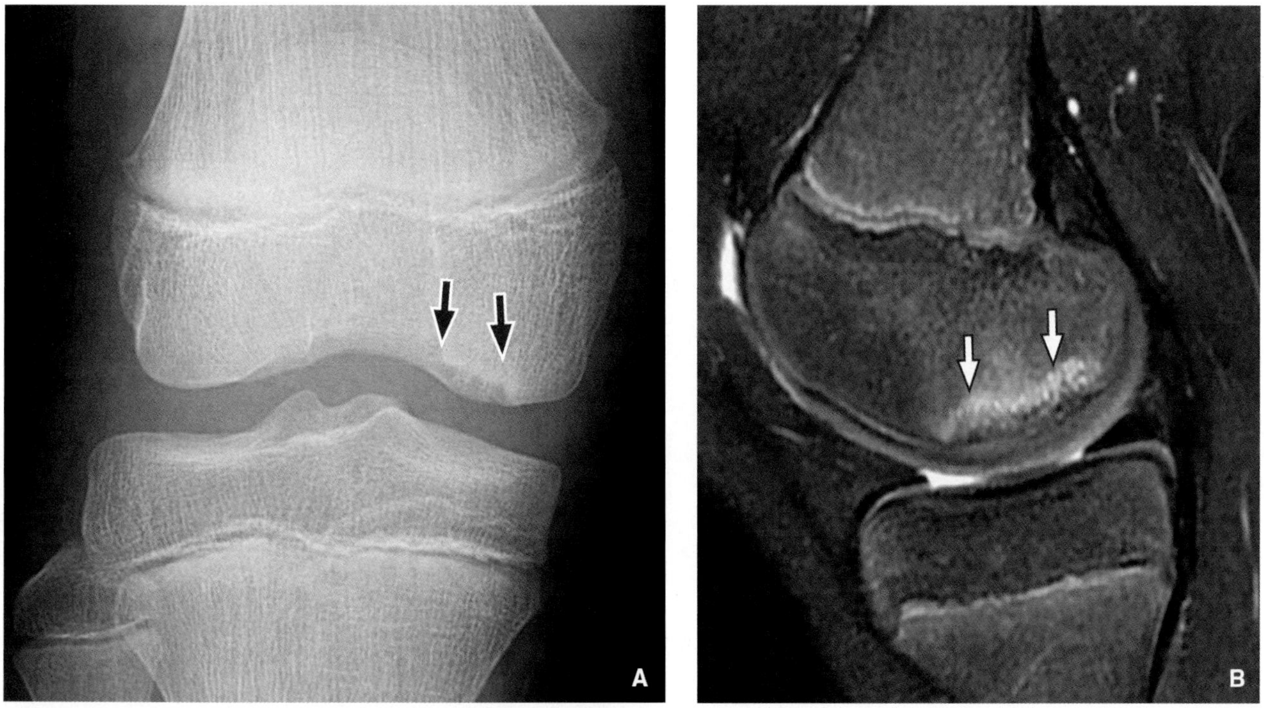

FIGURE 25.28 **Juvenile-type stable osteochondritis dissecans (OCD) in an adolescent football player. A:** Frontal tunnel view of the right knee shows well-circumscribed elliptical shape subchondral lucency (*arrows*) in the lateral aspect of the medial femoral condyle. This is the most common location for knee OCD. **B:** Sagittal fat-suppressed T2-weighted MR image of the right knee of the same patient shows an elliptical area of subchondral bone marrow edema (*arrows*) and indistinctness of the overlying developing subchondral plate. The overlying articular cartilage is intact.

indicate separation can be seen. In more advanced cases, the fragment may be incongruent or become a loose body. MRI is most helpful in evaluating lesion stability; determining the fluid interfaces, the integrity of the articular surface, and the displacement of fragments; and identifying loose bodies (Fig. 25.28B). MRI is also useful for further characterizing the extension of the lesion, thus providing accurate measurements, which is useful in candidates for chondroplasty.[111–113]

The criteria for stability on MRI depend on the type of OCD (i.e., juvenile vs. adult). MR imaging findings that suggest instability in the adult type include high T2 signal rim, cystic changes underlying the lesion, a high T2 (fluid) signal intensity fracture line that extends through the overlying articular cartilage or fluid-filled osteochondral defects. In the juvenile type, imaging features that suggest instability include a peripheral rim of fluid signal intensity, multiple breaks in the subchondral bone plate on fluid-sensitive sequences and a second outer rim of low T2 signal intensity. The presence of cysts that underlie the lesion is not as specific in juvenile OCD; however, the number (multiple tiny cysts) or the size (a single cyst >5 mm) has a low sensitivity but high specificity for instability.[115–119] Different from the adult type, a high T2 (fluid) signal intensity rim is not an equivocal sign of instability in juvenile OCD.[115,120]

The treatment and prognosis depend on the status of the physis and the stability of the lesion. Nonoperative treatment includes restricted weight bearing and activity modifications. For stable lesions that fail nonoperative measures, drilling of the lesion is an option in order to stimulate a healing response. For unstable lesions, operative management is usually performed with fragment excision (Fig. 25.29) and fixation or chondrocyte implantation. Most lesions in patients with open physes are stable, with a tendency to heal well with nonoperative treatment, leaving no sequelae. On the other hand, adult-type OCD is more frequently unstable and tends to become complicated with degenerative arthritis.[111,113]

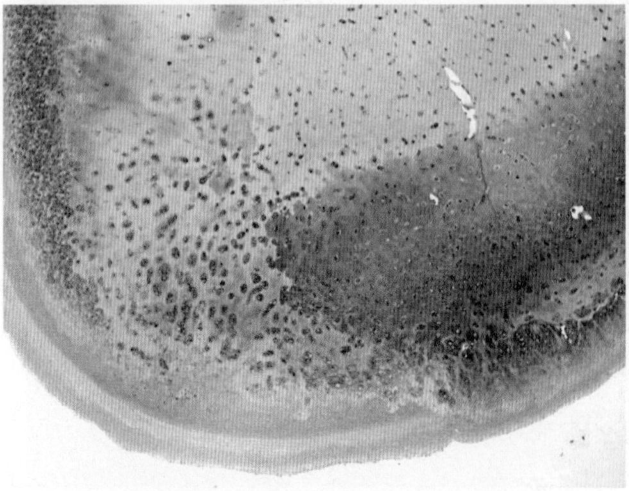

FIGURE 25.29 **Loose body, removed from the knee of a 14-year-old boy with medial femoral condyle osteochondritis dissecans.** The tissue is composed predominantly of hyaline cartilage, with focal ossification and a surrounding rim of synovium-lined perichondrium-like fibrous tissue (hematoxylin and eosin, original magnification, 40×).

Osteochondritis Dissecans of the Elbow and Panner Disease

Osteochondritis dissecans (OCD) of the elbow, less common than similar lesions in the knee and ankle, occurs in adolescence and in early adulthood. It involves the capitellum, and even though the etiology is unknown and probably multifactorial, there is a high association with overhead throwing injuries.[112] Chronic repetitive valgus stress leads to capitellar injury against the radial head, the so-called lateral compression injuries.[121]

On radiographs, focal trabecular rarefaction and an elliptical lucency are present in the subchondral bone of the anterior capitellum, the weight-bearing portion (Fig. 25.30 and **Schematic P**). Articular surface flattening and fissuring that lead to incongruity and loose body formation can be seen in more advanced cases. Hypertrophy, deformity, or irregularity of the radial head may also be seen as the disease progresses. MRI is useful in providing accurate measurements, characterizing the integrity of the articular surface and fluid interfaces and identifying loose bodies.[112,121,122]

Changes in the capitellum can also be seen in children between 4 and 8 years of age, representing another subset of patients. In these younger children, diffuse sclerosis and/or fragmentation of the entire capitellar ossification nucleus is present in the dominant extremity and is called Panner disease. It is speculated that OCD and Panner disease are a continuum of the same entity, but Panner disease tends to be self-limiting, leaving no sequelae with nonoperative treatment. Unlike OCD, Panner disease is not associated with loose bodies.[121–123]

The treatment of Panner disease is directed to alleviate the symptoms with activity modification. On the other hand,

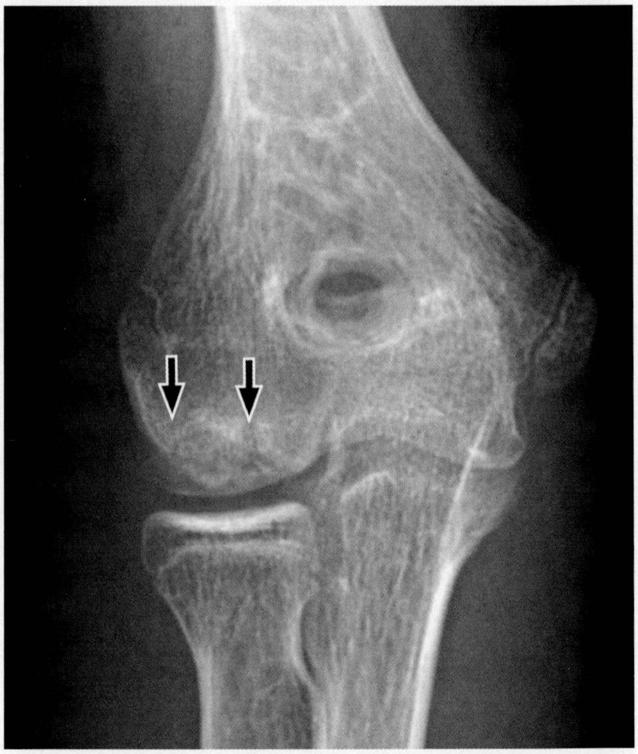

FIGURE 25.30 **A 14-year-old boy baseball pitcher with capitellar osteochondritis dissecans.** Frontal elbow radiograph shows large elliptical subchondral lucency in the capitellum with an irregular but sclerotic border (*arrows*).

treatment of pediatric patients with OCD is determined by the status of the articular cartilage. Affected pediatric patients with intact articular cartilage can be managed nonoperatively. Surgical indications include nonresponse to conservative management, symptomatic loose bodies, articular cartilage disruption, and displaced osteochondral fragments.[121,122] The prognosis of OCD is not as good as it is in Panner disease, because it frequently leads to impairment of the elbow function as well as degenerative arthritis.[121,122]

Musculoskeletal Disorders Due to Arthropathy

Juvenile Idiopathic Arthritis

JIA is the most common chronic childhood rheumatic disease.[124] JIA encompasses a heterogeneous group of disorders, which by definition must affect one or more joints with swelling, pain, or a limited range of motion that lasts for at least 6 weeks in a patient who is younger than 16 years of age.[3,125] JIA has a worldwide distribution with regional variations, in part due to the heterogeneity of the disease.[125,126] Among developed nations, JIA has a yearly incidence of two to 20 cases per 100,000 people and a prevalence of 16 to 150 cases per 100,000 people.[127] The pathogenesis of the disease is not fully understood; however, there are new theories involving interactions between both the innate and adaptive systems as a continuum.[128–130]

The pathogenesis of JIA has synovial inflammation or synovitis as the triggering point, which translates clinically as a painful and edematous joint with a limited range of motion. Acute synovitis progresses to chronic synovitis, resulting in synovial hypertrophy, periarticular soft tissue edema, and joint effusion. This is followed by pannus formation, which may result in articular cartilage erosions, and finally osseous erosions, representing irreversible changes (Fig. 25.31). Joint space narrowing develops early with a tendency to progress to ankylosis, which is less commonly seen now with the newer and more effective medications.[3]

The International League of Associations for Rheumatology (ILAR) group replaced the older terms "juvenile chronic arthritis" and "juvenile rheumatoid arthritis."[125,131,132] JIA is classified into seven mutually exclusive subgroups or categories according to its onset as systemic, polyarticular (more than four joints), and oligoarticular (up to four joints). It is further subclassified by clinical examination, the absence or presence of rheumatoid factor (RF), and the absence or presence of HLA B27 (Table 25.2).[3,131,133–135]

The three main imaging modalities currently used in the evaluation of JIA are radiographs, US, and MRI, with each modality playing a role in disease evaluation and featuring both advantages and disadvantages as discussed in the imaging technique section. MRI provides the most comprehensive evaluation of a joint in pediatric patients with JIA. The MR protocol in children with suspected JIA should include T1 and fluid-sensitive sequences, a gradient-echo sequence, and fat-suppressed T1-weighted MR images prior to and after intravenous gadolinium administration. Dynamic contrast-enhanced MRI (DCE-MRI) can be added as part of the protocol for a more accurate assessment of the disease activity based on the time of contrast enhancement.[136,137]

The main imaging findings of JIA include synovitis, erosions, periarticular soft tissue edema, enthesitis, and periarticular and generalized osteopenia. Synovitis, the earliest finding in JIA, is best identified with US (Fig. 25.32) and thickening of the synovium with or without nodularity with MRI (Fig. 25.33A). Increased vascularity on color Doppler US images and homogeneous and vivid enhancement on contrast MRI are suggestive of active inflammation (Fig. 25.33B).[3,124,125,132] Gradient-echo sequences should be routinely used to detect the presence of hemosiderin, which is virtually diagnostic of pigmented villonodular synovitis.[138]

Erosions, indicative of underlying articular cartilage and bone destruction, are not a constant finding in JIA but rather are a later manifestation of the disease, indicating irreversible changes; they are more frequently seen with positive rheumatoid factor (RF) polyarthritis. MRI is the best imaging modality for evaluating articular cartilage and detecting erosions as thinning or very focal defects of the articular cartilage and subchondral bone.[3,124,132,133,139,140] MRI also has the unique ability to detect potential pre-erosive changes, such as bone marrow edema.[124,139] T2 relaxation mapping holds potential for the identification of pediatric patients who are at risk because of its ability to evaluate

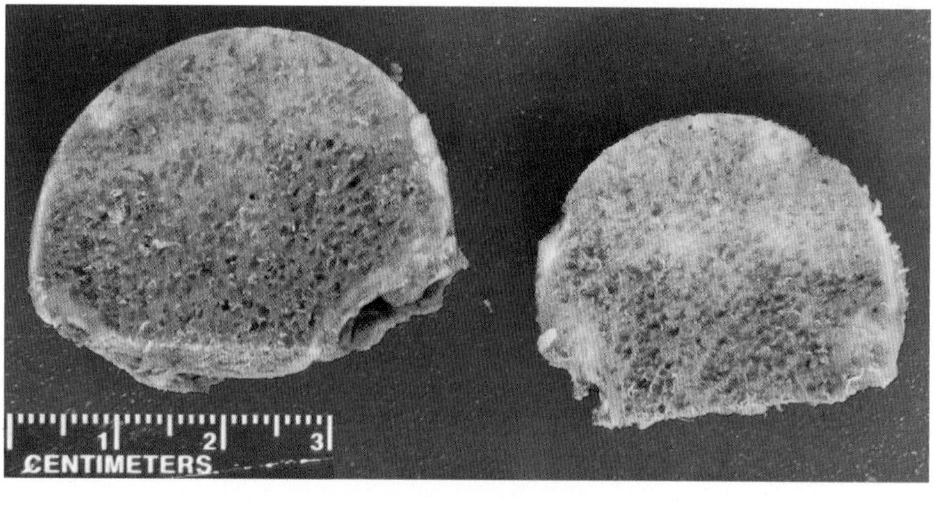

FIGURE 25.31 **Juvenile idiopathic arthritis in a 16-year-old girl with chronic polyarticular involvement.** The femoral head shows cartilage thinning (eburnation) and subchondral cyst formation. Histologically, fibrous overgrowth (pannus) was seen focally (not shown).

TABLE 25.2 Types of Juvenile Idiopathic Arthritis According to the International League of Associations for Rheumatology (ILAR)

Type of Arthritis	Number of Joints Involved	Diagnostic Criteria	Characteristic Features
Systemic	Variable	Fever for 2 wk plus one of the following: rash, myalgias, adenopathy, hepatosplenomegaly, serositis	No sex predilection Mean age of presentation: 4–6 y
Oligoarthritis	Variable	Persistent: less than four joints throughout the disease course Extended: less than four joints in the first 6 mo of disease; then four joints	Increased risk of iritis
Polyarthritis rheumatoid factor (RF) (−)	More than five joints	RF (−)	Symmetric, affects small and large joints
Polyarthritis RF (+)	More than five joints	RF (+) on two separate occasions at least 3 mo apart	Tends to start late in childhood Similar to adult rheumatoid arthritis
Psoriatic arthritis	Variable	Presence of psoriasis or arthritis and two of the following: history of psoriasis in a first degree relative, dactylitis, nail changes	Presence of RF (+) is an exclusion criterion. Two presentations: early onset between 2 and 3 y; late onset between 10 and 12 y
Enthesis-related arthritis (ERA)	Variable	Arthritis and enthesitis and two of the following: sacroiliac tenderness, inflammatory lumbosacral pain, (+) HLA-B27, anterior uveitis, onset of arthritis in a boy older than 8 y, ankylosing spondylitis, inflammatory bowel disease, Reiter syndrome	Presence of psoriasis or family history of psoriasis is an exclusion criteria Usually begins with hip or knee arthritis. Axial involvement later in the disease
Undifferentiated	Variable	Diagnosis of exclusion when arthritis does not meet the criteria for other types	

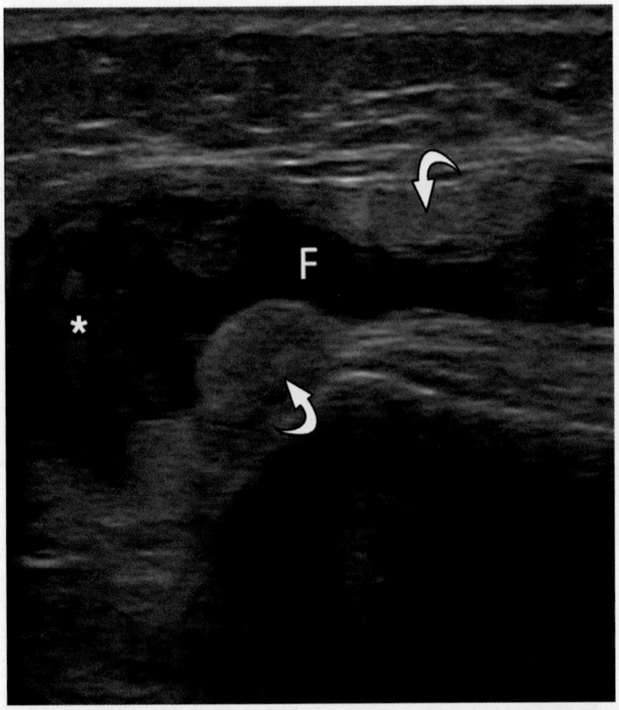

FIGURE 25.32 **A 5-year-old girl with positive rheumatoid factor oligoarthritis.** Sagittal gray-scale ultrasound image of the right knee shows a large effusion (*F*) with eccentric synovial thickening (*curved arrows*) and echogenic floating debris (*asterisk*).

the microstructure of the articular cartilage before visible erosions are present.[137,141] US can also demonstrate chondral erosions along the periphery of the joint, but it is less sensitive in evaluating the underlying bone, being more useful in younger, more cartilaginous joints.[140] In contrast, erosions are a late finding on radiographs (Figs. 25.31 and 25.34).[140] Joint space narrowing that can progress to ankylosis is more commonly seen in RF-positive patients (Fig. 25.35).[3,133] The 3D capabilities of US and MRI allow for a more accurate and comprehensive evaluation of the articular cartilage thickness.[3,124]

Periarticular soft tissue edema is an early but nonspecific finding that indicates inflammation. Synovial cysts and periarticular adenopathy are secondary findings that can be seen in JIA and occurs most commonly in the knee, the most frequently affected joint.[3,132,133] Joint effusions are accurately diagnosed with either US or MR (Figs. 25.32 and 25.33). These two modalities confirm the presence of fluid allowing its characterization. On US, effusions associated with JIA can be simple or complex with floating debris or echogenic avascular soft tissue (Fig. 25.32).[3,133] On MRI, low T2 signal synovial tissue with no enhancement on T1-weighted MR images inside the joint is a feature that supports the diagnosis of JIA early in the course of the disease.[142] Rice bodies are a rare but fairly characteristic finding in patients with JIA but can occur in chronic synovitis of other etiologies. When calcified, they can easily be detected on radiographs; however, when cartilaginous, these

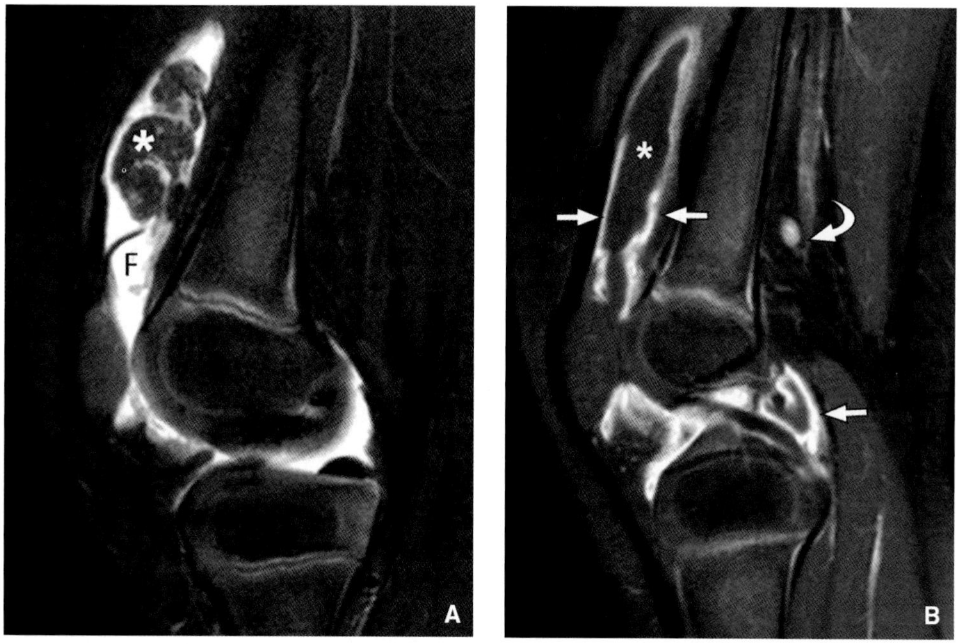

FIGURE 25.33 **A 5-year-old girl with positive rheumatoid factor oligoarthritis (same patient from Figure 25.32). A:** Sagittal fat-suppressed T2-weighted MR image shows the hyperintense joint effusion (*F*) and the hypointense debris (*asterisk*) in the suprapatellar recess. **B:** Sagittal contrast-enhanced fat-suppressed T1-weighted MR image shows diffuse synovial enhancement (*straight arrows*) indicative of synovitis not apparent on the T2-weighted sequence and a joint effusion (*asterisk*). An incidental popliteal lymph node (*curved arrow*) is present.

are better detected on MRI. Rice bodies are best detected on the fluid-sensitive sequences as slightly hypointense structures that are surrounded by the brighter fluid.[143]

Enthesitis, a feature of JIA, especially of the enthesitis-related arthritis (ERA) subtype, refers to inflammation that occurs at the sites of tendon and ligament insertion. On MRI, enthesitis produces an increased signal at the tendinous and ligament insertion sites on fluid-sensitive sequences (Fig. 25.36) and enhancement after gadolinium administration. Associated bursitis may be present. In the cervical spine, synovial proliferation around the C1-C2 articulation can lead to ligamentous laxity and spinal instability.[3,133]

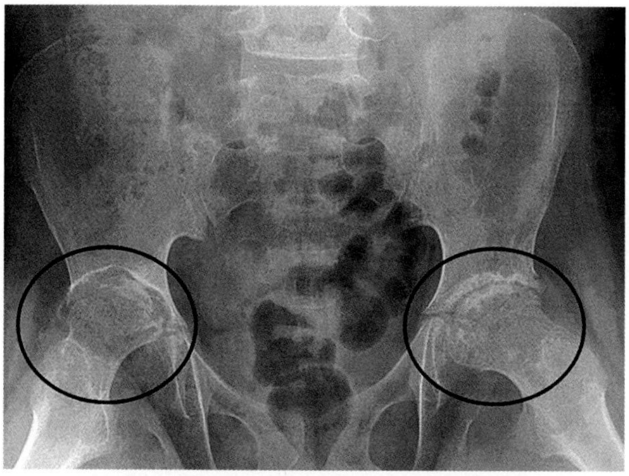

FIGURE 25.34 **A 16-year-old girl with enthesitis-related arthritis type of juvenile idiopathic arthritis.** Frontal radiograph of the pelvis shows severe bilateral symmetric hip joint space narrowing with erosions in the femoral head and acetabular roof (*circles*). No sacroiliac joint involvement is apparent on this radiograph.

Periarticular and generalized osteopenia are common early findings seen on radiographs. Periarticular osteopenia is the result of the localized hyperemia around the joint, whereas generalized osteopenia results from the chronicity of the disease, disuse, and therapy, for example, steroids.[132,133] Periosteal

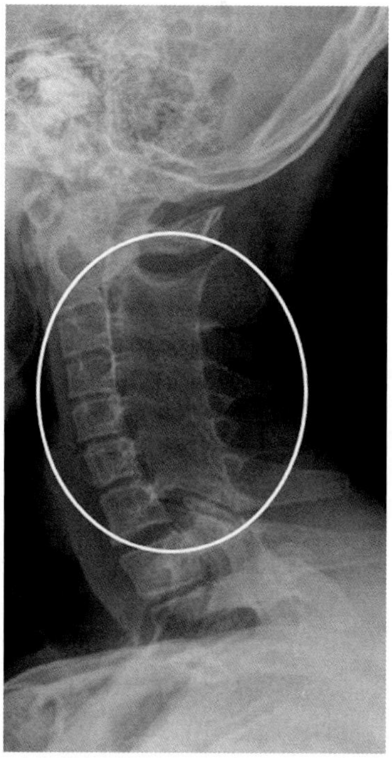

FIGURE 25.35 **A 14-year-old girl with long-standing positive rheumatoid factor juvenile idiopathic arthritis.** Lateral radiograph of the cervical spine shows ankylosis (*circle*) of every facet joint from C2 to C7 and secondary hypoplasia of the vertebral bodies of C3-C6.

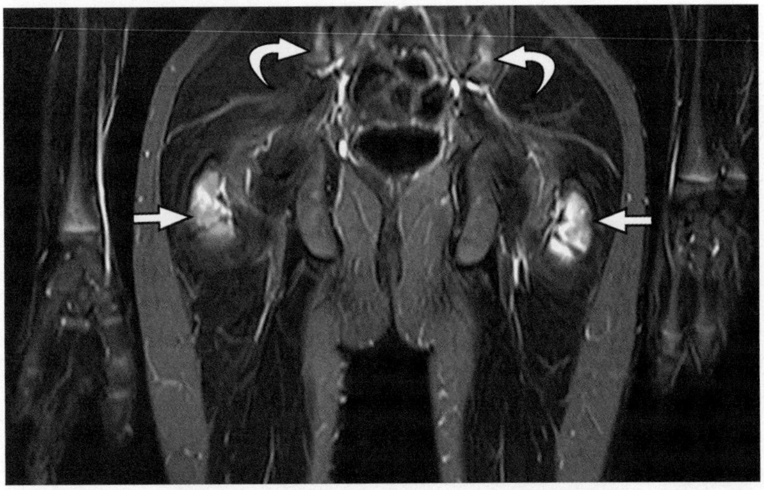

FIGURE 25.36 **A 12-year-old boy with enthesitis-related arthritis type of juvenile idiopathic arthritis.** High inversion recovery signal intensity (*curved arrows*) is noted along both sides of sacroiliac joints. Increased signal intensity (*straight arrows*) is also seen around the growth plates of greater trochanter apophyses and at the insertions of both gluteus medius muscles.

new bone formation is most commonly seen in the phalanges, metacarpals, and metatarsals. A fairly classic presentation of psoriatic arthritis is dactylitis, the so-called sausage finger or toe, seen as fusiform soft tissue edema with associated periosteal reaction.[3,144] Periarticular inflammation, epiphyseal destruction, and ligament laxity leading to joint subluxation can result in abnormal osseous development. Periarticular hyperemia induces accelerated growth and maturation with secondary epiphyseal enlargement that, if asymmetric, can result in limb length discrepancy.[133] The mandible is frequently affected with secondary micrognathia and antegonial notching.[133]

There has been a recent trend of using an earlier and more aggressive treatment in pediatric patients with JIA to prevent permanent joint damage. Nonsteroidal anti-inflammatory drugs are the first line of treatment not only for controlling the inflammation but also for pain control. Important advances in the disease's treatment include the earlier injection of intra-articular steroids in oligoarticular disease with less systemic effects and the use of disease-modifying drugs, such as methotrexate and cyclosporine, as well as biologic agents, such as antitumor necrosis factor (anti-TNF) medications.[125] The control of disease activity in the first months of disease has been proven to have prognostic value.[145]

Sacroiliitis

Juvenile spondyloarthritis (SpA) is a subset of childhood arthritis, characterized by an increased male–female ratio, relatively older age of onset, predilection for large-joint arthritis in the lower extremities, high frequency of enthesitis, risk of sacroiliitis, and frequent presence of the HLA-B27 antigen.[146] Under the ILAR classification system, most cases of spondyloarthropathies are clustered into ERA, psoriatic arthritis, or undifferentiated arthritis.[146,147] In general, sacroiliitis is one of the main manifestations of SpA, where affected pediatric patients usually complain of low back and/or buttock pain. However, children and adolescents rather tend to present with hip or large joint arthritis and enthesitis, at least in the initial stage of the disease.[146–148] Furthermore, the radiographic involvement of the sacroiliac joints may precede the symptoms by many years (silent sacroiliitis).[146–148]

Radiographic manifestations of sacroiliitis include widening of the sacroiliac joints, irregularity, sclerosis, and demineralization as well as erosions (Fig. 25.37).[11,149] A unique feature of spondyloarthropathies is that erosions are not permanent, and during healing, new bone formation would occur and ankylosis would develop.[150] MRI is a sensitive imaging modality for identifying early subtle changes (i.e., bone marrow edema) before radiographic findings are present and even before symptoms develop (silent sacroiliitis).[146,149,151] Findings of sacroiliitis on MRI include subchondral bone marrow edema that affects the ilium first (Fig. 25.38). As the disease progresses, erosions develop in the subchondral bone extending outward through the cortex into the joint, finally producing joint space widening. The involvement is almost always bilateral but not necessary symmetric.[150] Whole-body MRI can be used in the workup of pediatric patients with spondyloarthropathies using specific protocols (coronal short tau inversion recovery [STIR] multistation; sagittal STIR of spine; axial oblique STIR of sacroiliac [SI] joints; coronal oblique STIR of SI joints; sagittal STIR of knees; sagittal STIR

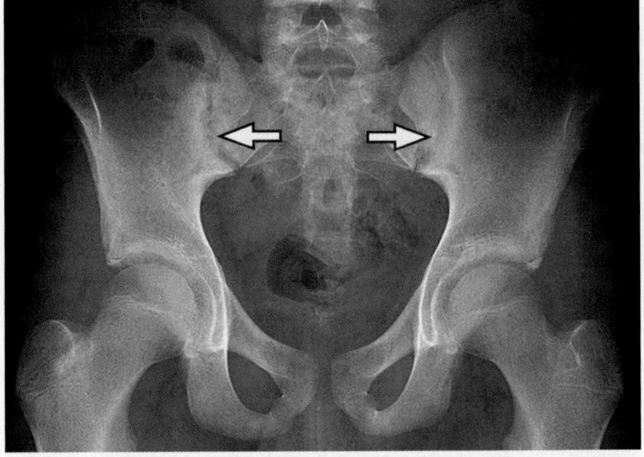

FIGURE 25.37 **A 13-year-old boy with bilateral sacroiliitis who presented with low back pain.** Frontal pelvis radiograph shows symmetric widening, irregularity, and erosions in both sacroiliac joints (*arrows*).

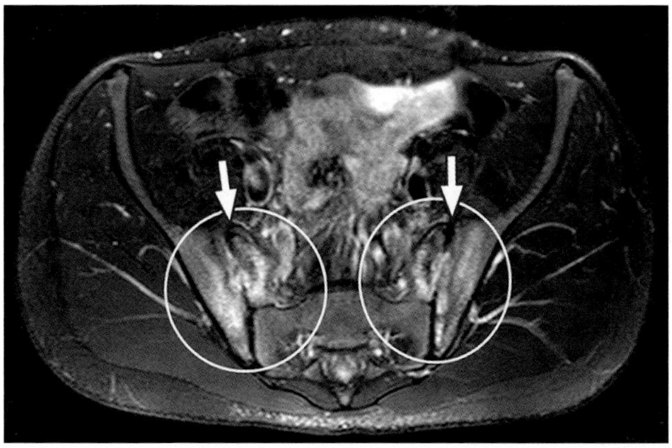

FIGURE 25.38 **A 13-year-old boy with bilateral sacroiliitis who presented with low back pain (same patient from Figure 25.37).** Axial fat-suppressed T2-weighted MR image shows bilateral symmetric widening of both sacroiliac joints (*arrows*) with erosions and marrow edema (*circles*) on both sides of the joint.

of ankles; scan time, about 30 minutes). This technique evaluates the extent of the disease, and if contrast is injected, it also evaluates disease activity, which is helpful when dealing with a disease that frequently involves areas that are difficult to assess clinically or complex joints, such as the ankle.[4]

Because of the diagnostic, therapeutic, and prognostic implications, some authors have suggested recognizing SpA as a distinct and independent disease. The diagnosis of SpA has significant therapeutic and prognostic implications: The risk of sacroiliitis and treatment does not prevent further radiographic progression. Risk factors for sacroiliitis and the future development of ankylosing spondylitis (AS) in children and adolescents that warrant routine MRI screening include acute anterior uveitis, limited mobility of the lumbar spine, elevated erythrocyte sedimentation rate, human leukocyte antigen (HLA)-B27 positivity, hip arthritis, prolonged disease duration, and male sex. Hip arthritis is a clear radiologic finding that is predictive of future development of AS in patients with JIA.[146–148]

The differential diagnosis of sacroiliitis in children is Behcet disease. SI joint tenderness and/or inflammatory lumbosacral pain along with anterior uveitis in a child who is HLA-B27 positive should raise the concern for Behcet disease. Sacroiliitis also is a feature of familial Mediterranean fever, especially with HLA-B27 positivity.[147] Pyogenic sacroiliitis is rare, accounting for 1% to 2% of osteoarticular infections in children. The diagnosis is difficult because of the lack of specific signs and symptoms. Affected pediatric patients may present with fever, radiculopathy due to nerve irritation, or even sepsis. The most common etiologic agent is *Staphylococcus aureus*. MRI is the imaging modality of choice for the diagnosis of pyogenic sacroiliitis. It shows enhancing bone marrow edema, fluid in the joint space, erosions, and bone destruction as well as periarticular soft tissue inflammations and abscesses.[152,153]

The treatment of SpA is different from that of JIA. The biologic agents, such as anti-TNF agents (the "workhorse" therapy), are effective for addressing axial disease in terms of pain control, spinal mobility, and quality of life. However, the impact of biologic agents on the progression of the disease is currently less clear.

Juvenile Dermatomyositis, Polymyositis, and Other Childhood Inflammatory Myopathies

Childhood idiopathic inflammatory myopathies (CIIM) can be divided into clinicopathologic or serologic subsets with distinctive epidemiology and clinical, pathologic, or prognostic features. Juvenile dermatomyositis (JDM) is the most common subtype, representing up to 85% of all CIIM.[154] The other two major subtypes of CIIM are juvenile polymyositis and overlap myositis syndrome.

The incidence of juvenile polymyositis is lower than that of JDM, representing 2% to 8% of all CIIM. Differentiating features are mainly clinical, with polymyositis lacking the skin rashes. The weakness in polymyositis is often proximal and distal with frequent muscle atrophy. Overlap myositis, accounting for 3% to 10% of all CIIM, is diagnosed when JDM or polymyositis is associated with another autoimmune disease, such as lupus, JIA, type 1 diabetes mellitus, or inflammatory bowel disease.[154] Amyopathic JDM, in which the characteristic skin rash is present in the absence of muscle involvement, can rarely occur.[154,155] The average age of onset is ~7 years, with girls being more frequently affected than boys.[155]

The etiology of JDM is not fully understood but is most likely related to an autoimmune reaction in genetically susceptible individuals to environmental triggers. The final mechanism that is responsible for muscular and extramuscular injury is better understood: microangiopathy mediated by the complement and the membrane attack complex, which triggers ischemic phenomena.[154–156]

The only validated tool for diagnosing JDM are the criteria of Bohan and Peter.[157] The most important criteria are the cutaneous manifestations, heliotrope, and Gottron papules, which very often are the first to appear. The remainder criteria include symmetric muscular weakness, muscular enzyme anomalies, electromyography (EMG) that shows denervation and myopathy, and a confirmatory muscle biopsy (Fig. 25.39). Other manifestations of JDM include nonerosive arthritis that predominantly involves the fingers, wrists, elbows, and knees

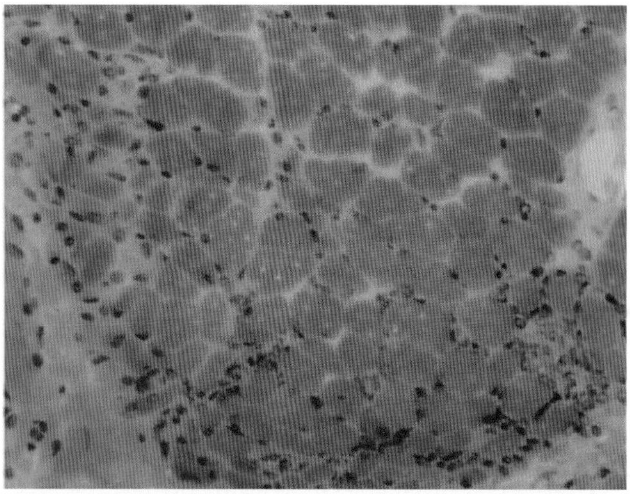

FIGURE 25.39 **A 5-year-old girl with dermatomyositis.** Skeletal muscle shows a perifascicular mononuclear inflammatory infiltrate as well as muscle fiber atrophy (hematoxylin and eosin, original magnification, 400×).

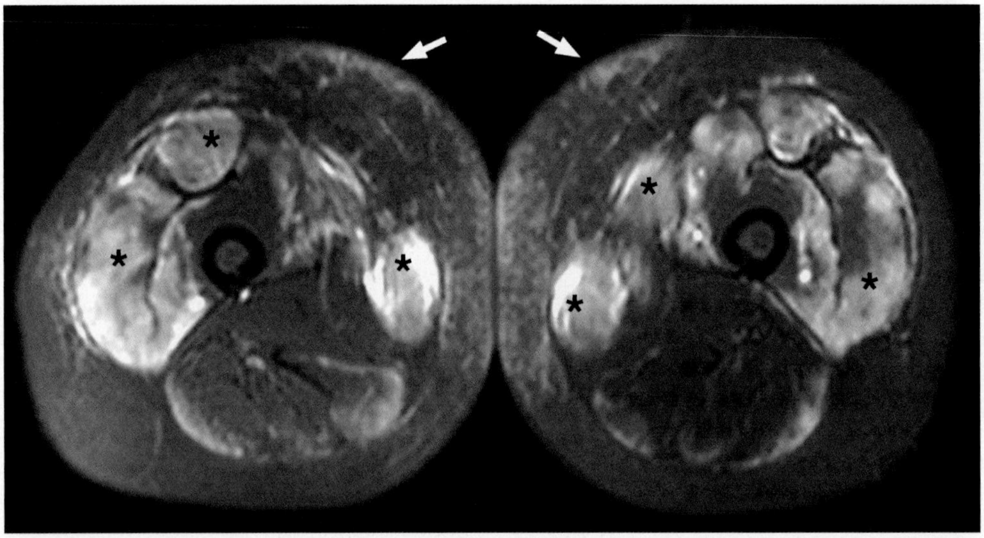

FIGURE 25.40 **A 10-year-old boy with biopsy-proven dermatomyositis who presented with lower extremity weakness and fever.** Axial fat-suppressed T2-weighted MR image shows bilateral fairly symmetric hyperintense appearance of "predominantly" the anterior muscle compartment of the thigh (*asterisks*). Also present are edema and stranding of the subcutaneous fat (*arrows*).

seen early in the course of the disease,[158] vasculopathy of the GI tract, and rarely pulmonary interstitial lung disease.[155] The presence of abnormal muscular enzymes is the most common paraclinical criterion used in the diagnosis. The sensitivity of this criterion is higher when the enzymes are analyzed all together, and it decreases as the disease progresses.

MRI, although not a criterion, has increasingly been used for diagnosis, localization, and monitoring disease activity, widely replacing the more invasive muscle biopsy and electromyography (EMG).[154–156] The most reliable finding on MR imaging is muscle edema on fluid-sensitive sequences seen as hyperintense areas. T1-weighted MR images are useful in assessing fatty muscle infiltration seen as increased muscle signal and decreased muscle bulk and are indicative of atrophy in chronic cases or as the sequelae of steroid therapy. This finding is bilateral and tends to be symmetrical (Fig. 25.40). The gluteal and thigh regions are the most commonly affected areas. Axial MR images are useful for evaluating the muscle group and subcutaneous tissue involvement whereas coronal MR images are helpful for determining the extent of the disease.[154,156,159,160] The routine use of gadolinium is not indicated for all cases but is rather patient specific: When the findings are obvious on the fluid-sensitive MR sequences, there is no need for intravenous contrast.[159] Subcutaneous edema seen as a streaky, irregular, high signal on fluid-sensitive sequences is usually seen in an early-stage, untreated disease. Thickened T2 hyperintense fascial planes following a distribution pattern similar to that of the involved muscle groups is indicative of fascial involvement on MRI.[156,159] Both US and MRI are useful in determining the potential sites of biopsy to avoid false-negative results.[159] More recently, T2 mapping provides an accurate assessment of disease activity based on the T2 relaxation time.[161]

Calcinosis is a complication of the disease that can occur despite a normal physiologic calcium/phosphate ratio. Calcinosis is easily detected on radiographs and occurs in the extensor surfaces of the joints and in areas that have been exposed to trauma (Fig. 25.41). On MRI, calcinosis has variable signal intensity depending on the degree of calcium or protein present.[154,155,159]

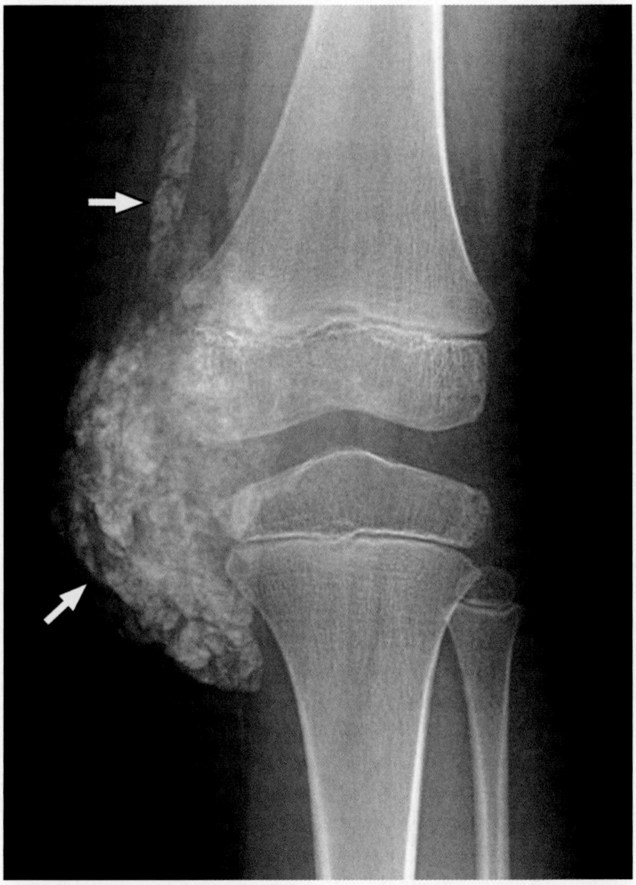

FIGURE 25.41 **Calcinosis in a 12-year-old boy with long-standing dermatomyositis.** Frontal knee radiograph shows confluent periarticular nodular calcium deposits (*arrows*) within the soft tissues around the knee.

The goals of treatment in JDM include control of the underlying inflammatory myositis and prevention and/or treatment of complications such as contractures and calcinosis. The most commonly used medications are steroids in combination with immunosuppressive medications such as methotrexate.[155,162] The prognosis of JDM and polymyositis depends on the variable course of the disease. Monocyclic disease, which typically progresses into permanent remission after ~2 years of activity, occurs in about one-third of patients. These patients tend to have a good response to standard treatment. Polycyclic disease, in which periods of remission are followed by relapse and chronic continuous disease, occurs in the other two-thirds of patients.[155]

References

1. Greenspan A. *Orthopedic Imaging. A Practical Approach*. 4th ed. Philadelphia, PA: Lippincott Williams & Wilkins; 2004.
2. States LJ. Imaging of metabolic bone disease and marrow disorders in children. *Radiol Clin North Am*. 2001;39(4):749–772.
3. Restrepo R, Lee EY. Epidemiology, pathogenesis, and imaging of arthritis in children. *Orthop Clin North Am*. 2012;43(2):213–225, vi.
4. Restrepo R, Lee EY, Babyn PS. Juvenile idiopathic arthritis: current practical imaging assessment with emphasis on magnetic resonance imaging. *Radiol Clin North Am*. 2013;51(4):703–719.
5. Dimeglio A, Canavese F. Imaging in Legg-Calvé-Perthes disease. *Orthop Clin North Am*. 2011;42(3):297–302.
6. Sabharwal S. Blount disease. *J Bone Joint Surg Am*. 2009;91(7):1758–1776.
7. Ejindu VC, Hine AL, Mashayekhi M, et al. Musculoskeletal manifestations of sickle cell disease. *Radiographics*. 2007;27(4):1005–1021.
8. Morishita K, Petty RE. Musculoskeletal manifestations of mucopolysaccharidoses. *Rheumatology (Oxford)*. 2011;50(suppl 5):v19–v25.
9. Weber U, Hodler J, Kubik RA, et al. Sensitivity and specificity of spinal inflammatory lesions assessed by whole-body magnetic resonance imaging in patients with ankylosing spondylitis or recent-onset inflammatory back pain. *Arthritis Rheum*. 2009;61(7):900–908.
10. Doria AS, Chaudry GA, Nasui C, et al. The use of parallel imaging for MRI assessment of knees in children and adolescents. *Pediatr Radiol*. 2010;40(3):284–293.
11. Resnick D. *Bone and Joint Imaging*. 2nd ed. Philadelphia, PA: W.B. Saunders Company; 1996.
12. Shore RM, Chesney RW. Rickets: part I. *Pediatr Radiol*. 2013;43(2):140–151.
13. Carroll DM, Doria AS, Paul BS. Clinical-radiological features of fractures in premature infants—a review. *J Perinat Med*. 2007;35(5):366–375.
14. States LJ. Imaging of rachitic bone. *Endocr Dev*. 2003;6:80–92.
15. Shore RM, Chesney RW. Rickets: part II. *Pediatr Radiol*. 2013;43(2):152–172.
16. Pettifor JM. Nutritional rickets: pathogenesis and prevention. *Pediatr Endocrinol Rev*. 2013;10(suppl 2):347–353.
17. Felger EA, Kandil E. Primary hyperparathyroidism. *Otolaryngol Clin North Am*. 2010;43(2):417–432.
18. Kollars J, Zarroug AE, van Heerden J, et al. Primary hyperparathyroidism in pediatric patients. *Pediatrics*. 2005;115(4):974–980.
19. Bhadada SK, Bhansali A, Dutta P, et al. Characteristics of primary hyperparathyroidism in adolescents. *J Pediatr Endocrinol Metab*. 2008;21(12):1147–1153.
20. Belcher R, Metrailer AM, Bodenner DL, et al. Characterization of hyperparathyroidism in youth and adolescents: a literature review. *Int J Pediatr Otorhinolaryngol*. 2013;77(3):318–322.
21. Cooke KM, Cowell C, Lam AH, et al. Imaging paediatric endocrine disorders. *Baillieres Clin Endocrinol Metab*. 1989;3(1):191–224.
22. Kataria R, Agarwala S, Mitra DK, et al. Primary hyperparathyroidism in children. *Pediatr Surg Int*. 1996;11(5–6):374–377.
23. Schmitt CP, Mehls O. Mineral and bone disorders in children with chronic kidney disease. *Nat Rev Nephrol*. 2011;7(11):624–634.
24. Ziółkowska H, Pańczyk-Tomaszewska M, Majkowska Z, et al. Imaging of bone in the diagnostics of renal osteodystrophy in children with chronic renal failure. *Med Sci Monit*. 2001;7(5):1034–1042.
25. Bacchetta J, Boutroy S, Delmas P-D, et al. New bone imaging techniques in children with chronic kidney disease. *Arch Pediatr*. 2009;16(11):1482–1490.
26. van Diemen-Steenvoorde R, Donckerwolcke RA, de Haas G. Generalized soft tissue calcification in children and adolescents with end stage renal failure. *Eur J Pediatr*. 1986;145(4):293–296.
27. Ross AJ. Parathyroid surgery in children. *Prog Pediatr Surg*. 1991;26:48–59.
28. Nieto J, Ruiz-Cuevas P, Escuder A, et al. Tertiary hyperparathyroidism after renal transplantation. *Pediatr Nephrol*. 1997;11(1):65–68.
29. Saengsuda Y. The accuracy of 99m Tc-MIBI scintigraphy for preoperative parathyroid localization in primary and secondary-tertiary hyperparathyroidism. *J Med Assoc Thai*. 2012;95(suppl 3):S81–S91.
30. de Andrade JSC, Mangussi-Gomes JP, da Rocha LA, et al. Localization of ectopic and supernumerary parathyroid glands in patients with secondary and tertiary hyperparathyroidism: surgical description and correlation with preoperative ultrasonography and Tc99m-Sestamibi scintigraphy. *Braz J Otorhinolaryngol*. 2014;80(1):29–34.
31. De Sanctis V, Soliman A, Fiscina B. Hypoparathyroidism: from diagnosis to treatment. *Curr Opin Endocrinol Diabetes Obes*. 2012;19(6):435–442.
32. Maeda SS, Fortes EM, Oliveira UM, et al. Hypoparathyroidism and pseudohypoparathyroidism. *Arq Bras Endocrinol Metabol*. 2006;50(4):664–673.
33. Rockman-Greenberg C. Hypophosphatasia. *Pediatr Endocrinol Rev*. 2013;10(suppl 2):380–388.
34. Mertens MT, Gertner E. Rheumatic manifestations of scurvy: a report of three recent cases in a major urban center and a review. *Semin Arthritis Rheum*. 2011;41(2):286–290.
35. Ratanachu-Ek S, Sukswai P, Jeerathanyasakun Y, et al. Scurvy in pediatric patients: a review of 28 cases. *J Med Assoc Thai*. 2003;86(suppl 3):S734–S740.
36. Pimentel L. Scurvy: historical review and current diagnostic approach. *Am J Emerg Med*. 2003;21(4):328–332.
37. Oestreich AE. The acrophysis: a unifying concept for understanding enchondral bone growth and its disorders. II. Abnormal growth. *Skeletal Radiol*. 2004;33(3):119–128.
38. Gongidi P, Johnson C, Dinan D. Scurvy in an autistic child: MRI findings. *Pediatr Radiol*. 2013;43(10):1396–1399.
39. Alissa EM, Ferns GA. Heavy metal poisoning and cardiovascular disease. *J Toxicol*. 2011;2011:870125.

40. Ibrahim D, Froberg B, Wolf A, et al. Heavy metal poisoning: clinical presentations and pathophysiology. *Clin Lab Med.* 2006;26(1):67–97, viii.
41. Ferrer A. Metal poisoning. *An Sist Sanit Navar.* 2003;26(suppl 1):141–153.
42. Chisolm JJ Jr. Poisoning from heavy metals (mercury, lead, and cadmium). *Pediatr Ann.* 1980;9(12):458–468.
43. Rusyniak DE, Arroyo A, Acciani J, et al. Heavy metal poisoning: management of intoxication and antidotes. *EXS.* 2010;100:365–396.
44. Almeida A, Roberts I. Bone involvement in sickle cell disease. *Br J Haematol.* 2005;129(4):482–490.
45. Lonergan GJ, Cline DB, Abbondanzo SL. Sickle cell anemia. *Radiographics.* 2001;21(4):971–994.
46. Ganguly A, Boswell W, Aniq H. Musculoskeletal manifestations of sickle cell anaemia: a pictorial review. *Anemia.* 2011; 2011:794283.
47. Jaramillo D. Whole-body MR imaging, bone diffusion imaging: how and why? *Pediatr Radiol.* 2010;40(6):978–984.
48. Pratesi A, Medici A, Bresci R, et al. Sickle cell-related bone marrow complications: the utility of diffusion-weighted magnetic resonance imaging. *J Pediatr Hematol Oncol.* 2013; 35(4):329–330.
49. Martinoli C, Bacigalupo L, Forni GL et al. Musculoskeletal manifestations of chronic anemias. *Semin Musculoskelet Radiol.* 2011;15(3):269–280.
50. Ballas SK, Gupta K, Adams-Graves P. Sickle cell pain: a critical reappraisal. *Blood.* 2012;120(18):3647–3656.
51. Goebel HH, Müller HD. Storage diseases: diagnostic position. *Ultrastruct Pathol.* 2013;37(1):19–22.
52. Stevenson DA, Steiner RD. Skeletal abnormalities in lysosomal storage diseases. *Pediatr Endocrinol Rev.* 2013;10(suppl 2):406–416.
53. Palmucci S, Attinà G, Lanza ML, et al. Imaging findings of mucopolysaccharidoses: a pictorial review. *Insights Imaging.* 2013;4(4):443–459.
54. Valayannopoulos V, Wijburg FA. Therapy for the mucopolysaccharidoses. *Rheumatology (Oxford).* 2011;50(suppl 5):v49–v59.
55. Wraith JE. *Hand Book of Clinical Neurology.* 3rd ed. Amsterdam, Netherlands: Elsevier; 2013: Vol. 113.
56. Lachman R, Martin KW, Castro S, et al. Radiologic and neuroradiologic findings in the mucopolysaccharidoses. *J Pediatr Rehabil Med.* 2010;3(2):109–118.
57. Tandon V, Williamson JB, Cowie RA, et al. Spinal problems in mucopolysaccharidosis I (Hurler syndrome). *J Bone Joint Surg Br.* 1996;78(6):938–944.
58. Manger B, Mengel E, Schaefer RM. Rheumatologic aspects of lysosomal storage diseases. *Clin Rheumatol.* 2007;26(3):335–341.
59. Wenstrup RJ, Roca-Espiau M, Weinreb NJ, et al. Skeletal aspects of Gaucher disease: a review. *Br J Radiol.* 2002;75(suppl 1):A2–A12.
60. Rohrbach M, Clarke JTR. Treatment of lysosomal storage disorders: progress with enzyme replacement therapy. *Drugs.* 2007;67(18):2697–2716.
61. Mikosch P, Hughes D. An overview on bone manifestations in Gaucher disease. *Wien Med Wochenschr.* 2010;160(23–24): 609–624.
62. Zerin JM, Hernandez RJ. Approach to skeletal maturation. *Hand Clin.* 1991;7(1):53–62.
63. Gilli G. The assessment of skeletal maturation. *Horm Res.* 1996; 45(suppl 2):49–52.
64. Bull RK, Edwards PD, Kemp PM, et al. Bone age assessment: a large scale comparison of the Greulich and Pyle, and Tanner and Whitehouse (TW2) methods. *Arch Dis Child.* 1999;81(2): 172–173.
65. Loder RT, Estle DT, Morrison K, et al. Applicability of the Greulich and Pyle skeletal age standards to black and white children of today. *Am J Dis Child.* 1993;147(12):1329–1333.
66. Mora S, Boechat MI, Pietka E, et al. Skeletal age determinations in children of European and African descent: applicability of the Greulich and Pyle standards. *Pediatr Res.* 2001;50(5):624–628.
67. Zafar AM, Nadeem N, Husen Y, et al. An appraisal of Greulich-Pyle Atlas for skeletal age assessment in Pakistan. *J Pak Med Assoc.* 2010;60(7):552–555.
68. Koc A, Karaoglanoglu M, Erdogan M, et al. Assessment of bone ages: is the Greulich-Pyle method sufficient for Turkish boys? *Pediatr Int.* 2001;43(6):662–665.
69. Ontell FK, Ivanovic M, Ablin DS, et al. Bone age in children of diverse ethnicity. *AJR Am J Roentgenol.* 1996;167(6):1395–1398.
70. Duthie RB, Houghton GR. Constitutional aspects of the osteochondroses. *Clin Orthop Relat Res.* 1981;158:19–27.
71. Atanda A, Jr, Shah SA, O'Brien K. Osteochondrosis: common causes of pain in growing bones. *Am Fam Physician.* 2011; 83(3):285–291.
72. Perry DC, Hall AJ. The epidemiology and etiology of Perthes disease. *Orthop Clin North Am.* 2011;42(3):279–283, v.
73. Barker DJ, Hall AJ. The epidemiology of Perthes' disease. *Clin Orthop Relat Res.* 1986;209:89–94.
74. Dillman JR, Hernandez RJ. MRI of Legg-Calve-Perthes disease. *AJR Am J Roentgenol.* 2009;193(5):1394–1407.
75. Kim HKW, Herring JA. Pathophysiology, classifications, and natural history of Perthes disease. *Orthop Clin North Am.* 2011;42(3):285–295, v.
76. Joseph B. Prognostic factors and outcome measures in Perthes disease. *Orthop Clin North Am.* 2011;42(3):303–315, v–vi.
77. Johnson C, May DA, McCabe KM, et al. Non-cartilaginous metaphyseal cysts in Legg-Calvé-Perthes disease: report of a case. *Pediatr Radiol.* 1997;27(10):824–826.
78. Doria AS, Guarniero R, De Godoy RM Jr, et al. Contrast-enhanced power Doppler imaging: comparison with scintigraphic phases of revascularization of the femoral head in Legg-Calvé-Perthes disease. *J Pediatr Orthop.* 2002;22(4):471–478.
79. Doria AS, Guarniero R, Cunha FG, et al. Contrast-enhanced power Doppler sonography: assessment of revascularization flow in Legg-Calvé-Perthes' disease. *Ultrasound Med Biol.* 2002; 28(2):171–182.
80. Joseph B, Price CT. Consensus statements on the management of Perthes disease. *Orthop Clin North Am.* 2011;42(3):437–440.
81. Nelitz M, Lippacher S, Krauspe R, et al. Perthes disease: current principles of diagnosis and treatment. *Dtsch Arztebl Int.* 2009; 106(31–32):517–523.
82. Duri ZAA, Patel DV, et al. The immature athlete. *Clin Sports Med.* 2002;21(3):461–482, ix.
83. Kodali P, Islam A, Andrish J. Anterior knee pain in the young athlete: diagnosis and treatment. *Sports Med Arthrosc.* 2011;19(1):27–33.
84. Iwamoto J, Takeda T, Sato Y, et al. Radiographic abnormalities of the inferior pole of the patella in juvenile athletes. *Keio J Med.* 2009;58(1):50–53.
85. Medlar RC, Lyne ED. Sinding-Larsen-Johansson disease. Its etiology and natural history. *J Bone Joint Surg Am.* 1978;60(8): 1113–1116.
86. Dupuis CS, Westra SJ, Makris J, et al. Injuries and conditions of the extensor mechanism of the pediatric knee. *Radiographics.* 2009;29(3):877–886.

87. Bradway JK, Klassen RA, Peterson HA. Blount disease: a review of the English literature. *J Pediatr Orthop.* 1987;7(4): 472–480.
88. Langenskiöld A. Tibia vara. A critical review. *Clin Orthop Relat Res.* 1989;246:195–207.
89. Sabharwal S, Wenokor C, Mehta A, et al. Intra-articular morphology of the knee joint in children with Blount disease: a case-control study using MRI. *J Bone Joint Surg Am.* 2012;94(10):883–890.
90. Craig JG, van Holsbeeck M, Zaltz I. The utility of MR in assessing Blount disease. *Skeletal Radiol.* 2002;31(4):208–213.
91. Thompson GH, Carter JR. Late-onset tibia vara (Blount's disease). Current concepts. *Clin Orthop Relat Res.* 1990;255:24–35.
92. Kujala UM, Kvist M, Heinonen O. Osgood-Schlatter's disease in adolescent athletes. Retrospective study of incidence and duration. *Am J Sports Med.* 1985;13(4):236–241.
93. Gholve PA, Scher DM, Khakharia S, et al. Osgood Schlatter syndrome. *Curr Opin Pediatr.* 2007;19(1):44–50.
94. Hirano A, Fukubayashi T, Ishii T, et al. Magnetic resonance imaging of Osgood-Schlatter disease: the course of the disease. *Skeletal Radiol.* 2002;31(6):334–342.
95. Weiss JM, Jordan SS, Andersen JS, et al. Surgical treatment of unresolved Osgood-Schlatter disease: ossicle resection with tibial tubercleplasty. *J Pediatr Orthop.* 2007;27(7):844–847.
96. DiGiovanni CW, Patel A, Calfee R, et al. Osteonecrosis in the foot. *J Am Acad Orthop Surg.* 2007;15(4):208–217.
97. Gillespie H. Osteochondroses and apophyseal injuries of the foot in the young athlete. *Curr Sports Med Rep.* 2010;9(5):265–268.
98. Borges JL, Guille JT, Bowen JR. Köhler's bone disease of the tarsal navicular. *J Pediatr Orthop.* 1995;15(5):596–598.
99. Carmont MR, Rees RJ, Blundell CM. Current concepts review: Freiberg's disease. *Foot Ankle Int.* 2009;30(2):167–176.
100. Katcherian DA. Treatment of Freiberg's disease. *Orthop Clin North Am.* 1994;25(1):69–81.
101. Cerrato RA. Freiberg's disease. *Foot Ankle Clin.* 2011;16(4): 647–658.
102. Herrera-Soto JA, Price CT. Core decompression for juvenile osteonecrosis. *Orthop Clin North Am.* 2011;42(3):429–436, ix.
103. Lowe TG, Line BG. Evidence based medicine: analysis of Scheuermann kyphosis. *Spine.* 2007;32(19 suppl):S115–S119.
104. Wenger DR, Frick SL. Scheuermann kyphosis. *Spine.* 1999; 24(24):2630–2639.
105. Rodriguez DP, Poussaint TY. Imaging of back pain in children. *AJNR Am J Neuroradiol.* 2010;31(5):787–802.
106. Summers BN, Singh JP, Manns RA. The radiological reporting of lumbar Scheuermann's disease: an unnecessary source of confusion amongst clinicians and patients. *Br J Radiol.* 2008; 81(965):383–385.
107. Ferlic RJ, Lee DH, Lopez-Ben RR. Pediatric Kienböck's disease: case report and review of the literature. *Clin Orthop Relat Res.* 2003;408:237–244.
108. Lutsky K, Beredjiklian PK. Kienböck disease. *J Hand Surg Am.* 2012;37(9):1942–1952.
109. Schuind F, Eslami S, Ledoux P. Kienbock's disease. *J Bone Joint Surg Br.* 2008;90(2):133–139.
110. Cross D, Matullo KS. Kienböck disease. *Orthop Clin North Am.* 2014;45(1):141–152.
111. Cahill BR. Osteochondritis dissecans of the knee: treatment of juvenile and adult forms. *J Am Acad Orthop Surg.* 1995; 3(4):237–247.
112. Schenck RC Jr, Goodnight JM. Osteochondritis dissecans. *J Bone Joint Surg Am.* 1996;78(3):439–456.
113. Detterline AJ, Goldstein JL, Rue J-PH, et al. Evaluation and treatment of osteochondritis dissecans lesions of the knee. *J Knee Surg.* 2008;21(2):106–115.
114. Doyle SM, Monahan A. Osteochondroses: a clinical review for the pediatrician. *Curr Opin Pediatr.* 2010;22(1):41–46.
115. Kijowski R, Blankenbaker DG, Shinki K, et al. Juvenile versus adult osteochondritis dissecans of the knee: appropriate MR imaging criteria for instability. *Radiology.* 2008;248(2): 571–578.
116. De Smet AA, Fisher DR, Graf BK, et al. Osteochondritis dissecans of the knee: value of MR imaging in determining lesion stability and the presence of articular cartilage defects. *AJR Am J Roentgenol.* 1990;155(3):549–553.
117. Nelson DW, DiPaola J, Colville M, et al. Osteochondritis dissecans of the talus and knee: prospective comparison of MR and arthroscopic classifications. *J Comput Assist Tomogr.* 1990;14(5):804–808.
118. De Smet AA, Ilahi OA, Graf BK. Reassessment of the MR criteria for stability of osteochondritis dissecans in the knee and ankle. *Skeletal Radiol.* 1996;25(2):159–163.
119. Mesgarzadeh M, Sapega AA, Bonakdarpour A, et al. Osteochondritis dissecans: analysis of mechanical stability with radiography, scintigraphy, and MR imaging. *Radiology.* 1987;165(3):775–780.
120. O'Connor MA, Palaniappan M, Khan N, et al. Osteochondritis dissecans of the knee in children. A comparison of MRI and arthroscopic findings. *J Bone Joint Surg Br.* 2002;84(2): 258–262.
121. Kobayashi K, Burton KJ, Rodner C, et al. Lateral compression injuries in the pediatric elbow: Panner's disease and osteochondritis dissecans of the capitellum. *J Am Acad Orthop Surg.* 2004;12(4):246–254.
122. Klingele KE, Kocher MS. Little league elbow: valgus overload injury in the paediatric athlete. *Sports Med.* 2002; 32(15):1005–1015.
123. Chen FS, Diaz VA, Loebenberg M, et al. Shoulder and elbow injuries in the skeletally immature athlete. *J Am Acad Orthop Surg.* 2005;13(3):172–185.
124. Magni-Manzoni S, Malattia C, Lanni S, et al. Advances and challenges in imaging in juvenile idiopathic arthritis. *Nat Rev Rheumatol.* 2012;8(6):329–336.
125. Jordan A, McDonagh JE. Juvenile idiopathic arthritis: the paediatric perspective. *Pediatr Radiol.* 2006;36(8):734–742.
126. Saurenmann RK, Rose JB, Tyrrell P, et al. Epidemiology of juvenile idiopathic arthritis in a multiethnic cohort: ethnicity as a risk factor. *Arthritis Rheum.* 2007;56(6):1974–1984.
127. Prakken B, Albani S, Martini A. Juvenile idiopathic arthritis. *Lancet.* 2011;377(9783):2138–2149.
128. McGonagle D, Aziz A, Dickie LJ, et al. An integrated classification of pediatric inflammatory diseases, based on the concepts of autoinflammation and the immunological disease continuum. *Pediatr Res.* 2009;65(5 pt 2):38R–45R.
129. Mellins ED, Macaubas C, Grom AA. Pathogenesis of systemic juvenile idiopathic arthritis: some answers, more questions. *Nat Rev Rheumatol.* 2011;7(7):416–426.
130. Stoll ML. Interactions of the innate and adaptive arms of the immune system in the pathogenesis of spondyloarthritis. *Clin Exp Rheumatol.* 2011;29(2):322–330.
131. Petty RE, Southwood TR, Manners P, et al. International League of Associations for Rheumatology classification of juvenile idiopathic arthritis: second revision, Edmonton, 2001. *J Rheumatol.* 2004;31(2):390–392.

132. Azouz EM. Juvenile idiopathic arthritis: how can the radiologist help the clinician? *Pediatr Radiol.* 2008;38(suppl 3): S403–S408.
133. Johnson K. Imaging of juvenile idiopathic arthritis. *Pediatr Radiol.* 2006;36(8):743–758.
134. Stoll ML, Punaro M. Psoriatic juvenile idiopathic arthritis: a tale of two subgroups. *Curr Opin Rheumatol.* 2011;23(5):437–443.
135. Colbert RA. Classification of juvenile spondyloarthritis: Enthesitis-related arthritis and beyond. *Nat Rev Rheumatol.* 2010;6(8):477–485.
136. Malattia C, Damasio MB, Basso C, et al. Dynamic contrast-enhanced magnetic resonance imaging in the assessment of disease activity in patients with juvenile idiopathic arthritis. *Rheumatology (Oxford).* 2010;49(1):178–185.
137. Damasio MB, Malattia C, Martini A, et al. Synovial and inflammatory diseases in childhood: role of new imaging modalities in the assessment of patients with juvenile idiopathic arthritis. *Pediatr Radiol.* 2010;40(6):985–998.
138. Hughes TH, Sartoris DJ, Schweitzer ME, et al. Pigmented villonodular synovitis: MRI characteristics. *Skeletal Radiol.* 1995;24(1):7–12.
139. Breton S, Jousse-Joulin S, Finel E, et al. Imaging approaches for evaluating peripheral joint abnormalities in juvenile idiopathic arthritis. *Semin Arthritis Rheum.* 2012;41(5):698–711.
140. Malattia C, Damasio MB, Magnaguagno F, et al. Magnetic resonance imaging, ultrasonography, and conventional radiography in the assessment of bone erosions in juvenile idiopathic arthritis. *Arthritis Rheum.* 2008;59(12):1764–1772.
141. Kim HK, Laor T, Graham TB, et al. T2 relaxation time changes in distal femoral articular cartilage in children with juvenile idiopathic arthritis: a 3-year longitudinal study. *AJR Am J Roentgenol.* 2010;195(4):1021–1025.
142. Kirkhus E, Flatø B, Riise O, et al. Differences in MRI findings between subgroups of recent-onset childhood arthritis. *Pediatr Radiol.* 2011;41(4):432–440.
143. Chung C, Coley BD, Martin LC. Rice bodies in juvenile rheumatoid arthritis. *AJR Am J Roentgenol.* 1998;170(3):698–700.
144. Lee EY, Sundel RP, Kim S, et al. MRI findings of juvenile psoriatic arthritis. *Skeletal Radiol.* 2008;37(11):987–996.
145. Minden K. Adult outcomes of patients with juvenile idiopathic arthritis. *Horm Res.* 2009;72(suppl 1):20–25.
146. Stoll ML, Bhore R, Dempsey-Robertson M, et al. Spondyloarthritis in a pediatric population: risk factors for sacroiliitis. *J Rheumatol.* 2010;37(11):2402–2408.
147. Scofield RH, Sestak AL. Juvenile spondyloarthropathies. *Curr Rheumatol Rep.* 2012;14(5):395–401.
148. Burgos-Vargas R. The assessment of the spondyloarthritis international society concept and criteria for the classification of axial spondyloarthritis and peripheral spondyloarthritis: a critical appraisal for the pediatric rheumatologist. *Pediatr Rheumatol Online J.* 2012;10(1):14.
149. Braun J, Sieper J, Bollow M. Imaging of sacroiliitis. *Clin Rheumatol.* 2000;19(1):51–57.
150. Lambert RGW, Dhillon SS, Jaremko JL. Advanced imaging of the axial skeleton in spondyloarthropathy: techniques, interpretation, and utility. *Semin Musculoskelet Radiol.* 2012;16(5):389–400.
151. Bollow M, Biedermann T, Kannenberg J, et al. Use of dynamic magnetic resonance imaging to detect sacroiliitis in HLA-B27 positive and negative children with juvenile arthritides. *J Rheumatol.* 1998;25(3):556–564.
152. Molinos Quintana A, Morillo Gutiérrez B, Camacho Lovillo MS, et al. Pyogenic sacroiliitis in children-a diagnostic challenge. *Clin Rheumatol.* 2011;30(1):107–113.
153. Ghedira Besbes L, Haddad S, Abid A, et al. Pyogenic sacroiliitis in children: two case reports. *Case Rep Med.* 2012;2012: 415323.
154. Feldman BM, Rider LG, Reed AM, et al. Juvenile dermatomyositis and other idiopathic inflammatory myopathies of childhood. *Lancet.* 2008;371(9631):2201–2212.
155. Batthish M, Feldman BM. Juvenile dermatomyositis. *Curr Rheumatol Rep.* 2011;13(3):216–224.
156. Zouagui A, Abourazzak S, Idrissi ML, et al. Actuality of juvenile dermatomyositis. *Joint Bone Spine.* 2011;78(3):235–240.
157. Bohan A, Peter JB. Polymyositis and dermatomyositis (first of two parts). *N Engl J Med.* 1975;292(7):344–347.
158. Tse S, Lubelsky S, Gordon M, et al. The arthritis of inflammatory childhood myositis syndromes. *J Rheumatol.* 2001;28(1): 192–197.
159. Gardner-Medwin JMM, Irwin G, Johnson K. MRI in juvenile idiopathic arthritis and juvenile dermatomyositis. *Ann N Y Acad Sci.* 2009;1154:52–83.
160. Johnson K, Davis PJC, Foster JK, et al. Imaging of muscle disorders in children. *Pediatr Radiol.* 2006;36(10):1005–1018.
161. Reed AM, Mason T. Recent advances in juvenile dermatomyositis. *Curr Rheumatol Rep.* 2005;7(2):94–98.
162. Martin N, Li CK, Wedderburn LR. Juvenile dermatomyositis: new insights and new treatment strategies. *Ther Adv Musculoskelet Dis.* 2012;4(1):41–50.

Index

Note: Page numbers in italics indicate figures; those followed by "t" indicates table.

B

E

F

J

K

M

O

T

RRS1707